Jablonski's
DICTIONARY
OF
DENTISTRY

Jablonski's
DICTIONARY
OF
DENTISTRY

by Stanley Jablonski

Krieger Publishing Company *9/ 96*
Malabar, Florida
1992

Original Edition 1982
Reprint Edition 1992 with new material
(Based on Illustrated Dictionary of Dentistry)

Printed and Published by
KRIEGER PUBLISHING COMPANY
KRIEGER DRIVE
MALABAR, FLORIDA 32950

Copyright © 1982
Transferred to Stanley Jablonski 1990
Reprinted by Arrangement.

Library of Congress Cataloging-In-Publication Data
Jablonski, Stanley.
    Jablonski's dictionary of dentistry / Stanley Jablonski.
       p.   cm.
    Reprint.
    ISBN 0-89464-477-7 (library bind. : acid free paper)
    1. Dentistry--Dictionaries. I. Title.
    [DNLM: 1. Dentistry--dictionaries. WU 13 J11i 1982a]
RK27.J3 1990
617.6'003--dc20
DNLM/DLC
for Library of Congress   90-4590
                                      CIP

10   9   8   7   6   5   4   3   2

Introduction

PURPOSE AND SCOPE This Dictionary has been compiled to gather in one place and define terminologies in all specialties of dentistry and allied fields of science and technology, health care (including dental practice management and health insurance), as well as some peripheral terms that are considered to be important or of potential interest to dental practitioners, researchers, educators, students, and auxiliary personnel. Some terms no longer in general use but of historical or etymological interest are also included.

FORMAT The style of the Dictionary follows that of most leading biomedical dictionaries as refined from traditional practices and adapted to modern needs, as in *Dorland's Illustrated Medical Dictionary.*

A typical main entry of a preferred term (as opposed to a synonym) consists of the name (in bold-face type), a phonetic respelling (in parentheses), an etymological source (in square brackets), a descriptive definition, and, finally, synonyms, trademarks (where applicable), and cross-references.

A compound entry, consisting of a noun and an adjective or modifier, is defined under the noun, according to traditional biomedical lexicographical style, which has its origin in the Latin custom of placing adjectives after nouns. Although there are now many non-Latin terms in biomedical (particularly dental) terminology, the inversion of terms under nouns permits clustering of terms on the same subject, thus allowing the reader to find related terms at one place and facilitating extensive browsing.

Many illustrations and tables complement the definitions, and are aimed at giving the user maximum information within the framework of a dictionary.

Information considered to be unsuitable for the standard dictionary format has been arranged in the frontmatter and in appendices. This includes The Language of Medicine and Dentistry (pp. xi–xiv), the organization and functions of the American Dental Association (Appendix 1), and the Canadian Dental Association (Appendix 6), directories of schools of dentistry in the United States (Appendices 2–5) and Canada (Appendices 7–9), and Laboratory Reference Values of Clinical Importance (Appendix 10).

ARRANGEMENT AND ALPHABETIZATION Entries will be found alphabetized on the sequence of the letters, regardless of space or hyphens that may occur between them. An exception to this occurs in the case of compound eponymic terms; for example, *Brown Kelly* and *Brown-Symmers disease* precede *brownian,* and *Caldwell projection* precedes *Caldwell-Luc operation.* In eponymic terms, the apostrophe s ('s) is ignored in determing the alphabetical sequence; thus *Barton's bandage* precedes *Bartonella* and *Addison's anemia* precedes *Addison-Biemer anemia,* both as a main entry and under *anemia.* Similarly, umlauts (ö, ü) are ignored in alphabetizing proper names. German proper names in which umlauts appear are sometimes Anglicized; for example, *Böck* may be written *Boeck* and *Müller* may be written *Mueller.* Proper names beginning with "Mc" and "Mac" are alphabetized as though spelled "mac" in every instance, the sequence being determined by the letter immediately following the *c.*

A proper name (capitalized entry) appears before a common noun (or lower case entry) with the identical spelling. Thus, *Bacteria* precedes *bacteria, Streptococcus* precedes *streptococcus.*

The plural of a word that is irregularly formed or of a foreign word is given following the phonetic respelling and often is given a separate bold-face listing in proper alphabetical order. Subentries appear in proper alphabetical order, determined by the subsequent modifying word or phrase, regardless of whether they are singular or plural. For example, under *arteria,* the entries *a. alveolaris inferior, arteriae alveolares superiores anteriores,* and *a. alveolaris superior posterior* appear in that order.

ETYMOLOGY Information on the derivation of a word appears in square brackets following the phonetic respelling, or following the plural form of the word, when that is given. The original foreign words from which the terms in this Dictionary are derived are reproduced in italic type, the language of their origin being indicated by the appropriate abbreviation (see list under the heading Abbreviations).

As a guide to related vocabulary, especially on anatomical terms, the Latin and/or Greek equivalent of a term may be given; for example, "liver [L. *jecur;* Gr. *hepar*]" and "kidney [L. *ren;* Gr. *nephros*]."

The Greek Alphabet

Capital	Small Letter	Sound	Name	Transcription
A	α	*aha*	alpha	a
B	β	*bet*	beta	b
Γ	γ	*get*	gamma	g
Δ	δ	*do*	delta	d
E	ε	*egg*	epsilon	e
Z	ζ	*adze*	zeta	z
H	η	*fête*	eta	ē
Θ	θ	*thin*	theta	th
I	ι	*it* / ma*chi*ne	iota	i
K	κ	*key*	kappa	k
Λ	λ	*let*	lambda	l
M	μ	*met*	mu	m
N	ν	*net*	nu	n
Ξ	ξ	*hex*	xi	x
O	ο	*oho*	omicron	o
Π	π	*pet*	pi	p
P	ρ	*r* (trilled)	rho	r
Σ	σ, ς*	*set*	sigma	s
T	τ	*tell*	tau	t
Υ	υ	ü (German)	upsilon	y
Φ	φ	*photo*	phi	ph
X	χ	*ach* (German)	chi	ch
Ψ	ψ	ti*ps*	psi	ps
Ω	ω	*oho*	omega	ō

* Sigma is written σ at the beginning or in the middle of a word and ς at the end of a word. E.g., σύνθεσις.

DEFINITIONS   An effort has been made to assign the descriptive definitions to those terms for which a preference has been shown or to which priority has been given in the scientific literature that we used as our reference sources. All synonyms and other secondary entries have been directed to these preferred terms. Certain descriptive definitions are more extensive and in-depth than is customary in standard dictionaries. An encyclopedic approach has been taken in areas of particular complexity. In keeping with the purposes of the Dictionary, particular attention is given to terms associated with dentistry.

Whenever possible, uniformity of definitions has been maintained within each specialty. In the case of anatomical structures, their definitions usually comprise information on systems to which they belong or organs from which they derive, descriptions of their form and topography, and descriptions of their structure (both gross anatomy and histology); anatomical terms listed in *Nomina Anatomica* are identified by the abbreviation NA. The definitions of diseases usually include descriptions of their clinical properties, etiology, symptomatology, pathology, and epidemiology. The chemical names, pharmacological class names, therapeutic and pharmacological properties, toxic effects, and trademarks of drugs are usually given. Enzymes are coded according to a numerical system (E.C. numbers), which is explained in the vocabulary under *enzyme*.

Terms that are no longer in common usage but are of historical interest are usually identified with an annotation, such as "formerly used" or "in the past."

SOURCES   Specialized dental glossaries were used as a primary source of information for the definitions. In instances in which the needed data were not available in glossaries or in which the information obtained from glossaries required augmentation or updating, textbooks and other forms of authoritative current monographic and serial literature were used as source material.

When authoritative sources differed about the meaning of a term, minor differences have been reflected in single definitions and major ones in separate definitions for the same term.

CROSS-REFERENCES   Cross-references direct the reader from synonyms, abbreviations, acronyms, trademarks, or other types of secondary entries to the preferred terms where descriptive definitions are found, omitting the word *see*.

A definition cross-referencing a synonym to a single-word preferred term appears as follows:

moniliasis (mon-ĭ-li′ah-sis) candidiasis.

When an entry sends the reader to a compound preferred term, the main entry is indicated by small capital letters and lower case letters indicate a subentry. For example:

acrodysplasia (ak"ro-dis-pla'se-ah) [*acro-* + *dysplasia*] Apert's SYNDROME.

or under *periodontitis*

suppurative apical p., chronic apical ABSCESS.

The reader is alerted to the existence in other parts of the Dictionary of related terms or additional important information by the cross-references *see also, see under,* and *cf.* (*compare*).

CAPITALIZATION   Standard rules for the capitalization of scientific terms is followed in the Dictionary. First letter capitalization has been used for proper names and the names of biological kingdoms, phyla, classes, orders, families, and genera; species are set in lower case letters.

An attempt has been made to identify and capitalize all trademarks, but the absence of capitalization does not always exclude the possibility that the name is a trademark or the subject of proprietary rights.

PRONUNCIATION   With the exception of proper names, trademarks, and combining forms, the pronunciation of words is indicated by a simple phonetic respelling in parentheses immediately following the main bold-face entry. As a rule, the most commonly heard pronunciation is given. Diacritical markings to distinguish vowel sounds are used only when necessary. The basic rules are:

An unmarked vowel ending a syllable is long (ba'be).

An unmarked vowel in a syllable ending with a consonant is short (ab'dukt).

A long vowel in a syllable ending with a consonant is indicated by a macron (ah-bāt, lēd, la'bĭl, tōōth).

A short vowel that constitutes or ends a syllable is marked with a breve (ĕ-de'mah, ĭ-mu'nĭ-te).

The syllable *ah* is used for the sound of *a* in open, unaccented syllables (ah-sis'tant, ah-bāt').

The primary accent in a word is indicated by a bold-face, single accent ('). The secondary accent is indicated by a light-face, double accent ("); an unstressed syllable is followed by a hyphen.

ABBREVIATIONS   Abbreviations used in the text are few and fairly obvious.

a.	artery (L. *arteria*)	i.e.	that is (L. *id est*)
Ar.	Arabic	It.	Italian
A.S.	Anglo-Saxon	L.	Latin
c.	about (L. *circa*)	l.	ligament (L. *ligamentum*)
cf.	compare (L. *confer*)	m.	muscle (L. *musculus*)
dim.	diminutive	n.	nerve (L. *nervus*)
e.g.	for example (L. *exempli gratia*)	pl.	plural
Fr.	French	Port.	Portuguese
gen.	genitive	sing.	singular
Ger.	German	Sp.	Spanish
Gr.	Greek	v.	vein (L. *vena*)

In elaboration of entries that are themselves abbreviations, the words "abbreviation for" have usually been omitted.

PROFESSIONAL REVIEW   In an effort to ensure the accuracy, completeness, and currency of the information and to make certain that it represents the thinking and knowledge of the scientific community, particularly, the profession of dentistry, the material presented in this Dictionary has been submitted to extensive review by our consultants (see p. ix), who are acknowledged authorities in their respective disciplines of dentistry and allied sciences.

Consultants

MAJOR M. ASH, JR., D.D.S., M.S., M.D.H.C.
Professor and Chairman, Department of Occlusion; Director, TMJ Clinic and Stomatognathic Physiology and EMG Laboratories; Research Scientist, Dental Research Institute — University of Michigan School of Dentistry, Ann Arbor.

NEVILLE J. BRYANT, A.R.T., F.A.C.B.S.
Chief Technologist — Toronto Western Hospital, Ontario, Canada.

SOTIROS D. CHAPARAS, M.S., PH.D.
Director, Mycobacterial and Fungal Antigens Branch — Bureau of Biologics, Food and Drug Administration, Bethesda, Maryland. Associate Professor, Department of Botany — Howard University, Washington, D.C. Faculty Chairman, Department of Microbiology and Immunology — Foundation for Advanced Education in the Sciences, National Institutes of Health, Bethesda, Maryland.

ANN EHRLICH, C.D.A., B.A., M.A.
Dental Management Consultant — Atlanta, Georgia. Former Faculty Member — University of North Carolina School of Dentistry, Chapel Hill.

AHMED H. EL-HOSHY, PH.D.
Computer Specialist — National Library of Medicine, Bethesda, Maryland.

JOHN P. FARKAS, M.D.
Medical Director, Radiologic Services — Roseville Community Hospital, Roseville, California. Adjunct Professor, Department of Pharmacology — University of the Pacific, Stockton, California.

R. E. GAENSSLEN, PH.D.
Professor and Director, Forensic Science Program — University of New Haven, West Haven, Connecticut. Formerly, Associate Professor, Department of Biochemistry — John Jay College of Criminal Justice, City University of New York.

ROBERT W. GARDIER, M.S., PH.D.
Professor, Department of Pharmacology, Director, Doctoral Program in Biomedical Sciences, School of Medicine and College of Science and Engineering — Wright State University, Dayton, Ohio.

ROBERT J. GORLIN, D.D.S., M.S.
Regents' Professor and Chairman, Department of Oral Pathology and Genetics; Professor, Departments of Pathology, Dermatology, Pediatrics, Obstetrics-Gynecology, Otolaryngology — University of Minnesota, Duluth. Consultant Staff — University Hospitals, Veterans' Administration Hospital, Minneapolis Children's Hospital, Hennepin County General Hospital, St. Paul Children's Hospital, Ramsey County Hospital, Gillette State Hospital for Crippled Children, Mt. Sinai Hospital.

LOUIS H. GUERNSEY, B.S., D.D.S., M.S.D., F.A.C.D., F.I.C.D.
Professor and Chief, Department of Oral/Maxillofacial Surgery — School of Dental Medicine and Hospital of the University of Pennsylvania, Philadelphia.

MICHAEL A. HEUER, D.D.S., M.S., F.A.C.D., F.I.C.D.
Professor and Chairman, Department of Endodontics — Dental School of Northwestern University, Chicago, Illinois. Secretary — American Association of Endodontists. Consultant — American Board of Endodontics. Diplomate — American Board of Endodontics. Northwestern University Dental Associates — Northwestern Memorial Hospital.

RONALD E. JORDAN, D.D.S., M.S.D.
Professor and Chairman, Department of Restorative Dentistry — University of Western Ontario, London, Canada.

ALETHA A. KOWITZ, B.S., M.S.
Director, Bureau of Library Services — American Dental Association.

WILTON MARION KROGMAN, PH.D., L.L.D.(H.C.), D.SC.(H.C.)
Director of Research — H. K. Cooper Clinic, Lancaster, Pennsylvania.

HOWARD K. KURAMITSU, PH.D.
Professor, Departments Microbiology and Immunology — Northwestern University Medical and Dental Schools, Chicago, Illinois.

EUGENE P. LAZZARI, B.S., M.A., PH.D.
Professor, Department of Biochemistry — University of Texas Dental Branch, Houston.

MORTIMER LORBER, D.M.D., M.D.
Associate Professor, Departments of Physiology and Biophysics — Georgetown University Schools of Dentistry and Medicine, Washington, D.C. Consultant — Naval Medical Research Institute, Dental Research Branch.

CLIFFORD H. MILLER, D.D.S.
Associate Dean, Administrative Affairs; Professor, Department of Operative Dentistry — Northwestern University Dental School, Chicago, Illinois.

KEITH L. MOORE, PH.D., F.I.A.C., F.R.S.M.
Professor and Chairman, Department of Anatomy; Faculty of Medicine — University of Toronto, Ontario, Canada.

RALPH W. PHILLIPS, M.S., D.Sc., F.A.C.D., F.I.C.D.
Associate Dean for Research; Research Professor of Dental Materials; Director, Oral Health Research Institute — Indiana University School of Dentistry, Indianapolis.

JOHN F. PRICHARD, D.D.S.
Private Practice of Periodontics.

D. VINCENT PROVENZA, PH.D., F.A.C.D.
Professor and Chairman, Department of Anatomy — Baltimore College of Dental Surgery, University of Maryland School of Dentistry.

ROBERT W. PUMPER, B.A., M.S.C., PH.D.
Professor, Departments of Microbiology and Immunology — University of Illinois College of Medicine, Chicago. Consultant, Department of Pathology — St. James Hospital, Chicago Heights, Illinois. Diplomate — American Society of Microbiology. Certified — Public Health Virology.

JOHN W. RIPPON, PH.D.
Associate Professor, Department of Medicine (Dermatology) — University of Chicago. Director, Mycology Service Laboratory — University of Chicago Hospitals.

JOSEPH I. ROUTH, PH.D.
Professor Emeritus, Department of Biochemistry — University of Iowa, Iowa City.

WILLIAM G. SHAFER, D.D.S., M.S.
Distinguished Professor and Chairman, Department of Oral Pathology — Indiana University School of Dentistry, Indianapolis.

RICHARD G. TOPAZIAN, D.D.S.
Professor and Chairman, Department of Oral and Maxillofacial Surgery, School of Dental Medicine; Professor of Surgery, School of Medicine — University of Connecticut, Farmington.

WILLIAM J. UPDEGRAVE, D.D.S.
Director, Department of Dental Radiology — The L. D. Pankey Institute for Advanced Dental Education, Miami, Florida. Professor Emeritus, Department of Radiology — Temple University School of Dentistry, Philadelphia, Pennsylvania.

ROBERT L. VANARSDALL, JR., B.A., D.D.S.
Director, Post Doctoral Orthodontics; Associate Professor, Departments of Orthodontics and Periodontics — University of Pennsylvania School of Dental Medicine, Philadelphia. Staff Member — Children's Hospital of Philadelphia, Albert Einstein Medical Center, Philadelphia, Pennsylvania.

*RUSSELL C. WHEELER, D.D.S., F.A.C.D.
Formerly, Visiting Professor and Research Professor in Dental Anatomy and Physiology — Washington University School of Dentistry, St. Louis, Missouri.

RUSSELL T. WOODBURNE, PH.D.
Professor Emeritus, Department of Anatomy — University of Michigan, Ann Arbor.

---

*Deceased.

The Language of Medicine and Dentistry — An Introductory Note

Western medicine had its origin in Greece in the fifth century B.C., in the Age of Pericles. When the Greek physician Hippocrates (430–370? B.C.) established the scientific and ethical principles of medicine basic elements of the language of medicine were already formulated. Thus, Greek was the original language of modern medicine, and, by extension, of dentistry.

With the Roman conquest of Greece, bringing to an end the Hellenic Era, Greek gave way to Latin. By the time Christ was born, Latin was already established in Europe and in parts of Asia and Africa — first, as the language of the Roman conquerors, and later, spreading to local populations.

During the fourth century A.D., Latin also replaced Greek as the official language of the Church. As Christianity spread gradually throughout Europe to become the principal religion, Latin became the first (and probably the last) universal language by means of which scholars of all nations of what was then known as the civilized world could communicate with each other. It served in this capacity for more than 1500 years, almost into the twentieth century.

This is not to say that everyone spoke the same Latin. The language of the streets of Rome, Vulgar Latin, was obviously different from that used by classical writers in many respects. And the speech of local populations in remote outposts of the Empire, who learned Latin from the Roman legionnaires, must have been different from that spoken in Rome. Also, similar to what occurs now, different branches of learning and technology developed jargons to suit their specific requirements. This was especially true with the language of medicine.

In ancient Rome, which had little medical tradition of its own, physicians were mostly itinerant Greek healers during the Hellenic Era and imported Greek slaves (*servi medici*) after the Roman conquest of Greece. One would assume that these reluctant immigrants learned Latin (called a language of barbarians by the Greek intellectuals of the time) without much enthusiasm. They borrowed heavily from Greek whenever the need arose, eventually developing a jargon that was a mixture of Latin and Greek words with superimposed Latin syntax, which was in many ways similar to the patois spoken by immigrant populations everywhere.

Although the basis for medical terminology was established during the Hellenic Era, and an impressive medical vocabulary (much of it still in use) existed before the fall of the Roman Empire, the development of the language of medicine, as we know it today, did not actually begin until the works of da Vinci, Vesalius, and other anatomists of the Renaissance identified and described parts of the human body; thus laying the foundation for a systematic anatomical nomenclature that is the base for modern medical and dental terminology.

As used in the United States and other English-speaking countries, anatomical terminology exists in two parallel forms: one that is official, composed of Latin and some Greek words, and one that is unofficial, composed of Latin, Greek, and English words, some of which are Anglicized forms of Latin and Greek.

The first, the official, internationally recognized terminology identifies preferred anatomical names (eliminating those that are erroneous, ambiguous, or duplicate), organizes anatomical nomenclature into accepted hierarchical classifications and schemes, and serves as the paradigm and authority for national anatomical terminologies. This official Latin and Greek terminology is maintained and controlled by the International Anatomical Committee and is listed in the publication *Nomina Anatomica.*These terms are usually identified in the literature, especially in dictionaries, with the abbreviation NA.

The second, unofficial terminology, is that which is commonly used in the medical and dental literature of individual countries. In English-speaking countries, older, gross anatomy terms are usually in English, whereas names of organs that were identified later, fine structures for which English equivalents are lacking, and parts of the body for which there are no "polite" English words are in Latin and Greek. Thus, names of organs such as the *skin, neck, liver, kidney,* or *tooth* are in English (their official NA equivalents are *cutis, cervix, hepar, ren,* and *dens,* respectively), whereas names for organs that were described relatively late, such as *reticulum, epithelium, cerebellum, sinus,* and *neuron,* are in Latin or Greek. Also, Latin or Greek is used for such terms as *penis, anus,* and *vagina,* which are considered "nicer" than their English counterparts. Terms in the last two categories are also in the official (NA) terminology.

Many older English anatomical terms, such as *sweetbread, gristle,* and *sinew,* have been either discarded or are now used only in connection with animal tissues and organs, and their sometimes Anglicized Latin counterparts (*pancreas, cartilage,* and *tendon,* respectively) are considered as proper terms in human anatomy.

The majority of Latin and Greek anatomical terms now in use had no original anatomical meaning; they have been borrowed from the general vocabulary. *Pons,* for instance, is Latin for bridge; *reticulum* is a diminutive for *rete,* a Latin word for net; nerve derives from Latin *nervus,* in turn Latinized from Greek *neuron,* bowstring; and *testis* is Latin for witness (believed to have originated from an ancient custom of a man taking an oath with his hand on his testicle).

The majority of Greek names are not recognized in *Nomina Anatomica* as official anatomical terms. Nevertheless, they are essential to the language of medicine, particularly in forming compound nonanatomical terms and adjectives, as in *odontalgia* (toothache) and *odontoid* (resembling a tooth), both terms deriving from Greek *odous* (a tooth), a non-NA term.

English nouns are often used to modify other nouns, as when referring to the breaking of a tooth, *tooth fracture.* The same concept can be also expressed as *dental fracture,* in which the NA term for tooth (*dens*) is used and is modified to the adjectival form by an appropriate suffix. Generally, Latin and Greek anatomical names are modified when used as adjectives in English sentences, but there are exceptions: one correctly refers to *maxillary injury* (instead of *maxilla injury*) and *cranial tumor* (instead of *cranium tumor*), but *sinus infection* is preferable to *sinusal infection,* and both *sternum fracture* and *sternal region* are acceptable.

Some adjectives are used alone as nouns — *canine, incisor,* and *molar teeth* are usually referred to as *canines, incisors,* and *molars,* respectively. The *musculus biceps femoris* (NA) is usually called *biceps.* And many dental writers refer to *centric occlusion* as simply *centric.* This practice has its dangers, however. While one could correctly conclude that *temporal fracture* applies to the temporal bone, referring to injury of the temporal bone as *temporal injury* would be ambiguous, for the injury could apply to the temporal artery, nerve, or region, as well as to the temporal bone. Perhaps, *temporal bone injury* would have been more appropriate.

Much of the language of medicine and dentistry consists of composite terms in which stems derived from Latin and Greek anatomical names are appended with prefixes and suffixes. Generally, although there are many exceptions, prefixes denote sites, locations, and orientation, and suffixes indicate conditions, states, techniques, and devices.

Names of pathological conditions of the tongue, as an example, are produced by appending the anatomical stems *gloss-* or *glosso-* (Greek *glōssa,* tongue) with suffixes, such as *-pathy* (Greek *pathos,* suffering), to denote general pathological conditions, *-itis* to denote inflammation, *-algia* (Greek *algos,* pain) to denote painful conditions, or *-plegia* (Greek *plēgē,* stroke) to denote paralysis.

Surgical terms may be formed by adding to the same stem suffixes, such as *-ectomy* (Greek *ektomē,* excision), *-tomy* (Greek *tomē,* a cutting), or *-rrhaphy* (Greek *rhaphē,* suture). Synonymous terms may be constructed when both Latin and Greek names for the same organ are used in the stem, as in *gingivitis* (Latin *gingiva* + Greek *-itis*) and *gingivectomy* (Latin *gingiva* + Greek *-ectomy*), which are also called *ulitis* (Greek *oulon,* gingiva + *-itis*) and *ulectomy* (*oulon* + *-ectomy*).

The name of the instrument *glossodynamometer* (for recording the power of the tongue to resist pressure) originates from *glosso-* + *dynamometer;* the latter, in turn, derives from Greek *dynamis,* power, and *metron,* measure.

Names of neoplasms are formed by combining anatomical or histological designations characteristic of tumors with the suffix *-oma,* as in *osteoma* (a tumor composed of bony tissue), which derives from Greek *osteon,* bone, + *-oma.*

Terms relating to several organs are built on stems constructed from several anatomical names. A disease involving the stomach, intestine, liver, and kidney, for example, would have a stem *-gastroenterohepatonephro-,* deriving from Greek *gastēr* (stomach), *enteron* (intestine), *hepar* (liver), and *nephros* (kidney), to which prefixes and suffixes may be appended as needed.

Not all pathological terms are formed by combining anatomical names with appropriate prefixes or suffixes. *Tetanus* (muscle spasm) has its origin in the time of Hippocrates, when it was known as *tetanos*, and *diabetes* derives from Greek *diabētēs* (a syphon, from *dia*, through, and *beinein* to go). Some terms derive from modern European languages, such as *jaundice* (French *jaune*, yellow). Many names identify diseases and their pathogenic organisms, such as salmonellosis (*Salmonella*, a bacterial genus, + *-osis*, a suffix denoting a process, often a disease), or by their symptoms, as in *pruritus* (Latin *prurire*, to itch).

Many terms in medicine and dentistry are eponymous; that is, they are named after persons or other proper nouns. A livid appearance of the face indicative of approaching death is known as *facies hippocratica*, named after Hippocrates, who is said to have been first to describe the condition. Other examples are *Begg appliance*, an orthodontic appliance named after its inventor, *Christmas disease*, a hemorrhagic condition named after the patient in whom it was first observed, and *Tangier disease*, named after an island in the Chesapeake Bay, where the disease was first reported. Often, eponyms are used with syndromes or other pathological conditions that cannot be readily defined with self-explanatory designations.

The term *syndrome* (Greek *syndromē*, concurrence) traditionally was defined as a set of symptoms, usually three or more, which occur together; but, in current usage, it is applied to any condition that cannot be easily defined and is characterized by complex etiology, involvement of several organs or systems, and varied symptomatology. *Otopalatodigital syndrome* is self-explanatory, but nothing about the nature of *Recklinghausen syndrome* can be discerned from its eponymic name (first described by the German physician Friedrich Daniel von *Recklinghausen*). *LEOPARD syndrome* is an acronym for an unmanageably long designation: *l*entigines, *e*lectrocardiographic abnormalities, *o*cular hypertelorism, *p*ulmonary stenosis, *a*bnormalities of genitalia, *r*etardation of growth, and *d*eafness. In addition, the term *syndrome* is now often appended to names of organs that are believed to be the source of complex pathological conditions (e.g., *brachial syndrome*) and to names of already well-known conditions that are believed to be more complex than originally suspected (e.g., *tuberculosis syndrome, hypertension syndrome, diabetes syndrome*).

Bacteriological nomenclature follows the method for naming plants and animals established in 1735 by the Swedish naturalist Karl von Linné (who Latinized his name to Linnaeus). Names of bacteria are created by Latinizing eponyms and Greek words and with the use of some original Latin names. For instance, the colon bacterium, *Escherichia coli*, is named after its discoverer, Theodor *Escherich*, and *Streptococcus* derives its name from Greek *streptos*, twisted, and Latin *coccus*, which is a Latinized form of Greek *kokkos*, a berry.

The kingdom, orders, and families of bacteria are always in the plural form, the genus in the singular form, and species in the genitive form — all according to the Latin rules of grammar.

Traditionally, plant and animal viruses were named after diseases that they cause, the term *virus* modifying the name of the condition, as in *smallpox virus*. Bacterial viruses, or bacteriophages, on the other hand, were named by attaching the suffix *-phage* (Greek *phagein*, to eat) to the name of the host organism, as in *coliphage* (*colibacillus* + *-phage*), and complemented by code symbols, such as T1, C16, S13, etc. Later, efforts were made to name viruses according to certain criteria, such as the characteristics of the host, properties of the virion, or the features of the reproductive cycle. Recently, plant pathologists proposed a taxonomy based on the Linnean method, whereby the order Virales would encompass all viruses. The order would be subdivided into families, genera, and species. At the same time, the International Committee on Nomenclature of Viruses proposed a taxonomic system for naming viruses with generic names appended with an ending *-virus* (e.g., *Rhinovirus*, from Greek *rhis*, nose, + *-virus*), complemented by a parallel method, whereby viruses would be designated with cryptograms describing each virus according to a conventional key. In spite of many proposals, the problem of virus nomenclature and taxonomy still remains in a state of flux.

Terms generated by combining word fragments drawn from the list of already existing anatomical names and standard prefixes and suffixes are self-explanatory, and precisely define complex concepts that otherwise would require whole sentences, or even paragraphs, in a manner that is readily understood by physicians and dentists across language barriers and millennia apart. The number of these combinations being almost infinite, the potential biomedical vocabularly is, thus, virtually limitless. Herein lies the genius of the Greek fathers of the language of medicine. They have created a language unsurpassed in its simplicity, utility, economy, even beauty, which, in its basic form, has survived two millennia of linguistic evolution, numerous changes in medical philosophy, and the enormous growth of terminology brought about by constantly expanding scientific discovery. It has also survived the decline of its parent tongues as universal languages of learning, continuing to grow even at a time when its practitioners no longer possess a basic classical background.

Since everything in the environment influences in some way our health and well-being, terminologies in all branches of science, technology, social and behavioral study, administration, etc., technically belong in the language of medicine and dentistry. Each of these terminologies has its own history, mechanism for growth, and other characteristics with which students of biomedical disciplines must have some familiarity. The space allotted in this Dictionary does not allow for discussion of the entire field of scientific and technical linguistics, only those aspects that influence directly human, particularly oral, health, or the core of the language of medicine and dentistry.

STANLEY JABLONSKI

Annandale, Virginia

Acknowledgments

This Dictionary represents an effort to which many have contributed. The total number of persons who have been helpful is far too great to be listed here, but I would like to acknowledge my gratitude for the most important contributions to this endeavor.

I am deeply indebted to the scientific consultants who, in spite of their crowded schedules, generously offered their services in the preparation of the manuscript and reviewed its contents for accuracy and to ensure that it represents the thinking of the profession of dentistry. I take great pleasure in presenting a complete list of the consultants on page ix.

It would have been impossible to write this Dictionary without my having access to collections of the National Library of Medicine. I am most grateful to its Director, Dr. Martin M. Cummings, for making these collections available to me. I also wish to acknowledge the support, encouragement, and help received from my former colleagues at the National Library of Medicine. I would especially like to express my appreciation to Estelle Abrams, Albert Berkowitz, Lois Blaine, Mary Hantzes, Dr. Joseph Leiter, Grace McCarn, Robert Mehnert, Theodore Webster, and members of the staff of the Circulation Control Section, who guided me expertly and with great patience through intricate pathways of the Library collections. My special thanks go to Dr. Maria Farkas, Daniel Carangi, Ruth Stander, and Geraldine Nowak.

Kind cooperation received from the American Dental Association throughout the many years of the preparation of this Dictionary is very much appreciated, and my thanks go to Aletha A. Kowitz, Director of the Bureau of the Library Services, Dr. Donald Washburne, former Director of the Bureau, Ruth D. Schultz, James Sweeney, the late Dr. George Timke, and Drs. Thomas Ginley, Richard Tiecke, and John Hafferen.

I am grateful to Heather Lang-Runtz of the Canadian Dental Association for her cooperation in providing me with the organization, functions, and objectives of the Association.

CONTENTS

A

A 1. subspinale. 2. accommodation. 3. Ångstrom UNIT. 4. mass NUMBER. 5. BLOOD GROUP A.

Å Ångström UNIT.

a. accommodation; ampere; anode; anterior; aqua; arteria; total acidity.

a- 1. [Gr.] an inseparable prefix signifying want or absence; appears as *an* before stems beginning with a vowel or with *h*. 2. [L.] a prefix signifying separation, or away from.

α the first letter of the Greek alphabet. See ALPHA.

ĀĀ, aa [Gr. *ana* of each] abbreviation used in prescription writing, following the names of two or more ingredients and signifying "of each."

AAAS American Association for the Advancement of Science.

AADE 1. American Association of Dental Editors. 2. American Association of Dental Examiners.

AADGP American Academy of Dental Group Practice (see under ACADEMY).

AADP American Academy of Denture Prosthetics.

AADPA American Academy of Dental Practice Administration (see under ACADEMY).

AADR American Academy of Dental Radiology (see under ACADEMY).

AADS American Association of Dental Schools (see under ASSOCIATION).

AAE American Association of Endodontists.

AAFP American Academy of Family Physicians.

AAGFO American Academy of Gold Foil Operators (see under ACADEMY).

AAGO American Academy of Gnathologic Orthopedics (see under ACADEMY).

AAGP American Academy of General Practice.

AAHD American Association of Hospital Dentists (see under ASSOCIATION).

AAID American Academy of Implant Dentistry (see under ACADEMY).

AAMC American Association of Medical Colleges.

AAMI Association for the Advancement of Medical Instrumentation.

AAMP American Academy of Maxillofacial Prosthetics (see under ACADEMY).

AAMRL American Association of Medical Record Librarians.

AAO American Association of Orthodontists (see under ASSOCIATION).

AAOGP American Academy of Orthodontics for the General Practitioner (see under ACADEMY).

AAOM American Academy of Oral Medicine (see under ACADEMY).

AAOP American Academy of Oral Pathology (see under ACADEMY).

AAP 1. American Academy of Pediatrics. 2. American Academy of Pedodontics (see under ACADEMY). 3. American Academy of Periodontology (see under ACADEMY).

AAPA American Academy of Physician Assistants.

AAPHD American Association of Public Health Dentists (see under ASSOCIATION).

Aarane trademark for *cromolyn sodium* (see under CROMOLYN).

Aaron of Alexandria [7th century A.D.] a physician who wrote medical works in the Syriac language, all of which are lost except fragments (e.g., on smallpox) preserved by Rhazes.

Aarskog's syndrome [D. *Aarskog*] see under SYNDROME.

Aarskog-Scott syndrome [D. *Aarskog*] Aarskog's SYNDROME.

AAS American Analgesia Society (see under SOCIETY).

Aasse's syndrome [J. M. *Aasse*] see under SYNDROME.

AAV adenoassociated VIRUS.

AAV, primate adenoassociated viruses isolated from primates.

AAV-2, AAV-3 types of primate adenoassociated viruses (see under VIRUS) found in man.

AB 1. BLOOD GROUP AB. 2. apiobuccal.

A.B. abbreviation for L. *Ar'tium Baccalau'reus,* Bachelor of Arts.

ab antibody.

ab- [L. *ab* of, off] a prefix signifying from, off, away from.

Abacin trademark for a mixture of sulfamethoxazole and trimethoprim.

abacterial (ab″ak-te′re-al) nonbacterial; free from bacteria.

abamp abampere.

abampere (ab-am′pĕr) in the centimeter-gram-second system, a unit of electromagnetic current equivalent to 10 amperes; absolute ampere. Abbreviated *abamp*.

abandonment (ah-ban′don-ment) 1. giving up; leaving completely; forsaking. 2. the unilateral severance by the dentist or physician of the professional relationship between himself or herself and the patient without reasonable notice and at a time when there is still the need for continuing professional care.

Abano Pietro d' see PETER OF ABANO.

abarticular (ab″ar-tik′u-lar) 1. not affecting the joint. 2. remote from a joint.

abarticulation (ab″ar-tik″u-la′shun) [*ab-* + L. *articulatio* joint] dislocation of a joint.

abasia (ah-ba′zhe-ah) [*a* neg + Gr. *basis* step + *-ia*] inability to walk.

abate (ah-bāt′) to lessen or decrease.

abatement (ah-bāt′ment) [Fr. *abatre* to throw down] decrease in the severity of symptoms or pain.

abaxial (ab-ak′se-al) [*ab-* + L. *axis*] not situated at the axis.

Abbé flap see under FLAP.

Abbé-Estlander operation see under OPERATION.

Abbe's condenser (illuminator) [Karl Ernst *Abbe,* German physicist, 1840–1905] see under CONDENSER.

Abbe-Zeiss counting chamber [K. E. *Abbe;* Carl *Zeiss,* German optician, 1816–1888] Thoma-Zeiss counting CHAMBER.

Abbocillin V trademark for *penicillin V hydrabamine* (see under PENICILLIN).

Abbot's paste [William *Abbot,* British physician, born 1831] see under PASTE.

ABC axiobuccocervical.

abcoulomb (ab-koo′lom) in the centimeter-gram-second system, a unit of electricity equivalent to 10 coulombs. Called also *absolute coulomb.*

Abderhalden-Fanconi syndrome [Emil *Abderhalden,* Swiss physiologist, 1877–1950; Guido *Fanconi,* Swiss biochemist, born 1892] see under SYNDROME.

Abderhalden-Kaufmann-Lignac syndrome [E. *Abderhalden;* G. O. E. *Lignac*] Abderhalden-Fanconi SYNDROME.

abdomen (ab-do′men) [L., possibly from *abdere* to hide] that portion of the body which lies between the thorax and the pelvis.

ABDPH American Board of Dental Public Health (see under BOARD).

abducens (ab-du′senz) [L. "drawing away"] an adjective used in conjunction with names of anatomical structures, such as nerves or muscles, which serve to abduct a part of the body.

abducent (ab-du′sent) [L. *abducens*] abducting, or effecting a separation, as an abducent nerve.

abduct (ab-dukt′) [*ab-* + L. *ducere* to draw] to draw away from the median plane or (in the digits) from the axial line of a limb.

abduction (ab-duk′shun) [L. *abductio*] drawing or leading away from the axis of the body.

abductor (ab-duk′tor) [L.] that which abducts or leads away from the axis of the body.

ABE American Board of Endodontics (see under BOARD).

Aberel trademark for *tretinoin.*

aberrant (ab-er′ant) [L. *aberrans,* from *ab* + *errare* to wander] 1. wandering. 2. deviating from the normal.

aberratio (ab″er-a′she-o) [L.] aberration.

aberration (ab″er-a′shun) [*ab-* + L. *errare* to wander] 1. any deviation from the normal. 2. unequal refraction or focalization of light rays by a lens. **angle of a.,** ANGLE of deviation. **chromatic a.,** unequal deviation of light rays of different wavelengths passing through a refractive medium, resulting in fringes of

color around the image produced. Called also *newtonian a.*
chromatic a., lateral, difference in magnification due to differences in position of the principal points for light of different wavelengths; also, a difference of focal point. **chromatic a., longitudinal,** difference in position along the axis for the focal points of light, produced by unequal deviation of light rays of different wavelengths by a lens. **chromosomal a.,** one affecting a single chromosome. **chromosome a.,** CHROMOSOME aberration. **dioptric a., spherical a. meridional,** unequal refraction of light rays as a result of variation of refractive power in different portions of the same meridian of a lens. **newtonian a.,** chromatic a. **penta-X chromosomal a.,** one in which there are five X chromosomes in a female. **spherical a.,** zonal aberration in relation to an axial point. Called also *dioptric a.* **spherical a., negative,** unequal refraction of light rays by a lens, those passing through the outer zones of the lens being focused farther from the lens than those passing through the central zones. **spherical a., positive,** unequal refraction of light rays by a lens, those passing through the outer zones of the lens being focused closer to the lens than those passing through the central zones. **tetra-X chromosomal a.,** one in which there are four X chromosomes in a female. **triple-X chromosomal a.,** one in which there are three X chromosomes in a female. **zonal a.,** unequal refraction of light rays by a lens, the rays passing through different zones being focused at different distances from the lens.

abetalipoproteinemia (a-ba″tah-lip″o-pro″te″in-e′me-ah) acanthocytosis.

ABG axiobuccogingival.

abient (ab′e-ent) avoiding the source of stimulation; said of a response to a stimulus or stimulation. Cf. ADIENT.

abiogenesis (ab″e-o-jen′ĕ-sis) [*a* neg. + Gr. *bios* life + Gr. *genesis* generation] the spontaneous generation of life. Cf. BIOGENESIS.

abiology (a″bi-ol′o-je) [*a* neg. + Gr. *bios* life + *-logy*] the study of nonliving things.

abionergy (ab″e-on′er-je) [*a* neg. + Gr. *bios* life + Gr. *ergon* work] abiotrophy; hypotrophy.

abiotrophy (ab″e-ot′ro-fe) [*a* neg. + Gr. *bios* life + Gr. *trophē* nutrition] trophic failure; loss of vitality; degeneration of vital functions. Called also *abionergy* and *hypotrophy*.

abirritant (ab-ir′rĭ-tant) [*ab-* + L. *irritans* irritating] 1. soothing; relieving irritation. 2. an agent which relieves irritation.

ABL axiobuccolingual.

ablastemic (a″blas-tem′ik) [*a* neg. + Gr. *blastēma* a shoot] not germinal.

ablate (ab-lāt′) [L. *ablatus* removed] to remove.

ablatio (ab-la′she-o) [L.] ablation.

ablation (ab-la′shun) [L. *ablatio*] 1. separation or detachment. 2. removal of a part; excision.

abluent (ab′lu-ent) [*ab-* + L. *luens* washing] 1. cleansing. 2. a cleansing agent.

ablution (ab-lu′shun) [L. *ablutio* washing] washing; cleansing.

abmortal (ab-mor′tal) situated or directed away from a dead or injured part.

abnerval (ab-ner′val) away from a nerve; specifically, passing of electric currents through a muscle away from the point of attachment of its nerve. Called also *abneural.*

abneural (ab-nu′ral) [*ab-* + Gr. *neuron* nerve] 1. away from the central nervous system; distant from the central nervous system. 2. abnerval.

abnormal (ab-nor′mal) [*ab-* + L. *norma* rule] not normal; differing from the usual.

abnormality (ab″nor-mal′ĭ-te) 1. any abnormal condition. 2. a defective quality of the body or an organ; a developmental anomaly; a malformation. See also ANOMALY, DEFORMITY, and MALFORMATION. **chromosome a.,** a CHROMOSOME aberration. **congenital a.,** a developmental anomaly present at birth. **dental a.,** dental ANOMALY. **dental a., eugnathic,** eugnathic ANOMALY. **dentofacial a.,** dentofacial ANOMALY. **drug-induced a.,** one caused in a fetus by maternal ingestion of toxic drugs. **dysgnathic a.,** dysgnathic ANOMALY. **eugnathic a., eugnathic dental a.,** eugnathic ANOMALY. **maxillofacial a.,** a deformity of the jaws and the facial structures, usually a developmental defect that may be genetically determined. See also dysgnathic ANOMALY. **multiple a.,** a developmental anomaly involving several organs or systems; co-occurrence of abnormalities involving several organs or systems, usually present at birth. **oral a.,** a defect, usually a developmental anomaly, involving oral structures other than the teeth. Called also *oral anomaly.*

ABO 1. see ABO blood groups, under BLOOD GROUP. 2. American Board of Orthodontics.

Abomacetin trademark for *erythromycin.*

ABOMS American Board of Oral and Maxillofacial Surgery (see under BOARD).

ABOP American Board of Oral Pathology (see under BOARD).

aborad (ab-o′rad) [*ab-* + L. *os* mouth] directed away from the mouth.

aboral (ab-o′ral) [*ab-* + L. *os* mouth] opposite to, away from, or remote from the mouth.

abortifacient (ah-bor″tĭ-fa′shent) [L. *abortio* abortion + *facere* to make] 1. causing abortion. 2. an agent which causes abortion; called also *abortient* and *aborticide.*

abortion (ah-bor′shun) [L. *abortio*] 1. the premature expulsion from the uterus of the products of conception. 2. premature stoppage of a natural or a morbid process.

abortive (ah-bor′tiv) [L. *abortivus*] 1. incompletely developed; premature. 2. incomplete; cut short. 3. abortifacient.

ABP 1. American Board of Pedodontics (see under BOARD). 2. American Board of Periodontology (see under BOARD). 3. American Board of Prosthodontics (see under BOARD). 4. arterial blood pressure; see blood PRESSURE.

abradant (ah-bra′dant) abrasive.

abrade (ah-brād′) [L. *abradere* to scrape off] to scrape, rub, or wear off; to rub away the external covering or layer of a part.

Abrami's disease [Pierre *Abrami,* French physician, 1879–1943] acquired hemolytic JAUNDICE.

abrasio (ah-bra′se-o) [L.] abrasion. **a. den′tium,** abrasion (2).

abrasion (ah-bra′zhun) [L. *abrasio*] 1. wearing away of a substance or structure through mechanical processes, such as grinding, rubbing, or scraping. 2. usually pathologic wearing away of the tooth substance by mastication, brushing, bruxism, clenching, and other mechanical causes. Called also *abrasio dentium.* See also ATTRITION, EROSION, and WEAR. 3. a denuded area on the body from which the skin or mucous membrane has been abraded. **betel nut a.,** excessive wearing of the crowns of teeth resulting from the chewing of betel nuts. **bobby pin a.,** notching in the incisal edges produced by the use of teeth to open bobby pins. **dentifrice a.,** abnormal wearing off of tooth substance, particularly the cementum and dentin of an exposed root, by brushing with an abrasive-containing dentifrice. **denture a.,** wearing away of a denture or its part due to improper finishing, faulty brushing, mastication, bruxism, or any other cause. **gingival a.,** a loss of gingiva due to injury caused by contact with coarse foods or other irritants, faulty brushing techniques, or any other physical cause, usually associated with inflammatory changes. **occupational a.,** excessive wearing away of the tooth substance due to any occupational cause, such as abrasive dust, holding nails between the teeth, the biting of thread, and similar causes. **tobacco a.,** excessive wearing of the crowns of teeth associated with tobacco chewing.

abrasive (ah-bra′siv) 1. causing abrasion. 2. an agent used for abrading, grinding, or polishing. In dentistry, abrasive particles are glued onto paper or plastic disks that are attached to a handpiece or bonded to grinding wheels and dental stones. Diamond chips are attached to steel wheels, disks, and cylinders which are driven by rotary instruments. Abrasive particles are graded on the basis of the fineness of the standard sieve through which they can pass, e.g., an abrasive graded as number 8 can pass through a sieve with eight meshes per inch. Some abrasives, e.g., silicon carbide, are graded as 8, 10, 12, 14, 16, 20, 24, 30, 36, 46, 60, 80, 90, 100, 120, etc. Finer abrasives are designated as powders or flours, and are graded in increasing fineness, as F, FF, FFF, etc., or in the case of impregnated papers, as 0, 00, 000, etc. Abrasives used most commonly in dentistry include ferric oxide (jeweler's rouge), stannic oxide (putty powder), pumice, and tripoli.

abrasor (ah-bra′zor) an instrument used for abrasion.

Abreu, Manoel de [1892–1962] a Brazilian physician who discovered the technique of photofluorography (sometimes called *abreuography* in his honor).

abreuography (ab″roo-og′rah-fe) photofluorography.

Abricycline trademark for *tetracycline* (1).

Abrikossoff, Aleksey Ivanovitch see ABRIKOSSOV.

Abrikossov's (Abrikossoff's) tumor [Aleksei Ivanovich *Abrikossov,* Russian pathologist, 1875–1955] myoblastoma.

abs- a prefix signifying away, from.

abs. feb. abbreviation for L. *absen′te feb′re,* while fever is absent.

abscess (ab′ses) [L. *abscessus,* from *ab* + *cedere* to go] a localized collection of pus in a tissue, organ, or confined space, commonly caused by infection with pyogenic bacteria. **acute a.,** one characterized by a short course, fever, and painful local inflammation. **alveolar a.,** apical a. **alveolar a., acute,** apical a., acute. **alveolar a., chronic,** apical a., chronic. **alveolar a., lateral,** lateral a. **apical a.,** inflammation of tissues surrounding the apical portion of a tooth, associated with the collection of pus, usually resulting from infection following pulp infection through a carious lesion, but sometimes also occurring as a result of an injury causing pulp necrosis. Severe pain and slight extrusion of the tooth from its socket are the principal symptoms. Complications may include lymphadenitis and extension to the bone marrow, resulting in osteomyelitis. Called also *alveolar a., dentoalveolar a., periapical a.,* and *apical pericementitis.* **apical a., acute,** an acute inflammatory reaction involving the tissues surrounding the apical portion of a tooth, characterized by rapid onset, acute pain, tenderness of the tooth to touch and pressure, pus formation, and swelling of tissues in a later stage. Pulpal necrosis may be a cause. Called also *acute alveolar a., acute dentoalveolar a.,* and *acute periapical a.* **apical a., chronic,** a chronic inflammatory reaction of the tissues surrounding the apical portion of a tooth, characterized by an intermittent discharge of pus through a sinus tract, with gradual onset, little or no swelling of the affected tissue, and slight discomfort, if any. Pulpal necrosis may be a cause. Called also *chronic alveolar a., chronic dentoalveolar a., chronic periapical a.,* and *suppurative apical periodontitis.* **Bezold's a.,** subperiosteal abscess of the temporal bone. **Bezold's a., internal,** a complication of acute suppurative otitis media, in which pus tracks anteriorly alongside the auditory tube to the pharynx, where a retropharyngeal abscess forms and eventually ruptures into the postnasal space. **bicameral a.,** one which has two chambers or pockets. See also *shirt-stud a.* **bone a.,** collection of pus in bone tissue. See OSTEOMYELITIS and suppurative PERIOSTITIS. **brain a.,** one affecting the brain, usually resulting from an extension of an infection, such as otitis media. **caseous a., cheesy a.,** one that contains cheesy matter. **circumscribed a.,** one limited by a layer of connective tissue. **circumtonsillar a.,** peritonsillar a. **cold a.,** one with little evidence of inflammation and fever; it is usually tuberculous. See also SCROFULA. **collar-button a.,** shirt-stud a. **cornual a.,** one in the coronal pulp tissue, usually associated with a pulp horn. See also suppurative PULPITIS. **deep a.,** one occurring below the deep fascia. **Delpech's a.,** a rapidly developing abscess accompanied by great prostration but little fever. **dental a.,** an abscess in or about a tooth. **dentoalveolar a.,** apical a. **dentoalveolar a., acute,** apical a., acute. **dentoalveolar a., chronic,** apical a., chronic. **dry a.,** one that disappears without pointing or breaking. **emphysematous a.,** tympanic a. **encysted a.,** one in which pus is circumscribed in a serous cavity. **epidural a.,** extradural a. **extradural a.,** a brain abscess situated between the dura and the cranial bone. Called also *epidural a.* **follicular a.,** one developing in a follicle. **frontal a.,** a brain abscess situated in the frontal lobe. **gangrenous a.,** one associated with gangrene of the surrounding tissue. **gas a.,** tympanic a. **gingival a.,** a localized, painful, inflammatory lesion of the gingiva, usually having a sudden onset and limited generally to the marginal gingiva or interdental papilla. In the early stages, occurring as a red swelling with a smooth shiny surface, but within 24 to 48 hours, it is usually fluctuant and pointed, with a surface orifice from which purulent exudate may be expressed. The adjacent teeth are often sensitive to percussion. If permitted to progress, the lesion generally ruptures spontaneously. The lesion consists of a purulent focus in the connective tissue surrounded by diffuse infiltration of polymorphonuclear leukocytes, edematous tissue, and vascular engorgement. The surface epithelium presents intra- and extracellular edema, invasion by leukocytes, and ulceration. Irritation from foreign substances, such as a toothbrush bristle or hard food particles forcefully embedded into the gingiva, are the usual causes. See also *periodontal a.* and acute inflammatory gingival ENLARGEMENT. **glandular a.,** one formed around or within a lymph node. **gravitational a., gravity a.,** one in which pus gravitates to a lower or deeper portion of the body. **hemorrhagic a.,** one which contains blood. **hot a.,** an acute abscess with symptoms of local inflammation. **hypostatic a.,** wandering a. **idiopathic a.,** one due to unknown causes. **interradicular a.,** an alveolar abscess characterized by the collection of pus between the roots of a tooth. **intramastoid a.,** one within the mastoid process of the temporal bone. **lateral a., lateral alveolar a.,** an alveolar abscess characterized by the collection of pus at a side of the root. See *periodontal a.* **lymphatic a.,** one of a lymph node. **mastoid a.,** one within the mastoid portion of the temporal bone. **mediastinal a.,** one within the tissues and organs of the mediastinum. **metastatic a.,** a secondary abscess, usually of embolic origin, in which organisms are carried by the circulation to a point distant from the primary lesion. **migrating a.,** wandering a. **miliary a.,** one of a group of small multiple abscesses. **mother a.,** a primary abscess from which other abscesses arise. **multiple a.,** one of a group of many abscesses. **ossifluent a.,** one dependent on a breaking down of bone tissue. **Paget's a.,** one recurring about the residue of a former abscess. **palatal a.,** an apical abscess of a maxillary tooth that erupts or extends toward the palate. **parietal a.,** periodontal a. **parotid a.,** one within the parotid gland. **periapical a.,** apical a. **periapical a., acute,** apical a., acute. **periapical a., chronic,** apical a., chronic. **pericoronal a.,** one around the crown of a partially erupted tooth. **peridental a.,** periodontal a. **periodontal a.,** a localized collection of purulent inflammatory material in the periodontal tissue, which may occur along the lateral aspect of the root, being a deep extension of infection from a periodontal pocket into the supporting tissue; in the cul-de-sac of a complex pocket with a tortuous course, being shut off from the surface; or in a pocket in which drainage is impaired. Common causes include incomplete removal of calculus during therapy of a periodontal pocket, where the gingival wall shrinks and occludes the pocket orifice, tooth injury, or perforation of the lateral wall of the root in endodontic therapy. Periodontal abscesses are classified according to their location as abscesses of the supporting periodontal tissue and abscesses of the soft tissue wall of a periodontal pocket; and according to their clinical course, as acute or chronic. Called also *lateral a., lateral alveolar a., parietal a.,* and *peridental a.* **periodontal infrabony a., acute,** a localized suppurative tissue infection in the gingival corium, infrabony pocket, or periodontal tissue, presenting an ovoid elevation of the gingiva along the lateral aspect of the root. The gingiva becomes edematous and red, with a smooth shiny surface. The shape of the lesion may vary, from domelike and relatively firm to pointed and soft. Pus may be expressed from the gingival margin. Throbbing radiating pain, tenderness of the gingiva to palpation, sensitivity of the tooth to percussion, tooth mobility, lymphadenitis, and systemic manifestations, such as fever, leukocytosis, and malaise, may be associated. Occasionally, an acute abscess may occur without notable symptoms. **periodontal infrabony a., chronic,** a localized collection of inflammatory material in the gingival corium, infrabony pocket, or periodontal tissue, usually presenting a sinus opening into the gingival mucosa near the gingival margin or, less frequently, an encapsulated lesion, characterized by a protracted, but largely asymptomatic, course. The pinpoint orifice of the sinus is usually covered by a minute pink, beadlike mass of granulation tissue. Some cases are characterized by episodes of dull gnawing pain, slight elevation of the tooth, and a desire to bite down and grind the affected tooth. Some chronic abscesses undergo acute exacerbation with all the associated symptoms. **peritonsillar a.,** one in the connective tissue of the tonsil capsule, resulting from suppuration of the tonsil. Called also *circumtonsillar a., angina phlegmonosa, angina tonsillaris,* and *quinsy.* **phlegmonous a.,** one associated with inflammation of the connective tissue. **phoenix a.,** a periodontal abscess which, after a period of latency, suddenly becomes symptomatic, the symptoms being identical to those of acute apical abscess. Symptoms may develop spontaneously following chronic apical periodontitis or, more commonly, after the initiation of endodontic treatment. Named after the phoenix of Egyptian mythology. **primary a.,** one developed at the seat of the infection. **pulp a., pulpal a.,** an acute or chronic inflammation of the dental pulp, associated with a circumscribed collection of necrotic tissue and pus arising from breakdown of leukocytes and bacteria, sometimes walled off with connective tissue. See also acute PULPITIS. **pyemic a.,** a constitutional abscess due to pyemia. **radicular a.,** one developing at the apex of the root of a tooth. **residual a.,** one seated near the residue of a former inflammation. **retropharyngeal a.,** a suppurative inflammation of the lymph nodes in the posterior and lateral walls of the pharynx. Called also *hippocratic angina.* **retrotonsillar a.,** one behind a tonsil, caused by any of the common pyogenic bacteria, usually occurring with or closely following acute tonsillitis or pharyngitis. **root a.,** a chronic or acute pustular condition affecting the supporting structures of the root of a tooth; when it is of endodontic origin, called *periapical abscess;* when periodontal in origin, called *periodontal abscess.* **satellite a.,** a secondary abscess arising from a primary one and situated near the latter. **scrofulous a.,** tuberculous a. **secondary a.,** one occurring as the result of another process. **septicemic a.,** one resulting from septicemia. **shirt-stud a.,** a superficial bicameral abscess in which a superficial pocket is connected with a deeper one by a passage. Called also *collar-button a.* **sterile a.,** one which contains no microorganisms. **stitch a.,** one which develops adjacent to a stitch or suture. **strumous a.,** tuberculous a. **subdural a.,** a brain abscess situated beneath the dura mater. **subfascial a.,** one situated beneath a fascia. **sudoriparous a.,** one arising in a sweat gland. **superficial a.,** one occurring near the surface. **sympathetic a.,** one arising some distance from the exciting cause. **thecal a.,** one arising in an enveloping sheath, such as a tendon sheath. **Tornwaldt's a.,** an abscess of the adenoids, usually associated with adenoid hyperplasia. **traumatic a.,** one caused by traumatic injury. **tuberculous a.,** one caused by infection with *Mycobacterium tuberculosis.* Called also *cold a., scrofulous a.,* and *strumous a.* **tympanic a.,** one that contains air or gas. Called also *emphysematous a.* and *gas a.* **tympanocervical a.,** one arising in the tympanum and extending to the neck. **tympanomastoid a.,** one involving the tympanum and the mastoid. **verminous a.,** one which contains insect larvae or other animal parasites. **von Bezold's a.,** Bezold's a. **wandering a.,** one that burrows in the tissues and finally points at a distance from the site of origin. Called also *hypostatic a.* and *migrating a.* **worm a.,** one caused by or containing worms.

abscessus (ab-ses'us) [L.] abscess.

abscissa (ab-sis'ah) [*ab-* + L. *scindere* to cut] one of two coordinates, the other of which is called *ordinate,* used as a frame of reference. The abscissa is usually horizontal and the ordinate vertical and, when suitable values have been assigned to them, corresponding data can be plotted.

abscission (ab-sish'un) [*ab-* + L. *scindere* to cut] removal by cutting.

absconsio (ab-skon'se-o) pl. *absconsio'nes* [L.] the cavity of a bone receiving and concealing the head of another bone.

abscopal (ab-sko'p'l) pertaining to the effect that irradiation of a tissue has on a nonirradiated tissue.

Absentil trademark for *disulfiram.*

Absidia (ab-sid'e-ah) a genus of true fungi of the class Zygomycetes, species of which may cause mucormycosis.

absolute (ab'sol-lūt) [L. *absolutus,* from *absolvere* to set free] free from limitations; unlimited; free from impurities; uncombined.

absorbefacient (ab-sor″bĕ-fa'shent) [L. *absorbere* to absorb + *facere* to make] 1. causing or promoting absorption. 2. an agent that promotes absorption.

absorbent (ab-sor'bent) [L. *absorbens,* from *ab* away + *sorbere* to suck] 1. able to take in, or suck up and incorporate. 2. a tissue structure involved in absorption. 3. a chemically inert substance capable of absorbing dissolved or suspended substances, such as gases, toxins, or bacteria. See also PROTECTIVE.

absorptiometer (ab-sorp″she-om'ĕ-ter) [L. *absorptio* + Gr. *metron* measure] 1. an instrument for measuring the solubility of gases. 2. a device for measuring the layer of liquid absorbed between two glass plates: used as a hematoscope.

absorption (ab-sorp'shun) [L. *absorptio*] 1. the uptake of substances into or across tissues. See also ADSORPTION and SORPTION. 2. in radiology, the taking up of energy by matter with which the radiation interacts. In the process, the number of particles (or photons) entering a body of matter is reduced by interaction with the matter. Similarly, there is a reduction of the energy of a particle while traversing a body of matter, resulting in a reduction of the intensity of a beam of radiation, and often producing secondary radiation. Sometimes used erroneously as a synonym of *capture.* See also absorbed DOSE, RAD, and RADIATION. 3. the use of reagents to remove antigens or antibodies from a mixture. **a. coefficient,** absorption COEFFICIENT. **external a.,** the absorption of foods, poisons, or other agents through the skin or mucous membranes. **internal a.,** the normal absorption of nutrients in digestion. **parenteral a.,** absorption otherwise than through the digestive tract. See also parenteral HYPERALIMENTATION. **pathologic a.,** the absorption into the blood of any bodily excretion or product, such as pus or urine.

absorptive (ab-sorp'tiv) 1. capable of absorbing; absorbent. 2. pertaining to absorption.

abstergent (ab-ster'jent) [L. *abstergere* to cleanse] 1. a cleansing application or medicine. 2. cleansing or purifying.

abstract (ab'strakt) [L. *abstractum,* from *abstrahere* to draw off] 1. a powder made from a drug or its fluid extract with lactose, and brought to twice the strength of the original drug or extract. 2. a condensation or summary of a book, report, or case history. **discharge a.,** a summary description prepared when the patient is discharged from a hospital or other health facility, containing selected data about the patient's stay in the hospital, including diagnoses, services received, length of stay, source of payment, and demographic information.

abstraction (ab-strak'shun) [L. *abstractio* a drawing away, separation] 1. a condition marked by the teeth or other maxillary and mandibular structures being lower than their normal position, away from the occlusal plane, thereby lengthening the face. Cf. ATTRACTION (2). 2. the withdrawal of any ingredient from a compound. 3. the letting of blood.

abterminal (ab-ter'mĭ-nal) [*ab-* + L. *terminus* end] moving away from the terminus toward the center; said of electric currents in muscular substance.

Abulcasis, Abulkasim see ALBUCASIS.

abuse (ah-būs') [L. *abusio* misuse] misuse, particularly excessive use. **child a.,** battered CHILD. **drug a.,** the use of drugs inconsistent with established or acceptable medical practices, including their excessive, unnecessary, or recreational use. See also drug ADDICTION, drug DEPENDENCE, and HABITUATION.

abut (ah-but') to touch, adjoin, or border on.

abutment (ah-but'ment) 1. a plate where abutting occurs. 2. a part of a structure that sustains thrust or pressure. 3. a tooth or root used as an anchorage for either a fixed or a removable dental prosthesis, or any other device, such as an implant, serving the same purpose. See also abutment TOOTH and IMPLANT. **auxiliary a.,** secondary a. **a. groove,** abutment GROOVE. **implant a.,** that part of a subperiosteal or intraperiosteal implant which protrudes into the oral cavity and serves as an abutment for retaining and stabilizing a denture. Called also *abutment post.* See also implant POST. **implant a., subperiosteal, implant structure a.,** the protruding post of a subperiosteal implant, which serves for the retention or support of a denture. See also IMPLANT denture, implant SUPERSTRUCTURE, and subperiosteal IMPLANT. **intermediate a.,** a natural tooth or root, without other natural teeth in proximal contact, which is used as an abutment, in addition to two terminal abutments. Called also *pier.* **isolated a.,** an intermediate abutment, particularly one used to support a removable partial denture. **a. locator,** abutment LOCATOR. **multiple a.,** one resulting from the fixed splinting of two or more adjacent natural teeth to serve as a unit in the support and retention of a fixed or removable partial denture. **multirooted a.,** a multirooted tooth used as an abutment, or an abutment formed by splinting two teeth into a single support (*multiple a.*). **a. post,** 1. implant a. 2. implant POST. **primary a.,** a tooth used for the direct support of a denture. **secondary a.,** a natural tooth used in addition to the primary abutments to provide support or indirect retention for a removable partial denture. Called also *auxiliary a.* **subperiosteal implant a.,** implant a., subperiosteal. **terminal a.,** a natural tooth located at an extremity of a fixed partial denture and used for the support and retention of the prosthesis.

abvolt (ab-vōlt') in the centimeter-gram-second system, a unit of electromotive force equivalent to 10^{-8} volt; absolute volt.

abwatt (ab-wot') in the centimeter-gram-second system, a unit of power equal to 10^{-7} watt; absolute watt.

AC 1. air CONDUCTION. 2. alternating CURRENT. 3. anodal CLOSURE. 4. axiocervical.

Ac actinium.

a.c. abbreviation for L. *an'te ci'bum,* before meals.

ACA 1. American College of Angiology. 2. American College of Apothecaries.

Acacia (ah-ka'shah) [L.; Gr. *akakia*] a genus of leguminous shrubs or trees containing several species that yield substances of importance in pharmacology, such as acacia (gum arabic).

acacia (ah-ka'shah) a dried, gummy exudate from the stems and branches of several species of *Acacia,* containing chiefly calcium, magnesium, and potassium salts of the polysaccharide arabic acid. It is soluble in water but not in alcohol. Used as a suspending agent for medicinal substances that are insoluble in water, in the preparation of emulsions, for making pills, and as a demulcent in the treatment of the throat and stomach. When used in blood substitutes and as a diuretic, it may cause various complications. Also used as an ingredient of denture adhesive powders. Called also *acacia gum, gum arabic,* and *senegal gum.*

academy (ah-kad'ah-me) [Gr. *Akadēmeia* the name of the gymnasium where Plato taught] 1. a school above the elementary level, usually supported by a private organization or a religious order. 2. a learned society of acknowledged leaders in their fields of endeavor, whose goal is advancement and excellence in the arts and sciences. See also COLLEGE. **American A. of Dental Group Practice,** an organization whose purpose is to improve the level of dental service provided by its members, limited to members of the American Dental Association, National Dental Association, or the organized national dental association of any foreign country. Its purposes include promotion of research; study and development of methods for the delivery of dental care; achievement of the proper recognition for the aims and goals of group practice; coordination of efforts with other organizations in order to further educational and philosophical advancements of the dental profession; and evaluation of the conduct, performance, and quality of dental practices through an accreditation system. Abbreviated *AADGP.* **American A. of Dental Practice Administration,** a professional organization of dentists whose objectives include encouragement and maintenance of the highest professional standard among its members; promotion of the study of all phases of dental practice administration; dissemination among its members and to the dental profession the knowledge thus gained; and acting as a guiding agency for the dissemination of dental education for the public welfare, in keeping with the principles of the American Dental Association. Abbreviated *AADPA.* **American A. of Dental Radiology,** a professional organization of dentists and professional workers in dental radiology, including nondentists and students, who are active in all aspects of dental radiology. Its purpose is the promotion and development of applications of the art and science of radiology in dentistry. Abbreviated *AADR.* **A. of Dentistry for the Handicapped,** a professional dental society whose goals and objectives include the education of professionals in the care of handicapped dental patients and the improvement of such care, and promotion and sponsoring of the literature dealing with the care for handicapped dental patients. Abbreviated *ADH.* **A. of Dentistry International,** a professional association of dentists established for the advancement of all phases of the science of dentistry on an international basis. Abbreviated *ADI.* **A. of General Dentistry,** a professional dental association established to represent the family dentist within the dental profession and to foster his or her continuing dental education. Abbreviated *AGD.* **American A. of Gnathologic Orthopedics,** a member of the Federation of Orthodontic Associations, open to dentists who have received certification from the Wiebrecht-Crozat Institute, Inc. Its purpose includes conducting programs, meetings, training, and advancing the Wiebrecht-Crozat science of developing functional occlusion. Abbreviated *AAGO.* **American A. of Gold Foil Operators,** a professional organization established for the promotion and use of compacted gold in restoring the hard structures of the mouth. Abbreviated *AAGFO.* **American A. of Implant Dentistry,** a professional organization of dentists who are engaged in implant dentistry, established to advance all phases of the science of dental implantology. Abbreviated *AAID.* **American A. of Maxillofacial Prosthetics,** a professional association having as its objective the accumulation and dissemination of knowledge and experience and the assistance in establishing and maintaining of research programs involving methods, techniques, and devices used in maxillofacial prosthetics. Abbreviated *AAMP.* **A. of Operative Dentistry,** a professional organization established to improve the standards of operative dentistry. Abbreviated *AOD.* **A. of Oral Dynamics,** a professional dental organization whose major objectives include teaching and promoting the use of the laws of nature, engineering principles, and their application to dentistry to acquire an optimum of force control in the human dentition in all phases of dentistry. Abbreviated *AOD.* **American A. of Oral Medicine,** a professional society of dentists having as its objectives the promotion of the study and dissemination of knowledge of the cause, prevention, and control of diseases of the teeth, their surrounding structures, and adnexa, and related subjects; the promotion of a closer medicodental relation to their studies; and the fostering and promotion of a better understanding between the fields of dentistry and medicine. Abbreviated *AAOM.* **American A. of Oral Pathology,** a professional organization whose objectives include promotion of the highest standards in education, research, and the practice of oral pathology; elevation of the scientific and professional status of those practicing this specialty of dentistry; advancement of the science of oral pathology and improvement of laboratory service to dentists, to hospitals, and to the public; encouragement of cooperation of oral pathologists with other dentists, with physicians, and with other pathology organizations and with medical technologists; helping to establish standards for the performance of laboratory procedures; improvement of the economic aspect of the practice of oral pathology; helping to maintain and strengthen the American Board of Oral Pathology; and helping in maintenance of the Registry of Dental and Oral Pathology of the American Registry of Pathology at the Armed Forces Institute of Pathology. Abbreviated *AAOP.* **American A. of Orthodontics for the General Practitioner,** a component society of the Federation of Orthodontic

Associations. Its major activities include: achieving, by mutual study and cooperative activities in the field of orthodontic research, a greater knowledge of the growth and development of the tissues of the teeth and adjacent parts from the point of view of the dentist in general practice; interchanging of ideas and stimulating interest in study and research among the fellow members; encouraging fellow dentists to plan a program of continuing education for better oral health and rehabilitation; aiding in maintaining a high standard of ethical practice for the control and prevention of malocclusion; promoting the ideals of the dental profession and all the professional groups allied with it for the advancement of the general welfare of the public; and carrying on all functions necessary to the successful operation of this organization. Abbreviated *AAOGP.* **American A. of Pedodontics,** a professional association of dentists whose primary concern is in the area of pedodontics, established for the advancement of the specialty of pedodontics. The Academy is the official sponsor of the American Board of Pedodontics. Abbreviated *AAP.* **American A. of Periodontology,** a professional dental association established to advance the art and science of periodontology. Abbreviated *AAP.* **International A. of Gnathology,** an international professional organization having objectives that include encouraging gnathologic research in institutions, or in foundations that may assist scientists to improve the education of dental students, dentists, physicians, and the laity in preventing and rectifying the ills and the faults of the organs of mastication. Abbreviated *IAG.*

acalcicosis (ah-kal″sĭ-ko′sis) a condition caused by dietary calcium deficiency.

Acamol trademark for *acetaminophen.*

acampsia (ah-kamp′se-ah) [a neg. + Gr. *kamptein* to bend + *-ia*] rigidity or inflexibility of a part or of a joint.

acanthesthesia (ah-kan″thes-the′ze-ah) [*acantho-* + Gr. *aisthēsis* sensation + *-ia*] perverted sensibility with a feeling as of pressure of a sharp point. See also PARESTHESIA.

acanthion (ah-kan′the-on) [Gr. *akanthion* little thorn] an osteometric landmark, being the tip of the anterior nasal spine. Abbreviated *ANS.*

acantho- [Gr. *akantha* a thorn or prickle] a combining form meaning thorny or spiny, or denoting a relationship to a sharp spine or thorn.

acanthocyte (ah-kan′tho-sīt) [*acantho-* + Gr. *kytos* cell] an abnormal erythrocyte showing irregularly spaced projections of various sizes and shapes; seen in acanthocytosis.

acanthocytosis (ah-kan″tho-si-to′sis) a hereditary syndrome, transmitted as a recessive trait, characterized by the presence of acanthocytes; retinitis pigmentosa; degenerative changes in the central nervous system involving the cerebellum and long tracts, with ataxia, areflexia, and demyelination; beta-lipoprotein deficiency; intestinal malabsorption; amaurosis; retarded growth; and crenation of the erythrocytes. Called also *abetalipoproteinemia* and *Bassen-Kornzweig syndrome.*

acanthoid (ah-kan′thoid) [*acantho-* + Gr. *eidos* form] resembling a spine; spinous.

acantholysis (ak″an-thol′ĭ-sis) [*acantho-* + Gr. *lysis* a loosening] detachment of the cells of the prickle layer of the skin, leading to the development of vesicles and bullae. **a. bullo′sa,** an old term for EPIDERMOLYSIS bullosa.

acanthoma (ak″an-tho′mah) [*acantho-* + *-oma*] a tumor composed of epidermal or squamous cells. **a. adenoi′des cys′ticum,** cystic adenoid EPITHELIOMA.

acanthosis (ak″an-tho′sis) [*acantho-* + *-osis*] hyperplasia or thickening of the prickle cell layer of the skin, such as is seen in a wart. **a. bullo′sa,** EPIDERMOLYSIS bullosa. **a. ni′gricans,** a rare disease characterized by hyperpigmentation and papillary hypertrophy, occurring most commonly on the neck, axillae, external genitalia, groin, face, inner thighs, hands, and breasts, which may involve the entire surface of the skin. When fully developed, the patches are deep black with shades of yellow and brown, and are more or less covered with nodules, papillomatous growths, and vegetating masses. It occurs in two forms: a juvenile form, which is usually benign, and an adult form, which is frequently associated with malignant tumors — usually adenocarcinoma of the stomach, less frequently of the gallbladder, ovary, pancreas, or other internal organs. The benign form may be genetically transmitted, dominant inheritance being the most common. Oral manifestations, which occur in about half the cases, include: hypertrophy and elongation of the papillae, which give the tongue a furrowed, shaggy, or prickly appearance and produce deep fissures; the lips may be covered by filiform or papillomatous growths, especially at the angles of the mouth; the gingivae may be enlarged, almost covering the teeth; the buccal mucosa, though usually less severely affected, may exhibit an uneven, velvety white appearance. Called also *keratosis nigricans.*

acapnia (ah-kap′ne-ah) [*a* neg. + Gr. *kapnos* smoke + *-ia*] absence or lack of carbon dioxide in the blood; commonly used to mean an abnormally decreased amount of carbon dioxide in the blood. See also HYPOCAPNIA. Cf. HYPERCAPNIA.

acarbia (ah-kar′be-ah) a condition in which the blood bicarbonate is lowered.

acaryote (ah-kăr′e-ōt) [*a* neg. + Gr. *karyon* kernel] akaryote.

acatalasemia (a″kat-ah-la-se′me-ah) [*a* neg. + *catalase* + Gr. *haima* blood + *-ia*] absence of catalase in the blood. See ACATALASIA.

acatalasia (a″kat-ah-la′ze-ah) a constitutional, congenital absence of the enzyme catalase, due to homozygosity for a mendelian gene. The condition has been observed in Japan and Switzerland. It may be asymptomatic, but is most commonly characterized by a relatively mild course and by the presence of small, painful, crateriform ulcers of the free gingiva, which appear in children as early as 2 to 3 years of age, and heal spontaneously. In a more severe form, there may be involvement of the entire gingiva, associated with recession and bone loss, resulting in loosening and exfoliation of teeth; lesions usually heal spontaneously after tooth extraction. In this form, the mandible or maxilla is affected, with gangrene, bony sequestration, and invasion of the nasal antrum. Called also *anenzymia catalasea* and *Takahara's syndrome.* Originally called *acatalasemia* because the absence of catalase was first detected in the red blood cells.

acatalepsia (ah-kat″ah-lep′se-ah) [*a* neg. + Gr. *katalēpsis* comprehension] 1. lack of understanding. 2. uncertainty of diagnosis.

acataposis (a-kat″ah-po′sis) [*a* neg. + Gr. *kata* down + *posis* drinking] an old term for DYSPHAGIA.

accelerant (ak-sel′er-ant) catalyst.

acceleration (ak-sel″er-a′shun) [L. *acceleratio*] quickening, hastening.

accelerator (ak-sel′er-a″tor) [L. "hastener"] 1. anything that hastens or increases the velocity of something or rate of a process. 2. any nerve or muscle which hastens the performance of a function. 3. any substance or agent which increases the rate of a chemical reaction. In vulcanization of rubber, it is usually an organic compound containing nitrogen and, sometimes, both nitrogen and sulfur, including amines, guanidines, thiazoles, thiuram sulfides, and dithiocarbamates, or inorganic substances, including lime, magnesium oxide, and lead oxide. The setting time of gypsum products is accelerated by substances such as sodium chloride, potassium sulfate, or syngenite. **a. factor, a. globulin,** FACTOR V. **linear a.,** an apparatus for the acceleration of subatomic particles, using alternating hollow electrodes in a straight vacuum tube, so arranged that when their high frequency potentials are properly varied the particles traveling through them receive successive increases in energy. It produces photons (x-rays) and electrons (negatively charged particles known as *beta rays*). **particle a.,** a device, such as a cyclotron, betatron, or linear accelerator, for imparting kinetic energy to electrically charged particles (electrons, protons, deuterons, and helium ions). **polysulfide a.,** a substance added to the polysulfide liquid to initiate its polymerization to form a rubber-like mass. Lead peroxide is the most commonly used polysulfide accelerator. Zinc oxide, zinc sulfide, titanium dioxide, calcium carbonate, and organic amines are sometimes added to base formulations as accelerators. Called also *polysulfide catalyst* and *polysulfide coreactant.* **prothrombin a.,** FACTOR V. **serum a., serum prothrombin conversion a.,** FACTOR VII.

accelerin (ak-sel′er-in) FACTOR VI.

acceptance (ak-sep′tans) 1. the act of taking or receiving something offered. 2. approval; assent. 3. an agreement whereby a dentist or physician, either expressly or by actions, offers to provide certain health services within his or her area of professional expertise to an individual, thus, assuming certain legal professional responsibilities to that person; and the patient agrees to compensate the dentist or physician for services rendered. A dentist or physician has no obligation to accept every individual who requests his or her services and retains freedom of being selective in choosing patients but, under the Civil Rights Acts, no person may be refused acceptance because of race, religion, sex, or national origin. 4. a program of the Council on Dental Materials and Devices of the American Dental Association for the evaluation of materials and devices used in dental practice, based on evidence of safety and usefulness established by biological, laboratory, and/or clinical evaluations. See also SEAL of Acceptance, and acceptable, provisionally acceptable, and unacceptable DEVICE and MATERIAL. 5. a program of the Council on Dental Therapeutics of the American Dental Association designed to evaluate drugs and therapeutics according to their safety and usefulness. See also accepted, provisionally accepted, and unaccepted dental THERAPEUTIC. **implied a.,** an acceptance interpreted by law from the acts or conduct of the patient.

acceptor (ak-sep′tor) a substance which unites with another substance; specifically, a substance which unites with hydrogen or oxygen, in an oxidoreduction reaction, and so enables the reaction to proceed. **proton a.,** a chemical compound which accepts protons; see BASE (3). See also Bronsted CONCEPT. **a. reductase,** dehydrogenase.

access (ak′ses) 1. the ability to enter or approach. 2. a way or means of approach. 3. the space or room required for adequate visualization and instrument handling in cavity preparation and insertion of restorative material. **root canal a.,** the cavity prepared in the crown of a tooth in order to obtain adequate access for cleansing, enlarging, shaping, and filling the root canal. Called also *access opening.*

accessory (ak-ses′o-re) [L. *accessorium*] supplementary or affording aid to another similar and generally more important thing.

accessorius (ak″ses-o′re-us) [L. "supplementary"] accessory; used in anatomical nomenclature in naming structures serving a supplementary function.

accident (ak′si-dent) [L. *accidens* a chance; a disastrous event] a sudden unforeseen occurrence or injury; a complication in the regular course of a disease. **cerebrovascular a.,** a condition with a sudden onset caused by an acute vascular lesion of the brain, such as hemorrhage, embolism, thrombosis, rupturing aneurysm, or spasm, which may be marked by hemiplegia or hemiparesis, vertigo, numbness, aphasia, and dysarthria. It may be followed by permanent neurologic damage and sometimes death. Called also *stroke* and *stroke syndrome.* **dental a.,** an unforeseen event resulting in injury to natural teeth or supporting structures. **radiation a.,** an accident resulting from the spread of radioactive material or from the exposure of individuals to ionizing radiations. **unavoidable a.,** an accident not occasioned, either remotely or directly, by the want of such care or skill as the law holds every person bound to exercise.

acclimation (ak″li-ma′shun) adaptation to changes in the environment, particularly a new climate.

acclimatization (ah-kli″mah-ti-za′shun) acclimation.

accommodation (ah-kom″o-da′shun) [L. *accommodere* to fit to] 1. adjustment to transient conditions. 2. adjustment of the eye for various distances. **histologic a.,** morphological and functional responses of cells to changed conditions.

accreditation (ah-kred″i-ta′shun) the process by which an agency or organization evaluates and recognizes an institution or program of study as meeting certain predetermined criteria or standards. The Commission on Accreditation of the American Dental Association is recognized by the United States Department of Education and the Council on Postsecondary Accreditation for accrediting educational programs in dentistry, i.e., dental schools, residency and postgraduate programs, dental assisting programs, dental hygiene programs, and dental laboratory technology programs. See also Joint Commission on Accreditation of Hospitals, under COMMISSION, and see also CERTIFICATION and LICENSURE. **hospital a.,** certification that a hospital has met the standards established by the Joint Commission on Accreditation of Hospitals for the quality of patient care and the operation of hospitals. See also Joint Commission on Accreditation of Hospitals, under COMMISSION.

accretio (ah-kre′she-o) [L.] abnormal adhesion of parts normally separate.

accretion (ah-kre′shun) [L. *ad* to + *crescere* to grow] 1. the normal increase in size of a tissue. 2. the adherence of parts normally separate. 3. a mass of foreign matter which has accumulated in a cavity. 4. accumulation on the teeth of foreign materials, such as plaque, materia alba, and calculus.

Accu-Cast trademark for a phosphate-bonded investment material for base-metal alloys.

Acculoy trademark for an *amalgam alloy* (see under AMALGAM).

Accusphere trademark for an *amalgam alloy* (see under AMALGAM).

ACD American College of Dentists (see under COLLEGE).

A.C.E. an anesthetic mixture containing alcohol, chloroform, and ether.

ace acentric (2).

-aceae [L. fem. pl. word ending] a word termination designating a family in microbiological taxonomy.

acellular (a-sel′u-lar) not made up of or containing cells.

acenesthesia (ah-sen″es-the′ze-ah) [*a* neg. + *cenesthesia*] abolition of the sense of well being.

acentric (ah-sen′trik) [Gr. *akentrikos* not centric] 1. not central or not in the center. 2. a chromosome or chromosome segment without a centromere. Abbreviated *ace.* See also DELETION (2).

ACEP American College of Emergency Physicians.

acephalia (ah″sĕ-fa′le-ah) [*a* neg. + Gr. *kephalē* head] congenital absence of the head.

acephalostomia (ah-sef″ah-lo-sto′me-ah) [*a* neg. + Gr. *kephalē* head + *stoma* mouth + *-ia*] a developmental anomaly characterized by absence of the head, with a a kind of mouth on the superior aspect.

acephalostomus (ah-sef″ah-los′to-mus) a malformed fetus exhibiting acephalostomia.

acephalus (ah-sef′ah-lus) [*a* neg. + Gr. *kephalē* head] a malformed fetus without a head.

acephaly (ah-sef′ah-le) acephalia.

acescence (ah-ses′ens) [L. *acescere* to become sour] 1. sourness. 2. the process of becoming sour.

acescent (ah-ses′ent) slightly acid.

acesodyne (ah-ses′o-dīn) [Gr. *akesis* cure + *odynē* pain] anodyne; allaying pain. See also ANALGESIC.

acetaldehyde (as″et-al′dĕ-hīd) an aldehyde, CH_3CHO, occurring as a flammable liquid with a characteristic pungent odor, which is miscible in water and organic solvents. Used in the production of perfumes, synthetic rubber, plastics, and other products. It has a general narcotic action similar to ethanol; large doses may cause respiratory paralysis and death. Called also *acetic aldehyde* and *ethanal.*

Acetalgin trademark for *acetaminophen.*

***p*-acetamidophenol** (as″et-am″i-do-fe′nol) acetaminophen.

acetaminophen (as″et-am′ĭ-no-fen) an analogue of phenacetin and acetanilid, N-(4-hydroxyphenyl)acetamide, occurring as a white, odorless, crystalline powder with a slightly bitter taste, which is soluble in boiling water, ethanol, and sodium hydroxide. It has analgesic and antipyretic properties similar to those of aspirin, but lacks aspirin's anti-inflammatory properties, also being less toxic. Used in the treatment of headache, toothache, neuralgia, myalgias, and other painful conditions, being particularly useful in persons who are sensitive to aspirin. Acetaminophen is believed to potentiate the action of oral anticoagulants. Adverse reactions may include methemoglobinemia, urticaria, laryngeal edema, and agranulocytosis. Hepatic necrosis and renal failure may follow overdosage. Called also p-*acetamidophenol, paracetamol,* and p-*hydroxyacetanilide.* Trademarks: Acamol, Acetalgin, Apamide, Dirox, Fininol, Paraspen, Tapar, Tylenol, Valadol.

Acetamox trademark for *acetazolamide.*

acetanilid (as″ĕ-tan′ĭ-lid) an analgesic and antipyretic, N-phenylacetamide, occurring as a white powder, crystals, or scales that are soluble in water, ethanol, chloroform, and glycerol. Used in the treatment of pain, particularly of the neuralgic type, and rheumatic disorders. It is prone to produce methemoglobinemia and is seldom used. Called also *acetylaminobenzene, acetylaniline,* and *antifebrin.*

acetate (as′ĕ-tāt) an ester or salt of acetic acid containing in its structure the CH_3COO radical. Acetates are decomposed by acids and heat. **mercuric a.,** $Hg(C_2H_3O_2)_2$, occurring as a white, crystalline powder that is soluble in water and alcohol. Used in the preparation of medicinal substances and organic synthesis. It is a strong poison. Called also *mercury acetate.* **methyl a.,** METHYL acetate. **phenylmercuric a.,** a local antibacterial agent, (acetato-O)phenylmercury, occurring as a white, odorless, crystalline powder or small white prisms or leaflets that are freely soluble in ethanol and acetone and slightly soluble in water. Used in treating abrasions, lacerations, and infections of the skin. Also used in contraceptive gels and foams, and as a preservative for drugs, as a herbicide, and as a fungicide. Abbreviated *PMA* and *PMAS.* Called also *acetoxyphenylmercury.* Trademarks: Gallotox, Liquiphen, Mersolite, Phix, Riogen. **salicylic acid a.,** aspirin. **vinyl a.,** VINYL acetate.

acetazolamide (as″et-ah-zol′ah-mīd) a carbonic anhydrase inhibitor, N-(5-sulfomoyl-1,3,4-thiadiazol-2-yl)acetamide, occurring as a white or yellowish, odorless powder that is slightly soluble in ethanol and hot water and very slightly soluble in cold water. Used in the treatment of congestive heart failure, epilepsy, glaucoma, and edematous diseases. The most frequent adverse reactions include drowsiness, paresthesia, fatigue, excitement, gastrointestinal disorders, disorientation, bone marrow depression, renal calculi, fever, and hypersensitivity. Systemic acido-

sis and tolerance occur with chronic use. Trademarks: Acetamox, Diamox, Fonurit, Glupax, Natrionex.

Acetexa trademark for *nortriptyline hydrochloride* (see under NORTRIPTYLINE).

acetic (ah-se′tik, ah-set′ik) pertaining to vinegar or acetic acid; sour.

Acetobacter (ah-se″to-bak′ter) [L. *acetum* vinegar + Gr. *baktērion* little rod] a genus of gram-negative, aerobic, nonsporogenous bacteria of uncertain affiliation, which are capable of oxidizing ethanol to acetic acid. The organisms are made up of nonmotile or motile by peritrichous flagella, ellipsoidal or rod-shaped straight or curved cells, 0.6 to 0.8 μm by 1.0 to 3.0 μm in size, occurring singly or in pairs or in short chains. They are found in fruits, vegetables, souring fruit juices, vinegar, and alcoholic beverages. Called also *Acetobacterium, Mycoderma,* and *Termobacterium.*

Acetobacterium (ah-se″to-bak-te′re-um) *Acetobacter.*

acetomorphine (as″ĕ-to-mor′fēn) diacetylmorphine.

acetone (as′ĕ-tōn) [*acetic* + *ketone*] an intermediate product of metabolism of fatty acids, eventually broken down into carbon dioxide and water, 2-propanone. It occurs as a yellow to amber, oily liquid with a faint characteristic odor and a warm bitter taste, which is soluble in water, ethanol, cottonseed and corn oils, ethyl acetate, methanol, and toluene, but not in mineral oils. Acetone is found in the body in high concentrations in certain pathological conditions, such as diabetes mellitus and starvation, with resulting specific odor detectable in the breath. Used as a solvent, e.g., for fatty bodies, resins, poroxylin, mercurials, rubber, and celluloid-like materials, and in the manufacture of various organic compounds, such as ascorbic acid, chlorobutanol, and chloroform. Also used as a dehydrating agent. Called also *dimethyl ketone, β-ketopropane,* and *pyroacetic ether.* See also ketone BODY. **a. body,** ketone BODY. **a. chloroform,** chlorobutanol.

acetonemia (as″ĕ-to-ne′me-ah) [*acetone* + Gr. *haima* blood + *-ia*] the presence of acetone bodies in the blood.

acetonuria (as″ĕ-to-nu′re-ah) excess of acetone bodies in the urine.

***p*-acetophenetide** (as″et-to-fĕ-net′tĭd) phenacetin.

acetophenetidin (as″et-to-fĕ-net′ĭ-din) phenacetin.

acetosoluble (as″ĕ-to-sol′u-b′l) soluble in acetic acid.

acetoxyphenylmercury (as″ĕ-tok″sĭ-fen″il-mer′ku-re) phenylmercuric ACETATE.

acetphenetidin (as″et-fĕ-net′ĭ-din) phenacetin.

acetrizoate sodium (as″ĕ-tri-zo′āt) a water-soluble contrast medium, 3-(acetylamino)-2,4,6-triiodobenzoic acid sodium salt, which is miscible with body fluids and saliva and rapidly eliminated from the body. Used in radiography, including sialography. Trademarks: Bronchoselectan, Cystokon, Diaginol, Iodopaque, Thixokon, Tri-Abrodil, Triopac, Urokon, Vesamin, Visotrast.

acetum (ah-se′tum) [L.] 1. vinegar. 2. a medicinal solution of a drug in dilute acid.

acetyl (as′ĕ-til) [L. *acetum* vinegar + Gr. *hylē* matter] the radical CH_3CO, the form in which acetic acid enters into various compounds.

acetylaminobenzene (as″ĕ-til-am″ĭ-no-ben′zēn) acetanilid.

acetylaniline (as″ĕ-til-an′ĭ-lin) acetanilid.

acetylation (ah-set″ĭ-la′shun) the introduction of an acetyl group (CH_3CO-) into the molecule of an organic compound having OH or NH_2 groups.

acetylcholine (as″ĕ-til-ko′lēn) the acetylated form of choline, 2-(acetoxy)-N,N,N-trimethylethanaminium, which is normally present in many parts of the body and serves as the chemical transmitter substance in conveying impulses in the nervous system at synapses. Its physiological function consists chiefly of acting on the postganglionic parasympathetic fibers to the autonomic effector cells, the preganglionic autonomic fibers to the sympathetic and parasympathetic ganglion cells and to the adrenal medulla; the somatic motor nerves to the skeletal muscles; and some parts of the central nervous system. Nerve endings secreting acetylcholine as the transmitter substance are known as *cholinergic* (as opposed to *adrenergic* which secrete norepinephrine). Pharmacologically, acetylcholine is a parasympathomimetic drug (see under DRUG), which produces vasodilatation, a decrease in heart rate, and a decrease in the force of cardiac contraction. It stimulates gastrointestinal and urinary activity. The administration of acetylcholine is contraindicated in asthma, hyperthyroidism, coronary diseases, and peptic ulcer. Abbreviated *ACh.* **a. hydrolase,** acetylcholinesterase.

acetylcholinesterase [E.C.3.1.1.7] (as"ĕ-til-ko"lin-es'ter-ās) a carboxylic ester hydrolase that catalyzes the hydrolysis of acetylcholine to choline and acetate, acting on a variety of acetic esters; it also catalyzes transacetylation. The enzyme is found in various tissues, including nerves, muscles, erythrocytes, saliva, and other tissues. Abbreviated *AChE*. Called also *acetylcholine hydrolase*, *choline esterase I*, *cholinesterase*, and *true cholinesterase*.

acetylene (ah-set'ĭ-lēn) a colorless gas, HC≡CH, with an ethereal odor, which is formed by the action of water on calcium carbide, being the type class of unsaturated triple-bonded hydrocarbons (see ALKYNE). It has been used as a general anesthetic. Acetylene burns with an intensely hot flame and, when mixed with oxygen, forms an explosive compound; it also forms explosive compounds with silver, mercury, and copper. Acetylene is a simple asphyxiant, also causing necrosis, dyspnea, and collapse. Called also *ethine* and *ethyne*.

Acetylin trademark for *aspirin*.

acetylmetacresol (as"ĕ-til-met-ah-kre'sol) METACRESYL acetate.

Ac-G accelerator globulin; see FACTOR V.

Ac-globulin accelerator globulin; see FACTOR V.

ACH index see under INDEX.

ACh acetylcholine.

ACHA American College of Hospital Administrators.

achalasia (ak"ah-la'ze-ah) [*a* neg. + Gr. *chalasis* relaxation + -*ia*] failure to relax of the smooth muscle fibers of the gastrointestinal tract at any point of junction of one part with another; especially the failure of the esophagogastric sphincter to relax with swallowing, due to degeneration of ganglion cells in the wall of the organ. Called also *cardiospasm*. **cricopharyngeal a.**, Asherson's SYNDROME.

Achatite trademark for a *silicate cement* (see under CEMENT).

AChE acetylcholinesterase.

ache (āk) a continuous, fixed pain. **head a.**, headache. **tooth a.**, toothache.

acheilia (ah-ki'le-ah) [*a* neg. + Gr. *cheilos* lip + -*ia*] a developmental anomaly characterized by the absence of one or both lips.

acheilous (ah-ki'lus) having no lips; pertaining to acheilia.

achlorhydria (ah"klor-hi'dre-ah) [*a* neg. + *chlorhydria*] absence of hydrochloric acid from gastric secretions; usually associated with anemia.

achloride (ah-klo'rīd) a salt which is not a chloride.

Acholeplasma (ah-ko"le-plas'mah) [*a* neg. + Gr. *cholē* bile + *plasma* something formed or molded] a genus of prokaryotic microorganisms of the family Acholeplasmataceae, order Mycoplasmatales. The organisms occur as gram-negative, nonmotile saprophytic and parasitic forms, possibly pathogenic to a variety of hosts. Contrary to *Mycoplasma*, they do not require sterol for growth. The cells are spherical, about 125 to 220 nm in diameter, or filamentous, about 2 to 5 μm in length, bounded by a triple-layered membrane about 7 nm in thickness. They are resistant to various antibiotics, including the penicillins ampicillin, cloxacillin, and methicillin. Called also *Sapromyces*.

Acholeplasmataceae (ah-ko"le-plas"mah-ta'se-e) [*Acholeplasma* + -*aceae*] a family of prokaryotic microorganisms of the order Mycoplasmatales, consisting of the genus *Acholeplasma*.

achondroplasia (ah-kon"dro-pla'ze-ah) [*a* neg. + Gr. *chondros* cartilage + *plassein* to form + -*ia*] a hereditary disorder, transmitted as an autosomal recessive trait, characterized by disorders of epiphyseal chondroblastic growth and maturation, resulting in short-limb dwarfism. Affected patients have short bodies with thick, muscular extremities and stubby fingers, often associated with limited motion of the joints, lumbar lordosis, prominent buttocks, protruding abdomen, and inability to straighten the elbows. Oral manifestations include a retruding maxilla with relative mandibular prognathism, malocclusion, and partial anodontia. Called also *chondrodystrophia fetalis*, *chondrogenesis imperfecta*, *congenital osteosclerosis*, and *Parrot's disease*.

Achor-Smith syndrome [Richard William Paul *Achor*, American physician, born 1922; Lucian S. *Smith*, American physician, born 1910] see under SYNDROME.

Achro trademark for *tetracycline hydrochloride* (see under TETRACYCLINE).

achroiocythemia (ah-kroi"o-si-the'me-ah) [Gr. *achroios* colorless + *kytos* hollow vessel + *haima* blood + -*ia*] deficiency or lack of hemoglobin in the erythrocytes.

achroma (ah-kro'mah) [*a* neg. + Gr. *chrōma* color] absence of color or of normal pigmentation.

Achromacin trademark for *tetracycline hydrochloride* (see under TETRACYCLINE).

achromacyte (ah-kro'mah-sīt) [*a* neg. + Gr. *chrōma* color + *kytos* hollow vessel] an erythrocyte lacking normal color.

achromasia (ak"ro-ma'se-ah) [*a* neg. + Gr. *chrōma* color + -*ia*] 1. lack of normal pigmentation of the skin. 2. absence of the normal staining reaction from a tissue or cell.

achromatic (ak"ro-mat'ik) [*a* neg + Gr. *chōmatikos* pertaining to color] 1. staining with difficulty. 2. containing achromatin. 3. refracting light without decomposing it into its component colors.

achromatin (ah-kro'mah-tin) [*a* neg. + Gr. *chrōma* color] the faintly staining ground substance of the cell nucleus.

achromatocyte (ak"ro-mat'o-sīt) [*a* neg. + Gr. *chrōma* color + *kytos* hollow vessel] a decolorized erythrocyte.

achromatolysis (ah-kro"mah-tol'ĭ-sis) [*a* neg + Gr. *chrōma* color + *lysis* dissolution] disorganization of the achromatin of a cell.

achromatophil (ah"kro-mat'o-fil) [*a* neg + Gr. *chrōma* color + *philein* to love] 1. having no affinity for stains. 2. an organism or tissue element that does not stain easily.

Achromycin trademark for *tetracycline* (1). **A. V**, trademark for *tetracycline hydrochloride* (see under TETRACYCLINE).

acid (as'id) 1. [L. *acidus*, from *acere* to be sour] sour; having properties opposed to those of the alkalies. 2. [L. *acidum*] any compound of an electronegative element with one or more hydrogen atoms that are readily replaceable by electropositive atoms; a compound which, in aqueous solution, undergoes dissociation with the formation of hydrogen ions. Acids have a sour taste, turn blue litmus red, and unite with bases to form salts. Acids are distinguished as *binary* or *hydracids*, and *ternary* or *oxacids*: the former contain no oxygen; in the latter the hydrogen is united to the electronegative element by oxygen. The hydracids are distinguished by the prefix *hydro-*. The names of acids end in "ic," except in the case in which there are two degrees of oxygenation. The acid containing the greater amount of oxygen has the termination -*ic*, the one having the lesser amount, the termination -*ous*. Acids ending in -*ic* form the salts with the termination -*ate*; those ending in -*ous* form the salts ending in -*ite*. The salts of hydracids end in -*ide*. Acids are called *monobasic*, *dibasic*, *tribasic*, and *tetrabasic*, respectively, when they contain one, two, three, or four replaceable hydrogen atoms. See also Bronsted CONCEPT (1) and Lewis CONCEPT (2). **acetic a.**, a carboxylic acid, CH₃COOH, occurring as a clear colorless liquid with a characteristic pungent odor. Pure acetic acid (99.8 percent) is known as *glacial acetic acid*. It is generally used in aqueous solution; a dilute solution of acetic acid is vinegar. Used as a solvent, reagent, and food additive, and in various chemical processes. It has bactericidal and bacteriostatic properties, *Pseudomonas aeruginosa* being particularly susceptible to its action, and it is used in 1 percent solution on the skin for surgical dressings. Also used in burn therapy. Called also *ethanoic a.*, *methanecarboxylic a.*, *metacarboxylic a.*, and *vinegar a.* **acetic a., dilute,** a 6 percent aqueous solution of acetic acid. **acetic a. ethynyl ester, acetic a. vinyl ester,** VINYL acetate. **acetic a., glacial,** pure acetic acid containing no less than 99.4 percent by weight of acetic acid, occurring as a clear liquid with a strong pungent odor. Used in various chemical processes and, pharmaceutically, as an acidifying agent. Ingestion may cause erosive lesions of the mouth and gastrointestinal tract, with hematemesis, diarrhea, uremia, shock, and death. Chronic exposure may cause bronchitis, eye irritation, and erosion of the dental enamel. **acetoacetic a.,** a colorless syrupy compound, CH₃—CO—CH₂—COOH, which is one of the ketone bodies. An intermediate substance of fat and ketogenic amino acid metabolism, which may be reduced to beta-hydroxybutyric acid and forms acetone and carbon dioxide. It may be found in excessively large amounts in the blood and urine in some pathological conditions, such as diabetes mellitus or starvation. See also ketone BODY. **acetylpropionic a.,** levulinic a. **acetylsalicylic a.,** aspirin. **aconitic a.,** an acid, 1-propene-1,2,3-tricarboxylic acid, occurring in various plants, particularly in sugar beets and sugar cane. In oxidative carbohydrate metabolism, the *cis-* form is an intermediate product in the conversion of citric acid to isocitric acid in the Krebs cycle. Used as a plasticizer. Called also *citridic a.* and *quisetic a.* **acroleic a., acrylic a.,** an oxidation product of acrolein, C₃H₄O₂, being a colorless, pungent, corrosive liquid that is miscible with water, alcohol, and ether, which polymerizes readily in the presence of oxygen. It is used as a monomer for acrylic polymers in acrylic resin production. The acid is highly toxic, irritant, and corrosive to the skin and, being highly flammable, is potentially explosive. Called also *acroleic a.*, *ethylenecarboxylic a.*, *propene a.*, *2-propenoic a.*, and *vinylformic a.* **adenosine diphosphoric a.,** ADENOSINE diphosphate. **adenosinephosphoric a.,** adenylic a. **5'-adenyldiphosphoric a.,** ADENOSINE triphosphate. **adenylic a.,** the monophosphoric ester of adenosine; the nucleotide containing adenine, D-ribose, and phosphoric acid, being a constituent of various coenzymes. It is one of the products of hydrolysis of nucleic acids, and occurs in various tissues, nuclear material, and yeast. Called also *adenine nucleotide, adenosine monophate, adenosine monophosphate, adenosine phosphate, adenosinephosphoric a.,* and *AMP.* See also ADENOSINE 3'5'-cyclic phosphate. **5'-adenylphosphoric a.,** ADENOSINE diphosphate. **alginic a.,** a colloidal carbohydrate acid obtained from seaweeds; a hydrophilic, tasteless, slightly soluble substance. Called also *polymannuronic a.* and *algin.* See also ALGINATE. **aliphatic a.,** an organic acid with an open carbon chain. **allomaleic a.,** fumanic a. **allylmercaptopenicillinic a.,** PENICILLIN O. **alphaaminobutyric a.,** α-aminobutyric a. **amino a.,** any of a class of organic compounds containing the amino (NH_2) group and the carboxyl (COOH) group. The amino acids form the chief structure of proteins, several being essential in human nutrition (see *amino a's, essential*) and many occur naturally. Except for glycine, all contain an asymmetric carbon atom and thus exist in the D or L form; naturally occurring mammalian amino acids have the L configuration. The amino acids behave both as weak acids and as weak bases, containing at least one carboxyl and one amino group, and their behavior is thus amphoteric. According to their chemical structure, they may be classified as aliphatic, acidic, heterocyclic, basic, sulfur-containing, and aromatic. See also PEPTIDE and PROTEIN. **α-amino a., primary,** an undissociated form of amino acids in which the α-carbon (the carbon atom next to the carboxyl group) attaches to an amino group; one in which the carboxyl and amino group are attached to the same carbon atom. Proteins yielding only α-amino acids on complete hydrolysis are known as *simple proteins.* **amino a., essential,** an amino acid that is essential for optimal growth in young animals or for nitrogen equilibrium in adults. Those essential for nitrogen equilibrium in humans are isoleucine, leucine, lysine, methionine, phenylalanine, threonine, tryptophan, and valine; histidine, in addition to these eight, is required by infants. **amino a., glucogenic,** any amino acid whose carbon skeleton may be converted to pyruvate or intermediates in the Krebs cycle, which can in turn be converted to glucose. **amino a., ketogenic,** an amino acid that may readily be converted to acetyl groups and acetoacetate and which then follow the degradative metabolic pathway of lipids and form ketone bodies. **amino a., secondary,** see *imino a.* **p-aminobenzoic a.,** an acid, 4-aminobenzoic acid, occurring as a white or yellowish, odorless, crystalline powder or crystals that become discolored on exposure to light and are freely soluble in ethanol and solutions of alkali hydroxides and carbonates and slightly soluble in water and ether. In bacterial cells, *p*-aminobenzoic acid is incorporated into folic acid, but its metabolism may be blocked by sulfonamides, hence its antibacterial activity; it is not converted to folic acid in certain mammalian cells. Being essential in bacterial metabolism, the acid has been designated as a member of the vitamin B complex; the lack of evidence that it is essential in human nutrition argues against this. Used chiefly as a sunscreen because of its ability to absorb ultraviolet rays in the region of 280 to 320 μ. Also proposed (as its potassium salt) for softening fibrotic tissue in scleroderma, dermatomyositis, morphea, and pemphigus, and in the treatment of lupus erythematosus. Abbreviated *PABA.* Called also *para-aminobenzoic a., anticantinic vitamin, vitamin H'* and *vitamin B_x.* **2-aminobutanoic a.,** α-aminobutyric a. **3-aminobutanoic a.,** β-aminobutyric a. **4-aminobutanoic a.,** γ-aminobutyric a. **α-aminobutyric a.,** an amino acid, $CH_3CH_2CH(NH_2)COOH$, found in the brain tissue. The DL-form occurs as water- and alcohol-soluble crystals, the ethyl ester of which forms a viscous liquid that is soluble in water and organic solvents; the L-form occurs as sweet leaflets, the hydrochloride of which is readily soluble in water. Called also *alphaaminobutyric a.* and *2-aminobutanoica.* **β-aminobutyric a.,** an amino acid, $CH_3CH(NH_2)CH_2COOH$. The DL-form occurs as tasteless crystals that are soluble in water, but not in ether and ethanol, the methyl ester of which is an odoriferous liquid that is soluble in water, ethanol, and ether; the D-form occurs as prisms. Called also *3-aminobutanoic a.* and *beta-aminobutyric a.* **γ-aminobutyric a.,** an amino acid, $H_2NCH_2CH_2CH_2COOH$, occurring as a water-soluble substance. It is an inhibitory transmitter in the central nervous system, producing inhibition accompanied by hyperpolarization through an increase in chloride conductance at cortical neurons and at cerebellar neurons. Used as an anticonvulsant agent. Abbreviated *GABA* and *gaba.* Called also *4-aminobutanoic a., gamma-aminobutyric a.,* and *piperidic a.* Trademarks: Gamarex, Gammalon. **aminocaproic a., ϵ-aminocaproic a.,** a nonessential amino acid, 6-aminohexanoic acid, occurring as a tasteless, odorless, white, crystalline powder that is readily soluble in water, acids, and alkalies, slightly soluble in ethanol and methanol, and insoluble

in ether and chloroform. It suppresses the formation of fibrinolysin (an enzyme destroying fibrinogen and fibrin), and is used in the treatment of hemorrhagic disorders due to excessive fibrinolysis brought about by either pathologic conditions or the administration of anticoagulants which inhibit fibrinolysis (fibrinolytic inhibitors). Diuresis, nausea, diarrhea, pruritus, erythema, skin rash, stuffy nose, thrombosis, and teratogenesis are some of its side reactions. Called also *epsilon-aminocaproic a., epicapramin,* and *epsicapramin.* Trademarks: Afibrin, Amicar, Caprocid, Capromol, Hemocaprol, Ipsilon. **4-aminofolic a.,** aminopterin. **6-aminohexanoic a.,** aminocaproic a. **α-aminopropionic a., 2-aminopropionic a.,** alanine. **β-aminopropionic a., 3-aminopropionic a.,** β-ALANINE. **4-aminopteroylglutamic a.,** aminopterin. **aminosalicylic a., p-aminosalicylic a.,** an acid, 4-amino-2-hydroxybenzoic acid, occurring as a white, almost odorless powder that darkens on exposure to light and air, and is slightly soluble in ether and alcohol, very slightly soluble in water, and insoluble in benzene. It is an antibacterial agent that suppresses both the growth and multiplication of *Mycobacterium tuberculosis.* It is a structural analogue of *p*-aminobenzoic acid and its action on bacteria is believed to be that of a competitive metabolic inhibitor. Abbreviated *PAS* and *PASA.* Called also *para-aminosalicylic a.* **aminosuccinic a.,** aspartic a. **amygdalic a.,** mandelic a. **antiscorbic a.,** ascorbic a. **arachic a.,** arachidic a. **arachidic a.,** a saturated fatty acid, *n*-eicosanoic acid, from the peanut, *Arachis hypogaea,* also occurring in vegetable and fish oils. Used in biochemical research and in various chemical processes. Called also *arachic a.* **arachidonic a.,** a polyunsaturated (essential) fatty acid, 5,8,11,14-eicosatetraenoic acid, associated with vitamin F, which occurs in the liver, brain, glands, and depot fats, and is a constituent of lecithin and a biosynthetic source of some prostaglandins. **argininosuccinic a.,** an amino acid synthesized from citrulline in the presence of adenosine triphosphate and argininosuccinate synthetase and, in turn, is converted to fumaric acid and arginine in the course of the formation of urea, being an intermediate product in protein metabolism. **arsenous a.,** 1. a monobasic acid that forms arsenites. 2. ARSENIC trioxide. **ascorbic a.,** a vitamin, L-threo-2,3,4,5,6-pentahydroxy-2-hexene-γ-lactone, occurring as a white or yellowish, odorless powder or crystals with an acidic taste, which darken on exposure to light and are soluble in water, slightly soluble in ethanol, and insoluble in benzene, ether, and chloroform. Ascorbic acid is present in plants, including fresh vegetables, such as green peppers and cabbage; fruits, particularly citrus fruits, and strawberries. It is also found in animal tissues; primates (including man), guinea pigs, and some other mammalian species being the only animals unable to synthesize ascorbic acid. The vitamin is believed to be involved in oxidation and cellular respiration, tyrosine metabolism, corticosteroid synthesis, and other metabolic and physiologic functions. Used chiefly in the treatment and prevention of scurvy. It has also been suggested for use in a wide variety of conditions, e.g., in dentistry for dental caries, gingivitis, and periodontal diseases. It is believed to be relatively nontoxic. For daily requirements of ascorbic acid, see table at NUTRITION. Called also *antiscorbutic a., avitamic a., cevitamic a., hexuronic a., antiscorbutic factor,* and *vitamin C.* Trademarks: Anti-Skorbutin, Cevalin. **aspartic a.,** an acidic, naturally occurring, nonessential, dibasic amino acid, aminosuccinic acid. It is widely distributed in proteins; also found in the saliva. Called also *aminosuccinic a.* Abbreviated *Asp.* See also *amino a.* **aurelic a., aureolic a.,** mithramycin. **auric s.,** the acid that forms salts called *aurates.* **avitamic a.,** ascorbic a. **azotic a.,** nitric a. **barbituric a.,** a cyclic ureide produced by the condensation of malonic acid ester with urea, forming salts with metals, 2,4,6(1*H*,3*H*,5*H*)-pyrimidinetrione, it occurs as white, efflorescent, odorless crystals that are slightly soluble in water and readily soluble in nonpolar solvents, such as chloroform and oil. Barbituric acid does not depress the central nervous system, but its salts have hypnotic and sedative properties. Called also *malonylurea* and *pyrimidinetrione.* See also BARBITURATE. **behenic a.,** a saturated fatty acid, *n*-decosanoic acid, occurring in milk fat, vegetable oils, and marine animal oils, being particularly plentiful in mustard and rape seed oils. Used in various chemical processes. **benzenecarboxylic a.,** benzoic a. **o-benzenedicarboxylic a., 1,2-benzenedicarboxylic a.,** phthalic a. **benzoic a.,** a compound, benzenecarboxylic acid, occurring as white needles or scales that are odorless or may have a slight odor, being soluble in water, alcohol, chloroform, ether, and benzene. It is an acid in the aromatic series, used chiefly as an antifungal agent. Its derivatives are widely used as anesthetics and preservatives and in other pharmaceutical preparations. Called also *phenylformic a.*, *flowers of Benjamin*, and *flowers of benzoin.* **beta-aminobutyric a.**, *β-aminobutyric a.* **binary a's**, a group of acids composed of hydrogen and one other element and containing no oxygen. Their names begin with the prefix *hydro-* and end with the suffix *-ic*, such as hydrochloric acid or hydrobromic acid. Called also *hydracids.* **boletic a.**, fumaric a. **boracic a.**, boric a. **boric a.**, a compound, H_3BO_3, occurring as colorless, odorless, white crystals or a white crystalline powder or scales, which are soluble in water, glycerol, and alcohol. Used as a mild topical antiseptic and astringent, chiefly in ophthalmology. In dentistry, used mainly as a component of mouthwashes. Ingestion may cause vomiting, diarrhea, nausea, rash of the skin and mucous membranes, convulsions, collapse, and death. Boric acid is particularly dangerous to infants. Called also *boracic a.* and *orthoboric a.* **botulinic a.**, an acid found in putrid sausages, believed to consist of allantotoxicon mixed with other substances. **bromauric a.**, a compound, $HAuBr_4 + 5H_2O$, that forms a brownish crystalline acid; used as a readily soluble form of gold and as a source of colloidal gold. See also BROMAURATE and colloidal GOLD. **butacarboxylic a.**, valeric a. **1,4-butanedioic a.**, succinic a. **butanoic a.**, butyric a. **butylacetic a.**, caproic a. **butyric a.**, a saturated fatty acid, $CH_3CH_2CH_2COOH$, found in butter, sweat, feces, and urine, and in traces in the spleen and in blood. It occurs as an oily, colorless liquid with a penetrating unpleasant rancid odor. Used as a flavoring agent and in various chemical and industrial processes. Called also *butanoic a.*, *n-butyric a.*, *ethylacetic a.*, and *propylformic a.* **n-butyric a.**, butyric a. **cannabinolic a.**, see CANNABINOID. **capric a.**, a saturated, crystalline fatty acid, $CH_3(CH_2)_8COOH$, with unpleasant rancid odor, found in butter, coconut oil, and other fats. Used as a flavoring agent and food additive and in various chemical processes. Called also *decanoic a.*, *decyclic a.*, and *decoic a.* **caproic a.**, a saturated fatty acid, $CH_3(CH_2)_4COOH$, occurring in milk fat, palm oil, and other vegetable oils as an oily, colorless or slightly yellow liquid with an odor of limburger cheese. Used in the manufacture of artificial flavors and in various chemical processes. Called also *butylacetic a.*, *hexanoic a.*, *hexoic a.*, and *hexylic a.* **caprylic a.**, a saturated fatty acid, $CH_3(CH_2)_6C-OH$, from goat's and cow's milk and some seed oils, occurring as an oily liquid with slightly rancid taste, which is soluble in organic solvents and very slightly soluble in water. Its salt, stannous octoate, is used as a catalyst in the polymerization of silicone. Called also *octanoic a.* **carbazotic a.**, picric a. **carbolic a.**, phenol (1). **carbonic a.**, 1. a weak acid, H_2CO_3, formed by dissolving carbon dioxide in water; it forms carbonates. 2. CARBON DIOXIDE. **carboxylic a.**, an organic compound containing one or more carboxyl groups ($-COOH$) in the molecule. Carboxylic acids are widely distributed in nature, especially in foods. **caryophyllic a.**, eugenol. **cellulosic a.**, oxidized CELLULOSE. **cephalosporanic a.**, a component of cephalosporin antibiotics, containing dihydrometathiazine ring, and being an analogue of penicillanic acid. **cerinic a.**, cerotic a. **cerotic a.**, **cerotinic a.**, a monobasic saturated fatty acid, *n*-hexacosanoic acid, obtained from beeswax and other insect and plant waxes. Called also *cerinic a.* **cetylacetic a.**, stearic a. **cetylic a.**, palmitic a. **cevitamic a.**, ascorbic a. **chlorhydric a.**, hydrochloric a. **cholic a.**, an acid, $3\alpha,7\alpha,12\alpha$-trihydroxy-5β-cholan-24-oic-acid, found in bile and derived from cholesterol. Upon combining with glycine and taurine, it forms glycocholic and taurocholic acids, the salts of which are bile salts. Used an as emulsifying and choleretic agent, and in various processes. **chromic a.**, 1. a dibasic acid, H_2CrO_4; its salts are called *chromates.* 2. an acid, CrO_3, occurring as dark red prismatic crystals, flakes, or granules; sometimes used in the treatment of acute necrotizing ulcerative gingivitis, and used in the past as an astringent, topical antiseptic, and corrosive preparation. Called also *chromic anhydride* and *chromium trioxide.* **cinnamic a.**, a compound, 3-phenyl-2-propenoic acid, occurring as a white, crystalline powder that is soluble in benzene, ether, glacial acetic acid, carbon dioxide, and oils, but is insoluble in water. Used in the production of some drugs and perfumes, and in various chemical processes. Used also as an anthelmintic. Its salts are used in sunscreens for protecting the lips. Called also *cinnamylic a.* and *β-phenylacrylic a.* **cinnamylic a.**, cinnamic a. **cis-butanedioic a.**, maleic a. **citric a.**, an acid, 2-hydroxy-1,2,3-propanetriocarboxylic acid;

$$CH_2-COOH$$
$$|$$
$$HOCCOOH$$
$$|$$
$$CH_2COOH$$

found in lemons and a variety of animal and plant tissues, and occurring as an odorless, sour, colorless, translucent powder or crystals that are soluble in water, alcohol, and ether, being available in both hydrated and anhydrous forms. In carbohydrate metabolism, citric acid is an intermediate product in the Krebs cycle, being produced from oxalacetic acid and, through the catalytic action of aconitase, is converted to *cis*-aconitic acid. Used as an acidulant for beverages and pharmaceutical preparations. Also used in a 50 percent solution as an etching agent. Therapeutically, used as an anticoagulant (incompatible with potassium tartrate, alkaline earths, bicarbonates, acetates, and sulfides). Formerly used to dissolve urinary calculi and in the treatment of rickets. Some citric acid preparations, such as Stohl's solution, may be irritating to the oral mucosa and cause necrotic and ulcerative lesions. **citric a. cycle**, Krebs CYCLE. **citridic a.**, aconitic a. **colistimethanesulfonic a.**, colistimethate. **conjugate a.**, an acid formed by a base which has gained a proton. **cresylic a.**, cresol. **crystallinic a.**, novobiocin. **cyclamic a.**, a compound, cyclohexylsufamic acid, occurring as white, odorless, crystalline solid with a sweet-sour taste, which is soluble in water and alcohol. Its salts, particularly sodium, potassium, and calcium cyclamates, have been used as nonnutritive, noncaloric sweeteners (see CYCLAMATE). Called also *cyclohexanesulfamic a.*, *cyclohexylsulfamic a.*, and *hexamic a.* **cyclohexanesulfamic a.**, **cyclohexylsulfamic a.**, cyclamic a. **decanoic a.**, **decoic a.**, capric a. **n-decosanoic a.**, behenic a. **decylic a.**, capric a. **dehydrocholic a.**, an acid, 3,7,12-trioxo-5β-cholan-24-oic acid, isolated from bile, which occurs as a white, odorless, bitter powder that is soluble in glacial acetic acid and solutions of alkali hydroxides and carbonates, slightly soluble in ether, methanol, chloroform, and ethanol, and is insoluble in water. Used as a hydrocholeretic in the treatment of constipation, flatus, and other gastrointestinal disorders. Its sodium salt is called *sodium dehydrocholate.* Trademarks: Acolen, Bilidren, Cholan-DH, Chologon, Decholin, Dehychol. **deoxycholic a.**, a substance, $3\alpha,12\alpha$-dihydroxy-5β-cholanic acid, which is derived from cholesterol and, upon combining with glycine and taurine, forms glycocholic and taurocholic acids, the salts of which are bile salts. Used as a choleretic agent. Also used as a detergent in studies of membrane-associated and other proteins. **deoxypentosenucleic a.**, **deoxyribonucleic a.**, **deoxyribose nucleic a.**, DNA. **dextronic a.**, gluconic a. **dextrotartaric a.**, ordinary tartaric acid, which turns the plane of polarization to the right. Called also D-*tartaric a.* **di-a.**, see *dicarboxylic a.* **dibasic a.**, an acid with two displaceable hydrogen atoms per molecule. **dicarboxylic a.**, an aromatic or aliphatic acid having two carboxyl ($-COOH$) groups. Written also *di-a.* **2,5-dihydroxybenzoic a.**, gentisic a. **2,3,3-dihydroxypropanoic a.**, glyceric a. **2,3-dihydroxysuccinic a.**, tartaric a. **diphosphoric a.**, pyrophosphoric a. **diprotic a.**, one that yields two hydrogen ions per molecule, such as sulfuric acid. **disulfuric a.**, sulfuric a., fuming. **djenkolic a.**, 3,3'-methylenedithiobis-(2-aminopropionic acid), a naturally-occurring nonessential amino acid obtained by hydrolysis of djenkol nuts. **n-dodecanoic a.**, lauric a. **edetic a.**, ethylenediaminetetraacetic a. **n-eicosanoic a.**, arachidic a. **elaidic a.**, an unsaturated fatty acid, *trans*-9-octadecenoic acid, the *cis* form of which is oleic acid. Used in biomedical research and as a standard in chroma-

$$O$$
$$\|$$

tography. **enanthic a.**, a saturated fatty acid, $CH_3(CH_2)_5C-OH$, not known to occur naturally, but produced by oxidation of fats, which occurs a clear, oily liquid with unpleasant odor. Used in organic synthesis and in various industrial processes. Called also *enanthylic a.*, *hepatoic a.*, *heptanoic a.*, and *heptylic a.* **enanthylic a.**, enanthic a. **engraver's a.**, nitric a. **epsilon-aminocaproic a.**, ϵ-aminocaproic a. **essential amino a.**, amino a., essential. **a. etchant**, acid ETCHANT. **a. etching**, acid ETCHING. **ethacrinic a.**, a compound, [2,3-dichloro-4-(2-methylene-1-oxobutyl)phenoxy]acetic acid, occurring as a white, odorless, bitter, crystalline powder, which is soluble in ethanol, ether, and chloroform and, slightly, in water. It is a diuretic agent used in treating fluid retention in conditions such as congestive heart failure, cirrhosis of the liver, and renal diseases. Side effects may include anorexia, abdominal discomfort, dysphagia, nausea, vomiting, diarrhea, gastrointestinal hemorrhage, pancreatitis, hyperuricemia, hypoglycemia, gout, agranulocytosis, neutropenia, thrombocytopenia, hematuria, jaundice, vertigo, deafness, tinnitus, headache, skin rashes, fatigue, and confusion and other disorders. Trademarks: Crinuryl, Edecril, Edecrin, Endecril, Hydromedin, Reomax. **ethanedioic a.,** oxalic a. **ethanoic a.,** acetic a. **o-ethoxybenzoic a.,** a substance used to reinforce zinc oxide–eugenol cement (see under CEMENT). Abbreviated *EBA.* Called also ortho-*ethoxybenzoic a.* **ethylacetic a.,** butyric a. **ethylamine sulfonic a.,** taurine. **ethylenecarboxylic a.,** acrylic a. **ethylenediaminetetraacetic a.,** a compound, *N,N′*-1,2-ethanediylbis[*N*-(carboxymethyl)glycine], occurring as colorless crystals that are soluble in water but not in common organic solvents. It is a chelating agent used in the treatment of lead and other heavy metal poisoning and various conditions associated with pathologic calcification. The acid interferes with blood calcium, thus serving as an anticoagulant. In dentistry, used for softening hard tissue around pulp stones constricted by calcific deposits, thus facilitating their removal, removing broken instruments that have become embedded in the tissues by producing local decalcification, and in preparing root canals. Also used as a stabilizer in some dental preparations to bind heavy metal ions, such as iron, thereby preventing them from interfering with the pharmacological action of the preparation. Rapid administration or excessive use may produce hypocalcemic convulsions and death. Abbreviated *EDTA.* Called also *edetic a.* Trademark: Havidote. **ethylformic a.,** propionic a. **ethylidenelactic a.,** lactic a. **eugenic a.,** eugenol. **fatty a's,** monobasic aliphatic acids containing only carbon, hydrogen, and oxygen and made up of an alkyl radical attached to the carboxyl group. Usually, they are monocarboxylic acids with hydrocarbon residues that are both acyclic and unbranched, found in animal or vegetable fat or oil. Naturally occurring fatty acids almost always have straight chains and an even number of carbon atoms, human sebum being an exception, having not only odd numbered, but also branched-chain fatty acids. Fatty acids may be saturated or may contain one or more double bonds. They represent the basic lipid moiety of both triglycerides and phospholipids; the sterol nucleus of cholesterol is synthesized from degradation products of fatty acid molecules. See also LIPID metabolism. **fatty a's, essential,** unsaturated fatty acids that cannot be formed in the body and, therefore, must be provided by the diet; the most important are linoleic, linolenic, and arachidonic acids. **fatty a's, long chain,** fatty acids having more than six carbon atoms in the chain. **fatty a's, nonesterified,** fatty acids which are not esterified to hydroxyl groups of glycerol to form triglycerides. Abbreviated *NEFA.* **fatty a's, normal,** fatty acids that have straight carbon chains, or at least ones that are not branched. **fatty a's, polyunsaturated,** unsaturated fatty acids having two or more double bonds. **fatty a's, saturated,** fatty acids with the general formula $C_2H_{2n}O_2$, in which the hydrocarbon chain is saturated. They are fewer in number than the unsaturated acids and their melting point is higher than that of unsaturated acids; many are derived from animal sources, although some are found also in plants. Increase in blood cholesterol due to high dietary intake of animal-derived saturated fatty acids is suspected as being related to arteriosclerosis. Some naturally occurring saturated fatty acids include acetic, propionic, *n*-butyric, caproic, caprylic, pelargonic, capric, lauric, myristic, palmitic, stearic, arachidic, behenic, lignoceric, cerotic, and montanic acids. **fatty a's, short chain,** fatty acids having fewer than six carbon atoms. In human digestion, they enter the blood directly from the intestine; in ruminants, they are the major end-products of microbial fermentation in the digestive tracts. Called also *volatile fatty a's.* See also LIPID metabolism. **fatty a's, unsaturated,** fatty acids with the general formula $C_nN_{2n}O_2$, usually consisting of alkyl chains containing 16, 18, or 22 carbon atoms with the characteristic end group −COOH and combining one or more double bonds. All the common unsaturated fatty acids are liquid at room temperature; their melting point generally being lower than that of the saturated acids. Most vegetable oils are mixtures of several unsaturated fatty acids or their glycerides. Safflower, peanut, olive, corn, and soybean oils are the most common sources of unsaturated fatty acids. Some naturally occurring unsaturated fatty acids include palmitoleic, oleic, elaidic, vaccenic, linoleic, α-linolenic, γ-linolenic, eleostearic, arachidonic, and nervonic acids. **fermentation lactic a.,** see *lactic a.* **fluohydric a.,** hydrofluoric a. **fluoric a.,** hydrofluoric a. **folic a.,** a vitamin of the B complex, *N*-[4-[[(2-amino-1,4-dihydro-4-oxo-6-pteridinyl)methyl]benzoyl]-L-glutamic acid, occurring as an orange, odorless crystalline powder that is slightly soluble in water, readily soluble in alkali hydroxide and carbonate solutions, hot diluted hydrochloric acid, and sulfuric acid, and insoluble in ethanol and organic solvents. It is an essential

vitamin that is reduced in the body to tetrahydrofolic acid, which is the coenzyme serving as an acceptor for one-carbon units, and other folate coenzymes which participate with vitamins B_6 and B_{12} in various metabolic reactions, including purine synthesis, pyrimidine nucleotide synthesis, amino acid conversion, and the generation of the formate pool. Occurring in nearly all foods, folates are most abundant in yeasts, liver, and fresh green vegetables. Used therapeutically in folate deficiency. Folic acid is not toxic in man, but it may reverse the effect of antiepileptic drugs, such as phenobarbital, primidone, and phenytoin. Called also *pteroylglutamic a. (PGA), folacin, vitamin B$_c$,* and *vitamin M.* Folic deficiency is caused by inadequate intake of folates or produced by the administration of folic acid antagonists, associated chiefly with glossitis, diarrhea, weight loss, and neurological disorders, such as forgetfulness, sleeplessness, and irritability, which may be due to cerebral metabolic disorders. Deficiency due to the administration of folate antagonists in pregnancy may result in fetal abnormalities. For daily requirements of folic acid, see folacin in table at NUTRITION. See also megaloblastic ANEMIA. **folic a. analogue,** folic acid ANALOGUE. **folic a. antagonist,** folic acid ANALOGUE. **folic a. inhibitor,** folic acid ANALOGUE. **folinic a.,** citrovorum

$$O$$
$$\|$$

FACTOR. **formic a.,** a carboxylic acid, H—C—OH, originally produced by the distillation of ants, now made synthetically, occurring as a colorless liquid with pungent odor. It is a strong reducing agent used as a decalcifier and in various chemical and industrial processes. Used therapeutically as a counterirritant and astringent. It is caustic to the skin and mucous membranes and absorption may cause albuminuria and hematuria. Called also *hydrogen carboxylic a.* and *methanoic a.* **fumaric a.,** the *trans*-isomer of maleic acid, *trans*-1,2-ethylenedicarboxylic acid, occurring as colorless, odorless crystals with a fruity acid taste, which are soluble in water and alcohol, but are insoluble in ether and chloroform. In oxidative carbohydrate metabolism, an intermediate product in the Krebs cycle, being formed from succinic acid through the action of succinic dehydrogenase in the presence of FAD and, in turn, being converted to malic acid. Used in food preservation and preparation as a drying, acidulant, and flavoring agent, to replace citric and tartaric acids, and in various industrial processes. Called also *allomaleic a., boletic a., licheninc a.,* and trans-*butanedioic acid.* See also ferrous FUMARATE. **galacturonic a.,** a uronic acid derivative isomeric with glucuronic acid, being an oxidized form of galactose. It is the principal component of pectin. **gamma-aminobutyric a.,** γ-aminobutyric a. **gentisic a.,** a compound, 2,5-dihydroxybenzoic acid, occurring as needle-like crystals that are soluble in water, ethanol, and ether, but not in carbon disulfide, benzene, and chloroform. Used as an analgesic and antirheumatic drug. Called also *5-hydroxysalicylic acid.* Its sodium salt is called *sodium gentisate.* **glacial phosphoric a.,** metaphosphoric a. **gluconic a.,** an acid, $C_6H_{12}O_7$, obtained by oxidation of glucose, occurring as a light brown syrupy liquid with a mild taste. Used in the pharmaceutical and food industries. Called also *dextronic a., glycogenic a., glyconic a.,* and *pentahydroxycaproic a.* **glucuronic a.,** a uronic acid derivative isomeric with galacturonic acid. It is a tetrahydroxy-aldehyde acid with the configuration of glucose, found in the urine, either united with phenols or with aromatic acids. D-Glucuronic acid is a component of hyaluronic acid, chondroitin-4-sulfate, chondroitin-6-sulfate, and heparin (the mucopolysaccharides). Preparations of D-glucuronic acid have been used in the treatment of arthritis. **glutamic a.,** an acidic, naturally occurring, nonessential amino acid, 2-aminoglutaric acid, which is also found in the saliva. Used as an experimental antiepileptic. The L-form is used as a meat flavoring agent; the magnesium salt hydrobromide as a tranquilizer; and the hydrochloride as a gastric acidifier. In biochemistry, the terms *glutamic acid* and *glutamate* are used interchangeably, even though glutamate technically refers to the negatively charged ion. Abbreviated *Glu.* See also amino ACID. **glyceric a.,** an acid, 2,3-dihydroxypropanoic acid, formed by oxidation of glycerol, active in the oxidative metabolism of carbohydrates (Embden-Meyerhof PATHWAY), in its phosphorylated form. **glycerophosphoric a.,** an acid occurring as a syrupy, clear, odorless liquid, produced by the interaction of glycerol and phosphoric acid. Called also *phosphoglyceric a.* and *phosphoric acid glycerol ester.* See also CALCIUM glycerophosphate. **glycocholic a.,** a conjugated form of cholic acid and glycine, the salt of which is one of the bile salts. **glycogenic a., glyconic a.,** gluconic a. **heparinic a.,** heparin. **hepatoic a., heptanoic a., heptylic a.,** enanthic a. **n-hexacosanoic a.,** cerotic a. **hexadecanoic a.,** palmitic a. **9-hexadecenoic a.,** palmitoleic a. **hexadecylic a.,** palmitic a. **2,4-hexadienoic a.,** sorbic a. **hexamic a.,** cyclamic a. **hexanoic a., hexoic a., hexylic a.,** caproic a. **hexuronic a.,** ascorbic a. **hyaluronic a.,** a mucopolysaccharide whose molecule consists of repeating units of D-glucuronic acid and *N*-acetyl-D-glucosamine joined in a β-1,3 linkage. It is a highly viscous substance with a molecular weight within the range of 50,000 to 8×10^6, occurring as a gel of the ground substance (intercellular cement of connective tissue). Hyaluronic acid is found in various tissues, especially the skin and has been isolated from the vitreous humor, umbilical cord, and synovial fluid, and has also been found in hemolytic streptococci group C. It is digested by the enzyme hyaluronidase. **hydriodic a.,** an aqueous solution of hydrogen iodide. *Diluted hydriodic acid* occurs as a colorless or pale yellow liquid that is miscible with water and ethanol, 100 ml of which contains 9.5 to 10.5 gm hydrogen iodide; hypophosphorous acid is added to prevent the formation of free iodine in the solution. Used as a reducing agent, disinfectant, and pharmaceutic necessity, and in various chemical and pharmaceutical processes. It is a strong irritant. *Hydriodic acid syrup* is a mixture of diluted hydriodic acid with dextrose, occurring as a transparent, colorless or yellowish, syrupy liquid with a sweet acidulous taste, and is used as a vehicle for expectorants. **hydriodic a., anhydrous, HYDROGEN** iodide. **hydro a's,** binary a's. **hydrobromic a.,** a solution of hydrogen bromide gas in water, marketed in various concentrations. It is a colorless or yellowish preparation that slowly darkens on exposure to air and light and is miscible with water and alcohol. It is a strong irritant. Used as a sedative. See also **BROMIDE. hydrochloric a.,** hydrogen chloride solution in water, HCl, occurring as a clear, colorless, highly corrosive acid. It is a normal component of the gastric juice. Called also *chlorhydric a.* and *muriatic a.* **hydrocyanic a.,** a compound, HCN, occurring as a light, colorless gas with the odor of almonds. It is a toxic substance that is lethal to most living things; used chiefly as a fumigant. Exposure usually causes tachypnea followed by dyspnea, unconsciousness, convulsions, respiratory arrest, and death. Sodium nitrite and sodium thiosulfate are the common antidotes. Called also *hydrogen cyanide.* **hydrofluoric a.,** a solution of hydrogen fluoride with water, occurring as a highly toxic, colorless, fuming liquid, whose salts form fluorides. Contact or inhalation may cause severe burns of the eyes, mucous membranes, and skin, and respiratory disorders; ingestion usually results in necrosis of the mouth, esophagus, and stomach, and death. Chronic inhalation of small amounts may produce fluorosis. Called also *fluohydric a.* and *fluoric a.* **hydrofluoric a. gas, anhydrous hydrofluoric a.,** hydrogen **FLUORIDE. hydrogen carboxylic a.,** formic a. **hydrohalic a's,** strong acids formed by hydrogen halides in aqueous solutions, such as hydrofluoric acid. **α-hydroxybenzeneacetic a.,** mandelic a. **2-hydroxybenzoic a.,** salicylic a. **o-hydroxybenzoic a.,** salicylic a. **hydroxybutanedioic a.,** malic a. **3-hydroxybutanoic a., β-hydroxybutyric a. β-hydroxybutyric a.,** an acid, 3-hydroxybutanoic acid, which is an intermediate product in fat metabolism, being one of the ketone bodies along with acetoacetic acid and acetone; found in large amounts in the blood and urine in some pathological conditions, such as diabetes mellitus or starvation. It occurs as a viscid, yellow mass, soluble in water, alcohol, and ether. See also ketone **BODY. 2-hydroxypropanoic a.,** lactic a. **α-hydroxypropionic a., 2-hydroxypropionic a.,** lactic a. **5-hydroxysalicylic a.,** gentisic a. **hydroxysuccinic a.,** malic a. **hypochlorous a.,** a compound, HClO, known only in aqueous solution as a greenish yellow liquid that deteriorates when exposed to light. It is a strong oxidizing agent whose salts and derivatives, such as oxychlorosene and calcium and sodium hypochlorite, are used in medicine as germicidal agents in wound irrigation. **hyponitrous a.,** An unstable acid of the composition HO−N=N−OH, formed by the action of nitrous acid on hydroxylamine. Hyponitrous acid anhydride is nitrous oxide (see under OXIDE). **hypoxanthylic a.,** inosinic a. **imino a's,** secondary amino acids having the imine group R—CH. Proline and hydroxyproline are the principal

$$\overset{\|}{\underset{NH}{}}$$

imino acids. **inosinic a.,** an acid, hypoxanthine riboside-5-phosphoric acid, which is a mononucleotide made up of hypoxanthine, ribose, and phosphoric acid, being one of the decom-

position products of nucleic acids in their metabolism. It occurs as a syrup with a sour taste, soluble in water and formic acid and, sparingly, in alcohol and ether. Used as a flavor enhancer. Called also *hypoxanthylic a.* **iodic a.,** a strong acid, HIO, with oxidizing properties, formed by oxidation of iodine with nitric acid, chlorates, or hydrogen peroxide. It occurs as orthorhombic crystals that darken on exposure to light and decompose at temperatures of 70 to 220° F. Used as an astringent and disinfectant. **iodoacetic a.,** an acid, CH_2ICOOH, whose sodium salt is used in the study of muscle physiology. **iodogorgoic a.,** 3,5-diiodotyrosine. **iodopanoic a.,** iopanoic a. **iopanoic a.,** a compound, 3-amino-α-ethyl-2,4,6-triiodohydrocinnamic acid, occurring as a cream-colored, tasteless, photosensitive powder with a faint characteristic odor, which is soluble in ethanol, chloroform, and ether but not in water. Used as a contrast medium in radiography. Called also *iodopanoic a.* Trademarks: Telepaque, Colepax. **iothalamic a.,** a compound, 3-(acetylamino)-2, 4, 6-triiodo-5-[(methylamino)carbonyl] benzoic acid, occurring as a white, odorless powder that is soluble in alkali hydroxide solutions and, slightly, water and ethanol. Its *N*-methylglucamine and sodium salts are used as contrast media. **isoamyl ethyl barbituric a.,** amobarbital. **isonicotinic a. hydrazide,** isoniazid. **isovaleric a.,** see *valeric a.* **keto a.,** a chemical compound containing the CO group along with the COOH. **α-ketoglutaric a.,** an acid, 2-oxopentanediotic acid; in oxidative carbohydrate metabolism, it is an intermediate product in the Krebs cycle, being produced from isocitric acid through oxalosuccinic acid by the action of isocitric dehydrogenase, and being converted in turn to succinate. Called also *α-oxoglutaric a.* **ketosuccinic a.,** oxalacetic a. **lactic a.,** a compound, α-hydroxypropionic acid, $C_3H_6O_3$, occurring as a colorless, odorless, yellowish hygroscopic liquid that is miscible with water, alcohol, and glycerol and soluble in organic solvents. It is known in three forms: DL(+)-lactic acid which occurs in the muscles and is produced by the action of *Micrococcus acidi paralactici* (hence the synonyms *paralactic a.* and *sarcolactic a.*); θD(−)-lactic acid produced by the action of *Bacillus acidi levolactica;* and DL-lactic acid, the inactive or racemic form (also known as *fermentation lactic a.,* found in the stomach, sour milk, and certain fermentation foods. Lactic acid is formed from pyruvic acid when glycolysis occurs under anaerobic conditions. In the oxidation of phosphoglyceraldehyde, coenzyme is reduced, NAD→NADU, and in the reduction of pyruvic acid to lactic acid the reverse occurs, NADU→NAD. In muscle contraction, lactic acid is the product of glycogen breakdown in the process of liberation of energy for contraction. Called also *ethylidenelactic a.* and *2-hydroxypropanoic a.* See also lactic acid **CYCLE. lauric a., laurostearic a.,** a naturally occurring saturated fatty acid, *n*-dodecanoic acid, from laurel seed oil, also occurring in various vegetable fats, such as the glyceride, especially in coconut oil and milk fat. Used as a food additive and in the production of cosmetics, detergents, and various chemical substances. **levotartaric a.,** L-tartaric acid, a form of tartaric acid which rotates plane polarized light to the left. **levulic a.,** levulinic a. **levulinic a.,** an acid of low toxicity, $CH_3COCH_2CH_2COOH$, occurring as yellow crystals that are soluble in water, alcohol, esters, ethers, and ketonic hydrocarbons, but not in aliphatic hydrocarbons. Used in the production of pharmaceutical preparations and other products. Called also *acetylpropionic a., levulic a.,* and *4-oxopentanoic a.* **lichenic a.,** fumaric a. **lignoceric a.,** a long chain saturated fatty acid *n*-tetracosanoic acid, found in small amounts in most natural fats. Obtained from kerasin and sphingomyelin on hydrolysis. **linoleic a.,** a polyunsaturated (essential) fatty acid, *cis*-9,12-octadecadienoic acid, having two double bonds. It is a component of vitamin F and a major constituent of various vegetable oils, including cottonseed, soybean, peanut, corn, sunflower seed, poppy seed, linseed, and other oils. **linolenic a.,** a polyunsaturated (essential) fatty acid, occurring as 9,12,15-octadecatrienoic (α-linolenic), or 6,9,12-octadecatrienoic (γ-linolenic) acids, having three double bonds. It occurs in many vegetable oils. **α-lipoic a.,** a member of the vitamin B complex, 1,2-dithiolane-3-valeric acid, occurring as crystals which are soluble in fat solvents but insoluble in water, which is found in the liver and in various microorganisms. It is a necessary cofactor in oxidative reactions of keto acids and oxidative decarboxylation, and is a growth factor for certain microorganisms. Called also *thioctic a.* and *pyruvate oxidation factor.* **lithic a.,** uric a. **lysergic a.,** a compound, 9,10-didehydro-6-methylergoline-8-β-carboxylic acid. A product of cleavage of ergot alkaloids, occurring as normal lysergic acid and in the *cis*-form. It is a potent psychomimetic drug, subject to government control. **lysergic a. diethylamide,** an acid, 9,10-didehydro-*N*,*N*-diethyl-6-methylergoline-8β-carboxamide, which is one of the principal ergot alkaloids with psychotomimetic properties (see psychotomimetic AGENT). It also counteracts the central effects of barbiturates and, in turn, is counteracted by supressants such as chloropromazine, and antagonizes the effect of serotonin. Clinical application of the drug is largely experimental. The drug is widely abused, and is subject to FDA regulations. Psychological dependence on lysergic acid diethylamide is rare and its acute toxicity is relatively low, but it commonly produces chromosomal aberrations and serious psychological disturbances in users. Abbreviated *LSD* and *LSD-25*. Called also *lysergide*. **maleic a.**, an acid, *cis*-1,2-ethylenedicarboxylic acid, occurring as colorless crystals with a faint odor and a strong astringent taste that are soluble in water and acetone and very slightly soluble in benzene. Used to retard the decomposition of fats and oils and in the production of antihistaminics and other drugs. It is a strong irritant. Called also *cis-butanedioic a.* and *maleinic a.* See also *fumaric a.* **maleinic a.**, maleic a. **malic a.**, an acid, hydroxybutanedioic acid, found in apples and other fruits. The naturally occurring L-form is a sour, colorless crystalline substance, readily soluble in water and alcohol and slightly soluble in ether. In carbohydrate metabolism, it is an intermediate product in the Krebs cycle, being the product of conversion of fumaric and converted in turn to oxalacetic acid. Called also *hydroxysuccinic a.* **mandelic a.**, an acid, α-hydroxybenzeneacetic acid, occurring as orthorhombic plates that darken on exposure to light and are soluble in water, ether, and isopropyl alcohol. Used as an antiseptic. Called also *amygdalic a., paramandelic acid, phenylglycolic a., phenylhydroxyacetic a.,* and *racemic mandelic a.* **mefenamic a.**, an acid, 2-[(2,3-dimethylphenyl)amino]benzoic acid, occurring as a white to off-white, odorless, tasteless with a bitter aftertaste, crystalline powder that darkens on exposure to light and is soluble in ethanol and dimethylformamide, but not in water. It is an analgesic used in the treatment of pain that persists for periods of less than 1 week, such as postextraction pain. Contraindicated in children, pregnancy, hypersensitivity, and gastrointestinal ulcerations. Adverse reactions may include diarrhea, autoimmune hemolytic anemia, thrombocytopenic purpura, leukopenia, eosinophilia, pancytopenia, agranulocytosis, bone marrow hypoplasia, drowsiness, vertigo, gastrointestinal discomfort, headache, vomiting, skin rash, urticaria, blurred vision, insomnia, sweating, and earache. Less commonly occurring side effects may include cardiac arrhythmia, facial edema, dyspnea, dysuria, hematuria, color blindness, renal and hepatic lesions, and increased insulin need by diabetic patients. Trademarks: Coslan, Lysalgo, Parkemed, Ponstan, Ponstel, Pontal, Tanston, Vialidon. **mesotartaric a.** (*meso*-tartaric a.), an optically inactive form of tartaric acid. **metacarboxylic a.**, acetic a. **metacresylic a.**, METACRESYL acetate. **metaphosphoric a.**, an acid, HPO₃, occurring as a transparent, hygroscopic solid. Used as a reagent for chemical analysis and as a test for albumin in the urine; also used for making zinc oxyphosphate cement. Called also *glacial phosphoric a.* **metasilicic a.**, a form of silicic acid, H_2SiO_3. **metavanadic a.**, vanadic a. **methacrylic a.**, α-methacrylic a., an acid occurring as long prisms which form a corrosive liquid with an acrid, pungent odor. It is soluble in warm water and miscible with alcohol and ether, and polymerizes easily, especially on heating or in the presence of hydrochloric acid, forming a ceramic-like solid. Called also *2-methylpropenoic a.* See also METHACRYLATE. **methanecarboxylic a.**, acetic a. **methanoic a.**, formic a. **methylacetic a.**, propionic a. **β-methylbutyric a.**, see valeric a. **2-methylpropenoic a.**, methacrylic a. **monamino a.**, monoamino a., an organic acid which contains an NH₂ group. **monobasic a.**, an acid with one displaceable hydrogen atom per molecule. **monoprotic a.**, one that yields one hydrogen ion per molecule, such as hydrochloric acid. **montanic a.**, a saturated fatty acid, *n*-octacosanoic acid. **muramic a.**, a condensation product of glucosamine and lactic acid, 3-O-lactyl ether of D-glucosamine; found in bacterial cell walls. See also PEPTIDOGLYCAN. **muriatic a.**, hydrochloric a. **mycolic a.**, a long-chain, branched fatty acid with a high molecular weight, characteristic of mycobacteria. **myristic a.**, a saturated fatty acid, *n*-tetradecanoic acid, occurring in nutmeg butter (*Myristica fragrans*), also found in palm oil, milk fats, and most other animal and vegetable fats. Used as a food additive and in the production of soaps, cosmetics, and other chemical substances. *n*-nanoic a., pelargonic a. **nervonic a.**, an unsaturated fatty acid, *cis*-15-tetracosanoic acid, occurring in sphingomyelin. **nicotinic a.**, a water soluble vitamin of the B complex, 3-pyridinecarboxylic acid, occurring as colorless, odorless, bitter crystals or as a white crystalline powder that is soluble in water, ethanol, and alkali but not in fat solvents. It is found in all cells where it is converted to nicotinamide, which is a constituent of coenzymes I and II that are involved in the anaerobic oxidation of carbohydrates, the coen-

zymes serving as a hydrogen acceptor in the oxidation of the substrate. Poultry, meats, fish, potatoes, cereals, and leafy vegetables are its principal dietary sources. Pharmacologically, nicotinic acid lowers cholesterol and triglyceride levels in the blood. Used in the treatment of hyperlipoproteinemias and pellagra. Adverse reactions may include cutaneous flushing, pruritus, liver disorders, hypoglycemia, and abnormal glucose tolerance. Called also *antipellagra vitamin, niacin,* and *pellagra, P.P.,* and *preventive factor.* For daily requirements of nicotinic acid, see niacin in table at NUTRITION. **nicotinic a. amide**, nicotinamide. **nicotinic a. diethylamide**, nikethamide. **nitric a.**, an acid, HNO_3, occurring as a transparent, colorless, or yellowish fuming, suffocating, and corrosive liquid, which decomposes most organic substances and attacks almost all metals. It is miscible with water and decomposes in alcohol. Sometimes used as a cauterizing agent for skin lesions such as warts. Also used as an acidifying agent in pharmaceutical preparations. Inhalation of its vapors may cause bronchitis and pneumonia; ingestion causes corrosive burns of the mouth, esophagus, and stomach, shock, and death; and contact causes burns of the skin and mucous membranes. Called also *aqua fortis, azotic a.,* and *engraver's a.* **nitric a., fuming,** *white fuming nitric acid* contains more than 97.5 percent nitric acid, less than 2 percent water, and less than 0.5 percent oxides of nitrogen. It is a colorless or pale yellow fuming liquid, readily decomposed in the presence of high temperatures or light, becoming red in color. *Red fuming nitric acid* contains more than 86 percent nitric acid, 6–15 percent oxides of nitrogen, and less than 5 percent water. **nitrous a.**, an unstable weak acid, HNO_2, which in aqueous solution changes into nitric oxide and nitric acid. Used in the determination of urea. **nitroxanthic a.**, picric a. **nonanoic a., nonoic a., nonylic a.**, pelargonic a. **nonulosaminic a.**, sialic a. **noradrenaline a. tartrate**, LEVARTERENOL bitartrate. **normal fatty a.**, see *fatty a.* **normal valeric a.**, see valeric a. **nucleic a's**, chainlike macromolecules composed of nucleoproteins that contain sugars, phosphate, and a nitrogen-containing base, purine or pyrimidine. They store and transfer genetic information and are major components of all cells, representing 5–15 percent of their dry weight. Nucleic acids are also present in viruses, infectious nucleic acid–protein complexes being capable of directing their own replication. See DNA and RNA. **n-octacosanoic a.**, montanic a. **octadecanoic a.**, stearic a. **cis-9-octadecenoic a.**, oleic a. **trans-9-octadecenoic a.**, elaidic a. **trans-11-octadecanoic a.**, vaccenic a. **octanoic a.**, caprylic a. **oleic a.**, a monounsaturated fatty acid, *cis*-9-octadecenoic acid, which is a constituent of common fats and oils, and is obtained from animal tallow or vegetable oils. Used as a solvent in drug preparations, food grade additive, and in various chemical processes. **organic a.**, any acid the radical of which is a carbon derivative; a compound in which a hydrocarbon radical is united to COOH (a carboxylic acid) or to SO₃H (a sulfonic acid). **orthoboric a.**, boric a. **ortho-ethoxybenzoic a.**, *o*-ethoxybenoic a. **ortho-hydroxybenzoic a.**, salicylic a. **orthophosphoric a.**, phosphoric a. **orthophosphorous a.**, phosphorous a. **orthosilicic a.**, the simplest form of silicic acid, H_4SiO_4, occurring as a white powder, insoluble in water and acids, except hydrofluoric acid. **osmic a.**, OSMIUM tetroxide. **oxalacetic a.**, an intermediate product in the Krebs cycle of carbohydrate metabolism, being formed from malic acid by the action of malic dehydrogenase in the presence of NAD and malate dehydrogenase, and being converted to citric acid by condensation with acetyl-CoA in the presence of condensing enzyme. Called also *ketosuccinic a., oxobutanedioic a.,* and *oxosuccinic a.* **oxalic a.**, an acid, $(COOH)_2 \cdot 2H_2O$, occurring as colorless crystals, which is present in various plants, especially those of the genera *Oxalis* and *Rumex*. Used as a reagent, in making glucose from starch, as a disinfectant, and in various chemical and industrial processes. It is caustic and corrosive to the skin and mucous membranes. Ingestion may cause vomiting, diarrhea, melena, gastroenteritis, and death. Excessive amounts of calcium oxalate may produce kidney damage. Some species of *Penicillium* and *Aspergillus* convert sugars to oxalates. Called also *ethanedioic a.* **α-oxoglutaric a.**, α-ketoglutaric a. **2-oxopentanedioic a.**, α-ketoglutaric a. **4-oxopentanoic a.**, levulinic a. **oxosuccinic a.**, oxalacetic a. **oxy a's**, ternary a's. **oxyphenylaminopropionic a.**, tyrosine. **palmitic a.**, a saturated fatty acid, $CH_3(CH_2)_{14}COOH$, found in palm and other vegetable oils and in animal fats, which occurs as white crystalline scales that are insoluble in water, sparingly soluble in cold alcohol, and soluble in hot alcohol, ether, chloroform, and propyl alcohol. Its metabolic degradation produces carbon dioxide, water, and energy. Called also *cetylic a., hexadecanoic a., hexadecylic a.* **palmitoleic a.,** an unsaturated fatty acid, 9-hexadecenoic acid, found in marine animals, reptilian, avian, amphibian, and, to a lesser extent, mammalian fats. Called also *physetoleic a.* **pantothenic a.,** a vitamin of the B complex, N-(2, 4-dihydroxy-3, 3-dimethylbutyryl-3, 3-dimethylbutyryl)-β-alanine, which is very hygroscopic, easily destroyed by acids, bases, and heat, and is soluble in water, ethyl acetate, dioxane, and glacial acetic acid, moderately soluble in ether and amyl alcohol, and insoluble in benzene and chloroform. The liver, kidneys, yeasts, crude molasses, milk, grain, cereals, and rice are principal sources of pantothenic acid. In its active form, it is a constituent of coenzyme A. Called also *vitamin B₅*. Pantothenic acid is required by all animals, being involved in the production of adrenocortical hormones from acetate and cholesterol and takes parts in metabolic processes, including acetyl or other group transfer, fatty acid synthesis, and oxidation. Human requirement for pantothenic acid is not known but recommended daily intake is 5 to 12 mg per 2500 Cal. Human pantothenic acid deficiency has not been recorded because of its wide natural occurrence in foods of animal and plant origin. Experimental deficiency may produce fatigue, nausea, gastric disorders, headache, lassitude, adrenal hyperfunction, and paresthesia; in rats, ulcerations and hyperkeratosis of the oral mucosa associated with gingival and periodontal necrosis may occur. *para-***aminobenzoic a.,** *p*-aminobenzoic a. *para-***aminosalicylic a.,** aminosalicylic a. **paralactic a.,** see *lactic a.* **paramandelic a.,** mandelic a. **parasilicic a.,** a form of silicic acid, H₆SiO₆. **paratartaric a. (DL-tartaric a.),** an optically inactive form of tartaric acid, being a mixture of dextrotartaric and levotartaric acids. Called also *racemic tartaric a.* and *uvic a.* **pelargonic a.,** a fatty acid, *n*-nanoic acid, CH₃(CH₂)₇COOH, occurring as a colorless or yellowish oil with slight odor, found in the garden geranium (*Pelargonium*) and other plants. Used in the manufacture of various chemicals and pharmaceuticals. It may be irritating to the skin and mucous membranes. Called also *nonanoic a., nonoic a.,* and *nonylic a.* **penicillanic a.,** a compound, 3,3-dimethyl-7-oxo-4-thio-1-azabicyclo[3,2,0]heptane-2-carboxylic acid. It is a basic component of penicillin, from which all penicillins derive, having no antimicrobial properties of its own. **penicillic a.,** an antibiotic, 3-methoxy-5-methyl-4-oxo-2,5-hexadienoic acid, elaborated by various species of *Penicillium* and *Aspergillus.* **penicilloic a.,** one of several inactive substances obtained by cleaving penicillins, as by the enzyme penicillinase. **pentahydroxycaproic a.,** gluconic a. **pentanoic a.,** normal valeric a.; see *valeric a.* **periodic a.,** any of a series of acids which can be thought of as being formed by the union of different amounts of water with periodic anhydride (I₂O₇), varying from HIO₄ to H₇IO₇. **pertechnetic a.,** a compound, HTeO₄, from which technecium salts are produced. See also PERTECHNETATE. **phenoxymethylenepenicillic a.,** PENICILLIN V. **β-phenylacrylic a.,** cinnamic a. **2-phenylcinchonimic a.,** cinchophen. **phenylformic a.,** benzoic a. **phenylglycolic a.,** phenylhydroxyacetic a., mandelic a. **phenylic a.,** phenol (1). **phocenic a.,** valeric a. **phosphatidic a.,** a compound formed by the esterification of the three hydroxyl groups of glycerol with two fatty acid groups and one phosphoric acid group; the characteristic group of the phospholipids. Originally isolated from plants, phosphatidic acids are probably intermediates in the synthesis of phospholipids and triglycerides in animal tissues. **phosphoglyceric a.,** glycerophosphoric a. **phosphoric a.,** an acid, H₃PO₄, occurring as a clear, odorless, syrupy liquid or as transparent, unstable crystals, formed by the oxidation of phosphorus, which are miscible with water and ethanol. When properly diluted, it has a pleasing acid taste; in concentrated solutions, the acid is irritating to the skin and mucous membranes. Used as a pharmaceutical solvent, an acidulant of fluoride solutions and beverages, a component of dental cements, and an enamel etching agent. When mixed with zinc oxide, it forms zinc phosphate cement (see under CEMENT). Formerly used in the treatment of lead poisoning. Called also *orthophosphoric a.* **phosphoric a., glacial,** metaphosphoric a. **phosphoric a. glycerol ester,** glycerophosphoric a. **phosphoric a. triethyleneimide,** triethylenephosphoramide. **phosphorous a.,** a compound, H₃PO₃, occurring as white, hygroscopic, water-soluble crystals with garlic-like taste, whose salts are called *phosphines;* used as a reagent and reducing agent. Called also *orthophosphorous a.* **phthalic a.,** an acid, 1,2-benzenedicarboxylic acid, occurring as colorless crystals that are readily soluble in alcohol but sparingly in water and ether. Used in the production of drugs and dyes, as a laboratory

reagent, and in various chemical processes. Called also *o-benzenedicarboxylic a.* and *o-phthalic a.* **o-phthalic a.,** phthalic a. **physetoleic a.,** palmitoleic a. **picric a.,** a compound, 2,4,6-trinitrophenol, occurring as pale yellow, odorless, bitter crystals that are soluble in water, alcohol, benzene, chloroform, and ether. It is a highly explosive substance used as a tissue fixative, dye, antiseptic, astringent, and stimulant of epithelialization. In a solution, used in the treatment of minor burns and exudative wounds. Called also *carbazotic a., nitroxanthic a.,* and *picronitic a.* **piperidic a.,** γ-aminobutyric a. **pivalic a.,** trimethylacetic a.; see *valeric a.* **polyacrylic a.,** a polymer of acrylic acid, occurring as a clear solid that is soluble in water. A 40 percent aqueous solution mixed with zinc oxide forms polycarboxylate cement. **polyanhydroglucuronic a.,** oxidized CELLULOSE. **polycarboxylic a.,** an organic acid having two or more carboxyl (COOH) groups. **polymannuronic a.,** alginic a. **primary α-amino a.,** α-amino a. **propanoic a.,** propionic a. **propene a., 2-propenoic a.,** acrylic a. **2-propenyl-acrylic a.,** sorbic a. **pro-**

$$\text{pionic a., a carboxylic acid, } CH_3CH_2\overset{\text{O}}{\overset{\|}{C}}—OH,$$ found in chyme and sweat, and one of the products of bacterial fermentation of wood pulp. It occurs as an oily liquid with a slightly pungent, rancid odor. Its salts are used as mold inhibitors in bread, in the production of pharmaceuticals, and in various chemical and industrial processes. Sodium proprionate is used in the treatment of dermatomycoses. Called also *ethylformic a., methylacetic a.,* and *propanoic a.* **propylacetic a.,** normal valeric a.; see *valeric a.* **propylformic a.,** butyric a. **pteroic a.,** a crystalline compound, *p*-[(2-amino-4-hydroxy-6-pteridylmethyl)-amino]-benzoic acid, which is a combination of *p*-aminobenzoic acid (PABA) and pteridine that, in combination with glutamic acid, forms folic acid. **pteroylglutamic a.,** folic acid. **pyrazinoic a. amide,** pyrazinamide. **4-pyridinecarboxylic a.,** isoniazid. **pyrophosphoric a.,** a compound, H₄P₂O₇, occurring as a viscous, syrupy liquid which solidifies after long standing at room temperature and, when diluted with water, is converted to orthophosphoric acid. Its salts are pyrophosphates. Called also *diphosphoric a.* **pyrosulfuric a.,** fuming sulfuric a.; see *sulfuric a.* **quisetic a.,** aconitic a. **racemic mandelic a.,** mandelic a. **racemic tartaric a.,** paratartaric a. **retinoic a.,** tretinoin. **ribonucleic a.,** ribose nucleic a., RNA. **saccharic a.,** 1. a dibasic acid, COOH·-(CHOH)₄COOH, formed by the action of nitric acid on dextrose or carbohydrates containing dextrose. 2. a monobasic acid, C₆H₁₂O₆, or tetraoxycaproic acid, not existing in nature. **salicylic a.,** a compound, 2-hydroxybenzoic acid, occurring as a white, odorless, crystalline powder or needles with a sweetish, acrid taste, that are soluble in water, ethanol, chloroform, ether, and benzene. Used as a keratolytic agent in the treatment of warts and eczematoid dermatitis. It has also some antifungal and antiseptic properties and is used in the treatment of ringworm and other fungal diseases. Its esters are used as analgesics, antipyretics, and anti-inflammatory agents. Called also ortho-*hydroxybenzoic a.* See also SALICYLATE. **salicylic a., acetate,** aspirin. **salicylic a. amide,** salicylamide. **sarcolactic a.,** see *lactic a.* **secondary amino a.,** see *imino a.* **sialic a.,** any one in a group of amino sugars containing nine or more carbon atoms; *N*- and *O*-substituted derivatives of neuraminic acid, occurring in mucoproteins, mucopolysaccharides, and mucolipids, and found in various animal tissues and bacteria. Called also *nonulosaminic a.* **silicic a.,** 1. an acid of which silicon is the base, forming silicates, and occurring in several forms, as orthosilicic acid, metasilicic acid, and parasilicic acid. 2. less correctly, silica, SiO₂, or silicic anhydride. **sorbic a.,** a compound, 2,4-hexadienoic acid, occurring as a crystalline powder with a specific odor, which is soluble in water, alcohol, and ether. Used as a fungistatic agent in food preservation, particularly cheese, and in various other processes. Called also *2-propenyl-acrylic a.* **stannic a.,** a colloidal or gelatinous compound, Sn(OH)₄, formed by the addition of alkalies to tin salts. It is amphoteric, forming tin salts with strong acids and alkali stannates with strong bases. **stearic a., stearophanic a.,** a compound, C₁₈H₃₆O₂, occurring as a hard, white or yellowish, glossy, crystalline solid or powder with the taste and odor of tallow, which is soluble in ethanol, chloroform, ether, acetone, carbon tetrachloride, and disulfide, but not in water. Commercial stearic acid is a mixture of stearic, palmitic, and oleic acids. Used for suppositories, coating bitter remedies and enteric pills, ointments, impregnatic plaster of Paris, cosmetics, and impression compounds. Called also *cetylacetic a.* and *octadecanoic a.* **strong a.,** an acid that dissociates in solution almost completely into ions at ordinary concentrations. **succinic a.,** an acid, 1,4-butanedioic acid, found in amber, lichens, fossils, and certain hydatid cysts. In the oxidative metabolism of carbohydrates, it is an intermediate product in the Krebs cycle. Used as a growth

retardant. Formerly used in the treatment of diabetic ketosis and, combined with salicylates, of rheumatic fever and arthritis. **sulfinic a.,** an organic compound containing the group SO · OH. *o*-**sulfobenzoic a.,** saccharin. **sulfonic a.,** a compound, SO_2OH, derived from sulfuric acid by replacing an OH group; used in the production of dyes and drugs. **sulfuric a.,** an acid, H_2SO_4, occurring as a dense, oily, colorless to dark brown (depending on purity) liquid. It is a very reactive substance that dissolves most metals (except the noble ones), oxidizes hydrates, and chars most organic compounds, being extremely corrosive to tissues. When combined with sulfur trioxide, it forms *fuming sulfuric acid.* Used in a wide variety of industrial processes, and, formerly, in the treatment of gastric hypoacidity and as a topical caustic. Called also *hydrogen sulfate* and *oil of vitriol.* **sulfuric a., fuming,** an acid, $H_2SO_4 \cdot SO_3$, occurring as a heavy, oily, colorless to dark brown (depending on purity) liquid with the strong suffocating odor of sulfur trioxide. It is formed by sulfuric acid and sulfur trioxide. Used as a sulfating and sulfonating agent in industrial processes. It is highly toxic, corrosive, and suffocating. Called also *disulfuric a.* and *oleum.* **sulfurous a.,** sulfur dioxide in aqueous solution, H_2SO_3, occurring as a colorless liquid with a strong pungent odor. Used as a disinfectant, bleaching agent, parasiticide, food preservative, and in other processes. Exposure, particularly ingestion or inhalation of fumes, may cause lesions of the eyes and mucous membranes. **tartaric a.,** an acid, 2,3-dihydroxysuccinic acid, occurring in four forms: (1) ordinary or dextrotartaric acid; (2) levotartaric acid; (3) paratartaric acid, a mixture of (1) and (2), hence optically inactive; and (4) mesotartaric acid, optically inactive from internal compensation. Used in baking and tanning, and as a chemical reagent. D-**tartaric a.,** dextrotartaric a. DL-**tartaric a.,** paratartaric a. L-**tartaric a.,** levotartaric a. **tartaric a., racemic,** paratartaric a. *meso*-**tartaric a.,** mesotartaric a. **taurocholic a.,** a conjugated form of cholic acid and taurine, the salt of which is one of the bile salts. **teichoic a's,** components of the cell wall of gram-positive bacteria, consisting of long chains of either glycerol or ribitol which are linked by means of phosphodiester bonds and which carry various substituents, including amino acids and monosaccharides. Fatty acylated forms of teichoic acids are believed to be associated with the cell membranes of gram-positive bacteria. **ternary a's,** a group of acids composed of oxygen and another element in addition to hydrogen, commonly being named after an element other than hydrogen or oxygen, and ending with the suffix -*ic*, such as sulfuric acid or nitric acid. Called also *oxy a's.* ***n*-tetracosanoic a.,** lignoceric a. ***n*-tetradecanoic a.,** myristic a. **tetraoxycaproic a.,** saccharic a. (2). **thio a.,** an organic acid in which divalent sulfur has replaced one or all of the oxygen atoms of the carboxyl group. **thioaminopropionic a.,** cysteine. **thioctic a.,** α-lipoic a. *trans*-**butenedioic a.,** fumaric a. *trans*-1,2-**ethylenedicarboxylic a.,** fumaric a. **tri-a.,** see *tricarboxylic a.* **tribasic a.,** an acid with three displaceable hydrogen atoms per molecule. **tricarboxylic a.,** an aromatic or aliphatic acid having three carboxyl (—COOH) groups in the compound. Written also *tri-a.* **trichloroacetic a.,** a caustic substance, occurring as a water-soluble, crystalline solid with a slight characteristic odor, $C_2HCl_3O_2$. Used in dental cavity preparation and as a cauterizing agent in apthous ulcers, warts, and verrucae. Contact with the skin or mucous membrane may cause severe burns. **trimethylacetic a.,** see *valeric a.* **triprotic a.,** one that yields three hydrogen ions per molecule, such as phosphorus acid. **tungstic a.,** a compound, H_2WO_4, occurring as a yellow or greenish yellow powder, insoluble in water and acids, except hydrofluoric acid, and slowly soluble in caustic alkalies. Used as a source of metallic tungsten and as precipitant for some nitrogenous substances. **uric a.,** a crystallizable acid, 8-hydroxyxanthine or 2,6,8-trioxypurine, which is insoluble in water and ether but is soluble in alkaline salts. In man, it is probably produced by the liver and excreted in the urine; its rate of excretion reflecting purine catabolism and being influenced by 11-oxygenated corticosteroids and ACTH. The blood level of uric acid increases in gout and in the Lesch-Nyhan syndrome; its salts (urates) are the principal components of calcareous concretions and tophi. Called also *lithic a.* **uridylic a.,** a nucleotide constituent of RNA, being a monophosphoric ester of uracil. Called also *uridine phosphoric a.* and *uridine monophosphate (UMP).* **uridine phosphoric a.,** uridylic a. **uronic a.,** an acid derived from simple sugar by oxidation of the primary group at the opposite end of aldose to a carboxyl group. Uronic acids are not found in nature in the free state, but some of their derivatives, such as glucuronic and galacturonic acids, are of biological importance. **uvic a.,** paratartaric a. **vaccenic a.,** an unsaturated fatty acid, *trans*-11-octadecanoic acid, isomeric with oleic acid; found in butterfat and in some animal fats. It contains a growth-promoting factor for rats. **valerianic a.,** see

valeric a. **valeric a.,** a carboxylic acid found in the roots of *Valeriana officinalis* and *Angelica archangelica*, and which may be produced synthetically. Called also *butacarboxylic a.* and *phocenic a.* It occurs in four forms: (1) *normal valeric acid* (pentanoic a., propylacetic a., valerianic a., and valeric a.); (2) *isovaleric acid*; (3) β-*methylbutyric acid*; and (4) *trimethylacetic acid (pivalic a.)*. It is a colorless liquid with a penetrating odor and taste that is moderately toxic and irritating. Used in various chemical, pharmaceutical, and industrial processes. Its salts were once considered medicinal and were used for their supposed antispasmodic and nerve stimulant effects. **vanadic a.,** a compound, HVO_3, occurring as golden scales. Used as an oxidizing and antiseptic agent. It may cause chronic poisoning. Called also *metavanadic a.* **vinegar a.,** acetic a. **vinylformic a.,** acrylic a. **vitamin A a.,** tretinoin. **weak a.,** an acid that dissociates in solution only slightly into ions at ordinary concentrations.

acidalbumin (as″id-al′bu-min) a protein which dissolves in acids and shows acid reaction.

Acidaminococcus (ah-sid″ah-min″o-kok′us) a genus of gram-negative, anaerobic bacteria of the family Veillonellaceae, occurring as oval or kidney-shaped diplococci, about 0.6 to 1.0 μm in diameter. Amino acids, especially glutamic acid, can serve as their sole source of energy. They have been isolated from the gastrointestinal tract of animals, including man.

acidaminuria (as″id-am″i-nu′re-ah) an excess of urinary amino acids.

acidemia (as″i-de′me-ah) [*acid* + Gr. *haima* blood + -*ia*] a decreased pH of the blood, irrespective of changes in the blood carbonates.

acid-fast (as′id-fast) not readily decolorized by acids when stained. See acid-fast bacteria, under BACTERIUM.

acidic (ah-sid′ik) of or pertaining to an acid; acid-forming; having a pH of less than 7.

acidifier (as-sid″i-fi′er) an agent that causes or increases acidity.

acidify (as-sid′i-fi) 1. to render acid. 2. to become acid.

acidimetry (as-i-dim′ĕ-tre) the determination of free acid in a solution.

acidity (ah-sid′i-te) 1. the state of being acid. 2. the acid content.

acidocyte (as″i-do-sīt″) eosinophil.

acidocytopenia (as″i-do-si″to-pe′ne-ah) [*acidocyte* + Gr. *penia* poverty] a condition characterized by an abnormally low number of eosinophil leukocytes in the blood.

acidocytosis (as″i-do-si-to′sis) a condition characterized by an abnormally large number of eosinophil leukocytes in the blood.

acidogenic (as″i-do-jen′ik) producing acid or acidity, or produced by acid or acidity.

acidophil (ah-sid′o-fil) [L. *acidum* acid + Gr. *philein* to love] 1. a cell or a histological structure staining readily in acids. 2. an organism that grows well in highly acid media. 3. a cell of the anterior pituitary characterized by a round or oval shape with cleanly defined boundaries, round or ovoid nucleus, and cytoplasmic granules that stain bright orange with orange-G counterstain.

acidophilic (as″i-do-fil′ik) 1. readily stained with acid dyes. 2. thriving in acid media; said of microorganisms.

acidoresistant (as″i-do-re-zis′tant) 1. resistant to acids. 2. resistant to decoloration by acids; said of certain microorganisms.

acidosis (as″i-do′sis) a pathologic condition resulting from the increase of the level of acids in body fluids and reduced alkali reserve, characterized by an increase in hydrogen ion content (decrease in pH). Cf. ALKALOSIS. **compensated a.,** metabolic or respiratory acidosis in which compensatory mechanisms have returned the pH toward normal. **congenital hyperchloremic a.,** Lightwood-Albright SYNDROME. **diabetic a.,** metabolic acidosis resulting from accumulation of ketones in uncontrolled diabetes mellitus. **hypercapnic a.,** respiratory a. **hyperchloremic a.,** metabolic acidosis in which there is an increase in plasma chlorides. **idiopathic renal a.,** Lightwood-Albright SYNDROME. **metabolic a., nonrespiratory a.,** that in which the acid-base equilibrium shifts toward the acid side because of loss of base or retention of noncarbonic, or fixed (nonvolatile), acids. **renal tubular a.,** metabolic acidosis secondary to renal disorders. **renal tubular a. with rickets,** Lightwood-Albright SYNDROME. **respiratory a.,** that associated with excess retention of carbon dioxide in the body. Called also *hypercapnic a.* **starvation a.,** metabolic acidosis in caloric starvation, associated with the accumulation of ketone bodies. **uremic a.,** that due to chronic kidney diseases associated with diminished ability to excrete acids in the urine.

acidulated (ah-sid′u-lāt″ed) rendered acid; acidified.

acidulous (ah-sid′u-lus) somewhat acid.

aciduria (as″ĭ-du′re-ah) the presence of acid in the urine.

aciduric (as″ĭ-du′rik) [L. *acidum* + *durare* to endure] acid-tolerant; said of bacteria able to withstand a degree of acidity usually fatal to nonsporulating bacteria.

acidyl (as′ĭ-dil) any acid radical.

acidylation (ah-sid″ĭ-la′shun) acylation.

Acinetobacter (ah-sĭ-ne′to-bak″ter) [*a* neg. + Gr. *kinēsis* motion + *baktērion* little rod] a genus of gram-negative, nonmotile, non-sporogenous, aerobic, penicillin-resistant bacteria of the family Neisserieaceae, occurring as short and plump rods, about 1.0 to 1.5 μm by 1.5 to 2.5 μm in size, approaching coccoid shape in the stationary phase. They have been isolated from animals, including man, under normal and pathological conditions, and from water and soil. **A. mal′lei,** *Pseudomonas mallei*; see under PSEUDOMONAS. **A. parapertus′sis,** *Bordetella parapertussis*; see under BORDETELLA.

aciniform (ah-sin′ĭ-form) [L. *acinus* grape + *forma* form] resembling an acinus, a grape, or a bunch of grapes.

acinotubular (as″ĭ-no-tu′bu-lar) tubuloacinar.

acinus (as′ĭ-nus), pl. *ac′ini* [L. "grape, berry"] a general anatomical term used in connection with a minute saclike dilatation, particularly in a gland. Often used as a synonym for *alveolus*.

AcK actinium K; see FRANCIUM.

Ackerman bar joint (bar) [H. *Ackerman*, Swiss dentist] see under JOINT.

Ackerman-Proffit classification [J. L. *Ackerman*, American dentist; William R. *Proffit*, American dentist] see MALOCCLUSION.

Acket trademark for *salicylamide*.

aclusion (ah-klu′zhun) absence of occlusion of the opposing surfaces of teeth. See OCCLUSION.

ACMA American Occupational Medical Association.

Acme articulator see under ARTICULATOR.

acne (ak′ne) [probably a corruption of Gr. *akmē* point or of *achnē* chaff] 1. any inflammatory disease of the sebaceous glands. 2. a. vulgaris. See also CHLORACNE. **a. rosa′cea,** a chronic disease of the face, especially of the nose and adjacent areas, usually observed among middle-aged patients with seborrhea, and characterized by erythema, acneiform lesions, telangiectasis, and in some instances hypertrophy. Called also *brandy nose* and *rosacea*. See also RHINOPHYMA. **a. vulga′ris,** an inflammatory condition of the sebaceous glands, usually occurring during puberty and adolescence, and characterized by an eruption of papules and pustules.

acneiform (ak-ne′ĭ-form″) resembling acne.

acocantherin (ak″o-kan′ther-in) ouabain.

Acolen trademark for *dehydrocholic acid* (see under ACID).

ACOMS American College of Oral and Maxillofacial Surgeons (see under COLLEGE).

aconitase (ah-kon′ĭ-tās) aconitate HYDRATASE.

ACORDE A Consortium on Restorative Dentistry Education; a project aimed at reaching a concensus on how various restorative procedures can be performed, organized jointly by the American Dental Association; the American Association of Dental Schools, Section on Operative Dentistry; the Division of Dentistry of the Bureau of Health Resources, Health Resources Administration, Public Health Service, Department of Health and Human Services; and the National Medical Audiovisual Center of the National Library of Medicine.

acoria (ah-ko′re-ah) [*a* neg. + Gr. *koros* satiety + *-ia*] a condition characterized by absence of satiety; a form of polyphagia.

acou- [Gr. *akouein* to hear] a combining form denoting relationship to hearing.

acoumetry (ah-koo′mĕ-tre) [*acou-* + Gr. *metrein* to measure] the testing of the accuracy or acuteness of hearing.

acoustic (ah-koōs′tik) [Gr. *akoustikos*] pertaining to sound or the sense of hearing.

ACP American College of Prosthodontists (see under COLLEGE).

ACPA American Cleft Palate Association (see under ASSOCIATION).

acquired (ah-kwīrd′) [L. *acquirere* to obtain] attained; not congenital; developed after birth: said of a pathological condition.

acquisitus (ah-kwis′ĕ-tus) [L.] acquired.

ACR American College of Radiology (see under COLLEGE).

acral (ak′ral) [Gr. *akron* extremity] pertaining to an extremity or apex.

acraldehyde (ak-ral′dĕ-hīd) acrolein.

acrania (ah-kra′ne-ah) [*a* neg. + Gr. *kranion* skull + *-ia*] a developmental abnormality characterized by complete or partial absence of the cranium.

acranius (ah-kra′ne-us) a malformed fetus exhibiting acrania.

acratia (ah-kra′she-ah) [*a* neg. + Gr. *kratos* power + *-ia*] 1. loss of strength; weakness. 2. incontinence.

Acremonium (ak″re-mo′ne-um) a genus of soil-inhabiting dermatomycetous fungi (Fungi Imperfecti), associated with eye infection (mycotic keratitis), a few species being involved in mycotic mycetoma. The genus is a source of cephalosporins. Formerly called *Cephalosporium*.

acrid (ak′rid) [L. *acer, acris* sharp] pungent, sharp, irritating.

acridine (ak′rĭ-dēn) a tricyclic, heterocyclic hydrocarbon, $C_{13}H_9N$, obtained from coal tar, which occurs as small, colorless needles that are soluble in alcohol, ether, and carbon disulfide, and sparingly in hot water. Used in the synthesis of dyes and drugs; its derivatives are mostly fluorescent yellow dyes (acridine dyes) and those used in medicine (as antiseptics) are acriflavine and proflavine. It is a strong irritant to the skin and mucous membranes and causes sneezing on inhalation. Called also *10-azaanthracene*.

acriflavine (ak″rĭ-fla′vin) a granular, odorless, deep orange powder, which is a mixture of 2,8-diamino-10-methylacridinium chloride and 2,8-diaminoacridine; used as a topical antiseptic. Called also *neutral a.* and *chromoflavine*. **acid a.,** a. hydrochloride. **a. hydrochloride,** a mixture of the hydrochlorides of 3,6-diamino-1-methylacridnium chloride and 3,6-diaminoacridine. Sometimes used as an antiseptic and germicide. Called also *acid a., acid flavine*, and *trypaflavine*. **neutral a.,** acriflavine.

Acrilan trademark for an acrylic resin obtained by polymerization of acrylonitrile, which is resistant to mineral acids, common solvents, weak alkalies, and other corrosive substances.

acro- [Gr. *akron* extremity; *akros* extreme] a combining form denoting relation to an extremity, top, or summit.

acroanesthesia (ak″ro-an″es-the′ze-ah) [*acro-* + *anesthesia*] loss of sensation in the extremities.

acrobaryte (ak″ro-bar′it) BARIUM sulfate.

acrobrachycephaly (ak″ro-brak″ĕ-sef′ah-le) [*acro-* + Gr. *brachys* short + *kephalē* head] a congenital abnormality characterized by fusion of the coronal suture and abnormal shortening of the anteroposterior diameter of the skull.

acrocentric (ak″ro-sen′trik) [*acro-* + Gr. *kentron*, L. *centrum* center] having the centromere near one end. See acrocentric CHROMOSOME.

acrocephalia (ak″ro-se-fa′le-ah) acrocephaly.

acrocephalic (ak″ro-sĕ-fal′ik) pertaining to or characterized by a skull with a highly arched cranial vault. Called also *acrocephalous*. See acrocephalic SKULL.

acrocephalopolydactyly (ak″ro-sef″ah-lo-pol″e-dak′tĭ-le) See Carpenter's SYNDROME.

acrocephalopolysyndactyly (ak″ro-sef″ah-lo-pol″e-sin-dak′tĭ-le) acrocephalosyndactyly with polydactyly as an additional feature; two types are known: type I inherited as an autosomal dominant trait (see Pfeiffer's SYNDROME) and type II inherited as an autosomal recessive trait (see Carpenter's SYNDROME).

acrocephalosyndactyly (ak″ro-sef″ah-lo-sin-dak′tĭ-le) [*acrocephaly* + *syndactyly*] a congenital malformation consisting of a pointed shape of the top of the head and syndactyly of the four extremities. Called also *acrosphenosyndactylia*. See also ACROCEPHALOPOLYSYNDACTYLY. **a. I,** Apert's SYNDROME. **a. III,** Saethre-Chotzen SYNDROME. **Noack's a.,** Pfeiffer's a., Pfeiffer's SYNDROME.

acrocephalous (ak″ro-sef′ah-lus) acrocephalic.

acrocephaly (ak″ro-sef′ah-le) [*acro-* + Gr. *kephalē* head] a condition characterized by a skull with a highly arched cranial vault. Called also *acrocephalia*. See acrocephalic SKULL and OXYCEPHALY.

acrocinesis (ak″ro-si-ne′sis) [*acro-* + Gr. *kinēsis* motion] excessive mobility; abnormal freedom of movement.

acrocranic (ak″ro-kra′nik) pertaining to a dry skull with a highly arched cranial vault. See ACROCEPHALIC and acrocephalic SKULL.

acrocraniodysphalangia (ak″ro-kra″ne-o-dis″fah-lan′je-ah) Apert's SYNDROME.

acrocrany (ak′ro-kra″ne) [*acro-* + *cranium*] a skull with a highly arched cranial vault. See also acrocephalic SKULL and ACROCEPHALY.

acrodermatitis (ak″ro-der″mah-ti′tis) [*acro-* + *dermatitis*] inflammation of the skin of the hands and feet; dermatitis of the extremities. **a. enteropath′ica,** a familial syndrome of early childhood, often with an onset at the time of weaning, consisting of diarrhea, steatorrhea, alopecia, paronychia with nail dystrophy, pustulous dermatitis, perferentially located around body orifices, perioral pustules, and frequently blepharitis and conjunctivitis. Defective tryptophan metabolism is the suspected etiologic factor. Called also *Brandt's syndrome* and *Danbolt-Closs syndrome*.

acrodynia (ak″ro-din′e-ah) [acro- + Gr. *odynē* pain + -*ia*] a disease of young children, believed to be caused by mercury poisoning, the source of which is usually a teething powder, ammoniated mercury ointment, calomel lotion, or mercury bichloride disinfectant. It is characterized by restlessness, insomnia, weight loss, anorexia, tachycardia, superficial sensory loss, paresthesia, photophobia with or without conjunctivitis, fever, leukocytosis, albuminuria, muscular hypotonia, and erythemic eruptions on the skin of the fingers, toes, nose, buttocks, and cheeks. Oral manifestations consist of profuse salivation; painful, sensitive gingivae, sometimes exhibiting ulcers; bruxism and premature shedding of teeth; and difficult mastication. Called also *dermatopolyneuritis, epidemic erythema, pink disease,* and *Swift's disease.*

acrodysplasia (ak″ro-dis-pla′se-ah) [acro- + *dysplasia*] Apert's SYNDROME.

acrolein (al-ro′le-in) [L. *acer* acrid + *oleum* oil] a flammable and unstable (thus, potentially explosive), volatile, acrid yellow to red liquid, $CH_2:CHCHO$, being a decomposition product of glycerol and glycerides, which on oxidation produces acrylic acid. It irritates the eyes and mucosa, causing lacrimation, and may cause asthmatic reaction and, in high concentrations, pulmonary edema. Called also *acraldehyde, acrylaldehyde, acrylic aldehyde,* and 2-*propenal.*

acromegaly (ak″ro-meg′al-le) [acro- + Gr. *megalē* great] a disorder due to hyperfunction of the anterior pituitary gland after maturity, usually caused by an adenoma, associated with hypersecretion of growth hormone, resulting in overgrowth of the bones, connective tissue, and viscera. Skeletal changes principally involve the skull and small bones of the hands and feet, resulting in prominent cheek bones; frontal bossing; grossly overdeveloped mandible pressing on the tongue and alveolar processes, with consequent relative mandibular prognathism; and broadening of the hands, fingers, and feet. Enlargement of the soft tissue is usually manifested by large ears and nose; thick lips; enlarged tongue with a lobulated margin and papillary hypertrophy, which fills the oral cavity and exerts pressure on the teeth, resulting in tipping of the teeth to the buccal or labial side; fleshy appearance of the hands and feet; widespread splanchnomegaly; and hypertrophy of the target organs for anterior pituitary hormones, including the adrenal cortex, thyroid gland, parathyroid glands, and gonads. Sexual disorders, diabetes mellitus, hemianopsia, and increased intracranial pressure may be associated. *Gigantism* is regarded as the childhood form of acromegaly.

acronym (ak′ro-nim) [acro- + Gr. *onoma* name] a word formed by the initial letters of the principal components of a compound term.

acro-osteolysis (ak″ro-os″te-ol′i-sis) [acro- + Gr. *osteon* bone + -*lysis* dissolution] osteolysis of the bones of the extremities. See Hajdu-Cheney SYNDROME.

acropetal (ah-krop′ĕ-tal) [acro- + L. *petere*, to seek] rising toward the summit.

acrosclerosis (ak″ro-skle-ro′sis) [acro- + *sclerosis*] a form of scleroderma with marked involvement of the fingers and face. The oral cavity is seldom affected, but involvement of the skin of the face may extend to the lips and cause difficulty in opening the mouth.

acrosphenosyndactylia (ak″ro-sfe″no-sin″dak-til′e-ah) acrocephalosyndactyly.

acrotism (ak′ro-tizm) [*a* neg. + Gr. *krotos* beat + -*ism*] absence or weakness of the pulse.

Acrowax C trademark for a synthetic *dental wax* (see under WAX).

acrybaryte (ak″rĭ-bar′it) BARIUM sulfate.

acrylaldehyde (ak″rĭl-al′dĕ-hĭd) acrolein.

acrylate (ak′rĭ-lāt) a salt of acrylic acid containing the $C_3H_3O_2$— radical; a monomer used in the production of thermosetting acrylic surface-coating resins. See also acrylic ACID and acrylic RESIN.

acrylic (ah-kril′ik) 1. derived from acrylic acid. 2. acrylic RESIN.

acrylonitrile (ak″rĭ-lo-ni′tril) a colorless, mobile liquid with a mild odor, $CH_2:CH·CN$, which is soluble in common organic solvents and miscible with water. It may polymerize spontaneously, particularly on exposure to light, sometimes explosively. Used in the production of certain acrylic resins and as a pesticide fumigant for grain. It is highly flammable and toxic through its cyanide component. Called also 2-*propenenitrile* and *vinyl cyanide.*

ACS 1. American Chemical Society. 2. antireticular cytotoxic SERUM.

ACS I acrocephalosyndactyly I; see Apert's SYNDROME.

ACS III acrocephalosyndactyly III; see Saethre-Chotzen SYNDROME.

act (akt) 1. something done; a performance or deed. 2. a formal decision or law by a governmental agency. **State Dental Practice A.,** a law which controls the practice of dentistry in individual states.

Actedron trademark for *amphetamine.*

ACTH adrenocorticotropic HORMONE.

Actidil trademark for *triprolidine.*

Actidilon trademark for *triprolidine.*

Actilin trademark for *neomycin B.*

actin (ak′tin) a contractile protein. Its molecule is formed by two strands of F-actin (polymeric form), each composed of G-actin (globular form) monomers, wound around each other in thin filaments. The assembled thin actin filaments also contain tropomyosin and troponin for making and breaking cross-bridges and for generation of mechanical energy during muscle contraction. Actin filaments are a part of the I bands of striated muscle, and their function in muscle contraction consists of sliding among the myosin filaments to reduce the size of the sarcomere. See also ACTOMYOSIN, I BAND, muscle CONTRACTION, MYOSIN, and ratchet THEORY. **F-a., fibrous a.,** the polymeric form of actin, forming a part of the actin molecule. Two strands of F-actin, each made up of G-actin monomers, are wound around each other, producing a coil about 6 nm in diameter in the I band of the sarcomere. **G-a., globular a.,** the monomeric form of actin, having a molecular weight of 46,000, which forms strands of F-actin. It consists of a single polypeptide chain, globular in shape, containing one residue of ε-*N*-methyllysine, seven cysteines, and a large number of proline residues in addition to the other amino acids. It is easily polymerized to form the fibrous form of actin, F-actin. Molecules of G-actin bind calcium ions, ATP, and ADP.

actinic (ak-tin′ik) [Gr. *aktis* ray] pertaining to the rays beyond the violet end of the spectrum.

actiniform (ak-tin′ĭ-form) [Gr. *aktis* ray + L. *forma* form] formed like a ray; radiate.

actinism (ak′tĭ-nizm) [Gr. *aktis* ray] the chemical action of radiant energy, as in photography or heliotherapy.

actinium (ak-tin′e-um) [Gr. *aktis* ray] a silvery white metal, being a trivalent element homologous with lanthanum. Symbol, Ac; atomic weight, 227, atomic number, 89; specific gravity, 10.07. It has 11 isotopes, ^{227}Ac being the principal one, emitting soft beta rays and alpha rays, and having half-life of 21.6 years. Neutron bombardment of radium and uranium ore are the principal sources of actinium. It is a radioactive poison of the bone-seeking type. See also actinium SERIES. **a. group, a. series,** actinide SERIES. **a. K,** see FRANCIUM.

actino- [Gr. *aktis, aktinos* a ray] a combining form denoting relation to a ray, as ray-shaped, or pertaining to some form of radiation.

Actinobacillus (ak″tĭ-no-bah-sil′us) [actino- + *bacillus*] a genus of nonmotile, gram-negative, facultatively anaerobic bacteria of uncertain affiliation, occurring as oval or rod-shaped cells, 0.4 by 0.4 μ in size, which do not form endospores. They are pathogenic to cattle, sheep, horses, and pigs. **A. equu′lis,** a species found in the oral cavity and tonsils of horses, which causes suppurative lesions of the kidneys and joints in pigs and foals and endocarditis in pigs. **A. ligniere′sii,** a species causing gastrointestinal granulomatous lesions, particularly of the tongue in cattle, and suppurative lesions of the skin and lungs in sheep. **A. mal′lei,** *Pseudomonas mallei;* see under PSEUDOMONAS. **A. mu′ris,** *Streptobacillus moniliformis;* see under STREPTOBACILLUS.

Actinobacterium (ak″tĭ-no-bak-te′re-um) [actino- + Gr. *baktērion* little rod] a term frequently used erroneously as a synonym for *Actinomyces.* **A. israe′li,** *Actinomyces israelii;* see under ACTINOMYCES. **A. liquefa′ciens,** *Propionibacterium acnes;* see under PROPIONIBACTERIUM.

actinochemistry (ak″tĭ-no-kem′is-tre) [actino- + *chemistry*] the branch of chemistry dealing with the action of rays; photochemistry.

Actinocladothrix (ak″tĭ-no-klad′o-thriks) *Actinomyces.*

actinodermatitis (ak″tĭ-no-der″mah-ti′tis) [actino- + Gr. *derma* skin + -*itis*] dermatitis caused by sunrays or other forms of radiation; radiodermatitis.

actinogenesis (ak″tĭ-no-je′ĕ-sis) [actino- + Gr. *genesis* production] the production of rays; radiogenesis.

actinometry (ak″tĭ-nom-ĕ-tre) [actino- + Gr. *metron* measure] the measurement of the photochemical power of light.

Actinomyces (ak″tĭ-no-mi′sēz) [actino- + Gr. *mykēs* fungus] a genus of bacteria of the family Actinomycetaceae, order Actinomycetales, made up of gram-positive, non–acid-fast, non–spore-forming, nonmotile organisms, occurring as diphtheroid cells or rods with branching filaments, 1 μm or more in diameter. Most species are facultative anaerobes, requiring CO_2 for growth. Species may be either catalase negative or positive and fermentative, glucose fermentation products including acetic, formic, lactic, and succinic acids. Some species are pathogenic for animals, including man. Many are inhabitants of the human oral cavity, being found abundantly in dental plaque and in the gingival margin. *Actinomyces* has been used erroneously as a generic name for aerobic streptomycetes. Called also *Actinocladothrix, Discomyces,* and, erroneously, *Actinobacterium.* **A. asteroi′des,** *Nocardia asteroides;* see under NOCARDIA. **A. bo′vis,** a species of facultative anaerobes, growing in the presence of CO_2, which is sensitive to penicillin, streptomycin, tetracyclines, cephalosporin, and lincomycin. It is the etiologic agent of actinomycosis in cattle, and reportedly has been isolated from the human mouth. **A. brasilien′sis,** *Nocardia brasiliensis;* see under NOCARDIA. **A. dentocario′sus,** *Rothia dentocariosa;* see under ROTHIA. **A. eppinge′ri,** *Nocardia asteroides;* see under NOCARDIA. **A. gonidiafor′mis,** *Fusobacterium gonidiaformans;* see under FUSOBACTERIUM. **A. israe′lii,** a species causing actinomycosis in man and, occasionally, in cattle, which is normally found in the human oral cavity, including the tonsillar crypts and in pathological conditions such as dental calculus. It is sensitive to penicillin, tetracyclines, chloramphenicol, cephalosporin, and lincomycin. Also called *Actinobacterium israeli, Corynebacterium israeli, Discomyces israeli, Nocardia israeli, Proactinomyces israeli,* and *Streptothrix israeli.* **A. lu′teus,** *Nocardia lutea;* see under NOCARDIA. **A. mu′ris, A. mu′ris rat′ti,** *Streptobacillus moniliformis;* see under STREPTOBACILLUS. **A. naeslun′dii,** a species inhabiting the oral cavity in man, occurring in high proportions in the tonsillar crypts and in pathological conditions such as dental calculus and plaque, cemental caries, and advanced dentinal lesions. Periodontal destruction was observed in experimental infection in the rat. **A. odontolyt′icus,** a species of filamentous, facultative anaerobes, isolated from deep dentinal caries in man. **A. pseudonecroph′orus,** *Fusobacterium necrophorum;* see under FUSOBACTERIUM. **A. visco′sus,** a species of facultative anaerobes that may grow aerobically with CO_2, isolated from the oral cavity of man, hamsters, and rats. In man, it occurs in high proportions in the tonsillar crypts and in pathological conditions such as dental calculus and plaque, cemental caries, and advanced dentinal lesions. Spontaneous subgingival plaque, periodontal lesions, and cemental caries develop in infected hamsters. Called also *Odontomyces viscosus.*

actinomyces (ak″tĭ-no-mi′sēz), pl. *actinomyce′tes.* Any microorganism of the genus *Actinomyces.*

Actinomycetaceae (ak″tĭ-no-mi″sĕ-ta′se-e) [*Actinomyces* + -*aceae*] a family of bacteria of the order Actinomycetales, comprising the genera *Actinomyces, Arachnia, Bacterionema, Bifidobacterium,* and *Rothia.*

Actinomycetales (ak″tĭ-no-mi″se-ta′lēz) [*Actinomyces* + -*ales*] an order of bacteria, ranging in diameter from 0.5 to 2.0 μm, most being less than 1.0 μm. They form branching filaments that, in some families, develop into a mycelium; fragmentation of the filaments results in the formation of coccoid, elongate, or diphtheroid elements. Some families form spores, which may be produced singly on hypha, in pairs, or in chains; a large number of spores produce chains that may be straight, looped, or spiral. These organisms are usually gram-positive but may change with age. They are generally found in soil and fresh water, and some are pathogenic to animals, including man, and various forms are normal inhabitants of the human oral cavity. The order includes the families Actinomycetaceae, Actinoplanaceae, Dermatophilaceae, Nocardiaceae, and Streptomycetaceae.

actinomycete (ak″tĭ-no-mi′sēt) any microorganism of the order Actinomycetales.

actinomycetes (ak″tĭ-no-mi-se′tēz) plural of actinomyces or actinomycete.

actinomycin (ak″tĭ-no-mi′sin) any of a family of antibiotics obtained from cultures of various species of bacteria of the genus *Actinomyces (Streptomyces).* **a. D,** dactinomycin.

actinomycosis (ak″tĭ-no-mi-ko′sis) [*actino-* + Gr. *mykēs* fungus] any infection with actinomycetes, particularly a chronic disease of cattle caused by *Actinomyces bovis* or of man caused by *A. israelii.* In man, it is characterized by multiple indurated abscesses about the face, neck, chest, and abdomen, which discharge through numerous sinuses. Cervicofacial actinomycosis is the most common form, the organism having gained entrance through soft tissue wounds, through the pulp of a broken-down tooth, or through ducts of the salivary glands. It presents a dark-red discoloration of the skin, slate-blue elevated lesions, multiple nodules with ridges and furrows in the creases of the skin and neck, distinct boardlike induration, and multiple sinuses with both macroscopic and microscopic granules in the purulent discharge. The tongue is occasionally the primary site; the lesion is a deep-seated, slow-growing, painless nodule that eventually breaks through the mucosa, discharging a yellowish, purulent material. Gingival lesions are somewhat similar. Called also *big jaw, clams, clyers, lumpy jaw, Rivalta's disease,* and *wooden tongue.*

actinophage (ak-tin′o-fāj) [*actino-* + *phage*] a bacteriophage destructive to actinomycetes.

Actinoplanaceae (ak″tin′o-pla-na′se-e) [*Actinoplanes* + -*aceae*] a family of soil bacteria of the order Actinomycetales, including the genera *Actinoplanes, Amorphosporangium, Ampullariella, Spirillospora,* and *Streptosporangium.*

Actinoplanes (ak″tĭ-no-pla′nēz) [*actino-* + Gr. *planēs* one who wanders] a genus of soil bacteria of the family Actinoplanaceae, order Actinomycetales.

actinotherapy (ak″tĭ-no-ther′ah-pe) [*actino-* + Gr. *therapeia* treatment] treatment of disease with rays of light, particularly sunrays or ultraviolet rays.

action (ak′shun) [L. *actio*] 1. the performance of a function of the body or any of its parts or organs. 2. the exertion of force or power. **buffer a.,** the action exerted by a buffer in regulating the change of pH. **calorigenic a.,** the total energy released in the body by food. **cumulative a.,** action of suddenly increased intensity, as may be evidenced after administration of several doses of drugs. **gliding a.,** gliding MOVEMENT. **hinge a.,** hinge MOVEMENT. **reflex a.,** one that results when some sensation or stimulation passes over a reflex arc to a peripheral organ which is thus stimulated to activity without the aid of volition. **specific a.,** the action of a drug exerted on a certain definite pathogenic organism. **specific dynamic a.,** the increase in metabolism over the basal rate brought about by the ingestion and assimilation of food. **thermogenic a.,** the action of a food or drug in increasing the production of heat or the temperature of the body. **trigger a.,** an action which releases energy, metabolic or physiologic processes, and the like, whose character has no relation to the process which caused the release.

activate (ak′tĭ-vāt) 1. to render active. 2. to adjust an orthodontic appliance so that it will exert effective force on the teeth and jaws.

activation (ak″tĭ-va-shun). 1. the act or process of rendering active. 2. acceleration of chemical or physical changes in a substance, molecule, or atom by the action of heat, radiation, or the presence of another substance.

activator (ak′tĭ-va″tor) 1. an agent that renders some other agent active, especially a substance that combines with an inactive substance to render it capable of effecting its proper action. 2. a substance that stimulates the development of a particular structure in the embryo. 3. functional a. **a. appliance,** functional a. **bow a.,** a functional activator the halves of which are connected by a bow or safety-pin loop made of 0.9- to 1.0-mm wire. Between the halves of the anterior area, a layer of rubber is attached as a shock absorber and to open the bite in front. Its purpose is to use the transverse movements of the lower jaw. The construction bite not being in a fixed relationship, the lower half of the appliance may be changed in its relation to the upper half, beginning with the small forward positioning and increasing this gradually. The application of the activator has an effect similar to that of intermaxillary elastics, although the action is pushing instead of pulling. Called also *Schwarz a.* See illustra-

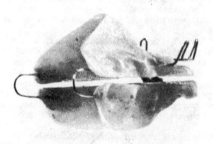

Bow activator. (From T. M. Garber and B. Neumann: Removable Orthodontic Appliances. Philadelphia, W. B. Saunders Co., 1977.)

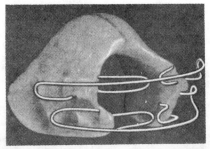

Open activator. (From T. M. Graber and B. Neumann: Removable Orthodontic Appliances. Philadelphia, W. B. Saunders Co., 1977.)

tion. **functional a.,** a removable orthodontic appliance which acts as a passive transmitter of the force produced by the function of the activated muscle, and applied to the teeth and alveolar processes. The weight of the appliance together with the guiding effect on the teeth during deglutition are believed to influence the position of the teeth and their contiguous alveolar

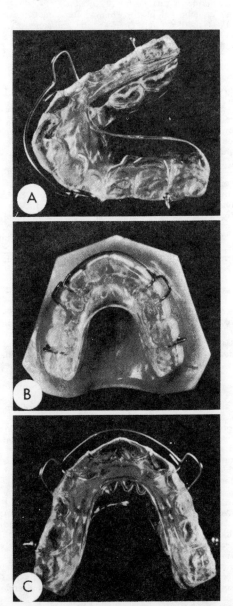

A to C, Different views of functional activator. (From A. M. Schwarz and M. Gratzinger: Removable Orthodontic Appliances. Philadelphia, W. B. Saunders Co., 1968; courtesy of Arne Bjork.)

bone. By guiding the mandible into a forward position with the appliance, the new reflexes thus created are expected to help to maintain this position. Simultaneously, the forces created by the muscles attempting to return to the original mandibular position are expected to act on the maxillary denture retruding the teeth. The activator, developed by Andresen, represents the original effort giving rise to the principles of functional jaw orthopedics. Called also *activator, activator appliance, Andresen appliance, Andresen monoblock, monoblock,* and *monoblock appliance.* See illustration. **Klammt a., open a. monoblock a.,** functional a. **open a.,** a functional activator having the anterior part open to allow easier breathing. Called also *Klammt a.* See illustration. **prothrombin a.,** PROTHROMBIN activator. **Schwarz a.,** bow a.

active (ak'tĭv) characterized by action. **optically a.,** having the power of rotating the plane of polarization.

activity (ak-tiv'ĭ-te) 1. the state or quality of exerting energy or of accomplishing an effect. 2. in physical chemistry, the ratio of the fugacity of a substance in a particular experimental state to the fugacity in the standard state at the same temperature. **enzyme a.,** the catalytic effect exerted by an enzyme, expressed as units per milligram of enzyme (specific a.) or as molecules of substrate transformed per minute per molecule of enzyme (molecular a.). **molecular a.,** see *enzyme a.* **specific a.,** 1. see *enzyme a.* 2. the radioactivity of a radioisotope of an element per unit weight of the element in a sample. The activity per unit mass of a pure radionuclide. The activity per unit weight of any sample of radioactive material.

Actocortin trademark for *hydrocortisone sodium phosphate* (see under HYDROCORTISONE).

actomyosin (ak″to-mi'o-sin) a complex of the proteins actin and myosin occurring in muscle. Cf. ACTIN and MYOSIN.

actuary (ak'choo-ar″e) a person who computes insurance premiums and risks according to statistical probabilities.

acu- [L. *acus* needle] a combining form denoting relationship to a needle.

acuclosure (ak″u-klo'zhur) arrest of hemorrhage by means of a needle.

acufilopressure (ak″u-fil'o-presh″er) [*acu-* + L. *filum* thread + *pressio* pressure] a combination of acupressure and ligation.

acuity (ah-ku'ĭ-te) [L. *acuitas* sharpness] acuteness or clearness, especially of the vision.

acuminate (ah-ku'mĭ-nāt) [L. *acuminatus*] sharp pointed; having a pointed apex.

acupressure (ak'u-presh″er) [*acu-* + L. *pressio* pressure] compression of a bleeding vessel by inserting needles into adjacent tissue.

acupuncture (ak″u-pungk'chur) [*acu-* + L. *punctura* a prick] a method of insertion of needles into specific exterior body locations for the purpose of treating diseases at various stages and obtaining regional analgesia. According to the original Chinese philosophy, insertion of needles prevents excessive accumulation or blocking of flow of vital forces, thus preventing diseases from progressing. In modern medicine, it is used primarily in producing analgesia. Acupuncture points for dental analgesia are located either on the hands, feet, ears, or temporomandibular joint.

acus (a'kus) [L.] a needle or needlelike process.

acusection (ak″u-sek'shun) [*acu-* + *section*] cutting by means of the electrosurgical needle.

acusector (ak″u-sek'tor) [*acu-* + L. *sectere* to cut] an electric needle used like a scalpel in dividing tissues.

acute (ah-kūt') [L. *acutus* sharp] 1. sharp; poignant. 2. having a short and relatively severe course; opposed to a chronic course which extends over a long period of time.

acutenaculum (ak″u-tĕ-nak'u-lum) [*acu-* + *tenaculum*] an instrument for holding a surgical needle; a needle holder. **Hullihen's a.,** an instrument used in staphylorrhaphy to faciliate the passage of the needle through the margins of the cleft in the soft palate.

acutorsion (ak″u-tor'shun) [*acu-* + L. *torsio* a twisting] the twisting of an artery with a needle to control hemorrhage.

acyanotic (ah-si″ah-not'ik) not characterized by cyanosis.

acyclic (ah-si'klik) 1. pertaining to organic compounds having an open-chain structure. See acyclic COMPOUND. 2. not occurring in cycles.

acyl (as'il) an organic acid radical in which the hydroxyl group is replaced by another group.

acylation (as″ĭ-la'shun) a chemical reaction whereby an acyl radical is introduced into the molecule. Called also *acidylation.*

acylglycerol (as″il-glis″er-ōl) glyceride.

Acylpyrin trademark for *aspirin*.

AD 1. axiodistal. 2. adenoid degeneration (agent); see human AD-ENOVIRUS.

A.D. abbreviation for L. *au′ris dex′tra*, right ear.

ad. abbreviation for L. *ad′de*, add, or *adde′tur*, let there be added: used in prescription writing.

ad- [L. *ad* to] a prefix expressing to or toward, addition to, nearness, or axiodistal.

-ad a suffix expressing direction toward, as in cephalad, caudad.

ADA 1. American Dental Association; see Appendix. 2. American Diabetic Association. 3. American Dietetic Association.

ADA Health Foundation Research Institute see American Dental Association in Appendix.

ADA procedure numbers see ADA Uniform Code on Dental Procedures and Nomenclature, under CODE.

ADA Uniform Code on Dental Procedures and Nomenclature see under CODE.

ADAA American Dental Assistants Association (see under ASSOCIATION).

adactylia (ah″dak-til′e-ah) [*a* neg. + Gr. *daktylos* finger + *-ia*] a developmental abnormality characterized by absence of digits on the hand or foot.

adamantine (ad″ah-man′tēn) [Gr. *adamantinos* very hard] pertaining to the enamel of the teeth.

adamantinoblastoma (ad″ah-man″tī-no-blas-to′mah) ameloblastoma.

adamantinoma (ad″ah-man″tī-no′mah) ameloblastoma. **pituitary a.**, craniopharyngioma. **a. polycys′ticum**, see cystic AMELOBLASTOMA.

adamantoblast (ad″ah-man′to-blast) [*adamas* + Gr. *blastos* germ] ameloblast.

adamantoblastoma (ad″ah-man″to-blas-to′mah) ameloblastoma.

adamanto-odontoma (ad″ah-man″to-o-don-to′mah) ameloblastic ODONTOMA.

adamas (ad′ah-mas) [Gr. "unconquerable"] anything fixed or unalterable. **a. den′tis**, dental ENAMEL.

Adams, William Milton [1905–1957] a distinguished American maxillofacial surgeon who developed the technique for treating facial fractures by internal fixation by wire.

Adams clasp see under CLASP.

Adams' saw [William *Adams*, English surgeon, 1801–1900] see under SAW.

Adams-Stokes disease [Robert *Adams*, Irish physician, 1791–1875; William *Stokes*, Irish physician, 1804–1878] see under DISEASE.

Adanon trademark for the *dl* form of *methadone hydrochloride* (see under METHADONE).

Adapin trademark for *doxepin hydrochloride* (see under DOXEPIN).

adaptation (ad″ap-ta′shun) [L. *adaptare* to fit] 1. the act or process of adapting or adjusting of bodily processes to meet new conditions or environment. 2. the condition in reflex activity marked by a decrease in responsiveness to repeated stimulation. 3. proper fitting of a denture. 4. the degree of proximity and interlocking of filling material to the cavity wall. 5. the exact adjustment of bands to teeth. **epithelial a.**, close approximation of the gingival epithelium to the tooth surface. **masticatory a.**, physiological, structural, and functional changes in the masticatory system to compensate for or to adjust to intrinsic or extrinsic factors.

adapter (ah-dap′ter) a device by which different parts of an apparatus or instrument are connected. **band a.**, an orthodontic instrument designed to assist in adapting an orthodontic band to a tooth. See illustration.

adaxial (ad-ak′se-al) located on the side of, or directed toward the axis.

Adazine trademark for *triflupromazine hydrochloride* (see under TRIFLUPROMAZINE).

ADC axiodistocervical.

ADCC antibody dependent cellular CYTOTOXICITY.

add. abbreviation for L. *ad′de* add, or *adde′tur* let there be added.

adde (ad′e) [L.] add.

addict (ad′ikt) an individual who cannot resist a habit, especially the use of drugs or alcohol, for physiological or psychological reasons. See also ADDICTION.

addiction (ah-dik′shun) the state of being unable to resist a habit, especially strong dependence on a drug. **alcohol a.**, alcoholism. **drug a.**, a state characterized by an overwhelming desire or need to continue use of a drug, with a tendency to increase the dosage and a physiological and psychological dependence on its effects. Cf. drug DEPENDENCE and drug HABITUATION. See also physical DEPENDENCE.

Addis count [Thomas *Addis*, San Francisco physician, 1881–1949] see under COUNT.

Addison's anemia, keloid [Sir Thomas *Addison*, English physician, 1793–1860] see pernicious ANEMIA and MORPHEA.

Addison-Biemer anemia [Sir Thomas *Addison*; Anton *Biemer*, German physician, 1827–1892] pernicious ANEMIA.

additive (ad′ī-tiv) 1. characterized or produced by addition. 2. something that is added. 3. food a. **food a.**, a substance added intentionally to food, generally in small quantities, to prevent spoilage, to stabilize or improve its keeping qualities, texture, flavor, or appearance, or to aid in processing.

adduct (ah-dukt′) [L. *adducere* to draw toward] to draw toward the median line of the body or toward a neighboring part.

adductor (ah-duk′tor) [L.] that which or one who adducts.

aden- see ADENO-.

adenalgia (ad″ĕ-nal′je-ah) [aden- + Gr. *algos* pain + *-ia*] pain in a gland; adenodynia.

adendric (ah-den′drik) [*a* neg. + Gr. *dendron* tree] lacking dendrons or branches.

adenectomy (ad″ĕ-nek′to-me) [aden- + Gr. *ektomē* excision] 1. excision of a gland. 2. excision of adenoid growths.

adenectopia (ad″ĕ-nek-to′pe-ah) [aden- + Gr. *ektopos* displaced + *-ia*] malposition or displacement of a gland.

adenia (ah-de′ne-ah) chronic enlargement of the lymphatic glands.

adeniform (ah-den′ī-form) [aden- + L. *forma* shape] resembling a gland, especially in shape; adenoid.

adenine (ad′ĕ-nēn) a substance, 6-aminopurine, widely distributed in animal and plant tissues and a constituent of DNA and RNA. It occurs as a white, odorless, microcrystalline powder that is readily soluble in water, acids, and alkalies and slightly soluble in alcohol. Used in medical research. Called also *vitamin B₄*. **a. nucleotide**, adenylic ACID. **a. riboside**, adenosine.

adenitis (ad″ĕ-ni′tis) [aden- + *-itis*] inflammation of a gland. **acute infectious a.**, infectious MONONUCLEOSIS. **cervical a.**, inflammation of the cervical lymph nodes; seen in certain diseases, such as scarlet fever. **inoculation a.**, cat-scratch DISEASE. **phlegmonous a.**, inflammation of a gland and the surrounding connective tissue; adenophlegmon.

adeno-, aden- [Gr. *adēn, adenos* gland] a combining form denoting relationship to a gland or glands.

adenoacanthoma (ad″ĕ-no-ak″an-tho′mah) an adenocarcinoma in which some or the majority of the cells exhibit differentiation. Called also *adenocancroid*.

adenoameloblastoma (ad″ĕ-no-ah-mel″o-blas-to′mah) [adeno- + *ameloblastoma*] adenomatoid odontogenic TUMOR.

adenoblast (ad′ĕ-no-blast″) [adeno- + Gr. *blastos* germ] an embryonic cell that gives rise to glandular tissue.

adenocancroid (ad″ĕ-no-kang′kroid) adenoacanthoma.

adenocarcinoma (ad″ĕ-no-kar″sī-no′mah) [adeno- + *carcinoma*] a neoplastic tumor containing epithelial cells with a glandular or glandlike pattern. Called also *glandular cancer* and *malignant adenoma*. **acinar a., acinous a.**, acinar cell a. **acinar cell a., alveolar a.**, a small, encapsulated salivary gland tumor, usually of the parotid gland, composed of polygonal cells resembling those of serous acini, and having a granular cytoplasm. It most commonly affects middle-aged women, and has a tendency to recur and is often metastatic. Called also *acinar a., acinous a., acinic cell adenoma, acinic cell carcinoma*, and *serous cell adenoma*. **papillary a.**, one in which the tumor elements are arranged as finger-like processes or as a solid spherical nodule projecting from an epithelial surface. Called also *polypoid a*. **pleomorphic a.**, pleomorphic adenoma, malignant; see under ADENOMA. **polypoid a.**, papillary a.

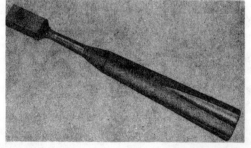

Band adapter. (From H. O. Torres and A. Ehrlich: Modern Dental Assisting. 2nd ed. Philadelphia, W. B. Saunders Co., 1980.)

adenocele (ad'ĕ-no-sēl") [*adeno-* + Gr. *kēlē* tumor] an adenomatous cystic tumor.

adenocellulitis (ad"ĕ-no-sel"u-li'tis) [*adeno-* + *cellulitis*] inflammation of a gland and the cellular tissue around it.

adenochondroma (ad"ĕ-no-kon-dro'mah) a tumor containing both adenomatous and chondromatous elements, as in a mixed tumor of the salivary gland. Called also *chondroadenoma*.

adenocyte (ad'ĕ-no-sīt) [*adeno-* + Gr. *kytos* hollow vessel] a mature secretory cell of a gland.

adenodynia (ad"ĕ-no-din'e-ah) [*adeno-* + Gr. *odynē* pain + *-ia*] pain in a gland; adenalgia.

adenofibrosis (ad"ĕ-no-fi-bro'sis) fibroid degeneration of a gland.

Adenogen trademark for *carbazochrome salicylate* (see under CARBAZOCHROME).

adenogenous (ad"ĕ-noj'ĕ-nus) [*adeno-* + Gr. *gennan* to produce] originating from glandular tissue.

adenohypophyseal (ad"ĕ-no-hi"po-fiz'e-al) pertaining to the adenohypophysis (anterior pituitary GLAND).

adenohypophysis (ad"ĕ-no-hi-pof'ĭ-sis) [*adeno-* + *hypophysis*] [NA alternative] pituitary gland, anterior; see under GLAND.

adenoid (ad'ĕ-noid) [*aden-* + Gr. *eidos* form] 1. resembling a gland; glandlike; adeniform. 2. [pl.] hypertrophy of the pharyngeal tonsil. 3. pharyngeal TONSIL.

adenoidectomy (ad"ĕ-noid-ek'to-me) [*adenoid* + Gr. *ektomē* excision] excision of the adenoids.

adenoiditis (ad"ĕ-noid-i'tis) [*adenoid* + *-itis*] inflammation of the adenoid tonsils. See also TONSILLITIS.

adenolymphocele (ad"ĕ-no-lim-fo'sēl) [*adeno-* + *lymphocele*] lymphadenocele.

adenolymphoma (ad"ĕ-no-lim-fo'mah) a benign salivary gland tumor found almost exclusively in the parotid glands, which occurs bilaterally, and is more common in men than in women. Typically, it is an encapsulated, smooth, round lesion with multiple communicating cysts. It has two components, lymphoid and epithelial, with two layers of cells; the surface row consists of tall columnar cells, and the deep row consists of cuboidal, rounded, or polygonal cells. Called also *Albrecht-Arzt-Warthin tumor, cystic papillary adenoma, orbital inclusion adenoma, papillary cystadenolymphoma, papillary cystadenoma lymphomatosum,* and *Warthin's tumor.*

adenoma (ad'ĕ-no'mah) [*adeno-* + *-oma*] an epithelial, benign tumor with a glandlike structure. **acidophilic a.,** oxyphil a. **acinic cell a.,** acinar cell ADENOCARCINOMA. **basophil a.,** Cushing's SYNDROME (1). **benign pleomorphic a.,** see *pleomorphic a.* **cystic papillary a.,** adenolymphoma. **lymphomatoid a.,** Mikulicz's DISEASE. **malignant a.,** adenocarcinoma. **malignant pleomorphic a.,** pleomorphic a., malignant. **orbital inclusion a.,** adenolymphoma. **oxyphil a., oxyphilic a., oxyphilic granular cell a.,** a rare, benign, slow-growing tumor of the salivary gland, usually of the parotid gland, which most frequently affects elderly patients of both sexes. Typically, it is a small, freely movable lesion, divided into lobules by strands of fibrous connective tissue, which is red on section. Histologically, the tumor is made up of large cells with an eosinophilic cytoplasm and distinct cell membranes, arranged in bands in a sparsely vascularized stroma. Called also *acidophilic a.* and *oncocytoma.* **pleomorphic a.,** a benign, slow-growing tumor of the salivary gland, occurring as a small, painless, firm nodule, usually of the parotid gland, but also found in any major or accessory salivary gland anywhere in the oral cavity. It is the most common tumor of the salivary glands and affects patients of both sexes and all ages, but is most often found in women in the fifth decade. The pleomorphic character of the tumor is due to its variety of cells: cuboidal, columnar, and squamous cells, showing all forms of epithelial growth. It is commonly called "mixed" tumor, but is not "mixed," in that it contains only epithelial cells. At different times, it has been known by more than 50 different names, e.g., *enchondroma, enclavoma,* and *endothelioma,* many of which are no longer considered as synonyms. **pleomorphic a., malignant,** a metastasizing salivary gland tumor that may be present as a benign lesion for several years and suddenly begins to grow. Histologically, it has most of the characteristics of the benign pleomorphic adenoma, but in addition contains large aggregates of large hyperchromatic cells and atypical nuclei and exhibits bizarre mitotic activity. Called also *malignant mixed tumor* and *pleomorphic adenocarcinoma.* **Plummer's a.,** adenoma of the thyroid gland. See also Plummer's DISEASE. **sebaceous a., sebaceous cell a.,** an extremely rare benign tumor of the salivary glands, believed to represent hyperplasia of heterotopic sebaceous glands. **serous cell a.,** acinar cell ADENOCARCINOMA.

adenomalacia (ad"ĕ-no-mah-la'she-ah) [*adeno-* + Gr. *malakia* softness] abnormal softening of a gland.

adenomatoid (ad"ĕ-no'mah-toid) resembling adenoma.

adenomatosis (ad"ĕ-no-mah-to'sis) a condition characterized by multiple adenomatous growths. **hereditary a.,** Gardner's SYN-

DROME. **a. o'ris,** enlargement of the mucous glands of the lip without secretion or inflammation.

adenomatous (ad"ĕ-nom'ah-tus) pertaining to adenoma or to nodular hyperplasia of a gland.

adenomyoepithelioma (ad"ĕ-no-mi"o-ep"ĭ-the-le-o'mah) adenoid cystic CARCINOMA.

adenopathy (ad"ĕ-nop'ah-the) [*adeno-* + Gr. *pathos* disease] any disease of the glands, especially the lymphatic glands.

adenopharyngitis (ad"ĕ-no-far"in-ji'tis) [*adeno-* + Gr. *pharynx* + *-itis*] inflammation of the tonsils and pharynx.

adenophlegmon (ad"ĕ-no-fleg'mon) [*adeno-* + *phlegmon*] inflammation of a gland and the surrounding connective tissue; phlegmonous adenitis.

adenosclerosis (ad"ĕ-no-skle-ro'sis) [*adeno-* + *sclerosis*] the hardening of a gland.

adenosine (ah-den'o-sēn) a nucleoside, 9-beta-D-ribofuranosyladine, occurring as a white, crystalline, odorless powder with a mild saline or bitter taste, which is soluble in hot water. Called also *adenine riboside.* **cyclic a. 3',5'-monophosphate, a. 3',5'-cyclic phosphate,** an adenine nucleotide (adenosine) in which the hydroxyl groups in the 3 and 5 position of ribose have formed a cyclic ester with phosphoric acid. It is a high-energy compound found in all cells, whose principal role is to serve as an effector of a series of events initiated by interaction of various hormones with specific receptor molecules that are components of the plasma membranes of the cell upon which these hormones exert a regulatory influence. Called also *cyclic a. 3',5'-monophosphate, cAMP, cyclic AMP,* and *second messenger.* See also LIPOLYSIS. **a. diphosphate (ADP),** a nucleotide formed from ATP on hydrolysis of a phosphate bond; when recombined with phosphoric acid with the use of energy derived from the cellular nutrients, it forms ATP. Called also *a. 5'-pyrophosphate, adenosine diphosphoric acid,* and *5'-adenylphosphoric acid.* **a. monophate, a. monophosphate (AMP),** adenylic ACID. **a. nucleotide,** adenylic ACID. **a. phosphate,** 1. adenylic ACID. 2. any of the three interconvertible compounds in which adenosine is attached through its ribose group to one (a. monophosphate), two (a. diphosphate), or three (a. triphosphate) phosphoric acid molecules. **a. 3'-phosphate,** adenylic acid derived from yeast nucleic acid; see adenylic ACID. **a. 5'-phosphate,** adenylic acid derived from muscle; see adenylic ACID. **a. 5'-pyrophosphate,** a. diphosphate. **a. triphosphate (ATP),** a nucleotide composed of a nitrogenous base, adenine, a pentose sugar, ribose, and three phosphate groups, the last two radicals being connected to the other phosphate of the molecule by high-energy phosphate bonds, each of which contain about 8000 calories of energy per mole of ATP. Its functions consist of supplying energy for the transport of sodium through membranes, permitting protein synthesis by the ribosomes, and supplying the energy needed during muscle contraction. In metabolic processes, ATP is spent and remade over again. First, energy released from nutrients is used to form ATP and, when ATP releases its energy, a phosphoric acid radical is split away and adenosine diphosphate (ADP) is formed, followed by the recombination of ADP and phosphoric acid with the use of energy derived from the cellular nutrients. Called also *adenylpyrophosphate* and *5'-adenyldiphosphoric acid.*

adenosinetriphosphatase [E.C.3.6.1.3.] (ah-den"o-sin-tri-fos'fah-tās) a hydrolase acting on acid anhydrides, which catalyzes the splitting of adenosine triphosphate with liberation of ADP and orthophosphate. These enzymes are associated with formed elements, such as intracellular structures and cell membranes; thus, myosin ATPase is concerned with muscle contraction, mitochondrial ATPase in securing energy from products of biological oxidation, and so on. Abbreviated *ATPase.* Called also *adenylpyrophosphatase, ATP monophosphatase,* and *triphosphatase.*

adenosis (ad"ĕ-no'sis) 1. any disease of the glands. 2. the development or formation of gland tissue.

adenotome (ad'ĕ-no-tōm") [*adeno-* + Gr. *tomē* cutting] 1. an instrument for cutting glands. 2. an instrument for excision of the adenoids.

adenotomy (ad"ĕ-not'o-me) [*adeno-* + Gr. *tomē* cutting] 1. the cutting or removal of a gland. 2. incision of the adenoids.

adenotonsillectomy (ad"ĕ-no-ton"sil-lek'to-me) removal of the tonsils and adenoids.

Adenoviridae (ad"ĕ-no-vi'rĭ-de) [*adeno-* + *virus* + *-idae*] a family of naked icosahedral viruses, having linear double-stranded DNA (molecular weight of the DNA is 20×10^6 to 30×10^6); isometric virions, 70 to 80 nm in diameter; and capsids made up of 252 capsomers with 12 vertices with filamentous structures projecting outward. The family is divided into two genera: *Mastadenovirus* (mammalian hosts) and *Aviadenovirus* (avian hosts). Most adenoviruses are associated with respiratory infections, many being latent; some multiply in the intestinal tract and are recovered in feces; and others occur in lymphoid tissues. Some strains cause malignant tumors in experimental animals. Hybrids between adenoviruses and *Polyomavirus* have been produced in the laboratory. See also human ADENOVIRUS.

adenovirus (ad″ĕ-no-vi′rus) any virus of the family Adenoviridae. **human a.**, any of the more than 30 strains of adenoviruses occurring in human hosts. The virus is associated with a variety of diseases, including minor respiratory infections in infants and children, febrile diseases in adolescents and young adults, conjunctivitis, keratoconjunctivitis, pharyngoconjunctivitis, pneumonia, diarrhea, and mesenteric enteritis. It is also suspected of being involved in neoplastic diseases and its strains are divided according to their oncogenic activity. Groups A (types 12, 18, and 31) and B (types 3, 7, 14, 16, and 21) being oncogenic, and groups C (types 1, 2, 5, and 6) and D (types 9, 10, 13, 15, 17, 19, and 26) being nononcogenic. The virus is probably airborne and may be isolated from feces and urine. Most excised human tonsils and adenoids contain adenoviruses. Called also *adenoid degeneration (AD) agent* and *adenoidal-pharyngeal-conjunctival (APC) agent.*

adenylpyrophosphatase (ad″ĕ-nil-pi″ro-fos′fah-tās) adenosinetriphosphatase.

adenylpyrophosphate (ad″ĕ-nil-pi″ro-fos′fāt) ADENOSINE triphosphate.

adephagia (ad″ĕ-fa′je-ah) [Gr. *adēn* enough + *phagein* to eat + *-ia*] insatiable hunger.

adeps (ad′eps) [L.] lard, the purified omental fat of the hog; used in the preparation of ointments. **a. la′nae**, wool FAT. **a. la′nae hydro′sus,** lanolin.

adequacy (ad′ĕ-kwah-se) the state of being sufficient for a specific purpose. **velopharyngeal a.,** sufficient functional closure of the velum against the postpharyngeal wall· so that air and hence sound cannot enter the nasopharyngeal and nasal cavities.

adequate and well-controlled studies *see under* STUDY.

Aderer "A" Soft trademark for a soft *dental casting gold alloy* (see under GOLD) with relatively low hardness.

Aderer "B" Medium trademark for a medium hard *dental casting gold alloy* (see under GOLD).

Aderer No. 3 Bridge Gold see under GOLD.

Aderer No. 16 trademark for a low noble metal dental wrought gold wire alloy.

Aderer No. 20 clasp see under CLASP.

ADG axiodistogingival.

ADH 1. Academy of Dentistry for the Handicapped (see under ACADEMY). 2. antidiuretic hormone; see VASOPRESSIN.

ADHA American Dental Hygienists' Association (see under ASSOCIATION).

AD/here trademark for *mecrylate.*

adhere (ad-hēr′) to cling together; to become fastened.

adherence (ad-hēr′ens) the act or quality of sticking together. **immune a.,** a complement-dependent phenomenon in which antigen-antibody complexes (e.g., bacteria coated with antibody), which have reacted with complement C3, adhere to particles having receptors for C3b, such as red blood cells and macrophages. Soluble complexes may cause the particles on which they adhere to agglutinate.

adherend (ad-hēr′end, ad′hī-rend) a material or an object bonded with the use of an adhesive.

adhesio (ad-he′ze-o) [L. "clinging together"] a connecting band or structure.

adhesion (ad-he′zhun) [L. *adhaesio* from *adhaerere* to stick to] 1. the force which causes two substances brought into intimate contact to attach with each other, when unlike molecules of one substance are attracted to another. See also COHESION (2) and WETTING. 2. the stable joining of parts to each other, which may occur abnormally. 3. a fibrous band or structure by which parts abnormally adhere. **palatopharyngeal a.,** usually, a congenital adherence of the posterior portion of the soft palate and the pharynx, often associated with other abnormalities. Sometimes such adherence results from scar formation after adenoidectomy or infection. **sublabial a.,** abnormal union of the sublabial mucosa of the upper lip to the alveolar process; usually present in cleft lip.

adhesiotomy (ad-he″ze-ot′o-me) the cutting or division of adhesions.

adhesive (ad-he′siv) 1. pertaining to, characterized by, or causing adherence of adjoining surfaces. 2. a substance that causes close adherence of adjoining surfaces. **Benefit denture a.,** trademark for a denture adhesive, 100 gm of which contains 74.85 gm hydroxyethyl cellulose, 25 mg methylcellulose, and 150 mg hexachlorophene. **Cora-Caine analgesic a.,** trademark for an adhesive analgesic ointment, 100 mg of which contains 14 gm benzocaine, 2 gm aluminum hydroxide, 0.5 gm zinc oxide, and the necessary amounts of petrolatum, gum karaya, and flavoring and coloring agents. **Co-Re-Ga denture a. powder,** see under POWDER. **dental a.,** a dental SEALANT. **denture a.,** a compound, either a powder or paste, used to stabilize dentures in the mouth. Denture adherent powders are prepared from fine vegetable gum powders, such as karaya, acacia, tragacanth, ethylene oxide, polymer, and other agents that become mucilaginous or gelatinous on adding water. Wintergreen, peppermint, and other flavoring agents, and borax, boric acid, and various antiseptics are sometimes added. Denture adherent pastes are usually prepared from karaya gum, petroleum, and coloring and flavoring agents.

adhesiveness (ad-he′siv-nes) the quality or state of being adhesive. **platelet a.,** PLATELET adhesiveness.

Adhib. abbreviation for L. *adhiben′dus*, to be administered.

ADI 1. axiodistoincisal. 2. Academy of Dentistry International (see under ACADEMY).

adiabatic (ah-di″ah-bat′ik) occurring without gain or loss of heat.

Adiaben trademark for *chlorpropamide.*

adiactinic (ah-di″ak-tin′ik) [*a* neg. + Gr. *dia* through + *aktis* ray] not permitting the passage of actinic rays.

adiadochokinesia (ah-di″ah-do″ko-ki-ne′se-ah) [*a* neg. + Gr. *diadochos* succeeding + *kinēsis* motion] inability to perform rapid alternating movements, such as opening and closing the jaws or lips, raising and lowering the eyebrows, or tapping the fingers. Called also *adiadochokinesis.*

adiadochokinesis (ah-di″ah-do″ki-ne′sis) adiadochokinesia.

adiaphoresis (ah-di″ah-fo-re′sis) [*a* neg. + Gr. *diaphorein* to perspire] deficiency or absence of perspiration.

adiastole (ah″di-as′to-le) absence of diastole.

adicillin (ad′ĭ-sil′in) penicillin N.

adient (ad′ĕ-ent) tending toward the source of stimulation; positive. Cf. ABIENT.

Adigal trademark for *lanatoside A.*

Adipan trademark for *amphetamine.*

adipectomy (ad″ĭ-pek′to-me) [L. *adeps* fat + Gr. *ektomē* excision] excision of excess adipose tissue.

Adipex trademark for *methamphetamine hydrochloride* (see under METHAMPHETAMINE).

adipo- [L. *adeps, adipis* fat] a combining form denoting relationship to fat.

adipocele (ad′ĭ-po-sēl) [*adipo-* + Gr. *kēlē* hernia] a hernia containing fat or fatty tissue.

adipocere (ad′ĭ-po-sēr″) [*adipo-* + L. *cera* wax] a waxy substance formed during the decomposition of animal bodies, and seen especially in human bodies buried in moist places. It consists principally of insoluble salts of fatty acids. Called also *grave wax.*

adipolysis (ad″ĭ-pol′ĭ-sis) [*adipo-* + Gr. *lysis* dissolution] lipolysis (1).

adipose (ad′ĭ-pōs) [L. *adiposus* fatty] fatty; fat; relating to fat.

adiposis (ad″ĭ-po′sis) [*adipo-* + *-osis*] 1. obesity; excessive accumulation of fatty tissue in the body. 2. fatty changes in an organ or tissue.

adipositas (ad″ĭ-pos′ĭ-tas) [L.] fatness; adiposity. **a. ex vac′uo,** fatty ATROPHY.

adiposity (ad″ĭ-pos′ĭ-te) the state of being fat; obesity.

adiposuria (ad″ĭ-po-su′re-ah) [*adipo-* + Gr. *ouron* urine + *-ia*] the occurrence of fats in the urine; lipuria.

adipsia (ah-dip′se-ah) [*a* neg + Gr. *dipsa* thirst + *-ia*] absence of thirst, or abnormal avoidance of drinking.

aditus (ad′ĭ-tus), pl. *ad′itus* [L.] a general anatomical term for the entrance or approach to an organ or part. **a. glot′tidis infe′rior,** the inferior opening of the glottis. **a. glot′tidis supe′rior,** the superior opening of the glottis. **a. laryn′gis** [NA], the aperture by which the pharynx communicates with the larynx. **a. or′bitae** [NA], orbital APERTURE.

adjunct (ad′junkt) an accessory or auxiliary agent or measure.

adjustment (ah-just′ment) 1. the act or process of modification of a physical state or revision of mental attitudes in response to changing conditions. 2. in chiropractic, manipulation of the spine, said to restore normal nerve function. 3. a modification made in a denture after its completion and insertion in the mouth. 4. in bookkeeping, an entry specifying that portion of the receivable account that is not collectable, as the amount of the fee which Medicaid will not pay and which cannot be collected from the patient. **incisal guide a.,** occlusal adjustment that produces a minimum of overbite (vertical overlap) and a maximum of overjet (horizontal overlap), eliminates fremitus and racking effects on the anterior segment of teeth in the protrusive glide, and attains maximal incisive group function. **occlusal a.,** selective grinding of occlusal surfaces of the teeth in an effort to eliminate premature contacts and occlusal interferences; to establish optimal masticatory effectiveness, stable occlusal relationship, direction of main occlusal forces, and efficient multidirectional patterns; to improve functional relations and to induce physiologic stimulation of the masticatory system; to eliminate occlusal trauma; to eliminate abnormal muscle tension, bruxism, and associated pain; to eliminate dysfunctional temporomandibular joint discomfort or pain; to establish optimal occlusal patterns prior to extensive restoration to reshape and recontour the teeth for masticatory efficiency and gingival protection; to aid in the stabilization of orthodontic results; and to recondition abnormal swallowing habits. Instruments used in occlusal adjustment include adhesive wax strips, a grease marking pencil, articulating paper, carborundum stones or diamond points, sandpaper disks, and rubber polishing wheels. Called also *occlusal equilibration.* See also GRINDING. **postretention a.,** after orthodontic therapy, minor shifting of teeth from the position into which they were moved. See also RETENTION (4).

adjuvant (ad'ju-vant) [L. *adjuvans* aiding] 1. aiding or assisting. 2. a substance or ingredient which assists or modifies the action of other substances or ingredients. 3. a substance or condition that results in an increased immune response to an antigen; the response may be related to the quantity of antibody or antigen, to the level of cell-mediated immunity, or to hypersensitivity. See also IMMUNOPOTENTIATION. **Freund's a., complete,** incomplete Freund's adjuvant to which killed mycobacteria or related organisms are added to further intensify the immune response. **Freund's a., incomplete,** a water-in-oil emulsion used as a vehicle for antigens and injected as a depot to increase the immune response, e.g., increase the titer of antibody or the degree of autoimmune disease.

ad lib. abbreviation for L. *ad lib'itum,* at pleasure, as desired.

admedial (ad-me'de-al) situated near the median plane.

administration (ad-min"is-tra'shun) 1. the act or process of managing or performing executive duties. 2. a body of persons or an agency responsible for managing certain tasks. 3. the act or process of giving a drug or a remedy. **local a.,** local APPLICATION. **Occupational Safety and Health A.,** a branch of the U.S. Department of Labor having the responsibility of enforcing all mandatory industrial safety and health standards. Abbreviated *OSHA.* **parenteral a.,** administration of a drug or any substance not through the alimentary canal, but by some other route, such as injection. **practice a.,** in dentistry, the management of all business and organizational aspects of a dental practice. **Social Security A.,** the administration within the Department of Health and Human Services which, in addition to administering the social security programs, has the responsibility for management and operation of the Medicare program. Abbreviated *SSA.* **topical a.,** topical APPLICATION.

admission (ad-mish'un) 1. the act of allowing to enter. 2. the acceptance of a person by a hospital or other health care facility as an in-patient for at least an overnight stay. 3. an acknowledgement of the truth; a point or statement acknowledged; concession. **a. against interest,** a statement made by an individual which serves to defeat his own interests.

admov. abbreviation for L. *ad'move, admovea'tur,* add, let there be added.

adnerval (ad-ner'val) [L. *ad* near + Gr. *neuron* nerve] 1. situated near a nerve. 2. toward a nerve. Called also *adneural.*

adneural (ad-nu'ral) adnerval.

adnexa (ad-nek'sah) [L., pl.] appendages or adjunct parts. See also APPENDAGE. **a. oc'uli,** the lacrimal apparatus and other appendages of the eye. **tooth a.,** structures associated with a tooth, i.e., the alveolus and the periodontal ligament.

ADO axiodisto-occlusal.

ADOD arthrodentosteodysplasia; see Hajdu-Cheney SYNDROME.

adolescence (ad"o-les'ens) [L. *adolescentia*] the period of life beginning with the appearance of secondary sex characteristics and terminating with the cessation of somatic growth; from about 13 to 18 years of age.

ADP ADENOSINE diphosphate.

ADP-60 trademark for a small capacity automatic film processor.

Adphen trademark for *phendimetrazine tartrate* (see under PHENDIMETRAZINE).

Ad pond. om. abbreviation for L. *ad pon'dus om'nium,* to the weight of the whole.

Adrenal trademark for *epinephrine.*

adrenal (ad-re'nal) [L. *ad.* near + *ren* kidney] 1. pertaining to the adrenal gland. 2. adrenal GLAND.

adrenalectomy (ad-re"nal-ek'to-me) [*adrenal* + Gr. *ektomē* excision] excision of the adrenal gland.

adrenalin (ad-ren'ah-lin) epinephrine.

adrenalinemia (ad-ren"ah-lin-e'me-ah) [*adrenalin* + Gr. *haima* blood + *-ia*] the presence of epinephrine in the blood.

adrenalinuria (ad-ren"ah-lin-u're-ah) [*adrenalin* + Gr. *ouron* urine + *-ia*] the presence of epinephrine in the urine.

adrenergic (ad"ren-er'jik) 1. pertaining to mediation of impulses in the autonomic nervous system by norepinephrine. 2. pertaining to drugs that mimic or block stimulation of nerves of the autonomic nervous system which are mediated by norepinephrine. 3. pertaining to nerves of the autonomic nervous system which are mediated by norepinephrine. 4. adrenergic DRUG. Cf. CHOLINERGIC.

adrenine (ah-dre'nēn) epinephrine.

adreno- [L. *ad* near + *ren* kidney] a combining form denoting relationship to the adrenal gland.

adrenoceptor (ad-re"no-sep'tor) adrenergic RECEPTOR.

adrenocortical (ad-re"no-kor'ti-kal) pertaining to the adrenal cortex.

adrenocorticosteroid (ad-re"no-kor"ti-ko-ste'roid) 1. pertaining to a steroid hormone of the adrenal cortex. 2. adrenal cortex HORMONE.

adrenocorticotropic (ad-re"no-kor"ti-ko-trop'ik) [*adrenal cortex* + *-tropic*] having an influence on the adrenal cortex, or pertaining to adrenocorticotropic hormone (see under HORMONE).

adrenocorticotropin (ad-re"no-kor"ti-ko-trop'in) adrenocorticotropic HORMONE.

adrenodontia (ad-ren"o-don'she-ah) [*adreno-* + Gr. *odous* tooth] a tooth form once thought to be indicative of adrenal predominance: the canines are large and sharp, and the occlusal surfaces of the teeth have a brownish coloration.

adrenolytic (ad"ren-o-lit'ik) [*adreno-* + Gr. *lytikos* dissolving] 1. opposing the effects of impulses mediated by adrenergic receptors. 2. adrenolytic DRUG. Cf. SYMPATHOLYTIC.

adrenomimetic (ad-ren"o-mi-met'ik) 1. sympathomimetic. 2. sympathomimetic DRUG.

adrenoreceptor (ad-re"no-re-sep'tor) adrenergic RECEPTOR.

Adrenosem trademark for *carbazochrome salicylate* (see under CARBAZOCHROME).

adrenotropic (ad-ren"o-trop"ik) [*adreno-* + Gr. *tropos* a turning] having specific affinity for or influence on the adrenal glands.

Adrestat-F trademark for *carbazochrome salicylate* (see under CARBAZOCHROME).

Adriamycin trademark for *doxorubicin hydrochloride* (see under DOXORUBICIN).

Adrian, Edgar Douglas [born 1889] an English physician; co-winner, with Sir Charles Scott Sherrington, of the Nobel prize for medicine and physiology in 1932.

Adrianol trademark for *phenylephrine hydrochloride* (see under PHENYLEPHRINE).

Adriblastina trademark for *doxorubicin hydrochloride* (see under DOXORUBICIN).

Adroyd trademark for *oxymetholone.*

Adson forceps see under FORCEPS.

Adson-Brown forceps see under FORCEPS.

adsorbent (ad-sor'bent) 1. pertaining to adsorption. 2. the substance which takes up another substance by adsorption.

adsorption (ad-sorp'shun) [*ad-* + L. *sorbere* to suck] the attachment of one substance to the surface of another; the concentration of a gas or a substance in solution in a liquid on a surface in contact with the gas or liquid, resulting in a relatively high concentration of the gas or solution at the surface. See also ABSORPTION and SORPTION.

adst. feb. abbreviation for L. *adstan'te feb're,* while fever is present.

ADT 1. Accepted Dental Therapeutics; see accepted dental THERAPEUTIC. 2. ADENOSINE triphosphate.

ADTA American Dental Trade Association.

ADTe tetanic CONTRACTION.

adult (ah-dult') [L. *adultus* grown up] 1. having attained full growth or maturity. 2. a living organism which has attained full growth or maturity. 3. under health plans, a subscriber or spouse. Also, any dependent who has reached the age at which eligibility as a child ceases.

adulteration (ah-dul"ter-a'shun) addition of an impure or unnecessary ingredient to cheat or falsify a preparation.

Adumbran trademark for *oxazepam.*

adumbration (ah"dum-bra'shun) giving forth a shadow; sometimes used incorrectly to mean geometric unsharpness.

advancement (ad-vans'ment) 1. surgical detachment, as of a muscle or tendon, followed by reattachment at an advanced point. 2. in dentistry, moving a retruded mandible forward to a normal position.

Adv. abbreviation for L. adver'sum, against.

adventitia (ad"ven-tish'e-ah) [L. adventicius from without, from ad to + venire to come] outermost; a general anatomical term used to designate the outer coat of a tubular structure; often used alone to denote the tunica adventitia.

adventitial (ad"ven-tish'al) 1. pertaining to the tunica adventitia. 2. adventitious.

adventitious (ad"ven-tish'us) 1. accidental or acquired. 2. found out of the normal or usual place. Called also adventitial.

Ad 2 vic. abbreviation of L. ad du'as vi'ces, at two times, for two doses.

adynamia (ah"di-na'me-ah) [a neg. + Gr. dynamis might + -ia] lack or loss of the normal or vital powers; asthenia.

AE [Ger.] antitoxineinheit (see antitoxic UNIT).

ae- for words beginning thus, see also those beginning E-.

Aeby's muscle, plane [Christopher Theodore Aeby, Swiss anatomist, 1835–1885] see depressor muscle of lower lip, under MUSCLE, and Huxley's PLANE.

Aeg. abbreviation for L. ae'ger, ae'gra, the patient.

aeluropsis (e"loo-rop'sis) [Gr. ailouros cat + opsis vision] a slanting palpebral fissure like that of a cat.

aer (a'er) [Gr. aēr] atmos.

aer- see AERO-.

aerated (a'er-āt"ed) [L. aeratus] 1. charged with air. 2. charged with a gas, such as carbon dioxide.

aeration (a"er-a'shun) 1. the charging or saturation of a material (usually a liquid) with air, or some similar gas. 2. the exchange of carbon dioxide for oxygen by the blood in the lungs.

aerial (a-e're-al) 1. pertaining to the air. 2. mycelial growth above the substrate.

aeriform (a-er'ĭ-form) [aer- + L. forma form] like the air; gaseous.

aero-, aer- [Gr. aēr; L. aer air or gas] a combining form denoting relation to air or gas.

Aerobacter (a"er-o-bak'ter) [aero- + Gr. baktērion little rod] a genus of the family Enterobacteriaceae, consisting of motile rods. The name is no longer used in bacteriological taxonomy and Aerobacter species have been assigned to the genus Enterobacter. A. aerog'enes, Enterobacter aerogenes, see under ENTEROBACTER. A. cloa'cae, Enterobacter cloacae; see under ENTEROBACTER.

aerobe (a'er-ōb) [aero- + Gr. bios life] a heterotrophic microorganism which can live and grow in the presence of free oxygen, using molecular oxygen as the ultimate acceptor of electrons from its organic electron donors. Called also aerobic cell, aerobic microorganism, and aerobic organism. See also heterotrophic CELL. Cf. ANAEROBE. facultative a., one that is able to live under either aerobic or anaerobic conditions, using oxygen when it is available, and when it is not, using organic compounds as electron acceptors. Cf. facultative ANAEROBE. obligate a., one that requires free access to molecular oxygen for growth.

aerobic (a-er-o'bik) growing only in the presence of molecular oxygen.

aerobioscope (a"er-o-bi'o-skōp) [aero- + Gr. bios life + skopein to view] an apparatus for analyzing the bacterial composition of air.

aerobiosis (a"er-o-bi-o'sis) [aero- + Gr. bios life] life in the presence of oxygen.

aerocele (a'er-o-sēl") [aero- + Gr. kēlē tumor] a tumor formed by air filling an adventitious pouch, such as a laryngocele or tracheocele.

Aerococcus (a"er-o-kok'us) [aero- + Gr. kokkos berry] a genus of bacteria of the family Streptococcaceae, consisting of gram-positive, nonmotile, spheroid coccoid cells, about 1.0 to 2.0 μm in diameter, with a tendency toward tetrad formation. A. vir'idans, a species isolated from human urinary infections and endocarditis; it may be pathogenic for lobsters. Called also Gaffkya homari and Pediococcus homari.

aerodontalgia (a"er-o-don-tal'je-ah) toothache experienced at lowered atmospheric pressure, as in an aircraft flight or in a decompression chamber, caused by the expansion of air in the maxillary sinuses. Called also aero-odontalgia and aero-odontodynia.

aerodontics (a"er-o-don'tiks) that branch of dentistry concerned with the effects on the teeth of high altitude flying.

aerodynamics (a"er-o-di-nam'iks) [aero- + Gr. dynamis might] the science of air and gases in motion.

aeroembolism (a"er-o-em'bo-lizm) gas EMBOLISM.

aerogen (a'er-o-jen") a gas-producing microorganism.

aerogenesis (a"er-o-jen'ĕ-sis) [aero- + Gr. genesis production] the production of gas.

aerogram (a'er-o-gram") [aero- + Gr. gramma mark] pneumogram (2).

Aerolin trademark for albuterol.

Aeromatt trademark for precipitated calcium carbonate (see CALCIUM carbonate).

Aeromonas (a"er-o-mo'nas) [aero- + Gr. monas unit] a genus of bacteria of the family Vibrionaceae, usually found in water. Some species are pathogenic for fish and amphibians.

aero-odontalgia (a"er-o-o"don-tal'je-ah) aerodontalgia.

aero-odontodynia (a"er-o-o-don"to-din'e-ah) aerodontalgia.

aero-otitis (a"er-o-o-ti'tis) [aero- + otitis] barotitis.

Aeropax trademark for simethicone.

aerophagia (a"er-o-fa'je-ah) [aero- + Gr. phagein to eat] spasmodic swallowing of air followed by eructations, occurring in some gastrointestinal disorders. Called also aerophagy and gastrospiry.

aerophagy (a"er-of'ah-je) [aero- + Gr. phagein to eat] aerophagia.

aerophilic (a"er-o-fil'ik) requiring air for proper growth.

aerosinusitis (a"er-o-si"nŭ-si'tis) [aero- + sinusitis] acute inflammation of the mucous membrane lining the paranasal sinuses, caused by rapid lowering of the barometric pressure and resulting expansion of air in the sinuses. Called also barosinusitis and sinus barotrauma.

aerosol (a'er-o-sol") 1. a colloid system in which the continuous phase (dispersion medium) is a gas. 2. a solution of a drug which can be atomized into a fine mist. 3. a suspension of fine particles in gas.

Aerosol OT trademark for a synthetic dental wax (see under WAX).

Aerosporin trademark for polymyxin B.

aerotitis (a"er-o-ti'tis) barotitis.

AES 1. American Endodontic Society (see under SOCIETY). 2. American Equilibration Society (see under SOCIETY).

Æsculapius [Gr. Askelēpios] the mythical god of healing, son of Apollo and the nymph Coronis and father of Hygeia and Panacea. See STAFF of Æsculapius.

Aetina trademark for ethionamide.

Aetios see AËTIUS.

Aëtius (Aetios) of Amida (Antiochenus) [6th century A.D.] a Byzantine Greek writer, whose Tetrabiblion gives details of the works of Rufus (of Ephesus), Leonides, Soranus (of Ephesus), and Philumenus, and good accounts of diseases of the eye, ear, nose, and throat, and also technical procedures (e.g., tonsillectomy, urethrotomy, and the treatment of hemorrhoids).

Afatin trademark for dextroamphetamine sulfate (see under DEXTROAMPHETAMINE).

AFDH American Fund for Dental Health (see under FUND).

afebrile (ah-feb'ril) without fever.

afferent (af'er-ent) [ad- + L. ferre to carry] centripetal; conveying toward a center.

affinity (ah-fin'ĭ-te) [L. affinitas relationship] 1. inherent likeness or relationship. 2. a special attraction for a specific element, organ, or structure. antibody a., ANTIBODY affinity. chemical a., the force that unites atoms into molecules. electron a., the energy released when an electron is added to a gaseous atom, the highest affinities being associated with the smallest atoms where the electrons enter an orbital near the nucleus. residual a., the force which enables molecules to combine into larger aggregates.

afflux (af'luks) [L. affluxus, affluxio] the rush of blood or liquid to a part.

affricate (af'rĭ-kit) a speech sound comprising occlusion, plosion, and frication, as either of the ch sounds in church, the j sound in joy, the ts sound in cats, and, often the tr sound in tree and the dr sound in dry. Called also affricative.

affrication (af"rĭ-ka'shun) the changing of a stop sound to an affricate.

affricative (a-frik'ah-tiv) 1. pertaining to or forming an affricate. 2. affricate.

Afibrin trademark for aminocaproic acid (see under ACID).

afibrinogenemia (ah-fi"brin-o-jĕ-ne'me-ah) a blood clotting disorder caused by absence of fibrinogen in the blood, resulting in excessive bleeding, ecchymoses, and hematomas. The acquired form, which is caused by the destruction of fibrinogen, is more common. Congenital afibrinogenemia is probably transmitted as a recessive trait and occurs in both sexes; it is due to an inability to produce fibrinogen. Spontaneous gingival bleeding and postextraction hemorrhage may occur. The term *hypofibrinogenemia* is used to denote the condition that occurs when the fibrinogen level is low; *dysfibrinogenemia* is used for afibrinogenemia or for hypofibrinogenemia. Called also *fibrinogenopenia*.

Afrin trademark for *oxymetazoline hydrochloride* (see under OXYMETAZOLINE).

Afsillin trademark for *penicillin G procaine* (see under PENICILLIN).

aftercare (af′ter-kār) the care and treatment of a convalescent patient. Called also *aftertreatment*.

aftercondensation (af″ter-kon″den-sa′shun) postcondensation.

afterdischarge (af″ter-dis′charj) a response to stimulation of sensory neurons which persists after the stimulus has ceased. It is directly related to a parallel circuit or the number of neurons in an oscillatory circuit and is usually related to synaptic fatigue; rapid fatigue decreases the period of afterdischarge.

aftergilding (af″ter-gild′ing) the histologic application of gold salts to nerve tissue after fixation and hardening.

afterglow (af′ter-glo″) screen LAG.

afterstain (af″ter-stān″) a stain used after another stain for the purpose of producing greater differentiation of details.

aftertaste (af″ter-tāst′) a taste continuing after the substance producing it has been removed.

aftertreatment (af″ter-trēt′ment) aftercare.

AG axiogingival.

Ag silver (L. *argentum*).

ag antigen.

agammaglobulinemia (a-gam″ah-glob″u-lĭ-ne′me-ah) [*a* neg. + *gamma globulin* + Gr. *haima* blood + *-ia*] a group of immunologic conditions characterized by deficient levels of immunoglobulins (gamma globulins) in the blood, leading to recurrent infection. Called also *antibody deficiency syndrome*. See also HYPOGAMMAGLOBULINEMIA. **autosomal recessive a.**, Swiss type a. **secondary a.**, that in which production of immunoglobulins is obstructed by an underlying disease, such as reticuloendothelial or lymphoid disorders. **sex-linked recessive a.**, an immunological condition usually affecting males up to five. or six months of age, characterized by a marked decrease of IgG, decrease or absence of IgM, and absence of IgA, associated with a failure to form antibody or with poor formation of antibody against a variety of antigens. Plasma cells are absent or reduced, and germinal centers in lymphoid tissue are absent. The sinusoids and reticuloendothelial cells of the sinusoids are prominent against an acellular background. The spleen is usually small and the thymus may be hypoplastic, but in most instances it is normal. Susceptibility to infection with *Staphylococcus aureus*, pneumococci, streptococci, and meningococci is common. Affected patients may have delayed-type hypersensitivity and reject primary allografts. The thymus-dependent lymphocytes seem to be intact. Called also *congenital hypogammaglobulinemia* and *sex-linked recessive hypogammaglobulinemia*. **Swiss type a.**, a genetically determined immunologic disorder, transmitted as a simple autosomal recessive trait, which is characterized by the inability of the body to produce humoral antibodies, resulting in a decrease or absence of all immunoglobulins. It is marked by a reduction in the number of lymphocytes, aplasia of the thymus, and absence of plasma cells, germinal centers in the lymph nodes, tonsils, adenoids, and Peyer's patches. Affected patients usually do not develop delayed-type hypersensitivity or cell-mediated immunity, and they do not reject allografts. Called also *autosomal recessive a.*

aganglionic (a-gang″gle-on′ik) pertaining to or characterized by absence of ganglion cells.

agar (ag′ar) a dried mucilaginous substance extracted from *Gelidium cartilagineum, Cracilaria confervoides*, and related red algae, used as a laxative, in making emulsions, and as a culture medium for bacteria. **a. impression material**, impression material, reversible hydrocolloid; see under MATERIAL.

agate (ag′it) a variegated stone showing curved, colored bands or other markings; a form of silicon dioxide.

Agathinus of Sparta [1st century A.D.] a Greek physician who was a pupil of Athenaeus and, like his master, a Pneumatist. See also PNEUMATIST.

age (āj) 1. the duration of individual existence measured in units of time. 2. the measure of some individual attribute in terms of the chronological age of an average normal individual showing the same degree of proficiency. **anatomical a.**, age expressed in terms of the chronological age of the average individual showing the same body development. **bone a.**, osseous development shown roentgenographically, stated in terms of the chronological age at which the development is ordinarily attained. **chronological a.**, the age expressed in terms of the period elapsed from the time of birth. **a. distribution**, age DISTRIBUTION. **a. hardening**, age HARDENING.

agency (a′jen-se) 1. an organization authorized to perform certain activities for another organization. 2. an administrative division of an organization. 3. the capacity or condition of exerting power. **home health a.**, an agency which provides home health care. Under Medicare, such an agency must provide skilled nursing services and at least one additional service, such as occupational therapy, medical social services, speech therapy, etc., in the home of the patient. **voluntary health a.**, any nonprofit, nongovernment agency, governed by lay and/or professional individuals, organized on a national, state, or local basis, whose primary purpose is health-related, such as the American Cancer Society, a visiting nurse association, or a nonprofit hospital.

agenesis (ah-jen′ĕ-sis) [*a* neg. + Gr. *genesis* production] absence of an organ; frequently used to designate such absence resulting from failure of the appearance of the primordium of an organ in embryonic development. See also APLASIA. **enamel a.**, enamel HYPOPLASIA. **gonadal a.**, Turner's SYNDROME. **unilateral facial a.**, first and second branchial arch SYNDROME.

agent (a′gent) [L. *agens* acting] 1. a person authorized by another to act on his or her behalf. 2. a representative of the insurer in negotiating, servicing, or effecting health insurance contracts. An agent may be an employee of the insurer or an independent contractor. See also CARRIER (5). 3. any power, principle, or substance capable of producing a physical, chemical, or biological effect. **adenoid degeneration (AD) a., adenoidal-pharyngeal-conjunctival (APC) a.**, human ADENOVIRUS. **adrenergic a.**, adrenergic DRUG. **adrenergic blocking a.**, adrenergic blocking DRUG. **α-adrenergic blocking a.**, α-adrenergic blocking DRUG. **adrenolytic a.**, adrenolytic drug; see adrenergic blocking DRUG. **adrenomimetic a.**, adrenomimetic drug; see sympathomimetic DRUG. **alkylating a.**, any of a group of substances capable of undergoing an electrophilic chemical reaction through the formation of carbonium ion intermediates or of transition complexes with target molecules, with the formation of covalent linkages (alkylation) with various nucleophilic substances, including those that are biologically active, such as phosphate, amino, sulfhydryl, hydroxyl, carboxyl, and imidazole groups. In biological systems, alkylating agents interfere with cell division in proliferating tissue; and their action is said to be cytotoxic; thus, they are used in the treatment of neoplasms. In addition, they are also cytolytic, mutagenic, carcinogenic, and teratogenic, and also inhibit glycolysis, respiration, and various biochemical processes. Their action is biologically similar to that of ionizing radiation. The DNA molecule is the primary target. Alkylating agents in this group include nitrogen mustards, ethyleneimines, alkyl sulfonates, nitrosoureas, and triazenes. **antiadrenergic a.**, adrenergic neuron blocking DRUG. **antianxiety a.**, antianxiety DRUG. **anticholinergic a.**, anticholinergic DRUG. **anticholinesterase a.**, cholinesterase INHIBITOR. **antineoplastic a.**, see ANTINEOPLASTIC (2). **antiparasympathetic a.**, antiparasympathetic DRUG. **antispasmodic a.**, see ANTISPASMODIC (2). **anxiolytic a.**, antianxiety DRUG. **atropine a., atropinelike a.**, antimuscarinic DRUG. **autonomic a.**, autonomic DRUG. **autopharmacological a.**, autacoid. **bactericidal a.**, see BACTERICIDE. **bacteriostatic a.**, an agent, usually a chemical, which inhibits the growth and reproduction of bacteria without actually killing them. **Bittner a.**, mammary tumor virus of mice; see under VIRUS. **bleaching a.**, any chemical substance used in removal of discoloration; in dentistry, usually of pulpless teeth. **cardiovascular a.**, cardiovascular DRUG. **cavity lining a.**, an agent applied to the floor and walls of the prepared cavity prior to placing a restoration to protect the pulp from irritation, thermal shock, trauma, and effects of microleakage, and/or to prime and cleanse the cavity in its preparation for the restoration. Cavity lining agents include cavity bases, liners, varnishes, primers, and cleaners. **cholinergic a., cholinomimetic a.**, parasympathomimetic DRUG. **cholinergic blocking a.**, cholinergic blocking DRUG. **cholinolytic a.**, see antimuscarinic DRUG. **competitive a.**, neuromuscular blocking a. (1). **coupling a.**, a chemical substance with which the surface of the filler material is coated to form a stable adhesive bond between the filler and the resin when the two are mixed to form a composite resin. Silanes are the principal coupling agents. **cross-linking a.**, a chemical substances which promotes the process of cross-linking. See also *vulcanizing a.*, CROSS-LINKING, and POLYMERIZATION. **curariform a.**, see *neuromuscular blocking a.* (1). **cytotoxic a.**, an agent capable of producing toxic effects on cells; see ANTINEOPLASTIC (2). **demelanizing a.,** an agent that inhibits the production of melanin, thereby enhancing depigmentation; used in the treatment of severe freckling and conditions characterized by hyperpigmentation. Monobenzone and hydroquinone are the principal demelanizing agents. Called also *hypopigmenting a.* and *demelaninizer.* Cf. *melanizing a.* **depolarizing a., depolarizing neuromuscular blocking a.,** a muscle relaxant that mimics the action of acetylcholine and depolarizes the nerve membrane, resulting in brief periods of firing manifested by transient muscular fasciculation, the phase being followed shortly by neuromuscular paralysis. Succinylcholine and decamethonium are the principal depolarizing agents. Called also *depolarizing drug.* See also *neuromuscular blocking a.* (2). **desiccating a.,** see DESICCANT (2). **desquamating a.,** keratolytic (2). **disclosing a.,** an agent used for disclosing plaque on the surface of the teeth; usually a selective dye solution which, on application, shows plaque to be of a different color than that of the surrounding tooth surface. Called also *disclosing solution.* **disinfectant a.,** see DISINFECTANT. **drying a.,** see DESICCANT (2). **Eaton a.,** *Mycoplasma pneumoniae;* see under MYCOPLASMA. **emulsifying a.,** see EMULSIFIER. **euphoriant a.,** any psychoactive agent capable of elevating or improving mood, such as marihuana. Some euphoriants, such as amphetamine, may exert psychotogenic effects in higher doses and are thus also classified as psychotomimetic agents. Called also *euphoriant* and *euphoriant drug.* **foamy a.,** Spumavirinae. **ganglionic blocking a.,** ganglionic blocking DRUG. **germicidal a.,** see GERMICIDE. **glazing a.,** a substance capable of giving a smooth, shiny surface to something, such as dimethacrylate when applied to the surface of the finished restoration. **H₁ blocking a.,** H₁ INHIBITOR. **H₂ blocking a.,** H₂ INHIBITOR. **hallucinogenic a.,** psychedelic a. **histamine blocking a.,** histamine INHIBITOR. **hydroalcoholic diluting a.,** a vehicle for alcohol- and water-soluble drugs, being an aqueous solution of ethanol and other components, such as aromatic, low-alcoholic, high-alcoholic, and iso-alcoholic elixirs (see under ELIXIR). **hyperpigmenting a.,** melanizing a. **hypopigmenting a.,** demelanizing a. **immunosuppressive a.,** any agent capable of inhibiting an immune response, including x-radiation, chemicals (e.g., mercaptopurine), antilymphocyte serum, or suppressor cells. Called also *immunosuppressive* and *immunosuppressant.* **insurance administrative a.,** CARRIER (5). **iodine disclosing a.,** a solution consisting of 7.7 percent iodine, 2.3 percent zinc iodide, 2.3 percent potassium iodide, 49 percent glycerol, and distilled water; used for disclosing dental plaque. Called also *iodine disclosing solution.* See also *disclosing a.* **luting a.,** a compound, such as wax, clay, or cement, used to seal and make tight joints or other connections of an apparatus or device. **Marburg a.,** Marburg VIRUS. **melanizing a.,** an agent that stimulates the production of melanin in the body, thereby enhancing skin pigmentation. Used to facilitate repigmentation in vitiligo, increase tolerance to sun rays, and enhance pigmentation. Trioxsalen and methoxsalen are the principal melanizing agents. Called also *hyperpigmenting a.* Cf. *demelanizing a.* **muscarinic a.,** muscarinic DRUG. **mysticomimetic a.,** any psychedelic agent of natural origin, such as mescaline or psilocybin. Called also *mysticomimetic* or *mysticomimetic drug.* **neuromuscular blocking a.,** a muscle relaxant that acts on the neuromuscular junction. Two basic types are recognized: (1) agents which act on the motor end-plate membrane of the myoneural junction, competing with acetylcholine for the receptor site of the membrane, so that the acetylcholine cannot increase sufficiently the permeability of the membrane to initiate a depolarizing wave; thus, preventing the passage of impulses from the end-plate to the muscle. Agents in this class are called *competitive, stabilizing, curariform,* and *nondepolarizing agents* or *drugs.* Tubocurarine is the principal competitive neuromuscular blocking agent. (2) Agents that prevent the transmission of impulses by completely depolarizing the muscle fibers, while the end-plates are allowed to act normally. Agents in this class are called *depolarizing agents* or *drugs.* **nicotinic a.,** nicotinic drug; see parasympathomimetic DRUG. **nondepolarizing a., nondepolarizing neuromuscular blocking a.,** neuromuscular blocking a. (2). **neuroleptic a.,** antipsychotic DRUG. **Norwalk a.,** an unclassified virus, about 27 nm in diameter, which is responsible for outbreaks of human gastroenteritis; initially isolated in Norwalk, Ohio. **opaquing a.,** opacifier. **oxidizing a.,** an element which gains electrons in an oxidation-reduction reaction. **oxygen-liberating a.,** a chemical agent that releases oxygen; used as a topical anti-infective, particularly against infections caused by anaerobic organisms, such as

acute ulcerative gingivitis. **papilloma, polyoma, and vacuolating a.,** Papovaviridae. **parasympathetic blocking a.,** parasympathetic blocking DRUG. **parasympatholytic a.,** parasympatholytic blocking DRUG. **phantasticant a.,** psychedelic a. **polishing a.,** an abrasive substance which produces a smooth glossy surface. See also ABRASIVE. **psychedelic a.,** any agent capable of inducing changes in psychic processes in normal persons (i.e., perception, thought, feeling, mood, and behavior) in doses which do not necessarily cause significant changes in metabolic, sensorimotor, and autonomic processes. The term comprises agents that produce hallucinations, visions, and illusions. Called also *hallucinogenic a., hallucinogen, hallucinogenic drug, phantasticant,* and *psychedelic.* **psychoactive a.,** any agent capable of modifying mood in doses which do not necessarily cause significant changes in metabolic, sensorimotor, and autonomic processes. Called also *psychogenic a., psychotropic a., psychoactive drug, psychogenic drug,* and *psychotropic drug.* **psychodysleptic a.,** psychotoxic a. **psychogenic a.,** psychoactive. **psychotherapeutic a.,** any psychoactive agent used for the treatment of abnormalities of mental function, including antipsychotic, mood-stabilizing, antidepressant, and antianxiety-sedative drugs. Called also *psychotherapeutic* and *psychotherapeutic drug.* **psychotogenic a.,** psychotomimetic a. **psychotomimetic a.,** any psychoactive or psychotoxic agent capable of producing abnormal states of altered perception, thought, and feeling, i.e., mimicking a psychosis, including psychedelic agents as well as those agents that have stimulant or depressant actions on the central nervous system, such as LSD and amphetamine. Some agents, such as marihuana, may exert euphoriant effects in small doses but act as psychotomimetics in higher doses. Called also *psychotogenic a., psychotogenic drug, psychotomimetic,* and *psychotomimetic drug.* **psychotoxic a.,** any psychoactive agent capable of producing abnormalities of mental function. Called also *psychodysleptic a., psychodysleptic drug, psychotoxic,* and *psychotoxic drug.* **psychotropic a.,** psychoactive a. **Pulpdent pulp capping a.,** trademark for a substance used in pulp capping, consisting of a 52.5 percent suspension of calcium hydroxide in an aqueous methyl cellulose solution. **radiomimetic a.,** alkylating a. **α-receptor blocking a.,** α-adrenergic blocking DRUG. **β-receptor blocking a.,** β-adrenergic blocking DRUG. **reducing a.,** the element which loses electrons in an oxidation-reduction reaction. **sclerosing a.,** a chemical irritant capable of causing tissue injury resulting in inflammation and eventual fibrosis, and of breaking down the intimal surface of blood vessels resulting in thrombosis. Used therapeutically to obliterate varicose veins and in other procedures in which formation of fibrous tissue is required, as in closing an opening and the like. Called also *sclerosant.* **separating a.,** separating MEDIUM. **spasmolytic a.,** SPASMOLYTIC (2). **stabilizing a., stabilizing neuromuscular blocking a.,** neuromuscular blocking a. (1). **surface-active a.,** surfactant. **sweetening a.,** sweetener. **sympatholytic a.,** see adrenergic blocking DRUG. **sympathomimetic a.,** sympathomimetic DRUG. **therapeutic a.,** THERAPEUTIC (2). **vulcanizing a.,** a chemical agent which promotes cross-linking in vulcanization. Sulfur and organic peroxides are the agents most commonly used in vulcanization of rubber, and ethyl orthosilicate in vulcanization of silicones. See also *cross-linking a.* **wetting a.,** a surfactant which, when added to water, lowers its surface tension and promotes wetting by causing the water to penetrate more easily into, or to spread over the surface of, another material. Soaps and alcohols are the principal wetting agents. In film processing, wetting agents are used after washing the film to accelerate the flow of water from the film surface, thus accelerating the drying process.

ageusia (ah-gu′ze-ah) [a neg. + Gr. *geusis* taste] impaired sense of taste.

agger (aj′er), pl. *ag′geres* [L.] eminence; a prominence or projection. See also EMINENCE and EMINENTIA. **a. na′si** [NA], a ridgelike elevation midway between the anterior extremity of the middle nasal concha and the inner surface of the dorsum of the nose. Called also *nasoturbinal concha* and *ridge of nose.*

agglomerated (ah-glom′er-āt″ed) [L. *agglomeratus,* from *ad* together + *glomus* mass] crowded into a mass.

agglutination (ah-gloo″tĭ-na′shun) [L. *agglutinatio*] 1. the action or process of uniting or adhering. 2. a mass of elements grouped together. 3. a process of union in the healing of a wound. 4. clumping together of a suspension of antigen-carrying cells, microorganisms, or particles in the presence of specific antibodies (agglutinins). **acid a.,** the agglutination of particles, e.g., microorganisms, due to low pH. **cold a.,** agglutination of red blood cells *in vivo* or *in vitro* by the presence of a cold agglutinin that is active at temperatures of less than 32° C. See also AUTOAGGLUTINATION (1). **cross a.,** group a. **intravascular a.,** agglutination of erythrocytes or other cells in the intact blood vessel occurring in response to injury, certain diseases, or antibody. Called also *sludging of blood*. **erythrocyte a.,** hemagglutination. **group a.,** agglutination of various members (cells) of a group of biologically related organisms or red cells by an agglutinin specific for one of the surface antigens of that group. Called also *cross a*. See also BLOOD GROUP. **O a.,** the agglutination of bacteria in the presence of antibody to the heat-stable somatic antigen. **platelet a.,** the clumping together of blood platelets.

agglutinin (ah-gloo′tĭ-nin) an antibody whose presence produces agglutination of microorganisms, blood cells, or antigen-coated particles. Serum agglutinins are immunoglobulins produced in response to stimulation by agglutinogens. Called also *agglutinating antibody* and *blood group antibody*. **a. anti-A,** one present in blood groups B and O that will cause agglutination of red cells having A antigen. Called also *antibody anti-A*. **a. anti-B,** one present in blood groups A and O that will cause agglutination of red cells having B antigen. Called also *antibody anti-B*. **anti-Rh a.,** one of the Rh specificities (often, anti-Rh₀) in Rh-negative mothers carrying an Rh-positive fetus or after transfusion of Rh-positive blood into an Rh-negative patient. See also Rh blood groups, under BLOOD GROUP. **chief a.,** the specific immune agglutinin in the blood of an animal immunized against an infectious disease agent; it is active at a higher dilution of the blood serum than is the partial agglutinin. Called also *haupt-a*. and *major a*. **cold a.,** one which acts only at low temperatures. See also AUTOAGGLUTININ. **complete a's,** agglutinating antibodies, e.g., IgM hemagglutinins, demonstrable by simple direct mixing with antigen-containing particles. **cross a.,** one which, although formed in response to a specific chemical grouping of one particulate antigen, also has specific action on a different particulate antigen with a similar chemical grouping. See also antigenic DETERMINANT. **group a.,** one which has a specific action on certain organisms or cells, but which will agglutinate other closely related strains and species as well. **haupt-a.,** chief a. **immune a.,** a specific agglutinin found in serum as a result of recovering from a disease or having been injected with microorganisms, cells, or antigens. **incomplete a.,** one that is unable to cause agglutination directly, which may be due to the property of the antibody, e.g., it may have only one combining site. The term is also applied to Rh antibodies that are demonstrable only when suspended in high-molecular-weight media or by the antiglobulin test. **leukocyte a.,** one which agglutinates leukocytes. **major a.,** chief a. **minor a.,** partial a. **normal a.,** a specific agglutinin found in the blood of an animal or of man that has neither had the associated disease nor been injected with the causative microorganism. **partial a.,** one present in an agglutinative serum which acts on organisms and cells that are closely related to the specific antigen, but in a lower dilution. Called also *minor a., coagglutinin,* and *para-agglutinin*. **platelet a.,** one which agglutinates blood platelets. **somatic a.,** one specific for the body of a microorganism, and is not, for example, flagellar or capsular.

agglutinogen (ag″loo-tin′o-jen) 1. any substance which, acting as an antigen, stimulates the production of agglutinins. 2. an antigen located on the erythrocytes which stimulates the production of specific antibodies (agglutinins) against the erythrocytes that were used to produce the antibodies, thus determining the blood group specificity of an individual. Blood group agglutinogens are nitrogenous, neutral, heteropolysaccharides, containing amino acids or peptides and lipids as well as carbohydrates. Rh antigens are thought to be lipids. Red cell ABO structures are glycolipids. They are used as genetic markers in the study of population genetics, anthropology, and medicolegal practice, such as establishment of paternity. Called also *blood group substance* (especially in soluble form [glycoprotein] as found in body fluids of secretors). See also BLOOD GROUP. **a. A,** 1. one present in blood groups A and AB. 2. a surface protein of some strains of coagulase-positive staphylococci, having a molecular weight of about 13,000, liberated from bacterial cells during their growth, being released by deoxyribonuclease. It elicits a hypersensitive reaction in guinea pigs and rabbits by reaction with the Fc fragment of IgG molecules, which then fixes complement. It also precipitates normal γ-globulin. Called also *antigen A* and *protein A*. **a. B,** one present in blood groups B and AB. **a. M,** one of the MNSs blood group system, which is present in the Ms, MS, MSs, MNs, MNS, and MNSs blood groups. **a. N,** one of the MNSs blood group system, which is present in the Ns, NS, NSs, MNS, MNs, and MNSs blood groups. **private a.,** one limited to one or several families. **public a.,** one found in large groups of a population. **a. rh, rh′, rh″, RH₀, Rh₁, Rh₂, Rhz, rhy** and **rhʷˡ** agglutinogens of the Rh blood group system. The term *agglutinogen* is used in the Wiener nomenclature and conceptualization of the Rh blood groups (see under BLOOD GROUP). **a. s,** one of the MNSs blood group system; which

is present in the MS, MSs, NS, NSs, MNS, and MNSs blood groups. **a. s,** one of the MNSs blood group system, which is present in the Ms, MSs, Ns, NSs, MNSs, and MNs blood groups.

aggred. feb. abbreviation for L. *aggredien′te feb′re,* while the fever is coming on.

aggregation (ag″rĕ-ga′shun) [L. *aggregare* to lead to a flock] 1. clustering; clumping; bringing together. 2. a clumped mass. **leukocyte a.,** LEUKOCYTE aggregation. **platelet a.,** PLATELET aggregation.

Ag₂Hg₃ α₁-phase of dental amalgam; see α-PHASE.

Agilene trademark for *polyethylene*.

aging (āj′ing) progressive changes produced with the passage of time. **alloy a.,** age HARDENING.

Agit. vas. abbreviation for L. *agita′to va′se,* the vial being shaken.

aglossia (ah-glos′e-ah) [*a* neg. + Gr. *glōssa* tongue   -*ia*] 1. congenital absence of the tongue. 2. absence of the power of speech.

aglossostomia (ah″glos-o-sto′me-ah) [*a* neg. + Gr. *glōssa* tongue + *stoma* mouth + -*ia*] congenital absence of the tongue and mouth opening.

aglycemia (ah″gli-se′me-ah) [*a* neg. + Gr *glykys* sweet + *haima* blood   -*ia*] absence of sugar from the blood.

aglycone (ah-gli′kōn) [*a* neg. + Gr. *glykys* sweet + -*on*] a hydroxy nonsugar component of glycosides.

angathia (ag-na′the-ah) [*a* neg. + Gr. *gnathos* jaw + -*ia*] a congenital condition characterized by total or partial absence of a jaw. See also CYCLOPIA hypognathus.

agnathus (ag-na′thus) a deformed fetus exhibiting agnathia.

agnogenic (ag″no-jen′ik) [Gr. *agnōs* unknown + *genesis* origin] of unknown origin or etiology.

agnosia (ag-no′ze-ah) [*a* neg. + Gr. *gnōsis* perception] loss of or impaired ability to recognize sensory stimuli. **gustatory a.,** impaired ability to taste.

-agogue [Gr. *agōgos* leading, inducing] a word termination meaning an agent which leads or induces.

agomphiasis (ag″om-fi′ah-sis) [*a* neg. + Gr. *gomphios* molar + -*ia*] 1. looseness of the teeth. 2. absence of the teeth; anodontia. Called also *agomphosis*.

agomphious (ah-gom′fe-us) without teeth.

agomphosis (ag″om-fo′sis) agomphiasis.

agonal (ag′o-nal) pertaining to the death agony; occurring at the moment of, or just before death.

agonist (ag′o-nist) a prime mover; an organ, such as a muscle, opposed in action to another organ, so that the action of one organ is controlled and checked automatically by action of the second organ. Cf. ANTAGONIST. 1. a prime mover. 2. a muscle opposed in action by another muscle (an antagonist). 3. a drug capable of combining with receptors to initiate drug action. **partial a.,** a drug that can elicit some but not a maximal effect.

agony (ag′o-ne) [Gr. *agōnia*] 1. severe pain or extreme suffering. 2. the death struggle.

-agra [Gr. *agra* a catching, seizure] a word termination meaning a seizure or acute pain.

agraffe (ah-graf′) [Fr.] a clamplike instrument for clamping together the edges of a wound.

agranulocyte (ah-gran′u-lo-sit′) [*a* neg. + *granular* + -*cyte*] a leukocyte which has no prominent granules in the cytoplasm, produced by the lymph nodes, spleen, tonsils, thymus, and beneath the epithelium of the gastrointestinal mucosa. See LYMPHOCYTE and MONOCYTE. Called also *lymphoid leukocyte* and *nongranular leukocyte*.

agranulocytosis (ah-gran″u-lo-si-to′sis) a frequently fatal disease occurring most commonly in middle-aged women, and characterized by the disappearance of granulocytes and a fall in the total leukocyte count. Paleness of the mucous membranes; jaundice; gangrenous ulceration of the gingivae, tonsils, palate, lips, pharynx, and oral mucosa; and regional adenopathy are the principal symptoms. Bacterial superinfection may occur in advanced stages. Drugs are believed to be the principal etiologic factor, and the following are suspected: aminopyrine, arsenic compounds, barbiturates, chloramphenicol, chlorpromazine, DDT, gold salts, imipramine, mepazine, methampyrone, methimazole, phenindione, phenothiazine, phenylbutazone, prochlorperazine, promazine, sulfonamides, thiouracil, and tolbutamide. Called also *agranulocytic angina, aneutrocytosis, aneutrophilia, granulocytic hypoplasia, idiopathic leukopenia, malignant leukopenia, malignant neutropenia, mucositis necroticans agranulocytica, pernicious leukope-*

nia, Schultz's angina, and Schultz's syndrome. **infantile genetic a.,** congenital NEUTROPENIA. **periodic a.,** a rare form characterized by periodic recurrence of symptoms similar to those seen in other forms of agranulocytosis, and including fever, malaise, regional lymphadenopathy, headache, arthritis, and skin infection. The cycle of recurrence commonly occurs every three weeks, although it may be longer. Oral manifestations consist of stomatitis, sore throat, gingivitis, and ulcers of the mucosa. The roentgenogram may show loss of superficial alveolar bone. In children, there may be loss of bone around multiple teeth, sometimes called *prepubertal periodontitis.* Hematologic studies show a low count of neutrophils, with their complete disappearance at the height of the disease, associated with an increase in monocytes and lymphocytes. Called also *cyclic agranulocytic angina, cyclic neutropenia,* and *periodic neutropenia.*

Agribon trademark for *sulfadimethoxine.*

Agrobacterium (ag″ro-bak-te′re-um) [Gr. *agros* field + *baktērion* a little rod] a genus of nitrogen-fixing, gram-negative, aerobic bacteria of the family Rhizobiaceae, made up of flagellated rods, found in soil and in the roots or stems of plants. With the exception of *R. radiobac′ter,* they produce stem hypertrophy of plants.

ague (a′gu) [Fr. *aigu* sharp] 1. malarial fever, or any other severe recurrent symptom of malarial origin. 2. a chill.

agyria (ah-ji′re-ah) [*a* neg. + Gr. *gyros* ring + -*ia*] a malformation in which the convolutions of the cerebral cortex are not normally developed and the brain is usually small. Called also *lissencephaly.* See also agyria-pachygyria SYNDROME.

AH-26 trademark for an epoxy type resin used as a root canal sealer.

AHA 1. American Heart Association. 2. American Hospital Association.

AHCA American Health Care Association.

AHEC area health education CENTER.

Ahern's knot enamel KNOT.

AHF antihemophilic factor; see FACTOR VIII.

AHG antihemophilic globulin; see FACTOR VIII.

Ai axioincisal.

aid (ād) help or assistance; any device or appliance by which a function an be improved or augmented. **first a.,** emergency assistance and treatment furnished in cases of accident, injury, or ilness. **pharmaceutic a., pharmaceutical a.,** pharmaceutic NECESSITY. **speech a., prosthetic,** an appliance used to close a residual traumatic or surgical cleft in the hard or sot palates, or both, and/or to restore other palatal continuity necessary to the production of vocal sounds.

aide (ād) one who assists; an assistant. **nurses' a.,** a member of the ancillary medical staff, whose duties include assisting nurses in taking care of patient's needs which do not require professional training, such as housekeeping tasks. Nurses' aides are usually trained on he job and are not subject to licensing.

ailment (āl′ment) any disease or affection of the body.

Aim see under DENTIFRICE.

Ainsworth's punch [George C. *Ainsworth,* Boston dentist, 1852–1948] see under PUNCH.

AIOB American Institute of Oral Biology (see under INSTITUTE).

air (ār) [L. *aer;* Gr. *aēr*] a gaseous mixture of one part oxygen, four parts nitrogen, and small amounts of carbon dioxide, ammonia, argon, nitrites, and organic matter, which makes up the earth's atmosphere. **a. embolism,** gas EMBOLISM. **factitious a.,** nitrous OXIDE.

airbrasive (ār′bra-siv) an instrument for cutting tooth structure or removing deposits from teeth by application of a mixture of sand and aluminum oxide by air blast.

Airdent trademark for a dental unit which utilizes abrasive particles applied by air blast for the preparation of dental cavities; no longer used.

airway (ār′wa) 1. the passage by which air enters and leaves the lungs. 2. a mechanical device used for securing unobstructed respiration during general anesthesia or other occasions in which the patient is not ventilating or exchanging gases properly. See *oral a.* **oral a., oropharyngeal a.,** a rubber or plastic hollow tube inserted into the mouth and back of the throat to prevent the tongue from slipping back into the throat and closing off the passage of air. See illustration. See also endotracheal TUBE.

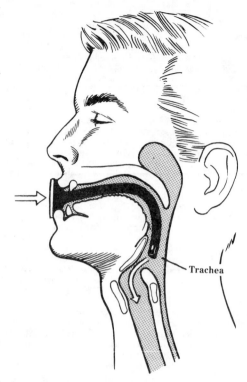

Oral airway. (From B. F. Miller and C. B. Keane: Encyclopedia and Dictionary of Medicine and Nursing. 2nd ed. Philadelphia, W. B. Saunders Co., 1978.)

Ajellomyces (ah″jĕ-lo-mi′sēz) a genus of ascomycetous fungi. **A. capsula′tus,** the perfect (sexual) stage of *Histoplasma capsulatum.* **A. dermatid′idis,** the perfect (sexual) stage of *Blastomyces dermatitis.*

akaryocyte (ah-kar′e-o-sīt″) [*a* neg. + Gr. *karyon* kernel + *kytos* hollow vessel] a non-nucleated cell, e.g., an erythrocyte. Written also *acaryote.*

akaryote (ah-kar′e-ōt) [*a* neg. + Gr. *karyon* kernel] akaryocyte.

akinesia (ah″ki-ne′ze-ah) [*a* neg. + Gr. *kinēsis* motion + -*ia*] abnormal absence or poverty of movement. **a. al′gera,** congenital facial DIPLEGIA. **O'Brien's a.,** paralysis of the orbicularis oculi muscle produced by injection of an anesthetic solution directly over the orbital branch of the seventh cranial nerve as it emerges from behind the ear and extends toward the orbital region along the ramus of the jaw. **reflex a.,** loss of reflex movement.

akinesthesia (ah-kin″es-the′zhe-ah) absence of kinesthesia; absence of the sense of movement.

Aktiven trademark for *chloramine-T.*

AL axiolingual.

Al aluminum.

-al in chemical nomenclature, a suffix used in forming the names of compounds, indicating the presence of the aldehyde group, −CHO, as *chloral.*

Ala alanine.

ala (a′lah), pl. *a′lae* [L. "wing"] a general term used in anatomy to designate any winglike structure or process. Called also *wing.* **a. cris′tae gal′li** [NA], frontal HAMULUS. **a. mag′na os′sis sphenoida′lis, a. ma′jor os′sis sphenoida′lis** [NA], great wing of sphenoid bone; see under WING. **a. mi′nor os′sis sphenoida′lis** [NA], small wing of sphenoid bone; see under WING. **a. na′si** [NA], the flaring cartilaginous process forming the outer side of each nostril. **a. par′va os′sis sphenoida′lis,** small wing of sphenoid bone; see under WING. **a. tempora′lis os′sis sphenoida′lis,** great wing of sphenoid bone; see under WING. **a. of vomer, a. vo′meris** [NA], one of the two lateral expansions on the superior border of the vomer, coming into contact with the sphenoidal process of the palate and the vaginal process of the medial pterygoid plate.

alabaster (al′ah-bas″ter) gypsum.

alae (a′le) [L.] plural of *ala.*

AlaG axiolabiogingival.

Alajouanine's syndrome [T. *Alajouanine*, French neurologist] see under SYNDROME.

alalia (ah-la′le-ah) [*a* neg. + Gr. *lalein* to speak + *-ia*] inability to speak.

Alamon trademark for *hydroxyzine hydrochloride* (see under HYDROXYZINE).

alanine (al′ah-nēn) an aliphatic, naturally occurring, nonessential amino acid, 2- or α-aminopropionic acid, which is also found in the saliva. Abbreviated *Ala*. See also amino ACID. **a. aminotransferase,** alanine AMINOTRANSFERASE. **β-a.,** a naturally occurring amino acid, 3-aminopropanoic acid, carnosine, and anserine. Called also *β-aminopropionic acid.* **a. carboxypeptidase,** alanine CARBOXYPEPTIDASE. **a. nitrogen mustard,** melphalan.

alastrim (ah-las′trim) VARIOLA minor.

alate (a′lāt) [L. *alatus* winged] having wings; winged; winglike.

Alathon trademark for *polyethylene.*

alba (al′bah) [L., fem. of *albus* white] white; used as an adjective in names of anatomical structures or tissues or of certain diseases.

Albacar trademark for *precipitated calcium carbonate* (see under CALCIUM carbonate).

Albacer trademark for a synthetic *dental wax* (see under WAX).

Albamycin trademark for *novobiocin.*

albation (al-ba′shun) [L. *albare* to whiten] the act of whitening; bleaching.

albefaction (al″bĕ-fak′shun) [L. *albus* white + *facere* to make] the process of making white or bleaching.

Albers-Schönberg's disease (marble bones) [Heinrich *Albers-Schönberg,* German roentgenologist] see under DISEASE.

Albertini, Ambrosius see Fanconi-Albertini-Zellweger SYNDROME.

albicans (al′bĭ-kanz) [L.] white.

albinism (al′bĭ-nizm) [L. *albus* white + *-ism*] congenital absence of pigment in the skin, hair, and eyes. Called also *albinismus.*

albinismus (al″bĭ-niz′mus) [L.] albinism.

albino (al-bi′no) an individual affected with albinism.

Albinus' muscle [Bernard Siegfried *Albinus*, anatomist and surgeon in Leyden, 1697–1770] risorius MUSCLE.

Albiotic trademark for *lincomycin.*

albite (al′bit) sodium FELDSPAR.

Albl's ring see under RING.

Albococcus epidermis (al″bo-kok′us ep″ĭ-der′mis) *Staphylococcus epidermidis;* see under STAPHYLOCOCCUS.

Albrecht's bone [Karl Martin Paul *Albrecht,* German anatomist, 1851–1894] basiotic BONE.

Albrecht-Arzt-Warthin tumor [Heinrich *Albrecht,* Vienna pathologist; L. *Arzt,* Vienna pathologist; Alfred Scott *Warthin,* American pathologist, 1866–1931] adenolymphoma.

Albright's syndrome [Fuller *Albright,* Boston physician, born 1900] 1. see under SYNDROME (1). 2. pseudopseudohypoparathyroidism.

Albright-Butler-Bloomberg syndrome [F. *Albright;* Allan May *Butler;* Esther *Bloomberg*] vitamin D–resistant RICKETS.

Albright-McCune-Sternberg syndrome [F. *Albright;* D. *McCune;* Karl *Sternberg,* German pathologist, 1872–1935] Albright's SYNDROME (1).

Albucasis [c. 936–1013] the most famous Arabic writer on surgery; the surgical part of his encyclopedic *Al tarsif* ("The Collection") greatly influenced medieval European medicine. His writings include the first illustration of surgical and dental instruments. In cauterization for toothache, he applied to the tooth a red-hot iron passed through an iron or copper tube to protect the adjacent tissues. Albucasis is considered to be the first author writing about dental calculus and its removal. He also listed rules for tooth extraction. Called also *Abulcasis* and *Abulkasim.*

albumin (al-bu′min) a simple protein found in nearly every animal and in many vegetable tissues, which is characterized by being soluble in water and coagulable by heat. It contains carbon, hydrogen, nitrogen, oxygen, and sulfur. On hydrolysis, it yields α-amino acids and their derivatives. Typical albumins are those found in egg white (ovalbumin), blood (serum albumin), milk (lactalbumin), and other naturally occurring substances. **a. A,** an albumin believed to exist in small amounts in the blood serum of cancer patients, but which accumulates in large amounts in cancer cells. **blood a.,** see *plasma a.* **coagulated a.,** albumin altered by heat or chemical action so as to be insoluble in water, neutral salt solutions, or dilute acid and alkaline solutions. **egg a.,** ovalbumin. **iodinated** ^{125}I **serum a.,** a sterile, buffered isotonic solution containing not less than 10 mg of radioiodinated normal human serum albumin per milliliter, and adjusted to provide not more than 1 millicurie of

radioactivity per milliliter; used as a diagnostic aid in determining blood volume and cardiac output. Called also *radioiodinated* (^{125}I) *serum a. (human).* **milk a.,** lactalbumin. **native a.,** any albumin normally present in the body. **plasma a.,** albumin found in blood plasma, which together with globulin represents two major classes of plasma proteins. It is precipitated from plasma with 100 percent ammonium sulfate, while 50 percent ammonium sulfate is used to precipitate globulin. It is the major component of fraction A (4S protein), but its molecules are the smallest in the blood protein group (molecular weight of 69,000). Plasma albumin is separated into three components by filter paper electrophoresis, α_1, α_2, and β. Its functions relate to osmotic pressure regulation and fatty acid transport. Preparations of plasma albumin are used as plasma expanders, in the treatment of shock, and in the correction of hypoproteinemia. **radioiodinated** (^{125}I) **serum a. (human),** iodinated ^{125}I serum a. **serum a.,** albumin found in blood serum. See *plasma a.* **serum a., radioiodinated,** human serum albumin iodinated with radioactive iodine (^{131}I) which emits beta and gamma rays. The preparation has a half-life of 8 days and is used in determining blood circulation time, blood volume, and cardiac output, and in the diagnosis of brain tumors.

albuminemia (al-bu″mĭ-ne′me-ah) [*albumin* + Gr. *haima* blood + *-ia*] the presence of an abnormally large amount of albumin in the blood plasma or serum.

albuminoid (al-bu″mĭ-noid″) [*albumin* + Gr. *eidos* form] 1. resembling albumin. 2. a group of simple proteins, including keratins, elastins, and collagens, that can be dissolved only by hydrolysis and by boiling in strong acids. On hydrolysis, they yield only α-amino acids. 3. scleroprotein.

albuminolysis (al-bu″mĭ-nol′ĭ-sis) the splitting up of albumins.

albuminous (al-bu′mĭ-nus) containing or of the nature of an albumin.

albuminuria (al″bu-mĭ-nu′re-ah) [*albumin* + Gr. *ouron* urine + *-ia*] the presence in the urine of excessive amounts of plasma albumin. See also PROTEINURIA. **Bence Jones a.,** Bence Jones PROTEINURIA.

albuterol (al-bu′tĕ-rōl) a β-adrenergic receptor agonist, α′-[(*tert*-butylamino)methyl]-4-hydroxy-*m*-xylene-α,α′-diol, occurring as a crystalline powder that is soluble in most organic solvents. Used chiefly as a bronchodilator. Called also *salbutamol.* Trademarks: Aerolin, Sultanol.

ALC axiolinguocervical.

Alcaine trademark for *proparacaine hydrochloride* (see under PROPARACAINE).

Alcaligenes (al″kah-lij′ĕ-nēz) [Arabic *al-qualy* potash + Gr. *gennan* to produce] a genus of gram-negative, aerobic, saprophytic bacteria of uncertain affiliation, made up of coccoid or rod-shaped cells, 0.5 to 1.2 μm by 0.5 to 2.6 μ in size, occurring singly. The organisms are motile with one to four (sometimes as many as eight flagella). Their metabolism is respiratory, O₂ being the electron acceptor. Some strains are capable of anaerobic respiration in the presence of nitrates or nitrites; most strains require nitrogen. They inhabit the intestines of vertebrates, and also occur in dairy products, rotting eggs and other foods, fresh water, and decomposing organic matter. Sometimes spelled *Alkaligenes.* **A. bronchisep′ticus,** *Bordetella bronchiseptica;* see under BORDETELLA. **A. faeca′lis,** a species found in the human intestinal tract and feces.

alcohol (al′ko-hol) [Arabic *al-koh′l* something subtle] 1. a class of organic compounds having the functional group —OH, formed from hydrocarbons by the substitution of one or more hydroxyl groups for an equal number of hydrogen atoms; the term is extended to various substitution products which are neutral in reaction and which contain one or more alcohol groups. Alcohols are distinguished as monohydric, dihydric, trihydric, etc., depending on the number of hydroxy groups present. Physically, alcohols are colorless liquids with a wide range of boiling points. All are strongly polar, many are flammable, and all are combustible. Methyl and allyl alcohols are toxic. The names of alcohols usually end in *-ol.* 2. ethyl a. **absolute a.,** dehydrated a. **β-aminoethyl a.,** ethanolamine. **amyl a.,** a colorless, oily liquid, $C_5H_{11}OH$, with a characteristic odor; miscible with ethyl alcohol, ether, and chloroform, and slightly soluble in water. **anhydrous a.,** dehydrated a. **aromatic a.,** any fatty alcohol in which a hydrogen of the alkyl chain is replaced by an aromatic group. **benzyl a.,** a clear oily liquid, $C_6H_5CH_2OH$, occurring in balsam of Peru, balsam of Tolu, and storax; used as a local anesthetic. **dehydrated a.,** a hygroscopic, clear, volatile liquid with characteristic odor and burning taste, containing not less than 99 percent by volume of ethyl alcohol. Called also *absolute a.* and *anhydrous a.* **a. dehydrogenase,** alcohol DEHYDROGENASE. **denatured a.,** alcohol which has been rendered unfit for internal or medicinal use by addition of methyl alcohol or acetone, but which may still be used for industrial purposes or as a solvent. **deodorized a.,** alcohol that contains 92.5 per cent of ethyl alcohol, and is free from fusel oil (amyl alcohol) and organic impurities. **dihydric a.,** dihydroxy a. **dihydroxy a.,** one containing two hydroxyl groups in its structure, such as a glycol. Called also *dihydric a.* **ethyl a.,** an alcohol, C_2H_5OH, occurring as a clear, mobile, flammable liquid with a characteristic odor and a biting taste. It is produced by fermentation of sugars and from ethylene, acetylene, synthetic gas, ethyl sulfate, methane, and other substances. Effects of alcohol may include irritation of denuded areas and mucosae, a burning sensation and redness of the skin on rubbing; dehydration of protoplasm; nerve degeneration and neuritis on injection near a nerve; depolarization of peripheral nerves and blocking of impulse conduction; depression of the action of the brain involved in integrated function, thus releasing the cortex from its integrating control and resulting in disorders of memory, discrimination, concentration, and coordination; general anesthesia of long duration; and influencing various physiological activities of the body. The effect of alcohol is enhanced by taking sedatives, hypnotics, and tranquilizers. Therapeutically, ethyl alcohol is applied topically as an astringent; counterirritant and rubefacient; to prevent bedsores and decubitus ulcer in bedridden patients; to reduce fever by virtue of its cooling effects by evaporation; and as a blocking agent injected in the proximity of sympathetic ganglia to peripheral nerves, as in relieving pain in trigeminal neuralgia or inoperative cancer. In dentistry, 70 to 77 percent alcoholic solutions are used as an antiseptic, particularly for cleansing of the operative area in surgery; as a desiccant in the preparation of cavities and in root canal therapy; for sponging shallow cavities and margins of deeper cavities; and in other procedures. In pharmacy, it is used as a solvent and vehicle for drugs. Ethyl alcohol is used in alcoholic beverages in various concentrations. Its internal use is contraindicated in liver and kidney diseases, peptic ulcer, epilepsy, urinary infection, and other diseases. Called also *ethanol.* **fatty a.,** any hydroxide of a hydrocarbon derived from the paraffin series. **hexahydric a.,** sorbitol. **isopropyl a.,** an alcohol, $CH_3CH(OH)CH_3$, occurring as a colorless liquid with a slight odor resembling that of a mixture of ethyl alcohol and acetone. It is miscible with water, ethyl alcohol, ether, and other solvents, and is used in antifreeze, as a solvent, in the production of cosmetics, as a denaturing agent for ethyl alcohol, and in various chemical and industrial processes. Pharmaceutically, it is used as a rubefacient and antiseptic, being more germicidal than ethyl alcohol. In dentistry, it serves as a substitute for ethyl alcohol. When used for cleansing the skin for surgery or injection, it tends to cause the wound to bleed more profusely than ethyl alcohol, because of its vasodilator properties. Ingestion or inhalation of its vapors may causing flushing, headache, vertigo, depression, nausea, vomiting, anesthesia, and coma; 100 ml may be fatal. Called also *secondary propyl a., dimethyl carbinol, isopropanol,* and *2-propanol.* **isopropyl rubbing a.,** a preparation containing between 68 to 72 percent isopropyl alcohol in water; used as a rubefacient. Formerly called *isopropyl alcohol rubbing compound.* **methyl a.,** a flammable, clear, colorless liquid with a characteristic odor, CH_3OH; miscible with water, alcohol, and ether, used as an industrial solvent. It is highly toxic and ingestion, inhalation, or percutaneous absorption may cause blindness, convulsions, acidosis, respiratory failure, and death. Called also *wood a.* and *methanol.* **monohydric a.,** one containing a single hydroxyl group. **phenylic a.,** PHENOL (1). **polyhydric a.,** one containing more than two hydroxyl groups. Called also *polyalcohol* and *polyol.* **propyl a., secondary,** isopropyl a. **n-propyl a.,** an alcohol, $CH_3CH_2CH_2OH$, occurring as a clear, colorless liquid with an odor similar to that of ethyl alcohol, which is miscible with water and most organic solvents. Used as a solvent for ethyl alcohol, waxes, vegetable oils, resins, cellulose, and various other organic substances. It is a highly flammable substance presenting a fire risk, which may be irritating to the eyes and mucous membranes and cause depression, lack of coordination, and other symptoms of ethyl alcohol intoxication. Called also *propylic a.* and *1-propanol.* **propylic a.,** *n*-proply a. **rubbing a.,** a rubefacient preparation containing acetone, methyl isobutyl ketone, and ethyl alcohol. **salicyl a.,** a compound,

o-hydroxybenzyl alcohol, occurring as a crystalline powder that is very soluble in ethyl alcohol, chloroform, and ether and readily soluble in water and benzene. Used as a local anesthetic in infiltration and topical anesthesia of the mucous membranes. Trademarks: Salicain, Saligenin, Saligenol. **secondary propyl a.,** isopropyl a. **trihydric a.,** alcohol containing three hydroxyl groups in its structure, such as glycerol. **wood a.,** methyl a.

alcoholic (al″ko-hol′ik) [L. *alcoholicus*] 1. pertaining to or containing alcohol. 2. a person suffering from alcoholism.

alcoholism (al′ko-hol-izm″) alcohol addiction disorder manifested by repeated excessive drinking of alcoholic beverages to an extent that it interferes with the drinker's health and his social and economic functioning. Alcoholics exhibit a high tolerance to anesthetics and sedatives. Called also *dipsomania.* See also fetal alcohol SYNDROME.

Alcophobin trademark for *disulfiram.*

Alcopon trademark for *caramiphen ethanedisulfonate* (see under CARAMIPHEN).

Aldactone A trademark for *spironolactone.*

Aldanil trademark for *sodium formaldehyde sulfoxylate* (see under SODIUM).

aldehyde (al′de-hīd) [*alcohol* + L. *de* away from + *hydrogen*] any

$$H$$
$$|$$

of a group of compounds having the functional group —C—O, which holds an intermediate position between the alcohols and the acids, a typical aldehyde being acetaldehyde. The names of aldehydes usually end in *-al.* **acetic a.,** acetaldehyde. **acrylic a.,** acrolein. **formic a.,** formaldehyde. **glyceric a.,** glyceraldehyde. **methyl a.,** formaldehyde. **a. reductase,** alcohol DEHYDROGENASE.

Alder's anomaly [Albert *Alder*] see under ANOMALY.

Alder-Reilly anomaly [A. *Alder;* William Anthony *Reilly*] Alder's ANOMALY.

Alderin trademark for *pronethalol.*

aldesulfone sodium (al′de-sul′fōn) SULFOXONE sodium.

Aldinamide trademark for *pyrazinamide.*

Aldo 33 trademark for a synthetic *dental wax* (see under WAX).

aldolase (al′do-lās) aldehyde LYASE.

Aldomet trademark for *methyldopa.*

Aldometil trademark for *methyldopa.*

Aldomycin trademark for *nitrofurazone.*

aldose (al′dōs) a carbohydrate containing an aldehyde group. Called also *aldehyde-containing sugar* and *aldose sugar.*

aldoside (al′do-sīd) a glycoside that on hydrolysis yields an aldose.

aldosterone (al″do-ster′ōn) a mineralocorticoid, 11β,21-dihydroxy-3,20-dioxypregn-4-en-18-al(11-18)-lactol. Its secretion is influenced slightly by adrenocorticotropic hormone and, to a larger degree, by angiotensin and reduction of intravascular volume after sodium restriction. It is the most potent mineralocorticoid and its main role is to maintain the water-electrolyte balance, chiefly through the mechanism of renal tubular reabsorption of sodium and the distribution of sodium, potassium, water, and hydrogen ions between the cellular and extracellular fluids. Used therapeutically in disorders of water-electrolyte metabolism. **a. inhibitor,** any substance that inhibits the action of aldosterone; see aldosterone inhibitor DIURETIC. **a. inhibitor diuretic,** aldosterone inhibitor DIURETIC.

Aldrich, Martha [American biochemist, born 1897] see Hench-Aldrich TEST.

Aldrich's syndrome [Robert A. *Aldrich*] see Wiskott-Aldrich SYNDROME.

Aleco trademark for a medium hard *dental casting gold alloy* (see under GOLD).

Aleco No. 4 trademark for a hard *dental casting gold alloy* (see under GOLD) for bridges.

Aleco No. 5 trademark for hard *dental casting gold alloy* (see under GOLD).

Aleco No. 9 trademark for an extra hard *dental casting dental gold alloy* (see under GOLD).

alembroth (ah-lem′broth) ammoniated MERCURY.

Alergicide trademark for *chlorcyclizine.*

-ales [L., fem. pl. word ending] a word termination denoting an order in microbiological taxonomy.

Aleudrin trademark for *isoproterenol.*

aleukemic (ah″lu-ke′mik) 1. marked by or pertaining to aleukemic leukemia. 2. not marked by leukemia.

aleukia (ah-lu′ke-ah) [*a* neg. + Gr. *leukos* white + *-ia*] absence of leukocytes from the blood; leukopenia. **a. hemorrha′gica,** aplastic ANEMIA.

aleukocytic (ah-lu″ko-sit′ik) showing no leukocytes.

aleukocytosis (ah-lu″ko-si-to′sis) [*a* neg. + *leukocyte* + *-osis*] deficiency in the leukocyte content of the blood; leukopenia.

aleuriospore (ah-lu′re-o-spōr) a terminal or lateral, asexual fungal spore similar to a conidium except that it is not shed (not deciduous), being released only by dissolution of its attachment to the mycelium.

Alexander attachment see under ATTACHMENT.

alexin (ah-lek′sin) [Gr. *alexein* to ward off] an early term for *complement; cytase.*

Alfacillin trademark for *phenethicillin.*

Alficetyn trademark for *chloramphenicol.*

Alflorone trademark for *fludrocortisone.*

ALG axiolinguogingival.

alga (al′gah) any individual organism of the algae.

algae (al′je) [L., pl., "seaweeds"] a group of cryptogamous plants, in which the body is unicellular or consists of a thallus; it includes the seaweeds and many unicellular fresh-water plants, most of which contain chlorophyll. Algae account for about 90 percent of the earth's photosynthetic activity. **blue-green a.,** a group of prokaryotic cells comprising the Cyanobacteria (kingdom Procaryotae), occurring singly or as chains of cells forming filaments, most of which are motile. They are enclosed by rigid, multilayered walls with inner peptidoglycan layers, and with gelatinous or fibrous sheaths surrounding the walls. Paired photosynthetic lamellae traverse the cytoplasmic region, and granules of aggregates of phycobiliprotein pigments are located on the surfaces of the cells. The organisms resemble bacteria in many respects, but differ primarily in that they are phototropic, using water as an electron donor and producing oxygen by photosynthesis. They contain the photopigments chlorophyll *a* and phycobiliproteins. Reproduction is by binary or multiple fission or by the serial release of exospores from sessile individuals. Filamentous forms reproduce by repeated intercalary cell division and by random fragmentation of the filament or by terminal release of short motile chains of cells.

Algafan trademark for *propoxyphene hydrochloride* (see under PROPOXYPHENE).

Algamon trademark for *salicylamide.*

alganesthesia (al-gan″es-the′ze-ah) [Gr. *algos* pain + *anesthesia*] absence of sense of pain; analgesia.

algesi-, alge-, algo- [Gr. *algos* pain] a combining form denoting relationship to pain.

algesia (al-je′ze-ah) sensitivity to pain; hyperesthesia.

algesic (al-je′zik) painful.

algesichronometer (al-je″ze-kro-nom′ĕ-ter) [*algesi-* + Gr. *chronos* time + *metron* measure] an instrument for recording the time required to produce a painful impression.

algesimeter (al″je-sim′ĕ-ter) [*algesi-* + Gr. *metron* measure] an instrument used in measuring the sensitiveness to pain as produced by pricking with a sharp point.

algesimetry (al″jĕ-sim′ĕ-tre) the measurement of sensitiveness to pain.

algesiogenic (al-je″ze-o-jen′ik) [*algesi-* + Gr. *gennan* to produce] producing pain.

algesthesia (al″jes-the′ze-ah) pain sensibility; algesthesis.

algesthesis (al″jes-the′sis) [*algesi-* + Gr. *aisthēsis* perception] the perception of pain; any painful sensation.

-algia [Gr. *algos* pain + *-ia* condition] a word termination indicating a painful condition.

Algiamida trademark for *salicylamide.*

Algident trademark for a fast setting *irreversible hydrocolloid impression material* (see under MATERIAL).

Algidon trademark for the *dl*-form of *methadone hydrochloride* (see under METHADONE).

Algil trademark for *meperidine hydrochloride* (see under MEPERIDINE).

algin (al′jin) alginic ACID.

alginate (al′ji-nāt) a salt of alginic acid, which is extracted from seaweeds. Calcium, sodium, and ammonium alginates have been used as foam, clot, or gauze for absorbable surgical dressings. Soluble alginates are generally linear polymers of the sodium or potassium salt of anhydro-*β*-*d*-mannuronic acid and, when mixed with water, form a sol. The greater the molecular weight of the alginate, the greater the viscosity of the sol. When mixed with a reactor such as gypsum, the sol solidifies irreversibly into a gel which is used as a dental impression material. **Coa a.,** trademark for an *irreversible hydrocolloid impression material* (see under MATERIAL). **Hydro-Jel a.,** trademark for a fast setting *irreversible hydrocolloid impression material* (see under MATERIAL). **a. impression material,** impression material, irreversible hydrocolloid; see under MATERIAL.

algiomotor (al″ji-o-mo′tor) producing painful movements, such as spasm.

algiomuscular (al″ji-o-mus′ku-lar) pertaining to muscular action resulting from painful stimulation.

algiovascular (al″ji-o-vas′ku-lar) pertaining to vascular action resulting from painful stimulation.

algo- see ALGESI-.

Algolysin trademark for the *dl*-form of *methadone hydrochloride* (see under METHADONE).

algometer (al-gom′ĕ-ter) [*algo-* + Gr. *metron* measure] an instrument for testing sensitivity to painful stimuli. **pressure a.,** an instrument for measuring sensitivity to pressure.

algometry (al-gom′ĕ-tre) the measurement of sensitivity to painful stimuli, as with an algometer.

algor (al′gor) [L.] a chill or rigor; coldness. **a. mor′tis** ["chill of death"], the gradual decrease of temperature of the body after death.

Ali Abbas [10th century A.D.] a celebrated Persian physician who wrote *Al-Maliki* (the "Royal Book"), a comprehensive treatise on medicine.

Alibert's disease [Louis *Alibert,* French dermatologist, 1768–1837] cutaneous LEISHMANIASIS.

alicyclic (al″ĭ-sik′lik) having the properties of both aliphatic and cyclic substances.

Alidine trademark for *anileridine.*

ali-esterase (al′ĭ-es′ter-ās) carboxylesterase.

alignment (ah-līn′ment) [Fr. *aligner* to put in a straight line] 1. the act of arranging in a line; the state of being arranged in a line. 2. bringing the natural or artificial teeth in a line, so that they may form two regular parabolic curves of the dental arches and reestablish a harmonious relationship with the supporting structures and with the opposite dentition. Spelled also *alinement.*

aliment (al′ĭ-ment) [L. *alimentum*] food.

alimentary (al″ĭ-men′tar-e) pertaining to food or nutritive material, or to the organs of digestion.

alimentation (al″ĭ-men-ta′shun) the act of giving or receiving nutriment. **artificial a.,** the giving of food or nourishment to persons who cannot take it in the usual way. Called also *artificial feeding.* See also parenteral FEEDING. **forced a.,** 1. the feeding of a person against his will. Called also *forced feeding.* 2. the giving of more food to a person than his appetite calls for. **parenteral a.,** parenteral FEEDING.

alimentology (al″ĭ-men-tol′o-je) the science of nutrition.

alinasal (al″ĭ-na′sal) pertaining to the ala nasi.

alinement (ah-līn′ment) alignment.

aliphatic (al″ĭ-fat′ik) [Gr. *aleiphar* oil] pertaining to organic compounds whose molecules have carbon atoms arranged in straight chains, rather than in a ring. See aliphatic COMPOUND.

alisphenoid (al-ĭ-sfe′noid) [*ala* + *sphenoid*] 1. pertaining to the great wing of the sphenoid bone. 2. a part of the postsphenoid on either side of the basisphenoid, which forms the greater part of the great wing of the sphenoid bone. Called also *alisphenoidal bone.*

alkalemia (al″kah-le′me-ah) [*alkali* + Gr. *haima* blood + *-ia*] increased pH of the blood, irrespective of changes in the blood bicarbonate.

alkalescence (ak″kah-les′ens) slight or incipient alkalinity.

alkali (al′kah-li) [Arabic *al-galīy* potash] any of a class of compounds which form soluble soaps with fatty acids, turn red litmus blue, and form soluble carbonates. Essentially, the hydroxides of cesium, lithium, potassium, rubidium, and sodium; they include also the carbonates of these metals and of ammonia. **volatile a.,** ammonia.

Alkaligenes (al″kah-lij′ĕ-nēz) *Alcaligenes.*

alkalimetry (al″kah-lim′ĕ-tre) the measurement of the alkalies present in any substance. **Engel's a.,** a method of determining the alkalinity of the blood by titrating a diluted specimen with normal tartaric acid solution until it reddens litmus paper. The amount of tartaric solution necessary to produce the result indicates the alkalinity of the blood.

alkaline (al′kah-līn) [L. *alkalinus*] having the reaction of an alkali; relating to alkali.

alkaloid (al′kah-loid″) [*alkali* + Gr. *eidos* form] one of a large group of basic nitrogenous organic compounds found in plants, usually having strong physiological or toxic effects on the animal body. They are usually derivatives of the nitrogen ring compounds, presenting colorless crystals that are bitter in taste, soluble in alcohol, and slightly soluble in water. Their names end in *-ine.* Examples are: atropine, caffeine, coniine, morphine, nicotine, quinine, and strychnine. **antineoplastic a.,** one that prevents or inhibits the growth of neoplasms, such as vinblastine and vincristine.

alkalosis (al″kah-lo′sis) a pathologic condition resulting from accumulation of base in, or loss of acid from, the body; it is characterized by a decrease in hydrogen ion concentration (increase in pH). Cf. ACIDOSIS. **compensated a.,** a condition in which compensatory mechanisms have returned the pH toward normal, while the blood bicarbonate is higher than normal. **metabolic a.,** a disturbance in which the acid-base status of the body shifts toward the alkaline side because of retention of base or loss of noncarbonic or fixed (nonvolatile) acids. **metabolic compensated a.,** a form in which the pH of the blood has been returned toward normal by retention of carbonic acid through pulmonary mechanisms. **respiratory a.,** that in which hyperventilation causes loss of carbonic acid. **respiratory compensated a.,** respiratory alkalosis in which the pH of the blood has been returned toward normal through retention of acid or excretion of base by renal mechanisms. **a. syndrome,** milk alkali SYNDROME.

alkane (al′kān) a group of straight-chain aliphatic hydrocarbons, whose names end in -ane, e.g., ethane. See also CYCLOALKANE and PARAFFIN (1).

Alkathene trademark for *polyethylene*.

alkene (al′kēn) a group of aliphatic unsaturated hydrocarbons, having the functional group C=C. The names of alkenes end in -ene, e.g., ethene. See also OLEFIN.

Alkeran trademark for *melphalan*.

Alkiron trademark for *methylthiouracil*.

alkyl (al′kil) a paraffin hydrocarbon radical which results when an aliphatic hydrocarbon loses one hydrogen atom.

alkylamine (al′kil-ah′mēn) an amine-containing alkyl group attached to aminonitrogen.

alkylation (al″kĭ-la′shun) the substitution of an alkyl group for an active hydrogen atom in an organic compound. See also alkylating AGENT.

alkyne (al′kīn) a group of hydrocarbons having the functional group C≡C, whose names end in -yne, e.g., ethyne (acetylene).

allachesthesia (al″ah-kes-the′ze-ah) [Gr. *allachē* elsewhere + *aisthēsis* perception + -ia] the sensation of touch experienced at a point remote from the point touched.

allantoic (al″an-to′ik) pertaining to the allantois.

allantoin (ah-lan′to-in) a crystallizable substance, 5-ureodohydantoin, found in the allantoic fluid, fetal urine, and plants, which is a product of purine metabolism in most mammals, except man and higher apes. Synthetic allantoin is produced by the oxidation of uric acid with alkaline potassium permanganate, and is used in the treatment of suppurating wounds, ulcers, and osteomyelitis. In dentistry, it is used in some medicated denture adhesives.

allantois (ah-lan′to-is) [Gr. *allantos* sausage + *eidos* form] a fetal membrane, being a primitive bladder which initiates as a tubular ventral diverticulum of the hindgut of embryos of reptiles, birds, and mammals. In eggs of reptiles and birds, it expands to a large sac for storing urine and, after fusing with the chorion lining the shell, provides for gas exchange. It is prominent in some mammals; in others, including man, it is vestigial except that its blood vessels give rise to those of the umbilical cord. See illustration at fetal membranes, under MEMBRANE.

Allbee with C trademark for a mixture of vitamins, one capsule of which contains 15 mg thiamine mononitrate, 10 mg riboflavin, 5 mg pyridoxine hydrochloride, 10 mg niacinamide, 10 mg calcium pantothenate, and 300 mg ascorbic acid.

Allbee-T trademark for a mixture of vitamins, each film-coated tablets containing 500 mg sodium ascorbate, 100 mg niacinamide, 25 mg calcium pantothenate, 10 mg pyridoxine hydrochloride, 10 mg riboflavin, 15 mg thiamine mononitrate, 5 mcg cyanocobalamin, and 150 mg desiccated liver.

Alledryl trademark for *diphenhydramine*.

allele (ah-lēl′) [Gr. *allēlōn* of one another] one of two or more genes situated at the same locus on homologous chromosomes, which determine the character of inheritance. Alleles segregate at meiosis, and an individual normally receives only one of each pair of alleles from each parent. The presence of an identical pair of alleles at a given locus or loci determines the homozygous state; two different alleles cause the heterozygous state. Called also *allelomorph* and *allelomorphic gene*. See also ISOALLELE. **autosomal dominant a.,** autosomal dominant CHARACTER. **autosomal recessive a.,** autosomal recessive CHARACTER. **codominant a.,** codominant CHARACTER. **dominant a.,** 1. autosomal dominant CHARACTER. 2. X-linked dominant CHARACTER. **multiple a's,** a group of more than two alleles at a single locus on homologous chromosomes, as those which determine the ABO blood groups. **recessive a.,** 1. autosomal recessive CHARACTER. 2. X-linked recessive CHARACTER. **sex-linked a.,**

sex-linked CHARACTER. **X-linked dominant a.,** X-linked dominant CHARACTER. **X-linked recessive a.,** X-linked recessive CHARACTER.

allelic (ah-le′lik) pertaining to alleles; produced by alternative genes.

allelo- [Gr. *allēlōn* of one another] a combining form denoting relationship to another.

allelomorph (ah-le′lo-morf) [*allelo-* + Gr. *morphē* form] allele.

Allemann's syndrome [Richard *Allemann*, Swiss physician, 1893–1958] see under SYNDROME.

Allen, Charles [17th century] a British surgeon whose book, *Curious Observations in that Difficult Part of Chirurgery Relating to the Teeth*, published in 1685, was the first dental book in the English language.

Allen, John [19th century] an American dentist who, in 1851, patented the continous-gum technique (see under TECHNIQUE).

Allen's root pliers [Albert Bromely *Allen*, American dentist, 1862–1943] see under PLIERS.

Allerclor trademark for *chlorpheniramine maleate* (see under CHLORPHENIRAMINE).

Allecur trademark for *climizole*.

Allergen trademark for *diphenylpyraline*.

allergen (al′er-jen) [*allergy* + Gr. *gennan* to produce] 1. any substance, frequently a protein, capable of inducing allergy or specific susceptibility. 2. extracts of certain foods, bacteria, or pollens used in the treatment of or testing for hypersensitivity to specific substances. Called also *allergic antigen*.

allergenic (al″er-jen′ik) acting as an allergen; inducing allergy.

allergic (ah-ler′jik) relating to allergy.

Allergin trademark for *diphenhydramine*.

Allergisan trademark for *chlorpheniramine maleate* (see under CHLORPHENIRAMINE).

allergoid (al′er-goid) an allergenic substance chemically altered so that its ability to trigger an allergic response is reduced or eliminated but which can still induce blocking antibody to the allergen and thus reduce allergic reactivity.

allergology (al″ler-gol′o-je) the science dealing with the problems of allergy and hypersensitivity.

allergy (al′er-je) [Gr. *allos* other + *ergon* work] a pathological condition resulting from the exaggerated reactivity of the body to exposure to a specific foreign substance having allergenic properties, involving the antigen-antibody reaction — the antibody having been produced by the host during an earlier exposure to the substance, and the antigen representing the foreign substance. Anaphylaxis, hay fever, asthma, Quincke's edema, stomatitis medicamentosa, and stomatitis venenata are specific forms of allergy. See also HYPERSENSITIVITY. **bacterial a.,** allergy to a specific bacterial antigen, preconditioned during an earlier contact with the same bacterial agent. **endocrine a.,** allergy to an endogenous hormone. **bronchial a.,** bronchial ASTHMA. **contact a.,** an allergic condition of the skin or mucous membranes resulting from contact with substances to which the patient is sensitive. See contact DERMATITIS and STOMATITIS venenata. **delayed a.,** an allergic response which appears hours or days after exposure to an allergen. **drug a.,** drug REACTION. **food a.,** hypersensitivity following ingestion of food containing allergens to which the patient is sensitized. Symptoms may include angioedema, vascular engorgement, urticaria, eczema, ecchymoses, erosions, excessive mucous secretion, spasmodic muscular contractions, abdominal pain, vomiting, diarrhea, mucoid stools, wheezing, and, in severe cases, hematemesis, melena, purpura, arthralgia, and anaphylactic shock. Oral manifestations that may occur include swelling of the lips, edema of the glottis and oral mucosa, perioral dermatitis, recurrent vesicles, erosion, ulcers, itching, and burning. See also *gastrointestinal a.* **gastrointestinal a.,** clinical phenomena resulting from antigen-antibody reactions in the intestinal wall, including disease entities that are not associated with ingestion of food. Symptoms may be similar to those in food allergy. Cf. food INTOLERANCE. **hereditary a.,** atopy. **immediate a.,** an allergic response which appears within a short time, i.e., from a few minutes up to an hour after exposure to an allergen. **spontaneous a.,** atopy.

alleviation (ah-le″ve-a′shun) the act or process of lessening, diminishing, or making more bearable, as the severity of suffering or pain.

Allis' inhaler [Oscar H. *Allis*, Philadelphia surgeon, 1833–1921] see under INHALER.

Allison retractor (forceps) see under RETRACTOR.

allo- [Gr. *allos* other] a combining form denoting a condition differing from the normal, or reversal, or referring to another.

alloantibody (al″o-an′tĭ-bod″e) isoantibody.

alloantigen (al″o-an′tĭ-jen) allogeneic ANTIGEN.

allochiria (al″o-ki′re-ah) [*allo-* + Gr. *cheir* hand + -ia] a condition in which if one extremity is stimulated, the sensation is referred to the opposite side.

Allocor trademark for *lanatoside C.*

allocortex (al″o-kor′teks) [*allo-* + *cortex*] the nonlaminated portion of the cerebral cortex, which represents the more primitive areas, such as the olfactory cortex.

allocytophilic (al″o-si″to-fil′ik) [*allo-* + Gr. *kytos* hollow vessel + *philein* to love] having an affinity for cells derived from the same species.

allodiploidy (al″o-dip′loid-de) the state of having two sets of chromosomes derived from different parental species.

allogeneic (al″o-jĕ-ne′ik) [*allo-* + Gr. *genos* kind] 1. having cell types that are antigenically distinct. 2. in transplantation, denoting individuals (or tissues) that are of the same species but antigenically distinct. Called also *homologous*. NOTE: In contrast, *syngeneic* (or *isogeneic*) refers to individuals having identical genotypes, and *xenogeneic* to individuals of different species, which by definition have different genotypes. Called also *allogenic.*

allogenic (al″o-jen′ik) allogeneic.

allograft (al′o-graft) allogenic GRAFT.

alloisomerism (al″o-i-som′er-izm) isomerism which does not appear in the formula.

allokinesis (al″o-ki-ne′sis) movement that is not performed voluntarily but is produced passively or occurs reflexly.

allolalia (al″o-la′le-ah) [*allo-* + Gr. *lalein* to speak + *-ia*] any defect of speech of central origin.

allomerism (ah-lom′er-izm) [*allo-* + Gr. *meros* part] change of chemical constitution without change in the crystalline form.

allometron (al″o-met′ron) [*allo-* + Gr. *metron* measure] an evolutionary change in bodily form or proportion as expressed in measurements and indices.

allometry (al-lom′ĕ-tre) the measurement of the changing shape of an organism with increase in size, i.e., the determination of the relationship of two varying dimensions, usually linear.

allomorphism (al″o-mor′fizm) [*allo-* + Gr. *morphē* form] change of the crystalline form without change in the chemical constitution.

alloplast (al′o-plast) [*allo-* + Gr. *plassein* to mold or shape] an inert material used for tissue implants.

alloplasty (al′o-plas″te) [*allo-* + Gr. *plassein* to mold or shape] an old term for plastic surgery in which use is made of material not from the human body.

alloploid (al′o-ploid) [*allo-* + *-ploid*] 1. having any number (two or more) of chromosome sets derived from different ancestral species. 2. an individual or cell having any number (two or more) of chromosome sets derived from different ancestral species.

alloploidy (al″o-ploi′de) the state of having any number (two or more) of chromosome sets derived from different ancestral species. See also ALLODIPLOIDY and ALLOPOLYPLOIDY.

allopolyploidy (al″lo-pol′e-ploi-de) the state of having more than two chromosome sets derived from different ancestral species.

allopurinol (al″o-pu′rin-ol) a compound, 1*H*-pyrazolol[3,4-*d*]-pyrimidin-4-ol, occurring as a white to off-white, tasteless powder that is soluble in alkali hydroxide solutions, slightly soluble in water and ethanol, and insoluble in chloroform and ether. It is hypoxanthine analog and a xanthine oxidase inhibitor that interferes with blood uric acid levels by blocking the reactions preceding uric acid formation. Used in the treatment of gout and uric acid nephropathy and in the prevention of uric acid calculi formation in patients under chemotherapy for cancer. It also relieves pain, owing to its inhibition of uric acid levels in the blood. Rash, fever, leukopenia, arthralgia, and hypersensitivity are the most common side reactions. Diarrhea, peripheral neuritis, bone marrow depression, cataract, and liver damage may occur. Trademarks: Epidropal, Foligan, Uricemil, Zyloprim.

allorhythmia (al″o-rith′me-ah) [*allo-* + Gr. *rhythmos* rhythm + *-ia*] irregularity in the rhythm of the heart beat or pulse that recurs in a regular fashion.

all or none (awl or nun) see all or none LAW.

allorphine (al′lor-fēn) nalorphine.

allotoxin (al′o-tok′sin) [*allo-* + *toxin*] any substance produced within the body which serves in its defense against toxins by neutralizing their toxic properties.

allotransplantation (al″o-trans″plan-ta′shun) [*allo-* + *transplantation*] transplantation of tissue from one individual into the body of another.

allotrio- [Gr. *allotrios* strange] a combining form denoting strange or foreign.

allotriodontia (ah-lot″re-o-don′she-ah) [*allotrio-* + Gr. *odous* tooth + *-ia*] 1. transplantation of teeth from one individual into the mouth of another. 2. presence of teeth in unusual places, such as in a dermoid tumor.

allotriogeustia (ah-lot″re-o-gu′ste-ah) [*allotrio-* + Gr. *geusis* taste + *-ia*] a perverted sense of taste.

allotriolith (al″o-tri″o-lith) [*allotrio-* + Gr. *lithos* stone] a calculus in an abnormal situation, or one composed of unusual materials.

allotrope (al′o-trōp) an allotropic form; see ALLOTROPISM (1).

allotrophic (al″o-trōf′ik) [*allo-* + Gr. *trophikos* nourishing] having an altered or perverted nutrient value.

allotropic (al″o-trōp′ik) [*allo-* + Gr. *tropikos* turning] exhibiting allotropism.

allotropism (ah-lot′ro-pizm) [*allo-* + Gr. *tropos* a turning] 1. the appearance of an element in two or more distinct forms (allotropic form), each exhibiting different physical properties, e.g., carbon appearing as coal. 2. a tropism between different structures, e.g., between spermatozoa and ova.

allotype (al′o-tīp) any of the alternative characters controlled by allelic genes. Inv a., Km ANTIGEN.

allotypy (al′o-ti′pe) [*allo-* + Gr. *typos* type] the genetically controlled property, in proteins, of existing in antigenically distinguishable forms in different members of the same species, i.e., as serum protein isoantigens; the condition of being an allotype.

allowance (ah-low′ans) a share or amount allotted or granted. In health insurance, a schedule of allowances lists covered hospital, medical, or dental services and assigns to each service a sum that represents the total obligation of the plan with respect to payment for such service, which does not necessarily represent the full fee for that service, the patient being required to pay the difference between the allowance and the actual fee. The schedule of allowances is also known as *table of a's, fee schedule,* and *indemnification schedule.* See also allowable costs, under COST. **charity a.,** the difference between gross-revenue charges at established rates and amounts to be received from an indigent patient or from a voluntary agency or the government on behalf of an indigent patient. **contractual a.,** the difference between billings at established charges and amounts received or due from third-party payers under contract agreement. **courtesy a.,** the difference between billings at established charges and amounts received from persons having special privileges, such as physicians or dentists or employees and their dependents. Called also *courtesy discount, professional courtesy,* and *professional discount.* **indemnity a.,** in insurance, the amount to be paid by the plan. See *allowance.* **maximum a.,** the maximum dollar amount a health insurance plan will pay toward the cost of a service. **a. schedule, schedule of a's,** see *allowance.* **table of a's,** see *allowance.*

alloxazine (ah-lok′sah-zēn) a heterocyclic compound obtained by condensation of aloxan and *o*-phenylenediamines, the isomer of which, isoalloxazine, is the nucleus of riboflavin, which is the cofactor in flavoproteins.

alloy (ah-loi′) [Fr. *aloyer* to mix metals] a solid mixture of metallic elements or compounds with other metallic or nonmetallic (metalloid) elements in various proportions, which are mutually soluble in the molten condition. Alloys are considered as solid solutions in which the foreign solute atoms are added to the pure metal and displace its atoms in the lattice (see also point DEFECT). When cooled to the solid state, the molten alloy may be transformed to one or more phases depending on temperature, pressure, cooling rate, or composition. Physical properties of an alloy may differ from those of component metals, as when the strength of a single-phase alloy is greater than that of a pure metal. An alloy containing mercury as one of its components is known as *amalgam.* See tables. **a. A,** a cobalt-chrome alloy. **a. aging,** age HARDENING. **amalgam a.,** AMALGAM alloy. **austenitic a.,** an iron-base alloy in the stainless steel group, containing nickel and chromium. **a. B,** a cobalt-chrome alloy. **Balanced a.,** trademark for an *amalgam alloy* (see under AMALGAM). **base metal crown and bridge a's,** platinum-colored, lightweight alloys, usually nickel-chromium, silver-tin, or tin-antimony systems, used in fixed prosthodontics, particularly with fused porcelain veneers. **Bean's a.,** an alloy of tin and silver. **binary a.,** one in which two elements are present. **a. C,** a cobalt-chrome alloy. **Caulk spherical a.,** trademark for an *amalgam alloy* (see under AMALGAM). **chromium base casting a.,** any alloy containing chromium; usually a cobalt-chrome alloy in which cobalt is totally or partially replaced by nickel. Used for casting dental appliances, such as denture bases, partial denture structures, and, occasionally, certain types of bridgework. **chromium-cobalt a.,** cobalt chrome a. **chromium-cobalt-nickel base a.,** a cobalt-chrome alloy, containing a minimum of 85 percent by weight of chromium, cobalt, and nickel; used for casting dental

PHYSICAL CONSTANTS OF THE ALLOY-FORMING ELEMENTS

Element	Symbol	Atomic Weight	Melting Point (°C.)	Boiling Point (°C.)	Density (gm/cc)	Linear Coefficient of Thermal Expansion (Per °C. $\times 10^{-4}$)
Aluminum	Al	26.98	660.2	2450	2.70	0.236
Antimony	Sb	121.75	630.5	1380	6.62	0.108
Bismuth	Bi	208.98	271.3	1560	9.80	0.133
Cadmium	Cd	112.40	320.9	765	8.37	0.298
Carbon	C	12.01	3700.0	4830	2.22	0.06
Chromium	Cr	52.00	1875.0	2665	7.19	0.062
Cobalt	Co	58.93	1495.0	2900	8.85	0.138
Copper	Cu	63.54	1083.0	2595	8.96	0.165
Gold	Au	196.97	1063.0	2970	19.32	0.142
Indium	In	114.82	156.2	2000	7.31	0.33
Iridium	Ir	192.2	2454.0	5300	22.5	0.068
Iron	Fe	55.85	1527.0	3000	7.87	0.123
Lead	Pb	207.19	327.4	1725	11.34	0.293
Magnesium	Mg	24.31	650.0	1107	1.74	0.252
Mercury	Hg	200.59	−38.87	357	13.55	0.40
Molybdenum	Mo	95.94	2610.0	5560	10.22	0.049
Nickel	Ni	58.71	1453.0	2730	8.90	0.133
Palladium	Pd	106.4	1552.0	3980	12.02	0.118
Platinum	Pt	195.09	1769.0	4530	21.45	0.089
Rhodium	Rh	102.91	1966.0	4500	12.44	0.083
Silicon	Si	28.09	1410.0	2480	2.33	0.073
Silver	Ag	107.87	960.8	2216	10.49	0.197
Tantalum	Ta	180.95	2996.0	5425	16.6	0.065
Tin	Sn	118.69	231.9	2270	7.298	0.23
Titanium	Ti	47.90	1668.0	3260	4.51	0.085
Tungsten	W	183.85	3410.0	5930	19.3	0.046
Zinc	Zn	65.37	420.0	906	7.133	0.397

(From R. W. Phillips: Skinner's Science of Dental Materials. 7th ed. Philadelphia, W. B. Saunders Co., 1973; compiled from T. Lyman: Metals Handbook. 8th ed., Vol. 1. Cleveland, American Society for Metals, 1961.)

COMPOSITION OF COBALT-CHROME ALLOYS

Alloy No.	Chromium	Cobalt	Nickel	Molybdenum	Tungsten	Manganese	Silicon	Iron	Carbon	Aluminum	Boron	Gallium	Copper	Beryllium	Niobium	Titanium
A	21.6	43.5	20.1	7	—	3.0	0.35	0.25	0.05	—	—	—	3.5	0.9	—	—
B	30	62.5	—	5	—	0.5	0.5	1.0	0.5	—	—	—	—	—	—	—
C	13	—	68	4.5	—	?	2.5	?		6	—	—	—	—	2	1
D	30	64	—	5	—	—	0.35	—	0.35	—	—	0.05	0.04	—	—	—
E	26.1	52	14.2	4.0	—	0.7	0.58	1.2	0.22	—	—	—	—	—	—	—
F	17	—	66	5	—	5	0.5	0.5	0.1	5	—	—	—	—	—	—
G	20	—	73.5	—	—	0.5	3.5	1	1	—	0.5	—	—	—	—	—
HS21	27	62.6	2	6	—	0.6	0.6	1.0	0.2	—	—	—	—	—	—	—
HS31	23	57.6	10	—	7	0.6	0.6	1.0	0.4	—	—	—	—	—	—	—

*Values under each element are percentages.

A from Taylor, Liebfritz and Adler, J. Amer. Dent. Ass., Mar., 1958.
B from Asgar and Allan, J. Dent. Res., March–April, 1968.
C from *Metals Handbook*, Vol. 1, 8th ed., 1961.
D and E from Asgar, Techow and Jacobson, J. Prosth. Dent., Jan., 1970.
F from Asgar. An overall study of partial dentures. USPHS Research Grant DE-02017. National Institutes of Health. Bethesda, Md., Sept., 1968.
G from Harcourt, Riddibough and Osborne. Brit. Dent. J., Nov., 1970.
HS21, HS31 from *Metals Handbook*, 1948.

(From R. W. Phillips: Skinner's Science of Dental Materials. 7th ed. Philadelphia, W. B. Saunders Co., 1973.)

appliances, such as denture bases, partial denture structures, and, occasionaly, certain types of bridgework. **chromium-iron a.**, see stainless STEEL. **cobalt-chrome a.**, a corrosion-resistant and relatively light alloy, being essentially a solid solution of 70 percent cobalt and 30 percent chromium. Molybdenum, tungsten, silicon, and small amounts of iron, copper, beryllium, and other elements may be added as hardeners. Cobalt may be replaced totally or partially with nickel (Haynes stellite). Boron acts as a deoxidizer and hardener, but also reduces ductility and increases hardness. Some cobalt-chrome alloys (such as Vitallium) are used in the production of orthodontic wires, denture clasps, dental implants, dental castings, surgical staples, orbital implants, nasal skeletal supports, tendon rods, tubes for blood vessel anastomosis, skull plates, fracture plates, screws, bolts, and nails. Called also *chromium-cobalt a., stellite a.,* and *stellite.* Available under numerous trademarks. See table. **cobalt-chromium-nickel a.**, alloy consisting of about 40 percent cobalt, 20 percent chromium, 15 percent nickel, 7 percent molybdenum, 2 percent manganese, 0.15 percent carbon, 0.4 percent beryllium, and the balance iron. Used extensively in the production of orthodontic appliances. Cobalt-chromium-nickel wrought wires are available in various degrees of hardness (soft, ductile, semispring temper, and spring temper), which may be softened by heat soaking at 1100 to 1200°C (2012–2192°F), followed by a quench. The age-hardening temperature range is 260 to 650°C (500–1202°F), e.g., holding at 482°C (900°F) for 5 hours. **contour a.**, a former term for an alloy especially suitable for creating anatomically shaped filling. **copper-rich a.**, high copper a. **cut a., cut amalgam a.**, a dental amalgam alloy that is cut from a cast ingot into small particles (filings) about average 35 μm in diameter. Called also *lathe-cut a.* and *filing.* **A. D,** a cobalt-chrome alloy. **dental amalgam a.**, AMALGAM alloy. **dental casting gold a.**, see under GOLD. **dispersion a., dispersion phase a., dispersion system a.**, an alloy in which the γ_2-phase is eliminated or minimized. One example is an alloy of about 10 percent silver with gold. Another type is a cut silver-tin alloy to which silver-copper eutectic spherical particles have been added to strengthen the alloy, the dispersed spheres acting as a filler. The copper in the spheres combines with the tin during trituration, the tin being occupied by the copper and the mercury having only silver available for reaction, thereby reducing or eliminating the γ_2-phase. See also *high copper a.* **A. E,** a cobalt-chrome alloy. **eutectic a.**, an alloy having a fusion temperature lower than those of its components. In the alloy, two or more phases may be present that are mutually insoluble when solidified; when solidifying, the components of the alloy separate, even though they were soluble in the molten state. Eutectic alloys are generally brittle and have low resistance to corrosion and tarnish; they are used in dentistry mainly in solders in order to decrease the fusion temperature. Called also *eutectic mixture.* **a. F,** a cobalt-chrome alloy. **ferrous a.**, an iron-containing alloy, such as steel. **a. G,** a cobalt-chrome alloy. **gallium a.**, an alloy in which gallium (having a melting point of 29.78°C) is used instead of mercury. When mixed with tin, it forms a eutectic system that is liquid at room temperature. The alloy thus formed can be mixed with some powdered metals, such as a silver-tin alloy, similarly to mercury. Mixing a palladium-gallium alloy powder with a liquid gallium-tin eutectic system produces a material that will harden at mouth temperature and has somewhat higher strength and lower flow characteristics than conventional alloys. Because of its low resistance to corrosion and bioincompatibility, the alloy is not used clinically. **gold a.**, GOLD alloy. **gold-copper a.**, a binary alloy containing various proportions of gold and copper. At temperatures greater than 400°C (752°F) the components form substitutional solid solutions in all proportions and, on slow cooling, solid-solid precipitations occur from the supersaturated condition, the disordered solid solution becoming a superlattice AuCu₃, while quenching always produces a substitutional solid solution. Alloys having a high gold content are resistant to corrosion and are used in dentistry. Called also *gold-copper system.* **high copper a.**, a dental amalgam alloy whose copper content has been increased to more than 6 percent with a corresponding decrease in the silver content. The addition of copper is expected to enhance the performance of the alloy by reducing or eliminating the γ_2-phase during trituration. Called also *copper-rich a.* and *low silver a.* Available under numerous trademarks. See also *dispersion a.* and *non-gamma II a.* **a. HS21,** a cobalt-chrome alloy which resembles Vitallium, also containing nickel molybdenum, manganese, silicon, iron, and carbon. Called also *Haynes stellite 21.* **a. HS31,** a cobalt-chrome alloy also containing nickel, tungsten, manganese, silicon, iron, and carbon. Called also *Haynes stellite 31.* **hypereutectic a.**, a eutectic alloy having composition

greater than eutectic (see under COMPOSITION); one being a solid solution whose solvent is low in proportion to the solute or one composed of the β-solid solution. See also phase DIAGRAM. **hypoeutectic a.**, a eutectic alloy having a composition less than eutectic (see under COMPOSITION); one being a solid solution whose solute concentration is low in proportion to the solvent or one composed of the α-solid solution. See also phase DIAGRAM. **iron-carbon a.**, see carbon IRON and carbon STEEL. **iron-chromium a.**, see stainless STEEL. **JD a.**, trademark for a high fusing cobalt-chrome casting alloy (see *cobalt-chrome a.*). **lathe-cut a.**, cut a. **LG a.**, trademark for a high fusing cobalt-chrome casting alloy (see *cobalt-chrome a.*). **Linc a.**, trademark for an *amalgam alloy* (see under AMALGAM). **low silver a.**, high copper a. **mercury a.**, see AMALGAM. **a.-mercury ratio,** alloy-mercury RATIO. **mixed type a.**, an alloy composed of combinations of two or more types of alloy systems. **nickel-chromium a.**, an alloy containing 80 percent nickel and 20 percent chromium, having a tensile strenth of 6650 kg/cm² (95,000 psi) in the annealed state and 11,540 kg/cm² (165,000 psi) in the hardened state. The extra spring alloy has a tensile strength of 14,000 kg/cm² (200,000 psi). Its modulus of elasticity is 2,170,000 kg/cm² (31,000,000 psi) and Bohn hardness number is 142 to 157 in the annealed state and 201 to 225 in the hardened state. Nickel-chromium wires are used in electrical units and in orthodontic appliances. **Nobillium a.**, trademark for a high fusing cobalt-chrome casting alloy (see *cobalt chrome a.*). **non–gamma II a.**, an alloy which, during trituration, does not form or forms minimal γ_2-phase. See *dispersion a.* and *high copper a.* **peritectic a.**, an alloy which solidifies, whereby an atomic diffusion occurs on slow cooling to change the β-phase to the α-phase. See also *eutectic a.* and peritectic REACTION. **platinum-silver a.**, a binary peritectic alloy of platinum and silver. Called also *platinum-silver system.* **preamalgamated a.**, a dental alloy containing some mercury, added to provide more rapid amalgamation. **quaternary a.**, one in which four elements are present. Called also *quaternary system.* **quinary a.**, one having five components. Called also *quinary system.* **Royal a.**, trademark for an *amalgam alloy* (see under AMALGAM). **Shofu spherical a.**, trademark for an *amalgam alloy* (see under AMALGAM). **Silver Crest a.**, trademark for an *amalgam alloy* (see under AMALGAM). **silver-copper a.**, a binary, eutectic alloy containing various proportions of silver. In one form, an alloy of 92.5 percent silver and 7.5 percent copper, it is known as *sterling silver.* Heat treatment may increase its tensile strength and yield point. Used rarely as an inlay material for deciduous teeth. Called also *silver-copper system.* **silver-palladium a.**, a type of white gold which may or may not contain relatively small amounts of gold. **silver-tin a.**, a peritectic alloy of silver and tin. Together with trace amounts of copper and zinc, it is a component of amalgam alloy. Called also *silver-tin system.* **solid solution a.**, one in which the atoms of the solute are randomly distributed throughout the space lattice of the solvent; dental alloys are usually of this type. **spherical a., spherical amalgam a.**, an amalgam alloy fabricated in small spheres, usually about 5 to 50 μm in diameter, generally formed by an atomizing procedure with the molten alloy. **stellite a.**, cobalt-chrome a. **a. system,** an aggregate of two or more metals in all possible combinations. **ternary a.**, one in which three elements are present. Called also *ternary system.* **tin-antimony a.**, a base-metal crown and bridge alloy occurring as a platinum-colored light-weight metal. **a. X-12,** trademark for a high fusing cobalt-chrome casting alloy (see *cobalt chrome a.*). **zinc-free a.**, an amalgam alloy without any zinc.

alloyage (ah-loi′ij) the combining of metals into alloys. See also AMALGAMATION.

All-Pro trademark for an automatic film developer used in dental practice for developing x-ray film.

allyl (al′il) [L. *allium* garlic + Gr. *hyle* matter] a univalent organic group CH₂:CH·CH₂. **a. isothiocyanate,** a volatile oil isolated from the seeds of black mustard, 3-isothiocyanato-l-propene, which occurs as a colorless or pale yellow, refractive liquid with a pungent odor and an acrid taste. It is miscible with ethanol and most organic solvents and slightly soluble in water. Used as a counterirritant in ointments and plasters and in the preparation of flavors; also used in the manufacture of war gases.

allylguaiacol (al″il-gwi′ah-kol) eugenol.

allylmercaptopenicillin (al″il-mer″kap-to-pen″i-sil′in) penicillin O.

***N*-allylnormophine** (al″il-nor-mor′fēn) nalorphine.

Almeida see DE ALMEIDA.

ALO axiolinguo-occlusal.

alopecia (al″o-pe′she-ah) [Gr. *alōpekia* a disease, like the mange of foxes, in which the hair falls out] loss of hair from any part of the body; baldness.

Aloperidine trademark for *haloperidol.*

Alpen trademark for *phenethicillin.*

alpha (al′fah) α, the first letter of the Greek alphabet; used as part of a chemical name to denote the first of a series of isomeric compounds, or the carbon atom next to the carboxyl group. The succeeding letters of the Greek alphabet, beta (β), gamma (γ), delta (δ), etc., are used to name, in order, succeeding compounds or carbon atoms.

Alphacaine trademark for *lidocaine hydrochloride* (see under LI-DOCAINE).

alphaprodine hydrochloride (al″fah-pro′dēn) a narcotic analgesic, *cis*-(+)-1,3-dimethyl-4-phenyl-4-piperidinol propanoate (ester) hydrochloride, occurring as a white, crystalline powder with a slight odor, which is soluble in water, ethanol, and chloroform, but not in ether. Used in moderate to severe pain, chiefly for analgesia of brief duration in minor surgery and outpatient practice. Its depressant action is potentiated by barbiturates, some general anesthetics, and phenothiazines. Adverse reactions include respiratory depression, vertigo, sweating, drowsiness, urticaria, and, less commonly, nausea, vomiting, restlessness, and confusion. Abuse leads to habituation or addiction; withdrawal produces symptoms similar to those of meperidine. Trademarks: Nisentil, Nisintel, Prisilidene.

Alphavirus (al″fah-vi′rus) [*alpha* + *virus*] a genus of mosquito-borne arboviruses of the family Togaviridae, consisting of viruses formerly classified as group A arboviruses. Alphaviruses cause inapparent infections of mammals, birds, and reptiles, but some strains may produce generalized infections associated with encephalitis in man. There are more than 20 individual alphaviruses.

alphavirus (al″fah-vi′rus) any virus of the genus *Alphavirus.*

ALS antilymphocyte SERUM.

Alserin trademark for *reserpine.*

Alt. dieb. abbreviation for L. *alter′nis die′bus,* every other day.

alternating (awl″ter-nāt″ing) [L. *alternatio*] occurring by turn in regular succesion.

a4Altherr, Franz [Swiss physician] see chronic atrophic POLYCHONDRITIS (Meyenburg-Altherr-Uehlinger syndrome).

Alt. hor. abbreviations for L. *alter′nis ho′ris,* every other hour.

Altmann-Gersh method [Richard *Altmann;* Isidore *Gersh,* American anatomist, born 1907] see under METHOD.

Aluctyl trademark for *aluminum lactate* (see under ALUMINUM).

Aludrine trademark for *isoproterenol.*

alum (al′um) 1. either of two compounds, potassium alum or ammonium alum, both of which are colorless, odorless, crystalline substances with a sweetish astringent taste, and are soluble in water and glycerol, but not in alcohol. Used as an astringent and styptic and sometimes added to mouthwashes. Also used as a hardener of emulsion in x-ray film processing. Ingestion of excessive amounts may cause burns of the mouth and pharynx. Called also *alumen.* 2. a generic term for any member of a class of double sulfates formed on potassium alum or ammonium alum. 3. any member of a class of double aluminum-containing compounds. **ammonium a.,** see *alum* (1). **burnt ammonium a.,** exsiccated ammonium alum; see *exsiccated a.* **concentrated a.,** incorrect name for ALUMINUM sulfate. **dried a.,** exsiccated a. **exsiccated a.,** either exsiccated ammonium alum or exsiccated potassium alum, both of which occur as a white odorless powder, with a sweetish, astringent taste, and containing at least 96.5 per cent of the labeled product. Used in water purification, dying and printing fabrics, and other industrial processes. Therapeutically, it is an astringent and styptic agent. Called also *burnt a., dried a.,* and *alumen exsiccatum.* **exsiccated ammonium a.,** see *exsiccated a.* **exsiccated potassium a.,** see *exsiccated a.* **potassium a.,** see *alum* (1).

alumen (ah-loo′men) [L.] alum. **a. exsicca′tum,** exsiccated ALUM.

alumina (ah-loo′mĭ-nah) ALUMINUM oxide. **α-a.,** corundum. **hydrate a.,** see ALUMINUM hydroxide. **levigated a.,** see ALUMINUM oxide.

aluminium (al″u-min′e-um) aluminum.

Aluminoid (ah-loo′mĭ-noid) trademark for a preparation of *aluminum hydroxide gel* (see ALUMINUM hydroxide).

aluminosilicate (ah-loo′mĭ-no-sil′ĭ-kāt) a compound of aluminum with metal oxides or other radicals; it is a component of

polycarboxylate cements. See also ALUMINUM silicate. **calcium a.,** calcium FELDSPAR. **potash a.,** potassium a., potassium FELDSPAR. **soda a.,** sodium a., sodium FELDSPAR.

aluminum (ah-loo′mĭ-num) [L. *alumen* alum] a light, whitish, lustrous metal that is ductile, malleable, and easily machined. Symbol Al; atomic number, 13; group IIIA of the period table; atomic weight, 26.982; specific gravity, 2.699; valence, 3. It is derived from bauxite, not occurring free in nature. Aluminum is resistant to corrosion, but tends to be oxidized by water and is attacked by hydrochloric acid, hot sulfate acid, perchloric acid, and strong alkalies. Its electrical conductivity is about two-thirds that of copper. Aluminum products are widely used in industry, particularly in the production of structures in which a high degree of the strength/weight ratio is of essence. In dentistry, it is used in the manufacture of dentures, obturators, and other prosthetic devices. Aluminum filters are used in radiology. Aluminum dust is flammable and explosive and, therefore, hazardous; its inhalation is suspected as a possible cause of lung disease, but it is generally considered to be a nontoxic metal. **a. acetate,** a compound, $Al(C_2H_3O_2)_3$; used in solution as an astringent and antiseptic. See Burow's SOLUTION. **a. acetylsalicylate,** aluminum ASPIRIN. **a. ammonium sulfate,** exsiccated ammonium alum (see exsiccated ALUM). **a. aspirin,** aluminum ASPIRIN. **basic a. carbonate,** a. carbonate, basic. **a. carbonate,** a compound, $Al_2(CO_3)_3$; used as a styptic agent. **a. carbonate, basic,** an aluminum oxycarbonate preparation containing about 5 percent aluminum oxide and about 2.4 percent carbonate, being a strong gastric antacid that binds more phosphate than aluminum hydroxide. Used in gastric hyperacidity, peptic ulcer, and phosphate nephrolithiasis. **a. chlorate,** a compound, $AlCl_3O_9$; used as an antiseptic and astringent agent. **a. chloride,** a compound, $AlCl_3$, occurring as a white or grayish or yellow crystalline odorless powder. The hexahydrate, $AlCl_3 + 6H_2O$, is used as a local astringent. Also used in deodorant and antiperspirant preparations. **colloidal a. hydroxide,** aluminum hydroxide gel (see *a. hydroxide*). **a. filter,** aluminum FILTER. **a. glycinate,** dihydroxyaluminum aminoacetate, an antacid preparation. **a. hydrate,** a. hydroxide. **a. hydroxide,** a compound, $Al(OH)_3$, occurring as a white, tasteless, and odorless powder with mildly astringent, antacid, and adsorbent properties. When ingested, it combines with the hydrochloric acid of gastric juice to form aluminum chloride, thus neutralizing gastric acidity. It is used in antacid, dentifrice, antiperspirant, and other pharmaceutic preparations. Also used as an adsorbent, emulsifier, ion-exchanger, and mordant. Therapeutic preparations of aluminum hydroxide are partly aluminum hydroxide and partly aluminum oxide hydrated. They are available as aluminum hydroxide gel, an aqueous suspension of aluminum hydroxide with flavoring agents and vehicles; dried aluminum hydroxide gel; and dried aluminum hydroxide tablets. Untoward effects may include phosphate depletion and osteomalacia and interference with the therapeutic effects of tetracyclines. Called also *a. hydrate, a. trihydrate,* and *hydrate alumina.* **a. lactate,** a compound, $Al(C_3H_5O_3)_3$, occurring as a water-soluble white powder; used in dental impression materials. Trademark: Aluctyl. **a. magnesium hydroxide,** magaldrate. **a. monostearate,** a combination of aluminum with various proportions of stearic and palmitic acids; used in preparation of a suspension of penicillin G procaine. **a. orthophosphate,** a. phosphate. **a. oxide,** a substance, Al_2O_3, occurring as a white crystalline powder, which is soluble in alkaline solutions, but not in water and organic solvents, melts at 2030°C, and has a Mohs hardness number of 8.8. Found in nature as the minerals bauxite, beyerite, boehmite, corundum, diaspore, and gibbsite, ruby and sapphire being its impure varieties. The mixed mineral bauxite is a hydrate aluminum oxide. Aluminum oxide can be produced in various grain sizes, usually from bauxite. Very fine particles can be obtained by a water flotation process, the product (levigated alumina) being used as a metal polishing agent. Used in the production of abrasives, refractories, ceramics, catalysts, laboratory wares, and fluxes, and in chromatography. Called also *alumina.* **a. oxide, hydrated,** see *a. hydroxide.* **a. phosphate,** a compound, $AlPO_4$, occurring as a white infusible powder with antacid properties, which is insoluble in water and acetic acid, but is slightly soluble in nitric and hydrochloric acid. Used in the treatment of gastric hyperacidity and peptic ulcer, and, with calcium sulfate and sodium silicate, as flux in dental cements, ceramics, and glass; available as gel or dried gel. Called also *a. orthophosphate.* **a. potassium sulfate,** potassium alum (see ALUM [1]). **a. silicate,** one of several clays having a common formula $Al_2(SiO_3)_3$; natural forms include andalusite, silimanite, and mullite. Used in ceramics. See also ALUMINOSILICATE, FELDSPAR, and KAOLIN. **a. silicate, hydrated,** bentonite. **a. subacetate,** a yellow liquid prepared by the interaction of aluminum sulfate, acetic acid, and precipitated calcium carbonate; used as an astringent wash when diluted with 20 to 40 volumes of water. **a. sulfate,** a compound, $Al_2(SO_4)_3$, occurring as a white, lustrous crystalline powder or granules with a sweet taste. In aqueous solution, used as an astringent, antiinfective, and antiperspirant agent. Also used as a deodorizing, decolorizing, pesticidal, and mordant agent. Incorrectly called *concentrated alum.*

alundum (ah-lun′dum) electrically fused alumina; used in making laboratory appliances that are to be subjected to intense heat.

Alupent trademark for *metaproterenol sulfate* (see under META-PROTERENOL).

Alutyl trademark for *cinchophen.*

Aluwax trademark for a wax wafer containing aluminum, which retains heat longer than when the metal is not present, so that a centric relation check bite (or registration) can be accomplished; used for registering the relationship of the mandible to the maxilla with the mandible in centric relation.

Alv. adst. abbreviation for L. *al′vo adstric′ta,* when the bowels are constipated.

alveolalgia (al″ve-o-lal′je-ah) [*alveolus* + *-algia*] pain occurring in the dental alveolus, sometimes observed after tooth extraction. See also dry SOCKET.

alveolar (al-ve′o-lar) [L. *alveolaris*] pertaining to an alveolus.

alveolate (al-ve′o-lāt) marked by honeycomb-like pits.

alveolectomy (al″ve-o-lek′to-me) [*alveolus* + Gr. *ektromē* excision] subtotal or complete excision of the alveolar process of the maxilla or mandible; usually performed in the treatment of neoplasms, prior to irradiation therapy of the jaws for malignancy, restoration of the contour of the jaws in cases of extreme protrusion of the alveolus, or for functional and esthetic purposes, such as in the treatment of maxillary or mandibular prognathism. **partial a.,** surgical excision of a portion of the alveolar process.

alveoli (al-ve′o-li) [L.] plural of *alveolus.*

alveolitis (al″ve-o-li′tis) inflammation of the alveolus. Called also *odontobothritis.* **a. sic′ca doloro′sa,** dry SOCKET.

alveolo- [L. *alveolus*] a combining form denoting relationship to an alveolus.

alveoloclasia (al-ve′o-lo-kla′ze-ah) [*alveolo-* + Gr. *klasis* breaking] destruction of the dental alveolus. See marginal PERIODONTITIS.

alveolocondylar (al-ve″o-lo″kon′dĭ-lar) pertaining to the alveolar process and condyle.

alveolodental (al-ve″o-lo-den′tal) pertaining to a tooth and its alveolus.

alveololabial (al-ve″o-lo-la′be-al) pertaining to the alveolar process and the lips.

alveololingual (al-ve″o-lo-ling′gwal) pertaining to the alveolar process and the tongue.

alveolomerotomy (al-ve″o-lo″mĕ-rot′o-me) [*alveolo-* + Gr. *meros* part + *tomē* a cutting] excision of a part of the alveolar process.

alveolonasal (al-ve″o-lo-na′sal) pertaining to the alveolar point of the nasion.

alveolopalatal (al-ve″o-lo-pal′ah-tal) pertaining to the alveolar process and the palate.

alveoloplasty (al-ve′o-lo-plas″te) [*alveolo-* + Gr. *plassein* to form] conservative contouring of the alveolar process, in the preparation for immediate or future denture construction. **interradicular a., intraseptal a.,** the surgical removal of the interradicular bone and the collapsing of the cortical plates on each other to achieve an acceptable or more desirable contour.

alveolotomy (al″ve-o-lot′o-me) [*alveolo-* + Gr. *tomē* a cutting] cutting into a dental alveolus; usually performed to expose or remove an embedded tooth, to expose a cyst or neoplasm, or for an apicoectomy.

alveolus (al-ve′o-lus) [L., dim of *alveus* hollow] a general term used in anatomical nomenclature to designate a small saclike dilatation. See also ACINUS. **buccal a.,** the buccal crypt of a dental alveolus that is divided by a septum into buccal and lingual components. **canine a.,** a dental alveolus investing a canine tooth. It is the third from the median line, and is a relatively large and deep socket, with an oval and regular form; its labial width being greater than the lingual. It extends distally and is flattened mesially, being somewhat concave distally. Its bony structure is frail at the canine eminence. **dental a., a. dent′alis,** one of the cavities or sockets in the alveolar process of the mandible or maxilla, in which the roots of the teeth are held by the fibers of the periodontal ligament. Called also *alveolar cavity, odontobothrion,* and *tooth socket.* **distobuccal a.,** the distobuccal crypt of a dental alveolus whose buccal component is divided by a septum into mesial and distal components. **first premolar a.,** a kidney-shaped dental alveolus investing the first premolar tooth, which is partially divided by a

bony spine that fits into the medial developmental groove of the root, dividing the socket into buccal and lingual portions. In instances when the root is not bifurcated for part of its length, the terminal portion of the cavity is separated into the buccal and lingual alveoli. It is flattened distally and is much wider buccolingually than mesiodistally. **lingual a.,** the lingual crypt of a dental alveolus that is divided by a septum into buccal and lingual components. **maxillary first molar a.,** a dental alveolus investing the maxillary first molar tooth, made up of three alveoli: lingual, mesiobuccal, and distobuccal; the lingual alveolus being the largest of the three. **mesiobuccal a.,** the mesiobuccal crypt of a dental alveolus whose buccal component is divided by a septum into mesial and distal components. **mucous a.,** a salivary gland alveolus secreting mucin. See *salivary gland a.* **salivary gland a.,** a dilated pocket ramifying from ducts in the salivary gland lobules, which is composed of cells secreting a viscid fluid containing mucin (mucous a.), or cells secreting a thin watery fluid (serous a.). **second premolar a.,** a dental alveolus investing the second premolar tooth, having a kidney-shaped form that is reverse to the one of the first premolar. It is partially divided by a bony spine situated in the distal part of the socket. The cavity usually accommodates a single broad root with a blunt end. **serous a.,** a salivary gland alveolus secreting a thin watery fluid. See *salivary gland a.*

Alvodine trademark for *piminodine esylate* (see under PIMIN-ODINE).

alymphocytosis (ah-lim″fo-si-to′sis) complete or nearly complete absence of lymphocytes from the circulating blood. See LYM-PHOPENIA.

Am 1. americium. 2. Am FACTOR.

AMA American Medical Association.

Amalcap trademark for a preproportioned *dental amalgam* (see under AMALGAM), available in disposable capsules containing 43.51 to 45.95 percent mercury.

amalgam (ah-mal′gam) [Gr. *malagma* poultice or soft mass] an alloy in which mercury is one of the components, presenting as a soft silvery paste, when freshly prepared, which hardens into a solid mass. **a. alloy,** a silver-tin alloy (Ag_3Sn), with trace amounts of copper with or without zinc, which is mixed (triturated) with mercury to form dental amalgam, and is prepared by melting its components and casting it into an ingot. The initial alloy melt is of pertectic composition, occurring as nonhomogenous grains of various sizes, made up of a mixture of β- and γ-phases. The equilibrium relationship is reestablished by a homogenizing heat treatment, whereby the ingot is heated in an oven at a temperature below the solidus (450°C or 840 F) for various periods, up to 24 hours. The ingot is then cut into small particles (filings) about 35 m or spheres 5 to 50 m in diameter. The microstresses induced during cutting and machining are reduced by a heat aging method by heat treatment at about 100°C (212 F) for a few hours. Available under numerous trademarks. Called also *dental amalgam alloy.* See table. **a. condensation,** amalgam CONDENSATION. **copper a.,** an amalgam available in the form of preamalgamated pellets containing 60 to 70 percent mercury and 30 to 40 percent copper. The pellets are heated in a test tube or in an iron spoon until the mercury appears in droplets, and the mass is then triturated. Used chiefly in restorations for deciduous teeth. The amalgam corrodes in the oral fluids, but the corrosion products are believed to have bactericidal properties which inhibit dental caries, the incidence of caries on the surface of the adjacent teeth which have been in contact with copper amalgam appear to be less frequent than when other types of amalgam are used. Seldom used now owing to the potential for corrosion and concern about dangers of mercury toxicity from vapor liberated in preparation. **cut a. alloy,** cut ALLOY. **dental a.,** an amalgam

TYPICAL COMPOSITION OF MODERN AMALGAM ALLOYS

Metal	Average (%)	Range (%)
Silver	69.4	66.7–74.5
Tin	26.2	25.3–27.0
Copper	3.6	0.0– 6.0
Zinc	0.8	0.0– 1.9

(From Guide to Dental Materials. 5th ed. Chicago, American Dental Association, 1970.)

used in restorative dentistry, containing mercury, silver, tin, copper, and possibly zinc. It is prepared by mixing (amalgamation or trituration) mercury with amalgam alloy (a silver-tin alloy) to form a silvery, soft paste for condensation into the prepared cavity where it hardens to form a dental restoration. Available under numerous trademarks. Formerly called *royal mineral succedaneum.* **gold a.,** a fusible and crumbling amalgam containing 40 percent gold and 60 percent mercury; no longer used. **a. mixer,** triturator. **pin-retained a., pin-supported a., pinned a.,** pin-supported RESTORATION. **retrograde a.,** retrograde FILLING. **scrap a.,** amalgam left over after the prepared cavity has been filled. **silver a.,** dental amalgam consisting of silver that forms a metallic compound with mercury, which usually contains 67 to 70 percent silver; 25 to 27 percent (but no less than 25 percent) tin; a maximum of 6 percent copper; and a maximum of 2 percent zinc. Some preamalgamated alloys may contain as much as 3 percent mercury. See also ARGYRIA. **spherical a. alloy,** spherical amalgam ALLOY.

amalgamation (ah-mal″gah-ma′shun) trituration (3). **manual a.,** mortar and pestle TRITURATION. **mechanical a.,** mechanical TRITURATION. **mortar and pestle a.,** mortar and pestle TRITURATION.

amalgamator (ah-mal″gah-ma′tor) triturator. **Baker a.,** trademark for a *mechanical triturator* (see under TRITURATOR), having an operational speed of 4400 rpm. **Crown a.,** trademark for a *mechanical triturator* (see under TRITURATOR), having an operational speed of 3000 rpm. **mechanical a.,** mechanical TRITURATOR.

amaurosis (am″aw-ro′sis) [Gr. *amaurōsis* darkening] partial or complete blindness, usually due to diseases of the brain or optic nerve, but without any apparent lesions of the eye itself. See also AMBLYOPIA.

Ambard's formula [Léon *Ambard,* Strassburg physiologist, born 1876] see under FORMULA.

amber (am′ber) a yellowish fossil resin, the gum of several species of coniferous trees, found in the coastal areas of the Baltic sea. Called also *succinum.*

Amberg's line [Emil *Amberg,* American physician, 1868–1948] see under LINE.

ambly- [Gr. *amblys* dull] a combining form denoting dullness.

amblygeustia (am″ble-gu′ste-ah) [ambly- + Gr. *geusis* taste + -ia] abnormal dullness of the sense of taste.

amblyopia (am″ble-o′pe-ah) [ambly- + Gr. *ops* eye + -ia] partial blindness without any apparent lesion of the eye itself. See also AMAUROSIS.

ambo- [L. *ambo* both] a combining form signifying both, or on both sides.

amboceptor (am″bo-sep′tor) [ambo- + L. *capere* to take] an antibody, particularly a hemolysin, capable of binding complement after it has combined with a red blood cell.

Amboclorin trademark for *chlorambucil.*

Ambodryl trademark for *bromodiphenhydramine hydrochloride* (see under BROMODIPHENHYDRAMINE).

ambulance (am″bu-lans) [Fr.] a vehicle for conveying the sick or injured, and equipped with an apparatus for rendering emergency treatment.

ambulant (am′bu-lant) [L. *ambulans* walking] walking or able to walk; ambulatory.

ambulatory (am″bu-lah-to′re) 1. pertaining to medical services rendered in a hospital or a clinic to persons who are not confined to the hospital bed or who are not confined overnight; outpatient. See also ambulatory CARE and ambulatory hospital CARE. 2. ambulant; able to walk; walking.

Amcill trademark for *ampicillin.*

Amcill-S trademark for *ampicillin sodium* (see under AMPICILLIN).

AMDS Association of Military Dental Surgeons.

ameba (ah-me′bah), pl. *ame′bae* or *ame′bas* [L., from Gr. *amoiba* change] a minute protozoon of the subphylum Sarcodina. It is a single-celled nucleated mass of protoplasm which changes shape by extending cytoplasmic processes, by means of which it moves about and absorbs nourishment. The majority of amebae are free-living in soil and water, but several are parasitic in man, including *Entamoeba gingivalis, E. coli, E. hartmanii,* and *E. histolytica.* Also written *amoeba.*

amebiasis (am″ē-bi′ah-sis) a condition resulting from the infection with amebae, especially *Entamoeba histolytica.*

amebic (ah-me′bik) pertaining to or of the nature of an ameba.

amebicide (ah-me′bĭ-sīd) [ameba + L. *caedere* to kill] an agent which is destructive to amebae.

ameboid (ah-me′boid) [ameba + Gr. *eidos* form] resembling an ameba in form or in movement. See also ameboid MOVEMENT.

Amechol trademark for *methacholine bromide* (see under METHACHOLINE).

amelification (ah-mel″ĭ-fi-ka′shun) [Old Fr. *amel* enamel + L. *facere* to make] the development of enamel cells into enamel.

amelo- [Old Fr. *amel* enamel] a combining form meaning enamel.

ameloblast (ah-mel′o-blast) [amelo- + Gr. *blastos* germ] a cylindrical epithelial cell in the innermost layer of the enamel organ; its functions include contribution to the development of the dentinoenamel junction by the deposition of a layer of the matrix, thus producing the foundation for the prisms, and production of the matrix for the enamel prisms and interprismatic substance. Subsequent to polarization, the elongated nucleus is basally located in the cell. A double-walled nuclear membrane delimits the karyoplasm, which contains fine suspended chromatin granules and nucleoli. The mitochondria occupy an area between the nucleus and cell membrane. The distal juxtanuclear area contains the endoplasmic reticulum, and the zone distal to this is occupied by the Golgi complex and secretory granules. Called also *adamantoblast, enamel builder, enamel cell, enameloblast,* and *ganoblast.*

ameloblastoma (ah-mel″o-blas-to′mah) [amelo- + Gr. *blastos* germ + -oma] a destructive odontogenic tumor derived from tissue of the type characteristic of the enamel organ, most commonly located in the mandible in the molar ramus area and, less commonly, in the maxilla, invading the antrum, and in the floor of the nose. Simple ameloblastoma is composed of clumps and nests of cells surrounded by a layer of cuboidal or columnar cells resembling ameloblasts; enclosed within this layer are cells resembling stellate reticulum. Ameloblastomas may grow to considerable size and are locally invasive; most are benign, but some may undergo malignant degeneration and metastasize. Called also *adamantinoblastoma, adamantinoma,* and *adamantoblastoma.* **acanthomatous a.,** one exhibiting squamous metaplasia of the epithelium, in which central cells assume squamatoid features. **cystic a.,** one in which stellate reticulum-like tissue has undergone cystic degeneration. Called also *adamantinoma polycepticum.* See also multilocular CYST. **pituitary a.,** craniopharyngioma. **melanotic a., pigmented a.,** melanoameloblastoma.

amelodentinal (am″ĕ-lo-den′tĭ-nal) pertaining to the enamel and dentin of a tooth.

amelogenesis (ah″mel-o-jen′ĕ-sis) [amelo- + Gr. *genesis* production] the elaboration of dental enamel by ameloblasts, beginning with its participation in the formation of the dentinoenamel junction to the production of the matrix for the enamel prisms and interprismatic substance. Steps of amelogenesis involve the formation of Tomes' process and prism space and the formation of the daily prism increment. **a. imperfec′ta,** a hereditary disease characterized by faulty development of the dental enamel, due to agenesis or hypoplasia of the dental enamel or its hypocalcification. It is marked by very thin and friable enamel that is frequently stained in various shades of brown. For amelogenesis imperfecta due to enamel hypoplasia or aplasia, see enamel HYPOPLASIA; for that due to hypocalcification or hypomineralization, see enamel HYPOCALCIFICATION. Called also *hereditary brown enamel, hereditary brown opalescent teeth,* and *hereditary enamel dysplasia.*

amelogenic (am″ĕ-lo-jen′ik) forming enamel, pertaining to amelogenesis.

Americaine trademark for *benzocaine.*

American Gold "B" Bridge see under GOLD.

American Gold "C" Partial Extra Hard see under GOLD.

American Gold "T" Bridge Hard see under GOLD.

americium (am″ĕ-ri′sĭ-um) [named after *America*] a synthetic element. Symbol, Am; atomic weight, 243; valences, 3, 4, 5, 6; atomic number, 95; specific gravity, 13.67. It occurs in an alpha-form, having a double close-packed hexagonal structure, and in a beta-form, having a face-centered cubic structure. It has isotopes 347 to 246, 243 being the most stable; all are radioactive poisons. The half-life of ^{241}Am is 470 years; that of ^{243}Am is 8.8 × 10^3. ^{241}Am is used as a diagnostic aid in bone mineral analysis.

Ames plastic porcelain see under PORCELAIN.

Ames Z-M trademark for a *zinc phosphate cement* (see under CEMENT).

Amethaine trademark for *tetracaine hydrochloride* (see under TETRACAINE).

Amethocaine trademark for *tetracaine hydrochloride* (see under TETRACAINE).

amethopterin (ah-meth-op′ter-in) methotrexate.

amethyst (am′ĭ-thist) a crystallized form of silicon dioxide.

Amicar trademark for *aminocaproic acid* (see under ACID).

amide (am'īd) [*ammonia* + *-ide*] an organic compound derived from ammonia by substituting an acyl radical for hydrogen, or from an acid by replacing the −OH group by −NH₂. **nicotinic acid a.**, nicotinamide. **salicylic acid a.**, salicylamide.

amidinase [E.C.3.5] (am″ĭ-din'ās) former name for a subclass of hydrolases acting on carbon-nitrogen bonds, other than peptide bonds. **arginine a.**, arginase.

amidine (am'ĭ-dēn) a compound containing the monovalent group −C(:NH) · NH₂. **insoluble a.**, **tegumentary a.**, amylopectin.

amidine-lyase [E.C.4.3.2] (am″ĭ-dēn-li'ās) a sub-subclass of carbon-nitrogen lyases, the enzymes of which catalyze the removal of an amidine group, as from L-argininosuccinate to form fumarate and L-arginine, by cleaving the C−N bonds.

amido- a chemical prefix indicating the presence of the radical NH₂ along with the radical CO.

amidobenzene (am″ĭ-do-ben'zēn) aniline.

Amidofebrin trademark for *aminopyrine.*

Amidon trademark for the *dl*-form of *methadone hydrochloride* (see under METHADONE).

Amidopyrazoline trademark for *aminopyrine.*

Amidryl trademark for *diphenhydramine.*

Amimycin trademark for *oleandomycin.*

amine (ah-mēn', am'in) an organic compound containing the functional group −NH₂; any member of the group of chemical compounds formed from ammonia by replacement of one or more of the hydrogen atoms by organic (hydrocarbon) radicals. Amines are basic, their base strength depending on the number of aryl or alkyl groups (R) that replace the hydrogen atoms on the nitrogen molecule, and are classified as *primary* −NF₂, *secondary* −NH₂, and *tertiary* −N−R. The lower molecular
|
R
weight amines are water-soluble gases; those of higher molecular weight are insoluble in water and soluble in organic solvents. Both types have an unpleasant odor that decreases with the decreased volatility. They occur widely in living cells, being a part of nucleic acids (pyrimidine and purine derivatives), amino acids, etc. The amines include allylamine, amylamine, ethylamine, methylamine, propylamine, and many other compounds. **quaternary a's**, organic derivatives of NH₄OH in which the hydroxyl group and the four H atoms are replaced by radicals. **sympathomimetic a's**, a group of amines which have sympathomimetic properties and mimic the action of epinephrine. See also CATECHOLAMINE. **vasoactive a.**, any amine capable of inducing vasomotor changes in the blood vessels, including histamine, serotonin, and catecholamines.

-amine a chemical suffix indicating the presence in the compound of the −NH₂ group.

amino (ah-me'no, am'ĭ-no) the monovalent chemical radical −NH₂.

amino- a chemical prefix indicating the presence in the compound of the −NH₂ group.

aminoacidemia (ah-me″no-, am″ĭ-no-as″ĭ-de'me-ah) [*amino acid* + Gr. *haima* blood + *-ia*] an excess of amino acids in the blood.

aminoaciduria (ah-me″no-, am″ĭ-no-as″ĭ-du're-ah) [*amino acid* + Gr. *ouron* urine + *-ia*] an excess of amino acids in the urine.

aminobenzene (ah-me″no-, am″ĭ-no-ben'zēn) aniline.

aminobenzoate (ah-me″no-, am″ĭ-no-ben'zo-āt) a salt of aminobenzoic acid. **ethyl a.**, benzocaine.

aminoethane (ah-me″no-, am″ĭ-no-eth'ān) ethylamine.

Aminoform trademark for *methenamine.*

aminoglycoside (ah-me″no-, am″ĭ-no-gli-ko'sīd) a glycoside in which the sugar moiety is substituted with one or more amino groups; see aminoglycoside ANTIBIOTIC.

2-aminoheptane (ah-me″no-, am″ĭ-no-hep'tān) tuaminoheptane.

aminomethane (ah-me″no-, am″ĭ-no-meth'ān) methylamine.

aminophylline (ah-me″no-fil'in, ah-mĭ-nof'ĭ-lēn) a central stimulant, theophylline ethylenediamine, occurring as white or yellowish granules or powder with a slightly ammoniacal odor and a bitter taste, which is soluble in water, but not in alcohol and ether. Its pharmacological effects include stimulation of the central nervous system and cardiac muscle, relaxation of smooth muscle, particularly the bronchial muscles, and diuretic action. Aminophylline therapy may counteract the action of sedatives in patients with bronchial asthma. Trademarks: Carena, Inophylline, Metaphyllin, Stenovasan.

aminopolypeptidase (ah-me″no-, am″ĭ-no-pol″e-pep'tĭ-dās) an enzyme that hydrolyzes polypeptides by cleaving the peptide linkage adjacent to the free amino group.

aminopterin (am'ĭ-nop'ter-in) a folic acid antagonist, N-{p-[(2, 4-diamino-6-pteridymmethyl-yl)amino]benzoyl}glutamic acid,

occurring as yellowish needles that are soluble in sodium hydroxide solution. It is used as an antineoplastic agent and, occasionally, as an abortifacient. Interference with folic acid utilization may cause folic acid deficiency (see folic ACID). Administration during pregnancy may cause fetal abnormalities (see fetal aminopterin SYNDROME). Called also 4-*aminofolic acid* and 4-*aminopteroylglutamic acid.*

aminopurine (ah-me″no-, am″ĭ-no-pu'rēn) a purine that is a component of nucleic acid and the nucleotides; the aminopurines include adenine and guanine.

aminopyrine (ah-me″no-, am″ĭ-no-pi'rēn) an analgesic and antipyretic agent, 4-dimethylamino-2,3-dimethyl-1-phenyl-3-pyrazolin-5-one, occurring as a white crystalline powder or crystals that are affected by light and are soluble in water, ethanol, benzene, chloroform, and ether. Used in the treatment of neuralgic pain, rheumatic disorders, and other painful conditions. Sometimes fatal agranulocytosis may occur in sensitive individuals. Trademarks: Amidofebrin, Amidopyrazoline, Amidopyrine, Novamidon, Pyradone, Pyramidon.

aminosalicylate (ah-me″no-, am″ĭ-no-sal″ĭ-sil'āt) a salt of aminosalicylic acid. **calcium a.**, a salt of aminosalicylic acid, 4-amino-2-hydroxybenzoic acid calcium salt, occurring as cream-colored crystals or powder with a slightly bitter-sweet taste, which is soluble in water, methanol, acetone, and, slightly, in alcohol. Used in the treatment of tuberculosis. It can cause hypercalcemia. Called also *calcium para-aminosalicylate*. Trademark: Pasara. **potassium a.**, a salt of aminosalicylic acid, 4-amino-2-hydroxybenzoic acid potassium salt, occurring as a white to cream-colored, odorless powder with a saline taste, which is soluble in water, sparingly soluble in alcohol, and very soluble in ether and chloroform. Used in the treatment of tuberculosis, particularly in cases when restriction of sodium intake is indicated. **sodium a.**, a salt of aminosalicylic acid, a dihydrate of 4-amino-2-hydroxybenzoic acid monosodium salt, occurring as a white to cream-colored, odorless, sweet and saline crystalline powder that is soluble in water, sparingly soluble in alcohol, and barely soluble in ether and chloroform. Used in the treatment of tuberculosis. Adverse reactions may include epigastric discomfort, anorexia, nausea, vomiting, diarrhea, renal lesions, drug fever, leukopenia, and hypokalemia. Called also *sodium para-aminosalicylate.*

aminotransferase [E.C.2.6.1] (ah-me″no-, am″ĭ-no-trans'fer-ās) a subclass of transferases, the enzymes of which catalyze the transfer of amino groups from α-amino acid to α-keto acid, usually ketoglutaric acid, to form the corresponding α-keto acid and glutamine. Most aminotransferases contain pyridoxal phosphate, i.e., they are pyridoxal-phosphate–proteins. Called also *transaminase* and *transaminating oxidoreductase*. See also TRANSAMINATION. **alanine a.** [E.C.2.6.1.2], an aminotransferase that contains pyridoxal phosphate, which catalyzes the conversion of L-alanine + 2-oxoglutarate to pyruvate + L-glutamate in the process of transamination. The human red cell enzyme exhibits genetically controlled multiple molecular forms (isoenzymes). A marked rise of the concentration of the enzyme in the blood is indicative of viral hepatitis. Called also *glutamic-alanine transaminase* and *glutamic-pyruvic transaminase.* **aspartate a.** [E.C.2.6.1.1], an aminotransferase that contains pyridoxal phosphate, which catalyzes the conversion of L-aspartate + 2-oxoglutarate to oxaloacetate + L-glutamate in the process of transamination. The enzyme exists in two major forms in humans: mitochondrial and soluble, the two being controlled by independent genetic loci. A marked rise in the concentration of the enzyme in the blood is indicative of myocardial infarction. Called also *glutamic-aspartic transaminase* and *glutamic-oxaloacetic transaminase.*

ammeter (am'me-ter) [ampere + Gr. *metron* measure] an instrument for measuring the strength of current in amperes.

ammoaciduria (am″o-as″ĭ-du're-ah) [*ammonia* + Gr. *ouron* urine + *-ia*] the presence of ammonia and amino acids in the urine. **aromatic spirit of a.**, SPIRIT of ammonia, aromatic. **spirit of a., aromatic**, SPIRIT of ammonia, aromatic.

ammonemia (ah″mo-ne'me-ah) [*ammonia* + Gr. *haima* blood + *-ia*] the presence of abnormally high amounts of ammonia in the blood.

ammonia (ah-mo'ne-ah) [named after Jupiter *Ammon,* near whose temple in Libya it was formerly obtained] a colorless, toxic gas with a pungent odor, NH₃, used as a refrigerant and fertilizer. Inhalation may cause edema of the respiratory tract, spasm of the glottis, asphyxia, and death. In venous blood, its content is about 75 to 200 μg/100 ml, the renal blood containing ammonia liberated from glutamine and certain amino acids. In the intestine, it is produced by bacteria from proteins and by converting urea into ammonia and carbon dioxide. Ammonia is also released by exercising muscles and the brain. The liver is the principal site of ammonia disposal, where it is converted into urea. It is synthesized by the epithelial cells in the kidney tubules and collecting ducts and reacts with hydrogen ions to form ammonium ions, which are then excreted with the urine. Ammonia is produced in the body by the dissociation of ammonium (NH_4) into hydrogen ions (H^+) and ammonia, being involved in controlling hydrogen-ion concentration. Blood ammonia may be elevated in severe liver diseases associated with portacaval shunt, being accompanied by loss of consciousness, tremor, hyperreflexia, and abnormal EEG. Called also *volatile alkali.* **aqua a.,** AMMONIUM hydroxide. **a. lyase,** ammonia-lyase. **a. water,** a 10 percent aqueous solution of ammonia, occurring as a colorless liquid with a pungent odor. Used as a reflex stimulant in syncope, weakness, or threatened faint. Its vapors are irritating to the eyes and mucous membranes. Diluted to 1 percent solution, used for cleansing dentures by immersion.

ammoniacal (am″o-ni′ah-kal) containing ammonia or treated with excess ammonia.

ammonia-lyase [E.C.4.3.1] (ah-mo′ne-ah-li′ăs) a sub-subclass of carbon-nitrogen lyases that catalyze the removal of ammonia (with the formation of a double bond) by cleaving the $C-N$ bond.

ammonirrhea (am″o-nĭ-re′ah) [*ammonia* + Gr. *rhoia* flow] the excretion of ammonia, as in the urine or sweat.

ammonium (ah-mo′ne-um) the radical NH^+_4, having the properties of and a resemblance to an alkali metal radical. In the body, the ammonium ion dissociates to the hydrogen ion (H^+) and ammonia (NH_3), thereby playing an important role in acid-base balance. Ammonia is excreted from the body in the urine by reacting with hydrogen ions to form ammonium ions, which are then excreted. Ammonium salts are used as expectorants, diuretics, and reflex stimulants, and also used in the treatment of metabolic alkalosis. **burnt a. alum,** exsiccated ammonium alum (see exsiccated ALUM). **a. hydrate,** a. hydroxide. **a. hydroxide,** NH_4OH, usually available as a 28 to 29 percent aqueous solution (*stronger ammonia water*), occurring as a colorless liquid with a strong pungent odor. It dissolves copper and zinc, fumes in the proximity of volatile acids, and reacts with mineral acids. Used as a detergent for removing stains and bleaching. When dissolved to a 10 percent solution (*ammonia water*), used as a reflex respiratory stimulant. Dissolved to 1 percent solution, used for cleansing dentures. It is highly toxic and extremely irritating, especially to the eyes and mucous membranes. Called also *a. hydrate, aqua ammonia,* and *spirit of hartshorn.* **a. ichthosulfonate,** ichthammol.

ammoniuria (ah-mo′ne-u′re-ah) [*ammonia* + Gr. *ouron* urine + *-ia*] an excess of ammonia in the urine.

amnion (am′ne-on) [Gr. "bowl"; "membrane enveloping the fetus"] the transparent, avascular, and thin but tough fetal membrane which lines the amniotic cavity, consisting of a single layer of ectodermal epithelium, and having a mesodermal connective tissue covering. It is the inner fetal membrane which contains the fetus and the amniotic fluid surrounding it. The growth of the fetus causes the amniotic cavity to expand, filling the entire chorionic cavity by the second month of pregnancy. In mammals, the amniotic tissue derives from the trophoblast by folding and splitting, its margin being attached during the early stages of embryonic development to the embryonic disk which later becomes the floor of the amniotic cavity. Called also *amniotic sac.* See also amniotic CAVITY and amniotic FLUID, and see illustration at fetal membranes, under MEMBRANE.

amniotic (am″ne-ot′ik) pertaining to or developing an amnion.

amobarbital (am″o-bar′bĭ-tal) an intermediate-acting barbiturate, hypnotic, and sedative, 5-phenyl-5-ethylbarbituric acid, occurring as white, crystalline, odorless powder with a bitter taste. It is used in epilepsy, psychoneurotic states, hypertension, gastrointestinal disorders, and coronary disease, and in preoperative and postoperative medication. It is an addictive drug subject to the regulation of the Controlled Substances Act. Adverse reactions and contraindications are similar to those of other barbiturates. Called also *amylbarbitone* and *isoamyl ethyl barbituric acid.* Trademark: Amytal. **a. sodium,** the sodium salt of amobarbital, occurring as a white, friable, hygroscopic, odorless, bitter granular powder, having the same uses, indications, contraindications, and side effects as the parent compound and other barbiturates. It is very soluble in

water and rapidly decomposes when exposed to air. Called also *amylbarbitone sodium.*

Amoeba (ah-me′bah) a genus of amebae of the order Amoebida, class Rhizopoda, including many free-living species in water and soil. Many species once included in this genus are now assigned to other taxonomic categories. **A. bucca′lis,** *Entamoeba coli* (see under ENTAMOEBA). **A. co′li,** *Entamoeba coli* (see under ENTAMOEBA). **A. denta′lis,** *Entamoeba gingivalis* (see under ENTAMOEBA). **A. dysente′riae, A. histolyt′ica,** *Entamoeba histolytica* (see under ENTAMOEBA).

amoeba (ah-me′bah) ameba.

Amoebida (ah-me′bĭ-dah) an order of protozoa of the class Rhizopoda, subphylum Sarcodina, comprising all the amebae symbiotic in animals, including man, but most are free-living and inhabit water, soil, and decaying matter.

Amoëdo y Valdés, Oscar [1865–1945] a professor of odontology in Paris, who published *L'Art Dentaire en Médecine Légale* in 1898, which is considered to be the foundation of modern forensic dentistry.

amorph (ah′morf) [*a* neg. + Gr. *morphē* form] an apparently inactive gene that has no detectable product. Called also *amorphic gene.* See also mutant GENE.

Amorphosporangium [*a* neg. + Gr. *morphē* form + *sporangium*] a genus of soil bacteria of the family Actinoplanaceae.

amorphous (ah-mor′fus) [*a* neg. + Gr. *morphē* form] 1. having no definite form; shapeless. 2. pertaining to material with a structure in which the molecules tend to be distributed at random, similar to molecules in a liquid; a solid substance which does not crystallize and is without definite shape. 4. any bacteria without visible differentiation in structure.

Amosyt trademark for *dimenhydrinate.*

Amotril trademark for *clofibrate.*

amount (ah-mownt′) the sum total of two or more quantities or sums. **deductible a.,** see deductible CLAUSE.

amoxicillin (ah-mok″sĭ-sil′in) a semisynthetic penicillin, [D(−)-6-[2-amino-2-(*p*-hydroxyphenyl)acetamidol]-3,3-dimethyl-7-oxo-4-thia-1-azabicyclo[3,2,0]heptane-2-carboxylic acid trihydrate. It is a bitter, white to off-white crystalline powder with a characteristic odor, which is slightly soluble in water, ethanol, and methanol. Effective against nonpenicillinase-producing strains of diplococci, staphylococci, streptococci, *Escherichia coli, Neisseria,* and *Haemophilus.* Adverse reactions may include nausea, vomiting, diarrhea, urticaria, erythema, hypersensitization, and other disorders common to other penicillins. Called also p-*hydroxy-ampicillin.* Trademarks: Amoxil, Larocin.

Amoxil trademark for *amoxicillin.*

AMP adenosine monophate or adenosine monophosphate; see adenylic ACID. **cyclic AMP,** ADENOSINE 3′,5′-cyclic phosphate.

amp ampere.

cAMP ADENOSINE 3′,5′-cyclic phosphate.

Ampazine trademark for *promazine.*

amperage (am′per-ij) the strength of an electric current expressed in amperes or milliamperes.

ampere (am′pēr) [named after A. M. *Ampère*] the unit of electric current in the SI system of measurement, being the current produced by 1 volt acting through a resistance of 1 ohm. The international ampere is the unvarying electrical current which, when passed through a solution of silver nitrate in accordance with certain specifications, deposits silver at the rate of 0.001118 gm per second. Abbreviated *A* or *amp.* See also SI. **absolute a.,** abampere.

Ampère, André Marie [1775–1836] a French mathematician and physicist, who is considered to be the "father of electrodynamics." See AMPERE.

Amperil trademark for *ampicillin.*

Amphedroxyn trademark for *methamphetamine hydrochloride* (see under METHAMPHETAMINE).

amphetamine (am-fet′ah-mēn) 1. synthetic racemic desoxynorephedrine, (+)-α-methylphenethylamine, occurring as a colorless liquid that is freely soluble in ether and ethanol and slightly soluble in water. It is a sympathomimetic drug that stimulates the central nervous system, which is used in the treatment of behavioral disorders in children, narcolepsy, parkinsonism, and depression; to counteract central depressants; and as an appetite depressant. Repetitive use may lead to drug dependence. Adverse reactions may include overstimulation of the central nervous system, agitation, restlessness, tremor, insomnia, headache, vertigo, euphoria, parasitosis, hallucinations, schizophrenia-like symptoms, exhaustion, ketosis, paresthesia, emaciation, dysphoria, mydriasis, tachycardia, hypertension, pallor, skin rash, chills, xerostomia, impotence, and diarrhea. Trademarks: Actedron, Adipan, Benzedrine, Norephedrane, Phendrine. 2. a term sometimes used to mean any compound that is chemically or pharmacologically related to amphetamine, including sympathomimetic amines used as appetite suppressants, phenylisopropylamine derivatives, and similar substances. Popularly called *speed.*

amphiarthrosis (am″fe-ar-thro′sis) [Gr. *amphi* on both sides + *arthrōsis* joint] cartilaginous JOINT.

amphitene (am′fi-tēn) see ZYGOTENE.

ampho- [Gr. *amphō* both] a combining form denoting both.

amphochromatophil (am″fo-kro-mat′o-fil) [*ampho-* + Gr. *chrōma, chromatos* color + *philein* to love] amphophilic CELL.

amphochromophil (am″fo-kro′mo-fil) [*ampho-* + Gr. *chrōma* color + *philein* to love] 1. amphophilic CELL. 2. amphophilic.

amphocyte (am′fo-sīt) [*ampho-* + *-cyte*] amphophilic CELL.

ampholyte (am′fo-līt) [*ampho-* + *electrolyte*] amphoteric ELECTROLYTE.

Ampho-Moronal trademark for *amphotericin B.*

amphophil (am′fo-fil) [*ampho-* + Gr. *philein* to love] 1. amphophilic CELL. 2. amphophilic.

amphophilic (am-fo-fil′ik) [*ampho-* + Gr. *philein* to love] stainable with either acid or basic dyes. Called also *amphochromophil* and *amphophil.* **a.-basophil**, staining with both acid and basic stains, but having a greater affinity for basic ones. **gram-a.**, tending to stain both positive and negative with Gram stain. **a.-oxyphil**, staining with both acid and basic dyes, but having a greater affinity for the acid ones.

amphoteric (am-fo-ter′ik) [Gr. *amphoteros* pertaining to both] having opposite character; pertaining to substances having both acid and basic properties; combining with both acids and bases; affecting red and blue litmus.

amphotericin B (am″fo-ter′ĭ-sin) a macrolide antibiotic, elaborated by *Streptomyces nodosus,* occurring as an odorless, yellow to orange powder that is soluble in dimethylformamide and dimethylsufoxide, slightly soluble in methyl alcohol, and insoluble in water, ethyl alcohol, ether, benzene, and toluene. It is a wide-spectrum antifungal antibiotic, used in a variety of mycoses, including coccidioidomycosis, cryptococcosis, candidiasis, histoplasmosis, aspergillosis, sporotrichosis, phycomycosis, and North American blastomycosis. Topical application may cause infrequent local irritation or allergic dermatitis, but parenteral use in systemic infections may produce a variety of adverse reactions, including chills, fever, nausea, vomiting, diarrhea, abdominal cramps, hemorrhagic gastroenteritis, headache, vertigo, thrombophlebitis, myalgia, arthralgia, anemia, purpura, and other complications. Trademarks: Ampho-Mononal, Fungilin, Fungizone.

ampicillin (amp″ĭ-sil′in) a semisynthetic penicillin, 6-(D-2-amino-2-phenylacetamido)-3,3-dimethyl-7-oxo-4-thia-1-azabicyclo-[3,2,0]heptane-2-carboxylic acid. The trihydrate is a stable, white, odorless crystalline powder that is soluble in dimethylcetamide and dimethylsulfoxide, slightly soluble in water and alcohol, and insoluble in various organic solvents. It is a wide-spectrum, acid- and penicillinase-resistant antibiotic, used in the treatment of diseases caused by enterobacteria, *Haemophilus influenzae, Neisseria, Bacillus pertussis, Shigella, Salmonella, Escherichia coli, Proteus, Aerobacter,* and other bacteria. It may cause nausea, vomiting, diarrhea, glossitis, stomatitis, and hypersensitivity reactions. Called also D-α-*aminobenzyl penicillin.* Trademarks: Amcill, Amperil, Ampicin, Ampifen, Divercillin, Pen-A, Viccillin. **a. sodium**, the monosodium salt of ampicillin, occurring as a white to off-white, hygroscopic crystalline powder that is very soluble in water and isotonic sodium chloride solution. Its properties are similar to those of the parent compound. Trademarks: Amcill-S, Cilleral, Pen A/N.

Ampicin trademark for *ampicillin.*

Ampifen trademark for *ampicillin.*

amplification (am″plĭ-fi-ka′shun) [L. *amplificatio*] the act or process of making something larger or stronger, as an increase in the strength of voltage, current, power, or sound intensity. **image a.**, image-tube INTENSIFICATION.

amplifier (am′plĭ-fi″er) something that enlarges or increases, especially an electronic device that increases the strength of an input signal, or an apparatus for increasing the magnification of a microscope. **image a.**, a device that increases the dim light from fluoroscopic screens through the use of mirrors.

amplitude (am′plĭ-tūd) [L. *amplitudo*] 1. largeness or fullness, wideness or breadth of range or extent. 2. in physics, maximum displacement of a wave from the zero or equilibrium position during one period of oscillation.

ampudontology (am″pu-don-tol′o-je) that aspect of dentistry concerned with the etiology, diagnosis, and treatment of teeth requiring the removal of one or more roots, or the sectioning and separation of roots. It includes root amputation, hemisection, and bicuspidization, as well as the alteration, reshaping, and final restoration of the involved teeth.

ampul (am′pul) ampule.

ampule (am′pul) [Fr. *ampoule*] a small glass container capable of being sealed so as to preserve its contents in a sterile condition; used principally for containing hypodermic solutions. Spelled also *ampul.*

ampulla (am-pul′lah), pl. *ampul′lae* [L. "a jug"] a general term used in anatomical nomenclature to designate a flasklike dilatation of a tubular structure.

ampullae (am-pul′le) [L.] plural of *ampulla.*

Ampullariella (am″pul-lar″ĭ-el′lah) a genus of soil bacteria of the family Actinoplanceae.

ampullate (am-pul′āt) flask-shaped.

amputation (am″pu-ta′shun) [L. *amputare* to cut off, or to prune] the removal or cutting off of an appendage or an outgrowth of the body, such as a limb, especially by surgery. **pulp a.**, pulpotomy. **root a.**, excision of one root of a multirooted tooth, or two roots of upper molars, usually associated with endodontic therapy of the remaining roots. Amputation of the root of a single-rooted tooth is called *apicoectomy,* and that of two roots of a two-rooted mandibular tooth is *hemisectomy.* Called also *radisectomy.* **spontaneous a.**, loss of a part which occurs without surgical intervention, as may occur in leprosy or diabetes mellitus.

amu atomic mass UNIT.

amygdala (ah-mig′dah-lah) [Gr. *amygdalē* almond] any almond-shaped structure, such as a tonsil. **accessory a., a. accesso′ria**, lingual TONSIL.

amygdalase (ah-mig′dah-lās) β-GLUCOSIDASE.

amygdalectomy (ah-mig″dah-lek′to-me) [*amygdalo-* + Gr. *ektomē* excision] 1. excision of the amygdaloid body. 2. excision of a tonsil; tonsillectomy.

amygdaline (ah-mig′dah-lin″) [L. *amygdalinus*] 1. like an almond. 2. pertaining to a tonsil; tonsillar.

amygdalitis (ah-mig″dah-li′tis) inflammation of a tonsil. See TONSILLITIS.

amygdalo- [Gr. *amygdalē* almond] a combining form denoting relationship to an almond-shaped structure or to the tonsil.

amygdaloid (ah-mig′dah-loid) [*amygdalo-* + Gr. *eidos* form] resembling an almond, or tonsil.

amygdalolith (ah-mig′dah-lo-lith″) [*amygdalo-* + Gr. *lithos* stone] a concretion or calculus in a tonsil; tonsillolith.

amygdalopathy (ah-mig″dah-lop′ah-the) [*amygdalo-* + Gr. *pathos* illness] any disease of a tonsil; tonsillopathy.

amygdalothrypsis (ah-mig″dah-lo-thrip′sis) [*amygdalo-* + Gr. *thrypsis* crushing] a procedure once used to remove a hypertrophied tonsil by crushing with a strong forceps.

amygdalotome (ah-mig′dah-lo-tōm″) [*amygdalo-* + Gr. *tomē* a cutting] tonsillotome.

amygdalotomy (ah-mig″dah-lot′o-me) [*amygdalo-* + Gr. *tomē* a cutting] 1. incision of the amygdaloid body. 2. tonsillotomy.

amyl (am′il) [Gr. *amylon* starch] the five-carbon aliphatic radical, C_5H_{11}, occurring in eight isomeric arrangements (exclusively of optical isomers). Called also *pentyl.* **a. nitrite**, amyl NITRITE.

amylase (am′ĭ-lās) a hydrolase that catalyzes the hydrolysis of starches into smaller molecules; it occurs in the saliva and pancreatic secretions. **α-a.** [E.C.3.2.1], an enzyme in the saliva and pancreatic juice (salivary and pancreatic α-amylase, respectively) that catalyzes the hydrolysis of starch, glycogen, and related polysaccharides and oligosaccharides, acting on the α-1,4-glycosidic linkages and breaking down carbohydrates into simpler structures during the process of digestion. Salivary and pancreatic amylases in humans are under the control of independent genetic loci. Called also *diastase* and *glycogenase.* **β-a.** [E.C.3.2.1.2], an enzyme found primarily in plants, which catalyzes the hydrolysis of starch, glycogen, and related polysaccharides and oligosaccharides by acting upon the α-1,4-glycosidic linkages and producing β-maltose by inversion. Called also *saccharogen a., diastase,* and *glycogenase.* **pancreatic a.**, α-amylase found in the pancreatic juice. **saccharogen a.**, β-a. **salivary a.**, α-amylase found in the saliva. Called also *ptyalase, ptyalin,* and *salivin.*

amylasuria (am″ĭ-lās-u′re-ah) [*amylase* + Gr. *ouron* urine + *-ia*] the presence of amylase in the urine.

amylbarbitone (am″il-bar′bĭ-tōn) British name for amobarbital. **a. sodium**, AMOBARBITAL sodium.

amylin (am′ĭ-lin) amylopectin.

amylo- [Gr. *amylon* starch] a combining form denoting relationship to starch.

amylogenic (am″ĭ-lo-jen′ik) [*amylo-* + Gr. *gennan* to produce] producing starch.

amyloid (am′ĭ-loid) [*amylo-* + Gr. *eidos* form] 1. resembling starch; characterized by a starchlike formation. 2. an abnormal complex material, most probably a glycoprotein, the exact biochemical composition of which has not been defined. Its protein component may be related to the immunoglobulins (gamma globulins), and its bears only a superficial resemblance to starch. 3. a substance produced by the action of sulfuric acid on cellulose; it gives a blue color when treated with iodine.

amyloidosis (am″ĭ-loi-do′sis) a systemic disease characterized by deposits of an eosinophilic glycoprotein in various tissues, particularly in small blood vessels and basement membranes, which causes weakness, dyspnea, weight loss, dysphagia, constipation, impotence, paresthesia, hypotension, purpura, and syncope. Oral symptoms include macroglossia and amyloid tumors, particularly in the tongue and gingivae. Generally, amyloidosis is classified as primary, secondary, familial, senile cardiac, associated with multiple myeloma, or associated with familial Mediterranean fever.

amylopectin (am″ĭ-lo-pek′tin) a polysaccharide (hexosan) which, together with amylose, makes up starch. It is a glucose polymer with both α-1,4 and α-1,6 linkages, representing the insoluble component of starch. Called also *amylin, α-amylose, insoluble amidine, starch cellulose,* and *tegumentary amidine.*

amylopectinosis (am″ĭ-lo-pek″tĭ-no′sis) GLYCOGENOSIS IV. **debrancher deficiency a.,** glycogenosis IV.

amylophosphorylase (am″ĭ-lo-fos-for′ĭ-lās) phosphorylase.

amylopsin (am″ĭ-lop′sin) [Gr. *amylon* starch + *pepsis* digestion] an enzyme in the pancreatic juice that catalyzes the hydrolysis of starches; it is similar to α-amylase.

amylorrhea (am″ĭ-lo-re′ah) [amylo- + Gr. *rhoia* flow] abnormal excretion of starches in the stools.

amylose (am′ĭ-lōs) [Gr. *amylon* starch] a polysaccharide (hexosan) which, together with amylopectin, makes up starch. It is a glucose polymer connected by α-1,4 linkages, representing the soluble component of starch. Microcrystalline amylose is available as a food ingredient and dietary energy source. **α-a.,** amylopectin.

amylosuria (am″ĭ-lo-su′re-ah) [amylo- + Gr. *ouron* urine + -ia] the presence of amylose in the urine.

amylosynthesis (am″ĭ-lo-sin′thĕ-sis) the synthesis of starch.

amyluria (am′ĭ-lu′re-ah) [amylo- + Gr. *ouron urine* + -ia] an excess of starch in the urine.

amyoplasia (ah-mi″o-pla′ze-ah) [a neg. + Gr. *mys* muscle + *plassein* to form + -ia] deficient muscle development. **a. congen′ita,** Guérin-Stern SYNDROME.

amyotonia (a″mi-o-to′ne-ah, ah-mi″o-to′ne-ah) [a neg. + Gr. *mys* muscle + *tonos* tension + -ia] atonic condition of the musculature of the body.

amyotrophic (ah-mi″o-trof′ik) pertaining to or characterized by amyotrophy.

amyotrophy (ah″mi-ot′ro-fe) [a neg. + Gr. *mys* muscle + *trophē* nourishment] atrophy of muscle tissue. Called also *muscular atrophy.*

Amytal trademark for *amobarbital.*

ANA American Nurses' Association.

ana- [Gr. *ana* up, back, again] a prefix indicating upward, backward, excessive, or again.

anabiosis (an″ah-bi-o′sis) [Gr. *anabiōsis* a reviving] restoration of vital processes after their apparent cessation.

anabiotic (an″ah-bi-ot′ik) apparently lifeless, but still capable of living.

Anabolex trademark for *stanolone.*

anabolic (an″ah-bol′ik) pertaining to or promoting anabolism.

anabolism (ah-nab′o-lizm″) [Gr. *anabolē* a thowing up] a biosynthetic phase of metabolism consisting of building up from simpler precursors of organic molecules, such as nucleic acids, proteins, polysaccharides, and lipids. The process consists of enzymatic synthesis and requires input of chemical energy which is supplied by the adenosine triphosphate generated during catabolism. Catabolism and anabolism take place concurrently in cells but they are usually regulated independently.

anabolite (ah-nab′o-līt) a product of anabolism.

Anacardone trademark for *nikethamide.*

anachoresis (an″ah-ko-re′sis) [Gr. *anachōrēsis* a retreating] the preferential collection or deposit of particles at a certain site, as of bacteria or of metals which have localized out of the blood stream in areas of inflammation. See also anachoretic PULPITIS.

anachoretic (an″ah-ko-ret′ik) pertaining to, characterized by, or resulting fron anachoresis.

anacidity (an″ah-sid′ĭ-te) [an neg. + acidity] lack of normal acidity.

Anadrol trademark for *oxymetholone.*

anaerobe (an-a′er-ōb) [an neg. + Gr. *aēr* air + *bios* life] a heterotrophic microorganism that lives and grows in the complete, or almost complete, absence of molecular oxygen, using organic compounds as electron acceptors. Called also *anaerobic cell, anaerobic microorganism,* and *anaerobic organism.* See also heterotrophic CELL. Cf. AEROBE. **facultative a.,** one capable of living under either anaerobic or aerobic conditions, using organic compounds as electron acceptors or oxygen, when it is present. Cf. facultative AEROBE. **obligate a., strict a.,** one capable of growing only in the complete absence of molecular oxygen, using organic compounds as electron acceptors, some being killed by oxygen.

anaerobic (an″a-er-o′bik) 1. lacking molecular oxygen. 2. growing in the absence of molecular oxygen.

Anaesthesin trademark for *benzocaine.*

analeptic (an″ah-lep′tik) [Gr. *analepsis* a repairing] a central nervous system stimulant.

analgesia (an″al-je′ze-ah) [an neg. + Gr. *algēsis* pain + -ia] loss of sensitivity to pain, which may affect the whole body or a part, without loss of consciousness. See also ANESTHESIA and HYPALGESIA. Cf. HYPERALGESIA and HYPERESTHESIA. **a. al′gera, a. doloro′sa,** spontaneous pain in a denervated part. Called also *anesthesia dolorosa.* **infiltration a.,** infiltration ANESTHESIA. **narcolocal a.,** local analgesia preceded by premedication. **paretic a.,** loss of the sense of pain accompanied by partial paralysis. **permeation a.,** permeation ANESTHESIA. **relative a.,** in dental anesthesia, a maintained level of conscious-sedation, short of general anesthesia, in which the pain threshold is elevated, usually induced by inhalation of nitrous oxide and oxygen. See also PSYCHOSEDATION. **surface a.,** topical ANESTHESIA. **unilateral a.,** hemianalgesia.

analgesic (an″al-je′sik) 1. relieving pain. 2. not sensitive to pain. 3. a chemical agent which relieves pain, usually by acting centrally to elevate the pain threshold without disturbing consciousness by interfering with pain impulses carried over nerve tracts at subcortical levels of the brain. Many analgesics act also as antipyretic and anti-inflammatory agents. They are usually classified as addicting and nonaddicting — addicting analgesics including opium derivatives (opiate analgesics) and nonopiates, while the nonaddicting agents are mostly salicylates and salicylate-like substances with acid side chains. Also classified under analgesics are endorphins and enkephalins, which are endogenous peptides with morphine-like action. Called also *acesodyne, analgetic,* and *anodyne,* and popularly *pain killer.* **addicting a., addictive a.,** one that is addictive or habit forming. Many are opium derivatives or opioids; they include morphine, codeine, ethylmorphine, hydrocodone, hydromorphone, levorphanol tartrate, oxymorphone, and benzylmorphine. Nonopiate addictive analgesics include alphaprodine, anileridine, fentanyl citrate, meperidine hydrochloride, methadone, pentazocine, phenazocine, and piminodine esylate. **narcotic a.,** any natural or synthetic drug that has morphine-like pharmacological properties, producing analgesia associated with drowsiness, mental clouding, and changes of mood, without loss of consciousness, and being to a greater or lesser degree addictive or habit-forming. Called also *opioid a.* and *opioid.* See also NARCOTIC. **opiate a.,** an addicting analgesic that is an opium derivative, such as morphine. See also OPIATE. **opioid a.,** narcotic a.

Analgesine trademark for *antipyrine.*

analgetic (an″al-jet′ik) analgesic.

analgia (an-al′je-ah) [an neg. + Gr. *algos* pain + -ia] absence of pain.

analgic (an-al′jik) insensible to pain.

analog (an′ah-log) analogue.

analogue (an′ah-log) 1. a part or organ having the same function as another, but of a different evolutionary origin. 2. a chemical compound with a structure similar to that of another, but differing from it in respect to a certain component. A compound with similar electronic structure but different atoms. Written also *analog.* **folic acid a.,** a substance structurally similar to folic acid, an essential dietary vitamin concerned with the metabolic transfer of one-carbon units into molecules, thus being its competitive inhibitor. Folic acid analogues are antimetabolites. Their site of action is the enzyme dihydrofolate dehydrogenase, which interferes with enzymatic reduction of folic acid to tetrahydrofolic acid and related compounds, such as folinic acid, which are coenzymes for metabolic reactions. The metabolic reactions include synthesis of the DNA constituent thymidylic acid and inhibition of formation of both DNA and RNA. Used chiefly in the treatment of neoplasms, methotrexate being the principal folic acid analogue. Called also *antifolate, folic acid antagonist,* and *folic acid inhibitor.* **purine a.,** a substance structurally similar to purine, purine bases being components of nucleotide subunits from which DNA and RNA molecules are formed. Purine analogues are antimetabolites which, by interfering with DNA and RNA synthesis, inhibit tissue proliferation; thus they are used in the treatment of cancer, chiefly leukemias. They are also used as immunosuppressive agents in tissue and organ transplantation. Mercaptopurine and thioguanine are the principal purine analogues used clinically. Called also *purine antagonist*. **pyrimidine a.**, a substance structurally similar to pyrimidine, including ones that have been altered by substitution in the ring, changes in the ring structure, or changes in the sugar moiety of the nucleoside. Pyrimidine analogues are antimetabolites which interfere with pyrimidine metabolism by competitive inhibition, pyrimidine bases being components of nucleotide subunits from which DNA and RNA molecules are formed. Because of their ability to inhibit the synthesis of nucleic acids in proliferating tissues, they are used as antineoplastic agents. Halogenated pyrimidines, such as fluorouracil, are typical analogues used in cancer therapy. The bone marrow and mucosa of the gastrointestinal system and oral cavity are the target tissue for their cytotoxic action. Anorexia, diarrhea, nausea, gastrointestinal necrosis, dysphagia, proctitis, susceptibility to infection, retrosternal burning, alopecia, hyperpigmentation, and bone marrow depression with leukopenia, thrombocytopenia, and anemia are the most common adverse reactions. Oral changes may include xerostomia, stomatitis and necrosis of the oral mucosa with patchy membranes, erythema, and ulcers. Called also *pyrimidine antagonist*.

analphalipoproteinemia (an-al″fah-lip″o-pro″te-in-e′me-ah) Tangier DISEASE.

analysis (ah-nal′ĭ-sis), pl. *anal′yses* [ana- + Gr. *lysis* dissolution] 1. separation of a substance into component parts in order to ascertain its nature and composition. 2. the process or method of studying the nature of something, or of determining its essential features. **bite a.**, occlusal a. **cephalometric a.**, a cephalometric analysis based on the tracing of the x-ray photograph of the living head, usually in the lateral view. **Downs' a.**, roentgenographic cephalometric criteria used for orthodontic diagnosis. **occlusal a.**, an analysis of the contact of the teeth in centric relation and during excursions of the mandible to determine if occlusal dysfunction is present. Called also *bite a.* **radiochemical a.**, determination of the content of an element in a chemical compound using a method of measuring the disintegration rate of radionuclides.

analyzer (an′ah-li″zer) 1. one who or that which analyzes. 2. a prism attached to a polarizing apparatus which extinguishes the ray of light polarized by the polarizer. 3. Pavlov's name for a specialized part of the nervous system which controls the reactions of the organism to changing external conditions. 4. a nervous receptor together with its central connections, by means of which sensitivity to stimulations is differentiated. **amino acid a.**, an analytical instrument that separates, identifies, and measures quantities of amino acids and related compounds. **blood gas a.**, an instrument for measuring partial pressure of oxygen, carbon dioxide, carbon monoxide, and nitrogen in the blood. **breath a.**, an instrument for determining the volume and composition of respired gases; some types are specifically designed for detecting alcohol in the breath. See also CAPNOGRAPH, OXIMETER, and SPIROMETER. **carbon dioxide a.**, capnograph. **oxygen gas a.**, an instrument for measuring the oxygen content of a gaseous mixture, or dissolved oxygen in a liquid, or saturation of blood hemoglobin with oxygen, or partial pressure of oxygen in blood.

anamnesis (an″am-ne′sis) [Gr. *anamnēsis* a recalling] 1. the faculty of memory. 2. the collected data concerning a patient, his family, previous environment, and experiences, past history of disease or injury based on the patient's own memory or recall at the time of dental and/or medical interview and examination, as well as any results of treatment.

anaphase (an′ah-fāz) [ana- + *phase*] that stage of mitosis or meiosis, following metaphase, in which the centromeres split and the chromatids that are lined up on the spindle begin to move apart toward the pole of the spindle to form the daughter chromosomes. See MEIOSIS and MITOSIS.

anaphylactic (an″ah-fi-lak′tik) pertaining to or possessing anaphylaxis.

anaphylactin (an″ah-fi-lak′tin) the antibody in anaphylaxis; it reacts with antigen on smooth muscles, and on blood vessels with the release of pharmacologically active mediators such as histamines. Called also *anaphylactic antibody*.

anaphylactogen (an″ah-fi-lak′to-jen) a substance capable of inducing anaphylaxis. See also ALLERGEN (1), ANAPHYLACTIN, and SENSITINOGEN.

anaphylactoid (an″ah-fi-lak′toid) resembling anaphylaxis.

anaphylatoxin (an″ah-fi″lah-tok′sin) a substance produced upon the activation of complement which serves as a mediator of inflammation. Injection into animals results in the development of signs and symptoms consistent with those of systemic anaphylaxis. Anaphylatoxin activity is a property of low-molecular-weight complement fragments C3a and C5a.

anaphylaxis (an″ah-fi-lak′sis) [ana- + Gr. *phylaxis* protection] an immediate allergic reaction exhibiting extreme sensitivity of the body to a foreign substance. It may be systemic (generalized) or localized (cutaneous). Called also *allergic shock, hypersusceptibility, protein sensitization,* and *Theobald Smith phenomenon.* See also immediate HYPERSENSITIVITY. **acquired a.**, that in which sensitization is known to have been produced by the administration of a foreign immunogen. **active a.**, the anaphylactic state triggered in an individual by the injection of a foreign immunogen; distinguished from passive anaphylaxis. **active cutaneous a.**, cutaneous a., active. **aggregate a.**, an anaphylactic reaction in which antigen may be injected immediately after the injection of antiserum, occurring after the release of mediators that is secondarily triggered by antigen-antibody complexes. **antiserum a.**, passive a. **cutaneous a., active**, localized anaphylaxis in the form of the wheal and flare reaction on injection of antigen into the skin of a sensitized subject. Used as a test for allergy to substances such as pollen. Occasionally seen as a cutaneous manifestation of generalized anaphylaxis. **cutaneous a., passive**, localized anaphylaxis passively transferred by intradermal injection of a cytotropic antibody and, after a latent period (about 24 to 72 hours), intravenous injection of the homologous antigen and Evans blue dye. Blueing of the skin at the site of the intradermal injection is evidence of increased local vascular permeability. Used in studies of antibodies causing immediate hypersensitivity reactions. Abbreviated PCA. **cytotoxic a.**, that following the injection of antibodies specific for natural antigenic constituents of the body cell surfaces. **cytotropic a.**, that induced by antigen reacting with antibody which has become fixed to mediator cells (e.g., mast cells, basophilic leukocytes) that release mediators of anaphylaxis when reacting with allergen. **generalized a.**, a widespread anaphylactic reaction. In the laboratory, it is produced by injecting a small dose of antigen (sensitizing dose) which leads to antibody production. Anaphylaxis is then induced by a secondary intravenous dose of antigen (challenging dose). In the guinea pig, the condition is characterized by scratching, sneezing, coughing, convulsions, collapse and death due to respiratory impairment resulting from constriction of smooth muscle in the bronchioles and bronchial edema. A sharp drop in blood pressure and increased vascular permeability may be associated. In the rabbit, the shock organ is the heart, and right-sided heart failure is the main cause of death. In man, the condition is characterized by itching, erythema, vomiting, abdominal cramps, diarrhea, and respiratory distress. In severe cases, laryngeal edema and vascular collapse may result in death. For localized anaphylactic phenomena, see *cutaneous a., active, cutaneous a., passive,* and Arthus REACTION. **heterologous a.**, passive anaphylaxis induced by the transference of serum antibody from a donor animal of a species different from that of the recipient. **homologous a.**, passive anaphylaxis induced by the transference of serum antibody from one animal to another of the same species. **indirect a.**, that induced by an animal's own antigen modified in some way. **inverse a.**, 1. that in which the shocking agent is antibody (anaphylactin) rather than antigen (anaphylactogen). 2. anaphylactic shock produced by a single intravenous injection into guinea pigs of Forssman antibody which interacts with Forssman antigen in their tissues. **local a.**, that confined to a limited area, e.g., cutaneous anaphylaxis. See also Arthus REACTION. **passive a.**, that occurring in a normal individual as a result of the transfer of serum antibody of a previously sensitized individual. Called also *antiserum a.* **passive cutaneous a.**, cutaneous a., passive. **reverse a., reverse passive a.**, that produced by the injection of antigen followed by the injection of antiserum; also, local reactions from the union of circulating antibodies with antigen fixed by tissue cells.

anaplasia (an″ah-pla′ze-ah) [ana- + Gr. *plassein* to form] a condition marked by regressive changes in adult cells toward more primitive (embryonic) cell types, considered as a criterion of malignancy of neoplasms. Called also *dedifferentiation, reversionary atrophy,* and *undifferentiation.* Cf. DYSPLASIA (2) and METAPLASIA.

Anaplasma (an″ah-plaz′mah) [Gr. *anaplasma* something without form] a genus of bacteria of the family Anaplasmataceae, order Rickettsiales, appearing in the erythrocytes as dense, homogeneous round bodies, 0.3 to 1.0 μm in size. The organisms of this genus are obligate parasites, which are transmitted to vertebrates by arthropods, and infecting ruminants only.

Anaplasmataceae (an″ah-plaz″mah-ta′se-e) [*Anaplasma* + *-aceae*] a family of gram-negative, non–acid-fast bacteria of the order Rickettsiales, made up of obligately parasitic organisms that are sometimes pathogenic (anemia being the principal symptom), which are generally found in the blood, particularly within or on erythrocytes of various wild and domestic vertebrates. The organisms are sensitive to tetracyclines. The family Anaplasmataceae includes the genera *Anaplasma* and *Haemobartonella*.

anaplasmosis (an″ah-plaz-mo′sis) infection with any organism of the genus *Anaplasma*.

Anapresin trademark for *guanethidine*.

Anarcon trademark for *nalorphine*.

Anarexol trademark for *cyproheptadine hydrochloride* (see under CYPROHEPTADINE).

anasarca (an″ah-sar′kah) [*ana-* + Gr. *sarx* flesh] the diffuse swelling of the subcutaneous tissue seen in edema.

anasterone (an″ah-ste′rōn) oxymetholone.

anastomosis (ah-nas″to-mo′sis), pl. *anastomo′ses* [Gr. *anastomō-sis* opening, outlet] 1. a communication or opening between two blood vessels. 2. an opening between two normally distinct spaces or organs, created by pathological processes, surgical procedures, or trauma. **arteriovenous a.,** direct interconnection between an artery and a vein, bypassing the capillary bed.

anat. anatomy; anatomical.

Anatensol trademark for *fluphenazine hydrochloride* (see under FLUPHENAZINE).

anatomical (an″ah-tom′ĭ-kal) pertaining to anatomy, or to the structure of the organism.

anatomist (ah-nat′o-mist) a specialist in the field of anatomy.

anatomy (ah-nat′o-me) [*ana-* + Gr. *temnein* to cut] 1. the science of the structure of an organism; morphology. 2. dissection of the body for the purpose of studying its various parts. **comparative a.,** a comparison of the structure of different animals and plants, one with another. **dental a.,** the study of the structure of the teeth and the relations of the dental organs toward each other and toward the adjoining parts, organs, and systems functionally related to the teeth. **descriptive a.,** the study and description of particular systems, organs, or parts of the body. Called also *systematic a.* **developmental a.,** anatomical changes taking place during the embryologic development of the organism. See also EMBRYOLOGY. **general a.,** the study of the structure and composition of the body and its tissues and fluids. **gross a., macroscopic a.,** the study of body structures that are visible to the naked eye. **medical a.,** application of anatomy to the study of the causes, manifestations, and treatment of diseases. **microscopic a., minute a.,** that which is studied only with the aid of a microscope. See HISTOLOGY. **morbid a., pathologic a.,** the anatomical study of diseased structures. Called also PATHOANATOMY. See HISTOPATHOLOGY and PATHOLOGY. **radiological a.,** the study of the anatomy of organs based on their x-ray visualization. Called also *x-ray a.* **regional a.,** the study of limited areas or portions of the body. **surgical a.,** the consideration of anatomy as applied to the diagnosis and treatment of surgical conditions. **systematic a.,** descriptive a. **x-ray a.,** radiological a.

Anautine trademark for *dimenhydrinate*.

Anavar trademark for *oxandrolone*.

Anayodin trademark for *sodium iodide* (see under SODIUM).

Ancef trademark for *cefazolin sodium* (see under CEFAZOLIN).

anchor (ang′ker) a means by which something is held securely. **endosteal implant a.,** a metal implant in the shape of a ship's anchor, usually made of a chromium-cobalt alloy, being a part of the substructure of an implant denture, which is placed deeply into the bone to provide retention for the prosthesis. See also endosseous IMPLANT, implant DENTURE, implant SUBSTRUCTURE, and subperiosteal IMPLANT. **a. molar,** anchor MOLAR.

anchorage (ang′ker-ij) 1. to keep hold or be firmly fixed. 2. fixation. 3. in operative dentistry, the fixation of fillings or of artificial crowns or bridges. 4. in orthodontics, the nature and degree of resistance to displacement offered by an anatomical unit when used for the purpose of effecting tooth movement. See illustration. **Baker a.,** an intermaxillary anchorage designed for the adjustment of jaw relationships and teeth through the use of rubber elastics from the maxilla to the mandible. See illustration. **cervical a.,** an orthodontic anchor-

age in which the back of the neck is used for resistance through a strap fitted around the neck. **compound a.,** an orthodontic

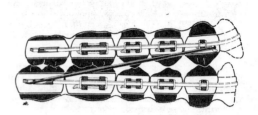

A

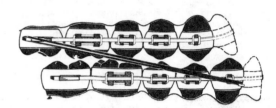

B

Baker anchorage. *A,* for Class II malocclusion; *B,* for Class III malocclusion. (From T. M. Graber: Orthodontics — Principles and Practice. 3rd ed., Philadelphia, W. B. Saunders Co., 1972.)

anchorage in which the resistance is obtained from two or more teeth. **extramaxillary a.,** extraoral a. **extraoral a.,** an orthodontic anchorage in which the resistance unit is outside the oral cavity, as in cranial, occipital, or cervical anchorage (headgear). Called also *extramaxillary a.* **intermaxillary a.,** an orthodontic anchorage in which the resistance units situated in one jaw are used to effect tooth movement in the other jaw. Called also *maxillomandibular a.* **intraoral a.,** an orthodontic anchorage in which the resistance units are all located within the oral cavity. **maxillomandibular a.,** intermaxillary a. **multiple a.,** an orthdontic anchorage in which more than one type of resistance unit is used. Called also *reinforced a.* **occipital a.,** an orthodontic anchorage in which the resistance is borne by the top and back of the head, and the force transmitted to the teeth by means of the headgear and heavy elastics connected with attachment on the teeth. **precision a.,** precision ATTACHMENT. **reciprocal a.,** an orthodontic anchorage in which the movement of one or more dental units is balanced against the movement of one or more opposing dental units. See also reciprocal FORCE. **reinforced a.,** multiple a. **simple a.,** an orthodontic anchorage in which larger teeth or groups of teeth and their location are used to move teeth of lesser size; the resistance to the movement comes solely from resistance to tipping movement of the anchored unit. **stationary r.,** an orthodontic anchorage in which the resistance to the movement of one or more dental units comes from the resistance to bodily movement of the anchorage unit.

ancillary (an′sil-lār′e) [L. *ancillaris* relating to a maid servant] assisting in the performance of a service; auxiliary. 2. ancillary PERSONNEL. **a. personnel,** ancillary PERSONNEL.

Ancobon trademark for *flucytosine*.

Ancorvis hinge see under HINGE.

Ancotil trademark for *flucytosine*.

ancylo- see ANKYLO-.

Andersch's ganglion [Carolus Samuel *Andersch,* German anatomist, 18th century] inferior ganglion of glossopharyngeal nerve; see under GANGLION.

Andersen's disease, syndrome (triad) [Dorothy Hansine *Andersen,* American physician, born 1901] see GLYCOGENOSIS IV, and see under SYNDROME.

Anderson's operation see under OPERATION.

Andramine trademark for *dimenhydrinate*.

Andresen appliance, Andresen monoblock appliance [V. *Andresen,* Norwegian orthodontist] functional ACTIVATOR.

Andrews bar (bridge) see under BAR.

TYPES OF ANCHORAGE

1. SIMPLE ANCHORAGE
2. STATIONARY ANCHORAGE
3. RECIPROCAL ANCHORAGE
4. INTRA—ORAL ANCHORAGE
5. EXTRA—ORAL ANCHORAGE
6. INTRAMAXILLARY ANCHORAGE
7. INTERMAXILLARY ANCHORAGE
8. MULTIPLE OR REINFORCED ANCHORAGE.

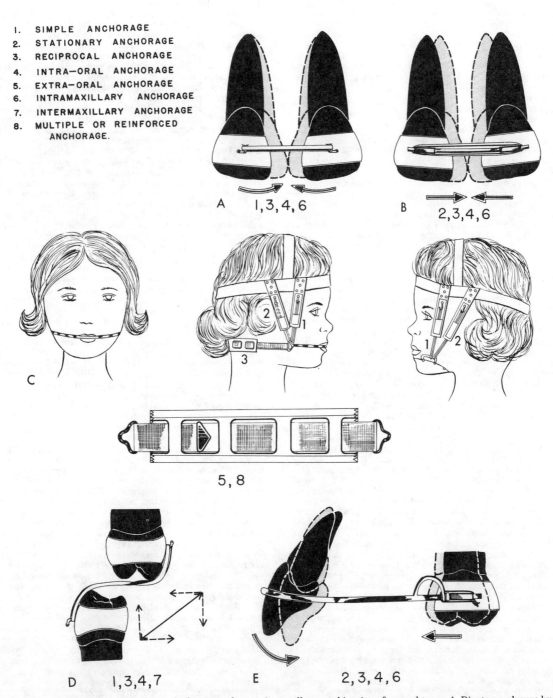

A 1,3,4,6

B 2,3,4,6

C

5, 8

D 1,3,4,7

E 2,3,4,6

Types of anchorage. Diagrams show that orthodontic anchorage is usually a combination of several types. *A*, Diastema closure by elastic action tipping crowns together. *B*, Bodily movement of incisors to close diastema. *C*, Extraoral force. *D*, Criss-cross elastics to correct cross-bite. *E*, Retraction of maxillary incisors by tipping them lingually. Molar resistance is of a bodily nature. Under *C*, you will note three directions of extraoral force pull: 1 is vertical for open bites; 2 is oblique for mandibular prognathism; 3 is horizontal for cervical traction. Direction is important with force magnitude within tooth moving range, less important with orthopedic force. (From T. M. Graber: Orthodontics — Principles and Practice. 3rd ed., Philadelphia, W. B. Saunders Co., 1972.)

Androcur trademark for *cyproterone acetate* (see under CYPRO-TERONE).

Androfluorene trademark for *fluoxymesterone.*

androgen (an'dro-jen) [Gr. *anēr, andros* man + *gennan* to produce] a male sex hormone produced chiefly by the testes and also by the adrenal cortices and ovaries, serving as the precursor for sex hormones. All natural androgens are steroids and derive from androstane. Generally, they are responsible for the development of male sex organs and the distinguishing characteristics of the masculine body. Testosterone is the prototype of androgens. There are numerous synthetic androgens.

Androlin trademark for *testosterone.*

Androlone trademark for *stanolone.*

Androsan trademark for *methyltestosterone.*

androstanazole (an"dro-stan'ah-zōl) stanozolol.

androstane (an'dro-stān) a class of steroid compounds having methyl groups at C-10 and C-13. See also STEROID.

Androsterolo trademark for *fluoxymesterone.*

Anectine trademark for *succinylcholine chloride* (see under SUC-CINYLCHOLINE).

Anel operation, probe [Dominique *Anel,* French surgeon, 1679–1730] see under OPERATION and PROBE.

anelasticity (an-e"las-tis'ĭ-te) viscoelasticity.

anemia (ah-ne'me-ah) [Gr. *an* neg. + *haima* blood + *-ia*] a condition characteristized by a decreased oxygen-carrying capacity of the blood with symptoms of hypoxia, caused by a reduced number of circulating erythrocytes or a reduced concentration of hemoglobin in the peripheral blood. See also OLIGEMIA, OLIGOCHROMEMIA, and OLIGOCYTHEMIA. **achlorhydric a.,** iron-deficiency a. **achlorhydric a., simple,** hypochromic a., essential. **Addison's a., Addison-Biermer a.,** pernicious a. **African a.,** sickle cell a. **aplastic a.,** a form of pancytopenia resulting from bone marrow aplasia, associated with faulty erythropoiesis, thrombocytopenia, and leukopenia. Pallor, fever, dyspnea, weakness, numbness and tingling of the extremities, and edema are the most common symptoms. Other symptoms include petechiae, purpura, and hematomas, with nasal, oral, and gastrointestinal bleeding, and gingival and pharyngeal ulcers. Hematological changes include a lowered hemoglobin level and packed red cells and the presence of circulating immature red cells. The bone marrow is composed typically of yellowish material containing fat, fibrous tissue, and lymphocytes. Extravasated blood may be present. The primary form is relatively rare, occurring mostly in young adults and ending in death. Secondary anemia may be produced by a variety of agents, including ionizing radiations, cytostatic agents, benzene derivatives, certain antibiotics, such as chloramphenicol, antimetabolites, arsenicals, insecticides, and a number of other chemical compounds; this form may occur at any age and improvement may be obtained by removing the cause. Called also *aregenerative a., bone marrow a., hypoplastic a., toxic a., toxic paralytic a., aleukia hemorrhagica, panmyelopthisis,* and *progressive hypocythemia.* **aplastic a. with congenital anomalies,** Fanconi's a. **aregenerative a.,** aplastic a. **Benjamin's a.,** Benjamin's SYNDROME. **Biermer's a.,** pernicious a. **congenital aplastic a.,** Fanconi's a. **congenital hemolytic a.,** hereditary SPHEROCYTOSIS. **congenital hypoplastic a.,** Diamond-Blackfan SYNDROME. **congenital a. of newborn,** ERYTHROBLASTOSIS fetalis. **Cooley's a.,** hereditary hemolytic anemia, which is the homozygous form of β-thalassemia, occurring in infancy and childhood, usually in persons of Mediterranean extraction. It is characterized by continued production of fetal hemoglobin and skeletal changes resulting from erythroid hyperplasia, which includes trabecular striation of the cortices of the long bones and the "hair-on-end" appearance of the skull. The hematologic changes consist of hypochromic microcytic anemia with anisocytosis, poikilocytosis, target cells, stippled cells, normoblastosis, reticulocytosis, and moderate leukocytosis. Pallor, prominent abdomen due to hepatosplenomegaly, fever, growth retardation, large head, frontal bossing, mongoloid facies, muddy color of the skin, and jaundice may occur. Oral manifestations usually include prominence of the premaxilla with malocclusion, pallor of the oral mucosa, trabecular pattern of the jaws on the roentgenogram, with coarsening of some trabeculae and the disappearance of others, resulting in a "salt-and-pepper effect," and mild osteoporosis. Some children die before reaching adolescence. Called also *erythroblastic a., Mediterranean a., target cell a., chronic familial erythremia, thalassemia major,* and *thalassemic syndrome.* Cf. THALASSEMIA minor. **Diamond-Blackfan a.,** Diamond-Blackfan SYNDROME. **erythroblastic a.,** Cooley's a. **Faber's a.,** hypochromic

a., essential. **Fanconi's a., Fanconi's refractory a.,** aplastic anemia associated with a wide spectrum of congenital disorders, consisting of generalized purpura present at birth or shortly thereafter, brown patchy pigmentation, dwarfism, microcephaly, hypogonadism, cryptorchism, hypospadias, strabismus, microphthalmia, ptosis, epicanthal folds, nystagmus, deafness, ear deformity, syndactyly, Sprengel's deformity, bone defects of the radial sides of the forearm and hand, obesity, exaggerated tendon reflexes, mental retardation, cleft palate, and splenic atrophy, together with symptoms typical of aplastic anemia. It is familial and is believed to be transmitted as an autosomal recessive trait. Called also *aplastic a. with congenital anomalies, congenital aplastic a., aplastic infantile funicular myelosis,* and *congenital pancytopenia.* **familial hemolytic hypochromic a., familial microcytic a.,** THALASSEMIA minor. **hemolytic a.,** any anemia, especially hereditary spherocytosis, hereditary elliptocytosis, the thalassemias, and sickle cell anemia, in which there is premature destruction of erythrocytes and hemolysis. The onset may be preceded by episodes of weakness and yellow discoloration of the skin. Abdominal pain, gallbladder disease, and leg ulcers are the principal symptoms of mild chronic cases. Acute cases may be marked by acute fever, weakness, irritability, pain in the extremities, nausea, vomiting, anorexia, and general malaise, and hemorrhagic manifestations may be present. In severe cases, there may be hemoglobinuria, hematuria, anuria, shock, splenomegaly, and skeletal abnormalities, including abnormalities of the skull, general underdevelopment, and supernumerary digits. See also HEMOLYSIS. **hemolytic a., autoimmune,** hemolytic anemia which, in addition to other features of hemolytic anemia, is also characterized by the presence of antibodies on the surface of the erythrocytes and a positive Coombs antiglobulin test. That occurring in association with other diseases, such as lupus erythematosus or lymphoma, is known as *secondary* or *symptomatic;* that occurring alone without associated diseases, is known as *primary* or *idiopathic.* The condition has further been divided into a variant involving cold hemagglutinins (0–4° C) and warm hemagglutinins (37 C). **hemolytic familial nonspherocytic a.,** a congenital familial form of chronic hemolytic anemia characterized by jaundice, hepatomegaly, splenomegaly, osseous changes, and a tendency toward the development of mongoloid facies. The erythrocytes are normochromic and normocytic to macrocytic and have normal osmotic and mechanical fragility. Called also *Zuelzer-Kaplan syndrome.* **hemolytic a. of Marchiafava,** Marchiafava-Micheli SYNDROME. **hypochromic a.,** anemia characterized by hypochromic erythrocytes, usually due to iron deficiency and also caused by impaired hemoglobin synthesis determined by genetic or acquired factors, such as lead poisoning. Hypochromic and iron-deficiency anemias are considered as being synonymous, but some types of hypochromic anemias are not associated with iron deficiency and some mild cases of iron deficiency are often not hypochromic. Clinical features and symptoms of hypochromic anemia are similar to those seen in iron-deficiency anemia. **hypochromic a., essential,** a chronic iron-deficiency anemia with a low corpuscular concentration of hemoglobin, characterized by small, pale-red erythrocytes, associated with achlorhydria, koilonychia, and glossitis. Called also *chronic microcytic a., Faber's a., simple achlorhydric a.,* and *chronic chlorosis.* **hypochromic familial hemolytic a.,** THALASSEMIA minor. **hypochromic microcytic a.,** iron-deficiency a. **hypoplastic a.,** aplastic a. **hypoplastic a. of childhood,** Diamond-Blackfan SYNDROME. **icterohemolytic a.,** acquired hemolytic JAUNDICE. **iron-deficiency a.,** anemia due to deficiency of iron in the blood, characterized by hypochromic and microcytic erythrocytes. Stained blood initially shows pale small red cells and a few elliptocytes and, as the condition progresses, hypochromia, anisocytosis, poikilocytosis, and microcytosis, with mean corpuscular volume being less than 80 cuμ, mean corpuscular hemoglobin less than 30 $\mu\mu$, and mean corpuscular hemoglobin concentration less than 30 percent. Craving for ice, pallor of the skin and mucosa, palpitation, dyspnea, vertigo, fatigability, epigastric pain, whiteness of the sclera, dryness of the hair, spoon-shaped nails, and achlorhydria are the most common symptoms. Oral symptoms may include fissuring at the angles of the mouth, stomatitis, atrophy of the papillae of the tongue, paleness of the tongue, giving it a shiny smooth appearance, a burning sensation of the tongue, sensitivity to hot or spicy foods, and dysphagia. Leukoplakia and carcinoma sometimes occur in areas of mucosal atrophy. Causes may include dietary iron deficiency (see also table under NUTRITION); faulty iron absorption, especially after gastrectomy; pregnancy, particularly when complicated by vaginal bleeding; hemorrhage, as in peptic ulcer; hiatal hernia; gastrointestinal cancer; vaginal bleeding; excessive blood donation; and intravascular hemolysis. Iron-deficiency and hypochromic anemias are sometimes considered as being synonymous, but some types of hypochromic anemia are not associated with iron deficiency and some mild cases of iron-deficiency anemia are often not hypochromic. Called also *achlorhydric a., hypochromic microcytic a.,* and *chlorosis.* See also Plummer-Vinson SYNDROME. **macrocytic a.,** anemia in which the erythrocytes are larger than normal, associated with a decrease in the number of erythrocytes, the amount of hemoglobin, and the volume of packed erythrocytes. **Marchiafava's hemolytic a.,** Marchiafava-Micheli SYNDROME. **Mediterranean a.,** Cooley's a. **megaloblastic a.,** one of several anemias, especially pernicious anemia, caused by deficiency, faulty utilization, or excessive requirement of vitamin B_{12} or folic acid, and the presence in the blood of megaloblasts. **microcytic a.,** anemia in which the erythrocytes are smaller than normal, associated with a decreased volume of hemoglobin; copper deficiency may be a cause. **microcytic a., chronic,** hypochromic a., essential. **microcytic a., hypochromic,** iron-deficiency a. **normocytic a.,** anemia in which there is a proportionate decrease in the number of erythrocytes, the quantity of hemoglobin, and the volume of packed cells, while the erythrocytes (normocytes) retain their normal size, shape, and hemoglobin content. **pernicious a.,** a chronic megaloblastic anemia caused by cyanocobalamin (vitamin B_{12}) deficiency and the lack of intrinsic factor, which is characterized by faulty maturation of the erythrocytes with the formation of abnormally large megaloblastic precursors, pathological changes in the gastric mucosa, degenerative changes in the spinal cord and white matter of the brain, and specific oral manifestations. It occurs most commonly in middle-aged and elderly individuals, and is associated with weakness, pallor, shortness of breath, digital paresthesias, numbness, lack of coordination, spasticity, difficulty in walking, decreased sense of taste and smell, mental dullness, apathy, and sometimes psychoses. Gastrointestinal changes include achylia gastrica, diarrhea, and constipation. The peripheral blood may show low red cell counts, oval spherocytosis, poikilocytosis, leukopenia with hypersegmented polymorphonuclear leukocytes, thrombocytopenia, and eosinophilia. The bone marrow is usually hypercellular and shows abnormal white and red cells. Oral symptoms include glossitis, glossodynia, and glossopyrosis associated with excoriation of the tongue, chiefly of the tip and edges, and beefy red lesions characteristic of Moeller's and Hunter's glossitis (see under GLOSSITIS). Periods of remission and exacerbation with parallel blood changes occur. Called also *Addison's a., Addison-Biermer a.,* and *Biermer's a.* **primary a.,** that due to diseases of the hematopoietic system. **primary refractory a.,** aplastic a. **pure red cell a.,** Diamond-Blackfan SYNDROME. **secondary a.,** that due to anemia resulting from diseases originating outside of the hematopoietic system. **sickle cell a.,** a hereditary form of hemolytic anemia, occurring almost exclusively in persons of Negro ancestry, transmitted as a dominant trait, and affecting women more often than men. Crystallization of sickle cell hemoglobin in the presence of low oxygen tension and reduced pH in the blood is responsible for the sickling phenomenon, resulting in the appearance of sickle-shaped erythrocytes in the blood and increased viscosity of capillary blood. The onset occurs early in life, after normal hemoglobin is replaced with sickle cell hemoglobin, characterized by arthralgia and abdominal cramps. Greenish-yellow sclera, blindness, nystagmus, pale mucosae, weakness, fatigability, sinus arrhythmia, prominent pulsation in the neck area, moderate hepatomegaly, hematuria, leg ulcers, kyphosis, scoliosis, oxycephaly, hemiplegia, epistaxis, coma, aphasia, stupor, cranial nerve palsies, headache, convulsions, and other symptoms may occur. Oral manifestations may include osteoporosis of the jaws, showing trabecular changes in the alveolar bones and large, irregular marrow spaces on the roentgenogram. Called also *African a., hemoglobin S disease,* and *sicklemia.* See also sickle cell TRAIT. **splenic a., familial,** Gaucher's DISEASE. **target cell a.,** Cooley's a. **toxic a., toxic paralytic a.,** aplastic a.

anencephaly (an″en-sef′ah-le) [*an* neg. + Gr. *enkephalos* brain] a congenital abnormality characterized by the absence of the cranial vault above the orbital ridges. Portions of the inferior edge of the parietal bones may persist; but the squamous part of the occipital bone is absent. The cerebral hemispheres are usually missing or consist of a formless, reddish mass, composed of thin-walled vascular channels.

anenzymia (an″en-zi′me-ah) [*an* neg. *enzyme* Gr. *haima* blood + *-ia*] deficiency of enzymes normally present in the blood. **a. catala′sea,** acatalasia.

anergy (an′er-je) the loss of a previous reactivity to specific antigen(s); the loss may include either immediate hypersensitivity or delayed hypersensitivity, or both.

anesthesia (an″es-the′ze-ah) [*an* neg. + Gr. *aisthēsis* sensation] 1.

partial or total absence of sensation to stimuli, such as cold, heat, touch, or painful irritation, usually resulting from pathologic disruption of nerve transmission. 2. lack of sensitivity to pain, especially insensitivity to pain induced by artificial means, such as drugs, for the purpose of performing surgery or other painful procedure. See also ANALGESIA and anesthetic TEST. Cf. HYPALGESIA and HYPERALGESIA. **angiospastic a.,** loss of sensibility dependent on spasm of the blood vessels. **balanced a.,** an anesthetic method with the use of a combination of drugs, each in an amount sufficient to produce its desired effect to the optimum degree and keep its undesirable effects to a minimum. See also *mixed a.* **basal a.,** that which acts as a basis for further and deeper anesthesia; a state of narcosis produced by preliminary medication so profound that the added inhalation anesthetic necessary to produce surgical anesthesia is greatly reduced. **Bier's local a.,** intravenous regional anesthesia produced by injecting 0.5 percent procaine solution into a vein of an extremity rendered bloodless by elevation and constriction. Called also *vein a.* **block a.,** peripheral nerve block a. **bulbar a.,** lack of sensation caused by a lesion of the pons. **caudal a.,** epidural anesthesia in which the anesthetic has been introduced into the caudal segment of the vertebral canal. **central a.,** lack of sensation caused by disease of the nerve centers. **cerebral a.,** lack of sensation caused by a cerebral lesion. **closed a.,** inhalation anesthesia maintained by the continuous rebreathing of a relatively small amount of the anesthetic gas, normally used with an absorption apparatus for the removal of carbon dioxide. **compression a.,** loss of sensation resulting from pressure on a nerve. **conduction a.,** regional a. **dissociated a., dissociation a.,** loss of certain sensations while others remain intact. **doll's head a.,** loss of sensation affecting the head, neck, and upper part of the thorax. **a. doloro′sa,** ANALGESIA algera. **electric a.,** that induced by passage of an electric current. **endobronchial a.,** that produced by introduction of a gaseous mixture through a slender tube placed into a large bronchus. **endotracheal a.,** that produced by introduction of a gaseous mixture through a wide-bore tube inserted into the trachea. **epidural a.,** regional anesthesia produced by the deposition of a local anesthetic into the extradural space within the vertebral canal. Depending on the level of the introduction of the anesthetic, it is known as caudal, sacral, or lumbar anesthesia. Called also *peridural a.* **facial a.,** loss of sensation caused by a lesion of the facial nerve. **field block a.,** regional anesthesia obtained by circumscribing the operative field with a continuous wall of local anesthetic, thereby the nerve fibers supplying the site of operation and traversing the barrier are blocked and the operative area is rendered insensitive to painful stimuli. Called also *field block.* **frost a.,** local anesthesia effected by topical refrigeration produced by a jet of highly volatile liquid. See also *refrigeration a.* and CRYOANESTHESIA. **general a.,** a reversible state of insensibility to pain with loss of consciousness, produced by chemical agents that act on the brain. Drugs producing general anesthesia can be administered by inhalation, or intravenously, intramuscularly, or rectally, or via the gastrointestinal system. **gustatory a.,** loss of the sense of taste. **high pressure a.,** regional anesthesia produced by controlled application of pressure to a nerve trunk or its branches. **hypnosis a.,** production of insensibility to pain during surgical procedures by means of hypnotism. **hypotensive a.,** that accompanied by the deliberate lowering of the blood pressure, a procedure said to reduce blood loss. See also induced HYPOTENSION. **hypothermic a.,** anesthesia accompanied by the deliberate lowering of the body temperature. **infiltration a.,** regional anesthesia in which an anesthetic solution is injected into the operative field so that the small terminal nerve fibers and their sensory receptors are rendered insensitive in the area to be operated on; local anesthesia. Called also *infiltration analgesia.* **inhalation a.,** general anesthesia produced by the inhalation of vapors of anesthetic volatile liquids or gases. See illustration. **insufflation a.,** that produced by introducing a mixture of anesthetic gases through a tube into the respiratory tract, as in endobronchial or endotracheal anesthesia. Called also *intubation a.* **intranasal a.,** local anesthesia produced by insertion into the nasal cavity of pledgets soaked in a solution of an anesthetic agent, which is effective after topical application, or by insufflation of a mixture of anesthetic gases through a tube introduced into the nose. Called also *intranasal block.* **intraoral a.,** anesthesia produced within the oral cavity by injection, spray, pressure, etc. **intraosseous a.,** local anesthesia produced by the administration of an anesthetic agent directly into the cancellous portion of bone. **intrapulpal a.,** local anesthesia produced

PATIENT

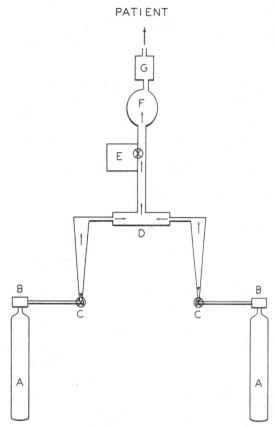

The components of an anesthetic machine. *A*, Source of anesthetic gases and oxygen. *B*, Reducing valves. *C*, Needle valves and flowmeters. *D*, Mixing manifold. *E*, Vaporizer for volatile anesthetic liquids. *F*, Reservoir bag. *G*, Delivery apparatus. (From D. C. Sabiston, Jr.: Davis-Christopher Textbook of Surgery. 12th ed. Philadelphia, W. B. Saunders Co., 1981.)

by the administration of an anesthetic agent directly into the dental pulp. **intravenous regional a.,** anesthesia produced by injecting a large volume of dilute local anesthetic solution into a vein of a bloodless extremity, the injected solution being confined to the extremity by a tourniquet. **intubation a.,** insufflation a. **local a.,** regional anesthesia confined to a specific limited part of the body without loss of consciousness; infiltration anesthesia. See also local ANESTHETIC. **lumbar a.,** epidural anesthesia in which the anesthetic has been introduced into the lumbar segment of the vertebral canal. **mixed a.,** anesthesia produced by the administration of more than one anesthetic agent. See also *balanced a.* **nerve block a.,** peripheral nerve block a. **olfactory a.,** lack of the sense of smell. Called also *anosmia.* **open drop a.,** inhalation anesthesia with the use of a cone, without provision for rebreathing. **paraneural a.,** regional anesthesia in which an anesthetic agent is infiltrated around a nerve. **partial a.,** anesthesia with retention of some degree of sensibility. **peridural a.,** epidural a. **perineural a.,** regional anesthesia produced by injection of an anesthetic agent close to a nerve. **peripheral a.,** loss of sensation due to changes in the peripheral nerves. **peripheral nerve block a.,** regional anesthesia produced by injecting a local anesthetic in the proximity of major nerve trunks, thereby rendering the area supplied by the trunk insensitive to painful stimuli. Called also *block a., nerve block a., nerve block,* and *peripheral nerve block.* **permeation a.,** analgesia of a body surface produced by the application of a local anesthetic, most commonly to mucous membranes. Called also *permeation analgesia.* See also *topical a.* **plexus a.,** regional anesthesia in which a local anesthetic is injected around a nerve plexus. **pressure a.,** regional anesthesia produced by a local anesthetic forced into the tissues by pressure. **refrigeration a.,** regional anesthesia produced by applying a tourniquet

and chilling the part near freezing temperature. Called also *crymoanesthesia.* See also *frost a.* **regional a.,** the production of reversible blockade of pain perception or transmission through the use of local anesthetic drugs or physical agents, such as cold or pressure. Anesthetic methods involving the sensory receptors include topical anesthesia and local infiltration anesthesia; anesthetic methods blocking nerve conduction consist of field block, peripheral nerve block, epidural anesthesia, and spinal anesthesia; the mechanism of action of intravenous regional anesthesia is unclear. Called also *conduction a.* **sacral a.,** epidural anesthesia in which the anesthetic has been introduced into the sacral segment of the vertebral canal. **segmental a.,** loss of sensation caused by lesions of nerve roots. **semiclosed a.,** inhalation anesthesia in which there is partial rebreathing of the expired gases, with a carbon dioxide absorber in the circuit. **semiopen a.,** inhalation anesthesia administered by the use of an open cone or a partially open circuit; there is partial rebreathing of the expired gases without a carbon dioxide absorber in the circuit. **spinal a., subarachnoid a.,** regional anesthesia produced by injecting a local anesthetic into the subarachnoid space and into the cerebrospinal fluid so that the drug is allowed to bathe the nerve roots and desensitize the area supplied by the nerves. Called also *rachianesthesia.* **surface a.,** topical a. **surgical a.,** that degree of anesthesia at which surgery may safely be performed; ordinarily used to designate such depth of general anesthesia. **tactile a.,** loss or impairment of the sense of touch. **thermal a., thermic a.,** loss of the temperature sense. **topical a.,** a regional anesthetic method for blockade of pain perception produced by applying local anesthetics to the skin or mucous membranes. Called also *surface a.* and *surface analgesia.* See also *permeation a.* and topical ANESTHETIC. **total a.,** loss of all sensibility in the affected part. **traumatic a.,** loss of sensation caused by injury to a nerve. **unilateral a.,** hemianesthesia. **vein a.,** Bier's local a.

anesthesimeter (an-es"the-sim'e-ter) [*anesthesia* + Gr. *metron* measure] 1. an instrument used to regulate the amount of an anesthetic administered. 2. an instrument for taking the degree of insensitiveness.

Anesthesin trademark for *benzocaine.*

anesthesiologist (an"es-the"ze-ol'o-jist) a physician specializing in anesthesiology. See also ANESTHETIST.

anesthesiology (an"es-the"ze-ol'o-je) [*anesthesia* + *-logy*] that branch of medicine concerned with anesthesia and anesthetics.

anesthesiophore (an"es-the'ze-o-for) [*anesthesia* + Gr. *phoros* bearing] 1. conveying anesthetic action. 2. the portion of the molecule of a chemical compound which is responsible for its anesthetic action.

anesthetic (an"es-thet'ik) 1. pertaining to, characterized by, or producing anesthesia. 2. a drug or agent used to induce anesthesia and render the body or its part insensitive to pain. **basal a.,** a central nervous system depressant producing unconsciousness that is not of sufficient depth to permit surgery but serves as a basis for further and deeper anesthesia. **Cetylite liquid topical a.,** trademark for a topical anesthetic preparation, containing 2 percent tetracaine hydrochloride, 14 percent benzocaine, 2 percent butyl aminobenzoate, 0.5 percent benzalkonium chloride, and 0.005 percent cetyldimethyl ethyl ammonium bromide, in a water-soluble base. **general a.,** an agent that produces insensitivity to pain in the entire body in association with the loss of consciousness. **inhalation a.,** an anesthetic agent existing at room temperature, either as a gas or as a volatile liquid, which must be vaporized prior to its administration. Gases, such as nitrous oxide or cyclopropane, are compressed in metal cylinders identified by a color code and administered through a respirator. Volatile gases, such as chloroform, halothane, enflurane, diethyl ether, and methoxyflurane, are administered through a special anesthetic machine. See illustration at inhalation ANESTHESIA. **intravenous a.,** one introduced intravenously for the induction of either general or regional anesthesia. **local a.,** an agent capable of reversibly blocking perception and transmission of pain in limited areas of the body, without loss of consciousness; used to prevent pain in surgery, injuries, diseases, and therapeutic procedures that may involve pain. Functionally, local anesthetics may be divided into those which produce anesthesia through the production of cold, such as ether and ethyl chloride; protoplasmic poisons, such as phenol; and agents which affect the sensory nerves or their endings, believed to act by preventing the depolarization of the nerve membrane and the propagation of the impulse by interference with the sodium-potassium ion exchange across the membrane. Local anesthetics are applied topically or they are injected into tissues, as in infiltration anesthesia, nerve block anesthesia, spinal anesthesia, and extradural anesthesia. Insoluble and some soluble anesthetics are applied topically to

Technique	Local Anesthetic	Duration of Action
Topical anesthesia (mucous membranes)	Lidocaine	15 minutes
	Cocaine	30 minutes
	Tetracaine	45 minutes
	Benzocaine*	Several hours
Local infiltration	Procaine	¼–½ hour
	Lidocaine	½–1 hour
	Mepivacaine	½–1 hour
	Tetracaine	2–3 hours
Major nerve block	Lidocaine	1–2 hours
	Mepivacaine	1–2¼ hours
	Tetracaine	2–3 hours
Epidural anesthesia	Procaine	½–1 hour
	Lidocaine	¾–1½ hours
	Mepivacaine	1–2¼ hours
	Tetracaine	2–3 hours
Spinal anesthesia	Procaine	½–1 hour
	Lidocaine	¾–1½ hours
	Tetracaine	1–2 hours
Intravenous regional anesthesia	Lidocaine	Varies

*As the base.
(Modified from D. C. Sabiston, Jr.: Davis-Christopher Textbook of Surgery. 12th ed. Philadelphia, W. B. Saunders Co., 1981.)

the skin and mucous membranes; the injectable anesthetics are always soluble. All anesthetics are toxic, their effects varying with the tolerance of the patient, and all are metabolized by the liver and excreted with the urine. See also *local anesthetic solution*. See table. **topical a.**, a local anesthetic applied directly to the area to be anesthetized, usually the skin or mucous membrane. Anesthetic ointments are effective on normal and inflamed tissue, while aqueous solutions are effective on inflamed skin and mucous membranes but not on intact skin because such solutions are unable to penetrate normal epidermis. Aqueous solutions of local anesthetics, such as salts of cocaine, lidocaine, or tetracaine, are used for topical anesthesia of the pharyngeal, nasal, and oral cavities and of the esophagus, larynx, and trachea.

anesthetist (ah-nes′thĕ-tist) a person, such as a nurse, trained in the administration of anesthetics. See also ANESTHESIOLOGIST. **nurse a.**, NURSE anesthetist.

anesthetization (ah-nes″thĕ-ti-za′shun) the production of insensibility to pain.

anesthetize (ah-nes′thĕ-tīz) to put under the influence of anesthetics.

aneuploid (an′u-ploid) [*an* neg. + *euploid*] 1. having a lesser or greater number of whole chromosomes than the normal diploid number of the species. 2. an individual or cell having a lesser or greater number of whole chromosomes than the normal diploid number of the species.

aneuploidy (an″u-ploi′de) [*an* neg. + *ploidy*] a chromosomal aberration, being a deviation from an exact multiple of the haploid number of chromosomes, whether fewer (hypoploidy) or more (hyperploidy). It occurs as a consequence of an error in a meiotic division, leading to unequal distribution of one pair of homologous chromosomes to the daughter cells so that one cell has both and the other has neither chromosome of a pair. See also CHROMOSOME aberration, EUPLOIDY, MONOSOMY, POLYPLOIDY, and TRISOMY.

aneurysm (an′u-rizm) [Gr. *aneurysma* a widening] a localized abnormal dilatation of a blood vessel, resulting in the development of a blood-filled sac. **arteriovenous a.**, an aneurysm which provides a direct communication between an artery and vein. See also arteriovenous FISTULA.

aneutrocytosis (ah-nu″tro-si-to′sis) [*a* neg. + *neutrocytosis*] agranulocytosis.

aneutrophilia (ah-nu″tro-fil′e-ah) [*a* neg. + *neutrophilia*] agranulocytosis.

ANF antinuclear FACTOR.

Angelman's syndrome [H. *Angelman*] happy puppet SYNDROME.

angi- see ANGIO-.

angialgia (an″je-al′je-ah) [*angi-* + Gr. *algos* pain + *-ia*] pain in a vessel or vessels, especially blood vessels. Called also *angiodynia*.

angiectasis (an″je-ek′tah-sis) [*angi-* + Gr. *ektasis* dilatation] dilatation and distention of a blood vessel.

angiectomy (an″je-ek′to-me) [*angi-* + Gr. *ektomē* excision] excision or resection of a vessel.

angiectopia (an″je-ek-to′pe-ah) [*angi-* + Gr. *ek* out + *topos* place + *-ia*] abnormal position or course of a vessel.

angiitis (an″je-i′tis), pl. *angii′tides* [*angi-* + *-itis*] inflammation of a vessel, particularly a blood or a lymph vessel; vasculitis. **necrotizing a.**, PERIARTERITIS nodosa.

angina (an-ji′nah, an′ji-nah) [L.] 1. any disease accompanied by spasmodic, choking, or suffocating pain; especially one that affects the throat. 2. **a. pectoris.** **a. acu′ta**, simple sore throat. Called also *a. simplex.* **agranulocytic a.**, agranulocytosis. **benign croupous a.**, PHARYNGITIS herpetica. **Bretonneau's a.**, diphtheria. **a. catarrha′lis**, acute PHARYNGITIS. **a. cor′dis**, a. pectoris. **cyclic agranulocytic a.**, periodic AGRANULOCYTOSIS. **a. epiglottide′a**, inflammation of the epiglottis. **exudative a.**, croup. **a. follicula′ris**, follicular TONSILLITIS. **a. gangreno′sa**, gangrenous inflammation of the fauces. Called also *malignant a.* **herpes a.**, **a. herpet′ica**, herpangina. **hippocratic a.**, retropharyngeal ABSCESS. **a. laryn′gea**, laryngitis. **a. ludovi′ci**, Ludwig's a. **Ludwig's a.**, **a. ludwig′ii**, a severe form of cellulitis of the submaxillary space and secondary involvement of the sublingual and submental spaces, usually resulting from an infection in the mandibular molar area or a penetrating injury of the floor of the mouth. The second and third molars are the most common source of infection, from where it perforates the bone, commonly the lingual plate, to establish drainage, thus spreading to other parts. The presenting lesion is a rapidly developing hard swelling of the floor of the mouth, spreading to the parapharyngeal spaces, carotid sheath, pterygopalatine fossa, and neck. Elevation of the tongue, difficulty in eating and swallowing, fever, edema of the glottis, rapid breathing, and moderate leukocytosis are the most common symptoms. Complications may include asphyxia and cavernous sinus thrombosis with subsequent meningitis. Streptococci are present in nearly all cases, but fusiform bacilli, staphylococci, and other bacteria are also found in most instances. Called also *a. ludovici, phlegmon of the floor of the mouth,* and *submaxillary cellulitis.* **malignant a.**, a. gangrenosa. **monocytic a.**, infectious MONONUCLEOSIS. **a. nosoco′mii**, PHARYNGITIS ulcerosa. **a. parotid′ea**, mumps. **a. pec′toris**, a coronary heart disease, consisting of severe paroxysmal chest pain, resulting from transient ischemia that falls short of inducing ischemic necrosis of the myocardium, almost always associated with marked coronary arteriosclerosis but without myocardial infarction. Called also *a. cordis, angor pectoris, Elsner's asthma, Heberden's asthma, Heberden's disease, Rougnon-Heberden disease,* and *stenocardia.* **a. phlegmono′sa**, peritonsillar ABSCESS. **Plaut's a.**, **pseudomembranous a.**, necrotizing ulcerative GINGIVOSTOMATITIS. **a. rheumat′ica**, pharyngitis associated with rheumatic diathesis. **a. scarlatino′sa**, pharyngitis associated with scarlet fever. **Schultz's a.**, agranulocytosis. **Senator's a.**, an acute and rapidly fatal pharyngolaryngeal infection. **a. sim′plex**, simple sore throat. Called also *a. acuta.* **streptococcal a.**, sore throat due to streptococcal infection. See septic sore THROAT. **a. tonsilla′ris**, peritonsillar ABSCESS. **a. trachea′lis**, croup. **Vincent's a.**, painful membranous ulceration with edema and hyperemic patches of the oropharynx and throat, caused by spreading of acute necrotizing gingivitis.

Anginal trademark for *dipyridamole*.

anginal (an-ji′nal, an′ji-nal) pertaining to angina.

angio-, angi- [Gr. *angeion* vessel] a combining form denoting relationship to a vessel.

angioataxia (an″je-o-ah-tak′se-ah) [*angio-* + *ataxia*] irregular tension of a blood vessel.

angioblast (an′je-o-blast″) [*angio-* + Gr. *blastos* germ] 1. the mesenchymal tissue of the embryo from which blood cells and blood vessels differentiate. Called also *angioderm.* 2. an individual vessel-forming cell.

angiocardiography (an″je-o-kar″de-og′rah-fe) [*angio-* + Gr. *kardia* heart + *graphein* to write] roentgenographic examination of the heart and great vessels following introduction of a contrast medium into the vascular system or a cardiac chamber.

angiocardiokinetic (an″je-o-kar″de-o-ki-net′ik) [*angio-* + Gr. *kardia* heart + *kinēsis* motion] 1. affecting the motions or movements of the heart and blood vessels. 2. an agent that affects the movements or motions of the heart and blood vessels.

angiocardiopathy (an″je-o-kar″de-op′ah-the) [*angio-* + Gr. *kardia* heart + *-pathy*] any disease of the heart and blood vessels.

angiocarditis (an″je-o-kar-di′tis) [*angio-* + Gr. *kardia* heart + *-itis*] any inflammatory disease of the heart and great vessels.

angiocheiloscope (an″je-o-ki′lo-skōp″) [*angio-* + Gr. *cheilos* lip + *skopein* to view] an instrument for observing blood circulation of the lips under magnification.

angioderm (an″je-o-derm) angioblast (1).

angiodynia (an″je-o-din′e-ah) [*angio-* + Gr. *odynē* pain + *-ia*] angialgia.

angiofibroma (an″je-o-fi-bro′mah) [*angio-* + *fibroma*] an angioma containing fibrous tissue; fibroangioma. **juvenile a., naso-pharyngeal a. nasopharyngeal a.,** a relatively rare benign, nonencapsulated, expansile, infiltrating tumor of the naso-pharynx of adolescent males, consisting chiefly of a vascular network and a connective tissue stroma with abundant endothelium-lined vascular spaces. Nasal obstruction, adenoid speech, discomfort in swallowing, and auditory tube obstruction are the principal clinical symptoms. Called also *juvenile a., juvenile nasopharyngeal fibroma,* and *nasopharyngeal fi-broangioma.*

angiogenesis (an″je-o-jen′ě-sis) [*angio-* + *genesis*] the development of the blood vessels.

angiogranuloma (an″je-o-gran″u-lo′mah) [*angio-* + *granuloma*] a tumor having the characteristics of both granuloma and angioma. **gingival a.,** pregnancy GINGIVITIS.

angiography (an″je-og′rah-fe) [*angio-* + Gr. *graphein* to write] the roentgenographic visualization of the blood vessels following introduction of contrast material. Called also *vasography.*

angiohemophilia (an″je-o-he″mo-fil′e-ah) [*angio-* + *hemophilia*] Willebrand-Jürgens SYNDROME.

angioid (an′je-oid) [*angio-* + Gr. *eidos* form] resembling a blood vessel.

angiologia (an″je-o-lo′je-ah) angiology; in Nomina Anatomica, *angiologia* encompasses the nomenclature relating to the heart, arteries, veins, lymphatic system, and spleen.

angiology (an″je-ol′o-je) [*angio-* + Gr. *logos* treatise] the scientific study of the vessels of the body; applied also to the sum of knowledge relating to the blood vessels and lymph vessels. Called also *angiologia.*

angioma (an″je-o′mah) [*angio-* + *-oma*] a tumor made up of blood vessel cells (hemangioma) or lymph vessel cells (lymphangioma). **a. caverno′sum, cavernous a.,** a sharply defined, unencapsulated hemangioma, made up of large, blood-filled cavernous vascular channels, among which capillary-like laminae are sometimes dispersed. Typically, it presents a reddish-blue spongy soft mass about 1 to 2 cm in diameter, found on the skin and mucous membranes, and also in some visceral organs, brain, and eye ground. It is the most common type of oral hemangioma. Called also *cavernous hemangioma, erectile tumor,* and *vascular nevus.* See also capillary HEMANGIOMA. **a. cor′poris diffu′sum, a. cor′poris diffu′sum universa′le,** Fabry's DISEASE. **cutaneocerebral a.,** Sturge-Weber SYNDROME. **a. hemorrha′gicum heredita′ria,** hereditary hemorrhagic TELANGI-ECTASIA.

angiomatosis (an″je-o-mah-to′sis) a condition characterized by the development of multiple angiomas. **encephalotrigeminal a.,** Sturge-Weber SYNDROME. **Kaposi's a.,** Kaposi's SARCOMA. **a. meningo-oculofacia′lis,** Sturge-Weber SYNDROME.

angioneurectomy (an″je-o-nu-rek′to-me) [*angio-* + *neuro-* + Gr. *ektomē* excision] excision of vessels and nerves.

angioneurosis (an″je-o-nu-ro′sis) [*angio-* + *neurosis*] a vascular disorder due to a neurological lesion. **cutaneous a.,** Quincke's EDEMA.

angiopathy (an-je-op′ah-the) [*angio-* + Gr. *pathos* disease] any disease of the vessels. **giant-cell hyalin a.,** pulse GRANULOMA.

angioplasty (an-′je-o-plas″te) [*angio-* + Gr. *plassein* to form] surgical repair of the blood vessels.

angiopsathyrosis (an″je-o-sath″ĭ-ro′sis) fragility of the blood vessels.

angioreticuloendothelioma (an″je-o-re-tik″u-lo-en″do-the-le-o′-mah) Kaposi's SARCOMA.

angiorrhaphy (an″je-or′ah-fe) [*angio-* + Gr. *rhaphē* suture] suture of a blood vessel or vessels.

angiosarcoma (an″je-o-sar-ko′mah) [*angio-* + *sarcoma*] a malignant neoplasm of vascular origin, found anywhere in the body, but most commonly in the skin, liver, spleen, lungs, bones, and retroperitoneal organs. It is made up of endothelial vascular cells that are largely undifferentiated and produce no blood vessels. Called also *hemangioendotheliosarcoma* and *malignant hemangioendothelioma.* **a. pigmento′sum,** Kaposi's SAR-COMA.

angiosclerosis (an″je-o-skle-ro′sis) [*angio-* + *sclerosis*] hardening of the blood vessels.

angioscope (an′je-o-skōp″) [*angio-* + Gr. *skopein* to view] a microscope for observing capillary blood vessels.

angiospasm (an′je-o-spazm″) [*angio-* + Gr. *spasmos* spasm] spasmodic contraction of the blood vessels.

angiostenosis (an″je-o-stě-no′sis) [*angio-* + *stenosis*] stenosis of a blood vessel, resulting in obstruction of its lumen.

angiostomy (an″je-os′to-me) [*angio-* + Gr. *stomoun* to provide with an opening or mouth] the operation of making an opening into a blood vessel and inserting a cannula therein.

angiostrophe (an″je-os′tro-fe) [*angio-* + Gr. *strophē* a twist] the twisting of a blood vessel to arrest hemorrhage.

angiotelectasis (an″je-o-tě-lek′tah-sis) [*angio-* + Gr. *telos* end + *ektasis* dilatation] dilatation of the minute arteries and veins.

angiotome (an′je-o-tōm″) [*angio-* + Gr. *tomē* a cutting] any one of the segments of the vascular system of the embryo.

angiotomy (an″je-ot′o-me) [*angio-* + Gr. *tomē* a cutting] the cutting or severing of a blood or lymph vessel.

angiotonic (an″je-o-ton′ik) [*angio-* + Gr. *tonos* tension] increasing the vascular tension.

angiotribe (an′je-o-trib″) [*angio-* + Gr. *tribein* to crush] a strong forceps in which pressure is applied by means of a screw, used to crush tissue containing an artery in order to check hemorrhage from the vessel. Called also *vasotribe.*

angiotripsy (an′je-o-trip″se) production of hemostasis by use of the angiotribe. Called also *vasotripsy.*

Angitrit trademark for *trolnitrate phosphate* (see under TROLNI-TRATE).

angle (ang′g'l) [L. *angulus*] 1. the area or point of junction of two intersecting borders or surfaces; angulus. 2. the degree of divergence of two intersecting lines or planes. 3. tooth a. **a. of aberration,** a. of deviation. **alveolar a.,** the angle between a line running through a point beneath the anterior nasal spine and the most prominent point on the lower border of the alveolar process of the maxilla and the cephalic horizontal (glabella to opisthocranion). **alveolar profile a.,** an angle formed by the nasospinale-prosthion line with the Frankfort Horizontal; used for measuring the degree of inclination of the upper facial skeleton and the degree of protrusion of the upper jaws. It may be used in classifying skulls as prognathous, mesognathous, and orthognathous. See also gnathic INDEX. **anterior a. of petrous portion of temporal bone,** a short area on the petrous part of the temporal bone consisting of two parts: one, adjoining the squamous part of the bone at the petrosquamous suture; the other, a free part articulating with the great wing of the sphenoid bone. Called also *angulus anterior pyramidis ossis temporalis.* **anterior inferior a. of sphenoid bone,** sphenoid a. of parietal bone. **anterior superior a. of parietal bone,** frontal a. of parietal bone. **a. of aorta,** angle of APERTURE. **a. of aperture,** angle of APERTURE. **auriculo-occipital a.,** an angle formed at the porion by the intersection of lines from the lambda and opisthion. **axial a.,** any angle, the formation of which is partially dependent on the axial wall of a tooth cavity preparation, as the axiodistal angle or buccoaxial angle. See table. **axial line a.,** any line angle which is parallel with the long axis of a tooth. **basal mandibular a.,** an angle formed at the gnathion by the intersection of lines from the right and the left gonion. **Bennett a.,** the angle formed by the midsagittal plane and the path of the advancing condyle during lateral movement of the mandible, as viewed in the horizontal plane. See also Bennett MOVEMENT. **beta a.,** the angle between the radius fixus and a line joining the bregma and hormion. **bevel a.,** the degree of an angle formed by a bevel. **biorbital a.,** an angle formed by the intersection of the posterior extensions of the axes of the two orbits. **a. bisection,** see bisecting angle TECHNIQUE. **a. board,** angle BOARD. **Broca's a.,** ophryospinal a. **buccal a's,** the angles formed between the buccal surface and the other surfaces of a posterior tooth, or between the buccal wall of a tooth cavity preparation and other walls, named according to the surfaces which participate in their formation. See table. **bucco-occlusal line a.,** the junction of the buccal and occlusal surfaces of the posterior teeth. See illustration. **cavity a's,** the angles formed by the junction of two or more walls of a cavity preparation in a tooth, designated according to the walls participating in their formation. G. V. Black's rules for designating the angles are as follows: (1) all line angles are formed by the junction of two walls along a line and are named by combining the names of these walls; (2) all point angles are formed by the junction of three walls; point angles are also named according to the walls of the anatomic surfaces involved and, thus, will include three terms; and (3) all angles of the cavity preparation are named for the specific walls that are joined to form the angle. See table. **cavosurface a.,** the angle formed by the junction of one of the walls of a cavity preparation and a surface of the crown of a tooth. **cephalic a.,** any of a variety of angles of the skull and face. See *craniofacial a.* **cephalometric a.,** any angle formed by intersecting craniometric and cephalometric lines; used for cephalometric measurements and orthodontic diagnosis. **chi a.,** an angle formed at the hormion by the intersection of lines from the staphylion and basion. **condylar a.,** the angle between the planes of the basilar

CAVITY ANGLES
Line Angles
(Formed by the junction of two walls)

axiodistal	gingivoaxial
axiogingival	labiogingival
axioincisal	linguoaxial
axiolabial	linguodistal
axiolingual	linguogingival
axiomesial	linguomesial
axio-occlusal	linguopulpal
axiopulpal	mesiobuccal
buccoaxial	mesiogingival
buccodistal	mesiolabial
buccogingival	mesiolingual
buccomesial	mesio-occlusal
buccopulpal	mesiopulpal
distobuccal	pulpoaxial
distogingival	pulpodistal
distolabial	pulpolabial
distolingual	pulpolingual
disto-occlusal	pulpomesial
distopulpal	

Point Angles
(Formed by the junction of three walls)

axiodistogingival	distopulpolingual
axiodisto-occlusal	gingivobuccoaxial
axiolabiogingival	gingivolinguoaxial
axiolinguogingival	mesiobuccopulpal
axiomesiogingival	mesiolinguopulpal
axiomesio-occlusal	mesiopulpolabial
distobuccopulpal	mesiopulpolingual
distolinguopulpal	pulpobuccoaxial
distopulpolabial	pulpolinguoaxial

(From Dorland's Illustrated Medical Dictionary. 26th ed. Philadelphia, W. B. Saunders Co., 1981.)

clivus and the foramen magnum. **condylar a. of mandible,** an angle formed by a tangent of the lower border and a tangent of the posterior border of the mandible; used for determining the degree of inclination of the condyle to the plane of the mandibular body. Called also *gonial a.*; popularly referred to as *jaw a.* **a. of convexity,** a roentgenographic cephalometric measurement, formed by connecting nasion, subspinale (point A), and pogonion, reflecting the convexity (or concavity) of the facial profile. Abbreviated *NAP.* **cranial a.,** any of a variety of angles of the dry skull. See also *craniofacial a.* **craniofacial a.,** the angle between the basifacial (Ba-N) and basicranial (Ba-S) axes at the

middle of the ethmoidosphenoid suture. **critical a.,** the angle of incidence at which a ray of light passing from one medium to another of different density changes from refraction to total reflection. Called also *limiting a.* **cusp a.,** 1. the angle made by the slopes of a cusp of a tooth with the plane that passes through the tip of the cusp, measured mesiodistally or buccolingually. 2. the angle made by the slopes of a cusp with a perpendicular line bisecting the cusp, measured mesiodistally or buccolingually. 3. one half of the included angle between the buccal and lingual or mesial and distal cusp inclines. **cusp-plane a.,** the incline of the cusp plane in relation to the plane of occlusion. **Daubenton's a.,** an angle formed at the opisthion by the intersection of lines from the nasion and basion. Called also *occipital a.* **a. of deviation,** the angle between a refracted ray and the incident ray prolonged. Called also *a. of aberration.* **distal a's,** the angles formed between the distal surface and other surfaces of a tooth, or between the distal wall of a tooth cavity and other walls; named according to the surfaces which participate in their formation. See table and illustration. **distal incisal a.,** see *incisal a.* **distobuccal line a.,** the junction of the distal and buccal surfaces of the posterior teeth. See illustration. **distobucco-occlusal point a.,** the junction of the distal, buccal, and occlusal surfaces of the posterior teeth. See illustration. **distolabial line a.,** the junction of the distal and labial surfaces of the anterior teeth. See illustration. **distolabioincisal point a.,** the junction of the distal, labial, and incisal surfaces of the anterior teeth. See illustration. **distolingual line a.,** the junction of the distal and lingual surfaces found on both the anterior and posterior teeth. See illustration. **distolinguoincisal point a.,** the junction of the distal, lingual, and incisal surfaces of the anterior teeth. See illustration. **distolinguo-occlusal point a.,** the junction of the distal, lingual, and occlusal surfaces of the posterior teeth. See illustration. **disto-occlusal line a.,** the junction of the distal and occlusal surfaces of the posterior teeth. See illustration. **ethmocranial a., ethmoid a.,** the angle formed by the plane of the cribriform plate of the ethmoid bone prolonged to meet the basicranial axis. **facial a.,** the angle formed by the junction of the Frankfort Horizontal plane and the nasion-pogonion line in the lateral roentgenographic cephalometric tracing. Used to express the degree of retrusion or protrusion of the chin. See also PROGNATHISM and RETROGNATHIA. **Frankfort–mandibular plane a.,** an angle formed by the intersection of the

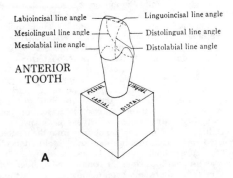

A

Labioincisal line angle — Linguoincisal line angle
Mesiolingual line angle — Distolingual line angle
Mesiolabial line angle — Distolabial line angle

ANTERIOR TOOTH

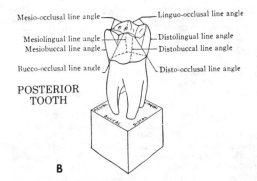

B

Mesio-occlusal line angle — Linguo-occlusal line angle
Mesiolingual line angle — Distolingual line angle
Mesiobuccal line angle — Distobuccal line angle
Bucco-occlusal line angle — Disto-occlusal line angle

POSTERIOR TOOTH

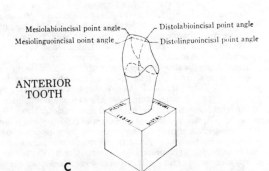

C

Mesiolabioincisal point angle — Distolabioincisal point angle
Mesiolinguoincisal point angle — Distolinguoincisal point angle

ANTERIOR TOOTH

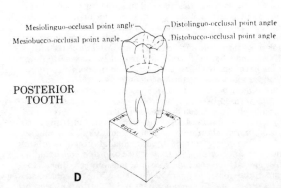

D

Mesiolinguo-occlusal point angle — Distolinguo-occlusal point angle
Mesiobucco-occlusal point angle — Distobucco-occlusal point angle

POSTERIOR TOOTH

Tooth angles: *A* and *B*, line angles; *C* and *D*, point angles. (From R. C. Wheeler: Dental Anatomy, Physiology and Occlusion. 5th ed. Philadelphia, W. B. Saunders Co., 1974.)

Frankfort Horizontal plane and the mandibular plane. Abbreviated *FMA*. **frontal a. of parietal bone,** the anterosuperior angle of the parietal bone, which is membranous at birth and forms part of the anterior fontanelle. Called also *anterior superior a. of parietal bone* and angulus frontalis ossis parietalis [NA]. **gonial a.,** 1. a. of mandible. 2. condylar a. of mandible. **horizontal a.,** the angle, measured within a horizontal plane, at which the central ray of the useful beam is projected relative to a vertical plane of reference. **impedance a.,** the ratio between the resistance of the body to an electric current and its condenser function. See also IMPEDANCE. **a. of incidence,** the angle made with the perpendicular by a ray of light which strikes a denser or a rarer medium. **incisal a.,** one of the angles formed by the junction of the incisal and the mesial or distal surfaces of an anterior tooth; called the *mesial* and the *distal incisal angle,* respectively. **incisal guide a.,** the angle formed with the horizonal plane by drawing a line in the sagittal plane between the incisal edges of the maxillary and mandibular central incisers when the teeth are in centric occlusion. See also *incisal a.* **incisal mandibular plane a.,** one of the three angles composing the Tweed triangle, designating the axial inclination of the lower incisor to the mandibular plane in the lateral cephalometric roentgenogram. Abbreviated *IMPA.* **Jacquart's a.,** ophryospinal a. **jaw a., a. of jaw,** 1. condylar a. of mandible. 2. a. of mandible. **labial a's,** the angles formed between the labial surface and other surfaces of an anterior tooth, or between the labial wall of a tooth cavity and other walls; named according to the surfaces participating in their formation. See table and illustration. **labioincisal line a.,** the junction of the labial and incisal surfaces of the anterior teeth. See illustration. **lateral a. of eye,** the angle formed by the lateral junction of the superior and inferior eyelids. Called also *angulus oculi lateralis* [NA]. **limiting a.,** critical a. **line a.,** an angle formed by the junction of two planes; used to designate the junction of two surfaces of a tooth, or of two walls of a tooth cavity preparation. Line angles of the posterior teeth include the mesio-occlusal, linguo-occlusal, mesiolingual, distolingual, mesiobuccal, distobuccal, bucco-occlusal, and disto-occlusal angles. Those of the anterior teeth include the labioincisal, linguoincisal, mesiolabial, distolabial, mesiolingual, and distolingual angles. See table and illustration. **lingual a's,** the angles formed between the lingual and other surfaces of a tooth, or between the lingual wall of a tooth cavity preparation and other walls; named according to the surfaces which participate in their formation, e.g., the linguopupal angle is formed at the junction of the lingual and pupal walls of a cavity preparation. See table and illustration. **linguoincisal line a.,** the junction of the lingual and incisal surfaces of the anterior teeth. See illustration. **linguo-occlusal line a.,** the junction of the lingual and occlusal surfaces of the posterior teeth. See illustration. **a. of mandible, mandibular a.,** the angle created at the junction of the posterior edge of the ramus and the lower edge of the mandible. Called also *gonial a., jaw a.,* and *angulus mandibulae* [NA]. See also *basal mandibular a., condylar a. of mandible,* and *mandibular profile a.* **mandibular profile a.,** an angle formed by a line connecting the interdentale inferius and the anteriorly most prominent chin point and the Frankfort Horizontal, when the occlusal position of the mandible is secured, and if this position cannot be established, between the line connecting the interdentale inferius and the anterior point on the chin and the tangent of the lower border of the mandible. It is used in measuring the degree of mandibular prognathism. **mastoid a. of parietal bone,** the posteroinferior angle of the parietal bone, which articulates with the posterior part of the temporal bone and the occipital bone. Called also *posterior inferior a. of parietal bone, angulus mastoideus ossis parietalis* [NA], and *mastoid margin of parietal bone.* **maxillary a.,** the angle between two lines extending from the point of contact of the upper and lower central incisors to the orphyron and the most prominent point of the lower jaw (pogonion). **mesial a's,** the angles formed between the mesial surface and other surfaces of a tooth, or between the mesial wall of a tooth cavity and other walls; named according to the surfaces participating with the mesial in their formation. See table and illustration. **medial a. of eye,** the angle formed by the medial junction of the superior and inferior eyelids. Called also *angulus oculi medialis* [NA]. **mesial incisal a.,** see *incisal a.* **mesiobuccal line a.,** the junction of the mesial and buccal surfaces of the poterior teeth. See illustration. **mesiobucco-occlusal point a.,** the junction of the mesial, buccal, and occlusal surfaces of the posterior teeth. See illustration. **mesiolabial line a.,** the junction of the mesial

and labial surfaces of the anterior teeth. See illustration. **mesiolabioincisal point a.,** the junction of the mesial, labial, and incisal surfaces of the anterior teeth. See illustration. **mesiolingual line a.,** the junction of the mesial and lingual surfaces of the anterior and posterior teeth. See illustration. **mesiolinguoincisal point a.,** the junction of the mesial, lingual, and incisal surfaces of the anterior teeth. See illustration. **mesiolinguoocclusal point a.,** the junction of the mesial, lingual, and occlusal surfaces of the posterior teeth. See illustration. **mesioocclusal line a.,** the junction of the mesial and occlusal surfaces of the posterior teeth. See illustration. **metafacial a.,** the angle between the base of the skull and the pterygoid process. Called also *Serres' a.* **a. of mouth,** the angle formed at either side of the mouth by the junction of the upper and lower lips. Called also *angulus oris* [NA]. **a. of Mulder,** an angle formed by the intersection of the facial line of Camper and a line from the root of the nose to the spheno-occipital suture. **nasal profile a.,** an angle formed by a line from the nasion to the nasospinale and the Frankfort Horizontal; used for measuring the inclination of the nasal and alveolar part of the upper facial skeleton and determining the degree of protrusion of the jaws. The degree of inclination may be used to classify skulls as prognathous, mesognathous, and orthognathous. See also gnathic INDEX. **occipital a.,** Daubenton's a. **occipital a. of parietal bone,** the posterosuperior angle of the parietal bone, which during fetal life participates in the formation of the posterior fontanelle. Called also *posterior superior a. of parietal bone* and *angulus occipitalis ossis parietalis* [NA]. **olfactive a., olfactory a.,** the angle formed by the palatal plane (ANS-PNS) and the os planum of the sphenoid bone. **ophryospinal a.,** the angle at the anterior nasal spine between lines from the porion to the glabella. Called also *Broca's a., Jacquart's a.,* and *Topinard's a.* **orifacial a.,** one of the facial angles formed by the junction of the Frankfort Horizontal with the nasion-pogonion plane. **parietal a.,** the angle formed by the junction of lines passing through the extremities of the transverse bizygomatic diameter and the maximum transverse frontal diameter. Called also *Quatrefage's a.* **parietal a. of sphenoid bone,** parietal margin of great wing of sphenoid bone; see under MARGIN. **a. of petrous portion of temporal bone,** the angle on the petrous portion of the temporal bone that separates the posterior from the inferior surface. Called also *angulus posterior pyramidis ossis temporalis* and *posterior border of petrous portion of temporal bone.* **point a.,** any angle formed by the junction of three surfaces of a tooth crown, or three walls of a tooth cavity preparation, named according to the tooth surfaces or the cavity walls participating in its formation. Point angles on the posterior teeth include the mesiolinguo-occlusal, mesiobucco-occlusal, distolinguo-occlusal, and distobucco-occlusal angles. Point angles on the anterior teeth include the mesiolabioincisal, mesiolinguoincisal, distolabioincisal, and distolinguoincisal angles. See table and illustration. **a. of polarization,** the angle at which light is most completely polarized. **posterior inferior a. of parietal bone,** mastoid a. of parietal bone. **posterior superior a. of parietal bone,** occipital a. of parietal bone. **profile a.,** see *alveolar profile a., mandibular profile a., nasal profile a., Rivet's a.,* and *total profile a.* **Quatrefage's a.,** parietal a. **Ranke's a.,** the angle formed by the (Gl-Op) plane of the skull and a line passing through the center of the nasofrontal suture and the center of the alveolar border. **Rivet's a.,** an angle formed at the prosthion by the intersection of lines from the nasion and basion; used for measuring the degree of inclination of the profile of the upper facial skeleton. It may be used for classifying skulls as prognathous, mesognathous, and orthognathous. **Serres' a.,** metafacial a. **somatosplanchnic a.,** the angle formed by junction of the somatic and splanchnic layers of the mesoblast in the embryo. **sphenoid a., sphenoidal a.,** 1. an angle at the top of the sella turcica between lines from the rhinion and from the tip of the rostrum of the sphenoid bone. 2. the anteroinferior angle of the parietal bone. Called also *Welcher's a.* **sphenoid a. of parietal bone,** the anteroinferior angle of the parietal bone, which articulates with the great wing of the sphenoid bone and the frontal bone. Called also *anterior inferior a. of sphenoid bone, angulus sphenoidalis ossis parietalis* [NA], and *sphenoidal margin of parietal bone.* **superior a. of parietal bone, posterior,** occipital a. of parietal bone. **superior a. of petrous portion of temporal bone,** the angle on the internal surface of the petrous portion of the temporal bone that separates its posterior and anterior surfaces. Called also *angulus superior pyramidis ossis temporalis* and *superior border of petrous portion of temporal bone.* **target a.,** the acute angle between the anode target and the electron stream emanating from the cathode. **tentorial a.,** the angle between the basicranial axis and the plane of the tentorium. **tooth a's,** the angles formed by the junction of two or more surfaces of a tooth, named according to the surfaces participating in their formation. See illustration. **Topinard's a.,** ophryospinal a. **total profile a.,** an angle between a line connecting the nasion and prosthion and the Frankfort Horizontal line; used for measuring the degree of protrusion of the jaws. Using the degree of the total profile angle, skulls may be classified as prognathous, mesognathous, and orthognathous. See also gnathic INDEX. **venous a.,** the angle formed by the junction of the internal jugular and subclavian veins. **a. of Virchow,** an angle formed at the nasion by the intersection of lines from the basion and subnasale. **Vogt's a.,** an angle between the nasobasilar and alveolonasal lines. **Weisbach's a.,** an angle formed at the alveolar point by the intersection of lines from the basion and from the middle of the frontonasal suture. **Welcher's a.,** sphenoid a.

Angle's band, classification, splint [Edward Hartley *Angle,* American dentist who contributed to orthodontics as a specialty, 1855–1930] see under BAND and SPLINT, and see OCCLUSION.

angor (ang′gor) [L. "a strangling"] angina. **a. pec′toris,** ANGINA pectoris.

Ångström's law, unit [Anders Jonas *Ångström,* Swedish physicist and pioneer in developing standards for spectroscopy, 1814–1874] see under LAW and UNIT.

angstrom (awng′strem) [named after A. J. *Ångström*] Ångström UNIT. **international a.,** Ångström UNIT.

angular (ang′gu-lar) [L. *angularis*] sharply bent; having corners or angles.

angulation (ang″gu-la′shun) [L. *angulatus* bent] 1. the formation of a sharp obstructive angle, as in the intestine or any other tubular structure. 2. deviation from a straight line. 3. the direction of the primary beam of radiation in relation to object and film. **horizontal a.,** the angle measured within the horizontal plane at which the central ray of the x-ray beam is projected relative to a reference in the vertical or sagittal plane. **vertical a.,** the angle measured within the vertical plane at which the central ray of the x-ray beam is projected related to a reference in the vertical or sagittal plane.

anguli (ang′gu-li) [L.] plural of *angulus.*

angulus (ang′gu-lus), pl. *an′guli* [L.] an angle; a general term used in anatomical nomenclature for a triangular area, or an angle of a particular body, structure, or part. **a. ante′rior pyram′idis os′sis tempora′lis,** anterior angle of petrous portion of temporal bone; see under ANGLE. **a. fronta′lis os′sis parieta′lis** [NA], frontal angle of parietal bone; see under ANGLE. **a. infectio′sus,** perlèche. **a. mandib′ulae** [NA], ANGLE of mandible. **a. mastoi′deus os′sis parieta′lis** [NA], mastoid angle of parietal bone; see under ANGLE. **a. occipita′lis os′sis parieta′lis** [NA], occipital angle of parietal bone; see under ANGLE. **a. oc′uli latera′lis** [NA], lateral angle of eye; see under ANGLE. **a. oc′uli media′lis** [NA], medial angle of eye; see under ANGLE. **a. o′ris** [NA], ANGLE of mouth. **a. parieta′lis os′sis sphenoida′lis,** parietal margin of great wing of sphenoid bone; see under MARGIN. **a. poste′rior pyram′idis os′sis tempora′lis,** angle of petrous portion of temporal bone; see under ANGLE. **a. sphenoida′lis os′sis parieta′lis** [NA], sphenoid angle of parietal bone; see under ANGLE. **a. supe′rior pyram′idis os′sis tempora′lis,** superior angle of petrous portion of temporal bone; see under ANGLE.

anhidrosis (an″hi-dro′sis) [*an* neg. + Gr. *hidrōs* sweat + *-osis*] inability to produce or secrete sweat; deficient sweating.

anhydrase (an-hi′drās) dehydratase. **carbonic a.,** carbonate DEHYDRATASE. **carbonic a. inhibitor,** see carbonic INHIBITOR and see carbonic anhydrase inhibitor DIURETIC.

anhydration (an″hi-dra′shun) dehydration.

anhydremia (an″hi-dre′me-ah) [*an* neg. + Gr. *hydōr* water + *haima* blood + *-ia*] deficiency of water in the blood.

anhydride (an-hi′drīd) [*an* neg. + Gr. *hydōr* water] a chemical compound, usually an acid, from which water has been removed. Anhydrides of bases are oxides; those of alcohols are ethers. **abietic a.,** rosin. **carbonic a.,** CARBON dioxide. **chromic a.,** chromic ACID (2). **hyponitrous acid a.,** nitrous OXIDE. **phthalic a.,** a compound, 1,3-isobenzofurandione, occurring as white, lustrous needles with a mild odor that are soluble in alcohol and slightly soluble in ether and hot water. Used in the production of drugs, dyes, insecticides, and other chemicals, and as a hardener for resins. See also CELLULOSE acetate phthalate. **silicic a.,** SILICON dioxide. **stannic a.,** stannic OXIDE. **sulfuric a., a. of sulfuric acid,** SULFUR trioxide. **sulfurous a.,** SULFUR dioxide. **titanic a.,** titanic ACID. **titanium dioxide. zirconic a.,** ZIRCONIUM oxide.

anhydrite (an-hi′drīt) the natural anhydrous form of calcium sulfate.

anhydrous (an-hi′drous) 1. deprived or destitute of water. 2. pertaining to a hydrate from which water of crystallization has been removed.

anicteric (an″ik-ter′ik) without icterus; not associated with jaundice.

anileridine (an″ĭ-ler′ĭ-dēn) an addictive nonopioid analgesic related to meperidine, 1-[2-(4-aminophenyl)ethyl]-4-phenyl-4-piperidinecarboxylic acid ethyl ester, occurring as a white to yellowish, odorless, slightly bitter, crystalline powder that darkens on exposure to light and is soluble in ethanol, chloroform ether, and, very slightly, water. Used to relieve moderate to severe pain. In dental practice, used chiefly to relieve postoperative pain. Adverse reactions may include respiratory depression, shock, and cardiac arrest. Less severe reactions may include sedation, nausea, vomiting, sweating, agitation, vertigo, weakness, tremor, hallucinations, euphoria, and disorientation. Its addictive properties are similar to those of morphine. Trademarks: Alidine, Apodol, Leritine, Nipecotan. **a. hydrochloride,** the hydrochloride salt of anileridine, occurring as a white, odorless, crystalline powder that is stable in air and is soluble in water, sparingly soluble in ethanol, and insoluble in ether and chloroform. Its pharmacological and toxicological properties are similar to those of the parent compound.

aniline (an′ĭ-lēn, an′ĭ-lin) [Arabic *an′nil* indigo, *nil* blue; L. *nil* indigo] a colorless oily liquid from coal tar and from indigo, made commercially by reducing nitrobenzene. It is slightly soluble in water and freely soluble in ether and alcohol. Combined with other substances, especially chlorine and the chlorates, it forms the aniline dyes that are derived from coal tar. Used as an antiseptic and in the preparation of medicinal substances, resins, varnishes, and other chemicals. Inhalation, ingestion, or cutaneous absorption may cause cyanosis, methemoglobinemia, anemia, anorexia, vertigo, headache, confusion, and other complications. Called also *amidobenzene* and *aminobenzene.*

animé (ah-ne′me) [Fr.] copal.

anion (an′i-on) [Gr. *ana* up + *ion* going] the negatively charged ion which travels to the anode or positive pole during electrolysis. The anions include all nonmetals, the acid radicals, and the hydroxyl ion. They are indicated by a minus sign, as Cl⁻ (formerly by a prime, as Cl′).

anionotropy (an″ĭ-on-ot′ro-pe) [*anion* + Gr. *tropē* a turning] a type of tautomerism in which the migrating group is a negative ion rather than the more usual hydrogen ion. Cf. PROTOTROPY.

Aniprime trademark for *flumethasone.*

aniso- [Gr. *anisos* unequal, uneven] a combining form denoting unequal or dissimilar.

anisochromia (an″ĭ-so-kro′me-ah) [*aniso-* + Gr. *chrōma* color + *-ia*] an abnormal variation in the color of erythrocytes caused by unequal hemoglobin content.

anisocytosis (an-i″so-si-to′sis) [*aniso-* + Gr. *kytos* hollow vessel + *-osis*] a condition characterized by the presence of erythrocytes showing abnormal variation in size.

anisodont (an-i′so-dont) [*aniso-* + Gr. *odous* tooth] 1. one who has unequal, asymmetric teeth. 2. an animal having irregular, asymmetric teeth, as in certain reptiles.

anisotonic (an-i″so-ton′ik) 1. showing a variation in tonicity or tension. 2. not isotonic; having an osmotic pressure differing from that of a solution with which it is compared.

ankle (ang′k′l) the region of the joint between the leg and foot. See TARSUS (1).

ankylo- [Gr. *ankylos* bent or crooked] a combining form meaning bent, or in the form of a noose or loop.

ankylocheilia (ang′kĭ-lo-ki′le-ah) [*ankylo-* + Gr. *cheilos* lip + *-ia*] adhesion of the lips to each other.

ankyloglossia (ang″kĭ-lo-glos′e-ah) [*ankylo-* + Gr. *glōssa* tongue + *-ia*] restricted movement of the tongue resulting in speech difficulty; adherent tongue. Called also *lingua fraenata* and *tonguetie.* See also glossopalatine ANKYLOSIS. **complete a.,** ankyloglossia resulting from fusion between the tongue and the floor of the mouth. **partial a.,** ankyloglossia resulting from a short lingual frenum or one which is attached too near the tip of the tongue.

ankylosed (ang′kĭ-lōsd) fused or obliterated, as a joint.

ankyloses (ang″kĭ-lo′sēz) plural of *ankylosis.*

ankylosis (ang″kĭ-lo′sis), pl. *ankylo′ses* [Gr. *ankylōsis*] abnormal immobility of a part or consolidation of a joint. See also SYNOSTOSIS. **bony a.,** that due to abnormal union of the bones of a joint. Called also *true a.* **cricoarytenoid joint a.,** complete fixation of the cricoarytenoid joint of the larynx, due to inflammation, characterized by hoarseness, cough, and difficulty in expectoration. **extra-articular a., extracapsular a.,** immobility or restricted mobility of a joint due to the development of abnormal bony or fibrous tissue outside the capsule of the joint. **false a.,** 1. that not due to abnormal union of the bones comprising the joint, but to some other cause. 2. inability to open the mouth, suggesting temporomandibular joint ankylosis, which is caused by trismus, rather than by disease of the joint. **fibrous a.,** that due to immobilization of a joint by the presence of abnormal fibrous tissue. **glossopalatine a.,** attachment of the tip of the tongue to the hard palate. See also ANKYLOGLOSSIA. **intra-articular a., intracapsular a.,** immobility or restricted mobility of a joint caused by the development of abnormal bony or fibrous tissue or union within the capsule of a joint. **ligamentous a.,** that resulting from rigidity of the ligaments. **temporomandibular joint a.,** immobility or hypomobility of the temporomandibular joint, which may be caused by congenital defects, birth injury, trauma, malunion of condylar fractures, loss of tissue with scarring, inflammation, infections, arthritis, congenital syphilis, and neoplasms. In the intra-articular type, there is progressive destruction of the meniscus with flattening of the mandibular fossa, thickening of the head of the condyle, and narrowing of the joint space; this type is basically fibrous, although ossification in the scar may result in a bony union, permitting little or no mobility of the joint. In the extra-articular type, there is fixation of the joint by a fibrous or bony mass external to the joint proper; movement is possible in this type when an attempt is made to thrust the chin forward. **tooth a.,** solid fixation of a tooth, resulting from fusion of the cementum and alveolar bone, with obliteration of the periodontal ligament. It is uncommon in the deciduous dentition and very rare in permanent teeth. **true a.,** bony a. **zygomatic-coronoid a.,** restricted opening of the jaws associated with hyperplasia of the inner surface of the malar bone with fibrous attachment to the coronoid process of the mandible.

ankylotic (ang″ki-lot′ik) pertaining to or marked by ankylosis.

ankylotomy (ang″ki-lot′o-me) [ankylo- + Gr. tomē cut] lingual frenotomy for relieving ankyloglossia.

anlage (ahn′lah-geh, an′lāj), pl. anla′gen [Ger. "a laying on"] the earliest or primary stage in the development of an organ or structure; primordium.

Annalin trademark for gypsum hemihydrate (see under HEMIHYDRATE).

annealing (ah-nēl′ing) 1. the heating of a material, such as glass or metal, followed by controlled cooling to remove internal stresses and induce a desired degree of toughness, temper, or softness of the material. See also metal a. 2. the hardening of amalgam by heating it in an oven. 3. the heating of a material, such as gold foil, in an electric annealing tray or by passing it through a cleanly burning alcohol flame to volatilize and drive off impurities from its surface. A foil of pure gold (24 carat), whose surface has been completely cleaned by annealing, is rendered cohesive and will weld at room temperature to surfaces of other gold foils. Annealing is effective for removing contaminants, such as oxygen or ammonia, but not sulfur (which does not volatilize on heating). Some recrystallization of gold may occur. Called also degassing. See also cohesive gold FOIL. **metal a.,** the heating of a cold-worked metal to about half its melting temperature in an effort to alter its tensile strength and ductility by removing internal stresses and restoring its undistorted crystalline structure. The process consists of three stages: Recovery, when cold-work properties begin to disappear without observable changes in the metal microstructure; recrystallization, when distorted grains are replaced by new strain-free grains; and grain growth, when small grains merge to form larger ones. The tensile strength and ductility are changed minimally during the recovery stage, the tensile strength is increased and ductility increased during the recrystallization, and only slight changes in ductile and tensile properties are observed during the grain growth stage.

annular (an′u-lar) [L. annularis] shaped like a ring.

annuli (an′u-li) [L.] plural of annulus.

annulus (an′u-lus), pl. an′nuli [L. "a ring"; dim. of anus ring, circle] a ring, or ringlike or circular structure. The spelling has been changed to anulus in official anatomical nomenclature.

anochromasia (an″o-kro-ma′ze-ah) 1. absence of the usual staining reaction from a tissue or cell. 2. a condition in which the erythrocytes show a piling up of hemoglobin at the periphery so that the center is pale.

anociassociation (ah-no″se-ah-so″se-a′shun) [a neg. + L. nocere to injure + association] the blunting of harmful association impulses; a method of anesthesia designed to minimize the effect of surgical shock. The mind of the patient is calmed by an injection of scopolamine and morphine 1 hour before the operation. The general anesthetic employed is usually nitrous oxide and oxygen. The field of operation is blocked by infiltration with procaine. Sharp dissection and gentle manipulations are em-

ployed. To minimize postoperative discomfort in serious cases, quinine and urea hydrochloride solution is injected at some distance from the wound. Called also anocithesia.

anocithesia (ah-no″se-the′ze-ah) anociassociation.

anode (an′ōd) [Gr. ana up + hodos way] 1. the positive pole or electrode to which negative ions are attracted. 2. in an x-ray tube, a solid copper device equipped with a tungsten insert, serving as a target for high-velocity electrons from the heated cathode, which on being suddenly arrested, give rise to x-rays. See also x-ray tube TARGET and x-ray tube, hot-cathode, under TUBE. **hooded a.,** the anode in an x-ray tube that incorporates a copper shield to overcome the emission of secondary x-rays. **rotating a.,** the anode in an x-ray tube on which the tungsten target constantly rotates.

anodontia (an″o-don′she-ah) [an neg. + Gr. odous tooth + -ia] absence of the teeth. Called also agomphiasis and anodontism. See also HYPODONTIA, OLIGODONTIA, and PSEUDOANODONTIA. **false a., induced a. induced a.,** that resulting from extraction of all teeth. Called also false a. **partial a.,** hypodontia. **total a.,** a rare condition characterized by congenital absence of all teeth, both deciduous and permanent, which is frequently associated with generalized deformities, such as hereditary ectodermal dysplasia. **true a., a. ve′ra,** total or partial congenital absence of teeth.

anodontism (an″o-don′tizm) anodontia.

anodyne (an′o-dīn) [an neg. + Gr. odynē pain] 1. relieving pain. 2. a medicine or drug that relieves pain. The anodynes include opium, morphine, codeine, aspirin, and others. Called also acesodyne. See also ANALGESIC.

anodynia (an″o-din′e-ah) [an neg. + Gr. odynē pain + -ia] freedom from pain.

Anodynine trademark of antipyrine.

Anodynon trademark for ethyl chloride (see under CHLORIDE).

anomalad (ah-nom′ah-lad) a group of morphological defects that stem from a single localized structural anomaly which resulted in a cascade of consequent defects. See also ABNORMALITY and SYNDROME. **Robin's a.,** brachygnathia and cleft palate, often associated with glossoptosis, backward and upward displacement of the larynx, angulation of the manubrium sterni, and pressure marks on the chest caused by the rami of the mandible. Cleft palate makes sucking and swallowing difficult and permits easy access of fluids to the larynx. Periodic inspiratory distress, exacerbated by feeding or lying the child on its back, is frequent and is initiated by choking. The condition may proceed to stridor, cyanosis, and rib retraction, and is often accompanied by vomiting. It may occur without associated abnormalities, but is more likely to be a component of various teratogenic syndromes or hereditary conditions, its mode of transmission being that of the syndrome with which it is associated. Called also micrognathia-glossoptosis syndrome, Pierre Robin's syndrome, and Robin's syndrome.

anomalo- [Gr. anōmalos irregular, from an neg + homalos even] a combining form meaning irregular or uneven.

anomalous (ah-nom′ah-lus) [Gr. anōmalos] not normal; deviating from the natural order.

anomaly (ah-nom′ah-le) [Gr. anōmalia] marked deviation from the normal standard; abnormality. **Alder's a., Alder-Reilly a.,** a leukocyte anomaly characterized by the presence of azurophilic granulation of the neutrophils, eosinophils, basophils, monocytes, and lymphocytes occurring in Hunter-Hurler syndrome. Called also leukocyte granulation a. **dental a.,** a congenital or acquired abnormality in which a tooth or teeth deviate from normal form, function, or position. Called also dental abnormality. **dental a., eugnathic.** eugnathic a. **dentofacial a.,** a congenital or acquired abnormality in which the dental and oral structures deviate from normal form, function, or position. Called also dentofacial abnormality. **dysnathic a.,** a congenital or acquired dental anomaly, also involving the mandible or the maxillae, or both jaws. Called also dysgnathic abnormality. **eugnathic a.,** a dental anomaly involving only the teeth and their alveolar supporting structures. Called also eugnathic dental a., eugnathic abnormality, and eugnathic dental abnormality. **Hegglin's a.,** May-Hegglin a. **Jordan's a.,** sudanophilic inclusions in the cytoplasm of granulocytes, present in some systemic diseases. **leukocyte granulation a.,** Alder's a. **May-Hegglin a.,** a cytoplasmic anomaly of the leukocytes, characterized by the presence of Döhle's bodies and giant blood platelets. It is inherited as a dominant trait and affected patients are usually clinically normal, but about one-fourth have a hemorrhagic tendency, which is related to thrombocytopenia and abnormal platelet function. The prothrombin consumption test, clot retraction, and other tests may show defective platelet function. Döhle's bodies are usually found in the neutrophils but they may also occur in eosinophils, basophils, monocytes, and lymphocytes. Called also Hegglin's and May-Hegglin syn-

drome. **oral a.,** oral ABNORMALITY. **Pelger-Hüet a.,** a hereditary anomaly of leukocyte maturation, characterized by decreased segmentation of the nuclei of granulocytes, giving the nuclei a rodlike or dumbbell shape and a coarse, lumpy structure; condensation of nuclear chromatin in granulocytes, lymphocytes, and monocytes; and normal cytoplasmic maturation. Döhle bodies may be present. Usually, there are no associated systemic abnormalities. It is believed to be transmitted as a simple dominant trait. See also *pseudo–Pelger-Hüet a.* **Peters' a.,** a congenital form of corneal opacity characterized by leukoma in association with the absence of Descemet's membrane and of the endothelium and anterior synechiae; it may be associated with cleft lip and palate. **pseudo–Pelger-Hüet a.,** an acquired form of Pelger-Hüet anomaly seen in some leukemias, myeloproliferative syndromes, malaria, myxedema, and other disorders. Morphologically, it is identical with the hereditary form (see *Pelger-Hüet a.*). **Rieger's a.,** Rieger's SYNDROME.

anonymous (ah-non′ĭ-mus) nameless; innominate.

anophthalmia (an″of-thal′me-ah) [*an* neg. + Gr. *ophthalmos* eye + *-ia*] a developmental disorder characterized by complete absence of the eyes or, more commonly, the presence of vestigial eyes.

anorexia (an″o-rek′se-ah) [Gr. "want of appetite"] lack or loss of appetite for food.

anosmia (an-oz′me-ah) [*an* neg. + Gr. *osmē* smell + *-ia*] lack of the sense of smell. Called also *olfactory anesthesia.*

anostosis (an″os-to′sis) [*an* neg. + Gr. *osteon* bone + *-osis*] defective development of bone.

anoxemia (an″ok-se′me-ah) [*an* neg. + *oxygen* + Gr. *haima* blood + *-ia*] absence or lack of oxygen in the blood; commonly used to mean abnormally decreased content of oxygen in the blood. See also ANOXIA.

anoxia (ah-nok′se-ah) [*an* neg. + *oxygen* + *-ia*] absence or lack of oxygen; commonly used to mean abnormally decreased oxygen content in the tissues. See also ANOXEMIA, HYPOXEMIA, and HYPOXIA.

Anparton trademark for *clofibrate.*

Anprolene trademark for *ethylene oxide* (see under ETHYLENE).

ANS acanthion.

ansa (an′sah), pl. *an′sae* [L. "handle"] a general anatomical term for a looplike structure. Called also *loop.* **a. cervica′lis** [NA], **a. hypoglos′si,** a nerve loop formed between the hypoglossal and second cervical nerves, running along the surface of the carotid sheath to the middle of the neck and actually constituting branches (inferior and superior rami) of the first three cervical nerves. It sends off branches that supply the omohyoid, sternohyoid, and sternothyroid muscles. Called also *loop of hypoglossal nerve.*

ansae (an′se) [L.] plural of *ansa.*

Ansbacher unit [Stefan *Ansbacher,* German-born biologist in the United States] see under UNIT.

ANSI American National Standards Institute (see under INSTITUTE).

Ansolysen trademark for *pentolinium tartrate* (see under PENTOLINIUM).

Anspor trademark for *cephadrine.*

Anstie's rule [Francis Edmund *Anstie,* English physician, 1833–1874] see under RULE.

ant. anterior.

ant- see ANTI-.

Antabuse trademark for *disulfiram.*

Antadol trademark for *phenylbutazone.*

Antagonate trademark for *chlorpheniramine maleate* (see under CHLORPHENIRAMINE).

antagonism (an-tag′o-nizm″) [Gr. *antagōnisma* struggle] opposition or contrariety between similar things, as between muscles, medicines, or organisms.

antagonist (an-tag′o-nist) [Gr. *antagōnistēs* an opponent] 1. an opponent; an adversary; one who opposes another. 2. a tooth in one jaw that opposes a tooth in the other jaw. 3. antagonistic MUSCLE.. **adrenergic a.,** see adrenergic blocking drugs, under DRUG. **α-adrenergic a.,** see -adrenergic blocking drugs, under DRUG. **β-adrenergic a.,** see β-adrenergic blocking drugs, under DRUG. **anticoagulant a.,** ANTICOAGULANT antagonist. **competitive a.,** 1. a drug which occupies a significant proportion of the receptors and thereby prevents them from reacting maximally with an agonist. 2. a substance that competes with a substrate or with an enzyme which ordinarily attacks the substrate, thus interfering with usual metabolic activity. The antagonist is usually a substrate analogue. **folic acid a.,** folic acid ANALOGUE. **H₁ a., H₁** INHIBITOR. **H₂ a., H₂** INHIBITOR. **histamine a.,** histamine INHIBITOR. **metabolite a.,** ANTIMETABOLITE. **morphine a.,** narcotic a. **narcotic a.,** a substance that antagonizes the action of narcotics, chiefly by competing with morphine-like compounds for opioid receptor sites. Additionally, some produce psycho-

tomimetic and other effects of morphine; act on severe but not mild forms of respiratory depression; cause withdrawal syndrome that differs from that produced by morphine; precipitate the withdrawal syndrome in patients on high levels of morphine, but act as its substitute at lower levels of dependence; and are required in lesser amounts to precipitate withdrawal symptoms or to antagonize effects as physical dependence develops. They are sometimes classified as pure antagonists (e.g., naloxone) when their action is limited to opioid inhibition, or partial agonists or agonist-antagonists of the nalorphine type (e.g., nalorphine, levallorphan) when the antagonism is associated with autonomic, endocrine, analgesic, and respiratory depressant effects, such as those which are typical of morphine. Drugs, such as pentazocine, which exert a morphine-like action, without precipitating withdrawal symptoms at high doses of morphine but suppressing withdrawal at low doses, are known as partial agonists of the morphine type. Used chiefly in the treatment of narcotic-induced respiratory depression and in the diagnosis and therapy of narcotic addiction. Called also *morphine a.* and *opioid a.* **noncompetitive a.,** a drug that may react with the receptor in such a way as not to prevent agonist-receptor combination, but to prevent the combination from initiating a response, or to inhibit some subsequent events in the chain of action that led to the final response. **opioid a.,** narcotic a. **pure narcotic a.,** see *narcotic a.* **purine a.,** purine ANALOGUE. **pyrimidine a.,** pyrimidine ANALOGUE. **thyroid a.,** any substance which interferes with the synthesis of thyroid hormone by interfering with the incorporation of iodine into an organic form. Principal thyroid antagonists include compounds containing a thiocarbamide group, such as thiourea, thiouracil, and related compounds, and those containing an aminobenzene group, such as aniline and sulfonamides. See also THYROXINE.

Antalin trademark for *calcium disodium edetate* (see under CALCIUM).

Antallergan trademark for *pyrilamine.*

Antalvic trademark for *propoxyphene hydrochloride* (see under PROPOXYPHENE).

antazoline phosphate (ant-az′o-lēn) an antihistaminic drug that acts on the H₁ receptor, 2-[*N*-benzylanilino)methyl]-2-imidazoline, occurring as a white crystalline powder with a bitter haste, which produces temporary numbness of the tongue, and is readily soluble in water, slightly soluble in methanol, and insoluble in benzene and ether. It is used in the treatment of allergic diseases, such as allergic conjunctivitis. Trademarks: Antihistal, Antistin.

ante- [L. *ante* before] a prefix signifying before in time or place.

antecedent (an″te-se′dent) [L. *antecedere* to go before, precede] 1. occurring or existing before but influencing or conditioning an issue or occurrence. 2. a condition or situation occurring or existing before but influencing or conditioning an issue or occurrence. **plasma thromboplastin a.,** FACTOR XI.

ante cibum (an′te si′bum) [L.] before meals; abbreviated *a.c.* in prescriptions.

antefebrile (an″te-feb′ril) [*ante-* + L. *febris* fever] before the onset of fever.

anteflexion (an-te-flek′shun) [*ante-* + L. *flexio* bend] an abnormal forward curvature of an organ or part; displacement in which the organ is actually bent forward. See also ANTERVERSION (1).

Antegan trademark for *cyproheptadine hydrochloride* (see under CYPROHEPTADINE).

antegrade (an′te-grād) anterograde.

anteriad (an-tēr′e-ad) toward the anterior surface of the body.

anterior (an-tēr′e-or) [L. "before"; neut. *anterius*] situated in front of or in the forward part of an organ; affecting the forward part of an organ; toward the head end of the body; in anatomical nomenclature, used in reference to the ventral or belly surface of the body.

antero- [L. *anterior* before] a prefix signifying before.

anteroclusion (an″ter-o-kloo′zhun) mesioclusion.

anteroexternal (an″ter-o-eks-ter′nal) situated on the front and to the outer side.

anterograde (an′ter-o-grād″) [*antero-* + L. *gredi* to go] moving or extending forward. Called also *antegrade.*

anteroinferior (an″ter-o-in-fēr′e-or) situated in front and below

anterointernal (an″ter-o-in-ter′nal) situated in front and to the inner side.

anterolateral (an″ter-o-lat′er-al) situated in front and to one side.

anteromedian (an″ter-o-me′de-an) situated in front and toward the median plane.

anteroposterior (an″ter-o-pos-te′re-or) extending from the front backward; in roentgenology, it denotes such direction of the beam.

anterosuperior (an″ter-o-su-pēr′e-or) situated in front and above.

anteroventral (an″ter-o-ven′tral) situated in front and toward the ventral surface.

anteversion (an″te-ver′zhun) [*ante-* + L. *versio* turning] 1. the forward tipping or tilting of an organ; displacement in which the organ is tipped forward, but is not bent at an angle, as occurs in anteflexion. 2. a form of malocclusion in which the teeth or other maxillary structures are further forward than normal. Cf. RETROVERSION.

anthelmintic (ant″hel-min′tik) [*anti-* + Gr. *helmins* worm] 1. destructive to worms. 2. an agent that is destructive to worms.

Anthiphen trademark for *dichlorophen.*

Anthisan trademark for *pyrilamine.*

Anthony see sinus BALLOON (Shea-Anthony antral balloon).

anthracene (an′thrah-sēn) 1. a tricyclic aromatic hydrocarbon $C_{14}H_{10}$, presenting yellow crystals with blue fluorescence that are soluble in alcohol and ether but are insoluble in water. It is derived from coal tar and is used in the production of dyestuffs.

anthracosis (an-thrah-ko′sis) [Gr. *anthrax* coal, carbuncle + *-osis*] a form of pneumoconiosis caused by the inhalation of coal dust, thus causing the lungs and the regional lymph nodes to become dark or even black in color. **a. lin′guae,** black TONGUE.

anthrax (an′thraks) [Gr. "coal, carbuncle"] a skin disease of sheep, horses, and cattle caused by *Bacillus anthracis,* which is sometimes contracted by veterinarians, butchers, farmers, and other workers exposed to contaminated animal products. After inoculation, lesions appear within 1 to 3 days, and consist of inflammatory papules which evolve into bullae containing blood or pus, surrounded by intense infiltrations. A ring of vesicles forms around the bullae, surmounting the infiltrated zone; the edematous zone may be extensive (malignant edema). The bullae rupture, leaving shallow ulcers which dry to form a tough, black eschar. The regional lymph nodes usually enlarge and sometimes suppurate. Severe cases may be associated with fever, prostration, headache, and septicemia. The face and neck are the common sites; involvement of the lips and tongue may lead to extension to the throat and upper respiratory tract, also causing phlegmon of the floor of the mouth and glottic edema. Involvement of the lungs and intestines may lead to death. Called also *malignant pustule.*

anthropo- [Gr. *anthrōpos* man] a combining form denoting a relationship to man, or to a human being.

anthropoid (an′thro-poid) [*anthropo-* + Gr. *eidos* form] resembling man. The anthropoid apes are the tailless apes, including the chimpanzee, gibbon, gorilla, and orangutan.

anthropology (an″thro-pol′o-je) [*anthropo-* + Gr. *logos* word, reason] the study of man, his origins, historical and cultural development, and races, usually subdivided into physical anthropology, cultural (social) anthropology, ethnology, archeology, and linguistics.

anthropometry (an″thro-pom′ĕ-tre) [*anthropo-* + Gr. *metron* measure] the measurement of the dimensions and proportions of the human body. In the living body, the measurement of the head is known as *cephalometry* and of the body as *somatometry;* in the dry skeleton, the measurement of the skull is known as *craniometry* and of the bones as *osteometry.*

anthropomorphism (an″thro-po-mor′fizm) [*anthropo-* + Gr. *morphē* form] the attribution of human behavior, form, or character to one who or that which is not human.

anti-, ant- [Gr. *anti* against] a prefix signifying counteracting, effective against, or opposing.

antiadrenergic (an″ti-ah-dren-er′jik) 1. opposing the effects of impulses mediated by the adrenergic receptors. 2. adrenergic neuron blocking DRUG.

antianemic (an″ti-ah-ne′mik) 1. counteracting or preventing anemia. 2. an agent that counteracts or prevents anemia.

antiantibody (an″ti-an′ti-bod″e) an immunoglobulin that is formed to passively administered antibody that is itself capable of acting as an immunogen, and that can interact with the newly formed antibody. The passively administered antibody is most often a heterologous protein.

antiantidote (an″ti-an′ti-dōt″) a substance that counteracts the action of an antidote.

antiarrhythmic (an″ti-ah-rith′mik) 1. preventing or alleviating cardiac arrhythmias. 2. an agent that prevents or alleviates cardiac arrhythmias.

antibacterial (an″ti-bak-te′re-al) 1. destroying or suppressing the growth or reproduction of bacteria. See also BACTERICIDAL and BACTERIOSTATIC. 2. an agent that destroys or suppresses the growth or reproduction of bacteria.

antibechic (an″ti-bek′ik) [*anti-* + Gr. *bēchikos* suffering from cough] 1. relieving cough. 2. an agent that relieves cough. Called also *antitussive.*

antibiosis (an″ti-bi-o′sis) [*anti-* + Gr. *bios* life] an association between two types or populations of organisms that is detrimental to one of them.

antibiotic (an″ti-bi-ot′ik) 1. of the nature of or pertaining to antibiosis. 2. a chemical substance produced by or obtained from living cells, especially bacteria, fungi, or actinomycetes, or an equivalent synthetic compound, which suppresses the growth of other organisms, frequently leading to their destruction. According to their antibiotic properties, antibiotics are sometimes classified as those which inhibit cell wall formation, including penicillins, cephalosporins, cycloserine, vancomycin, ristocetin, and bacitracin; those which affect the permeability of the cell membrane, including polymyxins, nystatin, and amphotericin; those which inhibit protein synthesis by their action on ribosomes, including chloramphenicol, tetracyclines, erythromycin, oleandomycin, and lincomycin; and those which inhibit nucleic acid function. **aminoglycoside a.,** any of a group of antibiotics containing one or more amino sugars, such as glucosamine or neosamine linked by glycoside linkages to a basic 6-membered carbon ring. They include gentamicin, kanamycin, neomycin, and streptomycin. These antibiotics are similar in their antibacterial effects; act at the ribosome, causing misreading of one or more codons; and have similar toxic effects, especially causing hearing disorders. **antifungal a.,** an antibiotic effective against fungi. **antineoplastic a.,** an antibiotic capable of arresting or inhibiting the growth of neoplastic cells. Dactinomycin, daunorubicin, doxorubicin, bleomycin, and mithramycin are the most commonly used antineoplastic antibiotics. **bactericidal a.,** one that kills bacteria. **bacteriostatic a.,** one that suppresses the growth or reproduction of bacteria. **broad-sprectrum a.,** one effective against a broad range of bacteria, such as tetracycline and chloramphenicol which are effective against both gram-negative and gram-positive bacteria. **cephalosporin a.,** see CEPHALOSPORIN. **macrolide a.,** an antibiotic characterized by a lactone ring, a ketone function, commonly an α-β-unsaturated system, and a deoxyamino sugar containing a dimethylamino group. See MACROLIDE. **narrow-spectrum a.,** one effective against a narrow range of bacteria, such as penicillin G which is effective only against gram-positive bacteria and *Neisseria,* or bacitracin whose effectiveness is limited to only gram-positive bacteria. **oral a.,** one effective when administered orally. **penicillin a.,** see PENICILLIN. **polyene a.,** one having the general structure $(CH = CH)_n$ and containing large lactone rings; usually effective against fungi. **polypeptide a.,** any of a group of antibiotics having polypeptide chains as the basis of their structure. The group includes bacitracin, capreomycin, colistimethate, colistin, gramicidin, polymyxin, and tyrothricin; only colistin and polymyxin are chemically and pharmacologically related to each other. **tetracycline a.,** see TETRACYCLINE (2).

antiblastic (an″ti-blas′tik) [*anti-* + Gr. *blastos* germ] retarding growth or multiplication, as of tumor or bacterial cells.

antibody (an″ti-bod″e) a plasma globulin, most predominantly a gamma globulin, which has a specific amino acid sequence by virtue of which it interacts specifically with the antigen that induced its synthesis in lymphocytes, or with antigen closely related to it. Antibodies are classified according to their mode of action as, for example, agglutinins, bacteriolysins, hemolysins, opsonins, and precipitins. Abbreviated *ab.* See also IMMUNO-GLOBULIN. **a. affinity,** the strength of binding between a single antigenic determinant (ag) and its corresponding antibody (ab), expressed in terms of the symbols in equilibrium constant (K) of the reaction, where [ ] indicates concentration:

$$K = \frac{[ab - ag]}{[ab]\,[ag]}$$

representing the reaction ab + ag $\rightleftharpoons$ ab − ag complex. Antibodies with high affinity constant bind strongly. **agglutinating a.,** agglutinin. **allocytophilic a.,** a cytotropic antibody derived from the same species; see *cytotropic a.* **anaphylactic a.,** anaphylactin. **a. anti-A,** AGGLUTININ anti-A. **anti-B a.,** AGGLUTININ anti-B. **antitissue a.,** cytotoxic a. **a. avidity,** the strength of binding of a full antigen molecule having more than one determinant with an antiserum containing the corresponding antibodies. The multivalence of most antigens results in a bonus effect, which is due to linkages by several antibodies to different determinants on the same antigen and results in a strength of binding of the entire antigen molecule that is greater than the sum of the individual links of determinants with homologous antibody. **blocking a.,** one having the same specificity as other antibodies but interferes with their action because of dissimilar associated properties. In atopic allergies blocking antibody reacts with and prevents allergen from reacting with sensitizing antibody in the tissues. **blood group a.,** agglutinin. **cross-reacting a.,** one that combines with an antigen other than the one that induced its production. **cytophilic a.,** cytotropic a. **cytotoxic a.,** one that causes damage to antigen-bearing cells, usually involving complement, either by cytolysis or by damaging the cell membrane without lysis. Cytotoxic antibodies play a role in immunologic diseases by activation of complement with the production of intermediate components that mobilize leukocytes, have anaphylatoxic properties, and produce structure damage to cell membranes. Called also *antitissue a.* **cytotropic a.,** a type of antibody which attaches to tissue cells (such as mast cells and basophils) through Fc segments to induce the release of histamine and other vasoconstrictor amines important in immediate hypersensitivity.reactions. In man, this antibody (also known as *reagin*) is primarily of the immunoglobulin class IgE. Called also *cytophilic a.* Cytotropic antibodies derived from the same species are called *homocytotropins,* or *allocytophilic* or *homocytotropic antibodies;* those from different species, *heterocytotropins,* or *heterocytotropic* or *xenocytophilic antibodies.* **a. dependent cellular cytotoxicity,** see under CYTOTOXICITY. **fluorescent a.,** see IMMUNOFLUORESCENCE. **Forssman a.,** one produced in response to the injection of tissue extracts containing Forssman antigen. **heat labile a.,** one whose ability to react with antigen is destroyed by heating to 56°C. **heterocytotropic a.,** a cytotropic antibody derived from a different species; see *cytotropic a.* **heterogenetic a.,** one capable of reacting with antigens phylogenetically unrelated to the antigen that stimulated its production as well as with the homologous antigen. **heterophile a.,** one produced by injection of a heterogenetic or heterophilic antigen. **homocytotropic a.,** a cytotropic antibody derived from the same species; see *cytotropic a.* **incomplete a.,** 1. one combining specifically with Rh-positive erythrocytes without causing visible agglutination but which, in the presence of antihuman globulin (Coombs) serum or high-molecular-weight media, e.g., albumin, will cause red cell clumping. Other red cell–coating proteins, not group specific, may demonstrate similar properties. 2. one with one antigen-binding site or one in which the two antigen-binding sites are so close together that the antibody behaves functionally as a univalent antibody. **Ku a., K5 a.,** see Ku ANTIGEN. **natural a's,** serum proteins present in low titer with the structural properties of immunoglobulins, which can react specifically with antigens, even though the individuals in which they are formed had no known previous exposure to those antigens. They may result from unknown exposure to naturally occurring antigens, e.g., food or bacterial flora. **neutralizing a.,** one that, on mixture with homologous toxin or infectious agent, detoxifies or reduces the infectious titer; components of the antigen-antibody complex can be dissociated and recovered in their original forms; reversibility of the association often decreases with time; the host cell influences effectiveness of interaction — e.g., a virus that is neutralized for one kind of host cell may be infectious for another. **PK a., Prausnitz-Küstner a.,** reagin (1). **reaginic a.,** reagin (1). **sensitizing a.,** a term applied to antibodies that attach to cells or particles and that "sensitize" them and render them susceptible to body defenses. *In vitro,* such antibodies permit the cells or particles to manifest an immunological reaction, e.g., agglutination, lysis by complement, or phagocytosis. **xenocytophilic a.,** a cytotropic antibody derived from a different species; see *cytotropic a.*

anticarcinogenic (an″ti-kar-sin″o-jen′ik) inhibiting or preventing the development of cancer.

anticariogenic (an″ti-kar″e-o-jen′ik) suppressing the development of caries; anticarious.

anticarious (an″ti-ka′re-us) anticariogenic.

anticatalyst (an″ti-kat′ah-list) a substance that retards the action of a catalyzer.

anticathode (an″ti-kath′ōd) the part in a vacuum tube opposite the cathode; the target.

antichlor (an″ti-klōr) SODIUM thiosulfate.

anticholinergic (an″ti-ko″lin-er′jik) 1. inhibiting the passage of impulses through the autonomic receptors mediated by acetylcholine. Cf. CHOLINERGIC. 2. a drug blocking autonomic effectors innervated by postganglionic cholinergic nerves mediated by acetylcholine. The term applies to blocking of media-

tion at both nicotinic and muscarinic receptors, but it is sometimes used as a synonym for antimuscarinic drugs (see under DRUG).

anticholinesterase (an″ti-ko-lin′es′ter-ās) see cholinesterase inhibitors, under INHIBITOR.

anticoagulant (an″ti-ko-ag′u-lant) 1. serving to prevent the coagulation of the blood. 2. any substance that suppresses, delays, or nullifies coagulation of the blood. The action of anticoagulants consists of binding or removing calcium from the blood, thus preventing its participation in blood coagulation; interfering with the hepatic synthesis of vitamin K–dependent clotting factors; interfering with the conversion of prothrombin to a thrombin and the action of thrombin on fibrinogen; thrombolytic action; and interfering with platelet function, with their aggregation. They are used chiefly in the treatment and prevention of thrombosis; their use may cause hemorrhage during oral surgery and cause spontaneous gingival bleeding. See also blood COAGULATION. **a. antagonist,** any substance that suppresses the action of anticoagulants; used in the treatment of hemorrhagic complications occurring during anticoagulant therapy. Prothrombopenic anticoagulants are inhibited mainly by vitamin K; heparin is antagonized by various amines, ammonium compounds, and proteins which precipitate polysulfate, such as protamine sulfate; and fibrinolytic anticoagulants (fibrinolytic inhibitors) are counteracted by aminocaproic acid. **calcium-sequestering a.,** any anticoagulant that binds calcium, thereby preventing it from participation in clotting processes (see blood COAGULATION). Citrates are the principal calcium-sequestering anticoagulants; they are used chiefly in preventing stored blood from coagulating. **circulating a.,** a substance developing in the circulating blood that inhibits blood coagulation. Circulating anticoagulants may be directed against a specific coagulation factor or against a particular stage of blood coagulation. **oral a.,** any anticoagulant taken orally; usually a prothrombopenic anticoagulant. Chemically, oral anticoagulants are derivatives of 4-hydroxycoumarin or indan-1,3-dione. **prothrombopenic a.,** any agent that inhibits the hepatic synthesis of the vitamin K–dependent production of prothrombin (factor II). Prothrombopenic anticoagulants are usually administered orally, and are also known to inhibit coagulation factors VII, IX, and X. Dicumarol is the prototype of this group.

anticomplement (an″ti-kom′plĕ-ment) a substance that inactivates, opposes, or counteracts the action of complement.

anticonvulsant (an″ti-kon-vul′sant) 1. preventing or relieving convulsions. 2. an agent that prevents or relieves convulsions.

antidepressant (an″ti-de-pres′sant) 1. preventing or relieving mental depression. 2. an agent that relieves or prevents mental depression; one that stimulates the mood of a mentally depressed person.

antidiabetic (an″ti-di″ah-bet′ik) 1. preventing or alleviating diabetes. 2. an agent that prevents or alleviates diabetes.

antidiarrheal (an″ti-di″ah-re′al) 1. counteracting diarrhea. 2. an agent that counteracts diarrhea.

antidiuretic (an″ti-di″u-ret′ik) [anti- + diuretic] 1. suppressing the secretion of urine. 2. an agent which suppresses urinary secretion.

antidote (an″ti-dōt) [L. antidotum, from Gr. anti against + didonai to give] a remedy for counteracting a toxin, poison, or harmful effect.

antidromic (an″ti-drom′ik) [Gr. antidromein to run in a contrary direction] conducting impulses in a direction opposite to the normal; said of neurons in the posterior roots of the spinal cord.

antidysenteric (an″ti-dis″en-ter′ik) 1. preventing or alleviating dysentery. 2. an agent that prevents or alleviates dysentery.

antiedemic (an″ti-e-dem′ik) 1. preventing or alleviating edema. 2. an agent that prevents or alleviates edema.

antielectron (an″ti-e-lek′tron) positron.

antiemetic (an″ti-e-met′ik) [anti- + Gr. emetikos inclined to vomit] 1. preventing or alleviating nausea and vomiting. 2. an agent that prevents or alleviates nausea and vomiting.

antiepileptic (an″ti-ep″ĕ-lep′tik) 1. counteracting epilepsy. 2. an agent that counteracts epilepsy.

antifebrile (an″ti-feb′ril) antipyretic.

antifebrin (an″ti-feb′rin) acetanilid.

antifibrinolysin (an″ti-fi″bri-nol′i-sin) an inhibitor of fibrinolysin.

antiflux (an″ti-fluks) a substance that inhibits the action of flux, thereby reducing the flow of a solder, used to confine the flow of the molten solder. Lead pencil or iron rouge or whiting in alcohol are commonly used as antiflux.

antifolate (an″ti-fo′lāt) folic acid ANALOGUE.

Antiformin trademark for an alkaline solution of *sodium hypochlorite* (see under SODIUM).

antifungal (an″ti-fung′gal) 1. destructive to fungi, or suppressing their reproduction or growth; effective against fungal infections. 2. an agent that is destructive to fungi, suppresses the growth or reproduction of fungi, or is effective against fungal infections. Called also *antimycotic*.

antigen (an′ti-jen) [*antibody* + Gr. *gennan* to produce] any substance which, under appropriate conditions, can induce the formation of antibodies or specifically sensitized lymphocytes and is capable of reacting specifically in some detectable manner with the antibodies or lymphocytes so induced. Antigens may be soluble substances, such as toxins and foreign proteins, or particulate, such as bacteria and tissue cells. Abbreviated *ag*. **a. A,** agglutinogen A. **allergic a.,** allergen. **allogeneic a., allotypic a.,** any of a group of antigens genetically controlled by antigenic determinants, which distinguish one individual of a given species from another, being different forms of an antigen coded for at the same locus in all individuals of a species. In man, antigenic determinants of allogeneic antigens are found on erythrocytes, leukocytes, blood platelets, serum proteins, and the surface of cells making up the fixed tissue of the body, including histocompatibility antigens. They are involved in the pathogenesis of hemolytic disease of the newborn, transfusion reactions, and transplantation immunity. Called also *homologous a., isophile a., alloantigen,* and *isoantigen.* **Australia (Au) a.,** the antigen associated with the coat of the hepatitis B virus, which is found in the sera of patients with acute and chronic serum hepatitis (hepatitis caused by the hepatitis B virus). It is found rarely in the sera of patients with infectious hepatitis (hepatitis caused by hepatitis A virus), but only if they are chronic carriers of the HB$_s$Ag. Au antigen is also found in the sera of large numbers of apparently normal people in the tropics and Southeast Asia. So named because it was first detected in the serum of an Australian aborigine. Called also *HB a. (HB,Ag), hepatitis a., hepatitis-associated (HAA) a., hepatitis B surface a., serum hepatitis a.,* and *SH a.* **autologous a.,** autoantigen. **a. B,** agglutinogen B. **blood group a.,** agglutinogen. **C a.,** a red cell antigen of the Rh blood group system. **carbohydrate a's,** numerous polysaccharides isolated from bacteria, other cells, and natural substances, which function as specific haptens or as complete antigens. **Cellano a.,** the blood group antigen K. Called also *K2 a.* and *Cellano factor.* See Kell blood groups, under BLOOD GROUP. **common a.,** an antigenic determinant present in two or more different antigen molecules and frequently leads to cross-reactions among them. See also antigenic DETERMINANT. **complete a.,** one that both stimulates the immune response and reacts with the products (e.g., antibody) of that response. Called also *functional a.* See also *immunogenic a.* **conjugated a.,** one produced by coupling through covalent bonds a hapten to a carrier molecule, such as a protein, carbohydrate, or synthetic polypeptide; when it induces immunization, the resultant immune response may be directed against the hapten, or both the hapten and the carrier. **cross-reacting a.,** one that combines with antibody produced in response to a different but related antigen, owing to similarity of antigenic determinants. **D a.,** the most important determinant of the Rh blood group system, important in the development of isoimmunization in Rh-negative persons exposed to the blood of Rh-positive persons. **Di^a a.,** a Diego antigen. Called also *Di^a factor.* **Di^b a.,** a Diego antigen. Called also *Di^b factor.* **Diego a.,** either of the blood group antigens Di^a or Di^b. See Diego blood groups, under BLOOD GROUP. Called also *Diego factor.* **Do^a a.,** a Dombrock antigen. **Do^b a.,** a Dombrock antigen. **Dombrock a.,** either of the blood group antigens Do^a or Do^b; see Dombrock BLOOD GROUP. **Duffy a.,** either of the blood group antigens Fy^a or Fy^b; see Duffy blood groups, under BLOOD GROUP. **E a.,** a red cell antigen of the Rh blood group system. **endogenous a's,** antigens found within the tissues, surfaces, or lumens of an individual. **envelope a's,** K a's. **exogenous a.,** one presented to the host from the exterior, such as in the form of microorganisms, drugs, pollen, or pollutants; responsible for infections and immunologically mediated diseases, such as asthma and other allergies. **F a.,** Forssman a. **fetal a's,** antigens demonstrable during fetal life but not normally in adults; their reappearance in adults is attributed to reactivation of genes associated with cellular transformation to the malignant state. See also FETOPROTEIN. **flagellar a.,** H a. **fluorescent a.,** see IMMUNOFLUORESCENCE. **Forssman a.,** a heterogenetic antigen (hapten) inducing the production of antisheep hemolysin, occurring in cells of various

unrelated animals, mainly in the organs but not in the erythrocytes (guinea pig, horse) but sometimes only in the erythrocytes (sheep), and occasionally in both (chicken). In the original and strict sense, the antigen is typified by that found in the guinea pig kidney and other tissues and characterized by heat stability and solubility in alcohol; the antigenic determinant is polysaccharide in nature. The term is sometimes used erroneously to refer to any antigen producing sheep hemolysin, but antibodies to it are not necessarily identical, as they are in the case of true Forssman antigen. Called also *F a.* **functional a.,** complete a. **Fy^a a.,** a Duffy antigen. Called also *Fy^a factor.* **Fy^b a.,** a Duffy antigen. Called also *Fy^b factor.* **Gm group a.,** one of more than 20 allotypic markers on the Fc or Fd portion of the heavy γ chains of human IgG immunoglobulin. **H a.** [Ger. *Hauch* film], antigen of the flagella of motile bacteria. Called also *flagellar a.* See also *O a.* **H-2 a.,** major histocompatibility complex (of mouse); see under HISTOCOMPATIBILITY. **HB a. (HB,Ag),** Australia a. **hepatitis a., hepatitis-associated a. (HAA), hepatitis B surface a.,** Australia a. **heterologous a., heterophile a., xenogeneic a.** **histocompatibility a's,** genetically determined isoantigens present on the lipoprotein membranes of some cells, which incite an immune response when grafted onto a genetically disparate individual and thus determine the compatibility of tissue in transplantation. See major histocompatibility complex, under HISTOCOMPATIBILITY. **HLA a., HL-A a.,** major histocompatibility complex (of man); see under HISTOCOMPATIBILITY. **homologous a.,** allogeneic a. **human leukocyte a.,** see major histocompatibility complex (of man), under HISTOCOMPATIBILITY. **H-Y a.,** a histocompatibility antigen which depends on a gene of the Y chromosome. **Ia a., I-A a.,** an allogeneic antigen controlled at the H-2 locus of the mouse chromosome 17 (region I). Ia antigens have a molecular weight between 28,000 and 32,000 daltons. They occur on surfaces of T- and B-lymphocytes, macrophages, epidermal cells, and sperm cells, and are involved in immune responses, stimulating antigen in the mixed lymphocyte reactions, graft versus host reactions, and immune supressor activity. See also major histocompatibility complex (of man), under HISTOCOMPATIBILITY. **immunogenic a.,** antigen capable of eliciting an immune response. See also complete a. and TOLEROGEN. **incomplete a.,** hapten. **Inv group a.,** Km a. **isogeneic a.,** one carried by an individual which is capable of eliciting an immune response in genetically different individuals of the same species, but not in the individual bearing it. **isophile a.,** allogeneic a. **Jk a.,** a rare silent Kidd antigen. **Jk^a a.,** a Kidd antigen. Called also *Jk^a factor.* **Jk^b a.,** a Kidd antigen. Called also *Jk^b factor.* **Js^a a.,** a blood group antigen of the Kell blood groups (see under BLOOD GROUP). Called also *K6 a., Sutter a., Js^a factor, K6 factor,* and *Sutter factor.* **Js^b a.,** a blood group antigen of the Kell blood groups (see under BLOOD GROUP), produced by the allele of Js^a. Called also *K7 a., Js^b factor,* and *K7 factor.* **K a.,** Cellano a. **K a's,** antigens found in bacteria that function as blocking antigens in that their presence interferes with agglutination by O antisera. Called also *envelope a's* and *somatic surface a's.* **K1 a.,** Kell a. **K2 a.,** Cellano a. **K3 a.,** Kp^a a. **K5 a.,** Ku a. **K6 a.,** Js^a a. **K7 a.,** Js^b a. **Kell a.,** the Kell blood group antigen in the Kell blood groups (see under BLOOD GROUP). Called also *K1 a., factor K1,* and *Kell factor.* **Kidd a.,** the blood group antigens Jk^a, Jk^b, or Jk; see Kidd blood groups, under BLOOD GROUP. **Km a.,** one of three alloantigens found in the constant region of the κ light chains in immunoglobulins of humans and other species. Called also *Inv group a.* and *Inv allotype.* **Kp^a a.,** a blood group antigen of the Kell blood groups (see under BLOOD GROUP). Called also *K3 a., Penny a., Kp^a factor,* and *Penny factor.* **Kp^b a.,** a blood group antigen of the Kell blood groups (see under BLOOD GROUP), produced by the allele of Kp^a. Called also *K4 a., Rautenberg a., K4 factor, Kp^b factor,* and *Rautenberg factor.* **Ku a.,** a blood factor in the Kell blood groups (see under BLOOD GROUP). The serum of persons who are K^0 contains an antibody which reacts with every Kell phenotype except K^0, and is referred to as *anti-Ku.* Called also *Peltz a., K5 a., Ku factor, K5 factor,* and *Peltz factor.* See also K^0 PHENOTYPE. **Le^a a.,** a Lewis antigen. Called also *Le^a factor.* **Le^b a.,** a Lewis antigen. Called also *Le^b factor.* **Lewis a.,** a either the Le^a or Le^b antigen; see Lewis blood groups, under BLOOD GROUP. Called also *Lewis factor.* **Lu^a a.,** a Lutheran antigen. Called also *Lu^1 factor.* **Lu^b a.,** a Lutheran antigen. Called also *Lu^b factor.* **Lutheran a.,** either of the blood group antigens Lu^a or Lu^b; see Lutheran blood groups, under BLOOD GROUP. Called also *Lutheran factor.* **Ly a's,** phenotypic antigen expressions of subpopulations of T-lymphocytes. An association has been found between certain Ly antigens and helper or suppressor activities of T-lymphocytes. **M a.,** a type-specific antigen that appears to be located primarily in the cell wall and is associated with virulence of *Streptococcus pyog-*

enes. **NP a.,** a nucleoprotein antigen present in the poxviruses. **O a.** [Ger. *ohne Hauch* without film], one occurring in the lipopolysaccharide layer of the wall of gram-negative bacteria, as opposed to flagellar H antigen. Called also *somatic a.* **organ-specific a.,** any antigen that occurs exclusively in a particular organ and serves to distinguish it from other organs. Two types of organ specificity have been proposed: (1) first-order of tissue specificity, attributed to the presence of an antigen characteristic of a particular organ in a single species; (2) second-order of organ specificity, attributed to an antigen characteristic of the same organ in many even unrelated species. **partial a.,** hapten. **particulate a.,** an antigen present on a particle, such as a microorganism, cell, or inert particle. **Peltz a.,** Ku a. **Penny a.,** Kp^a a. **private a's,** antigens of the low frequency blood groups; so called because they are found only in members of a single kindred, probably differing from ordinary blood group systems only in their incidence. **public a's,** antigens of the high frequency blood groups; so called because they are found in almost all persons tested. **R a.,** a type-specific antigen similar to M antigen of streptococci, except that it is resistant to tryptic digestion. **Rautenberg a.,** Kp^a a. **residue a's,** naturally occurring haptens split from the antigenic complex by autolysis or methods of preparation of purified antigen. **S a.,** a heat-stable, soluble viral antigen that is nucleoprotein in nature; it is found in influenza and the mumps group of viruses. **sequestered a's,** the subsurface cellular constituents of cells, such as those of the thyroid, not normally exposed to the lymphoreticular system. These antigens are not usually recognized as "self," and may lead to autoantibody production and possible autoimmune disease. **serum hepatitis (SH) a.,** Australia a. **shock a.,** specific antigen capable of eliciting characteristic immunological reaction (e.g., anaphylaxis, cell death) in a sensitized animal. **somatic a.,** O a. **somatic surface a's,** K a's. **species-specific a's,** antigens restricted to a single species but occurring in most members of that species. See also species SPECIFICITY. **Sutter a.,** Js^a a. **T a.,** a nonstructural, complement-fixing viral antigen synthesized in the early stage of the infectious cycle; it persists in cells that have been modified by oncogenic adenoviruses. **therapeutic a.,** any substance which, on injection into the body, stimulates the formation of protective antibodies; a vaccine. **Thy 1 a.,** cell-surface isoantigen of mice, found on T-lymphocytes, on brain cells, and on skin and fibroblasts in small amounts, occurring in two allelic forms: Thy 1.1. and Thy 1.2. Formerly called *theta* (Θ) a. **theta (Θ) a.,** Thy 1 a. **tolerogenic a.,** tolerogen. **tumor-specific a., tumor-specific tissue a.,** a cell-surface antigen of tumors that elicits a specific immune response in the host. Abbreviated *TSA* and *TSTA.* **V a., Vi a.,** virulence a., an antigen contained in the capsule of a bacterium, such as the typhoid bacillus, and thought to contribute to its virulence. **xenogeneic a.,** one found in a variety of phylogenetically-unrelated species, including Forssman antigens and various antigens that cross-react with exogenous antigens, such as renal and cardiac tissues and beta hemolytic streptococci. They are also involved in the pathogenesis of certain diseases, including glomerulonephritis and rheumatic fever, and give rise to antibody responses which are useful in the diagnosis of certain diseases, such as the cross-reaction of group A beta hemolytic streptococcal antigen and human heart tissue in rheumatic heart disease. Called also *heterologous a., heterophile a., heteroantigen,* and *xenoantigen.*

antigenic (an-tĭ-jen'ik) having the properties of an antigen.

antigenicity (an″tĭ-jĕ-nis'ĭ-te) the property of a substance (antigen) which allows it to induce the production of and to react with the products of the specific immune response, e.g., antibody or specifically sensitized T-lymphocytes. See also IMMUNOGENICITY.

antiglobulin (an″tĭ-glob'u-lin) an antibody produced against a globulin (usually another antibody) of a species. It may neutralize the antibody activity of the globulin or be used for its localization in tissue. See also antibody TEST and IMMUNOFLUORESCENCE.

Antihistal trademark for *antazoline phosphate* (see under ANTAZOLINE).

antihistaminic (an″tĭ-his″tah-min'ik) 1. counteracting the effect of histamine. 2. a drug that counteracts the effect of histamine. See also histamine INHIBITOR.

antihypertensive (an″tĭ-hi″per-ten'siv) 1. counteracting high blood pressure. 2. an agent that reduces high blood pressure or counteracts hypertension.

antihypnotic (an″tĭ-hip-not'ik) 1. preventing or hindering sleep. 2. an agent that prevents or hinders sleep.

anti-infective (an″tĭ-in-fek'tiv) 1. counteracting infection. 2. an agent that counteracts infection.

anti-inflammatory (an″tĭ-in-flam'ah-to″re) 1. countering or suppressing inflammation. 2. an agent that counteracts or suppresses inflammation.

anti-invasin I (an″tĭ-in-va'sin) an enzyme present in normal blood plasma that antagonizes hyaluronidase.

antilewisite (an″tĭ-lu'is-īt) dimercaprol.

antilipemic (an″tĭ-li-pe'mik) 1. counteracting high fat levels in the blood of hyperlipemia. 2. an agent that counteracts high fat levels in the blood of hyperlipemia.

antilithic (an″tĭ-lith'ik) [*anti-* + Gr. *lithos* stone] 1. preventing the formation of calculi. 2. an agent that prevents the formation of calculi.

antilytic (an″tĭ-lĭt'ik) inhibiting or suppressing lysis.

antimetabolite (an″tĭ-mĕ-tab'o-līt) a substance with a molecular structure similar to that of a particular natural metabolite and interferes with the function of the natural metabolite. It is a competitive inhibitor of a natural endogenous substrate of the enzyme, bearing a close structural resemblance to one required in normal physiological functioning, and exerting its effect by interfering with the utilization of the essential metabolite. Examples of antimetabolites are sulfonamides, which compete with *para*-aminobenzoic acid and, thus, interfere with its incorporation into folic acid; and methotrexate, which competes with folic acid for folic reductase and, thus, interferes with the formation of folinic acid. Antimetabolites which interfere with DNA and RNA synthesis in proliferating tissues are used as antineoplastic agents; they include folic acid, pyrimidine, and purine analogues. Called also *competitive inhibitor* and *metabolite antagonist.* See also Woods-Fildes THEORY.

antimicrobial (an″tĭ-mi-kro'be-al) 1. killing microorganisms, or suppressing their multiplication or growth. 2. an agent that kills microorganisms or suppresses their multiplication or growth.

antimitotic (an″tĭ-mi-tot'ik) inhibiting or preventing mitosis.

antimongolism (an″tĭ-mon'go-lizm) chromosome 21q SYNDROME.

antimongoloid (an″tĭ-mon'go-loid) opposite to that characteristic of mongolism (see Down's SYNDROME), as antimongoloid slant of the palpebral fissures, whereby the outer rims slant downward.

antimonial (an″tĭ-mo'ne-al) pertaining to or containing antimony.

antimonic (an″tĭ-mon'ik) pertaining to or containing pentavalent antimony.

antimonid (an″tĭ-mo'nid) a binary compound of antimony.

antimonious (an″tĭ-mo'ne-us) pertaining to or containing trivalent antimony. Called also *antimonous.*

antimonium (an″tĭ-mo'ne-um), gen. *antimo'nii* [L.] antimony.

antimonous (an″tĭ-mōn'us) antimonious.

antimony (an'tĭ-mo'ne) [L. *antimonium, stibium*] a silvery, lustrous, hard, brittle heavy metal. Symbol, Sb; atomic number, 51; atomic weight 121.74. It is caustic on contact and its salts, notably tartrates, have emetic effects through their action on the medulla oblongata, also causing nausea and coughing. The reflex action of antimony salts on the bronchial and salivary glands produces excessive production of bronchial mucus and sialorrhea. Sometimes used as parasiticides and in the treatment of protozoal and helminthic infections. In the past, antimony compounds were used extensively in various medicines and cosmetics but, because of their toxic effects, their use has been largely discontinued. Antimony compounds may cause keratitis, dermatitis, conjunctivitis, and nasal septum ulceration; symptoms of poisoning being similar to those of arsenic poisoning. In the presence of hydrogen, antimony may form stibine, which is extremely toxic. **a. hydride,** stibine. **tin-a. alloy,** tin-antimony ALLOY.

antimonyl (an-tim'o-nil″) the univalent radical SbO−.

antimuscarinic (an″tĭ-mus-kah-rin'ik) 1. opposing the action of muscarine. 2. antimuscarinic DRUG.

antimycotic (an″tĭ-mi-kot'ik) destructive to fungi, or suppressing their reproduction or growth; effective against fungal infections; antifungal.

antinatriuresis (an″tĭ-na″tre-u-re'sis) inhibiting the excretion of sodium in the urine.

antinauseant (an″tĭ-naw'ze-ant) 1. preventing or relieving nausea. 2. an agent that prevents or relieves nausea. See also ANTIEMETIC.

antineoplastic (an″tĭ-ne″o-plas'tik) 1. inhibiting or preventing the development of neoplasms; antioncotic. 2. an agent that inhibits or prevents the development of neoplasms. Antineoplastic agents, with the exception of hormones, are generally cytotoxic chemical substances which interfere with nuclear functions of cell division, thereby inhibiting mitosis in proliferating tissues, without being specific for cancer cells and affecting both neoplastic and nonneoplastic tissues. Acting on proliferating cell systems and genetic information transfer, they also interrupt immune processes, thus being immunosuppressive. They may be classified as alkylating agents, including nitrogen mustards, ethylenimines, alkyl sulfonates, nitrosoureas, and triazines; antimetabolites, including folic acid, pyrimidine, and purine analogues, antineoplastic alkaloids, antibiotics, enzymes, and hormones; and radioactive isotopes. All are toxic, but are used in tolerable doses. Dental patients receiving antineoplastics may exhibit susceptibility to infection, oral ulcers, mucosal sloughing, necrotic lesions, and blood dyscrasis due to suppressive effects of cytotoxic drugs on the hematopoietic system.

antineuralgic (an″ti-nu-ral′jik) 1. alleviating or counteracting neuralgia. 2. an agent that alleviates or counteracts neuralgia.

antiniad (an-tin′e-ad) toward the antinion.

antinial (an-tin′e-al) pertaining to the antinion.

antinion (an-tin′e-on) the frontal pole of the head; the median frontal point farthest from the inion.

antiodontalgic (an″ti-o′′don-tal′jik) relieving toothache.

antioncotic (an″ti-ong-kot′ik) [*anti-* + Gr. *onkos* bulk, mass] 1. inhibiting or preventing the development of tumors; antineoplastic. 2. an agent that inhibits or prevents the development of tumors.

antiotomy (an″ti-ot′o-me) [*Gr. antias* tonsil + *tomē* a cutting] excision of the tonsils; tonsillectomy.

antioxidant (an″ti-ok′si-dant) a substance that retards oxidation.

antiparasitic (an″ti-par″ah-sit′ik) 1. destructive to parasites or inhibiting parasitic infestation. 2. an agent that is destructive to parasites or inhibits parasitic infestation.

antiparasympathomimetic (an″ti-par″ah-sim″pah-tho-mi-met′ik) 1. opposing the action of the parasympathetic nervous system. 2. a substance inhibiting impulses of the parasympathetic nervous system. The term applies to blocking impulses mediated at both nicotinic and muscarinic receptors, but it is sometimes used as a synonym for an antimuscarinic drug (see under DRUG).

antiphlogistic (an″ti-flo-jis′tik) [*anti-* + Gr. *phlogos* flame] 1. counteracting inflammation and fever. 2. an agent that counteracts inflammation and fever.

antiplasmin (an″ti-plaz′min) a principle of the blood plasma, also found in the blood platelets, which inhibits plasmin. Two substances have been identified as plasmin: One is an α-globulin with a molecular weight of 55,000, having both slow and immediate antiplasmin activity; and the other is a heat and acid stable α-macroglobulin.

antiprotozoal (an″ti-pro-to-zo′al) 1. destroying protozoa, or checking their growth or reproduction. 2. an agent that destroys protozoa or checks their growth or reproduction.

antiputrefactive (an″ti-pu″tre-fak′tiv) 1. counteracting putrefaction. 2. an agent that counteracts putrefaction.

antipruritic (an″ti-proo-rit′ik) 1. relieving or preventing itching. 2. an agent that prevents or relieves itching.

antipsychotic (an″te-si-kot′ik) 1. favorably modifying psychotic behavior and symptoms. 2. antipsychotic DRUG.

antipyogenic (an″ti-pi″o-jen′ik) [*anti-* + Gr. *pyon* pus + *gennan* to produce] preventing the development of pus.

antipyretic (an″ti-pi-ret′ik) [*anti-* + Gr. *pyretos* fever] 1. relieving or reducing fever. 2. an agent that relieves or reduces fever. Called also *antifebrile, antithermic,* and *febrifuge.*

antipyrine (an″ti-pi′ren) [*anti-* + Gr. *pyr* fire] an analgesic, antipyretic, and anti-inflammatory agent, 2,3-dimethyl-1-phenyl-3-pyrazoline-5-one, occurring as a white, odorless, slightly bitter, crystalline powder or solid that is soluble in water, ethanol, chloroform, and ether. Used for measuring total body water and for assessing liver oxidase activity. Used in the past in the treatment of pain. The drug is toxic and may cause agranulocytosis. Called also *phenazone.* Trademarks: Analgesine, Anodyne, Parodyne, Sedatine.

antipyrotic (an″ti-pi-rot′ik) [*anti-* + Gr. *pyrōsis* a burning] 1. protective against burns. 2. an agent or drug used in the treatment of burns.

antiscorbutic (an″ti-skor-bu′tik) [*anti-* + L. *scorbutus* scurvy] effective in the prevention or relief of scurvy.

Antisep trademark for *dextromethorphan hydrobromide* (see under DEXTROMETHORPHAN).

antisepsis (an″ti-sep′sis) [*anti-* + Gr. *sēpsis* putrefaction] the prevention of sepsis by the inhibition or destruction of the causative organism. See also DISINFECTION and STERILIZATION.

antiseptic (an″ti-sep′tik) 1. preventing decay or putrefaction. 2. an agent capable of inhibiting the growth and development of pathogenic microorganisms without necessarily destroying them. See also DISINFECTANT and STERILIZATION.

antiserum (an″ti-se′rum) a serum that contains antibody or antibodies; it may be obtained from an animal that has been immunized either by injection of antigens into the body or by infection with microorganisms containing the antigens. See also immune SERUM. **polyvalent a.,** one containing antibodies against several antigens.

antisialagogue (an″ti-si-al′ah-gog) 1. counteracting the formation or secretion of saliva. 2. an agent that counteracts any influence that promotes the flow of saliva. See also antimuscarinic drugs, under DRUG.

antisialic (an″ti-si-al′ik) [*anti-* + Gr. *sialon* saliva] 1. checking the flow of saliva. 2. an agent that checks the flow of saliva.

Anti-Skorbutin trademark for *ascorbic acid* (see under ACID).

antispasmodic (an″ti-spaz-mod′ik) 1. relieving spasm, usually of smooth muscle, as in the arteries, bronchi, intestines, or sphincters, but also of voluntary muscle; spasmolytic. 2. an agent that relieves spasm. Usually pertaining to antimuscarinic drugs (see under DRUG).

antispastic (an″ti-spas′tik) antispasmodic with specific reference to skeletal muscle.

Antistin trademark for *antazoline phosphate* (see under ANTAZOLINE).

antistreptokinase (an″ti-strep-to-ki′nās) an antibody that inhibits streptokinase.

Antitanil trademark for *dihydrotachysterol.*

antithermic (an″ti-ther′mik) [*anti-* + Gr. *thermē* heat] antipyretic.

antithrombin (an″ti-throm′bin) a substance capable of neutralizing the action of thrombin and thus limiting or restricting blood coagulation.

antithrombotic (an″ti-throm-bot′ik) preventing thrombosis.

antitoxin (an″ti-tok′sin) [*anti-* + Gr. *toxicon* poison] antibody to toxin, whether of microbial, animal, or plant origin, which combines specifically with the toxin, usually with neutralization of toxicity. See also TOXIN.

antitrismus (an″ti-triz′mus) a spasm that prevents closure of the mouth.

antitrypsin (an″ti-trip′sin) a substance which inhibits the action of trypsin. α_1-a., a serum glycoprotein, being a major fraction of α_1-globulin. Its electrophoretic activity is in the α_1 field, sedimentation coefficient, 3.85S, and molecular weight, 50,000 to 68,000. It is synthesized in the liver, and its function includes inhibition of proteinase and thrombin activity.

antitussive (an″ti-tus′iv) 1. alleviating or preventing cough. 2. an agent that alleviates and prevents cough. Called also *antibechic.*

antivenene (an″ti-vĕ-nēn′) antivenin.

antivenin (an″ti-ven′in) [*anti-* + L. *venenum* poison] a substance used in the treatment of poisoning by animal venom. It may be an antibody. Called also *antivenene* and *antivenom.* See also antivenomous SERUM.

antivenom (an″ti-ven′om) antivenin.

Antodyne trademark for *phenoxypropanediol.*

antorphine (an-tor′fēn) nalorphine.

antra (an′trah) [L.] plural of *antrum.*

antral (an′tral) of or pertaining to an antrum.

antrectomy (an-trek′to-me) [*antrum* + Gr. *ektomē* excision] surgical excision of an antrum.

Antrenyl trademark for *oxyphenonium bromide* (see under OXYPHENONIUM).

antritis (an-tri′tis) inflammation of an antrum, chiefly the maxillary antrum (sinus).

antro- [L. *antrum;* Gr. *antron* cave] a combining form denoting relationship to an antrum (sinus); often used with specific reference to the maxillary antrum, or sinus.

antroatticotomy (an″tro-at′′i-kot′o-me) the surgical operation of opening the maxillary antrum (sinus) and the attic of the tympanum.

antrobuccal (an″tro-buk′al) pertaining to or communicating with the maxillary antrum (sinus), and buccal cavity, as an antrobuccal fistula.

antrocele (an″tro-sēl) [*antro-* + Gr. *kēlē* tumor] a cystic accumulation of fluid in the maxillary antrum (sinus).

antrodynia (an″tro-din′e-ah) [*antro-* + Gr. *odynĕ* pain] pain in an antrum; antronalgia.

antronalgia (an″tro-nal′je-ah) [*antro-* + Gr. *algos* pain] pain in an antrum; antrodynia.

antronasal (an″tro-na′zal) pertaining to the maxillary antrum (sinus) and the nose.

antroscope (an′tro-skōp″) [*antro-* + Gr. *skopein* to examine] an instrument for illuminating and examining the maxillary antrum (sinus).

antroscopy (an-tros′ko-pe) examination of an antrum (sinus) with the antroscope.

antrostomy (an-tros′to-me) [*antro-* + Gr. *stomoun* to provide with an opening, or mouth] the operation of making an opening into the maxillary antrum (sinus) through the medial wall of the nose or through the lateral wall into the oral cavity for purposes of providing drainage.

antrotome (an′tro-tōm) [*antro-* + Gr. *tomē* a cutting] an instrument used for performing antrotomy.

antrotomy (an-trot′o-me) [*antro-* + Gr. *tomē* a cutting] the operation of cutting into the maxillary antrum (sinus), as in antrostomy.

antrotympanic (an″tro-tim-pan′ik) pertaining to the mastoid antrum (sinus) and the tympanic cavity.

antrotympanitis (an″tro-tim″pah-ni′tis) inflammation of the mastoid antrum (sinus) and of the middle ear.

antrum (an′trum), pl. *antrums* or *an′tra* [L.; Gr. *antron* cave] a cavity or chamber; a general term for an anatomical cavity or chamber, especially within a bone. **ethmoid a., a. ethmoida′le,** ethmoid bulla of ethmoid bones; see under BULLA. **a. of Highmore, a. highmo′ri,** maxillary SINUS. **mastoid a., a. mastoi′deum** [NA], tympanic a. **a. maxilla′re, maxillary a.,** maxillary SINUS. **tympanic a., a. tympan′icum,** a large, irregular air cavity in the mastoid portion of the temporal bone, communicating with the tympanic cavity and the mastoid cells. A thin bony plate, the tegmen tympani, separates it from the middle fossa of the cranial cavity, and the lateral semicircular canal projects into its cavity; it opens into the tympanic cavity with the epitympanic recess. Called also *mastoid a., a. mastoideum* [NA], and *mastoid cavity.*

Antulcus trademark for *oxyphencyclimine hydrochloride* (see under OXYPHENCYCLIMINE).

Anturan trademark for *sulfinpyrazone.*

Antyllus [A.D. 2nd century] a noted Greek surgeon of antiquity, a Pneumatist, whose treatment of aneurysms by ligation above and below remained standard practice until the time of John Hunter (18th century). He also made contributions to plastic surgery, ophthalmology, and public health. His writings remain only in fragments and in the works of others (particularly Oribasius).

ANUG acute necrotizing ulcerative gingivitis; see acute necrotizing GINGIVITIS.

anulus (an′u-lus), pl. *an′uli* [L., dim of *anus* ring, circle] an anatomical term used to designate a ringlike anatomical structure. See also ANNULUS.

anuria (ah-nu′re-ah) [*a* neg. + Gr. *ouron* urine + *-ia*] suppression of urine to less than 100 ml in 24 hours.

anxiety (ang-zi′ĕ-te) a feeling of apprehension, uncertainty, and fear without apparent stimulus. See also antianxiety DRUG.

anxiolytic (ang″si-o-lit′ik) 1. dispelling or allaying anxiety. 2. antianxiety DRUG.

AOD 1. Academy of Operative Dentistry (see under ACADEMY). 2. Academy of Oral Dynamics (see under ACADEMY).

aorta (a-or′tah), pl. *aortas, aor′tae* [L.; Gr. *aortē*] [NA] the main trunk of the systemic arterial system. It arises from the left ventricle at the aortic valve, being at this point about 3 cm in diameter, and ascends for about 5 cm toward the neck and head (*ascending a.*), then bends to the left in an arch (*arch of a.*), to pass downward through the thorax (*thoracic a.*) and through the abdomen (*abdominal a.*). The head and neck are supplied through the arteries branching off the arch of the aorta (the brachiocephalic trunk and the left carotid and subclavian arteries). Called also *arteria a.* **abdominal a.,** see *aorta.* **arch of a.,** ARCH of aorta. **arteria a.,** aorta. **ascending a.,** see *aorta.* **thoracic a.,** see *aorta.* **transverse a.,** ARCH of aorta.

aortae (a-or′te) [L.] plural and genitive of *aorta.*

aortic (a-or′tik) of or pertaining to the aorta.

aortitis (a″or-ti′tis) [*aorta* + *-itis*] inflammation of the aorta.

aortography (a″or-tog′rah-fe) [*aorta* + Gr. *graphein* to write] roentgenography of the aorta after the introduction of a radiopaque medium.

AP anterior pituitary; see under GLAND.

A-P anteroposterior PROJECTION.

Ap apex (3).

ap- see APO-.

Apamide trademark for *acetaminophen.*

Aparkan trademark for *trihexyphenidyl hydrochloride* (see under TRIHEXYPHENIDYL).

apathism (ap′ah-thizm) the state of being slow in responding to stimuli.

apathy (ap′ah-the) [Gr. *apatheia*] lack of feeling of emotion; indifference.

apatite (ap′ah-tīt) a calcium phosphate compound, $Ca_5(PO_4)_3OH$, being one of the two mineral constituents of bones and teeth (the other, $CaCO_3$). See HYDROXYAPATITE.

APC 1. adenoidal-pharyngeal-conjunctival (agent); see human ADENOVIRUS. 2. a preparation containing acetylsalicylic acid, phenacetin, and caffeine, used as an analgesic and antipyretic agent.

Apert's syndrome [Eugène *Apert,* French pediatrician, 1868–1940] see under SYNDROME.

apertognathia (ah-per″tog-na′the-ah) [L. *apertus,* from *aperio* to open + Gr. *gnathos* jaw + *-ia*] open BITE. **compound a.,** open bite, compound; see under BITE. **infantile a.,** open bite, infantile; see under BITE. **simple a.,** open bite, simple; see under BITE.

apertura (ap″er-tu′rah), pl. *apertu′rae* [L.] aperture; a general anatomical term used to designate an opening or an orifice. **a. exter′na aqueduc′tus vestib′uli** [NA], external aperture of aqueduct of vestibule; see under APERTURE. **a. exter′na canalic′uli coch′leae** [NA], external aperture of canaliculus of cochlea; see under APERTURE. **a. infe′rior canalic′uli tympan′ici,** inferior aperture of tympanic canaliculus; see under APERTURE. **a. pirifor′mis** [NA], piriform APERTURE. **a. si′nus fronta′lis** [NA], APERTURE of frontal sinus. **a. si′nus sphenoida′lis** [NA], APERTURE of sphenoid sinus. **a. supe′rior canalic′uli tympan′ici,** superior aperture of tympanic canaliculus; see under APERTURE. **a. tympan′ica canalic′uli chor′dae tym′pani** [NA], tympanic aperture of canaliculus of chorda tympani; see under APERTURE.

aperturae (ap″er-tu′re) [L.] plural of *apertura.*

aperture (ap′er-chūr) [L. *apertura*] an opening or an orifice. Called also *apertura.* **angle of a., angular a.,** the angle formed at a luminous point between the most divergent rays that are capable of passing through the objective of a microscope. Called also *a. of lens.* **bony anterior nasal a.,** piriform a. **external a. of aqueduct of vestibule,** the external opening for the aqueduct of the vestibule, located on the internal surface of the petrous part of the temporal bone, lateral to the opening for the internal acoustic meatus. Called also *apertura externa, aqueductus vestibuli* [NA], and *fissure of aqueduct of vestibule.* **external a. of canaliculus of cochlea,** the external opening of the cochlear canaliculus on the margin of the jugular foramen in the temporal bone. Called also *apertura externa canaliculi cochleae* [NA] and *external opening of aqueduct of cochlea.* **external a. of tympanic canaliculus,** inferior a. of tympanic canaliculus. **a. of frontal sinus,** the external opening of the frontal sinus into the nasal cavity. Called also *apertura sinus frontalis* [NA]. **inferior a. of tympanic canaliculus,** the lower opening of the tympanic canaliculus on the inferior surface of the petrous part of the temporal bone. Called also *external a. of tympanic canaliculus, apertura inferior canaliculi tympanici,* and *opening for tympanic branch of glossopharyngeal nerve.* **internal a. of tympanic canaliculus,** superior a. of tympanic canaliculus. **a. of lens,** angle of a. **numerical a.,** a measure of the efficiency of a microscope objective, being the product of the sine of one-half the angle of the aperture times the lowest refractive index of any medium, between the objective and specimen. **orbital a.,** the opening to the orbit in the cranium. Called also *aditus orbitae* [NA], *anterior opening of orbital cavity,* and *orbital opening.* **piriform a.,** the anterior nasal opening in the skull. Called also *bony anterior nasal a., apertura piriformis* [NA], *nasal opening of facial skeleton,* and *piriform opening.* **a. of sphenoid sinus,** a round opening just above the superior nasal concha, interconnecting the sphenoid sinus and nasal cavity. Called also *apertura sinus sphenoidalis* [NA], *opening of sphenoidal sinus,* and *sphenoidal fossa.* **superior a. of tympanic canaliculus,** the upper opening of the tympanic canaliculus in the temporal bone, leading to the tympanum. Called also *internal a. of tympanic canaliculus, apertura superior canaliculi tympanici, opening for lesser superficial petrosal nerve, opening for smaller superficial petrosal nerve,* and *superior opening of tympanic canal.* **tympanic a. of canaliculus of chorda tympani,** the opening through which the chorda tympani enters the tympanic cavity. Called also *apertura tympanica canaliculi chordae tympani* [NA].

apex (a′peks), pl. *apexes, a′pices* [L.] 1. tip; summit; the point or extremity of a conical object; a general term for the tip or extremity of an anatomical structure. 2. a craniometric point on sagittal contour of the skull located by projection of a vertical to the Frankfort Horizontal, erected at the porion. Abbreviated *Ap.* 3. root a. **a. auric′ulae** [NA], darwinian a. **blunderbuss a.,** blunderbuss CANAL. **closed a.,** a root apex of a mature permanent tooth having undergone calcification, which gives the appearance of being closed, in spite of the presence of one or more foramina communicating with the outside. **a. cus′pidis** [NA], the apex of the cusp of a tooth. **darwinian a.,** a pointed protrusion sometimes observed on the upper border of the ear. Called also *a. auriculae* [NA]. **immature a., immature root a.,** root a., immature. **a. lin'guae** [NA], a. of tongue. **a. na'si** [NA], the most distal portion of the nose; the tip of the nose. **a. par'tis petro'sae os'sis tempora'lis** [NA], **a. of petrous portion of temporal bone, a. pyram'idis os'sis tempora'lis,** the truncated portion of the petrous part of the temporal bone that is directed anteriorly and medially and ends at the medial opening of the carotid canal. **a. rad'icis den'tis** [NA], **root a.,** the tip or the terminal end of the root of a tooth. **root a., immature,** a flaring open apex of an incompletely developed tooth. Called also *immature a.* **a. of tongue,** the most distal portion of the tongue. Called also *a. linguae* [NA].

apexification (a"peks-ĭ-fi-ka'shun) a method of inducing apical closure or the continued apical development of the root of an incompletely formed tooth in which the pulp is no longer vital, usually by the formation of osteodentin or a similar hard tissue. Calcium hydroxide pastes and mixtures are commonly used to induce apexification.

apexigraph (a-peks'ĭ-graf) a device for determining the position of the apex of a tooth root.

Apexo elevator see under ELEVATOR.

apexogenesis (a"peks-o-jen'ĕ-sis) normal development of the apex of a root of a tooth.

apexograph (a-peks'o-graf) a delicate, flexible broach used for exploring the apical portion of the root canal of a tooth.

APHA American Public Health Association.

aphagia (ah-fa'je-ah) [*a* neg. + Gr. *phagein* to eat + *-ia*] abstention from eating. **a. al'gera,** refusal of a person to take food because it gives pain.

aphasia (ah-fa'ze-ah) [*a* neg. + Gr. *phasis* speech] defect or loss of the power of expression by speech, writing, or sign, or of comprehending spoken or written language, due to injury or disease of the brain centers.

aphonia (ah-fo'ne-ah) [*a* neg. + Gr. *phōnē* voice] loss of the voice.

aphtha (af'thah), pl. **aph'thae** [L.; Gr. "thrush"] 1. small ulcer. 2. (pl.) recurrent aphthous STOMATITIS. See also foot-and-mouth DISEASE, HERPANGINA, PERIADENITIS mucosa necrotica recurrens, and Riga-Feda DISEASE. **Bednar's aphthae,** symmetric excoriation of the hard palate over the pterygoid plates in infants, thought to be due to the pressure of the nipple against the palate during nursing, or sucking of the thumb or foreign objects. **Behçet's aphthae,** Behçet's SYNDROME. **Cardarelli's aphthae,** Riga-Fede DISEASE. **Mikulicz's aphthae, recurring scarring aphthae,** PERIADENITIS mucosa necrotica recurrens. **Riga's aphthae,** Riga-Fede DISEASE.

aphthae (af'the) [L.] plural of *aphtha.*

aphthoid (af'thoid) [*aphtha* + Gr. *eidos* form] 1. thrushlike; resembling thrush. 2. an exanthema resembling that of thrush. **Pospischill-Feyrter a.,** a sometimes fatal form of primary herpetic gingivostomatitis affecting chiefly infants and young children who are in poor physical condition, which extends to organs other than the mouth, and involves the perioral areas, esophagus, genitalia, fingers, and other parts. The primary lesion presents as a vesicle with central invagination and with a thick surface. The rash extends, forming necrotic plaques, ulcers, and erosions. Painful lymphadenopathy is usually present. Called also *Pospischill-Feyrter disease.* See also primary herpetic GINGIVOSTOMATITIS.

aphthosis (af-tho'sis) any condition marked by aphthae. **a. generalisa'ta,** Stevens-Johnson SYNDROME. **generalized a.,** 1. Behçet's SYNDROME. 2. Stevens-Johnson SYNDROME. **Neumann's a.,** Stevens-Johnson SYNDROME. **Touraine's a.,** Behçet's SYNDROME.

aphthous (af'thus) pertaining to, characterized by, or affected with aphthae.

Aphthovirus (af'to-vi'rus) a provisional genus tentatively assigned to the family Picornaviridae, consisting of the hand, foot, and mouth disease virus. See RHINOVIRUS.

apical (ap'ĭ-kal) pertaining to or situated at the apex, as of a tooth root.

apicectomy (a"pĭ-sek'to-me) 1. excision of the apex of the petrous portion of the temporal bone. 2. apicoectomy.

apices (ap'ĭ-sēz) [L.] plural of *apex.*

apicitis (a"pe-si'tis) inflammation of an apex, as the apex of a tooth, the lung, or the petrous bone (petrositis).

apicoectomy (a"pĭ-ko-ek'to-me) [*apex* + Gr. *ektomē* excision] 1. excision of the apical portion of a tooth through an opening made in the overlying labial, buccal, or palatal alveolar bone; ordinarily performed in conjunction with apical curettage and

with or as an adjunct to root canal therapy. Called *apicectomy, root resection,* and *root end resection.* See also root AMPUTATION. 2. apicectomy.

apicostomy (a"pĭ-kos'to-me) [*apex* + Gr. *stomoun* to provide with an opening or mouth] dental TREPHINATION.

apicotomy (a"pĭ-kot'o-me) puncture of the apex of the petrous portion of the temporal bone.

aplasia (ah-pla'ze-ah) [*a* neg. + Gr. *plassein* to form] lack of development of an organ; frequently used to designate complete suppression or failure of development of a structure from the embryonic primordium. See also AGENESIS. **bone marrow a.,** aplastic ANEMIA. **condylar a.,** a failure of development of the mandibular condyle, interfering with articulation of the temporomandibular joint. It may occur unilaterally or bilaterally, and is often associated with other abnormalities, such as defects or absence of the external ear, hypoplasia of the mandible, or macrostomia. Unilateral aplasia usually results in facial asymmetry and malocclusion. **enamel a.,** see enamel HYPOPLASIA. **enamel and dentin a.,** faulty development of the dental enamel and dentin, which is different from amelogenesis imperfecta and dentinogenesis imperfecta. It is characterized by nearly complete aplasia of the enamel and dysplasia of the dentin, large pulp chambers, and failure of secondary dentin formation. The enamel is pale gray, the dentin has a sandy-brown discoloration, and the pulp is visible through the occlusal surface of the posterior teeth. **a. os'sea microplas'tica,** Vrolik's SYNDROME. **salivary gland a.,** absence of a salivary gland or of groups of salivary glands, characterized by xerostomia, cracking of the lips, fissuring of the corners of the mouth, and collection and stagnation of food debris around the teeth, resulting in dental caries, and often, loss of teeth.

aplastic (ah-plas'tik) [*a* neg. + Gr. *plassein* to form] pertaining to or characterized by aplasia.

apnea (ap-ne'ah) [*a* neg. + Gr. *pnoia* breath] 1. cessation of breathing. 2. asphyxia.

apneumatic (ap"nu-mat'ik) 1. free from air. 2. done with the exclusion of air.

apo-, ap- [Gr. *apo* from] a prefix denoting separation or derivation from.

apocrine (ap'o-krin) [Gr. *apokrinesthai* to be secreted] denoting secretion by the apocrine glands (see under GLAND).

Apodol trademark for *anileridine.*

apoferritin (ap"o-fer'ĭ-tin) a protein of molecular weight 460,000 which forms a compound with ferric hydroxide clusters, called *ferritin.*

Apollonia see ST. APOLLONIA.

Aponal trademark for *doxepin hydrochloride* (see under DOXEPIN).

aponeuroses (ap"o-nu-ro-sēz') plural of *aponeurosis.*

aponeurosis (ap"o-nu-ro'sis), pl. *aponeuro'ses* [Gr. *aponeurōsis*] [NA] a white, flattened or ribbonlike tendinous expansion, serving as the origin or insertion of a flat muscle. Called also *tendinous membrane.* **epicranial a.,** a tendinous structure which covers the skull like a cap. It attaches the occipital and frontal bellies of the occipitofrontal muscle and the temporoparietal muscle, and is closely connected to the integument by subcutaneous connective tissue. A fascial cleft separates it from the pericranium, thus permitting free sliding of the scalp over the skull. Called also *a. of occipitofrontal muscle* and *galea aponeurotica* [NA]. **a. lin'guae** [NA], **lingual a.,** the connective tissue framework of the tongue, supporting and giving attachment to the intrinsic and extrinsic muscles; composed of the connective tissue layer of the tunica mucosa, the lingual septum, and the posterior transverse expansion of the septum which attaches to the hyoid bone. **a. of occipitofrontal muscle,** epicranial a. **palatine a.,** a fibrous sheet in the anterior part of the soft palate, derived mainly from the tendons of the two tensor muscles, giving attachment to the uvular muscle and to the palatopharyngeal and levator veli palatini muscles. **pharyngeal a., a. pharyn'gis, pharyngobasilar a., a. pharyngobasila'ris,** pharyngobasilar FASCIA. **suprahyoid a.,** a broad fibrous band extending from the tendon of the digastric muscle and attaching to the body of the hyoid bone. **temporal a.,** temporal FASCIA.

aponeurositis (ap"o-nu-ro-si'tis) [*aponeurosis* + *-itis*] inflammation of an aponeurosis.

apophyses (ah-pof'ĭ-sēz) plural of *apophysis.*

apophysis (ah-pof'ĭ-sis), pl. *apoph'yses* [Gr. "an offshoot"] any outgrowth or swelling, especially a bony outgrowth that has never been entirely separated from the bone of which it forms a part. See also TUBERCLE and TUBEROSITY. **genial a.,** mental SPINE. **Ingrassia's a.,** a small wing of sphenoid bone; see under WING. **a. os'sium,** epiphysis.

apoplexia (ap"o-plek'se-ah) [L.] apoplexy. **a. u'vulae,** staphylohematoma.

apoplexy (ap′o-plek′se) [L. *apoplexia*] 1. a sudden neurologic disorder, limited by some to intracranial hemorrhage, extended by others to include occlusive lesions of the brain. 2. any massive extravasation of blood within an organ.

aposthema (ap″os-te′mah) [Gr. *apostēma*] an abscess.

apothecary (ah-poth′ĕ-ka″re) [Gr. *apothēke* storehouse] pharmacist.

apoxesis (ap″ok-se′sis) [Gr. *apoxein* to scrape off] a term used in the past to denote scaling of deposits on the root of a tooth. See also apical CURETTAGE, ODONTEXESIS, and SCALING. **subgingival a.,** subgingival SCALING.

apozem, apozema, apozeme (ap′o-zem, ap-oz′e-mah, ap′o-zēm) [Gr. *apozēma* decoction, from *apo* away + *zein* to boil] decoction.

apparatus (ap″ah-ra′tus), pl. *appara′tus* or *apparatuses* [L., from *ad* to + *parare* to make ready] 1. an arrangement of a number of parts acting together in the performance of some special function. 2. a collection of structurally different tissues or organs, which act cooperatively in execution of a body function, such as the masticatory apparatus. See also SYSTEM. 3. a collection of instruments, materials, etc., used together to execute a given procedure. **attachment a.,** the apparatus which attaches a tooth to its socket, consisting of the cementum, periodontal ligament, and alveolar bone. **digestive a., a. digesto′rius** [NA], digestive SYSTEM. **genitourinary a.,** urogenital SYSTEM. **Golgi a., internal reticular a.,** an intracellular component, consisting of lamellar membranous structures, each made up of curved parallel arrays of flattened saccules or cisternae that are often expanded at their ends. It is usually not visible in living cells or ordinary histological preparations, but it may be observed in negative image as an unstained juxtanuclear area. Its functions include concentration and packaging of the secretory products of cells producing protein-rich secretions, and of synthesis of secretory products rich in polysaccharides. Called also *Golgi complex.* **masticatory a.,** the structures involved in mastication, including the teeth, mandibular musculature, mandible, temporomandibular joints, accessory facial muscles, and tongue, together with their innervation. **a. respirato′rius** [NA], **respiratory a.,** respiratory SYSTEM. **urogenital a., a. urogenita′lis** [NA], urogenital SYSTEM.

appendage (ah-pen′dij) a part which is accessory to a main structure; appendix. **cornified a.,** keratinized skin a. **glandular skin a.,** the apocrine, eccrine, and sebaceous glands. **keratinized skin a.,** the hair and nails. Called also *cornified a.* **skin a.,** a structure situated within the skin, whose morphology and function differ from that of the skin, including the hair, nails, and the apocrine, eccrine, and sebaceous glands. **a. of ventricle of larynx,** APPENDIX of laryngeal ventricle.

appendices (ah-pen′di-sēz) plural of *appendix.*

appendix (ah-pen′diks), pl. *appendixes, appendices* [L., from *appendere* to hang upon] an appendage; an accessory, supplementary, or dependent part attached to a main structure. **a. of laryngeal ventricle, a. ventric′uli laryn′gis,** a sac or diverticulum extending upward from the anterior portion of the ventricle of the larynx, between the free edge of the vestibular fold and the thyroid cartilage, and having on its surface more than 60 openings for mucous glands. Muscular fasciculi on its surface attach the apex to the arytenoid cartilage, the thyroepiglotticus muscle separating it from the thyroid cartilage. It is enclosed in a fibrous capsule and is continuous with the vestibular ligament. Called also *appendage of ventricle of larynx, laryngeal sac, laryngeal saccule,* and *sacculus laryngis* [NA].

appetite (ap′ĕ-tīt) [L. *appetere* to desire] a natural longing or desire, especially for food.

apple (ap′l) the fruit of the tree *Pyrus malus;* also the tree itself. **Adam's a.,** laryngeal PROMINENCE.

Applebaum see HEMOCHROMATOSIS (Recklinghausen-Applebaum disease).

appliance (ah-pli′ans) 1. any device, instrument, or apparatus used for a particular purpose. 2. in dentistry, a general term referring to devices used to provide a function or therapeutic effect. Some use the term in connection with dental prostheses, fixation splints, removable occlusal overlays, or obturators; others restrict its use to only those devices which are worn by the patient in the course of treatment, such as splints, orthodontic appliances, and space maintainers, considering obturators, fixed partial dentures, or crowns as prostheses. See also DENTURE, PROSTHESIS, and RESTORATION. **acrylic resin and copper band a.,** a provisional appliance for splinting teeth, consisting of copper bands fitted over the cervical portions of the teeth, with acrylic resin applied over the bands and contoured so as to establish the relationship with the opposing and adjacent teeth. The appliance provides protection for the investing and supporting structures of the splinted teeth. **activator a.,** functional ACTIVATOR. **active plate a.,** a removable orthodontic appliance equipped with devices that are the source of an active force that moves the teeth. It is designed for interrupted or intermittent application of orthodontic forces in combination with the concepts of functional jaw orthopedics, which utilize the patient's own muscles and inherent growth and development patterns. The chief components of the appliance are the basic plate, clasps, labial bow, springs, screws, and elastics. Called also *active plate.* **Andresen a., Andresen monoblock a.,** functional

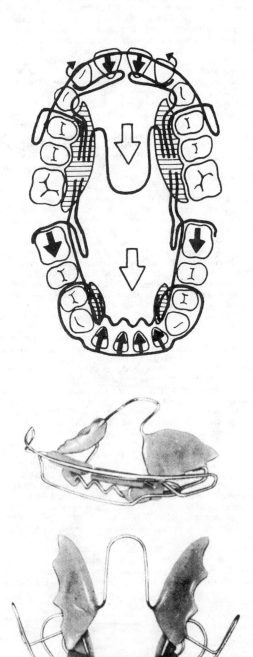

Bimler appliance with continuous labial arch in lower appliance and U-shaped connecting Coffin spring. (From T. M. Graber: Orthodontics — Principles and Practice. 3rd ed. Philadelphia, W. B. Saunders Co., 1972; courtesy of H. P. Bimler.)

ACTIVATOR. **Begg's a.,** an orthodontic appliance consisting of a light wire (a round austenitic stainless steel arch wire of 0.016 inch diameter) and brackets permitting the tipping of tooth crowns but horizontal buccal tubes on the anchor molars to prevent their tipping, together with elastics. The appliance is designed to use the optimum orthodontic force for moving teeth. Called also *light round wire a.* and *differential force a.* See also Begg's THEORY, Begg's TECHNIQUE, and differential FORCE. **Bimler a.,** a removable orthodontic appliance believed to stimulate reflex muscle activity, which in turn produces the desired tooth movement. Called also *Bimler stimulator.* See also functional jaw ORTHOPEDICS. See illustration. **Bowles mutliphase a.,** multiphase a. **Case a.,** an early type of orthodontic appliance designed for moving tooth roots. **Coffin a.,** Coffin PLATE. **craniofacial a.,** a device used to immobilize and/or reduce mandibular or midfacial fractures. The appliance is either external, using wires or bars to headcaps or skeletal pins, or internal, using circumzygomatic wires, cirummandibular wires, or wires passing through drill holes in the zygomatic process of the frontal bone, inferoanterior border of the zygomatic arch, infraorbital rim, anterior nasal spine, and the inferior rim of the bony nares. **Crozat a.,** a removable orthodontic appliance, originally developed and patented by W. W. Walker, used to align teeth during orthodontic therapy. It is the principal appliance used to encourage and guide the growth of the bony structure itself so that there will be room for all the teeth in their proper places, resulting in arch development. The appliance is usually made of precious metal rather than customary stainless steel. Sometimes called *crozat* and *Walker appliance.* See illustration. **Denholz a.,** an orthodontic appliance consisting of a wire assembly which contains a vestibular acrylic screen and open coil spring segments that fit over the wire arch. The appliance uses muscle anchorage to drive first permanent molars distally. Round buccal tubes on the first permanent molar bands (or full metal crowns) receive the arch wire. When the arch is inserted by the patient into the tubes, the labial screen stands well away from the anterior teeth. The coil spring is compressed as the lip resists the stretching, exerting a distal thrust on the molar teeth. The patient exercises 1 to 2 hours daily, forcibly closing the lips over the labial screen. See illustration. **differential force a.,** Begg a. **edgewise a.,** a fixed, multibanded orthodontic appliance developed by E. H. Angle, which uses a rectangular labial arch wire ligated to brackets on bands cemented to individual teeth. The term "edgewise" refers to the bracket being machined so that the rectangular arch wire is inserted with its long dimension horizontal, instead of vertical as in the ribbon arch bracket. Called also *edgewise attachment.* See also edgewise BRACKET. **expansion plate a.,** any orthodontic appliance equipped with an expansion plate. Called also *split plate a.* **extraoral a.,** an orthodontic appliance using the resistance unit outside the oral cavity. See extraoral ANCHORAGE. **finger-sucking re-education a.,** a habit-breaking fixed orthodontic appliance fitted over the anterior portion of the palate, designed to correct habitual finger-sucking. **fixed a.,** one cemented to the teeth or attached by means of adhesive material. Called also *permanent a.* **fracture a.,** any of the various devices used in fixation of fractures, such as pins, clamps, or screws. **Fränkel a.,** function CORRECTOR. **Griffin a.,** an orthodontic appliance having a resilient arch assembly. **habit-breaking a.,** an orthodontic appliance designed to correct faulty habits, such as finger-sucking, tongue-thrusting, infantile swallowing, or any other habit that may lead to malocclusion. **Hawley a.,** Hawley RETAINER. **hay rake a.,** a formerly used habit-controlling appliance employed to limit abnormal excursions of the tongue by

providing a stirrup that arrested tongue thrusts. It consisted of an acrylic palatal plate secured by spring clasps and a wire railing about 0.5 cm in height and 3 cm in length palatal to the upper incisors. **jackscrew a.,** an early orthodontic appliance used to expand the upper arch. It consists of two metal bands placed on the teeth to be moved, connected by shafts fitting into a centrally located nut. The thread of the shafts causes the bands to press against the teeth, when the nut is turned one way, and to release pressure, when it is turned the other way. **Jackson's a.,** a removable orthodontic appliance, capable of many variations. It is retained in position by crib-shaped wires, bent to follow the outline of the buccal and lingual contours of the bicuspid and molar teeth, and united by cross wires lying in the occlusal embrasures. Called also *Jackson crib.* **Johnston twin wire a.,** twin wire a. **jumping-the-bite a.,** Kingsley a. **Kesling a.,** an occlusal splint made of soft acrylic resin or latex rubber, which fits over the occlusal and incisal surfaces of the teeth. It is designed to hold the mandible in a certain relationship to the maxilla by grasping both the mandibular and maxillary teeth in the same appliance. It is used in treating bruxism. **Kingsley a.,** an active plate appliance having a bite plate with an inclined anterior plane to move the mandible forward by jumping the bite. Called also *jumping-the-bite a., jumping-the-bite plate,* and *Kingsley plate.* **labiolingual a.,** an orthodontic appliance for intermaxillary therapy. It consists of a maxillary labial arch, 0.036 to 0.040 inch in diameter, introduced into horizontal buccal tubes attached to the anchor bands and lingual arches of the same diameter fitted into vertical or horizontal tubes fastened to the lingual side of the anchor bands. The first permanent molar teeth serve as anchorage, and the mandibular lingual arch is attached to the molar bands to permit removal of the arch for cleaning and adjusting. Wires of smaller diameter are sometimes fashioned into loops attached to both the labial and lingual arches to initiate different types of movement. The original design used finger or auxiliary springs to move individual teeth in the lower arch, while the arch itself served as a base for elastic traction. The lingual arch serves best as a space maintainer or for use as part-time elastic traction. The appliance is now used in conjunction with a fixed guide plane and intermaxillary elastics to eliminate functional retrusion. Called also *labial and lingual arches* and *labiolingual technique.* **light round wire a.,** Begg a. **lip habit a.,** a fixed, habit-breaking orthodontic appliance, which is worn for long periods of time. It consists of a lingual arch that is usually soldered to a full metal crown on second deciduous or first permanent molars, and has an acrylic cushion (lip plumper) on the labial aspect of the canines to intercept lip-biting and lip-sucking habits. Called also *lip sucking habit crib.* **Mayne muscle control a.,** an orthodontic appliance consisting of a wire arch anchored to the molar teeth and an acrylic cushion (lip plumper), using the lip pressure to exert distal force on molars and to allow the tongue to position the lower incisor teeth labially, thus reducing overjet. It may also be used as anchorage. **monoblock a.,** functional ACTIVATOR. **mouthstick a.,** mouthstick. **Mühlemann a.,** propulsor. **multibanded a.,** an orthodontic appliance incorporating bands other than the molar anchor bands. **multiphase a.,** a multiband orthodontic appliance which incorporates the properties of the universal and edgewise appliances. Called also *Bowles multiphase a.* and *Bowles technique.* See also multiphase BRACKET. **Nord a.,** a removable orthodontic appliance equipped with a lowered expansion plate and an expansion screw. Called also *Nord plate* and *Nord expansion plate.* **obturator a.,** obturator. **orthodontic a.,** a device, either fixed to the teeth or removable, that provides a mechanism for application of force to the teeth and their supporting structures to produce changes in the relationship of the teeth to each other and to control their growth and development. Such an appliance is used in orthodontic therapy to move

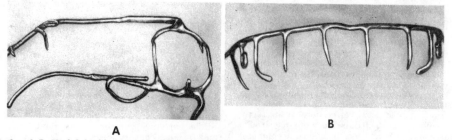

A   **B**

A, Crozat skeleton detail. *B,* High labial base wire with various spurs. (From T. M. Graber: Orthodontics — Principles and Practice. 3rd ed. Philadelphia, W. B. Saunders Co., 1972; courtesy of R. B. Smythe.)

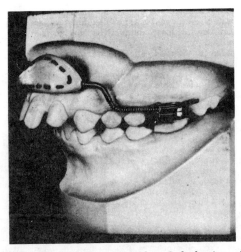

Denholz appliance. (From T. M. Graber: Orthodontics — Principles and Practice. 3rd ed. Philadelphia, W. B. Saunders Co., 1972; courtesy of the Rocky Mountain Dental Products Co.)

the teeth into esthetically desirable positions and physiologic alignment within the dental arch and into proper relationship with the opposing dentition. An orthodontic appliance is also used in the treatment of fractures and injuries of the maxillae to stabilize or immobilize the teeth and jaws. Called also *regulating a.* and *braces.* See also ANCHORAGE, arch WIRE, and BRACKET. **palatal expansion a.,** an orthodontic appliance equipped with a jackscrew, used to expand the upper arch. See *jackscrew a.* **permanent a.,** fixed a. **pin and tube a.,** an early orthodontic appliance developed by E. H. Angle, in which each band on the tooth has a vertical tube that parallels the long axis of the tooth, the arch wire having pins soldered in such a position as to influence the total position of each tooth. **prosthetic a.,** a device affixed to or implanted in the body, designed to take the place, or perform the function of a missing body part, such as an artificial arm or single or multiple teeth. See also DENTURE and PROSTHESIS. **regulating a.,** orthodontic a. **removable a.,** one that may be inserted into or removed from the mouth by the patient. Orthodontic removable appliances are generally classified as those that effect actual tooth movement through adjustment of springs or attachments within the appliance, and those that stimulate reflex muscle activity, which in turn produces the desired tooth movement. **retaining a.,** retainer. **ribbon arch a.,** an orthodontic appliance developed by E. H. Angle to replace the pin and tube appliance. It consists of a flattened wire inserted into a special bracket against the labial and buccal surfaces of the teeth, and usually intended for lateral movements of the teeth. The use of the rectangular or ribbon arch wire allows adjustment of the appliance to exert pressure on the apices of the teeth. Called also *ribbon arch.* See also ribbon arch BRACKET. **Schwarz a.,** a removable orthodontic appliance with a tissue-borne anchorage and appurtenances of wire for tooth movement. See also functional jaw ORTHOPEDICS. **space retaining a.,** space MAINTAINER. **split plate a.,** expansion plate a. **therapeutic a.,** therapeutic PROSTHESIS. **thumb-sucking a.,** any device that discourages thumb-sucking. **tongue-thrust a.,** a habit-breaking orthodontic appliance designed to correct the tongue-thrust habit. It is a tongue crib similar to the finger-sucking appliance, having the spurs bent down behind the lower incisors during full occlusal contact of the posterior teeth. The purpose of the crib is to prevent anterior tongue thrusts and plunger-like action during deglutition and to condition tongue posture so that the dorsum of the tongue approximates the palatal vault, and the tip of the tongue contacts the palatal rugae during deglutition, instead of moving through the incisal space. The appliance is used also for correcting the visceral deglutition habit. **twin wire a.,** an orthodontic appliance developed by J. Johnson, using fixed lingual arches and a labial arch consisting of a pair of 0.010 round wires attached to brackets on the anterior teeth. Called also *Johnson twin wire a.,* and *twin wire.* See also twin wire BRACKET. **universal a.,** an orthodontic appliance designed by S. R. Atkinson, which combines the edgewise and ribbon arch techniques, affording precise control of individual teeth in all planes of space. It consists of bands for all the teeth in both arches, each band being attached to a bracket with two transverse slots for labial or buccal wires,

whereby the cervical slot opens buccally and the incisal or occlusal slot opens superiorly. The wires for the cervical bracket are 0.008 to 0.015 inch in diameter and the flat wires for the occlusal bracket are 0.010 to 0.015 × 0.028 inch. The wires are held in place by a pin lock pin. A lingual arch with a 0.30-inch diameter fits into horizontal lingual molar sheaths. The round wire permits mesiodistal and intrusive and extrusive movements; the flat wire rotates and allows buccolingual tooth movement. See also universal BRACKET. **visceral deglutition a., visceral swallowing a.,** a habit-breaking orthodontic appliance designed to correct the visceral deglutition habit. See *tongue thrust a.* **Walker a.,** Crozat a.

application (ap″li-ka-shun) 1. applying or putting or laying something on; that which is applied. 2. a salve or a healing agent. 3. putting to a special use or purpose. **local a.,** application of a drug or any therapeutic substance directly to the site to be treated and affecting only the area to which it is applied; as opposed to the systemic administration. Called also *local administration.* **new drug a.,** an application that must be approved by the U.S. Food and Drug Administration before any new drug may be marketed and made available for prescriptions by physicians, dentists, and other health professionals. The application must include reports on animal and clinical studies, list of ingredients, description of manufacturing methods, quality control procedures, samples of the drug, and the proposed labeling. Abbreviated *NDA.* **topical a.,** local application to a particular surface area, as of an anti-infective agent to an infected area of the skin. Called also *topical administration.*

applicator (ap″li-ka″tor) an instrument for making local applications. **root canal a.,** a hand-operated, slender, tapering, flexible, pointed endodontic instrument, having a round cross section and a roughened surface with numerous projections at its working tip; used for holding cotton fibers or applying liquids into root canals. See illustration at root canal THERAPY.

Apponus, Petrus see PETER OF ABANO.

apposition (ap″o-zish′un) [L. *appositio*] 1. the placing of things in juxtaposition or proximity; specifically, the deposition of successive layers upon those already present. See also appositional GROWTH. 2. the condition of being in juxtaposition or proximity or of being placed or fitted together. 3. the fourth or calcification stage of odontogenesis, characterized by the differentiation of the peripheral mesenchymal cells into odontoblasts in the dental papilla, the establishment of the dentinoenamel junction, and the deposition and development of the dentin matrix. See illustration at ODONTOGENESIS.

approach (ah-prōch′) 1. to draw nearer or closer; approximate. 2. a surgical procedure by which an organ or part is exposed. **buttonhole a.,** surgical treatment of a periodontal abscess, consisting of making an incision in the fluctuant abscess, followed by curettage of the area adjoining the root and the fundus of the abscess through the destroyed portion of the alveolar plate or bone. **lingual a.,** invisible FOIL. **Risdon a.,** a surgical method of exposing the ascending ramus of the mandible by means of an incision made below and behind the angle of the mandible, for treatment of fractures, e.g., condylar fracture, or for reconstructive surgery.

approximal (ah-prok′si-mal) situated close together.

approximate (ah-prok′si-māt) 1. nearly correct or equal. 2. to draw nearer or closer; to approach.

appurtenance (ah-per′ten-nans) an accessory or adjunct to something; something added to another.

apraxia (ah-prak′se-ah) [Gr. "a not acting," "want of success"] inability to carry out purposeful movements in the absence of paralysis or other motor or sensory impairment, especially inability to make proper use of an object.

Apresoline trademark for *hydralazine.*

apron (a′prun) a piece of clothing worn as a protection for the body in front. **a. band,** apron BAND. **lead a., leaded a., leaded protective a.,** a lead-impregnated rubber apron used to protect both the patient and the operator and other personnel from the effects of radiation during radiological examination. The use of such an apron is mandatory in some states and is recommended by the American Academy of Dental Radiology, especially with children and pregnant women. Called also *protective a.* **lingual a.,** lingual PLATE. **protective a.,** lead a. **rubber dam a.,** a small strip of rubber dam, perforated to fit over an implant abutment; used to inhibit introduction of cement into the space around the implant.

aprosopia (ap″ro-so′pe-ah) [*a* neg. + Gr. *prosōpon* face] congenital absence of structures of the face.

APS American Prosthodontic Society (see under SOCIETY).

apselaphesia (ap″sel-ah-fe′ze-ah) [*a* neg. + Gr. *psēlaphēsis* touch] diminution of the sense of touch.

aptyalia, aptyalism (ap″tĭ-a′le-ah; ap-ti′ah-lizm) [*a* neg. + Gr. *ptyalizein* to spit] deficiency or absence of the saliva; xerostomia; asialia.

apyetous (ah-pi′ĕ-tus) [*a* neg. + Gr. *pyon* pus] showing no pus; not suppurating.

apyogenous (ah″pi-oj′ĕ-nus) not caused by pus.

apyous (ah-pi′us) [*a* neg. + Gr. *pyon* pus] having no pus; nonpurulent.

apyretic (ah″pi-ret′ik) [*a* neg. + *pyretic*] having no fever; afebrile.

Aq. abbreviation for L. *a′qua*, water.

aqua (ak′kwah, ah′kwah), pl. *a′quae* [L.] water. **a. ammo′nia,** AMMONIUM hydroxide. **a. for′tis,** nitric ACID.

Aquacillin trademark for *penicillin G procaine* (see under PENICILLIN).

Aquadrate trademark for a preparation of *urea*.

aquae (ak′we, ah′kwe) [L.] plural of *aqua*.

Aquamephyton trademark for a preparation of *phytonadione*.

Aquamox trademark for *quinethazone*.

Aquamycetin trademark for *chloramphenicol*.

Aquatensen trademark for *methyclothiazide*.

aqueduct (ak′wĕ-dukt″) [L. *aqueductus*] a passage or channel in a body structure or organ. Called also *aqueductus*. **a. of cochlea,** 1. perilymphatic DUCT. 2. CANALICULUS of cochlea. **a. of Cotunnius,** 1. a. of vestibule. 2. CANALICULUS of cochlea. **fallopian a., a. of Fallopius,** CANAL for facial nerve. **a. of Sylvius,** the narrow channel in the midbrain that connects the third and fourth ventricles. Called also *aqueductus cerebri* [NA]. **a. of vestibule,** a small canal extending from the vestibule of the inner ear to open onto the posterior part of the internal surface of the petrous part of the temporal bone. It lodges the endolymphatic duct, an arteriole, and a venule. Called also *a. of Cotunnius* and *aqueductus vestibuli* [NA]. 2. endolymphatic DUCT.

aqueductus (ak″wĕ-duk′tus) [L., from *aqua* water + *ductus* canal] aqueduct; a passage or channel in a body structure or organ. **a. cer′ebri** [NA], AQUEDUCT of Sylvius. **a. cochle′ae,** 1. NA alternative for perilymphatic DUCT. 2. CANALICULUS of cochlea. **a. endolymphat′icus,** endolymphatic DUCT. **a. perilymphat′ici,** perilymphatic DUCT. **a. vestib′uli,** 1. [NA] AQUEDUCT of vestibule. 2. NA alternative for endolymphatic DUCT.

aqueous (a′kwĕ-us, ak′wĕ-us) [L. *aqua* water] watery; prepared with water.

Aquinone trademark for *menadione*.

aquocobalamin (ak″kwo-ko-bal′ah-min) vitamin B$_{12b}$.

AR alloy RESTORATION.

Ar 1. argon. 2. articulare.

arabinose (ah-rab′ĭ-nōs) a pentose (aldose) obtained from gum arabic and the gum of the cherry tree, being of metabolic importance only to plants. Used in culture media for certain microorganisms. Called also *pectin sugar*. **cytosine a.,** cytarabine.

Arachnia (ah-rak′ne-ah) [Gr. *arachnion* cobweb] a genus of gram-positive, non–acid-fast, non–spore-forming, nonmotile, facultative bacteria of the family Actinomycetaceae, order Actinomycetales, which do not require CO$_2$ for growth. They occur as branched diphtheroid rods, 0.2 to 0.3 µm by 3.0 to 5.0 µm in size, and as branched filaments, 5.0 to 20.0 m in length. Swollen coccoid cells and/or spheroplasts develop during the stationary growth phase. They are a cause of human actinomycosis and are pathogens of laboratory mice.

arachnitis (ar″ak-ni′tis) [*arachno-* + *-itis*] inflammation of the arachnoid. Called also *arachnoiditis*.

arachnodactyly (ah-rak′no-dak′tĭ-le) [Gr. *arachnē* spider + *daktylos* finger] abnormally elongated fingers and toes, suggesting spider legs. Called also *spider fingers*. See Marfan's SYNDROME. **congenital contractural a.,** a hereditary syndrome, transmitted as an autosomal dominant trait, combining multiple congenital joint contractures, arachnodactyly, deformed ears, short neck, kyphoscoliosis, and craniofacial defects, including an oval shape of the skull, frontal prominence, flat nasal bridge, deeply set eyes, which have the appearance of having mild ptosis, possible mild hypertelorism, small nose with upturned tip, long philtrum, small mouth, mandibular retrognathia, mild protrusion of the auricles, and obliteration of the concha by the antihelix, giving the ear a crumpled appearance. Abbreviated CCA. Called also *CCA syndrome* and *congenital contractural arachnodactyly syndrome*.

arachnoid (ah-rak′noid) [Gr. *arachnoeidēs* like a cobweb] 1.

resembling a spider's web. 2. the intermediate of the three membranes (meninges) that envelop the brain and spinal cord; it is composed of loose connective tissue. Called also *arachnoidea* [NA].

arachnoidea (ar″ak-noi′de-ah) [Gr. *arachnoeidēs* like a cobweb] [NA] arachnoid (2).

arachnoiditis (ah-rak′noid-i′tis) [*arachnoid* + *-itis*] inflammation of the arachnoid. Called also *arachnitis*.

Aracytidine trademark for *cytarabine*.

Aralen trademark for *chloroquine*.

Aramine trademark for *metaraminol bitartrate* (see under METARAMINOL).

Aran's law [François Amilcar *Aran*, French physician, 1817–1861] see under LAW.

Arantius, canal of, duct of [Julius Caesar *Arantius,* Italian anatomist and physician, 1530–1589] DUCTUS venosus.

arbor (ar′bor), pl. *ar′bores* [L.] a treelike structure or part; a structure or system resembling a tree with its branches.

arbores (ar′bo-rēz) [L.] plural of *arbor*.

arborescent (ar″bo-res′ent) [L. *arborescens*] branching like a tree.

arborization (ar″bor-i-za′shun) 1. the branching termination of certain nerve cell processes. 2. a form of the termination of a nerve fiber when in contact with a muscle fiber. 3. the treelike appearance of capillary vessels in inflamed conditions.

arboroid (ar′bo-roid) [*arbor* + Gr. *eidos* form] branching like a tree.

arborvirus (ar″bor-vi′rus) [*arthropod-borne* + *virus*] the original name for an arthropod-borne virus, abbreviated to *arbovirus* to avoid the connotation of tree (arbor).

arbovirus (ar″bo-vi′rus) [*arthropod-borne* + *virus*] any of the some 200 strains of enveloped RNA viruses that can multiply in both arthopods and vertebrates, and are transmitted to vertebrates by bites of blood-sucking arthropods, usually mosquitoes and ticks. Most are icosahedral, but some strains have helical or complex structures, the particles being 20 to 100 nm in diameter. Arboviruses have been grouped together, chiefly because of their common mode of transmission through arthropod bites, without regard for their morphological and immunological properties. They are now assigned to the families Bunyaviridae, Reoviridae, Rhabodiviridae, and Togaviridae, and the term *arbovirus* has assumed an epidemiological rather than taxonomical connotation. Formerly called *arborvirus* (written also *arbor virus*). **a. group A,** a group of mosquito-borne viruses with a common serological cross-reactivity; assigned to the genus *Alphavirus*. **a. group B,** a group of arthropod-borne viruses, some transmitted by mosquitoes and others by ticks, exhibiting common serological cross-reactivity; assigned to the genus *Flavivirus*. **a. group C,** see C group of viruses, under VIRUS.

arc (ark) [L. *arcus* bow] a structure or projected path having a curved or bowlike outline; by extension, a visible electrical discharge generally taking the outline of an arc. **auricular a.,** a measurement from the center of one auditory meatus to that of the other. Called also *binauricular a.* **adjustive a's of closure,** arcs of jaw closure found in deflective malocclusion caused by an intercusping of the teeth that does not coincide with a centrically related jaw closure. **binauricular a.,** auricular a. **bregmatolambdoid a.,** the arc extending along the course of the saggital suture from the bregma to the lambda. **a's of mandibular closure,** circular or elliptic arcs created by closure of the mandible. **nasobregmatic a.,** the arc extending from the nasion to the bregma. **naso-occipital a.,** the arc extending from the nasion to the most inferior part of the external occipital protuberance. **neural a.,** a series of two or more neurons connecting certain receptors and effectors, and contituting the pathway for neural reactions and reflexes. Called also *sensorimotor a.* **reflex a.,** a complete arc traveled by an impulse in reflex action, from a peripherral receptor along the afferent fibers to the central nervous system, and back along the efferent nerve fibers to the effector organ. **sensorimotor a.,** neural a.

Arcacil trademark for *penicillin V potassium* (see under PENICILLIN).

arcade (ar-kād) an anatomical structure composed of a series of arches.

arch (arch) [L. *arcus* bow] a structure with a curved or bowlike outline. See also ARCUS. **alveolar a.,** an arch formed by the ridge of the alveolar process of the upper or lower jaw; the maxillary or mandibular arch. Called also *alveolar margin, arcus alveolaris,* and *margo alveolaris*. **alveolar a. of mandible,** the superior free border of the alveolar process of the mandible, forming an arch. Called also *alveolar border of mandible, alveolar limbus of mandible, alveolar margin of mandible, alveolar surface of mandible, arcus alveolaris mandibulae* [NA], and *limbus alveolaris mandibulae*. **alveolar a. of maxilla,**

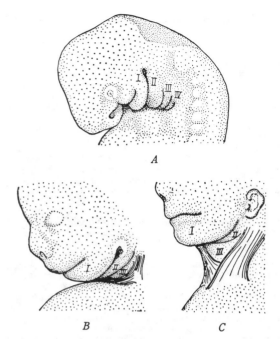

A

B   *C*

Human stages, illustrating the relation of the branchial arches (numbered) to the ventral surface of the neck. *A,* At 5 weeks (× 8); *B,* at 7 weeks (× 3.5); *C,* at 3 months (× 2). (From L. B. Arey: Developmental Anatomy. 7th ed., Philadelphia, W. B. Saunders Co., 1974.)

the inferior free border of the alveolar process of the maxilla, forming an arch. Called also *alveolar border of maxilla, alveolar limbus of maxilla, alveolar margin of maxilla, alveolar surface of maxilla, arcus alveolaris maxillae* [NA], and *limbus alveolaris maxillae.* **a. of aorta,** an arch formed by the curving of the ascending aorta to the left and continuing downward as the descending aorta. It gives rise to the arteries which supply the neck and head (brachiocephalic trunk and left common carotid and left subclavian arteries). Called also *arcus aortae* [NA] and *transverse aorta.* **aortic a's,** paired vessels arching from the ventral to the dorsal aorta through the branchial arches of fishes and amniote embryos. In mammalian development, arches 1 and 2 disappear; arch 3 joins the common to the internal carotid; the left arch 4 remains as the arch of the definitive aorta while the right arch 4 joins the aorta to the subclavian artery; arch 5 disappears; and the ventral halves of arch 6 form the pulmonary arteries while the connections to the dorsal aorta are lost, although the left half, or ductus arteriosus, serves until birth. **a. bar,** arch BAR. **basal a.,** apical BASE. **branchial a's,** paired arched barlike columns that bear the gills in lower aquatic vertebrates and, in the embryos of higher vertebrates, appear in comparable form before subsequent modification to structures of the ear and neck. They develop during the fourth week of embryonic life from the mesoderm around the foregut, being separated by the branchial grooves. Together with the somites, they participate in development of the structures of the neck, jaws, tongue, larynx, pharynx,

external ear, and other parts of the face and neck, including their muscles, cartilages, and bones (see table at SOMITE). The first arch (mandibular a.) bifurcates into maxillary and mandibular processes and during the sixth week, the second (hyoid a.) overlaps the next three; the more caudal sink into a depression (cervical sinus); the fourth and fifth are drawn into the cervical sinus; and by the end of the sixth week all branchial arches disappear. Called also *pharyngeal a's* and *visceral a's.* See illustration. **a. of cricoid cartilage,** a slender, convex arch, about 5 to 7 mm in length, forming the anterior part of the cricoid cartilage and giving attachment to the cricothyroid and the constrictor pharyngis muscles. Called also *arcus cartilaginis cricoideae* [NA]. **dental a.,** the curving structure formed by a line described by the buccal surfaces or through the central grooves of the molars and bicuspids of the teeth in their normal position, viewed from the incisal and occlusal aspects. Called also *arcus dentalis* [NA]. The *inferior dental arch* (arcus dentalis inferior [NA], or mandibular arch) is formed by the mandibular teeth, and the *superior dental arch* (arcus dentalis superior [NA], or maxillary arch) is formed by the maxillary teeth. A dental arch in which the curve from the incisor to the molar region is relatively abrupt, forming an angle at the cuspids, with the line through the bicuspids and molars being nearly straight is known as a *square arch.* One that is less angular at the cuspids than the square arch, but the bicuspid and molar line are nearly straight, is known as a *rounded square arch.* One in which the cuspid angle is lost and the curve, broad in the incisor region, continues to the molar, resembling a horseshoe, is known as a *rounded* or *horseshoeshaped arch.* One in which the arch is very narrow at the incisors, the sides diverging relatively straight backwood through the bicuspids and molars, is known as a *V-shaped arch.* One in which the arch curves continuously from the molars on

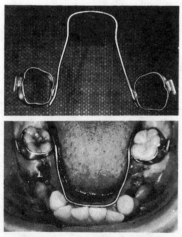

Fixed lingual arch. (From T. M. Graber: Orthodontics — Principles and Practice. 3rd ed. Philadelphia, W. B. Saunders Co., 1972; courtesy of W. R. Mayne.)

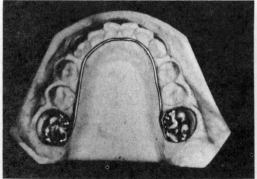 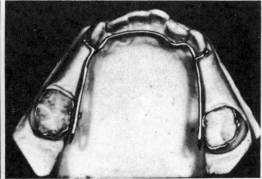

Mershon arch. (From T. M. Graber: Orthodontics — Principles and Practice. 3rd ed. Philadelphia, W. B. Saunders Co., 1972.)

one side to those of the opposite side in such a way that two such arches placed back-to-back form an oval is known as an *oval arch*. **dental a., inferior,** see *dental a.* **dental a., residual,** the curved contour of the maxillary or mandibular ridges remaining after tooth removal. **dental a., superior,** see *dental a.* **edentulous a.,** a dental arch characterized by the absence of some or all teeth. See also Kennedy, Bailyn, and Skinner CLASSIFICATION. **edentulous a., partially,** a dental arch from which one or more, but not all, teeth are missing. **glossopalatine a.,** palatoglossal a. **Gothic a. tracing,** needlepoint TRACING. **horseshoe-shaped a.,** see *dental a.* **hyoid a.,** the second branchial arch, from which are developed the styloid process, stylohyoid ligament, and lesser cornu of the hyoid bone. See table at SOMITE. **jugular venous a.,** a transverse venous trunk that provides communication between the two anterior jugular veins. Called also *arcus venosus juguli* [NA] and *horizontal jugular vein.* **labial and lingual a's,** labiolingual APPLIANCE. **lingual a.,** a wire appliance made to conform to the lingual aspect of the dental arch; used to promote or to prevent movement of the teeth in orthodontic therapy. **lingual a., fixed,** a space-retaining appliance consisting of an arch wire designed to fit the lingual surface of the teeth, and soldered to metal crowns or orthodontic bands. Called also *stationary lingual a.* See illustration. **lingual a., fixed-removable,** a space-maintaining appliance consisting of an arch wire designed to fit the lingual surface of the teeth, having an attachment which allows the dentist to remove and adjust the arch. The most commonly used attachment consists of a half-round tube soldered to the orthodontic band posts at both ends of the wire, which fit vertically into the tube and are locked in place by a spring mechanism. To remove the appliance, the dentist presses the appliance with a scaler to release the post. **lingual a., passive,** an orthodontic appliance for maintaining space and preserving arch length when bilateral primary molars are prematurely lost. **lingual a., stationary,** lingual a., fixed. **malar a.,** zygomatic a. **mandibular a.,** 1. the first branchial arch, from which are developed the bone of the lower jaw, the malleus, and the incus. See table at SOMITE. 2. inferior dental a.; see *dental a.* **maxillary a.,** 1. superior dental a.; see *dental a.* 2. palatal a. **Mershon a.,** a type of fixed lingual arch. See illustration. **nasal a.,** the arch formed by the nasal bones and by the nasal process of the maxilla. **oral a.,** palatal a. **oval a.,** see *dental a.* **palatal a.,** the arch formed by the roof of the mouth from the teeth on one side of the maxilla to the teeth on the other, or if the teeth are missing, from the residual dental arch on one side to that on the other. Called also *maxillary a., oral a.,* and *palatomaxillary a.* **palatine a., anterior,** palatoglossal a. **palatine a., posterior,** palatopharyngeal a. **palatoglossal a.,** the anterior of the two folds of mucous membrane on either side of the oropharynx, connected with the soft palate and enclosing the palatoglossal muscle. Called also *anterior palatine a., glossopalatine a., anterior column of fauces, anterior pillar of fauces, anterior pillar of soft palate, arcus glossopalatinus,* and *arcus palatoglossus* [NA]. **palatomaxillary a.,** palatal a. **palatopharyngeal a.,** the posterior of the two folds of mucous membrane on each side of the oropharynx, connected with the soft palate and enclosing the palatopharyngeal muscle. Called also *pharyngoepiglottic a., pharyngopalatine a., posterior palatine a., arcus palatopharyngeus* [NA], *arcus pharyngopalatinus, posterior column of fauces, posterior pillar of fauces,* and *posterior pillar of soft palate.* **palpebral a., inferior,** an arch derived from the lateral and medial palpebral anteries, supplying the lower eyelid. Called also *arcus palpebralis inferior* [NA] and *arcus tarseus inferior.* **palpebral a., superior,** an arch derived from the lateral and medial palpebral arteries, supplying the upper eyelid. Called also *arcus palpebralis superior* [NA] and *arcus tarseus superior.* **passive lingual a.,** lingual a., passive. **pharyngeal a's,** branchial a's. **pharyngoepiglottic a.,** pharyngopalatine a., palatopharyngeal a. **premandibular a's,** see branchial a's. **residual dental a.,** dental a., residual. **ribbon a.,** ribbon arch APPLIANCE. **rounded a.,** see *dental a.* **rounded square a.,** see *dental a.* **square a.,** see *dental a.* **stationary lingual a.,** lingual a. stationary. **superciliary a.,** a smooth elevation arching upward and laterally from the glabella, a little above the margin of the orbit. Called also *arcus superciliaris* [NA]. **supraorbital a. of frontal bone,** supraorbital margin of frontal bone; see under MARGIN. **tapering a.,** a dental arch that converges from molars to central incisors to such an extent that lines passing through the central grooves of the molars and premolars intersect within 1 inch anterior of the central incisiors. **thyrohyoid a.,** the third pharyngeal arch,

which becomes represented by the greater cornu of the hyoid bone. **trapezoidal a.,** a dental arch similar to the tapering arch but with a lesser degree of convergence, the anterior teeth being somewhat squared to abruptly rounded from canine tip to canine tip, and the canines acting as corners for the arch. **U-shaped a.,** a dental arch in which the arch width between the first premolars and the last molars are almost equal, the curves from canine to canine being abrupt so that the arch assumes the shape of the letter U. **V-shaped a.,** see *dental a.* **visceral a's,** branchial a's. **W a.,** a fixed maxillary orthodontic appliance with either bilateral or unilateral extension arms, for expanding the arches. **a. width,** see arch WIDTH. **zygomatic a.,** the arch formed by the articulation of the broad temporal process of the zygomatic bone and the slender zygomatic process of the temporal bone, giving attachment to the masseter muscle and serving as a line of demarcation between the temporal and infratemporal fossae. Called also *malar a., arcus zygomaticus* [NA], and *zygoma.*

arch-, arche- see ARCHI-.

archenteron (ar-ken′ter-on) [*arche-* + Gr. *enteron* intestine] the primitive digestive cavity of those embryonic forms whose blastula becomes a gastrula by invagination.

archi-, arch-, arche- [Gr. *archē* beginning] a combining form denoting first, beginning, or original.

Archigenes of Apamea [1st century A.D.] a celebrated Greek physician who practiced in Rome, a pupil of Agati Agathinus (and a Pneumatist). Portions of his several works are preserved. His surgical observations (e.g., on amputation and ligation) are noteworthy. Archigenes surmised that toothache often results from disease of the interior part of the tooth (pulpitis) and perforated the tooth with a small drill at the discolored part of the crown because he believed that a morbid substance in the tooth would find an outlet through the hole.

arciform (ar′sĭ-form) [L. *arcus* bow + *forma* shape] having a shape like an arc or bow.

Arcolano, Giovanni [died 1484] a physician-surgeon in Padova, whose work, *Pratica,* contains references to filling teeth with gold, has drawings of dental instruments, and 10 rules for dental health. Called also *Giovanni Ercolani, Ioannes Arculanus,* and *Ioannes de Arculis.*

arcon (ar′kon) [*articulator* + *con*dyle] see arcon ARTICULATOR.

Arcton 6 trademark for *dichlorodifluoromethane.*

arcuate (ar′ku-āt) [L. *arcuatus* bow-shaped] shaped like an arc or bow.

Arculanus see ARCOLANO.

arcus (ar′kus) [L. "a bow"] arch; a general term used in anatomical nomenclature to designate any structure having a curved or bowlike outline. **a. alveola′ris,** alveolar ARCH. **a. alveola′aris mandib′ulae** [NA], alveolar arch of mandible; see under ARCH. **a. alveola′ris maxil′lae** [NA], alveolar arch of maxilla; see under ARCH. **a. aor′tae** [NA], ARCH of aorta. **a. cartilag′inis cricoi′deae** [NA], ARCH of cricoid cartilage. **a. denta′lis** [NA], dental ARCH. **a. denta′lis infe′ior** [NA], inferior dental arch; see dental ARCH. **a. denta′lis supe′rior** [NA], superior dental arch; see dental ARCH. **a. glossopalati′nus, p. palatoglos′sus** [NA], palatoglossal ARCH. **a. palatopharyn′geus** [NA], palatopharyngeal ARCH. **a. palpebra′lis infe′rior** [NA], palpebral arch, inferior; see under ARCH. **a. palpebra′lis supe′ior** [NA], palpebral arch, superior; see under ARCH. **a. pharyngopalati′nus,** palatopharyngeal ARCH. **a. supercilia′ris** [NA], superciliary ARCH. **a. tar′seus infe′rior,** palpebral arch, inferior; see under ARCH. **a. tar′seus supe′rior,** palpebral arch, superior; see under ARCH. **a. veno′sus jug′uli** [NA], jugular venous ARCH. **a. zygomat′icus** [NA], zygomatic ARCH.

ARD acute respiratory DISEASE (of any undefined form).

Ardee trademark for a *denture reliner* (see under RELINER), probably prepared from ethyl alcohol plasticizers and acrylic resins.

Ardex trademark for *dextroamphetamine sulfate* (see under DEXTROAMPHETAMINE).

area (a′re-ah), pl. *a′reae, areas* [L.] a limited space; any space with boundaries; a general term used in anatomical nomenclature to designate a specific surface or functional region. See also REGION. **basal seat a.,** denture-bearing a. **bilaminar a. of articular disk,** retroarticular CUSHION. **catchment a.,** a geographic area defined and served by a health program or an institution, such as a hospital or community mental health center. The program usually serves all persons residing in the area or it may be restricted to only those persons who are enrolled in the program. **contact a.,** 1. any area at which bodies or materials touch. 2. the area where the mesial and distal surfaces of the teeth touch each other. Called also *interproximal contact a., centric stop, contact point, contact surface,* and *facies contactus dentis* [NA]. See also interproximal SPACE. **a. cribro′sa me′dia,** inferior vestibular a. of internal acoustic meatus. **a. cribro'sa supe'erior,** superior vestibular a. of internal acoustic meatus. **denture-bearing a., denture foundation a., denture-supporting a.,** the surface of the oral tissues (residual alveolar ridge) which supports a denture. Called also *basal seat a., stress-bearing a., stress-supporting a.,* and *denture foundation.* See also *rest a.* and denture-supporting STRUCTURE. **a. of facial nerve, a. ner'vi facia'lis** [NA], the part of the fundus of the internal acoustic meatus where the facial nerve enters the facial canal. **hinge a.,** a flexible, proline-rich area on the IgG molecule which acts as a hinge on the Fab fragment and permits the antibody molecule to adapt itself to bind with antigen. **a. hypoglos'si,** the portion of the mouth beneath the tongue. **impression a.,** the surface of the oral structures recorded in an impression. **interglobular a's,** the areas of dentin lying between the calcoglobules. **interproximal contact a.,** contact a. (2). **Kiesselbach's a.,** an area on the anterior part of the nasal septum above the intermaxillary bone, which is richly supplied with capillaries and is a common site of nosebleed. Called also *Little's a.* and *Kiesselbach's space.* **Little's a.,** Kiesselbach's a. **mesobranchial a.,** the pharyngeal floor, between the pharyngeal arches and pouches of each side. **olfactory a.,** a part of the olfactory organ; it is an area of the nasal cavity lined with mucous membrane rich in olfactory cells, located in the superior region of each nasal cavity, extending from the anterior limits of the superior concha posteriorly for about 1 cm, and confined to the part of the nasal fossa walled off by the ethmoid bone. It is distinguished by its tan color, in contrast with the pink color of the respiratory mucosa. Called also *olfactory epithelium* and *regio olfactoria* [NA]. **pear-shaped a.,** retromolar PAD. **post dam a.,** posterior palatal seal a. **posterior palatal seal a., postpalatal seal a.,** the soft tissues along the junction of the hard and soft palates on which pressure may be applied by a denture to aid in its retention. Called also *post dam a.* See also posterior palatal SEAL. **pressure a.,** an area beneath a denture which is subjected to excessive pressure, with consequent displacement of tissue. **recipient a.,** an area on the body on which a skin or bone graft or a tooth is implanted. **relief a.,** the portion of the surface of the mouth upon which pressures or forces are reduced or eliminated in prosthodontic therapy. See also RELIEF (3). **rest a.,** the prepared surface of a tooth or fixed restoration into which the rest fits, giving support to a removable partial denture. On the posterior teeth it is usually located in the marginal ridge portion of the occlusal surface and over the center of the residual alveolar ridge; on the anterior teeth it is usually located in the cingulum. Called also *rest seat.* See also denture base SADDLE. **retention a. of tooth,** see INFRABULGE. **retromylohyoid a.,** an area in the alveolingual sulcus just lingual to the retromolar pad, which extends lingually down to the floor of the mouth and back to the retromylohyoid curtain, being bounded anteriorly by the lingual tuberosity (the distal end of the mylohyoid ridge). **rugae a.,** the portion of the mouth in which rugae are found. Called also *rugae zone.* **saddle a.,** the edentulous portion of the dental arch on which a fixed or removable prosthesis rests. **self-cleansing a.,** an area on a tooth surface accessible to the scouring action of food and saliva and to movements of the tongue, lips, and cheeks. **stress-bearing a.,** 1. denture-bearing a. 2. the portion of the mouth capable of providing support for a denture. 3. surfaces of oral structures which resist forces, strains, or pressures brought upon them during function. **stress-supporting a.,** denture-bearing a. **supporting a.,** 1. the surface of the mouth available for support of a denture. 2. those areas of the maxillary and mandibular edentulous ridges which are considered best suited to carry the forces of mastication when dentures are in function. **treatment a.,** operatory. **vermilion a.,** vermilion BORDER. **vestibular a. of internal acoustic meatus, inferior,** the lower portion of the fundus of the internal acoustic meatus. Called also *a. cribrosa media* and *a. vestibularis inferior* [NA]. **vestibular a. of internal acoustic meatus, superior,** the upper portion of the fundus of the internal acoustic meatus. Called also *area cribrosa superior* and *a. vestibularis superior* [NA]. **a. vestibula'ris infe'rior** [NA], inferior vestibular a. of internal acoustic meatus. **a. vestibula'ris supe'rior** [NA], superior vestibular a. of internal acoustic meatus. **vocal a.,** the part of the glottis between the vocal cords.

areata, areatus (ar''e-a-tah; ar''e-a'tus) occurring in areas or patches.

Areca (ar'ĕ-kah) [East Indian] a genus of palm tree, chiefly Asiatic. *A. catechu* affords betel nut.

arecoline (ah-rek'o-lēn) an *Areca catechu* (betel nut) alkaloid, N-methyltetrahydronicotinite, occurring as a colorless, odorless, oily liquid that is soluble in water, alcohol, chloroform, and ether. It is a cholinomimetic drug that acts on the autonomic effector cells and stimulates postganglionic nerve impulses. Also used as an anthelmintic.

areflexia (ah''re-flek'se-ah) [*a* neg. + *reflex* + -*ia*] absence of the reflexes.

aregenerative (ah''re-jen'er-a''tiv) characterized by absence of regeneration.

Arenaviridae (ah-re''nah-vi'rĭ-de) [L. *arena* sand + *virus* + -*idae*] a family of enveloped viruses. The genome is (−)RNA. The nucleocapsid (the symmetry of which is unknown) is assembled in the cytoplasm and the envelope is acquired by budding through the cell membranes. In thin sections, electron-dense granules are apparent in the envelope; the granules are 20 to 30 nm across, resembling ribosomes or glycogen granules and are sometimes arranged in a circular pattern and connected by filaments in the interior of virions, giving an appearance of sand. The virion is round or pleomorphic with a diameter averaging 110 to 130 nm. Club-shaped projections on the surface are 10 nm long. The family consists of a single genus, *Arenavirus.*

Arenavirus (ah-re''nah-vi'rus) a genus of viruses of the family Arenaviridae, which includes lymphocytic choriomeningitis virus, American hemorrhagic fever viruses (comprising Junin, Tacaribe, Machupo, Amapari, Tamaini, Pichinde, Parana, and Latino viruses), and Lassa fever virus.

arenavirus (ah-re''nah-vi'rus) any virus of the family Arenaviridae or of the genus *Arenavirus.*

areola (ah-re'o-lah), pl. *are'olae* [L., dim. of *area* space] 1. any minute space or interstice in a tissue. 2. a circular area of a different color, such as the area surrounding the nipple of the breast. **vaccinal a.,** the ring of redness that surrounds a vaccinia pustule.

areolae (ah-re'o-le) [L.] plural or *areola.*

areolar (ah-re'o-lar) pertaining to or containing areolae; containing minute interspaces.

Arestocaine trademark for *mepivacaine hydrochloride* (see under MEPIVACAINE).

Aretaeus of Cappadocia [2nd century A.D.] a famous Greek Pneumatist who wrote on acute and chronic diseases. His clinical descriptions (e.g., diabetes, pleurisy, tetanus) are outstanding, and in the best Hippocratic tradition. See also PNEUMATIST.

Arfonad trademark for *trimethaphan camsylate* (see under TRIMETHAPHAN).

Arg arginine.

argentaffin (ar-jen'tah-fin) [L. *argentum* silver + *affinis* having affinity for] having affinity for or staining readily with silver and chromium salts.

argentaffinoma (ar''jen-taf''ĭ-no'mah) a tumor formed from the argentaffin cells, found in the gastrointestinal tract, usually in the appendix and small intestine. Called also *carcinoid.*

argentation (ar''jen-ta'shun) [L. *argentum* silver] staining with a silver salt.

argentic (ar-jen'tik) containing silver.

Argentum trademark for *dental mercury* (see under MERCURY). **A. "A,"** trademark for an *amalgam alloy* (see under AMALGAM).

argentum (ar-jen'tum) [L.] silver.

argilla (ar-jil'lah) kaolin.

argillaceous (ar''jĭ-la'shus) made up of clay.

arginase [E.C.3.5.3.1] (ar'jĭ-nās) a hydrolase acting on carbon-nitrogen bonds, other than peptide bonds. Found chiefly in the liver, but also in the mammary glands, testes, and kidneys, it catalyzes the conversion of arginine to urea and also to ornithine in protein metabolism. It also hydrolyzes α-*N*-substituted L-arginine and canavanine. Called also *arginine amidinase* and *canavase.*

arginine (ar'jĭ-nēn) a basic, naturally occurring, nonessential amino acid, 2-amino-5-guanidinovaleric acid. It contains the strongly basic guanidino group and provides the amidine group for the synthesis of creatine. Used as a detoxicant for ammonia in hepatic failure. Abbreviated *Arg.* See also amino ACID. **a. amidinase,** arginase. **a. succinase,** argininosuccinate LYASE.

arginosuccinase (ar''jĭ-no-suk'sĭ-nās) argininosuccinate LYASE.

argon (ar'gon) [Gr. *argos* inactive] a colorless, tasteless, and odorless gas found in the atmosphere, which has a monoatomic structure with its outer shell completely filled, thus being inert. Symbol, Ar; atomic weight, 39.948; atomic number, 18; group 0 of the periodic table. Argon has three stable isotopes (36, 38, 40) and six artificial radioactive ones (33, 35, 37, 39, 41, 42). It is considered to be nontoxic, but may act as a simple asphyxiant.

argyremia (ar''jĭ-re'me-ah) [Gr. *argyros* silver + *haima* blood + -*ia*] the presence of silver or silver salts in the blood.

argyria (ar-jir'e-ah) [Gr. *argyros* silver + *-ia*] bluish-gray discoloration of the skin and mucous membranes from prolonged exposure to silver, usually observed in individuals employed in the silver industry and patients using silver-containing drugs, especially ointments. Localized discoloration may occur from deposition of silver amalgam fragments in the tissue; the area around embedded amalgam fragments may appear as a bluishblack lesion, suggesting melanin pigmentation. In the generalized form, pigmentation is diffusely dispersed throughout the oral cavity and there are no other symptoms. Called also *argyrosis*.

argyrophil (ar-ji'ro-fil) [Gr. *argyros* silver + *philein* to love] staining or easily impregnated with silver.

argyrosis (ar"ji-ro'sis) argyria.

arhinencephaly (ah-rin-en"sef'ah-le) a congenital abnormality characterized by absence of the rhinencephalon, associated with malformations of the anterior part of the brain and skull, hypotelorism, and premaxillary agenesis.

arhinia (ah-rin'e-ah) [*a* neg + Gr. *rhis* nose + *-ia*] congenital absence of the nose.

Arias' syndrome [Irwin M. *Arias*, American physician, born 1926] see under SYNDROME.

ariboflavinosis (a-ri"bo-fla-vi-no'sis) a nutritional deficiency of riboflavin (vitamin B₂), characterized by perlèche, which may be the first sign; seborrheic dermatitis around the scrotum and nose, usually in the nasolabial folds and the alae nasi, and of the trunk and extremities; sore throat; glossitis; anemia; and vascularization of the cornea. Ariboflavinosis occurs usually in conjunction with other vitamin deficiencies, rarely alone. In growing mice, it may be associated with narrowing of the mandibular condyles.

Aristaloy trademark for an *amalgam alloy* (see under AMALGAM).

Aristaloy Cr trademark for a *high copper alloy* (see under ALLOY).

Aristamid trademark for *sulfisomidine*.

Aristocort trademark for *triamcinolone*.

Aristoderm trademark for *triamcinolone acetonide* (see under TRIAMCINOLONE).

Aristol trademark for *thymol iodide* (see under THYMOL).

Aristopan trademark for *triamcinolone hexacetonide* (see under TRIAMCINOLONE).

Aristotle [384–322 B.C.] a Greek philosopher, pupil of Plato, and tutor of Alexander the Great. His writings include a dental systematization of different classes of animals and express the beliefs that men have more teeth than women, teeth increase in length during life, individuals with more teeth live longer than those with fewer teeth, and teeth are generated after the body has already been constituted.

Arlidin trademark for *nylidrin hydrochloride* (see under NYLIDRIN).

arm (arm) [L. *armus*] 1. the part of the upper limb extending from the shoulder to the elbow. Called also *brachium* [NA]. 2. a slender part or extension, usually having mobility and independent function, which projects from the main structure. 3. an extension or projection by which a removable partial denture is retained in position in the mouth. See also CLASP. 4. CHROMOSOME arm. **bar clasp a.,** a clasp arm that serves as an extracoronal retainer, originating from the denture base, a major or minor connector, or the framework of a denture, traverses soft tissue, approaches the tooth undercut area from a gingival direction, and terminates in a retentive undercut lying gingival to the height of contour. It provides retention by the resistance of metal to deformation. **chromosome a.,** CHROMOSOME arm. **circumferential clasp a.,** a clasp arm that originates above the height of contour, traverses part of the suprabulge portion of the tooth, approaches the tooth undercut from an occlusal direction, and terminates in a retentive undercut lying gingival to the height of contour. It provides retention by the resistance of metal to deformation. Called also *retentive circumferential clasp a.* **endosteal implant a.,** an anterior or posterior extension of the framework of an implant substructure. Called also *implant anchor.* See also implant SUBSTRUCTURE. **engine a.,** an armlike adjustable extension of the dental engine, consisting of three sections connected to each other by flexible joints which allow free movement of the handpiece, and a system of pulley wheels and a belt for transmitting power. See illustration at dental UNIT. **moment a.,** the distance from the axis of rotation to the line of the force associated with the rotation, measured over the shortest distance from the axis to the line of the force, being a **parallel** line lying at a right angle to the line of the force.

reciprocal a., an arm of a clasp located in such a manner as to reciprocate any force arising from an opposing clasp arm on the same tooth. **retention a., retentive a.,** an arm of a clasp that is flexible and that engages the infrabulge area at the terminal end of the arm. Called also *retention terminal.* **retentive circumferential clasp a.,** circumferential clasp a. **stabilizing a.,** an arm of a clasp that is rigid and that contacts the tooth at or occlusal to the surveyed height of contour. **stabilizing circumferential clasp a.,** a circumferential clasp arm which is relatively rigid and contacts the height of contour of the tooth. **T clasp a.,** a T-shaped bar clasp arm that arises from the denture framework or a metal base and approaches the retentive undercut from a gingival direction. **Y clasp a.,** a Y-shaped bar clasp arm that arises from the denture framework or a metal base and approaches the retentive undercut from a gingival direction.

armamentarium (ar"mah-men-ta're-um) [L.] the total store of available resources. The equipment, such as instruments, drugs, and other things, used in a technique or specialty. See also INSTRUMENTARIUM. **endodontic a.,** endodontic instruments; see ENDODONTICS and root canal THERAPY. **occlusal adjustment a.,** occlusal ADJUSTMENT. **periodontal a.,** periodontal instruments; see PERIODONTICS.

Arndt's law [Rudoff *Arndt*, German neurologist, 1835–1900] Arndt-Schulz LAW.

Arndt-Gottron disease [G. *Arndt*; H. A. *Gottron*] see under DISEASE.

Arndt-Schulz law [R. *Arndt*; Hugo *Schulz*, German pharmacologist, 1853–1932] see under LAW.

Arning's carcinoid [E. *Arning*] see under CARCINOID.

Arnold see zygomaticoorbital FORAMEN (internal zygomatic foramen of Arnold).

Arnold's canal, canaliculus, ganglion, nerve [Philipp Friedrich *Arnold*, German anatomist, 1803–1890] see under CANAL, and see mastoid canaliculus for Arnold's nerve, under CANALICULUS; otic GANGLION; and auricular branch of vagus nerve, under BRANCH.

Arnold's neuralgia [Julius *Arnold*, German pathologist, 1835–1915] recurrent laryngeal NEURALGIA.

Arnold-Chiari deformity [J. *Arnold*, German pathologist, 1835–1915; Hans *Chiari*, German pathologist, 1851–1916] see under DEFORMITY.

aromatic (ar"o-mat'ik) [L. *aromaticus;* Gr. *aromatikos*] 1. pertaining to aromatic compounds, a large group of unsaturated cyclic hydrocarbons having one or more benzene rings. See aromatic HYDROCARBON. 2. having a spicy odor.

arrangement (ah-ranj'ment) 1. the disposal or positioning of parts. 2. an agreement, settlement, disposition, or understanding. **anterior tooth a.,** the arrangement of anterior teeth for esthetic or phonetic effects. **tooth a.,** 1. the positioning of teeth on a denture for specific purposes. 2. the setting of teeth on temporary bases.

arrest (ah-rest') stoppage; the act of stopping. **cardiac a., heart a.,** a sudden and often unexpected cessation of cardiac activity due to either cessation of periodic impulses which trigger the heart muscle contractions, heart muscle twitching, or ventricular fibrillation or flutter. Unless resuscitation is applied within minutes from the onset of the arrest, permanent tissue damage, especially in the brain, due to insufficient blood supply, or death results. See also cardiopulmonary RESUSCITATION.

Arrhenius' equation [Svante August *Arrhenius*, Swedish chemist, 1859–1927] see under EQUATION.

arrhythmia (ah-rith'me-ah) [*a* neg. + Gr. *rhythmos* rhythm] any condition characterized by abnormal rhythm of the heart.

arsenic (ar'se-nik) [L. *arsenicum, arsenium, arsenum,* from Gr. *arsen* strong] 1. a brittle, lustrous, silvery gray heavy metal that gives off a peculiar odor of garlic and turns dark on exposure to air. Symbol, As; atomic number, 33; atomic weight, 74.922; specific gravity, 5.73; group VA of the periodic table. Some arsenic compounds are used in the treatment of spirochetal infections, some hematological disorders, and skin diseases. Arsenic is capable of penetrating the epithelium and causing necrosis and sloughing. In agriculture, arsenic is used in parasiticides, fungicides, and pesticides. Most arsenic compounds are highly toxic, their toxic action being inhibition of sulfhydryl enzymes. Acute poisoning, due to ingestion of massive doses of arsenic, may result in death within 24 hours, usually without any significant morphologic changes. Less severe poisoning is characterized by the appearance after 24 hours of generalized visceral hyperemia, petechiae of the serous membranes and skin, necrotic capillary changes, gastric congestion and edema, usually followed by petechial hemorrhage and coagulation necrosis, thromboses, fatty changes in the liver and kidneys, fatty degeneration of the myocardium, and petechial hemorrhage and edema of the brain. Presenting symptoms include vomiting and severe diarrhea. Death is caused by vascular collapse and central nervous system depression. Chronic poisoning is due to progressive accumulation of small doses of arsenic, characterized by gastrointestinal, neurological, and cutaneous changes similar to, but less severe than, those found in acute poisoning; vascular lesions and petechial hemorrhage are not evident. Myelin degeneration and destruction of axis cylinders of the peripheral nerves are the principal neurological changes. Presenting symptoms include weakness, frequently associated with paralysis and anesthesia, diarrhea, and hepatic and renal changes. Oral symptoms include pain, massive inflammation of the mucosa, severe gingivitis, excessive salivation, ulcers, purpura, and sometimes mobility of the teeth. Recovery usually follows interruption of exposure to arsenic. (See also arsenical STOMATITIS.) Arsenic compounds are also suspected of having carcinogenic and teratogenic effects. 2. a. trioxide. **a. trihydride,** arsine. **a. trioxide, white a.,** a highly toxic white or glassy compound, AsO_3, with a sweetish taste; formerly used in the treatment of skin and lung diseases. Formerly, in dentistry, minute amounts of arsenic trioxide were sealed in the pulp chamber for the purpose of devitalizing the pulp; because of the high risk of poisoning, the method has been abandoned. Called also *arsenous acid* and *arsenous oxide*. See also *arsenic* (1).

arsenical (ar-sen′ĭ-kal) [L. *arsenicalis*] 1. pertaining to or containing arsenic. 2. an arsenic compound or a drug containing an arsenic compound. Chemically, arsenicals are grouped into inorganic and organic compounds; the presence or absence of substituents being a factor in determining the solubility of a compound and its ability to penetrate cell membranes.

arsenide (ar′sĕ-nīd) a binary compound of negative trivalent arsenic. **hydrogen a.,** arsine.

arsenite (ar′sĕ-nīt) a salt of arsenous acid.

arsenous (ar′sĕ-nus) containing arsenic in its lower or triad valency.

arsine (ar′sin) any member of a peculiar group of volatile arsenical bases, AsH_3, formed when arsenous acid is brought in contact with albuminous substances. It is a colorless neutral gas with a disagreeable garlic-like odor. Inhalation of even small amounts may be toxic, causing hemolytic jaundice, gastroenteritis, nausea, hematemesis, anorexia, headache, paresthesia, hemoglobinuria, anuria, and, sometimes, death. Called also *arsenic trihydride* and *hydrogen arsenide*.

Arsobal trademark for *melarsoprol*.

arsphenamine (ars-fen′ah-mēn) a compound, 4′4′-arsenobis-(2-aminophenyl) dihydrochloride, occurring as a light, yellow, odorless, hygroscopic powder. Used in the past as a spirocheticide in the treatment of syphilis and, sometimes, in the treatment of acute necrotizing ulcerative gingivitis. Called also *salvarsan*.

Artane trademark for *trihexyphenidyl hydrochloride* (see under TRIHEXYPHENIDYL).

arterenol (ar″te-re′nol) norepinephrine.

arteria (ar-te′re-ah), pl. *arte′riae* [L.; Gr. *artēria*] a tubular vessel which transports blood under high pressure away from the heart to the tissues. See also ARTERY. **a. alveola′ris infe′rior** [NA], alveolar artery, inferior; see under ARTERY. **arte′riae alveola′res superio′res anterio′res** [NA], alveolar arteries, anterior; see under ARTERY. **a. alveola′ris supe′rior poste′rior** [NA], alveolar artery, posterior superior; see under ARTERY. **a. angula′ris** [NA], angular ARTERY. **a. anon′yma,** brachiocephalic TRUNK. **a. aor′ta,** aorta. **a. auricula′ris poste′rior** [NA], auricular artery, posterior; see under ARTERY. **a. auricula′ris profun′da** [NA], auricular artery deep; see under ARTERY. **a. basila′ris** [NA], basilar ARTERY. **a. bucca′lis** [NA], **a. buccinato′ria,** buccal ARTERY. **a. cana′lis pterygoi′dei** [NA], ARTERY of pterygoid canal. **a. carot′is commu′nis** [NA], carotid artery, common; see under ARTERY. **a. carot′is exter′na** [NA], carotid artery, external; see under ARTERY. **a. carot′is inter′na** [NA], carotid artery, internal; see under ARTERY. **a. centra′lis ret′inae** [NA], central artery of retina; see under ARTERY. **a. cerebel′li infe′rior ante′rior** [NA], cerebellar artery, anterior inferior; see under ARTERY. **a. cerebel′li infe′rior poste′rior** [NA], cerebellar artery, posterior inferior; see under ARTERY. **a. cerebel′li supe′rior** [NA], cerebellar artery, superior; see under ARTERY. **a. cer′ebri ante′rior** [NA], cerebral artery, anterior; see under ARTERY. **a. cer′ebri me′dia** [NA], cerebral artery, middle; see under ARTERY. **a. cer′ebri poste′rior** [NA], cerebral artery, posterior; see under ARTERY. **a. cervica′lis ascen′dens** [NA], cervical artery, ascending; see under ARTERY. **a. cervica′lis profun′da** [NA], cervical artery, deep; see under ARTERY. **a. cervica′lis superficia′lis** [NA alternative], cervical artery, superficial; see under ARTERY. **arte′riae cilia′res,** ciliary arteries; see under ARTERY. **a. corona′ria (sinis′tra et dex′tra),** coronary ARTERY. **arte′riae dorsa′les lin′guae,** dorsal branches of lingual artery; see under BRANCH. **a. dorsa′lis na′si** [NA], dorsal artery of nose; see under ARTERY. **a. ethmoida′lis ante′rior** [NA],

ethmoidal artery, anterior; see under ARTERY. **a. ethmoida′lis poste′rior** [NA], ethmoidal artery, posterior; see under ARTERY. **a. facia′lis** [NA], facial ARTERY. **a. fronta′lis,** supratrochlear ARTERY. **a. infraorbita′lis** [NA], infraorbital ARTERY. **a. innomina′ta,** brachiocephalic TRUNK. **a. labia′lis infe′rior** [NA], labial artery, inferior; see under ARTERY. **a. labia′lis supe′rior** [NA], labial artery, superior; see under ARTERY. **a. labyrin′thi** [NA], labyrinthine ARTERY. **a. lacrima′lis** [NA], lacrimal ARTERY. **a. laryn′gea infe′rior** [NA], laryngeal artery, inferior; see under ARTERY. **a. laryn′gea supe′rior** [NA], laryngeal artery, superior; see under ARTERY. **a. lingua′lis** [NA], lingual ARTERY. **a. masseter′ica** [NA], masseteric ARTERY. **a. maxilla′ris** [NA], maxillary ARTERY. **a. maxilla′ris exter′na,** facial ARTERY. **a. maxilla′ris inter′na,** maxillary ARTERY. **a. menin′gea ante′rior** [NA], meningeal artery, anterior; see under ARTERY. **a. menin′gea me′dia** [NA], meningeal artery, middle; see under ARTERY. **a. menin′gea poste′rior** [NA], meningeal artery, posterior; see under ARTERY. **a. menta′lis** [NA], mental ARTERY. **arte′riae nasa′les posterio′res, latera′les et sep′ti** [NA], 1. nasal arteries, posterior lateral; see under ARTERY. 2. septal arteries, posterior; see under ARTERY. **a. occipita′lis** [NA], occipital ARTERY. **a. ophthal′mica** [NA], ophthalmic ARTERY. **a. palati′na ascen′dens** [NA], palatine artery, ascending; see under ARTERY. **a. palati′na descen′dens** [NA], palatine artery, descending; see under ARTERY. **a. palati′na ma′jor** [NA], palatine artery, greater; see under ARTERY. **arte′riae palati′nae mino′res** [NA], palatine arteries, lesser; see under ARTERY. **arte′riae palpebra′les latera′les** [NA], palpebral arteries, lateral; see under ARTERY. **arte′riae palpebra′les media′les** [NA], palpebral arteries, medial; see under ARTERY. **a. pharyn′gea ascen′dens** [NA], pharyngeal artery, ascending; see under ARTERY. **a. prin′ceps cervi′cis,** descending branch of occipital artery; see under BRANCH. **a. profun′da lin′guae** [NA], lingual artery, deep; see under ARTERY. **arte′riae pulmona′les,** pulmonary arteries; see under ARTERY. **a. sphenopalati′na** [NA], sphenopalatine ARTERY. **a. sternomastoi′dea,** one of the sternocleidomastoid branches of the occipital artery (see under BRANCH). **a. stylomastoi′dea** [NA], stylomastoid ARTERY. **a. subcla′via** [NA], subclavian ARTERY. **a. sublingua′lis** [NA], sublingual ARTERY. **a. submenta′lis** [NA], submental ARTERY. **a. supraorbita′lis** [NA], supraorbital ARTERY. **a. suprascapula′ris** [NA], suprascapular ARTERY. **a. supratrochlea′ris** [NA], supratrochlear ARTERY. **a. tempora′lis me′dia** [NA], temporal artery, middle; see under ARTERY. **arte′riae temporales profundae** [NA], temporal arteries, deep; see under ARTERY. **a. tempora′lis superficia′lis** [NA], temporal artery, superficial; see under ARTERY. **a. thyroi′dea i′ma** [NA], thyroid artery, lowest; see under ARTERY. **a. thyroi′dea infe′rior** [NA], thyroid artery, inferior; see under ARTERY. **a. thyroi′dea supe′rior** [NA], thyroid artery, superior; see under ARTERY. **a. transver′sa col′li** [NA], cervical artery, transverse; see under ARTERY. **a. transver′sa facie′i** [NA], facial artery, transverse; see under ARTERY. **a. tympan′ica ante′rior** [NA], tympanic artery, anterior; see under ARTERY. **a. tympan′ica infe′rior** [NA], tympanic artery, inferior; see under ARTERY. **a. vertebra′lis** [NA], vertebral ARTERY. **a. zygomaticoorbita′lis** [NA], zygomaticoorbital ARTERY.

arteriae (ar-te′re-e) [L.] plural of *arteria*.

arterial (ar-te′re-al) pertaining to an artery or to the arteries.

arteriectasis (ar″tĕ-re-ek′tah-sis) [*artery* + Gr. *ektasis* dilatation] dilatation and, usually, lengthening of an artery.

arteriectomy (ar″tĕ-re-ek′to-me) [*artery* + Gr. *ektomē* excision] excision of a portion of an artery.

arteriectopia (ar″tĕ-re-ek-to′pe-ah) [*artery* + Gr. *ektopos* out of place] displacement of an artery from its normal location.

arterio- [L. *arteria*; Gr. *artēria*] a combining form denoting relationship to an artery or arteries.

arteriogenesis (ar-te″re-o-jen′ĕ-sis) [*arterio-* + Gr. *genesis* production] the formation of arteries.

arteriogram (ar-te′re-o-gram″) [*arterio-* + Gr. *gramma* a writing] a roentgenogram of an artery after injection of a radiopaque medium.

arteriography (ar″te-re-og′rah-fe) [*arterio-* + Gr. *graphein* to write] roentgenography of arteries after injection of radiopaque material. See also ANGIOGRAPHY. **catheter a.,** radiography of vessels after introduction of contrast material through a catheter inserted into an artery.

arteriola (ar-te″re-o′lah), pl. *arterio′lae* [L. "a small artery"] a small arterial branch less than 0.3 mm in diameter. Called also *arteriole*.

arteriolae (ar-te″re-o′le) [L.] plural of *arteriola*.

arteriolar (ar″te-re′o-lar) pertaining to arterioles.

arteriole (ar-te′re-ōl) [L. *arteriola*] a small arterial branch less than 0.3 mm in diameter. Called also *arteriola*. **precapillary a.,** a terminal arteriole with incomplete investing coats that end in capillaries.

arteriolith (ar-te′re-o-lith″) [*arterio-* + Gr. *lithos* stone] a chalky concretion in an artery.

arteriolitis (ar-te″rĭ-o-li′tis) inflammation of the arterioles.

arteriopathy (ar″te-re-op′ah-the) [*arterio-* + Gr. *pathos* disease] any arterial disease.

arteriosclerosis (ar-te″re-o-sklĕ-ro′sis) [*arterio-* + Gr. *sklēros* hard] thickening and loss of elasticity of arterial walls due to fibrous and mineral deposits in the tunica media, or due to deposits of fatty substances in the inner lining of an artery. Called also *hardening of arteries*. **cerebral a.,** that in which the arteries of the brain are affected, due to mineral deposits in the media, or due to fatty deposits in the intima, resulting in loss of elasticity or occlusion of the artery. **coronary a.,** that associated was thickening of the coronary arteries, due to deposits of cholesterol on their walls and narrowing of the arterial lumen. Massive deposits may result in coronary occlusion with resulting myocardial infarction. See coronary OCCLUSION. See also arteriosclerotic heart DISEASE.

arteriosclerotic (ar-te″re-o-sklĕ-rot′ik) pertaining to or characterized by arteriosclerosis.

arteriospasm (ar-te′re-o-spasm″) spasm of an artery.

arteriostensis (ar-te″re-o-stĕ-no′sis) [*arterio-* + Gr. *stenos* narrow] the narrowing or stenosis of the lumen of an artery.

arteriostrepsis (ar-te″re-o-strep′sis) [*arterio-* + Gr. *streptos* twisted] the twisting of an artery for the arrest of hemorrhage.

arteriotomy (ar″te-re-ot′o-me) [*arterio-* + Gr. *tomē* cut] incision of an artery.

arteriovenous (ar-te″re-o-ve′nus) pertaining to or affecting an artery and a vein.

arteritides (ar″te-rit′ĭ-dēz) plural of *arteritis*.

arteritis (ar″tĕ-ri′tis), pl. *arterit′ides* [*artery* + *-itis*] inflammation of an artery. See also ENDARTERITIS and PERIARTERITIS. **cranial a., giant cell a.,** temporal a. **a. oblit′erans,** ENDARTERITIS obliterans. **senile a.,** temporal a. **temporal a.,** inflammation of the temporal and other cranial arteries of unknown etiology, usually occurring during the sixth and seventh decades of life. A pulseless, enlarged superficial temporal artery and a severe throbbing headache are the principal symptoms. Frequently, pain may be localized first in the teeth, temporomandibular joint, scalp, or occiput. Facial edema and neuralgia; visual disorders, including diplopia; hearing disorders; involvement of the third, fourth, and sixth cranial nerves; cerebral thrombosis; and mental disorders may occur. The diseased artery is narrowed by granulomatous lesions located at the junction between the media and intima. Histiocytes, lymphocytes, plasma cells, eosinophils, and giant cells are usually present in the tissue. The aorta, coronary artery, and other vessels may also be involved. Called also *cranial a.* and *senile a.*

artery (ar′ter-e) [L. *arteria*; Gr. *artēria*, from *aēr* air + *tērein* to keep, because the arteries were supposed by the ancients to contain air, or from Gr. *aeirein* to lift or attach] a tubular, elastic structure which transports blood under pressure away from the heart to the tissues. It has a strong wall, consisting typically of an outer fibroelastic coat (*tunica adventitia*), a middle coat made up of transverse elastic and muscle fibers (*tunica media*), and an inner coat made up of endothelial cells surrounded by longitudinal elastic fibers and connective tissue (*tunica intima*). Called also *arteria* [NA]. **accessory meningeal a.,** accessory meningeal branch of middle meningeal artery; see under BRANCH. **alveolar a's, anterior superior,** branches of the infraorbital artery that supply the incisor and canine regions of the upper jaw. They follow the canals in the anterior wall of the maxillary sinus to the alveolar process, where they anastomose with branches of the posterior superior alveolar artery; at the piriform aperture they anastomose with the nasal arteries. Their branches enter the apical foramina of roots to supply the dental pulp, giving off twigs to the periodontal ligament. The perforating arteries descend in the septa between the sockets, ending in the gingival papillae; the interradicular arteries descend between the roots, ending at their bifurcations. Called also *anterior dental a's* and *arteriae alveolares superiores anteriores* [NA]. **alveolar a., inferior,** usually a branch of the mandibular segment of the maxillary artery when that artery lies above the lateral pterygoid muscle but, when the maxillary artery runs a deep course, it is a branch of the posterior deep temporal artery by a common

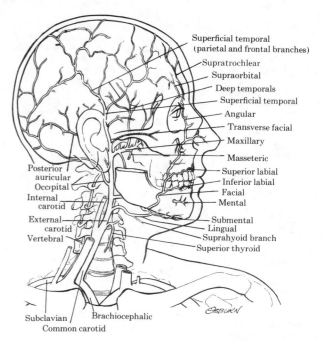

Arteries of the head and neck. (From Dorland's Illustrated Medical Dictionary. 26th ed. Philadelphia, W. B. Saunders Co., 1981.)

trunk which passes around the lower border of the lateral pterygoid muscle. From its origin, it turns downward toward the mandibular foramen and the mandibular canal. Once in the canal, it gives off branches into the marrow spaces of the bone and to the teeth and alveolar process, one group. of branches entering the root canals through the apical foramina and supplying the dental pulp (dental branches), and the other (alveolar or perforating branches) entering the interdental and interradicular septa. The alveolar branches ascend in marrow canals, while small branches, arising at right angles, enter the periodontal ligaments of adjacent teeth or adjacent roots. Called also *inferior dental a., mandibular a.,* and *arteria alveolaris inferior* [NA]. **alveolar a's, perforating,** branches of the alveolar arteries that are distributed in the septa between the sockets of adjacent teeth. Called also *alveolar perforating branches*. **alveolar a., posterior superior,** usually a branch of the pterygopalatine portion of the maxillary artery, frequently arising in conjunction with the infraorbital artery at the pterygopalatine fossa, but sometimes deriving from the buccal artery. It winds its way over the convexity of the maxillary tuber, running downward and forward and giving off several branches. Some branches enter the posterior superior alveolar canals to supply the molar and premolar teeth; the terminal or gingival branches continue on the outer surface of the bone and supply the mucous membrane on the outer surface of the alveolar process of the gingiva in the premolar and molar region; some supply maxillary sinuses; and some continue to the cheek. Called also *superior dental a.* and *arteria alveolaris superior posterior* [NA]. **angular a.,** the terminal segment of the facial artery, which ascends to the median angle of the orbit, supplies the lacrimal sac and the orbicularis oculi muscle, and anastomoses with the infraorbital artery and the dorsal nasal branch of the ophthalmic artery. Called also *arteria angularis* [NA]. **auditory a., internal,** labyrinthine a. **auricular a., deep,** a small branch of the mandibular segment of the maxillary artery; it passes through the parotid gland deep to the temporomandibular joint, and through the cartilaginous or bony wall of the external acoustic meatus to supply the skin of the auditory canal, tympanic membrane, and temporomandibular joint. Called also *arteria auricularis profunda* [NA]. **auricular a., posterior,** a small artery branching off the external carotid artery; it arises just opposite the styloid process and ascends under the parotid gland on the styloid process of the temporal bone to the groove between the cartilage of the ear and the mastoid process, where it divides. Its branches include the stylomastoid artery and the auricular and occipital branches. Called also *arteria auricularis posterior* [NA]. **basilar a.** one that arises from the junction of the right and left vertebral arteries at the base of the skull and supplies the brain and labyrinth. Called also *arteria basilaris* [NA]. **brachiocephalic a.,** brachiocephalic TRUNK. **buccal a., buccinator a.,** a small branch of the pterygoid portion of the maxillary artery; it may branch off just before the maxillary artery enters the slit between the two heads of the lateral pterygoid artery when the maxillary artery is located on the outer surface of the lateral pterygoid muscle, or pass laterally through the slit between the inferior and superior heads of the lateral pterygoid muscles when the maxillary artery runs a deep course. Thereafter, it turns downward and forward, crossing the temporal tendon obliquely and reaching the space between the masseter and buccinator muscles below the buccal fat pad. The terminal branches supply the buccinator muscle of the cheek and the mucous lining of the mouth, and anastomose with the facial artery and the infraorbital artery. Called also *arteria buccalis* [NA] and *arteria buccinatoria.* **caroticotympanic a.,** caroticotympanic branch of internal carotid artery; see under BRANCH. **carotid a., common,** either of the two principal arteries, one on each side of the neck, which supply the head and neck. The right begins from the brachiocephalic trunk, being confined to the neck; the left arises from the arch of the aorta, thus consisting of thoracic and cervical parts. Inferiorly, they are separated only by the trachea, but their courses diverge, being widely separated at the level of the superior border of the thyroid cartilage, where they subdivide into the external and internal carotid arteries. A sheath, derived from the deep cervical fascia, envelops each artery and also encloses the internal jugular vein and the vagus nerve. A small neurovascular structure in the bifurcation (carotid body) contains chemoreceptors which monitor the oxygen content of the blood and help to regulate respiration. A slight dilatation on the terminal portion of the common carotid artery and on the internal carotid artery just above the bifurcation (carotid sinus) contains pressoreceptors in its wall, which are stimulated by blood pressure changes. Called also *cephalic a.* and *arteria carotis communis* [NA]. **carotid a., external,** a major artery that begins at the bifurcation of the common carotid artery, just opposite the superior border of the thyroid cartilage and runs upward, curves anteriorly to the space behind the neck of the mandible, and continues up the neck, diminishing in size with each new branch. Its branches, which supply the head and neck, include the superior thyroid, ascending pharyngeal, lingual, facial, occipital, posterior auricular, superficial temporal, and maxillary arteries. Called also *arteria carotis externa* [NA]. **carotid a., internal,** a large artery that begins at the bifurcation of the common carotid artery, just opposite the thyroid cartilage, from where it ascends along the lateral wall of the pharynx, gradually diverging from the external carotid artery. At the base of the skull, it enters the carotid canal and, once inside the skull, is situated above the fibrocartilage of the foramen lacerum. After leaving the carotid canal, it enters the cavernous sinus and, in a tight S-shaped curve, passes toward the dura mater at the roof of the cavernous sinus to reach the intradural space and the brain. Sometimes, it is divided into the cervical and cranial parts, or into the petrous, cavernous, and cerebral parts; branches include the caroticotympanic, cavernous, hypophyseal, ganglionic, and anterior meningeal branches and the ophthalmic, anterior cerebral, middle cerebral, posterior communicating, and anterior choroidal arteries. Called also *arteria carotis interna* [NA]. **central a. of retina,** a. of retina, central. **cephalic a.,** carotid a., common. **cerebellar a., anterior inferior,** a branch of the basilar artery that supplies the anterior part of the inferior surface of the cerebellum. Called also *arteria cerebelli inferior anterior* [NA]. **cerebellar a., posterior inferior,** a branch of the vertebral artery that supplies the cerebellum, medulla oblongata, and choroid plexus of the fourth ventricle. Called also *arteria cerebelli inferior posterior* [NA]. **cerebellar a., superior,** a branch of the basilar artery that supplies the upper cerebellum, midbrain, pineal body, and choroid plexus of the third ventricle. Called also *arteria cerebelli superior* [NA]. **cerebral a., anterior,** an artery that arises from the internal carotid artery and divides into several branches which supply various structures of the brain. Called also *arteria cerebri anterior* [NA]. **cerebral a., middle,** the largest branch of the internal carotid artery, it supplies cerebral structures. Called also *arteria cerebri media* [NA]. **cerebral a., posterior,** an artery that arises from the basilar artery and divides into several branches which supply various structures of the brain. Called also *arteria cerebri posterior* [NA]. **cervical a., ascending,** a branch of the inferior thyroid artery that supplies the muscles of the neck and bodies of the vertebrae, and anastomoses with branches of the vertebral, ascending pharyngeal, and occipital arteries. Called also *arteria cervicalis ascendens* [NA]. **cervical a., deep,** a branch of the costocervical trunk supplying deep muscles of the neck. Called also

arteria cervicalis profunda [NA]. **cervical a., superficial,** a variant branch of the transverse cervical artery that supplies muscles of the scapula and neck. Called also *arteria cervicalis superficialis* [NA alternative], *ramus superficialis arteriae transversae colli* [NA], and *superficial branch of transverse cervical artery.* **cervical a., transverse,** a branch of the thyrocervical trunk of the subclavian artery that supplies a major part of the trapezius muscle. Called also *arteria transversa colli* [NA]. **ciliary a's,** a group of arteries arising from the ophthalmic artery, supplying the structures of the eye. Called also *arteriae ciliares.* **Cohnheim's a.,** terminal a. **conducting a's,** large arterial trunks, such as the aorta, subclavian artery, and common carotid artery, and the brachiocephalic and pulmonary trunks. **coronary a.,** either of the two large arteries (left and right coronary arteries) that arise from the aortic sinuses in the ascending aorta and supply all the heart muscles with blood. Obstruction by a thrombus (coronary thrombosis) or fatty deposits (coronary arteriosclerosis) may result in myocardial damage (myocardial infarction) and death, commonly referred to as *heart attack.* Called also *arteria coronaria (sinistra et dextra)* [NA] and *coronary vessel.* See also coronary OCCLUSION. **cricothyroid a.,** cricothyroid branch of superior thyroid artery; see under BRANCH. **dental a's, anterior,** alveolar a's, anterior superior. **dental a., inferior,** alveolar a., inferior. **dental a., superior,** alveolar a., posterior superior. **dorsal lingual a's,** dorsal lingual branches of lingual artery; see under BRANCH. **dorsal a. of nose,** a terminal branch of the ophthalmic artery; it emerges from the orbit and supplies a branch to the lacrimal sac and divides into two parts, one supplying the root of the nose and anastomosing with the angular artery, and the other supplying the outer surface of the dorsum of the nose and anastomosing with its fellow of the opposite side and with the lateral nasal branch of the facial artery. Called also *arteria dorsalis nasi* [NA]. **end a.,** one which undergoes progressive branching without development of channels connecting it to other arteries. **ethmoidal a., anterior,** a branch of the ophthalmic artery; it passes through the anterior ethmoidal canal to supply the anterior and middle ethmoidal air cells and the frontal sinus. Its nasal branches descend into the nasal cavity through the crista galli to supply the lateral wall and the septum and dorsum of the nose, while the meningeal branch supplies the dura mater. Called also *arteria ethmoidalis anterior* [NA]. **ethmoidal a., posterior,** a branch of the ophthalmic artery; it passes through the posterior ethmoidal canal to supply the posterior ethmoidal air cells, while its branches reach the nasal cavity through the cribriform plate to anastomose with the sphenopalatine artery. It also has a branch to the dura mater. Called also *arteria ethmoidalis posterior* [NA]. **facial a.,** a branch of the external carotid artery; it arises in the carotid triangle, and after passing under the ramus of the mandible, joins the facial vein on the posterior surface of the submandibular gland and winds around the inferior border of the mandible near the surface, crossing the cheek near the angle of the mouth, and passing alongside the nose until it ends near the eye. Its cervical branches include the ascending palatine artery, tonsillar branch, glandular branches, and submental artery. The facial branches include the inferior and superior labial arteries, lateral nasal branch, angular artery, and muscular branches. Called also *external maxillary a., arteria facialis* [NA], and *arteria maxillaris externa.* **facial a., transverse,** an artery arising from the superficial temporal artery at the parotid gland. It divides into numerous branches which supply the parotid gland and duct, masseter muscle, and integument and which anastomose with the facial, masseteric, buccal, and infraorbital arteries. Called also *transverse a. of face* and *arteria transversa faciei* [NA]. **frontal a.,** supratrochlear a. **hyoid a.,** suprahyoid branch of lingual artery; see under BRANCH. **infraorbital a.,** a branch of the pterygopalatine portion of the maxillary artery, arising close to the posterior superior alveolar artery, sometimes by a common trunk. It enters the orbit through the inferior orbital fissure and emerges through the infraorbital canal. Its branches supply the orbit, lacrimal gland, upper lip, muscles of the eye, nose, and teeth. The orbital branches arise in the infraorbital canal and supply the muscles of the eye. The anterior superior alveolar branches enter the anterior alveolar canal to supply the canine and incisor teeth and the maxillary sinus. Facial branches emerge at the infraorbital foramen and supply the lower eyelid and lacrimal sac, side of the nose, and upper lip. Anastomoses are made with the dorsal nasal and lacrimal branches of the ophthalmic artery, and with the labial and angular branches of the facial, transverse facial, and buccal arteries. Called also *arteria infraorbitalis* [NA]. **innominate a.,** brachiocephalic TRUNK. **interdental a's,** interradicular a's. **interradicular a's,** branches of the alveolar arteries distributed in the septa between the roots of adjacent teeth. Called also *interdental a's, interdental branches,* and *interradicular branches.* **labial a., inferior,** a facial branch of the facial artery; it arises near the angle of the mouth, passes along the edge of the lower lip, supplies the labial glands and the mucous membrane and the muscles of the lower lip, and anastomoses with its fellow of the opposite side and with the mental branch of the inferior alveolar artery. Called also *arteria labialis inferior* [NA]. **labial a., superior,** a facial branch of the facial artery, passing along the edge of the upper lip, supplying the upper lip and giving off the septal branch, which supplies the nasal septum, and the alar branch, which supplies the ala of the nose. Called also *arteria labialis superior* [NA]. **labyrinthine a.,** a branch of the basilar artery that supplies the internal ear. Called also *internal auditory a.* and *arteria labyrinthi* [NA]. **lacrimal a.,** a branch of the ophthalmic artery that supplies the lacrimal gland, giving off branches running to the eyelid (lateral palpebral arteries), the temporal region (zygomatic branches), cheek, supraorbital area, nose (dorsal nasal artery), retina, and muscles of the eye. Called also *arteria lacrimalis* [NA]. **laryngeal a., inferior,** a branch of the inferior thyroid artery; it supplies the muscles and mucous membrane of the larynx and trachea, anastomosing with its fellow of the opposite side and with the superior laryngeal branch of the superior thyroid artery. Called also *arteria laryngea inferior* [NA]. **laryngeal a., superior,** the largest of the branches of the superior thyroid artery, which accompanies the internal laryngeal branch of the superior laryngeal nerve. It pierces the thyrohyoid membrane to supply the larynx, and anastomoses with its fellow of the opposite side. In some instances, it branches off directly from the external carotid artery. Called also *arteria laryngea superior* [NA]. **lingual a.,** a branch of the external carotid artery, it arises opposite the tip of the greater cornu of the hyoid bone, passes at first obliquely toward the greater cornu, then loops under the hypoglossal nerve, passes deep to the digastricus and stylohyoideus muscles, toward the hyoglossus muscle, and finally ascends to the tongue and runs on its inferior surface to the tip as the *deep lingual artery*. It gives off four branches: suprahyoid branch and dorsal lingual, sublingual, and deep lingual arteries. Called also *arteria lingualis* [NA]. **lingual a., deep,** the terminal portion of the lingual artery, which runs a tortuous course under the surface of the tongue to its tip, and anastomoses with its fellow of the opposite side. Called also *ranine a.* and *arteria profunda linguae* [NA]. **lingual a's, dorsal,** dorsal lingual branches of lingual artery; see under BRANCH. **mandibular a.,** alveolar a., inferior. **masseteric a.,** a branch of the pterygoid portion of the maxillary artery; it arises from the lateral surface of the artery and, after passing through the mandibular notch and between the condylar process of the mandible and the posterior border of the tendon of the temporal muscle, reaches the masseter muscle. It anastomoses with the masseteric branches of the facial artery and with the transverse facial artery. A small branch also supplies the temporomandibular joint. Called also *arteria masseterica* [NA]. **maxillary a.,** the larger of the two terminal branches of the external carotid artery, which is distributed in the ear, meninges, nose, nasal sinuses, palate, both jaws, and muscles of mastication. It arises deep to the neck of the mandible and runs through the parotid gland and between the ramus of the mandible and the sphenomandibular ligament to the pterygopalatine fossa. The artery is sometimes divided for convenience into the mandibular, pterygoid, and pterygopalatine segments; its branches include the deep auricular, anterior tympanic, inferior alveolar, middle meningeal, and accessory meningeal arteries; deep temporal and pterygoid branches; messeteric, buccal, posterior superior alveolar, infraorbital, and descending palatine arteries; artery of the pterygoid canal; and sphenopalatine artery. Rami of some branches are mixed in. Called also *internal maxillary a., arteria maxillaris* [NA], and *arteria maxillaris interna.* **maxillary a., external,** facial a. **maxillary a., internal,** maxillary a. **medullary a.,** nutrient a. **meningeal a., anterior,** a small branch of the anterior ethmoidal artery that supplies the dura mater of the anterior cranial fossa. Called also *anterior meningeal branch of internal carotid artery* and *arteria meningea anterior* [NA]. **meningeal a., middle,** a branch of the mandibular part of the maxillary artery; it enters the cranium through the foramen spinosum of the sphenoid bone and divides in the groove on the great wing of the sphenoid bone into the anterior and posterior branches, both supplying the dura mater and cranial bones. Called also *arteria meningea media* [NA]. **meningeal a., posterior,** a branch of the ascending pharyngeal artery that supplies the dura mater and cranial bones. Called also *arteria meningea posterior* [NA]. **meningeal a., small,** accessory meningeal branch of middle meningeal artery; see under BRANCH. **mental a.,** the larger of the two terminal branches of the inferior alveolar artery, which emerges through the mental foramen, supplies the soft tissues of the chin, and anastomoses with branches of the inferior labial artery. Called also *arteria mentalis* [NA] and *mental branch of inferior alveolar artery.* **mylohyoid a.,** mylohyoid branch of inferior alveolar artery; see under BRANCH. **myomastoid a.,** occipital branch of posterior auricular artery; see under BRANCH. **nasal a's, posterior lateral,** branches of the sphenopalatine artery; they arise close to the roof of the nasal cavity and subdivide into smaller branches on the lateral wall of the nasal cavity to supply the middle and upper nasal conchae and the mucous membrane of the corresponding nasal passages, their smaller branches perforate the lateral nasal wall to reach the mucous membrane of the maxillary sinus. Called also *arteriae nasales posteriores laterales* and *posterior lateral nasal branches of sphenopalatine artery.* **nasopalatine a.,** sphenopalatine a. **a's of neck,** cervical a's (deep, superficial, and transverse). **Neubauer's a.,** thyroid a., lowest. **a. of nose, dorsal,** dorsal a. of nose. **nutrient a.,** any artery that supplies the bone marrow. Called also *medullary a.* **occipital a.,** a branch of the external carotid artery; it arises opposite the facial artery near the lower margin of the posterior belly of the digastric muscle, ending in the posterior part of the scalp. Its branches include the muscular branches, sternocleidomastoid artery, auricular, meningeal, descending, and terminal branches, and posterior auricular artery. Called also *arteria occipitalis* [NA]. **ophthalmic a.,** an artery that arises from the internal carotid artery at the point where it emerges from the cavernous sinus; it enters the orbital cavity through the optic canal to supply the eyeball, its muscles, and the lacrimal glands, some of its branches reaching other areas of the head. Its branches include the lacrimal, supraorbital, posterior and anterior ethmoid, medial palpebral, supratrochlear, dorsal nasal central artery of the retina, and muscular branches. Called also *arteria ophthalmica* [NA]. **palatine a., ascending,** an artery that arises from the facial artery near its origin, passes between the styloglossus and stylopharyngeus muscles to the side of the pharynx, and continues over the upper border of the constrictor pharyngis superior and pterygoideus medialis muscles to the base of the skull. It then divides near the levator veli palatini into two branches, one of which supplies the soft palate and the palatine gland and anastomoses with its fellow of the opposite side, and the other supplies the palatine tonsil and the auditory tube and anastomoses with the ascending pharyngeal arteries. Called also *arteria palatina ascendens* [NA]. **palatine a., descending,** one of the branches of the pterygopalatine portion of the maxillary artery; it arises in the pterygopalatine fossa, descends through the pterygopalatine canal, and gives rise to the greater palatine artery, which enters the oral cavity through the major palatine foramen, and to the minor palatine arteries, which arise inside the pterygopalatine canal and reach the oral cavity through the minor palatine foramina. Called also *arteria palatina descendens* [NA]. **palatine a., greater,** the major branch of the descending palatine artery; it emerges through the major palatine foramen and turns anteriorly in the submucosa of the hard palate in a groove between the horizontal palatine process of the maxilla and the inner plate of the alveolar process. Its branches supply the mucous membrane and the glands of the hard palate and the lingual surface of the upper alveolar process of the gingiva. The gingival branches anastomose with the gingival branches of the perforating arteries of the superior alveolar artery. The terminal branch (nasopalatine branch), reaches the incisive foramen and ascends through the incisive canal to the nasal cavity, where it anastomoses with the septal branches of the sphenopalatine artery. Called also *major palatine a.* and *arteria palatina major* [NA]. **palatine a's, lesser,** branches given off by the descending palatine artery inside the pterygopalatine canal; they enter the oral cavity through the minor palatine foramina to supply the soft palate and the palatine tonsils and anastomose with the branches of the ascending palatine artery. Called also *minor palatine a's* and *arteriae palatinae minores* [NA]. **palatine a., major,** palatine a., greater. **palatine a's, minor,** palatine a's, lesser. **palpebral a's, lateral,** branches of the ophthalmic artery that supply the eyelid and conjunctiva. Called also *arteriae palpebrales laterales* [NA]. **palpebral a's, medial,** branches of the ophthalmic artery that encircle the eyelids near their free margins. A branch passes to the nasolacrimal duct to supply the mucous membrane; others anastomose with the zygomatico-orbital branch of the temporal artery, lateral palpebral branches of the lacrimal artery, transverse facial artery, and angular artery. Called also *arteriae palpebrales mediales* [NA]. **perforating alveolar a's,** alveolar a's, perforating. **pharyngeal a., ascending,** the smallest artery branching off the external carotid artery; it usually arises from the posterior part of the external carotid artery near its origin, and ascends vertically in the neck between the internal carotid artery and the pharynx. It may also arise from the occipital artery. It supplies the pharynx, soft palate, ear, and meninges. Its branches include the pharyngeal, palatine, and prevertebral branches, inferior tympanic artery, and meningeal branches. Called also *arteria pharyngea ascendens* [NA]. **pterygoid a's,** pterygoid branches of maxillary artery; see under BRANCH. **a. of pterygoid canal,** a small terminal branch of the pterygopalatine segment of the maxillary artery; it arises in the pterygopalatine fossa and passes through the pterygoid canal to supply the upper part of the pharynx, auditory tube, and sphenoid sinus, one of its branches anastomosing with the tympanic arteries in the tympanic cavity. Called also *vidian a.* and *arteria canalis pterygoidei* [NA]. **pulmonary a's,** the right and left pulmonary arteries arising from the common pulmonary trunk, which convey unaerated blood from the heart to the lungs. Called also *arteriae pulmonales.* See also pulmonary CIRCULATION. **ranine a.,** lingual a., deep. **a. of retina, central,** a branch of the ophthalmic artery that supplies the retina. Called also *arteria centralis retinae* [NA]. **septal a's, posterior,** branches of the sphenopalatine artery that pass over the roof of the nasal cavity and take a diagonal course downward and forward along the nasal septum, supplying it with several branches. One of these branches (nasopalatine branch), passes through the incisive canal to anastomose with the nasopalatine branch of the greater palatine artery. Called also *arteriae nasales posteriores septi* and *posterior septal branches of sphenopalatine artery.* **sphenopalatine a.,** a terminal branch of the pterygopalatine portion of the maxillary artery that supplies the nasal cavity. It passes from the upper part of the pterygopalatine fossa through the sphenopalatine foramen into the nasal cavity, accompanying the pterygopalatine nerve, in which it divides into two branches: the posterior septal branch, which supplies the nasal septum, and the posterior lateral nasal branch, which supplies the middle and upper nasal conchae and the mucous membrane in the corresponding nasal passages, and assists in the supply to the frontal, ethmoidal, maxillary and sphenoidal sinuses. Called also *nasopalatine a.* and *arteria sphenopalatina* [NA]. **sternocleidomastoid a.,** one of the sternocleidomastoid branches of the occipital artery (see under BRANCH). **sternocleidomastoid a., superior,** sternocleidomastoid branch of superior thyroid artery; see under BRANCH. **sternomastoid a.,** one of the sternocleidomastoid branches of the occipital artery (see under BRANCH). **stylomastoid a.,** an artery branching off the posterior auricular artery that supplies the tympanic cavity, tympanic antrum, and mastoid cells. Called also *arteria stylomastoidea* [NA]. **subclavian a.,** either of two major arteries, one on each side, the right one deriving from the brachiocephalic trunk and the left from the arch of the aorta; each divides into several branches which supply the head, neck, upper limbs, thoracic wall, and spinal cord. Branches include the vertebral, thyrocervical, internal thoracic, costocervical, and dorsal scapular arteries. Called also *arteria subclavia* [NA]. **sublingual a.,** a branch of the lingual artery; it arises at the anterior margin of the hyoglossus muscle, supplies the sublingual gland, and gives off branches which, in turn, supply the mylohyoideus and neighboring muscles, oral mucosa, and gingivae. Called also *arteria sublingualis* [NA]. **submental a.,** the largest of the cervical branches of the facial artery; it arises at the submandibular gland and passes anteriorly superficial to the mylohyoideus muscle under the body of the mandible, and turns upward at the symphysis and divides over the border of the mandible into the superficial and deep branches. It supplies the muscles of the submental region, its superficial branch passing between the integument and levator labii inferioris muscle and anastomosing with the inferior labial artery, and its deep branch supplying the lip and anastomosing with the inferior labial and mental arteries. Called also *arteria submentalis* [NA]. **supraorbital a.,** a branch of the ophthalmic artery that supplies the muscles, integument, and pericranium of the forehead, and the rectus superior and levator palpebrae muscles. Called also *arteria supraorbitalis* [NA]. **suprascapular a.,** a branch of the inferior thyroid artery that supplies the clavicular, deltoid, and scapular regions. Called also *arteria suprascapularis* [NA]. **supratrochlear a.,** one of the terminal branches of the ophthalmic artery; it runs along with the supratrochlear nerve, and supplies the integument, muscles, and pericranium of the forehead, anastomosing with its fellow

of the opposite side and with the supraorbital artery. Called also *frontal a., arteria frontalis,* and *arteria supratrochlearis* [NA]. **temporal a's, deep,** branches of the pterygoid portion of the maxillary artery. The anterior branch (*anterior deep temporal a.*) and the posterior branch (*posterior deep temporal a.*) supply the temporalis muscle. Called also *arteriae temporales profundae* [NA]. **temporal a., middle,** an artery arising from the superficial temporal artery above the zygomatic arch; it gives off branches that supply the temporalis muscle and anastomose with the deep temporal branches of the maxillary artery. Called also *arteria temporalis media* [NA]. **temporal a., superficial,** the smaller of the two terminal arteries of the external carotid artery; it arises at the parotid gland, passes over to the zygomatic process of the temporal bone, continues upward for about 5 cm, and then divides. Its branches include the transverse facial, middle temporal, and zygomatico-orbital arteries, and anterior auricular, frontal, and parietal branches. Called also *arteria temporalis superficialis* [NA]. **terminal a.,** one that does not divide into branches, but is directly continuous with capillaries. Called also *Cohnheim's a.* **thyroid a., inferior,** a branch of the thyrocervical trunk that divides into the inferior laryngeal artery, tracheal, pharyngeal, and esophageal branches, ascending cervical artery, and muscle branches. Called also *arteria thyroidea inferior* [NA]. **thyroid a., inferior, of Cruveilhier,** cricothyroid branch of superior thyroid artery; see under BRANCH. **thyroid a., lowest,** an artery that varies considerably in size and has no branches, which arises either from the brachiocephalic trunk or from the aorta. It supplies the thyroid gland and appears to compensate for deficiency of other thyroid vessels. Called also *Neubauer's a.* and *arteria thyroidea ima* [NA]. **thyroid a., superior,** a branch of the external carotid artery beginning at the level of the greater cornu of the hyoid bone. Its branches, which supply the adjacent muscles and the ventral part and isthmus of the thyroid gland, include the infrahyoid and sternocleidomastoid branches, superior laryngeal artery, and cricothyroid branch. Called also *arteria thyroidea superior* [NA]. **tonsillar a.,** tonsillar branch of facial artery; see under BRANCH. **transverse a. of face,** facial a., transverse. **tympanic a., anterior,** a small branch of the mandibular segment of the maxillary artery that passes behind the temporomandibular joint and through the petrotympanic fissure, forming a vascular circle around the tympanic membrane, and anastomoses with the artery of the pterygoid canal and the caroticotympanic branch of the internal carotid artery. Called also *arteria tympanica anterior* [NA]. **tympanic a., inferior,** a branch of the ascending pharyngeal artery that supplies the tympanic cavity. Called also *arteria tympanica inferior* [NA]. **vertebral a.,** the first and largest branch of the subclavian artery; it supplies branches to the muscles of the neck, vertebrae, spinal cord, cerebellum, and interior of the cerebrum. Called also *arteria vertebralis* [NA]. **vidian a.,** a. of pterygoid canal. **zygomatico-orbital a.,** an artery arising from the superficial temporal artery that supplies the lateral side of the orbit, running between the layers of the temporal fascia to the lateral angle of the orbit. Called also *arteria zygomaticoorbitalis* [NA].

arthr- see ARTHRO-.

arthralgia (ar-thral'je-ah) [*arthr-* + *-algia*] pain in a joint or joints. **temporomandibular a.,** temporomandibular dysfunction SYNDROME.

arthrectomy (ar-threk'to-me) [*arthr-* + Gr. *ektomē* excision] excision of a joint.

arthrempyesis (ar″threm-pi-e′sis) [*arthr-* + Gr. *empyēsis* suppuration] suppuration in a joint.

arthresthesia (ar″thres-the′ze-ah) [*arthr-* + Gr. *aisthēsis* perception] joint sensibility; the perception of joint motions.

arthritic (ar-thrit'ik) 1. pertaining to or affected with arthritis. 2. a person affected with arthritis.

arthritis (ar-thri′tis), pl. *arthrit′ides* [Gr. *arthron* joint + *-itis*] any inflammatory condition of a joint or joints. **atrophic a.,** rheumatoid a. **blenorrhagic a.,** Reiter's DISEASE. **chronic infectious a.,** rheumatoid a. **chronic senescent a.,** osteoarthritis. **a. defor′mans,** rheumatoid a. **gonococcal a.,** infectious arthritis caused by *Neisseria gonorrhoeae;* a complication of gonorrhea. **hypertrophic a.,** osteoarthritis. **infectious a. of temporomandibular joint,** a relatively uncommon form of arthritis of the temporomandibular joint, due to infection with a variety of bacteria, including *Neisseria gonorrhoeae,* streptococci, staphylococci, and tubercle bacilli. Direct extension of infection into the joint from an adjacent cellulitis or osteomyelitis, which may follow dental, parotid gland, or facial or ear infection, is a common cause. It is usually associated with fever, edema, swelling, trismus, leukocytosis, and heat over the affected side. The acute form results in inflammation of the capsule and joint space; pus or exudate in the joint space may be associated with destruction of the disk and articular surface with formation of granulation tissue, eventually evolving to scar tissue. In the chronic type, there may be eburnation and excavation of articular surfaces. Ankylosis may occur in both the acute and chronic types. **a. nodo′sa, proliferative a.,** rheumatoid a. **rheumatic a.,** rheumatic FEVER. **rheumatoid a.,** a chronic constitutional disease considered to be one of the collagen diseases, which is characterized by inflammatory changes in the connective tissue and polyarthritis with special predilection for small joints. Lesions are usually symmetric and cause swelling and proliferative inflammation of the synovial membrane, often complicated by irreversible damage to the joint capsule and articular cartilage, accompanied by replacement of involved structures by granulation tissue and joint deformity. Its course is usually erratic with many remissions and exacerbations. The temporomandibular joint may be involved. There is usually bilateral swelling, tenderness, pain, and stiffening of the joint, sometimes associated with clicking and snapping of the joint and ankylosis. Malocclusion with anterior open-bite may be an early sign. Osteoporosis, limitation of condylar movement, flattening of the condyle, and condylar irregularities are the most common roentgenologic signs. Called also *atrophic a., chronic infectious a., a. deformans, a. nodosa, proliferative a., chronic articular rheumatism,* and *rheumatic gout.* **a. sic′ca,** arthritis without exudation into a joint cavity. **suppurative a.,** arthritis exhibiting suppurative inflammation within a joint space, usually due to bacterial infection, most commonly one caused by staphylococci or streptococci. Infrequently, it is caused by trauma, bleeding into a joint, or a metabolic disorder, such as gout, associated with leukocyte infiltration. Typhoid fever, influenza, measles, and scarlet fever are occasionally causative factors. **traumatic a. of temporomandibular joint,** inflammatory disease of the temporomandibular joint resulting from a blow to the mandible, particularly the chin, which may involve any part of the joint, especially the synovial tissues, ligaments, capsule, or meniscus. Pain and limitation of movement are the principal symptoms. Injury may cause involvement of the condyle and mandibular growth disorders in children. **tuberculous a.,** arthritis caused by infection with *Mycobacterium tuberculosis,* seen principally in children, and almost invariably associated with pulmonary tuberculosis. **urethral a.,** Reiter's DISEASE.

arthro-, arthr- [Gr. *arthron* joint] a combining form denoting relationship to a joint or joints.

Arthrobacter (ar″thro-bak′ter) [Gr. *arthron* a joint + *baktron* a rod] a genus of soil bacteria of the family Corynebacteriaceae, occurring as gram-positive, strictly aerobic, non–acid-fast, coccoid cells or rods.

arthrocele (ar″thro-sēl) [*arthro-* + Gr. *kēlē* tumor] a swelling of a joint.

arthrocentesis (ar″thro-sen-te′sis) surgical puncture or aspiration of a joint.

arthrochalasis (ar″thro-kal′ah-sis) [*arthro-* + Gr. *chalasis* relaxation] abnormal relaxation or flaccidity of a joint.

arthrochondritis (ar″thro-kon-dri′tis) inflammation of the cartilage of a joint.

arthrodentosteodysplasia (ar″thro-dent″os″te-o-dis-pla′se-ah) dysplasia involving the articular, dental, and osseous tissue. Abbreviated *ADOD.* See Hajdu-Cheney SYNDROME.

arthrodial (ar-thro′de-al) [Gr. *arthrodia* a particular type of articulation] pertaining to a gliding joint.

arthrodynia (ar″thro-din′e-ah) [*arthro-* + Gr. *odynē* pain] pain in a joint or joints.

arthroempyesis (ar″thro-em″pi-e′sis) [*arthro-* + Gr. *empyēsis* suppuration] suppuration from a joint.

arthroereisis (ar″thro-ĕ-ri′sis) [*arthro-* + Gr. *ereisis* a raising up] operative limiting of the motion in a joint that is abnormally mobile.

arthrogryposis (ar″thro-grī-po′sis) [*arthro-* + Gr. *grypōsis* a crooking] persistent flexure or contracture of the joints. **a. mul′tiplex congen′ita,** Guérin-Stern SYNDROME.

arthrometry (ar-throm′ĕ-tre) the measurement of the range of mobility of joints.

arthroneuralgia (ar″thro-nu-ral′je-ah) [*arthro-* + *neuralgia*] pain arising in or around a joint.

arthro-ophthalmopathy (ar″thro-of″thal-mop′ah-the) 1. any dis-

ease involving both the joints and the eyes. 2. Stickler's SYNDROME. **hereditary a.,** Stickler's SYNDROME.

arthropathology (ar″thro-pah-thol′o-je) [*arthro-* + *pathology*] the study of the structural and functional changes produced in the joints by disease.

arthropathy (ar-throp′ah-the) [*arthro-* + Gr. *pathos* disease] any disease of a joint or joints.

arthrophyma (ar″thro-fi′mah) [*arthro-* + Gr. *phyma* swelling] the swelling of a joint.

arthroplasty (ar″thro-plas′te) [*arthro-* + Gr. *plassein* to form] plastic surgery of a joint or of joints; the formation of movable joints. **gap a.,** surgical correction of dental ankylosis by creating a space by ostectomy between the ankylosed part and the portion to be made movable. **interposition a.,** surgical correction of ankylosis of the temporomandibular joint by separating the immobile fragment from the mobilized fragment and interposing a substance, such as fascia, cartilage, metal, or plastic, between them. **intracapsular temporomandibular joint a.,** operative recontouring of the articular surface of the mandibular condyle without the removal of the articular disk.

arthropneumoroentgenography (ar″thro-nu″mo-rent-gen-og′rah-fe) [*arthro-* + Gr. *pneuma* air + *roentgenography*] roentgenography of a joint after injection into it of air, oxygen, or carbon dioxide.

arthropyosis (ar″thro-pi-o′sis) [*arthro-* + Gr. *pyōsis* suppuration] the formation of pus in a joint cavity.

arthrosclerosis (ar″thro-sklĕ-ro′sis) [*arthro-* + Gr. *sklērōsis* hardness] stiffening or hardening of the joints.

arthrosis (ar-thro′sis) 1. [Gr. *arthrōsis* a jointing] a joint or articulation. 2. [*arthro-* + *-osis*] any disease of a joint or joints.

arthrospore (ar″thro-spōr) [*arthro-* + Gr. *sporos* seed] an asexual spore formed by the walling off of a preexisting hypha or branch to give a chain of spores.

arthrosteitis (ar″thros-te-i′tis) [*arthro-* + Gr. *osteon* bone + *-itis*] inflammation of the bony structures of a joint.

arthrostomy (ar-thros′to-me) [*arthro-* + Gr. *stomoun* to provide with a mouth or opening] surgical creation of an opening into a joint, as for the purpose of drainage.

arthrosynovitis (ar″thro-sin″o-vi′tis) [*arthro-* + *synovitis*] inflammation of the synovial membrane of a joint.

arthrotome (ar′thro-tōm) [*arthro-* + Gr. *tomē* cut] a knife for incising a joint.

arthrotomy (ar-throt′o-me) [*arthro-* + Gr. *tomē* cut] surgical incision of a joint.

arthrotropic (ar″thro-trop′ik) [*arthro-* + Gr. *tropos* a turning] having an affinity for or tending to settle in the joints.

arthroxesis (ar-throk′sĕ-sis) [*arthro-* + Gr. *xēsis* scraping] the scraping of an articular surface.

Arthur, Robert [1819–1880] a Baltimore dentist who was the first to make known the cohesive property of gold foil, as produced by annealing by the use of serrated, pointed instruments. See ARTHURIZING (Arthur's method).

arthurizing (ar′ther-īz-ing) [named after Robert *Arthur*] a method for the prevention of dental caries by separating the teeth by filing the interproximal surfaces, thereby allowing self-cleansing. No longer used. Called also *Arthur's method.*

Arthus reaction (phenomenon) [Nicolas Maurice *Arthus,* French physiologist, 1862–1945] see under REACTION.

article (ar′tĭ-k'l) [L. *articulus* a little joint] one of the portions or segments forming a jointed series.

articular (ar-tik′u-lar) [L. *articularis*] of or pertaining to a joint.

articulare (ar-tik″u-la′re) a craniometric landmark used in roentgenographic cephalometry, being the point of intersection of the posterior margin of the ascending ramus of the mandible and the shadow of the cranial base, as seen on the lateral x-ray of the head (Björk). Abbreviated *Ar.* Called also *point Ar.*

articulate (ar-tik′u-lāt) [L. *articulatus* jointed] 1. divided into or united by joints. 2. enunciated in words and sentences. 3. to divide into or to unite so as to form a joint. 4. to adjust or place the teeth in their proper relation to each other in making an artificial denture.

articulated (ar-tik′u-lāt″ed) connected by a movable joint; consisting of separate segments so joined as to be movable on each other.

articulatio (ar-tik″u-la′she-o), pl. *articulatio′nes* [L.] the union or junction between two or more separate structures, such as bones; an articulation. Called also *joint, junctura ossium,* and *osseous junction.* **a. bicondyla′ris,** a condylar joint with a meniscus between the articular surfaces, as in the temporomandibular joint. **a. compos′ita** [NA], composite JOINT. **a. condyla′ris** [NA], condylar JOINT. **a. cricoarytenoi′dea** [NA], cricoarytenoid ARTICULATION. **a. cricothyroi′dea** [NA], cricothyroid ARTICULATION. **a. mandibula′ris,** temporomandib′-

ular JOINT. **a. pla′na,** plane JOINT. **a. sella′ris** [NA], saddle JOINT. **a. sim′plex** [NA], simple JOINT. **a. spheroi′dea** [NA], spheroidal JOINT. **a. temporomandibula′ris** [NA], temporomandibular JOINT. **a. trochoi′dea** [NA], rotary JOINT.

articulation (ar-tik″u-la′shun) [L. *articulatio*] 1. the place of union or junction between two or more bones of the skeleton. Called also *articulatio, joint,* and *junctura.* 2. speech a. 3. (*a*) the contact relationship of the occlusal surfaces of the teeth while in action; (*b*) the arrangement of artificial teeth so as to accommodate the various positions of the mouth and to serve the purpose of the natural teeth which they replace. **anatomic a.,** a rigid or movable junction of bony parts. **articulator a.,** the use of a mechanical device that simulates the movements of the temporomandibular joint, permitting the orientation of casts in a manner duplicating or simulating various positions or movements of the mandible. **balanced a.,** the simultaneous contact between the upper and lower teeth as they glide over each other when the mandible is moved from centric relation to the various eccentric relations and back to centric relation again. **ball-and-socket a.,** spheroidal JOINT. **composite a., compound a.,** composite JOINT. **craniomandibular a.,** temporomandibular JOINT. **cricoarytenoid a.,** a synovial joint between the upper border of the cricoid cartilage and the base of the arytenoid cartilage. Called also *articulatio cricoarytenoidea* [NA]. **cricothyroid a.,** one between the lateral aspect of the cricoid cartilage and the inferior horn of the thyroid cartilage. Called also *articulatio cricothyroidea* [NA]. **dental a.,** the contact relationship of the maxillary and mandibular teeth when moving into and away from centric occlusion. **gliding a.,** plane JOINT. **laws of a.,** see under LAW. **mandibular a., maxillary a.,** temporomandibular JOINT. **pivot a.,** rotary JOINT. **saddle a.,** saddle JOINT. **simple a.,** simple JOINT. **speech a.,** enunciation of distinct speech. **spheroidal a.,** spheroidal JOINT. **temporomandibular a.,** 1. temporomandibular JOINT. 2. the articulation of the condyloid process of the mandible and the interarticular disk with the mandibular fossa of the temporal bone. **temporomaxillary a.,** temporomandibular JOINT. **trochoidal a.,** rotary JOINT.

articulationes (ar-tik″u-la″she-o′nēz) [L.] plural of *articulatio.*

articulator (ar-tik′u-la″tor) 1. a device for effecting a jointlike union. 2. dental a. **Acme a.,** trademark for a lightweight, easy to use adjustable dental articulator. The axles representing the condyles are mounted on the lower member and the guiding mechanism is located on the upper member. **adjustable a.,** 1. a dental articulator which may be adjusted to permit movement of the casts into recorded eccentric relationships. 2. a dental articulator capable of adjustment to more than one eccentric position. **arcon a.,** a dental articulator in which the condylar elements are attached to the lower member, thereby simulating the natural attachment. Called also *Bergström′s a.* **Balkwell a.,** a dental articulator providing for the downward movement and lateral shift of the condyles. **Bergström′s a.,** arcon a. **Bonwill a.,** a dental articulator based on the Bonwill triangle hypothesis (see under TRIANGLE), using an average distance of 4 inches between each condyle and the incisor point. **Christensen a.,** a dental articulator for determining positional relations of condylar paths. **Denar a.,** trademark for a "fully" adjustable in-

strument capable of simulating many mandibular movements or jaw positions. It can be programmed by a chew-in technique, checkbite, or through the use of a pantograph. **dental a.,** a mechanical device designed to represent the temporomandibular joint and the jaws and to simulate as accurately as possible their movements and relationships; used for diagnostic and restorative procedures, for matching upper and lower dentures with the casts, and for mounting artificial teeth in such a manner that optimum relations, occlusion, and articulation are obtained in restorations. Called also *occluding frame.* See illustration. **Dentatus a.,** trademark for a semiadjustable dental articulator, having a condylar guiding mechanism attached to it. Some models are so constructed that they will accept a hinge axis transfer mounting; others are used with a face-bow that relates the maxillary cast to the articulator from an arbitrarily selected axis. **Evans′ a.,** a dental articulator which first incorporated the capability for simulating protrusive and lateral movements. **Gariot′s a.,** a simple dental articulator, employing a hinge principle only, which was invented by Gariot in 1805; presumed to be the first articulator. **Granger a.,** trademark for an adjustable dental articulator; it has a variable intercondylar distance and a side shift setting which is made harmonious by grinding special guides to conform with it. Accessories include an extraoral tracing apparatus, interchangeable condylar paths with varying radii, hinge axis locator, and face-bow. Trademarks: Gnatholator, Gnathosimulator, Simulator. **Gysi′s a.,** a dental articulator designed to duplicate most movements of the mandible, including the paths of the condyle and incisors; used as a guide in the construction of full dentures. **Hanau a.,** trademark for a series of "fully" and semiadjustable articulators. Some models are so constructed that they will accept a hinge axis transfer mounting; others are used with a face-bow that relates the maxillary cast to the articulator from an arbitrarily selected axis. **Hanau 130–21 a.,** trademark for a modified Hanau articulator, having the guiding elements on the upper member of the instrument and the condylar spheres on the lower member. **hinge a.,** a dental articulator with only a hinge joint, permitting no lateral or gliding motion. Called also *plain-line a.* **Ney a.,** trademark for an adjustable dental articulator which allows complete adjustment of intercondylar distances, being equipped with interchangeable condyle paths with varying radii. It is designed to be set through the use of impression paste, intraoral registration obtained in conjunction with mandibular guide bars related to the patient's jaws with prefabricated plastic matrices. **nonarcon a.,** a dental articulator in which the condyles are attached to the upper member, as opposed to an arcon articulator in which they are attached to the lower member. **plain-line a.,** hinge a. **semiadjustable a.,** a dental articulator that may be adjusted so that at least one movement conforms with a mandibular movement of a patient. **Stuart a.,** an adjustable dental articulator that permits full adaptation of the intercondylar distance and accommodation of special guides to the lateral shift of the mandible. **Walker a.,** an adjustable dental articulator for individual mandibular movements, taking registration of the inclination of individual condylar paths. **Whip-Mix a.,** trademark for a semiadjustable dental articulator that allows special guides to be brought to a true relative position independently of the adjustment for the condylar inclination. The casts are related to the instrument by a face-bow which is fixed onto the skull by plastic plugs inserted into each external auditory meatus.

artifact (ar′ti-fakt) [L. *ars* art + *factum* made] 1. any man-made object. 2. in histology or microscopy, any structure or feature that has been introduced by processing a tissue. 3. any substance or structure not naturally present in living tissue, but of which an authentic image appears in a radiograph. 4. a blemish or an unintended radiographic image which is not an authentic appearance, such as one resulting from the faulty manufacture, manipulation, exposure, or processing of an x-ray film.

artificial (ar″ti-fish′al) [L. *ars* art + *facere* to make] made by art rather than by nature, not natural or pathological.

artifistulation (ar″ti-fist″u-la′shun) a surgical procedure whereby the alveolar plate of bone is perforated to relieve pressure and pain caused by accumulation of exudate.

Artriona trademark for *cortisone acetate* (see under CORTISONE).

Artz see ADENOLYMPHOMA (Albrecht-Artz-Warthin tumor).

Arusal trademark for *carisoprodol.*

aryepiglottic (ar″e-ep″i-glot′ik) arytenoepiglottic.

aryepiglotticus (ar″e-ep″i-glot′i-kus) aryepiglottic MUSCLE.

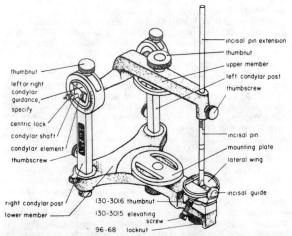

Hanau H2-PR articulator. (Modified from M. M. Ash, Jr. and S. R. Ramfjord: An Introduction to Functional Occlusion. Philadelphia, W. B. Saunders Co., 1981.)

thumbnut
left or right condylar guidance, specify
centric lock
condylar shaft
condylar element
thumbscrew
right condylar post
lower member

incisal pin extension
thumbnut
upper member
left condylar post
thumbscrew

incisal pin
mounting plate
lateral wing
incisal guide

130-3016 thumbnut
130-3015 elevating screw
96-68 locknut

aryl- chemical prefix indicating a radical belonging to the aromatic series.

arylsulfatase [E.C.3.1.6.1] (ar″il-sul′fah-tās) a sulfuric ester hydrolase that catalyzes the hydrolysis of a phenol sulfate to the phenol and sulfate. Called also *sulfatase*.

arytenoepiglottic (ar-it″ĕ-no-ep″ĭ-glot′ik) [Gr. *arytaina* ladle + *epiglottis*] pertaining to the arytenoid cartilage and to the epiglottis. Called also *aryepiglottic*.

arytenoid (ar″ĕ-te′noid) [Gr. *arytaina* ladle + *eidos* form] shaped like a jug or pitcher, as the arytenoid cartilage.

arytenoidectomy (ar″ĕ-te″noid-ek′to-me) [*arytenoid* + Gr. *ektomē* excision] excision of the arytenoid cartilage.

arytenoideus (ar″ĕ-te-noi′de-us) [L.] arytenoid muscle (oblique and transverse); see under MUSCLE. **a. obli′quus,** oblique arytenoid MUSCLE. **a. transver′sus,** transverse arytenoid MUSCLE.

arytenoiditis (ar″ĕ-te″noi-di′tis) inflammation of the arytenoid cartilage or muscle.

arytenoidopexy (ar″ĕ-tĕ-noi′do-pek″se) [*arytenoid* + Gr. *pēxis* fixation] surgical fixation of arytenoid cartilage or muscle. Called also *Kelly's operation* and *King's operation*.

Arzt, L. [Vienna pathologist] see ADENOLYMPHOMA (Albrecht-Arzt-Warthin tumor).

As arsenic.

A × s a symbol for *ampere per second;* see COULOMB.

ASAAD American Society for the Advancement of Anesthesia in Dentistry (see under SOCIETY).

asbestos (as-bes′tōs) [Gr. "unquenchable"] impure magnesium and calcium silicate minerals, occurring as fine, slender, flaxy fibers that are incombustible and resist most solvents. Used chiefly as a thermal insulator and as a plastic and rubber reinforcing agent. In dentistry, used as a binding medium in zinc oxide–eugenol packs. Exposure to asbestos dust can result in mesothelioma, squamous cell carcinoma, and adenocarcinoma of the lung after a long latent period. Called also *native calcium–magnesium silicate.*

Asboe-Hansen's disease [G. *Asboe-Hansen*] see under DISEASE.

Ascal trademark for *calcium acetylsalicylate* (see under CALCIUM).

ascending (ah-send′ing) [L. *ascensus*] rising upward; having an upward course.

Asch's splint [Morris Joseph *Asch,* American laryngologist, 1833–1902] see under SPLINT.

Asche forceps see under FORCEPS.

Ascher's syndrome [Karl W. *Ascher,* German ophthalmologist] see under SYNDROME.

Aschoff body, cell [Karl Albert Ludwig *Aschoff,* German pathologist, 1866–1942] see under BODY and CELL.

ascites (ah-si′tēz) [L.; Gr. *askitēs,* from *askos* bag] accumulation of excessive amounts of transudate within the peritoneal cavity. Called also *peritoneal cavity edema.*

Asclepiad [Gr. *Asklēpiadēs*] a member of an organized guild of physicians, followers of Æsculapius, who were the priests in the early Greek temples of healing (see ASCLEPION). The name is also applied to any devoted, high-minded physician.

Asclepiades [born in Bithynia (Asia Minor) in 124 B.C.] a celebrated physician who studied in Alexandria, and later popularized Greek medicine in Rome. Opposed to Hippocratic humoralism, he taught that disease resulted from a mechanical disturbance of the passage of atoms through the pores of the body. His followers, the Methodists, further simplified this concept.

asclepion, pl. *ascle′pia* [Gr. *Asklēpieion* temple of Asklepios (Æsculapius)] one of the early Greek temples of healing, the most celebrated of which were at Cos, Epidaurus, Cnidus, and Pergamos. Greek temple medicine flourished during the time of Hippocrates (late 5th century B.C.), but was quite independent of his school. See also ÆSCULAPIUS and ASCLEPIAD.

Ascodeen-30 trademark for an analgesic preparation containing 325 mg aspirin and 30 mg codeine phosphate.

ascomycete (as-ko′mi-sēt) any individual fungus of the Ascomycetes.

Ascomycetes (as″ko-mi-se′tēz) [Gr. *askos* bag + *mykēs* fungus] a class of true fungi (Eumycetes), the individual members of which form ascospores. The class consists of ascospore-forming yeasts, mildews, and molds of cheese, jelly, and fruits. Called also *sac fungus.*

ascomycetous (as″ko-mi-se′tus) of or pertaining to the Ascomycetes.

ascomycosis (as″ko-mi-ko′sis) European BLASTOMYCOSIS.

ascorbate (as-kor′bāt) a salt of ascorbic acid. **calcium a.,** CALCIUM ascorbate.

ascorbemia (as″kor-be′me-ah) the presence of ascorbic acid in the blood.

ascorburia (as″kor-bu′re-ah) the presence of ascorbic acid in the urine.

ascospore (as′ko-spōr) [Gr. *askos* bag + *sporos* seed] a sexual spore formed within a special sac (ascus), as in ascomycetous fungi.

ascoxal (as-kok′sal) a plaque and calculus inhibitor mixture containing ascorbic acid, sodium percarbonate, and copper sulfate.

Ascriptin trademark for an analgesic preparation, one tablet of which contains 325 mg aspirin, 150 mg magnesium-aluminum hydroxide, and various amounts of excipients and flavoring agents.

ASCP American Society of Clinical Pathologists.

ASDC American Society of Dentistry for Children (see under SOCIETY).

-ase a word ending denoting an enzyme.

asecretory (ah-se′kre-to″re) without secretion.

asepsis (a-sep′sis) [*a* neg. + Gr. *sēpesthai* to decay] 1. freedom from pathogenic microorganisms. 2. the prevention of contact with microorganisms. **integral a.,** an aseptic technique in which not only the instruments, drapes, and gloved hands of the surgical team are sterile, but also the entire operating room and the air are free of viable microorganisms.

Asepta-Klot B trademark for a surgical dressing, 100 gm of which contains 7.5 gm clove oil, 3.4 gm polyvinylpyrrolidone-iodine complex, and the necessary amounts of glycerol and alcohol in a petrolatum base.

Asepta-Klot S trademark for a surgical dressing, 100 gm of which contains 3.4 gm chlorobutanol, 7.0 gm clove oil, 3.2 gm polyvinylpyrrolidone-iodine, and various amounts of glycerol and alcohol in a petrolatum base.

aseptic (a-sep′tik) [*a* neg. + Gr. *sēpsis* decay] free from infection or septic material; sterile.

ASG American Society for Genetics.

ASH American Society for Hematology.

ash (ash) the incombustible residue remaining after a substance has been incinerated. **pearl a.,** POTASSIUM carbonate. **tin a.,** stannic OXIDE.

ASHA 1. American School Health Association. 2. American Speech and Hearing Association.

Asherson's syndrome [N. *Asherson,* English physician] see under SYNDROME.

ASHP American Society of Hospital Pharmacists.

asialia (ah″si-a′le-ah) [*a* neg. + Gr. *scialon* spittle] absence or deficiency of the secretion of the saliva; aptyalism; xerostomia.

ASII American Science Information Institute.

-asis a word termination denoting state or condition. See also -SIS.

Asn asparagine.

ASOS American Society of Oral Surgeons.

Asp aspartic ACID.

asparaginase [E.C.3.5.1.1] (as-par′ah-jin-ās″) a hydrolase that acts on carbon-nitrogen bonds other than peptide bonds, which is found in bacterial, fungal, and animal cells. In the purified form, it occurs as a white, crystalline powder that is soluble in water but not in organic solvents. Its function consists of hydrolysis of L-asparagine to L-asparate. When introduced into a tissue, it interferes with the synthesis of some proteins, such as plasma albumin, insulin, and clotting factors. It also inhibits antibody synthesis. Used in the treatment of acute lymphocytic leukemia, in which it affects cells which are incapable of converting aspartic acid to asparagine. Adverse reactions may include hepatic, pancreatic, and central nervous system disorders, elevation of blood ammonia, blood coagulation disorders, decreased insulin production, and graft rejection. Symptoms include fever, chills, nausea, depression, pancreatitis, and anaphylaxis. Called also *a. II* and *L-asparagine amidohydrolase.* Trademarks: Crasnitin, Elspar, Leunase. **a. II,** asparaginase.

asparagine (as-par′ah-jēn, as-par′ah-jin) [Gr. *asparagos* asparagus] an acidic nonessential amino acid, 2-amino-4-succinamic acid. It is the monoamide of aspartic acid, occurring in asparagus and other plants. Used as a diuretic and in bacterial culture media. Abbreviated *Asn.* Called also *alpha-aminosuccinamic acid* and *aspartamic acid.*

aspartame (ah-spar′tam) an artificial sweetener and flavor enhancer, 3-amino-N-(α-carboxyphenethyl)succinamic acid N-methyl ester, supplying about 1/180 of the calories in an equivalent amount of sucrose. It is hydrolyzed in the digestive tract to L-aspartic acid and L-phenylalanine, thus increasing blood phenylalanine and being contraindicated in patients with phenylketonuria. On cooking, it undergoes breakdown, losing sweetness in the process. Proposed for use as a sugar substitute in sweetened cereals, chewing gum, and some instant foods. Trademarks: Equa, Tri-Sweet.

aspartate (ah-spahr′tāt) a salt of aspartic acid, or aspartic acid in dissociated form. **a. aminotransferase,** aspartate AMINOTRANS-FERASE.

ASPD American Society of Psychosomatic Dentistry and Medicine (see under SOCIETY).

aspect (as′pekt) [L. *aspectus,* from *aspicere* to look toward] 1. that part of a surface facing in any designated direction. 2. the look or appearance. **dorsal a.,** the surface of a body as viewed from the back (human anatomy) or from above (veterinary anatomy). **tooth a's,** tooth surfaces; see under SURFACE. **ventral a.,** the surface of a body as viewed from the front (human anatomy) or from below (veterinary anatomy).

aspergillosis (as″per-jil-o′sis) a fungal disease caused by species of *Aspergillus,* and marked by inflammatory granulomatous lesions of the skin, ear, orbit, nasal sinuses, lungs, and sometimes of the bones and meninges. It is sometimes associated with leukemia, being a contributory factor in the death of leukemic patients.

Aspergillus (as″per-jil′us) [L. *aspergere* to scatter] a genus of dermatomycetous fungi (Fungi Imperfecti) that cause aspergillosis.

asphyxia (as-fik′se-ah) [*a* neg. + Gr. *sphyxis* pulse] suffocation; a condition due to lack of oxygen in respired air, resulting in impending or actual cessation of apparent life.

asphyxiant (as-fik′se-ant) a substance capable of producing asphyxia.

aspiration (as″pĭ-ra′shun) [L. *ad* to + *spirare* to breathe] 1. the act of inhaling; inspiration. 2. the removal of fluids or gases from a cavity by the application of suction.

aspirator (as″pĭ-ra′tor) an instrument, such as a syringe or tube connected to a suction-creating device, used for removal of fluids or gases contained within a cavity. See also SYRINGE. **dental a.,** one operating by means of a suction pump, and used for removal of water, blood, saliva, and debris from the oral cavity during dental operations. **Frazier a.,** one equipped with a stylet for removing entrapped tissue and debris from parts of the oral cavity.

aspirin (as′pĭ-rin) [*a* acetyl + *spiracic* acid, an obsolete name for salicylic acid] the prototype of salicylate analgesics and antipyretics, 2-(acetyloxy)benzoic acid, occurring as an odorless, acidic, crystalline, white powder or as tubular or needle-like crystals that are soluble in water, ethanol, chloroform, and ether. It is used chiefly to allay pain. Also used in the therapy of gout, rheumatic fever, and rheumatoid arthritis. Aspirin inhibits the synthesis of prostaglandins in inflamed tissues, thus preventing sensitization of pain receptors to stimuli, and is believed to exert analgesic and antipyretic effects by acting on the hypothalamus. It also tends to displace certain drugs, such as penicillins and anticoagulants, from binding sites in the blood and competes with certain substances, such as para-aminobenzoic acid and salicylamide for metabolic pathways. Toxic effects of aspirin are similar to those of other salicylates. When used locally by placing against a tooth, it may cause burns (see aspirin BURN). Aspirin is also suspected of having a pathogenic role in peptic ulcer. Called also *acetylsalicylic acid* and *salicylic acid acetate.* Trademarks: Acetylin, Acylpyrin, Aspro. Aspirin is also a constituent of many proprietary preparations, including Ascodeen-30, Bufferin, Codempiral, Empiral, Empirin, Phenaphen, and Sal-Fayne. **aluminum a.,** an aspirin preparation, hydroxybis(salicylic acid acetate)aluminum, occurring as a white powder or granules that are soluble in aqueous solutions of alkali hydroxides and carbonates, but not in water and organic solvents. Its therapeutic and toxicological properties are similar to those of aspirin and other analgesic salicylates. Called also *aluminum acetylsalicylate.* Trademark: Aspirin Dulcet. **calcium a.,** CALCIUM acetylsalicylate. **A. Dulcet,** trademark for *aluminum a.* **soluble a.,** CALCIUM acetylsalicylate.

Aspirol trademark for aromatic ammonia, each crushable tablet containing about 223 mg ammonium hydroxide in 36 percent alcohol with aromatic and coloring substances.

Aspro trademark for *aspirin.*

assault (ah-sawlt′) 1. a violent physical or verbal attack. 2. an unlawful attempt or threat to do physical violence to another. **technical a.,** a wrongful act, intentional or inadvertent, involving contact between people which is not consented to, nor permitted, by social usage (even without injury). Dental treatment performed without the patient's consent, even if it is beneficial, may be considered to be technical assault.

assay (ah-sa′) analysis; especially determining the amount or purity of a chemical substance in alloys, mixtures, living tissues, or any other system, by means of physical or biological methods. **biological a.,** bioassay.

Assézat's triangle [Jules *Assézat,* French anthropologist, 1832–1876] facial TRIANGLE.

assignment (ah-sīn′ment) in law, the transference of a claim, title, interest, property, or right; also the document by which this is accomplished. **benefit a., a. of benefits,** in health insurance, a procedure whereby the subscriber (insured) authorizes the insurance company (carrier) to make payment directly to the dentist or physician for allowable benefits.

assimilation (ah-sim″ĭ-la′shun) [L. *assimilatio,* from *ad* to + *similare* to make like] 1. the act or process of absorbing and incorporating. 2. to make similar or cause to resemble. 3. the transformation of nourishment into living tissue; anabolism.

assistant (ah-sis′tant) one who assists or aids, or provides support in performing certain tasks and duties; an aide. **coordinating a.,** dental a., coordinating. **dental a.,** a person who assists with the care of dental patients, including dental auxiliaries and ancillary personnel. The scope of the assistant's tasks and responsibilities vary, being determined by the needs of the employers, educational preparations of the assistant, and state regulations on dental practice. Usual duties consist of serving as a receptionist, secretary, office manager, chairside assistant, laboratory assistant, x-ray technician, or dental educator, working under the supervision of a dentist. Educational requirements vary, but many states require at least one academic year in an accredited dental assisting program and clinical training requirements. See also American Dental Assistants Association, under ASSOCIATION, ancillary PERSONNEL, dental assisting PROGRAM, and dental AUXILIARY. **dental a., administrative,** a dental assistant who aids the dentist by performing business office functions and managing the nonprofessional aspects of dental practice. **dental a., certified,** a dental assistant who has satisfactorily completed the educational requirements specified by the American Dental Association for dental assistants and who has passed a comprehensive written examination of the Certifying Board for Dental Assistants, and has thus been found to be competent in performing the tasks of a dental assistant. See also *dental a., currently certified.* **dental a., chairside,** a dental assistant who is responsible for chairside assisting, control of patients through the operatories, radiography, and preventive dentistry education of patients. See also four-handed DENTISTRY. **dental a., control,** a dental assistant whose responsibilities consist of conducting the preventive dentistry programs for the practice, including instruction in personal oral hygiene, nutritional counseling, and other aspects of preventive dentistry. **dental a., coordinating,** a dental assistant who is responsible for tray setups, sterilization of instruments, chairside assisting, radiographs, and control of patient flow through the operatories. **dental a., currently certified,** a certified dental assistant who, in addition to standard educational and certification requirements for the certified dental assistant, renews her or his certification annually and maintains current continuing education requirements. A currently certified dental assistant is entitled to use the initials *CDA* after her or his name and to wear the insignia of CDA. **dental a., expanded function,** former name for *dental d., extended function.* **dental a., extended function,** an auxiliary member of the dental health team who is specifically trained to perform direct patient care functions, including preliminary oral examination; exposing and processing radiographs; rubber dam application; preliminary impression taking; oral health education; topical fluoride application; matrix placement and removal; placement and removal of temporary restorations; placement, carving, and finishing amalgam restorations; and placement and finishing of resin, composite, and silicate restorations. Functions vary in accordance with the dental practice acts of individual states, but generally, they are limited to reversible procedures which are performed under the direct supervision of the dentist. Many states require them to be specially registered. Abbreviated *EFDA.* Formerly called *expanded function dental a., expanded duty dental auxiliary (EDDA),* and *expanded function dental auxiliary.* See also *dental a., registered,* DAU, and TEAM. **dental a., registered,** a dental assistant who is registered, or licensed, by the state to perform certain extended functions as permitted under the dental practice act of that state. Abbreviated *RDA.* See *dental a., extended function.* **foil a.,** foil HOLDER. **medical laboratory a.,** a person working under direct supervision of a medical technician, pathologist, physician, or qualified scientist in performing routine laboratory procedures requiring basic technical skills and some independent judgment in chemistry, hematology, and microbiology. The requirements for a certifying examination include a high school diploma or equivalent, either graduation from an American Medical Association approved school or completion of a basic military laboratory course, and a year of experience. Certification is awarded by the Board of Registry following successful completion of an examination. **medical specialty a.,** physician a. **physician a.,** one who has been trained in an accredited program and certified by an appropriate board to perform certain of a physician's duties, including history taking, physical examination, diagnostic tests, treatment, certain minor procedures, etc., all under the responsible supervision of a licensed physician. Abbreviated *PA.* Called also *medical specialty a.* and *physician's associate.* See also MEDEX.

ASSO American Society for the Study of Orthodontics (see under SOCIETY).

associate (ah-so'she-it, ah-so'se-it, ah-so'she-āt') [L. *ad* to + *socius* a fellow] one who performs equal tasks; a partner or a fellow. **physician's a.,** physician ASSISTANT.

association (ah-so"she-a'shun, ah-so"se-a'shun) [L. *associatio,* from *ad* to + *socius* a fellow] 1. the coordination of functions of similar parts. 2. a group or body of persons having similar interests or objectives. 3. the nonrandom occurrence of two or more phenotypic characteristics in members of a kindred. See also LINKAGE. 4. in epidemiology, a relationship between two variables, such as age and the incidence of diabetes. Several different types of associations are recognized, such as artifactual, causal, and chance. **American Cleft Palate A.,** a professional association having as its objectives encouragement of scientific research in the causes and nature of cleft palate and cleft lip; promotion of the science and art of rehabilitation of persons with cleft palate and associated deformities; encouragement of cooperation among those specialists who are interested in the rehabilitation of persons with cleft palate; and stimulation of public interest in and support of the rehabilitation of such persons. Abbreviated *ACPA.* **American Dental A.,** see Appendix. **American Dental Assistants A.,** an association whose major task is the representation of the profession of dental assistants on a national level. Through its Certifying Board, the association also conducts a series of national examinations to ascertain professional competency and proficiency (those who hold certificates for the current year may use the title *Certified Dental Assistant*). Registration by the Board is a credential recognized in some states instead of or in addition to certification. The title *Registered Dental Assistant* may be used for those assistants who have successfully completed an examination administered in their states. Abbreviated *ADAA.* See also dental ASSISTANT. **American A. of Dental Editors,** an association of dental editors, devoted to the professional aspects of dental journalism. Abbreviated *AADE.* **American A. of Dental Schools,** an organization which promotes the advancement of dental education, research, and services in all institutions that offer accredited programs of dental education in the United States. Abbreviated *AADS.* See Appendix. **American Dental Hygienists' A.,** the national association of dental hygienists, organized to cultivate, promote, and sustain the art and science of dental hygiene, to represent and safeguard the interest of the members of the dental hygiene profession, and to contribute toward the improvement of the health of the public. See also dental HYGIENIST. Abbreviated *ADHA.* **American A. of Hospital Dentists,** a professional association of dentists who practice and teach in the hospital environment, having as its objectives promotion of total comprehensive dental health care in hospitals; furtherment of the involvement of dentists in patient care, education, and research in hospitals; cooperation with and assistance of other health professions and agencies in the development of programs for total health care; provision of continuing education programs and training; service as a representative of dentists involved in hospital care; and provision of a liaison among medicine, the hospital, and the dental profession. Abbreviated *AAHD.* **American A. of Orthodontists,** a professional association of orthodontists in the United States and Canada. Its objectives include advancing the science and art of orthodontics, encouraging and sponsoring research, striving for higher standards of excellence in orthodontic instruction and practice, and contributing its part in health service. Abbreviated *AAO.* **American A. of Public Health Dentists,** an organization established to advance the understanding and appreciation of dental public health and preventive dentistry; to

serve as a liaison agency between public health dentistry and other elements of organized dentistry and public health; to provide a medium for the exchange and dissemination of scientific knowledge concerning preventive dentistry and oral health; and to promote the continued improvement in dental services provided to the public. Abbreviated *AAPHD.* **American Standards A.,** former name for the American National Standards Institute (see under INSTITUTE). **Blue Cross A.,** the national nonprofit organization to which more than 70 Blue Cross plans in the United States voluntarily belong. It administers programs of licensure and approval for Blue Cross plans, provides specific services related to the writing and administering of health care benefits across the country, and represents the Blue Cross plans in national affairs. Under contract with the Social Security Administration, it is intermediary in the Medicare program for most of the participating providers (hospitals, skilled nursing facilities, and home health agencies). Abbreviated *BCA.* See also Blue Cross PLAN. **A. of Blue Shield Plans,** the national nonprofit organization to which individual Blue Shield plans voluntarily belong; its functions consist of administration of health services and representation of the Blue Shield plans in national affairs. See also Blue Shield PLAN. **Canadian Dental A.,** see Appendix. **Delta Dental Plans A.,** a nationwide federation of dental service corporations providing dental care coverage insurance. Abbreviated *DDPA.* **individual practice a.,** a partnership, corporation, association, or other legal entity which has entered into an arrangement for provision of their services with persons who are licensed to practice dentistry, medicine, osteopathy, or with other health manpower. Abbreviated *IPA.* **International A. of Oral Myology,** a professional organization of dentists, dental hygienists, speech pathologists, and persons having university degrees in anatomy, physiology, child development, and health-related fields. Its objectives include basic scientific study of the processes of deglutition and dissemination of information and providing services concerning oral myofunctional disorders. Abbreviation *IAOM.* **International A. for Orthodontics,** an international professional association of orthodontists, having as its principal aim continuing education in orthodontics for general dentists and pedodontists and sponsoring the International Board of Orthodontics which presents certificates to qualified general dentists and pedodontists. Abbreviated *IAO.* **National A. of Seventh-Day Adventist Dentists,** a professional association of dentists established to encourage participation in activities of the Church; to foster missionary endeavor, including care of needy patients and donation of professional time to hospitals and clinics; and to emphasize the missionary possibilities of dentistry as a profession. Abbreviated *NASDAD.* **visiting nurse a.,** a voluntary health agency which provides nursing services in the home. Abbreviated *VNA.* Called also *visiting nurse service.*

astatine (as'tah-tēn) [Gr. *astatos* unstable] a very rare element, which is the heaviest member of the halogen family, having 20 isotopes, all radioactive. Symbol, At; atomic weight, 210; atomic number, 82; group VIIA of the period table. The longest lived and the most stable isotope is ^{210}At with a half-life of 8.3 hours. It is derived by alpha bombardment of bismuth. Naturally occurring astatine is believed to consist of less than 1 oz in the earth's crust. Like iodine, it has an affinity for the thyroid gland, but its use in medicine is still experimental. Astatine is a radioactive poison with strong carcinogenic properties.

aster (as'ter) [L.; Gr. *astēr* star] rays radiating from the centrosphere in mitosis. Sometimes called *astrosphere, cytaster,* and *kinosphere.*

asteria (as-te're-ah) [Gr.] plural of *asterion.*

asterion (as-te're-on), pl. *ast'eria* [Gr. "starred"] the point of union of the occipital, parietal, and temporal bones, or the point on the surface of the skull where the lambdoid, parietomastoid, and occipitomastoid sutures meet.

Asterococcus (as"ter-o-kok'us) *Mycoplasma.* **A. fermen'tans,** *Mycoplasma fermentans;* see under MYCOPLASMA. **A. hom'inis,** *Mycoplasma hominis;* see under MYCOPLASMA. **A. mu'ris,** *Streptobacillus moniliformis;* see under STREPTOBACILLUS. **A. saliva'rius,** *Mycoplasma salivarium;* see under MYCOPLASMA.

asteroid (as'ter-oid) [Gr. *astēr* star + *eidos* form] star-shaped; resembling a star.

asthenia (as-the'ne-ah) [Gr. *asthenēs* without strength + *-ia*] lack or loss of strength or energy; weakness.

asthma (az'mah) [Gr. "panting"] a disease marked by recurrent attacks of paroxysmal dyspnea, with wheezing, coughing, and a sense of constriction. 2. bronchial a. **allergic a.,** bronchial a. **bacterial a.,** that due to bacterial infection. Periodontal and periapical dental infection are suspected of having an aggravating effect on this type of asthma. **bronchial a.,** an allergic disease marked by recurrent attacks of paroxysmal dyspnea, with wheezing, coughing, and a sense of constriction, due to spasmodic contraction of the bronchi brought about by exposure to an allergenic substance. Called also *allergic a.* and *bronchial allergy.* **cardiac a.,** paroxysmal dyspnea occurring in association with some heart diseases. **Elsner's a., Heberden's a.,** ANGINA pectoris. **Millar's a., Wichmann's a.,** LARYNGISMUS stridulus.

ASTM American Society for Testing and Materials (see under SOCIETY).

Astonin-H trademark for *fludrocortisone.*

Astragalus (ah-strag'ah-lus) a genus of luguminous plants; the source of tragacanth.

astringent (ah-strin'jent) [L. *astringens,* from *ad* to + *stringere* to bind] 1. causing contraction, usually locally, after topical application. 2. an agent which causes tissues to contract locally by precipitating proteins, associated with limiting cell membrane permeability and reduction of mucous and other secretions and of capillary blood flow. Astringents are used to arrest hemorrhage by coagulating blood, reduce mucous membrane inflammation, promote healing, control perspiration, and toughen the skin. In dentistry, they are used to control capillary hemorrhage, reduce oral inflammation, and displace gingival tissue for taking impressions. Permanganates, tannins, acids, alcohols, and, chiefly, the salts of aluminum, zinc, manganese, iron, and bismuth are the principal astringents.

astro- [Gr. *astron* star] a combining form indicating relation to a star, or having the shape of a star.

astrocyte (as'tro-sīt) [*astro-* + Gr. *kytos* hollow vessel] a large neuroglial cell of ectodermal origin, having one or more elongated processes which contact the pia mater or blood vessels. Together with the pia mater, they invest the brain and spinal cord and form cuffs around penetrating blood vessels. Collectively, such cells are called *astroglia.* Together with the oligodendrocytes, they form the *macroglia.* See illustration at NERVE. **fibrous a.,** one found chiefly in the white substance, which shows filaments coursing through the cell body and processes, when stained. **protoplasmic a.,** one found chiefly in the gray substance, having a large, oval nucleus containing scattered chromatin granules but no nucleoli. It is believed to replace lost tissue by forming glial scars.

astroglia (as-trog'le-ah) [*astro-* + *neuroglia*] the astrocytes considered as tissue; see also MACROGLIA.

Astron 77 trademark for a heat-cured denture base acrylic polymer.

astrosphere (as'tro-sfēr) [*astro-* + Gr. *sphaira* sphere] 1. aster. 2. the central mass of an aster, exclusive of the rays.

Asucrol trademark for *chlorpropamide.*

asymmetrical (a″sim-met'rĕ-kal) not symmetrical; of different distribution on the two lateral halves of a structure.

asymmetry (a-sim'ĕ-tre) [*a* neg. + Gr. *symmetria* symmetry] lack or absence of symmetry; dissimilarity in corresponding lateral halves of a structure which are normally alike. In chemistry, lack of symmetry in the special arrangements of the atoms and radicals within the molecule.

asymptomatic (a″simp″to-mat'ik) showing or causing no symptoms.

asynergy (a-sin'er-je) [*a* neg. + Gr. *synergia* cooperation] lack of coordination among parts or organs normally acting in harmony.

asynovia (ah″sĭ-no've-ah) deficiency of the synovial secretion.

asystole (ah-sis'to-le) [*a* neg. + *systole*] cardiac standstill or arrest; absence of a heartbeat.

At astatine.

Atabrine trademark for *quinacrine hydrochloride* (see under QUINACRINE). See also Atabrine STOMATITIS.

atactic (ah-tak'tik) [Gr. *ataktos* irregular] 1. lacking coordination; irregular; pertaining to or characterized by ataxia. 2. pertaining to a polymer in which the radicals are randomly distributed. See also ISOTACTIC and SYNDIOTACTIC.

ataractic (at″ah-rak'tik) [Gr. *ataraktos* without disturbance, quiet] 1. pertaining to or capable of producing calmness or peace of mind. 2. an agent capable of producing such a condition; a tranquilizer.

ataralgesia (at″ar-al-je'ze-ah) [Gr. *ataraktos* without disturbance, quiet + *-algesia*] a method of combined sedation and analgesia designed to abolish the mental distress and pain attendant on surgical procedures, with the patient remaining conscious and alert.

Atarax trademark for *hydroxyzine hydrochloride* (see under HYDROXYZINE).

ataraxia (at″ah-rak'se-ah) [Gr. "impassiveness," "calmness"] perfect peace or calmness of mind; used especially to designate a detached serenity without depression of mental faculties or clouding of consciousness.

ataxia (ah-tak'se-ah) [Gr., from *a* neg. + *taxis* order] faulty

muscular coordination. **locomotor a.,** TABES dorsalis. **a. muscula'ris,** MYOTONIA congenita. **a. telangiecta'sia,** cerebellar ataxia of children, transmitted as an autosomal recessive trait, associated with oculocutaneous telangiectasia, frequent respiratory infections, and progressive mental deterioration. The ataxia becomes apparent when the child begins to walk. The telangiectasia becomes evident at about five years of age, appearing first on the bulbar conjunctiva and later on the ears, transnasal (butterfly) area of the face, palate, sternum, antecubital and popliteal fossae, and dorsae of the extremities. Choreoathetoid movements, dysarthria, drooling, growth retardation, slow slurred speech, jerky eye movements, fixation nystagmus, rapid spasmodic blinking, café-au-lait spots, and keratosis pilaris are the principal symptoms. Most patients die during adolescence. Called also *ataxia-telangiectasia* and *Louis-Bar's syndrome.*

-ate 1. a word termination forming a participial noun as the object of the process indicated by the root to which it is affixed, e.g., *hemolysate,* something hemolyzed; *homogenate,* something homogenized; *injectate,* something injected. Also forming adjectives, signifying possession of the quality indicated by the root, e.g., *dentate* and *corticate*; and verbs, signifying performance of the action indicated by the root, e.g., *decussate* and *pulsate.* 2. in organic chemistry, a suffix that replaces the *-ic* ending in names of acids (as in glycerate for glyceric acid), indicating that the acid involved is in dissociated form or combined with an ester.

Ateculon trademark for *clofibrate.*

atelectasis (at″ĕ-lek'tah-sis) [Gr. *ateles* imperfect + *ektasis* expansion] 1. incomplete expansion of the lungs at birth. 2. collapse or deflation of the adult lung due to impaired inflow caused by obstruction of the air passages by a foreign body, exudates, or a tumor. See also PNEUMOTHORAX.

Atensin trademark for *mephenesin.*

Ateriosan trademark for *clofibrate.*

Athenaeus of Attalia [1st century A.D.] a celebrated physician, latterly of Rome, and founder of the Pneumatist school of medicine. See also PNEUMATIST.

atherogenesis (ath″er-o-jen'ĕ-sis) the formation of atheromatous lesions in the arterial intima.

atheroma (ath″er-o'mah) [Gr. *athere* gruel + *-oma*] a mass of cholesterol-containing plaque of degenerated, thickened arterial intima occurring in atherosclerosis.

Atheropront trademark for *clofibrate.*

atherosclerosis (ath″er-o″sklĕ-ro'sis) a common form of arteriosclerosis in which deposits of yellowish plaques (atheromas) containing cholesterol are formed within the intima and inner media of large and medium-sized arteries.

athetosis (ath″ĕ-to'sis) [Gr. *athetos* not fixed + *-osis*] a form of dyskinesia characterized by slow, writhing, purposeless movements, usually affecting the hands and face, and caused by lesions of the midbrain, thalamic nuclei, pallidostriatum, and internal capsule of the cerebral cortex. The globus pallidus, nucleus ruber, and corticospinal tracts may also be involved. Called also *mobile spasm.*

Atrombine-K trademark for *warfarin.*

Athrombon trademark for *phenindione.*

athyreosis (ah-thi″re-o'sis) [*a* neg. + Gr. *thyreoid* thyroid + *-osis*] lack of the thyroid gland. See also CRETINISM.

atlas (at'las) [Gr. *Atlas* the Greek god who bears up the pillars of Heaven] 1. the first cervical vertebra, which articulates above with the occipital bone and below with the axis. 2. a collection of illustrations on one subject.

atm atmosphere (3).

atmo- [Gr. *atmos* steam or vapor] a combining form denoting relationship to steam or vapor.

atmos (at'mos) [Gr. "steam" or "vapor"] a unit of air pressure, being a pressure of 1°/cm²; equal to a column of mercury 760 mm high. Called also *aer.*

atmosphere (at'mos-fēr) [*atmo-* + Gr. *sphaira* sphere] 1. the gaseous envelope surrounding the earth. 2. any gaseous envelope or medium. 3. a unit of pressure equal to 101.325 newtons/m² and very nearly equal to the pressure exerted by a vertical column of mercury 760 mm high at a temperature of 0°C under standard gravity, being equivalent to the pressure of the air upon the earth at sea level, about 14.7 lb/in². Abbreviated *atm.*

atmospheric (at″mos-fēr'ik) of or pertaining to the atmosphere.

at no atomic NUMBER.

Atocin trademark for *cinchophen.*

atom (at'om) [Gr. *atomos* indivisible] the smallest particle of an

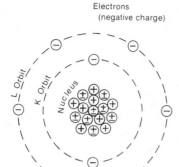

Electrons
(negative charge)

L Orbit
K Orbit
Nucleus

Diagram of an oxygen atom, representing the fundamentals of matter. Nucleus is composed of: (1) protons (positively charged); (2) neutrons (no charge); (3) other. (From H. O. Torres and A. Ehrlich: Modern Dental Assisting. 2nd ed. Philadelphia, W. B. Saunders Co., 1980.)

element which can enter into a chemical compound but itself is indivisible by chemical means. It comprises a dense inner core (nucleus) and a much less dense outer domain consisting of electrons which are in motion around the nucleus. The nucleus is positively charged; the amount of the charge corresponds to the atomic number of the atom. The number and arrangement of negatively charged electrons determine the chemical and physical properties of the atom, except its atomic weight and its radioactivity. See illustration. **activated a.**, 1. ionized a. 2. one in which some of the orbital electrons have been driven out into larger and less stable orbits; it is thus prepared to release its stored energy as these electrons return to their normal and stable orbits. Called also *excited a.* **Bohr a.**, the conception of a nuclear atom in which the orbital electrons are able to occupy only certain orbits, these orbits being determined by quantum limitations. **central a.**, in a coordination compound, an atom to which other atoms (*coordinating a's*) are attached. **coordinating a's**, in a coordination compound, atoms attached to the central atom. **excited a.**, activated a. (2). **ionized a.**, one from which one or more of the outer or valence electrons have been removed, or to which one or more electrons have been added (hence positive and negative ions). Called also *activated a.* **nuclear a.**, the conception or theory of the atom as composed of a small central nucleus surrounded by orbital electrons. Called also *Rutherford a.* **Rutherford a.**, nuclear a. **tagged a.**, one which has been made radioactive, so that its course in the body may be checked.

atomic (ah-tom'ik) of or pertaining to an atom. **a. percent**, the ratio of the number of atoms of the component to the number of atoms of the whole multiplied by 100, whereby the number of atoms is obtained by dividing the weight of the element by its atomic weight (AW) and multiplying by Avogardo's number (N):

$$\text{number of atoms} = \frac{\text{weight of component in grams}}{\text{AW}} \times N$$

atomizer (at'om-īz"er) an instrument for breaking a liquid up into spray.

atonia (ah-to'ne-ah) atony.

atony (at'on-ne) [*a* neg. + Gr. *tonos* tension] lack of normal tone or strength.

Atophan trademark for *cinchophen*.

atopy (at'o-pe) a clinical hypersensitivity state, or allergy, in persons with a hereditary predisposition to develop some form of allergy. Reagin, which is a specific immunoglobulin E (IgE), is involved. Called also *hereditary allergy* and *spontaneous allergy*.

Atosil trademark for *promethazine*.

ATP ADENOSINE triphosphate. **ATP gluconate transphosphatase,** glucokinase. **ATP glucose transphosphatase, ATP hexose transphosphatase,** hexokinase. **ATP monophosphatase,** adenosinetriphosphatase. **ATP phosphohydrolase,** adenosinetriphosphatase. **ATP pyrophosphatase,** ATP PYROPHOSPHATASE.

ATPase 1. adenosinetriphosphatase. 2. ATP PYROPHOSPHATASE.

atresia (ah-tre'ze-ah) [*a* neg. + Gr. *trēsis* a hole + *-ia*] the lack of closure of a normal body orifice or passage. **biliary a.**, a biliary tract abnormality due to arrested fetal development, consisting of obliteration or hypoplasia of one or more components of the bile ducts. Clinically, it is characterized by obstructive jaundice, dark urine, pale yellow stools, steatorrhea, hepatosplenomegaly, pruritus, skin xanthomas, and high-flow cardiac murmurs. Complications may include growth retardation, osteomalacia, portal hypertension with varices, hemorrhagic diathesis, hypersplenism, ascites, cyanosis of the digits, finger clubbing, and respiratory tract infections. Green-stained teeth due to hyperbilirubinemia is the principal dental feature. Life expectancy seldom exceeds 3 to 5 years.

atreto- [Gr. *atretos* not perforated] a combining form denoting absence of a normal opening; imperforate.

atretocephalus (ah-tre"to-sef'ah-lus) [*atreto-* + Gr. *kephalē* head] a fetus lacking the orifices normally present in the head.

atretolemia (ah-tre"to-le'me-ah) [*atreto-* + Gr. *laimos* gullet + *-ia*] lack of the normal opening into the larynx or the esophagus.

atretorrhinia (ah-tre"to-rin'e-ah) [*atreto-* + Gr. *rhis* nose + *-ia*] lack of the normal opening into the nose.

atretostomia (ah-tre"to-sto'me-ah) [*atreto-* + Gr. *stoma* mouth + *-ia*] lack of the normal opening into the oral cavity.

atria (a'tre-ah) [L.] plural of *atrium*.

atrium (a'tre-um), pl. *a'tria* [L.; Gr. *atrion* hall] 1. a chamber; used in anatomical nomenclature to designate a chamber affording entrance to another structure or organ. 2. an atrium of the heart. Called also *auricle.* See *left a.* and *right a.* **a. dex'trum** [NA], right a. **a. glot'tidis, a. of glottis,** VESTIBULE of larynx. **a. laryn'gis, a. of larynx,** VESTIBULE of larynx. **left a.**, the upper left chamber of the heart; it receives oxygenated blood from the lungs through the pulmonary vein, and delivers it into the left ventricle through the left atrioventricular valve. Called also *a. sinistrum* [NA]. **a. mea'tus me'dii** [NA], **a. of middle meatus of nose,** a shallow depression in front of the middle nasal meatus, between the agger nasi and the middle nasal concha. **right a.**, the upper right chamber of the heart; it receives venous blood from the venae cavae and coronary sinus, and delivers it into the right ventricle through the right atrioventricular valve. Called also *a. dextrum* [NA]. **a. sinis'trum** [NA], left a.

Atromid S trademark for *clofibrate*.

Atromidin trademark for *clofibrate*.

Atropa (at'ro-pah) [Gr. *Atropos* "undeviating," one of the Fates] a genus of solanaceous plants, from which various alkaloids are derived, including atropine, scopolamine, and *l*-hyoscyamine, which generally possess antimuscarinic properties. The genus includes *A. acuminata* and *A. belladonna.* See BELLADONNA.

atrophia (ah-tro'fe-ah) [L.; Gr., from *a* neg. + Gr. *trophē* nourishment] atrophy.

atrophic (ah-trof'ik) pertaining to or characterized by atrophy.

atrophied (at'ro-fēd) marked by atrophy; shrunken.

atrophy (at'ro-fe) [L.; Gr. *atrophia*] an acquired decrease in the size of a normally developed tissue or organ, resulting from a reduction in cell size or a decrease in the total number of cells, or both. **afunctional a.**, disuse a. (2). **alveolar a.**, atrophy of the alveolar process with bone resorption. See PERIODONTOSIS. **alveolar a., precocious advanced,** precocious advanced alveolar a. **arthritic a.**, atrophy of the muscles and bones surrounding a diseased joint. **blue a.**, a blue pigmentation that sometimes follows self-injection of drugs, found in addicts. **bone a.**, resorption of bone; physiologic bone atrophy. See also OSTEOPOROSIS. **compression a.**, atrophy of a part due to constant pressure. **concentric a.**, atrophy of a hollow organ in which the cavity is contracted. **degenerative a.**, the wasting of a part due to a degeneration of its cells. **denervated muscle a.**, atrophy of a muscle due to disruption of its innervation. **disuse a., a. of disuse,** 1. wasting caused by lack of normal exercise of a part. See also OSTEOPOROSIS of disuse. 2. periodontal atrophy occurring when the functional stimulation required for the maintenance of the periodontal tissue is lacking. It is characterized by thinning of the periodontal ligament, narrowing of the periodontal space, reduction in the number of periodontal fibers, disruption of the fiber bundle arrangement, thickening of cementum, reduction in the height of the alveolar bone, and osteoporosis. Called also *afunctional a.* **endocrine a.**, atrophy of an organ, tissue, or system due to disorders of the endocrine glands with resultant diminishing of the production of trophic hormonal stimulation necessary for its normal functioning. **exhaustion a.**, atrophy believed to be due to prolonged overwork of an endocrine organ. Continued demand on the adrenal, pituitary, or thyroid glands will be followed at first by enlargement of the organ, but eventually there results a progressive loss of parenchymal elements. **familial spinal muscular a.**, infantile muscular a. **fatty a.**, fatty infiltration following atrophy of the tissue elements of a part. Called also *adipositas ex vacuo.* **gingival a.,** gingival RECESSION. **hemifacial a.,** facial HEMI-ATROPHY. **hemilingual a.,** atrophy affecting one side of the tongue. **infantile muscular a.,** a familial form of progressive spinal muscular atrophy of infants, with hypotonia and wasting of the skeletal muscles, resulting from degeneration of the anterior horn cells of the spinal cord. The clinical picture is that of the floppy infant, with difficulty in holding the head up, sluggish movements, and flaccid paralysis. Dysphagia and fascicular twitching of the tongue are common. The facial muscles are not affected, and the expressivity of the face contrasts with the general flaccid appearance of the body. Several siblings may be affected. Most patients die within several months. Called also *familial spinal muscular a., progressive spinal muscular a., Werdnig's disease,* and *Werdnig-Hoffmann syndrome.* **Landouzy-Déjérine a.,** Landouzy-Déjérine DYSTROPHY. **muscular a.,** atrophy of muscle tissue. Called also *amyotrophy.* **neural a.,** neuropathic a. **neuropathic a.,** muscular atrophy due to neurological diseases. Called also *neural a.* **neurotrophic a.,** that due to disruption of the peripheral nervous system supplying the tissue. **pathologic a.,** that characterized by tissue changes more extensive than those due to normal aging processes or atrophy due to an abnormal or pathologic process in the body. **periodontal a.,** reduction of the size of the alveolar process, associated with recession of the gingiva with subsequent exposure of the root surface. Called also *senile a.* **physiologic a.,** senile a. (1). **physiologic bone a.,** the loss of bone tissue through physiological processes associated with aging. Called also *senile bone a., physiologic bone resorption,* and *senile bone resorption.* **pigmentary a.,** atrophy characterized by deposits of pigments in the atrophic tissues. **postmenopausal a.,** atrophy and thinning of various tissues, such as the oral or genital mucosa, occurring after menopause. **precocious advanced alveolar a.,** a type of periodontal bone loss in young patients who favor a high carbohydrate diet, usually associated with elevated serum cholesterol and calcium levels and a flat sugar tolerance curve. **presenile a.,** 1. premature atrophy of certain organs, occurring without any apparent cause. 2. premature periodontal atrophy associated with reduction of the size of the alveolar process and recession of the gingiva, occurring without any apparent cause. **pressure a.,** atrophy caused by persistent pressure on an organ or tissue, believed to be related to vascular atrophy. **progressive muscular a.,** amyotrophic lateral sclerosis in which there is massive involvement of the lower motor neurons with generalized muscular atrophy. **progressive spinal muscular a.,** infantile muscular a. **progressive unilateral facial a.,** progressive atrophy of the skin, tissues, and bones, affecting one side of the face. **pulp a.,** a degenerative process of the dental pulp, characterized by a diminution in size and wasting away of pulpal cells, usually associated with an interference with nutrition. Called also *atrophic pulp degeneration.* **reticular pulp a.,** atrophy of the pulp of a tooth, characterized by the development of large vacuolated spaces with a decrease in the number of cellular elements, and associated with disappearance of the odontoblasts. It is now thought to be a fixation artefact, a form of autolysis. **reversionary a.,** anaplasia. **rheumatic a.,** muscular atrophy in persons affected with rheumatic diseases. **senile a.,** 1. atrophy which affects certain organs in all individuals as part of the normal aging process; physiologic atrophy. 2. periodontal a. **senile bone a.,** physiologic bone a. **senile skin a.,** senile ELASTOSIS. **unilateral a.,** hemiatrophy. **vascular a.,** that due to reduced blood supply, as in arteriosclerosis.

atropine (at′ro-pēn) an alkaloid derived from belladonna, hyoscyamus, or strammonium, or produced synthetically, *endo*(±)-α-(hydroxymethyl)benzeneacetic acid 8-methyl-8-azabicyclo[3,2,1]oct-3-yl ester. It occurs as white crystals or as a crystalline powder that is soluble in water, alcohol, glycerol, chloroform, and ether. Atropine is a potent antimuscarinic drug and is used as an antispasmodic to relax smooth muscles; to relieve the tremor and rigidity of parkinsonism; to increase the heart rate by blocking vagus nerves; as a respiratory stimulant; to suppress sweating and salivation; to suppress gastrointestinal spasms; as an antidote for various toxic and anticholinesterase agents; and as a mydriatic and cycloplegic. In dentistry, it is used principally to control secretion of saliva before dental procedures and during anesthesia. The use of atropine may be contraindicated in some forms of prostatic diseases, glaucoma, diabetes mellitus, hyperthyroidism, and heart disease. Drying of the mouth and mucous membranes, increased intraocular pressure, restlessness, tremor, fatigue, motor disorders, skin rash, flushing, vomiting, disorientation, hallucinations, delirium, leukocytosis, respiratory and vascular collapse, and death include potential adverse reactions. **a. esterase,** carboxylesterase. **a. sulfate,** the sulfate salt of atropine, occurring as

colorless crystals or white, crystalline powder, having actions and uses similar to those of the parent drug.

attachment (ah-tach′ment) 1. a connection by which one thing is fixed to another. 2. a device for retention and stabilization of a dental prosthesis. See also RETAINER (2). **abnormal frenulum a., abnormal frenum a.,** aberrant insertion of labial, buccal, and lingual frena that may initiate periodontal disease by retracting gingival margins, creating diastemas, limiting lip and tongue movements, and the like. **Alexander a.,** an intracoronal attachment in which the male sections are joined to the crowns and the attachments are tapered and used with a buccolingual path of insertion. **a. apparatus,** attachment APPARATUS. **ASC 52 a.,** trademark for a *hinge stress-breaker* (see under STRESS-BREAKER). **ball-and-socket a.,** a precision stud attachment, in which the male part, a ball-type extension from a cast post and cap, engages the female part, a resin dome incorporated in an overlay denture. **Ballard stress equalizer a.,** a stress-breaker consisting of a ball-and-socket joint built into a partial removable denture, which permits free movement, without permitting separation of two major connectors. Called also *Ballard stress equalizer.* **bar a.,** one consisting of a bar spanning an edentulous area and joining together teeth or roots, the denture fitting over the bar and connecting it by one or more sleeves. Dentures having rigid sleeve-bar junctions do not allow any movement; those having bar joints allow some play between the denture and bar. See illustration. See also BAR. **Bowles a., Bowles multiphase a.,** multiphase BRACKET. **Ceka a.,** trademark for an extracoronal projection attachment, in which the female part, soldered to the abutment tooth, fits into a conical male part within the denture. The retaining pin in the male part is removable and may be unscrewed; one type allows some play between the abutment and the denture, the other being rigid. **channel shoulder pin a.,** channel shoulder pin TECHNIQUE. **Chayes a.,** an intracoronal entirely frictional precision attachment with a T-shaped male unit. **C & L a.,** trademark for a spring-clip semiprecision intracoronal attachment, having an L spring and a counterpoise C rest. Called also *C & L retainer* and *C & L unit.* **Clark a.,** an attachment making use of the Neurohr-Williams rest shoe, which provides a thin-gauge platinum box for the tapered Neurohr type rest. The rest shoes are placed in the several abutment castings with the aid of a master cast, differing from the Neurohr spring-lock attachment in that it uses a lingual clasp arm on the denture casting to engage an undercut created in the abutment casting on the side of the tooth away from the tapered rest. **C & M 637 a.,** trademark for a *hinge stress-breaker* (see under STRESS-BREAKER). **combined a.,** a precision attachment combining a hinge type of connecting element with stress-breaking capabilities outside the crown joined directly to an intracoronal attachment. Called also *combined unit.* **Conex a.,** trademark for a projection extracoronal attachment that provides a rigid union between the denture and the abutment. See illustration. **Crismani a.,** trademark for a precision intracoronal attachment whose retention is augmented by a spring clip. See illustration. **Crismani combined a.,** trademark for a combined precision attachment consisting of a hinge stress-breaker connector within the denture and a rigid intracoronal attachment; a spring-controlled hinge movement allowing the lateral play. Called also *Crismani combined unit.* **CSP a.,** channel shoulder pin TECHNIQUE. **Cu-Sil a.,** trademark for an attachment for overlay dentures, in which silicone rubber gaskets are processed around abutment teeth to reduce abutment stress and to provide an effective border seal. **Dalbo a.,** Dalbo stud a. **Dalbo extracoronal a.,** trademark for a projection unit, having the male part soldered to the surface of the

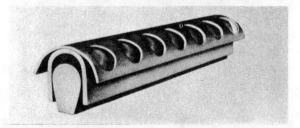

Dolder bar joint attachment. A well-tested example of a single sleeve joint allowing vertical and rotational units. (From H. W. Prieskel: Precision Attachments in Dentistry. 3rd ed. London, Henry Kimpton, Ltd., 1979.)

abutment crown to form a projection to which the female element within the prosthesis is joined. The male part has an L-shaped projection bar with a ball joint in the lower extremity. The female part fits over the bar and engages the sides of the ball connection of the male; the lock between the socket and the ball providing the direct retention. The attachment allows for some play between the male and female parts. Called also *Dalbo extracoronal unit.* See illustration. **Dalbo stud a.,** trademark for a stud attachment that is available in three different types: the resilient type, most commonly used in series, which has a spherical male unit that allows some alignment; the rigid type, which has a male unit that fits rigidly into the female unit; and the stress-broken unit, which has a spherical male unit resting against a coil spring in the female unit, which allows both vertical and rotational movement. Called also *Dalbo a.* and *Dalbo stud unit.* See illustration. **Dalla Bona a.,** trademark for a nonresilient stud attachment. **Dolder bar joint a.,** a bar attachment containing a flexible joint that allows play between the denture and bar. Called also *Dolder bar* and *Dolder bar joint.* See illustration. **Dolder bar unit a.,** a bar attachment with a rigid connection between the bar and sleeve, retention being entirely frictional owing to parallel vertical surfaces of both sections. Called also *Dolder bar unit.* See illustration. **dowel rest a.,** a modification of the Clark attachment, consisting of a boxlike rest seat in the abutment casting for support of the partial denture, and a dimple on the lingual surface of the abutment casting for retention, which is engaged by a boss on the lingual arm on the denture framework, thus providing retention without the use of a visible clasp arm. **edgewise a.,** edgewise BRACKET. **epithelial a. (of Gottlieb),** a band or wedge of epithelium, the external surface of which adheres to the crown and the internal surface to the lamina propria of the free gingiva. It extends from the base of the gingival sulcus to the upper limits of the periodontal ligament, its length being about 2 mm. Initially, the cuff is attached to the anatomic crown but, with the growth of the root, it becomes located on the slope of the crown and, later, on the cervix of the tooth. Late in life it may be attached entirely on the root. The cuff seals the periodontal tissue and protects it from foreign material in the oral cavity. Called also *gingival a., attached gingival cuff, epithelial cuff, gingival collar,* and *gingival cuff.* **extracoronal a.,** a precision attachment in which the retaining mechanism is outside the crown of an abutment tooth or restoration. Principal types of extracoronal attachments include the projection attachment, in which the male unit is soldered to the surface of the abutment crown, forming a projection to which the female unit within the denture is joined; the connecting attachment, which is used to join two sections of a prosthesis without the need for anchoring the restoration to the tooth; and the combined attachment, which consists of a hinge type of connecting element outside the tooth, which is joined directly to an intracoronal attachment. See illustration. See also CLASP (2) and extracoronal RETAINER. **friction a.,** intracoronal a. **Gerber a.,** a stud attachment in which the male unit is screwed on the base,

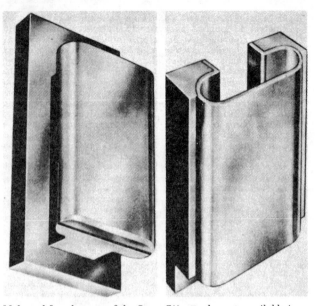

Male and female parts of the Stern G/A attachment; available in several sizes. (From H. W. Preiskel: Precision Attachments in Dentistry. 3rd ed. London, Henry Kimpton, Ltd., 1979.)

and retained by a spring clip in the female unit engaging a peripheral groove in the male unit. One type allows some vertical movement and the other is almost rigid. **gingival a.,** epithelial a. **gingival a. (of Gottlieb),** the attachment of the gingival epithelium to the tooth, consisting of a collar-like band of stratified squamous epithelium. It is three to four layers thick early in life, but the number of layers increases to 10 or more with age, its length ranging from 0.25 to 1.35 nm. It attaches to the enamel by a basal basement membrane, the lamina densa being its part adjacent to the enamel and the lamina lucida attaching to hemidesmosomes. Together with the gingival fibers, the gingival attachment forms the dentogingival junction. Called also *attached epithelial cuff.* **gingival latch a.,** Stern gingival latch a. **Hade-Ring a.,** trademark for a stud attachment, having a very low profile. **Hart-Dunn a.,** an attachment for a unilateral distal extension partial denture, being an embrasure hook of round wrought wires placed just beneath the contact areas in the mesial and distal areas of the selected abutment tooth, slightly curved to allow easy placement from the lingual direction and protection of the interdental papillae. **Hruska a.,** a screw-retaining system for joining a bridge to nonvital roots. Called also *Hruska unit.* **implant superstructure a.,** any device in an implant denture, such as a precision attachment, coping, or clasp, designed to fit onto the implant abutments. **internal a.,** intracoronal a. **intracoronal a.,** a precision attachment in which a cryptlike unit or slot (female part) is built entirely into the crown and an insert or flange (male part) extends from the prosthesis proper and fits into the slot when the denture is attached to the crown. The flange may be retained by friction between the parallel surfaces of the male and female parts together, or it may be augmented by mechanical locks, screws, or adjustable latches. Called also *friction a., internal a., key-and-keyway a., slotted a., intracoronal retainer,* and, sometimes, *precision a.* See illustration. **Ipsoclip a.,** trademark for a spring-loaded plunger attachment, in which the plunger in the removable part of the prosthesis slips into a slot in the abutment, thus locking the denture in place; used most commonly with bar attachments and overlay dentures. Called also *Ipsoclip unit.* See illustration. **key-and-keyway a.,** intracoronal a. **McCollum a.,** an intracoronal entirely frictional precision attachment with an H-shaped male unit. **multiphase a.,** multiphase BRACKET. **Neurohr spring-lock a.,** a spring-lock attachment that provides extracoronal retention for partial dentures, employing tapered vertical rests retained within the contours of the abutment tooth. A single buccal clasp arm, with a ball terminus, engages an undercut in the abutment casting and retains the denture in place. **new a.,** reattachment (3). **orthodontic a.,** orthodontic BRACKET. **parallel a.,** a device used for attaching a denture base to an abutment tooth. Retention is provided by friction between the parallel walls of the two parts of the attachment. See also *bar a.* **Pin-Dalbo a.,** trademark for a modified Dalbo extracoronal attachment, allowing the two sec-

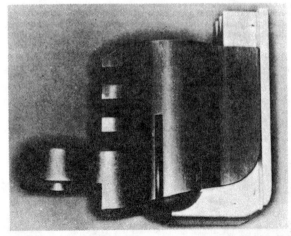

Dalbo extracoronal projection attachment. (From H. W. Preiskel: Precision Attachments in Dentistry. 3rd ed. London, Henry Kimpton, Ltd., 1979.)

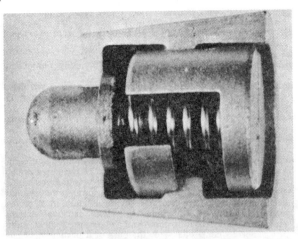

Cross sectional photograph of Ipsoclip attachment. The spring-loaded plunger mechanism may be dismantled by undoing the bayonet clip at the opposite end to the plunger. The Ipsoclip attachment is generally buried lingually in the outer, removable section of the prosthesis. (From H. W. Preiskel: Precision Attachments in Dentistry. 3rd ed. London, Henry Kimpton, Ltd., 1979.)

tions to be locked together during impression or rebasing. **pinledge a.,** an attachment having pins which extend into pinholes placed in a series of flattened ledges on the lingual surface of the prepared tooth. **precision a.,** 1. a precision device used for attaching fixed or removable partial dentures to the crown of an abutment tooth or a restoration. One type is the intracoronal attachment and the other type is the extracoronal attachment. Called also *precision anchorage.* See also *extracoronal a., intracoronal a.,* and *semiprecision a.* 2. intracoronal a. **Pressomatic a.,** trademark for an attachment in which a rubber cartridge in the removable part of the denture slips into a slot in the abutment, thus locking the prosthesis in place. Called also *Pressomatic unit.* **projection a.,** an extracoronal precision attachment in which the male unit, which is soldered

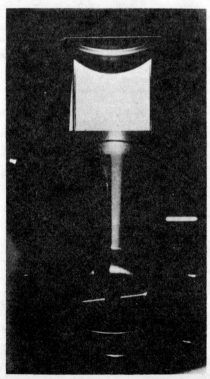

Removable section of the Conex attachment. Note the parallel walls that provide a precise path of insertion. (From H. W. Preiskel; Precision Attachments in Dentistry. 3rd ed. London, Henry Kimpton, Ltd., 1979.)

to the surface of the abutment crown, forms a projection that joins with the female unit built into the prosthesis, the lock between the two parts providing the direct retention. Called also *projection unit.* See illustration. **ribbon arch a.,** ribbon arch BRACKET. **Roach a.,** bar CLASP. **Rothermann a.,** a stud attachment in which the female clip engages the side of the male unit — one type allowing some movement and the other being rigid. **Schatzmann a.,** an intracoronal precision attachment whose retention is augmented by a spring-loaded plunger. **Schubiger a.,** an attachment system consisting of a threaded stud on a base, which is soldered to a post diaphragm; a sleeve fitting over the stud, to which a bar attachment is soldered; and a nut which attaches the sleeve to the stud. Called also *Schubiger system* and *Schubiger screw unit.* **Scott a.,** a projecting extracoronal precision attachment, being a removable telescopic unit with an axial-rotation joint with retention provided by parallel-sided steel pins. **semiprecision a.,** attachment of a denture to an abutment of a tooth or a restoration by a semiprecision rest, sometimes supplemented by a spring-loaded plunger or clip, fitting into a rest seat on the lateral surface of a crown, which is especially deepened to provide added retention. See illustration. **Sherer a.,** an indirect retainer which combines intracoronal attachment with extracoronal retention. Positive seating and support are attained through the dovetail-shaped key in its keyway in the abutment restoration. **slotted a.,** intracoronal a. **Stabilex a.,** trademark for a projecting extracoronal attachment that provides a rigid connection between the male and female parts, the retention being provided by adjustable pins which may be unscrewed and replaced. **Steiger's a.,** Steiger's JOINT. **Steiger-Boitel a.,** a single bar attachment, providing additional retention by parallel-sided pins in the sleeve, engaging holes in the bar. Called also *Steiger-Boitel bar.* **Stern a.,** trademark for a combined precision attachment, having a hinge stress-breaker in the connecting element outside the crown, which is joined directly to an intracoronal attachment unit. Called also *Stern stress-breaker a.* and *Stern stress-breaker unit.* **Stern G/A a.,** trademark for an intracoronal precision attachment whose retention is entirely frictional, having a T-shaped male unit. See illustration. **Stern gingival latch a., Stern G/L a.,** trademark for an intracoronal precision attachment whose retention may be adjusted by opening out the base of the male unit. Called also *gingival latch a.* **Stern stress-breaker a.,** Stern a. **stress-breaker a.,** a precision attachment which contains a stress-breaking device, as in the combined attachment. See also STRESS-BREAKER. **stud a.,** one in which the male portion, a stud-shaped projection soldered to the diaphragm of a post crown, fits into the female portion embedded within the prosthesis. Most commonly used in complete dentures. See illustration. **superstructure a.,** one which retains a superstructure onto the implant abutment, usually a precision coping, clasp, or combination of both devices. Similar to an attachment in removable partial dentures. **Tach-E-Z a.,** Tach-E-Z RETAINER. **twin wire a.,** twin wire BRACK-

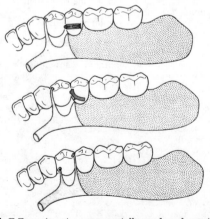

A, Tach-E-Z unit. A commercially-produced spring-loaded plunger used in conjunction with a mesially placed semiprecision rest. B, C and L unit. The commercially-produced spring clip provides additional retention to a mesially placed occlusal rest. C, laboratory-produced retaining system employing a distally placed semiprecision rest and a lingual retaining arm engaging a dimple in the crown. (From H. W. Preiskel: Precision Attachments in Dentistry. 3rd ed. London, Henry Kimpton, Ltd., 1979.)

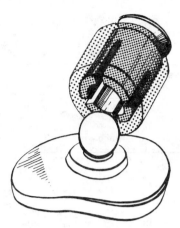

The Dalbo stud attachment. (From H. W. Preiskel: Precision Attachments in Dentistry. 3rd ed. London, Henry Kimpton, Ltd., 1979.)

ET. universal orthodontic a., universal BRACKET. **Zest Anchor system a.,** trademark for a stud attachment, in which a nylon male unit in the denture base fits into the female unit within the root canal below the gingival line. Called also *Zest Anchor system.*

attack (ah-tak′) an episode or onset of illness. **heart a.,** coronary OCCLUSION. **hypoglycemic a.,** hypoglycemic SHOCK.

attar (at′ar) [Persian "essence"] any essential or volatile oil of vegetable origin. **a. of roses,** OIL of roses.

attenuation (ah-ten″u-a′shun) [L. *attenuatio,* from *ad* to + *tenuis* thin] 1. the act or process of thinning or weakening. 2. weakening the virulence of pathogenic microorganisms by passage through an intermediate host, thus diminishing the virulence of the organism for the primary host. 3. reduction in energy in a beam of radiation during the process of passage through a tissue or other material.

attic (at′ik) a cavity situated on the tegmental wall of the tympanic cavity, just above the facial canal. Called also *attic of middle ear, recessus epitympanicus* [NA], and *epitympanum.* **a. of middle ear,** attic.

atticitis (at′ĭ-ki′tis) inflammation of the attic.

atticoantrotomy (at″ĭ-ko-an-trot′o-me) the surgical opening of the attic and the antrum of the middle ear.

atticotomy (at″ĭ-kot′o-me) the surgical opening of the attic.

attitude (at′ĭ-tud) [L. *attitudo* posture] 1. a posture or position of the body; habitus. 2. a tendency to respond positively or negatively to something.

atto- [Danish *atten* eighteen] in the metric system, a combining form denoting one quintillionth (10^{-18}) of the unit designated by the root with which it is combined. Abbreviated *a.* See also metric SYSTEM.

attraction (ah-trak′shun) [L. *attractio* a drawing together] 1. the process of drawing one body toward another. 2. a condition marked by teeth or other maxillary and mandibular structures being higher than their normal position, thereby causing shortening of the face. Cf. *abstraction* (1). **capillary a.,** the force that attracts the particles of a fluid into and along the caliber of a tube. **electric a.,** the tendency of bodies bearing opposite electric charges to move toward each other. **magnetic a.,** the tendency of bodies possessing circulating electric currents to move toward each other.

attrahens (at′rah-enz) [L.] drawing toward.

attrition (ah-trish′un) [L. *attritio* a rubbing against] the physiologic wearing away of a substance or structure; specifically, wearing away of a tooth as a result of tooth-to-tooth contact, as in mastication, occurring only on the occlusal, incisal, and proximal surfaces. It is chiefly associated with aging. See also ABRASION, EROSION, and WEAR. See illustration at ODONTOGENESIS.

Atumin trademark for *dicyclomine hydrochloride* (see under DICYCLOMINE).

at vol atomic VOLUME.

at wt atomic WEIGHT.

atypia (a-tip′e-ah) the condition of being irregular or not conformed to type.

atypical (a-tip′ĭ-kal) [*a* neg. + Gr. *typos* type or model] not conforming to the type; irregular.

AU 1. Ångström UNIT. 2. abbreviation for L. *au′res u′nitas,* both ears together.

Au gold (L. *aurum*).

audio- [L. *audire* to hear] a combining form denoting relationship to hearing.

audiogram (aw′de-o-gram″) [*audio-* + Gr. *gramma* a writing] a chart of the variations of the acuteness of hearing of an individual.

audiology (aw″de-ol′o-je) [*audio-* + *-logy*] the science of hearing, particularly the study of impaired hearing.

audiometry (aw″de-om′e-tre) [*audio-* + Gr. *metrein* to measure] the testing of the sense of hearing.

audit (aw′dit) [L. *auditus* act of hearing] examination and verification of accounts. **medical a.,** a detailed retrospective review and evaluation of selected medical records by a qualified professional staff performed in some hospitals, group practices, and occasionally in private practices for the evaluation of professional performance by comparing it with accepted criteria, standards, and current professional judgment. Medical audits are generally concerned with the care of a particular disease and are undertaken to identify deficiencies in applied care in anticipiation of educational programs for its improvement. **Medical A. Program (MAP),** one of the two programs of the Commission on Professional and Hospital Activities (see under COMMISSION). **Medicare a.,** the examination of financial and statistical records of a provider of medical services in an effort to ascertain that the costs claimed by the provider are in accordance with the law and the regulations promulgated by the Secretary of the Department of Health and Human Services. **a. of treatment,** the qualitative review of health care services rendered or proposed. In dental insurance, it may take the form of a comparison of a patient's records and claim form information, a patient's questionnaire, an examination of pre- or postoperative radiographs, or a pre- or post-treatment clinical examination of the patient.

auditory (aw′dĭ-to-re) [L. *auditorius*] pertaining to hearing.

Auer body [John *Auer,* American physician, 1875–1948] see under BODY.

Aufrecht's sign [Emanual *Aufrecht,* German physician, 1844–1933] see under SIGN.

Auger effect, electron see under EFFECT.

aura (aw′rah), pl. *au′rae* [L. "breath"] 1. a distinctive atmosphere surrounding an object. 2. a subtle sensory stimulus. 3. a luminous radiation surrounding an object. 4. a subjective sensation or motor phenomenon, such as voices, lights, or paresthesia, which precedes and marks the onset of paroxysmal attacks, such as an epileptic seizure.

aural (aw′ral) [L. *auralis*] 1. pertaining to the ear. 2. pertaining to, or of the nature of, an aura.

aurate (aw′rāt) a salt of auric acid.

Aureociclina trademark for *chlortetracycline hydrochloride* (see under CHLORTETRACYCLINE).

Aureocina trademark for *chlortetracycline.*

Aureomycin trademark for *chlortetracycline hydrochloride* (see under CHLORTETRACYCLINE).

Aureotan trademark for *aurothioglucose.*

aures (aw′rēz) [L.] plural of *auris.*

auric (aw′rik) pertaining to or containing trivalent gold, Au≡.

Auricidine trademark for *gold sodium thiosulfate* (see under GOLD).

auricle (aw′rĭ-k'l) [L. *auricula* a little ear] 1. the projecting part of the external ear; the flap of the ear. See PINNA. 2. a. of heart. **a. of heart,** 1. the ear-shaped appendage of either atrium of the heart. 2. an old term for atrium of the heart. See left ATRIUM and right ATRIUM.

auricula (aw-rik′u-lah), pl. *auric′ulae* [L., dim. of *auris*] a little ear; [NA] the portion of the external ear not contained within the head; the pinna, or flap of the ear. Applied also to the auricle of the heart, and sometimes mistakenly used as a synonym for an atrium of the heart.

auriculae (aw-rik′u-le) [L.] plural of *auricula.*

auricular (aw-rik′u-lar) [L. *auricularis*] pertaining to an auricle, or to the ear.

auriculare (aw-rik″u-la′re) [L. *auricularis* pertaining to the ear] a craniometric point at the top of the opening of the external auditory meatus.

auricularis (aw-rik″u-la′ris) [L.] 1. pertaining to the ear; auricular. 2. auricular MUSCLE.

aurinasal (aw″rĭ-na′zal) pertaining to the ear and the nose.

auris (aw′ris), pl. *au′res* [L.] [NA] the ear; the organ of hearing. **a. exter′na** [NA], external EAR. **a. inter′na** [NA], internal EAR. **a. me′dia** [NA], middle EAR.

aurochromoderma (aw″ro-kro″mo-der′mah) [L. *aurum* gold + Gr.

chrōma color + Gr. *derma* skin] a greenish-blue staining of the skin, sometimes occurring in conjunction with discoloration of the mucous membrane, particularly of the mouth, following the administration of a gold compound. Called also *chrysoderma*.

Aurocidin trademark for *gold sodium thiosulfate* (see under GOLD).

α-auromercaptoacetanilide (aw″ro-mer-kap″to-as″ĕ-tan′ĭ-lĭd) aurothioglycanide.

aurotherapy (aw″ro-ther′ah-pe) [L. *aurum* gold + *therapy*] therapy with the use of gold compounds; chrysotherapy.

aurothioglucose (aw″ro-thi″o-gloo′kōs) a gold compound, 1-*thio*-D-glucopyranosato gold, occurring as a yellow, odorless crystalline powder that is freely soluble in water, but not in alcohols and most other organic solvents. Used in the treatment of rheumatoid arthritis. It has the toxic properties of gold. Called also *gold thioglucose*. Trademarks: Aureotan, Aurumine, Oronol, Solganal.

aurothioglycanide (aw″ro-thi″o-gli′kah-nĭd) a gold derivative, [[(phenylcarbamoyl)methyl]thio]gold, occurring as a grayish yellow powder that is insoluble in water, benzene, and other organic solvents. Used in the treatment of rheumatoid arthritis. It has the toxic properties of gold. Called also α-*auromercaptoacetanilide* and *aurothioglycolanilide*. Trademark: Lauron.

aurothioglycolanilide (aw″ro-thi″o-gli″kōl-an′ĭ-lĭd) aurothioglycanide.

aurothiomalate disodium, aurothiomalate sodium (aw″ro-thi″o-ma′lāt) GOLD sodium thiomalate.

Aurothion trademark for a *gold sodium thiosulfate* (see under GOLD).

aurothiosulfate natrium, aurothiosulfate sodium (aw″ro-thi″o-sul′fāt) GOLD sodium thiosulfate.

aurous (aw′rus) pertaining to or containing monovalent gold, Au−.

aurum (aw′rum) [L.] gold. **a. paradox′um,** tellurium.

Aurumine trademark for *aurothioglucose*.

auscultation (aws″kul-ta′shun) [L. *auscultare* to listen to] the act of listening for sounds within the body, chiefly for ascertaining the condition of the lungs, heart, pleura, abdomen, and other organs, or for detecting crepitation in bone fractures.

Austenal No. 2 trademark for a medium hard *dental casting gold alloy* (see under GOLD).

Austenal No. 5 trademark for a hard *dental casting gold alloy* (see under GOLD).

austenite (o′stĕ-nīt) a solid solution of carbon (and possibly other elements) in γ-iron; maximum carbon content in the binary Fe−Fe₃C system is 2 percent.

Austin retractor see under RETRACTOR.

Austracol trademark for *chloramphenicol*.

Austrapine trademark for *reserpine*.

aut- see AUTO-.

autacoid (aw′tah-koid) [aut- + Gr. *akos* remedy] any of the endogenous substances, such as hormones, neurohumors, and other substances that are produced by the body and exert an effect on bodily functions. Called also *autopharmacological agent*.

authorization (aw″thor-i-za′shun) the act of giving permission to do something; permission. **prior a.,** in health insurance, approval by the carrier of treatment recommended by a participating dentist or physician before the provision of service. Called also *preauthorization, precertification, predetermination of benefits,* and *pretreatment*.

auto-, aut- [Gr. *autos* self] a prefix denoting relationship to self.

autoagglutination (aw″to-ah-gloo″tĭ-na′shun) 1. clumping or agglutination of an individual's cells by his own serum, as in autohemagglutination. Autoagglutination occurring at low temperatures is called *cold agglutination.* 2. agglutination of a particulate antigen, such as bacteria or erythrocytes, when suspended in physiological saline solution in the absence of specific antibody.

autoagglutinin (aw″to-ah-gloo″tĭ-nin) an autologous serum factor with the property of agglutinating the individual's own cellular elements; e.g., the red cells and blood platelets. An autoagglutinin that functions at low temperatures is called a *cold agglutinin.* **red cell a.,** autohemagglutinin.

autoallergic (aw″to-ah-ler′jik) pertaining to or characterized by autoallergy (autoimmunity); autoimmune.

autoallergy (aw″to-al′er-je) autoimmunity.

autoamputation (aw″to-am″pu-ta′shun) the spontaneous detachment from the body of an appendage or of an abnormal growth, such as a polyp.

autoanaphylaxis (aw″to-an″ah-fi-lak′sis) anaphylaxis from reactions within the body independent of the introduction of substances from without, and induced by substances derived from the individual himself; anaphylaxis induced by serum or other substance from the individual himself.

autoantibody (aw″to-an′tĭ-bod″e) an antibody (immunoglobulin) formed in response to, and reacting against, one of the individual's own normal antigenic endogenous body constituents.

autoanticomplement (aw″to-an″tĭ-kom′plĕ-ment) an anticomplement formed in the body against its own complement.

autoantigen (aw″to-an′tĭ-jen) an antigen that is a constituent of the tissue in the host. Under normal conditions, it is separated from the action of antibodies or immune cells by barriers, such as the membrane of a cell, but, under some abnormal conditions, the barrier may be breached through the effects of inflammation or acute infection with release of antigens that produce an immune response, triggering the host to mount an immunological attack against his own tissue. Called also *autologous antigen*. See also autoimmune DISEASE, AUTOIMMUNITY, and sequestered ANTIGEN.

autoantitoxin (aw″to-an″tĭ-tok′sin) an antitoxin produced actively by the body to protect it from injury by an endogenous homologous toxin.

autochthonous (aw-tok′tho-nus) [Gr. *autochtōn* sprung from the land itself] 1. found in the place of formation; not removed to a new site. 2. denoting a tissue graft to a new site on the same individual (autogenous graft); autoplastic. Cf. HETEROCHTHONOUS.

autoclave (aw′to-klāv) [auto- + L. *clavis* key] a steam sterilizer consisting of a hermetically closed container, in which the temperature of electrically heated water is allowed to raise to at least 121°C (250°F), at which point all living organisms are killed, with parallel increase in the steam pressure to more than 15 psi. Gauges are provided for controlling temperature and pressure levels. Dental and surgical instruments are placed in the autoclave after being thoroughly cleansed and wrapped or packed to permit easy penetration by the steam, and sterilized for no less than 20 minutes. Specially designed or adapted pressure cookers are sometimes used as autoclaves. See also CHEMICLAVE.

autoclaving (aw″to-klāv′ing) sterilization with the use of an autoclave.

Autoclip trademark for a stainless steel surgical clip inserted by means of a mechanical applier that automatically feeds a series of clips for wound closing.

autogeneic (aw″to-jĕ-ne′ik) autoplastic; autogenous; pertaining to an autograft.

autogenous (aw-toj′ĕ-nus) [auto- + *genesis*] 1. originated within; self-generated; autogeneic. 2. pertaining to tissue arising, transferred, or transplanted within an individual. 3. pertaining to a vaccine made from the patient's own bacteria, as opposed to stock vaccines which are made from standard cultures.

autograft (aw′to-graft) [auto- + *graft*] autogenous GRAFT.

autohemagglutination (aw″to-hem″ah-gloo″tĭ-na′shun) agglutination of the erythrocytes of the individual by his own serum.

autohemagglutinin (aw″to-hem″ah-gloo′tĭ-nin) an autoagglutinin which agglutinates the individual's own erythrocytes. Called also *red cell autoagglutinin*.

autohemolysin (aw″to-he-mol′ĭ-sin) a type of autoantibody or other self factor having the ability to lyse autologous erythrocytes.

autohemolysis (aw″to-he-mol′ĭ-sis) [auto- + *hemolysis*] hemolysis produced by agents present in a person's own serum.

autohemopsonin (aw″to-hem″op-so′nin) an opsonin that renders the red cells susceptible to phagocytosis and destruction by phagocytic cells of the patient's body.

autoimmune (aw″to-im-mun′) pertaining to or characterized by autoimmunity. Called also *autoallergic*.

autoimmunity (aw″to-im-mu′nĭ-te) a condition in which factors, such as inflammation, acute infections, or other factors, cause the host to mount an immunological attack against its own tissue, being either a specific humoral immune (autoantibody-mediated) response or cell-mediated immunity. Conditions in which the response results in tissue damage with or without clinical symptoms are referred to as *hypersensitivity;* those associated with clinical abnormalities as *autoimmune diseases*. Called also *autoallergy*. See also AUTOANTIBODY and AUTOANTIGEN.

autoimmunization (aw″to-im″u-ni-za′shun) The induction in an individual of an immune response to its own tissue constituents, which may lead to pathological sequelae, i.e., to autoimmune disease. Called also *autosensitization*. See also AUTOANTIBODY.

autoinfection (aw″to-in-fek′shun) [auto- + *infection*] infection by an agent already present in the body or transferred from one part of the body to another.

autointoxication (aw″to-in-tok″sĭ-ka′shun) [auto- + *intoxication*] intoxication by some poison generated within the body.

autokinesis (aw″to-ki-ne′sis) [*auto-* + Gr. *kinēsis* motion] voluntary motion.

autologous (aw-tol′o-gus) [*auto-* + Gr. *logos* relation] related to self- designating products or components of the same individual organism.

autolysate (aw-tol′ĭ-sāt) a substance or substances produced by autolysis.

autolysis (aw-tol′ĭ-sis) [*auto-* + Gr. *lysis* dissolution] the disintegration of tissue, especially individual cells or groups of cells, by the action of their own autogenous lysosomal enzymes. See also NECROSIS.

automatic (aw″to-mat′ik) [Gr. *automatos* self-acting] 1. spontaneous or involuntary; done by no act of the will. 2. self-moving; self-regulating.

automaton (aw-tom′ah-ton″) 1. any mechanical device designed to act as if by its own motive power. 2. a detachable, flexible instrument designed to stabilize the tongue, or to retract the tongue or the cheek. Some types are designed with interchangeable reflective mirrors on the side of the apparatus to be placed next to the restorative or operative area.

autonomic (aw″to-nom′ik) [*auto-* + Gr. *nomos* law] 1. independent, self-controlling. 2. pertaining to the autonomic nervous system.

autoplant (aw′to-plant) autogenous GRAFT.

autoplast (aw′to-plast) autogenous GRAFT.

autoplastic (aw″to-plas′tik) 1. pertaining to autoplasty. 2. autochthonous.

autoplasty (aw′to-plas″te) [*auto-* + Gr. *plassein* to form] plastic repair of injured or diseased tissue by transplanting tissue taken from another part of the patient's own body. See also autogenous GRAFT and autogenous TRANSPLANTATION.

autoprothrombin (aw″to-pro-throm′bin) an activation product of prothrombin. **a. C,** FACTOR X. **a. I,** FACTOR VII. **a. II,** FACTOR IX.

autopsy (aw′top-se) [*auto-* + Gr. *opsis* view] the postmortem examination of the body; necropsy.

autoradiography (aw″to-ra″de-og′rah-fe) the making of a radiograph of an object or tissue by recording on a photographic plate the radiation emitted by the examined object or tissue; used most commonly for studying DNA synthesis in chromosomes labeled with tritiated thymidine. Called also *radioautography*.

autosensitization (aw″to-sen″sĭ-ti-za′shun) autoimmunization.

autosite (aw′to-sīt) [*auto-* + Gr. *sitos* food] the larger more nearly normal component of asymmetrically conjoined twins, to which the parasite is attached.

autosomal (aw″to-so′mal) pertaining to an autosome.

autosome (aw′to-sōm) [*auto-* + Gr. *sōma* body] any chromosome other than a sex chromosome; in man there are 22 pairs of autosomes. See additional terms under CHARACTER.

autotransformer (aw″to-trans-for′mer) [*auto-* + *transformer*] an electrical device which controls the voltage of an alternating current. It consists of a single wire wrapped around a soft iron core; the selected voltage reflecting the number of windings around the core. In an x-ray machine, it serves as the kilovoltage selector. See also TRANSFORMER.

autotroph (aw′to-trōf) autotrophic CELL.

autotrophic (aw″to-trof′ik) [*auto-* + Gr. *trophē* nutrition] self-nourishing; said of cells which derive carbon directly from carbon dioxide. See autotrophic CELL. Cf. HETEROTROPHIC.

Auveloper trademark for a large capacity automatic film processor.

auxiliary (awk-sil′e-aře) [L. *auxiliaris*] 1. affording aid. 2. one who affords aid; ancillary. See also ancillary PERSONNEL. 3. an accessory device or appliance. **dental a.,** a person who assists a dentist in performing dental services. By general usage, dental auxiliaries include chairside assistants, dental hygienists, and laboratory technicians, but exclude the ancillary personnel. **dental a., expanded duty, dental a., expanded function,** former name for extended function dental assistant; see under ASSISTANT. **Dental A. Utilization,** see DAU. **torquing a.,** an accessory arch wire used to apply torsion on a tooth in any of the three planes of space; used in orthodontic therapy. **Women's A. to the American Dental Association,** an association of the wives of active and retired members of the American Dental Association and the widows of former members. Its purpose is to assist the American Dental Association in its objective of encouraging the improvement of the health of the public. Abbreviated *WAADA.*

auxo- [Gr. *auxē* increase] a combining form denoting relationship to growth.

A/V ampere/volt; see SIEMENS.

AV, A-V arteriovenous; atrioventricular; auriculoventricular.

Av average; avoirdupois (see under WEIGHT).

Avagal trademark for *methantheline bromide* (see under METHANTHELINE).

availability (ah-va″lah-bil′ĭ-te) 1. the state of being suitable, accessible, or ready for use; at hand. 2. a measure, in terms of type, volume, and location, of the supply of health resources and services relative to the need (or demand) of a given individual or community.

avascular (ah-vas′ku-lar) [*a* neg. + *vascular*] not supplied with blood vessels.

avascularization (ah-vas″ku-lar-i-za′shun) the diversion of blood from tissue, accomplished either by ligating vessels or by applying tight elastic bandages.

Avellis' syndrome [George *Avellis,* German laryngologist, 1864–1916] see under SYNDROME.

Avenzoar [1113–1162] a renowned Islamic physician born in Seville, Spain, whose principal writing was a compendium of practice, *al-Teïsir,* which contains many interesting clinical reports. Also in his writings he described the itch-mite (*Acarus scabiei*), and did not hesitate to criticize Galen. He taught Averroes. Called also *Ibn Zuhr.*

Averroes [1126–1198] a distinguished Islamic philosopher and physician, born at Cordoba. Better known as a philosopher, his chief philosophical work is his commentary on Aristotle; his chief medical work is the *Colliget,* a predominantly philosophical approach to a system of medicine. Called also as *Ibn Rushd.*

Aviadenovirus (a″vĭ-ad″ĕ-no-vi′rus) [L. *avis* bird + *adenovirus*] a genus of adenoviruses, producing a wide variety of diseases in birds and fowl.

Avicenna [980–1037] a celebrated Persian physician and philosopher, surnamed the "Prince of Physicians." His great encyclopedia, the *Canon,* written in Arabic, influenced medical thought and teaching for hundreds of years, its dogmatic, pontifical style having particular appeal for the medieval physician. He discussed the filing of elongated teeth and reported that "in order to have loosened teeth become firm again, one must avoid using same in mastication." He wrote on diseases of the gingiva, such as ulcers, suppuration, recession, and fissures. Called also as *Ibn Sina.*

avidin (av′ĭ-din) a basic protein in chicken egg white, which binds biotin, rendering it inactive. A diet consisting of large amounts of raw egg white may produce biotin deficiency.

avidity (a-vid′ĭ-te) eagerness; greediness. **antibody a.,** ANTIBODY avidity.

Avipoxvirus (a″vĭ-poks-vi′rus) [L. *avis* bird + *poxvirus*] a genus of poxviruses causing skin diseases in wild birds and domestic fowl.

avirulence (a-vir′u-lens) lack of virulence; lack of competence of an infectious agent to produce pathologic effect.

avitaminosis (a-vi″tah-mĭ-no′sis) a condition due to deficiency of vitamins. For specific types of vitamin deficiency, see the specific vitamin. **a. B₂,** Strachan-Scott SYNDROME.

avivement (ah-vev-mont′) [Fr.] the refreshing of the edges of a wound by surgical procedures.

AVLINE Audiovisuals Online; an acronym for computer-searchable data bank containing references to audiovisual teaching packages, used in health science education, sponsored by the National Library of Medicine.

Avlocardyl trademark for *propranolol.*

Avloprocil trademark for *penicillin G procaine* (see under PENICILLIN).

Avogadro's law, number (constant) [Amadeo *Avogadro,* Italian physicist, 1776–1856] see under LAW and NUMBER.

avogram (av′o-gram) one-septillionth (10^{-24}) of a gram, or 1 picopicogram; so named from Avogardo's number, 6.03×10^{23}. The mass of a molecule in avograms is therefore 1.66 times its conventional molecular weight.

avoirdupois (av″er-dŭ-poiz′) [Fr. *avoir* property + L. *de* of + *pois* weight] a system of weights; see avoirdupois WEIGHT.

avulsion (ah-vul′shun) [L. *avulsio,* from *a* away + *vellere* to pull] the tearing away of a part of a structure.

awu atomic weight unit; see atomic mass UNIT.

Axeropthol trademark for *vitamin A.*

axes (ak′sēz) [L.] plural of *axis.*

axial (ak′se-al) pertaining to an axis or any axis-like structure, as to the long axis of a tooth.

axifugal (ak-sif′u-gal) [*axis* + L. *fugere* to flee] directed away from an axon or axis.

axio- [L. *axis,* Gr. *axōn* axle] a combining form denoting relationship to an axis, especially the long axis of a tooth, as in the names of cavity angles.

axiobuccal (ak″se-o-buk′kal) [*axio-* + L. *buccalis,* from *bucca* cheek] pertaining to the axial and buccal walls of a tooth cavity.

axiobuccocervical (ak-se-o-buk″ko-ser′vĭ-kal) pertaining to or formed by the axial, buccal, and cervical walls of a tooth cavity preparation.

axiobuccogingival (ak"se-o-buk"ko-jin'ji-val) pertaining to or formed by the axial, buccal, and gingival walls of a tooth cavity preparation.

axiobuccolingual (ak"se-o-buk"ko-ling'gwal) pertaining to the long axis of the buccal and lingual surfaces of a posterior tooth.

axiocervical (ak"se-o-ser'vi-kal) axiogingival.

axiodistal (ak"se-o-dis'tal) pertaining to or formed by the axial and distal walls of a tooth cavity preparation.

axiodistocervical (ak"se-o-dis"to-ser'vi-kal) distoaxiogingival.

axiodistogingival (ak"se-o-dis"to-jin'ji-val) distoaxiogingival.

axiodistoincisal (ak"se-o-dis"to-in-si'zal) distoaxioincisal.

axiodisto-occlusal (ak"se-o-dis"to-o-kloo'zal) distoaxio-occlusal.

axiogingival (ak"se-o-jin'ji-val) pertaining to or formed by the axial and gingival walls of a tooth cavity preparation. Called also *axiocervical.*

axioincisal (ak"se-o-in-si'zal) pertaining to or formed by the axial and incisal walls of a tooth cavity preparation.

axiolabial (ak"se-o-la'be-al) pertaining to or formed by the axial and labial walls of a tooth cavity preparation.

axiolabiogingival (ak"se-o-la"be-o-jin'ji-val) labioaxiogingival.

axiolabiolingual (ak"se-o-la"be-o-ling'gwal) pertaining to the long axis and the labial and lingual surfaces of an anterior tooth.

axiolingual (ak"se-o-ling'gwal) pertaining to or formed by the axial and lingual walls of a tooth cavity preparation.

axiolinguocervical (ak"se-o-ling"gwo-ser'vi-kal) linguoaxiogingival.

axiolinguogingival (ak"se-o-ling"gwo-jin'ji-val) linguoaxiogingival.

axiolinguo-occlusal (ak"se-o-ling"gwo-o-kloo'zal) pertaining to or formed by the axial, lingual, and occlusal walls of a tooth cavity preparation.

axiomesial (ak"se-o-me'ze-al) mesioaxial.

axiomesiocervical (ak"se-o-me"ze-o-ser'vi-kal) mesioaxiogingival.

axiomesiodistal (ak"se-o-me"ze-o-dis'tal) pertaining to the long axis and the mesial and distal surfaces of a tooth.

axiomesiogingival (ak"se-o-me"ze-o-jin'-ji-val) mesioaxiogingival.

axiomesioincisal (ak"se-o-me"ze-o-in-si'zal) mesioaxioincisal.

axio-occlusal (ak"se-o-o-kloo'zal) pertaining to or formed by the axial and occlusal walls of a tooth cavity preparation.

axiopulpal (ak"se-o-pul'pal) pertaining to or formed by the axial and pulpal walls of a tooth cavity preparation.

axipetal (ak-sip'e-tal) [*axis* + L. *petere* to seek] directed toward or facing an axon or axis.

axis (ak'sis), pl. *ax'es* [L.; Gr. *axōn* axle] 1. a straight line about which a body or a geometric structure would rotate if it did revolve; used as a general term in anatomical nomenclature. See also BREADTH, HEIGHT, LENGTH, and PLANE. 2. the second cervical vertebra. **basibregmatic a.,** the vertical distance from basion to bregma, representing the maximum height of the cranium. **basicranial a.,** a line from basion to gonion. See also Huxley's PLANE. **basifacial a.,** a line joining the gonion and the subnasal point. Called also *facial a.* **binauricular a.,** a line joining the two porions. **cephalocaudal a.,** the long or vertical axis of the body. **condylar a.,** a line through the transverse axis of the two mandibular condyles around which the mandible may rotate during a part of the opening movement of the jaw. Called also *condylar chord.* **condylar a., condyle a.,** mandibular a. **craniofacial a.,** the axis of the bones at the base of the skull, including the mesethmoid, presphenoid, basisphenoid, and basioccipital. **a. cylinder,** axon. **dorsoventral a.,** any line in the sagittal plane at a right angle to the long axis of the body. **Downs' Y a., Y a. facial a.,** basifacial a. **hinge a.,** mandibular a. **horizontal a.,** mandibular a. **long a. of body,** the imaginary straight longitudinal line passing through the neck, thorax, abdomen, and pelvis. **longitudinal a.,** an imaginary anteroposterior line through a mandibular condyle around which the mandible may rotate in a rolling motion. **mandibular a.,** an imaginary line through two mandibular condyles around which the mandible rotates without translatory movement. Called also *condylar a., condyle a., hinge a., horizontal a.,* and *transverse a.* See also hinge axis POINT. **opening a.,** an imaginary line around which the condyles may rotate during opening and closing movements of the mandible. **a. of preparation,** the directional path taken by a dental restoration as it slides on or off the preparation. See also PATH of insertion. **sagittal a. of mandible,** an imaginary anteroposterior line through the mandibular condyle around which a mandible may rotate in a yawing or pitching motion. **thyroid a.,** thyrocervical TRUNK. **transverse a.,** mandibular a. **vertical a. (of mandible),** an axis about which the condyle rotates at the time of homolateral motion of the mandible. **Y a.,** the angle of a line connecting the sella turcica and the gnathion as related to the Frankfort Horizontal; it is an indicator of downward and forward growth of the mandible. Called also *Downs' Y a.*

axistyle (ak'si-stil) the pair of axial fibrils observed in bacteria of the genus *Leptospira,* which is the organ of locomotion. Called also *axial filament.*

axolemma (ak"so-lem'ah) [*axon* + Gr. *eilēma* a sheath] the plasma membrane of an axon. Called also *Mauthner's membrane* and *Mauthner's sheath.* See also NEURILEMMA.

axon (ak'son) [Gr. *axōn* axle, axis] 1. the axis of the body; the vertebral column. 2. a slender, elongated process extending from a neuron, which contains neurofibrils and mitochondria, has a smooth surface, and terminates with several twiglike branches (telodendrons), sometimes having collaterals running along its course. It transmits nerve impulses away from the cell body. Called also *axis cylinder.* See illustration at NERVE. **a. reflex,** axon REFLEX. **a. terminals,** synaptic terminals; see under TERMINAL.

axoplasm (ak'so-plazm) [*axon* + *plasma*] the cytoplasm of an axon. Called also *hyaloplasm.*

Ayala's quotient (equation index) [A. G. *Ayala,* Italian neurologist, 1878–1943] see under QUOTIENT.

Ayerza's syndrome [Abel *Ayerza,* Buenos Aires physician, 1861–1918] see under SYNDROME.

Ayfivin trademark for *bacitracin.*

Azachloramide trademark for *chloroazodin.*

azacyclopropane (ah"zah-si"klo-pro'pān) ethylenimine.

Azapen trademark for *methicillin.*

azaribine (ah-zar'i-bēn) the triacetyl derivative of 6-azauridine, 2-β-D-ribofuranosyl-*as*-triazine-3,5(2*H*,4*H*)-dione-2',3'6-triacetate, obtained from cultures of *Escherichia coli.* It is a pyrimidine analogue which becomes deacetylated in the blood to 6-azauridine and 6-azauridylic acid, inhibiting the formation of uridylic acid by blocking the enzyme orotidylate decarboxylase, thereby interfering with pyrimidine biosynthesis. Used in the treatment of psoriasis, mycosis fungoides, and polycythemia vera. The adverse reactions associated with azaribine are less severe than those of other pyrimidine analogues, but may include erythropoietic disorders, drowsiness, lethargy, vertigo, hyperreflexia, tremor, diplopia, aphagia, dysarthria, and thromboembolism. Trademark: Triazure.

Azaron trademark for *tripelennamine.*

6-azauridine (ah"zah-u'ri-dēn) a pyrimidine analogue obtained from *Escherichia coli* cultures, 2-β-D-ribofuranosyl-1,2,4-triazine-3,5 (2*H*, 4*H*)-dione. In the blood, it is converted to azauridylic acid, inhibiting the formation of uridylic acid by blocking the enzyme orotidylate decarboxylase, thereby interfering with pyrimidine biosynthesis. Used in the treatment of psoriasis, mycosis fungoides, and polycythemia vera. Its adverse reactions may include erythropoietic disorders, drowsiness, lethargy, vertigo, hyperreflexia, tremor, diplopia, aphagia, dysarthria, and thromboembolism. Called also *6-azauracil riboside* (AzUr). Trademark: Ribo-Azauracil.

aziridine (ah-zir'i-dēn) ethylenimine.

azo- a chemical prefix indicating the presence of the group $-N:N-$, as in azobenzene or azo dye.

azobenzene (az"o-ben'zēn) the parent substance of azo dyes and some pH indicators, $C_6H_5N_2C_6H_5$, occurring as yellow or orange crystals that are soluble in alcohol and ether, but not in water. Used as a fumigant, acaricide, and rubber accelerator. Exposure may cause liver lesions. Called also *benzeneazobenzene, diphenyldiazine,* and *diphenyldiimide.*

azole (az'ōl) pyrrole.

Azolmetazin trademark for *sulfamethazine.*

Azomonas (ah-zo-mo'nas) [Fr. *azote* nitrogen + Gr. *monas* unit] a genus of nitrogen-fixing bacteria of the family Azotobacteraceae.

azote (az'ōt) [*a* neg. + Gr. *zōe* life] nitrogen.

azotemia (az"o-te'me-ah) [*azote* + Gr. *haima* blood + *-ia*] excessive concentration of urea or other nitrogenous bodies in the blood. Called also *nitremia.*

Azotobacter (ah-zo'to-bak"ter) [Fr. *azote* + Gr. *baktērion* little rod] a genus of bacteria of the family Azotobacteraceae, found chiefly in soil and water.

Azotobacteraceae (ah-zo"to-bak"tĕ-re'se-e) [*Azobacter* + *-aceae*] a family of nitrogen-fixing, gram-negative, aerobic, rod-shaped bacteria, inhabiting chiefly water, soil, and some plants. It includes the genera *Azotobacter, Azomonas,* and *Beijerinckia.*

azoturia (az"o-tu're-ah) [*azote* + Gr. *ouron* urine] an excess of urea or other nitrogen compounds in the urine.

AzUr 6-azauridine.

B 1. point B (see SUPRAMENTALE). 2. Bolton POINT. 3. bregma. 4. blood group B (see under BLOOD GROUP). 5. boron. 6. gauss.

b 1. barn. 2. point B (see SUPRAMENTALE).

β the second letter of the Greek alphabet. See BETA.

β⁺ position.

Ba 1. barium. 2. basion.

ba basion.

Baader's dermatostomatitis, syndrome [Ernst *Baader*, German physician] Stevens-Johnson SYNDROME.

Babbit metal [Isaac *Babbitt*, American inventor, 1799–1862] see under METAL.

babbling (bab'ling) 1. foolish or meaningless chatter. 2. the random production of meaningless vocal sounds characteristic of infants from about the sixth week of age.

babe (bāb) a baby or child; infant. **battered b.**, battered CHILD.

Babinski-Nageotte syndrome [Joseph François Felix *Babinski*, French neurologist, 1857–1932; Jean *Nageotte*, French pathologist, 1866–1948] see under SYNDROME.

Bacarate trademark for *phendimetrazine tartrate* (see under PHENDIMETRAZINE).

Baciferm trademark for *bacitracin zinc* (see under BACITRACIN).

Bacillaceae (bas″il-la′se-e) [*bacillus* + *-aceae*] a family of rod-shaped, chiefly gram-positive bacteria, made up of cells capable of producing cylindrical, ellipsoidal, or spherical endospores, which are terminally, subterminally, or centrally located. The spores contain central cells enclosed by a cortex of peptidoglycan and an outer spore protein coat. Most are found in soil and dust. The family includes the genera *Bacillus, Clostridium, Desulfotomaculum, Sporolactobacillus,* and *Sporosarcina.*

bacilli (bah-sil′i) [L.] plural of *bacillus.*

Bacillus (bah-sil′us) [L. "little rod"] a genus of gram-positive, aerobic bacteria of the family Bacillaceae, including large (about 0.3 to 2.2 by 1.2 to 7.0 μm) organisms, separated into more than 30 species, of which only a few are actually or potentially pathogenic, the remainder being saprophytic soil forms. Bacilli are rod-shaped, straight or nearly straight cells, most of which are motile and have lateral flagella. They generally form catalase and their metabolism is respiratory, fermentative, or both. Many organisms historically classified in *Bacillus* have been now assigned to other genera. **B. ac′nes,** *Propionibacterium acnes;* see under PROPIONIBACTERIUM. **B. adeni′tis e′qui,** *Streptococcus equi;* see under STREPTOCOCCUS. **B. aegyp′tius,** *Haemophilus aegyptius;* see under HAEMOPHILUS. **B. aerog′enes,** *Enterobacter aerogenes;* see under ENTEROBACTER. **B. aerog′enes capsula′tus,** *Clostridium perfringens;* see under CLOSTRIDIUM. **B. aerugino′sus,** *Pseudomonas aeruginosa;* see under PSEUDOMONAS. **B. anaero′bius diphtheroi′des,** *Propionibacterium acnes;* see under PROPIONIBACTERIUM. **B. an′thracis,** the causative agent of anthrax. It is a large, nonmotile pathogenic bacterium (about 3 to 5 by 1 to 1.5 μm), which stains with aniline dyes. The members occur singly or in end-to-end pairs or short chains, forming spores which are most abundant at 32 to 35°C and under aerobic conditions, being either free or located centrally within the cell. Under ordinary conditions of culture, exotoxin is not produced, nor is the cell substance toxic; however, under special growth conditions exotoxin production occurs. Called also *B. cereus* var. *anthracis* and *anthrax bacillus.* **B. botuli′nus,** *Clostridium botulinum;* see under CLOSTRIDIUM. **B. bre′vis,** *Flavobacterium breve;* see under FLAVOBACTERIUM. **B. bronchica′nis, B. bronchisep′ticus,** *Bordetella bronchiseptica;* see under BORDETELLA. **B. bullo′sus,** *Fusobacterium bullosum;* see under FUSOBACTERIUM. **B. cadav′eris budayi′ricus,** *Eubacterium budayi;* see under EUBACTERIUM. **B. cana′lis par′vus,** *Flavobacterium breve;* see under FLAVOBACTERIUM. **B. capillo′sus,** *Bacteroides capillosus;* see under BACTEROIDES. **B. ce′reus,** a species that causes food poisoning in man. **B. ce′reus var. an′thracis,** *B. anthracis.* **B. chol′erae, B. chol′erae-asiat′icae.** *Vibrio cholerae;* see under VIBRIO. **B. chol′erae-su′is,** *Salmonella cholerae-suis;* see under SALMONELLA. **B. cloa′cae,** *Enterobacter cloacae;* see under ENTEROBACTER. **B. co′li,** *Escherichia coli;* see under ESCHERICHIA. **B. conjunctivit′idis,** *Haemophilus aegyptius;* see under HAEMOPHILUS. **B. diphthe′riae,** *Corynebacterium diphtheriae;* see under CORYNEBACTERIUM. **B. dysente′riae,** *Shigella dysenteriae;* see under SHIGELLA. **B. enterit′idis,** *Salmonella enteritidis;* see under SALMONELLA. **B. fluores′cens,** *Pseudomonas fluorescens;* see under PSEUDOMONAS. **B. foe′dans,** *Eubacterium foedans;* see under EUBACTERIUM. **B. frag′ilis,** *Bacteroides fragilis;* see under BACTEROIDES. **B. funduliform′mis,** *Fusobacterium necrophorum;* see

under FUSOBACTERIUM. **B. furco′sus,** *Bacteroides furcosus;* see under BACTEROIDES. **B. fusifor′mis,** *Fusobacterium nucleatum;* see under FUSOBACTERIUM. **B. gallina′rum,** *Salmonella gallinarum;* see under SALMONELLA. **B. glutino′sus,** *Fusobacterium glutinosum;* see under FUSOBACTERIUM. **B. helminthoi′des,** *Eubacterium helminthoides;* see under EUBACTERIUM. **B. hepatodystroph′icus,** *Propionibacterium acnes;* see under PROPIONIBACTERIUM. **B. histolyt′icus,** *Clostridium histolyticum;* see under CLOSTRIDIUM. **B. incon′stans,** *Proteus inconstans;* see under PROTEUS. **B. influenzaefor′mis,** *Fusobacterium russii;* see under FUSOBACTERIUM. **B. lacuna′tus,** *Moraxella lacunata;* see under MORAXELLA. **B. lep′rae,** *Mycobacterium leprae;* see under MYCOBACTERIUM. **B. lympho′philus,** *Propionibacterium lymphophilum; see under* PROPIONIBACTERIUM. **B. mal′lei,** *Pseudomonas mallei;* see under PSEUDOMONAS. **B. marces′cens,** *Serratia marcescens;* see under SERRATIA. **B. monilifor′me,** *Eubacterium moniliforme;* see under EUBACTERIUM. **B. mortif′erus,** *Fusobacterium mortiferum;* see under FUSOBACTERIUM. **B. muco′sus anaero′bius,** *Fusobacterium prausnitzii;* see under FUSOBACTERIUM. **B. muco′sus ozae′nae,** *Klebsiella ozaenae;* see under KLEBSIELLA. **B. multifor′mis,** *Eubacterium multiforme;* see under EUBACTERIUM. **B. necroph′orus,** *Fusobacterium necrophorum.* **B. necrot′icus,** *Fusobacterium mortiferum;* see under FUSOBACTERIUM. **B. no′vyi, B. oedemat′iens, B. oede′matis malig′ni No. II,** *Clostridium novyi;* see under CLOSTRIDIUM. **B. ozae′nae,** *Klebsiella ozaenae;* see under KLEBSIELLA. **B. parapertus′sis,** *Bordetella parapertussis;* see under BORDETELLA. **B. paraty′phi-al′vei,** *Hafnia alvei;* see under HAFNIA. **B. par′vus liquefa′ciens,** *Propionibacterium acnes;* see under PROPIONIBACTERIUM. **B. perfrin′gens,** *Clostridium perfringens;* see under CLOSTRIDIUM. **B. pes′tis,** *Yersinia pestis;* see under YERSINIA. **B. phleg′monis emphysemato′sae,** *Clostridium perfringens;* see under CLOSTRIDIUM. **B. plau′ti,** *Fusobacterium plauti;* see under FUSOBACTERIUM. **B. pneumo′niae,** *Klebsiella pneumoniae;* see under KLEBSIELLA. **B. pneumosin′tes,** *Bacteroides pneumosintes;* see under BACTEROIDES. **B. pola′ris sep′ticus,** *Pasteurella multocida;* see under PASTEURELLA. **B. pseudodiphtherit′icus,** *Corynebacterium pseudodiphtheriticum;* see under CORYNEBACTERIUM. **B. pseudomal′lei,** *Pseudomonas pseudomallei;* see under PSEUDOMONAS. **B. pseudotuberculo′sis,** *Corynebacterium pseudotuberculosis;* see under CORYNEBACTERIUM. **B. putre′dinis,** *Bacteroides putredinis;* see under BACTEROIDES. **B. pyocya′neus,** *Pseudomonas aeruginosa;* see under PSEUDOMONAS. **B. radiifor′mis,** *Bacteroides serpens;* see under BACTEROIDES. **B. rapa′zii,** *Eubacterium moniliforme;* see under EUBACTERIUM. **B. rhusiopa′thiae,** *Erysipelothrix rhusiopathiae;* see under ERYSIPELOTHRIX. **B. schottmuel′leri,** *Salmonella schottmuelleri;* see under SALMONELLA. **B. sep′ticus,** *Clostridium septicum;* see under CLOSTRIDIUM. **B. ser′pens,** *Bacteroides serpens;* see under BACTEROIDES. **B. shi′gae,** *Shigella dysenteriae;* see under SHIGELLA. **B. sporog′enes,** *Clostridium sporogenes;* see under CLOSTRIDIUM. **B. te′nuis spatulifor′mis,** *Eubacterium tenue;* see under EUBACTERIUM. **B. tet′ani,** *Clostridium tetani;* see under CLOSTRIDIUM. **B. tortuo′sus,** *Eubacterium tortuosum;* see under EUBACTERIUM. **B. tuberculo′sis,** *Mycobacterium tuberculosis;* see under MYCOBACTERIUM. **B. tuberculo′sis gallina′rum,** *Mycobacterium avium;* see under MYCOBACTERIUM. **B. ty′phi,** *Salmonella typhi;* see under SALMONELLA. **B. ty′phi mu′rium,** *Salmonella typhimurium;* see under SALMONELLA. **B. ventrio′sus,** *Eubacterium ventriosum;* see under EUBACTERIUM. **B. welch′ii,** *Clostridium tetani;* see under CLOSTRIDIUM. **B. xero′sis,** *Corynebacterium xerosis;* see under CORYNEBACTERIUM.

bacillus (bah-sil′us), pl. *bacil′li* [L.] 1. any microorganism of the genus *Bacillus.* 2. in general, any rod-shaped bacterium. **aerobic bacilli,** see BACILLUS. **anaerobic bacilli,** see CLOSTRIDIUM. **anthrax b.,** *Bacillus anthracis;* see under BACILLUS. **Bang's b.,** *Brucella abortus;* see under BRUCELLA. **Bordet-Gengou b.,** *Bordetella pertussis;* see under BORDETELLA. **botulism b.,** *Clostridium botulinum;* see under CLOSTRIDIUM. **coli b., colon b.,** *Escherichia coli;* see under ESCHERICHIA. **Ducrey's b.,** *Haemophilus ducreyi;* see under HAEMOPHILUS. **dysentery b.,** *Shigella dysenteriae;* see under SHIGELLA. **enteric b.,** any bacillus of the family Enterobacteriaceae. **Escherich's b.,** *Escherichia coli;* see under ESCHERICHIA. **Flexner's b.,** *Shigella flexneri;* see under SHIGELLA. **Frankel's b.,** *Clostridium perfringens;* see under CLOSTRIDIUM. **Friedländer's b.,** *Klebsiella pneumoniae;* see under KLEBSIELLA. **Ghon-Sacks b.,** *Clostridium septicum;* see under CLOSTRIDIUM. **glanders b.,** *Pseudomonas mal-*

lei; see under PSEUDOMONAS. **Hansen's b.,** *Mycobacterium leprae;* see under MYCOBACTERIUM. **hemolytic influenza b.,** *Haemophilus parahaemolyticus;* see under HAEMOPHILUS. **Hofmann's b.,** *Corynebacterium pseudodiphtheriticum;* see under CORYNEBACTERIUM. **influenza b.,** *Haemophilus influenzae;* see under HAEMOPHILUS. **Johne's b.,** *Mycobacterium paratuberculosis;* see under MYCOBACTERIUM. **Klebs-Loeffler b.,** *Corynebacterium diphtheriae;* see under CORYNEBACTERIUM. **Koch-Weeks b.,** *Haemophilus aegyptius;* see under HAEMOPHILUS. **leprosy b.,** *Mycobacterium leprae;* see under MYCOBACTERIUM. **leprosy b., rat,** *Mycobacterium lepraemurium;* see under MYCOBACTERIUM. **Novy's b.,** *Clostridium novyi;* see under CLOSTRIDIUM. **b. paratyphoid C,** *Salmonella hirschfeldii;* see under SALMONELLA. **plague b.,** *Yersinia pestis;* see under YERSINIA. **Preisz-Nocard b.,** *Corynebacterium pseudotuberculosis;* see under CORYNEBACTERIUM. **rat leprosy b.,** *Mycobacterium lepraemurium;* see under MYCOBACTERIUM. **Schmitz's b.,** *Shigella dysenteriae* (type 2); see under SHIGELLA. **Shiga's b.,** *Shigella dysenteriae* (type 1); see under SHIGELLA. **tetanus b.,** *Clostridium tetani;* see under CLOSTRIDIUM. **tubercle b.,** *Mycobacterium tuberculosis;* see under MYCOBACTERIUM. **Whitmore's b.,** *Pseudomonas pseudomallei;* see under PSEUDOMONAS. **yellow b.,** *Mycobacterium kansasii;* see under MYCOBACTERIUM.

bacitracin (bas″ĭ-tra′sin) a polypeptide antibiotic from a strain of *Bacillus subtilis,* believed to consist of at least nine components, *bacitracin A* being the principal one. It occurs as a white to buff, odorless, hygroscopic powder that is readily soluble in water, ethanol, methanol, and glacial acetic acid, but not in acetone, chloroform, or ether. Bacitracin inhibits bacterial cell synthesis, being active against gram-positive cocci and bacilli, including *Neisseria, Haemophilus influenzae, Treponema pallidum, Actinomyces,* and *Fusobacterium.* Also used in the treatment of amebiasis. Pain, induration, and petechiae at the site of injection, rash, malaise, anorexia, nausea, vomiting, and a peculiar taste are some of the side effects. Parenteral application may result in severe nephrotoxicity. Hypersensitivity may occur. Trademarks: Ayfivin, Penitracin, Topitracin, and Zutracin. **b. zinc,** the zinc salt of bacitracin, occurring as a white to pale tan, odorless powder that is sparingly soluble in water. It has actions similar to those of the parent drug, and is incorporated in various ointments and in postsurgical and periodontal dressings. Trademark: Baciferm.

back (bak) 1. the posterior aspect of any part. 2. the posterior part of the trunk from the neck to the pelvis.

back-cross (bak′kros) a mating of a heterozygote to a recessive homozygote (A/a × a/a) in which the progeny (½ A/a, ½ a/a) reveal the genotype of the heterozygous parent.

backing (bak′ing) in dentistry, a piece of metal that supports a porcelain or resin facing on a fixed or removable partial denture. **alloy b.,** one made of an alloy instead of pure platinum or gold.

backlog (bak′log) 1. an accumulation, as of work left undone. 2. accrued needs; see under NEED.

backscatter (bak′skat-er) radiation deflected by scattering processes at angles greater than 90 degrees to the original direction of the beam of radiation. See also backscatter FACTOR, scattered rays, under RAY, and SCATTERING.

bacteremia (bak″tĕr-e′me-ah) [Gr. *baktērion* little rod + *haima* blood + *-ia*] the presence of bacteria in the blood. **posttreatment b.,** appearance of bacteria in the blood following a therapeutic procedure, such as bacteremia following scaling, curettage, or gingivectomy. In most instances, bacteremia is transient, but it may persist, particularly when aseptic procedures are not observed, eventually leading to infection, septicemia, and endocarditis. Streptococci and diphtheroids are the bacteria found most often in the blood after therapeutic oral procedures.

Bacteria (bak-te′re-ah) [L.] a division of the kingdom Procaryotae, including all prokaryotic microorganisms that are not bluegreen algae. Sometimes, prokaryotic microorganisms lacking a true cell wall are considered to be unrelated to the Bacteria, and are placed in a separate class — the Mollicutes. See also BACTERIUM.

bacteria (bak-te′re-ah) [L.] plural of *bacterium.*

bacterial (bak-te′re-al) pertaining to or caused by bacteria.

bactericidal (bak-tēr″ĭ-si′dal) [*bacterium* + L. *caedere* to kill] causing death of bacteria; killing bacteria; capable of killing bacteria.

bactericide (bak-tēr′ĭ-sīd) an agent capable of destroying bacteria (but not necessarily the spores) within 10 minutes after application. See also DISINFECTANT.

bacterin (bak′ter-in) a bacterial vaccine.

bacteriology (bak-te″re-ol′o-je) the field of study dealing with bacteria. See also MICROBIOLOGY.

bacteriolysis (bak-te″re-ol′ĭ-sis) [*bacterium* + Gr. *lysis* dissolution] disruption of the structural integrity of a bacterial cell resulting in the release of its cytoplasmic contents.

bacteriolytic (bak-te″re-o-lit′ik) pertaining to or causing destruction of bacteria.

Bacterionema (bak-te″re-o-ne′mah) [*bacterium* + Gr. *nēma* thread] a genus of bacteria of the family Actinomycetaceae, order Actinomycetales, occurring as facultative anaerobic, gram-positive, non–acid-fast, nonmotile, pleomorphic organisms, comprising nonseptate and septate filaments (about 1.0 to 1.5 by 20 to 200 μm in size) and bacilli (1.5 to 2.5 by 3.0 to 10.0 μm in size). **B. matrucho′tii,** a species found in the oral cavity of man and other primates, particularly in dental calculus and plaque. Subcutaneous or intradermal injections of live suspensions into mice produce nodules or abscesses.

bacteriophage (bak-te′re-o-fāj″) [*bacterium* + Gr. *phagein* to devour] a virus that lyses bacteria. The virus particle attaches itself to the bacterial cell wall and viral nucleoprotein enters the cell, resulting in the synthesis of virus and its liberation on physical disruption of the cell. Bacteriophages are usually specific for bacterial species, but they may be strain-specific or may infect more than one species of bacteria. Called also *bacterial virus* and *phage.*

bacteriosis (bak-te″re-o′sis) any bacterial disease.

bacteriostasis (bak-te″re-os′tah-sis, bak-te″re-o-sta′sis) [*bacterium* + Gr. *stasis* stoppage] the inhibition or retardation of the growth, but not the killing, of bacteria, usually by chemical or biological methods.

bacteriostat (bak-te′re-o-stat″) an agent that causes bacteriostasis.

bacteriostatic (bak-te″re-o-stat′ik) 1. inhibiting or retarding the growth or multiplication of bacteria without actually destroying them. 2. an agent that inhibits or retards the growth or multiplication of bacteria; a bacteriostatic agent.

bacteriotoxemia (bak-te″re-o-tok-se′me-ah) the presence of bacterial toxins in the blood.

bacteriotoxic (bak-te″re-o-tok′sik) 1. toxic to bacteria. 2. pertaining to or caused by bacterial toxin.

bacteriotropic (bak-te″re-o-trop′ik) [*bacterium* + Gr. *tropos* a turning] turning toward or changing bacteria; opsonic.

Bacterium (bak-te′re-um) [L., Gr. *baktērion* little rod] a name formerly given a genus of microorganisms, consisting of non–spore-forming, rod-shaped bacteria, not necessarily related closely, which were not formally defined in other genera. Organisms that were placed in this genus have now been assigned to other genera. **B. abor′tus,** *Brucella abortus;* see under BRUCELLA. **B. aegypti′acum,** *Haemophilus aegyptius;* see under HAEMOPHILUS. **B. aerog′enes,** *Enterobacter aerogenes;* see under ENTEROBACTER. **B. aerugine′um, B. aerugino′sum,** *Pseu-*

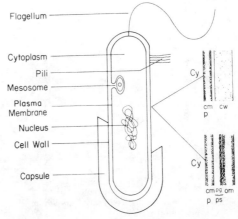

Diagrammatic representation of a typical bacterial cell. Not all structures are encountered in all cells. *Upper insert* shows structural details of the cell envelope of gram-positive cells; *lower insert* shows that of gram-negative cells. *Cy,* cytoplasm; *cm,* cell membrane; *cw,* cell wall of gram-positive bacteria; *om,* outer membrane of gram-negative cell envelope; *pg,* peptidoglycan layer; *ps,* periplasmic space. (Modified from B. A. Freeman: Burrows Textbook of Microbiology. 21st ed. Philadelphia, W. B. Saunders Co., 1979.)

domonas aeruginosa; see under PSEUDOMONAS. **B. bipol'are multo'cidum,** *Pasteurella multocida;* see under PASTEURELLA. **B. bre've,** *Flavobacterium breve;* see under FLAVOBACTERIUM. **B. buda'yi,** *Eubacterium budayi;* see under EUBACTERIUM. **B. cloa'cae,** *Enterobacter cloacae;* see under ENTEROBACTER. **B. co'li commu'ne,** *Escherichia coli;* see under ESCHERICHIA. **B. cylindroi'des,** *Eubacterium cylindroides;* see under EUBAC-TERIUM. **B. diphthe'riae,** *Corynebacterium diphtheriae;* see under CORYNEBACTERIUM. **B. dysente'riae,** *Shigella dysenteriae;* see under SHIGELLA. **B. fluores'cens,** *Pseudomonas fluorescens;* see under PSEUDOMONAS. **B. freun'dii,** *Citrobacter freundii;* see under CITROBACTER. **B. ga'yoni,** *Lactobacillus fermentum;* see under LACTOBACILLUS. **B. influen'zae,** *Haemophilus influenzae;* see under HAEMOPHILUS. **B. lac'tis,** *Streptococcus lactis;* see under STREPTOCOCCUS. **B. melaninogen'icum,** *Bacteroides melaninogenicus;* see under BACTEROIDES. **B. monocytog'enes, B. monocytog'enes hom'inis,** *Listeria monocytogenes;* see under LISTERIA. **B. multo'cidum,** *Pasteurella multocida;* see under PASTEURELLA. **B. ozae'nae,** *Klebsiella ozaenae;* see under KLEBSIELLA. **B. paraty'phi, B. paraty'phi ty'pus A,** *Salmonella paratyphi A;* see under SALMONELLA. **B. paraty'phi ty'pus B,** *Salmonella*

schottmuelleri; see under SALMONELLA. **B. pes'tis,** *Yersinia pestis;* see under YERSINIA. **B. pneumo'niae croupo'sae,** *Klebsiella pneumoniae;* see under KLEBSIELLA. **B. pneumosin'tes,** *Bacteroides pneumosintes;* see under BACTEROIDES. **B. pseudodiphtherit'icum,** *Corynebacterium pseudodiphtheriticum;* see under CORYNEBACTERIUM. **B. pseudotuberculo'sis,** *Yersinia pseudotuberculosis;* see under YERSINIA. **B. pullo'rum,** *Salmonella gallinarum;* see under SALMONELLA. **B. pyocya'neum,** *Pseudomonas aeruginosa;* see under PSEUDOMONAS. **B. rettge'ri,** *Proteus rettgeri;* see under PROTEUS. **B. rhinosclero-ma'tis,** *Klebsiella rhinoscleromatis;* see under KLEBSIELLA. **B. rhusiopa'thiae,** *Erysipelothrix rhusiopathiae;* see under ERYSIPELOTHRIX. **B. son'nei,** *Shigella sonnei;* see under SHIGELLA. **B. tuberculo'sis,** *Mycobacterium tuberculosis;* see under MYCOBACTERIUM. **B. tularen'sis,** *Francisella tularensis;* see under FRANCISELLA. **B. tus'sis-convulsi'vae,** *Bordetella pertussis;* see under BORDETELLA. **B. ty'phi,** *Salmonella typhi;* see under SALMONELLA. **B. whit'mori,** *Pseudomonas pseudomallei;* see under PSEUDOMONAS. **B. xero'sis,** *Corynebacterium xerosis;* see under CORYNEBACTERIUM. **B. zoogleifor'mans,** *Fusobacterium prausnitzii;* see under FUSOBACTERIUM.

bacterium (bak-te're-um), pl. *bacte'ria* [L.; Gr. *baktērion*] in general, any of the microorganisms comprising one of the divisions, the Bacteria, of the kingdom Procaryotae. Bacteria are unicellular prokaryotic organisms or simple associations of

DISTRIBUTION OF INDIGENOUS MICROORGANISMS IN MAN

Organism	Mouth	Oro-pharynx	Naso-pharynx	Intestine	Skin	Eye	External Genitalia	Vagina
α-Streptococcus	1	1	2	2	0	0	2	2
β-Streptococcus	tr	3	tr	2*	0	0	0	tr
γ-Streptococcus	2	2	tr	2	0	0	2	2
Anaerobic streptococcus	2	2	0	2	0	0	2	2
Pneumococcus	tr	3	tr	0	0	0	0	0
Staphylococcus epidermidis	2	tr	3	2	1	2	2	2
Staphylococcus aureus	2	2	3	2	0	0	0	tr
Other staphylococci	2	2	tr	2	tr	tr	tr	2
Corynebacterium†	1	2	2	2	1	1	2	2‡
Lactobacillus	2	0	0	2	0	0	0	1
Leptotrichia	2	0	0	0	0	0	0	0
Actinomyces	2	2	0	0	0	0	0	0
Bacteroides	2	tr	tr	1	0	0	tr	tr
Fusobacterium	2	tr	0	2	0	0	2	0
Spirochetes	2	tr	0	2	0	0	2	0
Anaerobic vibrios	2	tr	tr	0	0	0	0	tr
Neisseria meningitidis	0	3	3	0	0	0	0	0
Other neisseriae	2	1	1	0	0	0	tr	tr
Veillonella	1	2	2	0	0	0	0	2
Haemophilus	tr	3	3	0	0	0	0	0
Mycoplasmas	2	2	0	2	0	0	2	2
Coliform bacteria	tr	tr	tr	1	0	0	2	2
Proteus	0	0	0	2	0	0	tr	0
Pseudomonas	tr	0	0	tr	0	0	tr	0
Clostridium	0	0	0	2	0	0	0	0
Bacillus	0	0	0	0	0	0	0	0
Mycobacterium	0	0	0	tr	tr	0	3	0
Yeasts	2	2	0	2	2	0	2	2‡
Protozoa	2	tr	0	3	0	0	3	3

1 = Generally present and constituting a principal fraction of the regional microbial flora.
2 = Generally present but constituting a minor fraction of the regional microbial flora.
3 = Carriers found frequently, in whom the organisms may constitute a prominent fraction of the regional microbial flora.
tr = Often found, usually in small numbers, as a trace component or a transient.
0 = If found, may be assumed to be a transient.
* = Group D hemolytic enterococci.
† = A very small proportion of the populace acts as the reservoir of diphtheria, owing to the persistence of *C. diphtheriae* in the nasopharynx.
‡ = During the period of ovarian activity.

(From G. W. Burnett, H. W. Scherp, and G. S. Schuster: Oral Microbiology and Infectious Diseases. 4th ed. Baltimore, Williams and Wilkins, 1976.)

similar cells, ranging in size from minute (about 0.2 by 0.2 to 0.7 μm) to large (about 1.0 to 1.3 by 3 to 10 μm). Morphologically, they occur in three forms: spherical (coccus), rod-shaped (such as bacilli), and spiral (vibrio, spirillum, and spirochete). The principal structures of typical bacteria, from outermost inward, are the flagella (organelle of locomotion) fimbriae (pili), gelatinous capsular material, semirigid cell wall (with muramic acid as a unique constituent), and cytoplasmic membrane, and within the cytoplasm mesosomes, ribosomes, inclusion vacuoles, chromatophores, and prokaryotic nucleus (nucleoid or nuclear region). There is normally one nucleus per cell, but multiple nuclei (two to four) may occur in dividing cells. Bacteria contain large amounts of nucleic acids; DNA is contained mostly in the nucleus, while RNA (rRNA, tRNA, mRNA) is found in the surrounding cytoplasm. The simple cytoplasm displays no conspicuous endoplasmic reticulum, and may contain granules composed chiefly of high-molecular-weight polyphosphate, polysaccharide granules, and submicroscopic particulates. Some bacteria, especially bacilli, form spores within the cell body (see bacterial SPORE). Bacterial cell multiplication involves growth and division, usually binary, but occasionally unequal and by budding. Bacteria resemble the blue-green algae in many respects, but differ primarily in that they do not produce oxygen in the process of photosynthesis and contain no chlorophyll *a* or phycobiliproteins. See also BACTERIA. See illustration and table. For proportional distribution of prominent bacteria on various oral surfaces and in saliva, see table at MOUTH flora. **acid-fast bacteria**, bacteria which may be stained only with difficulty and which, after staining, are resistant to decoloration, even with highly effective agents such as acid-alcohol. The common characteristic of acid-fast bacteria is their high lipid content. They include the genus *Mycobacterium* and some species of actinomycetes and corynebacteria, bacterial spores also showing this characteristic. **acidogenic bacteria,** bacteria capable of producing acids. Principal acidogenic bacteria implicated in the production of dental caries include *Lactobacillus acidophilus*, *L. brevis*, *L. necrodentalis*, *Streptococcus mitis*, *S. mutans*, *S. pyogenes*, and certain other bacteria. See also acidogenic THEORY. **aciduric bacteria**, bacteria which are able to withstand a degree of acidity usually fatal to nonsporulating bacteria. Acidogenic bacteria involved in the development of dental caries are also aciduric. **coccal b.,** see COCCUS. **coryneform bacteria,** club-shaped bacteria; a group of bacteria that display coryneform shape during some stage of their growth on artificial media. Called also *corynebacteria*. See CORYNEBACTERIACEAE and PROPIONIBACTERIACEAE. **endospore-forming bacteria,** see BACILLACEAE. **gram-negative bacteria,** bacteria which are decolorized, usually with ethanol, and are lightly stained by the counterstain, being pink in color when safranin is used, after staining with Gram's method (see under STAINING). As a group, they are relatively resistant to antibacterial activity of basic dyes, anionic and cationic detergents, phenols, sulfonamides, and penicillin, but are susceptible to azides, tellurites, oxidizing agents, and streptomycin; are susceptible to digestion by proteolytic enzymes and the lytic action of alkali; are resistant to the lytic action of lysozyme; are susceptible to lytic action of antibody; have a low mechanical stability; contain lipopolysaccharides, large amounts of lipids, and all amino acids in their cell walls; and lack teichoic acids in their cell walls. See table. **gram-positive bacteria,** bacteria which retain the primary stain and are violet in color, when stained by Gram's method (see under STAINING). As a group, they are relatively susceptible to antibacterial activity of basic dyes, anionic and cationic detergents, phenols, sulfonamides, and penicillin, but are relatively resistant to azides, tellurites, oxidizing agents, and streptomycin; are resistant to digestion by proteolytic enzymes and the lytic action of lysozyme; are resistant to the lytic action of antibody; have high mechanical stability; lack lipopolysaccharides and some amino acids in their cell walls; often contain teichoic acids in their cell walls; and have a low lipid content in their cell walls. See table. **pioneer bacteria,** bacteria penetrating dental tissue in advance of carious processes; observed in the earliest stages of dental caries. **proteolytic bacteria,** bacteria capable of producing proteolysis; they have been implicated in the development of dental caries. See proteolysis-chelation THEORY and proteolytic THEORY. **rod-shaped bacteria,** collectively, bacteria having a bacillary form, some being long and slender, others short and thick; some having sides more or less parallel to one another, others with fusiform shape; or some having square ends, others rounded ones. Bacteria of the families Bacillaceae, Enterobacteriaceae, Lactobacillaceae, and Vibrionaceae are rod shaped. Called also *rods*. **spiral bacteria,** bacteria made up of spiral forms that, if straightened out, would resemble long, slender bacilli. They are differentiated as those in which the spirals are rigid (as in the genus *Spirillum*), and those in which they are flexible; among the latter, a further differentiation is made on the tightness of the coiling. The tightly coiled forms include several genera differentiated by finer morphological criteria, including differentiation of the outer sheath, a central filament about which the protoplasm is coiled, etc. *Treponema* is one of the genera in this category, and *Leptospira*, distinguished by sharp, hooklike bends at the ends of the cell, is another. The genus *Borrelia* is comprised of less tightly coiled spiral forms, which have the appearance of long, slender undulating bacillary forms. Together, the flexible spiral forms are referred to as the *spirochetes*.

bacteroid (bak′tĕ-oid) [*bacteria* + *eidos* form] 1. resembling the bacteria. 2. a structure resembling a bacterium.

Bacteroidaceae (bak″tĕ-roi-da′se-e) [*Bacteroides* + *-aceae*] a family of gram-negative, anaerobic bacteria, occurring as nonmotile or motile, nonsporogenous rods with peritrichous flagella. The organisms have been isolated from the natural cavities of man and other animals, and some have been isolated from infections. Some species are believed to be pathogenic. It consists of the genera *Bacteroides*, *Fusobacterium*, and *Leptotrichia*.

Bacteroides (bak″tĕ-roi′dēz) [Gr. *baktērion* little rod + *eidos* form] a genus of obligately anaerobic, gram-negative bacteria of the family Bacteroidaceae. They are primarily parasites of the intestinal tract and mucous membranes of animals, including man. Some species are pathogenic, and some have been implicated in periodontal disease. Called also *Ristella*. **B. aerofa′ciens,** *Eubacterium aerofaciens;* see under EUBACTERIUM. **B. a′vidus,** *Propionibacterium avidum;* see under PROPIONIBACTERIUM. **B. biacu′tus,** a species isolated from cases of appendicitis and infected wounds. Called also *Ristella biacuta*. **B. bullo′sus,** *Fusobacterium bullosum;* see under FUSOBACTERIUM. **B. capillo′sus,** a species isolated from cysts, wounds, and feces in man, from the intestine in swine and mice, and from sludge. Called also *Bacillus capillosus*, *Pseudobacterium capillosum*, and *Ristella capillosa*. **B. clostridiifor′mis,** a species isolated from abscesses in man, liver lesions in turkeys, and the rumen contents of calves. **B. coag′ulans,** a species isolated from human feces and lungs. Called also *Pasteurella coagulans* and *Pseudobacterium coagulans*. **B. constella′tus,** a species isolated from an inflamed human lacrimal sac. **B. corro′dens,** a species isolated from the human oral cavity, intestines, urogenital tract, and blood drawn after tooth extraction; also associated with respiratory and intestinal infections. Called also *Ristella corrodens*. **B. cylindroi′des,** *Eubacterium cylindroides;* see under EUBACTERIUM. **B. frag′ilis,** a species forming a part of the normal intestinal flora in animals, including man. Also isolated from the human oral cavity, and in cases of appendicitis, peritonitis, cardiac diseases, rectal abscesses, pilonidal cysts, surgical wound infections, urogenital lesions, and soft tissue infections. Called also *B. inaequalis*, *Bacillus fragilis*, *Pseudobacterium fragilis*, *P. inaequalis*, *P. incommunis*, and *P. uncatum*. **B. freun′dii,** *Fusobacterium mortiferum;* see under FUSOBACTERIUM. **B. furco′sus,** a species isolated in man from cases of appendicitis and pulmonary abscesses, and from feces. Called also *Bacillus furcosus*, *Pseudobacterium furcosum*, and *Ristella furcosa*. **B. glutino′sus,** *Fusobacterium glutinosum;* see under FUSOBACTERIUM. **B. inaequ′alis,** *B. fragilis*. **B. len′tus,** *Eubacterium lentum;* see under EUBACTERIUM. **B. limo′sus,** *Eubacterium limosum;* see under EUBACTERIUM. **B. melaninogen′icus,** a species requiring hemin for growth, and producing an olive-brown to jet-black hematin derivative if excess hemin is available; some strains also require menadione or a related naphthoquinone. All strains are proteolytic and produce collagenase. Most are nonfermentative, but produce lactic, acetic, propionic, isobutyric, formic, and isovaleric acids, probably from amino acids; some ferment glucose, galactose, and lactose; and a few ferment glucose, fructose, sucrose, maltose, and raffinose and hydrolyze starch. The species, which is believed to be pathogenic, inhabits the gingival sulcus of the human oral cavity, and also is found in the urine and feces and in infections of the soft tissue, mouth, and respiratory, urogenital, and intestinal tracts. Called also *Bacterium melaninogenicum*, *Fusiformis nigrescens*, and *Ristella melaninogenica*. **B. ochra′ceus,** a species isolated from the gingival crevices and infections of man. It closely resembles *Capnocytophaga*. Called also *Bacteroides oralis* subsp. *elongatus* and *Ristella ochraceus*. **B. ora′lis,** a species growing on blood sugar and forming round colonies (0.5 to 2 mm in diameter), which ferments glucose, galactose, fructose, mannose, maltose, sucrose, lactose, cellobiose, and raffinose; hydrolyzes starch; and produces iodophilic polysaccharide from glucose. Succinic and acetic acids, with small amounts of lactic, formic, isobutyric, and isovaleric acids, are the end products of glucose fermentation. Some strains are β-hemolytic. Hemin stimulates the growth of some strains. The gingival sulcus of man appears to be its principal habitat. It is also associated with infections, usually of the oral cavity and respiratory and genital tracts. Called also *Ristella oralis*. **B. ora′lis** subsp. **elongatus,** *B. ochraceus.* **B. pneumosin′tes,** a species isolated in man from the nasopharynx and lungs, from blood, and in cases of brain abscesses. It is believed to be involved in secondary infections of the upper respiratory tract. Called also *Bacillus pneumosintes, Bacterium pneumosintes,* and *Dialister pneumosintes.* **B. praeacu′tus,** a species isolated in man from gangrene, from blood, and from infantile intestines. Called also *Coccobacillus praeacutus* and *Fusobacterium praeacutum.* **B. putre′dinis,** a species isolated from abscesses and appendicitis in man. Called also *Bacillus putredinis, Pseudobacterium putredinis,* and *Ristella putredinis.* **B. recta′lis,** *Eubacterium rectale;* see under EUBACTERIUM. **B. rumini′cola,** a species isolated from the rumens of various animals, and from human abscesses and feces. **B. ser′pens,** a species isolated from contaminated sea water, and associated with infections of the intestines, respiratory tract, middle ear, and blood in man. Called also *Bacillus radiiformis, B. serpens,* and *Pseudobacterium serpens.* **B. symbio′sus,** *Fusobacterium symbiosum;* see under FUSOBACTERIUM. **B. te′nuis,** *Eubacterium tenue;* see under EUBACTERIUM. **B. tortuo′sus,** *Eubacterium tortuosum;* see under EUBACTERIUM. **B. va′rius,** *Fusobacterium varium;* see under FUSOBACTERIUM. **B. ventrio′sus,** *Eubacterium ventriosum;* see under EUBACTERIUM.

Bactocill trademark for *oxacillin.*

Bactopen trademark for *cloxacillin.*

baddeleyite (bad′el-e-īt″) the natural form of zirconium oxide.

badge (baj) any emblem or special identification, usually worn as a mark of distinction. Also, anything worn like a badge. **film b.,** a light-tight package of photographic film worn like a badge by persons likely to be exposed to ionizing radiations. The absorbed dose can be calculated by the degree of film darkening caused by the radiation. See also COUNTER.

Baelz's disease [Erwin von *Baelz,* German physician, 1849–1913] CHEILITIS glandularis apostematosa.

Baer's cavity [Karl Ernst *Baer,* Russian anatomist, 1792–1876] see under CAVITY.

Baer's plane see under PLANE.

Bäfverstedt's syndrome [Bo Erik *Bäfverstedt,* Swedish dermatologist] benign LYMPHADENOMATOSIS.

Bagodryl trademark for *diphenhydramine.*

Bailyn's classification [M. *Bailyn,* American dentist] see under CLASSIFICATION.

bainite (ba′nīt) a fine two-phase dispersion of iron carbide in ferrite. See also SPHEROIDITE.

bake (bāk) to expose to high temperature at low humidity, as in the hardening of porcelain.

Bakelite [named after L. H. *Baekeland,* its inventor] trademark for phenolformaldehyde resin, used in the construction of denture bases. Condensation polymerization involved in its formation is believed to consist of reactions between phenol and formaldehyde to form an alcohol, followed by the reaction of condensation to form the macromolecules.

Baker, John [c. 1732–1796] an American dentist born in England. He is considered to be the first professional dentist practicing in America, and believed to have introduced the use of gold for filling teeth.

Baker amalgamator see under AMALGAMATOR.

Baker anchorage see under ANCHORAGE.

Baker Inlay see under INLAY.

Baker Inlay Extra Hard see under INLAY.

Baker Inlay Hard see under INLAY.

Baker's velum [Henry *Baker,* Boston surgeon] see under VELUM.

baking (bāk′ing) firing (2). **high biscuit b.,** high biscuit FIRING. **low biscuit b.,** low biscuit FIRING. **medium biscuit b.,** medium biscuit FIRING.

Bakontal trademark for *barium sulfate* (see under BARIUM).

Bakwin-Eiger syndrome [Harry *Bakwin,* American physician, born 1894; Marvin *Eiger,* American physician] HYPEROSTOSIS corticalis deformans juvenilis.

BAL British anti-lewisite (see DIMERCAPROL).

balance (bal′ans) [L. *bilanx*] 1. an instrument for weighing. 2. something used to produce equilibrium. 3. the harmonious adjustment of a part; the harmonious performance of functions. **acid-base b.,** a condition in which the net rate of acid or alkali production by the body is balanced by the net rate of acid or alkali excretion from the body, resulting in a stable concentration of H^+ (hydrogen ions) in the body fluids. **calcium b.,** the balance between the calcium intake and its output through the body excretions. **enzyme b.,** in bacteria, a once-postulated steady state in relative enzyme and substrate concentrations in a bacterial culture that is altered in a different environment, thus accounting for bacterial adaptation. **fluid b.,** the state of the body in relation to ingestion and excretion of water and electrolytes. Called also *water b.* **nitrogen b.,** the state of the body in regard to ingestion and excretion of nitrogen, determined by simultaneous measuring of the rate of protein intake and the rate of protein utilization. If 8 gm of nitrogen are excreted into the urine each day, then the total excretion, including that in the feces (additional 10 percent), is calculated as being 8.8 gm. This value multiplied by 100/16 gives a calculated total protein metabolism of 55 gm per day. A *negative nitrogen balance* implies greater protein utilization than protein intake; a *positive nitrogen balance* implies a net gain of protein in the body. Factors that cause negative balance include malnutrition, debilitating diseases, and glucocorticoid hormones; positive nitrogen balance is caused by exercise, growth hormone, and testosterone. **occlussal b.,** balanced occLUSION. **water b.,** fluid b.

balanitis (bal″ah-ni′tis) [Gr. *balanos* an acorn + *-itis*] inflammation of the glans penis.

Balkwell articulator [F. H. *Balkwell,* English dentist, 19th century] see under ARTICULATOR.

ball (bawl) a spherical mass or body. **cotton b.,** a spherical mass of rolled cotton, commonly used for the topical application of medicinal substances; cotton balls smaller than ⅜ inch in diameter are known as *cotton pellets.* **fatty b. of Bichat,** buccal fat PAD.

Ballance, Sir Charles Alfred [British surgeon, 1856–1936] see Körte-Balance OPERATION.

Ballard stress equalizer attachment (stress equalizer) [Charles S. *Ballard,* American dentist] see under ATTACHMENT.

Baller-Gerold syndrome [F. *Baller;* M. *Gerold*] see under SYNDROME.

ballistics (bah-lis′tiks) [Gr. *ballein* to throw] the scientific study of the motion of projectiles in flight. **wound b.,** the scientific study of the speeds and direction of missiles (bullets and other projectiles) in relation to the injuries they produce.

ballistocardiograph (bah-lis″to-kar′de-o-graf) the apparatus used in ballistocardiography. See also MICROGRAPH (1).

ballistocardiography (bah-lis″to-kar″de-og′rah-fe) the graphic recording, by means of a ballistocardiograph, of the movements of the body caused by the heartbeat, used to determine the degree of elasticity or atheroma of the aorta, and, more rarely, to calculate cardiac output.

balloon (bah-loon′) 1. a sac that can be inserted into a body cavity or tube and distended with air or gas. 2. to distend with air or gas; to inflate. **Shea-Anthony antral b.,** sinus b. **sinus b.,** a hollow rubber structure, expandable with either liquid or air, used to support depressed fractures of the walls of the maxillary sinus; the balloon of a Foley catheter is frequently used for this purpose. Called also *Shea-Anthony antral balloon.*

ballooning (bah-loon′ing) 1. swelling or puffing out like a balloon. 2. distending any cavity of the body with air or gas for therapeutic purposes.

balm (bahm) [Fr. *baume*] a healing of soothing medicine. Called also *balsam.*

Balme's cough [Paul Jean *Balme,* French physician, born 1857] see under COUGH.

balsam (bawl′sam) [L. *balsamum;* Gr. *balsamon*] 1. a semifluid, resinous and fragrant juice from various species of evergreen trees or shrubs, having various components, chiefly oleoresins, terpens, and cinnamic and benzoic acids. Balsams are combustible and generally nontoxic; all are soluble in organic solvents, but not water. 2. balm. **black b.,** b. of Peru. **Canada b.,** a liquid oleoresin obtained from *Abies balsamea,* the balsam tree of North America, composed chiefly of pinene, bornyl acetate, and resin. It is a pale yellow or greenish yellow, viscous liquid with an odor of pine, which is soluble in ethanol, but not in water. It is a component of zinc oxide–eugenol type of dental materials and root canal sealers. Called also *b. of fir* and *Canada turpentine.* **b. of fir,** Canada b. **Honduras b.,** b. of Peru. **Indian b.,** b. of Peru. **b. of Peru, peruvian b.,** a liquid obtained from *Myroxylon pereirae,* containing chiefly a volatile oil and a resin and smaller amounts of vanillin, coumarin, dihydrobenzoic acid, farnesol (a sesquiterpene alcohol), styrol, and a phytosterol. The resin component is a mixture of benzoic and cinnamic acid esters of the alcohol peruresinotannol. The balsam occurs as a dark brown, viscid, transparent liquid with an acrid taste and a strong aftertaste and a vanilla-like odor, which is soluble in ethanol, chloroform, and glacial acetic acid, but not in water. Used chiefly as a local irritant to promote the growth of epithelial cells. Also used as a component of some cement liquids. Allergic reactions to balsam may occur. Called also *black b.*, *Honduras b.*, *Indian b.*, *Surinam b.*, and *China oil.* **Surinam b.**, b. of Peru.

Bamatter's syndrome [F. *Bamatter*] hereditary osteodysplastic GERODERMA.

band (band) 1. an object or appliance that confines or restricts while allowing a limited or desired degree of movement. 2. a strip that holds together or binds two or more separate objects. 3. a strip of thin metal, formed into a hoop, to encircle horizontally the crown of a natural tooth or its root. 4. an elongated area with parallel or roughly parallel borders, that is distinct from the surrounding surface by its color, texture, or other characteristics. See *chromosome b.* **A b's,** 1. chromosome bands obtained with Giemsa stain in lymphocytes three months or older, which are located near the centromeres and telomeres on several chromosomes. See also A-BANDING. 2. a dark transverse band in the middle of the sarcomere which, together with the adjacent lighter I bands, forms cross striations on the skeletal muscle. It is made up of myosin filaments as well as the ends of the actin filaments where they overlap the myosin. In the middle of the band is a lighter zone (H band), which is bisected by a dense transverse line (M band). Its length of about 1.6 μm is constant. The band is optically anisotropic, having the property of double refraction, hence the synonym *anisotropic band.* Called also *Q b.*, *A disk, anisotropic disk, Q disk,* and *transverse disk.* See illustration at MUSCLE. **absorption b.,** one of the dark bands in the spectrum due to absorption of light by the medium (a solid, a liquid, or a gas) through which the light has passed. Cf. absorption LINE. **b. adapter,** band ADAPTER. **adapter b.,** ADAPTER band. **anchor b.,** orthodontic b. **Angle b.,** an orthodontic clamp band tightened by a threaded screw on the lingual side. **anisotropic b.,** A b. (2). **apron b.,** a labial, incisal or gingival extension of an orthodontic band that aids in retention of the band and in proper positioning of the bracket. **BUdR (bromodeoxyuridine) b's,** chromosome bands showing after treatment of cultured lymphocytes with BUdR. They may be used in the identification and delineation of inactive X chromosomes and in sister chromatid exchanges in a variety of clinical syndromes. **C (constitutive heterochromatin) b's,** chromosome bands that show after staining on the pericentromeric areas of all chromosomes and, particularly, on the secondary constrictions of chromosomes 1, 9, and 16, and on the distal segments of the long arms of the Y chromosome (13–15, 21–22). Their size varies from person-to-person in relation to the amount of satellite DNA present and the staining technique used. C bands are usually transmitted unchanged from parents to offspring and constitute an example of polymorphism in man. See also C-BANDING. **canine b.,** an orthodontic band fitted over a canine tooth. **chromosome b's,** alternating dark and light or fluorescent transverse bands produced on chromosomes by differential staining; named according to the procedure used: C bands, F bands, G bands, etc. See chromosome BANDING. **clamp b.,** an anchor band held in place with a screw nut. **contoured b.,** an orthodontic band shaped to the contour of the tooth. **copper b.,** a band or tube made of copper, such as one fitted over a tooth in endodontic therapy to allow placement of the rubber dam for asepsis during root canal procedures. Copper bands are available in a variety of sizes, being suitable for trimming and contouring to fit individual teeth. **elastic b.,** see ELASTIC (3). **F b's, Feulgen b's,** chromosome bands produced by differential staining by the conventional Feulgen reaction; they resemble the C, R, and G bands. Most of the areas of negatively stained Q and G bands are also negative in the F bands, but some telomeric segments that are positively stained in the Q and G bands are negatively stained in the F bands. The distal half of the Y chromosome is brightly fluorescent with the Q band, intensively stained with the G bands, and appears negative under F-banding. See also F-BANDING. **G b's, Giemsa b's,** chromosome bands produced along the entire length of chromosomes after Giemsa staining, being the reverse of R bands whereby the dark R bands correspond to light G bands and vice versa. They are generally similar to Q bands but, in addition, show positively stained secondary constrictions of chromosomes 1, 9, and 16. G bands are often used as reference bands. See also G-BANDING. **H b.,** H ZONE. **Hunter-Schreger b's,** lines of Schreger; see under LINE. **I b.,** a light transverse band in the sarcomere which alternates with darker A bands and forms cross striations of skeletal muscle. It is made up of thin F-actin filaments and is about 1.0 μm long. The Z band bisects the I band in the middle and lengthens when the fiber is stretched

and shortens during contraction. It is isotropic or homogeneous to polarized light, hence the synonym *isotropic band.* Called also *I disk, isotropic disk,* and *J disk.* See illustration at MUSCLE. **isotropic b.,** *I b.* **lip furrow b.,** vestibular LAMINA. **M b.,** a narrow, dark, dense, transverse line in the sarcomere that bisects the H zone. Called also *Hensen's line, M disk, M line,* and *mesophragma.* See also INOPHRAGMA. **matrix b.,** a cylindrical copper band or a short tube filled with a softened impression compound and seated over a tooth, allowing the compound to flow into the prepared cavity, in obtaining impressions of single teeth which contain prepared cavities. Also used in the placement and contouring of certain restorative materials, e.g. resin and glass ionomer cement. **molar b.,** an anchor band applied on a molar tooth to serve in anchoring an orthodontic appliance. Attached to the band is a bracket which holds the arch wire of the appliance. **N b's, nuclear organizer b's,** chromosome bands produced by selective staining of very limited regions of chromosomes which coincide with those areas recognized as bearing the loci for ribosomal cistrons (nuclear organizers). They are produced by staining with Giemsa stain after extracting nucleic acids and histones from chromosome preparations. N bands form purplish-red spots restricted to the satellite region of an acrocentric chromosome, appearing in most nuclei of interphase lymphocytes as tiny spots clustering within the nucleolus. **orthodontic b.,** a band fitted over a tooth to serve to anchor a fixed orthodontic appliance. Most bands are seamless, but some may be pinched, welded, or soldered. The basic elements of orthodontic bands are precious metals or chrome-cobalt stainless alloys, especially fabricated to produce the greatest strength and durability with a minimum of bulk. A high polish prevents adhesion of food particles. Bands come in strips, rolls, or precut blanks, with the attachments in place, or are preformed, contoured, and seamless forms of varying sizes and shapes. Bands for the anterior teeth are usually 0.003 to 0.004 inch thick and 0.125 inch wide; canine and premolar bands are usually 0.004 inch thick and 0.150 inch wide; molar bands are 0.005 to 0.006 inch thick and 0.180 to 0.200 inch wide. Each band is supplied with an attachment or bracket to receive the arch wire and to transmit the adjustment force to

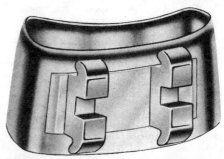

Twin edgewise bracket attached to preformed seamless orthodontic band. (From T. M. Graber: Orthodontics — Principles and Practice. 3rd ed. Philadelphia, W. B. Saunders Co., 1972; courtesy Rocky Mountain Dental Products Co.)

the tooth. See illustration. **Parham b.,** a metallic ribbon used to fix a fractured bone by encircling it at the site of the fracture. **phonatory b.,** the vocal cords, or an artificial substitute for them. **premolar b.,** an orthodontic band fitted over a premolar tooth. **b. pusher,** band PUSHER. **Q b.,** A b. (2). **Q b's, quinacrine b's,** chromosome bands showing distinctive fluorescence patterns after quinacrine mustard staining, being specific for each species and each chromosome pair. Intensive fluorescence of Q bands is observed in the distal half of the long arms of the Y chromosome and the pericentromeric region of chromosome 3 and the satellites of the acrocentric chromosomes. Q bands were formerly accepted as reference bands but are now replaced by the G and R bands. See also Q-BANDING. **R b's, reverse b's,** chromosome bands produced with Giemsa stain; they are the reverse to G and Q bands, whereby the light G and Q bands correspond to dark R bands and vice versa. The exceptions are the secondary constrictions of chromosome 9, which are negatively stained with both the Q- and R-banding and slightly stained with the G-banding. Phase contrast or fluorescence microscopy is usually required for the visualization of R bands. See also R-BANDING. **b. remover**, band REMOVER. **rubber b.**, see ELASTIC (3). **Schreger's b's**, lines of Schreger; see under LINE. **seamless b.**, an orthodontic band consisting of a continuous stip of metal forming a ring corresponding to the shape of the tooth. **b. seater**, band SEATER. **slip b.**, a band formed when a metal is placed under a load and one grain tends to slip or slide on another. **stainless steel b.**, a band or tube made of stainless steel, such as those fitted over a tooth to allow placement of the rubber dam for asepsis during root canal procedures. Stainless steel bands are available in a variety of sizes, both for molar and bicuspid teeth, being partially contoured. **Streeter's b's**, a syndrome combining amputations and constrictions of digits, microtia, cleft palate, cleft of mucosal portion of the lip, mandibular asymmetry, skin appendages, and isolated dextrocardia. **T b's, telomeric b's**, chromosome bands produced with Giemsa stain similarly to those in R-banding, but having some R bands removed with a salt solution; only the most resistant ones are retained in certain telomeric regions of the chromosome. See also T-BANDING. **Z b.**, a thin membrane bisecting the I band and seen on longitudinal sections of striated muscle as a dense transverse line which segments the sarcomere into units of dark and light bands (A and I bands). Called also *Amici's disk* or *line, Dobie's layer* or *line, intermediate disk, Krause's line* or *membrane, telophragma, thin disk,* and *Z disk, line,* or *membrane.* See also INOPHRAGMA. See illustration at MUSCLE.

bandage (ban′dij) 1. a strip or roll of gauze or other material for wrapping or binding any part of the body. 2. to cover by wrapping with a strip of gauze or other material. **Barton's b.**, a figure-of-eight bandage passing below the mandible and around the cranial bone to give upward support to the mandible. **extraoral b.**, a type of headgear used in the past to retard mandibular growth in orthodontic therapy of malocclusion. See also extraoral APPLIANCE. **intraoral adhesive b.**, an adhesive dressing used after intraoral surgery, such as one consisting of pectin, gelatin, sodium carboxymethyl cellulose, and polyisobutylene, coated on the outside with a polyethylene film. Used to secure periodontal grafts without suturing.

bandelette (ban′dĕ-let) see bandelette PLATE.

banding (band′ing) 1. the act of encircling and binding with a thin strip of material. 2. chromosome b. **A-b.**, differential staining of old (three months or older) slides of lymphocytes, consisting of treating the slides with sodium hydroxide, rinsing in distilled water, incubating in phosphate buffer, pH 6.8 at 60°C, and staining with Giemsa stain. See also A bands, under BAND. **C-b.**, differential staining of chromosomes through the use of an alkali denaturation and reassociation technique consisting of a series of treatments with hydrochloride and sodium hydroxide followed by incubation at 60–65°C. See also C bands, under BAND. **chromosome b.**, a cytogenetic method, based on Caspersson's method (see Q-b.), which allows visualization of differentially stained regions of a chromosome as a continuous series of light and dark bands specific for the chromosome and species, thus permitting identification of chromosome abnormalities. Known as C-banding, F-banding, etc., according to the staining technique used. See also CHROMOSOME nomenclature, and see illustration. **F-b.**, Feulgen b., differential staining of chromosomes through the use of conventional Feulgen technique reaction. Chromosomes are first treated with 0.14 M phosphate buffer, rinsed in saline-citrate solution, and held at 20°C or below in the solution. The slides are then rinsed with distilled water, post-fixed in methanol–acetic acid and stained with Feulgen reaction. Called also *Feulgen method* and *Feulgen staining.* See also F bands, under BAND. **G-b., Giemsa b.**, differential staining of chromosomes through the use of Giemsa solution following preliminary air-drying and oven-heating (60–65°C), or DNA denaturation. The same banding results may be obtained with Wright and other blood stains. Called also *Giemsa method* and *Giemsa staining.* See also G bands, under BAND. **N-b.**, chromosome staining with Giemsa stain after extracting nucleic acids and histones. See N bands, under BAND. **Q-b., quinacrine b., quinacrine mustard b.**, differential staining of chromosomes either directly with quinacrine mustard or first treated with different grades of alcohol and then stained with fluorochrome. The technique was first developed by Caspersson, and is considered the pioneering work in chromosome banding. It is most commonly used for the identification of the Y chromosome and chromosomal polymorphic variants; it is used largely for bone marrow studies. Called also *Caspersson meth-*

od, *Caspersson technique,* and *quinacrine staining.* See also Q bands, under BAND. **R-b., reverse b.** a chromosome staining method consisting of air drying the slide, immersing it in phosphate buffer for 10 minutes, rinsing with water, and staining with Giemsa reaction. Acridine orange staining may be used to obtain fluorescent bands. See also Giemsa STAIN and R bands, under BAND. **T-b., telomeric b., terminal b.**, a chromosome staining method consisting of heat treatment with the use of a salt solution maintained at pH 5.1–5.3 at 87°C, rinsing in distilled water, and staining with buffered Giemsa reaction. Acridine orange staining may be used to obtain fluorescent bands. See also R bands, under BAND. **tooth b.**, the technique of cementing stainless steel bands to the teeth to hold orthodontic attachments in position. See also tooth BONDING.

banewort (bān′wort) belladonna (1).

Bang's bacillus, disease [Bernhard Lauritz Frederik *Bang,* Danish physician, 1848–1932] see *Brucella abortus,* under BRUCELLA, and BRUCELLOSIS.

bank (bangk) a stored supply of human organs or tissues for future use by other individuals. **blood b.**, an organization, usually a hospital or other medical care institution, which collects, stores, labels, processes, and distributes blood for transfusion.

Bannister's disease [Henry Martyn *Bannister,* Chicago physician, 1844–1920] Quincke's EDEMA.

Bannwarth's syndrome [Alfred *Bannwarth*] see under SYNDROME.

Banthine trademark for *methantheline bromide* (see under METHANTHELINE).

Bantogen trademark for *penicillin V calcium* (see under PENICILLIN).

bar (bahr) 1. a metal segment of greater length than width that serves to connect two or more parts of a removable partial denture. See also BEAM (4). 2. a unit of pressure, being a pressure of 10^6 dyne/cm²; 1 bar = 0.987 atm. Sometimes used inaccurately for 1 dyne/cm². Called also *barye.* **Ackermann b.**, Ackermann bar JOINT. **Andrews b.**, a curved bar attachment made of a nonmagnetic austenitic metal. A single bar type is used for anterior gaps and the twin bar type is used posteriorly. Called also *Andrews bridge.* **arch b.**, any of several types of heavy wire bars shaped to the outer circumference of the dental arch and extending from one side to the other so that intervening teeth may be attached to it; used for the treatment of fractures of the jaws and/or stabilization of injured teeth. **arch b., Erich**, Erich arch b. **arch b., fixable-removable cross**, cross arch bar splint CONNECTOR. **buccal b.**, an orthodontic appliance consisting of a rigid metal wire extending from the buccal side to the molar band anteriorly. **b. clasp**, bar CLASP. **connecting b.**, connector b. **connector b.**, a connector unit of a removable partial denture, fabricated as parallel-sided bars (or rigid connectors and retainers), and round- or oval-sided bars, which serve to connect parts of dentures, splint or connect abutments (implant, natural, or a combination of these), connect and splint crowns, or splint teeth that have received root therapy, the bars being soldered to the root face covering or coping. Since they permit some movement, connector bars serve also as stress-breakers. Called also *connecting b.* and *minor connector.* See also CONNECTOR. **Dolder b.**, Dolder bar joint ATTACHMENT. **double lingual b.**, continuous CLASP. **Erich arch b.**, an arch bar made of soft, readily contoured wire; used for intermaxillary fixation. **fixable-removable cross arch b.**, cross arch bar splint CONNECTOR. **Gaerny b.**, a bridgelike bar attachment, being a modification of the channel shoulder pin technique, in which retention is provided by precise contact between parallel surfaces of the inner and outer copings and of the connecting bars and sleeves, fitted without pins over crowns about 5 mm in length. **Gilson fixable-removable b.**, cross arch bar splint CONNECTOR. **horseshoe b.**, a major connector, being a U-shaped bar that connects two or more bilateral parts of a maxillary partial denture to bypass a torus palatinus. **hyoid b's**, a pair of cartilaginous plates forming the second visceral arch, from which a part of the hyoid bone develops. **I b.**, an extracoronal, infrabulge, removable partial denture component that is smoothly tapered from origin to rounded tip, flexible, and usually provides retention at, but not directly at, its terminus. **b. joint**, bar JOINT. **Kazanjian T b.**, an appliance useful in reconstruction of the lip and jaw; it is fixed with an acrylic prosthesis to provide soft tissue support during reconstruction. Called also *T b. of Kazanjian.* **Kennedy b.**, 1. a metal bar usually resting on the lingual surfaces of teeth to aid in their stabilization and to act as an indirect retainer. 2. continuous CLASP. **labial b.**, a major connector located labial to the dental arch, joining two or more bilateral parts of a mandibular removable partial denture. **lingual b.**, continuous CLASP. **mesostructure b.**, an integral addition to the implant denture substructure, which intraorally connects the anterior and posterior abutments, being a rigid bar located well above the oral mucosa. It provides rigidity and strength to the substructure and distributes masticatory forces throughout the supporting bone. Called also *integral intraoral bilateral posterior mesostructure*. **occlusal rest b.**, a minor connector used to attach an occlusal rest to a major part of a removable partial denture. **palatal b.**, a major connector, being a bar which extends across the palate and unites two or more parts of a maxillary removable denture. A similar broad coverage of the palate is called *major palatal connector*. **palatal b., anterior**, a major connector uniting bilateral units of a maxillary removable partial denture, being a thin metal plate that is placed in the anterior palatal region. It gives rigidity to the denture by means of its own form imparted by the rugae and by lying in two planes. Called also *anterior major palatal connector*. **palatal b., beaded**, a major connector that has been beaded to provide positive contact with underlying tissue. **palatal b., posterior**, a major connector located in the posterior palatal region; used to assist in bilateral unification of the denture when the anterior bar alone would lack rigidity. Called also *posterior major palatal connector*. **Passavant's b.**, a horizontal ridge that appears on the posterior wall of the pharynx during swallowing, produced by contraction of the palatopharyngeal sphincter; it also occurs during speech in persons with cleft palate. Called also *Passavant's cushion*, *Passavant's pad*, *Passavant's ridge*, and *pharyngeal ridge*. **RP-I b.**, a variant of the I bar. **Steiger-Boitel b.**, Steiger-Boitel ATTACHMENT. **T b. of Kazanjian**, Kazanjian T b.

barbital (băr′bĭ-tal) the oldest of all barbiturates, 5,5-diethylbarbituric acid, occurring as colorless or white crystals or powder with a slightly bitter taste, which is soluble in water, alcohol, chloroform, and ether. Used as a long-acting hypnotic and sedative in the treatment of insomnia, convulsive disorders, psychoneurotic states, hypertension, gastrointestinal disorders, and heart diseases. Also used in pre- and postanesthetic medication and in allaying apprehension in dental patients. Also used as a buffer in *in vitro* biochemical reactions. Adverse reactions are those associated with barbiturate therapy. It is an addictive drug subject to the regulation of the Controlled Substances Act. Called also *barbitone* and *diethylmalonylurea*. Trademarks: Malonal, Veronal.

barbitone (bar′bĭ-tōn) British name for *barbital*.

barbiturate (bar-bit′u-rāt) a salt of barbituric acid that is classified as a cyclic ureide, occurring in either keto or enol form. Barbiturates depress the activity of all excitable tissues, being most active in producing depression of the cortical region of the central nervous system and having lesser effects on skeletal, cardiac, and smooth muscle. They are anticonvulsants, sedatives, and hypnotics, without having analgesic properties. In small doses, they have little effect on blood pressure and respiration, but in large doses, they produce a dramatic fall in blood pressure, body temperature, and respiration, resulting in collapse, coma, and death. Their action is classified by duration of their effects: long-acting (mephobarbital and phenobarbital), intermediate-acting (amobarbital and butabarbital sodium), short-acting (pentobarbital and secobarbital), and ultrashort-acting (methohexital sodium, thiamylal sodium, and thiopental sodium). Used in insomnia, psychoneurotic disorders, anxiety with hypertension and cardiac complications, and convulsive disorders. Also used as an adjunct in analgesia, in preanesthetic medication, basal anesthesia, and complete surgical anesthesia. In dentistry, barbiturates are used to allay apprehension before dental interventions. They are addictive and their side reactions may include lassitude, vertigo, headache, nausea, diarrhea, skin rash, eruptions of the oral mucosa, and peripheral nerve injury when injected. They are contraindicated in porphyria. Barbiturates are folic acid antagonists and may cause folic acid deficiency and blood dyscrasias. The barbiturates are popularly called *sleeping pills*.

Bardeleben see VON BARDELEBEN.

Barfurth's law see under LAW.

Baridol trademark for *barium sulfate* (see under BARIUM).

barium (ba′re-um, bar′e-um), gen. *ba′rii* [L.; Gr. *baros* weight] a pale, yellowish, slightly lustrous, soft metallic element belonging to the alkaline earth group. Symbol, Ba; atomic number, 56; atomic weight, 137.33; specific gravity, 3.5; valence, 2; group IIA of the periodic table. There are six stable isotopes (130, 132, 134, 136–138) and 13 radioactive ones. In metallic form, barium reacts with water, ammonia, halogens, oxygen, and most acids, and oxidizes readily when exposed to air. Barium is used as a carrier for radium, in the production of electronic tubes, as a lubricant for anode rotors in x-ray tubes, and in a variety of other products. All water- or acid-soluble barium

compounds are poisonous, causing chiefly very intense muscle stimulation. Symptoms, which are related to this stimulation, may include vomiting, colic, diarrhea, hemorrhage, hypertension, arrhythmias, arteriolar spasm, and muscle tremor; ingestion of gram quantities of soluble barium salts may produce fatal cardiac arrest. **b. sulfate**, the sulfate salt of barium, occurring as a bulky, fine, odorless, tasteless white powder, free from grittiness, and practically insoluble in water and alcohol. Used as a contrast medium in roentgenography of the digestive tract and as a radiopaque, inert material in dental products. Contrary to water-soluble barium compounds, which are poisonous, barium sulfate is nontoxic but, not being absorbed, may cause constipation and fecal impaction, and local granulomatous reactions. Called also *acrobaryte*, *acrybaryte*, *blanc fixe*, and *synthetic baryta*. Trademarks: Bakontal, Baridol, Citobaryum, Neobar, Unibaryt.

Barkann's technique [L. *Barkann*, American dentist] see under TECHNIQUE.

Barker's point see under POINT.

Barlow's disease [Sir Thomas *Barlow*, British physician, 1845–1945] infantile SCURVY.

barn (barn) a unit area used in expressing the cross sections of atoms, nuclei, electrons, and other particles, being, equal to 10^{-24} cm². Symbol *b*.

Barnum, Sanford Christie [1838–1885] a New York dentist who first devised the rubber dam.

baro- [Gr. *baros* weight] a combining form denoting relationship to weight or pressure.

barometer (bah-rom′ĕ-ter) [baro- + Gr. *metron* measure] an instrument for measuring atmospheric pressure. **Torricelli b.**, a barometer consisting of a glass tube more than 760 mm in length, sealed at one end, completely filled with mercury, and inverted in a mercury-filled beaker. When inverted, the mercury drops in the tube, creating a vacuum in the upper part of the tube, the extent of its drop being determined by the force per unit area which the earth's atmosphere exerts on the mercury in the beaker. The mercury drops until the pressure exerted by the atmosphere equals that exerted by the column of mercury at the level of the mercury surface in the beaker. The pressure is measured in atmospheres, 1 atmosphere being the average pressure exerted by the earth's atmosphere at sea level, being equivalent to 14.7 lb/in², or a pressure which will support a column of mercury 760 mm in height.

barosinusitis (bar″o-si″nu-si′tis) aerosinusitis.

barotitis (bar″o-ti′tis) [baro- + *otitis*] a disease of the ear produced by exposure to changes in the barometric pressure. Called also *aerotitis*. **b. me′dia**, a symptom complex produced by a difference between the atmospheric pressure of the environment and the air pressure in the middle ear. Called also *otitic barotrauma*. See also DYSBARISM.

barotrauma (bar″o-traw′mah) [baro- + Gr. *trauma* wound] injury caused by pressure; especially injury to the walls of the eustachian tube and the ear drum due to changes in the barometric pressure. **otitic b.**, BAROTITIS media. **sinus b.**, aerosinusitis.

Barr, Y. M. see Epstein-Barr VIRUS.

Barr body [Murray Llewellyn *Barr*, Canadian anatomist, born 1908] sex CHROMATIN.

Barrat see elfin facies SYNDROME (Williams-Barrat syndrome).

Barré, Jean Alexandre [French neurologist, born 1880] see Guillain-Barré SYNDROME.

Barré-Liéou syndrome [M. J. *Barré*; Young Choen *Liéou*] see under SYNDROME.

barrier (bar′e-er) a structure or mechanism which inhibits free flow between adjacent areas or systems; a barricade or obstruction. **blood-brain b.**, a barrier that prevents most substances in the blood from rapidly entering into the brain. The barrier is believed to exist in the capillary basement membrane of the brain parenchyma, except in several regions, such as the pineal, posterior pituitary, and median hypothalamic eminences. The ventral portion is highly permeable to water, carbon dioxide, and oxygen; slightly permeable to common electrolytes; but almost totally impermeable to arsenic, sulfur, gold, and large molecules. Called also *hematoencephalic b.* **blood–cerebrospinal fluid b.**, a barrier that prevents various substances in the blood from entering the cerebrospinal fluid. It is highly permeable to water, carbon dioxide, and oxygen; slightly permeable to electrolytes, but almost totally impermeable to sulfur, arsenic, and gold. **hematoencephalic b.**, blood-brain b. **protective b.**, a shield of radiation-absorbing material, such as lead, concrete, or plaster, used to protect against ionizing radiation. Called also *radiation b.* **protective b., primary,** one used to reduce a primary beam of radiation to a permissible exposure rate. **protective b., secondary,** one used to reduce stray or scattered radiation to a permissible exposure rate. **radiation b.,** protective b.

Bartenwerfer syndrome [Kurt *Bartenwerfer,* German physician, 1892–1946] see under SYNDROME.

Bartholin, duct of [Casper *Bartholin,* Jr., Danish anatomist, 1655–1738] major sublingual DUCT.

Barton, A. L. a Peruvian physician.

Barton's bandage [John Rhea *Barton,* American surgeon, 1794–1871] see under BANDAGE.

Bartonella (bar″to-nel′lah) [named after A. L. *Barton*] a genus of gram-negative bacteria of the family Bartonellaceae, order Rickettsiales, occurring as rounded or ellipsoidal cells or as slender, straight, curved, or bent rods, either singly or in chains of several segmenting organisms. The organisms have cell walls and reproduce by binary fusion. **B. bacillifor′mis,** the etiologic agent of bartonellosis, transmitted by the bites of sandflies, and occurring as rods, often curved, measuring 0.25 to 0.5 by 1.0 to 3.0 μm; in a coccoid form measuring about 0.75 μm in diameter; or as a ringlike variety. The species is generally found in the mountainous regions of Peru, Ecuador, and Colombia at elevations between 1,500 and 9,000 feet, owing to the ecology of its vector. It is seen in the blood and endothelial cells of the lymph nodes, spleen, and liver of infected humans; man is its reservoir host.

Bartonellaceae (bar″to-nel-la′se-e) [*Bartonella* + *-aceae*] a family of bacteria of the order Rickettsiales, consisting of gram-negative rods and coccoid, ring-, or disk-shaped organisms with cell walls, usually beaded or filamentous, and generally less than 3 μm in size. The members occur as pathogenic parasites in the erythrocytes in man and other vertebrates. It includes the genus *Bartonella.*

bartonellosis (bar″to-nel-lo′sis) infection with *Bartonella bacilliformis,* occurring most commonly in the mountainous regions of Peru, Ecuador, and Colombia at elevations between 1,500 and 9,000 feet, which is where its vector, the sandfly, propagates. During the initial phase (Oroya fever, Carrión's disease) the microorganisms invade the erythrocytes and endothelial cells of the blood and lymph capillaries, causing macrocytic anemia. As the condition progresses, the organisms form large masses in the infected cells, and the liver, spleen, and lymph nodes enlarge and become hemorrhagic. Pain in the bones, joints, and muscles, fever, sweating, petechiae and red papules of the skin, pallor of the skin and mucous membranes (including the oral mucosa), and progressive anemia follow. Some cases become fulminant and death usually follows in 10 days, but most continue for several months to recovery. About 1 month after recovery from the initial phase, a skin eruption (verruga peruana) may occur; it is characterized by wartlike, vascular, granulomatous lesions containing proliferating endothelial cells that are usually filled with microorganisms.

Bärtschi-Rochain's syndrome [Werner *Bärtschi-Rochain*] see under SYNDROME.

bary- [Gr. *barys* heavy] a combining form meaning heavy or difficult.

barye (bar′e) bar (2).

baryta (bah-ri′tah) any of several compounds of barium. **synthetic b.,** BARIUM sulfate.

basad (ba′sad) toward a base or basal aspect.

basal (ba′sal) pertaining to or situated near a base.

base (bās) [L.; Gr. *basis*] 1. the lowest part or foundation of anything. See also BASIS. 2. the main ingredient of a compound. 3. in chemistry, a compound that contains the hydroxyl group, – OH, and ionizes to form hydroxide ions in an aqueous solution. A compound which reacts with an acid to form water and salt. The most common bases are sodium hydroxide, potassium hydroxide, calcium hydroxide, and ammonia. See also Bronsted CONCEPT (2) and Lewis CONCEPT (1). 4. a unit of a removable prosthesis that supports the supplied tooth and any intermediary material and, in turn, receives support from the tissue of the basal seat. 5. base PASTE. 6. the chemical compound comprising the drug only and not its salt form. **acidifiable b.,** a chemical substance that will unite with water to form an acid. **acrylic resin b.,** a denture base made of acrylic resin. **apical b.,** that portion of the jaws giving support to the teeth. Called also *basal arch.* **b. of arytenoid cartilage,** the triangular inferior part of the arytenoid cartilage which bears the articular surface. Called also *basis cartilaginis arytenoideae* [NA]. **b. plate,** baseplate. **cavity b.,** a cavity lining agent used beneath perma-

nent restorations to enhance recovery of injured pulp or to protect it from thermal shock, galvanic shock, mechanical trauma, microleakage, and toxic substances in some restorations. Zinc phosphate, zinc oxide–eugenol, and calcium hydroxide cements are used commonly as cavity bases. Small amounts of rosin, fused silica, dicalcium phosphate, ethyl cellulose, and powdered mica may be added to provide smooth mixes. **cement b.,** a layer of insulated, sometimes medicated, dental cement placed in the deep portions of a cavity preparation to protect the pulp, reduce the bulk of the metallic restoration, or eliminate undercuts in a tapered preparation. **cement b., proximal,** a cement base placed in the deep area of the proximal surface of a cavity preparation for pulpal protection. **cheoplastic b.,** a denture base produced by casting molten metal in a mold. **cranial b.,** the endochondral bony support for the brain, separating the cranium from the facial skeleton. **conjugate b.,** a base which has lost its proton. **b. of cranium, external,** the outer surface of the inferior region of the skull. Called also *basis cranii externa* [NA]. **b. of cranium, internal,** the inner surface of the inferior region of the skull, constituting the floor of the cranial cavity. Called also *basis cranii interna* [NA]. **denture b.,** that part of a denture, made either of metal or resin or a combination of both materials, which supports the supplied teeth and/or receives support from the abutment teeth, the residual alveolar ridge, or both. See also denture base SADDLE. **denture b., processed,** that portion of a polymerized prosthesis covering the oral mucosa of the maxilla and/or mandible, to which artificial teeth are attached with a second processing. **denture b., tinted,** a denture base with coloring that simulates the natural color and shading of the oral tissue. **denture b. saddle,** denture base SADDLE. **film b.,** a thin, flexible, transparent sheet of cellulose acetate or similar material which carries the radiation- and light-sensitive emulsion of x-ray or photographic films. **extension b., free-end b.,** a unit of a removable denture that extends anteriorly or posteriorly, terminating without support by a natural tooth in a free end. **intermediary b.,** a nonmetallic material placed between the restoration and the tooth structure to protect the vital pulp from chemical irritants and to provide insulation from temperature changes. Zinc phosphate, polycarboxylate, and reinforced zinc oxide–eugenol are used most commonly as intermediary bases. Called also *dentin substitute.* See illustration at RESTORATION. **b. of mandible,** inferior border of mandible; see under BORDER. **metal b.,** a metallic portion of a denture base forming a part or all of the basal surface of the denture. It serves as a base for the attachment of the acrylic resin part of the denture base and the teeth. **nitrogenous b.,** an aromatic, nitrogen-containing molecule that serves as a proton acceptor, e.g., purine or pyrimidine. **nuclein b's, nucleinic b's,** purine b's. **ointment b.,** OINTMENT base. **plastic b.,** a denture base, baseplate, or record base made of a plastic material. **purine b's,** a group of chemical compounds of which purine is the base, including 6-oxypurine (hypoxanthine), 2,6-dioxypurine (xanthine), 6-aminopurine (adenine), 2-amino-6-oxypurine (guanine), 2,6,8-trioxypurine (uric acid), and 2,6-dioxypurine (xanthine). Called also *nuclein b's, nucleinic b's,* and *xanthine b's.* **pyrimidine b's,** a group of chemical compounds of which pyrimidine is the base, including 2,4-dioxy-pyrimidine (uracil), 2,4-dioxy-5-methylpyrimidine (thymidine), and 2-oxy-4-amino-pyrimidine (cytosine), which are constituents of nucleic acids. **record b.,** baseplate. **shellac b.,** resinous materials adapted to maxillary or mandibular casts to form baseplates. **sprue b.,** sprue FORMER. **stabilized b.,** stabilized BASEPLATE. **strong b.,** one that is highly dissociated in solution. **temporary b.,** baseplate. **tissue-supported b.,** the base of a denture which derives most of its support from tissues of edentulous areas beneath it, and not from the abutment teeth. **b. of tongue,** ROOT of tongue. **tooth-borne b.,** the base of a partial denture supported by the abutment teeth and not by the tissue beneath it. **tissue-tissue-supported b.,** the base of a denture supported by both the abutment teeth and tissue of edentulous areas beneath it. **trail b.,** baseplate. **weak b.,** one that dissociates in solution to a small extent into ions and furnishes relatively few hydroxide ions. **xanthine b's,** purine b's.

Basedow's disease [Carl Adolph von *Basedow,* German physician, 1799–1854] exophthalmic GOITER.

baseline (bās′līn) 1. a known quantity or a set of known quantities used as a reference point in evaluating similar data. 2. any line chosen as a base of registration for serial x-rays.

baseplate (bās′plāt) a temporary preformed shape fabricated of shellac, wax, or acrylic resin, representing the base of a denture and used for making maxillomandibular (jaw) relation records, for arranging artificial teeth, or for trial placement in the mouth. Called also *record base, temporary base, trial base.* **gutta-percha b.,** gutta-percha combined with fillers and coloring materials, rolled into sheets; used for temporary restorations, filling root canals, and separating teeth. **b. material,** baseplate MATERIAL. **permanent b.,** one that will ultimately become the base of the completed denture. **stabilized b.,** a baseplate lined with a plastic or other suitable material to improve its adaptation and stability. Called also *stabilized base.*

bases (ba'sēz) [L.] plural of *basis.*

basi-, basio- [L., Gr. *basis*] a combining form denoting relationship to a base or foundation.

basial (ba'se-al) pertaining to the basion.

basialveolar (ba"se-al-ve'o-lar) extending from the basion to the alveolar point.

basiarachnitis (ba"se-ar"ak-ni'tis) inflammation of the basal part of the arachnoid. Called also *basiarachnoiditis.*

basiarachnoiditis (ba"se-ah-rak"noi-di'tis) basiarachnitis.

basic (ba'sik) 1. pertaining to or having the properties of a base; having a pH greater than 7.2; capable fo neutralizing acids. 3. representing or used as a starting point.

basicranial (ba"se-kra'ne-al) [*basi-* + Gr. *kranion* cranium] pertaining to the base of the skull.

Basidiomycetes (bah-sid"e-o-mi-se'tēz) a class of true fungi (Eumycetes), in which the spores are borne on club-shaped organs, and comprising the basidiospore-forming yeasts, mushrooms, rusts, and smuts.

basidiospore (bah'sid'e-o-spōr) a spore formed on a basidium.

basidium (bah-sid'e-um), pl. *basid'ia.* The clublike organ of the fungal class Basidiomycetes which, following karyogamy and meiosis, bears a basiospore.

basifacial (ba"se-fa'shal) [*basi-* + L. *facies* face] pertaining to the lower part of the face.

basihyal (ba"se-hi'al) BODY of hyoid bone.

basihyoid (ba"se-hi'oid) BODY of hyoid bone.

basilar (bas'ĭ-lar) [L. *basilaris,* from *basis* base] pertaining to a base or basal part.

basilaris (bas'ĭ-la'ris) [L.] situated at the base. **b. cra'nii,** a composite of the numerous bones which serve the brain as a supportive floor and form the axis of the whole skull.

basinasial (ba"se-na'ze-al) pertaining to the basion and the nasion.

basio- see BASI-.

basioccipital (ba"se-ok-sip'ĭ-tal) pertaining to the basilar process of the occipital bone.

basioglossus (ba"se-o-glos'us) [*basio-* + Gr. *glōssa* tongue] the part of the hypoglossus muscle attached to the base of the hyoid bone.

basion (ba'se-on) [L.; Gr. *basis* base] a craniometric landmark located at the midpoint of the anterior border of the foramen magnum in the midsagittal plane. Abbreviated *Ba* or *ba.* Called also *point Ba* and *point ba.* See also OPISTHION. See illustration at CEPHALOMETRY.

basipetal (ba-sip'ĕ-tal) [*basi-* + L. *petere* to seek] descending or developing in the direction of the base.

basis (ba'sis), pl. *ba'ses* [L.; Gr.] the lowest part, the foundation; used in anatomical nomenclature to designate the base of a structure. See also BASE. **b. cartilag'inis arytenoi'deae** [NA], BASE of arytenoid cartilage. **b. cer'ebri,** inferior surface of cerebrum; see under SURFACE. **b. cra'nii exter'na** [NA], BASE of cranium, external. **b. cra'nii inter'na** [NA], BASE of cranium, internal. **b. enceph'ali,** inferior surface of cerebrum; see under SURFACE. **b. mandib'ulae** [NA], inferior border of mandible; see under BORDER. **b. na'si,** the portion of the nose opposite to the apex.

basisphenoid (ba"se-sfe'noid) [*basi-* + *sphenoid*] a part of the embryonic sphenoid bone between the great wings, developing into the back part of the body of the sphenoid bone.

basitemporal (ba"se-tem'po-ral) [*basi-* + *temporal*] pertaining to the lower part of the temporal bone.

basocyte (ba'so-sīt) basophil (2).

Basolan trademark for *methimazole.*

basophil (ba'so-fil) [Gr. *basis* base + *philein* to love] 1. any cell or histologic structure staining readily with basic dyes. 2. a granulocyte whose granules are basophilic. Basophils develop from metamyelocytes and are spherical cells about 7 to 9 μ in diameter, having nuclei which are elongated, often bent in the form of an S, and provided with one or more constrictions. The nucleoli are usually invisible and the chromatin network is loose and pale. The round, water-soluble granules are of various sizes, and stain dark red with neutral red stains. Basophils are usually present during the healing phase of inflammation, suggesting their reparative role. The presence of heparin in their metachromatic granules indicates their role in absorption or preventing clotting of the blood and lymph in the obstructed tissue. They are mediator cells, representing 0.5 percent of the leukocyte count, which contain vasoactive amines, such as histamine and serotonin, and are believed to be involved in immediate sensitivity. The release of mediators may be triggered in several ways: contact of cells with antigen-antibody complexes, through complement dependent or independent mechanisms, either directly by chemical agents or indirectly through the interaction of antigen with membrane-bound IgE; it may be modulated by cyclic AMP; or it may result from the deposition in tissues of circulating soluble antigen-antibody complexes and tissue injury. Called also *basocyte, basophilic cell, granulocyte,* or *leukocyte,* and *mast leukocyte.* See also table of *Reference Values in Hematology* in Appendix.

basophilia (ba"so-fil'e-ah) 1. presence in the circulating blood of basophilic normoblasts, either as a result of an abnormal condition or through retention in mature nonnucleated erythrocytes of the remnants of the cytoplasmic basophilic substance. Precipitation of the basic substance stained with methyl alcohol or a similar agent is roughly proportional in the intensity of the stain to the amount of substance present. 2. presence in the circulating blood of abnormally large numbers of basophilic leukocytes. **diffuse b.,** that in which the cells appear uniformly blue or gray after staining. **punctate b.,** that characterized by the presence of bluish or bluish black granules in stained erythrocytes, seen in various pathological conditions, such as anemias or heavy metal poisoning, as well as in some normal persons. Called also *basophilic stippling.*

basophilic (ba-so-fil'ik) staining readily with basic dyes.

basophilism (ba-sof'ĭ-lizm) abnormal increase of basophil cells. **Cushing's b., pituitary b.,** Cushing's SYNDROME (1).

Bass' method, technique, toothbrush (brush) [C. C. *Bass,* American physician, a pioneer in preventive dentistry] see TOOTHBRUSHING, and under TOOTHBRUSH.

Bassen-Kornzweig syndrome [Frank A. *Bassen*] acanthocytosis.

Bastedo's rule [Walter Arthur *Bastedo,* American physician, 1873–1952] see under RULE.

batch (bach) 1. a quantity or number coming at one time. 2. bringing a quantity or number of things together. 3. in computer technology, a group of similar sources of data that are processed in a single operation. 4. to group similar sources of data, for example, punched cards, for processing as a single unit.

bath (bath) 1. a conductive or convective medium, such as water, vapor, sand, or mud, with which the body is laved or in which the body is wholly or partly immersed for cleansing or therapeutic purposes. 2. an apparatus in which a body or object may be immersed. **acid b.,** 1. a bath with water medicated with a mineral acid. 2. in film processing, immersion of film in an acid bath of 28 percent solution of acetic acid to improve its radiographic quality, after development and water bath; used in place of the ordinary rinse bath for the purpose of arresting developing processes. Called also *shortstop* and *stop b.* or *stopbath.* **developing b.,** see film DEVELOPMENT. **electroplating b.,** a solution used for electroplating a compound or wax impression, consisting of 225 to 250 gm anhydrous copper sulfate, 75 ml concentrated sulfuric acid, 10 ml phenol, 25 to 50 ml ethyl alcohol, and 1000 ml distilled water. **fixing b.,** see film FIXATION. **rinse b.,** in film processing, the washing of residual developer from the film with water prior to placing it in the fixer. **silver cyanide b.,** a solution used for electroplating polysulfide rubber impressions, consisting of 36 gm silver cyanide, 60 gm potassium cyanide, 40 gm potassium carbonate, and 1000 ml distilled water. **stop b.,** acid b. **water b.,** 1. a vessel containing water for immersing bodies or for immersing liquid-containing vessels that are to be heated or cooled, or are to be held at a given temperature. 2. in film development, immersion in water of film after development to wash out the alkaline developer in the emulsion, or after fixation, to wash out excess fixer and to help prevent streaking of the film.

Batten, Frederic Eustace [English neurologist, 1865–1918] see myotonic DYSTROPHY (Curschmann-Batten-Steinert syndrome).

Battle's sign [William Henry *Battle,* British surgeon, 1855–1936] see under SIGN.

Baudens wiring [Jean Baptiste *Baudens,* French military surgeon, 1804–1857] circumferential WIRING.

Bauhin's glands [Gaspard (Caspar) *Bauhin,* Swiss anatomist, 1560–1624] anterior lingual glands; see under GLAND.

Baum's operation see under OPERATION.

Baumès, Pierre Prosper François [French physician, 1791–1871] see Colles-Baumès LAW.

bauxite (bok'sīt) [named after *Les Baux,* near Arles in southern France] a rock consisting of hydrous aluminum oxide or hydroxides (see ALUMINUM oxide).

bayonet (ba'o-nit, ba'o-net) a binangled offset instrument, the nib of which nevertheless extends in a straight line from the shaft.
b. forceps, bayonet FORCEPS.

bb Bolton POINT.

BCA Blue Cross Association; see under ASSOCIATION.

BCNU carmustine.

b.d. abbreviation for L. *bis di'e*, twice a day.

BDA British Dental Association.

Bdellovibrio (del″o-vib′re-o) [Gr. *bdella* leech + *vibrio*] a genus of bacteria of uncertain affiliation, made up of small rod-shaped or curved cells, 1.0 to 2.0 μm in length and 0.35 μm in width, which are motile by means of a single polar sheathed flagellum. They are found in soil and marine environments as obligate parasites on certain species of gram-negative bacteria, including *Pseudomonas, Salmonella,* and coliform bacteria.

BDG buccal developmental GROOVE.

BDS Bachelor of Dental Surgery.

BDSc Bachelor of Dental Science.

Be beryllium.

Beacillin trademark for *penicillin G benzathine* (see under PENICILLIN).

beam (bēm) 1. a long, slender piece of metal, wood, or other material, serving as a rigid member or support for a structure. 2. a group of parallel or nearly parallel rays. 3. a unidirectional, or approximately unidirectional, emission of electromagnetic radiation or particles. 4. any slender structure of a denture or orthodontic appliance designed to provide support to the structure and subjected to lateral stresses, such as a dental bar or an orthodontic arch wire whose curvature changes under load. See also BAR (1). **cantilever b.,** one supported by a fixed support at only one of its ends. **central b.,** central RAY. **continuous b.,** one that continues over three or more supports; those supports not at the beam being equally free supports. **b. deflection,** beam DEFLECTION. **homogeneous b.,** homogeneous RADIATION. **monochromatic b.,** monochromatic RADIATION. **primary b.,** primary RADIATION. **restrained b.,** one that has two or more supports; at least one of which permits some freedom of rotation to the point of support. **simple b.,** a straight beam that has two supports, one at either end. **useful b.,** that part of the primary radiation permitted to emerge from the tubehead assembly of an x-ray generator, as limited by the tubehead aperture or port and accessory collimating devices. Called also *useful radiation* and *useful rays.*

BEAR Committee on the Biological Effects of Atomic Radiation; see Committee on the Biological Effects of Ionizing Radiation, under COMMITTEE.

bearing (bār'ing) 1. a supporting surface or point. 2. reference or relation. **central b.,** the force between the maxilla and mandible at a single point located as near as possible to the center of the supporting areas of the jaws. Used in the distribution of closing forces evenly throughout the areas of the supporting structures during registration and recording of maxillomandibular jaw relations and during correction of occlusal errors. See also central-bearing tracing DEVICE.

beat (bēt) a throb or pulsation, as of the heart or of an artery. See also PULSE. **irregular b.,** arrhythmia. **premature b.,** extrasystole. **rapid b.,** tachycardia.

Beckwith's syndrome [John Bruce *Beckwith,* American physician, born 1933] Beckwith-Wiedemann SYNDROME.

Beckwith-Wiedemann syndrome [J. B. *Beckwith;* Hans Rudolph *Wiedemann,* German physician] see under SYNDROME.

Béclard's triangle [Pierre Augustin *Béclard,* French anatomist, 1785–1825] see under TRIANGLE.

Becort trademark for *bethamethasone.*

becquerel (bek-rel′) [named after Antoine Henri *Becquerel*] a unit of radiation established by the International Commission on Radiation Units and Measurements to replace the curie (Ci) as a standard unit. It is equal to the second to the power minus one (s^{-1}), and applies to the activity of a quantity of radioactive nuclide as measured by the rate of spontaneous nuclear transformation: $Bq = 1 \ s^{-1} = 2.703 \times 10^{-11}$ Ci. Symbol Bq.

Becquerel rays [Antoine Henri *Becquerel,* French physicist, 1852–1908; co-winner with M. S. Curie and P. Curie of the Nobel prize in physics for 1903, for studies on spontaneous radioactivity] see under RAY, and see BECQUEREL.

bed (bed) 1. a supporting structure or tissue. 2. a couch or support for the body during sleep.

Bednar's aphthae [Alois *Bednar,* physician in Vienna, 1816–1888] see under APHTHA.

Bedsonia (bed-so′ne-ah) a former genus of microorganisms now assigned to the genus *Chlamydia.*

beeswax (bēz′waks) 1. a substance secreted by bees for construction of the honeycomb. 2. a glossy, hard, brittle substance obtained by melting the honeycomb of the bee, consisting chiefly of cerotic acid and myricin, which is soluble in hot alcohol, chloroform, benzene, ether, and carbon disulfide, slightly soluble in cold alcohol, and insoluble in water. It melts at 62 to 65°C. In its natural state, beeswax is yellow (see yellow WAX), but on bleaching it becomes white (see white WAX). Used in dentistry for impression making. Also used in ointments and other pharmaceutic preparations. Called also *insect wax.* **bleached b.,** white WAX. **white b.,** white WAX. **yellow b.,** yellow WAX.

Befedon trademark for *nylidrin hydrochloride* (see under NYLIDRIN).

Begg's appliance, technique, theory (philosophy) [Peter Raymond *Begg,* Australian orthodontist, born 1898] see under APPLIANCE, TECHNIQUE, and THEORY.

Behçet's syndrome (aphthae, disease, triple symptom complex) [Halusi *Behçet,* Turkish dermatologist, 1889–1948] see under SYNDROME.

Behring's law [Emil Adolph von *Behring,* German bacteriologist, 1854–1917, who with Shibasaburo Kitasato, first described antitoxins; winner of the Nobel prize for medicine in 1901] see under LAW.

Beijerinck, M. W. a Dutch microbiologist.

Beijerinckia [named after M. W. *Beijerinck*] a genus of nitrogen-fixing, gram-negative, aerobic, rod-shaped bacteria of the family Azotobacteraceae, isolated from soil, particularly in tropical climates.

Beilby layer see metallographic POLISHING.

BEIR Committee on the Biological Effects of Ionizing Radiation; see under COMMITTEE.

Bekadid trademark for *hydrocodone.*

Bekhterev-Strümpell-Marie syndrome [Vladimir Mikhailovich *Bekhterev,* Russian physician, 1857–1927; Ernst Adolf Gustav Gottfried von *Strümpell,* German physician, 1853–1925; Pierre *Marie,* French physician, 1853–1940] see under SYNDROME.

bel (bel) the common logarithm of the ratio of two powers, usually electric or acoustic powers; such ratios are usually expressed in decibels. An increase of 1 bel in intensity approximately doubles the loudness of most sounds.

Belfacillin trademark for *methicillin.*

Belfene trademark for *diphenylpyraline.*

Bell's law, palsy, phenomenon [Sir Charles *Bell,* Scottish physiologist, 1774–1842] see under LAW, PALSY, and PHENOMENON.

Bell's suture see under SUTURE.

Bell-Magendie law [C. *Bell;* François *Magendie,* French physiologist, 1783–1855] Bell's LAW.

belladonna (bel″ah-don′ah) [Ital. "fair lady"] 1. *Atropa belladonna,* a solanaceous plant of Europe and Asia, which is a source of various alkaloids, including atropine, scopolamine, and *l*-hyoscyamine. Called also *banewort, deadly nightshade, death's herb* and *dwale.* 2. belladonna leaf; the dried leaves and flowering or fruiting tops of *Atropa belladonna,* yielding not less than 0.35 percent of belladonna alkaloids. **b. extract,** an alcoholic extract of belladonna leaves containing, in each 100 gm, 1.15 to 1.35 gm belladonna alkaloids. Used as an antimuscarinic, similarly to atropine. Xerostomia is a common adverse reaction. **b. tincture,** an alcoholic preparation of belladonna leaves containing, in each 100 ml, 27 to 33 mg of alkaloids of belladonna leaf. Used as an antimuscarinic, similarly to atropine. Xerostomia is a common adverse reaction.

belly (bel′e) 1. abdomen. 2. the fleshy part of a muscle. Called also *venter musculi* [NA]. **anterior b. of digastric muscle,** the smaller of the two fleshy bellies of the digastric muscle; it arises from the digastric fossa of the mandible and extends backward to join the posterior belly through an intermediate tendon attached to the hyoid bone. Called also *venter anterior musculi digastrici* [NA]. **frontal b. of occipitofrontal muscle,** the quadrilateral, flat belly of the occipitofrontal muscle which has no bony attachments and originates in the epicranial aponeurosis and inserts into the skin of the eyebrows and the root of the nose. Innervated by the temporal branches of the facial nerve, its functions include tightening the scalp, drawing back the skin of the temples, and wrinkling the forehead and widening the eyes in the production of facial expressions. Called also *frontalis, frontal muscle, musculus frontalis,* and *venter frontalis musculi occipitofrontalis* [NA]. **inferior b. of omohyoid muscle,** the lower belly of the omohyoid muscle; it runs obliquely upward and forward from the scapula, crossing the posterior triangle of the neck, and unites with the superior belly by a central tendon. Called also *venter inferior musculi omohyoidei* [NA]. **occipital b. of occipitofrontal muscle,** the quadrilateral, flat belly of the occipitofrontal muscle; it arises from the lateral two thirds of the superior nuchal line of the occipital bone and from the mastoid part of the temporal bone and inserts into the epicranial aponeurosis. Supplied by the posterior auricular branch of the facial nerve, its functions include drawing back the scalp, raising the eyebrows, and wrinkling the forehead in the production of facial expressions. Called also *musculus occipitalis, occipital muscle, occipitalis*, and *venter occipitalis musculi occipitofrontalis* [NA]. **posterior b. of digastric muscle,** the larger of the two fleshy bellies of the digastric muscle; it arises from the mastoid notch of the temporal bone and extends forward to join the anterior belly through an intermediate tendon attached to the hyoid bone. Called also *venter posterior musculi digastrici* [NA]. **superior b. of omohyoid muscle,** the upper belly of the omohyoid muscle; it runs upward and medially and inserts into the hyoid bone. Called also *venter superior musculi omohyoidei* [NA].

Benadryl trademark for *diphenhydramine*. **Bromo-B.,** trademark for *bromodiphenhydramine*.

Bence Jones protein, proteinuria (albuminosuria) [Henry *Bence Jones*, English physician, 1814–1875] see under PROTEIN and PROTEINURIA.

bend (bend) a turn or curve; a curved part. **first order b's,** in orthodontic therapy, adjustments made in a labial arch wire, incorporating offsets in the horizontal plane, which are usually made in the areas of the cuspids and premolar and molar teeth, accommodating differences in thickness in the labiolingual or buccolingual diameters of the teeth. **second order b's,** in orthodontic therapy, bends in the vertical plane of an arch wire. **third order b's,** in orthodontic therapy, bends in an arch wire to maintain or produce torsion (torque) of a tooth. **V b's,** in orthodontic therapy, V-shaped bends incorporated in an arch wire, usually placed mesial or distal to the cuspids and intended to improve the axial relationship of teeth.

Bendopa trademark for *levodopa*.

bends (bendz) 1. decompression SICKNESS. 2. see air EMBOLISM (2).

Beneckea (be-nek'e-ah) a genus incertae sedis, consisting of many vibrio-like organisms. One species, *B. parahaemolytica*, has been placed in the genus *Vibrio* (*V. parahaemolyticus*).

Benedetti, Alessandro [1460–1525] an Italian physician from Verona who first wrote about the harmful effects of mercury on the teeth and gingivae.

beneficiary (ben″ĕ-fish′e-er′e, ben″ĕ-fish′ĕ-re) a person who receives or is eligible to receive, either directly or on his or her behalf, payments or other benefits under an insurance program or from a health maintenance organization. Sometimes called *eligible individual, enrollee, first party, insured, member*, and *participant*.

benefit (ben′ĕ-fit) 1. anything that is advantageous. 2. in health insurance, the sum of money or services provided in a policy for certain types of procedures performed. 3. schedule of b's. **allowable b.,** any item of service or treatment covered, in whole or part, under an insurance program. See also ALLOWANCE. **b. assignment, assignment of b's,** ASSIGNMENT of benefits. **coordination of b's,** see coordination of benefits CLAUSE. **dental service b.,** a contract benefit paid directly to the provider of dental care for services rendered. **duplication of b's,** see coordination of benefits CLAUSE. **extension of b's,** coverage of charges incurred after a covered person's insurance terminates, usually to complete a plan of treatment commenced while the covered person was insured. Called also *extended coverage*. **indemnity b.,** indemnity PROGRAM. **maximum annual b.,** in health insurance, the maximum dollar amount the plan will pay in compensation for losses or services incurred by an individual or family in a specified policy year; the subscriber incurring the losses above the specified amount or being responsible for all charges for services above the maximum. Called also *annual policy maximum* and *maximum policy benefit*. See also indemnity ALLOWANCE. **b. period,** benefit PERIOD. **predetermination of b's,** prior AUTHORIZATION. **schedule of b's,** in a health insurance plan, a list of services covered under the contract. See also ALLOWANCE. **b. year,** see benefit PERIOD.

Benemid trademark for *probenecid*.

Benesal trademark for *salicylamide*.

benign (be-nīn′) [L. *benignus*] not malignant; a mild form of disease favorable for recovery.

benjamin (ben′jah-min) benzoin (1).

Benjamin's syndrome (anemia) [E. *Benjamin*, German physician] see under SYNDROME.

Bennett angle, movement (shift) see under ANGLE and MOVEMENT.

Benodin trademark for *diphenhydramine*.

benoxyl (ben-ok′sil) BENZOYL peroxide.

Bentelan trademark for *betamethasone sodium phosphate* (see under BETAMETHASONE).

bentonite (ben′ton-īt) a native colloidal, hydrated magnesium

silicate, occurring as a white to gray, odorless and tasteless powder that swells to 12 times its volume in the presence of water to form a translucent suspension with a pH of about 9. Used as a protective colloid to stabilize suspensions, as an emulsifying agent for oils, base for ointments, bulk laxative, and ingredient of dentifrices. Called also *mineral soap, soap clay*, and *wilkinite*.

Bentonyl trademark for *trolnitrate phosphate* (see under TROLNITRATE).

Bentyl trademark for *dicyclomine hydrochloride* (see under DICYCLOMINE).

Benvil trademark for *tybamate*.

Benylan trademark for *diphenhydramine*.

Benzalin trademark for *nitrazepam*.

benzalkonium chloride (ben″zal-ko′ne-um) a mixture of alkylbenzyldimethylammonium chloride, with a general formula [C₆H₅CH₂N(CH₃)₂R]Cl, occurring as a white or yellowish thick gel or gelatinous mass with an aromatic odor and bitter taste. It is soluble in water, alcohol, and benzene. Used as a topical local antibacterial agent applied to the skin and mucous membranes. Also used as an astringent, detergent, and emulsifying agent, and for the sterilization of surgical instruments. It is effective chiefly against gram-positive bacteria, but not against mycobacteria, gram-negative bacteria, and clostridial spores, and also ineffective against viruses. Some organisms, including *Pseudomonas*, can grow and reproduce in benzalkonium chloride solutions. Ingestion may cause poisoning. Also, it may cause skin and mucous membrane irritation and sensitization. Trademark: Zephiran.

Benzatin trademark for *diphenhydramine*.

Benzedrex trademark for *propylhexedrine*.

Benzedrine trademark for *amphetamine*.

benzene (ben′zēn) a hydrocarbon, C₆H₆, occurring as a colorless to light yellow, mobile liquid obtained mainly as a by-product in the destructive distillation of coal, along with coal tar and other products. Benzene has an aromatic odor, and burns with a light flame. It is used as a solvent in organic synthesis in the manufacture of medicinal compounds, dyes, and other substances. Benzene is toxic and when allowed to enter the body by any route, poisoning occurs, most commonly as a result of inhalation of vapors causing irritation of the mucous membrane, including the oral mucosa, convulsions, depression, and death due to respiratory failure. It may first stimulate leukocyte formation with resulting leukocytosis and, sometimes, myeloid leukemia, followed by inhibition of the precursors of all formed blood elements with resulting aplastic anemia. Called also *benzol*. **b. compound,** aromatic COMPOUND. **ethenyl b.,** styrene. **methyl b.,** toluene. **polyvinyl b.,** polystyrene. **b. ring,** benzene RING. **vinyl b.,** styrene.

benzeneazobenzene (ben″zēn-az″o-ben′zēn) azobenzene.

1,4-benzenediol (ben-zēn-di′ol) hydroquinone.

benzethonium chloride (ben″ze-tho′ne-um) a quaternary ammonium compound, benzyldimethyl 2[2-(*p*-(1,1,3,3-tetramethylbutyl)phenoxy]ethoxy]ethyl ammonium chloride, occurring as colorless crystals with a mild odor and bitter taste, which is soluble in water, alcohol, and chloroform and slightly soluble in ether. Used in aqueous solutions and tinctures as an antiseptic for topical application to wounds, lacerations, and infections of the surfaces of the skin and of the mucous membranes of the eye, nose, and oral cavity. Also used as a mild astringent. It is used in some cosmetics and antibacterial soaps. Ingestion may cause vomiting, convulsions, and coma. Trademarks: Phemerol, Quatrachlor, Solamin.

Benzidazol trademark for *tolazoline hydrochloride* (see under TOLAZOLINE).

benzoate (ben′zo-āt) a salt of benzoic acid.

benzocaine (ben′zo-kān) a topical anesthetic, *p*-aminobenzoic acid ethyl ester, occurring as a white, odorless, crystalline powder or solid that is soluble in alcohol, chloroform, fatty oils, and diluted mineral acids and almost insoluble in water. Used chiefly in ointments and a variety of proprietary sprays, powders, creams, and lozenges in the treatment of pain associated with abrasions, ulcers, and other lesions of the skin and mucous membranes. Localized allergic reactions may occur. It inhibits the antibacterial action of sulfonamides. Called also *ethyl aminobenzoate*. Trademarks: Americaine, Anaesthesin, Anesthesin.

Benzodent trademark for an analgesic adhesive ointment, 100 gm of which contains 20 gm benzocaine, 0.40 gm eugenol, 0.1 gm β-hydroxyquinoline sulfate, and the necessary amounts of petrolatum and sodium carboxymethylcellulose.

benzoin (ben′zoin) 1. a balsamic resin obtained from *Styrax* *benzoin* or *S. paralleloneurus* (known as *Sumatra b.*), or from *S. tonkinensis* or other species of *Styrax* (known as *Siam b.*). Siam benzoin contains chiefly the crystalline ester corniferyl benzoate and small amounts of corniferyl alcohol, benzoic acid, *d*-siaresinolic acid, cinnamyl benzoate, and vanillin. Sumatra benzoin is believed to contain the benzoic and cinnamic acid esters of the alcohol benzoresinol and, probably, coniferyl alcohol, free benzoic and cinnamic acids, styrene, cinnamyl cinnamate (styracin), phenylpropyl cinnamate, vanillin, benzaldehyde, benzyl cinnamate and the alcohol *d*-sumaresinol. It occurs as an amorphous solid of various colors, with a characteristic balsamic odor, which is soluble in ethanol and, slightly, in water. Used as a protective for irritation of the skin and mucous membranes. Mixed with glycerol and water, it is applied to skin ulcers, bedsores, cracked nipples, and fissures of the lips, and with sugar for bronchial and throat inflammation. Sometimes used in boiling water as a steam inhalant as an expectorant and soothing agent. In a 20 percent alcoholic solution, used as a soothing and protective agent in gingivitis and herpetic lesions. Also used for fixing or sealing drugs in gingival crevices. Called also *gum b., resin b., benjamin, gum benjamin,* and *resin benjamin.* 2. a white, crystalline compound, 2-hydroxy-1,2-diphenylethanone, prepared by condensation of benzaldehyde in potassium cyanide solution. Used chiefly in chemical synthesis. Called also *benzoylphenylcarbinol* and *bitter almond-oil camphor.* **gum b., resin b.,** benzoin (1).

benzol (ben′zŏl) benzene.

benzolin (ben′zo-lin) DIBUCAINE hydrochloride.

benzoquinone (ben″zo-kwĭ-nōn′) quinone.

benzosulfimide (ben″zo-sul′fĭ-mīd) saccharin.

benzothiazine (ben″zo-thi′ah-zēn) a two-ring heterocyclic analog of 1,2,4-benzothiadiazine-1,1-dioxide. See benzothiazine DIURETIC.

benzoxiquine (ben-zoks′ĭ-kwin″) a disinfectant, 8-quinolinol benzoate (ester), occurring as a crystalline substance that is soluble in ethanol and ether but not in water. Called also *benzoxyline.* Trademark: Dioxyline.

benzoxyline (ben″zo-zi′lēn) benzoxiquine.

benzoyl (ben′zo-il) the radical, $C_6H_5 \cdot CO$, of benzoic acid and of a number of other compounds. **b. hydrochloride,** COCAINE hydrochloride. **b. peroxide,** a white, granular or crystalline, tasteless substance, $(C_6H_5CO)_2O_2$, soluble in organic solvents and slightly soluble in water. Used as a keratolytic agent in the treatment of acne vulgaris and to promote skin peeling. Also used as a catalyst in the polymerization of acrylic resins. It decomposes rapidly at high temperatures and may be explosive. Called also *b. superoxide, benoxyl, dibenzoyl peroxide,* and *oxy-5.* **b. superoxide,** b. peroxide.

benzoylcholinesterase (ben″zo-il-ko″lin-es′ter-ās) cholinesterase (1).

benzoylmethylecgonine (ben″zo-il-meth″il-ek′go-nēn) cocaine.

benzoylphenylcarbinol (ben″zol-fen″il-kar′bĭ-nol) benzoin (2).

benzyl (ben′zil) the hydrocarbon radical, C_7H_7 or $C_6H_5 \cdot CH_2$, of benzyl alcohols and various other bodies.

benzylmorphine hydrochloride (ben″zil-mor′fēn) a semisynthetic opium alkaloid, $C_{24}H_{25}NO_3 \cdot HCl$, prepared from morphine and benzyl chloride in the presence of sodium ethalate, occurring as a white crystalline powder that is soluble in water, ethanol, chloroform, and methanol and is slightly soluble in acetone, ether, and amyl alcohol. It is an addictive analgesic and antitussive agent. Trademark: Peronine.

benzylpenicillin (ben″zil-pen-ĭ-sil′in) penicillin G. **b. potassium,** PENICILLIN G potassium. **b. procaine,** PENICILLIN G procaine. **b. sodium,** PENICILLIN G sodium.

Ber see BAER.

Berant's syndrome [M. *Berant*] see under SYNDROME.

Berdmore, Thomas a dentist of King George III, whose book, *A treatise on the disorders and deformities of the teeth and gums,* published in 1768, was the first English-language textbook of dentistry.

Bergen syndrome see under SYNDROME.

Bergonié-Tribondeau law [Jean Alban *Bergonié,* French physician, 1857–1925; Louis *Tribondeau,* French naval physician, 1872–1918] see under LAW.

Bergström's articulator arcon ARTICULATOR.

beriberi (ber″e-ber′e) [Singhalese, "I cannot," signifying that the person is too ill to do anything] a severe form of thiamine deficiency, formerly endemic in the Orient, usually caused by a diet consisting largely of white (polished) rice, and occurring elsewhere during periods of severe malnutrition. It is character-

ized by cardiovascular and neurological complications and, in some instances, edema (see *wet b.*). Neurological complications may include polyneuritis, hyperesthesia of feet or finger tips, tenderness of calf muscles, painful muscle cramps, muscle atrophy, decreased or absent patellar and achilles tendon reflexes, paralysis, foot drop, retrobulbar neuritis, myelin degeneration, and sometimes Wernicke's encephalopathy. Cardiovascular complications mainly include palpitation, dyspnea, cardiac hypertrophy and dilatation, and congestive heart failure. See also THIAMINE. **wet b.,** beriberi associated with edema, probably due to congestive heart failure.

berkelium (berk′le-um) [named after *Berkeley,* California, where it was produced] a man-made radioactive element. Symbol, Bk; atomic weight, 247; atomic number, 97; valences, 3, 4; specific gravity, 14. It was originally produced as ^{243}Bk with a half-life of 4.6 hours, by cyclotron bombardment of americium-241 with helium ions. Unavailability of sufficient amounts of the element in stable form made it impossible to perform extensive studies on its physical properties, but it is expected to be a metal with a grayish color, and having one of the lightest specific weights of all metals, the highest melting point resistance to nitric acid, good thermal conductivity, nonmagnetic properties, and high permeability to x-rays. Eight isotopes are now known, the most stable being ^{249}Bk with a half-life of 314 days.

Berkmycen trademark for *oxytetracycline.*

Berlin's syndrome [Chaim *Berlin*] see under SYNDROME.

Berman-Moorhead locator see under LOCATOR.

Bernard's syndrome [Jean *Bernard,* French hematologist] acute familial HEMOLYSIS.

Bernard-Horner syndrome [Claude *Bernard,* French physician, 1813–1878; Johann Friedrich *Horner,* Swiss ophthalmologist, 1831–1886] see under SYNDROME.

Bernays' sponge [Augustus Charles *Bernays,* American surgeon, 1854–1907] see under SPONGE.

Beromycin trademark for *penicillin V potassium* (see under PENICILLIN).

Berry's ligament [Sir James *Berry,* Canadian surgeon, 1860–1946] thyrohyoid LIGAMENT.

Bertin's bone, ossicle [Exupère Joseph *Bertin,* French anatomist, 1712–1781] sphenoidal CONCHA.

beryllium (ber-il′e-um) [Gr. *beryllos* beryl] a grayish, hard, brittle, flexible metal with a sweet taste. Symbol, Be; atomic weight, 9.01218; atomic number, 4; specific gravity, 1.848; valence, 2; group IIA of the periodic table. It has a single stable isotope. Beryllium is soluble in alkalies and acids, except for nitric acid, and resistant to oxidation at normal room temperature. It is used in nuclear reactors and various electric and space technology products. Because of its high permeability to x-rays, beryllium is used in x-ray machine windows. Contact dermatitis, eye lesions, ulcers of the skin and mucous membranes, pneumonia, granulomatous lesions, and death may follow exposure to even small quantities of beryllium. Called also *glucinum.*

Besecil trademark for *methylthiouracil.*

Besnier's prurigo [Ernest *Besnier,* French dermatologist, 1831–1909] see under PRURIGO.

Besnier-Boeck-Schaumann syndrome [E. *Besnier;* Caesar Peter Möller *Boeck,* Norwegian dermatologist, 1845–1913; Jörgen *Schaumann,* Swedish dermatologist, 1879–1953] sarcoidosis.

Bespaloff's sign see under SIGN.

beta (ba′tah) β, the second letter of the Greek alphabet, used in organic chemical nomenclature to denote the position of a substituent or radical on a carbon chain.

Beta-Cardone trademark for *sotalol.*

Betadine trademark for *povidone-iodine.*

Betafluorene trademark for *betamethasone.*

betamethasone (ba″tah-meth′ah-zōn) a synthetic glucocorticoid derived from 16-dehydropregnenolone, 9-fluoro-11β,17,21-trihydroxy-16β-methylpregna-1,4-diene-3,20-dione, occurring as a white, odorless, crystalline powder that is slightly soluble in acetone, ethanol, methanol, dioxane, chloroform, and ether and is insoluble in water. Used in the treatment of adrenocortical insufficiency and as an anti-inflammatory and antiallergic agent. In dentistry, used in the treatment of sensitive dentin, postoperative pulpal reactions, ulcers of the oral mucosa, and arthritic temporomandibular lesions, and in tissue transplantation. Side reactions are similar to those of other glucocorticoids, but sodium and water retention and potassium loss are rare. Trademarks: Becort, Betafluorene, Betasol, Celestone. **b. acetate,** betamethasone acetylated with acetic anhydride, occurring as a white, odorless powder that is soluble in ethanol, chloroform, and acetone, but is insoluble in water. **b. sodium phosphate,** a 21-disodium phosphate derivative of betamethasone. Trademarks: Bentelan, Betnesol. **b. valerate,** a 17-valerate derivative of betamethasone, occurring as a white, odorless, crystalline powder that is soluble in acetone, chloroform, and ethanol, slightly soluble in benzene and ether, and insoluble in water. Trademarks: Betnesol-V, Betneval, Celestan-V, Valisone.

beta-plus (ba′tah-plus) positron.

Betasol trademark for *bethamethasone.*

betatron (ba′tah-tron) an apparatus for accelerating electrons to millions of electron volts by means of magnetic induction. It produces electrons (negatively charged particles known as *beta rays*) and photons (x-rays).

betel (bēt′t′l) [Tamil *vettilei*] an East Indian masticatory, consisting of a piece of betel nut rolled up with lime in a betel leaf; it is tonic, astringent, and stimulant. Prolonged chewing of betel leaves (buyo leaves) may cause cancer (see buyo leaf CANCER).

Betnesol trademark for *betamethasone sodium phosphate* (see under BETAMETHASONE).

Betnesol-V trademark for *betamethasone valerate* (see under BETAMETHASONE).

Betneval trademark for *betamethasone valerate* (see under BETAMETHASONE).

Betz cell [Vladimir Aleksandrovich *Betz*, Russian anatomist, 1834–1894] see under CELL.

Beuren's syndrome [A. J. *Beuren*] elfin facies SYNDROME.

bevel (bev′el) 1. the slope of a surface from the horizontal or vertical; a slanting edge. 2. to produce a slanting of the enamel margins of a tooth cavity. **cavosurface b.,** the incline or slant of the cavosurface angle of a prepared cavity wall in relation to the plane of the enamel wall. **contra b.,** reverse b. **instrument b.,** the sloping sharp edge of a cutting instrument. **reverse b.,** the slant on the side reverse to the working side of an instrument, usually closer to the shaft or shank or toward the lesser angle with the shaft. Called also *contra b.* **standing b.,** an obtuse angle formed by one surface or line with another. **under b.,** an acute angle formed by one surface or line with another.

Bezold's abscess, mastoiditis, perforation, sign [Friedrich *Bezold*, Munich otologist, 1842–1908] see under ABSCESS, MASTOIDITIS, PERFORATION, and SIGN.

Bez-Thru trademark for floss threaders for threading dental floss under bridges and between connected jacket crowns.

bhang (bang) [Hindi] a cannabinoid substance prepared in India from a mixture of the dried leaves of young stems of uncultivated *Cannabis sativa,* usually ingested as a decoction with milk, sugar, and water, or sometimes smoked or chewed for its intoxicating properties. See also CANNABINOID.

BHI Bureau of Health Insurance; see under BUREAU.

BHN Brinell hardness number; see under HARDNESS.

Bi bismuth.

bi- [L. *bi* two] 1. a prefix signifying two or twice. 2. in chemical nomenclature, generally used in connection with molecules made up of two similar halves; the number of each type of monodentate ligand in a coordination compound. See also BIS- and DI-.

biangled (bi-ang′g′ld) having two angles or bends.

biarticular (bi″ar-tik′u-lar) pertaining to two joints.

bias (bi′as) 1. a particular tendency or inclination, especially one which inhibits impartial consideration; prejudice. 2. in statistics, a systematic, calculated (as opposed to random) deviation from the true value. 3. in electronics, a steady component of an electric potential difference. **grid b.,** the direct voltage in the grid circuit of an electron tube.

Bib. abbreviation for L. *bi′be,* drink.

bibasic (bi-ba′sik) doubly basic; having two hydrogen atoms that may react with bases.

bibeveled (bi′bev-eld) having a slanting surface on two sides, as some dental instruments; hatchet edged.

bicalcium (bi-kal′se-um) CALCIUM phosphate, basic.

bicarbonate (bi-kar′bo-nāt) any salt containing the HCO₃⁻ anion. **blood b.,** the bicarbonate of the blood; see alkali RESERVE. **b. of soda,** SODIUM bicarbonate.

Bichat, Marie François Xavier [1771–1802] an eminent French anatomist and physiologist, who founded the fields of scientific histology and pathological anatomy. See Henle's fenestrated MEMBRANE (Bichat's membrane), and buccal fat PAD (fatty ball of Bichat).

bichloride (bi-klo′rīd) any chloride that contains two equivalents of chlorine. **mercury b.,** mercuric CHLORIDE.

Bicillin trademark for *penicillin G benzathine* (see under PENICILLIN). **B. V,** trademark for *penicillin B benzathine* (see under PENICILLIN).

Bickerstaff's encephalitis [E. R. *Bickerstaff,* British physician] see under ENCEPHALITIS.

biconcave (bi-kon′kāv) [*bi-* + L. *concavus*] having two concave surfaces.

biconvex (bi-kon′veks) [*bi-* + L. *convexus*] having two convex surfaces, as the opposite sides of a structure.

Bicortone trademark for *prednisone.*

bicuspid (bi-kus′pid) [*bi-* + L. *cuspis* point] 1. having two cusps or points. 2. a bicuspid valve. 3. a tooth with two cusps. See premolar teeth, under TOOTH.

bicuspidal (bi-kus′pī-dal) 1. pertaining to a bicuspid tooth. 2. having two cusps.

bicuspidate (bi-kus′pī-dāt) having two cusps.

bicuspoid (bi-kus′poid) a figure in space resembling a bicuspid tooth, representing the space traversed in all its movements by a point in one jaw in relation to the other jaw.

b.i.d. abbreviation for L. *bis in di′e,* twice a day.

bidental (bi-den′tal) [*bi-* + L. *dens* tooth] having, pertaining to, or affecting two teeth.

bidentate (bi-den′tāt) 1. having two teeth or toothlike structures. 2. bidentate LIGAND.

Biederman's sign [Bear *Biederman,* American physician, born 1907] see under SIGN.

Bier's local anesthesia see under ANESTHESIA.

Biermer's anemia [Anton *Biermer,* German physician, 1827–1892] pernicious ANEMIA.

bifid (bi′fid) cleft into two parts or branches.

Bifidobacterium (bif″ī-do-bak-te′re-um) [L. *bifidus* cleft + Gr. *baktērion* little rod] a genus of gram-positive, non–acid-fast, non–spore-forming, nonmotile bacteria of the family Actinomycetaceae, order Actinomycetales. The organisms occur as rods with varied shapes, uniform or branched, bifurcated Y and V forms, and club or spatulate shapes, their morphology being influenced by nutritional conditions. Mostly anaerobic, some strains exhibit oxygen tolerance in the presence of CO_2. They stain irregularly; while some cells may be stained with methylene blue, others in the same culture remain unstained. **B. adolescen′tis,** a species isolated from human feces, the appendix, dental caries, and the vagina.

bifidus (bif′ī-dus) bifid.

biforate (bi-fo′rāt) [*bi-* + L. *fora* opening] having two foramina or openings.

bifunctional (bi-funk′shun-al) 1. having two functions. 2. in chemistry, having two reaction sites; said of a molecule.

bifurcate (bi-fur′kāt) [*bi-* + L. *furca* fork] forked; divided into two branches.

bifurcatio (bi″fur-ka′she-o), pl. *bifurcatio′nes* [L.] bifurcation.

bifurcation (bi″fur-ka′shun) [L. *bifurcatio,* from *bi-* + *furca* fork] 1. division into two branches. 2. the site where a single structure divides into two, as in the roots of a molar tooth.

bifurcationes (bi″fur-ka″she-o′nēz) [L.] plural of *bifurcatio.*

bigeminal (bi-jem′ī-nal) [L. *bigeminum* twin] occurring in twos; twin.

Bikadid trademark for *hydrocodone.*

bilabial (bi-la′be-al) a sound produced with the lips close together or touching; a consonant sound formed with the lips closed, as *p, b,* and *m.*

bilaminar (bi-lam′ī-nar) [*bi-* + L. *lamina* layer] pertaining to or having two laminae or layers.

bilateral (bi-lat′er-al) [*bi-* + L. *latus* side] having two sides, or pertaining to both sides.

bile (bīl) [L. *bilis*] fluid secreted by the liver and stored in the gallbladder before being discharged into the duodenum, where it plays an essential role in absorption by dissolving the products of fat digestion, thus assisting in fat absorption from the gastrointestinal system.

Bilevon trademark for *hexachlorophene.*

bili- [L. *bilis* bile] a combining form denoting relationship to the bile.

Bilidren trademark for *dehydrocholic acid* (see under ACID).

bilirubin (bil″ī-roo′bin) [*bili-* + L. *ruber* red] a bile pigment; it is a breakdown product of heme, mainly formed from the degradation of hemoglobin, but also formed by breakdown of other heme pigments. Bilirubin normally circulates in plasma as a complex with albumin, and is taken up by the liver and conjugated to form bilirubin diglucuroside and excreted in bile. See also HYPERBILIRUBINEMIA.

bilirubinemia (bil″ī-roo-bī-ne′me-ah) [*bilirubin* + Gr. *haima* blood + *-ia*] the presence of bilirubin in the urine.

bilirubinuria (bil″ī-roo-bī-nu′re-ah) [*bilirubin* + Gr. *ouron* urine + *-ia*] the presence of bilirubin in the urine.

billet (bil′et) pluglet.

Billroth's operation [Christian Albert Theodor *Billroth,* Austrian surgeon, 1829–1894] see under OPERATION.

bilobate (bi-lo′bāt) having two lobes.

bilobular (bi-lob′u-lar) having two lobules.

bilocular (bi-lok′u-lar) [bi- + L. *loculus* cell] having two compartments.

bilophodont (bi-lof′o-dont) [bi- + Gr. *lophos* ridge + *odous* tooth] having molariform teeth with two transverse ridges.

bimanual (bi-man′u-al) [bi- + L. *manualis* of the hand] with both hands; performed by both hands.

bimastoid (bi-mas′toid) pertaining to both mastoid processes.

bimaxillary (bi-mak′sĭ-ler″e) [bi- + *maxilla*] pertaining to or affecting both jaws.

bimethyl (bi-meth′il) ethane.

Bimler appliance (stimulator) [H. P. *Bimler*] see under APPLIANCE.

bimodal (bi-mo′dal) having two modes or peaks; said of a graphic curve.

bimolecular (bi″mo-lek′u-lar) relating to or formed from two molecules.

binangle (bin′ang-g'l) having two angles; a dental instrument having two angulations in the shank connecting the handle, or shaft, with the working portion of the instrument, known as the blade, or nib.

binary (bi′nah-re) 1. a numbering system based on twos rather than tens, in which the selective position of a number, expressed as 0 or 1, corresponds to a power of 2 multiplier. 2. in mathematics, of or pertaining to a binary system, or assigning a third quantity to two given quantities, as in the addition of two numbers. 3. in chemistry, pertaining to compounds containing only two elements with two or more atoms; a mixture of any two substances; as containing two bases or any combination of two metals. See also binary COMPOUND.

binder (bīnd′er) a substance that holds solid particles in a mixture together.

Binder's syndrome [K. H. *Binder*] see under SYNDROME.

Bindit trademark for a self-curing *repair resin* (see under RESIN).

Bing bridge [Benjamin *Bing*, American dentist in Paris, 19th century] see under BRIDGE.

bio- [Gr. *bios* life] a combining form denoting relationship to life.

bioassay (bi″o-as-sa′) [bio- + *assay*] determination of the active power of a sample of a drug by noting its effect on animals, as compared with the effect of a standard preparation. Called also *biological assay*. See also PHARMACOMETRICS.

bioavailability (bi″o-ah-vāl″ah-bil′ĭ-te) the degree to which a drug or other substance becomes available to the target tissue after administration, determined by the rate of absorption of a dose of the drug, measured by the time-concentration curve for appearance of the administered drug in the blood.

biochemistry (bi″o-kem′is-tre) [bio- + *chemistry*] the chemistry of living organisms and of vital processes. Called also *biological chemistry* and *physiological chemistry*.

biodegradable (bi″o-de-grād′ah-b'l) susceptible of degradation by biological processes.

Biodopa trademark for *levodopa*.

bioelectricity (bi″o-e″lek-tris′ĭ-te) [bio- + *electricity*] electricity produced by living cells.

bioequivalence (bi″o-e-kwiv′ah-lens) a condition existing when two different drugs have the same bioavailability. See also bioequivalent DRUG.

bioethics (bi″o-eth′iks) [bio- + *ethics*] the study of social and moral questions raised by developments in the fields of biology and medicine, including dentistry. See medical ETHICS.

BIOETHICSLINE an acronym for a computer-searchable data base containing references to the literature dealing with bioethical topics such as euthanasia and human experimentation, produced jointly by the National Library of Medicine and the Kennedy Institute of Ethics at the Georgetown University.

biofeedback (bi″o-fēd′bak) 1. the process of providing sensory, usually auditory or visual, information to a person on the status of autonomic functions of the body, as by sounding of a tone when blood pressure is at a desirable level, so that the person may eventually be conditioned to exert control over the function. 2. a technique of instrumentation intended to give a person immediate and continuing signals of change in bodily function of which the person is usually unaware.

biogenesis (bi″o-jen′e-sis) [bio- + Gr. *genesis* origin] 1. the origin of life, or of living organisms. 2. the theory that living organisms can originate only from organisms already living. Cf. ABIOGENESIS.

biologic (bi″o-loj′ik) pertaining to biology.

biological (bi″ol-loj′ĭ-kal) 1. biologic. 2. a medicinal preparation made from living organisms and their products, including a vaccine, toxin, antitoxin, or antigen. Called also *biological product*.

biology (bi-ol′o-je) [bio- + -*logy*] the science that deals with the study of life or living matter in all its forms and phenomena.

Biolux 521 trademark for a heat-cured denture base acrylic polymer.

biomechanics (bi″o-mē-kan′iks) [bio- + *mechanics*] the application of mechanical laws to living structures, specifically to the locomotor systems of the human body. See also BIONICS. **dental b.**, the relationship between the biologic behavior of oral structures and the physical influence of a dental restoration or appliance. Called also *dental biophysics*.

biometry (bi-om′ĕ-tre) [bio- + Gr. *metron* measure] 1. the science of the application of statistical methods to biological factors; analysis of biological data. 2. in insurance, the calculation of the expectation of life.

Biomioran trademark for *chlorzoxazone*.

Bio-Mycin trademark for *oxytetracycline hydochloride* (see under OXYTETRACYCLINE).

Biomycin trademark for *chlortetracycline hydrochloride* (see under CHLORTETRACYCLINE).

bion (bi′on) [Gr. *bioun* a living being] an individual living organism.

bionecrosis (bi″o-ne-kro′sis) necrobiosis.

bionics (bi-on′iks) the science concerned with study of the functions, characteristics, and phenomena found in the living world and application of the knowledge gained to new devices and techniques in the world of machines. See also BIOMECHANICS.

bio-osmotic (bi″o-oz-mot′ik) [bio- + *osmotic*] pertaining to osmotic processes in a living organism. See also DIFFUSION.

Biophedrin trademark for the *l*-form of *ephedrine hydrochloride* (see under EPHEDRINE).

biophysics (bi-o-fiz′iks) [bio- + *physics*] the science dealing with the application of physical methods and theories to biological problems. **dental b.**, dental BIOMECHANICS.

biopsy (bi′op-se) [bio- + Gr. *opsis* vision] the removal and examination of tissue or other material from the living body for purposes of diagnosis. See also surgical PATHOLOGY. **aspiration b.**, needle b. **endoscopic b.**, removal of tissue by appropriate instruments introduced through an endoscope. **excisional b.**, biopsy of tissue removed by incision; biopsy of an entire lesion, including a significant margin of contiguous normal-appearing tissue. **exploratory b.**, exploration combined with biopsy to determine the type and extent of neoplasms, both deep and superficial. **fractional b.**, histologic study of only fragments of a growth which have been removed for the purpose, before excision of the lesion in its entirety. **incisional b.**, biopsy of a selected portion of a lesion and, if possible, of adjacent normal-appearing tissue. **needle b.**, biopsy of material obtained by aspiration through a needle. Called also *aspiration b.* **punch b.**, biopsy of material obtained from body tissue by a punch. **sponge b.**, histological examination of material obtained by rubbing a sponge made of a suitable material over a lesion, and consequent fixing, sectioning, staining, and examination of the entire sponge. **surface b.**, examination of cells scraped from the surface of a suspected lesion. **surgical b.**, examination of tissue removed from the body by surgery. **total b.**, examination of tissue of a lesion that has been removed in its entirety.

biorhythm (bi″o-rith″m) biologic RHYTHM.

biose (bi′ōs) 1. a carbohydrate containing two hydroxyl groups. 2. former name for DISACCHARIDE.

Biostat trademark for *oxytetracycline*.

biosynthesis (bi″o-sin′thĕ-sis) [bio- + *synthesis*] the synthesis of a chemical compound by a living tissue.

Biotetraciclin trademark for *demeclocycline*.

Biotexin trademark for *novobiocin*.

biotin (bi′o-tin) a vitamin of the B complex, hexahydro-2-oxo-1*H*-thieno[3,4-*d*] imidazole-4-pentanoic acid, occurring as a colorless crystalline compound that is soluble in water, dilute alkali, and alcohol, but not in other organic solvents. It is a coenzyme for several carboxylation reactions catalyzed by enzymes and is involved in CO_2 fixation. It occurs in bacteria, yeasts, and fungi. Foods especially rich in biotin include egg yolk, liver, kidneys, milk, and yeast. Relatively large amounts of biotin may be administered without toxic effects. Human requirements are not known but a daily intake of 150 to 300 mg is considered adequate. Called also *coenzyme R* and *vitamin H*. Biotin deficiency is rare because of the wide availability of biotin in foods and because it is synthesized by intestinal bacteria. Experimental deficiency varies with species. Human subjects fed biotin-deficient diets and large amounts of raw egg white, which contains avidin, a biotin-binding protein, may develop dermatitis of the extremities, pallor of the skin and mucous membranes, depression, lassitude, somnolence, hyperesthesia, muscle pain, anorexia, nausea, slight anemia, and electrocardiographic changes. Oral symptoms may include pallor of the tongue and papillary atrophy similar to that seen in geographic tongue.

biotransformation (bi″o-trans″for-ma′shun) the series of chemical alterations of a compound (e.g., a drug) which occur within the body, as by enzymatic activity.

biparietal (bi″pah-ri′ĕ-tal) pertaining to the two parietal eminences or bones.

biperforate (bi-per′fō-rāt) [*bi-* + L. *perforatus* bored through] having two perforations.

bipolar (bi-pol′ar) 1. having two poles; having processes at both poles. 2. pertaining to both poles. 3. a two-poled nerve cell.

bird-face (bird′fās) a form of dyscephaly in which the skull is small and the facial bones are large, giving a birdlike appearance. See Seckel's SYNDROME.

birth (birth) the act or process of being born.

birthmark (birth′mark) nevus.

bis- [L. *bis* twice] 1. a prefix signifying two or twice. 2. in chemical nomenclature, meaning twice, generally used in connection with molecules made up of two similar halves; the number of each type of monodentate ligand in a coordination compound, particularly the number of chelate or complicated ligands. See also BI- and DI-.

biscuit (bis′ket) in dentistry, porcelain that has undergone the first (low biscuit) firing and assumes a surface texture resembling that of a cookie. Called also *bisque*. See FIRING (2). **hard b.,** dental porcelain during firing after shrinking but before vitrification. Called also *hard bisque*. **high, low, medium b. firing,** see under FIRING. **soft b.,** dental porcelain during firing while it undergoes stiffening but before shrinkage has begun. Called also *soft bisque*.

biscuiting (bis′ket″ing) the first (low biscuit) baking of porcelain. See FIRING (2).

bisection (bi-sek′shun) [*bi-* + L. *sectio* a cut] a division or cutting into two parts; hemisection.

biseptate (bi-sep′tāt) [*bi-* + L. *septum* partition] divided into two parts by a septum.

BIS-GMA dimethacrylate.

Bishop retractor see under RETRACTOR.

bishydroxycoumarin (bis″hi-drok″se-koo′mah-rin) dicumarol.

bis in die (bis in de′a) [L.] twice a day; abbreviated *b.d.* or *b.i.d.*

bismuth (biz′muth) [L. *bismuthum*] a brittle, silvery metal with a pinkish tinge. Symbol, Bi; atomic number, 83; atomic weight, 208.9808; specific gravity, 9.947; melting point, 271.3°C; valences, 2, 3, 4; group VA of the periodic table; Brinell hardness number, 7. Bismuth has one stable isotope. It is soluble in nitric and hydrochloric acids. It is not fabricable at room temperature, but is extrudable at 437°F. Bismuth-containing preparations are used in the treatment of skin disease but their application is diminishing; formerly used in the treatment of syphilis. Massive intake of bismuth may cause death. Mild poisoning produces necrosis of the gastric mucosa, liver, and kidneys. Presenting symptoms include foul breath, diarrhea, lack of appetite, weakness, and muscular pain. Oral manifestations include pigmentation of the oral mucosa, especially of the gingiva and buccal mucosa. A thin blue-black line (bismuth line) of the marginal gingiva, sometimes confined to the gingival papilla, is the most characteristic sign; the lips, ventral surface of the tongue, and any localized area of inflammation may be involved. The pigment represents precipitated granules of bismuth sulfide produced by the action of hydrogen sulfide on bismuth in the tissue. See also bismuth PIGMENTATION and bismuth STOMATITIS. **b. sulfide,** dark brown crystals or powder that may be produced by the action of hydrogen sulfide on bismuth in the tissue, representing the pigment in bismuth pigmentation (see under PIGMENTATION).

bisphenol (bis-fe′nol) a compound occurring in two forms: *Bisphenol A,* 4,4′-(1-methylethylidene)bisphenol, occurring as crystalline solids or flakes that are soluble in aqueous alkaline solutions, ethanol, acetone and, slightly, carbon tetrachloride, but not in water; used in the manufacture of epoxy resins and polycarbonates and as a fungicide; *Bisphenol B,* 4,4′-(1-methylpropylidene)bisphenol, occurring as crystalline granules that are soluble in acetone, benzene, carbon tetrachloride, methanol, ether, and water; used in the production of phenolic resins. **b. A glycidyl methacrylate,** see under METHACRYLATE.

bisque (bisk) [Fr.] biscuit. **hard b.,** hard BISCUIT. **soft b.,** soft BISCUIT.

bisulfide (bi-sul′fīd) disulfide.

bit (bit) 1. a small piece or quantity of anything. 2. binary DIGIT.

bite (bīt) 1. the forcible closure of the lower against the upper teeth. 2. the measure of force exerted in the closure of the teeth. 3. a record of the relationship of upper and lower teeth, in occlusion, obtained by biting into a mass of modeling substance. 4. the part of an artificial tooth on the lingual side between the shoulder and the incisal edge of the tooth. 5. a wound or puncture made by the teeth or other parts of the mouth. 6. a morsel of food. **balanced b.,** balanced OCCLUSION. **biscuit b.,** an interocclusal record made in soft wax, usually in centric position. **b. block,** bite BLOCK. **check b.,** a thin sheet of wax or a modeling compound placed between the teeth, in centric, eccentric, lateral, or protrusive occlusion, and pressed to their buccal or labial surfaces after the jaws have been closed; used to check dental occlusion in the articulator in properly aligning study models. Written also *check-bite*. **check b., lateral,** interocclusal record, lateral; see under RECORD. **closed b.,** malocclusion, being decreased occlusal vertical dimension with an abnormal overbite in which the mandible protrudes; that is, the incisal edges of the mandibular anterior teeth extend lingually past the incisal edges of the maxillary, approaching the lingual gingival margin, when the jaws are in habitual occlusion. Called also *deep b., closed-bite malocclusion, deep overbite,* and *deep vertical overlap.* **compound b.,** open b., compound. **cross b.,** crossbite. **deep b.,** closed b. **dual b.,** two positions for centric occlusion. **edge-to-edge b., end-to-end b.,** edge-to-edge OCCLUSION. **b. guard,** occlusal GUARD. **infantile open b.,** open b., infantile. **mush b.,** mushbite. **open b.,** a condition marked by failure of opposing teeth to establish occlusal contact when the jaws are closed. Called also *apertognathia, nonocclusion,* and *open-bite malocclusion.* **open b., compound,** lack of occlusion between the premolar areas. Called also *compound apertognathia.* **open b., infantile,** one from molar to molar that develops with the earliest growth of the alveolar process and eruption of the teeth. Called also *infantile apertognathia.* **open b., simple,** one involving the canine teeth. Called also *simple apertognathia.* **over b.,** overbite. **raising b.,** RAISING bite. **b. rim,** occlusion RIM. **scissors b.,** total lingual crossbite of the mandible, with the mandibular teeth completely contained within the maxillary dental arch in habitual occlusion. Written also *scissors-bite.* **simple open b.,** open b., simple. **skeletal open b.,** long face SYNDROME. **skeletal-type deep b.,** short face SYNDROME. **b. stick,** mouthstick. **underhung b.,** a bite characteristic of mandibular prognathism in which the incisal edges of the mandibular anterior teeth extend labially to the incisal edges of the maxillary anterior teeth when the jaws are in habitual occlusion. **wax b.,** an impression, made simultaneously, of both the upper and the lower jaw, by having the subject bite on a double layer of soft baseplate wax. **X-b.,** crossbite.

bite-block (bīt′blok) 1. occlusion RIM. 2. bite BLOCK.

bitegage (bīt′gāj) a device used in prosthodontics as an aid in securing proper occlusion of the maxillary and mandibular teeth.

bitelock (bīt′lok) occlusion RIM.

bitemporal (bī-tem′po-ral) pertaining to both temporal bones.

biteplane (bīt′plān) an orthodontic removable appliance, made of acrylic resin, covering all the maxillary teeth, and kept in place by orthodontic wrought wire clasps and labial wires; used in the diagnosis and treatment of pain of the temporomandibular joint and adjacent muscles. Written also *bite plane.*

biteplate (bīt′plāt) bite PLATE.

bite-wing (bīt′wing) a central tab or wing of a dental x-ray film, which is held between the upper and lower teeth during radiography of oral structures. See also bite-wing FILM and bite-wing RADIOGRAPH.

biting (bī′ting) [L. *morsicatio*] 1. the act or process of cutting or tearing with the teeth, as of food. 2. the act or process of causing a wound or puncture by the teeth or other mouth parts of a living organism. **cheek b.,** a habit of sucking and biting one's own cheek, sometimes during sleep, which may lead to maceration and milky white appearance of the buccal mucosa, malposition of the teeth, and muscular discomfort, thereby predisposing to traumatic occlusion. Called also *morsicatio buccarum* and *pathomimia mucosae oris.* See also Lesch-Nyhan SYNDROME. **lip b.,** a habit consisting of compulsive biting of one's own lip, which may lead to soft tissue injury, malposition of the teeth, and muscular discomfort, thereby predisposing to traumatic occlusion. Called also *cheilophagia.* See also Lesch-

Nyhan SYNDROME. **b. pressure,** occlusal PRESSURE. **tongue b.,** a habit consisting of biting the tip of one's own tongue, which may lead to soft tissue injury, malposition of the teeth, and muscular discomfort, thereby predisposing to traumatic occlusion.

bitumen (bi-tu′men) a mixture of hydrocarbons occurring both naturally and as residue from petroleum distillation. **sulfonated b.,** ichthammol.

bituminol (bi-tu′mĭ-nol) ichthammol.

bivalence (biv′ah-lens) [*bi-* + L. *valere* powerful] the property of an atom of certain chemical elements of forming chemical bonds with two other atoms or groups.

bivalent (bi-va′lent, biv′ah-lent) 1. having a valence of two; characterized by bivalence. 2. denoting homologous chromosomes associated in pairs, during the first meiotic phase. Called also *divalent*.

bizygomatic (bi″zi-go-mat′ik) [*bi-* + *zygoma*] pertaining to the two most prominent points on the two zygomatic arches.

Bk berkelium.

black (blak) 1. reflecting no light or true color; of the darkest hue. 2. a black pigment. **animal b., bone b.,** animal CHARCOAL. **carbon b.,** a form of amorphous carbon, composed of fine charcoal particles produced by incomplete combustion or thermal decomposition of natural gas or petroleum. Depending on the method of production, it is known as *channel b., furnance b., gas b.,* and *thermal b.,* **channel b., furnance b., gas b.,** types of carbon black. **ivory b.,** animal CHARCOAL. **lamp b.,** a form of amorphous carbon, produced by smoky flame of burning oils, rosin, or fats. **Paris b.,** animal CHARCOAL. **thermal b.,** a type of carbon black.

Black's formula, wiring [Greene Vardiman *Black,* American dentist, researcher, and educator, 1831–1915] see under FORMULA and WIRING, and see DENTISTRY.

Blackfan, Kenneth D. see Diamond-Blackfan SYNDROME.

blackhead (blak′hed) comedo.

blackout (blak′owt) a condition characterized by failure of vision and momentary unconsciousness, due to diminished circulation to the brain. See also COMA and UNCONSCIOUSNESS.

Bladan trademark for *tetraethyl pyrophosphate* (see under PYROPHOSPHATE).

bladder (blad′der) [L. *vesica, cystis;* Gr. *kystis*] a membranous sac, such as one serving as a receptacle for secretion; often used alone to designate the urinary bladder. Called also *vesica.* **urinary b.,** the musculomembranous sac, situated in the anterior part of the pelvic cavity that serves as a reservoir for urine, which it receives from the kidneys through the ureters and discharges through the urethra. Called also *vesica urinaria* [NA].

blade (blād) 1. the flat, cutting part of a knife. 2. the end portion of a dental instrument designed for cutting, probing, or scraping, connected by a shank to the handle. See illustration at DENTISTRY. **carving b.,** carver. **endosteal implant b.,** a metal part of an implant substructure, usually made of a chromium-cobalt alloy or titanium, forming a wedge-shaped blade with openings or vents for tissues to proliferate through, thus providing additional retention. See also endosseous IMPLANT, implant SUBSTRUCTURE, and subperiosteal IMPLANT. **b. implant,** blade IMPLANT. **knife b.,** an elongated or short pointed sharp blade of a surgical knife. See illustration at SCALPEL. **scalpel b.,** see SCALPEL.

Blaes see BLASIUS.

Blair, Vilray Papin [1871–1955] a distinguished American plastic and maxillofacial surgeon.

Blair knife see under KNIFE.

blanc (blaw) [Fr.] white. **b. fixe,** BARIUM sulfate.

bland (bland) [L. *blandus*] mild or soothing.

Blandin's ganglion, glands [Philippe Frédéric *Blandin,* French surgeon, 1798–1849] see submandibular GANGLION, and lingual glands, anterior, under GLAND.

Blandin-Nuhn cyst [P. F. *Blandin;* Anton *Nuhn,* German anatomist, 1814–1880] see under CYST.

Blasius' (Blaes') duct [Gerhard *Blasius,* Dutch anatomist, 17th century] parotid DUCT.

Blaskovics' operation see under OPERATION.

blast (blast) [Gr. *blastos* germ] 1. an immature stage in cellular development before appearance of the definitive characteristics of the cell. Used also as a word termination. See also BLASTO-. 2. [Anglo-Saxon *blœst* a puff of wind] the wave of air pressure produced by detonation or explosion.

blastema (blas-te′mah) [Gr. *blastēma* shoot] 1. the primitive substance from which cells are formed. 2. a group of cells that give rise to a new individual.

blasto- [Gr. *blastos* germ] a combining form denoting relationship to a bud or budding, particularly to an early embryonic stage, as to a primitive or formative element, cell, or layer.

blastocoele (blas′to-sēl) [*blasto-* + Gr. *koilos* hollow] the fluid-filled cavity of the mass of cells (blastula or blastocyst) produced by cleavage of a zygote. Called also *blastocyst cavity, cleavage cavity, segmentation cavity,* and *subgerminal cavity.*

blastocyst (blas′to-sist) [*blasto-* + Gr. *kystis* bladder] in embryonic development, a cellular capsule consisting of about 30 cells forming a wall around a hollow cavity filled with fluid, which evolves from the morula by about the fourth day after fertilization, and begins to burrow into the uterine wall in the process of implantation. It consists of the inner cell mass which forms the germinal disk composed of the columnar or cuboidal cells, and the enveloping layer (outer cell mass) made up of flattened cells. The inner cell mass becomes the embryo proper, whereas the outer cell mass will form an extraembryonic ectodermal layer (trophoblast). Called also *blastodermic vesicle.* See illustrations at CLEAVAGE and EMBRYO.

blastocyte (blas′to-sīt) [*blasto-* + Gr. *kytos* hollow vessel] an embryonic cell that has not yet become differentiated.

blastoderm (blas′to-derm) [*blasto-* + Gr. *derma* skin] in embryonic development, a thin cellular structure produced by cleavage of the zygote, forming the hollow sphere of the blastula, or the cellular cap above a floor of segmented yolk in the discoblastula of telolecithal eggs. When fully formed, it contains the three primary germ layers: the ectoderm, entoderm, and mesoderm. Called also *germinal membrane* and *membrana germinativa.* See also BLASTULA and BLASTOCYST, and see illustration at EMBRYO.

blastodisc (blas′to-disk) [*blasto-* + Gr. *diskos* disk] the convex structure formed by the blastomeres at the animal pole of an ovum undergoing incomplete cleavage.

blastomere (blas-to′mēr) [*blasto-* + Gr. *meros* a part] one of the cells produced by mitotic division of the zygote during cleavage. The increase of blastomeres follows the doubling sequence, 2, 4, 8, 16, etc., each new series of cells being smaller than the preceding one, and each daughter cell receiving the full double assortment of chromosomes, one set of which comes from each parent. By the third day, the blastomeres begin to cluster together to form the morula. Called also *cleavage cell* and *segmentation sphere.* See illustration at CLEAVAGE.

Blastomyces (blas″to-mi′sēz) [*blasto-* + Gr. *mykēs* fungus] a genus of deuteromycetous fungi (Fungi Imperfecti) growing in mycelial forms at room temperature and in yeastlike forms at body temperature. *B. dermatitis* is pathogenic to animals, including man, causing blastomycosis; its sexual stage is *Ajellomyces dermatitidis.* **B. brasilien′sis,** *Paracoccidioides brasiliensis;* see under PARACOCCIDIOIDES.

blastomycosis (blas″to-mi-ko′sis) any infection caused by organisms of the genus *Blastomyces.* See also COCCIDIOIDOMYCOSIS. **European b.,** a subacute or chronic *Cryptococcus neoformans* infection, chiefly affecting the central nervous system. It usually begins as a mild respiratory infection or granulomatous dermatitis, which may be followed by fever, visual disorders, stiffness of the neck, headache, vomiting, convulsions, and other symptoms and complications of meningoencephalitis. The pulmonary lesions may also occur alone or in combination with the central nervous system infection. The cutaneous lesions may appear as verrucoid granuloma, superficial acneiform lesions, or diffuse subcutaneous nodules which form draining sinuses and scars. Infrequently, there may be granulomatous and ulcerative lesions of the nasopharynx; the vaginal, conjunctival, and oral mucosa may be involved rarely. Soft, verrucous, dark-violet lesions may be found on the tonsils, tongue, and lips, resulting in necrosis and secondary ulcerating nodules. Called also *b. purulenta profunda, ascomycosis, Buschke's disease, Busse-Busche disease, cryptococcosis, Torula meningitis, torulopsis,* and *torulosis.* **North American b.,** a chronic progressive, cutaneous, or systemic, or combined systemic and cutaneous disease, caused by the fungus *Blastomyces dermatitidis,* which occurs almost exclusively in North America. The cutaneous lesions are characterized by papules or papulopustules which develop into crusted, warty eruptions and oozing sinuses. Areas of the face, particularly the facial orifices, are common sites. Oral lesions are not as prominent as cutaneous ones, with minute ulcers being the most prominent feature. The oral infection may represent spreading of facial lesions to the nasal, oral, and conjunctival mucous membranes, or it may be primary. Called also *blastomycetic dermatitis* and *Gilchrist's disease.* **b. purulen′ta profun′da,** European b. **South American b.,** a chronic granulomatous disease of the skin, mucous membranes, lymphatic system, and internal organs, caused by the fungus *Paracoccidioides (Blastomyces) brasiliensis,* occurring chiefly in South American farm laborers. Picking of the teeth with twigs or chewing leaves contaminated with the fungus is the suspected cause. Four types are recognized: (1) a mucocutaneous form, characterized by papules, chiefly of the oral region, which appear concurrently with lymphatic involvement; (2) a lymphangitic form, characterized by enlargement of regional lymph nodes; (3) a visceral form, involving the spleen, liver, pancreas, intestine, and other organs; and (4) a mixed form, involving the skin as well as the internal organs and lymphatic system. The gingiva is usually the site of the primary lesion. Initially, the lesion presents a circumscribed ulcer surrounding a tooth, which spreads to the rest of the oral mucosa, producing stomatitis and red-speckled erosions and ulcers. Edema and swelling of the lips, enlargement of the submandibular and cervical lymph nodes, and fistulation usually follow. Called also *de Almeida's disease, Lutz's disease, Lutz-Splenodore-de Almeida disease, paracoccidioidal granuloma,* and *paracoccidioidomycosis.*

blastopore (blas'to-pōr) [*blasto-* + Gr. *poros* opening] the opening of the archenteron to the exterior of the embryo, at the gastrula stage.

blastosphere (blas'to-sfēr) [*blasto-* + Gr. *sphaira* sphere] blastula.

blastospore (blas'to-spōr) [*blasto-* + Gr. *sporos* seed] a spore occurring at the end of aerial hyphae in acropetal succession.

blastula (blas'tu-lah), pl. *blas'tulae* [L.] in embryonic development, a structure consisting of a single layer of cells (blastoderm) surrounding a fluid-filled cavity (blastocoele), which develops during cleavage of the zygote. Further development of the blastula results in arrangement of the cells in the three germ layers: the ectoderm, mesoderm, and enteroderm. Called also *blastosphere.* See also BLASTOCYST, CLEAVAGE, DISCOBLASTULA, and germ LAYER, and see illustration at EMBRYO.

blastulae (blas'tu-le) [L.] plural of *blastula.*

bleacher (blēch'er) a chemical agent that removes stains or color. **skin b.,** demelaninizing AGENT.

bleaching (blēch'ing) the act or process of removing stains or color by chemical means. **coronal b.,** the act or process of removing discolorations from the crowns of pulpless teeth through the use of chemical agents, usually but not necessarily in combination with heat. Oxidizing agents, such as 30 percent hydrogen peroxide solution, are generally used.

bleb (bleb) a bulla or skin vesicle filled with fluid.

bleeder (blēd'er) 1. one who bleeds freely or is subject to hemorrhage. 2. any large blood vessel cut during a surgical procedure. 3. one who lets blood.

bleeding (blēd'ing) 1. the escape of blood from an injured vessel. See HEMORRHAGE. 2. the letting of blood. **gingival b.,** hemorrhage from the gingiva; gingival hemorrhage. **gingival b., acute,** an acute episode of hemorrhage from the gingival tissue, caused by trauma or occurring spontaneously in acute gingival disease. Laceration by toothbrushing, injury on biting hard food, or pricking with a toothpick are the most common causes. Acute necrotizing ulcerative gingivitis is one of the chief causes of spontaneous bleeding. **gingival b., chronic,** hemorrhage from the gingivae, usually occurring as a complication of a chronic disease, such as chronic gingivitis. It may be provoked by the irritating activity of toothbrushing, toothpicks, solid foods, or food impaction. It is associated commonly with engorgement of the capillaries, increased permeability and ulceration of the crevicular epithelium, exudation, and thinning of the gingival epithelium. **occult b.,** escape of very small amounts of blood.

Blegvad-Haxthausen syndrome [Olaf *Blegvad,* Danish ophthalmologist, 1888–1961; Holger *Haxthausen,* 1892–1958] see under SYNDROME.

blenn- see BLENNO-.

blennadenitis (ben″ad-ĕ-ni'tis) [*blenn-* + Gr. *adēn* gland + *-itis*] inflammation of mucous glands.

blenno-, blenn- [Gr. *blennos* mucus] a combining form denoting relationship to mucus.

blennogenic (blen″no-jen'ik) [*blenno-* + Gr. *gennan* to produce] producing mucus.

blennoid (blen'noid) [*blenn-* + Gr. *eidos* form] resembling mucus.

blennorrhagia (blen″no-ra'je-ah) [*blenno-* + Gr. *rhēgnynai* to break forth] excessive discharge of mucus; blennorrhea.

blennorrhea (blen″no-re'ah) [*blenno-* + Gr. *rhoia* flow] 1. excessive discharge of mucus; blennorrhagia. 2. gonorrhea.

blennostasis (blen-nos'tah-sis) [*blenno-* + Gr. *stasis* standing] the suppression of an abnormal flow of mucus.

blennostatic (blen″no-stat'ik) [*blenno-* + Gr. *histanai* to halt] correcting of excessive mucous secretion.

bleomycin (ble″o-mi'sin) a class of glycopeptide antibiotics isolated from cultures of *Streptomyces verticillus,* occurring as a colorless or yellowish powder that becomes blue on exposure to copper and is soluble in water and methanol, slightly soluble in ethanol, and insoluble in acetone, ether, and acetates. Bleomycins are cytotoxic drugs, capable of fragmenting the DNA molecule. Used in the treatment of Hodgkin's disease and other lymphomas and in squamous cell carcinoma of the head, neck, and other organs. Adverse reactions may include alopecia, hyperpigmentation, pruritic erythema, skin ulcers and vesiculation, and stomatitis. Bone marrow depression is minimal.

blephar- see BLEPHARO-.

blepharadenitis (blef″ar-ad″ĕ-ni'tis) [*blephar-* + Gr. *adēn* gland + *-itis*] inflammation of the meibomian glands. Called also *blepharoadenitis.*

blepharal (blef'ah-ral) pertaining to the eyelids.

blepharectomy (blef'ah-rek'to-me) [*blephar-* + Gr. *ektomē* excision] excision of the eyelid.

blepharism (blef'ah-rizm) [L. *blepharismus;* Gr. *blepharizein* to wink] spasm of the eyelids; continuous blinking.

blepharitis (blef'ah-ri'tis) [*blephar-* + *-itis*] inflammation of the eyelids.

blepharo-, blephar- [Gr. *blepharon* eyelid] a combining form denoting relationship to an eyelid or eyelash.

blepharoadenitis (blef'ah-ro-ad″ĕ-ni'tis) blepharadenitis.

blepharoatheroma (blef'ah-ro-ath″er-o'mah) an encysted tumor or sebaceous cyst of an eyelid.

blepharochalasis (blef'ah-ro-kal'ah-sis) [*blepharo-* + Gr. *chalasis* relaxation] abnormal relaxation of the skin of the eyelid.

blepharoclonus (blef'ah-rok'lo-nus) [*blepharo-* + *clonus*] clonic spasm of the orbicularis oculi muscle, appearing as an increased winking of the eye.

blepharodiastasis (blef'ah-ro-di-as'tah-sis) [*blepharo-* + Gr. *diastasis* separation] excessive separation of the eyelids, causing the fissure to be very wide.

blepharoncus (blef'ah-rong'kus) [*blepharo-* + Gr. *onkos* bulk, mass] a tumor on the eyelid.

blepharopachynsis (blef'ah-ro-pak-in'sis) [*blepharo-* + Gr. *pachynsis* thickening] abnormal thickening of an eyelid.

blepharophimosis (blef'ah-ro-fi-mo'sis) [*blepharo-* + Gr. *phimōsis* a muzzling] abnormal narrowness of the palpebral fissures.

blepharoplasty (blef'ah-ro-plas'te) plastic surgery of the eyelids.

blepharoplegia (blef'ah-ro-ple'je-ah) [*blepharo-* + Gr. *plēgē* stroke] paralysis of an eyelid; paralysis of both muscles of the eyelid.

blepharoptosis (blef'ah-ro-to'sis) [*blepharo-* + Gr. *ptōsis* a fall] drooping of the upper eyelid.

blepharorrhaphy (blef'ah-ror'ah-fe) [*blepharo-* + Gr. *rhaphē* suture] tarsorrhaphy.

blepharospasm (blef'ah-ro-spazm″) [*blepharo-* + Gr. *spasmos* spasm] spasm of the orbicularis oculi muscle, producing more or less complete closure of the eyelids.

blepharostenosis (blef'ah-ro-stē-no'sis) [*blepharo-* + *stenosis*] narrowing of the palpebral fissure.

blepharosynechia (blef'ah-ro-sĭ-ne'ke-ah) [*blepharo-* + Gr. *synecheia* a holding together] the growing together or adhesion of the eyelids.

blepharotomy (blef'ah-rot'o-me) [*blepharo-* + Gr. *tomē* a cut] surgical incision of an eyelid. Called also *tarsotomy.*

blindness (blīnd'nes) partial or complete lack of vision. See also AMAUROSIS and AMBLYOPIA. **legal b.,** blindness as defined by law; in most states of the United States, maximal visual acuity of the better eye, after correction, of 20/200 or less; with a total diameter of the visual field in that eye of 20 degrees or less.

blister (blis'ter) [L. *vesicula*] a localized collection of fluid in the epidermis causing elevation of the horny upper layer and its separation from the underlying parts. See also BULLA. **fever b's,** see HERPES simplex. **Marochetti's b.,** a small blister seen under the tongue in rabies.

Blk black; see color coding table at root canal THERAPY.

Blocain trademark for *propoxycaine hydrochloride* (see under PROPOXYCAINE).

Bloch-Sulzberger syndrome [Bruno *Bloch,* Swiss dermatologist, 1878–1933; Marion Baldur *Sulzberger,* American dermatologist, born 1895] see under SYNDROME.

block (blok) 1. an obstruction or stoppage. 2. an obstruction of nerve or muscle impulses. 3. see regional ANESTHESIA. **air b.,** interference with the normal inflation and deflation of the lungs and with the pulmonary blood flow, produced by the leakage of air from the pulmonary alveoli into the interstitial tissue of the lung and into the mediastinum. **bite b.,** 1. a film holder for intraoral radiography, which the patient bites and holds between the occlusal surfaces of the maxillary and mandibular teeth to provide stable retention of the film packet. 2. occlusion RIM. **cocaine b.,** see BLOCKING (1). **cryogenic b.,** local cooling of tissue. **dedicated time b.,** a term used to refer to scheduling an appointment for a period that is usually longer than a normal appointment for a special type of dental or medical procedure. Abbreviated DTB. **epidural b.,** spinal anesthesia produced by injection of an anesthetic agent between the vertebral spines into the extradural space. **field b.,** field block ANESTHESIA. **heart b.,** the block or impairment of the conduction mechanism in heart excitation. **intranasal b.,** intranasal ANESTHESIA. **nerve b.,** pheripheral nerve block ANESTHESIA. **paraneural b.,** regional anesthesia produced by injecting an anesthetic close to a nerve. See peripheral nerve block ANESTHESIA. **perineural b.,** regional anesthesia produced by injecting an anesthetic in the proximity of a nerve. See peripheral nerve block ANESTHESIA. **peripheral nerve b.,** peripheral nerve block ANESTHESIA. **sympathetic b.,** blocking of the sympathetic nerve trunk by paravertebral infiltration with an anesthetic agent.

blockade (blok-ād′) 1. the rendering of the reticuloendothelial cells of the body less capable of phagocytosis and destruction of harmful agents by overloading them with a heavy intravenous injection of harmless material. 2. the prevention by drugs of certain physiologic or enzymatic actions. 3. the prevention of the effects of certain drugs by other chemical agents.

blockage (blok′ij) the process of blocking or obstructing; the condition of being blocked or obstructed.

blocking (blok′ing) 1. the cutting off of an afferent nerve path, as by the injection of cocaine (cocaine block). 2. the inhibition of an intracellular biosynthetic process, as by the injection of actinomycin D. 3. the fastening of a histological or other suitable material which may be clamped in the microtome.

blockout (blok′owt) elimination in a master cast of undesirable undercut areas, including all areas that would offer interference to the placement of the denture framework and those areas which are not crossed by a rigid part of the denture, accomplished by filling in areas to be blocked out with materials such as a mixture of wax and clay, hard inlay wax, or other suitable materials. Called also wax out. See also blockout MATERIAL and RELIEF (4). **arbitrary b.,** a hard wax blockout applied to all gingival crevices, gross tissue undercuts situated below areas involved in design of denture framework, tissue undercuts distal to cast framework, and labial and buccal tooth and tissue undercuts not involved in denture design. **parallel b.,** blockout of tissue undercuts that would offer interference to the seating of a denture, trimmed parallel to the path of placement, and applied at the proximal tooth surfaces to be used as guiding planes, beneath all minor connectors, tissue undercuts to be crossed by rigid connectors and origin of bar clasps, deep interproximal spaces to be covered by minor connectors or lingual plates, and beneath bar clasp arms to gingival crevices. **shaped b.,** the shaping in the master cast of ledges or shelves on buccal and lingual surfaces to locate plastic or wax patterns for nonretentive reciprocal clasp arms that follow the height and convexity of a tooth, and for retentive clasp arms to be placed as low as tooth contour permits.

Blodi, Frederick C. [American physician, born 1917] see Reese's DYSPLASIA (Reese-Blodi syndrome).

blood (blud) [L. sanguis, cruor; Gr. haima] a fluid found in all higher animals and some invertebrates, whose function is to carry to the tissues oxygen and other substances necessary for sustaining life, and to remove from the tissues carbon dioxide and other waste materials. It represents about 7 percent of the body weight. Blood is transported to the tissues and circulated through the cardiovascular system, and is composed of the liquid medium, the blood plasma (see under PLASMA), and the formed elements (erythrocytes, leukocytes, and blood platelets). Hemoglobin gives blood its red color; arterial blood is bright red, while the venous blood is darker red. See table of Reference Values for Blood, Plasma and Serum in the Appendix. See also BLOOD GROUP and terms beginning HEMATO- and HEMO-. **central b.,** blood obtained from the pulmonary venous system; sometimes applied to splanchnic blood, or blood obtained from chambers of the heart or from bone marrow. **b. chemistry,** see table of Reference Values for Blood, Plasma and Serum in Appendix. **citrated b.,** blood treated with sodium citrate and/or citric acid to prevent clotting. **b. clotting, b. coagulation,** blood COAGULATION. **compatible b.,** blood which, after transfusion from one individual to another, will be accepted without undergoing or causing agglutination and hemolysis due to blood group incompatibility. **b. count,** determination of the number of formed elements of the blood, usually in a cubic millimeter. See

also ERYTHROCYTE count, LEUKOCYTE count, and blood platelet count, under PLATELET. **defibrinated b.,** whole blood from which fibrin has been removed, thus preventing formation of a red cell clot. **b. factor,** a factor which determines blood group specificity. See AGGLUTINOGEN. **b. fat,** blood LIPID. **b. glucose,** see blood SUGAR. **incompatible b.,** blood which, after transfusion from one individual to another with a different blood group, undergoes or causes agglutination and hemolysis. **b. lipid,** see under LIPID. **b. matching,** typing of the blood groups of the recipient and of the donor blood to insure compatibility, thereby preventing agglutination of the erythrocytes and hemolysis due to transfusion of incompatible blood. **occult b.,** blood present in such small quantities that it can be detected only by chemical tests of suspected material, or by microscopic or spectroscopic examination. **oxalated b.,** blood to which oxalate solution has been added to prevent coagulation. **peripheral b.,** blood obtained from acral areas, or from the circulation remote from the heart, as from the ear lobe, finger tip, or antecubital vein. **b. plasma,** blood PLASMA. **b. platelet count,** see under PLATELET. **b. pressure,** blood PRESSURE. **sludged b.,** blood in which erythrocytes have become aggregated into masses. **b. smear,** a specimen of the blood, stained and spread over a glass slide, used in determining the morphology, staining reaction, and maturity of the erythrocytes; morphology and maturity of various types of leukocytes; and the presence of parasites in the blood. **splanchnic b.,** a general term applied to blood in the thoracic, abdominal, and pelvic viscera. **b. sugar,** blood SUGAR. **b. transfusion,** blood TRANSFUSION. **b. turbidity,** blood TURBIDITY. **b. type,** see BLOOD GROUP. **b. volume,** the total amount of blood in the body, varying in relation to body weight and adipose tissue content and averaging about 79 ml/kg ± 10 percent in normal lean adults. In a person weighing 70 kg, the blood contains about 5 liters — 3 liters of plasma and 2 liters of erythrocytes, the total body fluids consisting of about 40 liters. Obese adults, whose fat tissue is less richly vascularized, have less blood in proportion to their body weight. See also HEMATOCRIT and total red cell VOLUME. **whole b.,** blood from which none of the elements have been removed.

blood group, blood group system (blud grup; blud grup sis′tim) a characteristic of blood in different individuals, which is genetically determined and has common antigenic properties. Blood groups are based on the presence of specific antigens (agglutinogens) on the erythrocytes that can stimulate production of antibodies in the blood plasma (agglutinins), acting against the erythrocytes which caused their production. The specificity of the antigens is controlled by allelic genes, which are given the same designation as the antigen whose production they stimulate. The ABO blood groups are the classical system, but a number of other blood groups are also recognized. The most commonly known blood groups include Diego, Dombrock, Duffy, Ii, Kell, Kidd, Lewis, Lutheran, MNSs, and Rh. **b. g. A,** a blood group phenotype in the ABO blood group system, characterized by the presence of A antigen on red cells and anti-B agglutinins in serum, and secretion of substance A in the body fluids (in secretors). About 41 percent of the white population has blood group A. **b. g. AB,** a blood group phenotype in the ABO blood group system, characterized by the presence of A and B antigens on the red cells and secretion of substances A and B in the body fluids (in secretors). About 3 percent of the white population has blood group AB. **ABO b. g's,** a blood group system consisting of blood groups (phenotypes) A, AB, B, and O. The system is transmitted as a genetic trait through three multiple alleles, O, A, and B, which form six genotypes: OO, AA, AO, BB, BO, and AB. Transmission follows the following rules: 1. agglutinogens A and B are present in a child only when they are also present in one or both parents. 2. the group AB is almost always transmitted only from A and B, but not O parents. 3. any agglutinogen may be present in a child only when it is also present in at least one parent. Group O has agglutinins anti-A and anti-B, but no agglutinogens; group A has agglutinogens A and agglutinins anti-B; group B has agglutinogens B and agglutinins anti-A; group AB has agglutinogens A and B, but no agglutinins. About 47 percent of the white population has group O; 41 percent has group A; 9 percent has group B; and 3 percent has group AB. Transfusion of incompatible ABO blood may lead to agglutination of the erythrocytes and hemolysis. Called also OAB blood groups. **b. g. B,** a blood group phenotype in the ABO blood group system, characterized by the presence of B antigen on red cells and anti-A agglutinins in serum, and secretion of substance B in the body fluids (in secretors). About 9 percent of white population has blood group B. **Diego b. g's,** a blood group system, a polymorphic variation of which occurs most commonly in South American Indians, Japanese, and Chinese, but very seldom in Europeans and blacks. Antigens Di^a and Di^b make up this group. Incompatibilities in this system may be sometimes implicated in post-transfusion complications and fetal erythroblastosis. **Dombrock b. g.**, a blood group system, discovered when the antibody was detected in a polytransfused female, found in about 53 percent of Caucasians. It consists of the Do^a and Do^b antigens. **Duffy b. g's,** a blood group system that in Caucasians appears to be dependent on alleles Fy^a and Fy^b; in blacks, about 68 percent fail to react with antiserum to either antigen, and are called Fy(a−b−). This is explained by a third (silent) allele, Fy. The system is sometimes involved in post-transfusion hemolytic complications and fetal erythroblastosis. **Ii b. g.,** a blood group system present on the erythrocytes of most adults, which is not present at birth but appears progressively during the first months of life. **Kell b. g's,** a blood group system named after the person in whose blood the antibody defining it was first discovered. Anti-Kell (anti-K) antibodies were first found in the serum of the mother of a child with probable erythroblastosis. Later, in the serum of another mother (whose surname was Cellano) of a child with the same disorder was found the expected antithetical antibody, first called *anti-Cellano* and later *anti-Kell*. Additional antigens belonging to the Kell group were later discovered: Kp^a (Penny), Kp^b (Rautenberg), Js^a (Sutter), Js^b, and at least nine others (which were designated by numbers). The serum of individuals who are of the K^o phenotype (see under PHENOTYPE) contains a rare antibody that reacts with every Kell phenotype except K^o and is called *anti-Ku* (anti-K5). After blood groups ABO and Rh, this system is the third most common cause of hemolytic complications after transfusion of incompatible blood and fetal erythroblastosis. **Kidd b. g's,** a blood group system implicated in isolated cases of post-transfusion hemolytic complications and fetal erythroblastosis. The system consists of three alleles: Jk^a, Jk^b, and a rare silent allele, Jk. **Landsteiner's nomenclature (classification) of b. g's,** a classification of the ABO blood group system in which the blood groups are designated A, AB, B, and O, depending on the presence or absence of agglutinogens A and B; see *ABO b. g's.* Called also *International classification (of blood groups).* **Lewis b. g's,** a blood group system characterized by the presence of Lewis substance(s) in saliva and other body fluids and absorption of the antigens onto erythrocytes from the blood plasma. After absorption, red cells will react with anti-Le^a or anti-Le^b. Naturally occurring anti–Lewis antibodies sometimes react best at temperatures below room temperature. The red cell Lewis antigens "develop" slowly after birth, since this is primarily a body fluid group system. The system's genetics and biosynthesis of Le^a and Le^b substances are now known to be closely related to the ABO and secretor systems. Lewis typing has some medicolegal use because of its relationship to the secretor system. The system is of little importance in blood transfusion. It is not used in paternity testing because of complexities in its mode of inheritance. **Lutheran b. g's,** a blood group system consisting of the Lu^a and Lu^b antigens, which are controlled by allelic genes. Most European and blacks are Lu(a−b+), fewer being Lu(a+b−). Lu(a+b−) is fairly rare. Lutheran antisera are extremely scarce. The system has little importance in blood transfusion. **b. g. M,** a blood group of the MNSs system, determined by genes allelic to N. The MN locus is closely linked to the Ss locus, and M phenotypes include MS, Ms, MNSs, MNS, and MNs. **b. g. MN,** a blood group of the MNSs system, consisting of the MNS, MNs, and MNSs phenotypes. **b. g. MNS,** see *b. g's MN.* **b. g. MNs,** see *b. g. MN.* **MNSs b. g's,** a blood group system consisting of blood groups M, N, and MN. The system is believed to be transmitted through at least four alleles. A parent M cannot have a child N; a parent N cannot have a child M; a child cannot be MN, unless M and N are present in one or both parents: a parent transmits a child MS, Ms, NS, or Ns as a unit, so that a child of an MS-Ns father receives either MS or Ns from him and will receive a similar pair from the mother. The MN and Ss loci are closely linked so that MN and Ss genes travel together on the same chromosome. About 28 percent of the white population has the M group, about 21 percent has the N group, and 59 percent has the MN group. The system has chiefly medicolegal and anthropological application, having little importance in post-transfusion complications. **b. g. Ms,** see *b. g. M.* **b. g. N,** a blood group of the MNSs system, consisting of NS, Ns, NSs, MNS, MNs, and MNSs phenotypes, all of which will react with anti-N. **b. g. NS,** see *b. g. N.* **b. g. Ns,** see *b. g. N.* **b. g. O,** a blood group in the ABO blood group system, characterized by the presence of anti-A and anti-B agglutinins, but no agglutinogens, and secretion of substance H in the saliva, tears, and other body fluids (in secretors). Having no agglutinogens, group O blood is considered safe for transfusion to persons with all groups from the ABO system. Persons with group O blood are considered as universal donors. About 47 percent of the white population have blood group O. Group O red cells can be

Rh BLOOD GROUP

Weiner Gene	Weiner Agglutinogen	Weiner Blood Factor	Fisher-Race Gene Complex	Fisher-Race Antigen
r	rh	**hr′, hr″**	cde	c, e
r'	rh′	**rh′, hr″**	Cde	C, e
r''	rh″	**hr′, rh″**	cdE	c, E
R^0	Rh$_0$	**Rh$_0$, hr′, hr″**	cDe	c, D, e
R^1	Rh$_1$	**Rh$_0$, rh′, hr″**	Cde	C, D, e
R^2	Rh$_2$	**Rh$_0$, hr′, rh″**	cDE	c, D, E
R^z	Rh$_z$	**Rh$_0$, rh′, rh″**	CDE	C, D, E
r^y	rh$_y$	**rh′, rh″**	CdE	C, E

agglutinated by specific agglutinins of plant or animal origin called *anti-H reagents.* **OAB b. g's,** ABO b. g's. **b. g. P,** a blood group system having several types, such as P$_1$, P$_2$, and P^k. The group is not known to cause post-transfusion complications. **Rh b. g's,** a blood group system based on the discovery that serum from rabbits that had been injected with erythrocytes of the rhesus monkey causes agglutination of erythrocytes in 85 percent of humans without relation to their other blood groups. According to one classification, there are eight basic Rh genes with eight corresponding agglutinogens, each of which is associated with more than one blood factor (see under FACTOR). Representing this classification is Weiner's nomenclature, and the system is called the *Rh-Hr blood group system* by Weiner. According to a second classification, there are three sets of allelic genes: C and c, D and d, and E and e; the d gene is silent. Every person inherits one gene from each pair, a total of three genes from each parent. Representing this classification is the C-D-E (Fisher-Race) nomenclature. The D(Rh$_0$) antigen is most potent in the system. See table. About 83 percent of the American white population and 93 percent of the black population are Rh-positive. Introduction of Rh-positive blood into a Rh-negative recipient or passage of erythrocytes from a Rh-positive fetus into a Rh-negative mother may produce isoimmunization. See also fetal ERYTHROBLASTOSIS. **Rh-Hr b. g's,** see *Rh b. g's.* **b. g. substances,** substances secreted in saliva, urine, tears, semen, gastric juice, and milk in about 85 percent of the population. They are stable and heat resistant, and consist of glycoproteins whose antigen structure is identical to that of the corresponding lyoprotein ABO antigen on the red cells. Common blood group substances include A, B, H, and Le^a substances. See also AGGLUTINOGEN.

Bloom's syndrome [David *Bloom*, American physician] see under SYNDROME.

Bloom-Torre-Machacek syndrome [D. *Bloom*; Douglas P. *Torre*, American physician, born 1919] Bloom's SYNDROME.

Bloomberg, Esther see vitamin D–resistant RICKETS (Albright-Butler-Bloomberg syndrome).

blowpipe (blo′pīp) a tube through which a stream of air or gas is forced into a flame to concentrate and intensify the heat.

Blu blue; see color coding table at root canal THERAPY.

blue (blu) 1. one of the principal colors of the spectrum, the color of the sky. 2. a dye that is blue in color. **methylene b.,** a dye, 3,7-bis(dimethylamino)phenazothionium chloride, occurring as dark green, odorless crystals with bronze luster or crystalline powder. Used as a stain in bacteriology, as a reagent for some chemicals, and as an oxidation-reduction indicator. It has bacteriostatic properties and is sometimes used in the treatment of acute necrotizing ulcerative gingivitis. In high concentrations, it oxidizes ferrous iron or reduced hemoglobin to the ferric form, producing methemoglobin, and is thus used as antidote in cyanide poisoning; in low concentrations, it hastens the conversion of methemoglobin to hemoglobin. Called also *Swiss b.* **Swiss b.,** methylene b.

Blue Cross (blu kros) see Blue Cross Association, under ASSOCIATION, and see Blue Cross PLAN.

Blue Shield (blu shēld) see Association of Blue Shield Plans, under ASSOCIATION, and see Blue Shield PLAN.

bluestone (blu′stōn) cupric SULFATE.

Blumenbach's plane, process [Johann Friederich *Blumenbach*, German physiologist, 1752–1840] see under PLANE, and see uncinate process of ethmoid bone, under PROCESS. See also CLIVUS (clivus blumenbachii).

blush (blush) a sudden, brief erythema of the face and neck, resulting from vascular dilatation due to emotion or heat. **dentin b.,** red discoloration of dentin due to pulpal hemorrhage, sometimes seen when increased intrapulpal pressure, resulting from a traumatic restorative procedure, causes extravasation in the subodontoblastic layer of the pulp and the erythrocytes are forced into the dentinal tubules.

BMR basal metabolic rate; see basal METABOLISM.

Bo Bolton POINT.

board (bord) 1. a long and flat piece of wood or other material. 2. a group or a body of persons serving a special function. **American B. of Dental Public Health,** an organization sponsored by the American Association of Public Health Dentists to protect and improve the public health by the study and creation of standards for the practice of dental public health in all of its aspects and relationships, and to grant and issue to dentists who have successfully completed the prescribed advanced training and experience in dental public health certificates of special knowledge and ability in preventive dentistry and dental public health. Abbreviated *ABDPH.* **American B. of Endodontics,** an organization sponsored by the American Association of Endodontists to meet an existing public need for recognition of those who have special knowledge and skill in the diagnosis and treatment of contiguous pulpal and periapical tissues; to maintain standards of excellence in endodontic practice and determine the competence of applicants who serve the public through limitation of their practice; to certify those who have given evidence of specialized knowledge, training, and skill in endodontic study and technique and have met qualifications set up by the Board; and to furnish the dental and medical profession with a directory of endodontists certified by the Board. Abbreviated *ABE.* **American B. of Oral and Maxillofacial Surgery,** a professional organization established to elevate the standards of oral surgery and to advance its causes in an effort to provide optimum health care to the patient, by establishing criteria and qualifications for the issuance of certificates by the Board in the specialty of oral and maxillofacial surgery and to conduct examinations to establish the fitness of applicants for such certificates. Formerly called *American Board of Oral Surgery.* Abbreviated *ABOMS.* **American B. of Oral Pathology,** an organization established to encourage the study, elevate the standards, and promote and improve the practice of oral pathology; to determine the competence of those wishing to practice as oral pathologists through evaluation of credentials and examination of individuals who apply for certification by the Board; to grant and issue certificates to those who apply, whose credentials are accepted, and who successfully complete the examination by the Board; to maintain a registry of holders of certificates and to make available to the public, the dental and medical professions, hospitals, and dental schools a list of those persons certified and registered by the Board; and to establish criteria and administer a program for the recertification of individuals who have been granted certificates. Abbreviated *ABOP.* **American B. of Oral Surgery,** former name for the *American B. of Oral and Maxillofacial Surgery.* **American B. of Orthodontics,** an organization created by the American Society of Orthodontists to elevate the standards of the practice of orthodontics through stimulating and promoting the spirit of self-improvement and research among students and practitioners of orthodontics; to encourage and promote the continual review and elevation of standards of orthodontic education and treatment; and to conduct examinations for the purposes of evaluating the qualifications and skills of practicing orthodontists and to confer certificates upon those who meet the established standards of the Board. Abbreviated *ABO.* **American B. of Pedodontics,** an organization established by the American Society of Dentistry for Children to encourage the study, improve the practice, elevate the standards, and advance the science of pedodontics. To fulfill these objectives, the Board issues to dentists a certificate of recognition of special knowledge in pedodontics. Abbreviated *ABP.* **American B. of Periodontology,** an organization established by the American Academy of Periodontology to elevate the standards and advance the science and art of periodontology by encouraging its study and improving its practice; to conduct examinations to determine the qualifications and competence of dentists who voluntarily apply to the Board for certification as diplomates; to grant and issue diplomate certificates in the field of periodontology to qualified applicants and to maintain a registry of holders of such certificates; and to serve the health professions and health institutions by preparing and furnishing on request lists of periodontists certified as diplomates by the Board. Abbreviated

ABP. **American B. of Prosthodontics,** an organization established jointly by the Council of Dental Education of the American Dental Association and the Federation of Prosthodontic Organizations, whose major tasks and objectives include establishing criteria covering qualifications for the issuance of certificates by the Board in the specialty of prosthodontics and to conduct examinations to establish the fitness of applicants for such certificates and to publish through the American Dental Association lists of certified practitioners (diplomates) for the protection of the public. Abbreviated *ABP.* **angle b.,** a device used to facilitate the establishment of reproducible angular relationships between a patient's head and the plane of an x-ray film. **b. certified,** a physician, dentist, or other health professional who, after successfully passing an examination given by a specialty board, is certified as being a specialist in his or her field or discipline. See also specialty BOARD. **Certifying B. of the American Dental Assistants Association,** the examining board of the American Dental Assistants Association, which ascertains professional competency and proficiency of dental assistants through a series of examinations. Those who meet the requirements may use the title *Certified Dental Assistant.* Abbreviated *CBADAA.* **b. eligible,** an applicant for certification by his or her respective specialty board after it has examined the applicant's academic record and the board committee has reviewed and approved the applicant's credentials. **licensing b.,** a board, usually at a state level, which is responsible for examination or other form of determination of eligibility of applicants for licenses, issuance of licenses, suspension of licenses, enforcing of licensing statutes, and approval and supervision of schools. The board is usually composed of representatives of groups with direct interest in areas regulated by the board, with state officials serving as *ex officio* members. **National B. of Medical Examiners,** an organization which includes among its members representatives from the Federation of State Medical Boards, Council of Medical Education of the American Medical Association, Association of American Medical Colleges, American Hospital Association, Armed Services, Public Health Service, and Veterans Administration, as well as members elected at large. Functions include: preparation and administration of qualifying examinations to be used by states for licensing purposes, consultation and cooperation with examining boards of the states, consultation and cooperation with medical schools and other institutions in advancing medical education, assisting medical specialty boards and societies with certification procedures, and development of methods of testing and evaluating medical knowledge and competence. Abbreviated *NBME.* **specialty b.,** an organization, usually sponsored by various professional groups, which certifies dentists and physicians as specialists in their respective fields of dental and medical practice. It establishes requirements and standards for certification, determines the length and type of training and experience required, and conducts appropriate examinations. See also board CERTIFIED. **State Board of Dental Examiners, State Board of Dentistry,** an agency which is responsible for the administration and enforcement of the Dental Practice Act in the state.

Bochdalek's duct, ganglion [Vincent Alexander *Bochdalek,* anatomist in Prague, 1801–1883] see thyroglossal DUCT, and dental plexus, superior, under PLEXUS.

Bock's ganglion, nerve [August Carl *Bock,* German anatomist, 1782–1833] see carotid GANGLION, and pharyngeal branch of pterygopalatine ganglion, under BRANCH.

BOD biochemical oxygen DEMAND.

body (bod′e) 1. the trunk, or animal frame, with its organs. 2. a cadaver or corpse. 3. the largest and most important part of any organ. Called also *corpus.* 4. any mass or collection of material. **acetone b.,** ketone b. **adipose b. of cheek,** buccal fat PAD. **amygdaloid b.,** a small mass of subcortical gray matter within the tip of the temporal lobe. Called also *corpus amygdaloideum* [NA] and *nucleus amygdalae.* **aortic b's,** small neurovascular structures on either side of the aortic arch, the right aortic body being situated at the junction of the right subclavian and the right common carotid arteries, and the left in the angle between the left subclavian artery and the aorta. They contain chemoreceptors that play a role in reflex regulation of respiration by responding to changes in oxygen, carbon dioxide, and hydrogen ion concentrations in the blood. Called also *corpora paraaortica* [NA] and *glomera aortica.* **Aschoff b.,** a lesion of the heart muscle in patients with rheumatic fever, consisting of a focus of fibrinoid degeneration containing ragged, swollen, acidophilic fibers, surrounded by a granulomatous zone of mononuclear leukocytes, fibroblasts, Anichkov's cells, and Aschoff giant cells. **Auer b.,** an elongated inclusion representing a large granule, globule, or slender rod of azurophilic substance, found in the cytoplasm of myeloblasts, myelocytes, monoblasts, and

granular histiocytes of leukemic patients. **Barr b.**, sex CHROMA-
TIN. **basal b.**, basal CORPUSCLE. **Cabot's ring b.**, Cabot's RING.
carotid b., a small oval body, about 2 to 5 mm in diameter, lying
in the bifurcation of the right and left carotid arteries at the side
of the neck, which consists of epithelioid cells and nerve fibers,
and is supplied with chemoreceptors that monitor the oxygen
content of the blood and assist in the regulation of respiration
and blood circulation. Called also *carotid gland, carotid
glomus, glandula intercarotica, glomus caroticum* [NA], and
intercarotid gland. **cell b.**, that part of a cell which houses the
nucleus. See also PERIKARYON. **chromophilous b's**, Nissl b's.
ciliary b., the thickened part of the vascular tunic of the eye,
connecting the iris with the choroid. **crystalline b's**, crystalline
particles; see under PARTICLE. **Döhle's b.**, a round, oval, or
spindle-shaped inclusion body, usually about 1 to 2 μ in diameter, but sometimes up to 5 μ, found most commonly in the
cytoplasm of neutrophils of patients with various infections and
burns and those exposed to cytotoxic drugs; also found in
May-Hegglin anomaly, Pelger-Huët anomaly, Chediak-Higashi
syndrome, and in small numbers of patients in pernicious
anemia, hemolytic anemia, and myeloproliferative syndromes.
It stains sky blue to blue gray with Romanovskii's stain and is
not considered to be a true inclusion, but an area free of specific
granules and rich in RNA. **Donovan's b.**, *Calymmatobacterium
granulomatis;* see under CALYMMATOBACTERIUM. **foreign b.**, a
mass or particle of material which is not normal to the place
where it is found. **Giannuzzi's b's**, crescents of Giannuzzi; see
under CRESCENT. **Heindenhain's b's**, crescents of Giannuzzi;
see under CRESCENT. **Heinz b.**, a highly refractile particle of
denaturated hemoglobin 1 to 3 μ in diameter that can be
visualized with supravital stains but not with Wright's stain,
occurring in peripheral blood after exposure to certain drugs,
such as primaquine, acetanilid, and acetylphenylhydrazine,
and after splenectomy. **Howell-Jolly b.**, a small, round or oval
structure, larger than the usual granule, pinkish or bluish in
color, occurring singly in erythrocytes, in anemias and leukemias, and after splenectomy. They are thought to be nuclear
particles because they take the nuclear stain. Called also
Howell's b. **b. of hyoid bone**, the square central portion of the
hyoid bone to which the greater and lesser cornua are attached.
Its convex ventral surface presents a transverse ridge which
provides attachment for the geniohyoideus, mylohyoideus, sternohyoideus, and omohyoideus muscles. The concave dorsal
surface is separated from the epiglottis by the thyrohyoid membrane. The cranial border gives attachment to the thyrohyoid
membrane and parts of the genioglossus muscle. The caudal
border gives attachment to the sternohyoideus and omohyoideus muscles, and sometimes, part of the thyrohyoideus muscle. The levator glandulae thyroideae, when present, also attaches to the caudal border. It is connected to the greater
cornua by synchondroses which ossify during middle life.
Called also *basihyal, basihyoid,* and *corpus ossis hyoidei* [NA].
inclusion b's, round, oval, or irregular bodies occurring in the
protoplasm and nuclei of cells of the body, as in diseases caused
by filterable virus infections. **ketone b.**, one of a group of
ketones, including acetoacetic acid, β-hydroxybutyric acid, and
acetone. Ketone bodies are normal metabolic products of lipid
(and pyruvate) metabolism via acetyl-CoA within the liver, and
are oxidized by the muscles. Acetoacetic acid is convertible to
fatty acids and to steroids. In normal conditions, ketone bodies
are present in the blood in small amounts, averaging 0.5
mg/100 ml of blood; about 100 mg of ketone bodies are excreted
per day in the urine. The concentration of ketone bodies may
increase in the blood during starvation, diabetes mellitus, and
conditions that result in a restriction of carbohydrate metabolism, with a subsequent increase in fat metabolism to
supply the energy requirements of the body and a specific odor
detectable in the breath. The increase of the ketone body level
in the body is known as *ketosis*. Called also *acetone*. **Kurlov's
(Kurloff's) b.**, a large spherical inclusion seen in lymphocytes
and monocytes of guinea pigs and other animals, which appears
in living cells as a homogeneous yellowish-green body but, in
dry smears, stains similarly to azurophilic granules. **Lipschütz
b's**, intranuclear inclusion bodies found in the lesions of herpes
simplex and in the affected nerve cells. **b. of mandible**, the
horizontal, horseshoe-shaped portion of the mandible, which
continues on either side upward and backward into the ramus,
consisting of two lateral halves joined at the median line by the
symphysis menti. The external surface shows the symphysis as
a faint ridge which splits inferiorly to form the mental protuberance with the mental tubercle at its base. Inferior to the second
premolar on the external surface is the mental foramen giving
passage to the mental vessels and nerve. The mentalis, orbicularis oris, depressor labii inferioris, and depressor anguli oris
muscles attach to the external surface. The internal surface

offers attachment to the genioglossus, geniohyoid, digastricus,
mylohyoideus, and constrictor pharyngis superior muscles and
to the pterygomandibular raphe. The sublingual and submandibular glands rest against the internal surface. The superior
(alveolar) border forms 16 sockets for the lower teeth, and offers
attachment for the buccinator muscle. The inferior border is
plump, smooth, and rounded, having a shallow groove for the
facial artery. Called also *corpus mandibulae* [NA]. **Maragliano
b.**, a round or elliptical body in the center of an erythrocyte; it
resembles a vacuole, results from degenerative processes, and
is not a true cell inclusion. **b. of maxilla**, the large, somewhat
pyramidal, central portion of the maxilla. It contains a large
cavity, the maxillary sinus; presents the zygomatic, nasal,
palatine, and alveolar processes; and has anterior, posterior,
orbital, and nasal surfaces. Called also *corpus maxillae* [NA].
b. modifier, body MODIFIER. **Nissl b's**, large granular bodies
staining with basic dyes, forming the substance of a reticulum
of cytoplasm in a nerve cell. Called also *chromophilous b's,
tigroid b's, chromatic granules, chromophil corpuscles, chromophil substance, Nissl granules,* and *Nissl substance.* See
also RIBOSOME. **pacchionian b's**, arachnoidal granulations; see
under GRANULATION. **pearly b's**, epidermal pearls; see under
PEARL. **pineal b.**, pineal GLAND. **polar b's**, 1. the small abortive
cells with a haploid chromosome complement formed during
the maturation of the oocyte. Called also *polar cells.* See also
oocyte and *oogenesis.* 2. metachromatic granules located at the
ends of bacteria. **b. of sphenoid bone**, the central, cuboidal part
of the sphenoid bone, hollowed out to form two large cavities,
the sphenoid sinuses, to which the great wings, small wings,
and pterygoid processes are attached. Called also *corpus ossis
sphenoidalis* [NA] and *corpus sphenoidale.* See illustration at
BONE. **b. temperature**, body TEMPERATURE. **tigroid b's**, Nissl b's.
wolffian b., mesonephros.
Boeck's itch, scabies [Kark Wilhelm *Boeck,* Norwegian physician,
1808–1875] Norwegian SCABIES.
Boeck's sarcoid [Caesar Peter Möller *Boeck,* Norwegian derma-
tologist, 1845–1913] sarcoidosis.
Bofors see under DENTIFRICE.
Bogaert see van BOGAERT.
Bogolax trademark for *methylcellulose.*
Bogomolets' serum [Aleksandr Aleksandrovich *Bogomolets,* Rus-
sian physiopathologist, 1881–1946] antireticular cytotoxic
SERUM.
Bogorad's syndrome, [F. A. *Bogorad,* Russian physician] gustatory LACRIMATION.
Bohn's nodules see under NODULE.
Bohr atom [Neils Hendrick David *Bohr,* Danish physicist, 1885–
1962; winner of the Nobel prize for physics in 1922] see under
ATOM.
boil (boil) a localized infection with pyogenic bacteria, forming a
painful nodule in the skin and subcutaneous tissues, around a
slough or "core"; a furuncle. **Aleppo b., Baghdad b., Delhi b.**,
cutaneous LEISHMANIASIS. **gum b.**, parulis. **oriental b.**, cutaneous LEISHMANIASIS.
boiling (boil'ing) the process of changing from a liquid to a
gaseous state, accompanied by the production of gas bubbles
that rise to the surface of the liquid; brought about by increased
temperature which causes a large number of molecules to
attain sufficient energy to escape the retaining forces of the
condensed phase and to pass into the gaseous phase. See also
boiling POINT and VAPORIZATION.
Boitel, R. H. see Steiger-Boitel ATTACHMENT.
Bol. abbreviation for *bolus,* pill.
Boley gauge see under GAUGE.
Bolinan trademark for *povidone.*
Bolk's paramolar root [Louis *Bolk,* Dutch anatomist, 1866–1930]
accessory buccal ROOT.
bolt (bōlt) 1. a sliding bar or rod that inserts into a socket. 2. a
strong rod, pin, or screw, usually with a head at one end and
thread at the other end to receive a nut. **denture b.**, a mechanical device used for locking together parts of a sectional denture,
using the action similar to that of a rifle bolt. **P. W. (Pullen-
Warner) b.**, trademark for a *denture bolt.*
Bolton plane, point, triangle see under PLANE, POINT, and TRIAN-
GLE.
Bolton-nasion plane Bolton PLANE.
bolus (bo'lus) [L.; Gr. *bolos* lump] 1. alimentary b. 2. a rounded
mass of a pharmaceutical preparation ready to swallow. 3. a
concentrated mass of pharmaceutical preparation given intravenously for diagnostic purposes, e.g., an opaque contrast
medium or radioactive isotope. 4. a mass of scattering material,

such as wax, paraffin, bags of water, or a rice-flour mixture, placed between the radiation source and the skin to achieve a precalculated isodose pattern in the tissue irradiated. **b. al′ba,** kaolin. **alimentary b.,** the mass of food in the oropharynx or the esophagus, comprising one swallow.

bomb (bom) a heavy metal-shielded apparatus containing a quantity of radium or other radioactive element for use in clinical teleradiation therapy.

bombard (bom-bard′) to expose a tissue, organ, or the whole body to the action of ionizing radiation.

Bonare trademark for *oxazepam.*

bond (bond) 1. the linkage between two atoms or radicals in a chemical compound. 2. a mark used to indicate the number and attachment of the valencies of an atom in a formula; it is represented by a pair of dots or a line between the atoms, e.g., H—O—H, H—C≡C—H, or H:O:H, H:C:::C:H. **atomic b.,** a chemical bond in which each atom contributes one electron. **bridge b.,** a bond bridging two molecules together, involving compounds of hydrogen in which the hydrogen is attached by a polar covalent bond to one molecule, attracting another molecule. **coordinate covalent b.,** a single covalent bond in which one of the bonded atoms furnishes both of the electrons which are shared. **covalent b.,** a chemical bond resulting when electrons are shared by two atoms, to form a stable electronic shell around each nucleus. Sharing of two electrons results in a single covalent bond; sharing four electrons, a double bond; and sharing six electrons, a triple bond. Covalent bonds may be nonpolar, involving electrons evenly shared by the two atoms, or polar bonds, when the electrons are unevenly shared. See also *primary b.* **disulfide b.,** covalently linked sulfide groups −S−S−, important in linking polypeptide chains, as the heavy and light chains in γ-globulins. The linking is accomplished by means of two molecules of cysteine through their SH groups to form −S−S− bridges. **double b.,** a chemical bond in compounds, such as unsaturated compounds, where two single valence bonds connect two atoms. **heteropolar b.,** polar b. **homopolar b.,** nonpolar b. **hydrogen b.,** a primarily electrostatic bond between a hydrogen atom bound to a highly electronegative element (such as oxygen or nitrogen) in a given molecule, or part of a molecule, and a secondary highly electronegative atom in another molecule or in a different part of the same molecule. The hydrogen bond is generally represented by three dots, e.g., X−H⋯Y, where X and Y are electronegative atoms. The abnormal physical properties of water, including high boiling point, high melting point, high heats of vaporization and fusion, high surface tension, and the density maximum at 4°C, are attributable to abnormally high intermolecular attractive interaction of hydrogen bonds. These interactions arise as a result of the very strong attraction between the nonbonding electrons of the oxygen and partially positively-charged hydrogen atoms on adjacent molecules. **ionic b.,** a chemical bond formed between atoms of strongly electropositive character (electron donors) and atoms of strongly electronegative character (electron receivers), as in sodium chloride in which Na^+ and Cl^- share the sodium valence electron with the chlorine to form NaCl. See also *primary b.* **metallic b.,** a primary bond being a system in which all the positive ions interact with all the valence electrons to bond the atoms within the metal together, whereby metal ions (atoms stripped of the valence electrons) are arranged in a geometric network of a crystallographic lattice and the valence electrons are free to move within the crystals. The attraction between the positive metal ions and the free electrons is the bonding force. **molecular b.,** a chemical bond in which one atom contributes both electrons. **multiple b's,** a chemical bond which involves sharing more than one pair of electrons. **nonpolar b.,** a chemical bond formed by a combination of two atoms to form a molecule by sharing a pair of electrons, both atoms having equal electron affinities and the binding pair of electrons occupying a position midway between the atoms. Called also *homopolar b.* **peptide b.,** a covalent bond

$$\overset{O}{\underset{\parallel}{}}$$

through substituted amide (−N−C−) linkages in a protein molecule, allowing the amino acid residues to form long unbranched polymers. See also PEPTIDE. **pi b.,** π-b., a covalent bond between adjacent atoms resulting from the overlap of p-orbitals in a side-by-side fashion. **polar b.,** a chemical bond formed by the electrostatic union of two atoms established by the passage of one or more electrons from one atom to the other. Called also *heteropolar b.* **primary b.,** forces responsible for holding atoms and molecules in the condensed (solid or liquid) state, including ionic, covalent, and metallic bonds. −S−S− **b.,**

disulfide b. **secondary b's,** van der Waals forces; see under FORCE. **sigma b.,** σ-b. a covalent bond resulting from increased electron density along the axis connecting the nuclei of adjacent atoms. **single b.,** a chemical bond involving one pair of electrons. **triple b.,** a chemical bond involving three pairs of electrons. **valence b.,** a pair of electrons consisting of one electron from each of the two atoms they unite. **van der Waals b's,** van der Waals forces; see under FORCE.

bonding (bond′ing) joining together securely with an adhesive substance, such as glue or cement. **tooth b.,** the technique of fixing orthodontic brackets and other attachments directly to the enamel surface with orthodontic adhesives. See also tooth BANDING.

bone (bōn) [L. *os;* Gr. *osteon*] a dense type of connective tissue with hardness and tensile strength almost equal to that of cast iron. It consists of a hard exterior layer (*substantia compacta*) covered by a fibrous sheath, the periosteum, and a spongy substance (*substantia spongiosa*), forming a lattice of branching trabeculae into hollow spaces occupied by bone marrow. The interior surface layer is known as the *endosteum.* The bone tissue consists of osteocytes surrounded by a fibrous intercellular material composed of collagen fibers and made rigid by inorganic salts, chiefly calcium phosphate (85 percent), calcium carbonate (10 percent), and calcium fluoride and magnesium chloride (5 percent). Together with joints, bones form the framework of the skeleton in most vertebrates, and they serve as a protective cover for vital organs, such as the brain and thoracic organs, house the bone marrow, and store calcium and phosphate deposits of the body. Called also *os.* For related terms see those beginning OSSEO- and OSTEO-. **alar b.,** sphenoid b. **Albers-Schönberg's marble b's,** Albers-Schönberg's DISEASE. **Albrecht's b.,** basiotic b. **alisphenoid b.,** great wing of sphenoid bone; see under WING. **alisphenoidal b.,** alisphenoid. **alveolar b.,** the thin layer of bone making up the bony processes of the maxilla and mandible, and surrounding and containing the teeth; it is pierced by many small openings through which blood vessels, lymphatics, and nerve fibers pass. See also alveolar PROCESS. **alveolar b. proper,** cribriform plate of alveolar process; see under PLATE. **basal b.,** the relatively fixed and unchangeable framework of the mandible and maxilla, which limits the extent to which teeth can be moved in the alveolar or supporting bone if the occlusion is to remain stable. **basihyal b.,** the body of the hyoid bone. **basilar b.,** basioccipital b. **basioccipital b.,** a bone developing from a separate ossification center in the fetus, which becomes the basilar process of the occipital bone. Called also *basilar b.* **basiotic b.,** a small bone of the fetus between the basisphenoid and basioccipital bones. Called also *Albrecht's b.* **basisphenoid b.,** an embryonic bone that becomes the back part of the body of the sphenoid bone. **Bertin's b.,** sphenoidal CONCHA. **bregmatic b.,** parietal b. **brittle b's,** OSTEOGENESIS imperfecta. **bundle b.,** one of the two types of bone comprising the alveolar bone, so called because of the continuation into the principal fibers of the periodontal ligament. It is restricted to the cribriform plate, being located in appreciable amounts on the distal surfaces of the sockets in which physiologic mesial drift is effected. It is characterized by lamellae that are less prominent than those in other types of mature bone, large numbers of Sharpey's fibers, paucity of collagen fibrils, and large amounts of more calcified cementing substance that render bundle bone more resistant to x-rays than the surrounding bones, appearing on dental radiographs as a thin radiopaque line, hence the synonym *lamina dura.* Called also *lamellated b.* **cancellated b., cancellous b.,** spongy b. **cartilage b.,** any bone that develops within cartilage (intracartilaginous), ossification occurring within a cartilage model, in contrast to membrane bone (intramembranous). Called also *endochondral b., replacement b.,* and *substitution b.* **chalk b's,** Albers-Schönberg's DISEASE. **cheek b.,** zygomatic b. **collar b.,** clavicle. **compact b.,** the hard external portion of bone appearing solid to the unaided eye but microscopically showing spaces (lacunae) and intercommunicating tunnels (canaliculi) occupied by osteocytes and their processes, respectively; the latter may contact and are generally oriented toward blood vessels in the bone or its sheath (periosteum). The matrix consists of layers (lamellae) separated by cementing substance; lamellae occur as the result of differences in fibril orientation in adjacent layers. Rest periods in bone formation or destruction may be recorded as resting and resorption lines. Called also *dense b., compact tissue, compact substance of bone,* and *substantia compacta ossium* [NA]. **cortical b.,** the compact bone of the shaft of a bone that surrounds the medullary cavity. **cranial b's,** bones of the cranial part of the skull, including the occipital, frontal, temporal, sphenoid, ethmoid, parietal, lacrimal, and nasal bones, the inferior nasal concha, and vomer. Called also *b's of skull* and *ossa cranii* [NA]. See also *facial b's.* **cribriform b.,** ethmoid b. **dense b.,** compact b. **dermal b.,**

membrane b. **ectethmoid b's,** the lateral masses of the ethmoid bone. **endochondral b.,** cartilage b. **epactal b's,** wormian b's. **epactal b., proper,** interparietal b. **ethmoid b.,** a cubical bone situated between the two orbits in the anterior portion of the base of the cranium. The bone is light and spongy and consists of four parts: the cribriform plate, the perpendicular plate, and two labyrinths. The cribriform plate forms the base of the cranium and roof of the nasal cavity; the perpendicular plate forms a part of the nasal septum; and the labyrinth forms part of the orbit and the medial part of the nasal cavity. At birth the bone consists of underdeveloped labyrinth. During the first year of life the crista galli and perpendicular plate begin to ossify; they are joined to the labyrinths during the second year of life. Development of the ethmoidal cells of the labyrinth also begins after birth. Called also *cribriform b.* and *os ethmoidale* [NA]. **ethmoidal b., supreme,** nasal concha, supreme; see under CONCHA. **exoccipital b.,** one of the two lateral portions of the occipital bone, developing from separate centers of ossification into the portions that bear the condyles. **facial b's,** the facial skeleton, consisting of bones situated between the cranial base and the mandibular region. While some consider the facial bones to comprise the hyoid, palatine, and zygomatic bones, mandible, and maxilla, others also include the lacrimal and nasal bones, inferior nasal concha, and vomer but exclude the hyoid bone. Called also *facial skeleton* and *ossa faciei* [NA]. See also *cranial b's.* **b. file,** bone FILE. **flat b.,** any bone whose thickness is slight, sometimes consisting of only a thin layer of compact bone, or two layers with intervening spongy bone and marrow; usually bent or curved rather than flat. Called also *os planum* [NA]. **frontal b.,** the bone that forms the frontal part of the skull, consisting of a vertical part (squama), which forms the forehead, and a horizontal part (pars orbitalis), which forms the roofs of the orbits and the nasal cavity. It articulates with the sphenoid, ethmoid, two parietal, two nasal, two maxillary, two lacrimal, and two zygomatic bones. At birth, the frontal bone consists of two parts separated by the frontal suture; by the eighth year of life most of the suture is obliterated, but sometimes the separation may persist throughout life. The frontal sinuses begin to develop during the first or second year of life and attain their full size at or after puberty. Called also *os frontale* [NA]. **Henle's trapezoid b.,** pterygoid PROCESS. **hyoid b.,** a U-shaped bone situated at the base of the tongue, just above the thyroid cartilage, and suspended from the tips of the styloid process of the temporal bone by the styloid ligaments, and made up of the body, two greater cornua, and two lesser cornua. The body is a square, flat bony plate with a sharp lower edge and a thick upper border; the geniohyoideus, mylohyoideus, sternohyoideus, and parts of the thyrohyoideus muscles attach to its caudal border. The greater cornua projects dorsally from the body on either side, and attaches the thyrohyoid ligament and the hypoglossus, constrictor pharyngis, digastricus, and stylohyoideus muscles. The lesser cornu is a small conical eminence attached at the junction of the body and the greater cornua by a synovial joint, which frequently persists through life but sometimes ossifies in adults; it gives attachment to the stylohyoid ligament and the chondroglossus muscle. The hyoid bone does not articulate with other bones, thus having the mobility necessary for swallowing and phonation. It ossifies from six centers, with ossification of the body and greater cornua taking place during the last stages of fetal life, the lesser cornua during the first and second year after birth. Called also *lingual b., tongue b.,* and *os hyoideum* [NA]. **incarial b.,** interparietal b. **incisive b.,** the portion of the maxilla that bears the incisor teeth, which is situated anterior to a delicate suture sometimes seen in the young skull, and which extends laterally and rostrally on either side of the incisive foramen to the interval between the lateral incisors and the canine teeth. Developmentally, it is the premaxilla, which in the human subsequently fuses with the maxilla proper to form the adult bone. In most other vertebrates it persists as an independent bone. Called also *os incisivum* [NA]. See also PREMAXILLA. **interparietal b.,** the part of the squama of the occipital bone lying superior to the highest nuchal line, when it fails to unite with the bones of the skull, and remains separate throughout life. Called also *incarial b., proper epactal b., os incae,* and *os interparietale* [NA]. **ivory b's,** Albers-Schönberg's DISEASE. **jaw b., lower,** mandible. **jaw b., upper,** maxilla. **jugal b.,** zygomatic b. **lacrimal b.,** a thin, fragile, scalelike bone at the anterior part of the medial wall of the orbit, which articulates with the frontal and ethmoid bones, maxilla, and inferior nasal concha. Its lateral or orbital surface is divided by the posterior lacrimal crest into the anterior part, forming the lacrimal sulcus, which joins with the frontal process of the maxilla to form the lacrimal fossa, and the posterior part, forming part of the medial wall of the orbit. Part of the

orbicularis oculi muscle attaches to the crest. The lacrimal hamulus, a hooklike structure at the end of the crest, articulates with the maxilla and forms the orifice of the lacrimal canal; it sometimes exists as a separate bone known as the *lesser lacrimal bone.* A furrow on the medial or nasal surface forms part of the middle nasal meatus. It ossifies from a single center which appears about the twelfth week of fetal life. Called also *os lacrimale* [NA]. **lacrimal b., lesser,** the lacrimal hamulus when it occurs as a separate bone. **lamellated b.,** bundle b. **lingual b.,** hyoid b. **malar b.,** zygomatic b. **masticatory b.,** a bone involved in the masticatory processes or housing the teeth. Some authorities consider any bone attaching the masticatory muscles as being a masticatory bone, including the hyoid bone. **mastoid b.,** the posterior portion of the petrous part of the temporal bone, bounded anteriorly by the external acoustic meatus and articulating superiorly with the parietal bone and posteriorly with the occipital bone; the anterior part is fused to the squama and forms the external acoustic meatus and the tympanic cavity. A part of the bone contains hollowed out spaces, the mastoid cells. Called also *mamillary part of temporal bone, mastoideum, os mastoideum,* and *pars mastoidea ossis temporalis.* **maxillary b.,** maxilla. **maxillary b., inferior,** mandible. **maxillary b., superior,** maxilla. **maxilloturbinal b.,** nasal concha, inferior; see under CONCHA. **membrane b.,** one that develops within a connective tissue membrane, in contrast to bone preformed in cartilage. Called also *dermal b.* Cf. *cartilage b.* **nasal b.,** either of the two small, irregularly quadrilateral bones that fit between the two frontal processes of the maxilla and form the bridge of the nose. They are usually asymmetrical and their size varies considerably, giving the face and nose specific characteristics. Racial differences are prominent. The thick and short upper border of each bone articulates with the frontal bone, and the sharp lower border forms the upper part of the piriform aperture. The posterolateral border articulates with the frontal process of the maxilla, and the anterolateral border joins the nasal bone of the opposite side. The convex external surface is perforated by a foramen for a vein and is covered by the procerus and nasalis muscles. The concave internal surface presents a groove for the nasociliary nerve. The bones are ossified from two separate centers. They articulate with the frontal, ethmoid, and maxillary bones. Called also *os nasale* [NA]. **nasal b., supreme,** nasal concha, supreme; see under CONCHA. **nonlamellated b.,** woven b. **occipital b.,** a cup-shaped bone, trapezoidal in outline, situated at the posterior and inferior part of the skull, which consists of two compact lamellae (the outer and inner tables), sandwiching the cancellous tissue (diploë). It is thin and destitute of diploë in the inferior fossae, but is thick at the ridges, protuberances, condyles, and anterior portion of the basilar part. The bone develops by the fusion of four bones around a large oval opening (foramen magnum): the curved plate posterior to the foramen (squama), the thick roughly quadrilateral bone anterior to the foramen (basilar part), and a pair of bones at the lateral areas (lateral parts); the occipital plane of the squama is developed in membrane, and may remain separate throughout life (interparietal b.); the remaining parts develop in cartilage. The squama and the lateral parts unite at about the fourth year of life. Union with the sphenoid bone occurs between 18 and 25 years of age. It articulates with the two parietal and two temporal bones, the sphenoid bone, and the atlas. The cranial cavity communicates with the vertebral canal through the foramen magnum. Called also *os basilare* and *os occipitale* [NA]. **orbital b.,** zygomatic b. **orbitosphenoidal b.,** orbitosphenoid. **palate b.,** palatine b. **palatine b.,** either of the two bones which resemble the letter L, consisting of a horizontal and a vertical plate joined at right angles, and which form the posterior part of the hard palate, lateral walls of the nasal fossa, and posterior part of the floor of the orbit. Each articulates with the sphenoid and ethmoid bones, the opposite palatine bones, and the maxilla, vomer, and inferior nasal concha. Called also *palate b.* and *os palatinum* [NA]. See illustration at PALATE. **parietal b.,** either of the two quadrilateral cup-shaped bones forming the roof and sides of the cranium, and joining each other in the midline at the sagittal suture. The bone articulates with the occipital, frontal, temporal, and sphenoidal bones and the opposite parietal bone. It is ossified in a membrane from a single center. Sometimes, the parietal bone is divided into two parts by the anteroposterior suture. Called also *bregmatic b.* and *os parietale* [NA]. **petrous b.,** one of the three parts of the temporal bone, made up of a pyramid of dense bone housing the organ of hearing and equilibrium, and wedged in between the sphenoid and occipital bones at the base of the skull. Its base is fused to the squama and the mastoid bone; its apex fits between the posterior border of the great wing of the sphenoid bone and the basilar part of the occipital and sphenoid bones; its anterior surface forms the posterior part of the middle cranial fossa and is continuous with the inner surface of the squama; its posterior surface forms the anterior part of the posterior cranial fossa; its inferior part forms the external portion of the base of the skull. The anterior surface of the bone presents depressions for the convolutions of the brain. Called also *pars petrosa ossis temporalis* [NA], *petrous pyramid*, and *pyramis ossis temporalis*. **b. phosphate,** CALCIUM phosphate. **pneumatic b.,** a bone that contains air-filled cavities or sinuses. Called also *os pneumaticum* [NA]. **postsphenoidal b.,** postsphenoid. **prefrontal b.,** nasal process of frontal bone; see under PROCESS. **prefrontal b. of von Bardeleben,** nasal process of frontal bone; see under PROCESS. **preinterparietal b.,** a wormian bone, sometimes observed, detached from the anterior part of the interparietal bone. **premaxillary b.,** premaxilla. **presphenoidal b.,** presphenoid. **primitive b.,** woven b. **pterygoid b.,** pterygoid PROCESS. **b. rasp,** bone FILE. **replacement b.,** cartilage b. **Riolan's b.,** Riolan's OSSICLE. **rudimentary b.,** a bone that has only partially developed. **b's of skull,** cranial b's. **sphenoid b.,** a single, irregular, wedge-shaped bone at the base of the skull, resembling a butterfly with its wings extended, which forms part of the orbits and nasal fossae, and consists of the median portion (body of sphenoid bone), two great wings and two small wings, and two pterygoid processes. It articulates with four single bones, the vomer and the ethmoid, frontal, and occipital bones, and four paired bones, the parietal, temporal, zygomatic, and palatine bones, and sometimes, with the maxilla. Embryologically, it is first formed in cartilage and, after ossification begins, divides into the anterior part (presphenoid) and a posterior part (postsphenoid), which are connected to each other by a synchondrosis. At about the seventh or eighth month of fetal life the bones unite. At birth it is made up of the body and small wings and two lateral parts, each consisting of the great wings and pterygoid processes. The great wings and the body unite during the first year of life, and the small wings extend toward each other and meet at the jugum sphenoidale. By the twenty-fifth year, the sphenoid and occipital bones fuse. Called also *alar b., suprapharyngeal b., os basilare,* and *os sphenoidale* [NA]. **sphenoturbinal b.,** sphenoidal CONCHA. **spongy b.,** a spongy substance found below the compact bone, as a labyrinthine system of bone trabeculae and intercommunicating spaces occupied by the bone marrow. In younger individuals, the spaces are filled by the red, or hematopoietic, marrow, and in adults by yellow marrow or mostly fat cells. In the jaws, the trabecular systems vary in size, number, and pattern in response to the masticatory forces. Called also *cancellated b., cancellous b., spongiosa, spongy substance of bone,* and *substantia spongiosa ossium* [NA]. **spongy b., inferior,** nasal concha, inferior; see under CONCHA. **spongy b., superior,** nasal concha, superior; see under CONCHA. **squamo-occipital b.,** the squamous portion of the fetal occipital bone, including the supraoccipital and interparietal bones. **squamous b.,** temporal SQUAMA. **substitution b.,** cartilage b. **superior maxillary b.,** maxilla. **suprainterparietal b.,** a wormian bone sometimes occurring at the posterior part of the sagittal suture. **supraoccipital b.,** a bone developing from a separate ossification center in the fetus; it becomes the squamous part of the occipital bone below the superior nuchal line. **suprapharyngeal b.,** sphenoid b. **sutural b's,** wormian b's. **temporal b.,** either of the two irregular bones forming part of the lateral surface and base of the skull, containing the organs of hearing and equilibrium. Each consists of three parts, the squama and the petrous tympanic bones. At birth the three parts are separated, but early in life they fuse to one another, although the styloid process may remain independent for some time. Boundaries between different parts of the bone nearly disappear in the adult. Called also *os temporale* [NA]. **tongue b.,** hyoid b. **trapezoid b. of Henle,** pterygoid PROCESS. **turbinate b., highest,** nasal concha, supreme; see under CONCHA. **turbinate b., inferior,** nasal concha, inferior; see under CONCHA. **turbinate b., middle,** nasal concha, middle; see under CONCHA. **turbinate b., superior,** nasal concha, superior; see under CONCHA. **tympanic b.,** a curved bony plate of the temporal bone situated below the squama and in front of the mastoid process. Called also *pars tympanica ossis temporalis* [NA]. **vomer b.,** vomer. **von Bardeleben's prefrontal b.,** nasal process of frontal bone; see under PROCESS. **wormian b's,** isolated bones found in the sutures between the bones of the skull. They occur most com-

monly in the lamboidal suture and, less frequently, at the fontanelle, as irregularly shaped, more or less symmetrical small bones, varying in number from two to three in normal skulls and up to a hundred in hydrocephalus. Called also *epactal b's, sutural b's, ossa Wormi,* and *ossa suturatum* [NA]. See also *suprainterparietal b.* and Riolan's OSSICLE. **woven b.,** bony tissue found in the embryo and young children and in various pathologic conditions in adults, in which the bone fails to show the oriented arrangement of collagen fibers characteristic of lamellated bone. Called also *nonlamellated b.* and *primitive b.* **zygomatic b.,** a roughly diamond-shaped bone on either side of the head that forms the prominence of the cheek, and the lateral wall and floor of the orbit and parts of the temporal and infratemporal fossae. It articulates with the frontal bone, maxilla, zygomatic process of the temporal bone, and great wing of the sphenoid bone. At birth the bone may be divided by a horizontal suture into an upper and lower part. Called also *cheek b., jugal b., malar b., orbital b., os zygomaticum* [NA], and *zygoma.*

bonelet (bŏn′let) a small bone or ossicle.

Bonfil primer see under PRIMER.

Bonnet's syndrome [Paul *Bonnet,* French physician] trigeminal nonsympathetic NEURALGIA.

Bonnevie-Ullrich syndrome [Kristine *Bonnevie,* Norwegian physician, 1872–1950; Otto *Ullrich,* German physician, 1894–1957] see under SYNDROME.

Bonnier's syndrome [Pierre *Bonnier,* French physician, 1861–1918] see under SYNDROME.

Bonwill articular, crown, mallet, triangle [William Gibson Arlington *Bonwill,* American dentist, 1833–1899; he invented the articulator, developed the first electromagnetic mallet for insertion of gold foil, and was the first to use the dry mouth technique by using bibulous paper] see under ARTICULATOR, CROWN, MALLET, and TRIANGLE.

Böök's syndrome [Jan Arvid Böök, Swedish geneticist] see under SYNDROME.

booster (boost′er) 1. something that lifts, raises, advances, or promotes. 2. booster DOSE.

BOR before time of operation.

borate (bo′rāt) any salt of boric acid. **sodium b.,** SODIUM borate.

borax (bo′raks) [L., from Arabic, Persian *būrah*] SODIUM borate.

border (bor′der) a bounding or surrounding line, edge, or surface. See also MARGIN and MARGO. **alveolar b. of mandible,** alveolar arch of mandible; see under ARCH. **alveolar b. of maxilla,** alveolar arch of maxilla; see under ARCH. **brush b.,** the presence on the free surfaces of certain types of cells of numerous minute projections (microvilli) that, under the electron microscope, appear as slender cylindrical processes. There may be several thousand microvilli on a single cell surface; on some cells they may be limited to the secreting surface, on others they may be found on all sides. Microvilli vary in length from one cell type to another, being finger-like on some and club-shaped on others, sometimes uniformly arranged and other times having an irregular arrangement. The function of the brush border is believed to be related primarily to increasing the surface area of the cell for absorption and secretion. Called also *striated b.* **denture b.,** 1. the limit, boundary, or circumferential margin of a denture base. 2. the margin of the denture base at the junction of the polished surface with the impression (tissue) surface. 3. the extreme edges of a denture base at the buccolabial, lingual, and posterior limits. 4. the extreme margins of a denture base. Called also *denture edge* and *denture periphery.* **frontal b. of parietal bone,** frontal margin of parietal bone; see under MARGIN. **inferior b. of mandible,** the lower margin of the body of the mandible, presenting a plump, smooth, and rounded edge with a shallow groove at the junction with the ramus for the facial artery. Called also *base of mandible* and *basis mandibulae* [NA]. **infraorbital b. of maxilla,** infraorbital margin of maxilla; see under MARGIN. **infraorbital b. of orbit,** infraorbital margin of orbit; see under MARGIN. **lacrimal b. of maxilla,** lacrimal margin of maxilla; see under MARGIN. **b. molding,** border MOLDING. **nasal b. of frontal bone,** nasal margin of frontal bone; see under MARGIN. **occipital b. of parietal bone,** occipital margin of parietal bone; see under MARGIN. **occipital b. of temporal bone,** occipital margin of temporal bone; see under MARGIN. **orbital b. of great wing of sphenoid bone,** orbital surface of great wing of sphenoid bone; see under SURFACE. **parietal b. of frontal bone,** parietal margin of frontal bone; see under MARGIN. **parietal b. of temporal bone, parietal b. of temporal squama,** parietal margin of temporal bone; see under MARGIN. **posterior b. of petrous portion of temporal bone,** ANGLE of petrous portion of temporal bone. **b. seal,** border SEAL. **sphenoidal b. of temporal bone, sphenoidal b. of temporal squama,** sphenoidal margin of temporal bone; see under MARGIN. **squamous b. of parietal bone,** squamous margin of parietal bone; see under MARGIN. **superior**

b. of petrous portion of temporal bone, superior angle of petrous portion of temporal bone; see under ANGLE. **striated b.,** brush b. **temporal b. of zygomatic bone,** temporal margin of zygomatic bone; see under MARGIN. **vermilion b.,** the red border of the lips, representing the transitional zone where the lips merge into mucous membrane. It is covered by translucent nonkeratinized epithelium that is rich in capillaries and papillae, giving the border the red color. Called also *marginal zone of lips, red zone of lips, vermilion area,* and *vermilion zone.*

Bordet, Jules Jean Baptiste Vincent [1870–1961] a Belgian bacteriologist who, with R. F. J. Pfeiffer, in 1894, elucidated the action of complement and antibody in cell lysis; winner of the Nobel prize for medicine and physiology in 1919. See complement FIXATION (Bordet-Gengou phenomenon or reaction).

Bordet-Gengou bacillus, phenomenon, reaction [J. J. B. V. *Bordet;* Octave *Gengou,* French bacteriologist, 1875–1957] see *Bordetella pertussis,* under BORDETELLA, and see complement FIXATION.

Bordetella (bor″dĕ-tel′lah) [named after J. J. B. V. *Bordet*] a genus of bacteria of uncertain affiliation, occurring as gram-negative, aerobic, minute coccobacilli (0.2 to 0.3 μm by 0.5 to 1.0 μm in size), found singly or in pairs and, rarely, in short chains. The cells are nonmotile or motile by lateral polytrichous flagella. They are parasitic in animals, including man, and pathogens of the respiratory tract. **B. bronchiesep′tica,** a species originally isolated from dogs ill with distemper; believed to be the cause of bronchopneumonia in animals. Called also *Alcaligenes bronchisepticus, Bacillus bronchicanis, B. bronchisepticus, Brucella bronchiseptica,* and *Haemophilus bronchisepticus.* **B. parapertus′sis,** a species occasionally found in whooping cough in man. Called also *Acinetobacter parapertussis, Bacillus parapertussis,* and *Haemophilus parapertussis.* **B. pertus′sis,** the etiologic agent of whooping cough, occurring as small ovoid rods (0.5 to 1.0 μm in length and 0.2 to 0.3 μm in diameter), having a capsule-like sheath, and found singly or in pairs or short chains. It produces a heat-labile toxin and a heat-stable endotoxin. It is sensitive to broad-spectrum antibiotics, such as chloramphenicol, ampicillin, and tetracyclines. Called also *Bacterium tussis-convulsivae, Bordet-Gengou bacillus,* and *Haemophilus pertussis.*

Bordier-Fränkel sign see under SIGN.

2-bornanone (bor′nah-nōn) camphor (1).

boron (bo′ron) [L. *borium*] a nonmetallic element occurring in the earth's crust in compounds, never as the element. Symbol, B; atomic weight, 10.81; atomic number, 5; valence, 3; melting point, 2079°C; Mohs hardness index, 9.3; group IIIA of the periodic table. Boron has two naturally occurring stable isotopes (10, 11) and three short-lived artificial ones (8, 12, 13). It is a dark brown to black, hard, amorphous crystalline powder, soluble in nitric and sulfuric acid, but not in water, alcohol, and ether. Used to harden other metals and, in nuclear chemistry, as a neutron absorber. Boron is relatively nontoxic. **b. carbide,** a compound, B_4C, occurring as a shiny black, hard crystalline powder, with a Mohs hardness index of 9.3, being softer than diamond, but harder than silicon carbide. It is resistant to the chemical action of acids and water and is made soluble by molten alkali. Boron carbide is produced by heating boron to very high temperatures to effect its union with carbon. It is used in nuclear reactors, and as an abrasive agent in industry and dentistry. Inhalation of boron carbide dust may cause respiratory disorders. Trademark: Norbide.

Borovskii's disease [P. F. *Borovskii,* Russian physician] cutaneous LEISHMANIASIS.

Borrel, Amédée [1867–1936] a French bacteriologist.

Borrelia (bo-rel′e-ah) [named after A. *Borrel*] a genus of spiral bacteria of the family Spirochaetaceae, order Spirochaetales, made up of gram-negative, anaerobic cells (about 0.2 to 0.5 μm in width and 3 to 5 μm in length), with 15 to 20 axial fibrils. They are generally parasitic on the mucous membranes of mammals, including man, and birds; some strains are pathogenic, causing relapsing fevers and spirochetoses in cattle and fowl. The organisms are also found in insect vectors of the disease, most often ticks and lice. **B. bucca′lis,** *Treponema buccale;* see under TREPONEMA. **B. dutton′ii,** an etiologic agent of relapsing fever in central and south Africa; transmitted by ticks. Called also *Dutton's spirochete, Spirillum duttoni,* and *Spirochaeta duttoni.* **B. herm′sii,** an etiologic agent of relapsing fever in western North America; transmitted by ticks. Called also *Spirochaeta hermsi.* **B. hispan′ica,** the etiologic agent of relapsing fever in the Iberian peninsula and southwest Africa; transmitted by ticks. Called also *Spirochaeta hispanica.* **B. phagede′nis,** *Treponema phagedenis;* see under TREPONEMA. **B. recurren′tis,** a species causing epidemic relapsing fever in man; transmitted by body lice. Called also *Spirochaeta obermeieri, S. recurrentis,* and *Spiroschaudinnia recurren-*

tis. **B. refrin′gens,** *Treponema refringens;* see under TREPONEMA. **B. vincen′ti,** *Treponema vincentii;* see under TREPONEMA.

Bose's operation [Heinrich *Bose,* German surgeon, 1840–1900] see under OPERATION.

boss (bos) a rounded eminence, as on the surface of a bone or tumor. **parietal b's,** sharp prominences on each side of the parietal bones.

Bosviel's disease [J. *Bosviel*] staphylohematoma.

botryoid (bot′re-oid) [Gr. *botrys* bunch of grapes + *eidos* form] resembling a bunch of grapes.

botulin (bot′u-lin) [L. *botulus* sausage] a toxin produced by *Clostridium botulinum,* sometimes found in imperfectly preserved or canned meats and vegetables, which can be fatal when ingested.

botulism (bot′u-lizm) [L. *botulus* sausage] an often fatal type of food poisoning caused by ingestion of improperly preserved food containing toxin produced by the bacterium *Clostridium botulinum.* Principal symptoms include gastrointestinal disorders, nausea, vomiting, dilated and nonreactive pupils, diplopia, blurred vision, flaccid paralysis, dryness of the oral mucosa, difficulty in speaking and swallowing, pharyngeal pain, weakness, and lassitude.

bouba (boo′bah) yaws. **b. brazilia′na,** mucocutaneous LEISHMANIASIS.

Boucher, Carl O. [1904–1975] an American prosthodontist, dental lexicographer, and writer.

Bouchut's tubes [Jean Antoine Eugène *Bouchut,* French physician, 1818–1891] see under TUBE.

bougie (boo-zhe′) [Fr. "wax candle"] a slender, flexible, hollow or solid, cylindrical instrument for introduction into tubular organs, usually for the purpose of calibrating or dilating constricted areas. **filiform b.,** one of very slender caliber; used for the gentle exploration of strictures or sinus tracts of small diameter with multiple false passages. **medicated b.,** one charged with a medicinal substance.

bougienage (boo-zhe-nahzh′) the passage of a bougie through a tubular structure or organ, to increase its caliber, as in the treatment of stricture of the esophagus.

boundary (bown′dre, bown′dĕ-re) something that forms a border or limit; also, the border or limit formed. **grain b.,** GRAIN boundary.

Bourdet, Étienne [18th century] a French dentist who advocated a dental prosthesis, the base of which was made of gold covered with a flesh-colored enamel (rose pearl); the teeth were attached to the base by pins.

Bourquin unit [Ann *Bourquin,* American nutritionist, born 1897] see under UNIT.

bouton (boo-taw′) [Fr.] button. **terminal b's,** synaptic terminals; see under TERMINAL.

Bovimyces pleuropneumoniae (bo″vĕ-mi′sēz ploor″o-nu-mo′ne-e) *Mycoplasma mycoides;* see under MYCOPLASMA.

bovine (bo′vīn) [L. *bos, bovis,* bullock, cow] pertaining to, characterized by, or derived from the ox (cattle).

bow (bo) any bow-shaped instrument, device, or apparatus. **hinge-b.,** adjustable axis FACE-BOW. **labial b.,** labial WIRE. **Logan b.,** an appliance used to prevent tension on sutures after surgery of cleft lip.

Bowditch's law [Henry Pickering *Bowditch,* Boston physiologist, 1840–1911] see under LAW.

bowel (bow′el) [Fr. *boyau*] the intestine.

Bowen's cavity primer [R. L. *Bowen,* American dentist] see under PRIMER.

Bowen's disease, epithelioma, precancerosis [John Templeton *Bowen,* American dermatologist, 1857–1941] CARCINOMA in situ.

Bowles multiphase appliance, multiphase attachment, technique [V. D. *Bowles,* American orthodontist] see multiphase APPLIANCE.

Bowman's capsule, gland, probe [Sir William *Bowman,* English physician, 1816–1892] see under CAPSULE and PROBE, and see olfactory GLAND.

box (boks) a rectangular structure. **endodontic b's,** metal or plastic containers used for the storage and/or sterilization of root canal instruments, absorbent points, and/or cotton pellets. Called also *P b's,* endodontic b's.

Box's technique [H. K. *Box*] see under TECHNIQUE.

boxing (bok′sing) 1. the material used to produce a box or casting. 2. a boxlike enclosure. 3. in the fabrication of dental restorations and appliances, the building up of vertical walls of wax or other suitable material to form a box around a dental impression into which the freshly mixed plaster or stone is poured, which is done to produce the desired size and form of the base of the cast and to preserve certain landmarks of the impression. The process consists of adapting a narrow strip or stick of wax around the impression below its peripheral height, followed by the application of a wider strip around the entire impression.

Boyd-Stearns syndrome [Julian Deigh *Boyd*, American physician, born 1894; Genevieve *Stearns*, American physician] see under SYNDROME.

Boyer's bursa, cyst [Alexis Baron de *Boyer*, French surgeon, 1757–1833] see under BURSA and CYST.

Boyle's law [Robert *Boyle*, British physicist, 1627–1691] see under LAW.

BP 1. blood PRESSURE;. 2. British Pharmacopoeia. 3. Bolton POINT.

b.p. boiling point.

BPh British Pharmacopoeia.

Bq becquerel.

BQA Bureau of Quality Assurance; see under BUREAU.

Br 1. bromine. 2. bregma.

brace (brās) 1. a device that holds parts together or in place. 2. an orthopedic appliance used to support, align, or hold parts of the body in correct position. 3. usually in the plural, an orthodontic appliance (see under APPLIANCE). **jaw b.,** mouth PROP.

brachia (bra′ke-ah) [L.] plural of *brachium*.

brachiocephalic (brak″e-o-sĕ-fal′ik) [Gr. *brachiōn* arm + *kephalē* head] pertaining to the arm and head, as in the brachiocephalic trunk.

brachiofaciolingual (brak″e-o-fa″she-o-ling′gwal) pertaining to or affecting the arm, the face, and the tongue.

brachium (bra′ke-um), pl. *bra′chia* [L.; Gr. *brachiōn*] 1. [NA] the arm; specifically the arm from shoulder to elbow. 2. a general anatomical term used to designate an armlike process or stricture.

Brachmann-de Lange syndrome [W. *Brachmann*; Cornelia *de Lange*, Dutch pediatrician, 1871–1950] de Lange's SYNDROME.

brachy- [Gr. *brachys* short] a combining form meaning short.

brachycephalia (brak″e-sĕ-fa′le-ah) brachycephaly.

brachycephalic (brak″e-sĕ-fal′ik) [*brachy-* + Gr. *kephalē* head] pertaining to or characterized by a short broad skull. Called also *brachycephalous*. See brachycephalic SKULL.

brachycephalism (brak″e-sef′ah-lizm) brachycephaly.

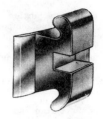
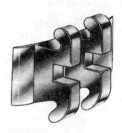
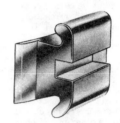

Edgewise bracket. (From T. M. Graber: Orthodontics — Principles and Practice. 3rd ed. Philadelphia, W. B. Saunders Co., 1972; courtesy Rocky Mountain Dental Products Co.)

brachycephalous (brak″e-sef′ah-lus) brachycephalic.

brachycephaly (brak″e-sef′ah-le) a condition characterized by a short broad skull. Called also *brachycephalia* and *brachycephalism*. See brachycephalic SKULL.

brachycheilia (brak″e-ki′le-ah) [*brachy-* + Gr. *cheilos* lip + *-ia*] a condition characterized by an abnormal shortness of the oral fissure. Called also *brachychily*. Cf. DOLICHOCHEILIA.

brachychily (brak-ik′ĭ-le) brachycheilia.

brachycranic (brak″e-kra′nik) pertaining to or characterized by a short broad cranium. See brachycephalic SKULL.

brachycrany (brak″e-kra′ne) a short broad cranium.

brachydont (brak″e-dont) [*brachy-* + Gr. *odous* tooth] an individual having teeth with short crowns. Cf. HYPSODONT.

brachyfacial (brak″e-fa′shal) characterized by or pertaining to a low broad face. See euryprosopic SKULL.

brachygnathia (brak″ig-na′the-ah) [*brachy-* + Gr. *gnathos* jaw +

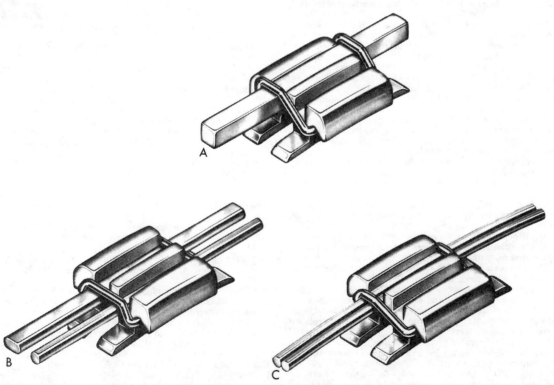

Multiphase bracket. *A,* Edgewise; *B,* universal; *C,* twin-wire. (From T. M. Graber: Orthodontics — Principles and Practice, 3rd ed. Philadelphia, W. B. Saunders Co., 1972; courtesy Unitek Corp.)

-ia] excessive shortness of the mandible. See also MICROGNA-THIA and RETROGNATHIA. Cf. PROGNATHISM.

brachygnathous (brak-kig'nah-thus) pertaining to or characterized by brachygnathia.

brachymetacarpalia (brak"e-met"ah-kar-pal'e-ah) [*brachy-* + *metacarpus* + *-ia*] abnormal shortness of the metacarpal bones.

cryptodontic b., a syndrome characterized by shortened metacarpals and metatarsals, short terminal thumbs, short straight clavicle, and multiple impacted teeth; it is transmitted as an autosomal dominant trait.

brachymorphic (brak"e-mor'fik) [*brachy-* + Gr. *morphē* form] a body build that is broad and stocky relative to stature. Called also *brachytypical* and *brevilineal*.

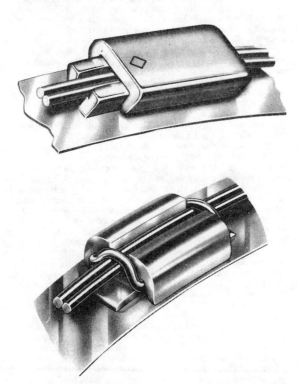

Twin-wire brackets. (From T. M. Graber: Orthodontics — Principles and Practice. 3rd ed. Philadelphia, W. B. Saunders Co., 1972; courtesy Unitek Corp.)

brachystaphyline (brak"e-staf'ĭ-lin) [*brachy-* + Gr. *staphylē* a bunch of grapes, uvula] pertaining to or characterized by a short, wide palate. See brachystaphyline SKULL.

brachytherapy (brak"e-ther'ah-pe) in radiotherapy, treatment with ionizing radiation whose source is applied to the surface of the body or is located a short distance from the body area being treated.

brachytypical (brak"e-tip'ĕ-k'l) brachymorphic.

bracing (brās'ing) 1. holding parts together or in place. 2. making something rigid or steady. 3. resistance to horizontal components of masticatory force.

bracket (brak'it) 1. a support, as of metal, wood, or any other material, projecting from the main structure to support something. 2. orthodontic b. **Bowles b.**, multiphase b. **edgewise b.**, one designed to accept a rectangular arch wire edgewise in an orthodontic appliance. Called also *edgewise attachment*. See illustration. See also edgewise APPLIANCE. **multiphase b.**, a bracket used with edgewise, universal, and twin-wire arch wires. Called also *Bowles b., Bowles attachment*, and *Bowles multiphase attachment*. See illustration. See also multiphase APPLIANCE. **orthodontic b.**, a small metal attachment soldered or welded to an orthodontic band or cemented directly to the teeth, serving to fasten the arch wire to the band or tooth. Called also *orthodontic attachment*. See also orthodontic APPLIANCE. **ribbon arch b.**, a bracket designed to accept a flattened wire in an orthodontic appliance. Called also *ribbon arch attachment*. See illustration. See also ribbon arch APPLIANCE. **twin-wire b.**, a bracket holding two fine-gauge arch wires in an orthodontic appliance. Called also *twin wire attachment*. See illustration. See also twin wire APPLIANCE. **universal b.**, a bracket for both the rectangular and flattened wire in an orthodontic appliance. Called also *universal orthodontic attachment*. See illustration. See also universal APPLIANCE.

Brackett's probe [Charles A. *Brackett*, American dentist, 1850–1927] see under PROBE.

brady- [Gr. *bradys* slow] a combining form meaning slow.

bradycardia (brad"e-kar'de-ah) [*brady-* + Gr. *kardia* heart] slowness of heart beat, as evidenced by a pulse rate of less than 60 beats per minute.

bradyglossia (brad"e-glos'e-ah) [Gr. *bradyglōssos* slow of speech] a speech disorder characterized by slowness of utterance; bradylalia.

bradykinesia (brad"e-kĭ-ne'se-ah) [*brady-* + Gr. *kinēsis* movement] abnormal slowness of movement; sluggishness of physical and mental responses.

bradykinin (brad"e-ki'nin) [*brady-* + Gr. *kinein* to move] a plasma kinin, which is a nonapeptide having the following amino acid sequence: Arg-Pro-Pro-Gly-Phe-Ser-Pro-Phe-Arg. It is formed by plasma kallikreins from plasma γ_2-globulin. Pharma-

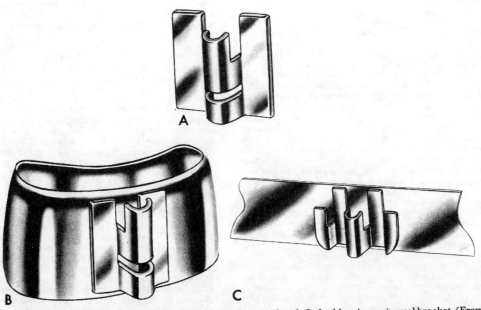

Universal bracket: *A*, ready to weld on band; *B*, welded to preformed incisor band; *C*, double-wing universal bracket. (From T. M. Graber: Orthodontics — Principles and Practice. Philadelphia, W. B. Saunders Co., 1972; courtesy Rocky Mountain Dental Products Co.)

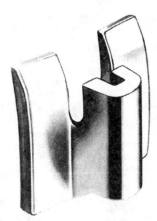

Modified ribbon arch bracket used in the light wire technique. (From P. R. Begg and P. G. Kesling: Begg Orthodontic Theory and Technique. 3rd ed. Philadelphia, W. B. Saunders Co., 1977.)

cologically, it causes vasodilation, increases capillary permeability, produces edema, evokes pain, and contracts and relaxes various extravascular smooth muscles. See also plasma KININ.

bradylalia (brad″e-la′le-ah) [*brady-* + Gr. *lalein* to talk] abnormally slow utterance of words; bradyglossia.

bradyphagia (brad″e-fa′je-ah) [*brady-* + Gr. *phagein* to eat] abnormal slowness of eating.

bradypnea (brad″e-ne′ah) [*brady-* + Gr. *pnoia* breath] slowness of breathing, as evidence by a respiration rate of less than 17 breaths per minute. See also RESPIRATION.

Brailsford, James Frederick [British physician] see Morquio's DISEASE (Brailsford-Morquio syndrome).

brain (brān) [Anglo-Saxon *braegen*] that part of the central nervous system contained within the cranium. Its largest part, the cerebrum, consists of an outer layer of gray matter, the cortex, and two hemispheres connected by the corpus callosum. The cortex is responsible for intellectual activities and association, interpretation, and integration of body functions. The hemispheres are subdivided into the occipital, parietal, frontal, and temporal lobes. Beneath the cortex, within the cerebral hemispheres, lies the thalamus, which is responsible for relaying sensory reflexes and for integrating sensations. Further below is the hypothalamus, which is responsible for vital metabolic processes and physiological functions, such as body temperature, hunger, thirst, digestion, sexual desire, and the reproductive cycle. Also below the thalamus is the midbrain, which contains a center for visual reflexes. Below the midbrain is the brain stem, connecting the spinal cord to the brain; it consists of the medulla oblongata, pons, and mesencephalon. In the medulla oblongata, the cerebrospinal tracts cross over, resulting in the control of the right side of the body by the left hemisphere and the left side by the right hemisphere. The medulla also contains centers regulating the activities of the cardiovascular and respiratory systems. Attached to the back of the brain stem is the cerebellum, which controls and coordinates the motion of various muscles involved in voluntary movements. The brain is protected by the skull and by three layers of meninges. Between the middle and inner layer is a space filled with cerebrospinal fluid, which acts as a shock absorber. Called also *encephalon.* See also terms beginning CEREBRO- and ENCEPHALO-. **electronic b.,** computer. **mechanical b.,** computer. **olfactory b.,** smell b., rhinencephalon. **b. stem,** brain STEM. **b. sugar,** cerebrose.

branch (branch) a division, or offshoot from a larger structure; a smaller structure given off by a larger one, or into which the larger structure divides. Called also *ramus.* **accessory meningeal b. of middle meningeal artery,** a branch arising from the middle meningeal artery, or directly from the maxillary artery, and entering the middle cranial fossa through the foramen ovale to supply the trigeminal ganglion, walls of the cavernous sinus, and neighboring dura mater. Called also *accessory meningeal artery, ramus meningeus accessorius arteriae meningeae mediae* [NA], and *small meningeal artery.* **alveolar b's, perforating,** alveolar arteries, perforating; see under ARTERY. **alveolar b's of inferior alveolar artery,** branches of the inferior

alveolar artery which enter the interdental and interradicular septa. Called also *perforating b's of inferior alveolar artery.* **alveolar b's of infraorbital artery, anterior superior,** branches which enter the anterior alveolar canals to supply the canine and incisor teeth and the maxillary sinus. **alveolar b's of infraorbital nerve, anterior superior,** large sensory branches of the maxillary division of the trigeminal nerve that originate from the infraorbital nerve in the infraorbital canal, either as a single common nerve or as two or three separate branches, coursing through a canal in the anterior wall of the maxillary sinus, and dividing into branches that supply the incisor and canine teeth. They communicate with the middle superior alveolar branch, and give off branches that pass through a canal in the lateral wall of the inferior meatus to supply the mucous membrane of the anterior part of the meatus and the floor of the nasal cavity, communicating with the nasal branches of the pterygopalatine nerve. Called also *anterior superior dental b's of infraorbital nerve, anterior superior alveolar nerve,* and *rami alveolares superiores anteriores nervi infraorbitalis* [NA]. **alveolar b. of infraorbital nerve, middle superior,** a sensory branch that leaves the infraorbital nerve in the infraorbital sulcus, from where it passes in the infraorbital canal first in the roof of the maxillary sinus and later in its lateral wall to supply the two premolar teeth and surrounding tissues and to join the alveolar plexus. Sometimes, the middle superior alveolar branch is absent and its fibers are incorporated into the anterior or posterior alveolar branches. Called also *middle superior dental b. of infraorbital nerve, middle superior alveolar nerve,* and *ramus alveolaris superior medius nervi infraorbitalis* [NA]. **alveolar b's of maxillary nerve, posterior superior,** two or three sensory branches of the maxillary division of the trigeminal nerve that arise from the maxillary nerve just before it enters the infraorbital groove. After crossing the tuberosity of the maxilla, they give off several twigs supplying the gingivae and mucous membrane of the cheek, and then enter the posterior alveolar canals on the infratemporal surface of the maxilla. In the canals, they give off three twigs which enter the foramina at the apices of each root of the molar teeth, provide branches to the maxillary sinus, and communicate with the middle superior alveolar nerve. Called also *posterior superior dental b's of maxillary nerve, posterior superior alveolar nerve,* and *rami alveolares superiores posteriores nervi maxillaris* [NA]. **anastomosing b's of auriculotemporal nerve with facial nerve,** communicating b's of auriculotemporal nerve with facial nerve. **anastomotic b.,** a branch connecting one nerve to another. Called also *ramus anastomoticus.* See *communicating b.* **anastomotic b's of lingual nerve with hypoglossal nerve,** communicating b's of lingual nerve with hypoglossal nerve. **anastomotic b. of middle meningeal artery with lacrimal artery,** a branch of the middle meningeal artery that is distributed to the orbit and anastomoses with the recurrent meningeal branch of the lacrimal artery. Called also *ramus anastomoticus arteriae meningeae mediae cum arteria lacrimali* [NA]. **anastomotic b. of otic ganglion with auriculotemporal nerve,** communicating b. of otic ganglion with auriculotemporal nerve. **anastomotic b. of otic ganglion with chorda tympani,** communicating b. of otic ganglion with chorda tympani. **anterior b. of great auricular nerve,** a general sensory branch that innervates the skin of the face over the parotid gland. Called also *ramus anterior nervi auricularis magni* [NA]. **anterior b. of superior thyroid artery,** a small branch that supplies the upper portion of the thyroid gland and joins its fellow of the opposite side along the upper border of the isthmus. Called also *ramus anterior arteriae thyroideae superioris* [NA]. **anterior auricular b's of superficial temporal artery,** branches that supply the lateral aspect of the pinna and the external acoustic meatus. Called also *rami auriculares anteriores arteriae temporalis superficialis* [NA]. **anterior meningeal b. of internal carotid artery,** meningeal artery, anterior; see under ARTERY. **articular b's of auriculotemporal nerve,** one or two sensory branches of the auriculotemporal nerve that supply the posterior part of the temporomandibular joint. **ascending b's of pterygopalatine ganglion,** orbital b's of pterygopalatine ganglion. **auricular b. of occipital artery,** an inconstant branch that helps supply the concha but, occasionally, gives rise to a secondary branch that supplies the dura mater, the diploë, and the mastoid cells. This secondary branch, when arising directly from the occipital artery, is known as the *mastoid branch.* Called also *ramus auricularis arteriae occipitalis* [NA]. **auricular b. of posterior auricular artery,** a branch that supplies the pinna and adjacent skin. Called also *ramus auricularis arteriae auricularis posterioris* [NA]. **auricular b. of vagus nerve,** a general sensory branch of the superior ganglion of the vagus nerve, one of its branches joining the posterior auricular nerve, and the other innervating the skin of the back of the auricle and posterior part of the external acoustic meatus. Called also *Arnold's nerve* and *ramus auricularis nervi vagi* [NA]. **buccal b's of facial nerve,** mixed motor and sensory branches distributed in the infraorbital and perioral areas of the face, supplying the lesser and greater zygomatic muscles, levator muscle of the upper lip, buccinator and orbicularis oris muscles, and small muscles of the nose. The superficial branches pass between the skin and the muscles and are reinforced by the infratrochlear and nasociliary branches of the ophthalmic nerve. The deep branches are reinforced by the zygomatic branches of the facial nerve and form an infraorbital plexus with the infraorbital branch of the maxillary nerve. Called also *infraorbital b's of facial nerve* and *rami buccales nervi facialis* [NA]. **caroticotympanic b. of internal carotid artery,** a small branch that supplies the tympanic cavity, entering it through a foramen in the carotid canal, and anastomoses with the anterior tympanic branch of the maxillary artery, and with the stylomastoid artery. Called also *tympanic b. of internal carotid artery, caroticotympanic artery,* and *ramus caroticotympanicus arteriae carotidis internae.* **cavernous b's of internal carotid artery,** small branches supplying the hypophysis, the trigeminal ganglion, and the walls of the cavernous and inferior petrosal sinuses. **cervical b. of facial nerve,** a motor branch that lies deep to and innervates the platysma, communicating with the mental branch of the inferior alveolar nerve. Called also *ramus colli nervi facialis* [NA]. **communicating b.,** a branch that communicates between two nerves or between two arteries. Called also *ramus communicans* [NA]. **communicating b's, gray,** grayish branches made up of predominantly unmyelinated fibers, which run from the sympathetic ganglia as visceral efferent fibers to supply the smooth muscles, blood vessels, and sweat glands. Called also *gray rami communicantes* and *postganglionic rami.* **communicating b's, white,** small whitish branches made up of predominantly myelinated fibers; they derive from the cell bodies in the lateral column of the gray matter of the spinal cord and emerge from the cord with the spinal nerves of the first twelve thoracic and two lumbar segments of the spinal cord. They contain primarily preganglionic fibers and thus are roots of the sympathetic ganglia. Called also *white b's, preganglionic rami, rami communicantes albae,* and *white rami communicantes.* **communicating b's of auriculotemporal nerve with facial nerve,** usually two branches containing sensory fibers from the auriculotemporal nerve which join, in the substance of the parotid gland, with sensory fibers of the zygomatic, buccal, and mandibular branches of the facial nerve, supplying the skin in the adjacent areas. Called also *anastomosing b's of auriculotemporal nerve with facial nerve, rami anastomotici nervi auriculotemporalis cum nervo faciali,* and *rami communicantes nervi auriculotemporalis cum nervo faciali* [NA]. **communicating b. of ciliary ganglion with nasociliary nerve,** a branch that connects the nasociliary nerve with the ciliary ganglion, consisting of sensory fibers that pass through the ganglion without synapses, and providing innervation to the cornea, iris, ciliary body, and choroid. It sometimes merges with filaments from the cavernous plexus of the sympathetic nerve, or from the anterior branch of the oculomotor nerve. Called also *long root of ciliary ganglion, radix longa ganglii ciliaris, ramus communicans ganglii ciliaris cum nervo nasociliari* [NA], and *ramus communicans ganglion ciliare.* **communicating b. of facial nerve with glossopharyngeal nerve,** a branch that interconnects the glossopharyngeal nerve with the facial nerve after emergence of the latter from the stylomastoid foramen. Called also *ramus anastomoticus nervi facialis cum nervo glossopharyngeo* and *ramus communicans nervi facialis cum nervo glossopharyngeo* [NA]. **communicating b. of facial nerve with tympanic plexus,** a branch that interconnects the facial nerve and the tympanic plexus of the glossopharyngeal nerve. Called also *ramus anastomoticus nervi facialis cum plexu tympanico* and *ramus communicans nervi facialis cum plexu tympanico* [NA]. **communicating b. of glossopharyngeal nerve with auricular branch of vagus nerve,** a small branch connecting the glossopharyngeal nerve with the auricular branch of the vagus nerve. Called also *ramus anastomoticus nervi glossopharyngei cum ramo auriculari nervi vagi* and *ramus communicans nervi glossopharyngei cum ramo auriculari nervi vagi* [NA]. **communicating b. of inferior laryngeal nerve with internal laryngeal branch,** a small branch interconnecting the inferior laryngeal nerve with the internal branch of the superior laryngeal nerve, behind or in the posterior cricoarytenoid muscle. Called also *ramus communicans nervi laryngei inferioris cum ramo laryngeo interno* [NA] and *ramus communicans nervi laryngei recurrentis cum ramo laryngeo interno.* **communicating b. of lacrimal nerve with zygomatic nerve,** a branch that carries parasympathetic postganglionic fibers origi-

nating in the pterygopalatine ganglion to the lacrimal gland. Called also *ramus anastomoticus nervi lacrimalis cum nervo zygomatico* and *ramus communicans nervi lacrimalis cum nervo zygomatico* [NA]. **communicating b. of lingual nerve with chorda tympani,** the chorda tympani as it joins the lingual nerve in the infratemporal fossa medial to the lateral pterygoid muscle, carrying parasympathetic and special sensory fibers. Called also *ramus communicans nervi lingualis cum chorda tympani* [NA]. **communicating b's of lingual nerve with hypoglossal nerve,** terminal branches forming a plexus at the anterior margin of the hypoglossal muscle; they interconnect the lingual and hypoglossal nerves. Called also *anastomotic b's of lingual nerve with hypoglossal nerve, rami anastomotici nervi lingualis cum nervo hypoglosso,* and *rami communicantes nervi lingualis cum nervo hypoglosso* [NA]. **communicating b. of nasociliary ganglion with nasociliary nerve,** a branch or branches carrying sensory fibers from the cornea, iris, ciliary body, and choroid, and passing through the ciliary ganglion to the nasociliary nerve. Called also *radix longa ganglii ciliaris* and *ramus communicans nervi nasociliaris cum ganglione ciliari* [NA]. **communicating b. of otic ganglion with auriculotemporal nerve,** a branch that carries postganglionic parasympathetic fibers from the otic ganglion to the auriculotemporal nerve for distribution to the parotid gland as secretory motor innervation. Called also *anastomotic b. of otic ganglion with auriculotemporal nerve, ramus anastomoticus ganglii otici cum nervo auriculotemporali,* and *ramus communicans ganglii otici cum nervo auriculotemporalis* [NA]. **communicating b. of otic ganglion with chorda tympani,** a small branch that interconnects the otic ganglion and the chorda tympani. Called also *anastomotic b. of otic ganglion with chorda tympani, ramus anastomoticus ganglii otici cum chorda tympani,* and *ramus communicans ganglii otici cum chorda tympani* [NA]. **communicating b. of otic ganglion with meningeal branch of mandibular nerve,** a branch that carries autonomic fibers destined for the meninges from the otic ganglion to the meningeal branch of the mandibular nerve. Called also *ramus anastomoticus ganglii otici cum ramo meningeo nervi mandibularis* and *ramus communicans ganglii otici cum ramo meningeo nervi mandibularis* [NA]. **communicating b's of spinal nerves,** branches connecting spinal nerves with sympathetic ganglia, each spinal nerve receiving a gray communicating ramus, and the thoracic and upper lumbar spinal nerves having in addition a white communicating ramus. Called also *rami communicantes nervorum spinalium* [NA]. **communicating b's of submandibular ganglion with lingual nerve,** two or more short nerves which interconnect the lingual nerve and the submandibular ganglion, and by which the ganglion is suspended from the nerve. The proximal nerves carry the preganglionic parasympathetic fibers from the ganglion to the chorda tympani, and the distal ones contain the postganglionic fibers which supply the sublingual gland. Called also *communicating b's of submaxillary ganglion with lingual nerve, motor roots of submandibular ganglion, rami communicantes ganglii submandibularis cum nervo linguali* [NA], and *rami communicantes ganglii submaxillaris cum nervo linguali.* **communicating b's of submaxillary ganglion with lingual nerve,** communicating b's of submandibular ganglion with lingual nerve. **communicating b. of superior laryngeal nerve with inferior laryngeal nerve,** a small branch interconnecting the internal branch of the superior laryngeal nerve with the inferior laryngeal nerve, behind or in the posterior cricoarytenoid muscle. Called also *ramus anastomoticus nervi laryngei superioris cum nervo laryngeo inferiore* and *ramus communicans nervi laryngei superioris cum nervo laryngeo inferiore* [NA]. **communicating b. of vagus nerve with glossopharyngeal nerve,** a small branch connecting the auricular branch of the vagus nerve with the glossopharyngeal nerve. Called also *ramus anastomoticus nervi vagi cum nervo glossopharyngeo* and *ramus communicans nervi vagi cum nervo glossopharyngeo* [NA]. **cricothyroid b. of superior thyroid artery,** a small artery which runs medially across the cricothyroid muscle and ligament, supplying the cricothyroid muscle and anastomosing with its fellow of the opposite side. Called also *cricothyroid artery, inferior thyroid artery of Cruveilhier,* and *ramus cricothyroideus arteriae thyroideae superioris* [NA]. **dental b's of anterior superior alveolar arteries,** branches that supply the incisor and canine teeth. Called also *rami dentales arteriarum alveolarium superiorum anteriorum* [NA]. **dental b's of inferior alveolar artery,** vessels arising from the inferior alveolar artery; they enter the root canals through the apical foramina and supply the dental pulp. Called also *rami dentales arteriae alveolaris inferioris* [NA]. **dental b's of inferior dental plexus, inferior,** sensory branches from the inferior alveolar nerve; they form a plexus within the bone of the mandible, sending filaments through the apical foramen to supply the pulp of the molar and premolar teeth. Called also *rami dentales inferiores plexus dentalis inferioris* [NA]. **dental b's of infraorbital nerve, anterior superior,** alveolar b's of infraorbital nerve, anterior superior. **dental b. of infraorbital nerve, middle superior,** alveolar b. of infraorbital nerve, middle superior. **dental b's of maxillary nerve, posterior superior,** alveolar b's of maxillary nerve, posterior superior. **dental b's of posterior superior alveolar artery,** branches that supply the molar and premolar teeth. Called also *rami dentales arteriae alveolaris superioris posterioris* [NA]. **dental b's of superior dental plexus, superior,** general sensory branches that innervate the maxillary teeth. Called also *rami dentales superiores plexus dentalis superioris* [NA]. **descending b. of occipital artery,** the largest branch of the occipital artery; it arises on the obliquus capitis superior muscle and divides into superficial and deep branches, supplying the trapezius and deep neck muscles. The superficial branch anastomoses with the ascending branch of the transverse cervical artery and the deep branch with the vertebral and deep cervical arteries. This latter anastomosis assists in establishing collateral circulation after ligation of the common carotid or subclavian artery. Called also *arteria princeps cervicis* and *ramus descendens arteriae occipitalis* [NA]. **descending b. of pterygopalatine ganglion, descending b. of sphenopalatine ganglion,** palatine nerve, greater; see under NERVE. **digastric b. of facial nerve,** a motor branch of the facial nerve; it arises near the stylomastoid foramen and innervates the posterior belly of the digastric muscle. Called also *digastric nerve* and *ramus digastricus nervi facialis* [NA]. **dorsal lingual b's of lingual artery,** two or three small arteries which arise beneath the hyoglossus muscle and ascend to the posterior part of the dorsum of the tongue, and supply the mucous membrane, the glossopalatine arch, tonsil, soft palate, and epiglottis, and anastomose with their fellows of the opposite side. Called also *arteriae dorsales linguae, dorsal lingual arteries,* and *rami dorsales linguae arteriae lingualis* [NA]. **dural b. of maxillary nerve,** meningeal nerve, middle; see under NERVE. **dural b. of occipital artery,** meningeal b. of occipital artery. **esophageal b's of inferior thyroid artery,** branches that supply the esophagus. Called also *rami esophagei arteriae thyroideae inferioris* [NA]. **ethmoidal b's of nasociliary nerve, anterior,** ethmoidal nerves, anterior; see under NERVE. **external b. of accessory nerve,** a branch of the accessory nerve that arises from the motor cells of the gray matter of the cervical spinal cord as the spinal roots of the accessory nerve, whose fibers run upward along the cord, enter the cranial cavity through the foramen magnum, and unite to form the external branch of the accessory nerve. It enters the jugular foramen where its nerves join those of the internal branch, thus forming the accessory nerve. Upon leaving the foramen, the external branch separates again and runs to the sternocleidomastoid and trapezius muscles, which it innervates. Called also *ramus externus nervi accessorii* [NA]. **external nasal b. of nasociliary nerve,** the nerve that emerges between the nasal bone and the lateral nasal cartilage to supply the skin of the ala and apex of the nose. **external b. of superior laryngeal nerve,** the smaller of the two branches of the superior laryngeal nerve, passing beneath the sternothyroid muscle, supplying motor innervation to the cricothyroid muscle and inferior pharyngeal constrictor. Called also *ramus externus nervi laryngei superioris* [NA]. **facial b's of infraorbital artery,** branches which descend through the infraorbital foramen. They supply the lacrimal gland, anastomosing with the angular artery; supply the nose, anastomosing with the dorsal branch of the ophthalmic artery; and pass between the levatores labii superioris muscles, anastomosing with the facial, transverse facial, and buccal arteries. **b. to frontal sinus from supratrochlear nerve,** a small branch piercing the bone in the supraorbital notch to supply the mucous membrane of the frontal sinus. **frontal b. of superficial temporal artery,** a tortuous terminal branch that supplies the forehead and frontal scalp. Called also *ramus frontalis arteriae temporalis superficialis* [NA]. **frontal b. of supraorbital nerve, medial b. of** supraorbital nerve. **ganglionic b's of internal carotid artery,** branches that supply the trigeminal ganglion. **gingival b. of greater palatine artery,** a vessel that supplies the lingual surface of the superior alveolar process of the gingiva and

anastomoses with the gingival branches of the perforating branch of the superior alveolar artery. **gingival b's of inferior dental plexus inferior,** general sensory branches from the inferior dental plexus that innervate the gingivae of the mandible. Called also *rami gingivales inferiores plexus dentalis inferioris* [NA]. **gingival b. of posterior superior alveolar artery,** a terminal branch which passes along the outer surface of the maxillary bone to supply the mucous membrane on the outer surface of the alveolar process of the gingiva in the premolar and molar region. **gingival b's of superior dental plexus, superior,** general sensory branches from the superior dental plexus that innervate the gingivae of the maxilla. Called also *rami gingivales superiores plexus dentalis superioris* [NA]. **glandular b's of facial artery, glandular b's of external maxillary artery,** three or four large branches of the facial artery as it passes over the lateral surface of the submandibular gland, some supplying the gland, others continuing to the lymph nodes, integument, and neighboring muscles. Called also *submaxillary b's of facial artery, rami glandulares arteriae facialis* [NA], and *rami glandulares arteriae maxillaris externae.* **glandular b's of submandibular ganglion,** short branches running from the submandibular ganglion to innervate the submandibular gland, bearing postganglionic parasympathetic (secretory) fibers from this ganglion and sympathetic fibers that are postganglionic from the superior cervical ganglion. Called also *rami glandulares ganglii submandibularis* [NA], *rami submaxillares ganglii submaxillaris,* and *submaxillary nerves.* **b. of glossopharyngeal nerve to carotid sinus,** a branch that arises from the glossopharyngeal nerve just as it emerges from the jugular foramen and terminates in the wall of the carotid sinus, supplying its pressure receptors with visceral afferent fibers. It communicates with the nodose ganglion or the pharyngeal branch of the vagus nerve. Called also *carotid sinus nerve, Hering's nerve, ramus sinus carotici nervi glossopharyngei* [NA], and *sinus nerve.* **gray communicating b's,** communicating b's, gray. **hyoid b. of lingual artery,** suprahyoid b. of lingual artery. **hyoid b. of superior thyroid artery,** infrahyoid b. of superior thyroid artery. **hypophyseal b's of internal carotid artery,** one or two minute branches that supply the hypophysis. **incisive b. of inferior alveolar nerve,** a terminal branch that continues anteriorly within the mandible and forms a plexus which supplies the canine and incisor teeth. **incisor b. of inferior alveolar artery,** the smaller of the two terminal branches of the inferior alveolar artery, which continues the course of the inferior alveolar artery beyond the mental foramen, running to the incisor teeth and anastomosing with its fellow of the opposite side. **infrahyoid b. of superior thyroid artery,** an artery running along the inferior border of the hyoid bone, into the thyrohyoideus muscle, supplying the infrahyoid region, and anastomosing with its fellow of the opposite side. Called also *hyoid b. of superior thyroid artery, ramus hyoideus arteriae thyroideae superioris,* and *ramus infrahyoideus arteriae thyroideae superioris* [NA]. **infraorbital b's of facial nerve,** buccal b's of facial nerve. **interdental b's,** interradicular arteries; see under ARTERY. **interganglionic b's,** the branches that interconnect the ganglia in the chain of the sympathetic trunk. Called also *rami interganglionares* [NA]. **internal b. of accessory nerve,** a branch of the accessory nerve that arises from the side of the medulla oblongata by four or five rootlets, from which it runs to the jugular foramen, interchanging filaments with or joining the external branch. It leaves the foramen separated from the external branch, carrying motor fibers to be distributed by branches of the vagus to the soft palate, pharyngeal constrictors, larynx, and esophagus. Called also *cranial part of accessory nerve* and *ramus internus nervi accessorii* [NA]. **internal nasal b's of nasociliary nerve,** fibers that supply the anterior part of the nasal septum and lateral wall of the nasal cavity. **internal b. of superior laryngeal nerve,** the larger of the two branches of the superior laryngeal nerve. It passes anteriorly and sends fibers to the epiglottis, base of the tongue, aryepiglottic fold, and larynx, supplying general sensory innervation to the mucous membrane and parasympathetic secretory motor innervation to the glands. Called also *ramus internus nervi laryngei superioris* [NA]. **interradicular b's,** interradicular arteries; see under ARTERY. **labial b's of infraorbital nerve, superior,** sensory branches that supply the skin of the upper lip, oral mucosa, and the labial glands, communicating with the branches of the facial nerve and jointly forming the infraorbital plexus. Called also *rami labiales superiores nervi infraorbitalis* [NA]. **laryngopharyngeal b's of superior cervical ganglion,** four to six sympathetic branches of the superior cervical ganglion that communicate with the glossopharyngeal branches of the glossopharyngeal and vagus nerves and form the pharyngeal plexus, innervating the larynx and pharynx. Called also *pharyngeal b's of superior cervical ganglion* and *rami laryngopharyngei ganglii cervicalis superioris* [NA]. **lateral b. of supraorbital nerve,** a sensory branch that supplies the frontal sinus, upper eyelid, and skin and subcutaneous tissue of the forehead and scalp laterally as far as the lambdoid suture. Called also *ramus lateralis nervi supraorbitalis* [NA]. **lingual b. of facial nerve,** an inconstant motor branch of the facial nerve, sometimes arising together with the stylohyoid branch, and helping to supply the styloglossal and glossopalatine muscles. Called also *ramus lingualis nervi facialis* [NA]. **lingual b's of glossopharyngeal nerve,** two general and special sensory branches of the glossopharyngeal nerve that innervate the tongue. One supplies the afferent sensory innervation for taste to the vallate papillae and general afferent fibers to the mucous membrane at the base of the tongue, the other innervates the mucous membrane of the posterior third of the tongue. It communicates with the lingual nerve. Called also *rami linguales nervi glossopharyngei* [NA]. **lingual b's of hypoglossal nerve,** motor branches of the hypoglossal nerve that supply both the intrinsic and extrinsic muscles of the tongue. Called also *rami linguales nervi hypoglossi* [NA]. **lingual b. of inferior alveolar artery,** a small artery that may arise from the inferior alveolar artery near its origin and descend with the lingual nerve to supply the mucous membrane of the mouth. **lingual b's of lingual nerve,** sensory branches of the lingual nerve that supply the anterior two-thirds of the tongue, adjacent areas of the mouth, and the gingivae. Called also *rami linguales nervi lingualis* [NA]. **b's from lingual nerve to isthmus of fauces,** general sensory branches from the lingual nerve that innervate the isthmus of the fauces. Called also *rami isthmi faucium nervi lingualis* [NA]. **malar b's of facial nerve,** zygomatic b's of facial nerve. **malar b. of zygomatic nerve,** zygomaticofacial b. of zygomatic nerve. **marginal mandibular b. of facial nerve,** a motor branch that passes forward from the front of the parotid gland along the border of the mandible, deep to the platysma and depressor anguli oris muscles, supplying the depressor anguli oris, risorius, depressor labii inferioris, and mentalis muscles, and communicating with the mental branch of the inferior alveolar nerve. Called also *ramus marginalis mandibulae nervi facialis* [NA]. **mastoid b. of occipital artery,** an inconstant branch that usually arises from the occipital artery and enters the cranial cavity through the mastoid foramen and supplies the dura mater, diploë, and mastoid cells. It may also originate from the auricular branch. Called also *ramus mastoideus arteriae occipitalis* [NA]. **mastoid b's of posterior auricular artery,** branches of the posterior auricular artery that supply the mastoid cells. Called also *rami mastoidei arteriae auricularis posterioris* [NA]. **medial b. of supraorbital nerve,** a small sensory branch that supplies the frontal sinus, upper eyelid, and skin and subcutaneous tissue of the forehead and scalp as far back as the parietal bone. Called also *frontal b. of supraorbital nerve* and *ramus medialis nervi supraorbitalis* [NA]. **meningeal b., anterior, of internal carotid artery,** meningeal artery, anterior; see under ARTERY. **meningeal b's of ascending pharyngeal artery,** small branches which supply the dura mater of the posterior cranial fossa. **meningeal b's of hypoglossal nerve,** filaments originating in the hypoglossal canal that pass back to the dura mater. **meningeal b. of mandibular nerve,** a branch of the mandibular division of the trigeminal nerve that arises from the trunk of the mandibular nerve and re-enters the skull through the foramen spinosum, accompanying the middle meningeal artery. It supplies the dura mater, sends filaments to the mucous membrane of the mastoid cells, and communicates with the meningeal branch of the maxillary nerve. Called also *recurrent b. of mandibular nerve, nervus spinosus,* and *ramus meningeus nervi mandibularis* [NA]. **meningeal b., middle, of maxillary nerve,** meningeal nerve, middle; see under NERVE. **meningeal b. of occipital artery,** one or more variable branches that enter the skull through the jugular foramen and condyloid canal and supply the dura mater. Called also *dural b. of occipital artery* and *ramus meningeus arteriae occipitalis* [NA]. **meningeal b. of vagus nerve,** a fiber from the superior ganglion of the vagus nerve; it supplies the dura mater of the posterior cranial fossa. Called also *ramus meningeus nervi vagi* [NA]. **mental b. of inferior alveolar artery,** mental ARTERY. **mental b's of mental nerve,** general sensory branches that supply the skin of the chin. Called also *rami mentales nervi mentalis* [NA]. **middle meningeal b. of maxillary nerve,** meningeal nerve, middle; see under NERVE. **muscular b's,** branches of peripheral nerves or vessels that supply muscle. Called also *rami musculares* [NA]. **muscular b's of hypoglossal nerve,** branches that supply the styloglossal, hyoglossal, genioglossal, and intrinsic muscles of the tongue. **muscular b's of inferior thyroid artery,** branches that supply the infrahyoid, longus colli, scalenus anterior, and constrictor pharyngis muscles. **muscular b's of occipital artery,**

branches which supply the digastricus, stylohyoideus, splenius, and longissimus capitis muscles. **muscular b's of ophthalmic artery,** branches that supply muscles of the upper eyelids and the eyes. **mylohyoid b. of inferior alveolar artery,** a branch of the mandibular segment of the maxillary artery; it branches off just before the artery enters the mandibular canal, following the mylohyoid nerve, to supply the mylohyoid muscle, where it anastomoses with branches of the submental artery. Called also *mylohyoid artery* and *ramus mylohyoideus arteriae alveolaris inferioris* [NA]. **nasal b's of anterior ethmoidal nerve,** the internal and external nasal branches of the anterior ethmoidal nerve, and their subdivisions. Called also *rami nasales anteriores nervi ethmoidalis anterioris* and *rami nasales nervi ethmoidalis anterioris* [NA]. **nasal b. of anterior ethmoidal nerve, external,** a general sensory branch, being a continuation of the anterior ethmoidal nerve, which supplies the skin of the dorsal part of the nose. Called also *ramus nasalis externus nervi ethmoidalis anterioris* [NA]. **nasal b's of anterior ethmoidal nerve, internal,** general sensory fibers that innervate the nasal septum and the mucosa of the lateral wall of the nasal cavity through the medial and lateral branches of the anterior ethmoidal nerve. Called also *rami nasales interni nervi ethmoidalis anterioris* [NA]. **nasal b's of anterior ethmoidal nerve, lateral,** general sensory branches from the internal nasal branches of the anterior ethmoidal nerve that supply the mucosa of the lateral wall of the nasal cavity. Called also *rami nasales laterales nervi ethmoidalis anterioris* [NA] **nasal b's of anterior ethmoidal nerve, medial,** general sensory branches from the internal nasal branches of the anterior ethmoidal nerve that innervate the nasal septum. Called also *rami nasales mediale nervi ethmoidalis anterioris* [NA] **nasal b. of facial artery, lateral,** a branch which supplies the ala and dorsum of the nose, anastomosing with its fellow of the opposite side, with the septal and alar branches, with the dorsal nasal branch of the ophthalmic artery, and with the infraorbital branch of the maxillary artery. **nasal b's of infraorbital nerve, external,** sensory branches that supply the skin of the side of the nose and the mobile septum of the nose, and join with branches of the nasociliary nerve. Called also *rami nasales externi nervi infraorbitalis* [NA]. **nasal b's of infraorbital nerve, internal,** general sensory branches that innervate the mobile septum of the nose. Called also *rami nasales interni nervi infraorbitalis* [NA]. **nasal b. of nasociliary nerve, external,** a branch that emerges between the nasal bone and the lateral nasal cartilage to supply the skin of the wing and apex of the nose. **nasal b's of nasociliary nerve, internal,** fibers that supply the anterior part of the nasal septum and lateral wall of the nasal cavity. **nasal b's, posterior lateral, of sphenopalatine artery,** nasal arteries, posterior lateral; see under ARTERY. **nasal b's of pterygopalatine ganglion, inferior [lateral] posterior,** sensory branches of the greater palatine nerve that supply the inferior concha and middle and inferior meatuses. Called also *rami nasales posteriores inferiores [laterales] ganglii pterygopalatini* [NA] and *rami nasales posteriores inferiors [laterales] ganglii sphenopalatini.* **nasal b's of pterygopalatine ganglion, superior [lateral] posterior,** sensory branches that supply the superior and middle nasal conchae and the posterior ethmoidal sinuses. Called also *rami nasales posteriores superiores [laterales] ganglii pterygopalatini* [NA] and *rami nasales posteriores superiores [laterales] ganglii sphenopalatini.* **nasal b's of pterygopalatine ganglion, superior [medial] posterior,** sensory branches that usually derive from the nasopalatine nerve, and supply the nasal septum. Called also *rami nasales posterior superiores mediales ganglii pterygopalatini* [NA] and *rami nasales posteriores superiores mediales ganglii sphenopalatini.* **nasopalatine b. of greater palatine artery,** the terminal branch of the greater palatine artery that ascends through the incisive canal and enters the nasal cavity, where it anastomoses with the septal branches of the sphenopalatine artery. **nasopalatine b. of posterior septal artery,** a branch of the posterior septal artery that passes through the incisive canal to anastomose with the nasopalatine branch of the greater palatine artery. **occipital b's of occipital artery,** medial and lateral branches of the occipital artery distributed to the scalp and, through the meningeal branch, to the dura mater. Called also *rami occipitales arteriae occipitalis* [NA]. **occipital b. of posterior auricular artery,** a branch that supplies the occipitalis muscle and the scalp, anastomosing with the occipital artery. Called also *myomastoid artery* and *ramus occipitalis arteriae auricularis posterioris* [NA]. **occipital b. of posterior auricular nerve,** a motor branch innervating the occipital belly of the occipitofrontal muscle. Called also *ramus occipitalis nervi auricularis posterioris* [NA]. **orbital b. of infraorbital artery,** a branch that arises in the infraorbital canal from the infraorbital artery and supplies some inferior muscles of the eye. **orbital b's of pterygopalatine ganglion,** branches consisting of two or three sensory and parasympathetic filaments that pass from the pterygopalatine ganglion through the orbital fissure to supply the orbital periosteum and the ethmoidal and sphenoidal sinuses. Called also *ascending b's of pterygopalatine ganglion* and *rami orbitales ganglii pterygopalatine* [NA]. **palatine b. of ascending pharyngeal artery,** a variable vessel which runs toward the constrictor pharyngis superior muscle and sends branches to the soft palate, tonsils, and auditory tube. **palpebral b's of infraorbital nerve, inferior,** sensory fibers of the infraorbital nerve that supply the skin and conjunctiva of the lower eyelids and join with the facial and zygomatic nerve. Called also *rami palpebrales inferiores nervi infraorbitalis* [NA]. **palpebral b's of infratrochlear nerve,** general sensory branches that innervate the eyelids. Called also *rami palpebrales nervi infratrochlearis* [NA]. **parietal b. of superficial temporal artery,** the posterior terminal branch, supplying the scalp and the parietal region. Called also *ramus parietalis arteriae temporalis superficialis* [NA]. **parotid b's of auriculotemporal nerve,** branches that communicate between the auriculotemporal nerve and the otic ganglion, and carry parasympathetic postganglionic fibers to the parotid gland. Called also *parotid nerve* and *rami parotidei nervi auriculotemporalis* [NA]. **parotid b's of facial vein,** small veins from the parotid gland which follow the parotid duct and open into the facial vein. Called also *anterior parotid veins, rami parotidei venae facialis* [NA], and *venae parotideae anteriores*. **parotid b's of superficial temporal artery,** branches that supply the parotid gland and the temporomandibular joint. Called also *rami parotidei arteriae temporalis superficialis* [NA]. **perforating alveolar b's,** alveolar arteries, perforating; see under ARTERY. **perforating b's of inferior alveolar artery,** alveolar b's of inferior alveolar artery. **petrosal b. of middle meningeal artery,** a branch arising in the region of the petrous part of the temporal bone, entering the hiatus for the greater petrosal nerve and anastomosing with the stylomastoid artery. Called also *ramus petrosus arteriae meningeae mediae* [NA] and *ramus petrosus superficialis arteriae meningeae mediae*. **pharyngeal b's of ascending pharyngeal artery,** three to four irregular vessels which descend from the ascending pharyngeal artery to supply the constrictor pharyngis medius and stylopharyngeus muscles. Called also *rami pharyngei arteriae pharyngeae ascendentis* [NA]. **pharyngeal b's of glossopharyngeal nerve,** three to four sensory branches which, together with the pharyngeal branches of the vagus nerve, form the pharyngeal plexus, which gives off branches innervating the mucous membrane of the oropharynx. Called also *rami pharyngei nervi glossopharyngei* [NA]. **pharyngeal b. of maxillary artery,** a small branch of the pterygopalatine portion of the maxillary artery; it passes posteriorly in the pharyngeal canal and supplies the auditory tube, upper part of the pharynx, and sphenoidal sinus. **pharyngeal b. of pterygopalatine ganglion,** a branch from the posterior part of the pterygopalatine ganglion, passing through the pharyngeal canal with the pharyngeal branch of the maxillary artery, to the mucous membrane of the nasal nasopharynx posterior to the auditory tube. Called also *Bock's nerve* and *ramus pharyngeus ganglii pterygopalatini* [NA]. **pharyngeal b's of vagus nerve,** usually two mixed branches containing sensory and motor fibers. They divide into several bundles that join branches of the glossopharyngeal, sympathetic, and external branch of the superior laryngeal nerve to form the pharyngeal plexus which, in turn, provides sensory innervation to the mucous membrane of the pharynx and motor innervation to muscles of the soft palate, except the tensor veli palatini muscle. Called also *rami pharyngei nervi vagi* [NA]. **posterior b. of great auricular nerve,** a general sensory branch that innervates the skin over the mastoid process and the back of the external ear. Called also *ramus posterior nervi auricularis magni* [NA]. **posterior b. of superior thyroid artery,** an artery that supplies the posterior part of the thyroid gland. Called also *ramus posterior arteriae thyroideae superioris* [NA]. **posterior lateral b's of sphenopalatine artery,** nasal arteries, posterior lateral; see under ARTERY. **prevertebral b's of ascending pharyngeal artery,** vessels which supply the longus capitis and colli muscles, sympathetic trunk, hypoglossal and vagus nerves, and lymph nodes, anastomosing with the ascending cervical artery. **pterygoid b's of maxillary artery,** branches of the pterygoid portion of the maxillary artery, irregular in number and origin depending on the relation of the maxillary artery to the lateral pterygoid muscle; they supply the pterygoid muscles. Called also *pterygoid arteries, rami pterygoidei arteriae maxillaris* [NA], and *rami pterygoidei arteriae maxillaris internae*. **recurrent b. of mandibular nerve,** meningeal b. of mandibular nerve. **sensory b's of tympanic plexus,** sensory fibers of the tympanic plexus; they innervate the mucous membranes of the tympanic cavity, auditory tube, and mastoid air cells, being a continuation of the tympanic nerve. **septal b's, posterior, of sphenopalatine artery,** septal arteries, posterior; see under ARTERY. **sternocleidomastoid b's of occipital artery,** branches, usually an upper and lower branch, which commonly arise from the occipital artery near its origin, but occasionally arise directly from the external carotid artery, and which supply the sternocleidomastoid and neighboring muscles. Called also *rami sternocleidomastoidei arteriae occipitalis* [NA]. **sternocleidomastoid b. of superior thyroid artery,** a branch of the superior thyroid artery that frequently arises directly from the external carotid artery. It runs caudally and laterally across the carotid sheath to supply the middle portion of the sternocleidomastoid and neighboring muscles and integument. Called also *sternomastoid b. of superior thyroid artery, ramus sternocleidomastoideus arteriae thyroideae superioris* [NA], and *superior sternocleidomastoid artery*. **sternomastoid b. of superior thyroid artery,** sternocleidomastoid b. of thyroid artery. **stylohyoid b. of facial nerve,** a motor branch that arises from the facial nerve just below the base of the skull to innervate the stylohyoid muscle. Called also *ramus stylohyoideus nervi facialis* [NA] and *stylohyoid nerve*. **stylopharyngeal b. of glossopharyngeal nerve,** the only motor branch of the glossopharyngeal nerve, which innervates the stylopharyngeal muscle. Called also *ramus musculi stylopharyngei nervi glossopharyngei* [NA], *ramus stylopharyngeus nervi glossopharyngei*, and *stylopharyngeal nerve*. **submaxillary b's of facial artery,** glandular b's of facial artery. **superficial b. of transverse cervical artery,** cervical artery, superficial; see under ARTERY. **b's of superior cervical ganglion,** laryngopharyngeal b's of superior cervical ganglion. **superior b. of oculomotor nerve,** the upper of the two motor branches of the oculomotor nerve; it innervates the superior rectus muscle and the levator palpebrae superioris. Called also *ramus superior nervi oculomotorii* [NA]. **suprahyoid b. of lingual artery,** an artery which passes along the upper border of the hyoid bone, supplying the suprahyoid muscles and anastomosing with its fellow of the opposite side. Called also *hyoid b. of lingual artery, hyoid artery, ramus hyoideus arteriae lingualis*, and *ramus suprahyoideus arteriae lingualis* [NA]. **temporal b's of auriculotemporal nerve, superficial,** sensory branches that accompany the superficial temporal artery and supply the skin of the temporal region of the scalp and communicate with the facial and zygomatic nerves. Called also *rami temporales superficiales nervi auriculotemporalis* [NA]. **temporal b's of facial nerve,** terminal motor branches that innervate the anterior and superior auricular muscles, the frontal belly of the occipitofrontal muscle, and the orbicularis oculi and corrugator muscles. Called also *rami temporales nervi facialis* [NA] and *temporal facial nerve*. **temporal b. of zygomatic nerve,** zygomaticotemporal b. of zygomatic nerve. **tentorial b. of ophthalmic nerve,** a sensory nerve branching off the ophthalmic nerve near its origin in the trigeminal ganglion and passing near the trochlear nerve and between the layers of the tentorium to innervate the dura mater of the tentorium cerebelli and falx cerebri. Called also *nervus tentorii, ramus tentorii nervi ophthalmici* [NA], and *tentorial nerve*. **terminal b's of occipital artery,** branches in the back of the head which supply the occipitalis muscle, pericranium, and integument, anastomosing with their fellows of the opposite side and with the posterior auricular and temporal arteries. **thyrohyoid b. of ansa cervicalis,** a motor branch from the superior root of the ansa cervicalis that innervates the thyrohyoid muscle. Called also *ramus thyreohyoideus nervi hypoglossi, ramus thyreohyoideus ansae cervicalis*, and *ramus thyrohyoideus ansae cervicalis* [NA]. **tonsillar b. of external maxillary artery,** tonsillar b. of facial artery. **tonsillar b. of facial artery,** an artery which ascends from the facial artery on the pharynx, between the pterygoideus medialis and styloglossus muscles, and supplies the palatine tonsil and the root of the tongue. Called also *tonsillar b. of external maxillary artery, ramus tonsillaris arteriae facialis* [NA], *ramus tonsillaris arteriae maxillaris externi*, and *tonsillar artery*. **tonsillar b's of glossopharyngeal nerve,** fibers from the glossopharyngeal nerve that form a network around the palatine tonsils, supplying them and the soft palate and fauces with general sensory innervation and communicating with the lesser palatine nerves. Called also *rami tonsillares nervi glossopharyngei* [NA] and *tonsillar nerves.* **tracheal b's of inferior thyroid artery,** branches that supply the trachea. Called also *rami tracheales arteriae thyroideae inferioris* [NA]. **tympanic b. of internal carotid artery,** caroticotympanic b. of internal carotid artery. **b. to tympanic membrane of auriculotemporal nerve,** a general sensory branch of the auriculotemporal nerve innervating the tympanic membrane. Called also *ramus membranae tympani nervi auriculotemporalis* [NA]. **white b's, white communicating b's,** communicating b's, white. **zygomatic b's of facial nerve,** sensory branches that run across the face in the region of the zygomatic bone and innervate the zygomaticus major and orbicularis oculi muscles, and communicate with branches of the lacrimal nerve and the zygomaticofacial branch of the maxillary nerve. Called also *malar b's of facial nerve* and *rami zygomatici nervi facialis* [NA]. **zygomatic b's of lacrimal artery,** branches of the lacrimal artery which pass through the zygomaticotemporal foramen to anastomose with the deep temporal arteries, and through the zygomaticofacial foramen to anastomose with the transverse facial artery. **zygomaticofacial b. of zygomatic nerve,** a sensory branch that passes along the inferior lateral angle of the orbit and leaves it through the zygomatico-orbital and zygomaticofacial foramina to supply the skin overlying the prominence of the cheek. It joins with the facial nerve and with the inferior palpebral branches of the infraorbital nerve. Called also *malar b. of zygomatic nerve, ramus zygomaticofacialis nervi zygomatici* [NA], and *zygomaticofacial nerve.* **zygomaticotemporal b. of zygomatic nerve,** a sensory branch that passes along the lateral wall of the orbit in the groove of the zygomatic bone and into the temporal fossa through a small foramen or the sphenozygomatic suture. Just above the zygomatic arch it pierces the temporal fascia to supply the skin of the anterior temporal region. It also gives off a branch to the lateral side of the orbit and communicates with the facial nerve and the auricular branch of the mandibular nerve. Called also *temporal b. of zygomatic nerve, ramus zygomaticotemporalis nervi zygomatici* [NA], and *zygomaticotemporal nerve.*

Brandt's syndrome [Thore Edvard *Brandt,* Swedish dermatologist] ACRODERMATITIS enteropathica.

Branhamella (bran″ham-el′ah) [named after Sara *Branham*] a genus of gram-negative bacteria of the family Neisseriaceae, occurring as nonmotile, nonsporogenous, aerobic cocci arranged in pairs with adjacent sides flattened. **B. catarrha′lis,** a species found in the oral cavity, including the lips, tongue, and cheeks, and in plaque and saliva, which may be responsible for mucosal inflammation, alone or in association with other organisms. It is occasionally found in venereal diseases, and is a possible pathogen of meningitis. The organism is susceptible to penicillin, streptomycin, tetracyclines, polymyxin B sulfate, and other antibiotics.

Branson trademark for an *ultrasonic denture cleanser* (see under CLEANSER).

Brassica (bras′ĕ-kah) [L.] a genus of cruciferous plants to which the cabbage, turnip, mustard, and related species belong. See MUSTARD.

breadth (bredth) the distance measured horizontally from side to side; lateral or transverse distance. **bicanine b.,** bicanine WIDTH. **bigonial b.,** b. of mandible. **bimolar b.,** bimolar WIDTH. **bizygomatic b.,** zygomatic b. **cranial b.,** the transverse distance between the two most prominent points on either side of the cranium (on the parietal bone). See also *b. of mandible.* **b. of mandible,** the distance between the right and left gonia. Called also *bigonial b.* **b. of mandible, anterior,** the distance measured along the inner borders of the right and left mental foramina. **b. of mandible, condylar,** the distance from the right to the left condylion laterale. **b. of mandibular ramus,** the smallest breadth of the ascending ramus of the mandible measured at the right angle to its height; also measured parallel to the lower border of the corpus of the mandible. **maxilloalveolar b.,** the transverse linear measurement of the outer surface of the upper alveolar process (excluding exostoses, if present). **midfacial b.,** the distance between the two zygomaxillaria. **b. of palate,** the transverse distance measured at the inner borders of the alveoli of the two upper second deciduous molars, and the two upper first permanent molars. **zygomatic b.,** the distance between the outer surfaces of the two zygomatic arches (zygion-zygion). Called also *bizygomatic b.*

break (brāk) 1. to interrupt the continuity, or an interruption in the continuity of a structure, especially bone. See FRACTURE. 2. the interruption of an electric circuit.

breaker (brāk′er) something that breaks or disrupts regularity, continuity, or arrangement. **stress b.,** stress-breaker.

breath (breth) [L. *spiritus halitus*] the air taken in and expelled from the lungs by expanding and contracting the thorax and diaphragm. See also HALITUS and RESPIRATION. **b. analyzer,** breath ANALYZER. **bad b., foul b.,** halitosis. **labored b.,** dyspnea. **lead b.,** the metallic odor of the breath in lead poisoning. Called also *halitus saturninus.* **liver b.,** FETOR hepaticus. **shortness of b.,** dyspnea.

breathing (brēth′ing) the alternate inspiration and expiration of air into and out of the lungs. See RESPIRATION. **frog b.,** glossopharyngeal b., respiration unaided by the primary or ordinary accessory muscles of respiration, the air being "swallowed" rapidly into the lungs by use of the tongue and muscles of the pharynx; used by patients with chronic muscle paralysis to augment their vital capacity. **intermittent positive pressure b.,** the active inflation of the lungs during inspiration under positive pressure from a cycling valve. Abbreviated *IPPB.* **mouth b.,** the inspiration and expiration of air primarily through the mouth, observed most commonly in obstruction and congestion of nasal passages.

Breen trademark for *polyvinyl chloride* (see under POLYVINYL).

bregma (breg′mah) [L.; Gr.] the point on the outer surface of the skull at the junction of the coronal and sagittal sutures; used as a craniometric landmark. Abbreviated *B* or *Br.* See illustrations at CEPHALOMETRY.

bregmatodymia (breg″mah-to-dim′e-ah) [*bregma* + Gr. *didymos* twin +′ *-ia*] an abnormality characterized by fusion at the bregmas of conjoined twins.

brei (bri) [Gr. "pulp"] tissue that has been ground to a pulp; homogenate.

Bremil trademark for *hydrochlorothiazide.*

bremsstrahlung (brem′strah-lung) [Ger. "braking radiation"] the continuous spectrum of x-ray produced as a result of rapid deceleration of high-speed electrons from the cathode, which penetrate the outer orbits of the tungsten atoms during their impact against the target in an x-ray tube. Called also *braking radiation.* See also heterogeneous RADIATION and white RADIATION.

brephoplastic (bref′o-plas′tik) [Gr. *brephos* embryo + *plassein* to form] formed from embryonic tissue or during embryonic development.

Breschet's sinus, veins [Gilbert *Breschet,* French anatomist, 1784–1845] see sphenoparietal SINUS, and diploic veins, under VEIN.

Brethine trademark for *terbutaline sulfate* (see under TERBUTALINE).

Bretonneau's angina, disease [Pierre *Bretonneau,* French physician, 1778–1862] diphtheria.

Brevais lattice space LATTICE.

brevi- [L. *brevis* short] a combining form meaning short.

Brevibacterium (brev″ĭ-bak-te′re-um) [*brevi-* + *bacterium*] a genus *incertae sedis,* the members of which have been assigned to the family Corynebacteriaceae.

Brevicidin trademark for *tyrocidine hydrochloride* (see under TYROCIDINE).

brevicollis (brev″ĭ-kol′is) [*brevi-* + L. *collum* neck] shortness of the neck. See Klippel-Feil SYNDROME.

brevilineal (brev″ĭ-lin′e-al) brachymorphic.

Brevital trademark for *methohexital sodium* (see under METHOHEXITAL).

brevium (bre′ve-um) prolactinium.

Brewer's operation see under OPERATION.

Bricanyl trademark for *terbutaline sulfate* (see under TERBUTALINE).

bridge (brij) 1. a structure that connects two distant points, including parts of an organ. Called also *pons.* 2. a prosthetic dental appliance which replaces lost teeth, being supported and held in position by attachments to adjacent teeth; the term is usually restricted to fixed nonremovable appliances. See also partial DENTURE. 3. see *intercellular b.* Aderer "C" B., trademark for a hard *dental casting gold alloy* (see under GOLD). **American Gold "B" B.,** see under GOLD. **American Gold "T" B. Hard,** see under GOLD. **Andrews b.,** Andrews BAR. **Bing b.,** an artificial porcelain tooth to which a platinum bar extends from each lateral side, the ends of the bar being anchored in fillings in adjacent natural teeth. Said to be one of the first efforts to insert a single tooth substitute by connecting it to adjoining teeth. **cantilever b.,** a fixed partial denture in which the pontic is cantilevered, being retained only on one side by the abutment tooth. Called also *cantilever fixed partial denture* and *fixed cantilever partial denture.* Sometimes called *extension b.* See illustration. **complex b.,** a bilateral bridge replacing any number of teeth, having more than one functional activity. **compound b.,** a fixed partial denture which incorporates the

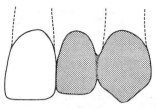

The cantilever bridge. In this design the pontic gains support from the tooth or teeth on one side of the gap only. (From D. H. Roberts: Fixed Bridge Prostheses. Bristol, England, John Wright & Sons Ltd., 1973.)

properties of two or more bridges, such as combining the properties of a fixed bridge with rigid connectors with those of a cantilever bridge or of a fixed bridge with rigid connectors with those of a fixed bridge with rigid and nonrigid connectors, thereby one end of the restoration uses retention of one type and the other of a different type. See illustration. **cross b.,** a projection extending from the myosin (thick) filament toward the actin (thin) filament in the sarcomere. See also muscle CONTRACTION and ratchet THEORY. **dental b.,** bridge (2). **dentin b.,** a scarlike deposit of reparative dentin or other calcific substance which reseals an exposed pulp or which forms across the excised surface of a pulp after pulpotomy. Bridge formation is believed to be enhanced by some chemical agents, such as calcium hydroxide paste. The presence of bridges does not necessarily indicate that the pulp apical to the bridges is vital and intact. **extension b.,** cantilever b. **fixed b.,** partial denture, fixed; see under DENTURE. **fixed-fixed b.,** a term sometimes used to refer to a fixed bridge with rigid connectors. **fixed-movable b.,** a term sometimes used to refer to a fixed bridge with rigid and nonrigid connectors. **fixed b. with rigid connectors,** a fixed partial denture in which all the components are rigidly soldered or cast in one piece. Sometimes called *fixed-fixed b.* See illustration. **fixed b. with rigid and nonrigid connectors,** a fixed partial denture that offers some stress-breaking. It consists of a major retainer, which is attached to a pontic and is supplied with a dovetail, and a minor retainer, which is supplied with a slot into which the dovetail of the major retainer fits. The attachment allows for some movement, thus providing stress-breaking. Sometimes called *fixed-movable b.* See illustration. **hydrogen b.,** a structure formed when a single water molecule intermingles with other water molecules, the hydrogen portion (positive) of one molecule being attracted to the oxygen portion (negative) of its neighboring molecule and the intermolecular van der Waals forces are established. **intercellular b.,** a structure formed by the meeting of short cytoplasmic projections from the cell surface of adjacent cells; formerly thought to constitute a bridge for cytoplasmic continuity between cells, but it has been demonstrated that the processes make contact at a desmonsome, hence each cell is independent. **Libra III Crown and B.,** see under LIBRA. **b. of the nose,** the upper portion of the external nose formed by the junction of the nasal bones. **removable b.,** partial denture, removable; see under DENTURE. **simplex b.,** an anterior or unilateral bridge that replaces one or two teeth, having one functional activity. It generally does not replace more than two teeth, the exception being the replacement of four incisors. **spring b.,** a fixed partial denture in which the pontic is connected to the retainer by a long, flexible palatal

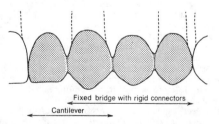

A compound bridge. Fixed with rigid connectors (1345) and cantilever (123) designs being combined. (From D. H. Roberts: Fixed Bridge Prostheses. Bristol, England, John Wright & Sons Ltd., 1973.)

bar. See illustration. **stationary b.,** partial denture, fixed; see under DENTURE.

Bridge III-C trademark for a hard *dental casting gold alloy* (see under GOLD).

Bridge Partial IV-D trademark for an extra hard *dental casting gold alloy* (see under GOLD).

Bridgett's line see under LINE.

bridgework (brij'work) a partial denture retained by attachments other than clasps. See DENTURE. **fixed b.,** partial denture, fixed; see under DENTURE. **removable b.,** partial denture, removable; see under DENTURE.

bridle (bri'd'l) 1. a frenum. 2. a loop or filament that crosses the lumen of a passage or the surface of an ulcer.

Brill-Symmers disease [Nathan Edwin *Brill,* New York physician, 1860–1925; Douglas *Symmers,* American pathologist, 1879–1952] giant cell LYMPHOMA.

brimstone (brim'stōn) sulfur.

Brinell hardness indenter point, hardness number, hardness scale, hardness test, see under POINT and HARDNESS.

brisement (brēz-maw') [Fr. "crushing"] the breaking up or tearing of anything, as of an ankylosis. **b. forcé,** the forcible breaking up or tearing of a bony ankylosis.

Brisfirina trademark for *cephapirin sodium* (see under CEPHAPIRIN).

Brissaud-Marie syndrome [Edouard *Brissaud,* French physician, 1852–1909; Pierre *Marie,* French physician, 1853–1940] hysterical glossolabial HEMISPASM.

Brissaud-Sicard syndrome [E. *Brissaud;* Jean Athanase *Sicard,* French neurologist, 1872–1929] see under SYNDROME.

Bristab trademark for *hydroflumethiazide.*

Bristacin trademark for *rolitetracycline.*

Bristamycin trademark for *erythromycin stearate* (see under ERYTHROMYCIN).

bristle (bris'l) a short, stiff, coarse hair or hairlike part. Bristles are used in making brushes, and may be either natural (*hog b.*) or manufactured (*nylon b.*). See TOOTHBRUSH. **hard b.,** one in a toothbrush, having a diameter of 0.014 inch. **natural b.,** hog bristle used in toothbrushes. **nylon b.,** an artificial bristle made of nylon, used in toothbrushes and other brushes. **soft b.,** one in a toothbrush, having a diameter of 0.007 inch.

Bristophen trademark for *oxacillin.*

British anti-lewisite dimercaprol.

brittle (brit'l) having hardness and rigidity but low ductility; friable; breaking readily.

brittleness (brit'l-nes) the quality of being brittle; fracturing or breaking readily.

broach (brōch) 1. an elongated, tapered and serrated cutting tool for shaping and enlarging holes. 2. root canal b. **barbed b.,** a thin, flexible, usually tapered and pointed, hand-operated or engine-driven endodontic instrument, made of soft iron, and having a series of sharply pointed barbs along the operative head. It is used for engaging and removing the dental pulp and other substances intact from the root canal or pulp chamber. A soft wire probe may be converted into a barbed broach by opening the cuts, thus extending the barbs. The identification symbol is an eight-pointed star. Called also *endodontic b.* and *root canal b.* See illustration at root canal THERAPY. **endodontic b.,** barbed b. **pathfinder b.,** root canal PROBE. **root canal b.,** a broach, usually barbed, used for removing the soft tissue contents of the root canal; see *barbed b.* **smooth b.,** root canal PROBE.

Broadbent registration point see under POINT.

Broca's angle, point [Pierre Paul *Broca,* French anatomist, anthropologist, and surgeon, 1824–1880] see ophryospinal ANGLE, and see under POINT.

Brocq's disease [Anne Jean Louis *Brocq,* French dermatologist, 1856–1928] see under DISEASE.

Brocq-Pautrier glossitis, syndrome [A. J. L. *Brocq;* Lucien M. *Pautrier,* French dermatologist, 1876–1959] median rhomboid GLOSSITIS.

Broders' index (classification) [Albert Compton *Broders,* American pathologist, 1885–1964] see under INDEX.

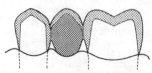

Fixed bridge with rigid connectors. All components are rigidly joined together. (From D. H. Roberts: Fixed Bridge Prostheses. Bristol, England, John Wright & Sons Ltd., 1973.)

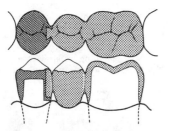

Fixed bridge with rigid and nonrigid connectors. The components are joined by a dovetail and slot. (From D. H. Roberts: Fixed Bridge Prostheses. Bristol, England, John Wright & Sons Ltd., 1973.)

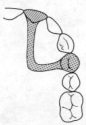

The spring bridge. In this design the pontic is connected to the retainer by means of a relatively long, flexible palatal bar and is largely tissue-borne. (From D. H. Roberts: Fixed Bridge Prostheses. Bristol, England, John Wright & Sons Ltd., 1973.)

bromanautine (bro″mah-naw′tēn) bromodiphenhydramine hydrochloride (see under BROMODIPHENHYDRAMINE).

bromaurate (brom′aw-rāt) GOLD bromide.

bromazine (bro′mah-zēn) bromodiphenhydramine hydrochloride (see under BROMODIPHENHYDRAMINE).

bromdiphenhydramine (brom″di-phen-hi′drah-mēn) bromodiphenhydramine hydrochloride (see under BROMODIPHENHYDRAMINE).

bromide (bro′mīd) any binary compound of bromine in which the bromine carries a negative charge (Br⁻); specifically, a salt (or organic ester) of hydrobromic acid (H + Br⁻). Bromides were formerly used as anticonvulsants and sedatives. Excessive drowsiness and, in large doses, neurological, dermatological, and gastrointestinal lesions have been associated with their use. The therapeutic and toxic effects of bromides derive from the replacement of chloride by bromide in body fluids. At present, bromides are used in certain over-the-counter drugs. See also BROMINISM. **aurous b.,** GOLD bromide. **hydrogen b.,** hydrobromide.

bromine (bro′mēn, bro′min) [L. *bromium, brominium, bromum;* Gr. *brōmos* stench] a halogen occurring as a dark, reddish brown, heavy, mobile, diatomic liquid that volatilizes at room temperature to produce a strong suffocating and irritating odor. Symbol, Br; atomic number, 35; atomic weight, 79.904; valences, −1, 1, 3, 5, 7; group VIIA of the periodic table. Bromine is soluble in water and carbon disulfide and unites readily with many elements. Its known isotopes range from 74 to 90; natural isotopes ⁷⁹Br and ⁸¹Br are stable. Isotopes 77, 80, and 82 are radioactive tracers. Inhalation of bromine vapors may produce serious irritation of the mucous membranes of the respiratory tract and mouth and ingestion of bromine solution may produce fatal gastroenteritis. Its compounds (bromides) are used in medicine. Fomerly used as a topical antiseptic and deodorant.

bromism (brōm′izm) brominism.

brominism (brōm′ĭ-nizm) a condition of poisoning produced by excessive use of bromine or a bromine compound; the symptoms produced are an eruption of acne upon the face and body, headache, coldness of the extremities, fetor oris, sleepiness, weakness, and impotence. Called also *bromism.*

5-bromo-2′-deoxyuridine (bro″mo-de-ok″se-u′rĭ-dēn) a thymidine analogue used as a selective stain of chromosomes. Abbreviated *BUdR.* Called also *broxuridine.* See also BUdR bands, under BAND.

bromodiphenhydramine hydrochloride (brom-di″fen-hi′drah-mēn) an antihistaminic, 2-[(p-bromo-α-phenylbenzyl)oxy]-N,N-dimethylethylamine hydrochloride, occurring as a white to pale buff crystalline powder with a faint odor and a bitter taste, which is stable in dry powder, but not in solution when exposed to direct sunlight, and is soluble in water, alcohol, and isopropyl alcohol. It acts on the H₁ receptor. Used in the treatment of mild local allergic reactions. Called also *bromanautine hydrochlo-*

ride, *bromazine hydrochloride,* and *bromdiphenhydramine hydrochloride.* Trademarks: Ambrodryl, Histabromamine.

brompheniramine maleate (brom-fen-ēr′ah-mēn) the bimaleate salt of the benzene analogue of chlorpheniramine, 2-[p-bromo-α-(2-dimethylaminother)benzyl]pyridine bimaleate, occurring as a white, odorless, crystalline powder that is readily soluble in water, alcohol, and chloroform and slightly soluble in ether and benzene. It is an antihistaminic drug acting on the H₁ receptor, which has anticholinergic and sedative properties. Used in the treatment of allergic diseases. Trademarks: Dimegan, Dimetane, Ebalin, Voltane.

bronchi (brong′ki) [L.] plural of *bronchus.*

bronchia (brong′ke-ah) [L.] plural of *bronchium.*

bronchial (brong′ke-al) [L. *bronchialis*] pertaining to one or more bronchi.

bronchiarctia (brong″ke-ark′she-ah) [*bronchus* + L. *arctare* to constrict] bronchostenosis.

bronchiectasis (brong″ke-ek′tah-sis) [*bronchus* + Gr. *ektasis* dilatation] chronic dilatation of the bronchi, which may affect only the small bronchi and cause sacculation or may produce dilatation of the entire bronchial tubes. Pooling of secretions, chronic inflammation, coughing, fetid breath, large amounts of sputum in the morning due to overnight collecting of the exudate, moist rales, breathing difficulty, and clubbing of the fingers are usually associated.

bronchiocele (brong′ke-o-sēl) [*bronchiole* + Gr. *kēlē* tumor] a dilatation or swelling of a bronchial branch.

bronchiole (brong′ke-ōl) [L. *bronchiolus*] one of the finer (1 mm or less) subdivisions of the branches of the bronchial tree, having no cartilage plates and having cuboidal epithelial cells.

bronchioli (brong-ki′o-li) [L.] plural of *bronchiolus.*

bronchiolitis (brong″ke-o-li′tis) [*bronchiole* + -*itis*] inflammation of the bronchioles. See also BRONCHOPNEUMONIA.

bronchiolus (brong-ki′o-lus), pl. *bronchi′oli* [L.] bronchiole; one of the finer subdivisions of the branched bronchial tree.

bronchitis (brong-ki′tis) [*bronchus* + -*itis*] inflammation of one or more bronchi. See also BRONCHOPNEUMONIA. **capillary b.,** bronchopneumonia.

bronchium (brong′ke-um), pl. *bron′chia* [L.] one of the subdivisions of the bronchus, smaller than a bronchus and larger than a bronchiole.

bronchocele (brong′ko-sēl) [*bronchus* + Gr. *kēlē* tumor] a localized dilatation of a bronchus.

bronchoconstriction (brong′ko-kon-strik′shun) bronchostenosis.

bronchoconstrictor (brong′ko-kon-strik′tor) 1. constricting or narrowing the lamina of the air passages of the lungs. 2. an agent that causes narrowing of the lamina of the air passages of the lungs.

bronchodilatation (brong″ko-dil-ah-ta′shun) a condition of the bronchi in which their caliber has been increased.

bronchodilation (brong″ko-di-la′shun) the act or process of increasing the caliber of bronchi.

bronchodilator (brong″ko-di-la′tor) 1. dilating or expanding the lumina of the air passages of the lungs. 2. an agent that dilates or expands the lumina of the air passages of the lungs by relaxing the smooth muscles of the air passages.

bronchopneumonia (brong″ko-nu-mo′ne-ah) [*bronchus* + *pneumonia*] an inflammatory disease of the lungs, occurring most commonly among the very young and the elderly, usually representing an extension of a pre-existing bronchitis or bronchiolitis. The terminal bronchioles become clogged with a mucopurulent exudate, forming consolidated patches in adjacent lobules. In the aged, particularly those suffering from another disorder such as a heart failure or a neoplastic disease, it is often fatal. Called also *bronchial pneumonia, capillary bronchitis, catarrhal pneumonia,* and *lobular pneumonia.* **hibernovernal b.,** Q FEVER.

Bronchoselectan trademark for *acetrizoate sodium* (see under ACETRIZOATE).

bronchosinusitis (brong″ko-si″nus-i′tis) coexisting inflammation of the paranasal sinuses and the lower respiratory passages.

bronchospasm (brong′ko-spazm) spasmodic contraction of bronchial muscles.

bronchostenosis (brong″ko-ste-no′sis) [*bronchus* + Gr. *stenōsis* a narrowing] stricture of cicatricial diminution of the caliber of a bronchial tube. Called also *bronchiarctia* and *bronchoconstriction.*

bronchus (brong′kus), pl. *bron′chi* [L.; Gr. *bronchos* windpipe] any of the large air passages within the lungs.

Bronsted concept see under CONCEPT.

Brooke's disease, epithelioma [Henry Ambrose Grundy Brooke, 1854–1919] cystic adenoid EPITHELIOMA.

Brophy's operation [Truman William *Brophy*, American oral surgeon, 1848–1928] see under OPERATION.

brow (brow) the forehead, or either lateral half of it. **olympic b.,** the overdeveloped forehead seen in congenital syphilis.

Brown see Adson-Brown FORCEPS.

brown (brown) 1. a dusky, reddish, yellow color. 2. a dye having a dusky, reddish, yellow color. **lead oxide b.,** LEAD dioxide.

Brown, James Barrett [born 1899] a distinguished American plastic and maxillofacial surgeon.

Brown, John [Scottish physician, 1735–1788] see BRUNONIANISM.

Brown, Robert [English botanist, 1773–1858] see brownian MOVEMENT.

Brown's syndrome [Jason W. *Brown*] see under SYNDROME.

Brown Kelly see KELLY, Adam Brown.

Brown-Symmers disease [Charles Leonard *Brown*, American physician, born 1899; Douglas *Symmers*, American pathologist, 1879–1952] see under DISEASE.

brownian (brow'ne-an) named after Robert *Brown*, as brownian movement (see under MOVEMENT).

brownism (brown'izm) brunonianism.

broxuridine (brok'su-ri-dēn) 5-bromo-2'-deoxyuridine.

Bruce, Sir David a British bacteriologist.

Brucella (broo-sel'ah) [named after Sir David *Bruce*] a genus of gram-negative, aerobic bacteria of uncertain affiliation, occurring as coccobacilli or short rods (0.5 to 0.7 μm by 0.6 to 1.5 μm in size), arranged singly and in short chains. The organisms are unencapsulated, nonmotile, and nonsporogenous, and are also catalase-positive and usually oxidase-positive. They are parasitic in various warm-blooded animals, including man. **B. abor'tus,** a species causing brucellosis in humans and contagious abortion in cattle. Called also *Bacterium abortus* and *Bang's bacillus*. **B. bronchisep'tica,** *Bordetella bronchiseptica;* see under BORDETELLA. **B. meliten'sis,** a species causing brucellosis, occurring primarily, although not exclusively, in goats as the reservoir of infection. Called also *Micrococcus melitensis.* **B. su'is,** a species occurring in four biotypes, being usually pathogenic for swine; it also infects humans, hares, reindeer, and other animals. **B. tularen'sis,** *Francisella tularensis;* see under FRANCISELLA.

brucella (broo'sel-ah) an individual microorganism of the genus *Brucella.*

brucellar (broo-sel'ar) pertaining to or caused by *Brucella.*

brucellosis (broo"sel-lo'sis) infection with *Brucella abortus, B. melitensis,* or *B. suis,* involving primarily the reticuloendothelial system, derived from contact with infected animals. Five types of human infection have been delineated: (1) the *intermittent* type with shifting articular rheumatism, weakness, night sweating, and body temperature near normal in the morning but rising to 101 to 104°F in the evening; (2) the *ambulatory* type with symptoms similar to those of the intermittent type, but to a milder degree; (3) the *undulant* type, generally due to *B. melitensis,* characterized by steplike increases in the temperature from day-to-day to a maximum, and, after a time, gradual decrease in temperature and possibly successive repetitions of this sequence of events; (4) the *malignant* type, almost always due to *B. melitensis,* in which the temperature is high and sustained with extreme hyperpyrexia before death; and (5) the *atypical chronic* type which may take the form of muscular stiffness, gastric disturbances, and neurological symptoms. Called also *Bang's disease* and *undulant fever.*

bruise (brōōz) subcutaneous accumulation of blood following a superficial injury produced by impact without laceration.

bruit (brwe, broot) [Fr.] a sound or murmur heard in auscultation, especially an abnormal one.

Brunn's membrane [Albert von *Brunn*, German anatomist, 1849–1895] see under MEMBRANE.

brunonianism (broo-no'ne-an-izm") [named after John *Brown*] the obsolete theory that all diseases are caused by excess (sthenia), or lack (asthenia) of stimulus. Called also *brownism* and *brunonian theory.* See also METHODIST (1).

brush (brush) tufts of bristles, hair, or other flexible materials set into a handle. **Bass' b.,** Bass TOOTHBRUSH. **bristle b.,** a cleansing and polishing instrument attached to the handpiece of the dental engine and used, with a paste, for polishing the teeth. Bristle brushes come as wheel and cup types. **b. condensation,** brush CONDENSATION. **denture b.,** one for cleaning dentures, adapted to the contour of the denture. **interproximal b.,** inter-

proximal TOOTHBRUSH. **polishing b.,** one consisting of a disk with natural, synthetic, or wire bristles, which may be mounted on a mandrel or a lathe; used for polishing functions in dentistry, within or outside the mouth (e.g., for dentures). **tooth b.,** toothbrush. **wire b.,** a polishing brush with wire bristles.

brushing (brush'ing) 1. the act of an application of a brush. 2. toothbrushing.

brush-on (brush-on) the application of resin to the prepared cavity by dipping a brush in the resin and transferring it drop-by-drop to the cavity.

bruxism (bruk'sizm) [Gr. *brychein* to gnash the teeth] an oral habit consisting of involuntary rhythmic or spasmodic nonfunctional gnashing, grinding, and clenching of the teeth in other than chewing movements of the mandible, usually performed during sleep, which may lead to occlusal trauma. It is believed to be related to repressed aggression, emotional tension, anger, and fear, with frustration being its principal cause. Occlusal interferences are considered to be a major etiologic factor. Increased tonus of the jaw muscles is a constant feature. Malocclusion, periodontal injury, crown damage, headache, temporomandibular joint disorders, and pain are the most common complications. Bruxism occurring in the daytime is called *bruxomania.* Called also *Karolyi effect, occlusal habit neurosis, odontoprisis, neuralgia traumatica, parafunction,* and *stridor dentium.* See also occlusal TRAUMA. **centric b.,** that characterized by clenching in centric occlusion. Called also *clamping habit* and *habitual clenching.* **eccentric b.,** that characterized by nonfunctional gnashing and grinding in eccentric excursions. Called also *habitual grinding, nonfunctional grinding, gnashing habit,* and *grinding habit.*

bruxomania (bruk"so-ma"ne-ah) [Gr. *brychein* + *mania*] bruxism occurring in the daytime, usually performed with the individual being unaware of it. See BRUXISM.

BTU British thermal UNIT.

Bu butyl.

bubo (bu'bo) [L. from Gr. *boubon* groin] the inflammatory swelling of a lymphatic gland, particularly of the axilla or groin. **climatic b., Frei's b., tropical b.,** LYMPHOGRANULOMA venereum.

bucca (buk'ah) [L.] [NA] the fleshy portion of the side of the face; the cheek. Called also *mala* [NA alternative]. **b. ca'vi o'ris** [NA], the fleshy portion of the side of the oral cavity, which is continuous with the commissure of the lips. Called also *cheek.*

buccal (buk'al) [L. *buccalis,* from *bucca* cheek] pertaining to the cheek; genal. In dental anatomy, the term is used to refer to the vestibular (or oral) surface of the premolars and molars that faces the cheek. Cf. LINGUAL. See illustration at SURFACE.

buccinator (buk'si-na"tor) [L. "trumpeter"] buccinator MUSCLE.

bucco- [L. *bucca* cheek] a combining form denoting relationship to the cheek.

buccoaxial (buk"ko-ak'se-al) [*bucco* + *axial*] pertaining to or formed by the buccal and axial walls of a tooth cavity preparation.

buccoaxiocervical (buk"ko-ak"se-o-ser'vi-kal) [*bucco-* + *axio-* + *cervical*] buccoaxiogingival.

buccoaxiogingival (buk"ko-ak"se-o-jin'ji-val) [*bucco-* + *axio-* + *gingival*] pertaining to or formed by the buccal, axial, and gingival walls of a tooth cavity. Called also *buccoaxiocervical.*

buccocervical (buk"ko-ser'vi-kal) [*bucco-* + *cervical*] 1. pertaining to the cheek and neck. 3. pertaining to the buccal surface of the neck of a tooth. 3. buccogingival.

buccoclusal (buk"ko-kloo'sal) 1. pertaining to buccocclusion. 2. bucco-occlusal.

buccocclusion (buk"ko-kloo'zhun) malocclusion in which the dental arch or a group of teeth is buccal to the normal position.

buccodistal (buk"ko-dis'tal) distobuccal.

buccogingival (buk"ko-jin'ji-val) [*bucco-* + *gingival*] 1. pertaining to the cheek and gingiva. 2. pertaining to or formed by the buccal and gingival walls of a tooth cavity preparation.

buccoglossopharyngitis (buk"ko-glos'o-far"in-ji'tis) inflammation involving the cheek, tongue, and pharynx. **b. sic'ca,** inflammation and dryness of the buccal mucosa, tongue, and pharynx. See also Sjögren's SYNDROME.

buccolabial (buk"ko-la'be-al) pertaining to the cheek and lip.

buccomaxillary (buk"ko-mak'si-ler"e) 1. pertaining to the cheek and maxilla. 2. communicating with the buccal cavity and the maxillary sinus, as a buccomaxillary fistula.

buccomesial (buk"ko-me'ze-al) mesiobuccal.

bucco-occlusal (buk"ko-o-kloo'zal) pertaining or formed by the buccal and occlusal surfaces of a tooth. Written also *buccoclusal.*

buccopharyngeal (buk"ko-fah-rin'je-al) [*bucco-* + *pharyngeal*] pertaining to the mouth and pharynx.

buccoplacement (buk″ko-plăs′ment) displacement of a tooth toward the cheek.

buccopulpal (buk″ko-pul′pal) pertaining to or formed by the buccal and pulpal walls of a tooth cavity preparation.

buccoversion (buk″ko-ver′zhun) the position of a tooth which lies buccally to the line of occlusion.

Buchner, Hans [1850–1902] a German bacteriologist who first described complement.

Buck wiring [Gurdon *Buck*, Jr., American surgeon, 1807–1877] interosseous WIRING.

buckling (buk′ling) 1. bending, warping, or bulging. 2. the crowding of anterior teeth in the dental arch.

Bucky's diaphragm, rays [Gustav P. *Bucky*, German-born roentgenologist in the United States] see under DIAPHRAGM, and see grenz rays, under RAY.

Bucky-Potter diaphragm [G. P. *Bucky*] Bucky's DIAPHRAGM.

bud (bud) any small part of the embryo or adult metazoan more or less resembling the bud of a plant and presumed to have potential for growth and differentiation. **gustatory b.**, taste b. **taste b.** any of the minute terminal organs of the gustatory nerve, presenting a spherical or ovoid nest of cells embedded in the stratified squamous epithelium of the tongue and sometimes the soft palate and the epiglottis, which has an opening at the surface and another at the basement membrane. The bud includes cover cells lined up on its outer shell, with the spindle-shaped cells having central nuclei (taste cells) occupying the center. Each taste cell protrudes through the gustatory pore in a hairlike process (taste hair). The buds located at the apex of the tongue are sensitive to sweet, those in the periphery to salt, those of the circumvallate papillae to bitter, and those of the peripheral foliate papillae to sour; there are no apparent differences between the various buds. Called also *gustatory b.*, *caliculus gustatorius* [NA], *gustatory bulb*, *Schwalbe's corpuscle*, and *taste bulb*. **tooth b.**, a knoblike tooth primordium developing into an enamel organ surrounded by a dental sac and encasing the dental papilla. Ten buds develop on each dental arch from the dental lamina (bud stage of odontogenesis), which differentiate into the deciduous teeth. Increased

mitotic activity and invagination of the inferior segment of the bud result in the bud becoming cap-shaped (cap stage). The connective tissue housed in the invagination is the dental papilla (future dental pulp) and that surrounding the primordium forms the dental sac (future periodontal ligament). By the fourth month, additional buds appear on the successional lamina (an extension of the dental lamina) for the first permanent molars and buds for the second permanent molars appear in infants of about 9 months of age and buds for the third molars by the fourth year of life. See illustration. See also dental GERM, dental LAMINA, enamel ORGAN, and successional LAMINA.

budding (bud′ing) 1. gemmation; a form of asexual reproduction in which the body divides into two unequal parts, the larger part being considered the parent and the smaller one the bud. 2. the process by which a new blood vessel arises from a preexisting vessel.

Budin's joint [Pierre Constant *Budin*, French physician, 1846–1907] see under JOINT.

BUdR 5-bromo-2′deoxyuridine; see BUdR bands, under BAND.

buffer (buf′er) any substance that tends to lessen the change in pH value, which otherwise would be produced by adding acids or alkalis. **acid-base b.**, a solution of two or more chemical substances that prevents significant changes in hydrogen ion concentration when either an acid or a base is added to the solution.

Bufferin trademark for an analgesic preparation containing aspirin, magnesium carbonate, and aluminum glycinate.

bug (bug) 1. any hemipterous insect. 2. a malfunction of a computer due to any mechanical or electrical failure or an error in a computer program. See also DEBUG.

builder (bil′der) one that builds. **enamel b.**, ameloblast.

build-up (bild′up) the gradual increase in strength, force, volume, number, etc. **radiation b.**, the increase in absorbed dose with depth below the surface of an irradiated object, due to an

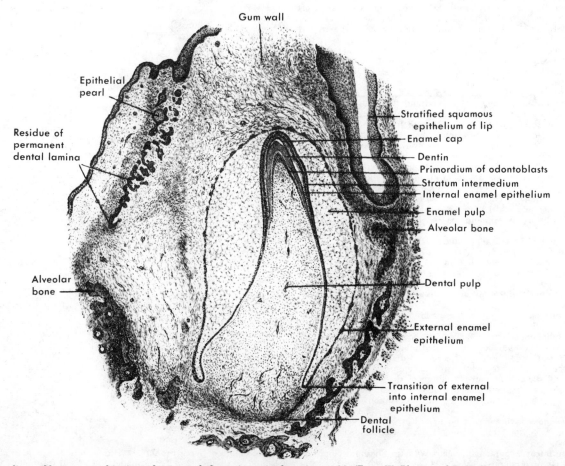

Primordium of lower central incisor of a 5-month fetus, in sagittal section. × 30. (From W. Bloom and D. W. Fawcett: A Textbook of Histology. 10th ed. Philadelphia, W. B. Saunders Co., 1975; after Schaffer.)

increasing production of secondary electrons in the material, as well as a build-up of scattered photons due to multiple scattering in broad beams of radiation.

Buist's method [Robert C. *Buist*, Scottish obstetrician, 1860–1939] see artificial RESPIRATION.

bulb (bulb) [L. *bulbus;* Gr. *bolbos*] any globelike, ovoid, or nearly spherical body. In anatomy, an enlargement on a tissue or organ; a rounded thing or enlarged part. **gustatory b.,** taste BUD. **hollow b.,** the part of a denture made hollow to minimize its weight. **inferior b. of jugular vein,** a slight dilatation of the internal jugular vein near its outlet into the brachiocephalic vein. Called also *bulbus venae jugularis inferior* [NA] and *inferior sinus of internal jugular vein.* **b's of Krause, Krause's end-b's,** small encapsulated nerve endings, consisting of cylindrical or oval bodies containing bulging connective tissue sheaths of myelinated fibers and semifluid cores in which axons terminate. They are found in various tissues, including the mucous membrane of the lips and tongue, and are associated with perception of cold. Called also *bulboid corpuscles, corpuscula bulbiformia, corpuscula bulboidea* [NA], and *Krause's corpuscles.* **olfactory b.,** a part of the rhinencephalon, forming a budlike expansion resting on the cribriform plate of the ethmoid bone, which communicates with the cerebral hemisphere through the olfactory tract and receives the fila olfactoria of the olfactory nerve. Called also *bulbus olfactorius* [NA]. **speech b.,** speech-aid PROSTHESIS. **superior b. of jugular vein,** a slight dilatation of the jugular vein near its origin. Called also *bulbus venae jugularis superior* [NA], *Heister's diverticulum,* and *superior sinus of internal jugular vein.* **taste b.,** taste BUD.

bulbar (bul'bar) pertaining to a bulb; formerly used alone with reference to the medulla oblongata.

bulbi (bul'bi) [L.] plural of *bulbus.*

bulbus (bul'bus), pl. *bul'bi* [L.] a bulb; a rounded mass, or enlargement. **b. caroti'cus,** carotid SINUS. **b. olfacto'rius** [NA], olfactory BULB. **b. ve'nae jugula'ris infe'rior** [NA], inferior bulb of jugular vein; see under BULB. **b. ve'nae jugula'ris supe'rior** [NA], superior bulb of jugular vein; see under BULB.

BULL Buccal or Upper Lingual of Lower; an acronym for Schuyler's rule for occlusal adjustment by grinding on the bucco-occlusal inclines (lingual inclines of the buccal cusps) or the maxillary teeth and the linguo-occlusal inclines (buccal inclines of the lingual cusps) of the mandibular teeth.

bulla (bul'ah), pl. *bul'lae* [L.] 1. a large vesicle, usually 2 cm or more in diameter. 2. a circumscribed, elevated lesion of the skin over 5 mm in diameter which contains fluid, such as seen in contact dermatitis. **ethmoid b.,** 1. ethmoid b. of nasal cavity. 2. ethmoid b. of ethmoid bone. **ethmoid b. of ethmoid bone,** a rounded projection of the ethmoid bone into the lateral wall of the middle nasal meatus just below the middle nasal concha, enclosing a large ethmoid air cell. Called also *ethmoid b., b. of ethmoidalis ossis ethmoidalis* [NA], *antrum ethmoidale,* and *ethmoid antrum.* **ethmoid b. of nasal cavity,** the large ethmoid air cell lodged in the ethmoid bulla of the ethmoid bone. Called also *ethmoid b.* and *b. ethmoidalis cavi nasi* [NA]. **b. ethmoida'lis ca'vi na'si** [NA], ethmoid b. of nasal cavity. **b. ethmoida'lis os'sis ethmoida'lis** [NA], ethmoid b. of ethmoid bone.

bullae (bul'e) [L.] plural of *bulla.*

bullous (bul'us) pertaining to or characterized by bullae.

bundle (bun'd'l) a collection of fibers or strands. **Korff's b's,** Korff's fibers; see under FIBER. **principal fiber b's,** preferentially arranged bundles of collagenous fibers suspending and anchoring the tooth in the alveolus. See also principal fibers, under FIBER.

bunodont (bu'no-dont) [Gr. *bounos* hill + *odous* tooth] a form of molar teeth of ungulates, having low, conic cusps.

bunolophodont (bu"no-lo'fo-dont) [Gr. *bounos* hill + *lophos* ridge + *odous* tooth] having cross-crested tuberculate teeth.

Bunon, Robert [18th century] a French dentist and writer who dispelled numerous popular misconceptions of his times, including the notion that extraction of the eye teeth may be injurious to the teeth and the role of the teeth and pregnancy. He is credited with the first accurate description of dental hypoplasia.

bunoselenodont (bu"no-sē-le'no-dont) [Gr. *bounos* hill + *selenē* moon + *odous* tooth] having teeth with rounded occlusal crests.

Bunsen burner, coefficient [Robert Wilhelm Eberhard von *Bunsen*, German chemist, 1811–1899] see under BURNER, and see absorption COEFFICIENT (2).

Bunyaviridae (bun"yah-vi-ri'de) a family of enveloped helical arboviruses containing single-stranded (−)RNA genomes that are segmented into three parts. The nucleocapsid is coiled and is assembled in the cytoplasm; the virion (diameter 100 nm; helix 2–3 nm) matures by budding from the Golgi apparatus and the endoplasmic reticulum. The family consists of a single genus, *Bunyavirus.*

Bunyavirus (bun"yah-vi'rus) the single genus of the family Bunyaviridae, including most of the arboviruses other than those belonging to the families Togaviridae, Reoviridae, and Rhabdoviridae. It comprises 87 members of the Bunyamwera supergroup (see under VIRUS), which is further subdivided into several groups, all members being antigenically related. Also, several groups of viruses have been tentatively assigned to this genus.

bur (ber) a rotary dental instrument made of steel or tungsten carbide, held and revolved in a handpiece, deriving power from the dental electric motor or air power. It consists of the *shank,* which may be tapered, notched, or elongated and smooth to fit into a handpiece; the *neck,* which connects the shank with the working part; and the *head,* which is the working part. A

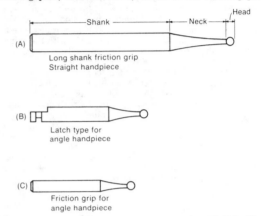

Basic designs of burs. (From H. O. Torres and A. Ehrlich: Modern Dental Assisting. 2nd ed. Philadelphia, W. B. Saunders Co., 1980.)

handpiece with a latched opening receives the notched bur; the latch is fastened into the bur notch. The longer shanks fit into a straight handpiece. Some burs have shanks designed to the correct diameter to fit into a handpiece by friction. The tapered- and latch-type bur shanks are designed to work with contra-angled handpieces. Burs are used to remove carious material

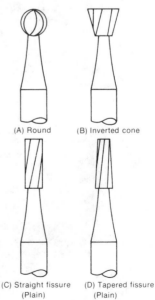

Basic shapes of burs. (From H. O. Torres and A. Ehrlich: Modern Dental Assisting. 2nd ed. Philadelphia, W. B. Saunders Co., 1980.)

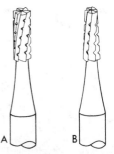

A, Straight fissure — cross-cut (dentate). *B,* Tapered fissure — cross-cut (dentate). (From H. O. Torres and A. Ehrlich: Modern Dental Assisting. 2nd ed. Philadelphia, W. B. Saunders Co., 1980.)

within decayed teeth, to reduce hard tissues that have been decayed or fractured, to form the design of the cavity preparation, and to finish and polish the teeth and restorations. They are available in a variety of sizes and shapes, including: round (¼–10), inverted cone (31¼–44), straight fissure (plain [55½–62] or dentate [556–563]), tapered fissure (plain [69–73] or dentate [699–703]), wheel (11½–16), bud (44½–51), pear (230–232), oval (218–221), cone (22½–33), and flame (242–246); low numbers in a series indicating small bur head sizes. Called also *drill.* See illustrations. **ACORDE b.,** an all-purpose bur for cavity preparation; no longer used. **barrel b.,** a dental bur with the head shaped like a barrel. See illustration. **bone b.,** surgical b. **bud b.** (nos. 44½–51), a dental bur with a bud-shaped head having a convexity in the center and a point at the end; used to remove excess restorative material and to provide concave form to a preparation. See illustration. **carbide b.,** a hard bur made of tungsten carbide, used with high-speed and ultra–high-speed equipment. **cone b.** (nos. 22½–33), a dental bur with a cone-shaped head; it is a finishing bur used on all margins and all surfaces in a crown preparation or for general polishing of metal restorations. See illustration. **cone b., inverted** (nos. 33¼–44), a dental bur with a head shaped like a truncated cone; used to provide a cavity preparation at the pulpal wall, to form retention grooves, including the base of an amalgam preparation, and for initial removal of large portions of carious material in posterior teeth. See illustration. **cross-cut b.,** dentate b. **cross-cut straight fissure b.,** straight fissure b. **cross-cut tapered fissure b.,** tapered fissure b. **cylinder b.,** a dental bur having a cylindrical head, such as those in straight fissure or

end-cutting fissure burs. See illustration. **dentate b.,** a dental bur having cross-cuts perpendicular to the linear cuts, as in the dentate tapered fissure and straight fissure burs. Called also *cross-cut bur.* **dentate straight fissure b.,** see *straight fissure b.* **dentate tapered fissure b.,** see *tapered fissure b.* **diamond b.,** a dental bur on which diamond chips have been bound. See also diamond rotary INSTRUMENT. **end-cutting fissure b.** (nos. 957–959), a dental bur with a cylindrical head, having the cutting portion placed on the end of the head only, the sides being smooth; used to reach inaccessible areas of the tooth preparation near the shoulder of the preparation, at the cementoenamel junction. **endodontic b.,** any bur used in shaping the pulp chamber of a tooth for access to the root canals. See illustrations. **excavating b.,** one used to remove dentin and debris from a tooth cavity. **Feldman b.,** a type of bibeveled surgical bur. Called also *Feldman drill.* See illustration. **finishing b.,** any dental bur with numerous, fine-cutting blades placed close together, such as oval or pear burs, used for finishing, smoothing, and shaping restorations. Called also *plug-finishing b.* **fissure b.,** any dental bur with a cylindrical or tapered head, such as straight fissure, tapered fissure, or end-cutting fissure burs. **flame b.** (nos. 242–246), a dental bur with a narrow head shaped like the flame of a candle; it is a finishing bur used primarily for polishing. See illustration. **Gates-Glidden b.,** Gates-Glidden DRILL. **inverted cone b.,** cone b., inverted. **Lindemann b.,** a surgical bur with spiral cutting edges, used to perform osteotomies of the jaws. See illustration. **oval b.** (nos. 218–221), a dental bur with an oval head; a finishing bur used for polishing amalgam restorations. See illustration. **pear b.** (nos. 230–232), a dental bur having a large bulbous head; a

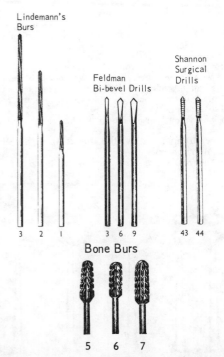

Assorted surgical burs. (From H. O. Torres and A. Ehrlich: Modern Dental Assisting. 2nd ed. Philadelphia, W. B. Saunders Co., 1980.)

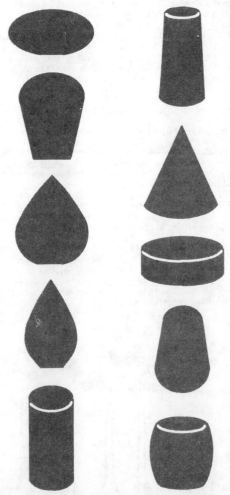

Shapes of bur heads. (From H. O. Torres and A. Ehrlich: Modern Dental Assisting. 2nd ed. Philadelphia, W. B. Saunders Co., 1980.)

finishing bur used to polish a large surface of restorative material. See illustration. **pear b., inverted,** a dental bur having the head shaped like a pear standing on its broad base. See illustration. **plain straight fissure b.,** see *straight fissure b.* **plain tapered fissure b.,** see *tapered fissure b.* **plug-finishing b.,** finishing b. **pointed cone b.,** cone b., pointed. **round b.** (nos. ¼–10), a dental bur with a spherical head; used for entry into and removal of carious enamel. See illustration. **Shannon b.,** a type of surgical bur. Called also *Shannon drill.* See illustration. **Starlite Omni-AT b.,** trademark for an hourglass-shaped diamond bur. **straight fissure b.,** a dental bur with a cylindrical head, which may be plain (nos. 55½–62) or dentate (those with cross cuts, nos. 556–563); used to form the axial walls of the cavity preparation and to provide axial retention grooves in the cavity preparation. Called also *cross-cut straight fissure b.* See illustrations. **straight fissure b., cross-cut,** straight fissure b. **straight fissure b., dentate,** see *straight fissure b.* **straight fissure b., plain,** see *straight fissure b.* **surgical b.,** a bur for cutting bone, normally used with low-speed handpieces. Called also *bone b.* See illustration. **tapered fissure b.,** a dental bur having a long head with sides that converge from the shank to a blunt end, which may be plain (nos. 69–73) or dentate (ones having cross cuts on linear cuts, nos. 699–703); used to form the axial walls of the cavity preparation and to provide axial retention grooves in the cavity preparation. Called also *cross-cut tapered fissure b.* See illustrations. **tapered fissure b., cross-cut,** tapered fissure b. **tapered fissure b., dentate,** see *tapered fissure b.* **tapered fissure b., plain,** see *tapered fissure b.* **wheel b.** (nos. 11½–16), a dental bur having a wheel-shaped head with the cutting edge placed perpendicular to the shank of the bur; used to provide access in developing retention for Class V amalgam preparations or other restorations in which slight retention is needed. See illustration. See also WHEEL.

Burckhardt's operation see under OPERATION.

burden (ber′den) a load; encumberance. **body b.,** the amount of radioactive material present in the body.

bureau (būr′o) [Fr. "a desk"] a specialized administrative unit. **b's of American Dental Association,** see American Dental Association in Appendix. **B. of Health Insurance,** an agency within the Social Security Administration responsible for administering the Medicare programs and for making contractual arrangements with individual carriers for the delivery of health care services. Abbreviated *BHI.* **Medical Impairment B.,** a clearing house of information on applicants for life insurance, which collects and distributes to its subscribers data derived from medical records of applicants, particularly those pertaining to adverse medical findings. Abbreviated *MIB.* **B. of Quality Assurance,** an agency within the Health Resources Administration of the Department of Health and Human Services which administers the Professional Standards Review Organization (PSRO) (see under ORGANIZATION). Abbreviated *BQA.*

buret, burette (bu-ret′) a graduated tube with a valve or stopcock at the bottom, used in chemistry to deliver a measured amount of liquid.

Bürger-Grütz syndrome [Max *Bürger;* O. *Grütz*] hyperlipoproteinemia I.

burimamide (ber-im′ah-mīd) a thiourea analog of histamine, *N*-[4-(1*H*-imidazol-4-yl)butyl]-*N'*-methyl thiourea. It is an antihistaminic that blocks the H_2 receptor, which inhibits gastric acid secretion. Together with the H_1 inhibitors, it blocks the hypotensive effect of histamine and histamine-induced edema.

Burkitt's lymphoma (tumor) [Denis Parsons *Burkitt,* British physician, born 1911] see under LYMPHOMA.

Burkitt lymphoma virus [D. P. *Burkitt*] see Epstein-Barr VIRUS.

Burlew wheel see under WHEEL.

burn (bern) 1. injury, usually involving surface structures of an organ, caused by exposure to heat, electricity, radiation, or chemical agents. 2. thermal b. **aspirin b.,** a chemical burn of the oral mucosa caused by the caustic properties of aspirin, and characterized by a burning sensation, followed by blanching and, sometimes, sloughing of the epithelium and bleeding. It is frequently observed when aspirin is used to alleviate toothache, by placing the tablet against the tooth and allowing the tongue or lip to hold it in position. **brush b.,** a wound caused by rubbing or friction. **chemical b.,** a lesion produced by a chemical irritant or corrosive substance. **electric b.,** one caused by passage of electricity through the body and transformation of electrical energy into heat, resulting from resistance of the body tissue. Injuries vary from superficial skin burns to deep visceral lesions. Exposure to low-intensity electric current, especially when there is good contact with moist skin, leaves minimal damage or no damage at all; exposure to high-intensity current, such as lightning, may cause death. In some instances, heat may produce steam which explodes solid organs, including bones. Electric burns of the oral mucosa in children are often caused by chewing on electrical cord, resulting in lesions of the lips and, sometimes, of the gingivae and tongue; destruction and necrosis of the tissue of developing tooth germs or buds is the common complication. See also electric INJURY and lightning MARK. **first degree b.,** thermal burn characterized by reddening of the skin and without deep lesions of the skin that may interfere with self-repair. **full thickness b.,** thermal burn characterized by destruction of the dermal appendages from which re-epithelialization occurs, thus preventing self-repair and requiring skin grafting. **partial b.,** thermal burns characterized by surface lesions that do not interfere with self-repair, thus not requiring skin grafting. **radiation b.,** 1. one caused by skin contact with or exposure to emitters of ionizing radiations, such as beta rays. 2. thermal b. **second degree b.,** thermal burn characterized by blistering and without deep lesions of the skin that may interfere with self-repair. **sun b.,** sunburn. **thermal b.,** an injury caused by exposure to heat, characterized by coagulation of tissue and localized vascular changes that permit loss of proteins and water, sometimes resulting in shock and death. Burns involving more than 20 percent of the total body surface are considered to be potentially fatal. Complications may include superinfection and sepsis, pulmonary edema, acute renal complications, and sometimes gastric ulcer. **third degree b.,** thermal burn characterized by destruction of deep structures of the skin.

burner (bern′er) a part of a fuel-burning device, such as a lamp or furnace, where the flame is produced. **Bunsen b.,** a gas burner in which gas is mixed with air in a perforated tube before ignition, in order to give efficient combustion; commonly used in laboratories.

Burnet, Sir Frank Macfarlane [born 1899] an Australian physician; co-winner, with Peter B. Medawar, of the Nobel prize for medicine and physiology in 1960, for the theoretical solution to the problem of transplanting tissues and organs from one animal to another.

Burnetia wolhynica (ber-ne′she-ah wol-hin′ĭ-kah) *Rochalimaea quintana;* see under ROCHALIMAEA.

Burnett's syndrome [Charles H. *Burnett,* American physician] milk alkali SYNDROME.

burnisher (ber′nish-er) an instrument with a blade or nib with a beveled margin, used for smoothing out roughness at the margin of the restoration and the enamel. See illustration. **agate b.,**

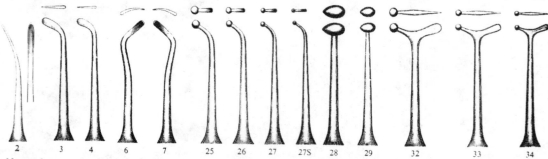

Assorted burnishers used to finish metal restorations. (From H. O. Torres and A. Ehrlich: Modern Dental Assisting. 2nd ed. Philadelphia, W. B. Saunders Co., 1980; courtesy of S. S. White Div. of Pennwalt Corp.)

one made of polished agate. **amalgam b.,** one used in burnishing the surface of amalgam restorations. **ball b.,** one with a nib in the shape of a ball. **beaver-tail b.,** straight b. **fishtail b.,** one resembling a fish's tail or a hammer, one end of the blade being flattened and the other ball-shaped. The flat end may be used in inverting the edges of a rubber dam around teeth. **fissure b.,** one with a head designed to fit into fissures. **flat b.,** one with a head that is flat on the sides. **gold b.,** one for burnishing direct filling gold and gold inlays. **straight b.,** one whose nib resembles a beaver's tail, having a broad, flat blade which is smoothly continuous with the shank and meets it in a slight curve, while the edges and the point are smoothly rounded. Called also *beaver-tail b.*

burnishing (ber′nish-ing) 1. the condensation and polishing under the sliding pressure of a smooth hard instrument, as in finishing the surface of a gold filling. See also POLISHING. 2. the adaptation of a thin, annealed sheet metal by means of a burnisher, as in forming a band about a tooth root or in fitting a matrix for porcelain.

burnout (bern′owt) 1. rendering something unserviceable or ineffectual by excessive heat. 2. radiographic b. 3. total destruction of something by fire. 4. wax b. Also written *burn-out.* **high heat b.,** burnout of invested wax with the use of a temperature of 597°C (1100°F) or higher. **inlay b.,** wax b. **radiographic b.,** overexposure of the plate to radiation with resulting black areas on the radiograph. **wax b.,** elimination through the use of heat of an invested wax pattern from a mold investment, thereby preparing the mold to molten casting metal. Called also *inlay b.*

burn-out (bern′owt) burnout.

Burns, space of [Allan *Burns,* Scottish anatomist, 1781–1813] jugular FOSSA.

Burow's solution [Karl August von *Burow,* surgeon in Koenigsberg, 1809–1874] see under SOLUTION.

bursa (ber′sah), pl. *bur′sae* [L.; Gr. "a wine skin"] a sac or a pocket in the fascia, whose inner surfaces are lubricated with a viscid fluid to prevent friction in areas where different structures rub against each other, as a tendon sliding over the periosteum of a bone. **Boyer's b.,** one situated beneath the hyoid bone. **b.-equivalent,** requiring interaction with human tissue analogous to the bursa of Fabricius in birds (bursal equivalent tissue). See B-lymphocytes, under LYMPHOCYTE, and see lymphoid SYSTEM. **b. of Fabricius,** an epithelial outgrowth of the cloaca in chick embryos, which develops in a manner similar to that of the thymus in mammals, atrophying after 5 or 6 months and persisting as a fibrous remnant in sexually mature birds. It contains lymphoid follicles, and before involution is a site of formation of lymphocytes associated with humoral immunity. See also *b.-equivalent.* **hyoid b.,** subcutaneous b. of prominence of larynx. **infrahyoid b., b. infrahyoi′dea** [NA], a bursa sometimes present below the hyoid bone at the attachment of the sternohyoid muscle. **b. muco′sa, mucous b.,** synovial b. **mus′culi tenso′ris ve′li palati′ni** [NA], b. of tensor veli palatini muscle. **b. mus′culi thyreohyoi′dei,** a bursa under the thyrohyoid muscle. **b. pharyn′gea** [NA], **pharyngeal b.,** an irregular, flask-shaped mucous blind sac of the nasopharynx, situated above the pharyngeal tonsil and sometimes extending up to the basilar process of the occipital bone; it represents persistence of an embryonic communication between the anterior tip of the notochord and the roof of the pharynx. Called also *Thornwaldt's (Tornwaldt's) b.* and *Thornwaldt's (Tornwaldt's) cyst.* **retrohyoid b., b. retrohyoi′dea** [NA], a bursa sometimes present behind the hyoid bone at the attachment of the sternohyoid muscle. **b. subcuta′nea prominen′tiae laryn′gea** [NA], subcutaneous b. of prominence of larynx. **subcutaneous b. of prominence of larynx,** a bursa over the anterior prominence of the thyroid cartilage of the larynx, under the skin. Called also *b. subcutanea prominentiae laryngeae* [NA], *hyoid b., subhyoid b.,* and *thyrohyoid b.* **subhyoid b.,** subcutaneous b. of prominence of larynx. **synovial b., b. synovia′lis** [NA], a closed synovial sac formed by clefts in the connective tissue between muscles, tendons, ligaments, and bones to facilitate the gliding of muscles and tendons over bony or ligamentous structures. It may be simple or multilocular in structure, and subcutaneous, submuscular, subfascial, or subtendinous in location. Called also *b. mucosa* and *mucous b.* **b. of tensor veli palatini muscle,** a bursa between the hamular process of the sphenoid bone and the tendon of the tensor veli palatini. Called also *bursa musculi tensoris veli palatini* [NA]. **Thornwaldt's (Tornwaldt's) b.,** pharyngeal b. **thyrohyoid b.,** subcutaneous b. of prominence of larynx.

bursae (ber′se) [L.] plural of *bursa.*

bursal (ber′sal) [L. *bursalis*] pertaining to a bursa.

bursitis (ber-si′tis). inflammation of a bursa. **nasopharyngeal b.,**

pharyngeal b. Thornwaldt's b. **Thornwaldt's (Tornwaldt's) b.,** chronic inflammation of the pharyngeal bursa (see BURSA pharyngea), attended with formation of a pus-containing cyst and nasopharyngeal stenosis. It is associated with persistent nasopharyngeal drainage, occipital headache and stiffness of the posterior cervical muscles, exacerbation of pain with movement of the head, sore throat, persistent low-grade fever, and halitosis. Called also *nasopharyngeal b., pharyngeal b., Thornwaldt's (Tornwaldt's) disease, Thornwaldt's (Tornwaldt's) syndrome, thornwalditis,* and *tornwalditis.*

Burton's line, sign [Henry *Burton,* English physician, 1799–1849] lead LINE.

Burton vitalometer see under VITALOMETER.

Buschke's disease [Abraham *Buschke,* German dermatologist, 1868–1943] 1. European BLASTOMYCOSIS. 2. SCLEREDEMA adultorum.

Busse-Buschke disease [Otto *Busse,* German physician, 1867–1922; Abraham *Buschke,* German dermatologist, 1868–1943] European BLASTOMYCOSIS.

busulfan (bu-sul′fan) an alkanesulfonic acid ester, 1,4-butanediol dimethanesulfonate, occurring as a white, crystalline powder that is slightly soluble in water, ethanol, and acetone. It is an alkylating agent with cytotoxic and myelosuppressive properties. Used in the treatment of granulocytic leukemia, polycythemia vera, and thrombocytosis. Adverse reactions may include thrombocytopenia with hemorrhagic tendency, lymphocytopenia, nausea, vomiting, diarrhea, impotence, amenorrhea, sterility, fetal abnormalities, renal damage, cheilosis, glossitis, anhidrosis, excessive pigmentation, and gynecomastia. Trademarks: Mielucin, Misulban, Mitosan, Myeleukon, Myelosan, Myleran, Sulfabutin.

butabarbital sodium (bu″tah-bar′bĭ-tal) an intermediate-acting barbiturate, 5-ethyl-5-(l-methylpropyl)-2,4,6(1H,3H,5H) pyrimidinetrione monosodium salt, which occurs as a white powder. Used as a sedative and hypnotic. Trademark: Butisol.

butacaine sulfate (bu″tah-kān′) a potent local anesthetic, 3-(dibutylamino-1-propanol-*p*-aminobenzoate) sulfate, occurring as a white, odorless, crystalline powder with a numbing taste, which is readily soluble in alcohol and chloroform, slowly soluble in water, and insoluble in ether, and is unstable when exposed to light. Applied to mucous membranes of the eye, ear, nose, and throat. Trademark: Butyn.

Butadion trademark for *phenylbutazone.*

Butalgin trademark for the *dl*-form of *methadone hydrochloride* (see under METHADONE).

butamben (bu-tam′ben) a local anesthetic, 4-aminobenzoic acid butyl ester, occurring as a white, odorless, tasteless, crystalline powder that is soluble in dilute acids, alcohol, ether, and chloroform. Called also *butyl aminobenzoate.* Trademarks: Butesin, Butoform. **b. picrate,** a picrate derivative of butamben, consisting of one molecule of trinitrophenol and two molecules of butamben (4-aminobenzoic acid butyl ester); used as a topical anesthetic for the treatment of burns, ulcers, and denuded areas of the skin.

butane (bu′tān) an aliphatic hydrocarbon, C_4H_{10}, derived from petroleum, occurring as a flammable gas; used as a fuel and in chemical synthesis. In high concentrations, butane is a simple asphyxiant and a potential narcotic.

Butazolidin trademark for *phenylbutazone.*

Butesin trademark for *butamben.*

Butethanol trademark for *tetracaine hydrochloride* (see under TETRACAINE).

Butisol trademark for *butabarbital sodium* (see under BUTABARBITAL).

Butler-Albright syndrome [Allan May *Butler;* Fuller *Albright,* Boston physician, born 1900] Lightwood-Albright SYNDROME.

Butler-Lightwood-Albright syndrome [A. M. *Butler;* Reginald *Lightwood;* F. *Albright*] Lightwood-Albright SYNDROME.

Butoform trademark for *butamben.*

butt (but) 1. to bring the surfaces of two distinct objects squarely or directly into contact with each other. 2. to place directly against the tissues covering the residual alveolar ridge.

butter (but′er) [L. *butyrum;* Gr. *boutyron*] the oily mass procured by churning cream; also a substance with a butter-like consistency. **cacao b., cocoa b.,** theobroma OIL.

button (but′n) 1. a knoblike elevation or structure. 2. a knoblike device used in surgery. Called also *bouton.* 3. a button-like formation, being excess metal remaining from casting and sprue, located at the end of the sprue, opposite the casting. **Biskra b.,** cutaneous LEISHMANIASIS. **implant b.,** intramucosal

INSERT. **lingual b.,** a round orthodontic attachment welded to the lingual side of bands bonded to the cuspid, bicuspid, or molar.

buttonhole (but′n-hōl) 1. a short straight incision into a cavity or organ. See also buttonhole APPROACH. 2. an abnormal narrowing of the caliber of a structure.

buttressing (but′tres-ing) building an external support to steady a structure. **b. bone formation,** buttressing bone FORMATION.

butyl (bu′til) a four-carbon hydrocarbon radical, $CH_3CH_2CH_2CH_3-$ or C_4H_9-. Abbreviated *Bu.* See also ISOBUTYL. **b. aminobenzoate,** butamben.

butylmercaptomethylpenicillin (bu″til-mer″kap-to-meth″il-pen″ĭ-sil′in) penicillin BT.

butylthiomethylpenicillin (bu″til-thi″o-meth″il-pen″ĭ-sil′in) penicillin BT.

Butyn trademark for *butacaine sulfate* (see under BUTACAINE).

butyrate (bu′tĭ-rāt) a salt or ester of butyric acid.

butyric (bu-tir′ik) derived from butter, as butyric acid.

Buzon trademark for *phenylbutazone.*

bypass (bi′pas) an auxiliary flow; a shunt.

byte (bīt) 1. a binary character serving as a unit of information, usually shorter than a computer word. 2. the representation of a character. 3. a unit of information for processing in certain types of computers, being a measurable portion of consecutive binary digits, e.g., an 8-bit or 6-bit byte.

C

C 1. cathode (or cathodal); Celsius or centrigrade (see under SCALE); complement. 2. carbon.

^{12}**C** carbon-12 (see under CARBON).

^{13}**C** carbon-13 (see under CARBON).

^{14}**C** carbon-14 (see under CARBON).

°**C** degree on the Celsius scale (see under SCALE).

C$_H$ see constant DOMAIN.

C$_L$ see constant DOMAIN.

c 1. curie. 2. centi-. 3. carat.

CA chronologic AGE.

Ca 1. cathode (or cathodal). 2. cancer. 3. calcium.

^{45}**Ca** calcium-45; a radioactive isotope of calcium; see RADIOCALCIUM.

ca. L. *cir′ca,* about.

cabinet (kab′ĭ-net) a small closet or place of enclosure.

Cabot's ring (ring body) [Richard C. *Cabot,* American physician, 1868–1939] see under RING.

cac- see CACO-.

cacao (kah-ka′o) 1. cocoa. 2. *Theobroma cacao.* **c. butter,** theobroma OIL.

cachexia (kah-kek′se-ah) [*cac-* + Gr. *hexis* habit + *-ia*] a profound and marked state of constitutional disorder; general ill health.

caco-, cac- [Gr. *kakos* bad] a combining form meaning bad, or ill.

cacodontia (kak″o-don′she-ah) [*caco-* + Gr. *odous* tooth + *-ia*] a term formerly used for a condition of having diseased or bad teeth.

cadaver (kah-dav′er) [L. from *cadere* to fall, to perish] a dead body; generally applied to a human body preserved for anatomical study. See also CORPSE.

Cadesco Premium trademark for a medium hard *dental casting gold alloy* (see under GOLD).

cadmium (kad′me-um) [L. *cadmia;* Gr. *kadmeia* ancient name for calamine, zinc carbonate] a metallic element. Symbol, Cd; atomic weight, 112.41; atomic number, 48; specific gravity, 8.65; valence, 2; group IIB of the periodic table. Its isotopes range in mass number from 103 to 121. Cadmium is a soft, blue-white, malleable metal that oxidizes readily in humid air, reacts slowly with hydrochloric acid, and is resistant to alkalies. It has a wide variety of industrial applications, and is used in easily fusible alloys, including a dental amalgam (1 Cd:4 Hg). Cadmium salts are toxic and ingestion of either metallic cadmium or its soluble compounds may cause intense salivation, vomiting, abdominal distress, renal disorders, headache, and anemia. Inhalation of cadmium dust or fumes may produce headache, vomiting, chest pain, restlessness, bronchopneumonia, and irritability. It sometimes is used as an agricultural anthelmintic.

caduceus (kah-du′se-us) the wand of Hermes or Mercury, the messenger of the gods. Used as a medical symbol and as the emblem of the Medical Corps, U.S. Army. The official symbol of the medical profession is the staff of Æsculapius (see under STAFF). See illustration.

caeno- [Gr. *kenos* empty] see CENO-(2).

caesium (se′ze-um) cesium.

Cafergot trademark for a preparation containing ergotamine tartrate and caffeine; used in the treatment of migraine.

caffeine (kah-fēn′, kaf′fe-in) [L. *caffeina*] a xanthine derivative, 1,3,7-trimethylxanthine, occurring as a bitter, odorless white crystalline powder that is readily soluble in chloroform and slightly soluble in water, alcohol, and ether. In solution, it is neutral to litmus. Coffee beans, tea leaves, kola nuts, maté, and by-products of decaffeinized coffee are its main sources, but it is also produced synthetically. Its pharmacological effects include stimulation of the central nervous system, action on the kidneys resulting in diuresis, stimulation of the cardiac muscle, and relaxation of the smooth muscles. It is used therapeutically in congestive heart failure to relieve paroxysmal dyspnea, in headache (in combination with analgesics), and in intoxication with central depressants. Death from caffeine overdosage is unlikely, but excessive intake may produce untoward reactions with insomnia, excitement, restlessness, and, in severe cases, tachycardia, tremor, diuresis, and sensory disturbances, such as tinnitus and flashes of light. In dental patients, it may counteract the action of sedatives. Central depressants, such as barbiturates, usually relieve the symptoms. Called also *coffeine, thein, guaranine,* and *methyltheobromine.* Trademark: No-Doz.

caffeinism (kaf′ēn-izm, kaf′e-in-izm″) a condition resulting from excessive intake of caffeine, either as a medicinal preparation or in the form of coffee or other caffeine-containing substances.

Caffey's syndrome [John *Caffey,* American pediatrician, born 1895] infantile cortical HYPEROSTOSIS.

Caffey-Kempe syndrome [J. *Caffey;* C. H. *Kempe,* American physician] battered CHILD.

Caffey-Silverman syndrome [J. *Caffey;* William A. *Silverman*] infantile cortical HYPEROSTOSIS.

Caffey-Smyth disease, syndrome [J. *Caffey;* Francis Scott *Smyth*] infantile cortical HYPEROSTOSIS.

cage (kāj) a box or enclosure.

caino- [Gr. *kainos* new, fresh] see CENO-(1).

cajeputol (kaj′ĕ-pu-tol) eucalyptol.

Cal large CALORIE.

cal small CALORIE.

calamine (kal′ah-mīn, kal′ah-min) 1. a native form of zinc silicate which is a source of metallic zinc, being unsuitable for making medicinal calamine. 2. a mixture of zinc oxide and ferric oxide, occurring as an odorless, tasteless, pink powder that is soluble in mineral acids, but not in water. Used chiefly as an astringent and protective and in the preparation of soothing ointments and lotions for sunburn, poison ivy poisoning, and other skin lesions. Called also *artificial c., prepared c., aerosus lapis,* and *lapis calaminaris.* **artificial c., prepared c.,** calamine (2).

Cal-Aspirin trademark for *calcium acetylsalicylate* (see under CALCIUM).

Calcamine trademark for *dihydrotachysterol.*

calcar (kal′kar) [L. "spur"] a spur, or a structure resembling a spur.

calcarea (kal-ka′re-ah) [L.] CALCIUM hydroxide or CALCIUM oxide.

calcareous (kal-ka′re-us) [L. *calcarius*] pertaining to or containing lime or calcium; chalky.

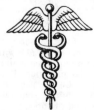

Caduceus. (From The Random House Dictionary of the English Language, © copyright, 1981 by Random House, Inc.)

calcarine (kal′kar-in) [L. *calcarinus* spur-shaped] 1. spur-shaped. 2. pertaining to calcar.

calcariuria (kal-ka″re-u′re-ah) [L. *calcarius* containing lime + Gr. *ouron* urine + *-ia*] the presence of calcium salts in the urine.

calcemia (kal-se′me-ah) [*calcium* + Gr. *haima* blood + *-ia*] the presence in the blood of excessive amounts of calcium; hypercalcemia.

calcic (kal′sik) of or pertaining to lime or to calcium.

calciferol (kal-sif′er-ol) vitamin D₂.

calcification (kal″sĭ-fĭ-ka′shun) [*calcium* + L. *facere* to make] the process by which organic tissue becomes hardened by a deposit of calcium salts within its substance. **diffuse pulp c.,** pulp c., diffuse. **dystrophic c.,** deposits of calcium salts in injured, degenerating, or dead tissues, which may occur with normal blood calcium levels. It may be encountered in any form of tissue injury, but especially in the presence of suppurative liquefaction, coagulation necrosis, fatty degeneration, and enzymatic necrosis. The most frequent types include calcification in tuberculous necrosis, arteriosclerosis, and scars. The gingivae, tongue, or cheeks are the most common sites of dystrophic calcification. Benign fibromas of the oral cavity and adjacent structures may also contain areas of calcification. See also *pulp c., diffuse.* **metastatic c.,** deposits of calcium salts in previously undamaged tissues, usually involving the kidneys, alveolar walls of the lungs, and gastric mucosa. Except for kidney stones, metastatic calcification does not appear to cause clinical dysfunction. **pathologic c.,** a condition characterized by abnormal deposits of calcium salts in the tissue, including dystrophic calcification, metastatic calcification, and calcinosis. **pulp c., c. of pulp, c. of pulp chamber,** mineralization of the dental pulp components due to deposits of calcium salts. It progresses as the affected person grows older, eventually leading to narrowing and sometimes obliteration of the pulp cavity. The process may be stimulated by trauma, deep fillings, carious lesions, traumatic occlusion, and other conditions. The condition may occur as diffuse calcific regression with hardening throughout the tissue or as a focal calcific regression with formation of calcified concretions. See also *pulp c., diffuse* and DENTICLE (2). **pulp c., diffuse, c. of pulp, diffuse,** dystrophic calcification in the root canals of teeth, characterized by formation of amorphous, unorganized linear strands or columns paralleling the blood vessels and nerves of the pulp. Called also *calcific degeneration.* **pulp c., fibrillar, c. of pulp, fibrillar,** a form of calcification of the dental pulp usually observed in older persons, which begins in the walls of the vascular channels or in the perineurium of the larger nerve trunks, and progresses along the blood vessels and nerves of the dental pulp, resulting in the formation of amalgamated spicules within the tissue. **root canal c.,** hardening and deposition of calcareous materials in the middle and apical portion of the root canal of a tooth, sometimes rendering the canal inaccessible for root canal therapy.

calcigerous (kal-sij′er-us) [*calcium* + L. *gerere* to bear] producing or carrying calcium.

calcination (kal″sĭ-na′shun) [L. *calcinare* to char] heating of a solid substance to bring about a state of thermal decomposition or dissociation, including polymorphic phase transition or thermal recrystallization, as in devitrification of glass and ceramics. Used to drive off gases from a substance or to remove water of crystallization, as in calcination of gypsum hemihydrate.

calcinosis (kal″sĭ-no′sis) a condition marked by the deposition of calcium salts in the skin and subcutaneous tissues. Deep structures, such as tendons and muscles, may also be involved. Calcium deposits may occur in apparently normal tissue, or in tissues damaged by a previous disorder, such as scleroderma or dermatomyositis. Blood calcium and phosphorus are usually normal. **c. circumscrip′ta,** local calcinosis usually confined to the skin and subcutaneous tissues of the extremities. **c. cu′tis,** a condition marked by deposition of calcium salts in the skin in the form of nodules or plaques. **c. infan′tum,** Lightwood-Albright SYNDROME. **c. interstitia′lis,** abnormal deposits of calcium in the connective tissue. **c. universa′lis,** a widespread form of calcinosis affecting the entire body.

Calciofon trademark for *calcium gluconate* (see under CALCIUM).

Calciopen K trademark for *penicillin V potassium* (see under PENICILLIN).

Calcipen V trademark for *penicillin V calcium* (see under PENICILLIN).

calcipenia (kal″sĭ-pe′ne-ah) [*calcium* + Gr. *penia* poverty] calcium deficiency. See HYPOCALCEMIA.

calcipexy (kal″sĭ-pek′se) [*calcium* + Gr. *pexis* fixation] fixation of calcium in the tissues.

calciphylaxis (kal″sĭ-fĭ-lak′sis) the formation of calcified tissue in response to administration of a challenging agent subsequent to induction of a hypersensitive state.

calciprivia (kal″sĭ-priv′e-ah) [*calcium* + L. *privus* without + *-ia*] deprivation or loss of calcium.

calcitonin (kal″sĭ-to′nin) a hormone of the thyroid gland, also produced in smaller amounts by the parathyroid glands. Calcitonin controls blood calcium levels by decreasing the renal tubular secretion of calcium, inhibiting calcium pumping in various cells, and decreasing the movement of calcium salts from bones to the blood. It also increases renal excretion of phosphates. Pharmacologically, it is isolated from pig thyroids and is used in the treatment of hypercalcemia, especially in hyperparathyroidism and in Paget's disease. Facial flushing and mild nausea may occur during calcitonin therapy. Called also *thyrocalcitonin.*

calcium (kal′se-um) [L. *calx* lime] a lustrous, silvery alkaline earth metal. Symbol, Ca; atomic number, 20; atomic weight, 40.08; valence, 2; group IIA of the periodic table. There are six stable isotopes of calcium: 40, 42–44, 46, 48. It reacts with water, alcohols, and acids with evolution of hydrogen. In finely powdered form, calcium ignites in air; contact with alkali hydroxides or carbonates may be explosive. It is found in nature only in compounds. Calcium is an essential component of bones and teeth, and is found in nearly all body tissues; 99 per cent of all body calcium being found in the skeleton as calcium carbonate or phosphate. In blood coagulation, calcium acts as a thrombokinase cofactor (known as factor IV) in conversion of prothrombin into thrombin. It is also essential in the regulation of membrane permeability and in the maintenance of the cardiac rhythm, muscle contraction, body function in newborn infants, lactation, and renal tubular function. It has been suggested that salivary calcium plays a role in dental caries etiology. For calcium deficiency, see HYPOCALCEMIA. See also HYPERCALCEMIA and HYPERCALCINURIA. For daily requirements of calcium, see table at NUTRITION. **c. acetylsalicylate,** a white powder that dissolves in water and alcohol, 2-(acetyloxy)benzoic acid calcium salt. Used as an analgesic, antipyretic, and antirheumatic. Called also *c. aspirin, acetylsalicylic acid calcium salt, salicylic acid acetate calcium salt,* and *soluble aspirin.* Trademarks: Ascal, Cal-Aspirin, Dispril, Disprin, Solprin, Tylcalsin. **c. aluminosilicate,** calcium FELDSPAR. **c. aminosalicylate,** calcium AMINOSALICYLATE. **c. aspirin,** c. acetylsalicylate. **c. ascorbate,** a white, yellowish, odorless crystalline powder that is soluble in water and slightly soluble in alcohol, but insoluble in ether. Used in the treatment of scurvy and as a food preservative and additive. Called also *ascorbic acid calcium salt.* **c. biphosphate,** c. phosphate, monobasic. **c. carbonate,** an odorless, tasteless, stable, noncombustible, nontoxic powder or crystals that are readily soluble in acids, with evolution of carbon dioxide, but only slightly soluble in water. Most of the calcium in the body occurs in the skeleton as calcium carbonate. Calcium is found in natural form in aragonite, oyster shells, calcite, chalk, limestone, marble, and travertine. Chemically produced preparations of calcium are known as *precipitated calcium carbonate* and *precipitated chalk* (trademarks: Aeromatt, Albacar, Purecal); in prepared form, they are known as *prepared calcium carbonate, prepared chalk, whiting, English white,* and *Paris white.* Calcium carbonate preparations are used in a variety of industrial products, and in dentifrices, insecticides, and drugs. They are also useful in dental laboratories as abrasive polishing material. Also used as an antacid. **chelated c.,** calcium forming a salt or complex with a chelating agent, such as ethylenediamine tetraacetic acid. See also CHELATION. **c. chloride,** CaCl₂; white, odorless, hygroscopic granules that are soluble in water (with heat liberation) and alcohol. Used in solution as an electrolyte replacement, in the treatment of hypocalcemic conditions, and as a diuretic, urinary acidifier, and antiallergic agent. Calcium chloride is relative nontoxic, but administration may cause gastrointestinal and cardiac disorders. Injections may produce irritation of veins accompanied by peripheral vasodilatation and a burning sensation. **c. diphosphate,** c. pyrophosphate. **c. disodium edetate, c. disodium ethylenediaminotetraacetate, c. disodium versenate,** a white, odorless, slightly hygroscopic, crystalline powder with a faint saline taste, disodium [[N,N′-1, 2-ethanediylbis[N-(carboxymethyl)glycinato]](4−)-N,N′,O,O′,Oᴺ,Oˣ]calciate(2−), which is soluble in water, but not in organic solvents. It is a chelating agent used chiefly in food preservation and in the treatment of heavy metal poisoning. Side reactions may include fever, malasie, fatigue, thirst, chills, myalgia, headache, vomiting, nasal congestion, lacrimation, glycosuria, anemia, dermatitis, and excessive urination. Called also *c. EDTA, edathamil calcium disodium, edetic acid calcium disodium salt,* and *sodium calcium edetate.* Trademarks: Antalin, Mosatil, Sormetal. **c. EDTA,** c. disodium edetate. **c. feldspar,** calcium FELDSPAR. **c. gluconate,** $C_{12}H_{22}CaO_{14}$; a white, colorless powder or granules that are tasteless, D-gluconic acid calcium salt. Used in solution in the treatment of hypocalcemic conditions. Trademarks: Calciofon, Calglucon, Glucal. **c. glycerophosphate,** odorless, almost tasteless, white crystalline powder with low toxicity, glycerophosphoric acid calcium salt, which is soluble in water, but not in alcohol. Used in the treatment of calcium and phosphorus deficiency, as a food stabilizer, and in dentifrices and baking powder. Called also *phosphoric acid glycerol esters calcium salt*. Trademark: Neurosin. **c. hydrate,** c. hydroxide. **c. hydroxide,** a white powder with a slightly bitter alkaline taste, produced by the action of calcium oxide with water. It readily absorbs CO_2 from air to form $CaCO_3$, and loses water when ignited to form calcium oxide. It is slightly soluble in water and readily dissolves in glycerin, acids, and syrup, but not in alcohol. Calcium hydroxide is used in pulp capping in which it is applied directly to the exposed areas before placing an overlay of zinc phosphate or other suitable material. It is effective in inducing continued root closure or apical bridging in immature permanent teeth which have lost their vitality before apical closure, but chronic pulpitis may persist after pulp capping and occasional internal absorption of the dentinal wall with pulp necrosis may occur. Calcium hydroxide suspensions are also used as cavity liners. Called also *c. hydrate, hydrated lime,* and *slaked lime.* Trademarks: Dycal, Hydroxyline, Hypo-Cal, Pulpdent cavity liner, Pulpdent pulp capping agent. **c. hydroxide cement,** calcium hydroxide CEMENT. **c. hypochlorite,** $Ca(OCl)_2$; a white crystalline solid that decomposes in water and alcohol. It is a chlorine carrier with algicidal, bactericidal, deodorant, disinfectant, fungicidal, and bleaching properties. Called also *c. oxychloride.* Trademark: Losantin. **c. iodide,** CaI_2; a hygroscopic yellowish-white crystalline powder that, when exposed to air, absorbs carbon dioxide and liberates iodine, and is soluble in water and ethyl and amyl alcohol. Used as an expectorant agent. **c. lactate,** white, almost odorless granules of powder, 2-hydroxypropanoic acid calcium salt, that is soluble in water, but not in alcohol. Used in the treatment of calcium deficiency, in the treatment of tetany (its absorption being enhanced by the simultaneous administration of lactose), and in the preparation of dentifrices. **c. levulinate,** $C_{10}H_{14}CaO_6$; a white powder with faint odor of burnt sugar and bitter salty taste, 4-oxopentanoic acid calcium salt, which is soluble in water and slightly soluble in alcohol, but insoluble in ether and chloroform. Used as a calcium replenisher in calcium deficiency. **c. monohydrogen phosphate,** c. phosphate, dibasic. **c. orthophosphate,** c. phosphate, tribasic. **c. orthotungstate,** c. tungstate. **c. oxide,** CaO; white hard lumps which crumble on exposure to moist air and react with water to form calcium hydroxide. Used to absorb carbon dioxide from air and as an industrial source of alkali. It is a strong caustic that may cause irritation of the exposed skin and mucous membrane. Called also *burnt lime, calx, quicklime,* and *unslaked lime.* **c. oxychloride,** c. hypochlorite. **c. para-aminosalicylate,** calcium AMINOSALICYLATE. **c. phosphate,** $CaPO_4$; a compound containing calcium and phosphate. Calcium phosphates are present in saliva, being partly bound to macromolecules, partly bound in inorganic ion pairs or complexes, and partly found in an unbound state, playing a role in cariogenesis. Therapeutically, the compound is used as a source of calcium and phosphate and as an antacid. Called also *bone phosphate.* See also APATITE. **c. phosphate, acid,** c. phosphate, monobasic. **c. phosphate, dibasic,** $CaHPO_4 \cdot 2H_2O$; a white, odorless, tasteless powder that is soluble in hydrochloric, nitric, and acetic acids, but not in alcohol, and slightly soluble in water. Used as an antacid and calcium and potassium replenisher. In anhydrous form, also used as a dental polishing agent. Called also *c. monohydrogen phosphate, secondary c. phosphate, bicalcium, dicalcium orthophosphate,* and *dicalcium phosphate.* **c. phosphate, monobasic,** $CaH_4(PO_4)_2$; colorless, pearly scales or powder that are soluble in water and acids. Used in fertilizers, baking powder, and food and feed supplements. Called also *acid c. phosphate, c. biphosphate, primary c. phosphate,* and *c. superphosphate.* **c. phosphate, precipitated,** c. phosphate, tribasic. **c. phosphate, primary,** c. phosphate, monobasic. **c. phosphate, secondary,** c. phosphate, basic. **c. phosphate, tertiary,** c. phosphate, tribasic. **c. phosphate, tribasic,** $Ca_3(PO_4)_2$; an amorphous, odorless, tasteless powder that is soluble in hydrochloric and nitric acid, but not in water, alcohol, and acetic acid. Used chiefly as a gastric antacid, but also given

orally to replenish calcium and phosphorus. Used also in fertilizers, dental powders, and feed supplements. Called also *c. orthophosphate, precipitated c. phosphate, tertiary c. phosphate, tricalcium orthophosphate,* and *tricalcium phosphate.* **precipitated c. carbonate,** see *c. carbonate.* **prepared c. carbonate,** see *c. carbonate.* **c. pyrophosphate,** $Ca_2P_2O_7$; a white powder or crystals that are soluble in hydrochloric and nitric acids, but not in water. Used as a fine polishing agent in dentifrices and for dentures. Also used as an abrasive, fertilizer, and feed supplement. It has a very low toxicity. Called also *c. diphosphate.* **radioactive c.,** an artificial radioactive isotope of calcium; namely, ^{41}Ca, ^{45}Ca, or ^{47}Ca. ^{45}Ca, with a half-life of 180 days, is the isotope used most commonly as a tracer in the study of calcium metabolism. Called also *radiocalcium.* **c. saccharin,** white crystals or a white crystalline powder with a faint aromatic odor and a very sweet taste, 1,2-benzisothiazolin-3-one 1,1-dioxide calcium salt. Used as a nonnutritive sweetener. **c. sulfate,** a compound occurring in the natural anhydrous form as anhydrite, $CaSO_4$, and in the natural hydrated form as gypsum, or gypsum dihydrate, $CaSO_4 \cdot 2H_2O$. **c. sulfate, dried,** GYPSUM hemihydrate. **c. sulfate hemihydrate,** GYPSUM hemihydrate. **c. sulfate, native,** c. sulfate, precipitated, gypsum. **c. superphosphate,** c. phosphate, monobasic. **c. tungstate,** $CaWO_4$; a white crystalline powder, occurring in nature as scheelite, which is insoluble in water, but dissolves in hot hydrochloric and other acids. It had been used for injection into malignant tumors to provide transillumination in x-ray treatment, and for coating radiographic intensifying screens to control fluorescence when struck by x-rays. Called also *c. orthotungstate* and *c. wolframate.* **c. wolframate,** c. tungstate.

calciuria (kal″sĭ-u're-ah) [*calcium* + Gr. *ouron* urine + *-ia*] the presence of calcium in the urine.

calcoglobulin (kal″ko-glob'u-lin) the form of globulin that occurs in calcifying tissue. See also CALCOSPHERITE.

calcospherite (kal″ko-sfēr'it) one of the small globular bodies formed during the process of calcification, by chemical union between the calcium particles and the albuminous organic matter of the intercellular substance. These particles coalesce to form calcoglobulin.

calculi (kal'ku-li) [L.] plural of *calculus.*

calculogenesis (kal″ku-lo-jen'ĕ-sis) [*calculus* + Gr. *genesis* production] the formation of calculi.

calculus (kal'ku-lus), pl. *cal'culi* [L. "pebble"] an abnormal concretion within the animal body, usually composed of mineral salts. **dental c.,** a hard, stonelike concretion, varying in color from creamy yellow to black, which forms on the teeth or dental prostheses through calcification of dental plaque. It is composed mostly of calcium phosphate, but also contains calcium carbonate, magnesium phosphate, water, and organic matter, having many chemical and physical similarities with dentin, cementum, enamel, and bone. Calculus is usually strongly attached to the tooth surface, but, in most instances, it may be scaled off without difficulty. According to its location, there are two general types: supragingival and subgingival. Called also *odontolith, tartar,* and *tophus.* See also *salivary duct c.* **hard c.,** dental calculus that is very dense and resistant to scaling; it contains a high percentage of calcium phosphate or calcium carbonate with relatively small amounts of organic matter. **c. index,** see oral hygiene INDEX. **c. inhibitor,** plaque and calculus INHIBITOR. **invisible c.,** subgingival c. **salivary c.,** 1. sialolith. 2. supragingival c. **serumal c.,** subgingival c. **subgingival c.,** calculus located below the crest of the marginal gingiva, usually in periodontal pockets. It is usually dense and hard, dark brown or green-black, flintlike in consistency, and firmly attached to the tooth surface. Called also *invisible c.* and *serumal c.* **supragingival c.,** calculus covering the coronal surface of the tooth to the crest of the gingival margin. It is usually white or white-yellow, having a claylike consistency, and can be easily detached from the tooth surface. It may occur on a single tooth or on a group of teeth, or be generalized throughout the mouth, being most frequent on the buccal surfaces of the maxillary molars, lingual surfaces of the mandibular anterior teeth, and central incisors. In extreme cases, it may form a bridgelike structure along adjacent teeth or cover the occlusal surface of teeth without functional antagonists. Called also *visible c.* and *salivary c.* **tonsillar c.,** a calcareous concretion found in a tonsil. **visible c.,** supragingival c.

Caldwell position see under POSITION.

Caldwell projection [Eugene W. *Caldwell*] see under PROJECTION.

Caldwell-Luc operation [George W. *Caldwell*, American physician, 1834–1918; Henry *Luc*, French laryngologist, 1855–1925] see under OPERATION.

Calglucon trademark for *calcium gluconate* (see under CALCIUM).

caliber (kal′ĭ-ber) [Fr. *calibre* the bore of a gun] the diameter of a tubular structure or organ.

calibration (kal″ĭ-bra′shun) determination or rectification of the accuracy of an instrument used for measuring, according to existing standards or by comparison with a similar instrument.

calices (kal′ĭ-sēz) [L.] plural of *calix.*

Caliciviridae (kal″ĭ-sĭ-vĭ′rĭ-de) a family of naked, icosahedral viruses developing and replicating in the cytoplasm. The virion is 30 to 40 nm in diameter and it has 32 capsomers. The viruses in this family contain single-stranded RNA with molecular weight of 3×10^6 and a single polypeptide of approximately 60,000. They infect cats, pigs, and sea lions, frequently causing oral lesions, but do not infect man. At present, the family does not include any genera, only two types: vesicular exanthema virus and feline calicivirus. These viruses formerly constituted a genus (*Calicivirus*) of the family Picornaviridae.

Calicivirus (kal″ĭ-sĭ-vi′rus) a former genus of the family Picornaviridae, which has been elevated to the status of a family; see CALICIVIRIDAE.

calicivirus (kal″ĭ-sĭ-vi′rus) any virus of the family Caliciviridae. **feline c.,** a calicivirus occurring only in the cytoplasm and forming irregular or paracrystalline aggregates or linear arrays. Its virion is 30 to 40 nm in diameter. Infection with different strains ranges from being asymptomatic to respiratory symptoms.

caliculi (kah-lik′u-li) [L.] plural of *caliculus.*

caliculus (kah-lik′u-lus), pl. *calic′uli* [L. dim. of *calix*] a small, cup-shaped structure or cavity; a small calix. **c. gustato′rius** [NA], taste BUD.

californium (kal″ĭ-for′ne-um) [named after *California* (University and state), where it was produced] a man-made radioactive element, originally produced by bombarding curium-242 with 35 MeV helium ions. Symbol, Cf; atomic weight, 251; atomic number, 98; valences, 2, 3. It has several isotopes, ^{251}Cf being the most stable; ^{252}Cf and ^{249}Cf are available in milligram amounts. ^{252}Cf is believed to be a potential source of radiation in radiotherapy.

calipers (kal′ĭ-perz) an instrument having two adjustable curved legs or jaws, used for measuring the thickness or diameter of an object.

calix (ka′liks), pl. *cal′ices* [L.] 1. any cup-shaped organ or cavity. 2. one of the renal calices. **renal calices,** the recesses of the renal pelvis; the major calices are the larger subdivisions, into which the minor calices open.

Callahan's method [John R. *Callahan,* American dentist, 1853–1918] 1. root canal filling method, Callahan's; see under METHOD. 2. see under METHOD.

callosity (kah-los′ĭ-te) [L. *callositas,* from *callus*] a circumscribed thickening of the skin, and hypertrophy of the horny layer, usually due to friction, pressure, or other irritation.

callus (kal′us) [L.] 1. a callosity. 2. a meshwork of fibrous tissue, cartilage, and bone, which unites the fractured ends of bone; it is ultimately replaced by hard adult bone. **central c.,** a provisional callus formed within the medullary cavity of a fractured bone. Called also *inner c., internal c., medullary c., myelogenous c.,* and *pin c.* **definitive c.,** an exudate formed between the fractured ends of the bone; it is permanent and becomes changed into true bone. Called also *intermediate c.* **ensheathing c.,** provisional callus forming a sheath about the ends of the fragments of a fractured bone. **external c.,** callus which forms around the outside of two fragments of a fractured bone. **inner c.,** central c. **intermediate c.,** definitive c. **internal c., medullary c., myelogenous c., pin c.,** central c. **provisional c.,** a callus which is formed within the medullary cavity and provides a fusiform, temporary bony union of the fracture, and which is absorbed after the repair is completed. Called also *procallus.*

Calmette's serum [Albert Léon Charles *Calmette,* French bacteriologist, 1863–1933] antivenomous SERUM.

Calmodid trademark for *hydrocodone bitartrate* (see under HYDROCODONE).

calor (ka′lor) [L.] heat; a localized increase in body temperature, being a cardinal sign of inflammation. See also FEVER and PYROGEN.

calorie (kal′o-re) [Fr.; L. *calor* heat] a unit of heat. The term is commonly used alone to designate the *small calorie* (abbreviated *cal*). See also British thermal UNIT. **gram c.,** small c. **I.T. c., International Table c.,** a unit of heat, equivalent to 4.1868 joules. **large c.,** the calorie used in metabolic studies, being the amount of heat required to raise the temperature of 1 kilogram of water 1°C, being equal to 1000 small calories. Abbreviated *Cal.* Called also *kilocalorie (kg-cal).* **mean c.,** ¹⁄₁₀₀ of the amount of heat required to raise the temperature of 1 gram of water from 0 to 100°C. **small c., standard c.,** the amount of heat required to raise the temperature of 1 gram of water 1°C. Abbreviated *cal.* Called also *gram c. (g-cal).*

calorigenic (kah-lor″ĭ-jen′ik) [L. *calor* heat + Gr. *gennan* to produce] producing heat or energy; increasing heat or energy production; increasing the consumption of oxygen.

calorimeter (kal″o-rim′ĕ-ter) [L. *calor* heat + Gr. *metron* measure] an instrument for measuring the amount of heat exchanged in any system. In physiology, an apparatus for measuring the amount of heat produced by an individual.

calvaria (kal-va′re-ah) [L. "skull"] the domelike structure at the top of the skull, usually oval, but sometimes nearly circular, which is made up of the frontal, parietal, and occipital bones, and is traversed by the coronal, sagittal, and lambdoidal sutures. Called also *concha of cranium, cranial vault,* and *skullcap.*

calvarium (kal-va′re-um) [L.] calvaria.

calx (kalks) [L.] 1. lime or chalk. 2. the hindmost part of the foot; the heel. 3. any residue obtained by calcination. 4. CALCIUM oxide.

calyces (kal′ĭ-sēz) plural of *calyx.*

Calymmatobacterium (kah-lim″ah-to″bak-te′re-um) [Gr. *kalymma* a hood or veil + *baktērion* little rod] a genus of gram-negative, facultatively anaerobic bacteria of uncertain affiliation, occurring as pleomorphic rods (1.0 to 2.0 μ in length) with rounded ends, and found singly and in clusters. Called also *Donovania.* **C. granulo′matis,** the etiologic agent of granuloma venereum in man. Called also *Donovan's body* and *Donovania granulomatis.*

calyx (ka′liks), pl. *cal′yces* [Gr. *kalyx* cup of a flower] calix.

cAMP ADENOSINE 3′,5′-cyclic phosphate.

Camper's plane (line) [Pieter *Camper,* Dutch physician, 1722–1789] see under PLANE.

2-camphanone (kam′phah-nōn) camphor (1).

camphidonium (kam″fĭ-do′ne-um) TRIMETHIDINIUM methosulfate.

camphor (kam′for) [L. *camphora;* Gr. *kamphora*] 1. a compound obtained from the leaves of *Laurus* species or *Cinnamomum camphora,* occurring as a crystalline solid, granules, or powder with a penetrating characteristic odor and a pungent taste. It slowly volatilizes at room temperature, is slowly soluble in water, and readily soluble in alcohol and other organic solvents. When applied to the skin, it produces a mild local anesthetic action, sometimes followed by numbness; when applied vigorously, it is a rubifacient. Systemically, it is a central nervous system stimulant; large doses may cause convulsions. A 1 to 3 percent lotion or ointment is used as a topical antipruritic and counterirritant. Called also *gum c., 2-bornanone,* and *2-camphanone.* See also camphorated PARACHLOROPHENOL and SPIRIT of camphor. 2. a general term applied to other compounds having characteristics similar to those of camphor. **bitter almond oil c.,** BENZOIN (2). **cantharides c.,** cantharidin. **gum c.,** camphor (1). **peppermint c.,** menthol. **spirit of c.,** SPIRIT of camphor. **thyme c.,** thymol.

Campylobacter (kam″pĭ-lo-bak′ter) [Gr. *kampylos* curved + *baktērion* little rod] a genus of gram-negative, microaerophilic to anaerobic, non–spore-forming, spirally curved bacteria of the family Spirillaceae, made up of slender rods (about 0.2 to 0.8 μm in width and 0.5 to 5.0 μm in length). The organisms occur as comma-like, S-shaped, and gull-winged cells with a single polar flagellum, being motile with a corkscrew-like motion, and are found in the oral cavity, intestines, and reproductive organs of animals, including man; some strains are pathogenic. **C. bub′ulus,** *C. sputorum* subsp. *bubulus.* **C. feca′lis,** a species, 0.3 to 0.6 μm in width and 2.0 to 4.0 μm in length, found in the feces of sheep and in the vagina and semen of cattle. **C. co′li,** *C. fetus* subsp. *jejuni.* **C. fe′tus,** a comma-like, S-shaped, or gull-winged microaerophilic species, also found in spheroid or coccoid forms in old cultures. It occurs in three subspecies: *C. fetus fetus, C. fetus intestinalis,* and *C. fetus jejuni.* Called also *Spirillum fetus, Vibrio fetus,* and *V. fetus* var. *venerealis.* **C. fe′tus** subsp. **fe′tus,** a subspecies causing abortion and infertility in cattle, which is transmitted venereally. **C. fe′tus** subsp. **intestina′lis,** a subspecies causing abortion in sheep and sporadic abortion in cattle, as well as human infection, which is transmitted orally. It is sensitive to antibiotics, including chloramphenicol, dihydrostreptomycin, erythromycin, neomycin, tetracyclines, and penicillin. Called also *Vibrio fetus* var. *intestinalis* and *V. foetus-ovis.* **C. fe′tus** subsp. **jeju′ni,** a subspecies isolated from the placenta and aborted fetuses of sheep and from the intestine of normal animals, including man. It causes an acute gastroenteritis of man, and is transmitted orally. Called also *C. coli, C. jejuni, Vibrio hepaticus,* and *V. jejuni.* **C. jeju′ni,** *C. fetus* subsp. *jejuni.* **C. sputo′rum,** a gull-winged or comma-like species, about 0.3 to 0.6 μm in width and 2.0 to 4.0 μm in length. Called also *Vibrio sputorum.* **C. sputo′rum** subsp. **bub′ulus,** a subspecies isolated from the genital tracts of male and female cattle and sheep. Called also *C. bubulus, Vibrio bubulus,* and *V. sputorum* var. *bubulum.* **C. sputo′rum** subsp. **sputo′rum,** a subspecies found in the gingival crevices of man, representing about 5 percent of the flora.

canal (kah-nal′) a relatively narrow tubular passage or channel. See also CANALICULUS, CANALIS, and SEMICANAL. **accessory palatine c's,** palatine c's, lesser. **alveolar c.,** mandibular c. **alveolar c's,** alveolar c's of maxilla. **alveolar c's of maxilla,** several canals in the maxilla for passage of the posterior superior alveolar vessels and nerves, each canal beginning on the infratemporal surface of the maxilla at an alveolar foramen. Called also *posterior dental c's* and *canales alveolares maxillae* [NA]. **c. of Arantius,** DUCTUS venosus. **archenteric c.,** neurenteric c. **archinephric c.,** pronephric DUCT. **Arnold's c.,** a channel in the petrous portion of the temporal bone for passage of the auricular branch of the vagus nerve. **accessory c.,** root c., accessory. **basipharyngeal c.,** vomerovaginal c. **bayonet c.,** root c., bayonet. **blastoporic c.,** neurenteric c. **blunderbuss c.,** a root canal of an incompletely formed root of a tooth in which the apical diameter of the root canal is greater than that of the coronal or cervical canal, having a shape similar to that of the flaring out barrel of a blunderbuss. Called also *everted c.* and *blunderbuss apex.* **branching c.,** root c., accessory. **Braun's c.,** neurenteric c. **C-shaped c.,** root c., C-shaped. **calciferous c's,** canals containing lime salts in cartilage that is undergoing calcification. **caroticotympanic c's,** caroticotympanic canaliculi; see under CANALICULUS. **carotid c.,** a passage in the petrous portion of the temporal bone, which lodges the internal carotid artery, beginning on the inferior surface just anterior to the jugular foramen, and running anteromedially for about 2 cm; it is seen interiorly in the floor of the middle cranial fossa, where it meets the carotid sulcus on the body of the sphenoid bone. Called also *canalis caroticus* [NA]. **c's of cartilage,** canals in an ossifying cartilage during its stage of vascularization. **c. of chorda tympani,** CANALICULUS of chorda tympani. **chordal c.,** notochordal c. **Civinini's c.,** CANALICULUS of chorda tympani. **collateral pulp c.,** a branch of a dental pulp canal emerging from the root at a position on the tooth surface, other than the apex. See *root c., accessory.* **condylar c.,** condyloid c. **condyloid c.,** a perforation sometimes present in the floor of the condyloid fossa, which provides a passage for the condylar emissaria, veins which connect the intracranial and extracranial veins. Called also *condylar c., canalis condylaris* [NA], *canalis condyloideus,* and *posterior condyloid foramen.* **condyloid c., anterior,** hypoglossal c. **craniopharyngeal c.,** an embryonic canal which connects the hypophyseal diverticulum with the buccal ectoderm in fetal life. It occasionally persists after birth, connecting the presphenoid and postsphenoid structures. **curved c.,** root c., curved. **c. of Cuvier,** DUCTUS venosus. **dental c., inferior,** mandibular c. **dental c's, posterior,** 1. alveolar c's of maxilla. 2. alveolar foramina of maxilla; see under FORAMEN. **dentinal c's,** dentinal tubules; see under TUBULE. **dilacerated c.,** root c., dilacerated. **Dorello's c.,** an opening sometimes found in the temporal bone, through which the abducens nerve and inferior petrosal sinus together enter the cavernous sinus. **ethmoid c., anterior,** a canal for transmission of the nasal branch of the nasociliary nerve and the anterior ethmoidal vessels. It begins at the anterior ethmoidal foramen in the frontoethmoidal suture of the medial wall of the orbit, traverses the ethmoidal labyrinth medially, and enters the anterior cranial fossa at the junction of the frontal and ethmoid bones. Called also *anterior ethmoid foramen, cribroethmoid foramen, ethmoidal sulcus of Gegenbaur,* and *foramen ethmoidale anterius* [NA]. **ethmoid c., posterior,** a canal for transmission of the posterior ethmoid vessels and nerves. It begins at the posterior ethmoid foramen in the frontoethmoidal suture of the medial wall of the orbit and ends at the foramen at the junction of the frontal and ethmoid bones in the anterior cranial fossa. Called also *foramen ethmoidale posterius* [NA] and *posterior ethmoid foramen.* **everted c.,** blunderbuss c. **facial c.,** c. for facial nerve. **c. for facial nerve, fallopian c.,** a canal in the temporal bone for the facial nerve, beginning in the internal acoustic meatus and passing anterolaterally dorsal to the vestibule of the inner ear for about 2 mm. Turning sharply backward at the genu of the facial canal, it runs along the medial wall of the tympanic cavity, then turns inferiorly and reaches the exterior of the petrous part of the bone at the stylomastoid foramen. Called also *facial c., spiroid c., aqueduct of Fallopius, canalis facialis* [NA], *canalis Fallopii,* and *fallopian*

aqueduct. **gubernacular c's,** four small openings in young crania, one behind each incisor tooth. **c. of Guidi,** pterygoid c. **haversian c.,** one of the freely anastomosing channels in compact bone which, together with haversian laminae, forms the haversian system. Called also *nutrient c. of bone, plasmatic c., canalis nutricius ossis* [NA], and *haversian space.* See also haversian CANALICULUS and haversian SYSTEM. **Hensen's c.,** a small canal leading from the saccule to the cochlear duct. Called also *Reichert's c., canalis reuniens, ductus reuniens* [NA], and *Hensen's duct.* **Hirschfeld's c.,** interdental c. **Huguier's c.,** CANALICULUS of chorda tympani. **Huschke's c.,** a passage formed by union of the tubercles of the tympanic ring; it commonly disappears during childhood. **hypoglossal c.,** a short canal through the lateral part of the occipital bone at the base of the occipital condyle, which provides the exit for the hypoglossal nerve and the entry for the meningeal branch of the ascending pharyngeal artery. It may be partially or completely divided by a horizontal bony bar. Called also *anterior condyloid c., anterior condyloid foramen,* and *canalis hypoglossi* [NA]. **incisive c.,** one of the small canals opening into the incisive fossa of the hard palate, and transmitting small vessels and nerves from the floor of the nose into the front part of the roof of the mouth. Called also *anterior palatine c., nasopalatine c., anterior palatine groove, canalis incisivus* [NA], and *foramen of Stensen.* **infraorbital c.,** a canal beneath the orbital surface of the maxilla, continuous posteriorly with the infraorbital sulcus, and opening anteriorly on the anterior surface of the body of the maxilla in the infraorbital foramen. It contains the infraorbital vessels and nerve. Called also *canalis infraorbitalis* [NA]. **interdental c.,** one of the channels in the alveolar process of the mandible, between the roots of the medial and lateral incisors, for the passage of anastomosing blood vessels between the sublingual and inferior dental arteries. Called also *Hirschfeld's c.* **Jacobson's c., c. for Jacobson's nerve,** tympanic CANALICULUS. **lacrimal c.,** nasolacrimal c. **lateral c.,** a lateral branch of the main root canal of a tooth which is approximately perpendicular to it. See *root c., accessory.* **lateral inferior vomerobasilar c.,** palatovaginal c. **mandibular c.,** a canal that pierces the ramus and the body of the mandible between the mandibular and mental foramina, running under the alveoli and communicating with them by small openings, and opening to the exterior at the bicuspid teeth through the mental foramen. It transmits the inferior alveolar vessels and nerve, from which branches are distributed to the teeth. Called also *alveolar c., inferior dental c.* and *canalis mandibulae* [NA]. **maxillary c., superior,** a round opening in the medial part of the great wing of the sphenoid bone that transmits the maxillary branch of the trigeminal nerve. Called also *foramen rotundum ossis sphenoidalis* [NA] and *superior maxillary foramen.* **maxillary c's, alveolar,** alveolar c's of maxilla. **medullary c.,** marrow CAVITY. **nasal c.,** nasolacrimal c. **nasolacrimal c.,** a canal formed by the lacrimal sulcus of the maxilla, lacrimal bone, and inferior nasal concha; it contains the nasolacrimal duct. Called also *lacrimal c., nasal c.,* and *canalis nasolacrimalis* [NA]. **nasopalatine c.,** incisive c. **neurenteric c.,** a temporary communication at the site of the primitive pit between the cavities of the yolk sac and amnion in an 18-day-old embryo. Called also *archenteric c., blastoporic c.,* and *Braun's c.* **notochordal c.,** a tunnel extending from the primitive pit into the notochordal process of the embryo during the third week of development. It forms by inpocketing of the blastopore into the notochordal process, followed by the development of minute ostia that provide access to the amniotic and yolk cavities. Called also *chordal c.* **nutrient c. of bone,** haversian c. **optic c.,** one of the paired openings in the sphenoid bone where the small wings are attached to the body of the bone at the apex of the orbit. Each transmits one of the optic nerves and the ophthalmic artery of its side. Called also *canalis opticus* [NA], *foramen opticum ossis sphenoidalis,* and *optic foramen of sphenoid bone.* **palatine c's, accessory,** palatine c's, lesser. **palatine c., anterior,** incisive c. **palatine c's, lesser,** openings in the palatine bone that branch off the great palatine canal to carry the lesser and middle palatine nerves and vessels to the roof of the mouth. Called also *accessory palatine c's, posterior palatine c's, canales palatini,* and *canales palatini minores* [NA]. **palatine c., major,** a passage in the sphenoid and palatine bones for the greater palatine vessels and nerve. Called also *palatomaxillary c., pterygopalatine c., sphenopalatine c., Tourtual's c., canalis palatinus major* [NA], and *canalis pterygopalatinus.* **palatine c's, posterior,** palatine c's, lesser. **palatomaxillary c.,** palatine c., major. **palatovaginal c.,** a narrow canal located in the roof of the nasal cavity between the inferior surface of the body of the sphenoid bone and the sphenoidal process of the palatine bone; it opens posteriorly into the nasal cavity and anteriorly into the pterygopalatine fossa. Called also *lateral inferior vo-*

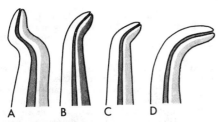

Various types of curved root canals. *A*, bayonet. *B*, curved. *C*, dilacerated. *D*, C-shaped. (From Warren T. Wakai: Case selection. *In* S. Cohen and R. C. Burns (eds.): Pathways of the Pulp. 2nd ed. St. Louis, The C. V. Mosby Co., 1980.)

merobasilar c., pharyngeal c., pterygopalatine c., sphenopalatine c., sphenopharyngeal c., canalis palatovaginalis [NA], and *canalis pharyngeus*. **perivascular c.,** a lymph space about a blood vessel. **pharyngeal c.,** palatovaginal c. **plasmatic c.,** haversian c. **pterygoid c.,** a horizontally running canal that passes forward through the base of the medial pterygoid plate of the sphenoid bone to open into the posterior wall of the pterygopalatine fossa just medial and inferior to the foramen rotundum; it transmits the pterygoid vessels and nerves. Called also *c. of Guidi, recurrent c., vidian c., canalis pterygoideus* [NA], and *canalis pterygoideus Vidii*. **pterygopalatine c.,** 1. palatine c., major. 2. palatovaginal c. **pulp c.,** root c. **pulp c., collateral,** collateral pulp c. **radicular c.,** root c. **recurrent c.,** pterygoid c. **Reichert's c.,** Hensen's c. **root c.,** the portion of the pulp cavity in the root of a tooth, extending from the pulp chamber to the apical foramen. More than one canal may be present in a single root, two commonly being present in the mesial root of the mandibular first molar. Dentin forms its inner wall, the wall usually being uninterrupted along its entire length. Occasionally, the canal may connect with smaller canals, the accessory root canals, apical foramina, and apical ramifications. Root canals are classified as follows: *class I, uncomplicated,* a mature root canal that is straight or gradually curved with constriction at the foramen; *class II, complicated,* a mature root canal that is severely curved or dilacerated, or with apical bifurcation, or auxiliary, lateral, or accessory canals, but with constriction of the foramen or foramina; *class III,* an immature root canal either flaring at the apex in blunderbuss apex, or having an open foramen; and *class IV,* a primary tooth undergoing resorption. Called also *pulp c., radicular c.,* and *canalis radicis dentis* [NA]. See also root canal THERAPY. **root c., accessory,** a lateral branching of the main root canal, which extends to the periodontal ligament. Any surface of the root, from the base of the coronal chamber to the apex, may open into an accessory canal. In the molar and the first bicuspid teeth the accessory canals may penetrate the interradicular fork and emerge from the floor of the pulp chamber. Accessory canals are most often found in the apical half of the roots and in furcation areas, although they may occur at any level. The tissue within the accessory and main root canals is basically the same. Called also *accessory c., branching c.,* and *secondary c.* See also apical FORAMEN and apical RAMIFICATION. **root c., bayonet,** a canal of the root of a tooth which is curved somewhat like a World War I bayonet. Called also *bayonet c.* and *double curve*. See illustration. **root c., C-shaped,** a root canal having a shape of the letter C, most commonly occurring in mandibular second molar teeth. Also called *C-shaped c., defalcated c., sickle-shaped c.,* and *defalcation*. See illustration. **root c., curved,** a root canal curving away from a lineal central axis; the tooth root having such a canal is likely to be curved as well. Called also *curved c.* See illustration. **root c., defalcated,** root c., C-shaped. **root c., dilacerated,** a canal of an abruptly curved root of a tooth. Called also *dilacerated c.* See illustration. **root c. disinfection, root c. sterilization,** root canal STERILIZATION. **root c. therapy,** root canal THERAPY. **secondary c.,** root c., accessory. **serous c.,** a minute lymph space. **sickle-shaped c.,** root c., C-shaped. **sphenopharyngeal c.,** palatovaginal c. **sphenopalatine c.,** 1. palatine c., major. 2. palatovaginal c. **spiroid c.,** c. for facial nerve. **sphenopharyngeal c.,** palatovaginal c. **c. of Steno, Stensen's c.,** parotid DUCT. **supraciliary c.,** a small opening sometimes present in or near the supraorbital notch; it transmits a nutrient artery and a branch of the supraorbital nerve to the frontal sinus. **supraoptic c.,** a minute canal which is the anterior continuation of the optic recess above the optic chiasma. **supraorbital c.,** supraorbital INCISURE. **Tourtual's c.,** palatine c., major. **van Hoorne's c.,** thoracic DUCT. **vidian c.,** pterygoid c. **Volkmann's c's,** minute cross channels, about 0.05 mm in diameter, for the passage of blood vessels through bone. **vomerine c.,** vomerovaginal c. **vomerobasilar c., lateral inferior,** palatovaginal c. **vomerobasilar c., lateral superior,** vomerovaginal c. **vomerovaginal c.,** an inconstant opening formed by the articulating margins of the wing of the vomer and the body of the sphenoid bone. Called also *basipharyngeal c., lateral superior vomerobasilar c., vomerine c., canalis basipharyngeus,* and *canalis vomerovaginalis* [NA]. **zygomaticofacial c., zygomaticotemporal c.,** zygomaticofacial FORAMEN.

canales (kah-na′lēz) [L.] plural of *canalis*.

canalicular (kan″ah-lik′u-lar) resembling or pertaining to a canaliculus.

canaliculi (kan″ah-lik′u-li) [L.] plural of *canaliculus*.

canaliculus (kan″ah-lik′u-lus), pl. *canalic′uli* [L., dim. of *canalis*] a very narrow tubular passage or channel. See also CANAL and CANALIS. **bone canaliculi,** slender, branching tubular passages radiating from the lacunae of compact bone, which penetrate the interstitial substance of the lamellae, and anastomose with the canaliculi of neighboring lacunae; believed to be essential in the nutrition of the bone cells. **canaliculi of true denticle,** minute canaliculi traversing irregularly through matrices of true denticles. **caroticotympanic canaliculi, canalic′uli caroticotympan′ici** [NA], numerous tiny passages in the temporal bone interconnecting the carotid canal and the tympanic cavity, and carrying communicating twigs between the internal carotid and tympanic plexuses. Called also *caroticotympanic canals* and *caroticotympanic foramina*. **cementum canaliculi,** minute tubular structures that house the protoplasmic extensions of cementocytes, which communicate with canaliculi from adjacent cells, although fusion of the cytoplasmic processes does not occur. **c. of chorda tympani, c. chor′dae tym′pani** [NA], a small canal that opens off the facial canal just before its termination, transmitting the chorda tympani nerve into the tympanic cavity. Called also *canal of chorda tympani, canalis chordae tympani, Civinini's canal,* and *Huguier's canal*. **c. of cochlea, c. coch′leae** [NA], a small canal in the petrous part of the temporal bone that interconnects the scala tympani of the inner ear with the subarachnoid cavity; it lodges the perilymphatic duct and a small vein. Called also *aqueduct of cochlea, aqueduct of Cotunnius,* and *aqueductus cochleae*. **dental canaliculi, canalic′uli denta′les** [NA], dentinal tubules; see under TUBULE. **haversian c.,** any one of a system of minute channels in compact bone connected with each haversian canal. See also haversian CANAL and haversian SYSTEM. **incisor c.,** incisive DUCT. **innominate c., c. innomina′tus,** SULCUS of lesser petrosal nerve. **lacrimal c.,** 1. the short passage in an eyelid, beginning at the punctum, which leads to the lacrimal sac. Called also *ductus lacrimalis* and *lacrimal duct*. 2. any passage for transmission of the secretion of the lacrimal glands. **mastoid c., mastoid c. for Arnold's nerve, c. mastoi′deus** [NA], a minute passaage beginning in the lateral wall of the jugular fossa of the temporal bone and passing into the temporal bone. The auricular branch of the vagus nerve passes through it to exit via the tympanomastoid fissure. **petrous c., c. petro′sus,** SULCUS of lesser petrosal nerve. **secretory canaliculi,** small intercellular spaces of the serous cells, which open into the acini. **Thiersch's c.,** one of the small channels in newly formed repair tissue through which the nutritive fluids circulate. **tympanic c., tympanic c. for Jacobson's nerve, c. tympan′icus** [NA], a small opening on the inferior surface of the petrous part of the temporal bone in the floor of the petrosal fossa; it transmits the tympanic branch of the glossopharyngeal nerve and a small artery. Called also *Jacobson's canal* and *canal for Jacobson's nerve*.

canalis (kah-na′lis), pl. *cana′les* [L.] a general anatomical term for a relatively narrow tubular passage or channel. Called also *canal*. See also SEMICANALIS. **cana′lis alveola′ris,** 1. alveolar canal of maxilla; see under CANAL. 2. mandibular CANAL. **cana′les alveola′res maxil′lae** [NA], alveolar canals of maxilla; see under CANAL. **c. basipharyn′geus,** vomerovaginal CANAL. **c. carot′icus** [NA], carotid CANAL. **c. chor′dae tym′pani,** CANALICULUS of chorda tympani. **c. condyla′ris** [NA], **c. condyloi′deus,** condyloid CANAL. **c. facia′lis** [NA], **c. Fallo′pii,** CANAL for facial nerve. **c. hypoglos′si** [NA], hypoglossal CANAL. **c. incisi′vus** [NA], incisive CANAL. **c. infraorbita′lis** [NA], infraorbital CANAL. **c. mandib′ulae** [NA], mandibular CANAL. **c. nasolacrima′lis** [NA], nasolacrimal CANAL. **c. nutri′cius os′sis** [NA], haversian CANAL. **c. op′ticus** [NA], optic CANAL. **cana′les palati′ni, cana′les palati′ni mino′res** [NA], palatine canals, lesser; see under CANAL. **c. palati′nus ma′jor** [NA], palatine canal, major; see under CANAL. **c. palatovagina′lis** [NA], palatovaginal CANAL. **c. pharyn′geus,** palatovaginal CANAL. **c. pterygoi′deus**

[NA], **c. pterygoi′deus Vi′dii,** pterygoid CANAL. **c. pterygopala-ti′nus,** palatine canal, major; see under CANAL. **c. rad′icis den′tis** [NA], root CANAL. **c. reu′niens,** Hensen's CANAL. **c. vomerovagina′lis** [NA], vomerovaginal CANAL.

canalization (kan″al-i-za′shun) 1. the formation of canals, natural, or morbid. 2. the surgical establishment of canals for drainage. 3. the formation of new canals or paths, especially blood vessels through an obstruction, such as a clot.

canavanine (kan-av′ah-nīn) a naturally occurring, nonessential amino acid, 2-amino-4-guanidinooxy-butyric acid, isolated from soy bean.

canavase (kan-av′ās) arginase.

cancellated (kan′sel-lāt-ed) having a latticelike structure, as the substantia spongiosa.

cancellous (kan′sĕ-lus) of a reticular, spongy, or lattice-like structure; said mainly of bony tissue.

cancer (kan′ser) [L. "crab"] the common name for a malignant tumor (see under TUMOR). Often used incorrectly as a synonym for carcinoma. **black c.,** malignant MELANOMA. **adenoid c.,** a malignant tumor made up of or containing cylindrical tubes lined with epithelium. **aniline c.,** cancer due to aniline dyes, occurring among those whose work requires exposure to aniline dyes. **apinoid c.,** scirrhous CARCINOMA. **c. atroph′icans,** scirrhous carcinoma surrounded by sclerosed and atrophied tissue. **betel c.,** buyo cheek c. **boring c.,** epithelioma of the skin of the face. **branchiogenous c.,** that originating in the superior cervical triangle, and supposed to be derived from an embryonal branchial cleft. **buyo cheek c.,** cancer of the cheek seen in natives of the Philippine Islands due to chewing buyo leaf or betel. Called also *betel c.* **cellular c.,** medullary CARCINOMA. **chondroid c.,** scirrhous carcinoma with a cartilage-like structure. **claypipe c.,** carcinoma of the lip due to irritation caused by a pipe stem. **colloid c.,** mucinous CARCINOMA. **contact c.,** that developing in a part of the body in contact with a previously existing malignant tumor. **cystic c.,** carcinoma that has undergone cystic degeneration. **dendritic c.,** papillary CARCINOMA. **c. a deux** [Fr. "cancer in two"], that attacking simultaneously or consecutively two persons who live together. **duct c.,** carcinoma arising from the epithelium of a duct. **endothelial c.,** endothelioma. **glandular c.,** adenocarcinoma. **hard c.,** scirrhous CARCINOMA. **pitch-worker's c.,** epithelioma of the face, neck, and scrotum seen in those who work in pitch. **retrograde c.,** a dormant atrophied malignant growth. **rodent c.,** rodent ULCER. **roentgenologists' c.,** a cancer, usually of the hands, in those whose work requires exposure to roentgen rays. **scirrhous c.,** scirrhous CARCINOMA. **smokers' c.,** epithelioma of the lip due to irritation by a pipe stem; also cancer of the oral cavity and throat, ascribed to injurious effects of smoking. **soft c.,** medullary CARCINOMA. **spindle cell c.,** a rare type of carcinoma affecting older persons, in which spindle-cell growth predominates, often associated with giant-cell cancer. These tumors may arise from any epithelial surface, but are found most often in sites that usually produce squamous or transitional cell carcinomas. **tubular c.,** an adenocarcinoma in which the cells are arranged in the form of tubules. **villous duct c.,** carcinoma with a villous growth pattern arising from the wall of a cyst.

canceremia (kan″ser-e′me-ah) the presence of cancer cells in the blood.

cancericidal (kan″ser-ĭ-si′dal) [*cancer* + L. *caedere* to kill] destructive to cancer or malignant cells.

cancerigenic (kan″ser-ĭ-jen′ik) [*cancer* + Gr. *gennan* to produce] giving rise to a malignant tumor; oncogenic.

CANCERLIT Cancer Literature; an acronym for a computer-searchable data base containing references dealing with neoplastic diseases, sponsored by the National Cancer Institute.

cancerology (kan″ser-ol′o-je) former name for ONCOLOGY.

cancerous (kan′ser-us) of the nature of or pertaining to cancer.

cancerphobia (kan″ser-fo′be-ah) 1. morbid dread of becoming affected with cancer. 2. delusion of being affected with cancer. Called also *carcinomatophobia* and *carcinophobia.*

CANCERPROJ Cancer Research Projects; an acronym for a computer-searchable data base containing references to descriptions of ongoing cancer research projects, collected by the Smithsonian Science Information Exchange and sponsored by the National Cancer Institute.

cancriform (kang′kri-form) resembling cancer; cancroid.

cancroid (kang′kroid) [*cancer* + Gr. *eidos* form] 1. resembling cancer; cancriform. 2. a skin cancer of a moderate degree of malignancy.

cancrum (kang′krum) [L.] canker. **c. o′ris,** noma.

candela (kan-del′ah) [L. *candela* candle] the SI unit of luminous intensity, being equal to 1/16 of the luminous intensity per square centimeter of a blackbody radiating at the temperature of the freezing point of platinum. Abbreviated *cd.* Called also *candle.* See also SI.

Candeptin trademark for candicidin.

candicidin (kan″dĭ-si′din) a broad-spectrum antifungal antibiotic produced by strains of *Streptomyces griseus,* occurring as a yellow to brownish powder with a fatty acid–like odor and a bitter taste. It is sensitive to light, humidity, and heat and is readily soluble in water, *n*-butanol solutions, and dimethyl sulfoxide, and slightly soluble in chloroform, acetone, and ethanol. Used especially in the treatment of candidiasis, and also of systemic mycoses, such as coccidioidomycosis, cryptococcosis, histoplasmosis, aspergillosis, sporotrichosis, phycomycosis, and North American blastomycosis. Rare hypersensitivity may occur. Trademarks: Candeptin, Vanobid.

Candida (kan′dĭ-dah) [L. *candidus* glowing white] a genus of dermatomycetous fungi (Fungi Imperfecti) characterized by the production of mycelia but not ascospores. *Candida* exists as a harmless inhabitant of both normal and abnormal mucous membranes, including that of the gastrointestinal tract and oral cavity, in symbiotic relation with many other microorganisms. Its growth is probably controlled by nutritional competition with other organisms and lactic acid–producing bacteria. The organism seeds itself in many preexisting pathologic processes, and may exaggerate the disease process. The use of antibiotics, to which *Candida* is relatively insensitive, often causes proliferation of its growth because of destruction of microorganisms living in symbiotic relation with the fungus. It is involved in a variety of opportunistic infections, ranging from temporary colonization of the buccal mucosa to disseminated fatal systemic mycosis. Formerly called *Monilia.* **C. al′bicans,** the most pathogenic species of *Candida.* The organism is a common harmless inhabitant of mucous membranes, but under certain conditions, such as a weakened state, poor hygiene, disruption of symbiotic relation, or preexisting pathologic condition, may cause infection. It has been implicated as the etiologic agent in perlèche, thrush, vaginitis, and various other infections.

candidal (kan′dĭ-dal) pertaining to or caused by fungi of the genus *Candida.*

candidiasis (kan″dĭ-di′ah-sis) any disease caused by infection with a fungus of the genus *Candida (Monilia),* especially *C. albicans.* The most common form of candidiasis involves the mucous membranes, including oral (see THRUSH) and vaginal and vulvovaginal candidiasis. Also relatively common are varieties of cutaneous candidiasis, including: candidal intertrigo, characterized by weeping, eroded lesions with a scalloped border, usually having a collar of overhanging scales and a red base, associated with satellite flaccid vesicopustules; candidal paronychia, characterized by ridges, furrows, and discoloration of the nails, sometimes associated with nail dystrophy; and candidiasis of the glabrous skin, in which the skin appears to have been immersed in water or exposed to occlusive wet dressings for a prolonged period, and characterized by maceration and erosion and redness of the skin, and the development of satellite pustules. Systemic candidiasis is relatively uncommon; bronchopulmonary and pulmonary forms being the most frequent. Called also *candidosis, moniliasis,* and *moniliosis.*

candidosis (kan-di-do′sis) candidiasis.

Candio-Hermal trademark for *nystatin.*

candle (kan′d'l) 1. a mass of wax or similar substance, usually cylindrical in shape, with a wick for burning, to furnish illumination or heat. 2. a cylindrical mass of material used as a filter in microbiology. 3. candela. See also *lumen* and *lux.* **international c.,** the unit of luminous intensity equal to the luminous intensity of 5 mm² of platinum at its solidification temperature. **meter c.,** lux.

Canesten trademark for *clotrimazole.*

canine (ka′nīn) [L. *canis* a dog] 1. pertaining to or like a dog. 2. canine TOOTH.

caninus (ka-ni′nus) 1. musculus caninus; see levator muscle of angle of mouth, under MUSCLE. 2. canine TOOTH.

canities (kah-nish′e-ēz) [L.] grayness or whiteness of the hair.

canker (kang′ker) [L. *cancrum*] ulceration, chiefly of the mouth and lips. Called also *cancrum.*

cannabicyclol (kah″nah-bī-si′klōl) a cannabinoid substance. See CANNABINOID.

cannabidiol (kah-nah′bī-dōl) a cannabinoid substance, (IR-*trans*)-2-[3-methyl-6-(1-methylethenyl)-2-cyclohexen-1-yl]-5-pentyl-1,3-benzenediol, occurring as a yellow resin or crystals that are soluble in ethanol, methanol, ether, benzene, chloroform, and petroleum ether, but not in water. It is a physiologically inactive component of cannabis. See also CANNABINOID.

cannabigerol (kah″nah-bi′jer-ōl) a cannabinoid substance. See CANNABINOID.

cannabinoid (kah-nab′ĭ-noid) [*Cannabis* + Gr. *eidos* form] any of the psychoactive substances obtained from the hemp plant (*Cannabis*), including cannabigerol, cannabicyclol, cannabinol, cannabidiol, cannabinolic acid, and other related substances; found in hashish, charas, bhang, ganja, dagga, and marihuana. The active substance is believed to be *l*-Δ⁹-tetrahydrocannabinol (Δ⁹-THC). Small doses may produce an increased sense of well-being, euphoria, feeling of relaxation, sleepiness, spontaneous laughter, and other behavioral changes. Decrease of muscle strength, impaired memory, and deterioration in capacity to carry out tasks requiring multiple mental steps usually takes place under the influence of higher doses. Still higher doses may induce hallucinations, delusions, paranoid feelings, altered sense of time, depersonalization, anxiety, and other symptoms of toxic psychoses. Increased heart rate and reddening of the conjunctivae are the principal physiologic effects. Investigated as a potential drug for allaying the symptoms of cancer chemotherapy.

cannabinol (kah-nah′bĭ-nōl) a cannabinoid substance, 6,6,9-trimethyl-3-pentyl-6H-dibenzol[*b,d*]pyran-1-ol, which is a physiologically inactive component of cannabis. See also CANNABINOID.

Cannabis (kan′ah-bis) [Gr. *kannabis* hemp] a genus of hemp plants. *C. sativa* contains psychoactive substances, such as cannabigerol, cannabicyclol, cannabinol, cannabidiol, cannabinolic acid, and other related esters that contain cannabinoid.

cannabis (kan′ah-bis) [Gr. *kannabis* hemp] the dried flowering tops of hemp plants, *Cannabis sativa*, which contain the active psychoactive substance *l*-Δ⁹-tetrahydrocannabinol, and is used for its euphoric and intoxicating effects. See also CANNABINOID.

Cannon's nevus [A. Benson *Cannon*] white sponge NEVUS.

cannula (kan′u-lah) [L. dim. of *canna* "reed"] a tube for insertion into a duct or cavity; during insertion its lumen is usually occupied by a trocar. Spelled also *canula*.

cannulation (kan″u-la′shun) the insertion of a cannula.

canon (kan′un) [L. "rule"] the working rule or formula for use in a scientific procedure. **C. of Medicine,** one of the oldest medical works, reputed to have been written about 2700 B.C. by Huang-Ti, the Yellow Emperor of China, containing two chapters on dentistry.

cant (kant) an inclination or slope. **c. of mandible,** the angle formed by the intersection of the mandibular (gonion–gnathion) plane with the sella–nasion or Frankfort Horizontal plane.

canthal (kan′thal) pertaining to a canthus.

cantharides (kan-thar′ĭ-dēz) [L.] a dried Spanish fly, *Lytta* (*Cantharis vesicatoria*), sometimes called "blister bug," the active substance of which is cantharidin. **c. camphor,** cantharidin.

cantharidin (kan-thar′ĭ-din) the active substance of cantharides, hexahydro-3αα,7αα-dimethyl-4β,7β-epoxyisobenzofuran-1,3-dione, occurring as white crystalline plates or scales that are soluble in acetone, chloroform, oils, ether, and hot water, but not in cold water. It is a rubefacient and vesicant drug to be applied only to the skin and mucous membranes. Following oral administration, the drug is absorbed from the gastrointestinal tract, causing vomiting, abdominal pain, and shock, and is excreted by the kidneys, causing irritation of the urinary tract with urgency of urination. Irritation of the urethra may cause priapism; hence, it is popularly known as an aphrodisiac. Called also *cantharides camphor.*

canthi (kan′thi) [L.] plural of *canthus.*

cantho- [Gr. *kanthos*] a combining form denoting relationship to the canthus.

cantholysis (kan-thol′ĭ-sis) [*cantho-* + Gr. *lysis* dissolution] surgical division of the canthus of an eye or of a canthal ligament.

canthoplasty (kan′tho-plas″te) [*cantho-* + Gr. *plassein* to form] plastic surgery of the medial and/or lateral canthus, especially section of the lateral canthus to lengthen the palpebral fissure; also, the surgical restoration of a defective canthus.

canthorrhaphy (kan-thor′ah-fe) [*cantho-* + Gr. *rhaphē* suture] the suturing of the palpebral fissure at either canthus.

canthotomy (kan-thot′o-me) [*cantho-* + Gr. *temnein* to cut] surgical division of the outer canthus.

canthus (kan′thus), pl. *can′thi* [Gr. *kanthos*] the angle at either end of the slit between the eyelids; the canthi are distinguished as outer or temporal, inner or nasal.

Cantil trademark for *mepenzolate bromide* (see under MEPENZOLATE).

cantilever (kan″tĭ-lev′er) a rigid construction or beam extending horizontally beyond its vertical support. A force directed against the unsupported end of the beam (a cantilever) acts as a lever,

in the same manner as pressure applied against a retainer engaged to an abutment tooth. See also cantilever BRIDGE.

Cantrex trademark for *kanamycin sulfate* (see under KANAMYCIN).

Cantril trademark for *mepenzolate bromide* (see under MEPENZOLATE).

canula (kan′u-lah) cannula.

caoutchouc (koo′chook) [Fr.] rubber (1).

cap (kap) a protective covering for the head or for a similar structure. **enamel c., germinal c.,** a caplike structure of the enamel organ developing during the cap stage of odontogenesis, and becoming a double-walled sac during the third month of fetal development. It is composed of an outer, convex wall (outer enamel layer) and an inner, concave wall (inner enamel layer); between the two is a filling of looser ectodermal cells which transforms into a stellate reticulum. See also cap STAGE and enamel ORGAN. **skull c.,** calvaria. **c. splint,** cap SPLINT.

capacitor (kah-pas′ĭ-tor) a device for holding and storing charges of electricity.

capacity (kah-pas′ĭ-te) [L. *capacitas,* from *capere* to take] 1. contents; volume. 2. the power and ability to receive, hold, retain, or contain, or the ability to absorb. 3. an expression of the measurement of material that may be held or contained. 3. the property by which a given body will take and hold an electric charge. 4. mental ability to receive, accomplish, endure, or understand. **cranial c.,** an expression of the amount of space within the cranium. **electrostatic c.,** the ratio of quantity of electricity to difference of potential. **functional residual c.,** the amount of air remaining at the end of normal quiet respiration. It is equal to the expiratory reserve volume plus residual air volume. Abbreviated *FRC.* **heat c.,** 1. specific HEAT. 2. thermal c. **inspiratory c.,** the volume of air that can be taken into the lungs on a full inspiration, starting from the resting inspiratory position; it is equal to the tidal volume plus the inspiratory reserve volume. Abbreviated *IC.* **maximum breathing c.,** the greatest volume of air that can be breathed in and out for a short time by voluntary effort. It is expressed as liters per minute. Abbreviated *MBC.* **maximum lung c.,** the total volume of air in the lungs after full inspiration, expressed as vital capacity plus residual volume. **thermal c.,** the amount of heat absorbed by a body in being raised from 15 to 16°C in temperature. Called also *heat c.* **total lung c.,** the total volume of air in the lungs after a forced inspiration. It represents the vital capacity plus the residual volume. Abbreviated *TLC.* **vital c.,** the volume of air that can be expelled from the lungs from a position of full inspiration, with no limit to the duration of either; it is equal to the inspiratory capacity plus the expiratory reserve volume.

Capastat trademark for *capreomycin sulfate* (see under CAPREOMYCIN).

Capazine trademark for *prochlorperazine.*

Capdepont syndrome [C. *Capdepont*] DENTINOGENESIS imperfecta.

Capdepont-Hodge syndrome [C. *Capdepont*] DENTINOGENESIS imperfecta.

capillarity (kap″ĭ-lār′ĭ-te) a manifestation of surface tension by which a liquid, when in contact with a solid, as in a capillary tube, is elevated or depressed, depending on the adhesive or cohesive properties of the liquid. Called also *capillary action.*

capillary (kap′ĭ-lar″e) [L. *capillaris* hairlike] 1. pertaining to or resembling a hair. 2. blood c. **arterial c.,** a blood capillary distal to the arterioles, which carries arterial blood. **blood c.,** a minute cylindrical vessel for carrying blood. In man, an average capillary has the diameter of an erythrocyte, or about 8 μ, and is made up of a single layer of endothelial cells in smaller capillaries, and of up to three layers of cells in large capillaries. The capillary wall acts as a semipermeable membrane between the blood and tissue fluid for the exchange of substances. Capillaries form a network in nearly all tissues, connecting the venules and the arterioles. Called also *capillary* and *vas capillare* [NA]. **erythrocyte c's,** capillaries in the bone marrow of early life which seem to produce erythrocytes. **lymphatic c.,** a small, thin-walled tubular structure of varying diameter; it ends blindly at one end and merges with other capillaries at the other end to form a network which collects excess tissue fluid and, together with lymph, empties it into larger lymphatic vessels. They often run parallel to the blood capillaries, absorbing leaked proteins and also allowing venous blood capillaries to reabsorb some materials. They are made of a single layer of flat endothelial cells and, in contrast to larger capillary vessels, do not have valves. **secretory c.,** one of the extremely fine canals situated between adjacent gland cells, being formed by the apposition of grooves in the surfaces of the cells. **sinusoidal c.,** sinusoid (2). **venous c's,** blood capillaries proximal to the venules, which carry venous blood.

capita (kap'ĭ-tah) [L.] plural of *caput.*

capitate (kap'ĭ-tāt) [L. *caput* head] head-shaped.

capitation (kap-ĭ-ta'shun) 1. in health insurance, fixed charges, assessed per capita or per family unit, for enrollment in a membership plan which provides health care services on a prepaid basis. 2. in health insurance, a fixed monthly or yearly charge paid to a doctor for health care services based on the number of patients assigned for treatment, whether the services are used or not.

capitonnage (kap″ĭ-to-nahzh') [Fr.] the surgical closure of a cyst cavity by applying sutures in such a way as to cause approximation of the opposing surfaces.

capitula (kah-pit'u-lah) [L.] plural of *capitulum.*

capitular (kah-pit'u-lar) pertaining to a capitulum or head of a bone.

capitulum (kah-pit'u-lum), pl. *capit'ula* [L. dim. of *caput* head] a general anatomical term for a little head, or a small eminence of a bone by which it articulates with another bone. **c. [process'sus condyloi'dei] mandib'ulae,** HEAD of mandible.

Capitus trademark for *ethosuximide.*

Capmaster trademark for a *mechanical triturator* (see under TRITURATOR).

capno- [Gr. *kapnos* smoke] a combining form signifying a sooty or smoky appearance; pertaining to carbon dioxide.

Capnocytophaga (kap″no-sĭ-tof'ah-gah) [*capno-* + Gr. *kytos* cell + *phagein* to eat] a genus of anaerobic, gram-negative, rod-shaped bacteria that have been implicated in the pathogenesis of periodontal disease. The organisms in this genus closely resemble *Bacteroides ochraceus.*

capnograph (kap'no-graf) [*capno-* + Gr. *graphein* to write] an instrument for measuring expiratory carbon dioxide level. Called also *carbon dioxide analyzer.* See also breath ANALYZER.

capnophilic (kap-no-fil'ik) [*capno-* + Gr. *philein* to love] growing best in the presence of carbon dioxide; said of bacteria.

Capostatin trademark for *capreomycin.*

capping (kap'ing) 1. the provision of a protective or obstructive covering. 2. in restorative dental procedures, the covering of cusps which have been weakened by caries with a protective metal overlay. See also RESTORATION. 3. in immunology, the formation of a cross-linked complex (cap) on the surface of a lymphocyte, produced by movement of the surface components toward one pole of the cell after reacting with antibody to these components or by reactivity with mitogen. Later, the cap disappears. 4. two-pour technique; see compression MOLDING. **pulp c.,** covering of an exposed or nearly exposed pulp with a protective dressing or cement to protect the pulp against further injury and to provide an environment for healing and repair processes. In direct capping, the dressing is placed directly over the pulp at the site of exposure. In indirect capping, it is placed over a thin partition of remaining dentin which, if removed, might expose the dental pulp. **pulp c., direct,** see *pulp c.* **pulp c., indirect,** see *pulp c.*

Capramol trademark for *aminocaproic acid* (see under ACID).

caprate (kap'rāt) a salt of capric acid, containing the radical $C_9H_{19}COO-$.

capreomycin sulfate (kap″re-o-mi'sin) an antibiotic produced by *Streptomyces capreolus,* occurring as a white or yellowish, odorless, amorphous powder that is soluble in water, but not in most organic solvents, and is sensitive to heat, moisture, and light. Used in the treatment of infections caused by acid-fast bacilli, especially tuberculosis. Hearing disorders, renal toxicity, pain and sterile abscesses at the site of injection, skin rashes, hypokalemia, eosinophilia, leukocytosis, leukopenia, and partial neuromuscular blockade are the potential side effects. Trademarks: Capastat, Caprolin, Capromycin, Capostatin.

Capripoxvirus (kah-prĭ″poks-vi'rus) [L. *caper* goat + *poxvirus*] a genus of poxviruses, causing poxlike disease in sheep, goats, and cattle.

caproate (kap'ro-āt) a salt of caproic acid, containing the radical $C_5H_{11}COO-$.

Caprocid trademark for *aminocaproic acid* (see under ACID).

Caprokol trademark for *hexylresorcinol.*

Caprolin trademark for *capreomycin sulfate* (see under CAPREOMYCIN).

Capromycin trademark for *capreomycin sulfate* (see under CAPREOMYCIN).

caprylate (kap'rĭ-lāt) a salt of caprylic acid. Called also *octoate.* **stannous c., tin c.,** stannous OCTOATE.

capsid (kap'sid) [L. *capsa* box] the protein shell that surrounds and protects the viral nucleic acid. In nonenveloped viruses, it contains the attachment proteins that interact with receptors on the host cell during viral attachment. It may have helical or cubic symmetry and is composed of structural units, or capsomers. According to the number of subunits possessed by capsomers, they are called dimers (2), trimers (3), pentamers (5), and hexamers (6). See illustration. **helical c.,** the capsid of a helical virus, resembling a cylinder with the RNA wound in a helix and encased by the structural units of the capsid. **icosahedral c.,** a capsid forming the icosahedron in a virion, capsomers on the faces of the icosahedron being surrounded by six neighboring capsomers and those on the vertices by five.

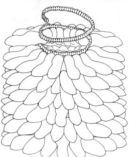

Schematic representation of a helical nucleocapsid. The RNA lies in a groove formed by the association of the structural units where it is protected from the environment. (From B. A. Freeman: Burrows Textbook of Microbiology. 21st ed. Philadelphia, W. B. Saunders Co., 1979; redrawn from Klug and Caspar: Adv. Virus Res. 7:274, 1960.)

capsomer (kap'so-mer) [L. *capsa* a box + Gr. *meros* part] the morphological unit of the capsid of a virus.

Capsul. abbreviation for L. *cap'sula,* capsule.

capsula (kap'su-lah), pl. *cap'sulae* [L.] a general anatomical term for a cartilaginous, fatty, fibrous, or membranous structure enveloping another structure, organ, or part. Called also *capsule.* **c. articula'ris** [NA], joint CAPSULE. **c. articula'ris articulatio'nis temporomandibula'ris** [NA], CAPSULE of temporomandibular joint. **c. articula'ris cricoarytenoi'dea** [NA], cricoarytenoid articular CAPSULE. **c. articula'ris cricothyroi'dea** [NA], cricothyroid articular CAPSULE. **c. articula'ris mandib'ulae,** CAPSULE of temporomandibular joint. **c. fibro'sa,** fibrous CAPSULE. **c. fibro'sa glan'dulae thyroi'deae** [NA], fibrous capsule of thyroid gland; see under CAPSULE. **c. glan'dulae thyroi'deae,** fibrous capsule of thyroid gland; see under CAPSULE.

capsulae (kap'su-le) [L.] plural of *capsula.*

capsular (kap'su-lar) pertaining to a capsule.

capsule (kap'sūl) [L. *capsula* a little box] 1. a structure in which something is enclosed. 2. an anatomical structure enclosing an organ or body part. Called also *capsula.* **articular c.,** joint c. **articular c., cricoarytenoid,** cricoarytenoid articular c. **articular c., cricothyroid,** cricothyroid articular c. **bacterial c.,** an envelope of gel surrounding a bacterial cell, usually polysaccharide but sometimes polypeptide in nature, which is associated with the virulence of pathogenic bacteria. **Bowman's c.,** the globular dilatations that form the beginning of a renal tubule of the kidney. Called also *glomerular c.* and *c. of glomerulus.* **cartilage c.,** a basophilic zone of cartilage matrix bordering on a lacuna and its enclosed cartilage cell. **cricoarytenoid articular c.,** a thin, loose, fibrous capsule surrounding the articulation between the cricoid and arytenoid cartilages. Called also *capsula articularis cricoarytenoidea* [NA]. **cricothyroid articular c.,** a capsule made of a fibrous tissue which encloses the articulation of the inferior horn of the thyroid cartilage with the cricoid cartilage. Called also *capsula articularis cricothyroidea* [NA]. **decavitamin c.,** a capsule containing not less than 1.2 mg vitamin A, 10 μg vitamin D, 70 mg ascorbic acid, 10 mg calcium pantothenate, 1 μg cyanocobalamin, 50 μg folic acid, 20 mg niacinamide, 2 mg riboflavin, 2 mg thiamine hydrochloride, or its equivalent as thiamine mononitrate, and a suitable form of α-tocopherol. Used as a dietary supplement. **fibrous c.,** one composed chiefly of fibrous elements. Called also *capsula fibrosa.* **fibrous c. of thyroid gland,** a fibrous sheath enclosing the thyroid gland; it is derived from the pretracheal cervical fossa. Called also *capsula fibrosa glandulae thyroideae* [NA] and *capsula glandulae thyroideae*. **glomerular c.,** Bowman's c. **c. of glomerulus,** Bowman's c. **hexavitamin c.,** a capsule containing not less than 1.5 mg vitamin A, 10 μg vitamin D, 75 mg ascorbic acid, 2 mg thiamine hydrochloride or an equivalent amount of thiamine mononitrate, 3 mg riboflavin, and 20 mg niacinamide. Used as a dietary supplement. **joint c.,** the saclike envelope of fibrous tissue which encloses the cavity of the synovial joint. Called also *articular c., capsula articularis* [NA], and *capsular ligament*. **salivary gland c.,** the capsule of a salivary gland, composed of fibrous connective tissue, and, when present, serves mainly in a delimiting capacity. Collagenous fibers predominate, but some elastic and reticular fibers are also present. Contained within the capsule are the vascular, lymphatic, and neural elements. **c. of temporomandibular joint,** an articular capsule surrounding the temporomandibular joint. Called also *capsula articularis articulationis temporomandibularis* [NA] and *capsula articularis mandibulae*. **tonsillar c.,** a connective tissue capsule which envelops the tonsils and separates them from the underlying connective tissue, thus facilitating enucleation of the tonsils in tonsillectomy. **tumor c.,** a fibrous membrane enclosing nearly all benign tumors.

capsulo- [L. *capsula* capsule] a combining form denoting relationship to a capsule.

capsuloplasty (kap′su-lo-plas″te) [*capsulo-* + Gr. *plassein* to form] plastic reconstruction of a capsule, especially a joint capsule.

capsulorrhaphy (kap″su-lor′ah-fe) [*capsulo-* + Gr. *raphē* suture] suturing of a capsule, especially a joint capsule.

capsulotomy (kap″su-lot′o-me) [*capsulo-* + Gr. *temnein* to cut] the incision of a capsule, such as a joint capsule.

capture (kap′chur) 1. to take by force. 2. a process in which an atomic or nuclear system acquires an additional particle, as the capture of electrons by positive ions. See also ABSORPTION (2).

capuride (kap′ur-īd) a monoureide hypnotic drug, *N*-(aminocarbonyl)-2-ethyl-3-methylpentanamide. Trademark: Pacinox.

caput (kap′ut), pl. *cap′ita* [L. "head"] 1. [NA] the superior extremity of the body; the head. 2. a general anatomical term applied to the expanded or chief extremity of an organ or part. **c. angula′re mus′culi quadra′ti la′bii superio′ris,** see levator muscle of upper lip and ala of nose, under MUSCLE. **c. infraorbita′le mus′culi quadra′ti la′bii superio′ris,** see levator muscle of upper lip, under MUSCLE. **c. mandib′ulae** [NA], HEAD of mandible. **c. mus′culi** [NA], HEAD of muscle. **c. natifor′me,** hot cross bun HEAD. **c. pla′num,** a flattened head. **c. proge′neum,** prognathism. **c. quadra′tum,** an abnormal squarely shaped head, sometimes occurring in rickets. **c. zygomat′icum mus′culi quadra′ti la′bii superio′ris,** see zygomatic muscle, lesser, under MUSCLE.

Carabelli cusp (tubercle) [Georg C. *Carabelli*, Austrian dentist, 1787–1842] see under CUSP.

Carachol trademark for *sodium dehydrocholate* (see dehydrocholic ACID).

caramiphen (kah-ram′ĭ-fen) a compound, 1-phenylcyclopentanecarboxylic acid 2-(diethylamino)ethyl. **c. ethanedisulfonate,** the 1,2-ethanedisulfonate ester of caramiphen. Used as an antitussive agent. Trademarks: Alcopon, Taoryl, Toryn. **c. hydrochloride,** the hydrochloride salt of caramiphen, occurring as white or nearly white crystals or crystalline powder, soluble in water and ethanol. Used as an anticholinergic. Trademarks: Panparnit, Parpanit.

carat (kar′at) 1. a measure of fineness of gold; pure gold being 24 carats or having 24 parts of gold and 18-carat gold having only 18 parts of gold and 6 parts of another metal. See also GOLD alloy. 2. a unit of weight of precious stones, being equivalent to 205 mg or 3.163 troy grains. Abbreviated *c* or *ct*. **international c.,** metric c. **metric c.,** an international unit of weight, being equivalent to 200 mg or 3.086 grains. It is subdivided into points, in which 1 point is equal to 0.01 carats, and pear grains, in which 1 pear grain equals 0.25 carats. Called also *international c.*

carbachol (kar′bah-kol) a cholinomimetic, 2-[(aminocarbonyl)-oxy]-*N,N,N*-trimethylethanaminium chloride, occurring as white or yellowish crystals or a crystalline hygroscopic, odorless powder with a faint amine-like odor, which is soluble in water and ethanol and insoluble in ether and chloroform. Used chiefly as a miotic. Sometimes also used in urinary retention, intestinal paresis, peripheral vascular diseases, and ozena. Headache, ciliary spasm, and decreased visual acuity are the principal side effects. Called also *carbamylcholine* and *carbamylmethylcholine*. Trademarks: Carcholin, Coletyl, Doryl, Lentin, Moryl.

carbamate (kar′bah-māt) a compound based on carbamic acid, NH₂COOH; used only in the form of its salts and derivatives.

carbamazepine (kar-bah-maz′ĕ-pēn) an anticonvulsant drug with

analgesic properties, 5*H*-dibenz[*b,f*]azepine-5-carboxamide, occurring as a white powder that is soluble in ethanol and acetone, but not in water. Used in the treatment of psychomotor epilepsy and trigeminal neuralgia, not being effective in other types of facial neuralgia. Side reactions may include aplastic anemia, agranulocytosis, thrombocytopenia, and leukopenia. Adverse reactions include fever, sore throat, ulcers of the mouth, petechiae, purpura, hemorrhagic disorders, vertigo, drowsiness, unsteadiness, nausea, and vomiting. Trademarks: Finlepsin, Tegretal, Tegretol.

Carbamidal trademark for *nikethamide*.

carbamide (kar-bam′īd) urea. **c. peroxide,** UREA peroxide.

carbaminohemoglobin (kar-bam″ĭ-no-he′mo-glo′bin) a combination of carbon dioxide with hemoglobin, CO₂HHb, being one of the forms in which carbon dioxide exists in the blood. Called also *carbohemoglobin*.

carbamoyl (kar′bah-moil) the radical NH₂CO−, from carbamic acid. Called also *carbamyl*.

carbamoyltransferase [E.C.2.1.3] (kar″bah-moil-trans′fer-ās) a sub-class of transferases, the enzymes of which catalyze the transfer of carbamoyl groups in protein metabolism. Called also *transcarbamoylase*. **ornithine c.** [E.C.2.1.3.3], a transferase that catalyzes the conversion of carbamyl phosphate and L-ornithine to citrulline orthophosphate and L-citrulline, being an early intermediate product in the formation of urea in protein metabolism. Called also *citrulline phosphorylase* and *ornithine transcarbamoylase*.

carbamyl (kar′bah-mil) carbamoyl. **c. phosphate,** a compound synthesized from adenosine triphosphate, carbon dioxide, and ammonia in the presence of the enzyme carbamyl phosphate synthetase and the cofactors *N*-acetylglutamate and magnesium. It reacts with ornithine in the formation of urea in protein metabolism.

carbamylcholine (kar″bah-mil-ko′lēn) carbachol.

carbamylmethylcholine (kar″bah-mil-meth″il-ko′lēn) carbachol.

Carbapen trademark for *carbenicillin disodium* (see under CARBENICILLIN).

carbazochrome salicylate (kar-baz′o-krōm) a hemostatic agent, 5*H*-dibenz[*b,f*]azepine-5-carboxamide, occurring as an orange-red, odorless powder with a sweetish saline taste, which is soluble in water and ethanol. Stinging may occur at the site of application. Trademarks: Adenogen, Adrenosem, Adrestat-F, Statimo.

carbenicillin (kar″ben-ĭ-sil′in) a semisynthetic penicillin, *N*-(2-carboxy-3,3-dimethyl-7-oxo-4-thia-1-azabicyclo[3,2,0]-hept-6-yl)-2-phenylmalonamic acid. It is effective against gram-positive bacteria, chiefly staphylococci, streptococci, pneumococci, and clostridia, and also against other bacteria, such as *Pseudomonas aeruginosa, Proteus, Escherichia coli, Enterobacter,* and *Serratia marscencens*. Generally, its toxic properties are similar to those of other penicillins. In large intravenous doses, it may produce nephrotoxicity. Blood coagulation disorders may occur in rare instances. Called also *carboxybenzylpenicillin*. **c. indanyl sodium,** the sodium salt of the indanyl ester of carbenicillin disodium, occurring as a white to off-white powder that is soluble in water and alcohol. It has the same actions as the parent drug. Used in the treatment of urinary tract infections due to susceptible strains of *Pseudomonas* and *Proteus* species, *Escherichia coli,* and enterococci. Trademark: Geocillin. **c. disodium,** the disodium salt of carbenicillin, occurring as a white to off-white, bitter, hygroscopic, odorless, crystalline powder that is soluble in water, ethanol, methanol, and dilute acids and alkali, but is insoluble in acetone, chloroform, and ether. It has the same actions as the parent drug, and is used in the treatment of severe systemic infections and septicemia, urinary and genitourinary tract infections, acute and chronic respiratory infections, and soft tissue infections. Trademarks: Carbapen, Pyopen.

carbide (kar′bīd) a binary compound of carbon with another element, including carbon monoxide, carbon disulfide, and carbon tetrachloride. **boron c.,** BORON carbide. **ditungsten c.,** a compound, W₂C, having physical properties similar to those of tungsten carbide. **metallic c.,** a binary carbon compound of a metal or metalloids. **silicon c.,** carborundum. **tungsten c.,** a compound, WC, occurring as a gray powder that is insoluble in water, but is attacked by a mixture of nitric and hydrofluoric acids, having a Mohs hardness number of 9+. Used in the production of drills and cutting instruments, being one of the principal materials in dental burs.

carbidopa (kar″bĭ-do′pah) a decarboxylase inhibitor, *S*-α-hydrazino-3,4-dihydroxy-α-methylbenzenepropanoic acid monohydrate. Used in combination with levodopa in the treatment of parkinsonism. Trademarks: Lodosin, Lodosyn.

Carbilazine trademark for *diethylcarbamazine*.

carbimazole (kar-bi′mah-zōl) a thyroid inhibitor, carbonothioic acid *O*-ethyl-*S*-(1-methyl-1*H*-imidazole-2-yl) ester, occurring as a crystalline powder with a characteristic odor and a bitter aftertaste, which is soluble in water, ethanol, ether, chloroform, and acetone. Used in the treatment of hyperthyroidism. Trademarks: Neo-Mercazole, Neo-Thyreostat.

carbinol (kar′bĭ-nol) 1. methyl ALCOHOL. 2. any aromatic or fatty alcohol containing the radical COH, which is formed by substituting one, two, or three hydrocarbon groups for hydrogen in methanol. **dimethyl c.,** isopropyl ALCOHOL. **ethynyl c.,** ethchlorvynol.

carbinoxamine maleate (kar″bin-ok′sah-mēn) an antihistaminic, 2-[*p*-chloro-*α*-]2-(dimethylamino)ethoxy[benzyl]pyridine maleate, occurring as a white, odorless crystalline powder with a bitter taste, which is readily soluble in alcohol, water, and chloroform and slightly soluble in ether. It acts on the H_1 receptor, with a weak atropine-like anticholinergic activity. Used in the treatment of mild allergic reactions. Trademarks: Ciberon, Clistin, Hislosine, Lergefin.

carbo (kar′bo) [L.] carbon; charcoal. **c. activa′tus,** activated CHARCOAL. **c. anima′lis,** animal CHARCOAL.

Carbocaine trademark for *mepivacaine hydrochloride* (see under MEPIVACAINE).

carbocyclic (kar″bo-si′klik) having or pertaining to a closed chain or ring formation which includes only carbon atoms. See carbocyclic COMPOUND.

carbohemia (kar″bo-he′me-ah) [*carbon dioxide* + Gr. *haima* blood + *-ia*] the presence of carbon dioxide in the blood.

carbohemoglobin (kar″bo-he-mo-glo′bin) carbaminohemoglobin.

carbohydrase (kar″bo-hi′drās) [*carbohydrate* + *-ase*] any of a group of enzymes that catalyze the hydrolysis of higher carbohydrates to lower forms, each enzyme being usually specific for one substrate only. See table at ENZYME.

carbohydrate (kar″be-hi′drāt) a class of organic compounds which, by classical definition, are those substances which contain carbon, hydrogen, and oxygen, whereby the hydrogen and oxygen are in the same proportion as in water, also contain-

$$H—\overset{|}{\underset{\underset{OH}{|}}{C}}—\overset{||}{\underset{O}{C}}—$$

ing the saccharose grouping or the first reaction product. As used currently, the term embraces: (*a*) aliphatic polyhydric alcohols in which either the primary alcohol function has been oxidized to aldehyde or the secondary alcohol function has been oxidized to ketone; and (*b*) condensation polymers of those partially oxidized polyalcohols. The fundamental structural units are the aldehyde-alcohols and ketone-alcohols. Simple carbohydrates, known as *monosaccharides* or *simple sugars,* are derivatives of straight-chain polyhydric alcohols and are classified according to the number of carbon atoms in the chain — those with two carbon atoms are diose; with three, triose; with four, tetrose; with five, pentose; and with six, hexose. The ending *-ose* identifies carbohydrates. When two monosaccharides are linked together, the resulting compound is a disaccharide and the combination of three is a trisaccharide. Oligosaccharides are those which are of two to five monosaccharides, and polymers of several monosaccharides are polysaccharides. Carbohydrates provide fuel for the animal body, their degradation to carbon dioxide and water representing a major source of energy. Some products of carbohydrate metabolism aid in the breakdown of certain foodstuffs, acting as catalysts in promoting oxidation. Carbohydrates are also used as starting material for the biological synthesis of other types of compounds, such as fatty acids and certain amino acids. They occur as white solids, sparingly soluble in organic liquids and, except for some polysaccharides, readily soluble in water. Fermentable carbohydrates are involved in the etiology of dental caries, but the mechanism is not fully understood. The terms *sugar, starch,* and *carbohydrate* are sometimes used synonymously. See table. **c. metabolism,** the process by which carbohydrates are absorbed and used by the body. It begins with the reduction of food particles into small fragments by mastication and moistening of these particles with saliva, which also lubricates the digestive passages, so that food may be swallowed as a bolus. The indigestible carbohydrates, such as celluloses and pentosans, pass through the digestive tract with-

---

CLASSIFICATION OF CARBOHYDRATES

I. Monosaccharides
    Trioses — $C_3H_6O_3$
        Aldose — Glyceraldehyde
        Ketose — Dihydroxyacetone
    Pentoses — $C_5H_{10}O_5$
        Aldoses — Arabinose
                Xylose
                Ribose
    Hexoses — $C_6H_{12}O_6$
        Aldoses — Glucose
                Galactose
        Ketoses — Fructose
    Ascorbic acid

II. Disaccharides — $C_{12}H_{22}O_{12}$
    Sucrose (glucose + fructose)
    Maltose (glucose + glucose)
    Lactose (glucose + galactose)

III. Polysaccharides
    Hexosans
        Glucosans — Starch
                 Glycogen
                 Dextrin
                 Cellulose

IV. Mucopolysaccharides
    Hyaluronic acid
    Chondroitin sulfate
    Heparin

(From J. I. Routh, D. P. Eyman, and D. J. Burton: Essentials of General, Organic, and Biochemistry. 3rd ed. Philadelphia, W. B. Saunders Co., 1977.)

out being absorbed, but disaccharides and polysaccharides are hydrolyzed by the digestive enzymes to their monosaccharide components, glucose, fructose, and galactose, and are absorbed from the intestine into the portal blood, beginning in the oral cavity where an enzyme in the saliva, salivary amylase (ptyalin), hydrolyzes starch to maltose. In the liver, fructose and galactose are converted to glucose. Glucose not immediately required for energy is stored in the liver in the form of glycogen and that to be used by cells is transported by blood to target cells. Before glucose can be used for energy, it is transported through the cell membrane into the cytoplasm by a carrier system, being made soluble in the membrane and, after passing through into the cell, becoming dissociated from the carrier. Insulin assists in the transport, increasing its rate as much as 10 times. Once in the cells, glucose undergoes glycolysis, combining with ATP to form ADP and glucose 6-phosphate, followed by a series of reactions in which energy is released, the end-product of reactions being pyruvic acid, and ADP controlling the rate of energy release in accordance with need for ATP by cells. Glycolysis can also occur under anaerobic conditions for brief periods, whereby the major portion of the pyruvic acid is converted to lactic acid. Some tissues, such as the myocardium, are capable of converting lactic acid to pyruvic acid for energy. In conditions of carbohydrate depletion, moderate quantities of glucose can be formed from amino acids and the glycerol portion of lipids by the process of gluconeogenesis. Conversely, when excessive amounts of carbohydrates are present and the glycogen storage capability of the liver has been exceeded, glucose transported by the portal system is converted to fatty acids to be stored in adipose tissue. See also Embden-Meyerhof PATHWAY, Krebs CYCLE, lactic acid CYCLE, and phosphogluconate PATHWAY.

carbon (kar′bon) [L. *carbo* coal, charcoal] 1. a nonmetallic tetrad element. Symbol, C; atomic number, 6; group IVA of the periodic table; atomic weight, 12.011; valence, +4 (both divalent and trivalent forms exist); its isotopes 12 and 13 are stable and 10, 11, 14, and 15 are radioactive. Carbon exists in two crystalline allotropic forms as diamond and graphite, and in various amorphous allotropic forms, as activated charcoal or coke. It is generally considered as metalloid, and is soluble in low percentages in iron and steel. Carbon is the principal constituent of all organic and a few inorganic compounds (carbon dioxide and carbon monoxide), being essential to life and the photosynthetic process. In elemental form, carbon is nontoxic, but exposure to its dust may produce lung disease. Breathing of air containing high concentrations of carbon monoxide results in saturation of the blood with gas and carboxyhemoglobinemia. The affinity of carbon monoxide for hemoglobin is 300 times that of oxygen and causes shifting of the oxyhemoglobin dissociation curve to the left so that the oxygen tension must fall before oxyhemoglobin can give up oxygen. Abnormal chest signs, edema, fever, hemorrhage, pinkish skin, sweating, anoxia, coma, increase in the respiratory and pulse rates, arrhythmia, vomiting, headache, peripheral neuritis, confusion, psychotic changes, and pain in extremities are the principal features of poisoning. Ulcers and suffusion of the oral mucosa may occur. Hematologic changes usually include eosinopenia, lymphocytopenia, and neutrophilia. Hematuria and urinary protein and sugar casts may be observed. 2. an electrode made of carbon shell in which medicaments may be enclosed. **activated c.,** activated CHARCOAL. **amorphous c.,** a quasigraphitic form of carbon, existing in various forms: *animal charcoal* from charred bones and other animal material; *carbon black* from incomplete combustion or thermal decomposition of natural gas; *lamp black* from burning fats, oils, and rosin; and *activated charcoal* from combustion of wood and other vegetable material. Generally used in deodorizing, filtering, and distillation, and in a variety of industrial processes. **c. black,** carbon BLACK. See also *amorphous c.* **c. bisulfide,** c. disulfide. **c.-12,** ^{12}C, a natural (nonradioactive) carbon isotope of mass number 12; used as the base to which the atomic weights are referred. **c.-13,** ^{13}C, a stable natural (nonradioactive) isotope of carbon, of atomic mass 13, used as a tracer in chemical reactions in living tissue. **c.-14,** ^{14}C, a radioactive isotope of carbon that emits beta radiation, having an atomic mass of 14 and a half-life of 5.750 years. It is produced by irradiation of calcium nitrate and serves as a source of labeled organic compounds, used as tracer compounds in metabolic studies and for dating geological and archeological specimens. **c. disulfide,** a flammable, toxic liquid with a characteristic odor, CS_2, which is slightly soluble in water, and serves as a solvent for rubber, sulfur, and iodine. It has local anesthetic properties, but is not used as such. Poisoning may occur through inhalation, ingestion, or skin absorption, causing mental disorders, vomiting, mucous membrane irritation, tremors, blood disorders, unconsciousness, and terminal convulsions. Contact may cause burning pain, erythema, and exfoliation. Called also *c. bisulfide.* **c. dioxide,** a colorless, noncombustible gas, CO_2, having a faint acid taste. It is soluble in hydrocarbons, most organic solvents, and in water, forming H_2CO_3. Carbon dioxide is usually stored and transported in the liquefied state under pressure. It occurs in the atmosphere, being necessary for the respiration cycle of plants and animals. It is produced by the body's metabolism and carried out of the system in the blood stream as bicarbonate ion, in chemical combination with hemoglobin (to a small extent) and plasma proteins, and in physical solution. Its rate of exhalation is the same as that of production. Depression of the carbon dioxide level in the blood stimulates the respiratory centers and increases respiration. A mixture of 5 to 10 percent carbon dioxide with oxygen is used in the treatment of various respiratory disorders, including respiratory depression, asphyxia, coma, carbon monoxide poisoning, hiccups, and other conditions in which respiratory stimulation is required. It is also used to increase the speed of induction and emergence from anesthesia and in negative contrast roentgenography. Called also *carbonic acid gas* and *carbonic anhydride.* **c. monoxide,** a poisonous, odorless, colorless, tasteless, nonirritating gas, CO, produced by incomplete combustion of organic matter. It occurs in the atmosphere, chiefly as a result of emission from internal combustion engines and other industrial sources. It is produced endogenously during the catabolism of hemoglobin and heme compounds; its concentration increasing during pregnancy, hemolytic diseases, burns, and anesthesia. The toxic properties of carbon monoxide are due to its ability to combine with hemoglobin to form carboxyhemoglobin, thereby preventing hemoglobin from being able to transport oxygen. Carbon monoxide is highly toxic when inhaled at high concentrations and it is the cause of many deaths. The symptoms of acute poisoning are closely correlated with the carboxyhemoglobin content of the blood and are those characteristic of hypoxia or anoxia. **radioactive c.,** a radioactive carbon isotope (^{10}C, ^{11}C, ^{14}C, and ^{15}C); the most important and most commonly referred to being ^{14}C. Called also *radiocarbon.* **c. tetrachloride,** a colorless, nonflammable, heavy liquid with a characteristic odor, CCl_4. Used therapeutically as an anthelmintic, and in industry as a degreasing agent, refrigerant, agricultural fumigant, drying agent, and dry solvent. Inhalation, ingestion, or skin absorption may cause nausea, vomiting, diarrhea, headache, stupor, kidney lesions with anuria and azotemia, liver injuries, and death. Liver lesions, kidney injury, and visual disorders may occur during chronic exposure. Contact may produce skin or mucous membrane lesions. Called also *perchlormethane* and *tetrachloromethane.*

carbonate (kar'bon-āt) an inorganic salt of the theoretical carbonic acid, containing the radical CO_3. Carbonates are soluble in acids; those of the alkali metals are soluble in water, and all others are insoluble. **calcium c.,** CALCIUM carbonate. **c. dehydratase,** carbonate DEHYDRATASE. **ferrous c.,** a compound, $FeCO_3$, used in the treatment of iron deficiency anemia. Called also *iron carbonate.* See IRON for toxic effects. **c. hydratase,** carbonate HYDRATASE. **c. hydro-lyase,** carbonate DEHYDRATASE. **iron c.,** ferrous c. **magnesium c.,** MAGNESIUM carbonate. **potassium c.,** POTASSIUM calcium. **sodium acid c., sodium hydrogen c.,** SODIUM bicarbonate.

carbonyl (kar'bo-nil) [*carbon* + Gr. *hylē* matter] the organic radical CO.

carbonyldiamide (kar″bo-nil-di-am'īd) urea.

Carboraffin trademark for *activated charcoal* (see under CHARCOAL).

carborundum (kar″bo-run'dum) a compound of carbon and silicon, silicon carbide, SiC, a substance which ranks next to the diamond in hardness, and is used as an abrasive and as a refractory. See also dental DISK and carborundum WHEEL.

Carbowax trademark for *polyethylene glycol* (see under GLYCOL).

carboxybenzylpenicillin (kar-bok″se-ben″zil-pen-ĭ-sil'in) carbenicillin.

carboxyhemoglobin (kar-bok″se-he″mo-glo'bin) a compound formed from combination of hemoglobin with carbon monoxide, usually seen in carbon monoxide poisoning. Abbreviated *HbCO.*

carboxyl (kar-bok'sil) a group or radical that determines the acidity of an organic acid, which may be written $-\overset{\displaystyle O}{\overset{\displaystyle \|}{C}}-OH$, $-COOH$, or $-CO_2H$. See also carboxylic ACID.

carboxylase [E.C.6.4] (kar-bok'sĭ-lās) a subclass of ligases, the enzymes of which form carbon-carbon bonds, mostly biotinylproteins, responsible for incorporating CO_2 into an organic molecule.

carboxylation (kar-bok″sĭ-la'shun) the addition of a carboxyl group (COOH).

carboxylesterase [E.C.3.1.1.1] (kar-bok″sil-es'ter-ās) a hydrolase acting on ester bonds, which catalyzes the hydrolysis of the esters of carboxylic acid, having wide specificity and also acting on vitamin A esters. Also found in the saliva. Called also *ali-esterase, atropine esterase, B-esterase, carboxyl esterase, cocaine esterase, methylbutyrase,* and *procaine esterase.*

carboxy-lyase [E.C.4.1.1] (kar-bok″sĭ-li'ās) a sub-subclass of lyases that catalyze the removal of chemical groups by cleaving carboxy groups with formation of carboxyl groups, resulting in formation of carbon dioxide.

carboxymethylcellulose (kar-bok″sĭ-meth″il-sel'u-lōs) a polymer in which CH_2COOH groups are substituted on the glucose units of the cellulose chain through another linkage. It is an odorless, colorless, nontoxic water-soluble powder that is insoluble in alcohol. In a 1 percent aqueous solution, it has a pH of 6.5 to 8.0 and viscosity varying from 5 to 200 centipoises, depending on the extent of esterification. Used in foods, detergents, cosmetics, and drugs as a thickening agent. Abbreviated *CMC.* Called also *CM cellulose.* See also METHYLCELLULOSE. **sodium c.,** the sodium salt of a polycarboxymethyl ether of cellulose, occurring as white granules or hygroscopic powder that is easily dispersed in water to form colloidal suspensions, but is insoluble in organic solvents. Used as a suspending agent and as a bulk laxative and gastric antacid. Also used in gels for dental topical application and in dentifrices. Called also *carboxymethylcellulose sodium* and *sodium cellulose glycolate.* Trademark: Thylose.

carboxypeptidase [E.C.3.4.12] (kar-bok″sĭ-pep'tĭ-dās) a subclass of hydrolases, being peptidylamino-acid or acylamino-acid enzymes, found in the pancreatic juice, which catalyze the hydrolysis of food proteins. The reaction results in the release of a C-terminal amino acid. Some exhibit broad specificities, while others require a specific C-terminal residue (e.g., alanine carboxypeptidase). **c. A** [E.C.3.4.12.2], one that catalyzes the hydrolysis of peptides by releasing C-terminal amino acids, with the exception of C-terminal arginine, lysine, and proline, cleaving peptidyl-L-amino acids into peptides and L-amino acids. It is a zinc protein found in the pancreas. Called also *carboxypolypeptidase*. **alanine c.** [E.C.3.4.17.6], an enzyme which, in the presence of water, splits peptidyl-L-alanine to peptide and L-alanine. **c. B** [E.C.3.4.12.3], one that catalyzes the hydrolysis of peptides, preferentially releasing C-terminal L-lysine or L-arginine. It is a zinc metalloprotein found in the pancreatic juice. Called also *protaminase*. **c. C** [E.C.3.4.12.1], one that catalyzes the hydrolysis of C-terminal amino acids from peptides, having a broad specificity and acting on peptides containing any C-terminal α-amino acid. **proline c.** [E.C.3.4.12.4], one that catalyzes the hydrolysis of proteins, releasing the C-terminal amino acid only if proline is in the penultimate position. It activates angiotensin II.

carboxypolypeptidase (kar-bok″sĭ-pol″e-pep′tĭ-dās) carboxypeptidase A.

Carcholin trademark for CARBACHOL.

carcinogen (kar-sin′o-jen) any carcinoma-producing substance.

carcinogenesis (kar″sĭ-no-jen′ĕ-sis) [Gr. *karkinos* cancer + *genesis* production] the production or development of cancer.

carcinogenic (kar″sĭ-no-jen′ik) producing cancer.

carcinogenicity (kar″sĭ-no-jĕ-nis′ĭ-te) the power, ability, or tendency to produce cancer.

carcinoid (kar′sĭ-noid) argentaffinoma. **Arning's c.**, a condition characterized by multiple, benign, flat tumors of the skin, manifested as whitish gray shiny lesions with brownish purple pigmented areas, usually seen on the face and trunk. Initial lesions are small rough spots which slowly expand. Although they heal spontaneously after several years, areas around old healed lesions usually become the sites of new crops of lesions. Arning compared this tumor to carcinoid; he classified it, however, with basal cell carcinoma. Called also *multiple cutaneous c.*, *carcinomatosis cutis disseminata*, *epithelioma pagetoide*, *erythemoid benign epithelioma*, and *pagetoid epithelioma*. **multiple cutaneous c.**, Arning's c.

carcinolysis (kar″sĭ-nol′ĭ-sis) destruction of cancer cells.

carcinolytic (kar″sĭ-no-lit′ik) pertaining to, characterized by, or causing carcinolysis.

carcinoma (kar″sĭ-no′mah) [Gr. *karkinōma*, from *karkinos* crab, cancer] a malignant neoplasm made up of epithelial cells tending to infiltrate the surrounding tissues and give rise to metastases. Often used incorrectly as a synonym for cancer. **acinic cell c.**, acinar cell ADENOCARCINOMA. **adenocystic c.**, **adenocystic basal cell c.**, adenoid cystic c. **adenoid cystic c.**, a slow-growing form of adenocarcinoma of the salivary glands that tends to metastasize and spread locally via the nerves. The tumor occurs most commonly in the parotid, submaxillary, and accessory glands of the palate and tongue, and may occur in the mucous glands of the respiratory tract and mammary glands. Local pain, swelling, and surface ulceration in intraoral tumors are the usual early symptoms. It is made up of small, deeply staining cells similar to basal cells, arranged in a Swiss cheese–like pattern in cords and ductlike structures, with mucoid material contained in the central parts. Hyalinized stromal connective tissue forms bands or cylinders around tumor cells (hence the original name *cylindroma*) separating or surrounded by nests or cords of small epithelial cells. When the cylinders occur within masses of epithelial cells, they give the tissue a perforated, sievelike, or cribriform appearance. Mitotic figures are rare. Called also *adenocystic c.*, *adenocystic basal cell c.*, *cribriform c.*, *pseudoadenomatous basal cell c.*, *adenomyoepithelioma*, and *basaloid mixed tumor*. **basal cell c.**, a neoplasm found usually in the skin of the scalp and face of middle-aged and elderly individuals who spend much time out-of-doors. It usually begins as a small, slightly elevated papule that may heal over and then reappear, eventually developing into a smooth tumor that spreads beneath the skin, infiltrating deeper tissues, including bones. It seldom metastasizes, but may spread to lymph nodes in rare instances. Common histological features include nests, islands, or sheets of cells showing indistinct cell membranes with large, deeply staining nuclei and a variable number of mitotic figures; the periphery of the cell nests is composed of cells resembling the basal layer of the skin. Basal cell carcinoma seldom occurs in the oral mucosa. **basosquamous cell c.**, carcinoma that histologically exhibits both basal and squamous elements; sometimes occurring in the oral cavity. **cribriform c.**, adenoid cystic c. **epidermoid c.**, carcinoma in which the cells tend to differentiate in the same way that the cells of the epidermis do, i.e., they tend to form

prickle cells and undergo cornification. It may occur in any organ having stratified squamous epithelium and is the most common malignant tumor of the oral cavity; the tongue, floor of the mouth, alveolar mucosa, palate, and buccal mucosa are the most common sites. A typical tumor presents an ulcerated and crusted lesion ranging from a few millimeters to several centimeters in size. It is usually well differentiated, although anaplastic lesions also occur, and is composed of sheets and nests of large cells from the squamous epithelium usually showing cell and intercellular bridges or tonofibrils. Keratinization and epithelial pearls are usually present; mitotic figures may be found. Predisposing lesions include burns, radiodermatitis, leukoplakia, and keratosis; other etiologic factors may include smoking, alcohol, syphilis, sunlight, and nutritional deficiencies. Called also *prickle cell c.* and *squamous cell c.* **exophytic c.**, carcinoma with marked outward growth like that of a wart or papilloma. **c. fibro′sum**, scirrhous c. **intraepidermal squamous cell c.**, **intraepithelial c.**, 1. c. *in situ.* 2. oral LEUKOPLAKIA. **medullary c.**, **c. medulla′re**, carcinoma composed mainly of epithelial elements with little or no stroma. Called also *cellular cancer* and *soft cancer*. **mucinous c.**, adenocarcinoma producing mucin in significant amounts. Called also *colloid cancer*, and sometimes erroneously called *colloid* or *gelatinous colloma*. **mucoepidermoid c.**, a malignant tumor of glandular tissue, especially the salivary glands, made up of sheets or nests of epidermoid and mucous cells arranged in a glandular pattern, sometimes showing microcysts that may rupture, producing pools of mucus and an inflammatory reaction. The parotid gland is the most common site, but other major or accessory salivary glands may be involved. Low-grade malignant tumors occur most commonly on the palate, buccal mucosa, tongue, and retromolar area as slow-growing lesions seldom exceeding 5 cm in diameter; they are not completely encapsulated and often contain cysts. High-grade malignant tumors are not encapsulated and produce pain, facial paralysis, infiltrate to adjacent tissues, and metastasize. **papillary c.**, carcinoma in which there are papillary excrescences. Called also *dendritic cancer*. **preinvasive c.**, c. *in situ.* **prickle cell c.**, epidermoid c. **pseudoadenomatous basal cell c.**, adenoid cystic c. **scirrhous c.**, carcinoma with a hard structure owing to the formation of dense connective tissue in the stroma. Called also *c. fibrosum*, *apinoid cancer*, *hard cancer*, and *scirrhous cancer*. **signet-ring cell c.**, a highly malignant, mucus-secreting tumor in which the mucus-secreting cells are anaplastic and appear rounded, with the nucleus displaced to one side by a globule of mucus in the cytoplasm. **c. sim′plex**, **spheroidal cell c.**, an undifferentiated carcinoma. **c. in si′tu**, carcinoma in which the tumor cells still lie within the epithelium of origin, without invasion of the basement membrane. It typically presents a crust-covered patch over a dull-red, moist, and granular or papillomatous undersurface, affecting the skin and mucous membrane. Oral tumors resemble leukoplakia and exhibit keratinization or erythematous, velvety plaques that may or may not be associated with whitish patches. Histologically, it shows hyperkeratosis, acanthosis, epithelial cell abnormalities of the spinous layer, bizarre mitotic figures, and multinucleated cells. Some authorities consider this condition to represent precancerous dyskeratosis; others think that the term applies to a laterally spreading intraepithelial superficial epithelioma or carcinoma. Carcinoma *in situ* of mucous membrane is similar to *Queyrat's erythroplasia.* The term is sometimes used to mean *leukoplakia.* Called also *intraepidermal squamous cell c.*, *intraepithelial c.*, *preinvasive c.*, *Bowen's disease*, *Bowen's epithelioma*, *Bowen's precancerosis*, and *dermatitis precancerosis.* **squamous cell c.**, epidermoid c. **c. telangiectat′icum**, **c. telangiecto′des**, carcinoma involving the cutaneous capillaries and producing telangiectatic changes. **transitional cell c.**, carcinoma arising from a transitional type of stratified epithelium in the mucosa of the nasopharynx, oropharynx, tongue, tonsils, nose, and paranasal sinuses, typically presenting a small, slightly elevated, ulcerated or eroded, indurated lesion. Histologically, it is characterized by strands and masses of polygonal to spindle cells growing within a fibrous stroma; the cell boundaries are poorly defined and masses of cells take the appearance of a syncytium. When associated with massive lymphoid infiltrate within the fibrous stroma, it is known as *lymphoepithelioma*. **verrucous c.**, epidermoid carcinoma having a predilection for the buccal mucosa, but also affecting other oral soft tissue, the larynx, and the genitalia. It is slow-growing, somewhat invasive, exophytic neoplasm, either papillary or verrucous in appearance.

carcinomata (kar″sĭ-no′mah-tah) plural of *carcinoma*.

carcinomatoid (kar″sĭ-nom′ah-toid) resembling carcinoma.

carcinomatophobia (kar″sĭ-no″mah-to-fo′be-ah) cancerphobia.

carcinomatosis (kar″sĭ-no-mah-to′sis) the condition of widespread dissemination of cancer; carcinosis. **c. cu′tis dissemina′ta,** Arning's CARCINOID.

carcinomatous (kar″sĭ-nōm′ah-tus) pertaining to, or of the nature of cancer; malignant.

carcinophobia (kar″sĭ-no-fo′be-ah) [*carcinoma + phobia*] cancerphobia.

carcinosarcoma (kar″sĭ-no-sar-ko′mah) a malignant tumor composed of carcinomatous and sarcomatous tissues.

carcinosis (kar″sĭ-no′sis) 1. widespread dissemination of cancer; carcinomatosis. 2. a cancer or malignant tumor.

carcinostatic (kar″sĭ-no-stat′ik) tending to check the growth of cancer.

card- see CARDIO-.

Cardamine trademark for *nikethamide.*

Cardarelli's aphthae [Antonio *Cardarelli,* Italian physician] Riga-Fede DISEASE.

Cardelmycin trademark for *novobiocin.*

cardia (kar′de-ah) [Gr. *kardia* heart] 1. the orifice between the stomach and the esophagus, and the upper (cardiac) portion of the stomach. Called also *ostium cardiacum* [NA]. 2. that part of the stomach surrounding the esophagogastric junction in which there are no acid- or pepsin-secreting cells. 3. formerly, a general term for the heart, or for the region of the heart.

cardiac (kar′de-ak) [L. *cardiacus,* from Gr. *kardiakos*] 1. pertaining to the heart. 2. a person with a heart disorder. 3. pertaining to the portion of the stomach close to the esophagus.

cardialgia (kar′de-al′je-ah) [*cardia + -algia*] 1. chest pain or pain in the region of the upper abdomen. 2. heart pain; cardiodynia.

Cardiamid trademark for *nikethamide.*

Cardigin trademark for *digitoxin.*

Cardilate trademark for *erythrityl tetranitrate* (see under ERYTHRITYL).

Cardiloid trademark for *erythrityl tetranitrate* (see under ERYTHRITYL).

cardio-, cardi- [Gr. *kardia* heart] a combining form denoting relationship to the heart or to the cardia.

Cardiobacterium (kar″de-o-bak-te′re-um) [Gr. *kardia* heart + *baktērion* little rod] a genus of gram-negative, facultatively anaerobic, rod-shaped bacteria of uncertain affiliation. **C. hom′inis,** a species occurring as non–acid-fast, pleomorphic (rods to oval) cells (about 0.5 to 0.75 by 1.0 to 3.0 μm in size) with swollen ends and occasional filaments, arranged singly, in pairs, short chains, or clusters. The organisms produce cytochrome oxidase and small amounts of indole, and are sensitive to penicillin, ampicillin, streptomycin, tetracyclines, chloramphenicol, and neomycin. The species has been isolated from the nose and throat in man, in whom it produces endocarditis, but has not been shown to be pathogenic to laboratory animals.

cardiodynia (kar″de-o-din′e-ah) [*cardio- + Gr. odynē* pain] heart pain; cardialgia.

cardioinhibitor (kar″de-o-in-hib′ĭ-ter) an agent that restrains the action of the heart.

cardioinhibitory (kar″de-o-in-hib′ĭ-to-re) restraining or inhibiting the movement of the heart.

cardiokinetic (kar″de-o-ki-net′ik) 1. stimulating the action of the heart. 2. an agent that stimulates the action of the heart.

cardiologist (kar″de-ol′o-jist) a physician who specializes in the diagnosis and treatment of diseases of the heart.

cardiology (kar″de-ol′o-je) the study of the heart, its functions, and diseases.

cardiopathia (kar″de-o-path′e-ah) cardiopathy. **c. ni′gra,** Ayerza's SYNDROME.

cardiopathy (kar″de-op′ah-the) [*cardio- + Gr. pathos* disease] any disease of the heart.

cardiospasm (kar′de-o-spasm″) achalasia.

cardiotonic (kar″de-o-ton′ik) [*cardio- + Gr. tonos* tonus] 1. having an effect on the tonus of the heart. 2. any substance that has a tonic effect on the heart, such as a cardiac glycoside.

Cardiovanil trademark for *ethamivan.*

Cardioxil trademark for *digoxin.*

Cardis trademark for *isosorbide dinitrate* (see under ISOSORBIDE).

carditis (kar-di′tis) [*cardio- + -itis*] inflammation of the heart. **rheumatic c.,** carditis in rheumatic fever.

Carditoxin trademark for *digitoxin.*

Cardoxin trademark for *dipyridamole.*

care (kār) attending to the needs or performing necessary services for a person, as in providing medical or nursing care to a patient. **acute c.,** medical care service of short duration, usually of less than 30 days, primarily oriented toward problems which require intensive attention and treatment to restore a previous state of health or to prevent the worsening of a present state, which may at times be emergent, and that may have related

long-term effects. It is most commonly given in hospitals, surgical centers, and clinics. **adequate c.,** 1. health care usually consisting of services that are most desirable in treating the condition. 2. the substitution of a less costly but satisfactory type of health care for a more costly type of service. **ambulatory c.,** 1. care provided to patients who are not confined to the hospital bed (outpatients), as opposed to services provided in the patient's home or to persons who are inpatients. Called also *outpatient c.* 2. ambulatory hospital c. **ambulatory hospital c.,** medical care sevices rendered in a hospital or a clinic to persons who are not confined overnight in a health care institution (outpatients). Called also *hospital outpatient c., hospital outpatient service,* and *outpatient service.* **community health c.,** activities, services, and programs intended to maintain and improve the general health status in a specified community. **dental c.,** the total of dental diagnostic, preventive, and restorative services. **dental c., adequate,** dental care consisting of repair of oral damage and the placing of the mouth in a condition to prevent deterioration. 2. dental care consisting of services that are the most desirable for an individual. 3. the substitution of a less costly but satisfactory type of dental care for a more costly type of service. **dental c., comprehensive,** dental care consisting of all services indicated for the restoration and maintenance of oral health, usually excluding purely cosmetic procedures. **dental c., emergency,** dental care consisting of dental services required for the treatment of unexpected and urgent conditions, such as acute infections, hemorrhage, toothache, or injury. See also *dental c., minimal.* **dental c., initial,** dental care consisting of services required for dental needs existing at the time of enrollment in an insurance plan for dental care or at the beginning of any dental treatment. See also *dental c., primary.* **dental c., incremental,** dental care consisting of services initiated at specific intervals of time to specified age groups in order to establish and maintain oral health. **dental c., maintenance,** dental care required to maintain oral health after initial care has been completed. **dental c., minimal,** dental care generally consisting of only those services which are required for the management of acute conditions of the teeth and gums; usually, emergency dental care. **dental c., primary,** the continuing management and coordination of health services provided by a dental care provider system of first contact and maintenance of health prevention of disease and injury, and restoration of health. It includes appropriate assessment of general and oral health status; provision of oral diagnostic, preventive, educational, and therapeutic services; and referral and coordination of episodic specialty care. Called also *primary care dentistry.* **emergency c.,** care for patients with severe, life-threatening, or potentially disabling conditions that require immediate intervention. **emergency c. facility,** emergency ROOM. **extended c. facility,** extended care FACILITY. **extended c. service,** extended care SERVICE. **health c.,** the promotion of health through preventive, diagnostic, and therapeutic services, as well as health maintenance, case-finding, and rehabilitation. **home health c.,** health services provided for aged, disabled, convalescent, or sick persons in their homes, usually by home health agencies, visiting nurse associations, hospitals, or other organized community groups. Under Medicare, such care may be provided only by a home health agency. Called also *home health service.* **hometown medical and dental c.,** a program, under the Veterans Administration, which compensates approved physicians and dentists for outpatient services provided to eligible veterans in their communities. **hospital outpatient c.,** see ambulatory hospital c. **intermediate c. facility,** intermediate care FACILITY. **long term c.,** care given to patients in a hospital, nursing home, rehabilitation center, or any medical care institution, for a period of no less than 30 days. Such care includes medical supervision and/or assistance. **outpatient c.,** 1. ambulatory c. 2. ambulatory hospital c. **primary c.,** the point of entry into the health system, consisting of the promotion and maintenance of health, prevention of disease, rehabilitation, health education services, and care of individuals with common health problems, uncomplicated illness, chronic latent illness, and certain aspects of complicated illness in the home or in an outpatient setting. Care is given on a family basis with professional medical personnel providing guidance in the use of health resources and referring to other levels of the health care system. **primary c., interdisciplinary,** all primary care provided by an interdisciplinary team or organization of health professionals and paraprofessionals who interact closely to deal with a combination of health problems that are beyond the competence of any individual team member. **progressive**

patient c., a system under which patients are grouped together in units depending on their need for care as determined by their degree of illness rather than by consideration of medical specialty, consisting of intensive care, intermediate care, and minimal care or self-care. **secondary c.,** health care, such as the general short term hospital, nursing home, emergency care facility, and the more highly specialized physician consultant services. **terminal c.,** care for a terminally ill patient. **tertiary c.,** specialized health care, such as select rehabilitation services and highly specialized technical medical procedures, such as open heart surgery, kidney dialysis, etc.

Carena trademark for *aminophylline.*

Caricide trademark for *diethylcarbamazine.*

caries (kar′ēz) [L. "rottenness"] 1. the molecular decay or death of a bone, in which it becomes softened, discolored, and porous. It produces a chronic inflammation of the periosteum and surrounding tissues, and forms a cold abscess filled with a cheesy, fetid, puslike liquid, which generally burrows through the soft parts until it opens externally by a sinus or fistula. 2. dental c. **arrested c.,** dental caries that becomes static or stationary and does not show any marked tendency for further progression. Formerly called *healed c.* **backward c.,** dental caries that progresses backward from the dentinoenamel junction into the enamel. Called also *internal c.* **cemental c., cementum c.,** dental caries involving the cementum of a tooth, usually observed in elderly persons with gingival recession. Carious lesions develop with the formation of plaque on the surface of cementum, followed by invasion of the cementum along calcified Sharpey's fibers or between the bundles of fibers, spreading laterally between various layers. Decalcification and proteolysis follow. **central c.,** a chronic abscess in the interior of a bone. **cervical c.,** dental caries, usually resulting from poor dental hygiene, characterized by a crescent-like cavity beginning as a slightly roughened chalky area on either the facial, lingual, or labial surface, extending from the area opposite the gingival crest occlusally to the height of convexity on the tooth surface. On occasion, the lesion extends beneath the free margin of the gingiva. **contact c.,** caries which develops on the surface of an adjacent tooth which has been in contact with the restorative material. **dental c.,** the most prevalent human disease, characterized by localized destruction of calcified tissue, initiated on the tooth surface by decalcification of the enamel, followed by enzymatic lysis of organic structures, leading to cavity formation that, if left unchecked, penetrates the enamel and dentin and may reach the pulp. Carious lesions develop most commonly in areas beneath dental plaque (see under PLAQUE) in which food stagnation occurs. Several theories on etiology have been proposed: The *acidogenic theory,* whereby acids produced by bacteria cause decalcification and softening of the residue; the *proteolytic theory,* whereby microorganisms destroy enamel protein; and the *proteolysis-chelation theory,* whereby keratolytic microorganisms cause formation of che-

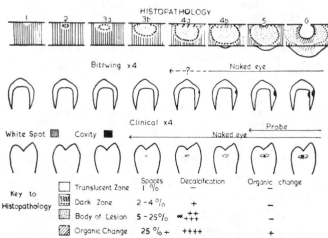

Diagrammatic representation of the stages of enamel caries as seen by histopathology, clinically, and radiographically. (From A. I. Darling: The pathology and prevention of caries. Br. Dent. J. 107:287, 1959. In G. W. Burnett, H. W. Scherp, and G. S. Schuster: Oral Microbiology and Infectious Diseases. 4th ed. Baltimore, Williams and Wilkins, 1976.)

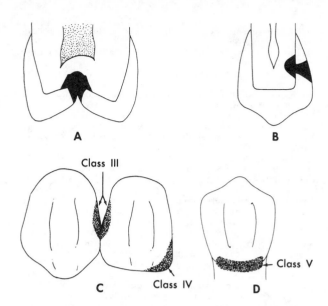

G. V. Black's classification of dental caries. *A,* Example of Class I carious lesion, occlusal decay. *B,* Class II caries, interproximal decay, illustrating the configuration with the spread observed commonly at the dentinoenamel junction. *C,* Examples of caries in anterior teeth. Class III lesions on the interproximal surfaces, but not involving the incisal surfaces. Class IV lesion on the interproximal surface and involving the incisal surface of the incisor or cuspid. *D,* Example of Class V carious lesion on the faciocervical area. (From H. W. Gilmore, M. R. Lund, D. J. Bales, and J. Vernetti: Operative Dentistry. 3rd ed. St. Louis, The C. V. Mosby Co., 1977.)

lates which, in turn, cause decalcification. *Lactobacillus acidophilus, Cladothrix placoides,* and *Leptothrix buccalis* are the most common microorganisms found in dental caries, but actinomycetes, streptococci, micrococci, *Neisseria,* and various other cocci are also present. Called also *tooth decay.* See illustration. See also CAVITY. G. V. Black's classification of dental caries (see illustrations) is as follows: *Class I:* Cavities occurring in the pit and fissure defects in the occlusal surfaces of the bicuspids and molars, the lingual surfaces of the upper incisors, and the facial and lingual grooves that are found occasionally on the occlusal surfaces of molar teeth. *Class II:* Cavities in the proximal surfaces of bicuspid and molar teeth. *Class III:* Cavities in the proximal surfaces of the incisor and cuspid teeth that do not involve the incisal angle. *Class IV:* Cavities in the proximal surfaces of incisor and cuspid teeth that do involve the incisal angle. *Class V:* Cavities in the gingival one-third of teeth (not in pits) and below the height of contour on the labial, facial, and lingual surfaces of the teeth. *Class VI:* Cavities in the incisal edges and smooth surfaces of teeth above the height of contour. (Not a true Black classification.) **dental c., acute,** dental caries usually involving several teeth and progressing rapidly, the lesion being light brown or gray and having caseous consistency. Pulp exposure and tooth sensitivity may be present. Called also *rampant c.* **dental c., chronic,** dental caries, usually occurring in adults, characterized by a slow course, long-standing involvement, relatively small number of teeth involved, relatively large point of entry, dark brown staining of decalcified dentin, leathery consistency of the lesion, deposition of secondary dentin, and relatively late involvement of the pulp. **dental c., initial,** dental c., primary. **dental c., primary,** dental caries in which the lesion constitutes the initial attack on the tooth surface. Called also *initial dental c.* **dental c., secondary,** dental caries occurring around the edges and under restorations, usually on the rough or overhanging margin and areas of fractured dental tissue. **healed c.,** former synonym for *arrested c.* **pit c.,** dental caries originating in pits or fissures, usually of the occlusal surfaces of molars and premolars or on the lingual surfaces of the maxillary incisors where food debris is most likely to accumulate, thus providing the terrain for microorganisms to grow and ferment. The pits or fissures may appear stained brown or black and become softened, and the enamel bordering them may become opaque bluish white. A typical lesion is usually a deep cavity with a narrow point of penetration. Called also *fissure c.* **dental c., postirradiation,** radiation c. **dentinal c.,** dental caries that spreads along the dentinoenamel junction and involves dentinal tubules, eventually reaching the pulp. Dentinal changes include transparent dentin, fatty degeneration of Tome's tubules, decalcification, bacterial invasion, and decomposition. **dry c.,** a form of tuberculosis of the joints and ends of bones. Called also *c. sicca.* **enamel c.,** dental caries that involves the enamel of a tooth. **fissure c.,** *pit c.* **incipient c.,** dental caries in an early stage of development, usually not requiring immediate restoration. **internal c.,** backward c. **lateral c.,** dental caries that extends internally at the dentinoenamel junction. **necrotic c.,** a disease in which pieces of bone lie in a suppurating cavity. **proximal c.,** dental caries usually beginning on a proximal surface (mesial or distal), just below the contact point of the teeth. In the early stages, the lesion appears as a faint white opacity of the enamel and, less frequently, as a yellow or brown pigmented area. As the process of decalcification progresses, the lesion becomes slightly roughened and, by the time it penetrates the enamel, the surrounding area assumes a bluish-white appearance. **radiation c.,** caries-like destruction of tooth substance, associated with xerostomia, produced by therapeutic x-radiation. The lesion resembles demineralization and begins at the cervical area of the tooth, resulting in brittleness of the tooth, fracture of the enamel, and sometimes amputation of the tooth crown at its neck. Called also *postirradiation dental c.* **rampant c.,** dental c., acute. **recurrent c.,** dental caries occurring beneath the marginal periphery of an existing dental restoration, usually due to retention of debris resulting from inadequate cavity restoration, or faulty sealing in the restoration, resulting in a "leaky margin," or improper cavity extension. **residual c.,** decayed material left in a prepared cavity and over which a restoration is placed. Called also *residual carious dentin.* **senile c.,** dental caries occurring in elderly persons whose supporting tissues have receded, being present primarily in the cementum, usually on proximal surfaces of the teeth. Called also *senile decay.* See also *cementum c.* **c. sic′ca,** dry c. **smooth surface c.,** dental caries originating on smooth surfaces of the teeth, usually on the proximal surfaces or on the gingival third of the facial and lingual surfaces.

cariogenesis (kăr″e-o-jen′ĕ-sis) development of caries.

cariogenic (kăr″e-o-jen′ik) [*caries* + Gr. *gennan* to produce] conducive to caries.

cariogenicity (kăr″e-o-jĕ-nis′ĭ-te) the quality of being conducive to the production of caries.

cariosity (kar″e-os′ĭ-te) [L. *cariosus*] affected with or of the nature of caries; carious.

carious (ka′re-us) [L. *cariosus*] affected with or of the nature of caries; cariosity.

carisoprodate (kar-i″so-pro′dāt) carisoprodol.

carisoprodol (kar-i″so-pro′dŏl) a sedative drug with skeletal muscle relaxant properties, N-isopropyl-2-methyl-2-propyl-1,3-propanediol dicarbamate, occurring as a slightly bitter crystalline substance that is soluble in organic solvents, sparingly soluble in water, and insoluble in vegetable oils. Used in alleviation of local muscle spasms and anxiety. Urticaria, weakness, lassitude, and excessive sedation are the potential side effects. Transient quadriplegia, ataxia, vertigo, diplopia, blindness, mydriasis, confusion, agitation, and euphoria may occur. The drug can be addicting. Called also *carisoprodate, isobamate,* and *isopropyl.* Trademarks: Arusal, Rela, Soma, Somadril.

carmustine (kar-mus′tin) a nitrogen mustard compound substituted with nitrosourea, N,N-bis(2-chloroethyl)-N-nitrosourea, occurring as a light-yellow powder that melts at room temperature to an oily liquid which is soluble in water and ethanol. It is an alkylating agent capable of inhibiting DNA, RNA, and protein synthesis. Used in the treatment of Hodgkin's disease and other lymphomas, brain tumors, melanomas, and other neoplasms. Delayed bone marrow depression with hematological complications, hepatotoxicity, lesions of the central nervous system, esophagitis, diarrhea, dyspnea, nausea, vomiting, and pain at the site of injection are the most common side reactions. Abbreviated *BCNU.*

carnitine (kar′nĭ-tin) a salt of 3-carboxy-2-hydroxy-N,N,N-trimethyl-1-propanaminium hydroxide. It is a constituent of striated muscle and the liver; believed to be involved in lipid transport to mitochondria. Injection causes excessive salivation, vomiting, and mydriasis. Used as a thyroid inhibitor. In the L-form, known as vitamin B_T.

Carnochan's operation [John Murray *Carnochan,* American surgeon, 1817–1887] see under OPERATION.

carnosine (kar′no-sin) a substance, N-β-alanyl-L-histidine, found in skeletal muscles of vertebrates. Because of its β-alanine content, sometimes referred to as a *pseudoprotein.*

carotene (kar′o-tēn) a yellow or red pigment, $C_{40}H_{56}$, found in carrots, sweet potatoes, leafy vegetables, milk, body fat, egg yolk, and other foods. It is a chromolipoid hydrocarbon and exists in several forms, α-, β-, and γ-carotene, which can be converted to vitamin A in the body. α-Carotene is widely distributed in nature but in small amounts; carrots, palm oil, and green leafy vegetables are the best sources. β-Carotene (Trademark: Solatene) is the most important provitamin A, being also largely distributed in nature, especially in chlorophyll-bearing plants. γ-Carotene is a rare carotenoid, found most commonly in *Penicillium sclerotiorum* and also occurring in small amounts in plants. See also VITAMIN A.

carotenemia (kar″o-tĕ-ne′me-ah) [*carotene* + Gr. *haima* blood + *-ia*] presence in the blood of excessive amounts of carotene, sometimes associated with yellowing of the skin resembling jaundice.

carotenoid (kah-rot′ĕ-noid) [*carotene* + Gr. *eidos* form] 1. any member of the group of red, orange, or yellow pigmented polyisoprenoid lipids found in carrots, sweet potatoes, green leaves, and some animal tissues; examples are the carotenes, lycopene, and xanthophyll. 2. marked by yellow color. 3. lipochrome.

caroticotympanic (kah-rot″ĭ-ko-tim-pan′ik) pertaining to the carotid canal and the tympanum.

carotid (kah-rot′id) [Gr. *karōtis* from *karos* deep sleep] pertaining to the carotid artery, body, or sinus.

carotodynia (kah-rot″o-din′e-ah) [*carotid* + Gr. *odynē* pain] tenderness along the course of the common carotid artery.

Carpenter's syndrome [George *Carpenter*] see under SYNDROME.

Carpue's operation, rhinoplasty [Joseph Constantine *Carpue,* English surgeon, 1764–1846] Indian RHINOPLASTY.

carrageenan, carragheenin (kar″ah-ge′nan, kar″ah-ge′nin) a galactan extracted from various species of red seaweeds, chiefly *Chondrus crispus,* consisting of a complex mixture of several polysaccharides. Carrageenan and its water-soluble calcium and sodium salts occur as a white to cream-white powder that is insoluble in alcohol and becomes viscous when dissolved in water. Used mostly as an emulsifying agent for liquid petrolatum and for cod liver oil and as a demulcent. Also used in denture adhesive powders. Called also *Irish moss.* Trademark: Viscarin.

Carrel-Dakin solution [A. *Carrel;* Henry Drysdale *Dakin,* American chemist, 1880–1952] sodium hypochlorite solution, diluted; see under SOLUTION.

carrier (kar′e-er) 1. an individual who harbors pathogenic organisms without manifest symptoms and thus may be responsible for spreading the infection. 2. a substance capable of accepting hydrogen and so be reduced and can then be re-oxidized. 3. an instrument or apparatus for carrying or transporting something. 4. an organization contracted by the Secretary of the Department of Health and Human Services for the administration of benefits under Part B of the Medicare program. 5. a company or organization that contracts an insurance plan, such as health or dental care plans, being responsible for collecting premiums, paying claims, and/or providing administrative services. Called also *insurance administrative agent, insurer, second party,* and *underwriter.* 6. carrier MOLECULE. 7. heterozygote. **amalgam c.,** an instrument for carrying freshly mixed amalgam to the prepared cavity. **female c.,** a woman who is heterozygous for a recessive X-linked trait; half of the sons of a female carrier show recessive X-chromosomal characteristics. **foil c.,** foil PASSER. **hemophilia c.,** the female transmitter of classical X-linked recessive hemophilia, who generally, but not always, demonstrates no overt manifestations of a hemorrhagic diathesis but in whom a coagulation factor deficiency may be detected by quantitative assay. **lentula c., lentulo paste c.,** lentulo. **c. molecule,** carrier MOLECULE. **not-for-profit c.,** a service corporation or prepayment plan organized under state not-for-profit statutes for the purpose of providing health care coverage. Called also *nonprofit insurer.* **paste c.,** lentulo. **primary c.,** a carrier who, under coordination of benefits, has the primary responsibility for paying benefits as if there were no additional coverage. Benefits received from the primary and secondary carriers may not together exceed the total amount of the fee charged for the service performed. **secondary c.,** a carrier who, under coordination of benefits, has the responsibility for paying additional (secondary) benefits after payment of benefits by the primary carrier. Benefits received from the primary and secondary carriers may not exceed the total amount of the fee charged for the service performed.

Carrión's disease [Daniel A. *Carrión,* a student in Peru who inoculated himself with bartonellosis and died of the disease, 1850–1885] bartonellosis.

Carter's intranasal splint, operation [William Wesley *Carter*, American surgeon, born 1869] see under SPLINT and OPERATION.

cartilage (kar′tĭ-lij) [L. *cartilago*] a specialized, fibrous connective tissue, forming most of the temporary skeleton of the embryo, providing a model in which most of the bones develop, and constituting a part of the growth mechanism. It consists of cells, chondrocytes, and extracellular fibers embedded in a gel-like matrix. Cartilage has no nerves or blood vessels of its own. Except where it is exposed to the synovial fluid in joints, cartilage is inclosed in perichondrium. Three types, hyaline, elastic, and fibrocartilage, are distinguished on the basis of the amount of amorphous matrix and the relative abundance of the collagenous and elastic fibers embedded in it. Called also *cartilago*. See also terms beginning CHONDR- and CHONDRO-. **accessory c's of nose,** alar c's, lesser. **alar c., greater,** either of the two thin, curved cartilages, one on each side at the apex of the nose, forming the medial and lateral crura. The part forming the medial crus is loosely attached to its fellow of the opposite side and assists in forming the mobile septum of the nose. The part forming the lateral crus curves laterally around the nostril, corresponding to the wing of the nose, and joins the frontal process of the maxilla. Called also *inferior c. of nose, lower lateral c. of nose,* and *cartilago alaris major* [NA]. **alar c's, lesser,** three or four small cartilaginous plates located in the fibrous tissue of the alae nasi, posterior to the greater alar cartilage. Called also *accessory c's of nose* and *cartilagines alares minores* [NA]. **annular c.,** cricoid c. **arthrodial c.,** articular c. **articular c.,** a thin layer of cartilage, usually hyaline, on the articular surfaces of bones in synovial joints. Called also *arthrodial c., diarthrodial c., investing c., obducent c.,* and *cartilago articularis* [NA]. **arytenoid c.,** one of the paired, pyramidal cartilages of the back of the larynx at the upper border of the cricoid cartilage. Its concave dorsal surface gives attachment to the arytenoidei obliquus and transversus muscles; the convex ventral surface gives rise to an elevation (*colliculus*), and to a ridge (*crista arcuata*); and the flat medial surface forms the lateral boundary of the intercartilaginous part of the rima glottidis. Called also *guttural c., pyramidal c., triquetral c., triquetrous c., cartilago arytaenoidea, cartilago arytenoidea* [NA], and *cartilago triquetra.* **auricular c.,** the internal plate of elastic cartilage in the external ear. Called also *conchal c.* and *cartilago auriculae* [NA]. **branchial c.,** one of the rods of cartilage in the branchial arches of the embryo. **calcified c.,** cartilage in which granules of calcium phosphate have been deposited in the interstitial substance. **cellular c.,** cartilage composed almost entirely of cells, with little interstitial substance. Called also *parenchymatous c.* **ciliary c.,** TARSUS palpebrae. **conchal c.,** auricular c. **connecting c.,** cartilage connecting the surfaces of an immovable joint. Called also *interosseous c.* **corniculate c.,** one of two small conical cartilaginous nodules at the apex of each arytenoid cartilage, situated in the posterior parts of the aryepiglottic folds of mucous membrane, and sometimes fused with the arytenoid cartilage. It consists of yellow elastic cartilage and articulates with the top of the arytenoid cartilage. Called also *c. of Santorini, supra-arytenoid c., cartilago corniculata* [NA], *cartilago corniculata* [*Santorini*], *cartilago santorini, corniculum,* and *corpora santoriana.* **cricoarytenoid c., posterior,** cricoarytenoid ligament, posterior; see under LIGAMENT. **cricoid c.,** a ringlike cartilage forming the caudal and dorsal parts of the wall of the larynx, consisting of a wide plate, the lamina of the cricoid cartilage, and a narrow, convex arch, the arch of the cricoid cartilage. The plate gives attachment to fibers of the esophagus and on its dorsal side provides a depression for the cricoarytenoideus posterior muscle. The arch provides attachment to the cricothyroidei and constrictor pharyngis muscles. Its caudal border gives attachment to the cricotracheal ligament, while its cranial border gives attachment to the cricothyroid ligament, and at the side of the conus elasticus, to the cricoarytenoidei laterales muscles. Called also *annular c., innominate c.,* and *cartilago cricoidea* [NA]. **cuneiform c.,** one of two small, elongated pieces of yellow elastic cartilage on either side of the aryepiglottic fold. Called also *c. of Wrisberg, cartilago cuneiformis* [NA], *cartilago cuneiformis* [*Wrisbergi*], and *cartilago wrisbergi.* **dentinal c.,** the substance remaining after the lime salts of dentin have been dissolved in an acid. **diarthroidal c.,** articular c. **elastic c.,** a flexible, elastic, yellowish type of cartilage found in the external ear, walls of the external auditory and eustachian tubes, epiglottis, and in parts of the corniculate and cuneiform cartilages. Its cells are round-

ed and encapsulated, and occur singly or in groups of two or four cells. The interstitial substance is permeated by frequently branching elastin fibers that form a dense network, being somewhat looser beneath the perichondrium. Like hyaline cartilage, it forms in the embryo by appositional growth. Called also *yellow c.* and *reticular c.* **epactal c's,** nasal c's, accessory. **epiglottic c.,** the plate of yellow elastic cartilage that constitutes the central part of the epiglottis. Called also *cartilago epiglottica* [NA]. **gingival c.,** the tissue covering the loculus, which contains an unerupted tooth. **greater alar c.,** alar c., greater. **guttural c.,** arytenoid c. **hyaline c.,** the most common and characteristic type of cartilage found in the adult on the ends of the ribs, in the tracheal rings of the larynx, and on the joint surfaces of the bones. It is a flexible, somewhat elastic, semitransparent substance with an opalescent bluish tint, composed of a basophilic, fibril-containing interstitial substance with cavities in which the chondrocytes occur. Called also *chondroid.* **inferior c. of nose,** alar c., greater. **innominate c.,** cricoid c. **interosseous c.,** connecting c. **intrathyroid c.,** a narrow, transparent strip of cartilage which joins the two laminae of the thyroid cartilage in infancy. **investing c.,** articular c. **Jacobson's c.,** vomeronasal c. **laryngeal c's,** the nine cartilages which form the larynx, including the thyroid, cricoid, epiglottis, two arytenoid, two corniculate, and two cuneiform cartilages. Called also *cartilagines laryngis* [NA]. **laryngeal c. of Luschka,** sesamoid c. of vocal ligament. **lesser alar c's,** alar c's, lesser. **lower lateral c. of nose,** alar c., greater. **Luschka's c.,** sesamoid c. of vocal ligament. **mandibular c.,** Meckel's c. **Meckel's c.,** the cartilaginous bar (in the embryo) into which the mesenchymal core of the mandibular process of the first mandibular arch is converted; from it or its sheath, the sphenomandibular ligament, the anterior malleolar ligament, the malleus, and the incus develop. Called also *mandibular c., tympanomandibular c.,* and *Meckel's rod.* **minor c's,** accessory nasal c's. **nasal c's,** the cartilaginous framework of the nose, consisting of one piece of septal cartilage which separates the nasal cavities from each other, two lateral cartilages which are lateral expansions of the septal cartilage, two greater alar cartilages which form thin curved plates on either side of the apex, and various lesser alar cartilages which are located in the fibrous membrane of the alae nasi. Called also *cartilagines nasi* [NA]. **nasal c's, accessory,** one or more small cartilages on either side of the nose between the greater alar and lateral nasal cartilages. Called also *epactal c's, minor c's, sesamoid c's of nose, cartilagines nasales accessoriae* [NA], and *cartilagines sesamoideae nasi.* **nasal c., lateral,** a part of the cartilaginous framework of the nose; it continues from the septal cartilage on either side of the nose just inferior to the nasal bone, but is separated from it by a narrow fissure. Its superior margin joins the nasal bone and the frontal process of the maxilla, and its inferior margin is connected with the greater alar cartilage. Called also *triangular c. of nose, upper lateral nasal c.,* and *cartilago nasi lateralis* [NA]. **nasal c., septal,** septal c. of nose. **nasal c., upper lateral,** nasal c., lateral. **obducent c.,** articular c. **ossifying c.,** temporary c. **palpebral c.,** TARSUS palpebrae. **parachordal c's,** the two cartilages at the sides of the occipital part of the notochord of the embryo. **parenchymatous c.,** cellular c. **permanent c.,** cartilage that remains unossified during life. **precursory c.,** temporary c. **pyramidal c.,** arytenoid c. **Reichert's c's,** cartilaginous bars in the outer side of the embryonic tympanum from which develop the styloid processes, stylohyoid ligaments, and lesser cornua of the hyoid bone. **reticular c.,** elastic c. **c. of Santorini,** corniculate c. **scutiform c.,** thyroid c. **septal c. of nose,** the hyaline cartilage forming the framework of the cartilaginous part of the nasal septum, and including the lateral nasal cartilages. Anteriorly, it is connected to the nasal bones; inferiorly, to the median crura of the greater alar cartilages; and posteriorly, to the perpendicular plate of the ethmoid. In some instances, especially in children, the sphenoidal process extends the cartilage posteriorly. Called also *septal nasal c.* and *cartilago septi nasi* [NA]. **sesamoid c. of larynx,** triticeal c. **sesamoid c's of nose,** nasal c's, accessory. **sesamoid c. of vocal ligament,** a small cartilage occasionally found within the vocal ligaments. Called also *laryngeal c. of Luschka, Luschka's c., cartilago sesamoidea laryngis, Luschka,* and *cartilago sesamoidea ligamenti vocalis* [NA]. **stratified c.,** fibrocartilage. **subvomerine c.,** vomeronasal c. **supra-arytenoid c.,** corniculate c. **tarsal c.,** TARSUS palpebrae. **temporary c.,** cartilage in the fetus that is destined to be replaced by bone. Called also *ossifying c.* and *precursory c.* **thyroid c.,** the largest cartilage of the larynx, consisting of two roughly rectangular plates which join in the midline, their posterior borders extending superiorly into long superior horns, and inferiorly into the shorter inferior horns. The lower horns articulate with the lower aspects of the cricoid cartilage. Its upper border is notched in the midline by the thyroid notch; below it there is the laryngeal prominence (Adam's apple), which is more pronounced in males than in females. Called also *scutiform c., cartilago thyroidea* [NA], and *cartilago thyreoidea*. **triangular c. of nose,** nasal c., lateral. **triquetral c., triquetrous c.,** arytenoid c. **triticeal c., triticeous c.,** a small cartilage in the thyrohyoid ligament. Called also cartilage of *sesamoid c. of larynx, cartilago triticea* [NA], *corpus triticeum,* and *corpusculum triticeum.* **tympanomandibular c.,** Meckel's c. **upper lateral nasal c.,** nasal c., lateral. **vomeronasal c.,** either of the two narrow, longitudinal strips of cartilage, one lying on either side of the anterior portion of the lower margin of the septal cartilage. Called also *Jacobson's c., subvomerine c., cartilago jacobsoni,* and *cartilago vomeronasalis* [NA]. **c. of Wrisberg,** cuneiform c. **yellow c.,** elastic c.

cartilagines (kar″tĭ-laj′ĭ-nēz) [L.] plural of *cartilago.*

cartilaginiform (kar″tĭ-lah-jin′ĭ-form) [*cartilage* + L. *forma* form] resembling cartilage. Called also *cartilaginoid.*

cartilaginoid (kar″tĭ-laj′ĭ-noid) [*cartilage* + Gr. *eidos* form] cartilaginiform.

cartilaginous (kar″tĭ-laj′ĭ-nus) consisting of or of the nature of cartilage.

cartilago (kar-tĭ-lah′go), pl. *cartilag′ines* [L.] cartilage. **c. ala′ris ma′jor** [NA], alar cartilage, greater; see under CARTILAGE. **cartilag′ines ala′res mino′res** [NA], alar cartilages, lesser; see under CARTILAGE. **c. articula′ris** [NA], articular CARTILAGE. **c. arytenoi′dea** [NA], **c. arytaenoi′dea,** arytenoid CARTILAGE. **c. auric′ulae** [NA], auricular CARTILAGE. **c. cornicula′ta** [NA], **c. cornicula′ta** [Santori′ni], corniculate CARTILAGE. **c. cricoi′dea** [NA], cricoid CARTILAGE. **c. cuneifor′mis** [NA], **c. cuneifor′mis** [Wrisber′gi], cuneiform CARTILAGE. **c. epiglot′tica** [NA], epiglottic CARTILAGE. **c. jacobso′ni,** vomeronasal CARTILAGE. **cartilag′ines laryn′gis,** laryngeal cartilages, see under CARTILAGE. **cartilag′ines nasa′les accesso′riae** [NA], nasal cartilages, accessory; see under CARTILAGE. **cartilag′ines na′si** [NA], nasal cartilages; see under CARTILAGE. **c. na′si latera′lis** [NA], nasal cartilage, lateral; see under CARTILAGE. **c. santori′ni,** corniculate CARTILAGE. **c. sep′ti na′si** [NA], septal cartilage of nose; see under CARTILAGE. **c. sesamoi′dea ligamen′ti voca′lis** [NA], **c. sesamoi′dea laryn′gis,** Luschka, sesamoid cartilage of vocal ligament; see under CARTILAGE. **cartilag′ines sesamoi′deae na′si,** nasal cartilages, accessory; see under CARTILAGE. **c. thyroi′dea** [NA], **c. thyreoi′dea,** thyroid CARTILAGE. **c. triquet′ra,** arytenoid CARTILAGE. **c. tritic′ea** [NA], triticeal CARTILAGE. **c. vomeronasa′lis** [NA], vomeronasal CARTILAGE. **c. wrisber′gi,** cuneiform CARTILAGE.

caruncle (kar′ung-k'l) a small fleshy eminence, whether normal or abnormal. Called also *caruncula.* **sublingual c.,** an eminence on each side of the frenulum of the tongue, at the apex of which are the openings of the major sublingual duct and the submandibular duct. Called also *caruncula sublingualis* [NA] and *sublingual papilla.*

caruncula (kah-rung′ku-lah), pl. *carun′culae* [L., dim of *caro* flesh] a small fleshy eminence. Called also *caruncle.* **c. sublingua′lis** [NA], sublingual CARUNCLE.

carunculae (kah-rung′ku-le) [L.] plural of *caruncula.*

carver (kar′ver) a knife or any other instrument used for carving or fashioning an object by cutting, such as one used for shaping artificial teeth and dental restorations. Called also *carving blade, carving instrument,* and *carving knife.* See illustration. **amalgam c.,** a small sharp blade of various shapes, made of hardened steel, used for contouring an amalgam interdental restoration. **wax c.,** any instrument used to carve wax patterns, generally a blunt blade of various size and shape, which can be heated for softening the wax while fashioning the pattern.

carving (kar′ving) 1. the act of fashioning or producing by cutting, as in shaping dental wax or amalgam. 2. a carved object. 3. the process of molding and shaping an artificial tooth or restoration to imitate the form, contour, and anatomy of natural teeth.

caryo- [Gr. *karyon* nucleus, or nut] a combining form denoting relationship to a nucleus. See also words beginning KARYO-.

Cascellius [1st century A.D.] a dentist, believed to be the first in Rome whose name has been recorded, and who extracted and repaired teeth.

case (kās) 1. a particular occurrence of disease or disorder. 2. a protective covering, or a structure which serves in that capacity. 3. one complete unit of replacement or restoration, as a denture or bridge. **borderline c.,** an instance of a disease in which the symptoms resemble those of a recognized condition but are not typical of it. **index c.,** 1. the first case of a contagious disease, as opposed to subsequent cases. 2. propositus; proband.

Case appliance, cleaver, obturator [Calvin S. *Case,* American dentist, 1847–1923, who introduced the use of rubber elastics in orthodontic therapy, developed a method for root movement,

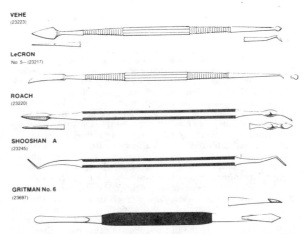

VEHE (23223)

LeCRON No 5— (23217)

ROACH (23220)

SHOOSHAN A (23245)

GRITMAN No. 6 (23697)

Porcelain and wax carvers. (From H. O. Torres and A. Ehrlich: Modern Dental Assisting. 2nd ed. Philadelphia, W. B. Saunders Co., 1980; courtesy of S. S. White Div. of Pennwalt Corp.)

and advocated extraction of teeth as an orthodontic method] see under APPLIANCE, CLEAVER, and OBTURATOR.

Case's enamel cleaver see under CLEAVER.

casebook (kās′book) a book in which a physician or dentist enters the records of his cases.

case-finding (kās-find′ing) that form of screening, the main object of which is to detect disease and bring patients to treatment.

casein (ka′se-in) [L. *caseus* cheese] a phosphoprotein, the principal protein of milk, the basis of curd of cheese.

caseous (ka′se-us) resembling cheese or curd; cheesy.

Caspersson's method [Torbjörn Oskar *Caspersson,* Swedish geneticist, born 1910] see Q-BANDING.

Casser's (Casserio's, Casserius') fontanelle [Giulio *Casser,* Italian anatomist, 1556–1616] mastoid FONTANELLE.

casserian (kah-ser′e-an) named after Giulio *Casser* (Casserio, Casserius), as casserian fontanelle (mastoid FONTANELLE).

Casserio, Casserius see CASSER.

cassette (kah-set′) [Fr. "little box"] a light-tight container in which films are placed for exposure to x-radiation, usually backed with lead to eliminate the effect of backscattered radiation. The back side is hinged for loading and is locked by metal clamps; the front side is placed toward the x-ray tube. It may have a built-in intensifying screen. Called also *exposure holder* and *film holder.* **cardboard c.,** a lightproof cassette made of cardboard, having a thin sheet of lead in the back to prevent backscatter radiation. **screen-type c.,** usually a metal cassette, with the exposure side of low atomic number material, such as Bakelite, aluminum, or magnesium, containing intensifying screens on both sides.

cast (kast) 1. an accurate reproduction or a replica of an object or part produced in a plastic material which has taken form in an impression or mold. 2. a rigid dressing, molded to the body while pliable, and hardening as it dries, to give firm support. 3. dental c. **blood c.,** a urinary cast that bears blood cells. **dental c.,** a positive reproduction of a maxillary or mandibular arch or a portion thereof made from an impression of that arch. Sometimes called *model.* **diagnostic c.,** a positive reproduction of the maxillary and/or mandibular arches, including the hard palate, mucobuccal, mucolabial, and sublingual folds and associated muscle and frenum attachments, pterygomaxillary notches, retromolar pads, and all teeth and edentulous ridge areas, made from impression material, and used for study and treatment planning. Called also *preextraction c., preoperative c., study c.,* and *study model.* **gnathostatic c.,** a cast of the teeth trimmed so that the occlusal plane is in its normal position in the mouth when the cast is set on a plane surface; used in orthodontic diagnosis. **implant c.,** a positive cast of exposed bony surfaces made in a surgical bone impression, which serves for designing and fabricating a subperiosteal or intraperiosteal implant framework. Called also *implant model.* **implant c., study,** a cast made from a mucosal impression which serves for the production of the wax trial denture and surgical impression trays, similar to other study casts. **investment c.,** refractory c. **c. investment,** investment. **master c.,** an accurate facsimile of oral structures, including the prepared tooth surfaces, residual alveolar ridge areas, and/or other parts of the dental arch, reproduced from an impression from which a prosthesis is to be fabricated. **c. material,** any material used for the production of a dental cast, including plaster of Paris and dental stone. **modified c.,** a master cast that is altered prior to processing a denture base. **preextraction c., preoperative c.,** diagnostic c. **refractory c.,** one made of heat resistant materials that will withstand high temperatures without disintegrating and which, when used in partial denture casting, has expansion to compensate for metal shrinkage. Called also *investment c.* **renal c.,** urinary c. **study c.,** diagnostic c. **working c.,** an accurate reproduction of the master cast employed in preliminary fitting of the casting, which is used instead of the master in order to prevent damage to the master cast. **urinary c.,** a cylindrical body found in the urinary sediment, representing an actual cast of the tubular lumen, made up of erythrocytes, epithelial cells, bacteria, hyaline material, or any other substance effused into the urinary passages and precipitated in the urine. They may be formed anywhere along the course of the nephron, but most are formed in the distal portion and in the collecting tubules. Called also *renal c.*

Castellani-Low symptom [Sir Aldo *Castellani,* Italian physician, 1877–1971; George Carmichael *Low,* English physician, 1872–1952] see under SYMPTOM.

casting (kast′ing) 1. any object formed by the solidification of plastic material, such as a gypsum product or molten metal, poured into an impression or mold, or the act of forming such an object. 2. the fabrication of a metallic dental restoration or appliance. The process involves the reproduction of the lost tooth structure or appliance in wax and surrounding the wax with an investment material which is a mixture of α-hemihydrate of gypsum and silica mixed with water. After the investment has hardened, the wax is removed and the molten metal is forced into the space vacated by the wax. 3. a metallic dental restoration or appliance fabricated by such a process. 4. a dental restoration of metal made to fit a cavity preparation and retained to or luted into it with a cementing medium. **dental c. gold alloy,** see under GOLD. **c. machine,** casting MACHINE. **c. ring,** casting RING. **superstructure c.,** a surgical alloy bar with clasps designed to telescope over the abutments to retain the superstructure in an implant denture. **vacuum c.,** the pouring of plastic material into an impression or mold, under conditions of lowered atmospheric pressure or vacuum.

Castle's factor [William Bosworth *Castle,* American physician, born 1897] see under FACTOR.

Castone trademark for a Class I *dental stone* (see under STONE).

Castorwax trademark for a synthetic *dent wax* (see under WAX).

cata- [Gr. *kata* down] a prefix signifying down, lower, under, against, along with, very.

catabasial (kat″ah-ba′ze-al) [*cata-* + *basion*] having the basion lower than the opisthion; said of certain skulls.

catabasis (kah-tab′ah-sis) [*cata-* + Gr. *bainein* to go] the stage of decline of a disease.

catabolic (kat″ah-bol′ik) pertaining to or of the nature of catabolism; retrograde or destructive.

catabolism (kah-tab′o-lizm) [Gr. *katabolē* a throwing down] the metabolic process consisting of the degradation of large and complex nutrient molecules, such as carbohydrates, lipids, and proteins, originating either in foods or derived from storage depots in the body, to smaller and simpler molecules, such as lactic acid, acetic acid, ammonia, carbon dioxide, or urea. The process is associated with the release of chemical energy inherent in the structure of nutrient molecules and its conservation in the form of energy transferring molecules of adenosine triphosphate (ATP). In turn, ATP supplies energy to anabolic processes. Catabolism and anabolism take place concurrently in cells, but they are regulated independently.

catabolite (kah-tab′o-līt) a product of catabolism.

catalase [E.C.1.11.1.6] (kat′ah-lās) an oxidoreductase acting on hydrogen peroxide as acceptor. It is a hemoprotein that specifically catalyzes the decomposition of hydrogen peroxide, and is found extensively in mammalian tissues and, in lesser amounts, in practically all cells except certain anaerobic bacteria. Used in food preservation by removing oxygen in packaged foods.

catalysis (kah-tal′ĭ-sis) [Gr. *katalysis* dissolution] increase in the velocity of a chemical reaction or process produced by the presence of a substance that is not consumed in the net chemical reaction or process. **contact c., heterogeneous c.,** that produced by the adsorbing power of contact surfaces; e.g., catalysis caused by colloidal platinum. **negative c.,** the slowing down or inhibition of a reaction or process due to presence of a catalyst. **surface c.,** that in which the reacting substances are adsorbed onto the surface of the catalyst and there react.

catalyst (kat′ah-list) any substance that brings about catalysis. Called also *accelerant.* **negative c.,** one that retards the velocity of a reaction. **polysulfide c.,** polysulfide ACCELERATOR. **silicone c.,** a sbstance that brings about the polymerization of silicone materials. Stannous octoate is a common catalyst.

catalytic (kat″ah-lit′ik) [Gr. *katalyein* to dissolve] 1. causing or pertaining to an alterative effect; causing catalysis. 2. an alterative or specific medicine.

catamnesis (kat″am-ne′sis) the history of a patient from the time he is discharged from treatment or from a hospital to the time of his death.

catapasm (kat′ah-pazm) [Gr. *katapasma*] a dusting powder applied to an injured surface.

cataphylaxis (kat″ah-fi-lak′sis) [*cata-* + Gr. *phylaxis* a guarding] 1. the movement of leukocytes and antibodies to the locality of infection. 2. a breaking down of the body's natural defense to infection.

Catapres trademark for *clonidine hydrochloride* (see under CLONIDINE).

Catapresan trademark for *clonidine hydrochloride* (see under CLONIDINE).

cataract (kat′ah-rakt) [L. *cataracta,* from Gr. *katarrhēgnynai* to break down] an opacity of the crystalline lens of the eye or of its capsule. **zonular c.,** the most common form of cataract in children, showing a gray disklike opacity in certain layers between the cortex and nucleus of the crystalline lens. It is either congenital or forms in infancy, usually affecting both eyes. It is also hereditary, and often associated with convulsions, rickets, dental abnormalities, and bone diseases. When associated with Lobstein's syndrome and atrophy of the skin, it is known as *Blegvad-Haxthausen syndrome.*

catarrh (kah-tahr′) [L. *catarrhus,* from Gr. *katarrhein* to flow down] inflammation of a mucous membrane, with a free discharge (Hippocrates); especially, such inflammation of the air passages of the head and throat. The term has been practically eliminated from the scientific vocabulary.

catechol (kat′ĕ-kol) pyrocatechol. **methyl c.,** guaiacol.

catecholamine (kat″ĕ-kol-am′in, kat″ĕ-kol′ah-mēn) a group of sympathomimetic amines, the aromatic portion of whose molecule is pyrocatechol and the aliphatic portion an amine. Catecholamines are derivatives of dopamine, epinephrine, norepinephrine, isoproterenol, and dopamine being of chief pharmacological interest. All, except isoproterenol, are endogenous substances which are stored in the body in special chromaffin cells, particularly of the adrenal medulla, postganglionic sympathetic neurons, and adrenergic neurons in the central nervous system. Pharmacologically, they are considered sympathomimetic drugs.

Catenabacterium (kat″ĕ-nah-bak-te′re-um) [L. *catena* chain + Gr. *baktērion* little rod] a genus made up of nonsporulating, anaerobic, gram-positive bacilli, the species of which have been assigned to the genus *Eubacterium.* **C. contor′tum,** *Eubacterium contortum;* see under EUBACTERIUM. **C. helminthoi′des,** *Eubacterium helminthoides;* see under EUBACTERIUM. **C. sabur′reum,** *Eubacterium saburreum;* see under EUBACTERIUM.

catenating (kat′ĕ-nāt′ing) [L. *catena* a chain] forming part of a chain or complex of symptoms.

catenoid (kat′ĕ-noid) [L. *catena* a chain] arranged like a chain or resembling a chain.

Cateudyl trademark for *methaqualone.*

catgut (kat′gut) an absorbable sterile strand obtained from collagen derived from healthy mammals, originally prepared from the submucous layer of the intestines of sheep; used as a surgical ligature. See also catgut SUTURE. **chromic c., chromicized c.,** catgut sterilized and impregnated with chromium trioxide to prolong its tensile strength in tissues. **formaldehyde c.,** catgut impregnated with a solution of formaldehyde by boiling in an alcohol-formaldehyde solution. **IKI c., iodine c.,** catgut treated with a solution of 1 part of iodine in 100 parts of a potassium iodide solution. **iodochromic c.,** catgut treated with a solution of iodine, potassium, iodide, and potassium dichromate. **silverized c.,** catgut impregnated with silver to give it increased strength and resisting qualities.

cathartic (kah-thar′tik) [Gr. *kathartikos*] 1. causing evacuation of the bowels. 2. an agent that causes evacuation of the bowels.

catheter (kath′ĕ-ter) [Gr. *kathetēr*] a tubular, flexible, surgical instrument for withdrawing fluids from (or introducing fluids into) a cavity of the body, especially one for introduction into the bladder through the urethra for the withdrawal of urine. **eustachian c.,** an instrument for inflating the eustachian tube, used in treating certain diseases of the middle ear. **faucial c.,** a eustachian catheter to be used through the fauces. **Foley c.,** an indwelling catheter retained in the bladder by a balloon which may be inflated with air or liquid. See also sinus BALLOON. **tracheal c.,** an instrument for removing mucus from the trachea by application of suction.

catheterization (kath″ĕ-ter-i-za′shun) the employment or passage of a catheter. **cardiac c.,** passage of a small catheter through a vein in an arm or leg or the neck and into the heart, permitting the securing of and detection of cardiac anomalies. **laryngeal c.,** insertion of a catheter into the larynx, for the evacuation of secretions or introduction of a gas.

catheterostat (kath-ĕ′ter-o-stat) a holder for containing and sterilizing catheters.

cathodal (kath′o-dal) of or pertaining to the cathode.

cathode (kath′ōd) [Gr. *kata* down + *hodos* way] the negative electrode or pole of a galvanic circuit; the electrode toward which positively charged ions (cations) or particles are attracted. Abbreviated *C, Ca,* or *Ka.* Cf. ANODE. **hot c.,** one having a heating filament, such as one found in an x-ray tube. See x-ray tube, hot-cathode, under TUBE.

cathodic (kah-thŏd′ik) pertaining to or emanating from a cathode.

catholicon (kah-thol′ĭ-kon) [Gr. *katholikos* general] that portion of an electrolyte that adjoins the cathode.

cation (kat′i-on) [Gr. *kata* down + *ion* going] a positively charged ion which travels to the cathode or negative pole during electrolysis. Cations include all the metals and hydrogen. In reaction, cations are indicated by a plus sign, as H⁺, or, rarely, by a dot, as H·.

cauda (kaw′dah), pl. *cau′dae* [L.] a tail, or tail-like appendage; used in anatomical nomenclature for such a structure.

caudad (kaw′dad) directed toward the tail; opposite to cranial or cephalad; cephalocaudad.

caudae (kaw′de) [L.] plural of *cauda.*

caudal (kaw′dal) [L. *cauda* tail] 1. pertaining to a cauda. 2. toward or nearer the cauda, or tail.

caudalis (kaw-da′lis) [L] pertaining to the cauda (tail), or to the inferior end of the body; an anatomical term used to denote relationship to the caudal or inferior extremity of an organ or part.

caudalward (kaw′dal-ward) toward the caudal end; in a direction away from the head.

caudate (kaw′dat) [L. *caudatus*] having a tail.

caudocephalad (kaw-do-sef′ah-lad) [L. *cauda* tail + Gr. *kephalē* head + L. *ad* toward] 1. proceeding in a direction from the tail toward the head. 2. in both a caudal and a cephalic direction.

Caulk impression paste see under PASTE.

Caulk Micro II trademark for a *high copper alloy* (see under ALLOY).

Caulk Optaloy trademark for an *amalgam alloy* (see under AMALGAM).

Caulk Optaloy II trademark for a *high copper alloy* (see under ALLOY).

Caulk spherical alloy see under ALLOY.

Caulk Syntrex F trademark for dental *silicate cement* (see under CEMENT).

causal (kaw′zal) pertaining to a cause; directed against a cause.

causalgia (kaw-zal′je-ah) [Gr. *kausos* heat + *-algia*] a syndrome characterized by continuous, burning pain, occurring as a result of injuries to peripheral nerves, most commonly, the sciatic and median nerves. The affected area is usually cool, hairless, and covered by a thin, smooth, shiny skin. Profuse sweating of both the affected and unaffected areas is usually present. In dentistry, causalgia may be produced by extraction of multirooted teeth, and is characterized by burning pain which begins within a few days to several weeks after injury. The pain may be evoked by contact, application of heat or cold, or by emotional stress. Called also *thermalgia.* See also NEURALGIA and PAIN (1). **facial c.,** atypical facial PAIN.

causative (kawz′ah-tiv) effective or responsible as a cause or agent.

cause (kawz) [L. *causa*] that which brings about any condition or produces any effect. **immediate c., precipitating c.,** a cause that is operative at the beginning of the specific effect. **predisposing c.,** anything that renders a person more liable to a specific condition without actually producing it. **primary c.,** the principal factor contributing to the production of a specific result. **remote c.,** any cause that does not immediately precede and produce a specific condition. **secondary c.,** one that is supplemental to the primary cause.

caustic (kaws′tik) [L. *causticus;* Gr. *kaustikos*] 1. burning or corrosive; destructive to living tissues. 2. having a burning taste. 3. an irritant that causes destruction of tissue at the site of contact. Used to destroy warts, condylomata, keratoses, moles, and hyperplastic tissue, and to induce desquamation of cornified epithelium (keratolytics). Some caustics are used in the treatment of fungal diseases and eczematoid dermatitis. When ingested, caustics cause chemical burns of the oral cavity and mucous membranes of the esophagus and stomach, leading to fibrosis and stenosis. Caustics which also precipitate cell proteins and produce an inflammatory exudate, resulting in formation of a scab, are known as *escharotics.* Called also CORROSIVE. **lunar c.,** toughened silver nitrate; see under SILVER.

cauterant (kaw′ter-ant) escharotic (2).

cauterization (kaw″ter-i-za′shun) the destruction of tissue with a hot instrument, electric current, or caustic substance.

cautery (kaw′ter-e) [L. *cauterium;* Gr. *kautērion*] 1. the application of a caustic substance, hot instrument, electric current, or other agent to destroy tissue. 2. a caustic substance or hot instrument used in cauterization. **galvanic c.,** galvanocautery.

cava (ka′vah) [L.] 1. plural of *cavum.* 2. a vena cava.

caval (ka′val) pertaining to a vena cava.

cavascope (kav′ah-skōp) [L. *cavum* hollow + Gr. *skopein* to examine] an instrument for illuminating and examining a cavity.

cave (kāv) [L. *cavum*] a small enclosed space within the body or an organ; a cavity or cavum.

cavern (kav′ern) [L. *caverna* cavity] a cavity caused by pathological processes.

caverna (ka-ver′nah), pl. *caver′nae* [L.] a general anatomical term used to designate a cavity.

cavernae (ka-ver′ne) [L.] plural of *caverna.*

cavernous (kav′er-nus) [L. *cavernosus*] containing caverns or hollow spaces; large chambered.

Cavidry trademark for a *cavity cleaner* (see under CLEANER) used for cleaning, drying, and degreasing the prepared cavity.

cavitary (kav′ĭ-ta″re) characterized by the presence of a cavity or cavities.

cavitas (kav′ĭ-tas), pl. *cavita′tes* [L. from *cavus* hollow] a hollow space or depression. See also CAVITY and CAVUM. **c. den′tis,** pulp CAVITY.

cavitates (kav″ĭ-ta′tēz) [L.] plural of *cavitas.*

cavitation (kav″ĭ-ta′shun) the formation of a cavity or cavities.

Cavitec trademark for *zinc oxide–eugenol cement* (see under CEMENT).

Cavi-Trol acidulated phosphate fluoride topical gel see under GEL.

cavity (kav′ĭ-te) [L. *cavitas*] 1. a hollow place or space, especially a space within a body or in one of its organs; it may be normal or pathological. See also CAVITAS and CAVUM. 2. the lesion or area of destruction of elements of a tooth; a carious cavity. See dental CARIES. 3. prepared c. **abdominal c.,** the cavity of the body, located between the diaphragm above and the pelvis below, which contains all the abdominal organs. Called also *cavum abdominis* [NA]. **access c.,** one produced to allow access to the pulp chamber for cleaning, shaping, and filling of the root canal. **alveolar c.,** dental ALVEOLUS. **amniotic c.,** the cavity of the closed amniotic sac (amnion) containing the embryo and the surrounding amniotic fluid. Early in pregnancy, it is relatively small but, as the embryo grows, it expands, eventually filling the entire chorionic sac (chorion). See illustration at fetal membranes, under MEMBRANE. **articular c.,** the space of a synovial joint, which is enclosed by the synovial membrane and articular cartilage. Called also *synovial c.* and *cavum articulare* [NA]. **axial surface c.,** one on a tooth surface where the general plane is parallel to the long axis of the tooth. **Baer's c.,** the cleavage cavity beneath the blastoderm. **c. base,** cavity BASE. **blastocyst c.,** blastocoele. **body c.,** 1. a visceral cavity, such as the thoracic, abdominal, or pelvic cavity. 2. coelom. **bony c. of nose,** nasal c., bony. **buccal c.,** 1. oral c. 2. that portion of the oral cavity bounded on one side by the teeth and gingivae (or the residual alveolar ridges), and on the other by the cheeks. 3. a carious lesion beginning on the buccal surface of a posterior tooth. **c. classification,** see dental CARIES. **c. cleaner,** cavity CLEANER. **cleavage c.,** blastocoele. **complex c.,** a carious lesion that involves three or more surfaces of a tooth. **complex c., compound c.,** a carious lesion involving two or more surfaces of a tooth, occurring through decay or through extension in the preparation. **compound c.,** a carious lesion that involves two surfaces of a tooth. **cranial c.,** the space enclosed by the bones of the cranium, its floor being formed by the cranial base and its roof by the calvaria. **c. débridement,** cavity TOILET. **dental c.,** a lesion produced by destruction of enamel and dentin in a tooth affected by caries. See dental CARIES. **distal c.,** a carious lesion beginning on the distal surface of a tooth. **DO c.,** a carious lesion involving the distal and occlusal surfaces of a tooth. **endodontic c.,** the preparation of the coronal portion of the tooth and pulp chamber so as to establish access to the orifices of the root canals for instrumentation and filling of the root canals. Sometimes called *access preparation.* See also convenience FORM and outline FORM. **faucial c.,** c. of pharynx. **fissure c.,** a carious lesion beginning in a fissure of a tooth. See pit CARIES. **gingival c., gingival third c.,** a carious lesion on the gingival third of the clinical crown of a tooth. **glandular c.,** a hollow sac formed by invagination of the epithelial sheath in a developing multicellular gland. **hemal c.,** coelom. **idiopathic bone c.,** traumatic CYST. **incisal c.,** a carious lesion beginning on the incisal surface of an anterior tooth. **infraglottic c.,** the lower part of the cavity of the larynx, extending from the rima glottidis to the trachea below. Its upper part near the rima is elliptical in shape, but its lower part assumes a circular form similar to that of the trachea. Called also *cavum infraglotticum* [NA]. **labial c.,** a carious lesion beginning on the labial surface of an anterior tooth. **laryngopharyngeal c.,** laryngopharynx. **c. of larynx,** the space enclosed by the walls of the larynx, extending from the entrance to the larynx to the cricoid cartilage. The rima glottidis divides the cavity into an upper part, the vestibule, and a lower part, the infraglottic cavity, which extends to the cavity of the trachea. Called also *cavum laryngis* [NA]. **lingual c.,** a carious lesion beginning on the lingual surface of a tooth. **lingual mandibular bone c.,** static bone CYST. **c. lining agent** cavity lining AGENT. **marrow c., medullary c.,** a spacious cavity of a long bone which contains the bone marrow. Called also *medullary canal* and *cavum medullare ossium* [NA]. **mastoid c.,** tympanic ANTRUM. **mesial c.,** a carious lesion beginning on the mesial surface of a tooth. **MO c.,** mesio-occlusal cavity; one on the mesial and occlusal surfaces of a tooth. **MOD c.,** mesio-occlusodistal cavity; one on the mesial, occlusal, and distal surfaces of a tooth. **c. of mouth,** oral c. **mouth c. proper,** oral c. proper. **nasal c.,** the proximal part of the respiratory system, situated below the cranial and above the oral cavities and between the orbits and the maxillary sinuses, communicating with the pharyngeal space through the choanae and with the outside through the nasal aperture. The nasal septum separates the right from the left cavity. The roof is formed by the nasal bone; the spine by the frontal bone; the cribriform plate by the ethmoid bone; the body by the sphenoidal bone, the sphenoidal concha, ala of the vomer, and sphenoidal process of the palatine bone; the floor by the palatine process of the maxilla and the palatine bone; the medial wall by the crest of the ethmoid bone, vomer, rostrum of the sphenoid bone, crest of the maxillae, and palatine bones; the lateral wall by the frontal process of the maxilla, lacrimal bone, ethmoid bone, maxilla, inferior nasal concha, vertical plate of the palatine bone, and medial pterygoid plate of the sphenoid bone. Called also *cavum nasi* [NA]. **nasal c., bony,** the space between the floor of the cranium and the roof of the mouth, extending between the pharynx posteriorly and the

external nose anteriorly, and divided by a median septum. Called also *cavum nasi osseum* [NA]. **nerve c.,** pulp c. **occlusal c.,** a carious lesion beginning on the occlusal surface of a posterior tooth. **oral c.,** an oval cavity situated at the entrance to the digestive tube, bounded anteriorly by the lips, laterally by the cheeks, and posteriorly by the isthmus faucium. It consists of an outer horseshoe-shaped part, the vestibule of the mouth, and an inner part, the oral cavity proper. Called also *buccal c., c. of mouth,* and *cavum oris* [NA]. See illustration. **oral c. external,** VESTIBULE of the mouth. **oral c. proper,** the inner part of the oral cavity, lined with mucous membranes and the lingual surfaces of the teeth, and bounded anteriorly and laterally by the alveolar arches with their contained teeth and posteriorly by the isthmus faucium, which communicates with the pharynx. The palate forms the roof; the tongue and the floor of the mouth provide the floor of the cavity. It receives secretions from the submandibular and sublingual glands. Called also *mouth c. proper* and *cavum oris proprium* [NA]. **orbital c.,** orbit. **pelvic c.,** the space bounded at the sides by the bones of the pelvis, above by the plane passing through arcuate lines, and below by the pelvic diaphragm. Called also *cavum pelvis* [NA]. **pharyngolaryngeal c.,** laryngopharynx. **pharyngonasal c.,** nasopharynx. **c. of pharynx, pharyngeal c.,** the space enclosed by the walls of the pharynx. Called also *faucial c.* and *cavum pharyngis* [NA]. **pharyngo-oral c.,** oropharynx. **pit c.,** a carious lesion beginning in a pit of a tooth. See also pit CARIES. **c. preparation,** cavity PREPARATION. **prepared c.,** one produced in a tooth to support and retain the filling material and protect the tooth structure remaining after removal of all carious tissue. **c. primer,** cavity PRIMER. **proximal c.,** a carious lesion beginning on a proximal (mesial or distal) surface of a tooth. See proximal CARIES. **pulp c.,** the natural cavity in the central portion of a tooth occupied by the dental pulp. It is divided into the pulp chamber, located in the crown portion of the tooth, and the root canal, located in the root portion. Called also *nerve c., cavitas dentis, cavum dentis* [NA], and *cavum pulpae.* **Rosenmüller's c.,** pharyngeal RECESS. **c. seal,** cavity SEAL. **segmentation c.,** blastocoele. **simple c.,** a carious cavity involving a single tooth surface. **smooth surface c.,** a carious lesion which has smooth-surfaced walls, without pits, fissures, or enamel faults. **somatic c.,** coelom. **spinal c.,** the cavity containing the spinal cord. **static bone c.,** static bone CYST. **subgerminal c.,** blastocoele. **synovial c.,** articular c. **synovial c., inferior, of temporomandibular joint,** the inferior cavity of the articular space of the temporomandibular joint, which is divided into a superior and an inferior cavity by the articular disk, and serves as the hinge joint of the temporomandibular articulation. Called also *lower temporomandibular joint.* See also interarticular disk of temporomandibular joint, under DISK, and see temporomandibular JOINT. **synovial c., superior, of temporomandibular joint,** the superior part of the articular space of the temporomandibular joint, which is divided into a superior and an inferior cavity by the articular disk, and serves as the gliding joint of the temporomandibular articulation. Called also *upper temporomandibular joint.* See also articular disk of temporomandibular joint, under DISK, and see temporomandibular JOINT. **thoracic c.,** the cavity bounded by the thoracic walls and the diaphragm. Called also *cavum thoracis* [NA]. **c. toilet,** cavity TOILET. **trigeminal c.,** a small cleft in the dura mater on the anterior surface of the petrous portion of the temporal bone, which lodges the trigeminal ganglion. Called also *cavum trigeminale* [NA]. **c. varnish,** cavity VARNISH. **visceral c.,** one of the great body cavities, such as the thoracic, abdominal, or pelvic cavity. Called also *body c.* **yolk c., yolk sac c.,** the space between the germ disk and the yolk in the developing zygote.

cavosurface (ka′vo-sur″fis) the surface of a cavity, as of a tooth.

cavum (ka′vum), pl. *ca′va* [L.] a general anatomical term used to designate a cavity or hollow space. See also CAVITAS and CAVITY. **c. abdom′inis** [NA], abdominal CAVITY. **c. articula′re** [NA], articular CAVITY. **c. infraglot′ticum,** infraglottic CAVITY. **c. den′tis** [NA], pulp CAVITY. **c. laryn′gis,** CAVITY of larynx. **c. medulla′re os′sium** [NA], marrow CAVITY. **c. na′si** [NA], nasal CAVITY. **c. na′si os′seum,** bony nasal CAVITY. **c. o′ris** [NA], oral CAVITY. **c. o′ris exter′num,** VESTIBULE of the mouth. **c. o′ris pro′prium** [NA], oral cavity, proper; see under CAVITY. **c. pel′vis** [NA], pelvic CAVITY. **c. pharyn′gis** [NA], CAVITY of pharynx. **c. pul′pae,** pulp CAVITY. **c. thora′cis** [NA], thoracic CAVITY. **c. trigemina′le** [NA], trigeminal CAVITY.

Cayler's syndrome cardiofacial SYNDROME.

Cazenave's disease [Pierre Louis Alphée *Cazanave,* French physician, 1795–1877] PEMPHIGUS foliaceus.

CB Bachelor of Surgery [L. *Chirur′giae Baccalaure′us*].

Cb columbium; see NIOBIUM.

CBADAA Certifying Board of the American Dental Assistants Association; see under BOARD.

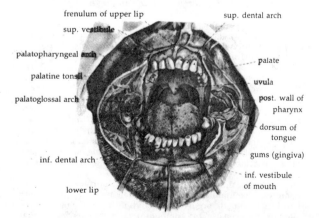

frenulum of upper lip — sup. dental arch
sup. vestibule
palatopharyngeal arch — palate
palatine tonsil — uvula
palatoglossal arch — post. wall of pharynx
— dorsum of tongue
— gums (gingiva)
inf. dental arch — inf. vestibule of mouth
lower lip

Oral cavity. (From J. Langman and M. W. Woerdeman: Atlas of Medical Anatomy. Philadelphia, W. B. Saunders Co., 1978.)

CBC, cbc complete blood COUNT.

CC chief COMPLAINT.

cc cubic CENTIMETER.

CCA congenital contractural ARACHNODACTYLY.

CCM cerebrocostomandibular SYNDROME.

CCME Coordinating Council on Medical Education; see under COUNCIL.

CCU coronary care UNIT.

CD$_{50}$ median curative dose.

Cd 1. condylion. 2. cadmium.

cd candela.

CDA 1. Canadian Dental Association; see Appendix. 2. certified dental ASSISTANT. 3. currently certified dental ASSISTANT.

CDC Center for Disease Control; see under CENTER.

CDG central developmental GROOVE.

CDS Christian Dental Society; see under SOCIETY.

CDT Certified Dental Technician; see under TECHNICIAN.

Ce cerium.

Cebefortis tablets see under TABLET.

cebocephaly (se"bo-sef'ah-le) [Gr. *kebos* monkey + *kephalē* head] a congenital abnormality characterized by a nose with a single nostril associated with hypotelorism, giving the head the appearance of that of a platyrrhine monkey.

cecum (se'kum) [L. *caecum*, blind, blind gut] 1. the dilated intestinal pouch into which open the ileum, the colon, and the appendix. 2. any blind pouch or cul-de-sac. **c. lin'guae,** FORAMEN caecum linguae.

Cedilanid trademark for *lanatoside C.*

Cedilanid D trademark for *deslanoside.*

Cedulamin trademark for *methenamine mandelate* (see under METHENAMINE).

Ceepryl trademark for *cetylpyridinium chloride* (see under CETYLPYRIDINIUM).

Cefadol trademark for *diphenidol hydrochloride* (see under DIPHENIDOL).

Cefadyl trademark for *cephapirin sodium* (see under CEPHAPIRIN).

Cefalotin trademark for *cephalothin sodium* (see under CEPHALOTHIN).

Cefamedin trademark for *cefazolin sodium* (see under CEFAZOLIN).

Cefamezin trademark for *cefazolin sodium* (see under CEFAZOLIN).

Cefatrexyl trademark for *cephapirin sodium* (see under CEPHAPIRIN).

cefazolin sodium (sef-a'zo-lin) a semisynthetic antibiotic, monosodium 3-[[(5-methyl-1,3,4-thiadiazol-2-yl)thio]methyl]-8-oxo-7-[2-(1H-tetrazol-1-yl) acetamido-5-thia-1-azabicyclo-4,2,0] oct-2-ene-carboxylate, derived from 7-aminocephalosporamic acid or obtained from the natural antibiotic cephalosporin C. It is effective against most pathogenic gram-positive bacteria, including *Staphylococcus aureus,* streptococci (other than enterococci), and pneumococci; somewhat less active against gram-negative bacteria, such as *Escherichia coli, Proteus mirabilis, Klebsiella, Enterobacter aerogenes,* and *Haemophilus influenzae.* Used in the treatment of infections of the respiratory and urogenital tracts, skin, soft tissues, bones, and joints, and in septicemias and endocarditis. Pain at the site of injection, phlebitis, skin rashes, eosinophilia, and elevated SGOT, SGPT, and alkaline phosphatase may occur during therapy. Trademarks: Ancef, Cefamedin, Cefamezin, Elzogram, Gramaxin, Tatacef.

Ceflorin trademark for *cephaloridine.*

Cefol trademark for a mixture of vitamins, each film-coated tablet containing 15 mg thiamine mononitrate, 10 mg riboflavin, 5 mg pyridoxine hydrochloride, 6 µg cyanocobalamin, 750 mg sodium ascorbate, 30 IU *d*-alpha-tocopherol acid succinate, 20 mg calcium pantothenate, 100 mg nicinamide, 0.5 mg folic acid, and various excipients.

Cefracycline trademark for *tetracycline* (1).

Ceglunat trademark for *lanatoside C.*

ceiling (se'ling) 1. the overhead interior lining of a room. 2. the upper limit of something. **income c.,** in health insurance, a specified level of individual or family income below which participating doctors have agreed to provide services to beneficiaries at a cost that does not exceed the amounts listed in a formal fee schedule. For beneficiaries with an income above the ceiling, the doctor may charge more than the scheduled fee and bill the individual for the difference.

Ceka attachment see under ATTACHMENT.

cel (sel) a unit of velocity, being the velocity of 1 cm per second.

cel- see CELO-.

Celadigal trademark for *lanatoside C.*

Celbenin trademark for *methicillin.*

-cele 1. [Gr. *kēlē* hernia] a word termination denoting relationship to a tumor or swelling. 2. [Gr. *koilia* cavity] a word termination denoting relationship to a cavity; sometimes spelled *-coele.*

Celestan-V trademark for *betamethasone valerate* (see under BETAMETHASONE).

Celestone trademark for *betamethasone.*

celiac (se'le-ak) [Gr. *koilia* belly] pertaining to the abdomen.

cell (sel) 1. the smallest unit that may exist either as an independent unit of life or, in association with other cells, form colonies (facultative association) or form body tissues (obligatory association), being the basic building block of all forms of life. A cell is basically a minute protoplasmic mass organized into the cytoplasm and cell nucleus in eukaryotes or a nucleotide in prokaryotes. It is enveloped by a plasma membrane and, in certain species, also by a cell wall. The cytoplasm is the site of biochemical activities of the cell and consists of an aqueous solution containing various salts, enzymes, and free molecules. Also contained in the cytoplasm are mitochondria, lysosomes, centrosomes, endoplasmic reticulum, microtubules, inclusions, Golgi apparatus and other organelles, and numerous membranes, which divide it into separate compartments. The nucleus, which is the site of cell division, is a spheroid body within the cell bounded by the nuclear envelope and containing nucleoli, chromatin granules, and a number of organelles. Chemically, it contains DNA, RNA, proteins, and lipids. See illustration. See also terms beginning CYTO-. 2. a small more or less closed space. **α-c's,** 1. cells of the islands of Langerhans which secrete glucagon. Similar to β-cells, they are enclosed in a continuous plasma membrane with nuclei surrounded by a double membrane. Their cytoplasm contains granular reticulum, mitochondria, secretory granules, and portions of the Golgi apparatus. They are smaller, have less granular reticulum, and their nuclei are more ovoid than in β-cells. 2. acidophils of the anterior pituitary gland. **accessory c's,** cells that cooperate with T- and B-lymphocytes in the initiation of the immune response. They have macrophage functions and process antigen for presentation to the antibody-forming cells. **acidophilic c.,** a cell having an affinity for acid dyes. Called also *acidocyte* and *acidophil.* **acinar c., acinic c.,** any secretory cells of an acinus. **adipose c.,** fat c. **adventitial c.,** a macrophage fixed along the bundles of collagen fibers along the walls of blood vessels. Called also *Marchand's c.* and *perivascular c.* See also MACROPHAGE. **aerobic c.,** aerobe. **agger nasi c's,** the cells of the anterior part of the ethmoid crest. **air c.,** one containing air, such as an alveolus of the lungs. **air c's of nose,** paranasal sinuses; see under SINUS. Cf. *heterotrophic c.* **albuminous c.,** serous c. **alpha c's,** α-c's. **ameboid c.,** any cell that is able to change its form and move about, such as a leukocyte. See also *migratory c.* and *wandering c.* **amphophilic c.,** one that stains readily with either acid or basic dyes. Called also *amphochromatophil, amphochromophil, amphocyte,* and *amphophil.* **anaerobic c.,** anaerobe. **Anichkov's c.,** Anichkov's MYOCYTE. **antipodal c's,** a group of four cells in the early embryo. **apocrine c.,** a cell of the apocrine glands in which the free or apical portion is cast off along with the secretory products that have accumulated therein. **Aschoff c.,** a giant cell with one or two nuclei or a folded multilobulate nucleus with prominent nucleoli and a basophilic cytoplasm, seen in an Aschoff body in the heart of patients with rheumatic fever. **Ashkenazy c's,** Hürthle c's. **autotrophic c.,** a relatively self-sufficient cell deriving energy directly from carbon dioxide as the sole source of carbon for its organic biomolecules. Called also *autotroph.* Cf. *heterotrophic c.* **B-c's,** B-lymphocytes; see under LYMPHOCYTE. **β-c's,** 1. cells of the islands of Langerhans which secrete insulin. Similarly to α-cells, they are enclosed in a continuous plasma membrane with nuclei surrounded by a double membrane. Their cytoplasm contains granular reticulum, mitochondria, secretory granules, and portions of the Golgi apparatus. They are larger, have more granular reticulum, and their nuclei are less ovoid than in α-cells. 2. basophilic cells of the anterior lobe of the pituitary gland. **band c.,** a granulocyte in which the nucleus forms a curved or coiled band. Called also *stab c.* and *staff c.* **basal c., basket c., basket c.,** 1. a cell of the cerebellar cortex whose axon gives off brushes of fibrils. 2. a basal slender spindle-shaped cell with a stellate body and processes containing darkly staining fibrils, found in various glands, such as mammary, lacrimal, and sweat glands, and in all the glands of the oral cavity in the epithelium of the terminal portion of the secretory ducts. It is believed to have contractile capacity and to facilitate movement of the glandular secretion into the ducts. Called also *basal c.* and *myoepithelial c.* **basophilic c.,** basophil

(2). **beaker c.,** goblet c. **beta c's, β-c's. Betz c.,** a large pyramidal ganglion cell forming one of the layers of the motor area of the gray matter of the brain. Called also *giant pyramidal c.* **bipolar c.,** a nerve cell with two processes. **blast c.,** the least differentiated blood cell without commitment as to its particular series. **bone c.,** osteocyte. **border c.,** see *supporting c.* **brood c.,** mother c. **burr c.,** an abnormal erythrocyte with numerous spinelike projections, seen in uremia, some types of hemolytic anemia, and thrombotic thrombocytopenic purpura. Called also *spur c.* and *spinous erythrocyte.* **caliciform c.,** goblet c. **cartilage c.,** chondrocyte. **caterpillar c.,** Anichkov's MYOCYTE. **cement c.,** cementocyte. **chalice c.,** goblet c. **chemolithotrophic c.,** a chemotrophic cell which derives energy from simple inorganic donors, such as hydrogen, hydrogen sulfide, ammonia, or sulfur. See also *photolithotrophic c.* **chemo-organotrophic c.,** a chemotrophic cell which derives energy from organic molecules as its electron donors, such as glucose. See also *photo-organotrophic c.* **chemotrophic c.,** a cell which derives energy through oxidation-reduction reactions. Cells using organic molecules as their electron donors, such as glucose, are known as *chemo-organotrophic cells;* those using simple inorganic donors, such as hydrogen, hydrogen sulfide, ammonia, or sul-

fur, are known as *chemolithotrophic cells.* See also *phototrophic c.* **chromaffin c's,** cells which have affinity to and stain with chromic acid. **ciliated c.,** any cell bearing cilia. **cleavage c.,** blastomere. **columnar c's,** cells of the columnar epithelium, being roughly rectangular in profile and hexagonal in surface view. In some tissues, they are very long (tall columnar c's) but in others their height is scarcely greater than their width (low columnar c's). Their nuclei are usually oval and often at the same level in the basal segment of the cells. The cell bases contact the basal lamina overlying the basement membrane. Most are found in areas of secretion or absorption, where they may be functionally modified by an increase in surface area by microvilli. **contractile fiber c's,** spindle-shaped and nucleated cells which may be collected into bundles to make up unstriated or smooth muscle. **connective tissue c.,** any of the cells of the fibrous and nonfibrous components of the various forms of connective tissue. **cover c.,** any cell that covers and protects other cells, especially epithelial cells which extend between the basement membrane and the surface of the taste buds and thus cover the taste cells. Called also *encasing* (or *incasing*) *c.* **crescent c's,** crescents of Giannuzzi; see under CRESCENT. **cuboid c., cuboidal c.,** an epithelial cell which in transverse and vertical diameters are approximately equal. **daughter c.,** any cell formed by the division of the mother cell; a newly formed cell in mitosis. **c. death,** necrosis. **Deiters' c.,** 1. an outer phalangeal cell; see *supporting c.* 2. neuroglial c. **demilune c's,**

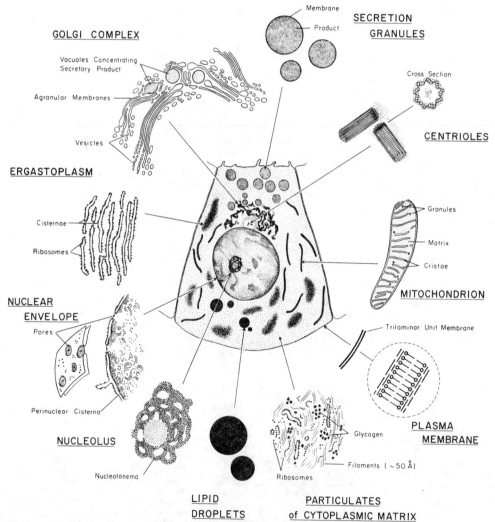

Diagram of a cell. The center illustrates the form of its organelles and inclusions as they appear by light microscopy. Around the periphery are representations of the finer structure of these same components as seen in electron micrographs. The ergastoplasm of light microscopy consists of aggregations of submicroscopic membrane-limited elements with granules of ribonucleoprotein adhering to their outer surface. This component is now also called the *granular endoplasmic reticulum.* The plasma membrane (encircled by an interrupted line) does not show structure that has been directly observed but represents one possible interpretation of the arrangement of lipid and protein molecules that may be related to the trilaminar appearance of cell membranes in electron micrographs. (From W. Bloom and D. W. Fawcett: A Textbook of Histology. 10th ed. Philadelphia, W. B. Saunders Co., 1975.)

crescents of Giannuzzi; see under CRESCENT. **dentin c.,** odontoblast. **elementary c's, embryonal c's,** small round cells produced by cleavage of the zygote. Called also *primordial c's.* **emigrated c.,** a leukocyte that has passed through the wall of a blood vessel into the neighboring tissue. **enamel c.,** ameloblast. **encasing c.,** cover c. **end c.,** one that is the end product of maturation. **endothelioid c's,** large protoplasmic cells frequently seen in disease of the blood-making organs, and believed by some to be derived from the endothelial lining of the blood and lymph vessels. **ependymal c's,** cells of the ependyma; cuboid cells which line the central cylinder of the spinal cord and the cavities of the brain. During embryonic development they are ciliated but lose their cilia on maturing. Called also *ependymocytes.* **epithelial c's,** cells covering the body surfaces and lining its cavities. See also EPITHELIUM. **epithelioid c.,** 1. a cell believed to derive from a monocyte, which is characterized by a somewhat larger size than that of a monocyte, ability to phagocytize, monocyte-like motility, indentation or oval shape of the nucleus, presence of a large rosette of dustlike vacuoles, abundance of cytoplasm, and absence or scarcity of mitochondria. It is characteristic of tuberculosis. 2. any of the connective tissue cells arranged so as to simulate epithelium. **erythroid c.,** an immature blood cell of the erythrocyte series. **ethmoidal c.,** one of numerous air-containing, thin-walled cellular cavities in the labyrinth of the ethmoid bone, which communicate with the nasal cavity and infundibulum and bulla of the ethmoid bone. They are partly open at the borders of the ethmoid bone and reach into neighboring bones, which complete their walls; the frontal bone forming the roof of the upper ethmoid cells, the sphenoid bone providing the roof for the posterior cells, the maxilla and palatine bones providing the roof for the inferior cells, and the thin plate of the lacrimal bone closing the anterior cells. Called also *cellula ethmoidalis* [NA]. See also ethmoidal SINUS. **eukaryotic c.,** a cell with a true nucleus (i.e., one bounded by a nuclear membrane), chromosomes that undergo mitotic division, and a variety of cellular organelles, including endocytoplasmic reticulum and Golgi complexes. Eukaryotic cells are characteristic of higher plants and animals, fungi, protozoa, and most algae, as opposed to prokaryotic cells (bacteria, blue-green algae, mycoplasmas). **fat c.,** a connective tissue cell storing varying amounts of lipids. Called also *adipose c.* and *lipocyte.* See also lipid METABOLISM. **ferment c.,** a cell that secretes an enzyme causing fermentation. **fiber c.,** any elongated and linear cell. **flagellate c.,** any cell having a flagellum, usually motile. **foam c's,** 1. cells with a peculiar vacuolated appearance owing to the presence of complex lipoids; such cells are seen notably in xanthoma; hence the synonym *xanthoma cells.* Called also *lattice c's.* 2. Mikulicz's c's. **ganglion c.,** a large nerve cell characteristic of ganglia. Called also *gangliocyte.* **Gaucher's c.,** a large cell with a small pyknotic nucleus and a granular or wrinkled cytoplasm resembling wrinkled tissue paper and an intracytoplasmic accumulation of cerebroside glycolipids; present in Gaucher's disease. **Gegenbaur's c.,** osteoblast. **germ c's,** the cells of an organism whose function is to reproduce the kind, i.e., an ovum or spermatozoon. Called also *initial c's.* **germ c's, primordial,** primordial germ c. **germinal c.,** a cell capable of dividing and differentiating. **ghost c.,** 1. one generally lacking in cytoplasmic organelles and inclusions and appearing only as a shadowy outline. 2. an erythrocyte having lost hemoglobin. Called also *shadow c.* **Giannuzzi's c's,** crescents of Giannuzzi; see under CRESCENT. **giant c.,** a very large cell frequently having several nuclei; the term is applied to the megakaryocytes of bone marrow and also to giant cells occurring in lesions of tuberculosis and other infectious granulomas and about foreign bodies. **giant pyramidal c.,** Betz c. **gitter c.,** microgliocyte. **goblet c.,** type of columnar epithelial cell, or unicellular gland, containing a large globule of mucin and bulged out like a goblet, which is found in various mucous membranes, especially the respiratory and intestinal epithelium. Called also *beaker c., caliciform c.,* and *chalice c.* See also *mucous c.* **granular c.,** a keratinocyte found mostly in the granular layer of the epidermis, which later becomes flattened and rhomboidal in shape, containing a dense collection of darkly staining granules, and finally dies and is desquamated. **gustatory c.,** taste c. **Hargraves' c.,** LE c. **heckle c.,** prickle c. **Heidenhain's c's,** crescents of Giannuzzi; see under CRESCENT. **HeLa c's,** cells of the first continuously cultured carcinoma strain, descended from a human cervical carcinoma; used in the study of life processes, including viruses, at the cell level. **helmet c.,** an abnormal erythrocyte form somewhat resembling a helmet, seen in hemolytic anemia. **helper c., helper T c.,** T helper c. **Hensen's c.,** the outermost supporting cell. See *supporting c.* **heterotrophic c.,** a cell that cannot obtain carbon directly from carbon dioxide and must obtain it in a complex reduced form, such as glucose. Cf. *autotrophic c.* **horn c's,**

epithelial cells that have lost their protoplasm, and have sharp edges and a horn-shaped contour. **Hortega c.,** microgliocyte. **Hürthle c's,** large eosinophilic cells sometimes found in the thyroid gland, which seem to be parathyroid nests (nidi) included by chance in thyroid tissue. Called also *Ashkenazy c's, interfollicular c's, oxyphil c's* and *parafollicular c's.* **hyperchromatic c.,** one that stains more intensely than is typical of its cell type. **incasing c.,** cover c. **c. inclusion,** cell INCLUSION. **indifferent c.,** a cell that has no characteristic structure, or that is not an essential part of the tissue in which it is found. Called also *unspecialized c.* **inflammatory c's,** cells participating in the inflammatory response to a noxious stimulus, including neutrophils, leukocytes, eosinophils, leukocytes, and macrophages. **initial c's,** germ c's. **interfollicular c's,** Hürtle c's. **islet c's,** cells composing the islands of Langerhans. See α-c. and β-c. **juvenile c.,** metamyelocyte. **K-c.,** killer c. **killer c.,** a cytotoxic cell involved in cell-mediated immune reactions, which is morphologically indistinguishable from a small lymphocyte, being Fc receptor–positive, surface immunoglobulin–negative, and C3b receptor–negative (i.e., a null cell). Killer cells have cytotoxic activity with target cells coated with specific IgG antibody in an antibody-dependent cellular cytotoxic reaction, in which an antibody molecule appears to form a bridge between the target cell and the effector cell. Called also *K-c.* **killer c., natural,** natural killer c. **Kupffer's c.,** one of the star-shaped or pyramidal, intensely phagocytic cells with a large ovial nucleus and a small prominent nucleolus, which line the walls of the sinusoids of the liver and form a part of the reticuloendothelial system. Called also *stellate c. of liver.* **lacrimoethmoid c's,** the ethmoid cells situated under the lacrimal bone. **large pyroninophyllic c's,** see B-lymphocytes, under LYMPHOCYTE. **lattice c.,** foam c's (1). **LE c.,** a neutrophilic leukocyte that has phagocytized globular homogenous nuclear material in the presence of the LE plasma factor (a component of γ-globulin); a characteristic of lupus erythematosus, but also found in other analogous connective tissue disorders. Called also *Hargraves' c.* and *lupus erythematosus c.* **lepra c.,** a vacuolated macrophage that contains masses of live bacilli, seen in leprous nodules. **Leydig's c.,** 1. one of the interstitial cells of the testis, which furnish the internal secretion of the testicle. 2. a mucous cell that does not secrete its products out over the surface of the epithelium. **littoral c's,** flattened cells lining the walls of lymph or blood sinuses. **lupus erythematosus c.,** LE c. **lymphoid c's,** mononuclear cells in lymphoid tissue, such as the lymph node, spleen, and tonsil, which are involved in immune responses by their ability to react specifically with antigen and to eleborate cell products. They include plasma cells and lymphocytes, and they trace their origin to the pluripotential stem cell that in the fetus is found in the yolk sac, bone marrow, and liver, and in the adult in the bone marrow. **malpighian c.,** keratinocyte. **Marchand's c.,** adventitial c. **marginal c's,** crescents of Giannuzzi; see under CRESCENT. **marrow c.,** any one of the immature blood cells that develop in the bone marrow. Called also *myeloid c.* **mast c.,** mastocyte. **mastoid c.,** one of the hollowed out air spaces in the mastoid process of the temporal bone, showing a wide variety in size, shape, and number in different parts of the process. Called also *cellula mastoidea* [NA], and *mastoid sinus.* **matrix c's,** flat cells found in the lobules of sebaceous glands, which undergo an abrupt transformation into the pale, foamy-looking, fat-containing cells of the alveoli. **mediator c's,** cells, such as mast cells, basophils, platelets, enterochromaffin cells, and neutrophils, which release in response to environmental stimulation macromolecular and low-molecular-weight substances (mediators) that are capable of amplifying the effect of phagocytic cells or may have a direct effect on target cells. Substances released by the mediator cells include histamine, serotonin, kinins, slow reactive substance of anaphylaxis, prostaglandins, eosinophilic chemotactic factors of anaphylaxis, lymphokines, and platelet activating factor. **memory c's,** lymphocytes which remain and may circulate in the blood after specific stimulation by antigen that results in clonal proliferation. These cells, after a further encounter with the same antigen, have the capacity to proliferate and differentiate into cell lines responsible for cell-mediated (T-lymphocytes) and humoral (B-lymphocytes) immunity. **Merkel's c's, Merkel-Ranvier c's,** melanoblasts of the skin. **mesenchymal c.,** the pluripotential, stellate cell of the mesenchyma, the protoplasmic processes of which meet those of adjacent cells, forming a cellular network. The intercellular spaces are occupied by a jelly-like ground substance and reticular fibers whose presence may be noted by the end of the second month of embryonic development. **mesothelial c's,** flattened epithelial cells of mesenchymal origin that line the serous cavities. **metallophil c's,** cells in which the cytoplasm has a great affinity for metal salts; these are cells of the reticuloendothelial system, and also a series of related cells that are not selectively stained by vital staining. **Mexican hat c.,** target c. (1). **migratory c.,** an ameboid cell found in the blood and tissue spaces. See also *wandering c.* **Mikulicz's c's,** the cells in rhinoscleroma that contain the bacillus of the disease (*Klebsiella rhinoscleromatis*). Called also *foam c.* **mitral c's,** the pyramidal cells forming one of the layers of the olfactory bulb. **mother c.,** any cell that divides so as to form new or daughter cells. Called also *brood c.* and *parent c.* **mouth c's,** squamous cells detached from the epithelium lining the oropharynx, found in the sputum. **mucoalbuminous c., mucoserous c.,** a cell having histologic characteristics between those of mucous cells and serous cells. **mucous c.,** a cell that secretes mucin or mucus. In salivary glands, mucous cells are concerned with secretion of the mucous substance of the glands. It may be either columnar or pyramidal, stains blue with hematoxylin and eosin dyes, and has a rounded nucleus located in the basal half of the cell. Preparatory to the active period, the organelles hypertrophy so that during the secretory phase the endoplasmic reticulum is capable of an increased production, while the Golgi apparatus refines and packages mucinogen (precursor of mucus). The rise of mucinogen droplets causes the nucleus and other organelles to decrease in number and be pushed downward with resulting distention of the bottom of the cell and the cell assumes a pear- or goblet-shaped form (see *goblet c.*). The surface membrane ruptures and the mucinogen is expelled in the lumen of the acinus. During the postsecretory phase, it resumes its original shape and the surface membrane is repaired. A mucous cell differs from a serous cell in that it has a better defined lateral cell membrane, secretory canaliculi are absent and the distal surface membrane is destroyed during the secretory phase. **muscle c.,** an elongated and nucleated contractile fiber cell peculiar to muscle. **myeloid c.,** marrow c. **myeloma c.,** a cell found in the bone marrow and occasionally in the peripheral blood of patients with multiple myeloma. In the more anaplastic form, the cell is large, has abundant blue-staining cytoplasm with no perinuclear pallor, and has one or more moderately large and vesicular nuclei that may be centrally or eccentrically placed and may contain nucleoli. In better differentiated tumors, the cell is smaller and, except for the finer chromatic structure, greatly resembles a plasmacyte. **myoepithelial c.,** basket c. **natural killer c.,** a naturally occurring cell of unknown identity, which does not contain known T- or B-lymphocyte markers and does not require prior sensitization for its generation. It is thought to be involved in nonspecific killing of virally transformed target cells, rejection of allogenic grafts, and tumor rejection. Called also *NK-c.* See also *killer c.* **nerve c.,** neuron. **Neumann's c's,** nucleated cells in the bone marrow developing into erythrocytes. **neuroepithelial c's, neuroglia c's,** neuroglial c's. **neuroglial c's,** the cells of the neuroglia, which is the supporting structure of nervous tissue, including astrocytes, oligodendrocytes, and microgliocytes. Called also *Deiters' c's, neuroepithelial c's,* and *neuroglia c's.* **neutrophilic c.,** a cell, particularly a leukocyte, stainable by neutral dyes. See NEUTROPHIL. **NK-c.,** natural killer c. **noble c's,** the differentiated cells of the organs and tissues of the body. **nucleated c.,** any cell having a nucleus. **nucleated red c., nucleated red blood c.,** any of the immature forms of a red blood cell, as a normoblast. **null c.,** a lymphocyte which lacks the surface antigens characteristic of B- and T-lymphocytes. **oat c's, oat-shaped c's,** cells shaped like oat grains, seen in certain kinds of carcinoma; also a characteristic of erythrocytes in sickle cell anemia. **olfactory c.,** a sensory cell of the olfactory organ. It is a bipolar cell, having a large spherical nucleus surrounded by a small amount of cytoplasm and two processes. The superficial or receptor process, a modified dendrite, protrudes to the surface of the epithelial membrane, ending as a minute spheroid body with six or more hairlike processes (olfactory hairs) which serve as active receptive structures. The central or deep process, an axon, extends through the basement membrane and joins the bundles of unmyelinated fibers of the olfactory nerve. Called also *Schultze's c.* **osseous c.,** osteocyte. **oxyphil c's,** Hürthle c's. **packed human blood c's, packed red blood c's (human),** whole blood from which plasma has been removed; used therapeutically in blood transfusion. **palatine c's,** those parts of ethmoid cells that extend into the palatine bone. **parafollicular c's,** Hürthle c's. **parent c.,** mother c. **pathologic c.,** any cell that results from a disease process or that belongs to or arises from a pathogenic microorganism. **pavement c's,** the flat cells composing pavement epithelium. **pericapillary c's,** perithelium. **perivascular c.,** adventitial c. **phalangeal c.,** see *supporting c.* **photolithotrophic c.,** a phototrophic cell deriving energy from light and using inorganic compounds, such as water, hydrogen sulfide, or sulfur, as electron donors. See also *chemolithotrophic c.* **photo-organotrophic c.,** a phototrophic cell which also uses organic compounds, such as glucose, as its electron donors. See also *chemo-organotrophic c.* **phototrophic c.,** a cell that derives energy from light. Cells which also use inorganic compounds, such as water, hydrogen sulfide, or sulfur, as electron donors are known as *photolithotrophic cells;* those which also use organic compounds, such as glucose as their electron donors, are known as *photo-organotrophic cells.* **plasma c.,** a spherical or ellipsoidal leukocyte with a single, eccentrically placed nucleus containing clumped, radially arranged chromatin, an area of perinuclear clearing, and a generally abundant, sometimes vacuolated cytoplasm, which is involved in the production of gamma globulin. Plasma cells are believed to originate from lymphocytes by some researchers, while others suggest that they arise from reticular or blast cells. Called also *plasmacyte.* **pneumatic c.,** the cell-like structure of the petrous bone. **polar c's,** polar bodies; see under BODY. **polychromatic c., polychromatophil c.,** an immature erythrocyte staining with both acid and basic stains so that its color is a diffuse mixture of blue-gray and pink. **polyhedral c.,** one having a polyhedral form. **polyplastic c.,** one made up of various structural elements; also one that passes through various modifications of form. **prickle c.,** a cell provided with delicate radiating processes which connect with similar cells; the name applied to one of the dividing keratinocytes present in the prickle-cell layer of the epidermis. Called also *heckle c.* **primitive reticular c.,** reticular c., primitive. **primordial c's,** elementary c's. **primordial germ c.,** the earliest germ cell, originating on the yolk sac but migrating early in embryonic development to the developing gonads (sex glands). **prokaryotic c.,** a cell without a true nucleus, the nuclear membrane being absent and the nuclear structures being collected in a nuclear region, or nucleoid, and, therefore, it does not divide by mitosis. Prokaryotic cells are usually enclosed in a semirigid cell wall. Each prokaryotic cell forms an individual organism (bacterium, blue-green alga, mycoplasma), as opposed to eukaryotic cells which have true nuclei and are characteristic of higher plants and animals, fungi, protozoa, and most algae. **red c. count,** ERYTHROCYTE count. **red c., red blood c.,** erythrocyte. **resting wandering c.,** wandering resting c. **reticular c.,** the cells forming the reticular fibers of connective tissue; those forming the framework of lymph nodes, bone marrow, and spleen are part of the reticuloendothelial system and under appropriate stimulation may differentiate into macrophages. **reticular c., primitive,** a reticular cell of blood-forming tissue, which is capable of forming reticular fibers, and is functionally similar to the fibroblast. **reticulum c.,** see *reticular c.* **rhagiocrine c.,** a macrophage fixed along the bundles of collagen fibers of connective tissue. **Rieder c.,** a myeloblast having a nucleus with several wide and deep indentations suggesting lobulations, which represent asynchronism. It is believed to be caused by excessively rapid maturation and is seen in pathological conditions, such as leukemia. **Rindfleisch's c.,** eosinophil. **Rouget c.,** pericyte. **Russell body c.,** a leukocyte which is similar to a plasma cell but also contains acidophilic hyaline bodies and granules. See also *plasma c.* **sarcogenic c.,** a cell that develops into muscle fiber. **satellite c.,** 1. neurilemmal elements encapsulating a ganglion cell. 2. free nuclei that accumulate around cells in certain diseases. **scavenger c.,** one which absorbs and removes irritant products. See MACROPHAGE. **Schultze's c.,** olfactory c. **segmented c.,** a neutrophil in which the nucleus is divided into definite lobes, as distinguished from a band cell. **semilunar c's,** crescents of Giannuzzi; see under CRESCENT. **sensory c.,** a cell of the neurons of the peripheral sense organs. **seromucous c.,** one that is essentially a serous cell but behaves like both a serous and mucous cell. **serous c.,** a cell that secretes a watery protein-rich fluid. In salivary glands, serous cells are concerned with secretion of the serous substance of the glands. It may be either columnar or pyramidal; stains blue, showing striations, with hematoxylin and eosin dyes; and has a rounded nucleus located in the basal half of the cell. Small intercellular spaces form secretory canaliculi which open into the acinus. During the secretory phase, the endoplasmic reticulum is abundant and forms a dense network at the bottom of the cell. The Golgi complex is also well developed, its function consisting of packaging the material to be liberated as secretion granules. The inclusion fills the top of the cell and stains pink to red. As the secretion granules accumulate at the top of the cell, its nucleus and other organelles become more basally confined. A serous cell differs from a mucous cell in that it has a better defined lateral cell membrane and contains secretory canaliculi. Called also *albuminous c.* **shadow c.**, ghost c. **sickle c.**, an abnormal erythrocyte shaped in the form of a sickle or crescent, owing to the presence of varying proportions of hemoglobin S, which in the deoxygenated state becomes insoluble. See also sickle cell ANEMIA. **skein c.**, reticulocyte. **skeletogenous c.**, osteoblast. **smudge c's**, disrupted leukocytes appearing during the course of preparation of peripheral blood smears. **somatic c.**, a cell of the somatoplasm; an undifferentiated body cell. **sphenoid c.**, sphenoidal SINUS. **spur c.**, burr c. **squamous c's**, thin, platelike cells of the squamous epithelium, having regular hexagonal or irregular wavy outlines, each containing a nucleus. **stab c., staff c.**, band c. **star c's**, cells with large vacuoles in their cytoplasm and cytoplasmic bridges; seen in ameloblastoma. **stellate c.**, any star-shaped cell, such as a Kupffer cell or astrocyte, having a large number of filaments extending from it in all directions. **stellate c. of liver**, Kupffer's c. **stem c's**, small cells found in the fetus in the yolk sac, bone marrow, and liver and in the adult in the bone marrow. They produce two classes of committed stem cells: (1) a committed hematopoietic stem cell that can give rise to the erythroid element, granulocytes, or megakaryocytes; and (2) a committed lymphoid stem cell precursor that can give rise to cells in the lymphoid series. The commitment of any of these pathways is dependent on the microenvironment in which the cells develop. **stipple c.**, a red blood cell containing granules of varying size and shape, taking a basic or bluish stain with Wright's stain, as in punctate basophilia. **supporting c.**, any of the cells that form a framework for supporting the organ of Corti; they include (1) the outer and inner pillar or rods, (2) the inner and outer phalangeal cells (c's of Deiters), (3) the border cells, and (4) the cells of Hensen. Called also *sustentacular c.* **suppressor c's**, lymphoid cells, especially T-lymphocytes, that inhibit humoral and cell-mediated immune responses to antigen. These cells play an integral role in immunoregulation and are believed to be operative in various autoimmune and other immunological disease states. **sustentacular c.**, supporting c. **syncytial c.**, one whose cytoplasm is confluent with that of an adjacent cell. **T-c's**, T-lymphocytes; see under LYMPHOCYTE. **T-helper c.**, a subtype of T lymphocytes that cooperates with B cells in antibody formation. Called also *helper c.* and *helper T c.* **tactile c's**, tactile corpuscles; see under CORPUSCLE. **tadpole c.**, one with an elongated cytoplasmic tail. **target c.**, 1. an abnormally thin erythrocyte which, when stained, shows a dark center and a peripheral ring of hemoglobin, separated by a pale unstained ring containing less hemoglobin, giving it the appearance of a "bull's eye." Target cells are a combination of poikilocytosis and hypochromia, and may occur in various forms of anemia and other disorders, such as jaundice and hypercholesterolemia. Called also *Mexican hat c.*, *leptocyte*, and *Mexican hat erythrocyte.* 2. an antigen-bearing cell which is the target of attack by primed lymphocytes or by specific antibody. **tart c.**, a macrophage or monocytoid reticuloendothelial cell that contains a second, characteristic nucleus, usually placed in the primary nucleus and showing a nuclear membrane and definitely visible chromatin in thick structural arrangement, with relatively sharp differentiation between chromatin and parachromatin. **taste c.**, one of the spindle-shaped cells that occupy the inferior part of a taste bud, having a large, central nucleus, its peripheral end protruding through the gustatory pore to form the taste hair, and its central end communicating with endings of the gustatory nerves. Called also *gustatory c.* and *taste corpuscle.* **tegmental c's**, cells that cover any delicate structure. **tendon c's**, flattened tissue cells of connective tissue occurring in rows between the primary bundles of the tendons. **touch c's**, tactile corpuscles; see under CORPUSCLE. **Türk c., Türk irritation c.**, a mononuclear cell having the characteristics of a plasma cell but the nuclear pattern of a myeloblast, seen in some pathological conditions, such as anemia, infections, and leukemias. It has been suggested that they occur as a result of the atypical maturation of hemocytoblasts, or that they are pathologic forms of lymphoid leukocytes. Called also *irritation leukocyte* and *Türk irritation leukocyte.* **unit c.**, the smallest portion of a crystal in the space lattice; the three dimensional extension of the unit cell resulting in the regular macroscopic properties of crystals, such as angles between faces. **unspecialized c.**, indifferent c. **vasofactive c's, vasoformative c's**, cells that join with other cells to form blood vessels. **wandering c.**, an ameboid cell, such as a free macrophage, lymphocyte, mastocyte, or plasma cell. See also *migratory c.* **wandering resting c.**, a macrophage fixed along the bundles of collagen fibers of connective tissue. Called also *resting wandering c.* **Warthin-Finkeldey c.**, a peculiar multinucleated giant

cell present in tonsillar, nasopharyngeal, and appendiceal tissue in measles. **water-clear c.**, a large clear cell found in the parathyroid gland; these cells have a ballooned appearance and are especially numerous in adenoma of the gland. **white c. count**, LEUKOCYTE count. **white c., white blood c.**, leukocyte. **xanthoma c's**, foam c's (1).

cella (sel'ah), pl. *cel'lae* [L.] an enclosure or compartment; a cell.

cellae (sel'le) [L.] plural of *cella.*

Cellano antigen (factor) [named after the mother of a child with probable erythroblastosis, in whom Cellano antigen was first discovered] see under ANTIGEN and see Kell blood groups, under BLOOD GROUP.

cellobiase (sel"lo-bi'ās) β-glucosidase.

cellobiose (sel"lo-bi'ōs) a disaccharide, $C_{12}H_{22}O_{11}$, composed of two glucose molecules joined in a carbon-1 to carbon-4 β-linkage, being thus similar to maltose. Called also *cellose.*

celloidin (sĕ-loi'din) a concentrated preparation of pyroxylin, employed in microscopy for embedding specimens for section cutting.

cellose (sel'ōs) cellobiose.

Cellothyl trademark for *methylcellulose.*

cellula (sel'u-lah), pl. *cel'lulae* [L.] a small cell; a general term used in anatomical nomenclature for a small, more or less enclosed space. **c. ethmoida'lis** [NA], ethmoidal CELL. **c. mastoi'dea** [NA], mastoid CELL.

cellulae (sel'u-le) [L.] plural of *cellula.*

cellular (sel'u-lar) pertaining to, or made up of, cells.

cellularity (sel"u-lar'ĭ-te) the state of a tissue or other mass as regards the number of constituent cells.

cellulitis (sel"u-li'tis) 1. any inflammation of cellular tissue. 2. a spreading, diffuse, edematous, sometimes suppurative, hot, inflammatory lesion, associated with infection with invasive bacteria, principally streptococci, capable or producing hyaluronidase and fibrinolysins. Unlike in an abscess, which is well defined and localized, in cellulitis infection tends to spread through tissue spaces and cleavage planes owing to breaking down of hyaluronic acid, the intercellular binding substance, and fibrin by hyaluronidase and fibrinolysins. Called also *phlegmon.* **facial and cervical c.**, cellulitis usually originating from dental infections, such as apical abscess, osteomyelitis, or periodontal infection, and spreading rapidly through facial tissue spaces and cleavage planes (see tissue spaces, under SPACE). It is characterized by fever and painful swelling showing a hard lesion covered by inflamed, sometimes purplish skin or normal skin in cases of internal spreading of infection. Perforation of the outer cortical plate of the bone above the buccinator attachment occurs in infections originating from the maxilla; perforation below the buccinator attachment occurs in infections originating from the mandible. In the maxillary form, the upper half is involved, eventually spreading to the entire face and to the cervical area; in the mandibular form, the swelling initially involves only the lower half of the face. Lymphadenitis is usually associated and, in advanced stages, discharging facial abscesses may occur. Leukocytosis is a common symptom. Exudation of polymorphonuclear leukocytes and, sometimes, lymphocytes, with the presence of serous fluid and fibrin, and a nonspecific inflammation are the common histological features. Called also *facial and cervical phlegmon.* **submaxillary c.**, Ludwig's ANGINA.

Cellulomonas (sel"lu-lo-mo'nas) [*cellulose* + Gr. *monas* a unit] a genus of microorganisms of the family Corynebacteriaceae, made up of pleomorphic, gram-variable microorganisms found in soil.

cellulose (sel'u-lōs) a nondigestible polysaccharide with the glucose units linked as in cellulobiose, consisting of anhydroglucose units joined by an oxygen linkage to form long molecular chains. It is the fundamental skeletal structure of all vegetable tissue, occurring as a colorless, transparent solid that is insoluble in water, alcohol, and most common solvents. Cellulose products include wood, cotton, and other products of vegetable origin. In medicine, cellulose compounds are used for a variety of purposes, including as absorbable hemostatic agents, in the production of artificial kidneys, and as vehicles for drugs. **absorbable c.**, oxidized c. **c. acetate**, partially acetylated cellulose occurring in various forms that differ from each other in the degree of acetylation. Used in various industrial processes. **c. acetate phthalate**, a reduction product of phthalic anhydride and cellulose acetate, occurring as a white powder. Used as a tablet-coating agent. **acid c.**, a combination of cellulose with carboxyl groups, such as pectinic acid. **carboxymethyl c.**, carboxymethylcellulose. **carboxymethyl c. sodium,** sodium CAR-BOXYMETHYLCELLULOSE. **CM c.,** carboxymethylcellulose. **c. methyl ester,** methylcellulose. **microcrystalline c.,** purified, partially depolymerized cellulose prepared by treating it with mineral acids. Used as a tablet diluent. **oxidized c.,** cellulose oxidized with nitrogen dioxide, having a varying content of carboxylic acid groups. It occurs as an off-white gauze or lint, having a slight charred odor, which is soluble in alkali solutions, but not in water or acid solutions. Oxidized cellulose is a hemostatic agent which forms an artificial clot by combining cellulosic acid with hemoglobin, being used in surgery (including tooth extraction) as an aid for controlling moderate bleeding. It is usually implanted or packed into the wound; absorption in the wound occurs between the second and seventh day after surgery. Not used for permanent packing in fracture fixation because of its interference with bone regeneration. Called also *absorbable c., cellulosic acid,* and *polyanhydroglucuronic acid.* Trademarks: Hemo-Pak, Novocell, Oxycel. See also absorbable GAUZE. **oxidized c., regenerated,** an oxidized cellulose preparation produced by mixing cellulose with alkali to form a viscous substance which is then spun into filaments and subsequently oxidized. Regenerated oxidized cellulose is considered to have greater purity, to be less friable, and to be less adhesive to surgical instruments than oxidized cellulose. Both types of cellulose are used similarly, but the regenerated type may cause delayed healing if it is placed deeply into the socket after tooth extraction. Trademark: Surgicel. **sodium c. glycolate,** SODIUM carboxymethylcellulose. **starch c.,** amylopectin.

Cellumeth trademark for *methylcellulose.*
CELO chicken-embryonal-lethal orphan (virus); see under VIRUS.
Celontin trademark for *methsuximide.*
Celsius scale, thermometer [Anders *Celsius,* Swedish astronomer, 1701–1744] see under SCALE and THERMOMETER.
Celsus, Aurelius Cornelium [1st century A.D.] a celebrated Roman medical encyclopedist — "the Cicero of medicine." Of his many writings, only his *De re medicina* (in eight books) survives; the four classical signs (*Celsus' quadrilateral*) of inflammation — *calor* (heat), *dolor* (pain), *rubor* (redness), and *tumor* (swell-

ing) — are mentioned in the third book of this work. His writings contain the earliest record of orthodontic treatment (by finger pressure). Celsus caused the painful tooth to fall to pieces by introducing into the cavity certain astringent substances, such as pared pepper berry, or by applying paste around the tooth. His works also contain reference to the removal of stains from the teeth, the treatment of ulcers of the tongue and mouth, and the surgical treatment of oral disease.
cement (se-ment′) [L. *cementum*] 1. a substance that serves to produce solid union between two surfaces. 2. a filling material, such as zinc phosphate, used in dentistry to assist in retaining gold castings in prepared teeth and to insulate the tooth pulp from metallic and other fillings. 3. dental c. 4. cementum. ASP

CLASSIFICATION OF DENTAL CEMENTS

Cement	Principal Uses	Secondary Uses
1. Zinc phosphate	Luting agent for fabricated restorations	Temporary restorations Thermal insulating base
2. Zinc phosphate with copper or silver salts added	Temporary restorations	Root canal restorations
3. Copper phosphate (red and black)	Temporary restorations	Luting agent for orthodontic bands
4. Zinc oxide–eugenol	Temporary restorations Thermal insulating base Pulp capping Luting agent for fabricated restorations	Root canal restorations
5. Calcium hydroxide	Pulp capping Thermal insulating base	
6. Silicate	Tooth restorations	
7. Silicophosphate	Luting agent for fabricated restorations	Posterior tooth restorations
8. Acrylic or BIS-GMA resin	Luting agent for fabricated restorations	Temporary restorations
9. Polycarboxylate	Luting agent for fabricated restorations	Luting agent for orthodontic bands or brackets
10. Glass ionomer	Coating for eroded areas Pit and fissure sealant	

(From R. W. Phillips: Elements of Dental Materials. 3rd ed. Philadelphia, W. B. Saunders Co., 1977.)

COMPRESSIVE STRENGTH AND SOLUBILITY OF CEMENTS

Class	Cement Type	Consistency	Compressive Strength 7-Day-Old Specimens Store in Distilled Water at 37°C		Solubility and Disintegration in Distilled Water for 7 Days at 37°C	Dimensional Changes on Setting
			kg/cm²	psi	% by wt.	μm/cm
I	Zinc oxide–eugenol	Filling	140– 390	2,000– 5,500	0.02–0.1	– 31 to – 85
	Zinc oxide–eugenol EBA	Various	700–1,050	10,000–15,000	00.4	– 12 to – 24
II	Zinc phosphate	Filling Cementing	1,340 900–1,460	19,000 12,800* 20,800	0.05 0.1 ± 0.1	– 5 to – 7
	Zinc phosphate water-settable	Cementing	850–1,520	12,100 21,600	0.21–0.36	Not available
III	Copper phosphate {Red}	Filling Cementing	1,480 980	21,000 14,000	0.05 0.3	— – 12
	Copper phosphate {Black}	Filling Cementing	630 420–1,500	9,000 6,000–22,000	3.7 0.3–3.5	— + 3 to – 28
IV	Silicate	Filling	1,630–1,910	23,200–27,200	0.7–1.3	+ 5 to – 26 + 30 to – 5
V	Zinc silicophosphate	Cementing	1,030–1,740	14,700 24,800	0.7–2.3	—
		Filling	1,370–1,790	19,500 25,500	0.2–2.0	– 12 to – 21
VI	Resin	Cementing	530–880	7,500 12,500	0.0–0.4	– 146 to – 275
VII	Polycarboxylate	Cementing	550–1,270	7,800–18,000*	0.04–0.08*	+ 50 to + 420

*Specimens 24 hours old. (Modified from Guide to Dental Materials. 8th ed. American Dental Association, 1976–1978.)

A c., a dental cement containing aluminum silicates, polyacrylic resins, and leachable fluorides. **black copper c.,** copper c., black. **calcium hydroxide c.,** a dental cement that promotes the formation of a protective layer of secondary dentin, which is particularly beneficial in aiding healing of the pulp. Aqueous or nonaqueous suspensions of calcium hydroxide are allowed to flow over the floor of the cavity preparation. Evaporation of the suspending medium leaves a thin, powdery layer of calcium hydroxide, which is often covered with a stronger cement, such as zinc phosphate cement. Used principally for capping the pulp and as a thermal insulating base. Trademark: Hydrex. **CBA No. 9080 c.,** trademark for a resin cement based on the adduct of diglycidyl ether of bisphenol A and methacrylic acid. **combination c.,** silicophosphate c. **copper c., black,** a dental cement produced by mixing a powder containing 9.1 percent cupric oxide and 8.4 percent cobalt oxide with a phosphoric acid liquid. Used in temporary restorations and as a luting agent for orthodontic bands. It may be irritating to the dental pulp. No longer used because of its poor biostability. **copper c., red,** a zinc phosphate cement, produced by the addition of small amounts of cuprous oxide for bactericidal purposes. Used in temporary restorations and as a luting agent for orthodontic bands. It may be irritating to the dental pulp. No longer used because of its poor biostability. Called also *pseudocopper c.* **dental c.,** a bonding substance used in restorative and orthodontic procedures. Cements are available in the form of a powder and liquid that are mixed together immediately before use, setting to a hard mass. Dental cement has cohesive properties, is strong and hard, is insoluble in oral fluids, is nonreactogenic, does not contract on setting, has a coefficient of thermal expansion similar to that of the tooth structure, is easy to manipulate, is nonporous, has chemical and physical properties that are not influenced by oral temperature and humidity, and has color that is harmonious with the tooth structure. See tables. **dimethacrylate c.,** a resin cement in which dimethacrylate is the major component. **Durelon c.,** trademark for a *polycarboxylate c.* **EBA c.,** a fortified zinc oxide–eugenol cement, having some of its eugenol replaced with *o*-ethoxybenzoic acid. **Elite c.,** trademark for a fine grain dental *zinc phosphate c.* **endodontic c.,** root canal SEALER. **Flecks c.,** trademark for a *zinc phosphate c.* **Fluoro-Thin c.,** trademark for a *silicophosphate c.* **glass ionomer c.,** a dental cement produced by mixing a powder prepared from a calcium aluminosilicate glass and a liquid prepared from an aqueous solution of prepared polyacrylic acid. It is a cement of low strength and toughness that cannot be used for restoration in high masticatory stress areas, such as the posterior teeth. Used chiefly for small restorations on the proximal surfaces of anterior teeth and for restoration of eroded areas at the gingival margin. It contains fluoride which slowly leaches, thereby contributing to the prevention of caries. The cement is sensitive to moisture and is soluble during the first several hours after setting and is usually protected by a sheet of wax, a matrix strip, and a cavity varnish. It is characterized by its biological kindness to the pulp and its potential for adhesion by reaction of the polyacrylic acid and calcium in the teeth. **Grip c.,** trademark for a *polymethyl methacrylate c.* **hydrophosphate c.,** a zinc phosphate cement, into which dihydrogen phosphate has been incorporated, which is activated with distilled water rather than phosphoric acid. **Justi Resin c.,** trademark for a *polymethyl methacrylate c.* **Kent zinc c.,** trademark for *zinc phosphate c.* **MQ c.,** trademark for a *silicate c.* **Mynol c.,** trademark for an iodoform preparation used as a therapeutic root canal sealer. **periodontal c.,** periodontal PACK. **PMMA c.,** polymethyl methacrylate c. **polycarboxylate c.,** a dental cement used as a luting agent for fabricating restorations and orthodontic bands or brackets and as a cavity lining. It is prepared by mixing a powder and a liquid, the powder being a mixture of zinc oxide with less than 10 percent magnesium sulfate and, more frequently, stannous fluoride, and the liquid being a 40 percent aqueous solution of polyacrylic acid. On mixing, the material sets through the formation of zinc. The cement adheres to the tooth surface and is essentially nonirritating to the dental pulp. It may be prepared as a fluid, rapidly setting material to a viscous, putty-like material, the liquid form being used for cementing purposes and the viscous substance for cavity lining. Called also *zinc polyacrylate c.* and *zinc polycarboxylate c.* Trademarks: Durelon c., Elite c. **polymethyl methacrylate c.,** a resin cement having polymethyl methacrylate mixed with acrylic polymers and mineral fillers. Called also *PMMA c.* Trademarks: Grip c., Justi resin c., and Smith's resin c. **porcelain c.,** former name for *silicate c.* **pseudocopper c.,** copper c., red. **red copper c.,** copper c., red. **resin c.,** a dental cement composed either of polymethyl methacrylate or dimethacrylate, produced by mixing an acrylic monomer liquid with acrylic polymers and mineral fillers. The cement is insoluble in

water and is thus resistant to fluids in the mouth, and is also irritating to the dental pulp. Used chiefly as a luting agent for fabricated and temporary restorations. **root canal c.,** root canal SEALER. **silicate c.,** a dental cement produced by mixing a buffered phosphoric acid liquid with a powder that is a mixture of acid soluble aluminosilicate glass made by fusing silica (SiO_2), alumina (Al_2O_3), calcium oxide (CaO), and other glass-forming substances, such as sodium, aluminum fluoride, and calcium fluoride. Metallic oxides are added for color. On mixing, the mass sets to a hard, translucent, porcelain-like solid. Used chiefly for temporary and semipermanent restorations of anterior teeth where the use of metals might be objectionable. The cement is relatively brittle and tends to disintegrate and discolor. It is neither adhesive nor used for luting purposes. Fluoride-containing silicate cements prevent the development of caries and reduce the solubility of adjacent enamel and dentin *in vitro.* Called also *synthetic porcelain;* formerly called *porcelain cement.* Trademarks: Achatite, Ames plastic porcelain, Caulk Syntrex F, MQ c., and S.S. White new filling porcelain. **silicate zinc c.,** silicophosphate c. **silicophosphate c.,** a mixture of silicate and zinc phosphate cements, primarily used as a temporary filling material and for cementation of orthodontic bands and cast restorations. The cement is acidic and may cause pulp irritation. Called also *combination c.,* *silicate zinc c.,* and *zinc silicophosphate c.* Trademark: Fluoro-Thin c. **Smith's resin c.,** trademark for a *polymethyl methacrylate c.* **Smith's zinc c.,** trademark for a *zinc phosphate c.* **zinc oxide c.,** a cement produced by the reaction of zinc oxide powder and a concentrated aqueous solution of zinc chloride. Zinc chloride has been replaced by eugenol, thus producing zinc oxide–eugenol cement. **zinc oxide–eugenol c.,** a dental cement used chiefly in temporary fillings, thermal insulating bases, and root canal fillings. Some formulations are used as luting agents for the permanent cementation of gold inlays and crowns. Its nearly neutral pH causes minimal pulpal irritation. The cement is produced by mixing zinc oxide powder with eugenol liquid in the presence of a small amount of water, first converting zinc oxide hydrates to its hydroxide, $ZnO + H_2O - Zn(OH)_2$, followed by reaction with the eugenol to form zinc eugenolate and water, $Zn(OH)_2 + 2\ HO\cdot\text{-}C_{10}H_{11}O_2 - Zn(O\cdot C_{10}\cdot H_{11}O_2)_2 + 2H_2O$. The cement consists of zinc oxide particles held together by zinc eugenolate crystals with some free eugenol being also present. It has low relative strength and poor resistance to abrasion and disintegration; its compression strength is 100 to 4000 psi. Trademarks: Cavitec, Temrex, Zebacem. Abbreviated ZOE. **zinc oxide–eugenol c., fortified, reinforced, modified, or improved,** any zinc oxide–eugenol cement that has been strengthened by the addition of fillers such as polymethyl methacrylate, polystyrene, zinc oxide, hydrogenated rosin, fused quartz, aluminum oxide, or *o*-ethoxybenzoic acid. Although strengthened, many of these cements retain their low resistance to abrasion and disintegration. **zinc phosphate c.,** a dental cement used as a luting agent for fabricated restorations and, secondarily, in temporary restorations and as a thermal insulating base. It is produced by mixing a powder, consisting chiefly of zinc oxide with magnesium oxide added as a modifier, and a liquid, which is a mixture of phosphoric acid, water, and metallic salts, such as aluminum and zinc phosphates. The metallic salts (buffering salts) are added to reduce the reaction rate and thus allow sufficient time for thorough mixing. On mixing the liquid and the powder, the cement is formed: $ZnO + 2H_3PO_4 \rightarrow Zn(H_3PO_4)_2 + H_2O$ with release of heat. The cement is crystalline in structure with the original undissolved powder particles suspended in crystals of zinc phosphate compound. Trademarks: Ames Z-M, Elite c., Flecks c., Kent zinc c., Lang crown, bridge and inlay, Modern Tenacin, S-C, Smith's Zinc c. **zinc phosphate c., modified,** zinc phosphate cement to which copper oxide or silver salts have been added to increase antiseptic properties. Copper-produced low pH may cause pulpal irritation. **zinc polyacrylate c., zinc polycarboxylate c.,** polycarboxylate c. **zinc silicophosphate c.,** silicophosphate c. **ZOE c.,** zinc oxide–eugenol c.

cementation (se"men-ta'shun) 1. the attachment of anything by the means of cement. 2. the attachment of a restoration to atural teeth by means of cement. 3. the attachment of a band or bands to the teeth by means of an adhesive material.

cementicle (se-men'tĭ-k'l) a small, discrete focus of calcified tissue that may or may not represent true cementum, found in the periodontal ligament, most commonly in the apical root area or in molar bifurcations. The exact cause is unknown, but calcification of epithelial cells, small hyalinized areas, or thrombosed vessels in the periodontal ligament, or by displacement of pieces of cementum are believed to be the most common causes. **adherent c., attached c.,** one firmly attached to the cementum. Free cementicles together in close association with the root surface on occasion fuse and become attached to the cementum of the root. **free c., interstitial c.,** one completely surrounded by the connective tissue of the periodontal ligament. Free cementicles may fuse together on occasion and also may become attached to the cementum of the root.

cementification (se-men″tĭ-fĭ-ka′shun) cementogenesis.

cementite (se-men′tīt) an intermetallic compound, Fe₃C, having an orthorhombic unit cell of 12 iron and 4 carbon atoms. It can decompose to form graphite and ferrite, usually occurrin in cast iron but not in steel. **spheroidized c.,** spheroidite.

cementitis (se″men-ti′tis) inflammation of the cementum of a tooth.

cementoblast (se-men′to-blast) [*cementum* + Gr. *blastos* germ] a large cell, about 8 to 12 μ in diameter, ranging in shape from squamous to cuboidal, which is active in the formation of cementum. It has a large central nucleus and usually a single nucleolus. Those active in the formation of cellular cementum exhibit long branching cell processes which, when cells become entrapped in the cementum, occupy canaliculi of the matrix. See also CEMENTOGENESIS.

cementoblastoma (se-men″to-blas-to′mah) cementoma. **benign c.,** true CEMENTOMA.

cementoclasia (se-men″to-kla′se-ah) dissolution and resorption of the cementum of a tooth, usually occurring as a complication of trauma, such as excessive masticatory force or excessive pressure during orthodontic treatment, and pathological conditions, such as infection, cysts, or tumors.

cementoclast (se-men′to-klast″) [*cementum* + Gr. *klasis* breaking] a cell, cytomorphologically the same as an osteoclast, which is involved in cementum resorption; the cavities produced by resorption being known as *resorption lacunae.*

cementocyte (se-men′to-sīt) [*cementum* + Gr. *kytos* hollow vessel] a cell found in the lacunae of cellular cementum, rom 8 μ to over 15 μ in diameter, having a wide variety of shapes, from round to oval or flattened. Numerous protoplasmic processes, about 1 μ in diameter and up to 12 to 15 μ in length, extend from its free surface; the extensions are often oriented toward the free surface of the cementum, but are frequently inclined laterally toward the dentin, or toward each other. Called also *cement cell.*

cementogenesis (se-men″to-jen′ĕ-sis) [*cementum* + Gr. *genesis* formation] the development of cementum on the root dentin of a tooth, beginning with disorganization and perforation of the root sheath, followed by formation of openings through which undifferentiated mesenchymal cells and fibroblasts emerge from the dental sac. As they approach the radicular dentin, the cells differentiate into cementoblasts and form the cementoblastic layer. Cells engaged in the production of cellular cementum develop branching cell processes that are more prominent than those of cells involved in the production of acellular cementum; the processes are destined to occupy the canaliculi when their parent cells become entrapped in the cementum. The fibrillogenic activity of cementoblasts contributes fibers in matrix formation. The next stage in the development of the cementum matrix consists of addition of the ground substance and, as the matrix matures, it becomes calcified through the deposition of hydroxyapatite crystals. Called also *cementification.*

cementoid (se-men′toid) the surface uncalcified layer of the cementum in areas of intact periodontal tissue, about 8 μ or less in width, except for areas of active cementogenesis where it may be more. When stained with hematoxylin and eosin, it becomes highly refractile and eosinophilic. It is believed to protect the cementum by resisting resorption. Called also *precementum* and *uncalcified cementum.*

cementoma (se″men-to′mah) [*cementum* + *-oma*]. 1. formation of circumscribed areas of fibrous connective tissue containing small masses of cementum, usually in or about the periodontal ligament around the apex of a tooth, most frequently a mandibular incisor. The calcified material lies usually unattached to the tissue of a tooth and the lesion is not considered neoplastic. Called also *cementoblastoma* and *periapical cemental dysplasia.* 2. true c. **gigantiform monstrous c.,** a form of multiple, extensive true cementoma. **true c.,** an odontogenic tumor presenting as a proliferating mass of tissue, continuous with the tissue of the root of a tooth, and having the histological structure of cementum. Called also *benign cementoblastoma.*

cementopathia (se-men″to-path′e-ah) periodontitis or periodontosis resulting from disease or defect of the cementum of a tooth.

cementoperiostitis (se-men″to-per″e-os-ti′tis) periodontitis.

cementosis (se″men-to′sis) hypercementosis. **aberrant c.,** aberrant CEMENTUM.

cementum (se-men′tum) [L.] [NA] the bonelike rigid connective tissue covering the root of a tooth from the cementoenamel junction to the apex and lining the apex of the root canal, also assisting in tooth support by serving as attachment structures for the periodontal ligament. The upper one-third to one-half of the root is covered by acellular cementum, and the remainder by cellular cementum. The width of cementum at the cementoenamel junction is about 10 μ, thickening progressively toward the apex; in some older individuals it may reach 600 to 700 μ. Its chief component is collagen; hydroxyapatite being the principal mineral component. The fibrillar collagen component is embedded in a ground substance of glycoprotein. Trace amounts of copper, fluorine, iron, lead, potassium, silicon, sodium, and zinc may be found. Called also *cement, crusta petrosa dentis,* and *substantia ossea dentis.* **aberrant c.,** the aberrant occurrence of cementum, usually on the crown (see *coronal c.*), and in the periodontal ligament (see CEMENTICLE). Called also *aberrant cementosis.* **acellular c.,** the part of the cementum covering one-third to one-half of the root of a tooth adjacent to the cementoenamel junction, which is usually apposed by a layer of cellular cementum. It consists of collagenous fibers and unformed ground (cementing) substance, but having no cellular components. Called also *primary c.* **afibrillar c.,** the outer layer of the cementum on the crown, to which epithelium attaches. **cellular c.,** the part of the cementum covering the apical one-half to two-thirds of the root of a tooth, which is usually apposed by a layer of acellular cementum. It contains cementocytes embedded in the calcified matrix. Called also *secondary c.* **coronal c.,** the aberrant occurrence of cementum on the crown of a tooth. It is found most commonly at the cervical region, where it projects as a spike extension (cementum spur), and, less commonly, at the occlusal fissure. **intermediate c.,** a layer of cementum at the cementodentinal junction, bordered on one side by dentin and on the other by acellular cementum. It exhibits a staining reaction more comparable to dentin than to cementum. Its presence is believed to be due to faulty cementogenesis in which connective tissue becomes entrapped between cellular elements of the cementum, where it becomes calcified. **primary c.,** acellular c. **root c.,** cementum of the root of a tooth. **secondary c.,** cellular c. **uncalcified c.,** cementoid.

cen centromere. See CHROMOSOME nomenclature.

ceno- 1. [Gr. *kainos* new, fresh] a combining form denoting new. Spelled also *caino-* and *kaino-.* 2. [Gr. *kenos* empty] a combining form denoting empty. Spelled also *caeno-* and *keno-.* 3. [Gr. *koinos* shared in common] a combining form denoting relationship to a common feature or characteristic. Spelled also *coeno-, coino-,* and *koino-.*

cenogenesis (se″no-jen′ĕ-sis) [*ceno-*(1) + Gr. *genesis* production] the appearance of a new feature in development, in adaptive response to environmental conditions.

Centedrin trademark for *methylphenidate.*

center (sen′ter) [Gr. *kentron;* L. *centrum*] 1. the middle point of the body. See also CENTRUM. 2. a collection of nerve cells concerned with a particular function. Also spelled *centre.* **area health education c.,** an organization or system of health, educational, and service institutions whose policy and programs are frequently under the direction of a medical school or university health science center and whose prime goals are to improve the distribution, supply, quality, utilization, and efficiency of health personnel in relation to the specific area having inadequate health care facilities. Abbreviated *AHEC.* **brain c.,** 1. an area of the brain having a specialized structure or function. 2. a group of cells in the brain having a specialized function. **cell c.,** centrosome. **community health c.,** an ambulatory health care center, usually serving a catchment area with scarce or nonexisting health services or a population with special health needs. **coughing c.,** a center in the medulla oblongata, situated above the respiratory center, which controls the act of coughing. **deglutition c.,** swallowing c. **dentary c.,** an ossification center of the mandible, giving origin to the lower border and outer plate. **dominating c.,** the principal or controlling center of a group having a common function. **C. for Disease Control,** a branch of the Department of Health and Human Services, which serves as a focal point for disease control and public health activities, by providing facilities and services for the investigation, prevention, and control of diseases; supporting quarantine and other activities to prevent introduction of communicable diseases from abroad, conducting research into the epidemiology, laboratory diagnosis, prevention, and treatment of infectious diseases; providing grants for various disease control programs; and setting standards for laboratories in related fields. Abbreviated *CDC*. **epiotic c.**, the center of ossification that forms the mastoid process. **facial c.**, a center for face movements, located in the lower part of the ascending frontal convolution of the brain. **Flemming's c.**, germinal c. **freedom in c.**, an occlusal relationship in which maximum intercuspation is provided for that is straight anterior to centric relation contact and that may be lateral to an existing centric occlusion, and in which there is freedom to move into centric relation contact as well as between centric occlusion and the retruded contact position without interference. **germinal c.**, the area in the lymphoid tissue in which mitotic figures are observed frequently, differentiation and formation of lymphocytes occur, and elements related to antibody formation are found. Called also *Flemming's c.* and *secondary nodules*. **glossokinetic c.**, the center in the posterior part of the left second frontal gyrus that controls movements of the tongue concerned with articulate speech. **gustatory c.**, the center in the cerebral cortex believed to control taste. Called also *taste c.* **inhibitory c.**, any nerve center that restrains any function or process of other centers. **nerve c.**, a collection of nerve cells in the central nervous system that are associated in the performance of some particular function. **c. of ossification**, a point at which the process of ossification begins; in the embryo, an area of accumulation of osteoblasts where bone development begins. Called also *ossification point*. **reflex c.**, any center in the brain or spinal cord in which a sensory impulse is changed into a motor impulse. **respiratory c.**, a center in the medulla oblongata and pons that coordinates respiratory movements, which comprises the medullary, apneustic, and pneumotopic centers. **rotation c.**, the point or axis about which a body rotates. **sphenotic c.**, a center of ossification in the sphenoid bone for the lingula. **swallowing c.**, a center on the floor of the fourth ventricle that controls the act of swallowing. Called also *deglutition c.* **taste c.**, gustatory c. **temperature regulating c.**, **thermoregulatory c.**, a center in the anterior hypothalamus responsible for regulating body temperature, which consists of a heat loss center and a heat conservation and production center. See also body TEMPERATURE. **vasoconstrictor c.**, a center in the medulla oblongata that controls contraction of the blood vessels; it is part of the vasomotor center. **vasodilator c.**, a center in the medulla oblongata that controls dilatation of the blood vessels; it is part of the vasomotor center. **vasomotor c's**, centers in the tuber cinereum, medulla oblongata, and spinal cord that regulate contraction (*vasoconstrictor c.*) and dilatation of the blood vessels (*vasodilator c.*).

centesimal (sen-tes'ĭ-mal) [L. *centesimus* hundredth] divided into hundredths or based on division into hundredths.

centesis (sen-te'sis) [Gr. *kentēsis*] perforation or tapping, as with an aspirator, trocar, or needle. Used also as a word termination, affixed to a root, indicating the part on which the operation is performed, as abdominocentesis, thoracocentesis, and the like.

centi- [L. *centum* a hundred] in the metric system, a combining form denoting one-hundredth (10^{-2}) of the unit designated by the root with which it is combined. Abbreviated *c*. See also metric SYSTEM and *Tables of Weights and Measures* at WEIGHT.

centigrade (sen'tĭ-grād) [*centi-* + L. *gradus* a step] consisting of or having 100 gradations (steps or degrees), as a Celsius (centigrade) temperature scale. Abbreviated C. See TEMPERATURE.

centigram (sen'tĭ-gram) [*centi-* + *gram*] a unit of mass (weight) in the metric system, being one-hundredth (10^{-2}) of a gram, or the equivalent of 0.1543 grain. Abbreviated *cg* or *cgm*.

centiliter (sen'tĭ-le"ter) [*centi-* + *liter*] a unit of volume in the metric system, being one-hundredth (10^{-2}) of a liter and consisting of 10 milliliters. It is equivalent to 2.7 fluid drams or 0.3315 fluid ounce. Abbreviated *cl*.

centimeter (sen'tĭ-me"ter) [*centi-* + *meter*] a unit of length in the metric system, being one-hundredth (10^{-2}) of a meter, or 0.3937 inch. One-tenth of a centimeter is the millimeter. Abbreviated *cm*. **cubic c.**, a unit of volume in the metric system, being equal to a cube each side of which measures 1 centimeter. It is equivalent to one-thousandth (10^{-3}) of a liter, 1000 cubic millimeters, or 0.0011 of a quart of fluid. Abbreviated *cc, cm³, cu. cm.* See also MILLILITER. **square c.**, a unit in the metric system used for measuring areas, being equal to a square both sides of which measure 1 centimeter. It is equivalent to 100 square millimeters (mm²) or 0.155 square inches. Abbreviated *cm²*.

centinormal (sen'tĭ-nor'mal) [*centi-* + L. *norma* rule] having a hundredth part of the standard strength; said of solutions.

centipoise (sen'tĭ-poiz) [*centi-* + *poise*] a unit of viscosity in the metric system, being one-hundredth (10^{-2}) of a poise.

centiunit (sen"tĭ-u'nit) [*centi-* + L. *unus* one] one-hundredth of the conventional unit.

centra (sen'trah) [L.] plural of *centrum*.

centrad (sen'trad) toward the center, especially toward the center of the body.

central (sen'tral) situated at or pertaining to a center; not peripheral. In the context of pathological literature, the term is often used to mean situated at or pertaining to the center of a bone, as within the jaw bone, as in central tumor.

centralis (sen-tra'lis) a general anatomical term denoting a centrally located structure.

centraxonial (sen"trak-so'ne-al) having the axis in a central median line.

centre (sen'ter) center.

centric (sen'trik) pertaining to or situated at the center; central. The term is sometimes used alone as a noun to mean centric relation, centric occlusion, centric position, or power centric. **acquired c.**, centric OCCLUSION. **broad c.**, centric resulting in increased lateral dimensions that may occur with an occlusal adjustment and in restorations made according to the principle of freedom in centric. See also *long c.* **habitual c.**, centric OCCLUSION. **long c.**, the occlusal contact relationship in which maximum intercuspation of the teeth is provided for (up to 0.5 mm) anterior to centric relation contact and in which there is freedom to move into centric relation from centric occlusion without interference and without a change in contact vertical dimension. Not found in the natural dentition, it is produced as a result of an occlusal adjustment or full-mouth reconstruction. **Myo-Monitor c.**, a centric occlusion position determined with the use of the Myo-Monitor. **c. occlusion**, centric OCCLUSION. **point c.**, maximum intercuspation of the teeth in centric relation, being coincident at a point of centric occlusion and centric relation contacts. **c. position**, centric POSITION. **power c.**, the position of the mandible during a forceful bite. **c. relation**, retruded c., centric RELATION. **slide in c.**, SLIDE in centric. **true c.**, centric RELATION.

centrifugal (sen-trif'u-gal) [*center* + L. *fugere* to flee] moving away from a center; efferent or exodic.

centrifugation (sen-trif'u-ga'shun) the process of separating the lighter portions of a solution, mixture, or suspension from the heavier portions by centrifugal forces.

centrifuge (sen'trĭ-fūj) [*center* + L. *fugere* to flee] 1. a machine by which centrifugation is effected. 2. to subject to centrifugation.

centrilobular (sen"trĭ-lob'u-lar) pertaining to the central portion of a lobule.

centriole (sen'trĭ-ōl) a small granule or short rod within the centrosome. It is a hollow cylinder about 150 mμ in diameter and 300 to 500 mμ in length, open at one end and closed at the other, filled with cytoplasm. In mammalian cells centrioles usually occur in pairs and are called *diplosomes*. They are self-duplicating bodies and, when they replicate early in cell division, the pairs produced take up positions at opposite poles of the nucleus. **double c.**, diplosome.

centro- [Gr. *kentron*; L. *centrum*] a combining form indicating relationship to a center, or to a central location.

centromere (sen'tro-mēr) the constricted portion of the chromosome, consisting of a small mass of heterochromatin which holds the two chromatids together. Variations in the shape of chromosomes are determined by the location of the centromere, which is thus used in their classification (see CHROMOSOME nomenclature). A chromosome without a centromere is said to be *acentric;* one having the centromere located medially is characterized by arms that are about equal in length and is said to be *metacentric* or V-shaped; one having the centromere in an eccentric or submedial location has arms of different lengths and is said to be *submetacentric* or J-shaped; one having the centromere in a quasi-terminal location has exaggeratedly long and short arms and is said to be *acrocentric* or I-shaped; and one having two centromeres is said to be *dicentric*. Called also *kinetochore* and *primary constriction*.

centron (sen'tron) a postulated preexisting spherical stromal structure in the lymph node cortex; cortical follicles result from the grouping of lymphoid cells in relation to the centron during antigen stimulation.

centrosome (sen'tro-sōm) [*centro-* + Gr. *sōma* body] a specialized hyaline zone in the cytoplasm, which contains the centrioles, and is considered to be associated with cell division. It is usually located adjacent to the cell nucleus and may occupy a shallow indentation on its surface, and is often partially surrounded by the Golgi apparatus, but it may also be located in the apical cytoplasm just beneath the cell surface away from the cell nucleus or the Golgi apparatus. Called also *attraction sphere, cell center, centrosphere, cytocentrum,* and *microcentrum.*

centrosphere (sen′tro-sfēr) [*centro-* + Gr. *sphaira* sphere] centrosome.

centrum (sen′trum), pl. *cen′tra* [L.; Gr. *kentron*] center; used in anatomical nomenclature to designate a central structure, or the central part of a structure. See also CENTER.

Cēpacol trademark for *cetylpyridinium chloride* (see under CETYLPYRIDINIUM).

Cepalorin trademark for *cephaloridine.*

cephal- see CEPHALO-.

cephalad (sef′ah-lad) [Gr. *kephalē* head] toward the head, rostrad; opposite of caudad.

cephalalgia (sef″ah-lal′je-ah) [Gr. *kephalalgia*] pain in the head; cephalgia; headache.

cephaledema (sef″al-ĕ-de′mah) [*cephal-* + Gr. *oidēma* swelling] edema of the head.

cephalexin (sef″ah-lek′sin) a cephalosporin antibiotic, D-7-(2-amino-2-phenylacetamido)-3-8-oxo-5-thia-1-azabicyclo[4,2,0]-oct-2-ene-2-carboxylic acid, occurring as a white, acid-fast, crystalline powder that is slightly soluble in water and insoluble in organic solvents. It is bacteriostatic at low and bactericidal at high concentrations, acting against both gram-positive and gram-negative bacteria, including strains of *Clostridium, Streptococcus, Pneumococcus, Corynebacterium, Bacillus anthracis, Listeria, Neisseria, Escherichia coli, Proteus, Salmonella,* and *Shigella.* It may be used in the treatment of most

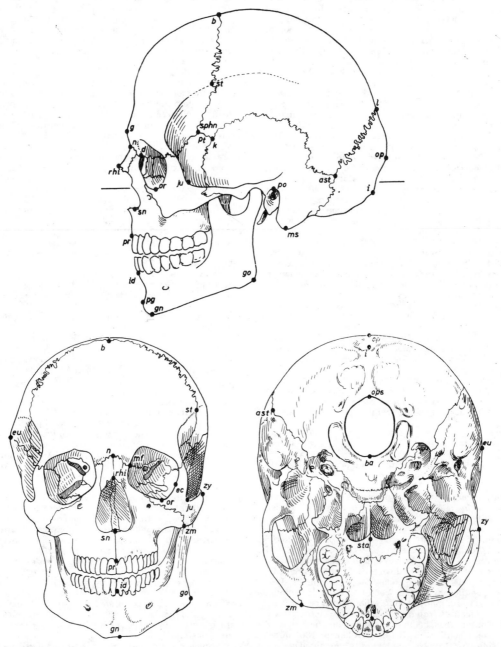

Ast, asterion. *Ba*, basion. *D*, dac, dacryon. *Ec*, ectoconchion. *Eu*, eurvon. *G*, glabella. *Gn*, gnathion. *Go*, gonion. *I*, inion. *Id*, intradentale. *L*, lambda. *Mf*, maxillofrontale. *Ms*, mastoidale. *N*, nasale. *O*, orale. *Op*, opisthocranion. *Ops*, opisthion. *Or*, orbitale. *Pg*, pogonion. *Po*, porion. *Pr*, prosthion. *Pt*, pterion. *Rhi*, rhinion. *Sn*, subnasale. *Sphn*, sphenoidale. *St*, stephanion. *Sta*, staphylion. *Zm*, zygomaxillare. *Zy*, zygion. (Modified from W. M. Krogman: The Human Skeleton in Forensic Medicine. 1961. Courtesy of Charles C Thomas, Publisher, Springfield, Illinois.)

odontogenic infections of multibacterial etiology, including penicillinase-producing strains of *Straphylococcus*. Side effects include hypersensitization, diarrhea, nausea, vomiting, abdominal cramps, skin rash, urticaria, neutropenia, eosinophilia, tinnitus, ataxia, diplopia, and changes in the intestinal and vaginal flora. Trademarks: Ceporexine, Keflex, Larixin, Sencephalin.

cephalgia (sĕ-fal′je-ah) pain in the head; cephalalgia; headache. **histamine c.**, cluster headache. **c. pharyngotympan′ica**, a peculiar form of headache related to diseases of the pharynx and middle ear, characterized by painful points in the regions of the temporal and occipital nerves. Called also *Legal's disease*.

cephalhematocele (sef′al-he-mat′o-sēl) [*cephal-* + Gr. *haima* blood + *kēlē* hernia] a hematocele under the pericranium, communicating with one or more sinuses of the dura mater through the cranial bones.

cephalhematoma (sef′al-he-mah-to′mah) [*cephal-* + Gr. *haima* blood +-*oma*] a hematoma beneath the pericranium.

cephalhydrocele (sef′al-hi′dro-sēl) [*cephal-* + *hydrocele*] a serous or watery accumulation under the pericranium.

cephalic (sĕ-fal′ik) [L. *cephalicus*; Gr. *kephalikos*] pertaining to the head, or to the head end of the body.

cephalin (sef′ah-lin) a phospholipid, being either phosphatidyl ethanolamine or phosphatidyl serine, in which two unsaturated fatty acids form ester linkages with hydroxyl groups of glycerophosphoric acid, the phosphate residue of which is esterified to either ethanolamine or serine. Found chiefly in the brain, but also occurring in various animals and plant tissues, including nerve tissue and egg yolk. It is a yellowish, amorphous substance with a characteristic odor and taste, which is soluble in most organic solvents, except acetone, and is insoluble in water, but can be dispersed in it in a colloidal state. Cephalins are involved in blood coagulation, being the principal component of thromboplastin. When hydrolyzed by enzymes, such as those in snake venoms, the unsaturated fatty acid residue is removed from the molecule, and the product becomes a lysocephalin, a potent hemolytic agent. A cephalin fraction, usually from brain tissue, is used in the partial thromboplastin time test (see under TIME).

cephalitis (sef′ah-li′tis) encephalitis.

cephalo-, cephal- [Gr. *kephalē* head] a combining form denoting relationship to the head.

cephalocaudad (sef′ah-lo-kaw′dad) 1. proceeding in a direction from the head toward the tail; caudad. 2. in both a cephalic and caudal direction.

cephalocaudal (sef′ah-lo-kaw′dal) [*cephalo-* + L. *cauda* tail] pertaining to the long axis of the body, in a direction from head to tail.

cephalocele (se-fal′o-sēl) [*cephalo-* + Gr. *kēlē* hernia] a protrusion of a part of the cranial contents. **orbital c.**, a protrusion of the cranial contents through a defect in the orbital wall.

cephalodymus (sef′ah-lod′i-mus) [*cephalo-* + Gr. *didymos* twin] a twin fetus with a single united head. See also CRANIOPAGUS.

cephaloglycin (sef′ah-lo-gli′sin) a cephalosporin antibiotic, 3-[(acetyloxy)methyl] - 7 - [(amino-phenylacetyl)amino] - 8 - oxo - 5-thia-1-azabicyclo[4,2,0]oct-2-ene-2-carboxylic acid. It is prepared from the natural antibiotic cephalosporin C, and occurs as a white crystalline powder that is slightly soluble in water, but is insoluble in most organic solvents. It is bacteriostatic at low and bactericidal at high concentrations, acting against both gram-positive and gram-negative bacteria, including strains of *Clostridium, Streptococcus, Pneumococcus, Corynebacterium, Bacillus anthracis, Listeria, Neisseria, Escherichia coli, Proteus, Salmonella,* and *Shigella*. Diarrhea, nausea, vomiting, and abdominal cramps, occasionally hypersensitization with urticaria, rashes, dermatitis, and eosinophilia may occur. Trademarks: Kafocin, Kefglycin.

cephalogram (sef′ah-lo-gram) cephalometric ROENTGENOGRAM.

cephalography (sef′ah-log′rah-fe) [*cephalo-* + Gr. *graphein* to write] roentgenography of the head.

cephalometer (sef′ah-lom′ĕ-ter) [*cephalo-* + Gr. *metron* measure] an instrument for measuring the head; an orienting device for positioning the head for radiographic examination and measurement.

cephalometric (sef′ah-lo-met′rik) pertaining to cephalometry.

cephalometry (sef′ah-lom′ĕ-tre) [*cephalo-* + Gr. *metron* measure] a branch of anthropometry, being the measurement of the dimensions of the head of living persons, taken either directly or by roentgenography. Certain combinations of linear and angular measurements developed from tracing the oriented lateral and frontal radiographic head film are used to study the growth of the skull and head under normal and abnormal conditions, to

analyze disharmonies in the pattern of craniofacial growth and development, and to determine the nature of abnormalities and the need for correction. See illustration. For specific measurements see BREADTH, HEIGHT, INDEX, LENGTH, LINE, and PLANE. **fetal c.**, measurement of the fetal skull *in utero* by means of x-ray films or by interpreting the echoes of ultrasonic waves received from each side of the skull. **radiologic c., roentgenographic c.**, cephalometry by the use of roentgenography, for identification of landmarks and making measurements.

cephalomotor (sef′ah-lo-mo′tor) [*cephalo-* + L. *motus* motion] moving the head; pertaining to motions of the head.

cephalopagus (sef′ah-lop′ah-gus) craniopagus.

cephalophore (sef′ah-lo-fŏr) a cephalostat for standardization in taking sequential facial photographs.

cephaloridine (sef′ah-lor′i-dēn) a cephalosporin antibiotic, (6R-*trans*) - 1 - [2-carboxy - 8 - oxo - 7 - [(2-thinylacetyl)amino] - 5 - thia-1-aza-bicyclo[4,2,0]oct-2-en-3-yl-methyl]pyridinium hydroxide inner salt. It is prepared from a mixture of cephalothin, thiocyanate, pyridine, and phosphoric acid, and occurs as a white crystalline powder that may become discolored when exposed to light and is soluble in water, but not in organic solvents. It is bacteriostatic at low and bactericidal at high concentrations. It is active against a wide spectrum of bacteria, its potency against gram-positive organisms being greater, including *Staphylococcus, Streptococcus, Pneumococcus, Neisseria, Haemophilus, Escherichia coli, Klebsiella, Aerobacter, Proactinomyces,* and *Treponema*. Nausea, vomiting, hypersensitization, skin rash, nephrotoxicity, azotemia, myoclonus, muscle twitching, and coma may occur. Trademarks: Cepalorin, Ceflorin, Ceporan, Keflodin, Loridine, Sefacin.

cephalosporin (sef′ah-lo-spor′in) any of a group of antibiotics elaborated by *Acremonium* (*Cephalosporium*) that contain cephalosporanic acid. Cephalosporins inhibit microbial cell formation and are active against a wide spectrum of gram-positive and gram-negative bacteria and certain fungi and viruses, including *Streptococcus, Staphylococcus, Clostridium, Listeria, Bacillus subtilis, Neisseria, Actinomyces, Salmonella, Shigella, Escherichia coli, Haemophilus influenzae, Klebsiella, Proteus,* and *Aerobacter*. Side effects include hypersensitization, fever, eosinophilia, serum sickness, urticaria, rashes, pain, neutropenia, anaphylaxis, and abscesses. The group includes cephalexin, cephaloglycin, cephaloridine, cephalothin, cephapirin, and cephradine. **c. C**, an antibiotic, 7-(D - 5 - amino - 5 - carboxyvaleramido) - 3 - (hydroxymethyl) - 8 - oxo - 5 - thia - 1 - azabicyclo[4,2,0]-oct-2-ene-2-carboxylic acid acetate. It acts against both gram-negative and gram-positive microorganisms. **c. N,** penicillin N. **c. P,** a steroid antibiotic, 6α, 16β-bis(acetyloxy)-$3\alpha,7\beta$-dihydroxy - 29 - nordammara-17(20),24-dien-21-oic acid. Chemically, it is related to helvolic and fusidic acids. In crude form, cephalosporin P contains at least five components, P_1, P_2, P_3, P_4, P_5. It is active only against gram-positive microorganisms.

cephalosporinase [E.C.3.5.2.8] (sef′ah-lo-spor′i-nās) a hydrolase acting on carbon-nitrogen bonds, other than peptide bonds, which inactivates cephalosporins by hydrolyzing the CO·NH bonds in the lactam ring, thus increasing resistance to the antibiotic. Called also β-lactamase II.

cephalosporiosis (sef′ah-lo-spor″re-o′sis) infection with the fungus *Cephalosporium* (now called *Acremonium*).

Cephalosporium (sef″ah-lo-spo′re-um) former name for *Acremonium*.

cephalostat (sef′ah-lo-stat″) a head-positioning device used in dental radiology, facial photography, cephalometry, and other procedures requiring exact positioning of the head. See also GNATHOSTAT.

cephalothin sodium (sef′ah-lo-thin) a cephalosporin antibiotic, 6R - *trans* - 3 - [(acetyloxy)methyl] - 8 - oxo - 7 - [(2 - thienylacetyl) - amino]-5-thia-1-azabicyclo[4,2,0]oct-2-ene-carboxylic acid monosodium salt. It is a semisynthetic derivative of cephalosporin C with the aminocephalosporanic acid nucleus, occurring as a white, odorless crystalline powder that is freely soluble in water, slightly soluble in dextrose, methanol, and ethanol, and insoluble in most organic solvents. It is a wide-spectrum antibiotic active against penicillinase-producing staphylococci, betahemolytic streptococci, pneumococci, *Escherichia coli, Aerobacter, Haemophilus, Klebsiella, Bacillus pertussis, Salmonella, Shigella,* and other bacteria. Induration, sterile abscesses, and irritation at the site of administration, and occasional hypersensitization associated with urticaria, fever, rash, eosinophilia, leukopenia, and neutropenia may occur. Trademarks: Cefalotin, Cepovenin, Keflin, Microtin.

cephalothoracopagus (sef″ah-lo-tho″rah-kop′ah-gus) a double monster consisting of two similar components united in the frontal plane, the fusion extending from the crown of the head to the middle abdominal region.

cephapirin sodium (sef-ah-pi′rin) a cephalosporin antibiotic, 3-[(acetyloxy)methyl] - 8 - oxo - 7[[(4 - pyridinylthio)acetyl]amino] - thia-1-azabicyclo[4,2,0]oct-2-ene-carboxylic acid monosodium salt. It is derived from cephalosporin C, and occurs as a white, odorless crystalline powder that dissolves in water and hydrochloric and glacial acetic acids and is insoluble in chloroform and ether. Active against strains of *Staphylococcus, Streptococcus, Diplococcus, Neisseria, Haemophilus, Shigella, Salmonella, Proteus, Klebsiella,* and other gram-positive and gram-negative organisms. Nausea, pallor, diarrhea, hypertension, tachycardia, chest pain, headache, visual disorders, syncope, agitation, arthralgia, and neurological complications may occur. Hypersensitization is rare. Trademarks: Brisfirina, Cefadyl, Cefatrexyl.

cephradine (sef′rah-dēn) a cephalosporin antibiotic, 7-[(amino-1,4-cyclohexanedien-1-ylacetyl)amino]-3-methyl-8-oxo-5-thia-1-azabicyclo[4,2,0]oct-2-ene-2-carboxylic acid monohydrate, occurring as a white, crystalline powder that is sparingly soluble in water, slightly soluble in alcohol, and insoluble in ether and chloroform. It is bacteriostatic at low and bactericidal at high concentrations, acting against both gram-positive and gram-negative bacteria, including strains of enterococci, clostridia, streptococci, pneumococci, corynebacteria, *Bacillus anthracis, Listeria, Neisseria, Escherichia coli, Proteus, Salmonella,* and *Shigella.* Nausea, vomiting, diarrhea, abdominal cramps, and heartburn are the most common side effects. Hypersensitization occurs infrequently. Trademarks: Anspor, Velosef.

Ceporan trademark for *cephaloridine.*

Ceporexine trademark for *cephalexin.*

Cepovenin trademark for *cephalothin sodium* (see under CEPHALOTHIN).

cera (se′rah) [L.] wax. **c. al′ba,** white WAX. **c. fla′va,** yellow WAX.

ceraceous (se-ra′shus) [L. *cera* wax] waxlike in appearance.

ceramic (sĕ-ram′ik) 1. of or pertaining to ceramics. 2. a product manufactured by the action of heat on earthy materials, in which silicon and silicates occupy a predominant position. Porcelain, glass, refractories, some cements, fused alumina, silicon carbide, aluminum silicate fibers, and clay products, such as brick, tile, and terra cotta, are the principal ceramics. It is a compound formed by direct oxidation of metals by agents such as oxygen or halogen gases or suitable acids. There is usually more than one atom at any given ceramic lattice point, the crystal containing more than one type of atoms in stoichiometric ratio to preserve electroneutrality. All the electrons are associated with bond formation and there are no relatively free electrons available for heat and electricity conduction. Ceramics occur usually as hard but brittle materials that may be opaque, translucent, or transparent, depending on the availability of free electrons to interact with incident light quanta. They absorb and reflect a wide variety of light wavelengths and are thus available in a variety of colors. The chemical properties of ceramics make them resistant to most chemical substances. Most have a high melting point. Densification of ceramic materials is usually accomplished by the agglomeration of compacted powder that may involve a solid state diffusion, known as sintering, the preservation of the liquid structure in the solidified state, vitrification, and diffusion between solid surrounded by liquid, liquid phase sintering. Hence, some ceramics, such as glass, are sometimes referred to as supercooled liquid. **dental c.,** any ceramic material used in dentistry, such as silicate cements and porcelains in dental restorations and dentures; zinc oxide–eugenol and zinc phosphate cements in cavity bases and cementing media; zinc oxide–eugenol pastes in impression materials; gypsum products in impression, modeling, and investment materials; and gypsum and silica in investment materials. The terms *dental porcelain* and *dental ceramic* are sometimes used synonymously.

ceramics (sĕ-ram′iks) [Gr. *keramos* potters' clay] 1. the modeling and processing of objects made of clay or similar material. 2. objects made of ceramic material. **dental c.,** the use of ceramic

materials (see dental CERAMIC) in dentistry. Called also *ceramodontics* and *ceramic dentistry.*

ceramide (ser′ah-mīd) the basic unit of most sphingolipids, an *N*-acyl derivative of sphingosine or its congeners, in which a long-chain fatty acid is attached to the amino group of carbon-2 through an amide linkage. It is a common structure of sphingolipids and glycolipids. **digalactosyl c.,** a glycosphingolipid which accumulates in the kidneys in Fabry's disease. **galactosyl c.,** cerebroside. **glucosyl c.,** a major sphingolipid which accumulates in large quantities in the reticuloendothelial cells in Gaucher's disease. Called also *glucocerebroside.* **c. trihexoside,** a sphingolipid which accumulates excessively in Fabry's disease.

Cerami-Gold trademark for a phosphate-bonded investment material for base-metal alloys.

ceramist (sĕ-ram′ist) one who is skillful in ceramics.

ceramodontics (sĕ-ram″o-don′tiks) dental CERAMICS.

cerate (se′rāt) [L. *cera* wax] a medicinal preparation for external application, made with a basis of fat or wax, or both, intermediate in consistency between an ointment and a plaster.

cerato- [Gr. *keras* horn] a combining form meaning horn or horny. See also words beginning KERATO-.

ceratocricoid (ser″ah-to-kri′koid) pertaining to the posterior horn of the thyroid cartilage and the cricoid cartilage.

ceratocricoideus (ser″at-o-kri-koi′de-us) ceratocricoid MUSCLE.

ceratohyal (ser″ah-to-hi′al) lesser horn of hyoid bone; see under HORN.

ceratopharyngeus (ser″at-o-fahr-in′je-us) ceratopharyngeal MUSCLE.

cerebellum (ser″ĕ-bel′um) [L. dim. of *cerebrum* brain] the part of the brain attached to the back of the brain stem, under the curve of the cerebrum, occupying the posterior cranial fossa. It is connected, by way of the midbrain, with the motor area of the cortex and with the spinal cord, and is concerned with the coordination of motion of muscles involved in voluntary movement.

cerebron (ser′ĕ-bron) phrenosin.

cerebrose (ser′ĕ-brōs) see GALACTOSE.

cerebroside (ser′ĕ-bro-sīd″) a general designation for a group of monohexosyl ceramides consisting of a sphingosine base, fatty acid, and either glucose or galactose in molar ratio of 1:1:1. It is abundant in the membranes of nervous tissue, especially the myelin sheath, and is a major component of the cell coat of higher organisms. A cerebroside containing lignoceric acid is known as *kerasin;* one containing hydroxylignoceric acid is *phrenosin;* one containing unsaturated lignoceric acid with one double bond (nervonic acid) is *nervon;* and one containing a hydroxy derivative of nervonic acid is *oxynervon.* Called also *galactosyl ceramide.*

cerebrum (ser′ĕ-brum; sĕ-re′brum) [L.] 1. the largest portion of the brain, consisting of an outer layer and two cerebral hemispheres separated by the corpus callosum. 2. a term sometimes applied to the postembryonic prosencephalon and mesencephalon together or to the entire brain.

cerelose (ser′ĕ-lōs) dextrose.

ceresin (ser′ĕ-sin) [L. *cera* wax] a mixture of complex hydrocarbons purified by treatment with sulfuric acid. It is a white or yellow, crumbly, tasteless waxy cake having a slight odor, which is soluble in ether, alcohol, benzene, chloroform, and other organic solvents, but is insoluble in water. Ceresin is combustible and nontoxic. Used as a substitute for beeswax for impression and inlay waxes and modeling compounds, for making bottles for hydrofluoric acid, and in various chemical products. Called also *ceresin wax, cerin, cerosin,* and *purified ozokerite.*

cerin (se′rin) ceresin.

cerium (se′re-um) [named after the asteroid *Ceres,* which was discovered shortly before the element] a rare earth of the lanthanide group of the periodic table. Symbol, Ce; atomic weight, 140.12; atomic number, 58; melting point, 799°C; specific gravity, 6.657; valences, 2, 3, 4. Cerium occurs in the form of four natural isotopes, 140, 142, 136, and 138, and a number of radioactive ones. The isotope ^{142}Ce has a half-life of 5 × 10^{15} years, ^{144}Ce has a half-life of 284.5 days and emits beta rays, and ^{141}Ce has a half-life of 32.5 days and emits beta and gamma rays, being used in medical and biological research. Artificial isotopes include 132–135, 137, 139, and 143–148. Cerium is a gray, ductile, and malleable metal, which oxidizes in the presence of moist air and decomposes in water. Its salts are used in various technologies.

cerosin (ser′o-sin) ceresin.

certificate (ser-tif′ĭ-kit, ser-tif′ĭ-kāt) a document serving as evidence or testifying to a fact, as of the status, qualifications, or truth of something. For example, a document awarded to an individual after completion of educational studies for which a diploma is not issued, which may certify that the person receiving the certificate is qualified to practice in certain professions. See also CERTIFICATION. **c. of eligibility,** a legal document certifying that the beneficiary is entitled or eligible to something, such as services under a prepaid health care program. Called also *proof of eligibility (POE).* **c. holder,** subscriber (3). **c. of insurance,** in group insurance, a statement issued to a member of a group certifying that an insurance contract covering the member has been written and containing a summary of the terms applicable to that member. **c. of necessity,** c. of need. **c. of need,** a certificate issued by a governmental representative to an organization or an individual, which proposes the construction or modification of a health facility or health service, with an understanding that such facility or service will be needed for those for whom it is intended. Called also *c. of necessity.*

certification (ser″tĭ-fĭ-ka′shun) 1. the act of attesting as certain the process by which a nongovernmental agency or association grants recognition to an individual who has met certain predetermined qualifications specified by that agency or association. Such qualifications may include: (*a*) graduation from an accredited or approved program; (*b*) acceptable performance on a qualifying examination or series of examinations; and/or (*c*) completion of a given amount of work performance. Called also *registration.* See also ACCREDITATION, CERTIFICATE, dental assistant, currently certified, under ASSISTANT, and LICENSURE. 2. a written statement or document attesting the truth of some statement or event. 3. the reporting to health officers of an infectious disease. 4. a program of the Council on Dental Materials and Devices of the American Dental Association whereby materials and devices used in dental practice are evaluated on appropriate physical standards or specifications. Materials and devices meeting these standards and specifications are listed in the *Guide to Dental Materials and Devices* and are awarded the Seal of Certification, which may be used in advertising, in brochures, and on packages. **admission c.,** a form of medical care review in which an assessment is made of the medical necessity of a patient's admission to a hospital or other inpatient institution. **antibiotic c.,** an FDA program whereby each batch of every antibiotic drug for human use is certified by the FDA as possessing the necessary characteristics of identity, strength, quality, and purity to adequately insure safety and effectiveness in use. **Seal of C.,** see *certification* (4). **c. of eligibility,** a document attesting the eligibility or qualification of an individual to a service or benefit. See also CERTIFICATE of eligibility.

certified (ser′tĭ-fīd″) 1. having, or proved by, a certificate; guaranteed in writing. 2. having a certificate. **board c.,** BOARD certified.

Cerubidin trademark for *daunorubicin.*

ceruloplasmin (se-roo″lo-plaz′min) a glycoprotein (MW = 151,000, sedimentation coefficient 1.26S) produced in the liver, which transports about 96 percent of all copper in the blood plasma.

cerumen (sĕ-roo′men) [L. from *cera* wax] the waxy secretion produced by the ceruminous glands in the external ear canal. Called also *earwax.*

cervical (ser′vĭ-kal) [L. *cervicalis,* from *cervix* neck] pertaining to the neck or to any cervix.

cervico- [L. *cervix* neck] a combining form denoting the neck or a necklike structure.

cervicodorsal (ser″vĭ-ko-dor′sal) pertaining to the neck and the back.

cervicodynia (ser″vĭ-ko-din′e-ah) [cervico- + Gr. *odynē* pain] pain in the neck.

cervicofacial (ser″vĭ-ko-fa′she-al) pertaining to the neck and face.

cervicolabial (ser″vĭ-ko-la′be-al) labiocervical.

cervicolingual (ser″vĭ-ko-ling′gwal) linguocervical.

cervico-occipital (ser″vĭ-ko-ok-sip′ĭ-tal) pertaining to the neck and occiput.

cervicoplasty (ser″vĭ-ko-plas′te) [*cervix* + Gr. *plassein* to form] plastic surgery of the neck.

cervix (ser′viks), pl. *cer′vices* [L.] neck; used in anatomical nomenclature to designate the lower front part connecting the head and trunk, or a constricted part of an organ. See also NECK and COLLUM. **c. den′tis,** NECK of tooth. **implant c.,** that part of the post of an implant which connects the infrastructure with the abutment.

cesium (se′ze-um) [L. *caesium,* from *caesius* blue] an alkali metal element. Symbol, Cs; atomic weight, 132.9054; atomic number, 55; melting point, 48.40°C; specific gravity, 1.873; valence, 1; Mohs hardness index, 0.2; group IA of the periodic table. Cesium has one natural isotope, ^{133}Cs, and several artificial ones, 123, 125–132, and 134–144. It is a silvery white soft metal, which is soluble in acids and alcohol and reacts explosively with water, oxygen, halogens, sulfur, and phosphorus; it has the lowest melting point of any metal and the lowest ionization potential of any element. Cesium has numerous applications in nuclear technology; its toxicity is relatively low. Written also *caesium.* **c. hydrate,** c. hydroxide. **c. hydroxide,** CsHO; a white, yellowish, fused, very deliquescent crystalline mass with strong alkaline reaction. It is known as the strongest base which attacks glass. Called also *c. hydrate.*

Céstan's paralysis [Etienne Jacques Marie *Céstan,* French physician, 1872–1932] Céstan-Chenais SYNDROME. See also Raymond-Céstan SYNDROME.

Céstan-Chenais syndrome [E. J. M. *Céstan;* L. *Chenais,* French physician] see under SYNDROME.

Cestoda (ses-to′dah) a subclass of Cestoidea comprising the true tapeworms. Adult tapeworms are endoparasitic in the alimentary tract of various vertebrates; their larval stages (cysticercus, coenurus, hydatid, sparganum) may be found in various organs or tissues. Called also *Eucestoda.*

cestode (ses′tōd) 1. any tapeworm or platyhelminth of the class Cestoidea, especially those of the subclass Cestoda. 2. cestoid.

cestoid (ses′toid) [Gr. *kestos* girdle + *eidos* form] resembling a tapeworm.

Cestoidea (ses-toi′de-ah) a class of tapeworms (platyhelminths) characterized by the absence of a mouth and digestive tract and by the presence of a noncuticular layer covering their bodies. It comprises two subclasses: Cestoda, parasitic in the intestinal tract of vertebrates, and Cestodaria, parasitic in the intestine and coelom of some primitive fishes and rarely in reptiles.

cetaceum (sĕ-ta′se-um) spermaceti.

Cetamium trademark for *cetylpyridinium chloride* (see under CETYLPYRIDINIUM).

Cethylose trademark for *methylcellulose.*

Cethytin trademark for *methylcellulose.*

cetyl (se′til) a univalent alcohol radical, $CH_3(CH_2)_{14}CH_2$.

cetyldimethylethylammonium bromide (se″til-di-meth″il-eth″il-ah-mo′ne-um) a quaternary ammonium cationic germicidal detergent, occurring as a white powder that is readily soluble in water and alcohol and slightly soluble in chloroform, benzene, and ether. Used in a 6.5 percent solution for the sterilization of surgical and dental instruments. Sometimes used as a topical antiseptic applied to mucous membranes in a 0.005 percent solution.

Cetylite liquid topical anesthetic see under ANESTHETIC.

cetylpyridinium chloride (se″til-pi″rĭ-din′e-um) a surface-active antiseptic drug which is effective against nonsporulating bacteria, 1-hexadecylpyridinium chloride, occurring as a white powder with a slight characteristic odor that is very soluble in water, alcohol, and chloroform and slightly soluble in benzene and ether. Used in preoperative disinfection of the surgical area, in the treatment of minor wounds, and for irrigation of or topical application to the mucous membranes; also included in some mouthwashes and antibacterial soaps and detergents. It has been tested as a plaque and calculus inhibitor. Trademarks: Ceepryl, Cēpacol, Cetamium, Dobendan, Pristacin, Pyrisept.

Cevalin trademark for *ascorbic acid* (see under ACID).

Cf californium.

cf. abbreviation for L. *con′fer,* bring together, compare.

cg centigram.

cgm centigram.

CGS centimeter-gram-second system; a system of measurements in which the units, e.g., the dyne and erg, are based on the centimeter as the unit of length, the gram as the unit of mass, and the second as the unit of time.

Chain, Ernst Boris [born 1906] a German biochemist; co-winner, with Sir Alexander Fleming and Sir Howard Walter Florey, of the Nobel prize for medicine in 1945, for his work on antibacterial substances produced by microorganisms.

chain (chān) a collection of objects linked together in linear fashion, or end-to-end, as the assemblage of atoms or radicals in a chemical compound, or an assemblage of individual bacterial cells. **α-c.,** a heavy chain of immunoglobulin A (IgA); see *heavy c.* **γ-c.,** a heavy chain of immunoglobulin G (IgG); see *heavy c.* **δ-c.,** a heavy chain of immunoglobulin D (IgD); see *heavy c.* **ε-c.,** a heavy chain of immunoglobulin E (IgE); see *heavy c.*

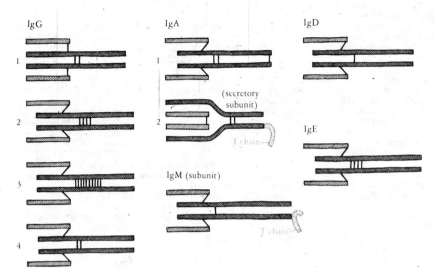

Arrangement of peptide chains in various subclasses of immunoglobulins. Disulfide bonds are represented by black bars. In the IgA and IgM subunits, the chain, in gray, indicates where it would appear in the respective polymeric forms. (From J. A. Bellanti: Immunology II. Philadelphia, W. B. Saunders Co., 1978.)

branched c., an open chain of atoms, usually carbon, with one or more side chains attached to it. **closed c.,** several atoms linked together so as to form a ring, as a ring formed by a chain of atoms in the benzene ring. See also benzene RING and cyclic COMPOUND. **F c.,** fast c. **fast c.,** a polypeptide chain representing a

fragment resulting from papain digestion of the γ-globulin molecule, which is characterized by a relatively fast electrophoretic mobility and a similarity with the heavy chain. Called also *F c.* and *fast chain protein.* **H c's,** heavy c's. **heavy c's,** the two larger polypeptide chains, having a molecular weight from 55,000 (IgG) to 70,000 (IgM), which together with the two smaller light chains comprise the basic unit of structure of an immunoglobulin molecule. They contain the determinant of the antigenic specificity for each of the immunoglobulins. Heavy chains are identified by lower case Greek letters corresponding to the capital English–letter equivalent of the immunologic class: γ (IgG), α (IgA), μ (IgM), δ (IgD), and ε (IgE). Called also *H c's* and *heavy chain proteins.* See illustration. See also heavy chain DISEASE and IMMUNOGLOBULIN. **J c.,** a glycopeptide component of polymeric immunoglobulins A and M, being a relatively small molecule (MW = 35,000) with a high sulfhydryl content and high capacity for cross-linking with heavy chains. In secretions, two IgA monomers are linked together by a J chain and a secretory component (a nonimmunoglobulin) to produce a complex of high molecular weight. **κ-c.,** see *light c's.* **L c's,** light c's. **λ-c.,** see *light c's.* **lateral c.,** side c. **light c's,** the two smaller polypeptide chains, having a molecular weight of about 22,000, which together with the two larger heavy chains comprise the basic unit of structure of an immunoglobulin molecule. They determine the gene specificity of the immunoglobulin. There are two light chains, κ (type I) and λ (type II), named after the investigators who made the original observation, Korngold and Lipari, respectively. Bence Jones protein is considered to be a protein fragment of antibody consisting solely of light chains, either single or joined together by pairs of disulfide bonds. Called also *L c's* and *light chain proteins.* See also Bence Jones PROTEINURIA and IMMUNOGLOBULIN. **μ-c.,** a heavy chain of immunoglobulin M (IgM); see *heavy c.* **open c.,** several atoms united to form an open chain; compounds of this series are

related to methane and are also called fatty, aliphatic, acyclic, or paraffin compounds. Called also *straight c.* **polypeptide c.,**

$$-\overset{|}{C}-\overset{|}{C}-\overset{|}{C}-$$

a structural unit of proteins, consisting of amino acids covalently bonded together and forming unbranched polymers that are united through peptide bonds. There may be more than one chain in a protein molecule, each chain having hundreds of amino acid units, and each type of protein molecule having a specific chemical composition, molecular weight, and sequential order of its amino acid building blocks. **S c.,** slow c. **side c.,** a chain of atoms attached to a larger chain or to a ring. Called also *lateral c.* **siloxane c.,** a straight chain having silicon atoms single-bonded to oxygen with each silicon atom being linked with four oxygen atoms. See SILOXANE. **slow c.,** a polypeptide chain representing a fragment resulting from papain digestion of a γ-globulin molecule, which is characterized by a

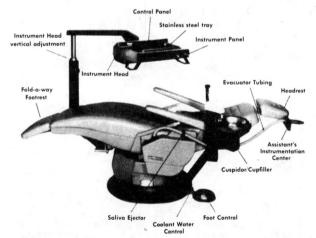

A chair-mounted dental unit. The compact, one-piece design provides convenient working areas for both the dentist and the dental assistant. (From V. R. Park, J. R. Ashman, and G. J. Shelly: A Textbook for Dental Assistants. 2nd ed. Philadelphia, W. B. Saunders Co., 1975; courtesy of Ritter Sybron Corp.)

relatively slow electrophoretic mobility and a similarity with the light chain. Called also *S c.* and *slow chain protein.* **straight c.,** open c.

chair (chār) a seat for one person, which has four legs and a back rest, and sometimes arm rests. **dental c.,** an adjustable chair in which the patient sits during dental procedures, which may be combined with a dental unit (see under UNIT), or be separate. See illustrations.

chairside (chār'sīd) at the side of the dental chair, as during the treatment of a dental patient. See also dental assistant, chairside, under ASSISTANT.

chalcedony (kal'sē-do'ne) a microcrystalline, translucent form of silicon dioxide.

chalk (chawk) [L. *calx, creta*] a natural calcium carbonate, being the amorphous remains of minute marine organisms deposited on the sea bottom and decomposed by the action of acids and heat. Used as a polishing agent in dentistry and frequently as an ingredient in dentifrices. **French c.,** native TALC. **precipitated c.,** precipitated calcium carbonate (see CALCIUM carbonate). **prepared c.,** prepared calcium carbonate (see CALCIUM carbonate).

challenge (chal'enj) 1. the administration of the second or later dose (challenge dose) in a previously sensitized individual in an effort to evoke an immunologic reaction or to determine an effect, such as susceptibility to or protection against a disease-producing agent. See also reacting DOSE. 2. the administration of a toxin, virulent pathogen, or tumor cell to a previously vaccinated or control individual to test the effectiveness of the vaccination.

chamaecephalic (kam"e-sě-fal'ik) chamecephalic.

chamaecephaly (kam"e-sef'ah-le) [Gr. *chamai* low + *kephalē* head] chamecephaly.

chamber (chām'ber) [L. *camera;* Gr. *kamara*] an enclosed space or antrum. **Abbe-Zeiss counting c.,** Thomas-Zeiss counting c. **air-equivalent ionization c., air-wall ionization c.,** an ionization chamber in which the materials of the wall and electrodes are such that ionizing radiations produce ionization essentially similar to that in an extrapolation ionization chamber. **extrapolation ionization c., free air ionization c.,** an ionization chamber with electrodes whose spacing can be adjusted and accurately determined to permit extrapolation of its reading to zero volume chamber. See also *standard ionization c.* **ionization c.,** a chamber filled with a gas, including air, and two electrodes of different electrical potentials, designed for measuring the quantity of ionizing radiation in terms of the charge of electricity associated with ions produced within a defined volume of gas. Photons entering the chamber produce ions that drift toward the electrodes, producing current which, after electronic amplification, is recorded on a meter. See also COUNTER and DOSIMETER. **monitor ionization c.,** an ionization chamber used for checking the constancy of the performance of an x-ray generator. **pocket ionization c.,** a pocket-sized ionization chamber used for monitoring exposure of personnel coming in contact with radiation sources. **pulp c.,** that portion of the pulp cavity located in the tooth crown and occupied by the dental pulp. See also root CANAL. **relief c.,** a recess in the impression surface of a denture to reduce or eliminate pressure or force from that area of the mouth. See also RELIEF (3, 4). **standard ionization c.,** an ionization chamber in which a delimited beam of radiation passes between the electrodes without striking them or other internal parts of the equipment. See also *extrapolation ionization c.* **thimble ionization c.,** a small thimble-shaped ionization chamber, usually with walls of organic material. **thin-wall ionization c.,** an ionization chamber having walls of sufficient thinness to permit the maximum corpuscular rays to enter the chamber through the wall from the outside. **Thoma-Zeiss counting c.,** a device placed in the bottom of a slide of a microscope, which is divided into minute squares, thereby facilitating the counting of cells. Called also *Abbe-Zeiss counting c.* **tissue-equivalent ionization c.,** an ionization chamber in which the walls, electrodes, and gas are selected as to produce ionization essentially equivalent to the characteristics of the tissue under consideration.

chamecephalic (kam"e-sě-fal'ik) pertaining to or characterized by a low flat cranial vault. Spelled also *chamaecephalic.* See chamecephalic SKULL.

chamecephaly (kam"e-sef'ah-le) [Gr. *chamai* low + *kephalē* head] a condition characterized by a low flat head. Spelled also *chamaecephaly.* See chamecephalic SKULL.

chamestaphyline (kam"e-staf'ĭ-lin) [Gr. *chamai* low + *staphylē* a bunch of grapes, uvula] pertaining to or characterized by a low-arched palate. See chamestaphyline SKULL.

chamfer (sham'fer) 1. pertaining to a marginal finish either curved or formed by a plane at an obtuse angle to the external

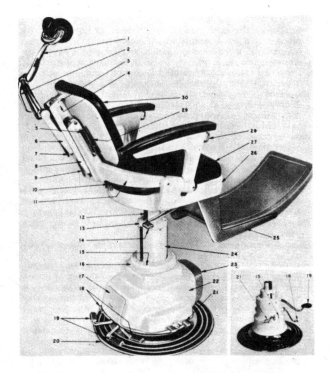

1. Headrest Assembly	11. Back Yoke	21. Rotation Lock Pedal
2. Headrest Locking Lever	12. Inner Elevating Tube	22. Base Cylinder
3. Backrest Connecting Pin	13. Elevating Tube Cover	23. Cover for Power Unit
4. Set Screw for Backrest Pin	14. Chair Tilt Release	24. Outer Elevating Tube
5. Back Tilt Release	15. Lowering Speed Adjusting Screw	25. Foot Platform
6. Headrest Elevation Slide	16. Base Upper Cover	26. Seat Frame
7. Headrest Slide Release	17. Cover for Switch Mechanism	27. Seat Cushion
8. Back Elevation Slide	18. Lowering Pedal	28. Arm Lock Release
9. Back Slide Release	19. Raising Pedal	29. Back Tilting Lock
10. Back Supporting Bar	20. Base Plate	30. Back Cushion

A typical dental chair and its parts. Ritter Model "C" Century Motor Chair. (From V. R. Park, J. R. Ashman, and G. J. Shelly: A Texbook for Dental Assistants. 2nd ed. Philadelphia, W. B. Saunders Co., 1975; courtesy of Ritter Co., Inc.)

surface of a prepared tooth. See illustration. See also chamfer EDGE. 2. pertaining to a marginal finish that produces a curve from an axial wall to the cavosurface in an extracoronal cavity preparation.

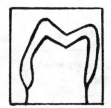

Chamfer.

CHAMPUS Civilian Health and Medical Program of Uniformed Services; a congressionally funded program administered by the Department of Defense, without premium but with cost-sharing provisions, which supplements for care delivered by civilian health providers to retired members and dependents of active and retired members of the uniformed services.

CHAMPVA Civilian Health and Medical Program of Veterans Administration; a congressionally funded program administered by the Department of Defense for the Veterans Administration, without premium but with cost-sharing provisions, which pays for health care provided by civilian providers to dependents of totally disabled veterans who are eligible for retirement pay from the uniformed services.

chancre (shang'ker) [Fr. "canker," from L. *cancer* crab] the primary lesion of syphilis developing at the site of infection, usually on the penis, vulva, cervix uteri, or the oral cavity, presenting a small nodule which erodes into a reddish ulcer covered with a yellowish exudation. See also primary SYPHILIS. **sporotrichotic c.,** a primary lesion in localized sporotrichosis, appearing at the site of inoculation after an incubation period of 3 weeks to 3 months, usually on the lips or in the mouth.

chancroid (shang'kroid) an infection caused by *Haemophilus ducreyi.* It begins as a painless macule on the genitalia, which enlarges and becomes pustular; an ulcer forms with a shaggy base and adjacent bubo formation.

channel (chan'el) [L. *canalis* a water pipe] a canal; a groove or deep furrow which serves as a trough for the conveyance of any flowing substance. **blood c.,** a narrow passage for the blood, which has no distinct walls. **central c.,** a long straight capillary that connects an arteriole to a venule. See also *thoroughfare c.* **lymph c.,** a small lymph sinus found in or around lymph nodes and lymphatic vessels. **thoroughfare c.,** one between terminal arterioles and venules, larger than a capillary. See also *central c.*

Chaoul tube [Henri *Chaoul*, Lebanese radiologist in Berlin, 1887–1964] see under TUBE.

Chapple's syndrome [Charles Culloden *Chapple*, American physician, died 1979] see under SYNDROME.

character (kar'ak-ter) 1. any attribute or feature that permits distinction of one thing from another. 2. a complex of mental and ethical traits typical of a person, group of persons, or society. 3. advanced stages, often end points, of the developmental sequences that are determined by gene action, sometimes associated with environmental factors, resulting in a special phenotype. Called also *characteristic, phene, phenotypic expression of gene,* and *trait.* 4. a symbol or a set of symbols representing a letter, numeral, punctuation mark, and the like, which a computer may read, store, and write. **auto-**somal dominant c., in mendelian inheritance, a normal or abnormal genetic trait transmitted from parents to progeny, whereby a trait of the parental generation (P_1) appears in all heterozygous, homozygous, heterokaryotic, or heterogenotic members of the first filial generation (F_1) and in three-quarters of the members of the second filial generation (F_2). The character is the result of transmitting genetic information coded in a single gene on an autosome brought about by genetic factors and environmental influences. It appears in every generation without skipping, and is transmitted by an affected person to about half his or her children, while unaffected persons do not transmit the dominant character to their children; both males and females are likely to have or transmit the trait. If the genetic information or mutant gene is located on the sex chromosome, it is a sex-linked dominant character. Called also *autosomal dominant allele, autosomal dominant gene, autosomal dominant inheritance,* and *autosomal dominant trait.* See also PEDIGREE. **autosomal recessive c.,** in mendelian inheritance, a normal or abnormal genetic trait transmitted from parents to progeny, which is expressed only when the allele is in the homozygous state, and appears only in siblings, not in their parents, offspring, or other relatives; on the average, one-fourth of the siblings of the propositus being affected. The parents of the affected offspring may be consanguineous, and males and females are affected equally. If the genetic information or mutant gene is located on a sex chromosome, it is a sex-linked recessive character. Called also *autosomal recessive allele, autosomal recessive gene, autosomal recessive inheritance,* and *autosomal recessive trait.* See also PEDIGREE. **codominant c.,** one in which both alleles of a pair of homologous chromosomes are expressed independently in the heterozygote, as in the AB blood group, where both A and B antigens are present. Called also *codominant allele, codominant gene,* and *codominant trait.* **dominant c.,** see *autosomal dominant c.* and *X-linked dominant c.* **recessive c.,** see *autosomal recessive c.* and *X-linked recessive c.* **sex-limited c.,** a trait which is autosomally transmitted but expressed in only one sex. Called also *sex-*

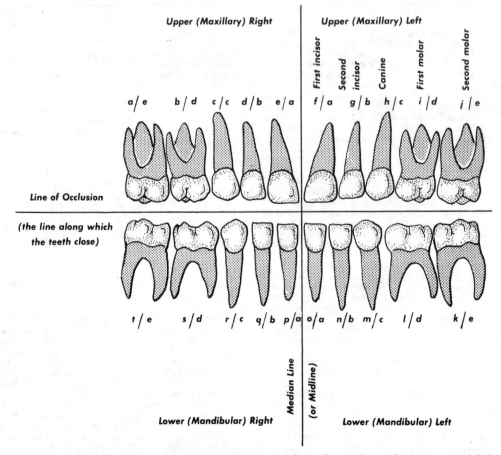

Quadrants of the deciduous dentition. The first letter of each pair designates the tooth according to the consecutive alphabetical notation and the second according to the Palmer notation. (From V. R. Park, J. R. Ashman, and G. J. Shelly: A Textbook for Dental Assistants. 2nd ed. Philadelphia, W. B. Saunders Co., 1975.)

limited trait. **sex-linked c.,** in mendelian inheritance, a normal or abnormal genetic trait transmitted from parents to progeny along the sex lines, whereby a sex-linked character may be X-linked or Y-linked, only X-linkage having clinical significance. Called also *sex-linked allele, sex-linked gene, sex-linked inheritance,* and *sex-linked trait.* See *X-linked dominant c., X-linked recessive c.,* and holandric INHERITANCE. **X-linked dominant c.,** in mendelian inheritance, an allele found on the X chromosome transmitted from parents to progeny, which is expressed in all offspring, whether homozygous or heterozygous. An affected male transmits the trait to all his daughters and none of his sons. An affected female who is heterozygous transmits the trait to half of her offspring of either sex, but a female who is homozygous transmits it to all her offspring. Disorders transmitted as X-linked dominant characters are rare, but they occur twice as often in females as in males. Called also *X-linked dominant allele, X-linked dominant gene, X-linked dominant inheritance,* and *X-linked dominant trait.* See also PEDIGREE. **X-linked recessive c.,** in mendelian inheritance, an allele found on the X chromosome transmitted from parents to progeny, which is expressed in all males who carry the allele (since they have only one X chromosome), and in females only if the allele is found on homologous chromosomes, as in hemophilia. It is passed from an affected man through all his daughters to half their sons, never being transmitted directly from father to son. An occasional heterozygous female may express the disorder due to lyonization (Lyon HYPOTHESIS). Called also *X-linked recessive allele, X-linked recessive gene, X-linked recessive inheritance,* and *X-linked recessive trait.* See also PEDIGREE.

characteristic (kar″ak-ter-is′tik) 1. character. 2. pertaining to a character.

charas (chahr′as) hashish.

charcoal (char′kōl) carbon prepared by charring wood and other organic material. **activated c.,** a form of amorphous carbon (see under CARBON) prepared from the residue after destructive distillation of wood and other vegetable material. Used as an adsorptive and antidote, especially in the emergency treatment of various types of poisoning, including that by drugs. Called also *carbo activatus.* Trademarks: Carboraffin, Norit, Nuchar, Ultracarbon. **animal c.,** a form of amorphous carbon (see under CARBON), which is charcoal prepared from bones and other animal matter. Called also *animal, bone, ivory,* and *Paris black,* and *carboanimalis.*

Charcot's sclerosis, syndrome, vertigo [Jean Martin *Charcot,* French neurologist, 1825–1893] see amyotrophic lateral SCLEROSIS, and see under VERTIGO. See also Souques-Charcot GERODERMA.

Charcot's sign see under SIGN.

charge (charj) 1. to fill or supply a thing with that which it is fitted to receive. 2. to supply with electricity; to energize. 3. to change the net amount of positive or negative electricity. 4. usually in the plural, prices assigned to units of services, such as a visit to a doctor, a day in a hospital, or a surgical procedure. **actual c's,** in health insurance, the amount a patient is actually billed for a particular service or procedure, which may differ from the customary, prevailing, and/or reasonable charges under Medicare or insurance programs. **allowable c.,** in health insurance, the maximum fee that a third party will use in reimbursing a provider for a given service. See also fixed FEE. **covered c's,** in health insurance, charges for services covered under the plan. **customary c's,** customary fees; see usual, customary, and reasonable fees, under FEE. **electrostatic c.,** see electrostatic units, under UNIT. **prevailing c.,** in health insurance, a fee most commonly charged for a specific service in a given area; a customary fee. See usual, customary, and reasonable fees, under FEE. **reasonable c's,** reasonable fees; see usual, customary, and reasonable fees, under FEE. **risk c.,** in health insurance, that part of a premium which the insurer uses to generate or replenish surpluses needed to protect against the possibility of excessive losses under his policies. See also RETENTION (6) and WITHHOLD (2). **space c.,** the effect of electrons emitted from the heated filament in the x-ray tube which tend to repel or hold back other electrons in the filament. **usual c's,** usual fees; see usual, customary, and reasonable fees, under FEE.

charlatan (shar′lah-tan) [Fr.] one who pretends to possess knowledge or skill or practices a profession without proper qualifications and credentials; in medicine, a quack. See also EMPIRIC (2).

Charles' law [Jacques Alexandre César *Charles,* French physicist, 1746–1823] see under LAW.

Charlin's syndrome [Carlos *Charlin,* Chilean ophthalmologist, born 1886] ciliary NEURALGIA.

Charpy's test [George *Charpy,* French engineer, who, in 1907, established the principles for evaluating materials according to their physical properties, independently of their composition] see under TEST.

Char-stem trademark for an interdental tip, being a counter-angle holder for the end of a toothpick for cleansing interdental spaces.

chart (chart) 1. a simplified graphic representation of the fluctuation of some variable, as of pulse, temperature, or respiration. 2.

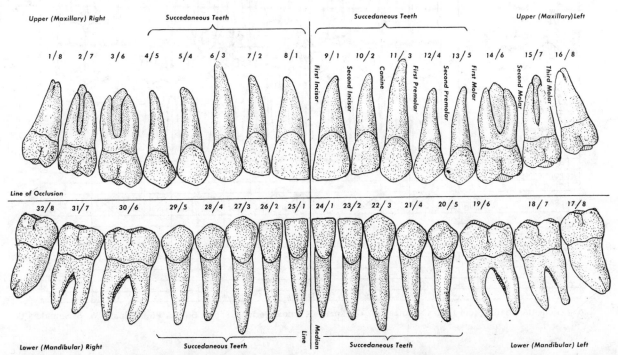

Upper and lower left and right quadrants of permanent dentition. Teeth are numbered consecutively beginning with the upper right quadrant (first numeral of each pair) and consecutively within each quadrant (second numeral of each pair). (From V. R. Park, J. R. Ashman, and G. J. Shelly: A Textbook for Dental Assistants. 2nd ed. Philadelphia, W. B. Saunders Co., 1975.)

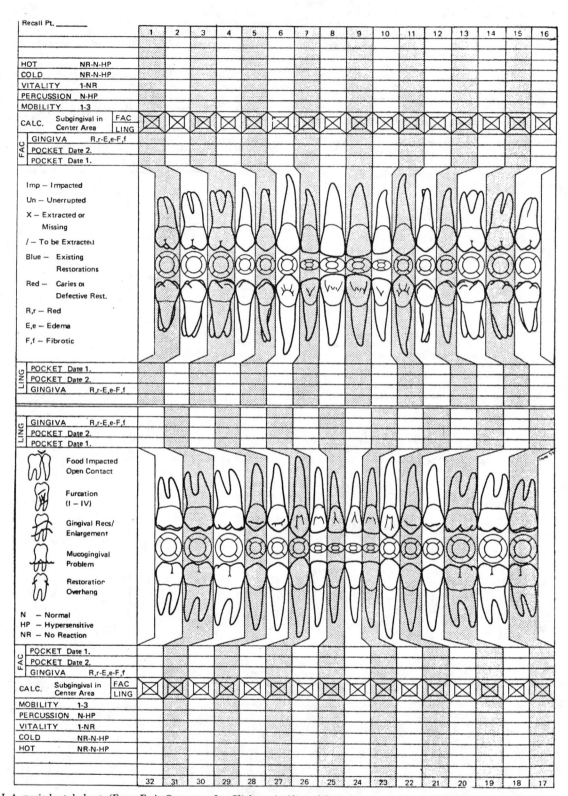

Recall Pt. _____				1	2	3	4	5	6	7	8	9	10	11	12	13	14	15	16
HOT	NR-N-HP																		
COLD	NR-N-HP																		
VITALITY	1-NR																		
PERCUSSION	N-HP																		
MOBILITY	1-3																		
CALC.	Subgingival in Center Area	FAC																	
		LING																	
GINGIVA	R,r-E,e-F,f																		
POCKET Date 2.																			
POCKET Date 1.																			

Imp — Impacted

Un — Unerrupted

X — Extracted or
  Missing

/ — To be Extracted

Blue — Existing
  Restorations

Red — Caries or
  Defective Rest.

R,r — Red

E,e — Edema

F,f — Fibrotic

POCKET Date 1.
POCKET Date 2.
GINGIVA R,r-E,e-F,f

GINGIVA R,r-E,e-F,f
POCKET Date 2.
POCKET Date 1.

Food Impacted
Open Contact

Furcation
(I – IV)

Gingival Recs/
Enlargement

Mucogingival
Problem

Restoration
Overhang

N — Normal
HP — Hypersensitive
NR — No Reaction

POCKET Date 1.
POCKET Date 2.
GINGIVA R,r-E,e-F,f

CALC.	Subgingival in Center Area	FAC																	
		LING																	
MOBILITY	1-3																		
PERCUSSION	N-HP																		
VITALITY	1-NR																		
COLD	NR-N-HP																		
HOT	NR-N-HP																		
				32	31	30	29	28	27	26	25	24	23	22	21	20	19	18	17

U.C.L.A. periodontal chart. (From F. A. Carranza, Jr.: Glickman's Clinical Periodontology. 5th ed. Philadelphia, W. B. Saunders Co., 1979.)

a chart or a record of the clinical data of a particular case. See also *dental c.* and *hospital c.* **dental c.,** 1. a diagrammatic chart of the teeth on which clinical, radiological, and forensic findings may be indicated. Most charts divide dentition into quadrants, the line of occlusion separating the upper (maxillary) teeth from the lower (mandibular) ones, and the median vertical line separating the right from the left teeth. According to one method of charting, the teeth are numbered consecutively starting from the upper extreme right tooth (the right third molar), proceeding to the left third molar, and continuing from the left lower third molar to the third molar on the opposite side. This method accounts for the full dentition of 32 teeth. According to another method, teeth in each quadrant are numbered separately, the count beginning from the central incisors and continuing posteriorly to the third molars. According to still another method, the teeth are identified, by either a consecutive alphabetical notation, or within each quadrant by lower case letters (Palmer notation). Combinations of Arabic and Roman numerals to indicate deciduous and permanent teeth have also been used in dental charts. See also two-digit tooth-recording SYSTEM and Universal Numbering SYSTEM. See illustration. 2. a patient's clinical records, usually including a health history, acquaintance form, examination and treatment records, and frequently x-rays. Called also *dental record.* **hospital c.,** a chart containing basic information about the hospitalized patient. Most hospital charts include: (1) patient information sheet, containing admission diagnosis, address, age, next of kin, insurance information, and other personal data; (2) a chart of the daily recording of vital signs; (3) nurses' notes; (4) history and physical examination; (5) order sheet; (6) consent form; (7) laboratory tests; (8) progress notes, including admission note, daily progress notes, and discharge note; (9) discharge summary. **periodontal c.,** a dental chart showing the status of periodontal tissue and health. See illustration.

Chart. abbreviation for L. *char'ta,* paper.

chartaceous (kar-ta'shus) like paper; papyraceous.

Charters' method, technique [W. J. *Charters,* American dentist] see TOOTHBRUSHING.

Chaudhry, Anand P. see Gorlin-Chaudhry-Moss SYNDROME.

Chauffard, Anatole Marie Émile [French physician, 1855–1932] see hereditary SPHEROCYTOSIS (Minkowski-Chauffard syndrome).

Chauliac, Guy de [1300–1368] an eminent French surgeon who practiced in Avignon. In his treatise on surgery (*Chirurgia magna*), which was regarded as a standard work until Paré's time, he discusses the quality of dental care and tooth extraction during his time.

Chayes attachment [Herman E. S. *Chayes,* American dentist, 1878–1933] see under ATTACHMENT.

ChE cholinesterase (1).

Cheadle's disease [Walter Butler *Cheadle,* English pediatrician, 1835–1910] infantile SCURVY.

Cheadle-Möller-Barlow disease [W. B. *Cheadle;* Julius Otto Ludwig *Möller,* 1819–1887; Sir Thomas *Barlow,* British physician, 1845–1945] infantile SCURVY.

check-bite (chek'bīt) check BITE. **lateral c.-b.,** interocclusal records, lateral; see under RECORD.

Chédiak-Higashi syndrome [Moisés *Chédiak;* Ototaka *Higashi*] see under SYNDROME.

cheek (chēk) a fleshy protuberance, especially the fleshy portion of the side of the face; called also *bucca* [NA]. Also applied to the fleshy mucous membrane–covered side of the oral cavity; called also *bucca cavum oris* [NA]. **c. biting,** cheek BITING. **cleft c.,** CLEFT cheek. **c. sucking,** cheek SUCKING.

Cheever's operation see under OPERATION.

cheil- see CHEILO-.

cheilectomy (ki-lek'to-me) [*cheil-* + Gr. *ektomē* excision] 1. excision of a lip. 2. the operation of chiseling off the irregular bony edges of a joint cavity that interfere with motion.

cheilectropion (ki"lek-tro'pe-on) [*cheil-* + *ectropion*] eversion of the lip.

cheilion (ki'le-ahn) the corner of the mouth.

cheilitis (ki-li'tis) [*cheil-* + *-itis*] inflammation of the lips. See also CHEILOSIS. **actinic c.,** painful swelling of the lip (usually the lower lip) and development of scaly crust and erosions on the vermilion border after overexposure to sunrays. Called also *solar c.* **angular c.,** perlèche. **apostematous c.,** c. glandularis apostematosa. **cigarette paper c.,** focal inflammatory lesions caused by pulling cigarette paper stuck to the surface of the lips. **commissural c.,** cheilitis affecting principally the angles (commissures) of the mouth. **c. exfoliati'va,** persistent exfoliation of the lip caused by inflammation of the mucous membrane, similar to but not identical with dermatitis seborrheica. It is characterized by the appearance of yellowish and somewhat darker crusts and scales, sometimes projecting a quarter

of an inch on the vermilion surface of the lips, which may exhibit constant exfoliation. **c. glandula'ris,** c. glandularis apostematosa. **c. glandula'ris apostemato'sa,** a rare disease characterized by enlargement, hardening, and finally eversion of the lip, usually the lower lip, leading to exposure of the openings of the accessory salivary glands, which themselves become enlarged and sometimes nodular, appearing as small red macules with dilated follicular orifices exudating mucoid or mucopurulent fluid. Called also *apostematous c., c. glandularis, Baelz's disease, myxadenitis labialis,* and *Volkmann's c.* **c. granulomato'sa,** inflammatory disease of the lip, especially the lower lip, characterized by nonpitting swelling scaling, fissuring, and vesicles or pustules on the vermilion border. It is similar to but not identical with cheilitis glandularis apostematosa. When associated with facial paralysis and fissured tongue, it is known as *Melkersson-Rosenthal syndrome.* Called also *Miescher's c.* and *essential granulomatous macrocheilitis.* **impetiginous c.,** impetigo of the lips. **Miescher's c.,** c. granulomatosa. **migrating c.,** perlèche. **solar c.,** actinic c. **c. vena'ta,** that caused by toxic substances. **Volkmann's c.,** c. glandularis apostematosa.

cheilo-, cheil- [Gr. *cheilos* lip; an edge or brim] a combining form denoting relationship to the lip, or to an edge or brim. See also terms beginning LABIO-.

cheiloangioscopy (ki"lo-an"je-os'ko-pe) [*cheilo-* + Gr. *angeion* vessel + *skopein* to examine] observation of the circulation in the blood vessels of the lip.

cheilocarcinoma (ki"lo-kar"sĭ-no'mah) carcinoma of the lip.

cheilognathopalatoschisis (ki"lo-na"tho-pal"ah-tos'kĭ-sis) cheilognathouranoschisis.

cheilognathoprosoposchisis (ki"lo-na"tho-pros"o-pos'kĭ-sis) [*cheilo-* + Gr. *gnathos* jaw + *prosōpon* face + *schisis* cleft] a developmental anomaly characterized by the presence of an oblique facial cleft continuing into the lip and upper jaw. Called also *cheilognathopalatoschisis.*

cheilognathoschisis (ki"lo-na-thos'kĭ-sis) [*cheilo-* + Gr. *gnathos* jaw + *schisis* cleft] a developmental anomaly characterized by the presence of a cleft in the lip and jaw.

cheilognathouranoschisis (ki"lo-na"tho-u-rah-nos'kĭ-sis) [*cheilo-* + Gr. *gnathos* jaw + *ouranos* palate + *schisis* cleft] a developmental anomaly characterized by the presence of a cleft in the lip, upper jaw, and palate; cheilognathopalatoschisis.

cheilophagia (ki"lo-fa'je-ah) [*cheilo-* + Gr. *phagein* to eat] biting of the lips. See lip BITING.

cheiloplasty (ki"lo-plas"te) [*cheilo-* + Gr. *plassein* to form] plastic surgery of the lip; labioplasty. **reduction c.,** surgical reduction of the size of the lip.

cheilorrhaphy (ki-lor'ah-fe) [*cheilo-* + Gr. *rhaphē* suture] the operation of suturing the lip, as in surgical repair of a congenitally cleft lip.

cheiloschisis (ki-los'kĭ-sis) [*cheilo-* + *schisis*] CLEFT lip.

cheilosis (ki-lo'sis) [*cheilo-* + *-osis*] a noninflammatory condition of the lips characterized by chapping and fissuring. See also CHEILITIS. **angular c.,** perlèche.

cheilostomatoplasty (ki"lo-sto-mat"o-plas"te) [*cheilo-* + Gr. *stoma* mouth + *plassein* to form] plastic restoration of the lips and mouth.

cheilotomy (ki-lot'o-me) [*cheilo-* + Gr. *tomē* a cutting] incision into the lip.

Cheladrate trademark for *edetate disodium* (see under EDETATE).

Chelaplex III trademark for *edetate disodium* (see under EDETATE).

chelate (ke'lāt) [Gr. *chēlē* claw] a molecular structure in which a central atom, usually a metal, is attached to two or more coordinating atoms by covalent bonds; a ligand having more than a single site which can furnish a lone pair of electrons. By extension, applied to chemical compounds in which metal ions are sequestered and firmly bound into a ring within the chelating molecule. Because of their ability to bind and neutralize heavy metals, chelates are used in the treatment of poisoning. Called also *polydentate ligand.* See also chelate COMPOUND and proteolysis-chelation THEORY.

chelation (ke-la'shun) 1. combination with a metal in complexes in which the metal is a part of a ring. 2. in dentistry, decalcification in which calcium ions are removed from the tooth structure by a chemical agent, such as ethylenediamine tetracetic acid, which then combines to form a new compound, calcium chelate.

Chelen trademark for *ethyl chloride* (see under CHLORIDE).

chem- see CHEMO-.

chemabrasion (kĕm-ah″brə′shun) [Gr. *chem* + L. *abrasio* abrasion] the superficial destruction and exfoliation of the epidermis and upper layers of the dermis with the use of chemical agents to remove scars, tattoos, pigmented nevi, wrinkles, etc. Called also *chemexfoliation*. See PLANNING.

chemamnesia (kem″am-ne′ze-ah) the controlled and reversible amnesia induced by a drug, as in certain anesthesia procedures.

Chémant, Nicholas Dubois [18th century] a French dentist who, in cooperation with Duchâteau, pioneered the use of ceramics in dental prostheses.

Chembar trademark for a calcium hydroxide cavity liner in a polystyrene-chloroform solution.

chemexfoliation (kem″eks-fo″le-a′shun) [*chem-* + *exfoliation*] chemabrasion.

chemical (kem′ĭ-kal) 1. of, or pertaining to, chemistry. 2. a substance composed of chemical elements, or obtained by chemical processes.

chemiclave (kem″ĭ-klāv) an autoclave which, in addition to steam, employs chemical disinfectants for the sterilization of instruments. **Harvey 500 c.,** trademark for an autoclave which employs a mixture of chemical disinfectants (ethyl alcohol and a mixture of alcohols and ketones, formaldehyde, and water) vaporized to about 30 psi at 132°C (270°F). **Harvey 6000 c.,** trademark for a larger version of the Harvey 500 chemiclave.

Chemictina trademark for *chloramphenicol*.

chemisorption (kem″ĭ-sorp′shun) the formation of bonds between substances with high surface energy, such as metals, and some other substance, such as gas or liquid, the bond being comparable in strength with ordinary chemical bonds.

chemist (kem′ist) 1. an individual skilled in chemistry. 2. a pharmacist (British).

chemistry (kem′is-tre) [Gr. *chēmeia*] the science that deals with the composition of substances and with the changes that they may undergo, including the study of elements, atomic relations of matter, and properties of substances and their energy relationships. **analytical c.,** that which deals with analysis of different elements in a compound. **biological c.,** biochemistry. **dental c.,** the chemistry of dental materials. **blood c.,** see table of *Reference Values for Blood, Plasma and Serum* in Appendix. **forensic c.,** the use of chemical knowledge in the solution of legal problems, such as chemical analysis of poisons and other substances suspected of being the cause of death or injury. **inorganic c.,** chemistry of inorganic compounds or polar substances which do not contain carbon. Called also *mineral c.* **medical c.,** chemistry as it relates to medicine. **mineral c.,** inorganic c. **organic c.,** originally, chemistry of compounds derived from living organisms (either animal or plants), generally being easily combustible and sensitive to heat and strong acids and bases. Currently, chemistry of carbon (nonpolar) compounds. **pharmaceutical c.,** chemistry dealing with the composition of pharmaceutical preparations. Called also *pharmacochemistry*. **physical c.,** that branch of chemistry which deals with the relationship of chemical and physical properties, including electrochemistry, thermochemistry, radiochemistry, photochemistry, etc. **physiological c.,** biochemistry. **structural c.,** chemical study of the structure of a molecule. See also structural FORMULA. **surface c.,** in the field of catalysis, the study of chemical reactions between the outermost layer of atoms of a solid and molecules brought to the solid surface in the liquid or gaseous state.

chemo-, chem- [Gr. *chēmeia* chemistry] a combining form denoting relationship to chemistry, or to a chemical.

Chemocide PK trademark for *propylparaben*.

Chemofuran trademark for *nitrofurazone*.

chemolithotroph (ke″mo-lith′o-trōf) [*chemo-* + Gr. *lithos* stone + *trophē* nutrition] chemolithotrophic CELL.

chemo-organotroph (ke″mo-or′gah-no-trōf) chemo-organotrophic CELL.

chemoprophylaxis (ke″mo-pro″fi-lak′sis) [*chemo-* + Gr. *prophylax* an advanced guard] the use of chemical agents as a means of preventing development of a specific disease.

chemoreceptor (ke″mo-re-sep′tor) 1. a sensory receptor adapted for excitation by chemical substances. Chemoreceptors detect taste and smell, as well as detecting oxygen and carbon dioxide levels in the arterial blood. There are also binding sites on the plasma membrane of cells for peptide hormones and on the nuclear membrane for steroid hormones. 2. a possible group of molecules in the cell protoplasm having the power of binding chemicals, including toxins of various types.

chemosurgery (ke″mo-ser′jer-e) the destruction of tissue by chemical agents for therapeutic purposes. See also chemosurgical GINGIVECTOMY.

chemotaxis (ke″mo-tak′sis) [*chemo-* + Gr. *taxis* arrangement] the movement of an organism in response to a chemical stimulus, such as the movement of leukocytes in the direction of inflammation, brought about by the release of a chemical substance by injured tissues. **leukocyte c.,** unidirectional migration of white blood cells from blood vessels toward the inflammatory focus. **negative c.,** orientation and movement of cells from a region of high to a region of low concentration of a specific chemical compound or element. **positive c.,** orientation and movement of cells from a region of low to a region of high concentration of a specific chemical compound or element. Neutrophil and eosinophil leukocytes, monocytes, and lymphocytes show positive chemotaxis toward various agents, including activated complement.

chemotherapy (ke″mo-ther′ah-pe) the treatment of disease by administering chemical compounds which adversely affect the causative agent but do not harm the patient.

chemotroph (ke′mo-trof) [*chemo-* + Gr. *trophē* nutrition] chemotrophic CELL.

Chenais, L. [French physician] see Céstan-Chenais SYNDROME.

Cheney's syndrome [W. D. *Cheney*] Hajdu-Cheney SYNDROME.

cheoplastic (ke″o-plas′tik) pertaining to cheoplasty.

cheoplasty (ke′o-plas″te) [Gr. *chein* to pour + *plassein* to form] a method once used to mold artificial teeth with an alloy of tin, silver, and bismuth.

cherubism (cher′u-bizm) a familial disease characterized by fullness of the cheeks and jaws, producing the typical chubby face suggestive of a cherub, associated with a white line on the sclera beneath the iris, swelling of the submandibular region, wide alveolar ridges, a narrow V-shaped palate, premature shedding of deciduous teeth, defective permanent dentition, absence of many teeth, and displacement and lack of eruption of some teeth. Multinucleate giant cells of the osteoclastic type, small hemorrhages, scattered deposits of granular hemosiderin, spindle cell fibroblasts, dilated capillary-like blood spaces lined with endothelium, lacunar absorption and replacement of the connective tissue in the cortical bone, replacement of the medulla and most of the cortex by dysplastic bone tissue, and collagenous intercellular deposits are the principal pathologic findings. It occurs in early childhood and is considered to be a form of fibrous dysplasia of the bone, with partial shift of the osteolytic phase of bone metamorphosis. Called also *disseminated fibrous dysplasia, familial fibrous dysplasia of jaws, familial multilocular cystic disease of jaws, familial fibrous swelling of jaws, fibrous dysplasia of jaws,* and *Jones' disease.*

chest (chest) the thorax.

Chevallier's glossitis posterior triangular GLOSSITIS.

chewing (choo′ing) the movements of the mandible during mastication. See also chew-in RECORD, masticating CYCLE, masticatory FORCE, and MASTICATION.

Cheyne-Stokes respiration [John *Cheyne,* Scottish physician, 1777–1836; William *Stokes,* Irish physician, 1804–1878] see under RESPIRATION.

CHF congestive heart FAILURE.

Chiari, Hans [German pathologist, 1851–1916] see Arnold-Chiari DEFORMITY.

chiasm (ki′azm) [L., Gr. *chiasma*] a decussation or X-shaped crossing. Called also *chiasma.* **optic c.,** the part of the hypothalamus formed by the crossing over of the fibers of the optic nerve from the medial half of each retina. Called also *chiasma opticum* [NA].

chiasma (ki-as′mah), pl. *chiasma′ta* [Gr., L.] chiasm; a decussation or X-shaped crossing. 1. in genetics, the point at which members of a chromosome pair are in contact during the prophase of meiosis and because of which recombination, or crossing over, occurs on separation. 2. in anatomical nomenclature, the crossing of two elements or structures, as the optic nerves. **c. op′ticum** [NA], optic CHIASM.

chiasmal (ki-az′mal) chiasmatic.

chiasmata (ki-as′mah-tah) [Gr., L.] plural of *chiasma.*

chiasmatic (ki-az-mat′ik) crosswise; resembling a chiasm. Called also *chiasmal.*

Chicago nomenclature see CHROMOSOME nomenclature, Chicago.

chickenpox (chik-en-poks) an acute, highly contagious, viral disease of young children, caused by the varicella-zoster virus. After an incubation period of 11 to 21 days, there is a characteristic rash, followed by fever, malaise, nasopharyngitis, and anorexia, sometimes associated with a scarlatiniform or morbilliform eruption. Typically, the rash begins as crops of small red papules that develop into clear teardrop vesicles surrounded by erythema, which are easily broken, followed by scab formation; the crops erupt for 3 to 4 days, starting on the trunk and spreading to the face and scalp and rarely to the extremities. Small, blistering, slightly raised vesicles surrounded by erythema may erupt on the buccal mucosa, palate, and pharynx; shortly after formation they rupture and form small eroded ulcers with red margins resembling aphthous lesions. Called also *varicella*.

Chiene's operation [John *Chiene*, Scottish surgeon, 1843–1923] see under OPERATION.

Chievitz's organ [John Henrik *Chievitz*, Danish anatomist, 1850–1901] see under ORGAN.

child (chīld) a young person between infancy and puberty. **c. abuse,** battered c. **battered c.,** a young child or infant who has suffered intentional injury, usually inflicted by a parent and, less commonly, a parent substitute. Fractures, often multiple but inflicted at different times, and subdural hematomas are the most common types of injuries. The skin may show scratches and scars, which may give an impression of healing burns, and numerous ecchymoses on various parts of the body. Oral examination may show lesions of the anterior pillar of the fauces and loss of tissue from the vault of the palate. The nose is often broken, giving it a flat appearance, such as seen in boxers. The principal radiographic signs include metaphyseal fragmentations and traumatic involucrums (external cortical thickenings) of the shafts of unfractured and otherwise healthy bones and trauma of the growing bones, such as metaphyseal cupping, traumatic bowing of the ends of the diaphyses due to metaphyseal infractions, and ectopic ossification of accessory epiphyseal centers in injured cartilaginous epiphyses, in which ossification centers do not normally develop. Called also *c. abuse, battered babe, battered babe syndrome, battered child syndrome, battered infant, Caffey-Kempe syndrome, parent-infant traumatic stress syndrome,* and *Silverman's syndrome.* **handicapped c.,** a child whose growth and development are impeded by a physical or mental defect or adverse environmental conditions. **puppet c.,** happy-puppet SYNDROME.

chilitis (ki-li′tis) cheilitis.

chill (chil) a shivering or shaking; an attack of involuntary contractions of the voluntary muscles, accompanied by a sense of cold and pallor of the skin. Called also *ague.*

chilo- see CHEILO-.

Chilomastix (ki″lo-mas′tiks) a genus of protozoa of the subphylum Mastigophora, the members of which have three anterior flagella and a fourth undulating within the cleft formed by the cytosome; the organisms are found in the intestine of vertebrates.

chimera (ki-me′rah) [Gr. *chimaira* a mythological fire-spouting monster with a lion's head, goat's body, and serpent's tail] an individual organism whose body contains cell populations derived from different zygotes, of the same or of different species, occurring spontaneously, as in twins (blood group chimeras), or produced artificially, as an organism which develops from combined portions of different embryos, or one in which tissues or cells of another organism have been transplanted. Cf. MOSAIC (2).

chin (chin) the lower anterior portion of the face in the region of the symphysis of the mandible. Called also *mentum* [NA]. See also terms beginning GENIO- and MENTO-.

chincap (chin′kap) an extraoral orthodontic appliance consisting of a caplike device fitted over the chin, which is connected to the headgear by elastics for the purpose of exerting upward and backward force on the mandible in the treatment of prognathism.

chinoline (chin′o-lēn) quinoline.

chip (chip) a small piece of something broken off. **bone c's,** small pieces of bone, usually cancellous, generally used to fill in bony defects to facilitate recalcification.

chiropractic (ki″ro-prak′tik) [Gr. *cheir* hand + Gr. *prattein* to do] a system of therapeutics based on the principle that disease is caused by abnormal function of the nervous system. It attempts to restore normal function of the system by manipulation and treatment of the structures of the human body, especially those of the spinal column.

chiropractor (ki″ro-prak″tor) a practitioner of chiropractic. Most states require graduation from an approved school of chiropractic with the degree of Doctor of Chiropractic (D.C.) and a state license by a board of chiropractic.

chisel (chis″l) 1. a wedge-like instrument with a cutting edge at the end of the blade. 2. a dental instrument, the cutting edge of which is in line with the center of the handle; used for planing or smoothing a surface, as during cavity preparation. See illustration. **binangle c.,** one with two angles in the shank; used

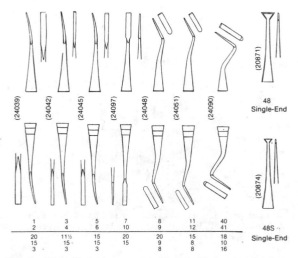

							48 Single-End
(24039)	(24042)	(24045)	(24097)	(24048)	(24051)	(24090)	(20871)

							48S Single-End
							(20874)

1 2	3 4	5 6	7 10	8 9	11 12	40 41	
20 15 3	11½ 15 3	15 15 3	20 15	20 9 8	15 8 8	18 10 16	

Chisels. (From H. O. Torres and A. Ehrlich: Modern Dental Assisting. 2nd ed. Philadelphia, W. B. Saunders Co., 1980; courtesy of S. S. White Div. of Pennwalt Corp.)

for accessing the proximal and cervical cavity walls of posterior preparations. **binangled c.,** one whose blade forms two angles before meeting with the shank. See illustration. **bone c.,** one for cutting bone, enamel, and dentin. **contra-angle c.,** a paired, binangled, chisel-like cutting instrument whose blade meets the shank at an angle greater than 12°. It is normally single-beveled; known as *reverse-beveled* when the bevel is on the mesial side of the blade. Called also *posterior c.* **curved c.,** one with a slightly curved shank; used for anterior proximal restorations. **enamel c.,** a hand-held cutting instrument, having a beveled edge at a right angle to the axis of the blade, a constricted shank, and a "shoulder" where the shank meets the blade; designed to be used in a push motion for breaking down tooth structures undermined by caries, smoothing cavity walls, and sharpening line and point angles. See illustration. **monangle c.,** a chisel having one angle in the shank; used with a push or pull motion for smoothing the shoulder and cervical cavity walls. **periodontal c.,** a straight instrument which curves slightly as the blade extends from the shank, the straight cutting

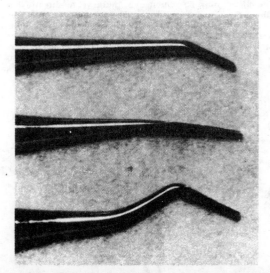

Types of dental chisels. Top to bottom: monangle chisel (hoe), curved chisel, and binangle chisel. (From H. W. Gilmore, M. R. Lund, D. J. Bales, and J. Vernetti: Operative Dentistry. 3rd ed. St. Louis, The C. V. Mosby Co., 1977.)

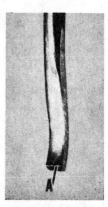

A straight chisel has a cutting edge formed by a bevel at the tip of the shank. (From P. F. Steele: Dimensions of Dental Hygiene. 2nd ed. Philadelphia, Lea & Febiger, 1975.)

edge at the end of the instrument being beveled at a 45° angle. Used chiefly for scaling the proximal surfaces of teeth too closely spaced to permit the use of other scalers, usually in the anterior part of the mouth. Called also *chisel scaler*. See illustration. **posterior c.,** contra-angle c. **Sorensen c.,** a single-bevel bone chisel made of carbon steel; used in maxillofacial surgery for splitting and removing bone over impacted teeth. See illustration. **straight c.,** a cutting instrument in which the shank is straight and the cutting edge is in line with the center of the handle; used on anterior teeth and cervical restorations. **Wedelstaedt c.,** one whose blade is continuous with the shank, without a constricting neck, and curving from the shank. The chisel is produced in various widths, having regular or contra-angle bevels.

Chlamydia (klah-mid′e-ah) [Gr. *chlamys* cloak] a genus of microorganisms of the family Chlamydiaceae, order Chlamydiales, occurring as small, nonmotile, gram-negative, spheroid organisms. Their developmental cycle consists of the development of an elementary body (infectious form), occurring as a small sporule (0.2 to 0.4 μm in diameter), which contains a nucleus and ribosomes surrounded by a multilaminated wall; an initial body (vegetative form), which divides intracellularly and occurs as a thin-walled reticulated spheroid (about 0.8 to 1.5 μm in diameter), contains nuclear fibrils and ribosomal elements; and an intermediate body, which is a transitional stage between the initial body and elementary body. Multiplication of *Chlamydia* may be inhibited by tetracyclines, penicillin, 5-fluorouracil, and other drugs. The members of this genus, which cause a wide variety of diseases in man and animals, were formerly identified with the genera *Bedsonia, Chlamydozoon,* and *Miyagawanella.* **C. psitta′ci,** a species, various strains of which cause psittacosis in man and ornithosis in

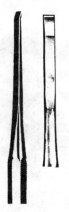

Shank and blade of Sorensen chisel. (From H. O. Torres and A. Ehrlich: Modern Dental Assisting. 2nd ed. Philadelphia, W. B. Saunders Co., 1980.)

nonpsittacine birds; pneumonitis in cattle, sheep, swine, cats, goats, and horses; epizootic bovine abortion and enzootic abortion of ewes; enteritis in calves; sporadic encephalomyelitis in calves; epizootic chlamydiosis of hares and muskrats; and conjunctivitis of cattle, sheep, and guinea pigs. Formerly called *Chlamydozoon psittaci, Ehrlichia psittaci,* and *Rickettsia psittaci.* See also MIYAGAWANELLA. **C. tracho′matis,** a species, various strains of which cause trachoma, inclusion conjunctivitis, nonspecific urethritis, proctitis, mouse pneumonitis, and lymphogranuloma venereum. The organism is parasitic in man, transmission occurring by contamination of the conjunctiva, oral or genital contact, during care of the young, during sexual contact, or by urogenital exudates during birth. Formerly called *Chlamydozoon trachomatis* and *Rickettsia trachomatis.* See also MIYAGAWANELLA.

chlamydia (klah-mid′e-ah), pl. *chlamyd′iae* [Gr. *chlamys* cloak] any microorganism of the genus *Chlamydia.*

Chlamydiaceae (klah-mid″e-a′se-e) a family of microorganisms of the order Chlamydiales (formerly assigned to the order Rickettsiales), consisting of coccoid organisms (about 0.2 to 1.5 μm in diameter), which multiply only within the cytoplasm of host cells by a developmental cycle characterized by changing of a small elementary body into a larger initial body that divides by fusion. Daughter cells reorganize and condense to become elementary bodies which survive outside the cell and infect other host cells. They are parasitic in birds and mammals (including man) and have been isolated from sanguivorous insects and arachnids, but the role of arthropods in their transmission is unclear. The family contains the genus *Chlamydia.*

chlamydiae (klah-mid′e-e) plural of *chlamydia.*

chlamydial (klah-mid′e-al) pertaining to or caused by *Chlamydia.*

Chlamydiales (klah-mid′e-al-ēz) an order of coccoid, gram-negative, parasitic microorganisms, which multiply only within the cytoplasm of the vertebrate host cell by a unique developmental cycle. It includes the family Chlamydiaceae.

chlamydiosis (klah-mid″e-o′sis) a disease caused by infection with microorganisms of the genus *Chlamydia.*

Chlamydozoaceae (klam″ĭ-do″zo-a′se-e) a former family of microorganisms now assigned to the family Chlamydiaceae.

Chlamydozoon (klam″ĭ-do-zo′on) a former genus of microorganisms now assigned to the genus *Chlamydia.* **C. psitta′ci,** *Chlamydia psittaci;* see under CHLAMYDIA. **C. tracho′matis,** *Chlamydia trachomatis;* see under CHLAMYDIA.

Chlo-Amine trademark for *dexchlorpheniramine maleate* (see under DEXCHLORPHENIRAMINE).

chloasma (klo-az′mah) [Gr. *chloazein* to be green] melasma. **c. periora′le virgin′ium,** brownish or blackish pigmentation, associated with macular seborrhea, situated chiefly around the mouth but also involving other parts of the face, and occurring in normal young women at the time of the first menstrual period.

chlor- see CHLORO-(2).

chloracne (klor-ak′ne) a disease of the follicular orifice associated with comedo formation, caused by contact with chlorine compounds, including certain chlorinated hydrocarbons, such as tars, oils, waxes, and greases. It usually occurs a month or more after exposure, in an area of direct contact with the offending substance, usually on the arms, neck, and face. Lesions represent follicular papules or small cysts. The oral mucosa may be involved, with reddening of the gingiva and swelling of the tonsils, and comedos and irregular scars may appear about the lips. See also ACNE.

chloral (klo′ral) [*chlorine + -al*] 1. a compound, trichloroacetaldehyde, occurring as a colorless, mobile, oily liquid with a pungent, irritating odor, produced by the chlorination of ethyl alcohol with addition of sulfuric acid. Used in the production of liniments, DDT, and chloral hydrate. It is a toxic substance that causes severe lesions on ingestion or inhalation. 2. c. hydrate. **c. hydrate,** a nonbarbiturate, nonanalgesic hypnotic and sedative, 2,2,2-trichloro-1,1-ethanediol, occurring as colorless or white crystals with an aromatic slightly acrid odor and a slightly caustic taste, which is soluble in water, alcohol, chloroform, and ether. It is slowly decomposed in aqueous solution and, in the presence of alkaline substances, breaks down into chloroform and formate. Used in nocturnal and preoperative sedation and, as an adjunct to opiates, in postoperative medication. Contraindicated in heart, kidney, and liver diseases. Gastric irritation with vomiting and nausea is the principal side effect. Its effects are augmented by ethyl alcohol. Called also *hydrated c.* Trademarks: Kessodrate, Noctec, Somnos. **hydrated c.,** c. hydrate.

chlorambucil (klo-ram′bu-sil) a nitrogen mustard, 4-[bis(2-chloroethyl)amino]benzenebutanoic acid, occurring as an off-

-white granular powder that is soluble in alkali and acetone and slightly soluble in water. It is an aromatic derivative of mechlorethamine that has cytotoxic properties. Used in the treatment of lymphocytic leukemia, primary macroglobulinemia, Hodgkin's disease and other lymphomas, and in other neoplasms. It is the least toxic nitrogen mustard, causing occasional gastrointestinal discomfort, dermatitis, hepatotoxicity, fetal abnormalities, and predisposition to infection. Principal toxic effects are bone marrow depression and cytotoxic effect on lymphoid organs and epithelial tissue, associated with anemias. Called also *chloraminophene*. Trademarks: Amboclorin, Leukeran.

chloramine-B (klo'rah-mēn) a topical antiseptic, *N*-chlorobenzenesulfonamide sodium, occurring as a white powder with a faint chlorine odor that is soluble in water and alcohol and, sparingly, in ether and chloroform.

chloramine-T (klo'rah-mēn) a topical antiseptic, *N*-chloro-*p*-toluenesulfonamide sodium salt, occurring as a white or yellowish crystalline solid with a faint chlorine odor, which is soluble in water and alcohol. Used in 1 to 2 percent aqueous solutions to treat wounds. When used externally, it is practically nontoxic. Trademarks: Aktiven, Chloraseptine, Chlorazone, Halamid.

chloraminophene (klo-ram'ĭ-no-fēn) chlorambucil.

chloramphenicol (klo'ram-fen'ĭ-kol) a broad-spectrum antibiotic originally isolated from cultures of *Streptomyces venezuelae* and later produced synthetically, 4-[bis(2-chloroethyl)-amino]benzenebutanoic acid. It occurs as white to grayish or yellowish, odorless, bitter needles or plates that are soluble in ethanol, acetone, butanol, and ethyl acetate and slightly soluble in ether, water, and chloroform. It inhibits protein synthesis by its action on bacterial ribosomes and acts on *Enterobacter aerogenes, Escherichia coli, Klebsiella pneumoniae, Bordetella, Haemophilus, Pasteurella, Pseudomonas, Bacteroides, Salmonella, Proteus, Neisseria, Shigella, Brucella,* and *Vibrio*. It also suppresses streptococci, staphylococci, *Actinomyces, Bacillus anthracis, Corynebacterium diphtheriae, Clostridium, Listeria, Bartonella,* and *Leptospira*. Toxic effects may include hypersensitivity with skin manifestations, angioedema, hemorrhage of the skin and mucosa of the intestinal and respiratory tracts, atrophic glossitis sometimes with black coating of the tongue, and bone marrow lesions that may result in leukopenia, thrombopenia, aplasia of the bone marrow, and sometimes fatal pancytopenia. Newborn infants are unable to metabolize the drug. Trademarks: Alficetyn, Aquamycetin, Austracol, Chemictina, Chlorasol, Chlorocid, Chloromycetin, Levomycetin, Novomycetin, Synthomycetine, Treomicetina. **c. palmitate,** a salt of chloramphenicol, occurring as a white, tasteless, crystalline powder with a faint odor, which is slightly soluble in water and freely soluble in methanol, ethanol, chloroform, and benzene. Lacking the bitter taste of chloramphenicol, it is better suited for oral use. It has the same antibacterial and toxic properties as the parent drug. Trademark: Clorolifarina. **c. pantothenate,** a pantothenic acid ester compounded with chloramphenicol; used as an antibacterial and antirickettsial agent. **c. sodium succinate,** chloramphenicol compounded with sodium succinate, occurring as a light yellow crystalline powder that is freely soluble in water and alcohol. Its antibacterial and toxic properties are the same as those of the parent compound.

Chloraseptine trademark for *chloramine-T*.

Chlorasol trademark for *chloramphenicol*.

chlorate (klo'rāt) any salt of chloric acid containing the radical ClO_3-.

Chlorazone trademark for *chloramine-T*.

chlorbutol (klor-bu'tol) chlorobutanol.

chlorcyclizine hydrochloride (klor-si'klĭ-zēn) an antihistaminic drug, 1-(*p*-chloro-α-phenylbenzyl)-4-methylpiperazine, occurring as a white, odorless, crystalline powder that is soluble in water and alcohol and is slightly soluble in benzene and ether. Chlorcyclizine inhibits histamine mediation at the H_1 receptor, with mildly sedative properties and a low incidence of side effects. It also exhibits slight anticholinergic and antispasmodic effects, some local anesthetic action, and enhances the effects of epinephrine. Used in the treatment of allergic diseases. Trademarks: Alergicide, Perazyl, Trihistan.

chlordiazepoxide (klor″di-a″zĕ-pok'sīd) a minor tranquilizer, 7-chloro-*N*-methyl-5-phenyl-3*H*-1,4-benzodiazepin-2-amine-4-oxide, occurring as a yellow, odorless, crystalline powder that is sensitive to sunlight and is soluble in chloroform and alcohol, but not in water. Used in managing withdrawal symptoms of acute alcoholism, skeletal muscle spasms, and anxiety states, and as a premedication agent in anesthesia. In dentistry, used chiefly as a sedative in general anesthesia premedication and in preparing patients for dental procedures. The drug may be

addictive and its adverse reactions include drowsiness, ataxia, confusion, rashes, edema, menstrual disorders, impotence, blood dyscrasias, jaundice, and hepatic lesions. Rage, excitement, hostility, and decreased tolerance to alcohol may occur. Trademark: Libritabs. **c. hydrochloride,** the hydrochloride salt of chlordiazepoxide, having indications and contraindications similar to those of the parent compound. Trademark: Librium.

Chlorethone trademark for *chlorobutanol*.

chlorguanide hydrochloride (klor-gwan'ĭd) CHLOROGUANIDE hydrochloride.

chlorhexidine (klor-heks'ĭ-dēn) a topical anti-infective agent, *N,N″* - bis(4 - chlorophenyl) - 3,12 - diimino - 2,4,11,13 - tetra-azatetradecanediimidamide. It has been tested as a potential plaque and calculus inhibitor.

chloride (klo'rīd) any salt of hydrochloric acid; any binary compound of chlorine in which the latter carries a negative charge of electricity (Cl^-). **aminomercuric c.,** ammoniated MERCURIC. **cobaltous c.,** a red crystalline hygroscopic compound, $CoCl_2$, occurring as leaflets that turn pink on exposure to moist air. It is soluble in water, acetone, alcohol, ether, glycerol, and pyridine. Similarly to cobalt, cobaltous chloride stimulates erythropoiesis and, in large doses, may produce toxic reactions consisting of cyanosis, coma, and death. Other toxic reactions may include cutaneous flushing, dermatitis, tinnitus, deafness, nausea, vomiting, anorexia, thyroid hyperplasia, myxedema, chest pain, congestive heart failure, weakness, and other complications. It is used in the production of vitamin B_{12} and in a variety of industrial processes. Radioactive cobaltous chloride ($^{57}CoCl_2$) has a half-life of 270 days and is a pure gamma ray emitter. Called also *cobalt dichloride*. **ethyl c.,** an anesthetic chloroethane (C_2H_5Cl), occurring as a flammable gas with an ethereal odor and a burning taste, which liquefies at 12°C and becomes a colorless, mobile, volatile liquid, and is slightly soluble in water and freely soluble in ethanol and ether. Used as a local anesthetic by freezing and rarely as an inhalation anesthetic. In topical application, ethyl chloride causes freezing of the tissue with painful thawing and tissue damage with delayed healing. In inhalation anesthesia, it may cause cardiac arrhythmias, hepatotoxicity, and irritation of the skin and mucous membranes. Called also *chloroethyl, ether chloratus, ether hydrochloric, ether muriatic* and *monochlorethane*. Trademarks: Anodynon, Chelen, Kelene, Narcotile. **ferric c.,** $FeCl_3$; occurring as orange yellow or brownish crystalline solids. Used as a reagent and topically as an astringent and styptic. Called also *iron chloride*. **ferrous c.,** $FeCl_2$; occurring as greenish-white crystals that are soluble in water and alcohol. Used in the treatment of iron deficiency anemia. Called also *iron chloride, iron dichloride,* and *iron protochloride*. For toxic effects see IRON. **o-HYDROXYPHENYLMERCURIC c.,** o-HYDROXYPHENYLMERCURIC chloride. **iron c.,** 1. ferrous c. 2. ferric c. **mercuric c.,** $HgCl_2$; occurring as odorless crystals or white powder. Used as a topical antiseptic and disinfectant. It is very poisonous and is corrosive to mucous membrane, and ingestion may cause abdominal pain, vomiting, nausea, hematemesis, diarrhea, melena, kidney damage, and sometimes death. Called also *mercury bichloride* and *mercury perchloride*. **mercury amide c.,** ammoniated MERCURY. **polyvinyl c.,** POLYVINYL chloride. **sodium c.,** SODIUM chloride. **vinyl c.,** VINYL chloride.

chlorine (klor'ēn, klo'rēn, klo'rin) [L. *chlorum, chlorinum,* from Gr. *chlōros green*] a heavy, yellowish green, gaseous halogen with a suffocating odor. Symbol, Cl; atomic number, 17; atomic weight, 35.453; melting point, 100.98°C; specific gravity, 1.56; valences, 1, 3, 4, 5, 7; group VIIA of the periodic table. In addition to two natural isotopes, ^{35}Cl and ^{37}Cl, chlorine has seven radioactive isotopes and two isomers. The radioactive trace elements include ^{36}Cl, emitting beta rays and having a half-life of 3.08×10^5 years and ^{38}Cl, emitting beta rays and having a half-life of 37.29 min. In nature, chlorine is always in a combined form. Its principal functions in the body include maintenance of water balance and osmotic pressure, acid-base balance, and neuromuscular irritability, sodium being the chief cation and chlorine the chief anion of extracellular fluids and potassium being the cation of intracellular fluids. Chlorine is believed to activate the salivary enzyme ptyalin. Used for disinfection, fumigation, and bleaching, either in an aqueous solution (chlorine water) or as chlorinated lime. It is a powerful irritant, either on contact or by inhalation, which may cause lesions of the skin and mucous membrane, including fatal pulmonary edema. **c. dioxide,** a strong oxidizing agent, ClO_2, occurring as a reddish yellow gas with irritating odor, which decomposes in water and alkalies, forming a mixture of chlorite and chlorate. Used as a bleaching, deodorizing, and antiseptic agent. It may be irritating to the skin and mucous membranes on contact or by inhalation. Called also *chlorine peroxide*. **c. peroxide,** c. dioxide.

Chlormene trademark for *chlorpheniramine maleate* (see under CHLORPHENIRAMINE).

chlormeprazine (klor-mep'rah-zēn) prochlorperazine.

chlormerodrin (klor-mer'o-drin) a mercurial diuretic drug, [3-[(aminocarbonyl)amino]-2-methoxypropyl]chloromercury, occurring as a white, odorless, bitter powder that is soluble in water, methanol, and ethanol, but not in acetone and ether. Used in the treatment of congestive heart failure, the nephrotic syndrome, glomerulonephritis, hepatic cirrhosis, portal obstruction, hypertension, and other conditions. Adverse reactions may include flushing of the face, gastrointestinal disorders, pruritus, urticaria, skin rashes, weakness, muscle pains, blood electrolyte imbalance, and potential secondary shock. Trademarks: Diureone, Katonil, Mercloran, Mercoral, Neohydrin, Percapyl.

chloro- [Gr. *chlōros* green] 1. a combining form meaning green. 2. pertaining to an organic compound which has chlorine atoms substituted for the hydrogen atom. *Chlor-* and *chloro-* are often used interchangeably, but *chlor-* indicates a closer relationship of chlorine to the compound.

chloroazodin (klo"ro-a'zo-din) an antibacterial substance that slowly liberates chlorine, N, N"-dichlorodiazenedicarboxylamide, occurring as yellow needles or plates with a burning taste and a slight chlorine odor, which are very soluble in water and sparingly soluble in alcohol, glycerol, chloroform, ether, and vegetable oils. In dentistry, used chiefly in the sterilization of dental pulp canals and periapical abscesses, in the treatment of fistulae, and in wet dressings for infected wounds. Trademark: Azochloramide.

chlorobutanol (klo"ro-bu'tah-nol) a topical anesthetic with germicidal and antibacterial properties, 1,1,1-trichloro-2-methyl-2-propanol, occurring as colorless to white crystals with a camphoraceous odor and taste that are soluble in water, alcohol, glycerol, chloroform, ether, and oils. Used in dentistry in combination with cinnamon and clove oil in the treatment of pain in pulpitis, in dressings for exposed pulp, and in treating postextraction sockets and bony lesions following surgery. Also used as a hypnotic and sedative, in the treatment of vomiting associated with gastritis, as a preservative in biological solutions, including those of epinephrine, posterior pituitary extracts, and alkaloids, and as a plasticizer. Excessive use may lead to habituation and addiction. Called also *acetone chloroform* and *chlorbutol*. Trademarks: Chlorethone, Methaform, Sedaform.

Chlorocid trademark for *chloramphenicol*.

chlorocobalamin (klo"ro-ko-bal'ah-min) a member of the vitamin B_{12} group in which the cyanide group is replaced by a chloride group. See VITAMIN B_{12}.

chloroethane (klo"ro-eth'ān) ethyl CHLORIDE.

chloroethene (klo"ro-eth'ēn) VINYL chloride. **c. homopolymer,** POLYVINYL chloride.

chloroethylene (klo"ro-eth'ĭ-lēn) VINYL chloride. **c. polymer,** POLYVINYL chloride.

chloroform (klo'ro-form) a compound, trichloromethane, occurring as a clear, colorless, mobile liquid with a sweetish taste and an ethereal odor, which is not flammable but very volatile. It is miscible with alcohol, ether, volatile oils, and organic solvents, and dissolves in water. Its use as an inhalation anesthetic is now limited because of toxic effects, especially on the heart and liver. When taken internally in small doses, it is a carminative, and when used externally, it is an irritant. Used chiefly as a solvent for fats, oils, rubber, alkaloids, waxes, gutta-percha, and resins; as a cleansing agent; and as a preservative and antibacterial agent in the preparation of drugs. Called also (incorrectly) *formyl trichloride*. **acetone c.,** chlorobutanol.

chloroformism (klo'ro-form"izm) 1. the habitual use of chloroform for its narcotic effect. 2. the anesthetic effect of the vapor of chloroform.

chloroguanide hydrochloride (klor"o-gwan'ĭd) a compound, N-(4-chlorophenyl)-N'-(1-methylethyl)imidocarbonimidic diamide hydrochloride, occurring as a white, crystalline powder that is soluble in water and ethanol, but not in chloroform and ether. It is a low-toxicity antimalarial agent that is converted in the body to a triazine derivative that inhibits dihydrofolate reductase in the malarial parasite, thus impairing nucleotide synthe-

sis such that schizogony cannot take place. Called also *chlorguanide hydrochloride* and *proguanil hydrochloride*. Trademark: Paludrine.

chloromercuriphenol *o*-(chloromercuri)phenol (klo"ro-mer"ku-rĭ-fe'nol) *o*-HYDROXYPHENYLMERCURIC chloride.

Chloromycetin trademark for *chloramphenicol*.

Chloronase trademark for *chlorpropamide*.

Chloronautine trademark for *dimenhydrinate*.

chloropercha (klo"ro-per'chah) gutta-percha dissolved in chloroform; used in root canal therapy. Trademark: Kloropercha N-Ø.

p-**chlorophenol** (par"ah-klo"ro-fe'nol) parachlorophenol.

chlorophenothane (klo"ro-fe'no-thān) a contact insecticide, 1,1,1-trichloro-2,2-bis(*p*-chlorophenyl)ethane, occurring as a colorless, bitter, almost odorless, off-white crystalline powder or white crystals that are soluble in ethanol, acetone, chloroform, and ether, but not in water. It is effective against a wide variety of insects and other arthropods. Mammalian poisoning produces chiefly neurological changes, including hyperexcitability, tremor, hypothermia, convulsions, respiratory failure, and death. Chronic intoxication may produce liver damage, central nervous system degeneration, agranulocytosis, weakness, cardiac failure, and death. Sensitization of myocardial catecholamines may result in sympathoadrenal discharge and cardiac arrhythmias. Vehicles, such as petroleum products, increase toxicity. Called also (incorrectly) *dichlorodiphenyltrichloroethane (DDT)*, *dicophane*, and *pentachlorin*. Trademarks: Gesarol, Neocid.

chlorophyll (klo'ro-fil) [*chloro-* + Gr. *phyllon* leaf] a proporphyrin derivative containing magnesium, which is located in the chloroplasts of green leaves, being a green plant pigment essential to photosynthesis. It is a photoreceptor up to wavelengths of 700 μ, transferring radiant energy to its chemical environment in plant cells, where the energy derived from the sunlight forms pentoses, trioses, fructose, and more complex sugars through the process of photosynthesis. Chlorophyll occurs in three forms: *a* — a blue-green microcrystalline wax which, in alcoholic solution, has deep-red fluorescence; *b* — a yellow-green microcrystalline wax which, in solution with organic solvents, has red fluorescence; and *c* — occurring in marine organisms. Used chiefly as a deodorant in dentifrices, soaps, cosmetics, mouthwashes, and perfumes. Also used as a colorant.

chloroplast (klo'ro-plast) [*chloro-* + Gr. *plastos* formed] a chlorophyll-bearing body of plant cells. Called also *chloroplastid*.

chloroplastid (klo"ro-plas'tid) chloroplast.

chloroprocaine hydrochloride (klo"ro-pro'kān) a local anesthetic having pharmacological and toxicological properties similar to those of procaine hydrochloride, 2-(diethylamino)ethyl 4-amino-2-chlorobenzoate monohydrochloride. It occurs as a white, odorless, crystalline powder with a numbing taste, which is soluble in water and ethanol, slightly soluble in chloroform, and insoluble in ether. Trademark: Nesacaine.

chloroquine (klo'ro-kwin) an antimalarial agent, 7-chloro-4-[(diethylamino-1-methylbutyl)amino]quinoline, occurring as an odorless, bitter, white or yellowish crystalline powder that is readily soluble in dilute acids, chloroform, and ether, and very slightly soluble in water. Also used in the treatment of lupus erythematosus, rheumatoid arthritis, and photoallergic reactions. Headache, visual disorders, gastrointestinal disorders, pruritus, myasthenia, myopathy, and lichenoid skin eruption may occur. Trademark: Aralen. **c. hydrochloride,** the hydrochloride salt of chloroquine, having actions and uses similar to those of the parent drug.

Chlorosal trademark for *chlorothiazide*.

chlorosis (klo-ro'sis) a disorder, generally of pubescent females, characterized by greenish color of the skin due to iron deficiency. See iron deficiency ANEMIA. **chronic c.,** hypochromic anemia, essential; see under ANEMIA.

chlorosulthiadil (klo"ro-sul-thi'ah-dil) hydrochlorothiazide.

chlorothiazide (klo"ro-thi'ah-zīd) the prototype of benzothiazine diuretics (see under DIURETIC), 6-chloro-2H-1,2,4-benzothiadiazine-7-sulfonamide 1,1-dioxide, occurring as an odorless, white, crystalline powder that is freely soluble in demethylformamide and dimethyl sulfoxide, slightly soluble in methanol and pyridine, very slightly soluble in water, and insoluble in ether, benzene, and chloroform. Adverse effects are similar to those associated with other benzothiazine diuretics. Trademarks: Chlorosal, Chlorurit, Diuresal, Diuril, Salunil, Saluric, Urinex.

chlorothymol (klo"ro-thi'mol) a powerful germicide, 6-chloro-4-isopropyl-1-methyl-3-phenol, occurring as white crystals or crystalline powder with a characteristic odor and an aromatic pungent taste, which becomes discolored when exposed to light and is soluble in alcohol, benzene, chloroform, and caustic soda, but not in water. It is incorporated in some dental preparations for application to the gingiva and oral mucosa in infection.

Chloro-Thymonol trademark for a preparation used in root canal dressing.

chlorpheniramine maleate (klor″fen-ir′ah-mēn) an antihistaminic drug which inhibits histamine mediation at the H_1 receptor, *dl*-2-[*p*-chloro-α-2-(dimethylamine)ethyl] pyridine maleate, occurring as a white, odorless, crystalline powder that is soluble in water, alcohol, and chloroform and is slightly soluble in ether and benzene. Used in the treatment of allergic diseases and insect bites, and as an adjunct in anaphylactic shock. Also widely used in antitussive preparations. Called also *chlorprophenpyridamine*. Trademarks: Allerclor, Allergisan, Antagonate, Chlor-Trimeton, Chlormene, Polaronil, Piriton.

chlorpromazine (klor-pro′mah-zēn) a phenothiazine derivative, 2-chloro-10-(3-dimethylaminopropyl)phenothiazine, occurring as a white, crystalline solid with an amine-like odor, which is soluble in alcohol, chloroform, ether, and dilute mineral acids, but not in water. It is a major tranquilizer, used as an antiemetic and in the management of psychoneurotic disorders, particularly those associated with anxiety; porphyria; hiccups; apprehension in surgical and cancer patients; and other conditions in which tranquilizer therapy is indicated. Adverse reactions may include drowsiness; extrapyramidal disorders, including parkinsonism-like disorders, dystonia, dyskinesia, torticollis, restlessness, and hyperreflexia; seizures; cardiovascular disorders, including postural hypotension, tachycardia, bradycardia, dizziness, and cardiac arrest; blood dyscrasias, including agranulocytosis, eosinophilia, leukopenia, hemolytic anemia, thrombocytopenic purpura, and pancytopenia; liver diseases; allergy, including urticaria, photosensitivity, and contact dermatitis; endocrine disorders, including ovulation and menstrual disorders, gynecomastia, and changes in libido; hypercholesterolemia; xerostomia; nasal congestion; increased appetite; edema; and constipation. Trademark: Thorazine. **c. hydrochloride,** the monohydrochloride salt of chlorpromazine, occurring as a white or creamy white, odorless, crystalline powder that is soluble in water, alcohol, and chloroform, but not in ether and benzene, which darkens on exposure to light. It has actions, uses, and side effects similar to those of the parent drug.

chlorpropamide (klor-pro′pah-mĭd) a sulfonylurea oral hypoglycemic agent, 1-(*p*-chlorophenylsulfonyl)-3-propylurea, occurring as a white, odorless, crystalline powder that is readily soluble in pyridine and alkali hydroxide solutions, slightly soluble in ethanol and chloroform, and insoluble in water. Used in the treatment of some types of diabetes mellitus. Gastrointestinal disorders, weakness, headache, tinnitus, paresthesias, hypersensitivity, skin rashes, alcohol intolerance, and occasional cholestatic jaundice, liver lesions, leukopenia, thrombocytopenia, pancytopenia, and agranulocytosis may occur. Trademarks: Adiaben, Asucrol, Chloronase, Diabenal, Diabinese, Oradian.

chlorprophenpyridamine maleate (klor′pro-fen-pī-rid′ah-mēn) CHLORPHENIRAMINE maleate.

chlortetracycline hydrochloride (klor″tet-rah-si′klēn) a natural tetracycline antibiotic elaborated by cultures of *Streptomyces aureofaciens*, 7-chloro-4-dimethylamino-1,4,4a,5,5a,6,11,12a-octahydro - 3,6,10,12,12,12a - pentahydroxy - 6 - methyl - 1,11 - dioxo-2-naphthacenecarboxamide monohydrochloride. It occurs as a yellow, odorless, crystalline powder that is slowly affected by light and is soluble in water, alcohol, carbonates, and hydroxides and is insoluble in acetone, chloroform, and ether. Its antimicrobial action and toxic properties are similar to those of other tetracyclines. Absorption in intramuscular administration is erratic. Milk and other calcium-containing substances should not be taken during therapy. Trademarks: Aureociclina, Aureocina, Aureomycin, Biomycin, Isphamycin.

chlorthalidone (klor-thal′ĭ-dōn) an oral diuretic, 3-hydroxy-3-(4-chloro-3-sulfamylphenyl)phthalamide, occurring as a white or yellowish crystalline powder that is soluble in methanol, slightly soluble in ethanol, and insoluble in water. Used in the treatment of congestive heart failure, some types of obesity, and the premenstrual syndrome. Also used as an adjunct to antihypertensive drugs. Electrolyte disorders and renal damage may occur. Trademarks: Hydroton, Hygroton.

Chlor-Trimeton trademark for *chlorpheniramine maleate* (see under CHLORPHENIRAMINE).

Chlorurit trademark for *chlorothiazide*.

Chlorylen trademark for *trichloroethylene*.

chlorzoxazone (klor-zok′sah-zōn) a centrally acting muscle relaxant, 5-chloro-2-benzoaxazolamine, occurring as a white or creamy white, odorless, glistening crystalline powder that is readily soluble in acetone and methanol and slightly soluble in

water. Used in the treatment of painful muscle spasm, fibrositis, bursitis, myositis, spondylitis, sprains, and strains. Side reactions include skin rashes, nausea, vomiting, vertigo, malaise, headache, drowsiness, gastrointestinal disorders, jaundice, and hypersensitivity. Trademarks: Biomioran, Paraflex, Solaxin.

choana (ko′a-nah), pl. *choa′nae* [L.; Gr. *choanē* funnel] 1. any funnel-shaped cavity or infundibulum. 2. [pl.] the paired openings between the nasal cavity and the nasopharynx. Called also *bony choanae, choanae osseae,* and *posterior nares.* **primary c.,** the opening of the embryonic olfactory sac into the mouth. **secondary c.,** the permanent or definitive choana after the formation of the palate.

choanae (ko-a′ne) [L.] plural of *choana.* **bony c., c. os′seae,** choana (2).

choanal (ko′ah-nal) pertaining to a choana.

choanoid (ko′ah-noid) [Gr. *choanē* funnel + *eidos* form] funnel-shaped.

choice (chois) 1. the act of choosing; selection. 2. that which is preferable above another or other things or persons. **dual c.,** dual OPTION.

choke (chōk) 1. to interrupt respiration by obstruction or compression, or the condition resulting from such interruption. 2. [pl.] a burning sensation beginning in the substernal region, with increasing uncontrollable urge to cough, and great apprehension and anxiety, leading to vasodepressor syncope, experienced during decompression.

chol- see CHOLE-.

cholagogue (ko′lah-gog) [chol- + Gr. *agogos* leading] an agent that stimulates the flow of bile into the duodenum.

Cholan-DH trademark for *dehydrocholic acid* (see under ACID).

cholane (ko′lān) a class of steroid compounds having a branched five-carbon side chain at C-17. See also STEROID.

Cholaxin trademark for *dextrothyroxine sodium* (see under DEXTROTHYROXINE).

Cholaxine trademark for *sorbitol.*

chol-, see CHOLE-.

chole-, chol-, cholo- [Gr. *cholē* bile] a combining form denoting relationship to the bile.

cholecalciferol (ko″lē-kal-sif′er-ol) vitamin D_3.

Choledyl trademark for *oxtriphylline.*

choleretic (ko″ler-et′ik) 1. stimulating the production of bile. 2. an agent which stimulates the production of bile or is used for replacement therapy in biliary deficiency states; bile, bile acids, and bile salts are the most common choleretics.

cholestane (ko′les-tān) a class of steroid compounds having a doubly-branched 8-carbon side chain at C-17. See also STEROID.

cholesterol (ko-les′ter-ōl) [chole- + *sterol*] a sterol, cholest-5-en-3β-ol, occurring as a fatlike, pearly substance in the form of acicular crystals. It is found in most animal tissues, but principally in the blood, central nervous system, bile, fats, liver, kidney, adrenals, milk, and egg yolk. It is present in certain glands and is believed to be the parent compound for steroid hormones and vitamin D. Cholesterol is also involved in the formation of gallstones and degenerative changes in the arterial wall leading to arteriosclerosis. The presence of excessively large amounts of cholesterol in the blood causes hypercholesterolemia.

choline (ko′lēn) a compound, 2-hydroxy-*N,N,N*-trimethylethanaminium hydroxide, sometimes considered a member of the vitamin B complex, occurring as a viscid, strongly alkaline substance, its crystals being soluble in water and alcohol, but not in ether. Choline is found in various plants and animal tissues, chiefly nerve tissue, egg yolk, kidneys, liver, and heart, and can also be synthesized in the human body. It absorbs carbon dioxide from the atmosphere. Choline is a component of lecithin and sphingomyelin, and serves as a precursor of acetylcholine, as a methyl donor in transmethylation, and as a lipotropic substance in the body, being essential for the utilization of fats by the liver. Pharmacologically, it has acetylcholine-like action, but is much less active. The human requirement for choline is not known, but a daily intake of 500 to 900 mg is considered adequate. Choline deficiency occurs very rarely in man. A choline-deficient diet in experimental animals may produce fatty liver degeneration, hemorrhagic necrosis of the liver, anemia, and hypoproteinemia. **carbamyl c.,** carbachol. **c. esterase I,** acetylcholinesterase. **c. esterase II,** cholinesterase. **phosphatidyl c., c. phosphoglyceride,** lecithin. **c. theophyllinate,** oxtriphylline.

cholineine (ko′li-nēn) quinoline.

cholinergic (ko″lin-er′jik) 1. pertaining to mediation of impulses in the autonomic nervous system by acetylcholine. 2. pertaining to drugs that mimic the stimulation of nerves of the autonomic nervous system that are mediated by acetylcholine; cholinomimetic. 3. pertaining to nerves of the autonomic system that are mediated by acetylcholine. 4. parasympathomimetic. See parasympathomimetic DRUG. Cf. ADRENERGIC.

cholinesterase [E.C.3.1.1.8] (ko″lin-es′ter-ās) 1. a hydrolase that catalyzes the hydrolysis of acylcholine into choline and carboxylic acid anion; it acts on a variety of choline esters, as well as other compounds. Found chiefly in the blood plasma. Abbreviated ChE. Called also *benzoylcholinesterase, butyrylcholine esterase, choline esterase II,* and *pseudocholinesterase.* 2. acetylcholinesterase. **c. inhibitor,** cholinesterase INHIBITOR. **c. reactivator,** cholinesterase REACTIVATOR. **true c.,** acetylcholinesterase.

cholinomimetic (ko″lī-no-mi-met′ik) 1. mimicking the action of acetylcholine on the autonomic nervous system and the effector systems; cholinergic. 2. parasympathomimetic. See parasympathomimetic DRUG.

cholo- see CHOLE-.

Chologon trademark for *dehydrocholic acid* (see under ACID).

chondr- see CHONDRO-.

chondrectomy (kon-drek′to-me) [*chondr-* + Gr. *ektomē* excision] surgical excision of cartilage.

chondric (kon′drik) cartilaginous; of or relating to cartilage.

chondrification (kon″drĭ-fi-ka′shun) [*chondr-* + L. *facere* to make] the act or process of formation of cartilage. In the embryo, the cartilage is formed when the mesenchymal cells congregate in the centers of chondrification when they differentiate and secrete a metachromatic hyaline matrix. The increase of interstitial material in the centers is associated with isolation of cells in separate compartments or lacunae where the cells mature and become chondrocytes.

chondrin (kon′drin) a protein, resembling gelatin, from cartilage; it is considered to be a mixture of gelatin and mucin.

chondrio- [Gr. *chondrion,* dim. of *chondros* (1) a granule (2) gristle or cartilage] a combining form denoting relationship (1) to a granule or (2) to cartilage.

chondriosome (kon′dre-o-sōm″) [*chondrio-* + Gr. *sōma* body] mitochondrion; see MITOCHONDRIA.

chondritis (kon-dri′tis) [*chondr-* + *-itis*] inflammation of cartilage. See also POLYCHONDRITIS.

chondro-, chondr- [Gr. *chondros* cartilage] a combining form denoting a relationship to cartilage.

chondroadenoma (kon″dro-ad″ĕ-no′mah) adenochondroma.

chondroangeopathia punctata (kon″dro-an″je-o-path′e-ah punk-ta′tah) Conradi-Hünermann SYNDROME.

chondroangioma (kon″dro-an″je-o′mah) benign mesenchymoma containing chondromatous and angiomatous elements.

chondroblast (kon′dro-blast) [*chondro-* + Gr. *blastos* germ] one of the large, plump, immature cells arranged in a single layer between the perichondrium and the matrix of the cartilage, which become trapped in the matrix during the processes of chondrogenesis. Called also *chondroplast.*

chondrocranium (kon″dro-kra′ne-um) [*chondro-* + Gr. *kranion* head] the cartilaginous cranial structure of the embryo.

chondrocyte (kon′dro-sīt) [*chondro-* + Gr. *kytos* hollow vessel] one of the mature cartilage cells found clustered in small groups beneath the perichondrium and free surface of articular cartilage. They are rarely visible under the light microscope, but under the electron microscope their shapes tend to be irregular. The nucleus is round or oval and contains from one to several nucleoli, depending on species, and there is a juxtanuclear cell center with a pair of centrioles and a well developed Golgi apparatus. Called also *cartilage cell.*

chondrodynia (kon″dro-din′e-ah) [*chondro-* + Gr. *odynē* pain] pain in a cartilage.

chondrodysplasia (kon″dro-dis-pla′ze-ah) [*chondro-* + *dysplasia*] faulty development of the diaphyseal ends of the long bones. **hereditary c., infantile hereditary c.,** Morquio's DISEASE. **c. puncta′ta, dominant,** Conradi-Hünermann SYNDROME.

chondrodystrophia (kon″dro-dis-tro′fe-ah) [*chondro-* + *dys-* + Gr. *trophē* nutrition] chondrodystrophy. **c. calcif′icans,** Conradi-Hünermann SYNDROME. **c. feta′lis,** achondroplasia. **c. tar′da,** Morquio's DISEASE.

chondrodystrophy (kon″dro-dis′tro-fe) abnormal development of cartilage. **atypical c.,** Morquio's DISEASE.

chondrogenesis (kon″dro-jen′ĕ-sis) [*chondro-* + Gr. *genesis* production] the formation of cartilage. **c. imper′fecta,** achondroplasia.

chondrogenic (kon″dro-jen′ik) giving rise to or forming cartilage.

chondroglossus (kon″dro-glos′us) chondroglossus MUSCLE.

chondroglucose (kon″dro-glu′kōs) a sugar formed by the action of hydrochloric acid on chondrin from cartilage.

chondroid (kon′droid) [*chondro-* + Gr. *eidos* form] 1. resembling cartilage. 2. hyaline CARTILAGE.

chondroitin (kon-dro′ĭ-tin) a mucopolysaccharide, $C_{18}H_{27}NO_{14}$, found in the cornea and differing from hyaluronic acid in that it contains acetylgalactosamine in place of acetylglucosamine. **c. sulfate,** a sulfate ester derivative of chondroitin, found in the cartilage, cornea, bone, and other types of connective tissue of vertebrates. It occurs in three forms: *c. sulfate A* (chondroitin-4-sulfate), which contains a sulfate ester group at carbon 4 of the *N*-acetylgalactosamine residue; *c. sulfate C* (chondroitin-6-sulfate), which contains a sulfate ester at atom 6; and *c. sulfate B* (see DERMATAN SULFATE), in which the uronic acid constituent is replaced by 1-iduronic acid. A copolymer of forms A and C is chondromucoid.

chondroitinuria (kon-dro″ĭ-tin-u′re-ah) the presence of chondroitic acid in the urine.

chondrolysis (kon-drol′ĭ-sis) [*chondro-* + Gr. *lysis* dissolution] dissolution or degeneration of cartilage.

chondroma (kon-dro′mah) [*chondro-* + *-oma*] a benign, painless, slow-growing tumor made up of a mass of hyaline cartilage with areas of calcification and necrosis. An increase in the rate of growth and the presence of multinucleated cells indicate a possibility of malignancy. When the jaws are involved, which occurs very rarely, the usual site is the anterior maxilla or the cuspid area of the mandible. A tumor occurring centrally in the substance of a cartilage or bone is known as an *enchondroma* (true c.); one developing on the surface of a cartilage is called *ecchondroma;* and malignant chondroma is *chondrosarcoma.* Called *enchondroma of jaws.* **malignant c.,** chondrosarcoma. **true c.,** enchondroma.

chondromalacia (kon″dro-mah-la′she-ah) [*chondro-* + Gr. *malakia* softness] softening of cartilage. **generalized c.,** chronic atrophic POLYCHONDRITIS.

chondromucin (kon″dro-mu′sin) [*chondro-* + *mucin*] chondromucoid.

chondromucoid (kon″dro-mu′koid) [*chondro-* + *mucoid*] the cartilaginous tissue mucoid. It is the principal constituent of the ground substance of the cartilage, consisting of a mucoprotein (or glycoprotein), which is a copolymer of chondroitin sulfate A and chondroitin sulfate C. Called also *chondromucin* and *chondromucoprotein.* See also PROTEOGLYCAN.

chondromucoprotein (kon″dro-mu″ko-pro′te-in) 1. chondromucoid. 2. proteoglycan.

chondromyxosarcoma (kon″dro-mik″so-sar-ko′mah) a malignant mesenchymoma containing sarcomatous and cartilaginous elements.

chondronecrosis (kon″dro-ne-kro′sis) [*chondro-* + *necrosis*] necrosis of cartilage.

chondro-osseous (kon″dro-os′e-us) [*chondro-* + *osseous*] composed of or pertaining to cartilage and bone.

chondropathia punctata (kon″dro-path′e-ah punk-ta′tah) Conradi-Hünermann SYNDROME.

chondropathology (kon″dro-pah-thol′o-je) [*chondro-* + *pathology*] the pathology of disease of cartilage.

chondropathy (kon-drop′ah-the) [*chondro-* + Gr. *pathos* disease] disease of a cartilage.

chondropharyngeus (kon″dro-fahr-in′je-us) chondropharyngeal MUSCLE.

chondroplast (kon′dro-plast) [*chondro-* + Gr. *plassein* to form] chondroblast.

chondrosarcoma (kon″dro-sar-ko′mah) [*chondro-* + *sarcoma*] a malignant form of chondroma whose rate of growth is increased. **central c.,** one developing in the interior of a bone. Called also *endochondrosarcoma.* **mesenchymal c.,** one in which there are areas of small anaplastic cells adjoining calcifying or ossifying zones of chondroid that do not appear to be malignant.

chondrosarcomatosis (kon″dro-sar″ko-mah-to′sis) the formation of multiple chondrosarcomas.

chord (kord) cord. **condylar c.,** condylar AXIS.

chorda (kor′dah), pl. *chor′dae* [L.; Gr. *chordē* cord] a cord or sinew. **c. dorsa′lis,** notochord. **c. spina′lis,** spinal CORD. **c. tym′pani** [NA], chorda tympani NERVE. **c. umbilica′lis,** umbilical CORD. **chor′dae voca′les,** vocal CORDS.

chordae (kor′de) [L.] plural of *chorda.*

chordal (kor′dal) pertaining to any chorda or cord.

chordectomy (kor-dek′to-me) [L. *chorda* cord + Gr. *ektomē* excision] excision of a cord, particularly a vocal cord.

chorditis (kor-di′tis) [L. *chorda* cord + *-itis*] inflammation of a cord, such as a vocal cord.

chorea (ko-re′ah) [L.; Gr. *choreia* dance] the occurrence of involuntary but well-coordinated jerky, rapid, and complex movements. **diaphragmatic c.,** laryngeal c. **laryngeal c.,** the utterance of a peculiar cry in cases of painless tic. Called also *diaphragmatic c.* and *Schrötter's c.* **Schrötter's c.,** laryngeal c.

chorion (ko′re-on) [Gr.] 1. in human embryology, the cellular outermost fetal membrane, composed of trophoblast lined with mesoderm. It develops villi about 2 weeks after fertilization of the ovum, is vascularized by allantoic vessels a week later, gives rise to the placenta, and persists until birth. Called also *chorionic sac.* See illustration at fetal membranes, under MEMBRANE. 2. in mammalian embryology, the cellular outermost fetal membrane, not necessarily developing villi. 3. in biology, the noncellular membrane covering eggs of various animals, including fish and insects.

chorionic (ko″re-on′ik) pertaining to the chorion.

choroid (ko′roid) [*chorion* + Gr. *eidos* form] the thin, dark brown, vascular coat investing the posterior five-sixths of the eyeball.

choroiditis (ko″roid-i′tis) [*choroid* + *-itis*] inflammation of the choroid.

Chotzen, F. [German psychiatrist] see Saethre-Chotzen SYNDROME.

CHP comprehensive health planning.

c-hr curie-hour.

Christ-Siemens-Touraine syndrome [J. *Christ,* German dentist; Hermann Werner *Siemens,* German dermatologist, born 1891; Henri *Touraine,* French dermatologist, 1883–1961] hypohydrotic ectodermal DYSPLASIA.

Christensen articulator [Carl *Christensen,* Danish dentist, 19th and 20th centuries] see under ARTICULATOR.

Christian, Henry Asbury [American physician, 1876–1951] see Hand-Schüller-Christian DISEASE.

Christian's syndrome [J. C. *Christian*] see under SYNDROME.

Christmas disease, factor [*Christmas,* the family name of the first patient with the disease who was studied in detail] see under DISEASE, and see FACTOR IX.

chrom- see CHROMO-.

chromaffin (kro-maf′in) [*chrom-* + L. *affinis* having affinity for] taking up and staining strongly with chromium salts; said of certain cells.

Chromargyre trademark for *merbromin.*

chromatid (kro′mah-tid) either of the two parallel strands joined at the centromere which make up a chromosome and which separate in cell division, each going to a different pole of the dividing cell and each becoming a chromosome of one of the two daughter cells.

chromatin (kro′mah-tin) [Gr. *chrōma* color] a substance in the cell nucleus having characteristic staining properties. It is a combination of DNA with histones and other proteins and serves as a carrier of genetic materials and information. In dividing cells, chromatin is condensed into elongated structures (euchromatin), being the interphase form of the chromosomes; in cells not in division, it is condensed (heterochromatin) into irregular clumps known as *karyosomes.* **sex c.,** the persistent mass formed by the X chromosome which is inactive in the metabolism of cells, appearing as a planoconvex, pyramidal, or spheroidal intranuclear body, usually at the periphery of the interphase nucleus just inside the nuclear envelope. Normal females have sex chromatin, hence they are chromatin-positive, whereas normal males lack it, hence they are chromatin-negative. Called also *Barr body.* See also Lyon HYPOTHESIS.

chromato- [Gr. *chrōma, chrōmatos* color] 1. a combining form denoting relationship to chromatin. 2. see CHROMO-.

chromatography (kro″mah-tog′rah-fe) [*chromato-* + Gr. *graphein* to write] a method of separating and identifying the components of a complex mixture by differential movement through a two-phase system, in which the movement is effected by a flow of a liquid or a gas (mobile phase) which percolates through an adsorbent (stationary phase) or a second liquid phase, based on the physicochemical principles of adsorption, partition, ion exchange, or exclusion, or a combination of these principles. Chromatographic techniques may be classified according to the nature of the adsorbent employed, the physical characteristics of the mobile and stationary phases, or the type of technique employed. **affinity c.,** immobilization of antibody or antigen to an insoluble matrix onto which has been coupled the complementary binding substance. For example, Au antibody coupled onto a matrix can selectively bind from a mixture the specific antigen complementary to it. **filter paper c.,** paper c. **gas c.,** that in which an inert gas is used to move the vapors of the materials to be separated through a column of inert material. **gas-liquid c.,** that in which the substances to be separated are moved by an inert gas along a long tube filled with a finely divided inert solid

coated with a nonvolatile oil; each component migrates at a rate determined by its solubility in oil and its vapor pressure. **paper c.,** that in which a sheet of blotting paper, usually filter paper, is substituted for the adsorption column. After separation of the components as a consequence of their differential migratory velocities, they are stained to make the chromatogram visible. Called also *filter paper c.* **partition c.,** a form of separation of solutes utilizing the partition of the solutes between two liquid phases, namely, the original solvent and the film of solvent on the adsorption column. **thin-layer c.,** chromatography through a thin layer of inert material, such as cellulose.

chromatophil (kro′mah-to-fil″) [*chromato-* + Gr. *philein* to love] a cell or element that stains easily.

chromatophore (kro′mah-to-fōr″) [*chromato-* + Gr. *pherein* to bear] any pigment cell or color-producing plastid, such as those of the cutis or deep layers of the epidermis. See also MELANOPHORE.

chrome (krōm) 1. a chromium-plated alloy. 2. a chromium-containing pigment. **c. green, c. ocher, c. oxide,** chromic OXIDE.

chromic (kro′mik) pertaining to or containing trivalent chromium, Cr≡.

chromium (kro′me-um) [L.; Gr. *chrōma* color] a steel-gray, lustrous metallic element. Symbol, Cr; atomic number, 24; atomic weight, 51.996; melting point 1900°C; specific gravity, 7.18; valences, 2, 3, 6; group VIB of the periodic table. Chromium has four naturally occurring isotopes and several artificial radioactive ones (46–49, 51, 55, 56), ^{51}Cr (gamma rays), being the longest-living with a half-life of 26.5 days. It is used in chrome-steel and chrome-nickel-steel alloys. The isotope ^{51}Cr is used as a radioactive tracer in the determination of blood volume, blood cell life, cardiac output, and other diagnostic and research procedures; it is a radioactive poison. Inhalation of chromium dust may cause a toxic reaction. **c.-cobalt alloy,** cobalt-chrome ALLOY. **cobalt-c.-nickel alloy,** cobalt-chromium-nickel ALLOY. **c.-iron alloy,** stainless STEEL. **nickel-c. alloy,** nickel-chromium ALLOY. **c. steel,** stainless STEEL. **c. trioxide,** chromic ACID (2).

chromo-, chrom-, chromato- [Gr. *chrōma, chrōmatos* color] a combining form denoting relationship to color.

Chromobacterium (kro″mo-bak-te′re-um) [*chromo-* + Gr. *baktērion* little rod] a genus of gram-negative, aerobic or facultatively anaerobic bacteria of uncertain affiliation, which characteristically produce a violet pigment that is soluble in alcohol but not in water or chloroform. They are usually found in soil and water in tropical countries, and sometimes produce pyogenic or septicemic infections in animals, including man.

chromocenter (kro′mo-sen″ter) 1. karyosome. 2. a fused mass of heterochromatin with spokelike extensions of euchromatin, representing the chromosomes in the salivary glands of some insects.

chromoflavine (kro″mo-fla′vin) acriflavine.

chromogen (kro′mo-jen) [*chromo-* + Gr. *gennan* to produce] any substance that may give origin to a coloring matter.

chromogenesis (kro″mo-jen′ĕ-sis) [*chromo-* + Gr. *genesis* production] the formation of pigments or colors.

chromogenic (kro″mo-jen′ik) producing a pigment or coloring matter.

chromomere (kro′mo-mēr) [*chromo-* + Gr. *meros* part] 1. any one of the beadlike granules of chromatin composing a chromosome. 2. granulomere.

chromonema (kro″mo-ne′mah), pl. *chromone′mata* [*chromo-* + Gr. *nēma* thread] a central threadlike core of the chromosone, bearing the genes which are arranged in a string, each gene occupying a specific location, the locus. See also GENOME.

chromonemata (kro″mo-ne′mah-tah) plural of *chromonema.*

chromophil (kro′mo-fil) [*chromo-* + Gr. *philein* to love] any cell, structure, or tissue that is easily stainable.

chromophobe (kro′mo-fōb) [*chromo-* + Gr. *phobein* to be affrighted by] 1. a cell or a histological structure which does not stain readily. 2. a cell of the anterior pituitary characterized by small size, a small ovoid nucleus containing dense chromatin, a scant and apparently agranular cytoplasm, and generally indistinct outlines.

chromoprotein (kro″mo-pro′te-in, kro″mo-pro′tēn) [*chromo-* + *protein*] a conjugated protein having a colored prosthetic group, usually a metal. Hemoglobin is the principal chromoprotein.

chromosome (kro′mo-sōm) [*chromo-* + Gr. *sōma* body] 1. in animal cells, a readily-stainable, rod-shaped organelle in the nuclei of dividing cells, which stores and transmits genetic

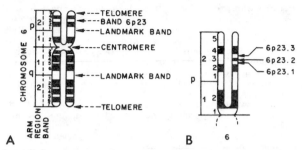

A, Diagrammatic representation of chromosome 6 in metaphase. B, Diagrammatic representation of chromosome 6 in an earlier stage of mitosis illustrating the presence of subbands in 6p23. (From J. J. Yunis: New Chromosomal Syndromes. New York, Academic Press, 1977.)

information. It is formed by condensed chromatin coiled into spiral filaments (chromatids) joined more or less in the center by the centromere, its location varying in different chromosomes, to form an irregular X. The DNA on the framework of protein associated with RNA and histones are its chief components. The lengths of DNA strands constituting the genes, or units of heredity, are arranged in a linear order, each gene having its precise location, or locus (see illustration at DNA). Replication of chromosomes results in the production of daughter chromosomes and each daughter cell in cell division has the same complement of genetic information as the parent cell. A specific chromosomal constitution (the karyotype), having the same number of chromosomes and the same length, shape, and

sequence of genes, is characteristic of each animal species. In man there are 46 chromosomes, including 22 pairs alike in males and females (autosomes) and a pair of sex chromosomes which differ in males and females (see X c. and Y c.). The human chromosomes are identified and classified on the basis of the size and centromere location, according to the rules of the Denver nomenclature (see c. nomenclature, Denver and illustration), each pair having been assigned a number from 1 to 23 and the entire complement having been divided into seven groups identified by letters A through G. See also c. nomenclature. 2. in bacterial cells, a closed circle of double-stranded DNA that contains the genetic material of the cell and is attached to the cell membrane. **c. aberration,** any deviation from the normal chromosome number or the structure of a chromosome, including aneuploidy. Called also c. abnormality. See c. abberation, numerical and c. abberation, structural, and see table. **c. aberration, numerical,** a deviation in the number of chromosomes, occurring chiefly through the failure of paired chromosomes to disjoin at anaphase either in a mitotic or meiotic division (nondisjunction). See also ANEUPLOIDY and DIPLOIDY. **c. aberration, structural,** any abnormal structure of a chromosome, including deletion, duplication, inversion, translocation, or an isochromosome. **c. abnormality,** c. aberration. **acentric c.,** see DELETION (2). **acrocentric c.,** one having the centromere in a quasi-terminal position and thus having exaggerately long and short arms. Called also I-shaped. **c. arm,** either of the two segments of the chromosome separated by the centromere. The arms are equal in length when the centromere is in the median position; they are of unequal length when the centromere is off-center. The symbol p indicates the short arm of the chromosome, and q the long arm. See also acrocentric c., metacentric c., and submetacentric c. **c. band,** see chromosome BAND. **c. banding,** chromosome BANDING. **daughter c.,** a chromatid when it reaches the pole of the cell in the anaphase stage of mitosis. **deletion c.,** see DELETION (2). **derivative c. (der),** see c. nomenclature. **dicentric c.,** a chromosome or its

TABLE OF CHROMOSOMAL ABERRATIONS

Chromosomal Aberration	Syndrome
chromosome 4, partial deletion of short arm chromosome 4p deletion chromosome 4p syndrome	Wolf-Hirschhorn SYNDROME
chromosome 4p trisomy	4p TRISOMY
chromosome 4, partial trisomy of long arm partial chromosome 4q trisomy	4q TRISOMY
chromosome 5p duplication	TRISOMY 5p
chromosome 7, partial duplication of long arm partial chromosome 7q duplication partial chromosome 7q trisomy	7q TRISOMY
chromosome 8 trisomy syndrome trisomy 8 mosaicism	TRISOMY 8
chromosome 8 trisomy due to distal segment of long arm	Warkang's SYNDROME
chromosome 8p deletion syndrome	see under SYNDROME
chromosome 9 syndrome	see under SYNDROME
chromosome 9 trisomy mosaicism	TRISOMY 9 mosaicism
chromosome 9 ring syndrome	see under SYNDROME
chromosome 9p monosomy	9p MONOSOMY
chromosome 9 trisomy syndrome	TRISOMY 9
chromosome 9p trisomy syndrome	9p TRISOMY
partial chromosome 9q trisomy syndrome	9q TRISOMY
chromosome 9p tetrasomy chromosome 9, tetrasomy of short arm	9p TETRASOMY
chromosome 9p syndrome	see under SYNDROME
chromosome 10, short arm deletion syndrome chromosome 10p deletion	see under SYNDROME
chromosome 10, duplication of short arm syndrome partial chromosome 10p duplication	10p TRISOMY
chromosome 10, duplication of long arm syndrome chromosome 10q duplication	10q TRISOMY
chromosome 10 trisomy	Cockayne's SYNDROME
chromosome 11, partial duplication of short arm partial chromosome 11p duplication	11p TRISOMY
chromosome 11, partial duplication of long arm partial chromosome 11q duplication	11q TRISOMY

longitudinal subunits (chromatids or subchromatids) having two centromeres. Dicentric chromosomes are produced directly or through asymmetrical reciprocal translation prior to replication of the chromosomes in the interphase nucleus. Abbreviated *dic.* **female sex c.,** X c. **gametic c.,** one in a haploid cell (gamete) consisting of a double strand of DNA. **homologous c.,** one of a matching pair in the diploid complement that contains the alleles of specific genes. **I-shaped c.,** acrocentric c. **J-shaped c.,** submetacentric c. **male sex c.,** Y c. **marker c. (mar),** see genetic MARKER and *c. nomenclature.* **metacentric c.,** one having the centromere located medially and thus having arms of about equal length. Called also *V-shaped.* **c. nomenclature,** the nomenclature recommended by the Chicago Conference in 1966 (Chicago nomenclature) and modified by the Paris Conference in 1971 (Paris nomenclature) for the identification of chromosomal bands and regions and for the location of structural chromosomal abnormalities. Bands and regions are designated through a code consisting of the following elements: the chromosome number, a symbol for the arm (p = short arm, q = long arm), and the region and band number. Sub-bands are identified by numbers following a decimal point after the original band designation. Designations for chromosomal abnormalities consist of the number of chromosomes, followed by the sex chromosome constitution, the symbol representing the abnormality, the numbers of involved chromosomes in the first parentheses, and the band composition in the second parentheses. According to the Chicago nomenclature, the designation 46,XY,t(2;6)(q34;p12) indicates a karyotype of 46 chromosomes, male, a reciprocal translation involving chromosome 2, region 3, band 4, and in the short arm of chromosome 6, region 1, band 2. The Paris nomenclature provides for detailed genetic information. A case in which a son received from his father the abnormal chromosome 2 and a normal chromosome 6, his karyotype would be designated as follows: 46,XY,der(2)t(2;6) (q34;p12)pat, indicating a karyotype of 46 chromosomes, an XY sex complement, abnormality in chromosome 2, being derived

from a balanced translation in the father that involved chromosomes 2 and 6 with the indicated break point. The boy has a partial trisomy for a segment of the short arm of chromosome 6 (from band 6p12 to 6pter, attached to the long arm of chromosome 2) and a monosomy for part of the long arm of chromosome 2 (from band 2q34 to 2qter, absent in the derivative chromosome 2, and attached, in the father, to the short arm of derivative chromosome 6). See *Table of Chromosomal Aberrations* and table of *Nomenclature Symbols.* See also chromosome BANDING. **c. nomenclature, Chicago,** genetic nomenclature recommended at the Chicago Conference in 1966. See *c. nomenclature* and table of *Nomenclature Symbols.* **c. nomenclature, Denver,** the classification of human chromosomes on the basis of size and centromere position, adopted in 1960 at a meeting of human geneticists in Denver, Colorado. See *c. nomenclature,* and see illustration. **c. nomenclature, Paris,** genetic nomenclature recommended at the Paris Conference in 1971. See *c. nomenclature* and table of *Nomenclature Symbols.* **Philadelphia c.,** a translocation involving the long arm of chromosome 22, usually to the long arm of chromosome 9, found in the megakaryocytic, granulocytic, and erythrocytic cells lines, but not in lymphoid elements of patients with chronic myelogenous leukemia. **ring c.,** a chromosome in which both ends have been lost (deletion) and the two broken ends have reunited to form a ring-shaped figure. Abbreviated *r.* **satellite c.,** satellite (3). **sex c.,** chromosomes that are associated with the determination of sex, in mammals constituting an equal pair, called the X and the Y chromosomes. See *X c.* and *Y c.* **submetacentric c.,** one having the centromere located in an eccentric or submedial location and thus having arms of different lengths. Called also *J-shaped c.* **V-shaped c.,** metacentric c. **X c.,** the female sex chromosome, being the differential sex

TABLE OF CHROMOSOMAL ABERRATIONS *(Continued)*

Chromosomal Aberration	Syndrome
chromosome 11, partial deletion of long arm partial chromosome 11q deletion	chromosome 11q SYNDROME, partial deletion
chromosome 12p monosomy syndrome partial chromosome 12p monosomy	chromosome 12p SYNDROME, partial deletion
chromosome 12p trisomy syndrome	12p TRISOMY
chromosome 13 syndrome trisomy 13 syndrome trisomy 13 trisomy D₁	Patau's SYNDROME
chromosome 13, partial deletion syndrome	see under SYNDROME
chromosome 13 ring syndrome chromosome D₁₃ ring syndrome	see under SYNDROME
chromosome 14, partial duplication of long arm	14q TRISOMY
chromosome 15, partial duplication of long arm	15q TRISOMY
chromosome 18, supernumerary isochromosome syndrome	see under SYNDROME
chromosome 18 syndrome chromosome E trisomy	TRISOMY 18
chromosome 18p deletion syndrome	chromosome 18p SYNDROME
chromosome 18q syndrome	see under SYNDROME
chromosome 18q deletion syndrome	see under SYNDROME
chromosome 19, duplication of long arm	TRISOMY 19q
chromosome 20 trisomy	TRISOMY 20
chromosome 20p, partial duplication syndrome chromosome 20p trisomy	20p TRISOMY
chromosome 21 trisomy	Down's SYNDROME
chromosome 21q syndrome	see under SYNDROME
chromosome 21q deletion syndrome	
chromosome 21 ring	dysplasia-epilepsy SYNDROME
chromosome 22 trisomy chromosome G₁ trisomy	TRISOMY 22
XXXX chromosome	XXXX SYNDROME
XXXXX chromosome	XXXXX SYNDROME

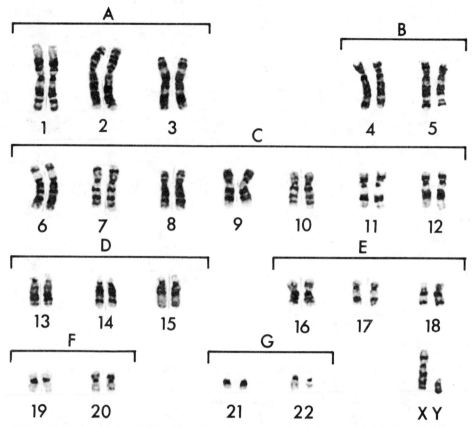

Normal male karyotype with Giemsa banding ("G banding"). The chromosomes are individually labeled, and the seven groups A to G are indicated. (From J. S. Thompson and M. W. Thompson: Genetics in Medicine. 3rd ed. Philadelphia, W. B. Saunders Co., 1980; photomicrograph courtesy of R. G. Worton.)

chromosome carried by half the male gametes and all female gametes in man and other male-heterogametic species; the female gamete is XX and male XY. See also Lyon HYPOTHESIS, X-linked dominant CHARACTER, and X-linked recessive CHARACTER. **c. XXXXY syndrome,** see Klinefelter's SYNDROME. **c. XXXY syndrome,** see Klinefelter's SYNDROME. **XXY syndrome,** see Klinefelter's SYNDROME. **c. XXYY syndrome,** see Klinefelter's SYNDROME. **Y c.,** the male sex chromosome, being the differential sex chromosome carried by half the male gametes and none of the female gametes in man and in some other male-heterogametic species in which the homologue of the X chromosome has been retained; the female gamete is XX and the male XY. See also holandric INHERITANCE and sex-linked CHARACTER.

chromous (kro'mus) pertaining to or containing divalent chromium, Cr=.

chron- see CHRONO-.

chronic (kron'ik) [L. *chronicus,* from Gr. *chronos* time] of long duration; occurring over a long period of time, as opposed to acute, which occurs over a short period of time.

chronicity (kro-nis'ĭ-te) the quality of being chronic.

chrono-, chron- [Gr. *chronos* time] a combining form denoting relationship to time.

chronobiology (kron″o-bi-ol'o-je) [*chrono-* + Gr. *bios* life + *-logy*] the scientific study of mechanisms of biologic time structure, including rhythmic manifestations of life. See also PERIODICITY and RHYTHM.

chryso- [Gr. *chrysos* gold] a combining form indicating relationship to gold.

chrysoderma (kris″o-der'mah) [*chryso-* + Gr. *derma* skin] aurochromoderma.

chrysotherapy (kris″o-ther'ah-pe) [*chryso-* + *therapy*] treatment with gold or its salts.

CHSS Cooperative Health Statistics System; see under SYSTEM.

churus (chur'us) hashish.

Chvostek's sign [Franz *Chvostek,* Austrian physician, 1835–1884] Chvostek-Weiss SIGN.

Chvostek-Weiss sign [F. *Chvostek;* Nathan *Weiss,* Austrian physician, 1851–1883] see under SIGN.

chyle (kīl) [L. *chylus* juice] lymph from the thoracic duct, having a milky appearance because of a high fat content, usually 5 to 15 percent.

chylomicron (ki″lo-mi'kron) a droplet consisting of colloidal particles composed of triglycerides, cholesterol, phospholipids, and proteins, found in the intestinal lymphatic system and blood after meals and having a half-life of 10 to 15 minutes. Chylomicrons are responsible for transporting lipids from the intestine to the liver, muscles, and adipose tissue. They are believed to be synthesized in the intestine and exhibit α_2 electrophoretic mobility. The turbidity of plasma in postalimentary hyperlipemia is due to the presence of chylomicrons in the blood. Particles found in hyperlipemic plasma in diabetic acidosis, also referred to as *chylomicrons,* are believed to be chemically different from chylomicrons in postprandial hyperlipemia. See also blood TURBIDITY, HYPERCHYLOMICRONEMIA, and LIPID metabolism.

chylothorax (ki″lo-tho'raks) [*chyle* + Gr. *thōrax* chest] the presence of chyle in the thoracic cavity, due to puncture of the thoracic duct and effusion of chyle. Called also *chylous hydrothorax.*

chymotrypsin [E.C.3.4.21.1] (ki″mo-trip'sin) a serine proteinase that catalyzes the hydrolysis of proteins to peptones, polypeptides, and amino acids by breaking the peptide linkages of the carboxyl groups of hydrophobic amino acids, preferentially tyrosine, tryptophan, phenylalanine, and leucine. Chymotrypsins A and B have similar specificity. The enzyme is produced in the form of inactive chymotrypsinogen by the acinous cells of the pancreas, and carried by the pancreatic juice into the duodenum where it is activated by trypsin. Once in the duodenum, chymotrypsin is involved in digesting food proteins. Chymotrypsin extracted from the animal pancreas is used thera-

CHROMOSOME NOMENCLATURE SYMBOLS

Chicago Conference

A–G	the chromosome groups
1–22	the autosome numbers
X, Y	the sex chromosomes
diagonal (/)	separates cell lines in describing mosaicism
?	questionable identification of chromosome or chromosome structure
*	chromosome explained in text or footnote
ace	acentric
cen	centromere
dic	dicentric
end	endoreduplication
h	secondary constriction or negatively staining region
i	isochromosome
inv	inversion
mar	marker chromosome
mat	maternal origin
p	short arm of chromosome
pat	paternal origin
q	long arm of chromosome
r	ring chromosome
s	satellite
t	translocation
repeated symbols	duplication of chromosome structure

Paris Conference

A. Recommended changes in Chicago Conference nomenclature

+   1. The + and − signs should be placed *before* the appropriate symbol where they mean additional or missing whole chromosomes.
−   They should be placed *after* a symbol where an increase or decrease in length is meant. Increases or decreases in the length of secondary constrictions, or negatively staining regions, should be distinguished from increases or decreases in length owing to other structural alterations by placing the symbol h between the symbol for the arm and the + or − sign (e.g., 16qh+).
    2. All symbols for rearrangements are to be placed before the designation of the chromosome(s) involved in the rearrangement, and the rearranged chromosome(s) always should be placed in parentheses, e.g., r(18), i(Xq), dic(Y).

B. Recommended additional nomenclature symbols

del	deletion
der	derivative chromosome
dup	duplication
ins	insertion
inv ins	inverted insertion
rcp	reciprocal translocation*
rec	recombinant chromosome
rob	Robertsonian translocation* ("centric fusion")
tan	tandem translocation*
ter	terminal or end ("pter" for end of short arm; "qter" for end of long arm)
:	break (no reunion, as in terminal deletion)
::	break and join
→	from − to

*Optional, where greater precision is desired than that provided by the use of t as recommended by the Chicago Conference.

(From G. G. Yunis: New Chromosomal Symbols. New York: Academic Press, 1977.)

peutically as a proteolytic enzyme. It also has esterase activity. **c. A,** see *chymotrypsin.* **c. B,** see *chymotrypsin.* **c. C,** a form of chymotrypsin that cleaves polypeptides preferentially at leucine, tyrosine, phenamine, methionine, tryptophan, glutamine, and asparagine residues.

chymotrypsinogen (ki-mo-trip-sin′o-jen) [*chymotrypsin* + Gr. *gennan* to produce] a precursor of chymotrypsin, produced in an inactive form by the acinous cells of the pancreas, and is activated by trypsin in the duodenum.

Ci curie.

Cib. abbreviation for L. *cibus,* food.

Cibazol trademark for *sulfathiazole.*

Ciberon trademark for *carbinoxamine maleate* (see under CAR-BINOXAMINE).

cicatrices (sik-ah-tri′sēz) [L.] plural of *cicatrix.*

cicatricial (sik″ah-trish′al) pertaining to or of the nature of a cicatrix.

cicatrix (sik-a′triks; sik′ah-triks), pl. *cicatri′ces* [L.] a new tissue which is formed in the healing of a wound; a scar. **Parrot's c's,** Parrot's scars; see under SCAR.

cicatrization (sik″ah-tri-za′shun) a healing process occurring through the formation of scar tissue and consequent excessive collgenization, resulting in the production of a cicatrix. Called also *epulosis.*

cicutine (sik′u-tēn) coniine.

Cidal trademark for *salicylamide.*

Cidex trademark for *glutaraldehyde.*

Cidomycin trademark for *gentamicin sulfate* (see under GEN-TAMICIN).

Cidrex trademark for *hydrochlorothiazide.*

Cieszynski's rule of isometry [Polish engineer] bisecting angle TECHNIQUE.

cilia (sil′e-ah) [L.] plural of *cilium.*

ciliated (sil′e-āt″ed) provided with cilia or with a fringe of hairs.

Ciliophora (sil″e-of′o-rah) a subphylum of protozoa characterized by the presence of cilia during some stage of development and usually possessing two kinds of nuclei (a micronucleus and a macronucleus). Most species are free-living but some are parasitic. Called also *Infusoria.*

cilium (sil′e-um), pl. *cil′ia* [L.] 1. an eyelid or its outer edge. 2. [pl.] [NA] the hairs growing on the edges of the eyelids. Called also *eyelashes.* 3. a minute vibratile, hairlike process projecting from the free surface of a cell, e.g., certain epithelial cells. Cilia beat rhythmically to move the cell or to move fluid or mucous films over the cell surface. Cf. FLAGELLUM.

Cillenta trademark for *penicillin G benzathine* (see under PENI-CILLIN).

Cilleral trademark for *ampicillin sodium* (see under AMPICIL-LIN).

Cillobacterium (sil″lo-bak-te′re-um) a genus made up of non-sporulating, aerobic, gram-positive bacilli formerly considered as a taxonomic unit; its species have been assigned to the genus

Eubacterium. **C. spatulifor′me, C. te′nue,** *Eubacterium tenue;* see under EUBACTERIUM.

CIM Cumulated Index Medicus; see under INDEX.

Cincaine trademark for *dibucaine hydrochloride (see under* DIBUCAINE).

Cinchocaine trademark for *dibucaine hydrochloride* (see under DIBUCAINE).

Cinchona (sin-ko′nah) [named after a countess of *Chincon*] a genus of rubiaceous trees, all natives of South America, the source of quinoline alkaloids, quinine, quinidine, cinchonine, and cinchonidine.

cinchonidine (sin-ko′nĭ-dēn) an alkaloid from the bark of the plant *Cinchona,* (8α,9R)-cinchonan-9-ol, occurring as a white crystalline powder. Used in the treatment of malaria.

cinchonine (sin′ko-nēn) an alkaloid from the bark of the plant *Cinchona,* (9S)-cinchonan-9-ol, occurring as white, crystalline crystals with a bitter taste. Used in the treatment of malaria.

cinchophen (sin′ko-fen) an analgesic, 2-phenyl-4-quinolinecarboxylic acid, occurring as white, odorless, slightly bitter needles that turn yellow on exposure to light and are soluble in chloroform, ether, and ethanol, but not in water. Used in the treatment of gout. Seldom used because of its ability to produce sometimes fatal toxic hepatitis. Called also *2-phenylcinchoninic acid.* Trademarks: Alutyl, Atocin, Atophan.

cinefluorography (sin″e-floo′or-og′rah-fe) cineradiography.

cinematography (sin″e-mah-tog′rah-fe) cineradiography.

cinematoradiography (sin″e-mah-to-ra″de-og′rah-fe) cineradiography.

cinemicrography (sin″e-mi-krog′rah-fe) the making of the successive images with the use of a motion picture camera of a small object through the lens system of a microscope.

cineole (sin′e-ol) eucalyptol.

cineradiography (sin″e-ra″de-og′rah-fe) the making of the successive images appearing on a fluoroscopic screen with the use of a motion picture camera. Called also *cinefluorography, cinematography, cinematoradiography, cineroentgenofluorography,* and *cineroentgenography.*

cineroentgenofluorography (sin″e-rent″gen-o-floo″or-og′rah-fe) cineradiography.

cineroentgenography (sin″e-rent″gen-og′rah-fe) cineradiography.

cinesi- see KINESI-.

cineto- see KINETO-.

cingula (sin′gu-lah) [L.] plural of *cingulum.*

cingule (sin′gul) cingulum.

cingulum (sin′gu-lum), pl. *cin′gula* [L. "girdle"] 1. a girdle, belt, or band that encircles a structure or part. Called also *cingule* and *girdle.* 2. a bundle of association fibers that partly encircles the corpus callosum. 3. the lingual lobe of an anterior tooth, making the bulk of the cervical third of its lingual surface. Called also *basal ridge, linguocervical ridge,* and *linguogingival ridge.*

cinnamate (sĭ-nam′āt) a salt of cinnamic acid. Used to screen out ultraviolet rays in preventing injuries of the lips by sunlight.

cinnamene (sin′ah-mēn) styrene.

cinnamic (sĭ-nam′ik) of or relating to cinnamon or cinnamic acid.

cinnomol (sin′ah-mōl) styrene.

CIOMS Council for International Organizations of Medical Sciences.

cion- [Gr. *kiōn* uvula] a combining form denoting relationship to the uvula.

cionitis (si″o-ni′tis) [*cion-* + *-itis*] uvulitis.

cionoptosis (si″on-op-to′sis) [*cion-* + Gr. *ptōsis* a falling] uvuloptosis.

cionorrhaphy (si″o-nor′ah-fe) [*cion-* + Gr. *raphē* suture] staphylorrhaphy.

cionotomy (si″o-not′o-me) [*cion-* + Gr. *tomē* cutting] uvulotomy.

Cipractin trademark for *cyproheptadine hydrochloride* (see under CYPROHEPTADINE).

circadian (ser″kah-de′an) [L. *circa* about + *dies* a day] pertaining to a period of about 24 hours. Applied especially to the rhythmic repetition of certain phenomena in living organisms at about the same time each day (circadian rhythm). For example, the level of circulating eosinophils in man peaks about 10 AM. The terms *circadian* and *diurnal,* which applies to activities during the daytime, are often used interchangeably.

circinate (ser′sĭ-nāt) resembling a ring or circle.

circle (ser′k′l) [L. *circulus*] a round figure, structure, or part. **centigrade c.,** a circle divided into 100°; used in Black's formula for measuring the angle of the blade and cutting edge in handcutting dental instruments. See illustration at DENTISTRY.

circuit (ser′kit) [L. *circuitus*] the path of an electric current in a system. **broken c., open c. closed c.,** a continuous circuit, allowing the current to pass through. **filament c., heating c.,** the circuit which supplies power to the heating filament of an x-ray tube. **interrupted c.,** open c. **open c.,** a circuit having a break in it so that the current cannot pass through it. Called also *broken c.,* and *interrupted c.* **primary c.,** the circuit which, in an x-ray generator, provides power to the autotransformer. **secondary c.,** the circuit which, in an x-ray generator, supplies power from the autotransformer for the production of x-rays. **short c.,** a usually unintentional condition existing when a conductor in a circuit establishes contact short of the terminal with another conductor, thereby preventing the current from reaching its destination.

circular (ser″ku-lar) [L. *circularis*] shaped like a circle; occurring in a circle.

circulation (ser″ku-la′shun) [L. *circulatio*] a movement or flow, especially of liquids, through a closed system, whereby the circulating material returns to its point of origin and retraces its previous course time after time. In biology, if not otherwise stated, the term refers to the course of the blood in the cardiovascular system. **arterial c.,** see *systemic c.* **assisted c.,** pumping that assists the natural activity of the heart. **blood c.,** see *systemic c.* **cardiovascular c.,** systemic c. **collateral c., compensatory c.,** the flow of blood through secondary or collateral channels after obstruction of principal blood vessels. **coronary c.,** the blood supply to, and drainage from, the heart, excluding its chambers. The term is applied usually to the vessels of the myocardium. **extracorporeal c.,** the circulation of blood outside the body, as through a heart-lung machine for carbon dioxide–oxygen exchange, or through an artificial kidney for removal of substances usually excreted in the urine. See also artificial HEART and heart-lung MACHINE. **greater c.,** systemic c. **lesser c.,** pulmonary c. **lymph c.,** the flow of lymph in the lymphatic system, involving the lymphatic capillaries, lymphatic vessels, lymph nodes, thoracic duct, and right lymphatic duct. See also lymphatic SYSTEM. **portal c.,** the circulation of the blood from the gastrointestinal system and spleen through capillaries of the liver via the portal vein. **pulmonary c.,** that part of the systemic circulation in which the blood is pumped from the heart through the pulmonary arteries to discharge carbon dioxide, is reoxygenated in the lungs, and is returned to the heart through the pulmonary vein. Called also *lesser c.* **c. rate,** circulation RATE. **systemic c.,** the flow of the blood through the cardiovascular system. Considered to begin when the blood in the left ventricle of the heart is pumped into the aorta to be distributed into the major arterial trunks, from where it flows into individual arteries, arterioles, and capillaries to deliver a fresh supply of oxygen and nutrients to the tissues. The head and neck are supplied through the brachiocephalic trunk branching from the aorta. Two of the three main branches of the trunk are the two carotid arteries, each dividing into an internal and external branch. After completing the arterial phase, the blood passes into the venous circulation, consisting of a network of capillaries, which collect waste materials, including carbon dioxide, venules, veins, and the venae cavae. The head and neck are drained through the superior vena cava. The venous blood enters the heart through the right atrium, from where it is pumped into the right ventricle to enter the pulmonary circulation — first into the pulmonary artery and, after discharging carbon dioxide and reoxygenation in the lungs, into the pulmonary vein which delivers it back into the heart through the left atrium. From the left atrium, the freshly oxygenated blood is pumped into the left ventricle, ready to be recirculated. Called also *cardiovascular c., greater c.,* and *vascular c.* **c. time,** circulation TIME. **vascular c.,** systemic c. **venous c.,** see *systemic c.*

circulatory (ser″ku-lah-to″re) pertaining to the circulation.

circulus (ser′ku-lus), pl. *cir′culi* [L. " a ring"] a circle or circuit; used in anatomical nomenclature to designate such an arrangement, usually of arteries or veins.

circum- [L.] a prefix signifying around.

circumduction (ser″kum-duk′shun) [L. *circumducere* to draw around] a circular movement, such as one of the head of a bone in the socket of a joint.

circumference (ser-kum′fer-ens) [*circum-* + L. *ferre* to bear] the outer boundary or surface of a rounded body.

circumferential (ser″kum-fer-en′shal) pertaining to or forming a circumference.

circumflex (ser′kum-fleks) [L. *circumflexus* bent about] 1. bent or curved like a bow. 2. wandering about, said of vessels or nerves with a wandering course.

circumoral (ser″kum-o′ral) [circum- + L. os mouth] around or near the mouth.

circumorbital (ser″kum-or′bĭ-tal) [circum- + L. orbita orbit] situated around or occurring near an orbit.

circumscribed (ser′kum-skrībd) [circum- + L. scribere to write] having a definite contour; bounded or limited.

circumvallate (ser″kum-val′āt) [circum- + L. vallare to wall] surrounded by a trench or by a ridge, as the vallate papilla.

cire perdue (seer′ per-du′) [Fr. "lost wax"] disappearing CORE.

cirrhosis (sir-ro′sis) [Gr. kirrhos orange yellow] 1. liver c. 2. chronic interstitial inflammation of any organ. **alcoholic c.,** liver cirrhosis in chronic alcoholics, believed to result from nutritional disturbances and the hepatotoxic effects of ethyl alcohol, particularly abnormal accumulation of triglycerides in the parenchymal cells, resulting in degenerative changes. Abdominal distention, hepatomegaly, ascites, and other symptoms of liver cirrhosis are also typical of alcoholic cirrhosis. Enlargement of the parotid glands is common. **biliary c.,** liver cirrhosis due to obstruction of the biliary tract, often occurring as a complication of bile duct abnormalities, carcinoma of the pancreas and extrahepatic ducts, or biliary calculi. The clinical course includes particularly severe jaundice, steatorrhea, and fever, in addition to other symptoms of liver cirrhosis. **liver c.,** chronic interstitial inflammation of the liver characterized by fibrosis, necrosis, and regeneration of the parenchymal cells, associated with an increase in the connective tissue, giving the liver a nodular or granular texture. Symptoms include anorexia, nausea, vomiting, pain, portal hypertension with ascites, esophageal varices, hydrothorax, hepatosplenomegaly, gastrointestinal hemorrhages with hematemesis, endocrine complications, neurologic complications, hepatic coma, and jaundice. Oral manifestations consist chiefly of enlargement of the parotid glands. Called also *chronic interstitial hepatitis*. **pigmentary c.,** hemochromatosis.

cirso- [Gr. kirsos varix] a combining form denoting relationship to a varix.

cirsoid (ser′soid) [cirso- + Gr. eidos form] resembling a varix.

CI-S simplified calculus index; see oral hygiene index, simplified, under INDEX.

cis- [L. "on the same side"] 1. a prefix denoting on this side, on the same side, on the near side. 2. in organic chemistry, a form of geometric isomerism in which the hydrogen atoms attached to two carbon atoms with double bonds are substituted adjacently on the same side of the molecule. Usually written in italics and disregarded in alphabetization. See cis-ISOMER. 3. in genetics, having the two mutant genes of a pseudoallele on the same chromosome. Cf. TRANS-.

cistern (sis′tern) [L. cisterna] a closed space serving as a reservoir for fluid. Called also *cisterna* [NA].

cisterna (sis-ter′nah), pl. cister′nae [L.] a closed spaced serving as a reservoir for fluid; cistern. **c. chy′li** [NA], the lower, dilated part of the thoracic duct in the lumbar region; it receives lymph from the lower part of the body and the abdomen, including the lower extremities, lower thoracic walls, viscera of the pelvis, kidneys, adrenals, intestines, abdominal wall, stomach, pancreas, and visceral surface of the liver. Called also *receptaculum chyli*.

cisternae (sis-ter′ne) [L.] plural of *cisterna*.

cistron (sis′tron) [L. cis on this side + trans on the other side + Gr. on neuter ending] a unit of genetic activity, being the smallest unit of genetic material (DNA or RNA) capable of transmitting genetic information in determining the sequence of amino acids in protein synthesis. As classically conceived, cistron is approximately synonymous with gene.

Citànest trademark for *prilocaine hydrochloride* (see under PRILOCAINE).

Citelli's syndrome [Salvatore Citelli, Italian scientist, 1875–1947] see under SYNDROME.

Citexal trademark for *methaqualone*.

Citnatin trademark for *sodium citrate* (see under SODIUM).

Citobaryum trademark for *barium sulfate* (see under BARIUM).

citrate (sit′rāt, si′trāt) any salt of citric acid. The citrate ion is an intermediary in carbohydrate metabolism, most citrates (about 70 percent) being found in the bones, where they are believed to play a role in calcium metabolism. Citrates bind calcium in the blood, thus preventing conversion of prothrombin to thrombin in clot formation, and serve as anticoagulants. Some are used in the treatment of renal acidosis. Whole blood in blood banks is prevented from coagulating by addition of citrate solutions. In dentistry, citrates are used to retard the setting of dental stone and plaster. Some citrate preparations have irritating effects on the oral mucosa and may cause necrotic and ulcerative lesions. See also citric acid CYCLE. **sodium c.,** SODIUM citrate. **trisodium c.,** SODIUM citrate.

Citricon trademark for a *silicone impression material* (see under MATERIAL).

Citrobacter (sit″ro-bak′ter) [L. citrus lemon + Gr. baktērion little rod] a genus of gram-negative, facultatively anaerobic bacteria of the family Enterobacteriaceae, occurring as motile peritrichously flagellated, nonencapsulated rods, which are of uncertain pathogenicity. The organisms are found in the normal intestinal tract; in infections of the gastrointestinal tract, urogenital system, gallbladder, meninges, and middle ear; in the urine and feces; and in food and water. The genus includes the species *C. fruendii* and *C. intermedius*.

Citrosodine trademark for *sodium citrate* (see under SODIUM).

citrulline (sit′ru-lēn) an amino acid, 2-amino-5-ureidovaleric acid. It is an arginine derivative isolated from watermelon juice. **c. phosphorylase,** ornithine CARBAMOYLTRANSFERASE.

Civatte's disease [Achille Civatte, French dermatologist, 1877–1956] reticulated pigmented POIKILODERMA.

Civinini's canal, process of external pterygoid plate, spine [Filippo Civinini, Italian anatomist, 1805–1844] see CANALICULUS of chorda tympani and pterygospinous PROCESS.

C & L attachment (retainer, unit) see under ATTACHMENT.

Cl chlorine.

cl centiliter.

Cladothrix asteroides (klad′o-thriks as″ter-oi′dēz) Nocardia asteroides; see under NOCARDIA.

claim (klām) 1. to demand by or as one's due. 2. a request by an insurer for payment due under the terms of an insurance plan. 3. a request by an insured person for benefits due under the terms of the plan. In health insurance, the claim usually consists of a statement listing services rendered, dates of services, and itemization of costs. **E-Z c.,** superbill. **c's incurred policy,** claims incurred POLICY. **instant c.,** superbill. **c's made policy,** claims made POLICY. **c's review,** claims REVIEW.

claimant (kla′mant) one who makes a claim; a beneficiary under an insurance plan.

clamp (klamp) 1. any device used to grip, join, compress, or fasten parts. 2. a surgical instrument for effecting compression. See also clamp FORCEPS. 3. a device used to stabilize dentures or orthodontic appliances. **cervical c., gingival c. cotton roll rubber dam c.,** a rubber dam clamp with a buccal and lingual wing or flange to hold cotton rolls in position in the mouth. **Crile's c.,** a rubber-shod clamp used to secure temporary hemostasis in suture of blood vessels. **Ferrier 212 gingival c.,** a purposely unbalanced gingival clamp for retracting gingival tissue from the field of operation, which is stabilized in position with a modeling compound; used for gold foil insertion in restorative dentistry. **gingival c.,** one for retracting gingival tissue; used for gold foil insertion in restorative dentistry. Called also *cervical c.* **Hatch c.,** a rubber dam clamp used for retaining the rubber dam in operating on gingival third cavities, in all teeth except the molars. **Ivory c.,** trademark for a rubber dam clamp. **Joseph's c.,** one used after a nasal operation for aligning the mobilized fragments of the bony framework of the nose. **pedicle c.,** clamp FORCEPS (1). **root rubber dam c.,** one whose jaws are designed to fit on the root surface of a tooth; used for the retention of a rubber dam. **rubber dam c.,** a device made of spring metal that is used to retain the rubber dam on a tooth, having beveled jaws that contact the tooth and a bow that connects the jaws. The material used is either plated metal or stainless steel to resist corrosion. Clamps are available in various shapes to match most teeth, the winged and wingless types being the two basic varieties. **S.S.W. c., S.S. White c. S.S. White c.,** trademark for a rubber dam clamp. Called also *S.S.W. c.*

clams (klamz) actinomycosis.

Clapton's line copper LINE.

Clarissimus Galenus see GALEN.

Clark attachment [E. B. Clark, American dentist] see under ATTACHMENT.

Clark's rule 1. see under RULE (1). 2. [C. A. Clark] see under RULE (2).

-clasia [Gr. klasis breaking] a word termination denoting a degenerative or destructive condition, as in periodontoclasia.

clasmatocyte (klaz-mat′o-sīt) [Gr. klasma a piece broken off + kytos hollow vessel] previously used to designate branched cells in connective tissue that allegedly detach portions of their processes as a means of discharging their secretions. The term is now used for macrophages fixed along the bundles of collagen fibers of connective tissue. See MACROPHAGE.

clasp (klasp) 1. a device, usually of metal, which holds things together. 2. a part of an extracoronal direct retainer that retains

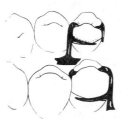

Half-and-half clasp. (From D. Henderson and V. L. Steffel: McCracken's Removable Partial Prosthodontics. 6th ed. St. Louis, The C. V. Mosby Co., 1981.)

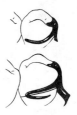

Reverse-action or hairpin clasp. (From D. Henderson and V. L. Steffel: McCracken's Removable Partial Prosthodontics. 6th ed. St. Louis, The C. V. Mosby Co., 1981.)

and stabilizes the denture by attaching it to the abutment teeth. It may be adapted about a tooth or in the embrassures of teeth or it may rest and surround the abutment teeth. See also extracoronal ATTACHMENT and extracoronal RETAINER. **c. No. 4,** trademark for a high noble metal dental wrought gold wire alloy. **c. No. 18,** trademark for a low noble metal dental wrought wire alloy. **Adams c.,** a formed wire clasp, of modified arrowhead design, utilizing the buccal, mesial, and distal proximal undercuts of a tooth for retention. See also *arrow c.* **Aderer No. 20 c.,** trademark for a high noble metal dental wrought gold wire alloy. **arrow c., arrowhead c.,** a clasp made by bending a single piece of stainless steel wire of high tensile strength in the shape of an arrowhead. It engages the mesial and distal proximal undercuts on the buccal aspects of adjacent teeth, and is used to stabilize an orthodontic appliance by taking hold or grasping the teeth in the interproximal areas. See also *Adams c.* **backaction c.,** one that originates on one surface of a tooth and traverses the suprabulge area to another surface, where it is supported by an occlusal rest; it then continues to encircle the tooth on the third surface, where it terminates in the infrabulge area beyond the opposite angle of the tooth surface where it originates. **bar c.,** one whose arms are bar-type extensions from major connectors or from within the denture base; the arms pass adjacent to the soft tissues and approach the point of contact on the tooth in the cervico-occlusal direction. Called also *Roach c.* See also bar clasp ARM. **cast c.,** one made of an alloy that has been cast into the desired form and that retains its crystalline structure. **circumferential c.,** one that encircles more than 180° of a tooth, including opposite angles, and usually contacts the tooth throughout the extent of the clasp, at least one terminal being in the infrabulge area (cervical convergence). See also *ring c.* and circumferential clasp ARM. **combination c.,** one that employs a wrought wire retentive arm and a cast reciprocal or stabilizing arm. **continuous c., continuous lingual c.,** one made of two or more stainless steel lingual clasps joined to each other and then joined to a major connector by two or more minor connectors. The clasp is used on the lingual lower anterior teeth, sometimes carried posteriorly to the bicuspids, and occasionally used on the upper anterior teeth for bracing. It is one of the earliest stressbreakers, whereby one arm supports the clasps and other components and the other supports and connects the distal extension bases. Called also *continuous bar rest, continuous bar retainer, continuous retainer, Kennedy bar,* and *lingual bar.* **Crozat c.,** a metal attachment of a removable appliance adapted to the embrassure. **embrassure c.,** one that passes through the embrassure, using two occlusal rests, clasping the two teeth with circumferential clasps that have a common body; used where no edentulous space exists. **formed c.,** wrought c. **c. guideline,** survey LINE (3). **hairpin c.,** reverse-action c. **half-and-half c.,** one consisting of a circumferential retentive arm arising from one direction and a reciprocal arm arising from another. See illustration. **infrabulge c.,** a bar clasp arm arising from the border of the base, either as an extension of a cast base or attached to the border of a resin base. **lingual c., continuous** continuous c. **mesiodistal c.,** one that embraces the distolingual and mesial surfaces of a tooth and takes its retention in either or both mesial and distal undercuts. **movable c., movable-arm c.,** a clasp whose arm is mounted in a spring-lock box, which allows adjustment of its tension. The movable-arm assembly may be made in acrylic resin base, with projecting portions of the

spring-lock finished flush with the resin base. **multiple c.,** one consisting of two opposing circumferential clasps joined at the terminal end of the two reciprocal arms. **reverse-action c.,** one in which one arm is circumferential, while on the other side, the arm is bent back to permit engaging a proximal undercut from an occlusal approach. Called also *hairpin c.* See illustration. **ring c.,** one with a long arm which encircles nearly all the circumference of the tooth, its free end almost reaching the point of origin. See also *circumferential c.* **Roach c.,** bar c. **wrought c.,** one made of an alloy that has been drawn into a wire, whereby the crystalline structure has been converted to one of a fibrous nature. Called also *formed c.*

class (klas) 1. a taxonomic category subordinate to a phylum (or subphylum) and superior to an order. 2. in statistics, a group of variables, all of which show a particular value or a value falling between certain limits. The frequency of class is the number of variables that it contains.

classic (klas′ik) of first class or rank; standard.

classification (kas′sĭ-fĭ-ka′shun) systematic arrangement into categories or classes according to common characteristics. **Ackerman-Proffit c.,** see under MALOCCLUSION. **American Cleft Palate Association c.,** see CLEFT palate. **Angle's c.,** see under MALOCCLUSION. **Bailyn's c.,** a method of classifying partially edentulous conditions and partial dentures, based on the location of the edentulous spaces in relation to the remaining teeth. See illustration. **Broders' c.,** Broders' INDEX. **caries c., cavity c.,** see dental CARIES. **chromosome c.,** CHROMOSOME nomenclature. **cleft palate c.,** see CLEFT palate. **enzyme c.,** ENZYME classification. **International c., (of blood groups),** Landsteiner's nomenclature of blood groups; see under BLOOD GROUP. **International C. of Diseases, Adapted,** a classification developed by the World Health Organization and adapted by the United States Public Health Service for use in the United States. It classifies diseases and operations for the purpose of indexing hospital records, diseases being grouped according to the problems they present, as in grouping together neoplastic or parasitic diseases. The three-digit code is used to number the disease categories, with subdivisions being numbered by a four-digit code. Abbreviated *ICDA.* **Kennedy c.,** a method of classifying partially edentulous conditions and partial dentures, based on the location of the edentulous spaces in relation to the remaining teeth. *Class I* — bilateral edentulous areas located posterior to the remaining teeth; *Class II* — a unilateral edentulous area located posterior to the remaining teeth; *Class III* — a unilateral edentulous area bounded by teeth anterior and posterior to the space; *Class IV* — an edentulous area located anterior to right and left remaining teeth and crossing the midline. See illustration. **Lansteiner's c. of blood groups,** Landsteiner's nomenclature of blood groups; see under BLOOD GROUP. **Papanicolaou's c.,** see Pap TEST. **Schwarz's c.,** a theoretical classification of the biological efficiency of orthodontic forces, based on the magnitude and duration of the force, but disregarding the histologic reactions. *First degree of efficiency:* forces below the threshold of stimulation required for actual orthodontic movement. *Second degree of efficiency:* forces causing orthodontic movement by continuous resorption of the alveolar bone in the pressure area, with concomitant apposition of bone in the areas of traction and without any root resorption. *Third degree of efficiency:* forces permanently interrupting the circulation of the periodontal ligament. *Fourth degree of efficiency:* forces of high magnitudes which mechanically destroy the periodontal ligament. **Skinner's c.,** a method of classifying partially edentulous conditions and partial dentures, based on the location of the edentulous spaces in relation to the remaining teeth. See illustration. **Stark c.,** see CLEFT palate. **Veau c.,** see CLEFT palate. **Wiener's c.,** see Rh blood groups, under BLOOD GROUP.

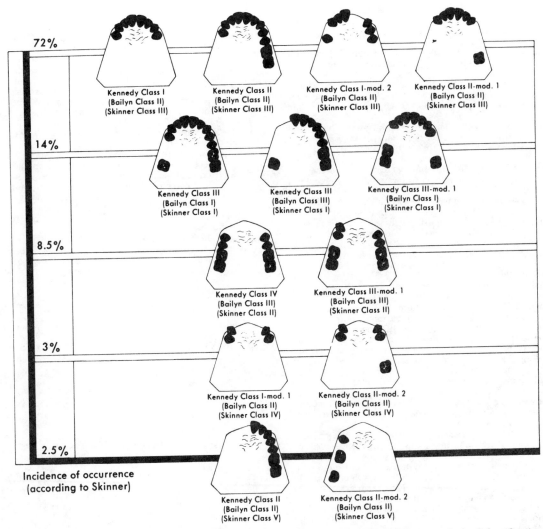

72%

Kennedy Class I
(Bailyn Class II)
(Skinner Class III)

Kennedy Class II
(Bailyn Class II)
(Skinner Class III)

Kennedy Class I-mod. 2
(Bailyn Class II)
(Skinner Class III)

Kennedy Class II-mod. 1
(Bailyn Class II)
(Skinner Class III)

14%

Kennedy Class III
(Bailyn Class I)
(Skinner Class I)

Kennedy Class III
(Bailyn Class III)
(Skinner Class I)

Kennedy Class III-mod. 1
(Bailyn Class I)
(Skinner Class I)

8.5%

Kennedy Class IV
(Bailyn Class III)
(Skinner Class II)

Kennedy Class III-mod. 1
(Bailyn Class III)
(Skinner Class II)

3%

Kennedy Class I-mod. 1
(Bailyn Class II)
(Skinner Class IV)

Kennedy Class II-mod. 2
(Bailyn Class II)
(Skinner Class IV)

2.5%

Incidence of occurrence
(according to Skinner)

Kennedy Class II
(Bailyn Class II)
(Skinner Class V)

Kennedy Class II-mod. 2
(Bailyn Class II)
(Skinner Class V)

Representative examples of partially edentulous arches classified by the Kennedy, Bailyn, and Skinner methods of classification. (From D. Henderson and V. L. Steffel: McCracken's Removable Partial Prosthodontics. 6th ed. St. Louis, The C. V. Mosby Co., 1981.)

Claude's syndrome [Henri *Claude,* French physician, 1869–1945] inferior nucleus ruber SYNDROME.

Claude Bernard's syndrome [*Claude* Bernard, French physician, 1813–1875] Bernard-Horner SYNDROME.

clause (klawz) an article, provision, or part of a formal document, such as an insurance contract. **coinsurance c.,** a provision in an insurance contract stipulating that the insured will pay a share for specified services, such as dental expenses, covered in the plan. See also COINSURANCE (2). **common deductible c.,** deductible c., common. **coordination of benefits c.,** a clause in a health insurance contract specifying that the insured person covered by more than one insurance plan will be limited to the amount that will be equal to the cost of the services received, after each deductible has been satisfied, thereby preventing over-insurance and duplication of benefits. Abbreviated *COB.* **deductible c., annual,** one that specifies the amount that must be satisfied each year before benefits become effective. Called also *annual deductible.* **deductible c., common,** one that specifies the amount deductible from each insured loss before insurance will respond. In health insurance, that portion of medical or dental care expenses which the insured must pay before the plan's benefits begin. Called also *deductible* and *dedutible amount.* See also COST-SHARING. **deductible c., family,** one specifying the amount which is satisfied by the combined expenses of all covered family members, as in a plan with a

$25.00 deductible amount which may limit its application to a maximum of three deductibles, or $75.00 for the family, regardless of the number of family members. Called also *family deductible.* **deductible c., lifetime,** one that specifies the amount which must be satisfied only once while the policy is in force before benefits become effective. Called also *lifetime deductible.* **deductible c., sliding scale,** one that does not set a fixed deductible amount but provides a sliding scale amount that varies according to income of the insured. **grandfather c.,** a provision of law that permits certain ongoing programs or operations to continue despite a change in the law which would otherwise prevent them from taking place, as the exemption of some drugs from premarket approval requirements on the basis of their longstanding use, or continuing of eligibility or coverage for individuals or organizations already receiving program benefits. Called also *grandfather provision.* **insurance c.,** one that indicates the parties to a health or other insurance contract, sets forth the type of losses, benefits, or services covered, and defines the benefits to be paid. **prorating c.,** one in a health insurance contract, whereby participating practitioners agree to accept a percentage reduction in their billings to offset the amount by which the total cost of services provided exceeds the total premium received. It is a method for spreading losses equitably among participating practitioners. **recurring c.,** a provision in a health insurance policy that specifies a period of time during which the recurrence of a condition is considered a continuation of a prior period of disability or hospitalization, rather than a separate spell of illness.

claustra (klaws'trah) [L.] plural of *claustrum*.

claustrum (klaws'trum), pl. *claus'tra* [L. "a barrier"] the thin layer of gray matter in the basal ganglia lateral to the external capsule of the brain.

clavicle (clav'ĭ-k'l) [L. *clavicle* dim. of *clavis* key] a bone that articulates with the sternum and scapula, forming the anterior half of the shoulder girdle on either side. Called also *collar bone*.

clawhand (klaw'hand) flexion and atrophy of the hand and fingers, occurring in diseases or conditions, such as leprosy or syringomyelia. Called also *main en griffe*. Also written *claw hand*.

clay (kla) a native hydrated aluminum silicate, produced by the decomposition of rocks due to weathering, having the general formula $Al_2O_3 \cdot SiO_2 \cdot xH_2O$. Chemically, clay has a sheet structure from a $(Si_2O_5)_n$ layer along with a layer of aluminum hydroxide $Al(OH)_3$ octahedra. It occurs as a reddish-brown to buff (depending on the iron oxide content), odorless substance, made up of fine, irregularly shaped crystals 1 to 150 μ in diameter, having a specific gravity of about 2.50, which is insoluble in water and organic solvents, but absorbs water to form a plastic, moldable mass, water serving as a lubricant between the colloidal particles. Used in ceramics, refractories, colloidal suspensions, rubber and plastic products, films, and other products. **China c.**, kaolin. **soap c.**, bentonite.

clean (klēn) 1. free of dirt. 2. the term is sometimes used to indicate absence of all matter in which microorganisms may find favorable conditions for continued life and growth.

cleaner (kle'ner) an agent used for cleaning. **cavity c.**, originally, any agent used to sterilize the prepared cavity before placing the restoration. With the development of air turbine handpieces, the term evolved to include agents for cleaning, degreasing, and drying the prepared cavity. Cavity cleaners used for these purposes before placing the restoration are various solutions of hydrogen peroxide, ethanol, acetone, and chloroform. Trademark: Cavidry. **dentin c., enamel c.**, acid ETCHANT. **denture c.**, denture CLEANSER.

cleanser (klen'zer) a preparation, usually a liquid or powder, used for cleansing or for removing stains. **denture c.**, any agent, substance, or device, used for removing stains and food particles from and deodorizing artificial dentures. Most proprietary cleansers are of the immersion or soak-in types, falling into the alkaline peroxide and alkaline hypochlorite groups, and are usually available as powders or tablets. Preparations similar to toothpastes, which are applied with a denture brush adapted to the contour of the denture, are also available commercially. Substances such as soap and water, bicarbonate of soda, precipitated calcium carbonate, salt, household cleansers, and vinegar are also used as cleansers. Household powder cleansers have an adverse abrasive action on dentures. Mechanical denture cleansers include: ultrasonic devices (see *dental c., ultrasonic*); magnetic stirrers consisting of a magnetic motor in the base of the unit that rotates a propeller-like apparatus; and devices consisting of a U-shaped electromagnet with a metal bar mounted close to the open face of the U causing vibration of the cleansing fluid. Called also *denture cleaner*. **denture c., abrasive**, a cleanser, usually a powder containing an abrasive agent, such as calcium phosphate, or a paste containing a dilute acid in addition to an abrasive agent, used for cleansing dentures through brushing. **denture c., alkaline hypochlorite**, a chemical immersion cleanser in which loosening of food debris and removal of stains and plaque is accomplished through the bleaching action of the cleanser on the organic matrix, causing dissolution of its polymer structure. This type has been reported to tarnish and corrode metal surfaces of the denture. **denture c., alkaline peroxide**, a chemical immersion cleanser containing sodium peroxide, sodium perborate or percarbonate, and an alkaline detergent to reduce surface tension. **denture c., dilute acid**, a dilute solution of hydrochloric, phosphoric, or acetic acid, which removes inorganic phosphates and stains from dentures. **denture c., enzyme**, a solution containing enzymes acting on glycoproteins, mucoproteins, and extracellular polysaccharide structures in the matrix of plaque formed on dentures, resulting in their breakdown. **denture c., immersion**, a chemical solution of hypochlorites, peroxides, acids or enzymes, in which dentures are immersed for removing stains and plaque and to loosen food debris. **denture c., magnetic**, see *denture c.* **denture c., ultrasonic**, a device that, through ultra-

sonic agitation, augments the cleansing action of various chemical cleansing solutions in which dentures are immersed.

cleansing (klenz-ing) making something clean. **interdental c.**, removal of food debris and bacterial plaque from the interdental areas that are often inaccessible to toothbrushes, but may be reached by floss and interdental instruments.

clearance (klēr'ans) 1. the act of clearing; especially, removal of a substance from the blood by an excretory organ. 2. the amount of space existing between opposed structures. **blood urea c.**, the volume of blood cleared of urea per minute by renal elimination, determined by measuring the quantity of urea entering the urine each minute divided by plasma urea concentration. Normal urea clearance is 70 ml of plasma per minute for the average adult; a lesser value indicates decreased renal function. Clinical symptoms of renal insufficiency usually begin to become apparent when the urea clearance falls below approximately 20 ml per minute. Called also *urea c.* **interocclusal c.**, interocclusal DISTANCE. **occlusal c.**, a condition in which the opposing occlusal surfaces may glide over one another without any interfering projection. **urea c.**, blood urea c.

cleat (klēt) a fixed point of anchorage, usually in the form of a metal spur or loop embedded in the acrylic resin base of a Hawley retainer or soldered onto an arch wire, to which a rubber dam elastic or other device is attached during orthodontic tooth movement.

cleavage (klēv'ij) the mitotic division of the fertilized ovum (zygote), consisting of segmentation of the zygote into 2, 4, 8, 16, etc., cleavage cells (blastomeres), each new series of cells

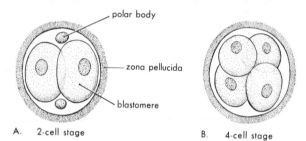

A.   2-cell stage   B.   4-cell stage

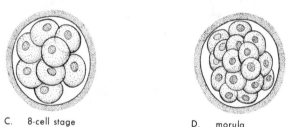

C.   8-cell stage   D.   morula

Cleavage of the zygote and formation of the blastocyst. A to D, various stages of cleavage (developmental stage 2). (From K. Moore: The Developing Human. 2nd ed. Philadelphia, W. B. Saunders Co., 1977.)

becoming smaller than the previous ones. By the third day, the blastomeres begin to cluster together to form the morula. See illustration.

cleaver (klēv-er) a heavy knife or hatchet. **Case's enamel c.**, a hand-operated instrument with a strong edge, used for removing enamel in the preparation of a root-end for a crown. **Orton's enamel c.**, an instrument for trimming tooth enamel, especially during crown preparation.

cleft (kleft) a longitudinal opening or fissure. See also FISSURA and FISSURE. **alveolar c.**, cleft of the alveolus, sometimes associated with cleft lip and cleft palate. **bilateral c.**, a double cleft, one on each side of the median line. **branchial c.**, one of the clefts between the branchial arches of the embryo, formed by rupture of the membrane separating the corresponding entodermal (pharyngeal) pouch and the ectodermal (branchial) groove. Called also *visceral c.* and *branchial fissure*. See also branchial cleft CYST, and see illustration and table at branchial arches, under ARCH. **c. cheek**, a developmental anomaly characterized by an abnormal fissure, caused by failure of union of some of the facial processes. **facial c.**, a cleft occurring along any plane where embryonic processes normally unite to form the face. **facial c., horizontal**, facial c., lateral. **facial c., lateral**, trans-

CLEFT PALATE ASSOCIATION	STARK	VEAU
	PRIMARY PALATE	
PRE PALATE	SUBTOTAL UNILATERAL	
PRE PALATE	SUBTOTAL UNILATERAL	
PRE PALATE	TOTAL UNILATERAL	
PRE PALATE	TOTAL BILATERAL	
	SECONDARY PALATE	
PALATE	SUBTOTAL	I
PALATE	TOTAL	II
PALATE (SUBMUCOUS)	SECONDARY SUBTOTAL	
	PRIMARY AND SECONDARY	
PRE PALATE AND PALATE	TOTAL UNILATERAL	III
PRE PALATE AND PALATE	TOTAL BILATERAL	IV

Classification of cleft lip and cleft palate. (From V. A. Chalian, J. E. Drane, and S. M. Standish: Maxillofacial Prosthetics. Baltimore, Williams & Wilkins, 1971.)

verse facial cleft extending from the angle of the mouth toward the ear. Called also *horizontal facial c.* and *transverse facial c.* See also MACROSTOMIA. **facial c., oblique,** rare form of facial cleft extending from the lip to the inner canthus of the eye. It may be superficial but usually separates the underlying bone and is associated with cleft lip, cleft palate, or lateral facial cleft. Called also *meloschisis* and *prosopoanoschisis.* **fascial c.,** a cleavage between two continuous fascial surfaces which allows the two surfaces to move over each other. **fascial c., perivisceral,** a fascial cleft that surrounds the visceral fascia and separates it from the middle cervical fascia, carotid sheath, and prevertebral fascia, and allows the esophagus and pharynx to move during the act of swallowing. The anterior part of the fascial cleft is known as the *previsceral cleft* and the posterior part as the *retropharyngeal cleft.* **gingival c.,** a narrow V-shaped recession or split in the marginal gingivae, most commonly on the labial aspect of the mandibular incisors and buccal gingivae of the maxillary molars, usually seen in pocket formation. Called also *gingival fissure.* **hyoid c.,** hypomandibular c. **hypomandibular c.,** the cleft between the mandibular and hyoid arches in the developing embryo. Called also *hyoid c.* **interdental c.,** diastema. **c. jaw,** a cleft between the median nasal and maxillary processes through the alveolus. Called also *gnathoschisis.* **c. lip,** a congenital defect of the lip, usually involving the upper lip, due to failure of the median nasal and maxillary processes to fuse, sometimes associated with cleft of the nose, alveolar process, hard palate, and velum. Called also *cheiloschisis, harelip,* and *stomatoschisis.* See illustration. **c. lip, mandibular,** a rare form of cleft lip usually involving only the soft tissue of the lower lip, occasionally both the lip and the jaw, due to failure of fusion of the mandibular process. **c. lip, maxillary,** c. lip. **c. palate,** congenital fissure of the palate due to faulty fusion that, typically, opens through the roof of the mouth into the nasal cavity and extends anteriorly to the premaxilla, where it deviates to the right or left, following the line of fusion. The soft palate alone or both the soft and hard palate may be involved. It is often associated with other abnormalities, including cleft lip, cleft jaw, defects of dental structures, and a wide variety of congenital systemic anomalies. There are numerous classifications of cleft palate, but the most common are those of the American Cleft Palate Association, Stark, and Veau. Called also *palatoschisis, palatum fissum, uraniscochasma, uranoschism,* and *uranostaphyloschisis* (cleft of both the hard and the soft palate). See illustration. **postalveolar c.,** cleft palate with normal alveolar process. **prealveolar c.,** cleft lip with normal alveolar process. **previsceral c.,** the anterior part of the perivisceral fascial cleft. **retropharyngeal c., retropharyngeal fascial c.,** retropharyngeal SPACE. **Stillman's c.,** a small apostrophe-shaped fissure extending apically from the gingival margin to a depth of 5 to 6 mm, usually on the vestibular surface of a tooth, considered to be ulcerative processes. Originally, such clefts were believed to be caused by trauma of occlusion, but recent research disproves this. **synaptic c.,** a narrow gap, about 200 Å in width, which separates the terminal portion of the presynaptic axon from the soma of the postsynaptic neuron or its dendrite(s). See illustration at SYNAPSE. **c. tongue,** bifid TONGUE. **transverse fascial c.,** facial c., lateral. **c. uvula,** bifid UVULA. **visceral c.,** branchial c.

Cléjat, C. [French dermatologist] see POIKILODERMATOMYOSITIS (Petges-Cléjat syndrome).

cleid- see CLEIDO-.

cleido-, cleid- [Gr. *kleis* that which serves for closing; the clavicle, so called because it locks the neck and breast together] a combining form denoting relationship to the clavicle, or to something barred.

cleidocranial (kli″do-kra′ne-al) [*cleido-* Gr. *kranion* head] pertaining to the clavicles and the head. See also cleidocranial DYSOSTOSIS.

clenching (klench′ing) the clamping and pressing of the jaws and teeth together in centric occlusion, frequently associated with acute nervous tension or physical effort, such as pushing or lifting a heavy object or performing a difficult task. See also BRUXISM. **habitual c.,** centric BRUXISM.

Cleocin trademark for preparations of *clindamycin.*

cleoid (kle′oid) [Anglo-Saxon *cle* claw + Gr. *eidos* form] a nib shaped like a claw, used frequently to carve amalgam restorations. See illustration at DISCOID.

clerk (klerk) a person who is responsible in an office or business for files, records, handling of correspondence, and the like. In a dental or medical office, an auxiliary member of the staff who is responsible for keeping patients' records, appointment records, and billings. **insurance c.,** an auxiliary member of the staff in a dental office who is responsible for handling and filing of insurance claims.

click (klik) a slight sharp sound. See also CREPITATION. **temporomandibular joint c.,** see temporomandibular joint SUBLUXATION.

clicking (klik′ing) 1. production of sharp, slight sounds. 2. a snapping, cracking or crepitant noise evident on excursions of the condyle of the temporomandibular joint. Called also *crepitus.*

climizole hydrochloride (klem′ĭ-zōl) an antihistaminic drug acting on the H_1 receptor, 1-*p*-chlorobenzyl-2-(1-pyrrolidinyl-methyl) benzimidazole monohydrochloride. It occurs as white crystals or powder with a bitter taste, which is soluble in ethanol and chloroform and slightly in water, but is insoluble in ether. Used in the symptomatic therapy of allergic reactions. Trademarks: Allercur, Histocuran, Klemidox, Reactrol.

clindamycin (klin″dah-mi′sin) a semisynthetic antibiotic, 7(S)-chloro-7-deoxylincomycin. A 7-deoxy-derivative of chlorinated lincomycin, it has similar pharmacological and toxic properties, being somewhat more potent than the parent compound. It inhibits protein synthesis by its action on bacterial ribosomes and acts against staphylococci, streptococci, actinomycetes, *Bacteroides, Fusobacterium,* and gram-negative bacilli. Diarrhea, abdominal pain, fever, blood and mucus in the stools, skin rash, exudative erythema multiforme, granulocytopenia, thrombopenia, and anaphylaxis are potential side reactions. Called also *clinimycin.* Trademarks: Cleocin, Dallacin C. **c. hydrochloride,** the monohydrochloride salt of clindamycin, occurring as a white, odorless, crystalline powder with a characteristic taste, which is soluble in water, methanol, and ethanol, but not in acetone. Trademark: Dalactine. **c. palmitate hydrochloride,** the palmitate ester of clindamycin hydrochloride, occurring as a white amorphous powder with a characteristic odor and taste, which is soluble in methanol, benzene, chloroform, ethanol, and water. It is an oral preparation for pediatric use, which is hydrolyzed to the active parent compound. **c. phosphate,** the phosphate ester of clindamycin, occurring as a white, odorless, hygroscopic, crystalline powder that decomposes to free clindamycin on exposure to high temperature, and is freely soluble in water, slightly soluble in ethanol, and insoluble in ether and chloroform. Following parenteral administration, it rapidly hydrolyzes to the active parent compound.

clinic (klin′ik) [Gr. *klinikos* pertaining to a bed] 1. a clinical lecture; examination of patients before a class of students;

instruction at the bedside. 2. an establishment where patients are admitted for special study and treatment by a group of medical specialists, sometimes including dentists, practicing together. 3. a facility, sometimes a part of a hospital, for diagnosis and treatment of outpatients. **ambulant c.,** one for patients not confined to bed. **dry c.,** a clinical lecture with the presentation of case histories but without the presence of the patients described. **table c.,** a teaching technique in continuing dental education, in which several clinicians repeatedly give short presentations and students move freely from one presentation to another.

clinical (klin′e-k'l) pertaining to a clinic or the bedside; pertaining to or founded on actual observation and treatment, as distinguished from theoretical or basic sciences.

clinician (klĭ-nish′an) one who is an expert in clinical medicine or dentistry. **nurse c.,** NURSE clinician.

clinimycin (klin′ĭ-mi′sin) clindamycin.

clinodactyly (kli″no-dak′tĭ-le) [Gr. *klinein* to bend + *daktylos* finger] permanent lateral or medial deviation or deflection of one or more fingers.

clinoid (kli′noid) [Gr. *klinē* bed + *eidos* form] resembling a bed; bed-shaped, as the clinoid process.

clinoidale (kli″noi-da′le) the most superior point on the contour of the anterior clinoid.

CLINPROT Clinical Cancer Protocols; an acronym for a computer-searchable data base containing summaries of clinical investigations on new anticancer agents and treatment techniques, sponsored by the National Cancer Institute.

clip (klip) 1. any device that grips or holds something tightly. 2. a metallic device for approximating the edges of a wound or for the prevention of bleeding from small individual blood vessels. See also clip FORCEPS.

clisis (kli′sis) [Gr. *klisis* inclination] attraction or inclination.

Clistin trademark for *carbinoxamine maleate* (see under CARBINOXAMINE).

clival (kli′val) pertaining to the clivus.

clivus (kli′vus) [L. "slope"] [NA] a bony surface in the posterior cranial fossa, sloping upward from the foramen magnum to the dorsum sellae, the lower part being formed by a portion of the basilar part of the occipital bone and the upper part by a surface of the body of the sphenoid bone. Called also *clivus blumenbachii*. **basilar c., c. basila′ris,** c. ossis occipitalis. **c. blumenbach′ii,** clivus. **c. os′sis occipita′lis,** the lower part of the clivus, formed by the basilar portion of the occipital bone. Called also *basilar c., c. basilaris* and *basilar groove of occipital bone*. **c. os′sis sphenoida′lis,** the upper part of the clivus, formed by a surface of the sphenoid bone. Called also *basilar groove of sphenoid bone.*

cloaca (klo-a′kah), pl. *cloa′cae* [L. "drain"] 1. in mammalian embryology, the terminal end of the hindgut before division into rectum, bladder, and genital primordia. 2. in pathology, an opening in the involucrum of a necrosed bone.

Cloaca cloacae (klo-a′kah klo-a′se) *Enterobacter cloacae*; see under ENTEROBACTER.

Clobren-SF trademark for *clofibrate.*

clofibrate (klo-fi′brāt) an anticholesteremic agent, ethyl-2-(p-chlorophenoxy)-2-methylpropionate, occurring as a colorless or pale yellow liquid with a characteristic odor and taste, which is soluble in acetone, chloroform, benzene, and ethanol, but not in water. Used to decrease blood cholesterol and triglyceride levels. It also increases the anticoagulant effects of thrombopenic drugs. Side effects may include urticaria, pruritus, stomatitis, alopecia areata, nausea, flatulence, headache, vertigo, asthenia, myalgia, and dermatitis. The hair of some women may become dry and brittle. Trademarks: Amotril, Anparton, Ateculon, Ateriosan, Atheropront, Atromid-S, Atromidin, Clobren-SF, Hyclorate, Lipavlon, Neo-Atromid, Normet, Regelan, Serotinex.

Clomid trademark for *clomiphene citrate* (see under CLOMIPHENE).

clomiphene citrate (klo-mi′fēn) an antiestrogenic drug, 2-[p-(2-chloro-1,2-diphenylvinyl)phenoxy]triethylamine citrate, occurring as a white to a pale yellow, odorless powder that is slightly soluble in ethanol, water, and chloroform, and is insoluble in ether. It blocks negative feedback of endogenous estrogen to the hypothalamus, acting selectively on luteotropic hormone, but not on follicle-stimulating hormone. Used to induce ovulation. Symptoms of menopause, breast enlargement, ovarian pain, and multiple pregnancies may occur. Trademarks: Clomid, Clomphid, Dyneric, Ikaklomine.

Clomphid trademark for *clomiphene citrate* (see under CLOMIPHENE).

clonic (klon′ik) [Gr. *klonos* turmoil] pertaining to or of the nature of clonus.

clonidine hydrochloride (klo′nĭ-dēn) an antihypertensive agent, 2-(2,6-dichloroanilino)-2-imidazoline monohydrochloride, occurring as a white, odorless, bitter, crystalline powder that is soluble in water, methanol, ethanol, and chloroform. It acts chiefly by decreasing vasodilation and bradycardia and stimulating α-adrenergic receptors in the vasomotor and cardioinhibitory centers. It also appears to reduce the release of norepinephrine from the sympathetic nerves. Also used in the treatment of migraine. Side effects may include xerostomia, orthostatic hypotension, salt and water retention, impotence, constipation, depression, and potentiation of the pressor actions of sympathomimetics and angiotensin and antagonism of the depressor action of isoproterenol. Trademarks: Catapres, Catapresan, Dixarit, Isoglaucon.

clonus (klo′nus) [Gr. *klonos* turmoil] a spasm characterized by alternate muscular contraction and relaxation in rapid succession. See also MYOCLONUS.

Clopane trademark for *cyclopentamine hydrochloride* (see under CYCLOPENTAMINE).

Cloquet's ganglion [Hippolyte *Cloquet,* French anatomist, 1787–1840] see under GANGLION.

Cloramin trademark for *mechlorethamine hydrochloride* (see under MECHLORETHAMINE).

clorazepate dipotassium (klo-raz′ĕ-pāt) a minor tranquilizer, 7-chloro-2,3-dihydro-2,2-dihydroxy-5-phenyl-1H-1,4-benzodiazepine-carboxylic acid dipotassium salt, occurring as a fine, light-yellow, odorless crystalline powder with a slightly burning taste, which is sensitive to light, heat, and moisture, and is readily soluble in water, slightly soluble in alcohol, and insoluble in organic solvents. Used in the treatment of anxiety conditions. In dentistry, the drug is used as a psychosedative to allay apprehension before dental procedures. It is potentially addictive and its adverse effects include drowsiness, dizziness, gastrointestinal disorders, blurred vision, xerostomia, headache, mental confusion, insomnia, rashes, fatigue, ataxia, irritability, genitourinary disorders, slurred speech, hypotension, liver and kidney dysfunction, depression, and nervousness. It is contraindicated in hypersensitive persons, in the elderly and young children, in pregnancy, and in nursing mothers. Trademark: Tranxene.

Clorolifarina trademark for *chloramphenicol palmitate* (see under CHLORAMPHENICOL).

Clorox trademark for an aqueous solution of *sodium hypochlorite* (see under SODIUM).

Clorpactin trademark for *oxychlorosene.*

Clortetrin trademark for *demeclocycline hydrochloride* (see under DEMECLOCYCLINE).

Close Up see under DENTIFRICE.

Closina trademark for *cycloserine.*

Closs, Karl [Norwegian physician] see ACRODERMATITIS enteropathica (Danbolt-Closs syndrome).

clostridia (klo-strid′e-ah) plural of *clostridium.*

clostridial (klo-strid′e-al) pertaining to or caused by clostridia.

Clostridium (klo-strid′e-um) [Gr. *klōstēr* spindle] a genus of rod-shaped, anaerobic, generally gram-positive bacteria of the family Bacillaceae, most members of which are motile by means of peritrichous flagella, while some are nonmotile. Most strains are obligatory anaerobes, but some may grow in the presence of air. They form spherical spores that usually distend the cells. The genus includes more than 300 species, commonly found in soil, marine and fresh water sediments, and in the intestinal tract of animals, including man. Several species are pathogenic, but their status as parasites is not fully understood; none of the pathogenic species have ability to invade the body tissue by itself, some are incapable of setting up infection, while others produce infection, but only when aided by traumatic injury or by other bacteria. **C. botuli′num,** a species causing botulism in man and various diseases in animals, occurring as a large (0.3 to 1.3 by 1.6 to 9.4 μm), pleomorphic, gram-positive, motile, sporulating rods with four to eight peritrichous flagella. They occur in pairs and in chains; spore formation varies, some strains producing abundantly, others sparsely. The species is subdivided into seven types: A, B, C (α and β), D, E, F, and G, according to the type of toxin produced and its immunological properties; the types are further subdivided into proteolytic and nonproteolytic strains. Toxins of all types are similar pharmacologically. Toxin A (a complex made up of a hemagglutinin portion [nontoxin] and a neurotoxin) is the most potent, having LD_{50} 5×10^{-9} mg N for the mouse; its lethal dose for man is about 1 μg. **C. histolyt′icum,** a species of obligate anaerobes, occurring singly or as paired gram-positive, motile short rods (about 0.5 to 0.7 by 3.0 to 5.0 μm), found in some cases of gas gangrene. It forms terminal spores and has peritrichous flagella, usually more than 20 in number. Numerous toxins are formed, including a lethal and necrotizing α-toxin and several proteolytic enzymes. One of these, the β-toxin, is a collagenase, and another, the γ-toxin, is a cysteine-activated enzyme which attacks altered collagen. A third, designated the δ-toxin, is a serologically distinct protease. Called also *Bacillus histolyticus.* **C. no'vyi,** a species found in 32 to 48 percent of cases of gas gangrene, occurring as gram-positive rods with subterminal oval spores, which range in size from 0.8 to 1.0 and 2.5 to 10.0 μm, and found singly or in chains. The organisms are nonmotile under normal conditions and have numerous spiral flagella that often become tangled. Six toxins have been identified: α, β, γ, δ, ε, ζ; the α-toxin is one of the most potent poisons known. The toxins are characterized by necrotizing, hemolytic, and lecithinase activity. Called also *C. oedematiens, Bacillus oedematiens, B. oedematis maligni No. II, B. novyi* and *Novy's bacillus.* **C. oedemat'iens,** *C. novyi.* **C. perfrin'gens,** a species occurring as plump, nonmotile, anaerobic, gram-positive rods of variable length (ranging in size from 0.9 to 1.3 by 3.0 to 9.0 μm), which are found singly or in chains. A polysaccharide capsule is usually present and spores are formed sparingly in the absence of fermentable carbohydrates. The species is divided into six types: A, B, C, D, E, and F. Several toxins are produced, most being hemolysins, proteolytic enzymes, and necrotic agents. During sporulation, types A and C produce a heat labile exotoxin (enterotoxin), believed to be involved in food poisoning. *C. perfringens* is the principal pathogen of gas gangrene, but may also occur in some gastrointestinal and other nongangrenous disorders, including food poisoning. In gas gangrene, once established at the site of an injury, the organisms proliferate and invade adjacent tissue, spreading along the interstitial tissues of muscle; large amounts of hyaluronidase are usually present at the site of infection. These bacteria are usually found in soil, marine sediment, wounds, and feces, and are also normal inhabitants of the human intestine. Called also *C. welchii, Bacillus perfringens, B. aerogenes capsulatus, B. phlegmonis emphysematosae,* and *Frankel's bacillus.* **C. sep'ticum,** a species occurring as gram-positive, sporulating, spindle-shaped, anaerobic rods, or filaments with slightly rounded and subterminal ends, which in young cultures are motile with peritrichous flagella. Spores are formed only in media with excess fermentable carbohydrates. The organisms produce α-toxin, an oxygen-labile hemolysin, and β-toxin, a deoxyribonuclease attacking the nuclei of leukocytes, and also form hyaluronidase (sometimes called γ-toxin). *C. septicum* is usually found in gas gangrene in association with other organisms, but it may also occur alone. On inoculation, *C. septicum* produces gas and serous edema and invades the adjacent tissues and circulation to cause usually fatal septicemia. Called also *Bacillus septicus, Ghon-Sacks bacillus, Vibrio septicus,* and *vibrion septique.* **C. sporog'enes,** a species widely distributed in nature, made up of harmless saprophytes in pure culture, but is associated with pathogenic anaerobes in mixed gangrenous infections; they have been confused frequently with the pathogenic forms. Spores are usually resistant and invariably survive with those of the pathogens or even after the pathogenic spore formers are killed in preliminary selected heating. These bacteria occur singly, in pairs, in short chains and, sometimes, in filaments as actively motile, gram-positive, slender, spore-forming rods with rounded ends and peritrichous flagella, ranging in size from 0.3 to 0.4 by 3.0 to 7.0 μm. *C. sporogenes* frequently occurs in the intestines of healthy humans and animals. Called also *Bacillus sporogenes.* **C. tet'ani,** a species found as a common inhabitant of soil and human and horse intestines, which is the causative agent of tetanus. They occur as slender, motile by several peritrichous flagella, gram-positive, sporulating rods with rounded ends, ranging in size from 0.3 to 0.5 μm by 2 to 5 μm, with larger filaments sometimes present. The spore of *C. tetani* has no exosporium, and is located near the end of the cell, being larger than the sporangium, thus giving the cell a drumstick-like appearance. Individual cells usually form short chains. Two toxins are produced: *tetanospasmin,* a potent soluble toxin that affects the nervous system, and *tetanolysin,* a hemolysin similar to streptolysin. The organisms usually gain entrance to the tissues by means of a deep dirty wound; they proliferate at the site of penetration only if favorable conditions exist, such as simultaneous inoculation with saprophytes, chemical irritation, or a low oxidation-reduction potential, producing toxins which then create intoxication. Bacillemia is rare. The optimum temperature for growth is 37°C, growth ceasing at 45°C.

Called also *Bacillus tetani, B. welchii,* and *tetanus bacillus.* **C. welch'ii,** *C. perfringens.*

clostridium (klo-strid'e-um), pl. *clostrid'ia.* Any microorganism of the genus *Clostridium.*

closure (klo'shur) the act of shutting, or of bringing together two parts, one or both of which may be movable. Abbreviated *C.* **flask c.,** the bringing together of the two halves or parts of a flask in which a denture base is formed. **flask c., final,** the last closure of a flask before curing the denture base material packed in the mold. **flask c., trial,** preliminary closure of a flask, to eliminate excess material and to ensure that the mold is completely filled. **maxillary antrum c.,** sinus c. **palatopharyngeal c.,** a sphincter action sealing the oral cavity from the nasal cavity by the synchronous movement of the soft palate superiorly, the lateral pharyngeal wall medially, and the posterior wall of the pharynx anteriorly. **sinus c.,** adapting surrounding tissue over an opening between the maxillary sinus and the oral cavity. Called also *maxillary antrum.* **velopharyngeal c.,** closure of nasal air escape by the elevation of the soft palate and contraction of the posterior pharyngeal wall.

clot (klot) a semisolidified mass, as of blood or lymph. **blood c.,** a coagulum formed of blood, either in or out of the body. See also blood COAGULATION, EMBOLUS, and THROMBUS.

cloth (kloth) a piece of material or fabric made from natural or synthetic fibers. **squeeze c.,** a piece of cloth used for squeezing out by hand pressure excess mercury from dental amalgam mix.

clotrimazole (klo-trim'ah-zōl) an antifungal agent, 1-(o-chloro-α,α-diphenylbenzyl)imidazole, occurring as a crystalline substance that is soluble in water, benzene, toluene, acetone solutions, chloroform, and ethyl acetate. Trademarks: Canesten, Lotrimin, Mycosporin.

clotting (klot'ing) the act or process of clot formation. **blood c.,** blood COAGULATION.

cloverleaf skull (klo'ver-lēf' skul) cloverleaf SKULL.

cloxacillin sodium (kloks"ah-sil'in) a broad-spectrum semisynthetic penicillin, 3-o-chlorophenyl-5-methyl-4-isoxazolyl penicillin monosodium monohydrate, occurring as a white, odorless, bitter, slightly hydroscopic, crystalline powder that is soluble in water and alcohol and slightly soluble in acetone and chloroform. It is a penicillinase-resistant antibiotic, acting against gram-positive and certain gram-negative bacteria. Its toxic properties are similar to those of other penicillins. Trademarks: Bactopen, Ekvacillin, Methocillin-S, Prostaphin-A, Tegopen.

clubbing (klub'ing) a proliferative change in the soft tissues about the terminal phalanges of the fingers or toes, with or without osseous changes.

clubhand (klub'hand) a deformity in which the hand is twisted out of shape or position, usually in strong flexion. Called also *talipomanus.* Also written *club hand.* See also MANUS valga and MANUS vara.

clumping (klump'ing) the aggregation of particles, such as bacteria or blood cells, into irregular masses; agglutination. **blood cell c.,** clumping of blood cells, especially erythrocytes, into irregular masses; hemagglutination.

clutch (klutch) 1. to grip or hold tightly or firmly. 2. a device for gripping the teeth in a dental arch. Also, one to which face-bow or tracing devices may be attached rigidly.

cluttering (klut'er-ing) hurried nervous speech, marked by the dropping of syllables.

clyers (kli'erz) actinomycosis.

CM crête manche; see endosseous implant, CM, under IMPLANT.

C & M 637 attachment see under ATTACHMENT.

Cm curium.

cm centimeter.

cm² square CENTIMETER.

cm³ cubic CENTIMETER.

CMC carboxymethylcellulose.

CME continuing medical education.

CMI cell-mediated IMMUNITY.

CN the cyanide radical.

CNS central nervous SYSTEM.

CO 1. CARBON monoxide. 2. centric OCCLUSION. 3. carbonyl.

CO₂ CARBON dioxide.

CO₃ carbonate.

Co cobalt.

⁵⁷Co an artificial radioactive cobalt isotope. See COBALT.

⁵⁸Co an artificial radioactive cobalt isotope. See COBALT.

⁶⁰Co an artificial radioactive cobalt isotope. See COBALT.

CoI coenzyme I; see nicotinamide-adenine DINUCLEOTIDE.

CoII coenzyme II; nicotinamide-adenine dinucleotide phosphate; see under DINUCLEOTIDE.

co- a prefix signifying with, together.

CoA coenzyme A.

coacervation (ko-as″er-va′shun) a phenomenon that involves both lyophilic and hydrophilic colloids, but particularly the latter, being the separation of microscopic liquid droplets when sols of two hydrophilic colloids of opposite electric charge are mixed. These droplets may later unite to form a viscous layer at the bottom of the container, constituting a new phase.

coagglutinin (ko″ah-gloo′tĭ-nin) partial AGGLUTININ.

coagula (ko-ag′u-lah) [L.] plural of *coagulum*.

coagulase (ko-ag′u-lās) an enzyme produced by bacteria, such as staphylococci, which accelerates blood clotting. It is a protein (therefore, readily inactivated by proteolytic enzymes), which is believed to react with prothrombin or with some form of modified prothrombin, to form a complex composed of coagulase and a coagulase-reacting factor; the complex has thrombin-like enzymatic activity and cleaves fibrinogen, producing the fibrin clot. Some authorities believe that it is the procoagulase which reacts with a serum factor similar to but not identical with prothrombin, to produce the actual coagulase which, in turn, brings about the clotting of blood. Only pathogenic strains of staphylococci produce coagulase, although its role in pathogenicity has not been established.

coagulation (ko-ag″u-la′shun) [L. *coagulatio*] 1. the process of transformation of a liquid to a gelatinous or semisolid mass. 2. the solidification of a sol into a gelatinous mass. 3. blood c. **blood c.,** the process by which a blood clot is formed, which may be initiated by interaction of substances in damaged tissue (extrinsic system), by trauma to the blood itself, as when blood is removed from the body (intrinsic system), or by snake venom. For convenience in classifying the hemorrhagic disorders and the tests used to study them, blood coagulation has been arbitrarily divided into four phases: *I*, the initiator (contact) reaction; *II*, thromboplastinogenesis; *III*, thrombogenesis; and *IV*, fibrin formation. See illustration. See also bleeding TIME, coagulation FACTOR, and HEMOSTASIS. **c. inhibitor,** see ANTICOAGULANT. **intravascular c.,** defibrination SYNDROME. **c. time,** measurement of the clotting time of whole blood, which consists of placing a sample of blood 5 min after withdrawal in a siliconized or uncoated test tube and tilting it until it is inverted

PHASE I: THE INITIATOR (CONTACT) REACTION

PHASE II: THROMBOPLASTINOGENESIS

PHASE III: THROMBINOGENESIS

PHASE IV: FIBRIN FORMATION

Schematic representation of the process of blood coagulation. (From J. B. Miale: Laboratory Medicine. Hematology. 5th ed. St. Louis, The C. V. Mosby Co., 1977.)

180° without blood flowing. Normal values for clotting in uncoated tubes is 6 to 17 min, and 19 to 60 min in siliconized tubes. Decreased coagulation time indicates digitalis therapy and increased time occurs in various conditions, including hemophilia and other coagulation disorders, anemias, leukemias, and acute febrile conditions, and in those persons in whom suppression of the clotting mechanism is being used therapeutically. Called also *clotting time*.

coagulopathy (ko-ag″u-lop′ah-the) [*coagulation* + Gr. *pathos* disease] any disease associated with abnormal blood coagulation. **consumptive c.,** defibrination SYNDROME.

coagulum (ko-ag′u-lum), pl. *coag′ula* [L.] a clot or curd.

Coakley's operation [Cornelius Godfrey *Coakley*, American surgeon, 1862–1934] see under OPERATION.

coalescence (ko″ah-les′ens) [L. *coalescere* to grow together] 1. the fusion or blending together, such as fusion of separate lesions into one, or growing together of the roots of a tooth. See also CONCRESCENCE. 2. in firing of dental porcelain, the last phase of the fusion when the porcelain assumes an overglazed surface and rounded form. See also high biscuit FIRING and MATURITY (3).

Coapt trademark for *mecrylate*.

coapt (ko′apt) [L. *coaptare*] to approximate, as the edges of a wound or the ends of a fractured bone.

coarctate (ko-ark′tāt) [L. *coarctare* to straighten or tighten] 1. to press close together; contract. 2. pressed together; restrained.

coarctation (ko-ark-ta′shun) [L. *coarctatio*, from *cum* together + *arctare* to make tight] a condition of stricture or contraction.

coat (kōt) [L. *cotta* a tunic] a membrane or other structure covering or lining a part or organ.

coating (kōt′ing) 1. covering something with a layer of a substance that adheres to its surface. 2. a substance, usually a liquid which hardens on application to the surface of an object, thus providing a superficial covering layer. **enteric c.,** a substance covering a tablet that resists the action of fluids and enzymes in the upper digestive tract, but dissolves readily in the upper intestine, thus preventing the contents of the tablet from being released before reaching its destination in the intestine. **tongue c.,** a condition in which the dorsum of the tongue gives the appearance of being covered with a whitish foreign matter.

COB coordination of benefits; see under CLAUSE.

cobalamin (ko-bal′ah-min) 1. a general term for any active compound containing the α-(5,6-dimethylbenzimidazoyl)corrin nucleus, depending on the group that replaces CN. The cobalamins include cyanocobalamin (vitamin B_{12}), hydroxycobalamin (vitamin B_{12a}), aquocobalamin (vitamin B_{12b}), and nitrocobalamin (vitamin B_{12c}). Collectively, the cobalamins are known as *carbamides*. 2. cyanocobalamin.

cobalt (ko′bawlt) [L. *cobaltum*] a gray, ductile, magnetic, malleable metal. Symbol, Co; atomic number, 27; atomic weight, 58.9332; melting point, 1495°C; specific gravity, 8.9; valences, 2, 3; group VIII of the periodic table. Cobalt has one stable isotope, ^{59}Co, and several artificial ones, 54–58 and 60–64. The isotope used most frequently in biomedical research and industry is ^{60}Co, which emits beta and gamma radiation and has a half-life of 5.3 years; it has largely replaced radium in cancer therapy. Other radioisotopes of biomedical importance are ^{57}Co (half-life of 267 days and emitting gamma and K rays) and ^{58}Co (half-life of 58 days and emitting positron, gamma, and K rays). Cobalt is resistant to water and air and dissolves in nitric acid and, more slowly, in hydrochloric and sulfuric acids. Its metabolic function is chiefly in hematopoiesis. Pharmacologically, cobalt stimulates erythropoietin production and improves hemoglobin and erythrocyte values in certain anemias, and it is an essential component of vitamin B_{12}. By blocking of some respiratory enzymes, such as cytochrome oxidase and succinic dehydrogenase, cobalt is believed to stimulate erythropoiesis by causing intracellular hypoxia, resulting in polycythemia. Cobalt and some of its compounds, such as cobaltous chloride, may cause intoxication by producing cyanosis, coma, and death. Other toxic reactions may include cutaneous flushing, dermatitis, anorexia, nausea, vomiting, weakness, tinnitus, nerve deafness, thyroid hyperplasia, myxedema, chest pain, congestive heart failure, and other complications. Cobalt deficiency is observed only in animals. Used chiefly in magnetic alloys. Also used as a blue pigment in dental ceramics. **chromium-c. alloy,** cobalt-chrome ALLOY. **c.-chromium-nickel alloy,** cobalt-chromium-nickel ALLOY. **c. dichloride,** cobaltous CHLORIDE.

cobaltic (ko-bawl′tik) pertaining to or containing trivalent cobalt, CO≡.

cobaltous (ko-bawl′tus) pertaining to or containing divalent cobalt, Co^{++}, as in cobaltous chloride.

cobamide (ko'bah-mīd) a general term including the cobalamins. Called also *vitamin B₁₂*.

Cobefrin trademark for *nordefrin hydrochloride* (see under NORDEFRIN).

coca (ko'kah) the dried leaves of *Erythroxylon coca*, a South American plant, which is the major source of cocaine and other alkaloids.

cocaine (ko'kån) an alkaloid from coca leaves, benzoylmethylecgonine, occurring as white crystals or crystalline powder. It is soluble in water, alcohol, chloroform, ether, turpentine, olive oil, liquid petrolatum, acetone, and carbon disulfide. Its most important clinical action is its ability to block nerve conduction when applied locally. Its most striking systemic effect is stimulation of the central nervous system. Some of the numerous side effects of cocaine after systemic administration are medullary stimulation with increased respiratory rate (followed by rapid shallow breathing and depression); in small doses, vagal stimulation with resulting slow heart rate and, in moderate doses, increased heart rate; initial rise in blood pressure, followed by a fall; rise in body temperature; and potentiation of both the excitatory and the inhibitory responses of the sympathetic nervous system to catecholamines and nerve stimulation. Cocaine is absorbed from all sites of application and most of it is metabolized by the liver with some cocaine being excreted unchanged. Cocaine, being addictive, is used in topical anesthesia. Cocaine solutions for surface anesthesia vary from 1.0 to 4.0 percent for application to the cornea and 5 to 10 percent for application to nose and throat. The preparation usually includes epinephrine. Dry cocaine moistened with epinephrine solution (cocaine mud) is sometimes used in surface anesthesia of the nose and throat. There is a potential hazard of interaction between cocaine and catecholamines. Absorption of an excessive dose of cocaine causes poisoning. Symptoms of acute poisoning include excitement, restlessness, anxiety, garrulousness, confusion, headache, tachycardia, respiratory disorders, chills, fevers, mydriasis, exophthalmos, formication, nausea, vomiting, convulsions, delirium, Cheyne-Stokes respiration, and death from respiratory arrest. Diazepam or barbiturates are the principal antidotes. See also COCAINISM. **c. esterase**, carboxylesterase. **c. hydrochloride**, the hydrochloride salt of cocaine, occurring as white crystals, granules, or powder with a saline, slightly bitter taste, which numbs the tongue and lips. It is soluble in water, alcohol, chloroform, glycerol, and acetone, but not in ether or oils. Similarly to the parent drug, it is used in solutions of 2 to 10 percent.

cocainism (ko'kăn-izm) cocaine intoxication; a condition resulting from chronic abuse of cocaine as a stimulant or narcotic. Symptoms include dilation of the pupils, exophthalmos, and tachycardia. See also COCAINE.

coccal (kok'al) resembling or pertaining to cocci.

cocci (kok'si) [L.] plural of *coccus*.

Coccidioides (kok-sid″e-oi′děz) a genus of deuteromycetous fungi (Fungi Imperfecti). **C. im′mitis**, a species that reproduces within the tissues exclusively by a process of endogenous spore formation within spherules. The newly liberated spores are small mononucleate cells, 1 to 3 μ in diameter. As it enlarges, the cell becomes multinucleate and reaches a diameter of 50 to 60 μ. It is the etiologic agent of coccidioidomycosis.

coccidioidomycosis (kok-sid″e-oi″do-mi-ko′sis) a disease caused by infection with the fungus *Coccidioides immitis*, occurring most commonly in the arid and hot zones of South and North America. It occurs in two forms: a primary form characterized by pulmonary lesions associated with cough, hemoptysis, arthralgia, pain in the chest, fever, malaise, and, sometimes, erythematous skin lesions; and a secondary form characterized by skin ulcers and subcutaneous abscesses, nodules, and tumors that metastasize from internal lesions, chiefly of the lungs and lymph nodes. Tumors are elastic and vary in size; they are not accompanied by an inflammatory reaction. The abscesses are accompanied by an inflammatory reaction and contain thick, mucoid pus which drains through sinuses and produces ulcers. The secondary lesions are usually found on the hands, neck, and face, particularly the perioral region. Papillomatous and verrucous lesions, chiefly of the face, neck, scalp, trunk, and upper extremities, may occur. The terms *California disease, San Joaquin disease, San Joaquin fever*, and *valley fever* refer to the primary, or pulmonary, form of the disease; *coccidioidal granuloma* refers to the secondary, or cutaneous, form.

coccobacilli (kok″o-bah-sil′li) plural of *coccobacillus*.

Coccobacillus (kok″o-bah-sil′us) a former genus of bacteria, the species of which have been assigned to other genera. **C. ducrey′i**, *Haemophilus ducreyi*; see under HAEMOPHILUS. **C. pfeif′feri**, *Haemophilus influenzae*; see under HAEMOPHILUS.

C. praeacu′tus, *Bacteroides praeacutus*; see under BACTEROIDES.

coccobacillus (kok″o-bah-sil′us), pl. *coccobacil′li*. An oval bacterial cell intermediate between the coccus and bacillus forms.

coccobacteria (kok″o-bak″te-re-ah) [Gr. *kokkos* berry + *baktērion* little rod] spheroid bacteria or cocci; see COCCUS.

coccoid (kok′oid) [Gr. *kokkos* berry + *eidos* shape] resembling a coccus; globose.

cocculin (kok′u-lin) picrotoxin.

coccus (kok′us), pl. *coc′ci* [L.; Gr. *kokkos* berry] a spherical bacterium about 0.6 to 1.0 μm in diameter. Cocci are differentiated on the basis of the arrangement of their cells with respect to one another; the relationship resulting from the plane in which cell division occurs and the tendency of daughter cells to remain attached or be close to one another after division is complete. Completely separated cocci are known as *micrococci*. Cocci occur in pairs when daughter cells remain attached and the cell division occurs in only one plane — these are termed *diplococci*. Some diplococci are elongated and are paired with long axes parallel; those with coffee bean shapes are known as *gonococci* and *meningococci*. A more marked tendency to remain attached results in the formation of chains of four to twelve cells — thus attached cocci are known as *streptococci*. A tendency of daughter cells to remain adjacent to one another associated with cell division in two or more planes and the occurrence of irregular groups is characteristic of *staphylococci*. Cell division occurring in two or more perpendicular planes associated with cells remaining together and the cocci being found in tetrads or in cubical pockets of eight cells is typical of the genus *Sarcina*.

-coccus a word termination signifying a spheroid bacterium, as a staphylococcus.

cochl. abbreviation for L. *cochlea′re*, a spoonful.

cochleare (kok″le-a′re) [L.] spoon or spoonful.

Cockayne's syndrome [Edward Alfred *Cockayne*, British physician, 1880–1956] see under SYNDROME. See also EPIDERMOLYSIS bullosa (Weber-Cockayne syndrome).

cocktail (kok′tāl) a beverage concocted of various ingredients. **lytic c.**, a concoction of various drugs used to block the function of the autonomic nervous system at every level, thus inhibiting the homeostatic defense reactions of the organism and producing the state known as artificial hibernation; used in various surgical procedures.

cocoa (ko′ko) a powder prepared from roasted, cured kernels of the ripe seed of *Theobroma cacao*. Called also *cacao*. **c. butter**, theobroma OIL.

Coct. abbreviation for L. *coc′tio*, boiling.

code (kōd) 1. a collection of the existing laws, rules, or regulations. 2. a system of symbols, such as letters, words, or other marks, to represent something, e.g., a system of symbols for representing information in a computerized data bank or information system. **ADA Uniform C. on Dental Procedures and Nomenclature**, a standard nomenclature of usual dental procedures developed by the American Dental Association for use in official reporting and in dental insurance claims. The nomenclature is complemented by a five-digit code: The first digit to the left is 0 and indicates dental services, as opposed to hospital, surgical, or other medical services, which are assigned specific numbers; the second designates a category of dental service;

DENTAL SERVICE CATEGORIES OF THE ADA UNIFORM CODE ON DENTAL PROCEDURES AND NOMENCLATURE

	Category of Service	Code Series
I.	Diagnostic	00100–00999
II.	Preventive	01000–01999
III.	Restorative	02000–02999
IV.	Endodontics	03000–03999
V.	Peridontics	04000–04999
VI.	Prosthodontics — removable (partial & complete denture prosthesis)	05000–05999
VII.	Prosthodontics — fixed (bridges)	06000–06999
VIII.	Oral surgery	07000–07999
IX.	Orthodontics	08000–08999
X.	Other services	09000–09999

(From J.A.D.A., 79:814–817. October 1969.)

the third designates the class of service within a given category; the fourth designates the subclass of the service; and the fifth is supplied for future expansion. Under this code system, the number 02150 would indicate a two-surface amalgam restoration on a permanent tooth — the first digit (0) indicating a dental procedure; the second (2) a restoration; the third (1) an amalgam restoration; the fourth (5) a permanent tooth and the number of surfaces involved; the fifth (0) not having any meaning. It is commonly referred to as *ADA procedure numbers*. **c. of ethics,** the standard of moral principles and practice to which a profession adheres. A series of principles used as a guide in assisting a dentist to fulfill the moral obligations of the professional dental practice. Called also *principle of ethics*. See Hippocratic oath at HIPPOCRATES, and medical ETHICS. **genetic c.,** the arrangement of nucleotides (nitrogenous bases) in the polynucleotide chain of a chromosome that governs the transmission of genetic information in protein synthesis. The sequence of four bases (adenine, thymine, cytosine, and guanine in DNA, and adenine, uracil, cytosine, and guanine in RNA) forms the genetic code, and each three-base sequence forms one triplet that is specific for an amino acid; the sequence of triplets, in turn, containing the code for one polypeptide. **C. of Hammurabi,** a legal code of the 20th century B.C., instituted by Hammurabi, a king of Babylonia, which dealt with criminal and civil matters, being the first document presenting the concept of the civil and penal responsibilities of the physician. It also contains the first reference to the therapeutic extraction of teeth.

codehydrogenase I (ko″de-hi′dro-jen″ās) nicotinamide-adenine DINUCLEOTIDE.

codehydrogenase II (ko″de-hi′dro-jen″ās) nicotinamide-adenine dinucleotide phosphate; see under DINUCLEOTIDE.

codeine (ko′dēn) [L. *codeina*] an opium alkaloid, 7,8-didehydro-4,5-α-epoxy-3-methoxy-17-methylmorphinan-6-α-ol, occurring as colorless or white crystals or powder that effloresces slowly in dry air and is affected by light. It is slightly soluble in water and readily soluble in alcohol and chloroform. Pharmacologically, codeine is an opiate analgesic resembling morphine, but its analgesic activity in humans is about one-sixth to one-fifteenth that of morphine, and it is about one-tenth as potent as morphine in depressing the cough and respiratory centers. Used as an analgesic, narcotic, and antitussive. Abuse leads to habituation and addiction. Called also *methyl ether of morphine, methylmorphine,* and *morphine monomethyl ether.* **DH-c.,** dihydrocodeine. **c. phosphate,** the phosphate salt of codeine, occurring as fine white, needle-shaped crystals or white crystalline, odorless powder that is affected by light and is soluble in water and alcohol. It is a narcotic analgesic used in dentistry to alleviate pain when drugs stronger than aspirin are required, frequently used in combination with aspirin; the combination enhances the analgesic effects of both drugs. It is also used as an antitussive agent. Called also *methylmorphine phosphate.* **c. sulfate,** the sulfate salt of codeine, occurring as a white crystalline solid or crystalline powder that is soluble in water, alcohol, and methanol, but insoluble in chloroform and ether. Used as an antitussive and narcotic analgesic agent.

Codempiral trademark for an analgesic preparation containing aspirin, phenacetin, phenobarbital, and codeine phosphate.

Codescaine trademark for *lidocaine hydrochloride* (see under LIDOCAINE).

Codesco Premium trademark for a hard *dental casting gold alloy* (see under GOLD).

Codesco Premium Type IV trademark for an extra hard *dental casting gold alloy* (see under GOLD).

Codesco topical fluoride phosphate anticaries gel see under GEL.

Codethyline trademark for *ethylmorphine hydrochloride* (see under ETHYLMORPHINE).

Codhydrine trademark for *dihydrocodeine.*

Codinovo trademark for *hydrocodone bitartrate* (see under HYDROCODONE).

Codman's triangle [Ernest Amory *Codman,* American surgeon, 1869–1940] see under TRIANGLE.

codon (ko′don) a series of three nitrogenous bases (nucleotides) in a polynucleotide of DNA or RNA, carrying the specific genetic information which is translated into a single amino acid in protein synthesis. Called also *triplet*. See also TRANSLATION and transfer RNA.

Coe alginate see under ALGINATE.

Coecal trademark for the Class I (Type III) *dental stone* (see under STONE).

Coe-Comfort trademark for a *denture reliner* (see under RELINER), believed to be prepared from ethyl alcohol plasticizers and acrylic resins.

Coe Cure trademark for a self-curing *repair resin* (see under RESIN).

coefficient (ko″ĕ-fish′ent) [*co-* + L. *efficiens* effecting, effective] 1. an expression of the change or effect produced by the variation in certain factors, or of the ratio between two different quantities. 2. in chemistry, a number or figure put before a chemical formula to indicate how many times the formula is to be multiplied. **absorption c.,** 1. the ratio of the rate of change of x-rays in a homologous material to the intensity at a given point. It is a fractional decrease in the intensity of a beam of x-rays per unit thickness (*linear absorption c.*), per unit mass (*mass absorption c.*), or per atom (*atomic absorption c.*) of the absorbing substance. The total absorption coefficient is the sum of the individual energy-absorbing processes (see Compton EFFECT, photoelectric EMISSION, and pair PRODUCTION). 2. a number indicating the volume of a gas absorbed by a unit volume of a liquid at 0°C, and a pressure of 760 mm Hg. Called also *Bunsen c.* **Ambard's c.,** Ambard's FORMULA. **atomic absorption (attenuation) c.,** the fractional reduction in x-ray intensity produced by a layer thickness of one atom per square centimeter. **Bunsen c.,** absorption c. (2). **c. of diffusion,** the amount of diffusion which takes place across a given unit area (e.g., 1 cm²) through 1 unit thickness (e.g., 1 cm) of a substance in 1 unit time (e.g., 1 sec). Symbol *D.* **c. of elasticity,** MODULUS of elasticity. **electronic absorption c.,** the fractional reduction in x-ray intensity produced by a layer thickness of one electron per square centimeter. **homogeneity c.,** the ratio of the half-value and the additional thickness of the material needed to reduce a radiation beam to one-fourth of its original exposure rate; it is unity for monoenergetic photons. See also half-value LAYER. **linear absorption c.,** a factor expressing the fraction of a beam of x-rays or gamma rays absorbed in unit thickness of material. **linear c. of thermal expansion,** the change in length per unit length of a material when its temperature is raised or lowered 1 degree. See thermal EXPANSION. **mass absorption c.,** the linear absorption coefficient per centimeter, divided by the density of the absorber in grams per cubic centimeter. **c. of thermal conductivity,** see thermal CONDUCTIVITY (2).

Coe Flex trademark for a *polysulfide impression material* (see under MATERIAL).

Coe-Flo trademark for a hard *zinc oxide–eugenol impression paste* (see under PASTE).

coel- [Gr. *koilia* cavity] a combining form denoting relationship to a cavity or space; sometimes spelled *cel-*.

-coele [Gr. *koilia* cavity] a word termination denoting relationship to a cavity or space; sometimes spelled *-cele*.

coelom (se′lom) [Gr. *koilōma*] the space between the split layers of lateral mesoderm of the embryo or between the somatopleure and the splanchnopleure. It develops during the fourth week of embryonic development, at first as a pair of bilaterally symmetrical chambers which join later. Within the embryo it becomes subdivided into separate compartments for the heart, lungs, and abdominal viscera. The surface of the mesoderm bound to the coelom forms the mesothelium. Called also *body cavity, coeloma, hemal cavity,* and *somatic cavity.* **extraembryonic c.,** the cavity bordered by chorionic mesoderm and the mesoderm of the amnion and yolk sac; it communicates temporarily at the umbilicus with the intraembryonic coelom.

coeloma (se-lo′mah) coelom.

coeno- [Gr. *koinos* shared in common] see CENO-(3).

coenzyme (ko-en′zīm) a low-molecular-weight organic substance which can attach itself to a specific protein to form an active enzyme system. Coenzymes generally act as acceptors or donors of a functional group or of atoms that are removed from or contributed to the substrate. Sometimes, they are readily dissociable from the enzyme protein. Called also *enzyme cofactor.* **c. A,** a substance essential for the formation of acetylcholine and for many acetylation reactions in the body, involved in acetyl or other acyl group transfer, fatty acid synthesis, and oxidation. It is built up from pantothenic acid, cysteamine, adenosine, and phosphoric acid. Abbreviated *CoA.* **c. I (CoI),** nicotinamide-adenine DINUCLEOTIDE. **c. II (CoII),** nicotinamide-adenine dinucleotide phosphate; see under DINUCLEOTIDE. **c. Q,** ubiquinone. **c. R,** biotin. **Warburg's c.,** nicotinamide-adenine dinucleotide phosphate; see under DINUCLEOTIDE.

Coe-Pack see under PACK.

Coe-Pak paste see under PASTE.

Coe-Soft trademark for a *denture reliner* (see under RELINER).

cofactor (ko′fak-tor) an element or principle with which another must unite in order to function. **enzyme c.,** coenzyme. **platelet c. I,** FACTOR VIII. **platelet c. II,** FACTOR IX.

coffeine (kof′fe-in) caffeine.

Coffin plate (appliance), spring [C. R. *Coffin*, American dentist, 1826–1891] see under PLATE and SPRING.

Coffin-Lowry syndrome [G. S. *Coffin*; R. B. *Lowry*] see under SYNDROME.

Coffin-Siris syndrome [G. S. *Coffin*; E. *Siris*] see under SYNDROME.

COFS cerebro-oculofacioskeletal SYNDROME.

cohesion (ko-he′zhun) [L. *cohaesio*, from *con* together + *haerere* to stick] 1. the act or process of sticking together. 2. the attractive force which holds the molecules of the same kind together. See also ADHESION (1).

cohesive (ko-he′siv) uniting together; characterized by cohesion.

Cohnheim's artery [Julius Friedrich *Cohnheim*, German pathologist, 1839–1884] terminal ARTERY.

CoI coenzyme I; see nicotinamide-adenine DINUCLEOTIDE.

CoII coenzyme II; nicotinamide-adenine dinucleotide phosphate; see under DINUCLEOTIDE.

coil (koil) anything wound in a spiral. See also HELIX.

coino- [Gr. *koinos* shared in common] see CENO-(3).

coinsurance (ko″in-shur′ans) 1. insurance jointly with another or others. 2. a means of sharing, dividing, or splitting the cost of health services between the health plan and the insured person; a form of cost-sharing insurance. In dental insurance, a common division is 80 percent–20 percent, the insurance company paying 80 percent of the cost of the dental service and the patient paying 20 percent. Percentages vary and may be applied to scheduled or usual, customary, and reasonable fee plans. Called also *copayment*. See also COST-SHARING.

coisogeneic (ko-i″so-jĕ-ne′ik) congeneic.

col (kol) a valley-like depression of the interdental gingiva, which connects the facial and lingual papillae, and conforms to the shape of the interproximal contact area. At the time of eruption and for a period thereafter, it is covered by reduced enamel epithelium derived from the approximating teeth, which is later replaced by stratified squamous epithelium from the adjacent interdental papillae.

Colace trademark for *dioctyl sodium sulfosuccinate* (see under DIOCTYL).

colamine (ko′lah-min) ethanolamine.

colation (ko-la′shun) [L. *colatio*] 1. the process of straining or filtration. 2. the product of such a process.

colchicine (kol′chĭ-sin) a very poisonous alkaloid obtained from trees of the genus *Colchicum*, (S)-N-(5,6,7,9-tetrahydro-1,2,3,10 - tetramethoxy - 9 - oxobenzo[a]heptalen - 7 - yl)acetamide, occurring as a pale yellow, odorless amorphous powder or scales that darken on exposure to light and are soluble in water, ether, ethanol, and chloroform. Used in the treatment of acute attacks of gouty arthritis.

Colchicum (kol′chĭ-kum) a genus of Old World liliaceous trees, the meadow saffron, from which colchicine is obtained.

cold (kōld) 1. a relatively low temperature or absence of heat. The effect of cold on tissues is characterized by a diminution of capillary blood flow and decreased metabolic rate, resulting in a decrease of exchange between blood and tissues and transient anemia, later followed by congestion. Cold is used to control bleeding and to minimize inflammation in early cases of trauma in which there is no acute infection, after tooth extraction or after surgical removal of impacted teeth, in cases of early fractures of the jaws or temporomandibular dislocation, and after other types of oral surgery. 2. common c.; see acute CORYZA. **allergic c.,** hay FEVER. **chest c., common c., head c.,** acute CORYZA. **June c.,** hay FEVER. **c. sores,** see HERPES simplex. **c. work,** cold WORK.

Coldan trademark for *naphazoline*.

Cole, H. N. [American physician] see DYSKERATOSIS congenita (Zinsser-Engman-Cole syndrome).

Colepax trademark for *iopanoic acid* (see under ACID).

Coletyl trademark for *carbachol*.

Colgate see under DENTIFRICE.

colibacillemia (ko″lĭ-bas-ĭ-le′me-ah) [*coli bacillus* + Gr. *haima* blood + *-ia*] the presence of coli bacilli (*Escherichia coli*) in the blood.

colibacillosis (ko″lĭ-bas-ĭ-lo′sis) infection with coli bacilli (*Escherichia coli*).

colibacilluria (ko″lĭ-bas″ĭ-lu′re-ah) [*coli bacillus* + Gr. *ouron* urine + *-ia*] the presence of coli bacilli (*Escherichia coli*) in the urine.

colibacillus (ko″lĭ-bah-sil′us) *Escherichia coli*; see under Escherichia.

colic (kol′ik) [Gr. *kōlikos*] 1. pertaining to the colon. 2. acute abdominal pain. **lead c.,** abdominal colic due to lead poisoning. Called also *painter's c.* See also LEAD. **painter's c.,** abdominal colic observed in painters exposed to lead-base paints. Called also *lead c.* See also LEAD.

Colimycin trademark for *colistin sulfate* (see under COLISTIN).

Colisticina trademark for *colistin sulfate* (see under COLISTIN).

colistimethate sodium (ko-lis″tĭ-meth′āt) a methane sulfonate derivative of colistin, colistimethanesulfonic acid, occurring as a white to yellowish, odorless powder that is readily soluble in water, slightly soluble in methanol, and insoluble in ether and acetone. Used in the treatment of infections caused by *Pseudomonas*, *Salmonella*, *Shigella*, and the coli-aerogenes group of bacteria. Transient paresthesias, pruritus, skin lesions, visual and speech disorders, drug fever, vertigo, gastrointestinal disturbances, leukopenia, agranulocytosis, leukopenia, pain at the site of injection, azotemia, and kidney disorders may occur. It is only partially as effective and toxic as colistin. Called also *colistin sulfomethate*.

colistin (ko-lis′tin) a polypeptide antibiotic isolated from cultures of *Bacillus colistinus*. It is a cyclopolypeptide composed of colistins A, B, and C, being identical with polymyxin B except for the substitution of a residue of D-leucine for that of D-phenylalanine. **c. sulfate,** the sulfate salt of colistin, occurring as a white to yellowish, odorless powder that is readily soluble in water, slightly soluble in methanol, and insoluble in acetone and ether. Used in the treatment of infections caused by *Pseudomonas*, *Salmonella*, *Shigella*, and the coli-aerogenes group of bacteria. It is less potent than polymyxin B, except against *Klebsiella pneumoniae* and *Serratia marcescens*. Transient paresthesias, pruritus, skin lesions, visual and speech disorders, drug fever, vertigo, gastrointestinal disorders, leukopenia, and agranulocytosis may occur. Called also *polymyxin E.* Trademarks: Colimycin, Coly-Mycin, Colisticina. **c. sulfomethate,** COLISTIMETHATE sodium.

colla (kol′lah) [L.] plural of *collum*.

collagen (kol′ah-jen) [Gr. *kolla* glue + *gennan* to produce] a scleroprotein serving as a supportive protein in the structure of bone, teeth, skin, tendons, cartilage, and all other connective tissues. Collagens are fibrous proteins, which contain about 33 percent glycine and about 20 percent both proline and hydroxyproline, but lack the sulfur-containing amino acid cysteine. They are soluble in the presence of dilute acidic buffers, pH 3 to 4, and are precipitated at neutral pH. Prolonged boiling in water converts collagens to soluble products termed *gelatins*. They are the principal protein of the dentin and cementum. In the periodontium, collagen fibers originate in the cementum and pass into the lamina propria or into periodontal ligament fibers, giving tonus to the gingiva and supporting the teeth in their bony sockets. Collagen loss occurs in periodontal diseases. See also collagen DISEASE.

collagenase [E.C.3.4.24.3] (kol-laj′ĕ-nas) [*collagen* + *-ase*] a metalloproteinase capable of causing hydrolytic scission of peptide bonds in the helical regions of undenatured collagen. It is present in higher organisms (including man) that have collagen as a major component of their tissues and in microorganisms that do not elaborate collagen, including bacterial strains present in dental plaque, such as *Clostridium, Mycobacterium, Pseudomonas,* and *Bacteroides*. The level of collagenase present in inflamed gingival tissue appears to be greater than in normal tissue.

collapse (kŏ-laps′) [L. *collapsus*] 1. a state of extreme prostration and depression, with failure of circulation. 2. abnormal falling in of the walls of any part or organ. **circulatory c.,** SHOCK.

collar (kol′ler) 1. an encircling band around any neckline structure. 2. a narrow metal band that fits over an abutment or a post in dental restoration. **gingival c.,** epithelial ATTACHMENT (of Gottlieb). **periosteal bone c.,** a band of spongy bone around the middle of the diaphysis of an early bone. It is made up of osteoblasts and serves as a peripheral ossification center in diaphyseal bone development.

collateral (ko-lat′er-al) [L. *con* together + *latus* side] 1. secondary or accessory; not direct or immediate. 2. a small side branch, as of a blood vessel or nerve.

college (kol′ij) 1. an institution of higher learning or a constituent unit of a university, furnishing courses of instruction in the liberal arts and sciences, usually leading to a Bachelor of Arts degree. 2. a group or body of persons having a common purpose. See also ACADEMY. **American C. of Dentists,** a professional association established to promote the highest ideals in health care, advance the standards and efficiency of dentistry, develop good human relations and understanding, and extend the benefits of dental health to the greatest number of persons. Abbreviated *ACD*. **American C. of Oral and Maxillofacial Surgeons,** a professional organization of certified oral and maxillofacial surgeons, having as its objective the preservation and promotion of the integrity of the specialty of oral and maxillofacial surgery and its advancement, pursuing the highest standards of professionalism of its members, and the advancement of the art and science of the specialty by encouraging and implementing continuing education. Abbreviated *ACOMS.* **American C. of Prosthodontists,** a professional dental organization established to foster interest in the specialty of prosthodontics with the objective of improving the quality of dental treatment for the prosthodontic patient through educational activities designed to bring new ideas, techniques, and research into clinical practice and to enhance the prosthodontic services received by the public. Abbreviated *ACP.* **International C. of Dentists,** an international society of dentists established to recognize those who have made professional contributions in a measure to warrant recognition and to encourage others to discharge more fully their obligations. The United States of America Section is open by invitation to outstanding members of the profession who belong to the American Dental Association or are dental officers in the Armed Forces, Public Health Service, and Veterans Administration and who are engaged in the practice of dentistry, are engaged in research, teach dental subjects, or write and edit dental literature. Four classes of membership exist: Fellows, Masters, Honorary Fellows, and Life Members.

Colles-Baumès law [A. *Colles;* Pierre Prosper François *Baumès,* French physician, 1791–1871] see under LAW.

Colles' law [Abraham *Colles,* Irish surgeon, 1773–1843] Colles-Baumès LAW.

Collet-Sicard syndrome [Frédéric Justin *Collet,* French physician, born 1870; Jean Athanase *Sicard,* French neurologist, 1872–1929] see under SYNDROME.

colliculus (kŏ-lik'u-lus), pl. *collic'uli* [L.] a small elevation or mound. **c. of arytenoid cartilage,** a small mound on the anterior margin of the anterolateral surface of the arytenoid cartilage, near its apex, which gives raise to a ridge, the crista arcuata. Called also *c. cartilaginis arytaenoideae* and *c. cartilaginis arytenoideae* [NA]. **c. cartilag'inis arytenoi'deae** [NA], **c. cartilag'inis arytenoi'deae,** c. of arytenoid cartilage. **facial c., c. facia'lis** [NA], an elevation of the medial eminence in the rhomboid fossa, caused by the internal genu of the facial nerve as it loops around the abducent nucleus. Called also *eminentia facialis, eminentia teres,* and *facial eminence of eminentia teres.*

collimation (kol"lĭ-ma'shun) 1. the bringing into line; a making parallel. 2. in microscopy, making the light rays parallel; the process of aligning the optical axis of the optical system to the reference mechanical axes or surfaces of the instrument, or the adjustment of two or more optical axes with respect to each other. 3. in radiology, the elimination of the peripheral (more divergent) portion of an x-ray beam by means of metal tubes, cones, or diaphragms interposed in the path of the beam.

collimator (kol"lĭ-ma'tor) a lead disk with an aperture of desired size or shape, serving as the diaphragm which defines and limits the size and shape of the primary beam of x-rays to the examined area.

Collimycin trademark for *lincomycin.*

Collin's law see under LAW.

Collins, Treacher see TREACHER COLLINS.

colliquation (kol"ĭ-kwa'shun) [L. *con* together + *liquare* to melt] liquefactive degeneration of tissue.

collision (ko-lizh'un) 1. the striking together or impact of objects or bodies traveling on converging courses. 2. a close approach of two or more particles, photons, atoms, or nuclei, during which quantities of energy, momentum, and charge may be exchanged. **elastic c.,** that in which there is no change either in the internal energy of each participating system or in the sum of their kinetic energies of translation. **inelastic c.,** that in which there are changes both in the internal energy of one or more of the colliding systems and in the sum of their kinetic energies of translation before and after the collision.

Colliver's symptom see under SYMPTOM.

collodion (ko-lo'de-on) [L. *collodium,* from Gr. *kollōdēs* glutinous] a substance consisting of pyroxylin, ether, and alcohol. It occurs as a clear, or slightly opalescent, viscous liquid with a slight ethereal odor, which dries to form a transparent, tenacious film. Used to protect small wounds or abrasions of the skin or mucous membranes from external irritation. **c. elastique, flexible c. flexible c.,** a preparation of camphor, castor oil, and collodion, forming a tenacious, flexible film over small wounds and abrasions. Called also *c. elastique.*

colloid (kol'oid) [Gr. *kollōdēs* glutinous] 1. glutinous or resem-

bling glue. 2. a state of matter in which the matter is dispersed in or distributed throughout some medium called the *dispersion medium.* The matter thus dispersed is called the *disperse phase* of the colloid system. The particles of the disperse phase are larger than an ordinary crystalloid molecule, but are not large enough to settle out under the influence of gravity; they range in size from $0.1\ \mu$ to $1\ \mu\mu$. There are two kinds of colloids: *suspension colloids* (suspensoids), in which the disperse phase consists of particles of any insoluble substance, as a metal, and the dispersion medium may be gaseous, liquid, or solid; and *emulsion colloids* (emulsoids), in which the dispersion medium is usually water and the disperse phase consists of highly complex organic substances, such as starch or glue, which absorb much water, swell, and become uniformly distributed throughout the dispersion medium in a manner not well understood. The former tend to be less stable than the latter. See also SOLUTION and SUSPENSION. 3. the translucent, yellowish, gelatinous substance resulting from colloid degeneration. **association c.,** one in which the dispersed particles are each made up of many molecules. **dispersion c.,** see *colloid* (2). **emulsion c.,** see *colloid* (2). **hydrophilic c.,** emulsion c.; see *colloid* (2). **hydrophobic c.,** suspension c.; see *colloid* (2). **c. impression material,** see impression material, irreversible hydrocolloid and impression material, reversible hydrocolloid, under MATERIAL. **irreversible c.,** one that cannot be dispersed. Cf. *reversible c.* **lyophilic c.,** emulsion c.; see *colloid* (2). **lyophobic c.,** suspension c.; see *colloid* (2). **lyotropic c.,** emulsion c.; see *colloid* (2). **protective c.,** one that is able to prevent the precipitation of another colloid. See also EMULSIFIER. **reversible c.,** one that can be dispersed after having been precipitated or a gel that can be converted into a sol. Called also *stable c.* Cf. *irreversible c.* **suspension c.,** see *colloid* (2). **thyroid c.,** the colloid found in the acini of the thyroid gland, consisting essentially of thyroglobulin.

colloma (ko-lo'mah) [Gr. *kolla* glue + *-oma*] see mucinous CARCINOMA.

collum (kol'lum), pl. *col'la* [L.] 1. [NA] the neck; the portion of the body connecting the head and trunk; the lower front portion of the collum is called the *cervix,* and the back is called the *nucha.* 2. a general anatomical term applied to any necklike part of a body, structure, or organ. **c. den'tis** [NA], NECK of tooth. **c. mandib'ulae** [NA], **c. proces'sus condyloi'dei mandib'ulae,** NECK of mandible.

collunaria (kol"u-na're-ah) [L.] plural of *collunarium.*

collunarium (kol"u-na're-um), pl. *colluna'ria* [L.] a nasal douche.

Collut. abbreviation for L. *colluto'rium,* mouth wash.

collutoria (kol"u-to're-ah) [L.] plural of *collutorium.*

collutorium (kol"u-to're-um), pl. *colluto'ria* [L.] collutory.

collutory (kol'u-to"re) [L. *collutorium*] a mouth wash or gargle. **Miller's c.,** a mouthwash containing benzoic acid, tincture of krameria, and oil of peppermint.

coloboma (kol"o-bo'mah), pl. *colobomas* or *colobo'mata* [L.; Gr. *kolobōma*] a mutilation or defect; especially a congenital fissure of any part of the eye.

colobomata (kol"lo-bo'mah-tah) [L.] plural of *coloboma.*

Cologel trademark for *methylcellulose.*

coloring (kol'or-ing) the act or method of applying color. **extrinsic c.,** coloring from without, as applying color to the external surface of a dental prosthesis. **intrinsic c.,** coloring from within, as the incorporation of pigment within the material of a dental prosthesis.

Coltirot trademark for *tyrothricin.*

columbium (ko-lum'be-um) niobium.

columella (kol"u-mel'lah), pl. *columel'lae* [L.] 1. a little column. 2. in molds, the central axis of a spore case, around which the spores are arranged. **c. na'si,** the fleshy distal margin of the nasal septum.

columellae (kol"u-mel'le) [L.] plural of *columella.*

column (kol'um) [L. *columna*] a pillarlike or a cylindrical structure; used in anatomical nomenclature for such a structure. See also COLUMNA and PILLAR. **enamel c's,** enamel prisms; see under PRISM. **fat c.,** one of the columns of fatty tissue extending from the cutaneous connective tissue to the hair follicles and sweat glands. Called also *Warren's fat c.* and *columna adiposa.* **c. of fauces, anterior,** palatoglossal ARCH. **c. of fauces, posterior,** palatopharyngeal ARCH. **c's of folds of tongue,** foliate papillae; see under PAPILLA. **Kölliker's c.,** a bundle of myofibrils. Called also *muscle c.* and *sarcostyle.* **muscle c.,** Kölliker's c. **c. of nose,** nasal SEPTUM. **spinal c.,** vertebral c. **vertebral c.,** the columnar assemblage of the vertebrae from the cranium through the coccyx. Called also *spinal c., columna vertebralis* [NA], and *spine.* **Warren's fat c.,** fat c.

columna (ko-lum'nah), pl. *colum'nae* [L.] column; a pillarlike or cylindrical structure; used in anatomical nomenclature to designate such a structure or part. **c. adipo′sa,** fat COLUMN. **c. na′si,** nasal SEPTUM. **c. vertebra′lis** [NA], vertebral COLUMN.

columnae (ko-lum′ne) [L.] plural of *columna.*

Coly-Mycin trademark for *colistin sulfate* (see under COLISTIN).

Coly-Mycin M trademark for *colistimethate sodium* (see under SODIUM).

coma (ko′mah) [L.; Gr. *kōma*] a state of unconsciousness from which the patient cannot be aroused, even by powerful stimuli. **diabetic c.,** a complication of diabetes mellitus, usually occurring in ketoaciduria and, less commonly, in elevation of blood sugar to such a degree that the hyperosmolality of the plasma causes unconsciousness. It is due to failure to take insulin or other antidiabetic drug, faulty dietary habits, or postoperative complications. Symptoms include rapid breathing, air hunger, weakness, anorexia, dry skin and mouth, fruity odor of the breath, drowsiness, abdominal pain, hypotension, tachycardia, dehydration, sunken eyeballs, glycosuria, hyperglycemia, high acetoacetic acid level, and loss of consciousness. See also hypoglycemic SHOCK. **hepatic c.,** coma in acute or chronic liver disease due to shunting of portal venous blood through collateral vessels into the peripheral circulation and metabolic changes, particularly alteration of brain ammonium metabolism. It is characterized by mental confusion, a characteristic flapping tremor of the fingers and hands, and loss of consciousness followed by deepening coma and death. **hyperosmolar nonketotic c.,** diabetic coma in which the level of ketone bodies is normal, owing to hyperosmolarity of extracellular fluid resulting in dehydration of intracellular fluid; often a consequence of overtreatment with hyperosmolar solutions. **irreversible c.,** coma in which for a period of 24 hours there is complete unreceptivity and unresponsivity even to the most intensely painful stimuli, nonspontaneous movement or breathing, absence of elicitable reflexes, and an isoelectric electroencephalogram. Called also *brain death syndrome.*

comatose (ko′mah-tōs) pertaining to or affected with coma.

Combetin trademark for *strophanthin.*

combination (kom′bĭ-na′shun) 1. the act of bringing or joining into a close union; to unite. Also, that which is formed by bringing or joining things together. 2. the union of two or more substances to form a new chemical substance. 3. a chemical reaction in which two elements combine and form a binary compound, or two binary compounds form a complex compound.

combustion (kom-bust′yun) [L. *combustio*] the act or process of burning. Chemically, it is a process of rapid oxidation with emission of heat. Combustion generally occurs when a substance rapidly unites with oxygen, but may also occur in the absence of oxygen.

Comfolax trademark for *dioctyl sodium sulfosuccinate* (see under DIOCTYL).

Comfortid trademark for *indomethacin.*

Commando's operation see under OPERATION.

comminuted (kom′ĭ-nūt′ed) [L. *comminutus,* from *com* together + *minuere* to diminish] broken or crushed into small pieces, as a comminuted fracture.

comminution (kom′ĭ-nu′shun) [L. *comminutio*] the act of breaking, or condition of being broken, into small fragments. **c. of food,** the reduction of food into small parts. See MASTICATION.

commission (kŏ-mish′un) a group or body of persons designated to take action on some matter. **c's of the American Dental Association,** see American Dental Association in Appendix. **Educational C. for Foreign Medical Graduates,** an organization sponsored by the American Medical Association, American Hospital Association, American Association of Medical Colleges, and other associations, which operates a program of educating, testing, and evaluating foreign medical graduates who seek internships and residencies in the United States. Certification of foreign medical graduates is granted by the commission after receiving documentation of their education and passage of examinations of their medical competence and comprehension of spoken English. Such certification is necessary for licensure of foreign graduates in most states and territories. Abbreviated *ECFMG.* **Joint C. on Accreditation of Hospitals,** a commission made up of representatives of the American College of Physicians, American College of Surgeons, American Hospital Association, American Medical Association, and American Dental Association. The Commission was formed to promote a high quality of health care by establishing guidelines and standards for the quality of patient care and for the operation of hospitals, and for the verification that these guidelines and standards are carried out by hospitals. Abbreviated *JCAH.* **C. on Professional and Hospital Activities,** a nonprofit organization sponsored by the American College of Physicians, American College of Surgeons, American Hospital Association, and Southwestern Michigan Hospital Council, which collects, processes, and distrib-

utes data on hospital utilization and management, evaluation, and research purposes and abstracts and classifies information obtained from medical records and makes information accessible through the computerized data library. The two branches of the program are the Professional Activity Study (PAS) and the Medical Audit Program (MAP). Abbreviated *CPHA.*

commissura (kom″mĭ-su′rah), pl. *commissu′rae* [L. "a joining together"] a site of union of corresponding parts. See also COMMISSURE. **c. labio′rum o′ris,** [NA], labial COMMISSURE. **c. palpebra′rum latera′lis,** [NA], lateral commissure of eyelids; see under COMMISSURE. **c. palpebra′rum media′lis** [NA], medial commissure of eyelids; see under COMMISSURE. **c. palpebra′rum nasa′lis,** medial commissure of eyelids; see under COMMISSURE. **c. palpebra′rum tempora′lis,** lateral commissure of eyelids; see under COMMISSURE.

commissurae (kom″mĭ-su′re) [L.] plural of *commissura.*

commissural (kom-mis′u-ral) pertaining to a commissure.

commissure (kom′ĭ-shūr) [L. *commissura* a joining together] a site of union of corresponding parts. Called also *commissura.* **labial c.,** the junction of the upper and lower lips at either side of the mouth; the corner of the mouth. Called also *commissura labiorum oris* [NA]. **lateral c. of eyelids,** the lateral junction of the superior and inferior eyelids. Called also *commissura palpebrarum lateralis* [NA] and *commissura palpebrarum temporalis.* **medial c. of eyelids,** the medial junction of the superior and inferior eyelids. Called also *commissura palpebrarum medialis* [NA] and *commissura palpebrarum nasalis.*

committee (kŏ-mit′e) a group of persons designated to study, take action on, or report on a particular matter. **American National Standards C. MD156 for Dental Materials and Devices,** a committee of the American National Standards Institute with the participation of various American governmental, professional, and industrial groups and the Fédération Dentaire Internationale, serving under the administrative sponsorship of the Council on Dental Materials and Devices of the American Dental Association. The Committee, which cooperates with the International Organization for Standardization, is organized into four groups: (1) subcommittees on restorative materials; (2) subcommittees on prosthetic materials; (3) subcommittees on terminology and special projects; and (4) subcommittees on instruments and equipment. **BEAR C.,** C. on the Biological Effects of Atomic Radiation; see *C. on the Biological Effects of Ionizing Radiation.* **C. on the Biological Effects of Atomic Radiation (BEAR C.),** C. on the Biological Effects of Ionizing Radiation. **BEIR C.,** C. on the Biological Effects of Ionizing Radiation. **C. on the Biological Effects of Ionizing Radiation,** a joint committee of the National Academy of Sciences, Division of Medical Sciences, and the National Research Council. Abbreviated *BEIR C.* Formerly called *C. on the Biological Effects of Atomic Radiation (BEAR C.).* **dental review c.,** one composed of dentists and administrative personnel which reviews questionable dental claims and which may recommend policy decisions regarding dental care. See also peer REVIEW. **hospital credentials c.,** one charged with the responsibility for reviewing qualifications of applicants for clinical privileges in a hospital and for delineation of their responsibilities. **hospital disaster planning c.,** one charged with the responsibility for formulating and updating a plan for the hospital's role in a community disaster. **hospital infection control c.,** one charged with the responsibility for surveying the incidence of infections in a hospital and for establishing procedures for infection control and patient isolation. **hospital joint conference c.,** one made up of representatives of the executive committee and of the governing body of a hospital, set up to serve as a forum for the discussion of matters of interest to the hospital in regard to policies and their implementation. **hospital medical records c.,** one charged with the responsibility for assuring high standards of medical records in a hospital. **hospital operating room c.,** one charged with the responsibility for reviewing all the activities in the operating room. **hospital pathology c.,** hospital tissue c. **hospital pharmacy and therapeutics c.,** one charged with the responsibility for the surveillance of all drug usage in a hospital. **hospital tissue c.,** one charged with the responsibility for reviewing of all tissues removed from patients in the operating room and for reconciling discrepancies between operative and pathologic diagnosis, whenever they occur. Called also *hospital pathology c.* and *hospital tissue c.* **hospital transfusion review c.,** one charged with the responsibility for reviewing all transfusion of blood and blood products and the rationale for the use of blood transfusion and of the choice of products used in a hospital. **hospital utilization review c.,** one charged with the responsibility for certification that a patient's extended hospital stay was necessary for medical reasons. See also utilization REVIEW. **C. F-4 on Medical and Surgical Materials and Devices,** a committee of the American Society for Testing and Materials, having as its objectives the development of definitions of terms and nomenclature, methods of test, and specifications for materials for surgical implants as well as the implants themselves. **C. F-8 on Protective Equipment for Sports,** a committee of the American Society for Testing and Materials, having as its objective the development of standards and definitions for protective equipment for sports, including mouthguards. **C. TC106,** a committee of the International Standards Organization, which is responsible for the standardization of terminology, test methods, and specifications for dental materials, instruments, appliances, and equipment on an international level. The American National Standards Institute is the American representative. **tissue c.,** hospital tissue c. **utilization review c. (URC),** see *hospital utilization review c.* and utilization REVIEW.

communicable (ko-mu′nĭ-kah-b'l) capable of being transmitted from one person to another or from one species to another.

comedo (kom′ĕ-do), pl. *comedo′nes* [L. "glutton"] a plug in an excretory duct of the skin, containing microorganisms, e.g., *Corynebacterium acnes*, and desquamated keratin, called also *blackhead.*

comonomer (ko-mon′o-mer) a monomer capable of reacting with another monomer. See also COPOLYMER. **surface-active c.,** Bowen's cavity PRIMER.

Comp. abbreviation for L. *compos′itus*, compound.

compact (kom′pakt) 1. compressed dense; firm. 2. to form by uniting or condensing particles by the application of pressure, as in the progressive condensation of direct filling gold and the building up of plastic amalgam in a prepared tooth.

compaction (kom-pak′shun) the act or process of joining or packing together. **direct filling gold c.,** compaction of direct filling gold, including pellets of powdered gold, mat gold, or gold foil (including its products, such as cylinders, rope, or pellets) in the prepared cavity. The first pieces are wedged into the cavity at the convenience point (a small depression at the edge of the cavity) and additional pieces are welded to the original one with a condenser, the face of which is placed against the gold, and the other end is struck sharply with a small mallet. Additional pieces are placed and the process is repeated until the cavity is filled. Each piece is carefully "stepped" by placing the condenser point against the rope or pellet in successive adjacent positions as the instrument is struck with the mallet. Compaction may also be accomplished with the use of mechanical condensers, which consist of points activated by light blows that are repeated with frequencies that range from 360 to 3600 per min. **gold foil c.,** compaction of gold foil (or any of its products) in the prepared cavity. See *direct filling gold c.*

compatibility (kom-pat″ĭ-bil′ĭ-te) [L. *compatibilis*] the quality of being compatible. **blood c.,** see compatible BLOOD.

compatible (kom-pat′ĭ-b'l) 1. capable of harmonious coexistence. 2. in pharmacology, suitable for simultaneous administration without nullification or aggravation of the effects of either. 3. in blood grouping and tissue typing, for transfusion or transplantation from one individual to another without causing immune reactions.

Compazine trademark for *prochlorperazine dimaleate* (see under PROCHLORPERAZINE).

compensation (kom″pen-sa′shun) [L. *compensatio*, from *cum* together + *pensare* to weigh] 1. the counterbalancing for any defect of structure or function. 2. something given or received as an equivalent or as reparation for services, debt, loss, injury, suffering, etc. **workmen's c.,** mandatory state social insurance programs which provide cash benefits to workers or their dependents injured, disabled, or deceased in the course, and as a result, of employment, including benefits for some or all of the medical services necessary for treatment and restoration to a useful life and possibly a productive job. See also disability income INSURANCE and employers' liability INSURANCE. **c. technique,** see compensation TECHNIQUE. **shrinkage c.,** compensation TECHNIQUE.

competence (kom′pĕ-tens) 1. the ability of an organ or part to perform adequately any function required of it. 2. the ability of embryonic cells to respond to inductors by a plurality of types of differentiation. **immunologic c.,** immunocompetence.

competition (kom″pĕ-tish′un) 1. the act of contending with another for something. 2. the phenomenon in which two structurally similar molecules strive for a single binding site on a third molecule. 3. antigenic c. **antigenic c.,** immunosuppression toward an antigen by an unrelated antigen injected simultaneously or shortly before.

complaint (kom-plănt′) a symptom, disease, or disorder. **chief c.,** the symptom or group of symptoms about which the patient first consults the physician or dentist; the presenting symptom. Abbreviated *C.C.*

complement (kom′plĕ-ment) an important effector mechanism of antigen-antibody interactions, which consists of a complex of nine sequentially activated components. The first component, C1, is a trimolecular complex (C1q, C1r, C1s), which recognizes a conformational change in IgG or IgM after it has reacted with antigen or on aggregation, and forms a C1 esterase. Thereafter, the other components become activated in the following sequence: 4, 2, 3, 5, 6, 7, 8, 9. Activated forms are indicated by a bar over the numeral (e.g., $\overline{C1}$), or over the numerals signifying a complex of components (e.g., $\overline{C567}$). Biologically active fragments of a component are designated by the lower case letters a or b (e.g., C3a). A number of activities occur in the process which result in immune adherence, conglutination, chemotaxis, generation of anaphylotoxin, cytolysis, opsonization, and inflammation. The sequence described involving the 1, 4, 2 components of complement constitute the *classical pathway;* the *alternative pathway* bypasses components 1, 4, and 2. Called also *alexin.* See also complement activation PATHWAY

CONGENITAL ABNORMALITIES OF COMPLEMENT

DEFECT	ASSOCIATED DISEASE
C1q	Combined immunodeficiency disease
C1s	Systemic lupus erythematosus (SLE)
C1r	SLE-like
C2	Some normal
	Some with glomerulonephritis
	Some with SLE-like diseases
C4	SLE-like
C3	Recurrent pyogenic infections
C5	SLE-like disease
C5 dysfunction	Syndrome in infants with diarrhea,
	Dermatitis, infections
C6	Gonococcemia
C7	Raynaud's phenomenon
C8	Gonococcemia
C1s inhibitor deficiency	Hereditary angioneurotic edema
C3b inactivator deficiency	Recurrent infections (also known as Type 1
	C3 hypercatabolism)
C3 hypercatabolism, Type 2	Partial lipodystrophy, glomerulonephritis

(From J. A. Bellanti: Immunology II. Philadelphia, W. B. Saunders Co., 1978.)

and complement FIXATION. **deficiency of c.,** abnormalities of the complement system, divided into (a) congenital deficiencies of complement components or inhibitors, and (b) acquired deficiencies of complement components, usually associated with various clinical diseases and abnormalities. See table. **c. fixation,** complement FIXATION. **c. priming,** see complement activation PATHWAY.

Complemix trademark for *dioctyl sodium sulfosuccinate* (see under DIOCTYL).

complex (kom′pleks) [L. *complexus* woven together] 1. complicated; not simple. 2. the sum, combination, or a collection of various things. **antigen-antibody c.,** immune c. **Behçet's triple symptom c.,** Behçet's SYNDROME. **dextran iron c.,** a sterile, colloidal solution of ferric hydroxide in complex with partially hydrolyzed dextran of low molecular weight; used in the treatment of iron deficiency anemias. Called also *iron dextran c.* and *iron-dextran.* Trademarks: Fenate, Imferon. **glucitol iron c.,** IRON sorbitex. **Golgi c.,** Golgi APPARATUS. **H-2 c.,** major histocompatibility c. (of mouse); see under HISTOCOMPATIBILITY. **histone-DNA c.,** *see* NUCLEOHISTONE. **HLA c., HL-A c.,** major histocompatibility c. (of man); see under HISTOCOMPATIBILITY. **hyperkeratosis c.,** oral LEUKOPLAKIA. **immune c.,** a combination of an antigen bound specifically to an antibody, which may occur in soluble form or as a precipitate. Soluble immune complexes may become deposited on tissues, such as the endothelium lining small blood vessels, which may cause complement components to be activated and induce inflammation. Called also *antigen-antibody c.* **iodine-polyvinylpyrrolidone c.,** povidone-iodine. **iron dextran c.,** dextran iron c. **Lazarus c.,** a condition observed among survivors of cardiac arrest, characterized by anxiety, depression, recurrent nightmares, and a feeling of alienation. Most patients eventually overcome mood disturbances and adjust to the memory of their traumatic experience. Named after Lazarus, who was brought to life by Jesus three days after death. **major histocompatibility c.,** see under HISTOCOMPATIBILITY. **major histocompatibility c. (of man),** see under HISTOCOMPATIBILITY. **periodontitis c.,** periodontosis. **QRS c.,** see ELECTROCARDIOGRAPHY. **vitamin B c.,** VITAMIN B complex.

complexion (kom-plek′shun) [L. *complexio* combination] the natural color and appearance of the skin, especially of the face.

complication (kom″pli-ka′shun) [L. *complicatio,* from *cum* together + *plicare* to fold] 1. the act or process of becoming involved, intricate, or complex. 2. the concurrence of two or more diseases or pathologic processes in the same person. See also SEQUELA. 3. a disease co-occurring with another disease or diseases.

Compocillin trademark for *penicillin G hydrabamine* (see under PENICILLIN).

Compocillin-V trademark for *penicillin V hydrabamine* (see under PENICILLIN).

Compocillin-VK trademark for *penicillin V potassium* (see under PENICILLIN).

component (kom-po′nent) a constituent element or part. **anterior c.,** a forward propelling force which is the result of meshing and pounding of the occlusal inclined planes of the teeth and the mesial inclination of the teeth. **plasma thromboplastin c.,** FACTOR IX. **secretory c., T c., transport c.,** secretory PIECE.

composite (kom-poz′it) 1. made up of disparate or separate parts. 2. a substance made up of disparate or separate parts; a composite material (see under MATERIAL).

composition (kom″po-zish′un) 1. the act of making or forming something by combining parts or elements. 2. an aggregate material formed from two or more components. **eutectic c.,** a composition of an eutectic alloy, having its components in exact proportions at which the alloy has its lowest melting point, depicted on the phase diagram at the point where the solidus and liquidus curves merge. Called also *eutectic.* **modeling c.,** impression COMPOUND.

compound (kom-pownd′) [L. *componere* to place together] 1. made of two or more parts or ingredients. 2. any substance made up of two or more kinds of materials. 3. in chemistry, a substance whose molecules consist of unlike atoms, and whose constituents cannot be separated by physical means. 4. to mix drugs, or make up a prescription. 5. a mixture of resins and oils with added coloring and flavoring agents, which softens on heating and solidifies on cooling. Used as a nonelastic molding or impression material to stabilize clamps and separators on the teeth and in making dental impressions. 6. in genetics, a genotype in which two different mutant alleles are present. Also, an individual having different mutant alleles at a locus. See also HETEROZYGOTE and HOMOZYGOTE. **c. 42,** warfarin. **acyclic c.,** an organic compound whose structure is characterized by an open chain. **addition c.,** one formed by the union of

two or more compounds or elements. **aliphatic c.,** an organic compound characterized by an open chain arrangement of the constituent carbon atoms. See also aliphatic HYDROCARBON. **anhydrous c.,** a hydrate from which water of crystallization has been removed. **aromatic c.,** a compound having one or more closed chains or benzene rings in its structure. Called also *benzene c.* See aromatic HYDROCARBON. **benzene c.,** aromatic c. **binary c.,** one containing only two elements with two or more atoms, such as sodium chloride. **carbocyclic c.,** an organic compound whose structure is characterized by a closed chain, having carbon atoms in the ring. **chelate c.,** a compound which will inactivate a metallic ion with the formation of an inner ring structure in the molecule, the metallic ion becoming a member of the ring. Chelate compounds form stable, soluble complexes with calcium and heavy metals. The most widely used chelating agent is ethylenediaminetetra-acetic acid disodium salt (see under ACID). **closed-chain c.,** a compound having several atoms linked together so as to form a ring, as in the benzene ring. See closed CHAIN. **composite c.,** composite MATERIAL. **c. cone,** compound CONE. **coordination c's,** compounds consisting of molecules or ions in which atoms (coordinating ions) are clustered around and are attached to the central atom, being bound by coordinate covalent bonds. The atoms or ions surrounding the central metal ion are known as *ligands.* **cyclic c.,** an organic compound whose structure is characterized by a closed chain. **Darvon c.,** see DARVON compound. **deliquescent c.,** a term used in the past to designate a hygroscopic compound capable of dissolving in moisture absorbed from the air at room temperature. **desoxy c's,** organic compounds in which the hydroxyl (OH) group has been replaced by hydrogen. **duplicating c.,** a compound, usually a hydrocolloid, used to duplicate dental casts or models. A representative formula for a reversible hydrocolloid duplicating compound consists of the following ingredients: agar 2.6 percent, borax 0.2 percent, potassium sulfate 2.0 percent, a preservative 0.2 percent, glycerol 35.0 percent, and water 60.0 percent. Called also *duplicating material.* **efflorescent c.,** a term used in the past to designate a substance (hydrate) which gives up water of crystallization on exposure to air at room temperature and, consequently, becoming anhydrous. **endothermic c.,** a term used in the past to designate a compound whose formation is attended with absorption of heat. **exothermic c.,** a term used in the past to designate a compound whose formation is attended with loss of heat. **c. heater,** compound HEATER. **heterocyclic c.,** a compound having a cyclic or ring structure, often in the shape of a pentagon, containing one or more atoms other than carbon, such as pyrrole, furan, and pyridine. **hydrated c.,** hydrate. **hygroscopic c.,** a term used in the past to designate a compound which takes up water on exposure to air at room temperature. A compound taking up sufficient water to finally dissolve is said to be deliquescent. **impression c.,** a thermoplastic impression material believed to contain beeswax, Burgundy pitch, shellac, gutta-percha, stearin compounds, kauri resin, and fillers, such as French chalk, but whose exact formulation is a trade secret of the manufacturer. Two basic types are in use: *Type I* (or true impression c.) which is used for sectional impressions of partially edentulous jaws, either for preparing working gypsum casts on which dentures are constructed or for preparing casts on which impression trays are formed. Also used to obtain impressions of single teeth in which cavities have been prepared, whereby a matrix band is filled with the compound and then pressed over a tooth, allowing the compound to flow into the prepared cavity. *Type II* (or tray c.) which is used in constructing dentures to form a tray used for reproducing the mouth tissue (primary impression). Called also *modeling c., modeling composition,* and *modeling plastic.* **inorganic c.,** one that contains both an electropositive and an electronegative element or radical and does not contain carbon, but including oxides of carbon and carbonates. **intermetallic c.,** a compound of two metals, the metals being only partially soluble in one another. **ionic c.,** one in which the atoms are held together by ionic bonds. **isopropyl alcohol rubbing c.,** isopropyl rubbing ALCOHOL. **modeling c.,** impression c. **open-chain c.,** one having atoms arranged in an open chain. See open CHAIN. **organic c.,** any compound having carbon atoms, excluding oxides of carbon and carbonates; any nonpolar compound consisting of carbon and hydrogen, with or without oxygen, nitrogen, or other compounds, not including oxides and carbonates. **organophosphorus c.,** organophosphate. **paraffin c.,** a hydrocarbon compound having an open chain; an open-chain compound (see open CHAIN). **quaternary c.,** one in which an atom, such as nitrogen, is substituted by four groups. **quaternary ammonium c's,** organic nitrogen compounds having a molecular structure in which a central nitrogen atom is joined to four organic groups as well as to an acid radical. Quaternary ammonium compounds are generally cationic surface-active compounds and tend to be adsorbed on the surface. Called also *quaternary ammonium salts.* **ring c.,** one having a closed chain or ring. See closed CHAIN. **saturated c.,** one in which all available valence bonds of an atom, especially carbon, are attached to other atoms; paraffin compounds with their straight chains are an example. **substitution c.,** one formed by replacement of elements of a molecule by other elements. **c. tracing stick,** one dispensed in stick form. **tray c.,** one similar to impression compound, but characterized by less flow and more viscosity in the soft state and more rigidity in the solid state. See *impression c.* **true impression c.,** see *impression c.* **c. Type I,** see *impression c.* **c. Type II,** see *impression c.* **unsaturated c.,** one in which all the available valence bonds are not satisfied (saturated), the extra bonds being held as double bonds, chiefly by carbon. The unsaturated compounds are more reactive than those which are saturated, the other elements readily adding to the unsaturated linkages.

compress (kom'pres) [L. *compressus*] a pad or bolster of folded linen or other material, applied with pressure; it is sometimes medicated. See also PACK (2). **cribriform c.,** one perforated with holes, like a sieve, to permit the escape of fluids from an underlying wound. **fenestrated c.,** one pierced with a hole for the discharge of purulent material or to permit inspection of the underlying wound. **graduated c.,** one composed of layers of gradually decreasing size.

compression (kom-presh'un) [L. *compressio* from *comprimere* to squeeze together] 1. the act or process of pressing together or squeezing. See also compression FRACTURE. 2. a form of mechanical stress, whereby external forces (the load) exert pressure against a body and tend to diminish its volume in the direction parallel to that of the stress. Called also *compressive force* and *compressive stress.* **digital c.,** compression of a blood vessel by the fingers for the purpose of checking hemorrhage. **instrumental c.,** compression of a blood vessel by an instrument. **c. molding,** compression MOLDING.

compressor (kom-pres'or) [L.] 1. any device, instrument, or agent by which compression may be achieved. 2. a muscle that compresses. **air c.,** a device for building up air pressure in a tank; used to supply compressed air for the air syringe, spray syringe, and air turbine handpieces. **c. na'ris,** transverse part of nasal muscle; see under PART.

Compton effect, photon, scattering [Arthur Holly Compton, American physicist, 1892–1962; winner of the Nobel prize for physics in 1927] see under EFFECT and PHOTON, and see incoherent SCATTERING.

compulsion (kom-pul'shun) an irresistible impulse to perform some act contrary to one's better judgment or will. Oral habits, such as bruxism and clenching, are considered by some as compulsive acts.

computer (kom-pu'ter) an electronic device capable of carrying out repetitious and complex mathematical or character manipulations at high speeds. A typical computer consists of input and output devices; storage, arithmetic, and logical units; and a control unit. Formerly called *electronic brain* and *mechanical brain.* **analogue c.,** one that solves mathematical problems by using physical analogues, such as electric voltages or shaft rotations, of the numerical variables occurring in the problem. **digital c.,** one that processes information represented by combinations of discrete or discontinuous data, being a device capable of performing operations controlled by sequences of internally stored instructions.

con- [L. *con* along with] a prefix signifying with.

Conadil trademark for *sulthiame.*

concave (kon'kāv) [L. *concavus*] having a rounded, somewhat depressed surface.

concentration (kon"sen-tra'shun) [L. *concentratio*] 1. bringing or directing toward the center. 2. rendering a solution less dilute by evaporating the solvent or by adding more substance. 3. gathering together that which is diffused. **c. difference,** diffusion GRADIENT. **hydrogen ion c.,** the degree of concentration of hydrogen ions (the acid element) in solution, used to indicate or express the reaction of that solution; see pH. Symbol [H⁺]. **ionic c.,** the number of moles of an ion contained in the unit volume of a solution or in the unit mass of solvent. **maximum urinary**

concentration (MUC), see under SOLUTION. **mean corpuscular hemoglobin c.,** see MCHC.

concentric (kon-sen'trik) [L. *concentricus*, from *con* together + *centrum* center] having a common center; extending out equally in all directions from a common center.

concept (kon'sept) the image of a thing as held in the mind. **Bronsted c.,** 1. an acid is any molecular or ionic species which can give up a proton — proton donor. 2. a base is any molecular or ionic species which can take up a proton — proton acceptor. **Lewis c.,** 1. a base is any molecular or ionic species which has available an unshared pair of electrons. 2. an acid is a species which could attach itself to such a pair of electrons.

concha (kong'kah) pl. *conchae* [L.; Gr. *konchē*] a shell; used in anatomical nomenclature to designate a shell-shaped structure or part. **c. bullo'sa,** a cystic distention of the middle nasal concha, sometimes seen in chronic rhinitis. **c. of cranium,** calvaria. **ethmoidal c., inferior,** nasal c., middle. **ethmoidal c., superior,** nasal c., superior. **nasal c., inferior, c. nasa'lis infe'rior** [NA], a thin bony plate with curved margins, articulating with the ethmoid, maxilla, and lacrimal and palatine bones, and forming the lower part of the lateral wall of the nasal cavity, together with its mucous membrane. Called also *inferior spongy bone, inferior turbinate bone,* and *maxilloturbinal bone.* **nasal c., middle, c. nasa'lis me'dia** [NA], the lower of two bony plates projecting from the inner wall of the ethmoid labyrinth and separating the superior from the middle meatus of the nose, and the mucous membrane covering the plate. Called also *inferior ethmoidal c., ethmoid cornu,* and *middle turbinate bone.* **nasal c., superior, c. nasa'lis supe'rior** [NA], the upper of two bony plates projecting from the inner wall of the ethmoid labyrinth and forming the upper boundary of the superior meatus of the nose, and the mucous membrane covering the plate. Called also *superior ethmoidal c., superior spongy bone,* and *superior turbinate bone.* **nasal c., supreme, c. nasa'lis supre'ma** [NA], a thin bony plate occasionally found projecting from the inner wall of the ethmoid labyrinth above the bony superior nasal concha, and the mucous membrane covering the plate. Called also *highest turbinate bone, supreme ethmoidal bone,* and *supreme nasal bone.* **nasoturbinal c., AGGER nasi. sphenoidal c., c. sphenoida'lis** [NA], one of two thin, curved bony plates at the anterior and lower part of the body of the sphenoid bone, on either side, partially closing the bony sphenoidal sinuses and forming part of the roof of the nasal cavity. Called also *Bertin's bone, Bertin's ossicle, sphenoturbinal bone,* and *sphenoturbinal ossicle.*

conchae (kong'ke) [L.] plural of *concha.*

concomitant (kon-kom'i-tant) [L. *concomitans,* from *cum* together + *comes* companion] accompanying; joined with another.

Concordin trademark for *protriptyline hydrochloride* (see under PROTRIPTYLINE).

concrescence (kon-kres'ens) [con- + L. *crescere* to grow] 1. a growing together; a union of parts originally separate. 2. in embryology, the flowing together and piling up of cells. 3. a form of fusion of two adjacent teeth occurring after root formation has been completed, whereby the teeth are united by cementum only. It is thought to arise as a result of traumatic injury or crowding of the teeth with resorption of the interdental bone so that the two roots are in approximate contact and become fused by the deposition of cementum. It may occur before or after the teeth have erupted, generally involving only two teeth but fusion of three teeth has been also reported. Called also *tooth c.* See also FUSION (4) and GEMINATION. **tooth c.,** see *concrescence* (3).

concrete (kon-krēt') [L. *concretus*] 1. solid, tangible. 2. a mass of coalesced particles, solidified or hardened after having been more or less fluid.

concretio (kon-kre'she-o) [L.] concretion.

concretion (kon-kre'shun) [L. *concretio,* from *cum* together + *crescere* to grow] 1. a calculus or inorganic mass in a natural cavity or in the tissue of an organism. 2. abnormal union of adjacent parts. 3. a process of becoming harder or more solid.

concussion (kon-kush'un) [L. *concussio*] violent jar or shock, or the condition which results from such an injury.

condensation (kon"den-sa'shun) [L. *condensare* to make thick or dense, to press close together] 1. any act or process of condensing or becoming more compact; gas liquefaction. 3. the packing of filling material into a prepared tooth cavity. **amalgam c., hand,** packing freshly mixed amalgam into the prepared cavity with the use of a hand condenser, usually contra-angled toward its working end. The amalgam is packed in small increments, usually 3 to 5 mm in diameter, starting in the center of the cavity, followed by slightly tipping the condenser toward the cavity walls, each increment being packed tightly to force the alloy particles together, working the excess mercury to the surface. Only amalgam less than 3½ min old is used, otherwise lamination and rough surfaces may occur. **amalgam c., mechanical,** condensation of freshly mixed dental amalgam through the use of a mechanical device, operated by providing an impact type of force by rapid vibration or use of ultrasonic energy for the condenser. As in the manual technique, the amalgam is placed in the prepared cavity in small increments, usually 3 to 5 mm in diameter, working from the center toward the walls of the cavity. Mechanical condensers are then used to pack the amalgam and to bring the excess mercury to the surface. **brush c.,** in condensation of porcelain in the matrix prior to firing, sprinkling dry porcelain powder on the surface with a brush and placing the wet powder in the matrix. Water is absorbed by capillary action and the drying powder is pushed off with the end of the brush. **filling material c.,** packing of filling materials in a prepared cavity with the use of a manual or mechanical condenser. A brush-on technique may be used for resins. **gold foil c.,** see direct filling gold COMPACTION. **c. polymerization,** condensation POLYMERIZATION. **porcelain c.,** the application of porcelain paste to the matrix or die made from an impression of the prepared tooth, the surface of which has been covered with a thin platinum sheet, using various methods designed to cause the particles to settle and become closely packed, while displacing air bubbles and excess water to the surface from where it is blotted out. Vibration, spatulation, whipping, gravitation, pressure, and brush application are some of the methods used. **pressure c.,** pressure applied with an absorbent material to the surface of porcelain paste during its condensation with mechanical vibrators. **c. resin,** condensation RESIN. **spatulation c.,** spatulation (2). **vibration c.,** in packing porcelain paste in a matrix for firing, moving of the serrated handle of a carver lightly in one direction across the projection of the die or cast, thereby producing vibrations. Excess water coming to the surface is blotted out and the process is repeated until vibration brings no more water to the surface. Various mechanical vibrators and molds are also available. **whipping c.,** in condensation of porcelain paste prior to firing, the building up of the paste in the matrix with a brush or blade, the brush or blade being used with a whipping motion to produce a gentle vibration. The excess water brought to the surface by the motion is blotted out.

condenser (kon-den'ser) [L. *condensare* to make thick, press close together] 1. a vessel or apparatus for condensing gases or vapors. 2. a device on a microscope used to supply illumination of the degree necessary for the specimen under study to be easily visible, and under the conditions necessary for the full resolving power of the instrument to be realized. 3. a manual or mechanical instrument designed to pack and condense restorative material within a prepared cavity. Its working end is called the *nib* or *point;* the end of the nib, which may be smooth or serrated, is termed the *face.* Called also *plugger.* See illustration. **Abbe's c.,** a condenser placed below the stage of a microscope, having two or three lenses that may be moved downward or upward, thereby controlling the concentration of light on the specimen. Called also *Abbe's illuminator.* **amalgam c.,** a condenser for packing and condensing plastic amalgam in a prepared tooth cavity. Called also *amalgam plugger.* **automatic c.,** mechanical c. **back-action c.,** one having the shank bent into a U shape so that the direction of the force applied is toward the operator. Called also *reverse c., back-action plugger,* and *reverse plugger.* **bayonet c.,** a condenser with the nib of various angles, lengths, and diameters, in which the offset of the nib and the approximately right-angled bends in the shank permit an improved line of force for condensation of direct filling gold. **electromallet c.,** a mechanical condenser for compacting direct filling gold, in which condensing points are held in either a straight or a right-angled handpiece; frequency of blows varying from 200 to 3600 strokes/min. An electronic device controls the force of blows. Called also *McShirley's electromallet.* **foil c.,** gold c. **foot c.,** one having a long, angled, foot-shaped nib. Called also *foot plugger.* **gold c.,** an instrument for compacting direct filling gold (either gold foil, mat gold, or pellets of powdered gold) into the prepared cavity in dental restorations. Manual compaction is accomplished with a condenser, the head of which is placed against the gold filling, and the other end is struck sharply with a small mallet. Some condensers having spring-loaded mechanisms which drive their heads against the gold filling, once the instrument is pressed down. Originally, gold condensers had single pyramidal faces but those in use currently have a series of small pyramids or serrations on their faces. These act as swagers, exerting lateral force on their inclines, in addition to providing direct compressive force as the load is applied to the condenser. Called also *foil c., foil plugger,* and *gold plugger.* **gold c., mechanical,** a mechanically-driven condenser for compacting direct filling gold in the prepared cavity. It consists of an engine, either pneumatic or electric, which drives the condensing points, held in a straight or right-angled handpiece, producing comparatively light blows that are repeated with frequencies ranging from 360 to 3600 per min. An electronic device controls the force of the blows. An electrically driven mechanical gold condenser is called an *electromallet.* **hand c.,** one in which muscular effort, with or without the use of a mallet, provides the compacting force. **Hollenback c.,** pneumatic c. **mechanical c.,** a condenser equipped with a spring-activated, pneumatic, or electronic mechanism for compacting the restorative material in a prepared cavity through repeated blows, such as the S.S. White spring-loaded instrument. Called also *automatic c., automatic mallet,* and *automatic plugger.* **parallelogram c.,** one with the face shaped liked a rectangle or a parallelogram. **pneumatic c.,** a mechanical condenser, in which pneumatic pressure supplies the compacting or condensing force at speeds up to 360 strokes/min. The instrument has a straight and right-angled handpiece. Called also *Hollenback c.* **c. point,** nib. **reverse c.,** back-action c. **root canal filling c.,** one designed specifically for root canal therapy, being a smooth, flat-ended, and slightly tapered metal hand-operated instrument used to vertically condense filling material in a root canal. Called also *endodontic plugger* and *root canal plugger.* See illustration at root canal THERAPY. See also root canal filling SPREADER. **round c.,** one whose face has a circular outline.

condensor (kon-den'sor) condenser.

condition (kon-dish'un) 1. an essential part of stipulation of an agreement. 2. a requirement. 3. a state of health. 4. to train; to subject to conditioning. **basal c.,** a condition of the body at rest when minimal energy is expanded for the maintenance of respiration, glandular activity, and other vegetative functioning. See basal METABOLISM. **pathological c.,** a disease or illness. **pre-existing c.,** in health insurance, any pathologic condition of an insured person which existed before his or her enrollment in the plan.

conditioner (kon-dish'o-ner) a substance added to another substance to increase its usability. **hydrocolloid c.,** a device for conditioning hydrocolloids by bringing them to the proper temperature to liquefy and keeping them ready for instant use, accomplished by thermostatically controlled circulating hot water. **Nuva-System Tooth c.,** trademark for a 50 per cent

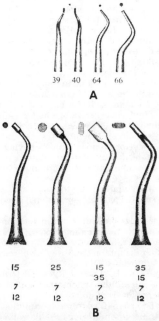

A, Gold foil pluggers or condenser points. *B,* Amalgam pluggers or condensers. (From H. O. Torres and A. Ehrlich: Modern Dental Assisting. 2nd ed. Philadelphia, W. B. Saunders Co., 1980; courtesy of S. S. White Div. of Pennwalt Corp.)

phosphoric acid solution buffered with 7 percent zinc oxide; used as an etching agent. **tissue c.,** a soft resin insert which, when attached to the denture base, cushions its impact on the underlying tissue and provides protection to tissues that may have lost their tonus and suffer a general lack of blood supply, and is also believed to have a massaging activity. Polyethyl methacrylate (a copolymer), and an aromatic ester, such as butyl phthalate butyl glycolate (a monomer), are used in the production of tissue conditioners. **tooth c.,** acid ETCHANT.

conditioning (kon-dish′un-ing) learning in which a response is elicited by a neutral stimulus that previously has been repeatedly presented in conjunction with the stimulus that originally elicited the response. See also conditioned REFLEX.

conduction (kon-duk′shun) [L. *conductio*] the act or process of transmission of sound, electricity, or heat through a conductor. **air c.,** the conduction of sound waves to the sensorium through the auditory canal and middle ear to the inner ear. **bone c.,** the conduction of sound to the cochlea through the bones of the skull, particularly the temporal bone. Called also *cranial c.* See also dentoaural HEARING. **cranial c.,** bone c. **ephaptic c.,** electric transmission of impulses directly through the membrane from one nerve fiber alongside another. The physical junction is an ephapse, as in the outer cerebral cortex.

conductivity (kon″duk-tiv′ĭ-te) the capacity of a body of conducting heat, electricity, or sound. **electrical c.,** 1. the ability of a material to conduct electricity. 2. the quantity of electricity transferred across a unit area, per unit potential, per unit time. **heat c.,** thermal c. **thermal c.,** 1. the ability of a substance to transmit heat (heat transfer). 2. the amount of heat that passes, per unit time, through a unit volume of a substance. A coefficient of thermal conductivity may be expressed as BTU $\times$ ft [°F $\times$ hr $\times$ ft², or cal $\times$ cm]°C $\times$ sec $\times$ cm². The magnitude is calculated by multiplying the coefficient by appropriate dimensional units and temperature gradient to obtain the value in BTU per hour or calories per second. For the thermal conductivity of dental material, see under MATERIAL.

conductor (kon-duk′tor) [L.] 1. a body, object, or substance capable of transmitting heat, electricity, or sound. 2. a grooved director for surgical use. 3. a healthy individual who may transmit some hereditary condition, as the daughter of a hemophiliac.

conduplicato (kon-du″pli-ka′to) [L. *conduplicare* to double up] doubled up.

condylar (kon′dĭ-lar) pertaining to a condyle; condylicus.

condyle (kon′dīl) a round eminence or protuberance at the articular extremity of a bone. **aplastic c.,** condylar APLASIA. **balancing c.,** former name for *orbiting c.* **c. chord,** hinge AXIS. **double c.,** a rare congenital condition usually characterized by unilateral duplication of the head of the condyle, rarely of the neck. **idling c.,** former name for *orbiting c.* **mandibular c.,** the posterior process on the ramus of the mandible; it is composed of two parts: a superior part, the articular portion, and an inferior part, the condylar neck. The articular portion forms a rounded head covered with cartilage, which fits into the glenoid fossa of the temporal bone, forming the temporomandibular articulation. The neck forms the constricted portion below the articular part of the condyle. Called also *condyloid process, little head of mandible,* and *processus condylaris mandibulae* [NA]. **occipital c.,** one of the two oval processes for articulation with the atlas, which project from the anterior surfaces of the lateral parts of the occipital bone, encroaching on the basilar parts of the occipital bone. The articular portion, a convex surface facing laterally and caudally, is attached to the capsule of the atlanto-occipital articulation. On the median side of each condyle there is a tubercle for the alar ligament. A short canal through the base of the condyle (the hypoglossal canal) provides an exit for the hypoglossal nerve and an entry for the meningeal branch of the ascending pharyngeal artery. Called also *condylus occipitalis* [NA]. **orbiting c.,** one that arcs around the vertical axis of the rotating condyle. Formerly called *balancing c.* and *idling c.*

condylectomy (kon″dil-ek′to-me) [condyle + Gr. *ektomē* excision] excision of a condyle; the surgical excision of all or a portion of the mandibular condyle from the condyloid process of the mandible.

condyli (kon′dĭ-li) [L.; Gr] plural of *condylus.*

condylicus (kon-dil′ĭ-kus) pertaining to a condyle; condylar.

condylion (kon-dil′ĭ-on) [Gr. *kondylion* knob] an osteometric landmark, being the most lateral point on the surface of the mandibular condyle. Abbreviated Cd. Called also *condylar point, con-*

dyle summit, and *point Cd.* See illustration at CEPHALOMETRY.

condyloid (kon′dĭ-loid) [condyle $\times$ Gr. *eidos* form] resembling a condyle or knuckle.

condyloma (kon″dĭ-lo′mah), pl. *condylo′mata* [Gr. *kondylōma,* knuckle, knob] 1. a wartlike excrescence. 2. rarely, c. latum. **c. la′tum,** a papular syphilitic lesion localized to moist skin folds, especially about the anogenital areas, which may hypertrophy and erode to form a soft, red cauliflower-like mass, usually with a moist weeping surface.

condylomata (kon″dĭ-lo′mah-tah) [Gr.] plural of *condyloma.*

condylomatoid (kon″dĭ-lo′mah-toid) resembling a condyloma.

condylomatosis (kon″dĭ-lo″mah-to′sis) a condition characterized by the presence of multiple condylomas. **c. pemphigoi′des malig′na,** PEMPHIGUS vegetans.

condylomatous (kon″dĭ-lo′mah-tus) of the nature of a condyloma.

condylotomy (kon″dĭ-lot′o-me) [condyle + Gr. *tomnein* to cut] surgical incision or division of a condyle; usually the removal of a portion, such as the articular surface, of the mandibular condyle.

condylus (kon′dĭ-lus), pl. *con′dyli* [L.; Gr. *kondylos* knuckle] a rounded projection on a bone, usually for articulation with another. **c. occipita′lis** [NA], occipital CONDYLE.

cone (kōn) [Gr. *konos;* L. *conus*] 1. a solid figure or body with a circular base tapering to a point. 2. in radiology, a conical or open-ended cylindrical structure attached over the portal of the x-ray tube housing. Used as an aid in centering the radiation beam on the target field and as a guide to source-to-film distance; also often designed to collimate primary and/or scattered radiation, and/or to retain disks for added filtration. Called also *pointer cone.* 3. in root canal therapy, a solid substance, usually gutta-percha or silver, having a tapered form, and fashioned to conform to the shape of the root canal. **bifurcation c.,** the cone-shaped structure at the bifurcation of a root. **elastic c. of larynx,** the lower (caudal) portion of the fibroelastic membrane of the larynx, composed of yellow elastic tissue, and consisting of an anterior part (middle cricothyroid ligament) and two lateral parts. The anterior part connects the thyroid and cricoid cartilages, and the lateral parts are situated beneath the mucous membrane of the larynx, extending from the cricoid cartilage to the vocal ligaments. Called also *conus elasticus laryngis* [NA], *cricothyroarytenoid ligament, cricothyroid membrane,* and *cricovocal membrane.* **compound c.,** one formed from impression compound; used for making impressions of individual preparations. **felt c.,** a cone-shaped attachment made up of compressed felt, mounted onto a stationary motor and used for polishing dentures. See also felt WHEEL. **growth c.,** a bulbous enlargement of the growing tip of a nerve axon. **gutta-percha c.,** a plastic, radiopaque cone produced from gutta-percha combined with various other ingredients and available in various standard sizes that conform with the dimensions of root canal reamers and files; used to fill and seal root canals in conjunction with root canal sealer cements. Called also *gutta-percha point.* See also root canal filling methods, under METHOD. **implantation c.,** a cone-shaped elevation serving for insertion of the axon into its neuron. Called also *axon hillock.* **long c.,** in radiology, a tubular "cone" designed to establish an extended anode-to-skin distance, usually within a range of 10–25 cm or more. See also cone distance, long, under DISTANCE. **retinal c's,** the specialized outer ends of the visual cells which, together with retinal rods, form the light-sensitive elements of the retina. **short c.,** in radiology, a conical or tubular "cone" having as one of its functions the establishment of an anode-to-skin distance up to 10–25 cm. See also cone distance, short, under DISTANCE. **silver c.,** silver POINT.

Conex attachment see under ATTACHMENT.

conexus (ko-nek′sus) [L. "connection, union"] a connecting structure.

conference (kon′fĕ-renz) a meeting for consultation or discussion, or to settle differences between individuals, organizations, etc. **Dental Laboratory C.,** a trade organization established to advance and further the interest and welfare of the dental laboratory industry. Abbreviated *DLC.*

configuration (kon-fig″u-ra′shun) the general form of a body or anything. **electronic c.,** the schematic tabulation of the electrons at the energy levels of an atom.

confluence (kon′floo-ens) [L. *confluens* running together] the meeting of streams; in embryology the flow of cells, a component process of gastrulation. Called also *confluens.* **c. of sinuses,** the point of junction of the superior saggital, straight, occipital, and two transverse sinuses of the dura mater, lodged in a depression at one side of the internal occipital protuber-

confluens (kon'floo-ens) [L.] confluence; the meeting of streams. **c. sin'uum** [NA], CONFLUENCE of sinuses.

confluent (kon'floo-ent) [L. *confluens* running together] becoming merged; arranged in close proximity, with coalescence of lesions.

cong. abbreviation for L. *con'gius*, gallon.

congelation (kon"jě-la'shun) [L. *congelatio*] frostbite or freezing.

congeneic (kon"jě-ne'ik) having identical genotypes except for substitution at one histocompatibility locus of a foreign allele; pertaining to strains of animals developed from inbred (isogenic) strains by repeated mating with animals from another stock that have a foreign gene, the final congeneic strain then presumably differing from the original inbred strain by the presence of this gene. Called also *coisogenic*.

congener (kon'jě-ner) something closely related to another thing, as a muscle having the same function as another, or a chemical compound closely related to another in composition and exerting similar or antagonistic effects, or something derived from the same source or stock.

congenital (kon-jen'ĭ-tal) [L. *congenitus* born together] present at birth; said of conditions which develop *in utero*.

congestion (kon-jest'yun) [L. *congestio*, from *congerere* to heap together] an excess of blood in a part; hyperemia.

congestive (kon-jes'tiv) pertaining to, characterized by, or resulting in congestion.

conglutination (kon-gloo"ti-na'shun) agglutination of antigenantibody-complement complexes by conglutinin.

conglutinin (kon-gloo'tĭ-nin) a beta globulin with an affinity for the polysaccharide portion of the C3 component of complement.

coni (ko'ni) [L.] plural of *conus*.

conical (kon'ĭ-kal) cone-shaped.

conicine (ko'nĭ-sēn) coniine.

conidia (ko-nid'e-ah) plural of *conidium*.

conidial (ko-nid'e-al) pertaining to or of the nature of conidia; bearing conidia.

conidiophore (ko-nid'e-o-fōr) [L. *conidium* + Gr. *phoros* bearing] the branch of the mycelium of a fungus that bears conidia.

conidiospore (ko-nid'e-o-spōr) [Gr. *konidion* a particle of dust + *spore*] conidium.

conidium (ko-nid'e-um), pl. *conid'ia* [Gr. *konidion* a particle of dust] an asexual spore shed at maturity and formed by splitting off from the summit of a conidiophore. Called also *conidiospore* and *exospore*.

coniine (ko'nĭ-ēn) an alkaloid, 2-propylpiperidine; the poisonous principle of hemlock, *Conium maculatum* L., occurring as a colorless alkaline liquid that undergoes darkening and polymerization on exposure to light and air. Ingestion causes drowsiness, weakness, nausea, vomiting, respiratory disorders, paralysis, and death. It has been used therapeutically as a sedative. Called also *cicutine* and *conicine*.

coniotomy (ko"ne-ot'o-me) superior TRACHEOTOMY.

conjugation (kon"ju-ga'shun) [L. *conjugatio* a blending] the act of blending. In bacterial genetics, a form of sexual reproduction in which a donor bacterium (male) contributes DNA to a recipient (female), which then incorporates differing genetic information into its own chromosome by recombination, and passes the recombined set on to its progeny by replication. In chemistry, the joining together of two compounds to produce another compound.

conjunctiva (kon"junk-ti'vah) [L.] the delicate membrane that lines the eyelids and covers the exposed surface of the sclera.

conjunctivitis (kon-junk"tī-vi'tis) inflammation of the conjunctiva.

connatal (kon-na'tal) [con-+ L. *natus* birth] occurring at the time of birth; acquired at birth.

connector (ko-nek'tor) 1. anything serving as a link between two separate objects or units. 2. the part of a partial denture that connects its components. 3. the part of a fixed partial denture that unites the retainer and the pontic; it may be rigid or nonrigid. **c. bar**, connector BAR. **cross arch bar splint c.**, a removable cross arch connector used to stabilize weakened abutments that support a fixed prosthesis by attachment to teeth on the opposite side of the dental arch, which may be removed by the dentist but not by the patient. Called also *fixable-removable cross arch bar* and *Gilson fixable-removable bar*. **implant superstructure c.**, any of the rigid bars that unite the superstructure attachment into one strong element in an implant denture. **major c.**, a rigid unit of a removable partial denture, serving as its chassis, which joins the parts of the prosthesis on one side of the dental arch to those on the other

side, and to which all other components are attached. The lingual, palatal, or labial bars or plates are the most common major connectors. Called also *saddle c.* **major c., double,** one having two parts, such as a double lingual bar. **major palatal c.,** a broad palatal coverage which unites parts of a maxillary removable denture. A narrow bar serving the same purpose is called the *palatal bar*. **major c., split,** one that is divided into parts, such as the continuous clasp. **minor c.,** connector BAR. **nonrigid c.,** a precision or nonprecision connector used in dentures having retainers and/or pontics which are united by joints permitting limited movement. **palatal c., major,** major palatal c. **palatal c., anterior major,** palatal bar, anterior; see under BAR. **palatal c., posterior major,** palatal bar, posterior; see under BAR. **rigid c.,** one used in dentures having retainers and/or pontics which are united by a soldered cast or welded joint (in metallic fixed restorations) or are fused (in ceramic restorations). **saddle c.,** major c. **Steiger's c.,** Steiger's JOINT. **superstructure c.,** a rigid bar joining superstructure attachments into a single rigid unit of the subperiosteal implant. **subocclusal c.,** a nonrigid connector positioned gingivally to the occlusal plane.

conoid (ko'noid) [Gr. *kōnoeidēs*] resembling or shaped like a cone.

conotomy (ko-not'o-me) intercricothyrotomy.

Conradi-Hünermann syndrome [Erich *Conradi;* Carl *Hünermann*] see under SYNDROME.

CONS consultation.

Cons. abbreviation for L. *conser'va*, keep.

consanguineous (kon"san-gwin'e-us) [con- + L. *sanguinis* of blood] related by blood; of common parentage.

consanguinity (kon"san-gwin'ĭ-te) [con- + L. *sanguinis* of blood] blood relationship; kinship through common parentage. See also INBREEDING.

consciousness (kon'shus-nes) [con- + L. *scio* to know, to perceive] the ability to perceive and usually to respond to sensory stimuli; awareness of objects or activities.

consent (kon-sent') a voluntary approval or permission for an action to be carried out by another person, such as a permission to perform a therapeutic procedure or experiment by a physician or a dentist. **implied c.,** consent presumed in certain actions by the patient, as when the patient enters the dental office and sits in the dental chair; the consent implying only an examination, diagnosis, and consultation. Called also *presumed c.* **informed c.,** consent given by a patient or volunteer who has proper understanding of the nature of the medical procedure or experiment and has full knowledge of the possible risks involved. See also informed consent FORM. **partially informed c.,** consent given by a patient or volunteer who is familiar with the technical aspects of the medical procedure or experiment and understands the description of the side effects but is not fully aware of possible medical or social consequences. **presumed c.,** implied c.

conservative (kon-ser'vah-tiv) [L. *conservare* to preserve] designed to preserve health, restore function, and repair structures by nonradical methods, as in conservative surgery in which organs are preserved whenever possible. Cf. RADICAL.

console (kon'sōl) a desklike structure by means of which devices or systems, such as power plants, organs, or computers, are controlled or operated. A computer console usually contains a keyboard, start and stop keys, sense switches, and other switches and register displays.

consolidation (kon-sol"ĭ-da'shun) [L. *consolidatio*] solidification; the process of becoming or the condition of being solid.

consonant (kon'so-nant) 1. a speech sound produced by occluding with or without releasing (p, b; t, d; k, g), diverting (m, n), or obstructing (f, v; s, z) the flow of air from the lungs. Cf. VOWEL. 2. in a syllable, any sound other than the sound of greatest sonority.

constant (kon'stant) [L. *constans* standing together] 1. not failing; remaining unaltered. 2. a datum, fact, or principle that is not subject to change. **Ambard's c.,** Ambard's FORMULA. **Avogadro's c.,** Avogadro's NUMBER. **decay c.,** a fraction of the number of atoms of a radionuclide which decay in unit time. Symbol λ. Called also *disintegration c.* and *radioactive c.* **disintegration c.,** decay c. **dissociation c.,** the equilibrium constant for the dissociation of a weak acid into hydrogen ion and its conjugate base in solution. **equilibrium c.,** a number that relates the concentrations of starting materials and products of a reversible chemical reaction to one another. Symbol K. **Faraday's c.,** 1. the quantity of electricity contained in 1 mole of electrons;

the value of the constant is 96,493.5 coulombs per mole of electrons. 2. the minimum amount of electricity necessary to electrodeposit 1 mole of a univalent metal. **c. h,** Planck's c. **heat c., Planck's c., quantum c.,** a constant, h, which represents the ratio of the energy of any quantum of radiation to its frequency; the value of h is 6.625×10^{-27} erg seconds. Called also *quantum unit*. See also quantum THEORY. **radioactive c.,** decay c. **thermal c.,** the heat in calories evolved during a particular reaction.

constipation (kon″stĭ-pa′shun) [L. *constipatio* a crowding together] infrequent or difficult evacuation of the feces.

constitution (kon″stĭ-tu′shun) [L. *constitutio*] the make-up or functional habit of the body, determined by the genetic, biochemical, and physical endowment of the individual, and modified by environmental factors. See also TYPE.

constriction (kon-strik′shun) [L. *con* together + *stringere* to draw] 1. a drawing together; a contraction, as of a vessel or duct. 2. a constricted organ or part. **primary c.,** centromere. **secondary c.,** in genetics, the narrowed heterochromatic area of the short arms of acrocentric autosomes by which a satellite is attached.

constrictor (kon-strik′tor) [L.] that which constricts, such as a muscle or an instrument by which a part may be constricted. **c. pharyn′gis infe′rior,** constrictor pharyngis inferior MUSCLE. **c. pharyn′gis me′dius,** constrictor pharyngis medius MUSCLE. **c. pharyn′gis supe′rior,** constrictor pharyngis superior MUSCLE.

consultant (kon-sul′tant) [L. *consultare* to counsel] someone, such as a dental or medical specialist, called in for advice and counsel. **dental c.,** in health insurance, an employee of a dental health insurance carrier, usually a dentist, who is responsible for reviewing and making decisions on questionable or unusual dental claims.

consultation (kon″sul-ta′shun) [L. *consultatio*] 1. a deliberation of two or more dentists or physicians who are seeking, through an exchange of information, to arrive at a decision with respect to the diagnosis or treatment of any particular case. In the course of this process the advice or opinion of specialists may be required. 2. a deliberation between a practitioner, such as a dentist or physician, and his patient on the diagnosis and treatment plan.

consumption (kon-sump′shun) [L. *consumptio* a wasting] 1. the act or process of expending by use. 2. the act or process of eating or drinking. 3. a wasting away of the body. 4. a former popular name for pulmonary tuberculosis (see under TUBERCULOSIS).

contact (kon′takt) [L. *contactus* a touching together] 1. the mutual touching of two objects or persons. 2. the junction of two conductors of electric current. 3. an individual known to have been sufficiently near an infected individual to have been exposed to the transfer of infectious material. See also *direct c., immediate*. 4. contactant. 5. contact AREA. **c. area,** contact AREA. **balancing c.,** the contact between the upper and lower occlusal surfaces of the natural or artificial teeth on the side opposite to the working contact. **complete c.,** contact of the entire proximal surface of one tooth with the entire proximal surface of the adjacent tooth. **deflective c., deflective occlusal c.,** occlusal c., deflective. **direct c., immediate,** the touching by a healthy person of a person having a communicable disease, the disease being transmitted as a result. **faulty c., faulty interproximal c.,** imperfections in the contact between adjacent teeth, often leading to food impaction between the teeth with subsequent development of periodontal complications. **indirect c.,** contact achieved through some intervening medium, as the propagation of a communicable disease through the air or by means of fomites. Called also *mediate c*. **initial c., initial occlusive c.,** occlusive c., initial. **interceptive occlusal c.,** occlusal c., interceptive. **mediate c.,** indirect c. **occlusal c.,** the contact between the upper and lower teeth when the jaws are closed in habitual occlusion. **occlusal c., deflective,** a form of occlusal interference in which the mandible is diverted from its normal path of closure to central jaw relation or the denture slides or rotates on its basal seat. Called also *deflective c*. and *cuspal interference*. **occlusal c., initial,** the initial normal, noninterfering occlusal contact and intercuspation occurring when the mandibular and maxillary teeth are brought together. In ideal occlusion, it takes place in centric occlusion. Called also *initial c*. **occlusal c., interceptive,** an initial contact of the teeth that stops or deviates from the normal movement of the mandible. **c. point,** contact AREA. **premature c.,** an occlusal contact or interference that occurs before a balanced and stable jaw-to-jaw relationship is reached in either centric relation or centric occlusion, or in the area between the two positions.

Premature contacts are sometimes classified as Classes I, II, and III. *Class I:* The buccal surfaces of the buccal cusps of the mandibular molars and premolars are against the lingual inclines of the buccal cusps of the maxillary molars and premolars; and the facial surfaces of the mandibular anterior teeth are against the lingual surfaces of the maxillary antagonists. *Class II:* The lingual surfaces of the lingual cusps of the maxillary molars and premolars are against the buccal inclines of the lingual cusps of the mandibular molars and premolars. *Class III:* The buccal inclines of the lingual cusps of the maxillary molars and premolars are against the lingual inclines of the buccal cusps of the mandibular molars and premolars. Called also *prematurity*. **proximal c., proximate c.,** touching of the proximal surfaces of two adjoining teeth. **weak c.,** contact in which the proximal surface on one tooth barely touches that of the adjacent tooth, enhancing the packing of food between the teeth. **working c.,** the contact between the upper and lower natural or artificial teeth on the side toward which the mandible has been moved in mastication.

contactant (kon-tak′tant) an allergen capable of inducing delayed contact–type hypersensitivity after one or more episodes of contact.

contagion (kon-ta′jun) [L. *contagio* contact, infection] 1. contagium. 2. transmission of a disease by contact with the sick. 3. a contagious disease.

contagious (kon-ta′jus) [L. *contagiosus*] capable of being transmitted; denoting certain types of infectious diseases.

contagium (kon-ta′je-um), pl. *conta′gia* [L.] any morbid matter which may transmit a disease. Called also *contagion*.

contaminant (kon-tam′ĭ-nant) something that causes contamination.

contamination (kon-tam″ĭ-na′shun) [L. *contaminatio*, from *con* together + *tangere* to touch] rendering something impure or unsuitable for human or animal use, as by introduction of microorganisms into a wound, discharging sewage into a stream, or introducing unedible substances into foodstuffs. **radioactive c.,** 1. presence of unwanted radioactive matter in substances and products, thus making them unusable or harmful to animal or plant life. 2. deposition of radioactive material at any site where it may harm persons, animals, plants, or the environment, or where it may hamper operation or experiment or render materials and equipment unoperable or unsafe.

contiguity (kon″tĭ-gu′ĭ-te) [L. *contiguus* in contact] contact or close proximity; the quality of being contiguous.

contiguous (kon-tig′u-us) [L. *contiguus*] in contact or nearly so.

continence (kon′tĭ-nens) [L. *continentia*] the ability to refrain; self-restraint. Cf. INCONTINENCE.

continuant (kon-tin′u-ant) a consonant, such as f or s, that may be prolonged without change of quality.

continuity (kon″tĭ-nu′ĭ-te) [L. *continuitas*, uninterrupted succession] the quality of being without interruption or separation.

contour (kon′toor) [Fr.] 1. a shape or outline of something. 2. to shape or form something. **buccal c.,** the shape of the buccal aspect of a posterior tooth, normally showing an occlusocervical convexity, with its greater prominence at the gingival third of the clinical buccal surface, thus providing protection for the margin of the gingivae. **gingival c.,** a festooning of the gingiva with slightly raised but still knifelike edge, rounding off toward the attached gingiva. Called also *gingival denture c*. **gingival denture c.,** 1. the form of the denture base or other material around the interproximal and cervical surfaces of artificial teeth. 2. gingival c. **proximal c.,** the form or outline of the mesial or distal surface of a tooth. **restoration c.,** restored proper contour in areas where surfaces of the teeth have been destroyed because of disease processes or excessive wear.

contouring (kon-toor′ing) the process of forming a contour; shaping. **occlusal c.,** correction by grinding of gross disharmonies of the occlusal tooth forms. See also occlusal ADJUSTMENT.

contra- [L. "against"] a prefix signifying against, opposed.

contra-angle (kon″trah-ang′g'l) an angulation by which the working part of a surgical instrument is brought to the desired angle in relation to the long axis of its shaft through the use of two or more bends, or angles. See also contra-angle HANDPIECE.

contra-aperture (kon″trah-ap′er-chŭr) [*contra* + L. *apertura* opening] a second opening made in an abscess to facilitate the discharge of its contents.

contraceptive (kon″trah-sep′tiv) 1. diminishing the likelihood of, or preventing conception. 2. an agent that diminishes the likelihood of, or prevents conception. **oral c.,** any substance that, when taken orally, diminishes the likelihood of, or prevents conception. Commonly, an estrogenic or progestational hormone, or their combination, which causes changes in the endocrine system that mimic those occurring in pregnancy, usually preventing ovulation. Adverse reactions may include nausea, vomiting, dizziness, headache, weight gain, breast discomfort, and other conditions similar to those occurring in early pregnancy; irregular menses; depression; fatigability; visual disorders, including retinal thrombosis, diplopia, and optic neuritis; skin rash; alopecia; hirsutism; brown macules on the face; biliary lithiasis and jaundice; blood pressure disorders; thromboembolism; galactorrhea; and oral disorders similar to those seen in pregnancy, including gingival changes, such as inflammation, hyperemia, swelling, loss of tissue tone, tenderness, ulceration, and bleeding.

contract (kon'trakt, kon-trakt') an agreement, enforceable by law, between two or more parties for doing or not doing something specified. In health insurance, an agreement between the beneficiary, or another party on his behalf, and the carrier to provide specified health care services in exchange for a specified compensation. **cancelable c.,** one that may be discontinued by notice from either party or by mutual consent. **open-end c.,** in health insurance: (1) a contract which permits periodic re-evaluation of the plan during the contract period. If indicated by the re-evaluation, services may be deleted or added to achieve a balance between premiums and cost of service provided; or (2) a contract which sets no dollar limits on the total services to be provided to beneficiaries but does list the particular services which will be included in the plan. **c. period, c. year,** benefit PERIOD.

contractility (kon"trak-til'ĭ-te) the capacity for shortening length, as of muscle under the influence of a nerve impulse.

contraction (kon-trak'shun) [L. *contractus* drawn together] 1. a shortening or reduction in size. 2. muscle c. 3. abnormal approximation of mandibular and maxillary structures to the median plane. See also DISTRACTION. **cicatricial c.,** the contraction which occurs in the tissues of a healing wound as a cicatrix (scar) is formed. **clonic c.,** muscle contraction rapidly alternating with periods of relaxation. It is associated with tapping the stretched muscle of a hyperreflexive patient, and often accompanies spasticity. **galvanotonic c.,** a sustained muscular contraction produced by a continuous electric current. The individual contractions fuse into a continuous response termed *tetanus*. **idiomuscular c.,** abnormally long contraction produced by direct mechanical stimulation of a wasted muscle. **irregular heart c.,** arrhythmia. **isometric c.,** muscle contraction that develops tension without appreciable shortening or change in distance between its origin and insertion. Thus, no external work is performed. Clenching of already occluded jaws is an example of isometric contraction involving the masticatory musculature. **isotonic c.,** muscle contraction in which the distance between the muscle's origin and insertion becomes less. Thus, work is accomplished. In chewing, the masticatory muscles contract isotonically. **muscle c.,** usually, the act or process of shortening the muscle length (isotonic muscle contraction), thereby providing the power for bodily motor activities. The process is explained by the sliding filament theory, in which the thin actin filaments slide inward between the thick myosin filaments, thus reducing the length of the sarcomere. The contraction mechanism is turned on by the release of calcium ions from the sarcoplasmic reticulum that activates ATPase, splitting ATP to ADP, and releasing energy for the sliding filaments. Energy is released by the heavy meromyosin part of myosin-splitting ATP. Removal of calcium by pumping it back into the sarcoplasmic reticulum turns off the process. See also ratchet THEORY. **myotatic c.,** contraction or irritability of a muscle brought into play by sudden passive stretching or by tapping on its tendon. The physiologic effect is to oppose changes in muscle length. **postural c.,** that state of muscular tension and contraction which just suffices to maintain the posture of the body. It is accomplished by alternating groups of fibers maintaining tonic contraction with minimal energy expenditure so that the maintenance of posture is not fatiguing. **premature c., premature heart c.,** extrasystole. **rapid heart c.,** tachycardia. **tetanic c.,** sustained contraction of a muscle without intervals of relaxation. Called also *tonic*. Symbol ADTe. **tone c.,** a weak, sustained muscular contraction present in resting muscle. **tonic c.,** tetanic c. **twitch c.,** the all-or-none response of a muscle cell to a single brief stimulus, which is followed by relaxation.

contracture (kon-trak'chŭr) [L. *contractura*] a condition of fixed high resistance to passive stretching of a muscle, resulting from fibrosis of the tissues supporting the muscles or the joints, or from disorders of the muscle fibers.

contrafissure (kon"trah-fish'ur) a fracture in a part opposite the site of a blow.

contraindication (kon"trah-in"dĭ-ka'shun) a condition, especially a disease, symptom, sign, or manifestation, the appearance of which renders a particular method of treatment improper or undesirable.

contralateral (kon"trah-lat'er-al) [*contra-* + L. *latus* side] situated on, pertaining to, or affecting the opposite side, as opposed to homolateral or ipsilateral.

contrast (kon'trast) 1. comparison in order to distinguish differences. 2. the visual differentiability of variability in photographic or film density produced on a radiograph by structural composition of the object or objects radiographed. See also DENSITY (4). **high c.,** short-scale c. **long-scale c., low c.,** that degree of contrast which limits visual differentiation to image densities produced by relatively disparate structural features. It increases the range of grays between the blacks and whites on a radiograph; lower kilovoltages decrease the range. **c. medium,** contrast MEDIUM. **short-scale c.,** that degree of contrast which favors visual differentiation of image densities produced by objects or object components relatively comparable in structure. It increases the range of grays between the blacks and whites on a radiograph; higher kilovoltages increase the range. Called also *high c.* **subject c.,** the relative differences in density and thickness of the components of the examined subject as shown by the variations in radiographic densities caused by the differences in absorbing power of the different kinds of material traversed by an x-ray beam.

contrastimulant (kon"trah-stim'u-lant) [*contra-* + *stimulant*] 1. counteracting or opposing stimulation. 2. a depressant drug.

contrastimulus (kon"trah-stim'u-lus) [*contra-* + *stimulus*] a remedy, force, or agent that opposes stimulation.

Contravul trademark for *sulthiame*.

contrecoup (kon-tr-koo') [Fr. "counterblow"] injury resulting from a blow on another site, such as a fracture of the skull caused by a blow on the opposite side. See also contrecoup CONTUSION.

Cont. rem. abbreviation for L. *continue'tur reme'dium*, let the medicine be continued.

control (kon-trōl') [Fr. *contrôle* a register] 1. to exercise restraint or discretion. 2. the governing or limitation of something. 3. to test or verify. 4. a standard against which experimental observations may be evaluated, as a procedure identical in all respects to the experimental procedure except for absence of the one factor that is being studied. **dead man's c.,** a control, such as an electric switch, that requires constant pressure to keep the power supply open, which is used on some types of equipment, such as x-ray machines, to prevent their inadvertent operation. Called also *dead man's switch*. **drug c.,** a national law or international agreement governing and restricting production, movement, and use of a drug to medical and scientific needs in the interest of public health and for the prevention of drug abuse. **plaque c.,** prevention of the accumulation of bacterial plaque and other deposits on the teeth and adjacent gingival surface through the use of mechanical cleansing with toothbrushes, dental floss, dentifrice, special interdental instruments, chemical plaque and calculus inhibitors, and other aids. **quality c.,** 1. A system for maintaining performance at a desired level of quality through continued inspection, verification, and corrective actions as required. 2. In dental health insurance, a procedure for checking the quality of dental care provided by participating dentists and for correcting any irregularities discovered. Called also *quality evaluation*. See also peer REVIEW, POSTSCREENING, and PRESCREENING. **stress c.,** a process by means of which the stress load generated by occlusal contact is eliminated or diminished.

contrusion (kon-troo'zhun) a crowding together, as malposed teeth pushed together.

contusion (kon-tu'zhun) [L. *contusio,* from *contudere* to bruise] an injury without breaking the skin; bruise. **contrecoup c.,** a contusion resulting from a blow on one side of the head with damage to the cerebral hemisphere on the opposite side by transmitted force.

conus (ko'nus), pl. *co'ni* [L.; Gr. *kōnos*] a cone; a general anatomical term denoting a structure resembling a cone. **c. elas'ticus laryn'gis** [NA], elastic cone of larynx; see under CONE.

convalescence (kon"vah-les'ens) [L. *convalescere* to become strong] the stage of recovery following an attack of disease, a surgical operation, or an injury.

convalescent (kon"vah-les'ent) 1. pertaining to or characterized by convalescence. 2. a patient who is recovering from a disease, surgical operation, or injury.

convection (kon-vek'shun) [L. *convectio,* from *convehere* to convey] transmission of heat in liquids or gases by a circulation carried on by the heated particles.

convergence (kon-ver'jens) 1. inclination toward a common point. 2. in embryology, the movement of cells from the periphery toward the midline during gastrulation. 3. in physiology, the coordinated movement of the two eyes toward fixation of the same near point. 4. in evolution, development of similar structures or organisms in unrelated taxa. 5. the point of meeting of convergent lines. **cervical c.,** the angle formed between the cervicoaxial inclination of a tooth surface on the one side and a diagnostic stylus of a dental cast survèyor in contact with the tooth at its height of contour.

convergent (kon-ver′jent) [L. *con* together + *vergere* to incline] meeting at or tending toward a common point.

convertase (kon-ver′tās) an enzyme that converts a substance to its active state. **C3 proactivator c., C3PA c.,** factor D̄.

converter (kon-ver′ter) one who or that which changes something into another form, product, state, frequency, etc. **rotary c.,** a device which, when operated by one type of current, produces another, as one which converts alternating to direct current.

convex (kon′veks) [L. *convexus*] curved or rounded like the exterior surface of a sphere.

convexity (kon-vek′sĭ-te) [L. *convexitas*] the quality of being convex; curved like the exterior of a sphere.

convexobasia (kon-vek″so-ba′se-ah) [*convex* + *base* of the skull] a deformity of the occipital bone, which is bent forward by the spine: seen in osteitis deformans.

convexoconcave (kon-vek″so-kon′kāv) convex on one surface and concave on the other.

convexoconvex (kon-vek″so-kon′veks) convex on each of two opposite surfaces.

convolution (kon″vo-lu′shun) [L. *convolutus* rolled together] a tortuous irregularity or elevation caused by a structure being infolded upon itself.

convulsion (kon-vul′shun) [L. *convulsio,* from *convellere* to pull together] a sudden, violent involuntary contraction or series of contractions of the voluntary muscles. Called also *spasm.* See also EPILEPSY.

convulsive (kon-vul′siv) pertaining to, characterized by, or of the nature of a convulsion.

cooker (kook′er) an appliance or utensil for cooking. **pressure c.,** a sturdy container that is hermetically closed to allow steam pressure to raise to a predetermined level. Specially adapted pressure cookers are used as autoclaves.

coolant (koo′lant) a substance, such as a liquid or gas, used to reduce the temperature or overheating of an object or system exposed to a source of heat or to friction. **tooth c.,** a fine stream of water ejected from the tip of the handpiece during operation on a tooth with a high-speed rotary instrument, with the use of the washed field technique, or a jet of air from the tip of the handpiece, with the use of the dry field technique, for the prevention of overheating of the tooth.

Cooley's anemia [Thomas Benton *Cooley,* American pediatrician, 1871–1945] see under ANEMIA.

Coolidge tube [William David *Coolidge,* American physicist, born 1873] x-ray tube, hot-cathode; see under TUBE.

cooling (kool′ing) the process of reducing the temperature, as in reducing fever in febrile patients or reducing heat in an overheated instrument or tissue.

Coombs' test [R. R. A. *Coombs,* British immunologist] antiglobulin TEST.

coordination (ko-or″dĭ-na′shun) 1. the process or action of organizing or arranging something in proper order or harmonious combination. 2. a proper order or relationship. 3. the harmonious functioning of interrelated organs and parts; applied especially to the process of the motor apparatus of the brain which provides for the coworking of particular groups of muscles for the performance of definite adaptive useful responses. **c. of benefits,** see coordination of benefits CLAUSE. **c. compound,** see coordination COMPOUND.

copal (ko-pal′) an odorless and tasteless, yellowish to yellowish brown resin obtained from various tropical trees or dug from the ground as a fossil. *Zanzibar copal* contains 80 percent trachylolic acid, 4 percent isotrachylolic acid, 6 percent resene, and volatile oil. *Kaurie copal* contains dammaric acid, dammaran, and a resin. *Hard copal* is insoluble in common solvents, but *soft copal* is partly soluble in ethanol, chloroform, and glacial acetic acid; both after having been fused are soluble in linseed oil and oil turpentine. Used in dentistry for modeling compounds and cavity varnishes. Also used in various chemical and industrial processes. Called also *gum c., resin c., animé,* and *courie.* **gum c., resin c.,** copal.

Copalite trademark for *copal varnish* (see under VARNISH).

copayment (ko-pa′ment) 1. the sharing of payment for something between two or more individuals or organizations. 2. coinsurance (2).

cope (kōp) 1. the upper half of a flask used in the casting art; applied in prosthetic dentistry to the upper or cavity side of a denture flask. 2. coping.

coping (kōp′ing) a truncated metal cone-shaped cap or a thimble which fits over the prepared natural tooth and serves as an abutment for dentures. A denture may be applied directly to the coping or it may incorporate a secondary coping which telescopes over the primary coping. Called also *primary c., cope, coping retainer, primary thimble,* and *thimble.* See also telescopic CROWN and overlay DENTURE. **paralleling c.,** a casting placed over an implant abutment to make it parallel to other natural or implant abutments. **primary c.,** coping. **secondary c.,** telescopic c. **telescopic c.,** a secondary coping which is incorporated into a denture and fits over the primary coping in its retention. Called also *secondary thimble* and *telescopic thimble.* See also telescopic CROWN. **transfer c.,** a covering or cap of metal, acrylic resin, or other suitable material, used to position a die in an impression.

copolymer (ko-pol′ĭ-mer) [*co-* + *polymer*] a polymer containing monomers of usually two, sometimes more, kinds. It is a product of polymerization occurring at the same time of two or more monomers which are soluble in each other, representing a molecular structure formed with all monomer units appearing in a chain, linked together. **block c.,** a copolymer in which blocks of identical monomers exist within the chain: ···−M−M−M−···−M−Y−Y−Y−···−Y−Y−Y−M−M−···. Called also *block polymer.* **graft c.,** copolymer in which monomers of one species are grafted onto a chain of monomers of another species:

Called also *graft polymer.* **random c.,** one in which no definite sequential pattern of units exists, the different monomers being randomly distributed among the chain: ···−M−M−Y−M−Y−M−Y−···. Called also *random polymer.* **vinyl acetate–vinyl chloride c.,** see VINYL chloride–vinyl acetate copolymer. **vinyl chloride–vinyl acetate c.,** see under VINYL.

copolymerization (ko-pol″ĭ-mer″ĭ-za′shun) polymerization in which two or more chemically different monomers are used as starting material, the polymer thus formed containing units of all of the original monomers.

copper (kop′er) [L. *cuprum;* Gr. *kypros*] a reddish, lustrous, ductile, malleable metal: Symbol, Cu; atomic number, 29; atomic weight, 63.64; melting point, 1083°C; specific gravity, 8.96; valences, 1, 2; group IB of the periodic table. It occurs in two natural isotopes, 63 and 65, and nine artificial ones, 58–62, 64, and 66–68. Copper is insoluble in water, but soluble in nitric acid and hot hydrobromic acid, and is attacked by acetic and other organic acids. It is essential in animal and plant metabolism, being necessary in bone formation and in hemopoiesis in which it acts as a catalyst in the transformation of inorganic iron into hemoglobin. A copper intake of 2 to 5 mg per day is provided in an average daily diet; liver, kidney, nuts, and raisins are the principal sources. Its normal serum level is 120 to 145 μg/l. It is found in most tissues, chiefly the liver, kidneys, heart, bone marrow, brain, hair, and blood, the liver being the apparent storage site. Copper deficiency is believed to be rare in man; when it occurs it may be associated with microcytic anemia and Menkes' syndrome; excessive accumulation occurs in hepatolenticular degeneration. Copper is relatively nontoxic, but it may destroy vitamin C on contact, and poisoning is caused by ingestion of copper salts, chiefly copper sulfate. Massive ingestion causes acute poisoning, characterized by violent vomiting (sometimes with bluish-green vomitus, hematemesis, colic, diarrhea, bloody stools, jaundice, melena, hemorrhagic gastritis, hemolytic anemia, hypotension, and, in severe cases, coma and death. Kidney and liver damage is usually present. Contact with copper salts, particularly copper sulfate, may result in eczematous and papulovesicular lesions of the skin and mucous membranes, ulceration and sloughing of the mucous membranes, conjunctivitis, and edema of the eyelids. Inhalation of copper dust may produce rhinitis and lesions of the nasal mucosa, including ulcers. Oral symptoms of copper poisoning usually include discoloration of the tongue and gingivae in the form of a greenish, reddish, or purplish line (copper line). See also terms beginning CUPR-. **c. amalgam,** copper AMALGAM. **c. cement,** copper CEMENT. **gold-c. system,** gold-copper ALLOY. **silver-c. system,** silver-copper ALLOY. **c. sulfate,** cupric SULFATE.

copperas (kop′er-as) commercial ferrous sulfate; used as a disinfectant and deodorizer. See ferrous SULFATE.

coprecipitin (ko″pre-sip′ĭ-tin) 1. a precipitin in the same serum with one or more other precipitins. 2. a univalent or nonprecipitating antibody that adds to the precipitate formed by an antigen and precipitating antibody with the same specificity.

copro- [Gr. *kopros* dung] a combining form denoting relationship to feces.

coproantibody (kop″ro-an′tĭ-bod″e) [*copro-* + *antibody*] an antibody, usually secretory immunoglobulin A, formed by lymphoid cells of the intestinal mucosa and submucosa, and released into the intestinal tract. It may be important in immunity to intestinal disease.

coproporphyrin (kop″ro-por′fĭ-rin) [*copro-* + *porphyrin*] a porphyrin occurring in the feces, but also found in the urine. Chemically, coproporphyrins are tetramethyl, tetrapropionic porphins.

copula (kop′u-lah) [L.] any connecting part or structure. **c. lin′guae,** hypobranchial EMINENCE.

cor (kor) [L.] [NA] heart.

Cora-Caine analgesic adhesive see under ADHESIVE.

Corbadrin *nordefrin hydrochloride* (see under NORDEFRIN).

Corbasil trademark for *nordefrin hydrochloride* (see under NORDEFRIN).

corchorin (kor-ko′rin) strophanthidin.

cord (kord) [L. *chorda;* Gr. *chordē* string] a long, round, flexible structure; a string. Called also *chorda.* **dental c.,** a cordlike mass of cells from which the enamel organ develops. **enamel c.,** an epithelial oblique spiral extension from the cell concentration at the base of the cap of a developing tooth, roughly dividing the cap into two halves. It is a temporary structure present briefly during the cap stage of odontogenesis. Called also enamel SEPTUM. **Ferrein's c.,** vocal c., true. **nephrogenic c.,** a cord formed from the intermediate mesoderm of the embryo, which gives rise to the mesonephric and metanephric tubules of the mesonephros and metanephros (permanent kidney), respectively. **nerve c.,** any nerve trunk or bundle of nerve fibers. **spinal c.,** the part of the central nervous system which conducts impulses to and from the brain, and controls many automatic muscular activities. It is an elongated cylindrical structure about 42 to 45 cm in length, extending from the foramen magnum at its cranial end, where it is continuous with the medulla oblongata, to about the level of the third lumbar vertebra at its lower end, where it tapers to a point. It is enclosed in three protective membranes, or meninges: the dura mater, the arachnoid, and the pia mater, and is composed of an inner core of gray substance, consisting chiefly of nerve cells, and a white substance, made up chiefly of myelinated nerve fibers. Thirty-one spinal nerves originate from the spinal cord and extend to various structures of the body. Called also *chorda spinalis* and *medulla spinalis* [NA]. **umbilical c.,** a flexible tubular sheath connecting the umbilicus with the placenta and giving passage to the umbilical arteries and veins. First formed during the fifth embryonic week from the connecting stalk, it contains the yolk stalk and the allantois. Called also *chorda umbilicalis* and *funiculus umbilicalis* [NA]. **vocal c's.** thin, reedlike bands which vibrate to make vocal sounds during speaking. One end of each cord is attached to the front of the laryngeal wall, and the opposite ends are connected to two small cartilages near the posterior wall of the larynx. The cartilages can be rotated so as to swing the cords apart or bring them together. When the cords are apart, the breath passes through silently; when they are close together, the passing air forces them to vibrate, thus producing sound. The superior pair is called the *vestibular folds,* or the false vocal cords, and the inferior pair the *true vocal cords.* Called also *chordae vocales.* **vocal c., false,** vestibular FOLD. **vocal c., inferior,** vocal c., true. **vocal c., superior,** vestibular FOLD. **vocal c., true,** a fold of mucous membrane of the larynx, enclosing two yellow elastic ligaments, the vocal ligaments, which are attached ventrally to the angle of the thyroid cartilage and dorsally to the vocal process of the arytenoid. Called also *Ferrein's c., inferior vocal c., Ferrein's ligament, plica vocalis* [NA], and *vocal fold.*

cordal (kor′dal) pertaining to a cord; used specifically in referring to the vocal cord.

cordate (kor′dāt) [L. *cor* heart] heart-shaped.

cordectomy (kor-dek′to-me) [*cord* + Gr. *ektomē* excision] excision of a cord, as a vocal cord.

cordopexy (kor′do-pek″se) [*cord* + Gr. *pēxis* fixation] the operation of displacing outward the vocal cord for laryngeal stenosis.

Cordran trademark for *flurandrenolide.*

core (kor) 1. the central part of anything, such as the central mass of necrotic matter in a boil. 2. a bar of iron around which a wire is wound to form an induction coil or electromagnet. 3. a sectional record, usually of plaster of Paris or one of its derivatives, of the relationships of parts, such as teeth, metallic

restorations, or copings. 4. **cast c. cast c.,** a metal casting, usually with a post in the canal of a root, designed to support and retain an artificial crown. **disappearing c.,** a method of constructing a mold for casting metal by encasing a wax model in plaster or other investing material, and when the latter is set, removing the wax by melting and burning out. Called also *cire perdue, lost wax technique,* and *Taggard's method.* **ionic c.,** atoms stripped of the valence electrons. **pulp c.,** PULP proper. **viral c.,** the internal part of the viral particle, which consists of nucleic acid and closely associated proteins.

coreactant (ko″re-ak′tant) one of two substances which react with each other. **polysulfide c.,** polysulfide ACCELERATOR.

corepressor (ko″re-pres′sor) a substance which binds with a repressor, thus activating it. See also REPRESSOR.

Cori, Carl F. [born 1896] a Prague-born biochemist in America; co-winner, with Gerty Theresa Cori and Bernardo Alberto Houssay, of the Nobel Prize for medicine and physiology in 1947, for discovery of how glycogen is catalytically converted.

Cori's disease [Gerty Theresa *Cori,* a Prague-born biochemist in America, 1896–1957; co-winner, with Carl F. Cori and Bernardo Alberto Houssay, of the Nobel Prize for medicine and physiology in 1947, for discovery of how glycogen is catalytically converted] GLYCOGENOSIS II.

coring (kor′ing) 1. the removal of a core; the cutting out of the central part of something. 2. in solidification, the induction of a nonhomogenous structure, as a solid solution solidifies, the first solid form, or the nucleus, having a different composition from that of the remainder of the crystal. In the solidification of alloys, the cores consist of the dendrites of the higher melting components of the alloy, suspended in the matrix containing the lower melting components.

corium (ko′re-um) [L. "hide"] [NA] the true skin; the layer of the skin beneath the epidermis which makes up the bulk of the skin, being about 4 mm in thickness. It represents the subcutaneous connective tissue of the body, and is composed of cellular elements (fibrocytes, histiocytes, and mastocytes), fibrous elements (reticular, collagenous, and elastics fibers), and a ground substance making up the interfibrillar matrix. The corium is the second barrier after the epidermis against injury and provides support for the vascular and nervous systems of the skin and for the cutaneous appendages. In addition, it is a potential reservoir for blood, electrolytes, and water. Called also *dermis.* **c. of gingiva, gingival c.,** a term used in the past for the connective tissue situated between the periosteum and the lamina propria of the gingival mucosa. **c. of tongue,** a term used in the past for the connective tissue of the tongue.

Corlan trademark for *hydrocortisone sodium succinate* (see under HYDROCORTISONE).

Cormed trademark for *nikethamide.*

Cormid trademark for *nikethamide.*

corn (korn) [L. *cornu* horn] 1. a horny induration and thickening of the stratum corneum of the skin, produced by friction and pressure; it forms a conical mass pointing down into the corium, producing pain and irritation. 2. a tall, annual, cereal plant, *Zea mays,* having a jointed, solid stem and bearing the grain seeds, or kernels, on large ears. **c. sugar,** dextrose. **c. oil,** corn OIL. **c. syrup,** glucose (1).

cornea (kor′ne-ah) [L. *corneus* horny] the transparent structure forming the anterior part of the fibrous tunic of the eye.

Cornelia de Lange's syndrome [*Cornelia de Lange,* Dutch pediatrician, 1871–1950] de Lange's SYNDROME.

corner (kor′ner) a point at which lines, sides, or walls meet. See also ANGLE. **c. of the mouth,** the junction at which the upper and lower lips meet, at either side of the mouth. See labial COMMISSURE.

corniculate (kor-nik′u-lāt) shaped like a small horn.

corniculum (kor-nik′u-lum) [L. dim. of *cornu*] corniculate CARTILAGE.

cornification (kor″nĭ-fi-ka′shun) [L. *cornu* horn + *facere* to make] 1. conversion into keratin or horn. 2. conversion of epithelium to the stratified squamous type.

Cornil, Lucien [French physician] see Lhermitte-Cornil-Quesnel SYNDROME.

Cornocentin trademark for *ergonovine maleate* (see under EROGONOVINE).

cornu (kor′nu) [L.] a horn; a pointed projection or excrescence on the body. Used as a general term in anatomical nomenclature for structures resembling such a projection or structure. **cor′nua cartilag′inis thyroi′deae,** horns of thyroid cartilage; see under HORN. **c. cuta′neum,** cutaneous HORN. **ethmoid c.,** middle nasal CONCHA. **greater c. of hyoid bone,** greater horn of hyoid bone; see under HORN. **c. infe′rius cartilag′inis thyroi′deae** [NA], inferior horn of thyroid cartilage; see under HORN. **lesser c. of hyoid bone,** lesser horn of hyoid bone; see under HORN. **c. ma′jus os′sis hyoi′dei** [NA], greater horn of hyoid bone; see under HORN. **c. mi′nus os′sis hyoi′dei** [NA], lesser horn of hyoid bone; see under HORN. **c. supe′rius cartilag′inis thyroi′deae** [NA], superior horn of thyroid cartilage; see under HORN.

cornua (kor′nu-ah) [L.] plural of *cornu.*

corona (ko-ro′nah), pl. *coro′nas,* or *coro′nae* [L.; Gr. *korōnē*] a crown. **c. cli′nica** [NA], clinical CROWN. **c. den′tis** [NA], dental CROWN.

coronad (kor′o-nad) toward the crown of the head or any corona.

coronae (ko-ro′ne) [L.] plural of *corona.*

coronal (ko-ro′nal) [L. *coronalis*] 1. pertaining to the crown of the head or to any corona. 2. situated in the direction of the coronal suture; said of a longitudinal plane or section passing through the body at right angles to the median plane. Called also *coronalis* [NA]. See under PLANE.

coronale (kor-o-na′le) 1. the point of the coronal suture at the end of the maximum frontal diameter. 2. frontal BONE.

coronalis (kor″o-na′lis) [L.] coronal (2).

coronary (kor′ŏ-na-re) [L. *corona;* Gr. *korōnē*] encircling in the manner of a crown; a term applied to vessels, nerves, etc. Sometimes used alone to mean coronary occlusion (see under OCCLUSION).

Coronaviridae (kor″o-nah-vi′rĭ-de) [L. *corona* crown + *virus* + *-idae*] a family of viruses having approximately spherical virions (60 to 160 nm in diameter) and lipid-containing envelopes covered with clublike projections that give them the appearance of crowns. The nucleocapsid is assembled in the cytoplasm and acquires an envelope by budding into the cytoplasmic vacuoles. The genome consists of single-stranded RNA. The family comprises a single genus, *Coronavirus.*

Coronavirus (kor″o-nah-vi′rus) the single genus of the family Coronaviridae, including human respiratory coronaviruses and human intestinal coronaviruses.

coronavirus (kor″o-nah-vi′rus) any virus of the family Coronaviridae or of the genus *Coronavirus.* **human intestinal c.,** a viral particle isolated from stools of adult patients during an epidemic of gastroenteritis. **human respiratory c.,** a virus associated with human acute upper respiratory disease, sometimes also causing lower respiratory tract infection in infants. Experimental infection of volunteers produces the common cold.

corone (kŏ-ro′ne) [Gr. *korōnē* anything hooked or curved] coronoid process of mandible; see under PROCESS.

coroner (kor′o-ner) an officer of the law who holds inquests in regard to violent, sudden, or unexplained deaths. See also medical EXAMINER.

coronion (kŏ-ro′ne-on) the tip of the coronoid process of the mandible.

coronoid (kor′o-noid) [Gr. *korōnē* anything hooked or curved + *eidos* form, shape] 1. shaped like a crow's beak. 2. crown-shaped. 3. coronoid process of mandible; see under PROCESS.

coronoidectomy (kor″o-noi-dek′to-me) surgical removal of the coronoid process of the mandible.

corpora (kor′po-rah) [L.] plural of *corpus.*

corporal (kor′po-ral) corporeal.

corporation (kor″pŏ-ra′shun) a group of persons united and regarded as an entity that, under law, exists independently of its membership, which may be reduced, enlarged, or exchanged in accordance with the bylaws of the corporation, and has power and liabilities distinct from those of its members. **dental service c.,** a professional sponsored nonprofit organization legally constituted to contract with groups of consumers to administer dental care plans on a prepaid basis. See also Delta Dental Plan, under PLAN.

corporeal (kor-po′re-al) [L. *corpus* body] pertaining to the body. Called also *corporal.*

corps (kor) 1. a subdivision of the armed forces. 2. a group of persons associated together or having a common activity. **National Health Service C.,** an organization under the United States Public Health Service, made up of physicians, dentists, nurses, and other personnel who serve in areas with a critical shortage of health manpower for the purpose of improving health care delivery to persons residing in such areas. Abbreviated *NHSC.*

corpse (korps) [L. *corpus* body] a dead body; used to refer specifically to a human body in the early period after death. See also CADAVER.

corpus (kor′pus), pl. *cor′pora* [L. "body"] any discrete mass of material, as of specialized tissue. Used in anatomical nomenclature to designate the entire organism, and applied also to the main portion of an anatomical part, structure, or organ. **c. adipo′sum buc′cae** [NA], buccal fat PAD. **c. amygdaloi′deum** [NA], amygdaloid BODY. **c. callo′sum** [NA] an arched mass of white matter, found in the depths of the longitudinal fissure separating the two cerebral hemispheres, which interconnects the two hemispheres. **c. lin′guae** [NA], the corpus of the tongue; the larger anterior part of the tongue, in the floor of the mouth. **c. mandib′ulae** [NA], BODY of mandible. **c. maxil′lae** [NA], BODY of maxilla. **c. os′sis hyoi′dei** [NA], BODY of hyoid bone. **c. os′sis sphenoida′lis** [NA], BODY of sphenoidal bone. **cor′pora paraaor′tica** [NA], aortic bodies; see under BODY. **c. pinea′le** [NA], pineal GLAND. **cor′pora santoria′na,** corniculate CARTILAGE. **c. sphenoida′le,** BODY of sphenoidal bone. **c. stria′tum** [NA], one of the components of the basal ganglia; specifically, a subcortical mass of gray and white substance in front of and lateral to the thalamus in each cerebral hemisphere. The gray substance is arranged in two principal masses, the caudate nucleus and the lentiform nucleus; the striate appearance on section of the area being produced by connecting bands of gray substance passing from one nucleus to the other through the white substance. The corpus striatum is associated with coordination of muscle movements; its other areas being presumed to inhibit the activity of the globus pallidum. **c. of tongue,** c. linguae. **c. tritic′eum,** triticeal CARTILAGE. **c. Wol′ffi,** mesonephros.

corpuscle (kor′pus'l) any small mass or body. See also CORPUSCULUM. **articular c's,** encapsulated nerve endings found within joints. Called also *corpuscula articularia* [NA] and *corpuscula nervorum articularia.* **axile c., axis c.,** the central part of a tactile corpuscle. **basal c.,** a small barrel-like thickening at the base of each cilium of ciliated cells, consisting of triplets of microtubules peripherally arranged. Called also *basal body.* **blood c.,** a formed blood element: erythrocyte, leukocyte, or blood platelet. **bone c.,** osteocyte. **bulboid c's,** bulbs of Krause; see under BULB. **chromophil c's,** Nissl bodies; see under BODY. **Dogiel's c.,** a sensory end-organ found in the mucous membrane of the eyes, nose, mouth, and genitals. **Golgi c.,** any of the encapsulated end-organs found in a tendon at its junction with the muscular fibers, which mediate tension differences to the innervating nerve fibers. **Grandry's c's, Grandry-Merkel c's, Merkel's c's, Krause's c's,** bulbs of Krause; see under BULB. **lamellar c's, lamellated c's,** large encapsulated nerve endings made up of bulbs about 2 to 4 mm in diameter, which consist of concentric lamellae, arranged somewhat like layers of an onion, and of a core in which the nerve fibers lose first their myelin sheath and later their neurilemma among the specialized layers. They are concerned with the perception of sensations, and are found in various parts of the body, including the deeper layers of the skin and the submucous membrane, including that of the lips and nose. Called also *corpuscula lamellosa* [NA]. See also *Pacini's c's* and *Ruffini's c's.* **Meissner's (oval, tactile, or touch) c's,** tactile c's. **Merkel's c's,** tactile corpuscles in the submucosa of the tongue and mouth, each consisting of a sheath continuous with the sheath of Henle of the nerve. Enclosed within the sheath are two flattened epithelial cells between the opposed surfaces of which is a biconvex disk continuous with the end of the neurofibrils. Called also *Grandry's c's, Grandry-Merkel c's,* and *Merkel's disks.* **oval c's of Meissner,** tactile c's. **Pacini's c's, pacinian c's,** lamellar corpuscles concerned with the perception of pressure. Called also *Vater's c's* and *Vater-Pacini c's.* **red c.,** erythrocyte. **Ruffini's c's,** lamellar corpuscles concerned with the perception of pressure and temperature. **salivary c.,** a white blood cell that has migrated through the oral epithelium and is mixed in the saliva. **Schwalbe's c.,** taste BUD. **tactile c's,** medium-sized encapsulated nerve endings, consisting of connective tissue capsules and tiny plates stacked one above the other; the nerve fiber penetrates the capsule and ends in globular enlargements. They are found chiefly in the corium of the hands and feet, but also in the skin of the lips and the mucous membranes of the lips and tongue, and other tissues. Called also *Meissner's (oval, tactile, or touch) c's, corpuscula tactus* [NA], *tactile cells,* and *touch cells.* **taste c.,** taste CELL. **terminal nerve c's,** nerve endings characterized by fibrous capsules of varying thickness that are continuous with the endoneurium. Called also *corpuscula nervosa terminalia* [NA], *corpuscula nervorum terminalia,* and *encapsulated nerve endings.* **Vater's c's, Vater-Pacini c's,** Pacini's c's. **white c.,** leukocyte.

corpuscula (kor-pus′ku-lah) [L.] plural of *corpusculum.*

corpuscular (kor-pus′ku-lar) pertaining to or of the nature of corpuscles.

corpusculum (kor-pus′ku-lum), pl. *corpus′cula* [L. dim. of *corpus*] any small mass or body. Used in anatomical nomencla-

ture to designate certain small discrete masses. See also COR-
PUSCLE. **corpus′cula articula′ria** [NA], articular corpuscles; see
under CORPUSCLE. **corpus′cula bulbifor′mia, corpus′cula bul-
boi′dea** [NA], bulbs of Krause; see under BULB. **corpus′cula
lamello′sa** [NA], see lamellar corpuscles; see under CORPUSCLE.
corpus′cula nervo′rum articula′ria, articular corpuscles; see
under CORPUSCLE. **corpus′cula nervo′sa termina′lia** [NA],
corpus′cula nervo′rum termina′lia, terminal nerve corpuscles;
see under CORPUSCLE. **corpus′cula tac′tus** [NA], tactile corpuscles; see under CORPUSCLE. **c. tritic′eum,** triticeal CARTILAGE.

correction (ko-rek′shun) 1. the act or process of correcting, improving, or setting right. 2. that which is used to correct a
mistake or abnormality. **occlusal c.,** correction of faulty occlusion or malocclusion.

corrector (kor-rek′tor) something that corrects or sets right. **function c.,** a removal orthodontic appliance utilizing oral and facial
muscle forces to move teeth and possibly change the relationship of dental arches. Called also *Fränkel appliance.*

correspondence (kor′ĕ-spon′dens) 1. the condition of being in
agreement, or conformity. 2. a written communication.

Corrigan's line, sign [Sir Dominic John *Corrigan,* Irish physician,
1802–1880] copper LINE.

corrosion (ko-ro′zhun) [L. *corrosio*] 1. the slow destruction of the
texture or substance of a tissue, as by the action of a corrosive
substance. 2. a gradual disintegration of a substance, such as
metal, by chemical or electrochemical factors in its environment. In dental restorations and dentures, it is due to chemical
reaction of metals with nonmetallic elements. See also TARNISH
(2). **aqueous c.,** electrochemical c. **chemical c.,** that due to a
chemical reaction. In the oral environment, a direct combination of the metallic and nonmetallic elements, bringing about
chemical reactions, such as oxidation, sulfuration, and halogenation, causing corrosive deterioration of metal components
of dentures and dental restorations. Electrochemical corrosion
almost always accompanies chemical corrosion. Called also *dry
c.* **concentration cell c.,** see *electrochemical c.* **dry c.,** chemical
c. **electrochemical c., electrolytic c.,** corrosion of a metal caused
by chemical reactions associated with the flow of electric
current. The process involves the wet-battery mechanism,
whereby one of the two dissimilar metals (one having a higher
number on the periodic table) immersed in an electrolyte solution undergoes hydrolysis and liberates electrons which are
transported in the solution to the metal having a lower number
on the periodic table, thereby generating galvanic current. The
metal giving up its electrons is an anode and the one accepting
the electrons is the cathode. Two mechanisms involving dissimilar metals include: the use of dissimilar metals in separate
restorations and heterogeneous combination of metal surfaces,
as the use of eutectic and peritectic alloys or dissimilar alloy-
solder combinations. Other mechanisms include the use of a
nonhomogeneous surface structure in amalgam restorations, in
which the polished area becomes an anode to the unpolished
one. In *concentration cell corrosion,* there are variations in the
electrolyte or in the composition of the given electrolyte within
the system, as in the presence of debris which produces one type
of electrolyte and the normal saliva which provides another.
Called also *aqueous c.* and *wet c.* **wet c.,** electrochemical c.

corrosive (ko-ro′siv) [L. *con* together + *rodere* to gnaw] 1. destructive to tissue. 2. an agent that destroys tissue. See also
CAUSTIC.

corrugator (cor′u-ga″tor) [L. *con* together + *ruga* wrinkle] a
muscle that produces wrinkles. **c. supercil′ii,** corrugator supercilii MUSCLE.

Cortalone trademark for *prednisolone.*

Cort-Dome trademark for *hydrocortisone.*

cortex (kor′teks) [L. "bark, rind, shell"] the outer layer of an organ
or other body structure, as distinguished from the underlying
substance. **adrenal c.,** the outer layer of the adrenal gland, the
inner part of which is the adrenal medulla. Its hormones are
divided into glucocorticoids (cortisol, cortisone, and corticosterone), mineralocorticoids (aldosterone and desoxycorticos-
terone), and androgens. Small amounts of progesterone are also
found in the adrenal cortex. It is divided into three zones: *zona
glomerulosa,* producing mostly mineralocorticoids, and *zona
fasciculata* and *zona reticularis,* producing mostly glucocorticoids and 17-ketosteroids. Called also *c. glandulae suprarenalis* [NA]. See also GLUCOCORTICOID and MINERALOCORTICOID,
and see Addison's DISEASE, adrenogenital SYNDROME, Cushing's
SYNDROME, general adaptation SYNDROME, and Waterhouse-
Friderichsen SYNDROME. **cerebral c., c. cer′ebri** [NA], **c. of
cerebrum,** the thin layer of gray matter on the surface of the
cerebral hemispheres, folded into gyri; its surface is divided by
a deep fissure from the front to the back into symmetrical right
and left hemispheres. Each of the halves is further subdivided
by shallower fissures, separating each hemisphere into four

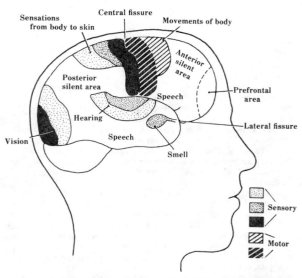

Projection areas of the brain. (From B. F. Miller and C. B. Keane:
Encyclopedia and Dictionary of Nursing. 2nd ed. Philadelphia, W.
B. Saunders Co., 1978.)

principal lobes: the occipital, parietal, frontal, and temporal. At
the bottom of the longitudinal fissure are the fibers of the white
matter of the corpus callosum, which connects the hemispheres. It reaches its highest development in man, where it is
responsible for higher mental functions, general movement,
visceral functions, perception, and behavioral reactions, and
for association and integration of these functions, different
parts of the cortex having responsibility for different functions
(see illustration). Called also *pallium.* **c. glan′dulae su-
prarena′lis** [NA], adrenal c. **c. no′di lymphat′ici,** cortical substance of lymph nodes; see under SUBSTANCE.

Cortexilar trademark for *flumethasone.*

cortical (kor′tĭ-kal) [L. *corticalis*] pertaining to or of the nature of
a cortex or bark.

corticalosteotomy (kor″tĭ-kal-os″te-ot′o-me) osteotomy through
the bone cortex at the base of the dentoalveolar segment, which
serves to weaken the resistance of the bone to the application of
orthodontic forces.

cortices (kor′tĭ-sēz) [L.] plural of *cortex.*

corticoid (kor′tĭ-koid) adrenal cortex steroid HORMONE.

corticosteroid (kor″tĭ-ko-ste′roid) adrenal cortex HORMONE.

corticotropin (kor″tĭ-ko-tro′pin) adrenocorticotropic HORMONE.

Cortiden trademark for *paramethasone.*

Cortifoam trademark for *hydrocortisone.*

Cortilet trademark for *fluorometholone.*

Cortiphate trademark for *hydrocortisone phosphate* (see under
HYDROCORTISONE).

cortisol (kor′tĭ-sol) hydrocortisone. **c. acetate,** HYDROCORTISONE
acetate.

cortisone (kor′tĭ-sōn) a natural glucocorticoid with some mineralocorticoid activity, produced in the zona fasciculata of the
adrenal cortex, its production being controlled by ACTH. Conversely, through a feedback mechanism, cortisone controls
ACTH secretion. Cortisone is involved in protein, lipid, and
carbohydrate metabolism and in immune and inflammatory
responses of the body. **c. acetate,** a salt of cortisone, occurring as
a white or almost white, odorless crystalline powder that is
soluble in alcohol, chloroform, dioxane, and acetone. Used in
the treatment of adrenocortical insufficiency and as an anti-
inflammatory and antiallergic agent. In dentistry, used in the
treatment of sensitive dentin, pulpal reactions to surgery, oral
ulcers in skin diseases, arthritic temporomandibular joint disorders, and in tissue transplantation. Side reactions may include euphoria, mental depression, psychoses, hypertension,
anorexia, peptic ulcer, susceptibility to infection, abnormal fat
distribution, moon face, edema, potassium loss, alkalosis, and
osteoporosis. Trademarks: Artriona, Cortistab, Cortisyl, Cortogen, Cortone, Incortin.

Δ¹-cortisone (del″tah-kor′tĭ-sōn) prednisone.

Cortistab trademark for *cortisone acetate* (see under CORTI-
SONE).

Cortisyl trademark for *cortisone acetate* (see under CORTI-SONE).

Cortogen trademark for *cortisone acetate* (see under CORTI-SONE).

Cortone trademark for *cortisone acetate* (see under CORTI-SONE).

corundum (ko-run′dum) a hard native or artificial aluminum oxide; transparent varieties being used as gems and other varieties as abrasives. In dentistry, used as an abrasive in grinding wheels and for points mounted on mandrels for the dental engine. Called also *α-alumina* and *oriental topaz.*

Corvisart's facies [Jean Nicolas de *Corvisart* des Marets, French physician, 1755–1821] see under FACIES.

corymbiform (ko-rim′bĭ-form) [Gr. *korymbos* the cluster of ivy flower + L. *forma* form] clustered; said of lesions grouped around a single, usually larger, lesion, as in late secondary syphilis.

corynebacteria (ko-ri″ne-bak-te′re-ah) plural of *corynebacterium.*

Corynebacteriaceae (ko-ri″ne-bak-te″re-a′se-e) [*Corynebacterium* + -*aceae*] a family of coryneform bacteria, related to the actinomycetes, consisting of the genera *Arthrobacter, Cellulomonas, Corynebacterium,* and *Kurthia.* The genera *incertae sedis Brevibacterium* and *Microbacterium* have also been assigned to this family.

Corynebacterium (ko-ri″ne-bak-te′re-um) [Gr. *korynē* club + *baktērion* little rod] a genus of bacteria of the family Corynebacteriaceae, the strains of which are divided generally into those pathogenic to man and other animals, those pathogenic to plants, and those not pathogenic. Strains pathogenic to man and animals are straight to slightly curved rods with irregularly staining segments, sometimes granules, often showing coryneform swellings. The organisms are usually gram-positive, nonmotile, and non–acid-fast. **C. ac′nes, C. anaero′bium,** *Propionibacterium acnes;* see under PROPIONIBACTERIUM. **C. a′vidum,** *Propionibacterium avidum;* see under PROPIONIBACTERIUM. **C. bo′vis,** a species found in aseptically drawn milk. **C. conjuncti′vae,** *C. xerosis.* **C. diphthe′riae,** a pathogenic species that is the etiologic agent of diphtheria, which also has been isolated from the nasopharynx of healthy carriers. The members occur as non–acid-fast, gram-positive, but easily decolorized, straight or slightly curved rods, which are frequently swollen at both ends, and are about 0.3 to 0.8 by 1.0 to 8.0 μm in size. According to the clinical severity of cases in which they are isolated, the strains are separable into three types — *mitis* (long, curved pleomorphoric rods with many granules); *intermedius* (long, barred forms with few granules); and *gravis* (short, irregular rods, with metachromatic granules). Most strains produce a lethal exotoxin, the ability to produce the toxin being determined by the presence of a prophage carrying a specific determinant called *tox*⁺. Many strains carry bacteriophage lytic for other strains. Called also *Bacillus diphtheriae, Bacterium diphtheriae, Klebs-Loeffler bacillus, Microsporon diphtheriticum, Mycobacterium diphtheriae,* and *Pacinia loeffleri.* **C. e′qui,** a species isolated from pneumonia in foals, the genital tract of mares, aborted equine fetuses, and the submaxillary lymph glands of swine. Called also *C. purulentus* and *Mycobacterium equi.* **C. fusifor′me,** *Fusobacterium nucleatum;* see under FUSOBACTERIUM. **C. granulo′sum,** *Propionibacterium granulosum;* see under PROPIONIBACTERIUM. **C. hofman′nii,** *C. pseudodiphtheriticum.* **C. infantisep′ticum,** *Listeria monocytogenes;* see under LISTERIA. **C. israe′li,** *Actinomyces israelii;* see under ACTINOMYCES. **C. lympho′philum,** *Propionibacterium lymphophilum;* see under PROPIONIBACTERIUM. **C. necro′phorum,** *Fusobacterium necrophorum.* **C. o′vis,** *C. pseudotuberculosis.* **C. par′vulum,** *Listeria monocytogenes;* see under LISTERIA. **C. par′vum, C. par′vum infectio′sum,** *Propionibacterium acnes;* see under PROPIONIBACTERIUM. **C. preisz-nocar′di, C.** *pseudotuberculosis.* **C. pseudodiphtherit′icum,** a nonpathogenic and nontoxigenic species, morphologically similar to *C. diphtheriae,* isolated from the nasopharyngeal mucosa of a normal man. Called also *C. hofmannii, Bacillus pseudodiphthericus, Bacterium pseudodiphthericum, Hofmann's bacillus,* and *Mycobacterium pseudodiphthericum.* **C. pseudotuberculo′sis,** a weakly toxigenic species, morphologically similar to *C. diphtheriae,* causing ulcerative lymphangitis, abscesses, and other suppurative infections in sheep, goats, horses, and other warm-blooded animals, and occasional infections in man. Called also *C. ovis, C. preisz-nocardi, Bacillus pseudotuberculosis, Mycobacterium tuberculosis-ovis,* and *Preisz-Nocard bacillus.* **C. purulen′tus,** *C. equi.* **C. pyog′enes bo′vis,** *Propionibacterium granulosum;*

see under PROPIONIBACTERIUM. **C. xero′sis,** a strain, believed to be nonpathogenic, originally isolated from the conjunctival sac in man, also inhabiting the skin and mucous membranes, including those of the oral cavity. Also called *C. conjunctivae, Bacillus xerosis, Bacterium xerosis, Mycobacterium xerosis,* and *Pacinia neisseri.*

corynebacterium (ko-ri″ne-bak-te′re-um), pl. *corynebacte′ria.* [Gr. *korynē* club + *baktērion* little rod] 1. any member of the family Corynebacteriaceae or of the genus *Corynebacterium.* 2. a bacterium that displays coryneform shape during some stage of its development on artificial media. See coryneform bacteria, under BACTERIUM.

coryneform (ko-ri′nĕ-form) [Gr. *korynē* + L. *forma* form] club-shaped. See coryneform bacteria, under BACTERIUM.

coryza (kŏ-ri′zah) [L.; Gr. *koryza*] a catarrhal condition of the nasal mucous membrane; acute coryza. **acute c.,** a symptom complex of viral infection of the upper respiratory tract, marked by congestion of the nasal mucous membrane, profuse nasal discharge, sneezing, sore or dry throat, malaise, postnasal discharge, headache, cough, feverishness, chilliness, burning eyes, and muscle aching. Fever is usually absent. Rhinoviruses comprise the largest single etiologic group, but influenza, parainfluenza, respiratory syncytial, coxsackie, and echoviruses and adenoviruses are sometimes associated. The terms *acute catarrhal rhinitis, chest cold, head cold, laryngitis,* and *pharyngitis* are sometimes used to designate the principal anatomic sites of infection. Called also *common cold.* **allergic c.,** hay FEVER. **syphilitic c.,** a condition of young infants symptomatic of congenital syphilis, characterized by redness and swelling of the nostrils and adjacent parts of the upper lip, and a purulent, hemorrhagic foul-smelling nasal discharge, leading to gummatous or ulcerative necrosis and perforation of the nasal septum, and in turn, to saddle nose. Called also *syphilitic rhinitis.*

coryzavirus (ko-ri″zah-vi′rus) common cold VIRUS.

Coschwitz's duct [Georgius Daniel *Coschwitz,* German physician, 1679–1729] see under DUCT.

Coslan trademark for *mefenamic acid* (see under ACID).

Cosmegen trademark for *dactinomycin.*

Cosmos denture corrective trademark for a temporary *denture reliner* (see under RELINER).

cost (kawst) the price paid for something. **acquisition c.,** in insurance, the cost of placing a new group program on the books, including clerical and other peripheral expenses. **administrative c's,** all overhead expenses incurred in the administration of an organization or a program, which are not directly related to the product or objectives but pertain to clerical, administrative, promotional, educational, and other not directly productive activities. In dental insurance, the overhead expenses incurred in the operation of a dental plan, exclusive of costs of dental service provided. In some instances, promotional or educational costs are separated from this category. **allowable c's,** in health insurance, the amount the insurer will reimburse under a hospital payment formula for health care services, the patient being required to pay the difference between the allowable costs and the actual fee. See also ALLOWANCE. **maximum allowable c. program,** maximum allowable cost PROGRAM.

costa (kos′tah), pl. *cos′tae* [L.] [NA] rib.

costae (kos′te) [L.] plural of *costa.*

Costen's syndrome [James Bray *Costen,* American otolaryngologist, born 1895] temporomandibular dysfunction SYNDROME.

cost-sharing (kawst shār′ing) in insurance, provisions which require the insured to pay some portion of expenses. Deductible clauses and coinsurance are two of several forms of cost-sharing.

co-thromboplastin (ko″throm″bo-plas′tin) FACTOR VII.

COTRANS Coordinated Transfer Application System; see under SYSTEM.

cotton (kot′n) [L. *gossypium*] a textile material derived from the seeds of one or more species of cultivated varieties of tropical and subtropical plants of the genus *Gossypium;* used as a dressing. **absorbent c.,** purified cotton from which natural wax has been removed so that it will absorb moisture. **purified c.,** the hair of the seed of cultivated varieties of *Gossypium hirsutum,* or other species of *Gossypium,* freed from impurities, deprived of fatty matter, bleached, and sterilized; used as a surgical aid. Called also *gossypium asepticum, gossypium depuratum,* and *gossypium purificatum.* **salicylated c.,** purified cotton charged with salicylic acid; used as an antiseptic dressing. **styptic c.,** cotton impregnated with a styptic solution and dried.

Cotugno see COTUNNIUS.

Cotunnius (Cotugno), aqueduct of [Domenico *Cotunnius,* Italian anatomist, 1736–1822] 1. AQUEDUCT of vestibule. 2. CANALICULUS of cochlea.

cough (kawf) [L. *tussis*] a sudden noisy expulsion of air from the lungs. **Balme's c.,** coughing when in the recumbent position, due to nasopharyngeal obstruction. **trigeminal c.**, a cough due to irritation of the fibers of the trigeminal nerve distributed to the throat, nose, and external meatus of the ear. **whooping c.**, an infectious disease of infants and young children, caused by infection with *Bordetella pertussis*. After an incubation period of two weeks, there is slight fever, sneezing, running at the nose, and dry cough. The second phase, in a week or two, is characterized by a paroxysmal cough, consisting of a deep inspiration followed by a series of quick short coughs. Ulceration of the lingual frenum, produced by pressing the tongue against the incisal edges of the mandibular anterior teeth during proxysms of cough, is pathognomonic for whooping cough. Called also *pertussis*.

coul coulomb.

Coulomb's laws [Charles Augustin de *Coulomb*, French physicist, 1736–1806] see under LAW. See also COULOMB.

coulomb (koo′lom) [named after C. A. de *Coulomb*] the SI unit of electrical charge, defined as the quantity of electrical charge transferred by 1 ampere in 1 second (symbol A × s). Abbreviated *coul.* **absolute c.**, abcoulomb. **international c.**, the former standard of electrical charge, equal to 0.999835 of an absolute coulomb.

Coumadin trademark for *warfarin*.

coumarin (koo′mah-rin). 1,2-benzopyrone; a fragrant, colorless crystalline preparation from tonka bean, sweet clover, and other plants, and also prepared synthetically. Various derivatives are used as anticoagulants. See also BISHYDROXYCOUMARIN, ETHYL biscoumacetate, and WARFARIN.

council (kown′sil) [L. *concilium*] a group appointed or elected to serve as an administrative or advisory body. For councils of the American Dental Association, see Appendix. **ADA c's**, see American Dental Association in Appendix. **Coordinating C. on Medical Education**, a supervisory body established to coordinate policy matters and accreditation at all levels of medical education, sponsored among others by the American Association of Medical Colleges, American Hospital Association, and Council of Medical Specialty Societies. Abbreviated *CCME*. **Health Insurance Benefits Advisory C.**, an advisory council of the Department of Health and Human Services whose primary role is to provide advice and recommendations on matters of general policy in the administration of Medicare and Medicaid. Abbreviated *HIBAC*. **National C. for Radiation Protection and Measurements**, the national body concerned with the standards for radiation protection in the United States. The Council, together with the American Dental Association, American College of Radiology, American Academy of Dental Radiology, and American National Standards Institute, sponsors programs for establishing and observing x-ray protection standards in dentistry. Abbreviated *NCRP*. **United States Adopted Name C.**, see USAN.

count (kownt) [L. *computare* to reckon] a numerical computation. **Addis c.**, a count of the cells in 10 ml of urinary sediment for the purpose of calculating the total urinary sediment of the 12-hour specimen. **blood c.**, BLOOD count. **blood platelet c.**, see under PLATELET. **complete blood c.**, a series of tests of the peripheral blood, including the hematocrit (percent), the amount of hemoglobin (grams percent), the white cell count (per cubic millimeter), and the proportions of the different white cells as they appear on a blood smear. Abbreviated *CBC* or *cbc*. **erythrocyte c.**, ERYTHROCYTE count. **gingival-bone c.**, an index for recording the gingival condition and the level of condition of the crest of the alveolar bone, where: In the gingival score, 0 = negative finding, 1 = mild gingivitis; 2 = moderate gingivitis; 3 = severe gingivitis. In the bone score, 0 = no bone loss; 1 = incipient bone loss or notching of the alveolar crest; 2 = bone loss approximating one-fourth of the root length or pocket formation, one side not over one-half root length; 3 = bone loss approximately one-half of root length or pocket formation, one side not over three-fourths root length, and slight mobility; 4 = bone loss approximately three-fourths of root length or pocket formation, one side to apex, and moderate mobility; 5 = bone loss complete and marked tooth mobility; 8 = maximum possible count per person. One score is assigned to each tooth studied. A mean is then computed for the whole mouth. Also called *Dunning-Leach index, gingival-bone index*, and *gingival-bone count index*. **leukocyte c.**, LEUKOCYTE count. **leukocyte c., differential**, LEUKOCYTE count, differential. **lymphocyte c.**, see table of *Reference Values in Hematology* in Appendix. **monocyte c.**, see table of *Reference Values in Hematology* in Appendix. **myelocyte c.**, see table of *Reference Values in Hematology* in Appendix. **neutrophil c.**, see table of *Reference Values in Hematology* in Appendix. **platelet c.**, blood platelet count; see under PLATELET. **red cell c.**, ERYTHROCYTE count. **white blood c.**, LEUKOCYTE count.

counter (kown′ter) an instrument or apparatus by which numerical value is computed; in radiology, a device for enumerating

ionizing events. **Geiger c.**, Geiger-Müller c. **Geiger-Müller c., GM c.**, an instrument for detecting and measuring ionizing radiation. It consists of a gas-filled tube (Geiger-Müller tube) containing two electrodes, between which there is an electrical voltage but no current flowing. Passage of ionizing radiation produces a short, intense pulse of current from the negative to the positive electrodes; the number of pulses per second indicating the intensity of radiation. Called also *Geiger c.* See also *proportional c.*, ionization CHAMBER, and Geiger PLATEAU. **proportional c.**, a gas-filled tube with two electrodes, one of which is a cylinder with a very fine wire. Passage of ionizing radiations produces secondary ions which result in pulses of electric current from the negative to the positive electrodes; the pulses produced being proportional to the number of ions formed in the gas by the primary radiation. See also *Geiger-Müller c.* **scintillation c.**, an instrument for indicating the emission of ionizing particles, making possible the determination of the concentration of radioactive isotopes in the body or other substance; the radiation is absorbed by a phosphor crystal, which emits minute flashes of light that are detected and amplified by a photomultiplier tube.

counterdie (kown′ter-di) the reverse image of a die, usually made of a softer and lower fusing metal than the die.

counterextension (kown″ter-eks-ten′shun) traction in a proximal direction coincident with traction in the opposite direction.

counterincision (kown″ter-in-sizh′un) a second incision usually made to promote drainage, but occasionally to relieve tension on the edges of a clean wound during closure. See also COUNTEROPENING.

counterirritant (kown″ter-ir′ĭ-tant) 1. producing counterirritation. 2. any agent which causes counterirritation.

counterirritation (kown″ter-ir″ĭ-ta′shun) a superficial irritation; an irritation that is intended to relieve some other irritation.

counteropening (kown″ter-o′pen-ing) a second incision made across an earlier one to promote drainage. See also COUNTERINCISION.

counterpuncture (kown′ter-punk″chur) a second opening made opposite another.

counterstain (kown′ter-stān) a stain applied to render the effects of another stain more discernible.

countertraction (kown′ter-trak″shun) traction opposed to another traction; employed in the reduction of fractures.

coup (koo) [Fr.] stroke. **en c. de sabre** (ahn-koo-duh-sahb′) [Fr. "saber stroke"], resembling the scar of a saber wound; used to designate such a lesion of linear scleroderma on the forehead and scalp. **c. sur coup** (koo-ser-koo′) [Fr. "blow on blow"], the administration of a drug in small doses at short intervals, to secure rapid, complete, or continuous action. Abbreviated *CSC*.

couple (kup″l) 1. a combination of two; a pair. 2. two equal forces operating on an object in parallel, but in opposite directions. It has a purely rotating effect which can be expressed as a movement, equal to the value of one of the forces multiplied by the distance between their lines of action. 3. an area of contact between two dissimilar metals, producing a difference in electrical potential.

coupling (kup′ling) 1. the act or process of combining or joining two separate parts together. See also coupling AGENT. 2. the occurrence on the same chromosome in a double heterozygote of the two mutant alleles of interest. Cf. REPULSION.

Cournand, André Frédéric [born 1895] a French-born American physiologist; co-winner, with Werner Theodor Otto Forssmann and Dickinson W. Richards, of the Nobel prize for medicine and physiology in 1956, for developing a technique in the diagnosis and treatment of heart disease.

courtesy (ker′tĕ-se) a considerate act, favor, or generosity. **c. allowance, c. discount, professional c.**, courtesy ALLOWANCE.

Coutard's law [Henri *Coutard*, French radiologist in America, 1876–1950] see under LAW.

covalence (ko-va′lens) [*co- + valence*] the process of joining atoms to form molecules by the sharing of electrons. See also covalent BOND. **dative c.**, covalence in which one atom in the compound contributes both electrons. **normal c.**, covalence in which both atoms in the compound contribute one electron each.

covariance (ko-var′e-ans) the expected value of the product of the deviations of corresponding values of two random variables from their respective means.

coverage (kov′er-ij) 1. the extent to which something is covered. 2. the guarantee against specific losses provided under the terms of an insurance policy. Often used interchangeably with benefit or protection, or to mean insurance or an insurance contract. **denture c.,** the extent to which the oral tissue is covered by the denture base. **extended c.,** extension of benefits; see under BENEFIT. **first dollar c.,** coverage under an insurance policy which begins with the first dollar of expense incurred by the insured for the covered benefits, having no deductible clause. **last dollar c.,** insurance coverage without upper limits or maximums on the amount of benefits payable to the insured person. **occlusal c.,** in a denture, the protection of the entire occlusal surface or incisal edge against the forces of mastication.

Cowden's syndrome see under SYNDROME.

Cowdria (kow'dre-ah) a genus of rickettsiae of the tribe Ehrlichieae; nonpathogenic for man.

Cowling's rule see under RULE.

cowpox (kow'poks) an eruptive disease of the skin, udders, and teats of cows, caused by the vaccinia virus, which is transmissible to man (see VACCINIA). The lesions of artificially infected bovine calves are the source of live viruses used in producing smallpox vaccine.

cowrie (kow're) copal.

Coxiella (kok"se-el'ah) [named after H. R. *Cox*] a genus of bacteria of the tribe Rickettsieae, family Rickettsiaceae. **C. burnet'ii,** a species that is the etiologic agent of Q fever, occurring as rods (ranging in size from 0.2 to 0.4 by 0.4 to 1.0 μm), sometimes as diplococci (1.0 to 1.6 μm long), or as spores (0.3 to 0.4 μm in diameter), lacking flagella or capsules. Normally, the organisms are gram-negative, but under certain conditions they may be gram-positive, being relatively resistant to heat and some chemical agents, more so than other rickettsiae. *C. burnetii* occurs worldwide in various domestic and wild animals. Human infection is most often airborne, but the organisms appear to enter the body by a variety of routes. Called also *Rickettsia burnetii* and *R. diaporica.*

coxsackievirus (kok-sak'e-vi'rus) [named after *Coxsackie,* a town in New York State where the virus was first isolated] a picornavirus of the genus *Enterovirus,* first isolated from patients with a paralytic poliomyelitis-like disease, occurring as particles, 28–30 nm in diameter, having RNA as a central core. Coxsackieviruses are divided into groups A and B and subdivided numerically into subgroups. Written also *Coxsackie virus* or *coxsackie virus.* See table.

cozymase (ko-zi'mās) nicotinamide-adenine DINUCLEOTIDE.

CP central PIT.

C3PA C3 proactivator; see FACTOR B.

C3PA-convertase C3 proactivator convertase; see FACTOR $\overline{\text{D}}$.

CPC clinicopathological conference.

CPHA Commission on Professional and Hospital Activities; see under COMMISSION.

Cpiron trademark for a preparation of *ferrous fumarate* (see under FUMARATE).

CPR cardiopulmonary RESUSCITATION.

cps cycles per second.

CPT Current Procedural Terminology; see under TERMINOLOGY.

CR centric RELATION.

Cr chromium.

CLINICAL SYNDROMES ASSOCIATED WITH COXSACKIEVIRUSES

Clinical Syndrome	Group
Aseptic meningitis	A
	B
Paralytic disease	A
	B
Herpangina	A
Fever, exanthema	A
	B
Acute upper respiratory infection	A
	B
Epidemic pleurodynia or myalgia	B
Myocarditis of the newborn	B
Interstitial myocarditis and valvulitis in infants and children	B
Pericarditis	B
Undifferentiated febrile illness	All

(Modified from B. D. Davis, et al.: Microbiology. 2nd ed. Hagerstown, Harper & Row, 1973.)

Craig Martin see under DENTIFRICE.

craniad (kra'ne-ad) [L. *cranium* head + *ad* toward] toward the cranium; toward the anterior (in animals) or superior (in humans) end of the body.

cranial (kra'ne-al) [L. *cranialis*] pertaining to the cranium, or to the anterior (in animals) or superior (in humans) end of the body.

cranio- [L. *cranium;* Gr. *kranion* the upper part of the head] a combining form denoting relationship to the skull.

craniocerebral (kra"ne-o-ser'e-bral) pertaining to the cranium and the brain.

craniofacial (kra"ne-o-fa'shal) pertaining to the cranium and the face.

craniograph (kra'ne-o-graf") [*cranio-* + Gr. *graphein* to write] an instrument for outlining the skull.

craniography (kra"ne-og'rah-fe) the act or process of producing an outline of the skull from craniometric data.

craniolacunia (kra"ne-o-lah-ku'ne-ah) [*cranio-* + L. *lacuna* a hollow + *-ia*] defective development of the fetal skull marked by depressed areas on the inner surface of the bones. Called also *lacuna skull.*

craniomalacia (kra"ne-o-mah-la'she-ah) [*cranio-* + Gr. *malakia* softness] a condition characterized by abnormal softening of the skull.

craniomeningocele (kra"ne-o-mĕ-nin'go-sēl) [*cranio-* + Gr. *mēninx* membrane + *kēlē* hernia] protrusion of the cerebral membranes through a defect of the skull. See also CRANIUM bifidum.

craniometer (kra"ne-om'ĕ-ter) [*cranio-* + Gr. *metron* measure] an instrument for measuring the skull in craniometry.

craniometric (kra"ne-o-met'rik) pertaining to craniometry.

craniometry (kra"ne-om'ĕ-tre) [*cranio-* + Gr. *metron* measure] a branch of anthropometry, being the measurement of the dimensions and angles of a bony skull. For specific measurements see BREADTH, HEIGHT, INDEX, LENGTH, LINE, and PLANE. See illustration at CEPHALOMETRY.

craniopagus (kra"ne-op'ah-gus) [*cranio-* + Gr. *pagos* a thing fixed] a double monster united by the heads. Called also *cephalopagus.* See also CEPHALODYMUS.

craniopathy (kra"ne-op'ah-the) [*cranio-* + Gr. *pathos* disease] any disease of the skull.

craniopharyngeal (kra"ne-o-fah-rin'jĕ-al) pertaining to the cranium and the pharynx.

craniopharyngioma (kra"ne-o-fah-rin"je-o'mah) a usually benign but sometimes malignant pituitary tumor arising from vestigial remnants of the craniopharyngeal anlage, presenting a solid or cystic lesion, occasionally of considerable size. Histologically, it may contain a wide variety of cell types, recalling the cells of tooth enamel (hence the synonyms *pituitary adamantinoma* and *pituitary ameloblastoma*). Calcification and anaplastic bone formation are common. Called also *craniopharyngeal duct tumor, Rathke's pouch tumor,* and *suprasellar cyst.*

craniophore (kra'ne-o-fōr) [*cranio-* + Gr. *phoros* bearing] a device for holding the skull during measurements of its diameters and angles.

cranioplasty (kra'ne-o-plas"te) [*cranio-* + Gr. *plassein* to mold] plastic surgery of the skull; surgical correction of defects of the skull.

craniopuncture (kra'ne-o-punk"chūr) [*cranio-* + *puncture*] surgical puncture of a bone of the skull.

craniorachischisis (kra"ne-o-rah-kis'ki-sis) [*cranio-* + Gr. *rhachis* spine + *schisis* fissure] congenital fissure of the skull and spinal column.

craniosacral (kra"ne-o-sa'kral) 1. pertaining to the skull and the sacrum. 2. pertaining to the craniosacral (parasympathetic) nervous system. See nervous SYSTEM.

cranioschisis (kra"ne-os'ki-sis) [*cranio-* + Gr. *schisis* fissure] a fissure of the skull, usually congenital.

craniosclerosis (kra"ne-o-sklĕ-ro'sis) [*cranio-* + Gr. *sklēros* hard] thickening of the bones of the skull.

craniostenosis (kra"ne-o-stĕ-no'sis) [*cranio-* + Gr. *stenōsis* narrowing] deformity of the skull caused by premature fusion of the cranial sutures, with consequent cessation of growth.

craniostosis (kra"ne-os-to'sis) [*cranio-* + Gr. *osteon* bone] congenital ossification of the cranial sutures.

craniosynostosis (kra"ne-o-sin"os-to'sis) [*cranio-* + Gr. *syn* together + *osteon* bone] premature closure of the cranial sutures. See also SYNOSTOSIS.

craniotabes (kra"ne-o-ta'bēz) [*cranio-* + L. *tabes* a wasting] reduction in the mineralization of the skull, with abnormal craniomalacia, usually located in the occipital and parietal bones along the lambdoidal sutures.

craniotopography (kra"ne-o-to-pog'rah-fe) [*cranio-* + *topography*] the study of the relations of the surface of the skull to the various parts of the brain beneath.

cranitis (kra-ni'tis) inflammation of the cranial bones; cranial osteitis.

cranium (kra'ne-um), pl. *cra'nia* [L.; Gr. *kranion* the upper part of the head] the upper part of the skull, made up of the occipital, frontal, sphenoidal, ethmoidal, two parietal, and two temporal bones. See also SKULL. **c. bif'idum,** a congenital abnormality characterized by cleft of the cranium, usually in the midline of the skull. When associated with protrusion of dura mater, the condition is known as *meningocele;* when the brain and meninges protrude, it is known as *meningoencephalocele.* **c. bif'idum occul'tum,** congenital cleft of the cranium without associated abnormalities of the brain or meninges, detectable only roentgenographically. **cerebral c., c. cerebra'le,** those portions of the bones of the head that contribute to the brain case. **visceral c., c. viscera'le,** those portions of the cranial bones that form the skeleton of the face, including the mandible and the hyoid bone.

Crasnitin trademark for *asparaginase.*

crater (kra'ter) [L. "bowl"] 1. a circular area of depression surrounded by an elevated margin. 2. an interdental depression in the gingival tissue and/or subjacent bone, often associated with the destructive effects of necrotizing ulcerative gingivitis. The buccal and lingual tissues are most commonly affected. **alveolar process c., bone c.,** a concavity in the crest of the interdental bone, confined within the vestibular and oral walls and, less frequently, between the tooth surface and the cortical bony plate. **gingival c.,** an excavation in the interproximal gingiva due to destruction of the papilla by necrosis. **interalveolar bone c.,** a periodontal bony defect consisting of a wide-mouthed cup- or bowl-shaped depression in the interalveolar bone, accompanied by a similar defect on the root of the root of the contiguous tooth. The side walls of the crater are formed by marginal bone on the vestibular and oral surfaces, and these walls may be of unequal height.

crateriform (kra-ter-i-form) [L. *crater* bowl + *forma* form] shaped like a crater; depressed or hollowed, like a bowl.

crazing (kra'zing) the appearance of minute cracks on the surface of artificial or natural teeth, porcelain, and resin denture bases. **resin c.,** the formation of small cracks in a resin, varying from microscopic to readily visible, under the influence of mechanical stress or as the result of the action of a solvent. In polymethyl methacrylate, cracks occur only as the result of tensile stress, appearing on the surface in a region in which the polymer molecules are oriented at right angles to the direction of the applied stress, gradually penetrating inward. Crazing of other resins through the action of solvents is marked by cracks that are randomly oriented, V- or Y-shaped cracks being the most common.

crease (krēs) a line or a well-defined depression, usually on the skin, formed in zones of folding, such as those on the palms of the hands. **simian c.,** a single transverse palmar crease formed by fusion of the proximal and distal palmar creases, observed in some chromosomal disorders, such as Down's syndrome, and in one to two percent of the normal population. Called also *simian line.*

creatine (kre'ah-tin) [Gr. *kreas* flesh] a compound, *N*-(aminoiminomethyl)-*N*-methylglycine, produced by the liver and kidneys by the transfer of the guanidine moiety of arginine to glycine, the product being methylated. It is present in muscles and, in lesser amounts, in the blood. In muscles, it combines with phosphoric acid to form creatine phosphate, which is a major source of energy in muscle contraction. Commercially (obtained from meat extracts) occurring as an anhydrous substance that is soluble in water, but not in ether. **c. phosphate,** a compound, *N*-(imino[phosphonoamino]-methyl)-*N*-methylglycine, found chiefly in muscles where it serves as a source of energy. Its high energy bond (a direct N – P linkage) has a free energy of hydrolysis of about 8500 calories per mol under standard conditions, the process of glycolysis supplying ATP, and the creatine phosphate and ATP acting jointly in muscle contraction. During recovery, when more ATP is formed from glycolysis, the creatine phosphate is regenerated. The ATP is the direct source of energy for muscle contraction, and the function of creatine phosphate and glycolysis is to supply ATP. The reversible interrelationship between ATP and creatine phosphate is shown in the following equation:

$$\text{creatine phosphate} + \text{ADP} \rightleftharpoons \text{ATP} + \text{creatine.}$$

Called also *phosphocreatine.*

creatinine (kre-at'i-nin, kre-at'i-nēn) a nitrogen-containing anhydride of creatine, 2-amin-1,5-dihydro-1-methy-4*H*-imidazol-4-one, present in tissues, but mostly in the urine, formed from either creatine phosphate or creatine, being the end-product of creatine metabolism in muscle tissue. It occurs as plae yellow

needles that are readily soluble in alcohol, benezene, chloroform, ether, and acetic acid and slightly soluble in water.

Credo Lidocaine-5 trademark for a topical anesthetic ointment, 100 gm of which contains 5 gm lidocaine in an ointment consisting of polyethylene glycol 4000 and polyethylene glycol 400 and various amounts of coloring and flavoring agents.

Credo topical gel see under GEL.

creep (krēp) 1. to shift or slide gradually. 2. the slow flow causing permanent deformation of materials held for long periods of time at stresses well below their conventional yield strength, usually occurring at temperatures near the softening point of the material. Waxes, rubbers, certain plastics, and certain other dental materials with a low melting point are subject to creep at room temperatures or in the mouth. See also FLOW (4). **dynamic c.,** that occurring in the presence of fluctuating stress. **static c.,** that occurring in the presence of constant stress.

Cremesone trademark for *hydrocortisone.*

crena (kre'nah), pl. *cre'nae* [L.] a notch or cleft.

crenae (kre'ne) [L.] plural of *crena.*

crenate (kre'nāt) [L. *crenatus*] scalloped or notched.

crenation (kre-na'shun) the formation of abnormal notching in the edge of an erythrocyte; the notched appearance of an erythrocyte caused by its shrinkage after suspension in a hypertonic solution. **c. of tongue,** scalloping along the lingual periphery of the tongue caused by its lying against the lingual surface of the mandibular teeth.

crenocyte (kre'no-sīt) a crenated erythrocyte; an erythrocyte having a notched appearance caused by shrinkage after suspension in a hypertonic solution. See also HEMOLYSIS.

creosote (kre'o-sōt) a mixture of phenols obtained by distilling wood tar, mainly beech, consisting mainly of guaiacol, cresol, methylcreosol, and phlorol, and occurring as an almost colorless or yellowish, refractive oily liquid with a penetrating smoky odor and a burning caustic taste. It is slightly soluble in water and is miscible with alcohol, ether, oils, and alkalies. Used externally as an antiseptic and internally as an expectorant in chronic bronchitis. Topical application to the cavity of a carious tooth is used to relieve toothache temporarily. Also used in the sterilization of root canals. Undiluted, it is a strong poison which will cause vascular collapse and death if ingested.

crepitation (krep'i-ta'shun) [L. *crepitare* to crackle] a crackling or clicking noise. Crepitation in the temporomandibular joint may be caused by roughness or cracks on the meniscus and the articulating joint surface, subluxation of the condyle over the edge of the meniscus, neuromuscular disorders, or stickiness of joint surfaces.

crepitus (krep'i-tus) [L.] 1. a discharge of gases from the bowel; flatus. 2. crepitation. 3. clicking (2). **articular c.,** joint c. **bony c.,** the crackling sound produced by the rubbing together of fragments of a fractured bone, or by air moving in soft tissues, as in subcutaneous emphysema. Sometimes also used to mean a sensation perceived by palpating fingers. **joint c.,** the grating sensation caused by the rubbing together of dry synovial surfaces of joints. Called also *articular c.* See also CREPITATION and temporomandibular joint SUBLUXATION.

Cresanol root canal dressing see under DRESSING.

Cresantin trademark for *metacresyl acetate* (see under METACRESYL).

crescent (kres'ent) [L. *crescens*] 1. shaped like a new moon. 2. a crescent-shaped structure. **articular c.,** a crescent-shaped articular fibrocartilage. **c's of Giannuzzi,** groups of cells, forming crescent-like structures, which partially surround portions of mucous acini, appearing in sections of mixed (seromucous) salivary glands when the mucous cells predominate. They are formed by the outnumbered serous cells pushed to the blind ends of the terminal portions or into saccular outpocketings. Called also *crescent cells, demilune cells, demilunes of Giannuzzi, demilunes of Heidenhain, Giannuzzi's bodies, Giannuzzi's cells, Heidenhain's bodies, Heidenhain's cells, marginal cells,* and *semilunar cells.* **sublingual c.,** the crescent-shaped area on the floor of the mouth, formed by the lingual wall of the mandible and the adjacent part of the floor of the mouth. **traumatic c.,** a crescent-shaped, small bluish-red area sometimes observed on the marginal gingivae. Traumatic crescents have been attributed to trauma from occlusion but, currently, they are believed to represent chronic inflammatory lesions caused by local irritants.

Cresilver trademark for an *amalgam alloy* (see under AMALGAM).

cresol (kre'sol) a mixture of three isomeric cresols, the *m*-isomer being the principal component, obtained from coal tar and from petroleum, and containing not more than 5 percent phenol. It is a colorless or yellowish highly refractive liquid with a phenol-like odor, which darkens on exposure to light and with aging, dissolves in water, and is miscible with glycerol, alcohol, benzene, and other solvents. Used as an antiseptic and disinfectant, particularly against vegetative bacteria and fungi, chiefly for the disinfection of dishes, utensils, hospital floors, and other objects. Formerly used, often in a formaldehyde solution, for the disinfection of dental instruments, in the treatment of periapical infections, and in root canal therapy. Chronic ingestion or percutaneous absorption may cause gastrointestinal disorders, vertigo, mental disorders, rash, jaundice, and oliguria. Ingestion of large doses may cause vascular collapse and death. Called also *cresylic acid, cresylol,* and *tricresol.*

Crest see under DENTIFRICE.

crest (krest) [L. *crista*] a projection or projecting structure, or ridge, especially one surmounting a bone or its border. See also CRISTA and RIDGE. **alveolar c.,** a thin margin of compact bone forming the coronal edge of a dental alveolus. **arcuate c. of arytenoid cartilage,** a ridge on the external surface of the arytenoid cartilage between the triangular pit and the oblong pit. Called also *crista arcuata cartilaginis arytenoideae* [NA]. **basilar c. of occipital bone,** pharyngeal TUBERCLE. **buccinator c.,** a ridge running from the base of the coronoid process of the mandible to a point near the last molar tooth, giving attachment to the buccinator muscle. Called also *crista buccinatoria.* **cerebral c's of cranial bones,** cerebral ridges of cranial bones; see under RIDGE. **conchal c. of maxilla,** an oblique ridge on the nasal surface of the body of the maxilla, just anterior to the lacrimal sulcus, which articulates with the inferior nasal concha. Called also *inferior turbinal c. of maxilla* and *crista conchalis maxillae* [NA]. **conchal c. of palatine bone,** a sharp transverse ridge, near the posterior edge of the palatine bone, which articulates with the inferior concha. Called also *inferior turbinal c. of palatine bone* and *crista conchalis ossis palatini* [NA]. **dental c.,** the maxillary ridge passing along the alveolar process of the fetal maxillary bones. **ethmoid c. of maxilla,** a low, oblique ridge on the medial surface of the frontal process of the maxilla, which articulates with the middle nasal concha. Called also *superior turbinal c. of maxilla* and *crista ethmoidalis maxillae* [NA]. **ethmoid c. of palatine bone,** a ridge near the upper end of the medial surface of the palatine bone, which articulates with the middle concha. Called also *superior turbinal c. of palatine bone* and *crista ethmoidalis ossis palatini* [NA]. **fimbriated c.,** fimbriated FOLD. **frontal c.,** a median ridge on the internal surface of the frontal bone, extending upward from the foramen cecum to unite with the sulcus for the superior sagittal sinus. Called also *crista frontalis* [NA] and *internal frontal crest.* **frontal c., external,** temporal line of frontal bone; see under LINE. **frontal c., internal,** frontal c. **gingival c.,** the coronal border of the gingiva. **glandular c. of larynx,** vestibular LIGAMENT. **infratemporal c.,** a crest separating the temporal surface of the great wing of the sphenoid bone into a temporal portion above and an infratemporal portion below. Called also *crista infratemporalis* [NA] and *pterygoid ridge.* **jugular c. of great wing of sphenoid bone,** zygomatic margin of great wing of sphenoid bone; see under MARGIN. **lacrimal c., anterior,** the lateral margin of a groove on the posterior border of the frontal process of the maxilla. Called also *crista lacrimalis anterior* [NA]. **lacrimal c., posterior,** a vertical ridge dividing the lateral or orbital surface of the lacrimal bone into two parts, and forming one margin of the fossa for the lacrimal sac. Called also *crista lacrimalis posterior* [NA]. **malar c. of great wing of sphenoid bone,** zygomatic margin of great wing of sphenoid bone; see under MARGIN. **mental c., external,** mental PROTUBERANCE. **mitochondrial c's,** complex infoldings in the mitochondrial cavity which originate in a membrane outside the cavity. **nasal c. of maxilla,** a ridge, raised along the medial border of the palatine process of the maxilla, with which the vomer articulates. Called also *crista nasalis maxillae* [NA]. **nasal c. of palatine bone,** a thick ridge projecting upward from the medial part of the horizontal plate of the palatine bone and articulating with the posterior part of the vomer. Called also *crista nasalis ossis palatini* [NA]. **neural c.,** a band of cells, dorsolateral to the neural tube. Its derivatives include cells of the cranial, spinal, and autonomic ganglia and adrenal medulla. See also neural TUBE, and see illustration at EMBRYO. **occipital c., external,** nuchal line, median; see under LINE. **occipital c., internal,** the inferior division of the cruciate eminence; it bifurcates near the foramen magnum and gives attachment to the falx cerebelli. Called also *crista occipitalis*

interna [NA]. **orbital c.,** supraorbital margin of frontal bone; see under MARGIN. **palatine c.,** a transverse crest often seen on the inferior surface of the horizontal plate of the palatine bone a short distance anterior to the posterior border. Called also *crista palatina* [NA]. **pharyngeal c. of occipital bone,** pharyngeal TUBERCLE. **sphenoidal c.,** a median ridge on the anterior surface of the body of the sphenoid bone, articulating with the perpendicular plate of the ethmoid and forming part of the septum of the nose. Called also *crista sphenoidalis* [NA], *ethmoidal process of Macalister,* and *ethmoidal spine of Macalister.* **supramastoid c.,** the superior border of the posterior root of the zygomatic process of the temporal bone. **temporal c. of frontal bone,** temporal line of frontal bone; see under LINE. **transverse c. of internal acoustic meatus,** a horizontal crest of bone that divides the fundus of the internal acoustic meatus into a superior and an inferior fossa. Called also *crista falciformis* and *crista transversa* [NA]. **turbinal c. of maxilla, inferior,** conchal c. of maxilla. **turbinal c. of maxilla, superior,** ethmoidal c. of maxilla. **turbinal c. of palatine bone, inferior,** conchal c. of palatine bone. **turbinal c. of palatine bone, superior,** ethmoid c. of palatine bone. **zygomatic c. of great wing of sphenoid bone,** zygomatic margin of great wing of sphenoid bone; see under MARGIN.

m-cresyl (met″ah-kre′sil) metacresyl.

cresylol (kre′sĭ-lol) cresol.

cretin (kre′tin; kret′in) [Fr.] a person affected with cretinism.

cretinism (kre′tin-izm) a congenital disease of infants and children caused by deficiency of thyroid hormone owing to insufficiency or lack of the thyroid gland, characterized by mental deficiency, dwarfism with disproportionately long trunk in relation to legs, epiphyseal dysgenesis, large head, delayed closure of the fontanelles, broad nose with wide flaring nostrils, open mouth, coarse features, puffy lips, deep husky voice, constipation, and protruding abdomen. Oral manifestations include delayed tooth eruption, delayed shedding of the primary dentition, underdeveloped jaws, especially the mandible, and a tongue enlarged by edema fluid, protruding and leading to malocclusion. Called also *congenital hypothyroidism, congenital myxedema,* and *infantile myxedema.* **adult c.,** myxedema. **athyreotic c.,** cretinism associated with agenesis of the thyroid gland. **endemic c.,** cretinism occurring in regions where goiter is common. **goitrous c.,** cretinism associated with goiter. **hypoparathyroid c.,** pseudohypoparathyroidism. **spontaneous c., sporadic c.,** cretinism in persons not descended from cretins, and who have not lived in regions where cretinism prevails.

Creveld see VAN CREVELD.

crevice (krev′is) [Fr. *crever* to split] a longitudinal fissure. See also FISSURE and GROOVE. **gingival c.,** a shallow trough or fissure, about 1.5 to 2.5 nm in depth, surrounding the anatomic crown, one wall of which is formed by the cuticle, the other by the gingival epithelium, and the bottom by the uppermost part of the epithelial cuff. The terms *gingival crevice* and *gingival sulcus* are sometimes used synonymously, but most authorities consider them to be two separate and distinct entities. Called also *subgingival space.* See illustration at gingival SULCUS.

crevicular (krĕ-vik′u-lar) pertaining to a crevice, especially the gingival crevice.

Creyx-Lévy syndrome [Maurice *Creyx;* Robert *Lévy*] see under SYNDROME.

crib (krib) 1. any racklike structure. 2. a removable anchorage for an orthodontic appliance. 3. a habit-breaking orthodontic appliance. **Jackson c.,** Jackson APPLIANCE. **lip-sucking habit c.,** lip habit APPLIANCE. **tongue c.,** a habit-breaking orthodontic appliance used to eliminate the visceral swallowing and tongue-thrusting habits and to stimulate the natural or somatic tongue posture and function.

cribra (krib′rah) [L.] plural of *cribrum.*

cribral (krib′ral) pertaining to the cribrum, or any sievelike structure.

cribrate (krib′rāt) [L. *cribratus*] perforated, as a sieve.

cribration (krib-ra′shun) 1. the quality of being cribrate. 2. the process or act of sifting or passing through a sieve, as a drug.

cribriform (krib′rĭ-form) [*cribrum* + L. *forma* form] perforated like a sieve; sievelike; ethmoid.

cribrum (kri′brum), pl. *cri′bra* [L. "sieve"] cribriform plate of ethmoid bone; see under PLATE.

Crick, Francis Harry Compton [born 1916] an English biologist; co-winner, with Maurice H. F. Wilkins and James Dewey Watson, of the Nobel prize for medicine and physiology in 1962, for discovery of the molecular structure of deoxyribonucleic acid. See also double HELIX (Watson-Crick helix or model).

crico- [Gr. *krikos* ring] a combining form denoting relationship to a ring.

cricoarytenoid (kri″ko-ar″ĭ-te′noid) pertaining to the cricoid and arytenoid cartilages.

cricoarytenoideus (kri″ko-ar″e-te-noi′de-us) cricoarytenoid MUS-CLE (lateral and posterior).

cricoid (kri′koid) [crico- + Gr. *eidos* form] 1. resembling a ring; ring-shaped. 2. cricoid CARTILAGE.

cricoidectomy (kri″koi-dek′to-me) [crico- + Gr. *ektomē* excision] excision of the cricoid cartilage.

cricoidynia (kri″koi-din′e-ah) [crico- + Gr. *odynē* pain] pain in the cricoid cartilage.

cricopharyngeal (kri″ko-fah-rin′je-al) pertaining to the cricoid cartilage and the pharynx.

cricopharyngeus (kri″ko-fahr-in′je-us) cricopharyngeal MUSCLE.

cricothyreotomy (kri″ko-thi″re-ot′o-me) [crico- + *thyroid* + Gr. *tomē* a cutting] incision through the cricoid and thyroid cartilages.

cricothyroid (kri-ko-thi′roid) [crico- + *thyroid*] pertaining to the cricoid and thyroid cartilages.

cricothyroideus (kri″ko-thi-roi′de-us) cricothyroid MUSCLE.

cricothyrotomy (kri″ko-thi-rot′o-me) [*cricothyroid* + Gr. *tomē* cutting] superior TRACHEOTOMY.

cricotomy (kri-kot′o-me) [crico- + Gr. *tomē* a cutting] incision of the cricoid cartilage.

cri du chat (kre du-shah) [Fr. "cat's cry"] see crying cat SYN-DROME.

Crile's clamp see under CLAMP.

Crinuryl trademark for *ethacrinic acid* (see under ACID).

crisis (kri′sis), pl. *cri′ses* [L., Gr. *krisis*] 1. a decisive moment or point. 2. the turning point in an acute disease, marked by a sudden increase or decrease in the severity of symptoms indicating imminent deterioration or improvement in the condition of the patient. **aplastic c.,** hemolytic c. **febrile c.,** an attack of chilliness, fever, and sweating. **hemolytic c.,** an acute aplastic condition observed in hemolytic anemia, and marked by complete cessation of the formation of erythrocytes, disappearance of the reticulocytes from the blood, decrease to normal values of serum bilirubin with urobilinuria, increase in the level of blood iron, leukopenia, and thrombocytopenia. Spontaneous recovery is a result of rapid regeneration of the erythropoietic tissue, which causes marked reticulocytosis, leukocytosis, and increase in thrombocytes, and a rapid fall in the level of serum iron. Called also *aplastic c.* and *Owren's syndrome.* **laryngeal c.,** paroxysmal spasm of the larynx, in the earlier course of tabes dorsalis. **pharyngeal c.,** a sudden attack occurring in tabes dorsalis, marked by peculiar sensations in the pharynx and involuntary swallowing movements. **spontaneous thyrotoxic c.,** Waldenström's DISEASE. **thyroid c., thyrotoxic c.,** a sudden and dangerous increase of the symptoms of thyrotoxicosis.

Crismani attachment, combined attachment (combined unit) see under ATTACHMENT.

crista (kris′ta), pl. *cris′tae* [L.] crest; a projection or projecting structure, a ridge, especially one surmounting a bone or its border. See also CREST and RIDGE. **c. arcua′ta cartilag′inis arytenoi′deae** [NA], arcuate crest of arytenoid cartilage; see under CREST. **c. buccinato′ria,** buccinator CREST. **c. concha′lis maxil′lae** [NA], conchal crest of maxilla; see under CREST. **c. concha′lis os′sis palati′ni** [NA], conchal crest of palatine bone; see under CREST. **cris′tae cu′tis** [NA], dermal ridges; see under RIDGE. **c. div′idens,** LIMBUS foraminis ovalis. **c. ethmoida′lis maxil′lae** [NA], ethmoidal crest of maxilla; see under CREST. **c. ethmoida′lis os′sis palati′ni** [NA], ethmoid crest of palatine bone; see under CREST. **c. falcifor′mis,** transverse crest of internal acoustic meatus; see under CREST. **c. fronta′lis** [NA], frontal·CREST. **c. gal′li** [NA], a triangular process resembling a cockscomb, which projects superiorly into the cranial fossa from the middle line of the cribriform plate of the ethmoid bone. Its slender posterior border serves for attachment of the falx cerebri. **c. infratempora′lis** [NA], infratemporal CREST. **c. lacrima′lis ante′rior** [NA], anterior lacrimal CREST. **c. lacrima′lis poste′rior** [NA], posterior lacrimal CREST. **c. margina′lis** [NA], marginal RIDGE. **cris′tae mitochondria′les,** the projections of the inner membrane of the mitochondria. **c. nasa′lis maxil′lae** [NA], nasal crest of maxilla; see under CREST. **c. nasa′lis os′sis palati′ni** [NA], nasal crest of palatine bone; see under CREST. **c. occipita′lis exter′na** [NA], nuchal line, median; see under LINE. **c. occipita′lis inter′na** [NA], occipital crest, internal; see under CREST. **c. palati′na** [NA], palatine CREST. **c. sphenoida′lis** [NA], sphenoidal CREST. **c. tempora′lis,** temporal line of frontal bone; see under LINE. **c. transver′sa** [NA], transverse crest of internal acoustic meatus; see under CREST. **c. transversa′lis** [NA], transverse RIDGE. **c. triangula′ris** [NA], triangular RIDGE.

cristae (kris′te) [L.] plural of *crista.*

cristobalite (kri-sto′bah-lit″) a colorless translucent allotropic form of silicon dioxide; used as a component of dental investments, and sometimes used in dental porcelain to control the thermal coefficient.

criteria (kri-te′re-ah) [Gr.] plural of *criterion.*

criterion (kri-te′re-on), pl. *crite′ria* [Gr. *kritērion* a means for judging] a standard by which something may be judged. **medical care criteria,** predetermined elements against which the quality of medical services are compared, based on professional experience of peers and on information derived from current medical literature.

Crohn's disease [Burrill Bernard *Crohn,* American physician, born 1884] see under DISEASE.

cromolyn sodium (kro′mo-lin) an antihistaminic and bronchodilator drug which inhibits histamine release, disodium 5,5′-[(2-hydroxytrimethylene)dioxy]bis[oxo - 4H - 1 - benzopyran - 2 - carboxylate]. It is a white, odorless, hygroscopic powder with a slightly bitter aftertaste, which is soluble in water, but not in alcohol and organic solvents. It is believed to act primarily on the mucosa and prevent the degranulation of sensitized mast cells after exposure to antigen. Used chiefly in the treatment of bronchial asthma. Transient maculopapular rash, urticaria, cough, occasional eosinophilic pneumonia, and arterial lesions are infrequent side effects. Called also *disodium cromoglycate.* Trademarks: Aarane, Frenasma, Intal, Nasmil.

Crookes' space, tube [Sir William *Crookes,* English physicist, 1832–1919] see under SPACE and TUBE.

cross (kros) 1. any structure consisting of an upright with a transverse beam, or anything resembling such a structure. 2. any organism produced by crossbreeding; a method of crossbreeding. **Blue C.,** see Blue Cross Association, under ASSOCIATION, and Blue Cross PLAN.

crossbite (kros′bit) malocclusion in which the mandibular teeth are in buccal version (or in complete lingual version in posterior segments) to the maxillary teeth, bilaterally, unilaterally, or involving only a pair of opposing teeth, so that opposing occlusal surfaces are not in contact in habitual occlusion. Called also *X-bite.* Written also *cross bite.* **anterior c.,** that in which one or more primary or permanent maxillary incisors is lingual to the mandibular incisors. **buccal c.,** that in which the maxillary molar is buccal to its mandibular antagonist. **lingual c.,** one in which the maxillary or mandibular molar is lingual to its antagonist. **posterior c.,** that in which one or more primary or permanent posterior teeth are locked in an abnormal relation with their antagonists; it may be buccal or lingual crossbite and may be accompanied with a shift of the mandible. **scissors-bite c., telescoping c.,** that in which the mandibular arch is entirely lingual to the maxillary arch.

crossing over (kros′ing o′ver) the exchange of genetic material between the chromosomes of a homologous pair during the diplotene stage of the first meiotic division, resulting in new combinations of genes. The exchange of genetic material takes place at the chiasmata of homologous chromosomes.

cross-linking (kros-link′ing) the union of high-polymer molecules by a system involving primary chemical bonds, occurring most commonly during the process of vulcanization or polymerization. The process may be initiated by heat, high-energy radiation, or cross-linking agents. See also cross-linked POLYMER, cross-linking AGENT, POLYMERIZATION, and VULCANIZATION.

crossmatching (kros-mach′ing) cross MATCHING.

croup (kroop) a condition resulting from acute obstruction of the larynx, occurring chiefly in infants and children, resulting in a resonant barking cough, hoarseness, and persistent stridor. Called also *angina trachealis* and *exudative angina.* **catarrhal c.,** croup accompanied by a catarrhal discharge. **diphtheric c.,** croup associated with infection by *Corynebacterium diphtheriae.* Called also *diphtheric laryngitis.* See also *membranous c.* **membranous c., pseudomembranous c.,** croup associated with a fibrinous exudate forming a membrane-like deposit, usually caused by *Corynebacterium diphtheriae.* Called also *laryngeal diphtheria.* See also membranous LARYNGITIS. **spasmodic c.,** LARYNGISMUS stridulosus.

croupous (kroo′pus) of the nature of croup, or attended with an exudation like that of croup.

Crouzon's disease, syndrome [Octave *Crouzon,* French neurologist, 1874–1938] craniofacial DYSOSTOSIS.

Crovaril trademark for *oxyphenbutazone.*

crowding (krowd′ing) filling to excess; excessively close together. **c. of teeth,** a condition in which teeth assume altered position, such as bunching, overlapping, displacement in various directions, or torsiversion.

Crown trademark for *dental mercury* (see under MERCURY).

crown (krown) [L. *corona*] 1. the uppermost part of an organ or structure, such as the top of the head. See also CORONA. 2. dental c. 3. an artificial crown replacing the natural dental crown. **anatomical c.,** the portion of a tooth that is covered by

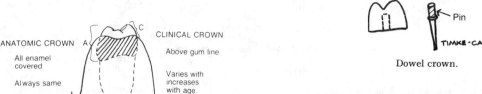

Anatomical crown (A) vs. clinical crown (C). (From H. O. Torres and A. Ehrlich: Modern Dental Assisting. 2nd ed. Philadelphia, W. B. Saunders Co., 1980.)

enamel, the true dental crown. It remains the same throughout life. See illustration. **artificial c.,** a restoration that reproduces the entire surface anatomy of the clinical crown of a tooth. It may be a metal casting alone, a metal casting with a veneer of tooth-colored porcelain or resin, or a jacket crown constructed of porcelain or resin. The crown may be attached to a prepared tooth stump or one that is partially rebuilt by a cast metal core alone or a cast core and a post, or it may be cemented to the remaining tooth structure. **basket c.,** an artificial gold crown that is fitted over a natural tooth with minimal removal of tissue, so-called because added retention is provided by a thin band of labial metal which is similar in shape to the handle of a basket. It is usually applied on the anterior teeth and the damaged incisal surface is filled in or veneered with acrylic resin. See illustration. **bell c.,** a tooth crown whose proportionate occlusal circumference is usually larger in relationship to its cervical circumference. **Bonwill c.,** a porcelain crown, held to the tooth root by means of a threaded metal dowel, which extends through a hole in the porcelain, and upon which a nut is screwed. **cap c.,** shell c. **celluloid c.,** a temporary crown made of celluloid which facilitates the fabrication of a temporary crown during fixed prosthodontic procedures. See also *temporary acrylic c.* **clinical c.,** that portion of the tooth above the clinical root, that is, the portion exposed beyond the gingiva and thus visible in the oral cavity. With advancing age, as the gingivae recede, more of the tooth is exposed, and thus the clinical crown becomes longer. Called also *extra-alveolar c.* and *corona clinica* [NA]. See illustration. **collar c.,** an artificial crown attached by a metal ferrule to a natural tooth root. **complete c.,** full c. **Davis c.,** a rarely used artificial porcelain crown produced in stock shapes, shades, and sizes, which is attached by a pin inserted into both the crown and the natural root of the tooth. Called also *post c.* See also overlay DENTURE. **dental c.,** the upper part of the tooth, which joins the lower part of the tooth, the root, at the cervix at a line called the cementoenamel junction, and terminates as the grinding surface of molar or bicuspid teeth, or the cutting edge of incisors. The entire surface of the crown is covered with enamel, which is thicker at the extremity and becomes progressively thinner toward the cervix. Called also *corona dentis* [NA]. See also *anatomical c.* and *physiological c.* **dowel c.,** an artificial crown that replaces the entire coronal portion of a tooth and is retained by a dowel extending into a filled root canal. **extra-alveolar c.,** clinical c. **c. flask,** denture FLASK. **full c., full veneer c.,** a dental restoration that completely reproduces the clinical crown of a natural tooth, usually made of gold casting with or without a baked porcelain or resin veneer. Called also *complete c.* **gold shell c.,** a prefabricated crown from plate gold from which a shell crown is produced. **half c.,** a modified three-quarter crown in which only half the surface of an anatomic crown is restored. **half-cap c.,** open-face c. **jacket c.,** a porcelain or acrylic resin restoration of the clinical crown which usually terminates at or under the gingiva. **jacket c., shoulderless,** a jacket crown designed to fit a tooth prepared without a shoulder type finish line. **c. length,** see tooth MEASUREMENT. **Libra II inlay and c.,** see under LIBRA. **Libra III c. and bridge,** see under LIBRA. **metal-ceramic c.,** a metallic restoration in which a thin veneer of porcelain is fused

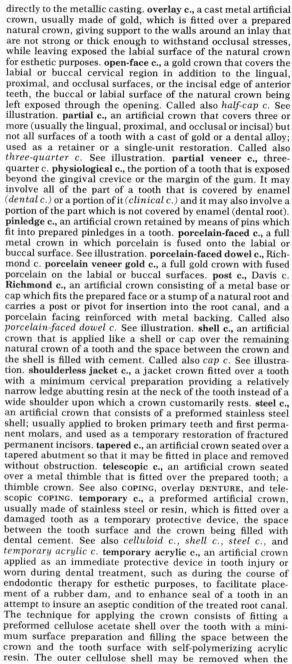

Dowel crown.

directly to the metallic casting. **overlay c.,** a cast metal artificial crown, usually made of gold, which is fitted over a prepared natural crown, giving support to the walls around an inlay that are not strong or thick enough to withstand occlusal stresses, while leaving exposed the labial surface of the natural crown for esthetic purposes. **open-face c.,** a gold crown that covers the labial or buccal cervical region in addition to the lingual, proximal, and occlusal surfaces, or the incisal edge of anterior teeth, the buccal or labial surface of the natural crown being left exposed through the opening. Called also *half-cap c.* See illustration. **partial c.,** an artificial crown that covers three or more (usually the lingual, proximal, and occlusal or incisal) but not all surfaces of a tooth with a cast of gold or a dental alloy; used as a retainer or a single-unit restoration. Called also *three-quarter c.* See illustration. **partial veneer c.,** three-quarter c. **physiological c.,** the portion of a tooth that is exposed beyond the gingival crevice or the margin of the gum. It may involve all of the part of a tooth that is covered by enamel (*dental c.*) or a portion of it (*clinical c.*) and it may also involve a portion of the part which is not covered by enamel (dental root). **pinledge c.,** an artificial crown retained by means of pins which fit into prepared pinledges in a tooth. **porcelain-faced c.,** a full metal crown in which porcelain is fused onto the labial or buccal surface. See illustration. **porcelain-faced dowel c.,** Richmond c. **porcelain veneer gold c.,** a full gold crown with fused porcelain on the labial or buccal surfaces. **post c.,** Davis c. **Richmond c.,** an artificial crown consisting of a metal base or cap which fits the prepared face or a stump of a natural root and carries a post or pivot for insertion into the root canal, and a porcelain facing reinforced with metal backing. Called also *porcelain-faced dowel c.* See illustration. **shell c.,** an artificial crown that is applied like a shell or cap over the remaining natural crown of a tooth and the space between the crown and the shell is filled with cement. Called also *cap c.* See illustration. **shoulderless jacket c.,** a jacket crown fitted over a tooth with a minimum cervical preparation providing a relatively narrow ledge abutting resin at the neck of the tooth instead of a wide shoulder upon which a crown customarily rests. **steel c.,** an artificial crown that consists of a preformed stainless steel shell; usually applied to broken primary teeth and first permanent molars, and used as a temporary restoration of fractured permanent incisors. **tapered c.,** an artificial crown seated over a tapered abutment so that it may be fitted in place and removed without obstruction. **telescopic c.,** an artificial crown seated over a metal thimble that is fitted over the prepared tooth; a thimble crown. See also COPING, overlay DENTURE, and telescopic COPING. **temporary c.,** a preformed artificial crown, usually made of stainless steel or resin, which is fitted over a damaged tooth as a temporary protective device, the space between the tooth surface and the crown being filled with dental cement. See also *celluloid c., shell c., steel c.,* and *temporary acrylic c.* **temporary acrylic c.,** an artificial crown applied as an immediate protective device in tooth injury or worn during dental treatment, such as during the course of endodontic therapy for esthetic purposes, to facilitate placement of a rubber dam, and to enhance seal of a tooth in an attempt to insure an aseptic condition of the treated root canal. The technique for applying the crown consists of fitting a preformed cellulose acetate shell over the tooth with a minimum surface preparation and filling the space between the crown and the tooth surface with self-polymerizing acrylic resin. The outer cellulose shell may be removed when the

Basket crown.

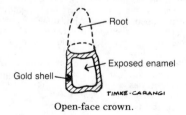

Open-face crown.

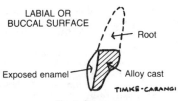

LABIAL OR
BUCCAL SURFACE
— Root
Exposed enamel — — Alloy cast
TIMKE·CARANGI

Partial crown.

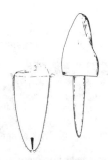

Richmond crown preparation with adjacent typical crown. (From L. B. Baum: Advanced Restorative Dentistry. Philadelphia, W. B. Saunders Co., 1973; courtesy of Hugh Cooper, Jr.)

acrylic crown is set or it may be retained as desired. **thimble c.,** an artificial crown supplied with a telescopic coping (secondary thimble), which telescopes over the coping (primary thimble); a telescopic crown. See also COPING. **three-quarter c.,** an artificial crown that covers mainly three surfaces of anterior teeth (mesial, distal, and lingual) and four surfaces of posterior teeth (mesial, distal, lingual, and occlusal). Three-quarter crowns may be constructed with or without a shoulder, with an incisal groove, proximal grooves, lingual pin-ledge, or any combination thereof. It is used as a retainer for a bridge or as a single unit restoration on a carious fractured tooth. Called also *partial veneer c.* **veneer c., complete,** a restoration of metal, porcelain, or acrylic resin that reproduces the entire surface anatomic form of the clinical crown and fits over a prepared tooth or root. **veneer c., partial,** three-quarter c. **veneered c.,** an artificial crown that bears a thin layer of tooth-colored resin or porcelain on the buccal or labial surface, attached or bonded to the metal casting. Called also *veneer metal c.* and *window c.* **veneer metal c.,** veneered c. **Weston c.,** an artificial crown used in the past, which consisted of a porcelain facing with two pins curved around a threaded dowel in the root, amalgam being packed around the pins, dowel, and root, and shaped as desired. **window c.,** veneered c.

Crown No. 1 trademark for a medium hard *dental casting gold alloy* (see under GOLD).

Crown amalgamator see under AMALGAMATOR.

Crown Hylastic trademark for a high noble metal dental wrought gold wire alloy.

Crown K inlay see under INLAY.

Crown Knapp No. 3, No. 9, Supreme, TT trademark for a hard *dental casting gold alloy* (see under GOLD).

crozat (kro′zat) Crozat APPLIANCE.

Crozat appliance, clasp, dental orthopedics, philosophy [G. B. *Crozat*] see under APPLIANCE, CLASP, and PHILOSOPHY, and see gnathologic ORTHOPEDICS.

CRP C-reactive PROTEIN.

CRST calcinosis, Raynaud phenomenon, sclerodactyly, telangiectasia; see CRST SYNDROME.

cruces (kroo′sēz) [L.] plural of *crux.*

cruciate (kroo′she-āt) shaped like a cross.

crucible (kroo′sĭ-b′l) 1. a vessel of metal or refractory material for heating substances to high temperatures. 2. a concave area on the top of a dental mold into which molten metal or alloy is poured. See also illustration at MOLD. **c. former,** crucible FORMER.

cruciform (kroo′sĭ-form) [L. *crux* cross + *forma* form] shaped like a cross.

cruor (kroo′or), pl. *cruo′res* [L.] a blood clot.

cruores (kroo-o′rēz) [L.] plural of *cruor.*

crura (kroo′rah) [L.] plural of *crus.*

crus (krus), pl. *cru′ra* [L.] 1. [NA] the leg, from knee to foot. 2. any leglike structure. **internal c. of greater alar cartilage,** medial c. of greater alar cartilage. **lateral c. of greater alar cartilage, c. latera′le cartilag′inis ala′ris majo′ris** [NA], the part of the greater alar cartilage that curves laterally around the nostril and helps maintain its contour. **medial c. of greater alar cartilage, c. media′le cartilag′inis ala′ris majo′ris** [NA], the part of the greater alar cartilage, loosely attached to its fellow of the opposite side, and helping to form the mobile septum of the nose. Called also *internal c. of greater alar cartilage.*

crust (krust) [L. *crusta*] an outer layer of solid matter formed by the drying of a bodily exudate or secretion. Called also *scab.*

crusta (krus′tah), pl. *crus′tae* [L. shell] a crust. **c. petro′sa den′tis,** cementum.

Cruveilhier, navicular fossa of, inferior thyroid artery of see scaphoid fossa of sphenoid bone, under FOSSA, and cricothyroid branch of superior thyroid artery, under BRANCH.

crux (kruks), pl. *cru′ces* [L.] cross; any structure resembling a cross.

cry (kri) 1. a sudden loud involuntary vocal sound. 2. to utter such a sound. See also crying cat SYNDROME.

cryalgesia (kri″al-je′ze-ah) [*cryo-* + Gr. *algēsis* pain + *-ia*] pain due to the application of cold.

cryanesthesia (kri″an-es-the′ze-ah) loss of power of perceiving cold.

Cryer elevator, forceps [Mathew H. *Cryer,* American oral surgeon, 1840–1921] see under ELEVATOR, and see FORCEPS No. 150 and No. 151.

cryesthesia (kri″es-the′ze-ah) [*cryo-* + Gr. *aisthēsis* perception] abnormal sensitivity to cold.

crymo- [Gr. *krymos* frost] a combining form denoting relationship to cold. See also words beginning CRYO-.

crymoanesthesia (kri″mo-an″es-the′ze-ah) [*crymo-* + *anesthesia*] refrigeration ANESTHESIA.

crymodynia (kri″mo-din′e-ah) [*crymo-* + Gr. *odynē* pain] rheumatic pain coming on in cold or damp weather.

cryo- [Gr. *kryos* cold] a combining form denoting relationship to cold. See also words beginning CRYMO-.

cryoanesthesia (kri″o-an″es-the′ze-ah) refrigeration ANESTHESIA.

cryobiology (kri″o-bi-ol′o-je) [*cryo-* + Gr. *bios* life + *-logy*] the science dealing with the effect of low temperatures on biological systems.

cryofibrinogen (kri″o-fi-brin′o-jen) a fibrinogen precipitating out of plasma at 4°C and subsequently redissolving at 37°C. Its precipitate dissolves in saline solution, but not in distilled water. Cryofibrinogens are most commonly found in multiple myeloma but may be also present in diseases that exhibit cryoglobulins.

cryofibrinogenemia (kri″o-fi-brin″o-jen-e′me-ah) a condition characterized by the presence of cryofibrinogens in the blood.

cryogammaglobulin (kri″o-gam″ah-glob′u-lin) cryoglobulin.

cryogenic (kri″o-jen′ik) pertaining to or causing the production of low temperatures.

cryoglobulin (kri″o-glob′u-lin) an abnormal globulin that precipitates out of serum at a temperature below 37°C, found in various diseases, such as plasma cell myeloma and other neoplastic diseases, infectious diseases, such as kala-azar or subacute infectious endocarditis, and systemic diseases, such as rheumatoid arthritis. Cryoglobulins may have the immunologic characteristics of immunoglobulins A, G, or M. Called also *cryogammaglobulin.*

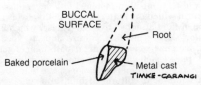

BUCCAL
SURFACE
— Root
Baked porcelain — — Metal cast
TIMKE·CARANGI

Porcelain-faced crown.

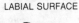
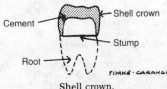

LABIAL SURFACE

Cement — — Shell crown
— Stump
Root — TIMKE·CARANGI

Shell crown.

cryoglobulinemia (kri″o-glob″u-lin-e′me-ah) a condition characterized by the presence of cryoglobulins in the blood.

cryoprecipitate (kri′o-pre-sip′ĭ-tāt) a precipitate that results from cooling.

cryoprobe (kri′o-prōb) a partially insulated tube which delivers extreme cold to the tissues in cryosurgery.

cryostat (kri′o-stat) [cryo- + Gr. histanai to halt] 1. a device by which temperature can be maintained at a very low level. 2. in pathology and histology, a chamber containing a microtome for sectioning frozen tissue.

cryosurgery (kri″o-ser′jer-e) [cryo- + surgery] destruction of tissue by application of extreme cold, usually by delivering the refrigerant to the tissues by means of a partially insulated tube (cryoprobe), either by employing liquid nitrogen or the expansion of a compressed gas, such as nitrous oxide. The liquid nitrogen equipment provides a temperature approximating −195°C; nitrous oxide in the vicinity of −70°C. It is used chiefly for destroying cancerous tissue, and is also used in producing anesthesia in neuralgias by nerve destruction.

cryotherapy (kri″o-ther′ah-pe) [cryo- + Gr. therapeia treatment] therapeutic use of cold.

crypt- see CRYPTO-.

crypt (kript) [L. crypta, from Gr. kryptos hidden] a blind pit or pitlike depression on a free surface. See also CRYPTA. **bony c.,** a crypt in the body of a jaw which encloses an erupting tooth. **dental c.,** an alveolar space filled by a developing tooth. **enamel c.,** a developmental space bounded by the dental ledges on either side and usually by the enamel organ; it is filled with mesenchyma. **tonsillar c's of palate, tonsillar c's of palatine tonsil,** blind pits in the surface of the nonkeratinized stratified squamous epithelium covering the palatine tonsil, varying from shallow invaginations to deep cavities with many branching terminals, which have about 35 craters opening on the surface of the gland at the tonsillar fossulae. The ducts of the glossopalatine glands empty near the openings of the crypts. Their obstruction by cellular debris is considered to be the principal cause of infection and tonsillitis. Called also *cryptae tonsillares tonsillae palatinae* [NA]. **c's of tongue, deep,** tonsillar c's of tongue, deep. **tonsillar c's of pharynx, tonsillar c's of pharyngeal tonsil,** the blind ends of the tonsillar fossulae of the pharyngeal tonsils. Called also *cryptae tonsillares tonsillae pharyngeae* [NA]. **tonsillar c's of tongue, deep,** irregular invaginations on the surface of the lingual tonsil with occasional bifurcations at their basal terminals, which open to the surface as raised craters located on the tongue surface posterior to the vallate papillae. The region immediately subjacent to the epithelium of the free surface of the crypts is occupied by a layer of nodules of lymphoid tissue; the epithelium of the crypts is interrupted occasionally by excretory ducts whose secretory terminals are situated deep within the tissue. Secretions of the mucous glands flush out the crypts of cellular and other debris; accumulation of debris is relatively rare. Called also *c's of lingual tonsil* and *deep c's of tongue*.

crypta (krip′tah), pl. *cryp′tae* [L.] crypt; a blind pit or pitlike depression on a free surface. See also CRYPT. **cryp′tae tonsilla′res tonsil′lae pharyn′gae** [NA], tonsillar crypts of pharyngeal tonsil; see under CRYPT. **cryp′tae tonsilla′res tonsil′lae palati′nae** [NA], tonsillar crypts of palatine tonsil; see under CRYPT.

cryptae (krip′te) [L.] plural of *crypta*.

cryptectomy (krip-tek′to-me) [crypt- + Gr. ektomē excision] excision or obliteration of a crypt.

cryptic (krip′tik) [Gr. kryptikos hidden] concealed, hidden, larval.

cryptitis (krip-ti′tis) inflammation of a crypt.

crypto-, crypt- [Gr. kryptos hidden] a combining form meaning hidden or concealed, or denoting relationship to a crypt.

Cryptocillin trademark for *oxacillin*.

cryptococcosis (krip″to-kok-o′sis) European BLASTOMYCOSIS.

Cryptococcus (krip′to-kok′us) [crypto- + Gr. kokkos a berry] a genus of dermatomycetous fungi (Fungi Imperfecti). Formerly called *Torula*. **C. histolyt′icus,** *C. neoformans*. **C. hom′inis, C. meningit′idis,** *C. neoformans*. **C. neofor′mans,** a species causing European blastomycosis. Formerly called *C. histolyticus, C. hominis,* and *C. meningitidis*.

cryptogenic (krip″to-jen′ik) [crypto- + Gr. gennan to produce] of obscure, doubtful, or unascertainable origin. Cf. PHANEROGENIC.

crystal (kris′al) [Gr. krystallos ice] 1. a homogenous and angular solid, having a definite form characterized by geometric plane surfaces and a symmetrical internal structure, whereby atoms,

ions, or molecules are arranged in a definite pattern known as the space lattice (see under LATTICE). 2. a clear, transparent, mineral or glass resembling ice. 3. a glass with a high degree of brilliance. **apatite c.,** hydroxyapatite c. **cementum c.,** a hydroxyapatite crystal formed in the cementum during its mineralization. **dentin c.,** a hydroxyapatite crystal, being the principal mineral component of the dentin. **c. grain,** crystal GRAIN. **hydroxyapatite c.,** one in the dental enamel and cementum, deposited as hydroxyapatite during tooth mineralization. Called also *apatite c.* **c. lattice,** space LATTICE. **c. nucleus,** solidification NUCLEUS.

crystalline (kris′tah-lin) 1. resembling a crystal in nature or clearness. 2. pertaining to a crystalline structure, the individual atoms of which have a regular arrangement with respect to one another, in a definite pattern and rows of atoms.

crystallization (kris″tah-li-za′shun) the transition from a dissolved, molten, liquid, or gaseous state to a solid state with the assumption of a crystalline form. The process involves atomic diffusion in a supercooled liquid beginning with the aggregation of atoms to form crystal embryos (homologous nucleation), or in the melt, which is not necessarily supercooled, where the nuclei are formed around clusters of atoms coming in contact with foreign particles or surfaces which they can wet (heterogeneous nucleation). The nuclei thus formed give rise to dendrites and, in turn, grains, the nucleus being the first structure to have the crystalline space lattice structure. The growth of the grains continues until the entire space is filled with crystals and the substance has achieved the solid phase. See also FREEZING. **nucleus of c.,** solidification NUCLEUS.

Crystallose trademark for *soluble saccharin* (see under SACCHARIN).

Crysticillin trademark for *penicillin G procaine* (see under PENICILLIN).

Crystoserpine trademark for *reserpine*.

Crytion trademark for a preparation of *gold sodium thiosulfate* (see under GOLD).

Cs cesium.

CSC COUP sur coup.

CSF cerebrospinal FLUID.

CSP channel should pin; see under TECHNIQUE.

ct carat.

Cu copper (L. *cuprum*).

cu cm cubic CENTIMETER.

cuff (kuf) a small collar-like structure encircling a part. **attached epithelial c., attached gingival c.,** epithelial ATTACHMENT (of Gottlieb). **epithelial c.,** a band of epithelial tissue surrounding an abutment post, extending through the mucoperiosteal layer from a subperiosteal implant into the oral cavity. Called also *gum cuff*. 2. epithelial ATTACHMENT (of Gottlieb). **gingival c.,** the most coronal portion of the gingiva immediately surrounding the tooth, coronal to its attachment in the tooth. Sometimes, the term is used synonymously with gingival attachment (of Gottlieb); see under ATTACHMENT. **gum c.,** epithelial c. (1)

cu in cubic INCH.

cul-de-sac (kul′de-sahk) [Fr.] a blind pouch.

cultivation (kul″tĭ-va′shun) [L. *cultivatio*] the propagation of living organisms, applied especially to the propagation of cells in artificial media.

culturable (kul′chur-ah-b'l) capable of being cultured.

cultural (kul′chŭr-ral) pertaining to a culture.

culture (kul′chŭr) [L. *cultura*] 1. the propagation of microorganisms or of living tissue cells in special media capable of sustaining life and growth. 2. a growth of microorganisms or other living cells. 3. to induce the propagation of microorganisms or living tissue cells in culture media. **attenuated c.,** a culture of microorganisms that have altered virulence. **bacterial c.,** growth of bacteria on an artificial culture medium. **cell c.,** a growth of cells *in vitro*; although the cells proliferate they do not organize into tissue. **continuous flow c.,** the cultivation of bacteria in a continuous flow of fresh medium to maintain bacterial growth in logarithmic phase. **direct c.,** one made by direct transfer from a natural source to an artificial medium. **endodontic c.,** growth of microorganisms isolated from the dental pulp chamber or periapical tissue. **fractional c.,** a technique for obtaining a single species of microorganisms from a culture containing more than one. **hanging-block c.,** one grown on a block of agar medium fastened to a coverglass. **hanging-drop c.,** one in which the material to be cultivated is inoculated into a drop of fluid attached to a coverglass, which is inverted over a hollow slide. **c. medium,** culture MEDIUM. **needle c.,** *stab c.* **plate c.,** one grown on a medium, usually agar or gelatin, on a Petri dish. **pure c.,** one of a single species of cells, without the presence of any contaminants. **shake c.,** one made by inoculating warm liquid agar culture medium in a tube to allow the development of separated colonies in the solidified medium on incubation; especially applicable to obligate anaerobes. **slant c.,** one made on a slanting surface of a solidified medium in a tube, the tube being tilted to provide a greater surface area for growth. **stab c.,** one in which the medium is inoculated by a needle thrust deeply into its substance. Called also *needle c.* and *thrust c.* **stock c.,** a permanent culture from which transfers may be made. **thrust c.,** stab c. **tissue c.,** the cultivation of tissue cells *in vitro* in an artificial medium.

cu mm cubic millimeter.

cumulative (ku'mu-la"tiv) [L. *cumulus* heap] increasing by successive additions.

cuneiform (ku-ne'ĭ-form) [L. *cuneus* wedge + *forma* form] shaped like a wedge.

cuniculi (ku-nik'u-li) [L.] plural of *cuniculus.*

cuniculus (ku-nik'u-lus), pl. *cunic'uli* [L. "rabbit," "rabbit-burrow"] a burrow, such as one produced by mites in scabies.

cup (kup) 1. a small, open container. 2. any cup-shaped part or structure. **chin c.,** an orthodontic device that directs a posterior and/or vertical force to the mandible through the attachment of a cup fitting over the chin to a headcap. **rubber c.,** a cleansing and polishing instrument, consisting of a rubber shell with or without web-shaped conformation in the hollow interior, used in a handpiece with a special contra-angle. The cup is used in conjunction with cleansing and polishing pastes. **suction c.,** 1. a cup-shaped object of rubber, glass, plastic, or other material which, by producing a partial vacuum, can be made to adhere to or draw something to a surface. 2. a thin rubber disk, usually with a hole in its center to fit over a button that is larger than the hole; when applied on the tissue surface of a denture, the cup adheres to the mucous membrane by suction.

Cupralloy trademark for a *high copper alloy* (see under ALLOY).

cupremia (ku-pre'me-ah) [L. *cuprum* copper + Gr. *haima* blood + *-ia*] the presence of copper in the blood.

cupric (ku'prik) pertaining to or containing divalent copper, Cu^{++}, ions in aqueous solution.

cupriuria (ku"pre-u're-ah) [L. *cuprum* copper   Gr. *ouron* urine + *-ia*] the presence of copper in the urine.

cuprous (ku'prus) pertaining to or containing monovalent copper, C^{+}.

cupruresis (ku"proo-re'sis) [L. *cuprum* copper + Gr. *ourēsis* making water] the urinary excretion of copper.

cupruretic (ku"proo-re'tik) [L. *cuprum* + Gr. *ourētikos* promoting urine] 1. pertaining to or promoting the urinary excretion of copper. 2. an agent that promotes the urinary excretion of copper.

cupula (ku'pu-lah), pl. *cu'pulae* [L.] a small inverted cup or dome-shaped cap over some structure.

cupulae (ku'pu-le) [L.] plural of *cupula.*

curage (ku-rahzh') [Fr.] curettage, especially when a finger, rather than curet, is used.

Curantyl trademark for *dipyridamole.*

curare (koo-rah're) any of various toxic extracts from numerous South America plants, including *Strychnos* and *Chondodendron*; used originally as arrow poisons, and considered to be the prototype of the competitive neuromuscular blocking agents. Three types of curare have been available, distinguished by the kind of containers in which they were packed: tube curare (bamboo c.), pot curare, and gourd curare (calabash c.). Currently, only purified preparations from *Chondodendron tomentosum* are available, occurring as substances that are soluble in water and dilute ethanol. Called also *ourari, urari, woorali,* and *woorari.* See also TUBOCURARINE chloride.

curaremimetic (koo-rah"re-mi-met'ik) having an action similar to that of curare, or producing similar effects, as by a competitive neuromuscular blocking agent.

curariform (ku-rah'rĭ-form) resembling curare; having pharmacological properties similar to those of curare. See neuromuscular blocking AGENT.

Curatin trademark for *doxepin hydrochloride* (see under DOXEPIN).

curative (kūr-ah-tiv) [L. *curarare* to take care of] tending to overcome disease and promote recovery.

cure (kūr) [L. *curatio,* from *cura* care] 1. the course of treatment of any disease, or of a special case. 2. the successful treatment of a disease or wound. 3. a system of treating diseases. 4. a medicine effective in treating disease. 5. the preservation of a product, such as tobacco, meat, or fish. 6. the hardening of a material by the process of curing. 7. a procedure for polymerization of the resinous denture base material.

curet (ku-ret') [Fr. *curette* scraper] an instrument with a fine blade, used in curettage. In periodontics, curets are used for cutting the soft tissue wall of periodontal pockets, to remove the inner lining and epithelial attachment, and for removing periodontal fibers from the walls of osseous defects associated with intrabony pockets. Curets are also used to remove calculus

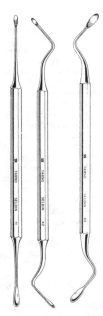

Curets (assorted) for access into the socket of an extracted tooth. (From H. O. Torres and A. Ehrlich: Modern Dental Assisting. 2nd ed. Philadelphia, W. B. Saunders Co., 1980.)

fragments and to smooth root surfaces. Spelled also *curette.* **Columbia c.,** trademark for a periodontal curet. **Gracey c's,** a set of curets which are available as paired (one blade and shank being a mirror image of the other) or double-ended instruments. They differ in the angulation of the shank to the hand, having fine blades which consist of thin rounded bends with two cutting edges formed by the junction of the outer and inner surfaces. They are designed and angled to adapt to specific anatomical areas of the dentition, and to be utilized with a push stroke, although they may be used with a pull stroke. Gracey curets are used for removing minute fragments of calculus and smoothing root surfaces and in curettage of soft tissues. See illustration. **McCall c.,** a type of periodontal curet. **surgical c.,** a straight or an acute-angled curette with a spoonlike blade that has a continuous sharp edge around the margin. In oral surgery, used to remove infectious material at the apex of the socket after tooth extraction. See illustration. **universal c.,** one with an angulated offset shank and a straight blade, the inner surface being flat and the outer rounded, with two cutting edges formed where they meet. Designed so that by altering and

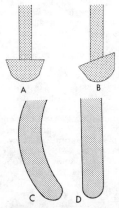

Principal types of curets. *A* and *B*, as seen from the toe of the instrument — *A*, universal curet; *B*, Gracey curet (note the offset blade angulation). *C* and *D*, as seen from the blade — *C*, universal curet; *D*, Gracey curet (the blade is curved; only the convex cutting edge is used). (From F. A. Carranza: Glickman's Clinical Periodontology. 5th ed. Philadelphia, W. B. Saunders Co., 1979.)

adapting the finger rest, fulcrum, and hand position of the operator most areas of the dentition can be reached. See illustration. **Younger-Goode c.**, a type of periodontal curet.

curettage (ku"re-tahzh') [Fr.] 1. the removal of granulation tissue growths or other material from the wall of a cavity or other surface. In tooth extraction, the removal of tooth particles or debris from sockets at the time of extraction, the enucleation cysts, dental granulomas, or cystic neoplasms, and the removal of small sequestrae from sockets during healing after the extraction. Called also *curettement*. See also DÉBRIDEMENT. 2. gingival c. **apical c.** periapical c. **gingival c.**, removal of degenerated and necrotic epithelium and underlying connective tissue of a periodontal pocket in an effort to convert a chronic ulcerated wound to an acute surgical wound, thereby insuring wound healing and attachment or epithelial adhesion, and shrinkage of the marginal gingiva. Gingival curettage is usually performed in edematous and fibroedematous processes, periodontal pockets of moderate depths, and horizontal alveolar bone loss in which osseous correction is not required. The term is sometimes used in connection with smoothing of root surface. Called also *soft tissue c.* and *subgingival c.* **periapical c.**, removal with a curet of diseased pathological soft tissues in the bony crypt surrounding a tooth root apex and smoothing of the apical surface of a tooth without excision of the tooth tip. Called also *apical c.* **soft tissue c., subgingival c.**, gingival c. **ultrasonic c.**, removal of mineralized deposits and bits of inflamed tissue from the tooth surface and the wall of the gingival crevice with an ultrasonic scaler. See ultrasonic SCALING.

curette (ku-ret') [Fr.] curet.

curettement (ku-ret'ment) curettage.

Curie, Marie Sklodowska [1867–1934] a Polish chemist in Paris who was the discoverer of radium; co-winner, with Pierre Curie and Antoine Henri Becquerel, of the Nobel prize for physics in 1903, for studies on spontaneous radioactivity; Mme. Curie also received the Nobel prize for chemistry in 1911 for the discovery and isolation of radium. See also CURIE.

curie (ku're) [named after Marie S. *Curie* and Pierre *Curie*] a unit of radioactivity, defined as the quantity of any radioactive nuclide in which the number of disintegrations per second is 3.700×10^{10}. It equals 0.663 mm^3 or 6.56×10^{-6} gm of emanation (radon) and maintains an air ionization of 2.75×10^4 csu (0.92 mg). Currently, it is based on the number of alpha particles emitted, by comparing the number emitted by a sample with the emission from 1 gm of radium or the emanation in equilibrium with it, or 3.6×10^{10} alpha particles per second. Symbol *c* or *Ci*. See also RUTHERFORD.

Curie's law [Pierre *Curie*, a French physicist, 1859–1906; co-winner, with Marie Sklodowska Curie and Antoine Henri Becquerel, of the Nobel prize for physics in 1903, for studies on spontaneous radioactivity] under LAW, and see CURIE and CURIETHERAPY.

curiegram (ku're-gram) [*curie* Gr. *gramma* a written record] a print made by radium emanation on a sensitized plate.

curie-hour (ku're-owr") a unit of dose equivalent to that obtained by exposure for one hour to radioactive material disintegrating at the rate of 3.7×10^{-10} atoms per second. Abbreviated *c-hr*.

curietherapy (ku"re-ther'ah-pe) [*curie* + *therapy*] originally, radium or radon therapy; but now applied to therapy given by emanations from any radioactive source. Written also *Curie therapy*.

curing (kūr'ing) a method for promoting and accelerating hardening processes through the use of dampness, heat, cold, or chemical or any other agent. See also POLYMERIZATION. **c. cycle**, curing CYCLE. **denture c.**, the process by which resinous denture base materials are polymerized or hardened. **rubber c.**, vulcanization.

curium (ku're-um) [named after Pierre Curie and Marie S. *Curie*] a synthetic radioactive element originally produced by helium-ion bombardment of plutonium-239. Symbol, Cm; atomic number, 96; atomic weight, 247; specific gravity, 13.51; valences 3, 4. There are 13 isotopes of curium, the most stable being ^{247}Cm with a half-life of 16 million years. It is a silvery white, brittle metal available in gram quantities, which is a radioactive poison of the bone-seeking type.

current (kur'ent) [L. *currens* running] 1. a flow or stream. 2. anything that flows. 3. electric c. **alternating c.**, electric current in which the flow of electrons in one direction is immediately followed by a flow in the opposite direction. Abbreviated *AC*. **direct c.**, electric current in which the electrons flow in a single direction. Abbreviated *DC*. **eddy c.**, an induced electric current circulating wholly within a mass of metal. **electric c.**, the flow or

movement of electric charge between two points. The electromotive power of electric current is measured in volts; its flow against the resistance is measured in amperes; the quantity of current is measured in coulombs. **coagulating c.**, an electric current applied by a needle, ball, or other type of electrode to coagulate tissue. **full-wave rectified c.**, current rectified through a full-wave rectifier. See full-wave RECTIFICATION. **galvanic c.**, a steady direct current produced by a chemical reaction, as in the presence of two dissimilar metals in a liquid medium, of the electric battery. See also GALVANISM. **half-wave rectified c.**, current rectified by a half-wave rectifier. See *half-wave* RECTIFICATION. **induced c.**, electricity in a circuit generated by proximity to another current, i.e., by induction. **rectified c.**, current converted from alternating to direct through a rectifier. **saturation c.**, the maximum current across an x-ray which utilizes for the production of x-rays all the electrons available at the cathode.

Curschmann-Batten-Steinert syndrome [Hans *Curschmann*, German physician, 1875–1950; Frederic Eustace *Batten*, English neurologist, 1865–1918; Hans *Steinert*, German physician] myotonic DYSTROPHY.

curvatura (kur"vah-tu'rah), pl. *curvatu'rae* [L.] any nonangular deviation from a straight line or surface. Called also *curvature*.

curvaturae (kur"vah-tu're) [L.] plural of *curvatura*.

curvature (kur'vah-tūr) [L. *curvatura*] any nonangular deviation from a straight line. **c. of cementoenamel junction on distal**, a curvature measured from the crest of the curvature of the cementoenamel junction on the labial and lingual surfaces, to the crest of the curvature of the cementoenamel junction on the distal surface of the anterior teeth. See tooth MEASUREMENT. **c. of cementoenamel junction on mesial**, a curvature measured from the crest of curvature at the cementoenamel junction and the labial and lingual surfaces, to the crest of curvature at the cementoenamel junction on the mesial surface in anterior teeth. See tooth MEASUREMENT. **compensating c.**, compensating CURVE. **occlusal c.**, CURVE of occlusion. **primary c. (of dentinal tubules)**, in longitudinal sections of dentin, a sigmoidally curvilinear curve, having outer convex and inner concave segments. **secondary c. (of dentinal tubules)**, in longitudinal sections of dentin, areas of lesser curvature of the dentinal tubules extending from the pulp chamber. **c. of Spee**, CURVE of Spee. **spinal c.**, deviation of the spine from its normal direction or position.

curve (kurv) [L. *curvum*] 1. a bending or flexure. 2. a line that is continuously bent. **alignment c.**, the dental curve determined by a line passing through the center of the teeth and paralleling with the dental arch. **anti-Monson c.**, reverse c. **apical c.**, the curving of the root canal at the apex of the tooth root. See also root CANAL. **bayonet c.**, a double curve of the root canal, somewhat in the form of a World War I bayonet. Called also *double curve*. See root canal, bayonet, under CANAL. **buccal c.**, the portion of the curve of occlusion from the mesial surface of the first premolar to the distal surface of the third molar. **compensating c.**, the curve introduced in the construction of artificial dentures to compensate for the opening influence produced by the condylar and incisal guidances during lateral and protrusive mandibular excursive movements. Called also *compensating curvature*. **defalcated c.**, sickle-shaped c. **dental c., c. of occlusion. dilacerated c.**, an abrupt curving of the root canal. See root canal, dilacerated, under CANAL. **dromedary c.**, a temperature or other curve showing two phases of elevation separated by a phase of depression. **dose-effect c., dose-response c.**, one indicating the relationship between a dose of radiation and the degree of a particular biological effect produced. **double c.**, bayonet c. **elastic c.**, see stress-strain DIAGRAM. **frequency c.**, one representing graphically the probabilities of different numbers of recurrences of an event. Called also *probability c.* **gradual c.**, curving of the root canal, gradually throughout its length from the cervical line to the apex of the tooth root. **isodose c.**, a diagram delimiting body areas receiving equal quantities of radiation in radiotherapy. **labial c.**, that portion of the curve of occlusion between the distal surfaces of the two canine teeth in the dental arch. **liquidus c.**, liquidus. **milled-in c.**, milled-in PATH (1). **Monson c.**, a curve of occlusion conforming to a segment of the surface of a sphere 8 inches in diameter, with its center in the region of the glabella. See also *compensating c.* **normal c. of distribution**, the symmetrical bell-shaped curve that is usually produced by plotting a single variable. **c. of occlusion**, 1. a curved surface which makes simultaneous contact with major portions of the incisal and occlusal prominences of the existing teeth. Called also *dental c.* and *occlusal curvature*. 2. the curve of a dentition on which the occlusal surfaces lie. **Pleasure c.**, reverse c. **probability c.**, frequency c. **reverse c.**, in excessive wear of the teeth, the obliteration of the cusps and formation of either flat or cupped-out occlusal surfaces, associated with reversal of the occlusal plane of the premolar and first and second molar teeth (the third molars being generally unaffected), whereby the occlusal surfaces of the mandibular teeth slope facially instead of lingually, and those of the maxillary teeth incline lingually. Called also *anti-Monson c.* and *Pleasure c.* **sine c.,** the wave form of an alternating current characterized by a rise from zero to maximum positive potential, descending back through zero to its maximum negative value, and then rising back to zero. **solidus c., solidus. sickle-shaped c.,** curving of the root canal in the form of the blade of a sickle. Called also *defalcated c.* See root canal, C-shaped, under CANAL. **c. of Spee,** anatomic curvature of the occlusal alignment of teeth, beginning at the tip of the lower canine, following the buccal cusps of the natural premolars and molars, and continuing to the anterior border of the ramus. Called also *curvature of Spee.* **stress-strain c.,** one representing the relation between stress and strain of materials, such as orthodontic wire, measured under progressively increasing loads, with stress and strain being determined and plotted under each load change. **temperature c.,** a graphic tracing showing variations in body temperature over a period of time. **tension c's,** lines observed in the arrangement of the cancellous tissue of bones, depending on the directions of tension exerted on the bones. **c. of Wilson,** in the theory that occlusion should be spherical, the curvature of the cusps as projected on the frontal plane expressed in both arches; the curve in the lower arch being concave and the one in the upper arch being convex. The curvature in the lower arch is affected by an equal lingual inclination of the right and left molars so that the tip points of the corresponding cross-aligned cusps can be placed into the circumference of a circle. The transverse cuspal curvature of the upper teeth is affected by the equal buccal inclinations of their long axes.

Cushing's syndrome [Harvey Williams *Cushing,* Boston surgeon, 1869–1939] see under SYNDROME.

cushion (koosh'un) a padlike mass of soft material. See also PAD. **c. of epiglottis,** 1. epiglottic PETIOLE. 2. epiglottic TUBERCLE. **Ezo dental c's,** trademark for a denture cushion, consisting chiefly of a fibrous gauze impregnated with wax. **Passavant's c.,** Passavant's BAR. **retroarticular c.,** a loose vascular areolar connective tissue which attaches the posterior part of the articular disk of the temporomandibular articulation to the articular capsule, the upper layer attaching to the temporal bone, and the lower layer to the condyle. Called also *bilaminar area of articular disk* and *retrodiscal pad.* See also *interarticular disk of temporomandibular joint,* under DISK. **sucking c.,** buccal fat PAD.

cusp (kusp) [L. *cuspis* point] 1. a tapering eminence. 2. one of the triangular segments of a cardiac valve. 3. a conical-shaped pointed or rounded eminence on or near the masticating surface of a tooth which occludes with the antagonizing tooth of the opposite dental arch. Called also *cuspis dentis* [NA], *dental tubercle, tubercle of crown of tooth,* and *tuberculum coronae dentis.* **accessory buccal c.,** paramolar. **Carabelli c.,** an accessory cusp on the lingual aspect of the mesiolingual cusp of an upper molar, which may be unilateral or bilateral and may vary considerably in size. It is present in some form in the majority of Caucasians, but is virtually never present in Eskimos and others of the Mongolian race. Called also *Carabelli's tubercle.* **central c.,** an additional cusp in the middle of the occlusal surface, usually of molars. The presence of central cusps may prevent normal articulation of the teeth, and forceful pressure during mastication may cause their fracture, resulting in pulpitis. It was believed by some to be a form of dens invaginatus, but invagination does not appear to be involved. Called also *interstitial c.* **c. height,** cusp HEIGHT. **interstitial c.,** central c. **c. plane,** cusp PLANE. **plunger c.,** a cusp, usually one which is worn and has either a broad flat or pointed surface, which tends to forcibly wedge food interproximally. See also food IMPACTION. **c. restoration,** cusp RESTORATION. **shoeing c.,** cusp RESTORATION. **stamp c.,** a cusp which, in a tooth-to-tooth occlusion, fits a fossa of its antagonist in a manner somewhat similar to that of a pestle fitting a mortar. The maxillary lingual cusps are considered as stamp cusps and the lower teeth may be regarded as flattened stamps. See also cusp-fossa RELATION. **supporting c's,** the lingual cusps of the maxillary molars and bicuspids, the buccal cusps of the mandibular molars and bicuspids, and the incisal edges of the mandibular anterior teeth, which in normal adult dentition maintain contact areas with the opposing fossae and interproximal embrasures and determine the occlusal vertical dimension of the face. See also contact AREA (2). **talon c.,** margoid DIFFERENTIATION. **tipping of c.,** cusp RESTORATION.

cuspid (kus'pid) 1. having a cusp or point. 2. cuspid tooth; see canine TOOTH.

cuspidate (kus'pĭ-dāt) [L. *cuspidatus*] having a cusp or cusps.

cuspides (kus'pĭ-dēz) [L.] plural of *cuspis.*

cuspidor (kus'pĭ-dor) a round glass or stainless steel bowl attached to the dental unit, into which the patient may expectorate. A water valve allows flushing of the cuspidor and washes away blood, debris, etc.

cuspis (kus'pis), pl. *cus'pides* [L.] cusp. **c. den'tis,** cusp (3).

cutaneous (ku-ta'ne-us) [L. *cutis* skin] pertaining to the skin.

cuticle (ku'tĭ-k'l) [L. *cuticula,* from *cutis* skin] 1. a layer of a strandlike accelular structure with a homogeneous matrix, sometimes enclosed within clearly demarcated linear borders, which covers the free surface of an epithelial cell. 2. eponychium. **acquired c.,** acquired PELLICLE. **attachment c.,** secondary c. **dental c.,** secondary c. **enamel c.,** primary c. **hair c.** a layer of cells lining the hair follicles. Called also *c. of root sheath.* **primary c.,** a film on the enamel of unerupted teeth, considered to be the final product of degenerating ameloblasts after completion of enamel formation. It is calcified and slightly more resistant to acid and alkali than the enamel, and tends to be worn away after eruption, particularly in areas exposed to abrasive foods. It persists at the gingival third of the enamel, especially on the interproximal aspects, and, to a lesser degree, on the occlusal surfaces of the posterior teeth in the developmental grooves. It is colorless initially, but becomes stained by food debris and bacteria, sometimes becoming green. Electron microscopy shows it to consist primarily of ameloblasts of the reduced enamel epithelium attached to the enamel by a basal lamina. Called also *enamel c., adamantine membrane, enamel membrane, enamel organ remnant, membrana adamantina,* and *Nasymth's membrane.* **c. of root sheath,** hair c. **secondary c.,** a film occuring on some teeth on both the enamel and the cementum, external to the primary cuticle, with which it combines, being deposited by the epithelial attachment as it migrates along the tooth and separates from the crown and root. It is not present on cementum to which the periodontal ligament is not attached. Electron microscopy shows it to have a coarsely granular structure (0.5 μ) adherent to the enamel and cementum. The epithelial attachment is attached to it by a basal lamina (0.1 μ). Some authorities consider it to be a nonkeratinized product of the epithelial attachment cells, probably contributed by the gingival fluid and saliva; others consider it as a pathologic product of inflamed gingiva, or a conglutinate of erythrocytes. Called also *attachment c., cuticula dentis* [NA], *dental c.,* and *transposed crevicular c.* **transposed crevicular c.,** secondary c.

cuticula (ku-tik'u-lah), pl. *cutic'ulae* [L. "little skin"] a horny secreted layer. See CUTICLE. **c. den'tis** [NA], secondary CUTICLE.

cuticulae (ku-tik'u-le) [L.] plural of *cuticula.*

cutie pie (ku'te pi) a battery-powered portable ionization chamber used as a monitor in radiation protection.

cutis (ku'tis) [L.] [NA] the skin; the outer integument or covering of the body, which provides the anatomical boundary between the body and the environment. **c. elas'tica,** Ehlers-Danlos SYNDROME. **c. lax'a,** abnormal laxity of the skin characterized by the presence of folds of pendulous skin, usually about the face, neck, arms, and other parts of the body. Called also *c. pendula,* and *lax skin.* **c. marmora'ta,** a bluish or purplish mottling of the skin, due to congestion of the blood, usually as a result of exposure to cold. **c. pen'dula,** c. laxa. **c. ver'ticis gyra'ta,** a skin disorder characterized by furrows occurring in the scalp, over the crown and back of the head, resembling convolutions of the brain.

cutter (kut'er) a device used for cutting. **pin and ligature c.,** an orthodontic instrument designed for cutting orthodontic pins and ligatures. See illustration.

cutting (kut'ing) separating, severing, or shearing from a main body. **cone c.,** failure to cover or expose the entire area of a radiograph with the useful beam, thereby only partially exposing the film.

Cuvier, canals of, ducts of (sinuses, veins) [Baron Georges Leópold Chrétien Frédéric Dagobert de *Cuvier,* French naturalist, 1769–1832] see DUCTUS venosus, and see under DUCT.

CV cardiovascular.

CVA cardiovascular ACCIDENT.

CVS cardiovascular SYSTEM.

cyan- see CYANO-.

cyanide (si'ah-nīd) any compound containing the radical CN. **hydrogen c.,** hydrocyanic ACID. **mercuric c.,** a very poisonous mercury salt, occurring as colorless, odorless, tetragonal crystals; used in solution as a topical antiseptic in the treatment of

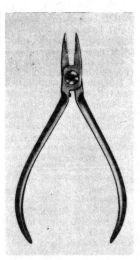

Pin and ligature cutter (From H. O. Torres and A. Ehrlich: Modern Dental Assisting. 2nd ed. Philadelphia, W. B. Saunders Co., 1980.)

diseases of the skin and mucous membranes, including those of oral mucosa, such as acute necrotizing ulcerative gingivitis. **vinyl c.,** acrylonitrile.

cyano-, cyan- [Gr. *kyanos* blue] a combining form denoting blue.

cyanoacrylate (si″ah-no-ak′rĭ-lāt) an acrylate monomer or polymer which is substituted by one or more cyano groups. Some cyanoacrylates are used as adhesives and pit and fissure sealants. See also cyanoacrylate RESIN. **ethyl c.,** an ethyl derivative of α-2-cyanoacrylate. **methyl c.,** a methyl derivative of α-2-cyanoacrylate.

Cyanobacteria (si″ah-no-bak-te′re-ah) [*cyano-* + *bacterium*] one of the two divisions of the kingdom Procaryotae, which comprises the blue-green algae.

cyanobacterium (si″ah-no-bak-te′re-um), pl. *cyanobacte′ria.* Any of the microorganisms of the Cyanobacteria.

cyanocobalamin (si″ah-no-ko-bal′ah-min) 1. vitamin B$_{12}$, α-(5,-6-dimethylbenzimidazolyl)cobamide cyanide, occurring as odorless, hygroscopic, dark red crystals that are soluble in water and ethanol. It is involved in various metabolic processes and is essential for normal growth, hematopoiesis, production of epithelial cells, maintenance of the myelin sheath, nucleic acid synthesis, conversion of homocysteine to methionine, maintenance of SH groups, synthesis of fats, carbohydrates, and proteins, and other metabolic processes. Cyanocobalamin combines with intrinsic factor for absorption, which is needed for maturation of erythrocytes. Widely distributed in nature, including milk, seafood, egg yolks, meat, and dairy products, it is synthesized by microorganisms, including fecal bacteria, in the human bowel, but without being absorbed into the system. Used therapeutically in numerous conditions, but proved to be effective only in cyanocobalamin deficiency. In pure forms, the vitamin is not believed to be toxic, but impurities may cause hypersensitivity, fever, chills, dyspnea, flushing, urticaria, and other adverse reactions. Called also *antipernicious anemia principle, Dorner factor, extrinsic factor,* and *LLD factor.* Cyanocobalamin deficiency usually results from lesions of the stomach, where the intrinsic factor is secreted, or the ileum, where intrinsic factor facilitates absorption of the vitamin, and is usually associated with pernicious anemia. Lesions that may cause inadequate secretion of intrinsic factor include corrosive burns of the gastric mucosa, linitis plastica, gastric neoplasms, and other diseases associated with atrophy of the stomach. Deficiency may also occur in strict vegetarians and in their breast-fed infants, and in competition for cyanocobalamin by intestinal parasites or bacteria. Glossitis, weight loss, diarrhea, and neurological disorders are the most prominent syndromes. For daily requirements for cyanocobalamin, see vitamin B$_{12}$ in table at NUTRITION. 2. cobalamin.

Cyano-Dent trademark for ethyl 2-cyanoacrylate; used for cementation of pins to retain restorations.

cyanosis (si″ah-no′sis) [Gr. *kyanos* blue] a bluish color of the skin, mucous membranes, or internal organs, most commonly observed on the lips, tip of the nose, ears, cheeks, and digital extremities. It is due to impaired oxygen-carrying capacity of the blood and excessive concentration of reduced hemoglobin in the blood. See under ANEMIA.

cybernetics (si″ ber-net′iks) [Gr. *kybernētēs* helmsman] the study of communications systems in machines and also in the human brain; or the controlling of an activity or a set of activities to keep them directed towards a particular goal.

Cyclaine trademark for *hexylcaine hydrochloride* (see under HEXYLCAINE).

cyclamate (si′klah-māt) a salt of cyclamic acid, including sodium, potassium, and calcium cyclamates. Cyclamates were formerly used as nonnutritive, noncaloric sweeteners, particularly in sugar-free soft drinks, but were found to produce bladder tumors in laboratory animals fed large amounts of cyclamates, calculated to be equivalent in human consumption to 138 to 553 bottles of cyclamate-sweetened drink per day. Cyclamates are now available in the U.S. only by prescription.

Cyclamin trademark for *troleandomycin.*

Cyclamycin trademark for *troleandomycin.*

cycle (si′k'l) [Gr. *kyklos* circle] a round or succession of observable phenomena, recurring in the same sequence and perhaps at regular intervals. See also PERIODICITY and RHYTHM. **carbon c.,** the process by which carbon is extracted from the air by plants in the form of carbon dioxide, then is converted to carbohydrates in the plant tissue, through photosynthesis, followed by animal consumption, and ultimately returning to the atmosphere in the decomposition of plant or animal tissue or through exhalation. **chewing c.,** masticating c. **citric acid c.,** Krebs c. **c's per second,** see HERTZ. **curing c.,** the heating process employed to control the initial propagation of resin polymerization in the denture mold. **Krebs c.,** a cycle of carbohydrate metabolism in which pyruvate is oxidized in animal and plant tissues and in bacteria to yield energy. Called also *citric acid c.* and *tricarboxylic acid c.* See illustration. **lactic acid c.,** a cycle of carbohydrates in energy metabolism, in which glucose is broken down through a series of events to lactic and pyruvic acids and regenerated back again. See also *Krebs c.,* carbohydrate METABOLISM, Embden-Meyerhof PATHWAY, and phosphogluconate PATHWAY. See illustration. **masticating c., masticatory c.,** the complete pathway of the mandible performed in mastication of food. It is usually of a teardrop shape when viewed from the frontal or lateral planes; the average jaw opening being 18.2 mm. In the early stages of mastication, the closing strokes usually terminate short of the occlusal contact but, as food softens and is reduced in size, the strokes approach the occlusal contact more closely than before, the duration of the average chewing contact being 0.1 to 0.15 second, while the average duration of the cycle is 1.046 seconds. The closing stroke ends in intercuspation (terminal functional orbit), followed by the opening stroke and the beginning of the new cycle. Called also *chewing c.* **nitrogen c.,** the steps by which nitrogen is extracted from the nitrates of soil and water, incorporated as amino acids and proteins in living organisms, and ultimately reconverted to nitrates: (1) conversion of nitrogen to nitrates by bacteria; (2) the extraction of the nitrates by plants and the building of amino acids and proteins by adding an amino group to the carbon compounds produced in photosynthesis; (3) the ingestion of plants by animals; and (4) the return of nitrogen to the soil in animal excretions or on the death and decomposition of plants and animals. See illustration. **tricarboxylic acid c.,** Krebs c.

cyclic (sik′lik) [Gr. *kyklikos*] 1. pertaining to or occurring in a cycle or cycles. 2. in chemistry, pertaining to organic chemical compounds whose structure is characterized by a ring of atoms in a nucleus. Three major groups of cyclic compounds include alicyclic, aromatic, and heterocyclic (see under COMPOUND). See also closed CHAIN.

cyclitis (sik-li′tis) [*ciliary body* + *-itis*] inflammation of the ciliary body. **heterochromic c.,** Fuchs' HETEROCHROMIA.

cyclizine (si-kli-zen) an antihistaminic drug, with antiemetic properties, 1-diphenylmethyl-4-methylpiperazine, occurring as a white, odorless, crystalline powder that is readily soluble in ethanol and chloroform and is slightly soluble in water. Used in the prevention and treatment of motion sickness and in postoperative control of nausea and vomiting. Large doses may cause drowsiness and xerostomia. Trademark: Marzine, Merezine, Nautazine, Neo-Devomit. **c. hydrochloride,** the monohydrochloride salt of cyclizine, occurring as a white crystalline powder or as small colorless crystals that have practically no odor and a bitter taste. Readily soluble in water, ethanol, chloroform, but not in ether. Its pharmacological properties are similar to those of the parent compound. Trademark: Valoid.

cyclo- [Gr. *kyklos* circle] 1. a combining form denoting round or

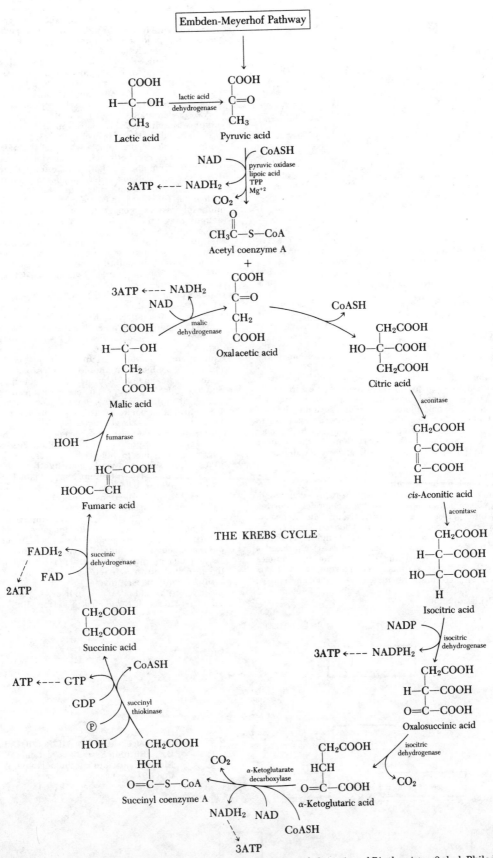

Krebs cycle. (From J. I. Routh, D. P. Eyman, and D. J. Burton: Essentials of General, Organic and Biochemistry. 3rd ed. Philadelphia, W. B. Saunders Co., 1977.)

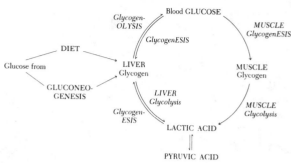

Lactic acid cycle. (From J. I. Routh, D. P. Eyman, and D. J. Burton: Essentials of General, Organic and Biochemistry. 3rd ed. Philadelphia, W. B. Saunders Co., 1977.)

recurring. Often used with particular reference to the eye. 2. in chemistry, a prefix denoting a ring compound.

cycloalkane (si″klo-al′kān) an alkane, the ends of the carbon chain of which are joined together in a ring, as in cyclopropane.

Cyclodol trademark for *trihexyphenidyl hydrochloride* (see under TRIHEXYPHENIDYL).

Cyclogyl trademark for *cyclopentolate hydrochloride* (see under CYCLOPENTOLATE).

cyclo-ligase [E.C.6.3.3] (si″klo-li′gās) a subclass of ligases, the enzymes of which catalyze the formation of C − N bonds, the breakdown of the terminal phosphate bonds of ATP.

cyclomethycaine sulfate (si″klo-meth′ĭ-kān) a topical anesthetic, 3-(2-methylpiperidino)-propyl *p*-cyclohexylbenzoate sulfate, occurring as a white, odorless, crystalline powder that is sparingly soluble in water, ethanol, chloroform, and isopropanol, and very slightly soluble in acetone, ether, and dilute acids. Used in treating lesions of the skin and mucous membranes, being more effective on the genitourinary mucosa than on the mucous membranes of the mouth, nose, bronchi, and eye. Trademarks: Surfacaine, Topocaine.

Cyclomycin trademark for *tetracycline* (1).

Cyclonal trademark for *hexobarbital*.

cyclopentamine hydrochloride (si″klo-pen′tah-mēn) a compound, *N*,α-dimethylcyclopentaneethylamine hydrochloride, occurring as a white, bitter, crystalline powder with a mild characteristic taste, which is soluble in water, ethanol, benzene, and chloroform, and slightly soluble in ether. It is an indirectly acting sympathomimetic with vasoconstrictor and pressor properties that relaxes the bronchioles and the intestine and induces mydriasis. Used chiefly as a nasal decongestant. Side effects include elevated blood pressure and excitability. Formerly used to maintain blood pressure during anesthesia. Trademarks: Clopane, Cyklosal, Sinos.

cyclopentane (si″klo-pen′tān) a cyclic hydrocarbon, C_5H_{10}, occurring in petroleum. Used as a solvent and in various chemical processes. **c. ring**, cyclopentane RING.

cyclopentolate hydrochloride (si″klo-pen′to-lāt) an antimuscarinic drug, 2-dimethylaminoethyl-1-hydroxy-α-phenylcyclopentaneacetate hydrochloride, occurring as a white, crystalline powder that is soluble in water and ethanol, but not in ether. Used chiefly in ophthalmology. Adverse reactions are similar to those of atropine, and may include vertigo, restlessness, tremor, fatigue, disorders of locomotion and orientation, convulsions, excessive thirst, xerostomia, visual disorders, anhidrosis, hyperpyrexia, nausea, vomiting, constipation, hallucinations, skin rash, flushing, leukocytosis, respiratory disorders, and shock. Trademarks: Cyclogyl, Mydplegic, Mydrilate, Zyklolat.

cyclophosphamide (si″klo-fos′fah-mīd) a nitrogen mustard, *N*,*N*-bis(2-chloroethyl)tetrahydro-2*H*-1,3,2-oxazaphosphorin-2-amine 2-oxide, occurring as a white, crystalline powder that is soluble in water and ethanol. It is a cytotoxic drug used in the treatment of lymphocytic leukemia, Burkitt's tumor of the jaw, Hodgkin's disease and other lymphomas, multiple myeloma, neuroblastoma, and other neoplasms. Also used in the treatment of mycosis fungoides and lupus erythematosus and as an immunosuppressive agent in tissue transplantation. Adverse reactions may include alopecia, nausea, vomiting, anorexia, mucosal ulcers, vertigo, nail ridging, cutaneous pigmentation, sterility in males, hepatic dysfunction, predisposition to infections, and bone marrow depression with leukopenia, thrombocytopenia, and hypoprothrombinemia. Called also *cyclophosphane* and *cytophosphane*. Trademarks: Cytoxan, Endoxan, Procytox, Sendoxan.

cyclophosphane (si″klo-fos′fān) cyclophosphamide.

cyclopia (si-klo′pe-ah) [*cyclo*- + Gr. ṓpo eye + -*ia*] a developmental defect characterized by the presence of a single median eye caused by merging of the orbital fossae into a single cavity. **c. hypogna′thus,** cyclopia associated with agnathia or hypognathia.

cyclopropane (si″klo-pro′pān) an inhalation anesthetic, C_3H_8, occurring as a highly flammable, colorless gas with a pungent taste and a hexane-like odor, which is soluble in water, ethanol, and fixed oils. It is the most potent of all anesthetic gases, used chiefly in major surgery. A hazard of explosion and cardiac irregularities associated with its use are the major disadvantages. Called also *trimethylene*.

cycloserine (si″klo-ser′ēn) a broad-spectrum antibiotic produced by *Streptomyces orchidaceus*, D-4-amino-3-isoxazolidone, occurring as a white to yellowish, odorless, crystalline powder that is freely soluble in water and slightly soluble in methanol and propylene glycol. It inhibits both gram-negative and gram-positive bacteria, being used chiefly against *Mycobacterium tuberculosis* and infections caused by streptococci, staphylococci, *Escherichia coli*, *Aerobacter aerogenes*, and *Chlamydia*. In *in vitro* studies, the presence of D-alanine blocks the antibacterial activity of cycloserine. Somnolence, headache, tremor, dysarthria, vertigo, confusion, irritability, suicidal tendencies, paranoia, depression, muscular twitching, hyperreflexia, paresis, convulsions, and other central nervous system disorders are the principal adverse reactions. Trademarks: Closina, Micoserina, Oxamycin, Seromycin.

cyclosilane (si″klo-si-lān′) a silicon hydride, SiH_2; see SILANES.

cyclosis (si-klo′sis) [Gr. *kyklōsis* a surrounding, enclosing] the

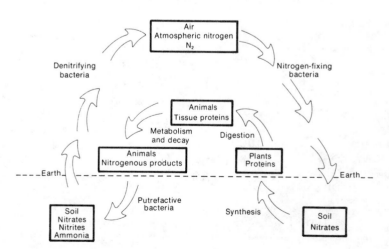

Nitrogen cycle. (From J. I. Routh, D. P. Eyman, and D. J. Burton: Essentials of General, Organic and Biochemistry. 3rd ed. Philadelphia, W. B. Saunders Co., 1977.)

movement of cytoplasm within the cell. Called also *cytoplasmic streaming* and *protoplasmic streaming*.

cyclotron (si'klo-tron) an apparatus for accelerating protons or deuterons to high energies by a combination of a constant magnet and an oscillating electric field.

Cyklosal trademark for *cyclopentamine hydrochloride* (see under CYCLOPENTAMINE).

cylinder (sil'in-der) [Gr. *kylindros* a roller] a solid body shaped like a column. **axis c.,** axon. **foil c., gold foil c.,** a cylinder of gold foil formed by repeatedly folding a sheet of foil into a narrow ribbon, which is then rolled into a cylindrical form. Used in a noncohesive state to line the surrounding walls of the prepared cavity or to fill the gingival portion of a proximal cavity.

cylindroma (sil"in-dro'mah) adenoid cystic CARCINOMA.

cymarigenin (si"mar-ĭ-gen'in) strophanthidin.

cynicism (sin-ĭ'sizm) [Gr. *kynikos* like a dog] the principle of Diogenes, who rejected all conventions and tried to live on nothing (like a dog), thus receiving the nickname *kyŏn*, a dog. It is based on the view that virtue is the only good aspect of human life and that its essence lies in self-control and independence.

cynodont (si'no-dont) [Gr. *kyŏn* dog + *odous* tooth] canine TOOTH.

cynotoxin (si"no-tok'sin) strophanthidin.

cyproheptadine hydrochloride (si"pro-hep'tah-dēn) an antihistaminic and antiserotonic agent, 4-(5*H*-dibenzo[*a,d*]cyclohepten-5-ylidene)-1-methylpiperidine hydrochloride, occurring as a white to yellowish, odorless, crystalline powder that is soluble in ethanol, methanol, chloroform, and water, but not in ether. Used in the treatment of pruritus, hay fever, angioedema, urticardia, and other allergic diseases. Sometimes used as an appetite stimulant. Side effects may include drowsiness, somnolence, xerostomia, dizziness, faintness, headache, and hypersensitivity. Rare central nervous system stimulation may occur. Trademarks: Anarexol, Antegan, Cipractin, Nuran, Periactin, Peritol, Vimicon.

cyproterone acetate (si-pro'ter-ōn) a potent antiandrogenic agent that also has progestational, androgenic, and antiestrogenic properties, 6-chloro-1β,2β-dihydro-17-hydroxy-3'*H*-cyclopropa-[1,2]pregna-1,4,6-triene-3,20-dione acetate. Trademark: Androcur.

Cys cysteine.

Cys-Cys cystine.

cyst (sist) [Gr. *kystis* sac, bladder] a sac or pouch without an opening, lined with epithelium, especially an abnormal sac containing gas, liquid, or semisolid material, formed in a natural cavity or in the substance of an organ. See also KERATOCYST and PSEUDOCYST. **adventitious c.,** a false cyst formed about a foreign body or an exudate. **aneurysmal bone c.,** a pseudocyst found in various bones, including the mandible; it is not lined with epithelium (hence *pseudocyst*) but presents a cavernous lesion filled with a fibrous connective tissue containing spongelike material with many cavernous or sinusoidal blood-filled spaces. **Blandin-Nuhn c.,** mucocele of the salivary gland near the tip of the tongue. **apical c.,** an epithelium-lined cyst in the bone at the apex of a pulpless tooth. **apical periodontal c.,** periapical c. **blood c.,** a cyst containing extravasated blood. Called also *sanguineous c.* **Boyer's c.,** a painless and gradual enlargement of the subhyoid bursa. **branchial cleft c.,** a usually superficial cyst situated on the lateral aspect of the neck; typically presenting a circumscribed movable mass near the anterior border of the sternocleidomastoid muscle, although some cysts have been found at the angle of the mandible, in the submandibular, parotid, and preauricular areas, and in the floor of the mouth. Believed by some to originate from the remnants of the branchial arches or pharyngeal pouches, but evidence suggests cystic transformation of epithelium entrapped in cervical lymph nodes. Called also *lymphoepithelial c.* **craniobuccal c.,** a cyst of Rathke's pouch. **craniopharyngeal duct c.,** one originating in the vestiges of the craniopharyngeal duct, being closely related to craniopharyngioma. **daughter c.,** a small cyst developed from a larger one. Called also *secondary c.* **dental c.,** one derived from any part of the odontogenic apparatus. **dental root c.,** periapical c. **dentigerous c.,** a fluid-containing odontogenic cyst surrounding the crown of an unerupted tooth, usually involving the crowns of normal permanent teeth. It is associated with a breakdown of the stellate reticulum during amelogenesis, after the crown of the tooth has been formed, and results in hypoplastic enamel. Called also *follicular c.* **dentoalveolar c.,** periodontal c. **dermoid c.,** a cyst of developmental origin, lined by a thin layer of stratified squamous epithelium, usually keratinized, and containing hair follicles, sweat glands, and sebaceous glands, probably resulting from entrapment of the ectoderm during uterine development. Most involve the ovary, occurring only rarely in the oral cavity. The oral lesion presents a bulge in the floor of the mouth and

submaxillary and sublingual areas, often causing eating and talking difficulty. Some become infected; some may develop sinus tracts to the skin and oral mucosa; and a few undergo malignant degeneration. See also *epidermoid c.* **developmental c.,** inclusion c. **dilatation c.,** one formed by dilation of a previously existing cavity. **distention c.,** a collection of watery fluid in a normal, but distended cavity. **end root c.,** periapical c. **endothelial c.,** one whose sac has an endothelial lining. **epidermoid c.,** a dermoid cyst composed only of a connective tissue wall lined by keratinized stratified squamous epithelium, without any other specialized structures showing. **eruption c.,** a dentigerous cyst presenting a dilatation of the follicular space about the crown of the erupting deciduous or permanent teeth in children, caused by the accumulation of tissue fluid or blood. Called also *eruption hematoma* because the presence of the blood in the cavity gives the cyst a purple or deep blue color. **extravasation c.,** traumatic c. **exudation c.,** one formed by the collection of exudate in a cavity. **false c.,** one in which the cavity is not lined by epithelium; a pseudocyst. **fissural c.,** inclusion c. **follicular c.,** dentigerous c. **gas c.,** one filled with gas. **gingival c.,** an odontogenic cyst of the soft tissue of either the free or attached gingiva, presenting a small, well-circumscribed, painless swelling, sometimes resembling a superficial mucocele. **globulomaxillary c.,** an inclusion cyst of the maxillary bone, located in the globulomaxillary fissure, usually between the lateral incisor and cuspid teeth, which, unless it becomes infected, seldom presents any clinical manifestation. It is lined by either stratified squamous or ciliated columnar epithelium. Called also *premaxillary-maxillary c.* **granddaughter c.,** one seen within a daughter cyst. **hemorrhagic c.,** traumatic c. **hydatid c.,** the larval cyst stage of the tapeworm *Echinococcus*. See ECHINOCOCCOSIS. **implantation c.,** one formed from tissue that has become implanted. **incisive canal c.,** median anterior maxillary c. **inclusion c.,** one formed by inclusion of a small portion of epithelium or mesothelium within connective tissue. Various inclusion cysts of bone occur in the jaws, arising along lines of fusion (e.g., *globulomaxillary c., median anterior maxillary c., median mandibular c., median palatal c.,* and *nasoalveolar c.*). They usually contain fluid or semisolid material, and are lined by epithelium derived from cells that are entrapped between embryonic processes of bones at union lines. Called also *development c.* and *fissural c.* See also Bohn's nodules, under NODULE and Epstein's pearls, under PEARL. **Klestadt's c.,** ñasoalveolar c. **latent bone c.,** static bone c. **lateral periodontal c.,** a cyst of the lateral periodontal membrane of an erupted tooth, usually occurring in the bicuspid region of the mandible. **lymphoepithelial c.,** branchial cleft c. **lateral c.,** a periodontal cyst along the lateral surface of the root of a tooth. See also *periapical c.* **mandibular median c.,** median mandibular c. **maxillary median anterior c.,** median anterior maxillary c. **maxillary sinus retention c.,** a form of mucous retention cyst of the maxillary sinus, characterized by accumulation of fluid within connective tissue spaces and by absence from the cavity of a definite lining, although some cysts may be lined by a respiratory type of epithelium. Called also *secretory c. of maxillary antrum* and *maxillary sinus mucocele.* **median anterior maxillary c.,** the most common of inclusion cysts of the maxilla, located in or near the incisive canal. It is usually lined by stratified squamous epithelium, pseudostratified ciliated columnar epithelium, or both, indicating the origin of the cyst from the proliferation of epithelial remnants of the nasopalatine duct. Called also *incisive canal c.* and *nasopalatine duct c.* **median mandibular c.,** a rare inclusion cyst occurring in the midline of the mandible, believed to be caused by inclusion of the epithelium trapped in the central groove of the mandibular process, or by cystic degeneration of a supernumerary tooth germ. It presents an oval round, irregular lesion, lined by a thin stratified squamous epithelium, often with folds and projections. **median palatal c.,** an inclusion cyst located in the midline of the hard palate between the lateral palatal processes, lined by stratified squamous epithelium overlying a dense fibrous connective tissue. **mother c.,** one enclosing other cysts. Called also *parent c.* **mucous c.,** mucous retention c. **mucous retention c.,** a retention cyst presenting a cavity dilated with accumulated mucus, usually located in the connective tissue and submucosa of the lower lip, caused by traumatic rupture of a salivary duct. It is usually lined by compressed fibrous connective tissue and fibroblasts, rather than epithelium. Called also *mucocele.* See also RANULA. **multilocular c.,** one containing many loculi or spaces. See also cystic AMELOBLASTOMA. **nasoalveolar c., nasolabial c.,** an inclusion cyst arising from epithelial remnants at the junction of the globular process, the lateral nasal process, and the maxillary process, which may be lined by columnar or squamous epithelium. Clinically, it may cause a swelling in the mucolabial fold and in the floor of the nose and superficial erosion of the outer surface of the maxilla. Called also *Klestadt's c.* **nasopalatine duct c.**, median anterior maxillary c. **necrotic c.**, one containing necrotic matter. **odentogenic c.**, one derived from epithelium, usually containing fluid or semisolid material, which develops during various stages of odontogenesis. Nearly all odentogenic cysts are enclosed within bone. Primordial cyst, dentigerous cyst, periodontal cyst, and gingival cyst are the specific types. **palatal c., median**, median palatal c. **palatine papilla c.**, a rare variant of median anterior maxillary cyst, which arises from epithelial rests in the incisive papilla, rather than in the bone. **parent c.**, mother c. **periapical c.**, a periodontal cyst involving the apex of an erupted tooth. It is the most common odontogenic cyst and is frequently a result of infection via the pulp chamber and root canal through carious involvement of the tooth. Called also *apical root c., dental root c., end root c.,* and *radicular c.* **periodontal c.**, one in the periodontal ligament and adjacent structures, usually at the apex of a tooth *(periapical c.)*, but sometimes along the lateral surfaces of the root. Called also *dentoalveolar cyst.* **periodontal c., apical**, periapical c. **pilonidal c.**, a hair-containing sacrococcygeal dermoid cyst or sinus. **premaxillary-maxillary c.**, globulomaxillary c. **primordial c.**, a relatively uncommon type of odontogenic cyst that develops through cystic degeneration and liquefaction of the stellate reticulum in an enamel organ before any calcified enamel or dentin has been formed. They may originate from supernumerary teeth, and are found in place of a tooth rather than being associated with one. **radicular c.**, periapical c. **residual c.**, a periodontal cyst which remains after or develops subsequent to extraction of a tooth. **retention c.**, one caused by retention of glandular secretion. See also *mucous retention c.* **retention c. of maxillary sinus**, maxillary sinus retention c. **salivary gland c.**, one caused by retention of salivary gland secretions. See also *mucous retention c.* and RANULA. **sanguineous c.**, blood c. **secondary c.**, daughter c. **secretory c.**, one caused by retention of glandular secretions; a retention cyst. **secretory c. of maxillary antrum**, maxillary sinus retention c. **solitary bone c.**, traumatic c. **Stafne's c.**, static bone c. **static bone c.**, a developmental inclusion of salivary glandular tissue within or, more commonly, adjacent to the lingual surface of the body of the mandible, forming a deep, circumscribed depression. It is sometimes bilateral, and is believed to be congenital, although it is rarely observed in children, occurring more commonly in males than in females. On the radiograph, it appears as an ovoid radiolucency situated between the mandibular canal and the inferior border of the mandible, just anterior to the angle. Called also *latent bone c., Stafne's c., lingual mandibular bone cavity, Stafne's mandibular defect,* and *static bone cavity.* **sublingual c.**, ranula. **suprassellar c.**, craniopharyngioma. **traumatic c.**, a cavity in a bone that is not lined by epithelium (hence not a true cyst), containing either a small amount of fluid, shreds of necrotic blood clot, or nothing. It occurs most commonly in young persons, and may be found in any bone, including the jaws, with the mandible being more frequently affected than the maxilla. Trauma is the suspected cause. Called also *extravasation c., hemorrhagic c., solitary bone c., unicameral bone c.,* and *idiopathic bone cavity.* **Thornwaldt's (Tornwaldt's) c.**, pharyngeal BURSA. **thyroglossal c., thyroglossal duct c., thyroglossal tract c.**, a firm, usually movable tender cyst varying in size from a few millimeters to several centimeters, usually located anywhere along the embryonic thyroglossal tract between the foramen cecum of the tongue and the thyroid gland. It apparently arises from remnants of the thyroglossal duct which do not become obliterated; its appearance is precipitated by infections. They occur usually in young persons, but they may develop at any age; some are congenital. Rupture may result in a thyroglossal fistula leading from the cyst to the skin or mucous membranes. These cysts usually grow slowly and are asymptomatic, unless they are located near the tongue, where they may cause dysphagia. **true c.**, one in which the cavity is lined by epithelium. **unicameral bone c.**, traumatic c.

cyst- see CYSTO-.

cystadenolymphoma (sis-tad″ĕ-no-lim-fo′mah) a tumor of epithelial and lymphoid tissue. **papillary c., papillary c. lymphomatosum**, adenolymphoma.

cystadenoma (sis″tad-ĕ-no′mah) [*cyst-* + *adenoma*] a benign

tumor of epithelial and lymphoid tissues, combining the properties of adenoma and cystoma.

Cystamin trademark for *methenamine*.

cysteine (sis-te′in) a sulfur-containing, naturally occurring nonessential amino acid, 2-amino-3-mercaptopropionic acid. Cysteine is oxidized to cystine, and is sometimes found in the urine. It has been used as a detoxicant. Abbreviated *Cys*. Called also *thioaminopropionic acid.* See also amino ACID.

cysti- see CYSTO-.

cystic (sis′tik) [Gr. *kystis* bladder] 1. pertaining to a cyst. 2. pertaining to the urinary bladder or to the gallbladder.

cysticerci (sis″tĭ-ser′si) plural of *cysticercus.*

cysticercosis (sis″tĭ-ser-ko′sis) infection with tapeworms due to ingestion of cysts (*Cysticercus cellulosae*) of the pork tapeworm (*Taenia solium*) or beef tapeworm (*Taenia saginata*). The larvae invade the walls of the small intestine and are transported with the blood and lymph to various sites, including the skin, mucous membranes, heart, liver, lungs, eyes, muscles, and brain. The larvae develop in the soft tissue into small translucent cysts, leading to inflammatory reaction. Dead larvae evoke further inflammation associated with fibroblastic proliferation, giant cells, formation of granulomas, and calcification. The nodules may be palpated in the soft tissue, and are especially notable in the tongue.

Cysticercus (sis″tĭ-ser′kus) [Gr. *kystis* bladder + *kerkos* tail] a former genus of larval forms of tapeworms. **C. cellulo′sae**, the larva of *Taenia solium* or *T. saginata.*

cysticercus (sis″tĭ-ser′kus), pl. *cysticer′ci.* A larval tapeworm.

cystido- see CYSTO-.

cystine (sis′tēn) a sulfur-containing, natural, nonessential amino acid, 3,3″-dithiobis-(2-aminopropanoic) acid. It is sometimes found in the urine and in the kidneys in the form of minute hexagonal crystals, frequently forming a cystine calculus in the bladder, and is also found in the saliva. Cystine is the chief sulfur-containing compound of the protein molecule, and is readily reduced to two molecules of cysteine. Abbreviated *Cys-Cys.* Called also *dicysteine.* See also amino ACID.

cystinosis (sis″tĭ-no′sis) Abderhalden-Fanconi SYNDROME.

cystis (sis′tis), pl. *cys′tides* [Gr. *kystis*] a pouch or sac; a cyst.

cysto-, cyst-, cysti-, cystido- [Gr. *kystis, kystides* a sac or bladder] a combining form denoting a relationship to a sac, cyst, or bladder; most frequently used in reference to the urinary bladder.

cystoid (sis′toid) [*cysto-* + Gr. *eidos* form] 1. resembling a cyst. 2. a cystlike, circumscribed collection of softened material, differing from a true cyst in having no enclosing capsule.

Cystokon trademark for *acetrizoate sodium* (see under ACETRIZOATE).

cytarabine (si-tar′ah-bēn) a pyrimidine analogue, 4-amino-1β-D-arabinofuranosyl-2(1*H*)-pyrimidinone, occurring as a white, odorless, crystalline powder that is soluble in water and slightly soluble in ethanol, chloroform, and methanol. It competitively interferes with the incorporation of uridine into deoxycytidine nucleotides. Used in the treatment of leukemias and other cancers. Also used in the treatment of megaloviral infections, particularly those caused by *Herpesvirus simplex.* Adverse reactions are similar to those of other pyrimidine analogues, and include lesions of the oral mucosa. Called also *cytosine arabinose.* Trademarks: Aracytidine, Cytosar.

cytase (si′tās) [Gr. *kytos* hollow vessel + *-ase*] 1. complement regarded as an enzyme; alexin. 2. an enzyme occurring in the seeds of various plants, having the power of making soluble the material of the cell wall.

cytaster (si′tas-ter) [*cyto-* + Gr. *aster* star] see ASTER.

-cyte [Gr. *kytos* hollow vessel, anything that contains or covers] a word termination denoting a cell, the type of which is designated by the root to which it is affixed, as erythrocyte, leukocyte, etc.

cytidine (si′tĭ-din) a nucleoside, 1-β-D-ribofuranosylcytosine, consisting of D-ribose and cytosine.

cyto- [Gr. *kytos* hollow vessel] a combining form denoting relationship to a cell.

cytocentrum (si″to-sen′trum) [*cyto-* + *centrum*] centrosome.

cytochrome (si′to-krōm) [*cyto-* + Gr. *chrōma* color] an electron-transferring protein (hemoprotein) that contains iron-porphyrin groups, found chiefly in the mitochondria of aerobic cells. Its function consists of transporting electrons in biological oxidation processes, by means of reversible valence changes, F(II)-Fe(III), during their catalytic cycles. Some types (c. oxidase) serve as the terminal catalyst in effecting the direct union of oxygen with electrons initially derived from oxidizable substances; other cytochromes are involved in transferring electrons from other enzymes to cytochrome oxidase. Cytochromes differ from each other by their prosthetic groups, and are classified as a, b, c, and d. **c. a,** that in which heme in the prosthetic group contains a formyl side chain. **c. b,** that in which proheme or related heme in the prosthetic group does not contain a formyl group and the prosthetic group is not bound convalently to the protein. **c. c,** that in which the side chain of the heme is bound covalently to the protein. **c. d,** that in which the prosthetic group contains a tetrapyrolic chelate of iron. **c. oxidase,** the enzyme that catalyzes the terminal reaction of electron transport in the process of biological oxidation, in which molecular oxygen is reduced to water.

cytodendrite (si″to-den′drīt) [*cyto-* + *dendrite*] dendrite.

cytogenetics (si″to-jĕ-net′iks) [*cyto-* + Gr. *gennan* to produce] the branch of genetics concerned with the study of cytological problems, especially the action of chromosomes in cell division, their origin, and their relation to the transmission and recombination of genes. See also molecular GENETICS.

cytoid (si′toid) [*cyto-* + Gr. *eidos* form] resembling a cell.

cytology (si-tol′o-je) [*cyto-* + *-logy*] the study of the composition and function of cells under normal and pathological conditions. **exfoliative c.,** microscopic examination of cells obtained by scraping the surface of the suspected area, or by rinsing the oral cavity; used in the diagnosis of malignant neoplasms.

cytolymph (si′to-limf) [*cyto-* + *lymph*] hyaloplasm (1).

cytolysis (si-tol′ĭ-sis) [*cyto-* + Gr. *lysis* dissolution] the dissolution of cells.

cytomegalia infantum (si″to-me-ga′le-ah in-fan′tum) cytomegalic inclusion DISEASE.

cytomegalovirus (si″to-meg″ah-lo-vi′rus) a highly host-specific herpesvirus that infects man, monkeys, rodents, and other animals. Infection with cytomegalovirus produces unique large cells, bearing intranuclear inclusions, in the salivary glands, kidneys, circulating leukocytes, and urine. The virus is transmitted sometimes by blood transfusion (posttransfusion syndrome) or transnatally or transplacentally. Called also *salivary gland virus*. **guinea pig c.,** a cytomegalovirus specific for the guinea pig, isolated from the submaxillary glands. Infection is usually inapparent, but is associated with inclusions in the salivary ducts. Called also *guinea pig salivary gland virus, salivary gland virus of guinea pig,* and *submaxillary virus*. **human c.,** cytomegalovirus that is specific for man, causing inapparent infections, especially of the salivary glands; cytomegalic inclusion disease; chronic cytomegalovirus infection, often in association with neoplastic diseases; localized granulomas; heterophile antibody–negative infectious mononucleosis; and other diseases. Infection is characterized by the presence of large cells up to 40 μm in diameter, bearing intranuclear inclusions 8 to 10 μm in diameter. **mouse c.,** cytomegalovirus causing usually a latent infection of the salivary glands in mice, with inclusions present in various cells. **rat c.,** one isolated from the salivary glands in the rat.

cytomorphosis (si″to-mor-fo′sis) [*cyto-* + Gr. *morphōsis* a shaping] the series of events in cell development. Four stages of cytomorphosis are recognized: *Stage I* — undifferentiated or young cells, including embryonal cells; *Stage II* — differentiated or completely specialized cells; *Stage III* — degenerating or older cells; *Stage IV* — moribund or dead cells.

cytopathology (si″to-pah-thol′o-je) [*cyto-* + Gr. *pathos* disease + *-logy*] the study of cells in disease; cellular pathology.

cytopenia (si″to-pe′ne-ah) [*cyto-* + Gr. *penia* poverty] deficiency in the cellular elements of the blood.

cytophil (si′to-fil) [*cyto-* + Gr. *philein* to love] having an affinity for cells.

cytophosphane (si″to-fos′fān) cyclophosphamide.

cytoplasm (si′to-plazm″) [*cyto-* + Gr. *plasma* plasm] the part of the protoplasm of a cell exclusive of the nucleus and the cell wall, in which the definite subcellular components are embedded and which is responsible for metabolic and synthetic activities of the cell. It is surrounded by the cell membrane and separated from the nucleus in eukaryotic cells by the nuclear membrane. Cytoplasm may be subdivided into the ground substance or cytoplasmic matrix and the cytoplasmic organelles. Its constituents include the centriole, endoplasmic reticulum, Golgi apparatus, mitochondria, and inclusions. Many soluble enzymes are found in the cytoplasm, particularly those associated with the conversion of glucose to pyruvic or lactic acid. See also NUCLEOPLASM.

cytoplasmic (si″to-plaz′mik) pertaining to or contained in the cytoplasm.

Cytosar trademark for *cytarabine*.

cytosine (si′to-sin) a pyrimidine base, 2-oxo-4-aminopyrimidine, found in DNA and RNA and in certain coenzymes. It occurs as lustrous platelets that are slightly soluble in water and alcohol. Used in biochemical research. **c. arabinose,** cytarabine.

cytotaxis (si-to-tak′sis) [*cyto-* + Gr. *taxis* arrangement] The movement and arrangement of cells with respect to a specific source of stimulation. See also LEUKOTAXIS.

cytotoxic (si″to-tok′sik) 1. capable of producing a toxic action in cells. 2. an agent that is capable of producing a toxic effect on cells. See also ANTINEOPLASTIC (2).

cytotoxin (si″to-tok′sin) [*cyto-* + *toxin*] a toxin or antibody that has a specific toxic action on cells of special organs.

cytotoxicity (si″to-tok-sis′ĭ-te) the quality of being capable of producing a specific toxic action on cells of special organs. **antibody dependent cellular c.,** cytotoxicity of cells coated with antibody by mononuclear cells which appear to be killer cells. Abbreviated *ADCC.*

cytotrophoblast (si″to-trof′o-blast) [*cyto-* + Gr. *trophē* nutrition + *blastos* germ] a thin inner cellular layer located next to the cavity of the blastocyst, formed by the trophoblast about seven to eleven days after fertilization. It gives rise to the syncytiotrophoblast. Called also *Langhan's layer.* See also TROPHOBLAST.

cytotropic (si″to-trop′ik) [*cyto-* + Gr. *tropos* a turning] attracting cells; possessing an affinity for cells; said especially of the antibodies responsible for immediate-type allergic reactions. See also cytotropic EFFECT.

Cytoxan trademark for *cyclophosphamide*.

cytozyme (si′to-zīm) [*cyto-* + Gr. *zymē* ferment] thromboplastin.

D

D 1. deuterium. 2. deciduous. 3. density. 4. diopter. 5. distal. 6. dorsal. 7. symbol for the units of vitamin D potency. 8. COEFFICIENT of diffusion. 9. dacryon.

D. abbreviation for L., *do′sis*, dose; *da*, give; *de′tur*, let it be given; *dexter*, right.

D- 1. a prefix signifying dextrorotatory. 2. a chemical prefix (small capital) which specifies that the substance corresponds in configuration to the standard substance D-glyceraldehyde, i.e., belongs to the same configurational family. In carbohydrate nomenclature, D refers to the configurational family of the *highest numbered* asymmetric carbon atom. In amino acid nomenclature, under rules adopted in 1947, D refers to the configurational family to which the *lowest numbered* asymmetric carbon atom, i.e., the 2-carbon or α-carbon belongs. Opposite of L-.

d deci-.

d- 1. a prefix signifying dextrorotatory. 2. a prefix used with one of the additional symbols .(+) or (−), especially in amino acid nomenclature in the literature from 1923 until approximately 1947, with reference to the configurational family to which the 2-carbon or α-carbon atom in the amino acid belongs, the actual direction of the rotation in a specific solvent being indicated by the plus or minus sign, as in *d*(−)alanine; opposed to *l*(+) or *l*(−), as in *l*(+)alanine or *l*(−)cystine. Now replaced by D-.

Δ the capital of the Greek letter delta.

δ the fourth letter of the Greek alphabet; see DELTA.

D-860 tolbutamide.

DA developmental AGE.

dac dacryon.

dacarbazine (dah-kar′bah-zēn) a triazene that functions as an alkylating agent, 5-(3,3-dimethyl-1-triazenyl)-1*H*-imidazole-4-carboxamide. Used principally in the treatment of malignant melanoma. Side effects include nausea, vomiting, bone marrow suppression with leukopenia and thrombocytopenia, and liver lesions. Called also *DIC* and *DTIC.*

dacry- see DACRYO-.

dacryo-, dacry- [Gr. *dakryon* tear] a combining form denoting relationship to tears.

dacryocyst (dak′re-o-sist″) [*dacryo-* + Gr. *kystis* sac] lacrimal SAC.

dacryocystorhinostenosis (dak″re-o-sis″to-ri″no-stĕ-no′sis) narrowing of the duct leading from the lacrimal sac to the nasal cavity.

dacryocystorhinostomy (dak″re-o-sis″to-ri-nos′to-me) [*dacryocyst*

+ Gr. *rhis* nose + *stomoun* to provide an opening, or mouth] surgical creation of a communication between the lacrimal sac and the nasal cavity. Called also *dacryorhinocystotomy* and *Toti's operation.*

dacryon (dak're-on) [Gr. *dakryon* tear] the craniometric point of junction of the anterior border of the lacrimal bone with the frontal bone and the maxilla on the medial orbital wall. Abbreviated *D* or *dac*. See illustration at CEPHALOMETRY.

dacryorhinocystotomy (dak"re-o-ri"no-sis-tot"o-me) dacryocystorhinostomy.

dacryosialoadenopathia (dak"re-o-si"ah-lo-ad"ĕ-nop'ah-the"ah) [*dacryo-* + Gr. *sialon* saliva + *adēn* gland + *pathos* disease + *-ia*] Sjögren's SYNDROME.

dacryosialocheilopathy (dak"re-o-si"ah-lo-ki-lop'ah-the). [*dacryo-* + Gr. *sialon* saliva + *cheilos* lip + *pathos* disease] Sjögren's SYNDROME.

dactinomycin (dak"tĭ-no-mi'sin) a cytotoxic antibiotic obtained from cultures of various species of *Streptomyces*, occurring as a bright red, photosensitive, crystalline powder that is soluble in ethanol and slightly soluble in water and ether. Used in the treatment of choriocarcinoma, Wilms' tumor, melanoma, and other cancers. The drug is locally toxic and cellulitis, phlebitis, and blood extravasation may occur at the site of injection. Other side effects may include anorexia, abdominal pain, diarrhea, gastrointestinal ulceration, proctitis, malaise, fatigue, lethargy, muscle pain, fever, skin eruptions, hyperpigmentation, erythema, anaphylaxis, susceptibility to infection, alopecia, and bone marrow depression with agranulocytosis, leukopenia, pancytopenia, thrombocytopenia, and anemia. Pharyngitis, esophagitis, and oral lesions, such as cheilitis, stomatitis, and ulcers, are common. Called also *actinomycin D* and *meractinomycin*. Trademarks: Cosmegen, Lyovac.

dactyl (dak'til) [Gr. *daktylos* a finger] a digit; a finger or toe.

dactyl- see DACTYLO-.

dactylo-, dactyl- [Gr. *daktylos* a digit] a combining form denoting relationship to a digit, usually referring to a finger but sometimes to a toe.

Dadex trademark for *dextroamphetamine sulfate* (see under DEXTROAMPHETAMINE).

Dagenan trademark for *sulfapyridine.*

dagga (dag'ah) a cannabinoid substance prepared from the plant *Cannabis sativa.*

Daguet ulceration see under ULCERATION.

Dagutan trademark for *soluble saccharin* (see under SACCHARIN).

Dakin's fluid, modified solution, solution [Henry Drysdale *Dakin,* American chemist, 1880–1952] sodium hypochlorite solution, diluted; see under SOLUTION.

Dalactine trademark for *clindamycin hydrochloride* (see under CLINDAMYCIN).

Dalbo attachment see under ATTACHMENT.

Dalbo extracoronal attachment (extracoronal unit) see under ATTACHMENT.

Dalbo stud attachment (stud unit) see under ATTACHMENT.

Dalla Bona attachment see under ATTACHMENT.

Dallacin C trademark for *clindamycin.*

Dalmane trademark for *flurazepam hydrochloride* (see under FLURAZEPAM).

dalton (dawl'ton) [named after John *Dalton*] a unit of mass, being one-sixteenth of the mass of the oxygen atom, or approximately 1.65×10^{-24} gm. See also MASS (3).

Dalton's law, atomic theory [John *Dalton,* English chemist and pharmacist, 1766–1844] see under LAW and THEORY. See also DALTON.

Dalzic trademark for *practolol.*

Dam, Charles Peter Henrik [born 1895] a Danish biochemist; co-winner, with Edward Adelbert Doisy, of the Nobel prize for medicine and physiology in 1945, for the isolation and synthesis of vitamin K.

dam (dam) 1. a barrier to obstruct the flow or water or other fluid. 2. rubber d. **rubber d.,** a sheet of latex rubber punched and placed over the teeth during dental procedures to isolate the field of operation from the rest of the oral cavity. Rubber dams are available in either rolls or precut sheets of various sizes, thickness, and color.

damar (dam'ar) dammar.

Dameshek, William [American physician, born 1900] see Estren-Dameshek SYNDROME.

dammar (dam'ar) a resinous exudate of *Dammara orientalis* and other varieties of pine trees in the East Indies and Philippines,

occurring as semitransparent, yellowish-white, friable masses with a melting point of about 120°C. It is soluble in alcohol, chloroform, ether, carbon disulfide, and oil of rosemary, partly soluble in turpentine, and insoluble in water. Used in dentistry in inlay casting to improve the smoothness of paraffin in molding and to render it more resistant to cracking and flaking, and to increase the toughness of dental waxes and to enhance their smoothness and luster. Also used in varnishes and for the preservation of tissue specimens for microscopy. Written also *damar*. Called *d. resin* and *gum d.* **gum d., d. resin,** dammar.

Danabol trademark for *methandrostenolone.*

Danantizol trademark for *methimazole.*

Danbolt-Closs syndrome [Niels Christian *Danbolt,* Norwegian dermatologist; Karl *Closs,* Norwegian physician] ACRODERMATITIS enteropathica.

Dane particle see under PARTICLE.

Danilone trademark for *phenindione.*

Danlos, Henri Alexandre [French dermatologist, 1844–1912] see Ehlers-Danlos SYNDROME.

Danten trademark for *phenytoin sodium* (see under PHENYTOIN).

Dantrium trademark for *dantrolene sodium* (see under DANTROLENE).

dantrolene (dan'tro-lēn) a skeletal muscle relaxant, 1-[[5-(p-nitrophenyl)furfurylidene]amino]hydantoin. **d. sodium,** the hemiheptahydrate sodium salt of dantrolene, occurring as a white or creamy, odorless, crystalline powder that is moderately soluble in acetone and methanol and slightly soluble in water. It is a skeletal muscle relaxant, used in the treatment of muscle spasms with pain in conditions such as fibrositis, bursitis, myositis, spondylitis, sprains, and other types of muscle diseases. Side effects are usually mild and include skin rashes, petechiae, nausea, vomiting, vertigo, malaise, headache, drowsiness and, rarely, hypersensitivity, jaundice and gastrointestinal bleeding. Trademark: Dantrium.

Danysz's phenomenon [Jan DANYSZ, Polish pathologist in Paris, 1860–1928] see under PHENOMENON.

Dapotum trademark for *fluphenazine hydrochloride* (see under FLUPHENAZINE).

dapsone (dap'sōn) the parent compound of the sulfones, 4,4'-sulfonyldianiline, occurring as a white or creamy white, odorless, slightly bitter crystalline powder that is slightly soluble in water and freely soluble in alcohol, acetone, and dilute mineral acids. It has bacteriostatic properties, being most effective against *Mycobacterium tuberculosis* and *M. leprae.* Used with limited success in the treatment of tuberculosis and, more effectively, of leprosy. Untoward effects may include hemolytic reaction, methemoglobinemia, anorexia, nausea, vomiting, headache, nervousness, insomnia, blurred vision, paresthesia, reversible neuropathy, pruritus, rash, and drug fever. Called also *diaminodiphenylsulfone (DDS).* Trademark: Eporal.

d'Arcet's metal [Jean *d'Arcet,* French physician and chemist, 1727–1801) see under METAL.

Daricon trademark for *oxyphencyclimine hydrochloride* (see under OXYPHENCYCLIMINE).

Darier's disease [Jean Ferdinand *Darier,* French dermatologist, 1856–1938] 1. KERATOSIS follicularis. 2. PSEUDOXANTHOMA elasticum.

darkroom (dark'room) dark ROOM.

Darling's disease [Samuel Taylor *Darling,* American physician, 1872–1925] histoplasmosis.

Darvocet-N trademark for analgesic preparations containing chiefly propoxyphene napsylate and acetaminophen.

Darvon trademark for analgesic preparations containing *propoxyphene hydrochloride* (see under PROPOXYPHENE). *Darvon with A.S.A.* is a mixture of propoxyphene hydrochloride and aspirin. *Darvon compound* contains 32 mg propoxyphene hydrochloride, 227 mg aspirin, 162 mg phenacetin, and 32.4 mg caffeine; *Darvon compound-65* has the same formulation except that it contains 65 mg propoxyphene hydrochloride.

Darvon-N trademark for analgesic preparations containing *propoxyphene napsylate* (see under PROPOXYPHENE). *Darvon-N with A.S.A.* is a mixture of propoxyphene napsylate and aspirin.

Darwin's theory [Charles Robert *Darwin,* English naturalist, 1809–1882] darwinism.

darwinian (dar-win'e-an) named for Charles Robert *Darwin,* as darwinian apex (see under APEX) or darwinian theory (see DARWINISM).

darwinism (dar'wĭ-nizm) [named after C. R. *Darwin*] the theory of evolution according to which higher organisms have been developed from lower ones through the influence of natural selection. Called also *Darwin's theory* and *darwinian theory.*

DAT dental aptitude test.

data (da'tah) [L.] plural of *datum*.

DATE dental auxiliary teacher education.

datum (da'tum), pl. *da'ta* [L.] 1. a term usually used in the plural form (*data*) to denote any or all facts, information, statistics, and the like either historical or derived by calculation or experimentation. 2. in computer technology, basic element of information that can be processed or produced by a computer. **d. symptom,** datum SYMPTOM.

Datura (da-tu'rah) a genus of solanaceous plants, the best known of which is *D. stramonium*. Its chief constituents are alkaloids hyoscyamine and scopolamine.

DAU Dental Auxiliary Utilization; a program sponsored by the Division of Dental Health, Department of Health and Human Services, designed to aid dental schools in training dental students to utilize trained, full-time chairside assistants, a practice referred to as "four-handed dentistry." See also dental assistant, extended function. under ASSISTANT, and TEAM.

Daubenton's angle, plane (line) [Lous Jean Marie *Daubenton*, French physician and naturalist, 1716–1800] see under ANGLE and PLANE.

daughter (daw'ter) 1. a female offspring. See also PEDIGREE. 2. daughter CELL. 3. decay PRODUCT.

daunomycin (daw-no-mi'sin) daunorubicin.

daunorubicin (daw-no-ru'bĭ-sin) a cytotoxic antibiotic isolated from cultures of *Streptomyces peucetius*, (8*S-cis*)-8-acetyl-10-[(3-amino- 2,3,6-trideoxy-α-L-lyxo-hexopyranosyl) oxy]-7,8,9,10-tetrahydro- 6,8,11 - trihydroxy - 1 - methoxy - 5,12 - naphthacenedione. It occurs as thin red needles that are soluble in alcoholic solutions and water, but not in nonpolar organic solvents. Used chiefly in the treatment of leukemias. Adverse reactions may include bone marrow depression with leukopenia and thrombocytopenia; hemorrhagic tendency; predisposition to infection; cardiovascular disorders, including arrhythmias, tachycardia, hypotension, and congestive heart failure; gastrointestinal disorders, such as hemorrhagic enterocolitis, vomiting, nausea, and abdominal pain; phlebitis; fever; anorexia; skin rash; and stomatitis. Called also *daunomycin* and rubidomycin. Trademark: Cerubidin.

da Vinci, Leonardo [1452–1519] an eminent Italian painter, inventor, sculptor, architect, musician, engineer, mathematician, scientist, and anatomist. He gave the first accurate representation of the skull, teeth, and related structures and the earliest description of articulation of the teeth, and established that the head is one-eighth the height of the body.

Davis crown see under CROWN.

Davosin trademark for *sulfamethoxypyridazine*.

Davoxin trademark for *digoxin*.

DAW dispense as written.

Day, Richard Lawrence [American physician, born 1905] see Riley-Day SYNDROME.

Dazzle trademark for an aqueous solution of *sodium hypochlorite* (see under SODIUM).

db decibel.

DBDG distobuccal developmental GROOVE.

DC 1. direct CURRENT. 2. Doctor of Chiropractic (see CHIROPRACTOR).

DD developmental DISABILITY.

o,p'-DDD mitotane.

DDM dichlorophen.

DDPA Delta Dental Plans Association (see under ASSOCIATION).

DDS 1. Doctor of Dental Surgery (see under DOCTOR). 2. dapsone.

DDSc Doctor of Dental Science.

DDT dichlorodiphenyltrichlorothane; see CHLOROPHENOTHANE.

DE dose EQUIVALENT.

de- [L. *de* down, from] a prefix signifying down or from; it is sometimes negative or primitive, and is frequently intensive.

deactivation (de"ak-tĭ-va'shun) the act or process of rendering or becoming inactive.

dead (ded) 1. destitute of life; deceased. See also DEATH. 2. numb.

deaf (def) lacking the sense of hearing or not having the full power of hearing.

deafferentate (de-af'er-en-tāt") to eliminate or interrupt afferent nerve impulses, as by destruction of the afferent pathway.

deaf-mutism (def-mut'izm) the absence of both of the sense of hearing and of the faculty of speech.

deafness (def'nes) lack or loss, complete or partial, of the sense of hearing. Moderate loss of hearing is often called *hearing loss* or *hypoacusis*. See also DYSACUSIS. **central d.,** that due to causes in the auditory pathways or in the auditory center of the brain. **conduction d.,** that due to a defect of the sound-conducting apparatus. Called also *transmission d.* **nerve d., neural d.,** that which is due to a lesion of the auditory nerve or the central neural pathways. **postlingual d.,** that acquired after the development of speech. **prelingual d.,** that acquired before the development of speech. **transmission d.,** conduction d.

dealer (de'ler) one who buys and sells articles. **dental d.,** a distributor of dental equipment and materials.

de Almeida's disease [Floriano Paulo *de Almeida*, Brazilian physician] South American BLASTOMYCOSIS.

deamination (de-am"ĭ-na'shun) the removal of the amino group (−NH₂) from a compound. Cf. TRANSAMINATION. **oxidative d.,** the splitting off of the amino group (NH₂) of an amino acid with the formation of ammonia and a keto acid. It is a catabolic process that is catalyzed by amino acid oxidase, as shown in the formula:

$$R-\underset{\underset{\text{amino acid}}{NH_2}}{\underset{|}{CH}}-COOH \xrightarrow[\text{FAD FADH}]{\overset{\text{amino acid}}{\text{oxidase}}} R-\underset{\underset{\text{imino acid}}{NH}}{\overset{\|}{C}}-COOH \xrightarrow[H_2O]{\text{hydrolysis}}$$

$$R-\underset{\underset{O}{\|}}{C}-COOH + NH_3$$

keto acid

See also TRANSAMINATION.

Dean and Webb titration see under TITRATION.

deaquation (de"ah-kwa'shun) [L. *de*, from *aqua* water] dehydration.

de Arculis see ARCOLANO.

death (deth) the cessation of life. **brain d.,** irreversible cessation of all vital activities of the brain, as determined by stoppage of brain waves on the electroencephalograph; used to establish the time of somatic death. **cell d.,** cessation of vital processes in a cell, due to irreversible damage to structural and metabolic integrity. The terms *cell death* and *necrosis* are often used interchangeably, but *necrosis* is also used in connection with morphologic changes that follow cell death. Called also *necrocytosis*. **pulp d.,** see necrotic PULP. **somatic d.,** permanent cessation of all vital activities in the body. Traditionally, the legal time of death was established with the cessation of respiratory functions; recently, the cessation of heart function was used as the determining factor of death; and more recently, the cessation of brain activities (brain death) was established as the determining factor. **time of d.,** see *somatic d.*

debanding (de-band'ing) the removal of the bands of a fixed orthodontic appliance.

De Barsy-Moens-Dierckx syndrome [A. M. *De Barsy*; E. *Moens*; L. *Dierckx*] see under SYNDROME.

Debenal trademark for *sulfadiazine*.

Debenal M trademark for *sulfamerazine*.

debility (dĕ-bil'ĭ-te) lack or loss of strength.

débouchement (da-boosh-maw') [Fr.] an opening out.

de Boyer see BOYER.

Debré's syndrome [Robert *Debré*, French physician] cat-scratch DISEASE. See also Abderhalden-Fanconi SYNDROME (Fanconi-De Toni-Debré syndrome).

débridement (da-brĕd'maw) [Fr.] 1. removal of foreign matter, including devitalized tissue in or around a wound. 2. progressive elimination of organic and inorganic debris within the root canal by mechanical instrumentation and/or chemical means. **canal d.,** root canal d. **cavity d.,** cavity TOILET. **chemical d.,** irrigation of a cavity with a disinfecting solution capable of dissolving organic matter to remove necrotic tissue and other debris, as in the preparation of the endodontic cavity in root canal therapy. **epithelial d.,** removal of the entire inner lining and the epithelial attachment from a gingival or periodontal pocket in gingival curettage. Called also *de-epithelization*. **root canal d.,** the elimination of debris and other foreign matter present in the root canal by mechanical or chemical means, including extirpation of diseased dental pulp and cleaning and sterilization of the empty canal in root canal therapy. Called also *canal d.* See also PULPECTOMY and PULPOTOMY. **surgical d.,** that done with the use of a surgical instrument. **wound d.,** cleaning of a wound by removing the superficial layer of tissue that has been contaminated, traumatized, or necrotized.

debris (dĕ-bre') [Fr.] accumulated fragments; rubbish. **d. index,** see oral hygiene INDEX. **organic d.,** remnants and breakdown products from degeneration of necrotic tissue or microorganisms, such as those found in the root canal. **food d.,** accumulated food particles in various recesses of the oral cavity or loosely attached to mucous membranes and tooth surfaces, providing a terrain for the development of dental plaque.

debug (de-bug') to locate and correct an error in a computer program or an electrical or mechanical defect in the computer. See also BUG.

Dec. abbreviation for L. *decan'ta,* pour off.

deca- [Gr. *deka* ten] see DEKA-.

decacurie (dek"ah-ku're) [Gr. *deka* ten + *curie*] a unit of radioactivity, being 10 curies.

decagram (dek'ah-gram) dekagram.

decalcification (de"kal-sĭ-fi-ka'shun) 1. the loss of calcium salts from a bone or tooth. See also CHELATION (2). 2. the process of removing calcareous matter.

decaliter (dek'ah-le"ter) dekaliter.

decameter (dek'ah-me"ter) dekameter.

decamethonium bromide (dek"ah-mĕ-tho'ne-um) a muscle relaxant, decamethylenebis (trimethyl ammonium bromide), occurring as a crystalline substance that is freely soluble in water and ethanol, slightly soluble in chloroform, and insoluble in ether. Initially, it produces nicotinic depolarization at the motor end-plate membrane, followed by spontaneous firing by muscle fibers, causing muscular fibrillation and fasciculation. Used chiefly during short surgical procedures and in manipulation. Side effects may include muscle pain, respiratory depression, apnea, potassium loss, excess salivation, hypertension or hypotension, bradycardia or tachycardia, hypothermia, paralysis, hypermagnesemia, and cardiac arrest. Trademark: Syncurine.

decane (dek'an) a ten-carbon straight chain hydrocarbon of the methane series, $C_{10}H_{22}$, occurring as a colorless, flammable liquid. Used in organic synthesis, as a solvent, and in various chemical processes. Inhalation of fumes may cause narcosis.

decanormal (dek"ah-nor'mal) dekanormal.

decantation (de"kan-ta'shun) [*de-* + L. *canthus* tire of a wheel] the pouring of a clear supernatant liquid from a sediment.

decapeptide (dek"ah-pep'tīd) [*deca-* + *peptide*] a polypeptide containing 10 amino acids.

Decapryn trademark for *doxylamine succinate* (see under DOXYLAMINE).

decarboxylase [E.C.4.1.1] (de"kar-bok'sĭ-lās) [*de-* + *carboxyl* + *-ase*] a subclass of lyases, and a subclass of carbon-carbon lyases, including enzymes that catalyze the removal of the carboxyl group of alpha-keto acids yielding carbon dioxide.

decarboxylation (de"kar-bok'sĭ-la'shun) removal of the carboxyl group from a compound.

decay (de-ka') [*de-* + L. *cadere* to fall] 1. the gradual decomposition of dead organic matter. 2. the process or stage of decline; old age and its effects on the mind and body. **aerobic d.,** decomposition of organic matter by bacteria in the presence of oxygen. **anaerobic d.,** decomposition of organic matter by microorganisms in the absence of oxygen. **beta d.,** disintegration of the nucleus of an unstable radionuclide in which the mass number is unchanged, but the atomic number is increased by 1, as result of emission of a negatively or positively charged (beta) particle and a neutrino. **d. constant,** decay CONSTANT. **natural d.,** the process whereby radioactive elements lose nuclear particles and energy and become stable elements, ranging from a few minutes to several billion years. **d. product,** decay PRODUCT. **radioactive d.,** the spontaneous transformation of one nuclide into a different nuclide or into a different energy state of the same nuclide, involving the emission from the nucleus of alpha particles, beta particles (or electrons), or gamma rays; or the nuclear capture or ejection of orbital electrons. Called also *radioactive disintegration.* **senile d.,** senile CARIES. **tooth d.,** dental CARIES.

Decentan trademark for *perphenazine.*

Decholin trademark for *dehydrocholic acid* (see under ACID).

Decholin Sodium trademark for *sodium dehydrocholate* (see dehydrocholic ACID).

deci- [L. *decem* ten] in the metric system, a combining form denoting one-tenth (10^{-1}) of the unit designated by the root with which it is combined. Abbreviated *d.* See also metric SYSTEM and *Tables of Weights and Measures* at WEIGHT.

decibel (des'ĭ-bel) [*deci-* + *bel* unit of sound] a unit used to express the ratio of two powers, usually electric or acoustic powers, equal to one-tenth the common logarithm of the ratio of the powers. One decibel is equal approximately to the smallest difference in acoustic power that the human ear can detect. Abbreviated *db.* See also BEL.

Decicain trademark for *tetracaine hydrochloride* (see under TETRACAINE).

decidua (de-sid'u-ah) [L., from *deciduus* falling off] the endometrium of the pregnant uterus, all of which, except the deepest layer, is shed at parturition. For implantation through the first three months of pregnancy, it is divided into the basal, capsular, and parietal decidua. Called also *membrana deciduae* [NA]. **basal d., d. basa'lis** [NA], the portion of the decidua directly underlying the chorionic vesicle and attached to the myometrium. **capsular d., d. capsula'ris** [NA], the portion of the decidua directly overlying the chorionic vesicle and facing the uterine cavity. **parietal d., d. parieta'lis** [NA], the portion of the decidua lining the uterus elsewhere than at the site of attachment of the chorionic vesicle.

deciduous (de-sid'u-us) [*de-* + L. *cedere* to fall] that which will fall off or shed; pertaining to an organ or part which serves a temporary purpose, such as deciduous teeth (see under TOOTH).

decigram (des'ĭ-gram) [*deci-* + *gram*] a unit of mass (weight) in the metric system, being one-tenth (10^{-1}) of a gram, or the equivalent of 1.544 grains. Abbreviated *dg.* See also metric SYSTEM and *Tables of Weights and Measures* at WEIGHT.

deciliter (des'ĭ-le"ter) [*deci-* + *liter*] a unit of volume in the metric system, being one-tenth (10^{-1}) of a liter and consisting of 10 centiliters. It is equivalent to 3.38 fluid ounces or 6.1028 cubic inches.

decimal (des'ĭ-mal) pertaining to tenths or the number 10. See decimal SYSTEM. See also METRIC.

decimeter (des'ĭ-me"ter) [*deci-* + *meter*] a unit of length in the metric system, being one-tenth (10^{-1}) of a meter and equal to 3.937 inches.

decinem (des'ĭ-nem) [*deci-* + *nem*] the unit of nutrition, being one-tenth (10^{-1}) of a nem. Abbreviated *dn.* See also NEM.

decinormal (des"ĭ-nor'mal) [*deci-* + L. *norma* rule] having one-tenth of the normal strength; said of solutions.

Declomycin trademark for *demeclocycline.*

decoagulant (de"ko-ag'u-lant) 1. reducing the amount of existing coagulants or precoagulants in the blood. 2. a substance which inhibits coagulation of blood by reducing the amount of existing coagulants or procoagulants.

Decoct. abbreviation for L. *decoc'tum,* a decoction.

decoction (de-kok'shun) [L. *decoctum,* from *de* down + *coquere* to boil] 1. the act or process of boiling. 2. a medicine or other substance prepared by boiling. Called also *apozem.*

decoctum (de-kok'tum) [L.] a decoction.

decoloration (de-kul"or-a'shun) 1. removal of color; bleaching. 2. lack or loss of color.

decompensation (de"kom-pen-sa'shun) 1. inability to compensate for a defect. 2. heart failure, congestive; see under FAILURE. **cardiac d.,** heart failure, congestive; see under FAILURE.

decomposition (de"kom-po-zish'un) [*de-* + L. *componere* to put together] 1. the separation of compound bodies into their constituent principles. 2. the breaking down of a chemical substance into simpler constituents.

decompression (de"kom-presh'un) 1. the removal of pressure. 2. the slow lessening of pressure on deep-sea divers to prevent the onset of the bends. See also decompression SICKNESS. **explosive d.,** a sudden decrease of atmospheric pressure as occurs in an aircraft when there is a loss of cabin pressure. Explosive decompression from sea level pressure to barometric pressure equaling that at above 50,000 feet in humans and to an almost complete vacuum in animals produces few clinical symptoms, except for the sudden increase of gases in the gastrointestinal tract. See also decompression SICKNESS. **nerve d.,** the relief of pressure on a nerve by the surgical widening of the bony canal or by removal of the constricting fibrous or bony tissue. **subtemporal d.,** cerebral decompression after removal of a portion of the temporal bone.

Decomycin trademark for *demeclocycline.*

decongestant (de"kon-jes'tant) 1. tending to reduce congestion or swelling. 2. an agent that reduces congestion or swelling.

decontamination (de"kon-tam-ĭ-na'shun) the freeing of a person or an object of contaminating substances, such as gases, radioactive material, etc.

decortication (de"kor-tĭ-ka'shun) [*de-* + L. *cortex* bark] 1. the removal of the bark, hull, husk, or shell from a plant, seed, or root, as in pharmacy. 2. removal of portions of the cortical substance of a structure or organ.

Decortin trademark for *prednisone.*

decrudescence (de"kroo-des'ens) diminution or abatement of the intensity of symptoms.

Decub. abbreviation for L. *decu'bitus,* lying down.

decubation (de″ku-ba′shun) [*de-* + L. *cubare* to lie down] the period in the course of an infectious disease from the disappearance of the symptoms to complete recovery and the end of the infectious period. Cf. INCUBATION.

decubitus (de-ku′bĭ-tus) [L. "a lying down"] an act of lying down; also the position assumed by lying down.

decuspation (de″kusp-a′shun) removal or complete reduction of the cusp of a tooth.

decussate (de-kus′āt) [L. *decussare* to cross in the form of an X] 1. to cross or intersect in the form of the letter X. 2. crossing in the form of the letter X.

decussation (de″kus-sa′shun) [L. *decussatio*] a general anatomical term for the intercrossing of fellow parts or structures in the form of an X.

dedentition (de″den-tish′un) [*de-* + L. *dens* tooth] the shedding or loss of teeth.

dedifferentiation (de-dif″er-en″she-a′shun) reverse differentiation; loss of differentiation. See also ANAPLASIA.

de d. in d. abbreviation for L. *de di′e in di′em*, from day to day.

deductible (de-duk′tĭ-b′l) 1. that which can be or is capable of being deducted. 2. deductible clause, common; see under CLAUSE. **d. amount,** deductible clause, common; see under CLAUSE. **annual d.,** deductible clause, annual; see under CLAUSE. **family d.,** deductible clause, family; see under CLAUSE. **lifetime d.,** deductible clause, lifetime; see under CLAUSE.

Dee-Eighteen trademark for an extra hard *dental casting gold alloy* (see under GOLD).

Deelastic trademark for *reversible hydrocolloid impression material* (see under MATERIAL).

Deeone trademark for a soft *dental casting gold alloy* (see under GOLD).

Deepep-Hard trademark for a high noble metal dental wrought gold wire alloy.

de-epithelization (de″ep″ĭ-the″li-za′shun) epithelial DÉBRIDEMENT.

Deesix trademark for a hard *dental casting gold alloy* (see under GOLD).

Deetwo trademark for medium hard *dental casting gold alloy* (see under GOLD).

DEF see DEF RATE.

defalcation (de″fal-ka′shun) 1. misappropriation. 2. root canal, C-shaped; see under CANAL.

defecation (def′ē-ka′shun) [L. *defaecare* to deprive of dregs] the evacuation of feces from the intestine.

defect (de′fekt) [L. *defectus* lack, failure] an imperfection, lack, or failure. **acquired d.,** an imperfection arising secondarily, after birth; not congenital. **birth d.,** congenital d. **bone d.,** 1. any abnormal structural bony change; osseous defect. 2. periodontal bony d. **congenital d.,** one present at birth, having developed

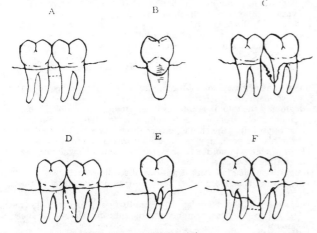

Osseous defects. *A* and *B*, An interproximal crater, a cup-shaped defect in the interalveolar bone. *C*, An interproximal hemiseptum, interalveolar bone destroyed on one tooth without affecting bone on the contiguous tooth. Loss of marginal bone caused a deep V-shaped inconsistent margin. *D*, An intrabony defect, a hemiseptum, and marginal bone on the vestibular and lingual surfaces form three bony walls; the tooth root is the fourth wall. *E*, A furca invasion with destruction of marginal bone causing an inconsistent margin. *F*, A periodontal defect in marginal bone with interalveolar bone destruction forming a crater apical to the margin. (From J. Prichard: Advanced Periodontal Disease. 2nd ed. Philadelphia, W. B. Saunders Co., 1972.)

during intrauterine life. Called also *birth d.* **Frenkel d.,** a point defect in which an ion leaves its normal site, leaving a vacancy, and forms an interstitial defect (see *point d.*). **interstitial d.,** see *point d.* **intrabony d.,** a defect produced by bone resorption around the teeth in the vicinity of those which are affected with destructive periodontitis caused by bacterial plaque. Called also *periodontal intrabony d.* See also intrabony POCKET. See illustration. **Laki-Lórand d.,** see FACTOR XIII. **line d.,** dislocation (2). **osseous d.,** 1. any abnormal structural bony change; bony defect. 2. periodontal bony d. **periodontal bony d.,** an abnormal change in the form or contour of the bony structures of the tooth socket (alveolus), caused by periodontal disease. The most common periodontal bony defects include crater formation and hemiseptum of the interalveolar bone, intrabony defects, defects in marginal bone, and interradicular defects, including furca invasion. Called also *bone* and *osseous d.* See illustration. **periodontal interradicular d.,** a periodontal bone defect occurring in the furcae of multirooted teeth, including furca invasion. **periodontal intrabony d.,** intrabony d. **periodontal d. in marginal bone,** an osseous defect in the tooth socket (alveolus) in the marginal bone, usually a vertical defect caused by uneven resorption of marginal bone; an inconsistent margin. See illustration. **point d.,** a defect in the atomic structure of a crystallographic solid, due to the presence of foreign atoms or to the absence of atoms in the space lattice. One due to the substitution of original atoms in the structure with foreign atoms is known as a *substitutional defect;* one in which foreign atoms occur in interstitial spaces is known as an *interstitial defect;* and one in which atoms are absent in the lattice is known as a *vacancy defect.* Each structure has a limit for the maximum amount of foreign atoms and, when this limit is reached, the structure is said to have reached the solubility limit (the crystallographic solid being considered a solution in which foreign atoms are the solute) and the solid undergoes a phase change. The presence of foreign atoms results in hardening of the solid. Point defects are produced artificially in alloying metals. **Prower d.,** FACTOR X deficiency. **Schottky d.,** a point defect in which equal numbers of anion and cation vacancies occur to preserve electrical neutrality. **septal d.,** a congenital heart defect consisting of an anomalous communication between the heart chambers through a septum, thereby diverting the blood from its circulatory routes. **speech d.,** any deviation of speech which is outside the range of acceptable variation in a given environment. **Stafne mandibular d.,** static bone CYST. **Stuart d.,** FACTOR X deficiency. **substitutional d.,** see *point d.* **vacancy d.,** see *point d.*

deferent (def′er-ent) [L. *deferens* carrying away] conveying anything away, as from a center.

deferoxamine (de″-fer-oks′ah-mēn) a chelating agent for iron mobilization isolated from *Streptomyces pilosus*, N - [5 - 3 [[(5-aminopentyl) hydroxycarbamoyl] propionamido] pentyl - 3 - [[5-(N - hydroxyacetamido) pentyl] carbamoyl] propionohydroxamic acid. **d. mesylate, d. methanesulfonate,** the methanesulfonate salt of deferoxamine, occurring as water-soluble white crystals. It is a chelating agent specific for iron, used in the treatment of severe iron poisoning and iron storage disease. Side effects may include pain and induration at the site of intramuscular injection, flushing, diarrhea, erythema, visual disorders, gastrointestinal disorders, itching, muscle spasm, anaphylaxis, tachycardia, and fever. Trademark; Desferal.

defervescence (def″er-ves′ens) [L. *defervescere* to cease boiling] the period of abatement of fever.

defibrillation (de-fib″rĭ-la′shun) 1. termination of atrial or ventricular fibrillation, usually by electroshock. 2. separation of fibers of a tissue by blunt dissection.

defibrination (de-fi″brĭ-na′-shun) deprival of fibrin.

deficiency (de-fish′en-se) a lack or defect. See also INSUFFICIENCY. For specific deficiencies, see the essential factor, as FACTOR XII, IRON, RIBOFLAVIN, etc. **Ac-globulin d.,** parahemophilia. **antibody d.,** immunodeficiency. **antibody d. syndrome,** agammaglobulinemia. **ascorbic acid d.,** scurvy. **beta-lipoprotein d.,** acanthocytosis. **calcium d.,** hypocalcemia. **d. of complement,** deficiency of COMPLEMENT. **copper d.,** 1. Menkes' SYNDROME. 2. microcytic ANEMIA. **factor I d.,** see AFIBRINOGENEMIA and HYPOFIBRINOGENEMIA. **factor II d.,** hypoprothrombinemia. **factor V d.,** hypoprothrombinemia. **factor V d., congenital,** see de Vries' SYNDROME and PARAHEMOPHILIA. **factor VII d.,** hypoprothrombinemia. **factor VII d., congenital,** see FACTOR VII. **factor VIII d.,** HEMOPHILIA A. **factor X d.,** see FACTOR X. **factor XI d.,** see FACTOR XI. **factor XII d.,** see FACTOR XII. **factor**

XIII d., see FACTOR XIII. **familial HDL d.,** Tangier DISEASE. **fibrinogen d.,** see AFIBRINOGENEMIA and HYPOFIBRINOGENEMIA. **Hageman d.,** see FACTOR XII. **iron d. anemia,** see iron deficiency ANEMIA. **labile factor d.,** parahemophilia. **mental d.,** former name for mental RETARDATION. **nicotinamide, nicotinic acid d.,** pellagra. **plasma thromboplastin antecedent d.,** see FACTOR XI. **potassium d.,** hypophosphatasia. **prothrombin d.,** hypoprothrombinemia. **proaccelerin d.,** parahemophilia. **PTA d.,** see FACTOR XI. **PTC d.,** Christmas DISEASE. **PTF-A d.,** HEMOPHILIA A. **PTF-B d.,** Christmas DISEASE. **PTF-C d.,** see FACTOR XI. **vertical maxillary d.,** short face SYNDROME. **vitamin C d.,** scurvy. **vitamin D d.,** rickets. **maxillary d., vertical,** short face SYNDROME.

deficit (def'ĭ-sit) a lack or deficiency.

definition (def'ĭ-nish'un) 1. the clear determination of the limits of anything. 2. image d. **image d.,** the distinctness or sharpness of fine detail on an image, as that of a radiograph. See also PENUMBRA, RESOLUTION (2), and UMBRA.

deflection (de-flek'shun) 1. a bending or turning aside. 2. a turning from a true course or straight line. 3. the deviation of an indicator of an instrument from the position taken as zero. **beam d.,** the distance which at a given point on a beam moves as the beam is under load, usually measured at the point where deflection is greatest (maximum deflection). **maximum d.,** the greatest degree of deflection under a given load.

deformation (de"for-ma'shun) 1. deformity. 2. the process of adaptation of material to stresses. At stresses below the proportional limit, the atoms in the crystal lattice are displaced in amount only so that, when the stress is relieved, they can return to their original position; once the proportional limit is exceeded, a permanent deformation takes place and the structure does not return to its original dimensions when the load is released, eventually resulting in displacement of atoms that is sufficiently extensive to produce a fracture. **elastic d.,** a temporary change of shape brought about by a mechanical force within the elastic (proportional) limit of the material under stress, with recovery to the original shape and dimension on removing the deforming force. The stress, being below the proportional limit, causes the atoms in the crystal lattice to be displaced in amount only so that, when it is relieved, they return to their original position. See also STRESS. **inelastic d.,** plastic d. **permanent d.,** plastic d. **plastic d.,** a permanent change of shape or dimension brought about by a mechanical force greater than the elastic (proportional) limit of the material under stress; the material will not recover its original shape on removing the deforming force. The stress, exceeding the proportional limit, causes the atoms in the crystal lattice to be displaced to the extent where they can no longer return to their original position in the crystal lattice. Should the stress continue, the displacement of atoms may become sufficiently extensive to result in a fracture. Called also *permanent d., inelastic d.,* and *permanent d.* See also mechanical STRESS.

deformity (de-for'mĭ-te) [L. *deformitas*] a misshapen form or condition; a disfigurement; a distortion of any part of the body. Called also *deformation.* See also ABNORMALITY and MALFORMATION. **Arnold-Chiari d.,** protrusion of the cerebellum and medulla oblongata through the foramen magnum into the cervical spinal canal; it may result in stenosis of the aqueduct of Sylvius, obstructive hydrocephalus, and atrophy of brain tissue. Deformity of the occipital bone and cervical vertebrae, platybasia, Klippel-Feil anomaly, softening and deformity of the cranial bones, meningocele, meningomyelocele, spina bifida, nystagmus, diplopia, papilledema, adhesive arachnoiditis, hemianopia, and cerebellar ataxia are the principal complications. **Sprengel's d.,** a congenital disorder, often associated with other abnormalities characterized by elevation of the scapula with rotation of its lower angle toward the spine, scoliosis, and sometimes an accessory bone between the scapula and the cervical spine. The arm on the affected side cannot be raised above a right angle.

Deg. degeneration; degree.

degassing (de-gas'ing) 1. to free from gas. 2. the volatilization of foreign matter from the surface of metals, as in the heat treatment of gold foil in rendering it cohesive. See ANNEALING (3).

degeneratio (de-jen"er-a'she-o) [L.] degeneration.

degeneration (de-jen"er-a'shun) [L. *degeneratio*] 1. reversible cell injuries. 2. change from a higher to a lower form; especially change of tissue to a lower or less functionally active form. When there is chemical change of the tissue itself, it is *true*

degeneration; when the change consists of the deposit of abnormal matter in the tissues, it is *infiltration.* Continuous degenerative processes over a prolonged period lead to cell death or necrosis. Called also *retrogression.* **adipose d.,** fatty d. **calcareous d.,** degeneration with infiltration of calcareous materials into the tissue. Called also *earthy d.* **calcific d.,** diffuse pulp CALCIFICATION. **colloid d.,** that in which the tissues assume a gummy gelatinous nature. Called also *gelatiniform d.* **dystrophic d.,** that arising from defective nutrition. **earthy d.,** calcareous d. **fatty d.,** that caused by the accumulation of fat within cells, due to incapacity of the cells to metabolize or mobilize normal amounts of lipids as a result of prior injury to the cell. Called also *adipose d.* See also fatty INFILTRATION. **fibrinoid d.,** accumulation in connective tissue or blood vessel walls of substances similar to precipitated fibrin, being a variety of plasma proteins, including fibrin, albumin, globulins, immunoglobulins, and complement. It appears most often in foci of immunologic injury. **fibrous d.,** fibrosis. **fibrous pulp d.,** pulp FIBROSIS. **gelatiniform d.,** colloid d. **hepatolenticular d.,** a hereditary syndrome, transmitted as an autosomal recessive trait, in which a decrease of ceruloplasmin produces accumulation of copper, chiefly in the brain, but also in the liver, kidneys, and cornea. Intellectual deterioration, dystonia, abnormal posturing, tremor at rest, clumsiness and, later, flapping tremor, rigidity, dysarthria, high-pitched voice, intermittent incoherence, and facial symptoms, including a set expression of the face with an open drooling mouth and the teeth exposed in a grimacing smile, are the principal symptoms. Called also *Kinnier Wilson's disease* and *Wilson's disease.* **hyaline d.,** regressive cellular changes in which the cytoplasm takes on a homogenous glassy, eosinophilic appearance. Called also *vitreous d.* and *hyalinosis.* **mucoid d.,** degeneration characterized by extracellular accumulation of mucopolysaccharide ground substance within connective tissue; not considered by some pathologists as a true form of degeneration. **mucous d.,** that in which mucus accumulates in epithelial tissue. **myxomatous d.,** accumulations of ground substance containing a variety of mucopolysaccharides synthesized by mesenchymal cells; not considered by some pathologists as a true form of degeneration. **progressive pyramidopallidal d.,** Lhermitte-Cornil-Quesnel SYNDROME. **pulp d.,** a progressive pathologic change in the dental pulp to a less functionally active form. **pulp d., atrophic,** pulp ATROPHY. **pulp d., calcific,** pulp d., dystrophic. **pulp d., diffuse calcific,** a degenerative condition of the dental pulp, associated with irregular calcific deposits that usually follow collagenous fiber bundles or blood vessels. Some deposits form large bodies but they also may form fine spicules. The deposits are usually located in the radicular portion of the pulp, generally being amorphous in structure. **pulp d., dystrophic,** a dystrophic condition of the dental pulp associated with calcific deposits in the pulp. Called also *calcific pulp d.* **sclerotic d.,** a variety of hyaline degeneration affecting connective tissue, especially the intima of arteries. **senile d.,** widespread degenerative changes, principally fibroid and atheromatous, which occur in old age. **true d.,** see DEGENERATION (2). **vitreous d.,** hyaline d.

degenerative (de-jen'er-ah-tive) of or pertaining to degeneration.

de Gimbard's syndrome [Martin Jules Louis Alexander *de Gimbard,* born 1858] see under SYNDROME.

degloving (de-gluv'ing) intra-oral surgical exposure of the bony mandibular structures, as by rolling the lower lip and vestibular soft tissue over the chin to expose the symphysis. The operation can also be performed in the posterior region if necessary.

Deglut. abbreviation for L. *deglutia'tur,* let it be swallowed.

deglutible (de-gloo'tĭ-b'l) capable of being swallowed.

deglutition (deg"loo-tish'un) the act of swallowing.

deglutitory (de-gloo'tĭ-to"re) pertaining to or promoting deglutition.

degradation (deg"rah-da'shun) the reduction of a chemical compound to one less complex, as by splitting off one or more groups.

degree (de-gre') 1. a grade or rank awarded scholars by a college or university. 2. a unit of measure of temperature. Symbol, °. 3. a unit of measure or arcs and angles. **d. of polymerization,** degree of POLYMERIZATION.

degustation (de"gus-ta'shun) [L. *degustatio*] the act or function of tasting.

dehiscence (de-his'ens) [L. *dehiscere* to gape] a splitting open. **alveolar d.,** root d. **root d.,** an isolated area in which the root of a tooth is denuded by bone, the denuded area extending from the margin to near the apex. The condition is known to occur more commonly on the vestibular than the oral surface, the anterior teeth being affected more frequently than the posterior ones.

wound d., separation of the layers of a surgical wound. **Zuckerkandl's d's,** small gaps occasionally seen in the papyraceous layer of the ethmoid bone.

Dehistin trademark for *tripelennamine*.

Dehychol trademark for *dehydrocholic acid* (see under ACID).

dehydratase (de-hi′drah-tās) any of the enzymes (lyases) that catalyze the elimination of the elements of water, often leaving double bonds. Called also *anhydrase*. **carbonate d.,** [E.C.4.2.1.1], a hydro-lyase that catalyzes the breakage of carbon-oxygen bonds with resulting elimination of water. It causes catalytic reversible hydration of carbon dioxide and dehydration of carbonic acid, playing a role in the transport of carbon dioxide in the erythrocytes and its exchange in the pulmonary parenchyma, also found in the renal cortex, gastric mucosa, pancreas, eye, and central nervous system. In renal tubular cells, the enzyme converts carbon dioxide to carbonic acid. When the enzyme is inhibited, the amount of hydrogen ions for exchange with sodium decreases, the excess sodium ions in the tubules combines with bicarbonate and is excreted from the kidneys with an increased volume of water, carbonate dehydrase inhibitors thus acting as diuretics. There are two genetic loci in humans responsible for carbonic anhydrase in red cells, CA_I and CA_{II}. Called also *carbonate hydro-lyase* and *carbonic anhydrase*.

dehydration (de″hi-dra′shun) [L. *de* away + Gr. *hydōr* water] 1. removal of water from a substance. 2. the condition that results from excessive loss of body water or inadequate fluid intake. Called also *anhydration, deaquation,* and *hypohydration*. See also dehydration FEVER.

dehydroandrosterone (de-hi″dro-an-dros′ter-ōn) dehydroepiandrosterone.

7-dehydrocholesterol (de-hi″dro-ko-les′ter-ōl) a sterol found in animal tissue which, when irradiated, is converted to vitamin D_3. **activated 7-d.,** cholecalciferol.

Δ¹-dehydrocortisone (del″ta-de-hi″dro-kor′tĭ-sōn) prednisone.

dehydroemetine (de-hi″dro-em′ĕ-tin) an amebicide, 2,3-didehydro-6′,7′,10,11-tetramethoxyemetan.

dehydroepiandrosterone (de-hi″dro-ep″ĭ-an-dros′ter-ōn) an androgenic steroid synthesized from cholesterol, 3β-hydroxyandrost-5-en-17-one, occurring as needles or leaflets that are readily soluble in ethanol and ether and sparingly soluble in chloroform and petroleum. Used in the treatment of certain endocrine diseases. Abbreviated *DHA*. Called also *dehydroisoandrosterone*.

dehydrogenase (de-hi′dro-jen-ās) any of a group of oxidoreductases that catalyze an oxidation reaction in which hydrogen is transferred from a substrate to an acceptor, often NAD(P) or FAB. Called also *reductase*. **aeroglucose d.,** glucose OXIDASE. **alcohol d.** [E.C.1.1.1.1.], an oxidoreductase that catalyzes the dehydrogenation of ethyl alcohol to acetaldehyde. Called also *aldehyde reductase*. **dihydrofolate d.** [E.C.1.5.1.4.], an oxidoreductase that acts on the CH—NH group of donors, being the primary target of folic acid analogues in their interference with folic acid metabolism. See also folic acid ANALOGUE. **isocitrate d.,** an oxidoreductase that acts on the CH—OH group of isocitric acid with NAD^+ and $NADP^+$ as the acceptor. In one form [E.C.1.1.1.41], it catalyzes, in the presence of NAD^+, the conversion of *threo*-D-isocitrate to 2-oxoglutarate, carbon dioxide, and NADH. In another form [E.C.1.1.1.42], it catalyzes, in the presence of $NADP^+$, the conversion of threo-D-isocitrate to 2-oxoglutarate, carbon dioxide, and NADPH. In oxidative carbohydrate metabolism (Krebs cycle), the enzyme is involved in converting isocitric acid to oxalosuccinic acid. Called also *decarboxylating isocitrate–PN transhydrogenase*. **lactic d., lactic acid d.,** an oxidoreductase that catalyzes the dehydrogenation of the alpha-hydroxy group of lactic acid to form pyruvic acid. Some forms oxidize other 2-hydroxymonocarboxylic acids. Enzymes in this group are classified in the subsubclass of oxidoreductases acting on the CH—OH group of donors and with NAD or NADP as acceptors [E.C.1.1.1.]. **malate d., malic d.** [E.C.1.1.1.37], an oxidoreductase acting on the CH—OH group of donors, which catalyzes the dehydrogenation of malic acid to oxaloacetic acid, also oxidizing some other 2-hydroxydicarboxylic acids. Called also *L-malate–NAD transhydrogenase*. **succinate d., succinic d.** [E.C.1.3.99.1], an oxidoreductase acting on the CH—CH group of donors, which is an iron-containing flavoprotein that catalyzes the conversion of succinic to fumaric acid in the Krebs cycle in carbohydrate metabolism. Called also *fumarhydrogenase, fumarate reductase,* and *fumaric hydrogenase*.

dehydroisoandrosterone (de-hi″dro-i″so-an-dro′ster-ōn) dehydroepiandrosterone.

3-dehydroretinol (de-hi″dro-ret′ĭ-nol) VITAMIN A₂.

Deiters' cell [Otto Friedrich Carl *Deiters*, German anatomist,

Dehistin / delitescence   233

1834–1863] 1. an outer phalangeal cell; see supporting CELL. 2. neuroglial CELL.

Dejean's syndrome [M. C. *Dejean*, French physician] orbital floor SYNDROME.

Déjérine's syndrome [Joseph Jules *Déjérine*, French physician, 1849–1917] alternating hypoglossal HEMIPLEGIA. See also Landouzy-Déjérine DYSTROPHY.

deka- [Gr. *deka* ten] in the metric system, a combining form denoting a quantity 10 times the unit designated by the root with which it is combined. Abbreviated *dk*. Written also *deca-*. See also metric SYSTEM and *Tables of Weights and Measures* at WEIGHT.

Dekacort trademark for *dexamethasone*.

dekagram (dek′ah-gram) [*deka-* + *gram*] a unit of mass (weight) in the metric system, being 10 grams or equivalent to 154.32 grains troy. Written also *decagram*.

dekaliter (dek′ah-le″ter) [*deka-* + *liter*] a unit of volume in the metric system, being 10 liters or equivalent to 2.64 gallons or 610.28 cubic inches. Written also *decaliter*.

dekameter (dek′ah-me″ter) [*deka-* + *meter*] a unit of length in the metric system, being of 10 meters or equivalent to 10.9361 yards. Written also *decameter*.

dekanem (dek′ah-nem) [*deka-* + *nem*] a unit of nutrition equivalent to 10 nems (10 gm of breast milk). Abbreviated *Dn*. See also NEM.

dekanormal (dek″ah-nor′mal) [*deka-* + L. *norma* rule] having ten times the strength of normal; said of solutions. Written also *decanormal*.

del deletion (2).

delacrimation (de-lak″rĭ-ma′shun) [L. *de* from + *lacrima* tear] excessive or abnormal flow of tears.

Delacurarin trademark for *tubocurarine chloride* (see under TUBOCURARINE).

delamination (de″lam-ĭ-na′shun) [L. *de* apart + *lamina* layer] separation into layers.

de Lange's syndrome [Cornelia *de Lange*, Dutch pediatrician, 1871–1950] see under SYNDROME.

de-lead (de-led′) to remove lead from a tissue, as from the bones in lead poisoning, by administration of edetate disodium calcium.

deleterious (del″e-te′re-us) [Gr. *deleterios*] injurious; hurtful.

deletion (de-le′shun) [L. *deletio* destruction] 1. elimination, especially by erasing or blotting out. 2. a structural chromosome aberration, consisting of the loss of a portion of a chromosome, either at one end following a single break, or more often internally following a break at two different points, resulting in the loss of genetic material. If the deleted portion includes a centromere, the information will be lost in subsequent cell division; if the deleted portion does not involve the centromere, the chromosome will replicate and divide, but the acentric fragment will fail to move at anaphase and probably will be lost. A deletion chromosome having lost both ends may unite at the two broken ends and form a ring (see ring CHROMOSOME). Abbreviated *del*. See also CHROMOSOME aberration. **partial d. of short arm of chromosome 4, partial d. 4p,** Wolf-Hirschhorn SYNDROME. **partial d. of short arm of chromosome 5, partial d. 5p,** crying cat SYNDROME. **d. of short arm of chromosome 8,** chromosome 8p deletion SYNDROME. **partial d. of short arm of chromosome 9,** MONOSOMY 9p. **partial d. of short arm of chromosome 10, partial d. 10p,** chromosome 10 short arm deletion SYNDROME. **partial d. of long arm of chromosome 11,** chromosome 11q syndrome, partial deletion; see under SYNDROME. **partial d. of short arm of chromosome 12,** chromosome 12p syndrome, partial deletion; see under SYNDROME. **partial d. of chromosome 13,** chromosome 13, partial deletion SYNDROME. **partial d. of chromosome D₁,** chromosome 13, partial deletion SYNDROME.

delimitation (de-lim′ĭ-ta′shun) [*de-* + L. *limitare* to limit] 1. the process of limiting or of becoming limited. 2. ascertainment of the limits and extent of some diseased tissue or process, or the spread of a disease in a host or a community.

delinquency (de-lin′kwen-se) antisocial, illegal, or criminal conduct.

deliquescence (del″ĕ-kwes′ens) [L. *deliquescere* to grow moist] the condition of becoming moist or liquefied as a result of absorption of water from the air.

deliquescent (del″ĕ-kwes′ent) having a tendency to form an aqueous solution or become liquid by the absorption of moisture from the air.

delitescence (del″ĭ-tes′ens) [L. *delitescere* to lie hidden] 1. sudden disappearance of symptoms or of objective signs of a disease or of a lesion. 2. the period of latency or incubation of a poison or morbific agent.

Delmeson trademark for *fluorometholone*.

Delpech's abscess [Jacques Mathieu *Delpech,* French surgeon, 1777–1832] see under ABSCESS.

delta (del'tah) [Gr. letter *delta* δ, Δ] 1. the fourth letter of the Greek alphabet. 2. any triangular space. **apical d.,** the apical ramification of the main root canal, usually at the dentinocemental junction of the root apex. **Delta Dental Plan,** see under PLAN.

Delta-Cortef trademark for *prednisolone*.

Deltacortenoio trademark for *prednisolone acetate* (see under PREDNISOLONE).

deltacortisone (del'tah-kor'tĭ-sōn) prednisone.

Deltacortril trademark for *prednisolone*.

delta E (del'tah e) prednisone.

Delta Prenovis trademark for *prednisone*.

Deltasone trademark for *prednisone*.

Delta-Stab trademark for *prednisolone*.

Deltisolone trademark for *prednisolone*.

Deltisone trademark for *prednisone*.

deltoid (del'toid) [L. *deltoides* triangular] triangular in outline, as the deltoid muscle.

Deltra trademark for *prednisone*.

Deltracortril trademark for *prednisolone*.

Deltrasone trademark for *prednisone*.

delusion (de-lu'zhun) [L. *delusio,* from *de* from + *ludus* a game] a false belief that cannot be corrected by argument or persuasion.

demand (de-mand') 1. requirement or claim. 2. to call or require. **biochemical oxygen d.,** the amount of dissolved oxygen required to bring about aerobic decay of dissolved organic matter. Abbreviated *BOD*.

demarcation (de″mar-ka'shun) [L. *demarcare* to limit] the marking off or ascertainment of boundaries.

Demarquay-Richet syndrome [J. N. *Demarquay;* Didier Dominique Alfred *Richet,* French surgeon, 1816–1891] van der Woude's SYNDROME.

Demarquay's sign [Jean Nicholas *Demarquay,* French surgeon, 1811–1875] see under SIGN.

demecarium bromide (dem'ĕ-ka're-um) a quaternary ammonium anticholinesterase drug, 3,3′-[1,10-decanediylbis[(methyliminocarbonyloxy]]bis[*N,N,N* - trimethyl - benzeneaminum]dibromide, occurring as a white, slightly hygroscopic powder that is freely soluble in water and ethanol, sparingly soluble in acetone, and insoluble in ether. Used chiefly in ophthalmology. Adverse effects may include myopia, photophobia, and other ocular disorders. Contact dermatitis, excessive salivation, nausea, vomiting, diarrhea, abdominal cramps, dyspnea, and convulsions may occur. Trademarks: Humorsol, Tomsilen.

demeclocycline (dem″ĕ-klo-si'klēn) a semisynthetic tetracycline antibiotic elaborated by a mutant strain of *Streptomyces aureofaciens,* 7-chloro-4-dimethylamino-1,4-4a,5,5a,6,11,12a-octahydro-3,6,10,12,12a-pentahydroxy-1,11-dioxo-2-naphthacenecarboxamide. It occurs as a yellow, odorless, bitter, crystalline powder that is soluble in water and alcohol, sparingly soluble in carbonates and alkali hydroxides, and insoluble in acetone and chloroform. Its antimicrobial properties and toxicity are similar to those of other tetracyclines. It should not be taken with milk, antacids, and calcium-containing substances. Trademarks: Bioterciclin, Declomycin, Decomycin, Ledermycin. **d. hydrochloride,** the monohydrochloride salt of demeclocycline, the description, uses, and toxicity of which are the same as those of the parent compound. Trademarks: Clortetrin, Meciclin, Mexocine.

demelanizer (de-mel'ah-ni″zer) demelanizing AGENT.

dementia (de-men'she-ah) [*de-* + L. *mens* mind] any condition characterized by mental deterioration. **d. paralyt'ica,** one of the most serious forms of neurosyphilis, involving the neurons and blood vessels of the meninges. The symptoms, which usually become evident several years after the primary infection, include progressive mental deterioration, apathy, emotional instability, euphoria, agitation, depression, disorientation, delusions, poor concentration, motor excitement, and Magnan's movement (forward and backward movement of the tongue when it is drawn out). Called also *cerebral tabes, general paralysis,* and *general paresis.*

Demerol trademark for *meperidine hydrochloride* (see under MEPERIDINE).

demethyldopan (de-meth″il-do'pān) uracil MUSTARD.

demi- [Fr. *demi;* L. *demidius* half] a prefix signifying half.

demifacet (dem″ĭ-fas'et) a small plane surface on either of two bones which both articulate with a third bone.

demilune (dem'ĭ-lōōn) 1. a half moon, or crescent. 2. shaped like a crescent; crescentic. **d's of Giannuzzi, d's of Heidenhain,** crescents of Giannuzzi; see under CRESCENT.

demineralization (de-min″er-al-i-za'shun) excessive loss of mineral or inorganic salts from tissues.

demography (de-mog'rah-fe) [Gr. *dēmos* people + *graphein* to write] the study of mankind collectively; especially of their geographical distribution and physical environment.

demorphan hydrobromide (de-mor'fan) DEXTRAMETHORPHAN hydrobromide.

demorphine (de-mor'fēn) diacetylmorphine.

Demotil trademark for *diphemanil methylsulfate* (see under DIPHEMANIL).

demucosation (de″mu-ko-sa'shun) removal of the mucous membrane from a part.

demulcent (de-mul'sent) 1. soothing; bland; allaying the irritation of inflamed or abraded surfaces. 2. compound, usually of high molecular weight, that soothes and alleviates irritation, especially of mucous membranes or abraded skin surfaces. Demulcents are used in aqueous solution in the form of lotions, ointments, or wet dressings, when applied to the skin; or in drinks or enemas, when applied to the gastrointestinal tract; or in lozenges or gargles, when applied to the throat. They are also used as vehicles for drugs with unpleasant taste or as emulsions or suspensions for those which are not soluble in water. Chemically, most demulcents are gums, mucilages, or starches, and include glycerol, acacia, tragacanth, and propylene glycol. Called also *lenitive.*

demyelination (de-mi'ĕ-lin-a'shun) loss of myelin without a proportionate loss of axis cylinders, occurring in some diseases of the central nervous system.

Denar articulator see under ARTICULATOR.

denasality (de″na-sal'ah-te) lack of adequate nasal resonance during speech due to obstruction of the nasal passages.

denaturation (de-na″chur-a'shun) the destruction of the usual nature of a substance. **alcohol d.,** the addition of methanol or acetone to alcohol to render it unfit for drinking. **protein d.,** treatment of proteins with heat, acid, alkali, urea solutions, or detergents in an effort to cause the proteins to lose their native properties as antigens, enzymes, etc. The process is believed to consist of unwinding the polypeptide chains without breaking the amino acid residues. The process may be reversible (see RENATURATION).

Dendrid trademark for *idoxuridine*.

dendrite (den'drīt) [Gr. *dendron* tree] 1. one of the threadlike branched prolongations of the cytoplasm of a neuron, which contain Nissl bodies, mitochondria, fibrillae, pigment, and other components of the perikaryon, but lack myelin or other sheath. Their size, shape, and number of branches and gemmules (short processes) vary with types of different neurons. Dendrites comprise most of the receptive surface of a neuron. Called also *cytodendrite, dendron, neurodendrite,* and *neurodendron.* 2. a treelike branching spreading out from the nucleus during the process of crystallization.

dendron (den'dron) [Gr.] dendrite.

denervation (de″ner-va'shun) resection or removal of the nerves of an organ or part.

dengue (deng'e; Spanish, dān-ga) an infectious, eruptive, febrile disease, marked by severe pains in the head, eyes, muscles, and joints, sore throat, catarrhal symptoms, and sometimes a cutaneous eruption and painful swellings of the parts. The disease comes on suddenly after an incubation period of from three to six days. The symptoms increase in severity for two or three days, then decrease somewhat, only to increase again on the fourth or fifth day, at which time the eruption appears. It occurs epidemically and sporadically in India, Egypt, Iran, the West Indies, and the South Pacific, and epidemics have occurred in Greece. It is caused by a virus, and is transmitted by the bite of the mosquitoes *Aedes aegypti, A. albopictus, A. polynesiensis,* and *Desvoidea obturans.*

Denholz appliance see under APPLIANCE.

Dennie's sign Morgan's LINE.

Denonvilliers' operation [Charles Pierre *Denonvilliers,* French surgeon, 1808–1872] see under OPERATION.

dens (dens), pl. *den'tes* [L.] a tooth or toothlike structure; used in official anatomical nomenclature to designate the small bonelike structures of the jaws, serving in the mastication of food. See also TOOTH. **d. acu'tus,** incisor TOOTH. **den'tes cani'ni** [NA], canine teeth; see under TOOTH. **dentes de Chiaie,** mottled ENAMEL. **den'tes decid'ui** [NA], deciduous teeth; see under

TOOTH. **d. in den'te, d. invagina'tus,** a developmental defect resulting from invagination of the crown before it is calcified; so named because severe invagination of enamel and dentin gives the appearance of a "tooth within a tooth." Called also *dilated odontoma, gestant odontoma, radix in radice,* and *tooth within a tooth.* **d. evagina'tus,** a condition most often found in persons of Oriental descent, characterized by a pulpal horn extending into a dentinal core on the occlusal surface of both maxillary and mandibular first and second premolars. Through abrasion or trauma the surface of the core may be reduced, resulting in pulpal exposure and necrosis. **den'tes incisi'vi** [NA], incisor teeth; see under TOOTH. **den'tes mola'res** [NA], molar teeth; see under TOOTH. **den'tes permanen'tes** [NA], permanent teeth; see under TOOTH. **den'tes premola'res** [NA], premolar teeth; see under TOOTH. **d. sa'piens,** molar tooth, third; see under TOOTH. **d. seroti'nus** [NA], molar tooth, third; see under TOOTH.

Densene 33 trademark for a denture base acrylic polymer.

densimeter (den-sim'ĕ-ter) [L. *densus* dense + Gr. *metron* measure] densitometer.

Densite trademark for Class II *dental stone* (see under STONE).

densitometer (den″sĭ-tom'ĕ-ter) 1. an apparatus for determining the density of a liquid. 2. an instrument for determining the degree of darkening of developed photographic or x-ray film by means of a photocell which measures light transmission through a given area of film. Called also *densimeter.*

densitometry (den″sĭ-tom'ĕ-tre) 1. determination of variations in density by comparison with that of another material, or with a certain standard. 2. determination of the degree of darkening of developed photographic or x-ray film by means of a densitometer. Called also *densography.*

density (den'sĭ-te) [L. *densitas*] 1. the quality of being compact or crowded. 2. the quantity of matter in a given space, calculated as weight per unit volume. Common units for expressing density include gram/milliliter (for solids and liquids), gram/liter (for gases), or pounds/cubic feet. 3. the quantity of electricity in a given area or in a given volume or in a given time. 4. the degree of darkening of exposed and processed photographic or x-ray film, expressed as the logarithm of the capacity of a given area of the film. In radiography, density is controlled by the milliampere-second, or variations in either amperage or time in seconds. See also CONTRAST (2). **background d.,** the density of a processed film due to factors other than the radiation exposure received through the recorded objects or structures, e.g., inherent film density, scatter, radiation, or fogging. **inherent d.,** the density of a processed film due to inherent factors, such as the density of film base, emulsion, gelatin, etc. **ionization d.,** the number of ion pairs per unit volume. **object d.,** the resistance of an object or material to the passage of x-rays. **tissue d.,** the resistance of a tissue to the passage of x-rays.

densography (den-sog'rah-fe) densitometry (2).

Densovirus (den″so-vi'rus) a genus of parvoviruses which infect invertebrates.

DENT Dental Exposure Normalization TECHNIQUE.

Dent Gold No. 1 see under GOLD.

dent-, denta- see DENTO-.

dentagra (den-tag'rah, den'tah-grah) [*deni-* + Gr. *agra* seizure] 1. a forceps for extracting teeth. 2. toothache.

dental (den'tal) [L. *dentalis*] 1. pertaining to a tooth or teeth. 2. a letter or sound made by or in part by the front teeth.

Dental H topical fluoride gel see under GEL.

dentaphone (den'tah-fōn) [*denta-* + Gr. *phōnē* sound] an instrument by means of which deaf persons are enabled to hear sounds propagated through the medium of the teeth.

dentate (den'tāt) [L. *dentatus*] serrated; resembling a structure or having an edge with teeth projecting like those of a saw.

Dentatus articulator see under ARTICULATOR.

dentes (den'tēz) [L.] plural of *dens.*

denti-, dentia- see DENTO-.

dentia (den'she-ah) [L.] a condition relating to development or eruption of the teeth; used also as a combining form denoting relationship to the teeth. **d. prae'cox,** premature eruption of the teeth, or the presence of teeth at birth. See also premature teeth, under TOOTH. **d. tar'da,** delayed DENTITION.

dentibuccal (den-ti-buk'al) [*denti-* + *buccal*] pertaining to the teeth and cheek.

Denticator trademark for a device used for gingival massage. It is a slender rod having a sharp rubber tip on one end and a blunt rubber tip at the other end.

denticle (den'tĭ-k'l) [L. *denticulus* little tooth] 1. a small toothlike process. 2. a calcified concretion ranging in size from a microscopic particle to up to 3 mm in diameter, which develops in the dental pulp as a part of aging processes. Called also *focal calcific regression of pulp, pulp nodule,* and *pulp stone.* See

also pulp CALCIFICATION. **adherent d.,** attached d. **attached d.,** a calcified formation in a pulp chamber partially attached to the dentin. Called also *adherent d.* **embedded d.,** interstitial d. **false d.,** a calcified formation in the pulp chamber of a tooth, which does not show the structure of true dentin. Instead of exhibiting dentinal tubules, the denticle is made up of concentric layers or lamellae deposited around a central nidus of calcified organic detritus, such as pulp cells or thrombi. **free d.,** a calcified formation in the pulp chamber lying entirely within the pulp tissue and not attached to the dentinal walls. **interstitial d.,** a calcified formation within the pulp chamber completely surrounded by dentin. Called also *embedded d.* **true d.,** a denticle usually developing from the floor or the lateral walls of the pulp chamber through the calcification of odontoblasts, and containing dentin and traces of dentinal tubules. True denticles are commonly of the adherent variety.

denticulated (den-tik'u-lāt″ed) [L. *denticulatus*] having minute teeth.

dentification (den″tĭ-fi-ka'shun) the formation of dentin or tooth substance.

dentiform (den'tĭ-form) [L. *dens* tooth + *forma* form] shaped like a tooth.

dentifrice (den'tĭ-fris) [L. *dentifricium*] a preparation, usually a paste, gel, or powder, used with a toothbrush for cleaning the accessible surfaces of the teeth. It usually contains mild abrasives, detergents, humectants, binders, flavoring agents, and sometimes antiseptics, deodorants, and caries-preventing agents. **accepted d.,** any dentifrice that has been evaluated by the Council on Dental Therapeutics of the American Dental Association and found to be safe and effective. Accepted products may use the Council's Seal of Acceptance or an authorized statement, and are listed in the publication *Accepted Dental Therapeutics.* **Aim d.,** trademark for a dentifrice containing stannous fluoride for the prevention of dental caries and hydrate silica as the abrasive agent. **Bofors d.,** trademark for a dentifrice containing sodium fluoride, acrylic particles, sorbitol, flavoring agents, wetting agents, cellulose, coloring agents, and water. **Close Up d.,** trademark for a cosmetic dentifrice; it is a gel with a moderate abrasion level, containing a mixture of silica gels as the abrasive agent. **Craig Martin d.,** trademark for a cosmetic dentifrice; it is a paste with a low abrasion level, containing tricalcium phosphate and calcium carbonate as abrasive agents. **Crest d.,** trademark for a dentifrice containing 0.4 percent stannous fluoride, 1 percent stannous pyrophosphate, 39 percent calcium pyrophosphate, 10 percent glycerol, 20 percent sorbitol in a 70 percent aqueous solution, 29.6 percent water, and miscellaneous formulating agents. Used in dental caries prevention. **Colgate II with MFP fluoride,** trademark for a toothpaste containing 0.76 percent sodium monofluorophosphate, 39.35 percent insoluble sodium metaphosphate, 5 percent anhydrous dicalcium phosphate, 11.9 percent sorbitol, 9.9 percent glycerol, 1.5 percent sodium lauryl sulfate, 27.39 percent water, and 4.2 percent miscellaneous agents. Said to be effective in dental caries control. **Extar d.,** trademark for a toothpaste containing polyphosphate as its active ingredient; used to remove calculus and retard its formation. **Fed-Mart d.,** trademark for a dentifrice containing stannous fluoride for the prevention of dental caries and insoluble sodium metaphosphate as the abrasive agent. **fluoride d.,** one contain-

COMPOSITION OF FLUORIDE DENTIFRICES

Component	Function	Concentration
Fluoride Agent	Reduce dental decay	1000 ppm F
Abrasive System	Remove plaque, stains and polish tooth surfaces	35–50%
Water		10–25%
Humectants	Retain moisture	10–30%
Detergent	Aid in cleaning of tooth surface	1–3%
Flavoring	To motivate dentifrice use	1–4%
Binder	To prevent separation of dentifrice components during storage and use	0.5–1%

(From Dentifrices — Then and Now. Dent. Outlook, 7:1, 1981.)

ing a fluoride, usually stannous or sodium fluoride, for the purpose of preventing dental caries. **K-Mart d.,** trademark for a dentifrice containing stannous fluoride as a caries-preventing agent and insoluble sodium metaphosphate as an abrasive. **Listerine d.,** trademark for a cosmetic dentifrice; it is a paste with a low abrasion level, containing dicalcium phosphate dihydrate as the abrasive agent. **Macleans fluoride d.,** trademark for a toothpaste containing 0.76 percent sodium monofluorophosphate, 38 percent calcium carbonate, 26 percent glycerin, 28.8 percent water, 1.15 percent sodium lauryl sulfate, and 5.3 percent various binding, flavoring, and preservative agents. **monofluorophosphate d.,** one containing monofluorophosphate as its active caries-preventing agent. **New Concept d.,** trademark for a cosmetic dentifrice; it is a paste with a moderate abrasion level, containing powdered egg shell and dicalcium phosphate dihydrate as abrasive agents. **Peak d.,** trademark for a cosmetic dentifrice. It is a paste with a low to moderate abrasion level, containing sodium bicarbonate and calcium carbonate as abrasive agents. **Pearl Drops d.,** trademark for a cosmetic dentifrice. It is a liquid suspension with a moderate abrasion level containing a mixture of hydrated aluminum and dibasic calcium phosphate dihydrate as abrasive agents. **Pepsodent c.,** trademark for a dentifrice containing aluminum oxide, hydrated silica, and dicalcium phosphate as the abrasive agents. **Protect d.,** trademark for a dentifrice used to protect against dental hypersensitivity; it is a paste containing sodium citrate in surface-active pluronic gel as the active component. **provisionally accepted d.,** one that has been evaluated by the Council on Dental Therapeutics of the American Dental Association, for which there is reasonable but limited evidence of dental usefulness and safety. **Pycopay d.,** trademark for a dentifrice used to retard calculus formation; it is a powder containing pancreatin in an abrasive agent, chiefly sodium chloride and sodium bicarbonate. **Safeway d.,** trademark for a dentifrice containing stannous fluoride as a caries-preventing agent and calcium pyrophosphate as an abrasive. **Sensodyne d.,** trademark for a toothpaste containing 10 percent strontium chloride as the active ingredient; used for treating hypersensitive dentin. **sodium fluoride d.,** one containing sodium fluoride as its active caries-preventing agent. **stannous fluoride d.,** one containing stannous fluoride as its active caries-preventing substance. **Thermodent d.,** trademark for a toothpaste containing as active ingredients sodium bicarbonate, sodium chloride, sodium sulfate, potassium sulfate, and formaldehyde; used in the treatment of hypersensitive dentin. **Topco d.,** a trademark for a dentifrice containing stannous fluoride as a caries-preventing agent and insoluble sodium metaphosphate as an abrasive. **Ultra Brite d.,** trademark for a dentifrice containing hydrated silica and aluminum oxide as abrasive agents. **Walgreen d.,** trademark for a dentifrice containing stannous fluoride as a caries-preventing agent and insoluble sodium metaphosphate as an abrasive. **Woolco d.,** trademark for a dentifrice containing stannous fluoride as a caries preventing agent and dicalcium phosphate dihydrate as an abrasive.

dentigerous (den″tij′er-us) [*denti-* + L. *gerere* to carry] bearing or containing teeth, as a dentigerous cyst.

dentilabial (den″tĭ-la′be-al) [*denti-* + L. *labium* lip] pertaining to the teeth and lips.

dentilingual (den″tĭ-ling′gwal) [*denti-* + L. *lingua* tongue] pertaining to the teeth and tongue.

Dentillium CB trademark for an iron-chromium alloy (see stainless STEEL).

dentimeter (den-tim′ĕ-ter) [*denti-* + Gr. *metron* measure] an instrument for measuring teeth.

dentin (den′tin) [L. *dens* tooth] the hard portion of the tooth surrounding the pulp, covered by enamel on the crown and cementum on the root, which is harder and denser than bone but softer than enamel, and is thus readily abraded when left unprotected. It consists of an organic matrix (92.3 percent collagen, 1.03 percent insoluble protein residue, 1.03 percent mucopolysaccharide, 1.03 percent lipid, and 4.61 percent citric acid), upon which mineral salts are deposited, forming hydroxyapatite crystals. Inorganic matter represents about 67 percent dentin, organic substances 20 percent, and water 13 percent. The hydroxyapatite crystals making up dentin range in diameter from 35 Å to 1,000 Å. Dentin is generally transparent, having usually yellowish coloration in primary dentin, which may vary in color from yellowish to that of the enamel. Dentin is permeated by numerous branching spiral canaliculi or tubules (dentinal tubules), which contain processes of connective tissue

cells (odontoblasts) that line the pulp cavity. Spelled also *dentine.* Called also *dentinum* [NA], *ebur dentis, intertubular substance of tooth, ivory, ivory membrane, ivory substance, membrana eboris of Kölliker, proper substance of tooth, substantia dentalis propria, substantia eburnea,* and *substantia fundamentalis dentis.* **adventitious d.,** secondary irregular d. **calcified d.,** see transparent d. **circumpulpar d.,** the inner portion of the dentin, adjacent to the pulp chamber, consisting of thinner fibrils. See also PREDENTIN. **d. cleaner,** acid ETCHANT. **coronal d.,** that portion of the dentin located in the anatomic crown. **cover d.,** mantle d. **developmental d.,** dentin formed during the various periods of tooth development to the time when the tooth takes its anatomic position in the oral cavity. **hereditary opalescent d.,** DENTINOGENESIS imperfecta. **functional d.,** secondary regular d. **interglobular d.,** imperfectly calcified dentinal matrix situated between the calcified globules near the periphery of the dentin. In ground sections, it appears as a darkened area shaped like a holly leaf intervening between the globules. It is usually found in the periphery of the coronal dentin subjacent to the mantle dentin, forming a band which corresponds to the incremental lines. **intertubular d.,** the dentin located between the dentinal tubules, which is less mineralized than the peritubular dentin. **irregular d.,** secondary irregular d. **mantle d.,** the peripheral portion of the dentin, adjacent to the enamel or cementum, consisting mostly of coarse fibers (Korff's fibers). Called also *cover d.* **opalescent d.,** dentin giving an unusual translucent or opalescent appearance to the teeth, as in dentinogenesis imperfecta. **peritubular d.,** the calcified dentin surrounding the dentinal tubules, which is more mineralized than the intertubular dentin. **primary d.,** dentin formed subsequently to the time when the tooth takes its anatomic position in the oral cavity. The amount of primary dentin produced is relatively small and uniformly distributed; there is no change in the structure or properties in developmental and primary dentin. It is separated from secondary dentin by a demarcation line, formed by a change in the directional path of the dentinal tubules. **radicular d.,** dentin confined to the root portion of a tooth. **reparative d.,** secondary irregular d. **residual carious d.,** residual CARIES. **sclerotic d.,** transparent d. **secondary d.,** dentin formed and deposited in response to a normal or slightly abnormal stimulus, after the complete formation of the tooth. See *secondary irregular d.* and *secondary regular d.* **secondary irregular d.,** dentin formed in response to stimuli associated with pathologic processes, such as caries or injury, or cavity preparation. Such dentin is usually irregular in nature, being composed of few tubules which may be tortuous in appearance, and it often demonstrates cellular inclusions. Called also *adventitious d., irregular d., reparative d.,* and *tertiary d.* **secondary regular d.,** dentin formed in response to stimuli associated with normal body processes. Called also *functional d.* **d. substitute,** intermediate BASE. **tertiary d.,** secondary irregular d. **transparent d.,** dentin in which dentinal tubules have become sclerotic or calcified, producing the appearance of translucency, usually resulting from injury, abrasion, and normal aging processes. Called also *calcified d., sclerotic d.,* and *dentinal sclerosis.*

dentinal (den′tĭ-nal) pertaining to dentin.

dentinalgia (den″tĭ-nal′je-ah) [*dentin* + *-algia*] pain in the dentin.

dentine (den′tēn) dentin.

dentinification (den-tin″ĭ-fĭ-ka′shun) the formation of dentin.

dentinoblast (den′tĭ-no-blast) [*dentin* + Gr. *blastos* germ] a cell that forms dentin.

dentinoclast (den′tĭ-no-klast″) [*dentin* + Gr. *klastos* broken] a cell, cytomorphologically the same as the osteoclast, which is involved in dentin resorption, the cavities produced by resorption being known as *resorption lacunae.*

dentinogenesis (den″tĭ-no-jen′ĕ-sis) [*dentin* + Gr. *genesis* formation] dentin formation. Dentin first appears in the layer between the ameloblasts and odontoblasts (basement membrane) and becomes calcified immediately. Formation progresses from the tip of the papilla over its slope to form a calcified cap becoming thicker by the apposition of new layers pulpward. Collagen fibrils of the initial dentin (mantle dentin), formed in the basement membrane, are arranged into fan-shaped bundles (Korff's fibers). The matrix of the remaining dentin (circumpulpal dentin) is mostly composed of smaller more delicate fibrils. A layer of uncalcified dentin intervenes between the calcified tissue and the odontoblast and its processes. **d. hypoplas′tica heredita′ria,** d. imperfecta. **d. imperfec′ta,** a hereditary disorder of tooth development, transmitted as an autosomal dominant trait, and characterized by discoloration of the teeth, ranging from dusky blue to brownish, poorly formed dentin with an abnormally low mineral content, obliteration of the pulp canal, and normal enamel. The teeth usually wear down rapidly, leaving short, brown stumps. Called also *d. hypoplastica hereditaria, Capdepont-Hodge syndrome, Capdepont's syndrome, Fargin-Fayelle syndrome, hereditary dark teeth, hereditary opalescent dentin, hereditary opalescent teeth, odontogenesis imperfecta, Stainton-Capdepont syndrome,* and *Stainton syndrome.* See also hereditary opalescent DENTIN and OSTEOGENESIS imperfecta.

dentinoid (den'tĭ-noid) [*dentin* + Gr. *eidos* form] 1. resembling dentin. 2. a former name for dentinoma. 3. predentin.

dentinoma (den″tĭ-no'mah) a benign odontogenic neoplasm composed only of dentin, which may be termed dentinoid or osteodentin tissue, undifferentiated odontogenic epithelium, and connective tissue. It occurs most frequently in the molar area of the mandible in association with an impacted tooth. Swelling, pain, mucosal perforation, and infection are the common symptoms. Formerly called *dentinoid.*

dentinum (den-ti'num) [L.] [NA] dentin.

dentist (den'tist) a person who has received a degree from an accredited school of dentistry and is licensed to practice dentistry by a state board of dental examiners. His degree may be that of Doctor of Dental Surgery (DDS) or Doctor of Dental Medicine (DMD). Called also *odontologist.* **nonparticipating d.,** in health insurance, one with whom the underwriter (carrier) does not have an agreement to render care to members of the plan. **participating d.,** in health insurance, a dentist with whom a dental plan has an agreement to render care to subscribers.

dentistry (den'tis-tre) 1. The science and art of preventing, diagnosing, and treating diseases, injuries, and malformations of the teeth, jaws, and mouth. 2. the practice of the dental profession collectively. Called also *odontoiatria, odontology, oral medicine,* and *stomatology.* Dental instruments may be classified as handcutting instruments, condensing (see CONDENSER), and miscellaneous. A handcutting or condensing instrument consists of a handle (shaft) that is held in the hand during use, a blade (cutting part of a handcutting instrument), or a nib (working part of a condenser), and a shank (connects the blade or the nib to the handle). Black's formulae permit precise identification of instruments according to length, width, and angles of their blades. In the three-number (basic) formula, the first number indicates the width of the blade in 1/10 mm; the second, its length in mm; and the third, the angle of the blade with the long axis of the handle in hundredths or a centigrade circle (100°). The number 15-8-12 describes a handcutting instrument whose blade is 1.5 mm in width, 8 mm in length, and whose angle with the long axis is 12°. In the four-number formula, the first number indicates the width of the blade in 1/10 mm; the second, the angle formed by the cutting edge and the axis of the instrument handle in degrees of a centigrade circle; the third, the length of the blade in mm; and the fourth, the angle of the blade and the long axis of the handle in degrees of a centigrade circle. The number 13-80-8-14 of the gingival margin trimmer indicates the width of the blade of 1.3 mm, the angle of the blade to the axis of the handle of 80°, the length of the blade of 8 mm, and the angle formed by the blade and long axis of the handle of 14°. See illustrations. **ambulatory hospital d.,** outpatient hospital d. **ceramic d.,** dental CERAMICS. **d. for children,** pedodontics. **community d.,** that branch of dentistry concerned with the distribution of dental and associated oral diseases, their causes,, and the management of resources for their prevention and treatment. **cosmetic d.,** that aspect of dental practice concerned with the repair and restoration of carious, broken, or defective teeth in such a manner as to improve their appearance. Called also *esthetic d.* See also esthetic DENTURE. **dry field d.,** see dry field TECHNIQUE. **esthetic d.,** cosmetic d. **forensic d.,** that branch of dentistry which deals with the application of the art and science of dentistry to the purposes of law. *Dental jurisprudence* and *forensic dentistry* are sometimes used synonymously, but some authorities consider dental jurisprudence as a branch of law and forensic dentistry as a branch of dentistry. Called also *legal*

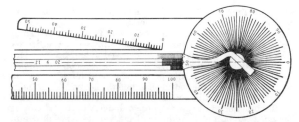

Centigrade circle with the long axis of a handcutting instrument placed on the center of the circle. Note angle of the blade of the instrument. (From Sturdevant, Barton, and Brauer: The Art and Science of Operative Dentistry. Copyright 1968. Used with permission of McGraw-Hill Book Company, New York.)

d. **four-handed d.,** the practice of dentistry with the help of a chairside assistant. Cf. *solo d.* (2). **geriatric d.,** gerodontics. **group d.,** see group PRACTICE. **hospital d.,** the practice of dentistry in a hospital wherein the dentist is called on to act as an integral part of the health care team in providing total health care for the patient. **industrial d.,** 1. that branch of dentistry concerned with the dental health in an industrial setting 2. dental service provided in an industrial establishment, usually restricted to emergency care. **interceptive restorative d.,** preventive use of simple dental restorations to correct conditions responsible for early periodontal breakdown, in an effort to avoid massive complicated restorative procedures to salvage dentitions mutilated by advanced periodontal disease. Called also *restorative interceptive d.* See also *preventive* PERIODONTICS. **legal d.,** forensic d. **operative d.,** that phase of clinical dentistry concerned with the restoration of parts of existing teeth that are defective through disease, trauma, or abnormal development to the state of normal function, health, and esthetics, including preventive, diagnostic, biological, mechanical, and therapeutic techniques, as well as material and instrument science and application. **outpatient hospital d.,** the practice of dentistry in a hospital without the need for admitting the patient. Called also *ambulatory hospital d.* **pediatric d.,** pedodontics. **preventive d.,** that phase of dentistry concerned with the preservation of healthy teeth and the maintenance of oral structures in a state of optimal health for the longest period of time possible. It comprises: (1) *primary prevention,* which includes fluoride therapy, diet control, plaque control, sealants, and pulp protection; (2) *secondary prevention (intervention),* which includes operative dentistry, periodontics, orthodontics, and other fields; and (3) *tertiary prevention (replacement),* which includes fixed and removable prosthodontics. See also *interceptive restorative d.,* oral PROPHYLAXIS, and preventive PERIODONTICS. **primary care d.,** dental care, primary; see under CARE. **prophylactic d.,** *oral* PROPHYLAXIS. **prosthetic d.,** prosthodontics. **psychosomatic d.,** that phase of dentistry which considers the mind-body relationship. **public health d.,** dental public HEALTH. **restorative d.,** that phase of clinical dentistry concerned with the restoration of existing teeth that are defective through disease, trauma, or abnormal development to the state of normal function, health, and esthetics, including crown and bridgework. See also RESTORATION. **restorative interceptive d.,** interceptive restorative d. **seat-down d.,** the practice of dentistry wherein the patient is placed in a reclining position and the dentist and the assistant are seated at the patient's side. See

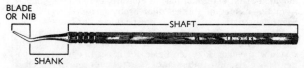

BLADE OR NIB — SHAFT — SHANK

Basic parts of handcutting instruments — handle or shaft, blade, shank, and nib. (From H. O. Torres and A. Ehrlich: Modern Dental Assisting. 2nd ed. Philadelphia, W. B. Saunders Co., 1980; courtesy of the Colwell Co.)

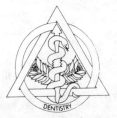

Symbol for dentistry. (From H. O. Torres and A. Ehrlich: Modern Dental Assisting. 2nd ed. Philadelphia, W. B. Saunders Co., 1980.)

also *four-handed d.* Cf. *stand-up d.* **solo d.,** 1. the practice of dentistry wherein the dentist maintains his or her own practice, and may work alone or may employ any number of dental auxiliaries. 2. the practice of dentistry in which the dentist operates on the patient alone, as opposed to four-handed dentistry in which the dentist works with the help of a chairside assistant. **stand-up d.,** the practice of dentistry wherein the patient is seated in the dental chair and the dentist stands up by the patient's side. Cf. *seat-down d.* **TEAM d.,** see TEAM. **team d.,** the practice of dentistry wherein delivery of dental care is provided through teamwork, involving various types of dental auxiliaries, working under the supervision or direction of a dentist, who also performs tasks requiring a high degree of professional competence and judgment. See also *four-handed d.* and dental AUXILIARY. **washed field d.,** see washed field TECHNIQUE.

dentition (den-tish′un) [L. *dentitio*] the teeth in the dental arch; ordinarily used to designate the natural teeth in position in their alveoli. **artificial d.,** denture. **chronology of d.,** see table of *Chronology of Human Dentition* at TOOTH. **deciduous d.,** deciduous teeth; see under TOOTH. **delayed d.,** eruption of the first deciduous teeth after the end of the thirteenth month of life or eruption of the first permanent teeth after the seventh year of life. Called also *retarded d., delayed eruption,* and *dentia tarda.* **diphyodont d.,** one characterized by the formation of two successive sets of teeth, a deciduous and a permanent one, as in man. Cf. *monophyodont d.* **first d.,** deciduous teeth; see under TOOTH. **heterodont d.,** one characterized by morphologically different teeth, such as incisors, molars, etc., as in man. **homodont d.,** one characterized by morphologically similar teeth. **mixed d.,** the complement of teeth in the jaws after eruption of some of the permanent teeth, before all of the deciduous teeth are shed. Called also *transitional d.* **monophyodont d.,** one characterized by the formation of only one set of teeth, all teeth being permanent. Cf. *diphyodont d.* **natural d.,** the natural teeth, considered collectively; it may comprise deciduous, permanent, or mixed dentition. **neonatal d.,** neonatal teeth; see under TOOTH. **permanent d.,** permanent teeth; see under TOOTH. **polyphyodont d.,** having several sets of teeth developing successively through life. **postpermanent d.,** postpermanent teeth; see under TOOTH. **precocious d.,** premature teeth; see under TOOTH. **predeciduous d.,** predeciduous teeth; see under TOOTH. **premature d.,** premature teeth; see under TOOTH. **primary d.,** deciduous teeth; see under TOOTH. **retarded d.,** delayed d. **secondary d.,** permanent teeth; see under TOOTH. **temporary d.,** deciduous teeth; see under TOOTH. **terminal d.,** dentition in extremely poor condition, requiring that all remaining teeth must be extracted and a complete denture inserted in their place. **third d.,** postpermanent teeth; see under TOOTH. **transitional d.,** mixed d.

dento-, dent-, denta-, denti-, dentia- [L. *dens* tooth] a combining form denoting relationship to a tooth or to the teeth. See also ODONTO-.

dentoalveolar (den″to-al-ve′o-lar) pertaining to a tooth and its alveolus.

dentalveolitis (den″to-al″ve-o-li′tis) periodontal DISEASE.

dentoaural (den″to-aw′ral) [*dento-* + *aural*] pertaining to or perceived by a tooth or the teeth and the ear, as dentoaural hearing.

dentode (den′tōd, den-tōd′) an exact reproduction of a tooth on a gnathographically mounted cast.

dentofacial (den″to-fa′shal) [*dento-* + L. *facies* face] pertaining to both the teeth and the face.

dentoform (den′to-form) a mock-up of the dentition and alveolar structures.

dentography (den-tog′rah-fe) odontography.

dentoid (den′toid) odontoid.

dentoidin (den-toi′din) a former term for the organic or albuminous ground substance of a tooth.

dentolegal (den″to-le′gal) pertaining to dental jurisprudence.

Dentomat trademark for a *mechanical triturator* (see under TRITURATOR), having an operational speed of 3300 rpm.

dentomechanical (den″to-mē-kan′ĭ-k'l) pertaining to the mechanics or biomechanics of dentistry.

dentonomy (den-ton′o-me) dental NOMENCLATURE.

Dentorium trademark for a high fusing cobalt-chrome casting alloy (see cobalt-chrome ALLOY).

dentosurgical (den″to-sur′jĭ-k'l) pertaining to or used in dentistry and oral surgery.

dentotropic (den″to-trop′ik) turning toward or having an affinity for tissues composing the teeth.

dentulous (den′tu-lus) possessing natural teeth.

denture (den′chur) [Fr.; L. *dens* tooth] a set of teeth; ordinarily used to designate an artificial or prosthetic replacement for missing natural teeth and adjacent tissues. Called also *dental prosthesis.* See also BRIDGE and RESTORATION. **acrylic resin d.,** a dental prosthesis made of acrylic resin. **d. adhesive,** denture ADHESIVE. **articulated partial d.** partial d., articulated. **bar d., bar joint d.,** an artificial denture retained through the use of a bar attachment. See bar ATTACHMENT. **d. base,** denture BASE. **d. base saddle,** denture base SADDLE. **d. border,** denture BORDER. **broken-stress partial d.,** partial d., articulated. **d. brush,** denture BRUSH. **cantilever fixed partial d.,** cantilever BRIDGE. **clasp d.,** a partial denture which is retained with a clasp. See also CLASP and direct RETAINER. **d. classification,** see Bailyn, Kennedy, and Skinner classifications, under CLASSIFICATION. **d. cleaner,** denture CLEANER. **complete d.,** a dental prosthesis replacing all the natural teeth and associated mandibular and maxillary structures, which is completely supported by the tissues, including mucous membrane, connective tissues, and underlying bone. Called also *full d., complete dental prosthesis,* and *complete denture prosthesis.* **conditioning d.,** a temporary denture used to condition the patient to wearing a denture, serving as a training aid, permitting him to gradually become accustomed to the presence of a denture in his mouth and to overcome problems of gagging, excessive salivation, decreased taste sensation, and other complaints. See also *interim d.* **continuous gum d.,** an artificial denture consisting of porcelain teeth, tinted porcelain denture base material, and a platinum bar, the gum portion of which is of fused porcelain. **d. curing,** denture CURING. **distal extension d.,** partial d., distal extension. **duplicate d.,** a second artificial denture intended to be a copy of the first denture. **d. edge,** denture BORDER. **esthetic d.,** an artificial denture which enhances the appearance of a patient. **d. esthetics,** denture ESTHETICS. **extension partial d.,** partial d., distal extension. **fixed partial d.,** partial d., fixed. **d. flask,** denture FLASK. **full d.,** complete d. **d. heel,** *distal end of denture;* see under END. **hidden-lock d.,** Ticonium hidden-lock d. **hinge d.,** hinge STRESS-BREAKER. **immediate d.,** immediate-insertion d., a complete or removable denture made before all teeth are extracted, so constructed that it may be inserted immediately following the removal of the natural teeth. **implant d.,** an artificial denture retained and stabilized through the use of a subperiosteal or intraperiosteal implant, consisting of the framework (substructure) implanted in contact with the bone, and the overlying structure (superstructure). Called also *implant restoration.* See also intraperiosteal IMPLANT and subperiosteal IMPLANT. **interim d.,** a temporary dental prosthesis to be used for a short interval of time for reasons of esthetics, mastication, occlusal support, and convenience, or for conditioning of the patient to the acceptance of an artificial substitute for missing natural teeth until more definite prosthetic dental treatment can be provided. Called also *provisional d.* See also *conditioning d.* and *transitional d.* **Lee d.,** a sectional partial metal denture incorporating an internal locking bolt. **d. magnet,** denture MAGNET. **metal base d.,** a dental restoration with a base of gold, chromium-cobalt alloy, aluminum, or other suitable metal. **model wax d.,** trial d. **mucosa-borne d.,** an artificial denture supported wholly by the mucous membranes; usually used in dental arches that lack teeth which could serve as abutments. **onlay d.,** overlay d. **overlay d.,** a removable tooth-supported partial or complete denture whose built-in secondary copings overlay or telescope over the primary copings fitting over the prepared natural crowns, posts, or studs. Called also *onlay d., telescopic d., overdenture, overlay, overlay prosthesis, overlay restoration,* and *telescopic prosthesis.* See also COPING, Davis CROWN, stud ATTACHMENT, and telescopic CROWN. **partial d.,** a prosthetic appliance replacing one or more missing teeth in one jaw, and receiving its support and retention from the underlying tissues and/or some or all of the remaining teeth. It may be fixed or removable. See also BRIDGE (2). **partial d., articulated,** a partial denture equipped with a stress-breaker. Called also *broken-stress partial d.* **partial d., broken-stress,** partial d., articulated. **partial d., class I,** a removable distal extension partial denture, deriving its support from the tissues of the residual arch, designed for class I edentulous patients. See also illustration at CLASSIFICATION. **partial d., class II,** a removable partial denture, deriving its support from the abutment teeth and from the tissue of the residual alveolar ridge, designed for class II edentulous patients. See also illustration at CLASSIFICATION. **partial d., class III,** a removable partial denture, deriving its support from the abutment teeth, designed for class III edentulous patients. See also illustration at CLASSIFICATION. **partial d., distal extension,** a removable partial denture that is retained by natural teeth only at the anterior end of the denture base segments, a portion of the functional load being carried by the residual alveolar ridge. Called also *distal extension d., extension partial d.,* and *distal extension restoration.* See also *partial d., class I.* **partial d., extension,** partial d., distal extension. **partial d., fixed,** a dental restoration of one or more missing teeth, which is attached to the prepared natural teeth, roots, or implants by means of cementation. Types include cantilever bridge, compound bridge, fixed bridge with rigid connectors, fixed bridge with rigid and nonrigid connectors, and spring bridge (see under BRIDGE). Called also *fixed bridge, fixed bridge prosthesis, fixed bridgework, fixed prosthesis,* and *stationary bridge.* **partial d., fixed cantilever,** cantilever BRIDGE. **partial d., removable,** a denture replacing one or more, but less than all, natural teeth, which is so constructed that it may be readily removed from the mouth. It may be entirely supported by the residual teeth, deriving its support from abutment teeth at each end of the edentulous area, or it may be supported from both the teeth and the tissue of the residual area, having at least one denture base extending anteriorly or posteriorly, terminating in a denture base portion that is not tooth supported; the last type is called *distal extension partial denture.* Called also *partial denture prosthesis, removable bridge,* and *removable bridgework.* See illustration. **partial d., sectional,** a denture consisting of two or more components, each having a different path of insertion, which engage in different undercuts, being locked together by various means or devices, such as hinges or mechanical locks, or through the use of frictional resistance. **partial d., tissue-borne,** tissue-borne partial d. **partial d., unilateral,** a partial denture designed to restore the missing teeth on one side of the dental arch. **d. periphery,** denture BORDER. **polished surface d.,** the part of the denture base which is usually polished, consisting of the buccal and lingual surfaces of the teeth and extending in the occlusal direction from the border of the denture, including the palatal surface. **precision d., precision retained d.,** a denture retained through the use of a precision attachment. **d. prosthetics,** prosthodontics. **provisional d., interim d. removable d.,** a dental restoration, complete or partial, that can be removed from the mouth at will. See also removable PROSTHODONTICS. **sectional partial d.,** partial d., sectional. **spoon d.,** see *tissue-borne partial d.* **d. sore mouth, d. stomatitis,** denture STOMATITIS. **swing-lock d.,** an artificial denture having a hinged labial flange. Called also *swing-lock prosthesis.* **telescopic d.,** overlay d. **temporary d.,** an artificial denture intended to serve a very short time in a temporary or emergency situation. See *conditioning d., interim d., transitional d.,* and *trial d.* **Ticonium hidden-lock d.,** an articulated denture provided with a device which prevents major connectors from coming apart but allows some freedom of movement of the denture base. The hidden-lock and split bar are built into the denture during the second casting, leaving an almost imperceptible junction between the two sections of the restoration. Called also *hidden-lock d.* **tissue-borne d.,** one that derives its support from the tissue of the residual alveolar ridge. See also *partial d., class I.* **tissue-borne partial d.,** a tissue-borne denture for the upper arch, which derives its support from a spoon-shaped section of plastic covering a large area of the palate. Sometimes called *spoon denture,* especially outside of North America. **tooth-borne d.,** one that is supported wholly by abutment teeth. See also *partial d., class III.* **tooth- and mucosa-borne d.,** a denture supported by both the mucosa and abutment teeth, e.g., partially edentulous arches in which there are no distal natural teeth and the denture bases are free-ended

and totally tissue or mucosa supported at their distal or terminal extensions. **transitional d.,** a removable partial denture that serves as a temporary prosthesis to which teeth will be added as more teeth are lost and that will be replaced after postextraction tissue changes have occurred. It may become an interim denture when all the teeth have been removed from the dental arch. **treatment d.,** a dental prosthesis used for the purpose of treating or conditioning the tissues that are called on to support and retain a denture base. **trial d.,** a temporary denture, usually made of wax on a baseplate, fabricated for placement in the patient's mouth for verification of its esthetic qualities, the making of records, or other procedures before the final denture is completed. Called also *model wax d.* **wax d., model,** trial d.

denturism (den′chur-ism) the practice of fabrication and fitting of dentures by dental technologists without benefit of a dentist's expertise.

denturist (den′chur-ist) a dental technologist who fabricates and fits dentures for patients without benefit of a dentist's expertise. Denturists practice in parts of Canada and the United States but in many states denturism is illegal.

denudation (den″u-da′shun) [L. *denudare* to make bare] the act or process of removal of the covering from any surface, thereby uncovering the structures beneath the surface. **interdental d.,** a periodontal surgical technique that includes excision of all soft tissue in the interproximal region, leaving the interalveolar crestal bone bare; used in the treatment of periodontal diseases. Called also *interdental excision* and *interdental resection.* See also GINGIVECTOMY.

Denver nomenclature see CHROMOSOME nomenclature, Denver.

deodorant (de-o′der-ant) [L. *de* from + *odorare* to perfume] 1. removing undesirable or offensive odors. 2. an agent capable of removing, obscuring, or preventing undesirable or offensive odors.

deoxy- in chemical nomenclature, a prefix used in naming compounds, to designate a compound containing one less atom of oxygen than the reference substance. For words beginning thus, see also those beginning DESOXY-.

deoxycorticosterone (de-ok″se-kor″te-ko′ster-ōn) a mineralocorticoid that is somewhat less powerful than aldosterone, 11-hydroxypregn-4-ene-3,20-dione. Used therapeutically in disorders of water metabolism. Side effects may include fluid and salt retention, hypertension, and hypokalemia. Called also *11-desoxycorticosterone.*

deoxygenation (de-ok″se-jen-a′shun) the act or process of depriving of oxygen.

deoxyribonucleoprotein (de-ok″se-ri″bo-nu″kle-o-pro′te-in) a nucleoprotein consisting of a deoxyribose (DNA) and a protein.

dexyribonucleotide (de-ok″se-ri″bo-nu′kle-o-tīd) a nucleotide of DNA, in which a nitrogenous base combines with deoxyribose and a phosphate group.

deoxyribose (de-ok″se-ri′bōs) a pentose (aldose), $CH_2OH \cdot (CHOH)_2 \cdot CH_2 \cdot CHO$, which is a constituent of DNA and certain coenzymes. See also RIBOSE.

Dep. abbreviation for L. *depura′tus,* purified.

department (de-part′ment) a division or part of an organization or institution. **D. of Health, Education, and Welfare (DHEW),** former name for *D. of Health and Human Services.* **D. of Health and Human Services (HHS),** a federal agency estab-

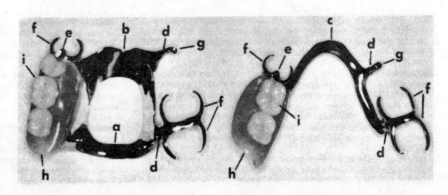

Maxillary and mandibular removable partial dentures with the components labeled. *a,* Posterior palatal bar. *b,* Anterior palatal bar (maxillary major connectors). *c,* Lingual bar — mandibular major connector. *d,* Minor connectors (or struts). *e,* Occlusal rests. *f,* Direct retainers. *g,* Indirect retainers — in this case auxiliary occlusal rests. *h,* Bases. *i,* Artificial teeth. (From R. W. Dykema, D. M. Cunningham, and J. F. Johnston: Modern Practice in Partial Prosthodontics. Philadelphia, W. B. Saunders Co., 1969.)

lished for furthering good health and providing essential human services in the United States. Its component departments include: (1) The National Institutes of Health (NIH), which consist of 11 institutes established to conduct and support research on cancer, heart diseases, environmental health, stroke, the aging processes, cell biology, dental disorders, and other important diseases and to provide library and information services for the biomedical community. (2) The Food and Drug Administration (FDA), which regulates safety of various products, such as drugs, foods, cosmetics, radiation-emitting devices (such as television), etc. (3) The Center for Disease Control, whose functions include communicable disease control, occupational safety, health information and education, family planning, and various preventive programs. (4) The Health Resources Administration, which recruits and trains the personnel and provides facilities to insure adequate health resources for the population. (5) The Health Services Administration, which funds community health centers and administers The National Health Service Corps, composed of physicians, dentists, nurses, and other health professionals, to provide quality health services to underserved areas. (6) The Alcohol, Drug Abuse, and Mental Health Administration, whose responsibilities include the prevention and eradication of problems related to alcohol and drug abuse and mental and emotional disorders. HHS also administers Medicare, in providing free health insurance for the aged, and, jointly with state agencies, Medicaid, in providing free health insurance for those who are unable to do so. Other departments of HHS include: The Office of Human Development Services, which manages the following programs: The Administration of Children, Youth, and Families (services for children, adolescents, and their families, abused children, battered women, runaway or homeless youth, and working parents); The Administration for native Americans (services for American Indians, Alaska Natives, and Native Hawaiians); The Administration on Aging (services for needy elderly persons); The Administration on Developmental Disabilities (services for disabled persons); and the President's Committee on Mental Retardation, which is located in the Office of Human Development Services, but advises the President and works with other government agencies for the prevention of mental retardation. Through the Social Security Administration, HHS operates the national social insurance programs. The Work Incentive Program (WIN) provides training employment and social services designed to shift families from welfare agencies to productive occupations. The Office of Child Support Enforcement programs pays state and local governments 75 percent of the costs incurred in establishing parent responsibility and child support. The Department of Health and Human Services was known previously as the Department of Health, Education, and Welfare (DHEW). **hospital emergency d.,** emergency ROOM.

dependence (de-pend′ens) the state of being dependent on or requiring another person or object in order to exist or act satisfactorily. **drug d.,** a state, psychic and sometimes also physical, resulting from the interaction between the living organism and a drug, characterized by behavioral and other responses that always include a compulsion to take the drug on a continuous or periodic basis in order to experience its psychic effects, and sometimes to avoid the discomfort of its absence. Tolerance may or may not be present. Cf. drug ADDICTION and drug HABITUATION. **physical d.,** drug dependence manifested by intense physical disturbances when the administration of the drug is suspended, including withdrawal or abstinence syndromes. The term is roughly equated with drug addiction (see under ADDICTION). **psychic d., psychological d.,** drug dependence in which a drug produces a feeling of satisfaction and a psychic drive that requires periodic or continuous administration of the drug to produce pleasure or to avoid discomfort. The term is roughly equated with drug habituation (see under HABITUATION).

dependent (de-pen′dent) 1. requiring or relying on someone or something else. 2. any person who is financially supported by another. 3. in insurance, persons other than a subscriber, such as a spouse, children, and certain other family members, as defined in the contract, who may receive benefits under the insurance policy. See also SUBSCRIBER (3).

depigmentation (de″pig-men-ta′shun) disappearance or removal of pigment.

depletion (de-ple′shun) [L. *deplere* empty] 1. the act or process of emptying; removal of a fluid, as the blood. 2. an exhausted state which results from excessive loss of blood.

depolarization (de-po″lar-i-za′shun) 1. the process or act of neutralizing polarity. 2. in neurophysiology, the reversal of the resting potential in excitable cell membranes when stimulated, i.e., the tendency of the cell membrane potential to become positive with respect to potential outside the cell.

Depo-Medrate a trademark for *methylprednisolone acetate* (see under METHYLPREDNISOLONE).

Depo-Medrol trademark for *methylprednisolone acetate* (see under METHYLPREDNISOLONE).

Depo-Medrone trademark for *methylprednisolone acetate* (see under METHYLPREDNISOLONE).

depo-preparation (de″po-, dep′o-prep″ah-ra′shun) a pharmaceutical preparation deposited in tissues by injection for slow absorption into blood for the purpose of giving long-term action.

deposit (de-poz′it) [L. *de* down + *ponere* to place] 1. sediment or drugs. 2. extraneous inorganic matter connected in the tissue or in a viscus or cavity. 3. tooth d. **calcareous d.,** deposition in the tissues of calcareous material. See dental CALCULUS. **tooth d.,** a hard or soft material deposited on the surface of a tooth. See dental CALCULUS, dental PLAQUE, and MATERIA alba.

depot (de′po, dep′o) [Fr. *dépôt*, from L. *depositum*] a body area in which a substance, e.g., a drug, can be accumulated, deposited, or stored and from which it can be distributed. **fat d.,** a site in the body in which large quantities of fat are stored, as in adipose tissue.

Depovernil trademark for *sulfamethoxypyridazine.*

depressant (de-pres′ant) 1. diminishing functional activity. 2. an agent that reduces functional activity and the vital energies in general by producing muscular relaxation and diaphoresis.

depression (de-presh′un) [L. *depressio;* from *de* down + *premere* to press] 1. a hollow or depressed area. See also FOSSA, FOVEA, and PIT. 2. the act or process of downward or inward displacement. 3. a lowering or decrease of functional activity. 4. a psychiatric syndrome consisting of dejected mood, psychomotor disorders, insomnia, and weight loss, sometimes associated with guilt feelings and somatic preoccupations. **pacchionian d's,** granular foveolae; see under FOVEOLA. **pterygoid d.,** pterygoid fossa of mandible; see under FOSSA. **tooth d.,** intrusion (3).

depressor (de-pres′or) [L.] 1. any device, instrument, or agent which depresses a part of the body (e.g., a tongue depressor), or an afferent nerve whose stimulation causes a fall of blood pressure. 2. a muscle that depresses. 3. a drug that alters mood to sadness or, if the mood is abnormally elevated, toward normal; or reduces the frequency of nerve impulses to reduce the strength of various bodily functions. **d. an′guli o′ris,** depressor muscle of angle of mouth; see under MUSCLE. **d. la′bii inferio′ris,** depressor muscle of lower lip; see under MUSCLE. **d. sep′ti na′si,** depressor muscle of nasal septum; see under MUSCLE. **d. supercil′ii,** depressor muscle, superciliary; see under MUSCLE.

Depridol trademark for the *dl*-form of *methadone hydrochloride* (see under METHADONE).

Depromic trademark for *propoxyphene hydrochloride* (see under PROPOXYPHENE).

de Quatrefage see QUATREFAGE.

der derivative chromosome; see CHROMOSOME nomenclature.

Deracil trademark for *thiouracil.*

de Reynier, J. P. see DYSOSTOSIS mandibularis (Nager-de Reynier syndrome).

derivation (der″i-va′shun) [L. *derivatio*, from *derivare* to draw off] 1. the origin or source of something. 2. a lead in electrocardiography.

derivative (dĕ-riv′ah-tiv) 1. producing or causing a derivation. 2. a chemical substance derived from another substance either directly or by modification or partial substitution.

derma (der′mah) [Gr.] skin.

derma- see DERMATO-.

dermabrasion (der-mah-bra′shun) [Gr. *derma* skin + L. *abrasio* abrasion] surgical removal of the frozen epidermis and as much of the dermis as necessary, by mechanical means, such as low- or high-speed wire brushes, emery paper cylinders, sand paper, etc., to remove scars, tattoos, pigmented nevi, wrinkles, and other irregularities of the skin. See also PLANING.

Dermacentroxenum sibericus (der″mah-sen-trok-se′num si-ber′i-kus) *Rickettsia sibirica;* see under RICKETTSIA.

dermad (der′mad) toward the integument.

Dermadex trademark for *hexachlorophene.*

dermal (der′mal) of or pertaining to the skin; cutaneous.

Dermalar trademark for *fluocinolone acetonide* (see under FLUOCINOLONE).

dermatan sulfate (der′mah-tan sul′fāt) an acid mucopolysaccharide made up of recurring units of iduronic acid and N-acetyl-D-galactosamine 4-sulfate; occurring in the skin. Called also *chondroitin sulfate B* and *β-heparin.*

dermatitis (der″mah-ti′tis) [dermato- + -itis] any inflammatory disease of the skin. **atopic d.**, an inflammatory skin disease that tends to occur in atopic individuals, and often begins in infancy as a manifestation of a food allergy, and may continue into childhood, adolescence, and adulthood; it sometimes lasts for a year or two and disappears partially or completely, or there may be a quiescent period with subsequent recurrence. The infantile form commonly begins as erythematous weepy patches on the cheeks, followed by extension to other parts of the body, such as the rest of the face, scalp, neck, cubital and popliteal areas, and buttocks. In older children, adolescents, and adults, it is characterized by intense pruritus, lichenification, excoriations, and crusting, and is frequently associated with asthma and hay fever. Called also *allergic eczema, atopic eczema, infantile eczema,* and *Besnier's prurigo.* **blastomycetic d.**, North American BLASTOMYCOSIS. **d. bullo′sa heredita′ria**, EPIDERMOLYSIS bullosa. **chronic atrophic lichenoid d.**, LICHEN sclerosus et atrophicus. **contact d.**, contact hypersensitivity manifested as an acute inflammatory disease of the skin, characterized by redness, swelling, vesicles, bullae, burning, and itching; it is caused by exposure, usually repeated, to a substance to which the patient is sensitive. Called also *dermatitis venenata.* See also drug REACTION and STOMATITIS venenata. **d. exfoliati′va generalisa′ta**, Leiner's d. **d. exfoliati′va infan′tum**, Ritter's DISEASE. **Kaposi's d.**, Kaposi's varicelliform ERUPTION. **Leiner's d.**, an exfoliative skin disease occurring in newborn and older infants, affecting usually those who are breast fed, which begins as seborrheic eczematoid lesions of the scalp and face or the gluteal region and eventually spreads to other areas. The lesions may consist of dry desquamative areas or seborrheic scales, which are usually associated with gastrointestinal disorders, including diarrhea. Called also *d. exfoliativa generalisata* and *erythrodermia desquamativa in infants.* **d. medicamento′sa**, dermatitis due to allergic reaction to drugs taken internally, characterized by erythema, urticaria, vesicles, bullae, pustules, ulcers, and gangrene. Called also *drug rash.* See also drug ALLERGY, drug eruption, fixed, under ERUPTION, drug REACTION, and STOMATITIS medicamentosa. **mucosynechial d.**, benign mucosal PEMPHIGOID. **d. precancero′sa**, CARCINOMA *in situ.* **d. pustula′ris**, d. vegetans. **seborrheic d.**, **d. seborrhe′ica**, a chronic skin disease characterized by moderate erythema, itching, yellow crusty patches, and scaling. In mild cases, the scalp may be the only area affected, dandruff being the sole manifestation. In more severe cases, the dermatitis may spread to portions of the skin adjacent to the hairline, eyebrows, nasal folds, retroauricular areas, and trunk. The cause is unknown but sweat retention, trauma, infections, antibiotic therapy, sebaceous dysfunction, nutrition, and emotional factors are believed to contribute to the occurrence and intensity of the disorder. Called also *eczema seborrheicum, seborrhea,* and *seborrheic eczema.* See also DANDRUFF. **d. veg′etans**, a skin disorder believed to be caused by a staphylococcal superinfection, characterized by miliary pustules surrounded by a hyperemic base on the axillae, scalp, groin, genitalia, lips, and oral mucosa. Coalescing pustules form crust-covered patches with vegetating surfaces beneath. The oral ulcers are caused by ruptured pustules. Histologically, the disorder is similar to pemphigus vulgaris. Called also *d. pustularis, Hallopeau's syndrome, pyoderma vegetans, pyoderma verrucosum,* and *pyodermatitis vegetans.* See also PEMPHIGUS vegetans. **d. venena′ta**, contact d.

dermato-, derma-, dermo- [Gr. *derma* skin] a combining form denoting relationship to the skin.

dermatoarthritis (der″mah-to-ar-thri′tis) skin disease associated with arthritis. **lipid d.**, multicentric RETICULOHISTIOCYTOSIS.

dermatodysplasia (der″mah-to-dis-pla′ze-ah) abnormal development of the skin.

dermatofibrosarcoma (der″mah-to-fi″bro-sar-ko′mah) a fibrosarcoma of the skin. **d. protub′erans**, a usually benign tumor of the skin, sometimes occurring about the head and neck, but very rarely on the oral mucosa, which typically begins as a plaquelike thickening, often associated with superficial discoloration. It gives the appearance of being encapsulated but, characteristically, invades and destroys the surrounding connective tissue. The most common pathological feature is the presence of radially arranged fibroblasts. The lesion sometimes metastasizes; there is a high recurrence rate.

dermatology (der″mah-tol′o-je) the medical specialty concerned with the diagnosis and treatment of skin diseases.

dermatome (der′mah-tōm) [derma- + Gr. *tomnein* to cut] 1. an instrument for cutting thin layers of skin for grafting. 2. the lateral portion of a mesodermal somite; see SOMITE.

dermatomyositis (der″mah-to-mi″o-si′tis) [dermato- + Gr. *mys* muscle + -itis] an acute or chronic collagen disease of the skin and skeletal muscles of unknown etiology. Initial symptoms include fever, malaise, and edema, tenderness, and weakness, usually of the extremities and about the shoulder girdle, eventually spreading to the intercostal muscles, diaphragm, and muscles of the larynx and pharynx leading to dysphagia, respiratory failure, and death. Skin lesions (more pronounced in acute cases) include pigmentation and depigmentation, thinning of the epidermis, and erythema with desquamation and rash. The face, especially the eyelids, ears, and anterior neck, are most commonly affected. Oral lesions usually consist of stomatitis, pharyngitis, and lesions of the masticatory muscles. Pathologically, the involved muscles and skin, and sometimes the heart, blood vessels, and serous membranes, are pale or yellowish brown and are either edematous or atrophic. The muscle cells show swelling followed by hyaline degeneration and necrosis, with diffuse interstitial infiltration of lymphocytes and plasma cells. Edema and erythema with perivascular lymphocytic and plasma cell infiltrates are the most significant pathologic skin changes.

Dermatophilaceae (der″mah-to-fi-la′se-e) [*Dermatophilus* + -aceae] a family of bacteria of the order Actinomycetales. It consists of both pathogenic and nonpathogenic, gram-positive, aerobic microorganisms, characterized by mycelial filaments or muriform thalli that divide transversely in at least two longitudinal planes to form masses of coccoid or cuboid motile cells. It consists of the genera *Dermatophilus* and *Geodermatophilus.*

Dermatophilus (der″mah-tof′ĭ-lus) [dermato- + Gr. *philus* loving] a genus of gram-positive, aerobic and facultatively anaerobic, non–acid-fast bacteria of the family Dermatophilaceae, order Actinomycetales. Some species are pathogenic and invade the uncornified epidermis. They have substrate mycelia consisting of long tapering filaments, which branch laterally at right angles, and septa formed in transverse and in horizontal and vertical longitudinal planes, giving rise to eight or less parallel rows of coccoid cells (spores), which become motile tufts of flagella. **D. congolen′sis**, a species causing infection in cattle, sheep, horses, goats, deer, and other herbivores. It is sometimes pathogenic to man, causing nonpainful pustules on the hands and arms, which break down to form ulcers, and eventually regress spontaneously.

dermatophyte (der′mah-to-fīt″) [dermato- + Gr. *phyton* plant] a fungus parasitic on the skin; the term embraces fungi of the form-class Deuteromycetes, including the genera *Microsporum, Epidermophyton,* and *Trichophyton.*

dermatopolyneuritis (der″mah-to-pol″e-nu-ri′tis) acrodynia.

dermatosclerosis (der″mah-to-skle-ro′sis) [dermato- + Gr. *sklērōsis* hardening] scleroderma.

dermatoses (der″mah-to′sēz) plural of *dermatosis.*

dermatosis (der″mah-to′sis), pl. *dermato′ses* [dermato- + -osis] any skin disease, especially one not characterized by inflammation.

dermatostomatitis (der″mah-to-sto-mah-ti′tis) [dermato- + stomatitis] inflammation of the skin and mucous membranes of the mouth. **Baader's d.**, Stevens-Johnson SYNDROME.

dermis (der′mis) the skin; sometimes used to mean the true skin or corium. See CORIUM.

dermo- see DERMATO-.

dermoid (der′moid) [derma- + Gr. *eidos* form] 1. resembling the skin. 2. dermoid CYST.

Dermotricine trademark for *tyrothricin.*

Deronil trademark for *dexamethasone.*

DES diethylstilbestrol.

Desace trademark for *deslanoside.*

Desacetyllanatoside C trademark for *deslanoside.*

desalivation (de″sal-ĭ-va′shun) the depriving of saliva.

De Salle's line nasal LINE.

descending (de-send′ing) [L. *descendere*] extending downward.

Deschamp's needle [Joseph François Louis *Deschamps*, French surgeon, 1740–1824] see under NEEDLE.

deschlorobiomycin (des-klo″ro-bi″o-mi′sin) tetracycline (1).

Desdemin trademark for *furosemide.*

desensitization (de-sen″sĭ-ti-za′shun) the prevention or reduction of recurrences of immediate hypersensitivity reactions by the administration of graded doses of allergen. The allergen causes the production of specific "blocking" IgG, thereby inhibiting further specific IgE synthesis or combining with the allergen and preventing the latter from combining with IgE on the surface of mast cells.

Desfedrin trademark for *methamphetamine hydrochloride* (see under METHAMPHETAMINE).

Desferal trademark for *deferoxamine mesylate* (see under DEFEROXAMINE).

desiccant (des'ĭ-kant) 1. promoting dryness; causing to dry up. 2. a chemical agent capable of taking up water from other substances, thus promoting their dryness; usually a hygroscopic compound, such as calcium chloride. Called also *desiccating agent*, *drying agent*, and *exsiccant*.

desiccation (des''ĭ-ka'shun) the act or process of drying up. **electric d.**, an electrosurgical technique in which deep-penetrating cellular dehydration of tissue is produced by a single electrode placed into tissue, using a highly damped high-frequency alternating current; a small pointed electrode without a conductive pad is used most commonly. Used in the treatment of tumors or other diseases. See also ELECTROSURGERY.

desipramine hydrochloride (des-ip'rah-mēn) an antidepressant drug with anticholinergic and epinephrine-potentiating properties, 10,11-dihydro-5-[3-(methylamino)propyl-5H-dibenz[b,f] azepine monohydrochloride, occurring as a white to off-white, odorless, crystalline powder with a bitter taste, which is sensitive to light and is soluble in chloroform, water, ethanol, and methanol, but not in ether. Contraindicated in severe coronary heart disease, glaucoma, and epilepsy. Trademarks: Irene, Norpramin, Pertofrane.

-desis [Gr. "binding"] a word termination indicating a binding or fusion.

deslanoside (des-lan'o-sīd) a cardiac glycoside from the leaves of *Digitalis lanata* ($C_{47}H_{74}O_{19}$), occurring as hygroscopic, odorless, white crystalline powder or colorless or white crystals that are slightly soluble in water, ethanol, methanol, and chloroform. Used similarly to digitalis in the treatment of congestive heart failure. It may cause cardiac arrhythmias, nausea, vomiting, neuralgic pains, headache, fatigue, drowsiness, and convulsions. Trademarks: Cedilanid D, Desace, Desacetyllanatoside C, Lanimerck.

desmethyldopan (des-meth''il-do'pan) uracil MUSTARD.

desmo- [Gr. *desmos* band, ligament] a combining form denoting relationship to a band, bond, or ligament.

desmocyte (des'mo-sīt) [*desmo-* + Gr. *kytos* hollow vessel] fibroblast.

desmoid (des'moid) [*desmo-* + Gr. *eidos* form] a fibromatous, unencapsulated tumor arising from a muscle sheath, usually of the abdominal wall, but also of other sites, including the head and neck; it is identified histologically in the intermediate zone between benign fibromas and slowly growing, well-differentiated fibrosarcomas. Called also *desmoid tumor*.

desmodont (des'mo-dont) periodontal LIGAMENT.

desmosome (des'mo-sōm) [*desmo-* + Gr. *sōma* body] a bipartite structure that forms the site of attachment between cells. It is a dense plaque formed by tonofibrils of adjacent cell membranes. Called also *macula adherens*. See also intercellular BRIDGE. **half d.**, hemidesmosome.

Desone trademark for a soft *dental casting gold alloy* (see under ALLOY).

desoxy- in chemical nomenclature, a prefix used in naming compounds, indicating the removal of oxygen. For words beginning thus, see also those beginning DEOXY-. See also desoxy COMPOUND.

11-desoxycorticosterone (des-ok''se-kor''te-ko'ster-ōn) deoxycorticosterone.

desoxyephedrine (des''ok-sĕ-ef'ĕ-drin) methamphetamine.

2-desoxyphenobarbital (des-ok''sĕ-fe''no-bar'bĭ-tal) primidone.

desquamation (des''kwah-ma'shun) [*de-* + L. *squama* scale] the shedding of epithelial elements, chiefly of the skin or mucous membranes.

desquamative (des-kwam'ah-tiv) pertaining to or characterized by desquamation.

dest. abbreviation for L. *destil'la*, distil, and *destilla'tus*, distilled.

destil. abbreviation for L. *destil'la*, distil.

Det. abbreviation for L. *de'tur*, let it be given.

detachment (de-tach'ment) [Fr. *detacher* to unfasten, to separate] the condition of being unfastened, disconnected, or separated.

detector (de-tek'tor) a device by which the presence of something, or the existence of a certain condition, is discovered. **radiation d.**, any device or substance that is sensitive to radiation and can produce a response signal suitable for its detection, measurement, or analysis. See also COUNTER.

detergent (de-ter'jent) [L. *detergere* to cleanse] 1. purifying; cleansing. 2. a substance capable of reducing the surface tension of water, specifically, a surface-active agent which concentrates at oil-water interfaces, exerting an emulsifying action, and thus aids in the removal of dirt and soil.

determinant (de-ter'mĭ-nant) [L. *determinare* to bound, limit, or fix] a factor that establishes the nature of an entity or event. **antigenic d.**, the structural component of an antigen molecule responsible for specific interaction with antibody (immunoglobulin) molecules elicited by the same or related antigen. It is the site on the antigen to which antibody becomes attached by its combining site, the determinant forming a three-dimensional fit with the antibody and being bound to it by a noncovalent link. Antigenic determinants consist of chemically active surface groupings of amino acids in globular proteins and sugar side chains in polysaccharides; called *antigenic determinant group*, or *epitope*. A small portion of the determinant group critical to establishing specificity is called *immunodominant point*. Antibodies produced in response to immunization with a carrier protein to which specific chemical groups (haptens) have been introduced artificially by conjugation show active specificity for antigenic determinant groups that are frequently identical or nearly identical in structure to the hapten.

determination (de-ter''mĭ-na'shun) establishment of the exact nature of an entity or event.

Dethyrona trademark for *dextrothyroxine sodium* (see under DEXTROTHYROXINE).

De Toni-Fanconi syndrome [Guido *De Toni*; Guido *Fanconi*, Swiss biochemist, born 1892] Abderhalden-Fanconi SYNDROME.

detorque (de-tork') an orthodontic technique used to reduce a root moving adjustment that has been placed in the arch wire, which usually will result in a more vertical inclination of the maxillary teeth.

detorsion (de-tor'shun) 1. the correction of a curvature or twisting. 2. a deficiency in a normal twisting.

detoxification (de-tok''sĭ-fi-ka'shun) 1. reduction of the toxic properties of poisons. 2. treatment designed to free an addict from his drug habit.

detrition (de-trish'un) [L. *de* away + *terere* to wear] a wearing away, as of the teeth, by friction. See also ABRASION.

detritus (de-tri'tus) [L. from *deterere* to rub away] particulate matter produced by or remaining after the wearing away or disintegration of a substance or tissue.

Detyroxin trademark for *dextrothyroxine sodium* (see under DEXTROTHYROXINE).

deuterium (doo-te're-um) [Gr. *deuteros* second] a stable, nonradioactive isotope of hydrogen, with a nucleus containing one neutron and one proton, having an atomic weight of 2.014, thus being twice as heavy as hydrogen. It is a colorless, odorless, noncorrosive, flammable gas that is considered nontoxic. Deuterium is used as a tracer element or indicator in studying fat and amino acid metabolism. When replacing hydrogen in water, it produces heavy water. Symbol ^{2}H or D. Called also *heavy hydrogen*. **d. oxide**, heavy WATER.

deutero-, deuto- [Gr. *deuteros* second] a combining form meaning second.

deuterohemophilia (doo''ter-o-he''mo-fil'e-ah) Christmas DISEASE.

deuteromycete (doo''ter-o-mi'sēt) any individual fungus of the Deuteromycetes; an imperfect fungus.

Deuteromycetes (doo''ter-o-mi-se'tēz) a form-class of true fungi (Eumycetes), consisting of organisms that have no known sexual stage and reproduce by asexual spore formation; the Fungi Imperfecti. It includes a few of the pathogenic fungi. Single-celled round forms are known as *imperfect yeasts*.

deuteromycetous (doo''ter-o-mi-se'tus) of or pertaining to the Deuteromycetes (Fungi Imperfecti).

deuteron (doo'ter-on) the nucleus of deuterium, or heavy hydrogen; deuterons are used as bombing particles for nuclear disintegration.

deuto- see DEUTERO-.

developer (de-vel'o-per) an agent that allows something to reach a more advanced or effective state. **film d.**, developing SOLUTION. **rapid d.**, developing solution, rapid; see under SOLUTION.

development (de-vel'op-ment) 1. the act or process of making something more advanced or effective. 2. the process of growth and differentiation. **film d.**, the first step in film processing, consisting of converting the latent image on the exposed film into the manifest image through the process of reduction of the exposed silver salts to metallic silver grains, thus rendering them black and giving shape to the image. It is an oxidation-reduction process, having the following formula: $2AgBr + C_6H_4(OH)_2 \rightarrow 2Ag^+ + 2Br^- + C_6H_4O_2 + 2H^+$. The process occurs in the developing solution which contains Metol and hydroquinone, Metol acting as the activator and hydroquinone as the developer. The developer removes bromine ions from silver bromide, thus leaving black metallic silver grains in emulsion. Other components of the developing solution include sodium carbonate which produces a pH of about 11.0, accelerates the reducing action, and softens the emulsion; potassium bromide which acts as a restrainer; and sodium sulfite which acts as a preservative and slows down oxidation. See also developing SOLUTION, film FIXATION, and film PROCESSING.

deviation (de″ve-a′shun) [L. *deviare* to turn aside] a departure or turning away from accepted standards. **angle of d.,** ANGLE of deviation. **standard d.,** in standardized tests, a measure of deviations from a central value, determined as the square root of the average of the squares of all deviations from the mean. Symbol σ. Abbreviated S.D.

device (de-vīs′) something contrived for a specific purpose. **acceptable d.,** any dental device which has been evaluated under the provisions of the acceptance program of the Council on Dental Materials and Devices of the American Dental Association, based on evidence of safety and usefulness established by biological, laboratory, and/or clinical evaluations. Products found both useful and safe are listed in the *Guide to Dental Materials and Devices* and are awarded the Seal of Certification, which may be used in advertising, in brochures, and on packages. **central-bearing d.,** one that provides a central point of bearing, or support, between upper and lower occlusion rims, consisting of a contracting point *(central-bearing point)* attached to one occlusion rim and a plate that provides the surface on which the bearing point rests or moves. **central-bearing tracing d.,** one for determining the central bearing or support between maxillary and mandibular occlusion rims or dentures. It consists of a contacting point attached to one occlusion rim or denture and a plate attached to the opposing occlusion rim or denture which provides the surface on which the bearing point rests or moves. Used to distribute closing forces evenly throughout the areas of the supporting structures during the recording of maxillomandibular relations and/or correcting disharmonious occlusal contacts. **compression d.,** in radiography, a device for reducing the thickness of an organ or part for x-ray examination. **provisionally acceptable d.,** a dental device which, after investigation and evaluation by the Council on Dental Materials and Devices of the American Dental Association, was found to lack sufficient evidence to justify classification as acceptable, but for which there is reasonable evidence of safety and usefulness, including clinical feasibility. **unacceptable d.,** a dental device which, after investigation and evaluation by the Council on Dental Materials and Devices of the American Dental Association, was found to be dangerous to the health of the user, obsolete, markedly inferior, or useless.

devitalization (de-vi″tal-i-za′shun) the deprivation of life, as of a tissue. **pulp d.,** the destruction of vitality of the dental pulp.

devitalize (de-vi′tal-īz) [de- + L. *vita* life] to deprive of vitality or of life.

De Vries syndrome [André *De Vries*] see under SYNDROME.

Dexacortal trademark for *dexamethasone.*

Dexameth trademark for *dexamethasone.*

dexamethasone (dek″sah-meth″ah-sōn) a synthetic glucocorticoid prepared from prednisolone, 9-fluoro-11β,17,21-trihydroxy-16α-methylpregna-1,4-diene-3,20-dione, occurring as a white, odorless, crystalline powder that is insoluble in water and slightly soluble in acetone, ethanol, dioxane, methanol, chloroform, and ether. Used in the treatment of adrenocortical insufficiency and as an anti-inflammatory and antiallergic agent. In dentistry, used in the treatment of sensitive dentin, pulpal reactions to surgery, oral ulcers, arthritic temporomandibular lesions, and in tissue transplantation. Side reactions are those of other glucocorticoids. Trademarks: Decacortin, Dekacort, Deronil, Dexacortal, Dexameth, Fluormone, Hexadrol, Oradexon, Maxidex, Policort.

Dexamphetamine trademark for *dextroamphetamine sulfate* (see under DEXTROAMPHETAMINE).

dexbrompheniramine maleate (deks″brom-fen-i′rah-mēn) the dextro isomer of brompheniramine, [p-bromo-α-(2-dimethylamino) ethyl] benzyl] pyridine, occurring as a white, odorless, crystalline powder that dissolves in water, alcohol, and chloroform. It is an antihistaminic agent that acts on the H₁ receptor. Used in the treatment of allergic diseases. Trademark: Disomer.

dexchlorpheniramine maleate (deks″klor-fen-i′rah-mēn) the dextrorotatory isomer of chlorpheniramine, *d*-2-[p-chloro-α-(2-dimethylaminoethyl)benzyl]pyridine maleate, occurring as a white, odorless, crystalline powder that is readily soluble in water, alcohol, and chloroform and slightly soluble in benzene and ether. It is a potent antihistaminic agent that acts on the H₁ receptor. Used in the treatment of allergic diseases. Trademarks: Chlo-Amine, Fortamine, Isomerine, Phendextro, Polaramine.

Dexedrine trademark for *dextroamphetamine sulfate* (see under DEXTROAMPHETAMINE).

Dexephrin trademark for *methamphetamine hydrochloride* (see under METHAMPHETAMINE).

Dexoval trademark for *methamphetamine hydrochloride* (see under METHAMPHETAMINE).

Dexten- trademark for *dextroamphetamine sulfate* (see under DEXTROAMPHETAMINE).

dexter (dek′ster) [L.] right; an anatomical term denoting the right-hand one of two similar structures, or the one situated on the right side of the body. Cf. SINISTER.

dextrad (deks′trad) toward the right side.

dextral (deks′tral) 1. right. 2. a right-handed person.

dextrality (deks-tral′ĭ-te) [L. *dexter* right] the preferential use, in voluntary motor acts, of the right member of the major paired organs of the body, as the right eye, hand, or foot. Cf. SINISTRALITY.

dextran (dek′stran) a water-soluble polysaccharide of glucose, produced by the action of a bacterium, *Leuconostoc mesenteroides,* on sucrose. Specific dextran preparations are designated according to their average molecular weight divided by 1000, as dextran 40, dextran 45, etc. Used as a plasma expander in hypovolemias and as a vehicle in dextran iron complex.

dextran-iron (dek″stran-i′ern) see dextran-iron COMPLEX.

dextriferron (deks″tri-fer′on) a complex of ferric hydroxide and partially hydrolized dextrin; used in the treatment of iron deficiency.

dextrin (deks′trin) a dextrorotatory product formed by the hydrolysis of starches, occurring as a white or yellow powder that is soluble in water and precipitated by alcohol. Used in the production of dry extracts and pills, for preparing emulsions and dry bandages, as a substitute for natural gum, and in various industrial products and processes. Called also *British* or *starch gum* and *gommelin.*

dextrinosis (deks″tri-no′sis) accumulation in the tissues of an abnormal polysaccharide. **debrancher deficiency limit d., limit d.,** GLYCOGENOSIS III.

dextro- [L. *dexter* right] 1. a combining form denoting relationship to the right. 2. a chemical prefix indicating dextrorotatory.

dextroamphetamine (dek″stro-am-fet′ah-min) the dextrorotatory isomer of amphetamine, (+)-α-methylphenethylamine, which is a sympathomimetic drug with weak peripheral and strong central stimulant action. Used in the treatment of narcolepsy, parkinsonism, and epilepsy. Also used to counteract the side effects or overdose of hypnotic and sedative drugs, to maintain blood pressure in surgery, as an appetite depressant, and in the treatment of hyperkinetic children and orthostatic hypotension. It is a habit-forming drug widely used by addicts. Side reactions may include restlessness, hyperactivity, insomnia, euphoria, dysphoria, headache, tremor, hypertension, tachycardia, arrhythmia, xerostomia, nausea, diarrhea, urticaria, skin rash, hypersensitivity, impotence, and various neurological and endocrine disorders. **d. phosphate,** the phosphate salt of dextroamphetamine, occurring as a white, bitter, odorless, crystalline powder that is soluble in water, slightly soluble in ethanol, and insoluble in organic solvents. **d. sulfate,** the sulfate salt of dextroamphetamine, occurring as a white, odorless, crystalline powder that is soluble in water and ethanol, but not in ether. Trademarks: Afatin, Ardex, Dadex, Dexamphetamine, Dexedrine, Dexten, Maxiton, Obesedrin, Simpamin.

dextrocompound (deks″tro-kom′pownd) see dextrorotatory ISOMER.

dextroglucose (deks″tro-gloo′kōs) dextrose.

dextromethorphan hydrobromide (deks″tro-meth′or-fan) a synthetic morphine derivative, D-3-methoxy-N-methylmorphinan hydrobromide, occurring as a white crystalline powder or crystals with a faint odor, which are soluble in water, ethanol, and chloroform, but not in ether. Used as an antitussive agent. Side effects may include drowsiness and gastrointestinal disorders. It is suspected of causing habituation or addiction. Called also *demorphan hydrobromide.* Trademarks: Antisep, Romilar, Sacophan, Supressin, Testamin, Tusilan.

dextropropoxyphene (deks″tro-pro-pok′sē-fen) propoxyphene.

dextroposition (deks″tro-po-zish′un) displacement to the right.

dextrorotatory (deks″tro-ro′tah-to-re) [*dextro*- + L. *rotare* to turn] turning to the right; pertaining to the property of chemical compounds, when in solution, of rotating the plane of polarized light to the right or clockwise. The prefix D- (formerly *d*-) and the symbol + are used in organic chemistry to distinguish dextrorotatory from levorotatory isomers.

dextrose (deks′trōs) a sugar, D(+)-glucose, similar to that found in animal blood, occurring as an odorless, colorless, crystalline or granular powder with a sweet taste that is soluble in water and alcohol. Dextrose solutions of varying concentrations, 2.5 to 25 percent, or in sodium chloride solutions, 0.11 to 0.9 percent, are used as body fluid replenishers and to reestablish blood sugar following blood loss, as after hemorrhage, shock, or surgical trauma. Commonly called *glucose*. Called also *anhydrous d., d. monohydrate, cerelose, dextroglucose, medicinal glucose, purified glucose,* and *bread, corn, grape,* or *starch sugar*. **anhydrous d., d. monohydrate,** dextrose.

dextrosinistral (deks″tro-sin′is-tral) [*dextro-* + L. *sinister* left] extending from right to left. Also applied to a person naturally left-handed but trained to use the right hand in certain performances.

dextrosuria (deks″tro-su′re-ah) [*dextrose* + Gr. *ouron* urine + *-ia*] the presence of dextrose in the urine. Called also *glucosuria*.

dextrothyroxine sodium (deks″tro-thi-rok′sin) the dextrorotatory isomer of thyroxine, 3,3′,5,5′-tetraiodothyronine sodium, occurring as a light yellow to buff, odorless, tasteless powder that assumes a slightly pink discoloration on exposure to light, and is soluble in solutions of alkali hydroxides, hot solutions of alkali carbonates, slightly soluble in water, and insoluble in acetone, chloroform, and ether. Used to lower blood cholesterol and lipids. Side effects may include increased metabolic rate, tachycardia, anginal pain in persons with coronary insufficiency, and other disorders. It also augments the action of anticoagulants. Called also D-*thyroxine sodium salt*. Trademarks: Cholaxin, Dethyrona, Detyroxin, Dynothel.

dextrotropic (deks″tro-trop′ik) [*dextro-* + Gr. *tropos* a turning] turning to the right.

dextroverted (deks″tro-vert′ed) turning to the right.

DF distribution FACTOR.

dg decigram.

DHA dehydroepiandrosterone.

DH-codeine dihydrocodeine.

DHE-45 trademark for *dihydroergotamime mesylate* (see under DIHYDROERGOTAMINE).

DHEW Department of Health, Education and Welfare; see Department of Health and Human Services, under DEPARTMENT.

di- [Gr. *dis* twice, double] 1. a prefix meaning twice. 2. a variant spelling of *de-, dia-,* and *dis-*. 3. a chemical prefix meaning two or twice; the number of each type of monodentate ligand in a coordination compound. See also BI- and BIS-.

dia- [Gr. *dia* through] a prefix meaning through, between, apart, across, or completely.

Diabenal trademark for *chlorpropamide*.

diabetes (di″ah-be′tēz) [Gr. *diabētēs* a syphon, from *dia* through + *bainein* to go] 1. a deficiency condition marked by habitual discharge of an excessive quantity of urine. 2. d. mellitus. **bronze d., bronzed d.,** hemochromatosis. **d. insip′idus,** a disease caused by deficiency of vasopressin, characterized by failure to reabsorb water by the distal renal tubules with resulting excretion of large volumes of urine, unrelenting thirst, and compensatory polydipsia. Oral complications include decreased salivary secretion. **lipoatrophic d.,** a disorder marked by generalized lipoatrophy, hepatosplenomegaly, enlargement of the parotid glands, disturbed carbohydrate metabolism, high metabolic rate, accelerated growth, intense lipemia, and diabetes mellitus. Pathologic findings include absence of subcutaneous and retroperitoneal depot fat, portal cirrhosis, proliferation of the parotid ducts, and dilatation of the sinuses of the lymph nodes. Called also *Lawrence's syndrome*. **d. melli′tus,** a metabolic disease caused by deficiency of insulin, manifested by faulty utilization of carbohydrates and compensatory catabolism of proteins and fats to supply the energy needs of the body, which result in hyperglycemia, ketosis, and glycosuria. Vascular changes, including arteriosclerosis and degenerative vascular changes, affecting the kidneys, eyes, heart, and nervous system, frequently leading to blindness, neuritis, congestive heart failure, and hypertension, are frequently associated. Symptoms include accelerated aging, weakness, lassitude, loss of weight, and specific odor of the breath due to ketosis. Oral complications may include fulminating periodontitis with abscesses, gingivitis with hemorrhagic gingival papillae, and xerostomia. It is commonly believed that diabetes mellitus is, in some way, transmitted as an inherited disease. Dental treatment, particularly subgingival curettage and surgical procedures, are performed only as emergency measures in uncontrolled diabetes mellitus. **phosphate d.,** vitamin D–resistant RICKETS.

Diabewas trademark for *tolazamide*.

Diabinese trademark for *chlorpropamide*.

Diabuton trademark for *tolbutamide*.

diacetylmorphine (di″ah-se″til-mor′fēn) an opium alkaloid, 7,8-didehydro-4,5α-epoxy-17-methylmorphinan-3,6α-diol diacetate, occurring as a white, bitter, crystalline powder that dissolves in water, alcohol, fats, and chloroform. Pharmacologically, diacetylmorphine is similar to morphine, but is a more potent analgesic and has less peripheral and more central effects. It is also an effective cough depressant, but its strong central effects, particularly on the respiratory center, render it relatively unsafe in clinical use. Owing to its ready solubility in water, it is very rapidly absorbed and because it is lipid soluble it easily penetrates the blood-brain barrier. In the body, diacetylmorphine is converted to monoacetylmorphine and then to morphine. Like morphine, it is extremely addictive. Called also *acetomorphine, demorphine, diamorphine,* and *heroin*.

di-acid (di-as′id) [Gr. *dis* twice + *acid*] dicarboxylic ACID.

Diacycline trademark for *tetracycline hydrochloride* (see under TETRACYCLINE).

diacylglycerol (di-as′il-glis″er-ōl) diglyceride.

diadochokinesia (di-ad″o-ko-ki-ne′se-ah) [Gr. *diadochos* succeeding + *kinesis* motion] The function of arresting one motor impulse and substituting for it one that is diametrically opposite, as in lowering and raising the mandible, occluding and opening the lips, and tapping with the finger. Called also *diadochokinesis*.

diadochokinesis (di-ad″o-ko-ki-ne′sis) diadochokinesia.

Diafen trademark for *diphenylpyraline*.

Diaginol trademark for *acetrizoate sodium* (see under ACETRIZOATE).

diagnosis (di″ag-no′sis) [*dia-* + Gr. *gnōsis* knowledge] 1. the art of distinguishing one disease from another. 2. the determination of the nature of a case of disease. In dentistry, the process may involve the evaluation of data obtained from dental and medical history, extraoral and intraoral examinations, a roentgenographic survey, pulp testing, exploration of all associated teeth and others with questionable restorations or carious lesions, articulated diagnostic casts, and a survey analysis. **biological d.,** diagnosis by tests performed on animals. **clinical d.,** diagnosis based on objective symptoms and laboratory findings during life. **cytohistologic d.,** cytologic d. **cytologic d.,** the use of cytologic or histologic examination of tissues and cells removed from the focus of disease, as in the diagnosis of a malignant tumor. Called also *cytohistologic d.* **differential d.,** differentiation of a disease from closely related or similar disease or diseases through the process of systematic comparison and contrasting of clinical, pathological, and laboratory data. **final d.,** the diagnosis arrived at through the examination and analysis of all pertinent data. **laboratory d.,** the diagnosis arrived at through the analysis and interpretation of laboratory data, such as chemical composition of body fluids and tissues. **oral d.,** the art and science of gathering, recording, and evaluating information that contributes to the identification of abnormalities of the head and neck regions which relate to the total health of the patient. **pathologic d.,** diagnosis by determining cytopathologic, histopathologic, and pathoanatomic changes in the affected tissues and organs. **physical d.,** determination of disease by inspection, palpation, percussion, and auscultation. **radiographic d., roentgen d.,** the diagnosis arrived at through the interpretation of radiographic findings.

diagram (di′ah-gram) 1. a figure, usually a line drawing, made to illustrate a geometrical theory, an operational plan, or a system. 2. the musculomembranous partition separating the abdominal and thoracic cavities. 3. a disk with one or more openings, or with an adjustable opening, mounted in relation to a lens or source of radiation by which a part of light or radiation may be excluded. **constitutional d.,** phase d. **equilibrium d.,** phase d. **phase d.,** a diagram depicting the solid and liquid phases of an alloy, as it relates to proportions of component metals, plotted against temperature. The liquidus is indicated by *AED* and the solidus *ABEGD*, *E* indicating the eutectic temperature for the silver-copper system; at this point the alloy is said to have a eutectic composition. Lines *BC* and *GF* indicate the changes in solid solubility of copper and silver and silver copper, respectively, as the temperature of the totally solid phase decreases, the solid solution of copper in silver being the α-solid solution and the solid solution of silver in copper being the β-solid solution. Called also *constitutional d.* and *equilibrium d.* See also eutectic ALLOY. See illustration. **stress-strain d.,** a diagram showing the relationship of stress and strain in response to

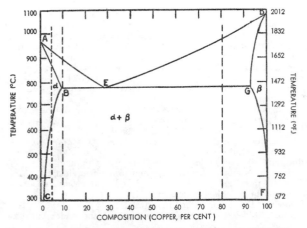

Phase diagram for the silver-copper system. (From R. W. Phillips: Skinner's Science of Dental Materials. 7th ed. Philadelphia, W. B. Saunders Co., 1973.)

increasing loads, usually plotted with stress as the ordinate and strain as the abscissa. The curve thus produced is called the *elastic curve*. **Venn d.,** one that uses overlapping circles to represent sets and their logical relationships. See Ackerman-Proffit classification, under MALOCCLUSION.

Diakarmon trademark for *sorbitol*.

Diaket trademark for an organic polyketone compound used as a root canal sealer (see under SEALER).

diakinesis (di″ah-ki-ne′sis) [*dia-* + Gr. *kinēsis* motion] the fifth and final stage of the prophase in the first division of meiosis, characterized by maximum contraction of the chromosomes.

dial (di′al) [L. *dialis* daily, from *dies* day] a circular area with graduations around the circumference and a centrally fixed pointer for indicating values of time, pressure, etc.

Dialister pneumosintes (di″ah-lis′ter nu″mo-sin′tēz) *Bacteroides pneumosintes*; see under BACTEROIDES.

dialysis (di-al′ĭ-sis) [*dia-* + Gr. *lysis* dissolution] the process of filtration through a semipermeable membrane (dialyzing membrane), whereby, depending on molecular weight, electrical charge, configuration, etc., dissolved substances and some crystalloids will pass readily through the membrane but colloids will pass slowly or not at all. **extracorporeal d.,** the process of

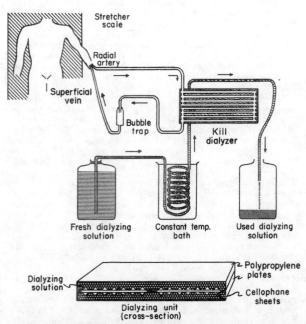

Schematic diagram of artificial kidney. (From A. C. Guyton. Textbook of Medical Physiology. 6th ed. Philadelphia, W. B. Saunders Co., 1981.)

removing toxic substances from the blood employing an artificial kidney machine situated outside of the body. It is used to remove waste products from the blood in uremia due to a renal shutdown or in some forms of poisoning. The blood is passed through minute blood channels bounded by thin sheets of cellophane (dialyzing membrane) that are permeable to all plasma constituents, except plasma proteins. On the other side of the membrane is an isotonic solution (dialyzing fluid) into which toxic substances in the blood diffuse. The concentration of toxic substances being greater in the blood plasma than in the dialyzing fluid, there will be a net transfer of them from the plasma into the fluid. To prevent blood from coagulating, heparin is infused into it as it enters the machine; to prevent bleeding in the patient as a result of heparin, the heparin is neutralized as the blood is returned to the patient. See illustration. **peritoneal d.,** the process of removing toxic substances from the blood through the use of an isotonic solution (dialyzing fluid) introduced into the peritoneal cavity. Toxic substances diffuse through the peritoneum which serves as the dialyzing membrane and enter into the fluid in the peritoneal cavity which is then removed.

diamagnetic (di″ah-mag-net′ik) 1. pertaining to or having the property of being repelled by a magnet. 2. pertaining to a substance that has magnetic properties weaker than those of air; a magnetic permeability under 1. See also PARAMAGNETIC.

diameter (di-am′ĕ-ter) the length of a straight line passing through the center of a circle and connecting opposite points on its circumference; hence the distance between two specified opposite points on the periphery of a structure such as the cranium or a tooth. **anteroposterior d.,** any distance between two points located on the anterior and posterior aspects, respectively, of the structure being measured. **bigonial d.,** the distance between the two gonia of the maxilla. **biparietal d.,** the distance between the two parietal eminences. **bitemporal d.,** the maximum distance between the right and left coronal sutures. **buccolingual d.,** the distance from the buccal to the lingual surface of a tooth crown at its widest point or greatest curvature. **buccolingual d. of crown,** measurement from the crest of curvature on the buccal surface to the crest of curvature on the lingual surface of posterior teeth. See table of *Measurements of the Permanent Teeth of Man* at TOOTH. **buccolingual d. of crown at the cervix,** measurement of the crown of the posterior teeth from the junction of the crown and root on the buccal surface to the junction of the crown and root on the lingual surface. **cranial d.,** a distance measured between certain landmarks of the skull, such as the biparietal, bitemporal, frontomental, occipitofrontal, occipitomental, and suboccipitobregmatic diameters. **craniometric d.,** any transverse line connecting two craniometric points of the same name, such as bigonial or biparietal diameter. **ectocanthic d.,** the distance between the lateral points of junction of the upper and lower eyelids of the two eyes. Called also *extracanthic d.* Cf. *endocanthic d.* **endocanthic d.,** the distance between the medial points of junction of the upper and lower eyelids of the two eyes. Called also *intercanthic d.* Cf. *ectocanthic d.* **extracanthic d.,** ectocanthic d. **frontomental d.,** the distance from the forehead to the chin, most often measured from the glabella to the gnathion and sometimes from the glabella to the pogonion. **fronto-occipital d.,** occipitofrontal d. **intercanthic d.,** endocanthic d. **labiolingual d. of crown,** measurement of the crown of anterior teeth from the crest of curvature on the labial surface to the crest of curvature on the lingual surface. See table of *Measurement of the Permanent Teeth of Man* at TOOTH. **labiolingual d. of crown at the cervix,** measurement of the crown of anterior teeth from the junction of the crown and root on the labial surface to the junction of the crown and root on the lingual surface. See table of *Measurements of the Permanent Teeth of Man* at TOOTH. **longitudinal d., intracranial,** the distance from the foramen cecum to the internal occipital protuberance. **mento-occipital d.,** occipitomental d. **mesiodistal d. of crown,** measurement of the crown of the posterior teeth from the crest of curvature on the mesial surface to the crest of curvature on the distal surface. See table of *Measurements of the Permanent Teeth of Man* at TOOTH. **mesiodistal d. of crown at the cervix,** measurement of the crown of posterior teeth from the junction of the crown and root on the mesial surface to the junction of the crown and root on the distal surface. See table of *Measurements of the Permanent Teeth of Man* at TOOTH. **occipitofrontal d.,** the distance from the external occipital protuberance to the most prominent midpoint of the frontal bone. Called also *fronto-occipital d.* **occipitomental d.,** the distance from the external occipital protuberance to the most forward point of the chin. Called also *mento-occipital d.* **parietal d.,** the distance between tuberosities or eminences of the parietal bones. **sagittal d.,** the distance from the glabella to the external occipital protuberance (glabella-inion); most often measured from the glabella to the.opisthocranion. **suboccipito-bregmatic d.,** the distance from the lowest posterior point of the occiput to the center of the anterior fontanelle. **temporal d.,** the distance between the tips of the alae magnae. **transverse d.,** the distance between two points located on opposite sides of the body part being measured, such as the biparietal diameter. **vertical d.,** the distance between two points situated on the upper and lower aspects of the structure being measured, such as the distance between the porion and the vertex of the skull.

diamide (di-am′ĭd) [*di-* + *amide*] 1. a compound having two amide groups (CONH₂). 2. hydrazine.

diamidine (di-am′ĭ-dēn) [*di-* + *amidine*] a compound containing two amidine groups (—C • : NH) • NH₂).

diamido- a chemical prefix indicating the presence in a compound of two amide groups (CONH₂).

diamine (di′ah-mēn″, di″ah-min′) a compound containing two amino groups (NH₂).

diaminoacridine (di-am″ĭ-no-ak′rĭ-dēn) proflavine.

diaminodiphenylsulfone (di-am′ĭ-no-di-fen″il-sul′fōn) dapsone.

diamond (di′mond, di′ah-mond) 1. a pure or nearly pure allotropic form of carbon crystallized isometrically, consisting of carbon atoms covalently bound by single bonds in a predominantly octahedral structure, forming a face-centered cubic crystal lattice. It is an extremely hard substance (Mohs hardness number, 10) used for polishing and cutting hard materials, such as glass, in making jewelry, in bearings for delicate instruments, and in other products. Diamond chips, impregnated in a binder to form diamond stones and disks, are the hardest, most effective abrasive for cutting tooth enamel. See also diamond rotary INSTRUMENT. 2. an equilateral quadrilateral, especially as placed with its diagonals vertical and horizontal.

Diamond-Blackfan syndrome (anemia) [Louis K. *Diamond*; Kenneth D. *Blackfan*] see under SYNDROME.

diamorphine (di-ah-mor′fēn) diacetylmorphine.

Diamox trademark for *acetazolamide.*

Dianabol trademark for *methandrostenolone.*

Diaparene trademark for *methylbenzethonium chloride* (see under METHYLBENZETHONIUM).

diapedesis (di″ah-pē-de′sis) [*dia-* + Gr. *pēdan* to leap] the migration through a vascular wall of cellular elements of the blood, such as leukocytes. See also EMIGRATION (2) and LEUKOCYTE migration. See also MIGRATION.

diaphanoscope (di-af′ah-no-skōp″) [Gr. *diaphanēs* transparent + *skopein* to examine] an instrument for transilluminating a body cavity. See also TRANSILLUMINATION.

diaphanoscopy (di-af″ah-nos′ko-pe) examination with the diaphanoscope; transillumination.

diaphragm (di′ah-fram) [Gr. *diaphragma*] 1. a separating membrane or structure. 2. a disk with one or more openings, or with an adjustable opening, mounted in relation to a lens or source of radiation by which part of the light or radiation may be excluded from the area. See also COLLIMATOR. 3. the musculomembranous partition separating the abdominal and thoracic cavities. Called also *diaphragma* [NA]. **Bucky's d., Bucky-Potter d.,** a diaphragm consisting of thin lead strips interspaced with a radiolucent material, placed in the direction of the short axis of the x-ray table in such a way that grid lines are prevented on the radiograph. Called also *Bucky-Potter grid.* **epithelial d.,** an epithelial structure evolving from Hertwig's root sheath, which narrows the opening into the pulp chamber, diminishing its caliber. It is made up of tall columnar cells, their intracellular spaces being occupied mostly by the elongated nuclei. It is situated across the base of the dental papilla, being in close contact with the bone forming the fundus of the developing alveolus; a thin layer of connective tissue (dental sac) separating the two structures. **d. of mouth, oral d., d. o′ris,** mylohyoid MUSCLE.

diaphragma (di″ah-frag′mah), pl. *diaphrag′mata* [Gr. "a partition-wall," "barrier"] 1. a separating membrane or structure; a diaphragm. 2. [NA] the musculomembraneous partition separating the abdominal and thoracic cavities.

diaphragmata (di″ah-frag′mah-tah) [Gr.] plural of *diaphragma.*

diaphysis (di-af′ĭ-sis), pl. *diaph′yses* [Gr. "the point of separation between stalk and branch"] 1. [NA] the elongated cylindrical portion (the shaft) of a long bone between the ends of extremities (the epiphyses), which are usually articular and wider than the shaft; it consists of a tube of compact bone, enclosing the medullary (marrow) cavity. Called also *shaft.* 2. the portion of a long bone formed from a primary center of ossification.

diarrhea (di″ah-re′ah) [*dia-* + Gr. *rhein* to flow] a condition characterized by frequent and watery fecal discharge. **Cochin-China d.,** tropical SPRUE.

diarthrodial (di″ar-thro′di-al) [Gr. *diarthrōsis* a movable articulation] pertaining to a diarthrosis or synovial joint.

diarthroses (di″ar-thro′sēz) plural of *diarthrosis.*

diarthrosis (di″ar-thro′sis), pl. *diarthro′ses* [Gr. *diarthrōsis* a movable joint] synovial JOINT.

diascope (di′ah-skōp) [*dia-* + Gr. *skopein* to examine] a piece of clear glass or plastic which, when pressed against the skin, causes the blood vessels to empty, and allows visual observation of the blanched underlying skin.

diascopy (di-as′ko-pe) transillumination.

Diasone trademark for *sulfoxone sodium* (see under SULFOXONE).

diastase (di′ah-stās) [Gr. *diastasis* separation] 1. α-AMYLASE. 2. β-AMYLASE.

Diastatin trademark for *nystatin.*

diastema (di″ah-ste′mah), pl. *diastem′ata* [Gr. *diastēma* an interval] 1. a space or cleft, such as one between two adjacent teeth in the same dental arch. 2. a narrow zone in the equatorial plane through which the cytosome divides in mitosis. **anterior d.,** a space between the incisor teeth, usually one between the maxillary central incisors. **frenum d.,** diastema associated with a heavy frenum attachment in the interdental space, considered to occur sometimes as a hereditary condition.

Diasulfa trademark for *sulfadimethoxine.*

diastereoisomer (di″ah-ster″e-o-i′so-mer) a compound exhibiting, or capable of exhibiting, diastereoisomerism.

diastereoisomeric (di″ah-ster″e-o-i″so-mer′ik) exhibiting diastereoisomerism.

diastereoisomerism (di″ah-ster″e-o″i-som′er-izm) a special type of optical isomerism in which the respective molecules of the compounds do not, at any time, exhibit a mirror-image (or enantiomorphic) relationship to one another. For example, the relationship between either *dextro-* or *levo-*tartaric acid and *meso-*tartaric acid is called diastereoisomeric. Diastereoisomers, in contrast to enantiomorphs, differ in both physical and chemical properties. Cf. ENANTIOMORPHISM.

diastole (di-as′to-le) [Gr. *diastolē* a drawing asunder; expansion] the dilation, or period of dilation, of the heart, especially of the ventricles, when the heart expands and blood enters to be pumped into the aorta and pulmonary artery during systole. See also systemic CIRCULATION. Cf. SYSTOLE.

diathermy (di′ah-ther″me) [*dia-* + Gr. *thermē* heat] heating of the body tissues due to their resistance to the passage of high-frequency electromagnetic radiation. In *medical diathermy,* the tissues are warmed·but not damaged; in *surgical diathermy* (electrocoagulation) tissue is destroyed. **short wave d.,** medical diathermy whereby the body is heated by means of an oscillating electromagnetic field of high frequency; the frequency varies from 10 million to 100 million cps and the wavelength from 30 to 3 m.

diathesis (di-ath′ĕ-sis) [Gr. "arrangement," "disposition"] a constitution or disposition of the body which makes the tissues react in special ways to certain extrinsic stimuli and thus tends to make the person more than usually susceptible to certain diseases. See also CONSTITUTION. **cystine d.,** Abderhalden-Fanconi SYNDROME. **hemorrhagic d.,** a tendency to bleed spontaneously, usually due to a blood clotting disorder. **infantile hemorrhagic d.,** infantile SCURVY.

diatomic (di″ah-tom′ik) [*di-* + Gr. *atomos* indivisible] 1. made up of two atoms or pertaining to a diatomic molecule, as in O₂ (diatomic or molecular oxygen). 2. pertaining to a substance containing two replaceable H atoms.

diatrizoate sodium (di″ah-tri-zo′ăt) 3,5-diacetamido-2,4,6-triiodobenzoic acid sodium salt; used as a water-soluble contrast medium in radiography, including angiocardiography and sialography. It is miscible with body fluids and saliva and rapidly eliminated from the body. Trademark: Hypaque.

diazepam (di-az′ĕ-pam) a minor tranquilizer, 7-chloro-1,3-dihydro-1-methyl-5-phenyl-2*H*-1,4-benzodiazepin-2-one, occurring as an off-white to yellow, odorless crystalline powder that is soluble in water, alcohol, chloroform, and ether. Used to manage acute alcohol withdrawal symptoms, skeletal muscle spasms, convulsions, and anxiety conditions. In dentistry, used chiefly as a sedative in general anesthesia premedication, in preparing patients for dental procedures, and as a sole agent for dental therapy lasting less than 1 hour. It is a potentially addicting agent; its adverse reactions include drowsiness, confusion, ataxia, and salivation. Diazepam has been reported to produce cleft palate in experimental animals and isolated cases of blood dyscrasias and jaundice have been reported. Trademark: Valium.

Diazil trademark for *sulfamethazine.*

diazine (di-az'in) any compound containing a ring of four carbon and two nitrogen atoms.

diazo- a chemical prefix indicating possession of the group —N₂-.

Diazon trademark for *sulfoxone sodium* (see under SULFOXONE).

diazone (di'ah-zōn) one of the dark bands, alternating with light bands (parazones), which form the lines of Schreger, seen under reflected light in a ground section of a tooth. It is believed that it is an area in which the enamel prisms have been cut in cross section.

diazoxide (di-az-ok'sīd) a vasopressor agent, 7-chloro-3-methyl-2*H*-1,2,4-benzothiadiazine 1,1-dioxide, occurring as a white to creamy, odorless, crystalline powder or solid that is soluble in dilute alkali solutions, but not in water. Used in the treatment of hypertensive crises. Side effects may include congestive heart failure, hyperglycemia, nausea, vomiting, gastrointestinal discomfort, burning sensation along the vein of injection, tachycardia, substernal pain, orthostatic hypotension, hyperuricemia, headache, drowsiness, hirsutism, hyperosmolar nonketotic coma, skin lesions, neutropenia, thrombocytopenia, and eosinophilia. Overdosage may cause shock. Trademarks: Hyperstat, Hypertonalum, Mutabase, Proglicem.

Diazyl trademark for *sulfadiazine.*

dibasic (di-ba'sik) [*di*- + Gr. *basis* base] containing two hydrogen atoms replaceable by bases, and thus yielding two series of salts, as H₂SO₄.

Dibendrin trademark for *diphenhydramine.*

Dibenyline trademark for *phenoxybenzamine.*

dibenzoyl- a chemical prefix indicating two benzoyl radicals. **d. peroxide,** BENZOYL peroxide.

Dibenzyline trademark for *phenoxybenzamine.*

3,5-dibromotyrosine (di-bro″mo-ti-ro'sin) 2-amino-3-(3,5-dibromo-4-hydroxyphenyl)propionic acid, a naturally-occurring nonessential amino acid. See also amino ACID.

dibucaine (di'bu-kān) a quinoline derivative, 2-butoxy-*N*-[2-(diethylamino) ethyl] cinchoninamide, occurring as a white, slightly hygroscopic crystalline powder with a slight characteristic odor, that darkens on exposure to light and is readily soluble in hydrochloric acid solutions and, slightly, in water. It is the most potent, most toxic, and longest acting of the commonly used local anesthetics. **d. hydrochloride,** the monohydrochloride salt of dibucaine, occurring as a white, odorless, bitter, slightly hygroscopic crystalline powder or solid that is freely soluble in water, ethanol, acetone, and chloroform, and slightly soluble in cold benzene, ethyl acetate, and toluene. Its pharmacological and toxicological properties are similar to those of the parent compound. Called also *benzolin.* Trademarks: Cincaine, Cinchocaine, Percaine, Sovacaine, Nupercaine.

DIC dacarbazine.

dic dicentric (2). See dicentric CHROMOSOME.

dicalcic (di-kal'sik) having in each molecule two atoms of calcium.

dicalcium orthophosphate (di-kal'se-um or″tho-fos'fāt) calcium phosphate, basic; see CALCIUM phosphate.

dicalcium phosphate (di-kal'se-um fos'fāt) calcium phosphate, dibasic; see CALCIUM phosphate.

dicaptol (di-kap'tol) dimercaprol.

dicelous (di-se'lus) [*di*- + Gr. *koilos* hollow] 1. hollowed on both sides. 2. having two cavities.

dicentric (di-sen'trik) 1. pertaining to, developing from, or having two centers. 2. pertaining to a dicentric chromosome. Abbreviated *dic.* See dicentric CHROMOSOME.

Dicestal trademark for *dichlorophen.*

Dichloran trademark for *dichlorobenzalkonium chloride* (see under DICHLOROBENZALKONIUM).

Dichloren trademark for *mechlorethamine hydrochloride* (see under MECHLORETHAMINE).

dichlorobenzalkonium chloride (di-klo″ro-ben″zal-ko'ne-um) an antiseptic, germicidal, algicidal, and fungicidal drug, (3,4-dichlorobenzyl)dodecyldimethylammonium chloride, occurring as bitter crystals that are soluble in water and alcohol. Used primarily for the disinfection of instruments. Also used as a deodorant and sensitizer. Trademarks: Dichloran, Tetrosan.

dichlorodifluoromethane (di-klo″ro-di-floor″o-meth'ān) a clear, colorless gas with a faint ethereal odor, CCl₂F₂. It is moderately toxic by inhalation. Used as a solvent, refrigerant, and aerosol

propellant. Suspected of being harmful to the environment, its use is regulated by the Food and Drug Administration. Trademarks: Arcton 6, Freon 12, Halon.

dichlorodiphenyltrichlorothane (DDT) (di-klor″o-di-fen″il-tri-klo″ro-eth'ān) chlorophenothane.

dichloroisoproterenol (di-klo″ro-i″so-pro-ter'ē-nōl) an isoproterenol derivative, 3,4-dichloro-α-(isopropylaminomethyl)benzyl alcohol; used as a β-adrenergic blocking drug.

dichlorophen(e) (di-klo'ro-fen, di-klo'ro-fēn) a moderately toxic fungicidal, bactericidal, and anthelmintic, 2,2'-dihydroxy-5,5'-dichlorodiphenylmethane. It occurs as a tan powder with a phenolic odor, which is readily soluble in acetone and ethanol, slightly soluble in benzene, toluene, and carbon tetrachloride, and insoluble in water. Abbreviated *DDM.* Trademarks: Anthiphen, Dicestal, Hyosan, Teniatol.

Dichlorosal trademark for *hydrochlorothiazide.*

dichlorotetrafluoroethane (di-klo″ro-tet″rah-floor″o-eth'ān) a clear, colorless gas with a faint ethereal odor, 1,2-dichlortetrafluoroethane. It is moderately toxic by inhalation. Suspected of being harmful to the environment, its use is regulated by the Food and Drug Administration. Called also *fluorocarbon-114.*

Dickens, Frank [English biochemist, born 1899] see phosphogluconate PATHWAY (Warburg-Dickens-Lipmann pathway).

Diclotride trademark for *hydrochlorothiazide.*

dicloxacillin sodium (di-kloks″ah-sil'in) a semisynthetic penicillin, 6[3-(2,6-dichlorophenyl)-5-methyl-4-isozazolecarboxamido]-3,3-dimethyl-7-oxo-4-thia-1-azabicyclo-[3,2,0] heptane-2-carboxylic acid monosodium monohydrate, occurring as a white to off-white crystalline powder with a characteristic faint odor, which dissolves in water and alcohol. It is a penicillinase-resistant antibiotic with a spectrum that is somewhat narrower than and toxicity similar to that of other penicillins. Used chiefly in the treatment of infections caused by penicillinase-producing bacteria. Trademarks: Dycill, Dynapen, Noxaben, Pathocil, Pen-Sint, Syntarpen, Veracillin.

Dico trademark for *dihydrocodeine bitartrate* (see under DIHYDROCODEINE).

Dicodid trademark for *hydrocodone.*

Dicodrine trademark for *hydrocodone bitartrate* (see under HYDROCODONE).

dicophane (di'ko-fān) chlorophenethane.

Dicortol trademark for *prednisolone.*

Dicoumarin trademark for *dicumarol.*

Dicoumarol trademark for *dicumarol.*

dictyospore (dik'te-o-spōr) a muriform spore; one having both longitudinal and transverse septations.

dictyotene (dik'te-o-tēn) [Gr. *diktyon* net + Gr. *tainia* ribbon] the state of suspended prophase of the first meiotic division in the primary oocyte of the developing ovary, which extends from late fetal life to sexual maturation. See also OOCYTE and OOGENESIS.

dicumarol (di-koo'mah-rol) a prothrombopenic anticoagulant, 3,3'-methylenebis-4-hydroxycoumarin, occuring as a white, crystalline powder with a faint odor and a slightly bitter taste, which is soluble in alkali hydroxide solution, slightly soluble in chloroform, and insoluble in water, alcohol, and ether. Used in the treatment and prevention of thromboembolic diseases. Occasional anorexia, nausea, vomiting, purpura, urticaria, and alopecia may occur. Spontaneous gingival bleeding and hemorrhagic complications in surgical patients are the principal adverse reactions. Called also *bishydroxycoumarin.* Trademarks: Dicoumarin, Dicoumarol, Melitoxin.

dicyclomine hydrochloride (di-si'klo-mēn) an antimuscarinic drug, 2-(diethylamino)ethyl(bicyclohexyl)-1-carboxylate hydrochloride, occurring as a white, odorless, bitter, crystalline powder that is soluble in water, ethanol, chloroform, and ether, but not in alkaline solutions. It has atropine-like effects on the gastrointestinal tract without suppressing gastric secretions. Used in the treatment of various gastrointestinal disorders. Side effects may include xerostomia, vertigo, constipation, visual disorders, fatigue, sedation, nausea, vomiting, headache, impotence, urinary retention, and skin rash. Trademarks: Atumin, Bentyl, Diocyl, Mamiesan, Procyclomin.

dicysteine (di'sis-te'in) cystine.

Didandin trademark for *diphenadione.*

die (di) a form to be used in the construction of something, e.g., a positive reproduction of the form of a prepared tooth in a suitable hard substance, such as a metal or a specially prepared artificial stone. Most dies are constructed of Class II (Type IV) dental stone, with dental amalgam and resins, usually filled acrylic or epoxy resins, being sometimes used as die material. See also COUNTERDIE. **amalgam d.,** a model of a tooth or other object made of amalgam; used in making dental prostheses. **counter-d.,** counterdie. **electroplated d.,** one formed by electroplating an impression, thereby forming a metallic positive reproduction of the form of a prepared tooth from an impression. Most impressions, which are made of materials such as wax or elastomers that do not conduct electricity, must be first metallized, whereby a thin layer of material is burnished onto their surfaces. The metallized impression is then placed in an electroplating bath and an electric contact is made between the copper matrix band or the metal tray and the surface of the impression, which is the cathode in the bath; a piece of copper is used for an anode. Called also *plated d.* **plated d.,** electroplated d. **d. stone,** Class II (Type IV) dental stone (see under STONE). **waxing d.,** a mold to which wax is adapted for the fabrication of a wax pattern.

Dieb. alt. abbreviation for L. *die'bus alter'nis,* on alternate days.

Dieb. tert. abbreviation for L. *die'bus ter'tiis,* every third day.

Diego antigen (factor), blood groups [named after the person in whom Diego antigen was first discovered] see under ANTIGEN and BLOOD GROUP.

diencephalon (di"en-sef'ah-lon) [*dia-* + Gr. *enkephalos* brain] the posterior part of the forebrain, consisting of the thalamus, metathalamus, subthalamus, hypothalamus, and epithalamus.

-diene chemical suffix denoting an unsaturated hydrocarbon containing two double bonds.

dienestrol (di"en-es'trol) an estrogen, 4,4'-(1,2-diethylidene-1,2-ethanediyl)diphenol, occurring as a colorless or white, odorless crystalline powder or crystals that are readily soluble in ethanol, acetone, ether, and methanol, slightly soluble in chloroform and fatty acids, and insoluble in water. Used in postovariectomy and postmenopausal replacement therapy. Side effects may include nausea, vomiting, and mild diarrhea. Trademarks: Dienoestrol, Synestrol.

Dienoestrol trademark for *dienestrol.*

Dierckx, L. see De Barsy-Moens-Dierckx SYNDROME.

Diergotan trademark for *dihydroergotamine mesylate* (see under DIHYDROERGOTAMINE).

diet (di'et) [Gr. *diaita* way of living] the customary allowance of food and drink taken by any person from day to day, particularly one especially planned to meet specific requirements of the individual, and including or excluding certain items of food. See also FOOD, MALNUTRITION, and NUTRITION. **adequate d.,** one that provides food in such a quantity and quality that will enable an individual to grow, mature, reproduce, and maintain optimum health. Called also *normal d.* **bland d.,** one free from irritating or stimulating foods. **clear liquid d.,** one consisting of clear liquids without residue; it is nonstimulating, non-gas-forming, and nonirritating. **general d.,** one containing practically all foods. **high-calorie d.,** one containing more calories than required to maintain normal body weight, usually more than 3500 to 4000 calories per day. **high-fat d.,** one containing large amounts of fat. Called also *ketogenic d.* **high-protein d.,** one containing large amounts of proteins, consisting chiefly of meat, fish, milk, vegetables, and nuts. **hospital d.,** one routinely provided in a hospital, which includes general, soft, and liquid diets or their modifications to suit individual patients. **ketogenic d.,** high-fat d. **liquid d.,** one limited to liquids or to foods that can be changed to a liquid state. **low-calorie d.,** one containing fewer calories than needed to maintain normal body weight, usually less than 1200 calories. See *reducing d.* **low-fat d.,** one containing limited amounts of fat. **low-fiber d.,** low-residue d. **low-purine d.,** one restricting foods rich in purines, such as meat, fowl, and fish and substituting milk, eggs, cheese, and vegetable proteins. Called also *purine-free d.* **low-residue d.,** one with a minimum of cellulose and fiber and restriction of connective tissue found in certain cuts of meats. Called also *low-fiber d.* **normal d.,** adequate d. **protein-sparing d.,** one consisting only of liquid protein or a liquid mixture of proteins, vitamins, and minerals, and containing no more than 600 calories. Used for maintaining a favorable nitrogen balance. **purine-free d.,** low-purine d. **reducing d.,** one specifically designed to reduce body weight, usually containing a large proportion of proteins and low amounts of carbohydrates and fats. See *low-calorie d.* **sodium restricted d.,** one containing minimal amounts of sodium compounds, such as monosodium glu-

tamate, baking powder, and sodium chloride, bicarbonate, cyclamate, saccharin, alginate, propionate, benzoate, sulfide, and hydroxide. Used chiefly in heart diseases, particularly congestive heart disease, hypertension, head injuries with sodium metabolism disorders, kidney diseases, ascites, and various body fluid disorders, especially those associated with fluid accumulation in tissues and swelling. **soft d.,** a regular diet modified in consistency to have no roughage; liquids and semisolid foods that are easily digested.

diethylcarbamazine (di-eth"il-kar-bam'ah-zen) an anthelmintic, *N,N* - diethyl - 4 - methyl - l - piperazinecarboxamide. Trademarks: Carbilazine, Caricide, Spatonin. **d. citrate,** the hydrogen citrate salt of diethylcarbamazine, occurring as a white, odorless, slightly hygroscopic powder that is soluble in water and ethanol, but not in acetone, chloroform, and ether. Used in the treatment of certain types of helminthiases. Side effects may include headache, malaise, weakness, arthralgia, anorexia, nausea, and vomiting. Leukocytosis, eosinophilia, and lymphatic swellings are believed to be caused by allergic reaction to disintegrating helminths. Trademarks: Dihydrogen Citrate, Hetrazan.

diethylene (di-eth'il-ēn) a compound containing two ethylene radicals. **d. glycol,** diethylene GLYCOL.

diethylmalonylurea (di-eth"il-mal"o-nil-u-re'ah) barbital.

diethylstilbestrol (di-eth"il-stil-bes'trol) a synthetic estrogen not related to natural estrogens containing the phenanthrene ring, 4,4' - (1,2 - diethyl - 1,2 - ethienediyl)bisphenol, occurring as a white, odorless, crystalline powder that is soluble in ethanol, ether, oils, and dilute alkali hydroxides, but not in water. Used in substitution therapy of postmenopausal and postovariectomy symptoms and various gynecological disorders. Nausea and vomiting are its principal side effects. Formerly used to prevent threatened or habitual abortion. Women exposed *in utero* to diethylstilbestrol show characteristic cervical and vaginal changes and are subject to increased risk of cervical and vaginal cancer. Abbreviated *DES.* Called also *stilbestrol.* Trademarks: Stilbetin, Stilboestrol, Synestrin.

dietotherapy (di"ĕ-to-ther'ah-pe) dietetic treatment, including counseling with recommendations on food selection and dietary habits.

difference (dif'er-enz) 1. the condition of being dissimilar or unlike. 2. that which makes something different. **potential d.,** voltage.

differential (dif'er-en'shal) [L. *differre* to carry apart] 1. pertaining to a difference or differences. 2. the difference of two or more motions or pressures. See also differential FORCE.

differentiation (dif'er-en"she-a'shun) 1. the distinguishing of one thing from another. 2. the act or process of acquiring individual characteristics, such as in the process of diversification of cells and tissues in an embryo. 3. increase in morphological or chemical heterogenicity. 4. the degree to which neoplastic cells morphologically resemble normal cells. **margoid d.,** a tooth anomaly, usually occurring in the upper lateral incisors and in mesiodentes, in which a very high accessory cusp connects with the incisal edge, producing a T form or, if lower, a Y-shaped crown contour. Called also *talon cusp.*

diffraction (di-frak'shun) [L. *dis* apart + *frangere* to break] the bending or breaking up into its component parts of a ray of light. **x-ray d.,** a method of histochemical analysis based on diffraction and scattering of x-rays by the analyzed specimen and observation of the scattered rays on a photographic film. **x-ray d., large-angle,** a method that allows observation of fine details of interatomic relationships in a molecule. **x-ray d., small-angle,** a method that allows observation on widely-spaced repetitions of groups of atoms in a molecule.

diffuse [L. *dis* apart + *fundere* to pur] 1. (di-fūs') not definitely limited or localized; widely distributed. 2. (di-fūz') to pass through, or to spread widely through a tissue or structure.

diffusion (di-fu'zhun) 1. the process of becoming diffused, or widely spread; the spreading or scattering of a material or energy. 2. the movement of molecules in a gas or liquid medium from the region of high concentration to the region of low concentration. In solids, the displacement in a space lattice of atoms with low energy levels by those with higher energy. Atoms and molecules diffuse in the solid state or solution in an attempt to produce equilibrium. An excess of a solute will produce supersaturation, resulting in crystallization or precipitation of the excess solute. See also OSMOSIS, RELAXATION (3), SELF-DIFFUSION, and SOLUTION (1). 3. the transport of substances across the cell membrane. Lipid-soluble substances, such as oxygen, carbon dioxide, fatty acids, or alcohols become dissolved in the lipid on coming in contact with the membrane and diffuse through the membrane in the same manner that diffusion occurs in water; other substances pass through minute pores in the membrane; while still other substances require a carrier (see *facilitated d.*). See also active TRANSPORT (2). **coefficient of d.,** COEFFICIENT of diffusion. **double d.,** see double diffusion TEST. **exchange d.,** the process in which diffusion of a molecule across a membrane in one direction brings about diffusion of another moleducle in the opposite direction. **facilitated d.,** diffusion of substances that are not soluble in lipids (such as sugars) and thus can not diffuse through the cell membrane in the regular way, through the use of a carrier molecule. After being bound to the carrier, a substance becomes soluble in lipid, and is transported through the membrane. After assisting the substance, the carrier releases it and is ready to combine with another molecule of the substance. Alternatively, diffusion of a substance through a membrane pore. Called also *mediated transport*. See also *carrier molecule*. **d. factor,** hyaluronidase. **free d.,** that in which there is no obstacle, such as a membrane; diffusion of substances in a homogeneous medium. **gel d.,** see gel diffusion TEST. **impeded d.,** that in which the rate is slowed down by the difficulty of passing through a membrane.

Digacin trademark for *digoxin*.

digastric (di-gas′trik) [*di-* + Gr. *gastēr* belly] having two bellies.

DiGeorge's syndrome [Angelo M. *DiGeorge*] see under SYNDROME.

digestant (di-jes′tant) 1. assisting or stimulating digestion. 2. an agent or drug which assists in the stimulation of digestion. The most commonly used digestants are choleretics (bile, bile acids, and bile salts) and hydrochloric acid.

digestion (di-jest′yun) [L. *digestio*, from *dis* apart + *gerere* to carry] 1. the act or process of converting food into chemical substances that can be absorbed and assimilated by the body. The oral phase consists of the reduction of the particle size of ingested food first by cutting with the incisors and then by the crushing and grinding action of the premolars and the molars. The saliva moistens the food and lubricates the passages so that it may be swallowed as a bolus. The saliva also provides the enzyme ptyalin, which catalyzes the hydrolysis of starch to maltose. See also INGESTION, carbohydrate METABOLISM, and protein METABOLISM. 2. the subjection of a body to prolonged heat and moisture, so as to disintegrate and soften it. **salivary d.,** the conversion of starch into maltose by salivary amylase.

Digifortis trademark for *digitalis*.

digilanide lanatoside.

digit (dij′it) [L. *digitus*] 1. a finger or toe. 2. any of the numerals 0 through 9. **binary d.,** in computer technology, a numeral in the binary scale, which may be 0 or 1. It is a single character in a binary number, a single pulse in a group of pulses, and a unit of information capacity of a computer storage device. Abbreviated *bit*.

digital (dij′ĭ-tal) 1. of, pertaining to, or performed with, a finger. 2. resembling the imprint of a finger. 3. using or involving numerical digits expressed in a scale of notation to represent discretely all variables occurring in a problem.

Digitaline trademark for *digitoxin*.

digitalis (dij″ĭ-tal′is) the dried leaf of *Digitalis purpurea* (purple foxglove), containing several glycosides, including digitoxin and gitoxin, which occurs as a dark green, bitter powder when ground. It is a cardiotonic drug used in the treatment of congestive heart failure and cardiac arrhythmias, acting directly on the myocardium to increase its force of contraction and cardiac tone. Slowing of the cardiac rate occurs when the rate was originally rapid due to failure. Nausea, vomiting, neuralgia, headache, drowsiness, fatigue, and, rarely, hallucinations may occur. Patients receiving the drug may exhibit hyperexcitability of pharyngeal and emetic reflexes during dental procedures. Called also *foxglove* and *Digitalis leaf*. Trademarks: Digifortis, Digitora. See also cardiac GLYCOSIDE.

digitate (dij′ĭ-tāt) having several finger-like processes.

digiti (dij′ĭ-ti) [L.] plural of *digitus*.

digitiform (dij′ĭ-tĭ-form) [L. *digitus* digit + *forma* form] resembling a finger; finger-like.

digitizing (dij″ĭ-tīz′ing) a method of marking tracings of lateral and p-a x-ray headfilms by numbers devised by G. F. Walker, B.M.D., a New Zealand orthodontist (now in the United States). Each craniometric landmark is located and numbered and additional numbers identify structural points. The tracings so digitized provide dimensions, angles, and ratios which are registered on punch-cards and stored in computer banks. There are 170 numbers in the lateral headfilm, in the p-a headfilm. M. Mazoheri, D.D.S., of Lancaster, Pennsylvania, has adapted the Walker method to the soft tissues of the facial profile and nasopharynx.

digitophyllin (dij″ĭ-tof′ĭ-lin) digitoxin.

Digitora trademark for *digitalis*.

digitoxin (dij″ĭ-tok′sin) a cardiac glycoside, 3β - [(*O* - 2,6 - dideoxy-β - D - ribo - hexopyranosyl - (1→4) - *O* - 2,6 - dideoxy - β - D - ribo-hexopyranosyl - (1→4) - 2,6 - dideoxy - β - D - ribo - hexopyranosyl)oxy] - 14 - hydroxy - card - 20(22) - enolide. It is isolated from leaves of *Digitalis purpurea* and other species of *Digitalis*, and occurs as a white or buff, odorless, crystalline powder that is soluble in ethanol and chloroform, very slightly soluble in ether, and insoluble in water. Used alone or as a component of digitalis in the treatment of cardiac arrhythmias and congestive heart failure. Associated adverse reactions are the same as those of digitalis. Called also *digitophyllin*. Trademarks: Cardigin, Carditoxin, Digitaline, Lanatoxin.

digitus (dij′ĭ-tus), pl. *dig′iti* [L.] digit; a finger or a toe.

diglossia (di-glos′e-ah) [*di-* + Gr. *glōssa* tongue + *-ia*] bifid TONGUE.

diglyceride (di-glis′er-īd) [*di-* + *glyceride*] a glyceride in which two hydroxyl groups of glycerol are esterified with fatty acids. Called also *diacylglycerol*.

digoxin (di-goks′in) a cardiac glycoside 3β - [(*O* - 2,6 - dideoxy - β - D - ribo - hexopyranosyl - (1→4) - *O* - 2,6 - dideoxy - β - D - ribo-hexopyranosyl - (1→4) - 2,6 - dideoxy - β - D - ribo - hexapyranosyl)oxy] - 12β - 14 - didhydroxy - 5β - card - 20(22) - enolide. It is isolated from leaves of *Digitalis lanata* and other species of *Digitalis*, and occurs as an odorless crystalline powder or clear to white crystals that are soluble in pyridine, slightly soluble in ethanol and chloroform, and insoluble in water and ether. Used alone or as a component of digitalis in the treatment of cardiac arrhythmias and congestive heart failure. Associated adverse reactions are the same as those of digitalis. Trademarks: Cardioxil, Davoxin, Digacin, Lanoxin, Vanoxin.

Dihidral trademark for *diphenhydramine*.

Dihydan Soluble trademark for *phenytoin sodium* (see under PHENYTOIN).

Dihydergot trademark for *dihydroergotamine mesylate* (see under DIHYDROERGOTAMINE).

Dihydral trademark for *dihydrotachysterol*.

dihydrate (di-hi′drāt) [*di-* + Gr. *hydōr* water] a hydrate containing two molecules of water for every molecule of other substance in the compound. **gypsum d.,** the native hydrated form of calcium sulfate; gypsum.

dihydrocodeine (di-hi″dro-ko′dēn) a synthetic narcotic analgesic, 4,5α-epoxy-3-methoxy-17-methylmorphinan-6α-ol, which is related to codeine, and has actions and drug dependence liability similar to those of codeine. Used as an analgesic and antitussive. Nausea, vomiting, lassitude, respiratory depression, sleepiness, and mental confusion have been reported. Called also *DH-codeine* and *drocode*. Trademarks: Codhydriene, Hydrocodin, Novicodin, Paracodin, Rapacodin. **d. bitartrate,** the bitartrate salt of dihydrocodeine, having the actions, uses, and side effects of the parent drug. Used as an analgesic and antitussive. Trademarks: Dico, Fortuss.

dihydrocodeinone (di-hi″dro-ko-de′ĭ-nōn) hydrocodone. **d. bitartrate,** HYDROCODONE bitartrate. **d. tartrate,** HYDROCODONE bitartrate.

dihydrocoenzyme I (di-hi″dro-ko-en′zīm) nicotinamide-adenine DINUCLEOTIDE.

dihydroergotamine (di-hi″dro-er-got′ah-mēn) a smooth muscle stimulant and vasoconstrictive agent, 9,10-dihydro-12′-hydroxy-2′-methyl-5′α-(phenylmethyl)ergotaman-3,6′18-trione, produced by the catalytic hydrogenation of ergotamine. It is sparingly soluble in methanol, ethanol, chloroform, and benzene, and insoluble in water. **d. mesylate,** the methanesulfonate salt of dihydroergotamine, occurring as a white to yellowish to reddish powder that is slightly soluble in water and chloroform and is readily soluble in alcohol. Similarly to its parent compound, it is a smooth muscle stimulant, having α-adrenergic–blocking and serotonin-inhibiting properties. Used in the treatment of migraine and as an oxytocic drug. Side effects may include precordial discomfort, nausea, vomiting, tachycardia, bradycardia, hypotension, myalgia, numbness and tingling of the digits, localized edema, and itching. Gangrene, especially of the extremities, can occur with chronic use or after large overdosage. Called also *DHE-45*. Trademarks: Diergotan, Dihydergot, Ergotex, Orstanorm.

Dihydrogen Citrate trademark for *diethylcarbamazine citrate* (see under DIETHYLCARBAMAZINE).

dihydrohydroxymorphinone (di-hi″dro-hi-drok″se-mor′fi-nōn) OXYMORPHONE hydrochloride.

dihydromethiazide (di-hi″dro-me-thi′ah-zīd) hydroflumethiazide.

dihydromorphinone (di-hi″dro-mor′fi-nōn) hydromorphone.

Dihydrone trademark for *oxycodone*.

dihydrotachysterol (di-hi″dro-tak-is′tĕ-rol) a chemical analogue of vitamin D₂ that is sometimes classified as a vitamin D, 9,10-seco-5,7-ergostratrien-3β-ol. It occurs as an odorless, white crystalline powder or colorless or white crystals that are soluble in ethanol, ether, and chloroform, sparingly soluble in vegetable oils, and insoluble in water. Because of its calcemic properties, used in the treatment of hypocalcemia and hypoparathyroidism. Hypercalcemia, anorexia, weight loss, nausea, vomiting, diarrhea, languor, osteoporosis, metastatic calcifications, renal lesions, anemia, and convulsions are its most common side reactions. Trademarks: Antitanil, Calcamine, Dihydral, Hygratyl, Hytakerol, Parterol.

dihydroxyacetone (di″hi-drok″se-as′ĕ-tōn) a ketose (triose), 1,3-dihydroxy-2-propanone, occurring in the form of phosphate esters as an intermediate in the fermentation and glycolysis of carbohydrates. It is also the precursor of the glycerol, which the organism synthesizes and incorporates into lipids. Produced by the oxidation of glycerin with nitric acid in the form of a colorless crystalline, hygroscopic solid that is soluble in water and alcohol. Used in the production of drugs, fungicides, cosmetics, and ointments that promote an artificial suntan. Called also *dihydroxypropanone*.

dihydroxyaluminum aminoacetate (di-hi-drok″se-ah-lu″mĭ-num am″ĭ-no-as′ĕ-tāt) and antacid preparation; aluminum glycinate.

dihydroxyfluorane (di″hi-drok″se-floo′o-rān) fluorescein.

3,4-dihydroxyphenylalanine (di″hi-drok″se-fen″il-al′ah-nēn) a nonessential naturally occurring amino acid, 2-amino-3-3,4-(dihydroxyphenyl)propionic acid.

dihydroxypropanone (di″hi-drok″se-pro-pan′ōn) dihydroxyacetone.

3,5-diiodotyrosine (di″i-o″do-ti′ro-sēn) 2-amino-3-(3,5-diiodo-4-hydroxyphenyl)propionic acid, a naturally-occurring amino acid. Called also *iodogorgoric acid*.

dil. abbreviation for L. *di′lue*, dilute or dissolve.

Dilabron trademark for *isoetharine*.

dilaceration (di-las″er-a′shun) [L. *dilaceratio*] a tearing apart. In dentistry, abnormal curvature in the root or crown of a formed tooth, believed to be the result of an injury to a tooth during its developmental period. A tooth so affected is called a *dilacerated*, *kinked*, or *sickle tooth*.

Dilantin trademark for *phenytoin*.

Dilatal trademark for *nylidrin hydrochloride* (see under NYLIDRIN).

dilatation (dil-ah-ta′shun) 1. the condition of being dilated or stretched. 2. dilation.

dilation (di-la′shun) 1. the action of dilating or stretching. 2. dilatation. See also VASODILATATION.

dilator (di-la′tor) [L.] 1. a device or instrument used in enlarging an orifice or canal by stretching. 2. a muscle that dilates. **d. na′ris**, alar part of nasal muscle; see under PART.

Dilaudid trademark for *hydromorphone hydrochloride* (see under HYDROMORPHONE).

Dilavase trademark for *isoxsuprine hydrochloride* (see under ISOXSUPRINE).

Dilosyn trademark for *methdilazine*.

Diluc. abbreviation for L. *dilu′culo*, at daybreak.

diluent (dil′u-ent) [L. *diluere* to wash] 1. an inert solid or liquid substance used to increase the bulk of another substance. 2. an inert agent that dilutes or renders another substance less potent, irritant, etc.

Dilurgen trademark for *meralluride*.

dilut. abbreviation for L. *dilu′tus*, diluted.

dilution (di-lu′shun) 1. the act or state of rendering something, usually a solution, less concentrated, weaker, less irritating, etc., by increasing its bulk by the addition of another substance (usually a liquid) that may or may not be a solvent for the solute. 2. rendering a medicine weaker by mixing it with another (inert) substance, which may be a liquid, powder, etc.

dim. abbreviation for L. *dimid′ius*, one half.

Dimarin trademark for *dimenhydrinate*.

Dimegan trademark for *brompheniramine maleate* (see under BROMPHENIRAMINE).

dimelia (di-me′le-ah) [*di-* + Gr. *melos* limb] an abnormality characterized by duplication of a limb.

dimenhydrinate (di″men-hi′drĭ-nāt) an H₁-blocking antihistaminic agent with anticholinergic properties, 2-(diphenylmethoxy)-*N*,*N*-dimethylethylamine-8-chlorotheo-phyllinate, occurring as a white, odorless, crystalline powder that is freely soluble in ethanol and chloroform and slightly soluble in water and ether. Used as an antinauseant and antiemetic agent, usually in combination with other drugs, such as diphenhydramine, in motion sickness, Meniere's disease, radiation sickness, and vestibular disorders associated with streptomycin therapy. Side reactions may include drowsiness, hallucinations, confusion, disorientation, dystonia, akathisia, and dysphasia. Trademarks: Amosyt, Anautine, Andramine, Chloronautine, Dimarin, Dramamine, Emedyl, Feston, Menhydrinate, Novamin, Travelin, Vomex A.

dimension (di-men′shun) [L. *dimensio* a measuring] 1. a numerical expression of a linear measurement of an object, using its length, breadth, thickness, or circumference, as of a square (two-dimensional object) or a cube (three-dimensional object). 2. the magnitude or size of an object or body. **contact vertical d.**, vertical d., contact. **occlusal vertical d. (OVD)**, vertical d., contact. **postural vertical d.**, vertical d., contact. **rest vertical d.**, vertical d., rest. **vertical d.**, the length of the face determined by the distance of separation of jaws. Called also *vertical opening*. **vertical d., contact**, the lower face height with the teeth in centric occlusion. Called also *occlusal vertical dimension (OVD)*. **vertical d., occlusal**, vertical d., contact. **vertical d., postural (PVD)**, the vertical height of the face when the mandible is suspended in postural resting position. **vertical d., rest**, the lower face height measured from a chin point to a point just below the nose, with the mandible in rest position.

dimer (di′mer) [*di-* + Gr. *meros* part] 1. a chemical compound consisting of two monomer molecules reacting to join together to form a single molecule containing two mers. See also POLYMER. 2. a capsomer having two structural subunits.

dimercaprol (di″mer-kap′rol) a clear, viscous, oily liquid with pungent disagreeable odor, 2,3-dimercapto-1-propanol, which is soluble in water, vegetable oils, alcohol, and various organic solvents. Originally developed in Great Britain as an antidote to lewisite, a vesicant arsenic war gas, it is now used as a chelating agent in the treatment of heavy metal poisoning by preventing inhibition of sulfhydryl enzymes in the tissue. Called also *British anti-lewisite (BAL)*, *dicaptol*, and *sulfactin*.

dimeric (di′mer-ik) 1. pertaining to, made of, or affecting two segments, as distinguished from monomeric, polymeric, etc. 2. exhibiting the characteristics of a dimer.

Dimerin trademark for *methyprylon*.

Dimetane trademark for *brompheniramine maleate* (see under BROMPHENIRAMINE).

dimethacrylate (di″meth-ak′rĭ-lāt) the reaction product of bisphenol A and glycidyl methacrylate, being the principal resin component of composite restorative materials and resin cements. It occurs as a sticky, viscous fluid that requires fillers to render it suitable for specific restorative techniques, with modifiers being used to control viscosity. Polymerization may be accomplished by means of peroxide-amine systems or also visible light or ultraviolet rays. A peroxide initiator is placed in the paste and an amine activator in either the second paste or the liquid. Dimethacrylate is also available with low filler content to be used on the surface of finished restorations as a glazing agent. It is used as a pit and fissure sealant, for covering enamel defects, in repairing fractured incisors and cervical erosions, for attaching orthodontic brackets and bands, for splinting teeth, for small anterior restorations, and as a cement for cast restorations. Called also *BIS-GMA*. **d. cement**, dimethacrylate CEMENT.

dimethicone (di-meth′ĭ-kōn) simethicone.

dimethindene maleate (di″meth-in′dēn) a potent antihistaminic acting on the H₁ receptor, 2-[1-[2-[2-(dimethylamino)ethyl]-inden-3-yl]ethyl]pyridine maleate, occurring as a white or off-white crystalline powder with a characteristic odor, which is sensitive to light, and is soluble in water, methanol, and chloroform. Used in the treatment of allergic diseases. Trademarks: Fenistil, Forhistal, Triten.

dimethisoquin hydrochloride (di″me-thi′so-kwin) a local anesthetic, 3-butyl-1-(2-dimethylaminoethoxy)isoquinoline hydrochloride, occurring as a white to off-white, odorless, crystalline powder that is soluble in water, chloroform, ethanol and, very slightly, ether. Used topically in pruritus, skin irritation, sunburn, and other cutaneous disorders. Trademarks: Isochinol, Pruralgan, Pruralgin, Quotane.

dimethisterone (di″meth-is′ter-ōn) a progestogen with estrogenic and androgenic actions, 17β-hydroxy-6α-methyl-17-(1-propyl)-androst-4-en-3-one, occurring as a white, odorless, tasteless, crystalline powder that is soluble in chloroform, pyridine, ethanol, and acetone, but not in water. Used in progestational therapy and as a component of some oral contraceptives. Side effects are similar to those of other oral contraceptives. Trademark: Secrosteron.

dimethyl (di-meth′il) ethane.

dimethylamine (di-meth″il-am′in) a gas, $(CH_3)_2NH$, with a strong ammoniacal odor, which is toxic and irritant and causes lesions of the mucous membranes and skin. It is used in chemical procedures.

dimethylbenzene (di-meth″il-ben′zēn) xylene.

dimethylketone (di-meth″il-ke′tōn) acetone.

dimethylmethane (di-meth″il-meth′ān) propane.

Dimezathine trademark for *sulfamethazine.*

Dimipressin trademark for *imipramine.*

Dimorphone trademark for *hydromorphinone.*

dimoxyline (di-mok′sĭ-lēn) a peripheral vasodilator, 1-(4-ethoxy-3-methoxybenzyl)-6,7-dimethoxy-3-methylisoquinoline. Called also *dioxyline.* Trademark: Paveril.

Dinarkon trademark for *oxycodone hydrochloride* (see under OXYCODONE).

dineric (di-ner′ik) [*di-* + Gr. *nēros* liquid] denoting a solution made up of two immiscible solvents with a single solute soluble in each.

Dingwall, Mary M. see Cockayne's SYNDROME (Neill-Dingwall syndrome).

dinitrosorbide (di-ni″tro-sor′bĭd) ISOSORBIDE dinitrate.

D. in p. aeq. abbreviation for L. *div′ide in par′tes aequa′les,* divide into equal parts.

dinucleotide (di-nu′kle-o-tīd) one of the cleavage products into which a polynucleotide may be split; a dinucleotide itself may be split into two mononucleotides. **flavin-adenine d.,** a coenzyme that is a condensation product of riboflavin phosphate and adenylic acid; it forms the prosthetic group of certain enzymes, including D-amino acid oxidase and xanthine oxidase, and is important in electron transport in mitochondria. Abbreviated *FAD.* **nicotinamide-adenine d.,** the dinucleotide of nicotinamide and of adenine, a coenzyme found in nature and involved in various enzymatic oxidoreductase reactions; the products of hydrolysis are 1 molecule of adenine, 1 of nicotinamide, 2 of D-ribose, and 2 of phosphoric acid. Called also *codehydrogenase I, coenzyme I (CoI), cozymase, dihydrocoenzyme I,* and *diphosphopyridine nucleotide (DPN).* Abbreviated *NAD.* **nicotinamide-adenine d. phosphate,** a coenzyme required for a limited number of reactions, similar to nicotinamide-adenine dinucleotide, except for the inclusion of 3 phosphate units. Called also *codehydrogenase II, coenzyme II (CoII), triphosphopyridine nucleotide (TPN),* and *Warburg's coenzyme.* Abbreviated *NADP.*

dioctyl sodium sulfosuccinate (di-ok′til so′de-um sul″fo-suk′sĭ-nāt) a surface-active agent, sulfobutanedioic acid 1,4-bis(2-ethylhexyl) ester sodium salt, occurring as a white, waxlike, plastic solid with a characteristic octyl alcohol-like odor, which is soluble in ethanol, glycerol, and hexene, and slowly soluble in water. Used chiefly in managing constipation and fecal impaction. Also used as an emulsifying, wetting, and dispersing agent in pharmaceutical preparations. It is a component of some dental preparations for surface application and, in small quantities, in preparations for oral administration. Abbreviated *DSS.* Called also *sodium dioctyl sulfosuccinate.* Trademarks: Colace, Comfolax, Complemix, Dio-Medicone, Diotilan, Diovac, Doximate, Doxol.

Diocyl trademark for *dicyclomine hydrochloride* (see under DICYCLOMINE).

Diogenes syndrome [named after *Diogenes,* a Greek philosopher and probably the founder of Cynicism, c. 412 B.C.–c. 323 B.C.] see under SYNDROME.

-dioic a chemical suffix indicating a dicarboxylic acid.

Dio-Medicone trademark for *dioctyl sodium sulfosuccinate* (see under DIOCTYL).

Dionin trademark for *ethylmorphine hydrochloride* (see under ETHYLMORPHINE).

Diopal trademark for *methscopolamine bromide* (see under METHSCOPOLAMINE).

Dioscorides of Anazarbos [1st century A.D.] a noted botanist and pharmacologist whose encyclopedia of materia medica was widely used for centuries after his death. Extracts of his works appear in an encyclopedia of medicine of Oribasius.

diose (di′ōs) a monosaccharide containing two carbon atoms in the molecule, $C_2H_4O_2$.

Diotilan trademark for *dioctyl sodium sulfosuccinate* (see under DIOCTYL).

Diovac trademark for *dioctyl sodium sulfosuccinate* (see under DIOCTYL).

dioxide (di-ok′sīd) a compound having two oxygen atoms. **carbon d.,** CARBON dioxide. **lead d.,** LEAD dioxide. **nitrogen d.,** NITROGEN dioxide. **silicon d.,** SILICON dioxide.

Dioxyline trademark for *benzoxiquine.*

dioxyline (di-ok′sĭ-lēn) dimoxyline.

Dipar trademark for *phenformin hydrochloride* (see under PHENFORMIN).

Dipaxin trademark for *diphenadione.*

dipeptidase [E.C.3.4.13.11] (di″pep′tĭ-dās) a dipeptide hydrolase that catalyzes the hydrolysis of dipeptides into two amino acids.

dipeptide (di-pep′tīd) [*di-* + *peptide*] a peptide which, on hydrolysis, yields two amino acids.

Diphantine trademark for *diphenhydramine.*

diphasic (di-fa′zik) [*di-* + Gr. *phasis* phase] occurring in two phases or stages. Cf. MONOPHASIC and TRIPHASIC.

diphemanil methylsulfate (di-fem′ah-nil) a quaternary ammonium antimuscarinic agent, 4 - (diphenylmethylene) - 1,1 - dimethyl - piperidinium methyl sulfate, occurring as white, bitter crystals with a faint odor, which are soluble in water and, sparingly, in ethanol and chloroform. Used in the treatment of hyperhidrosis, peptic ulcer, gastric hyperacidity, hypertrophic gastritis, and gastric hypermotility. Trademarks: Demotil, Diphenatil, Prantal, Nivelona.

diphenadione (di-fen″ah-di′ōn) a long-acting prothrombopenic oral anticoagulant, 2 - (diphenylacetyl) - 1H - indene - 1,3(2H) - dione, occurring as an odorless crystalline powder or crystals that are readily soluble in benzene, ether, and glacial acetic acid, slightly soluble in acetone and ethanol, and insoluble in water. Used in the treatment and prevention of thromboembolic diseases. Occasional nausea and vomiting may occur; spontaneous gingival bleeding and hemorrhagic complications in surgical patients are the principal complications. Trademarks: Didandin, Dipaxin, Solvan.

Diphenatil trademark for *diphemanil methylsulfate* (see under DIPHEMANIL).

diphenhydramine (di″fen-hi′drah-mēn) an antihistaminic agent that inhibits histamine mediation at the H_1 receptor, 2-(diphenylmethoxy-N,N-dimethylethylamine, occurring as a white, odorless, crystalline powder that darkens on exposure to light, is soluble in water, alcohol, chloroform, and acetone, and very slightly soluble in benzene and ether. It also possesses anticholinergic, antispasmodic, antitussive, antiemetic, and sedative effects. Used therapeutically, as the hydrochloride, in allergic diseases and motion sickness. It has potentially adverse effects in hypertension and heart disease. Trademarks: Alledryl, Allergin, Amidryl, Bagodryl, Benadryl, Benodin, Benylan, Benzantin, Dibendrin, Dihidral, Diphantine, Syntedril.

diphenidol (di-fen′ĭ-dol) an antiemetic and antinauseant, α,α-diphenyl-1-piperidinebutanol, occurring as a white, odorless, slightly bitter, crystalline powder that is soluble in chloroform, ether, and cyclohexane, slightly soluble in ethanol, and insoluble in water. Used in nausea and vomiting associated with infectious diseases, cancer chemotherapy, radiation sickness, and vertigo of vestibular origin. Side reactions may include xerostomia, hallucinations, drowsiness, confusion, dizziness, skin rashes, heartburn, headache, and visual disorders. Trademark: Vontrol. **d. hydrochloride,** the hydrochloride salt of diphenidol, which is freely soluble in methanol, water, and chloroform, but not in ether and benzene. Its pharmacological and toxic properties are similar to those of the parent compound. Trademark: Cefadol.

Diphentoin trademark for *phenytoin sodium* (see under PHENYTOIN).

Diphenylan trademark for *phenytoin sodium* (see under PHENYTOIN).

diphenyldiazene (di-fe″nil-di′ah-zēn) azobenzene.

diphenyldiimide (di-fe″nil-di′ĭ-mīd) azobenzene.

diphenylhydantoin (di-fe″nil-hi-dan′to-in) phenytoin.

diphenylpyraline (di-fen″il-pi′rah-lēn) an antihistaminic drug acting upon the H_1 receptor, 4-diphenylmethoxy-1-methylpiperidine, used therapeutically as the hydrochloride salt, occurring as crystals that are soluble in water, ethanol, and isopropanol. Used in the treatment of allergic diseases. Trademarks: Allergen, Belfene, Diafen, Hispril, Histyn, Mepiben.

diphosphate (di-fos′fāt) a salt with two phosphate groups. **calcium d.,** CALCIUM pyrophosphate. **ditin d.,** stannous PYROPHOSPHATE.

diphosphotransferase (di-fos″fo-trans′fer-ās) pyrophosphotransferase.

diphtheria (dif-the′re-ah) [Gr. *diphthera* membrane + *-ia*] an acute, contagious disease usually affecting young children, transmitted by direct contact and caused by the bacillus *Corynebacterium diphtheriae.* The incubation period is 2 to 5 days. Symptoms include fever, prostration, myocarditis, headache, vomiting, and restlessness. Diphtheritic membranes, which are patchy, grayish, thick pseudomembranes, usually of the tonsils, represent the principal symptom. Bronchopneumonia, paralysis, and cardiac failure may be associated. Polymorphonuclear leukocytosis is a hematologic symptom. Called also *Bretonneau's angina, Bretonneau's disease,* and *diphtherial tonsillitis.* **cutaneous d.,** a sometimes fatal form, occurring most often in the tropics, and usually characterized by skin ulcers and, less commonly, by nondescript lesions, such as an eczematous eruption. The usual cause is the reservoir of *Corynebacterium diphtheriae* in the throat, with poor hygiene as a contributing factor. It usually originates at the site of a pre-existing lesion, such as an insect bite, burn, or an eczematous eruption; the eruption sometimes spreads to the face around the ears, nares, and upper lip, most commonly being carried with nasal secretions. **false d.,** pseudodiphtheria. **faucial d.,** a mild form of diphtheria, with or without soreness of the throat, associated usually with low grade fever. During the first day there is congestion and swelling of the tonsillar and pharyngeal tissue, followed by small yellowish-white spots on the tonsils that coalesce and spread to the pillars, uvula, soft palate, pharynx, and sometimes to the nares. Rapid pulse, prostration, hypotension, difficulty in breathing and swallowing due to obstruction, and palatal paralysis may follow. **gangrenous d.,** that attended with gangrene of the skin or mucous membrane, or both. **d. gra'vis,** malignant d. **laryngeal d.,** membranous CROUP. **laryngotracheal d.,** that in which the infection invades the larynx and trachea, with edema, congestion, and pseudomembranes. Hoarseness, noisy breathing, brassy cough, and cyanosis are the common complications due to laryngeal obstruction. **latent d.,** that without membranous exudation or pseudomembranes. **malignant d.,** an often fatal form beginning with rigors, and marked by massive swelling of the neck (bull neck), tonsillar enlargement, and sometimes purpura. Called also *d. gravis.* **nasal d.,** an uncommon form in which the infection is mainly in the nasal passages, but may extend to the throat, nasopharynx, and larynx. Constitutional symptoms are usually absent or slight. **pharyngeal d.,** that which is especially manifested on the mucous membrane of the pharynx. Called also *diphtheric pharyngitis.* **wound d.,** infection of a wound with *Corynebacterium diphtheriae,* sometimes occurring as a postoperative complication, leading to the development of a false membrane on the surface of the wound.

diphyodont (dif'ĭ-o-dont) [*di-* + Gr. *phyein* to produce + *odous* tooth] having two dentitions, a deciduous and a permanent, as in man. Cf. MONOPHYODONT.

diplegia (di-ple'je-ah) [*di-* + Gr. *plēgē* stroke] symmetric paralysis affecting both sides of the body. **congenital facial d.,** congenital paralysis, usually bilateral, of the external rectus and facial muscles due to aplasia of the nuclei of the abducens and facial nerves, with inability to abduct the eyes beyond the midline and masklike facies being the principal features. Other important symptoms are drooling from the corners of the mouth, speech impairment because of difficulty in using the lips, Bell's phenomenon (upward movement of the eyes during attempted closure of the eyelids), and poor eyelid closure, resulting in exposure keratitis. Atrophy of the tongue, paralysis of the masticatory muscles and soft palate, and prominent everted lips are the principal oral symptoms. Clubfoot, syndactyly or absence of the fingers and toes, aplasia of the pectoral and sternocleidomastoid muscles, congenital hip dislocation, and other abnormalities may be present. Called also *akinesia algera, congenital abducens-facial paralysis, congenital facial paralysis, congenital oculofacial paralysis,* and *Möbius' syndrome.*

diplo- [Gr. *diploos* double] a combining form meaning double, twin, twofold, or twice.

Diplobacillus (dip"lo-bah-sil'us) former name for *Moraxella.* **D. moraxax'enfeld,** *Moraxella lacunata;* see under MORAXELLA.

diplococci (dip"lo-kok'si) plural of *diplococcus.*

Diplococcus (dip"lo-kok'us) [*diplo-* + Gr. *kokkos* a berry] a former genus made up of spherical or elongate cells dividing in one plane, and occurring in pairs or chains; its species are now assigned to various other genera. **D. constella'tus,** *Peptococcus constellatus;* see under PEPTOCOCCUS. **D. glycinoph'ilus,** *Peptococcus anaerobius;* see under PEPTOCOCCUS. **D. gonorrhoe'ae,** *Neisseria gonorrhoeae;* see under NEISSERIA. **D. mag'nus anaero'bius,** *Peptococcus anaerobius;* see under PEPTOCOCCUS. **D. muco'sus,** *Neisseria mucosa;* see under NEISSERIA. **D. pneumo'niae,** *Streptococcus pneumoniae;* see under STREPTOCOCCUS. **D. sic'cus,** *Neisseria sicca;* see under NEISSERIA.

diplococcus (dip"lo-kok'us), pl. *diplococci.* 1. a spherical bacterium occurring predominantly in pairs as a consequence of incomplete separation following cell division in a single plane; the organism may also be lanceolate (pneumococcus) or coffee-bean–shaped (gonococcus). 2. any microorganism of the former genus *Diplococcus.*

diploë (dip'lo-e) [Gr. *diploē* fold] the loose spongy bone between the two plates of the cranial bones.

diploid (dip'loid) [*diplo-* + *-ploid*] 1. having two homologous chromosome sets (one maternal and one paternal), found in most somatic cells, being double the number found in the gametes. In man the diploid chromosome number is 46. 2. an individual having two homologous chromosome sets. Cf. HAPLOID.

diploidy (dip'loi-de) the state of having two full sets of homologous chromosomes.

diplomate (dip'lo-māt) a person who has received a diploma or certificate. In medicine, the term refers particularly to a holder of a certificate of the National Board of Medical Examiners or of one of the American Boards in the Specialties.

diplopia (dĭ-plo'pe-ah) [[*diplo-* + Gr. *ōpē* sight + *-ia*] the perception of two images of a single object.

diplosome (dip'lo-sōm) [*diplo-* + Gr. *soma* body] a pair of centrioles in a mammalian cell, whose axes are perpendicular. Called also *double centriole.*

diplotene (dip'lo-tēn) [*diplo-* + Gr. *tainia* ribbon] the fourth stage of the first division of meiosis, characterized by longitudinal separation of the paired bivalent chromosomes. The two chromatids, though separated, remain in contact through the chiasmata throughout this phase and there is a continuous exchange of materials between them. See also CROSSING OVER.

dipole (di'pōl) 1. a system of two electrically or magnetically charged particles of opposite sign which are separated by a very small distance. 2. a molecule having a + (plus) and a − (minus) pole, said to possess a dipole moment. Designated +→, the pointed end corresponding to the negative end of the dipole. **fluctuating d.,** the electrical symmetry in which the electrons, which are distributed around the nucleus and produce an electrostatic field around the atom, fluctuate so that the field becomes momentarily plus and minus. A fluctuating dipole will attract other similar dipoles, but such interatomic form forces are weak.

Diprazin trademark for *promethazine.*

dipsomania (dip"so-ma'ne-ah) [Gr. *dipsa* thirst + *mania* madness] alcoholism.

dipstick (dip'stik) a strip of cellulose chemically impregnated to render it sensitive to protein, glucose, or other substances in the urine.

dipyridamole (di"pi-rid'ah-mōl) a coronary vasodilator, 2,6 - bis - (diethanolamino) - 4, 8 - dipiperidinopyramido (5, 4 - *d*) pyrimidine, occurring as a yellow crystalline powder that is soluble in ethanol and, slightly, in water. Trademarks: Anginal, Cardoxin, Curantyl, Persantine.

dipyrone (di'pi-rōn) methampyrone.

direct (di-rekt') [L. *directus*] 1. straight. 2. accomplished immediately in the shortest manner without the intervention of subsidiary means.

director (di-rek'tor) [L. *dirigere* to direct] any person, thing, or device that guides or directs. **grooved d.,** a grooved instrument used to guide the direction and depth of a surgical incision.

directoscope (di-rek'to-skōp) an instrument for the direct examination of the larynx.

dirhinic (di-ri'nik) pertaining to both nasal cavities.

Dirox trademark for *acetaminophen.*

Dir. prop. abbreviation for L. *directio'ne pro'pria,* with a proper direction.

DI-S simplified debris index; see oral hygiene index, simplified, under INDEX.

dis- a prefix denoting (1) [L. *dis* apart] reversal or separation, or (2) [Gr. *dis* twice, doubly] duplication.

disability (dis"ah-bil'ĭ-te) 1. any limitation of physical, mental, or social activity in an individual as compared with other individuals of similar age, sex, and occupation. The term frequently refers to limitation of principal activities, most commonly vocational. 2. legal incapacity; legal disqualification. **adjunct d.,** in the Veterans' Administration health care program, a non-service-connected disability associated with or held to be aggravating a service-connected disability. **developmental d.,** one which originates before the age of 18; can be expected to continue indefinitely; constitutes a substantial handicap to a person's ability to function normally in society; and may be attributable to mental retardation, cerebral palsy, epilepsy, autism, or any other condition closely related to mental retardation because it results in similar impairment of general intellectual functioning or adaptive behavior or requires similar treatment and services, or dyslexia resulting from one of the conditions listed. Abbreviated *DD*. **long-term d.,** one in which the patient is unable to function normally for 3 or more months due to chronic conditions or impairment. **nonservice-connected d.,** in the Veterans' Administration health care program, a disability which was not incurred or aggravated in the line of duty during active military service. **service-connected d.,** in the Veterans' Administration health care program, a disability incurred or aggravated in the line of duty in active military service; it may occur as a result of an injury or a disabling disease. **short-term d.,** one in which the patient is unable to function normally for less than 3 months.

disacidify (dis″ah-sid′ĭ-fi) to remove an acid from, or to neutralize an acid in, a mixture.

disaccharide (di-sak′ah-rīd) [*di-* + *saccharide*] a class of carbohydrates made up of two monosaccharides whose combination involves the splitting out of a molecule of water, having the general formula $C_n(H_2O)_{n-1}$ or $C_{12}H_{22}O_{11}$. It includes sucrose, lactose, and maltose. Formerly called *biose, disaccharose,* and *hexabiose.*

disacchariduria (di-sak″ah-ri-du′re-ah) [*disaccharide* + Gr. *ouron* urine + *-ia*] presence of a disaccharide (lactose or sucrose) in the urine.

disaccharose (di-sak′ah-rōs) former name for *disaccharide.*

Disadine trademark for *povidone-iodine.*

disarticulation (dis″ar-tik″u-la′shun) [*dis-(1)* + L. *articulus* joint] amputation or separation of a joint.

disc (disk) [L. *discus*] disk.

disc- see DISCO-.

discharge (dis-charj′) 1. a setting free, or liberation. 2. a matter or force set free. 3. an excretion or substance evacuated. 4. to release, send away, or allow to go. **hospital d.,** the departure from a hospital of a patient who has previously gone through the admission procedure and for whom a bed is no longer retained, whether the patient returned to his home, was transferred to another hospital or institution, or died.

disci (dis′ki) [L.] plural of *discus.*

disciform (dis′ĭ-form) [L. *discus* disk + L. *forma* shape] shaped like a disk.

disclosing (dis-klōz′ing) 1. the act or process of making known, revealing, or causing to appear. 2. a process which allows visualization of dental plaque through staining with a selective dye. See also disclosing AGENT.

disco-, disc- [L. *discus;* Gr. *diskos*] a combining form denoting relationship to a disk, or disk-shaped.

discoblastula (dis″ko-blas′tu-lah) [*disco-* + *blastula*] the specialized blastula formed by cleavage of a fertilized telolecithal ovum, consisting of a cellular cap — the germinal disk, or blastoderm — separated by the blastocoele from a floor of uncleaved yolk.

discoid (dis′koid) [*disco-* + Gr. *eidos* form] 1. shaped like a disk. 2. a disklike medicated tablet. 3. a dental instrument with a circular blade around the entire periphery, except where it meets the shank; used for carving dental restorations. See illustration.

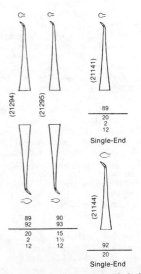

Discoid-cleoid. (From H. O. Torres and A. Ehrlich: Modern Dental Assisting. 2nd ed. Philadelphia, W. B. Saunders Co., 1980; courtesy of S. S. White Div. of Pennwalt Corp.)

4. A disk-shaped excavator designed to remove the carious dentin of a decayed tooth. See also EXCAVATOR.

discoloration (dis-kul″o-ra′shun) the act or process of altering color, including becoming faded or stained. **tooth d.,** any change in the hue, color, or translucency of a tooth due to any cause. Restorative filling materials, effect of drugs, both topical and systemic, pulpal necrosis, or hemorrhage may be responsible for discoloration.

Discomyces (dis″ko-mi′sēz) [*disco-* + Gr. *mykēs* fungus] *Actinomyces.* **D. brasilien′sis,** *Nocardia brasiliensis;* see under NOCARDIA. **D. israe′li,** *Actinomyces israelii;* see under ACTINOMYCES.

discount (dis-kownt′, dis′kownt) the amount deducted from the charge or bill. **courtesy d., professional d.,** courtesy ALLOWANCE.

discrepancy (dis-krep′an-se) disagreement or inconsistency. **tooth size d.,** lack of harmony of size of individual or groups of teeth when related to those within the same arch or the opposing arch.

discrete (dis-krēt′) [L. *discretus; discernere* to separate] distinct; having separate parts; especially characterized by separate lesions; not confluent.

discrimination (dis-krim″i-na′shun) noting or observing a difference. **auditory d.,** the ability to differentiate sounds of different frequencies, intensity, and pressure-pattern components; the ability to distinguish one speech sound from another.

discus (dis′kus) pl. *dis′ci* [L.; Gr. *diskos*] a circular or rounded flat plate; used as a general term in anatomical nomenclature to designate such a structure. Called also *disc* or *disk.* See also MENISCUS. **d. articula′ris** [NA], interarticular DISK. **d. articula′ris articulatio′nis mandibula′ris,** interarticular disk of temporomandibular joint; see under DISK. **d. articula′ris articulatio′nis sternoclavicula′ris** [NA], interarticular disk of sternoclavicular joint; see under DISK. **d. articula′ris articulatio′nis temporomandibula′ris** [NA], interarticular disk of temporomandibular joint; see under DISK.

disease (dĭ-zēz′) [Fr. *dès* from + *aise* ease] a morbid process having a characteristic train of symptoms. **Abrami's d.,** acquired hemolytic JAUNDICE. **acute d.,** one having a short and relatively severe course. Called also *acute illness.* **Adams-Stokes d.,** sudden syncopal attacks, with or without convulsions, in severe bradycardia or prolonged asystole, which accompany heart block. Called also *Adams-Stokes syndrome.* **Addison's d.,** a syndrome of adrenal hypofunction, bronzed pigmentation of the skin, anemia, diarrhea, and digestive disorders, sometimes associated with heart failure. Bronzed pigmentation of the oral mucosa may be the first symptom; the color of the mucosa may vary from pale to a deep chocolate color, spreading from the angles of the mouth toward the buccal mucosa. In some instances, pigmentation may develop on the gingivae, tongue, and lips. Called also *bronzed disease* and *suprarenal melasma.* **Albers-Schönberg's d.,** a congenital hereditary abnormality of bone growth characterized by density of the bones. Failure of resorption of cartilaginous intercellular ground substance causes the growth of cartilage and primitive bone to continue, while the cores of calcified cartilage and unlamellated osteoid persist, interfering with bone formation. Growth retardation and predisposition to fractures are the principal symptoms. Visual disorders, cataracts, hearing disorders, hypochromic anemia, facial paralysis, hepatosplenomegaly, enlargement of lymph nodes, osteomyelitis, and bone deformities secondary to fractures are the most common complications. Osteosclerosis and osteomyelitis of the jaws, retarded tooth eruption, fractures during tooth extraction, arrested root development, high incidence of dental caries, enamel hypoplasia, and dentinal defects are the chief oral manifestations. Some believe that there are possibly two independent forms of this disease: a congenital or malignant form, transmitted as an autosomal recessive trait, and a benign form, transmitted as an autosomal dominant trait. Called also *marble bone d., marble d., Albers-Schönberg's marble bones, chalk bones, disseminated condensing osteopathy, ivory bones, osteopetrosis,* and *osteosclerosis.* **Alibert's d.,** cutaneous LEISHMANIASIS. **Andersen's d.,** GLYCOGENOSIS IV. **Andes d.,** Monge's d. **Arndt-Gottron d.,** a disorder characterized by primary paraproteinemia associated with hardening and thickening of the skin. Hematologic changes include an increase of gamma globulin and elevated blood hexoses and hexosamines. Cutaneous changes appear suddenly as a reddish or grayish brown discoloration and hardening and thickening of the skin about the neck, joint flexures, and back, with formation of thick folds in the affected areas; masklike coarse facies with difficulty in opening the mouth is usually observed. Pale reddish of whitish multiple lichenoid nodules are often found on the neck, arms, and trunk. The skin changes are believed to be caused by infiltration of paraproteins into the connective tissue. Histologic findings include deposits of abnormal material rich in acid mucopolysaccharides that are intermixed with collagen fibers, chiefly in the reticular layer of the skin, and connective tissue cells and some mast cells may be also found. Called also *scleromyxedema.* **arteriosclerotic heart d.,** a coronary heart disease evolving from slow, progressive narrowing of the coronary arteries by deposits of atherosclerotic plaques in the lumen of the arteries, leading to slow deprivation of the myocardium of an adequate arterial supply, resulting in atrophy with necrosis of the individual fibers and small areas of scattered fibrosis. The heart valves, particularly on the left side, may simultaneously become thickened, fibrotic, and calcified. Angina pectoris is a common manifestation; myocardial infarction is a frequent complication. See also congestive heart FAILURE. **Asboe-Hansen's d.,** a skin disease of newborn girls characterized by bullous, keratogenic, pigmented dermatitis; it is inherited as an X-linked dominant trait lethal in the male. The lesions begin as blisters over red infiltrates on the trunk and extremities, but after several weeks or months, the bullae dry out and verrucous and keratogenic lesions appear; a few months later, slate-gray pigmentation develops, forming bizarre figures, which may persist for years. The bullous phase is associated with eosinophilia. *Bloch-Sulzberger syndrome* is considered to be the end phase of this disease, involving the skin, eyes, nails, central nervous system, and hair. Called also *incontinentia pigmenti of Asboe-Hansen.* **autoimmune d's,** traditionally, any condition in which an abnormal factor causes the host to mount an immunological attack against its own tissues. Currently, the term has been restricted to only protracted, self-perpetuating conditions in which there is clinical tissue damage. Autoimmune diseases are grouped into systemic diseases, in which the major involvement is seen in more than one organ (e.g., systemic lupus erythematosus, which expresses itself as vasculitis involving many organs); and organ-specific diseases, (e.g., Addison's disease, which involves the endocrine system, and rheumatic fever, which involves the heart). See also AUTOANTIGEN and HYPERSENSITIVITY. **Baelz's d.,** CHEILITIS glandularis apostematosa. **Bang's d.,** brucellosis. **Bannister's d.,** Quincke's EDEMA. **Barlow's d.,** infantile SCURVY. **Basedow's d.,** exophthalmic GOITER. **Behçet's d.,** SYNDROME. **bleeder's d.,** HEMOPHILIA A. **Borovskii's d.,** cutaneous LEISHMANIASIS. **Bosviel's d.,** staphylohematoma. **Bowen's d.,** CARCINOMA *in situ.* **Bretonneau's d.,** diphtheria. **Brill-Symmers d.,** giant follicle LYMPHOMA. **Brocq's d.,** a combination of erythema and diffuse brownish pigmentation of the perioral region, often extending to other parts of the face; it develops in apparently normal females at puberty and disappears and reappears during the menstrual cycle. A photosensitive substance in cosmetics is the suspected cause. Called also *erythrose péribuccale pigmentaire* and *erythrosis pigmentata faciei.* **bronzed d.,** Addison's d. **Brooke's d.,** cystic adenoid EPITHELIOMA. **Brown-Symmers d.,** a rapidly fatal form of encephalitis in children, marked by the sudden onset of symptoms, which include irritability, lack of appetite, vomiting, diarrhea, sore throat, fever, respiratory difficulties, ptosis, strabismus, nystagmus, papilledema, retraction of the angles of the mouth, muscular twitching, rigidity of the neck and jaws, coma, hemiplegia, and convulsions. It is characterized by extreme enlargement of the brain with splotchy hemorrhages, flattening of the convolutions, obliteration of the sulci, and softening of the brain. Called also *acute serous encephalitis.* **Buschke's d., Busse-Buschke d.,** European BLASTOMYCOSIS. **Caffey-Smyth d.,** infantile cortical HYPEROSTOSIS. **caisson d.,** decompression SICKNESS. **California d.,** coccidioidomycosis. **Carrión's d.,** see BARTONELLOSIS. **cat-scratch d.,** a syndrome characterized by lymphadenopathy, fever, red suppurative papules at the site of inoculation, fever, nausea, and malaise, occurring from one to several weeks after being scratched or bitten by a cat. The preauricular, submaxillary, or cervical chain of lymph nodes may be involved. The role of *Chlamydia* or a virus as possible etiologic agents is still unclear. Called also *benign reticulosis, Debré's syndrome, inoculation adenitis, nonbacterial regional lymphadenitis,* and *regional lymphadenitis.* **Cazenave's d.,** PEMPHIGUS foliaceus. **celiac d.,** a gastrointestinal disease of both children and

adults, caused by a genetically transmitted inborn error of protein metabolism with secondary faulty assimilation of fat. In the infantile form, diarrhea with bulky, foul-smelling stools and steatorrhea, abdominal distention, failure to gain weight, growth retardation, dehydration, acidosis, and oral symptoms are the principal features. Vomiting and diarrhea may be present shortly after birth, but other symptoms appear later. In the adult form, vomiting is rare, distension is less prominent, and weight loss is the major symptom. Ingestion of gluten exacerbates the condition. The intestinal mucosa usually shows deficiency of a peptidase. Oral symptoms include severe glossitis; atrophy of the filiform papillae with persistence of the fungiform papillae on the atrophic surface; burning sensation of the oral and lingual mucosa; and, sometimes, painful vesicular erosions. Called also *Gee-Herter d., gluten enteropathy, Herter's infantilism, intestinal infantilism,* and *nontropical sprue.* **α chain d.,** see *heavy chain d.* **Cheadle's d., Cheadle-Möller-Barlow d.,** infantile SCURVY. **Christmas d.,** a genetically determined blood coagulation disorder, similar to but somewhat milder than hemophilia A, caused by factor IX (Christmas factor) deficiency, and transmitted as a sex-linked recessive trait through female carriers. It occurs mostly in males, but the incidence in females is somewhat greater than in hemophilia A. For oral manifestations see HEMOPHILIA A. Named for the first patient with the disorder who was studied in detail. Called also *deuterohemophilia, factor IX deficiency, hemophilia B, hemophilia II, hemophiloid state C, PTC deficiency,* and *PTF-B deficiency.* **chronic d.,** a disease which is slow in its progress and of long continuance; it involves an impairment of bodily structure and/or function that necessitates a modification of the patient's life style, and persists or may be expected to persist over an extended period of time. Called also *chronic illness.* **Civatte's d.,** reticulated pigmented POIKILODERMA. **collagen d.,** any of a group of conditions showing common involvement of the collagenous connective tissue throughout many organs and systems of the body, but with varied etiologies. The group includes lupus erythematosus, dermatomyositis, scleroderma, polyarteritis nodosa, thrombotic purpura, rheumatoid fever, and rheumatoid arthritis. See also collagen SIALADENITIS. **communicable d.,** a disease the causative agent of which may pass or be carried from one person to another either directly or through a vector. **contagious d.,** a disease that is transmissible by contact with the sick. **Cori's d.,** GLYCOGENOSIS III. **coronary heart d.,** an ischemic heart disease, acute or chronic, arising from reduction or arrest of the blood supply to the myocardium in association with disease processes in the coronary arterial system. In most instances, it is due to atherosclerotic narrowing of the coronary ostia; dissecting aneurysms extending back into the coronary vessels; rheumatic temporal arteritis, and polyarteritis nodosa involving coronary vessels; or embolic occlusion and direct trauma to the heart inducing coronary thrombosis. The cardiac ischemia may induce asymptomatic diffuse atrophic fibrotic changes in the myocardium, often associated with valvular deformities, or acute crises of chest pain with or without infarction of the myocardium. Three forms are recognized: arteriosclerotic heart disease, myocardial infarction, and angina pectoris. See also congestive heart FAILURE. **Crohn's d.,** a disease of the terminal portion of the ileum, occurring mainly in young adults, characterized by disproportionate reaction of the connective tissue in the remaining walls of the intestine, leading frequently to stenosis and multiple fistulae. Oral lesions may include granulomatous lesions similar to those of the intestine, having a coarsely nodular or cobblestone mucosal surface, miliary ulceration, and linear fissures, with a patchy distribution. Swelling of the underlying submucosal connective tissue, proliferation in the sulci forming well-defined ridges, and aphthous ulcers or glossitis may be associated. Called also *regional enteritis, regional ileitis,* and *terminal ileitis.* **Crouzon's d.,** craniofacial DYSOSTOSIS. **cystine d., cystine storage d.,** Abderhalden-Fanconi SYNDROME. **cytomegalic inclusion d.,** a systemic disorder of the neonatal period due to infection with a cytomegalovirus (a virus of the herpesvirus group) presumably acquired before birth. Adults are rarely affected. Hepatosplenomegaly, microcephaly, mental retardation, motor disability, hemorrhage, and jaundice are the principal symptoms. Intranuclear and cytoplasmic inclusions in the cells of the salivary glands are the constant feature. Called also *protozoan cell d., salivary gland virus d., salivary gland virus inclusion d., cytomegalia infantum,* and *generalized salivary gland virus infection.* **Darier's d.,** 1. keratosis FOLLICULARIS. 2. PSEUDOXANTHOMA elasticum. **Darling's d.,** histoplasmosis. **de Almeida's d.,** South American BLASTOMYCOSIS. **deficiency d.,** one due to inadequate availability of essential factors, such as vitamins, proteins, or minerals. For specific deficiency diseases, see the essential factor, as CALCIUM, RIBOFLAVIN, etc. **Durand-Nicolas-Favre d.**, LYMPHOGRANULOMA venereum. **Ehrenfried's d.**, a hereditary congenital disorder characterized by multiple, more or less symmetrical cartilaginous and osteocartilaginous exostoses with secondary scoliosis, disproportionate dwarfism, enlarged joints, and other bone deformities. Called also *cancellous exostoses, chondral dysplasia, exostotic dysplasia,* and *multiple cartilaginous exostoses.* **English d.**, rickets. **Epstein's d.**, Epstein's pearls; see under PEARL. **Eulenburg's d.**, congenital PARAMYOTONIA. **Fabry's d.**, an inborn error of glycolipid metabolism, transmitted as an X-linked recessive trait, and characterized by cutaneous papules and macules with hyperkeratotic surfaces of the thighs and genitalia and other parts of the body. Pain and burning sensation in the extremities, corneal opacities, fever, kidney lesions, edema, hyperhidrosis, albuminuria, and deposits of abnormal glycolipids in the blood vessels, kidney glomeruli, ganglion cells, heart, eyes, and other tissues are present. Small, blood-filled cavities may be seen on the skin and oral mucosa, most commonly on the lower lip, near the mucocutaneous junction, palate near the soft palate junction, and, rarely, on the buccal and gingival mucosa. Called also *angioma corporis diffusum universale, glycolipid lipidosis,* and *hereditary dystrophic lipoidosis.* **familial multilocular cystic d. of jaws,** cherubism. **Fauchard's d.,** marginal PERIODONTITIS. **fifth venereal d.,** LYMPHOGRANULOMA venereum. **Filatov's d.,** infectious MONONUCLEOSIS. **fish-skin d.,** ichthyosis. **Følling's d.,** phenylketonuria. **foodborne d.,** any infectious or toxic disease which may be transmitted or conveyed by food; a disease which may be traced to a specific food, substance in the food, or dish which has been contaminated by noxious organisms or substance, or to a particular food-producing, food-dispensing, or food-processing procedure. **foot-and-mouth d.,** an infectious disease of hogs, sheep, and cattle, which may be transmitted to man through contact or through the use of contaminated milk, caused by a picornavirus (see foot-and-mouth disease VIRUS). Fever, nausea, vomiting, malaise, and ulcers of the pharynx, oral mucosa, and skin, especially of the soles and palms, are the principal symptoms. Oral lesions usually present as small vesicles of the lips, tongue, palate, and oropharynx; they rapidly rupture, but heal within about two weeks. Called also *aphthobullous stomatitis, aphthous fever, aphthous stomatitis, epidemic stomatitis,* and *epizootic stomatitis.* **Forbes' d.,** GLYCOGENOSIS III. **Fordyce's d.,** Fordyce's granules; see under GRANULE. **Fothergill's d.,** 1. trigeminal NEURALGIA. 2. SCARLATINA anginosa. **Fox's d.,** EPIDERMOLYSIS bullosa. **Francis' d.,** tularemia. **Franklin's d.,** see *heavy chain d.* **Frei's d.,** LYMPHOGRANULOMA venereum. **Friedreich's d.,** hemifacial HYPERTROPHY. **Gaucher's d.,** any of a group of hereditary cerebroside metabolism disorders characterized by the presence of Gaucher's cells (see under CELL), inherited as an autosomal recessive or autosomal dominant trait. Many cases occur in persons of Jewish ancestry. It may be detected at any age. In the infantile form, it is usually malignant with an early onset of symptoms consisting of hepatosplenomegaly, delayed development, strabismus, retroflexion of the head, dysphagia, bulbar palsy, respiratory disorders, and early death. When the onset is in early childhood, it progresses more slowly and there is a longer life expectancy. In the chronic (adult) form, the symptoms include hepatosplenomegaly with hypersplenism, thrombocytopenia with hemorrhage, rheumatic joint swelling, pathological fractures, scleral pingueculae, skin pigmentation, anemia, and jaundice; this form may be complicated by persistent hemorrhage after tooth extraction, osteoporosis of the jaws, thinning of the cortex, and tooth root resorption. Called also *cerebroside lipidosis* and *familial splenic anemia.* **Gee-Herter d.,** celiac d. **Gilchrist's d.,** North American BLASTOMYCOSIS. **Glisson's d.,** rickets. **glycogen d.,** glycogenosis. **glycogen heart d.,** GLYCOGENOSIS II. **glycogen storage d.,** glycogenosis. **Goldscheier's d.,** EPIDERMOLYSIS bullosa. **Greenfield's d.,** metachromatic LEUKODYSTROPHY. **Graves' d.,** exophthalmic GOITER. **Grisel's d.,** nasopharyngeal TORTICOLLIS. **d. of the Hapsburgs,** HEMOPHILIA A. **Hb SC d.,** sickle cell-hemoglobin C d. **H d.,** heavy chain d. **Hallopeau's d.,** LICHEN sclerosus et atrophicus. **hand-foot-and-mouth d.,** a viral disease of children, usually under 10 years of age, caused by coxsackieviruses, especially those of Group A, type 16. Symptoms appear after an incubation period of 2 to 6 days, consist of superficial vesicles on the borders of the palms and soles and ventral surfaces of the fingers and toes; they first appear as red papules, about 2 to 10 mm in diameter, which change to flaccid gray vesicles that resolve in about 10 days. The oral lesions consist of 5 to 10 painful aphthae, under 2 mm in diameter, involving any part of the oral and labial mucosa; they subside and heal within a week or ten days. Mild anorexia, fever,

malaise, and cervical adenitis may be present. **Hand-Schüller-Christian d.,** the chronic disseminated form of histiocytosis X, occurring most often in children and young adults, characterized by dissemination of histiocytes and a triad of clinical symptoms: exophthalmos, diabetes insipidus, and osteolytic bone lesions. The histiocytes contain little lipid, hence the disorder has been classified as a nonlipid reticuloendotheliosis. Tumorlike masses of cholesterol-loaded histiocytes cause exophthalmos by pushing against the eyeball; they may also compress the pituitary and hypothalamus. Principal symptoms include eczematous eruption, xanthomata, lymph node enlargement, hepatosplenomegaly, and pulmonary infiltrations. Oral lesions include red, soft, spongy gingivae, loose or shedding teeth, and mandibular erosion. Roentgenographically, the affected teeth appear to "float"; bone destruction is marked by radiolucent areas of various shapes and degrees; and rarefaction in the medullary spaces is indicated by poorly outlined "lacunae." The skull may assume an irregular or serpiginous pattern. The lesions present yellow areas with dark patches of old hemorrhages. Histologically, the lesion is a mass of granulation tissue made up mostly of proliferating histiocytes, with some eosinophils present. Called also *cholesterol granulomatosis* and *craniohypophyseal xanthoma.* **Hansen's d.,** leprosy. **Hashimoto's d.,** chronic thyroiditis characterized by progressive goiter with or without pressure symptoms, occurring most commonly in menopausal women, and believed to be caused by autoimmune processes of the body; it may be associated with other autoimmune conditions, such as rheumatoid arthritis or Sjögren's syndrome. Pathologically, it presents lymphocytic infiltration heavily admixed with plasma cells, leading to atrophy of the parenchyma. Called also *Hashimoto's thyroiditis* and *struma lymphomatosa.* **heavy chain d.,** a disorder of γ-globulin in patients with malignant lymphoma. The γG type (also known as *Franklin's d.*) is characterized by a protein antigenically related to the Fc fragment of the heavy chain of γG. Clinical symptoms include lymphadenopathy, splenomegaly, fever, anemia, and sometimes, hepatomegaly, leukopenia, and thrombocytopenia. Excessive susceptibility to bacterial infection is common. Oral manifestations may include erythema and edema of the palate, which usually subside after a few days. The bone marrow and lymph nodes contain atypical immature plasma cells with an admixture of atypical lymphocytes, reticulum cells, and eosinophils. The abnormal serum and urine protein shows fast γ and slow β mobility; its molecular weight is about 53,000; it is immunologically related to γG globulin and is similar to the fast chain. The level of normal immunoglobulins is usually depressed. The γA type (also known as *α chain d.*) was originally described in a young Arab woman with malignant lymphoma of the intestine. The abnormal protein found in serum, urine, and saliva was closely related to γA₁ and devoid of light chains. Some normal γA was present; γG and γA₁ and devoid of light chains. Some normal γA was present; γG and γM were abnormally low. The γM type is characterized by the presence of a heavy chain fragment related to the μ chain of IgM, and is devoid of light chains. Clinical symptoms in the original case included amyloid deposits, bone pain, lymphoproliferative disorders, and carpal-tunnel syndrome, but no eosinophilia, lymphadenopathy, or recurrent infection present in other forms of heavy chain disease. Called also *H d.* **Heberden's d.,** ANGINA pectoris. **Hebra's d.,** a mild form of erythema multiforme. **Heck's d.,** hyperplasia of the buccal, labial, and lingual mucosae, characterized by multiple, soft, sessile papules, with the lower lip seeming to be affected most frequently. The first observations were made in a group of American Indian children, and later commonly found among Greenland Eskimos. Called also *focal epithelial hyperplasia.* **Heine-Medin d.,** poliomyelitis. **Helwig's d.,** a benign epithelial tumor occurring most frequently as a single lesion on the face in older persons. Histologically, it is characterized by invaginating cup-shaped and finger-like tumors consisting of peripheral cells that resemble basal cells but are smaller, and squamoid cells in the center, which form various structures. Called also *inverted follicular keratosis.* **hemoglobin S d.,** sickle cell ANEMIA. **hemolytic d.,** one characterized by an abnormally short survival time of erythrocytes. **hemolytic d. of newborn,** ERYTHROBLASTOSIS fetalis. **Henoch's d.,** purpura associated with abdominal disorders; see Schönlein-Henoch SYNDROME. **Hers' d.,** GLYCOGENOSIS VI. **Hodgkin's d.,** a malignant condition of unknown etiology, considered by many to be a form of malignant lymphoma. It usually begins as a painless enlargement of the cervical lymph nodes, followed by splenomegaly, abdominal pain, weakness, anorexia, loss of weight, cough, dyspnea, and sometimes itching. Lesions present a wide variety of histological patterns — from almost pure lymphocytic infiltrates to histiocytic giant cells. A constant feature is the presence of Reed-Sternberg cells, giant tumor cells measuring up to 40 μ in diameter and having abundant cytoplasm that is irregular in shape and varies in staining reaction from acidophilic to basophilic. Cell nuclei are large, sometimes occupying half a cell, with some cells having two or more nuclei. The oral and nasal cavities are rarely involved. Called also *Hodgkin's granuloma, lymphogranuloma, lymphogranulomatosis maligna, malignant granuloma, malignant granulomatosis, malignant lymphogranulomatosis,* and *multiple lymphadenoma.* **homozygous C d.,** a condition characterized by the presence in the blood of hemoglobin C, associated with recurrent pain, abdominal cramps, convulsions, anemia, and hemorrhagic disorders. Osmotic fragility of the erythrocytes is decreased and their survival rate seems to be lowered. Thrombocytopenia, anisocytosis, poikilocytosis, and polychromatophilia are usually present. It is most common in Negroes but other ethnic groups may also be affected. **Horton's d.,** cluster HEADACHE. **hydatid d.,** echinococcosis. **iatrogenic d.,** one occurring as the result of treatment by a physician or, by extension, a dentist. **immune-complex d.,** serum SICKNESS. **infectious d.,** one due to organisms ranging in size from viruses to parasitic worms; it may be contagious in origin, result from nosocomial organisms, or be due to endogenous microflora from the nose and throat, skin or bowel. See also INFECTION. **International Classification of D., Adapted,** see under CLASSIFICATION. **iron storage d.,** hemochromatosis. **ischemic heart d.,** a disease of the heart, acute or chronic, arising from reduction or arrest of the blood supply to the myocardium. Called also *cardiac ischemia, heart ischemia,* and *myocardial ischemia.* See *coronary heart d.* **Jacob's d.,** permanent constriction of the mandible with inability to open the mouth. **Jacobi's d.,** POIKILODERMA atrophicans vasculare. **Jones' d.,** cherubism. **Kahler's d.,** multiple MYELOMA. **d. of kings,** HEMOPHILIA A. **kinky hair d.,** Menkes' SYNDROME. **Kinnier Wilson's d.,** hepatolenticular DEGENERATION. **Kniest's d.,** a form of bone dysplasia, transmitted as an autosomal dominant or X-linked chromosomal dominant trait, characterized by peculiar facies with flat mid-face and depressed nasal bridge, sometimes shallow orbits with protuberant eyes; short trunk with dorsal kyphosis, lumbar lordosis, short and broad thorax with sternal protrusion, and sometimes thoracic scoliosis; short extremities with prominent joints and restricted joint mobility; hearing loss; occasional myopia and retinal detachment; sometimes club feet; and cleft palate in about half of the cases. Called also *Kniest's syndrome.* **Legal's d.,** CEPHALALGIA pharyngotympanica. **legionnaires' d.,** a highly fatal disease caused by a gram-negative bacillus, *Legionella pneumophila,* which is not spread by person-to-person contact and is characterized by high fever, gastrointestinal pain, headache, and pneumonia; there may also be involvement of the kidneys, liver, and nervous system. An outbreak occurred in the summer of 1976 at an American Legion convention in Philadelphia, Pennsylvania. **Letterer-Siwe d.,** an acute, highly fatal, rapidly progressive form of histiocytosis X, usually occurring in early life, and characterized by widespread histiocytic proliferation of the reticuloendothelial system. The histiocytes contain little lipid, hence the disorder has also been classified as a nonlipid reticuloendotheliosis. Early symptoms include red to brown firm skin nodules resembling insect bites, followed by a maculopapular rash or multiple nodules that sometimes ulcerate and hemorrhage. Other symptoms consist of persistent spiking fever, hepatosplenomegaly, lymphadenopathy, nodular or diffuse involvement of visceral organs, anemia, leukopenia, thrombocytopenia, and hemorrhagic diathesis. Bone lesions are destructive and invade the bone marrow. Jaw involvement is usually manifested by alveolar bone loss simulating osteomyelitis and by ill-defined radiolucent areas on the roentgenogram, and is often associated with loosening and exfoliation of the teeth. Called also *aleukemic reticulosis, Letterer's reticulosis,* and *malignant reticulosis.* **light chain d.,** Bence Jones PROTEINURIA. **Lignac's d.,** Abderhalden-Fanconi SYNDROME. **liver glycogen d.,** GLYCOGENOSIS I. **Lortat-Jacob's d.,** benign mucosal PEMPHIGOID. **Lutz's d., Lutz-Splenodore-de Almeida d.,** South American BLASTOMYCOSIS. **Lutz-Miescher d.,** perforating ELASTOSIS. **McArdle's d.,** GLYCOGENOSIS V. **Magitot's d.,** periodontoclasia. **marble d., marble bone d.,** Albers-Schönberg's d. **Ménière's d.,** a disorder of unknown etiology, characterized by

sudden attacks of vertigo, tinnitus, prostration, vomiting, and progressive deafness, associated with distention of the endolymphatic system and degenerative changes of the sensory elements of the internal ear. Called also *auditory vertigo, aural vertigo, recurrent labyrinthine vertigo, endolymphatic hydrops,* and *Ménière's syndrome.* **Meyer's d.,** adenoid vegetations of the pharynx. **Mibelli's d.,** a chronic disease, usually developing early and persisting during life, which is inherited as a simple dominant trait. Originally, it was believed to consist of an abnormal keratinization and hyperkeratosis of the eccrine sweat pores (hence the synonym *porokeratosis*), but was shown to occur throughout the epidermis and/or mucous membranes. It is characterized by small collar-like keratotic ridges surrounded by grooves; the lesions begin as small keratotic papules and gradually expand, leaving clear, atrophic, depressed centers. Called also *hyperkeratosis excentrica, keratoma excentricum, parakeratosis annularis, parakeratosis centrifugata atrophicans,* and *porokeratosis centrifugata atrophicans.* **Miescher's d.,** perforating ELASTOSIS. **Mikulicz's d.,** a disease characterized by bilateral painless hypertrophy of the salivary glands and sometimes the lacrimal glands, associated with xerostomia. It is believed to be an incomplete form of Mikulicz's syndrome. Called also *benign lymphoepithelial lesion* and *lymphomatoid adenoma.* **Milton's d.,** Quincke's EDEMA. **Möller's d., Möller-Barlow d.,** infantile SCURVY. **Monge's d.,** a group of disorders produced by maladaptation to high altitudes. In less severe forms, anoxia produces absolute polycythemia, cyanosis, headache, decrease in mental and physical capacities, drowsiness, sensation of asphyxia, digestive disorders, nausea, vomiting, loss of weight, and visual disorders. In severe forms, the polycythemia is more pronounced and the other symptoms more severe and, in addition, there is discoloration of the sclerae, puffy eyelids, temporary blindness and deafness, epistaxis, bronchitis, dryness of the skin with excessive perspiration of the hands and forehead, opaque and striated nails, fatigue, anorexia, algesia, impotence, behavior and mental disorders, doubling of the second cardiac sound, and oral symptoms, including wine-red oral and nasal mucosae and macroglossia. Called also *Andes d.* and *high altitude erythremia.* See also ERYTHROCYTOSIS. **Morquio's d.,** a systemic mucopolysaccharidosis, inherited as an autosomal recessive trait, marked by early dwarfism followed, at the time the infant begins to walk, by vertebra plana, fusion of the cervical vertebrae, platybasia, enlarged wrists, disproportionately long arms, genu valgum, flat feet, waddling gait, flaccid muscles, barrel chest, pigeon breast, short neck, prominent abdomen, and a peculiar facies characterized by a wide mouth, protruding maxilla, and short nose. The teeth are usually widely spaced and have thin flaky enamel. Both the deciduous and permanent teeth have dull, gray crowns with pitted enamel. The cusps are small, flattened, and poorly formed. The palate is usually high and elongated. Caries are frequent. All patients excrete large amounts of keratosulfate in the urine, and some excrete chondroitin sulfate A. The eponym *Morquio-Ullrich syndrome* is used to designate the disease in which, in addition to skeletal changes, there is corneal opacity. *Bartenwerfer's syndrome* is a variant. Called also *atypical chondrodystrophy, Brailsford-Morquio syndrome, chondrodystrophia tarda, dysostosis enchondralis metaepiphysaria, eccentro-osteochondrodysplasia, familial osseous dystrophy, hereditary chondrodysplasia, hereditary osteochondrodystrophy, infantile hereditary chondrodysplasia, Morquio's syndrome, Morquio-Ullrich syndrome, mucopolysaccharidosis IV, osteochondrodystrophia, osteochondrodystrophia deformans, osteochondrodystrophy,* and *spondyloepiphyseal dysplasia.* **Neumann's d.,** PEMPHIGUS vegetans. **Nicolas-Favre d.,** LYMPHOGRANULOMA venereum. **Niemann-Pick d.,** a rare form of familial lipidosis with massive accumulation of foam cells in the reticuloendothelial system, liver, spleen, lungs, kidneys, pancreas, and heart, believed to be transmitted as an autosomal recessive trait. It occurs chiefly in children, is rare in adults, and is most common in persons of Jewish ancestry. Deposits of sphingomyelin, gangliosides, and cholesterol are found in the brain and spinal cord. Storage of lipids in the choroid plexus and cerebral atrophy, gliosis, and demyelination are present. Hepatosplenomegaly, pulmonary complications, mental and growth retardation, cachexia, anemia, progressive blindness, a cherry red spot of the macula lutea, and mongoloid facies are the principal clinical manifestations. Called also *lipid histiocytosis* and *sphingomyelin lipidosis.* **notifiable d.,** one which must be reported to federal, state, or local health authorities on diagnosis, because of its infectiousness, severity, or frequency. **occupational d.,** one due to one's employment. See table. **Ohara's d.,** a Japanese form of tularemia characterized by a primary lesion, an ulcer of the thumb or an ocular and tonsillar lesion. Called also *yato-byo.* See also TULAREMIA. **Osler's d.**, POLYCYTHEMIA vera. **Paget's d.**, OSTEITIS deformans. **Paget's d., juvenile,** HYPEROSTOSIS corticalis deformans juvenilis. **Parkinson's d.**, see PARKINSONISM. **Parrot's d.**, 1. osteochondritis with severe pain on movement, occurring in infants with congenital syphilis. Called also *Parrot's paralysis, Parrot's pseudoparalysis, syphilitic osteitis of newborn, syphilitic osteochondritis,* and *syphilitic pseudoparalysis.* 2. achondroplasia. **periodontal d.**, any of a group of pathological conditions that affect the surrounding and supporting tissues of the teeth, generally classified as inflammatory (gingivitis and periodontitis), dystrophic (periodontal trauma and periodontosis), and anomalies. Called also *dentoalveolitis.* **Pfeiffer's d.**, infectious MONONUCLEOSIS. **pink d.**, acrodynia. **pink spot d.**, tooth resorption, internal; see under RESORPTION. **Pinkus' d.**, LICHEN nitidus. **Pleasant's d.**, advanced alveolar bone destruction in the jaws of children with deciduous dentition and subsequent repair with normal growth of alveolar bone, normal eruption of permanent teeth, and normal growth and development of the child. **Plummer's d.**, hyperthyroidism due to toxic adenoma of the thyroid gland (Plummer's adenoma). **Pospischill-Feyrter d.**, Pospischill-Feyrter APHTHOID. **Potter's d.**, a rare condition characterized by multiple abnormalities combining Potter's facies (flattened palpebral fissures, prominent epicanthus, flattened bridge of the nose, mandibular micrognathia, low-set malformed ears) with renal agenesis or hypoplasia and other defects. Pulmonary hypoplasia, oligohydramnios, amnion nodosum, and skeletomuscular abnormalities, such as clubbing of the hands and feet and contractures, frequently occur. Called also *dysplasia renofacialis, Potter's syndrome,* and *renofacial syndrome.* **protozoan cell d.**, cytomegalic inclusion d. **Puente's d.**, CHEILITIS glandularis apostematosa. **Pyle's d.**, metaphyseal DYSPLASIA. **Quincke's d.**, Quincke's EDEMA. **Recklinghausen's d.**, 1. a hereditary disorder transmitted as an autosomal dominant trait, characterized by multiple neurofibromas and cafe-au-lait spots. The neurofibromas, varying in size from that of a small pea to a giant pendulous tumor, may appear on any part of the skin and in the oral cavity, and may undergo malignant degeneration. Epilepsy and other involvements of the nervous system; bone complications, including erosions and cystic lesions, scoliosis, kyphosis, lordosis, pseudoarthrosis; mental retardation; and sexual underdevelopment may be associated. Oral involvement

may include nodules of the oral mucosa; diffuse masses of tissue involving the palate, buccal tissue, and alveolar ridges; macroglossia; and neurofibromas of the jaws. Called also *von Recklinghausen's d., fibroma molluscum, neurinofibrolipomatosis, neurinomatosis centralis et peripherica,* and *neurofibromatosis.* 2. a generalized rarefying bone disorder seen in advanced hyperparathyroidism, characterized by cysts or by brown tumors in the form of deeply pigmented foci consisting of fibrous scarring of the bone with pseudocysts, hemorrhages, and collection of osteoclasts. Bone destruction is often associated with gross deformities, osteomalacia, fractures, tissue resorption, and replacement of destroyed bone with fibrous tissue. The pathogenesis is attributed to excessive production of parathyroid hormone with secondary calcium and phosphorus metabolism disorders. Called also *von Recklinghausen's d., osteitis fibrosa cystica, osteitis fibrosa generalisata, osteodystrophia generalisata,* and *osteopathia fibrosa generalisata.* **Recklinghausen-Applebaum d.**, hemochromatosis. **Reclus' d.**, ligneous PHLEGMON. **Reiter's d.**, a triad of arthritis, conjunctivitis, and urethritis, occurring predominantly in young males and rarely in females. Urethritis usually appears first, followed by conjunctivitis and then by arthritis, which dominates the clinical picture. The triad may be associated with fever, ulceration of the glans penis and oral mucosa, lesions of the palms and soles, nausea, anorexia, and occasionally erythema. Oral lesions consist of aphthous ulcers and bloody crusting of the lips. The etiology is unclear, but *Shigella,* pleuropneumonia-like organisms, and agents of venereal infection are suspected as possible factors. Called also *blennorrhagic arthritis, oculourethroarticular syndrome, urethral arthritis,* and *urethral rheumatism.* **rheumatic heart d.**, cardiac complication of rheumatic fever. See rheumatic FEVER. **Riga-Fede d.**, a small sublingual ulceration in infants with natal or neonatal teeth, caused by rubbing the lower incisors, most frequently observed in whooping cough. Called also *Cardarelli's aphthae, Riga's aphthae, Riga's papilloma, subglossitis diphtheroides,* and *sublingual fibrogranuloma.* **Rigg's d.**, marginal PERIODONTITIS. **Ritter's d.**, an exfoliative skin disease of infants beginning as plaques of the lower half of the face, which

ORAL MANIFESTATIONS OF OCCUPATIONAL DISEASE ACCORDING TO THE ETIOLOGIC AGENT

PHYSICAL STATE	PRINCIPAL ACTION	SPECIFIC FACTOR	OCCUPATION	POSSIBLE ORAL MANIFESTATIONS
Solid	Physical	Instruments for prehension	Cobblers, carpenters, glass blowers, musicians (wind instruments), seamstresses	Localized abrasion
	Chemical	Tar	Fishermen, asphalt and coal tar workers, pavers, pitch roofers, wood preservers	Stomatitis, carcinoma of lip and mucosa
Dust	Physical	Inorganic — Copper, iron, nickel, chromium, coal, etc.	Bronzers, cement workers, electrotypers, grinders (metal), miners, stone cutters	Staining of teeth, pigmentation of gingiva, generalized abrasion, calculus, gingivostomatitis, hemorrhage
		Organic — Bone, celluloid, sawdust, flour, tobacco	Bone, celluloid, flour, sawmill, textile, and tobacco workers	Staining of teeth, pigmentation of gingiva, generalized abrasion, calculus, gingivostomatitis, hemorrhage
	Chemical	Inorganic — Arsenic	Chemical workers, electroplaters, metal refiners, rubber mixers, lead smelters, insecticide makers	Necrosis of bone
		Bismuth	Bismuth handlers, dusting powder makers	Blue pigmentation of gingiva, oral mucosa, gingivostomatitis
		Chromium	Aniline compound, chrome, photographic and steel workers, blue printers, rubber mixers	Necrosis of bone, ulceration of oral tissue
		Fluorine	Cryolite workers	Osteosclerosis
		Lead	Electrotypers, insecticide and storage battery makers, lead refiners, printers, rubber compounders	Blue-black pigmentation of gingiva, gingivostomatitis
		Mercury	Bronzers (gun barrels), battery and paint makers, dentists, detonators, explosives and mercury salts workers	Gingivostomatitis, osteomyelitis, ptyalism
		Phosphorus (white, yellow)	Brass founders, match factory, phosphor bronze workers, fertilizer and fireworks makers	Gingivostomatitis, ulceration of oral tissues, osteomyelitis
		Organic — Sugar	Refiners, bakers, candy makers	Caries
Liquid	Physical	Hot food (coffee, tea, soup)	Tasters	Stomatitis, leukoplakia
		Aniline	Aniline, coal tar, explosives workers, painters, tannery workers, vulcanizers	Blue coloration of lips and gingiva
	Chemical	Benzene	Coke oven and lacquer workers, dry cleaners, vulcanizers, smokeless powder makers	Hemorrhage from gingiva, stomatitis, blue coloration of lips
		Cresol	Coal tar, rubber, tar, distillery and surgical dressing workers, disinfectant makers	Stomatitis
		Wine and liquor	Tasters	Anesthesia and paresthesia of tongue
Gas	Physical	Atmosphere — Increased pressure	Divers, caisson workers	Bleeding from gingiva
		Decreased pressure	Aviators	Bleeding from gingiva
	Chemical	Acids: H_2SO_4, HNO_3, HCl, HF	Acid and cartridge dippers, petroleum refiners, explosives and gun cotton workers, galvanizers	Bleeding, stomatitis, decalcification of enamel and dentin
		Amyl acetate	Alcohol, distillery, explosives, shellac, smokeless powder and shoe factory workers	Stomatitis
		Acrolein	Bone grinders, lard, soap, linoleum makers, varnish boilers	Stomatitis
		SO_2, NH_3, BR, Cl_2	Acetylene, dye, photographic film, phosgene makers, sugar refiners, refrigerating plant, disinfectant, laundry workers	Stomatitis
		CO, CO_2	Miners, smelters, gasoline motor workers	Coloration of lips (cherry red, blue)
Ray	Physico-chemical	Radium, x-ray	Technicians, watch dial painters, research men	Gingivitis, periodontitis, osteomyelitis and necrosis, xerostomia, osteosclerosis
		Actinic	Sailors, fishermen	Carcinoma of lip

eventually spread over the entire surface of the body, often involving the nasal and oral mucosae and conjunctivae. A bacterial, especially a staphylococcal, agent is suspected. Called also *dermatitis exfoliativa infantum* and *keratolysis neonatorum*. **Rivalta's d.,** actinomycosis. **Robinson's d.,** hidrocystoma. **Rougnon-Heberden d.,** ANGINA pectoris. **Rust's d.,** lesions of the atlanto-occipital region secondary to tuberculosis, syphilis, neoplasms, fractures, or rheumatism. Symptoms include suboccipital pain and swelling, drooping of the head, trigeminal neuralgia, hypoglossal paralysis, tongue atrophy, and vagus nerve paralysis with cardiac arrhythmia. Called also *malum rusti, malum suboccipitale, Rust's syndrome,* and *suboccipital vertebral d.* **salivary gland virus d.,** cytomegalic inclusion d. **San Joaquin d.,** coccidioidomycosis. **SC d.,** sickle cell–hemoglobin C d. **Schaumann's d.,** sarcoidosis. **Schenck's d.,** sporotrichosis. **Scheuermann's d.,** osteochrondrosis of the vertebral epiphyses in juveniles. It may be associated with multiple mucosal neuromas (see under NEUROMA). **Schönlein's d.,** purpura associated with articular symptoms; see Schönlein-Henoch SYNDROME. **serum d.,** serum SICKNESS. **sickle cell–hemoglobin C d.,** a condition in which both sickle cell hemoglobin and hemoglobin C are present. Symptoms are similar to those seen in sickle cell anemia, except for cardiac complications, but are milder. They include arthralgia, abdominal cramps, greenish-yellow sclerae, pale mucosae, weakness, hemorrhage, and oral manifestations. Anemia is sometimes more severe than in sickle cell anemia. Superinfection, especially with gram-negative bacteria complicated by osteomyelitis may occur. Bone marrow infarction and fat embolism are common. Called also *Hb SC d.* and *SC d.* **Spira's d.,** mottled ENAMEL. **storage d.,** a metabolic disorder in which some substance accumulates or is stored in certain cells in unusually large amounts; the stored substances may be lipids, proteins, carbohydrates, or other substances. See also THESAUROSIS. **suboccipital vertebral d.,** Rust's d. **Sutton's d.,** PERIADENITIS mucosa necrotica recurrens. **Swift's d.,** acrodynia. **Talma's d.,** MYOTONIA acquisita. **Tangier d.,** a hereditary disease, probably transmitted as an autosomal recessive trait, originally observed in inhabitants of Tangier Island in the Chesapeake Bay. It is characterized by severe deficiency or absence of α-lipoprotein (high-density lipoprotein [HDL]), hypocholesterolemia and enlarged liver, spleen, and lymph nodes. The principal oral manifestation is a characteristic orange-yellow coloration and enlargement of the tonsils. Called also *analphalipoproteinemia* and *familial HDL deficiency.* **Tay-Sachs d.,** a disease characterized by progressive mental deterioration, blindness, cherry-red spot in the retina, optic atrophy, and convulsions, occurring predominantly, although not exclusively, in children of Jewish ancestry, and having its onset shortly after birth; by the age of 3 to 4 years it is usually fatal. It is completely expressed in children homozygous for a mutant autosomal allele. Growth retardation, hyperacusis, listlessness, and weakness are the initial signs. Pathologically, there is an excess of gangliosides in the ganglion cells, also involving the gray and white matter, with consecutive proliferation and lipid loading of glial cells in the brain and extensive myelin degeneration. Called also *amaurotic familial idiocy* and *ganglioside lipidosis.* **terminal d.,** terminal ILLNESS. **thalassemia–hemoglobin C d.,** a condition, occurring chiefly in blacks, in which thalassemia is associated with the presence in the blood of hemoglobin C, attributed to the interaction of the hemoglobin C gene with the thalassemia gene. It is characterized chiefly by the presence in the blood of large, thin target cells and microcytes, erythroid hyperplasia of the bone marrow, and decreased osmotic fragility of the erythrocytes. Hb C represents about 75 to 80 percent of the total hemoglobin. Severe bone pain may occur. Called also *thalassemia C, C-thalassemia d.,* and *Zuelzer-Kaplan syndrome.* **C-thalassemia d.,** thalassemia–hemoglobin C d. **Thom-**

sen's d., MYOTONIA congenita. **Thornwaldt's (Tornwaldt's) d.,** Thornwaldt's (Tornwaldt's) BURSITIS. **Vaquez's d., Vaquez-Osler d.,** POLYCYTHEMIA vera. **venereal d.,** a contagious disease, acquired most commonly in sexual intercourse or other genital contact, including syphilis, gonorrhea, lymphogranuloma venereum, and chancroid. Abbreviated *VD.* **von Recklinghausen's d.,** Recklinghausen's d. (1,2). **von Zambusch's d.,** LICHEN sclerosus et atrophicus. **Waldenström's d.,** an acute form of thyrotoxicosis with muscular and cerebral complications, usually observed in elderly patients, and suspected of being due to iodine deficiency. The symptoms are varied and may include goiter, exophthalmos, and thyrotoxic crisis; severe vomiting, diarrhea, and weight loss; increased basal metabolism; slight fever in most instances and severe terminal hyperpyrexia in fatal cases; dyspnea; atrial fibrillation and low diastolic pressure; bulbar paralysis and paralysis of the sixth, seventh, and twelfth cranial nerves, with resultant deglutition disorders; psychotic behavior and hallucinations; lethargy and general asthenia or agitation and insomnia; coma; profuse perspiration; and apraxia, acalculia, dysarthria, choreiform movements, and amimia. Called also *acute thyrotoxic encephalopathy* and *spontaneous thyrotoxic crisis.* **Werdnig's d.,** infantile muscular ATROPHY. **wasting d.,** see WASTING. **Werlhof's d.,** thrombocytopenic purpura, idiopathic; see under PURPURA. **Wernicke's d.,** Wernicke's ENCEPHALOPATHY. **White's d.,** KERATOSIS follicularis. **white spot d.,** LICHEN sclerosus et atrophicus. **Wilson's d.,** hepatolenticular DEGENERATION. **Zahorsky's d.,** herpangina. **Zumbusch's d.,** LICHEN sclerosus et atrophicus.

dish (dish) a shallow vessel of glass or other material for laboratory work. **culture d.,** a shallow glass vessel for making microbial cultures. **dappen d.,** a small, heavy, solid glass, octagonal dish with a shallow depression to hold a few drops of medicaments or filling material. **evaporating d.,** a laboratory vessel, usually wide and shallow, in which material is evaporated by exposure to heat. **Petri d.,** a shallow glass receptacle for growing bacterial cultures.

disharmony (dis-har'mo-ne) lacking harmony; discordant. **occlusal d.,** a condition in which contacts of opposing occlusal surfaces of teeth are not in harmony with other tooth contacts, or occlusions do not coincide with their respective jaw relations. See MALOCCLUSION. Cf. occlusal HARMONY.

dish-face (dish'fās) see under FACE.

disilanyl (di-sil'ah-nil) a silicon hydride, Si_2H_5; see SILANES.

disinfectant (dis"in-fek'tant) 1. freeing from infection. 2. an agent, usually a chemical, capable of destroying within 10 minutes all vegetative bacteria, animal parasites, and all viruses except the hepatitis virus; spores are not destroyed. See also BACTERICIDE and bacteriostatic AGENT.

disinfection (dis"in-fek'shun) the act or process of destroying microbial life, but not resistant bacterial spores, through the use of heat or chemical agents. In dentistry, disinfection is commonly used on instruments, equipment, and supplies that are not used on living tissue. See also STERILIZATION. **boiling water d.,** disinfection by boiling of instruments, equipment, and supplies which do not penetrate into body tissue for at least 30 minutes (or 15 minutes after the water has again come to the boiling point). Cutting instruments are sterilized. **root canal d.,** root canal STERILIZATION.

disintegration (dis"in-te-gra'shun) [*dis-* + L. *integer* entire] the process of breaking up or decomposition. **d. constant,** decay CONSTANT. **radioactive d.,** radioactive DECAY.

disjunction (dis-junk'shun) the act or state of being disjoined. **craniofacial d.,** Le Fort III fracture: see Le Fort FRACTURE.

disk (disk) [L. *discus;* Gr. *diskos*] a circular or rounded flat plate. Called also *discus,* and spelled also *disc.* See also MENISCUS. A d., A BAND (2). **abrasive d.,** a thin, flat, oval, or concave circular plate with abrasive materials bonded to its surface and/or edge, either the inside (safe outside) or the outside (safe inside). A hole in the center is provided for the mandrel, the disk being held in place by a screw and a threaded end or a snap-on attachment. Abrasive disks are used with straight or contra-angled handpieces for low revolutions in polishing and finish-

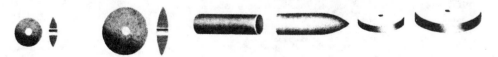

Assorted abrasive disks. (From H. O. Torres and A. Ehrlich: Modern Dental Assisting. 2nd ed. Philadelphia, W. B. Saunders Co., 1980; courtesy of S. S. White Div. of Pennwalt Corp.)

ing a cavity preparation and for cutting or polishing dental restorations. See illustration. See also grinding WHEEL. **Amici's d.,** Z BAND. **anisotropic d.,** A BAND (2). **articular d.,** interarticular d. **articular d. of sternoclavicular joint,** interarticular d. of sternoclavicular joint. **articular d. of temporomandibular joint,** interarticular d. of temporomandibular joint. **blastodermic d.,** the early embryonic disk formed during the blastocyst period of cleavage. **blood d.,** blood PLATELET. **carborundum d.,** a dental disk with carborundum as the abrading medium. **cloth d.,** rag WHEEL. **cutting d.,** a dental disk with abrasive material attached to its surfaces or edge, used for grinding or reducing teeth. **cuttlefish d.,** a dental disk having powdered cuttlefish bone bonded to its surfaces and edge. **Damascus d.,** trademark for a very thin and brittle abrasive dental disk of carbide for cutting metallic restorations and castings. Called also *Jo Dandy d.* **dental d.,** a disk with abrasive material bonded to its surface, used in dentistry for cutting, smoothing, or polishing; an abrasive disk. **diamond d.,** a steel dental disk with diamond chips bonded to its surface and/or edge. See also diamond rotary INSTRUMENT. **embryonic d.,** germinal d. **emery d.,** a steel dental disk with emery powder attached to its surfaces and/or edge. **Engelmann's d.,** H ZONE. **floppy d.,** a small, pliable magnetic disk. **garnet d.,** a steel dental disk with garnet particles bonded to its surfaces and/or edge. **Hensen's d.,** H ZONE. **I d.,** I BAND. **germinal d.,** a flattish area in the blastocyst in which the first traces of the embryo are seen. It forms during the second week of human development. **interarticular d.,** an oval, round, triangular, or sickle-shaped plate of interarticular fibrocartilage, found in certain synovial joints, including the temporomandibular, clavicular, wrist, knee, and sternoclavicular joints, which extends from a marginal attachment at the articular capsule and may completely divide the joint cavity into two separate compartments. It serves to fill in the space between the surfaces of articular cartilage and to increase the variety of movements of a joint. It is free on both surfaces, usually being thinner toward the center than at the circumference, and is held in position by a ligament. Called also *articular d., articular meniscus, discus articularis* [NA], and *meniscus articularis.* **interarticular d. of sternoclavicular joint,** a pad of interarticular fibrocartilage, the circumference of which is connected to the articular capsule of the sternoclavicular joint; it is attached superiorly to the clavicle and inferiorly to the first costal cartilage near its union with the sternum, and divides the joint into two compartments. Called also *articular d. of sternoclavicular joint, discus articularis articulationis sternoclavicularis* [NA], and *meniscus of sternoclavicular joint.* **interarticular d. of temporomandibular joint,** a thin, biconcave plate made of dense fibrous connective tissue interposed between the temporal bone and mandible, which divides the articular space into upper and lower compartments. Its superior concavoconvex surface accommodates itself to the form of the mandibular fossa and the articular tubercle, and its concave inferior surface accommodates itself to the condyle. It attaches to the articular capsule by a connective tissue structure, the bilaminar area, the upper stratum of which attaches to the temporal bone, while the lower stratum attaches to the condyle. The retroarticular cushion, a loose vascular areolar connective tissue, attaches the posterior segment, and the upper part of the disk, being loosely attached to the capsule, allows the gliding movement, while limiting attachment of the lower part allows the hinge movement. Called also *articular d. of temporomandibular joint, discus articularis articulationis temporomandibularis* [NA], *discus articulationis mandibularis, interarticular fibrocartilage of temporomandibular joint,* and *meniscus of temporomandibular joint.* **intermediate d.,** Z BAND. **isotropic d.,** I BAND. **J d.,** I BAND. **Jo Dandy d.,** Damascus d. **M d.,** M BAND. **magnetic d.,** in computer technology, a flat, circular, metal plate that has magnetized surfaces on which data can be stored. **d. mandrel,** disk MANDREL. **Merkel's d's,** see Merkel's corpuscles; see under CORPUSCLE. **polishing d.,** a dental disk with a very fine abrasive material, used for finishing and polishing of surfaces. **Q d.,** A BAND (2). **safe-side d.,** a dental disk having the abrading material bonded to only one side, for the protection of healthy teeth during the cutting, smoothing, or polishing of proximal teeth. **sandpaper d.,** an abrasive disk with pulverized silica as the abrading medium. **separating d.,** a dental disk made of steel or hard rubber. **thin d.,** Z BAND. **transverse d.,** A BAND (2). **Z d.,** Z BAND.

dislocatio (dis″lo-ka′she-o) [L.] dislocation.

dislocation (dis″lo-ka′shun) [*dis-* + L. *locare* to place] 1. the displacement of a part, especially a bone. Called also *luxation.* 2. a plastic deformation in the space lattice of a crystalline structure associated with a slip of atom planes, forming a line about which there is a discontinuity of the lattice structure.

Most dislocations are combinations of edge and screw types. Called also *line defect.* **complete d.,** one in which there is displacement of an articulating surface of a joint from its intended opposing surface. **complicated d.,** one which is associated with another important injury. **compound d.,** one in which the joint communicates with the external air. Called also *open d.* **congenital d.,** one which exists from or before birth. **consecutive d.,** one in which the luxated bone has changed its position since its first displacement. **edge d.,** dislocation in which the unit slip is always perpendicular to the dislocation line in a crystalline structure. **fracture d.,** one complicated by fracture of, or adjacent to, a joint. **habitual d.,** one which often recurs. **d. line,** dislocation LINE. **mandibular d.,** non–self-reducing dislocation of the condyle from the glenoid fossa. See *temporomandibular joint d.* **open d.,** compound d. **partial d.,** subluxation. **pathologic d.,** one which results from paralysis, synovitis, infection, or other disease. **primitive d.,** one in which the bones remain as originally displaced. **recent d.,** one in which there is no complicating inflammation. **recurrent temporomandibular joint d.,** temporomandibular joint d., recurrent. **screw d.,** one in which the unit slip is always parallel to the dislocation line in a crystalline structure. **simple d.,** one in which the joint is not penetrated by a wound. **temporomandibular joint d.,** displacement of the condyle in the glenoid fossa into a position anterior to the articular tuberculum of the temporomandibular joint, where it is held by sustained muscle spasm. The disorder may occur as a result of extrinsic injury, but it is usually due to muscle tonus disorders, being frequently triggered by the jaw-jerk reflex when the muscles are relaxed, as during sleep. It occurs most commonly among young women as a bilateral dislocation. Sprain of the joint is a common complication. Called also *mandibular d.* See also temporomandibular joint SUBLUXATION. **temporomandibular joint d., recurrent,** temporomandibular joint dislocation that recurs at frequent intervals. Called also *habitual temporomandibular joint luxation.* **traumatic d.,** one due to an injury or to violence.

dislodgment (dis-loj′ment) to remove, displace, or drive something from a particular place, as in displacing a dental prosthesis from its proper position.

disocclude (dis″o-klood′) loss of contact between opposing teeth as a result of tooth guidance, occlusal interferences, or occlusal adjustment.

disodium (di-so′de-um) having two atoms of sodium in each molecule. **d. aurothiomalate,** GOLD sodium thiomalate. **d. edetate,** EDETATE disodium. **d. cromoglycate,** CROMOLYN sodium.

Disomer trademark for *dexbrompheniramine maleate* (see under DEXBROMPHENIRAMINE).

disopyramide (di″so-per′ah-mīd) an antiarrhythmic cardiac depressant, α-[2-[bis(1-methylethyl)aminoethyl]-α-phenyl-2-pyridineacetamide. Trademarks: Ritmodan, Rythmodan.

disorder (dis-or′der) a derangement or abnormality of function; a morbid condition.

disorganization (dis-or″gan-i-za′shun) the process of destruction of any organic tissue; any profound change in the tissues of an organ or structure which causes the loss of most or all of its proper character.

Disotate trademark for *edetate disodium* (see under EDETATE).

dispar (dis′par) [L.] unequal.

disparate (dis′pah-rāt) [L. *disparatus, dispar* unequal] not situated alike; not exactly paired; dissimilar in kind.

dispensary (dis-pen′sah-re) [L. *dispensarium,* from *dispensare* to dispense] 1. traditionally, an outpatient clinic offering the services of a general practitioner for ambulatory consultation, with the assistance of a pharmacist (or dispenser) to provide elementary and standard medicines according to the physician's prescription. 2. an outpatient institution which may or may not be attached to a hospital, sometimes dealing with specific disease groups or age or social categories. Dispensaries of this type are characteristic of the health services of some countries, particularly the Soviet Union.

dispensatory (dis-pen′sah-to-re) [L. *dispensatorium*] a treatise on the qualities and composition of medicines. **D. of the United States of America,** a collection of monographs on unofficial drugs and drugs recognized by the United States Pharmacopoeia, the British Pharmacopoeia, and the National Formulary, and on general tests, processes, reagents, and solutions of the USP and NF as well as drugs used in veterinary medicine.

dispense (dis-pens′) [L. *dispensare,* from *dis* out + *pensare* to weigh] 1. to deal out in portions. 2. to prepare and distribute medicines to those who are to use them.

dispenser (dis-pen′ser) 1. one who or that which dispenses. 2. a container or mechanical device that delivers a controlled portion or unit. **mercury d.,** a device for delivering a controlled weight of mercury; used in mixing dental amalgam.

Dispersalloy·trademark for an *amalgam alloy* (see under AMALGAM).

dispersate (dis′per-sāt) a suspension of finely divided particles.

disperse (dis-pers′) [*dis*-(1) + L. *spargere* to scatter] to scatter components apart, as of a tumor or the fine particles in a colloid system; also the particles so dispersed.

dispersion (dis-per′shun) [L. *dispersio*] 1. the act of scattering or separating; the condition of being scattered. 2. the incorporation of the particles of one substance into the body of another, comprising solutions, suspensions, and colloids. See also disperse PHASE. 3. a colloid solution; see COLLOID (2). **d. alloy,** dispersion ALLOY. **colloid d.,** a colloid solution; see COLLOID (2).

dispersoid (dis-per′soid) a colloid in which the dispersity is relatively greater.

displaceability (dis-plās″ah-bil′ĭ-te) the quality of being susceptible to movement from an initial position, or the degree to which such movement is possible. **tissue d.,** the quality of tissue, particularly oral tissues, of being susceptible to displacement from its resting position, or the degree to which tissue displacement is possible.

displacement (dis-plās′ment) 1. removal from the normal position or place; ectopia. 2. the malposition of the crown and root of one or more teeth from the normal line of occlusion; also, the deflection of the mandible from its normal path of closure, i.e., posterior displacement. **condylar d.,** an abnormal position of the head of the condyle in the glenoid fossa due to a deviation or shift of the mandible, which is often the result of malocclusion.

display (dis-pla′) 1. to show, make visible, or exhibit. 2. in computer technology, a visible representation of data on a cathode ray tube screen, in a printed form, graph, or drawing.

Dispos-A-Cap trademark for proportioned amalgam alloy (see under AMALGAM) in disposable capsules, containing 49.60 to 50.40 percent mercury.

disposition (dis″po-zish′un) 1. a natural inclination. 2. a natural tendency, either physical or mental, toward a certain disease. 3. a distribution; an apportionment; an arrangement.

Dispril trademark for CALCIUM acetylsalicylate.

Disprin trademark for CALCIUM acetylsalicylate.

disproportion (dis″pro-por′shun) a lack of the proper relationship between two elements or factors.

disruption (dis-rup′shun) the act of separating forcibly, or the state of being abnormally separated.

dissect (dĭ-sekt′, di-sekt′) [L. *dissecare* to cut up] 1. to divide by cutting; to cut in pieces. 2. to separate and expose the various parts and structures of a cadaver in such a way that their characteristics and relations may be studied.

dissection (di-sek′shun) [L. *dissectio*] 1. the act of cutting apart, especially in tracing out and disclosing the individual tissues, parts, and organs of a cadaver for anatomical study. 2. the separation of tissues, especially in surgical procedures. **blunt d.,** separation of tissues along natural lines of cleavage, by means of a blunt instrument or finger. **neck d.,** the removal of the lymph nodes and contiguous tissues in the neck along the line of lymphatic drainage as treatment for malignant neoplasms that have involved the regional cervical lymphatic system, stemming from a primary malignant site in the mandibular and/or maxillofacial area. **sharp d.,** separation of tissues by means of the sharp edge of a knife or scalpel, or with scissors.

dissector (di-sek′tor) 1. one who dissects. 2. a handbook used as a guide for the act of dissecting.

disseminated (dis-sem′ĭ-nāt″ed) [*dis*-(1) + L. *seminare* to sow] scattered; distributed over a considerable area.

dissociation (dis-so″she-a′shun) [*dis*-(1) + L. *sociatio* union] 1. the act of separating or state of being separated. 2. the breaking up of chemical combinations into simpler constituents. The process may be the result of either added energy, as of gaseous molecules being dissociated by heat, or the effect of a solvent on a dissolved substance. All electrolytes dissociate in polar solutions.

dissolution (dis″so-lu′shun) [L. *dissolutio, dissolvere* to dissolve] 1. separation of a compound into its elements. 2. liquefaction. 3. the process of loosening, or of relaxing.

dissolve (diz-zolv′) 1. to bring to an end; terminate. 2. to cause a substance to pass into solution. 3. to pass into solution.

Dist. abbreviation for L. *distil′la,* distil.

distad (dis′tad) in a distal direction.

distal (dis′tal) [L. *distans* distant] farthest from any point of reference, as the surfaces of teeth more distant from the median line. Cf. PROXIMAL.

distalis (dis-ta′lis) [L.] distal; an anatomical term denoting remoteness from the point of origin or attachment of an organ or part.

distance (dis′tans) the measure of separation between two objects or points of reference. See also MEASUREMENT. **anode-film d.,** target-film d. **cone d.,** that measured along the central beam from the distal end of the cone to the surface of the radiographed object. Called also *cone-surface d.* **cone d., long,** that from the distal end of the long cone (usually 10–25 cm or more) to the surface of the radiographed object. See also long CONE. **cone d., short,** that from the distal end of the short cone (usually under 10–25 cm) to the surface of the radiographed object. See also short CONE. **cone-surface d.,** cone d. **diaphragm-surface d.,** that measured along the central beam from the distal end of the collimating diaphragm to the surface of the irradiated object. **focal-film d.,** target-film d. **interarch d.,** 1. the vertical distance between the maxillary and mandibular arches (alveolar or residual) under certain conditions of vertical dimension that must be specified. 2. the vertical distance between the maxillary and mandibular ridges. Called also *interridge d.* **interatomic d.,** that between individual atoms in a molecule or any other structure, the equilibrium interatomic distance being the distance at which the force of attraction between the atoms is equal to the force which tends to repel them. See also space LATTICE. **intercondylar d.,** that between the rotational centers of each condyle. **interocclusal d.,** that between the occlusal surfaces of the maxillary and mandibular teeth when the mandible is in its physiological rest position. The width of the space varies with the type of occlusion and with the tonus of the masticatory muscles, but it is commonly found in the anterior part of the mouth to be 1 to 3 mm, and it may be as much as 8 to 10 mm in the absence of occlusal disorders. Called also *freeway space, interocclusal clearance, gap* or *space,* and *interocclusal rest space.* **interridge d.,** interarch d. (2). **object-film d.,** that between the object being radiographed and the film, measured along the central ray, unless otherwise specified. **source-collimator d.,** that measured along the central beam from the front surface of the source to the distal end of the collimating diaphragm. **source-cone d.,** that measured along the central beam from the front surface of the source of radiation to the distal end of the cone. **source-film d.,** that measured along the central beam from the front surface of the focal spot in the tube to the surface of the film on which a radiographic exposure is being made. **source-surface d.,** that measured along the central beam from the front surface of the focal spot in the tube to the surface of the irradiated object. Abbreviated SSD. Called also *target-skin d.* **target-film d.,** that measured along the central beam from the focal spot in the tube to the film. Called also *anode-film d.* and *focal-film d.* **target-skin d.,** source-surface d.

distensibility (dis-ten″sĭ-bil′ĭ-te) capability of being distended.

distention (dis-ten′shun) [L. *distentio* stretching] the act or process of stretching out or enlarging; the state of being enlarged or distended.

distichiasis (dis″tĭ-ki′ah-sis) [Gr. *distichia* a double line] the presence of a double row of eyelashes on an eyelid, one or both of which are turned in against the eyeball.

distillate (dis′til-lāt) material that has been obtained by distillation.

distillation (dis″til-la′shun) the process of purification of liquids by first evaporating and then cooling the gas to condense it back to a liquid, thereby removing nonvolatile substances. **destructive d., dry d.,** decomposition of a solid by heating in the absence of air, which results in volatile liquid products. **fractional d.,** that attended by a successive separation of volatilizable substances in order of their respective volatility. **molecular d.,** a process of purification applied to drugs and pharmaceuticals, during which the crude material is evaporated under high vacuum of about one-millionth of an atmosphere, and the condensate is caught on a cooled surface held close in front of the evaporating layer. The process is applied to vitamins A, D, and E, to animal and vegetable sterols and hormones, and to drugs and intermediates. **vacuum d.,** distillation under reduced pressure to avoid the decomposition which might occur at atmospheric pressure.

disto- [L. *distans* distal, remote] a combining form denoting relationship to a distal or remote site.

distoaxiogingival (dis″to-ak″se-o-jin′jĭ-val) pertaining to the angle formed by the axial and gingival walls of a cavity preparation on the distal aspect of a tooth. Called also *axiodistocervical* and *axiodistogingival.*

distoaxioincisal (dis″to-ak″se-o-in-si′zal) pertaining to or formed by the distal, axial, and incisal walls of a tooth cavity preparation. Called also *axiodistoincisal*.

distoaxio-occlusal (dis″to-ak″se-o-o-kloo′zal) pertaining to or formed by the distal, axial, and occlusal walls of a tooth cavity preparation. Called also *axiodisto-occlusal*.

distobuccal (dis″to-buk′al) [*disto-* + *buccal*] pertaining to or formed by the distal and buccal surfaces of a tooth, or the distal and buccal walls of a cavity preparation in a tooth. Called also *buccodistal*. See illustration at tooth ANGLE.

distobucco-occlusal (dis″to-buk″o-o-kloo′zal) pertaining to or formed by the distal, buccal, and occlusal surfaces of a tooth. See illustration at tooth ANGLE.

distobuccopulpal (dis″to-buk″o-pul′pal) pertaining to or formed by the distal, buccal, and pulpal walls of a cavity preparation in a tooth.

distocervical (dis″to-ser′vǐ-kal) 1. pertaining to the distal surface of the neck of a tooth. 2. distogingival.

distoclination (dis″tok-lǐ-na′shun) deviation of a tooth from the vertical, in the direction of the tooth next distal (posterior) to it in the dental arch.

distoclusal (dis″to-kloo′zal) disto-occlusal.

distoclusion (dis″to-kloo-zhun) malocclusion in which the mandibular arch is in a posterior (distal) position in relation to the maxillary arch. Generally considered as identical with Class II in Angle's classification of malocclusion (see MALOCCLUSION). Called also *disto-occlusion, posterior occlusion, posteroclusion,* and *retrusive occlusion*.

distogingival (dis″to-jin′jǐ-val) [*disto-* + *gingival*] pertaining to or formed by the distal and gingival walls of a tooth cavity preparation. Called also *distocervical*.

distolabial (dis″to-la′be-al) [*disto-* + *labial*] pertaining to or formed by the distal and labial surfaces of a tooth, or the distal and labial walls of a cavity preparation in a tooth. See illustration at tooth ANGLE.

distolabioincisal (dis″to-la″be-o-in-si′zal) pertaining to or formed by the distal, labial, and incisal surfaces of a tooth. See illustration at tooth ANGLE.

distolingual (dis″to-ling′gwal) pertaining to or formed by the lingual and distal surfaces of a tooth, or the lingual and distal walls of a tooth cavity preparation. Called also *linguodistal (LD)*. See illustration at tooth ANGLE.

distolinguoincisal (dis″to-ling″gwo-in-si′zal) pertaining to or formed by the distal, lingual, and incisal surfaces of a tooth. See illustration at tooth ANGLE.

distolinguo-occlusal (dis″to-ling″gwo-o-kloo′zal) pertaining to or formed by the distal, lingual, and occlusal surfaces of a tooth. See illustration at tooth ANGLE.

distolinguopulpal (dis″to-ling″gwo-pul′pal) pertaining to or formed by the distal, lingual, and pulpal walls of a cavity preparation in a tooth.

distomolar (dis″to-mo′lar) a supernumerary molar distal to the third molar. Called also *fourth molar* and *retromolar*.

disto-occlusal (dis″to-o-kloo′zal) pertaining to or formed by the distal and occlusal surfaces of a tooth, or the distal and occlusal walls of a cavity preparation in a tooth. See illustration at tooth ANGLE. Called also *distoclusal*.

disto-occlusion (dis″to-o-kloo′zhun) distoclusion.

distoplacement (dis-to-plās′ment) displacement of a tooth distally.

distopulpal (dis″to-pul′pal) pertaining to or formed by the distal and pulpal walls of a cavity preparation in a tooth.

distopulpolabial (dis″to-pul″po-la′be-al) pertaining to or formed by the distal, pulpal, and labial walls of a cavity preparation in a tooth.

distopulpolingual (dis″to-pul″po-ling′gwal) pertaining to or formed by the distal, pulpal, and lingual walls of a cavity preparation in a tooth.

distortion (dis-tor′shun) [L. *dis* apart + *torsio* a twisting] 1. the state or act of twisting out of a natural or normal shape or position. 2. deviation of a radiographic image from the true outline or shape of an object or structure. **horizontal d.,** disproportional change in size and shape in the horizontal plane of a radiograph, due to oblique horizontal angulation. **magnification d.,** proportional enlargement of a radiographic image that may be minimized with increased source-film distance or decreased object-film distance. **vertical d.,** disproportional change in size, either elongation or foreshortening, of a radiographic image, due to incorrect vertical angulation or improper film placement.

distoversion (dis″to-ver′zhun) the position of a tooth which is farther than normal from the median line of the face along the dental arch.

distraction (dǐ-strak′shun) [L. *dis* apart + *tractio* a drawing] 1. a state in which the attention is diverted from the main portion of an experience. 2. the drawing apart. 3. a form of dislocation in which the joint surfaces have been separated without rupture of their binding ligaments and without displacement. 4. excessive space between fracture fragments due to interposed tissue or too forceful traction. 5. unusual width of the dental arch; placement of the teeth or other maxillary or mandibular structures further than normal from the median plane. See also CONTRACTION.

distress (dǐ-stres′) [L. *distringere* to draw apart] physical or mental anguish or suffering.

distribution (dis″trǐ-bu′shun) [L. *distributio*] 1. the specific location or arrangement of continuing or successive objects or events in space or time. 2. the branching, as of an artery. 3. the geographical range of an organism or disease. 4. in statistics, a set of numbers representing instances of a variable arranged according to their value. **age d.,** distribution of population by age groups, usually surveyed in 5- or 10-year intervals, frequently expressed as a percentage distribution of the entire population. Most often used in describing the make-up or composition of an insured group. **dose d.,** in radiology, a representation of the variation of dose with position in any region of an irradiated object.

disturbance (dis-tur′bans) a disruption of a normal condition or order of things; a disorder. **occlusal d.,** a faulty occlusion, or derangements in the patterns of occlusion. See MALOCCLUSION.

disulfide (di-sul′fīd) a compound containing two sulfides. Called also *bisulfide*.

disulfiram (di-sul′fǐ-ram) a compound, bis-(diethylthiocarbamyl)-disulfide, occurring as a white, odorless, crystalline powder that is soluble in ethanol, ether, acetone, benzene, chloroform, carbon disulfide and slightly in water. It blocks the oxidation of alcohol at the acetaldehyde stage, causing it to accumulate in the body with resulting flushing, palpitation, dyspnea, hyperventilation, increased pulse rate, nausea, vomiting, cyanosis, drowsiness, and hypotension. Excessive use may produce collapse. Used in the treatment of alcoholism by producing aversion to alcoholic beverages. Called also *tetraethylthiuram disulfide*. Trademarks: Absentil, Alcophobin, Antabuse, Etabus, Ethyl Thiurad, Noxal.

Disyncran trademark for *methdilazine*.

ditch (dich) 1. a long narrow excavation. 2. ditching.

ditching (dich′ing) 1. the formation of a long and narrow excavation or trench. 2. amalgam failure in a dental restoration in which marginal areas have become chipped and frayed. 3. undesirable loss of tooth substance in the region of a restorative margin.

ditin diphosphate, ditin pyrophosphate (di′tin) stannous PYROPHOSPHATE.

Dittrich's plug [Franz *Dittrich*, German pathologist, 1815–1859] see under PLUG.

Diucardin trademark for *hydroflumethiazide*.

Diucardyn trademark for *mercaptomerin sodium* (see under MERCAPTOMERIN).

Diural trademark for *furosemide*.

Diureone trademark for *chlormerodrin*.

Diuresal trademark for *chlorothiazide*.

diuresis (di″u-re′sis), pl. *diure′ses* [Gr. *diourein* to urinate] secretion of urine.

diuretic (di″u-ret′ik) 1. increasing the secretion of urine. 2. an agent or substance that increases the volume of urine excreted by the kidneys. Diuretics act by either increasing the glomerular filtration rate or by decreasing the rate of reabsorption of fluids from the renal tubules. Diuretics are also believed to have extrarenal sites of action, and are classified as those that increase glomerular filtration, those that increase the tubular osmotic load, and those that inhibit the secretion of antidiuretic hormone. They are used to reduce the amount of fluid in the body in the treatment of ascites, edema, and hypertension. **aldosterone inhibitor d.,** any substance that competes with aldosterone for receptor sites in the tubular epithelial cells and blocks the sodium reabsorption action of aldosterone, the sodium remaining in the tubules acting as an osmotic diuretic. Spironolactone is the principal aldosterone inhibitor. **antidiuretic hormone inhibitor d.,** any substance the inhibits the secretion of antidiuretic hormone. When large amounts of water are ingested, the body fluids become diluted and the antidiuretic hormone is no longer secreted by the pituitary system. **benzothiazine d.,** any of the diuretic analogues of 1,2,4-ben-zothiadiazine-1,1-dioxide, which block sodium reabsorption in the proximal renal tubules, resulting in sodium diuresis, and also acting as carbonic anhydrase inhibitors. Side effects may include azotemia, anorexia, gastric irritation, nausea, vomiting, stomach cramps, diarrhea, jaundice, pancreatitis, vertigo, paresthesia, headache, leukopenia, agranulocytosis, thrombocytopenia, aplastic anemia, orthostatic hypotension, hypersensitivity, anaphylaxis, hyperglycemia, glycosuria, muscle spasms, weakness, visual disorders, hematuria, hyponatremia, hypokalemia, hypochloremic alkalosis, and sialadenitis. Called also *thiazide d.* **carbonic anhydrase d.,** a substance which inhibits in the renal tubules the action of carbonic anhydrase (carbonate dehydratase), thus decreasing the amount of hydrogen ion for exchange with sodium; the excess of sodium ions in the tubules combine with carbonates and are excreted by the kidneys with an increased volume of water. **high-ceiling d.,** one that acts at a peak diuresis, also being characterized by a prompt onset of action, inhibition of sodium and chloride transport in the ascending limb of the loop of Henle, and independence of action from acid-base balance. Used chiefly in the treatment of edema of hepatic, cardiac, and renal origin. Fluid electrolyte balance disorders, hyperuricemia, precipitation of attacks of gout, gastrointestinal, hepatic, and hearing disorders, anemia, skin rash, paresthesias, and allergic reactions are the side reactions. Called also *loop d.* **loop d.,** high-ceiling d. **mercurial d.,** any mercury derivative that depresses the tubular reabsorption of sodium and fixed anion, chiefly chloride, water excretion occurring secondarily to the decrease of electrolyte reabsorption. Excessive dehydration, hyponatremia, hypokalemia, hypochloremia, blood dyscrasias, flushing of the face, fever, chills, gastrointestinal disorders, skin eruptions, pruritus, urticaria, weakness, somnolence, muscle pain, and symptoms of mercury poisoning are potential side reactions. Oral complications may include acute stomatitis and other orodental symptoms of mercurialism. **osmotic d.,** any of various electrolytes and nonelectrolytes that through their action on the osmotic pressure inhibit water reabsorption in the renal tubules, thus causing large amounts of tubular fluid to be flushed out into the urine. Used chiefly to reduce cerebrospinal and intraocular pressures, to prevent renal failure, and to treat various edematous diseases. Osmotic diuretics are freely filterable at the glomerulus, undergo limited reabsorption by the renal tubules, and are pharmacologically inert; they include urea, mannitol, sucrose, and sodium and potassium salts. Toxicity is related to the load of solute administered. **potassium-sparing d.,** one that increases the volume of urine excreted by the kidneys, without also promoting the excretion of potassium. **thiazide d.,** benzothiazine d.

Diuril trademark for *chlorothiazide.*

diurnal (di-er′nal) [L. *dies* day] 1. occurring during the daytime. Applied especially to the activities of living organisms that occur during the daylight hours. 2. daily; having a daily cycle (as a *diurnal rhythm*). The terms *diurnal* and *circadian,* which applies to the regular recurrence of activities in cycles of approximately 24 hours, are often used interchangeably.

divalent (di-va′lent) [Gr. *dis* twice + L. *valere* powerful] 1. bivalent. 2. carrying an electronic charge of two units.

Divercillin trademark for *ampicillin.*

divergence (di-ver′jens) a spreading or tending apart.

diverticula (di″ver-tik′u-lah) [L.] plural of *diverticulum.*

diverticulum (di″ver-tik′u-lum), pl. *divertic′ula* [L. *divertere* to turn aside] a hollow sac or pouch occurring normally or produced by herniation through the wall of a tubular organ. **Heister's d.,** superior bulb of jugular vein; see under BULB. **laryngeal d.,** a diverticulum of the laryngeal mucous membrane. **Meckel's d.,** an occasional sacculation or appendage of the ileum, derived from an unobliterated yolk stalk. **Pertik's d.,** an unusually deep recessus pharyngeus. **pharyngoesophageal d.,** a diverticulum at the junction of the pharynx and esophagus. Called also *Zenker's d.* **salivary d.,** a diverticulum of a salivary duct, usually occurring as a congenital abnormality. **thyroid d.,** an outpouching of the ventral floor of the embryonic pharynx that becomes the thyroid gland. **Zenker's d.,** pharyngoesophageal d.

divider (di-vi′der) one who or that which divides or separates into parts, groups, or sections. **stress d.,** stress-breaker.

Divinelle, W. A. [19th century dentist] a pioneer in the development of bridgework techniques, including the development of coping in denture retention.

divinylenimine (di-vi″ni-len′ĭ-mĭd) pyrrole.

division (di-vizh′un) [L. *divisio*] 1. the act or process of separating or sectioning into two or more parts. 2. a section or part of a larger structure. **cell d.,** see MEIOSIS and MITOSIS. **first meiotic d.,** see MEIOSIS. **mandibular d. of trigeminal nerve,** mandibular NERVE. **maxillary d. of trigeminal nerve,** maxillary NERVE. **meiotic d.,** meiosis. **mitotic d.,** mitosis. **ophthalmic d. of trigeminal nerve,** ophthalmic NERVE. **second meiotic d.,** see MEIOSIS.

Dixarit trademark for *clonidine hydrochloride* (see under CLONIDINE).

dizziness (diz′ĭ-nes) a sensation of unsteadiness associated with a whirling sensation in the head. When associated with a loss of equilibrium, the condition is called *vertigo.*

dk deka-.

DL- a chemical prefix denoting that the substance is an equimolecular mixture of the dextrorotatory and levorotatory enantiomorphs, such as is produced by chemical synthesis without resolution or by the process of racemization. Also written ±.

DLC Dental Laboratory Conference (see under CONFERENCE).

DLG distolingual GROOVE.

DMD Doctor of Dental Medicine (see under DOCTOR).

DMF see DMF RATE.

Dn dekanem.

dn decinem.

DNA deoxyribonucleic acid; a nucleic acid that serves to store and transfer genetic information. It is a macromolecule consisting of two long polynucleotide chains running in opposite directions and twisted into a double helix *(Watson-Crick helix),* regularly spaced hydrogen bonds holding the two chains together. Deoxyribonucleotides, the monomeric units of DNA, are composed of a sugar (deoxyribose), a nitrogenous heterocyclic base (purine or pyrimidine), and a phosphate. The backbone of the nucleotide is provided by alternating sugars and phosphates, with each sugar-phosphate unit representing one nucleotide. There are four different bases, hence four different types of nucleotides — those containing adenine being equal to the number containing thymidine and the number containing guanine being equal to the number containing cytosine. The sequence of four nitrogenous bases forms the genetic code, each three-base sequence forms one triplet that is specific for an amino acid, and a sequence of triplets contains the code for one polypeptide. A DNA-histone complex forms the basic fiber of the chromosome. DNA reproduces itself through the process of replication and produces RNA through transcription, which, in turn, produces proteins through the process of translation. Called also *deoxypentosenucleic acid, deoxyribose nucleic acid,* and *desoxyribonucleic acid.* See also REPLICATION and RNA, and see illustration. **DNA nucleotidyltransferase,** DNA NUCLEOTIDYLTRANSFERASE. **DNA polymerase,** DNA NUCLEOTIDYLTRANSFERASE. **DNA virus,** see under VIRUS.

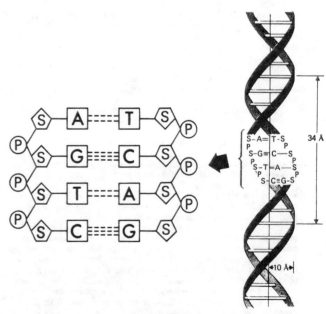

Double helix of DNA. Here P means phosphate diester, S means deoxyribose, A=T is the adenine-thymine pairing, and G≡C is the guanine-cytosine pairing. (After Conn and Stumpf: Outlines of Biochemistry. 2nd Ed. New York, Wiley, 1963.)

DNB Diplomate of the National Board (of Medical Examiners).

DO 1. Doctor of Osteopathy (see OSTEOPATH). 2. Doctor of Optometry (see OPTOMETRIST). 3. distal and occlusal.

Dobendan trademark for *cetylpyridinium chloride* (see under CETYLPYRIDINIUM).

doctor (dok′tor) [L. "teacher," from *docere* to teach] a holder of a diploma of the highest degree from a university; often used to refer to the practitioners of the healing arts, who have received degrees from schools of medicine, osteopathy, dentistry, or veterinary medicine, and are licensed to practice. The degree was created in the 12th century by the Holy Roman Emperor and German king Lothair II, and was awarded by the University of Bologna to Irnerius, a professor of law. The first doctor of medicine degree was conferred in 1329 by the College of Asti. In the United States, the first doctor of dentistry degree was conferred by the Baltimore College of Dental Surgery in 1842. Abbreviated *DR* or *Dr.* See also PHYSICIAN and PRACTITIONER. **D. of Chiropractic (DC)**, a person who has received a degree from an approved school of chiropractic. See CHIROPRACTOR. **D. of Dental Surgery (DDS)**, a degree established at the Baltimore College of Dental Surgery and conferred on graduates of dental schools in the United States since 1842. See DENTIST. **D. of Dental Medicine (DMD)**, a degree established by the founders of the Harvard Dental School in 1869 and conferred on graduates of the Harvard Dental School· and other schools of dentistry in the United States. See DENTIST. **D. of Medicine (MD)**, a degree conferred in the United States on graduates of medical schools. **D. of Naturopathy (ND)**, a person who has received a degree from an approved school of naturopathy. See NATUROPATH. **D. of Optometry (DO)**, a graduate of an approval school of optometry. See OPTOMETRIST. **D. of Osteopathy (DO)**, a person who has received a degree from a school of osteopathy. See OSTEOPATH.

doctrine (dok′trin) a theory supported by authorities and having general acceptance.

Dogiel's corpuscle see under CORPUSCLE.

Döhle's body [Paul *Döhle*, German pathologist, 1855–1928] see under BODY.

Doisy, Edward Adelbert [born 1893] an American biochemist; co-winner with Carl Peter Henrik Dam, of the Nobel prize for medicine and physiology in 1945, for the isolation and synthesis of vitamin K. See also Thayer-Doisy UNIT.

dol (dōl) [L. *dolor* pain] a unit of pain intensity.

Dolantin trademark for *meperidine hydrochloride* (see under MEPERIDINE).

Dolder bar joint attachment (bar, bar joint), bar unit attachment (bar unit) [E. J. *Dolder*] see under ATTACHMENT.

Dolenal trademark for *meperidine hydrochloride* (see under MEPERIDINE).

Dolene trademark for *propoxyphene hydrochloride* (see under PROPOXYPHENE).

dolicho- [Gr. *dolichos* long] a combining form meaning long.

dolichocephalia (dol″ĭ-ko-sĕ-fa′le-ah) dolichocephaly.

dolichocephalic, dolichocephalous (dol″ĭ-ko-sĕ-fal′ik; dol″ĭ-ko-sef′ah-lus) [*dolicho-* + Gr. *kephalē* head] characterized by or having a long narrow head. Called also *mecocephalic*. See dolichocephalic SKULL and LEPTOCEPHALY.

dolichocephalism (dol″ĭ-ko-sef′ah-lizm) dolichocephaly.

dolichocephaly (dol″ĭ-ko-sef′ah-le) a condition characterized by a long narrow head. Called also *dolichocephalia* and *dolichocephalism*. See dolichocephalic SKULL and LEPTOCEPHALY.

dolichocheilia (dol″ĭ-ko-ki′le-ah) [*dolicho-* + Gr. *cheilos* lip + *-ia*] a condition characterized by an abnormal length of the oral fissure. Cf. BRACHYCHEILIA.

dolichocranial (dol″ĭ-ko-kra′ne-al) [*dolicho-* + *cranium*] pertaining to or characterized by a long narrow cranium. See dolichocephalic SKULL.

dolichofacial (dol″ĭ-ko-fa′shal) having a long face.

dolichostenomelia (dol″ĭ-ko-ste″no-me′le-ah) [*dolicho-* + Gr. *stenos* narrow + *melos* limb + *-ia*] excessive slenderness of the extremities. See Marfan's SYNDROME.

Dolipol trademark for *tolbutamide*.

Dolophine trademark for the *dl*-form of *methadone hydrochloride* (see under METHADONE).

dolor (do′lor), pl. *dolo′res* [L.] pain. **d. cap′itis**, headache. **d. va′gus**, wandering PAIN.

dolores (do-lo′rēz) [L.] plural of *dolor*.

dolorific (do″lor-if′ik) producing or causing pain.

dolorimetry (do″lor-im′ĕ-tre) [L. *dolor* pain + Gr. *metrein* to measure] the measurement of pain.

dolorogen (do-lor″o-jen) a substance or agent which causes pain.

Doloxene trademark for *propoxyphene napsylate* (see under PROPOXYPHENE).

Dolvanol trademark for *meperidine hydrochloride* (see under MEPERIDINE).

Domain trademark for *sulfisomidine*.

domain (do-mān′) 1. a region having specific characteristics, as an immunobuin domain. 2. in physics, a connected region with uniform polarization in a twinned ferroelectric crystal. 3. in mathematics, a set of values assigned to the independent variables of a function. C_H **d.**, C_L **d.**, see *constant d.* **constant d.**, the C-terminal domain of the light chains (C_L) or the three or four domains of the C-terminal end of heavy chains (C_H) of an immunoglobulin having a relatively constant sequence of amino acids. Called also *constant region.* **variable d.**, the N-terminal domain of the light (V_L) or heavy chains (V_H) of an immunoglobulin molecule, having the variable primary sequence of amino acids that accounts for the specificity associated with each antibody. It contains the antigen binding properties of the molecule. Called also *variable region.* **immunoglobulin d.**, polypeptide chains of immunoglobulins folded into globular regions as the result of intrachain disulfide linkages, which are arranged symmetrically in immunoglobulins for each of approximately 110 amino acids. They have functional autonomy, e.g., binding of complement or cytophilic site, and share some amino acid sequence homology. An immunoglobulin chain is composed of linked domains — two in light chains; four in the γ, , and δ chains; and five in the μ and ε chains. In heavy chains, a nonhomologous stretch, the hinge region, separates the first two domains of the heavy chain from the other heavy chain domains. Called also *immunoglobulin region.* V_H **d.**, V_L **d.**, see *variable d.*

DOMF 2′7′-dibromo-4′-(hydroxymercuri)fluorescein; see MERBROMIN.

dominance (dom′ĭ-nans) 1. supremacy, or superior manifestation. 2. in mendelian inheritance, the appearance of one of two alternative parental characteristics in a heterozygote. See autosomal dominant CHARACTER and X-linked dominant CHARACTER.

dominant (dom′ĭ-nant) 1. exerting a ruling or controlling influence. 2. Pertaining to a dominant character; see autosomal dominant CHARACTER and X-linked dominant CHARACTER.

Donders, space of see under SPACE.

Doner factor VITAMIN B_{12}.

donor (do′nor) an individual who supplies living tissue or material to be used by another living body, such as a person who furnishes blood for transfusion or organs for transplantation. **d. site**, donor SITE. **universal d.**, a person having blood group O; such blood may be transfused to persons with other blood groups without causing agglutination or hemolysis.

Donovan's body [Charles *Donovan*] *Calymmatobacterium granulomatis;* see under CALYMMATOBACTERIUM.

Donovania (don″o-va′ne-ah) [named after Charles *Donovan*] *Calymmatobacterium.* **D. granulo′matis**, *Calymmatobacterium granulomatis;* see under CALYMMATOBACTERIUM.

Dopal trademark for *levodopa*.

L-dopa see LEVODOPA.

dopamine (do′pah-mēn) a catecholamine, 3,4-dihydroxyphenylethylamine, which is an endogenous sympathomimetic amine, being the immediate precursor of the adrenergic transmitter substance norepinephrine. Used therapeutically as the hydrochloride salt, which occurs as a white, crystalline powder that is soluble in water, methanol, and hot ethanol, but not in organic solvents. Dopamine acts on the β-adrenergic receptors and increases peripheral vascular resistance and cardiac output and raises arterial blood pressure. Not being able to cross the blood-brain barrier, it has no central effect. Used in the treatment of shock. Trademarks: Dynatra, Intropin.

Dopamet trademark for *methyldopa*.

Dopar trademark for *levodopa*.

Dopasol trademark for *levodopa*.

dope (dōp) a common name for a narcotic drug or any stupefying substance used chiefly to satisfy an addiction.

Dopom trademark for *guanethidine*.

Doppler effect [Christian Johann *Doppler*, Austrian physicist and mathematician, 1803–1853] see under EFFECT.

Dopram trademark for *doxapram hydrochloride* (see under *doxapram*).

Dorcate trademark for *silicophosphate cement* (see under CEMENT).

Dorello's canal see under CANAL.

Doriden trademark for *glutethimide*.

dormant (dor′mant) [L. *dormire* to sleep] sleeping; inactive; quiescent.

Dorme trademark for *promethazine*.

dormifacient (dor″mĭ-fa′shent) [L. *dormire* to sleep + *facere* to make] producing sleep.

Dormigen trademark for *methaqualone*.

Dormin trademark for *methapyrilene hydrochloride* (see under METHAPYRILENE).

dorsa (dor′sah) [L.] plural of *dorsum*.

dorsad (dor′sad) toward the back or dorsal aspect.

dorsal (dor′sal) [L. *dorsalis,* from *dorsum* back] 1. pertaining to the back or to any dorsum. 2. denoting a position more toward the back surface than some other object of reference; same as posterior in human anatomy.

Dorsalin trademark for *penicillin G procaine* (see under PENICILLIN).

dorsalis (dor-sa′lis) [L.] dorsal; an anatomical term denoting a position closer to the back surface. See also POSTERIOR.

dorsi- see DORSO-.

dorso-, dorsi- [L. *dorsum* back] a combining form denoting relationship to a dorsum or to the back (posterior) aspect of the body.

dorsocephalad (dor″so-sef′ah-lad) [dorso- + Gr. *kephalē* head] directed toward or facing the back of the head.

dorsolateral (dor″so-lat′er-al) pertaining to the back and to the side.

dorsomedian (dor″so-me′de-an) [dorso- + L. *medianus* middle] pertaining to the median aspect of the back.

dorsomesial (dor″so-me′se-al) pertaining to the mesial or median aspect of the back.

dorsonasal (dor″so-na′sal) pertaining to the bridge of the nose.

dorsonuchal (dor″so-nu′kal) pertaining to the back of the neck.

dorsoventrad (dor″so-ven′trad) [dorso- + L. *venter* belly] directed from or facing away from the dorsal toward the ventral aspect.

dorsoventral (dor″so-ven′tral) 1. pertaining to the back and belly surfaces of the body. 2. passing from the back to the belly surface.

dorsum (dor′sum), pl. *dor'sa* [L.] [NA] 1. the back. 2. the aspect of an anatomical part or structure corresponding in position to the back; posterior, in the human. **d. na'si** [NA], **d. of the nose,** that part of the external surface of the nose formed by junction of the lateral surfaces. **d. lin'guae** [NA], dorsum of TONGUE. **d. sel'lae** [NA], a square plate of bone forming the posterior boundary of the sella turcica; the posterior clinoid processes project from its superior extremity, and it is continuous inferiorly with the clivus. **d. of tongue,** dorsum of TONGUE.

Doryl trademark for *carbachol*.

dosage (do′sij) the determination and regulation of the size, frequency, and number of doses.

dose (dōs) [Gr. *dosis* a giving] a quantity to be administered at one time, such as a specified amount of medication, or a given quantity of x-rays or other radiation. **absorbed d.,** the amount absorbed per unit mass of irradiated material, measured in rems and rads. **absorbed d., integral,** integral absorbed d., **peak,** the maximum value of the absorbed dose which occurs along the central ray. **absorbed d., surface,** surface absorbed d. **air d.,** radiation exposure measured in a small mass of air under conditions of electronic equilibrium with the surrounding air, i.e., excluding backscatter from irradiated parts or objects; expressed in roentgens. Called also *exposure d.* and *air exposure.* **average d.,** the quantity of an agent which will usually produce the therapeutic effect for which it is administered. **average erythema d.,** erythema d., average. **booster d.,** an amount of an immunogen, such as vaccine, usually smaller than the amount given originally, injected at an appropriate time after primary immunization to sustain the immune response. **challenging d.,** 1. see CHALLENGE (2). 2. reacting d. **cumulative d., cumulative radiation d.,** cumulative EXPOSURE. **curative d., median,** one that abolishes symptoms in 50 per cent of the test subjects. Abbreviated CD_{50}. **daily d.,** the total amount of a drug administered in a 24-hour period. **depth d.,** the intensity of radiation at a given depth in an irradiated body, usually expressed as percentage of that at the surface of the body nearest the portal of entry. See also *percentage depth d.* **d. distribution,** dose DISTRIBUTION. **divided d.,** a fraction of the total quantity of the drug prescribed, to be given at intervals, usually during a 24-hour period. **doubling d.,** the dose of ionizing radiation which will result in a doubling of the current rate of spontaneous biological changes, such as mutations or cancers in the population. **effective d.,** that quantity of a drug that will produce the effects for which it is administered. Abbreviat-

ed *ED.* **effective d., median,** the amount of pathogenic bacteria, bacterial toxin, or other poisonous substance, required to kill or produce some characteristic symptom or lesion in 50 percent of uniformly susceptible animals inoculated with it. Abbreviated ED_{50}. **entrance d.,** ionizing radiation, including the primary radiation and backscatter, measured at the surface of the entrance point of the beam into the body, part, or object. Called also *entrance exposure* and *surface exposure.* **d. equivalent,** dose EQUIVALENT. **erythema d.,** that amount of radiant energy which, when applied to the skin, will cause slight, temporary redness. Abbreviated *ED.* Called also *erythema exposure.* **erythema d., average,** the average dose that will produce an erythemic reaction in the majority of individuals. **erythema d., maximum,** one that will produce erythema in even the most radioresistant person. **erythema d., threshold,** the single skin dose that will produce in 80 percent of those tested a faint but definite erythema within 30 days and in the other 20 percent no visible reaction. Abbreviated *TED.* **exit d.,** the intensity of radiation emerging from the body at the surface opposite the portal of entry. **exposure d.,** air d. **fractional d.,** the amount of an agent less than usually administered, given at shorter intervals than usual. **fractional d., fractionation d.,** 1. amounts of an agent less than that usually administered, given at shorter intervals than usual. See FRACTIONATION (1). 2. a dose of radiation given by a number of shorter exposures over a longer period than would be required if the dose was given by a continuous exposure in one session at the same dose rate. **genetically significant d.,** the amount of ionizing radiation which, if received by the gonads of every member of the population, would be expected to produce the same total genetic injury to the population as do the actual doses received by the various individuals. Abbreviated *GSD.* **gonadal d.,** the dose of ionizing radiation which is absorbed by the gonads. See also *genetically significant d.* **immunizing d.,** that dose of a vaccine needed to immunize 50 percent of animals tested. Abbreviated ImD_{50}. **infective d.,** that amount of pathogenic microorganisms that will cause infection in susceptible subjects. Abbreviated *ID.* **infective d., median,** the amount of pathogenic microorganisms that will cause infection in 50 percent of the test subjects. Abbreviated ID_{50}. **integral d., integral absorbed d.,** the total energy absorbed by an individual or other biological object during exposure to ionizing radiation, expressed in gram-rads (100 ergs). Called also *volume d.* **lethal d.,** the amount of an agent, such as radiation, which will or may be sufficient to cause death. Abbreviated *LD.* **lethal d., median,** one which is lethal for 50 percent of the test subjects. In radiology, the dose required to kill within a specified period of time (usually 30 days) half of the individuals in a large group of organisms similarly exposed. The median lethal dose for man is about 400–500 R. Abbreviated LD_{50} and *MLD.* See also $LD_{50/30}$. **lethal d., minimum,** 1. the amount of toxin which will just kill the experimental animal. Abbreviated *MLD.* 2. the smallest quantity of diphtheria toxin which will kill a guinea pig of 250-gm weight in 4 to 5 days when injected subcutaneously. **maintenance d.,** a dose (often a daily dose or dosage regimen) sufficient to maintain at the desired level the influence of a drug achieved by earlier administration of larger amounts. **maximum d.,** the largest quantity of an agent that may be safely administered to the average patient. **minimal d., minimum d.,** the smallest quantity of an agent that is likely to produce an appreciable effect. **nominal single d.,** an empirical quantitative method used for determining the isobiologic effect in comparing fractionation schedules and overall treatment time with a single fraction, accounting for the number of fractions and the total time separately: TD = NSD × $N^{0.24}$ × $T^{0.11}$, where *TD* is total dose; *N,* number of fractions; *T,* overall time course of treatment in days; *NSD,* nominal single dose. The unit expressing NSD is the ret. **optimal d., optimum d.,** the quantity of an agent which will produce the effect desired without unfavorable effects. **percentage depth d.,** the intensity of radiation expressed as a percentage at a given depth in an irradiated body, using as the point of reference the intensity of radiation at the surface of the body nearest the portal of entry. See also *depth d.* **permissible d.,** that amount of ionizing radiation which, in the light of current knowledge, is not expected to lead to appreciable bodily injury and is allowable according to current radiation protection guides. Called also *tolerance d.* **permissible d., maximum,** the largest amount of ionizing radiation that a person may receive safely. The present recommended maximum weekly dose for occupational workers is 0.1 R in a 48-hour work week, and in any 13-week period it must be no greater than 25 rems to the hands, forearms, feet, head, neck, and ankles, and no greater than 3 rems to the skin, gonads, eye, and erythropoietic organs. Abbreviated *MPD.* **priming d., a** quantity several times larger than the maintenance dose, used at the initiation of therapy to rapidly establish blood and tissue levels of the drug. **radiation absorbed d.,** the unit of absorbed dose, with a value of 100 ergs per gram. See RAD. **d. rate,** dose RATE. **reacting d.,** the second dose of sensitizing antigen, administered to an animal; it is followed by an immediate hypersensitive (anaphylactic or allergic) response. Called also *challenging d.* See also *sensitizing d.* and CHALLENGE (1). **sensitizing d.,** the first dose of sensitizing antigen in the induction of a hypersensitive (anaphylactic or allergic) response. See also *reacting d.* and ANAPHYLAXIS. **skin d.,** surface absorbed d. **surface-absorbed d.,** the absorbed dose delivered by a radiation beam at the point where the central ray passes through the superficial layer of the phantom or patient. Called also *skin d.* **threshold d.,** the minimum dose of ionizing radiation that will produce a detectable degree of any given effect. Called also *threshold exposure.* **tissue d.,** the absorbed dose of ionizing radiation in a tissue or organ, expressed in rads. **tolerance d.,** permissible d. **toxic d.,** the amount of an agent which will cause toxic symptoms in the majority of persons receiving the agent. **transit d.,** a measure of the primary radiation transmitted through the patient and measured at a point on the central beam some point beyond the patient. **unit skin d.,** see HED. **volume d.,** integral d.

dosimeter (do-sim′ĕ-ter) an instrument used to measure exposure to radiation. Called also *dosage meter, dose meter,* and *radiation meter.* See also COUNTER, ELECTROSCOPE, ionization CHAMBER, and SPECTROSCOPE. **integrating d.,** a measuring instrument consisting of an ionization chamber continuously feeding responses to an integrating system, determining the total accumulated radiation exposure. **d. pencil,** a small ionization chamber, being a tube worn like a pencil in the breast pocket by persons likely to be exposed to ionizing radiations. It is a small Lauritzen electroscope consisting of a fine fiber loop attached to an insulated electrode inclosed in a tube with a built-in graduated scale for viewing by placing one end of the tube to the eye, the opposite end facing a light.

dosimetry (do′sim′ĕ-tre) [Gr. *dosis* dose + *metron* measure] the determination of the amount, rate, and distribution of a radiation emitted from a source of ionizing radiation. **thermoluminescent d.,** measurement of radiation by heating a thermoluminescent material and determining its luminescence; the degree of luminescence is related to the amount of radiation exposure.

dosis (do′sis) [L., Gr. "a giving"] dose.

dossier (dos′e-a) [Fr.] a collection of documents concerning the same subject or individual, such as the accumulated records of patient's case history.

dot (dot) a small spot or speck.

double blind (dub′l blīnd) see double blind STUDY.

douche (dōōsh) [Fr.] a stream of water directed against a part of the body or into a cavity.

Douglas' graft sieve GRAFT.

dovetail (duv′tāl) a widened or fanned-out portion of a prepared cavity, usually established to increase the retention form and the resistance form. **lingual d.,** one established as a step portion, with lingual approach, in Classes III and IV preparations; used to supplement the retention and resistance form. **occlusal d.,** one established at the terminal or the occlusal step of a proximal cavity.

dowel (dow′l) a post or a pin, usually of metal, which is fitted into a prepared posthole within the root canal and cemented in place, serving to retain a dental restoration, such as a crown. Called also *post.* **Thompson d.,** a dowel for a semiprecision intracoronal attachment, which fits into a specially recessed well in the restoration of the abutment tooth, being free to rotate out of the well. Retention is provided by a metal projection on the lingual snubber arm of the partial denture that fits into a recess on the lingual surface of a restoration of the abutment tooth. The retainer is stress-broken to allow displacement of the denture base toward the ridges. Now rarely used in clinical procedures.

Dowicide 1 trademark for *orthophenylphenol.*

Dowmycin E trademark for *erythromycin stearate* (see under ERYTHROMYCIN).

Down's syndrome [John Langdon Haydon *Down,* English physician, 1828–1896] see under SYNDROME.

Downs' analysis, Y axis [W. B. *Downs,* American orthodontist] see under ANALYSIS, and see Y AXIS.

downtime (down′tīm) the period during which a computer is not operable.

doxapram hydrochloride (dok′sah-pram) a nonspecific analeptic, 1 - ethyl - 4 - (2-morpholinoethyl)-3,3-diphenylpyrrolidinone monohydrochloride, occurring as a white to off-white, odorless,

crystalline powder that is readily soluble in water and chloroform, sparingly soluble in ethanol, and insoluble in ether. Used as a respiratory stimulant. Convulsions, hypertension, tachycardia, arrhythmias, hypertension, cough, nausea, and vomiting are some of its adverse effects. Contraindicated in epilepsy. Trademarks: Dopram, Stimulexin.

doxepin hydrochloride (dok′sĕ-pin) an antidepressant agent, N, N - dimethyl - 3 - dibenz [b, e] oxepin - 11 - (6 H) - ylidene - 1 - propanamine, occurring as white, odorless, bitter, photosensitive crystals that are soluble in ethanol, chloroform, and water. Used in certain types of mental disorders. Xerostomia, visual disorders, constipation, hypotension, tachycardia, drowsiness, gastrointestinal disorders, sweating, vertigo, fatigability, edema, flushing, paresthesias, tinnitus, photophobia, impotence, skin rashes, and pruritus may occur. Trademarks: Adapin, Aponal, Curatin, Novoxapin, Sinequan.

Doximate trademark for *dioctyl sodium sulfosuccinate* (see under DIOCTYL).

Doxol trademark for *dioctyl sodium sulfosuccinate* (see under DIOCTYL).

doxorubicin hydrochloride (dok″so-ru″bĭ-sin) a cytotoxic antibiotic isolated from cultures of *Streptomyces peucetius,* (8S-cis)-10-[(3 - amino - 2,3,6 - trideoxy - α - L - lyxo - hexopyranosyl)oxy]-7,8,9,10 - tetrahydro - 6,8,11 - trihydroxy - 8 - (hydroxyacetyl)-methoxy - 5,12 - naphthacenedione hydrochloride. It occurs as a red-orange, odorless, hygroscopic, crystalline powder that is soluble in water and ethanol. Used in the treatment of certain neoplastic diseases. Trademarks: Adriamycin, Adriblastina.

Doxychol trademark for *doxycycline.*

doxycycline (dok″se-si′klēn) a broad-spectrum, semisynthetic tetracycline, 4α S - (dimethylamino) - 1, 4a α, 5, 5a α, 6, 11, 12a-octahydro - 3, 5α, 10, 12, 12a α - pentahydroxy - 6α - methyl - 1,11 - dioxo-2-naphthacenecarboxamide monohydrate. It occurs as a yellow, crystalline powder that is soluble in water, dilute acid and alkali hydroxide solutions, sparingly soluble in alcohol, and insoluble in chloroform and ether. It has similar antimicrobial and toxic properties to those of other tetracyclines, except that it is more potent and toxic. Used orally, absorption is delayed in the presence of milk and iron preparations. Called also Doxychol, Liviatin, Vibramycin. **d. hyclate,** a hydrochloride hemihydrate hemiethanolate derivative of doxycycline, occurring as a yellow, crystalline powder that is soluble in water and alkali hydroxide and carbonate solution, slightly soluble in alcohol, and insoluble in chloroform and ether. Trademarks: Ecodox, Hydramycin, Liomycin, Nivocillin, Novodox, Retens, Vibradox.

doxylamine succinate (dok″sil-am′ēn) an antihistaminic drug that acts on the H₁ receptor, 2-[α-[2-(dimethylamino)ethoxy]-α-methylbenzyl]pyridine succinate, occurring as a white powder with a characteristic odor, which readily dissolves in water, alcohol, and chloroform and slightly in ether and benzene. Used in the treatment of allergic diseases. Called also *mereprine.* Trademark: Decapryn.

DP 1. distal PIT. 2. degree of POLYMERIZATION.

DPN diphosphopyridine nucleotide; see *nicotinamide-adenine* DINUCLEOTIDE.

Dr doctor.

dr dram.

drachm (dram) [Gr. *drachmē*] dram.

draft (draft) 1. a potion; dose. 2. draw.

drag (drag) the lower or cast side of a denture flask to which the cope is fitted. The base of the cast is embedded in plaster of Paris or stone with the remainder of the denture pattern exposed to be engaged by the plaster of Paris or stone in the cope.

dragée (drah-zha′) [Fr. "sugar-plum"] a sugar-coated pill, or medicated preparation.

drain (drān) 1. to withdraw or draw off a liquid or fluid slowly or by degrees. 2. a device, such as a tube, which facilitates drawing off fluids from body organs, cavities, or tissues, as from a wound or infected area. See illustration. 3. any device by which a channel or open area may be established for the exit of fluids or purulent material from any cavity, wound, or infected area. **cigarette d.,** a Penrose drain with a piece of gauze placed inside to provide capillary action, thus improving the suction of the drain. **controlled d.,** one made by pressing a square of gauze into the wound and then packing with gauze strips, the ends of which, together with the corners of the square, are left projecting from the wound. **double-lumen d.,** see *sump d.* **Penrose d.,** a very thin rubber tube, usually ½ to 1 inch in diameter. **stab**

PENROSE

CIGARETTE

TUBE

SUMP

SUMP

TRIPLE LUMEN

Most commonly used drains. Ties are placed on the triple-lumen drain to hold the outer Penrose drain in place. (From D. C. Sabiston, Jr.: Davis-Christopher Textbook of Surgery. 12th ed. Philadelphia, W. B. Saunders Co., 1981.)

wound d., drainage accomplished by bringing out the drain through a small separate wound adjacent to the major operative incision. **sump d.,** a double- or triple-lumen drain that allows air to enter the drained area with the object of displacing fluid into the drain. **triple-lumen d.,** a sump drain in which a double-lumen tube is placed inside a Penrose drain.

drainage (drān′ij) the systematic withdrawal of fluids and discharges from a wound, sore, or cavity. **capillary d.,** drainage effected by strands of hair, catgut, spun glass, or other material of small diameter which induces capillary attraction. **suction d.,** closed drainage of a cavity, with a suction apparatus attached to the drainage tube. **through d.,** drainage achieved by passing a perforated tube or other type of drain through a cavity, so that irrigation may be effected by injecting fluid into one aperture and letting it escape through another.

dram (dram) [Gr. *drachmē*] a unit of weight. In the avoirdupois weight, it consists of 27.34 grains, 0.0625 ounces, or 1.772 grams. In the apothecaries weight, it consists of 60 grains, 3 scruples, 0.125 ounces, or 3.888 grams. Symbol ℨ . Abbreviated *dr.* Written also *drachm.* See also *Tables of Weights and Measures* at WEIGHT. **fluid d.,** a unit of capacity (liquid or wine measure) equivalent to 60 minims, 0.0078 pints, or 3.6966 cubic centimeters. Abbreviated *fl. dr.* Written sometimes *fluiddram.*

Dramamine trademark for *dimenhydrinate.*

Draper's law see under LAW.

draught (draft) 1. draft (1). 2. draw.

draw (draw) in dentistry, the taper or divergence of the walls of a cavity preparation for a cemented restoration. Called also *draft* and *draught.*

Drenison trademark for *flurandrenolide.*

Drenusil trademark for *polythiazide.*

dresser (dres′er) a surgical assistant who dresses wounds.

dressing (dres′ing) any of various materials used for covering and protecting a wound. **adhesive absorbent d.,** a sterile individual dressing consisting of a plain absorbent compress affixed to a film or fabric coated with a pressure-sensitive adhesive substance. **antiseptic d.,** one of gauze impregnated with an antiseptic substance. **bolus d.,** tie-over d. **Chloro-Thymonol root canal d.,** trademark for a germicidal preparation used in root canal therapy, consisting of 6 percent parachlorophenol, 5 percent thymol, 1 percent phenacaine hydrochloride, and a polyethylene glycol base. **cocoon d.,** a gauze dressing affixed to the surrounding skin by collodion or other liquid adhesive in such fashion that its elevated appearance resembles a cocoon. **Cresanol root canal d.,** a germicidal dressing used in root canal therapy, containing 25 percent parachlorophenol, 25 percent metacresyl acetate, and 50 percent camphor. **dry d.,** dry gauze or absorbent cotton applied to a wound. **fixed d.,** one impregnated with plaster of Paris, starch, or silicate of soda, used to secure fixation of the part when the material dries. **Getz Surgical D.,** trademark for an ointment used in surgical dressings, 100 gm of which contains 6 gm benzocaine, 5 gm chlorobutanol, 1 gm guaiacol, and various amounts of oil of wintergreen in an ointment base of lanolin, beeswax, and petrolatum. **Lister's d.,** gauze impregnated with phenol; used in the past for covering or packing a wound. **occlusive d.,** one which seals a wound from contact with air or microorganisms. **paraffin d.,** a gauze dressing impregnated with paraffin. **periodontal d.,** periodontal PACK. **pressure d.,** one by which pressure is exerted on the area covered to prevent the collection of fluids in the underlying tissues; most commonly used after skin or mucous tissue grafting and in the treatment of burns. **protective d.,** a light dressing

to prevent exposure to injury or infection. **root canal d.,** a medicated absorbent paper point or wisp of cotton sealed in the root canal or pulp chamber of a tooth for therapeutic purposes. **stent d.,** one in which is incorporated a mold or stent, to maintain the position of a graft. **tie-over d.,** one placed over a skin graft or other sutured wound, and tied on by the sutures which have been made of sufficient length for that purpose. Called also *bolus d.*

drift (drift) the act or process of moving under external influence; an aimless motion. See also drifting TOOTH. **genetic d.,** a chance variation, as in gene frequency, from one generation to another; the smaller the population, the greater the random variations. Called also *random genetic d.* **mesial d.,** the movement of a tooth in the mesial direction, occurring as a consequence of natural approximal wearing of the teeth. Called also *mesial movement.* See tooth migration, physiologic, under MIGRATION. **physiologic d.,** tooth migration, physiologic; see under MIGRATION. **random genetic d.,** genetic d.

drifting (drift′ing) moving, proceeding, or wandering from a set course, point, or position without resistance; straying. **tooth d.,** the moving of a tooth that does not result from destruction of the periodontal ligament, but consists of migration of the tooth into a space created by an unreplaced missing tooth. It occurs generally in the mesial direction, combined with tilting or extrusion beyond the occlusal plane; the premolars frequently drift distally.

drill (dril) a rotating cutting instrument for making holes in hard substances, such as bones or teeth. See also BUR. **bibeveled d.,** one with two flattened sides and the end cut in two beveled planes. **diamond d.,** one having a diamond chip at the cutting edge, used for drilling porcelain and other hard materials. **Feldman d.,** Feldman BUR. **Gates-Glidden d.,** an engine-driven endodontic instrument, having a small, nearly flame-shaped head set on a long attenuated noncutting shaft for mounting in a contra-angle handpiece; used in root canal preparation, being intended to cut with minimum pressure and, when pressure is applied, to break near the contra-angle. Called also *Gates-Glidden bur* and *G-type reamer.* See illustration at root canal THERAPY. **Peeso d.,** an engine-driven root canal reamer having a long, narrow, tapering head with side-cutting blades spiraling slightly with a wide rake angle, connected to the shank by a short neck. Used with a contra-angle handpiece for funneling the coronal half of the root canal and for establishing a dowel space after obturation of the canal in root canal therapy. Called also *P-type reamer.* See illustration at root canal THERAPY. **Shannon d.,** Shannon BUR. **spear-point d.,** one with a tribeveled, or three-planed, point. **twist d.,** one the blades of which are twisted like a corkscrew, used for drilling metals or holes in teeth for the placement of retentive pins.

drilling (dril′ing) the act or process of boring holes with a rotary instrument; the term is sometimes used in connection with cavity preparation.

drink (drink) a quantity of liquid taken in one swallow or in a series of successive swallows; to take a drink.

drip (drip) the slow, drop-by-drop, infusion of a liquid. **intravenous d.,** continuous intravenous instillation, drop-by-drop, of saline or other solution. **nasal d.,** a method of giving fluid slowly to dehydrated infants through a catheter inserted into the nose and pushed down into the esophagus. **postnasal d.,** the dripping of discharges from the postnasal region into the pharynx due to hypersecretion of mucus in the nasal or nasopharyngeal mucosa or to chronic sinusitis.

drocode (dro′kōd) dihydrocodeine.

Drocort trademark for *flurandrenolide.*

Drolban trademark for *dromostanolone propionate* (see under DROMOSTANOLONE).

dromostanolone propionate (dro″mo-stan′o-lōn) an androgenic anabolic steroid, 17β-hydroxy-2α-methyl-5α-androstan-3-one propionate, occurring as a white to creamy white, almost odorless, crystalline power that is soluble in methanol, ether, and chloroform, but not in water. Used in the treatment of certain neoplasms. Virilization is its chief side effect. Called also *drostanolone propionate.* Trademarks: Drolban, Masterone, Permastril.

drop (drop) [L. *gutta*] 1. a small quantity of liquid forming a sphere as its hangs or falls. 2. a minute quantity of anything. 3. in the plural form, a medicinal solution administered in minute quantities into the eyes, nose, or ears. **enamel d.,** enameloma. **Flura-D's,** see under *F.* **Luride d's,** trademark for a solution, 10 drops of which contain 2.2 mg sodium fluoride, being equivalent to 1 mg of fluoride ion; used in dental caries prevention. **Pearl D's,** see under DENTIFRICE. **toothache d's,** a preparation containing chlorobutanol dissolved in clove oil; applied topically to the aching teeth.

droperidol (drop-per′ĭ-dol) a potent tranquilizer, 1-[1-[3-(3-*p*-

fluorobenzoyl)propyl]-1,2,3,6-tetrahydro-4-pyridyl]-2-benzimidazolinone, occurring as a white to light tan, hygroscopic, odorless and tasteless, amorphous or microcrystalline powder, which is soluble in chloroform, alcohol, and water, and is slightly soluble in ether. Used as an adjunct to anesthesia to produce sedation. Trademark: Inapsine.

droplet (drop′let) a diminutive drop, such as the particles of moisture expelled from the mouth in coughing, sneezing, or speaking, which may carry infection. **enamel d.,** enameloma.

dropper (drop′er) a pipet or tube for dispensing liquid in drops.

dropsy (drop′se) [L. *hydrops*] presence of abnormal fluids in the cellular tissue or in a body cavity. Called also *hydrops.* See also EDEMA.

drostanolone propionate (dro-stan′o-lōn) DROMOSTANOLONE propionate.

drowning (drown′ing) suffocation and death resulting from filling of the lungs with water or other fluid, so that gas exchange becomes impossible. **secondary d.,** delayed death from drowning, due to such complications as pulmonary alveolar inflammation.

DrPH Doctor of Public Health.

drug (drug) any chemical substance or biological preparation, used for its chemical properties, which may be administered for the purpose of diagnosis, prevention, or treating of diseases or relief of pain, or for the purpose of improving or modifying any physiological or pathological condition. **d. abuse,** drug ABUSE. **accepted dental d.,** see accepted dental THERAPEUTIC. **d. addiction,** drug ADDICTION. **adrenergic d.,** an autonomic drug that mimics or blocks impulses mediated by the adrenergic transmitter (norepinephrine). Drugs that stimulate impulses are termed *sympathomimetic* (sometimes *adrenomimetic) drugs* and those that block norepinephrine-mediated impulses are known as *adrenergic blocking* (sometimes *adrenolytic* or *sympatholytic) drugs.* They are further subdivided into drugs that act on the α-adrenergic receptor and subserve smooth muscle stimulation and some intestinal relaxant function, adrenergic sweating, and adrenergic salivation; and those that act on the β-adrenergic receptors and subserve smooth muscle function, except some veins, and cause stimulation of the heart, lipolysis, and glycolysis. Called also *adrenergic* and *adrenergic agent.* **adrenergic blocking d.,** an agent that interferes with the activity of adrenergic mediators, including drugs that block catecholamines (including epinephrine and norepinephrine) or the effect of sympathomimetic drugs on the neuroeffector receptors. All known adrenergic blocking drugs are capable of inhibiting responses to both circulating sympathomimetics and to sympathetic activity. In the past, all known adrenergic blocking agents were known to be effective chiefly against α-adrenergic receptors and were unable to prevent myocardial stimulation, bronchial muscle relaxation, and vasodilation in skeletal muscles; newer drugs act also on β-adrenergic receptors. The adrenergic blocking drugs have been called *sympatholytics* or *adrenolytics,* because of their ability to lyse or abolish the response to the stimulation of the sympathetic nerves. Called also *adrenergic blocking agent.* See also *adrenergic neuron blocking d.* and *ganglionic blocking d.* **α-adrenergic blocking d.,** any of a group of agents which block the activity of α-adrenergic receptors, although most are also effective against other types of receptors, except β-receptors. They include most older adrenergic blocking drugs and are involved in vasoconstriction, salivation, gastrointestinal motility, uterine contractions, splenic contractions, sweating, and pancreatic secretion. Called also *α-receptor blocking d., α-receptor blocking agent,* and *α-adrenergic antagonist.* See also *α-adrenergic* RECEPTOR. **β-adrenergic blocking d.,** any of a group of substances which block the activity of the β-adrenergic receptors, sometimes differentiated as those acting on the heart (β_1) and those acting on smooth muscles (β_2). They are competitive antagonists, being mostly derivatives of isoproterenol, the side chain with an isopropyl-substitute secondary amine appearing to interact with the receptors. N-Tertiary butyl substituents have the same properties. Their pharmacological effects include decrease of heart rate and output, being more active during exercise than at rest; penetration of the blood-brain barrier, but having little effect on the central nervous system; inhibition of the increase of blood fatty acids induced by sympathomimetic amines and of the lipolytic action of catecholamines; blocking histamine release; antitremor activity; and inhibition of the release of renin induced by sympathomimetic amines. Used chiefly in the treatment of cardiac arrhythmias, angina pectoris, and hypertension. Cardiac depression and failure, increase of airway resistance, hypoglycemia, nausea, vomiting, diarrhea, insomnia, constipation, nightmares, lassitude, hallucinations, depression, and allergic diseases are the chief side effects. Called also *β-receptor blocking d., β-receptor blocking*

agent, and *adrenergic antagonist.* See also β-adreneric RECEPTOR. **adrenergic neuron blocking d.,** an adrenergic blocking drug that prevents the delivery of catecholamines (including epinephrine and norepinephrine) to the adrenergic receptors. Called also *antiadrenergic d.,* and *antiadrenergic* and *antiadrenergic agent.* See under *adrenergic blocking agent.* **adrenolytic d.,** one that blocks or lyses the responses mediated by the adrenergic receptors; the term is sometimes applied to adrenergic blocking drugs. Called also *adrenolytic.* Cf. *sympatholytic d.* **adrenomimetic d.,** sympathomimetic *d.* **d. allergy,** see drug REACTION. **antagonistic d.,** one that tends to counteract or neutralize the effect of another drug. **antiadrenergic d.,** adrenergic neuron blocking d. **antianxiety d.,** one that allays anxiety; a hypnotic or sedative. Called also *anxiolytic d., anxiolytic, anxiolytic agent, antianxiety agent,* and *minor tranquilizer.* **anticholinergic d.,** any of a group of drugs that block autonomic effectors innervated by postganglionic cholinergic nerves mediated by acetylcholine. The term applies to drugs blocking mediation at both nicotinic and muscarinic receptors, but it is sometimes used as a synonym for antimuscarinic drugs. Called also *anticholinergic agent.* **anticholinesterase d.,** cholinesterase INHIBITOR. **antihistaminic d.,** histamine INHIBITOR. **antihypertensive d.,** ANTIHYPERTENSIVE (2). **antimuscarinic d.,** any of a group of drugs which antagonize the action of acetylcholine, inhibiting its influences on autonomic effectors innervated by postganglionic cholinergic nerves mediated by muscarinic receptors, as well as some smooth muscles lacking cholinergic innervation. Generally, they have little effect at nicotinic receptors, but high doses of certain substances, such as atropine, may produce partial block of nicotinic receptors and some atropine analogues produce varying degrees of nicotinic blocking activity. They have some central effect, cholinergic transmission being predominantly nicotinic in the spinal cord and muscarinic at subcortical and cortical levels of the brain. Decreased gastrointestinal motility and secretion, xerostomia, drying of mucous membranes, mydriasis, loss of visual accommodation, urinary retention, hypohidrosis, cutaneous flush, bronchial and biliary dilatation, and antitremor action are the principal side effects of antimuscarinics. Natural antimuscarinic drugs are obtained from solaceous plants, but there are various synthetic preparations. Called also *atropine d.,* and *atropine-like drug* and *agent.* Some nonspecific terms are also used as synonyms, including *anticholinergic, antiparasympathetic, parasympatholytic, antispasmodic, spasmolytic, cholinolytic, parasympathetic blocking, cholinergic blocking drugs,* or *agents.* **antiparasympathetic d.,** one inhibiting impulses of the parasympathetic nervous system. The term applies to blocking impulses mediated at both nicotinic and muscarinic receptors, but the term is sometimes used as a synonym for antimuscarinic drugs. Called also *antiparasympathetic agent.* **antipsychotic d.,** one that favorably modifies psychotic behavior or symptoms. Called also *neuroleptic d., neuroleptic, neuroleptic agent,* and *major tranquilizer.* **antispasmodic d.,** see ANTISPASMODIC (2). **antithyroid d.,** thyroid ANTAGONIST. **anxiolytic d.,** antianxiety d. **atropine d., atropine-like d.,** antimuscarinic d. **autonomic d.,** any of a group of drugs which influence the activity of effector systems innervated by the autonomic nervous system. They are classified according to the chemical mediator which they mimic or block, a drug being *cholinergic* if it mimics or blocks stimulation of nerves mediated by the cholinergic transmitter (acetylcholine), or *adrenergic* if it mimics or blocks stimulation of nerves mediated by the adrenergic transmitter (norepinephrine). Those which stimulate nerves mediated by the adrenergic transmitter are termed *adrenomimetic* or *sympathomimetic;* those which stimulate nerves mediated by the cholinergic transmitter are termed *cholinomimetic* or *parasympathomimetic.* Drugs which block receptors are known as *blocking agents,* according to the chemical mediator with which they compete; drugs blocking the adrenergic mediator are *adrenergic blocking drugs;* those which block the cholinergic mediator at the neuroeffector receptor are *antimuscarinic drugs;* and those blocking acetylcholine at the ganglionic synapse are *ganglionic blocking drugs.* Their counterparts blocking somatic motor activity are known as *neuromuscular blocking agents* or *curarimimetics.* Called also *autonomic agents.* **bioequivalent d's,** two or more drugs that have the same bioavailability; therapeutically equivalent drugs. **blocking d.,** any drug that blocks the activity of neural receptors. See also *ganglionic blocking d.* **cardiovascular d.,** any of a group of drugs which, through direct or indirect action, affect the heart and blood vessels. The group includes vasodilators, vasoconstrictors, antihypertensive and hypotensive drugs, coronary vasoactive drugs, cardiac glycosides, antiarrhythmic drugs, cardiac stimulants, and other similar drugs. Most autonomic drugs are considered as members of the group, because of their action on the cardiovascular system. Called also *cardiovascular agent.* **chemically equivalent d's,** drug products from different sources which contain essentially identical amounts of the identical active ingredients in identical dosage forms; meet existing physiochemical standards in official compendia; and are considered to be indistinguishable. See also *therapeutically equivalent d's.* **cholinergic d.,** parasympathomimetic d. **cholinergic blocking d.,** any of a group of drugs which block autonomic effectors innervated by postganglionic cholinergic nerves mediated by both muscarinic and nicotinic receptors. The term is sometimes used as a synonym for antimuscarinic drugs. Called also *cholinergic blocking agent.* **cholinomimetic d.,** parasympathomimetic d. **clinically equivalent d's,** two or more drugs that are not necessarily chemically equivalent, but have the same therapeutic effect in treating the same disease. **competitive d., competitive neuromuscular blocking d.,** neuromuscular blocking AGENT. **d. control,** drug CONTROL. **crude d.,** the whole drug with all its ingredients, not purified to isolate the active principle. **curariform d., curariform neuromuscular blocking d.,** neuromuscular blocking AGENT. **d. dependence,** drug DEPENDENCE. **depolarizing d., depolarizing neuromuscular blocking d.,** neuromuscular blocking AGENT. **d. eruption,** DERMATITIS medicamentosa. **established name d.,** a name given to a drug or pharmaceutical product by the United States Adopted Names Council (USAN), being usually shorter and simpler than the chemical name; it is the one most commonly used in the scientific literature. **ethical d.,** one advertised only to physicians, dentists, and other health professionals. See also *prescription d.* **euphoriant d.,** euphoriant AGENT. **galenic d's,** galenicals. **ganglionic blocking d.,** any autonomic drug which acts by competing with acetylcholine for the cholinergic receptors of the autonomic postganglionic neurons. Like acetylcholine, most ganglionic blocking drugs are quaternary ammonium compounds, with some amines having similar properties. Called also *ganglionic blocking agent.* **hallucinogenic d.,** psychedelic AGENT. **generally recognized as effective d.,** one considered by experts qualified by scientific training and experience as safe and effective, which has been used to a material extent or for a material time, being a requirement that every drug must fulfill if it is not to be considered a new drug and thus be exempted from the premarket approval requirements for new drugs established by the Federal Food, Drug, and Cosmetic Act and administered by the Food and Drug Administration. Abbreviated *GRAE.* **generally recognized as safe d.,** a drug considered by experts qualified by scientific training and experience as being generally safe in therapeutic use, being a requirement that every drug must fulfill if it is not to be considered as a new drug and thus be exempted from the premarket approval requirements for new drugs established by the Federal Food, Drug, and Cosmetic Act and administered by the Food and Drug Administration. Abbreviated *GRAS.* **generic name d.,** the established, official, or nonproprietary name assigned to each drug by the United States Adopted Names Council (USAN), under which it is licensed. Generic names are assigned to drugs irrespective of their chemical or proprietary names given to the products by the manufacturers. See also *generically equivalent d's.* **generically equivalent d's,** drug products with the same active chemical ingredients sold under the same generic name, but with different brand names (trademarks). Generically equivalent drugs are sometimes assumed to be, but are not necessarily, therapeutically equivalent. **H$_1$-blocking d.,** H$_1$ INHIBITOR. **H$_2$-blocking d.,** H$_2$ INHIBITOR. **habit-forming d.,** any drug that produces dependence, whether physical or psychic, including drugs used therapeutically, as well as alcohol, tobacco, morphine, cocaine, or opium. **d. habituation,** drug HABITUATION. **hallucinogenic d.,** psychedelic AGENT. **histamine-blocking d.,** histamine INHIBITOR. **d. hypersensitivity,** see drug REACTION. **d. interaction,** drug INTERACTION. **investigational new d.,** any recently introduced drug that is not generally recognized among experts qualified by scientific training and experience as being safe and effective and thus is subject to the new drug application and premarket approval process under the Federal Food, Drug, and Cosmetic Act. Abbreviated *IND.* See also new drug APPLICATION. **magistral d.,** a medicine prepared by a pharmacist to a doctor's prescription, as distinguished from one that is kept in stock in pharmacies. Cf. *officinal d.* **d. monograph,** drug MONOGRAPH. **multi-source d.,** one available from more than one manufacturer or distributor, often under different brand names (trademarks). **muscarinic d.,** a parasympathomimetic drug mimicking the action of muscarine and acting on the muscarinic receptors in the postganglionic parasympathetic impulses; called also *muscarinic agent.* Cf. *antimuscarinic d.* **mysticomimetic d.,** mysticomimetic AGENT. **narcotic d.,** narcotic (2). **neuroleptic d.,** antipsychotic d. **neuromuscular blocking d.,** neuromuscular blocking AGENT. **New and Nonofficial Drugs,** a former annual publication of the Council of Drugs of the American Medical Association, containing descriptions of agents proposed for use in or on the human body in the prevention, diagnosis, or treatment of disease, which had been evaluated by the Council. Abbreviated *NND.* **nicotinic d.,** a parasympathomimetic drug acting on the autonomic ganglion cells and neuromuscular junctions, simulating the action of nicotine. Called also *nicotinic agent.* **nondepolarizing d., nondepolarizing neuromuscular blocking d.,** neuromuscular blocking AGENT. **nonofficial d.,** one that is not listed in the United States Pharmacopeia or the National Formulary. **nonproprietary d.,** one marked otherwise than under a trademark. **official d.,** one recognized by the United States Pharmacopeia or the National Formulary, having met the standards established by the respective authority. **officinal d.,** one kept in stock in pharmacies, as distinguished from one that is prepared to a doctor's prescription. Cf. *magistral d.* **OTC d.,** over-the-counter d. **over-the-counter d.,** one advertised and sold directly to the public without prescription. Called also *OTC d.* **parasympathetic blocking d.,** one which blocks impulses of the parasympathetic nervous system. The term applies to drugs blocking impulses mediated at both nicotinic and muscarinic receptors, but it is sometimes used as a synonym for antimuscarinic drugs. Called also *parasympathetic blocking agent.* Cf. *parasympatholytic d.* **parasympatholytic d.,** one which blocks impulses of the parasympathetic nervous system. The term applies to blocking of impulses mediated at both nicotinic and muscarinic receptors, but it is sometimes used as a synonym for antimuscarinic drugs. Called also *parasympatholytic agent.* Cf. *parasympathetic blocking d.* **parasympathomimetic d.,** an autonomic drug that produces excitation or inhibition of effector cells innervated by postganglionic parasympathetic nerves and is mediated by cholinergic receptors, mimicking the action of acetylcholine (hence the synonyms *cholinergic* and *cholinomimetic drug*). Drugs acting on the postganglionic parasympathetic impulses, simulating the effect of muscarine, are termed *muscarinic* and those acting on the autonomic ganglion cells and neuromuscular junction, simulating the action of nicotine, are known as *nicotinic drugs.* Acetylcholine is liberated not only in the parasympathetic postganglionic nerve endings, but also in somatic motor nerve endings and probably in central synapses, muscarinic receptors being present on ganglion cells and some neurons of the central nervous system; the action of cholinomimetic and parasympathomimetic drugs is not always parallel, but the terms have been considered to be synonymous. Functions of parasympathomimetic drugs include contraction of the iris; decrease of heart rate and contractility; dilatation of the arterioles of the skin, coronary bed, skeletal muscles, brain, lungs, abdominal viscera, and salivary glands; contraction of bronchial muscles; stimulation of bronchial glands; stimulation of gastric and intestinal motility and secretion; stimulation of contractions of the gallbladder, bile ducts, and urinary bladder; stimulation of erection of the penis; stimulation of secretions of the sweat, salivary, and nasopharyngeal glands; stimulation of secretion by the islands of Langerhans; and stimulation of secretion of epinephrine and norepinephrine. **phantasticant d.,** psychedelic AGENT. **prescription d.,** one available to the patient only by prescription, being potentially harmful unless used under doctor's supervision. Called also $R_x d.$ See also *ethical d.* **proprietary d.,** one marketed under a trademark. **provisionally accepted dental d.,** see provisionally accepted dental THERAPEUTIC. **psychedelic d.,** psychedelic AGENT. **psychoactive d.,** psychoactive AGENT. **psychodysleptic d.,** psychotoxic AGENT. **psychogenic d.,** psychoactive AGENT. **psychotherapeutic d.,** psychotherapeutic AGENT. **psychotogenic d.,** psychotomimetic AGENT. **psychotomimetic d.,** psychotomimetic AGENT. **psychotoxic d.,** psychotoxic AGENT. **psychotropic d.,** psychoactive AGENT. **d. rash,** DERMATITIS medicamentosa. **R$_x$ d.,** prescription d. **d. reaction,** drug REACTION. **d. receptor,** drug RECEPTOR. **α-receptor blocking d.,** α-adrenergic blocking d. **β-receptor blocking d.,** β-adrenergic blocking d. **d. sensitivity,** see drug REACTION. **spasmolytic d.,** one that relieves spasm; usually pertaining to an antimuscarinic drug. Called also *spasmolytic* and *spasmolytic agent.* **stabilizing d., stabilizing neu-**

romuscular blocking d., neuromuscular blocking AGENT. **sulfa d.**, any of a group of compounds containing both nitrogen and sulfur; see SULFONAMIDE. **surface-active d.**, surfactant. **sympathetic d.**, any drug acting on the sympathetic nervous system; see *sympathomimetic d.* and *adrenergic blocking d.* **sympatholytic d.**, one that blocks or lyses the response to the stimulation of the sympathetic nerves; the term is sometimes applied to adrenergic blocking drugs. Called also *sympatholytic.* Cf. *adrenolytic d.* **sympathomimetic d.**, an adrenergic drug that mimics the action of epinephrine and stimulates the effector organs mediated by the adrenergic transmitter substance (norepinephrine), or induces the release of norepinephrine from the postganglionic adrenergic nerves (indirectly acting sympathomimetic). Sympathomimetics are chiefly characterized by vasodilation at low concentrations, occurring mainly in the skeletal muscles and the coronary vascular bed, and vasoconstriction at higher concentrations, occurring mainly in the skin and the renal vascular beds. Elevation of blood glucose and lactates and stimulation of the central nervous system are their secondary features. Called also *adrenomimetic, adrenomimetic agent, sympathomimetic,* and *sympathomimetic agent.* See also CATECHOLAMINE. **therapeutically equivalent d's,** two or more drugs having essentially identical therapeutic effects in the same disease. Drugs differing chemically but having the same therapeutic effects are known as *clinically equivalent d's.* **unaccepted dental d.,** see unaccepted dental THERAPEUTIC.

drug-fast (drug′fast) drug-resistant.

druggist (drug′ist) 1. pharmacist. 2. a person who operates or manages a drug store; drug store operators, especially those who do not dispense drugs, are not required to be licensed pharmacists.

drug-resistant (drug′re-zis″tant) resistant to the action of drugs; said of microorganisms. Called also *drug-fast.*

Dry-Foil trademark for a tinfoil used in dental restoration, which is supplied with an adhesive powder or coating on one side.

DSP dibasic sodium PHOSPHATE.

DSS DIOCTYL sodium sulfosuccinate.

DTB dedicated time block; referring to scheduling an appointment for a period that is usually longer than a normal appointment for a special type of medical or dental care procedure.

DTD abbreviation for L. *da′tur ta′lis do′sis,* give of such a dose.

DTIC dacarbazine.

dubium [named after *Dubna,* the site of the Joint Nuclear Research of the U.S.S.R.] a proposed name for element 104 (see under ELEMENT).

Dubovitz's syndrome [Victor *Dubovitz*] see under SYNDROME.

Dubreuil-Chambardel's syndrome [L. *Dubreuil-Chambardel*] see under SYNDROME.

Dubreuilh's melanosis [M. W. *Dubreuilh*] Hutchinson's FRECKLE.

Duchâteau [18th century] a French chemist who, with Nicholas Dubois Chemant, pioneered the use of ceramics in dental prostheses.

Duchenne's dystrophy, paralysis [Guillaume Benjamin Amand *Duchenne,* French neurologist, 1806–1875] see under DYSTROPHY, and see bulbar PARALYSIS.

duckling (duk′ling) a young duck. **ugly d.,** see ugly duckling STAGE.

duct (dukt) [L. *ductus,* from *ducere* to draw or lead] a passage with well-defined walls, especially a tube for the passage of excretions or secretions. Called also *ductus.* **adipose d.,** an elongated sac in the cellular tissue filled with fat. **alimentary d.,** thoracic d. **d. of Arantius,** DUCTUS venosus. **archinephric d.,** pronephric d. **d. of Bartholin,** sublingual d., major. **Blasius' (Blaes') d.,** parotid d. **Bochdalek's d.,** thyroglossal d. **chyliferous d.,** thoracic d. **Coschwitz's d.,** a supposed salivary duct forming an arch over the dorsum of the tongue, proved by von Haller to be a vein. **craniopharyngeal d.,** hypophyseal d. **d's of Cuvier,** two short venous trunks which form by fusion of the precardinal and postcardinal veins and open into the atrium of the primitive heart; the right trunk becomes the superior vena cava. Called also *common cardinal veins of Cuvier* and *Cuvier's sinuses.* **efferent d.,** one that gives outlet to a glandular secretion. **endolymphatic d.,** a canal connecting the membranous labyrinth with the endolymphatic sac. Called also *aqueductus vestibuli* [NA alternative], *aqueductus endolymphaticus,* and *ductus endolymphaticus* [NA]. **excretory d.,** one that is merely conductive and not secretory. **frontonasal d.,** one in the lateral wall of the nasal cavity extending from the infundibulum of the ethmoid bone to the frontal air cells. Called also *nasofrontal d.* **Hensen's d.,** Hensen's CANAL. **d. of His,** thyroglossal d. **hypophyseal d.,** an embryonic structure composed of the elongated Rathke's pouch joining the infundibulum of the embryonic

hypophysis (pituitary gland). Called also *craniopharyngeal d.* **incisive d., incisor d.,** a passage sometimes found in the incisive canal that interconnects the nasal and oral cavities during embryonic development; it occasionally remains open in the adult. Called also *incisor canaliculus* and *ductus incisivus* [NA]. **intercalated d.,** a slender initial portion of the duct system interposed between an acinus of a gland and a secretory duct. **interlobular d.,** one existing between the lobules of a gland. **intralobular d.,** one within the lobule of a gland. **lacrimal d.,** lacrimal CANAL. **lacrimonasal d.,** nasolacrimal d. **lingual d.,** a depression on the dorsum of the tongue at the apex of the terminal sulcus. Called also *ductus lingualis.* **lymphatic d., left,** thoracic d. **lymphatic d., right,** a lymphatic vessel about 1.25 cm in length, located at the border of the scalenus anterior at the root of the neck, which collects lymph from the right side of the head, neck, and thorax, right upper arm, right lung, right side of the heart, and upper surface of the liver, and drains it into the blood at the junction of the right subclavian vein and the right internal jugular vein. It is provided with a nonreturn valve at the junction with the veins. Called also *ductus lymphaticus dexter* [NA]. **male d.,** mesonephric d. **mesonephric d.,** an embryonic duct initiated in association with rudiments of the pronephric kidney, taken over as an excretory duct by the mesonephros, and developed into various ducts of the reproductive system in the male and into vestigial structures in the female. Called also *male d., wolffian d.,* and *ductus mesonephricus* [NA]. **nasal d.,** nasolacrimal d. **nasofrontal d.,** frontonasal d. **nasolacrimal d.,** the passage that conveys the tears from the lacrimal sac into the interior nasal meatus. Called also *lacrimonasal d., nasal d.,* and *ductus nasolacrimalis* [NA]. **nasopharyngeal d.,** the lumen of the nasopharynx. **omphalomesenteric d.,** yolk STALK. **papillary d's,** straight renal tubules; see under TUBULE. **parotid d.,** one about 7 cm long, originating in the anterior part of the parotid gland, which drains the parotid gland into the oral cavity. It crosses the masseter muscle, a furrow of the buccal fat pad, and the buccinator muscle, and opens opposite the second upper molar at the parotid papilla. Called also *Blasius' (Blaes') d., d. of Steno, Stensen's d., canal of Steno, Stensen's canal,* and *ductus parotideus* [NA]. **d. of Pecquet,** thoracic d. **perilymphatic d.,** a small canal that connects the scala tympani with the subarachnoid space. Called also *aqueduct of cochlea, aqueductus of cochlea* [NA alternative], *aqueductus perilymphatici,* and *ductus perilymphatici* [NA]. **pronephric d.,** a segmental duct formed by the merging of the pronephric tubules, which opens into the cloaca; it later serves as the mesonephric duct. Called also *archinephric d.* and *archinephric canal.* **d. of Rivinus,** sublingual d., minor. **salivary d's,** the ducts that convey the saliva, including the parotid, submandibular, and sublingual (major and minor) ducts. **secretory d.,** a small duct that is tributary to an excretory duct of a gland and that also has a secretory function. **d. of Steno, Stensen's d.,** parotid d. **striated d.,** a secretory duct characterized by striations due to the presence of mitochondria arranged in rows parallel with the long axis of the cell. **sublingual d., larger,** sublingual d., major. **sublingual d., major,** one that drains the anterior part of the sublingual gland, and opens at the sublingual caruncula. Called also *d. of Bartholin, larger sublingual d.,* and *ductus sublingualis major* [NA]. **sublingual d., minor,** one of five to twenty small ducts that drain the sublingual gland. Some, especially those situated on the superior surface of the gland, open separately into the mouth on the elevated crest of mucous membrane on both sides of the frenum of the tongue. Called also *d. of Rivinus, small sublingual d.,* and *ductus sublingualis minor* [NA]. **sublingual d., small,** sublingual d., minor. **submandibular d.,** one about 5 cm in length, beginning deep in the submandibular gland, which discharges secretions of the submandibular gland. It passes between the mylohyoid and hyoglossal muscles, then between the submandibular gland and the genioglossal muscle, and opens at the sublingual caruncle, at the side of the frenulum linguae. Called also *submaxillary d., Wharton's d.,* and *ductus submandibularis* [NA]. **submaxillary d.,** submandibular d. **suderiferous d.,** sweat d. **sweat d.,** one that leads from the body of a sweat gland to the surface of the skin. Called also *suderiferous d.* and *ductus sudoriferus* [NA]. **thoracic d.,** a lymphatic trunk which serves as a channel for lymph from the left side of the body above the diaphragm and from all of the body below the diaphragm, discharging it into the venous circulation through the subclavian vein. In adults, it is a vessel about 3 to 5 mm in diameter and about 38 to 45 cm in length. It begins in the abdomen as an occasional dilatation, the *cisterna chyli*, passes through the thoracic cavity, and ends by opening into the angle of junction of the left subclavian vein with the left internal jugular vein. Its tributaries include the left subclavian, left jugular, and left bronchomediastinal trunks, the lumbar and intestinal trunks, and the intercostal lymph trunks. Called also *alimentary d., chyliferous d., left lymphatic d., d. of Pecquet, ductus thoracicus* [NA], and *van Hoorne's canal.* **thyroglossal d., thyrolingual d.,** a hollow narrow embryonic duct connecting the anlage of the median lobe of the thyroid gland to the base of the tongue. It usually becomes a solid stalk and fragments during the sixth week of intrauterine life, its point of origin on the tongue marked by an enlarged pit called the *foramen cecum.* Failure of obliteration of the stalk may result in formation of a thyroglossal duct cyst (see under CYST) and fistula. Called also *Bochdalek's d., d. of His, ductus thyroglossus* [NA], and *thyroglossal tract.* **umbilical d.,** yolk STALK. **d. of Vater,** thyroglossal d. **vitelline d.,** yolk STALK. **Wharton's d.,** submandibular d. **wolffian d.,** mesonephric d.

ductal (duk'tal) pertaining to a duct.

ductile (duk'til) [L. *ductilis,* from *ducere* to draw, to lead] susceptible of being hammered thin, or of being fashioned in a new form.

ductility (duk-til'ĭ-te) 1. the quality of a material of being capable of being drawn out into wire. 2. the ability of a material to withstand permanent deformation under tensile stress without fracturing. Ductility may be calculated by determining the percentage of elongation after the tested material has been fractured under tension. Material, such as orthodontic wire, is fixed in a testing device and, after placing two marks to indicate the original length of the wire (gauge length), it is stretched until it fractures. After placing the two broken ends together, the increase in the gauge length is measured and the percentage of elongation is calculated: percent elongation = $(\Delta l_{max})/l_o \times 100$, where Δl_o = maximum (increased) length and Δl_o = gauge (original) length. See MALLEABILITY.

ductless (dukt'les) having no excretory duct.

ductule (dukt'ūl) a minute duct. Called also *ductulus.* **excretory d's of lacrimal gland,** numerous ductules that traverse the palpebral part of the lacrimal gland and open into the superior fornix of the conjunctiva. Called also *ductuli excretorii glandulae lacrimalis* [NA].

ductuli (duk'tu-li) [L.] plural of *ductulus.*

ductulus (duk'tu-lus), pl. *duc'tuli* [L.] ductule. **duc'tuli excreto'rii glan'dulae lacrima'lis** [NA], excretory ductules of lacrimal gland; see under DUCTULE.

ductus (duk'tus), pl. *duc'tus* [L.] a general term for a passage with well-defined walls, especially a tube for the passage of excretions or secretions. Called also *duct.* **d. endolymphat'icus** [NA], endolymphatic DUCT. **d. inci'sivus** [NA], incisive DUCT. **d. lacrima'lis,** lacrimal CANAL. **d. lingua'lis,** lingual DUCT. **d. lymphat'icus dex'ter** [NA], lymphatic duct, right; see under DUCT. **d. mesoneph'ricus** [NA], mesonephric DUCT. **d. nasolacrima'lis** [NA], nasolacrimal DUCT. **d. paroti'deus** [NA], parotid DUCT. **d. perilymphat'ici** [NA], perilymphatic DUCT. **d. reu'niens** [NA], Hensen's CANAL. **d. sublingua'lis ma'jor** [NA], sublingual duct, major; see under DUCT. **d. sublingua'lis mino'res,** sublingual duct, minor; see under DUCT. **d. submandibula'ris** [NA], submandibular DUCT. **d. sudorif'erus** [NA], sweat DUCT. **d. thora'cicus** [NA], thoracic DUCT. **d. thyroglos'sus** [NA], thyroglossal DUCT. **d. veno'sus,** a major blood channel or bypass that develops through the embryonic liver from the left umbilical vein to the inferior vena cava. It shunts well-oxygenated blood from the placenta through the liver. In the adult; it persists as the ligamentum venosum. Called also *canal of Arantius, canal of Cuvier,* and *duct of Arantius.*

Duffy antigen (factor), blood groups [named after the person in whom the first antigen of the Duffy blood groups was discovered] see under ANTIGEN and BLOOD GROUP.

Duke method see bleeding TIME.

dull (dul) not resonant on percussion.

Dulong and Petit law [Pierre Louis *Dulong,* French chemist, 1745–1838; Alexis Therése *Petit,* French physicist, 1791–1820] see under LAW.

Dumacyclin trademark for *tetracycline hydrochloride* (see under TETRACYCLINE).

Duncaine trademark for *lidocaine.*

Dunlop see Hirschfeld FILE (Hirschfeld-Dunlop file).

Dunn, A. L. [American dentist] see Hart-Dunn ATTACHMENT.

Dunning, Edwin James [1821–1901] a New York dentist who developed a method for manipulating noncohesive gold foil and who was the first to use plaster to take impressions of the oral structures.

Dunning-Leach index gingival-bone COUNT.

duodenum (du"o-de'num, du-od'ĕ-num) [L. *duodeni* twelve at a time] the first or proximal portion of the small intestine, extending from the stomach to the jejunum; so called because it is about 12 fingerbreadths in length.

Duodin trademark for *hydrocodone bitartrate* (see under HYDROCODONE).

Duovirus (du"o-vi'rus) *Rotavirus.*

dup duplication (2). See also CHROMOSOME nomenclature.

duplication (du"plĭ-ka'shun) 1. doubling; the act or process of creating something that is a replica of something else, such as a dental cast. 2. a structural chromosome aberration, consisting of the presence of an extra fragment of chromosome. It usually occurs as a result of unequal crossing over. Abbreviated *dup.* See also CHROMOSOME aberration and see TRISOMY. **d. of benefits,** see coordination of benefits CLAUSE. **chromosome arm d.,** partial TRISOMY. **partial d. of short arm of chromosome 5,** 5p TRISOMY. **partial d. of long arm of chromosome 7,** 7q trisomy, partial; see under TRISOMY. **partial d. of long arm of chromosome 10,** 10q TRISOMY. **partial d. of short arm of chromosome 10,** 10p TRISOMY. **partial d. of short arm of chromosome 11,** 11p TRISOMY. **partial d. of long arm of chromosome 11,** 11q TRISOMY. **partial d. of long arm of chromosome 14,** 14q TRISOMY. **partial d. of long arm of chromosome 15,** 15q TRISOMY. **partial d. of short arm of chromosome 20,** 20p TRISOMY.

Dupuytren's phlegmon [Guillaume *Dupuytren,* French surgeon, 1777–1835] see under PHLEGMON.

Duraflow trademark for a heat-cured denture base acrylic polymer.

dura mater (du'rah ma'ter) [L. "hard mother"] dura MATER.

Durand-Nicolas-Favre disease [J. *Durand,* French surgeon; Joseph *Nicolas,* French physician, born 1869; Maurice *Favre,* French physician, 1876–1954] LYMPHOGRANULOMA venereum.

Duran-Reynals factor [Francisco *Duran-Reynals,* American bacteriologist, 1899–1958] hyaluronidase.

Duraphat trademark for a fluoride-containing pit and cavity varnish, consisting of an alcoholic solution of a natural varnish containing sodium fluoride.

Durawax 1032 trademark for a synthetic *dental wax* (see under WAX).

Dur. dolor. abbreviation or L. *duran'te dolo're,* while the pain lasts.

Durelon cement see under CEMENT.

Duretic trademark for *methyclothiazide.*

Durham, Herbert [1866–1945] an English bacteriologist who, with Max von Gruber, described, in 1896, the agglutination test for bacteria. He also devised the fermentation tests used to speciate bacteria and yeasts.

Duroc trademark for a high strength Class II (Type IV) *dental stone* (see under STONE).

durometer (du"rom'ĕ-ter) an instrument for measuring hardness.

duty (doo'te, du'te) 1. action or behavior expected or required by moral or legal obligations. 2. action or performance required by one's position or occupation. 3. a task or chore which one is expected to perform. **legal d.,** the obligation, under law, of one person to another, as that of a dentist to a person whom he or she has accepted as his patient.

Duvadilan trademark for *isoxsuprine hydrochloride* (see under ISOXSUPRINE).

d.v. double vibrations (a unit for the measurment of sound waves).

dwale (dwāl) belladonna (1).

dwarf (dwarf) an abnormally undersized person. **Amsterdam d.,** de Lange's SYNDROME. **Russell d.,** see Russell's SYNDROME. **Seckel d.,** see Seckel's SYNDROME.

dwarfism (dwarf'izm) underdevelopment of the body; the state of being a dwarf. See also NANISM. **bird-headed d.,** Seckel's SYNDROME. **campomelic d.,** campomelic SYNDROME. **Lenz-Majewski d., Lenz-Majewski hyperostotic d.,** a syndrome combining progressive skeletal dysplasia with multiple congenital abnormalities, including dwarfism, mental retardation, emaciation, delayed closure of the fontanelles, hypertelorism, nasal obstruction, dental enamel hypoplasia, hyperextensible joints, proximal symphalangism, interdigital webbing, cryptorchidism, loose and atrophic skin, prominent cutaneous veins, progressive sclerosis of the skull, facial bones, and vertebrae, broad clavicles and ribs, short middle phalanges, diaphyseal undermodeling and mid-shaft cortical thickening, metaphyseal and epiphyseal hypostosis, and retarded skeletal maturation.

Called also *Lenz-Majewski syndrome*. **mesomelic d.,** dwarfism in which the midportions of the arms and legs are most severely affected. **nanocephalic d.,** Seckel's SYNDROME. **pituitary d.,** dwarfism characterized by the development of a diminutive but well-proportioned body, occurring more often in males than in females and frequently due to hypothalamopituitary lesions and fetal anoxia, but most cases are idiopathic. Symptoms include delayed growth, retarded sexual maturation, fine silky, sparse hair, and dental manifestations, including delayed tooth eruption resulting from retained deciduous teeth with unresorbed roots, widely opened apical foramina, small crowns, retarded osseous development of the jaws, especially of the mandible, associated with malposition of teeth and malocclusion, small dental arches with crowding of the teeth, and short roots. **primordial d.,** Seckel's SYNDROME. **Robinow's d.,** Robinow's SYNDROME.

dwt pennyweight.

Dy dysprosium.

dyad (di'ad) a double chromosome resulting from the halving of a tetrad.

Dycal trademark for a calcium hydroxide preparation which consists of a base: titanium dioxide (13.8 per cent), calcium sulfate (31.4 percent), calcium tungstate (15.2 percent), and glycol salicylate base; and a catalyst: calcium hydroxide (51.0 percent), zinc oxide (9.23 percent), zinc stearate (0.29 percent), and ethylene toluene sulfonamide. Used in dental pulp capping.

Dycholium trademark for *sodium dehydrocholate* (see dehydrocholic ACID).

Dychon trademark for *sodium dehydrocholate* (see dehydrocholic ACID).

Dycill trademark for *dicloxacillin sodium* (see under DICLOXACILLIN).

Dyclone trademark for *dyclonine hydrochloride* (see under DYCLONINE).

dyclonine hydrochloride (di'klo-nēn) a slow-acting local anesthetic, 1-(4-butoxyphenyl)-3-(1-piperidinyl)-1-propanone hydrochloride, occurring as a white crystalline powder or mass with a slight odor and a numbing effect on the tongue, which is soluble in water, acetone, alcohol, and chloroform. Used chiefly for topical application. Also used to allay pain in certain dental and medical procedures. Irritation at the site of application may occur. Called also *Dyclone*.

dye (di) any of various colored substances that contain auxochromes and, thus, are capable of coloring substances to which they are applied. Used for staining tissues and cells, in functional tests, in vital staining, and as antiseptics. **acid d., acidic d.,** one acidic in reaction and usually unites with positively charged ions of the material acted on. Called also *anionic d.* **acridine d.,** any fluorescent yellow dye derived from acridine. Acridine dyes are used as topical antiseptics, being most active against gram-positive bacteria. Proflavine and acriflavine are the principal ones. **amphoteric d.,** one containing both reactive basic and reactive acidic groups, and staining both acidic and basic elements. **anionic d.,** acid d. **azo d.,** a synthetic dye having —N≡N— as a chromophore group and produced from amino compounds by the process of diazotization and coupling. Used in the past as antiseptics and wound-healing agents, being more active against gram-positive than gram-negative bacteria. Also used in selective culture media and in some diagnostic procedures. **basic d.,** one basic in reaction and unites with negatively charged ions of material acted on. Called also *cationic d.* **cationic d.,** basic d. **metachromatic d.,** one that stains tissues two or more colors. **occlusal registration d.,** a water-soluble dye used in determining deflective occlusal contacts or interferences. **orthochromatic d.,** one that stains tissues a single color. **vital d.,** one that penetrates living cells and colors certain structures, without serious injury to the cells.

Dylene trademark for *polystyrene.*

dynamic (di-nam'ik) [Gr. *dynamis* power] pertaining to or manifesting force.

dynamics (di-nam'iks) that phase of mechanics which deals with the motions of material bodies taking place under different specific conditions.

dynamo- [Gr. *dynamis* power] a combining form denoting relationship to power or strength.

Dynapen trademark for *dicloxacillin sodium* (see under DICLOXACILLIN).

Dyna-Set trademark for a self-curing *repair resin* (see under RESIN).

Dynatra trademark for *dopamine.*

dyne (dīn) in the centimeter-gram-second system, a unit of force, being that amount of force which, when acting continuously upon a mass of 1 gm, will impart to it an acceleration of 1 cm per second.

Dynel trademark for an acrylic resin obtained by copolymerization of acrylonitrile and vinyl chloride, which is resistant to many chemical corrosive substances and solvents.

Dyneric trademark for *clomiphene citrate* (see under CLOMIPHENE).

-dynia see -ODYNIA.

Dynothel trademark for *dextrothyroxine sodium* (see under DEXTROTHYROXINE).

dys- [Gr. *dys*] a combining form signifying difficult, painful, bad, disordered, etc.; the opposite of EU-.

dysacusis (dis"ah-koo'sis) [*dys*- + Gr. *akousis* hearing] 1. a hearing impairment in which the loss is not measurable in decibels, as in disturbances in discrimination of speech or tone quality, pitch, or loudness, or in central auditory imperception, etc. See also DEAFNESS. Cf. HYPOACUSIS. 2. a condition in which certain sounds produce discomfort. Called also *auditory dysesthesia*.

dysallilognathia (dis-al"il-lo-na'the-ah) a condition characterized by disproportion of the maxilla and mandible.

dysarthria (dis-ar'thre-ah) [*dys*- + Gr. *arthroun* to utter distinctly + -*ia*] impaired ability to produce articulate speech.

dysautonomia (dis"aw-to-no'me-ah) [*dys*- + Gr. *autonomia* freedom to use its own laws] a disorder of the autonomic nervous system. **familial d.,** Riley-Day SYNDROME.

dysbarism (dis'bar-izm) [*dys*- + Gr. *baros* weight + -*ism*] any condition caused by differences between the surrounding atmospheric pressure and the total gas pressure in the tissues and body fluids, including barosinusitis, barotitis media, decompression sickness, and explosive decompression.

dyscephaly (dis-sef'ah-le) malformation of the skull and facial bones. **François d.,** Hallermann-Streiff SYNDROME.

dyschromia (dis-kro'me-ah) [*dys*- + Gr. *chrōma* color + -*ia*] a disorder of pigmentation of the skin or hair.

dyscrasia (dis-kra'ze-ah) [Gr. *dyskrasia* bad temperament] a term formerly used to indicate a depraved state of the humors, now used generally to indicate a morbid condition, especially one which involves an imbalance of component elements. **blood d.,** an abnormal condition of the blood. **plasma cell d.,** paraproteinemia.

dysentery (dis'en-ter"e) [L. *dysenteria*, from Gr. *dys* + *enteron* intestine] any intestinal disorder marked by inflammation and attended by pain and frequent stools.

dyseresthesia (dis"er-ĕ-the'ze-ah) [*dys*- + Gr. *erethizein* to irritate] impairment of sensibility to stimuli.

dysesthesia (dis"es-the'ze-ah) [*dys*- + Gr. *aisthēsis* perception] 1. impairment of any sense, especially of that of touch. 2. painful and persistent sensation induced by a gentle touch of the skin. **auditory d.,** dysacusis (2). **oral d.,** altered oral sensation, such as burning of the tongue (glossopyrosis).

dysfibrinogenemia (dis-fi"brin-o-je-ne'me-ah) see AFIBRINOGENEMIA.

dysfunction (dis-funk'shun) impaired functioning; called also *malfunction*. **familial autonomic d.,** Riley-Day SYNDROME. **temporomandibular d. syndrome,** see under SYNDROME.

dysgenesis (dis-jen'ĕ-sis) [*dys* + Gr. *gennan* to generate] faulty development. **d. iridodenta'lis,** iridodental DYSPLASIA.

dysgnathia (dis-na'the-ah) [*dys*- + Gr. *gnathos* jaw + -*ia*] an abnormality of the oral cavity and teeth, also involving the jaws. Cf. EUGNATHIA.

dysgnathic (dis-nath'ik) [*dys*- + Gr. *gnathos* jaw] pertaining to or characterized by an abnormality of the jaws. See under ANOMALY.

dyskaryosis (dis-kar"e-o'sis) atypical changes in cell nuclei.

dyskeratosis (dis"ker-ah-to'sis) [*dys*- + Gr. *keras* horn + -*osis*] a condition characterized by abnormal, premature, or imperfect keratinization. In dental literature, the term is often used alone to mean *malignant dyskeratosis*. **d. congen'ita,** a hereditary disorder probably transmitted as an autosomal recessive trait, characterized by nail dystrophy, atrophy and irregular pigmentation of the skin, and premalignant epithelial dysplasia of the oral, anal, genitourinary, and gastrointestinal mucosa, which may undergo malignant degeneration. The age of onset ranges from 5 to 50 years. Called also *Zinsser-Engman-Cole syndrome*. **d. follicula'ris veg'etans,** KERATOSIS follicularis. **hereditary benign intraepithelial d.,** a hereditary disease, transmitted as an autosomal dominant trait, originally described among members of a triracial isolate group of mixed Caucasian, American Indian, and Negro ancestry in North Carolina. Symptoms include leukoplakia-like lesions of the oral mucosa, presenting white spongy, macerated lesions, varying from delicate opalescent white membranous areas to a rough shaggy mucosa, frequently involving the corners of the mouth. Ocular symptoms include pterygium-like lesions, presenting superficial, foamy, gelatinous white plaques overlying the cornea, leading to blindness. Called also *Witkop-Von Sallmann syndrome.* **malignant d.,** abnormal keratinization associated with cellular atypia, dyskaryosis, hyperchromatism, changes in cell polarity, increased nuclear-cytoplasmic ratio, and abnormal mitosis.

dyskinesia (dis'ki-ne'ze-ah) [Gr. *dyskinēsia* difficulty of moving] impairment of the power of voluntary movement, resulting in fragmentary or incomplete movements.

dyslalia (dis-la'le-ah) [*dys-* + Gr. *lalein* to talk + *-ia*] impairment of utterance due to defects of the external speech organs or faulty learning and not due to lesions of the central nervous system.

dysmetria (dis-me'tre-ah) [*dys-* + Gr. *metron* measure + *-ia*] a condition associated with cerebellar damage, characterized by an inability to measure distance accurately when performing muscular acts; disturbance of the power to control the range of movement in muscular action. In *hypermetria,* voluntary muscular movement overreaches the intended goal, and in *hypometria,* voluntary muscular movement falls short of reaching the intended goal. In occlusion, the affected person is apt to occlude with greater force than necessary, causing abrasion of the teeth and periodontal disorders. Dysmetria should not be diagnosed as a disorder of occlusion without accompanying evidence of cerebellar damage. Cf. EUMETRIA.

dysmorphia (dis-mor'fe-ah) [*dys-* + Gr. *morphē* form + *-ia*] the condition of appearing under different forms. **mandibulofacial d.,** Hallermann-Streiff SYNDROME.

dysodontiasis (dis"o-don-ti'ah-sis) [*dys-* + Gr. *odous* tooth + *-iasis*] imperfect or difficult dentition; defective, delayed, or difficult eruption of teeth.

dysosmia (dis-oz'me-ah) [*dys-* + Gr. *osmē* smell + *-ia*] impaired sense of smell.

dysostosis (dis"os-to'sis) [*dys-* + Gr. *osteon* bone + *-osis*] defective ossification; defect in the normal ossification of fetal cartilages. **acrofacial d.,** a syndrome transmitted as an autosomal dominant trait, consisting of hexadactylia and metacarpal synostoses of the hands and feet, associated with mandibular cleft and faulty dentition. Called also *Weyers' syndrome.* **cleidocranial d.,** cleidocranial DYSPLASIA. **congenital metaphyseal d.,** metaphyseal d. **craniofacial d.,** a syndrome transmitted as an autosomal dominant trait. Approximately 30 percent of the cases represent new dominant mutations. It is characterized by acrocephaly, exophthalmos, strabismus, parrot-beaked nose, maxillary hypoplasia, relative mandibular prognathism, short upper lip, protruding lower lip, and hypertelorism. Called also *Crouzon's disease* and *Crouzon's syndrome.* **d. enchondra'lis metaepiphysa'ria,** Morquio's DISEASE. **hereditary d.,** Hajdu-Cheney SYNDROME. **hereditary metaphyseal d.,** metaphyseal d. **mandibular d. and peromelia,** aglossia-adactylia SYNDROME. **d. mandibula'ris,** hypoplasia of the mandible with abnormal implantation of the teeth combined with deformities of the pinna and atresia of the external auditory meatus, and associated with agenesis or hypoplasia of the thumbs and/or radii. Called also *Nager's acrofacial d.* and *Nager-de Reynier syndrome.* **mandibulofacial d.,** an autosomal dominantly inherited syndrome characterized by abnormal (antimongoloid) palpebral fissures, hypoplasia of the mandible and malar bones; lower lid defects, including coloboma, and absence of cilia and the lacrimal points; obliteration of the nasofrontal angle; and deformities of the external auditory meatus. Other abnormalities may include high palate, hearing loss, malocclusion, and macrostomia. Called also *bilateral facial agenesis, Franceschetti's syndrome* and *Treacher Collins syndrome.* **mandibulofacial d., unilateral,** oculovertebral DYSPLASIA. **mandibulofacial d. with epibulbar dermoids,** oculoauriculovertebral SYNDROME. **maxillofacial d.,** a variant of the first and second arch syndrome, transmitted as an autosomal dominant trait, characterized by anteroposterior shortening of the maxilla, occasionally resulting in a relative mandibular prognathism, antimongoloid slanting of the eyes and palpebral fissures, malformations of the auricles, and delayed speech development. Called also *maxillofacial syndrome.* **maxillonasal d.,** Binder's SYNDROME. **metaphyseal d.,** an extremely rare form of dysplasia characterized by radiolucent knobby metaphyseal segments, which on biopsy are seen to consist chiefly of proliferating cartilage with an irregular attempt at forming hypertrophic cartilage. The symptoms include mental retardation, dwarfism with extremely short lower extremities, immature facies and widely spaced exophthalmic eyes, contractures, reduced flexion of the hips and

knees, muscular atrophy, and funnel chest. Patients usually die during childhood. Abnormal intrauterine pressure, renal rickets, and hereditary and biochemical factors have been considered as possible etiologic factors by various authors. Called also *congenital metaphyseal d., hereditary metaphyseal d., Jansen's syndrome, Murk Jansen's syndrome,* and *osteochondritis subepiphysaria.* **Nager's acrofacial d.,** d. mandibularis. **orodigitofacial d.,** oral-facial-digital SYNDROME (1). **otomandibular d.,** first and second branchial arch SYNDROME.

dyspepsia (dis-pep'se-ah) [*dys-* + Gr. *peptein* to digest] impairment of the power or function of digestion; usually applied to epigastric discomfort following meals.

dysphagia (dis-fa'je-ah) [*dys-* + Gr. *phagein* to eat + *-ia*] difficulty in swallowing. **sideropenic d.,** Plummer-Vinson SYNDROME. **vallecular d.,** that caused by the lodgment of food above the epiglottis. **d. valsalvia'na,** that due to subluxation of the major cornu of the hyoid bone.

dysphasia (dis-fa'ze-ah) [*dys-* + Gr. *phasis* speech + *-ia*] impairment of speech, consisting of lack of coordination and failure to arrange words in their proper order, due to a central lesion.

dysphonia (dis-fo'ne-ah) [*dys-* + Gr. *phōnē* voice + *-ia*] any impairment of voice; a difficulty in speaking.

dysphrasia (dis-fra'ze-ah) [*dys-* + Gr. *phrasis* speech + *-ia*] imperfection of utterance due to a central or cerebral defect.

dyspigmentation (dis"pig-men-ta'shun) a disorder of pigmentation.

dysplasia (dis-pla'se-ah) [*dys-* + Gr. *plassein* to form + *-ia*] 1. any abnormal development. 2. an alteration in adult cells characterized by variation in their size, shape, and organization. Called also *atypical metaplasia.* Cf. ANAPLASIA and METAPLASIA. **acrocephalopolydactylous d.,** Carpenter's SYNDROME. **anteroposterior facial d.,** defective development resulting in abnormal anteroposterior relationship of the maxilla and mandible to each other or to the cranial base with secondary malocclusion. **branchio-otorenal d.,** a hereditary syndrome, transmitted as an autosomal dominant trait, and consisting of malformed external ears, preauricular pits, branchial cleft cysts, and deafness, which may be sensorineural, conductive, or mixed. Asthenic habitus, long narrow facies, constricted palate, deep overbite, cup-shaped anteverted pinnas, bilateral prehelical pits, cochlear defect, stapes fixation, renal dysplasia, aplasia of the lacrimal ducts, and myopia are associated. **cerebrofaciothoracic d.,** cerebrofaciothoracic SYNDROME. **chondral d.,** Ehrenfried's DISEASE. **chondroectodermal d.,** a congenital syndrome transmitted as an autosomal recessive trait, occurring commonly in the Amish population in Lancaster county, Pennsylvania. The syndrome is characterized by acromelic dwarfism, with thick and short bones of the extremities, defects of the proximal part of the tibia resulting in knock-knee; accelerated maturation of bones; fusion of the hamate and capitate bones of the wrist, polydactyly, dystrophic fingers and toes; dystrophy of the fingernails; eye abnormalities, congenital heart defects, usually septal defects or a single atrium; and oral changes consisting of defects of the upper lip (partial harelip, lip-tie) and dysplasia of the teeth. Called also *mesoectodermal d.* and *Ellis-van Creveld syndrome.* **cleidocranial d.,** a syndrome inherited as an autosomal dominant trait, marked by aplasia or hypoplasia of the clavicle permitting a remarkable range of shoulder movements, and delayed ossification of the skull, associated with excessively large fontanelles and delayed closing of the sutures. The fontanelles may remain open until adulthood, but the sutures often close with interposition of wormian bones. Large bosses of the frontal, parietal, and occipital regions give the skull a globular shape. Other abnormalities may include hypoplasia of the facial bones, absence of paranasal sinuses, high arched palate, cleft palate, congenital hip dislocation, underdeveloped pelvis, and various osseous defects. The maxilla is smaller than normal in relation to the mandible. The lacrimal and zygomatic bones may be hypoplastic. Delayed tooth eruption, short, thin, and deformed roots, absence of cementum on the roots of permanent teeth, and the presence of numerous unerupted supernumerary teeth are usually associated. Partial anodontia may occur. Called also *cleidocranial dysostosis, Marie-Sainton syndrome,* and *Scheuthauer-Marie-Sainton syndrome.* **craniocarpotarsal d.,** craniocarpotarsal DYSTROPHY. **craniodiaphyseal d.,** a hereditary condition, transmitted as an autosomal recessive trait, in which progressive cranial and facial hyperostosis results in striking distortion. The tubular bones of the skeleton are grossly modeled. **craniofacial d.,** any dysplastic disease of the craniofacial structures, usually associated with dysharmonies between the jaws with resulting malocclusion. **craniometaphyseal d.,** a hereditary syndrome transmitted as an autosomal dominant trait with variability of expression, particularly in the degree of cranial involvement, and sometimes as an autosomal recessive characteristic. The principal craniofacial defects consist of thick bony wedges over the bridge of the nose and glabella, ocular hypertelorism, wide alveolar ridges, and narrow nasal passages resulting in mouth breathing. Hyperostosis of the frontal and occipital bones, sclerosis of the base of the skull, hyperostosis of the facial bones with obliteration of the paranasal sinuses, and frequent hyperostosis of the mandible are the chief radiologic signs. Deafness, visual disorders, and facial paralysis are frequently associated. Called also *craniometaphyseal dysplasia syndrome*. See also *metaphyseal d*. **cranioskeletal d.**, Hajdu-Cheney SYNDROME. **craniotubular d.**, an abnormality characterized by symmetrical thickening of the craniofacial bones with secondary pressure on the nerves in the bony canals; it results in loss of vision, nystagmus, peripheral facial nerve palsy, nasal obstruction, and hearing difficulty, associated with metaphyseal and diaphyseal abnormalities of the tubular bones. **dental d.**, dentoalveolar d. **dentinal d.**, an apparently hereditary disorder of dentin formation marked by a normal appearance of coronal dentin associated with pulpal obliteration, faulty root formation, and a tendency for peripheral lesions without obvious cause. The tubular arrangement may be atypical, with dentin filling the pulp chamber exhibiting a globular, whorl-like arrangement with disorganized dentinal tubules. The teeth become loose and are exfoliated prematurely, probably because of the short pointed roots and periapical granulomas and cysts which are a common complication. Called also *rootless teeth*. **dentoalveolar d.**, abnormal development of two or more teeth within one or both jaws, producing disharmonious relationships between the teeth and their immediate supporting bone and periodontal structures, and resulting in malocclusion. A genetic mechanism is the most common cause, but the condition may also occur as a result of lack of space to accommodate all the teeth in the dental arches, due to premature loss of deciduous teeth, prolonged retention of deciduous teeth, or improper dental restoration. Clinically, the incisors may be rotated; canines may have insufficient room to erupt into their normal places; premolars may be partially impacted or may erupt buccally or lingually to their normal positions; and molar segments may drift mesially, forcing teeth anterior to them into positions of malocclusion. **d. dentofacia′lis**, a syndrome combining multiple oculodentofacial abnormalities, including hypoplasia of the dental root and premature eruption (dentes natales) and early loss of teeth; congenital cataract, microphthalmia, and glaucoma; and peculiar facies, including short philtrum, nasal deformities, relative micrognathia, and incomplete closure of the frontozygomatic suture. Called also *Weyers-Fülling syndrome*. **dentolabial d.**, a form of ectodermal dysplasia probably inherited as an autosomal dominant trait. Abnormalities present at birth usually include numerous cysts and fistulae, causing the vestibulum to have an uneven surface with elevations and depressions, and causing the lower lip to be split and have an atypical contour. Fissures of the soft palate and uvula may give an impression of cleft palate. Oligodontia or anodontia may become evident later, about the time of puberty. Hypertrophy of the lingual and labial frenum, medial diastema, and persistent embryonal lamina dentaria may be also present. **disseminated fibrous d.**, cherubism. **epiphyseal d., punctate**, Conradi-Hünermann SYNDROME. **exostotic d.**, Ehrenfried's DISEASE. **faciocardiomelic d.**, a syndrome characterized by polyhydramnios, low birth weight, dwarfism, epicanthal folds, abnormal ears, microretrognathia, microstomia, microglossia, glossoptosis, webbed neck, cardiac defects, radial and ulnar hypoplasia, radial deviation of the hands, brachymetacarpalia, thumb hypoplasia, simian creases, fibular and tibial hypoplasia, talipes varus, heel hypoplasia, delayed bone age, and early death. Parental consanguinity suggests an autosomal recessive pattern of inheritance. **familial fibrous d. of jaws**, cherubism. **familial metaphyseal d.**, metaphyseal d. **familial white folded d. of mucous membrane**, white sponge NEVUS. **fibrous d. of bone**, Jaffe-Lichtenstein SYNDROME. **fibrous d. of jaw**, cherubism. **frontometaphyseal d.**, a syndrome of prominent supraorbital ridges, joint limitations, and splayed metaphyses. Craniofacial abnormalities include coarse facies with a wide nasal bridge and prominent supraorbital ridges, incomplete sinus development, partial anodontia, high arched palate, micrognathia with a decreased angle of the mandible, and prominent antegonial notch. Limb defects consist of partial ankylosis of the fingers, wrist, elbow, knee, and ankle; arachnodactyly; Erlenmeyer-flask metaphyses of the femur and tibia; partial fusion of the carpal and tarsal bones; other skeletal and cardiac abnormalities; wide foramen magnum; flared pelvis; cardiac murmur; deafness; cryptorchidism; and hirsutism. Called also *Gorlin-Holt syndrome*. **frontonasal d.**, a syndrome

consisting of ocular hypertelorism; broadening of the nasal root; anterior cranium bifidum occultum; median facial clefting involving the nose or both the nose and upper lip and, in some cases, the palate; unilateral or bilateral clefting of the ala nasi; lack of formation of the nasal tip; and widow's peak. Called also *median cleft face syndrome*. **hereditary ectodermal d.**, hypohidrotic ectodermal d. **hereditary enamel d.**, AMELOGENESIS imperfecta. **hypohidrotic ectodermal d.**, a congenital developmental defect of ectodermal and mesodermal structures characterized by hypohidrosis, hypotrichosis, and anodontia or hypodontia. The combination of prominent frontal bones, wide, high, scanty eyebrows, saddle nose, thick lips, hypognathia, and pointed chin gives affected persons strikingly similar facies. Affected patients are usually small and delicately proportioned with soft, white, dry skin; fine, stiff, short, blond hair; and absent or scanty eyebrows and eyelashes. Intolerance to heat and hyperpyrexia after only mild exertion are caused by the absence or decreased number of sweat glands. There is frequent eczema, especially during childhood. Teeth are usually absent with frequent conical crown formation of teeth present. Absence of nipples and mammary glands and other defects are occasionally associated. It occurs predominantly in males and is transmitted usually as an X-linked recessive trait, and rarely as an autosomal recessive trait. Called also *anhidrosis-hypotrichosis-anodontia syndrome, Christ-Siemens-Touraine syndrome*, and *Weech's syndrome*. **iridodental d.**, a hereditary syndrome characterized by an association of iris abnormalities, corneal disorders, and anomalous tooth development. Individual abnormalities include dysplasia and minute perforations of the iris, pupillary synechiae, microphthalmos, corneal opacities, microdontia, oligodontia, enamel hypoplasia, and virilization. Dwarfism and myotonic dystrophy may occur. Called also *dysgenesis iridodentalis* and *Weyers' syndrome*. **lateral facial d. (LFD)**, first and second branchial arch SYNDROME. **d. linguofacia′lis**, oral-facial-digital SYNDROME (1). **mesoectodermal d.**, chondroectodermal d. **metaphyseal d.**, a hereditary disorder, transmitted as an autosomal recessive trait, and characterized by obtuse mandibular angle; mild mandibular prognathism; genua valga; thickening of the ribs, pubic bone, ischium, and clavicle; marked Erlenmeyer-flasklike appearance of the femur and proximal tibia with cortical thickening and osteoporosis; osteoporosis of distal long bones, distal metacarpals, and proximal phalanges; limited elbow extension; and occasionally, muscle weakness, arthralgia, scoliosis, and spontaneous fractures. Called also *familial metaphyseal d., Pyle's disease*, and *Pyle's syndrome*. **occipitofacial-cervicothoracic–abdominodigital d.**, Jarcho-Levin SYNDROME. **oculoauricular d., oculoauriculovertebral d.**, oculoauriculovertebral SYNDROME. **oculodentodigital d.**, oculodento-osseous d. **oculodento-osseous d.**, a syndrome inherited as an autosomal dominant trait, combining a thin nose with hypoplastic alae and thin anteverted nostrils; microphthalmos with iris anomalies; syndactyly and camptodactyly of the fourth and fifth fingers and bony anomalies of the middle digits of the fifth fingers and toes; and enamel hypoplasia. Microdontia, amelogenesis imperfecta, yellow discoloration of the teeth, partial anodontia, wide alveolar ridges, pulp stones, a parrot beak facies due to a small nose, and hypertelorism may be present. Called also *oculodentodigital d., oculodentodigital syndrome, oculodentodigital dysplasia syndrome, oculodento-osseous dysplasia syndrome, Meyer-Schwickerath and Weyers syndrome*, and *microphthalmos syndrome*. Abbreviated ODD. **oculovertebral d.**, a combination of microphthalmia and colobomas or anophthalmia with small orbit; facial scoliosis resulting from unilateral maxillary dysplasia and dysplastic soft tissue, macrostomia, alveolar malformations, and dental malocclusion; malformations of the vertebral column consisting of half-developed cleft and wedgelike vertebrae without synostosis, chiefly of the lumbothoracic region; and costal anomalies, such as branched and hypoplastic ribs. Called also *unilateral mandibulofacial dysostosis* and *Weyers-Thier syndrome*. **odontogenic d.**, odontodysplasia. **ophthalmomandibulomelic d.**, a syndrome characterized by corneal opacities; limb abnormalities, including aplasia of the lateral humeral condyle, radial head, and lower third of the ulna; and agenesis of the angle and the coronoid process of the temporomandibular joint. It appears to be transmitted as an autosomal dominant trait. **otodental d.**, a hereditary syndrome, transmitted as an autosomal dominant trait, characterized by progressive hearing deficit and abnormalities of the teeth (globodontia) and hypodontia. The crowns of the primary and secondary molars and the primary canines are large and bulbous; the developmental grooves on the occlusal surfaces are absent; the roots are short and tapered and some are taurodont in configuration; and the premolars are usually absent but, when present, are decreased in size. Called also *otodental syndrome*. **periapical cemental d.,** cementoma. **posterior marginal d.,** Rieger's SYNDROME. **progressive diaphyseal d.,** a progressive developmental disorder characterized by hyperostoses of the long bones, osteosclerosis, and muscular dystrophy. Typically, the onset is in early childhood with a peculiar waddling gait as the first symptom. The thickening starts in the diaphyseal cortex, usually of the tibia and femur, and spreads toward the metaphyses; later there may be thickening of many flat bones of the skull, face, and trunk and fusiform transformation of the short cylindrical bones. Enlargement of the head with frontal bossing, anemia, hepatosplenomegaly, neurological complications, proptosis, enophthalmia, optic atrophy, deafness, nystagmus, dental caries, genital infantilism, bowing of the tibia, kyphosis, lordosis, valgus deformities, poor nutrition, thick and dry skin, and flabby weak muscles are usually present in advanced stages. Called also *diaphyseal sclerosis, periostitis hyperplastica,* and *Camurati-Engelmann syndrome.* **punctate epiphyseal d.,** Conradi-Hünermann SYNDROME. **radiation d.,** radiation injury characterized by delayed bone growth and frequently associated with necrosis and osteomyelitis. **Rapp-Hodgkin ectodermal d.,** a hereditary syndrome characterized by growth retardation, thin skin with hypohidrosis and sparse fine hair, dysplastic nails, hypodontia with conical teeth, low nasal bridge, narrow nose, maxillary hypoplasia, small mouth, cleft lip and palate, cleft uvula, and hypospadias. It is transmitted as an autosomal dominant trait, but X-linked dominant inheritance is not excluded. **Reese's d.,** congenital, bilateral, retinal dysplasia occurring in the form of rosettes, usually associated with microphthalmia, cerebral agenesis, and other abnormalities. The anterior chamber is shallow and synechiae, persistent pupillary membrane, a white vascularized retrolental membrane, elongated ciliary processes, corneal opacities, and cataracts may be present. Associated abnormalities may include cleft lip, cleft palate, encephalocele, meningocele, pulmonary abnormalities, cardiac defects, urogenital anomalies, and skeletal deformities. Some authorities consider this syndrome to be a form of trisomy 13 (see Patau's SYNDROME). Called also *Reese-Blodi syndrome* and *Reese's syndrome.* **d. renofacia′lis,** Potter's DISEASE. **spondyloepiphyseal d.,** Morquio's DISEASE. **spondylothoracic d.,** Jarcho-Levin SYNDROME. **trichorhinophalangeal d.,** 1. a hereditary syndrome transmitted as an autosomal dominant (rarely recessive) trait with variable phenotypic expression, characterized by sparse hair of fine texture, prominent nose with bulbous end and narrow alae, long and wide philtrum, brachydactyly, and small stature. Called also *trichorhinophalangeal syndrome.* 2. an apparently nonhereditary syndrome characterized by somatic and mental retardation, microcephaly, sparse hair, large protruding ears, distinctively shaped nose, wide philtrum, micrognathia, multiple nevi, muscular hypotonia at birth, and bony exostoses. Called also *trichorhinophalangeal multiple exostoses d., Giedion-Langer syndrome, Langer-Giedion syndrome,* and *trichorhinophalangeal syndrome.* **trichorhinophalangeal multiple exostoses d.,** trichorhinophalangeal d. (2).

dyspnea (disp′ne-ah) [Gr. *dyspnoia* difficulty in breathing] difficult or labored breathing; shortness of breath.

dysprosium (dis-pro′se-um) [Gr. *dysprositos* hard to get at] a rare earth or lanthanide element; symbol, Dy; atomic number, 66; atomic weight, 162.50; melting point, 1412° C; valence, 3. It occurs in seven natural isotopes: 156, 158, 160–164, and several artificial radioactive isotopes: 149–155, 157, 159, 165–167. Dysprosium is a silvery-white metal that does not corrode in moist air, reacts slowly with water and halogen gases, is soluble in dilute acids, and is of relatively low toxicity. Used in nuclear technology.

dysrhythmia (dis-rith′me-ah) [*dys-* + Gr. *rhythmos* any regularly occurring motion + *-ia*] disturbance of rhythm, as abnormality of rhythm of speech: *d. pneumophrasia* is defective breath grouping; *d. prosodia* is defective placement of stress; *d. tonia* is defective inflection.

dyssebacea (dis″se-ba′she-ah) a disorder of sebaceous follicles; specifically, a condition seen (but not exclusively) in riboflavin deficiency, marked by greasy, branny seborrhea on the midface,

with erythema in the nasal folds, canthi, or other folds of the skin, or in all three.

dyssecretosis (dis″se-kre-to′sis) [*dys-* + L. *secretio* secretion + *-osis*] a disorder of secretion. **mucoserous d.,** Sjögren's SYNDROME.

dyssomnia (dis-som′ne-ah) [*dys-* + L. *somnus* sleep + *-ia*] any disorder of sleep.

dyssynergia (dis″sin-er′je-ah) [*dys-* + Gr. *synergia* cooperation + *-ia*] disturbance of muscular coordination.

dystaxia (dis-tak′se-ah) [*dys-* + Gr. *taxis* arrangement + *-ia*] difficulty in controlling voluntary movements; partial ataxia.

dystonia (dis-to′ne-ah) [*dys-* + Gr. *tonos* tension + *-ia*] a disorder of muscle tonus.

dystopia (dis-to′pe-ah) [*dys-* + Gr. *topos* place + *-ia*] malposition; faulty placement of an organ.

dystrophia (dis-tro′fe-ah) [*dys-* + Gr. *trephein* to nourish] dystrophy. **d. brevicol′lis congen′ita,** Nielsen's SYNDROME. **d. periosta′lis hyperplas′tica familia′ris,** Dzierzynsky's SYNDROME.

dystrophy (dis′tro-fe) [L. *dystrophia*] a disorder arising from defective or faulty nutrition. A general term used to indicate disorders resulting from faulty supply of nutrients or any element necessary for the development or maintenance of an organ or system. **congenital mesodermal d.,** Marfan's SYNDROME. **congenital muscular d.,** MYOTONIA congenita. **craniocarpotarsal d.,** a congenital deformity characterized by stiff masklike facies with flattened facial bones; blepharophimosis, blepharoptosis, deep-set eyes, ocular hypertelorism, and epicanthus; arched alae nasi forming colobomas; asymmetric deformed ears; and high arched palate, small tongue, and microstomia with thin protruding lips, giving the appearance of "whistling face." Usually there is ulnar deviation of the hands with finger contractures and severe talipes equinovarus. Scoliosis and hernia have been observed in other cases. Called also *craniocarpotarsal dysplasia, Freeman-Sheldon syndrome,* and *whistling face syndrome.* **Duchenne's d., Duchenne's muscular d.,** a genetically determined pseudohypertrophic form of progressive muscular dystrophy which occurs predominantly in boys, and is transmitted as an X-linked recessive trait. The clinical onset is usually between the ages of two and six years, beginning with atrophic changes in the muscles of the pectoral girdle and trunk, extending to the extremities. As their size increases, the muscles become firm and resilient, but their strength diminishes and, eventually, atrophy takes place. Inability to rise to an upright position without turning to the side, waddling gait, and progressive weakness are characteristic features. Usually, the extremities become flaccid and loose; shortening and contractures may occur. Kyphoscoliosis, pes equinus, loss of tendon reflexes, bone demineralization, and cardiac failure are frequent. The blood shows an increase of enzymes, notably aldolase and creatine phospokinase. Orofacial features include involvement of the masticatory, facial, ocular, laryngeal, and pharyngeal muscles in the late stages. Few patients survive past the second decade of life. Called also *pseudohypertrophic muscular dystrophy* and *pseudohypertrophic muscular paralysis.* **facioscapulohumeral progressive muscular d.,** Landouzy-Déjérine d. **familial osseous d.,** Morquio's DISEASE. **fibrous pulp d.,** pulp FIBROSIS. **Landouzy-Déjérine d., Landouzy-Déjérine muscular d.,** a hereditary form of progressive muscular dystrophy, transmitted as an autosomal dominant trait, in which the onset usually occurs during childhood and adolescence with atrophic changes of the muscles of the shoulder girdle and face. Inability to raise the arms above the head, myopathic facies, eyelids that remain partly open in sleep, and inability to whistle or to purse the lips (tapir mouth) due to weakness of facial muscles are the principal symptoms. Called also *facioscapulohumeral progressive muscular d.* and *Landouzy-Déjérine atrophy.* **myotonic d.,** a dominantly inherited, degenerative disorder occurring at any age from infancy to the forties, characterized by myotonia, especially of the lingual and thenar muscles, frontal baldness, cataracts, testicular atrophy, myopathic facies (hatchet facies), atrophy of the sternocleidomastoid muscle resulting in the "swan neck" deformity, and occasionally endocrine deficiencies, such as hypothyroidism and diabetes. Retarded motor and speech development, mental retardation, facial weakness and diplegia, and talipes are the principal signs. Called also *atrophic myotonia* and *Curschmann-Batten-Steinert syndrome.* **pseudohypertrophic muscular d.,** Duchenne's d. **unilateral d.,** hemidystrophy.

Dzierzynsky's syndrome [W. *Dzierzynsky*] see under SYNDROME.

E

E* a symbol indicating a lesion on the cell membrane of a red cell, at the site of complement fixation.

e⁻ electron.

-eae [L. fem. pl. ending] a word termination designating a tribe in microbiological taxonomy.

Eagle's syndrome [Watt Weems *Eagle,* American physician, born 1898] see under SYNDROME.

EAMES European Association for Maxillo-Facial Surgery.

Eames' technique [W. B. *Eames,* American dentist] see alloy-mercury RATIO.

ear (er) [L. *auris;* Gr. *ous*] The organ of hearing and equilibrium, consisting of the external ear, the middle ear (or tympanic cavity), and the internal ear (or labyrinth). Called also *auris* [NA]. See also terms beginning AURI- and AURO-. **external e.,** the part of the ear consisting of the projecting portion lying outside of the head (pinna or auricula), and the narrow passage leading to the tympanic membrane (external acoustic meatus). Called also *auris externa* [NA]. **e. drum,** tympanic MEMBRANE. **internal e., inner e.,** the central part of the ear, which comprises the vestibule, cochlea, and semicircular canals, and receives acoustic stimuli and serves as the terminal for the acoustic nerve. Called also *auris interna* [NA] and *labyrinth.* **middle e.,** the part of the ear which is situated in a space of the temporal bone, and contains a chain of movable bones which serve to transmit vibrations to the tympanic membrane. Called also *auris media* [NA], *tympanic cavity,* and *tympanum.*

earache (ēr'āk) pain in the ear; otalgia.

eardrum (ēr'drum) tympanic MEMBRANE.

earth (erth) 1. the soil and other pulverulent substances forming the ground. 2. any amorphous, easily pulverizable mineral. **diatomaceous e., infusorial e. infusorial e.,** a silicious earth composed mostly of the frustules and fragments of diatoms. By boiling with dilute hydrochloric acid, washing, and calcining, it can be so purified as to be a very pure form of silica, SiO₂. Used as an inert filler for some dental materials, such as impression materials. Called also *diatomaceous e.* and *silicious e.* **rare e.,** any of the 15 chemically related elements, belonging to group IIIB of the periodic table, and starting with lanthanum (at no. 57), and followed by cerium (58), praseodymium (59), neodymium (60), promethium (61), samarium (62), europium (63), gadolinium (64), terbium (65), dysprosium (66), holmium (67), erbium (68), thulium (69), ytterbium (70), and lutetium (71). Called also *lanthanide, lanthanoid,* and *lanthanum group* or *series, rare earth element,* and *rare element.* **silicious e.,** infusorial e.

earwax (ēr'waks) cerumen.

Eastman 910 trademark for *methyl 2-cyanoacrylate.*

Eastman Kodak 910 trademark for *mecrylate.*

eating (e'ting) the act or process of taking food by mouth, including mastication and swallowing. **clay e., dirt e., earth e.,** geophagia.

Eaton agent [M. D. *Eaton*] *Mycoplasma pneumoniae;* see under MYCOPLASMA.

EBA *o*-ethoxybenzoic ACID; see also EBA CEMENT.

Ebalin trademark for *brompheniramine· maleate* (see under BROMPHENIRAMINE).

Eberth, Karl Joseph [1835–1926] a German pathologist.

Eberthella (e″ber-thel'ah) [named after K. J. *Eberth*] a former genus of bacteria of the family Enterobacteriaceae; its species now have been assigned to other genera. **E. shi'gae,** *Shigella dysenteriae;* see under SHIGELLA. **E. ty'phi,** *Salmonella typhi;* see under SALMONELLA.

Ebner's fibril, glands, lines (imbrication lines of, incremental lines of) [Victor von *Ebner,* Vienna histologist, 1842–1925] see under FIBRIL and LINE, see von Ebner's glands, under GLAND.

ebonation (e″bo-na'shun) [L. *e* out + *bone*] the removal of fragments of bone after injury.

ébranlement (e-brahnl-maw') [Fr.] removal of a polyp by twisting the pedicle of the tumor.

ebullition (eb-u-lish'un) [L. *ebullire* to boil] 1. the process or condition of boiling. 2. the motion of a boiling liquid.

ebur (e'ber) [L.] ivory. **e. den'tis,** dentin.

eburnation (e″ber-na'shun) [L. *ebur* ivory] the hardening or ossification resulting in the transformation of bone into a dense, hard substance resembling ivory. See also OSTEOSCLEROSIS. **e. of dentin,** a condition observed in arrested dental caries, characterized by a large open cavity, usually on the occlusal surface of the deciduous and permanent teeth, in which decalcified dentin is burnished and takes a brown-stained, polished appearance.

eburneous (e-ber'ne-us) [L. *ebur* ivory] resembling ivory.

eburnitis (e″ber-ni'tis) [L. *eburnus* of ivory + *-itis*] increased hardness and density of dentin, generally occurring in exposed dentin, which may also undergo gradual discoloration, to yellow, to brown, and eventually, to black.

E.C. ENZYME classification.

Ec ectochonchion.

écarteur (a-kar-ter') [Fr.] a retractor.

ECC emergency cardiac care.

eccentric (ek-sen'trik) 1. situated or occurring away from a center. 2. proceeding from a center.

eccentro-osteochondrodysplasia (ek-sen″tro-os″te-o-kon″dro-displa'se-ah) [Gr. *ekkentros* from the center + *osteon* bone + *chondros* cartilage + *dys-* + *plassein* to form] Morquio's DISEASE.

ecchondroma (ek″kon-dro'mah) [Gr. *ek* out + *chondros* cartilage + *-oma*] a hyperplastic growth (chondroma) developing on the surface of the cartilage. Called also *ecchondrosis.*

ecchondrosis (ek″kon-dro'sis) ecchondroma.

ecchondrotome (ek-kon'dro-tōm) [Gr. *ek* out + *chondros* cartilage + *tomē* a cutting] a knife for excising cartilaginous tissue.

ecchymoma (ek-ĭ-mo'mah) a swelling due to a bruise.

ecchymoses (ek″ĭ-mo'sēz) [Gr.] plural of *ecchymosis.*

ecchymosis (ek″ĭ-mo'sis), pl. *ecchymo'ses* [Gr. *ecchymōsis*] a relatively large, about 1–5 cm in diameter, flat or slightly raised purplish red spot caused by extravasation of blood under the skin, which later turns blue or yellow. Cf. PETECHIA. **cadaveric e.,** one of the stains seen on the more dependent portions of the body after death, giving the appearance of bruises.

ecchymotic (ek-ĭ-mot'ik) pertaining to or of the nature of an ecchymosis.

Eccles, John Carew [born 1903] an Australian physiologist; co-winner, with Alan Lloyd Hodgkin and Andrew Fielding Huxley, of the Nobel prize for medicine and physiology in 1963, for discoveries concerning the ionic mechanisms involved in excitation and inhibition in the peripheral and central portions of the nerve cell membrane.

eccrine (ek'rin) [Gr. *ekkrinein* to secrete] pertaining to secretion; as in eccrine sweat gland (see under GLAND). See also ENDOCRINE and EXOCRINE.

eccrinology (ek-rĭ-nol'o-je) [Gr. *ekkrinein* to secrete + *-logy*] the study or science of secretions and excretions.

ecdemic (ek-dem'ik) [Gr. *ekdēmos* gone on a journey] not endemic; applied to a disease caused by a factor originating far from the place in which the disease is observed.

ECF 1. extracellular FLUID. 2. extended care FACILITY.

ECF-A eosinophil chemotactic factor of anaphylaxis; see under FACTOR.

ECFMG Educational Commission for Foreign Medical Graduates; see under COMMISSION.

ECG electrocardiogram.

echino- [Gr. *echinos* a prickly husk, hedgehog] a combining form denoting relationship to a spine, or spiny.

echinococcosis (e-ki″no-kok-o'sis) infestation with tapeworms of the genus *Echinococcus.* In humans, the disease is caused by the larval stage (hydatid cyst) of *Echinococcus granulosus* and *E. multilocularis.* The liver is most commonly affected, but other organs, such as bone, kidneys, brain, lungs, thyroid gland, and parotid glands also may be affected. A slowly growing tumor containing larval cysts is the most common symptom. The dog, whose excreta provide the source of human exposure, is the most important host, but other animals, including cattle and a wide variety of domestic and wild animals, provide a reservoir for the parasite. Called also *hydatid disease.*

Echinococcus (e-ki″no-kok'us) [echino- + Gr. *kokkos* berry] a genus of small tapeworms of the family Taeniidae. **E. granulo'sus,** a small tapeworm, measuring 3 to 6 mm in length. Called also *Taenia visceralis socialis granulosus.* See ECHINOCOCCOSIS. **E. multilocula'ris,** a small tapeworm, measuring 1.2 to 3.7 mm in length. Called also *Taenia echinococcus multilocularis.* See ECHINOCOCCOSIS.

echinovirus (ek″ĭ-no-vi'rus) see SPUMAVIRINAE.

ECHO enteric cytopathic human orphan (virus); see ECHOVIRUS.

echo (ek'o) [Gr. *ēchō* a returned sound] repetition of a sound as a result of reverberation of sound waves; also the reflection of ultrasonic, radio, and radar waves.

echothiophate iodide (ek″o-thi'o-fāt) a long-acting organophosphate and quaternary ammonium anticholinesterase, 2-

[(diethoxyphosphinyl)-thio]-*N*,*N*,*N*-trimethylethanaminium iodide, occurring as white, hygroscopic crystals with a slight mercaptan-like odor, which are soluble in water, methanol, and ethanol, but not in other organic solvents. Used chiefly in ophthalmology. Side reactions may include excessive salivation, nausea, vomiting, diarrhea, abdominal cramps, and hypersensitivity. Trademark: Phospholine.

echovirus (ek″o-vi′rus) [*enteric cytopathic human orphan + virus*] a picornavirus of the genus *Enterovirus,* occurring as a particle 24 to 30 nm in diameter, with an RNA central core. Originally isolated from human feces, the virus was believed to be unassociated with any specific disease, but was found to produce cytopathic changes in human cell cultures, hence its name. Echoviruses are believed to be involved in various clinical conditions, ranging from respiratory infection to aseptic meningitis. They are common inhabitants of the intestinal tract in man, entering the body through the oral cavity; the infections they produce being limited mostly to the upper respiratory tract. In some cases, the infection may spread, causing rashes and central nervous system infections. Written also *ECHO virus* or *echo virus.* **e. 4,** a strain causing aseptic meningitis associated with gastrointestinal disorders. **e. 6,** a strain causing aseptic meningitis in children, associated with muscle weakness, maculopapular rashes, and gastrointestinal disorders. **e. 8,** a strain causing respiratory and intestinal disorders. **e. 9,** a strain causing aseptic meningitis, sometimes associated with maculopapular rash. **e. 10,** *Orthoreovirus.* **e. 11,** a strain causing respiratory disorders and skin rash. Called also *virus U.* **e. 16,** a strain causing exanthematous disease, aseptic meningitis, and maculopapular rash. **e. 18,** a strain isolated from feces in infantile diarrhea. **e. 20,** a strain isolated from feces of children with coryza, fever, and diarrhea. Called also *JVI virus.* **e. 22,** a strain isolated in respiratory diseases. **e. 25,** a strain causing pharyngitis, cervical adenitis, fever, and skin rash in infants. **e. 28,** common cold VIRUS.

eclecticism [Gr. *eklegein* to pick out] an ancient system of medicine which treats diseases by the application of single remedies to known pathologic conditions, without reference to nosology, special attention being given to developing indigenous plants.

Ecodox trademark for *doxycycline hyclate* (see under DOXYCYCLINE).

ecoid (e′koid) the colorless framework of a red blood corpuscle.

ecology (e-kol′o-je) [Gr. *oikos* house + *-logy*] the science of organisms as affected by the factors of their environments; study of the environment and life history of organisms. See also ENVIRONMENT and environmental MEDICINE.

economics (e″ko-nom′iks, ek″o-nom′iks) [Gr. *oikos* house + *nemein* to manage] the study of processes involved in producing, distributing, and sharing resources, particularly their organization and effectiveness. **health e.,** the expenditure of time and resources in health services delivery, particularly their organization and financing; the efficiency with which resources are allocated and used for health purposes; and the effects of preventive, curative, and rehabilitative health services on the individual and society.

ecosystem (ek″o-sis′tem) the fundamental unit in ecology, comprising the living organisms and the nonliving elements interacting in a certain defined area. Sometimes written *eco system.* Called also *ecologic system.*

ectasia (ek-ta′ze-ah) [Gr. *ektasis* + *-ia*] dilatation or distention. Called also *ectasis.*

ectasis (ek′tah-sis) see ECTASIA.

ectatic (ek-tat′ik) distended or stretched; distensible.

ectental (ek-ten′tal) [Gr. *ektos* without + *entos* within] pertaining to the ectoderm and entoderm, and to their line of junction.

ectethmoid (ek-teth′moid) [Gr. *ektos* without + *ethmoid*] pertaining to the ectethmoid bone.

ecto- [Gr. *ektos* outside] a prefix denoting situated on, without, or on the outside.

ectochonchion (ek″to-kon′chi-on) the craniometric point on the lateral margin of the orbit marking the greatest breadth, measured either from the maxillofrontale or from the dacryon. Abbreviated *Ec.* See illustration at CEPHALOMETRY.

ectocondyle (ek″to-kon′dil) the external condyle of a bone.

ectoderm (ek′to-derm) [*ecto-* + Gr. *derma* skin] the outermost of the three primary germ layers of the embryo. From it are developed the epidermis and epidermal tissues, such as glands, hair, and nails; the epithelium of the sense organs, nasal cavity, sinuses, mouth, including the oral glands, and enamel; and the nervous tissue. See also GASTRULATION and germ LAYER, and

see illustration at EMBRYO. **blastodermic e., primitive e.,** the external layer of a blastula or blastodisc.

ectodermosis (ek″to-der-mo′sis) a disorder based on congenital maldevelopment of the organs of ectodermal derivation, such as nervous system, eye, and skin. **e. erosi′va pluriorificia′lis,** Stevens-Johnson SYNDROME.

ectogenous (ek-toj′ĕ-nus) [*ecto-* + Gr. *gennan* to produce] introduced from without; arising or originating outside the body.

ectomesenchyme (ek″to-mes′eng-kīm) [*ecto-* + *mesenchyme*] see MESENCHYMA.

-ectomize [Gr. *ektomē* excision + *izein* to render] a word termination meaning to deprive by excision. By extension, used in terms to designate destruction or deprivation by other methods as well.

ectomorph (ek′to-morf) [*ectoderm* + Gr. *morphē* form] an individual having a type of body build in which tissues derived from the ectoderm predominate; there is a preponderance of linearity and fragility, with large surface area, thin muscles and subcutaneous tissue, and slightly developed digestive viscera, as contrasted with endomorph and mesomorph.

ectomy (ek′to-me) [Gr. *ektomē*] excision of an organ or part. Used as a word termination to indicate excision of a structure or organ designated by the root to which it is affixed, as *tonsillectomy* or *odonectomy.* By extension, used in terms to designate destruction or deprivation by other methods as well.

ectoparasite (ek″to-par′ah-sīt) [*ecto-* + Gr. *parasitos* parasite] a parasite that lives on the outside of the body of the host.

ectopia (ek-to′pe-ah) ectopy.

ectopic (ek-top′ik) located away from the normal position. Cf. EUTOPIC.

ectopy (ek′to-pe) [Gr. *ektopos* displaced] displacement or malposition, especially if congenital. Called also *ectopia.*

ectosteal (ek-tos′te-al) [*ecto-* + Gr. *osteon* bone] pertaining to or situated on the outside of a bone.

ectostosis (ek″to-sto′sis) [*ecto-* + Gr. *osteon* bone] ossification beneath the perichondrium of a cartilage or the periosteum of a bone.

ectropion (ek-tro′pe-on) [Gr. "an everted eyelid," from *ektropē* a turning aside] the eversion or turning outward of an edge or margin, as of the eyelid.

eczema (ek′zĕ-mah) [Gr. *ekzein* to boil out] an inflammatory skin disease, characterized by lesions varying in character, with vesiculation, infiltration, watery discharge, and development of scales and crusts. **allergic e., atropic e.** atopic DERMATITIS. **herpetic e.,** Kaposi's varicelliform ERUPTION. **infantile e.,** 1. atopic dermatitis in infants. 2. any eczematous condition in infants, such as atopic dermatitis, diaper dermatitis, and seborrheic dermatitis. **seborrheic e., e. seborrhe′icum,** an old term for seborrheic DERMATITIS. **e. vaccina′tum,** Kaposi's varicelliform ERUPTION.

ED 1. emergency department (see emergency ROOM). 2. effective DOSE. 3. erythema DOSE.

ED₅₀ effective dose, median; see under DOSE.

edathamil (e-dath′ah-mil) edetate. **e. calcium disodium,** CALCIUM disodium edetate.

EDDA expanded duty dental auxiliary; see dental assistant, extended function, under ASSISTANT.

Edecril trademark for *ethacrinic acid* (see under ACID).

Edecrin trademark for *ethacrinic acid* (see under ACID).

edema (ĕ-de′mah) [Gr. *oidēma* swelling] the accumulation of abnormally large amounts of fluids in the interstitial spaces or body cavities, sometimes associated with diffuse swelling of the subcutaneous tissue (anasarca). It is caused by excessive drainage of fluids from the blood capillaries associated with the inability of lymphatic capillaries to absorb excess fluid, usually associated with increased hydrostatic pressure of the blood in conditions such as heart diseases, decreased osmotic pressure of the blood in conditions such as renal diseases, increased osmotic pressure of the interstitial fluid, or increased permeability of the blood capillaries. See also DROPSY and HYDROPS. **acute circumscribed e., acute essential e., angioneurotic e.,** Quincke's e. **cardiac e.,** systemic edema, often of the legs, due to increased venous and capillary pressure in congestive heart failure, often associated with sodium retention. **inflammatory e.,** edema due to inflammation, and attended with redness and pain. **lymphatic e.,** lymphedema. **malignant e.,** edema marked by rapid extension and destruction of tissue, such as seen in anthrax. **migratory e.,** Quincke's e. **nonpitting e.,** edema in which the tissue cannot be pitted by pressure. **passive e.,** edema occurring because of obstruction of vascular or lymphatic drainage from the area. **pericardial e.,** hydropericardium. **peritoneal cavity e.,** ascites. **pitting e.,** edema in which the tissues show prolonged existence of the pits produced by pressure.

pleural e., hydrothorax. **purulent e.,** a swelling due to the effusion of a purulent fluid. **Quincke's e.,** a disorder of the skin and subcutaneous and submucosal tissues, characterized by increased vascular permeability and the sudden appearance of painless, circumscribed nonpitting swellings of the face (around the eyes, chin, and lips), tongue, feet, genitalia, and trunk, which persist for a few hours to 2 or 3 days and then fade, although they may reappear, often at the same sites. It occurs in two forms: the hereditary form, probably transmitted as an autosomal dominant trait, which normally involves the larynx and viscera; and the sporadic form, which may be caused by allergy, infection, or emotional stress. Called also *acute circumscribed e., acute essential e., angioneurotic e., migratory e., wandering e., Bannister's disease, cutaneous angioneurosis, giant urticaria, Milton's disease, Milton's urticaria, Quincke's disease,* and *urticaria gigantea.* **Reinke's e.,** subepithelial edema of the vocal cords produced by drugs, sometimes associated with malignant degeneration. **venous e.,** that in which the effused liquid comes from the blood. **wandering e.,** Quincke's e.

edematogenic (ĕ-dem″ah-to-jen′ik) [Gr. *oidēma* swelling + *gennan* to produce] causing edema.

edematous (ĕ-dem′ah-tus) pertaining to or affected by edema.

edentate (e-den′tāt) edentulous.

edentia (e-den′she-ah) [L. *e* without + *dens* tooth] a condition characterized by absence of some or all teeth in the dental arch. See also Kennedy's CLASSIFICATION and Skinner's CLASSIFICATION.

edentics (e-den′tiks) that branch of dentistry concerned with the art, science, and technique of treating edentulous patients.

edentulate (e-den′tu-lāt) edentulous.

edentulous (e-den′tu-lus) [L. *e* without + *dens* tooth] without teeth; having lost some or all natural teeth. Called also *edentate* and *edentulate.*

edetate (ed′ĕ-tāt) a salt of edetic (ethylenediaminetetraacetic) acid; ethylenediaminetetraacetate (EDTA). Called also *edathamil.* **disodium e., e. disodium,** a water-soluble crystalline powder, (ethylenedinitrilo)tetraacetic acid disodium salt. It readily chelates calcium, and is used as an anticoagulant, to terminate the effect of injected calcium in digitalis tolerance tests, to decrease digitalis toxicity, and to suppress tachyarrhythmias. Side effects include nausea, vomiting, diarrhea, paresthesias, headache, and transient hypotension. Occasional fever, exfoliative dermatitis, and various lesions of the skin and mucous membranes may occur. A rapid injection may be fatal. Trademarks: Cheladrate, Chelaplex III, Disotate, Endrate.

edge (ej) a margin or border. **beam e.,** the lines joining the center of the anterior face of the source of the radiation beam to the diaphragm edges farthest from the source. **bevel e.,** a cutting edge produced by beveling. **chamfer e.,** a margin finished to an obtuse or blunt edge. See also CHAMFER (1). **cutting e.,** a beveled angle of an object or device by which something may be cut, such as the blade of a knife, or the incisal surface of an anterior tooth. **denture e.,** denture BORDER. **incisal e.,** the junction of the labial surfaces of an anterior tooth with a flattened linguoincisal surface creased by occlusal wear.

edge-strength (ej′strength) the ability of fine edges to resist fracture or abrasion, applied especially to such resistance in dental restorations.

edgewise (ej′wīz) with the edge forward, as in an edgewise appliance.

Edinger's law [Ludwig *Edinger,* German neurologist, 1855–1918] see under LAW.

Edlan-Mejchar operation [A. *Edlan;* B. *Mejchar*] see under OPERATION.

EDNA Emergency Department Nurses Association.

edrophonium chloride (ed′ro-fo′ne-um) an anticholinesterase drug, *N* - ethyl - 3 - hydroxy - *N, N* - dimethylbenzenaminium chloride, occurring as a white, odorless, crystalline powder that is soluble in water and ethanol, but not in ether and chloroform. It has direct nicotinic stimulant action at the neuromuscular junction. Used to abolish neuromuscular paralysis produced by *d*-tubocurarine and other similarly acting drugs and as a diagnostic agent in myasthenia gravis. Sometimes also used in the treatment of myasthenic crises. Side effects may include lacrimation, visual disorders, sweating, and vertigo. Trademark: Tensilon.

EDTA 1. ethylenediaminetetraacetic ACID. 2. ethylenediaminetetraacetate. **calcium EDTA,** CALCIUM disodium edetate.

education (ej″u-ka′shun) the act or process of imparting or acquiring knowledge. **continuing e.,** formal education at the postgraduate level, after completing requirements for a degree. Various states require a specified number of hours of recognized, continuing education per year as a condition for continued licensure in some health professions. See also *graduate e.* **dental assisting e.,** see dental assisting PROGRAM, and see Accredited Dental Assisting Programs in the Appendix. **dental health e.,** educational activities concerned with informing individuals and communities how dental health contributes to general health, how it should be attained and preserved, and how dental and oral diseases may be prevented, and with encouraging individuals and communities to transform knowledge into action. **graduate e.,** in general education, graduate school education given after receipt of a Bachelor of Arts (BA) degree, leading to a Master of Arts (MA) degree, Doctor of Philosophy (PhD), or equivalent degree. In dentistry, dental education given after receipt of the DDS or equivalent dental degree. In medicine, medical education given after receipt of the MD or equivalent medical degree, including the education received as an intern, resident, or fellow, and continuing education. See also *continuing e.* **undergraduate d.,** in general education, education leading to a Bachelor of Arts (BA) degree. In dentistry, dental education given before receipt of the DDS or equivalent dental degree, usually the 4 years of study in a dental school leading to a degree. In medicine, medical education given before receipt of the MD or equivalent medical degree, usually the 4 years of study leading to a degree.

educationally qualified (ed″u-ka′shun-al″le kwal′ĭ-fīd) in dentistry, the status of a specialist who has completed an educational program that has met the minimal guidelines for specialty training set forth by the Council on Dental Education of the American Dental Association.

Edwards' syndrome [J. H. *Edwards*] see TRISOMY 18.

Edwardsiella [named after P. R. *Edwards*] a genus of bacteria of the family Enterobacteriaceae, occurring as gram-negative, facultatively anaerobic, nonencapsulated, motile, peritrichously flagellated rods. *E. tar'da* has been isolated from the urine, blood, and feces of normal human subjects and in cases of diarrhea, and is also considered a normal inhabitant of the intestine in snakes.

EEC ectrodactyly-ectodermal dysplasia-clefting SYNDROME.

EEE eastern equine encephalomyelitis (virus); see under VIRUS.

EEG electroencephalogram.

EENT eye-ear-nose-throat.

Eez-Thru trademark for floss threaders for threading dental floss under bridges and between connected jacket crowns.

EFDA extended function dental assistant; see dental assistant, extended function, under ASSISTANT.

effect (ĕ-fekt′) the result produced by an action. **adverse e.,** see *side e.* **anode heel e.,** *heel e.* **Auger e.,** the emission of an electron from the extranuclear portion of an excited atom when the atom undergoes a transition to a less-excited state. It is an alternative process to the emission of an x-ray photon in the process of fluorescence. The ejected electron (Auger electron) has kinetic energy equal to the difference between the energy of the corresponding fluorescent x-ray photon and the binding energy of the ejected electron. **bonus e.,** see ANTIBODY avidity. **Compton e.,** an interaction between a photon and an electron. It consists of collision between a high-energy photon and an electron, the photon giving off some of its energy to the electron and ejecting it from the atom, thus producing the recoil electron. The recoil electron may strike other orbital electrons and the photon, having also been deflected and having lost some of its energy (Compton photon), may strike other electrons in the orbit, both producing additional ionization. See also photoelectric EMISSION and SCATTERING (2). **cytotropic e.,** a property of some classes of antibody of binding a limited number of mediator cells of the body, such as IgE, which binds to mast cells and basophils, and certain IgG molecules, which bind to receptors on macrophages of most mammalian species, including man. **Doppler e.,** the relationship of the apparent frequency of waves, as of sound, light, and radio waves, to the relative motion of the source of the waves and the observer, the frequency increasing as the two approach each other and decreasing as they move apart. **genetic e.,** any effect produced by radiation on the genes and chromosomes; any effect on male or female gonads with potential genetic consequences. **heel e.,** a slightly greater intensity of radiation in an x-ray beam on the cathode side than on the anode side, due to the angle at which x-rays emerge from beneath the surface of the focal spot, resulting in a more penetrated image on the cathode side. The effect is greater when shorter focal-film distance is used; it is seldom visible to the naked eye. Called also *anode heel.* **Karolyi e.,** bruxism. **photoelectric e.,** photoelectric EMISSION. **pleiotropic e.,** see

PLEIOTROPY. **secondary e.,** an indirect effect of the administration of a drug or another agent, as in superinfection occurring after long-term administration of broad-spectrum antibiotics. **side e.,** undesired effect produced by a drug or another agent administered for therapeutic purposes in a standard dose and form, usually eliciting an adverse reaction in the body. **toxic e.,** an adverse response elicited by a drug or agent in overdose. **Tyndall e.,** Tyndall PHENOMENON. **untoward e.,** an adverse or undesired effect elicited by a drug or agent, usually administered for therapeutic purposes; see *side e.* **wedging e.,** one produced by food impaction that forces the teeth apart.

effectiveness (e-fek′tiv-nes) the ability to produce a specific result or to exert a specific measurable influence. **relative biological e.,** an expression used to compare the biological effectiveness of different types of ionizing radiation. It is the inverse ratio of the amount of absorbed radiation required to produce a given effect to a standard (or reference) radiation required to produce the same effect. Abbreviated *RBE.* See also absorbed DOSE.

effector (ef-fek′tor) effector ORGAN.

efferent (ef′er-ent) [L. *ex* out + *ferre* to bear] centrifugal; conveying away from a center.

efficacy (ef′ĭ-kah-se) 1. capacity for serving to produce effects. 2. in health care delivery, the benefit or usefulness to the individual of preventive, therapeutic, or diagnostic services delivered.

efficiency (e-fish′en-se) ability to accomplish a desired effect or to perform a certain action.

efflorescence (ef′lo-res′ens) a rash or eruption; any skin lesion, especially numerous and conspicuous lesions.

efflorescent (ef′lo-res′ent) [L. *afflorescere* to bloom] pertaining to substances (hydrates) which give up water of crystallization on exposure to air at room temperature and become anhydrous.

effusion (e-fu′zhun) [L. *effusio* a pouring out] 1. the escape of fluid into a part or tissue. 2. an effused material. **pleural e.,** the accumulation of escaped fluid in the pleural cavity between the visceral and parietal pleura, usually in the presence of an infection or a neoplasm.

Efudex trademark for *fluorouracil.*

Ehlers-Danlos syndrome [Edvard *Ehlers,* Danish dermatologist, 1863–1937; Henri Alexandre *Danlos,* French dermatologist, 1844–1912] see under SYNDROME.

Ehrenfried's disease [Albert *Ehrenfried,* American physician] see under DISEASE.

Ehrenritter's ganglion [Johann *Ehrenritter,* Austrian anatomist, died 1790] superior ganglion of glossopharyngeal nerve; see under GANGLION.

Ehrlich's biochemical theory [Paul *Ehrlich,* German bacteriologist, 1854–1915; co-winner, with Elie Metchnikoff, of the Nobel prize for medicine and physiology in 1908, in recognition of his work in immunology] see under THEORY, and see side-chain THEORY. See also EHRLICHIA and EHRLICHIEAE.

Ehrlichia (ār-lik′e-ah) [named after Paul *Ehrlich*] a genus of bacteria of the tribe Ehrlichieae, family Rickettsiaceae, occurring as small, often pleomorphic, coccoid to ellipsoidal microorganisms, found singly or in compact colonies intracytoplasmically in the circulating leukocytes of infected animals, including cattle, sheep, goats, dogs, and probably horses. It is not pathogenic for man. **E. psitta′ci,** *Chlamydia psittaci;* see under CHLAMYDIA.

Ehrlichieae (ār′lĭ-ki′e-e) [named after Paul *Ehrlich*] a tribe of bacteria of the family Rickettsiaceae, order Rickettsiales, occurring as nonmotile, gram-negative, minute organisms, which are pathogenic for certain mammals but not for man. It includes the general *Cowdria, Ehrlichia,* and *Neorickettsia.*

Eiger, Marvin Sheldon [American physician, born 1930] see HYPEROSTOSIS corticalis deformans juvenilis (Bakwin-Eiger syndrome).

eiloid (i′loid) [Gr. *eilein* to roll up + *eidos* form] having a coiled appearance.

einstein [named after Albert *Einstein*] a unit of energy, being the amount of absorbed radiation needed to activate 1 mole of matter: E = 6.06 × 10²³ quanta, analogous to the faraday (6.06 × 10²³ electrons).

Einstein, Albert [1879–1955] German physicist and mathematician in the United States; formulator of the theory of relativity and winner of Nobel Prize in 1921. See Einstein-Starck LAW, and see EINSTEIN and EINSTEINIUM.

Einstein-Starck law [Albert *Einstein*] see under LAW.

einsteinium (īn-sti′ne-um) [named after Albert *Einstein*] an artificial radioactive element first discovered in the debris of a hydrogen bomb explosion and subsequently produced by cyclo-

tron bombardment of uranium with nitrogen ions and by irradiating plutonium or californium with neutroms. Symbol, Es; atomic weight, 254; atomic number, 99. Isotopes are known with mass numbers ranging from 246 to 253.

eisanthema (īs-an′the-mah) [Gr. *eis* into + *anthein* to bloom] an eruption on a mucous membrane.

eisodic (i-sod′ik) [Gr. *eis* into + *hodos* way] afferent or centripetal.

ejector (e-jek′tor) an apparatus for effecting the forcible expulsion or removal of a material or body. **apical fragment e.,** a type of small elevator, either straight or angular, used to remove roots, or parts of roots, fractured at their apical third. **saliva e.,** an apparatus for removal of saliva and water from the mouth of the patient during operations on the teeth.

eka- [Sanscrit *eka* one, first] a prefix added to the name of a known chemical element as a provisional designation of the unknown element which should occur next in the same group in the periodic table.

eka-aluminum (e″kah-ah-loo′mĭ-num) [*eka-* + *aluminum*] gallium.

eka-silicon (e″kah-sil′ĭ-kon) [*eka-* + *silicon*] germanium.

eka-tantalum (e″kah-tan′tah-lum) [*eka-* + *tantalum*] a proposed name for element 105 (see under ELEMENT).

EKG electrocardiography.

Ekvacillin trademark for *cloxacillin.*

elaborate (ĕ-lab′o-rāt) [L. *elaborare* to work out] to produce complex substances out of simpler materials.

elastic (ĕ-las′tik) [L. *elasticus*] 1. being able to return to the original dimensions or shape after stretching, compressing, and otherwise distorting. Also, an object or material having such an ability. 2. an elastic band, usually of rubber, used in orthodontic therapy. See illustration. **intermaxillary e.,** an elastic band used

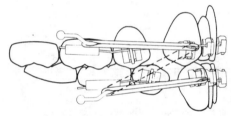

Horizontal (intramaxillary) space closing elastics in place. Intermaxillary elastics are represented by dotted lines. (From P. R. Begg and P. C. Kesling: Begg Orthodontic Theory and Technique. 3rd ed. Philadelphia, W. B. Saunders Co., 1977.)

to produce traction between the upper and lower teeth in orthodontic therapy. Called also *maxillomandibular e.* **intramaxillary e.,** an elastic band applied within the same dental arch in space closure. **maxillomandibular e.,** intermaxillary e. **rubber dam e.,** an elastic band of rubber dam latex used in orthodontic therapy. **vertical e.,** an elastic applied in a direction perpendicular to the occlusal plane, connecting one arch wire to the other and usually used for approximating teeth to improve intercuspation.

elastica (ĕ-las′tĭ-kah) [L.] 1. a general term for any elastic tissue in the body. 2. elastic MEMBRANE. 3. rubber (1). **e. exter′na,** elastic membrane, external; see under MEMBRANE. **e. inter′na,** elastic membrane, internal; see under MEMBRANE.

elasticity (e″las-tis′ĭ-te) the property of a body of being susceptible of being stretched, or being deformed under stress, and then assume its original configuration when the stress is removed. See also Hooke's LAW and mechanical STRESS. **coefficient of e.,** MODULUS of elasticity. **physical e. of muscle,** the physical quality of muscle of being elastic, returning to its resting length after passive stretch. It is a property of the connective tissue components and the tendons. **physiologic e. of muscle,** the biologic quality, unique to muscle, of being able to change and resume resting length under neuromuscular control. It is not true elasticity as it involves contractile as well as noncontractile (connective tissue) elements. **total e. of muscle,** the combined effect of physical and physiologic elasticity of muscle.

Elasticon trademark for a *silicone impression material* (see under MATERIAL).

elastin (ĕ-las′tin) a yellow scleroprotein, the essential constituent of yellow elastic connective tissue, especially in the ligaments and arterial walls. When moist, it is flexible and elastic; when dry, it becomes brittle. Elastin is insoluble in water and is resistant to acids, alkalies, and proteolytic enzymes. Contrary to other scleroproteins, it does not convert to gelatin in boiling water.

elastoma (e″las-to′mah) a condition, usually a tumor, characterized by the proliferation of elastic tissue fibers or abnormal collagen fibers of the skin. **Miescher's e.,** perforating ELASTOSIS.

elastomer (ĕ-las′to-mer) a polymer, being a soft, rubber-like material, containing large molecules with weak interaction among them, cross-linked at certain points to form a three-dimensional structure. Elastomers may be stretched when chains are pulled apart and uncoiled but, on removal of the stress, they snap back to their relaxed state and original dimensions. Under room temperature, elastomers are noncrystalline but may crystallize under tensile stress. Elastomers are considered to be synthetic rubbers. See also elastomeric impression MATERIAL.

elastometer (e″las-tom′ĕ-ter) [*elasticity* + Gr. *metron* measure] an instrument for measuring elasticity of tissue. If applied to the skin, the presence of edema could be quantitated, but its presence would interfere with the accurate measurement of the elasticity of deeper tissues.

elastometry (e″las-tom′ĕ-tre) the measurement of elasticity.

elastopathy (e″las-top′ah-the) a disease or deficiency of elastic tissue.

elastorrhexis (e-las″to-rek′sis) rupture of fibers composing elastic tissue.

elastosis (e″las-to′sis) a degenerative condition due to changes in the elastic connective tissue fibers of the skin. **actinic e.,** degeneration of the elastic connective fibers of the skin due to excessive exposure to sunrays, affecting most commonly the face, neck, and other exposed areas of the body. Called also *solar e.* **e. intrapapilla′re**, **e. perfo′rans serpigino′sa**, perforating **e. perforating e.**, **reactive perforating e.**, an elastic tissue defect that usually affects young males in their twenties, characterized by keratotic pale to red papules arranged in an arciform serpiginous pattern and forming a ringed eruption on the face and nape, usually on the posterior or lateral portion of the neck near the hairline, and less frequently, on the arms. Removal of adherent keratinized caps often reveals bleeding craters. The presence of elongated tortuous channels in the epidermis, in which abnormal elastic tissue perforates and is extruded, is the most significant pathological feature. Called also *e. intrapillare, e. perforans serpiginosa, keratosis follicularis serpiginosa, Lutz-Miescher disease, Miescher's disease,* and *Miescher's elastoma*. **senile e., e. sini′lis,** a degenerative condition of the skin peculiar to old age, in which the skin exhibits discoloration in various shades of brown, wrinkling, and distinct pea- to bean-sized maculations over the face, dorsum of the hands, genitalia, anus, and lower extremities. The oral mucosa is seldom affected but the lips may become mildly keratotic, occasionally bleeding at the vermilion edge. Called also *senile skin atrophy*. **solar e.,** actinic e.

Elbrecht splint see under SPLINT.

elective (e-lek′tiv) 1. tending to combine with or act on one substance rather than another. 2. subject to the choice or decision of the patient or physician; applied to procedures that are advantageous to the patient but not urgent.

Electraloy trademark for an alloy containing an electrolytic precipitate of pure (99.995 percent) gold with small amounts of calcium, the product being sandwiched between two sheets of pure gold. Used as a direct filling alloy in dental restorations.

electricity (ĕ-lek-tris′ĭ-te) motion of electrons, protons, and other charged particles, manifesting itself as attraction, repulsion, heat, light, and other forms of energy. **static e.,** the electricity contained or produced by charged bodies; electricity in motionless charges, as on the terminals of an open-circuit battery or on hard rubber after it has been rubbed, or considered without reference to motion. See also static marks, under MARK.

electro- [Gr. *ēlektron* amber] a combining form denoting relationship to electricity.

electroanesthesia (ĕ-lek″tro-an″es-the′ze-ah) anesthesia, either local or general, induced by electricity.

electrocardiogram (ĕ-lek″tro-kar′de-o-gram″) [*electro-* + Gr. *kardia* heart + *gramma* mark] a graphic tracing of the voltage preceding the contraction of the heart muscle. The normal electrocardiogram shows deflections resulting from atrial and ventricular electrical activity. The first deflection, P, is due to excitation of the atria. The QRS deflections are due to excitation (depolarization) of the ventricles. The T wave is due to recovery of the ventricles (repolarization). The U wave is a potential undulation of unknown origin immediately following the T wave, seen in normal electrocardiograms and accentuated in hypokalemia. Abbreviated *ECG* or *EKG*. See also LEAD¹. See illustration.

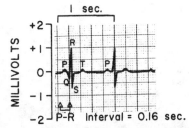

Normal electrocardiogram. (From A. C. Guyton: Textbook of Medical Physiology. 6th ed. Philadelphia, W. B. Saunders, 1981.)

electrocardiography (ĕ-lek″tro-kar″de-og′rah-fe) [*electro-* + *cardio-* + Gr. *graphein* to record] the making of graphic records of the voltage preceding contraction of the heart muscle. See ELECTROCARDIOGRAM. Abbreviated *ECG* or *EKG*. See illustration.

electrocautery (ĕ-lek″tro-kaw′ter-e) an apparatus for cauterizing tissue, consisting of a platinum wire in a holder, which is heated to a red or white heat when the instrument is activated by an electric current.

electrochemistry (ĕ-lek″tro-kem′is-tre) chemical reactions involving either the consumption or generation of electrical current.

electrocoagulation (ĕ-lek″tro-ko-ag″u-la′shun) a method of coagulation and hemostasis through dehydration, using a moderately or highly damped high frequency alternating current. A ball or loop electrode is used with a conductive pad, usually for hemostasis or localized tissue destruction. See also ELECTROSURGERY.

electrocryptectomy (ĕ-lek″tro-krip-tek′to-me) [*electro-* + *crypt* + Gr. *ektomē* excision] diathermic destruction of a tonsillar crypt.

electrode (ĕ-lek′trōd) [Gr. *ēlektron* amber + *hodos* way] a medium used between an electric conductor and the object to which the current is applied; an instrument with a point or surface from which to transmit an electric current to the body of a patient or to another instrument. **negative e.,** see CATHODE. **positive e.,** see ANODE.

electrodeposition (ĕ-lek″tro-de″po-zish′un) the deposition of metal by electric action (electroplating), sometimes employed in dentistry for the copper or silver coating of impressions, etc.

electrodermatome (ĕ-lek″tro-der′mah-tōm) an electrical dermatome for cutting off even layers of the skin in a short time; used in skin grafting, shaving scars, etc.

electrodessication (ĕ-lek″tro-des″ĭ-ka′shun) dehydration of tissue by the use of a high frequency electric current. See FULGURATION.

electrodiagnosis (ĕ-lek″tro-di″ag-no′sis) the use of electrical devices in the diagnosis of pathologic conditions.

electroencephalography (ĕ-lek″tro-en-sef″ah-log′rah-fe) [*electro-* + *encephalo-* + Gr. *graphein* to record] the recording of the potentials on the skin of the skull generated by currents emanating spontaneously from nerve cells in the brain. The dominant frequency of these potentials is about 8 to 10 cycles per second and the amplitude about 10 to 100 microvolts. Variations in wave characteristics correlate well with neurological conditions and so have been useful as diagnostic criteria. Abbreviated *EEG*.

electroexcision (ĕ-lek″tro-ek-siz′zhun) excision performed by electrosurgical means.

electroformer (ĕ-lek″tro-for′mer) a device for the electrolytic deposition (electroplating) of copper or silver upon an impression, usually for an inlay or crown, in order to produce an accurate model or die with a hard, tough, and smooth surface.

electrogalvanism (ĕ-lek″tro-gal′vah-nizm) galvanism.

electrography (e″lek-trog′rah-fe) [*electro-* + Gr. *graphein* to record] the graphic recording of changes in electric potential, as in electrocardiography, electroencephalography, etc.

electrokinetic (ĕ-lek″tro-ki-net′ik) [*electro-* + Gr. *kinēsis* motion] pertaining to motion produced by an electric current.

electrokymograph (ĕ-lek″tro-ki′mo-graft) the instrument used in electrokymography.

electrokymography (ĕ-lek″tro-ki-mog′rah-fe) the graphic recording of the motion of or changes in density of organs by registering variations in intensity of a small beam of roentgen rays on an electrokymograph, consisting of a fluoroscope, a pick-up unit, and a recording instrument; used especially for showing motion of the cardiac silhouette.

electrolysis (e″lek-trol′ĭ-sis) [*electro-* + Gr. *lysis* dissolution] 1. the chemical decomposition of an electrolyte by the passage of an electric current. See also IONTOPHORESIS. 2. removal of excessive hair from the body by means of an electric current.

electrolyte (ĕ-lek′tro-līt) [*electro-* + Gr. *lytos* that may be dissolved] a substance that dissociates into ions when fused or in solution, and thus becomes capable of conducting electricity; an ionic solute. **amphoteric e.,** a compound which dissociates into both hydrogen (H⁺) and hydroxyl (OH⁻) ions. Called also *ampholyte*. **strong e.,** an ionic compound and hydrolyzable covalent polar compound that dissociates completely into ions when in dilute solution. **weak e.,** a compound that dissociates only slightly into ions when in solution and exists essentially as undissociated molecules.

electrolyzer (ĕ-lek′tro-lī″zer) an electric device for use in the root canal to break down by direct current a chemical substance used in root canal therapy into its various ions. Called also *ionizer*.

electromagnet (ĕ-lek″tro-mag′net) a temporary magnet made by passing electric current through a coil of wire surrounding a core of soft iron.

electromallet (ĕ-lek″tro-mal′et) an electronically controlled mechanical condenser for packing and condensing direct filling gold in a prepared cavity. See electromallet CONDENSER. **McShirley's e.,** electromallet CONDENSER.

electromedication (ĕ-lek″tro-med″ĭ-ka′shun) iontophoresis.

electrometer (e″lek-trom′ĕ-ter) [*electro-* + Gr. *metron* measure] an electrostatic instrument for measuring the potential difference between two points; used to measure changes in the potential of charged electrodes due to ionization occasioned by radiation.

electromotive (ĕ-lek″tro-mo′tiv) pertaining to motion of or produced by electricity. See also electromotive FORCE.

electromyogram (ĕ-lek″tro-mi′o-gram) the record obtained by electromyography.

electromyography (ĕ-lek″tro-mi-og′rah-fe) [*electro-* + Gr. *mys* muscle + *graphein* to record] the recording and study of the intrinsic electrical properties of skeletal muscle: (1) by means of surface or needle electrodes to determine merely whether the muscle is contracting or not (useful in kinesiology); or (2) by insertion of a needle electrode into the muscle and observing by cathode-ray oscilloscope and loud-speaker the action potentials spontaneously present in a muscle (abnormal) or induced by voluntary contractions, as a means of detecting the nature and location of motor unit lesions; or (3) recording the electrical activity evoked in a muscle by electrical stimulation of its nerve (called also *electroneuromyography*), a procedure useful for study of several aspects of neuromuscular function, neuromuscular conduction, extent of nerve lesion, reflex responses, etc. Abbreviated *EMG*.

electron (ĕ-lek′tron) a negatively charged fundamental particle of the atom, which has a mass approximately $1/1840$ of that of a proton. Negative electrons surround the positively charged nucleus, forming the atomic shell; their number and arrangement determine the valence and other chemical characteristics of the atom. On an isolated conductor, they produce static electricity; when flowing along the conductor, they constitute an electric current. Electrons ejected from a radioactive substance form beta rays. Symbol e^-. **Auger e.,** see Auger EFFECT. **bonding e.,** one involved in bonding one atom to another in a molecule. **emission e.,** one of the electrons which give radioactivity to the atom. **free e.,** one not bound to the nucleus of an atom, but may move from one atom nucleus to another. **positive e.,** positron. **recoil e.,** one which, after colliding with a high-energy photon (Compton photon), impairs some of its energy and is ejected from the atom, sometimes striking along the way other electrons, thus producing additional ionization. See also Compton EFFECT. **valence e's,** electrons in the outermost quantum level, or shell of an atom, which determine chemical properties of the atom and are involved in its binding to other atoms. **e. volt,** electron VOLT.

electronegative (ĕ-lek″tro-neg′ah-tiv) [*electro-* + *negative*] 1. bearing a negative charge or excess of electrons. 2. capable of capturing electrons, as an electronegative element.

electronegativity (ĕ-lek″tro-neg″ah-tiv′ĭ-te) the attraction for valence electrons from element to element; the tendency to become negatively charged.

electroneuromyography (ĕ-lek″tro-nu″ro-mi-og′rah-fe) electromy-

ography in which the nerve of the muscle under study is stimulated by application of an electric current.

electronics (ĕ″lek-tron′iks) the science and technology which deals with the conduction of electricity through gases, solids, or a vacuum.

electrophoresis (ĕ-lek″tro-fo-re′sis) the migration of colloidal or suspended particles in a liquid medium toward electrodes having charges that are opposite to those of the particles; negative particles migrating toward the positive electrode and positive particles toward the negative electrode. Most solids, being negatively charged, migrate to the anode, with the exception of basic dyes, hydroxide solutions, and colloids that have adsorbed hydroxide ions, which being positively charged, migrate toward the cathode. The phenomenon of electrophoretic migration is used for analytic purposes, particularly in the study of proteins which act in the manner of colloidal particles.

electrophysiology (ĕ-lek″tro-fiz″ĕ-ol′o-je) the study of the electric reactions associated with body functions such as nerve conduction, muscle contraction, and gland secretion.

electroplating (ĕ-lek″tro-plāt-ing) plating or coating of an object with a layer of metal through the use of electrolytic processes. When electroplating with copper, the object is placed in an electroplating bath and an electrical contact is made between the copper matrix band or the metal tray and the surface of the object (such as a dental impression), which is the cathode in the bath. A piece of copper is used for the anode. In electroplating objects which do not conduct electricity, as when a wax impression is used, the object is first metallized, whereby a thin layer of metal is burnished onto its surface. See also electroplated DIE. **e. bath,** electroplating BATH.

electropolishing (ĕ-lek″tro-pol′ish-ing) removal of a minute layer of metal by electrolysis to produce a bright, shiny surface.

electropositive (ĕ-lek″tro-poz′ĭ-tiv) [*electro-* + *positive*] 1. bearing a positive charge or a deficiency of electrons. 2. capable of losing electrons, as an electropositive element.

electroresection (ĕ-lek″tro-re-sek′shun) resection of tissue with fully rectified undamped high frequency biterminal current. The concentration of current causes molecular disintegration and volatilization of the tissue without coagulation and is considered self-limiting. See also ELECTROSURGERY.

electrosalivogram (ĕ-lek″tro-sah-li′vo-gram) [*electro-* + *saliva* + Gr. *gramma* that which is written] a graphic record or curve showing the action potential of the salivary glands, obtained with an electrically operated instrument.

electroscission (ĕ-lek″tro-sizh′un) cutting tissue by use of the electric cautery.

electroscope (ĕ-lek′tro-skōp) [*electro-* + Gr. *skopein* to examine] an instrument for measuring the intensity of radiation by detecting the motion imparted to charged strips suspended from a conductor. See also DOSIMETER. **Lauritzen e.,** DOSIMETER pencil.

electrosection (ĕ-lek″tro-sek′shun) an incision made by electrosurgical means.

electrosol (ĕ-lek′tro-sol) a colloidal solution (sol) of a metal obtained by passing an electrical discharge between metal electrodes in distilled water.

electrostatic (ĕ-lek″tro-stat′ik) pertaining to static electricity; pertaining to electric charges at rest. See also electrostatic CAPACITY.

electrosterilization (ĕ-lek″tro-ster″ĭ-li-za′shun) sterilization with the use of an electric, usually galvanic, current to dissociate a chemical substance into positive and negative ions, thus achieving a greater germicidal effect. It may be used within the root canal. **root canal e.,** see *electrosterilization*.

electrosterilizer (ĕ-lek″tro-ster″ĭ-li′zer) an electric apparatus used for electrosterilization.

electrosurgery (ĕ-lek″tro-ser′jer-e) the use of high-frequency electric currents for cutting or destroying tissue. One type of electrosurgical device consists of a spark-gap generator which produces a current characterized by surging peaks with intervals of highly reduced or damped-out energy; another type utilizes electronic circuitry to convert alternating current into high frequency radio current, and includes instruments which produce both partially rectified and undamped fully rectified current (multiple circuit units). In partially rectified currents, the alternating surging peaks are partially reduced or "damped" before peak cycles recur, and is used for coagulation, desiccation, and fulguration; in fully rectified current the alternating cycles are filtered out, producing an undamped current, which is used for cutting tissue without coagulation. The current is applied into the tissues through an electrode (active electrode); a conductive pad of flat metal or metallized rubber (passive electrode) in contact with the patient, but not necessarily in contact with the skin, is used to complete the circuit (biterminal circuit). Most electrodes are single ended or monopolar and are used in a biterminal circuit, with the passive electrode in contact with the patient. See also electric DESICCATION, ELECTROCOAGULATION, ELECTRORESECTION, and FULGURATION.

electrosyneresis (ĕ-lek″tro-sin-ĕ-re′sis) immunofiltration.

electrotherm (ĕ-lek′tro-therm) [electro- + Gr. thermē heat] an electrosurgical appliance used for cutting.

electrotome (ĕ-lek′tro-tōm) [electro- + Gr. tomē a cut] an electrosurgical cutting instrument.

electrotomy (ĕ-lek-trot′o-me) electroexcision with low current, high voltage, and high frequency; a procedure in which the tissues are not coagulated.

electrotrephine (ĕ-lek″tro-tre′fin) a form of trephine operated by electricity.

element (el′ĕ-ment) [L. elementum] 1. any of the primary parts or constituents of a thing. 2. in chemistry, a simple substance that cannot be decomposed by chemical means and that is made up of atoms alike in their nuclei and therefore in their atomic weight and in their radioactive properties. Ninety-two of the at least 106 currently recognized chemical elements occur naturally. Chemical elements may be grouped into an ascending series according to their atomic numbers. They also may be arranged in the form of a chart (periodic table, Mendeleev's table) according to the periodic law, in which corresponding elements from the several periods form groups with similar properties. See Periodic Table of Selected Elements. **e. 104,** an artificial element reported to have been discovered as the isotope $^{260}104$, produced by bombarding plutonium with accelerated 113 to 115 MeV neon ions, which decays by spontaneous fission and has a half-life of 0.3 ± 0.1 sec. Subsequently discovered isotopes include: $^{257}104$ (half-life 4–5 sec), $^{253}104$ (half-life 105 sec), $^{258}104$ (half-life 1/100 sec), $^{249}104$ (half-life 3–4 sec), $^{255}104$ (half-life 185 sec), and $^{259}104$. The names dubium, kurchatorium (symbol Ku), and rutherfordium (symbol Rf) have been proposed. **e. 105,** an artificial element produced by bombardment of americium-243 with neon-22, occurring in three isotopes: 260 (half-life 1.6 sec), 261 (half-life 1.8 sec), and 262 (half-life 40 sec). The names hahnium and ekatantalum have been proposed. **e. 106,** an artificial element produced by bombarding californium-249 with oxygen-18 ions; it has one isotope: 263 (half-life 0.9 sec). **alkaline e.,** an element in group IA of the periodic table, including lithium, sodium, potassium, rubidium, and cesium. **alloy-forming e.,** see table at

ALLOY. **anatomic e.,** morphological e. **biogenic e.,** a chemical element contained in living tissue. **electronegative e.,** any chemical element that adds electrons (or tends to add electrons) during chemical combination. These are the elements with more than three valences, especially the nonmetals. **electropositive e.,** any of the chemical elements that lose electrons (or tend to lose electrons) during chemical combination, especially the light metals. **formed blood e.,** one of the cellular components of the blood: an erythrocyte, leukocyte, or blood platelet. **haloid e's,** elements in group VII of the periodic table, including fluorine, chlorine, bromine, and iodine. **inert e.,** an element that does not combine with other elements. Inert elements are found in group 0 of the periodic table and include the noble gases: helium, argon, krypton, xenon, and radon. See also noble GAS and noble METAL. **morphological e.,** any cell, fiber, or other of the ultimate structures which make up tissues and organs. Called also anatomic e. and tissue e. **nonmetallic e.,** nonmetal (1). **radioactive e.,** a chemical element which spontaneously transmutes into another element with emission of corpuscular or electromagnetic radiations. The natural radioactive elements are all those with atomic numbers above 83, and some other elements, such as potassium (atomic no 19) and rubidium (atomic no 37), which are very weakly radioactive. **rare e.,** rare EARTH. **tissue e.,** morphological e. **trace e's,** chemical elements distributed throughout the tissues of the body in very small amounts (traces). Traces of manganese, iron, copper, cobalt, and zinc, found in all organisms, are essential in nutrition; barium, aluminum, vanadium, molybdenum, iodine, silicon, and strontium are essential for only certain species. **tracer e.,** radioactive TRACER. **transcalifornium e's,** the elements with atomic numbers higher than that of californium (at no 98), which were discovered subsequent to the discovery of californium in 1950. They are einsteinium (99), fermium (100), mendelevium (101), nobelium (102), lawrencium (103), and elements 104, 105, and 106. **transuranic e's, transuranium e's,** the elements with atomic numbers higher than that of uranium (at no 92). Applied originally to neptunium (93), plutonium (94), americium (95), curium (96), berkelium (97), and californium (98), the term now, by definition, includes the transcalifornium elements as well.

PERIODIC TABLE OF SELECTED ELEMENTS

(From R. W. Phillips: Skinner's Science of Dental Materials. 7th ed. Philadelphia, W. B. Saunders Co., 1973; modified after A. W. Grosvenor (ed.): Basic Metallurgy Principles. Vol. I. Cleveland, American Society for Metals, 1954.)

elementary (el″ĕ-men′tah-re) 1. simple or fundamental. 2. not resolvable or divisible into simpler parts or components.

eleo- [Gr. *elaion* oil] a combining form denoting relationship to oil.

eleoma (el″e-o′mah) [*eleo-* + *oma*] a tumor or swelling caused by the injection of oil into the tissues.

elephantiasis (el″ĕ-fan-ti′ah-sis) abnormal thickening or swelling of any organ or tissue; especially massive swelling of the legs, which assume the appearance of elephant's legs, such as seen in filariasis due to subcutaneous edema caused by obstruction of lymphatic vessels by filarial parasites. **e. gingi′vae,** fibromatosis GINGIVAE. **e. graeco′rum,** leprosy.

elevation (el″ĕ-va′shun) 1. a raised area, or point of greater height. 2. the height to which something is raised. 3. the act of moving or raising to a higher position; lifting. **frontonasal e.,** frontonasal PROCESS. **nasolateral e.,** nasolateral PROCESS. **periosteal e.,** the separation of a mucoperiosteal flap from the bone, usually performed with a periosteal elevator. **tooth e.,** EXTRUSION (3).

elevator (el′ĕ-va″tor) [L. *elevare* to lift] 1. an instrument for elevating tissue, for removing osseous fragments, or for extracting teeth or their fragments. 2. dental e. **angular e.,** one in which the blade angles from the shank to the right or to the left. **Apexo E.,** trademark for a *wedge elevator.* **apical e.,** an instrument for removing fractured root tips retained in the apex of the tooth socket following tooth extraction. The shank of the instrument has an angle to provide access within the socket; an added barb on the tip is provided for reaching a fractured root tip. Called also *apical pick* and *root pick.* See illustration. **cross bar e.,** one in which the handle is at a right angle to the shank. Called also T-*bar e.* **Cryer e.,** an instrument used as a lever in tooth extraction to remove portions of the root of a tooth. **dental e.,** an instrument having a blade that engages the teeth or their roots and extracts teeth by elevating them from their alveoli through leverage applied to the handle. Elevators are used to luxate and remove teeth which cannot be engaged by the beaks or forceps, such as impacted or malposed teeth; to remove fractured or carious roots; to loosen teeth prior to application of forceps; to split teeth which have been grooved; and to remove intraradicular bone. A typical elevator consists of a handle, which may be a continuation of the shank or be placed at a right angle to it, a shank, and a blade. Elevators are generally classified as those used to remove the entire tooth (No. 1R-1L); to remove roots broken off at the gingival line (No. 81-4-5); to remove roots broken off halfway to the apex (No. 81-4-5, 14R-14L, or 11R-11L); to remove the apical third of the root

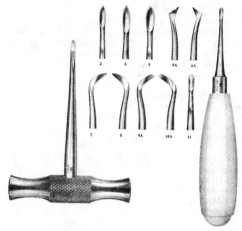

Tooth elevators. (From H. O. Torres and A. Ehrlich: Modern Dental Assisting. 2nd ed. Philadelphia, W. B. Saunders Co., 1980; courtesy of S. S. White Co.)

(apical fragment ejectors Nos. 1, 2, and 3); and to lift the mucoperiosteum. They may also be classified as straight, wedge, angular (right and left), and cross bar elevators. Called also *exolever.* See illustration. **Hu-Friedy E.,** trademark for a *dental elevator* or *periosteotome.* **malar e.,** an instrument used to elevate or reposition the malar or zygomatic bone and/or zygomatic arch. **Miller's e.,** a dental elevator having a slight curve at the end of the shank, which allows the blade to be inserted into the soft maxillary bone between the distal root of the second molar and the crown of the third. It is normally used for the removal of impacted maxillary third molar teeth. See also *Potts' e.* **Miller Apexo E.,** trademark for a *dental elevator.* **Molt e.,** a type of periosteotome. **Ohl e.,** a type of periosteotome. **periosteal e.,** periosteotome. **Potts' e.,** a variant of Miller's elevator that is smaller and weaker and has a T-bar. **root e.,** a dental elevator for extracting a fractured root of a tooth. Root elevators may be designed in pairs, a right and left, and as single, straight, mitered, or double ended. See illustration. **screw e.,** one designed to be screwed into a root canal for subsequent removal of the root, usually of the fractured apical third. **straight e.,** one in which the shank continues in a straight line with the handle. Straight elevators usually are available in various blade sizes and are gauged by the number given to the elevator, e.g., 301. **subperiosteal e.,** periosteotome. **T-bar e.,** cross bar e. **tooth e.,** see *dental e.* **wedge e.,** one used as a lever

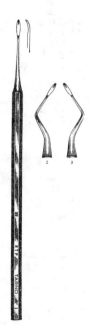

Apical elevator. (From H. O. Torres and A. Ehrlich: Modern Dental Assisting. 2nd ed. Philadelphia, W. B. Saunders Co., 1980; courtesy of S. S. White Co.)

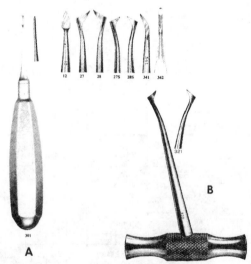

A, Assorted sizes and designs of root elevators. *B,* Alternate design of handle. "T" shape provides leverage when removing fractured roots. (From H. O. Torres and A. Ehrlich: Modern Dental Assisting. 2nd ed. Philadelphia, W. B. Saunders Co., 1980; courtesy of S. S. White Co.)

in tooth extraction, being placed in a hole drilled into the root of the tooth below the investing bony tissue to rework a tooth. **Woodson e.,** a type of periosteotome.

Elgiloy trademark for an iron-cobalt-chromium-nickel alloy (containing 16 percent iron), originally developed for watch springs; used in the production of orthodontic wires.

eligible (el′ĭ-jĕ-b′l) qualified; worthy of being chosen, accepted, adopted, etc. **board e.,** BOARD eligible.

eligibility (el″ĭ-jĕ-bil′ĭ-te) the state or quality of being eligible. **certificate of e., proof of e.,** CERTIFICATE of eligibility. **certification of e.,** CERTIFICATION of eligibility.

Elinol trademark for *fluphenazine.*

Elisal trademark for *sulthiame.*

Elite cement see under CEMENT.

elixir (ĕ-lik′ser) [L., from Arabic] a clear, sweetened, usually hydroalcoholic liquid containing flavoring substances and sometimes active medicinal agents, used orally as a vehicle or for the effect of the medicinal agent contained. **aromatic e.,** a solution containing 2.4 ml orange oil, 0.6 ml lemon oil, 0.24 ml coriander oil, 0.24 ml anise oil, 375 ml syrup, 30 gm talcum, 22 percent ethanol, and sufficient quantity of water to make 1000 ml. Used as a flavored vehicle for drugs. Called also *simple e.* **high-alcoholic e.,** a solution containing 4 ml compound orange spirit, 3 saccharin, 200 ml glycerol, and a sufficient quantity of ethanol to make 1000 ml. Used as a vehicle for drugs. **iso-e., iso-alcoholic e.,** a mixture of low- and high-alcoholic elixirs. When iso-elixir is specified, the proportion of its components is that which will produce a solution of the required alcohol strength. Used as a vehicle for drugs. **low-alcoholic e.,** a solution containing 10 ml compound orange spirit, 100 ml ethanol, 200 ml glycerol, 330 gm sucrose and a sufficient quantity of purified water to make 1000 ml. Used as a vehicle for drugs. **simple e.,** aromatic e.

Elkosin trademark for *sulfisomidine.*

ellipsoid (ĕ-lip′soid) having a spindle-shaped form; a structure with a spindle-like shape.

elliptocyte (ĕ-lip′to-sīt) an abnormal elliptical erythrocyte, such as is seen in elliptocytosis.

elliptocytosis (ĕ-lip″to-si-to′sis) a condition characterized by the presence of elliptocytes in the blood; especially hereditary elliptocytosis, which is a form of hemolytic anemia transmitted as a simple dominant trait, often associated with the Rh blood type. It occurs most commonly in families of Dutch, German, and Italian ancestry. Symptoms are usually mild but in some cases there may be splenomegaly, leg ulcers, and maxillofacial, dental, and cranial abnormalities.

Ellis-van Creveld syndrome [Richard White Bernhard *Ellis*, English pediatrician; S. *van Creveld*, Dutch pediatrician] chondroectodermal DYSPLASIA.

Elmex Protector trademark for a polyurethane pit and fissure sealant; see POLYURETHANE.

Elon trademark for a reducing substance in film-developing solution, which controls the detail of the film and brings up its image. See also developing SOLUTION and film PROCESSING.

elongation (e″long-ga′shun) 1. the act, process, or condition of increasing in length. 2. the ratio of the increase in length after fracture to the original gauge length, expressed in percent, in the ductility test (see DUCTILITY [2]). Called also *percentage e.* 3. pathologic migration of a tooth in the occlusal or incisal direction. See pathologic tooth MIGRATION. 4. a form of distortion in which a radiographic image is proportionally longer than the x-rayed subject. **percentage e.,** elongation (2). **tooth e.,** EXTRUSION (3).

Elschnig's syndrome [Anton *Elschnig*, German ophthalmologist, 1863–1939] see under SYNDROME.

Elspar trademark for *asparaginase.*

eluate (el′u-āt) the substance separated out by, or the product of, elution or elutriation.

eluent (e-lu′ent) a solution used in elution.

elution (e-lu′shun) [L. *e* out + *luere* to wash] in chemistry, the separation of material by washing, as in the freeing of an enzyme from its absorbent.

elutriation (e-lu″tre-a′shun) [L. *elutriare* to wash out] the operation of pulverizing substances and mixing them with water to separate the heavier constituents, which settle out in solution, from the lighter constituents.

Elzogram trademark for *cefazolin sodium* (see under CEFAZOLIN).

emaciation (e-ma″se-a′shun) [L. *emaciare* to make lean] excessive thinness due to undernourishment.

emanation (em-ah-na′shun) [L. *e* out + *manare* to flow] that which is given off, such as a gaseous disintegration product given off from radioactive substances or an affluvium.

embalming (em-bahm′ing) treating a corpse with various pre-servatives and antimicrobial preparations, to prevent decay and putrefaction.

embarrass (em-bar′as) to impede the function of; to obstruct.

Embden-Meyerhof pathway [Gustav *Embden*, German biochemist] see under PATHWAY.

embedding (em-bed′ing) 1. the fixation of a tissue specimen in a firm medium, in order to keep it intact during the cutting of thin sections. 2. implantation. 3. occurrence deep within surrounding structures.

embolectomy (em″bo-lek′to-me) [*embolus* + Gr. *ektomē* excision] surgical excision of an embolus from a blood vessel.

emboli (em′bo-li) [L.] plural of *embolus.*

embolic (em-bol′ik) pertaining to an embolus or to an embolism.

embolism (em′bo-lizm) [L. *embolismus*, from Gr. *en* in + *ballein* to throw] the formation of a blood clot (embolus) within a blood vessel, which is carried away by the blood stream from its point of origin to distant sites, producing occlusion of vessels and impairing the flow of the blood, and resulting in ischemic necrosis and infarction of tissue. Embolism differs from *thrombosis* in that in thrombosis the clot is stationary. **air e.,** gas e. **bacillary e.,** obstruction of a vessel by an aggregation of bacilli. **bone marrow e.,** embolism caused by material from a fractured bone. **cerebral e.,** embolism of a cerebral artery. **coronary e.,** embolism of one of the coronary arteries. **fat e.,** embolism due to the presence in the circulation of fat microglobules, occurring as a consequence of severe traumatic injuries to fat-laden tissues, such as fractures of bones containing fatty marrow or damage to the subcutaneous fat depots. **gas e.,** 1. embolism caused by bubbles of air that have entered the circulation. It may occur during delivery or abortion, being forced into ruptured venous system by uterine contractions; in pneumothorax during the rupture of a vein or artery; or during an injury to the lung or the chest wall with opening of a large vein into which air is forced during the negative pressure of inspiration. Air bubbles may occlude major vessels, including those of the lungs and brain, causing respiratory distress, neurological disorders, such as convulsions or coma, and sudden death. 2. minute bubbles formed by oxygen, carbon dioxide, and nitrogen liberated from solution in the blood during a rapid ascent from high to low pressure; while oxygen and carbon dioxide are rapidly reabsorbed, nitrogen may form bubbles within blood vessels and tissues. Called also *aeroembolism* and *air embolism.* See also decompression SICKNESS. **pantaloon e.,** saddle e. **pulmonary e.,** obstruction of the pulmonary artery or one of its branches by an embolus, often associated with pulmonary infarction. Most cases are caused by an embolus migrating from the veins in the left leg in phlebitis, particularly in patients recovering from surgery, but some instances result from fat emboli in bone injuries or valvular vegetation in the right atrium in chronic heart diseases. Sudden drop in blood pressure, pain in the chest, tightness across the chest, and dyspnea are the common signs. Death may follow when a massive embolus obstructs the flow in the pulmonary artery. See also pulmonary INFARCTION. **saddle e.,** an embolism lodging at the bifurcation of the aorta, causing sudden severe pain in the legs, abdomen, and back, with numbing and coldness. Called also *pantaloon e.* **systemic e.,** embolism in which emboli arise almost always in thrombi within the left ventricle, in myocardial infarction or other myocardioses, or within the left atrium, in rheumatic heart disease or surgical complications, and travel through the arterial circulation to lodge in smaller vessels of the brain, lower extremities, spleen, and kidneys.

embolus (em′bo-lus), pl. *em′boli* [Gr. *embolos* plug] a plug or clot in a blood vessel or in one of the heart cavities, formed by coagulation of the blood, and carried from the point of its formation to a distant site. The most common source of an embolus is a dislodged *thrombus.*

embrasure (em-bra′zhur) a space continuous with an interproximal space, produced by curvatures of teeth that are in contact in the same arch, which widen out from the contact area labially or bucally and lingually. Embrasures serve to provide a spillway for the escape of food during mastication, allow the flow of food away from the occlusal surfaces, over the gingival tissue, and toward the vestibular area, and make the teeth more self-cleansing because the rounded surfaces of the enamel of the crowns are more exposed to the cleansing action of foods, fluids, and the friction of the tongue, lips, and cheeks. Called also *spillway* and *interdental spillway.* See also interproximal SPACE. **buccal e.,** one that widens out from the area of contact toward the cheek between the molar and premolar teeth. **incisal**

e., occlusal e. **interdental e.**, the space formed by the interproximal contours of adjoining teeth, beginning at the contact area and extending lingually, facially, occlusally, and apically. **labial e.**, one that widens out from the area of contact toward the lips between the canine and incisor teeth. **lingual e.**, one that widens out from the area of contact toward the lingual sides of the teeth. **occlusal e.**, the space bounded by the marginal ridges as they join the cusps and incisal ridges. Called also *incisal e.*

embryo (em-bre-o) [Gr. *embryon*] 1. in plants, the element of the seed that develops into a new individual. 2. in animals, those derivatives of the fertilized ovum (zygote) that develop into offspring. Embryonic development begins with fertilization of an oocyte by a spermatozoon. The developing human is called an embryo until the end of the eighth week. Through the sexual reproduction and birth. It is primarily concerned with the study of development occurring during the first eight weeks after fertilization. In some animals, it extends beyond the incident of birth or hatching into the postnatal period, and it may include the larval development of some animals. See also ONTOGENY and PHYLOGENY. **comparative e.**, a comparison of the embryonic development of different animals one with another.

embryonal (em′bre-o-nal) pertaining to the embryo.

embryonic (em″bre-on′ik) of or pertaining to the embryo.

embryopathy (em″bre-op′ah-the) [*embryo* + Gr. *pathos* disease] a morbid condition or disease having its origin in a disorder occurring during embryonic development.

E/MC Ultrasonic trademark for an *ultrasonic denture cleanser* (see under CLEANSER).

Emedyl trademark for *dimenhydrinate.*

emergency (e-mer′jen-se) [L. *emergere* to raise up] an unlooked

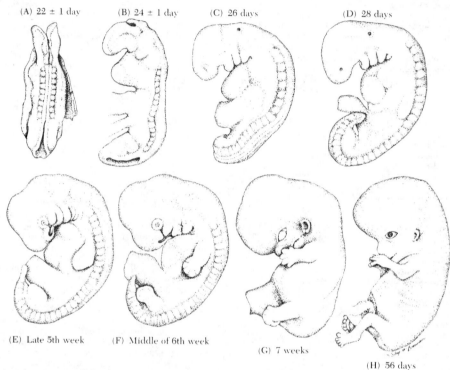

(A) 22 ± 1 day   (B) 24 ± 1 day   (C) 26 days   (D) 28 days

(E) Late 5th week   (F) Middle of 6th week   (G) 7 weeks   (H) 56 days

Human embryo at various stages of development. The relative size has been distorted to better show correspondence of parts. (From Dorland's Illustrated Medical Dictionary. 26th ed. Philadelphia, W. B. Saunders Co., 1981; adapted as follows: *A* and *D*, from photograph by Nislimura; *B*, from a drawing by Key; *C, E, F, G*, from Carnegie Collection.)

process of cell division, it becomes organized into primary embryonic layers (ectoderm, mesoderm, and entoderm), each differentiating into specialized tissues which form all organs of the body. The orofacial structures begin developing during the fifth week at the time when the embryo is about 5 mm in length, with the development of the branchial arches. Formation of the palate begins during the sixth week; the primary teeth begin to form during the seventh week when the embryo is about 12 mm in length; palatal shelves begin to develop during the eighth week, the tongue lying between the shelves; mandibular growth accelerates during the ninth week, followed by the tongue falling into space and the beginning of closure of the palate. See illustration. 3. in crystal formation, an unstable atomic aggregate forming in a supercooled liquid which gives rise to solidification nuclei in the process of crystallization, after having reached the critical radius when the volume-free energy balances the surface-free energy.

embryogenesis (em″bre-o-jen′ĕ-sis) [*embryo* + *genesis*] the process of embryonic development.

embryologist (em″bre-ol′o-jist) an expert in embryology.

embryology (em″bre-ol′o-je) [*embryo* + *-logy*] the science dealing with the origin and embryonic development of the body, including the study of the series of events taking place between the for or sudden occasion; an accident; an urgent or pressing need. **e. care**, emergency CARE. **e. care facility**, emergency ROOM. **e. dental care**, dental care, emergency; see under CARE. **medical e.**, any condition in which there is a danger of serious complications or death, and requiring immediate attention. See also artificial RESPIRATION, cardiac MASSAGE, emergency CARE, and RESUSCITATION.

emery (em′er-e) impure crystalline corundum mixed with iron oxides, used as an abrasive. See also dental DISK and grinding WHEEL.

Emeside trademark for *ethosuximide.*

emesis (em′ĕ-sis) [Gr. *emein* to vomit] vomiting.

emetic (ĕ-met′ik) [Gr. *emetikos*; L. *emeticus*] 1. bringing on or causing the act of vomiting. 2. an agent that causes vomiting.

emetine (em′ĕ-tin) the principal alkaloid of ipecac, 6′,7′,10,11-tetramethoxymetan, occurring as a white, light- and heat-sensitive powder that is soluble in methanol, ethanol, acetone, ethyl acetate, ether, and chloroform and sparingly soluble in water and petroleum ether. It has expectorant, emetic, and amebicidal properties. **e. hydrochloride**, the dihydrochloride salt of emetine, occurring as a white to yellowish, odorless, photosensitive, crystalline powder that is freely soluble in water and ethanol. Used chiefly in the treatment of amebiasis. Side effects may include diarrhea, nausea, vomiting, muscle weakness, stiffness, muscle pain, hypotension, precordial pain, dyspnea, and tachycardia.

Emetiral trademark for *prochlorperazine*.

emf electromotive FORCE.

EMG 1. electromyography. 2. exomphalos-macroglossia-gigantism. See Beckwith-Wiedemann SYNDROME.

emigration (em″ĭ-gra′shun) [L. *e* out + *migrare* to wander] 1. the act or process of leaving a region. 2. the escape of motile leukocytes from the blood vessels to reach the perivascular tissue, occurring during inflammatory and reparative processes in tissues; diapedesis.

eminence (em′ĭ-nens) [L. *eminentia*] a prominence or projection, especially one upon the surface of a bone. See also AGGER and EMINENTIA. **arcuate e.,** an arched prominence on the internal surface of the petrous bone in the floor of the middle cranial fossa, marking the position of the superior semicircular canal; it is particularly prominent in young skulls. Called also *e. of superior semicircular canal* and *eminentia arcuata* [NA]. **articular e. of temporal bone,** articular tubercle of temporal bone; see under TUBERCLE. **canine e.,** a prominent bony ridge overlying the root of either canine tooth on the labial surface of both the maxilla and the mandible. **e. of concha,** an eminence on the medial surface of the auricle that corresponds to the concha on the lateral surface. Called also *eminentia conc~ae* [NA]. **cruciate e.,** the cross-shaped bony prominence which divides the internal surface of the squama of the occipital bone into four fossae. It is formed by the intersection of the ridges associated with the sulci of the superior sagittal sinus and the transverse sinuses. The inferior division of the eminence is known as the *internal occipital crest.* Called also *cruciate line, eminentia cruciata,* and *eminentia cruciformis* [NA]. **facial e. of eminentia teres,** facial COLLICULUS. **frontal e.,** one of the slight rounded prominences on the frontal bone on either side above the eyes, forming the most prominent portions of the forehead. Called also *frontal tuber* and *tuber frontale* [NA]. **hypobranchial e.,** a median ventral elevation on the embryonic tongue formed by union of the second branchial arches; it represents the future root of the tongue. Called also *copula linguae.* **jugular e.,** jugular tubercle of occipital bone; see under TUBERCLE. **nasal e.,** the prominence above the root of the nose. **occipital e.,** a ridge in the lateral ventricle of the embryonic brain, corresponding to the occipital fissure in the adult. **parietal e.,** the somewhat laterally bulging prominence on either side of the sagittal suture, just superior to the superior temporal line of the external surface of the parietal bone. Called also *parietal tuber* and *tuber parietale* [NA]. **e. of superior semicircular canal,** arcuate e. **thyroid e.,** laryngeal PROMINENCE. **vagal e.,** TRIGONE of vagus nerve.

eminentia (em″ĭ-nen′she-ah), pl. *eminen′tiae* [L.] a general term used in anatomical nomenclature to designate a prominence or projection, especially one on the surface of a bone. See also AGGER and EMINENCE. **e. arcu′ata** [NA], arcuate EMINENCE. **e. articula′ris oss′sis tempora′lis,** articular tubercle of temporal bone; see under TUBERCLE. **e. con′chae** [NA], EMINENCE of concha. **e. crucia′ta, e. crucifor′mis** [NA], cruciate EMINENCE. **e. facia′lis,** facial COLLICULUS. **e. hypoglos′si,** TRIGONE of hypoglossal nerve. **e. jugula′ris,** jugular tubercle of occipital bone; see under TUBERCLE. **e. later′alis cartilag′inis cricoi′deae,** articular surface of cricoid cartilage; see under SURFACE. **e. sym′physis,** the prominent lower border of the middle of the chin. **e. te′res,** facial COLLICULUS. **e. va′gi,** TRIGONE of vagus nerve.

emissaria (em″ĭ-sa′re-ah) [L.] plural of *emissarium.*

emissarium (em″ĭ-sa′re-um), pl. *emissa′ria* [L. "drain"] emissary VEIN. **e. condyloi′deum,** emissary vein, condylar; see under VEIN. **e. mastoi′deum,** emissary vein, mastoid; see under VEIN. **e. occipita′le,** emissary vein, occipital; see under VEIN. **e. parieta′le,** emissary vein, parietal; see under VEIN.

emissary (em′ĭ-sa″re) [L. *emissarium* drain] affording an outlet, referring especially to the venous outlets from the dural sinuses through the skull. See emissary VEIN.

emission (e-mish′un) [L. *emissio* a sending out] the act or process of giving off or discharging. **photoelectric e.,** emission of secondary radiations following collision of an atom with high-energy photons of an x-ray beam, with resulting ejection of electrons (photoelectrons) from the atomic orbit and transfer of energy from the photon to photoelectrons. Called also *photoelectric effect.* See also coherent SCATTERING and Compton EFFECT. **radioactive e.,** the emission of particles or radiations from atoms of radioactive substances. See alpha PARTICLE, beta PARTICLE, and gamma rays, under RAY. **thermionic e.,** the release of electrons from an incandescent material, as the release of electrons in an x-ray tube when the tungsten cathode filament is heated by a low-voltage current.

Emivan trademark for *ethamivan*.

Emmo endomolare.

Emodin trademark for *ibuprofen*.

emollient (e-mol′ent) [L. *emolliens* softening, from *e* out + *mollis* soft] 1. softening or soothing. Called also *malactic.* 2. an agent, usually a fatty or oleaginous substance, which is applied to the skin or mucous membranes as a protective and for softening the skin and rendering it more pliable. Emollients protect inflamed or injured tissues from outside irritants or airborne bacteria and provide an occlusive film to prevent the protected tissues from drying by evaporation, but are used chiefly as vehicles for active drugs. The most commonly used emollients are vegetable and mineral oils, animal fats, and waxes.

Emp. abbreviation for L. *emplas′trum*, a plaster.

e.m.p. abbreviation for L. *ex mo′do prescrip′to*, as directed.

emphraxis (em-frak′sis) [Gr.] a stoppage or obstruction.

emphysema (em″fĭ-se′mah, em″fĭ-ze′mah) [Gr. "an inflation"] abnormal accumulation of air in tissues or organs, particularly in the lungs. **cervicofacial e.,** interstitial emphysema of the cervicofacial area, characterized by a unilateral swelling of the face and/or neck, which occurs rapidly and is generally associated with pain, particularly during the first few days. A variety of dental procedures may be the cause, including tooth extraction, blowing of compressed air into a root canal or into a periodontal pocket, or blowing of air from a high-speed air-rotor machine. It may also occur after middle-face fractures or, spontaneously, as a result of breathing actions following some types of surgical procedures, or any type of a tissue break permitting air to enter connective tissue spaces. **interstitial e.,** the presence of air in the connective tissue stroma, usually of the lungs, mediastinum, or subcutaneous tissue.

Empiral trademark for an analgesic preparation containing aspirin, phenacetin, and phenobarbital.

Empiric [Gr. *empeirikos* experienced] 1. the second of the post-hippocratic schools of medicine, which arose in the second century B.C., under the leadership of Philinos of Cos and Serapion of Alexandria. As opposed to Dogmatists, the Empirics declared that the search for the ultimate causes of phenomena was vain, but they were active in endeavoring to discover the immediate causes. They paid particular attention to the totality of symptoms. In their search for a line of treatment to benefit a particular set of symptoms they employed the "tripod of Empirics": (1) their own chance observations — their own experience; (2) learning obtained from contemporaries and predecessors — the experience of others; and (3) in cases of new diseases, the formation of conclusions from other diseases which they resembled — analogy. The Empirics paid great attention to clinical observation, and were guided in their methods of treatment almost entirely on experience. Called also *empiricism.* 2. a believer in or practitioner of the Empiric school of medicine.

empiric (em-pir′ik) 1. empirical. 2. a practitioner whose skill is based on experience and observation, rather than formal education. See also CHARLATAN.

empirical (em-pir′ĕ-kal) based on experience and observation.

empiricism (em-pir′ĭ-sizm) [Gr. *empeirikos* experienced] 1. the Empiric school of medicine. See EMPIRIC (1). 2. reliance on experience and observation. 3. quackery.

Empirin trademark for an analgesic preparation, one tablet of which contains 230 mg aspirin, 150 mg phenacetin, 30 mg caffeine, and excipients.

empyema (em″pi-e′mah) [Gr. *empyēma*] accumulation of pus in a body cavity. **mastoid e.,** suppurative inflammation of the mucous lining of the cavities of the mastoid process.

EMS Emergency Medical Service.

emul. abbreviation for L. *emul′sum*, emulsion.

emulgent (ĕ-mul′jent) emulsifier.

emulsifier (ĕ-mul″sĭ-fi′er) a substance used for rendering an emulsion more stable by reducing the surface tension or protecting the drops with a film, as a protective colloid which causes globules in an emulsion to remain suspended for an indefinite period, such as a phosphoric acid attaching itself to the protein molecule and counteracting the hydrophobic character of fat, thus stabilizing an emulsion and converting one that is temporary into the permanent state. Called also *emulgent* and *emulsifying agent.*

emulsify (ĕ-mul′sĭ-fi) To convert or to be converted into an emulsion.

emulsion (ĕ-mul′shun) [L. *emulsion, emulsum*] 1. any colloidal suspension of one liquid in another. 2. an emulsion for which official pharmaceutic standards have been promulgated, including cod liver oil emulsion, cod liver oil emulsion with malt, liquid petrolatum emulsion, and phenolphthalein in liquid petrolatum emulsion. **double e.**, a photographic emulsion of silver halide salts impregnated in gelatin and coated on both sides of a radiographic film base. **exposed film e.**, see film DEVELOPMENT. **e. ointment**, emulsion OINTMENT. **permanent e.**, one, such as milk and cream, in which globules remain suspended permanently. **photographic e.**, a light- and radiation-sensitive gelatinous coating incorporating silver halide, which is applied to film. Called also *silver e.* **silver e.**, photographic e. **single e.**, a photographic emulsion of silver halide salts impregnated in gelatin and coated only on one side of a radiographic film base. **temporary e.**, one, such as oil and water, in which globules remain suspended for a short time and the two liquids separate. Addition of some types of colloids, emulsifying agents, will coat the globules of the fat or oil and prevent them from running together, thereby converting a temporary emulsion to a permanent one. **x-ray film e.**, an emulsion of dehydrated suspension of silver bromide in gelatin coated on both sides of x-ray film. See x-ray FILM.

emulsoid (ē-mul′soid) emulsion colloid; see COLLOID (2).

E-Mycin trademark for *erythromycin estolate* (see under ERYTHROMYCIN).

enamel (en-am′el) 1. the glazed surface of baked porcelain, metal, or pottery. 2. any hard, smooth, glossy coating or enamel-like surface. 3. dental e. **aprismatic e.**, the outer stratum of the dental enamel, a few microns in thickness, believed by some to consist of a solid layer without enamel prisms; others believe that the initial deposits (layers) of enamel are also aprismatic. **ceramic e.**, porcelain or glass fused directly to a cast alloy crown shell that fits the prepared tooth. See also metal-ceramic RESTORATION. **cervical e.**, that part of the dental enamel which envelops the cervical portion of a tooth. It is characterized by short enamel prisms, better definition of the incremental lines and the perikymata than in other parts of the tooth, and the horizontal orientation of the enamel prisms in the deciduous teeth. **e. cleaner**, acid ETCHANT. **curled e.**, dental enamel in which the columns are bent and are wavy and intertwined with one another. Called also *gnarled e.* Cf. *straight e.* **dental e.**, a hard thin translucent layer of calcified substance which envelops and protects the dentin of the crown of the tooth. It is the hardest substance in the body and is almost entirely composed of calcium salts (95–96 percent); organic content, mostly protein (0.2–1.0 percent); and water (3.9–4.3 percent). Under the microscope, it is composed of thin rods (enamel prisms) held together by cementing substance, and surrounded by an enamel sheath. Called also *adamantine layer, adamantine substance, adamas dentis, enamelum* [NA], *stratum adamantinum*, and *substantia adamantina dentis.* **dwarfed e.**, nanoid e. **e. excrescence**, 1. enamel SPUR. 2. enameloma. **e. fissure**, FISSURE (2). **gnarled e.**, curled e. **hereditary brown e.**, AMELOGENESIS imperfecta. **hypoplastic e.**, enamel HYPOPLASIA. **mottled e.**, a chronic endemic form of hypoplasia of the dental enamel caused by drinking water with a high fluorine content during the time of tooth formation, and characterized by defective calcification that gives a white chalky appearance to the enamel, which gradually undergoes brown discoloration. Called also *dentes de Chiaie, fluorosis, mottled teeth*, and *Spira's disease.* **nanoid e.**, imperfectly formed dental enamel which is thinner than normal. Called also *dwarfed e.* **opaque e.**, see enamel HYPOCALCIFICATION. **e. spur**, enamel SPUR. **straight e.**, dental enamel having straight rods, as distinguished from those in gnarled enamel. Cf. *curled e.* **white e.**, see enamel HYPOCALCIFICATION.

enameloblast (en-am″el-o-blast) ameloblast.

enameloma (en-am″el-o′mah) [*enamel + -oma*] a non-neoplastic excrescence sometimes found at the bifurcation of a multirooted tooth, at the end of an enamel spur, or on the root surface, which may be composed only of enamel, contain a small dentin nucleus or core, or contain a minute strand of dentin and pulp. Called also *enamel drop, enamel droplet, enamel excrescence, enamel nodule*, and *enamel pearl.*

enameloplasty (en-am″el-o-plas′te) the contouring of the enamel surface of a tooth performed with a fine-finish diamond point in the air turbine handpiece, as in smoothing the cavosurface margin or in removing developmental grooves or defects that are less than 1/3 the enamel thickness.

enamelum (en-am′el-um) [NA] dental ENAMEL.

enanthem (en-an′them) enanthema.

enanthema (en″an-the′ma), pl. *enanthemas, enanthem′ata* [Gr. *en* in + *anthema* a blossoming] a lesion of or eruption on a mucous membrane. Called also *enanthem.*

enantiomorph (en-an′te-o-morf′) [Gr. *enantios* opposite + *morphē* form] a compound exhibiting, or capable of exhibiting, enantiomorphism; an enantiomorphic isomer.

enantiomorphic (en-an″te-o-mor′fik) pertaining to or exhibiting enantiomorphism.

enantiomorphism (en-an″te-o-mor′fizm) [Gr. *enantios* opposite + *morphē* form] a special type of optical isomerism in which a nonsuperimposable, mirror-image relationship exists at all times between the respective molecules of the compounds. Enantiomorphic isomers always rotate the plane of polarized light to the same degree, but in opposite directions; otherwise most of their chemical and physical properties are identical. The molecules are always asymmetric, very often as the result of possession of one or more asymmetric carbon atoms. Thus, lactic acid, $CH_3CHOHCOOH$, possessing one such carbon atom, exists in both a *dextro* and a *levo* form. The molecules of some enantiomorphic compounds (e.g., certain biphenyl or spirane compounds) are asymmetric as a whole, but do not possess any asymmetric carbon atoms. Cf. DIASTEREOISOMERISM.

en bloc (ahn blok′) [Fr.] in a lump; as a whole.

encapsulation (en-kap″su-la′shun) 1. any act of inclosing in a capsule. 2. a physiologic process of inclosure in a sheath made up of a substance not normal to the part.

encephalitides (en″sef-ah-lit′ĭ-dēz) plural of *encephalitis*.

encephalitis (en″sef-ah-li′tis), pl. *encephalit′ides* [*encephalo-* + *-itis*] inflammation of the brain tissue. Sometimes called *cephalitis.* **acute primary hemorrhagic e.**, Strümpell-Leichtenstern e. **acute serous e.**, Brown-Symmers DISEASE. **Bickerstaff's e.**, **brain stem e.**, a syndrome consisting of a prodromal malaise followed by a downward progression of midbrain disturbances with almost complete suppression of all functions related to brain stem innervation, but without cardiac or respiratory disorders. Clinically, it is manifested by drowsiness, headache, defective conjugate movements, diplopia, and nystagmus. Most cases are associated with ophthalmoplegia, deafness, and palsy of the trigeminal nerve, and facial palsy is almost always present. Herpes simplex virus is suspected as a pathogenic agent. Called also *brain stem e.* **Strümpell-Leichtenstern e.**, acute hemorrhagic encephalitis characterized by necrosis, hemorrhage, and demyelination of the white matter. Symptoms include fever, headache, and cough; stupor, confusion, disorientation, and hallucinations; hemihypesthesia, hemiparesis, quadriplegia, facial palsy, and nuchal rigidity; diplopia and papilledema; and dysphasia. Viral infection, allergy, and toxic reaction have been suggested as possible etiologic factors. Called also *acute primary hemorrhagic e.*

encephalo- [Gr. *enkephalos* brain] a combining form denoting relationship to the brain.

encephalocele (en-sef′ah-lo-sēl″) [*encephalo-* + Gr. *kēlē* hernia] protrusion of the dura mater through a cranium bifidum or a traumatic opening in the cranium. See also MENINGOENCEPHALOCELE. **sincipetal e.**, encephalocele with protrusion of the brain substance through a cranial defect in the superior and anterior part of the skull, usually located between the nasal and frontal bones.

encephalography (en-sef′ah-log′rah-fe) [*encephalo-* + Gr. *graphein* to write] roentgenographic examination of the brain. See also PNEUMOENCEPHALOGRAPHY.

encephalon (en-sef′ah-lon) [Gr. *enkephalos*] the brain.

encephalopathy (en-sef′ah-lop′ah-the) [*encephalo-* + Gr. *pathos* disease] any disease of the brain. **acute thyrotoxic e.**, Waldenström's DISEASE. **Wernicke's e.**, a syndrome consisting of listlessness, disorientation, hallucinations, restlessness, and other symptoms of delirium tremens; oculomotor paralysis; and ataxia. The brain lesions, which are bilateral, involve the gray matter around the third and fourth ventricles and the aqueduct of Sylvius, marked by pinhead-sized petechial hemorrhages, congested capillaries, and proliferation of the capillaries. It is caused by a thiamine deficiency with chronic alcoholism as a contributing factor, but it may occur as a complication of other disorders, such as pernicious vomiting of pregnancy and gastric carcinoma. Called also *Wernicke's disease.*

enchondroma (en″kon-dro′mah) [Gr. *en* in + *chondros* cartilage + *-oma*] a benign chondromatous tumor made up of mature hyaline cartilage, occurring within the interior of small bones, usually of the hands and feet, but sometimes also in the long bones, and less commonly in the skull and pelvis. It is a firm, slightly lobulated, round, glassy, grayish-blue translucent lesion embedded within the spongiosa, and is composed of small masses or nodules of hyaline cartilage, separated by a scant fibrous stroma. Called also *true chondroma.* 2. see pleomorphic ADENOMA. **e. of jaws**, chondroma.

enchylema (en″ki-le′mah) [Gr. *en* in + *chylos* juice] hyaloplasm (1).

enchyma (en'kĭ-mah) [Gr. *en* in + *chymos* juice] the substance elaborated from absorbed nutritive materials; the formative juice of the tissues.

enclave (en'klāv, ahn-klahv') [Fr.] a tissue detached from its normal connection and enclosed within another organ or tissue.

Encorton trademark for *prednisone*.

encranius (en-kra'ne-us) [Gr. *en* in + *kranion* skull] a teratoid parasitic twin located within the cranium of the autosite.

encysted (en-sist'ed) [Gr. *en* in + *kystis* sac, bladder] encapsulated, enclosed within the walls of a cyst, sac, or bladder.

end (end) 1. either extremity or edge of anything that has length. 2. endoreduplication; see also CHROMOSOME nomenclature. **distal e. of denture,** the most posterior part of a removable dental restoration. Called also *denture heel* and *heel of denture*. See also FLANGE (2).

end- see ENDO-.

endarteritis (end″ar-ter-i'tis) [end- + Gr. *artēria* + -*itis*] arteritis characterized by inflammation of the intima of an artery. **e. oblit'erans,** narrowing of the small arteries caused by an increase in the fibrous tissue of the intima. Called also *arteritis obliterans*.

Endecril trademark for *ethacrinic acid* (see under ACID).

endemic (en-dem'ik) [Gr. *endēmos* dwelling in a place] a disease of low morbidity that is constantly present in a human community.

endemiology (en-de″me-ol'o-je) [*endemic* + -*logy*] the field of study dealing with the occurrence of endemic diseases.

endemy (en'de-me) an endemic disease.

endergonic (end″er-gon'ik) characterized by or accompanied by the absorption of energy; pertaining to processes which involve energy flowing into the system. Cf. EXERGONIC.

enderon (en'der-on) [Gr. *en* in + *deros* skin] the deeper part of the skin (corium) or mucous membrane, as distinguished from the epithelium or epidermis.

Enders, John Franklin [born 1897] an American microbiologist; co-winner, with Frederick C. Robbins and Thomas H. Weller, of the Nobel prize for medicine and physiology in 1954, for the discovery that poliomyelitis viruses multiply in human tissue.

end-feet (end'fēt) synaptic TERMINAL.

ending (end'ing) the terminal portion of something; the termination. **annulospiral e's,** wide, ribbon-like sensory nerve endings, which are wrapped around the fibers of a nerve fiber ending in the vertebrate central nervous system. **encapsulated nerve e's,** terminal nerve corpuscles; see under CORPUSCLE. **epilemmal e's,** sensory nerve endings in striated muscle in which the nerve endings are in close contact with the muscle fibers but do not penetrate the sarcolemma. **flower-spray e's,** branched, slender sensory nerve endings on the sarcolemma of muscle spindles. **free nerve e's,** neural receptors consisting of small knobs or disks formed by anastomoses of fine fibrillae branching off nerve fibers, which loose their myelin sheath near their endings and their neurilemma at their endings, terminating as free, branching endings. They are found in the epidermis and in the epithelium covering certain mucous membranes, and are believed to serve as receptors for temperature and pain. Called also *terminationes nervorum liberae* [NA]. **grape e's,** sensory nerve endings in muscle which have the form of terminal swellings. **nerve e.,** a fine branchlike termination of an axon. **synaptic e's,** synaptic terminals; see under TERMINAL.

endo-, end- [Gr. *endon* within] a prefix denoting an inward situation, within. See also terms beginning ENTO-.

endoblast (en'do-blast) [*endo-* + Gr. *blastos* germ] entoblast. See ENTODERM.

endocarditis (en″do-kar-di'tis) [*endocardium* + -*itis*] inflammation of the endocardium, usually a complication of rheumatic fever and, sometimes, of other febrile diseases.

endocardium (en″do-kar'de-um) [*endo-* + Gr. *kardia* heart] the inner endothelial lining of heart cavities and the connective tissue bed on which it lies.

endoceliac (en″do-se'le-ak) [*endo-* + Gr. *koilia* cavity] inside a body cavity.

endocellular (en″do-sel'u-lar) within a cell.

endochondral (endo″kon'dral) occurring inside or within cartilage.

endochondrosarcoma (en″do-kon″dro-sar-ko'mah) central CHONDROSARCOMA.

endocranial (endo-kra'ne-al) situated within the cranium.

endocranium (en″do-kra'ne-um) [*endo-* + Gr. *kranion* skull] the endosteal outer layer of the dura mater of the brain.

endocrine (en'do-krin) [*endo-* + Gr. *krinein* to separate] 1. secreting internally. 2. pertaining to internal secretions. 3. pertaining to endocrine glands (see under GLAND). Cf. EXOCRINE.

endocrinology (en″do-krĭ-nol'o-je) [*endocrine* + -*logy*] the study of the endocrine system and its role in the functioning and in the diseases of the body.

endocyte (en'do-sīt) [*endo-* + Gr. *kytos* hollow vessel] any cell inclusion.

endocytosis (en″do-si-to'sis) [*endo-* + Gr. *kytos* hollow vessel] 1. the uptake by a cell of particles that are too large to diffuse through its wall; the opposite of exocytosis. 2. the process whereby a phagocytic cell contacts a foreign body, invaginates at the site of plasma membrane contact with the foreign body, becomes pinched-off, and results in the containment of the foreign body in a vacuole within the cytoplasm. See also PHAGOCYTOSIS.

endoderm (en'do-derm) [*endo-* + Gr. *derma* skin] See entoderm.

endodontia (en″do-don'she-ah) a former synonym of *endodontics*.

endodontic (en″do-don'tik) of or pertaining to endodontics.

endodontics (en″do-don'tiks) [end- + Gr. *odous* tooth + -*ics*] that branch of dentistry concerned with the etiology, prevention, diagnosis, and treatment of diseases and injuries that affect the dental pulp, tooth root, and periapical tissue. In current terminology, the term *endodontics* is used in a more restrictive sense than the term *endodontology*, which comprises the scientific study of the dental pulp and associated processes in health and disease. But, sometimes, the terms are used interchangeably. Formerly called *endodontia*. The endodontic armamentarium includes root canal instruments (see root canal THERAPY) and various other instruments and equipment, including mirrors, pliers, syringes, incubators, and sterilization devices. **pedodontic e.,** endodontic diagnosis and therapy as applied to the mixed dentition (primary and permanent) of children and adolescents. **surgical e.,** treatment of diseases and injuries of the dental pulp through the use of surgical methods, including trephination, marsupialization, apicoectomy, retrofilling, root fracture fixation, hemisection, and root amputation.

endodontist (en″do-don'tist) a dentist who specializes in or limits his practice to endodontics. Called also *endodontologist*.

endodontium (en″do-don'she-um) [end- + Gr. *odous* tooth] dental PULP.

endodontologist (en″do-don-tol'o-jist) endodontist.

endodontology (en″do-don-tol'o-je) the scientific study of the dental pulp and associated processes in health and disease. In current terminology, the term *endodontology* is used in a broader sense than the term *endodontics*, which is restricted to the etiology, prevention, diagnosis, and treatment of disease and injuries of the dental pulp and associated processes. But, sometimes, the terms are used interchangeably.

endodontoma (en″do-don-to'mah) tooth resorption, internal; see under RESORPTION.

endogenous (en-doj'ĕ-nus) [*endo-* + Gr. *gennan* to produce] 1. growing from within. 2. developing or originating within the organism, or arising from causes within the organism.

endognathion (en″do-na'the-on) [*endo-* + Gr. *gnathos* jaw] the inner segment of the incisive bone.

endointoxication (en″do-in-tok″sĭ-ka'shun) poisoning caused by an endogenous toxin.

endolaryngeal (en″do-lah-rin'je-al) [*endo-* + Gr. *larynx*] situated on or occurring within the larynx.

endolarynx (en'do-lar″inks) the interior or cavity of the larynx.

endolymph (en'do-limf) [*endo-* + *lymph*] the fluid contained in the membranous labyrinth of the ear.

endolysis (en-dol'ĭ-sis) [*endo-* + Gr. *lysis* dissolution] dissolution or breaking up of the cytoplasm of a cell.

endomastoiditis (en″do-mas″toi-di'tis) inflammation within the mastoid cavity and cells.

endomesenchyme (en″do-mes'eng-kīm) [*endo-* + *mesenchyme*] see MESENCHYME.

endomesoderm (en″do-mes'o-derm) [*endo-* + Gr. *mesos* middle + *derma* skin] see MESENCHYMA.

Endometer trademark for an electronic device for root canal measurement, determining the length of the canal by reading the electropotential of the periodontal ligament.

endometria (en″do-me'tre-ah) [Gr.] plural of *endometrium*.

endometrium (en-do-me'tre-um), pl. *endom'tria* [*endo-* + Gr. *metra* uterus] [NA alternative] the inner mucous membrane of the uterus. Its thickness varies with the phases of the menstrual cycle. From implantation through the first three months of pregnancy, it is divided into the basal, capsular, and parietal decidua (see DECIDUA). Called also *tunica mucosa uteri* [NA].

endometry (en-dom'ĕ-tre) [*endo-* + Gr. *metron* measure] the measurement of the capacity of a cavity.

endomolare (en″do-mo-la're) in cephalometry, the most lingual or palatal margins of the alveoli of the permanent upper second molars.

endomorph (en'do-morf) [*endo*derm + Gr. *morphē* form] an individual having the type of body build in which tissues derived from the endoderm predominate. There is relative preponderance of soft roundness throughout the body, with large digestive viscera and accumulations of fat, and with large trunk and thighs and tapering extremities, as contrasted with ectomorph and mesomorph.

endomysium (en″do-mis′e-um) [endo- + Gr. *mys* muscle] a sheath of delicate reticulum which surrounds individual muscle fibers.

endonasal (en″do-na′zal) within the nose.

endoneurium (en″do-nu′re-um) [endo- +Gr. *neuron* nerve] the interstitial connective tissue in a peripheral nerve, separating the individual nerve fibers.

endonuclear (en″do-nu′kle-ar) within a nucleus.

endoparasite (en″do-par′ah-sīt) [endo- + Gr. *parasitos* parasite] a parasite that lives within the body of its host.

endopeptidase (en″do-pep′tī-dās) [endo- + *peptide* + -ase ending denoting an enzyme] proteinase.

endophasia (en″do-fa′ze-ah) the silent reproduction of a word or words.

endophlebitis (en″do-fle-bi′tis) [endo- + Gr. *phleps* vein + -itis] inflammation of the intima of a vein.

endophyte (en′do-fīt) [endo- + Gr. *phyton* plant] a microorganism living in symbiosis with plants; a parasitic organism living within the body of its host.

endoplasm (en′do-plazm) [endo- + Gr. *plasma* something formed] the central portion of the cytoplasm of a cell.

endoplasmic (en″do-plas′mik) composed of or pertaining to endoplasm.

endoplast (en′do-plast) [endo- + Gr. *plassein* to form] the cell nucleus.

endoradiosonde (en″do-ra″de-o-sond′) a small radio transmitter inserted within a body cavity or tube, as within the intestinal lumen to measure the pressure.

endoreduplication (en″do-re-du″plī-ka′shun) replication of the chromosomes without subsequent cell division. Abbreviated *end.*

end-organ (end′or-gan) one of the larger, encapsulated endings of the sensory nerves.

endorhinitis (en″do-ri-ni′tis) [endo- + Gr. *rhis* nose + -itis] inflammation of the lining membrane of the nasal passages.

endorphin (en-dor′fin, en′dor-fin) an endogenous peptide which mimics the action of morphine in the nervous system. Found in the brain, cerebrospinal fluid, pituitary gland, and other vertebrate organs. Believed to be a neurological modular or transmitter. A specific pentapeptide endorphin is known as an *enkephalin.*

endorsement (en-dors′ment) 1. approval or sanction. 2. the placing of one's signature on a contract or other document to signify approval of it. 3. in licensure of health professions, the recognition by a state of a license given by another state, when the qualifications and standards required by the original licensing state are equivalent to or higher than those of the endorsing state. See also RECIPROCITY (2).

endoskeleton (en″do-skel′ĕ-ton) [endo- + *skeleton*] the bony and cartilaginous skeleton of the body, exclusive of that part of the skeleton which is of dermal origin. Called also *neuroskeleton.*

endosmosis (en″dos-mo′sis) [end- +Gr. *ōsmos* impulsion] a movement in liquids separated by a membranous or porous septum, by which one fluid passes through the septum into the cavity which contains another fluid of different density.

endospore (en′do-spōr) [endo- +Gr. *sporos* seed] a resting spore produced endogenously by bacteria, which is usually characterized by fine structures and resistance to heat, chemicals, and adverse environmental factors.

endosteal (en-dos′te-al) pertaining to the endosteum; occurring or located within a bone.

endosteitis (en-dos″te-i′tis) inflammation of the endosteum.

endosteum (en-dos′te-um) [endo- + Gr. *osteon* bone] a layer of vascular areolar tissue lining the wall of the bone marrow cavity and the haversian canals of compact bone and covering the trabeculae of spongy bone. During the developmental quiescence, the tissue is similar to the bone marrow but during the active periods, it is characterized by the presence of osteoclasts and osteoblasts. It has both hematopoietic and osteogenic capabilities and takes an active part in depositing new bone, eroding the existing one, and in healing fractures. Called also *medullary membrane.*

endothelia (endo-the′le-ah) [Gr.] plural of *endothelium.*

endothelial (en″do-the′le-al) pertaining to or made up of endothelium.

endothelialization (en″do-the″le-al-i-za′shun) the healing of the inner surfaces of vessels or grafts by endothelial cells.

endothelioma (en″do-the″le-o′mah) [*endothelium* + -oma] a tumor which originates from the endothelium. Called also *endothelial cancer.* See pleomorphic ADENOMA.

endothelium (en″do-the′le-um), pl. *endothe′lia* [endo- + Gr. *thēlē* nipple] [NA] a layer of epithelial cells of mesodermal origin, which lines the cavities of the heart and of the blood and lymph vessels, and the serous cavities of the body.

endothermic (en″do-ther′mik) [endo- + Gr. *thermē* heat] characterized by or accompanied by the absorption of heat. Cf. EXOTHERMIC.

endotoxin (en″do-tok′sin) a heat-stable toxin present in the bacterial cell but not in cell-free filtrates of cultures of intact bacteria. Endotoxins are found primarily in gram-negative organisms, in which they are identical with the somatic antigen. They occur in the cell wall as a lipopolysaccharide complex extractable in trichloracetic acid and glycols. Endotoxins are pyrogenic and increase capillary permeability, their activity being substantially the same regardless of the species of bacteria from which they are derived. Called also *bacterial pyrogen.* Cf. EXOTOXIN.

endovenous (en″do-ve′nus) intravenous.

Endoxan trademark for *cyclophosphamide.*

end-piece (end′pēs) in early immunological theory, the pseudoglobulin fraction of guinea pig serum, which remains soluble when electrolytes are removed from serum; it does not combine directly with antibody-coated erythrocytes and corresponds to the C2 component of complement.

end-plate (end′plāt) end PLATE.

end point, end-point (end point) end POINT.

Endrate trademark for *edetate disodium* (see under EDETATE).

end-section (end-sek′shun) end SECTION.

Enduron trademark for *methyclothiazide.*

-ene a chemical suffix used to indicate an unsaturated hydrocarbon containing one double bond.

energy (en′er-je) [Gr. *energeia*] the ability to do work. Energy exists in various forms, each of which may be converted into any of the other forms; heat, light, motion, sound, and electricity being forms of energy. To measure the amount of energy in any of its forms, it is ordinarily converted to heat energy and expressed in calories. The accepted SI unit of energy is the joule. See also tables at SI. **activation e.,** the energy required to displace atoms with a low energy level with those with a higher energy. See also DIFFUSION (2). **atomic e.,** 1. the internal energy of the atom which was absorbed when it was formed. 2. energy that can be liberated by changes in the nucleus of an atom (as by fission of a heavy nucleus or fusion of light nuclei into heavier ones with accompanying loss of mass). Called also *nuclear e.* **binding e.,** the minimum energy required to dissociate the nucleus, or to displace its components. Binding energy of a nucleus is the energy required to dissociate into its component neutrons and protons; neutron and/or proton binding energies are those required to remove a neutron or proton, respectively, from a nucleus; electron binding energy is that required to remove an electron from an atom or a molecule. **biologic e., biotic e.,** the form of energy peculiar to living matter, i.e., energy produced by biologic processes. See illustration. **chemical e.,** the energy that is stored up in chemical substances and is released or consumed during chemical changes. See also *endothermic e.* and *exothermic e.* **endothermic e.,** a thermodynamic process in a chemical reaction which consumes heat. **exothermic e.,** a thermodynamic process in a chemical reaction which yields heat to the surroundings. **free e.,** the energy equal to the maximum amount of work that can be obtained from a

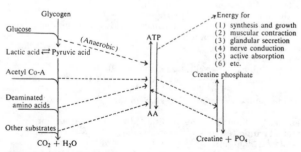

Overall schema of energy transfer from foods to the adenylic acid (AA) system and then to the functional elements of the cells. (From A. C. Guyton: Textbook of Medical Physiology. 6th ed. Philadelphia, W. B. Saunders Co., 1981.)

process occurring under conditions of fixed temperature and pressure. See also ENTROPY (2). **ionizing e.,** the average energy lost by ionizing radiation in producing an ion pair in a gas. **kinetic e.,** energy in action or actually performing a task. **lattice e.,** the forces which hold the atoms together in a crystal. See also metallic BOND. **nuclear e.,** atomic e. **photon e.,** electromagnetic energy in the form of photons, with a value in ergs equal to the product of their frequency in cycles per second and Planck's constant (E = hν). Symbol hν. **e. of position, potential e.,** available energy at rest, which is not involved in actual work. **radiant e.,** the energy of electromagnetic waves, such as radio waves, visible light, x-rays, or gamma rays. **stabilization e.,** the variation of the force of interaction, or the energy of interaction, between the atoms in a molecule, being related to the internuclear separation of the atoms. **surface e.,** the product of multiplication of surface tension by the two-thirds power of the molecular weight and specific volume. One of the parameters that influence the ability of an adhesive to bond to the surface of an adherent. The higher the surface energy, the more likely adhesion will occur and vice versa.

enflurane (en′floo-rān) a nonflammable, nonvolatile inhalation anesthetic, 2-chloro-1,1,2-trifluoroethyl difluoromethyl ether, occurring as a clear liquid with a sweetish ethereal odor, which is soluble in water and miscible with organic solvents. It is contraindicated in patients with liver and biliary tract diseases. Central nervous system excitation may occur in deep anesthesia. The flow of saliva is not increased by enflurane anesthesia. Trademark: Enthrane.

Engel's alkalimetry [Rodolphe Charles *Engel*, Alsatian chemist, 1850–1916] see under ALKALIMETRY.

Engelmann's disk [Theodor Wilhelm *Engelmann*, German physiologist, 1843–1909] H ZONE.

engine (en′jin) a machine by which energy is converted into mechanical motion. **e. arm,** engine ARM. **dental e.,** a machine operated by electricity, water, or compressed air, which provides power for rotary dental instruments. **high-speed e.,** a machine that provides power to a high-speed handpiece which operates at speeds above 12,000 rpm. **surgical e.,** a machine that provides power for rotary surgical instruments. **ultraspeed e.,** a machine that provides power for ultra–high-speed handpieces operating at speeds of 100,000 to 300,000 rpm.

engineering (en′ji-nēr′ing) 1. the practical application of sciences such as physics, chemistry, mathematics, etc. 2. the action, work, or profession dealing with designing, constructing, or operating mechanical devices and structures. **dental e.,** the application of engineering principles in dentistry, particularly in the design and construction of dental prostheses, instruments, and equipment.

Engman, Martin Feeney [dermatologist in St. Louis, 1869–1953] see DYSKERATOSIS congenita (Zinsser-Engman-Cole syndrome).

engorged (en-gorjd′) distended or swollen with fluids.

engorgement (en-gorj′ment) hyperemia, local congestion; excessive fullness of any organ, vessel, or tissue due to accumulation of fluids, especially that due to accumulation of blood.

Engstler see West's lacuna SKULL (West-Engstler skull).

enhancement (en-hans′ment) an immune response resulting in prolonged survival of tumor cells in a host due to the production of blocking factors, T-suppressor cells, or some other factor.

Enidrel trademark for *oxazepam*.

enkephalin (en-kef′ah-lin) an endogenous pentapeptide in the brain and pituitary gland, which mimics the action of morphine in the nervous system. Suspected of being synthesized from larger peptides called *endorphins*.

enlargement (en-larj′ment) an increase in size of an organ or part. **gingival e.,** hyperplastic enlargement of the gingival tissue. It may occur as a result of inflammatory or fibrous lesions resulting from irritation or injury brought about by mechanical or chemical factors or systemic or localized pathologic processes. See also FIBROMATOSIS gingivae and gingival HYPERPLASIA. **gingival e., acute inflammatory,** an acute expansive inflammatory lesion, such as a gingival or periodontal abscess. **gingival e., chronic inflammatory,** a form of inflammatory enlargement, usually due to prolonged irritation, which originates as a slight ballooning of the interdental papilla, marginal gingiva, or both. It begins as a bulge around the involved teeth and increases in size until it covers part of the crown, and progresses slowly and painlessly unless it is complicated by acute infection or trauma. Its chief histological features consist of the presence of inflammatory fluid and cellular exudate, degeneration of the epithelium and connective tissue, new capillary formation, vascular engorgement, hemorrhage, proliferation of the epithelium and connective tissue, and new collagen fibers. **gingival e., combined,** gingival hyperplasia complicated by secondary inflammatory changes. **gingival e., diffuse,** that involving the marginal and attached gingivae and papillae. **gingival e., discrete,** an isolated sessile or pedunculated tumor-like enlargement of the gingivae. Called also *tumor-like gingival*. See also pregnancy TUMOR. **gingival e., generalized,** that involving the gingiva throughout the mouth. **gingival e., inflammatory,** gingival enlargement due to inflammatory changes. See *gingival e., acute inflammatory,* and *gingival e., chronic inflammatory.* **gingival e., localized,** that limited to the gingiva adjacent to a single tooth or group of teeth. **gingival e., marginal,** that confined to the marginal gingiva. **gingival e., papillary,** that confined to the interdental papilla. **gingival e. in puberty,** enlargement, usually of the interdental and marginal tissue of the vestibular gingivae, while the oral surfaces remain unaltered, occurring during puberty. Typically, it presents a bulbous lesion of the interproximal papillae, which is predominantly inflammatory, with edema and degenerative changes. Local irritants are the principal cause and the lesion does not disappear until they are removed, although the enlargement tends to undergo spontaneous reduction after puberty. **tumor-like gingival e.,** gingival e., discrete.

enol (e′nol) one of two tautomeric forms of a substance, the other being the keto form. The enol is formed from the keto by migration of hydrogen from the adjacent carbon atom to the carbonyl group:

$$\begin{array}{ccc} \text{R·CH} & & \text{R·CH}_2 \\ \parallel & & | \\ \text{R·C·OH} & & \text{R·C:O} \\ \text{enol form} & & \text{keto form} \end{array}$$

enolase [EC.4.2.1.11] (e′no-lās) a hydrolyase that is active in carbohydrate metabolism, in the Embden-Meyerhof pathway, and catalyzes the conversion of 2-phosphoglyceric acid to phosphoenol pyruvic acid. Called also *2-phosphoglycerate hydratase* and *phosphopyruvate hydratase.*

enophthalmos (en-of-thal′mos) [Gr. *en* in + *ophthalmos* eye] abnormal retraction of the eye into the orbit.

enostosis (en″os-to′sis) [Gr. *en* in + *osteon* bone] a morbid bony growth developed within the cavity of a bone or on the internal surface of the bone cortex.

en plaque (ahn-plak′) [Fr.] in the form of a plaque or plate.

enrollee (en-ro-le′, en-ro′le) 1. a person who enrolls, or has enrolled, in a class, school, course of study, etc. 2. beneficiary.

enrollment (en-rōl′ment) 1. the act or process or registering or entering one's name in a roll, record, or register, as in applying for and being accepted for participation in an insurance plan. See also enrollment PERIOD. 2. the number enrolled, as the number of persons in an insurance plan. **open e.,** a period when new subscribers may elect to enroll in a health insurance plan or prepaid group practice.

ensiform (en′si-form) [L. *ensis* sword + *forma* form] shaped like a sword; xiphoid.

Enslin's triad see under TRIAD.

ENT ear, nose, and throat.

ent- ENTO-.

entad (en′tad) toward the center; inwardly.

ental (en′tal) [Gr. *entos* within] inner; central.

Entamoeba (en″tah-me′bah) a genus of amebae of the order Amoebida, class Rhizopoda, parasitic in vertebrates, and distinguished by a more or less spherical nucleus with a relatively small chromosome near its center, and numerous chromatic granules lining the nuclear membrane. *E. bucca′lis, E. gingiva′lis. E. gingiva′lis,* a species found in the mouth, about the human gingivae. About 25 to 33 percent of healthy persons are carriers of *E. gingivalis* and the percentage increases to about 60 in patients with periodontal disease. Called also *E. buccalis, Amoeba buccalis,* and *Amoeba dentalis. E. hartman′ni,* a species that is somewhat smaller than but otherwise similar to *E. histolytica;* it is a nonpathogenic organism found in the human intestine. *E. histolyt′ica,* a species which causes amebic dysentery and tropical abscess of the liver. Called also *E. troplicalis, Amoeba histolytica,* and *Amoeba dysenteriae. E. tropicalis, E. histolytica. E. co′li,* a species that resembles *E. histolytica* but is nonpathogenic and is found in the human intestinal tract. Called also *Amoeba coli.*

enter- see ENTERO-.

enteramine (en″ter-am′in) 5-hydroxytryptamine.

Enterfram trademark for *neomycin B.*

enteritis (en″ter-i′tis) [*enter-* + *-itis*] inflammation of the intestine, particularly the small intestine. **regional e.,** Crohn's DIS-EASE.

entero-, enter- [Gr. *enteron* intestine] a combining form denoting relationship to the intestine.

Enterobacter (en″ter-o-bak′ter) [*entero-* + *baktērion* little rod] a genus of gram-negative, facultatively anaerobic, rod-shaped bacteria of the family Enterobacteriaceae, made up of motile, peritrichously flagellated cells, some being encapsulated. The organisms ferment glucose with the production of acid and gas. **E. aerog′enes,** a species isolated from feces, sewage, soil, and dairy products. Called also *Aerobacter aerogenes, Bacillus aerogenes,* and *Bacterium aerogenes.* **E. aerog′enes** subsp. **haf′niae,** *Hafnia alvei;* see under HAFNIA. **E. al′vei,** *Hafnia alvei;* see under HAFNIA. **E. cloa′cae,** a species found in feces, soil, and water, and less commonly, in urine pus, and pathological material. Called also *Aerobacter cloacae, Bacillus cloacae, Bacterium cloacae,* and *Cloaca cloacae.*

Enterobacteriaceae (en″ter-o-bak-te″re-a′se-e) [*Enterobacter* + *-aceae*] a family of gram-negative, facultatively anaerobic, rod-shaped bacteria, occurring as small, motile or nonmotile, capsulated or unencapsulated, non–spore-forming, non–acid-fast cells. Their metabolism is respiratory and fermentative, with acid being produced from fermentation of glucose. All strains, except for one serotype of *Shigella,* are oxidase-negative. It includes the genera *Citrobacter, Edwardsiella, Enterobacter, Erwinia, Escherichia, Hafnia, Klebsiella, Salmonella, Serratia, Proteus,* and *Yersinia,* some of which are pathogenic.

enterokinase (en″ter-o-ki′nās) enteropeptidase.

enteropathy (en″ter-op′ah-the) [*entero-* + Gr. *pathos* illness] any disease of the intestine. **gluten e.,** celiac DISEASE.

enteropeptidase [E.C.3.4.21.9] (en″ter-o-pep′tĭ-dās) a serine proteinase that activates trypsinogen to trypsin and also acts on benzoyl-arginine ethyl ester. Called also *enterokinase.*

Enterosalicyl trademark for *sodium salicylate* (see under SALICYLATE).

Enterosalil trademark for *sodium salicylate* (see under SALICYLATE).

enterotoxin (en″ter-o-tok′sin) 1. a toxin specific for the cells of the intestinal mucosa. 2. an exotoxin that is protein in nature and relatively heat stable, being usually involved in food poisoning after ingestion of contaminated food; produced by microorganisms such as *Bacillus cereus, Clostridium perfringens, Escherichia coli, Staphylococcus aureus,* and *Vibrio cholerae.*

Enterovirus (en″ter-o-vi′rus) [Gr. *enteron* intestine + *virus*] a genus of picornaviruses, occurring as acid-stable (pH 3) particles 20 to 30 nm in diameter. Most enteroviruses reside in the intestinal tract of vertebrates and most of their infections are inapparent. Some strains cause intestinal disorders or myocarditis, while others produce generalized infections involving the central nervous system, causing diseases such as poliomyelitis and aseptic meningitis associated with heart damage. Human enteroviruses include poliovirus, coxsackievirus, and echovirus. Enteroviruses also infect monkeys, cattle, swine, mice, and other animals. Some newly discovered enteroviruses are numbered sequentially from 68, regardless of subgroups.

enterovirus (en″ter-o-vi′rus) any virus of the genus *Enterovirus.*

Entexidin trademark for *phthalylsulfathiazole.*

enthalpy (en′thal-pe) [Gr. *en* within + *thalpein* to warm] the state of heat consumption or release during a process of constant pressure. See also endothermic ENERGY and exothermic ENERGY. **e. of fusion,** the amount of heat (thermal energy) required to bring about melting of a given amount of a solid. **e. of solution,** the amount of heat (thermal energy) released or consumed upon dissolution. **e. of sublimation,** the amount of heat (thermal energy) required to bring about sublimation of a given amount of a solid. **e. vaporization,** the amount of heat (thermal energy) which must be supplied to a given quantity of a liquid to bring about vaporization.

entity (en′tĭ-te) [L. *ens* being] an independently existing thing; a reality.

ento-, ent- [Gr. *entos* inside] a prefix signifying within, or inner. See also terms beginning with ENDO-.

entoblast (en′to-blast) [*ento-* + Gr. *blastos* germ] 1. entoderm. 2. a cell nucleolus.

entoderm (en′to-derm) [*ento-* + Gr. *derma* skin] the innermost of the three primary germ layers of the embryo. From it are derived the epithelium of the pharynx, respiratory tract (except the nose), digestive tract, bladder, and urethra. Called also

*e*ndoblast, endoderm, entoblast, trophic layer, and *vegetative layer.* See also GASTRULATION and germ LAYER, and see illustration at EMBRYO.

entomo- [Gr. *entomon* insect] a combining form denoting relationship to insects.

Entomophthora coronata (en″to-mof′thor-ah kor″o-na′ta) a phycomycetous fungus, which is the etiologic agent of rhinophycomycosis.

Entomopoxvirus (en-to″mo-poks-vi′rus) [*entomo-* + *poxvirus*] a genus of poxviruses that parasitize insects.

entropion (en-tro′pe-on) [Gr. *en* in + *tropein* to turn] the turning inward (eversion) of an edge or margin, as of the margin of the eyelid.

entropy (en′tro-pe) 1. diminished capacity for spontaneous change, as occurs in aging. 2. the unavailable energy of a substance due to the internal motion of the molecules. See also free ENERGY.

Entusil trademark for *sulfisoxazole.*

enunciation (ĕ-nun′se-a′shun) the act or the matter of uttering or pronouncing words or sentences.

enucleation (ĕ-nu″kle-a′shun) [L. *e* out + *nucleus* kernel] the removal of an organ, tumor, tooth, or another body in such a way that it comes out clean and whole, like a nut from its shell.

enuresis (en″u-re′sis) [G. *enourein* to void urine] involuntary discharge of the urine.

envelope (en′vĕ-lōp) 1. an encompassing structure or membrane. 2. viral e. **e. of border movements,** the limit of jaw movements in the horizontal or sagittal plane. **cell e.,** the outer limiting structure of a cell. In mycoplasmas, which lack a true cell wall, it is only a simple membrane (about 7.5 nm in thickness), combining the function of both the cell wall and the plasma membrane, which it resembles. In gram-positive bacteria, in addition to the cytoplasmic membrane enclosing the cytoplasm and appearing as a "double-tract" membrane under the electron microscope, the cell is surrounded by an amorphous cell wall, about 15 to 50 nm in thickness, sometimes reaching 80 nm. In gram-negative cells, the envelope, about 15 nm in thickness, is made up of two parallel, multilayered membranes: an inner, or plasma, membrane, which is similar to that seen in gram-positive cells, and the cell wall, which is composed of a second or outer membrane. See also cell WALL. **nuclear e.,** nuclear MEMBRANE. **viral e.,** the limiting membrane surrounding the nucleocapsid in certain viruses, characterized by the presence of spike proteins at the outer surface.

environment (en-vi′ron-ment) [Fr. *environner* to surround, to encircle] the sum total of all the conditions and elements which make up the surroundings and influence the development of an individual. See also ECOLOGY and environmental MEDICINE.

enzymatic (en″zi-mat′ik) relating to, caused by, or of the nature of an enzyme.

enzyme (en′zĭm) [Gr. *en* in + *zymē* leaven] a protein which catalyzes reactions of other substances by combining with substrate molecules (reactants) in such a way that the active site of the enzyme molecule fits the substrate with a kind of lock and key correspondence, the combination assuming a new configuration in which the substrate is so modified that it undergoes reaction and is released from the enzyme and the enzyme assumes its original form. About 2000 enzymes are known, many of which may coexist in a single cell. Hundreds of chemical reactions in cells are catalyzed by enzymes, usually being linked into sequence of consecutive reactions having common intermediates. See also *e. classification.* For salivary enzymes, see table. **antineoplastic e.,** one that is capable of arresting or inhibiting the growth of neoplasms, such as asparaginase. **e. classification,** a system by which enzymes are assigned to groups or classes within categories. The classification adopted by the Enzyme Commission of the International Union of Biochemistry is the one currently in use. In this scheme, enzymes are coded according to the reaction catalyzed, the root indicating the reaction being followed by the suffix *-ase,* except for certain proteolytic enzymes, such as pepsin, trypsin, papain, and others. Both systematic names (ones specifying, precisely as possible, catalytic reaction of enzymes) and trivial names (ones which are less precise but are short and convenient for use) are used. The classification is based on the system of numerical codes (*E.C.* numbers), the first number of which indicates one of the six major classes of enzymes; the second indicates the sub-class; the third gives the sub-sub-class, and the fourth is the serial number of the enzyme in its sub-sub-class. The six major classes of enzymes are: 1. *Oxidoreductases:* Enzymes involved in catalyzing oxidation-reduction in cells. The second number indicates the group in the hydrogen donor which undergoes oxidation; the third the type of acceptor

SALIVARY ENZYMES

Enzyme	Source		
	Glands	Micro-organ-isms	Leuko-cytes
Carbohydrases			
Amylase	+		
Maltase		+	+
Invertase		+	
β-Glucuronidase	+	+	+
β-D-Galactosidase		+	+
β-D-Glucosidase		+	
Lysozyme	+		+
Hyaluronidase		+	
Mucinase		+	
Esterases			
Acid phosphatase	+	+	+
Alkaline phosphatase	+	+	+
Hexosediphosphatase		+	
Aliesterase	+	+	+
Lipase	+	+	+
Acetylcholinesterase	+		+
Pseudo-cholinesterase	+	+	+
Chondrosulfatase		+	
Arylsulfatase		+	
Transferring enzymes			
Catalase		+	
Peroxidase	+		+
Phenyloxidase		+	
Succinic dehydro-genase	+	+	+
Hexokinase		+	+
Proteolytic enzymes			
Proteinase		+	+
Peptidase		+	+
Urease		+	
Other enzymes			
Carbonic anhydrase	+		
Pyrophosphatase		+	
Aldolase	+	+	+

(From H. H. Chauncey: Salivary enzymes. J.A.D.A., 63: 360, 1961. Copyright by the American Dental Association. Reprinted by permission.)

involved; the fourth is the serial number. 2. *Transferases:* Enzymes which catalyze the transfer of a chemical group from one substrate to another. The second number indicates the group transferred; the third the nature of the acceptor group; and the fourth is the serial number. 3. *Hydrolases:* Enzymes which catalyze hydrolytic reactions and includes digestive enzymes. The second number indicates the nature of the bond hydrolyzed; the third gives the nature of the substrate, with the exception of peptidyl-peptide hydrolase, where the third number is based on the catalytic mechanism; the fourth is the serial number. 4. *Lyases:* Enzymes which catalyze the removal of chemical groups without hydrolysis. The second number indicates the position where the bond is broken; the third shows the group eliminated; and the fourth is the serial number. 5. *Isomerases:* Enzymes which catalyze geometric or steroisomeric changes within a molecule. The second number gives the type of isomerism; the third the type of substrate; and the fourth is the serial number. 6. *Ligases:* Enzymes which catalyze the linking together of two molecules with the breaking of a pyrophosphate bond of ATP or a similar triphosphate. The second number indicates the bond formed; the third number is only in use in the CN ligases; and the fourth is the serial number. **e. cofactor,** see coenzyme. **debranching e.,** in carbohydrate metabolism, any of several enzymes which hydrolyze the branch linkages in branched polysaccharide chains, e.g., hydrolyze

glucosidic bonds at the branch points which are different from the glucosidic bonds in the main chains. **e. inhibitor,** see enzyme INHIBITOR. **inorganic e.,** see metal SOL. **e. precursor,** PRECURSOR (3). **proteolytic e.,** peptide HYDROLASE. **salivary e's,** see table. **e. unit,** enzyme UNIT. **Warburg's e.,** nicotinamide-adenine dinucleotide phosphate; see under DINUCLEOTIDE. **yellow e's,** see FLAVOPROTEIN.

enzymology (en″zi-mol′o-je) the study of enzymes.
enzymolysis (en″zi-mol′ĭ-sis) [*enzyme* + Gr. *lysis* dissolution] the disintegrative action or reaction produced by an enzyme.
enzymopathy (en″zi-mop′ah-the) inborn error of METABOLISM.
enzymopenic (en″zi-mo-pen′ik) characterized by or caused by a lack of an enzyme in the blood.
enzymuria (en″zi-mu′re-ah) [*enzyme* + Gr. *ouron* urine + *-ia*] the presence of an enzyme or enzymes in the urine.
EOS European Orthodontic Society.
eosin (e′o-sin) [Gr. *eos* dawn] a coal tar dye; specifically the potassium and sodium salts of tetrabromfluorescein. Used as a dye for histological specimens, especially for plasma cells, for microscopic study.
eosinocyte (eo″sin′o-sīt) eosinophil.
eosinophil (e″o-sin′o-fil) [*eosin* + Gr. *philein* to love] 1. any cell or histologic structure staining readily with eosin. 2. a granulocyte, about 9 in diameter, whose granules are eosinophilic and stain a bright red, with a nucleus that usually has two oval lobes connected by a slender thread of chromatin, and cytoplasm containing coarse, round granules of uniform size that stain with acid dyes. Eosinophils make up about 2 to 5 percent of the leukocyte count in adult humans. They arise in the bone marrow from metamyelocytes, maturing there in 1 to 6 days before entering the blood, where they have a half-life of about 30 min. With maturation of the cells, there occurs a transition from primary (azurophilic) granules to large cytoplasmic granules that have a crystalloid substructure. In the tissues, they have a half-life of about 12 days, and are eliminated through the mucosal surfaces of the respiratory and gastrointestinal tracts. These cells have the capacity to phagocytose microorganisms and soluble antigen-antibody complexes, but their function is not fully understood; major roles postulated include the ingestion of immune complexes and their involvement in limiting inflammatory reactions, presumably by antagonizing the effect of certain mediators. Eosinophils have also been found to participate in an antibody-mediated cytotoxicity reaction in the clearance of certain parasitic organisms. Called also *acidocyte, acidophilic granulocyte, eosinocyte, eosinophilic granulocyte* or *leukocyte,* and *Rindfleisch's cell.* See also *table of Reference Values in Hematology* in Appendix.
eosinophilia (e″o-sin″o-fil′e-ah) [*eosin* + Gr. *philein* to love + *-ia*] 1. the condition of being readily stained with eosin. 2. presence in the blood of abnormally large numbers of eosinophils (above 250 per cmm), usually seen in allergic conditions, skin diseases, parasitic diseases, infections, some diseases of the hematopoietic system, and after irradiation. It may also occur as a primary condition, either congenital or acquired. Called also *eosinophilic leukocytosis.*
eosinophilic (e″o-sin″o-fil′ik) readily stainable with eosin.
epactal (e-pak′tal) [Gr. *epaktos* brought in] 1. supernumerary. 2. pertaining to an epactal bone. See wormian bones, under BONE.
ependymocyte (e-pen′di-mo-sīt′) [*ependyma* + Gr. *kytos* hollow vessel] an ependymal cell.
ephapse (e-faps′) [Gr. *ephapsis* a touching] a point of lateral contact (other than synapse) between nerve fibers, across which impulses are conducted directly through the nerve membranes from one fiber to the other.
ephaptic (e-fap′tik) denoting the conduction of nerve impulse across an ephapse.
Ephedral trademark for *the l-form of ephedrine hydrochloride* (see under EPHEDRINE).
ephedrine (ĕ-fed′rin) a sympathomimetic amine, having also a central nervous stimulant action, (—)-erythro-α-[1-(methylamino)ethyl]benzyl alcohol. Isomeric forms include *d-, dl-,* and *l-*forms. It occurs as an almost colorless solid and as white crystals or granules that are soluble in water, ethanol, chloroform, ether, and liquid petrolatum. Used in the treatment of the after-effects of overdosage of hypnotics and sedatives, and in myasthenia gravis, postural hypotension, shock, bronchial asthma and other forms of bronchial spasms, hay fever, paranasal sinusitis, and allergic diseases, and to support blood pressure in spinal anesthesia. Side effects may include agita-

tion, insomnia, headache, tachycardia, arrhythmias, hypotension, precordial pain, nausea, vomiting, and urinary problems. Overdosages may cause euphoria, confusions, delirium, and hallucinations. The *dl*-form is called also *racemic e.* and *racephedrine*. **e. hydrochloride,** the hydrochloride salt of ephedrine, occurring as a white, crystalline powder or crystals that are soluble in water and ethanol, but not in ether. Its pharmacological and toxicological properties are similar to those of the parent compound. The *dl*-form is called also *racephedrine hydrochloride*; Trademark: Ephetonin. Trademarks for the *l*-form: Biophedrine, Ephedral, Ephedrosst, Sandedrine. **racemic e.,** the *dl*-form of ephedrine. **e. sulfate,** the sulfate salt of ephedrine, occurring as a white, odorless powder or crystals that are photosensitive when in aqueous solution, and are soluble in water and ethanol but not in ether. Its pharmacological and toxicological properties are similar to those of the parent compound.

Ephedrosst trademark for the *l*-form of *ephedrine hydrochoride* (see under EPHEDRINE).

ephelides (e-fel′ĭ-dēz) [Gr.] plural of *ephelis*.

ephelis (e-fe′lis), pl. *ephel′ides* [Gr. *ephēlis*] freckle.

ephemeral (ĕ-fem′er-al) [Gr. *ephēmeros* short-lived] transient; short-lived.

Ephetonin trademark for the *dl*-form of *ephedrine hydrochloride* (see under EPHEDRINE).

epi- [Gr. *epi* on] a prefix denoting on or upon.

epibulbar (ep″ĭ-bul′bar) upon the eyeball.

epicanthus (ep″ĭ-kan′thus) [epi- + Gr. *kanthos* canthus] a vertical fold of skin on either side of the nose, sometimes covering the inner canthus. It is present as a normal characteristic in persons of certain races and sometimes occurs as a congenital anomaly in others. Called also *epicanthic fold, palpebronasal fold,* and *plica palpebronasalis* [NA].

epicapramin (ep″ĭ-kap′rah-min) aminocaproic ACID.

Epicort trademark for *hydrocortisone*.

epicranium (ep″ĭ-kra′ne-um) [epi- + Gr. *kranion* skull] the integument, aponeurosis, and muscular expansion of the scalp.

epicrisis (ep″ĭ-kri′sis) [epi- + *crisis*] 1. a second or supplementary crisis. 2. a critical analysis or discussion of a case of disease after its termination.

epicritic (ep″ĭ-krit′ik) [Gr. *epikrisis* determination] of or pertaining to epicritic sensibility, the ability of the skin to differentiate fine tactile and thermal changes.

epidemic (ep″ĭ-dem′ik) [Gr. *epidēmios* prevalent] 1. pertaining to a disease, especially one that is communicable, having a potential for spreading to or infecting a large segment of the human and/or animal population. 2. a condition in which a large number of people and/or animals have been infected by a communicable disease.

epidemiologist (ep″ĭ-de″me-ol′o-jist) one who is an expert and specializes in epidemiology.

epidemiology (ep″ĭ-de″me-ol′o-je) [epidemic + -logy] the study of the distribution of disease and disability in human populations and of the factors which influence that distribution, applying to all types of diseases, whether acute or chronic, physical or mental, communicable or noncommunicable. **analytical e.,** that aspect of epidemiology concerned with investigating, by means of retrospective and prospective studies, hypotheses formulated to explain these observations. **descriptive e.,** that aspect of epidemiology concerned with observing the distribution of a disease or diseases in populations. **experimental e.,** that aspect of epidemiology concerned with experiments which attempt to measure the effect of controlled trials of the manipulation of suspected harmful influences or of preventive measures in populations.

epidermatoplasty (ep″ĭ-der-mat′o-plas″te) [epidermis + Gr. *plassein* to form] skin grafting done with pieces of epidermis with the underlying outer layer of the corium.

epidermis (ep″ĭ-der′mis), pl. *epider′mides* [epi- + Gr. *derma* skin] [NA] the outermost nonvascular layer of the skin, made up of solidly cellular tissue with a high metabolic rate and self-restorative powers, composed mostly of keratinocytes and some melanocytes. It is attached to the corium, and is usually about 0.1 mm thick, but on the palms and soles may become 0.8 and 1.4 mm thick, respectively. The epidermis on the palms and soles exhibits maximal cellular layerings and differentiation, and is comprised of a *malpighian*, or *germinative, layer*, which includes the *basal* and *prickle-cell layers;* a *granular layer;* a *clear layer;* and a *horny layer.* In the thinner epidermis of the general body surface only the malpighian layer and the horny layer are present constantly.

epidermoid (ep″ĭ-der′moid) [epi- + Gr. *derma* skin + *eidos* form] 1. resembling the epidermis. 2. epidermoid CYST.

epidermolysis (ep″ĭ-der-mol′ĭ-sis) [epidermis + Gr. *lysis* dissolution] a condition characterized by destruction of the epidermis, usually associated with formation of blebs and bullae. **e. bullo′sa,** a rare hereditary skin disease characterized by bullous and vesicular eruptions precipitated by slight trauma, in which the onset usually occurs during infancy. The disease is seen in two forms: the simple nonscarring form of Weber and Cockayne, transmitted as an autosomal dominant trait; and the dystrophic form of Goldscheier, transmitted as an autosomal recessive trait. In the simple form, bullae arise on any part of the skin. In the dystrophic form the lesions occur chiefly on the extremities, and the bullae, often hemorrhagic, are associated with scarring, pigmentation or depigmentation, atrophic changes over the denuded areas, scaling, hyperemia, miliumlike cysts, nail dystrophy, leukoplakia, thickening of the skin, claw-hand, and a glovelike epidermal sac. The scars may damage the bone and interfere with growth, producing dwarfism. Oral lesions are common, especially in the dystrophic form. The appearance of bullae may be preceded by white spots or patches of inflammation, and may be precipitated by minor irritation, such as nursing or simple dental procedures in the oral cavity. Dental operations may result in denudation of large areas of mucous membranes. Hoarseness, dysphagia, and dental defects, including rudimentary teeth, anodontia, hypoplastic teeth, and crowns denuded of enamel, may be present. *Herlitz's syndrome* is the fatal form of this disease. Called also *e. hereditaria tarda, acantholysis bullosa, acanthosis bullosa, bullous recurrent eruption, dermatitis bullosa hereditaria, Fox's disease, Goldscheier's disease, keratolysis bullosa hereditaria,* and *Weber-Cockayne syndrome.* **e. bullo′sa leta′lis,** Herlitz SYNDROME. **e. heredita′ria tar′da,** e. bullosa.

Epidermophyton (ep″ĭ-der-mof′ĭ-ton) [epidermis + Gr. *phyton* plant] a genus of dermatophytes that causes tinea corporis and infection of the feet and nails, and the perineal region in males.

Epidione trademark for *trimethadione*.

Epidropal trademark for *allopurinol*.

epidural (ep″ĭ-du′ral) situated upon or outside the dura mater.

epifascial (ep″ĭ-fash′e-al) upon a fascia.

epiglottic (ep″ĭ-glot′ik) pertaining to the epiglottis.

epiglottidectomy (ep″ĭ-glot″ĭ-dek′to-me) [epiglottis + Gr. *ektomē* excision] excision of the epiglottis.

epiglottiditis (ep″ĭ-glot″ĭ-di′tis) inflammation of the epiglottis.

epiglottis (ep″ĭ-glot′is) [epi- + Gr. *glottis* glottis] [NA] a leaflike cartilaginous structure made up of a thin plate of yellow elastic cartilage (epiglottic cartilage), situated behind the root of the tongue, at the entrance to the larynx and trachea. Its narrow part is attached to the thyroepiglottic ligament and the broad part is free, the caudal part connecting it to the body of the hyoid bone by the hyoepiglottic ligament. The curved anterior surface is covered on its free portion by mucous membrane which forms the glossoepiglottic folds, the lateral one being attached to the pharynx. The valleculae form depressions between the root of the tongue and the epiglottis. Muscular action during deglutition pushes the larynx against the epiglottis, thus preventing food from entering the larynx and air passages and directing it into the esophagus.

epiglottitis (ep″ĭ-glot-ti′tis) inflammation of the epiglottis. **cherry-red e.,** Kleinschmidt's SYNDROME.

epignathus (e-pig′nah-thus) [epi- + Gr. *gnathos* jaw] congenital oral TERATOMA.

epihyoid (ep″ĭ-hi′oid) situated upon the hyoid bone.

epilamellar (ep″ĭ-lah-mel′ar) situated upon the basement membrane.

epilation (ep″ĭ-la′shun) [L. *e* out + *pilus* hair] the removal of hair.

epilepsy (ep′ĭ-lep″se) [Gr. *epilēpsia* seizure] a group of neurological conditions marked by paroxysmal transient disturbances of brain function that may be manifested as episodic impairment or loss of consciousness, resulting from disorders of electrical activity of the brain. The term includes disorders associated with convulsions and unconsciousness as well as those which are not. **continuous e.,** Kozhevnikov's e. **cortical e.,** Jackson's e. **focal e.,** Jackson's e. **Jackson's e.,** seizures involving one or several parts of the body on the same side, which may begin as spasm of a single part, usually the angle of the mouth, index finger, great toe, or thumb, and "march" to other areas. Consciousness is retained, unless seizures spread to the opposite side of the body. The condition indicates focal lesions of the contralateral side of the brain, usually in the area of the motor cortex. Called also *cortical e., focal e.,* and *jacksonian seizures.* **Kozhevnikov's e., partial e.,** clonic muscular twitching repeated at fairly regular intervals in one part of the body for a period of days or weeks. Each twitch is an abrupt jerk lasting one-fourth of a second, usually involving one muscle group but occasionally including other related muscles on the same side of the body, without relation to consciousness. The muscles involved are chiefly the flexors of the limbs, lateral flexors of the neck, and facial muscles. Kozhevnikov thought that the essential lesions were located in the cortex, but structures other than the cortex may also be involved. Called also *continuous e.*

epileptiform (ep″ĭ-lep′tĭ-form) [Gr. *epileptikos* + L. *forma* form] 1. resembling epilepsy or its manifestations. 2. occurring in severe or sudden paroxysms.

epimandibular (ep″ĭ-man-dib′u-lar) [*epi-* + L. *mandibulum* jaw] situated upon the lower jaw.

epimer (ep′ĭ-mer) an isomer differing from the compound with which it is compared in the arrangement of hydrogen and hydroxyl on the last asymmetric carbon atom of a chain.

epimerase [E.C.5.1.1] (e-pim′ĕ-rās) a subclass of isomerases, the enzymes of which catalyze the inversion of one of the asymmetric groups in substrates having more than one center of asymmetry, converting the substrate to its epimer.

epimysium (ep″ĭ-mis′e-um) [*epi-* + Gr. *mys* muscle] a sheath of fibrous connective tissue which encloses an entire muscle. Called also *perimysium externum.*

epinephrine (ep″ĭ-nef′rin) a catecholamine, 3,4-dihydroxy-α-[(methylamino)methyl]benzyl alcohol. It is a hormone found in the chromaffin cells of the adrenal medulla, which acts pharmacologically as a sympathomimetic, being mediated through the adrenergic receptors. Epinephrine occurs as a white, microcrystalline, odorless powder that darkens on exposure to light and air, and is slightly soluble in water and alcohol and insoluble in organic solvents. In moderate doses, it constricts the blood vessels of the skin, mucous membranes, and viscera, producing a rapid rise of blood pressure; this is associated with a reflex inhibition of the heart rate, while causing the blood vessels of the skeletal muscles and the coronary bed to dilate, and also increasing the blood flow through the muscles and the liver. Vasoconstriction may be followed by vasodilatation and a rapid fall of blood pressure. Epinephrine is also a central nervous system stimulant inducing a feeling of anxiety and tremor. Increased respiration and oxygen consumption, high blood sugar and lactate levels, decreased liver and glycogen levels, profuse sweating, and release of ACTH by the anterior pituitary are among other effects of epinephrine. Clinically, it is used as a local vasoconstrictor agent, hemostatic agent, adjunct in local anesthesia, and in the treatment of allergic diseases and anaphylactic shock. Formerly used in the treatment of traumatic shock. Side effects may include tachycardia, arrhythmia, vertigo, tremor, restlessness, anxiety, and fear. Excessive doses may cause hypertension and ventricular fibrillation. Usually used therapeutically as the *l*-form. Called also *adrenalin* and *adrenine.* Trademarks: Adrenal, Hemostatin, Levorenine, Suprarenin, Vasotonin.

epineurium (ep″ĭ-nu′re-um) [*epi-* + Gr. *neuron* nerve] the outer layer of a sheath which surrounds and holds together nerve trunks, composed of connective tissue and collagenous fibers.

epipalatus (ep″ĭ-pal-ah′tus) congenital oral TERATOMA.

epipharynx (ep″ĭ-far′inks) nasopharynx.

epiphyses (ĕ-pif′ĭ-sēz) [Gr.] plural of *epiphysis.*

epiphysis (ĕ-pif′ĭ-sis), pl. *epiph′yses* [Gr. "an outgrowth, excrescence"] [NA] 1. the end of a long bone, usually wider than the shaft, and either entirely cartilaginous or separated from the shaft by a cartilaginous disk. 2. part of a bone formed from a secondary center of ossification, commonly found at the ends of long bones, on the margins of flat bones, and at tubercles and processes; during the period of growth, epiphyses are separated from the main portion of the bone by cartilage. Called also *apophysis ossium* and *epiphyseal process.* **e. cer′ebri,** pineal GLAND. **stippled epiphyses,** Conradi-Hünermann SYNDROME.

episphenoid (ep″ĭ-sfe′noid) [*epi-* + *sphenoid*] congenital oral TERATOMA.

epistasis (ĕ-pis′tah-sis) [*epi-* + Gr. *stasis* a standing] 1. suppression of a secretion or excretion. 2. the interaction between the products of two genes at different loci, in which the one gene prevents the phenotypic expression of the other. See also dominant CHARACTER.

epistaxis (ep″ĭ-stak′sis) [Gr.] nosebleed; hemorrhage from the nose. **hereditary e.,** hereditary hemorrhagic TELANGIECTASIA.

epithalamus (ep″ĭ-thal′ah-mus) [NA] the part of the diencephalon superior and posterior to the thalamus.

epithelia (ep″ĭ-the′le-ah) [Gr.] plural of *epithelium.*

epithelial (ep″ĭ-the′le-al) pertaining to or made up of epithelium.

epithelialization (ep″ĭ-the″le-al-i-za′shun) epithelization.

epithelio- a combining form denoting relationship to the epithelium.

epithelioma (ep″ĭ-the″le·o′mah) [*epithelium* + *-oma*] an epithelial

neoplasm; a tumor consisting mainly of epithelial cells and primarily derived from the skin or mucous surfaces. **adenoid e.,** cystic adenoid e. **benign calcifying e.,** a sharply defined, firm, benign tumor of the face, neck, or arms. The typical lesion is inclosed in a fibrous capsule, and is situated deep in the dermis and covered by normal skin, with varying degrees of erythema and discoloration overlying the tumor area. Aggregates of darkly staining cells, foreign body giant-cell reaction, calcification, and, rarely, ossification in calcified patches are the principal pathological features. Called also *Malherbe's e.* **Bowen's e.,** CARCINOMA *in situ.* **Brooke's e.,** cystic adenoid e. **cystic adenoid e.,** an uncommon, benign, familial skin disease believed to be transmitted as a dominant trait, in which masses of basal cells in the corium originate from the basal cell layer of the epidermis and hair follicles. The lesions form firm, flesh-colored, translucent papules with slight surface telangiectasia, which are largely confined to the eyelids, with a symmetrical distribution of virtually hundreds of lesions, although solitary lesions may be found; small lesions may coalesce to form a solid sheet of tumor. The tumors usually appear near puberty and become stationary after enlarging for several years, but regression and, rarely, malignant degeneration may occur. Called also *Brooke's e., adenoid e., acanthoma adenoides cysticum, nevus follicularis,* and *Brooke's disease.* **erythemoid benign e.,** Arning's CARCINOID. **Malherbe's e.,** benign calcifying e. **multiple primary self-healing squamous e.,** primary pseudoepitheliomatous HYPERPLASIA. **pagetoid e., e. pagetoide,** Arning's CARCINOID.

epithelium (ep″ĭ-the′le-um), pl. *epithe′lia* [*epi-* + Gr. *thēlē* nipple] [NA] the covering of internal and external body surfaces, including the lining of vessels and other small cavities, which consists of cells joined by small amounts of cementing substances. It is classified into types on the basis of the number of layers deep and the shape of the superficial cells. See illustration. **ciliated e.,** a type bearing vibratile cilia on the free surface. **columnar e.,** that made up of tall prismatic cells. See *simple columnar e.* and *stratified columnar e.* **cornified e.,** keratinized e. **crevicular e.,** that covering the inner soft tissue wall of the gingival crevice. **cubical e., cuboidal e.,** that composed of cells which have a cubical shape. **enamel e.,** in the developing tooth, the inner layer of cells (ameloblasts) of the enamel organ that deposit the organic matrix of enamel, plus the outer layer of cubical cells. The reduced enamel epithelium is the remains of

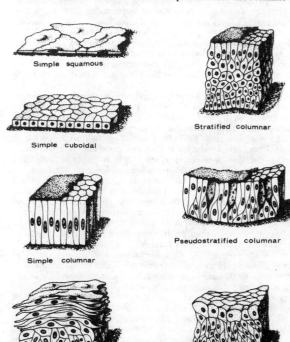

Shape and arrangement of cells in the principal types of epithelia. (From W. Bloom and D. W. Fawcett: A Textbook of Histology. 10th ed. Philadelphia, W. B. Saunders Co., 1975.)

both layers after enamel formation is complete. **enamel e., inner,** in the bell stage of odontogenesis, the single layer of cells adjacent to the dental papilla, which become differentiated into ameloblasts. Called also *preameloblast.* **enamel e., reduced,** a layer of the enamel organ appearing after the formation of the dental enamel, at which time the ameloblasts assume the shape of the cells of the stratum intermedium. **gingival e.,** squamous epithelium covering the underlying connective tissue stroma of the gingivae. It is made up of cells connected to each other by desmosomes, each having two dense attachment plaques about 150 Å thick. Between the plaques there is a lamellated structure, consisting of four layers of low density, as seen with the electron microscope, separated by three darker osmophilic layers. The space between the cells is filled with a granular and fibrillar cement substance and cytoplasmic projections of the cell wall resembling microvilli; tonofibrils radiating from the attachment plaques into the cytoplasm of the cells. In the stratum corneum of highly keratinized gingiva (palate), the desmosomes are modified, and the cell membranes are thickened and separated by a three-layered structure. Sometimes, epithelial cell connections are tight junctions (zonula occludens), areas where the outer membranes of adjoining cells are fused; and intermediate junctions (zonula adherens), areas in which the cell membranes are parallel and separated by a space (200–300 Å wide) filled with amorphous material. In the female, large Feulgen-positive particles are found adjacent to the nuclear membrane in most cases; rarely, similar structures are found in the male. **glandular e.,** that made up of glandular or secreting cells. **hornified e.,** keratinized e. **hyperkeratinized e.,** that which is completely keratinized. See also *keratinized e.* **junctional e.,** that adhering to the tooth surface at the base of the gingival crevice, consisting of one or several layers of nonkeratinizing cells. **keratinized e.,** stratified epithelium in which the superficial cells accumulate keratin in their cytoplasm and are reduced to scalelike cell residues; in the oral cavity, found chiefly in the gingiva and the hard palate. It is classified as completely keratinized (hyperkeratinized) and incompletely keratinized (parakeratinized). Called also *cornified e.* and *hornified e.* **laminated e.,** stratified e. **masticatory e.,** the keratinized stratified squamous epithelium covering the masticatory mucous membrane. **noncornified e., nonhornified e.,** nonkeratinized e. **nonkeratinized e.,** stratified epithelium in which the superficial cells do not accumulate keratin. In the oral cavity, it lines areas such as the vestibular mucosa, undersurface of the tongue, floor of the mouth, and soft palate. Called also *noncornified e.* and *nonhornified e.* **olfactory e.,** olfactory AREA. **oral e.,** that lining of the oral cavity, consisting of the keratinized (masticatory) epithelium lining the hard palate, gingivae, and tongue, and the nonkeratinized epithelium lining the sheltered regions, such as the base of the tongue, sublingual region, lips, cheeks, soft palate, and tonsils. **parakeratinized e.,** that which is incompletely keratinized. See also *keratinized e.* **pavement e.,** that composed of a single layer of flat cells. **pigmentary e., pigmented e.,** that containing granules of pigment. **pocket e.,** that part of the sulcal epithelium lining periodontal pockets, characterized by the presence of hyperplasia and ulceration. **protective e.,** that which forms a protective covering, as the epidermis. **pseudostratified e.,** a nonstratified columnar epithelium which lines the respiratory tract (nasal passage, pharynx, trachea, bronchi, and bronchioles), having spindle and polyhedral cells mixed with the columnar cells, so arranged that the nuclei occur at two or more levels, thus giving the epithelium a false appearance of stratification. **respiratory e.,** the pseudostratified epithelium that lines all but the finer divisions of the respiratory tract. **rod e.,** that in which the cells are rod-shaped. **simple e.,** that composed of a single layer of cells. **simple columnar e.,** that composed of a single layer of tall prismatic cells. **simple squamous e.,** that composed of a single layer of flat cells. **squamous e.,** epithelium composed of flattened platelike cells. See *simple squamous e.* and *stratified squamous e.* **stratified e.,** that composed of two or more layers of cells. Called also *laminated e.* **stratified columnar e.,** a multilayered epithelium in which the more superficial cells are of the prismatic and cuboidal or columnar type. **stratified squamous e.,** a multilayered epithelium in which the more superficial cells are flattened. **sulcal e., sulcular e.,** the parakeratinized part of the gingival epithelium that covers the soft tissue wall of the gingival sulcus, extending from the gingival margin to the line of attachment of the epithelium to the tooth surface. It may become hyperplastic and ulcerative in the presence of periodon-

tal pockets (pocket e.). **vestibular e.,** the nonkeratinized stratified squamous epithelium of the mucous membrane of the vestibule of the mouth, which lines the lips and the cheeks. Its superficial desquamating layer is composed of several layers of loosely bound cells that are easily dislodged by abrasive forces; cells in this layer are approaching death, being deprived of the source of nutrition, since the epithelium is avascular. In the malpighian layer, the basal layer is more prominent than the prickle-cell layer, having a single layer of columnar cells.

epithelization (ep″ĭ-the″lĭ-za-shun) healing by the growth of epithelium over a denuded area. In the oral epithelium, the process begins within 24 hours after injury by mitotic activity of cells around the clot, followed by converging of cells at the center of the wound and walling it off from the outside. After tooth extraction, the converging epithelial cells make contact with one another and cover the clot-filled alveolar crater in about 2 weeks. Called also *epithelialization.*

epitope (ep′ĭ-tōp) see antigenic DETERMINANT.

epitympanic (ep″ĭ-tim-pan′ik) 1. situated upon or above the tympanum. 2. pertaining to the attic (epitympanum).

epitympanum (ep″ĭ-tim′pah-num) attic.

epitype (ep′ĭ-tīp) a group of related epitopes. See antigenic DETERMINANT.

épluchage (a″ploo-shahzh′) [Fr. "cleaning," "picking"] removal of the contused and contaminated tissues of a wound.

Epolene N-10 trademark for a synthetic *dental wax* (see under WAX).

eponychium (e″o-nik′e-um) [*epi-* + Gr. *onyx* nail] 1. [NA] the narrow band of epidermis extending from the nail wall onto the nail surface; the cuticle. 2. the horny part of the periderm at the site of the future nail.

eponym (ep′o-nim) [Gr. *epōnymos* named after] one for whom or which something is named. Traditionally, eponymic names were given to medical entities, such as pathological conditions, diagnostic signs, or anatomical structures, after persons who first described them, as in *Hodgkin's disease* named after Thomas Hodgkin, an 18th century English physician. The practice has been extended to naming pathological conditions after persons in whom they were first observed, as in *Christmas disease* or *Johnie McL. disease*, or geographic areas or localities in which conditions were first reported, as in *Tangier disease*, named after an island in the Chesapeake Bay. The practice has been further extended to giving names of mythological characters, as in *Ulysses syndrome*, related to the legend of Ulysses, the Greek epic hero.

eponymic, eponymous (ep″o-nim′ik; ĕ-pon′ĭ-mus) pertaining to an eponym.

Eporal trademark for *dapsone.*

epoxide (ĕ-pok′sĭd) an organic compound containing a reactive group resulting from the union of an oxygen atom with two other atoms, usually carbon. Commonly referred to as *epoxy.* See also epoxy RESIN.

epoxy (e-pok′se) 1. epoxy RESIN. 2. epoxide.

Epoxylite 9070 trademark for a polyurethane pit and fissure sealant; see POLYURETHANE.

Epoxylite 9075 trademark for *bisphenol A glycidyl methacrylate* (see under METHACRYLATE).

EPSDT Early Periodic Screening Diagnosis Treatment; a federally-sponsored preventive care program specifically designed for children and adolescents up to 21 years of age, also including, by referral, dental care.

epsicapramin aminocaproic ACID.

Epsom salts (ep′som) MAGNESIUM sulfate.

epsomite (ep′so-mīt) the natural form of magnesium sulfate heptahydrate; see MAGNESIUM sulfate.

Epstein, Emile see van Bogaert-Scherer-Epstein SYNDROME.

Epstein's pearls (disease) [Alois *Epstein,* Prague physician, 1849–1918] see under PEARL.

Epstein-Barr virus [M. A. *Epstein;* Y. M. *Barr*] see under VIRUS.

Eptoin trademark for *phenytoin sodium* (see under PHENYTOIN).

epulides (ep-u′lĭ-dēz) [Gr.] plural of *epulis.*

epulis (ep-u′lis), pl. *epu′lides* [Gr. *epoulis* a gum boil] 1. a nonspecific term applied to tumors and tumorlike masses of the gingiva. 2. peripheral ossifying FIBROMA. **congenital e.,** a benign, nonencapsulated soft, pedunculated tumor of the mucosa of the jaws, usually the maxilla, of newborn infants. It is usually found in the incisor region, arising on the crest of the alveolar ridge or process, and is composed of large, closely packed cells showing granular, eosinophilic cytoplasm. Congenital epulis is quite similar to myoblastoma but is believed that these are two separate entities. Called also *e. of newborn.* **e. fibromato′sa,** a fibroma arising from the alveolar periosteum and the periodontal ligament. **e. fissura′tum,** fibrous inflammatory HYPERPLASIA. **giant cell e., e. gigantocellula′ris,** a sessile or pedunculated lesion of the gingiva, or less frequently, the mucous membrane covering edentulous ridges, which represents inflammatory reactions to injury or hemorrhage, and is not considered a true neoplasm. It presents a smooth spherical or an irregularly shaped multilobulated protuberance varying in color from pink to purplish blue, sometimes covering several teeth. Its consistency varies from spongelike to firm. Histologically, it is composed of a spindle cell stroma punctuated by multinucleate giant cells. Called also *osteoclastoma, peripheral giant cell granuloma, peripheral giant cell lesion, peripheral giant cell reparative granuloma, peripheral giant cell tumor,* and *peripheral reparative granuloma.* **e. granuloma-to′sa,** a pyogenic granuloma on the gingiva resulting from mechanical or other irritation. **e. of newborn,** congenital e. **ossifying fibroid e.,** peripheral ossifying FIBROMA.

epulofibroma (ep″u-lo″fi-bro′mah) a fibroma of the gingiva.

epuloid (ep′u-loid) resembling an epulis.

epulosis (ep″u-lōsis) [Gr. *epoulo′sis*] cicatrization.

epulotic (ep″u-lot′ik) [Gr. *epoulōtikos*] pertaining to, characterized by, or promoting cicatrization.

Equa trademark for *aspartame.*

equalization (e″kwah-li-za′shun) making equal or uniform. **pressure e.,** the act or process of equalizing or evenly distributing pressure.

equalizer (e″kwah-li′zer) one who or that which equalizes or makes things equal or uniform. **Ballard stress e.,** Ballard stress equalizer ATTACHMENT. **stress e.,** stress-breaker.

Equanil trademark for *meprobamate.*

equate (e′kwāt) to make equal or equivalent.

equation (e-kwa′zhun) [L. *aequatio,* from *aequare* to make equal] an expression made up of two members connected by the sign of equality, =. See also INDEX and QUOTIENT. **Ambard's e.,** Ambard's FORMULA. **Arrhenius'e.,** an equation describing the temperature dependence of a reaction rate constant, $k = Ae^{-E_aRT}$, where k is the rate constant, Ae the activation energy, R the gas constant, T the absolute temperature, A the preexponential factor. **Ayala's e.,** Ayala's QUOTIENT. **balanced e.,** see *chemical e.* **chemical e.,** a quantitative and qualitative statement expressing a chemical reaction, the reacting substances being placed on the left side of the formula and those of the reaction products on the right with the equality sign between. The equation must obey the law of conservation of mass in that the reactants and products must contain the same total mass of each type of atom in the system; when this requirement is met, the equation is said to be balanced. To represent the formation of water, the equation is written:

$$2H_2 + O_2 = 2H_2O$$

Called also *reaction e.* See also OXIDATION-REDUCTION. **Henderson-Hasselbalch e.,** a formula for calculating the pH of a buffer solution, such as blood plasma, pH = pK' + log (BA)/(HA), where HA is the concentration of a weak acid, BA the concentration of a weak salt of this acid, and pK' the buffer system. **reaction e.,** chemical e.

equator (e-kwa′tor) [L. *aequator* equalizer] an imaginary line encircling a globe, equidistant from the poles. Used in anatomical nomenclature to designate such a line on a spherical organ, dividing the surface into two approximately equal parts. Called also *aequator.*

equatorial (e″kwah-to′re-al) pertaining to an equator; occurring at the same distance from each extremity of an axis.

equi- [L. *aequus* equal] a combining form meaning equal.

equiaxial (e″kwe-ak′se-al) [*equi-* + Gr. *axōn* axle] having axes of the same length.

equilateral (e″kwī-lat′er-al) having sides that are equal or identical. Called also *isolateral.*

equilibration (e″kwi-li-bra′shun) the achievement of a balance between opposing elements or forces. **mandibular e.,** 1. the act(s) performed to place the mandible in equilibrium. 2. a condition in which all of the forces acting upon the mandible are neutralized. 3. a term applied to adjustive grinding of an interfering tooth structure during the functional stroke. **occlusal e.,** occlusal ADJUSTMENT.

equilabrator (e″kwi-li-bra′tor) an apparatus used to produce or maintain a state of balance between opposing forces.

equilibria (e″kwi-lib′re-ah) [L.] plural of *equilibrium.*

equilibrium (e″kwi-lib′re-um) [L. *aequus* equal + *libra* balance] a state of balance or equipoise; a condition in which opposing forces exactly counteract each other. **chemical e.,** a balanced state reached when a chemical reaction apparently stops and decomposition and recombination proceed at equal speed. Called also *dynamic chemical e.* See also reversible REACTION. **e. constant,** equilibrium CONSTANT. **e. diagram,** phase DIAGRAM.

dynamic e., the condition of balance between varying shifting, and opposing forces which is characteristic of living processes. **dynamic chemical e.,** chemical e. **functional e.,** the equalization of the counteraction of antagonistic forces acting on a system, such as the masticatory apparatus, where the forces from the facial and labial muscles are equalized by the forces exerted by the tongue. **Hardy-Weinberg e.,** Hardy-Weinberg LAW. **radioactive e.,** a fixed ratio between a radioactive element and one of its disintegration products that results after the lapse of a suitable time, owing to their half-value periods. That of uranium and radium is 2,380,000 to 1.

equivalence (ĕ-kwiv′ah-lens) 1. the condition of being equivalent. 2. the ratio of antigen to antibody concentration which results in total incorporation of both reagents to form a maximal antigen-antibody combination, yielding a precipitate or aggregate. 3. see equivalent WEIGHT.

equivalent (ĕ-kviv′ah-lent) [L. *aequivalens,* from *aequus* equal + *valere* to be worth] 1. having the same value. 2. chemical e. 3. a symptom that replaces one that is usual in a given disease. **aluminum e.,** the thickness of pure aluminum affording the same radiation attenuation, under specified conditions, as the material or materials being considered. See also aluminum FILTER and FILTRATION (2). **bursa-e.,** BURSA-equivalent. **bursal e. tissue,** bursal equivalent TISSUE. **chemical e.,** 1. gram e. 2. drug products from different sources which contain essentially identical amounts of the identical active ingredients in identical dosage forms; meet existing physiochemical standards in official compendia; and are considered to be indistinguishable. **clinical e.,** see clinically equivalent drugs, under DRUG. **concrete e.,** the thickness of concrete having a density of 2.35 gm/cm³, which would afford the same radiation attenuation, under specified conditions, as the material or materials being considered. **dose e.,** the product of absorbed radiation dose in rads and modifying factors, namely the quality factor (QF), distribution factor (DF), and any other necessary factors. The unit of dose equivalent is the rem. Abbreviated *DE.* **generic e.,** see generically equivalent drugs, under DRUG. **gram e.,** that quantity in grams of the active reagent which will bring into reaction 1 gram of hydrogen. Called also *chemical e.* See also NORMALITY. **lead e.,** the thickness of pure lead affording the same radiation attenuation, under specified conditions, as the material or materials being considered. **lethal e.,** a gene carried in the heterozygous state, which, if homozygous, would be lethal, or any combination of genes which would be lethal to 100 percent of homozygotes; for example, a combination of two genes in the heterozygous state, either of which in the homozygous state would be lethal to 50 percent of the carriers. **neutralization e.,** the equivalent weight of an acid as determined by neutralization with a base regarded as a primary standard. **rad e. therapeutic,** see RET. **therapeutic e.,** see therapeutically equivalent drugs, under DRUG. **tissue e.,** a term used to describe a material whose absorbing and scattering properties for a given radiation simulate as closely as possible those of a given biological material, such as bone, fat, or muscle. For muscle and soft tissue, water is usually the best tissue-equivalent material. **toxic e.,** the amount of poison per kilogram of body weight necessary to kill an animal.

Er erbium.

Eraldin trademark for *practolol.*

Erantin trademark for *propoxyphene hydrochloride* (see under PROPOXYPHENE).

erasion (e-ra′zhun) [L. *erasio*] removal by scraping, or curettage.

Erb, Werner [German physician] see Rotter-Erb SYNDROME.

Erb-Goldflam syndrome [Wilhelm Heinrich *Erb,* German physician, 1840–1921; Samuel *Goldflam,* Polish physician, 1852–1932] MYASTHENIA gravis.

erbium (er′be-um) [named after *Ytterby,* a town in Sweden] a rare earth occurring as a dark gray metallic, soft, malleable solid. Symbol, Er; atomic number, 68; atomic weight, 167.26; melting point, 159°C; specific gravity, 9.066; valence, 3. Erbium has six naturally occurring isotopes (162, 164, 166–168, 170), and a number of artificial radioactive ones (152–154, 157–161, 163, 165, 169, 170–171). It is insoluble in water, but soluble in acids. Used in nuclear and laser technology. Its toxicity is low.

Erco-Fer trademark for *ferrous fumarate* (see under FUMARATE).

Ercolani see ARCOLANO.

erector (e-rek′tor) [L.] a general anatomical term for a structure that erects, as a muscle which raises or holds up a part.

erg (erg) [Gr. *ergon* work] in the centimeter-gram-second system, a unit of work or energy, being the work performed when the force of 1 dyne moves its point of operation through a distance of 1 cm; equivalent to 2.4×10^{-8} gram calories, or 0.624×10^{12} electron volts.

ergasia (er-ga′se-ah) [Gr. "work"] a hypothetical substance which stimulates the activity of body cells.

ergastoplasm (er-gas′to-plazm) [Gr. *ergasia* work + *plasm*] granular reticulum; see endoplasmic RETICULUM. See also RIBOSOME.

Ergate trademark for *ergotamine tartrate* (see under ERGOTAMINE).

ergo- [Gr. *ergon* work] a combining form denoting relationship to work.

Ergobasine trademark for *ergonovine*.

ergocalciferol (er-go-kal-sif′er-ol) VITAMIN D₂.

ergocornine (er″go-kor′nēn) a natural ergot alkaloid derived from lysergic acid, 12′-hydroxy-2′,5′α-bis(1-methylethyl)ergotaman-3′,6′,18-trione. It is soluble in acetone, chloroform, ethyl acetate, ethanol, and methanol, but not in water. Similarly to other ergot alkaloids, it is a smooth muscle stimulant with vasoconstrictor properties. Used in the treatment of migraine.

ergocristine (er″go-kris′tēn) a natural ergot alkaloid derived from lysergic acid, 12 - hydroxy - 2′ - (1 - methylethyl) - 5′α - (phenyl-methyl)ergotaman-3′,6′,18-trione. It is soluble in ethanol, methanol, acetone, chloroform, ethyl acetate, slightly soluble in ether, and insoluble in water. Similarly to other ergot alkaloids, it is a smooth muscle stimulant with vasoconstrictor properties. Used chiefly in the treatment of migraine.

Ergomar trademark for *ergotamine tartrate* (see under ERGOTAMINE).

Ergometrine trademark for *ergonovine*.

ergonomics (er″go-nom′iks) [ergo- + Gr. *nomos* law] the science relating to man and his work, embodying the anatomic, physiologic, psychologic, and mechanical principles affecting the efficient use of human energy. When applied to dentistry, it is the science encompassing all factors that relate to the quality and quantity of dental care delivered (work output) in comparison to the amount of work input and the amount of physical and mental fatigue generated in the process, its objective being to seek means by which an equal or greater work output may be achieved with less mental or physical fatigue experienced by the dentist, the assistant, or the patient.

ergonovine (er″go-no′vēn) a natural ergot alkaloid, 9,10-didehydro - N - (2 - hydroxy - 1 - methylethyl) - 6 - methylergoline - 8β (S)-carboxamide; it may also be produced synthetically. It occurs as a crystalline substance that is soluble in alcohol, ethyl acetate, acetone, and water. Used chiefly as an oxytocic drug and in the treatment of migraine. Trademarks: Ergobasine, Ergometrine, Ergotrate, Ergotocine, Syntometrine. **e. maleate,** the maleate salt of ergonovine, occurring as a white or yellowish, odorless, microcrystalline, photosensitive powder that is soluble in water and ethanol, but not in ether and chloroform. It is a smooth muscle stimulant and vasoconstrictor agent, used chiefly as an oxytocic and in the treatment of migraine. Nausea, vomiting, and hypertensive episodes are principal side effects. Gangrene of the hands and feet due to pathological changes in the peripheral blood vessels may be associated with too large doses or prolonged use. Trademarks: Cornocentin, Ermetrine.

ergosome (er′go-sōm) [ergo- + Gr. *sōma* body] polyribosome.

ergosterol (er-gos′tĕ-rol) a compound, ergosta-5,7,22-trien-3β-ol, occurring as colorless crystals that are soluble in ethanol, benzene, and ether, but not in water. On exposure to light and air, the crystals turn yellow. It is an antirachitic drug and a vitamin D precursor which is converted to vitamin D₂ (see under VITAMIN) after ultraviolet irradiation. **activated e.,** VITAMIN D₂.

ergot (er′got) [Fr.; L. *ergota*] the dried sclerotium of *Claviceps purpurea*, which develops on rye plants. It is a source of several alkaloids, divided into two series of optically active, isomeric groups: the pharmacologically active *l* forms (designated by the suffix *-ine*), and the pharmacologically inactive *d* forms (designated by the suffix *-inine*). The former are naturally occurring alkaloids and the latter result from chemical manipulation. The *l* forms are characterized by their stimulant effects on the smooth muscle and vasoconstrictor properties, and are used in the treatment of migraine and as oxytocics.

ergotamine (er-got′ah-mēn) an ergot alkaloid, 12′-hydroxy-2′-methyl - 5α-(phenylmethyl)ergotaman - 3′,6′,18 - trione, hav-

ing smooth muscle-stimulating and vasoconstrictor properties. Used chiefly as an oxytocic and in the treatment of migraine. **e. tartrate,** the tartrate salt of ergotamine, occurring as a white to yellowish crystalline powder or colorless crystals that are slightly soluble in water and ethanol; an excess of tartaric acid increases their solubility. It is smooth muscle stimulant with vasoconstrictor properties, used chiefly in the treatment of migraine and as an oxytocic. Nausea, vomiting, epigastric discomfort, diarrhea, bradycardia or tachycardia, paresthesia, myalgia, edema (especially of the face and extremities), dermatitis, and occasional hypertension are the principal side effects. Prolonged administration may produce severe vasoconstriction, gangrene, and endarteritis. Trademarks: Ergate, Ergomar, Ergotartrat, Exmigra, Femergin, Lingraine, Lingran.

Ergotartrat trademark for *ergotamine tartrate* (see under ERGOTAMINE).

Ergotex trademark for *dihydroergotamine mesylate* (see under DIHYDROERGOTAMINE).

Ergotocine trademark for *ergonovine*.

Ergotrate trademark for *ergonovine*.

Erich, John Bernhardt [born 1907] a distinguished American plastic and maxillofacial surgeon.

Erich arch bar see under BAR.

erinitrit (er″i-ni′trīt) SODIUM nitrite.

Erlenmeyer flask [Emil Richard August Carl *Erlenmeyer,* German chemist, 1825–1909] see under FLASK.

Ermetrine trademark for *ergonovine maleate* (see under ERGONOVINE).

Eromycin trademark for *erythromycin estolate* (see under ERYTHROMYCIN).

erosion (e-ro′zhun) [L. *erosio,* from *erodere* to erode] 1. an eating away; destruction of the surface of a tissue. 2. progressive loss of the hard substance of a tooth by chemical processes that do not involve bacterial action. See also ABRASION and ATTRITION. 3. the act or process of gradual destruction of something; the attacking of the surface of an object, such as a metal restoration, by electrolytic and chemical processes, particularly when two dissimilar metals are present. **dish-shaped e.,** a dish-shaped shallow concavity, confined mainly to the gingival half of the tooth, its border frequently touching the gingiva. It occurs most commonly on the incisor teeth, the deepest part of the lesion being in the center of the concavity, the walls radiating upward to sound tooth structure. If allowed to develop unchecked, the erosion usually assumes a ∪ shape. Called also *saucer-shaped e.* notch-shaped e., wedge-shaped e. **saucer-shaped e.,** dish-shaped e. **V-shaped e.,** wedge-shaped e. **wedge-shaped e.,** a V-shaped lesion occurring most commonly on the mesial aspect of the facial surfaces of bicuspid and molar teeth. It usually starts at the level of the gingival border, spreading rapidly, and involving tooth structure below the gingivae. The wedge develops along the gingival wall perpendicularly to the surface of the tooth and the facial wall and at a right angle to the base of the lesion. Tooth sensitivity is usually associated. Called also *notch-shaped e.* and V-*shaped e.*

erosive (e-ro′siv) 1. causing, characterized by, or producing erosion. 2. an agent that produces erosion.

erratic (ĕ-rat′ik) [L. *errare* to wander] 1. deviating from the proper or expected course or conduct. 2. wandering.

error (er′or) a defect in structure or function; a deviation. **inborn e. of metabolism,** inborn error of METABOLISM.

eructation (e-ruk-ta′shun) [L. *eructatio*] the act of belching.

eruption (e-rup′shun) [L. *eruptio* a breaking out] 1. a prominent lesion of the skin marked by redness. 2. the process of breaking out, appearing, or becoming visible. 3. tooth e. **active e.,** the continued eruption of the teeth after complete formation of their dentinal roots, consisting of the movement of the teeth in the direction of the occlusal plane, being coordinated with attrition. The teeth erupt to compensate for tooth substance worn away by attrition and attrition reduces the clinical crown and prevents it from becoming disproportionately long in relation to the clinical root. Ideally, the rate of active eruption keeps pace with tooth wear, preserving the vertical dimension. As the teeth erupt, cementum is deposited at the apices and furcations of the roots, and bone is formed along the fundus of the alveolus and at the crest of the alveolar bone; part of the tooth substance lost by attrition is replaced by lengthening of the root and socket depth is maintained to support the root. See also attritional OCCLUSION. **bullous e.,** an eruption of large blebs or blisters. **bullous recurrent e.,** EPIDERMOLYSIS bullosa. **continuous e.,** a concept that tooth eruption continues throughout life and does not cease when teeth meet their functional antagonists. See also *active e.* and *passive e.,* and see attritional OCCLUSION. **delayed e.,** delayed DENTITION. **drug e., fixed,** a cutanous manifestation in drug hypersensitivity, characterized by the appearance of skin eruptions on the same areas of the body, regardless of the drug or the route of its administration. See also drug REACTION. **ectopic e.,** eruption of a maxillary first permanent molar mesial to its normal position, resulting in the resorption of the roots of the second primary molar. It also occurs occasionally in the mandibular permanent lateral incisor area, causing premature resorption of the root of the adjacent primary cuspid. **fixed e.,** a circumscribed inflammatory skin lesion(s) that recurs at the same site(s) over a period of months or years; each attack lasts only a few days but leaves residual pigmentation which is cumulative. **fixed drug e.,** a drug eruption that recurs at the same site. **Kaposi's varicelliform e.,** a diffuse eruption of umbilicated vesicles and pustules resembling varicella, occurring on the skin of the upper trunk, neck, scalp, and face, in patients with pre-existing active dermatitis, particularly atopic dermatitis. High fever may accompany the eruption, which may last for several days to a week. Both the vaccinia virus and the herpes simplex virus have been isolated. Called also *eczema vaccinatum, herpetic eczema, Kaposi's dermatitis,* and *pustulosis herpetica infantum.* **macular e.,** an eruption in the form of spots, due to hemorrhage, congestion, or increased or diminished pigmentation. **maculopapular e.,** an eruption that consists of both maçules and papules; the term is sometimes used loosely when only one or the other is present. **passive e.,** the apparent eruption of a tooth that is actually the exposure of the crown of the tooth by separation of the epithelial attachment from the enamel and migration to the cementoenamel junction. **passive e., altered, passive e., delayed,** passive eruption taking place at the time when the gingiva remains on the bullous portion of the enamel instead of receding to the cementoenamel junction. **petechial e.,** an eruption in the form of very minute spots, due to hemorrhage; a purpura. **premature e.,** see premature teeth, under TOOTH. **polymorphous e.,** an eruption characterized by lesions in many different stages of evolution, from incipient through mature to healing. **recurrent summer e.,** HYDROA aestivale. **surgical e.,** surgical removal of tissue blocking an unerupted tooth, to permit eruption. **tooth e.,** the final stage of odontogenesis, whereby a tooth breaks out from its crypt through surrounding tissue. It occurs when the growth of the root has begun, and is accomplished through the appositional activity in radicular dentinogenesis and cementogenesis. Contributing to tooth eruption are the organizational and proliferative activity of the primitive pulp, the activity of the vascular channels in the dental pulp, and the reorganization of the body crypt and the periodontal connective tissue. See illustration at ODONTOGENESIS and *Table of Chronology of Human Dentition* at TOOTH.

eruptive (e-rup'tiv) pertaining to or characterized by eruption.

Erwinia (er-win'e-ah) [named for *Erwin* F. Smith] a genus of gram-negative, facultatively anaerobic bacteria of the family Enterobacteriaceae, occurring as single, straight rods, 0.5 to 1.0 μm in length by 1.0 to 3.0 μm in width. They are generally saprophytic organisms causing diseases in plants or constituting the epiphytic flora, with the exception of one strain that has been isolated from animals.

Erycin trademark for *erythromycin.*

erysipelas (er"ĭ-sip'ĕ-las) [Gr. *erythros* red + *pella* skin] a contagious disease of the skin and occasionally of the mucous membranes, caused by infection with group A hemolytic streptococci. A local lesion, fever, malaise, irritability, vomiting, and lack of appetite are the common symptoms. The butterfly type lesion extending from one cheek to the other across the nose is usually present in facial involvement; it may be hot, red, and tender, sometimes associated with vesiculation. Leukocytosis is usually present. Oral involvement may include a hard, painful swelling of the pharynx, nose, and larynx, sometimes leading to suffocation. Complications may include bronchopneumonia, septicemia, peritonitis, abscesses, thrombosis of the dural sinuses, and meningitis or brain abscesses. Called also *St. Anthony's fire* and *St. Francis' fire.*

Erysipelothrix (er"ĭ-sip'ĕ-lo-thriks") [erysipelas + Gr. *thrix* hair] a genus of rod-shaped bacteria of uncertain affiliation, including gram-negative, aerobic, nonsporing, nonmotile organisms with a tendency to form long filaments that may thicken to show granules. They are parasitic in mammals, birds, and fish. **E. monocytog'enes,** *Listeria monocytogenes;* see under LISTERIA. **E. rhusiopa'thiae,** a species occurring as short, slender, straight or slightly curved rods, about 0.2 to 0.4 by 0.5 to 2.5 μm in size. It is the causative agent of swine erysipelas, and also infects sheep, turkeys, and rats. An erythematous-edematous lesion, commonly on the hand, resulting from contact with infected meat, hides, or bones, represents the usual type of infection in man. It is resistant to polymyxin B and sulfonamides, but is sensitive to penicillin, streptomycin, neomycin, and other antibiotics. Called also *Bacillus rhusiopathiae* and *Bacterium rhusiopathiae.*

erythema (er"ĭ-the'mah) [Gr. *erythēma* flush] redness of the skin or mucous membranes due to hyperemia, inflammation, or denudation. **e. annula're,** see *e. multiforme.* **e. bullo'sum,** see *e. multiforme.* **e. bullo'sum veg'etans,** PEMPHIGUS vegetans. **epidemic e.,** acrodynia. **e. dose, e. exposure,** erythema DOSE. **e. figura'tum,** see *e. multiforme.* **e. i'ris,** see *e. multiforme.* **e. margina'tum,** see *e. multiforme.* **e. mi'grans,** benign migratory GLOSSITIS. **e. multifor'me,** an acute, inflammatory disease of the skin and mucous membranes, marked by multiform reddish macules, papules, and vesicles with a symmetric distribution over the sides of neck and face, dorsal surfaces of hands, forearms, feet, legs, and mucous membranes. The lesions develop rapidly, usually within days, and attacks last about 2 to 3 weeks; they may appear as separate rings (*e. annulare*), vesicles or bullae (*e. bullosum*), and concentric rings (*e. iris*), or in round patches with elevated edges (*e. marginatum*), or in variously figured arrangements (*e. figuratum*). It has also been classified according to severity of symptoms into a mild form (*Hebra's disease*) and a severe form (*Stevens-Johnson syndrome*). Oral lesions, similar to those of the skin, consist of hyperemic macules, papules, or vesicles that erode and are painful. Ocular complications consisting of conjunctivitis leading to corneal ulcers occur. It is believed to have an allergic etiology. A form consisting of stomatitis, conjunctivitis, and a macular eruption is known as *Fuch's syndrome.* **e. multiforme, bullous malignant,** Stevens-Johnson SYNDROME. **e. multifor'me exudati'vum ma'jor,** Stevens-Johnson SYNDROME. **e. streptog'enes,** PITYRIASIS alba.

erythematous (er"ĭ-them'ah-tus) of the nature of erythema.

erythemogenic (er"ĭ-the'mo-jen'ik) [erythema + Gr. *gennan* to produce] causing erythema.

erythralgia (er"ĭ-thral'je-ah) [erythro- + -algia] redness and pain of the skin.

erythremia (er"ĭ-thre'me-ah) [erythro- + Gr. *haima* blood + -ia] presence in the blood of excessive numbers of erythrocytes; POLYCYTHEMIA vera. **chronic familial e.,** Cooley's ANEMIA. **high altitude e.,** Monge's DISEASE.

erythremoid (er"ĭ-thre'moid) resembling erythremia.

erythrite (ĕ-rith'rīt) erythritol.

erythritol (ĕ-rith'ri-tol) a compound that is twice as sweet as sucrose, 1,2,3,4-butanetetrol, found in algae, lichens, grasses, and fungi, which is also produced synthetically. It occurs as tetragonal prisms that are soluble in water, pyridine, and ethanol, but not in ether. Used as a coronary vasodilator. Called also *erythrite, erythroglucin, erythrol, phycide,* and *tetrahydroxybutane.* **e. tetranitrate,** ERYTHRITYL tetranitrate.

erythrityl tetranitrate (e-rith'rī-til) a powerful explosive, 1,2,3,4-butanetetrol tetranitrate, occurring as a white, bitter powder with a nitric oxide–like odor, which is soluble in acetone and ethanol, but not in water. Used only in solution as a vasodilator. Headache, dizziness, and nausea may occur. Called also *erythritol tetranitrate, erythrol tetranitrate,* and *tetranitrol.* Trademarks: Cardilate, Cardioid.

erythro- [Gr. *erythros* red] a combining form meaning red, or denoting a relationship to red.

erythroblast (e-rith'ro-blast) [erythro- + Gr. *blastos* germ] an immature nucleated erythrocyte. See also ERYTHROPOIESIS. **basophilic e.,** basophilic NORMOBLAST. **early e.,** basophilic NORMOBLAST. **late e.,** polychromatic NORMOBLAST. **polychromatic e.,** polychromatic NORMOBLAST.

erythroblastosis (ĕ-rith"ro-blas-to'sis) presence of erythroblasts in the circulating blood. **fetal e., e. fetalis. e. feta'lis,** a fetal hemolytic disease characterized by excessive destruction of erythrocytes, associated with active erythropoiesis and the presence of circulating erythroblasts. It is transmitted from Rh-positive fathers whose blood factor acts as an antigen to Rh-negative mothers, thus causing isoimmunization with consequent destruction of fetal erythrocytes. A similar condition may be caused by ABO incompatibility. Principal symptoms include nonpitting edema, jaundice, thoracic and abdominal distention, hepatosplenomegaly, above-average birth weight, short neck, pallor, and purpura, occurring singly or in various combinations. Deposition of blood pigment in the enamel and dentin may cause the teeth to assume a green, brown, or bluish discoloration. Many affected infants are stillborn; those which are born alive show symptoms within the first days of life. First-born infants of Rh-incompatible parents are not affected. Called also *congenital anemia of newborn, hemolytic disease of newborn, hydrops fetalis,* and *icterus gravis neonatorum.*

Erythrocin trademark for *erythromycin.*

erythrocyte (ĕ-rith'ro-sīt) [erythro- + Gr. *kytos* hollow organ] a red cell or red blood cell; a biconcave disk about 7.2 μ in diameter and 2.2 μ in thickness, concerned mainly with transporting oxygen, and also with the reaction between carbon dioxide and water through the use of carbonic anhydrase, which allows the blood to react with carbon dioxide, and with acid-base equilibrium of the body. Erythrocytes are produced by the bone marrow (see ERYTHROPOIESIS) after birth. During their development they are known as *pronormoblasts, erythroblasts, normoblasts,* and *reticulocytes.* Their life-span is about 120 days, and worn out cells are destroyed mainly by the spleen, with hemoglobin being digested by the reticuloendothelial cells and iron being released into the blood and transported to the bone marrow to produce new erythrocytes, while heme is converted into the bile pigment. Deficiency of erythrocytes or their ability to carry oxygen causes anemia; excessive numbers of erythrocytes is known as *polycythemia.* Erythrocytes are destroyed in hypotonic solutions (see HEMOLYSIS) and in hypertonic solutions shrivel or crenate. Called also *red corpuscle.* See also table of *Reference Values in Hematology* in Appendix. **e. count,** determination of the number of erythrocytes in a measured volume of blood. A lowered erythrocyte count (oligocythemia) is present in such conditions as pernicious anemia, hemolytic jaundice, iron deficiency anemia, acute aplastic anemia. An increased erythrocyte count indicates polycythemia. Called also *red cell count.* See also table of *Reference Values in Hematology* in Appendix. **e. half-life,** the time at which 50 percent of a given number of erythrocytes have been destroyed. **e. membrane,** erythrocyte STROMA. **Mexican hat e.,** target CELL (1). **e. sedimentation rate, e. sedimentation time,** an expression of the extent of settling of erythrocytes, per unit time, in a column of fresh citrated or otherwise treated blood. The average rate is 0 to 15 mm/hr in adult males; 0 to 20 mm/hr in adult females; and 0 to 10 mm/hr in children. An increase in the sedimentation rate occurs in diseases characterized by widespread tissue injury, as in rheumatoid arthritis, rheumatic fever, tuberculosis, myocardial infarction, or neoplasms. **spinous e.,** burr CELL. **e. stroma,** erythrocyte STROMA.

erythrocytosis (ĕ-rith″ro-si-to′sis) an absolute form of polycythemia which occurs as a secondary condition following stimulation of erythropoiesis by some external factor. Common etiologic factors include faulty oxygen saturation due to lowered atmospheric pressure or impaired pulmonary ventilation, cardiopulmonary defects, such as congenital heart diseases, production of abnormal hemoglobins by various toxic substances and drugs, and various tumors which stimulate erythropoiesis. Called also *secondary polycythemia.* See also Monge's DISEASE and Ayerza's SYNDROME.

erythroderma (ĕ-rith″ro-der′mah) [*erythro-* + Gr. *derma* skin] abnormal redness of the skin, especially over large areas of the body. **e. desquamativa in infants,** Leiner's DERMATITIS.

erythrodontia (ĕ-rith″ro-don′she-ah) [*erythro-* + Gr. *odous* tooth] reddish brown discoloration of the teeth.

erythroglucin (ĕ-rith′ro-gloo′sin) erythritol.

erythrol (ĕ-rith′rol, er′ith-rol) erythritol. **e. tetranitrate,** ERYTHRITYL tetranitrate.

erythromycin (ĕ-rith″ro-mi′sin) a broad-spectrum macrolide antibiotic, 14-ethyl - 7,12,13 - trihydroxy - 3,4,7,9,11,13-hexamethyl-2,10 - dioxo - 6 - [[3,4,6 - trideoxy - 3 - (dimethylamino) - β - D - xylo-hexopyranosyl]oxy] - oxacyclotetradec - 4 - yl - 2,6 - dideoxy-3 -*C* - methyl-3-*O*-methyl-α-L-ribo-hexopyranoside, elaborated by *Streptomyces erythreus.* It occurs as a white or yellowish powder or crystals that are odorless and slightly hygroscopic and are soluble in alcohol, chloroform, ether, and acetone, moderately soluble in amyl acetate and ethylene chloride, and slightly soluble in water. Erythromycin is active against bacteria, rickettsiae, and viruses, also having shown *in vivo* activity against amebae, treponemas, and pinworms. Gram-positive cocci are particularly sensitive; they include staphylococci, streptococci, and pneumococci. Strains of gram-negative bacilli, *Haemophilus, Mycoplasma, Neisseria, Clostridium, Treponema, Fusobacterium nucleatum, Borrelia vincenti, Corynebacterium,* and other organisms are also sensitive. Used mainly in penicillin-resistant infectious diseases, including necrotizing ulcerative stomatitis. Called also *e. A.* Trademarks: Abomacetin, Erycin, Erythrocin, Ilotycin, Retcin. **e. A,** erythromycin. **e. estolate,** the 2′ -propionate dodecyl sulfate salt of erythromycin, occurring as a white, odorless, tasteless powder that is soluble in alcohol, acetone, and chloroform, but not in water. Its properties are similar to those of erythromycin, except that it may cause jaundice. This salt is converted to

erythromycin in the intestine. Called also *e. propionate lauryl sulfate.* Trademarks: E-Mycin, Eromycin, Ilosone, Lauromicina, Neo-Erycinum. **e. ethylsuccinate,** the 2′-ethyl succinate salt of erythromycin, occurring as a white or yellowish, odorless, tasteless, crystalline powder that is readily soluble in acetone, chloroform, ethanol, and benzene, slightly soluble in ether, and very slightly soluble in water. It has properties similar to those of erythromycin. Trademarks: Pediamycin. **e. glucoheptonate, e. gluceptate, e. glucoheptonic acid salt,** the glucoheptonate salt of erythromycin, occurring as a white, odorless, slightly hygroscopic powder that is readily soluble in water, ethyl and methyl alcohol, slightly soluble in acetone and chloroform, and insoluble in ether. Its properties are similar to those of erythromycin. Trademark: Ilotycin. **e. lactobionate,** an antibiotic prepared from erythromycin base and lactobiono-δ-lactone in water-acetone, and occurring as a white or yellowish powder or crystals with a faint odor, which is freely soluble in water and ethyl and methyl alcohol, slightly soluble in chloroform and acetone, and insoluble in ether. Its properties are similar to those of erythromycin. **e. octadecanoate,** e. stearate. **e. propionate lauryl sulfate,** e. estolate. **e. stearate,** the stearic acid salt of erythromycin, occurring as a white or yellowish, odorless, slightly bitter powder or crystals that are soluble in chloroform, ether, and ethyl and methyl alcohol, but insoluble in water. It is hydrolyzed in the small intestine to yield erythromycin. Called also *e. octadecanoate.* Trademarks: Bristamycin, Dowmycin E, Gallimycin, Pantomicina.

erythron (er′ĭ-thron) [Gr. *erythros* red] the circulating erythrocytes and the bone marrow from which they arise.

erythroplakia (ĕ-rith″ro-pla′ke-ah) ERYTHROPLASIA of Queyrat. **speckled e.,** see ERYTHROPLASIA of Queyrat.

erythroplasia (ĕ-rith″ro-pla′ze-ah) a condition of the mucous membrane characterized by erythematous papular or macular lesions. **e. of Queyrat,** a chronic disease of the mucous membranes, histologically characterized by epithelial changes ranging from mild dysplasia to carcinoma *in situ* or invasive carcinoma. The lesions are moist and shiny and, in the original description, occurred on the glans penis; they also affect the female genitalia and the lips of the oral mucosa. Three different types of lesions of the oral cavity have been described: (1) a bright, soft lesion with straight or scalloped well-demarcated margins, often very extensive, usually found on the buccal mucosa, sometimes on the soft palate, and rarely on the tongue and floor of the mouth; (2) erythroplasia interspersed with patches of leukoplakia in which the erythematous areas are irregular and not as bright as in the first type; most commonly occurring on the tongue and floor of the mouth; and (3) soft, slightly elevated, red lesions with an irregular outline and a granular or finely nodular surface speckled with tiny white plaques, sometimes referred to as *speckled leukoplakia* or *speckled erythroplakia,* occurring anywhere in the oral cavity. Called also *erythroplakia.*

erythropoiesis (ĕ-rith″ro-poi-e′sis) [*erythro-* + Gr. *poiesis* making] the production of erythrocytes, occurring during early embryogenesis in the yolk sac, during midpregnancy in the liver, spleen, and lymph nodes, and during the latter part of gestation and after birth, in the bone marrow. The erythrocytes derive from the bone marrow elements after birth and undergo gradual changes first to become pronormoblasts, which have large nuclei; there follows the basophil erythroblast stage, when the nucleoli disappear and the cytoplasm assumes a basophilic appearance; the polychromatophil erythroblast stage, when hemoglobin begins to appear; the orthochromatic erythroblast stage, when the cytoplasm possesses almost its full complement of hemoglobin and the nucleus undergoes pyknotic degeneration. The mature erythrocyte has no nucleus and its cytoplasm is filled with hemoglobin. Some circulating erythrocytes retain some basophilic reticulum; they are known as *reticulocytes.* Erythropoiesis is controlled by the oxygen content of the blood through the medium of erythropoietin which is synthesized and acts in response to anoxia.

erythropoietin (ĕ-rith″ro-poi′ĕ-tin) [*erythro-* + Gr. *poein* to make] a nondialyzable, relatively heat-stable glycoprotein with a molecular weight between 25,000 and 45,000, produced by the tissues, especially in the kidneys and liver, in response to hypoxia, which stimulates the production of erythrocytes (see ERYTHROPOIESIS). Called also *erythropoietic stimulating factor* and *hemopoietin.*

erythrose (er′ĭ-thros) [Fr.] erythrosis. **e. péribuccale pigmentaire,** Brocq's DISEASE.

erythrosis (er′ĭ-thro′sis) [*erythro-* + *-osis*] any condition marked by reddish discoloration of the skin and mucous membranes. **e. pigmenta′ta fa′ciei,** Brocq's DISEASE.

Es einsteinium.

Escat's phlegmon see under PHLEGMON.

eschar (es'kar) [Gr. *eschara* scab] a slough, such as one produced by burns or by gangrene.

escharotic (es-kah-rot'ik) 1. corrosive; capable of producing scab or eschar. 2. a caustic agent that precipitates the proteins of the cell and produces inflammatory exudate, resulting in the formation of a scab or eschar. Used to cauterize cutaneous and aphthous ulcers, minor wounds, and other lesions. Called also *cauterant*.

Escherich's bacillus [Theodor *Escherich*, German physician, 1857–1911] *Escherichia coli*; see under ESCHERICHIA.

Escherich's sign [Theodor *Escherich*] see under SIGN.

Escherichia (esh″er-i′ke-ah) [named after Theodor *Escherich*] a genus of bacteria of the family Enterobacteriaceae, occurring as gram-negative, facultatively anaerobic, straight rods, 1.1 to 1.5 by 2.0 to 6.0 μm in size (live organisms), or 0.4 to 0.7 by 1.0 to 3.0 μm (stained or dried organisms). **E. co′li,** a species constituting the greater part of the intestinal flora of man and other animals. *E coli* is characteristically positive to indol and methyl red tests, and negative to the Voges-Proskauer and citrate tests. The members are divided into physiological types on the basis of sucrose and salicin fermentation by some workers. They are separable into serotypes on the basis of distribution of heat-stable O antigens, envelope antigens of varying heat stability, and heat-labile flagellar antigens. Usually nonpathogenic, but pathogenic strains, often hemolytic, and predominantly certain serotypes are common. Pathogenic strains, which cause scours in calves and a hemorrhagic septicemia in newborn infants (Winckel's disease), are one of the most frequently encountered causes of human urinary tract infection and epidemic diarrheal disease, especially in children, and are found infrequently in localized suppurative processes. They often become the predominant bacteria in the flora of the mouth and throat during antibiotic therapy. Called also *Bacillus coli, Bacterium coli commune, coli bacillus, colibacillus, colon bacillus,* and *Escherich's bacillus.* **E. freun′dii,** *Citrobacter freundii;* see under CITROBACTER.

ESE abbreviation for Ger. *elektrostatische Einheit;* see electrostatic units, under UNIT.

Esidrex trademark for *hydrochlorothiazide.*

-esis a word termination denoting state or condition. See -SIS.

Eskacillin trademark for *penicillin G potassium* (see under PENICILLIN).

Eskazine trademark for *trifluoperazine hydrochloride* (see under TRIFLUOPERAZINE).

Esmarin trademark for *trichlormethiazide.*

eso- [Gr. *eso* inward] a combining form meaning within.

esoethmoiditis (es″o-eth″moi-di′tis) [*eso-* + *ethmoiditis*] inflammation within the sinuses of the ethmoid bone.

esophagus (e-sof′ah-gus) [Gr. *oisophagos,* from *oisein* to carry + *phagema* food] [NA] a musculomembranous tube which conveys food from the pharynx to the stomach by means of peristaltic waves and the force of gravity. Spelled also *oesophagus.*

Esopin trademark for *homatropine methylbromide* (see under HOMATROPINE).

esosphenoiditis (es″o-sfe-noi-di′tis) [*eso-* + *sphenoiditis*] osteomyelitis of the sphenoid bone.

esotropia (es″o-tro′pe-ah) [*eso-* + Gr. *tropein* to turn] deviation of a visual axis toward that of the other eye when fusion is a possibility.

Esparin trademark for *promazine.*

Espril trademark for *nialamide.*

espundia (es-poon′de-ah) mucocutaneous LEISHMANIASIS.

esquillectomy (es″kwil-lek′to-me) [Fr. *esquille* fragment + Gr. *ektome* excision] excision of fragments of bone following fractures caused by projectiles.

essence (es′ens) [L. *essentia* quality or being] 1. the most significant property of something. 2. a solution of a volatile or essential oil in alcohol. 3. the active principle of a plant.

essential (ĕ-sen′shal) [L. *essentialis*] 1. indispensable; necessary; constituting the necessary or inherent part of a thing. 2. pertaining to an essence. 3. having no apparent external cause; idiopathic.

Esser operation epithelial INLAY.

Essig-type splint see under SPLINT.

ester (es-ter) a class of compounds formed from alcohols and acids by the removal of water, having a functional group

$$O \atop \|$$

—C—O—C and a name ending in *-ate.* Called also *compound ether* and *ethereal salt.* **acetic acid ethynyl e., acetic acid vinyl e.,** VINYL acetate.

esterase [E.C.3.1] (es′ter-ās) [*ester* + *-ase*] a subclass of hydrolases, the enzymes of which catalyze the hydrolysis of ester linkages. Included in this group are some lipases that hydrolyze triglycerides, nucleases, and phosphatases that hydrolyze phosphoric acid ester bonds and other enzymes. **B-e., ali-e., atropine e.,** carboxylesterase. **butyrylcholine e.,** cholinesterase (1). **carboxyl e.,** carboxylesterase. **choline e. I,** acetylcholinesterase. **choline e. II,** cholinesterase (1). **cocaine e., procaine e.,** carboxylesterase.

esterification (es-ter″i-fi-ka′shun) the conversion of an acid into an ester by the addition of an alcohol.

esthesia (es-the′ze-ah) [Gr. *aisthēsis* perception] perception, feeling, or sensation.

esthesic (es-the′sik) [Gr. *aisthēsis* perception] pertaining to perception of sensations.

esthesio- [Gr. *aisthēsis* perception] a combining form denoting relationship to feeling or to the perceptive faculties.

esthesioneuroblastoma (es-the″ze-o-nu″ro-blas-to′mah) olfactory NEUROBLASTOMA.

esthesioneuroepithelioma (es-the″ze-o-nu″ro-ep″ĭ-the″le-o′mah) olfactory NEUROBLASTOMA.

esthetic (es-thet′ik) [Gr. *aisthēsis* sensation] 1. pertaining to sensation. 2. pertaining to beauty, or the improvement of appearance.

esthetics (es-thet′iks) 1. the branch of philosophy dealing with beauty. 2. in dentistry, a philosophy concerned with the appearance of a dental restoration, as achieved through its color and/or form. **denture e.,** the effect produced by a dental prosthesis on the cosmetic appearance of the patient. See also esthetic DENTISTRY and esthetic DENTURE.

estimate (es′tĭ-māt′) 1. to calculate or make a judgment as to the approximate quantity, extent of, or cost of something. 2. statement of the approximate charge for work or services to be performed, as an approximation of the anticipated cost of the recommended dental procedures, which may include information as to the amount that the patient's insurance may be expected to cover.

Estlander flap [Jakob August *Estlander,* Finnish surgeon, 1831–1881] see under FLAP. See also Abbé-Estlander OPERATION.

estradiol (es″trah-di′ol, es-tra′de-ol) an estrogen, estra-1,3,5(10)-triene-3,17-β-diol, occurring in three forms: α-, β-, and *cis-* (see under ESTROGEN).

estrane (es′trān) a class of steroid compounds, having a methyl group at C–13. See also STEROID.

Estren-Dameshek syndrome [Solomon *Estren,* American physician, born 1918; William *Dameshek,* American physician, born 1900] see under SYNDROME.

estriol (es′tre-ol) an estrogen, estra-1,3,5(10)-triene-3,1α,17β-triol; see ESTROGEN.

estrogen (es′tro-jen) a group of female sex hormones produced by nonpregnant females chiefly by the ovaries and, in lesser amounts, by the adrenal cortices; in pregnancy they are also produced by the placenta. Estrogens are synthesized from acetate, which is converted to cholesterol and, eventually, to androgens (male sex hormones also produced by the female endocrine glands), which are the immediate precursors of estrogens. All estrogens are steroids (see STEROID), containing 18 carbon atoms, substituted with oxygen or hydroxy groups at carbon 3 and 17, ring A being aromatic. At least six natural steroids are known, but only β-estradiol, estrone, and estriol occur in significant amounts. There are also several synthetic estrogens. The functions of estrogens consist of causing cellular proliferation and growth of tissue of the female sex organs, including that of the vagina, uterus, and fallopian tubes; enlargement of the breasts; growth of axillary and pubic hair, regional pigmentation; and shaping of the body contours. Under the influence of estrogens, the endometrial surface of the uterus is reepithelialized during the proliferative phase of menstruation and, during the secretory phase, they cause additional cell proliferation in the endometrium. Estrogens are used in the treatment of menopausal and menstrual disorders, functional uterine bleeding, acne, and osteoporosis; in preventing heart attacks; as oral contraceptives; in suppressing post-partum lactation; and in certain neoplastic diseases. Adverse reactions may include nausea and vomiting similar to that seen in early pregnancy, weight gain, fatigability, depression, brownish macules on the face, biliary calculi and jaundice, and thromboembolism. An increased incidence of cancer is suspected of being associated with estrogen use in certain women. Oral symptoms similar to changes in pregnancy, including gingival changes, such as mild inflammation, hyperemia, swelling, loss of tissue tone, tenderness, ulceration, and bleeding, may occur.

estrone (es'trōn) an estrogen, 3-hydroxyestra-1,3,5(10)-trien-17-one; see ESTROGEN.

esu electrostatic units; see under UNIT.

Et ethyl.

Etabus trademark for *disulfiram*.

Etambro trademark for *tetraethylammonium bromide* (see under TETRAETHYLAMMONIUM).

etchant (ech'ant) an agent used for etching. **acid e.,** a 30 to 50 percent solution of phosphoric acid, used in the technique of acid etching. Called also *dentin cleaner, enamel cleaner,* and *tooth conditioner.*

etching (ech'ing) 1. the application to the surface of metal or glass of a corrosive substance, such as an acid, for the purpose of creating a design or picture. 2. acid e. **acid e.,** the application of an acid, usually a 30 to 50 percent phosphoric acid solution, to the surface of the enamel for about 2 minutes to produce a rough surface (etch), the depth of which should not exceed 30 μ. The etching increases mechanical retention and provides added bonding to the resin to the tooth, also cleansing the enamel and providing improved wetting of the resin.

ethambutol hydrochloride (ĕ-tham'bu-tol) a bacteriostatic drug, −(+)2,2′-(ethylenediimino)-di-l-butanol hydrochloride, occurring as a white, bitter, crystalline powder that is soluble in water and propylene glycol, slightly soluble in alcohol, and insoluble in chloroform. It is used in the treatment of tuberculosis, being particularly effective in isoniazid- and streptomycin-resistant cases. Its pharmacological effect is believed to be due to its interfering with the RNA synthesis. Visual disorders, dermatitis, pruritus, anaphylaxis, anorexia, nausea, vomiting, abdominal pain, pyrosis, fever, headache, vertigo, malaise, confusion, hallucinations, paresthesia, leukopenia, gout, and liver disorders may occur. Trademark: Myambutol.

ethamivan (eth-am'ĭ-van) an analeptic, *N,N*-diethylvanillamide, occurring as a white crystalline powder with a faint, characteristic odor, which is freely soluble in ethanol, acetone, benzene, and chloroform and sparingly soluble in water and ether. Used as a respiratory stimulant in the treatment of barbiturate poisoning, to shorten postanesthetic recovery, and to relieve symptoms of hypoventilation. Side effects may include excessive stimulation of the central nervous system, coughing, sneezing, laryngospasm, muscle twitching, pruritus, flushing, and, in excessively large doses, hyperexcitability and convulsions. Trademarks: Cardiovanil, Emivan, Vandid.

ethanal (eth'ah-nal) acetaldehyde.

ethanamine (eth'an-am'in) ethylamine.

ethane (eth'ān) a hydrocarbon (alkane) of the methane series, C_2H_6, occurring as a colorless, odorless, relatively inactive, flammable gas, used in organic synthesis, as a fuel, and as a refrigerant. It is a simple asphyxiant, which, in high concentrations, is narcotic. Called also *bimethyl, dimethyl,* and *ethyl hydride.*

ethanol (eth'ah-nol) ethyl ALCOHOL.

ethanolamine (eth″ah-nol′ah-mēn) a substance, 2-aminoethanol, occurring as a colorless, viscous liquid with strong taste and ammoniacal odor, which is soluble in carbon tetrachloride, alcohol, and chloroform and miscible with water. It is used as an accelerator in the production of antibiotics and in various chemical processes. Ethanolamine occurs as a component of phospholipids, especially lecithins. The oleate is used as a sclerosing agent. Called also *β-aminoethyl alcohol, colamine, ethyloamine,* and *monoethanolamine.* **phosphatidyl e.,** cephalin.

ethchlorvynol (eth-klor'vĭ-nol) a mild hypnotic, 1-chloro-3-ethyl-1-penten-4-yn-3-ol, occurring as a colorless to yellowish liquid with a pungent odor, which is miscible with organic solvents, but not with water, and darkens on exposure to light and air. Used in insomnia, sleep disorders, anxiety, tension, and excitement. Prolonged use may lead to habituation or addiction; side reactions may include drowsiness, nausea, confusion, headache, dermatitis, hypotension, dizziness, blurring of vision, facial numbness, and allergic reactions. It is contraindicated in patients with a history of drug addiction, hypersensitivity, and porphyria, and in concomitant use of alcohol and central nervous system depressants. Called also *ethynyl carbinol.* Trademark: Placidyl.

ethene (eth-ēn') ethylene. **e. homopolymer,** polyethylene.

ethenylbenzene (eth″en-il-ben′zēn) styrene.

ether (e'ther) [L. *aether*, Gr. *aither* the upper and purer air] 1. ethyl e. 2. a compound in which an oxygen atom is interposed between two carbon atoms in the molecular structure, derived from alcohol by elimination of water. The lowest member of the series (methyl ether) is gaseous; others are liquid but rapidly vaporize. 3. hypothetical medium in the universe for the transmission of radio waves. **anesthetic e., ethyl e. e. chlora'tus, ethyl** CHLORIDE. **compound e.,** ester. **diethyl e., ethyl e. ethyl e.,** a colorless, mobile liquid with a sweetish taste and a burning odor, 1,1′-oxybisethane which is highly flammable and volatile, dissolving in water and being miscible with alcohol, benzene, chloroform, oils, and solvent hexane. It is the oldest inhalation anesthetic still widely used in spite of the danger of explosion. Also used as a surface antiseptic and cleansing agent, in expectorant and cough mixtures, in liniments, and as a solvent. It is mildly irritating to the skin and respiratory and oral mucosae, and inhalation of high doses may cause necrosis, coma, and death. Called also *ether, anesthetic, diethyl,* or *sulfuric e., ethoxyethane,* and *ethyl oxide.* **e. hydrochloric,** ethyl CHLORIDE. **e. muriatic,** ethyl CHLORIDE. **pyroacetic e.,** acetone. **salicylic e.,** ethyl SALICYLATE. **sulfuric e.,** ethyl e.

ethics (eth'iks) [Gr. *ethos* the manner and habits of man or of animals] the rules or principles which govern right conduct; the science of moral obligation, a system of moral principles, and the morality of one's conduct toward others. **medical e.,** the rules or principles governing the professional conduct of physicians. See also BIOETHICS and hippocratic oath, at HIPPOCRATES.

ethimide trademark for *ethionamide.*

ethinamate (ĕ-thin'ah-māt) a short-acting hypnotic, 1-ethynylcyclohexyl carbamate, occurring as white, odorless powder that is soluble in water, alcohol, chloroform, and ether. Used in the management of insomnia and in allaying apprehension before dental procedures. Drowsiness, skin rashes, paradoxical excitement in children, and habituation are some of the adverse reactions. It should not be used concurrently with other depressants and alcohol, and in patients with a history of drug abuse. Trademarks: Valamin, Valmid.

ethine (e'thēn) acetylene.

ethinyl (eth'ĭ-nil) ethynyl. **e. trichloride,** trichloroethylene.

Ethiodan trademark for *iophendylate.*

Ethiodol trademark for *ethiodized oil* (see under OIL).

ethionamide (eth″ĭ-on'ah-mīd) an antibacterial drug, 2-ethyl-4-pyridinecarbothioamide, occurring as a bright yellow powder with a faint sulfide-like odor, which is readily soluble in methanol and sparingly soluble in water, chloroform, ether, ethanol, and propylene glycol. Used in the treatment of tuberculosis. Side reactions may include nausea, vomiting, liver lesions, purpura, gynecomastia, inner ear lesions, drowsiness, depression, peripheral nervous system disorders, acne, and allergic dermatitis. It may also enhance toxicity of other drugs. Trademarks: Aetina, Ethimide, Iridocin, Nisotin, Thio-Mid, Trecator, Trescatyl.

ethmocephaly (eth″mo-sef'ah-le) [Gr. *ĕthmos* sieve + *kephalē* head] a congenital abnormality characterized by absence of the nasal bone, premaxilla, and turbinate bones, associated with fusion of the lacrimal, ethmoid, and frontal bones.

ethmofrontal (eth″mo-fron'tal) [*ethmoid* + *frontal*] pertaining to the ethmoid and frontal bones.

ethmoid (eth'moid) [Gr. *ēthmos* sieve + *eidos* form] sievelike; cribriform; pertaining to the ethmoid bone.

ethmoidectomy (eth″moi-dek'to-me) [*ethmoid* + Gr. *ektomē* excision] excision of the ethmoid cells or of a portion of the ethmoid bone.

ethmoiditis (eth″moi-di'tis) inflammation of the ethmoid bone.

ethmoidotomy (eth″moi-dot'o-me) surgical incision into the ethmoid sinus.

ethmolacrimal (eth″mo-lak'rĭ-mal) pertaining to the ethmoid and the lacrimal bones.

ethmomaxillary (eth″mo-mak'sĭ-lār-e) pertaining to the ethmoid and maxillary bones.

ethmonasal (eth″mo-na'zal) pertaining to the ethmoid and nasal bones.

ethmopalatal (eth″mo-pal'ah-tal) pertaining to the ethmoid and palatine bones.

ethmosphenoid (eth″mo-sfe'noid) pertaining to the ethmoid and sphenoid bones.

ethmoturbinal (eth″mo-tur'bĭ-nal) pertaining to the superior and middle nasal conchae.

ethmovomerine (eth″mo-vo'mer-in) pertaining to the ethmoid bone and the vomer.

Ethnine trademark for *pholcodine.*

Ethocaine trademark for *procaine hydrochloride* (see under PROCAINE).

ethoheptazine citrate (eth″o-hep'tah-zēn) an analgesic agent, ethyl hexahydro-1-methyl-4-phenylazepinecarboxylate citrate salt, occurring as a white, odorless powder that is sparingly soluble in water and alcohol and insoluble in ether. Used in relieving mild to moderate pain. Nausea, vomiting, epigastric pain, vertigo, and pruritus are the principal side effects.

ethosuximide (eth″o-suk′sĭ-mīd) an antiepileptic agent, 3-ethyl-3-methyl-2,5-pyrrolidinedione, occurring as a white crystalline powder or waxy solid with a characteristic odor, which is soluble in alcohol, ether, water, and chloroform and slightly in hexane. Side effects may include anorexia, nausea, vomiting, cramps, epigastric distress, abdominal pain, leukopenia, agranulocytosis, pancytopenia, aplastic anemia, eosinophilia, drowsiness, headache, vertigo, euphoria, hyperactivity, gingival enlargement, and hirsutism. Trademarks: Capitus, Emeside, Ethymal, Mesentol, Pemal, Pentinimid, Petnidan, Pyknolepsinum, Succimal, Suximal, Zarotin.

ethotoin (e-tho′to-in) an antiepileptic agent 3-ethyl-5-phenyl-2,4-imidazolidinedione, occurring as a white crystalline powder that is soluble in ethanol, benzene, ether, and alkali hydroxide solutions. Side reactions may include nausea, vomiting, fatigue, vertigo, headache, diplopia, nystagmus, rashes, numbness, fever, diarrhea, lymphadenopathy, and gingival enlargement. Trademark: Peganone.

***p*-ethoxyacetanilide** (par″ah-eth-ok′se-as″ĕ-tan″ĭ-lĭd) phenacetin.

ethoxyethane (eth-ok″se-eth′ān) ethyl ETHER.

Ethrane trademark for *enflurane.*

ethyl (eth′il) [*ether* + Gr. *hylē* matter] a radical of the two-carbon hydrocarbon, CH₃CH₂− or C₂H₅−. Abbreviated *Et.* **e. alcohol,** ethyl ALCOHOL. **e. aminobenzoate,** benzocaine. **e. biscoumacetate,** a coumarin derivative, bis(4-hydroxy-oxo-2*H*-1-benzopyran-3-yl) acetic acid ethyl ester, occurring as a crystalline dimorphous preparation, soluble in acetone and benzene, but not in water. Used as an anticoagulant in the treatment of thrombosis. It may predispose patients toward hemorrhage after oral surgery and cause spontaneous hemorrhage from the gingivae. Called also *tromexan, pelentan, ethyldicoumarol acetate, pelenton,* and *tromexan.* See also ANTICOAGULANT and COUMARIN. **e. chloride,** ethyl CHLORIDE. **e. ether,** ethyl ETHER. **e. hydride,** ethane. **e. oxide,** ethyl ETHER. **E. Parasept,** trademark for *ethylparaben.* **sal e.,** ethyl SALICYLATE. **e. salicylate,** ethyl SALICYLATE. **E. Thiurad,** trademark for disulfiram.

ethylamine (eth″il-am′ēn) an irritant, colorless, volatile liquid or gas with a strong ammoniacal odor, CH₃CH₂NH₂, which causes lesions of the skin and mucous membranes. Used in the production of drugs, dyes, and other chemical products. *E. oleate* is used as a sclerosing agent. Called also *aminoethane, ethanamine,* and *monoethylamine.*

ethylation (eth″il-a′shun) the act or process of introducing an ethyl group (C₂H₅) into a compound.

ethylbenzene (eth″il-ben′zēn) styrene.

ethyldicoumarol acetate (eth″il-di-koo′mah-rol) ETHYL biscoumacetate.

ethylene (eth′ĭ-lēn) [L. *aethylenum*] a colorless, flammable gas, somewhat lighter than air, H₂C=CH₂, which has a sweet taste and odor. Used in general anesthesia. It is potentially explosive, and inhalation of high concentrations may cause asphyxia and unconsciousness. Also used in the manufacture of ethyl alcohol and various chemicals; ethylene is a monomer in the production of polyethylene. Called also *ethene* and *olefiant gas.* **e. glycol,** ethylene GLYCOL. **methyl e.,** propylene. **e. oxide,** a colorless, flammable gas, C₂H₄O, which is soluble in water, alcohol, and ether. It is an alkylating agent with a broad germicidal spectrum, including spores and, probably, viruses. Used chiefly (usually mixed with CO₂ to reduce fire and explosion hazard) as a hospital disinfectant, as a fumigant, and as an argicultural fungicide. Also used to sterilize surgical and dental instruments, usually for 3 hours at 30°C. Airing of sterilized objects for 5 days at room temperature or 8 hours at 120°C prevents exposure to gas residues which may cause nausea, vomiting, and neurological disorders; severe exposure may result in death. Chemical burns can result from wearing inadequately aired articles of clothing, gloves, or shoes. Trademarks: Anprolene, Oxirane.

ethylenediaminotetraacetate (eth″ĭ-lēn-di″ah-mĭ-no-tet″rah-as′ĕ-tāt) a salt of ethylenediaminotetraacetic (edetic) acid; edetate. Abbreviated *EDTA.*

ethylenimine (eth″ĭ-lēn-im′ēn) an explosive, very poisonous chemical compound, C₂H₅N, occurring as a clear liquid with a strong odor of ammonia, which polymerizes easily and is miscible with water and most organic solvents. It causes cancer and irritation of the eyes, mucous membranes, and skin. Used in various chemical processes. Some ethylenimine derivatives (triethylenemelamine and triethylenethiophosphoramide) have alkylating properties and are used as cytotoxic drugs in cancer therapy. Called also *azacyclopropane* and *aziridine.*

ethylmorphine hydrochloride (eth″il-mor′fēn) a semisynthetic

opium alkaloid, 7,8-didehydro-4,5α-epoxy-3-ethoxy-17-methyl-morphinan-6α-ol hydrochloride, occurring as a white or yellowish, fine, odorless, crystalline powder that is soluble in water and ethanol and slightly soluble in chloroform and ether. It is an addicting analgesic and sedative with pharmacological properties similar to those of codeine. Because it is less likely to cause nausea and depression than morphine, it is used as a morphine substitute. When applied topically to abraded skin and mucous membranes, it produces hyperemia. Adverse reactions may include vertigo, headache, nausea, respiratory depression, vomiting, and constipation. Trademarks: Codethyline, Dionin.

ethyloamine (eth″il-o-ah′mēn) ethanolamine.

ethylparaben (eth″il-par′ah-ben) an antibacterial agent, 4-hydroxybenzoic acid ethyl ester, occurring as a white powder or colorless crystals that are soluble in glycerol, acetone, ethanol, ether, propylene glycol and slightly in water. Used in ointments and cosmetic preparations. Also used as a pharyngeal antiseptic. It may cause occasional hypersensitivity. Trademarks: Ethyl Parasept, Nipagin A, Solbrol A.

Ethymal trademark for *ethosuximide.*

ethyne (e′thin) acetylene.

ethynyl (eth′ĭ-nil) the group —C≡CH, when it occurs in organic compounds. Called also *ethyinyl.* **e. carbinol,** ethchlorvynol.

etiologic, etiological (e″te-o-loj′ik; e″te-o-loj′e-kal) pertaining to etiology, or to the causes of disease.

etiology (e″te-ol′o-je) [Gr. *aitia* cause + *-logy*] the study or sum of knowledge regarding causes of diseases. See also PATHOGENESIS.

etiotropic (e″te-o-trop′ik) [Gr. *aitia* cause + *tropos* turning] directed against the cause of a disease.

etorphine (et′or-fēn) a narcotic analgesic, 4,5α-epoxy-3-hydroxy-6-methoxy-α,17-dimethyl-α-propyl-6,14-ethenomorphinan-7α(R)-methanol, which has potentially habituating or addicting properties.

Etylon trademark for *tetraethylammonium bromide* (see under TETRAETHYLAMMONIUM).

Eu 1. europium. 2. euryon.

eu- [Gr. *eu* well] a combining form signifying well, easily, good; the opposite of DYS-.

Eubacterium (u″bak-te′re-um) [*eu-* + Gr. *baktērion* little rod] a genus of coryneform bacteria of the family Propionibacteriaceae, occurring as gram-positive, obligately anaerobic, non-spore-forming, nonmotile or motile, uniform or pleomorphic rods, which produce organic acids from carbohydrates or peptone, including butyric, acetic, or formic acids. They are found in the body cavities of animals, including man, soft tissue infections, vegetable products, and soil. Some species may be pathogenic. **E. aerofa′ciens,** a species isolated from various infections, including pleurisy, infected postoperative wounds, peritonitis, and furuncles, and from human feces and the intestinal contents of chickens, dogs, and swine. Called also *Bacteroides aerofaciens* and *Pseudobacterium aerofaciens.* **E. alactolyt′icum,** a species isolated from dental calculus, and from various infections, including pleurisy, infected postoperative wounds, and abscesses of the brain, lungs, intestines, and mouth. Called also *Ramibacterium alactolyticum* and *R. dentium.* **E. buda′yi, E. cadav′eris,** a species isolated from a cadaver, poorly sterilized catgut, and soil. Called also *Bacillus cadaveris butyricus, Bacterium budayi,* and *Pseudobacterium cadaveris.* **E. combe′sii,** a species isolated from human infection and from soil in Africa. **E. contor′tum,** a species isolated from various infections of humans, including appendicitis, salpingitis, rectocolitis, and pleurisy, and from human feces. Called also *Catenabacterium contortum.* **E. cylindroi′des,** a species isolated from human feces. Called also *Bacterium cylindroides, Bacteroides cylindroides,* and *Pseudobacterium cylindroides.* **E. endocardi′tidis,** a species isolated from a patient suffering from endocarditis and from soil and water. **E. foe′dans,** a species originally isolated from putrefied ham. Called also *Bacillus foedans.* **E. helminthoi′des,** a species occurring as nonmotile, straight or curved cells, about 0.7 to 1.0 by 3.0 to 20.0 μm in size, which are gram-positive in young cultures and gram-negative in older ones. Isolated from the mouth of infants, intestines of mollusks, and mud. Called also *Bacillus helminthoides* and *Catenabacterium helminthoides.* **E. len′tum,** a species isolated from various infections, including infected postoperative wounds and abscesses and from human blood and feces. Called also *Bacteroides lentus* and *Pseudobacterium lentum.* **E. limo′sum,** a species isolated from human feces, various human infections, including abscesses, the intestinal contents of rats, poultry, and fish, and mud. Called also *Bacteroides limosus* and *Mycobacterium limosum.* **E. monilifor'me,** a species isolated from various infections and from blood. Called also *Bacillus moniliforme* and *Bacillus rapazii.* **E. multifor'me,** a species isolated from dog feces and from soil. Called also *Bacillus multiformis.* **E. nitritog'enes,** a species isolated from human infections, cheese, peptic digest of meat, intestinal contents of a fish, and Antarctic soil. **E. par'vum,** a species occurring in pairs or chains of cells, isolated from various human infections, including appendicitis, pleurisy, brain abscesses, tonsillitis, and bronchitis, and from feces of foals. **E. recta'le,** a species isolated from feces and rectal abscesses. Called also *Bacteroides rectalis* and *Pseudobacterium rectale.* **E. sabur'reum,** a species isolated from materia alba on teeth. Called also *Catenabacterium saburreum* and *Leptotrichia aerogenes.* **E. te'nue,** a species isolated from various pathological conditions, including pleural fluid in malignant lymphogranuloma, breast cancer, and abscess, and from dog feces. Called also *Bacillus tenuis spatuliformis, Bacteroides tenuis, Cillobacterium spatuliforme,* and *C. tenue.* **E. tortuo'sum,** a species isolated from human infections and feces, mouse intestines, turkey liver lesions and enteritis, soil, and fresh water. Called also *Bacillus tortuosus, Bacteroides tortuosus,* and *Mycobacterium flavum* var. *tortuosum.* **E. ventrio'sum,** a species isolated in man from oral and pulmonary abscesses, neck infection, pleurisy, and bronchiectasis, and from human and dog feces. Called also *Bacillus ventriosus, Bacteroides ventriosus,* and *Pseudobacterium ventriosum.*

Eubine trademark for *oxycodone hydrochloride* (see under OXYCODONE).

eucalyptol (u″kah-lip′tol) a flavoring agent having also expectorant and antiseptic properties, 1,8-epoxy-*p*-methane, obtained from *Eucalyptus;* it is the principal component of eucalyptus oil. Eucalyptol occurs as a colorless liquid with a characteristic aromatic camphoraceous odor and a cooling spicy taste, and is soluble in ethanol and miscible with ethanol, chloroform, ether, glacial acetic acid, and volatile oils, but not with water. Used in the treatment of bronchitis and in inflammatory conditions of the nose and throat and in certain dermatoses. In dentistry, used as a solvent for gutta-percha for root canal filling and in the liquid portion of certain root canal sealers. It may cause burns of the mucous membranes on contact. Formerly used in the treatment of the root canal in preparation for filling. Called also *cajeputol* and *cineole.*

eucapercha (u″kah-per′chah) gutta-percha dissolved in eucalyptus oil; used in root canal therapy.

Eucaryotae (u-kar″e-o′te) [*eu-* + Gr. *karyon* nucleus] a kingdom of organisms made up of eukaryotic cells, including animals, higher plants, fungi, protozoa, and most algae (except bluegrass algae). Cf. PROCARYOTAE.

eucaryote (kar′e-ōt) eukaryote.

eucaryotic (u″kar-e-ot′ik) eukaryotic.

Eucestoda (u-ses-to′dah) Cestoda.

euchromatin (u-kro′mah-tin) the condensed state of chromatin with partially or fully uncoiled strands, being the interphase form of the chromosomes.

Eucodal trademark for *oxycodone hydrochloride* (see under OXYCODONE).

Eucoran trademark for *nikethamide.*

Eudatin trademark for *pargyline.*

eugenics (u-jen′iks) [*eu-* + Gr. *gennan* to produce] the study and control of procreation as a means of improving the hereditary characteristics of a race.

eugenol (u′jen-ol) a colorless or pale yellow liquid, 4-allyl-2-methoxyphenol, with a characteristic odor of cloves (from which it is extracted, being the active ingredient of oil of cloves), and a pungent, spicy taste, which darkens and thickens on exposure to air. It is slightly soluble in water and miscible with ethanol, ether, chloroform, and fixed oils. Used chiefly as an antiseptic and analgesic. In periodontology, used in a solution with oil or in a mixture with rosin and zinc oxide as a protective pack after gingival excision. In endodontics, used as an antiseptic in root canal therapy. Eugenol may cause burns of the mucous membranes on contact. When mixed with zinc oxide and water, eugenol forms zinc oxide–eugenol cement (see under CEMENT). Called also *allylguaiacol, caryophyllic acid,* and *eugenic acid.* **e. pack,** eugenol PACK.

euglobulin (u-glob′u-lin) a class of globulins that are insoluble in water but soluble in saline solutions. Cf. PSEUDOGLOBULIN.

eugnathia (u-na′the-ah) [*eu-* + Gr. *gnathos* jaw + -*ia*] an abnormality of the oral cavity, which is limited to the teeth and their immediate alveolar supports, and does not include the jaws. Cf. DYSGNATHIA.

eugnathic (u-nath′ic) [*eu-* + Gr. *gnathos* jaw] pertaining to or characterized by a normal state of the jaws.

eugnosia (u-no′se-ah) [*eu-* + Gr. *gnōsis* perception] ability to perceive and synthesize sensory stimuli into normal perception.

eukaryote (u-kar′e-ōt) an organism made up of eukaryotic cells (cells with true nuclei), including higher plants and animals, fungi, protozoa, and most algae. Written also *eucaryote.* Cf. PROKARYOTE.

eukaryotic (u″kar-e-ot′ik) [*eu-* + Gr. *karyon* nucleus] pertaining to eukaryotic cells or to organisms having eukaryotic cells (eukaryotes), such as higher plants and animals, fungi, protozoa, and most algae. Written also *eucaryotic.* Cf. PROKARYOTIC.

Eulenburg's disease [Albert *Eulenburg,* German neurologist, 1840–1917] congenital PARAMYOTONIA.

eumetria (u-me′tre-ah) [*eu-* + Gr. *metron* measure] a normal condition in which there is a proper measuring of distance in muscular acts so that a voluntary movement precisely achieves the intended goal: the proper range of movement. Cf. DYSMETRIA.

eumorphism (u-mor′fizm) [*eu-* + Gr. *morphē* form] retention of the normal form of a cell.

Eumycetes (u″mi-se′tēz) one of the two mycological divisions consisting of the proper or true fungi, which includes the perfect fungi (Ascomycetes, Zygomycetes, and Basidiomycetes), and a form-class of imperfect fungi (Deuteromycetes).

Eunoctin trademark for *nitrazepam.*

euphoria (u-fo′re-ah) [Gr. "the power of bearing easily"] bodily comfort; well-being; absence of pain or distress. In psychiatry, an abnormal or exaggerated sense of well-being, particularly common in the manic state.

euphoriant (u-fo′re-ant) 1. pertaining to, characterized by, or producing a condition of euphoria. 2. euphoriant AGENT.

Euphozid trademark for *iproniazid.*

euploid (u′ploid) [*eu-* + Gr. -*ploid*] 1. having a balanced set or sets of chromosomes. 2. an individual or cell having a balanced set or sets of chromosomes.

euploidy (u-ploi′de) the state of having a balanced set or sets of chromosomes.

eupnea (up-ne′ah) [*eu-* + Gr. *pnein* to breathe] normal breathing. See RESPIRATION.

Eurinol trademark for *trichlormethiazide.*

europium (u-ro′pe-um) [named after *Europe*] one of the rarest of the rare earths. Symbol Eu; atomic number, 63; atomic weight, 151.96; melting point 822°C; specific gravity, 5.243; valences, 2, 3. It is the most reactive of all rare earths, occurring as a steel-gray, malleable, soft metal, which oxidizes rapidly in air and may burn spontaneously. Europium has two naturally occurring isotopes (151 and 153) and many artificial radioactive ones (143–150, 152, 154–160). Used in electronic and nuclear technology. Its toxicity is unknown.

eury- [Gr. *eurys* wide] a combining form meaning wide or broad.

eurycephalic (u″re-sĕ-fal′ik) [*eury-* + Gr. *kephalē* head] pertaining to or characterized by a wide head. (The term is rarely used; *brachycephalic* is used more commonly.)

eurycranial (u″re-kra′ne-al) [*eury-* + *cranium*] pertaining to or characterized by a wide skull. (The term is rarely used; *brachycranial* is used more commonly.)

eurygnathic (u″rig-nath′ik) [*eury-* + Gr. *gnathos* jaw] pertaining to or characterized by a wide jaw.

eurygnathism (u-rig′nah-thizm) [*eury-* + Gr. *gnathos* jaw] the state of having a wide jaw.

euryon (u′re-on) [Gr. *eurys* wide] the point on the right and left parietal bones marking the greatest transverse diameter of the skull or head. Abbreviated *Eu.* See also entries under POINT and illustration at CEPHALOMETRY.

euryopia (u″re-o′pe-ah) [*eury-* + Gr. *ōps* eye] the state of having a wide opening of the eyes.

euryprosopic (u″re-pro-sop′ik) [*eury-* + Gr. *prosōpon* face] pertaining to or characterized by a low and wide face. See euryprosopic SKULL.

eurythermic (u″re-ther′mik) [*eury-* + Gr. *thermē* heat] able to grow through a wide range of temperature; said of bacteria capable of growing at 28°C to 50°C and above.

Eustachio (Eustachius), Bartolommeo [1524–1574] an Italian anatomist whose *Libellus de Dentibus,* published in 1563, was the first treatise of its kind of any consequence. He accurately described the number of roots of molar teeth and all the variations occurring in their number, length, and form.

Eustachius see EUSTACHIO.

Eustigmin trademark for *neostigmine.*

Eustrophinum trademark for *strophanthin.*

eutectic (u-tek′tik) [Gr. *eutēktos* easily melted or dissolved] 1. melting readily; said of a mixture that melts at a lower temperature than any of its ingredients. See also eutectic ALLOY. 2. eutectic COMPOSITION.

Eutensol trademark for *guanethidine.*

euthanasia (u″thah-na′zhe-ah) [eu- + Gr. *thanatos* death] 1. an easy or painless death. 2. mercy killing; the deliberate ending of life of a person suffering from an incurable and painful disease. **active e.,** that involving the use of methods designated to promote death sooner than would otherwise be expected. Called also *positive e.* **active involuntary e.,** active euthanasia without the patient's consent. **active voluntary e.,** active euthanasia with the patient's consent. Called also *assisted suicide.* **negative e.,** passive e. **passive e.,** that involving a failure to use therapies that would prolong life in a patient with a terminal illness. Called also *negative e.* **positive e.,** active e.

euthyroid (u-thi′roid) having a normally functioning thyroid gland.

Eutonyl trademark for *pargyline.*

eutopic (u-top′ik) [eu- + Gr. *topos* place] situated normally. Cf. ECTOPIC.

evacuator (ĕ-vak′u-a-tor) an instrument for removing fluid or small particles from a body cavity or container; formerly applied to an instrument for compelling evacuation of the bowels or bladder. **oral e.,** a suction device used for removing fluids, tooth fragments, and other debris from the field of operation.

evagination (ĕ-vaj″ĭ-na′shun) an outpouching of a layer or part. See also INVAGINATION.

evaluation (ĕ-val′u-a′shun) the act or process of appraising or determining a set of values. **quality e.,** quality CONTROL.

Evans' articulator [Daniel T. *Evans,* Philadelphia dentist, 19th century] see under ARTICULATOR.

Evans' syndrome [Robert S. *Evans,* American physician, born 1912] see under SYNDROME.

evaporation (ĕ-vap″o-ra′shun) vaporization. **heat of e.,** HEAT of evaporation.

Everbest Prosonic trademark for a vibrating type of *denture cleanser* (see under CLEANSER).

Ev, ev electron VOLT.

Eve's method [Frank Cecil *Eve,* English physician, 1871–1952] see artificial RESPIRATION.

eversion (e-ver′zhun) [L. *eversio*] a turning outward or inside out.

évidement (a-vĕd-maw′) [Fr.] the operation of scooping out a cavity or diseased portion of an organ.

evidence (ev′ĭ-dens) something that makes plain or clear or proves a fact. **e. of insurability,** a statement or proof of a person's physical condition or occupation affecting his acceptability for insurance.

évideur (a-ve-dur′) [Fr.] an instrument for performing évidement.

Evipal trademark for *hexobarbital.*

Evipan trademark for *hexobarbital.*

evolution (ev″o-lu′shun) [L. *evolutio,* from *e* out + *volvere* to roll] 1. an unrolling. 2. the process of development in which an organ or organism becomes more and more complex by the differentiation of its parts; a continuous and progressive change according to certain laws and by means of resident force.

evulsio (ĕ-vul′se-o) [L., from *e* out + *vellere* to pluck] evulsion.

evulsion (ĕ-vul′shun) [L. *evulsio*] extraction by force. See AVULSION.

Ewing's sarcoma (tumor) [James *Ewing,* New York pathologist, 1866–1943] see under SARCOMA.

Ewing's sign see under SIGN.

ex- [L. *ex;* Gr. *ex* out, away from] a prefix meaning away from, without, or outside, and sometimes used to denote completely, as in *exacerbation.*

exacerbation (eg-zas″er-ba′shun) [ex- + L. *acerbus* harsh] increase in the severity of symptoms or disease.

Exal trademark for *vinblastine sulfate* (see under VINBLASTINE).

examination (eg-zam″ĭ-na′shun) [L. *examinare*] 1. inspection or investigation, especially as a means of diagnosing disease, qualified according to the methods employed, as physical, roentgen, cystoscopic examination, etc. 3. the act or process of testing the level of knowledge, competency, or qualifications. **national board e.,** an examination developed and administered by a national board of examiners to test dental or medical students, usually, during the second and final year of dental or medical school and during the internship year. In most states the examination is required for licensure as a dentist or physician.

examiner (eg-zam′ĭ-ner) one who performs examination. **medical e.,** a physician who is knowledgeable in pathology, toxicology, diagnostic methods, and other fields of medical sciences as they apply to law and justice. His duties include investigation of the circumstances surrounding crimes resulting in death, including performing the necessary autopsies, and testifying in court as the medicolegal expert. See also CORONER.

exanthem (eg-zan′them) [Gr. *exanthēma*] any eruptive disease. Called also *exanthema.*

exanthema (eg″zan-the′mah), pl. *exanthemas, exanthem′ata* [Gr.] exanthem.

exanthemata (eg″zan-them′ah-tah) plural of *exanthema.*

exanthematous (eg″zan-them′ah-tus) of the nature of exanthem.

exarticulation (eks″ar-tik-u-la′shun) [ex- + L. *articulus* joint] amputation of a joint; removal of a portion of a joint.

excavatio (eks″kah-va′she-o), pl. *excavatio′nes* [ex- + L. *cavus* hollow] a general term used in anatomical nomenclature to designate a hollowed-out space. Called also *excavation.*

excavation (eks″kah-va′shun) [L. *excavatio*] 1. the act of hollowing out. 2. a hollowed-out space. Called also *excavatio.* **dental e.,** removal of carious material from a tooth in preparation for restoration.

excavator (eks′kah-va″tor) 1. an instrument for hollowing out something by removing the center or inner part, or for making a hole or cavity. 2. a scoop or gauge for surgical use. **dental e.,** a handcutting instrument designed for removing the carious dentin of a decayed tooth. See also DISCOID (4). **hatchet e.,** hatchet (2). **spoon e.,** a dental excavator having a spoonlike blade with the entire margin tapered and sharpened to cut carious dentin out of tooth cavities. Called also *spoon.* See illustration.

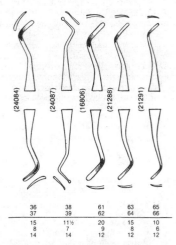

36	38	61	63	65
37	39	62	64	66

15	11½	20	15	10
8	7	9	8	6
14	14	12	12	12

Spoon excavators. (From H. O. Torres and A. Ehrlich: Modern Dental Assisting. 2nd ed. Philadelphia, W. B. Saunders Co., 1980.)

excementosis (ek-se″men-to′sis) hyperplasia of the cementum of the root of a tooth.

exception (ek-sep′shun) 1. something left out or excluded. 2. the act or process of leaving out or excluding something. 3. exclusion (3).

excess (ek′ses) a condition or state of surpassing or going beyond the bounds, limits, or expected amount or level. **marginal e.,** the contour of a restoration being greater than desired in the region of its margin. **vertical maxillary e.,** long face SYNDROME.

excipient (ek-sip′ĕ-ent) [L. *excipiens,* from *ex* out + *capere* to take] an inert substance added to a prescription in order to give a suitable consistency or form to the drug; a vehicle.

excise (ek-sīz′) to cut out or off.

excision (ek-sizh′un) [L. *excisio,* from *ex* out + *caedere* to cut] removal, as of an organ, by cutting. **conservative e.,** see conservative SURGERY. **interdental e.,** interdental DENUDATION. **local e.,** that limited to the immediate area of the lesion. See local SURGERY. **radical e.,** that involving not only the lesion but also tissues and organs that may be remote from the site. See radical SURGERY. **wide e.,** that involving the lesion and immediate adjacent tissues and parts.

excitability (ek-sīt″ah-bil′ĭ-te) susceptibility or readiness to respond to a stimulus.

excitant (ek-sīt′ant) an agent that produces excitation of the vital functions, or of those of the brain.

excitation (ek″si-ta′shun) [L. *excitatio*, from *ex* out + *citare* to call] 1. stimulation of physical or mental processes or actions. 2. the act of irritation or stimulation. 3. the addition of energy, as the excitation of a nucleus, atom, or molecule by absorption of photons or from inelastic collision with other particles.

exclusion (eks-kloo′zhun) [L. *exclusio*, from *ex* out + *claudere* to shut] 1. the act or instance of shutting or keeping out. 2. a surgical operation in which a portion of an organ is separated from the remainder but is not removed from the body. 3. in health insurance, perils or conditions listed in an insurance or medical care coverage policy for which the policy will not provide benefit payment. Common exlusions may include pre-existing conditions, such as heart disease or hypertension which began before the policy was in effect. In dental insurance, orthodontic treatment is a frequent exclusion. Called also *exception* and *limitation*.

excoriation (eks-ko″re-a′shun) [L. *excoriare* to flay, from *ex* out + *corium* skin] any superficial loss of substance marked by "dug out" lesions, such as one produced by scratching.

excrescence (eks-kres′ens) [*ex-* + L. *crescere* to grow] any abnormal outgrowth or projection. **enamel e.,** see enamel SPUR and enamel PEARL.

excretion (eks-kre′shun) [L. *excretio*] 1. the act or process of discharging waste products. Cf. SECRETION (1). 2. any waste substance or material which is discharged.

excursion (eks-ker′zhun) [L. *excursio*, from *ex* out + *currere* to run] movements occurring from a normal, or rest, position of a movable part in performance of a function, as those of the mandible to attain functional contact between the cusps and the mandibular and maxillary teeth in mastication, or of the chest wall in respiration. Called also *excursive movement*. See also masticatory MOVEMENT. **lateral e.,** sideward movement of the mandible between the position of closure and that in which the tips of the cusps of opposing teeth are in vertical proximity. See also lateral RELATION. **protrusive e.,** movement of the mandible between the position of closure and that in which the incisal edges of the anterior teeth are in vertical approximation. See also jaw relation, protrusive, under RELATION. **retrusive e.,** the slight backward and return movement of the mandible between the position of closure and one slightly posterior, more often present with mandibular overclosure. See also centric RELATION.

excursive (eks-ker′sive) pertaining to or characterized by excursion.

exercise (ek′ser-sīz) the performance of physical exertion for improvement of physical condition or health or for the correction of a physical deficiency or defect.

exerciser (ek′ser-si′zer) 1. a device used for exercise. 2. a nipple-shaped rubber or plastic device for infants to suck on, designed to stimulate a normal nursing motion. The primary, smaller exerciser is for infants under 1 year of age; the secondary, larger version is for infants over 1 year of age. Improperly designed exercisers are responsible for faulty dental development leading to malocclusion. Called also *pacifier*. See also SUCKLING. **primary e.,** see *exerciser* (2). **secondary e.,** see *exerciser* (2). **temporomandibular joint e.,** trismus STENT.

exeresis (eks-er′ĕ-sis) [Gr. *exairesis* a taking out] surgical removal or excision.

exergonic (ek″ser-gon′ik) characterized or accompanied by the release of energy; pertaining to processes which involve energy flowing out of the system. Cf. ENDERGONIC.

exesion (eg-ze′shun) [L. *exedere* to eat out] the gradual destruction of superficial parts of a tissue.

exfoliatin (eks-fo′le-ah-tin) a powerful toxin produced by staphylococci, primarily *Staphylococcus aureus*, which causes scalded skin syndrome (see under SYNDROME). It is a simple protein of about 24,000 daltons molecular weight, being antigenic and inducing both neutralizing and precipitating antibody; it converts to toxoid by treatment with formaldehyde. Two serologically unrelated types have been distinguished: *A* is relatively heat-stable and its biological activity is retained after heating to 100°C for 20 minutes, and *B*, produced by strains other than those of phage group II, is heat-labile and its biological activity is destroyed by heating to 60°C for 30 minutes. Called also *exfoliative toxin*.

exfoliatio (eks″fo-le-a′she-o) [L., from *ex* + *folium* leaf] exfoliation. **e. aera′ta lin′guae,** benign migratory GLOSSITIS.

exfoliation (eks″fo-le-a′shun) [L. *exfoliatio*] the shedding of something, as of scales from the surface of the body.

exfoliative (eks-fo′le-a″tiv) characterized by exfoliation.

exhalation (eks″hah-la′shun) [L. *exhalatio*, from *ex* + *halare* to breathe] 1. the act of breathing out (see also HALITUS). 2. the giving off of watery or other vapor. 3. a vapor or other substance exhaled or given off.

exhaustion (eg-zawst′yun) [*ex-* + L. *haurire* to drain] 1. privation of energy with consequent inability to respond to stimuli. 2. withdrawal. 3. a condition of emptiness caused by withdrawal. **heat e.,** a form of stroke or shock occurring as the result of prolonged exposure to excessive heat.

Exhib. abbreviation for L. *exhibea′tur*, let it be given.

exhibition (ek″si-bish′un) administration of a drug.

exhumation (eks″hu-ma′shun) [*ex-* + L. *humus* earth] disinterment; removal of the dead body from the earth after burial.

exitus (ek′sĭ-tus), pl. *ex′itus* [L. "a going out"] 1. an exit or outlet. 2. death.

Exmigra trademark for *ergotamine tartrate* (see under ERGOTAMINE).

exo- [Gr. *exo* outside] a prefix meaning outside, or outward.

exoccipital (eks″ok-sip′ĭ-tal) [*exo-* + *occipital*] pertaining to the exoccipital bone.

exocrine (ek-so′krin) [*exo-* + Gr. *krinein* to separate] secreting outwardly, as in exocrine gland. Cf. ENDOCRINE.

exocytosis (eks″o-si-to′sis) [*exo-* + Gr. *kytos* a hollow vessel] 1. the discharge from a cell of particles that are too large to diffuse through its wall; the opposite of endocytosis. 2. the process of expulsion from the phagocytic cell of the digested residual body. See also PHAGOCYTOSIS.

exodic (eks-od′ik) [*ex-* + Gr. *hodos* way] away from a center; centrifugal, efferent.

exodontia (ek″so-don′she-ah) exodontics.

exodontics (ek″so-don′tiks) [L. *ex* out + Gr. *odous* tooth] that branch of dentistry dealing with extraction of teeth. Called also *exodontia*.

exodontist (ek″so-don′tist) a dentist who practices exodontics.

exogenic (ek″so-jen′ik) exogenous.

exogenous (eks-oj′ĕ-nus) [*exo-* + Gr. *gennan* to produce] produced or originating outside the organism; growing by additions to the outside.

exognathia (ek″sog-na′the-ah) prognathism.

exognathion (ek″sog-na′the-on) [*exo-* + Gr. *gnathos* jaw] the maxilla exclusive of the premaxilla.

exolever (ek″so-le′ver) dental ELEVATOR.

exopeptidase (ek′so-pep′tĭ-dās) [*exo-* + *peptide* + *-ase*) peptidase.

Exophene trademark for *hexachlorophene*.

exophthalmic (ek-sof-thal′mik) of or pertaining to or characterized by exophthalmos.

exophthalmos (ek″sof-thal′mos) [*ex-* + Gr. *ophthalmos* eye] abnormal protrusion of the eyeball. See also exophthalmic GOITER.

exophytic (ek″so-fit′ik) [*exo-* + Gr. *phyein* to grow] 1. growing outward. 2. pertaining to the proliferation on the outside or surface epithelium of an organ or tissue from which a tumor originates.

exospore (ek′so-spōr) conidium.

exostosis (ek″sos-to′sis) [*ex-* + Gr. *osteon* bone] a hyperplastic bony growth projecting outward from the surface of a bone. See also TORUS mandibularis and TORUS palatinus. **cancellous exostoses,** Ehrenfried's DISEASE. **ivory e.,** a bony growth of great density. **e. luxu′rians,** progressive myositis ossificans; see under MYOSITIS. **multiple cartilaginous exostoses,** Ehrenfried's DISEASE. **mu..tiple exostoses of jaws,** bony growths, usually of the buccal surface of the maxilla below the mucobuccal fold in the molar region, which sometimes interfere with prosthetic appliances.

exothermic (ek″so-ther′mik) [*exo-* + Gr. *thermē* heat] characterized or accompanied by release of heat. Cf. ENDOTHERMIC.

exotic (eg-zot′ik) of foreign origin; not native.

exotoxin (ek″so-tok′sin) a toxic substance formed by bacteria found outside the bacterial cell, or free in the culture medium. Exotoxins are heat-labile, and protein in nature. They are detoxified with retention of antigenicity by treatment with formaldehyde (formol toxoid), and are the most poisonous substances known to man; the LD_{50} of crystalline botulinum type A toxin for the mouse is 4.5×10^{-9} mg. Cf. ENDOTOXIN.

expansion (eks-pan′shun) [L. *expandere* to spread out] 1. the process or state of being increased in extent, surface, or bulk. 2. the region or area of increased bulk or surface. **e. of the arch,** maxillary e. **cubical e.,** increase in volume by an increase in all dimensions. **delayed e.,** expansion occurring in an amalgam restoration due to the presence of moisture. Called also *secondary e.* **effective setting e.,** the linear dimensional change in a material, such as plaster, occurring under the conditions of its practical usage. **hygroscopic e.,** an increase in the dimensions of a body or substance as a result of absorption of moisture. **hygroscopic setting e.,** expansion in a hemihydrate-water mixture occurring when it is allowed to set when immersed in water, being several times greater than the normal setting expansion. It is a continuation of the setting expansion because the immersion water replaces the water of hydration and, thus, prevents the confinement of the growing crystals by the surface tension of the excess water. **maxillary e.,** an orthodontic method used for correcting narrow or collapsed maxillary arches and functional posterior cross-bite, whereby increased maxillary arch width is obtained with the use of various appliances which provide laterally expansive force resulting in orthopedic movements (bony separation and remodeling at sutural articulations) and orthodontic movements (tooth tipping and bodily translation). Rapid maxillary expansion (RME) is accomplished with appliances generating forces from 3 to more than 20 lbs. In slow palatal expansion, the forces are usually about 2 lbs. The RME normally causes midpalatal suture opening; some suture opening also occurs with slow expansion. Called also *e. of the arch* and *palatal e.* **mercuroscopic e.,** expansion of dental amalgam during its setting as the tin is released from the γ_2-phase, free mercury being left behind, which then diffuses back into the amalgam and reacts with the residual alloy particles to form additional γ_1- and γ_2-phases. This results in unilateral expansion in or near the amalgam-tooth interface and produces a protrusion of the restoration away from the supporting tooth structure. The protrusion, being unsupported, is easily fractured. **normal setting e.,** the linear dimensional change in a material, such as plaster, occurring during its setting under normal conditions. **palatal e.,** maxillary e. **secondary e.,** delayed e. **setting e.,** an increase in the dimension of a body or material, such as plaster of Paris, dental stone, or dental plaster, taking place concurrently with its hardening, and sometimes resulting in warping of the dental impression. Normally, setting expansion of dental plaster and other gypsum products is 0.3 to 0.4 percent, some stronger gypsum products, such as Types III and IV (see dental STONE), having a setting expansion as low as 0.8 percent. Expansion may be controlled in dental stone and plaster by additives, such as potassium sulfate. **rapid maxillary e. (RME),** see *maxillary e.* **slow maxillary e.,** see *maxillary e.* **thermal e.,** the increase of the volume of a body or substance as a result of an increase in its temperature, being greater in gases than in solids or liquids. A few substances actually contract slightly when heated, their coefficient of thermal expansion being negative. In materials, thermal expansion is measured in terms of the linear coefficient of thermal expansion, which is the increase in length of a material per unit length when the temperature is increased 1°C. See table at dental MATERIAL. **wax e.,** increase in the dimensions of a wax pattern for a dental restoration to compensate for shrinkage of the gold during the casting process.

expectancy (ek-spek′tan-se) the probability of occurrence of a specific event. **life e.,** the number of years, based on statistical averages, which a given person of a specific age or class may reasonably expect to continue living.

expectorant (ek-spek′to-rant) [*ex-* + L. *pectus* breast] 1. promoting the ejection, by spitting, of mucus or other fluids from the lungs and trachea. 2. an agent that promotes the ejection of mucus or exudates from the lungs, bronchi, and trachea. Sometimes extended to all remedies that quiet cough (antitussives).

expectoration (ek-spek″to-ra′shun) 1. the act or process of coughing up and spitting out materials from the lungs, bronchi, and trachea. 2. sputum.

expense (ek-spens′) 1. cost or charge. 2. charges incurred in the execution of an undertaking or commission, as the cost to the insurer of conducting his business. See also BENEFIT. **allowable e's,** the dollar amount allowable for each dental procedure covered by a dental insurance policy. **blanket medical e.,** a provision, usually included as an added feature of an insurance policy, primarily providing some other type of coverage, which entitles the insured to collect, up to a maximum established in the policy, for all hospital and medical expenses incurred. **catastrophic e.,** in health insurance, any large and unexpected expenditure for health services which would impose a financial burden on the patient.

experiment (ek-sper′ĭ-ment) [L. *experimentum* proof from experience] a procedure done in order to discover or to demonstrate some fact or general truth.

experimentation (ek-sper′ĭ-men-ta′shun) conducting an experiment. **human e.,** experimental studies performed under clinical conditions on human subjects, usually volunteers or, less commonly, patients. Called also *clinical research.*

expiration (eks″pĭ-ra′shun) [*ex-* + L. *spirare* to breathe] 1. the act of breathing out, or expelling air from the lungs. 2. termination, or death.

explant 1. (eks-plant′) to take from the body and place in an artificial medium for growth. 2. (eks′plant) tissue taken from its original site and transferred to an artificial medium for growth.

explode (eks-plōd′) [L. *explodere,* from *ex* out + *plaudere* to clap the hands] 1. to undergo sudden and violent decomposition or combustion. 2. to burst; to spread rapidly, as an epidemic.

exploration (eks″plo-ra′shun) [L. *exploratio,* from *ex* out + *plorare* to cry out] the act or process of examining, studying, or exploring, as of an organ for diagnostic purposes.

explorer (eks-plor′er) 1. an instrument used in exploring for foreign bodies. 2. a slender steel instrument with a fine, flexible, sharp point, used to examine the minute indentations of the anatomical developmental grooves of the crown of a tooth for minute breaks in the pits or fissures on the surface. 3. in periodontology, an instrument used to locate subgingival deposits before scaling and to check for smoothness of the root surface after scaling. See illustration. See also periodontal PROBE. **cowhorn e.,** a slender explorer.

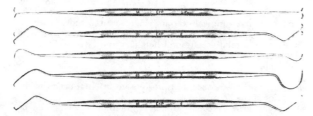

Explorers. (From H. O. Torres and A. Ehrlich: Modern Dental Assisting. 2nd ed. Philadelphia, W. B. Saunders Co., 1980.)

exponent (eks′po-nent) a symbol placed above and at the right of another symbol to indicate the power to which the letter is to be raised, as, x^2.

exposure (eks-po′zhur) 1. the act of lying open, as surgical exposure. 2. the condition of being subjected to something, as to an infectious agent or extremes of weather or radiation, which may have a harmful effect. 3. in radiology, a measure of the amount of ionizing radiation at the surface of the irradiated object, e.g., the body. See also air DOSE and exposure DOSE. 4. the number of persons eligible for benefits of a dental plan in any given period; most frequently expressed in man-years. For example, three persons covered for 4 months each would equal 1 man-year exposure. **acute e.,** a short duration exposure to ionizing radiation, usually of relatively high intensity. **air e.,** air DOSE. **chronic e.,** a prolonged exposure to usually low intensity ionizing radiation that is continuous (protracted e.) or intermittent (fractionation e.). **cumulative e., cumulative radiation e.,** the total accumulated exposure resulting from repeated radiation exposures of the whole body or of a particular region. Called also *cumulative dose* and *cumulative radiation dose.* See also whole-body IRRADIATION. **e. dose,** air DOSE. **double e.,** the superimposed exposures on the same radiographic or photographic film. **entrance e.,** entrance DOSE. **erythema e.,** erythema DOSE. **fractionation e.,** see *chronic e.* **e. holder,** cassette. **protracted e.,** see *chronic e.* **protraction e.,** see *chronic e.* **pulp e.,** see exposed PULP. **e. rate,** exposure RATE. **surface e.,** entrance e. **threshold e.,** threshold DOSE. **whole-body e.,** whole-body IRRADIATION.

expression (eks-presh′un) [L. *expressio*] 1. the appearance of the face as determined by the physical or emotional state. 2. the act or process of evacuating or squeezing out by pressure. See also EXTRUSION. 3. gene e. **gene e., genetic e.,** the act or process of translating or converting the genetic code (genotype) into observable characteristics including the physical, biochemical, and physiological nature of an individual (phenotype). See also CHARACTER, GENOTYPE, PHENOTYPE, TRANSCRIPTION, and TRANSLATION. **phenotypic e. of gene,** character (3).

expressivity (eks″pres-siv′ĭ-te) [L. *expressus*] the degree of expression of a genotype in a phenotype. See also PENETRANCE.

exsanguination (eks-sang″wĭ-na′shun) extensive loss of blood.

exsiccant (ek-sik′ant) desiccant.

exstrophy (ek′stro-fe) [*ex-* + Gr. *strephein* to turn oneself] eversion or turning inside out of an organ, as the bladder.

exsufflation (ek″suf-fla′shun) [ex- + L. *sufflatio* a blowing up] the act or process of forcing discharge of the breath by artificial or mechanical means.

ext. extract.

Extar see under DENTIFRICE.

extender (ek-sten′der) [ex- + L. *tendere* to stretch] something which enlarges or prolongs. **artificial plasma e.,** a substance which can be transfused to maintain the fluid volume of the blood in event of great necessity, supplemental to the use of whole blood and plasma.

extension (ek-sten′shun) [L. *extensio*] 1. the act or process of drawing parts away from each other; elongation; prolongation; stretching out. 2. the act or process of increasing an angle between two ends of a joined part, such as the arm and forearm, until they attain a straight line. See also HYPEREXTENSION. **e. of benefits,** see under BENEFIT. **groove e.,** enlargement of a cavity preparation outline to include a developmental groove. **nail e.,** extension exerted on the distal fragment of a fractured bone by means of a nail or pin (Steinmann pin) driven into the fragment. Called also *Steinmann's e.* **e. for prevention,** the principle of cavity preparation laid down by G. V. Black, whereby the boundaries of a cavity are extended to surfaces that are normally free of caries, thereby reducing the probability of recurrence of decay. The additional extension provides smoothly finished margins that may be readily cleaned, or they are placed under the free gingival margin. **ridge e.,** an intraoral surgical procedure for deepening the vestibular and oral sulci so as to increase the relative intraoral height of the ridge to facilitate denture retention. **Steinmann's e.,** nail e. **vestibular e.,** vestibuloplasty.

exterior (eks-te′re-or) situated on or near the outside; outer.

exteriorize (eks-te′re-or-īz) to transpose an internal organ to the exterior of the body.

extern (eks′tern) a medical student or graduate in medicine who assists in the care of patients in a hospital, but does not reside in the hospital.

external (eks-ter′nal) [L. *externus* outside] situated on the outside.

exteroceptor (eks″ter-o-sep′tor) any of the specialized nerve endings that are scattered throughout the body and are concerned with perceiving external stimuli and relaying them to the central nervous system, e.g., tactile, sound, visual, temperature, or olfactory stimuli. Often used to denote those receptors for adjacent, rather than distant, stimuli, thereby omitting visual and auditory stimuli. See also RECEPTOR (6).

extirpation (ek″ster-pa′shun) [L. *extirpare* to root out, from *ex* out + *stirps* root] complete removal of something. **cyst e.,** the total removal of a cyst lining and primary closure of the cavity. See also MARSUPIALIZATION. **dental pulp e.,** pulpectomy.

extra- [L. *exter* outward] a prefix meaning outside of, beyond, or in addition.

extra-articular (eks″trah-ar-tik′u-lar) [extra- + L. *articulus* joint] outside of a joint.

extrabuccal (eks″trah-buk′al) outside of the mouth or cheek.

extracapsular (eks″trah-kap′su-lar) outside of a capsule.

extracoronal (eks″trah-ko-ro′nal) outside the crown of a tooth.

extracorporeal (eks″trah-kor-po′re-al) [extra- + L. *corpus* body] situated or occurring outside the body.

extracorpuscular (eks″trah-kor-pus′ku-lar) outside of the corpuscles.

extracranial (eks″trah-kra′ne-al) outside of the cranium.

extract (eks′trakt) [L. *extractum*] a concentrated preparation of a vegetable or animal drug obtained by removing the active constituents therefrom with a suitable menstruum, evaporating all or nearly all the solvent, and adjusting the residual mass or powder to a prescribed standard. Extracts are prepared in three forms: semiliquid or of syrupy consistency, pilular or solid, and as dry powder. **belladonna e.,** BELLADONNA extract.

extraction (eks-trak′shun) [L. *ex* out + *trahere* to draw] 1. the process or act of luxating or drawing out. 2. the preparation of an extract. 3. tooth e. **elevator e.,** extraction of a tooth with the use of elevators. **forceps e.,** extraction of a tooth with the use of forceps. **painless e.,** a term coined by Gardner Q. Colton for tooth extraction performed under nitrous oxide analgesia. **progressive e.,** serial e. **rubber band e.,** extraction accomplished by placing a rubber band around a tooth and allowing it to work itself toward the root. The method is bloodless and is sometimes used in patients with hemorrhagic disorders. **selected e.,** serial e. **serial e.,** the selective extraction of deciduous teeth during the period of mixed dentition in accordance with the shedding and eruption of the teeth. The extraction is accomplished over an extended period of time to allow autonomous adjustment to relieve crowding of the dental arches during eruption of the lateral incisors, canines, and premolars, eventually involving the extraction of the first premolar teeth. Called also *selected e.* and *progressive e.* **tooth e.,** the surgical removal of a tooth, accomplished with the use of forceps and elevators or by splitting or sectioning the tooth with chisels and burs and removing individual segments separately.

extractor (eks-trak′tor) an instrument used for removing a calculus or foreign body.

extractum (eks-trak′tum), pl. *extrac′ta* [L., from *ex* out + *trahere* to draw] an extract.

extradental (eks″trah-den′tal) [extra- + *dental*] outside a tooth or teeth.

extramural (eks″trah-mu′ral) [extra- + L. *murus* wall] situated or occurring outside the wall of an organ or structure.

extraneous (eks-tra′ne-us) [L. *extraneous* external] existing or belonging outside the organism.

extraoral (eks″trah-o′ral) [extra- + L. *oral*] outside the mouth; outside the oral cavity.

extrasystole (eks″trah-sis′to-le) a premature contraction of the heart that is independent of the normal rhythm and arises in response to an impulse in some part of the heart other than the sinoatrial node. Called also *premature beat, premature contraction,* and *premature-heart contraction.*

extravasation (eks-trav″ah-sa′shun) [extra- + L. *vas* vessel] 1. a discharge or escape, as of blood, from a vessel into the tissue. See also ECCHYMOSIS and PETECHIA. 2. the process of being extravasated. 3. blood or other substance which has been extravasated.

extravascular (eks″trah-vas′ku-lar) situated or occurring outside a vessel or the vessels.

extraversion (eks″trah-ver′zhun) in orthodontics, malocclusion in which the teeth or other maxillary structures are further from the median plane than normal, resulting in a wide dental arch. Called also *extroversion.* Cf. INTRAVERSION.

extremity (eks-trem′ĭ-te) 1. a distal or terminal portion. 2. an arm or leg.

extrinsic (eks-trin′sik) [L. *extrinsecus* from without] derived from or situated on the outside; external.

extro- [L. *extra* outside of, beyond] a prefix meaning outward, outside.

extroversion (eks″tro-ver′zhun) 1. a turning inside out; exstrophy. 2. extraversion.

extrude (eks-trōōd) 1. to force out, or to occupy a position mesial, distal, labial or buccal, or lingual or palatal to that normally occupied. 2. to occupy a position occlusal to that normally occupied, said of an over-erupted tooth.

extrusion (eks-troo′zhun) 1. thrusting or pushing out; expulsion by force. 2. the over-eruption or movement of a tooth beyond its normal occlusal plane in the absence of opposing occlusal force, as when the contacting tooth in the opposite arch has been lost. See also tooth migration, pathologic, under MIGRATION. 3. an orthodontic technique for the elongation or elevation of a tooth. Cf. INTRUSION (3).

extubation (eks″tu-ba′shun) the removal of a previously inserted tube.

exuberant (eg-zu′ber-ant) [L. *exuberare* to be very fruitful] copious or excessive in production; showing excessive proliferation.

exudate (eks′u-dāt) [L. *exsudare* to sweat out] a fluid of high specific gravity (usually over 1.020), rich in plasma proteins and cellular elements and debris, usually present in inflammatory conditions. Noninflammatory edema fluid is known as *transudate.* **fibrinous e.,** an exudate having an abundance of fibrinogen, resulting in subsequent fibrin formation at the site of injury. **hemorrhagic e.,** sanguineous e. **purulent e.,** pus. **sanguineous e.,** an exudate having an abundance of red blood cells. Called also *hemorrhagic e.* **serous e.,** an exudate characterized by an abundance of serous fluid and the presence of very few cellular blood elements. **suppurative e.,** pus.

exudation (eks″u-da′shun) 1. the escape of fluid, cells, and cellular debris from blood vessels and their deposition in or on the tissue, usually as a result of inflammation. 2. an exudate. **fibrinous e.,** exudation in which there is the outpouring of large amounts of plasma proteins, including fibrinogen, associated with the precipitation of masses of fibrin, seen in severe forms of inflammation with marked increase of vascular permeability. **gingival e.,** exudation from the gingiva, usually of the ulcerated crevicular epithelium in an inflammatory focus. **hemorrhagic e.,** exudation associated with extravasation of large numbers of red cells, occurring in the inflammatory focus at the site of severe injury. **purulent e.,** exudation characterized by the production of large amounts of pus (purulent exudate), due to the presence of pyogenic organisms in the inflammatory focus.

Called also *suppurative e*. **serous e.**, one in which there is the extensive outpouring of watery, low-protein fluid which, according to the site of injury, may be derived from the blood serum or the secretions of serous mesothelial cells, i.e., the cells lining the body cavities and the joint spaces, as in the skin blister from a burn, in which the fluid is derived from the blood serum. **suppurative e.**, purulent e.

exuviation (eks-u″ve-a′shun) [L. *exuere* to divest oneself of] the shedding of any epithelial structure, as of the deciduous teeth.

eye (i) [L. *oculus;* Gr. *ophthalmos*] the organ of vision. It is a sphere composed of three coats: the clear transparent layer on the front of the eyeball (cornea), which is a continuation of the sclera (white of the eye); the middle layer (choroid), which contains blood vessels and the retina, containing rods and cones, which are specialized light-sensitive cells. The light is transmitted through the lens, as the iris widens or narrows the pupil to allow for different light conditions. The light is focused on the retina and the image is transmitted to the brain through the optic nerve. Called also *oculus* [NA]. See also terms beginning OCULO-. **cat e.**, see cat-eye SYNDROME. **crossed e's,** strabismus.

eyebrow (i′brow) 1. the transverse elevation at the junction of the forehead and the upper eyelid, consisting of five layers: skin, subcutaneous tissue, a layer of interwoven fibers of the orbicularis oculi and occipitofrontalis muscles, a submuscular areolar layer, and pericranium. Called also *supercilium* [NA]. 2. the hairs growing on the transverse elevation at the junction of the forehead and the upper lid of either eye. Called also *supercilia* [NA].

eyelash (i′lash) one of the hairs growing at the edge of an eyelid; collectively called *cilia* [NA].

eyelet (i′let) an orthodontic attachment, normally used in conjunction with the edgewise appliance, welded or soldered for better rotational control.

eyelid (i′lid) either of the two movable folds (upper and lower) that protect the anterior surface of the eye. Called also *palpebra* [NA]. See also words beginning BLEPHAR- and PALPEBR-. **lower e.**, the lower of the two eyelids. Called also *palpebra inferior* [NA]. **upper e.**, the upper of the two eyelids. Called also *palpebra superior* [NA].

eyepiece (i′pēs) the lens or system of lenses in a microscope (or telescope) that is nearest to the eye of the user and that serves to further magnify the image produced by the objective. **comparison e.**, one which presents, as though in juxtaposition, the image produced by the objective. See also comparison MICROSCOPE. **huygenian e.**, a negative eyepiece consisting of two planoconvex lenses, the convexities being directed toward the objective. **negative e.**, a combination of two lenses, one of which is below the plane in which the real image from the objective is formed. **Ramsden's e.**, a positive eyepiece consisting of two planoconvex lenses with the convexities turned toward each other. **positive e.**, a lens combination, consisting of two planoconvex lenses or of an achromatic doublet or triplet, the combination being above the plane in which the real image from the objective is formed. **widefield e.**, a positive eyepiece consisting of a doublet and a single element, giving a wider field of view than that afforded by other eyepieces.

eyepoint (i′point) a point above the eyepiece in which all the beams of light emerging from the microscope intersect.

F

F 1. Fahrenheit (see under SCALE). 2. field of VISION. 3. formula. 4. farad. 5. gilbert. 6. fluorine. 7. designation for the degree of fineness of abrasive particles used in dentistry; see ABRASIVE (2).

°F degree on the Fahrenheit scale (see under SCALE).

F₁, F-one first filial GENERATION.

F₂, F-two second filial GENERATION.

F-4 see Committee F-4 on Medical and Surgical Materials and Devices, under COMMITTEE.

F-8 see Committee F-8 on Protective Equipment for Sports, under COMMITTEE.

f femto-.

FA fatty ACID.

Fab [fragment, antigen-binding] one of two segments of an immunoglobulin molecule cleaved by papain, which retains the ability to combine wih antigen. It contains one of the two binding sites and one Fc piece. Fab can be further cleaved by disrupting the −S−S− bond, leaving a free light chain and the N-terminal portion of the heavy chain. Called also *FAb fragment* and *Fab piece*. See also Fc.

F(ab′)₂ a fragment obtained by pepsin digestion of immunoglobulin molecules on the C-terminal side of the disulfide link which holds the two heavy chains together. The resultant fragment has a molecular weight of about 90,000 and consists of the remaining undigested portion of the two heavy chains, each still held together and containing both Fab fragments. F(ab′)₂ behaves as a divalent antibody, having two antibody combining sites, but does not contain the sites for complement fixation.

Faber's anemia [Knud Helge *Faber,* Danish physician, 1862–1952] hypochromic essential ANEMIA.

fabrication (fab″ri-ka′shun) in dentistry, construction or building up, as of a dental restoration.

Fabricius 1. see FABRIZIO. 2. see FABRY, Wilhelm.

Fabrizio, Girolamo (Hieronymus Fabricius of Aquapendente) [1537–1619] an Italian anatomist and surgeon who was the pupil and successor (at Padua) of Gabriele Fallopio and was the teacher of William Harvey. Fabrizio was the first to demonstrate the valves of the veins. In his works, he described forced opening of the dental arches in cases of prolonged constriction, cleaning of the teeth, treatment of dental caries, filling of teeth with gold leaf, removal and resection of abnormal teeth, and tooth extraction.

Fabry, Wilhelm (Hildanus Fabricius) [1560–1634] German surgeon who wrote extensively on dental surgery.

Fabry's disease [Johannes *Fabry,* German dermatologist, 1860–1930] see under DISEASE.

Facb [fragment, antigen and complement binding] a residue of the IgG molecule remaining after the pFc′ fragment has been removed from the Fc fragment portion by the action of plasmin.

FACD Fellow of the American College of Dentists.

face (fās) [L. *facies;* Gr. *prosōpon*] 1. the anterior aspect of the head from the forehead to the chin. 2. any presenting aspect, or surface. See also FACIES. 3. the end portion of the nib of a condensing instrument, which comes into contact with the restorative material during its packing and condensation in a prepared cavity. **adenoid f.**, adenoid FACIES. **bovine f.**, FACIES bovina. **bird f.**, bird-face. **cleft f.**, macrostomia. **concave f.**, dish f. **cow f.**, FACIES bovina. **dish f., dished f.**, a facial type in which the middle third of the face appears retruded in relation to the remainder of the craniofacial complex. It is characterized by a prominence of the forehead, a recession of the midface and lower half of the nose, a lengthening of the upper lip, and a prognathic chin. Called also *concave f., concave facial type,* and *facies scaphoidea.* **euryprosopic f.**, euryprosopic SKULL. **f. form,** face FORM. **frog f.**, flatness of the face due to intranasal disease. **hippocratic f.**, FACIES hippocratica. **hyperdivergent f., idiopathic long f.**, long face SYNDROME. **hypereuryprosopic f.**, hypereuryprosopic SKULL. **hyperleptoprosopic f.**, hyperleptoprosopic SKULL. **hypodivergent f., idiopathic short f.**, short face SYNDROME. **leptoprosopic f.**, 1. LEPTOPROSOPIA. 2. leptoprosopic SKULL. **long f.**, long face SYNDROME. **mesoprosopic f.**, mesoprosopic SKULL. **moon f., moon-shaped f.**, the peculiar rounded face, such as seen in Cushing's syndrome, or following administration of adrenal corticoids. Called also *moon facies.* **narrow f.**, 1. LEPTOPROSOPIA. 2. leptoprosopic SKULL. **short f.**, short face SYNDROME. **wide f.**, euryprosopic SKULL.

face-bow (fās′bo) 1. a caliper-like device used to record the positional relationship of the maxillary arch to the temporomandibular joint (or opening axis of the jaw) and to orient dental casts in the same relationship to the opening axis of the articulator. See also face-bow FORK and PANTOGRAPH. See illustration. **adjustable axis f.**, a face-bow with caliper ends (condyl ends) that can be adjusted in such a way as to permit location of

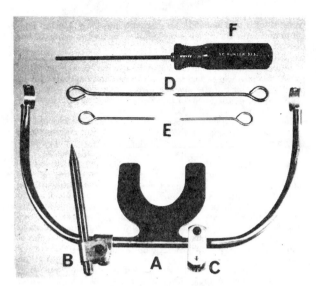

Armamentarium for face-bow: *A*, bow with bite plate attached; *B*, toggle for positioning orbital pointer; *C*, adaptor for mounting stand; *D*, pair of hinge axis pointers (heavy); *E*, pair of hinge axis pointers (light); *F*, wrench. (From H. C. Kilpatrick: Work Simplification in Dental Practice. 3rd ed. Philadelphia, W. B. Saunders Co., 1974.)

the hinge axis of rotation of the mandible. Called also *kinematic f.* and *hinge-bow.* **kinematic f.**, adjustable axis f. **f. record**, face-bow RECORD.

faceometer (fãs-om′ĕ-ter) an instrument for measuring the dimensions of the face.

facer (fa′ser) a device used in covering or lining with different material the front surface of something, or in preparing the surface for such a lining. **root f.**, an engine-driven rotating instrument used in facing the exposed root surface of a crownless tooth, having a wheel-shaped end and/or side-cutting head in the center of which is a cylindrical, truncated cone or pointed projection with smooth surfaces that enters the root canal. See illustration at root canal THERAPY.

facet (fas′et) [Fr. *facette*] a small plane surface on a hard body, as on a bone. **articular f.**, a small plane surface on a bone at the site where it articulates with another structure; see terms beginning FACIES articularis. **occlusal f.**, a flattened plane produced by wear on a convex tooth surface.

facette (fah-set′) [Fr.] facet.

facial (fa′shal) [L. *facialis*] pertaining to or toward the face. In dental anatomy, the term is used to refer to the surface of a tooth directed toward the face (including the buccal and labial surfaces) and opposite the lingual (or oral) surface. Used synonymously with *vestibular.* See illustration at SURFACE.

facies (fa′she-ēz), pl. *fa′cies* [L.] 1. a term used in anatomical nomenclature to designate (*a*) the anterior aspect of the head, from forehead to chin, inclusive, and also (*b*) a specific surface of a body structure, part, or organ. 2. the expression or appearance of the face. **f. abdomina′lis**, the expression characterized by a pinched, anxious, and furrowed face with the nose and upper lip drawn up, seen in abdominal diseases. **adenoid f.**, the dull expression, with open mouth, sometimes seen in children with adenoid growths. **f. ante′rior**, 1. anterior SURFACE (1). 2. the mesial surface of a tooth, especially a molar or bicuspid. **f. ante′rior den′tium premola′rium et mola′rium**, anterior surface of premolar and molar teeth; see under SURFACE. **f. ante′rior maxil′lae** [NA], anterior surface of maxilla; see under SURFACE. **f. ante′rior palpebra′rum** [NA], anterior surface of eyelids; see under SURFACE. **f. ante′rior par′tis petro′sae os′sis tempora′lis** [NA], anterior surface of petrous part of temporal bone; see under SURFACE. **f. ante′rior pyram′idis os′sis tempora′lis**, anterior surface of petrous part of temporal bone; see under SURFACE. **f. anterolatera′lis cartilag′inis arytenoi′deae**, the external surface of the arytenoid cartilage which bears the triangular pit, oblong pit, and arcuate crest. **f. articula′ris**, articular SURFACE. **f. articula′ris arytenoi′dea cartilag′inis cricoi′deae**, the surface of the cricoid cartilage that articulates with the arytenoid cartilage. **f. articula′ris cartilag′inis aryte-**

noi′dea, the surface of the arytenoid cartilage that articulates with the cricoid cartilage. **f. articula′ris fos′sae mandibula′ris, f. articula′ris os′sis tempora′lis** [NA], articular surface of mandibular fossa; see under SURFACE. **f. articula′ris os′sium** [NA], see articular SURFACE. **f. articula′ris thyroi′dea cartilag′inis cricoi′deae** [NA], articular surface of cricoid cartilage; see under SURFACE. **f. bovi′na**, the facial expression sometimes seen in craniofacial dysostosis. Called also *bovine face* and *cow face.* **f. bucca′lis den′tis**, buccal SURFACE. **f. cerebra′lis a′lae mag′nae, f. cerebra′lis a′lae majo′ris** [NA], cerebral surface of great wing; see under SURFACE. **f. cerebra′lis os′sis fronta′lis**, internal surface of frontal bone; see under SURFACE. **f. cerebra′lis os′sis parieta′lis**, internal surface of parietal bone; see under SURFACE. **f. cerebra′lis par′tis squamo′sae os′sis tempora′lis** [NA], **f. cerebra′lis squa′mae tempora′lis**, cerebral surface of temporal squama; see under SURFACE. **f. contac′tus den′tis** [NA], contact AREA (2). **Corvisart′s f.**, the peculiar facies seen in aortic regurgitation, characterized by a swollen and purplish blue face, shiny eyes, and puffy eyelids. **crying f., asymmetric**, a condition in which the face appears asymmetrical at rest, the mouth being pulled downward to one side when crying due to unilateral partial weakness involving the lip depressor muscle. It is usually associated with a wide variety of congenital defects, e.g., cardiofacial syndrome. **f. dista′lis den′tis** [NA], distal SURFACE. **f. doloro′sa**, the facial expression of a patient experiencing pain or severe sickness. **f. dorsa′lis**, posterior SURFACE (1). **elfin f.**, a peculiar facies giving the affected person a small, merry, or mischievous appearance. See elfin facies SYNDROME. **f. exter′na os′sis fronta′lis** [NA], external surface of frontal bone; see under SURFACE. **f. ex′terna os′sis parieta′lis** [NA], external surface of parietal bone; see under SURFACE. **f. facia′lis den′tis**, NA alternative for vestibular SURFACE. **fetal f.**, see Robinow′s SYNDROME. **f. fronta′lis os′sis fronta′lis**, external surface of frontal bone; see under SURFACE. **f. hippocra′tica**, a drawn, pinched, and pale appearance of the face, indicative of approaching death. Called also *hippocratic face.* **f. infe′rior**, inferior SURFACE. **f. infe′rior cer′ebri** [NA], inferior surface of cerebrum; see under SURFACE. **f. infe′rior hemisphe′rii cerebel′li** [NA], inferior surface of cerebellar hemisphere; see under SURFACE. **f. infe′rior hemisphe′rii cer′ebri** [NA], inferior surface of cerebral hemisphere; see under SURFACE. **f. infe′rior lin′guae** [NA], inferior surface of tongue; see under SURFACE. **f. infe′rior par′tis petro′sae os′sis tempora′lis** [NA], inferior surface of petrous part of temporal bone; see under SURFACE. **f. infe′rior pyram′idis os′sis tempora′lis**, inferior surface of petrous part of temporal bone; see under SURFACE. **f. infratempora′lis maxil′lae** [NA], posterior surface of maxilla; see under SURFACE. **f. inter′na os′sis fronta′lis** [NA], internal surface of frontal bone; see under SURFACE. **f. inter′na os′sis parieta′lis** [NA], internal surface of parietal bone; see under SURFACE. **f. labia′lis den′tis**, labial SURFACE. **f. latera′lis**, lateral SURFACE (1). **f. latera′lis den′tium incisivo′rum et canino′rum** [NA], lateral SURFACE (2). **f. latera′lis os′sis zygomat′ici** [NA], lateral surface of zygomatic bone; see under SURFACE. **f. leonti′na** [L. "lion's face"], a peculiar, lion-like appearance of the face, seen in certain cases of advanced lepromatous leprosy and in fibrous dysplasia of the jaws. See also LEONTIASIS. **f. lepro′sa**, Bergen SYNDROME (1). **f. lingua′lis den′tis** [NA], lingual SURFACE. **f. mala′ris os′sis zygomat′ici**, lateral surface of zygomatic bone; see under SURFACE. **Marshall Hall′s f.**, the facies of hydrocephalus; a triangular face with a broad forehead and prominent frontal bones. **f. masticato′ria den′tis**, occlusal SURFACE (1). **f. maxilla′ris a′lae majo′ris** [NA], maxillary surface of great wing; see under SURFACE. **f. maxilla′ris lam′inae perpendicula′ris os′sis palati′ni** [NA], **f. maxilla′ris par′tis perpendicula′ris os′sis palati′ni**, maxillary surface of perpendicular plate of palatine bone; see under SURFACE. **f. media′lis cartilag′inis arytenoi′deae**, the surface of the arytenoid cartilage that faces medially, toward the opposite arytenoid cartilage. **f. media′lis cer′ebri** [NA], medial surface of cerebrum; see under SURFACE. **f. media′lis den′tium incisivo′rum et canino′rum**, the contact surface of the incisor and canine teeth that is directed toward the midline of the dental arch. **f. media′lis hemisphe′rii cer′ebri** [NA], medial surface of cerebral hemispheres; see under SURFACE. **f. mesia′lis den′tis** [NA], mesial SURFACE. **mitral f., mitrotricuspid f.**, the appearance of the face seen in mitral disease of long duration, marked by rosy, flushed cheeks and dilated capillaries. **moon f., moon FACE. myasthenic f.**, the characteristic facial expression in myasthenia gravis, caused by ptosis and weakness of the facial muscles. **myopathic f.**, the peculiar facial expression produced by relaxation of the facial muscles. **f. nasa′lis lam′inae horizonta′lis os′sis palati′ni** [NA], nasal surface of horizontal part of palatine bone; see under SURFACE. **f. nasa′lis lam′inae perpendicula′ris os′sis palati′ni** [NA], nasal surface of perpendicular

plate of nasal bone; see under SURFACE. **f. nasa'lis maxil'lae**
[NA], nasal surface of maxilla; see under SURFACE. **f. nasa'lis
par'tis horizonta'lis os'sis palati'ni,** nasal surface of horizontal
part of palatine bone; see under SURFACE. **f. nasa'lis par'tis
perpendicula'ris os'sis palati'ni,** nasal surface of perpendicular
plate of nasal bone; see under SURFACE. **f. occlusa'lis den'tis**
[NA], occlusal SURFACE (1). **f. orbita'lis a'lae mag'nae, f. orbita'lis a'lae majo'ris** [NA], orbital surface of great wing of
sphenoid bone; see under SURFACE. **f. orbita'lis maxil'lae** [NA],
orbital surface of maxilla; see under SURFACE. **f. orbita'lis os'sis
fronta'lis** [NA], orbital surface of frontal bone; see under SUR-
FACE. **f. orbita'lis os'sis zygomat'ici** [NA], orbital surface of
zygomatic bone; see under SURFACE. **f. [os'sea] cra'nii,** the bony
skeleton of the face. **f. palati'na lam'inae horizonta'lis os'sis
palati'ni** [NA], **f. palati'na par'tis horizonta'lis os'sis palati'ni,**
palatine surface of horizontal part of palatine bone; see under
SURFACE. **f. parieta'lis os'sis parieta'lis,** external surface of
parietal bone; see under SURFACE. **Parkinson's f.,** a masklike
facies with a wide-eyed unblinking expression, sialorrhea, and
greasy skin, pathognomonic of parkinsonism. **f. poste'rior,** posterior SURFACE (1). **f. poste'rior den'tium premola'rium et
mola'rium** [NA], posterior SURFACE (2). **f. poste'rior par'tis
petro'sae os'sis tempora'lis** [NA], posterior surface of petrous
part of temporal bone; see under SURFACE. **f. poste'rior
pyram'idis os'sis tempora'lis,** posterior surface of petrous part
of temporal bone; see under SURFACE. **Potter's f.,** flattened
palpebral fissures, prominent epicanthus, flattened bridge of
the nose, mandibular micrognathia, and low-set malformed
ears; a diagnostic sign of Potter's disease. **f. scaphoi'dea,** dish
FACE. **f. sphenomaxilla'ris a'lae mag'nae,** maxillary surface of
great wing; see under SURFACE. **f. tempora'lis a'lae mag'nae, f.
tempora'lis a'lae majo'ris** [NA], temporal surface of great wing;
see under SURFACE. **f. tempora'lis os'sis fronta'lis** [NA], temporal surface of frontal bone; see under SURFACE. **f. tempora'lis
os'sis zygomat'ici** [NA], temporal surface of zygomatic bone;
see under SURFACE. **f. tempora'lis par'tis squamo'sae** [NA],
tempora'lis squa'mae tempora'lis, temporal surface of temporal squama; see under SURFACE. **typhoid f., f. typho'sa,** the
vacant and bewildered, often wild and defiant expression, with
face flushed and a dusky, leaden hue, seen in the early stages of
typhoid fever. **f. vestibula'ris den'tis** [NA], vestibular SUR-
FACE.

facilitation (fah-sil"ĭ-ta'shun) [L. *facilis* easy] the promotion or
hastening of any natural process; the reverse of inhibition.
Specifically, the effect of a subthreshold nerve impulse resulting in an increase in the excitability of a neuron from other
convergent nerve fibers. A rapidly applied series of subthreshold stimuli can generate an excitatory postsynaptic potential
which, due to the added neurotransmitter, will let an all or none
impulse be discharged in the postsynaptic neuron. See also LAW
of facilitation.

facility (fah-sil'ĭ-te) 1. the quality of being easily performed. 2.
something that is established to serve a particular purpose, or to
facilitate a special type of activity. **emergency care f.,** emergency ROOM. **extended care f.,** an institution or a part of an
institution primarily engaged in providing skilled nursing care
and/or rehabilitation services to injured, disabled, or sick inpatients. Abbreviated *ECF*. See also extended care SERVICE and
nursing HOME. **intermediate care f.,** an institution recognized
under the Medicaid program which is licensed under state law
to provide, on a regular basis, health-related care and services
to individuals who do not require the degree of care or treatment
which a hospital or skilled nursing facility is designed to
provide, but who because of their mental or physical condition,
require care and services above the level of room and board that
can be made available only through institutional facilities.
Abbreviated *ICF*. **nursing f.,** an institution, such as an extended
care facility, a nursing home, or an old age institution, which
provides nursing care, either by a registered nurse or licensed
practical nurse, for patients and residents. **skilled nursing f.,** an
institution that provides skilled nursing care and rehabilitation
services to patients who do not require hospitalization.

facing (fās'ing) 1. a covering in front, as an outer layer of stone on
a masonry wall. 2. a porcelain reproduction of the labial or
buccal surface of a tooth, constructed either with or without
pins and soldered or cemented to a metal backing. **interchangeable f.,** a facing equipped with a standard slot in the porcelain to
fit a backing, baked in a mold that will also serve to produce
replacements of the same size, color, or shape. Called also
Thom's f. and *Steele's f.* **Steele's f., Thom's f.,** interchangeable f.

facio- [L. *facies* face] a combining form denoting relationship to
the face.

faciobrachial (fa"she-o-bra'ke-al) [*facio-* + Gr. *brachiōn* arm]
pertaining to the face and arm.

faciocephalalgia (fa"she-o-sef"ah-lal'je-ah) [*facio-* + Gr.: *kephalē*
head + *-algia*] neuralgic pain in the face and neck.

faciocervical (fa"she-o-ser've-kal) [*facio-* + L. *cervix* neck] pertaining to the face and neck.

faciolingual (fa"she-o-ling'gwal) [*facio-* + L. *lingua* tongue] pertaining to the face and tongue.

facioplasty (fa"she-o-plas'te) [*facio-* + Gr. *plassein* to form] plastic surgery of the face.

facioplegia (fa"she-o-ple'je-ah) [*facio-* + Gr. *plēgē* stroke] facial
PARALYSIS.

faciostenosis (fa"she-o-ste-no'sis) failure of the midface to grow.

facsimile (fak-sim'ĭ-le) an exact copy of something.

factitial (fak-tish'al) produced by artificial means; unintention-
ally produced.

factor (fak'tor) [L. "maker"] an agent or element that contributes
to the production of a result. **f. I,** fibrinogen. **f. II,** prothrombin. **f.
III,** tissue THROMBOPLASTIN. **f. IV,** calcium. **f. V,** a blood coagulation factor functioning in both the extrinsic and intrinsic
pathways of prothrombin activator (see under PROTHROMBIN)
formation, complexing with activated factor X and phospholipids. Factor V is destroyed by heating or by increasing the pH; it
is also destroyed by oxalates but not citrates. It is not adsorbed
by aluminum hydroxide or barium sulfate. Electrophoretically,
it migrates between β- and γ-globulin. Acquired factor V deficiency leads to hypoprothrombinemia; congenital deficiency
produces parahemophilia and de Vries' syndrome. Called also
*accelerator f., labile f., plasma converting f., Ac-globulin
(AC-G), accelerator globulin, proaccelerin, prothrombin accelerator* and *thrombogen.* See also blood COAGULATION. **f. VI,**
one previously thought to be an activated form of factor V. It no
longer is considered in the scheme of hemostasis. Called also
accelerin and *serum Ac globulin.* **f. VII,** a blood coagulation
factor synthesized in the liver, found in the serum but not in
plasma, which is adsorbed by aluminum hydroxide and barium
sulfate. In the extrinsic pathway, factor VII complexes with
thromboplastin and, in the presence of phospholipids, activates
factor X in the process of prothrombin activator formation.
Electrophoretically, it migrates between α- and β-globulin. Congenital deficiency of this factor, inherited as an autosomal
recessive trait, is characterized by bleeding tendency, gastrointestinal hemorrhage, cerebral hemorrhage, menorrhagia, epistaxis, and hemarthrosis. Hemorrhage may follow tonsillectomy
or tooth extraction. Factor VII deficiency also may be acquired
and is associated with vitamin K deficiency (see HYPO-
PROTHROMBINEMIA). Called also *stable prothrombin F, autoprothrombin I, co-thromboplastin, proconvertin-convertin,
serum accelerator,* and *serum prothrombin conversion accelerator (SPCA).* **f. VIII,** a blood coagulation factor functioning in
the intrinsic pathway that, together with activated calcium and
platelet factor 3, activates factor X complexed with phospholipids and factor V to form prothrombin activator (see under
PROTHROMBIN). It is a relatively labile protein found in plasma
but not in serum, which is not adsorbed by aluminum hydroxide
and barium sulfate. Factor VIII migrates electrophoretically
within the β₂-globulin range. Deficiency of this factor results in
hemophilia A. Called also *antihemophilic f. A (AHG), antihemophilic globulin (AHG), platelet cofactor I,* and *thromboplastinogen.* See also blood COAGULATION. **f. IX,** a blood
coagulation factor functioning in the intrinsic pathway. Activated by factor XII, factor IX in turn activates factor X
together with activated factor VII and platelet factor 3, which
then complexes with phospholipids and factor V to form
prothrombin activator (see under PROTHROMBIN). It is a relatively stable protein found in serum but not in plasma, which
migrates in the α₂-globulin range, and is adsorbed by aluminum
hydroxide and barium sulfate. Deficiency of this factor results
in Christmas disease (hemophilia B). Called also *antihemophilic f. B, Christmas f., plasma f. X, autoprothrombin II,
plasma thromboplastin component (PTC),* and *platelet cofactor II.* See also blood COAGULATION. **f. X,** a blood coagulation
factor functioning in both the extrinsic and intrinsic pathways
of prothrombin activator formation (see under PROTHROMBIN),
complexing with phospholipids and factor V in the final stages
of the process. It is a heat-labile protein found in serum but not
in plasma, which migrates in the α-globulin range. A ge-
netically-determined deficiency of factor X (known as *Prower* or
Stuart defect) occurs in both males and females, probably
transmitted as an autosomal recessive trait, and is characterized by moderate to severe bleeding following injury, with rare
spontaneous epistaxis, hemarthroses, and gingival hemorrhage. Prothrombin time and prothrombin utilization are defi-

cient. Called also *Prower f., Stuart f., autoprothrombin C,* and *thrombokinase.* See also PROTHROMBIN activator and blood COAGULATION. **f. XA,** prothrombinase. **f. XI,** a blood coagulation factor acting in the intrinsic pathway. Activated by factor XII, factor XI in turn activates factor IX which, together with factor VII and platelet factor 3, activates factor X in producing prothrombin activator (see under PROTHROMBIN). It is a stable protein found in both plasma and serum, which migrates between the β- and γ-globulin ranges, and is adsorbed only partially or not at all by aluminum hydroxide and barium sulfate. A deficiency of this factor causes a disorder similar to, but milder than, hemophilia (known as *hemophilia C, hemophiloid state D,* and *PTF-C deficiency*). It is transmitted as an incompletely recessive autosomal trait, occurs in both sexes, and is characterized by prolonged coagulation time, poor prothrombin utilization, and inadequate thromboplastin generation. Spontaneous bleeding is rare in the disorder, but hemorrhage may follow injury and tooth extraction; occasionally, hemostasis appears to be satisfactory at the time of intervention. Called also *antihemophilic f. C* and *plasma thromboplastin antecedent (PTA).* See also blood COAGULATION. **f. XII,** a blood coagulation factor functioning in the intrinsic pathway. After a vascular injury, contact with collagen in the blood vessel wall causes factor XII to be converted into a proteolytic enzyme (tissue thromboplastin), being the first step in forming prothrombin activator (see under PROTHROMBIN). It is a stable protein found in plasma and serum, which is poorly adsorbed by alkaline earths, and migrates between the β- and γ-globulin ranges. A congenital abnormality of this factor (known as *Hageman deficiency* or *trait*) is transmitted as an autosomal recessive trait, and is characterized by a prolonged coagulation time, but no hemorrhagic tendency. Called also *contact f., glass f.,* and *Hageman f.* See also blood COAGULATION. **f. XIII,** a blood coagulation factor that polymerizes fibrin monomers so that they become stable and insoluble in urea, thus enabling fibrin to form a firm clot. It migrates in the β₂-globulin range. A hereditary disorder of this factor, which is usually present at birth, is characterized by a bleeding tendency after even a minor injury. Faulty wound healing, cerebral hemorrhage, ecchymoses, and hematomas are common. Spontaneous bleeding and bleeding from mucous membranes are rare. The disorder occurs in both males and females, and is probably transmitted as an autosomal recessive trait. Acquired factor XIII deficiency may occur in hypofibrinogenemia, liver diseases, and acute myeloblastic leukemia. Called also *fibrin-stabilizing f. (FSF)* and *Laki-Lórand f. (LLF).* See also blood COAGULATION. **accelerator f.,** f. V. **Am f.,** a genetically-transmitted allotypic antigen associated with the heavy chain of IgA. **antihemophilic f. A,** f. VIII. **antihemophilic f. B,** f. IX. **antihemophilic f. C,** f. XI. **antinuclear f.,** an autoantibody against constituents of cell nuclei that may be demonstrated by immunofluorescence and is present in the sera of patients with systemic lupus erythematosus and occasionally in rheumatoid arthritis and other collagen diseases. Abbreviated *ANF.* **antiscorbutic f.,** ascorbic ACID. **antixerophthalmia f.,** VITAMIN A. **f. B,** a heat-labile component of the alternative pathway of complement activation, which is activated by factor D̄ to cleave the C3 component. Called also *C3 proactivator (C3PA)* and *glycine-rich glycoprotein (GRG).* **backscatter f.,** the ratio of the exposure at the point of intersection of the central ray with the surfaces of the phantom, to the exposure at the same point in space under similar conditions of irradiation in the absence of the phantom. **beam direction f.,** the fraction of the workload during which the useful beam of radiation is directed at a barrier. Called also *use f.* **blood f.,** according to Wiener, the actual surface structure of the red cells with which specific antibodies react; certain blood factors are associated with the presence of certain agglutinogens, but the two are not identical in Wiener's conception. See also AGGLUTINOGEN. **bone f.,** a clinical guide for determining the diagnosis and prognosis of periodontal disease, based on the alveolar response to local injurious factors. In the presence of *positive bone factor,* new bone is formed constantly in an effort to compensate for the increased resorption due to harmful local factors, associated with bone loss that is maintained at a minimum. When the amount and rate of bone loss are in excess of what could be expected, taking into account the patient's age and the presence of local factors, a diagnosis of *negative bone factor* is made. This procedure is considered by some authorities as being obsolete. **Castle's f's,** factors responsible for the assimilation of vitamin B₁₂, failure of any of which is responsible for the development of pernicious anemia (see under ANEMIA). The

normal gastric mucosa and gastric juice contain a mucoprotein (*intrinsic factor*), which elaborates the absorption of the *extrinsic factor* (vitamin B₁₂). **Cellano f.,** Cellano ANTIGEN. **chemotactic f's,** factors released during the reaction of specific antigen with sensitized lymphocytes, being also generated by nonspecific mitogens, which induce chemotactic migration of monocytes, some factors being selectively chemotactic for neutrophils, eosinophils, and basophils. Their molecular weights range from 40,000 to 60,000. Other chemotactic factors may be produced by complement activation. **Christmas f.,** f. IX. **citrovorum f.,** the physiologically active form of folic acid, *N-p-*[(2 - amino - 5 - formyl - 5, 6, 7, 8 - tetrahydro - 4 - hydroxy - 6 - pteridinyl)methyl]-amino-benzoyl glutamic acid, the conversion of which is catalyzed by ascorbic acid. Citrovorum factor is essential for the growth of the bacterium *Leuconostoc citrovorum* and for certain other microorganisms and animals by taking a part in the transfer of 1-carbon, in the synthesis and transfer of methyl groups, and in the synthesis of DNA. Called also *folinic acid* and *leucovorin.* See also folic ACID. **coagulation f.,** a substance in the blood that is essential to the maintenance of normal hemostasis; the absence, diminution, or excess of which may lead to abnormality of the clotting mechanisms. Coagulation factors are designated by Roman numerals. See FIBRINOGEN (f. I), f. II, THROMBOPLASTIN (f. III), CALCIUM, PROTHROMBIN (f. IV), *f. V, f. VII, f. VIII, f. IX, f. X, f. XI, f. XII,* and *f. XIII;* factor VI is no longer considered in the scheme of hemostasis. Platelet factors, designated by Arabic numerals, also play a role in coagulation. See also blood COAGULATION and HEMOSTASIS. **complement f.,** see COMPLEMENT. **contact f.,** f. XIII. **Curling f.,** griseofulvin. **f. D,** an inactive precursor of factor D̄. **f. D̄,** a component of the alternative pathway of complement activation, which is a globulin (molecular weight about 25,000) that cleaves factor B into two fragments. Called also *C3 proactivator convertase (C3PA-convertase).* **Diᵃ f.,** Diᵃ ANTIGEN. **Diᵇ f.,** Diᵇ ANTIGEN. **Diego f.,** Diego ANTIGEN. **diffusion f.,** hyaluronidase. **distribution f.,** in radiology, the modification of biological effect due to nonuniform distribution of internally deposited isotopes. Abbreviated *DF.* See also dose EQUIVALENT. **Dorner f.,** cyanocobalamin. **Duffy f.,** see Duffy ANTIGEN. **Duran-Reynals f.,** hyaluronidase. **eosinophil chemotactic f. of anaphylaxis,** an acidic peptide mediator that is selectively chemotactic for eosinophils. It is a mixture of at least two tetrapeptides with a molecular weight of less than 500, which is stored in mast cells and basophils and is released in anaphylaxis following the reaction of antigen with cell-bound IgE. Abbreviated *ECF-A.* **erythropoietic stimulating f.,** erythropoietin. **extrinsic f.,** cyanocobalamin. **fibrin-stabilizing f.,** f. XIII. **Fyᵃ f.,** Fyᵃ ANTIGEN. **Fyᵇ f.,** Fyᵇ ANTIGEN. **f. Fyᵃ; Fyᵇ,** factors in the Duffy blood group. See Duffy GROUP. **glass f.,** f. XII. **Gm f.,** a genetically-transmitted allotypic antigen associated with the heavy chain of IgG. **growth hormone-release inhibiting factor (GH-RIF),** somatostatin. **Hageman f.,** f. XII. **initiating f.,** a component found in trace amounts in normal human serum, which seems to be similar to the nephritic factor of patients with hypocomplementemic nephritis, believed to initiate the activation of the alternative pathway of complement. Abbreviated *IF.* See also *nephritic f.* **intrinsic f.,** see Castle's f's. **Inv f.,** a genetically transmitted allotypic antigen associated with the kappa light chain of all immunoglobulins. Named in abbreviated form after the first patient in whom it was discovered. Called also *Km f.* **Jkᵃ f.,** Kidd ANTIGEN. **Jkᵇ f.,** Kidd ANTIGEN. **Jsᵃ f.,** Jsᵃ ANTIGEN. **Jsᵇ f.,** Jsᵇ ANTIGEN. **k f.,** k ANTIGEN. **f. Kᵒ,** a blood group factor. See Kell GROUP. **f. K1,** Kell ANTIGEN. **K2 f.,** K2 ANTIGEN. **K3 f.,** Kpᵃ ANTIGEN. **K4 f.,** Kpᵇ ANTIGEN. **K5 f.,** Ku ANTIGEN. **K6 f.,** Jsᵃ ANTIGEN. **K7 f.,** Jsᵇ ANTIGEN. **Kell f.,** Kell ANTIGEN. **Kidd f.,** Kidd ANTIGEN. **Km f.,** Inv f. **Kpᵃ f.,** Kpᵃ ANTIGEN. **Kpᵇ f.,** Kpᵇ ANTIGEN. **Ku f.,** Ku ANTIGEN. **labile f.,** f. V. **Laki-Lorand f.,** f. XIII. **lard f.,** vitamin A. **LE plasma f.,** a γ-globulin fraction in lupus erythematosus patients which induces the formation of LE cells (see under CELL). **Leᵃ f.,** Leᵃ ANTIGEN. **Leᵇ f.,** Leᵇ ANTIGEN. **Lewis f.,** Lewis ANTIGEN. **LLD f.,** cyanocobalamin. **Luᵃ f.,** Luᵃ ANTIGEN. **Luᵇ f.,** Luᵇ ANTIGEN. **Lutheran f.,** Lutheran ANTIGEN. **McLeod f.,** a blood group factor. See Kell GROUP. **migration inhibitory f.,** a lymphokine protein released from the interaction of sensitized lymphocytes with antigen or with mitogen, which inhibits the migration of macrophages. Abbreviated *MIF.* **milk f.,** see mammary tumor virus of mice; under VIRUS. **mitogenic f.,** a heat-stable substance (molecular weight about 25,000) released by sensitized lymphocytes stimulated with specific antigen or mitogens, having the capacity to cause blast cell transformation and increase tritiated thymidine uptake into cellular DNA. Together with transfer factor, it is believed to play a role in augmenting or amplifying the cell-mediated response by recruiting uncommitted lymphocytes. **mouse antialopecia f.,** inositol. **nephritic f.,** a 7S γ-globulin of normal serum, capable of cleaving the C3 component of complement to C3b directly, which was first seen in patients with renal disease characterized by low serum levels of complement (hypercomplementemic nephritis or glomerulonephritis). See also *initiating f.* **Oz f.,** a genetically transmitted allotypic antigen associated with the lambda chain of immunoglobulins. **pellagra preventive f.,** nicotinic ACID. **Peltz f.,** Ku ANTIGEN. **Penny f.,** Kp^a ANTIGEN. **phagocytosis promoting f. (P.P.F.),** opsonin (2). **plasma f. X, f. IX. plasma converting f.,** f. V. **platelet f. 1,** adsorbed factor V from the plasma. **platelet f. 2,** an accelerator of the thrombin-fibrinogen reaction, attached to platelets. **platelet f. 3,** in blood coagulation, a phospholipid released by blood platelets in response to blood injury, being the first step in the intrinsic pathway of the formation of prothrombin activator (see under PROTHROMBIN). Called also *platelet phospholipid.* See also blood COAGULATION. **platelet f. 4,** an intracellular protein component of blood platelets, capable of neutralizing the antithrombic activity of heparin in the fibrinogen-fibrin reaction and the inhibitory effect of heparin in the thromboplastin generation test. **platelet-activating f.,** a very basic low-molecular-weight (1,000) phospholipid, which induces platelet aggregation and the release of histamine. It has been found in man and in the rabbit and rat, and may serve as a potent amplifying agent for acute allergic and anaphylactic reactions. Abbreviated *PAF.* **P.P. f.,** nicotinic ACID. **Prower f.,** f. X. **pyruvate oxidation f.,** α-lipoic ACID. **quality f.,** in radiology, the linear energy transfer dependent factor by which absorbed doses are multiplied to obtain for radiation protection purposes a quantity that expresses the effect of the absorbed dose on a common scale for all ionizing radiations. Abbreviated *QF.* See also dose EQUIVALENT. **Rautenberg f.,** Kp^b ANTIGEN. **Rh f., f. Rh, rhesus f.,** any one of a series of blood factors specific antibodies to which can cause agglutination of human erythrocytes. The first one was found in the serum of rabbits that had been injected with erythrocytes of rhesus monkeys. See Rh blood groups, under blood GROUP. **rheumatoid f.,** an antibody against slightly denatured IgG, appearing most frequently on IgM in the serum of patients with rheumatoid arthritis and detectable by serological tests. **skin-reactive f.,** a lymphokine produced by the interaction of specifically sensitized lymphocytes with antigen and mitogens. When introduced into the skin of guinea pigs, it produces an indurated and erythematous lesion similar to that caused by the delayed-type cutaneous lesion, which disappears spontaneously in about 30 hours. **somatotropin release inhibiting f. (SRIF),** somatostatin. **spreading f.,** hyaluronidase. **stable prothrombin f., f. VII. stable prothrombin conversion f.,** f. VII. **Stuart f.,** f. X. **Sutter f.,** ANTIGEN Js^a. **f. T,** vitamin T. **tissue f.,** tissue THROMBOPLASTIN. **transfer f.,** a factor or substance produced by sensitized lymphocytes that has the capacity to transfer specific delayed hypersensitivity to another nonsensitive individual. It has been used to restore cellular immunity with varying degrees of success. **use f.,** beam direction f.

facultative (fak'ul-ta"tiv) not obligatory; pertaining to or characterized by the ability to adjust to particular circumstances or to assume a particular role.

faculty (fak'ul-te) [L. *facultas*] any normal power or function, especially a mental one. 2. the corps of professors and instructors of a college or university.

FAD flavin-adenine DINUCLEOTIDE.

Fahrenheit's scale, thermometer [Gabriel Daniel *Fahrenheit*, German physicist, 1686–1736] see under SCALE and THERMOMETER.

failure (fāl'yer) inability to perform. **heart f.,** a condition resulting from disorders of heart output or from increased venous pressure, most often applied to myocardial failure with increased pressures distending the ventricle and a cardiac output inadequate for the body needs. **heart f., congestive,** a clinical syndrome occurring either because of a decreased myocardial capacity to contract or because of an increased pressure-volume load is imposed on the heart. It is caused by primary damage to the heart muscle or is secondary to chronic excessive workload, as in severe valvular heart disease. Heart enlargement, diminished stroke volume, and damming back of blood in the venous system resulting in edema and congestion are the usual consequences. Dyspnea and undue fatigability are the common subjective symptoms. Abbreviated *CHF.* Called also *cardiac decompensation.*

faint (fānt) syncope.

Fajans' law [Kasimir *Fajans,* a physicist, born 1887] see under LAW.

Fajans-Soddy law [K. *Fajans*] see under LAW.

falces (fal'sēz) [L.] plural of *falx.*

falcial (fal'shal) pertaining to a falx.

falciform (fal'si-form) [L. *falx* sickle + *forma* form] sickle-shaped.

fallopian (fah-lo'pe-an) named for or described by Gabriele *Fallopio (Fallopius),* as fallopian aqueduct or canal (see CANAL for facial nerve) and fallopian hiatus (see HIATUS of canal for greater petrosal nerve).

Fallopius see FALLOPPIO.

Falloppio (Fallopius), Gabriele [1523–1562] an outstanding Italian anatomist, pupil of Vesalius, and later professor at Padua. He conducted research on the development of the teeth and accurately described the dental follicle. See also FALLOPIAN.

fallout (fawl'owt) the settling to the earth's surface of radioactive fission produces that have been projected into the atmosphere by the explosion of a nuclear device. See also SCAVENGING (3).

false (fawls) [L. *falsus*] not true; apparent but not real.

false negative (fawls neg'ah-tiv) in a diagnostic test, a negative reaction in the presence of disease.

false positive (fawls pos'ĭ-tiv) in a diagnostic test, a positive reaction in absence of disease.

falx (falks), pl. *fal'ces* [L. "sickle"] any sickle-shaped organ or part; used in anatomical nomenclature to designate such a structure.

familial (fah-mil'e-al) [L. *familia* family] occurring in or affecting more members of a family than would be expected by chance.

family (fam'ĭ-le) [L. *familia*] 1. a group of individuals descended from a common ancestor. 2. a taxonomic subdivision subordinate to an order (or suborder) and superior to a tribe (or subfamily). 3. in census statistics, a group of two or more persons related by blood, marriage, or adoption who are living together in the same household. 4. in group insurance, a group consisting of an individual and his dependents who are not necessarily related by blood or who are living in the same household.

Fanconi's anemia (refractory anemia), syndrome [Guido *Fanconi,* Swiss biochemist, born 1892] see under ANEMIA and SYNDROME, and see Abderhalden-Fanconi SYNDROME.

Fanconi-Albertini-Zellweger syndrome [G. *Fanconi;* Ambrosius *Albertini;* H. *Zellweger*] see under SYNDROME.

Fanconi-De Toni-Debré syndrome [G. *Fanconi;* Guido *De Toni;* Robert *Debré,* French physician] see Abderhalden-Fanconi SYNDROME.

Fanconi-Petrassi syndrome [G. *Fanconi;* G. *Petrassi*] see under SYNDROME.

Fanconi-Schlesinger syndrome [G. *Fanconi;* B. *Schlesinger*] elfin facies SYNDROME.

fang (fang) 1. a long sharp tooth having a conical crown and a single root, used to tear flesh; canine TOOTH. 2. an elongated hollow or grooved tooth through which poisonous snakes inject venom. 3. any elongated, pointed fanglike object. 4 a root of a tooth (now used infrequently)

Farabeuf's saw, triangle [Louis Hubert *Farabeuf,* French surgeon, 1841–1910] see under SAW and TRIANGLE.

farad (far'ad) [named after Michael *Faraday*] the SI unit of electric capacitance, being the capacity of a condenser which, charged with 1 coloumb, gives a difference of potential of 1 volt. Abbreviated *F.* See also SI.

faraday (far'ah-da) [named after Michael *Faraday*] the quantity of electrical charge associated with 1 gram equivalent of an electrochemical reaction, equal to about 96.510 coulombs.

Faraday's constant, dark space, law [Michael *Faraday,* English physicist, 1791–1867] see under CONSTANT, SPACE, and LAW. See also FARAD and FARADAY.

Farber's syndrome (lipogranulomatosis) [Sidney *Farber,* American physician, born 1903] see under SYNDROME.

Fargan trademark for *promethazine.*

Fargin-Fayolle syndrome DENTINOGENESIS imperfecta.

Farrar, John Nutting [1839–1913] an American dentist who developed the theory of the movement of teeth by intermittent forces, being the first to advocate the need of keeping the movements of the teeth within physiological limits.

fascia (fash'e-ah), pl. *fas'ciae* [L. "band"] [NA] a sheet or band of fibrous tissue, such as lies deep to the skin or forms an investment for muscles and various organs of the body. See illustration. **alar f.,** a delicate layer of cervical fascia that extends from the buccopharyngeal fascia at the midline to the carotid sheath laterally. **aponeurotic f.,** deep f. **buccinator f., f. buccopharyn'gea** [NA], **buccopharyngeal f.,** the portion of the cervical visceral fascia forming the external covering of the buccinator muscle, the pterygomandibular raphe, and the constrictor muscles of the pharynx. **cervical f., f. cervica'lis** [NA], the fascia which covers the region of the neck, variously divided according to its location as the infrahyoid and suprahyoid fasciae; the deep and superficial layers; the pretracheal, prever-

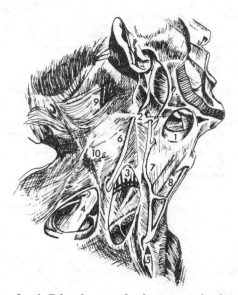

Fasciae of neck. Tela subcutanea has been removed and openings made in investing layer of deep fascia to show deeper fascia. Sternocleidomastoid muscle has been partly removed; submandibular gland, almost wholly removed; and parotid gland, removed as far as its duct. Submandibular space, 1; parotid space, 2; sternocleidomastoid, 3; supraclavicular fossa, 4; suprasternal space, 5; external jugular vein, 6; communicating vein, 7; anterior jugular vein, 8; nervus occipitalis minor, 9; n. auricularis magnus, 10. (From E. L. Granite: Anatomic considerations in infections of the face and neck. Review of the literature. J. Oral Surg., 34(1):34–44.)

tebral, and investing fasciae; the buccopharyngeal fascia; the alar fascia; etc. Called also *f. colli, f. of neck, proper f. of neck,* and *f. propria colli.* **cervical f., deep,** the fascia which invests the muscles in the dorsal region of the neck, forming numerous compartments and fascial clefts. Called also *infrahyoid f., f. of nape, f. nuchae* [NA], and *nuchal f.* **cervical f., investing,** investing layer of cervical fascia, see under LAYER. **cervical f., middle,** the part of the cervical fascia that invests the two layers of the infrahyoid muscles, consisting of three sheets which attach to the hyoid bone at one end, and to the sternum at the other. **cervical visceral f.,** a tubular fascial structure that continues from the visceral fascia of the mediastinum and envelops the trachea and esophagus at the point of their entrance to the neck, and the pharynx, larynx, and thyroid gland. It attaches to the pharyngeal tubercle, pterygoid hamulus, and mandible. Called also *visceral cervical f.* and *lamina pretrachealis fasciae cervicalis* [NA]. See also *buccinator f.* and *pretracheal f.* **f. col′li,** cervical f. **deep f.,** the gray, dense, firm, fibrous membrane covering the muscles, holding individual muscles, their groups, and other structures in their relative positions. Called also *aponeurotic f.* **extrapleural f.,** a prolongation of the endothoracic fascia sometimes found at the root of the neck. **infrahyoid f.,** cervical f., deep. **masseteric f.,** the portion of the parotideomasseteric fascia which encloses the lateral surface of the masseter muscle. **muscular fasciae of eye, fas′ciae muscula′res bul′bi** [NA], **fas′ciae muscula′res oc′uli,** the sheets of fascia investing the extraocular muscles, continuous with the vagina bulbi. **f. of nape,** cervical f., deep. **f. of neck,** cervical f. **nuchal f., f. nu′chae** [NA], cervical f., deep. **orbital fasciae, fas′ciae orbita′les** [NA], fibrous tissue surrounding the posterior part of the eyeball, supporting and binding together the structures within the orbit. **palpebral f., f. palpebra′lis,** orbital SEPTUM. **parotid f., f. parotide′a** [NA], the portion of the parotideomasseteric fascia which encloses the parotid gland. **parotideomasseteric f., f. parotideomasseter′ica,** the fascia enclosing the parotid gland and the lateral surface of the masseter muscle, which attaches to the zygomatic arch and is continuous with the cervical fascia. The parotid portion *(parotid f.)* is fused with the parotid gland through numerous septa extending into the capsule and fusing with the subcutaneous fascia. The masseteric portion *(masseteric f.)* attaches to the border of the

mandible, forming a compartment for the muscle. It encircles the ramus of the mandible and is continuous with the fascia of the pterygoid muscle. **pharyngobasilar f., f. pharyngobasila′ris** [NA], a strong fibrous membrane in the wall of the pharynx, lined internally with mucous membrane and incompletely covered on its outer surface by the overlapping constrictor muscles of the pharynx. It blends with the periosteum at the base of the skull. In the embryo, the buccopharyngeal membrane is formed at the end of the primitive gut where the ectoderm comes in contact with the entoderm, forming the floor of an external depression (the stomodeum). During the fourth week it ruptures and allows the stomodeum and the foregut to merge. Called also *aponeurosis pharyngis, aponeurosis pharyngobasilaris, buccopharyngeal membrane, oral plate, pharyngeal aponeurosis, pharyngeal plate, pharyngeal tunic, pharyngobasilar aponeurosis,* and *pharyngobasilar tunic.* **pretracheal f.,** the part of the cervical visceral fascia that covers the trachea, larynx, and thyroid gland. **prevertebral f., f. prevertebra′lis,** the layer of the cervical fascia which envelops the vertebral column and its muscles, continuous behind with the deep cervical fascia. It is separated from the subserous fascia by the retropharyngeal fascial cleft. A fibrous formation near the scalenus muscles is known as *Sibson's fascia.* Called also *lamina prevertebralis fasciae cervicalis* [NA]. **proper f. of neck, f. pro′pria col′li,** cervical f. **pterygoid f., f. pterygoi′dea,** a fascia that envelops the medial and lateral pterygoid muscles; one sheet attaches to the mandible at both borders and invests the medial pterygoid muscle. The superficial sheet attaches to the skull at the origin of the muscle and invests the lateral pterygoid muscle. The part between the two muscles attaches to the skull between the lateral pterygoid plate and the spine of the sphenoid bone; the part near the spine forms a band that attaches to the mandible, forming the sphenomandibular ligament. Another band, the pterygospinous ligament, situated between the two muscles, at times becomes ossified, forming the pterygospinous foramen and giving passage to mandibular branches of the trigeminal nerve. **Sibson's f.,** a fibrous formation on the prevertebral fascia near the scalenus muscles. **subcutaneous f.,** the subcutaneous layer of connective tissue that is continuous over the entire body, sometimes considered as the innermost part of the corium of the skin. Called also *superficial f., hypoderm, subcutaneous tissue,* and *tela subcutanea* [NA]. **subserous f.,** a connective tissue layer situated between the body wall and the serous membrane, which lines the body cavities. It may be very thin, as is the part which lines the pleura, or very thick and made up of adipose tissue, as is the part surrounding the kidneys. Called also *visceral f., subserous layer,* and *tela subserosa* [NA]. **superficial f.,** subcutaneous f. **suprahyoid f.,** the part of the cervical fascia that attaches to the border of the mandible at one end and to the hyoid bone at the other, forming the suprahyoid compartment. The investing or superficial layer covers the anterior belly of the digastric muscle, submandibular gland, stylohyoid muscle, intermediate tendon of the digastric muscle, and sternocleidomastoid muscle. **temporal f., f. tempora′lis** [NA], a strong fibrous sheet which covers the temporal muscle and gives attachment to many of its fibers. The upper part presents a thin, single-layer sheet and the lower part, near its attachment to the zygomatic arch, is formed by two layers, the lamina profunda (inner layer), and the lamina superficialis (outer layer). The orbital branch of the superficial temporal artery and some fatty tissue are located between the layers. It is an extension of the deep fascia; cranially it is continuous with the pericranium. Called also *temporal aponeurosis.* **thyrolaryngeal f.,** fascia investing the thyroid cartilage and attaching to the cricoid cartilage. **visceral f.,** subserous f. **visceral cervical f.,** cervical visceral f.

fasciae (fash′e-e) [L.] plural of *fascia.*

fascial (fash″e-al) pertaining to or of the nature of fascia.

fascicle (fas′ĭ-k′l) [L. *fasciculus*] a small bundle or cluster, especially of nerve or muscle fibers.

fasciculi (fah-sik′u-li) [L.] plural of *fasciculus.*

fasciculus (fah-sik′u-lus), pl. *fascic′uli* [L., dim. of *fascis* bundle] a small bundle or cluster; used in anatomical nomenclature to designate a small bundle of nerve or muscle fibers. Called also *fascicle.* **f. anterolatera′lis superficia′lis,** spinocerebellar tract, anterior; see under TRACT. **f. cerebellospina′lis,** spinocerebellar tract, posterior; see under TRACT.

fasciectomy (fas″e-ek′to-me) [*fascia* + Gr. *ektomē* excision] excision of fascia.

fasciitis (fas″e-i′tis) inflammation of fascia. Called also *fascitis.* **infiltrative f., nodular f., pseudosarcomatous f.,** pseudosarcomatous FIBROMATOSIS.

fasciodesis (fas″e-od′ĕ-sis) [L. *fascia* + Gr. *desis* binding] the operation of suturing a fascia to skeletal attachment.

fascitis (fah-si′tis) fasciitis.

Fastcure trademark for a self-curing *repair resin* (see under RESIN).

Fastidio Plain trademark for a heat-cured denture base acrylic resin.

Fastin trademark for *phentermine hydrochloride* (see under PHENTERMINE).

fat (fat) 1. adipose tissue; a white or yellowish tissue which forms soft pads between various organs of the body. 2. an ester of glycerol with fatty acids, usually oleic acid, palmitic acid, or stearic acid. **blood f.,** blood LIPID. **neutral f.,** glyceride. **wool f.,** lanolin.

fatal (fa′tal) causing death; deadly; mortal.

fatigue (fah-tēg) [Fr.; L. *fatigatio*] 1. the state of increased discomfort and decreased efficiency resulting from prolonged or excessive exertion; loss of power or capacity to respond to stimulation. 2. material f. **material f.,** the breaking or fracturing of a material caused by repeated cyclic or applied loads below the yield strength, usually beginning with minute cracks in a small region of high stress concentration, followed by enlargement of the cracks and, finally, brittle failure or fracture.

fatty (fat′e) pertaining to fat.

fauces (faw′sēz) [L., pl. of *faux* a gorge, narrow pass] [NA] the passage from the mouth to the pharynx, including both the lumen and its boundaries; the throat. Its isthmus is bounded superiorly by the soft palate, inferiorly by the dorsum of the tongue, and on both sides by the palatoglossal arch. Situated at the side of the fauces, between the palatoglossal and palatopharyngeal arches, are the palatine tonsils. Called also *vestibule of pharynx*. See also DEGLUTITION and ISTHMUS faucium.

Fauchard's disease [Pierre *Fauchard*, French dentist, 1678–1761; he is generally considered the founder of modern dentistry, and is responsible for the separation of dentistry from general medicine and surgery. His celebrated book, *Le chirurgien dentiste*, published in 1728, is considered a landmark in the history of dentistry. He pioneered the use of thread, silver and gold plates, files, and pelican and straight forceps; the replacement of teeth with human teeth and teeth made from hippotamus tusks, ivory, and bone; and the use of artificial dentures. Fauchard is believed to be the first to use the term *caries* and he refuted the idea that caries was caused by "worms of the teeth."] marginal PERIODONTITIS.

faucial (faw′shal) pertaining to the fauces.

faucitis (faw-si′tis) inflammation of the fauces. See also ANGINA, LARYNGITIS, and PHARYNGITIS.

Favistan tradement for *methimazole*.

Favre, Maurice [1876–1954] a French physician. See LYMPHOGRANULOMA venereum (Durand-Nicolas-Favre disease, Nicolas-Favre disease).

favus (fa′vus) [L. "honeycomb"] a form of tinea capitis characterized by the formation of yellow, cuplike crusts composed of dense mats of mycelia and epithelial debris, which enlarge to form prominent honeycomb-like masses. It is caused by *Trichophyton schoenleinii*. Called also *tinea favosa*.

Fayolle see DENTINOGENESIS imperfecta (Fargin-Fayolle syndrome).

Fc [*f*ragment, *c*rystallizable] a crystallizable fragment which, together with two Fab pieces, is obtained when an immunoglobulin molecule is cleaved by papain. It consists of the C-terminal portions of the heavy chains joined together by one or more $-S-S-$ bonds. Fc has no antibody activity, but includes that part of the heavy chain which determines its properties, such as the ability to fix complement and most of the antigenic determinants. Called also *Fc fragment* and *Fc piece*. See also FAB.

Fc′ a fragment of an immunoglobulin molecule produced by papain digestion. It is a noncovalently bonded dimer of most of the C-terminal half of the two Fc fragments without the terminal 13 amino acids. Called also *Fc′ fragment*.

Fd the amino-terminal portion of the heavy chain of an immunoglobulin molecule which lies to the N-terminal side of the site, being the half of the. heavy chain located in the Fab and representing the region that shares in the antigen-binding site of the immunoglobulin. Called also *Fd fragment* and *Fd piece*.

FDA Food and Drug Administration, a division of the Department of Health and Human Services; see under DEPARTMENT.

FDI Fédération Dentaire Internationale; a voluntary international federation of national dental associations and individual supporting members, founded in 1900 in Paris. Its primary objective is promotion of groups that contribute to the advancement of dentistry throughout the world.

Fe iron (L. *ferrum*).

Fe²⁺ ferrous.

Fe³⁺ ferric.

Fe(II) ferrous.

Fe(III) ferric.

Feb. dur. abbreviation for L. *feb′re duran′te*, while the fever lasts.

febricant (fe′brĭ-kant) causing fever.

febricide (feb′rĭ-sīd) [*febris* + L. *caedere* to kill] 1. lowering bodily temperature in fever. 2. an agent that reduces fever.

febrifacient (feb″rĭ-fa′shent) [*febris* + L. *facere* to make] producing fever.

febrifuge (feb′rĭ-fūj) [*febris* + L. *fuga* a flight] an agent that reduces body temperature in fever; antipyretic.

febrile (feb′ril) [L. *febrilis*] pertaining to or characterized by fever.

febris (fe′bris) [L.] fever. **f. uveoparotide′a subchron′ica,** Heerfordt's SYNDROME.

fecal (fe′kal) pertaining to or of the nature of feces.

feces (fe′sēz) [L. *faeces*, pl. of *faex* refuse] the excrement discharged from the intestine. See also DEFECATION.

Fechner's law [Gustav Theodor *Fechner*, German philosopher, 1801–1887] see under LAW.

Fede, Francesco [Italian physician 1832–1913] see Riga-Fede DISEASE.

Fédération Dentaire Internationale see FDI.

Fed-Mart see under DENTIFRICE.

fee (fe) a charge or payment for performed services. **capitation f.,** see CAPITATION. **customary f's,** see *usual, customary, and reasonable f's*. **fixed f.,** in health insurance, a compensation arrangement in which a participating doctor agrees to accept a prescribed sum as the total fee for one or more covered services. Called also *maximum f., fixed fee schedule,* and *maximum fee schedule*. See also allowable CHARGE. **maximum f.,** fixed f. **prefiled f.,** in dental health delivery and insurance, the submission of a participating dentist's schedule of usual fees to a dental service corporation or prepayment plan for the purposes of establishing a customary range of fees for that geographic area, and the payment of participating dentists on a usual, customary, and reasonable basis. See also *usual, customary, and reasonable f's*. **prevailing f.,** in health insurance, a fee paid by the carrier, based on a profile of usual and customary fees of the area, as determined by the carrier. See also *usual, customary, and reasonable f's*. **reasonable f's,** see *usual, customary, and reasonable f's*. **reduced f. plan,** reduced fee PLAN. **f. schedule,** see ALLOWANCE. **UCR f's,** usual, customary, and reasonable f's. **usual f's,** see *usual, customary, and reasonable f's*. **usual, customary, and reasonable f's,** in health insurance, fees for professional services: *Usual* fees are those usually charged for a given service, by an individual practitioner to his private patients, i.e., his own usual fees; *customary* fees are those in the range of the usual fees charged by practitioners of similar training and experience, for the same services within the specific and limited geographic area (socioeconomic area); *reasonable* fees are those within the usual and customary range or, in the opinion of the responsible professional association's review committee, are justifiable considering the special circumstances of the particular care in question. Abbreviated *UCR*.

feeblemindedness (fe″b′l-mind′ed-nes) former name for mental RETARDATION.

feedback (fēd′bak) the flow of information from a later phase of a process to an earlier phase; the return of some of the output of a system as input so as to exert some control in the process.

feeding (fēd′ing) the taking or giving of food. **artificial f.,** artificial ALIMENTATION. **forced f.,** forced ALIMENTATION. **parenteral f.,** introduction of nutrients into the body other than by the oral route, usually by introducing solutions rich in nutrients, such as glucose, lipids, proteins, vitamins, and other substances, into the venous system or the subclavian artery. Rectal instillation of nutrients was used in the past as a form of parenteral feeding. Called also *parenteral alimentation* and *parenteral nutrition*. See also enteral HYPERALIMENTATION and parenteral HYPERALIMENTATION.

fee-splitting (fe-split′ing) the division of moneys received by a specialist between himself and the practitioner who referred the patient to him.

Fegeler's syndrome [Ferdinand *Fegeler*, German physician] posttraumatic nevus flammeus; see under NEVUS.

FEHBP Federal Employees Health Benefits Program; see under PROGRAM.

Feichtiger, H. see Ullrich-Feichtiger SYNDROME.

Feil, André [French neurologist, born 1884] see Klippel-Feil SYNDROME.

Fe-In-Sol trademark for a ferrous sulfate solution, containing 25 mg iron in each ml; used in the treatment of iron deficiency anemia.

Feldman bur (drill) see under BUR.

feldspar (feld'spar) 1. igneous crystalline rocks, chiefly aluminosilicates with soda, potash, and lime. Most, chiefly potassium feldspar, are used in ceramics, being one of the principal components of porcelain. Also used in glasses, soaps, abrasives, and as bonding material for abrasive wheels. Called also *felspar*. 2. potassium f. **calcium f.**, one of several varieties of feldspar, $CaO \cdot Al_2O_3$. Called also *calcium aluminosilicate*. **potassium f.**, the principal form of feldspar used in ceramics, $K_2O \cdot Al_2O_3 \cdot 6SiO_2$, representing 27 percent of industrial porcelain and 70 to 90 percent of dental porcelain. It is the first component of the porcelain powder to melt during firing, forming a glassy matrix for the quartz and giving dental porcelain its translucency. In some types of dental porcelain, potassium feldspar is substituted with nepheline syenite. Called also *potash f., microline, orthoclase, potash aluminosilicate*, and *potassium aluminosilicate*. **soda f.**, sodium f. **sodium f.**, a compound, $Na_2O \cdot Al_2O_2 \cdot 6SiO_2$; used chiefly as a component of nepheline syenite in dental porcelain. Called also *soda f., albite, pericline, soda aluminosilicate*, and *sodium aluminosilicate*.

Feldstein, E. [French physician] see Klippel-Feldstein SYNDROME.

Fellowship trademark for an *amalgam alloy* (see under AMALGAM).

felspar (fel'spar) feldspar (1).

Felty's syndrome [Augustus Roi *Felty*, American physician, born 1895] see under SYNDROME.

Femadol trademark for *propoxyphene hydrocholoride* (see under PROPOXYPHENE).

Femergin trademark for *ergotamine tartrate* (see under ERGOTAMINE).

femto- [Danish *femten* fifteen] in the metric system, a combining form denoting one-quadrillionth (10^{-15}) of the unit designated by the root with which it is combined. Abbreviated *f*. See also metric SYSTEM.

Fenacilin trademark for *penicillin V*.

Fenadone trademark for the *dl*-form of *methadone hydrochloride* (see under METHADONE).

Fenate trademark for *dextran iron complex* (see under COMPLEX).

Fenazil trademark for *promethazine*.

Fenergan (fen'er-gan) trademark for *promethazine*.

fenestra (fe-nes'trah), pl. *fenes'trae* [L. "window"] 1. any window-like opening. 2. a general anatomical term for an opening or open area. 3. an opening in a bandage or cast, or in the blade of a forceps. 4. an opening found over the roots of teeth covered with thin bone.

fenestrae (fe-nes'tre) [L.] plural of *fenestra*.

fenestrate (fen'es-trāt) to pierce with one or more openings; sometimes applied to the walls of bony defects to stimulate repair.

fenestrated (fen'es-trāt"ed) [L. *fenestratus*] pierced with one or more openings.

fenestration (fen"es-tra'shun) [L. *fenestratus* furnished with windows] 1. the act or process of perforation. 2. the surgical procedure designed for the creation of an opening, such as an opening in the labyrinth of the ear. See also TREPHINATION. 3. an opening not usually present in a normal structure, such as the absence of bone over the apex of a tooth. **alveolar plate f., apical f. apical f.**, perforation of the cortical plate with round or oval openings, involving the cortical plate of bone overlying a portion of a pulpless primary tooth. Secondary ulcerations and proliferation of the vestibular tissues are often associated. The condition occurs in children and may involve all the primary teeth, but the plate overlying the upper primary incisors appears to be affected most commonly. Called also *alveolar plate f*. See also root DEHISCENCE. **cyst f.**, marsupialization. **dental f.**, dental TREPHINATION.

Feneticilline trademark for *phenethicillin*.

fenfluramine hydrochloride (fen-floor'ah-mēn) an amphetamine derivative, N-ethyl-α-methyl-m-(trifluoromethyl)phenethylamine hydrochloride, occurring as a white powder with a characteristic odor, which is sparingly soluble in water and methanol. It is a sympathomimetic drug with a mild sedative action. Used as an anorexic drug. Side effects may include drowsiness, insomnia, nausea, diarrhea, constipation, abdominal discomfort, xerostomia, vertigo, headache, and skin rashes. High doses may cause hypertension, tachycardia, and arrhyth-

mias. Trademarks: Gonal, Obedrex, Ponderax, Pondimin, Rotondin.

Fenibutol trademark for *phenylbutazone*.

Finimal trademark for *acetaminophen*.

Fenistil trademark for *dimethindene maleate* (see under DIMETHINDENE).

fenoterol (fen-o-ter'ol) a bronchodilator, 3,5-dihydroxy-α-[[(p-hydroxy-α-methylphenethyl)amino]methyl]benzyl alcohol.

Fenoxypen trademark for *penicillin V potassium* (see under PENICILLIN).

fentanyl (fen'tah-nil) a potent narcotic analgesic, N-(1-phenethyl-4-piperidyl)propionanilide. Used therapeutically as the citrate salt, which occurs as a white tasteless and odorless crystalline powder or crystals that are soluble in water, alcohol, and chloroform. It has a rapid onset but short duration, and is used in preanesthetic and postoperative medication in general or regional anesthesia. Respiratory depression, apnea, muscular rigidity, hypotension, nausea, vomiting, laryngospasm, and bronchospam are the most common adverse reactions. Abuse may lead to habituation and addiction.

Fentazin trademark for *perphenazine*.

Fergon trademark for a ferrous gluconate preparation.

Fergusson's incision (operation) [Sir William *Fergusson*, British surgeon, 1808–1877] see under INCISION.

Ferlucon trademark for a ferrous gluconate preparation.

fermentation (fer"men-ta'shun) [L. *fermentatio*] 1. enzymatic decomposition, especially of carbohydrates as used in the production of alcohol, bread, vinegar, and other products. 2. the anaerobic conversion of foodstuffs to a particular product, as in lactic fermentation. In contrast to respiration, it is a energy-yielding metabolic process that does not involve net oxidation or electron transport to oxygen or other electron acceptors. 3. glycolysis.

Fermi, Enrico [1901–1954] an Italian physicist; winner of the Nobel prize for physics in 1938.

fermium (fer'me-um) [named after Enrico *Fermi*] a transuranic element originally discovered in the debris of a thermonuclear explosion, which may be produced by irradiation or bombardment of plutonium, californium, einsteinium, and uranium. Symbol, Fm; atomic number, 100; atomic weight, 257. It occurs in the form of several isotopes, 244 to 258; ^{255}Fm has a half-life of 20.1 hrs and emits alpha particles, and ^{257}Fm has a half-life of 80 days and also emits alpha particles. Used in tracer studies.

ferrated (fer-āt'ed) charged with iron.

ferredoxin (fer"e-dok'sin) an iron-containing protein, also having a high sulfide content, which serves as an acceptor molecule in electron transport from chlorophyll during the formation of NADPH in photosynthesis.

Ferrein's cord, foramen, ligament [Antoine *Ferrein*, French physician, 1693–1769] see HIATUS of canal for greater petrosal nerve, and vocal cord, true, under CORD.

ferric (fer'ik) [L. *ferrum*] Containing iron in its plus-three oxidation state, Fe(III) (sometimes designated Fe^{3+}).

Ferrier 212 gingival clamp, separator [W. I. *Ferrier*] see under CLAMP and SEPARATOR.

ferrite (fer'īt) 1. an unstable compound of ferric oxide with a strong base, as in $NaFeO_2$. 2. a solid solution of carbon (and possibly other elements) in α-iron, the maximum solubility of carbon in α-iron being 0.02 percent. Δ**-f.**, Δ-IRON. **proeutectoid f.**, free ferrite formed during the cooling of iron alloys containing less than 0.8 percent carbon (hypoeutectoid steel), between the critical and eutectoid temperatures.

ferritin (fer'ī-tin) the primary iron storage protein in the body, which is composed of apoferritin held to ferric hydroxide clusters to the extent that 20 to 23 percent of crystallized ferritin is iron. It is found in the gastrointestinal mucosa, liver, spleen, bone marrow, and reticuloendothelial system. Ferritin may be also involved in the vasoconstrictor action of epinephrine and may play a role in hypotension, antidiuresis, and irreversible shock.

Ferronat trademark for a preparation of *ferrous fumarate* (see under FUMARATE).

Ferrone trademark for a preparation of *ferrous fumarate* (see under FUMARATE).

Ferronicum trademark for a preparation of *ferrous gluconate* (see under GLUCONATE).

ferroprotoporphyrin (fer"o-pro"to-por'fī-rin) a chelate complex of protoporphyrin with iron. A complex with Fe in the ferrous state is called *heme;* a complex with Fe in the ferric state is called *hematin*.

ferrous (fer'us) containing iron in its plus-two oxidation state, Fe(II) (sometimes designated Fe^{2+}). **f. fumarate**, ferrous FUMARATE.

-ferrous [L. *ferre* to bear] a word termination meaning bearing or producing.

ferrum (fer'um) [L.] iron.

fertilization (fer'tĭ-li-za'shun) the act of rendering gametes fertile or capable of further development, consisting of the spermatozoon penetrating the ovum to form the male pronucleus, thus initiating the process that completes the second meiotic division and production of the female pronucleus. The two pronuclei, having lost their membranes, combine to form the total of 46 chromosomes which replicate through mitotic processes to form two 46-chromosome daughter cells, followed by the long series of divisions of the new zygote, eventually leading to the development of the mature individual. See also OOGENESIS and SPERMATOGENESIS.

Ferv. abbreviation for L. *fer'vens*, boiling.

fervescence (fer-ves'ens) [L. *fervescere* to become hot] increase of body temperature; fever.

fester (fes'ter) to suppurate superficially.

Feston trademark for *dimenhydrinate*.

festoon (fes-tōōn') a carving in the base material of a denture that simulates the contours of the natural tissue being replaced by the denture. **gingival f.**, contour of the gingiva and oral mucosa over the roots of teeth with a thin alveolar process. **McCall's f.**, a rimlike enlargement of the gingival margin occurring on the vestibular surface, most commonly in the canine and premolar areas.

festooning (fes-tōōn'ing) the process of carving the base material of a denture or denture pattern to simulate the contours of the natural tissue to be replaced by the denture.

festschrift (fest'shrift) [Ger.] a memorial volume; a book made up of articles contributed by pupils or associates and friends of a scientist or leader, published usually to honor some special occasion, such as a birthday or other anniversary.

fetal (fe'tal) pertaining to a fetus.

feticide (fe'tĭ-sīd) [*fetus* + L. *caedere* to kill] the destruction or killing of the fetus.

fetid (fe'tid) [L. *foetidus*] having an unpleasant smell.

fetoglobulin (fe"to-glob'u-lin) fetoprotein. **α-f.**, α₁-FETOPROTEIN.

fetoprotein (fe"to-pro'te-in, fe"to-pro'tēn) a globulin with antigenic properties found in newborn infants and in older persons in the presence of certain diseases, especially neoplasms. Called also *fetoglobulin*. **α₁-f.**, a fetoprotein synthesized by fetal hepatocytes and found in the blood serum up to 2 weeks after birth. It is a protein with chemical properties similar to that of serum albumin, molecular weight of about 70,000, and sedimentation quotient of 4.5 to 5.0 S. Its presence in older patients may indicate liver carcinoma, malignant teratomas, and embryonal carcinoma of the gonads. Called also *αf.*, *α-fetoglobulin*, *α₁-fetospecific serum protein*, *α₁-globulin*, and *postalbumin*. **α-f.**, α₁-f. **β-f.**, a fetoprotein found in the fetal liver and in a variety of liver diseases. Chemically, it is similar to the protein portion of normal liver ferritin.

fetor (fe'tor) [L.] stench, or offensive odor. **f. ex o're; f. o'ris**, halitosis. **f. hepat'icus**, the characteristic odor of the breath in liver diseases. Called also *liver breath*.

fetus (fe'tus) [L.] the unborn offspring of any viviparous animal, specifically, the unborn offspring in the postembryonic period, after major structures have been outlined; in man 9 weeks after fertilization until birth.

Feulgen banding, bands, method, stain [Robert *Feulgen*, German chemist, 1884–1955] see F-BANDING and F bands, under BAND, and see under STAIN.

fever (fe'ver) [L. *febris*] 1. an abnormally high body temperature, above 98.6°F or 37.0°C, being a manifestation of infectious diseases, burns, trauma, lesions of the brain that affect the hypothalamus, as well as of the presence in the body of pyrogens and some drugs, such as thyroxine. Fever is considered by some as a protective mechanism of the body that destroys certain pathogenic microorganisms and enhances the metabolic rate, thus allowing the cells to increase their production of immune substances. Called also *fire*, *hyperthermia*, and *pyrexia*. See also CALOR and PYROGEN. See *Body Temperature Chart* at TEMPERATURE. 2. any disease characterized by abnormally elevated body temperature. **aphthous f.**, foot-and-mouth DISEASE. **black f.**, visceral LEISHMANIASIS. **f. blisters**, see HERPES simplex. **Choix f.**, Rocky Mountain spotted f. **Colorado tick f.**, a tickborne disease caused by a reovirus of the genus *Orbivirus*, and characterized by headache, fever, chills, and back and leg pain. It occurs in the Rocky Mountain regions where the tick vector is prevalent. **continuous f.**, persistently elevated body temperature, showing little or no variation and never falling to normal during any 24-hour period. **deer fly f.**, tularemia. **dehydration f.**, fever resulting from a loss of body water or inadequate intake of fluids, sometimes occurring as a

postoperative complication. **drug f.**, elevated body temperature seen during the course of administration of drugs, usually antibiotics, which may be associated with multiple small vessel inflammation. See also drug REACTION. **five-day f.**, trench f. **glandular f.**, infectious MONONUCLEOSIS. **Haverhill f.**, the bacillary form of rat-bite fever, caused by *Streptobacillus moniliformis*, and transmitted by contaminated raw milk and its products. It was first reported in Haverhill, Massachusetts. See also *rat-bite f.* **hay f.**, an allergic condition brought about by exposure to certain plant pollens, characterized by rhinitis, watering eyes, sneezing, coughing, itching of the affected parts, and congestion and edema of mucous membranes. Called also *allergic cold, allergic coryza, allergic rhinitis*, and *June cold*. See also nonseasonal allergic RHINITIS and vasomotor RHINITIS (1). **herpetic f.**, primary infection with herpes simplex virus, with diffuse involvement of the mucous membranes of the mouth and lips and the surrounding skin; sometimes associated with chills. **Kew Gardens spotted f.**, rickettsialpox. **Meuse f.**, trench f. **Oroya f.**, see BARTONELLOSIS. **pinta f.**, Rocky Mountain spotted f. **quintan f.**, trench f. **Pontiac f.**, a self-limited disease first noted in an outbreak in 1968 in a single building in Pontiac, Michigan, marked by fever, cough, muscle aches, chills, headache, chest pain, confusion, and pleuritis; it is now known to be caused by a strain of *Legionella pneumophilia*. **Q f., query f.**, a severe but seldom fatal, febrile rickettsial infection caused by *Coxiella burnetii*, characterized by influenza-like symptoms and pneumonia, and occasionally associated with subacute endocarditis. It is usually airborne, but may occur as a result of drinking contaminated and inadequately pasteurized milk, or may be transmitted by tick bites. Originally reported in Australia, the disease is now believed to occur worldwide. Called also *hibernovernal bronchopneumonia*. **rabbit f.**, tularemia. **rat-bite f.**, either of two clinically similar but etiologically distinct acute infectious diseases, usually transmitted through the bite of a rat, and occurring in a bacillary form caused by *Streptobacillus moniliformis*, and in a spirillary form caused by *Spirillum minor*. In the bacillary form, usually after a latent period of less than 10 days, the initial wound heals promptly without inflammation, but after a week or 10 days the bite site becomes inflamed, painful, and indurated, followed by adenitis, chills, vomiting, headache, high fever, morbilliform eruption, especially on the hands and feet, and polyarthritis that is often severe. This form also may be associated with ingestion of contaminated raw milk or its products (*Haverhill fever*), in which case there is no initial wound, the first symptoms being systemic. In the spirillary form, the latent period is most commonly greater than 10 days, inflammation recurs at the primary wound site, the rash is less evident than in the bacillary form, arthritis is rare, and the fever is commonly of the relapsing type. **remittent f.**, a fever in which the diurnal variation is 2°F or more, but in which the temperature never falls to a normal level. **rheumatic f.**, a systemic inflammatory disease, considered to be one of the collagen diseases, characterized by acute attacks of fever spaced by remissions lasting from months to years, even to decades. The onset may follow scarlet fever, streptococcal sore throat, and tonsillitis, infection with the group A hemolytic streptococci being considered as the principal etiologic factor. Serious complications include cardiac lesions characterized by Aschoff bodies, a collection of cells and leukocytes in the interstitial tissue, fibrosis, inflammatory reaction, thickening of the mural endocardium and valvulitis often associated with fibrous scarring and stenosis. Subcutaneous nodules (large areas of fibrinoid necrosis), fibrosis and scarring of the synovia, joint capsules, tendons, fasciae, and muscle sheaths, acute inflammatory exudative changes in the blood vessels, and pneumonia may be associated. Called also *acute articular rheumatism, polyarthritis rheumatica acuta*, and *rheumatic arthritis*. **Rocky Mountain spotted f.**, an infection due to *Rickettsia rickettsii*, transmitted by the bite of various ticks, and occurring in most of the United States. A reservoir of rickettsiae is maintained in rabbits and other small rodents. A few days after the tick bite, the disease begins with fever, muscle pain, and weakness, with headache followed in 2 to 4 days by a macular petechial eruption that starts on the hands and feet and spreads centripetally to the trunk and face. The sensorium is clouded. Mortality is generally high, being greater in adults than in children. Called also *Choix f., pinta f.*, and *tickborne typhus*, and also known by various names according to geographic area. **San Joaquin f.**, coccidioidomycosis. **scarlet f.**, an acute contagious and exanthematous disease of young children, caused by group A hemolytic streptococci, and usually transmitted by direct contact with an infected person and sometimes indirectly, as by contaminated milk. After an incubation period of about 2 to 7 days there is eruption of bright red, punctate lesions on the neck and, to a lesser degree, on the face, spreading downward to the chest and other areas; after about a week, there is severe desquamation, especially of the hands and feet. Sore throat, fever, nausea, vomiting, and headache are the earliest symptoms. Leukocytosis is usually present, and otitis, adenitis, arthritis, nephritis, and cardiac involvement may be associated. The chief oral manifestation is stomatitis scarlatina, usually presenting punctate scarlet enanthem, tonsillar exudate, strawberry tongue in the early stages, and raspberry tongue later. Called also *scarlatina*. **shin bone f. trench f. trench f.**, a relapsing fever occurring with as many as 10 to 12 febrile paroxysms, each lasting 20 to 40 hours, with chills, fever, sweating, various rashes, and splenomegaly. It is caused by *Rochalimaea quintana*, transmitted by the human louse. More than one million cases of trench fever occurred during World War I and somewhat fewer cases occurred during World War II, mostly on the Russian front. Called also *five-day f., Meuse f., quintan f., shin bone f.,* and *Wolhynian f.* **typhoid f.**, a contagious disease caused by *Salmonella typhi* infection, transmitted by contaminated water and foods. Fever, diarrhea, and characteristic red spots on the abdomen and chest are the principal symptoms. A dry, brown tongue (baked tongue) is the main oral manifestation. Osteomyelitis is sometimes a complication (see typhoid OSTEOMYELITIS). **undulant f.**, brucellosis. **uveoparotid f.**, Heerfordt's SYNDROME. **valley f.**, coccidioidomycosis. **Wolhynian f.**, trench f.

Fèvre-Languepin syndrome [Marcel *Fèvre;* Anne *Languepin*] see under SYNDROME.

Feyrter, F. see Pospischill-Feyrter APHTHOID.

FF designation for the degree of fineness of abrasive particles used in dentistry; see ABRASIVE (2).

FFF designation for the degree of fineness of abrasive particles used in dentistry; see ABRASIVE (2).

FH Frankfort Horizontal PLANE.

F.H. family HISTORY.

fiber (fi'ber) an elongated, threadlike structure. Called also *fibra.* Written also *fibre.* **A f's**, myelinated fibers of the somatic nervous system, including alpha, beta, and gamma fibers. **accelerating f's, accelerator f's**, adrenergic fibers transmitting the impulses that accelerate the heart beat. Called also *augmentor f's* and *cardiac accelerator f's.* **adrenergic f's**, postganglionic sympathetic nerve fibers that liberate norepinephrine when nerve impulses cross the synapse. Such fibers innervating the sweat glands are cholinergic. **alpha f's**, large, myelinated, fast motor or proprioceptive fibers of the A type. **alveolar f's**, fibers of the periodontal ligament extending from the cementum of the root of a tooth to the walls of the alveolus, distinguished as alveolar crest, horizontal, oblique, and apical fibers. See also *principal f's.* **alveolar crest f's**, fibers of the periodontal ligament extending obliquely from the cementum just beneath the epithelial attachment to the alveolar crest; they counterbalance the coronal thrust of the more apical fibers, thus helping to anchor the tooth to the alveolus and oppose lateral stresses. See also *principal f's.* **anastomosing f's, anastomotic f's**, nerve fibers extending from one muscle bundle or nerve trunk to another. **aperiodic f's**, aperiodic fibrils; see under FIBRIL. **apical f's**, fibers of the periodontal ligament extending from the cementum to the fundus of the alveolus; they prevent vestibulo-oral tipping of the tooth. See also *principal f's.* **argentaffin f's, argentophilic f's, argyrophilic f's**, reticular f's. **augmentor f's**, accelerating f's. **axial f.**, the axon of a nerve fiber. **B f's**, myelinated preganglionic autonomic axons. **beta f's**, touch fibers of the A type. **bone f's**, Sharpey's f's (1). **C f's**, unmyelinated postganglionic fibers of the autonomic nervous system, also the unmyelinated fibers found at the dorsal roots. They transmit slow (protopathic) pain impulses. **cardiac accelerator f's**, accelerating f's. **cardiac depressor f's**, vagal fibers to the heart which when stimulated cause a slowing in cardiac beat. Called also *depressor f's.* **cardiac pressor f's**, sympathetic nerve fibers to the heart which when activated cause an increase in cardiac beat. Called also *pressor f's.* **cemental f's**, the fibers of the periodontal ligament extending from the cementum to the zone of the intermediate plexus, where their terminations are interspersed with the terminations of the alveolar group of the periodontal fibers. **cholinergic f's**, nerve fibers that liberate acetylcholine at the synapse. They comprise the postganglionic parasympathetic fibers and the postganglionic sympathetic fibers to the sweat glands. **collagen**

f., collagenous f., a soft, flexible fiber about 1 to 12 μ in thickness and of indefinite length, forming a bundle of smaller collagen fibrils and often being cemented to other fibers to form larger bundles, which offer great resistance to pulling force and are present in all types of connective tissue. They are the principal components of the periodontal ligament (see *principal f's*). They stain red with hematoxylin and eosin. In fresh tissue they are almost colorless and are referred to as *white fibers.* **definite f's**, principal f's. **dentinal f.**, PROCESS of odontoblast. **dentinogenic f's**, Korff's f's. **depressor f's**, 1. nerve fibers which when stimulated at their central end cause a slow heart rate and diminished vasomotor tone, thereby decreasing arterial pressure. 2. cardiac depressor f's. **elastic f.**, one of the thin yellowish fibers, often branched and of elastic quality, which traverse the intercellular substance of connective tissue. When found in the periodontal ligament, they are usually associated with the afferent blood vessels. Called also *yellow f.* **f. A**, Orlon. **gamma f's**, efferent fibers of the A type that innervate the infrafusal fibers of the muscle spindle. **gingival f's**, the collagen fibers which make up the gingival corium, being attached on one end to the cementum and the alveolar periosteum of the gingiva on the other. They support the vestibular and oral gingivae, brace the marginal gingiva against the tooth, provide the rigidity necessary to withstand the forces of mastication without being deflected away from the tooth surface, and unite the free marginal gingiva with the cementum of the root and the adjacent gingiva. They comprise the gingivodental, circular, and transseptal fibers. **gingival f's, circular**, fibers which pass through the connective tissue of the marginal and interdental gingivae and encircle the tooth in a ringlike fashion. **gingival f's, transseptal**, interproximal gingival fibers which form horizontal bundles extending between the cementum of approximating teeth into which they are embedded. They lie in the area between the epithelium at the base of the gingival crevice and the crest of the interdental bone, and are sometimes classified with the principal fibers of the periodontal ligament. **gingivodental f's**, the gingival fibers of the vestibular, oral, and interproximal surfaces, being embedded in the cementum just beneath the epithelium at the base of the gingival crevice. On the vestibular and oral surfaces, they fan out toward the crest and outer surface of the marginal gingiva and terminate short of the epithelium. They also extend external to the periosteum of the vestibular and oral cortical plates of bone and terminate in the attached gingiva or blend with the periosteum. Interproximally, they extend toward the crest of the interdental gingiva. **gray f's**, unmyelinated nerve fibers, found largely, but not exclusively, in the sympathetic nerves. Called also *f's of Remak.* **Henle's f's**, the fibers of the fenestrated membrane which exist in certain arteries between the external and middle coats. **horizontal f's**, fibers of the periodontal ligament coursing longitudinally from the cementum to the occlusal third of the alveolus; they resist tooth displacement by lateral pressure. See also *principal f's.* **intermediate f's**, fibers located between the alveolar and cemental fibers of the periodontal ligament, which are especially well defined during tooth eruption. **interradicular f's**, fibers of the periodontal ligament extending from the cementum to the crest of the interradicular septum, which assist the tooth in resisting tipping and torque. **intrafusal f's**, modified narrow muscle fibers with abundant sarcoplasm and central nuclei. Each fiber is enclosed in a connective tissue capsule, and each contains sensory nerves ending in annulospiral or flower-spray endings and are supplied by efferent gamma fibers. Two to 10 of these fibers compose the muscle spindle. **Korff's f's**, collagen fibrils extending from fibroblasts (preodontoblasts), which project their processes toward the inner enamel epithelium (preameloblasts). From there, they reach the area of aperiodic fibrils and basal lamina, where they form bundles and make up the matrix for dentin, particularly the mantle dentin. The matrix area becomes occupied by ground substance to form predentin, followed by calcification to produce dentin. They are reticular argyrophilic fibers, about 0.1 to 0.2 μ in diameter, arranged in fan-shaped bundles perpendicularly to the prospective dentinoenamel junction. Small fibrils (beta fibrils) fill the space between individual bundles (Korff's bundles). Called also *dentinogenic f's, von Korff's f's, Korff's fibrils,* and *von Korff's fibrils.* **lattice f's**, reticular f's. **medullated nerve f.**, myelinated f. **motor f.**, a fiber in a mixed nerve which transmits impulses to a muscle fiber. **muscle f.**, a fiber of the skeletal muscle, about 10 to 100 μ in diameter, which may extend through the entire length of the muscle; it makes up the contractile mechanism of the muscle. Most fibers are innervated by a neuromuscular junction in the middle, and consist of several thousand myofibrils. **myelinated f., myelinated nerve f.**, a nerve fiber whose axon is encased in a myelin sheath, which in turn may be enclosed by a neurilemma. Called also *medullated f.* and *medullated nerve f.* Cf. *unmyelinated f.* **nerve f.,** a slender process of a neuron, especially the prolonged axon which conducts nerve impulses, varying in length from less than an inch to several feet. Most are covered by a myelin sheath, except at their origin from the cell body and near their terminations, and are classified on the basis of the presence or absence of the sheath as myelinated or unmyelinated. Those covered by a myelin sheath form the white substance of the central nervous system; both myelinated and unmyelinated fibers of the peripheral nerves are protected by neurilemma. See also *A f's, B f's,* and *C f's.* See illustration at NERVE. **nonmedullated f., nonmedullated nerve f.,** unmyelinated f. **oblique f's,** the largest fibers of the periodontal ligament extending from the cementum in a coronal direction obliquely to the apical two-thirds of the alveolus; they suspend and anchor the tooth in its socket and resist surface tooth pressures. See also *principal f's.* **odontogenic f's,** fibers of connective tissue (periodontium and pulp) contributing to the matrix of dentin and cementum. **osteocollagenous f's,** fibers gathered together into bundles, united by a special binding substance in the interstitial substance of bone. **osteogenic f's,** precollagenous fibers becoming the fibrous components of bone matrix. **oxytalan f.,** a connective tissue fiber, resistant to acid hydrolysis, found in structures subjected to mechanical stress, such as tendons, ligaments, adventitia, and connective tissue sheaths that surround the skin appendages. In the periodontal ligament, they are inserted, along with the collagen bundles, into either the cementum or the bone. **perforating f's,** Sharpey's f's. **postganglionic f's,** axons arising from postganglionic neurons when the cell bodies are in autonomic ganglia. **precollagenous f's,** see *reticular f's.* **preganglionic f's,** fibers constituting a preganglionic neuron. **pressor f's,** 1. nerve fibers which, when stimulated, cause or increase vasomotor tone. 2. čardiac pressor f's. **principal f's,** collagen fibers of the periodontal ligament, which follow a wavy course and are organized in bundles along the length of the root of a tooth, and function to suspend and anchor the tooth to the alveolus. They consist of the transseptal, alveolar crest, horizontal, oblique, and apical fibers. Terminal portions of the principal fibers that insert into the cementum and bone are known as *Sharpey's fibers.* Called also *definite f's* and *tooth attachment f's.* **f's of Remak,** gray f's. **reticular f's, reticulum f's,** delicate, immature connective tissue fibers, 0.2 to 1.0 μ in diameter, each representing a bundle of reticular fibrils, which form a network of lymphoid and myeloid tissue; they occur also in the interstitial tissue of glandular organs, papillary layer of the skin, and elsewhere. When found in the periodontal ligament, they are usually associated with the perithelium of vascular channels. They stain readily with silver (hence the synonym *argyrophilic fibers*) and weakly with hematoxylin and eosin. Considered by some to be forerunners of collagen fibers (hence the synonym *precollagenous fibers*), the principal difference between the two types being in the carbohydrate content; reticular fibers are carbohydrate rich and collagen fibers are carbohydrate poor. Called also *argentaffin f's, argentophilic f's, lattice f's,* and *Gitterfasern.* **Sappey's f's,** smooth muscle fibers in the check ligaments of the eye near their orbital attachments. **Sharpey's f's,** 1. bone fibers; collagenous fibers that pass from the periosteum into the outer circumferential and interstitial lamellae of bone. 2. terminal portions of principal fibers that insert into the cementum of a tooth (see also *principal f's*). Called also *perforating f's.* **spindle f's,** minute, straight, contractile, tubular organelles, often of different lengths, forming achromatic filaments extending between the poles of a dividing cell and, as a whole, making a spindle-shaped configuration. Their functions have not been precisely defined, but it has been suggested that they form an internal framework that helps cells keep their shape and assists the cells in changing shape and moving. **T f.,** a nerve fiber that branches at right angles from the axon of a nerve cell. **tooth attachment f's,** principal f's. **transseptal f's,** fibers of the periodontal ligament extending interproximally over the alveolar crest and embedding in the cementum of adjacent teeth; they support the interproximal gingiva and secure the adjacent tooth. See also *principal f's.* **ultraterminal f.,** a thin unmyelinated twig given off from the ramifications of the axons in the motor plate. **unmyelinated f., unmyelinated nerve f.,** a nerve fiber whose axon lacks a myelin sheath, but may be enclosed by a neurilemma. Called also *nonmedullated f.* and *nonmedullated nerve f.* Cf. *myelinated f.* **von Korff's f's,** Korff's f's. **white f.,** a collagen fiber in fresh tissue, so-called because of its almost colorless appearance. **yellow f.,** elastic f.

Fibiger, Johannes Andreas Grib [Danish pathologist, 1867–1928] winner of the Nobel prize for physiology and medicine in 1926.

fibra (fi′brah), pl. *fi′brae* [L.] a general term designating an elongated, threadlike structure. Called also *fiber.*

fibrae (fi′bre) [L.] plural of *fibra.*

fibre (fi′ber) fiber.

fibril (fi′bril) [L. *fibrilla*] a minute fiber or filament; often a component of a compound fiber. **anchoring f's,** minute fibrils which pass from the basement membrane through the basal lamina to the hemidesmosomes, and anchor the basement membrane to the epithelial cells. **aperiodic f's,** fine fibrils of connective tissue lacking markings, located between the connective tissue of the dental papilla and the inner enamel epithelium of the tooth germ. **argyrophilic f's,** reticulum f's. **axial f.,** in spirochetal bacteria, a long, slender, threadlike process which intertwines with the protoplasmic cylinder, being probably responsible for cell motility. Called also *axial filament.* **beta f's,** small fibrils of periodicities less than collagen, which occupy the space between Korff's fiber bundles. **collagen f's,** delicate fibrils, each about 0.3 to 0.5 μ in diameter, usually cemented together in wavy bundles to form larger collagen fibers; found in connective tissue. **dentinal f's,** component fibrils of the dentinal matrix. **Ebner's f.,** a term used in the past for a threadlike fibril in the dentin and in the cementum of a tooth. **Korff's f's,** Korff's fibers; see under FIBER. **precollagenous f's,** reticulum f's. **reticulum f's,** minute fibrils, bundles of which form the reticular fibers. Called also *argyrophilic f's* and *precollagenous f's.* **von Korff's f's,** Korff's fibers; see under FIBER.

fibrilla (fi-bril′ah), pl. *fibri′llae* [L.] fibril.

fibrillae (fi-bril′e) [L.] plural of *fibrilla.*

fibrillar, fibrillary (fi′bri-lar, fi′bri-lar″e) pertaining to a fibril or to fibrils.

fibrillated (fi′bri-lāt″ed) made up of fibrils.

fibrillation (fi″bri-la′shun) 1. a small, local, involuntary contraction of muscle, invisible under the skin, resulting from spontaneous activation of single muscle cells or muscle fibers. 2. the initial degenerative changes in osteoarthritis, characterized by softening of the articular cartilage and development of vertical clefts between groups of cartilage cells. **atrial f., auricular f.,** a cardiac arrhythmia characterized by rapid, continuous, uncoordinated, vermicular contraction of the atrial myocardium, which is dynamically functionless. It is the most common of all major arrhythmias and may occur as a complication of myocardial infarction. It may also occur in the absence of organic heart diseases during high fever or severe infection or following pulmonary embolism and after some types of surgery. The atria do not contract as a whole, small areas of the muscle tissue being stimulated at different times, hence the absence of the P waves in the electrocardiogram. The QRS and T complexes may be normal but are unevenly spaced owing to irregularity of the ventricular rate. **ventricular f.,** a cardiac arrhythmia characterized by fibrillary contractions of the ventricular muscle due to rapid repetitive excitation of the myocardial fibers without coordinated contraction of the ventricle. It may occur in coronary diseases as the terminal event, or, in relatively healthy persons, after minor myocardial infarction, after electric shock, or during general anesthesia in which certain drugs, such as cyclopropane or halothane, have been used, and particularly, with the use of epinephrine. If uncorrected immediately, ventricular fibrillation usually ends in cardiac arrest and death.

fibrilloblast (fi-bril″o-blast) [*fibril* + Gr. *blastos* germ] odontoblast.

fibrillogenesis (fi-bril″o-jen′ĕ-sis) [*fibril* + Gr. *genesis* formation] the formation of fibrillae. In dentinogenesis, the elaboration of beta fibrils leading to the formation of predentin.

fibrin (fi′brin) a whitish, insoluble protein component of the blood plasma, forming the principal substance of the blood clot, after being converted from fibrinogen through the action of thrombin. See also blood COAGULATION.

fibrinase (fi′brin-ās) plasmin.

fibrinogen (fi-brin′o-jen) [*fibrin* + Gr. *gennan* to produce] a blood protein which, during the process of coagulation, is converted to fibrin through the action of thrombin. It is a high-molecular-weight protein (340,000) occurring in the plasma in quantities of 100 to 700 mg/100 ml, most of it being formed in the liver; liver disease occasionally decreases the concentration of circulating fibrinogen. Its half-life is about 109 hours. Fibrinogen contains negatively charged peptides repelling molecules from each other so that clotting cannot take place spontaneously without fibrinogen being converted to fibrin. Fibrinogen deficiency results in afibrinogenemia or hypofibrinogenemia. Called also *factor I.* See also BLOOD coagulation.

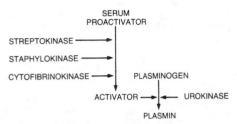

Fibrinolytic system of blood. Not shown are the inhibitors, one of which (antifibrinolysis) inhibits plasmin, whereas others (antistreptokinase, etc.) inhibit bacterial activators. Chloroform extraction of plasma destroys or removes antifibrinolysin. (From J. B. Miale: Laboratory Medicine. Hematology. 5th ed., St. Louis, The C. V. Mosby Co., 1977.)

fibrinogenase (fi″brin-oj′ĕ-nās) thrombin (1).

fibrinogenopenia (fi-brin″o-jen″o-pe′ne-ah) [*fibrin* + Gr. *gennan* to produce + *penia* poverty] afibrinogenemia.

fibrinolysin (fi″bri-nol′ĭ-sin) plasmin. **streptococcal f.,** streptokinase.

fibrinolysis (fi″bri-no-li′sis) [*fibrin* + Gr. *lysis* dissolution] dissolution of the blood clot occurring as a mechanism controlling intravascular clotting and preventing whole-body thrombosis in tissue repair processes. See illustration. See also blood COAGULATION.

fibro- [L. *fibra* fiber] a combining form denoting relationship to fibers.

fibroadamantoblastoma (fi″bro-ad″ah-man″to-blas-to′mah) ameloblastic FIBROMA.

fibroangioma (fi″bro-an″je-o′mah) [*fibro-* + *angioma*] an angioma containing much fibrous tissue; angiofibroma. **nasopharyngeal a.,** nasopharyngeal ANGIOFIBROMA.

fibroblast (fi′bro-blast) [*fibro-* + Gr. *blastos* germ] a connective tissue cell; a flat elongated cell with cytoplasmic processes at each end, having an oval, vesicular nucleus. They form and maintain the fibrous components of the body, such as tendons, aponeuroses, and supporting and binding tissues of all sorts. Called also *fibrocyte* and *desmocyte.*

fibroblastoma (fi″bro-blas-to′mah) a tumor arising from a fibroblast; such tumors are now differentiated as fibromas or fibrosarcomas. **perineural f.,** neurilemmoma.

fibrocartilage (fi″bro-kar′tĭ-lij) [*fibro-* + *cartilage*] a type of cartilage made up of typical cartilage cells (chondrocytes), with parallel thick, compact collagenous bundles forming the interstitial substances, separated by narrow clefts enclosing the encapsulated cells. Fibrocartilage unites the opposed bones in joints with slight movement, where strength of the union is required. Called also *fibrocartilago* and *stratified cartilage.* **basal f.,** the cartilage that fills the foramen lacerum of the skull. Called also *fibrocartilago basalis.* **basilar f.,** spheno-occipital SYNCHONDROSIS (1). **circumferential f.,** white fibrocartilage that forms a rim around some articular cavities and provides protection of bony edges. **connecting f.,** a disk of fibrocartilage that attaches opposing bones to each other by synchondrosis. Called also *spongy f.* **interarticular f.,** white fibrocartilage, forming flattened disks or oval, round, triangular, or sickle-like shapes, which are located between the surfaces of articular cartilage in certain joints which are exposed to frequent movements and jolts. They serve to fill in the space between the surfaces and to increase the variety of movements of a joint. Disks made of interarticular fibrocartilage are found in the temporomandibular, clavicular, wrist, knee, and sternoclavicular joints. See also interarticular DISK. **interarticular f. of temporomandibular joint,** articular disk of temporomandibular joint; see under DISK. **spongy f.,** connecting f. **stratiform f.,** white fibrocartilage that lines some bony grooves through which tendons glide, and is also found in some tendons and muscles where they glide over bones. It provides strength and support to the organs of which it is a part. **white f.,** a flexible and tough cartilage consisting of a mixture of white fibrous tissue and cartilaginous tissues, which is made up of fibrous connective tissue arranged in bundles, the cells being situated between the bundles. Four types of white fibrocartilage are recognized: interarticular, connecting, circumferential, and stratiform.

fibrocartilagines (fi″bro-kar″tĭ-laj′ĭ-nēz) [L.] plural of *fibrocartilago.*

fibrocartilago (fi″bro-kar″tĭ-lah′go), pl. *fibrocartilag′ines* [L.] fi-

brocartilage. **f. basa′lis,** basal FIBROCARTILAGE. **f. basila′ris,** spheno-occipital SYNCHONDROSIS (1).

fibrocyte (fi′bro-sīt) [*fibro-* + Gr. *kytos* hollow vessel] fibroblast.

fibrogranuloma (fi″bro-gran″u-lo′mah) a tumor having the properties of fibroma and granuloma. **sublingual f.,** Riga-Fede DISEASE.

fibrohemangioma (fi″bro-he-man″je-o′mah) a tumor combining the characteristics of a fibroma and hemangioma. **gingival f.,** pregnancy GINGIVITIS.

fibroid (fi′broid) [*fibro-* + Gr. *eidos* form] 1. having a fibrous structure. 2. fibroma. **ossifying f.,** peripheral ossifying FIBROMA.

fibroma (fi-bro′mah) [*fibro-* + *-oma*] a benign, usually small encapsulated connective tissue tumor, composed mainly of regular, well-formed fibrocytes and fibroblasts, which may occur at any age and in any site of the body. It is the most common benign tumor of the oral cavity, affecting most frequently the gingivae, buccal mucosa, tongue, lips, and palate. The tumor occurs as an elevated smooth, slow-growing lesion of normal color with a sessile or pedunculated base, which sometimes becomes irritated and inflamed and may show superficial ulceration. See also FIBROMATOSIS gingivae. **ameloblastic f.,** a relatively rare, slow-growing mixed odontogenic tumor, occurring most commonly in children and young adults, composed of embryonal fibrous connective tissue and primitive odontogenic epithelium. It is usually located in the molar region of the mandible, and is characterized by the proliferation of both epithelial and mesenchymal tissues without the formation of enamel or dentin. Called also *fibroadamantoblastoma, soft mixed odontogenic tumor,* and *soft mixed odontoma.* See also ameloblastic SARCOMA. **ameloblastic f., malignant,** ameloblastic SARCOMA. **f. caverno′sum,** a cavernous hemangioma containing an excess of fibrous tissue. **cystic f.,** one which has undergone cystic degeneration. **diffuse f. of gingiva,** FIBROMATOSIS gingivae. **f. du′rum,** hard f. **hard f.,** one characterized by the presence of hard, unyielding nodules. Called also *f. durum.* **juvenile nasopharyngeal f.,** nasopharyngeal ANGIOFIBROMA. **malignant f.,** odontogenic FIBROSARCOMA. **f. mol′le,** soft f. **f. mollus′cum,** Recklinghausen's DISEASE (1). **nonosteogenic f.,** a degenerative and proliferative lesion of the medullary and cortical tissue of bone, occurring most frequently near the ends of the diaphyses of a long bone and, less commonly, on the jaws, usually the mandible. It is a slow growing, painless growth, with a well-defined radiographic picture. **odontogenic f.,** a rare benign central tumor of the jaw, usually the mandible, originating from the embryonic structures of the tooth germ, dental papilla, or dental follicle. It is usually in close proximity to either the root or, in cases of unerupted teeth, the crown. Histologically, it is composed of stellate fibroblasts in a moderately fibrillar matrix with the occasional presence of some epithelial cells of dental origin. **ossifying f.,** a benign central tumor of the jaw, usually the mandible, consisting of fibrous connective tissue with foci of bone formation. It is a slow-growing tumor and is frequently asymptomatic, mild swelling and teeth displacement being the early signs. The tumor is not usually encapsulated and does not undergo malignant changes. **perineural f.,** a fibroma originating in nerve sheaths or perineural connective tissue. **peripheral odontogenic f.,** peripheral ossifying f. **peripheral ossifying f.,** a fibroma, usually of the gingiva, showing areas of calcification or ossification. Called also *peripheral odontogenic f., epulis,* and *ossifying fibroid.* **f. sarcomato′sum,** fibrosarcoma. **soft f.,** a fibroma characterized by the presence of soft, rubbery, pliable masses. Called also *f. molle.*

fibromatosis (fi″bro-mah-to′sis) a tendency to the development of fibromas; the formation or presence of multiple fibromas. **f. gingi′vae, gingival f.,** diffuse fibrous overgrowth of the gingival tissue. In the generalized form, there is overgrowth of both the maxillary and mandibular tissue, which may be transmitted as an autosomal dominant trait, be produced by drugs, especially anticonvulsant therapy with phenytoin (see Dilantin GINGIVITIS), or be of the idiopathic type. In the localized form (called also *fibroma*), there is unilateral or bilateral overgrowth of the gingival tissue of the maxillary tuberosity, occurring in two principal forms: the hereditary type, transmitted as an autosomal dominant trait, and the idiopathic type. The enlarged gingiva is pink, firm, almost leathery in consistency, and presents a minutely pebbled surface. In severe cases the teeth are almost completely covered, and the enlargement projects into the oral vestibule; the jaws appear distorted because of the bullous enlargement. Secondary inflammatory changes are common at the gingival margin. Called also *diffuse fibroma of gingiva, elephantiasis gingivae, fibrous hyperplasia of gingiva, gingivitis hypertrophica, keloid of gums,* and *macrogingivae.* See also gingival ENLARGEMENT. **pseudosarcomatous f.,**

an uncommon subcutaneous tumorous nodule having a firm, gray to pink hard surface, which may occur in any part of the body, including the lips and oral cavity. The lesion, which resembles fibrosarcoma histologically, is composed of plump or spindle-shaped connective tissue cells with nuclei that are often hyperchromatic or in mitosis. It lacks a capsule, and sometimes appears to infiltrate adjacent fascia or muscle and to surround nerves and blood vessels. Called also *infiltrative fasciitis*, *nodular fasciitis*, and *pseudosarcomatous fasciitis*.

fibromyxoma (fi″bro-mik-so′mah) a fibroma containing myxomatous tissue; myxofibroma.

fibro-osteoma (fi″bro-os″te-o′mah) a benign central tumor of the jaws, consisting of fibrous connective tissue with foci of bone formation that occupy the major portion of the tumor mass.

fibropapilloma (fi″bro-pap″ĭ-lo′mah) a papilloma containing fibrous tissue.

fibrosarcoma (fi″bro-sar-ko′mah) [L. *fibra* fiber + Gr. *sarkos* flesh + *-oma*] a malignant form of fibroma, which may originate as a benign fibroma, but more often arises as a primary malignancy. Oral fibrosarcoma may arise at any location, but is most common in the maxillary sinus, pharynx, lips, and periosteum of the maxilla and mandible. It usually presents a bulky, unencapsulated mass composed of soft, gray-white tissue with the consistency and appearance of raw fish flesh, with foci of necrosis and hemorrhage. All degrees of differentiation may be present, from good to extreme anaplasia. The cells are spindle-shaped with elongated nuclei, and the associated fibers are usually arranged in interlacing bands or fascicles. Mitotic activity in poorly differentiated lesions is prominent; in well differentiated ones it is almost absent. Called also *fibroma sarcomatosum* and *malignant fibroma*. **ameloblastic f.**, ameloblastic SARCOMA. **odontogenic f.**, a malignant form of odontogenic fibroma, presenting as a fleshy bulky lesion, which originates from the embryonic structures of the tooth germ, the dental papilla, or the dental follicle. Histologically, it contains cells resembling immature fibroblasts that are elongated and contain ovoid nuclei, situated in a fibrous meshwork which may or may not have foci of odontogenic epithelium. There is considerable mitotic activity in the cellular components of the tumor.

fibrosclerosis (fi″bro-skle-ro′sis) fibrosis associated with sclerosis.

fibrosis (fi-bro′sis) [L. *fibra* fiber + *-osis*] the formation of fibrous tissues; fibrous degeneration. **cystic f. of pancreas**, mucoviscidosis. **oral submucous f.**, a disease of the oral mucosa, pharynx, and esophagus. It is characterized by an insidious onset marked by a burning sensation followed by hardening of the mucous membrane, accompanied by blanching and formation of fibrous bands in the buccal mucosa, pterygomandibular raphe, and labial mucosa. Hardening and formation of scarlike tissue causes inability to protrude the tongue or whistle and involvement of the retromolar tissue produces trismus, dysphagia, and referred pain to the ears and deafness. The scarlike tissue is firmly attached to the underlying tissue, and the papillae of the tongue may undergo atrophy. Leukoplakia may follow. **pulp f.**, fibrotic changes in the dental pulp, occurring as a normal aging process, which is significantly accelerated by degenerative changes in the pulp. Called also *fibrous pulp dystrophy*.

fibrositis (fi″bro-si′tis) [L. *fibra* fiber + *-itis*] inflammatory hyperplasia of the fibrous tissue of the body. **f. ossif′icans**, progressive myositis ossificans; see under MYOSITIS.

fibrous (fi′brus) composed of or containing fibers.

FICA Federal Insurance Contributions Act.

FICD Fellow of the International College of Dentists.

fiduciary (fi-du′she-er″e) 1. a person entrusted with property or power for the benefit of another. 2. pertaining to the relationship between a person who has been entrusted with something for the benefit of another (fiduciary) and his principal, such as may exist between a doctor and his patient or a hospital trustee and the hospital.

field (fēld) 1. an area or open space. 2. in embryology, the condition or group of factors to which any living system owes its typical organization. **dry f.**, see dry field TECHNIQUE. **image f.**, the limits of a radiographic image on an image receptor. **magnetic f.**, that part of space about a magnet, or coil of current-carrying wire, in which its action is perceptible. **penumbra f.**, the region of free space which is irradiated by primary photons coming from only part of the radiation source. See PENUMBRA. **f. of radiation**, the geometrical projection on a plane perpendicular to the central rays of the distal end of the limiting diaphragm as seen from the center of the front surface of the source. The field is thus the same shape as the aperture of the collimator and it can be defined at any distance from the source. **visual f.**, **f. of vision**, that portion of space

which the fixed eye can see. **washed f.**, see washed field TECHNIQUE.

figure (fig′yer) [L. *figura*, from *fingere* to shape or form] 1. an object of a particular form. 2. a number, or numeral.

fila (fi′lah) [L.] plural of *filum*.

filament (fil′ah-ment) [L. *filamentum*] 1. a delicate fiber or thread. 2. in an x-ray machine, a coiled tungsten wire which when heated to incandescence, emits electrons. **actin f.**, myofilament. **axial f.**, 1. axial FIBRIL. 2. axistyle. **muscle f.**, **myosin f.**, myofilament.

filamenta (fil″ah-men′tah) [L.] plural of *filamentum*.

filamentous (fil-ah-men′tus) composed of long, threadlike structures; said of bacterial colonies.

filamentum (fil″ah-men′tum), pl. *filamen′ta* [L.] filament.

Filaria (fi-la′re-ah) [L. *filum* thread] a former loosely applied generic name for members of the superfamily Filarioidea. **F. labia′lis**, *Gongylonema pulchrum*; see under GONGYLONEMA.

filaria (fi-la′re-ah), pl. *fila′riae* [L. *filum* thread] a nematode worm of the superfamily Filarioidea.

filariae (fi-la′re-e) [L.] plural of *filaria*.

filarial (fi-la′re-al) pertaining to, caused by, or denoting filariae.

filariasis (fil″ah-ri′ah-sis) infection with filariae.

Filarioidea (fi-lar″e-oi′de-ah) a superfamily or order of nematode parasites, the adults being threadlike worms which invade the tissues and body cavities where the female deposits embryonated eggs (prelarvae) known as microfilariae. The microfilariae are ingested by blood-sucking insects in whom they pass their developmental stage and are returned to man by the bites of such insects.

Filatov's disease, spots [Nil Fedorovich *Filatov*, Russian physician, 1847–1902] see infectious MONONUCLEOSIS, and Koplik spots, under SPOT.

Fildes, P. see Woods-Fildes THEORY.

file (fil) a surgical or a dental instrument with a finely serrated surface, for reducing surplus hard substance, such as bone or materials used in dental restorations, or for smoothing roughened surfaces. **bone f.**, a cutting instrument having a narrow straight blade with transverse serrations for removing bone substance through a push-pull grating action. In oral surgery, used to file down the rough margins of the alveolus following tooth extraction. Called also *bone rasp*. See illustration. **endodontic f.**, root canal f. **finishing f.**, a thin, delicate file useful in finishing the margins of restorative materials. **gold f.**, a file with fine serrations for shaping gold or platinum restorations. **Hirschfeld f.**, **Hirschfeld-Dunlop f.**, a small, flat periodontal file designed with various blade angulations for reaching different surfaces of the tooth in removing calculus. **H-type f.**, **Hedström f.**, root canal f., H-type. **Kerr f.**, trademark for a K-type root

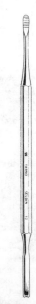

Bone file. Serrations on the tip are used to reduce sharp fragments of bone following tooth extraction. (From H. O. Torres and A. Ehrlich: Modern Dental Assisting. 2nd ed. Philadelphia, W. B. Saunders Co., 1980; courtesy of S. S. White Co.)

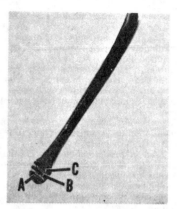

Periodontal file with three cutting edges: A, B, C. (From P. F. Steele: Dimensions of Dental Hygiene. 2nd ed. Philadelphia, Lea & Febiger, 1975.)

canal file. **Orban f.,** a relatively large periodontal file. **periodontal f.,** one with three cutting edges, designed for removing difficult to dislodge calculi from the tooth surface. See illustration. **rat-tail f.,** a hand-operated or engine-driven root canal file made of very flexible and soft steel, having spurlike projections fixed at right angles to the shaft, and tapering to the extremity like a rat's tail. Used with a pulling stoke for débridement of narrow, curved root canals, and in prosthetics to prepare and smooth the impression trays. The identification symbol is an octahedron. Called also *R-type rasp.* See illustrations at root canal THERAPY. **root canal f.,** an endodontic instrument for cleaning and shaping the root canals of a tooth. Called also *endodontic f.* See also BROACH and REAMER. **root canal f., H-type,** a hand-operated or engine-driven root canal file consisting of a series of tapered cone-shaped sections, successively larger from the tip toward the handle, the cutting edge being at the base of the cone so that the cutting occurs on a pulling stroke only during the rasping motion. Used to enlarge the root canal by either a cutting or abrasive action. The identification symbol is a circle. Called also *H-type f.* and *Hedström f.* See illustration at root canal THERAPY. **root canal f., K-type,** a hand-operated or engine-driven root canal file made of a carbon or stainless steel blank, usually square in cross-section, which is twisted so as to produce a series of spirals having from 1.97 to 0.88 cutting flutes per mm of operating head. It is quite similar to a root canal reamer, except for the number of cutting flutes. The identification symbol is a square. Called also *Kerr f.* See illustration at root canal THERAPY. **rubber f.,** vulcanite f. **scaler f.,** one used for the removal of calculi from the tooth surface. **Star root canal f.,** trademark for a carbon steel or stainless steel root canal file. **vulcanite f.,** a double-ended file, generally half-round, with coarse teeth. Called also *rubber f.*

filiform (fil′ĭ-form, fī′lĭ-form) [L. *filum* thread + *forma* form] 1. shaped like a thread. 2. pertaining to a very slender bougie.

filing (fīl′ing) 1. an act or instance of using a file. 2. a particle produced by rubbing something, such as a metal, with a file. 3. cut ALLOY.

filler (fil′er) any substance or material used to fill gaps, cavities, cracks, and the like, to increase the bulk or weight of another substance, or as a reinforcing agent. The principal purpose of a filler in dental restorations is to increase certain properties of the matrix material, i.e., strength, hardness, etc. In a composite material containing a filler and a matrix, interatomic or molecular bonds usually exist between the two. **resin f.,** any resin material, such as fused silica, crystalline quartz, lithium aluminum silicate, borosilicate glass, or glass containing barium fluoride, representing 70 to 80 percent of a composite resin.

filling (fil′ing) 1. the material inserted into a prepared tooth cavity, usually gold, amalgam, cement, or synthetic resin. 2. The process of inserting, condensing, shaping, and finishing filling substance in a prepared tooth cavity or root canal. **bead technique f., brush technique f.,** a nonpressure method of direct filling of the prepared cavity, accomplished by the application of a monomer-polymer resin mixture in increments, whereby the cavity is first moistened with the monomer, followed by dipping the tip of a small hair brush into the monomer and then touching it to the **polymer so** that a few particles cling to it to form a small bead **of powder** particles and monomer. The bead thus formed is **placed in** contact with the cavity floor and allowed to flow **over the** floor already dampened with the monomer. The **process is** repeated until the cavity is filled. Called also *bead technique* and *nonpressure technique.* **complex f.,** a filling for a complex cavity. **composite f.,** a filling that consists of a composite resin. **compound f.,** a filling for a cavity that involves two or more surfaces of a tooth. **direct f.,** one that is inserted and **completed** directly in the prepared cavity. See also direct filling RESIN and direct filling GOLD. **direct resin f.,** a direct filling made from a synthetic resin. See *bead technique f., flow technique f.,* and *pressure technique f.* **ditched f.,** the marginal failure **of an** amalgam restoration due to fracture of either the material **or the** tooth structure itself in the affected area. **flow technique f.,** a method of direct filling of the prepared cavity, whereby a **thin mix of a** polymer and monomer is carried into the cavity by means of a plastic instrument or small brush, the fluidity of the resin flowing into the cavity and adapting to its contours. After the cavity is filled, a matrix band is applied, without being held under pressure. **indirect f.,** a filling constructed on a die that has been made from an accurate impression of the tooth and that is inserted into the tooth cavity. **f. material,** filling MATERIAL. **Mosetig-Moorhof f.,** Mosetig-Moorhof bone WAX. **permanent f.,** a filling intended to provide complete function while the tooth remains in the oral cavity. **postresection f.,** retrograde f. **pressure technique f.,** a method of direct filling of the prepared cavity, whereby a dough formed by a monomer-polymer mixture is inserted into the cavity and held under pressure by a plastic strip over the material and between the adjacent teeth. Called also *bulk technique, bulk pack technique,* and *pressure technique.* **retrograde f.,** an amalgam or other type of filling placed in the apical portion of tooth to seal the root canal following surgical removal of a periapical lesion, which is performed through the apex of a tooth, approached through the alveolar bone. Called also *postresection f., retrograde amalgam,* and *retrograde obturation.* **reverse f.,** retrofilling. **root canal f.,** 1. a material or a combination of various materials placed inside a root canal for the purpose of obturating or sealing it. 2. a method of obturating and sealing root canals. See also canal OBTURATION and root canal filling methods, under METHOD. **root-end f.,** retrofilling. **temporary f.,** a filling placed in a tooth cavity with the intention of removing it within a short period of time. See also *treatment f.* **treatment f.,** a filling used to allay sensitive dentin prior to the final preparation of the cavity; said of a temporary filling when the extent of the carious process cannot be determined until the demineralized dentin is first hardened to facilitate its removal with a minimal chance of pulp exposure.

film (film) 1. a thin layer or coat. 2. a thin transparent sheet of cellulose acetate or similar material coated on one or both sides with an emulsion that is sensitive to light or radiation. **f. badge,** film BADGE. **bite-wing f.,** one used in radiography of oral structures, with a central protruding tab or wing to be used held between the upper and lower teeth. Used chiefly to detect interproximal decay and to determine the height of the alveolar crest of the bone which supports the teeth. Called also *interproximal f.* See also bite-wing RADIOGRAPH. **dental f.,** x-ray film especially designed and packaged for use in dental practice. It is prepared in a light-proof envelope with an inner lining of sheets of black paper and a sheet of lead foil on the tongue (or palate) side of the film to protect the exposed film from secondary radiation and to provide protection for the surrounding tissue from excessive exposure beyond the film packet. The surface of the envelope is identified with a tab opening on the side placed away from the radiographed tooth, the pebbly or solid side of the envelope being placed next to the lingual surface of the tooth, on the side opposite the x-ray unit. A small bump or dot is placed on the tissue surface of the film that has been exposed, thus helping to identify the tissue side when mounting the processed radiograph. The dot side of the radiograph identifies the upper right of the patient's mouth as the upper left on the patient's chart. **f. developer,** developing SOLUTION. **f. development,** film DEVELOPMENT. **direct exposure f.,** one that is highly sensitive to the direct action of x-rays, but has low sensitivity to screen fluorescence. **exposed f.,** one that has been exposed to x-rays and contains a latent image, but has not yet been processed. See also film PROCESSING. **extraoral f.,** a relatively large film, ranging in size from 5 to 7 inches up to 10 to 12 inches or more, which is placed outside the cavity in detecting large areas of pathological involvement, such as fractures of the facial bones, temporomandibular lesions, and impacted teeth or conditions associated with the patient's inability to open his mouth. **f. fixation,** film FIXATION. **fixed blood f.,** a thin film of blood spread on a slide, dried quickly, and fixed.

f. gamma, film GAMMA. **f. holder,** cassette. **interproximal f.,** bite-wing f. **intraoral f.,** a relatively small film that is placed in the patient's mouth in oral radiography, including the occlusal, bite-wing, and periapical film. **lateral jaw f.,** a radiograph showing either the ramus or the body of the mandible. **non-screen f.,** an x-ray film used without intensifying screens. Its emulsion is generally thicker and contains a greater silver content than that of a screen film, thus causing the film to be very sensitive to x-rays. It offers a fine detail of image and is used in the examination of relatively thin organs and structures. **occlusal f.,** film, which may be placed intra- or extraorally, used in topographic and cross-sectional radiography of the maxillary or mandibular dental structure and adjacent tissues. It is employed in determining the location of cystic lesions, impacted teeth, salivary duct calculi, bone fractures, and other lesions affecting large parts of the oral cavity. **passivating f.,** passivating LAYER. **periapical f.,** one used in radiography of the root apex of a tooth and the surrounding structures. **f. processing,** film PROCESSING. **screen f.,** one sensitive to both fluorescent light and x-rays; used with an intensifying screen. **single-emulsion f.,** one coated with emulsion on one side only. **f. speed,** film SPEED. **spot f.,** see spot-film RADIOGRAPHY. **sulfa f.,** one made from an emulsion of sulfadiazine, sulfanilamide, and methyl cellulose; used as a dressing for burns, cuts, and skin grafts. **ultraspeed f.,** one that is very sensitive to radiation or to light, thereby requiring less exposure than other types. It has the emulsion on both sides of the cellulose base. **x-ray f,** a sheet of cellulose acetate about 0.0075 inch thick or other synthetic material about 0.0073 inch thick, coated on both sides with a dehydrated suspension of silver bromide in gelatin, each coat about 0.001 inch thick. For increased sharpness of the image, the cellulose is usually tinted blue. Most film is coated with a scratch-deterring substance. The passage of x-rays causes silver bromide crystals to separate into positive silver ions (Ag+) and negative bromine ions (Br⁻) in the affected areas, thus producing a latent image. The film processing converts the latent image into the manifest image by selective reduction of silver halide salts to metallic silver grains in the affected areas (development), followed by the removal of silver halide in the unaffected areas (fixation). See also film PROCESSING.

filopodia (fi″lo-po′de-ah) plural of *filopodium.*

filopodium (fi″lo-po′de-um), pl. *filopo′dia* [L. *filum* thread + Gr. *pous* foot] 1. a slender, pointed pseudopodium composed of ectoplasm. 2. one of the minute processes, about 1 μ in diameter, which stem from the major odontoblastic processes, generally found in small dentinal tubules, being located mostly near the dentinoenamel junction.

filter (fil′ter) [L. *filtrum*] 1. a device for the straining of water or other liquids. 2. in radiology, material placed in the useful beam to filter out less penetrating radiation. See *aluminum f.* and FILTRATION (2). **aluminum f.,** a filter made of an aluminum plate of a desired thickness, which is placed in an x-ray generator in the pathway of the x-ray beam. It absorbs rays of longer wavelengths but allows passage of other radiations. **6B f.,** a safe light filter for screening out those rays in the spectrum to which x-ray films are sensitive. **built-in f.,** a nonremovable filter built into the tube-head assembly of an x-ray generator, which adds to the inherent filtration. **compensating f.,** in radiology, one designed to shield less dense areas so that a more uniform image may be produced on the radiograph. **external f.,** one placed in the pathway of the x-ray beam, externally to the tube-head assembly. **inherent f.,** one built into a shockproof x-ray tube, such as refined oil occupying the space between the glass tube and the shielding or any other structural element in the path of the useful beam of radiation; its filtering effect being equivalent to that of a minimum of 0.5 mm of aluminum. **MI-2 f.,** a safe light filter for screening out those rays in the spectrum to which x-ray films are sensitive, giving low level red-orange illumination to dark rooms. **Thoraeus f.,** one consisting of varying thicknesses of tin, copper, and aluminum, tin being usually next to the tube and aluminum forming the external layer.

filterable (fil′ter-ah-b′l) capable of passing through the pores of a filter; said of elements that can pass through a filter which will not permit the passage of the usual microorganisms.

filtrate (fil′trāt) a liquid that has passed through a filter.

filtration (fil-tra′shun) 1. the passage of a liquid through a filter to remove suspended particles or impurities. 2. in radiology, the use of substances that absorb radiations, such as aluminum, lead, or other metals, or oil, to eliminate radiations of certain wavelengths from a useful primary beam of x-radiation. **added f.,** supplemental radiation filtration obtained by means of a filter inserted in addition to inherent filtration, usually positioned before or at the base of the collimating device. **built-in f.,** radiation filtration achieved through built-in or nonremovable

absorbers installed into the tube-head assembly. **external f.,** radiation filtration achieved by added filtration absorbers and the attenuating effects of materials in the housing that are external to the tube-head assembly, such as a closed-end pointer cone. **inherent f.,** radiation filtration achieved by components installed in the tube-head assembly that are in the path of the useful beam, such as the glass wall of the x-ray tube, oil, or any other material permanently situated between the target and the collimator. **total f.,** the sum total of radiation filtration produced by built-in, external, and inherent filters expressed in aluminum equivalents.

filum (fi′lum), pl. *fi′la* [L.] a threadlike structure or part. **fi′la olfacto′ria,** bundles of olfactory nerve fibers which pass through the cribriform plate of the ethmoid bone. See also olfactory NERVE.

fimbria (fim′bre-ah) [L. *fimbriae* (pl.) a fringe] 1. a fringe, border, or edge; a general anatomical term for such a structure. 2. in microbiology, one of the minute filamentous appendages of certain bacteria. **fim′briae of tongue, fim′briae lin′guae,** fimbriated FOLD.

fimbriated (fim′bre-āt-ed) [L. *fimbriatus*] fringed.

finding (find′ing) an observation; a condition discovered.

fineness (fin′nes) 1. the state or quality of being superior or best grade. 2. the state of being composed of very small particles; not being coarse; see ABRASIVE (2). 3. the amount or proportion of a precious metal in an alloy, usually expressed in parts per thousand; in a gold alloy, pure gold (24 carat) is said to be 1000 fine, a gold alloy having ¾ gold and ¼ other metal(s), 750 fine gold, etc.

finger (fing′ger) a terminal extremity of the hand. **spider f.,** an abnormally elongated finger having the appearance of a leg of the spider. Called also *arachnodactyly.* See Marfan's SYNDROME.

finger-sucking (fing″ger-suk′ing) finger SUCKING.

Finimal trademark for *acetaminophen.*

finish (fin′ish) 1. to bring or come to an end or to completion. 2. to give something (e.g., a denture) a desired or particular surface texture. **denture f.,** the final perfection of the form of the polished surface of a denture. **satin f.,** the degree of finish of a polished surface, as of a denture, that has been made very smooth but without a high sheen.

Finkeldey see Warthin-Finkeldey CELL.

Finlepsin trademark for *carbamazepine.*

fire (fir) 1. a phenomenon of combustion producing heat and light. 2. fever. **St. Anthony's f., St. Francis' f.,** erysipelas.

firing (fir′ing) 1. the act of causing fire. 2. the fusing of porcelain paste (a mixture of a powder containing feldspar, kaolin, and other substances with distilled water), in the process of producing porcelain. During the firing, the baked material undergoes gradual changes; see *high biscuit f., low biscuit f.,* and *medium biscuit f.* Called also *baking.* 3. fritting. **air f.,** firing of dental porcelain with air being retained in the muffle. **diffusible gas f.,** the replacement of the air in the porcelain furnace with a gas, such as helium or water vapor, thus replacing the air between the powder particles during firing. When the porcelain matures, the gas, having a small atomic diameter, will diffuse and spread out between the atoms that compose the porcelain. **high biscuit f., high bisque f.,** the third and final stage of firing dental porcelain, whereby the glass flows freely and fills in the pores to the maximum, the shrinkage is complete, and color inherent in the porcelain develops, the surface of the porcelain assuming a mattelike finish. At this stage, the porcelain is said to have reached maturity (vitrification), which is divided into low, medium, and high stages. It is followed by the glaze stage when the material acquires luster, divided into low, medium, and high. The last stage is coalescence when the overglazed surface assumes a rounded form. True color and translucency and sheen on its surface are the signs of maturity of fired porcelain. Called also *high biscuit baking.* **low biscuit f.,** the first stage of firing dental porcelain, whereby the glass melts and flows just enough to cause the particles to adhere, but not enough to fill in spaces between the particles. At this stage, the porcelain remains white, opaque, porous, and rough, and there is little shrinkage. Called also *low biscuit baking.* **medium biscuit f., medium bisque f.,** the second stage of firing dental porcelain, whereby the glass flows freely and the porcelain exhibits a definite amount of shrinkage. The porcelain is still porous and opaque. Called also *medium biscuit baking.* **pressure f.,** increase of atmospheric pressure in the porcelain furnace after the porcelain has reached its maturation temperature and continuing until the porcelain has hardened. Air bubbles in the porcelain are thus compressed and reduced in size. **vacuum f.,** removal of the air from the muffle of the porcelain furnace during firing; the vacuum thus created causes the air to be pulled out from between the particles and allows the glass to flow into the vacated spaces.

Firmilay trademark for a hard *dental casting gold alloy* (see under GOLD).

first aid (ferst′ ād) first AID.

fission (fish′un) [L. *fissio*] 1. the act or process of splitting. 2. a form of asexual reproduction in which the cell divides into two parts. 3. nuclear f. **nuclear f.,** a nuclear reaction in which a nucleus of a heavy atom is split into two approximate equal masses, representing the nuclei of lighter new elements. The sum of the masses of the two new atoms is less than the mass of the parent heavy atom, and the reaction is thus associated with the emission of large amounts of energy. See also nuclear FUSION and nuclear REACTION.

fissula (fis′u-lah) [L., dim. of *fissum*] a little cleft.

fissura (fis-su′rah), pl. *fissu′rae* [L.] a general anatomical term for a cleft or groove. See also FISSURE, GROOVE, SULCUS, SUTURA, SUTURE, and SYNCHONDROSIS. **f. au′ris congen′ita,** preauricular fistula, congenital; see under FISTULA. **f. orbita′lis infe′rior** [NA], orbital fissure, inferior, see under FISSURE. **f. orbita′lis supe′rior** [NA], orbital fissure, superior; see under FISSURE. **f. petrooccipita′lis** [NA], petro-occipital FISSURE. **f. petrosquamo′sa** [NA], petrosquamous FISSURE. **f. petrotympan′ica** [NA], petrotympanic FISSURE. **f. pterygoi′dea,** pterygoid FISSURE. **f. pterygomaxilla′ris** [NA], pterygomaxillary FISSURE (1). **f. sphenooccipita′lis,** spheno-occipital FISSURE. **f. sphenopetro′sa** [NA], sphenopetrosal FISSURE. **f. tympanomastoi′dea** [NA], tympanomastoid FISSURE.

fissurae (fis-su′re) [L.] plural of *fissura*.

fissural (fish′u-ral) pertaining to a fissure.

fissure (fish′ur) [L. *fissura*] 1. any cleft or groove, normal or otherwise. Called also *fissura*. See also CLEFT, GROOVE, SULCUS, SUTURE, and SYNCHONDROSIS. 2. a deep ditch or cleft in the surface of a tooth; a developmental linear fault found most often in the occlusal or the buccal surface of a tooth, usually the result of the imperfect fusion of the enamel of the adjoining dental lobes. Considered as belonging to Class I cavities in Black's classification of dental caries (see dental caries classification, under CARIES). To be distinguished from a groove or sulcus. Called also *enamel f.* See also PIT (3). **angular f.,** sphenopetrosal f. **f. of aqueduct of vestibule,** external aperture of aqueduct of vestibule; see under APERTURE. **auricular f. of temporal bone,** tympanomastoid f. **basilar f.,** spheno-occipital f. **branchial f.,** branchial CLEFT. **craniofacial f.,** a vertical fissure separating the mesoethmoid into two parts. **enamel f.,** fissure (2). **entorbital f.,** a sulcus occasionally seen between the orbital and olfactory sulci. **ethmoid f.,** superior nasal MEATUS. **gingival f.,** vertical fissure of the gingiva. See gingival CLEFT. **glaserian f.,** petrotympanic f. **globulomaxillary f.,** the junction of the globular portion of the median nasal process and the maxillary process and the site of the globulomaxillary cyst. **f. of glottis,** RIMA glottidis. **lacrimal f.,** lacrimal sulcus of lacrimal bone; see under SULCUS. **mandibular f's,** the lowest facial fissure of the embryo. **maxillary f.,** a groove on the maxilla for the maxillary process of the palatal bone. **occipitosphenoidal f.,** spheno-occipital f. **oral f.,** ORIFICE of the mouth. **orbital f., inferior,** an opening in the posterolateral wall of the orbit, which joins the pterygomaxillary fissure at right angles, and is bounded by the inferior border of the orbital surface of the great wing of the sphenoid bone, lateral border of the orbital surface of the maxilla and the orbital process of the palatine bone, and zygomatic bone. Through it the temporal, infratemporal, and pterygopalatine fossae transmit the infraorbital and zygomatic nerves and the infraorbital nerves, including the maxillary nerve, its zygomatic branch, and the ascending branches from its sphenopalatine branch. Called also *inferior sphenoidal f., sphenomaxillary f.,* and *fissura orbitalis inferior* [NA]. **orbital f., superior,** an elongated cleft between the small and great wings of the sphenoid bone, which separates the lateral wall from the roof of the orbit. It transmits the oculomotor, trochlear, ophthalmic division of the trigeminal, and abducent nerves, and filaments of the cavernous plexus and the orbital branches of the middle meningeal artery to the orbit, and the superior ophthalmic vein and the recurrent branch of the lacrimal artery to the dura mater from the orbit. Called also *sphenoidal f., superior sphenoidal f., anterior lacerate foramen, foramen lacerum anterius,* and *fissura orbitalis superior* [NA]. **palpebral f.,** the longitudinal opening between the eyelids. Called

also *rima palpebrarum* [NA]. **parietosphenoid f.,** parietal notch of temporal bone; see under NOTCH. **petrobasilar f.,** petrooccipital f. **petromastoid f.,** tympanomastoid f. **petro-occipital f.,** a fissure extending backward from the foramen lacerum to the jugular foramen, between the basioccipital and the posterior or inner border of the petrous portion of the temporal bone. Called also *petrobasilar f., fissura petrooccipitalis* [NA], and *petrospheno-occipital suture of Gruber.* **petrosal f., superficial,** HIATUS of canal for greater petrosal nerve. **petrosphenoidal f.,** sphenopetrosal f. **petrosquamous f., petrosquamosal f.,** a slight fissure of varying distinctness in the floor of the middle cranial fossa, marking the line of fusion between the squamous and petrous portions of the temporal bone. Called also *fissura petrosquamosa* [NA]. **petrotympanic f.,** a narrow transversely running slit just posterior to the articular surface of the mandibular fossa of the temporal bone; an arteriole and the chorda tympani nerve pass through it, and it lodges a portion of the malleus. Called also *glaserian f., pterygotympanic f., tympanic f., tympanosquamous f.,* and *fissura petrotympanica* [NA]. **pterygoid f.,** an angular cleft on the inferior portion of each pterygoid process, the margins of which articulate with the pyramidal process of the palatine bone; it is inserted between the diverging medial and lateral pterygoid plates. Called also *fissura pterygoidea, palatine incisure, palatine notch, pterygoid incisure,* and *pterygoid notch.* **pterygomaxillary f.,** 1. a triangular cleft at right angles to the medial end of the inferior orbital fissure, formed by the divergence of the maxilla from the pterygoid process of the sphenoid bone; it transmits the terminal parts of the maxillary artery and veins. Called also *pterygopalatine f.* and *fissura pterygomaxillaris* [NA]. 2. an anthropometric landmark, being the projected contour of the fissure; the anterior wall represents closely the retromolar tuberosity of the maxilla, and the posterior wall represents the anterior curve of the pterygoid process of the sphenoid bone. Abbreviated *Ptm.* Called also *point Ptm.* **pterygopalatine f.,** pterygomaxillary f. (1). **pterygopalatine f. of palatine bone,** greater palatine sulcus of palatine bone; see under SULCUS. **pterygotympanic f.,** petrotympanic f. **retrocuticular f.,** a fissure in the oral epithelium made by a tooth at the time of eruption. **f. sealant,** pit and fissure SEALANT. **sphenoidal f.,** orbital f., superior. **sphenoidal f., inferior,** orbital f., inferior. **sphenoidal f., superior,** orbital f., superior. **sphenomaxillary f.,** orbital f., inferior. **spheno-occipital f.,** the fissure between the basilar part of the occipital bone and the body of the sphenoid bone. Called also *basilar f., occipitosphenoidal f., fissura sphenooccipitalis, basilar suture, occipitosphenoidal suture,* and *spheno-occipital suture.* **sphenopetrosal f.,** a fissure in the floor of the middle cranial fossa between the posterior edge of the great wing of the sphenoid bone and the petrous part of the temporal bone. Called also *angular f., petrosphenoidal f.,* and *fissura sphenopetrosa* [NA]. **tympanic f.,** petrotympanic f. **tympanomastoid f.,** an external fissure of the inferior and lateral aspect of the skull between the tympanic portion and the mastoid process of the temporal bone; the auricular branch of the vagus nerve often passes through it. Called also *auricular f. of temporal bone, petromastoid f.,* and *fissura tympanomastoidea* [NA]. **tympanosquamous f.,** petrotympanic f. **zygomatic f.,** infratemporal FOSSA. **zygomaticosphenoid f.,** a fissure between the orbital surface of the great wing of the sphenoid bone and the zygomatic bone.

fistula (fis′tu-lah), pl. *fistulas, fis′tulae* [L. "pipe"] an abnormal passage or communication, usually between two internal organs, or leading from an internal organ to the surface of the body, often draining fluids, such as pus from an abscess. **arteriovenous f.,** an abnormal communication between an artery and a vein; it may result from injury (*traumatic arteriovenous f.*). See also arteriovenous ANEURYSM. **f. au′ris congen′ita,** preauricular f., congenital. **blind f.,** one which opens at one end only; it may open only upon the cutaneous surface of the body (*external blind f.*) or on an internal mucous surface (*internal blind f.*). Called also *incomplete f.* Cf. *complete f.* **branchial f.,** a congenital fistula of the neck resulting from failure of closure of a branchial cleft. See also *cervical f.* **cervical f.,** one which communicates with the cavity of a thyroglossal cyst and opens in the midline of the neck. See also *branchial f.* **f. col′li congen′ita,** a congenital fistula in the neck, opening into the pharynx. **complete f.,** one which opens at both ends on a mucous surface or on the cutaneous surface of the body. Cf. *blind f.* **craniosinus f.,** one between the intracranial space and one of the paranasal sinuses, permitting the escape of cerebrospinal fluid into the nose. **external f.,** one which communicates with a hollow space and opens on the external surface of the body. **external blind f.,** see *blind f.* **incomplete f.,** blind f. **internal f.,** one communicating between two internal organs. **internal blind f.,** *see blind f.* **lacrimal f.,** one which opens into the lacrimal sac or duct. **lip f's, congenital,** usually symmetrical fistulas on either side of the midline of the transitional area of the mucous membrane of the lip, exuding clear mucoid fluid. It is a rare congenital abnormality, probably transmitted as an autosomal dominant trait. **lymphatic f.,** one which opens into a lymphatic vessel and discharges lymph. **oroantral f.,** one between the maxillary sinus and the oral cavity, sometimes through the tooth socket. **orofacial f.,** one from the oral cavity, opening on the cutaneous surface of the face. **oronasal f.,** one connecting the oral and nasal cavities. **pharyngeal f.,** one which opens into the pharynx. **preauricular f., congenital,** an epidermal-lined tract communicating with a pitlike depression just in front of the helix and above the tragus (ear pit), resulting from imperfect fusion of the first and second branchial arches in the formation of the auricle. Called also *f. auris congenita* and *fissura auris congenita.* **salivary f.,** one between a salivary duct and/or gland and the cutaneous surface, or into the oral cavity through other than a normal pathway. **submental f.,** a salivary fistula opening below the chin. **traumatic arteriovenous f.,** see *arteriovenous f.*

fistulae (fis′tu-le) [L.] plural of *fistula.*

fistulectomy (fis″tu-lek′to-me) [*fistula* + Gr. *ektomē* excision] excision of a fistulous tract.

fistulization (fis″tu-li-za′shun) 1. the act or process of becoming fistulous. 2. surgical opening into a hollow organ, cavity, or abscess; the creation of a communication between two structures which were not previously connected.

fistulotomy (fis″tu-lot′o-me) incision of a fistula.

fistulous (fis′tu-lus) [L. *fistulosus*] pertaining to or of the nature of a fistula.

fit (fit) the adaptation of one structure into another, as the adaptation of any dental restoration to its site in the mouth.

fixation (fik-sa′shun) [L. *fixatio*] 1. the act or operation of holding, suturing, or fastening in a fixed position. 2. the condition of being held in a fixed position. 3. in microscopy, the treatment of material so that its structure may be examined in greater detail with minimal alteration of the normal state, and also to provide information concerning the chemical properties (as of cell constituents) by interpretation of fixation reactions. 4. in chemistry, the process whereby a substance is removed from the gaseous or solution phase and localized. 5. film f. **alexin f.,** complement f. **complement f.,** the combination of antigen with specific IgG or IgM induces a conformational change on the Fc component of the heavy chain, which permits the complex to activate the complement sequence and causes its reduction in a mixture. The decrease of complement in a mixture can be detected by the addition of sensitized red blood cells. If free complement is present, hemolysis occurs; if not, no hemolysis is observed. This reaction is the basis of many serologic tests for infection, including the Wassermann test for syphilis, and reactions for gonococcus infection, glanders, typhoid fever, tuberculosis, amebiasis, etc. Called also *alexin fixation, Bordet-Gengou phenomenon,* and *Bordet-Gengou reaction.* **elastic band f.,** the stabilization of fractured segments of the jaws by means of intermaxillary elastic bands applied to splints or appliances. **external pin f.,** a method for stabilizing fractures by means of pins drilled into the bony parts through the overlying skin and connected by metal bars. **external pin f., biphase,** external pin fixation in which the rigid metal bar connector is replaced with an acrylic bar adapted at the time of the reduction. **film f.,** in film processing, the chemical removal of all of the undeveloped salts of the film emulsion, so that only the developed (reduced) silver will remain as a manifest image. It involves immersion in the fixing solution, consisting of sodium thiosulfate, which dissolves the excess silver bromide salts; potassium alum, which hardens the emulsion by shrinking and tanning action on the gelatin; acetic acid, which acts as a neutralizer and removes fats from the gelatin; and sodium sulfite, which acts as a preservative. See also film DEVELOPMENT, film PROCESSING, and fixing SOLUTION. **internal f.,** the fastening together of the ends of a fractured bone by means of wires, plates, screws, or nails applied directly to the fractured bone. **intramedullary f.,** intramedullary NAILING. **intraosseous f.,** the open reduction and stabilization of fractured bony parts by direct fixation to one another with surgical wires, screws, pins, and/or plates. **maxillomandibular f.,** the fixation of fractures of the maxilla or mandible in a functional relationship with the opposing dental arch, through the use of elastics, wire ligatures, arch bars, or other splints. **medullary f.,** intramedullary NAILING. **nasomandibular f.,** mandibular immobilization, especially for edentulous jaws, using maxillomandibular splints; a circummandibular wire is connected with an intraoral interosseous wire passed through a hole drilled into the anterior nasal spine of the maxilla. **nitrogen f.,** extraction of elementary nitrogen from the atmosphere and uniting it with

various compounds to form such compounds as ammonia or nitrates; accomplished by some plants (legumes), certain soil micoorganisms, or through artificial processes. **skeletal f.,** immobilization of the ends of a fractured bone by metal wires or plates applied directly to the bone (*internal skeletal f.*) or on the body surface (*external skeletal f.*).

fixer (fik′ser) 1. an agent that allows something to be held in a fixed position or state. 2. fixing SOLUTION.

Fl. fluid.

F.l.a. abbreviation for L. *fi′at le′ge ar′tis,* let it be done according to rule.

flabby (flab′e) without firmness, hanging loosely or limply, as skin; flaccid.

flaccid (flak′sid) lacking body or stiffness; soft, flabby, weak.

flagella (flah-jel′ah) [L.] plural of *flagellum.*

Flagellata (flaj″e-la′tah) Mastigophora.

flagellate (flaj′ĕ-lāt) 1. any microorganism having flagella as organs of locomotion. 2. any protozoan organism of the subphylum Mastigophora (Flagellata). 3. having flagella.

flagellum (flah-jel′um), pl. *flagel′la* [L. "whip"] a mobile, whiplike projection from the free surface of a cell, serving as a locomotor organelle. Flagella are common to certain protozoa and certain bacteria and are also found in other cells, such as epithelial cells. Cf. CILIUM (3).

Flagg, Josiah Foster [1789–1853] a Boston dentist who contributed to the development of the field of dental ceramics, and was a pioneer in the development of the field of pedodontics.

flame (flām) 1. the luminous elongated or piriform, mobile appearance of burning gas or vapor, as from wood, coal, etc., which is undergoing combustion, caused by the light emitted from energetically excited chemical species, or something having a flamelike appearance. The flame obtained with the gas-air blowpipe is characterized by conical zones; the first emanating directly from the nozzle is the zone in which the air and gas are mixed before combustion; the green one surrounding it, known as the combustion zone, is the zone in which the gas and air are in partial combustion; the next is dimly blue, and is known as the reducing zone; and the outer zone, known as the oxidizing zone, is the one in which combustion occurs with the oxygen in the air. Little heat is given off by the inner zone and the hottest part of the flame is the reducing zone just beyond the tip of the green combustion zone. Exposure of alloys and metals to the combustion and oxidizing zones causes oxidation. 2. to render an object sterile by exposure to a flame.

flaming (flām′ing) 1. emitting flame. 2. heating by flame, as in flame sterilization (see under STERILIZATION).

flange (flanj) 1. a projecting rim, collar, or ring on a shaft, pipe, or machine housing. 2. that part of the denture base which extends from the cervical ends of the teeth to the border of the denture. Called also *denture f.* **buccal f.,** the portion of the flange of a denture that occupies the buccal vestibule of the mouth and extends distally from the buccal notch. **denture f.,** flange (2). **labial f.,** the portion of the flange of a denture which occupies the labial vestibule of the mouth. **lingual f., mandibular lingual f.,** the portion of the flange of a mandibular denture which occupies the space adjacent to the residual alveolar ridge and next to the tongue.

flap (flap) 1. a section of tissue, such as skin or mucous membrane, partially detached from a part of the body, to be implanted at a new site or repositioned in its original position, having uninterrupted blood supply through its intact base. Called also *surgical f.* See also GRAFT. 2. an uncontrolled movement. **Abbé f.,** a triangular surgical flap taken from the median portion of the lower lip, and used to correct defects of the upper lip. **advancement f.,** sliding f. **bilobed f.,** Zimany's bilobed f. **bipedicle f.,** a pedicle flap with two vascular attachments. Called also *double-end f.* and *double pedicle f.* **circular f.,** a surgical flap of somewhat circular outline. **delayed transfer f.,** a surgical flap that is partially raised from its bed and then later replaced; done to force the flap to develop further collateral circulation through the pedicle. **direct transfer f.,** immediate transfer f. **distant f.,** a pedicle flap brought from a distant area and transplanted by bringing the donor area and the recipient site into close approximation. Called also *Italian f.* **double-end f., double pedicle f.,** bipedicle f. **envelope f.,** a mucoperiosteal flap retracted from a horizontal linear incision, as along the free gingival margin, with no vertical component of that incision. **Estlander f.,** a surgical flap cut from the corner of the upper lip, and used for repair of lateral defects of the lower lip. **full thickness f.,** 1. one containing a full thickness of tissue, such as the skin and subcutaneous tissue. 2. mucoperiosteal f. **full thickness perio-**

dontal f., a periodontal flap all of the soft tissue, including the periosteum, which is reflected to expose the underlying bone. Called also *mucoperiosteal periodontal f.* **full thickness skin f.,** skin f. **gauntlet f.,** pedicle f. **Gillies' f.,** rope f. **immediate transfer f.,** a surgical flap that is applied to the recipient site immediately after it is elevated from its bed. Called also *direct transfer f.* **Indian f.,** interpolated f. **interpolated f.,** a pedicle flap that is twisted or rotated on its base and placed into a contiguous area. Called also *Indian f.* **island f.,** a skin flap consisting of the skin and subcutaneous tissue with a pedicle made up of only the nutrient vessels. **Italian f.,** distant f. **lingual tongue f.,** a combination flap used to repair fistulae of the hard palate; a palatal flap forms the floor of the nose, and a flap taken from the back or edge of the tongue forms the palatal surface. **local f.,** surgical flap cut from the tissue neighboring the defect. **mucoperiosteal f.,** a flap of mucosal tissue, including the periosteum, reflected from bone. Called also *full thickness f.* **mucoperiosteal periodontal f.,** full thickness periodontal f. **mucosal f.,** partial thickness f. **mucosal periodontal f.,** split thickness periodontal f. **musculocutaneous f.,** a surgical flap cut from skin and muscle. **partial thickness f.,** one consisting of only the epithelium and a layer of underlying connective tissue. In periodontology, a flap of mucosa and connective tissue but not including the periosteum. Called also *mucosal f.* and *split thickness f.* **partial thickness periodontal f.,** split thickness periodontal f. **pedicle f.,** one consisting of full thickness of the skin or periodontal tissue, attached to the donor site by a pedicle with a nutrient blood supply. Called also *gauntlet f.* and *pedicle graft.* **periodontal f.,** a section of soft tissue surgically separated from the underlying bone; used chiefly to eliminate periodontal pockets, treat mucogingival defects, restore tissue destroyed by disease, and arrest gingival recession. **periodontal f., simple,** unpositioned f. **positioned f.,** a periodontal flap that is moved to a new position; it may be positioned mesially, distally, coronally, or apically. **repositioned f.,** one replaced to its original position; the term was used formerly in connection with a flap placed in a new position (see *positioned f.*). **rope f.,** a bipedicle flap made by elevating a long strip of tissue from its bed except at the two extremities, the cut edges then being sutured together to form a tube. Called also *Gillies' f., tube f., tubed pedicle f., tunnel f., Gillies' graft,* and *rope graft.* **rotation f.,** a pedicle flap whose width is increased by transforming the edge of the flap distal to the defect into a curved line; the flap is then rotated and a

counterincision is made at the base of the curved line, which increases the mobility of the flap. **skin f.,** a full-thickness mass or flap of tissue containing epidermis, dermis, and subcutaneous tissue. Called also *full thickness skin f.* **simple periodontal f.,** unpositioned f. **sliding f.,** one carried to its new position by a sliding technique of surgical advancement. Called also *advancement f.* **split thickness f.,** partial thickness f. **split thickness periodontal f.,** a periodontal flap including only the epithelium and a layer of the underlying connective tissue. Called also *mucosal periodontal f.* and *partial thickness periodontal f.* **surgical f.,** flap (1). **tube f., tubed pedicle f., tunnel f.,** rope f. **unrepositioned f.,** a periodontal flap which is replaced to the presurgical location at the end of the operation. Called also *simple periodontal f.* **von Langenbeck's pedicle mucoperiosteal f.,** a bipedicle flap of the conjoined mucoperiosteal tissues, used for closure of a cleft palate. **V-Y f.,** one in which the incision is made in the shape of a V and is sutured in the shape of a Y so as to lengthen an area of tissue; or conversely the incision is Y-shaped and the closure V-shaped to shorten an area of tissue. **Widman f.,** one created by a sectional incision starting at one end of the operative site in the center labial, buccal, or lingual surface of the tooth proceeding apically, obliquely, and distally, extending 2 to 4 mm on to the alveolar process and penetrating the gingiva, alveolar mucosa, and periosteum but avoiding penetration of the granulation tissue. A similar incision is made at the other end of the site. From the starting point of the first incision, a gingival incision is made following the gingival margin and extending interproximally to the next until reaching the other sectional incision. The gingiva is then dissected from the underlying granulation tissue and a mucoperiosteal flap is elevated exposing 2 to 3 mm of the alveolar process. The granulation tissue and calcareous deposits are removed. Rough bone projections are rounded off. The flaps are readapted and held in place by interproximal sutures but the interproximal bone is left exposed. **Widman f., modified,** one for reattachment or readaptation created by a scalloped reverse bevel incision to elevate a minimal mucoperiosteal flap. The collar of tissue proximal to the tooth is removed to the alveolar process. There is no correction of bone defects beyond that which may be needed to achieve adequate flap adaptation, including the interproximal area. Access is provided for root instrumentation and the soft tissues are readapted to the teeth and alveolar process without intentional apical positioning. **Z-f.,** one in which the incision is made in the shape of a Z so as to distribute the contraction into more than one direction; used to correct scars. **Zimany's bilobed f.,** a surgical flap consisting of a large lobe that is transposed into the primary defect and a smaller

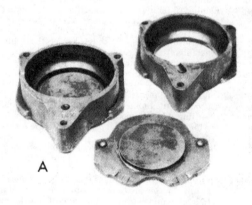

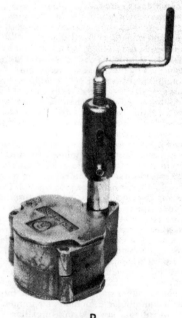

Denture flasks. *A,* For compression molding. *B,* For injection molding. (From R. W. Phillips: Skinner's Science of Dental Materials. 7th ed. Philadelphia, W. B. Saunders Co., 1973.)

A

B

second lobe that is transposed to fill the secondary defect produced by mobilization of the large lobe. Called also *bilobed f.*

flare (flār) 1. the red outermost zone of the "triple response" (Sir Thomas Lewis) urticarial wheal reaction, a manifestation of immediate, as opposed to delayed, allergy or hypersensitivity. 2. a spreading flush or area of redness on the skin, spreading out around an infective lesion or extending beyond the main point or reaction to an irritant. 3. sudden exacerbation of a disease.

flash (flash) excess material extruded from a mold, as in the packing of a denture by the compression technique.

flask (flask) 1. a small bottle or container. 2. a metal case in which the materials used in the fabrication of artificial dentures are placed for processing. 3. to place a denture in a flask for processing. **casting f.,** refractory f. **f. closure,** flask CLOSURE. **crown f.,** denture f. **f. culture,** one for growing cultures of bacteria or of other cells. **denture f.,** a sectional, boxlike case of metal which can be tightly closed, and with which sectional molds of plaster of Paris or dental stone are used to compress and form a resinous denture base or crown material during curing. Called also *crown f.* See illustration. See also compression MOLDING. **Erlenmeyer f.,** a glass flask with a conical body, broad base, and narrow neck. **injection f.,** one designed to permit the filling of the mold after the flask is closed or to permit the addition of denture base material to that in the flask after the flask is closed. **injection molding f.,** one into which a material, such as softened resin, is forced under pressure. See illustration. **refractory f.,** a metal tube in which a refractory mold is made for casting metal dental restorations. Called also *casting f.* and *casting ring.* **volumetric f.,** a narrow-necked vessel of glass calibrated to contain or deliver an exact volume at a given temperature.

flasking (flask'ing) 1. the act of investing in a flask. 2. the process of investing the cast and a wax denture in a flask preparatory to molding the denture base material into the form of the denture.

flatworm (flat'werm) any worm belonging to the phylum Platyhelminthes.

flav- see FLAVO-.

flavin (fla'vin) [L. *flavus* yellow] 1. a group of water-soluble pigments characterized by green fluorescence and the isoalloxazine nucleus (obtained by condensation of alloxan and monoalkyl-*o*-phenylenediamines), which are widely distributed in animal and plant tissues, including riboflavin and flavoprotein. 2. a yellow dye derived from oak bark. 3. flavoprotein.

flavine (fla'vin) ACRIFLAVINE hydrochloride.

Flavivirus (fla"vĭ-vi'rus) [L. *flavus* yellow + *virus*] a genus of arboviruses of the family Togaviridae, consisting of more than 30 viruses formerly classified in arbovirus group B. They may be transmitted by either mosquitoes or ticks, some by ingestion of contaminated milk. The name is associated with inclusion in the genus of the yellow fever virus (type species).

flavivirus (fla"vĭ-vi'rus) any virus of the genus *Flavivirus.*

flavo-, flav- [L. *flavus* yellow] a combining form meaning yellow.

Flavobacterium (fla"vo-bak-te're-um) [*flavo-* + Gr. *baktērion* little rod] a genus of gram-negative, facultatively anaerobic bacteria of uncertain affiliation, made up of motile (with peritrichous flagella) or nonmotile, coccoid or rod-shaped cells that characteristically produce orange, red, or yellow-brown pigmentation. Their metabolism is respiratory, and they are found in soil, fresh and sea water, on vegetables, and in dairy products. Some strains are suspected of being pathogenic. **F. bre've,** a species of nonmotile rods, ranging in size from 0.8 to 1.0 μm in width and 1.0 to 2.5 μm in length, which produce a light yellow pigment. They have been isolated from sewage, and are pathogenic to animals. Called also *B. brevis, B. canalis parvus,* and *Bacterium breve.* **F. meningosep'ticum,** a species of slender slightly curved rods with rounded ends, some encapsulated, which produce a yellow pigment. It has been isolated from the cerebrospinal fluid, blood, and throats of healthy human adults and infants, and also has been associated with meningitis and septicemia, particularly in infants.

flavone (fla'vōn) a plant pigment, 3-phenyl-4*H*-1-benzopyran-4-one, occurring as colorless, crystalline needles that are insoluble in water, which gives plants their yellow color. Numerous dyes are derived from it.

flavoprotein (fla"vo-pro'te-in) [*flavo-* + *protein*] a conjugated protein, being an oxidative enzyme, made up of a protein linked to coenzymes which are mono- or dinucleotides containing riboflavin. Because of their color, they are called *yellow enzymes.* Called also *flavin.*

Flavurol trademark for *merbromin.*

fld fluid.

fl dr fluid DRAM.

Flecks Cement see under CEMENT.

Fleming, Sir Alexander [1881–1955] a Scottish bacteriologist; co-winner, with Ernst Boris Chain and Sir Howard Walter Florey, of the Nobel prize for medicine and physiology in 1945, for the discovery of penicillin.

Flemming's center, interfibrillar substance [Walther *Flemming,* German anatomist, 1843–1905] see germinal CENTER and HYALOPLASM (1).

flesh (flesh) the soft, muscular tissue of the animal body. **proud f.,** excessive proliferation of granulation tissue associated with edema. See also exuberant GRANULATION.

flexibilitas (flek-sĭ-bil'ĭ-tas) [L.] flexibility.

flexibility (flek"sĭ-bil'ĭ-te) [L. *flexibilitas*] the ability to bend without a tendency to break. The term is sometimes used to indicate low brittleness, low stiffness, or low strength. **maximal f.,** the strain which occurs when a material is stressed to its proportional limit.

flexible (flek'sĭ-b'l) [L. *flexibilis, flexilis*] readily bent without a tendency to break.

Flexicon trademark for a *silicone impression material* (see under MATERIAL).

fleximeter (fleks-im'ĕ-ter) an instrument for measuring the amount of flexion of a joint.

flexion (flek'shun) [L. *flexio*] the act or process of bending.

Flexner's bacillus [Simon *Flexner,* American pathologist, 1863–1946] *Shigella flexneri;* see under SHIGELLA.

flexor (flek'sor) [L.] any muscle that flexes a joint.

Flexowax C trademark for a synthetic *dental wax* (see under WAX).

flexura (flek-shoo'rah), pl. *flexu'rae* [L.] flexure; a bending; a general anatomical term for a bent portion of a structure or organ.

flexurae (flek-shoo're) [L.] plural of *flexura.*

flexure (flek'sher) [L. *flexura*] a bending; a bent portion of a structure or organ. **f. strength,** flexure STRENGTH.

flocculation (flok"u-la'shun) a colloid phenomenon in which the dispersed phase separates into coarse, discrete, macroscopically visible particles rather than into a continuous mass, as in coagulation. See also flocculation TEST.

Flogoril trademark for OXYPHENBUTAZONE.

floor (floor) the lower part of a hollow structure. See also PARIES, ROOF, TECTUM, TEGMEN, and WALL. **axial f.,** axial WALL. **cavity f.,** the bottom or enclosing base wall of a prepared cavity upon which rests the restorative material. One on the axial plane is known as the *axial wall* and on the horizontal plane as the *pulpal wall.* **f. of nasal cavity,** palate. **f. of oral cavity,** sublingual SULCUS. **f. of orbit,** the inferior wall of the orbit, formed by the orbital surface of the maxilla, the orbital process of the zygomatic bone, and a small portion of the orbital process of the palatine bone. It lodges the lacrimal sulcus for the nasolacrimal canal and the infraorbital groove, which leads into the infraorbital canal and transmits the infraorbital nerve and vessels, and gives attachment to the obliquus inferior oculi muscle. Called also *inferior wall of orbit* and *paries inferior orbitae* (NA). **pulpal f.,** pulpal WALL.

flora (flo'rah) [L. *Flora,* the goddess of flowers] the plant life present in or characteristic of a special location. **mouth f., oral f.,** MOUTH flora.

flores [flo'rēz] [L., pl. of *flos* flower] 1. the blossoms or flowers of a plant. 2. a drug after sublimation. See also FLOWERS.

Florey unit [Sir Howard Walter *Florey,* English pathologist, born 1898; co-winner, with Ernst Boris Chain and Sir Alexander Fleming, of the Nobel prize for medicine and physiology in 1945, for the discovery of penicillin] Oxford UNIT.

florid (flor'id) [L. *floridus* blossoming] 1. in full bloom; occurring in fully developed form. 2. having a bright red color.

Florocid trademark for a sodium fluoride preparation.

floss (flos) any soft thread, usually of silk or cotton. **dental f.,** soft nylon or silk thread, waxed or unwaxed, used for cleaning the interdental spaces and dislodging loose debris, to carry a rubber dam through contact areas, or for testing contacts. **f. tape,** floss TAPE.

flour (flowr, flow'er) 1. finely ground meal of grain. 2. any fine, soft powder. **f. of pumice,** see PUMICE.

flow (flo) 1. to run or move smoothly in a manner characteristic of a fluid. 2. a smooth, uninterrupted movement characteristic of a fluid. 3. to circulate, as the blood. 4. a permanent deformation of materials under load, as the slow bending of a glass rod under its own weight when it is supported only at its two ends. The flow of dental materials, such as amalgams or waxes, is measured under compressive stress, whereby a cylinder of the material is placed under a certain compressive stress for a certain time, the flow being measured by the percent of shortening in length of the cylinder at the end of the test. See also CREEP (2). **gene f.,** gradual diffusion of genes from one population group to another. **f. technique filling,** flow technique FILLING.

flowers (flow'erz) 1. the blossoms of a plant. 2. a sublimed drug, as sulfur or benzoin. **f. of Benjamin,** benzoic ACID. **f. of benzoin,** benzoic ACID. **f. of tin,** stannic OXIDE.

flowmeter (flo'me-ter) an apparatus for measuring the rate of flow of liquids or gases.

floxacillin (flok"sah-sil'in) a penicillinase-resistant penicillin, 6-[3-(2-chloro-6-fluorophenyl)-5-methyl-4-isoxazolecarboxamido]-3,3-dimethyl-7-oxo-4-thia-1-azabicyclo[3,2,0]heptane-2-carboxylic acid. Trademarks: Floxapen, Flucloxacillin.

Floxapen trademark for *floxacillin.*

floxuridine (floks-ur'ĭ-den) a pyrimidine analogue, 2'-deoxy-5-fluorouridine, occurring as a white, odorless solid that is soluble in water, isopropanol, methanol, ether ethanol, and acetone, but not in chloroform, ether, and benzene. It competitively inhibits DNA synthesis by converting into a false nucleotide. Used as an antineoplastic agent in the treatment of cancer of the oropharynx, breast, colon, stomach, ovary, pancreas, and other organs, the use being restricted to cancers incurable by other means. Adverse reactions are similar to those of other pyrimidine analogues, and include lesions of the oral mucosa. Abbreviated *FUDR.* Called also *fluorodeoxyuridine.*

fl oz fluid OUNCE.

flu (floo) popular name for INFLUENZA.

Flucloxacillin trademark for *floxacillin.*

Flucort trademark for *flumethasone.*

fluctuation (fluk"tu-a'shun) [Lat. *fluctuatio*] 1. a variation, as about a fixed value or mass. 2. A wavelike motion, as of a fluid in a cavity of the body after succussion.

flucytosine (floo-si'to-sēn) an antifungal drug, 4-amino-5-fluoro-2(1*H*)-pyrimidinone, occurring as a white, odorless, crystalline powder that is soluble in water and ethanol, but not in chloroform and ether. It acts as an antimetabolite which interferes with nucleoprotein synthesis. Used in the treatment of infections caused by *Cryptococcus, Candida, Trulopsis glabrata, Sporotrichum schenckii,* and *Aspergillus,* and in other mycoses. Side effects may include nausea, vomiting, diarrhea, skin rashes, sedation, confusion, hallucinations, headache, vertigo, azotemia, and bone marrow depression with anemia, leukopenia, and thrombocytopenia. Called also *5-fluorocytosine.* Trademarks: Ancobon, Ancotil.

fludrocortisone (floo"dro-kor'tĭ-sōn) a synthetic mineralocorticoid with some glucocorticoid activity, 9-fluoro-11β,17,21-trihydroxypregn-4-ene-3,20-dione. Used chiefly for replacement therapy in adrenal insufficiency. Also used in the treatment of inflammatory, allergic, neoplastic, and other disorders. Side effects may include euphoria, paradoxical mental depression, hypertension, anorexia, peptic ulcer, colonic ulcers, increased susceptibility to infections, suppression of ACTH release, fat redistribution in the body, hypoglycemia, hypopotassemia, alkalosis, osteoporosis, myopathy, purpura, ecchymoses, and fractures. Called also *fludocortisone.* Trademarks: Alflorone, Astonin-H, Fluorocortone. **f. 21-acetate,** the 21-acetate salt of fludrocortisone, occurring as a white to yellowish, odorless powder that is soluble in ether, ethanol, and chloroform, but not in water. Its pharmacological and toxicological properties are similar to those of the parent compound. Trademark: Scherofluron.

fludroxycortide (floo-drok'sĭ-kor'tĭd) flurandrenolide.

fluid (floo'id) [L. *fluidus*] a substance that flows readily, being composed of elements or particles which freely change their relative position without their separating, such as liquid or gas. **amniotic f.,** fluid within the amniotic cavity produced by the amnion at the very earliest period of fetation and later by the lungs and kidneys; at first crystal clear, it later becomes cloudy. Its role consists of providing a protective water cushion for the fetus, absorbing jolts, equalization of pressure, and prevention of adherence to the amnion. It circulates and late in pregnancy replaces its water component at the rate of 500 ml each hour. The normal amount of amniotic fluid varies from 1/3 liter to 2 liters. **body f.,** a fluid necessary in the physiology of bodily functions. Principal normal body fluids are divided into intracellular fluids and extracellular fluids, including the interstitial fluid, cerebrospinal fluid, intraocular fluid, digestive fluids, blood plasma, lymph, urine, and synovial fluid. Body fluids represent about 50 to 57 percent of the total body weight. See also body water VOLUME and body WATER. **cerebrospinal f.,** a

clear, colorless liquid having small amounts of protein, glucose, and potassium and relatively large amounts of sodium chloride, contained within the four ventricles of the brain, subarachnoid space, choroid plexus, and brain parenchyma; it is circulated through the ventricles into the subarachnoid space, and is absorbed into the venous system. Abbreviated *C.S.F.* Called also *liquor cerebrospinalis* [NA]. **crevicular f.,** gingival f. **Dakin's f.,** sodium hypochlorite solution, diluted; see under SOLUTION. **dialyzing f.,** an isotonic aqueous solution used in extracorporeal or peritoneal dialysis, containing concentrations of sodium, potassium, calcium, magnesium, bicarbonate, lactate, and glucose that are identical with those of normal plasma, but containing no urea, creatinine, or urates. In chemical processes, the fluid is not always isotonic. **extracellular f.,** a general term for all the body fluids outside the cells, which circulates with the fluid of the blood through the capillary walls and supplies the cells with the needed nutrients and other substances. Abbreviated *ECF.* See illustration. See also active TRANSPORT and DIFFUSION. **gingival f.,** a fluid occurring in minute amounts in the gingival crevice, believed by some authorities to be an inflammatory exudate and by others to cleanse material from the crevice, contain sticky plasma proteins which improve adhesion of the epithelial attachment, have antimicrobial properties, and exert antibody activity. Its composition is similar to blood serum except in the proportions, containing electrolytes, amino acids, plasma proteins, fibrolytic factors, gamma globulins, albumin, lysozyme, fibrinogen, and acid phosphatase. Its amount increases by inflammation, chewing coarse foods, toothbrushing, massage, ovulation, and administration of hormonal contraceptives. Called also *crevicular f.* **inflammatory f.,** exudate. **interstitial f.,** the extracellular fluid that bathes the cells of most tissues but which is not within the confines of the blood or lymph vessels and is not a transcellular fluid; it is formed by filtration through the blood capillaries and is drained away as lymph. It is the extracellular fluid volume minus the lymph volume, the plasma volume, and the transcellular fluid volume. Called also *tissue f.* **intracellular f.,** the fluid inside the cells of the body, which contains dissolved solutes of substances necessary to cells for growth, repair, and carrying on their various functions. See illustrations. See also active TRANSPORT and DIFFUSION. **lymphatic f.,** lymph. **noninflammatory edema f.,** transudate. **oral f.,** saliva. **silicone f.,** SILICONE fluid. **synovial f.,** a clear, yellowish, viscous liquid, resembling the white of an egg, which serves to lubricate the joints and is contained in joint cavities, bursae, and tendon sheaths. It is supplied by a network of capillaries of the synovial membrane and is considered to be a dialysate of blood plasma containing albumin, globulin, and mucin. Called also *synovia.* **tissue f.,** interstitial f. **transcellular f.,** that portion of the extracellular fluid produced by active cellular secretion.

fluiddram (floo"id-ram') fluid DRAM.

fluidounce (floo-id-ouns') fluid OUNCE.

	EXTRACELLULAR FLUID	INTRACELLULAR FLUID
Na+	142 mEq/l.	10 mEq/l.
K+	5 mEq/l.	141 mEq/l
Ca++	5 mEq/l.	<1 mEq/l
Mg++	3 mEq/l.	58 mEq/l
Cl–	103 mEq/l.	4 mEq/l
HCO3–	28 mEq/l.	10 mEq/l
Phosphates	4 mEq/l.	75 mEq/l
SO4– –	1 mEq/l.	2 mEq/l
Glucose	90 mgm.%	0 to 20 mgm.%
Amino acids	30 mgm.%	200 mgm.%?
Cholesterol Phospholipids Neutral fat	0.5 gm.%	2 to 95 gm.%
Po2	35 mm.Hg	20 mm.Hg ?
Pco2	46 mm.Hg	50 mm.Hg ?
pH	7.4	7.0

Chemical compositions of extracellular and intracellular fluids. (From A. C. Guyton: Textbook of Medical Physiology. 6th ed. Philadelphia, W. B. Saunders Co., 1981.)

fluke (flōōk) 1. the triangular part of an anchor that catches the ground. 2. a structure or device that resembles the fluke of an anchor. 3. a trematode worm. **endosteal implant f.,** the end portion of the arm of an endosteal implant that rises to the most superficial portion within the bone.

flumethasone (floo-meth′ah-sōn) a potent anti-inflammatory glucocorticoid, 6 α, 9 - difluoro - 11β, 17α, 21 - trihydroxy - 16 α-methylpregna-1,4 diene-3,20-dione. Used chiefly in the topical therapy of skin diseases. Because of its rapid metabolic rate, side effects are minor. Trademarks: Aniprime, Cortexilar, Flucort. **f. 21-pivalate,** the 21-pivalate salt of flumethasone, occurring as a white crystalline powder that is slightly soluble in methanol, chloroform, and methylene chloride and insoluble in water. Its pharmacological and toxicological properties are similar to those of the parent compound. Trademarks: Locacorten, Locorten.

Flumethone trademark for *paramethasone*.

Fluocinil trademark for *fluocinolone acetonide* (see under FLUOCINOLONE).

fluocinolone acetonide (floo″o-sin′o-lōn) a potent glucocorticoid with anti-inflammatory and metabolic actions, 6α,9-difluoro-11β,21-dihydroxy-16α, 17-[(1-methylethylidene)bis(oxy)-pregna]-1,4-diene-3,20-dione, occurring as a white, odorless, crystalline powder that is soluble in ethanol, acetone, and methanol, slightly soluble in chloroform, and insoluble in water. Used in the treatment of nummular dermatitis, psoriasis, and neurodermatitis. It suppresses the inflammatory defenses to infection, sometimes leading to superinfection. Folliculitis or striae may occur under occlusive dressings. Topical preparations of fluocinolone acetonide often include neomycin to suppress secondary infections. Trademark: Dermalar, Fluocinil, Fluovitef, Jellin, Localyn, Synalar, Synamol, Synsac.

fluodrocortisone (floo″o-dro-kor′tĭ-sōn) fludrocortisone.

Fluomazina trademark for *triflupromazine hydrochloride* (see under TRIFLUPROMAZINE].

Fluon trademark for *polytetrafluoroethylene*.

fluorandrenolone (floo″or-an-dren′o-lōn) flurandrenolide.

fluorescein (floo″o-res′e-in) a fluorane dye and the parent compound of eosin, 2-(3,6-dihydroxy-9H-xanthen-9-yl)-benzoic acid. It occurs as a bright yellow powder that is soluble in alkali hydroxides or carbonates, alcohol, and ether, but not in water, and readily oxidizes in the presence of air. Used intravenously in fluorescent antibody technique. Also used to assess by its fluorescence the adequacy of circulation and combined with radioactive iodine in localization of brain tumors and other pathological conditions. Called also *dihydroxyfluorane* and *resorcinolphthalein*.

fluorescence (floo″o-res′ens) the property of emitting energy as an electromagnetic photon after absorbing energy, such as x-rays or ultraviolet light, the wavelength of the emitted energy being longer than that of the energy absorbed. Fluorescent radiation is a part of secondary radiation in roentgenography, and it is sometimes responsible for distortion of x-ray images. See also fluorescent RADIATION, LUMINESCENCE, PHOSPHORESCENCE, and secondary rays, under RAY.

fluoridation (floo-or″ĭ-da-shun) treatment with fluorides; specifically, the addition of about 1 ppm fluorine (as sodium fluoride, sodium fluorosilicate, stannous fluoride, or other fluoride) to the public water supply as part of the public health program to prevent or reduce the incidence of dental caries.

fluoride (floo′o-rīd) a salt of hydrofluoric acid, containing the radical F; it is a bound form of fluorine occurring in many tissues, notably the bones, teeth, thyroid gland, skin, aorta, and kidneys. Fluorides are absorbed from the gastrointestinal tract, lungs, and skin, the degree of absorption being determined by their solubility, and are excreted with the urine, sweat, saliva, and milk. Topical application of fluorides and their presence in drinking water prevent the development of dental caries. The F ion displaces the OH group in hydroxyapatite to form fluoroapatite in the hard tooth tissue, which is resistant to acids and carbohydrate decomposition products, thereby inhibiting cariogenesis. Fluorides also inhibit metabolism of oral bacterial enzymes, enzymes involved in tissue respiration and anaerobic glycolysis, and enzymes requiring calcium, manganese, magnesium, and copper, e.g., enolase, esterases, and alkaline phosphatases. Fluorides are used in the treatment of osteoporosis, Paget's disease of bone, and multiple myeloma, their action being that of calcium retention. In dentistry, fluorides are used in various topical preparations, dentrifices, and mouthwashes. Acute fluoride poisoning usually results from the accidental ingestion of an insecticide or rodenticide containing fluorides, usually characterized by excessive salivation, nausea, abdominal pain, vomiting, diarrhea, irritability, hyperreflexia, convulsions, hypocalcemia, hypoglycemia, and hypotension, with death occurring due to cardiac arrest and initial respiratory stimulation followed by depression. Chronic poisoning may result from prolonged exposure, such as when drinking water with high concentrations of fluorides. Osteosclerosis, calcifications of ligaments, and mottled enamel are the principal complications of chronic poisoning. **acidulated f.,** a fluoride preparation that has been acidified, usually with orthophosphoric acid; used in dental caries control. **f. dentrifice,** fluoride DENTRIFICE. **hydrogen f.,** a highly toxic gas, HF, which, in aqueous solution, forms hydrofluoric acid. Contact or inhalation may produce corrosive lesions of the skin, eyes, and mucous membranes; chronic inhalation of small amounts may produce fluorosis. Used in small amounts, particularly with other fluorides, in dental caries control. Called also *anhydrous hydrofluoric acid* and *hydrofluoric acid gas*. **sodium f.,** a compound, NaF, occurring as white crystals which are soluble in water, but not in alcohol; used in dentistry in dental caries prevention. Its mechanism of action on the tooth tissue is not fully understood, but it is believed to harden the outer layers of the enamel, thus reducing its solubility, through forming calcium fluoride or calcium fluoropatite. In aqueous solution, sodium fluoride has a neutral reaction, but tends to change to alkaline in a glass container; in a polyethylene bottle, it remains neutral. Sodium fluoride is used as tablets for oral administration, in solution for topical application, and in water fluoridation. It is also used as an agricultural insecticide and pesticide. Excessive intake of sodium fluoride may cause poisoning (see FLUORIDE). Trademarks: Florocid, Karidium, Lemoflur, Ossalin, Ossin, Villaumite, Zymafluor. **stannous f.,** a compound SnF₂, occurring as an odorless, white, crystalline solid with a bitter salty taste, which is soluble in water, but not in alcohol, ether, and chloroform. On exposure to air, it forms oxyfluoride. In aqueous solution, it is slightly acidic and deteriorates with formation of a white precipitate. Used as a topical agent in dental caries control, either in an aqueous solution or in dentifrices. Similarly to other fluorides, it is highly toxic by ingestion and on contact, causing irritation and necrotic changes in the mucous membranes and the skin. Called also *tin difluoride*. Trademark: Fluoristan. **topical f.,** a fluoride preparation, usually a 2 percent aqueous solution of sodium, stannous, or other fluorides, which is applied directly to the teeth of growing children in dental caries prevention programs. The use of fluoride-containing dentifrices and mouth rinses (usually a 0.02 to 0.1 percent fluoride solution) is also considered as a form of topical application.

Fluorident liquid see under LIQUID.

Fluorigard mouthrinse see under MOUTHRINSE.

fluorine (floo′o-rēn) [L. *fluere*, flow, flux] a gaseous halogen, occurring as a pale yellow gas with a pungent odor. Symbol, F; atomic number, 9; atomic weight, 18.998; group VIIA of the periodic table; valence, 1. It has one artificial radioactive isotope, ¹⁸F (half-life of 109.7 min). Fluorine is the most electronegative and reactive of all elements, reacting with all organic and most inorganic substances, violently with oxidizable substances. Because of its reactivity, it does not occur in a natural state, but is always found in a combined form. Fluorine occurs in many tissues as fluorides, notably the bones, teeth, thyroid gland, and skin. Used in the prevention of dental caries, also as a fluoride. It is a strong corrosive irritant; inhalation or contact with may cause lesions of the skin, eyes, and mucous membranes. Chronic absorption may cause mottled enamel, osteosclerosis, and calcification of ligaments.

Fluoristan trademark for a preparation of *stannous fluoride* (see under FLUORIDE).

Fluoritab trademark for a preparation of *sodium fluoride* (see under FLUORIDE).

Fluormone trademark for *dexamethasone*.

fluoroapatite (floor″o-ap′ah-tīt) a compound formed in the tooth enamel when a fluoride ion replaces the OH ion of hydroxyapatite, which is resistant to carbohydrate fermentation products and, thus, renders the teeth resistant to acid decay.

fluorocarbon (floo″o-ro-kar′bon) an organic fluorine and carbon compound, being similar to a hydrocarbon in which all or nearly all the hydrogen has been replaced by fluorine. Fluorocarbons are generally characterized by chemical inertness, nonflammability, heat stability, and low refractive indices, solubility, and surface tension. Used as aerosol propellants, refrigerants, solvents, fire-extinguishing agents, and lubricants, and in a variety of industrial processes. Fluorocarbons are suspected of destroying ozone in the stratosphere, and their use is regulated by the Food and Drug Administration. Trademark: Freon. **f. 11,** trichlorofluoromethane. **f. 114,** dichlorotetrafluoroethane.

5-fluorocytosine (floo′or-o-si′to-sēn) flucytosine.

fluorodeoxyuridine (floo″or-de-ok″se-ur′ĭ-dēn) floxuridine.

Fluorofen trademark for *triflupromazine hydrochloride* (see under TRIFLUPROMAZINE).

Fluoroflex trademark for *polytetrafluoroethylene.*

fluorography (floo″or-og′rah-fe) photofluorography.

Fluor-O-Kote topical fluoride gel see under GEL.

Fluoromar trademark for *fl
uroxene.*

fluorometer (floo″or-om′ĕ-ter) 1. an apparatus for measuring the quantity of rays given out by an x-ray tube. 2. an attachment for the fluoroscope, enabling the operator to secure the correct and undistorted shadow of the object and to locate exactly the position of the object.

fluorometholone (floor″o-meth′o-lōn) an anti-inflammatory glucocorticoid 9 - fluoro - 11β, 17 - dihydroxy - 6α - methylpregna - 1, 4 - diene - 3, 20 - dione, occurring as a white or yellowish, odorless, crystalline powder that is slightly soluble in ethanol, chloroform, and ether, and insoluble in water. Used chiefly in topical therapy of skin diseases. Trademarks: Cortilet, Delmeson, Loticort, Oxylone.

Fluoroplex trademark for *fluorouracil.*

fluoroentgenography (floo″o-ro-rent″gen-og′rah-fe) photofluorography.

fluoroscope (floo′o-ro-skōp) [*fluorescence* + Gr. *skopein* to examine] an instrument for immediate indirect examination of deep structures by means of x-rays, with or without contrast media. It consists of a screen suitably mounted with respect to an x-ray tube, on which the effect of radiation produces a fluorescent image of the examined organ. The screen is sealed to protect it from dirt and sandwiched between a protective cover mounted on the x-ray tube and a leaded glass on the viewing side — the lead partially protecting the operator from direct radiation. Called also *roentgenoscope.* See also fluorescent SCREEN (1).

fluoroscopy (floo″or-os′ko-pe) examination by means of the fluoroscope.

fluorosis (floo″or-os′sis) mottled ENAMEL.

Fluoro-Thin Cement see under CEMENT.

Fluoro-Uracil trademark for *fluorouracil.*

fluorouracil (floo″o-ur′ah-sil) a pyrimidine analogue, 5-fluoro-2,4(1*H*,3*H*)-pyrimidinedione, occurring as a white, odorless, crystalline powder that is soluble in water, ethanol, and methanol, and is insoluble in ether, benzene, and chloroform. It is a congener of uracil, which blocks the synthesis of thymidilic acid and deoxyribonucleic acid. Used as an antineoplastic agent in the treatment of cancers of the oropharynx, breast, colon, stomach, ovary, pancreas, and other organs. Also used in precancerous skin lesions and as an immunosuppressive agent in tissue and organ transplantation. Adverse reactions are similar to those of other pyrimidine analogues, and include lesions of the oral mucosa. Called also *5-FU.* Trademarks: Fluoracil, Fluril, Fluoroplex, Fluoro Uracil.

Fluotestin trademark for *fluoxymesterone.*

Fluothane trademark for *halothane.*

Fluovitef trademark for *fluocinolone acetonide* (see under FLUOCINOLONE).

fluoxymesterone (floo-ok″se-mes′ter-ōn) an anabolic androgen, 9 α - fluoro - 11 β, 17 β - hydroxy - 17 - methylandrost -4- en - 3 - one; occurring as a white, odorless, tasteless solid that is soluble in ethanol, slightly soluble in chloroform, and insoluble in water. Used in substitutional therapy of testicular insufficiency and in the palliative treatment of cancer. Sometimes used with estrogens in the treatment of postmenopausal osteoporosis. Side effects may include hirsutism, deepening of the voice, precocious puberty and epiphyseal closure, increased libido, priapism, flushing, acne, hypercalcemia, weight gain, and edema. Trademarks: Androfluorene, Androsterolo, Fluotestin, Halotestin, Testoral.

fluphenazine (floo-fen′ah-zēn) a major phenothiazine tranquilizer, 4-[3-[2-(trifluoromethyl)-10*H*-phenothiazin-10-yl]propyl]-1-piperazineethanol. Used in the treatment of psychotic disorders. Side effects may include parkinsonism, dystonia, dyskinesia, akathisia, oculogyric crises, opisthotonos, hyperreflexia, liver lesions, itching, erythema, urticaria, exfoliative dermatitis, endocrine disorders, and blood dyscrasias, including leukopenia, agranulocytosis, thrombocytopenic purpura, eosinophilia, and pancytopenia. Trademarks: Elinol, Pacinol, Prolixin, Siqualine, Siqualon, Tensofin, Valamina, Vespazine. **f. decanoate,** a salt of fluphenazine, occurring as a light-sensitive, yellow or yellowish orange viscous liquid with a characteristic odor, which is soluble in ethanol, acetone, benzene, and ether, but not in water. Its pharmacological and toxicological properties are similar to those of the parent compounds. **f. enanthate,** a salt of fluphenazine, occurring as a pale-yellow to orange-yellow, light-sensitive, turbid, viscous liquid that is soluble in ethanol, ether, benzene, and chloroform, but not in water. Its pharmacological and toxicological properties are similar to those of the parent compound. **f. hydrochloride,** the dihydrochloride salt of fluphenazine, occurring as a white, odorless, crystalline powder that is soluble in water, slightly soluble in acetone, ethanol, and chloroform, and insoluble in benzene and ether. Its pharmacological and toxicological properties are similar to those of the parent compound. Trademarks: Anatensol, Dapotum, Lyogen, Moditen, Omca, Trancin.

Fluracil trademark for *fluorouracil.*

Flura-Drops trademark for a solution, four drops of which contain 2.21 mg sodium fluoride, being equivalent to 1 mg fluoride ion; used in the prevention of dental caries.

Flura-Loz see under LOZENGE.

flurandrenolide (floor″an-dren′o-līd) a glucocorticoid, 6α-fluoro-11 β, 21 - dihydroxy - 16 α, 17 - [(1 - methylethylidene) bis (oxy)]-pregn-4-ene-3,20-dione, occurring as a white, odorless, crystalline powder that is soluble in chloroform and methanol, sparingly soluble in ethanol, and insoluble in water and ether. Used in the treatment of contact, atopic, and seborrheic dermatitis, pruritus, and neurodermatitis. It has a high potency topically, but low potency systemically. It suppresses the inflammatory defenses to infection, sometimes leading to superinfection. Topical preparations of flurandrenolide often include Neomycin to suppress secondary infections. Called also *fludroxycortide, fluorandrenolone, flurandrenolone,* and *flurandrenolone acetonide.* Trademarks: Cordran, Drenison, Drocort.

flurandrenolone, flurandrenolone acetonide (floor″an-dren′o-lōn) flurandrenolide.

Flura-Tablets see under TABLET.

flurazepam (floor-az′ĕ-pam) a hypnotic 7-chloro-1-[2-(diethylamino)ethyl] - 5 - (*o* - fluorophenyl) - 1, 3 - dihydro-2*H* -1,4-benzodiazepin-2-one, occurring as an off-white to yellowish crystalline powder with a slight odor, which is soluble in water and alcohol and slightly soluble in chloroform. Used chiefly in insomnia and sleep disorders, being contraindicated in hypersensitivity, pregnancy, children under 12 years of age, depression in elderly patients, liver and kidney disorders, and patients with a history of drug addiction. Abuse of flurazepam may lead to habituation or addiction. Adverse reactions that may be associated with its use include excessive salivation, xerostomia, headache, chest pains, and a wide variety of other disorders. Trademark: Dalmane.

Fluril trademark for *fluorouracil.*

Fluorocid trademark for a preparation of *sodium fluoride* (see under FLUORIDE).

Flurocortone trademark for *fludrocortisone.*

flurothyl (floor′o-thil) a central nervous system stimulant and convulsant, 1,1′-oxybis[2,2,2-trifluoroethane], occurring as a clear, colorless, volatile liquid with a mild ethereal odor, which is slightly soluble in water and miscible with ethanol, ether, propylene glycol, and halogenated solvents. Trademark: Indoklon.

fluroxene (floor-oks′ēn) a general inhalation anesthetic, (2,2,2-trifluoroethoxy)ethene, occurring as a clear, colorless, volatile liquid with an ethereal odor, which is soluble in water, and miscible with ethanol, ether, acetone, and halogenated solvents. Used in dental and other types of surgical procedures requiring only the first or upper second plane of anesthesia. Toxic effects are believed to be minimal. Trademark: Fluoromar.

flush (flush) 1. a redness of the face and neck; blushing. 2. a sudden increase of flow. 3. a sudden flow of liquid. **atropine f.,** flushing and dryness of the skin of the face and neck from overdosage with atropine. **carcinoid f.,** extensive blotchy red or bluish flushing on the face or trunk, often associated with diarrhea and abdominal pain, and sometimes with bronchospasm; it is possibly due to vasoactive kinins or other peptides associated with carcinoid tumor. **hectic f.,** a persistent or chronic flush of the skin associated with a chronic debilitating disease, usually febrile, such as pulmonary tuberculosis. **histamine f.,** sudden symmetric erythema of the face and upper trunk, usually associated with throbbing headache and bounding pulse, and histaminuria; seen in urticaria pigmentosa, it may also occur a few minutes after eating fish of the scombroid family (red snapper or mahimahi) contaminated by *Proteus* during cold storage prior to cooking. **mahogany f.,** a deep red or mahogany-colored, circumscribed spot seen on one cheek in some cases of lobar pneumonia. **malar f.,** hectic flush at the malar eminence.

Flutra trademark for *trichlormethiazide*.

flutter (flut′er) a rapid vibration or pulsation. **atrial f.**, a form of cardiac arrhythmia characterized by a rapid atrial contraction in the presence of a regular or irregular ventricular rate. The electrocardiogram shows a typical saw-tooth arrangement of the P waves and absent P-R interval. The ventricles not being able to respond to each atrial impulse, a partial block is usually present.

flux (fluks) 1. an excessive flow or discharge. 2. any substance that promotes the fusing of minerals or metals and prevents the formation of oxides. 3. any substance applied to metals that are to be united which, on application of heat, aids the flow of solder and prevents formation of oxides. 4. any fusible glass or enamel used as a base in ceramic processing. 5. the rate of flow or transfer of electricity, water, heat, energy, etc., determined in quantities that cross a unit area of a given surface in a unit of time. 6. the intensity of neutron radiation, expressed as the number of neutrons passing through 1 cm² in 1 sec. **casting f.**, a flux that increases fluidity of the metal and helps in preventing oxidation. **ceramic f.**, a flux used in the manufacture of porcelain and silicate powders. The fluorides, melting at a lower temperature than other ingredients, and aluminum phosphate are types of ceramic flux. **ionic f.**, the number of mols per second passing through an area of 1 cm² oriented perpendicularly to the direction of flow of the substance, expressed in ergs/cm². **luminous f.**, the rate of passage or radiant energy evaluated by reference to the luminous sensation produced by it. **magnetic f.**, magnetic field lines passing through a surface. **neutral f.**, a fusible material, usually an inorganic salt, which does not unite with the combined oxygen in the metal but merely dissolves the metal oxide. **neutron f.**, a measure of the intensity of neutron radiation. It is the number of neutrons passing through 1 square centimeter of a given target in 1 second. See also radiation INTENSITY. **oxidizing f.**, a material which, when heated, gives up oxygen but may unite with the base metals and form oxides. **radiant f.**, the rate of flow of radiant energy. **reducing f.**, a flux which contains powdered charcoal and unites with the oxygen of metallic oxides to free the metal impurities. **soldering f.**, a flux used for enhancing the flow of molten solder and to provide a tarnish-free surface in soldering. A typical soldering flux is a mixture of 55 parts borax glass, 35 parts boric acid, and 10 parts silica.

fly (flī) a dipterous, or· two-winged, insect. **Spanish f.**, cantharides.

Fm fermium.

F.M. abbreviation for L. *fi′at mistu′ra*, make a mixture.

FMA Frankfort–mandibular plane ANGLE.

FMG foreign medical graduate; see Educational Commission for Foreign Medical Graduates, under COMMISSION.

F.O.A. Federation of Orthodontic Associations.

Foamaseptic trademark for an antibacterial foam containing 0.25 percent benzethonium chloride, 15.3 percent isopropanol, and various amounts of methanol, ethoxylated lanolin, vegetable oil, and other emollients.

focal (fo′kal) pertaining to or occupying a focus.

foci (fo′si) [L.] plural of *focus*.

focus (fo′kus), pl. *fo′ci* [L. "fire-place"] 1. the point of convergence of light rays or of the waves of sound. 2. the chief center of a morbid process. **Ghon's f.**, a calcified nodule surrounded by a cluster of calcium deposits, resulting from healing processes involving the primary focus of tuberculous infection and the surrounding regional lymph node; usually in the hilar nodes. Called also *calcified primary lesion*. See also primary LESION. **f. of infection**, a circumscribed area of tissue infected with exogenous pathogenic microorganisms, which is the primary site of infection spreading to other sites, and is usually located near a mucous or cutaneous surface. Principal oral foci of infection include infected periapical lesions, teeth with infected root canals, and periodontal diseases. See also focal INFECTION. **line f.**, a principle employed in the design of an x-ray tube, by which the effective focal spot is sharply reduced relative to the actual (larger) focal spot desirable to deal with the heat generated. It involves focusing the cathode stream, in the pattern of a thin rectangle, onto an anode truncated at about 20 degrees to the transverse axis of the tube. **real f.**, the point at which convergent rays intersect.

fog (fog) 1. a colloid system in which the dispersion medium is a gas and the dispersed particles are liquid, e.g., a cloudlike mass of water droplets dispersed in air. 2. film f. **chemical f.**, darkening of film due to imbalance, contamination, or deterioration of processing solutions. **dichroic f.**, chemical fog of film characterized by a pinkish· hue under transmitted light or greenish appearance under reflected light, due to exhaustion of acid in the fixing solution. **film f.**, undesirable cloudiness or partial opacity of a radiographic image, produced by sources other than

the primary beam to which the film was exposed. **light f.**, darkening of the film due to its unintentional exposure to light, either before or after processing. **radiation f.**, darkening of film due to unintentional exposure to radiation during unprotected storage or to scatter radiation.

fogging (fog′ing) 1. the production of fog. 2. enveloping with fog. 3. the production of fog on a photographic or x-ray film (see film FOG).

foil (foil) metal in the form of a very thin, pliable sheet. **adhesive f.**, a tin foil coated on one side with powdered gum arabic or karaya gum, which is moistened and applied over the teeth, gingival tissue, or postoperative periodontal surgical dressing to provide protection to the covered area. **f. assistant**, foil HOLDER. **f. carrier**, foil PASSER. **cohesive gold f.**, a foil of pure gold (24 carat) having impurities, such as sulfur dioxide, oxygen, ammonium, and other contaminants removed from its surface by annealing or degassing. Two pieces of foil, whose surfaces have been thus completely cleaned, will weld to each other when brought together at room temperature, forming a single piece of gold that may be hammered, rolled, or otherwise fashioned into a desired shape or thinness. **f. condenser**, gold CONDENSER. **corrugated gold f.**, ropes of gold foil with superior welding properties, produced by placing the foil between sheets of paper which are ignited in a closed container; used as a direct filling material in restorative procedures. The method of preparing corrugated gold foil was discovered by accident during the great Chicago fire in 1871 when a dental dealer left books of gold foil in a safe, which became corrugated during the fire. **f. cylinder**, foil CYLINDER. **gold f.**, pure gold (24 carat) rolled into sheets and beaten with a mallet on a granite block to the thickness of about 6.4 μ, being sufficiently thin to transmit light. Structurally, the sheets have a fibrous appearance and their crystals are grossly elongated. The foil is available in sheets 4 in², their thickness being designated by numbers, whereby foil No. 2 has a thickness of 1/40,000 in, weighing 2 gr, No. 4 is 1/20,000 in, weighing 4 gr, etc. The sheets may be cut into 1/8, 1/16, 1/64, etc., and then compressed into pellets or cylinders. A number of sheets may be placed on top of each other to form laminated gold foil, which can then be cut into pellets or formed into cylinders. A platinum sheet may be sandwiched between two gold foils to form platinized foil. The foil also can be made into ropes, or corrugated, by placing it between sheets of paper which can be ignited in a closed container. Gold foil and its products are used as direct filling materials in dental restorations. **gold f., cohesive**, cohesive gold f. **gold f., corrugated**, corrugated gold f. **gold f., laminated**, laminated gold f. **gold f., noncohesive**, noncohesive gold f. **gold f., semicohesive**, semicohesive gold f. **gold f. condensation**, direct filling gold COMPACTION. **f. holder**, foil HOLDER. **invisible f.**, a cavity restoration technique in which all the foil is placed in the cavity from the lingual surface of a tooth and its labial outline is restricted to prevent visibility of the metal from the front. Called also *lingual approach*. **laminated gold f.**, a foil produced by placing a number of sheets of gold foil on top of each other. The laminated foil may be cut into pellets or formed into cylinders to be used as a direct filling material in restorative procedures. **mat f.**, a foil of mat gold sandwiched between two sheets of cohesive gold foil; used similarly to mat gold in building up the internal bulk of the restoration. **noncohesive gold f.**, gold foil, the surfaces of which have been contaminated by foreign matter, such as sulfur dioxide, oxygen, ammonia, or other impurities, and thus will not weld to another gold foil at room temperature. A foil of pure gold (24 carat) may be rendered cohesive by removing impurities from its surface (see *cohesive gold f.*). One not composed of pure gold or one contaminated by substances such as sulfur by exposure to rubber or matches, which does not volatilize when exposed to heat, is said to be permanently noncohesive. Gold may be rendered permanently noncohesive by treating its surface with various gases, such as ammonia. **f. passer**, foil· PASSER. **f. pellet**, foil PELLET. **platinized f.**, a foil for dental restoration made of cohesive gold foil interleaved with a platinum sheath, producing an alloy with a 15 percent platinum content, which is harder than the sheath made of the gold used in the foil. Available in 1/4 pellets. Called also *platinized gold*. **platinum f.**, a very thin foil of pure platinum with a high fusing point, thus being suitable for use as a matrix for soldering procedures. Also used to provide internal forms for porcelain restorations during their fabrication. **f. plugger**, gold CONDENSER. **f. rope**, foil ROPE. **semicohesive gold f.**, a foil which is not completely cohesive, the degree of cohesiveness being controlled by annealing or degassing. See also *cohesive gold f.* **tin f.**, a thin sheet rolled from tin or an alloy of tin and lead, used for wrapping various objects, such as drugs; also used as a separating material between the cast and denture base material during flasking and curing. Written also *tinfoil*. **tin f. substitute,** see separating MEDIUM.

Foix's syndrome [Charles *Foix*, French neurologist, 1882–1927] cavernous sinus SYNDROME.

Fol. abbreviation for L. *fo'lia*, leaves.

folacin (fŏl'ah-sin) folic ACID.

folate (fo'lāt) a salt of folic acid; a general term for a group of substances whose molecules are made up of a form of pteroic acid conjugates with L-glutamic acid. See folic ACID.

fold (fōld) a thin, recurved margin, or doubling. Called also PLICA. **aryepiglottic f.,** a fold of mucous membrane extending on each side between the lateral border of the epiglottis and the summit of the arytenoid cartilage. On the posterior margin of the fold, the cuneiform cartilage forms the cuneiform ventricle. Called also *arytenoepiglottic ligament* and *plica aryepiglottica* [NA]. **epicanthic f.,** epicanthus. **fimbriated f.,** a fold of mucous membrane with a fimbriated margin that extends outward from the frenum to the apex of the tongue. Called also *fimbriae linguae, fimbriae of tongue, fimbriated crest,* and *plica fimbriata* [NA]. **glossoepiglottic f.,** one of the three folds of mucous membrane extending from the root of the tongue to the epiglottis. Called also *plica glossoepiglottica.* **glossoepiglottic f., lateral,** either of two folds of mucous membrane extending, one on either side, between the base of the tongue and the epiglottis. Called also *plica glossoepiglottica lateralis.* **glossoepiglottic f., median,** a single fold of mucous membrane between the two lateral glossoepiglottic folds, connecting the base of the tongue to the epiglottis. Called also *plica glossoepiglottica mediana.* **Hasner's f.,** lacrimal f. **lacrimal f.,** a fold of mucous membrane at the lower opening of the nasolacrimal duct. Called also *Hasner's f., Hasner's valve, plica lacrimalis* [NA], and *plica lacrimalis Hasneri.* **f. of laryngeal nerve,** a fold of mucous membrane in the larynx, overlying the laryngeal nerve. Called also *plica nervi laryngei.* **marginal f's,** cellular structures which are modifications of surface membranes, believed to engulf particles to be taken into the cell. **medullary f.,** neural f. **mucobuccal f.,** the cul-de-sac formed where the mucous membrane is reflected from the upper or lower jaw to the cheek. Called also *mucosobuccal f.* **mucolabial f.,** the line of flexure of the oral mucous membrane as it passes from the mandible or maxilla to the lip. **mucosobuccal f.,** mucobuccal f. **neural f.,** one of the paired thickenings, lying one on each side of the neural groove, which continue to grow until they fuse, thus forming the neural tube during embryonic development of parts of the brain and spinal cord. Called also *medullary f.* See also neural TUBE. **palatine f's, palatine f's, transverse,** several irregular, sometimes branching wrinkles (rugae) on the anterior part of the hard palate, formed by a core of dense connective tissue covered by the oral mucosa. In man, rugae represent vestiges of highly developed folds in some animals, in which they play an auxiliary role in mastication. Called also *palatine rugae, plicae palatinae transversae* [NA], *rugae palatinae,* and *transverse palatine ridges.* **palpebronasal f.,** epicanthus. **pharyngoepiglottic f.,** a fold of mucous membrane running backward from the epiglottis. **pterygomandibular f.,** a fold of mucous membrane stretching from the region of the hamulus to the retromolar pad; it is especially prominent when the mouth is open. **salpingopalatine f.,** the mucosal fold passing caudally from the auditory tube to the lateral pharyngeal wall and the palate. Called also *plica salpingopalatina* [NA]. **salpingopharyngeal f.,** a vertical fold of mucous membrane passing caudally from the posterior lip of the pharyngeal orifice of the auditory tube of the lateral pharyngeal wall, and containing the salpingopharyngeus muscle. Called also *plica salpingopharyngea, salpingopharyngeal ligament,* and *tubopharyngeal ligament of Rauber.* **semilunar f.,** a curved fold of mucous membrane interconnecting the palatoglossal and palatopharyngeal arches and forming the upper boundary of the supratonsillar fossa. Called also *plica semilunaris* [NA]. **sublingual f.,** the elevation on the floor of the mouth under the tongue, covering part of the sublingual gland and containing its excretory ducts. Called also *plica sublingualis* [NA]. **transverse palatine f's,** palatine f's. **triangular f.,** a fold of mucous membrane extending backward from the palatoglossal arch and covering the anteroinferior part of the palatine tonsil. Called also *plica triangularis* [NA]. **ventricular f., vestibular f. vestibular f.,** one of two thick folds of mucous

membrane in the larynx, separating the ventricle from the vestibule, which is connected by the vestibular ligament to the thyroid cartilage. Called also *ventricular f., false vocal cord, plica ventricularis, plica vestibularis* [NA], and *superior vocal cord.* **vocal f.,** vocal cord, true; see under CORD.

Foley catheter see under CATHETER.

folia (fo'le-ah) plural of *folium.*

foliaceous (fo"le-a'shus) [L. *folia* leaves] pertaining to or resembling a leaf or leaves.

Foligan trademark for *allopurinol.*

folium (fo'le-um), pl. *fo'lia* [L. "leaf"] a general term used in anatomical nomenclature to designate a leaflike structure.

follicle (fol'li-k'l) a small sac, crypt, or gland. Called also *folliculus.* **dental f.,** the structure within the substance of the jaws enclosing the tooth before its eruption; the dental sac and its contents. **lingual f's,** lymphatic f's of tongue. **lymph f.,** FOLLICULUS lymphaticus. **lymphatic f's, laryngeal,** lymphatic aggregations in the mucosa of the ventricle of the larynx and on the posterior surface of the epiglottis. Called also *folliculi lymphatici laryngei* [NA] and *noduli lymphatici laryngei.* **lymphatic f's of tongue,** projections on the mucosa of the root of the tongue, caused by underlying nodular masses of lymphoid tissue, making up the lingual tonsil. Called also *folliculi linguales* [NA] and *lingual follicles.*

follicular (fo-lik'u-lar) [L. *follicularis*] of, pertaining to, or similar to a follicle or follicles.

folliculitis (fo-lik"u-li'tis) inflammation of a follicle or follicles; usually hair follicles. **deep f.,** folliculitis in which infection extends deeply into the follicle, usually also involving the surrounding tissue (see PERIFOLLICULITIS), and is marked by a pronounced inflammatory reaction. It is a form of pyoderma, usually caused by infection with coagulase-positive staphylococci. The face is the most frequent site, the upper lip being affected most commonly. **superficial f.,** a form of folliculitis in which superficial structures of the follicle are involved.

folliculus (fo-lik'u-lus), pl. *follic'uli* [L., dim. of *follis* a leather bag] a general term used in anatomical nomenclature to designate a small sac, crypt, or gland. Called also *follicle.* **follic'uli linguα'les** [NA], lymphatic follicles of tongue; see under FOLLICLE. **follic'uli lymphat'ici laryn'gei** [NA], laryngeal lymphatic follicles; see under FOLLICLE. **f. lymphat'icus,** 1. [NA] a small collection of lymphoid tissue found in such places as the mucosa of the gut. 2. a small transient collection of actively proliferating lymphocytes in the cortex of a lymph node, expressing the cytogenetic and defense functions of the lymphatic tissue. Called also *lymph f., lymphatic nodule,* and *nodulus lymphaticus.*

Følling's disease [Ivar Asbjörn *Følling*] phenylketonuria.

fomes (fo'mēz), pl. *fo'mites* [L. "tinder"] an object that is not in itself harmful, but is able to harbor pathogenic microorganisms and thus may serve as an agent of transmission of an infection. Called also *fomite.*

fomite (fo'mīt) fomes.

fomites (fo'mit-tēz) plural of *fomes.*

Fones' method (technique) [American dentist; in 1906, he trained his office assistant to perform prophylactic work, and is therefore considered to be the father of dental hygiene] see TOOTHBRUSHING.

fontanel (fon"tah-nel') fontanelle.

fontanelle (font"tah-nel') [Fr., dim. of *fontaine* spring, filter] a soft spot, such as one of the membrane-covered spaces remaining in the incompletely ossified skull. Spelled also *fontanel.* Called also *fonticulus.* **anterior f.,** an unossified, membranous, diamond-shaped area on the top of the skull in newborn infants up to a year and a half after birth, situated in the midline between the anterior corners of the parietal bones and the posterior corners of the paired frontal bones. Called also *bregmatic f., frontal f., quadrangular f., fonticulus anterior* [NA], *fonticulus frontalis,* and *fonticulus major.* **anterolateral f.,** sphenoidal f. **bregmatic f.,** anterior f. **Casser's f., casserian f.,** mastoid f. **frontal f.,** anterior f. **Gerdy's f.,** a fontanelle occasionally occurring in the sagittal suture. Called also *sagittal f.* **mastoid f.,** an unossified, membranous area on the skull of newborn infants, situated at the posterolateral corner of the parietal bone, between it and the temporal and occipital bones. Called also *casserian f., Casser's f., posterolateral f., posterotemporal f.,* and *fonticulus mastoideus* [NA]. **occipital f.,** posterior f. **posterior f.,** an unossified, membranous triangular area on the top of the skull in newborn infants through the first few months after birth, situated at the point where the two parietal bones and the occipital bone meet. Called also *occipital f., triangular f., fonticulus minor, fonticulus occipitalis,* and *fonticulus posterior* [NA]. **posterolateral f., posterotemporal f.,** mastoid f. **quadrangular f.,** anterior f. **sagittal f.,** Gerdy's f. **sphenoidal f.,**

an unossified, membranous area on the top of the skull in newborn infants, situated at the anterolateral corners of the parietal bone, between it and the frontal, temporal, and sphenoid bones. Called also *anterolateral f.* and *fonticulus sphenoidalis* [NA]. **triangular f.,** posterior f.

fonticuli (fon-tik′u-li) [L.] plural of *fonticulus.*

fonticulus (fon-tik′u-lus), pl. *fontic′uli* [L., dim. of *fons* fountain] fontanelle; a soft spot; one of the unossified, membranous spaces in the skull of the fetus or infant. **f. ante′rior** [NA], **f. fronta′lis, f. ma′jor,** anterior FONTANELLE. **f. mastoi′deus** [NA], mastoid FONTANELLE. **f. mi′nor, f. occipita′lis, f. poste′rior** [NA], posterior FONTANELLE. **f. sphenoida′lis** [NA], sphenoidal FONTANELLE.

Fonurit trademark for *acetazolamide.*

food (food) anything which, when taken into the body, serves to nourish or build up the tissues or to supply body heat; aliment; nutriment. **f. additive,** food ADDITIVE. **f. allergy,** food ALLERGY. **f. intolerance,** food INTOLERANCE. **isodynamic f.,** any food which generates equal amounts of energy in heat units. **f. preservative,** food PRESERVATIVE. **f. poisoning,** food POISONING.

foot (foot) [L. *pes*] 1. the distal portion of the vertebrate leg, upon which an individual stands and walks. Called also *pes* [NA]. 2. a unit of length, being 12 inches, or one-third of a yard, or equivalent to 30.48 centimeters. Abbreviated *ft.* See also *Tables of Weights and Measures* at WEIGHT.

foot-pound (foot-pownd′) a unit of work, representing the energy required to raise a mass of 1 pound 1 foot vertically against the force of gravity at sea level; 7.2 foot-pounds equal 1 kilogram-meter. Abbreviated *fp.* See also *Tables of Weights and Measures* at WEIGHT.

foramen (fo-ra′men), pl. *foram′ina* [L.] a natural opening or passage; used as a general term in anatomical nomenclature to designate such a passage, especially one into or through a bone. **accessory f.,** a lateral or accessory orifice, other than the main apical foramen, opening into the root canal of a tooth. Called also *lateral f.* **accessory palatine foramina,** lesser palatine foramina. **alveolar foramina of maxilla,** openings of the alveolar canals at the deepest portion of the tooth sockets in the maxilla. Called also *dental f., foramina alveolaria maxillae* [NA], and *posterior dental canals.* **alveolar f. of maxilla, posterior,** one of two or more openings on the infratemporal surface of the maxilla. **anterior condyloid f.,** hypoglossal CANAL. **anterior ethmoid f.,** ethmoid canal, anterior; see under CANAL. **anterior maxillary f.,** mental f. **anterior palatine f.,** incisive f. **apical f. of tooth, f. a′picis dentis** [NA], a minute aperture usually at or near the apex of a root of a tooth but on occasion located on a side of a root, which gives passage to the vascular, lymphatic, and neural structures supplying the pulp. In some instances, the main foramen branches near the apex to form two or more apical ramifications. Called also *f. radicis dentis, pulpal f.,* and *root f.* **Arnold's internal zygomatic f.,** zygomatico-orbital f. **caroticotympanic foramina,** caroticotympanic canaliculi; see under CANALICULUS. **carotid f.,** the inferior aperture of the carotid canal, giving passage to the carotid vessels. **cecal f.,** cecal f. of frontal bone. **cecal f. of frontal bone, f. ce′cum,** a blind opening formed between the frontal crest and the crista galli; it sometimes transmits a vein from the nasal cavity to the superior sagittal sinus. Called also *cecal f.* and *f. cecum ossis frontalis* [NA]. **f. ce′cum lin′guae** [NA], f. cecum of tongue. **f. ce′cum os′sis fronta′lis** [NA], cecal f. of frontal bone. **f. cecum of tongue,** a median pit on the dorsum of the posterior part of the tongue, marking the point of origin of the stalk of the thyroglossal duct. Called also *f. cecum linguae* [NA]. See also thyroglossal DUCT. **conjugate f.,** a foramen formed by a notch in each of two opposed bones. **cribroethmoid f.,** ethmoid canal, anterior; see under CANAL. **dental f.,** 1. alveolar f. of maxilla. 2. mandibular f. **ethmoid f., anterior, f. ethmoida′le ante′rius** [NA], anterior ethmoid CANAL. **ethmoid f., posterior, f. ethmoida′le poste′rius** [NA], posterior ethmoid CANAL. **facial zygomatic f.,** zygomaticofacial f. **Ferrein's f.,** HIATUS of canal for greater petrosal nerve. **foram′ina alveola′ria maxil′lae** [NA], alveolar foramina of maxilla. **frontal f., f. fronta′le** [NA], frontal INCISURE. **frontoethmoidal f.,** a foramen lying on the line of the frontoethmoidal suture. **great f., great occipital f.,** f. magnum. **greater palatine f.,** the inferior opening of the great palatine canal, found laterally on the horizontal plate of each palatine bone opposite the root of each third molar tooth; it transmits a palatine nerve and artery. Called also *f. palatinum majus* [NA], *posterior palatine f., pterygopalatine f.,* and *sphenopalatine f.* **f. of Huschke,** a small aperture in the thin central portion of the tympanic portion of the temporal bone; it is usually closed about the fifth year of life, but occasionally may persist into adult life. **incisive f.,** one of the openings in the incisive fossa of the hard palate that transmit the nasopalatine nerves. Called also an-

terior palatine f. and f. of Stensen. **incisor f., median,** f. of Scarpa. **infraorbital f., f. infraorbita′le** [NA], an opening on the anterior surface of the maxilla, above the canine fossa and below the infraorbital ridge, leading to the infraorbital canal, and giving passage to the infraorbital nerve and vessels. Called also *suborbital f.* **innominate f.,** an occasional opening in the temporal bone for passage of the small superficial petrosal nerve. **jugular f., f. jugula′re** [NA], the opening formed by the jugular notches on the temporal and occipital bones. Called also *posterior lacerate f.* **lacerate f., anterior,** orbital fissure, superior; see under FISSURE. **lacerate f., middle,** f. lacerum. **lacerate f., posterior,** jugular f. **f. lac′erum,** an irregular opening of variable size appearing at the base of the medial pterygoid plate of the great wing of the sphenoid bone, the tip of the petrous part of the temporal bone, and the basilar part of the occipital bone. It presents an opening in dried skulls but in the intact body is covered over by the fibrocartilaginous plate containing the auditory tube. The carotid artery traverses the carotid canal within the anterior aspect of the foramen lacerum, and lateral to the opening to the carotid canal is the sulcus tubae auditivae. Called also *f. lacerum medium, middle lacerate f.,* and *sphenotic f.* **f. lac′erum ante′rius,** orbital fissure, superior; see under FISSURE. **f. lac′erum me′dium,** f. lacerum. **lateral f.,** accessory f. **lesser palatine foramina,** the openings of the palatine canals at the base of the pyramidal process near its junction with the horizontal plate of the palatine bone, behind the palatine crest and the greater palatine foramina, for the transmission of the lesser palatine nerves. Called also *accessory palatine foramina* and *foramina palatina minora* [NA]. **f. mag′num** [NA], a large, oval opening in the inferior and anterior part of the occipital bone, bounded by the squama, the basilar part, and the lateral parts of the occipital bone, which serves as a communication between the cranial cavity and the vertebral canal. It transmits the medulla oblongata and its membranes, accessory nerves, vertebral arteries, anterior and posterior spinal arteries, and membrana tectoria and alar ligaments. Called also *great f., great occipital f.,* and *f. occipitale magnum.* **malar f.,** zygomaticofacial f. **mandibular f., f. mandib′ulae** [NA], **f. mandibula′re,** an opening on the medial surface of the ramus of the mandible, providing an entrance for the inferior alveolar vessels and nerve, and leading into the mandibular canal. The margin of this entrance presents a ridge with a sharp spine, the lingula mandibulae, for attachment of the sphenomandibular ligament. Called also *dental f., internal maxillary f.,* and *posterior maxillary f.* **mastoid f., f. mastoi′deum** [NA], an opening in the temporal bone posterior to the mastoid process and near its occipital articulation; an artery and vein usually pass through it. **maxillary f.,** maxillary HIATUS. **maxillary f., anterior,** mental f. **maxillary f., inferior,** oval f. of sphenoid bone. **maxillary f., internal, maxillary f., posterior,** mandibular f. **maxillary f., superior,** maxillary canal, superior; see under CANAL. **Meckel's internal zygomatic f.,** zygomaticotemporal f. **mental f., f. menta′le** [NA], an opening on the lateral part of the body of the mandible, inferior to the second premolar tooth, for the passage of the mental vessels and nerve. Called also *anterior maxillary f.* **multiple foramina,** two or more apical foramina leading to the main root canal. Most root canals of fully formed teeth terminate in an apical delta resulting in one or more collateral exits at or near the apex. This condition is more frequently found in multirooted than in single-rooted teeth. **f. occipita′le mag′num,** f. magnum. **olfactory f.,** one of the many perforations on either side of the crista galli in the cribriform plate of the ethmoid bone, for passage of the olfactory nerves. **optic f. of sphenoid bone, f. op′ticum os′sis sphenoida′lis,** optic CANAL. **orbital zygomatic f., orbitomalar f.,** zygomatico-orbital f. **oval f. of sphenoid bone, f. ova′le ba′sis cra′nii** [NA], **f. ova′le os′sis sphenoida′lis,** an opening in the posterior part of the medial portion of the great wing of the sphenoid bone; it transmits the mandibular nerve, the accessory meningeal artery, and sometimes the lesser petrosal nerve. Called also *inferior maxillary f.* **f. palati′num ma′jus** [NA], greater palatine f. **foram′ina palati′na mino′ra** [NA], lesser palatine foramina. **foramina of palatine tonsil,** tonsillar fossulae of palatine tonsil; see under FOSSULA. **parietal f., f. parieta′le** [NA], an opening on the posterior part of the superior portion of the parietal bone near the sagittal suture, for passage of a vein and arteriole. **posterior condyloid f.,** condyloid CANAL. **posterior ethmoidal f.,** ethmoid canal, posterior; see under CANAL. **posterior palatine f., pterygopalatine f.,** greater palatine f. **pterygospinous f.,** an opening between the upper border of the pterygospinous ligament and the skull, produced by an occasional ossification of the ligament; it transmits the branches of the mandibular division of the trigeminal nerve. **pulpal f.,** apical f. of tooth. **f. rad′icis den′tis,** apical f. of tooth. **rivinian f., Rivinus′ f.,** tympanic NOTCH. **root f.,** apical f. of tooth. **f. rotun′dum os′sis sphenoida′lis** [NA], maxillary canal, superior; see under CANAL. **f. of Scarpa,** one of the two foramina in the palatine process of the maxilla, one behind either upper medial incisor, for transmission of the nasopalatine nerves. Called also *median incisor f.* **sphenopalatine f.,** 1. an opening on the medial wall of the pterygopalatine fossa, formed by the continuation of the sphenopalatine notch by the under surface of the sphenoid bone, which interconnects the fossa with the nasal cavity, and transmits the sphenopalatine artery and nasal nerves. Called also *f. sphenopalatinum* [NA]. 2. greater palatine f. **f. sphenopalati′num** [NA], sphenopalatine f. (1). **sphenotic f.,** f. lacerum. **spinous f.,** f. spino′sum [NA], a sometimes double opening in the great wing of the sphenoid bone, near its posterior angle, for the transmission of the middle meningeal vessels and the (recurrent) meningeal branch of the mandibular nerve. **Spöndel′s f.,** a small transient foramen in the cartilaginous base of the developing skull between the ethmoid bone and the lower wings of the sphenoid bone. **f. of Stensen,** 1. incisive f., 2. incisive CANAL. **stylomastoid f., f. stylomastoi′deum** [NA], a foramen on the inferior part of the temporal bone between the styloid and mastoid processes, for passage of the facial nerve and the stylomastoid artery. **suborbital f.,** infraorbital f. **superior maxillary f.,** maxillary canal, superior; see under CANAL. **supraorbital f., f. supraorbita′le, f. supraorbita′lis** [NA], see supraorbital INCISURE. **teardrop f.,** the apical foramen having assumed the form of a teardrop through a faulty root canal shaping technique. Called also *zip f.* See also root canal SHAPING. **temporal zygomatic f., temporomalar f.,** zygomaticotemporal f. **thyroid f., f. thyroi′deum** [NA], an inconstantly present opening in the upper part of the lamina of the thyroid cartilage, resulting from incomplete union of the fourth and fifth branchial cartilages. **tonsillar foramina,** 1. tonsillar fossulae of pharyngeal tonsil. 2. tonsillar fossulae of palatine tonsil. See under FOSSULA. **f. of Vesalius, f. Vesa′lii,** an opening occasionally found medial to the oval foramen of the sphenoid bone, for passage of a vein from the cavernous sinus. **zip f.,** teardrop f. **zygomatic f., anterior, zygomatic f., external, zygomatic f., facial,** zygomaticofacial f. **zygomatic f., inferior,** zygomatic f., **internal, of Arnold,** zygomatico-orbital f. **zygomatic f., internal, of Meckel,** zygomaticotemporal f. **zygomatic f., orbital,** zygomatico-orbital f. **zygomatic f., posterior,** zygomaticotemporal f. **zygomatic f., superior,** zygomatico-orbital f. **zygomatic f., temporal,** zygomaticotemporal f. **zygomaticofacial f., f. zygomaticofacia′le** [NA], a small opening near the center of the lateral surface of the zygomatic bone, for passage to the zygomaticofacial nerve and vessels. Called also *anterior zygomatic f., external zygomatic f., facial zygomatic f., malar f.,* and *zygomaticofacial canal.* **zygomatico-orbital f., f. zygomaticoorbita′le** [NA], either of the two openings on the orbital surface of the zygomatic bone, which transmit branches of the zygomatic branch of the trigeminal nerve and branches of the lacrimal artery. Called also *inferior zygomatic f., internal zygomatic f. of Arnold, orbital zygomatic f., orbitomalar f.,* and *superior zygomatic f.* **zygomaticotemporal f., f. zygomaticotempora′le** [NA], the opening near the center of the temporal surface of the zygomatic bone, for passage of the zygomaticotemporal nerve. Called also *Meckel′s internal zygomatic f., posterior zygomatic f., temporal zygomatic f., temporomalar f.,* and *zygomaticotemporal canal.*

foramina (fo-ram′ĭ-nah) [L.] plural of *foramen.*

Forane trademark for *isoflurane.*

Forbes′ disease [Gilbert B. *Forbes*] GLYCOGENOSIS III.

force (fors) [L. *fortis* strong] strength, power, or pressure. **anchorage f.,** reciprocal f. **biting f.,** masticatory f. **chewing f.,** masticatory f. **compressive f.,** compression (2). **condensing f.,** the force required to compress materials, such as direct filling gold, amalgam, or wax in cavity filling. **constant f.,** continuous force or pressure, such as that applied to the teeth. **denture-dislodging f.,** the force required to displace a denture from its intended position on supporting structures. **denture-retaining f.,** the force required to retain a denture in its intended position on its supporting structures. **differential f., differential orthodontic f.,** a differential of orthodontic force, such as a relatively light force needed for moving an incisor tooth, especially by tipping its crown, as opposed to the greater force that would be

required to move a molar tooth used for anchorage. The principle of differential force is used in Begg′s theory (see under THEORY). See also Begg′s TECHNIQUE. **dynamic f.,** dynamic STRESS. **electromotive f.,** the potential energy difference between electrons on the anode and electrons on the cathode; the force which, by reason of differences across or between two points or electric terminals, causes flow of electricity from one place to another, giving rise to an electric current; it is measured in volts. Abbreviated *emf.* Called also *cell potential.* **extraoral f.,** in an extraoral orthodontic appliance, force applied from anchorage units outside the oral cavity, such as calvarial, occipital, or cervical. **impact f.,** the dynamic force during the striking or impact of one body against another. Called also *impact load.* **intermittent f.,** a force or pressure alternating with periods of rest. **masticatory f.,** the degree of force applied against the occlusal surfaces of the teeth by the muscles of mastication during the chewing of food. The average masticatory force exerted against the teeth in the posterior part of the mouth in a normal adult with natural dentition is approximately 77 kg (170 lbs); the force exerted on a single cusp of a molar tooth is approximately 1970 kg/cm^2 or $28,000 \text{ lbs/in}^2$. Called also *biting f.,* and *chewing f.* **occlusal f.,** the force on opposing teeth when the jaws are brought into approximation. See also *masticatory f.,* occlusal LOAD, and tactile sensibility THRESHOLD. **optimum orthodontic f.,** an orthodontic force that moves teeth the most rapidly, with least discomfort to the patient, and with least damage to the teeth and their investing tissue. **orthodontic f.,** the amount of force required to move a tooth during orthodontic therapy. It is believed that this force should not exceed the force of the systolic pressure of the capillary blood, or about 20 gm per 1 cm^2 of root surface; the excessive force producing compression of the blood vessels with subsequent necrosis of the periodontal tissue. The effective periodontal force needed to move a tooth may range from 60 gm or less for a canine tooth to 500 gm for a molar tooth. Called also *tooth-moving f.* **reciprocal f.,** anchorage force, whereby the resistance of one or more dental units is utilized to move one or more opposing dental units. See also reciprocal ANCHORAGE. **SI unit of f.,** newton. **tensile f.,** tension (3). **tooth-moving f.,** orthodontic f. **torsive f.,** torsion (2). **van der Waals f′s,** the weak forces between atoms and molecules which are responsible for crystallization of inert gases at low temperature and formation of soft crystals of low melting temperature. Called also *secondary bonds* and *van der Waals bonds.*

forceps (for′seps) [L.] 1. an instrument with two blades and a handle for compressing or grasping tissues in surgical operations, and for handling sterile dressing and other surgical supplies. 2. any forcipate organ or part. **f. No. 16,** universal forceps having beaks resembling the horns of a cow, designed to reach into the bifurcation of the roots of the mandibular molar tooth, compress the interseptal bone, and elevate the tooth from its socket. Called also *cow horn f.* and *horn beak f.* See illustration. **f. No. 18,** one for extracting the maxillary molar teeth. The 18-R is for the right first and second molars and the 18-L for the left first and second molars. **f. No. 24,** universal forceps for extracting the maxillary molars, having beaks designed to fit into the bifurcation of the buccal roots and a sharply curved handle to stabilize the fingers. See illustration. **f. No. 88,** one for the extraction of the maxillary first and second molar teeth, the 88R-2 being used for the right side and the 88L-2 for the left. The single-pointed beak is placed on the facial surface of the tooth, between the bifurcation of the roots. See illustration. **f. No. 99-A,** one used for extraction of the bicuspid, cuspid, and incisor teeth, having a sharply curved handle to stabilize the little finger. See illustration. **f. No. 99-C,** one with straighter lines than 99-A used for extraction of maxillary bicuspid, incisor, and cuspid teeth. See illustration. **f. No. 103,** universal lower forceps for the extraction of erupted mandibular premolars, incisors, and fractured roots. See illustration. **f. No. 150,** universal upper forceps for extracting maxillary incisor and bicuspid teeth and the roots. Also called *Cryer f.* See illustration. **f. No. 151,** universal lower forceps for the extraction of mandibular teeth and fractured roots. Called also *Cryer f.* See illustration. **f. No. 222,** universal forceps for the extraction of the mandibular third molar teeth, which has an extended tip that provides access of the beaks over and onto the crown of the tooth. See illustration. **f. No. 286,** upper forceps of bayonet design with an offset to provide access to the teeth and roots for their extraction. See illustration. **f. No. 287,** universal lower molar forceps for extracting the mandibular teeth, which may be placed in the bifurcation of the mesial and distal roots. A sharply curved handle is provided for leverage. See illustration. **Adson f.,** a type of straight tissue forceps, either plain, serrated, or provided with teeth at both tips for grasping tissue. **Adson-**

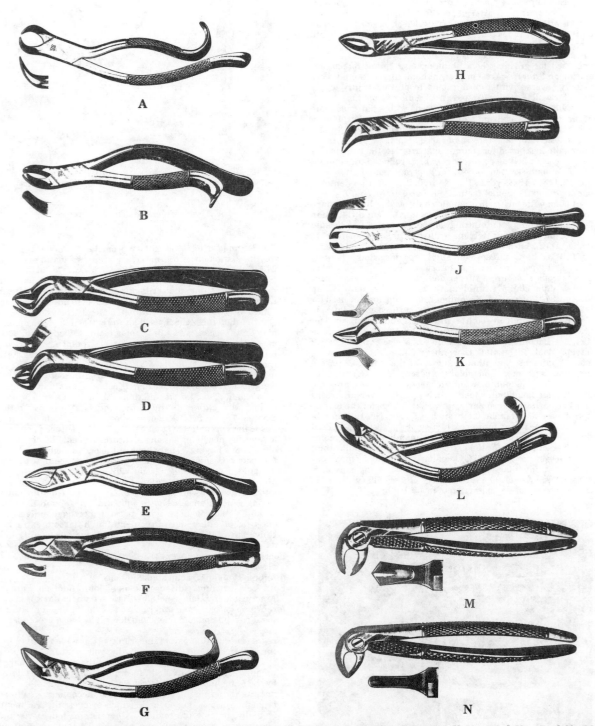

Dental forceps. *A*, No. 16; *B*, **No. 24**; *C*, **No. 88L-2**; *D*, No. 88R-2; *E*, No. 99-8; *F*, No. 99-C; *G*, No. 103; *H*, No. 150; *I*, No. 151; *J*, No. 222; *K*, No. 286; *L*, No. 287; *M*, **Mead 4**; *N*, **Mead 3**. (From H. O. Torres and A. Ehrlich: Modern Dental Assisting. 2nd ed. Philadelphia, W. B. Saunders Co., 1980. *A–L* **courtesy of S. S. White Co.**; *M* and *N* courtesy of Hu-Friedy Mfg. Co.)

Brown, straight tissue forceps provided with serrated teeth for grasping tissue. **alligator f.,** strong toothed forceps having a double clamp. **Allison f.,** Allison RETRACTOR. **apical fragment f.,** one with long, thin, sharp beaks, resembling those of a hemostat, used to remove apical root fragments in tooth extraction. Also called *splinter f.* **artery f.,** one for grasping and compressing an artery. See also HEMOSTAT (2). **Asch f.,** one especially designed for intranasal use. **Ash f.,** a type of rubber dam clamp forceps. **bayonet f.,** one whose blades are offset from the axis of the handle to aid in direct visualization, see *f. No. 286.* **bone f.,** one used for grasping bone. **bulldog f.,** a spring forceps for seizing an artery to arrest or prevent hemorrhage; the jaws are usually covered with rubber tubing to prevent injury to the vascular wall. See also HEMOSTAT (2). **bullet f.,** one for extracting bullets. **chalazion f.,** a tissue forceps with a flattened plate at the end of one arm and a matching ring on the other; it is an ophthalmologic instrument, also used for isolation of lip and cheek lesions to facilitate removal. **clamp f.,** 1. one with an automatic lock, used for compressing arteries, the pedicle of a tumor, etc. Called also *pedicle clamp.* 2. rubber dam clamp f. **clip f.,** a double-action forceps for applying wound clips. **cow horn f.,** f. No. 16. **Cryer f.,** 1. f. No. 150. 2. f. No. 151. **dental f.,** one for the extraction of teeth. Called also *extracting f.* **dressing f.,** one with scissor-like handles for grasping lint, drainage tubes, etc., in dressing wounds. **extracting f.,** dental f. **fixation f.,** one for holding a part during an operation. **Fox f.,** a locking type of curved tissue forceps with fine tips. **hemostatic f.,** hemostat (2). **horn beak f.,** f. No. 16. **Hu-Friedy f.,** trademark for a curved tissue forceps with sturdy tips. **insertion f.,** *point f.* **Ivory f.,** a type of rubber dam forceps used for placing rubber dam clamps to secure a rubber dam in the oral cavity. **Ivory rubber dam clamp f.,** trademark for a rubber dam clamp forceps. See illustration. **Kazanjian f.,** a cutting forceps used for resection of the nasal dorsal hump. **L f.,** one used on the left side of the dental arch in tooth extraction. **Laborde's f.,** one for grasping the tongue in Laborde's method of stimulating respiration. See Laborde's METHOD. **Liston's f.,** a type of bone cutting forceps. **lock f.,** point f. **Löwenberg's f.,** one for removing adenoid growths. **mandibular f.,** one for the extraction of mandibular premolar and molar teeth; see *f. No. 103, f. Mead 3,* and *f. Mead 4.* **mandibular anterior teeth f.,** one for extracting the anterior mandibular teeth, such as the universal forceps No. 151. **mandibular molar f.,** universal forceps for the extraction of mandibular molar teeth, such as forceps No. 16. **mandibular posterior f.,** one for the extraction of the posterior teeth of the mandible, such as forceps No. 287. **mandibular third molar f.,** universal forceps for the extraction of the mandibular third molar teeth; see *f. No. 222.* **maxillary bicuspid f.,** maxillary premolar f. **maxillary incisor f.,** one for extracting maxillary incisors; see *f. No. 99-A* and *f. No. 150.* **maxillary molar f.,** sturdy forceps for the extraction of molar teeth; see *f. No. 18, f.*

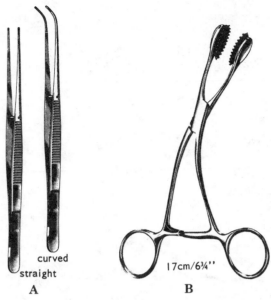

A, Tissue forceps. *B,* Tongue-forceps.

No. 24, and *f. No. 88.* **maxillary premolar f.,** universal forceps for the extraction of the maxillary premolar teeth; see *f. No. 286.* Called also *maxillary bicuspid f.* **f. MD3,** f. Mead 3. **f. MD4,** f. Mead 4. **f. Mead 3,** universal forceps for the extraction of the mandibular canine, incisor, and premolar teeth and fractured roots, with a right-angle offset to the beaks to provide leverage. Called also *f. MD3.* See illustration. **f. Mead 4,** one similar to but sturdier than the Mead 3, used for the extraction of the mandibular first, second, and third molar teeth. Called also *f. MD4.* **mosquito f.,** a small hemostatic forceps. **point f.,** one used in filling root canals, which securely holds the filling cones during their placement. Called also *insertion f.* and *lock f.* **R f.,** one used on the right side of the dental arch in tooth extraction. **rongeur f.,** rongeur. **rubber dam f.,** rubber dam clamp f. **rubber dam clamp f.,** one for placing rubber dam clamps into position. Called also *clamp f.* and *rubber dam f.* See illustration. **Semken-Taylor f.,** a slender type of either straight or curved tissue forceps. **splinter f.,** apical fragment f. **suture f.,** one used to hold the needle in passing a suture; a needle holder. **tenaculum f.,** one having a sharp hook at the end of each jaw. **thumb f.,** tissue f. **tissue f.,** one with or without fine teeth at the tips, designated for handling tissue with minimal trauma. Called also *thumb f.* See illustration. **tongue f.,** one for grasping the tongue, generally used to prevent aspiration of the tongue during general anesthesia. See illustration. **torsion f.,** one for making torsion on an artery to arrest hemorrhage. **universal f.,** one used on either side of the dental arch in tooth extraction. **University of Washington rubber dam clamp f.,** a type of rubber dam clamp forceps.

Forchheimer's spots (sign) [Frederick *Forchheimer,* Cincinnati physician, 1853–1913] see under SPOT.

forcipate (for′sĭ-pāt) shaped like forceps.

Fordyce's granules (disease, spots) [John Addison *Fordyce,* American dermatologist, 1858–1925] see under GRANULE.

forebrain (fōr′brān) the anterior part of the brain, consisting of the diencephalon and telencephalon. Called also *prosencephalon.*

foregut (for′gut) that part of the primitive gut which derives from the infolded cranial portion of the yolk sac and forms the epithelial lining of the digestive tube of the embryo cephalic to the junction of the yolk stalk. Its cranial part is limited laterally by the branchial arches and ventrally by the pericardial cavity; its anterior terminal part contains the buccopharyngeal membrane and a pit (stomodeum), which evolves into the mouth. Medially, it joins the midgut. It consists of four parts: oral, pharyngeal, esophageal, and gastric. The endodermal outpouchings of the pharyngeal part form the pharyngeal pouches, and the segmented intermediate mesoderm forms the branchial arches. The branchial arches, corresponding in number to the somites, form during the fourth week of embryonic life from the midventral evaginations of the foregut.

forehead (for′hed) the part of the face above the eyes. Called also *brow* and *frons.* **bony f.,** the frontal part of the skull; the frontal bone. Called also *frons cranii* [NA] and *frons of cranium.*

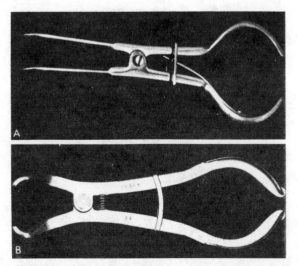

A, University of Washington rubber dam clamp forceps. *B,* Ivory rubber dam clamp forceps. (From S. Cohen and R. C. Burns: Pathways of the Pulp. 2nd ed. St. Louis, The C. V. Mosby Co., 1980.)

forensic (fo′ren-sik) [L. *forensis* public] pertaining to or used in the courts or legal processes. See also forensic DENTISTRY and forensic MEDICINE.

foreshortening (for-shor′ten-ing) in radiography, a form of distortion in which the image is shorter than the object. It is caused in the angle bisection technique by misdirecting the x-ray beam perpendicular to the plane of the film instead of the plane of the bisector, the vertical angulation being too steep.

Forhistal trademark for *dimethindene maleate* (see under DIMETHINDENE).

fork (fork) an instrument having two or more prongs. **bite f., face-bow f. face-bow f.,** the portion of the face-bow assembly used to attach an occlusion rim or transfer record of maxillary teeth to the face-bow proper. It consists of a horseshoe-shaped appliance coated with a suitable material, such as wax, to receive indentations of the teeth, which is placed against the maxillary teeth and a stud that fits a bracket of the face-bow. Called also *bite f.* and *transfer f.* See illustration at FACE-BOW. **transfer f.,** face-bow f.

form (form) [L. *forma*] 1. the character of a structure or entity, generally determined by its shape and size, or other external or visible features. 2. a procedure according to a set order or method. 3. to produce. 4. to construct a frame. 5. a standardized document with blank spaces for required information. **anatomic f.,** 1. the natural form of an anatomical structure. 2. the surface form of the edentulous ridge at rest or when it is not supporting a functional load. 3. the contour of the crown of a tooth. **arch f.,** the shape and contour of a dental arch. **claim f.,** uniform report f. **convenience f.,** 1. a modification of the access cavity form, performed in order to establish greater convenience in the placement of intracoronal interim restorations as well as instrumentation and filling of the root canal. See also endodontic CAVITY. 2. the modification necessary beyond basic outline form to facilitate proper instrumentation for the preparation of the cavity of a tooth or insertion of the restorative material. Also, the placing of starting points or slight undercuts to retain the first portions of restorative material while succeeding portions are placed. **face f.,** the geometric outline form of the face from an anterior view, sometimes described geometrically as square, tapering, or ovoid and by various combinations of basic geometric forms. See also facial PROFILE and FACIES. **informed consent f.,** a form designed to fully inform the patient in nontechnical terms about the nature and potential risks of the specific therapeutic or research procedure to be performed. Generally, it includes the name of the doctor, name of the patient, record number, date, description of the procedure, purpose of the procedure, expected benefits, possible risks and discomforts, fee, patient's right to accept or reject the procedure or to withdraw consent, consultant's comments, and the statement indicating that the patient understands the nature of the procedure and the risks involved. The form is signed by the doctor, patient, and consultant(s) (if any). In the case of a minor patient or one who is incapable of understanding or communicating, consent must be obtained from a close adult relative, such as a parent, or a legal guardian. See also informed CONSENT. **juvenile f.,** metamyelocyte. **occlusal f.,** the form of the occlusal surface of a tooth, row of teeth, or dentition. **outline f.,** 1. the outline of the form of the endodontic access cavity on the tooth surface, so shaped as to establish complete access for instruments in root canal therapy, and determined by extending the shape of the pulp lying internally onto the tooth enamel. See also endodontic CAVITY. 2. the shape of the area of the tooth surface included within the cavosurface margins of a prepared cavity, located on smooth enamel and refined to eliminate the discrepancies. **racemic f.,** racemate. **resistance f.,** the shape given to a prepared cavity to enable the restoration and remaining tooth structure to withstand masticatory forces. **retention f.,** adaptation of the form of a tooth cavity in such a way as to help maintain the filling material in the cavity. Retention forms include those required to meet the forces applied during the insertion of the restorative material, and those made to resist displacement in restorations exposed to functional forces. **spherical f. of occlusion,** an arrangement of teeth which places their occlusal surfaces on the surface of an imaginary sphere (usually 8 inches in diameter) with its center above the level of the teeth. **tooth f.,** the characteristic contour of a tooth, with its curves, lines, and angles, which permits the tooth to be differentiated from other teeth and its identity to be established. See also dental CHART. **uniform report f.,** a standardized statement which serves as a report and as the basis for payment of benefits under an insurance plan. A standardized dental health insurance claim form developed by the American Dental Association and the Health Insurance Council, accepted by many dental health insurance carriers, includes a certification signed by the benefi-

ciary and the dentist that services have been rendered, listing services rendered, and dates of services, and itemization of costs, requiring that the procedures be coded according to the ADA Uniform Code on Dental Procedures and Nomenclature (see under CODE). Called also *claim f.* and *attending dentist's statement.* **young f.,** metamyelocyte.

formaldehyde (for-mal′dĕ-hīd) a readily polymerizable, flammable gas, HCHO, with a strong, pungent, suffocating odor, which is soluble in water and alcohol. A 37 percent aqueous solution of formaldehyde with 10 to 15 percent methanol added to prevent polymerization is used as a fixing agent for histological specimens and as a disinfectant, antiseptic, and astringent. Disinfection of buildings, clothing, utensils, and other objects is the principal use for formaldehyde. A 3 to 4 percent solution of formaldehyde in isopropyl alcohol is used as a disinfectant for vegetative cells; mixtures of various amounts of formaldehyde in isopropyl alcohol have been used in the disinfection of dental instruments. Mixed with cresol, it is used in root canal therapy; also used to desensitize hypersensitive dentin. Contact may cause dermatitis; ingestion may result in hematemesis, hematuria, proteinuria, anuria, acidosis, and death. In the gaseous state, called also *formic aldehyde, methanal, methyl aldehyde, methylene oxide, oxomethane,* and *oxymethylene.* In aqueous solution, called also *formalin* and *formol;* trademark: Morbicid. **f. sodium sulfoxylate,** SODIUM formaldehyde sulfoxylate.

formalin (for′mah-lin) formaldehyde.

Formally trademark for an *amalgam alloy* (see under AMALGAM).

formatio (for-ma′she-o), pl. *formatio′nes* [L.] formation; a structure of definite shape.

formation (for-ma′shun) [L. *formatio*] 1. the act or process of giving shape or form; the creation of an entity. 2. a structure of definite shape. **central buttressing bone f.,** bone formation within the jaw in an attempt to buttress bone trabeculae weakened by resorption. **peripheral buttressing bone f.,** bone formation on the external surface of the jaw in an attempt to buttress bone trabeculae weakened by resorption, sometimes causing bulging of the bone contour or lipping. **reticular f.,** the portion of the brain stem and cervical spinal cord which contains centers regulating respiration, blood pressure, heart rate, and other functions. It is capable of modifying or integrating impulses from sensory receptors and is known to be related to arousal and wakefulness following stimulation of the reticular activating system. Through efferent pathways, it appears to facilitate or inhibit the response of motor neurons. **spore f.,** sporulation. **twin f.,** see GEMINATION.

formationes (for-ma′she-o-nēz) [L.] plural of *formatio.*

form-class (form-klas) an artificial taxonomic category comparable to a class, to which organisms are provisionally assigned, as are imperfect fungi until their perfect (sexual) stages are identified. Form-classes are subdivided into form-orders, form-families, and so on.

forme (fōrm), pl. *formes* [Fr.] form. **f. fruste** [Fr. "defaced"], a very mild or incomplete expression of a pathological condition. **f. fruste of Hurler's syndrome,** Scheie's SYNDROME.

former (for′mer) 1. preceding in time; prior or earlier. 2. something used for shaping or forming something else. **angle f.,** a paired right and left hoe-shaped handcutting instrument, having the blade sharpened on three sides, the extremes and the nib; used for finishing cavity margins, beveling or planing where necessary, sharpening line and point angles, and increasing retention in cavity preparation. See illustration. **crucible f.,** sprue f. **glass f.,** ions which combine with small mul-

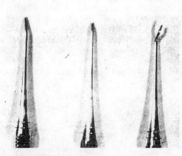

Angle formers. (From V. R. Park and J. R. Ashman: A Textbook for Dental Assistants. 2nd ed. Philadelphia, W. B. Saunders Co., 1975.)

tivalent atoms, such as silicon, boron, germanium, or phosphorus, forming stable bonds and structural units, such as SiO_4 tetrahedron or BO_3 triangle, organizing the random network in glass. **sprue f.,** a short piece of metal wire or a wax or plastic rod attached to the pattern by melting the wax at the point of attachment, used to provide the sprue in the investment through which the molten alloy can reach the mold after the wax has been eliminated. Called also *crucible f., sprue base,* and *sprue pin.*

form-family (form-fam′ĭ-le) see FORM-CLASS.

formication (for″mi-ka′shun) [L. *formica* ant] a form of paresthesia characterized by a sensation that ants are crawling over the skin.

formocresol (for″mo-kre′sol) a preparation containing formaldehyde and cresol; used in vital pulpotomy.

formol (for′mol) formaldehyde.

form-order (form-or′der) see FORM-CLASS.

formula (for′mu-lah), pl. *formulas* or *for′mulae* [L., dim of *forma* form] 1. a prescribed or set form or method. 2. a specific statement, using numerals and other symbols, of the composition of, or of the directions for preparing, a compound, such as a medicine, or of a procedure to follow for obtaining a desired value or result; a simplified statement, using numerals and symbols, of a single concept. 3. chemical f. **Ambard's f.,** a formula for finding the urea index (K) in kidney disease:

$$\frac{Ur}{\sqrt{D \times (70/P)} \times \sqrt{C/25}} = K,$$

in which *Ur* represents the proportion of the urea in the blood; *D,* the total urea for 24 hours in grams; *P,* the body weight in kilograms; *C,* the proportion of urea in the urine. **basic f.,** three-number f. **Black's f.** (G. V. Black), three- or four-number formulae for the identification of handcutting instruments according to length, width, and sizes and angles of their blades. See DENTISTRY. **chemical f.,** a combination of symbols used to express the chemical constitution of a substance; in practice, different types of formulas are employed. See *empirical f., molecular f., spatial f.,* and *structural f.* **constitutional f.,** structural f. **dental f.,** an expression in symbols of the number of and arrangement of teeth in the jaws. Letters represent the various types of teeth: I, *incisor;* C, *canine;* P, *premolar;* M, *molar.* Each letter is followed by a horizontal line. Numbers above the line represent maxillary teeth; those below, mandibular teeth. The human dental formula is $I\frac{2}{2} C\frac{1}{1} M\frac{2}{2} = 10$ (one side only) for deciduous teeth and $I\frac{2}{2} C\frac{1}{1} P\frac{2}{2} M\frac{3}{3} = 16$ (one side only) for permanent teeth. See also dental CHART. **empirical f.,** a chemical formula which expresses the proportions of the elements present in a substance. For substances composed of molecules, it expresses the relative numbers of atoms present in a molecule of the substance in the smallest whole numbers. For example, the empirical formula for ethane is written CH_3, whereas the actual molecular formula is C_2H_6. **four-number f.,** a four number formula indicating the width, length in mm, and angle (in degrees of a centigrade circle) of the blade and cutting edge of handcutting dental instruments, devised by G. V. Black. See DENTISTRY. **graphic f.,** structural f. **Hardy-Weinberg f.,** Hardy-Weinberg LAW. **molecular f.,** a chemical formula giving the number of atoms of each element present in a molecule of a substance, without indicating how they are linked. For example, the molecular formula for ethyl alcohol is written CH_3CH_2OH. **official f.,** one officially established by a pharmacopeia or other recognized authority. **spatial f.,** a chemical formula giving the numbers of atoms of each element present in a molecule of a substance, which atom is linked to which, the types of linkages involved, and the relative position of the atoms in space. For example, the spatial formula for glucose is

Called also *stereochemical f.* **stereochemical f.,** spatial f. **structural f.,** a chemical formula telling how many atoms of each element are present in a molecule of a substance, which atom is linked to which, and the type of linkages involved. For example, the structural formula for ethyl alcohol is

Called also *constitutional f.* and *graphic f.* **Thielemann's f.,** Thielemann's PRINCIPLE. **three-number f.,** a three-number formula indicating the width, length, and angle of a handcutting dental instrument, devised by G. V. Black. Called also *basic f.* See DENTISTRY.

formulary (for′mu-lar″e) a listing of drugs, usually by their generic names. **hospital f.,** a list of all the drugs routinely stocked by the hospital pharmacy. **National F.,** a compendium of standards for certain drugs and preparations that are not included in the United States Pharmacopeia. It is revised every 5 years, and recognized as a book of official standards by the Pure Food and Drugs Act of 1906. Abbreviated *NF.*

formyl (for′mil) [L. *formic* + Gr. *hylē* matter] the radical, HCO or $H \cdot C{:}O$ —, of formic acid. **f. trichloride,** chloroform.

fornix (for′niks), pl. *for′nices* [L. "arch"] any archlike or domelike structure; used in anatomical nomenclature to designate such structures. See also VAULT. **f. pharyn′gis** [NA], **f. of the pharynx,** VAULT of the pharynx.

Forssman antibody, antigen [John *Forssman,* Swedish pathologist, 1868–1947] see under ANTIBODY and ANTIGEN.

Forssmann, Werner Theodor Otto [born 1904] a German surgeon; co-winner, with André F. Cournand and Dickinson W. Richards, of the Nobel prize for medicine and physiology in 1956, for developing a technique in the diagnosis and treatment of heart disease.

Fortal trademark for *pentazocine.*

Fortalgesic trademark for *pentazocine.*

Fortalin trademark for *pentazocine.*

Fortamine trademark for *dexchlorpheniramine maleate* (see under DEXCHLORPHENIRAMINE).

Fortuss trademark for *dihydrocodeine bitartrate* (see under DIHYDROCODEINE).

fossa (fos′ah), pl. *fos′sae* [L. "a ditch"] 1. shallow depression or concavity; a hollow or depressed area. See also FOSSULA. 2. rounded or angular depression of varying size on the surface of a tooth. **amygdaloid f.,** the depression between the pillars of the fauces, on either side, which lodges the tonsil. **articular f. of mandible,** articular f. of temporal bone, mandibular f. **canine f., f. cani′na** [NA], a wide depression on the anterior surface of the maxillary body, formed in part by the projecting zygomatic process and situated superolaterally to the canine tooth socket, serving as attachment for the levator anguli oris muscle. Called also *maxillary f.* **f. carot′ica,** carotid TRIANGLE. **central f.,** a shallow depression on the occlusal surfaces of molars, formed by the converging of ridges terminating at a central point in the bottom of the depression. **cerebral f.,** any one of the depressions on the floor of the cranial cavity, such as the anterior, middle, and posterior cranial fossae. **condylar f., f. condyla′ris** [NA], condyloid f. **condyloid f.,** either of two pits situated on the lateral portions of the occipital bone, one on either side of the foramen magnum, posterior to the occipital condyle. Called also *condylar f., f. condylaris* [NA], *f. condyloidea, postcondyloid f.,* and *posterior condyloid f.* **condyloid f. of mandible, condyloid f. of temporal bone,** mandibular f. **f. condyloi′dea,** condyloid f. **cranial f., anterior, f. cra′nii ante′rior** [NA], the anterior subdivision of the floor of the cranial cavity, supporting the frontal lobes of the brain, and composed of the ethmoid, frontal, and sphenoid bones. **cranial f., middle, f. cra′nii me′dia** [NA], the middle subdivision of the floor of the cranial cavity, supporting the temporal lobes of the brain and the pituitary gland, and composed of the body and the greater wings of the sphenoid bone and the squamous and petrous parts of the temporal bone. **cranial f., posterior, f. cra′nii poste′rior** [NA], the posterior subdivision of the floor of the cranial cavity, lodging the cerebellum, pons, and medulla oblongata, and formed by portions of the sphenoid, temporal, parietal, and occipital bones. **Cruveilhier's f., navicular,** scaphoid f. of sphenoid bone. **digastric f.,** 1. a small roughened depression on the internal surface of the body of the mandible on each side of the symphysis, to which is attached the anterior belly of the digastric muscle. Called also *f. digastrica* [NA], *f. musculi biventeris, digastric fovea,* and *digastric impression.* 2. mastoid NOTCH. **f. digas′trica** [NA], digastric f. (1). **ethmoid f.**, a groove situated in the cribriform plate of the ethmoid bone; it lodges the olfactory bulb of the brain. Called also *olfactory f.* and *olfactory groove*. **f. of eustachian tube**, scaphoid f. of sphenoid bone. **floccular f.**, subarcuate f. of temporal bone. **f. of gasserian ganglion**, trigeminal impression of temporal bone; see under IMPRESSION. **Gerdy's hyoid f.**, carotid triangle, superior; see under TRIANGLE. **f. glan'dulae lacrima'lis** [NA], f. of lacrimal gland. **glenoid f.**, **glenoid f. of temporal bone**, mandibular f. **f. hel'icis**, scapha. **hypophyseal f.**, **f. hypophys'eos**, **f. hypophysia'lis** [NA], pituitary f. **incisive f.**, a shallow depression on the anterior surface of the body of the maxilla, mesial to the canine eminence, and overlying the roots of the incisor teeth, which gives origin to the depressor septi muscle. **incisive f. of mandible**, a shallow depression on the body of the mandible, immediately posterior to the symphysis and above the mental protuberance, situated below the alveolar border of the central and lateral incisors and anterior to the canines. **incisive f. of maxilla**, a slight depression on the anterior surface of the maxilla above the incisor teeth. Called also *myrtiform f.*, *f. praenasalis*, and *prenasal f.* **infratemporal f.**, **f. infratempora'lis** [NA], a shallow depression on the side of the cranium bounded superiorly by the infratemporal crest, posteriorly by the mandibular fossa, anteriorly by the posterior surface of the zygomatic process of the maxilla, and laterally by the inner surface of the zygomatic arch and the upper part of the ascending ramus of the mandible. A medial wall exists only in the anterior part and is formed by the lateral pterygoid plate of the sphenoid bone and the pyramidal process of the palatine bone. The pterygopalatine suture separates these two parts in young persons; a variably sharp line exists in older persons. It contains the pterygoid muscles, maxillary artery, pterygoid venous plexus, and branches of the mandibular nerve. The infraorbital nerve and artery and the zygomatic nerves enter the orbit through the inferior orbital fissure; the mandibular nerve enters through the oval foramen; the meningeal artery enters through the foramen spinosum; and the middle maxillary artery enters through the pterygopalatine fissure. Called also *zygomatic fissure*. **jugular f.**, **f. jugula'ris**, a shallow space between two laminae of the investing layer of the cervical fascia, located at the base of the neck just above the sternum. It is filled with fat and contains portions of the jugular veins and their branches, the sternal head of the sternocleidomastoid muscle, and some lymph nodes. Called also *space of Burns*. **jugular f. of temporal bone**, **f. jugula'ris os'sis tempora'lis** [NA], a prominent depression on the inferior surface of the petrous part of the temporal bone, forming the major part of the jugular notch; it forms the anterior and lateral wall of the jugular foramen and lodges the superior bulb of the internal jugular vein. Called also *suprasternal space*. **f. of lacrimal gland**, a shallow depression in the orbital part of the frontal bone, above the orbit, lodging the lacrimal gland. Called also *f. glandulae lacrimalis* [NA]. **f. of lacrimal sac**, lacrimal GROOVE. **lingual f.**, a shallow depression on the lingual surface of the incisors. **Malgaigne's f.**, carotid triangle, superior; see under TRIANGLE. **mandibular f.**, **f. mandibula'ris** [NA], a prominent depression in the inferior surface of the squamous part of the temporal bone at the base of the zygomatic process, in which the condyloid process of the mandible rests, divided by the petrotympanic fissure into posterior and anterior halves, with the anterior half being included in the temporomandibular articulation. Called also *articular f. of mandible*, *articular f. of temporal bone, condyloid f. of mandible, condyloid f. of temporal bone, glenoid f., glenoid f. of temporal bone,* and *articular fovea of temporal bone*. **mastoid f. of temporal bone**, suprameatal TRIANGLE. **maxillary f.**, canine f. **f. mus'culi biven'teris**, digastric f. (1). **mylohyoid f. of mandible**, sublingual f. **myrtiform f.**, incisive f. of maxilla. **nasal f.**, the portion of the nasal cavity anterior to the middle meatus. **navicular f. of Cruveilhier**, navicular f. of sphenoid bone, scaphoid f. of sphenoid bone. **olfactory f.**, ethmoid f. **oral f.**, stomodeum. **parietal f.**, the deepest portion of the inner surface of the parietal bone. **petrosal f.**, **f. for petrosal ganglion**, petrosal FOSSULA. **pituitary f.**, a deep depression in the middle of the sella turcica, lodging the pituitary gland. Called also *hypophyseal f.*, *f. hypophyseos, f. hypophysia'lis* [NA], and *suprasphenoidal f.* **postcondyloid f.**, posterior condyloid f., condyloid f. **f. praenasa'lis, prenasal f.**, incisive f. of maxilla. **pterygoid f. of inferior maxillary bone**, pterygoid f. of mandible. **pterygoid f. of mandible**, a pit on the inner side of the neck of the condyle of the mandible, for attachment of the lateral pterygoid muscle. Called also *pterygoid f. of inferior maxillary bone, fovea of condyloid process, fovea pterygoidea mandibulae* [NA], *fovea pterygoidea processus condyloidei, pterygoid depression, pterygoid fovea,* and *pterygoid pit*. **pterygoid f. of sphenoid bone**, **f. pterygoi'dea os'sis sphenoida'lis** [NA], a V-shaped fossa formed by the

divergence of the medial and lateral pterygoid plates of the sphenoid bone; it lodges the medial pterygoid muscle and tensor veli palatini muscle. **pterygomaxillary f.**, pterygopalatine f. **pterygopalatine f.**, **f. pterygopalati'na** [NA], a small, funnel-shaped space at the junction of the inferior orbital and pterygomaxillary fissures, bounded anteriorly by the medial part of the maxillary tuber, posteriorly by the anterior surface of the pterygoid process of the sphenoid bone, medially by the lateral surface of the vertical plate of the palatine bones, and superiorly by the greater sphenoid wing. It communicates with the orbit by the inferior orbital fissure, with the nasal cavity by the sphenopalatine foramen, and with the infratemporal fossa by the pterygomaxillary fissure. The posterior wall contains the foramen rotundum, pterygoid canal, and pharyngeal canal; the medial wall contains the sphenopalatine foramen and pterygopalatine canal. It narrows downward and continues into the pterygopalatine canal between the maxilla and the palatine bone and opens into the oral cavity through the greater and lesser palatine foramina, and contains the maxillary nerve, pterygopalatine ganglion, and terminal part of the maxillary artery. Called also *pterygomaxillary f.* and *sphenomaxillary f.* **retromandibular f.**, **f. retromandibula'ris**, the depression behind the angle of the jaw, on either side, beneath the auricle. **Rosenmüller's f.**, pharyngeal RECESS. **f. sac'ci lacrima'lis** [NA], lacrimal GROOVE. **scaphoid f.**, **f. scaphoi'dea**, 1. scapha. 2. triangular f. of auricle. **scaphoid f. of sphenoid bone**, **f. scaphoi'dea os'sis sphenoida'lis** [NA], 1. a small oval depression on the superior part of the posterior portion of the medial plate of the pterygoid process of the sphenoid bone; it gives origin to the veli palatini muscle. Called also *f. of eustachian tube, navicular f. of Cruveilhier,* and *navicular f. of sphenoid bone*. **sellar f.**, pituitary f. **sigmoid f.**, SULCUS of transverse sinus of occipital bone. **sigmoid f. of temporal bone**, SULCUS of sigmoid sinus of temporal bone. **sphenoidal f.**, APERTURE of sphenoid sinus. **sphenomaxillary f.**, pterygopalatine f. **f. subarcua'ta os'sis tempora'lis** [NA], subarcuate f. of temporal bone. **subarcuate f. of temporal bone**, a small fossa on the internal surface of the petrous part of the temporal bone just below the arcuate eminence, most prominent in the fetus. In the adult, it lodges a piece of dura and transmits a small vein. Called also *floccular f., f. subarcuata ossis temporalis* [NA], and *subarcuate hiatus*. **sublingual f.**, a smooth depression on the inner surface of the body of the mandible, immediately posterior to the median line and above the anterior part of the mylohyoid ridge, lodging a portion of the sublingual gland. Called also *mylohyoid f. of mandible, fovea sublingualis* [NA], and *sublingual fovea*. **submandibular f.**, submaxillary f., a smooth oblong depression on the medial aspect of the body of the mandible, between the mylohyoid ridge and the lower border of the bone, lodging a small portion of the submandibular gland. Called also *submaxillary f., fovea submandibularis* [NA], *fovea submaxillaris,* and *submandibular fovea*. **suprasphenoidal f.**, pituitary f. **supratonsillar f.**, **f. supratonsilla'ris** [NA], the space between the palatoglossal and palatopharyngeal arches above the tonsil. **temporal f.**, **f. tempora'lis** [NA], a shallow depression on the side of the cranium outlined posteriorly and superiorly by the temporal line; anteriorly, where the fossa is the deepest, by the temporal surface of the ascending or frontal process of the zygomatic bone; laterally by the zygomatic arch; and inferiorly by the parietal bone, squama of the temporal bone, temporal surface of the greater wing of the sphenoid bone, and temporal surface of the frontal bone. It serves as the attachment for the temporal muscle, and continues into the infratemporal fossa. **tonsillar f.**, **f. tonsilla'ris** [NA], the depression between the palatoglossal and palatopharyngeal arches in which the palatine tonsil is located. Called also *sinus interarcualis, sinus tonsillaris,* and *tonsillar sinus*. **triangular f.**, a shallow depression on the occlusal surfaces mesial or distal to the marginal ridges of the molar and premolar teeth. Triangular fossae may be sometimes found on the lingual surfaces of maxillary incisors at the cervical extremity of the lingual fossa at the junction of the marginal ridge and cingulum. **triangular f. of auricle**, **f. triangular'is auric'ulae** [NA], the cavity just above the concha of the ear between the crura of the antihelix. Called also *scaphoid f.* and *f. scaphoidea*. **trochlear f.**, **f. trochlea'ris**, trochlear FOVEA.

fossae (fos'e) [L.] plural of *fossa*.

fossula (fos'u-lah), pl. *fos'sulae* [L., dim. of *fossa*] a small fossa; a small depression in the surface of an organ or structure. **f. of cochlear window**, **f. fenes'trae coch'leae** [NA], f. of round window. **f. petro'sa** [NA], petrosal f. **f. fenes'trae vestib'uli**

[NA], f. of oval window. **f. of oval window,** a depression on the medial wall of the tympanic cavity, at the bottom of which is the fenestra vestibuli. Called also *fossula fenestrae vestibuli* [NA]. **petrosal f., f. of petrous ganglion,** a small depression on the under surface of the petrous portion of the temporal bone, on a small ridge separating the jugular fossa from the external carotid foramen. Called also *f. petrosa* [NA], *petrosal fossa, fossa for petrosal ganglion,* and *vallecula for petrosal ganglion.* **f. of round window,** a depression on the medial wall of the tympanic cavity, at the bottom of which is the fenestra cochleae. Called also *f. of cochlear window* and *f. fenestrae cochleae* [NA]. **tonsillar fossulae of palatine tonsil, fos′sulae ton-silla′res tonsil′lae palati′nae** [NA], the mouths of the tonsillar crypts of the palatine tonsil. Called also *foramina of palatine tonsil* and *tonsillar foramina.* **tonsillar fossulae of pharyngeal tonsil, fos′sulae tonsilla′res tonsil′lae pharyn′geae** [NA], the mouths of the tonsillar crypts of the pharyngeal tonsil. Called also *tonsillar foramina.*

fossulae (fos′u-le) [L.] plural of *fossula.*

fossulate (fos′u-lāt) marked by a small fossa; hollowed or grooved.

Fothergill's disease [John *Fothergill,* English physician, 1712–1780] 1. trigeminal NEURALGIA. 2. SCARLATINA anginosa.

foundation (foun-da′shun) 1. the structure or basis on which something is built. 2. a nonprofit organization established for a specific task. **denture f.,** denture-bearing AREA. **ADA Health F.,** see *American Dental Association* in Appendix. **medical f.,** an independent organization of physicians, usually sponsored by a local or state medical association, which is concerned with the delivery of medical services at reasonable cost. Some foundations are organized solely for peer review purposes or other specific functions, but some operate as prepaid group practices or as an individual practice association for a health maintenance organization.

Fournier teeth [Jean Alfred *Fournier,* French dermatologist, 1832–1914] Moon's teeth; see under TOOTH.

fovea (fo′ve-ah), pl. *fo′veae* [L.] a pit or depression; a general anatomical term for a small pit in the surface of a structure or organ. **articular f. of temporal bone,** mandibular FOSSA. **f. of condyloid process,** pterygoid fossa of mandible; see under FOSSA. **digastric f.,** digastric FOSSA (1). **oblong f. of arytenoid cartilage,** oblong pit of arytenoid cartilage; see under PIT. **f. oblon′ga cartilag′inis arytenoi′deae** [NA], oblong pit of arytenoid cartilage; see under PIT. **pterygoid f., f. pterygoi′dea mandib′ulae** [NA], **f. pterygoi′dea proces′sus condyloi′dei,** pterygoid fossa of mandible; see under FOSSA. **sublingual f., f. sublingua′lis** [NA], sublingual FOSSA. **submandibular f., f. submandibula′ris** [NA], **f. submaxilla′ris, submaxillary f.,** submandibular FOSSA. **f. triangula′ris cartilag′inis arytenoi′deae** [NA], triangular pit of arytenoid cartilage; see under PIT. **trochlear f., f. trochlea′ris** [NA], a depression on the anteromedial part of the orbital surface of the frontal bone for attachment of the trochlea of the superior oblique muscle; it is often replaced by a small trochlear spine. Called also *trochlear fossa* and *fossa trochlearis.*

foveate (fo′ve-āt) [L. *foveatus*] pitted.

foveation (fo″ve-a′shun) a pitted condition.

foveola (fo-ve′o-lah), pl. *fove′olae* [L., dim. of *fovea*] a small pit; a general anatomical term for a very small pit. **granular foveolae, fove′olae granula′res** [NA], **fove′olal granula′res Pacchioni,** small depressions on the internal surface of the parietal bone near the sulcus for the superior sagittal sinus, occupied by the arachnoidal granulations; they are best marked in the skulls of older persons. Called also *pacchionian depressions.* **palatine f. of Stieda,** a small pit on the surface of the soft palate, close to the midline and immediately behind the boundary between the hard and soft palate, found in most persons, into which some ducts of the palatine glands empty.

foveolae (fo-ve′o-le) [L.] plural of *foveola.*

foveolate (fo-ve′o-lāt) characterized by the presence of small pits or foveolae; pitted.

Foville's syndrome [Achille Louis François *Foville,* French neurologist, 1831–1887] see under SYNDROME.

Fowler's position [George Ryerson *Fowler,* American surgeon, 1848–1906] see under POSITION.

Fox's disease, [William Tilbury *Fox,* English dermatologist, 1836–1879] EPIDERMOLYSIS bullosa.

Fox forceps, scissors see under FORCEPS and SCISSORS.

Fox-Williams probe see under PROBE.

foxglove (foks′gluv) digitalis.

FP 1. abbreviation for L. *fi′at po′tio,* let a potion be made. 2. freezing POINT.

fp foot-pound.

F. pil. abbreviation for L. *fi′at pil′ulae,* let pills be made.

FPO Federation of Prosthodontic Organizations.

Fr 1. francium. 2. French (see under SCALE).

Fracastorius, Hieronymus [It. *Girolamo Fracastoro*] an Italian physician, poet, and geologist, born in Verona in 1475 or 1483 and died 1553, who published in 1530 a medical poem, *Syphilis sive morbus gallicus,* in which syphilis was first mentioned.

Fract. dos. abbreviation for L. *frac′ta do′si,* in divided doses.

fraction (frak′shun) in chemistry, one of the separable constituents of a substance. **f. A,** a fraction of plasma proteins separable by filter electrophoresis. It consists chiefly of albumin (see plasma ALBUMIN), having the smallest molecules of any plasma proteins; its molecular weight is 70,000. Fraction A corresponds to 4S protein. **filtration f.,** the portion of the plasma that is filtered through the renal glomerular membranes, calculated as the ratio of the plasma flow through both kidneys to the glomerular filtration rate per minute. **mole f.,** the number of moles of a component (solute) of a solution divided by the total number of moles of all components. **plasma f., plasma protein f.,** the various proteins separated from blood plasma. A sterile preparation of selected proteins from the blood plasma of adult human donors is used as a blood volume supporter.

fractional (frak′shun-al) [L. *fractio* a breaking] accomplished by repeated divisions.

fractionation (frak″shun-a′shun) 1. in radiology, division of the total dose of radiation into small doses administered at intervals; radiation given in this manner usually causes less biological damage than the same total dose given at once. Called also *dose f.* 2. in chemistry, separation of a substance into components, as by distillation or crystallization. **dose f.,** fractionation (1).

fracture (frak′chur) [L. *fractura,* from *frangere* to break] the breaking of a part, especially of a bony structure. **articular f.,** one of the joint surface of a bone. Called also *intra-articular f.* and *joint f.* **atrophic f.,** a pathologic fracture resulting from atrophy of the bone. **avulsion f.,** an indirect fracture caused by avulsion. **blow-out f.,** fracture of the orbital floor caused by a sudden increase of intraorbital pressure due to traumatic force; the orbital contents herniate into the maxillary sinus so that the interior rectus or inferior oblique muscle may become incarcerated in the fracture site, producing diplopia on looking up. In the pure type, there is a fracture of the orbital floor without involvement of the orbital rim. **brittle f.,** fracture of a material occurring as the result of bending or twisting, without prior stretching, in which the tensile strength of a structure may increase with the rate of stress application because there is less time for plastic flow to occur near the microcrack, thus relieving the stress concentration, being more common in plastic than elastic materials. See also *ductile f.* **buttonhole f.,** one in which the bone is perforated by a missile. Called also *perforating f.* **capillary f.,** one that appears in the roentgenogram as a fine hairlike line, the segments of bone not being separated; sometimes seen in fractures of the skull. **cemental f., cementum f.,** cemental TEAR. **closed f.,** one that does not produce an open wound in the skin. In simple fractures of the jaws, which involve most commonly the neck of the condyle of the mandible, the broken bone surface is not in contact with the secretions of the oral cavity, nor does it open on the surface of the face. Called also *simple f.* and *subcutaneous f.* **comminuted f.,** one in which the bone is fragmented, splintered, or crushed. When occurring in the jaws, it usually involves the region of the symphysis of the mandible or the anterior maxilla. **complete f.,** one in which the bone is entirely broken across. **complex f.,** one in which the break occurs in several directions. In complex fractures of the jaws the break may continue into the temporomandibular joint. **compound f.,** open f. **compression f.,** one produced by compression. **condylar process f.,** fracture of the condylar process, usually occurring as the result of indirect force. **condylar process f., high,** one occurring above the level of insertion of the lateral pterygoid muscle. **condylar process f., low,** one occurring at the base of the condylar process. **condylar process f., middle,** one occurring immediately below the lateral pterygoid muscle attachment. **depressed f.,** one of the skull in which a fragment is depressed below the surface. **direct f.,** one at the point of injury. **dislocation f.,** one of a bone near an articulation with its concomitant dislocation from that joint. **double f.,** one of a bone in two places. **ductile f.,** one of a material after it had been stretched under stress to maximum, in which plastic deformation of the grains can occur before fracture during a slow loading, being more common in elastic rather than plastic materials. See also *brittle f.* **dyscrasic f.,** one due to a weakening of the bone from debilitating disease. See also *pathologic f.* **endocrine f.,** one of a bone weakened by an endocrine disorder, such as hyperparathyroidism. See also *pathologic f.* **fissure f., fissured f.,** a linear fracture extending partially through a bone with no displacement of the bony fragments. Called also *linear f.* **greenstick f.,** an incomplete fracture in which one side of a bone is broken, the other being bent. Called also *hickory-stick f.* and *willow f.* **Guérin's f.,** Le Fort I f. **gunshot f.,** one produced by a bullet or other missile. See also *buttonhole f.* and *resecting f.* **gutter f.,** one of the skull in which the depression is elliptic in form. **hickory-stick f.,** greenstick f. **horizontal maxillary f.,** Le Fort I f. **impacted f.,** one in which one fragment is firmly driven into the other. **incomplete f.,** one which does not entirely destroy the continuity of the bone; an infraction. **indirect f.,** one at a point distant from the site of injury. **inflammatory f.,** one of a bone weakened by inflammatory disease. See also *pathologic f.* **intergranular f.,** one of a material having a crystalline structure, occurring along grain boundaries; it usually takes place at elevated temperatures. See also *transgranular f.* **intra-articular f.,** articular f. **intracapsular f.,** one within the capsule of a joint. **joint f.,** articular f. **Le Fort's f.,** bilateral horizontal fracture of the maxilla. Le Fort fractures are classified as follows: *Le Fort I f.,* a horizontal segmented fracture of the alveolar process of the maxilla, in which the teeth are usually contained in the detached portion of the bone; called also *Guérin's f.* and *horizontal maxillary f. Le Fort II f.,* unilateral or bilateral fracture of the maxilla, in which the body of the maxilla is separated from the facial skeleton and the separated portion is pyramidal in shape; the fracture may extend through the body of the maxilla down the midline of the hard palate, through the floor of the orbit, and into the nasal cavity. Called also *pyramidal f. Le Fort III f.,* a fracture in which the entire maxilla and one or more facial bones are completely separated from the craniofacial skeleton; such fractures are almost always accompanied by multiple fractures of the facial bones; called also *craniofacial dysjunction* and *transverse facial f.* **linear f.,** fissure f. **loose f.,** one in which the bone is completely broken so that the broken ends have free play. **multiple f.,** one in which the bone is fractured in two or more places without communication between the lines of fracture. It is the most common type of jaw fracture, usually occurring bilaterally in both the mandible and the maxilla, but may also occur unilaterally, the bone being fractured into several segments on one side only. **neoplastic f.,** a pathologic fracture due to weakening of the bone as a result of a malignant process. **open f.,** one in which there is an external wound leading to the break of the bone. In open fractures of the jaws, the broken bone fragments penetrate the mucosa into the oral cavity or perforate the facial skin. Fractures which communicate with a tooth socket are also termed *open fractures.* They generally occur anterior to the angle formed by the vertical ramus with the horizontal ramus. Called also *compound f.* **pathologic f.,** one due to the weakening of bone structure by pathologic processes, such as osteomalacia, osteomyelitis, tumors, osteogenesis imperfecta, and other diseases. In instances of severe destruction of bone, fractures of the jaws may occur spontaneously during eating, yawning, or talking. Called also *spontaneous f.* **perforating f.,** buttonhole f. **periarticular f.,** one extending close to, but not into, a joint. **ping-pong f.,** an indented fracture of the skull, resembling the indentation that can be produced with the finger in a ping-pong ball; when elevated it resumes and retains its normal position. **pond f.,** one of the skull in which a fissure circumscribes the radiating lines, giving the depressed area a circular form. **pressure f.,** one caused by pressure on the bone from an adjoining tumor. **pyramidal f.,** Le Fort II f. **resecting f.,** one in which a piece of the bone is removed by violence, as by a bullet. **secondary f.,** pathologic f. **simple f.,** closed f. **simple f., complex,** a closed fracture in which there is considerable injury to adjacent soft tissue. **single f.,** one in which the bone is fractured in only one place. Single fractures occur infrequently in the jaws, usually unilaterally, involving only the mandible. **splintered f.,** a comminuted fracture in which the bone is splintered into thin, sharp fragments. **spontaneous f.,** pathologic f. **stellate f.,** one with a central point of injury, from which radiate numerous fissures. **subcutaneous f.,** closed f. **tooth f.,** breaking of a tooth. **transgranular f.,** one of a material having a crystalline structure, occurring through the granules; it usually takes place at room temperature. See also *intergranular f.* **transverse f.,** one at right angles to the axis of the bone. **transverse facial f.,** Le Fort III f. **transverse maxillary f.,** a term sometimes used for horizontal maxillary fracture. See *Le Fort I f.* **traumatic f.,** one occurring as the result of external trauma; accidents, falls, gunshot injuries, or complications of tooth extraction being the

most common causes. **vertical tooth f.,** split TOOTH. **willow f.,** greenstick f.

fracture-dislocation (frak′tur dis″lo-ka′shun) a fracture near a joint associated with a dislocation.

Frademicina trademark for *lincomycin.*

Fradiomycin trademark for *neomycin.*

fragilitas (frah-jil′ĭ-tas) [L.] susceptibility, or lack of resistance, to factors capable of causing disruption of continuity or integrity; fragility. **f. os′sium,** abnormal brittleness of the bones. See OSTEOGENESIS imperfecta. **f. os′sium congen′ita,** Vrolik's SYN-DROME. **f. os′sium heredita′ria tar′da,** van der Hoeve's SYN-DROME. **f. os′sium tar′da,** Lobstein's SYNDROME.

fragility (frah-jil′ĭ-te) [L. *fragilitas*] susceptibility, or lack of resistance, to factors capable of causing disruption of continuity or integrity. See also *fragilitas.* **capillary f.,** susceptibility, or lack of resistance, of capillaries to disruption under conditions of increased stress. See also tourniquet TEST (1). **erythrocyte f.,** osmotic f. **osmotic f.,** the lack of resistance of the erythrocyte to hemolysis in a hypotonic solution, whereby the cell absorbs water and swells, resulting in bursting of the stroma. Called also *erythrocyte f.* See also osmotic HEMOLYSIS.

fragment (frag′ment) a part broken off a larger body. **antigen-binding f.,** Fab. **crystallizable f.,** Fc. **Fab f.,** Fab. **f. F(ab′)₂,** F(ab′)₂. **Fc f.,** Fc. **Fc′ f.,** Fc′. **Fd f.,** Fd. **pFc′ f.,** pFc′.

fragmentation (frag″men-ta′shun) a division into fragments.

fraise (frāz) [Fr. "strawberry"] a conical or hemispherical burr for cutting osteoplastic flaps or enlarging trephine openings.

frambesia (fram-be′ze-ah) [Fr. *framboise* raspberry] yaws.

frame (frām) a structure, usually rigid, designed for giving support to or for immobilizing a part. **implant superstructure f.,** superstructure f. **N-O f.,** Nygaard-Otsby f. **Nygaard-Otsby f., Otsby f.,** a radiolucent rubber dam frame made of plastic, curved to fit a patient's face, which may be positioned so that the patient breathes behind the dam and not into the operative field. Called also *N-O f.* **occluding f.,** dental ARTICULATOR. **radiolucent f.,** a rubber dam frame made of nylon or other radiolucent material that does not interfere with the roentgeno-graphic image. **ramus f.,** a horseshoe-shaped implant, serving as a stabilizing ridge for a full lower denture, especially in cases of severe bone resorption, which is designed for use with the two rami and the symphysis of the mandible as support. **rubber dam f.,** a U-shaped frame, made of metal or plastic material, for stretching and holding the rubber dam in position on the face during dental operations. **subperiosteal f., peripheral,** the labi-al, buccal, lingual, and distal portions of the subperiosteal implant substructure. **superstructure f.,** a metal frame of the superstructure of a subperiosteal implant, consisting of attach-ments and connectors. Called also *implant superstructure f.* **Wizard f.,** trademark for a type of metal rubber dam frame, which includes elastic straps encircling the patient's head. **Young f.,** a type of metal or plastic rubber dam frame used in endodontic therapy.

framework (frām′werk) the basic structure about which some-thing is formulated or built; as the metallic skeletal portion of a prosthesis to which are attached the resin flange and base components of the partial denture and the artificial teeth. **implant f.,** implant SUBSTRUCTURE.

Framycetin trademark for *neomycin B.*

Franceschetti's syndrome [Adolphe *Franceschetti*, Swiss physi-cian] mandibulofacial DYSOSTOSIS.

Franceschetti-Jadassohn syndrome [A. *Franceschetti*; Josef *Jadassohn*, German dermatologist in Bern, 1863–1936] Naege-li's SYNDROME.

Francis' disease [Edward *Francis*, American physician, born 1872] tularemia.

Francisella (fran″sĭ-sel′ah) [named after E. *Francis*] a genus of gram-negative, aerobic bacteria of uncertain affiliation, poten-tially pathogenic to man, which occur as coccoid to ellipsoidal, pleomorphic, nonmotile, minute rods; found in water. **F. novi′cida,** a species producing lesions similar to those occurring in tularemia in animals. Called also *Pasteurella novicida.* **F. tularen′sis,** a species made up of minute cells (0.2 μm in breadth and 0.3 to 0.7 μm in length), occurring as cocci in young cultures and as rods in older ones. It is the etiologic agent of tularemia in man, being transmitted from wild animals to man by drinking water, by blood-sucking insects, or by contact, and also causes a severe form of conjunctivitis. The species was originally isolated from California ground squirrels, now found in a wide variety of animals, and also isolated from water. The organisms are sensitive to streptomycin and, to a lesser degree, to tetracyclines and chloramphenicol. Called also *Bacterium tularensis*, *Brucella tularensis*, and *Pasteurella tularensis*.

francium (fran′se-um) [named after *France*] the heaviest element in the alkali metals, occurring as a result of alpha disintegration of actinium. Symbol, Fr; atomic number, 87; atomic weight, 223; melting point, 27°C; valence, 1; group IA of the periodic table. The isotope ²²³Fr (actinium K, symbol AcK) is the most stable of 20 francium isotopes now recognized; its half-life is 21 minutes and it emits beta rays. Francium occurs naturally in uranium ore and is produced artificially by bombarding thorium with protons. No weighable quantity of the element is available.

François' dyscephaly [Jules *François*, Belgian ophthalmologist] Hallermann-Streiff SYNDROME.

Franke's triad [Gustav *Franke*] see under TRIAD.

Fränkel appliance [R. *Fränkel*] function CORRECTOR.

Frankfort Horizontal, Frankford Horizontal plane see under PLANE.

Franklin's disease [E. C. *Franklin*] heavy chain DISEASE.

Fraser's syndrome [C. R. *Fraser*] cryptophthalmos SYNDROME.

FRC functional residual CAPACITY.

freckle (frek″l) a brownish pigmented spot on the epidermis or oral mucosa due to discrete accumulation of melanin as a result of the stimulant effect of a factor, such as sunlight, acting on clusters of melanocytes which have higher than normal tyrosinase activity. Called also *ephelis*. Cf. LENTIGO. **Hutchinson's f.,** a precancerous condition, occurring chiefly during middle and old age, and usually starting on the facial skin as a small dark brown or sepia spot. Among the various macules there may be simultaneous expansion and regression, but eventually they coalesce to form irregular pigmented areas, often reaching 10 cm in diameter. Thickening, induration, papules, verrucae, and ulceration signal the onset of malignancy. The average period from onset to development of malignant melanoma is about 10 years. Called also *infective senile f.*, *melanotic f.*, *dermoepidermal nevus*, *Dubreuilh's melanosis*, *precancerous melanosis*, and *tardive nevus*. **infective senile f., melanotic f.,** Hutchinson's f.

Freeman-Sheldon syndrome [E. A. *Freeman*, British physician; J. H. *Sheldon*, British physician] craniocarpotarsal DYSTROPHY.

freezing (frēz′ing) 1. solidification; the act or process of changing a liquid, such as water, to a solid, such as ice, with lowering of temperature. See also crystallization and freezing POINT. **f. temperature,** freezing TEMPERATURE.

Frei's bubo (disease) [Wilhelm Siegmund *Frei*, German dermatologist, 1885–1940] LYMPHOGRANULOMA venereum.

fremitus (frem′ĭ-tus) [L.] a vibration perceptible on palpation.

frena (fre′nah) [L.] plural of *frenum*.

Frenasma trademark for *cromolyn sodium* (see under CROMOLYN).

frenectomy (fre-nek′to-me) [*frenum* + Gr. *ektomē* excision] the excision of the frenum (frenulum).

Frenkel defect see under DEFECT.

frenoplasty (fre″no-plas′te) [*frenum* + Gr. *plassein* to form or shape] the correction of an abnormally attached frenum by surgically repositioning it.

frenotomy (fre-not′o-me) [*frenum* + Gr. *tomē* a cutting] the cutting of the frenum (frenulum), especially for release of a tongue-tie (ankyloglossia). **lingual f.,** incision of the lingual frenum; ankylotomy.

Frentirol trademark for *methimazole*.

frenula (fren′u-lah) [L.] plural of *frenulum*.

frenulum (fren′u-lum), pl. *fren′ula* [L., dim. of *fraenum* bridle] a small bridle; used in anatomical nomenclature as a general term to designate a small fold of integument or mucous membrane that checks, curbs, or limits the movements of an organ or part. See also FRENUM. **abnormally attached f.,** abnormal frenulum ATTACHMENT. **hypertrophied f.,** hypertrophied frenulum SYNDROME. **f. of inferior lip, f. la′bii inferio′ris** [NA], the fold of mucous membrane on the inside of the middle of the lower lip, connecting the lip to the corresponding gingiva and anchoring it to the alveolar process. **f. la′bii superio′ris** [NA], f. of superior lip. **f. lin′guae** [NA], lingual FRENUM. **f. of superior lip,** the fold of mucous membrane on the inside of the middle line of upper lip, connecting the lip to the corresponding gum. Called also *frenulum labii superioris* [NA]. **f. of superior lip, f. la′bii superio′ris** [NA], the fold of mucous membrane on the inside of the middle of the upper lip, connecting the lip to the gingiva and anchoring it to the alveolar process. **f. of tongue,** lingual FRENUM.

frenum (fre′num), pl. *fre′na* [L. *fraenum* bridle] a restraining structure or part; a fold of integument or mucous membrane that checks, curbs, or limits the movements of an organ or part. See also FRENULUM. **abnormally attached f.,** see abnormal frenulum ATTACHMENT. **labial f., f. labio′rum,** a fold of mucous membrane which connects each lip to the corresponding gingiva at the midline. **lingual f., f. of tongue,** a vertical fold of mucous membrane under the tongue, attaching it to the floor of the mouth and anchoring it to the mandibular alveolar process. Called also *frenulum linguae* [NA] and *sublingual ridge*.

Freon a trademark for a group of fluorocarbons. **F. 11,** trademark for *trichlorofluoromethane*. **F. 12,** trademark for *dichlorodifluoromethane*.

frequency (fre′kwen-se) 1. in statistics, the number of occurrences of a determinable entity per unit of time or of population. 2. the number of vibrations made by a particle or ray in 1 second. 3. the rate of oscillation or alternation in an alternating current; a complete cycle including the half cycle flowing in the positive direction and the half cycle flowing in the negative direction. **audio f.,** any frequency corresponding to a normally audible sound wave. **infrasonic f.,** any frequency below the audio frequency range. Called also *subsonic f*. **low f.,** an alternating current where frequency in cycles per second is low in reference to a certain standard, such as the pitch frequency of middle C. **SI unit of f.,** hertz. **subsonic f.,** infrasonic f. **supersonic f.,** ultrasonic f. **ultrasonic f.,** any frequency above the audio frequency range (see ULTRASONICS). Called also *supersonic f*.

fressreflex (fres′re-fleks) [Ger. "eating reflex"] rhythmic sucking, chewing, and swallowing movements elicited by stroking of the lips and cheeks.

Freund's adjuvant [Jules *Freund*, Hungarian-born bacteriologist in the U.S., 1890–1925] see under ADJUVANT.

Frey's syndrome [Lucie *Frey*, Polish physician] auriculotemporal SYNDROME.

Frias, J. L. see G SYNDROME (Opitz-Frias syndrome).

fricative (frik′ah-tiv) a speech sound produced by forcing an air stream through a narrow opening and resulting in audible high-frequency vibrations, such as *f* or *s*.

friction (frik′shun) [L. *frictio*] the action of rubbing; the resistance offered to sliding motion by rubbing. **internal f.,** the resistance to bending of some materials, particularly those with low elasticity, due to their crystalline structure, occurring when the stresses are changed rapidly and continually in a material, with the resulting conversion of excess energy into heat. **internal fluid f.,** viscosity.

Friderichsen, Carl [Danish physician, born 1886] see Waterhouse-Friderichsen SYNDROME.

Fried's rule see under RULE.

Friedländer's bacillus [Carl *Friedländer*, German pathologist, 1847–1887] *Klebsiella pneumoniae*; see under KLEBSIELLA.

Friedman splint cast bar SPLINT.

Friedreich's disease hemifacial HYPERTROPHY.

frit (frit) a fused mass produced by firing ceramic powder (a mixture of quartz, kaolin, pigments, opacifiers, a suitable flux, and other substances), which is ground to form a fine powder for use in fabricating dental porcelain restorations and artificial teeth.

fritting (frit′ing) plunging into water of a hot mass of fused material, such as glass. The sudden cooling produces a cracking and crazing which facilitates grinding of the material into a powder. Called also *firing*.

frons (fronz) [L. "the front, forepart"] the forehead; the region of the face above the eyes. **f. cra′nii** [NA], **f. of cranium,** bony FOREHEAD.

frontal (frun′tal) [L. *frontalis*] 1. pertaining to the forehead; metopic. 2. pertaining to a frontal plane. 3. pertaining to the anterior aspect of an organ of the body.

frontalis (frun-ta′lis) [L.] 1. frontal; used in anatomical nomenclature to designate relationship to the frontal or coronal plane. 2. frontal muscle; see frontal belly of occipitofrontal muscle, under BELLY.

frontipetal (frun-tip′ĕ-tal) [*frontalis* + L. *petere* to seek] directed to the front; moving in a frontal direction.

fronto- [L. *frons* forehead] a combining form signifying anterior position or denoting relationship to the forehead.

frontomalar (frun″to-ma′lar) [*fronto-* + *malar*] pertaining to the frontal and malar bones.

frontomaxillary (frun″to-mak′sĭ-lār′e) [*fronto-* + *maxillary*] pertaining to the frontal bone and the maxilla or the upper jaw.

frontonasal (frun″to-na′zal) [*fronto-* + *nasal*] pertaining to the frontal sinus and the nose.

fronto-occipital (frun″to-ok-sip′ĭ-tal) [*fronto-* + *occipital*] pertaining to the forehead and the occiput.

frontoparietal (frun″to-pah-ri′ĕ-tal) [*fronto-* + *parietal*] pertaining to the frontal and parietal bones.

frontotemporal (frun"to-tem"po-ral) [*fronto-* + *temporal*] pertaining to the frontal and temporal gones.

frontotemporale (frun"to-tem"po-ra'le) a craniometric landmark located in the most anterior point of the temporal line at the zygomatic process of the frontal bone. See illustration at CEPHALOMETRY.

frostbite (frost'bīt) damage to tissue resulting from excessive exposure to cold and freezing. The damage ranges from vasoconstriction and pallor with later desquamation and vesiculation of the skin to the loss of all cutaneous sensation followed by necrosis and damage to the corium. Rarely, the lips become disproportionately swollen with blisters and covered with crusts and ulcerations with regional lymph node enlargement; even less frequently the tongue may be involved.

β-fructofuranosidase [E.C.3.2.1.26] (ba'tah-fruk"to-fu"rah-no'sĭ-dās) a hydrolase that acts on glycosyl compounds, and catalyzes the hydrolysis of sugars possessing terminal nonreducing β-D-fructofuranoside residues. Reportedly, it is absent at birth in the intestine in some animals (including man) but its level rises thereafter. It is also found in the saliva. Called also *invertase, invertin, saccharase,* and *sucrase.* See also carbohydrate METABOLISM.

fructopyranose (fruk"to-pi'rah-nōs) fructose.

fructose (fruk'tōs) [L. *fructus* fruit + *-ose*] a hexose (ketose), which is a digestible monosaccharide that becomes converted to glucose in the intestine and serves as a source of energy in the animal body, and is provided in the human diet from fruits, honey, and some vegetables. It also occurs in bull and human semen. Fructose is prepared from inulin, occurring as white crystals with a sweet taste that are soluble in water, alcohol, and ether. Sterile fructose in aqueous solution (10 percent) is used as a fluid replenisher and to reestablish blood sugar levels following blood loss after hemorrhage, shock, or surgical trauma. It may be used in diabetic patients with ketosis. Called also *fructopyranose, fruit sugar, grape sugar,* and *levulose.* Trademarks: Laevosan, Levugen.

fructoside (fruk-to'sīd) a glucoside which on hydrolysis yields fructose and a hydroxy nonsugar component (aglycone).

fructosuria (fruk"to-su're-ah) [*fructose* + Gr. *ouron* urine + *-ia*] the presence of fructose in the urine.

fructosyl (fruk'to-sil) a radical of fructose.

fructosyltransferase [E.C.2.4] (fruk"to-sil-trans'fer-ās) a subsubclass of glycosyltransferases that catalyze the transfer of a fructosyl group, as from fructan to D-glucose to form sucrose. Called also *transfructosylase.*

Frusemin trademark for *furosemide.*

FSF fibrin stabilizing factor; see FACTOR XIII.

FSH follicle stimulating HORMONE.

ft foot.

Ftorocort trademark for *triamcinolone.*

5-FU fluorouracil.

Fuadin trademark for *stibophen.*

Fuchs' heterochromia, syndrome [Ernst *Fuchs,* German ophthalmologist, 1851–1930] see under HETEROCHROMIA and SYNDROME.

Fuchs' position see under POSITION.

FUDR floxuridine.

fugacity (fu-gas'ĭ-te) [L. *fugacitas,* from *fugere* to flee] a measure of the escaping tendency of a substance from one phase to another phase, or from one part of a phase to another part of the same phase. The logarithm of the fugacity is proportional to the chemical potential.

-fugal 1. [L. *fugare* to put to flight] a word termination implying banishing, or driving away, affixed to a stem designating the object of banishment, as *febrifugal,* relieving or dispelling fever. 2. [L. *fugere* to flee from] a word termination implying traveling away from, affixed to a stem designating the object from which flight is made, as *centrifugal,* traveling away from a center.

Fulcin trademark for *griseofulvin.*

fulcrum (ful'krum) [L. "bedpost"] the support upon which a level rests while force intended to produce motion is exerted. See also fulcrum LINE. **f. of tooth,** the axis of lateral movement of a tooth, considered to be situated at the middle third of the portion of root embedded in the alveolus and, thus, moving apically as the bone resorbs in periodontal diseases.

fulguration (ful"gu-ra'shun) [L. *fulgur* lightning] destruction of living tissue by electric sparks generated by a high frequency current, which may be direct or indirect. *Direct:* An insulated fulguration electrode with a metal point is connected to the uniterminal of the high frequency apparatus and a spark of electricity is allowed to impinge on the area to be treated. *Indirect:* The patient is connected directly by a metal handle to the uniterminal and the operator utilizes an active electrode to complete an arc from the patient. Fulguration may be used for destroying fistulous orifices, for eliminating tissue tabs, and for hemostasis. See also ELECTROSURGERY.

Fuller Albright's syndrome [Fuller *Albright,* Boston physician, born 1900] Albright's SYNDROME (1).

Fülling, Georg see DYSPLASIA dentofacialis (Weyers-Thier syndrome).

fulminant (ful'mĭ-nant) [L. *fulminare* to flare up] sudden, severe; occurring suddenly and with great intensity.

fulminate (ful'mĭ-nāt) to occur suddenly with great intensity.

Fulvicin trademark for *griseofulvin.*

fumarase (fu'mah-rās) fumarate HYDRATASE.

fumarate (fu'mar-āt) a salt of fumaric acid. **ferrous f.,** a compound, $FeC_4H_2O_4$; occurring as an odorless, almost tasteless, reddish granular anhydrous powder that is insoluble in alcohol and slightly soluble in water. Used in the treatment of iron deficiency. Excessive intake may cause poisoning (see IRON). Trademarks: Cpiron, Erco-Fer, Ferronat, Ferrone, Ircon, One-Iron. **f. hydratase,** fumarate HYDRATASE. **f. reductase,** succinate DEHYDROGENASE.

fumarhydrogenase (fu"mar-hi'dro-jen-ās) succinate DEHYDROGENASE.

fumigation (fu"mĭ-ga'shun) [L. *fumus* smoke, steam, vapor] disinfection through the use of poisonous fumes.

functio (funk'she-o) [L.] function. **f. lae'sa,** loss of function, being one of the cardinal signs of inflammation.

function (funk'shun) [L. *functio* performance] 1. an action or activity proper to a person or something. 2. Normal or proper action of a part or organ. **group f.,** multiple contact relations between the maxillary and mandibular teeth in lateral and protrusive movements, whereby simultaneous contact of several teeth act as a group to distribute occlusal forces.

functional (funk'shun-al) of or pertaining to function; affecting the function, but not structure; said of disorders of function with no organic cause.

fund (fund) money or other resource accumulated for some purpose; also, an organization that administers and allocates such a fund. **American F. for Dental Health,** an independent, nonprofit agency that raises and allocated funds to support dental education, dental research, and the delivery of dental health care. Abbreviated *AFDH.*

fundal (fun'dal) pertaining to a fundus.

fundamental (fun"dah-men'tal) pertaining to a base or foundation.

fundi (fun'di) [L.] plural or *fundus.*

fundiform (fun'dĭ-form) [L. *funda* sling + *forma* form] shaped like a sling.

fundus (fun'dus), pl. *fun'di* [L.] the bottom or base of anything; an anatomical term for any structure forming the bottom or base of an organ, or the part of a hollow organ farthest from its mouth.

fungal (fung'gal) pertaining to a fungus or fungi; mycotic.

fungemia (fun-je'me-ah) [*fungus* + Gr. *haima* blood + *-ia*] the presence of fungi in the blood.

fungi (fun'ji) [L.] plural of *fungus.* **F. Imperfec'ti,** see under FUNGUS.

fungicidal (fun"jĭ-si'dal) [*fungus* + L. *caedere* to kill] destructive to fungi.

fungicide (fun'jĭ-sīd) an agent capable of destroying fungi.

Fungicidin trademark for *nystatin.*

fungiform (fun'jĭ-form) [*fungus* + L. *forma* form] shaped like a fungus or mushroom; fungoid.

Fungilin trademark for *amphotericin B.*

fungistasis (fun"jĭ-sta'sis) [*fungus* + Gr. *stasis* a stopping] inhibition of the growth of fungi; mycostasis.

fungistatic (fun"jĭ-stat'ik) inhibiting the growth of fungi.

fungitoxic (fun"jĭ-tok'sik) exerting a toxic effect on fungi.

fungitoxicity (fun"jĭ-tok-sis'ĭ-te) the quality of exerting a toxic effect on fungi.

Fungizone trademark for *amphotericin B.*

fungoid (fung'goid) [*fungus* + Gr. *eidos* form] resembling a fungus, or mushroom; fungiform.

fungous (fung'gus) [L. *fungosus*] of the nature of, caused by, or resembling a fungus.

fungus (fung'gus), pl. *fun'gi* [L.] an organism living in water, soil, or decaying vegetable matter. Of more than 100,000 species, fewer than 100 are pathogenic to animals and, even these, are misplaced saprophytes, rather than obligate parasites. Fungi are generally nonmotile and nonphotosynthetic and may exist only as saprophytes or parasites. They occur as yeasts, molds, and mushrooms. Yeasts are single cells and molds are either single cells or multicellular filamentous colonies. The uninucleated cell can differentiate into sexually distinct cells, single yeast cells, multinucleated filamentous strands, or sporogenous bodies. Some pathogenic fungi exist only as yeast or monomorphic forms, but others exist only as mold forms; most pathogenic strains are dimorphic. Fungal cells resemble those of other eukaryotes, and consist of a nucleus, with limiting membrane, an endoplasmic membrane, mitochondria, and chromosomes. The cell wall is external to a cytoplasmic membrane and is made up of polymers of hexoses and hexosamines, containing chitin. Also found in the wall are insoluble glucans, soluble mannans, and protein-carbohydrate complexes. Snail and bacterial enzymes can digest the cell wall. Fungi are classified as a separate kingdom, comprising three divisions: Zygomycota, Ascomycota, and Basidiomycota, together with one form-division Deuteromycota (the members of which reproduce asexually). Most fungi pathogenic to humans are ascomycetes. **f. disease,** mycosis. **Fun′gi Imperfec′ti, imperfect fungi,** the Deuteromycetes; a group of true fungi (Eumycetes) assumed to have no sexual phase. They include a few of the pathogenic fungi. Single-celled round forms are called also *imperfect yeasts*. **perfect fungi,** fungi for which both sexual and asexual types of spores are known; they include Ascomycetes, Zygomycetes, and Basidiomycetes. **proper fungi,** Eumycetes. **sac fungi,** Ascomycetes. **true fungi,** Eumycetes.

funiculi (fu-nik′u-li) [L.] plural of *funiculus.*

funiculus (fu-nik′u-lus), pl. *funic′uli* [L.] a cord; a general anatomical term for a cordlike structure or part. **f. umbilica′lis** [NA], umbilical CORD.

funiform (fu′nĭ-form) [L. *funis* rope + *forma* shape] resembling or shaped like a rope or cord.

funis (fu′nis) [L. "cord"] any cordlike or ropelike structure.

Funk, Kazimierz [born 1884] a Polish biochemist who coined the word "vitamine" (later changed to *vitamin*) and who made one of the earliest attempts to isolate vitamin B₁.

funnel (fun′l) a conic, hollow structure with a narrow opening at the apex, generally used for pouring liquids into containers with narrow necks.

F.U.O. fever of undetermined origin.

Furacin trademark for *nitrofurazone.*

Furadantin trademark for *nitrofurantoin.*

furan (fu′ran) a heterocyclic compound, C_4H_4O, occurring as a colorless, flammable liquid that turns brown on standing. It is soluble in ether and alcohol, but not in water. On exposure to air, it forms peroxides. Furan is used in organic synthesis. Its derivatives are antibacterial and act against a wide spectrum of gram-positive and gram-negative organisms, presumably by interference with essential enzymatic activity; they are also active against some pathogenic protozoa and yeasts. Furans with antimicrobial properties include nitrofurantoin, nitrofurazone, furazolidone, and nifuroxime. The compound is toxic and absorbable through the skin; its vapors are narcotic. Called also *furfuran, oxole,* and *tetrole.*

Furantoin trademark for *nitrofurantoin.*

furazolidone (fu″rah-zol′ĭ-dōn) a furan derivative, 3-[(5-nitrofurfurylidene)amino]-2-oxazolidinone, occurring as a yellow crystalline powder that darkens on exposure to strong light, and is soluble in water. Used as an antibacterial and antitrichomonal agent. Trademarks: Furoxane, Giardil, Nifulidone, Topazone.

furca (fer′kah), pl. *fur′cae* [L.] furcation. **denuded f.,** see denuded FURCATION. **invaded f.,** see invaded FURCATION. **f. invasion,** furca INVASION.

furcal (fer′kal) [L. *furca* fork] shaped like a fork; forked.

furcation (fer-ka′shun) [L. *furca* fork] the anatomical area of a multirooted tooth where the roots divide. Called also *furca.* **denuded f.,** furca INVASION. **invaded f.,** a furcation that is affected by marginal periodontitis associated with resorption of bone. See furca INVASION.

furcula (fer′ku-lah) [L. "little fork"] a horseshoe-shaped ridge in the embryonic larynx, bounding the pharyngeal aperture in front and laterally.

Furesol trademark for *nitrofurazone.*

furfur (fer′fer), pl. *fur′fures* [L. "bran"] an old term for a branlike scale, such as dandruff.

furfuraceous (fer″fu-ra′shus) [L. *furfur* bran] resembling or exhibiting numerous branlike scales, such as dandruff.

furfuran (fer″fu-ran) furan.

furnace (fer′nis) a device or apparatus in which heat is generated. **inlay f.,** a furnace for burning off the wax from an inlay mold and for establishing the proper condition and temperature of the

investment to receive the molten casting alloy. **porcelain f.,** a furnace for firing dental porcelain. A typical unit contains a heating chamber (muffle), temperature indicator, and control mechanism. Dental laboratory furnaces are usually heated with electricity and industrial ones with electricity or gas. Most units are designed to generate temperatures for fusing porcelain in all ranges, 870 to 1370°C (1600–2500°F), although laboratory units are usually employed for low- and medium-fusing porcelain, while the commercial units are also used for high-fusing types. The muffle consists of a chamber made of a refractory material, about 3½ × 3½ × 2 inches in size, the chamber being smaller in units for firing jacket crowns, about which is wound a resistance type heating element. The temperature indicator, a combination of a pyrometer and a thermocouple, operates by the difference in potential generated between hot and cold junctions of two dissimilar metals or alloys; the hot one is placed in the muffle and the cold one at the terminal of the millivoltmeter. The dial, indicating millivolts, is graduated to read in °C or °F. Pumps for producing a vacuum, increasing the atmospheric pressure, or replacing the air with a gas in the chamber may also be attached. See also FIRING. **vacuum f.,** a porcelain furnace having a pump for evacuation of air from the muffle and to produce vacuum in the chamber. See also vacuum FIRING.

furosemide (fu-ro′sĕ-mīd) a diuretic drug, 4-chloro-N-furfuryl-5-sulfamoyl-anthranilic acid, occurring as a white to yellowish, odorless, tasteless, light-sensitive, crystalline powder that is freely soluble in acetone, dimethylformamide, alkali hydroxide solutions, and methanol, sparingly soluble in ethanol, ether, and chloroform, and insoluble in water. Used in the treatment of edema associated with heart, kidney, and liver diseases. Also used in the treatment of hypertension. Side effects may include reduced blood flow, particularly in cardiac, cerebral, and renal circulations, hyperglycemia, hyperuricemia, hypersensitivity, exfoliative dermatitis, pruritus, thrombocytopenia, leukopenia, paresthesias, visual disorders, orthostatic hypotension, nausea, vomiting, diarrhea, weakness, fatigue, vertigo, thirst, and excessive urination. Trademarks: Desdemin, Diural, Frusemin, Lasix, Profemin, Urosemide.

Furoxane trademark for *furazolidone.*

furrow (fer′o) a shallow depression; a groove. See also GROOVE and SULCUS. **branchial f.,** branchial GROOVE. **Jadelot's f.,** Jadelot's LINE. **mentolabial f.,** labiomental GROOVE. **skin f's,** fine depressions on the surface of the skin which vary in arrangement and size according to their situation. They are formed by the attachment of the skin to the deeper structures, by the movement to which the part is subjected, and by fibrous structures of the corium. Between these furrows are ridges dotted with sweat pores.

furuncle (fu′rung-k'l) [L. *furunculus*] a localized infection with pyogenic bacteria, forming a painful nodule in the skin and subcutaneous tissues, around a slough or "core"; a boil.

furuncular (fu-rung′ku-lar) pertaining to or of the nature of a furuncle or boil.

furunculoid (fu-rung′ku-loid) [furuncle + Gr. *eidos* form, shape] resembling a furuncle or boil.

furunculosis (fu-rung″ku-lo′sis) the persistent occurrence of furuncles or boils over a period of time of weeks or months.

furunculus (fu-rung′ku-lus), pl. *furun′culi* [L.] furuncle.

fusi (fu′si) [L] plural of *fusus.*

fusible (fu′zĭ-b'l) capable of being melted or fused.

fusicellular (fu″sĭ-sel′u-lar) fusocellular.

fusiform (fu′sĭ-form) [L. *fusus* spindle + *forma* form] spindle-shaped.

Fusiformis (fu″sĭ-for′mis) former name for *Fusobacterium.* **F. fusifor′mis,** *Fusobacterium nucleatum;* see under FUSOBACTERIUM. **F. nigres′cens,** *Bacteroides melaninogenicus;* see under BACTEROIDES. **F. nuclea′tus,** *Fusobacterium nucleatum;* see under FUSOBACTERIUM.

fusimotor (fu″sĭ-mo′tor) denoting motor nerve fibers (of gamma motoneurons) that innervate intrafusal fibers of the muscle spindle.

fusion (fu′zhun) [L. *fusio*] 1. the act or process of melting. 2. the abnormal coherence of adjacent parts or bodies. 3. the operative formation of an ankylosis. 4. union of two normally separated, adjacent tooth germs, either throughout their entire lengths or only at their crowns or roots. If the contact occurs before calcification begins, the two teeth may be completely united to form a single large tooth; if the contact occurs later, when a portion of the tooth crown has completed its formation, there may be union of the root only. The dentin is always confluent in cases of true fusion. The tooth may have separate or fused root canals. The deciduous as well as the permanent dentition may be affected. In addition to affecting two normal teeth, fusion may occur between a normal and supernumerary tooth. Called also *tooth f.* See also CONCRESCENCE (3) and GEMINATION. 5. The coordination of separate images of the same object in the two eyes into one. 6. nuclear f. **centric f.**, robertsonian TRANSLOCATION. **latent heat of f.**, see under HEAT. **nuclear f.**, the formation of a heavier nucleus from two lighter ones (such as hydrogen isotopes), with the attendant release of energy, as in the explosion of a hydrogen bomb. See also nuclear FISSION and nuclear REACTION. **tandem f.**, tandem TRANSLOCATION. **tooth f.**, see *fusion* (4).

Fusobacterium (fu"zo-bak-te′re-um) [L. *fusus* spindle + Gr. *baktērion* little rod] a genus of gram-negative, anaerobic, non-sporogenous bacteria of the family Bacteroides, occurring as nonmotile or motile (with peritrichous flagella) rods. They metabolize peptone or carbohydrates, producing butyric acid and, often, acetic and lactic acids, and lesser amounts of propionic, succinic, and formic acids. The organisms are found in cavities of man and other animals; some species may cause gingival disease. Formerly called *Fusiformis.* **F. bullo′sum**, a species isolated from human intestinal contents and bone marrow, and in cases of actinomycosis. Called also *Bacillus bullosus, Bacteroides bullosus,* and *Sphaerocillus bullosus.* **F. fusifor′me**, *Leptotrichia buccalis;* see under LEPTOTRICHIA. **F. glutino′sum**, a species isolated from pleurisy, pulmonary gangrene, perinephritis, and brain abscess of man. Called also *Bacillus glutinosus, Bacteroides glutinosus,* and *Ristella glutinosa.* **F. gonidiafor′mans**, a species isolated from human infections of the respiratory, urogenital, and gastrointestinal tracts, and from a lamb with pneumonia. Called also *Actinomyces gonidiaformis.* **F. mortif′erum**, a species isolated from the human oral cavity, intestines, and feces, and from cases of necrotic abscesses, septicemia, pleurisy, and urinary tract infection. Called also *F. ridiculosum, Bacillus mortiferus, B. necroticus, Bacteroides freundii, Pseudobacterium freundii, P. mortiferum,* and *P. necroticum.* **F. necroph′orum**, a species found in the body cavities of man and other animals; isolated from necrotic lesions, abscesses, and from the blood. Called also *Actinomyces pseudonecrophorus, Bacillus funduliformis, B.*

necrophorus, and *Corynebacterium necrophorum.* **F. nuclea′tum**, a species producing 1 to 2 mm circular to irregular convex, translucent colonies on horse blood agar, being usually nonhemolytic. It is found in the oral cavity in acute necrotizing gingivitis in association with *Treponema vincentii* and other microorganisms, and has been isolated from the pleural cavities and respiratory tract, and from infected wounds and other pathological conditions. Called also *F. plauti-vincenti, Bacillus fusiformis, Corynebacterium fusiforme, Fusiformis fusiformis, F. nucleatus,* and *Sphaerophorus fusiformis.* **F. plau′ti**, a species originally isolated from the human oral cavity and from cultures of *Entamoeba histolytica.* Called also *Bacillus plauti* and *Zuberella plauti.* **F. plau′ti-vincen′ti**, *F. nucleatum.* **F. praeacu′tum**, *Bacteroides praeacutum;* see under BACTEROIDES. **F. prausnit′zii**, a species isolated from feces and in cases of purulent pleurisy. Called also *Bacillus mucosus anaerobius* and *Bacterium zoogleiformans.* **F. ridiculo′sum**, *F. mortiferum.* **F. rus′sii**, a species isolated from human feces, and in cases of abscesses and actinomycosis in cats. Called also *Bacillus influenzaeformis* and *Sphaerophorus influenzaeformis.* **F. sta′bile**, a species isolated in cases of salpingitis, peritonitis, and septicemia following appendicitis. **F. symbio′sum**, a species isolated from human blood and feces and in cases of soft tissue infections. Called also *Bacteroides symbiosus* and *Zuberella pedipedis.* **F. va′rium**, a species isolated from human feces and from infected wounds, peritonitis, sinusitis, and pleurisy. Called also *Bacteroides varius.*

fusus (fu′sus), pl. *fu′si* [L.] a spindle-like object.

fusocellular (fu"so-sel′u-lar) [L. *fusus* spindle + *cellular*] having spindle-shaped cells.

fusospirillary (fu"so-spi′ri-lar"e) pertaining to or caused by fusiform bacilli and spirillae, as in acute necrotizing gingivitis.

fusospirillosis (fu"so-spi"ri-lo′sis) acute necrotizing GINGIVITIS.

FY fiscal YEAR.

G

G 1. gram. 2. giga-. 3. gingival. 4. glucose. 5. glabella (2).

g gram.

γ the third letter in the Greek alphabet. See GAMMA. Symbol for *microgram* and *immunoglobulin.*

Ga gallium.

GABA, gaba γ-aminobutyric ACID.

Gaddesden, John [14th century] an English writer whose work, *Rosa Anglica,* reviews medicine, mostly from the Roman and Arabian sources, with commentaries on the status of medicine in England. His comments deal with the treatment of toothache, purgation, bloodletting, scarification of the labial and sublingual mucosae, leeching, fumigation, cauterization, and the application of plasters, powders, and ointments.

Gadolin, Johann [1760–1852] a Finnish chemist and mineralogist.

gadolinite (gad′o-li-nīt″) [named after Johann *Gadolin*] a silicate ore from which gadolinium, holmium, and rhenium are extracted.

gadolinium (gad″o-lin′e-um) [named after Johann *Gadolin*] a rare earth derived from gadolinite as a magnetic, lustrous metal that tarnishes in moist air and is soluble in dilute acids, but not in water. Symbol, Gd; atomic number, 64; atomic weight, 157.25; valence, 1; specific gravity, 7.9004; melting point, 1313°C; group IIIA of the periodic table. It has seven natural isotopes, 152, 154, 155–158, and 160, and one radioactive isotope, ^{152}Gd, which has a half-life of 1.1×10^{14} years and emits alpha rays. Artificial radioactive isotopes include 145–151, 153, 159, 161, and 162. Gadolinium has the highest neutron absorption of any element. Its compounds are used in nuclear technology.

Gaduol trademark for *cod liver oil* (see under OIL).

Gaerny bar [A. *Gaerny*] see under BAR.

Gaffky, Georg Theodor [1850–1918] a German bacteriologist.

Gaffkya (gaf′ke-ah) [named after G. T. *Gaffky*] a former genus of gram-positive cocci; its species have been now assigned to other genera. **G. hom′ari**, *Aerococcus viridans;* see under AEROCOCCUS.

gag (gag) 1. a device used for holding the jaws open during oral or dental surgical intervention. 2. to retch; to strive to vomit associated with contraction of the constrictor muscle of the pharynx. **Molt mouth g.**, a device for holding the mouth open. See illustration.

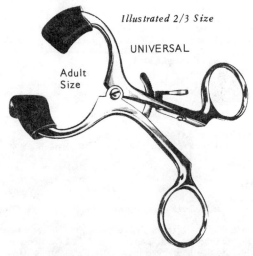

Molt mouth gag. (From H. O. Torres and A. Ehrlich: Modern Dental Assisting. 2nd ed. Philadelphia, W. B. Saunders Co., 1980.)

gait (gāt) the manner and style of walking.

Gaius Plinius Secundus see PLINY THE ELDER.

gal gallon.

galact- see GALACTO-.

galacto-, galact- [Gr. *gala, galaktos* milk] a combining form denoting relationship to milk.

galactosamine (gah-lak″to-sam′in) an amino sugar.

galactose (gah-lak′tōs) [*galact-* + *-ose*] a hexose (aldohexose), which is a constituent of various oligo- and polysaccharides occurring in pectins, gums, and mucilages. Obtained from lactose by enzymatic action or by boiling with a mineral acid. It is a white crystalline substance resembling glucose in most of its properties, but is less soluble, less sweet, and forms mucic acid when oxidized with nitric acid. D-Galactose is found in milk sugar, in the cerebrosides of the brain (cerebrose, brain sugar), in the raffinose of the sugar beet, and in gums and seaweeds, and L-galactose is found in flaxseed mucilage.

galactosemia (gah-lak″to-se′me-ah) the presence in the blood of galactose; a hereditary disorder of galactose metabolism, transmitted as an autosomal recessive trait, and characterized by hepatomegaly, cataracts, and mental retardation, with vomiting, diarrhea, jaundice, poor weight gain, and malnutrition in early infancy.

galactosidase (gah-lak″to-si′dās) a hydrolase occurring as α- and β-galactosidase. **α-g.** [E.C.3.2.1.22], a form of galactosidase that catalyzes the hydrolysis of α-D-galactoside to D-glucose. Called also *melibiase*. See also carbohydrate METABOLISM. **β-g.** [E.C.3.2.1.23], a form of galactosidase that catalyzes the hydrolysis of β-D-galactoside to D-galactose, occurring in the kidneys, intestine, liver, and saliva. Called also *lactase*. See also carbohydrate METABOLISM.

galactoside (gah-lak′to-sīd) a glycoside, which on hydrolysis, yields galactose and a hydroxy-nonsugar component (aglycone).

galactosuria (gah-lak″to-su′re-ah) [*galactose* + Gr. *ouron* urine + -*ia*] presence of galactose in the urine.

galea (ga′le-ah) [L.] a helmet; a general anatomical term for any helmetlike or caplike structure. **g. aponeurot′ica** [NA], epicranial APONEUROSIS.

Galen's ventricle [Claudius (Clarissimus Galenus), Greek physician and medical writer, c. A.D. 129–199; he was born at Pergamum (Asia Minor), and practiced in Rome, where he became physician to Emperor Marcus Aurelius. Although he did not dissect the human cadaver, he made many valuable anatomical and physiological observations on animals, and his writings on these and other subjects are extensive. His influence on medicine was profound in many centuries — his teleology ("nature does nothing in vain") being particularly attractive to the medieval mind, although it was stultifying as regards advances in medical thought and practice. Galen was the first to write of nerves of the teeth. He believed that the teeth are continually worn down by the effect of mastication and that nutrition repairs the losses and the teeth preserve the same size: when a tooth has no antagonist, it grows gradually longer; and dental caries is produced by the internal action of acrid and corroding humors] VENTRICLE of larynx.

galenic (gah-len′ik) pertaining to the ancient system of medicine taught and practiced by Galen.

galenicals (gah-len′ĭ-kalz) medicines prepared according to the formulas of Galen; the term is now used to denote standard preparations containing organic ingredients, as contrasted with pure chemical substances. Called also *galenics*. See also galenic PHARMACY.

galenics (gah-len′iks) galenicals.

gall (gawl) [L. *galla*] 1. the bile. 2. nutgall. **pistachia g's**, mastic.

gallbladder (gawl′blad-der) a small pear-shaped sac located on the posteroinferior surface of the liver, between the right and quadrate lobes; it serves as a storage place for bile. Called also *vesica felea* [NA].

Gallimycin trademark for *erythromycin stearate* (see under ERYTHROMYCIN).

gallium (gal′e-um) [L. *Gallia* France] a metallic element. Symbol, Ga; atomic number, 31; atomic weight, 69.72; valences, 2, 3; melting point, 29.78°C; specific gravity, 5.904; group IIIA of the periodic table. Gallium occurs as the natural isotopes 69 and 71; artificial radioactive isotopes are 63–68, 70, and 72–76. It is a silvery liquid that may be undercooled to almost 0°C without solidifying, which is soluble in acids, alkali, and mercury. Exposure to gallium may cause skin rashes and bone marrow depression. Its compounds are used as semiconductors. A gallium-tin eutectic, mixed with powdered metals, such as palladium, gold, nickel, and copper to form alloys, hardens at mouth temperature. A gallium-copper-tin alloy is reported to have strength properties superior to those of silver-tin amalgams and gallium alloys are believed to be more resistant to corrosion than other alloys. Mixing of gallium and palladium powder may produce a violent exothermic reaction. Called also *eka-aluminum*. **g. alloy**, gallium ALLOY.

gallon (gal′on) [L. *congius*] a measure of capacity (liquid or solid), being equal to 4 quarts. Abbreviated *gal*. See also *Tables of Weights and Measures at* WEIGHT. **British imperial g.**, a gallon consisting of 4 British imperial quarts, (277.420 cubic inches), or 4.545 liters. **U.S. g.**, a gallon consisting of 4 U.S. quarts (231 cubic inches), or 3.785 liters.

Gallotox trademark for *phenylmercuric acetate* (see under ACETATE).

GALT gut-associated lymphoid TISSUE.

Galvani, Luigi [1737–1798] an Italian physician and physiologist whose research led to the discovery that electricity may produce chemical changes.

galvanism (gal′vah-nizm) [named after Luigi *Galvani*] 1. production of electric current through a chemical reaction, as in the presence of two dissimilar metals in a liquid medium. See also galvanic CURRENT. 2. dental g. **dental g.**, production of galvanic current in the oral cavity due to the presence in dental restorations of two or more dissimilar metals that are bathed in saliva, thus producing a wet-cell battery. When touching each other, the current flowing from one restoration to another may irritate the dental pulp and cause sharp pain (galvanic shock). The flow of electric current may also be responsible for electrolysis and resulting electrochemical corrosion of restorations.

galvanocautery (gal″vah-no-kaw′ter-e) cautery accomplished by application of a wire heated with a galvanic current. Called also *galvanic cautery*.

galvanometer (gal″vah-nom′ě-ter) [*galvanism* + Gr. *metron* measure] an instrument for measuring current by electromagnetic action.

galvanosurgery (gal″vah-no-sur′jer-e) the application of galvanocautery for surgical purposes. Called also *galvanic surgery*.

galvanotherapeutics, galvanotherapy (gal″vah-no-ther″ah-pu′-tiks, gal″vah-no-ther′ah-pe) the therapeutic use of galvanic current. **root canal g.**, electrosterilization.

Gamarex trademark for γ-*aminobutyric acid* (see under ACID).

gamete (gam′ēt) [Gr. *gametē* wife, *gametēs* husband] 1. the reproductive element; one of two cells, male (spermatozoon) and female (ovum), whose union is necessary, in sexual reproduction, to initiate the development of a new individual. 2. the malarial parasite in its sexual form in the stomach of a mosquito.

gameto- [Gr. *gametē* wife, *gametēs* husband] a combining form denoting relationship to a gamete.

gametogenesis (gam″ēto-jen′ě-sis) [*gameto-* + Gr. *genesis* production] the production of gametes (spermatozoa and ova). See OOGENESIS and SPERMATOGENESIS.

gamma (gam′ah) 1. the third letter in the Greek alphabet, γ, used as part of chemical name to distinguish the position of the third carbon atom of an aliphatic chain or the position opposite the alpha position on the naphthalene ring. 2. microgram. 3. a numerical expression of the degree of development of a photographic film. 4. a unit of intensity of magnetic field, γ = 0.00001 gauss. **film g.**, the maximum slope of the plot of the density versus log exposure plot of a film.

gammaglobulinopathy (gam″ah-glob″u-lin-op′ah-the) gammopathy.

Gammalon trademark for γ-*aminobutyric acid* (see under ACID).

gammopathy (gam-op′ah-the) an immunoproliferative disorder characterized by abnormal proliferation of the lymphoid cells producing immunoglobulins. It may be *monoclonal*, in which there is an excess of one class of heavy chain (gamma, alpha, mu, delta, or epsilon) and one type of light chain (kappa or lambda) immunoglobulin subunits produced by a single clone of cells; the monoclonal gammopathies include multiple myeloma, macroglobulinemia, and heavy-chain disease. Or it may be *polyclonal*, which involves an excess of two or more classes of immunoglobulins and of both types of light chains. Polyclonal gammopathies include Hodgkin's disease and lymphatic leukemia. Called also *gammaglobulinopathy* and *immunoglobulinopathy*. See also PARAPROTEINEMIA.

Gamophen antibacterial soap see under SOAP.

Gamophen hand cleansing leaves see under LEAF.

Gangesol trademark for *trichlormethiazide*.

ganglia (gang′gle-ah) [L.] plural of *ganglion*.

gangliocyte (gang′gle-o-sīt″) [*ganglion* + Gr. *kytos* hollow vessel] ganglion CELL.

ganglion (gang′gle-on), pl. *gan′glia* or *ganglions* [Gr. "knot"] 1. a knot, or knotlike mass. 2. a general anatomical term for a group of nerve cell bodies located outside the central nervous system; occasionally applied to certain nuclear groups within the brain or spinal cord. 3. a form of cystic tumor occurring on an aponeurosis or tendon, as in the wrist. **Andersch's g.**, inferior g. of glossopharyngeal nerve. **Arnold's g.**, **auricular g.**, otic g. **ganglia of autonomic plexuses**, groups of nerve cell bodies found in the autonomic plexuses, composed primarily of sympathetic postganglionic neurons. Called also *ganglia plexuum autonomicorum* [NA], *ganglia plexuum sympathicorum,* and *ganglia of sympathetic plexuses.* **basal ganglia,** masses of gray matter of the brain that comprise the corpus striatum, amygdaloid body, and claustrum. Sometimes the thalamus and all subcortical nuclei are also considered as part of basal ganglia. They represent the second highest (after the cerbral cortex) centers for facilitating motor function; the globus pallidum sometimes being referred to as the motor center of the extrapyramidal system. **Blandin's g.,** submandibular g. **Bochdalek's g.,** dental plexus, superior; see under PLEXUS. **Bock's g.,** carotid g. **carotid g.,** a ganglion of the internal carotid plexus in the cavernous sinus. Called also *Bock's g.* and *Laumonier's g.* **carotid g., inferior,** a ganglion of the internal carotid plexus in the lower part of the carotid canal. Called also *Laumonier's g.* and *Schmiedel's g.* **carotid g., superior,** a ganglion of the internal carotid plexus in the upper part of the carotid plexus. **cephalic ganglia,** parasympathetic ganglia in the head, consisting of the ciliary, otic, pterygopalatine, and submandibular ganglia. **cervical g., inferior,** a ganglion at the level of the seventh cervical vertebra, usually a part of the cervicothoracic ganglion. Called also *g. cervicale inferius.* **cervical g., middle,** the smallest of the cervical ganglia, contributing branches to the heart, cervical region, and thyroid gland. Called also *ganglion cervicale medium* [NA], *inferior thyroid ganglion,* and *superior thyroid ganglion.* **cervical g., superior,** the uppermost ganglion of the cervical portion of the sympathetic trunk, being the largest ganglion of the sympathetic chain. It is buried in the connective tissue between the carotid sheath and the prevertebral fascia in front of the second and third cervical vertebrae. Its branches include the internal carotid nerve, communications with the cranial nerves, branches to the spinal nerves, pharyngeal branches, nerves to the external carotid artery, branches to the intercarotid plexus, and a nerve to the heart. Called also *ganglion cervicale superius* [NA]. **g. cervica'le infe'rius,** cervical g., inferior. **g. cervica'le me'dium** [NA], cervical g., middle. **g. cervica'le supe'rius** [NA], cervical g., superior. **cervicothoracic g., g. cervicothora'cium** [NA], a ganglion on the sympathetic trunk at the level of the seventh cervical and first thoracic vertebra, consisting of the inferior cervical and first thoracic ganglia, which are usually fused. It contributes branches to the head and neck, heart, and upper limbs. Called also *stellate g.* and *g. stellatum* [NA alternative]. **g. cilia're** [NA], **ciliary g.,** a parasympathetic ganglion in the posterior part of the orbit, containing postganglionic fibers, which supply the ciliary muscle, and sensory and postganglionic sympathetic fibers which pass through it without synapses. **Cloquet's g.,** an enlargement of the nasopalatine nerve in the anterior palatine canal. **dorsal root g.,** spinal g. **Ehrenritter's g.,** superior g. of glossopharyngeal nerve. **false g.,** an enlargement of a nerve that does not contain synaptic connections. **Gasser's g., gasserian g.,** trigeminal g. **geniculate g., g. genic'uli ner'vi facia'lis** [NA], a sensory ganglion situated on a U-shaped bend of the facial nerve *(geniculum of facial nerve).* It is a ganglion of the intermediate portion of the facial nerve, and its central processes supply the taste buds on the anterior part of the tongue through the chorda tympani and lingual nerves; soft palate through the greater superficial petrosal and lesser palatine nerves; and skin of the external acoustic meatus and mastoid process through fibers that join the auricular branch of the vagus nerve. **hypoglossal g.,** a ganglion of the hypoglossal nerve; rarely seen in man, except in the embryo. **inferior g. of glossopharyngeal nerve,** the lower of two ganglia on the glossopharyngeal nerve as it passes through the jugular foramen; both contain cell bodies for the afferent fibers of the nerve. Called also *Andersch's g., inferior jugular g., g. inferius nervi glossopharyngei* [NA], *lower g. of glossopharyngeal nerve, petrosal g., g. petrosum,* and *g. petrosum.* **g. inferior g. of vagus nerve,** a fusiform ganglion, about 25 mm in length, which lies on the vagus nerve just as it leaves the jugular foramen, about 10 mm distal to the superior ganglion. The central processes of its sensory cells pass through the superior ganglion without synaptic connections and enter the medulla oblongata near the rootlets of the superior ganglion. Its peripheral processes form a ramus of the superior laryngeal nerve and contribute fibers to branches of the vagus nerve to the larynx, trachea, bronchi, and thoracic and abdominal viscera. Called also *g. inferius nervi vagi* [NA], *inferior vagal g., lower g. of vagus nerve, nodose g.,* and *g. nodosum.* **g. infe'rius ner'vi glossopharyn'gei** [NA], inferior g. of glossopharyngeal nerve. **g. infe'rius ner'vi va'gi** [NA], inferior g. of vagus nerve. **jugular g. of glossopharyngeal nerve,** superior g. of glossopharyngeal nerve. **jugular g., inferior,** inferior g. of glossopharyngeal nerve. **jugular g. of vagus nerve, g. jugula're ner'vi va'gi,** superior g. of vagus nerve. **Küttner's g.,** a large lymph node on the internal jugular vein immediately beneath the posterior belly of the digastric muscle, forming the principal lymphatic terminus of the tongue. Called also *hauptganglion of Küttner, jugulodigastric node, nodus jugulodigastricus* [NA], and *nodus lymphaticus jugulodigastricus.* **Langley's g.,** a collection of nerve cells in the hilus of the submandibular gland in some animals. **Laumonier's g.,** 1. carotid g. 2. carotid g., inferior. **lower g. of glossopharyngeal nerve,** inferior g. of glossopharyngeal nerve. **lower g. of vagus nerve,** inferior g. of vagus nerve. **g. lymphat'icus,** lymph NODE. **Meckel's g.,** pterygopalatine g. **Müller's g.,** superior g. of glossopharyngeal nerve. **nodose g., g. nodo'sum,** inferior g. of vagus nerve. **olfactory g.,** a mass of tissue in the embryo which develops into the olfactory nerves. **otic g., g. o'ticum** [NA], a flat, oval, or stellate ganglion, about 2 to 4 mm in diameter, located in the infratemporal fossa, medial to the mandibular nerve and just inferior to the foramen ovale. It derives its preganglionic fibers from the glossopharyngeal nerve via the tympanic nerve and tympanic ganglion, the lesser petrosal nerve serving as its parasympathetic root. The postganglionic fibers, passing mainly through a communication with the auriculotemporal nerve, innervate the parotid gland. Called also *Arnold's g.* and *auricular g.* **petrosal g., g. petro'sus, petrous g.,** inferior g. of glossopharyngeal nerve. **gan'glia plex'uum autonomico'rum** [NA], **gan'glia plex'uum sympathico'rum,** ganglia of autonomic plexuses. **pterygopalatine g., g. pterygopalati'num** [NA], a triangular parasympathetic ganglion, about 5 mm in length, in the pterygopalatine fossa just below the maxillary nerve, being attached to the pterygopalatine branches of the maxillary nerve. Its preganglionic fibers derive from the facial nerve through the greater petrosal nerve and the nerve of the pterygopalatine canal. Its postganglionic fibers supply the lacrimal, nasal, and palatine glands, being concerned chiefly with the secretory motor activities of the glands. Called also *Meckel's g., sphenomaxillary g., sphenopalatine g.,* and *g. sphenopalatinum.* **Schmiedel's g.,** carotid g., inferior. **semilunar g., g. semiluna're,** trigeminal g. **sensory g.,** one that transmits sensory impulses in the peripheral nervous system. Also, a mass of nerve cell bodies in the brain subserving sensory functions. **sphenomaxillary g., sphenopalatine g., g. sphenopalati'num,** pterygopalatine g. **spinal g., g. spina'le** [NA], the ganglion found on the dorsal root of each spinal nerve, composed of unipolar nerve cell bodies of the sensory neurons of the nerve. Called also *dorsal root g.* **stellate g., g. stella'tum,** cervicothoracic g. **submandibular g., g. submandibula're** [NA], **g. submaxilla're, submaxillary g.,** a small parasympathetic ganglion, about 2 to 5 mm in diameter, suspended from the lingual nerve by two filaments, and located superior to the deep part of the submandibular gland on the lateral surface of the hyoglossus muscle. The preganglionic fibers are received from the intermediate nerve through the chorda tympani and the proximal filament connecting the submandibular gland to the lingual nerve (parasympathetic root); the postganglionic fibers innervate the sublingual and lingual glands and small glands in the floor of the mouth. Sympathetic fibers are derived through the second filament (sympathetic root) but they merely pass through having no synapses in the ganglion. Called also *Blandin's g.* **superior g. of glossopharyngeal nerve,** the upper of two ganglia on the glossopharyngeal nerve as it passes through the jugular foramen; both contain cell bodies for afferent fibers of the nerve. It may be absent and is considered as a detached part of the inferior ganglion. Called also *Ehrenritter's g., jugular g. of glossopharyngeal nerve, Muller's g., g. superius, g. superius nervi glossopharyngei* [NA], and *upper g.* **superior g. of vagus nerve,** a small, spherical ganglion, about 4 mm in diameter, which lies on the vagus nerve in the jugular foramen, giving off meningeal and auricular branches, the central processes of its sensory cells entering the medulla oblongata as three or four separate rootlets. Called also *jugular g. of vagus nerve, g. jugulare nervi vagi, superior vagal g.,* and *g. superius nervi vagi.* **g. supe'rius, g. supe'rius ner'vi glossopharyn'gei** [NA], superior g. of glossopharyngeal nerve. **g. supe'rius ner'vi va'gi** [NA], superior g. of vagus nerve. **ganglia of sympathetic plexuses,** ganglia of autonomic plexuses. **terminal g., g. termina'le** [NA], a group of nerve cells found along the terminal nerves, medial to the olfactory bulb. **thyroid g., inferior, thyroid g., superior,** old terms for cervical g., middle. **trigeminal g., g. of trigeminal nerve, g. trigemina'le** [NA], a flat, semilunar ganglion, about 1 by 2 cm in diameter, situated on the sensory root of the trigeminal nerve in a cleft within the dura mater (trigeminal cavity) on the anterior surface of the petrous portion of the temporal bone. It contains cells of origin of most of the sensory fibers of the trigeminal nerve and its peripheral fibers form the opththalmic and maxillary nerves and part of the mandibular nerve. Called also *gasserian g.*, *Gasser's g.*, *semilunar g.*, and *g. semilunare.* **tympanic g., g. tympan′icum** [NA], an enlargement on the tympanic branch of the glossopharyngeal nerve. **tympanic g. of Valentin,** a ganglion on a superior dental nerve. Called also *Valentin's g.* **upper g.,** superior g. of glossopharyngeal nerve. **vagal g., inferior,** inferior g. of vagus nerve. **vagal g., superior,** superior g. of vagus nerve. **Valentin's g.,** 1. tympanic g. of Valentin. 2. INTUMESCENTIA tympanica.

ganglioside (gang′gle-o-sīd) a galactose cerebroside found in the central nervous system.

gangosa (gang-go′sah) [Sp. "muffled voice"] mutilating RHINO-PHARYNGITIS.

gangrene (gang′grēn) [L. *gangraena;* Gr. *gangraina*] an eating sore, which ends in mortification] death and putrefaction of tissue, usually in considerable mass and usually associated with loss of vascular supply. The initial event may be a bacterial infection, causing vascular obstruction because of swelling or clotting, followed by invasion by saprophytes capable of surviving only in ischemic tissue. Called also *gangrenous necrosis.* See also NECROSIS and NECROBIOSIS. **dry g.,** gangrene without subsequent bacterial infection, characterized by dry and shriveled tissue. Called also *mummification* and *mummification necrosis.* **moist g.,** wet g. **pulp g.,** gangrenous pulp NECROSIS. **wet g.,** gangrene accompanied by bacterial invasion of the ischemic tissue, usually occurring as the result of sudden stoppage of the blood supply, due to an accident, freezing, burns, or prolonged use of a tourniquet. The tissue assumes the appearance of a bruise and may be swollen and blistered but the lesion later spreads rapidly. Called also *moist g.*

ganja (gan′jah) a cannabinoid substance prepared in India from *Cannabis sativa,* in which an infusion is made from the female plant. It may also be smoked and, when incorporated into sweet meats, is known as *majoon.* See also CANNABINOID.

ganoblast (gan′o-blast) ameloblast.

Gantanol trademark for *sulfamethoxazole.*

Gantrim trademark for a sulfamethoxazole-trimethoprim mixture.

Gantrisin trademark for *sulfisoxazole.*

gap (gap) an unoccupied interval in time; an opening or hiatus. **interocclusal g.,** interocclusal DISTANCE.

Garamycin trademark for *gentamicin sulfate* (see under GENTAMICIN).

Garasol trademark for *gentamicin sulfate* (see under GENTAMICIN).

Garcin's syndrome [Raymond *Garcin,* French physician] see under SYNDROME.

Gardette, James [1756–1831] a French-born American dentist who contributed to the development of dentistry in the United States.

Gardinal trademark for *phenobarbital.*

Gardner's needle holder see under HOLDER.

Gardner's syndrome [Eldon J. *Gardner*] see under SYNDROME.

Gardol trademark for *sodium lauroyl sarcosinate* (see under SODIUM).

Garg. abbreviation for L. *gargaris′mus,* gargle.

gargoylism (gar′goil-izm) [*gargoyle* a grotesquely carved figure] Hunter-Hurler SYNDROME.

Gariot's articulator [J. B. *Gariot,* French dentist, 18th and 19th centuries; inventor of the articulator] see under ARTICULATOR.

garnet (gar′net) a silicate of any combination of aluminum, cobalt, magnesium, iron and manganese. In dentistry, garnet particles are usually coated on paper or cloth with glue, being one of the common abrasives used in denture abrasive disks as operated with the handpiece.

Garré's osteomyelitis [Carl *Garré,* Swiss surgeon, 1857–1928] see under OSTEOMYELITIS.

Garretson, James Edmund (1828–1895) an American oral surgeon credited with having been the originator of the specialty of oral surgery.

gas (gas) 1. an elastic aeriform fluid. 2. a state of matter having no fixed shape or volume, but occupying the entire space afforded within the walls of its container, in which the molecules are practically unrestricted by cohesive forces. The densities of gases are much lower than those of liquids and solids. **carbonic acid g.,** CARBON dioxide. **hydrofluoric acid g.,** hydrogen FLUORIDE. **laughing g.,** nitrous OXIDE. **marsh g.,** methane.

noble g., an inert gas that does not combine with another element, found in group 0 of the periodic table; helium, argon, krypton, xenon, and radon are the noble gases. See also inert ELEMENT. **olefiant g.,** ethylene. **sweet g.,** CARBON monoxide.

gaseous (gas′e-us, gash′us) of the nature of a gas.

gasometry (gas-om′e-tre) [*gas* + Gr. *metron* measure] the determination of the amount of gas present in a mixture.

Gasser's ganglion, [Johann Laurentius *Gasser,* professor in Vienna from 1757 to 1765] trigeminal GANGLION. See also GASSERIAN.

gasserian (gas-se′re-an) named after or described by Johann Laurentius *Gasser,* as gasserian ganglion (see trigeminal GANGLION).

gastr- see GASTRO-.

gastric (gas′trik) [L. *gastricus;* Gr. *gastēr* stomach] pertaining to, affecting, or originating in the stomach.

gastrin (gas′trin) a polypeptide (heptadecapeptide) hormone secreted by the gastric cells of the antral mucosa of the pyloric glands, whose activity is related to the terminal tetrapeptide. Its secretion is stimulated by distention of the stomach by the bulk of food entering the stomach, and by certain chemical substances, such as food extractives, partially digested proteins, alcohol, caffeine, and other substances.

gastro-, gastr- [Gr. *gastēr* stomach] a combining form denoting relationship to the stomach.

gastrospiry (gas′tro-spi″re) [*gastro-* + L. *spirare* to breathe] aerophagia.

gastrula (gas′troo-lah) that early embryonic stage which follows the blastula. The simplest type consists of two layers (ectoderm and mesoderm), and of two cavities, one lying between the ectoderm and the entoderm, and the other (archenteron) formed by invagination so as to lie within the entoderm and having an opening (blastopore).

gastrulation (gas″troo-la′shun) a series of events that presage the characteristic body plan, consisting of moving of specific regions of the blastula into certain positions. The process results in an immediate evolution of the three germ layers (ectoderm, mesoderm, and entoderm), which further give rise to specific tissues and organs. See also germ LAYER, and see illustration at EMBRYO.

Gaucher's cell, disease [Phillippe Charles Ernest *Gaucher,* French physician, 1854–1918] see under CELL and DISEASE.

gauge (gāj) an instrument for determining physical properties of anything, including caliber, dimensions, pressure, etc. **Boley g.,** a watchmaker's gauge used in dentistry to measure accurately tooth, arch, and facial dimensions. See illustration. See also

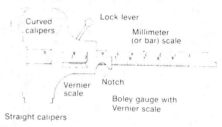

Components of the Boley gauge. (From H. O. Torres and A. Ehrlich. Modern Dental Assisting. 2nd ed. Philadelphia, W. B. Saunders Co., 1980.)

tooth MEASUREMENT. **BW g.,** a device for measuring the root canal, being a transparent gauge, and with a pin of known length luted to the surface of the tooth parallel to its long axis, which compares the length of the pin with that of the canal on the radiograph. **Starret wire g.,** a trademark for a metal disk with slots of different sizes, used for measuring the diameters of

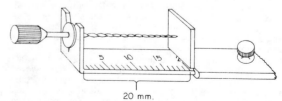

The working length of the tooth (21 mm) is set on the endodontic measuring gauge; all instruments inserted subsequently in the canal are set at this length. (From J. I. Ingle: Endodontics. Philadelphia, Lea & Febiger, 1965.)

wire. Also used for comparing the diameter of a silver point with a corresponding size root canal file. **test file g.,** a gauge for holding and measuring the length of files, reamers, or broaches, comparing the length of the instrument with that of the root canals represented on a radiograph of a tooth. See illustration. See also test HANDLE. **undercut g.,** an instrument for measuring the depth of an undercut in a dental cast, such as one used with dental surveyors.

Gaultheria (gawl-the're-ah) a genus of ericaceous plants; the leaves of *G. procumbens* of North America (wintergreen) are rich in methyl salicylate (see under SALICYLATE).

Gauss, Johann Karl F. [1777–1855] a German physicist. See GAUSS.

gauss (gows) [named after J. K. F. *Gauss*] the unit of magnetic flux density, equal to a force of 1 dyne on a unit magnetic pole, or 1 B (emu) = ⅓ × 10^{-10} esu. Symbol *B*. Replaced in SI by the tesla.

gauze (gawz) a light, open-meshed fabric of muslin or similar material. Before use in surgery, it is usually sterilized and frequently impregnated with various antiseptics. **absorbable g.,** gauze made from oxidized cellulose. **absorbent g.,** a well-bleached cotton cloth of plain weave, of various thread counts (20–44 per inch warp, 12–36 filling) and various weights (17.2–44.5 gm per yd). **absorbent g., sterile,** absorbent gauze which has been sterilized and subsequently protected from contamination. **petrolatum g.,** absorbent gauze saturated with white petrolatum; used as a protective covering for wounds.

gavage (gah-vahzh') [Fr. "cramming"] 1. forced feeding especially through a tube passed into the stomach. 2. the therapeutic use of very full diet; superalimentation.

Gay-Lussac's law [Joseph Louis *Gay-Lussac*, French naturalist, 1778–1850] Charles' LAW.

g-cal gram calorie; see small CALORIE.

Gd gadolinium.

Ge germanium.

gear (gēr) equipment. **cervical g.,** an extraoral orthodontic appliance that uses the back of the neck for anchoring or as a base of traction. See also ANCHORAGE. **head g.,** headgear.

Gee-Herter disease [Samuel Jones *Gee*, London physician, 1839–1911; Christian Archibald *Herter*, American physician, 1865–1910] celiac DISEASE.

Gegenbaur's cell, ethmoidal sulcus of [Carl *Gegenbaur*, German anatomist, 1826–1903] see OSTEOBLAST, and ethmoid canal, anterior, under CANAL.

Geiger counter, plateau [Hans *Geiger*, German physicist in England, 1882–1945] see Geiger-Müller COUNTER, and see under PLATEAU.

Geiger-Müller counter, tube [H. *Geiger*; W. *Müller*] see under COUNTER.

gel (jel) a colloidal solution of a liquid in a solid. **aluminum hydroxide g.,** ALUMINUM hydroxide. **Cavi-Trol acidulated phosphate fluoride topical g.,** trademark for a fluoride gel used topically in dental caries control, 100 gm of which contain 2 gm sodium fluoride, 0.34 gm hydrogen fluoride, and various amounts of thickening, flavoring, and coloring agents, which is acidulated with 0.98 gm phosphoric acid. **Codesco topical fluoride phosphate anticaries g.,** trademark for a fluoride gel used topically in dental caries control, 100 gm of which contain 2 gm sodium fluoride, 0.35 gm hydrogen fluoride, and various amounts of thickening, flavoring, and coloring agents, which is acidulated with 0.98 gm phosphoric acid. **Credo topical g.,** trademark for a fluoride gel used topically in dental caries control, 100 gm of which contain 2 gm sodium fluoride, 0.35 gm hydrogen fluoride, and various amounts of thickening, flavoring, and coloring agents, which is acidulated with 0.98 gm phosphoric acid. **Dental H topical fluoride g.,** trademark for a fluoride gel used topically in dental caries control, 100 gm which contain 2 gm sodium fluoride, 0.34 gm hydrogen fluoride, and various amounts of flavoring, thickening, and coloring agents, which is acidulated with 0.98 gm phosphoric acid. **Fluor-O-Kote topical fluoride g.,** trademark for a fluoride gel used topically in dental caries control, 100 gm of which contain 2 gm sodium fluoride, 0.35 gm hydrogen fluoride, and various amounts of flavoring, thickening, and coloring agents, which is acidulated with 0.98 gm phosphoric acid. **Healthco topical fluoride g.,** trademark for a fluoride gel used topically in dental caries control, 100 gm of which contain 2 gm sodium fluoride, 0.35 gm hydrogen fluoride, and various amounts of thickening, flavoring, and coloring agents, which is acidulated with 0.98 gm phosphoric acid. **Hurricane g.,** trademark for an ointment, 100 gm of which contains 20 gm benzocaine and various flavoring agents in a polyethylene glycol base. **Karidium phosphate fluoride topical g.,** trademark for a fluoride gel used topically in dental caries control, 100 gm of which contain 1.36

gm sodium fluoride, 0.65 gm hydrogen fluoride, 1.22 gm sodium dihydrogen phosphate monohydrate, and various amounts of thickening, flavoring, and coloring agents, which is acidulated with 0.012 gm phosphoric acid. **Kerr topical Flura-G.,** trademark for a fluoride gel used topically in dental caries control, 100 gm of which contain 2 gm sodium fluoride, 0.35 gm hydrogen fluoride, and various amounts of thickening, flavoring, and coloring agents, which is acidulated with 0.98 gm phosphoric acid. **Luride topical g.,** trademark for a fluoride gel used topically in dental caries control, 100 gm of which contain 2 gm sodium fluoride, 0.35 gm hydrogen fluoride, and various amounts of thickening and flavoring agents, which is acidulated with 1.2 gm phosphoric acid. **Nufluor g.,** trademark for a fluoride gel used topically in dental caries control, 100 gm of which contain 2 gm sodium fluoride, 0.34 gm hydrogen fluoride, and various amounts of preservative, thickening, flavoring, and coloring agents, which is acidulated with 0.98 gm phosphoric acid. **Pacemaker topical fluoride g.,** trademark for a fluoride gel used topically in dental caries control, 100 gm of which contain 2 gm sodium fluoride, 0.34 gm hydrogen fluoride, and various amounts of thickening, flavoring, and coloring agents, which is acidulated with 0.98 gm phosphoric acid. **Predent topical fluoride treatment g.,** trademark for a fluoride gel used topically in dental caries control, 100 gm of which contain 2.6 gm sodium fluoride, 0.16 gm hydrogen fluoride, and various amounts of thickening, flavoring, and coloring agents, which is acidulated with 0.98 gm phosphoric acid. **Rafluor topical g.,** trademark for a fluoride gel used topically in dental caries control, 100 gm of which contain 2 gm sodium fluoride, 0.35 gm hydrogen fluoride, and various amounts of thickening, flavoring, and coloring agents, which is acidulated with 1.05 gm phosphoric acid. **Rescue Squad topical g.,** trademark for a fluoride gel used topically in dental caries control, 100 gm of which contain 2 gm sodium fluoride, 0.34 gm hydrogen fluoride, and various amounts of thickening, flavoring, and coloring agents, which is acidulated with 0.98 gm phosphoric acid. **sodium fluoride–orthophosphoric acid g.,** a preparation used topically in dental caries control, containing 1.23 percent sodium fluoride, which is acidulated with 1 percent phosphoric acid in an aqueous medium with carboxymethylcellulose sodium. Its pH is between 3.0 and 3.4. **So-Flo phosphate topical g.,** trademark for a fluoride gel used topically in dental caries control, 100 gm of which contain 2 gm sodium fluoride, 0.35 gm hydrogen fluoride, and various amounts of thickening, flavoring, and coloring agents, which is acidulated with 0.98 gm phosphoric acid. **Sultan topical fluoride g.,** trademark for a fluoride gel used topically in dental caries control, 100 gm of which contain 2 gm sodium fluoride, 0.35 gm hydrogen fluoride, and various amounts of thickening, flavoring, and coloring agents, which is acidulated with 0.98 gm phosphoric acid. **Super-Dent topical fluoride g.,** trademark for a fluoride gel used topically in dental caries control, 100 gm of which contain 2 gm sodium fluoride, 0.35 gm hydrogen fluoride, and various amounts of thickening, flavoring, and coloring agents, which is acidulated with 0.98 gm phosphoric acid.

gelatin (jel'ah-tin) [L. *gelatina,* from *gelare* to congeal] a product obtained by partial hydrolysis of collagen derived from the skin, white connective tissue, and bones of animals; used as a suspending agent. It is also used pharmaceutically in the manufacture of capsules and suppositories, and has been suggested for intravenous use as a plasma substitute, and has been used as an adjuvant protein food. In x-ray film manufacture, it serves as a medium for suspending the silver halide crystals in the film emulsion.

gelation (jĕ-la'shun) the conversion of a sol into a gel.

Gelfoam trademark for *absorbable gelatin sponge* (see under SPONGE).

Gemella (jem'ē-lah) [L., dim. of *gemellus* a twin] a genus of bacteria of the family Streptococcaceae, occurring as gram-positive, aerobic or facultatively anaerobic, nonendosporogenic, nonmotile cocci, found singly or in pairs with adjacent sides flattened. **G. haemoly'sans,** a species isolated from human bronchial secretions and respiratory mucus, occurring as facultatively anaerobic or aerobic, fermentative cocci, 0.5 to 0.6 μm in diameter, which produce β-hemolysis on solid medium with rabbit or horse blood. It is sensitive to penicillin, streptomycin, tetracyclines, sulfathiazole, chloramphenicol, vancomycin, and other drugs. Called also *Neisseria haemolysans.*

geminate (jem'i-nāt) [L. *geminatus*] paired; occurring in pairs.

gemination (jem-ĭ-na'shun) a doubling; a form of fusion of two teeth which results in the formation of two teeth or of a double crown formed on a single root with a single pulp canal. The term is usually applied to fusion of two supernumerary teeth or union of one supernumerary with a regular tooth. Called also *twin formation, twin teeth,* and *twinning.* See also CONCRESCENCE (3), FUSION (4), and SCHIZODONTISM.

Gemini II trademark for a nickel-chromium base-metal crown and bridge alloy, also containing beryllium. Inhalation of dust during melting, milling, or grinding may cause beryllium poisoning.

gemma (jem′ah) [L. "bud"] 1. a budlike body or structure. 2. micelle (1).

gemmation (jĕ-ma′shun) [L. *gemmare* to bud] reproduction by budding; a kind of reproduction in cells in which a portion of the cell body is thrust out and then becomes separated, forming a new individual.

gemmule (jem′ŭl) [L. *gemmula,* dim. of *gemma* bud] 1. a reproductive bud; the immediate product of gemmation. 2. a short process branching out from a dendrite. 3. one of the hypothetical units assumed to be thrown off by the somatic cells, to be stored in the germ cells, and to determine the development of certain characteristics.

Gemonil trademark for *metharbital.*

-gen [Gr. *gennan* to produce] a word termination denoting an agent productive of the object or state indicated in the word stem to which it is affixed.

genal (je′nal) [L. *gena* cheek] pertaining to the cheek; buccal.

gender (jen′der) sex; the category to which an individual is assigned on the basis of sex.

gene (jēn) [Gr. *gennan* to produce] a unit of self-reproducing genetic material localized at a definite position (locus) on the chromosome. It represents a specific sequence of nucleotides, being a functional unit that determines the sequence of amino acids in protein synthesis, thus regulating development of the body and its metabolism. The genetic constitution of an individual (genotype), being the sum total of the genetic information contained in the linkage of chromosomes, determines the character of the individual (phenotype). Genes occur in diploid organisms as pairs of alleles, each pair segregating during cell division (see MEIOSIS), so that an offspring receives only one member of a pair from each parent. Functionally, genes are considered as *structural, operator,* and *regulator genes.* They are also considered as *cistrons, mutons,* and *recons.* As classically construed, the gene is approximately synonymous with cistron. See also CHROMOSOME. **allelic g's,** genes situated at corresponding loci on a pair of chromosomes. See also ALLELE. **allelomorphic g.,** allele. **amorphic g.,** amorph. **autosomal dominant g.,** autosomal dominant CHARACTER. **autosomal recessive g.,** autosomal recessive CHARACTER. **codominant g.,** codominant CHARACTER. **complementary g's,** two independent pairs of nonallelic genes, neither of which will produce its effect in the absence of the other. Called also *reciprocal g's.* **cumulative g's,** polygene. **dominant g.,** see autosomal dominant CHARACTER and X-linked dominant CHARACTER. **g. expression,** gene EXPRESSION. **g. flow,** gene FLOW. **immune response g's,** genes which control the immune responses to thymus-dependent antigens, including (*a*) the histocompatibility-linked immune response genes that are in close association with genes coding for the major histocompatibility antigens, and (*b*) the immunoglobulin allotype-linked response genes that appear to determine the structure of the immunoglobulin receptor on B-lymphocytes. **leaky g.,** one in which a switch in the sequence of bases in a nucleotide results in the production of a mutant protein, which, because of a single amino acid replacement, has only partial enzymatic activity; a hypomorph. **lethal g.,** a gene the presence of which brings about the death of the organism, or permits its survival only under certain conditions. **multifactorial g's,** a group of nonallelic genes which individually have little effect but act in conjunction with nongenetic factors, such as environment, in exerting phenotypic effect. See also POLYGENE. **mutant g.,** a gene that has undergone mutation, resulting in the loss, gain, or exchange of material and a permanent transmissible change in function. Such a gene may have become practically inactive (*amorph*), may act to antagonize or inhibit normal activity (*antimorph*), or may show only a slight reduction in its effectiveness (*leaky g.*). See also MUTATION (2). **nonstructural g's,** the operator and regulator genes, i.e., those not concerned in the formation of templates for messenger RNA. **operator g.,** a gene that serves as a starting point for reading the genetic code and that, through interaction with a repressor, controls the activity of the structural genes. The operator gene, together with the adjacent structural gene or genes controlled by it,

constitutes an operon. It is not regarded as a whole gene but as a site within a gene or gene complex. Called also *operator.* **quantitative g's,** polygene. **recessive g.,** see autosomal recessive CHARACTER and X-linked dominant CHARACTER. **reciprocal g's,** complementary g's. **regulator g.,** one that controls the rate of production of other genes by synthesizing a substance which inhibits the action of an operator gene. **sex-conditioned g.,** one that is fully expressed in one sex only; a sex-limited gene. See also PEDIGREE and sex-linked CHARACTER. **sex-linked g.,** one that is carried only on the X or Y chromosome. See sex-linked CHARACTER. **structural g.,** a gene that determines the amino acid sequence of a specific polypeptide chain. Messenger RNA is its primary product. **wild-type g.,** the normal allele of a rare mutant gene, sometimes symbolized by +. **X-linked g.,** one that is carried on the X chromosome. See X-linked dominant CHARACTER and X-linked recessive CHARACTER. **X-linked dominant g.,** X-linked dominant CHARACTER. **X-linked recessive g.,** X-linked recessive CHARACTER.

generation (jen″ĕ-ra′shun) [L. *generatio*] 1. the act or process of reproduction. 2. a class composed of all individuals removed by the same number of successive ancestors from a common predecessor, or occupying positions on the same level in a genealogical chart. See also PEDIGREE. **filial g., first,** all of the offspring produced by the mating of two individuals. Symbol F_1. **filial g., second,** all of the offspring produced by the mating of two individuals of the first filial generation. Symbol F_2. **parental g.,** the generation with which a particular genetic study is begun. Symbol P_1. **spontaneous g.,** a belief held in the past that living organisms could arise from nonliving material, such as the appearance of lice in human sweat or mice in decomposing fodder.

generator (jen′ĕ-ra″tor) any device that converts one type of energy into another. **electric g.,** one that converts mechanical energy into electrical energy. **x-ray g.,** an apparatus for the diagnostic or therapeutic use of x-rays. A typical medical unit usually consists of a table for the patient; a tube for generating x-rays mounted over the table; a film holder (cassette) placed under the table; and a panel for controlling kilovoltage, milliamperage, and exposure time. In a dental unit, the tube is mounted in a head connected to the unit through a flexible arm, so that it may be brought to a desired position, while the patient remains in the dental chair. The film, rather than being contained in the cassette, is placed intraorally directly under the area to be x-rayed. Called also *x-ray machine* and *x-ray unit.* See illustrations. See also x-ray TUBE.

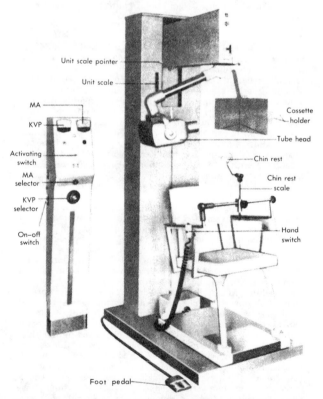

Panoramic x-ray unit. (From R. C. O'Brien: Dental Radiography. 4th ed.., Philadelphia, W. B. Saunders Co., 1981; courtesy of the S. S. White Dental Mfg Co., X. R. M. Division.)

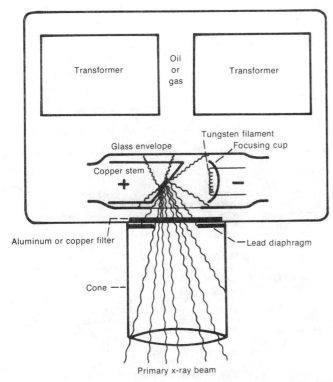

Transformer

Oil or gas

Transformer

Tungsten filament

Glass envelope

Focusing cup

Copper stem

+

−

Aluminum or copper filter

Lead diaphragm

Cone

Primary x-ray beam

Schematic drawing of the tube head. (From R. C. O'Brien: Dental Radiography. 4th ed., Philadelphia, W. B. Saunders Co., 1981.)

genesis (jen′ĕ-sis) [Gr. "production, generation"] the coming into being of anything; the process of originating. Often used as a word termination to denote production, formation, or development.

geneticist (jĕ-net′ĭ-sist) a specialist in genetics.

genetics (jĕ-net′iks) [Gr. *gennan* to produce] the study of heredity, including the mechanisms involved in storage, replication, mutation, recombination, and translation of genetic material in transmitting parental characteristics and traits to progeny. See also CHROMOSOME, HEREDITY, and INHERITANCE. **biochemical g.,** a branch of genetics concerned in the chemical aspects of heredity, particularly the genetic control of protein synthesis, either enzymes or structural components of cells and tissue, and in turn, all the developmental and metabolic processes of the body. **clinical g.,** the study of the possible genetic factors in the occurrence of pathological conditions. **molecular g.,** the branch of genetics concerned in the study of genetic systems and processes on the molecular level, including genetic mechanisms and the control of metabolic processes, replication of DNA, its transcription into RNA, and the translation of RNA to form proteins. See also CYTOGENETICS. **population g.,** the study of the distribution of genes in populations and of how genes and genotype frequencies are maintained or changed. See also Hardy-Weinberg LAW.

Gengou, Octave [French bacteriologist, 1875–1957] see *Bordetella pertussis,* under BORDETELLA (Bordet-Gengou bacillus), and complement FIXATION (Bordet-Gengou phenomenon or reaction).

genial, genian (jĕ-ni′al; jĕ-ni′an) [Gr. *geneion* chin] pertaining to the chin. See also MENTAL.

-genic [Gr. *gennan* to produce] a word termination meaning producing, or productive of.

genicula (jĕ-nik′u-lah) [L.] plural of *geniculum.*

genicular (jĕ-nik′u-lar) pertaining to the knee.

geniculate (jĕ-nik′u-lāt) [L. *geniculatus*] bent, like a knee.

geniculum (jĕ-nik′u-lum), pl. *genic′ula* [L., dim. of *genu* knee] a sharp, kneelike bend in a small structure or organ, such as a nerve. **g. cana′lis facia′lis** [NA], g. of facial canal. **g. of facial canal,** the U-shaped bend in the facial canal which lodges the geniculum of the facial nerve. Called also *g. cana′lis facia′lis* [NA], *genu of facial canal, and knee of aqueductus fallopii.* **g. of facial nerve, g. ner′vi facia′lis** [NA], the part of the facial nerve at the lateral end of the internal acoustic meatus, where the fibers bend into a U-shaped structure and where the roots of the facial nerve fuse and become swollen by the presence of the geniculate ganglion. Called also *external genu of facial nerve.*

genio- [Gr. *geneion* chin] a combining form denoting relationship to the chin. See also words beginning MENTO-.

geniocheiloplasty (je″ne-o-ki′lo-plas″te) [*genio-* + Gr. *cheilos* lip + *plassein* to form] plastic surgery of the chin and lip.

genioglossus (je″ne-o-glos′us) genioglossus MUSCLE.

geniohyoglossus (je″ne-o-hi″o-glos′us) genioglossus MUSCLE.

geniohyoid (je″ne-o-hi′oid) pertaining to the chin and hyoid bone.

geniohyoideus (je″ne-o-hi-oi′de-us) geniohyoid MUSCLE.

genioplasty (jĕ-ni′o-plas″te) [*genio-* + Gr. *plassein* to shape] plastic surgery of the chin.

geno- [Gr. *gennan* to produce] a combining form denoting relationship to reproduction or to sex.

genodermatosis (jen″o-der-mah-to′sis) [*geno-* + *dermatosis*] any of a wide variety of genetically determined skin disorders, ranging from aplastic defects to nevoid overgrowths, often associated with defects of other systems.

genome (je′nōm) [*gene* + chromos*ome*] a complete chromosome set that contains the sum total of its genes.

genotype (jen′o-tīp) [*geno-* + Gr. *typos* type] 1. the entire genetic constitution of an individual, being the sum total of the genetic information (genes) contained in the chromosomes, as distinguished from the phenotype, which represents the physical, biochemical, and/or physiological characteristics. Also, the alleles present at one or more specific loci. 2. the type species of a genus. Called also *idiotype.*

genous [Gr.] a word termination signifying arising or resulting from, or produced by.

gentamicin (jen″tah-mi′sin) an aminoglycoside antibiotic that acts on the bacterial ribosome, which is elaborated by fungi of the genus *Micromonospora,* and occurs as a white to buff, odorless powder that is soluble in water, but not in alcohol and organic solvents. It is active against gram-negative bacteria, including *Klebsiella, Enterobacter, Aerobacter, Escherichia coli, Shigella, Salmonella, Serratia marcescens,* and certain strains of *Pseudomonas* and *Proteus.* Used topically in the treatment of burns, impetigo, infected bed sores, pyoderma, and ear infections, and in the staphylococcal carrier state. Auditory and vestibular impairment, nephrotoxicity, and neuromuscular disorders may occur. **g. sulfate,** the sulfate salt of gentamicin. Trademarks: Cidomycin, Garamycin, Garasol, Genticin, Refobacin.

Genticin trademark for *gentamicin sulfate* (see under GENTAMICIN).

Gentinatre trademark for *sodium gentisate* (see under SODIUM).

gentiobiase (jen″she-o-bi′ās) β-GLUCOSIDASE.

gentisate (jen′ti-sāt) a salt of gentisic acid.

Gentisod trademark for *sodium gentisate* (see under SODIUM).

genu (je′nu), pl. *gen′ua* [L.] 1. the knee. 2. a general anatomical term used to designate any structure bent like the knee. **external g. of facial nerve,** GENICULUM of facial nerve. **g. of facial canal,** GENICULUM of facial canal.

genua (jen′u-ah) [L.] plural of *genu.*

geny- [Gr. *genys* jaw] a combining form denoting relationship to the jaw.

genyantralgia (jen″e-an-tral′je-ah) [*geny-* + *antrum* + *-algia*] pain in the maxillary sinus.

genyantritis (jen″e-an-tri′tis) [*geny-* + *antrum* + *-itis*] inflammation of the maxillary sinus.

genyantrum (jen″e-an′trum) [*geny-* + Gr. *antron* cave] maxillary SINUS.

geo- [Gr. *gē* earth] a combining form denoting relationship to the earth, or to soil.

Geocillin trademark for *carbenicillin indanyl sodium* (see under CARBENICILLIN).

geode (je′ōd) [Gr. *geōdes* earthlike, so called from a fancied resemblance to a mineral geode] a dilated lymph space.

Geodermatophilus (je″o-der″mah-tof′i-lus) a genus of soil bacteria of the family Dermatophilaceae, order Actinomycetales, occurring as aerobic, gram-positive organisms, which produce a muriform, tuber-shaped, noncapsulated, holocarpic, multilocular thallus containing cuboid cells.

geometry (je-om′ĕ-tre) that branch of mathematics which deals with the deduction of the properties, measurement, and relationships of points, lines, and angles in space. **x-ray beam g.,** the effect of various factors on the spatial distribution of radiation emerging from an x-ray generator or source. See also geometric UNSHARPNESS.

Geomycin trademark for *oxytetracycline hydrochloride* (see under OXYTETRACYCLINE).

Geon trademark for *polyvinyl chloride* (see under POLYVINYL).

geophagia (je-o-fa′je-ah) [*geo-* + Gr. *phagein* to eat] compulsive eating of clay or earth, most commonly observed in patients suffering from iron-deficiency anemia. The habit may lead to abrasion of the incisal edges of the anterior teeth and occlusal surfaces of the posterior teeth and wearing out of dentures. Iron therapy of anemia usually eliminates the craving. Called also *clay eating*, *dirt eating*, and *earth eating*. See also PICA.

geotrichosis (je″o-tri-ko′sis) a very rare infection caused by the fungus *Geotrichum candidum*, involving the lungs and oral cavity, and less commonly, the skin and gastrointestinal tract. The pulmonary involvement produces symptoms of pneumonia and bronchitis. Oral manifestations are similar to those seen in thrush, including the development on the oral mucosa of creamy, white, slightly elevated plaques made up of soft creamy or crumbled material resembling milk curds; the difference lies mainly in the microscopic picture of the lesion. The course of the disease and its clinical picture are also similar to those seen in candidiasis.

Geotrichum (je-ot′rĭ-kum) [*geo-* + Gr. *thrix* hair] a genus of deuteromycetous fungi (Fungi Imperfecti), the members of which form a true mycelium and reproduce by arthrospores only. Its sexual stage is an ascomycete.

geotropism (je-ot′ro-pizm) [*geo-* + Gr. *tropos* a turning] a tendency of growth or movement toward or away from the earth; the influence of gravity on growth. A tendency to grow toward the earth is *positive geotropism;* to grow away from the earth, *negative geotropism.*

Gerber attachment, hinge [A. *Gerber*] see under ATTACHMENT and HINGE.

Gerber space maintainer see under MAINTAINER.

Gerdy's fontanella, hyoid fossa [Pierre Nicholas *Gerdy,* French physician, 1797–1856] see under FONTANELLE, and see superior carotid TRIANGLE.

gereology (jer″e-ol′o-je) [Gr. *gēras* old age + *-logy*] the science which deals with old age and its phenomena.

Gerhardt's syndrome [Carl Adolf Christian Jakob *Gerhardt,* German physician, 1833–1902] see under SYNDROME.

Gerhardt-Semon law [C.A.C.J. *Gerhardt;* Sir Felix *Semon,* German laryngologist in London, 1849–1921] see under LAW.

geriatrics (jer″e-at′riks) [Gr. *gēras* old age + *iatrikē* surgery, medicine] the branch of medicine which treats all problems peculiar to old age and the aging. Called also *geriatric medicine.* **dental g.,** gerodontics.

germ (jerm) [L. *germen*] 1. a pathogenic microorganism. 2. living substance capable of developing into an organ, part, or organism as a whole; a primordium. **dental g.,** the collective tissues from which an entire tooth is formed, including the dental sac, dental organ, and dental papilla. See tooth BUD. **enamel g.,** the epithelial rudiment of the enamel organ.

germanium (jer-ma′ne-um) [L. *Germania* Germany] a nontoxic, grayish white metallic element. Symbol, Ge; atomic number, 32; atomic weight, 72.59; melting point, 937.4°C; specific gravity, 5.323; valences, 2, 4; Mohs hardness index, 6; group IVA on the periodic table. It has five natural isotopes (70, 72–74, 76) and several artificial radioactive ones (65–69, 71, 75, 77, 78). Germanium is attacked by nitric acid and aqua regia, but is stable in water, acids, and alkalies in the absence of dissolved oxygen. Used chiefly in electronic technology and in the production of glass capable of transmitting infrared radiation. Also used in certain dental alloys. Called also *eka-silicon.*

Germa-Medica liquid surgical soap see under SOAP.

germ-free (jerm′fre) free of microorganisms, said of an experimental animal reared under completely sterile conditions.

germicidal (jer″mĭ-si′dal) [L. *germen* germ + *caedere* to kill] lethal to pathogenic microorganisms.

germicide (jer″mĭ-sīd) a disinfectant which kills pathogenic microorganisms within 10 minutes, except the hepatitis virus and not necessarily the spores. Called also *germicidal agent.*

Gernebcin trademark for *tobramycin.*

gero-, geronto- [Gr. *gēras* old age; *gerōn, gerontos* old man] a combining form denoting relationship to old age or to the aged.

geroderma (jer-o-der′mah) [*gero-* + Gr. *derma* skin] dystrophic skin, giving the appearance of old age. Called also *gerodermia.* See also *progeria.* **hereditary osteodysplastic g.,** an X-linked syndrome characterized by generalized hyperlaxity, atrophy, and aging of the skin, hyperlaxity of joints, predisposition to fracture of bones, growth retardation, and muscle hyposomia. Called also *Bamatter's syndrome.* **Souques-Charcot g.,** a variant of Hutchinson-Gilford syndrome, consisting of loose, shiny, dry skin, subcutaneous atrophy, eunuchoid condition in males, and intellectual deficiency. Called also *gerodermia infantilis.*

gerodermia (jer-o-der′me-ah) [*gero-* + Gr. *derma* skin + *-ia*] geroderma. **g. infantil′is,** Souques-Charcot GERODERMA.

gerodontia (jer″o-don′she-ah) gerodontics.

gerodontic (jer″o-don′tik) [*gero-* + Gr. *odous* tooth] 1. pertaining to dental changes related to aging and old age. 2. pertaining to the practice of gerodontics.

gerodontics (jer″o-don′tiks) [Gr. *gēras* old age + *odous* tooth] the delivery of dental care to aging persons; the diagnosis, prevention, and treatment of problems peculiar to advanced age. Called also *dental geriatrics, geriatric dentistry,* and *gerodontia.*

gerodontist (jer″o-don′tist) a dentist who specializes in gerodontics.

gerodontology (jer″o-don-tol′o-je) the study of dentition and dental problems in the aged or aging.

Gerold, M. see Baller-Gerold SYNDROME.

geronto- see GERO-.

gerontologist (jer″on-tol′o-jist) a specialist in gerontology.

gerontology (jer″on-tol′o-je) [*geronto-* + *-logy*] the study of the problems of aging in all their aspects — clinical, biological, historical, and sociological.

Gersh, Isidore [American anatomist, born 1907] see Altmann-Gersh METHOD.

Gesarol trademark for *chlorophenothane.*

gestation (jes-ta′shun) [L. *gestatio,* from *gestare* to bear] the period of development of the young in viviparous animals. In humans, the gestation period is 9¼ calendar or 10 lunar months, each lunar month having 28 days. Birth occurs, on the average, 38 weeks after conception or 40 weeks after the beginning of the last menstrual period. See also PREGNANCY.

Getz Perfection trademark for a heat-cured denture base acrylic.

Getz surgical dressing see under DRESSING.

Ghon's focus, lesion, tubercle [Anton *Ghon,* Prague pathologist, 1866–1936] see under FOCUS and see primary (tuberculous) LESION.

Ghon-Sacks bacillus [A. *Ghon;* Anton *Sacks*] *Clostridium septicum;* see under CLOSTRIDIUM.

GH-RIF growth hormone-release inhibiting factor; see SOMATOSTATIN.

GI 1. gingival INDEX. 2. gastrointestinal SYSTEM.

gi gill.

Giannuzzi, crescents of (bodies, cells, demilunes) [Giuseppe *Giannuzzi,* Italian anatomist, 1839–1876] see under CRESCENT.

Giardia (je-ar′de-ah) [named after Alfred *Giard,* French biologist; 1846–1908] a genus of protozoa of the subphylum Mastigophora, found as an intestinal parasite in man and animals, causing diarrhea and other gastrointestinal disorders. Called also *Lamblia.*

Giardil trademark for *furazolidone.*

Giedion, A. see trichorhinophalangeal DYSPLASIA (2) (Langer-Giedion syndrome).

Giemsa banding (method, staining), bands, stain [Gustav *Giemsa,* German chemist and bacteriologist, 1867–1948] see G-BANDING, see G-bands, under BAND, and see under STAIN.

Gierke see VON GIERKE.

giga- [Gr. *gigas* mighty] a combining form designating gigantic size; in the metric system, used in naming units of measurement to indicate a quantity 1 billion (10^9) times the unit designated by the root with which it is combined. Symbol *G.* See also metric SYSTEM.

gigantism (ji′gan-tizm; ji-gan′tizm) [Gr. *gigas* giant] abnormal overgrowth, or excessive size and stature; a condition of abnormally high growth resulting from excessive secretion of growth hormone by the pituitary gland before closure of the epiphyses, brought about by a pituitary adenoma. It is regarded as the childhood form of acromegaly. The growth is usually symmetrical and patients lack the coarse features seen in acromegaly, but thickening of soft tissue and facial bones may occur after some years' duration. Teeth are proportional to the size of the jaws. **cerebral g.,** Sotos' SYNDROME. **unilateral g.,** hemigigantism.

giganto- [Gr. *gigas, gigantos* huge] a combining form meaning huge.

gigantosoma (ji-gan″to-so′mah) [*giganto-* + Gr. *sōma* body] great size and stature; gigantism.

Gigli's wire saw [Leonardo *Gigli,* Italian surgeon, 1866–1908] see under SAW.

Gilbert, W. [1544–1603] an English physicist. See GILBERT.

gilbert (gil′bert) [named after W. *Gilbert*] a unit of magnetomotive force, $1F = 10/\pi$ ampere-turns. Symbol *F.*

Gilchrist's disease [Thomas Casper *Gilchrist,* American dermatologist, 1862–1927] North American BLASTOMYCOSIS.

gildable (gil′dah-b'l) susceptible of being colored with gold stains.

Gilford's syndrome [Hastings *Gilford*, British physician, 1861–1941] Hutchinson-Gilford SYNDROME.

gill (jil) a unit of capacity (liquid or wine), being one-quarter of a pint. Abbreviated *gi.* See also *Tables of Weights and Measures* at WEIGHT. **British imperial g.**, one-quarter of a British imperial pint, being equivalent to 5 fluid ounces (8.669 cubic inches), or 142.066 cubic centimeters. **U.S. g.**, one-quarter of a U.S. pint, being equivalent to 4 fluid onces (7.218 cubic inches), or 118.291 cubic centimeters.

Gillies' flap, graft, operation [Sir Harold Delf *Gillies*, plastic and maxillofacial surgeon in New Zealand, 1882–1960; founder of the British Association of Plastic Surgeons] see rope FLAP, and see under OPERATION.

Gillmore initial and Gillmore final setting time see setting TIME.

Gillmore needle see under NEEDLE.

Gilmer's splint, wire, wiring [Thomas Lewis *Gilmer*, American oral surgeon, 1849–1931; he was the first to use wiring of the upper and lower teeth to obtain immobilization of fractured jaws] see under SPLINT, WIRE, and WIRING.

Gilson fixable-removable bar cross arch bar splint CONNECTOR.

Gimbard see DE GIMBARD.

Gingicaine trademark for a solution for topical application, 100 ml of which contain 22 gm benzocaine and various flavoring agents in polyethylene glycol.

gingiva (jin-ji′vah, jin′ji-vah), pl. *gingi′vae* [L. "gum of the mouth"] that part of the oral mucosa overlying the crowns of unerupted teeth and encircling the necks of those that have erupted, serving as the supporting structure for subadjacent tissues. It is formed by pale pink tissue immovably attached to the bone and the teeth, which joins the alveolar mucosa at the mucogingival junction. The loosely attached part, the free gingiva, joins the attached gingiva at the gingival groove. The wavy margin band is referred to as the *marginal gingiva*, and the interproximal area as the *interdent l gingiva*. The surface of the gingiva is covered by smooth epithelial tissue, having a stratum spinosum containing cells rich in keratohyalin, which degenerates and is responsible for keratinization, and a basal stratum resting on the basement membrane. Adjacent to the cell nuclei is sex chromatin, which is present only in females. Branches of the gingival artery and interdental alveolar arteries provide the blood supply and branches of the alveolar, buccal, and lingual nerves provide the innervation. Called also *gum*. See illustration. See also terms beginning ULA- and ULO-. **al-**

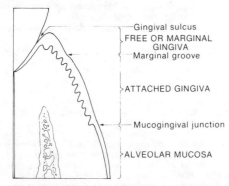

Anatomical landmarks of the gingiva. (From F. A. Carranza, Jr.: Glickman's Clinical Periodontology. 5th ed. Philadelphia, W. B. Saunders Co., 1979.)

veolar g., that part of the nonkeratinized oral mucosa which overlies the alveolar process. **areolar g.**, the oral mucous membrane lying beyond the keratinized mucosa over the alveolar process, being continuous with the buccal and labial mucosa. **attached g.**, that portion of the gingiva which is firm and resilient and is bound to the underlying cementum and the alveolar bone, thus being immovable. Its facial aspect extends to the relatively loose and movable alveolar mucosa, from which it is demarcated by the mucogingival line, its width varying from less than 1 mm to 9 mm. On the lingual aspect, it terminates at the junction with the mucous membrane lining the sublingual sulcus in the floor of the mouth. The palatal surface blends with the palatal mucosa. The attached gingiva is continuous with the marginal gingiva, and consists of stratified squamous epithelium and an underlying connective tissue stroma. The epithelium is differentiated into a cuboidal basal layer, a spinous layer comprising polygonal cells, a multiple-layered granular component consisting of flattened cells with prominent basophilic keratohyalin granules in the cytoplasm and

shrunken hyperchromic nucleus, and a cornified layer that may be keratinized or parakeratinized, or both. **buccal g.**, that portion of the gingiva located on the buccal aspect of the teeth. **cemental g.**, that portion of the attached gingiva attached to the cementum. **free g.**, the unattached portion of the gingiva forming the wall of the gingival crevice. Called also *unattached g.* and *free gum.* See also *marginal g.* **interdental g., interproximal g.**, that portion of the gingiva occupying the interproximal space beneath the area of tooth contact, the gingival embrasure; consisting of two papillae, one facial and one lingual, and a valley-like depression (col), which connects the papillae and conforms to the shape of the interproximal contact area. Called also *papillary g.* and *septal g.* **labial g.**, that portion of the gingiva found on the labial aspect of the teeth. **marginal g.**, the crest of the free gingiva surrounding the teeth in a collar-like fashion and separated from the adjacent attached gingiva by a shallow linear depression, the free gingival groove. It is usually slightly more than 1 mm wide, and forms the soft tissue v ll f the gingival sulcus. It consists of a central core of connective tissue covered by stratified squamous epithelium that is keratinized, parakeratinized, or both, on the crest and outer surface. The marginal gingiva contains prominent rete pegs and is continuous with the epithelium of the attached gingiva. The epithelium along the inner surface is devoid of rete pegs and is not keratinized, forming the lining of the gingival crevice. Called also *gingival margin.* **papillary g., septal g.**, interdental g. **unattached g.**, free g.

gingivae (jin-ji′ve, jin′ji-ve) [L., plural of *gingiva*] [NA] the gums: the mucous membrane, with the supporting fibrous tissue, which overlies the crowns of unerupted teeth and encircles the necks of those that have erupted. See also GINGIVA.

gingival (jin′ji-val, jun-ji′val) pertaining to the gingivae.

gingivalgia (jin″ji-val′je-ah) [*gingiva* + Gr. *algos* pain + *-ia*] pain in the gingivae. Called also *ulalgia.*

gingivectomy (jin″ji-vek′to-me) [*gingiva* + Gr. *ektomē* excision] surgical excision of the gingiva at the level of its attachment, thus, creating new marginal gingiva; used to eliminate gingival or periodontal pockets or to provide an approach for extensive surgical interventions, and to gain access necessary to remove calculus within the pocket. The procedure is indicated when the pockets are suprabony and there is an adequate zone of attached gingivae so that a sufficient amount will remain after eradication of the pocket. See also Kirkland instruments, under INSTRUMENT, and Kirkland KNIFE. **chemosurgical g.**, removal of diseased gingivae with a chemical agent, consisting of zinc oxide, zinc acetate, zinc stearate, rosin, paraformaldehyde, cottonseed oil, and eugenol. The mixture is applied on the tooth at the marginal gingiva and into the pocket. After 2 days the mixture is removed and the wound surface is cauterized with a mixture of silver nitrate, zinc chloride, or trichloroacetic acid to prevent excessive granulation. After the necrotic tissue has sloughed off, the acidity is neutralized with bicarbonate of soda.

gingivitis (jin-ji-vi′tis) [*gingiva* + *-itis*] inflammation of the gingivae. Gingivitis associated with bony changes is referred to as *periodontitis.* Called also *ulitis.* **acute g.**, gingival inflammation with a sudden onset and a relatively short duration, characterized by diffuse puffiness and softening, sloughing with grayish flakelike particles of debris adhering to the eroded surface, and vesicle formation. Pathological features include diffuse edema, fatty infiltration, xanthomatosis, necrosis with the formation of a pseudomembrane, and inter- and intracellular edema with degeneration of the nuclei and cytoplasm and rupture of the cell wall. **acute necrotizing g., acute necrotizing ulcerative g. (ANUG), acute ulcerative g., acute ulceromembranous g.**, a progressive painful infection marked by crateriform lesions of the interdental papillae that are covered by pseudomembranous slough and circumscribed by linear erythema. Fetid breath, increased salivation, and spontaneous gingival hemorrhage are additional features. It is usually observed in young adults and middle aged persons. Epidemics may occur in groups in close contact, such as military troops, hence the names *trench gums* and *trench mouth.* A spiral bacterium *Treponema vincentii* coexisting in symbiotic relationship with a fusiform bacillus (*Fusobacterium nucleatum*) is considered as a possible etiologic agent, but various other spirochetes, filamentous organisms, vibrios, cocci, and other bacteria have been isolated from infected patients. When lesions spread to the soft palate and oropharynx, the condition is known as *Vincent's angina.* Called also *fusospirillosis, fusospirillary marginal g., fusospirochetal g., necrotizing ulcerative g., phagedenic g., ulcerative g., Vincent's g., acute* *infectious gingivostomatitis, Plaut's ulcer, Plaut-Vincent stomatitis, putrid sore mouth, putrid stomatitis, Vincent's infection,* and *Vincent's stomatitis.* **allergic g.,** gingivitis due to allergic reaction to substances, such as pollen, food, or chemicals, characterized by acute inflammation with pronounced vascular response. **atrophic senile g.,** inflammation of the gingiva and the oral mucosa occurring in menopausal and postmenopausal patients. Principal features include a dry, burning sensation, associated with extreme sensitivity to temperature changes; abnormal taste sensation, variously described as "salty," "peppery," or "sour"; dryness and shiny appearance of the mucosa, whose color may vary from paleness to redness; and readily bleeding gums. Edentulous patients may experience difficulty with removable prostheses. Microscopically, the gingiva presents atrophy of the germinal and prickle cell layers of the epithelium and, in some instances, areas of ulceration. The condition is similar to chronic desquamative gingivitis; atrophic and diminished keratinization of the oral mucosa, due to altered estrogen metabolism, is considered as the etiologic factor of both conditions. Called also *chronic atrophic·senile g.* and *menopausal gingivostomatitis.* **bismuth g.,** bismuth STOMATITIS. **catarrhal g.,** a transitory form of gingivitis, sometimes associated with stomatitis, accompanied by erythema, swelling, and, occasionally, epithelial desquamation. It is believed to be caused by changes in the oral bacterial flora. See also catarrhal STOMATITIS. **chronic g.,** gingival inflammation with a protracted, usually fluctuating course. It is characterized by soggy puffiness that pits on pressure, softness and friability, ready fragmentation on exploration with a probe, and pinpoint surface areas of redness and desquamation. Principal pathologic features include inflammatory exudate infiltration, connective tissue and epithelium degeneration, edema, leukocyte infiltration, areas of rete peg elongation into the connective tissue, fibrosis, and epithelial proliferation. **chronic atrophic senile g.,** atrophic senile g. **combined g.,** chronic gingivitis associated with various dermatoses. **cotton-roll g.,** secondary infection of denuded areas of the gingivae caused by adherence of epithelium to cotton rolls placed in the mouth during dental procedures. **cyclic recurrent g.,** menstruation g. **desquamative g.,** inflammation of the gingivae characterized by a tendency of the surface epithelium to desquamate, associated with extreme sensitivity to citric acids and spicy foods, which is allayed by cool or tepid fluids. The gingivae present extensive bullae with a grayish epithelium that may be easily peeled off. Removal of the epithelium exposes a red and hypersensitive corium of connective tissue. Pathologically, a typical lesion presents thinning of epithelium, decreased keratinization of the epithelium surface, lytic processes of the epithelium, superficial erosion, hyperplasia surrounding zones of ulceration, and inflammatory reaction. **desquamative g., chronic,** a rare form of gingivitis occurring more often in females than in males. The mild form presents erythema of the gingivae, and usually affects females aged 17 to 23 years. The moderate form is manifested as patchy red and gray discoloration of the marginal and attached gingivae; a smooth, shiny surface; softness; slight pitting; peeling of the epithelium and exposure of bleeding underlying tissue on brushing; pain on inhalation of air; and smoothness and shiny appearance of the whole oral mucosa. This form occurs most often during the fourth decade of life. In the severe form, there are scattered areas of denudation and redness with grayish speckling, usually involving the labial surface, and the surface vessels may rupture and ooze clear watery fluid. A blast of air will cause elevation of the epithelium and bubble formation. This form is extremely painful and is associated with intolerance to coarse foods, condiments and temperature changes and with a constant dry, burning sensation. The condition is similar to atrophic senile gingivitis; atrophy and diminished keratinization of the oral mucosa due to altered estrogen metabolism is considered as the etiologic factor of both conditions. Called also *gingivosis.* **diffuse g.,** inflammation involving the marginal gingivae, attached gingivae, and interdental papillae. **Dilantin g.,** generalized hyperplasia, usually of the gingiva, but may rarely also involve other areas of the oral mucosa, resulting from overgrowth of the fibrous tissue following anticonvulsant therapy with Dilantin (phenytoin); it may begin from 2 weeks to 3 months after instituting drug therapy. Initially, it is manifested by painless enlargement of one or two interdental papillae, followed by stippling of the surface of the gingivae, eventually giving it a cauliflower-like, warty, or pebbled appearance. İn advanced stages, the gingivae become lobulated with clefts separating each enlarged gingiva, and the gingival tissue be-

comes dense, resilient, and insensitive. Edentulous regions usually remain normal. **Extragingival hyperplasia** may occur as a result of irritation by prosthetic appliances or other sources. Histologically, the tissue is made up of large bundles of collagen fibers interspersed with fibroblasts and fibrocytes. The covering stratified squamous epithelium is thick and has a thin keratinized layer. Called also *dilantin hyperplasia.* See also FIBROMATOSIS gingivae. **eruptive g.,** gingivitis occurring at the time of eruption of the teeth, particularly of the permanent teeth. Food impaction and accumulation of debris may be associated. **g. expulsi'va,** marginal PERIODONTITIS. **fusospirillary marginal g., fusospirochetal g.,** acute necrotizing g. **generalized g.,** inflammation of the gingivae of the entire mouth. **generalized diffuse g.,** inflammation of the entire gingiva and the alveolar mucosa, associated with obliteration of the demarcation between the tissues, bleeding, and exudates in the affected tissues. **g. gravida'rum,** pregnancy g. **hemorrhagic g.,** gingivitis associated with profuse bleeding, as in ascorbic acid deficiency. **herpetic g.,** that caused by herpesviral infection. **hormonal g.,** that associated with endocrine imbalance; see *atrophic senile g., chronic desquamative g.,* and *plasma cell g.* **hyperplastic g.,** that associated with proliferation of the gingival cells. See also gingival ENLARGEMENT and gingival HYPERPLASIA. **g. hypertroph'ica,** FIBROMATOSIS gingivae. **idiopathic g.,** that of unknown cause. **localized g.,** that confined to the gingivae of a single tooth or a group of teeth. **marginal g.,** inflammation of the marginal gingivae. **marginal g., generalized,** inflammation of the marginal gingivae in all the teeth, frequently extending to the interdental papillae. **marginal g., simple,** hyperemia of the gingivae with edema of the margins and gingival papillae, resulting from slight trauma or neglected dental hygiene. **marginal g., suppurative, g. margina'lis-suppurati'va,** that with formation of a purulent discharge. **menstruation g.,** that characterized by periodic recurrent hemorrhage with bright red and rose-colored proliferations of the interdental papillae, and persistent ulceration of the tongue and buccal mucosa that worsens just before the onset of menstruation, associated with desquamation of epithelial cells from the stratum granulosum and the surface. Called also *cyclic recurrent g.* See also MENOGINGIVITIS. **necrotizing ulcerative g. (NUG),** see acute necrotizing g. **nephritic g.,** uremic STOMATITIS. **nonspecific g.,** gingivitis, with or without ulceration, caused by local irritation, usually chemical, mechanical, or thermal. **papillary g.,** inflammation of the interdental papillae. **phagodenic g.,** acute necrotizing g. **plasma cell g.,** an association of cheilitis, glossitis, and gingivitis, believed to be caused by hypersensitivity associated with cyclic hormonal imbalance. The gingiva appears uniformly inflamed and deeply pink, but remains stippled, with edema of the free and attached gingiva. Histological studies show intense plasma cell infiltration in the lamina propria. Called also *atypical gingivostomatitis, cheilitis-glossitis-gingivitis syndrome, gingival plasmocytosis, gingivostomatitis syndrome,* and *idiopathic gingivostomatitis.* **pregnancy g.,** a discrete, semifirm, dusky red or purplish red mushroom-like mass with a smooth glistening surface with red pinpoint markings, which occurs on the marginal gingiva or on the interproximal space, being attached by a sessile or pedunculated base. It usually appears during the third month of pregnancy and is painless, unless there is ulceration on the surface, bleeds easily, and sometimes discharges pus. The lesion consists of a central mass of connective tissue with peripheral stratified squamous epithelium, the central mass consisting of diffusely arranged newly formed and engorged capillaries lined by cuboidal and endothelial cells. Edema and leukocytic infiltrations occur between the capillaries. Numerous rete pegs are present in the epithelium, and its surface is generally keratinized. The lesion is believed to be caused by tissue reaction to nonspecific infection precipitated by trauma and is clinically and histologically similar to pyogenic granuloma. Lesions that are clinically and histologically identical are also seen in nonpregnant women and in men. Called also *g. gravidarum, gingival angiogranuloma, gingival fibrohemangioma,* and *pregnancy tumor.* **pseudomembranous g.,** a transitory inflammation of the gingiva and oral mucosa, accompanied by erythema, swelling, and, occasionally, epithelial desquamation, which together with inflammatory products, forms a pseudomembrane overlying the affected area. **puberty g.,** that characterized by hyperemia and edema, seen during puberty. Endocrine changes occurring during puberty and drying of the mucosa because of mouth-breathing due to lymphoid hyperplasia of the tonsils and adenoids have been suggested as possible causes. **recurrent g.,** that characterized by the reappearance of inflammation after its apparent disappearance. **scorbutic g.,** that associated with vitamin C deficiency. **senile atrophic g.,** atrophic senile g. **streptococcal g.,** gingivitis of the marginal gingivae caused by streptococcal infection. **tuberculous g.,** tuberculous infection of the gingiva, characterized by diffuse, hyperemic, nodular or papillary proliferation of the gingival tissue. See also oral TUBERCULOSIS. **ulcerative g.,** acute necrotizing g. **uremic g.,** uremic STOMATITIS. **Vincent's g.,** acute necrotizing g.

gingivo- [L. *gingiva* gum] a combining form denoting relationship to the gingivae.

gingivobuccoaxial (jin″jĭ-vo-buk″ko-ak′se-al) pertaining to or formed by the gingival, buccal, and axial walls of a cavity preparation of a tooth.

gingivoglossitis (jin″jĭ-vo-glos-si′tis) [*gingivo-* + *glossitis*] inflammation of the gingivae and tongue.

gingivolabial (jin″jĭ-vo-la′be-al) [*gingivo-* + *labial*] pertaining to the gingivae and lips.

gingivolinguoaxial (jin″jĭ-vo-ling″gwo-ak′se-al) pertaining to or formed by the gingival, lingual, and axial walls of a cavity preparation of a tooth.

gingivoplasty (jin′jĭ-vo-plas″te) [*gingivo-* + Gr. *plassein* to form] surgical reshaping of the gingivae and papillae for correction of deformities (particularly enlargements) and to provide the gingivae with a normal and functional form, the incision creating an external bevel.

gingivosis (jin″jĭ-vo′sis) [*gingivo-* + *-osis*] 1. a chronic inflammation of the gingiva. 2. chronic desquamative GINGIVITIS.

gingivostomatitis (jin″jĭ-vo-sto″mah-ti′tis) inflammation involving both the gingivae and the oral mucosa. **acute herpetic g.,** primary herpetic g. **acute infectious g.,** acute necrotizing GINGIVITIS. **allergic g.,** plasma cell g. **atypical g.,** plasma cell GINGIVITIS. **bismuth g.,** bismuth STOMATITIS. **herpetic g.,** an infection of the oral mucosa, including the gingivae, by the herpes simplex virus, characterized by redness of the oral tissues, formation of multiple vesicles and painful ulcers, and fever. **herpetic g., acute, herpetic g., primary. herpetic g., primary,** a herpetic infection of the oral cavity in infants and children, usually under the age of 6 years. Early symptoms include fetor oris, dysphagia, painful lymphadenopathy, fever, dehydration, malaise, nausea, somnolence, convulsions, and excessive salivation followed by development of vesicles or erosions on the oral mucosa, usually on the gingiva and tongue. Typically, the lesion is about 2 to 4 mm in diameter, has well-defined borders with a red margin, and is covered by a yellowish pseudomembrane. Initially, it is characterized by discrete spherical gray vesicles, which may occur on the gingival, labial and buccal mucosae, soft palate, pharynx, sublingual mucosa, and tongue. After about 24 hours, the vesicles rupture and form painful small ulcers with a red, elevated halo-like margin and a depressed yellowish or grayish white central portion. Occasionally, disease may occur without overt vesiculation; diffuse erythematous shiny discoloration and edematous enlargement of the gingivae with a tendency toward bleeding being the principal symptoms. The infection usually subsides in about 7 to 14 days, without scar formation, and recurrences are very rare. Called also *acute herpetic g.* See also Popschill-Feyrter APHTHOID. **idiopathic g.,** plasma cell GINGIVITIS. **menopausal g.,** atrophic senile GINGIVITIS. **necrotizing ulcerative g.,** that caused by extension to the oral mucosa of necrotizing ulcerative gingivitis, characterized by ulceration, pseudomembrane, and odor, with lesions involving the palate or pharynx as well as the oral mucosa. Called also *fusospirochetal stomatitis, Plaut's angina,* and *pseudomembranous angina.* **plasma cell g., plasma cell g., idiopathic,** a condition characterized by cheilitis, glossitis, and erythematous gingivitis, occasionally associated with bleeding and diffuse dense plasma cell infiltrates. The etiology is unclear, but hypersensitivity, possibly to a microorganism or to some chewing gum constituent, is suspected. Called also *allergic g.* **white folded g.,** white sponge NEVUS.

ginglyform (jin′glĭ-form) ginglymoid.

ginglymoarthrodial (jin″glĭ-mo-ar-thro′de-al) partly ginglymoid and partly arthrodial.

ginglymoid (jin′glĭ-moid) [*ginglymus* + Gr. *eidos* form] resembling a ginglymus; ginglyform.

ginglymus (jin′glĭ-mus) [L.; Gr. *ginglymos* hinge] [NA] a joint that allows only backward and forward, but no side movement, as the hinge of a door. Called also *ginglymoid joint* and *hinge joint.*

girdle (ger′d'l) an encircling structure, or part; anything that encircles a body, cingulum. **shoulder g.,** the bony structure supporting the upper limbs.

gitalin (jit′ah-lin) an extract of *Digitalis purpurea,* containing gitoxin, gitaloxin, and digitoxin, occurring as a white to buff powder that is soluble in acetone, ethanol, chloroform, and ether and slightly in water. Used chiefly in the treatment of congestive heart failure.

gitoxin (jĭ-tok′sin) a cardiac glycoside, 3β-[(O - 2,6 - dideoxy-β-D-ribo-hexopyranosyl-(1→4)-O -2,6-dideoxy-β-D-ribo-hexopyranosyl-(1→4)-2,6-dideoxy-β-D-ribohexopyranosyl)oxy]-14,16β-dihydroxy-5β-card-20(22)-enolide, isolated from the leaves of *Digitalis purpurea.* It occurs as prism-like crystals that are soluble in a mixture of chloroform and ethanol or pyridine or in dilute ethanol, and is almost insoluble in chloroform, ethyl acetate, and acetone.

Gitterfasern (git′er-fas″ern) [Ger.] reticular fibers; see under FIBER.

Gl 1. glucinium; see BERYLLIUM. 2. glabella (2).

glabella (glah-bel′ah) [L. *glaber* smooth] 1. the area on the frontal bone between the two superciliary ridges and above the root of the nose. 2. in cephalometry, the most anterior point on the midsagittal plane, seen in lateral view above the supraorbital ridges. Abbreviated *Gl.* Called also *metopic point* and *point Gl.* See illustration at CEPHALOMETRY.

glabellad (glah-bel′ad) toward the glabella.

glabellum (glah-bel′um) glabella.

glabrous (gla′brus) [L. *glaber* smooth] smooth and bare.

glacial (gla′shal) [L. *glacialis*] pertaining to or resembling ice; vitreous; solid.

gland (gland) [L. *glans* acorn] a specialized organ of secretion. Called also *glandula.* See also terms beginning ADENO-. **accessory g.,** a detached mass of glandular tissue situated near or at some distance from a gland of similar structure. **acinar g., acinous g. acinotubular g.,** tubuloacinar g. **acinous g.,** one made up of one or more acini. Called also *acinar g.* and *alveolar g.* **admaxillary g.,** PAROTID G., ACCESSORY. **adrenal g.,** a flattened gland situated on the superior pole of each kidney, consisting of two physiologically distinct organs, the adrenal cortex, the outer layer, and the adrenal medulla, the inner part. It produces steroid hormones responsible for mineral metabolism, including maintenance of sodium, potassium, and chloride balance; carbohydrate, protein, and lipid metabolism; and tissue reactions, including hypersensitivity. Called also *suprarenal g.* and *glandula suprarenalis* [NA]. See also adrenal CORTEX and adrenal MEDULLA. **albuminous g., serous g. alveolar g.,** acinous g. **apocrine g.,** a coiled tubular exocrine gland that accumulates secretion in its cell apices and ruptures the surface membrane during the secretory activity. They are considered to be vestigial organs in man and include the apocrine sweat glands, ceruminous glands in the external auditory canal, ciliary glands, and in a highly specialized form, the mammary glands. **apocrine sweat g.,** a large sweat gland consisting of a secretory part, which is a coiled portion having numerous secretory cells encompassed by a mesh of myoepithelium which, in turn, is covered by a hyaline basement membrane; and an excretory duct, lined with two layers of epithelial cells and emptying into the hair follicle. They are located in the anogenital and axillary regions and around the nipples and in the ear canal; those in the auditory canal form cerumen (ear wax). Apocrine secretions are sterile but they are rapidly decomposed by bacterial action, resulting in odor. They serve no known useful purpose. Their secretion results from pain, fear, anger, or sexual stimulation; heat does not influence apocrine secretion. **arytenoid g's,** mucous glands in the posterior wall of the larynx. Called also *glandulae laryngeae posteriores.* **Avicenna's g.,** an encapsulated tumor. **Bauhin's g., Blandin's g.,** lingual g's, anterior. **Bowman's g's,** olfactory g's. **branched g.,** an exocrine gland in which the excretory unit is branched. **buccal g's,** minor serous or mucous glands situated in the submucosa of the cheek, continuing posteriorly from the labial glands. Those at the lower posterior corner of the cheek are called the *molar* or *retromolar glands.* Called also *cheek g's, genal g's, malar g's,* and *glandulae buccales* [NA]. **carotid g.,** carotid BODY. **ceruminous g's,** apocrine sweat glands of the external auditory canal that secrete the cerumen, a waxy secretion. Called also *glandulae ceruminosae* [NA]. **cheek g's.** buccal g's. **ciliary g's,** apocrine glands on the free margin of the eyelid near the eyelashes; modified sweat glands. Called also *glandulae ciliares conjunctivae* [NA] and *Moll's g's.* **compound g., conglomerate g.,** one composed of a number of small units whose excretory ducts combine to form ducts of a progressively higher order. **cutaneous g's,** the glands of the skin, including the sweat glands, sebaceous glands, and ceruminous glands. Called also *g's of skin* and *glandulae cutis* [NA]. **duct g.,** exocrine g. **ductless g.,** endocrine g. **Ebner's g's,** von Ebner's g's. **eccrine sweat g.,** small sweat glands, each consisting of a coiled tubule located in the corium, the secretory part of the gland, and an excretory duct emptying onto the skin surface.

The secretory part is a simple coiled tubule made up of a single truncated pyramidal cell, surrounded by a poorly developed mesh of myoepithelium. They are distributed over the entire surface of the body, with the forehead and soles and palms being most richly supplied. Their chief function is to provide evaporative cooling of the body. The central control of eccrine sweating is in the hypothalamus; an increase in the skin or blood temperature produces sweating. **endocrine g.,** any ductless gland which secretes specific substances (hormones) directly into the blood stream, including the adrenal, pituitary, thyroid, parathyroid, and pineal glands, and the islands of Langerhans of the pancreas, gonads, and paraganglia. Called also *ductless g.* and [pl.] *glandulae sine ductibus* [NA]. See also endocrine SYSTEM. **excretory g.,** any gland that excretes waste products from the system. **exocrine g., g. of external secretion,** any gland that discharges its secretions through ducts opening on external or internal surfaces of the body. Exocrine glands include the salivary, sweat, prostatic, intestinal, mammary, and lacrimal glands, and the liver and the pancreas. They are classified according to the mode of their secretory activity and the degree of damage occurring during the secretion: the *halocrine glands* expel secretions together with cell remnants; the *merocrine glands* release secretions without incurring damage to their cells; and the *apocrine glands* accumulate secretions in the cell apices and rupture the surface membrane during secretion. They may be further classified according to the shape of their ducts: the *simple glands* have ducts without any branches; the *branched glands* have ramified ducts; and the *compound glands* have branching units which combine with excretory ducts of progressively higher orders. Or, they may be classified according to their morphological character: the *acinous glands* are composed of acini and the *tubular glands* are made up of tubules. Called also *duct g.* **extraparotid lymph g's,** auricular lymph nodes, anterior; see under NODE. **genal g's,** buccal g's. **gingival g's,** glandlike infoldings of epithelium at the junction of gingiva and tooth. **Gley's g's,** thyroid g's, accessory. **globate g.,** lymph NODE. **glossopalatine g's,** mucous glands at the posterior end of the smaller sublingual glands, found chiefly in the area of the isthmus and the glossopalatine folds, and extending into the soft palate to communicate with the palatine glands, or into the lingual aspect of the mandibular retromolar region. **gustatory g's,** von Ebner's g's. **guttural g.,** one of the mucous glands of the pharynx. **haversian g's,** synovial villi; see under VILLUS. **heterocrine g's,** seromucous g's. **holocrine g.,** an exocrine gland which forms its secretions through disintegration of the whole glandular cell, such as a sebaceous gland. **incisive g.,** one of a small group of salivary glands situated symmetrically on the floor of the mouth near the insertion of the frenum of the tongue behind the lower incisors. Called also *glandula incisiva.* **intercarotid g.,** carotid BODY. **intramuscular g's of tongue,** lingual g's, anterior. **labial g's,** numerous small mucous or mixed glands in the lamina propria of the upper and lower lips. The spherical bodies of individual glands appear as protuberances but toward the midline of the lip they tend to concentrate and present a glandular mass. They have poorly defined capsule acini that are composed of both serous and mucous cells, with occasional seromucous cells being present, and striated and intercalated ducts. Called also *glandulae labiales oris* [NA]. **lacrimal g.,** one that lies at the upper outer angle of the orbit and secretes the tears. Called also *glandula lacrimalis* [NA]. **laryngeal g's,** mucous glands in the mucosa of the larynx. Called also *glandulae laryngeae* [NA]. **laryngeal g's, anterior,** mucous glands in the anterior part of the larynx. Called also *glandulae laryngeae anteriores.* **laryngeal g's, middle,** mucous glands located in the aryepiglottic fold. Called also *glandulae laryngeae mediae.* **laryngeal g's, posterior,** arytenoid g's. **lingual g's,** the salivary glands of the tongue. Called also *glandulae linguales* [NA]. **lingual g's, anterior,** seromucous salivary glands clustered under a thin mucous membrane close to the apex and the midline of the tongue; they drain through several ducts on the inferior surface of the tongue. Called also *Bauhin's g's, Blandin's g's, intramuscular g's of tongue, Nuck's g's, Nuhn's g's,* and *glandulae linguales anteriores* [NA]. **lingual g's, dorsal,** lingual g's, posterior. **lingual g's, posterior,** salivary glands situated on the dorsal part of the tongue, consisting of the serous group, or von Ebner's glands, which discharge most of their secretions into the bottom of the circular trough of the vallate papillae, and the mucous group, which discharge into the lingual crypts. Called also *dorsal lingual g's.* **lymph g.,** lymph NODE. **lymph g's, extraparotid,** auricular lymph nodes, anterior; see under NODE. **lymph g's,**

subparotid, subparotid lymph nodes; see under NODE. **malar g's,** buccal g's. **mandibular g.,** submandibular g. **merocrine g.,** an exocrine gland which releases secretions without incurring damage to its cells, such as a sweat gland. **molar g's,** buccal glands on the external aspect of the buccinator muscle whose ducts pierce it to open on the internal aspect of the cheek. Called also *retromolar g's* and *glandulae molares* [NA]. **Moll's g's,** ciliary g's. **mucilaginous g's,** synovial villi; see under VILLUS. **muciparous g.,** mucous g. **mucous g.,** a salivary gland that secretes a viscous semigelatinous secretion. Called also *muciparous g.* and *glandula mucosa* [NA]. **multicellular g.,** one made up of many cells, as opposed to a unicellular gland. **nasal g's,** numerous large mucous and serous glands in the respiratory part of the nasal cavity. Called also *glandulae nasales* [NA]. **g. of neck,** pharyngeal TONSIL. **Nuck's g's, Nuhn's g's,** lingual g's, anterior. **olfactory g's,** numerous branched tubuloacinar glands in the olfactory mucosa of the nasal cavity, which produce serous secretions. Called also *Bowman's g's* and *glandulae olfactoriae* [NA]. **palatine g's,** glands forming a composite group of several hundred individual glandular masses in the connective tissue of the lamina propria of the posterolateral regions of the hard palate and distributed throughout the submucosa of the soft palate and the uvula. The glands lack well defined capsules or septa and are separated from each other by bundles of collagen fibers. Their ducts tend to be long and narrow, wandering through the lamina propria before discharging on the epithelial surface, being lined by simple columnar or pseudostratified columnar cells. Their secretory terminals are both tubular and alveolar in form and are composed entirely of mucous cells. Called also *glandulae palatinae* [NA] and *staphyline g's.* **parathyroid g's,** four small glands disposed as two pairs near the lateral lobes of the thyroid gland, whose product, the parathyroid hormone, is concerned with calcium and phosphate metabolism. Called also *glandulae parathyroideae* [NA]. See also HYPERPARATHYROIDISM and HYPOPARATHYROIDISM. **parotid g.,** the largest of the salivary glands, situated symmetrically between the ear and the ascending ramus of the mandible, in the retromandibular fossa. It is composed of two partly overlapping parts: the larger, a somewhat flattened and quadrilateral part, is located between the ramus of the mandible and the mastoid process; the other, an irregular wedge-shaped part, extends toward the pharyngeal wall. Emanating from the anterior border are the branches of the parotid duct. The arteries of the parotid gland derive from the external carotid; the veins empty into the external jugular; the lymphatic vessels drain into deep cervical nodes; and the nerves derive from the sympathetic plexus on the external carotid artery and from the auriculotemporal nerve. It is classified as a serous gland, but its secretions are both serous and mucous. Called also *external salivary g.* and *glandula parotis* [NA]. **parotid g., accessory,** a more or less detached portion of the parotid gland that is frequently present. Called also *admaxillary g., glandula parotis accessoria* [NA], and *socia parotidis.* **pharyngeal g's,** mucous glands beneath the mucous membrane of the pharynx. Called also *glandulae pharyngeae* [NA]. **pineal g.,** a small, flattened, cone-shaped body, a part of the epithalamus, resting deep in the brain in a groove between the superior quadrigeminate bodies. It contains large amounts of histamine, acetylcholine, norepinephrine, melatonin, serotonin, and other biochemically-active substances but its physiological function in man is not understood. Called also *corpus pinale* [NA], *epiphysis cerebri,* and *pineal body.* **pituitary g.,** a small organ located in the sella turcica, a bony cavity in the sphenoid bone at the base of the skull. Its hormones regulate the activity of most of the endocrine system and growth of the body. Functionally and anatomically, it is composed of two main parts: an anterior lobe (see *pituitary g., anterior*) and a posterior lobe (see *pituitary g., posterior*). The anterior lobe includes the pars infundibularis (pars tuberalis), pars distalis, and pars intermedius (assigned in some systems of nomenclature to the posterior lobe). The posterior lobe includes the pituitary stalk and the pars nervosa. Called also *glandula pituitaria* [NA alternative], *hypophysis* [NA], and *hypophysis cerebri.* See also HYPERPITUITARISM and HYPOPITUITARISM. **pituitary g., anterior,** the anterior lobe of the pituitary gland, representing about 75 percent of the gland, composed of acidophils, basophils, amphophils, and chromophobes, which are arranged around vascular channels into which they secrete hormones. Hormones of the anterior lobe include adrenocorticotropic hormone, probably produced by the basophils, which influences the activity of the zonae fasciculata and reticularis of the adrenal cortex and the secretion of glucocorticoids; gonadotropic hormones, which influence the activity of the ovaries and testes; thyrotropin, probably secreted by the amphophils, which influences function of the thyroid gland; and somatotropin, probably produced by the eosinophils, which is the only anterior pituitary hormone that does not act on an end organ, but influences growth. Called also *adenohypophysis* [NA alternative], *anterior lobe of hypophysis, anterior lobe of pituitary gland, lobus anterior hypophyseos* [NA], and *prehypophysis*. See also *pituitary g.* **pituitary g., posterior,** the posterior lobe of the pituitary gland, connected to the hypothalamus, made up of tissue rich in neural material, and producing the hormones oxytocin and vasopressin. Called also *lobus posterior hypophyseos* [NA], *neurohypophysis* [NA alternative], and *posthypophysis*. See also *pituitary g.* **Poirier's g.,** one of the lymph nodes on the conoid ligament at the upper border of the isthmus of the thyroid gland. **prehyoid g's,** accessory thyroid glands found in the prehyoid area. See *thyroid g's, accessory.* **prostatic g.,** prostate. **retromolar g's,** molar g's. **Rivinus' g.,** sublingual g. **Rosenmüller's g.,** palpebral part of lacrimal gland; see under PART. **saccular g.,** one consisting of a sac or sacs, lined with glandular epithelium. **salivary g's,** the exocrine glands of the oral cavity that secrete saliva, which are made up of secretory units (parenchyma) and the framework (stroma). Larger glands are partitioned into lobules by septa or trabeculae which also house the blood vessels, lymphatics, and nerves; each lobule represents a ramification of a single duct, branching into numerous alveoli. Larger glands also contain the pacinian corpuscles, encapsulated nerve endings responsible for pressure reception. Major salivary glands include the parotid, submandibular, and sublingual glands; minor glands include the labial, buccal, palatine, tonsillar, molar, and lingual glands. Functionally, they are divided into serous, mucous, and mixed; the serous secretion decreasing from the anterior oral to the posterior pharyngeal region. See illustration and table. See also SALIVA, and terms beginning PTYALO- and SIALO-. **salivary g., external,** parotid g. **salivary g's, extrinsic,** salivary g's, major. **salivary g., internal,** 1. sublingual g. 2. submandibular g. **salivary g's, intrinsic,** salivary g's, minor. **salivary g's, major,** a group of larger salivary glands, including the parotid, submandibular, and sublingual glands. Called also *extrinsic salivary g's.* **salivary g's, minor,** a group of smaller salivary glands, including the labial, buccal, palatine, tonsillar, molar, and lingual glands. Called also *intrinsic salivary g's.* **salivary g., mixed,** seromu-

cous g. **Sandström's g's,** thyroid g's, accessory. **sebaceous g's,** numerous holocrine glands that secrete an oily substance and furnish a thin lipoidal film over the stratum corneum of the skin and hair, thus retarding evaporation. They are located in the corium of the skin between the smooth muscle (erector pili) and the hair follicle and open into the terminal portion of the hair follicle. Ectopic sebaceous glands may be present on the oral and labial mucosa. Called also *glandulae sebaceae* [NA]. **sentinel g.,** an enlarged lymph node, considered to be pathognomonic of some pathological condition elsewhere. **seromucous g.,** one that produces both serous and mucous secretions, such as the anterior lingual, buccal, labial, and submandibular glands. Called also *heterocrine g., mixed salivary g.,* and *glandula seromucosa* [NA]. **serous g.,** one that secretes a thin, nonviscous, watery fluid, which may or may not contain digestive ferments, including the parotid gland and Ebner's glands. Called also *albuminous g.* and *glandula serosa* [NA]. **Serres' g.,** a pearly mass of epithelial cells near the surface of the gum of an infant. Called also *epithelial pearls.* **simple g.,** an exocrine gland with a nonbranching excretory duct. **g's of skin,** cutaneous g's. **Stahr's g.,** Stahr's NODE. **staphyline g's,** palatine g's. **sublingual g.,** the smallest of the three principal paired salivary glands, classified as being essentially a mucous gland, which is a flattened, elongated structure situated in the floor of the mouth, on each side of the lingual frenum, its outer edge touching the sublingual depression on the inner surface of the mandible. Its superior surface is covered by mucous membrane and projects an elevation, the salivary eminence. It empties through five to fifteen ducts, some opening directly into the oral cavity, others joining the mandibular duct, and still others forming the duct of Bartholin. Called also *internal salivary g., Rivinus' s.,* and *glandula sublingualis* [NA]. **submandibular g., submaxillary g.,** a major salivary gland, the size of a walnut, irregularly shaped and situated symmetrically partly above and partly below the posterior half of the base of the mandible in the submandibular triangle. Its forward part borders on the an-

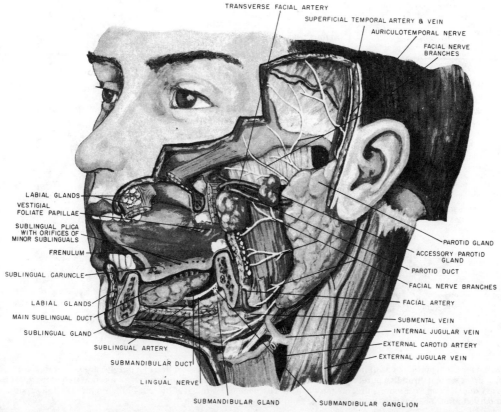

Lateral view of head, dissected to show relationship of paraoral structures. Vascular and nerve supply of the salivary glands and the muscles of mastication are indicated. (From D. V. Provenza: Oral Histology: Inheritance and Development. Philadelphia, Lippincott, 1964; after Frank H. Netter, M.D., The Ciba Collection of Medical Illustrations.)

CLASSIFICATION OF SALIVARY GLANDS

Location	Name	Type of Secretion	Size
Lip	Superior labial	Mixed (predominantly mucous)	Minor
	Inferior labial	Mixed (predominantly mucous)	Minor
Cheek	Buccal glands	Mixed (predominantly mucous)	Minor
	Parotid	Pure serous	Major
Palate			
Hard	Posterolateral palatines	Pure mucous	Minor
Soft	Palatine	Pure mucous	Minor
Tongue			
Corpus	Blandin-Nuhn (anterior lingual)	Mixed (predominantly mucous)	Minor
Root	Von Ebner (posterior lingual)	Pure serous	Minor
	Tonsil, Lingual (posterior lingual)	Pure mucous	Minor
Sublingual Sulcus (floor of mouth)			
	Submandibular	Mixed (predominantly serous)	Major
	Sublingual (extrinsic)	Mixed (predominantly mucous)	Major
	Sublinguals (intrinsic)	Mixed (predominantly mucous)	Minor
	Glossopalatine	Pure mucous	Minor

(From D. V. Provenza: Oral Histology: Inheritance and Development. Philadelphia, Lippincott, 1964.)

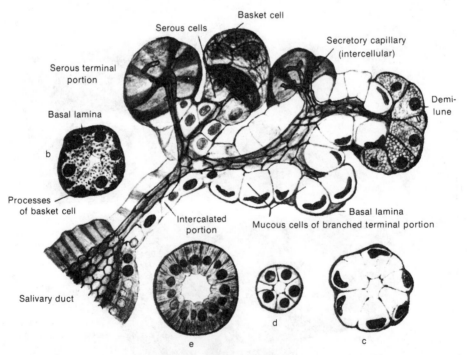

Reconstruction of a terminal portion of a submandibular gland with its duct. b, Cross section of a purely serous terminal portion, showing basal lamellae; c, cross section through a purely mucous terminal portion; d, cross section through an intercalated portion; e, cross section through a salivary duct. (From W. Bloom and D. W. Fawcett: A Textbook of Histology. 10th ed. Philadelphia, W. B. Saunders Co., 1975; redrawn and modified after a reconstruction by Vierling, from Braus.)

terior belly of the digastric muscle and its back rests against the stylomandibular ligament. Its secretions are discharged through the submandibular duct, whose orifice lies at the side of the lingual frenum. The submandibular gland is considered as being essentially a serous gland, but its secretions also contain mucus. See illustration. Called also *internal salivary g., mandibular g., glandula submandibularis* [NA], and *glandula submaxillaris.* **subparotid lymph g's,** subparotid lymph nodes; see under NODE. **sudoriferous g's,** sweat g's. **suprarenal g.,** adrenal g. **Suzanne's g.,** a mucous gland of the mouth, beneath the alveololingual groove. **sweat g's,** numerous exocrine merocrine glands that secrete sweat. Called also *sudoriferous g's* and *glandulae sudoriferae* [NA]. See also *apocrine sweat g.* and *eccrine sweat g.* **synovial g's,** synovial villi; see VILLUS. **thyroid g.,** the largest of the endocrine glands, consisting of two lobes situated just below the thyroid cartilage, in front and on either side of the trachea; the lobes are connected by a narrow band of tissue, the isthmus, and both the lobe and the isthmus are composed of numerous follicles filled with colloid. It serves as a storehouse of iodine and maintains control over growth and metabolism through its hormones thyroxine and triiodothyronine. The production and secretion of these hormones is regulated by thyrotropin, a hormone of the anterior pituitary gland; their synthesis is inhibited by the administration of iodine, thiocyanate, and various antithyroid agents (see thyroid ANTAGONISTS). Called also *glandula thyroidea* [NA] and *thyroid.* See HYPERTHYROIDISM, HYPOTHYROIDISM, and THYROID (1). **thyroid g's, accessory,** small exclaves of the thyroid gland, which may be found any place along the course of the thyroglossal duct, as well as in the thorax. Called also *Gley's g's, prehyoid g's, Sandstrom's g's,* and *glandulae thyroideae accessoriae* [NA]. **g. of tongue,** lingual g. **g. of tongue, intramuscular,** lingual g., anterior. **tubular g.,** an exocrine gland made up of or containing a tubule or tubules. **tubuloacinar g.,** one that is both tubular and acinous. Called also *acinotubular g.* **unicellular g.,** a cell which performs a secretory function, as a goblet cell. **von Ebner's (Ebner's) g's,** the serous group of the posterior lingual glands, which discharge most of their secretions into the troughs surrounding the vallate papillae. Their secretions flush debris from the troughs and dissolve substances to be tasted. Called also *gustatory g's.* **Weber's g.,** one of the tubular mucous glands of the tongue.

glanders (glan'derz) [L. *malleus*] an infectious bacterial disease of horses, mules, and donkeys caused by *Pseudomonas mallei,* which may be transmitted to man. It may be characterized by cutaneous cellulitis, vesiculation, and ulceration at the site of inoculation, associated with lymphangitis and nodular abscesses, or by nasal cellulitis that may lead to perforation of the septum and palatal and pharyngeal ulcers. Malaise, anorexia, and arthralgia are the early symptoms, followed by formation of a primary lesion or nodule which usually breaks down and forms an ulcer with an irregular bluish red border, often destroying the nasal septum and involving the oral cavity. Septicemia and papulopustular exanthem usually follow. Called also *malleus.*

glandilemma (glan''dǐ-lem'ah) [*gland* + Gr. *lemma* sheath] the capsule or outer envelope of a gland.

glandula (glan'du-lah), pl. *glan'dulae* [L.]. [NA] a gland: an aggregation of cells, specialized to secrete or excrete materials not related to their ordinary metabolic needs. **glan'dulae bucca'les** [NA], buccal glands; see under GLAND. **g. cerumino'sae** [NA], ceruminous glands; see under GLAND. **glan'dulae cilia'res conjuncti'vae** [NA], ciliary glands; see under GLAND. **glan'dulae cu'tis** [NA], cutaneous glands; see under GLAND. **g. incisi'va,** incisive GLAND. **g. intercarot'ica,** carotid BODY. **glan'dulae labia'les o'ris** [NA], labial glands; see under GLAND. **g. lacrima'lis** [NA], lacrimal GLAND. **g. lacrima'lis**

infe'rior, palpebral part of lacrimal gland; see under PART. **g. lacrima'lis supe'rior,** orbital part of lacrimal gland; see under PART. **glan'dulae laryn'geae** [NA], laryngeal glands; see under GLAND. **glan'dulae laryn'geae ante'riores,** laryngeal glands, anterior; see under GLAND. **glan'dulae laryn'geae me'diae,** laryngeal glands, middle; see under GLAND. **g. laryn'geae poste'riores,** arytenoid glands; see under GLAND. **glan'dulae lingua'les** [NA], lingual glands, see under GLAND. **glan'dulae lingua'les anterio'res** [NA], lingual glands, anterior; see under GLAND. **glan'dulae mola'res** [NA], molar glands; see under GLAND. **g. muco'sa** [NA], mucous GLAND. **glan'dulae nasa'les** [NA], nasal glands; see under GLAND. **glan'dulae olfacto'riae** [NA], olfactory glands; see under GLAND. **glan'dulae palati'nae** [NA], palatine glands; see under GLAND. **glan'dulae parathyroi'deae** [NA], parathyroid glands; see under GLAND. **g. paro'tis** [NA], parotid GLAND. **g. paro'tis accesso'ria** [NA], parotid gland, accessory; see under GLAND. **glan'dulae pharyn'geae** [NA], pharyngeal glands; see under GLAND. **g. pituita'ria** [NA alternative], pituitary GLAND. **g. seba'ceae** [NA], sebaceous glands; see under GLAND. **g. seromuco'sa** [NA], seromucous GLAND. **g. sero'sa** [NA], serous GLAND. **glan'dulae si'ne duc'tibus** (*ductless glands*) [NA], endocrine glands; see under GLAND. **g. sublingua'lis** [NA], sublingual GLAND. **g. submandibula'ris** [NA], submandibular GLAND. **g. submaxilla'ris,** submandibular GLAND. **glan'dulae sudorif'erae** [NA], sweat glands; see under GLAND. **g. suprarena'lis** [NA], adrenal GLAND. **g. thyroi'dea** [NA], thyroid GLAND. **glan'dulae thyroi'deae accesso'riae** [NA], thyroid glands, accessory; see under GLAND.

glandulae (glan'du-le) [L.] plural of *glandula.*

glandular (glan'du-lar) pertaining to a gland.

glandule (glan'dūl) [L. *glandula*] a small gland.

glans (glanz) [L. "acorn"] a general anatomical term for any small rounded mass, or glandlike body.

Glanzmann's syndrome (thrombasthenia) [Edouard *Glanzmann,* 1887–1959] see under SYNDROME.

Glaser (Glaserius), Johann Heinrich [1629–1675] a Swiss anatomist. See GLASERIAN.

glaserian (glah-se're-an) named after or described by Johann Heinrich *Glaser,* as glaserian fissure (see petrotympanic FISSURE).

Glaserius see GLASER.

glass (glas) [L. *vitrum*] 1. a hard but brittle and usually transparent ceramic material obtained by fusing a uniformly dispersed mixture of amorphous silica (sand), soda ash, and lime, sometimes combined with oxides of calcium, lead, lithium, cerium, and other metallic elements, which is heated to about 2000°F and then cooled gradually. Technically, it is an undercooled liquid of high viscosity. Some types of glass are used as a constituent of dental porcelain. See table. See also VETRIFICATION. 2. a container, usually cylindrical in shape, made of glass. **g. former,** glass FORMER. **g. ionomer cement,** see under CEMENT. **leaded g.,** a lead-impregnated glass mounted into booth windows and shields, which is used to protect the operator from radiation during the operation of the x-ray machine. **Pyrex g.,** trademark for glass that has a high degree of resistance to heat and chemical corrosion. Used in cooking utensils, laboratory and pharmaceutical glassware, and various other products. Also used as a component of some dental porcelains. **g. transition temperature,** see under TEMPERATURE. **Vycor G.,** trademark for glass produced in such a manner that all ingredients other than silica are removed. It is characterized by a high softening point when fired and a very low expansion coefficient.

TYPICAL GLASSES USED IN DENTAL PORCELAIN

GLASS	SiO_2 %	Al_2O_3 %	K_2O %	Na_2O %	CaO %	B_2O_3 %	ZnO %	ZrO_2 %
I	68.7	15.3	11.0	5.0				
II	58.4	15.1	6.1	15.6			0.8	4.0
III	41.2	36.2	1.0	3.6	7.1	10.9		
IV	65.2	15.1	7.4	4.2		8.1		

(From R. W. Phillips: Skinner's Science of Dental Materials. 7th ed. Philadelphia, W. B. Saunders Co., 1973; courtesy of R. W. Batchelor. Harrison and Son (Hanley) Ltd., England.)

Used in pharmaceutical and laboratory glassware and other products. Also used as a component of some dental porcelains.

Glastone trademark for a Class II (Type IV) *dental stone* (see under STONE).

Glauber's salt [Johann Rudolph *Glauber,* Dutch chemist, 1603–1668] SODIUM sulfate decahydrate.

glaze (glāz) 1. to cover with a glossy, smooth surface or coating. 2. a ceramic veneer added to a dental porcelain restoration after it has been fired, to give a completely nonporous, glossy or semiglossy surface. 3. the critical stage in the final firing of dental porcelain when complete fusion takes place, with the formation of a thin, vitreous, glossy surface. **high g.,** in firing of dental porcelain, a glaze in which the glass has very freely flowed out onto the surface, almost to the point of giving it a rounded form. A high glaze is close to coalescence and is undesirable, except when the crown or veneer will support a clasp arm. **low g.,** in firing of dental porcelain, an extension of maturity, or just beyond maturity, to the degree that glass has flowed out onto the surface, presenting a moderately glossy appearance. **medium g.,** in firing of dental porcelain, a glaze in which glass has freely flowed out into the surface, giving it a very glossy appearance.

glenoid (gle′noid) [Gr. *glēnē* socket + *eidos* form] resembling a pit or socket.

Gley's gland [Eugène Emile *Gley,* French physiologist, 1857–1930] thyroid gland, accessory; see under GLAND.

glia (gli′ah) [Gr. "glue"] 1. neuroglia. 2. a word termination denoting a gluelike structure or tissue.

Glickman's periodontal probe [Irving *Glickman,* American periodontologist, 1914–1972] see under PROBE.

glide (glīd) a smooth continuous movement without resistance. **acentric g.,** a condition in centric premature contact which makes the mandible glide into habitual occlusion on complete closure. **mandibular g.,** the side-to-side protrusive and intermediate movement of the mandible occurring when the teeth or other occluding surfaces are in contact. **occlusal g.,** the movement induced by deflective tooth contact that diverts the mandible from a normal path of closure to a centric relation.

glio- [Gr. *glia* glue] a combining form denoting relationship to a gluey substance or specifically to the neuroglia.

Glisson's disease [Francis *Glisson,* English physician and anatomist, 1597–1677] rickets.

Gln glutamine.

globi (glo′bi) [L.] plural of *globus.*

globin (glo′bin) an animal protein (molecular weight 61,992) insoluble in water but soluble in acids and alkali, which is the protein component of hemoglobin. It is composed of two amino acid chains, α and β; the first consists of 141 amino acids, the second of 146.

globodontia (glob′o-don″she-ah) an autosomal dominant disorder characterized by globe-shaped canine and posterior teeth; it may be associated with sensorineural deafness, forming otodental dysplasia.

globose (glo′bōs) [L. *globus* a ball] globe-shaped, spherical.

globular (glob′u-lar) 1. like a globe or globule. 2. pertaining to red blood cells.

globule (glob′ūl) [L. *globulus* a globule] 1. a small spherical mass; a little globe or pellet, as of medicine. 2. a lymph corpuscle; a fat corpuscle in milk. **dentin g's,** small spherical bodies in the peripheral dentin, created by beginning calcification of the matrix about discrete foci.

globulin (glob′u-lin) [L. *globulus* globule] a class of simple globular proteins with a molecular weight of about 150,000, which are characterized by being precipitated easily by neutral salts and being insoluble in ammonium sulfate solutions. Globulins are subdivided into *euglobulins,* which are insoluble in water, and *pseudoglobulins,* which are soluble. They are easily coagulated by heat and all are insoluble in alcoholic solutions. See also IMMUNOGLOBULIN. **g. A,** IMMUNOGLOBULIN A (IgA). **Ac-g.,** FACTOR V. **accelerator g.,** FACTOR V. **acute phase g.,** C-reactive PROTEIN. **α-g.,** the fastest moving globulin components found in the blood plasma and serum, further separated into fractions α_1 and α_2 on the basis of electrophoretic mobility. See IMMUNOGLOBULIN. **α₁-g.,** α_1-FETOPROTEIN. **antihemophilic g.,** FACTOR VIII. **g. D,** IMMUNOGLOBULIN D (IgD). **g. E,** IMMUNOGLOBULIN E (IgE). **fast g.,** 1. a fraction of a γ-globulin (immunoglobulin) believed to exist in the blood of cancer patients and pregnant women at delivery. Called also $\gamma_f g, g.\ T,$ and $T\ g.$ 2. a γ-globulin component with an electrophoretic mobility faster than most

IgG's and slower than most IgA's. **g. G,** IMMUNOGLOBULIN G (IgG). **gamma g.,** γ-g., immunoglobulin. γ_1-g., fast g. (1). γA g., *see* IMMUNOGLOBULIN A (IgA). γ_1A g., an allotypic subclass of immunoglobulin A (IgA). γ_2A g., an allotypic subclass of immunoglobulin A (IgA). γD g., IMMUNOGLOBULIN D (IgD). γ_1D g., an allotypic subclass of immunoglobulin D (IgD). γ_2D g., an allotypic subclass of immunoglobulin D (IgD). γE g., IMMUNOGLOBULIN E (IgE). γ_1E g., a subclass of immunoglobulin E (IgE). γG g., IMMUNOGLOBULIN G (IgG). γ_1G, a subclass of immunoglobulin G (IgG). γ_2G, a subclass of immunoglobulin G (IgG). **IgA g.,** IMMUNOGLOBULIN A. **iron-binding β-g.,** transferrin. γLg., an antibody having the electrophoretic mobility of γ-globulins, a molecular weight ranging from 10,000 to 40,000, and a sedimentation constant from 1.6 to 5.7S. γL globulins were originally discovered in the urine and are believed to represent the normal counterparts of Bence Jones proteins. Called also *microglobulin.* γM g., IMMUNOGLOBULIN M (IgM). γ_1M g., a subclass of immunoglobulin M (IgM). **19S γ-g.,** IMMUNOGLOBULIN M (IgM). **immune g.,** immunoglobulin. **g. M,** IMMUNOGLOBULIN M (IgM). **metal binding g.,** transferrin. **plasma g.,** a globulin found in blood plasma, which together with albumin represents two major classes of plasma proteins. Globulin is precipitated from plasma with 50 percent ammonium sulfate, while 100 percent ammonium sulfate is used for albumin. In an electrical field globulin may be separated into three fractions: α-globulin, β-globulin, and γ-globulin. **secretory γA g.,** see IMMUNOGLOBULIN A (IgA). **serum Ac-g.,** FACTOR VI. **T g., g. T,** fast g. (1).

globulinemia (glob″u-lin-e′me-ah) [*globulin* + Gr. *haima* blood + *-ia*] the presence of globulins in the blood.

globulinuria (glob″u-lin-u′re-ah) [*globulin* + Gr. *ouron* urine + *-ia*] the presence of globulin in the urine.

globus (glo′bus) pl. *glo′bi* [L.] a sphere or ball; a general anatomical term denoting a spherical structure. **g. hyster′icus,** a morbid sensation of a lump or ball in the throat, sometimes seen in hysteria; spheresthesia. **g. pal′lidus** [NA], the smaller and more medial part of the lentiform nucleus in the basal ganglia of the brain. It is believed to serve as the motor center of the extrapyramidal system, being inhibited by the corpus striatum. The globus pallidus connects to the muscles of mastication through the motor nucleus of the trigeminal nerve.

glomera (glom′er-ah) [L] plural of *glomus.*

glomeruli (glo-mer′u-li) [L.] plural of *glomerulus.*

glomerulitis (glo-mer″u-li′tis) inflammation of the glomeruli of the kidney.

glomerulonephritis (glo-mer″u-lo-ne-fri′tis) nephritis characterized by inflammation of the capillary loops of the glomeruli of the kidney.

glomerulus (glom-mer′u-lus), pl. *glomer′uli* [L., dim. of *glomus* ball] a tuft or cluster, used in anatomical nomenclature as a general term to designate such a structure, as one composed of blood vessels or nerve fibers. **nonencapsulated nerve g.,** a nerve ending in the connective tissue of various organs in which the terminal branches of the nerve form spherical or elongated structures resembling glomeruli. **olfactory g.,** one of the small globular masses of dense neuropil in the olfactory bulb containing the first synapse in the olfactory pathway.

glomoid (glo′moid) resembling a glomus.

glomus (glo′mus), pl. *glom′era* [L. "a ball"] a small body composed primarily of fine arteries connecting directly with veins, and possessing a rich nerve supply. **glom′era aor′tica** [NA], aortic bodies; see under BODY. **carotid g., g. carot′icum** [NA], carotid BODY. **g. jugula′re,** an aggregation of chemoreceptors in the dome of the bulb of the jugular vein.

gloss- see GLOSSO-.

glossa (glos′ah) [Gr. *glōssa*] the tongue.

glossagra (glos-sag′rah, glos′ag-rah) [*gloss-* + Gr. *agra* seizure] gouty pain of the tongue.

glossal (glos′al) pertaining to the tongue; lingual.

glossalgia (glos-sal′je-ah) [*gloss-* + *-algia*] pain in the tongue; glossodynia.

glossanthrax (glos-san′thraks) [*gloss-* + *anthrax*] carbuncle of the tongue.

glossectomy (glos-sek′to-me) [*gloss-* + Gr. *ektomē* excision] surgical excision of the tongue or its parts.

glossitis (glos-si′tis) [*gloss-* + *-itis*] inflammation of the tongue. **g. area′ta exfoliati′va,** benign migratory g. **atrophic g.,** Hunter's g. **benign migratory g.,** an inflammatory disease of the tongue of unknown etiology, characterized by multiple annular areas of desquamation of the filiform papillae on the dorsal surface of the tongue, usually presenting pinkish-red central lesions, outlined by thin, yellowish lines or bands, which change patterns and shift from one area to another every few days. Called also *g. areata exfoliativa, g. migrans, erythema migrans, exfoliatio aerata linguae, geographic tongue, lingua geographica, mappy tongue, pityriasis linguae,* and *wandering rash.*

Brocq-Pautrier **g.,** median rhomboid g. **Chevallier's g.,** posterior triangular g. **chronic superficial g.,** Möller's g. **diffuse interstitial g.,** a condition occurring in tertiary syphilis, almost exclusively in males, that may cause squamous cell carcinoma. It is characterized by nonulcerating irregular indurations forming asymmetric grooves on the dorsal surface of the tongue, alternating with leukoplakia. The tongue is initially enlarged but eventually undergoes shrinkage. **g. exfoliati'va,** Möller's g. **Hunter's g.,** a condition of the tongue seen in pernicious anemia, similar to Möller's glossitis, characterized by glossitis, glossodynia, glossopyrosis, and altered sense of taste, which may undergo spontaneous remission but invariably reappears. The pain and burning sensation are usually confined to the tongue but may also extend to other parts of the oral mucosa. Ultimately, the tongue becomes atrophic and assumes a beefy red color and a smooth shiny appearance, sometimes with small ulcers spreading over its surface. Called also *atrophic g.* and *bald tongue of pernicious anemia.* **idiopathic g.,** inflammation of the substance of the tongue and its mucous membrane. Called also *parenchymatous g.* **median rhomboid g.,** a congenital disorder of noninflammatory origin, characterized by a somewhat rhomboid reddish, smooth, and shiny lesion with some opalescent spots, occurring at about the middle third of the dorsal surface of the tongue, immediately anterior to the circumvallate papillae. It is similar to posterior triangular glossitis. Called also *g. rhomboidea mediana, Brocq-Pautrier g.,* and *Brocq-Pautrier syndrome.* **g. mi'grans,** benign migratory g., **Möller's, Moeller's g.,** a condition of the tongue, similar to Hunter's glossitis, characterized by superficial excoriation of the tongue, principally of the tip and edges. The lesions are beefy red, well-defined, irregular patches, in which the filiform papillae are thinned or absent and the fungiform papillae are swollen. The surface between the lesions may be smooth, whitish, or opalescent. Called also *bald tongue, chronic lingual papillitis, chronic superficial glossitis, glazed tongue, glossitis exfoliativa, glossodynia exfoliativa, glossy tongue, pallagrous tongue, slick tongue, smooth tongue,* and *varnished tongue.* **parasitic g., g. parasit'ica,** black TONGUE. **parenchymatous g.,** idiopathic g. **pellagrous g.,** Möller's g. **posterior triangular g.,** a disease of the tongue occurring in gastritis and other inflammatory diseases of the gastrointestinal system, characterized by triangular lesions of the posterior third of the tongue. The surface of the lesion is glossy red with nipple-like structures which often form agglomerates of isolated small plaques with well-defined borders. It is transitory, but usually recurs with exacerbation of gastrointestinal disorders. Except for the presence of gastrointestinal inflammatory lesions, it is similar to *median rhomboid glossitis.* Called also *Chevallier's g.* **g. rhomboi'dea media'na,** median rhomboid g. **unilateral g.,** hemiglossitis.

glosso-, gloss- [Gr. *glōssa* tongue] a combining form denoting relationship to the tongue. See also words beginning LINGUO-.

glossocele (glos'o-sēl) [*glosso-* + Gr. *kēlē* tumor] swelling and protrusion of the tongue.

glossocinesthetic (glos"o-sin-es-thet'ik) glossokinesthetic.

glossocoma (glŏ-sok'o-mah) retraction of the tongue.

glossodynamometer (glos"o-di"nah-mom'ĕ-ter) [*glosso-* + *dynamometer*] an instrument for recording the power of the tongue to resist pressure.

glossodynia (glos"o-din'e-ah) [*glosso-* + Gr. *odynē* pain] painful condition of the tongue; glossalgia. See GLOSSOPYROSIS. **g. exfoliati'va,** Möller's GLOSSITIS.

glossoepiglottic (glos"o-ep-ĭ-glot'ik) glossoepiglottidean.

glossoepiglottidean (glos"o-ep-ĭ-glo-tid'e-an) pertaining to the tongue and epiglottis; glossoepiglottic.

glossograph (glos'o-graf) [*glosso-* + Gr. *graphein* to record] an apparatus for recording tongue movements.

glossohyal (glos"o-hi'al) [*glosso-* + *hyoid*] pertaining to the tongue and hyoid bone.

glossokinesthetic (glos"o-kin"es-thet'ik) [*glosso-* + *kinesthetic*] pertaining to the subjective perception of the movements of the tongue.

glossology (glŏ-sol'o-je) [*glosso-* + *-logy*] 1. the sum of knowledge regarding the tongue. 2. a treatise on nomenclature.

glossomantia (glos"o-man-ti'ah) [*glosso-* + Gr. *manteia* divination] prognosis based on the appearance of the tongue.

glossoncus (glŏ-song'kus) [*glosso-* + Gr. *onkos* mass] a swelling of the tongue.

glossopalatinus (glos"o-pal"ah-ti'nus) palatoglossus MUSCLE.

glossopathy (glo-sop'ah-the) [*glosso-* + Gr. *pathos* disease] a disease of the tongue.

glossopexy (glos"o-pek'se) [*glosso-* + Gr. *pēxis* a fixing, putting together] lip-tongue adhesion.

glossopharyngeal (glos"o-fah-rin'je-al) [*glosso-* + *pharynx*] pertaining to the tongue and pharynx.

glossopharyngeum (glos"o-fah-rin'je-um) [*glosso-* + *pharynx*] the tongue and pharynx together.

glossopharyngeus (glos"o-fah-rin'je-us) glossopharyngeal MUSCLE.

glossophytia (glos"o-fit'e-ah) [*glosso-* + Gr. *phyton* plant] black TONGUE.

glossoplasty (glos'o-plas"te) [*glosso-* + Gr. *plassein* to mold] plastic surgery of the tongue.

glossoplegia (glos"o-ple'ge-ah) [*glosso-* + Gr. *plēgē* a stroke] paralysis of the tongue.

glossoptosis (glos"op-to'sis) [*glosso-* + Gr. *ptōsis* fall] retraction or downward displacement of the tongue.

glossopyra (glos"o-pi'rah) glossopyrosis.

glossopyrosis (glos"o-pi-ro'sis) [*glosso-* + Gr. *pyrōsis* burning] form of paresthesia characterized by pain, burning, itching, and stinging of the mucous membranes of the tongue without apparent lesions of the affected areas. It occurs most frequently in women past the menopause, sometimes in men, and infrequently in children. A variety of disorders and conditions have been implicated in its etiology, including: deficiency conditions such as pernicious anema and pellagra; diabetes mellitus; gastric hyperacidity or hypoacidity; referred pain; angioneurotic edema; electrogalvanic current generated by dissimilar metals in restorations; temporomandibular joint disturbances; and a variety of other conditions. Called also *burning tongue, glossodynia, glossopyra, painful tongue,* and *painful burning tongue.*

glossorrhaphy (glŏ-sor'ah-fe) [*glosso-* + Gr. *rhaphē* suture] suture of the tongue.

glossoscopy (glŏ-sos"ko-pe) [*glosso-* + Gr. *skopein* to examine] examination of the tongue.

glossospasm (glos'o-spasm) [*glosso-* + Gr. *spasmos* spasm] spasm of the tongue.

glossotilt (glos'o-tilt) [*glosso-* + Gr. *tillein* to pull] a lever which holds the tongue during one of the processes for artificial respiration.

glossotomy (glŏ-sot'o-me) [*glosso-* + Gr. *temnein* to cut] incision of the tongue.

glossotrichia (glos"o-trik'e-ah) [*glosso-* + Gr. *thrix* hair] hairy tongue; see black TONGUE.

glottides (glot'ĭ-dēz) plural of *glottis.*

glottis (glot'is), pl. *glot'tides* [Gr. *glōttis*] the vocal apparatus of the larynx, consisting of the true vocal cords and the opening between them. **intercartilaginous g., g. respirato'ria,** RIMA glottidis cartilaginea. **true g.,** RIMA glottidis. **g. voca'lis,** RIMA glottidis membranacea.

Glu glutamic ACID.

glucagon (gloo'kah-gon) a hormone produced by the α-cells of the islands of Langerhans. It is a polypeptide (molecular weight about 3500) that causes a rise in the blood sugar level by increasing the activity of liver phosphorylase, which is involved in the conversion of liver glycogen to glucose.

Glucal trademark for *calcium gluconate* (see under CALCIUM).

glucan (gloo'kan) a homopolysaccharide made up of recurring units of glucose, including glycogen and starch. Their formula is $(C_6H_{10}O_5)_x$, where x represents the number of glucose molecules. Frequently called *hexosan.*

Glucid trademark for *saccharin.*

glucinium (gloo-sin'e-um) [Gr. *glykys* sweet] beryllium.

D-glucitol (glu'sĭ-tol) sorbitol.

gluco- [Gr. *gleukos* sweetness] a combining form denoting relationship to glucose. See also words beginning GLYCO-.

glucocerebroside (gloo"ko-ser'ĕ-bro-sīd") glucosyl CERAMIDE.

glucocorticoid (gloo"ko-kor'tĭ-koid) any of a group of adrenal cortex hormones concerned with organic metabolism and response of the body to stress. It is a steroid with an O or OH substituent at C_{11} and an OH at C_{17} (see under STEROID). The chief functions of the glucocorticoids include acceleration of catabolism and inhibition of anabolism of proteins, increase of gluconeogenesis from protein and reduction of carbohydrate utilization, lipogenic metabolism of foodstuffs, immune response, and inflammatory response. Glucocorticoids are produced in the zona fasciculata of the adrenal cortex from cholesterol, and their secretion is controlled by ACTH. They are used as anti-inflammatory and immunosuppressant agents. In dentistry, used chiefly in the treatment of oral ulcers, arthritic temporomandibular joint lesions, postoperative edema, sensitive dentin and pulp, and inflammatory conditions. Also used in tissue transplantation. Side reactions may include euphoria, depression, psychoses, hypertension, anorexia, peptic ulcer, susceptibility to infection, abnormal fat distribution, moon face, edema, potassium loss, alkalosis, and osteoporosis. The group includes cortisone, cortisol, prednisolone, and 11- and 17-hydroxycorticosteroids.

glucoinvertase (gloo″ko-in-ver′tās) α-GLUCOSIDASE.

glucokinase [E.C.2.7.1.12] (gloo′ko-ki′nās) a hexokinase with an alcohol group as acceptor, which is involved in the conversion of glucose to glucose-6-phosphate in glycogenesis, occurring under the influence of insulin and in the presence of ATP and ADP. Called also *ATP gluconate transphosphatase.*

gluconate (gloo′ko-nāt) a salt of gluconic acid, containing the radical $HOCH_2(CHOH)_5COO-$. **ferrous g.,** a salt of gluconic acid, $Fe(C_{12}H_{22}O_{14})$, occurring as a yellowish gray or pale greenish yellow powder or granules with slight odor, which is soluble in water and glycerol, but not in alcohol. Used in the treatment of iron deficiency anemia. Excessive intake may cause poisoning (see IRON). Called also *iron gluconate.* Trademarks: Fergon, Ferlucon, Ferronicum, Iromon, Irox, Nionate. **iron g., ferrous g.**

Gluconobacter (gloo″ko-no-bak′ter) [*gluconic acid* + Gr. *baktērion* little rod] a genus of gram-negative, aerobic, rod-shaped bacteria of the family *Pseudomonadaceae,* found in flowers, souring fruits, vegetables, beer, cider, wine, baker's yeasts, and soil.

glucosaminopeptide (gloo″ko-sam″in-o-pep′tīd) peptidoglycan.

glucose (gloo′kōs) [Gr. *gleukos* sweetness, *glykys* sweet] 1. a hexose (aldose), which is a carbohydrate of plant origin that is used by the animal body as a source of energy. About 80 percent of the monosaccharides in foodstuffs is glucose; digestible disaccharides and polysaccharides, as well as other monosaccharides, such as fructose and galactose, are converted to glucose after ingestion. From the intestine, glucose is transported to the liver, from where it enters the systemic circulation to be distributed to all cells. Glucose not immediately needed for energy is converted into glycogen in the liver to be reconverted to glucose when the need arises. From the blood, glucose passes through the cell membrane with the aid of a carrier system and undergoes glycolysis, first combining with adenosine triphosphate to form adenosine diphosphate and glucose 6-phosphate, followed by a series of reactions until it releases energy, the end-product being pyruvic and lactic acids. Called also *corn syrup* and *starch syrup.* See also carbohydrate METABOLISM. 2. dextrose. D(+)-**g.,** dextrose. **g. oxidase,** glucose OXIDASE. **blood g.,** the concentration of glucose in the blood. Except immediately after meals, glucose is the only monosaccharide present in significant quantities in the blood and interstitial fluid, its level being controlled by insulin and glucagon. The normal glucose concentration in a person who has not eaten a meal within the past 3 or 4 hours is approximately 0 to 100 percent, rarely rising above 140 mg percent after meals, unless the patient has diabetes mellitus. The terms *blood sugar* and *blood glucose* are sometimes used synonymously. D-**g.,** D(+)-**g.,** dextrose. **medicinal g.,** dextrose. **g. phosphomutase,** phosphoglucomutase. **g.-6-phosphate,** an intermediate in carbohydrate metabolism, being the principal compound in the metabolism of glucose. In glycogenesis, it is made from glucose by the enzyme glucokinase by phosphorylation under the control of insulin, in the presence of ATP, and is in turn converted to glucose-1-phosphate by phosphoglucomutase. Once formed, it may be converted either to glycogen or to free glucose, or it may be metabolized by several mechanisms or pathways, e.g., the Embden-Meyerhof (anaerobic) pathway, followed by the Krebs (aerobic) cycle, or by the pentose phosphate pathway. **purified g.,** dextrose. **renal threshold for g.,** see under THRESHOLD.

glucosidase (gloo-ko′si-dās) [*glucoside* + *-ase*] a hydrolase that splits glucoside. **α-g.** [E.C.3.2.1.20], a glucosidase acting on glycosyl compounds, which catalyzes the hydrolysis of oligosaccharides by splitting terminal, nonreducing 1,4-linked α-D-glucose residues with release of α-glucose. The enzyme occurs in the small intestine and in yeast, molds, and malt, usually being associated with the enzyme amylase. It is also found in the saliva. Called also *glucoinvertase, glucosidosucrase,* and *maltase.* See also carbohydrate METABOLISM. **β-g.** [E.C.3.2.1.21], a glucosidase acting on glycosyl compounds, which catalyzes the hydrolysis of β-D-glucosides, β-D-galactosides, α-L-arabinosides, and β-D-xylosides and splits terminal nonreducing β-D-glucose residues with release of β-glucose. Called also *amygdalase, cellobiase,* and *gentiobiase.* See also carbohydrate METABOLISM.

glucoside (gloo′ko-sīd) 1. a glycoside, which on hydrolysis, yields glucose and a hydroxy nonsugar component (aglycone). 2. former name for *glycoside.*

glucosidosucrase (gloo″ko-si″do-su′krās) α-GLUCOSIDASE.

glucosuria (gloo″ko-su′re-ah) [*glucose* + Gr. *ouron* urine + *-ia*] 1. a condition in which glucose is present in the urine. 2. dextrosuria.

glucosyl (gloo′ko-sil) a glucose radical.

β-glucuronidase [E.C.3.2.1.32] (gloo″ku-ron′ĭ-dās) a hydrolase that attacks glycosidic linkages in gluruconides and is implicated in estrogen metabolism and cell division. Found in the spleen, liver, endocrine glands, and saliva.

glue (gloo) any substance used as an adhesive, particularly a preparation in the form of impure gelatin derived from boiling certain animal substances, such as hoofs, in water.

Glupax trademark for *acetazolamide.*

Gluside trademark for *saccharin.*

glutamate (gloo′tah-māt) a salt of glutamic acid. In biochemistry, the terms *glutamate* and *glutamic acid* are used interchangeably, even though glutamate technically refers to the negatively charged ion.

glutamine (gloo-tam′in) an acidic, naturally occurring, nonessential amino acid, 2-amino-5-glutaric acid, which is an amide of glutamic acid that yields ammonia on hydrolysis. Abbreviated *Gln.* See also amino ACID.

glutaraldehyde (gloo″tah-ral′dĕ-hīd) a disinfectant with bactericidal properties, which is also effective against some fungi and viruses. $CHO \cdot (CH_2)_3 \cdot CHO$. It occurs as a colorless liquid with a pungent odor, which is soluble in water and alcohol and oxidizes on exposure to air. Used as a 2 percent solution for cold sterilization of surgical and dental instruments. Immersion for 10 hours or more may be required to destroy sporogenous bacteria; immersion for more than 24 hours may cause corrosion of carbon steel instruments. Glutaraldehyde aerosols are also used to sterilize hospital and operating rooms. Irritation of the skin and mucous membrane may be caused by contact with the solution. Trademark: Cidex.

glutelin (gloo′tĕ-lin) a simple protein occurring in plant seeds, which is insoluble in all neutral solvents but is soluble in dilute acids and alkali and is coagulable by heat.

gluten (gloo′ten) [L. "glue"] the protein of wheat and other grains which gives the dough its tough elastic character.

glutenin (gloo′tĕ-nin) a prolamin obtained from wheat, which is soluble in dilute alcohol but not in water and absolute alcohol.

glutethimide (gloo-teth′ĭ-mīd) a hypnotic, 3-ethyl-3-phenyl-2,6-piperidinedione, occurring as a white crystalline powder that is soluble in ethyl acetate, acetone, ether, chloroform, alcohol, and methanol, but insoluble in water. Used in insomnia and sleep disorders, being contraindicated in patients with a history of drug abuse. Use may lead to habituation or addiction; adverse reactions may include drowsiness, interference with coumarin therapy, skin rash, exfoliative dermatitis, nausea, and, sometimes, blood dyscrasias. Trademark: Doriden.

Gly glycine.

glycan (gli′kan) see PEPTIDOGLYCAN.

glycemia (gli-se′me-ah) [Gr. *glykys* sweet + Gr. *haima* blood + *-ia*] the presence of glucose in the blood. See blood GLUCOSE and blood SUGAR, and see HYPERGLYCEMIA and HYPOGLYCEMIA.

glyceraldehyde (glis″er-al′de-hīd) an aldose (triose) produced by the oxidation of sugars in the body, designated as the reference standard for D- and L-carbohydrates and their derivatives. D-Glyceraldehyde occurs in the form of phosphate esters, as an intermediate in the fermentation and glycolysis of carbohydrates, being also the precursor of glycerol, which the organism synthesizes and incorporates into various lipids. Glyceraldehyde occurs as tasteless crystals from an alcohol-ether mixture that is soluble in water but not in benzene and organic solvents. Used in nutrition, biochemical research, and various chemical processes. Called also *glyceric aldehyde.*

glyceride (glis′er-īd) any of the fatty acid esters of glycerol. Glycerides are the principal component of storage fats in plant and animal tissues, especially of adipose tissue. Their melting point is determined by the fatty acid composition — generally increasing with the number and length of the saturated fatty acid composition. They undergo hydrolysis when boiled with acids or bases or by the action of lipases. Hydrolysis with alkali (saponification) produces a mixture of fatty acid soaps and glycerol. Compounds in which all three hydroxyl groups of glycerol are esterified with fatty acids are *triglycerides;* those with two hydroxyl group esterified are *diglycerides;* and those with a single hydroxyl group esterified are *monoglycerides.* Called also *acylglycerol* and *neutral fat.*

glycerin (glis′er-in) [L. *glycerinum*] glycerol.

glycerinum (glis″er-i′num) [L.] glycerin; see GLYCEROL.

glycerol (glis′er-ōl) [Gr. *glykeros* sweet + *-ol*] a trihydric sugar alcohol, 1,2,3-propanetriol, occurring as a clear, colorless, syrupy liquid with a sweet taste and a slight characteristic odor, which is miscible with water, ethanol, methanol, ethyl acetate, and acetone and is insoluble in ether, mineral and vegetable oils, and chloroform. Glycerol absorbs moisture from the air. Its metabolism is closely related to lipids, many of which contain glycerol. It is prepared by the hydrolysis of animal fats or vegetable oils. Used as a solvent, humectant, emollient, sweetener, demulcent, and lubricant, in the manufacture of nitroglycerin, as a vehicle for drugs, and in suppositories. In dentistry, used in mouthwashes and toothpastes. Called also *glycerin*. See also lipid METABOLISM. **g. phosphatide,** 1. phosphoglyceride. 2. phospholipid.

glycerophosphatase (glis″er-o-fos′fah-tās) phosphatase.

glyceryl (glis′er-il) The trivalent radical C_3H_5 of glycerol. **g. trinitrate,** nitroglycerin. **g. trioleate,** triolein. **g. tristearate,** tristearin.

glycinate (gli′sin-āt) any salt of glycine.

glycine (gli′sēn) an aliphatic, naturally occurring, nonessential amino acid, aminoacetic acid, with a sweet taste. It is also found in the saliva. Glycine has been synthesized and is used as a gastric antacid and dietary supplement. It has also been used in the treatment of muscle diseases. Abbreviated *Gly.* See also amino ACID.

glyco- [Gr. *glykys* sweet] a combining form denoting relationship to sugar. See also words beginning GLUCO-.

glycocalyx (gli″ko-kal′iks) the glycoprotein and polysaccharide coat of variable thickness and density found on certain types of cells, such as fibroblasts, muscle cells, pericytes, and epithelial cells. It may serve as a medium through which ions and molecules may be exchanged between the cell and its environment, provide a barrier that prevents the passage of large particles, supply a structure that strengthens intercellular bonds, or, being resistant to some proteolytic substances, serve as a protective layer for the cell. Called also *boundary layer, cement substance, cementing substance, external lamina, gap substance,* and *glycoprotein mantle.*

glycogen (gli′ko-jen) [*glyco-* + Gr. *gennan* to produce] a polysaccharide (hexosan) of high molecular weight (average 2.5 to 4.5 million), consisting of a single building block α-D-glucose, which serves as a reserve material in animal carbohydrate metabolism and in maintaining normoglycemic hemostasis. Glycogen is the only carbohydrate of animal origin. It is stored in the liver and in muscles, comprising less than 0.1 to 1 percent of the body weight. About 25 percent of dietary carbohydrate is stored in the liver as glycogen, being converted from glucose transported to the liver through the portal system, from where it is released into the systemic circulation as glucose. Glycogen in tissues other than liver and muscles serves as a source of hexose phosphate, which is used in various metabolic processes. Liver glycogen has a biologic half-life of 1 day; glycogen from other tissues has a 3- to 4-day half-life. Called also *animal starch* and *liver starch.* See also carbohydrate METABOLISM.

glycogenase (gli′ko-je′nās) 1. α-AMYLASE. 2. β-AMYLASE.

glycogenesis (gli″ko-jen′ē-sis) [*glycogen* + Gr. *gennan* to produce] the formation or synthesis of glycogen; the conversion of glucose to glycogen. The process includes: the conversion of glucose to glucose-6-phosphate by glucokinase, influenced by insulin and in the presence of ATP and ADP; the conversion of glucose-6-phosphate to glucose-1-phosphate by phosphoglucomutase; reaction of glucose-1-phosphate with uridine triphosphate to form an active nucleotide, uridine diphosphate glucose; and joining in glucosidic linkages of activated glucose molecules of uridine diphosphate glucose in the presence of a branching enzyme and uridine diphosphate glucose-glycogentransglucosylase, to form glycogen. See also lactic acid CYCLE.

glycogenolysis (gli″ko-je-nol′ĭ-sis) [*glycogen* + Gr. *lysis* dissolution] the breakdown of glycogen to re-form glucose in the cells, whereby each succeeding glucose molecule on each branch of the glycogen polymer is split away by a process of phosphorylation, catalyzed by the enzyme phosphorylase. See also carbohydrate METABOLISM, Krebs CYCLE, and lactic acid CYCLE.

glycogenosis (gli″ko-je-no′sis) [*glycogen* + -*osis*] any disease characterized by abnormal deposits of glycogen in various tissues. Called also *glycogen disease* and *glycogen storage disease.* **g. I,** a syndrome of faulty glycogen metabolism, transmitted as a recessive trait, which is usually present at birth or appearing shortly thereafter. Symptoms include abdominal rotundity, adiposity marked by fatty accumulation in the cheeks, breasts, buttocks, and back of extremities; growth retardation; swinging gait; hepatomegaly; pallor with peculiar yellowish color of the skin; pinkish xanthomas of the elbows, knees, and buttocks; mild anemia; glycogen deposits in the kidneys and liver; glucose-6-phosphatase deficiency; hypercholesterolemia; hyperlipemia; hypoglycemia; ketosis; acetonemia; acetonuria;

glycosuria; and hypophosphatemia. Called also *hepatorenal g., liver glycogen disease, von Gierke's syndrome,* and *Von Gierke-van Creveld syndrome.* **g. II,** a syndrome of faulty glycogen deposition, transmitted as a recessive trait, which does not seem to be associated with any specific enzymatic defect. Symptoms may be present at birth but, more often, they appear between the second and sixth month of life. Glycogenosis is usually generalized but the neuromuscular system and the heart are most severely affected with frequent involvement of the nervous system. Symptoms include cyanosis, mongoloid-like facies, growth retardation, hepatosplenomegaly, drooling, vomiting, anorexia, muscular hypotonia, and glycogen deposits in the heart, reticuloendothelial system, kidneys, liver, adrenals, pancreas, bone marrow, lymph nodes, thymus, and especially muscles, including the diaphragm and tongue. Cardiovascular symptoms may include dyspnea, cardiomegaly, cardiac edema, atypical systolic murmur, tachycardia, and inverted T waves and high-spiked T waves. The most common oral symptom is macroglossia. Called also *generalized g., glycogen heart disease,* and *Pompe's syndrome.* **g. III,** a syndrome of faulty glycogen metabolism, transmitted as a recessive trait, and associated with amylo-1,6-glucosidase deficiency. Its course is similar to that of glycogenosis I, except for the mildness of symptoms. Abdominal rotundity, hepatomegaly, appetite for sweets and breadstuffs, hypoglycemia, and muscular hypotonia are the principal symptoms. Pathologic features include glycogen deposits in the muscles and liver; glycogen isolated from these organs is characterized by short external chains. Called also *Cori's disease, debrancher deficiency limit dextrinosis, Forbes' disease,* and *limit dextrinosis.* **g. IV,** a rare disorder of glycogen metabolism characterized by glycogen deposits, chiefly in the liver, but also in the spleen, lymph nodes, intestinal mucosa, and muscles. Nodular liver cirrhosis and portal hypertension are usually associated. It is believed to be transmitted as a recessive trait and, presumably, is due to low amylo-(1,4)-(1,6)-transglucosidase activity. Called also *amylopectinosis, Andersen's disease,* and *debrancher deficiency amylopectinosis.* **g. V,** a syndrome of glycogen metabolism, probably transmitted as a recessive trait, associated with myophosphorylase deficiency. It may be present in childhood but symptoms may not be evident until adulthood. Symptoms include intermittent myoglobinuria associated with dark urine, weakness and wasting of muscles, muscle cramping on exertion, inability to perform physical work over long periods of time, tachycardia on exertion, diminished electromyographic activity, and excessive deposition of glycogen in muscles. Called also *glycolysis myopathy syndrome* and *McArdle's disease.* **g. VI,** a syndrome of faulty glycogen metabolism, transmitted as a recessive trait, and associated with liver phosphorylase deficiency. Symptoms are usually mild; they include growth retardation, hepatomegaly, mild hypoglycemia, mild ketosis, and glycogen deposition in the liver. Called also *hepatophosphorylase deficiency g.* and *Hers' disease.* **generalized g.,** g. II. **hepatophosphorylase deficiency g.,** g. VI. **hepatorenal g.,** g. I.

glycol (gli′kol) any of a group of aliphatic dihydric alcohols, having marked hygroscopic properties and useful as solvents and plasticizers. **diethylene g. monoethyl ether,** a compound, 2-ethoxyethoxyethanol, occurring as a slightly hygroscopic, colorless liquid with a slight pleasant odor, which is miscible with water and ethanol. Used as a dispersing agent for immiscible materials such as oils and water. It may cause liver damage. **ethylene g.,** a compound, 1,2-ethanediol, occurring as a clear, colorless, syrupy, hygroscopic fluid with a sweet taste, which is soluble in water, alcohol, and ether. It lowers the freezing point of water. Used chiefly as an antifreeze compound and in various industrial processes. Ingestion may cause central nervous system stimulation, followed by depression, vomiting, drowsiness, coma, respiratory failure, convulsions, renal damage, anuria, and death. **methyl g.,** propylene g. **polyethylene g.,** a polymer of ethylene glycol, α-hydro-ω-hydroxy(oxy-1,2-ethanediyl), occurring in several forms, from a liquid to a hard solid, being soluble or miscible in water and organic solvents. *Polyethylene glycol 300* is a clear, colorless, viscous liquid; *400* is a clear, colorless, viscous liquid; *600* is a clear, viscous, slightly hygroscopic liquid; *1500* is a hygroscopic soft, waxy solid similar in consistency to petrolatum; *1540* is a hygroscopic solid similar to beeswax; *4000* is a nonhygroscopic soft solid; and *6000* is a nonhygroscopic, hard, translucent solid. Polyethylene glycols are used as solvents and dispersing agents and, chiefly, water soluble bases, for ointments. Also used as water-soluble lubricants for rubber molds, in food packaging, and in various industrial processes. Trademarks: Carbowax, Macrogol, PEG, Poly-G, Polyglycol E, Solbase. **propylene g.,** a compound, 1,2-propanediol, occurring as a clear, viscous, odorless, liquid with a slightly acrid taste that is miscible with water, ethanol, acetone, and chloroform, is soluble in ether, and dissolves volatile oils. Used as a nontoxic antifreeze in the food industry, solvent for drugs, substitute for ethylene glycol and glycerol, diluent or binder, inhibitor of fermentation and mold growth, and propellant for air disinfectant aerosols. Called also *methyl g.* **sodium cellulose g.,** SODIUM carboxymethylcellulose.

glycolipid (gli″ko-lip′id) a lipid containing carbohydrate groups, usually galactose but also glucose, inositol, or others. Phosphate may or may not be present, and glycerol or sphingosine may occur. Glycolipids include cerebrosides and gangliosides.

glycolysis (gli-kol′ĭ-sis) [*glyco-* + Gr. *lysis* dissolution] the degradation of sugars into simpler compounds, chiefly pyruvic and lactic acids. Called also *fermentation.* See also carbohydrate METABOLISM.

glyconeogenesis (gli″ko-ne″o-jen′ĕ-sis) [*glyco-* + Gr. *neos* new + *gennan* to produce] the formation of carbohydrates from molecules which are not themselves carbohydrates, as in the formation of glucose from amino acids and from the glycerol portion of fat. See also carbohydrate METABOLISM.

glycoprotein (gli″ko-pro′te-in) a conjugated protein containing a protein and a carbohydrate, chiefly hexosamine. Glycoproteins are found in all forms of life, occurring in various tissues and having different functions: in the blood (as fetuin, fibrinogen, immunoglobulins, blood group proteins, and thyroxin-binding protein); in the urine (as hormones — chorionic gonadotropin and follicle- and thyroid-stimulating hormones); as enzymes (as ribonuclease B, β-glucuronidase, pepsin, and serum cholinesterase); in egg white; in mucous secretions (as submaxillary and gastric glycoproteins); in connective tissue (as collagen); in cell membranes; and in extracellular membranes. According to some authorities, compounds containing less than 4 percent carbohydrates are classified as glycoproteins, whereas those having more than 4 percent are mucoproteins. In other classifications, mucins, mucoids, chondroproteins, and various plasma proteins containing hexoses and other carbohydrates are known as either glycoproteins or mucoproteins. **acid g.,** orosomucoid. **glycine-rich g. (GRG),** FACTOR B.

glycoptyalism (gli″ko-ti′ah-lizm) [*glyco-* + *ptyalism*] glycosialia.

glycosaminoglucuronoglycan (gli-kōs′ah-mī″no-gloo″ku-ron″o-gli′kan) mucopolysaccharide.

glycosialia (gli″ko-si-a′le-ah) [*glyco-* + Gr. *sialon* saliva + *-ia*] the presence of glucose in saliva. Called also *glycoptyalism.*

glycosialorrhea (gli″ko-si″ah-lo-re′ah) [*glyco-* + Gr. *sialon* saliva + *rhoia* flow] excessive flow of saliva containing glucose.

glycoside (gli′ko-sīd) a compound, usually of plant origin, that contains a carbohydrate and another compound. Chemically, glycosides are acetals which, on hydrolysis, yield sugars and hydroxy nonsugar components (aglycones), being named for their sugar components as glucosides (yielding glucose), fructosides (yielding fructose), galactosides (yielding galactose), etc. Formerly called *glucoside.* **cardiac g.,** any of a group of chemically and pharmacologically similar glycosides occurring in certain plants, such as *Digitalis* and *Strophanthus,* which have a similar aglycone component and exhibit cardiotonic effect, increasing the strength of the myocardium. Used in the treatment of congestive heart failure and cardiac arrhythmias. Cardiac glycosides may cause nausea, vomiting, neuralgia, headache, drowsiness, fatigue, and, in rare instances, hallucinations. Patients receiving cardiac glycosides may show hyperexcitability of pharyngeal and emetic reflexes during dental procedures. See also DIGITALIS.

glycosuria (gli″ko-su′re-ah) [*glyco-* + Gr. *ouron* urine + *-ia*] the presence in the urine of an abnormally elevated concentrations of sugar, considered as one of the principal symptoms of diabetes mellitus.

glycosyl (gli′ko-sil) a radical derived from a carbohydrate.

glycosyltransferase [E.C.2.4] (gloo″ko-sil-trans′fer-ās) a subclass of transferases, the enzymes of which catalyze the transfer of glycosyl groups, some having also hydrolytic activities (transfer of glycosyl group from the donor to water). Called also *transglucosylase.*

Glycyrrhiza (glis″ir-ri′zah) [Gr. *glykys* sweet + *rhiza* root] a genus of leguminous plants.

glycyrrhiza (glis″ir-ri′zah) the dried rhizome and roots of *Gly-*

cyrrhiza glabra, used in a fluid extract or syrup as a sweetening agent for drugs. Called also *licorice, licorice root, liquorice,* and *sweet root.*

gm gram.

GMT gingival margin trimmer; see margin TRIMMER.

Gn gnathion.

gnashing (nash′ing) the grinding of the teeth together. See BRUXISM and BRUXOMANIA.

gnath- see GNATHO-.

gnathalgia (nath-al′je-ah) [*gnath-* + *-algia*] pain in the jaw; gnathodynia.

gnathic (nath′ik) pertaining to the jaw or cheek.

gnathion (nath′e-on) an anthropometric landmark indicating the lowest point on the median line of the mandible. Abbreviated *Gn.* Called also *point Gn.* See illustration at CEPHALOMETRY.

gnathitis (nath-i′tis) inflammation of the jaw.

gnatho-, gnath- [Gr. *gnathos* jaw] a combining form denoting relationship to the jaw.

gnathocephalus (nath″o-sef′ah-lus) [*gnatho-* + Gr. *kephalē* head] an abnormality characterized by absence of the head except for the jaws.

gnathode (nah-thōd′) a gnathographically mounted dental cast.

gnathodynamics (nath″o-di-nam′iks) [*gnatho-* + Gr. *dynamis* power] the study of the physical forces in mastication.

gnathodynamometer (nath″o-di″nah-mom′ĕ-ter) [*gnatho-* + *dynamometer*] an instrument used in measuring the force exerted in closing the jaws. Called also *occlusometer.* **bimeter g.,** a gnathodynamometer equipped with a central-bearing point of adjustable height.

gnathodynia (nath″o-din′e-ah) [*gnatho-* + Gr. *odynē* pain] pain in the jaw; gnathalgia.

Gnathograph (nath′o-graf) trademark for an adjustable dental articulator. The instrument resembles the Hanau articulator, except for having a provision for increasing the intercondylar distance.

gnathography (nath-og′rah-fe) [*gnatho-* + Gr. *graphein* to record] the recording of the strength of the patient's bite by a tracing of the changes in the flow of an electric current through a bite gauge.

gnathokin (nath′o-kin) an instrument used in the study of the articulation of certain cusps in protrusive balance with various slants and curvatures of the condyle paths.

Gnatholator trademark for a *Granger articulator* (see under ARTICULATOR).

gnathology (nath-ol′o-je) [*gnatho-* + *-logy*] a science that deals with the anatomy, histology, physiology, and pathology of the jaws and the masticatory system as a whole, including the applicable diagnostic, therapeutic, and rehabilitative procedures. See also gnathologic ORTHOPEDICS.

gnathoplasty (nath′o-plas″te) [*gnatho-* + Gr. *plassein* to mold] plastic surgery of the jaw.

gnathoschisis (nath-os′ki-sis) [*gnatho-* + *schisis*] CLEFT jaw.

gnathoscope (nath″o-skōp) a dental articulator having tiltable remnant hinge axles that are set in stirrup mounts so that they may be swiveled and turned and, thus, allow the setting of each condylar element in a way that it would provide an approximate path of travel for the condyles.

Gnathosimulator trademark for a *Granger articulator* (see under ARTICULATOR).

gnathostat (nath′o-stat) a jaw-positioning device used in dental radiology, facial photography, cephalometry, and other procedures requiring exact positioning of the jaws. See also CEPHALOSTAT.

gnathostatics (nath″o-stat′iks) [*gnatho-* + Gr. *statike* the art of weighing] a method of prosthodontic and orthodontic diagnosis based on determination of the basal and osteometric relationships between the teeth and their supporting bony structures.

gnotobiota (no″to-bi-o′tah) the specifically and entirely known microfauna and microflora of a specially reared laboratory animal.

gnotobiotic (no′to-bi-ot′ik) pertaining to a gnotobiote or to gnotobiotics.

gnotobiotics (no″to-bi-ot′iks) [Gr. *gnotos* known + *biota* the fauna and flora of a region] the science of rearing laboratory animals the microfauna and microflora of which are specifically known in their entirety.

Go gonion.

Godtfredsen's syndrome [Erik *Godtfredsen*] see under SYNDROME.

goiter (goi′ter) [L. *struma*] enlargement of the thyroid gland. See also HYPERTHYROIDISM. **exophthalmic g.,** a disorder due to hyperplasia of the thyroid gland, most commonly affecting adult and middle-aged women. It is characterized by hyperthyroidism, goiter, and exophthalmos, accompanied by cardiac arrhythmia, elevated basal metabolic rate, increased pulse rate, elevated protein-bound iodine level, weight loss, intolerance to heat, sweating, apprehensiveness, weakness, increased appetite, tremor, increased bowel activity, eyelid retraction, and stare. Periapical radiolucency may occur. Called also *Basedow's disease* and *Graves' disease*.

goitrogen (goi′tro-jen) a substance capable of producing goiter.

gold (gōld) [L. *aurum*] a noble metal. Symbol, Au; atomic number, 79; atomic weight, 196.9665; melting point, 1064.43°C; specific gravity, 19.32; valences, 1, 3; Mohs hardness number 2.5–3.0; group IB of the periodic table. It occurs as a single natural isotope (197) and several artificial radioactive ones (177–179, 181, 183, 185–196, 198–203). Gold is a yellow, very ductile metal that is resistant to water, air, oxygen, and acids, but reacts with aqua regia and mixtures containing chlorides, bromides, or iodides and some oxidizing agents. Similarly to other precious metals, it is measured in troy weight. When alloyed, in carats, pure gold has 24 parts (or carats). Gold compounds are used in the treatment of rheumatoid arthritis and some forms of synovitis. Their pharmacological effects consist of suppressing the release of histamine, preventing prostaglandin synthesis, and decreasing the binding of tryptophan to plasma proteins. The most toxic reactions to gold involve the skin and the mucous membrane, usually of the mouth, with exfoliative dermatitis, erythema, stomatitis, pharyngitis, tracheitis, gastritis, colitis, glossitis, and vaginitis being the principal manifestations. Gray to blue pigmentation of the mucous membrane may occur. Hematological complications may include thrombocytopenia, leukopenia, agranulocytosis, proteinuria, and albuminuria. Encephalitis, neuritis, and hepatitis may occur. In dentistry, gold is widely used in pure form or in alloys (see *g. alloy*) as filling material and in the preparation of dentures, crowns, inlays, orthodontic appliances, splints, and the like. It is also used for soldering (see gold SOLDER). See also terms beginning with AURO- and CHRYSO-. **Aderer No. 3 Bridge G.,** trademark for an extra hard *dental casting gold alloy.* **g. alloy,** any alloy which contains gold. Most gold used in dentistry (except for direct filling gold) is an alloy. Gold alloys are used principally in the production of gold wire for partial denture clasps and orthodontic wire and in dental casting. Copper, added to strengthen the gold, is the basic component of most alloys, and silver, platinum, palladium, and zinc are sometimes also added. The gold content of an alloy is rated according to the carat or parts of pure gold in 24 parts of the alloy, where pure gold is said to be 24 carat gold, an alloy with 18 parts of gold and 6 parts of other metal(s), 18 carat gold, etc. In dentistry, gold is usually rated by the fineness of the alloy, the fineness being parts per thousand of pure gold, where pure gold is said to be 1000 fine, an alloy with ¾ gold and ¼ other metals is 750 fine gold, etc. The carat rating can be converted to the fineness rating and vice versa by the following proportion: carat/24 = fineness/1000. **g. amalgam,** gold AMALGAM. **American G. "B" Bridge,** trademark for hard *dental*

casting gold alloy. **American G. "C" Partial Extra Hard,** trademark for an extra hard *dental casting gold alloy.* **American G. "T" Bridge Hard,** trademark for a hard *dental casting gold alloy.* **annealed g.,** gold which has been heated in a flame to remove impurities from its surface. Usually referring to pure (24 carat) gold foil with oxides and other impurities removed from its surface by a flame, thus increasing its cohesive properties. See also cohesive gold FOIL. **g. bromide,** a gold compound, AuBr, occurring as a yellowish gray mass. Called also *aurous bromide.* See also BROMAURATE and bromauric ACID. **24 carat g.,** pure g. **cohesive g., cohesive g. foil,** cohesive gold FOIL. **colloidal g.,** a purplish suspension of minute particles of metallic gold, made by reducing a solution of bromauric acid or other acid or salt of gold. The radioactive form, made by exposure to neutron bombardment, is used for intracavitary treatment of cancer. **g.-copper system,** gold-copper ALLOY. **Dent G. No. 1,** trademark for a medium hard *dental casting gold alloy.* **Dent G. No. 2,** trademark for a hard *dental casting gold alloy.* **dental g.,** gold, either in its pure form or in alloys, used in restorative and prosthetic dentistry, pure gold foil, mat, and powder being used as a direct filling material and gold alloys in the production of restorations, such as crowns. **dental casting g. alloy,** a gold alloy used in the fabrication of dental castings. It is classified as Types I (soft), II (medium hard), III (hard), and IV (extra hard), each type being available under numerous trademarks. See tables. **direct g., direct filling g.,** pure gold (24 carat), usually available in the form of gold foil, mat gold, or powdered gold, which is used as a direct filling material and can be compacted directly into the prepared cavity in restorative dentistry. **direct filling g. condensation,** direct filling gold COMPACTION. **Dutch g.,** an alloy of copper and zinc. **electrolytic g.,** pure gold (24 carat) powder formed by electrolytic precipitation from gold solution, which is compressed into strips and sintered, during which the self-diffusion of the powder causes the particles to conglomerate while retaining their dendritic structure (see *mat g.*). An alloy of electrolytic gold and calcium (calcium content is 0.1 to 0.5 percent by weight) is also available, which is usually sandwiched between two layers of gold foil for ease in handling. **encapsulated powdered g.,** powdered gold wrapped in gold foil. Trademark: Goldent. **g. foil,** gold FOIL. **g. foil condensation,** direct filling gold COMPACTION. **g. inlay,** gold INLAY. **g. knife,** gold KNIFE. **mat g.,** spongy strips of pure gold (24 carat) produced by compressing and sintering electrolytic gold powder (see *electrolytic g.*). The strips may be formed into ropes and cylinders and used as a direct filling material, chiefly in building up the internal bulk of the restoration, being easily compacted and adapted to the retentive parts of the prepared cavity. But more often, they are used in the base of restorations and then veneered over or overlaid with cohesive gold foil. A layer of mat

CLASSIFICATION OF DENTAL CASTING GOLD ALLOYS

Type	Gold and Platinum Group Metals (Min. %)	Vickers Hardness Number (Softened) Min.	Max.	Fusion Temp. °C	°F
I (soft)	83	50	90	930	1700
II (medium hard)	78	90	120	900	1650
III (hard)	78	120	150	900	1650
IV (extra hard)	75	150	—	870	1600

(Modified from R. W. Phillips: Elements of Dental Materials, 3rd ed. Philadelphia, W. B. Saunders Co., 1977.)

RANGE OF PERCENTAGE COMPOSITION OF DENTAL CASTING GOLD ALLOYS

Type	Gold	Silver	Copper	Palladium	Platinum	Zinc
I (soft)	80.2–95.8	2.4–12.0	1.6–6.2	0.0–3.6	0.0–1.0	0.0–1.2
II (medium hard)	73.0–83.0	6.9–14.6	5.8–10.5	0.0–5.6	0.0–4.2	0.0–1.4
III (hard)	71.0–79.8	5.2–13.4	7.1–12.6	0.0–6.5	0.0–7.5	0.0–2.0
IV (extra hard)	62.4–71.9	8.0–17.4	8.6–15.4	0.0–10.1	0.2–8.2	0.0–2.7

(Modified from American Dental Association. Council on Dental Materials and Devices. Guide to Dental Materials and Devices, 5th ed., Chicago. American Dental Association. 1971.)

gold sandwiched between layers of gold foil is known as *mat foil.* Called also *sponge g.* **MF-Y g.,** a gold alloy with a fusion temperature of 1204° (2200°F). **noncohesive g., noncohesive g. foil,** noncohesive gold FOIL. **Nürnberg g.,** an alloy containing 2.5 percent gold, 7.5 percent aluminum, and 90 percent copper. **1000 fine g.,** pure g. **g. plating,** gold PLATING. **platinized g., platinized** FOIL. **g. plugger,** gold CONDENSER. **powdered g.,** a fine granular form of pure gold (24 carat), obtained either by atomizing the metal from its molten state or by chemical precipitation. Its particles average about 15 μ in diameter, the largest being up to 74 μ. The powder is slightly precondensed into pellets about 1 to 3 mm in diameter, each pellet wrapped with gold foil. The ratio of foil to powder is 1 to 19. Used as a direct filling material in dental restorations. Formerly, gold powders were available in agglomerated form, furnished with a liquid, such as an alcohol or dilute carbolic acid, to hold the agglomerate together until it was placed and compaction begun. **pure g.,** gold that does not contain impurities or admixtures; 24 carat or 1000 fine gold. **radioactive g.,** a radioactive isotope of gold, usually ^{195}Au, ^{198}Au, or ^{199}Au; ^{198}Au is the most commonly used, either in solid form or colloidal solution. Radioactive gold emits gamma (0.411 MeV) as well as beta radiation (E max = 0.96 MeV) and has a half-life of 2.7 days. The gamma rays contribute from 6 to 10 percent of the total dose. Used as a diagnostic scintiscanning agent and as a therapeutic agent in the treatment of cancer. Called also *radiogold.* **g..sodium thiomalate,** a gold compound, [(1,2-dicarboxyethyl)thio] gold disodium salt, occurring as an odorless, fine, white to yellowish white powder with a metallic taste, which is soluble in water, but not in alcohol and ether. Used in the treatment of rheumatoid arthritis. It has the toxic properties of the parent compound. Called also *disodium aurothiomalate* and *sodium aurothiomalate.* Trademarks: Myochrysine, Myocrisin, Tauredon. **g. sodium thiosulfate,** a gold compound, $Na_3Au(S_2O_3)_2+2H_2O$, occurring as white needle-like or prismatic small glistening crystals that darken on exposure to light and are soluble in water, but not in alcohol and most organic solvents. Used in the treatment of rheumatoid arthritis. It has the toxic properties of the parent compound. Called also *aurothiosulfate natrium, aurothiosulfate sodium,* and *hyposulfite of gold and sodium.* Trademarks: Auricidine, Aurocidin, Aurothion, Crytion. **g. solder,** gold SOLDER. **sponge g.,** mat g. **g. thioglucose,** aurothioglucose. **white g.,** a gold alloy rendered white or silver-colored by the presence of platinum, palladium, silver, or nickel. The addition of about 10 percent palladium causes gold to become gray-white, while 25 percent platinum is needed to achieve the same effect. White gold alloys generally have relatively high melting points, are hard (Brinell hardness numbers of over 100 in the softened state), have a low ductility in comparison to gold-colored alloys, and have a comparatively low resistance to tarnishing. Alloys containing palladium and platinum are used in Types II, III, and IV dental casting gold alloys (see tables). See also silver-palladium ALLOY. **yellow g.,** any alloy containing sufficient gold to impart a yellow color, such as an alloy containing 41.67 percent gold, 38.5 percent copper, 5.83 percent silver, 12.83 percent zinc, and 1.17 percent nickel.

Goldenhar's syndrome [Maurice *Goldenhar*] oculoauriculovertebral SYNDROME.

Goldent trademark for *encapsulated powdered gold* (see under GOLD).

Goldflam, Samuel [Polish physician, 1852–1932] see MYASTHENIA gravis (Erb-Goldflam syndrome).

Goldman-Fox knife see under KNIFE.

Goldscheier's disease [Johannes Karl August Eugen Alfred *Goldscheier,* German physician, 1858–1935] EPIDERMOLYSIS bullosa.

Goldsmith I inlay see under INLAY.

Goldstein's rays [Eugene *Goldstein,* German physician, 1850–1930] see under RAY.

Golgi apparatus (complex), corpuscle, organ [Camillo *Golgi,* Italian histologist; co-winner, with Santiago Ramon y Cajal, of the Nobel prize for medicine and physiology in 1906, in recognition of their work on the structure of the nervous system] see under APPARATUS, CORPUSCLE, and ORGAN.

Goltz's syndrome [Robert W. *Goltz,* American physician, born 1923] Goltz-Gorlin SYNDROME. See also Gorlin's SYNDROME (Gorlin-Goltz syndrome).

Goltz-Gorlin syndrome [Robert W. *Goltz;* R. J. *Gorlin,* American dentist, oral pathologist, and geneticist] see under SYNDROME.

gommelin (gom'ĕ-lin) dextrin.

Gompertz's law see under LAW.

gomphosis (gom-fo'sis) [Gr. *gomphōsis* a bolting together] a type of fibrous joint in which a conical process is inserted into a socketlike portion, such as the styloid process of the temporal bone, or the teeth in the dental alveoli. Called also *socket joint of tooth.*

gonad (gon'ad) [L. *gonas,* from Gr. *gonē* seed] a gamete-producing gland; an ovary or testis.

gonadotropin (gon"ah-do-tro'pin) [*gonad* + Gr. *tropē* a turn] gonadotropic HORMONE. **chorionic g.,** a gonadotropic hormone produced by the placenta, which sustains the corpus luteum.

Gonal trademark for *fenfluramine hydrochloride* (see under FENFLURAMINE).

gonane (go'nān) a class of parent steroid compounds without any methyl groups attached to the cyclopenta-perhydrophenanthrene ring. See also STEROID.

Gongylonema (gon"ji-lo-ne'mah) [Gr. *gongylos* round + *nema* thread] a genus of nematodes. **G. pul'chrum,** a threadlike nematode found in the esophageal mucosa of humans, ruminants, and pigs. In humans, the worms have been found in the esophagus and oral cavity. Called also *Filaria labialis.*

gongylonemiasis (gon"ji-lo-ne-mi'ah-sis) infection with the nematode *Gongylonema pulchrum.* It is characterized by the presence of maturing and adult worms in the submucous tissues of the esophagus and oral cavity, which migrate through beneath the mucosa, causing mild irritation and apprehension but no apparent physical damage. The worms have been recovered from the lips, gingivae, palate, tonsils, and angle of the mouth. Human infection is apparently due to ingestion of infected insects, such as cockroaches or dung beetles, which are the intermediate hosts, or to drinking contaminated water.

gonia (go'ne-ah) plural of *gonion.*

gonial (go'ne-al) pertaining to the gonion.

gonio- [Gr. *gōnia* angle] a combining form denoting relationship to an angle.

goniometer (go"ne-om'ĕ-ter) [*gonio-* + Gr. *metron* measure] an instrument for measuring angles.

gonion (go'ne-on), pl. *go'onia* [Gr. *gōnia* angle] an anthropometric landmark located at the most inferior, posterior, and lateral point on the external angle of the mandible, being the apex of the maximum curvature of the mandible, where the ascending ramus becomes confluent with the corpus. Abbreviated *Go.* Called also *point Go.* See illustration at CEPHALOMETRY.

gono- [Gr. *gonē* seed] a combining form denoting relationship to semen or seed.

gonococcal (gon"o-kok'al) pertaining to gonococci.

gonococcemia (gon"o-kok-se'me-ah) [*gonococcus* + Gr. *haima* blood + *-ia*] the presence of gonococci in the blood.

gonococci (gon"o-kok'si) plural of *gonococcus.*

gonococcide (gon"o-kok'sīd) [*gonococcus* + L. *caedere* to kill] an agent that kills gonococci.

Gonococcus (gon"o-kok'us) [*gono-* + Gr. *kokkos* berry] *Neisseria gonorrhoeae;* see under NEISSERIA. **G. neisse'ri,** *Neisseria gonorrhoeae;* see under NEISSERIA.

gonococcus (gon"o-kok'us), pl. *gonococ'ci* [*gono-* + Gr. *kokkos* berry] any microorganism of the species *Neisseria gonorrhoeae,* the organism causing gonorrhea.

gonorrhea (gon"o-re'ah) [*gono-* + Gr. *rhein* to flow] an inflammatory bacterial disease of the mucous membrane of the urethra and genital tract caused by *Neisseria gonorrhoeae,* usually transmitted by sexual contact. In the male, the incubation period is about two to eight days, followed by dysuria and mucoid discharge from the urethra, which becomes purulent and profuse; symptoms subside after several weeks but a small amount of discharge persists. Urethral stricture, epididymitis, and sterility may follow. In females, the incubation period may be followed by an almost symptomless course, associated with minimal discharge. Advanced cases may be characterized by cervicitis with profuse discharge, abscesses, burning pain, blood and pus in the stools, salpingitis, adnexitis, and sterility. Complications may include perihepatitis, endocarditis, bacteremia, joint lesions, skin eruption, gonorrheal stomatitis, and gonococcal pharyngitis. Called also *blennorrhea.*

Good Samaritan a person who, like the Biblical Good Samaritan [Luke 10:30–37], compassionately renders assistance to the unfortunate. See also Good Samaritan LAW.

Goode see Younger-Goode CURET.

Gork (gork) originally, an acronym for "God only really knows," used by the hospital staff in connection with patients whose conditions defied diagnosis; now most commonly used in connection with patients who are comatose and are likely to remain so.

Gorlin's syndrome [Robert J. *Gorlin,* American dentist, oral pathologist, and geneticist] see under SYNDROME.

Gorlin-Chaudhry-Moss syndrome [R. J. *Gorlin;* Anand P.

Chaudhry; Melvin L. *Moss,* American dentist, born 1921] see under SYNDROME.

Gorlin-Goltz syndrome [R. J. *Gorlin;* Robert W. *Goltz,* American physician, born 1923] Gorlin's SYNDROME.

Gorlin-Holt syndrome [R. J. *Gorlin;* M. *Holt*] frontometaphyseal DYSPLASIA.

Goslee tooth [Hart J. *Goslee,* American dentist, 1871–1930] see under TOOTH.

gossypium (go-sip'ĕ-um) [L.] cotton. **g. asep'ticum, g. depura'tum, g. purifica'tum,** purified COTTON.

Gottinger's line see under LINE.

Gottlieb, Bernhard [Vienna dentist, 1885–1950] see epithelial ATTACHMENT (of Gottlieb).

Gottron, H. A. see Arndt-Gottron DISEASE.

Gougerot-Houwer-Sjögren [Henri *Gougerot,* French dermatologist, 1881–1955; A. W. M. *Houwer;* Henrik Samuel Conrad *Sjögren,* Swedish ophthalmologist, born 1899] Sjögren's SYNDROME.

Gougerot-Sjögren syndrome [H. *Gougerot;* Henrik Samuel Conrad *Sjögren,* Swedish ophthalmologist, born 1899] Sjögren's SYNDROME.

goundou (gōōn'doo) osteoplastic periosteitis of the nose, occurring as a sequal of yaws and seen most commonly in Central Africa and South America. It is characterized by headache, purulent nasal discharge, and the formation of symmetrical painless bony exostoses at the sides of the nose.

gout (gowt) [L. *gutta* a drop, because of the ancient belief that the disease was due to a "noxa" falling drop by drop into the joint] a metabolic disease caused by faulty uric acid metabolism, transmitted as a genetic trait (primary gout), or associated with certain hematopoietic disorders (secondary form). Attacks of painful arthritis due to deposits of urates in the joints, sometimes also involving the temporomandibular joint, are the principal feature. The characteristic gross lesion is a tophus, a focal deposit of chalky white urate, usually surrounded by a zone of inflammatory hyperemia. **juvenile g.,** Lesch-Nyhan SYNDROME. **rheumatic g., rheumatoid** ARTHRITIS.

GP general PRACTITIONER.

gr grain (2).

Gracey curets see under CURET.

Grad. abbreviation for L. *grada'tim,* by degrees.

Gradenigo syndrome [Giuseppe *Gradenigo,* Italian physician, 1859–1926] see under SYNDROME.

gradient (gra'dĕ-ent) the rate of increase or decrease of a variable magnitude; also the curve which represents it. **diffusion g.,** the gradient of the net rate of diffusion from the area of high concentration to the area of low concentration of a substance, being directly proportional to the larger concentration minus the lower concentration. Called also *concentration difference.*

graduate (grad'u-it) [L. *graduatus*] 1. a person who has received a degree from a university or college. 2. a measuring vessel marked by a series of lines.

GRAE generally recognized as effective; see under DRUG.

graft (graft) 1. to join, unite, or fasten by grafting. 2. to perform an operation of grafting. 3. any material or tissue that is not normally a part of an organ or tissue, implanted for the purpose of reconstructing or repairing. See also FLAP and IMPLANT. **accordion g.,** a full-thickness skin graft in which multiple slits have been made to allow it to be stretched to cover a larger area. **activated g.,** one in which the nerves and blood vessels have grown to nourish it, after a period of denervation and tenuous vascularity. **allogenic g., allogeneic g.,** a graft of tissue transplanted from a donor of the same species as the recipient, but having a different genotype. Called also *allograft* and *allogenic* or *allogeneic transplant.* See also *homologous g.* **allostatic g.,** a tissue graft intended to serve a temporary or mechanical function after transplantation so that continued viability of the tissue is not required. **allovital g.,** a tissue graft, e.g., kidney or skin, which must maintain its vitality to function normally after a transplantation. **autochthonous g., autogenous** g. **autodermic g., autoepidermic g.,** a skin graft taken from the patient's own body. **autogenous g., autologous g.,** a tissue graft transplanted from one site to another in the same individual. Called also *autochthonous g., autogenous transplant, autograft, autologous transplant, autoplast, autoplast,* and *autoplastic transplant.* See also AUTOPLASTY. **avascular g.,** a tissue graft in which not even transient vascularization is achieved. **bone g.,** a section of bone transplanted from one site to another in the same individual or from one individual (including cadaver) to another. Called also *osseous g.* and *bone transplant.* **bone g., onlay,** onlay bone g. **cartilage g's, diced,** diced cartilage g's. **congeneic g.,** isologous g. **cutis g.,** dermal g. **delayed g.,** a skin graft which is sutured back into its bed and subsequently

shifted to a new recipient bed. **dermal g., dermic g.,** skin from which epidermis and subcutaneous fat have been removed; used instead of fascia in various plastic procedures. Called also *cutis g.* **dermal-fat g.,** a composite graft of skin from which epidermis has been removed, and attached fat is used in various plastic procedures. **diced cartilage g's,** numerous small segments of cartilage that can be packed or molded into any desired contour like wet grains of sand; used to repair faulty cartilage of bone structure. **double papilla pedicle g.,** the use of the papillae on the mesial and distal sides of a tooth as a sliding graft that is joined over the tooth root with suture. **Douglas g.,** sieve g. **epidermic g.,** a piece of epidermis implanted upon a raw surface. Called also *Reverdin's g.* **fascia g.,** one taken from the fascia. **fascicular g.,** a nerve graft in which the bundles of nerve fibers are approximated and sutured separately. **fat g.,** a graft of fatty tissue completely freed from its bed; used in filling depressions. See also *filler g.* **filler g.,** one used for the filling of defects, as the filling of depressions with fatty tissue or of a bony cyst cavity with bone chips or diced cartilage. **free g.,** a tissue graft completely freed from its bed, in contrast with a flap. Called also *free transplant.* **full thickness g.,** a skin graft consisting of the full thickness of the skin, with little or none of the subcutaneous tissue. **full thickness periodontal g.,** a free graft consisting of the surface epithelium and connective tissue and the periosteum of the underlying bone. Called also *mucoperiosteal periodontal g.* See full thickness periododontal FLAP. **Gillies' g.,** rope FLAP. **graft-vs-host reaction,** graft-vs-host REACTION. **heterodermic g.,** a skin graft taken from a donor of a different species. **heterogenous g., heterologous g., heteroplastic g.,** a tissue graft transplanted from a donor of a different species than the host. Called also *xenogenic g., heterogenous transplant, heterograft, heterologous transplant,* and *xenograft.* **heterospecific g.,** a graft from or having specificity for a different species. **heterotopic g.,** a tissue graft transplanted into an anatomical site not normal for the tissue. **homogenous g., homologous g. homologous g., homoplastic g.,** a tissue graft transplanted from a donor of the same species as the recipient. A graft from a genetically identical donor is known as *isologous;* one from a genetically dissimilar donor of the same species is referred to as allogenic. Called also *homogenous g., homograft, homologous transplant, homoplast,* and *homoplastic transplant.* **homostatic g.,** a transplant which is progressively revitalized by the recipient tissue. Called also *homostatic transplant.* **homovital g.,** a vital transplant which retains its vitality after being grafted. Called also *homovital transplant.* **hyperplastic g.,** a skin graft which is in a state of active repair, as in recovery from inflammation. **iliac g.,** a bone graft whose donor site is the crest of the ilium, and may include associated portions of the lateral and superior aspects of the ilium. **implantation g.,** one in which small pieces of skin are embedded in granulation tissue of the same individual. Called also *seed g.* **isogeneic g.,** isologous g. **isologous g.,** 1. a tissue graft transplanted between genetically identical individuals, such as twins; transplantation of syngeneic or isogeneic tissue. See also *homologous g.* 2. a tissue graft transplanted between highly inbred animals, or between the F_1 hybrids produced by crossing inbred strains; transplantation of congeneic tissue. Called also *congeneic g., isogeneic g., syngeneic g., isogenic transplant, isograft, isologous transplant, syngenetic transplant,* and *syngraft.* **Kiel g.,** denatured calf bone used to fill defects or restore facial contour; used for chin and nasal augmentation. **mucosal g.,** one of mucosal tissue, usually comprising the entire mucosal thickness. **mucoperiosteal periodontal g.,** full thickness periodontal g. **mucosal periodontal g.,** split thickness periodontal g. **nerve g.,** replacement of an area of defective nerve with a segment from a sound one. **onlay bone g.,** bone used as a graft that is laid on or over cortical bone. **orthotopic g.,** a tissue graft transplanted into an anatomical site normal for the tissue. Called also *orthotopic transplant.* **osseous g.,** bone g. **papillary pedicle g.,** a sliding graft employing the gingival papilla as the graft material. **partial thickness periodontal g.,** split thickness periodontal g. **pedicle** FLAP. **periosteal g.,** a piece of periosteum applied to a denuded area of a bone. **pinch g.,** a piece of skin about ¼ in in diameter, obtained by elevating the skin with a needle and excising it with a knife. **g. rejection,** graft REJECTION. **Reverdin's g.,** epidermic g. **rope g.,** rope FLAP. **seed g.,** implantation g. **sieve g.,** a skin graft from which very small circular islands of skin are removed so that a larger denuded area can be covered, the sievelike portion being placed over one area, and the individual islands over surrounding or other denuded areas. Called also *Douglas' g.* **skin g.,** a piece of skin transplanted to replace a lost portion of the body skin surface; it may be a full thickness, thick-split, or split-skin graft. **split-skin g.,** a skin graft consisting of only a portion of the skin thickness. **split thickness g.,** a graft, varying in thickness, containing only mucosal elements and no subcutaneous tissues. **split thickness periodontal g.,** a free periodontal graft consisting of epithelium and a thin layer of the underlying connective tissue. Called also *mucosal periodontal g.* and *partial thickness periodontal g.* See also split thickness periodontal FLAP. **sponge g.,** a piece of sponge inserted into a wound to promote the formation of granulations. **syngeneic g.,** isologous g. **xenogenic g.,** heterogenous g.

grafting (graft'ing) the implanting or transplantation of a tissue or organ. See also TRANSPLANTATION.

Graham's law [Thomas *Graham,* Scottish chemist, 1805–1869] see under LAW.

grain (grān) [L. *granum*] 1. a seed, especially of a cereal plant. 2. a unit of weight in the metric system, being equivalent to 0.64789 grams. Abbreviated *gr.* See also *Tables of Weights and Measures* at WEIGHT. 3. crystal g. **apothecaries' g.,** a grain equivalent to 0.05 scruple, 0.0167 dram, or 0.0021 ounce. **avoirdupois g.,** a unit of weight, being 0.0366 dram or 0.00023 ounce. **g. boundary,** in the process of crystallization, a region of transition between the differently oriented space lattices of two neighboring grains which originate from two different nuclei and grow toward each other. The boundary region is more readily attacked by chemicals and is more prone to harbor impurities than the grain proper. See also *crystal g.* **columnar g.,** in the process of crystallization, a grain formed by heterogeneous nucleation, growing from the wall toward the center, such as one of a metal which had been cast in a cylindrical mold. **crystal g.,** a granular structure of a crystalline solid which forms from a solidification nucleus in a supercooled liquid and grows until the space is completely filled with crystals and the solid phase is achieved, collisions between the grains arresting their growth. Grains in a solid are separated from each other by grain boundaries, each grain having a separate space lattice. They are finer when the liquid to be crystallized is cooled rapidly than when it is cooled at a slower rate. Metals having smaller grains are stronger and more ductile than those with large grains; a large grain size increases the brittleness of a metal and reduces its strength. **equiaxial g.,** in the process of crystallization, a grain having the same diameter in all dimensions. **g. growth,** 1. in the process of crystallization, increase in the size of the grains through the process of dendrite development for crystal nuclei. See CRYSTALLIZATION. 2. in annealing, the merging of small grains to form larger ones. See metal ANNEALING. **pearl g.,** a unit of weight of precious stones, being equal to 0.25 metric carat. **radial g.,** in the process of crystallization, a grain formed by heterogeneous nucleation, growing perpendicularly in relation to the wall, such as one of a metal that had been cast in a square mold. **troy g.,** a grain equivalent to 0.042 pennyweight, or 0.002 ounce.

gram (gram) [Fr. *gramme*] a unit of mass (weight) in the metric system, being one-thousandth (10^{-3}) of a kilogram and equivalent to 0.03527 avoirdupois or 0.03215 troy and apothecary ounces, and 15.432 grains; 1000 milligrams make 1 gram. Abbreviated *g* or *gm.* See also *Tables of Weights and Measures* at WEIGHT. **g. calorie,** small CALORIE. **g. equivalent,** gram EQUIVALENT.

-gram [Gr. *gramma* that which is written, record] a word termination meaning that which is written or recorded.

Gram's method (staining) [Hans Christian *Gram,* Danish physician, 1853–1938] see under STAINING; see also gram-negative and gram-positive bacteria, under BACTERIUM.

Gramaxin trademark for *cefazolin sodium* (see under CEFAZOLIN).

gramicidin (gram″ĭ-si'din) a polypeptide antibiotic isolated from cultures of *Bacillus brevis,* believed to exist as chains of 15 amino acids, alternating D- and L- forms, comprising a mixture of gramicidins A, B, C, and D. Gramicidin A is the principal component, occurring as a white to off-white, odorless, crystalline powder that is soluble in alcohol, but not in water. It is active against gram-positive bacteria (except bacilli) and some gram-negative organisms, chiefly *Neisseria.* Used chiefly, in combination with polymyxin B and neomycin, in the treatment of wounds, ulcers, pyoderma, furuncles, conjunctivitis, rhinopharyngitis, and other superficial infections. Irrigation of para-

nasal sinuses with gramicidin solution may cause potentially fatal meningitis. It is a potent hemolytic agent, and, occasionally, anosmia and parosmia occur. Tyrothricin is a combination of gramicidin and tyrocidine. Trademarks: Gramoderm. **g. S, Soviet g.,** a cyclic decapeptide antibiotic isolated from cultures of a thermophilic strain of *Bacillus brevis,* having pharmacological and toxic properties similar to those of gramicidin.

gram-ion (gram-i'on) that quantity of an ion whose weight in grams is numerically equal to the atomic weight of the ion.

gram-meter (gram'me-ter) a unit of work representing the energy expended in raising 1 gm of weight 1 meter vertically against gravitational force at sea level. It is one-thousandth (10^{-3}) of a kilogram-meter, or about 98.000 ergs.

grammole (gram'mol) gram-molecule.

gram-molecule (gram-mol'ĕ-kūl) as many grams of a substance as are numerically equal to its molecular weight. Called also *grammole* and *molugram.* See also MOLE (3).

gram-negative (gram-neg'ah-tiv) see gram-negative bacteria, under BACTERIUM, and Gram's method, under STAINING.

Gramoderm trademark for *gramicidin.*

gram-positive (gram-poz'ĭ-tiv) see gram-positive bacteria, under BACTERIUM, and Gram's method, under STAINING.

gram-rad (gram'rad) a unit of work or energy equal to 100 ergs.

Grandry's corpuscles [French anatomist, 19th century] Merkel's corpuscles; see under CORPUSCLE.

Grandry-Merkel corpuscles [Friedrich Sigmund *Merkel,* German anatomist, 1845–1919] Merkel's corpuscles; see under CORPUSCLE.

Granger articulator see under ARTICULATOR.

Granger's line sign [Amedee *Granger,* New Orleans radiologist, 1879–1939] see under LINE and SIGN.

Grant's operation see under OPERATION.

granulatio (gran″u-la'she-o), pl. *granulatio'nes* [L.] [NA] a general term denoting a granule, or granular mass. **granulatio'nes arachnoidea'les** [NA], **granulatio'nes cerebra'les, granulatio'nes pacchio'ni,** arachnoidal granulations; see under GRANULATION.

granulation (gran″u-la'shun) [L. *granulatio*] 1. the formation in wounds of small, rounded, fleshy masses; also a mass so formed. 2. a small, round, abnormal mass of lymphoid tissue, as on the conjunctiva of the eyelids or within the pharynx. 3. the division of hard or metallic substances into small particles. **arachnoidal g's,** enlarged arachnoid villi, visible to the naked eye, projecting into the venous sinuses and creating slight depressions on the inner surface of the cranium. Called also *granulationes arachnoideales* [NA], *granulationes cerebrales, granulationes pacchioni,* and *pacchionian bodies.* **exuberant g.,** excessive proliferation of granulation tissue in the healing of a wound, which may protrude above the level of the skin. When the tissue becomes edematous, it is known as *proud flesh.*

granulationes (gran″u-la″she-o'nēz) [L.] plural of *granulatio.*

granule (gran'ul) [L. *granulum*] 1. a small particle or grain. 2. a small pill made from sucrose. **acidophil g's,** granules staining with acid dyes. **albuminous g's,** granules seen in the cytoplasm of many normal cells, which optically disappear on the addition of acetic acid, but are not affected by ether or chloroform. Called also cytoplasmic *g's.* **alpha g's,** 1. the coarse, highly refractive, eosinophil granules of leukocytes, which are composed of albuminous matter. Called also *eosinophil g's* and *oxyphil g's.* 2. acidophil granules in the cells of the pituitary gland. **amphophil g's,** beta g's. **azur g., azurophil g.,** a granule which stains easily with azure dyes; a coarse reddish granule seen in lymphocytes. Called also *hyperchromatin* and *kappa g.* **basophilic g.,** granules staining with basic dyes. **beta g's,** presecretion granules found in the pituitary gland and islands of Langerhans. Called also *amphophil g's.* **chromatic g's,** Nissl bodies; see under BODY. **cytoplasmic g's,** albuminous g's. **delta g's,** fine basophilic granules occurring in the lymphocytes. **eosinophil g's,** alpha g's (1). **epsilon g's,** neutrophil granules found in the protoplasm of polynuclear leukocytes. **fat g.,** lipid g. **Fordyce's g.,** ectopic sebaceous glands found on the lips and gums and in the mucosa of the cheeks in the form of yellowish-white milia. Called also *Fordyce's disease* and *Fordyce's spots.* **gamma g's,** basophilic granules found in the blood and marrow, and in the tissues. **glycogen g's,** irregularly shaped particles of glycogen, about 150 to 300 Å in diameter, which may be found individually or accumulated into groups of different sizes and shapes. Those found in groups form rosette configurations and are known as *alpha particles;* those occurring individually are known as *beta particles.* They may be stained with lead to intensify the color of glycogen. **Gravitz's g's,** minute granules seen in the erythrocytes in the basophilia of lead poisoning. **hyperchromatin g.,** azur g. **iodophil g's,** granules staining brown with iodine, seen in polymorphonuclear leukocytes in various acute infectious diseases. **kappa g.,** azur g. **keratohyalin g's, keratohyaline g's,** irregularly shaped granules of keratohyalin, found in the granular layer of the epidermis, which stain deeply with basic dyes and form keratin complexes with tonofilaments. See also KERATOHYALIN. **lipid g.,** a granule of fat that may be present in most cell types, usually occurring as a round and homogeneously textured particle of various size, usually being coalesced with adjacent ones when crowded. Called also *fat g., fat particle,* and *lipid particle.* **lipofuscin g.,** an irregularly shaped, yellow to bronze granule of variable size found in some muscle and nerve fibers; its membrane forms an outer boundary of the granule, adhering closely to the material it houses. **melanin g's,** coarse yellowish-brown to black pigment granules containing melanin, found in the melanocytes. **Nissl g's,** Nissl bodies; see under BODY. **oxyphil g's,** alpha g's (1). **pigment g's,** small pigment-bearing granules occurring in pigment cells, such as melanin granules. **protein g's,** microscopically observable particles of various proteins found in a variety of cells. See also crystalline PARTICLE. **secretory g's, secretion g's,** granules consisting of materials formed by the ribosomes and routed to the Golgi apparatus for further processing. They are usually spheroid but may be misshapen when closely packed and their size and density are variable, smaller ones being close to the Golgi component and the larger ones being nearer the secreting surface. Release of the granule is accomplished by a simultaneous fusion and rupture of the limiting membrane at the contact point of the granule with the cell membrane. The process involves the incorporation of the granule's membrane with that of the cell so that the continuity of the latter is not lost. See also *zymogen g's.* **sphere g.,** a large granular cell or corpuscle seen in serous exudation. **toxic g's,** basophilic, cytoplasmic granules originally thought to be present in leukocytes only during infections or other toxic states, but later found to occur in the absence of systemic toxicity, probably representing developmentally anomalous lysosomes. **zymogen g's,** secretory granules in certain cells, containing the precursors of enzymes that become active after they have left the cell.

granuliform (gran′u-lĭ-form) in the form of, or resembling, small grains.

granulo- [L. *granulum* granule] a combining form denoting a relationship to a granule(s).

granuloadipose (gran″u-lo-ad′ĭ-pōs) pertaining to fatty or lipid granules.

granuloblast (gran′u-lo-blast) an embryonic blood cell developing into a granulocyte.

granulocyte (gran′u-lo-sīt) [*granulo-* + Gr. *kytos* hollow vessel] 1. any cell containing granules. 2. a leukocyte produced by the bone marrow and containing granules in the cytoplasm. An immature granulocyte is known as a *myeloblast* and contains fewer than 10 granules. Later, when the centrosome becomes filled with granules, it is known as a *myelocyte.* At this stage, the cell undergoes mitosis and its nucleus shows polymorphism, assuming a horseshoe or sausage shape and dividing into two lobes. The average maturation time is about 3 to 4 days. Mature granulocytes with heterophilic (neutrophilic in man) granules are known as *heterophils* and *neutrophils;* those with basophilic granules are known as *basophils;* and those with eosinophilic granules are known as *eosinophils.* **acidophilic g.,** eosinophil. **basophilic g.,** basophil (2). **eosinophilic g.,** eosinophil. **neutrophilic g.,** neutrophil (1).

granuloma (gran″u-lo′mah) [L. *granulatio* granulation + *-oma*] a tumor-like mass or nodule of granulation tissue (actively growing fibroblasts and capillary buds), due to an inflammatory reaction to an infection, such as syphilis or tuberculosis, or invasion by a nonliving foreign body. The term is often restricted to a small (1 to 2 mm) collection of modified macrophages or histiocytes almost invariably surrounded by a rim of mononuclear cells. **g. annula′re,** a granuloma consisting of hard, reddish nodules arranged in a circle which enlarge until they form a ring. **apical g.,** a slowly expanding, spherical, granulomatous lesion adjacent to the root apex of a tooth, usually occurring as a complication of pulpitis. It consists of a proliferating mass of chronic inflammatory tissue made up of new blood vessels, proliferating connective tissue with predominance of plasma cells along with lymphocytes, histiocytes, and polymorphonuclear leukocytes, enclosed within a fibrous capsule which is an extension of the periodontal ligament. Hyperemia, edema, and inflammation of the apical periodontal ligament are its principal features, and increased vascularity and resorption of the supporting bone, sometimes also involving the root, may be associated. Mild pain on biting and sensitivity to percussion are the chief symptoms, but many cases are asymptomatic. Bone resorption may cause the radiographic appearance of localized apical radiolucency. Called also *chronic apical g., dental g., periapical g., apical periodontitis, apical chronic periodontitis,* and *chronic apical periodontitis.* **benign g. of thyroid,** chronic inflammation of the thyroid gland that changes into a bulky tumor which later becomes very hard. **beryllium g.,** a local sarcoid-like reaction in the skin caused by accidental implantation of a beryllium compound. **candida g.,** a horny or heavily crusted nodule on the scalp, face, finger, mucous membrane, and other parts of the body, seen in persistent cases of candidiasis. **central giant cell g., central giant cell reparative g., and central reparative g.,** a controversial lesion of the jaws considered by some authorities to be a giant cell tumor occurring in both benign and malignant forms, and by others as a form of osteogenic sarcoma, varying in degree of malignancy. Most authorities consider it to be a central lesion of the bone of the jaws, presenting an inflammatory reaction of injury or hemorrhage, which is not regarded as a true neoplasm. The affected bone may be enlarged and deformed, but penetration of the cortical plate is uncommon. Loosening and resorption of the teeth may be associated. The lesion is composed of a spindle cell stroma punctuated by multinucleate giant cells. Foci of old extravasated blood hemosiderin pigment and foci of trabeculae of osteoid bone are often present. Called also *central giant cell lesion.* **cholesterol g.,** a granulomatous lesion in which crystals of cholesterol esters are surrounded by foreign body giant cells in a mass of fibrotic granulation tissue. **chronic apical g.,** apical g. **coccidioidal g.,** coccidioidomycosis. **dental g.,** apical g. **eosinophilic g.,** a nonlipid reticuloendotheliosis, a form of histiocytosis X, usually occurring in the late teens and early adult life, marked by the accumulation of histiocytes and eosinophils. Typically, it is characterized by a solitary or, less frequently, multiple lesions, usually arising in the bone marrow. The jaws and the skull are the most common sites, but the ribs and other bones also may be involved. Lesions are destructive and perforate the cortex; destroyed areas are replaced by soft tissue. Early lesions are soft and brown, without necrosis; later the tissue becomes fibrous and grayish. Swelling and ulceration of the gingivae around loose teeth are the most common oral symptoms. General malaise and fever may occur. Roentgenologically, the lesion may appear as irregular radiolucent areas and the involved teeth appear to "float" in soft tissue. Multiple areas of rarefaction, sometimes suggesting cysts of the jaws, periapical granulomas, or periodontal diseases, are common. Pathological fractures may be present. Sheets of histiocytes, some containing drops of fat or debris are the principal histiological features. The early lesions contain large numbers of eosinophils; mature lesions are marked by fibrosis and, sometimes, xanthomatosis, with a smaller number of eosinophils. **g. fissura′tum,** a circumscribed, firm, reddish, fissured, fibrotic granuloma of the gum and buccal mucosa, occurring on an edentulous alveolar ridge and in the fold between the ridge and cheek; it is caused by an ill-fitting denture. **foreign-body g.,** a localized histiocytic reaction of the skin to a foreign body in the tissue, such as starch, talc, or oil. **g. gangraenes′cens,** a condition beginning with the formation of proliferating granulations in the nasal mucous membrane which invade the adjacent tissue and soon become gangrenous. **giant cell reparative g., central,** central giant cell g. **giant cell reparative g., peripheral,** giant cell EPULIS. **Hodgkin's g.,** Hodgkin's DISEASE. **infectious g.,** one caused by infection with pathogenic microorganisms. **g. inguin′ale,** g. venereum. **internal pulp g.,** tooth resorption, internal; see under RESORPTION. **laryngeal g.,** a firm nodule on the larynx due to trauma, particularly from endotracheal intubation or from excessive use of the voice. **lethal g.,** lethal midline g. **lethal midline g.,** a disease considered to be a variant of polyarteritis nodosa, characterized by granulomatous lesions of the nasal mucosa, sinuses, and pharynx. Massive, progressive, ulcerative lesions that destroy the involved tissue, including bones, are typical; they sometimes extend to the brain, and result in death. Histologically, it is characterized by minimal vascular changes, and by the presence of lymphocytes and bizarre reticulum cells. Thrombosis and necrosis are usually associated. Considered by some to be identical with *Wegener's granulomatosis.* Called also *lethal* and *midline lethal g.* **lipoid g.,** a granuloma containing lipoid cells; xanthoma. **malignant g.,** Hodgkin's DISEASE. **midline lethal g.,** lethal midline g. **paracoccidioidal g.,** South American BLASTOMYCOSIS. **periapical g.,** apical g. **periapical tuberculous g.,** periapical TUBERCULOMA. **peripheral giant cell g., peripheral giant cell reparative g.,** giant cell EPULIS. **plasma cell g.,** one in which other inflammatory cells are greatly outnumbered by plasma cells. **pulse g.**, a foreign body granuloma of the alveolar ridge caused by food fragments entering tissue through a postextraction socket, especially of the mandible, or through other defects, such as an open root canal or a periodontal pocket. Its principal components are circular or slightly ellipsoid bodies about 100 μ in diameter, each of which is made up of a cluster of several starch granules. Called also *giant-cell hyalin angiopathy.* **pyogenic g., g. pyogen'icum,** a solitary, soft, raised, sometimes pedunculated, dull red nodule that occurs as a response to a nonspecific infection precipitated by trauma, and usually reaches a size ranging from ½ to 2 cm in diameter in about a week. It may appear anywhere on the body but is most common on the skin and mucous membrane at the site of trauma. Oral lesions arise most frequently at the gingiva, but may be found on the lips, tongue, and buccal mucosa. A typical lesion is made up of newly formed capillaries, endothelial proliferation, and a nonspecific inflammatory infiltrate, often containing neutrophilic leukocytes, presenting a benign tumor of blood vessels or an overgrowth of granulation tissue. Some lesions show a tendency to hemorrhage. In spite of the name, pus formation is not a constant feature. Called also *septic g.* See also EPULIS granulomatosa, pregnancy GINGIVITIS, and pregnancy TUMOR. **reparative g.,** peripheral, giant cell EPULIS. **septic g.,** pyogenic g. **g. telangiectat'icum,** one characterized by numerous dilated blood vessels. **tuberculous g.,** tuberculoma. **g. vene'reum,** a granulomatous venereal disease caused by *Calymmatobacterium granulomatis,* which is most prevalent in the tropics, and affects chiefly the genital area, but extragenital organs, including the oral cavity, may be involved. Typical primary lesions are papules or nodules that ulcerate to form granular masses with rolled margins, which tend to enlarge and metastasize through the lymphatics. Inguinal ulcerations are the most common secondary lesions. Oral lesions may result as a secondary infection through autoinoculation or as a result of genital-oral contact, and may occur on any part of the mucosa of the mouth or lips, and are usually of the ulcerative, exuberant, or cicatricial type; they may include painful, sometimes bleeding, ulcers, proliferative granular masses with an intact epithelial covering, or edematous inflamed lesions covered by extensive fibrous scars. Histologically, the disease is marked by granulation tissue with infiltration of polymorphonuclear leukocytes and plasma cells. Typically, there are large mononuclear phagocytes containing minute intracytoplasmic cysts within which profuse numbers of the etiologic agent are found. Called also *g. inguinale* and *pudendal ulcer.*

granulomatosis (gran"u-lo"mah-to'sis) the formation of multiple granulomas. **g. benig'na,** sarcoidosis. **cholesterol g.,** Hand-Schüller-Christian DISEASE. **malignant g.,** Hodgkin's DISEASE. **necrotizing respiratory g.,** Wegener's g. **Wegener's g.,** a disease considered to be a variant of polyarteritis nodosa, characterized by the presence of granulomatous lesions in the larynx, trachea, kidneys, and lungs. Pathologic changes include necrotizing vasculitis, granulomatous masses, inflammatory cell infiltrates, and eosinophilic infiltrates. Oral lesions are not common, but when present include painful granulomatous lesions of the gingivae that involve the interdental papillae. Considered by some to be identical with *lethal midline granuloma.* Called also *necrotizing respiratory g.* and *rhinogenic polyarteritis.*

granulomere (gran'u-lo-mēr) [*granulo-* + Gr. *meros* part] the center portion of a blood platelet in dry smears stained with Romanovskii's stain, filled with purple granules. Called also *chromomere.* See also HYALOMERE.

granulosis (gran"u-lo'sis) the formation of a mass of granules. See also GRANULOMA. **g. ru'bra na'si,** a skin disease of the nose, which sometimes extends to the cheeks, marked by a bright red color of the part, over which are scattered reddish specks and papules. It is associated with hyperhidrosis of the area, and is due to chronic inflammation around the sweat glands.

grape (grāp) the fruit of numerous woody vines of the genus *Vitis.* **g. sugar,** dextrose.

graph (graf) [Gr. *graphein* to write, or record] 1. a diagram or curve representing varying relationships between sets of data. 2. a word termination denoting an instrument for writing or recording.

graphic (graf'ik) [Gr. *graphein* to write] written down; pertaining to representation by diagrams.

grapho- [Gr. *graphein* to record] a combining form denoting relationship to writing or to a record.

-graphy [Gr. *graphein* to write] a word termination meaning the act of writing or recording, or a method of recording.

GRAS generally recognized as safe; see under DRUG.

Gräsbeck, Ralph [Finnish physician] see Imerslung-Gräsbeck SYNDROME.

grasp (grasp) 1. to seize and hold firmly with or as if with the hand. 2. the act of seizing and holding; clasping. **modified pen g.,** a method of holding a dental instrument in which the thumb and second finger engage it at a point approximately 1 inch above the shank-handle junction. The shank rests against the side of the third finger opposite the ball of the finger, which is used as a finger rest and fulcrum and to guide the direction of the instrument. **palm and thumb g.,** a method of holding a dental instrument in which its handle is held in the cupped second, third, and fourth fingers, with the ball of the thumb at the junction of the handle and the shank. The thumb acts as a fulcrum as the blade engages the tooth surface, and the handle of the instrument is activated by a coordinated movement of the forearm, wrist, and cupped fingers. **pen g.,** a method of holding a dental instrument as if it were a pen, between the thumb and second and third fingers, at the junction of the shank and the handle of the instrument. The shank rests against the side of the pad of the third finger and the instrument is activated by a rolling motion by rotating the forearm and wrist with a steady finger rest as a fulcrum.

grave (grāv) [L. *gravis*] severe or serious.

gravel (grav'el) a term applied to fairly coarse concretions of mineral salts, as from the kidneys or bladder, of smaller size than the so-called stones. See also SIALOLITHIASIS.

Graves' disease [Robert James *Graves,* Irish physician, 1796–1853] exophthalmic GOITER.

gravida (grav'ĭ-dah) [L.] a pregnant woman. Called *gravida I* or *primigravida* during the first pregnancy, *gravida II* or *secundigravida* during the second pregnancy, and *gravida III* or *tertigravida* during the third pregnancy.

gravity (grav'ĭ-te) 1. the attractive force of the earth by which the terrestrial bodies are attracted to or tend to fall toward the center of the earth. 2. weight. **specific g.,** the weight of a substance compared with that of an equal volume of another substance, such as water, taken as a standard. It is calculated as the ratio of the density of the material to the density of water.

Gravitz's granules [Paul Albert *Gravitz,* German pathologist, 1850–1932] see under GRANULE.

gray (gra) a proposed unit of absorbed radiation dose equal to 1 joule/k or to 100 rads. Symbol *gy.*

green (grēn) 1. having the color of fresh leaves or of grass, between yellow and blue in the spectrum. 2. a green coloring matter or dye. **anadonis g., chrome g., g. cinnabar, leaf g., oil g., g. oxide of chromium, g. rouge, ultramarine g.,** chromic OXIDE.

Greene-Vermillion index oral hygiene index, simplified; see under INDEX.

Greenfield's disease [J. G. *Greenfield*] metachromatic LEUKODYSTROPHY.

Greenwood, Isaac, Sr. [1730–1803] the first American-born dentist, who was the first to use the dental foot engine made from a spinning wheel, and was the first in America to use models in dental prostheses. He served as a dentist to George Washington.

Greenwood, John [1760–1817] an American dentist who observed that dental decay is due to chemical and bacteriological factors. He served as a dentist to George Washington.

Greppi, Enrico see THALASSEMIA minor (Rietti-Greppi-Micheli syndrome).

GRG glycine-rich glycoprotein; see FACTOR B.

grid (grid) 1. a grating. 2. a chart with horizontal and perpendicular lines for plotting. 3. in radiology, a device consisting of thin lead strips interspaced with radiolucent material, used to reduce (absorb) scattered radiation that causes undesired density of the x-ray image. **aligned g.,** focused g. **Bucky-Potter g.,** Bucky's DIAPHRAGM. **crossed g's,** in radiology, grids usually constructed as two parallel grids, one being placed directly above the other so that the lead strips of the upper grid are at right angles to those of the lower one. **focused g.,** in radiology, one in which the lead foils are placed at an angle so that they all point toward a focus at a specified distance. Called also *aligned g.* **linear g.,** parallel g. **moving g.,** one which is moved continuously or oscillated throughout the making of a radiograph. **parallel g.,** in radiology, one in which lead strips are oriented parallel to each other. Called also *linear g.* **g. ratio,** grid RATIO. **stationary g.,** one placed in apposition to a roentgenographic film for its accentuation of detail, the grid lines being visible on the resultant image.

Griffin appliance [E. M. *Griffin,* American dentist] see under APPLIANCE.

Grifulvin trademark for *griseofulvin.*

grinding (grīnd'ing) 1. rubbing together with force; wearing away or polishing by rubbing. 2. in mastication, crushing of food by the posterior teeth, especially by molars. 3. bruxism. 4. shaping of a tooth contour through the use of abrasive tools. See also occlusal ADJUSTMENT. **habitual g., nonfunctional g.,** eccentric BRUXISM. **selective g.,** the modification of the occlusal forms of teeth by grinding at selected places marked by spots made by articulating paper. See also MILLING-IN. **spot g.,** elimination of high spots or occlusal interferences on natural dentitions or dentures by grinding.

grinding-in (grind'ing-in) the process of correcting errors in the centric and eccentric occlusion of natural or artificial teeth. See also MILLING-IN.

Grip cement see under CEMENT.

Grisactin trademark for griseofulvin.

Grisel's disease [P. Grisel] nasopharyngeal TORTICOLLIS.

griseofulvin (gris"e-o-ful'vin) a fungistatic antibiotic, (2S-trans)-7 - chloro - 2', 4, 6 - trimethoxy - 6' - methylspiro [benzofuran-2(3H),1' - [2]cyclohexene] - 3,4' - dione, elaborated by Penicillium griseofulvum and other species of fungi. It occurs as a white, odorless powder that is soluble in acetone and chloroform, sparingly soluble in alcohol, and very sparingly soluble in water. Used in the treatment of superficial infections with certain fungi. Infrequent side reactions, including skin rash, leukopenia, granulocytopenia, serum sickness, angioneurotic edema, and other hypersensitivity reactions may occur. Called also Curling factor. Trademarks: Fulcin, Fulvicin, Grifulvin, Grisactin, Spirofulvin, Sporostatin.

Grn green; see color coding table at root canal THERAPY.

Grob's syndrome [Max Grob, Swiss physician] see oral-facial-digital SYNDROME (1).

groove (grōōv) 1. a shallow linear depression; a furrow, especially one appearing during embryonic development or persisting in definitive bones. See also FISSURE, FURROW, and SULCUS. 2. a developmental linear channel or furrow on a tooth surface. See illustration at TOOTH. **abutment g.,** a transverse groove cut in the bone across the remnants of the alveolar ridge under the abutment to countersink the primary strut level with the bone surface. It is provided to furnish positive lateral seating for a subperiosteal implant and thus increase lateral resistance. **alveolingual g.,** the groove between the lower jaw and the tongue. **anterior palatine g.,** incisive CANAL. **arterial g's,** arterial sulci; see under SULCUS. **basilar g. of occipital bone,** CLIVUS ossis occipitalis. **basilar g. of sphenoid bone,** CLIVUS ossis sphenoidalis. **branchial g.,** any of the ectodermal inpocketings of the pharyngeal portion of the foregut that separate the branchial arches. They appear during the fourth week of life and are drawn into the branchial ducts during the sixth week. Called also branchial furrow. See illustration and table at branchial arches, under ARCH. **buccal g., buccal developmental g.,** a groove on the buccal surface of a posterior tooth. Abbreviated BDG. See also distobuccal g. and mesiobuccal g. **carotid g. of sphenoid bone, cavernous g. of sphenoid bone,** carotid SULCUS. **central g., central developmental g.,** a groove in the central part of the occlusal surface of bicuspid and first molar teeth. Abbreviated CDG. **chiasmatic g.,** optic g. **dental g., primitive,** a groove in the border of the jaw of the embryo. **developmental g's,** fine grooves or lines marking the fusion area between adjacent cusps, named according to the portion of the crown which they connect. Called also developmental lines and segmental lines. **digastric g.,** mastoid NOTCH. **distobuccal g., distobuccal developmental g.,** the distal of the two buccal grooves ordinarily found on the mandibular first molar. Abbreviated DBDG. **distolingual g., distolingual developmental g.,** the distal of the lingual grooves of the bicuspid and maxillary molar teeth. Abbreviated DLG. **ethmoidal g.,** ethmoidal sulcus of nasal bone; see under SULCUS. **g. for eustachian tube,** SULCUS of auditory tube. **gingival g., free,** a shallow groove on the vestibular surface of the gingiva, running parallel to the margin of the gingiva at a distance of 0.5 to 1.5 mm and usually at the level of, or somewhat apical to, the bottom of the gingival crevice. **g. of great superficial petrosal nerve,** SULCUS of greater petrosal nerve. **hamular g.,** SULCUS of pterygoid hamulus. **infraorbital g. of maxilla,** infraorbital sulcus of maxilla; see under SULCUS. **interdental g.,** a linear, vertical depression on the surface for the egress of food from the interproximal areas. **labial g.,** an embryonic groove produced by degeneration of the central cells of the vestibular lamina, which later becomes the vestibule of the oral cavity. **labiomental g.,** a horizontal furrow just above the chin; it separates the lower lip from the chin. Called also mentolabial furrow. **lacrimal g.,** a notch on the median edge of the orbital surface of the maxilla, formed by the lacrimal sulcus of the lacrimal bone, which lodges the lacrimal sac. Called also fossa of lacrimal sac and fossa sacci lacrimalis [NA]. **g. of lacrimal bone,** lacrimal sulcus of lacrimal bone; see

under SULCUS. **lingual g., lingual developmental g.,** a groove on the lingual surface of a posterior tooth. Abbreviated LDG. See also distolingual g. and mesiolingual g. **mesiobuccal g., mesiobuccal developmental g.,** the mesial of the two buccal grooves ordinarily found on the mandibular first molar. Abbreviated MBDG. **mesiolingual g., mesiolingual developmental g.,** a groove marking the junction of the fifth cusp with the palatal surface on upper molar tooth. Abbreviated MLG. **occlusal g.,** one of the developmental grooves on the occlusal surface of the posterior teeth. **lacrimal g. of Verga,** Verga's lacrimal g. **laryngotracheal g.,** a furrow at the caudal end of the embryonic pharynx that develops into the respiratory tract. **lateral g. for lateral sinus of occipital bone,** SULCUS of transverse sinus of occipital bone. **lateral g. for lateral sinus of parietal bone,** SULCUS of sigmoid sinus of parietal bone. **lateral g. for sigmoidal part of lateral sinus,** SULCUS of sigmoid sinus of temporal bone. **medullary g.,** neural g. **g. for middle temporal artery,** SULCUS for middle temporal artery. **mylohyoid g. of inferior maxillary bone, mylohyoid g. of mandible,** mylohyoid sulcus of mandible; see under SULCUS. **nasal g., g. for nasal nerve,** ethmoidal sulcus of nasal bone; see under SULCUS. **nasolabial g.,** nasolabial SULCUS. **nasolacrimal g.,** an epithelial ingrowth parallel with but medial to the nasomaxillary groove of the embryo, which marks the site of later development of the nasolacrimal duct. **nasomaxillary g.,** a furrow located between the maxillary and the lateral nasal process of the same side in the embryo. **nasopalatine g.,** a furrow on the lateral surface of the vomer which lodges the nasopalatine nerve and vessels. **nasopharyngeal g.,** a faint line between the nasal cavity and the nasopharynx. **neural g.,** the groove produced by the folding of the neural plate. It is bounded on each side by elevated neural folds which continue to thicken until they fuse, thus forming the neural tube which evolves into the brain and the spinal cord in the embryonic development. Called also medullary g. **occipital g.,** SULCUS of occipital artery. **olfactory g.,** ethmoid FOSSA. **optic g.,** a furrow on the intracranial surface of the body of the sphenoid bone, located just anterior to the tuberculum sellae, ending on either side of the optic foramen. It lodges the optic chiasm. Called also chiasmatic g., sulcus of chiasm, sulcus chiasmatis [NA], and optic sulcus. **palatine g. of maxilla,** palatine sulcus of maxilla; see under SULCUS. **palatine g. of palatine bone, palatomaxillary g. of palatine bone,** greater palatine sulcus of palatine bone; see under SULCUS. **postmental g.,** one running below the chin; it is observed more commonly in women than in men and becomes more pronounced with age. **primitive g.,** a narrow trench or furrow along the midline of the primitive streak of the embryo, which appears during the third week of development. **pterygopalatine g. of pterygoid plate,** a small groove situated in the line of fusion of the medial and lateral pterygoid plates of the sphenoid bone. Called also sulcus pterygopalatinus processus pterygoidei [NA]. **retention g.,** one formed by opposing vertical constriction in the tooth, providing a horseshoe-shaped grip on the tooth. **sigmoid g. of temporal bone,** SULCUS of sigmoid sinus of temporal bone. **g. of small superficial petrosal nerve,** SULCUS of lesser petrosal nerve. **g. for superior longitudinal sinus,** sagittal sulcus of parietal bone; see under SULCUS. **supplemental g.,** one on the surface of a tooth, which is supplemental to the developmental groove and does not mark the junction between the primary lobes. **venous g's,** venous sulci; see under SULCUS. **Verga's lacrimal g.,** a groove running downward from the lower orifice of the nasal duct. Called also lacrimal g. of Varga.

grooving (grōōv'ing) in occlusal adjustment, the restoration of the depth of developmental grooves made shallow by occlusal wear, usually done with a tapered diamond point.

gross (grōs) [L. grossus rough] coarse or large; visible to the naked eye, as gross pathology; macroscopic; taking no account of minutiae.

Grotthus' law see under LAW.

ground (grownd) 1. the solid surface of the earth. 2. earth or soil. 3. an electrical connection with the earth or any large conducting body used as a common return for the electrical circuit, and as an arbitrary zero of potential.

group (grōōp) 1. an assemblage of objects having certain things in common. 2. a number of persons being together or having something in common. **actinide g., actinium g., actinoid g.,** actinium SERIES. **antigenic determinant g.,** see antigenic DETERMINANT. **contracting g.,** a group of persons who are eligible to receive certain benefits, such as dental health services under a health insurance plan. **functional g.,** in chemistry, the atom or group of atoms that defines the structure of a particular class of compounds and determines its properties. **haptophore g.,** see HAPTOPHORE. **g. insurance,** group INSURANCE. **lanthanide g., lanthanoid g., lanthanum g.,** rare EARTH. **receptor g.,** that portion of the receptor molecule with which an agonist acts and which is vital to its function. See also drug RECEPTOR.

growth (grōth) 1. in multicellular organisms, a normal process of increase in size as a result of cellular proliferation and development accompanying extracellular structures. 2. an abnormal formation, such as a tumor. 3. the proliferation of cells, as in a bacterial or tissue culture. **appositional g.,** growth by apposition of new layers of tissues or cells on the surface of an organ or part. In bone growth, this is accomplished by the perichondrium which constantly differentiates into chondrocytes and secretes a matrix, thus building new layers on the surface of a cartilage. See also APPOSITION. **condylar g.,** the growth of the condyle of the temporomandibular joint, usually reflected in a downward and forward positioning of the mandible and teeth. **grain g.,** GRAIN growth. **interstitial g.,** growth occurring in the interior of parts or structures already formed. **new g.,** a neoplasm.

Gruber, petrospheno-occipital suture of [V. L. *Gruber,* Russian anatomist, 1814–1890] petro-occipital FISSURE.

Gruenberg symmetroscope see under SYMMETROSCOPE.

Grutz, O. see HYPERLIPOPROTEINEMIA I (Burger-Grutz syndrome).

GSD genetically significant DOSE.

gt. abbreviation for L. *gut'ta,* drop.

gtt. abbreviation for L. *gut'tae,* drops.

guaiac (gwi′ak) a resin from the wood of *Guajacum officinale* and *G. sanctum,* trees of Haiti and the Dominican Republic; used as a reagent in tests for occult blood and formerly in the treatment of rheumatism. It is a source of guaiacol.

guaiacol (gwi′ah-kol) a phenolic compound, 2-methoxyphenol, isolated from guaiac resin. It occurs as a white or yellowish crystalline solid or a yellowish refractive liquid with a characteristic aromatic odor, which darkens on exposure to light or air, and is slightly soluble in water, readily soluble in alcohol and glycerol, and miscible with chloroform, ether, oils, and glacial acetic acid. Used as an expectorant and as an antiseptic and germicidal agent in alleviation of postextraction pain and in some analgesic ointments. Called also *methylcatechol.*

guanethidine (gwan-eth′ĭ-dēn) an adrenergic neuron blocking agent, [2-(hexahydro-1(2*H*)-azocinyl)ethyl]guanidine, which partially depletes the adrenergic nerves of their norepinephrine and prevents the release of the remainder. It occurs as a white, crystalline powder with a strong odor, which is soluble in water, slightly soluble in alcohol, and insoluble in chloroform. Usually used in the form of the sulfate or monosulfate salt, most commonly used as an antihypertensive drug. In dentistry, it is used chiefly as a vasoconstrictor agent in local anesthesia, in gingival retraction, and to control postoperative bleeding. Orthostatic hypotension, vertigo, weakness, nausea, syncope, bradycardia, stuffy nose, xerostomia, diarrhea, urinary incontinence, failure of ejaculation, fatigue, and dyspnea are the principal side effects. Trademarks: Anapresin, Dopom, Eutensol, Ismelin, Octatensine, Oktadin, Sanotensin.

guanine (gwan′ēn) a purine constituent of DNA and RNA, 2-amino-6-oxypurine, occurring as colorless rhombic crystals that are readily soluble in ammonia water, potassium hydroxide solution, alcohol, and ether. It is found in guano, fish scales, leguminous seedlings, and animal tissues. Used in biochemical research. **g. riboside,** guanosine.

guanosine (gwan′o-sēn) a nucleoside, 2-amino-9-β-D-ribofuranosyl-9-*H*-purine-6(1*H*)-one, which is a component of nucleic acids and may be obtained from yeast nucleic acids. Used in biochemical research. Called also *guanine riboside.* **g. triphosphate,** an energy-rich compound similar to adenosine triphosphate, involved in several metabolic reactions, e.g., the formation of peptide bonds in protein synthesis and of an intermediate in purine synthesis.

guaranine (gwah-rah′nēn) caffeine.

guard (gahrd) a protective device. **bite g.,** occlusal g. **mouth g.,** an intraoral appliance, made of a soft plastic, which covers all occlusal surfaces and the palate and extends to the border of the attached gingiva on the vestibular surface of the teeth. Used for preventing lacerations of the lips and cheeks during contact sports. **night g.,** occlusal g. **occlusal g.,** a removable dental appliance usually constructed of plastic, which covers one or both dental arches, designed to minimize the damaging effect of bruxism and other occlusal habits, being usually worn at night. Called also *bite g.* and *night g.* See also occlusal SPLINT.

Gubler's line, hemiplegia, paralysis [Adolphe Marie *Gubler,* French physician, 1821–1879] see under LINE, and see Millard-Gubler SYNDROME.

Guérin's fracture [Alphonse François Marie *Guérin,* French surgeon, 1816–1895] Le Fort fracture I; see under FRACTURE.

Guérin-Stern syndrome [Jules René *Guérin,* 1811–1896; W. G. *Stern*] see under SYNDROME.

guidance (gīd′ans) the process of leading or directing a person toward a desired goal, or controlling or steering an object on a predetermined course or tract. **anterior g.,** incisal GUIDE. **condylar g.,** the path that the horizontal rotation axis of the condyles travels during normal mandibular opening, measured in degrees as related to the Frankfort Horizontal plane. It also influences mandibular movements from the temporomandibular joint, articular guidance, or condylar elements. Called also *condylar guide.* See also condylar guidance INCLINATION. **cuspid g.,** the occlusal contact relationship of the cuspid teeth in eccentric relationships, being the contact guidance between the cuspid teeth in lateral mandibular movements and between the maxillary cuspid and the first mandibular premolar teeth in protrusive movements. Complete bilateral cuspid guidance occurs only in a small segment of the population. **incisal g.,** the influence on mandibular movements of the lingual surfaces of the maxillary anterior teeth.

guide (gīd) a device by which another object is led in its proper course. **adjustable anterior g.,** anterior g., adjustable. **anterior g.,** that part of an articulator on which the anterior guide pin rests to maintain the vertical dimension of occlusion. It influences the degree of separation of the casts in eccentric relationship. **anterior g., adjustable,** an anterior guide, the superior surface of which may be varied to provide desired separation of the casts in various eccentric relationships. **condylar g.,** condylar GUIDANCE. **G. to Dental Materials and Devices,** a publication of the Council on Dental Materials and Devices of the American Dental Association, containing descriptions, evaluations, and standards for materials and devices, as well as some techniques, used in dental practice. Listed in the Guide are those products which have been evaluated and found as safe and useful and conforming to standards, as determined under the acceptance and certification programs of the Council. **incisal g.,** that part of an articulator which maintains the incisal guide angle. Called also *anterior guidance.* See also incisal guide ADJUSTMENT.

guideline (gīd′līn) 1. any line used as a marker or indicator. 2. a set of standards or criteria to be followed in performing certain tasks. **clasp g.,** survey LINE (3). **health care g's,** flexible models designed for the use and application of norms, standards, and criteria by individual organizations involved in the evaluation and enforcement of the quality of health care delivery.

Guidi, canal of [Guido *Guidi* (L. *Vidius*), Italian physician, 1500–1569] pterygoid CANAL. See also VIDIAN.

Guillain-Barré syndrome [Georges *Guillain,* French neurologist, 1876–1961; Jean Alexandre *Barré,* French neurologist, born 1880] see under SYNDROME.

guillotine (gil′o-tēn) [Fr.] an instrument for excising a tonsil or the uvula.

Guldberg and Waage law [Cato *Guldberg,* Norwegian chemist, 1836–1902; Peter *Waage,* Norwegian chemist, 1833–1900] see under LAW.

L-gulitol sorbitol.

gum (gum) [L. *gummi*] 1. gingiva. 2. a mucilaginous excretion from various plants; on hydrolysis, gums yield hexoses, pentoses, and uronic acids. **acacia g.,** acacia. **g. arabic,** acacia. **Australian g.,** wattle g. **g. benjamin,** benzoin (1). **g. benzoin,** benzoin (1). **British g.,** dextrin. **g. camphor,** camphor. **g. dammer,** dammar. **free g.,** free GINGIVA. **ghatti g.,** a gum from the dhava tree in India; used as a substitute for acacia. **karaya g.,** sterculia g. **g. lac,** shellac. **mesquite g.,** a gum from the plant *Prosopis juliflora,* of Texas; used as a substitute for acacia. **g. opium,** opium. **senegal g.,** acacia. **starch g.,** dextrin. **sterculia g.,** a dried gummy exudation of the plant *Sterculia,* occurring as a finely ground white powder with a faint odor, which is insoluble in alcohol, but rapidly absorbs water to form a viscous mucilage. Used as a cathartic and as a constituent of denture adhesive powders. Atopic coryza, eczema, atopic dermatitis, and gastrointestinal distress may occur in sensitive individuals. Called also *karaya g., Indian tragacanth,* and *sterculia.* **g. tragacanth,** tragacanth. **trench g's,** acute necrotizing GINGIVITIS; so called because it occurred in troops in the trenches in World War I. **wattle g.,** the gum of several Australian species of *Acacia;* used as a substitute for acacia. Called also *Australian g.*

gumboil (gum′boil) parulis.

gumma (gum′ah), pl. *gum'mata* or *gummas* [L. *gummi* gum] a soft, gummy, grayish tumor appearing as a single or as multiple lesions, usually of the liver, testes, or bones in tertiary syphilis.

Intraoral gummata most commonly involve the tongue and palate. A typical lesion varies in size from 1 mm to several cm and forms a nodular mass composed of inflammatory nonsuppurative tissue undergoing ulceration and necrosis. Called also *syphiloma.*

gummata (gum'ah-tah) [L.] plural of *gumma.*

gummi (gum'i) [L.] gum (of plants).

gun (gun) any gunlike device used for propelling, administering, or applying something under pressure. **Messing g.,** trademark for a metal root canal gun used as a carrier for root canal filling materials in endodontic therapy. See illustration. **root canal g.,**

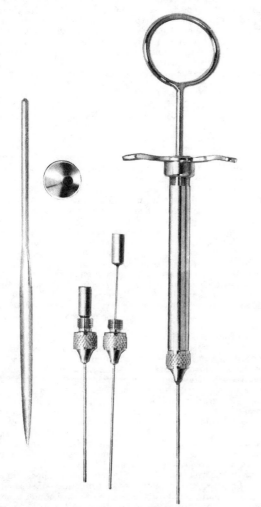

Messing gun for retrofilling of apex. (From H. O. Torres and A. Ehrlich: Modern Dental Assisting. 2nd ed. Philadelphia, W. B. Saunders Co., 1980; courtesy of Union Broach Co.)

a syringe type endodontic instrument. See *Messing g.* and endodontic irrigating SYRINGE. **ultraviolet light g.,** a generator capable of producing a narrow directional beam of ultraviolet light; used for the polymerization of synthetic resins. See also ultraviolet light-cured RESIN.

Gunn's syndrome (phenomenon) [Robert Marcus *Gunn,* English ophthalmologist, 1850–1909] see under SYNDROME.

Gunning's splint [Thomas Brian *Gunning,* American dentist, 1813–1889] see under SPLINT.

Günther's syndrome [Hans *Günther,* 1884–1956] erythropoietic PORPHYRIA.

gustation (gus-ta'shun) [L. *gustatio,* from *gustare* to taste] the sense of taste or the act or process of tasting or the sense of taste. See also TASTE and taste BUD. **colored g.,** the association of colors with tastes.

gustatism (gus'tah-tizm) a sensation of taste produced indirectly by other than gustatory stimuli.

gustatory (gus'tah-to"re) [L. *gustatorium*] pertaining to the sense of taste.

gustometer (gus-tom'ĕ-ter) [L. *gustare* to taste + Gr. *metron* measure] an apparatus used in the quantitative determination of taste thresholds.

gustometry (gus-tom'ĕ-tre) determination of thresholds of taste.

gut (gut) 1. the intestine or bowel. 2. primitive g. 3. catgut. **primitive g.,** an embryonic tubular structure that becomes the digestive tract and the respiratory system; the pits on both extremities of the structure, the stomodeum and proctodeum, developing into the mouth and anus, respectively. It is formed by folding inwardly of the splanchnopleure or roof of the yolk sac along the central axis of the embryo during the fourth week of development. The portion deriving from the cranial part of the yolk sac forms the foregut; the tail portion forms the hindgut; and the portion between the foregut and hindgut is known as the midgut.

gutta (gut'ah), pl. *gut'tae* [L.] a drop.

guttae (gut'e) plural of *gutta.*

gutta-percha (gut"tah-per'chah) the purified, coagulated, milky sap of various tropical trees of the genus *Sapotaceae,* found in the Malayan Archipelago. It is a *trans* isomer of rubber that becomes pliable at 25 to 30°C, plastic at 60°C, and molten at 100°C with partial decomposition. It is slightly soluble in eucalyptol and freely soluble in ether, chloroform, or xylol, but not in water, and becomes brittle on exposure to air and sunlight. Used for temporary sealing of dressings in cavities; also used in the form of cones for filling the root canal and in the form of sticks for sealing cavities over treatment. Gutta-percha is the least toxic, least tissue-irritating, and least allergenic root canal filling material, but its toxicity may be altered by the additive. It is available in standardized and nonstandardized (or regular) cones; standardized cones being used as primary cones and nonstandardized cones, more tapered in shape, as secondary or auxiliary cones in lateral and vertical condensation. Gutta-percha dissolved in chloroform is known as *chloropercha,* and in eucalyptol oil as *eucapercha.* **g. baseplate,** gutta-percha BASEPLATE. **g. cone,** gutta-percha CONE. **g. point,** gutta-percha CONE.

Guttat. abbreviation for L. *gutta'tim,* drop by drop.

guttate (gut'at) of the shape of a drop of water; said of certain lesions of the skin.

guttatim (gut-ta'tim) [L.] drop by drop.

guttering (guter-ing) the operation of cutting a gutter-like excision in a bone.

Gutt. quibusd. abbreviation for L. *gut'tis quibus'dam,* with a few drops.

guttur (gut'er) [L.] throat (1).

guttural (gut'er-al) pertaining to the throat.

gutturophony (gut"er-of'o-ne) [*guttur* + Gr. *phōnē* voice] a throaty quality of the voice.

gutturotetany (gut"ter-o-tet'ah-ne) [*guttur* + *tetany*] a guttural spasm, resulting in a kind of stutter.

Guy de Chauliac see CHAULIAC.

Gy gray.

gypsum (jip'sum) [L.; Gr. *gypsos* chalk] the natural hydrated form of calcium sulfonate, CaSO₄·2H₂O; gypsum dihydrate. On heating, it gives off part of its water and forms a fine white powder which, when rehydrated, produces gypsum hemihydrate. Called also *rock g., alabaster, light spar, mineral white, native calcium sulfate, precipitated calcium sulfate, satinite, satin spar,* and *terra alba.* **g. dihydrate,** gypsum. **dried g., g. hemihydrate. g. hardener,** gypsum HARDENER. **g. hemihydrate,** gypsum from which water of crystallization has been driven off by heating, occurring as a white chalky powder which, when rehydrated, sets in rapidly to re-form hard crystalline gypsum. The process is as follows: $2CaSO_4 \cdot 2H_2O + \text{heat} \rightarrow (CaSO_4)_2 \cdot H_2O + 3H_2O$. When calcined under steam pressure in an autoclave at temperatures of 120 to 130°C (250 to 265°F), dehydrated in an autoclave in the presence of sodium succinate, or dehydrated in a boiling solution of 30 percent calcium hydrochloride, dense prismatic crystals result. This form of the hemihydrate is known as α-hemihydrate, and it is used in the production of dental stone and is an essential ingredient of dental investments. When gypsum hemihydrate is subjected to temperatures of 110 to 120°C (230 to 250°F) and is allowed to set open to the air, irregular, spongy crystals, which are softer than those of the α-hemihydrate, are obtained. This form is known as β-hemihydrate, or plaster of Paris (see under PLASTER). Called also *dried g.* **g. retarder,** gypsum RETARDER. **rock g.,** gypsum.

gyrate (ji'rāt) [L. *gyratus* turned around] having or characterized by a ring or spiral shape.

gyri (ji'ri) [L.] plural of *gyrus.*

gyrus (ji'rus), pl. *gy'ri* [L.; Gr. *gyros* ring or circle] one of the tortuous elevations (convolutions) on the surface of the brain caused by infolding of the cortex.

Gysi's articulator [Alfred *Gysi,* Swiss dentist, 20th century] see under ARTICULATOR.

H

H 1. henry. 2. oersted. 3. SUBSTANCE H. 4. hydrogen. 5. Holz-kneckt UNIT.

h 1. a symbol for a secondary constriction or negatively staining region of a chromosome. See also CHROMOSOME nomenclature. 2. hectogram. 3. abbreviation for L. *ho'ra*, hour.

H⁺ hydrogen ION.

[H⁺] hydrogen ion CONCENTRATION.

¹H protium; also written *H1*. See HYDROGEN.

H₁ see H₁ histamine RECEPTOR; see also H₁ INHIBITOR.

²H deuterium; also written *H2*. See HYDROGEN.

H₂ see H₂ histamine RECEPTOR; see also H₂ INHIBITOR.

³H tritum; also written *H3*. See HYDROGEN.

H-2 see major histocompatibility complex of man, under HISTO-COMPATIBILITY.

Ha chemical symbol for *hahnium;* see ELEMENT 105.

HA2 hemadsorption (virus) 2; see parainfluenza virus type 1, under VIRUS.

HAA hepatitis-associated antigen; see Australia ANTIGEN.

habit (hab'it) [L. *habitus*, from *habere* to hold] 1. a fixed or constant practice established by frequent repetition. 2. predis-position or bodily temperament. See TYPE. 3. oral h. **apoplectic h.**, HABITUS apoplecticus. **clamping h., clenching h.**, centric BRUXISM. **drug h.**, a habitual use of drugs. See drug HABITUA-TION. **gnashing h.**, eccentric BRUXISM. **grinding h.**, eccentric BRUXISM. **masticatory h.**, the sequence and distribution of chewing activity and jaw movement in an individual, being influenced by the type of food chewed, occlusal interferences, restorations, absence of teeth, and personal habits. Most per-sons with a full complement of teeth have an alternating bilateral masticatory pattern, some chew bilaterally simultane-ously, and a small number chew unilaterally on one side. The bicuspid-molar segments of the dental arches appear to be used most frequently during the masticatory activity. **occupational h.**, one associated with a vocation and that is formed and performed either by necessity or for convenience; e.g., the holding of nails between the teeth by carpenters or the biting of thread by seamstresses and tailors. **oral h.**, one that causes changes in occlusal relationships, e.g., finger and thumb suck-ing, tongue thrusting, reverse swallowing, lip sucking, and the like. See also habit-breaking APPLIANCE. **physiologic h.**, an acquired modification of behavior or response to stimulation brought about and permanently fixed by constant repetition. **tongue h.**, conscious or unconscious movements of the tongue, not related to purposeful functions, which may produce maloc-clusion or injuries to tissues of the tongue or the attachment apparatus of the teeth. See also tongue THRUSTING.

habitual (hah-bich'u-al) of the nature of a habit; recurrent; chron-ic.

habituation (hah-bich"u-a'shun) 1. the gradual adaptation to a stimulus or to the environment. 2. a condition resulting from the repeated consumption of a drug, with a desire to continue its use. See *drug h.* **drug h.**, development of psychological (but not physiological) dependence on a drug with a desire to continue its use. See also drug ADDICTION.

habitus (hab'i-tus) [L. "habit"] 1. attitude. 2. physique. See also HABIT and TYPE. **h. apoplec'ticus**, a full, heavy, thick-set body build indicating a possible tendency to apoplexy. Called also *apoplectic habit.* **marfanoid h.**, a bodily habit that is charac-teristic of the Marfan syndrome, e.g., a tall and thin stature, arachnodactyly, scoliosis, pectus excavatum, and subluxated lenses.

Hade-Ring attachment see under ATTACHMENT.

haem-, haemo- see HEMO-.

Haemobartonella (he"mo-bar"to-nel'lah) a genus of gram-negative bacteria of the family Anaplasmataceae, order Rick-ettsiales, occurring as coccoid or rod-shaped organisms found on or within erythrocytes of many vertebrates; rods appear to be chains of coccoid forms. The organisms occur singly, in pairs, or in groups. They have single or double limiting membranes but do not appear to possess cell walls or nuclei. Most species are pathogenic, but anemia is usually not evident unless the animal is splenectomized. Most are transmitted by arthropods, except for *H. fe'lis,* parasitic in cats, which may be also transmitted by ingestion of contaminated blood. *H. mu'ris* is a parasite of rats, mice, and hamsters, and *H. ca'nis* is parasitic in dogs. Growth is inhibited by tetracyclines and arsenicals.

Haemodyn trademark for a solution of *povidone.*

Haemophilus (he-mof'i-lus) [Gr. *haima* blood + *philein* to love] a genus of gram-negative, facultatively anaerobic bacteria of uncertain affiliation, occurring as minute or medium-sized, coccobacillary to rod-shaped cells, which sometimes form threads and filaments and show pleomorphism. The organisms

are strict parasites and require in culture growth factors pres-ent in the blood. Some species are pathogenic. Sometimes written *Hemophilus.* **H. aegyp'tius**, a species *incertae sedis* causing acute mucopurulent human conjunctivitis. Called also *Bacillus aegyptius, B. conjunctivitidis, Bacterium aegyptia-cum, hemophilus of Koch-Weeks,* and *Koch-Weeks bacillus.* **H. aphro'philus**, a species isolated from the blood and heart valves in a patient with endocarditis and from the pharynx in dogs. **H. bo'vis**, *Moraxella bovis;* see under MORAXELLA. **H. bronchi-sep'ticus**, *Bordetella bronchiseptica;* see under BORDETELLA. **H. gallina'rum**, a species isolated from the nasal sinuses of fowl affected with coryza. **H. ducrey'i**, the etiologic agent of chan-croid in man. Called also *Coccobacillus ducreyi* and *Ducrey's bacillus.* **H. haemolyt'icus**, a species causing hemolysis in blood media. It is found normally in small numbers in the human upper respiratory tract, but may cause sore throat when present in profusion. **H. influen'zae**, a species indiginous to the human upper respiratory tract, occurring as coccobacilli or sometimes as cocci, about 0.2 to 0.3 by 0.5 to 2.0 μm in size. The virulent strains are encapsulated and form small, mucoid, transparent colonies which show iridescence on transparent media under oblique light; iridescence disappears in older cultures due to cell autolysis. It was isolated originally from cases of influenza and at the time was thought to be its etiologic agent (thus its name). *H. influenzae* is the leading cause of bacterial meningi-tis in the United States. It is sometimes isolated from the paranasal sinuses, sputum, conjunctivae, cerebrospinal fluid, and blood in conditions such as pharyngitis, sinusitis, otitis media, pneumonia, empyema, endocarditis, pyroarthrosis, laryngotracheal infection, and bacteremia. Called also *H. men-ingitides, Bacterium influenzae, Coccobacillus pfeifferi, in-fluenza bacillus,* and *Mycobacterium influenzae.* **H. in-fluen'zae su'is**, *H. suis.* **H. meningi'tidis**, *H. influenzae.* **H. parahaemolyt'icus**, a species found in the upper respiratory tract in man, often in association with acute pharyngitis. It occasionally causes endocarditis in man and pleuropneumonia and septicemia in swine. Called also *H. pleuropneumoniae* and *hemolytic influenza bacillus.* **H. parainfluen'zae**, a species isolated from the human upper respiratory tract, which is essentially nonpathogenic, except for rare cases of subacute endocarditis. It occurs as pointed rods, capsulated strains being homogeneous and noncapsulated heterogeneous. Called also *influenza-like hemophilus.* **H. paraphro'philus**, a potentially pathogenic species isolated from the human fauces and vagina, from urine, and from cases of subacute endocarditis, maxillary osteomyelitis, brain abscesses, paronychia, and appendicitis. **H. parapertus'sis**, *Bordetella parapertussis;* see under BORDE-TELLA. **H. paraphrohaemolyt'icus**, a species inhabiting the human mouth, which is a potential cause of sore throat; it has also been found in oral ulcers, in sputum, and in urethral discharge of male adults. **H. pertus'sis**, *Bordetella pertussis;* see under BORDETELLA. **H. pleuropneumo'niae**, *H. parahaemo-lyticus.* **H. su'is**, a species isolated from the respiratory tract, serous cavities, blood, meninges, and joints in swine. In associ-ation with a virus it causes swine influenza. Called also *H. influenzae suis.* **H. vagina'lis**, a species *incertae sedis* isolated from the human genital tract; a suspected cause of nonspecific vaginitis and urethritis. Called also *Hemophilus hemolyticus vaginalis.*

Hafnia (haf'ne-ah) [L. *Hafnia* Copenhagen] a genus of gram-negative bacteria of the family Enterobacteriaceae, made up of motile, peritrichously flagellated, unencapsulated, facultative-ly anaerobic rods. *H. al'vei* is found in feces, sewage, soil, water, and dairy products. Called also *Bacillus paratyphi-alvei, Enterobacter aerogenes* subsp. *hafniae,* and *E. alvei.*

hafnium (haf'ne-um) [L. *Hafnia* Copenhagen] a metallic element, occurring as a ductile metal with a brilliant silver luster, which is usually found in zirconium ore. Symbol, Hf; atomic number, 72; atomic weight, 178.49; melting point, 2227°C; specific gravity, 13.31; valences, 2, 3, 4; group IVB of the periodic table. It has six natural isotopes (174, 176–180) and several artificial ones (157, 158, 168–173, 175, 181–183). Used in nuclear and electronic technologies.

Hagedorn needle [Werner *Hagedorn*, German surgeon, 1831–1894] see under NEEDLE.

Hageman deficiency, factor, trait [named after the person in whom the coagulation factor was first seen] see FACTOR XII.

Hahn, Otto [1879–1968] a German scientist. See HAHNIUM.

Hahnemann, Christian Friedrich Samuel [1755–1843] the found-er of homeopathy.

hahnium (hahn'i-um) [named after Otto *Hahn*] a proposed name for element 105 (see under ELEMENT).

hair (har) [L. *pilus;* Gr. *thrix*] a long slender filament. Applied chiefly to such filamentous appendages of the skin. See also terms beginning PILI- and PILO-. **gustatory h.,** taste h. **h's of nose,** vibrissae. **olfactory h.,** one of six or more delicate protoplasmic processes which project from the olfactory cells located on the surface of the olfactory mucosa and which serve as active receptive structures in the process of olfaction. **sensory h's,** hairlike projections on the surface of sensory epithelial cells. **tactile h's,** hairs which are sensitive to touch, as the vibrissae of certain animals. **taste h.,** one of the short hairlike processes protruding from the taste cell through the gustatory pore. Called also *gustatory h.*

Hajdu-Cheney syndrome, [Nicholas *Hajdu;* W. D. *Cheney*] see under SYNDROME.

Halamid trademark for *chloramine-T.*

Haldol trademark for *haloperidol.*

Haldrate trademark for *paramethasone.*

Haldrone trademark for *paramethasone acetate* (see under PARA-METHASONE).

half-life (haf′līf) the time in which half the atoms of a particular radioactive substance disintegrate to another nuclear form, varying from millionths of a second to billions of years. **antibody h.,** the time required for the elimination of 50 percent of a measured dose of antibody from the body of the animal. **biological h.,** the time required for a biological system to eliminate by natural processes half the amount of a substance (such as a radioactive material) which has been introduced into it. **effective h.,** the time required for a radionuclide contained in a biological system to reduce its activity by half as a combined result of radioactive decay and biological elimination. **erythrocyte h.,** ERYTHROCYTE half-life. **radioactive h.,** see *half-life.*

halide (hal′īd) a binary compound of a halogen and a metal, always having −1 as an oxidation number, and having high ionic character as indicated by its high melting point. **hydrogen h.,** a compound prepared by the direct interaction of hydrogen gas and a halogen. In aqueous solutions, hydrogen halides behave as strong acids (hydrohalic acids).

halisteresis (hah-lis″tē-re′sis) [Gr. *hals* salt + *sterēsis* privation] a loss or lack of calcium salts in bone, as in osteolysis or osteomalacia.

halite (hal′it) SODIUM chloride.

halitosis (hal-ĭ-to′sis) [L. *halitus* exhalation] offensive breath. Called also *bad breath, fetor ex ore, fetor oris, foul breath, halitus oris fetidus,* and *stomatodysodia.*

halituous (hah-lit′u-us) [L. *halitus* exhalation] covered with moisture or vapor.

halitus (hal′ĭ-tus) [L.] the expired air; exhalation. See also BREATH and RESPIRATION. **h. or′is feti′dus,** halitosis. **h. saturni′nus,** lead BREATH.

Hall, Marshall see MARSHALL HALL.

Hallermann-Streiff syndrome [Wilhelm *Hallermann;* E. B. *Streiff*] see under SYNDROME.

Hallopeau's disease, syndrome [François Henri *Hallopeau,* French dermatologist, 1842–1919] see LICHEN sclerosus et atrophicus and DERMATITIS vegetans.

hallucination (hah-lu″sĭ-na′shun) [L. *hallucinatio;* Gr. *alyein* to wander in the mind] a sense perception without a source in the external environment; a perception of an external stimulus object in the absence of such an object.

hallucinogen (hah-lu″sĭ-no-jen″) [*hallucination* + Gr. *gennan* to produce] psychodelic AGENT.

hallucinog.nic (hah-lu″sĭ-no-jen′ik) 1. producing hallucinations. 2. hallucinogenic agent; see psychedelic AGENT.

halo (ha′lo) [L.; Gr. *halōs*] a luminous or colored circle surrounding an object.

halo- [Gr. *hals* salt] a combining form denoting relationship to a salt.

Halobacteriaceae (hal″o-bak-te″re-a′se-e) [*Halobacterium* + *-aceae*] a family of gram-negative, aerobic bacteria, occurring as rods or cocci, found in an environment in which an adequate supply of sodium chloride is available, such as sea water and proteinaceous material with salts, such as salted fish, meat, and hides. It consists of the genera *Halobacterium* and *Halococcus.*

Halobacterium (hal″o-bak-te″re-um) [Gr. *hals* salt + *baktērion* a little rod] a genus of halophilic, rod-shaped bacteria of the family Halobacteriaceae, found in salt lakes and heavily salted proteinaceous materials.

Halococcus (hal″o-kok″us) [Gr. *hals* salt + *kokkos* berry] a genus of halophilic coccoid bacteria of the family Halobacteriaceae.

halogen (hal′o-jen, ha′lo-jen) [*halo-* + Gr. *gennan* to produce] the group of nonmetallic elements, including fluorine, chlorine, bromine, iodine, and astatine, found in nature in bound forms, being too reactive to occur in the free state. The first two elements exist as gases, bromine is a liquid, and iodine a solid.

The melting and boiling points and the size of atoms increase gradually from fluorine to iodine; the tendencies of atoms to attract electrons decrease with increasing size. Each element has seven electrons in its outer shell. All possess a high electronegativity and readily form negative halide ions, commonly found in ionic salts.

halogenation (hal″o-jĕ-na′shun) introduction of a halogen, usually chlorine or bromine, into a chemical compound.

haloid (hal′oid) [*halo-* + Gr. *eidos* form] resembling or derived from a halogen.

Halon trademark for *dichlorodifluoromethane.*

haloperidol (hah-lo-per′ĭ-dol) a tranquilizer, 4-[4-(*p*-chlorophenyl)-4-hydroxypiperidino]-4′-fluorobutyrophenone, occurring as a white to yellowish, odorless, light-sensitive powder that is readily soluble in chloroform, methanol, acetone, benzene, and dilute acids, slightly soluble in ether and ethanol, and insoluble in water; the hydrochloride salt is water-soluble. Used in the treatment of various mental disorders. Side effects may include parkinsonism, dystonia, dyskinesia, oculogyric disorders, and akathisia. Blood dyscrasias, postural hypotension, tachycardia, hypersensitivity, cholestatic jaundice, and photosensitivity sometimes occur. Trademarks: Aloperidine, Haldol, Serenase.

halophilic (hal″o-fil′ik) [Gr. *hals* salt + *philein* to love] pertaining to or characterized by an affinity for salt; applied to microorganisms which require a high concentration of salt for optimal growth.

Halotestin trademark for *fluoxymesterone.*

halothane (hal′o-thān) an inhalation anesthetic of moderate potency, 2-bromo-2-chloro-1,1,1-trifluoroethane, occurring as a colorless, mobile, nonflammable (but volatile) liquid with a characteristic ethereal odor, which is slightly soluble in water and miscible with alcohol, chloroform, ether, and oils. In oral surgery, usually used in conjunction with nitrous exide. Sedative premedication prolongs the recovery time. Halothane reduces the flow of saliva and sensitizes the heart to the action of epinephrine and levarterenol. Hypotension is usually present during halothane-produced anesthesia. Contraindicated in patients with liver and biliary tract diseases. Trademark: Fluothane.

Halsted's mosquito hemostat, suture [William Stewart *Halsted,* American surgeon, 1852–1922] see under HEMOSTAT and SUTURE.

hamarto- [Gr. *hamartia* defect, sin] a combining form denoting relationship to a defect.

hamartoma (ham″ar-to′mah) [*hamarto-* + *-oma*] a benign tumorlike nodule composed of an overgrowth of mature cells and tissues that normally occur in the affected part, but often with one element predominating.

hamartomatosis (ham″ar-to-mah-to′sis) the development or presence of multiple hamartomas.

hamate (ham′āt) hooked.

Hamberger's schema [Georg Erhard *Hamberger,* German physician, 1697–1755] see under SCHEMA.

hammer (ham′er) 1. a tool or instrument consisting of a weighted head of metal or other appropriate material, attached to a handle, which is used for pounding or striking blows. 2. malleus (1). **dental h.,** a mallet used for condensing direct filling gold or amalgam during the insertion of fillings in teeth. It may be operated either by hand or be motor-driven. See also MALLET. **horn h.,** a hammer with the head made of horn, being relatively soft but tough; used in the past for pounding and adapting sheet metal to dies without indentation or injury of the surface. **sledge h.,** a dental hammer with a heavy, broad head and a short handle; used in the past in the laboratory for swaging and in the adaptation of sheet metal bases for dentures between die and counter die.

Hammond's splint see under SPLINT.

Hammurabi [18th century B.C. or earlier] a King of Babylonia, who was the author of the *Code of Hammurabi* (see under CODE).

Hampson unit see under UNIT.

hamster (ham′ster) a ratlike rodent, the most common of which is *Cricetus cricetus* bred and used extensively as a laboratory animal. Other species include *Cricetus larabensis,* the Chinese hamster, and *Mesocretus auratus,* the Syrian hamster.

hamular (ham′u-lar) shaped like a hook.

hamulus (ham′u-lus), pl. *ham′uli* [L. "little hook"] a general anatomical term denoting a hook-shaped process. **frontal h., h. fronta′lis,** a small winglike process on the anterior part of the crista galli of the ethmoid bone. Called also *ala cristae galli*

[NA] and *processus alaris ossis ethmoidalis.* **h. of ethmoid bone,** uncinate process of ethmoid bone; see under PROCESS. **lacrimal h., h. lacrima′lis** [NA], a hooklike projection on the anterior part of the inferolateral border of the lacrimal bone, which articulates with the lacrimal tubercle of the maxilla, and completes the orifice of the lacrimal canal. It may appear as a separate bone, and is then known as the *lesser lacrimal bone.* Called also *hamular process of lacrimal bone* and *uncinate process of lacrimal bone.* **pterygoid h., h. pterygoi′deus** [NA], a hooklike process curving laterally on the inferior extremity of the medial pterygoid plate of the sphenoid bone, around which the tendon of the tensor veli palatini muscle glides. Called also *hamular process of sphenoid bone.*

hamycin (hah-mi′sin) an antifungal antibiotic isolated from cultures of *Streptomyces pimprina,* occurring as a yellow amorphous powder that is soluble in pyridine, collidine, and some alcohols and is almost insoluble in water, benzene, and chloroform. Used in infections caused by *Candida, Curvularia lanata,* and *Aspergillus,* and in other mycoses. Trademark: Primamycin.

Hamy's line, plane see under LINE and PLANE.

Hanau's articulator, law, quint [R. L. *Hanau,* American dentist, 20th century] see under ARTICULATOR and LAW, and see Thielemann's PRINCIPLE.

hand (hand) [L. *manus*] the terminal portion of the arm below the wrist. Called also *main* and *manus* [NA]. **claw h.,** clawhand. **club h.,** clubhand. **flat h.,** MANUS plana.

Hand-Schüller-Christian disease [Alfred *Hand,* Jr., American pediatrician, 1868–1949; Artur *Schüller,* Vienna neurologist, born 1874; Henry Asbury *Christian,* American physician, 1876–1951] see under DISEASE.

Handi-Liner trademark for a *cavity varnish* (see under VARNISH).

handle (han′d'l) the elongated part of something, such as an instrument, made to be grasped. In dental instruments, it is usually mitered in a hexagonal shape for stability in gripping, and may serrated or smooth. It is connected to the working part (a blade or nib) by a shank. Called also *shaft.* See DENTISTRY. **test h.,** a patented handle that is fitted over a root canal intrument to limit its insertion into a root canal. See illustration. **Unigauge h.,** trademark for an adjustable test handle,

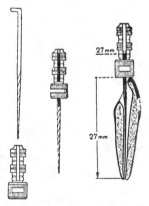

Test handle. (From L. I. Grossman: Endodontic Practice. 8th ed.. Philadelphia, Lea & Febiger, 1974.)

which can be positioned at any point along the shaft of the root canal instrument so as to vary the length of the instrument as measured from the handle to the tip.

handpiece (hand′pēs) a hand-held device which engages rotary instruments used for removing tooth structures, cleaning teeth, and polishing dental restorations, connected to the dental engine by an adjustable arm in the case of a belt driven instrument or by flexible tubing if air driven. See illustration and table. **air-bearing turbine h.,** a modified air turbine handpiece, using air bearings and operating at speeds of 400,000 rpm. **air turbine h.,** one with a turbine in the head of the handpiece and powered by compressed air. **contra-angle h.,** one in which the shaft of the rotary instrument is set at a desired angle through the use of two, or sometimes more, bends or angles; used to reach areas in the oral cavity that are difficult to access. **Giromatic h.,** trademark for an engine-driven contra-angle

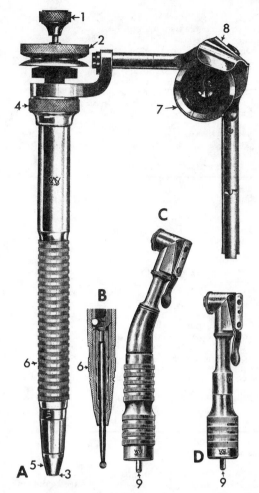

A, Conventional dental handpiece, showing tightening nut (1), drive pulley (2), open end of handpiece (3), rear end of handpiece (4), nose (5), outer sheath (6), pulley wheel (7), and wrist joint (8). *B,* Cross section of handpiece, showing a dental bur in position. *C,* Contra-angle attachment. (9) Shank. *D,* Right angle attachment. (From V. R. Park, J. R. Ashman, and G. J. Shelly: A Textbook for Dental Assistants. 2nd ed. Philadelphia, W. B. Saunders Co., 1975; courtesy of S. S. White Dental Mfg. Co.)

handpiece designed for endodontic use, operating by rotary reciprocal action through a 90° arc. Quarter-turn root canal reamers are used with this handpiece as are several other types of Group II root canal instruments. See also root canal THERAPY. **high-speed h.,** one which operates at speeds above 12,000 rpm. **Racer h.,** trademark for an engine-driven contra-angle handpiece designed for endodontic use, operating by vertical and rotary oscillation within the root canal. Quarter-turn root canal

PROGRESSIVE DEVELOPMENT OF DENTAL HANDPIECES

Date	Type	Rotational Speed (rpm)
1800	Hand Rotation	100
1870	Foot Drive	1,000
1900	Electric Motor Drive	5,000
1952	Pulley Modification	12,000
1953	Ball Bearings	20,000
1954	Water Turbine	40,000
1955	Modified Gear Ratio	125,000
1956	Belt in Handpiece	150,000
1957	Air Turbine	300,000
1963	Air Bearing Turbine	400,000

(From American Dental Association: Guide to Dental Materials and Devices. 8th ed. 1976–1978.)

reamers are used with this handpiece as are several other types of Group II root canal instruments. See also root canal THERAPY.
right-angle h., one in which the shaft of the rotary instrument is at a right angle (90°) to the long axis of the handpiece. **straight h.,** a conventional handpiece with an axis in line with the rotary instrument, as opposed to right-angle and contra-angle handpieces. **ultra–high-speed h.,** one which operates at speeds of 100,000 to 450,000 rpm. **ultrasonic h.,** a tooth-cutting instrument which sends aluminum oxide slurry against a tip which vibrates at ultrasonic frequency of 29,000 cps. **water-turbine h.,** one in which the rotary instrument is driven by a turbine powered by water under pressure.

hanger (hang′er) any device used for hanging something. **film processing h.,** one to which film is attached for immersion in film processing solutions. See film PROCESSING.

Hanhart's nanism (syndrome), syndrome [Ernest *Hanhart,* Swiss physician] see under NANISM, and see aglossia-adactylia SYNDROME.

Hannover's intermediate membrane enamel MEMBRANE (2).

Hansen's bacillus, disease [Gerhard Armauer *Hansen,* Norwegian physician, 1841–1912] see *Mycobacterium leprae,* under MYCOBACTERIUM, and see LEPROSY.

haplo- [Gr. *haploos* simple, single] a combining form meaning simple or single.

haploid (hap′loid) [Gr. *haploos* simple, single + *-ploid*] 1. having a single set of chromosomes, as normally carried by a gamete, or having one complete set of nonhomologous chromosomes. 2. an individual or cell having only one member of each pair of homologous chromosomes. Cf. DIPLOID.

haploidy (hap′loi-de) the state of having only one member of each pair of homologous chromosomes.

Hapsburg jaw, lip [named after the *Hapsburgs,* a German-Austrian royal family, including among its members many rulers of European states, such as Austria (1278–1918) and Spain (1504–1700)] see under JAW and LIP. See also HEMOPHILIA (disease of the Hapsburgs).

hapt-, hapte- see HAPTO-.

hapten (hap′ten) a specific substance whose chemical configuration is such that it can interact with specific combining groups of an antibody, but which, unlike an antigen, does not itself induce the formation of a detectable amount of antibody. When coupled with a carrier protein, haptens do elicit the immune response. In humoral immunity, the antibody specificity is directed primarily to the hapten; in cell-mediated immunity, to both the hapten and a portion of the carrier protein. Most haptens are of a low–molecular-weight (less than 5000) and carry only one or two antigenic determinants but some macromolecules, such as pneumococcal polysaccharides, are also considered as haptens. Called also *incomplete antigen* and *partial antigen.*

hapto-, hapt-, hapte- [Gr. *haptein* to touch, seize upon or hold fast] a combining form denoting relationship to touch or to seizure.

haptoglobin (hap″to-glo′bin) [*hapto-* + *globin*] a glycoprotein in the α_2-globulin fraction of serum which binds the globin portion of hemoglobin but not the heme. Three major genetically determined types are identified: Hp^{1-1}, Hp^{2-1}, and Hp^{2-2}. Haptoglobins consist of two kinds of polypeptide chains, α and β; three different α chains and one β chain have been distinguished by electrophoresis. They are synthesized in the liver; molecular weight about 85,000; sedimentation coefficient, 4.1–4.4 S.

haptophore (hap′to-fōr) [*hapto-* + Gr. *phoros* bearing] the specific group of the molecule of toxins, agglutinins, precipitins, opsonins, and lysins by which they become attached to their antibodies, antigens, or the receptors of cells, thus making possible their specific activity.

hardener (hard′en-er) a substance added to another substance to increase its hardness or to produce a harder surface or finish. **gypsum h.,** any substance added to a gypsum mix to increase its hardness upon setting, such as solutions containing aqueous colloidal silica or soluble resins, which harden the surface of dental stone.

hardening (hard′en-ing) the act or process of rendering something firm or hard. See also SCLEROSIS. **age h.,** the increase in hardness and strength of an alloy, occurring as a function of time. The process involves the formation in the solid state of discontinuities in the space lattice that will impede the production of dislocations under stress, the process being proportional to the temperature. Called also *alloy aging.* See *precipitation h.* and *order-disorder h.* **h. of arteries,** arteriosclerosis. **order-disorder h.,** hardening of an alloy having a random configuration of atoms in its lattice by heat treatment (tempering), followed by slowly decreasing the temperature. During the cooling process, atoms from a single lattice interpenetrate

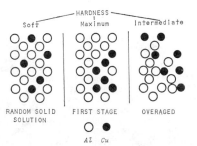

Atom movements in Al-Cu system producing age hardening. (From E. H. Greener, J. K. Harcourt, and E. P. Lautenschlager: Materials Science in Dentistry. Elmsford, New York, Pergamon Press, 1972.)

adjoining lattices and form superlattices. The presence of superlattices in a solid solution impedes dislocations and slipping from developing in the lattices, thereby increasing hardness and strength of the alloy. **precipitation h.,** a form of age hardening in which the atoms precipitate in a solid solution under the influence of heat treatment (tempering), thereby increasing the hardness and strength of an alloy. See illustration. **strain h.,** the hardening of a metal by cold work, as by repeated flexing or hammering at room temperature, whereby changes in the internal structure of the material are brought about by plastic deformation. Dislocations tend to build up at the grain boundaries, the barrier action slipping at the boundaries, causing the slip to occur on other intersecting slip planes. As point defects increase, the entire grain may become distorted. The distortions cause the metal to become stronger and harder, since the atoms in the lattice become more difficult to displace. The proportional limit is also increased, but the ductility is decreased. The ultimate result of cold work and strain hardening is fracture. Called also *work h.* **work h.,** strain h.

hardness (hard′nes) 1. the quality of firmness produced by cohesion of the particles composing a substance, as evidenced by resistance to penetration, abrasion, scratching, cutting, or

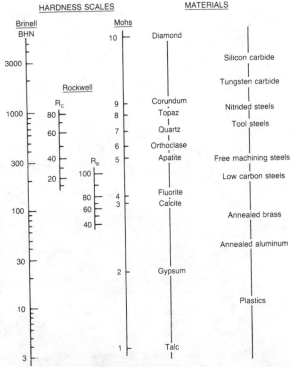

Comparison of hardness scales. (From L. H. VanVlack: Elements of Materials Science. 2nd ed., Reading, Mass., Addison-Wesley Publishing Co., Inc., 1964.)

shaping. It may denote strength, stiffness, brittleness, resilience, or toughness, or combinations of these qualities, its meaning depending on the material and on the use to which the material is to be subjected. See table. 2. a quality of water produced by soluble salts of calcium and magnesium or other substances which form an insoluble curd with soap and thus interfere with its cleansing power. 3. the penetrating power of x-rays depending on their wavelength; the shorter the wavelength the harder the rays and the greater their penetrating power. 4. the degree of refraction of the residual gas in a glass tube; the higher the vacuum the shorter the wavelength of the resulting x-rays. **Brinell h. number (BHN),** a number indicating the degree of hardness of materials, determined by pressing a hardened steel ball (Brinell hardness indenter point) into the surface of the material being tested under a load of 12.6 kg (27.8 lbs) and dividing the load by the area of the spherical indentation remaining after the load is removed; the number being inversely proportional to the size of the area of indentation. In the case where the area of indentation is 0.2 mm², for example, the Brinell hardness number is determined as follows:

$$\frac{load}{area\ of\ indentation} \quad \frac{12.6\ kg}{0.2\ mm} = 63\ BHN$$

See illustration. **Brinell h. scale,** a scale used to determine the relative hardness of materials. See *Brinell h. number.* Called also *Brinell scale.* **Brinell h. test,** a test in which the hardness of a material is calculated from the diameter of the impression made by a hardened steel ball pressed into the surface of the material being tested. Called also *Brinell test.* See *Brinell h. number.* **Knoop h. number (KHN),** a number indicative of the degree of relative hardness of materials, determined by pressing against the surface of the material being tested an indenter, consisting of a diamond ground to pyramidal form with a ratio of diagonals of 7.11 to 1 (Knoop hardness indenter point), and determining of the ratio of the load to the projected area of the resultant indentation. The Knoop method produces an impression without ridging or sinking in near the edge of the indentations; therefore, it is used most commonly in dental practice. Also, it is not influenced by the elastic recovery of the material. **Knoop h. scale,** a scale used to determine the relative hardness of materials. Called also *Knoop scale.* See *Knoop h. number.* **Knoop h. test,** a test in which the hardness of a material is calculated from the length of the long axis of the impression made by the rhomboidal pyramid of a diamond pressed into the surface of the material being tested. See *Knoop h. number.* **Mohs h. number (MHN),** a number of an arbitrary mineralogical scale of hardness in which a mineral will scratch other minerals that are lower on the scale (smaller hardness number) and will in turn be scratched by minerals higher on the scale. Called also *Mohs index.* See illustration and table. **Mohs hardness t.,** a

test for the hardness of minerals. Called also *Mohs test.* See *Mohs h. number.* **h. number,** a number indicative of the degree of relative hardness of materials. See *Brinell n., Knoop n., Mohs n., Rockwell n., Vickers n.,* and *scleroscope n.* See illustration and table. **Rockwell h. number (RHN),** a number indicative of the degree of relative hardness of materials. It is determined by pressing against the surface of the material being tested a steel ball or diamond conical point (Rockwell hardness indenter point) under a static load of a given magnitude (minor load); the load is then increased by a given amount (major load) and maintained for a certain period of time; and after the major load is again reduced to the minor load, the depth of the impression made by the indenter is measured. The number is designated according to the type of indenter and load employed, e.g., Rockwell B, Rockwell C, or Rockwell M. See illustration. **Rockwell h. scale,** a scale used to determine the relative hardness of materials. Called also *Rockwell scale.* See *Rockwell h. number* and illustration. **Rockwell h. test,** a test in which the hardness of a material is calculated by measuring the depth of the impression made by a steel or diamond conical point pressed into the surface of the material being tested. Called also *Rockwell test.* See also *Rockwell h. number* and table. **h. scale,** a number scale, such as the Brinell, Knoop, Mohs, Rockwell, or Vickers scales, indicative of the degree of relative hardness of materials. See illustration and table. **h. test,** a test designed to determine the relative hardness of a material. See *Brinell h. test, Knoop h. test, Mohs h. test, Rockwell h. test, Vickers h. test,* and scleroscope TEST. **Vickers h. number (VHN),** a number indicative of the degree of relative hardness of a material, determined by measuring the long diagonals of the indentations made by pressing a diamond in the shape of a square-based pyramid (Vickers hardness indenter point) into the surface of the material being tested under a specified load. **Vickers h. scale,** a scale used to determine the relative hardness of materials. Called also *Vickers scale.* See *Vickers h. number.* **Vickers h. test,** a test in which the relative hardness of materials is determined by measuring the long diagonals of indentations made by pressing the pyramidal point of a diamond into the surface of the material being tested. Called also *Vickers test.* See also *Vicker's h. number.*

hardware (hard'wār) 1. metal objects, such as tools, hinges, and the like. 2. in computer technology, electrical and mechanical components of a computer. Cf. SOFTWARE.

Hardy-Weinberg law (equilibrium, formula, ratio) [G. H. *Hardy,* English mathematician; Wilhelm *Weinberg,* German physician, 1862–1937] see under LAW.

harelip (har'lip) CLEFT lip.

Hargraves' cell LE CELL.

harmony (har'mo-ne) the state of working together smoothly. **occlusal h.,** proper occlusion of the teeth occurring in various positions of the mandible. Cf. occlusal DISHARMONY. **occlusal h., functional,** such occlusion of the teeth in all positions of the mandible during mastication as will provide the greatest masticatory efficiency without imposing undue strain or trauma on the supporting tissues.

Harris, Chapin Aaron [1806–1860] an American dentist, writer,

SCRATCH HARDNESS — MINERALOGICAL BASIS

Mohs Scale		Extension of Mohs Scale		
Hardness No.	Reference Mineral	Hardness No.	Reference Mineral	Metal Equivalent
1	Talc	1	Talc	
2	Gypsum	2	Gypsum	
3	Calcite	3	Calcite	
4	Fluorite	4	Fluorite	
5	Apatite	5	Apatite	
6	Feldspar orthoclase	6	Orthoclase	
		7	Vitreous pure silica	
7	Quartz	8	Quartz	Stellite
8	Topaz	9	Topaz	
		10	Garnet	
		11	Fused zirconia	Tantalum carbide
9	Sapphire or corundum	12	Fused alumina	Tungsten carbide
		13	Silicon carbide	
		14	Boron carbide	
10	Diamond	15	Diamond	

educator, and lexicographer. Co-founder with Hayden of the College of Dental Surgery in Baltimore, the first dental college in America.

Harris' neuralgia [W. *Harris*] cluster HEADACHE.

Hart-Dunn attachment [A. L. *Dunn*] see under ATTACHMENT.

Hartley-Krause operation [Frank *Hartley*, American surgeon, 1857–1913; Fedor *Krause*, German surgeon, 1857–1937] see under OPERATION.

Hartman's solution [Leroy Leo *Hartman*, born 1893] see under SOLUTION.

Harvey chemiclave see under CHEMICLAVE.

Hashimoto's disease (thyroiditis) [Hakaru *Hashimoto*, Japanese surgeon, 1881–1934] see under DISEASE.

hashish (hash-esh′) [Arabic "herb"] a cannabinoid substance of the unadulterated resin from the flowering tops of female *Cannabis sativa*, which is smoked or chewed for its intoxicating effects. Called also *charas* or *churus*. See also CANNABINOID.

Hasner's fold (valve) [Joseph Ritter von Artha *Hasner*, ophthalmologist in Prague, 1819–1892] lacrimal FOLD.

Hasselbalch, Karl A. [Danish scientist, born 1892] see Henderson-Hasselbalch EQUATION.

Hatch clamp see under CLAMP.

Hatchcock's sign see under SIGN.

hatchet (hach′it) a cutting dental instrument having its cutting edge in line with the axis of its blade; used for breaking down tooth structure undermined by caries, smoothing cavity walls, and sharpening line and point angles. It may be bibeveled or single beveled like a chisel. Called also *hatchet excavator*. See illustration. **enamel h.**, a handcutting instrument in which the

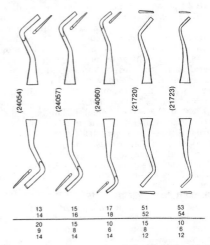

| 13 | 15 | 17 | 51 | 53 |
| 14 | 16 | 18 | 52 | 54 |

20	15	10	15	10
9	8	6	8	6
14	14	14	12	12

Hatchets. (From H. O. Torres and A. Ehrlich: Modern Dental Assisting. 2nd ed., Philadelphia, W. B. Saunders Co., 1980; courtesy of S. S. White Div. of Pennwalt Corp.)

broad side of the blade is parallel with the angle of the shank, which may be bibeveled or single beveled; used with a chipping or a lateral scraping stroke in developing an internal cavity form.

haupt-agglutinin (howpt′ah-gloo′ti-nin) chief AGGLUTININ.

haustra (hows′trah) [L.] plural of *haustrum*.

haustrum (hows′trum), pl. *haus′tra* [L. *haustor* drawer] a general anatomical term denoting a recess.

Haverhill fever [named after *Haverhill*, Massachusetts, where an epidemic first occurred] see under FEVER.

Haverhillia (ha′ver-il′e-ah) [named after *Haverhill*, Massachusetts where it was first isolated] *Streptobacillus*. **H. moniliform'mis, H. multifor'mis,** *Streptobacillus moniliformis;* see under STREPTOBACILLUS.

Havers, Clopton [1650–1702] an English physician and anatomist, known mainly for his researches on the minute structure of bone, which were recorded in his *Osteologia nova* published in 1691. See HAVERSIAN.

haversian (ha-ver′se-an) named after or described by Clopton *Havers*, as the haversian canal, canaliculus, glands (see synovial villi, under VILLUS), lamella, space, and system.

Havidote trademark for *ethylenediaminetetraacetic acid* (see under ACID).

Hawley bite plate, retainer (appliance) [C. A. *Hawley*, American dentist] see under PLATE and RETAINER.

Haxthausen, Holger [1892–1958] see Blegvad-Haxthausen SYNDROME.

Hayden, Horace H. [1769–1844] an eminent American dentist, educator, and organizer. Founder of the American Society ·of Dental Surgeons and co-founder, with Chapin Aaron Harris, of the College of Dental Surgery in Baltimore, the first dental college in America. He was also a well known botanist and geologist.

Hayem-Widal syndrome [George *Hayem*, French physician, 1841–1933] acquired hemolytic JAUNDICE.

Haynes stellite 21, stellite 31 [Elwood *Haynes*, American engineer] see ALLOY HS21 and ALLOY HS31.

Hb hemoglobin. **Hb A,** adult HEMOGLOBIN. **Hb C,** HEMOGLOBIN C. **Hb F,** fetal HEMOGLOBIN. **Hb S,** sickle cell HEMOGLOBIN.

25-HCC 25-hydroxycholecalciferol.

HCl hydrochloric ACID.

HCM health care management.

HD$_{50}$ a hemolyzing dose of complement that lyses 50 percent of a suspension of sensitized red blood cells.

HDL high-density lipoprotein; see α-LIPOPROTEIN.

He helium.

head (hed) [L. *caput;* Gr. *kephale*] 1. the upper part of the human body, which contains the brain, eyes, nose, ears, and mouth; and the corresponding anterior part of various animals. Called also *caput* [NA]. See also terms beginning CEPHALO-. 2. that end of an organ, particularly of a muscle or a bone, which is proximal to the cerebrospinal axis. 3. that part of anything which forms or is regarded as forming the top, summit, or upper end. **angular h. of quadratus labii superioris muscle,** see levator muscle of upper lip and ala of nose, under MUSCLE. **bur h.,** the working part of the bur. See BUR. **condylar h., h. of condyle,** the articular portion of the condyle, forming a rounded knob covered with cartilage, which fits into the glenoid fossa of the temporal bone, forming the temporomandibular articulation. **h. of condyloid process of mandible, h. of mandible. elongated h.,** dolichocephalic SKULL. **high h.,** see acrocephalic SKULL, hypsicephalic SKULL, and OXYCEPHALY. **hot cross bun h.,** in rickets, a head in which the eminences of the frontal and parietal bones form elevations separated by depressions which mark the lines of the cranial sutures. Called also *caput natiforme.* **hourglass h.,** one in which the coronal suture is depressed. **infraorbital h. of levator muscle of upper lip, infraorbital h. of quadratus labii superioris muscle,** see levator muscle of upper lip, under MUSCLE. **little h. of mandible,** mandibular CONDYLE. **long h.,** dolichocephalic SKULL. **low h.,** chamecephalic SKULL. **low-arched h.,** tapeinocephalic SKULL. **h. of mandible,** the articular surface of the condyloid process of the mandible. Called also *h. of condyloid process of mandible, capitulum [processus condyloidei] mandibulae,* and *caput mandibulae* [NA]. **h. of muscle,** the end of a muscle at the site of its attachment to a bone or other fixed structure (origin). Called also *caput musculi* [NA]. **nasal h. of levator muscle of upper lip, alaeque nasi muscle,** see levator muscle of upper lip and ala of nose, under MUSCLE. **short h.,** brachycephalic SKULL. **steeple h., tower h.,** oxycephaly. **tube h.,** a part of the x-ray generator consisting of the x-ray tube surrounded by a metal shield and suspended in oil which fills the space between the glass bulb and the shield, connected to the main unit by a flexible arm that allows the head to be brought to a desired position in relation to the patient. See also x-ray TUBE. See illustration at x-ray GENERATOR. **zygomatic h. of levator muscle of upper lip, zygomatic h. of quadratus labii superioris muscle,** see zygomatic muscle, lesser, under MUSCLE.

headache (hed′āk) pain in the head; cephalgia. Called also *dolor capitis.* See also MIGRAINE. **blind h.,** migraine. **cluster h.,** a condition characterized by unilateral headaches occurring in clusters, particularly in middle-aged males, in which severe pain is centered behind or close to the eye, but may extend to the cheek or to the occipital area. Ipsilateral nasal congestion, suffusion of the eye, excessive lacrimation, and facial redness and swelling may accompany or precede the headache. The duration is usually less than 30 minutes, but it may persist for several hours. The recurrent attacks often appear within a period of 24 hours, sometimes during sleep, and are similar to those induced by subcutaneous injection of histamine diphosphate. Called also *histamine h., Horton's h., Harris' neuralgia, histamine cephalgia, histamine neuralgia, Horton's disease, Horton's neuralgia,* and *periodic migrainous neuralgia.* **congestive h.,** one ascribed to congestion or hyperemia. Called also *hyperemic h.* **dental h.,** one occurring in association with toothache, after a tooth extraction, and various other dental conditions; it is believed to be a form of referred pain. **extracranial h.,** one due to any extracranial cause. **functional h.,** one due to tension or other emotional upset. See also MIGRAINE. **helmet h.,** pain involving the upper half of the head. **hemiplegic**

h., hemiplegic MIGRAINE. **histamine h., Horton's h.,** cluster h. **hyperemic h.,** congestive h. **intracranial h.,** one due to any intracranial cause. See also *organic h.* **leakage h.,** puncture h. **lower half h.,** a group of neuralgias which involve the lower half of the face, probably of vascular origin, and including sphenopalatine neuralgia and vidian neuralgia. **lumbar puncture h.,** puncture h. **muscle-contraction h., nervous h.,** one characterized by a steady ache in the temporal, occipital, parietal, or frontal regions, associated with a feeling of tightness and cramps of muscles in the neck and upper back. The pain may vary in severity and change from one site to another. It may persist from several days to several years. Called also *psychogenic h.* and *tension h.* **ophthalmoplegic h.,** hemiplegic MIGRAINE. **organic h.,** one due to intracranial or other organic disease. **postspinal h.,** puncture h. **psychogenic h.,** muscle-contraction h. **puncture h.,** a dull, usually pulsating headache, most often in the occipital region, occurring 12 to 24 hours following lumbar puncture, observed in patients who assume the erect posture, and usually subsiding if the patient lies flat. It has been speculated that leakage of the cerebrospinal fluid permits pressure on the unprotected pain-sensitive tissues of the posterior cranial fossa. Called also *leakage h., lumbar puncture h., postspinal h.,* and *spinal h.* **sick h.,** migraine. **Sluder's h.,** sphenopalatine NEURALGIA. **spinal h.,** puncture h. **tension h.,** muscle-contraction h. **traction h.,** one, usually of the vascular type, resulting from pulling on the intracranial structure by masses. **vacuum h.,** one due to obstruction of the outlet of the frontal sinus. **vascular h.,** one caused by dilatation and distention of branches of the carotid artery, associated with perivascular edema. The pain usually occurs in the temples and forehead. See also MIGRAINE and occipital NEURALGIA.

headcap (hed′kap) headgear. **plaster h.,** a cap fitting over the head, made of plaster of Paris, which incorporates points for applying fixation and traction appliance in the treatment of mandibular and maxillofacial injuries.

headdress (hed′dres) a covering for the head, such as a protective covering for the patient's head.

headgear (hed′gēr) 1. any covering for the head. 2. a harness-like device fitting over the top and back of the head, serving as a source of resistance for extraoral anchorage for an orthodontic appliance. Called also *headcap.* See also extraoral APPLIANCE. **high-pull h.,** an orthodontic device for giving an upward pull on the face-bow. **radiologic h.,** a covering for the head used in protecting the head from radiation injury.

HEADSTART (hed′start) a federally-sponsored program designed to provide educational, health, and social services to preschool children of poor families so that they may enter school having equal opportunity as less deprived children. Dental care is intended to be a part of the program.

healing (hēl′ing) a process of cure; the restoration of wounded parts. See also EPITHELIZATION and UNION. **h. by first intention,** primary UNION. **fibrous h.,** an uncommon complication which usually follows difficult tooth extraction associated with bone loss. The lesion is essentially a fibrous scar tissue with little or no evidence of ossification or inflammatory cell infiltration, which consists of dense bundles of collagen fibers with occasional fibrocytes and few blood vessels. It has few presenting symptoms, except for radiographic features, where it appears as a well circumscribed radiolucent area in the site of a previous extraction, suggesting residual infection. See also fibrous UNION. **h. by granulation,** secondary UNION. **primary h.,** primary UNION. **secondary h., h. by second intention,** secondary UNION.

health (helth) the state of optimal physical, mental, and social well-being and not merely the absence of disease and infirmity. **community h.,** all the personal health and environmental services in any human community. Sometimes used as a synonym for *public* or *environmental health.* See also community health CARE. **dental h.,** a state of complete normality and functional efficiency of the teeth and supporting structures and also of the surrounding parts of the oral cavity and of the various structures related to mastication and the maxillofacial complex. **dental public h.,** the prevention and control of dental diseases and promotion of dental health through organized community efforts, including dental health education of the public, applied dental research, the administration of group dental care programs, and the prevention and control of dental diseases on a community basis. Called also public health dentistry. **environmental h.,** that branch of public health concerned with the control of physical, chemical, and biological processes, influences, and factors that exercise or may exercise, by direct or indirect means, a significant effect on the physical and mental health and social well-being of man and his society. See also *community h.* **h. maintenance,** preventive health MAINTENANCE. **public h.,** preventing disease, prolonging life, and promoting mental and physical health and efficiency through organized community efforts for the sanitation of the environment, control of communicable infections, education of the individual in personal hygiene, organization of medical and nursing services for the early diagnosis and preventive treatment of diseases, and development of social mechanisms to ensure to every individual a standard of living adequate for the maintenance of health. See also *community h.*

HEALTH PLANNING & ADMIN Health Planning and Administration; a computer-searchable data base containing references from journals indexed for the MEDLARS system, *Hospital Literature Index,* and other publications dealing with topics pertaining to health planning, organization, financing, management, manpower, and related subjects. It is produced jointly by the National Library of Medicine and the American Hospital Association.

Healthco topical fluoride gel see under GEL.

hearing (hēr′ing) [L. *auditus*] the process or function of perceiving sound. **bone conduction h.,** bone CONDUCTION. **dentoaural h.,** bone conduction hearing, with a tooth or teeth serving as a sound-receptor. **h. loss,** deafness.

heart (hart) [L. *cor;* Gr. *kardia*] a hollow muscular organ located slightly to the left of the midline of the chest, which pumps

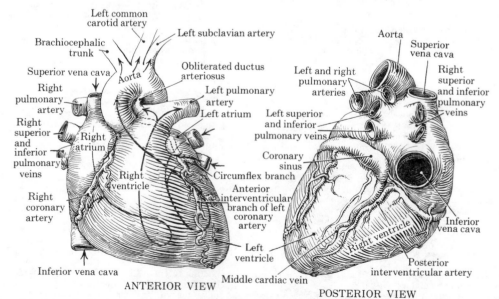

Structure of the heart. (From Dorland's Illustrated Medical Dictionary. 26th ed. Philadelphia, W. B. Saunders Co., 1980.)

blood through the body by its rhythmic contractions. It is enclosed in a muscular sac, consisting of an outer layer (pericardium), a middle layer (myocardium), and an inner lining (endocardium). The heart consists of four chambers and a system of valves: the *left ventricle*, which receives blood from the left atrium through the left atrioventricular (bicuspid or mitral) valve, and pumps it into the aorta through the aortic valve; the *right atrium*, which receives venous blood from the venae cavae and pumps it into the right ventricle through the right atrioventricular (tricuspid) valve; the *right ventricle*, which pumps blood into the pulmonary artery through the pulmonary valve; and the *left atrium*, which receives oxygenated blood from the lungs through the pulmonary vein and pumps it into the left ventricle. Called also *cor* [NA]. See illustration. See also terms beginning CARDIO-. **artificial h.**, a pumping mechanism that duplicates the output, rate, and blood pressure of the natural heart. It may replace the function of the entire heart or a portion of it. See also heart-lung MACHINE. **h. attack**, coronary OCCLUSION. **h. block**, heart BLOCK. **h. failure**, heart FAILURE. **h. failure, congestive**, see under FAILURE. **h. rate**, heart RATE.

heat (hēt) [L. *calor*; Gr. *thermē*] 1. the sensation of an increase in temperature. 2. increased body temperature. See CALOR and FEVER. 3. the energy which produces the sensation of heat. It exists in the form of molecular or atomic vibration (thermal agitation). Body heat may be transferred by conduction through a substance, by convection of a substance, by radiation, as electromagnetic waves, and by evaporation which cools the skin. 4. energy that is transferred as a consequence of a gradient in temperature. **h. of activation**, heat involved in catalytic processes. **h. capacity**, 1. specific h. 2. thermal CAPACITY. **h. of evaporation**, h. of vaporization. **h. of fusion**, the quantity of heat required to convert unit weight of a solid to the liquid state. **latent h. of fusion**, energy released in the form of heat during the transformation of a liquid to a solid state, measured in calories of heat liberated from 1 gm of a substance when it changes from the liquid to the solid state. **recovery h.**, that part of the heat developed by muscular contraction which is evolved after shortening. It follows the heat of activation. Called also *h. of shortening*. **sensible h.**, the heat which, when absorbed by a body, produces a rise in temperature unless an equal number of calories were lost concomitantly. **h. of shortening**, recovery h. **specific h.**, the amount of heat required to raise the temperature of unit mass of a substance 1 degree. Called also *h. capacity*. See also British thermal UNIT and CALORIE. **h. transfer**, heat TRANSFER. **h. treatment**, heat TREATMENT. **h. of vaporization**, the amount of heat required to convert a definite amount of a liquid at its boiling point into the gaseous state, e.g., 540 cal/gm water at 100° C. Called also *h. of evaporation*.

heater (hēt′er) a heat-producing apparatus. **compound h.**, a device for heating modeling compound and other impression materials that are softened by hot water, which is equipped with a thermometer and its holders, a lift, and two cloth covers to prevent the compound from adhering to the basin.

Heath's operation [Christopher *Heath*, English surgeon, 1835–1905] see under OPERATION.

Hebra's disease [Ferdinand von *Hebra*, Austrian dermatologist, 1816–1880] see under DISEASE.

Heck's disease [John W. *Heck*, American dentist, born 1923] focal epithelial HYPERPLASIA.

hecto- [Fr., from Gr. *hekaton* one hundred] in the metric system, a combining form denoting a quantity 100 (10^2) times the unit designated by the root with which it is combined. Abbreviated *h*. See also metric SYSTEM and *Tables of Weights and Measures* at WEIGHT.

hectogram (hek′to-gram) [*hecto-* + *gram*] a unit of mass (weight) in the metric system, being 100 (10^2) grams; the equivalent of 3.527 ounces avoirdupois weight, or 3.215 ounces apothecaries' weight. Abbreviated *h*.

hectoliter (hek′to-le″ter) [*hecto-* + *liter*] a unit of volume in the metric system, being 100 liters (10^2) or the equivalent of 26.418 U.S. gallons.

hectometer (hek-tom′ē-ter) a unit of linear measure in the metric system, being 100 (10^2) meters, or the equivalent, roughly, of 328 feet, 1 inch.

HED abbreviation for Ger. *Haut-Einheits-Dosis* (unit skin dose), a unit of roentgen-ray dosage established by Seitz and Wintz.

Hedström file root canal file, H-type; see under FILE.

Hedulin a trademark for *phenindione*.

heel (hēl) the hindmost part of the foot or a similar structure. **h. of denture**, distal end of denture; see under END.

Heerfordt's syndrome [Christian Frederik *Heerfordt*, Danish ophthalmologist] see under SYNDROME.

Hegglin's anomaly [Robert *Hegglin*] May-Hegglin ANOMALY.

Heidelberg jaw [named after *Heidelberg*, a German city] see under JAW.

Heidenhain's bodies, cells, demilunes [Rudolf Peter *Heidenhain*, German physiologist, 1834–1908] crescents of Giannuzzi; see under CRESCENT.

height (hīt) the vertical measurement of an object or body. In measurements of the human body, *height* and *length* are sometimes used interchangeably. **alveolar h., upper**, the distance between the nasospinale and interdentale superius. **basiobregmatic h.**, the distance measured from the basion to the bregma. **h. of contour**, the line encircling a tooth at its greatest bulge with reference to a predetermined part of insertion for a removable partial denture. See illustration at buccal SURFACE. **h. of contour, surveyed**, a line scribed or marked on a cast that designates the greatest bulge or diameter with respect to a selected path of denture placement or removal. **cusp h.**, 1. the shortest distance between the tip of a cusp of a tooth and its base plane. 2. the shortest distance between the deepest part of the central fossa of a posterior tooth and a line connecting the points of the cusps of the tooth. **excessive vertical maxillary h.**, long face SYNDROME. **facial h., anterior**, the height of the face measured from the nasion to the menton, gnathion, or pogonion. **facial h., lower**, the distance from interdentale inferius to gnathion. The ANS-Gn distance is used by some orthodontists in determining lower facial height. Called also *mental h.* and *symphyseal h. of mandible*. **facial h., posterior**, 1. a linear measure of a perpendicular line from the sella-nasion plane intersecting the mandibular plane; also measured from the sella to the gonion. 2. in orthodontics, the ramus height, i.e., from condylare to gonion. **facial h., upper**, the distance measured from nasion to interdentale superius; sometimes also measured from the nasion to the anterior nasal spine or to the prosthion. **h. of mandibular ramus**, the distance from the gonion to the highest point of the condyle; sometimes also measured from the gonion to the articulare. **mental h.**, facial h., lower. **h. of palate**, the distance of the maximum arching of the palate measured from the line connecting the inner borders of the alveoli of the two upper second molars, on both sides. **sitting h.**, sitting vertex h. **sitting vertex h.**, the distance from the highest point of the head in the sagittal plane to the surface on which the subject is seated; commonly called *sitting h.*; equivalent to *crown-rump length* in embryos, fetuses, and infants. **standing h., stature h.**, the distance from the highest point of the head in the sagittal plane to the surface on which the individual is standing; equivalent to *crown-heel length* in fetuses, embryos, and infants. **symphyseal h. of mandible**, facial h., lower.

Heimlich maneuver [Henry *Heimlich*, American physician] see under MANEUVER.

Heine-Medin disease [Jacob *Heine*, German physician, 1800–1879] POLIOMYELITIS.

Heinz body [Robert *Heinz*, German pathologist, 1865–1924] see under BODY.

Heister's diverticulum [Lorenz *Heister*, German anatomist, 1683–1758] superior bulb of jugular vein; see under BULB.

HeLa cells [derived from the name of the patient from whose carcinoma of the cervix uteri the parent carcinoma cells were isolated in 1951 at Johns Hopkins Hospital by Dr. George O. Gey] see under CELL.

helcoid (hel′koid) [Gr. *helkos* ulcer + *eidos* form] resembling an ulcer.

helcosis (hel-ko′sis) [Gr. *helkosis*] ulceration; the formation of an ulcer.

helico- [Gr. *helix* coil] a combining form denoting relationship to a coil, or to a snail.

helicoid (hel′i-koid) [*helico-* + Gr. *eidos* form] resembling or shaped like a coil or helix.

helion (he′le-on) helium.

helium (he′le-um) [Gr. *helios* sun] a colorless, odorless, tasteless, nontoxic, inert gas, first detected in the sun, and obtained from natural gas. Symbol, He; atomic number, 2; atomic weight, 4.003; melting point, below 272.2°C; density, 0.1785; valence, 0 (it is not known to combine with any other element); group 0 of the periodic table. It occurs as a natural isotope, ^{4}He, and has three short-lived artificial isotopes, 5, 6, and 8. Helium nuclei are alpha particles in radiations. Helium is produced in the decay of radioactive elements and by bombardment with radiations of beryllium, lithium, and other light elements. Used in a mixture with oxygen in the treatment of respiratory obstruction, as a diluent in anesthetic mixture, and, also mixed with oxygen, in heart surgery. The principal use for helium is in deep-sea diving to avoid toxic effects of oxygen on the lungs and central nervous system. Also called *helion*.

helix (he′liks) [Gr. "snail," "coil"] 1. a coil; anything wound in a spiral. 2. the superior and posterior free margin of the pinna of the ear. **double h., Watson-Crick h.,** a model of DNA formed by two long polynucleotide chains that run in opposite directions and are held together by regularly spaced hydrogen bonds, and that coil around each other into the double-stranded helical structure. Called also *Watson-Crick model*. See illustration at DNA.

helminth (hel′minth) [Gr. *helmins* worm] any parasitic worm.

helminthemesis (hel″min-them′ĕ-sis) [*helminth* + Gr. *emesis* vomiting] the vomiting of worms.

helminthiasis (hel″min-thi′ah-sis) an infection with helminths.

helo- [Gr. *hēlos* nail] a combining form denoting relationship to a nail, or to a wart or callus.

helper (help′er) one who or that which helps, aids, or assists. **lymphocyte h.,** helper CELL. **T-h. cell,** T-helper CELL.

Helwig's disease [E. B. *Helwig,* American physician] see under DISEASE.

hem-, hema- see HEMO-.

hemadsorption (hem″ad-sorp′shun) the adherence of red cells to other cells, particles, or surfaces. See also hemadsorption TEST.

hemagglutination (hem″ah-gloo″tĭ-na′shun) agglutination of erythrocytes by antibodies (hemagglutinins) or by viruses. **cold h.,** hemagglutination occurring in a mixture of erythrocytes and serum from the same individual at low temperatures (0° to 5°C), which is reversible by warming. **viral h.,** the agglutination of erythrocytes in the presence of hemagglutinating antibodies produced against specific receptors (antigens) on the erythrocyte stroma.

hemagglutinin (hem″ah-gloo″tĭ-nin) an antibody that agglutinates erythrocytes. **cold h.,** an antigen that reacts with its own specific antibody at low temperatures (i.e., below room temperature). **warm h.,** an antigen that reacts with its own specific antibody at warm temperatures (i.e., 30 to 37°C).

hemal (he′mal) pertaining to the blood.

hemangioameloblastoma (he-man″je-o-ah-mel″o-blas-to′mah) an ameloblastoma exhibiting large engorged capillaries. Called also *ameloblastic hemangioma*.

hemangioendothelioma (he-man″je-o-en″do-the″le-o′mah) [*hemangioma* + *endothelioma*] a benign neoplasm composed predominantly of masses of endothelial cells growing in and about vascular channels. It is an intermediate neoplasm between the well-differentiated hemangioma and anaplastic, cellular angiosarcoma. Its distribution pattern follows that of hemangioma, occurring most frequently in the skin, subcutaneous tissues, and mucous membranes, including that of the oral cavity. Typically, it presents a well-defined, pale gray to grayish red, firm tumor up to 4 to 5 cm in diameter, made up of masses and sheets of spindle endothelial cells, which may grow in whorls or undifferentiated sheets. The term is sometimes used to mean *hemangioendotheliosarcoma* (see ANGIOSARCOMA). **malignant h.,** angiosarcoma.

hemangioendotheliosarcoma (he-man″je-o-en″do-the″le-o-sar-ko′mah) [*hem-* + Gr. *angeion* vessel + *endothelium* + *sarcoma*] angiosarcoma.

hemangiofibroma (he-man″je-o-fi-bro′mah) a hemangioma characterized by proliferation of fibrous tissues.

hemangioma (he-man″je-o′mah) [*hem-* + *angioma*] a benign tumor made up of blood vessels, which may occur in any organ or tissue, but is most commonly located in the skin, subcutaneous tissues, and mucous membranes of the oral cavity and lips. Most are congenital and are present at birth. Oral tumors present a flat or raised, poorly defined, usually deep red or bluish red, lesion of the mucous membrane. According to some authorities, it is not a true neoplasm, but rather a developmental anomaly. See also ANGIOMA cavernosum. Cf. LYMPHANGIOMA. **ameloblastic h.,** hemangioameloblastoma. **capillary h.,** a hemangioma composed of blood vessels that, for the most part, have the caliber of the capillaries, usually located in the skin, subcutaneous tissue, and mucosa of the mouth and lips, but visceral organs may be also affected. Typically, it is a bright red to blue lesion ranging in diameter from a few millimeters to several centimeters; the covering epithelium is usually intact, but in exposed positions, it may ulcerate and be covered by oozing lesions. It is usually well defined but unencapsulated, and is made up of closely packed aggregations of thin-walled capillaries. The channels are lined with normal endothelial

cells and are filled with blood. Malignant degeneration is very rare. See also ANGIOMA cavernosum and NEVUS FLAMMEUS. **central h. of jaws,** a hemangioma that may occur either on the mandible or the maxilla. It is a bone-destroying lesion, varying in size and appearance, often suggestive of a cyst. **cavernous h.,** ANGIOMA cavernosum. **hypertrophic h.,** a cellular form of capillary hemangioma. **sclerosing h.,** a cellular tumor, believed to be a capillary hemangioma, which has been transformed from a vascularized tumor by the progressive proliferation of endothelial cells and connective tissue stroma.

hemangiopericytoma (he-man″je-o-per″ĭ-si-to′mah) a usually benign but sometimes metastasizing neoplasm of vascular origin, which may occur in any part of the body wherever there are capillaries, including the oral cavity. A typical tumor is found in the superficial soft tissues as a small, firm, circumscribed, sometimes nodular lesion composed of numerous capillary channels enclosed by round or spindle-shaped endothelial cells, resembling cells found in the glomangioma, identified as pericytes. Most tumors appear to be encapsulated at operation, but this is not often confirmed microscopically.

hemangiosarcoma (he-man″je-o-sar-ko′mah) a malignant tumor formed by proliferation of endothelial and fibroblastic tissue.

hematemesis (hem″ah-tem′ĕ-sis) [*hemat-* + Gr. *emesis* vomiting] the vomiting of blood.

hematin (hem′ah-tin) a complex of protoporphyrin with iron in the ferric state. See also HEME.

hemato- see HEMO-.

hematocele (hem′ah-to-sēl″) [*hemato-* + Gr. *kēlē* tumor] bloody effusion into a cavity.

hematocrit (he-mat′o-krit) [*hemato-* + Gr. *krinein* to separate] the volume of erythrocytes calculated in percent, as determined by centrifuging blood in specially graded tubes until the cells become packed in the bottom. In severe anemias, the percentage may fall to 10; in polycythemias, it may reach more than 60 percent. **body h.,** hematocrit calculated from samples taken from both the large and small vessels.

hematoencephalic (hem″ah-to-en″sĕ-fal′ik) [*hemato-* + Gr. *enkephalon* brain] pertaining to the blood and the brain, as in blood-brain barrier.

hematogenous (hem″ah-toj′ĕ-nus) [*hemato-* + *genesis*] produced by or derived from the blood; disseminated by the circulation or through the blood stream.

hematoma (hem″ah-to′mah) [*hemato-* + *-oma*] a localized lesion containing extravasated blood that is usually clotted, resulting from trauma or other factors causing rupture of blood vessels. It is normally circumscribed and in time assumes a dark discoloration. **eruption h.,** eruption CYST. **ossifying h.,** traumatic myositis ossificans; see under MYOSITIS.

hematopoiesis (hem″ah-to-poi-e′sis) [*hemato-* + Gr. *poiein* to make] the formation and development of blood cells. Called also *hemopoiesis*. See also ERYTHROPOIESIS, LEUKOPOIESIS, and THROMBOCYTOPOIESIS.

hematoscope (hem′ah-to-skōp) [*hemato-* + Gr. *skopein* to examine] 1. a photometric device used for determining the number of erythrocytes suspended in the blood, by means of measuring light dispersion. 2. a spectrophotometer for determining the blood hemoglobin level.

hematuria (hem″ah-tu′re-ah) [*hemat-* + Gr. *ouron* urine + *-ia*] the presence in the urine of blood.

heme (hēm) a protein-free constituent of the pigment portion of hemoglobin and various vegetable and animal cells, forming a chelate complex of protoporphyrin with iron in the ferrous state. Heme serves as coenzyme for proteins involved in oxygen transfer, for enzymes involved in oxidation reactions, and for enzymes catalyzing cleavage peroxides.

hemi- [Gr. *hēmi* half] a prefix signifying one-half.

hemialgia (hem″e-al′je-ah) [*hemi-* + *-algia*] pain affecting one side of the body or part; unilateral pain.

hemianalgesia (hem″e-an″al-je′ze-ah) [*hemi-* + *analgesia*] insensitivity to pain on one side of the body or part; unilateral analgesia.

hemianencephaly (hem″e-an″en-sef′ah-le) [*hemi-* + *an* neg. + Gr. *enkephalos* brain] a congenital defect characterized by absence of one side of the brain.

hemianesthesia (hem″e-an″es-the′ze-ah) [*hemi-* + *anesthesia*] anesthesia affecting one side of the body; unilateral anesthesia.

hemianopia (hem″e-ah-no′pe-ah) [*hemi-* + *an* neg. + Gr. *ōpē* vision + *-ia*] blindness affecting one half of the visual field.

hemianosmia (hem″e-an-oz′me-ah) [*hemi-* + *anosmia*] loss of sense of smell in one of the nostrils.

hemiatrophy (hem″e-at′ro-fe) [*hemi-* + *atrophy*] atrophy affecting one side of the body or of one half of an organ; unilateral atrophy. **facial h.,** progressive atrophy of some or all tissues on one side of the face, occasionally extending to other parts of the body and may involve the tongue, gingiva, soft palate, the cartilages of the nose, ear, and larynx, and the palpebral tarsus. The wasting usually begins during the second decade of life, but has been observed at birth as well as during middle age. Frequently pigmentation disorders, such as heterochromia, vitiligo, and pigmented facial nevi; trigeminal neuralgia; ocular complications, including strabismus, enophthalmos, ptosis, trichiasis, miosis, uveitis, and optic atrophy; jacksonian epilepsy and ataxia are associated. The immediate pathogenesis is not known, but local trauma and infection are considered to be predisposing factors. Called also *progressive facial h.*, *facial trophoneurosis*, *hemifacial atrophy*, *Parry-Romberg syndrome*, *progressive hemifacial paralysis*, *prosopodysmorphia*, and *Romberg's syndrome*. **progressive facial h.**, facial h. **progressive lingual h.**, progressive atrophy of one lateral half of the tongue.

hemicrania (hem″ĭ-kra′ne-ah) [*hemi-* + Gr. *kranion* skull] 1. pain involving only one part of the brain. See also MIGRAINE. 2. a birth defect characterized by lack of development of a part of the skull.

hemicraniectomy (hem″ĭ-kra″ne-ek′to-me) [*hemi-* + Gr. *kranion* skull + *ektomē* excision] sectioning the vault of the skull from before backward, near the median line, and forcing the entire side outward, thus exposing half of the brain.

hemicraniosis (hem″e-kra″ne-o′sis) a condition marked by hyperostosis of one half of the cranium or face.

hemidecortication (hem″ĭ-de-kor″tĭ-ka′shun) [*hemi-* + *decortication*] excision of one half of the cortex.

hemidesmosome (hem″e-des′mo-sōm) [*hemi-* + *desmosome*] a structure similar to a desmosome but representing only half of it, found on the basal surface of some epithelial cells, forming the site of attachment between the basal surface of the cell and the basement membrane. Called also *attachment plaque* and *half desmosome*.

hemidysesthesia (hem″e-dis″es-the′ze-ah) [*hemi-* + *dys-* + Gr. *aisthēsis* feeling] a disorder of sensation affecting one side of the body only.

hemidystrophy (hem″ĭ-dis′tro-fe) [*hemi-* + *dystrophy*] unequal development of two sides of the body; unilateral dystrophy.

hemiencephalus (hem″e-en-sef′ah-lus) [*hemi-* + Gr. *enkephalos* brain] a monster lacking one cerebral hemisphere.

hemifacial (hem″ĭ-fa′shal) pertaining to or affecting one half of the face.

hemigeusia (hem″ĭ-gu′se-ah) [*hemi-* + Gr. *geusis* taste + *-ia*] absence of the ability of taste perception on one side of the tongue.

hemigigantism (hem″ĭ-ji′gan-tizm) [*hemi-* + *gigantism*] overgrowth of one side of the body or part, as of the face; unilteral gigantism.

hemiglossal (hem″ĭ-glos′sal) [*hemi-* + Gr. *glōssa* tongue] pertaining to or affecting one side of the tongue; hemilingual.

hemiglossectomy (hem″ĭ-glos-sek′to-me) [*hemi-* + Gr. *glōssa* tongue + *ektomē* excision] resection of one side of the tongue.

hemiglossitis (hem″ĭ-glos-si′tis) [*hemi-* + *glossitis*] inflammation of one side of the tongue; unilateral glossitis.

hemignathia (hem″ĭ-nath′e-ah) [*hemi-* + Gr. *gnathos* jaw + *-ia*] a partial or complete unilateral lack of the mandible.

hemihidrosis (hem″ĭ-hi-dro′sis) [*hemi-* + Gr. *hidrōs* sweat] sweating on one side of the body only.

hemihydrate (hem″e-hi′drāt) a hydrate containing one molecule of water for every two molecules of other substance in the compound. **α-h.**, see GYPSUM hemihydrate. **α-h., modified**, Class I dental stone; see under STONE. **β-h.**, see GYPSUM hemihydrate. **calcium sulfate h.**, GYPSUM hemihydrate. **gypsum h.**, GYPSUM hemihydrate.

hemihypalgesia (hem″ĭ-hi′pal-je′ze-ah) [*hemi-* + *hypalgesia*] diminished capacity to perceive pain affecting one side of the body; unilateral hypalgesia.

hemihyperesthesia (hem″ĭ-hi″per-es-the′ze-ah) [*hemi-* + *hyperesthesia*] excessive sensitiveness of the skin or of organs of special sense, affecting one side of the body or part; unilateral hyperesthesia.

hemihyperplasia (hem″ĭ-hi″per-pla′ze-ah) [*hemi-* + *hyperplasia*] overdevelopment of one side of the body or part; unilateral hyperplasia.

hemihypertrophy (hem″ĭ-hi-per′tro-fe) [*hemi-* + *hypertrophy*] asymmetric overdevelopment of one half of the body or unilateral hypertrophy of a part. **facial h.**, hemifacial HYPERTROPHY.

hemihypoplasia (hem″ĭ-hi″po-pla′ze-ah) [*hemi-* + *hypoplasia*] underdevelopment of one side of the body or part; unilateral hypoplasia.

hemihypotonia (hem″ĭ-hi″po-to′ne-ah) [*hemi-* + *hypo-* + Gr. *tonos* tension + *-ia*] reduced tone of one side of the body or part; unilateral hypotonia.

hemilaryngectomy (hem″ĭ-lar″in-jek′to-me) [*hemi-* + *laryngectomy*] excision of one half of the larynx.

hemilateral (hem″ĭ-lat′er-al) [*hemi-* + *lateral*] affecting one half of one side.

hemilingual (hem″ĭ-ling′gwal) [*hemi-* + *lingual*] pertaining to or affecting one side of the tongue; hemiglossal.

hemimacroglossia (hem″ĭ-mak″ro-glos′e-ah) [*hemi-* + *macroglossia*] enlargement of one side of the tongue; unilateral macroglossia.

hemimandible (hem″ĭ-man′di-b'l) one of the lateral halves of the mandible.

hemimandibulectomy (hem″ĭ-man-dib-u-lek′to-me) [*hemi-* + *mandibulectomy*] surgical excision of one half of the mandible; unilateral mandibulectomy.

hemimaxillectomy (hem″ĭ-mak″sĭ-lek′to-me) [*hemi-* + *maxillectomy*] excision of half or part of the maxilla. Called also *partial maxillectomy*.

hemiparalysis (hem″ĭ-pah-ral′ĭ-sis) [*hemi-* + *paralysis*] hemiplegia.

hemiparaplegia (hem″ĭ-par″ah-ple′je-ah) [*hemi* + *paraplegia*] paralysis of the lower half of one side of the body; unilateral paraplegia.

hemiparesis (hem″ĭ-par′e-sis) [*hemi-* + *paresis*] muscular weakness of one side of the body or part; unilateral paresis.

hemiparesthesia (hem″ĭ-par″es-the′ze-ah) [*hemi-* + *paresthesia*] perverted sensation affecting one side of the body or part; unilateral paresthesia.

hemiparkinsonism (hem″ĭ-par′kin-son′izm) [*hemi-* + *parkinsonism*] parkinsonism affecting one side of the body; unilateral parkinsonism.

hemiplegia (hem″ĭ-ple′je-ah) [*hemi-* + Gr. *plēgē* stroke] paralysis of the muscles on one side of the body, affecting most commonly the face, arm, and leg. It is usually caused by a brain lesion, such as a tumor or cerebrovascular accident, and occurs on the side opposite the lesion. Called also *hemiparalysis* and *unilateral paralysis*. **abducens-facial h. alternans**, Millard-Gubler SYNDROME. **h. abducentofacia′lis**, Foville's SYNDROME. **h. al′ternans hypoglos′sica**, Jackson-MacKenzie SYNDROME. **h. al′ternans infe′rior**, 1. Millard-Gubler SYNDROME. 2. Foville's SYNDROME. **h. al′ternans infe′rior pon′tina**, Foville's SYNDROME. **h. al′ternans supe′rior peduncula′ris**, Leyden's PARALYSIS. **alternate h.**, that which affects a part on one side of the body and another part on the side opposite. Called also *crossed h.* and *h. cruciata.* **alternating hypoglossal h.**, hemorrhage or thrombosis of the anterior spinal artery producing ipsilateral paralysis of the tongue, contralateral pyramidal paralysis of the arm and leg, and occasionally contralateral loss of the proprioceptive and tactile senses. Called also *anterior bulbar syndrome*, *Déjérine's syndrome*, and *pyramidohypoglossal syndrome*. **capsular h.**, that due to a lesion of the internal capsule. **cerebral h.**, that caused by a brain lesion. **contralateral h.**, that on the side opposite the brain lesion. **crossed h., h. crucia′ta**, alternate h. **facial h.**, that in which the muscles of the face are affected. **faciobrachial h.**, that affecting the face and the arm on the same side. **faciolingual h.**, that affecting the face and tongue. **glossolaryngoscapulopharyngeal h.**, Collet-Sicard SYNDROME. **Gubler's h.**, Millard-Gubler SYNDROME. **middle alternating h.**, Millard-Gubler SYNDROME. **h. oculomotor′ica**, Leyden's PARALYSIS. **puerperal h.**, that which occurs shortly after childbirth. **Wernicke-Mann h.**, partial hemiplegia of the extremities characterized by typical posture and gait disorders. It is caused by lesions of the central nervous system which result in contralateral spastic paralysis of the muscles of upper and lower extremities and of the face. Called also *Wernicke-Mann type*.

hemiplegic (hem″ĭ-ple′jik) 1. pertaining to or affected with hemiplegia. 2. a person affected with hemiplegia.

hemisection (hem″ĭ-sek′shun) [*hemi-* + L. *sectio* a cut] a division or cutting into two parts; bisection. **tooth h.**, the surgical separation of a multirooted tooth through the furcation area in such a way that the blocked, defective, or periodontally affected root or roots may be removed along with the associated portion of the crown; used most commonly on lower molars, but may be performed on any multirooted tooth.

hemisectomy (he″me-sek′to-me) [*hemi-* + Gr. *ektomē* excision] amputation of one of two roots of a two-rooted mandibular tooth. See also root AMPUTATION.

hemiseptum (hem″e-sep′tum) 1. a half of a septum. 2. the remaining portion of the interdental septum after the mesial or distal portion has been destroyed by disease. See illustration at periodontal bony DEFECT. **h. of interalveolar bone**, a septum of the interalveolar bone that has been partially destroyed by periodontitis.

hemisotonic (hem″i-so-ton′ik) [*hem-* + *isotonic*] having the same osmotic pressure as the blood.

hemispasm (hem′ĭ-spazm) [*hemi-* + *spasm*] spasm affecting one side of the body or part; unilateral spasm. **hysterical glossolabial h.,** Brissaud-Marie SYNDROME.

hemisphere (hem′ĭ-sfēr) [*hemi-* + Gr. *sphaira* a ball, a globe] half of any spherical or roughly spherical structure or organ, such as the cerebral hemispheres. **cerebral h.,** either of two symmetrical parts of the cerebrum, separated from each other by a longitudinal fissure, and covered by a layer of gray matter, the cerebral cortex. Called also *hemispherium* [NA]. See BRAIN.

hemispherectomy (hem″ĭ-sfer-ek′to-me) [*hemisphere* + Gr. *ektomē* excision] excision of a hemisphere; usually a cerebral hemisphere.

hemispherium (hem″ĭ-sfe′re-um), pl. *hemisphe′ria* [L.] 1. a general anatomical term denoting half of a spherical or spheroid structure. 2. [NA] cerebral HEMISPHERE.

hemitetany (hem″ĭ-tet′ah-ne) [*hemi-* + *tetany*] tetany affecting only one side of the body; unilateral tetany.

hemizygosity (hem″ĭ-zi-gos′ĭ-te) the state of possessing only one of a pair of genes that influence the determination of a particular trait, as the male has no alleles on the Y chromosome for those on the X, so that his X-linked genes are expressed whether they are dominant or recessive. See also sex-linked CHARACTER.

hemizygous (hem″ĭ-zi′gus) exhibiting hemizygosity.

hemo-, haemo, hem-, haem-, hema-, haema-, hemato-, haemato- [Gr. *haima, haimatos* blood] a combining form denoting relationship to the blood.

hemoblast (he′mo-blast) [*hemo-* + Gr. *blastos* germ] hemocytoblast. **lymphoid h.,** pronormoblast.

Hemocaprol trademark for *aminocaproic acid* (see under ACID).

hemochromatosis (he″mo-kro″mah-to′sis) a disorder of iron metabolism characterized by a triad of hemosiderosis, liver cirrhosis, and diabetes mellitus, although all three components are not invariably present. The disorder may occur in a hereditary form (*idiopathic* or *classic h.*), or a exogenous form due to an external cause, such as massive blood transfusion or iron overload. It occurs most commonly in males over the age of 40, and is characterized by bronze-tan discoloration, chiefly of the face, arms, genitals, and skin folds, associated with iron deposits in the pancreas, liver, endocrine glands, skin, spleen, lymph nodes, and reticuloendothelial cells (see systemic HEMOSIDEROSIS). Liver disorders, anorexia, sexual impotence, gynecomastia, gastrointestinal disorders, weight loss, portal hypertension, and osseous and articular changes may occur. Pigmentation of the oral mucosa may be present. Called also *bronze diabetes, bronzed diabetes, iron storage disease, pigmentary cirrhosis,* and *Recklinghausen-Applebaum disease.*

hemocyanin (he″mo-si′ah-nin) [*hemo-* + Gr. *kyanos* blue] a chromoprotein containing copper, whose function is oxygen transport in mollusks and arthropods; it is a blue respiratory pigment corresponding to hemoglobin in higher animals.

hemocyte (he′mo-sīt) [*hemo-* + Gr. *kytos* hollow vessel] a blood cell, or formed element of the blood.

hemocytoblast (he″mo-si′to-blast) [*hemocyte* + Gr. *blastos* germ] a free stem cell believed to be the precursor of blood cells. Called also *hemoblast.*

Hemodal trademark for *menadione sodium bisulfite* (see under MENADIONE).

Hemodent trademark for an astringent solution, 1 gm of which contains 250 mg aluminum chloride. Used to stop gingival bleeding and to retract gingival tissue in impression taking.

hemoglobin (he″mo-glo′bin) [*hem-* + *globin*] the oxygen-carrying pigment of the blood, which gives it its red color. Hemoglobin is the principal protein of erythrocytes, forming a combination of globin and a pigment, heme. Hemoglobin has the property of combining with certain gases; combination with oxygen forms *oxyhemoglobin* and combination with carbon monoxide (seen in carbon monoxide poisoning), forms *carboxyhemoglobin.* Its function is to provide transport for oxygen from the lungs to the tissues. Abbreviated *Hb.* **h. A,** adult h. **adult h.,** hemoglobin that replaces fetal hemoglobin by the end of the first year of life. Its globin contains two pairs of peptide chains, the α-chain consisting of 141 amino acids and the β-chain of 146 amino acids. Abbreviated *Hb A.* Called also *h. A.* **h. C,** an abnormal adult hemoglobin in which lysine replaces glutamic acid in the β-chain. It is more soluble and more stable than normal hemoglobin A, but tends to crystallize under certain conditions and causes the erythrocytes to assume rigid, rod-shaped forms.

Hemoglobin C occurs most frequently in blacks in West Africa and, less commonly, American blacks, American Indians, and certain other ethnic groups. Abbreviated *Hb C.* See also hemoglobin C TRAIT, homozygous C DISEASE, sickle cell–hemoglobin C DISEASE, and thalassemia-hemoglobin C DISEASE. **extracorpuscular h.,** free hemoglobin; hemoglobin found outside of the erythrocytes, usually due to destruction of the erythrocyte stroma in hemolysis. **h. F,** fetal h. **fetal h.,** hemoglobin present in the blood of newborn infants, which is replaced by adult hemoglobin by the end of the first year of life, but is sometimes retained in some types of hereditary blood diseases, such as thalassemias. It is more resistant to alkali and its globin possesses a pair of α peptide chains which are similar to those in adult hemoglobin, but in addition, a pair of peptide chains designated γ which differ from β-chains. Abbreviated *Hb F.* Called also *h. F.* **free h.,** hemoglobin not contained within the erythrocytes. See *extracorpuscular h.* **h. M,** any of several hemoglobins having amino acid substitutions either in the alpha or beta chains and all associated with methemoglobinemia. **mean corpuscular h.,** see MCH. **mean corpuscular h. concentration,** see MCHC. **muscle h.,** myoglobin. **h. S,** sickle cell h. **sickle cell h.,** an abnormal hemoglobin in which valine replaces glutamine in the β-chain of the globin portion. When deoxygenated, sickle cell hemoglobin becomes insoluble owing to formation of tactoids (doubly-refracting rodlike particles), causing the erythrocyte to assume the shape of a sickle. Seen in sickle cell anemia and sickle cell trait (see under ANEMIA and TRAIT, respectively). Abbreviated *Hb S.* Called also *h. S.*

hemoglobinemia (he″mo-glo″bĭ-ne′me-ah) [*hemoglobin* + *-ia*] the presence in the blood plasma of extracorpuscular hemoglobin, usually due to hemolytic conditions.

hemoglobinometry (he″mo-glo″bĭ-nom′ĕ-tre) the measurement of the hemoglobin of the blood. Using the spectrophotometric method, an average content for adult males is 16 ± 2.0 gm/100 ml, and for adult females is 14 ± 2.0 gm/100 ml of blood.

hemoglobinopathy (he″mo-glo″bĭ-nop′ah-the) [*hemoglobin* + Gr. *pathos* disease] a hematologic disease, usually determined as a genetic trait, caused by the presence of an abnormal hemoglobin in the blood.

hemoglobinuria (he″mo-glo″bĭ-nu′re-ah) [*hemoglobin* + Gr. *ouron* urine + *-ia*] the presence of free hemoglobin in the urine; usually a sign of a hemolytic condition. **paroxysmal cold h.,** hemoglobinuria characterized by the sudden passage of dark brownish to black urine following exposure to cold, often associated with leg pains, abdominal cramps, malaise, chills, fever, vasomotor disorders, paleness of the skin, and blanching of the ears and lips. It is believed to be caused by the presence of autohemolysins in the blood which causes the erythrocytes to unite at low temperature, followed by hemolysis after the blood is rewarmed. It was classically seen in patients with syphilis, but it is also seen in the absence of syphilis, and is encountered following viral infections. **paroxysmal nocturnal h.,** Marchiafava-Micheli SYNDROME.

hemolysin (he-mol′ĭ-sin) [*hemo-* + Gr. *lysis* dissolution] any substance which enhances hemolysis by destroying the erythrocyte stroma, thus allowing for the hemoglobin to escape from the cell. **staphylococcal h.,** staphylolysin.

hemolysis (he-mol′ĭ-sis) [*hemo-* + Gr. *lysis* dissolution] rupture of the erythrocyte stroma resulting in the escape of hemoglobin from the cell. It may be caused by various conditions, including exposure to bacterial poisons, snake venoms, certain drugs, transfusion of incompatible blood, or exposure to cold in patients with paroxysmal cold hemoglobinuria. Hypertonic and hypotonic solutions produce hemolysis in vitro. See also *autohemolysis* and hemolytic ANEMIA. **acute familial h.,** a familial syndrome characterized by a sudden attack of acute anemia, jaundice, hemoglobinuria, and severe hemolysis. Generalized malaise, fever, abdominal pain, vomiting, and arthralgia may precede the onset of the acute symptoms. Called also *Bernard's syndrome.* **immune h.,** hemolysis resulting from changes in the erythrocyte membrane by immune complexes in the presence of complement. **osmotic h.,** hemolysis of erythrocytes in solutions with lower osmotic pressure than that of plasma (a 0.9 percent sodium chloride solution is isotonic with plasma), caused by swelling of the membrane resulting in its rupture and escape of hemoglobin and other cell components into the surrounding medium. See also osmotic FRAGILITY.

hemolytic (he″mo-lit′ik) pertaining to, characterized by, or causing hemolysis.

Hemo-Pak trademark for *oxidized cellulose* (see under CELLULOSE).

hemopericardium (he″mo-per″ĭ-kar′de-um) [*hemo-* + *pericardium*] hemorrhage associated with collection of blood within the pericardium.

hemoperitoneum (he″mo-per″ĭ-to-ne′um) [*hemo-* + *peritoneum*] hemorrhage associated with collection of blood in the peritoneal cavity.

hemopexin (he″mo-pek′sin) [*hemo-* + Gr. *pexis* fixation] a protein found in small quantities in human serum, which is synthesized by the liver, and contains a single polypeptide chain and about 30 percent carbohydrate. Hemopexin has a molecular weight of about 80,000 to 97,000 and a sedimentation coefficient of 4.8S to 4.3S. It is believed to be involved in heme removal from the blood by binding heme but not hemoglobin. Hemopexin often disappears from the blood in some hemolytic diseases.

hemophilia (he″mo-fil′e-ah) [*hemo-* + Gr. *philein* to love + *-ia*] 1. a genetically determined blood coagulation disorder, especially one which is caused by inadequate prothrombin utilization due to lack of plasma thromboplastin in factor VIII, IX, or XI deficiency. 2. h. A. **h. A,** the most common form of hemophilia, due to coagulation factor VIII deficiency, characterized generally by a prolonged coagulation time and a bleeding tendency that may result in hemarthroses, deep tissue hemorrhage, and uncontrolled hemorrhage even after a minor injury or surgical intervention. It is transmitted as a sex-linked recessive trait: parents transmitting the gene to daughters who, in turn, transmit it to one half of their daughters and to one half of their sons; as a rule, only males are affected but some cases have been reported in females. The disorder is usually present at birth but may go unrecognized for many years. Spontaneous periodic remissions and exacerbations are common. Oral manifestations include oozing of the blood from many sites in the oral cavity, which may persist for several days or weeks, and hematomas, usually of the tongue and floor of the mouth. Tooth extraction and tonsillectomy may produce fatal hemorrhage. Rubber band extraction (see under EXTRACTION) is sometimes used in hemophiliacs to prevent hemorrhage. Called also *classical h., h. I, bleeder's disease, disease of the Hapsburgs, disease of kings,* and *PTF-A deficiency.* **h. B,** Christmas DISEASE. **h. C,** hemophilia that may resemble hemoph lia A, but due to deficiency of coagulation factor XI (see under FACTOR). **classical h., h. A. h. I, h. A. h. II,** hemophilia B; see Christmas DISEASE. **vascular h.,** Willebrand-Jürgens SYNDROME.

hemophiliac (he″no-fil′e-ak) an individual exhibiting hemophilia.

hemophilic (he-mo-fil′ik) 1. having an affinity for blood; living in blood. In bacteriology, growing especially well in culture media containing blood. 2. pertaining to or characterized by hemophilia.

Hemophilus (he-mof′i-lus) *Haemophilus.* **H. hemolyt′icus vagina′lis,** *Haemophilus vaginalis;* see under HAEMOPHILUS.

hemophilus (he-mof′i-lus) any microorganism of the genus *Haemophilus.* **influenza-like h.,** *Haemophilus parainfluenzae;* see under HAEMOPHILUS. **h. of Koch-Weeks,** *Haemophilus aegyptius;* see under HAEMOPHILUS.

hemopoiesis (he″mo-poi-e′sis) hematopoiesis.

hemopoietin (he″mo-poi-e′tin) [*hemo-* + Gr. *poein* to make] erythropoietin.

hemoprotein (he″mo-pro′te-in, he″mo-pro′tēn) a conjugated protein containing heme as the prosthetic group.

hemoptysis (he-mop′ti-sis) [*hemo-* + Gr. *ptyein* to spit] the expectoration of blood or of blood-stained sputum.

hemorrhage (hem′or-ij) [*hemo-* + Gr. *rhēgnynai* to burst forth] the escape of blood from vessels, usually due to a rupture. Hemorrhage into a serous cavity is known as *hemothorax, hemopericardium,* and *hemoperitoneum.* That with accumulation of blood within a tissue with clot formation is known as *hematoma.* Small hemorrhages, usually in the skin, mucous membranes, and serosal surfaces, are known as *petechiae, purpura,* and *ecchymoses.* **alveolar h.,** hemorrhage from a dental alveolus. **arterial h.,** the escape of blood from an artery, as in a ruptured aneurysm. **essential h.,** that not attributable to an established cause. **gingival h.,** gingival BLEEDING. **internal h.,** that in which the extravasated blood remains within the body. **massive h.,** loss of blood so rapid and profuse that shock supervenes unless appropriate replacement is instituted promptly. **nasal h.,** epistaxis. **parenchymatous h.,** capillary hemorrhage into the substance of an organ. **h. per rhexin,** hemorrhage from rupture of a blood vessel. **petechial h.,** that occurring in minute points beneath the skin. See also *punctate h.* **plasma h.,** the loss of the fluid portion (plasma) of the blood. **postextraction h.,** that occurring after tooth extraction. **primary h.,** that occurring immediately following injury. **punctate h.,** spots of blood effused into the tissues from capillary hemorrhage. See also *petechial h.* **recurring h.,** intermittent episodes of bleeding. **secondary h.,** bleeding which follows an accident or injury after a lapse of time. **spontaneous h.,** that occurring without any apparent cause. **venous h.,** the escape of blood from the venous system. Called also *phleborrhagia.* **vicarious h.,** the

loss of blood from any area in consequence of the suppression of a bleeding in another area.

hemorrhagenic (hem″o-rah-jen′ik) [*hemórrhage* + Gr. *gennan* to produce] causing hemorrhage.

hemorrhagic (hem″o-raj′ik) pertaining to or characterized by hemorrhage; descriptive of any tissue into which bleeding has occurred.

hemosiderin (he″mo-sid′er-in) [*hemo-* + Gr. *sidēros* iron] a protein-iron complex, consisting of a water-insoluble protein and ferric hydroxide clusters, found in the cells of the reticuloendothelial system. It comprises almost one-half of the total body storage iron.

hemosiderinuria (he″mo-sīd″er-in-u′re-ah) the presence of hemosiderin in the urine.

hemosiderosis (he″mo-sīd″er-o′sis) deposition of iron in various tissues of the body resulting in a bluish-black or bronze pigmentation of affected areas, due to hemorrhage with subsequent release of the red cell iron or excessive iron intake. See also HEMOCHROMATOSIS. **hepatic h.,** systemic hemosiderosis characterized by excessive deposits of iron in the liver, usually in Kupffer cells. **localized h.,** a localized form that may occur in any tissue following a hemorrhage associated with a local release of the red cell iron. **pulmonary h.,** systemic hemosiderosis characterized by excessive deposits of iron in the lungs. **systemic h.,** a form associated with the excessive breakdown of red cells, most commonly encountered in hemolytic anemia, sickle cell anemia, hemolytic reactions to poisoning, excessive blood transfusion, and excessive iron intake, as in heavy drinkers of wine containing iron-rich sediments. Pigmentation is found first in the reticuloendothelial system of the bone marrow, lymph nodes, and spleen, progressing to the skin, kidneys, and pancreas. Massive cell destruction may cause release of pigment into the intercellular spaces, causing fibrous proliferation. Oral manifestations may include deposits of pigment in the salivary glands and pigmentation of the oral mucosa. Hemosiderosis is the principal component of hemochromatosis.

hemostasis (he-mos′tah-sis, he″mo-sta′sis) [*hemo-* + Gr. *stasis* halt] the arrest or checking of bleeding through natural processes or through the use of artificial means. Natural hemostasis involves: (1) constriction of the injured vessel, bringing about the reduction of blood flow through the damaged part; (2) formation of the platelet plug, whereby platelets, upon coming in contact with the wettable surface of the collagen fibers of the vascular wall, begin to swell, assume irregular forms with irradiating processes protruding outwardly, become sticky, and secrete large amounts of ADP which activates other platelets and causes them to stick together, thus forming a plug that keeps blood from escaping; (3) blood clotting; (4) growth of fibrous tissue into the blood clot to close the hole in the vessel permanently; (5) clot retraction. The clot may be dissolved by plasmin, once the repair is complete. Artificial hemostasis is accomplished by arresting the escape of blood by compression, tourniquet, application of bandages or adhesive tape, suturing the injured vessel, and administration of hemostatic drugs. See illustration. See also blood COAGULATION. **intravascular h.,** the

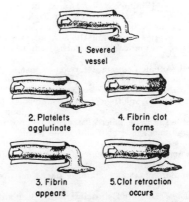

1. Severed vessel

2. Platelets agglutinate

3. Fibrin appears

4. Fibrin clot forms

5. Clot retraction occurs

The clotting process in the traumatized blood vessel. (From A. C. Guyton: Textbook of Medical Physiology. 6th ed. Philadelphia, W. B. Saunders Co., 1981; redrawn from Seegers: Hemostatic Agents. Charles C Thomas.)

arrest of bleeding through the formation of a fibrin plug which seals the broken vessel. **vascular h.,** the arrest of bleeding through vascular constriction following an injury to a blood vessel.

hemostat (he′mo-stat) 1. an agent that checks hemorrhage when applied to a bleeding point. 2. a small straight or curved scissors-like surgical instrument with grooved or serrated blades and a mechanical lock on the handles to prevent accidental opening; used for constricting blood vessels during surgery to prevent bleeding. Also used to hold dental film in the mouth. Called also *hemostatic forceps.* **Halsted's mosquito h.,** a delicate type of either straight or curved hemostat. See illustration. **Kelly h.,** a curved or straight type of a hemostat for holding material and tissue. See illustration.

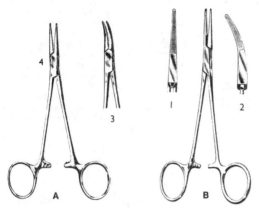

A, Kelly hemostats. *B,* Halsted mosquito hemostats. (From H. O. Torres and A. Ehrlich: Modern Dental Assisting. 2nd ed. Philadelphia. W. B. Saunders Co., 1980; courtesy of Hu-Friedy Mfg. Co., Inc.)

hemostatic (he″mo-stat′ik) [hemo- + Gr. *statikos* standing] 1. checking the flow of blood. 2. any agent, chemical or mechanical, that arrests bleeding. Mechanical devices include hemostatic forceps, bandages and packs, sutures, or tourniquets. Chemical hemostatic agents are those which arrest bleeding by producing rapid blood coagulation, formation of an artificial clot, providing a matrix that facilitates clotting, or constricting the blood vessel. See also ASTRINGENT. **adsorbable h.,** a substance used to control hemorrhage from minute vessels by arresting bleeding by formation of an artificial clot or providing an artificial matrix that facilitates clotting. Absorbable hemostatics are absorbed from the site of application after varying periods of time. Oxidized cellulose, absorbable gelatin sponge, and fibrinogen and thrombin preparations are the principal absorbable hemostatics.

Hemostatin trademark for *epinephrine.*

hemothorax (he″mo-tho′raks) [hemo- + *thorax*] hemorrhage associated with collection of blood in the pleural cavity.

Hench-Aldrich test [Philip S. *Hench,* American physician, 1896–1965, co-winner, with Edward Calvin Kendall and Tadeus Reichstein, of the Nobel prize for medicine and physiology in 1950, for discoveries concerning the adrenal cortex hormones; Martha *Aldrich,* American biochemist, born 1897] see under TEST.

Henderson-Hasselbalch equation [Lawrence Joseph *Henderson,* American chemist, 1878–1954; Karl A. *Hasselbalch,* Danish scientist, born 1892] see under EQUATION.

Henle's elastic membrane (fenestrated membrane), fibers, loop [Friedrich Gustav Jakob *Henle,* German anatomist and histologist, 1809–1885] see under MEMBRANE, FIBER, and LOOP; see also pterygoid PROCESS (trapezoid bone of Henle), sphenomandibular LIGAMENT (medial accessory ligament of Henle), sphenopalatine notch of palatine bone, under NOTCH (palatine incisure of Henle), supramalatine SPINE (spine of Henle), and temporomandibular LIGAMENT (lateral accessory ligament of Henle).

Henoch's disease [Edouard Heinrich *Henoch,* German physician, 1820–1910] Schönlein-Henoch SYNDROME.

henry (hen′re) [named after Joseph *Henry*] the SI unit of electric inductance, being the inductance in which an induced electromotive force of 1 volt is produced when the inducing current

is changed at the rate of 1 ampere per second. Abbreviated *H.* See also SI.

Henry, John [1797–1836] an American physicist. See HENRY.

Henry's law [William *Henry,* English chemist, 1774–1836] see under LAW.

Hensen's canal (duct), cell, disk, line, node (knot) [Victor *Hensen,* German anatomist and physiologist, 1835–1924] see under CANAL and NODE, and see supporting CELL, H BAND, and M BAND.

hepar (he′par) [Gr. *hēpar*] [NA] liver (1).

heparan sulfate (hep′ah-ran) a monosulfuric acid ester of an acetylated (*N*-acetyl) **heparin.**

heparin (hep′ah-rin) a sulfated dextrorotatory mucopolysaccharide, containing a repeating unit of α-1,3 linked glucuronic acid and glucosamine, with sulfate groups on some of the hydroxyl and amino groups. It occurs in various tissues, being most abundant in the liver and lungs. Pharmacologically, heparin is an anticoagulant, preventing the clotting of blood by inhibiting the conversion of prothrombin to thrombin (thrombin acting as a catalyst in converting plasma fibrinogen into the fibrin clot). Used in the treatment and prevention of thrombosis. Side effects may include predisposition toward hemorrhage after surgery and the development of spontaneous hemorrhage from the gingiva. Called also *heparinic acid.* See also ANTICOAGULANT. β-**heparin,** DERMATAN sulfate. **h. sulfate,** HEPARAN sulfate.

hepat- see HEPATO-.

hepatic (he-pat′ik) [L. *hepaticus;* Gr. *hepatikos*] pertaining to the liver.

hepatitides (hep″ah-tit′ĭ-dēz) plural of *hepatitis.*

hepatitis (hep″ah-ti′tis), pl. *hepati′tides* [hepat- + -itis] inflammation of the liver. **anicteric h.,** a form of infectious hepatitis that is not accompanied by jaundice. **chronic interstitial h.,** liver CIRRHOSIS. **epidemic h.,** infectious h. **homologous serum h.,** a form of infectious hepatitis transmitted by contaminated syringes, hypodermic needles, dental and surgical instruments, tattoo needles, razors, and, most commonly, transfusion of blood from infected persons. Professional personnel and laboratory workers are subject to occupational infection and drug addicts who share infected needles are particularly prone. It is characterized by hepatitis with or without jaundice (*anicteric h.*). In young patients the course is usually mild and is seldom accompanied by jaundice; in older persons it is often acute or subacute and is complicated by jaundice and liver necrosis. Called also *serum h., virus B h.,* and *homologous serum jaundice.* **infectious h.,** a viral disease usually transmitted by the fecal-oral route. Epidemics occur most commonly in institutions that house small children, owing to ingestion of contaminated beverages and food, such as drinking water, milk, or shellfish; poor hygienic conditions being the contributing factor. It is characterized by hepatitis with or without jaundice (*anicteric h.*) and liver necrosis. In young patients the course is usually mild and often is unaccompanied by jaundice; in older persons it has frequently an acute or subacute course and is complicated by jaundice and liver necrosis. Called also *epidemic h., virus A h., catarrhal jaundice,* and *epidemic jaundice.* See also *homologous serum h.* **serum h.,** homologous serum h. **virus A h.,** infectious h. **virus B h.,** homologous serum h.

hepato-, hepat- [Gr. *hēpar* liver] a combining form denoting relationship to the liver.

hepatomegaly (hep″ah-to-meg′ah-le) [hepato- + Gr. *megas* large] enlargement of the liver.

hepatosplenomegaly (hep″ah-to-sple″no-meg′ah-le) [hepato- + Gr. *splēn* spleen + *megas* big] enlargement of the liver and spleen.

hepatotoxicity (hep″ah-to-tok-sis′ĭ-te) the quality of exerting a destructive or poisonous effect upon the liver.

hepatotropic (hep″ah-to-trōp′ik) [hepato- + Gr. *tropos* a turning] having a special affinity for or exerting a specific effect upon the liver.

hepta-, hept- [Gr. *hepta* seven] a combining form meaning seven.

heptad (hep′tad) any element having a valence of seven.

Heptadon trademark for the *dl* form of *methadone hydrochloride* (see under METHADONE).

Heptadrine trademark for *tuaminoheptane.*

heptahydrate (hep″tah-hi′drāt) [hepta- + *hydrate*] a hydrate containing seven molecules of water for every molecule of other substance in the compound.

Heptalgin trademark for *phenadoxone hydrochloride* (see under PHENADOXONE).

Heptalin trademark for *phenadoxone hydrochloride* (see under PHENADOXONE).

Heptamine trademark for *tuaminoheptane.*

heptane (hep′tān) *n*-heptane; a seven-carbon straight chain hydrocarbon of the methane series, C_7H_{16}, obtained by distillation of petroleum, occurring as a highly volatile liquid. Used as a solvent, in the preparation of laboratory reagents, and in petroleum technology. Inhalation of fumes may cause mucosal irritation. In high concentrations, it may be narcotic.

heptazone hydrochloride (hep′tah-zōn) PHENADOXONE hydrochloride.

Heptin trademark for *tuaminoheptane*.

heptose (hep′tōs) a monosaccharide containing seven carbon atoms in a molecule, $C_7H_{14}O_7$.

herb (erb, herb) any leafy plant without a woody stem, especially one used as a household remedy or as a flavoring agent. **death's h.,** belladonna (1). **Nicot's h.,** *Nicotiana*.

herbicide (her′bĭ-sīd) [L. *herba* herb + *caedere* to kill] an agent that is destructive to weeds and plants.

heredity (he-red′ĭ-te) [L. *hereditas*] the genetic transmission of biological characteristics from parent to progeny, including the storage, replication, mutation, recombination, and translation of genetic material in chromosomes. See also GENETICS and INHERITANCE. **autosomal h.,** in mendelian inheritance, the transmission of a trait by a gene located on an autosome. See autosomal dominant CHARACTER and autosomal recessive CHARACTER. **sex-linked h.,** in mendelian inheritance, the transmission of a trait by a gene located on a sex chromosome. See holandric INHERITANCE, X-linked dominant CHARACTER, and X-linked recessive CHARACTER.

Hering's nerve [Heinrich Ewald *Hering*, German physiologist, 1866–1948] BRANCH of glossopharyngeal nerve to carotid sinus.

Herlitz syndrome [Gillis *Herlitz*, Swedish physician] see under SYNDROME.

hermaphroditism (her-maf′ro-dit′izm) [Gr. *Hermaphroditus*, a son of Hermes and Aphrodite, who became joined in one body with a nymph] a condition characterized by the presence of both ovarian and testicular tissue; originally, a state characterized by the presence of both male and female sex organs.

hernia (her′ne-ah) [L.] the protrusion of a loop or knuckle of an organ or tissue through an abnormal opening.

heroin (her′o-in) diacetylmorphine.

Herophilus of Chalcedon [c. 300 B.C.] a renowned Greek physician and anatomist of Alexandria who performed dissection of the human body, and whose important anatomical observation (e.g., on the brain, duodenum, and genitalia, and on the differentiation between nerves and blood vessels) have led many to regard him as the "Father of Anatomy." For torcular *Herophili*, see CONFLUENCE of sinuses.

herpangina (herp′an-ji′nah) [*herpes* + *angina*] an acute infectious disease, caused by coxsackie viruses group A, seldom lasting more than three to four days, usually occurring in young children during the warm months. It is characterized by abrupt fever and the appearance of numerous small vesicles, which are shortly replaced by small painful ulcers, each showing a gray base and an inflamed periphery, on the anterior faucial pillars and sometimes on the palate and tongue. Other manifestations may include anorexia, dysphagia, vomiting, headache, and pain and tenderness in the neck, abdomen, and extremities. Called also *angina herpetica, aphthous pharyngitis, herpes angina, pharyngitis vesicularis, vesicular pharyngitis,* and *Zahorsky's disease.*

herpes (her′pēz) [L., Gr. *herpēs*] 1. any inflammatory skin disease characterized by the presence of grouped vesicles on an inflammatory base, especially such diseases caused by a herpesvirus. 2. h. simplex. **h. catarrha′lis, h. simplex. h. facia′lis,** herpes simplex of the face. **h. febri′lis, h. labia′lis,** see *h. simplex.* **h. generalisa′tus,** herpetic inflammation scattered over the body. **h. genita′lis,** see *h. simplex.* **h. menstrua′lis,** a form of herpes simplex that occurs at the time of menstruation. **h. menta′lis,** herpes simplex of the submental region, caused by the herpes simplex virus type 1. **nasal h.,** herpes simplex associated with febrile rhinitis and eruption of vesicles around the nostrils and ulcerative lesions of the nasal mucous membranes, caused by the herpes simplex virus type 1. **h. progenita′lis,** see *h. simplex.* **h. sim′plex,** a common, acute viral disease marked by groups of vesicles, each vesicle about 3 to 6 mm in diameter, on the skin and mucous membranes, often on the border of the lips or the nares (h. labialis, cold sores), usually caused by herpes simplex virus type 1, or on the genitals (h. progenitalis, h. genitalis), usually caused by herpes simplex virus type 2. The lesions usually become covered with scabs and heal within a few days without scarring. It may accompany fever (h. febrilis, fever blisters), although there are other precipitating factors, such as exposure to cold or ultraviolet rays, menstruation, sunburn, cutaneous or mucosal abrasions, emotional stress, nerve injury, etc. Complications may include **conjunctivitis, meningoencephalitis, herpetic stomatitis,** and **Kaposi's** varicelliform erup-

tion. Called also *herpes* and *h. catarrhalis.* See also Pospischill-Feyrter APHTHOID and primary herpetic GINGIVOSTOMATITIS. **h. simplex, inoculation,** herpes simplex sometimes transmitted to dentists, physicians, dental hygienists, and other medical personnel by the saliva of an infected patient, penetrating through an abrasion of the skin. **h. sim′plex recur′rens,** recurrent episodes of herpes simplex at the same site. **h. ton′surans macu-lo′sus,** PITYRIASIS rosea. **traumatic h.,** a self-limited cutaneous herpesviral infection following trauma, the virus entering through burns or other wounds; the temperature rises moderately, and vesicles appear around the wound. Called also *wrestler's h.* **wrestler's h.,** traumatic h. **h. zos′ter,** an acute inflammatory disease of the cerebral ganglia and ganglia of the posterior nerve roots, caused by the varicella-zoster virus, and having an incubation period of from 7 to 14 days. It is characterized by groups of vesicles situated on an inflamed base, associated with fever, general malaise, and neuralgia, tenderness, and itching along the involved nerves, usually unilaterally. Oral and facial involvement occurs through the infection of the trigeminal nerve, and is characterized by the development of painful vesicles on the buccal mucosa, tongue, uvula, pharynx, and larynx. Called also *shingles, zona,* and *zoster.* **h. zos′ter auricula′ris, h. zos′ter o′ticus,** Hunt's SYNDROME.

Herpesvirus (her′pēz-vi′rus) [*herpes* + *virus*] a genus of DNA viruses of the family Herpetoviridae. The principal herpesviruses include herpes simplex viruses, which cause labial and genital lesions, and, possibly, cervical cancer; varicella-zoster group, the etiologic agents of chickenpox and herpes zoster; Epstein-Barr virus, responsible for infectious mononucleosis and associated with Burkitt's lymphoma and, possibly, nasopharyngeal carcinoma; and cytomegalovirus, the cause of cytomegalic inclusion disease. Herpesviruses cause many and various diseases and neoplasms in animals, including infectious bovine rhinotracheitis, pseudorabies, equine abortion, and infectious laryngotracheitis. **H. hom′inis type 1,** herpes simplex virus type 1; see under VIRUS. **H. hom′inis type 2,** herpes simplex virus type 2; see under VIRUS.

herpesvirus (her″pēz-vi′rus) a virus of the family Herpetoviridae or of the genus *Herpesvirus*. Written also *herpes virus.* **human h. type 1,** herpes simplex virus type 1; see under VIRUS. **human h. type 2,** herpes simplex virus type 2; see under VIRUS.

herpetiform (her-pet′ĭ-form) [L. *herpes* + *forma* form] resembling herpes.

Herpetoviridae (her″pĕ-to-vi′rĭ-de) [*herpes* + *virus* + *-idae*] a family of enveloped icosahedral viruses with linear double-stranded DNA contained in multilayered capsids that are about 100 nm in diameter. There are 162 capsomers in the virion lattice. The nucleocapsid is assembled in the cell nucleus and the envelope is acquired by budding. All viruses in the family infect vertebrate hosts. They are normally cytocidal for the cells they infect, but have a tendency to become dormant in infected hosts, as persistent or latent infections. *Herpetovirus* is the only genus in the family, but there is little agreement on the taxonomy of the Herpetoviridae.

herpetovirus (her″pĕ-to-vi′rus) any virus of the family Herpetoviridae.

Herplex trademark for *idoxuridine*.

Herrmann-Opitz syndrome [J. *Herrmann*; John M. *Opitz*, American physician, born 1935] see under SYNDROME.

Herrmann-Pallister-Opitz syndrome [J. *Herrmann*; P. D. *Pallister*; J. M. *Opitz*] see under SYNDROME.

Hers' disease [H. G. *Hers*] GLYCOGENOSIS VI.

Herter's infantilism [Christian Archibald *Herter*, American physician, 1865–1910] celiac DISEASE.

Hertwig, sheath of [Richard *Hertwig*, German zoologist, 1850–1937] root SHEATH (1).

Hertz, Heinrich Rudolf [1857–1894] a German physicist. See HERTZ.

hertz (hertz) [named after Heinrich Rudolf *Hertz*] the SI unit of frequency, being 1 cycle per second. Abbreviated *Hz*. See also SI.

Heryng's sign [Teodor *Heryng*, Polish physician, 1847–1925] see under SIGN.

Hess capillary test tourniquet TEST (1).

hetacillin (het′ah-sil′in) a penicillin antibiotic, 6-(2,2,-dimethyl-5-oxo-4-phenyl-1-imidazolidinyl)-3,3-dimethyl-7-oxo-4-thia-1-azabicyclo[3,2,0]heptane-2-carboxylic acid, occurring as rectangular plates that are soluble in sodium hydroxide solution, pyridine, and methanol, but not in most organic solvents and water. Hetacillin is converted in the body to ampicillin, and is used in the treatment of urinary tract infections caused by gram-negative organisms, *Escherichia coli* bacteremia, *Shigella* infections, *Salmonella* infections (including typhoid fever), and other bacterial diseases. The drug is destroyed by penicillinase. Side reactions may include hypersensitivity, stomatitis, glossitis, diarrhea, nausea, and vomiting. Called also *phenazacillin.* Trademarks: Penplenum, Versapen, Versatrex. **h. potassium,** the potassium salt of hetacillin, occurring as a white to buff, odorless, bitter, slightly hygroscopic crystalline powder that is freely soluble in water and ethanol. Its pharmacological and toxicological properties are similar to those of the parent compound. Trademarks: Natacillin, Hetacin K, Uropen, Versapen.

Hetacin K trademark for *hetacillin potassium* (see under HETACILLIN).

heter- see HETERO-.

heteresthesia (het″er-es-the′ze-ah) [*heter-* + Gr. *aisthēsis* perception] variation in the degree of cutaneous sensibility on adjoining areas of the body surface.

hetero-, heter- [Gr. *heteros* other] a combining form meaning other, or denoting relationship to another.

heteroantibody (het″er-o-an″ti-bod′e) an antibody (autoantibody) capable of reacting with antigen derived from another species.

heteroantigen (het″er-o-an′ti-jen) xenogeneic ANTIGEN.

heterochromatin (het″er-o-kro′mah-tin) that state of chromatin in which it is dark-staining and tightly coiled, forming irregular clumps (karyosomes) in the nuclei of cells that are not in division. See also C bands, under BAND.

heterochromia (het″er-o-kro′me-ah) [*hetero-* + Gr. *chrōma* color + *-ia*] diversity of color in a part that should normally be of one color. **h. cyc′lica,** Fuchs' h. **Fuchs' h.,** heterochromia and cyclitis, usually unilateral, associated with depigmentation and atrophy of the iris, secondary cataract, vitreous opacities, uveitis, and discrete keratic precipitates. Glaucoma and ipsilateral hemiatrophy may occur. Called also *h. cyclica* and *heterochromic cyclitis.*

heterochthonous (het″er-ok′tho-nus) [*hetero-* + Gr. *chthōn* a particular land or country] 1. originating in a region other than that in which it is found. 2. denoting a tissue graft from a donor of a phylogenetically different species (heterogenous graft). Cf. AUTOCHTHONOUS.

heterocrine (het′er-o-krin) [*hetero-* + Gr. *krinein* to separate] secreting more than one kind of matter.

heterocyclic (het″er-o-sik′lik) [*hetero-* + Gr. *kyklos* circle] pertaining to a closed chain structure in which one or more of the atoms is other than carbon. See also heterocyclic COMPOUND.

heterocytotropic (het″er-o-si″to-trop′ik) [*hetero-* + Gr. *kytos* hollow vessel + *tropos* a turning] having an affinity for cells of different species.

heterocytotropin (het″er-o-si″to-trōp′in) a cytotropic antibody derived from different species; see cytotropic ANTIBODY.

heterodont (het′er-o-dont) [*hetero-* + Gr. *odous* tooth] having teeth which are morphologically different, such as incisors and molars in man. Cf. HOMODONT.

heterodromous (het″er-od′ro-mus) [*hetero-* + Gr. *dromos* running] moving, acting, or arranged in the opposite direction.

heterodymus (het″er-od′i-mus) [*hetero-* + Gr. *didymos* twin] a monster with a second head, neck, and thorax implanted in the anterior thoracic or abdominal wall.

heterogeneic (het″er-o-jĕ-ne′ik) [*hetero-* + Gr. *genos* kind] xenogeneic.

heterogeneity (het″er-o-jĕ-ne′i-te) [*hetero-* + Gr. *genos* kind] 1. the state or quality of being heterogeneous. 2. the production of certain phenotypes by different genetic mechanisms or genotypes; genetic heterogeneity.

heterogeneous (het″er-o-je′ne-us) [*hetero-* + Gr. *genos* kind] 1. made of dissimilar components. 2. pertaining to a phenotype produced by genes located at more than one locus.

heterogenesis (het″er-o-jen′ĕ-sis) [*hetero-* + Gr. *genesis* generation] alternation of generations; reproduction that differs in character in successive generations. Cf. HOMOGENESIS.

heterogenous (het″er-oj′ĕ-nus) [*hetero-* + Gr. *genos* kind] having dissimilar origin.

heterograft (het′er-o-graft) [*hetero-* + *graft*] heterogeneous GRAFT.

heterohemolysin (het″er-o-he-mol′i-sin) 1. a hemolysin occurring spontaneously in the blood of an untreated animal that will hemolyze the blood of an animal of another species. 2. hemolysin established in one species by deliberate immunization with blood cells of an animal of another species.

heteroimmunity (het″er-o-im-mu′ni-te) 1. an immune state that results from the immunization of an animal belonging to one species with cells of an animal of a different species. 2. a state in which immunological response by the body to exogenous antigens, which include drugs and infectious agents, results in pathological changes.

heteroinfection (het″er-o-in-fek′shun) infection from outside the body; exogenous infection.

heterointoxication (het″er-o-in-tok″si-ka′shun) poisoning by material introduced from outside of the body.

heterokaryon (het″er-o-kar′e-on) [*hetero-* + Gr. *karyon* nucleus] a cell or hypha containing two or more nuclei of different genetic constitutions.

heterolateral (het″er-o-lat′er-al) [*hetero-* + L. *latus* side] relating to the opposite side; contralateral.

heterologous (het″er-ol′o-gus) [*hetero-* + Gr. *logos* due relation, proportion] 1. made up of tissue not normal to the part. 2. derived from an individual of a different species or from one having a different genetic constitution. 3. xenogeneic.

heterology (het″er-ol′o-je) 1. abnormality in structure, arrangement, or manner of formation. 2. in chemistry, the relationship between substances of partial identity of structure but of different properties.

heterolysis (het″er-ol′i-sis) [*hetero-* + Gr. *lysis* dissolution] dissolution of cell lysins or lysosomal enzymes originating outside of the injured cell. See also NECROSIS.

heterophosphatase (het″er-o-fos′fah-tās) hexokinase.

heteroplasia (het″er-o-pla′ze-ah) [*hetero-* + Gr. *plassein* to mold] the replacement of normal by abnormal tissue.

heteroploid (het′er-o-ploid″) 1. pertaining to or characterized by heteroploidy. 2. an individual or cell with an abnormal number of chromosomes.

heteroploidy (het′er-o-ploi″de) the state of having an abnormal number of chromosomes.

heteropolysaccharide (het″er-o-pol″e-sak′ah-rīd) a polysaccharide made up of two or more different monomeric units, as in hyaluronic acid, which consists of alternating residues of D-glucuronic acid and N-acetyl-D-glucosamine. Called also *mixed polysaccharide.* See also MUCOPOLYSACCHARIDE.

heterotopic (het″er-o-top′ik) [*hetero-* + Gr. *topos* place] occurring at an abnormal place or upon the wrong part of the body.

heterotrophic (het″er-o-trof′ik) [*hetero-* + Gr. *trophē* nutrition] feeding on others; not self-sustaining; said of cells which cannot derive carbon directly from carbon dioxide but must obtain it in a complex reduced form, such as glucose. See heterotrophic CELL. Cf. AUTOTROPHIC.

heterozygosity (het″er-o-zi-gos′i-te) [*hetero-* + *zygosity*] the state of possessing two different alleles at a given locus on a pair of homologous chromosomes. Cf. HOMOZYGOSITY.

heterozygote (het″er-o-zi′gōt) [*hetero-* + *zygote*] an individual having two different alleles at a given locus on a pair of homologous chromosomes. Called also *carrier.* See also COMPOUND (4). Cf. HOMOZYGOTE.

heterozygous (het″er-o-zi′gus) having two different alleles at a given locus on a pair of homologous chromosomes. Cf. HOMOZYGOUS. **double h.,** having different alleles at each of two separate loci.

Hetrazan trademark for *diethylcarbamazine citrate* (see under DIETHYLCARBAMAZINE).

Heuser's membrane [Chester *Heuser*, American embryologist, born 1885] see under MEMBRANE.

HEW Department of Health, Education, and Welfare; see Department of Health and Human Services, under DEPARTMENT.

hex-, hexa- [Gr. *hex* six] 1. a combining form meaning six. 2. in chemical nomenclature, generally used in connection with molecules made up of six similar parts; the number of each type of monodentate ligand in a coordination compound. The number of chelate or complicated ligands is indicated with the prefix *hexakis-*.

hexabasic (hek″sah-ba′sik) having six atoms replaceable by a base.

hexabiose (hek″sah-bi′ōs) former name for disaccharide.

hexachlorophene (hek″sah-klo′ro-fēn) an anti-infective agent for external use, 2,2′-methylenebis-(3,4,6-trichlorophenol), occurring as a white to tan crystalline powder that is insoluble in water, but is readily soluble in acetone, alcohol, ether, chloroform, and dilute alkalies. It is particularly effective against gram-positive bacteria. Used chiefly in germicidal soaps for surgical scrubs. Also used in the past in deodorant soaps, but was removed from over-the-counter preparations because of a potential neurotoxic effect. In a 1 percent solution, used to disinfect dental instruments. Trademarks: Bilevon, Dermadex, Exofene, pHisoHex, Surgi-Cen, Surofene. **h. liquid soap,** hexachlorophene liquid SOAP.

hexad (hek′sad) 1. a group or combination of six similar or related entities. 2. any element having a valence of six.

Hexadrol trademark for *dexamethasone*.

hexafluorenium bromide (hek″sah-flur-en′ĭ-um) a neuromuscular blocking agent, N,N' - Di - $9H$ - fluoren - 9 - yl - N,N,N',N' - tetramethyl-1,6-hexanediaminium dibromide, occurring as a white, crystalline powder that is soluble in ethanol, sparingly soluble in water, and insoluble in ether and chloroform. Its pharmacological properties are sometimes paradoxical, exerting weak neuromuscular blocking activity, potentiating neuromuscular blockage by tubocurarine, but antagonizing that by decamethonium, acting erratically on blockade by gallamine, potentiating and prolonging the neuromuscular actions of succinylcholine, and acting as a pseudocholinesterase inhibitor. Used chiefly to potentiate and prolong the effects of succinylcholine in surgical operations of long duration. Trademark: Mylaxen.

hexakis- in chemical nomenclature, a prefix indicating the presence of six similar chelate or complicated ligands in a coordination compound. See also HEX-(2).

hexamer (heks′ah-mer) [*hexa-* + Gr. *meros* part] 1. a chemical compound (polymer) having a combination of six simpler molecules (monomers). 2. a capsomer having six structural subunits.

hexamine (hek′sah-mēn) methenamine.

Hexanal trademark for *hexobarbital sodium* (see under HEXOBARBITAL).

Hexanastab trademark for *hexobarbital sodium* (see under HEXOBARBITAL).

hexane (hek′sān) *n*-hexane: a six-carbon straight chain hydrocarbon of the methane series, C_6H_{14}, obtained by distillation of petroleum, occurring as a colorless, volatile liquid with a faint peculiar odor. Used as a solvent, alcohol denaturant, and paint diluent, and in low-temperature thermometers and various industrial processes. Hexane is potentially toxic in high concentrations, causing irritation of the respiratory mucosa. Inhalation of its vapors may cause narcosis.

Hexenal trademark for *hexobarbital*.

hexestrol (hek-ses′trōl) a synthetic estrogen, 4,4′-(1,2-diethylethylene)diphenol, occurring as a white, crystalline powder that is soluble in ether, acetone, ethanol, and methanol, slightly soluble in benzene and chloroform, and insoluble in water.

hexobarbital (hek″so-bar′bĭ-tal) a barbiturate hypnotic and sedative drug, 5-(1-cyclohexen-1-yl)-1,5-dimethylbarbituric acid, occurring as a white, odorless, tasteless, crystalline powder that is soluble in methanol, hot ethanol, ether, chloroform, acetone, benzene, and alkali hydroxide solutions, and practically insoluble in water. Used in the treatment of insomnia, hyperthyroidism, delirium tremens, psychoneurotic disorders, and anxiety and tension associated with hypertension, coronary diseases, and gastrointestinal disorders. Also used as an anticonvulsant in tetanus, eclampsia, epilepsy, and poisoning by convulsant drugs. Abuse may cause acute and chronic poisoning and lead to habituation or addiction. Called also *hexobarbitone* and *methylhexabital*. Trademarks: Cyclonal, Evipal, Evipan, Hexenal. **h. sodium, h. soluble,** the sodium salt of hexobarbital, occurring as a white, hygroscopic, slightly bitter, light-sensitive, crystalline powder that is soluble in water and ethanol, but not in ether. It is a short-acting intravenous anesthetic. Called also *hexobarbitone sodium*. Trademarks: Hexanastab, Hexenal, Privenal.

hexobarbitone (hek″so-bar′bĭ-tōn) hexobarbital. **h. sodium,** HEXOBARBITAL sodium.

hexocyclium methylsulfate (hek″so-sil′kle-um) a quaternary ammonium antimuscarinic drug, 4-(β-cyclohexyl-β-hydroxyphenyl-ethyl)-1,1-dimethyl piperazinium methyl sulfate, occurring as a crystalline substance that is soluble in water, slightly soluble in chloroform, and insoluble in ether. Used to suppress gastric secretion. Side effects may include drying of mucous membranes (including xerostomia), decreased gastrointestinal motility, urinary retention, decrease in sweating, mydriasis, loss of visual accommodation, increase in intraocular pressure, cutaneous flush, bronchial dilatation, and tachycardia. Overdosage may produce paralysis. Trademarks: Tral, Tralin.

hexokinase [E.C.2.7.1.1] (hek″so-ki′nās) a phosphotransferase that catalyzes the transfer of a high-energy phosphate group of a donor (ATP) to D-hexose, producing ADP and D-hexose-6-phosphate. Called also *ATP glucose transphosphatase, ATP-hexose transphosphatase,* and *heterophosphatase*. See also GLUCOKINASE and carbohydrate METABOLISM.

hexosan (hek′so-san) any polysaccharide composed of hexoses; a hexose polymer. Frequently used as a synonym for *glucan*.

hexose (hek′sōs) a monosaccharide containing six carbon atoms in a molecule, $C_6H_{12}O_6$.

hexosediphosphatase [E.C.3.1.3.11] (hek″sos-di-fos′fah-tās) a phosphatase found in the liver, saliva, and elsewhere in the body, which catalyzes the hydrolysis of diphosphate esters in the biosynthesis of carbohydrates. It has at least three binding sites for AMP and contains four or more subunits; it is most active in the formation of glucose when the concentration of various glucose precursors is high and the AMP concentration is low.

hexosyltransferase [E.C.2.4.1] (hek″so-sil-trans′fer-ās) a subsubclass of glycosyltransferases, the enzymes of which catalyze the transfer of hexose group. Called also *transhexosylase*.

hexylcaine hydrochloride (hek′sil-kān) a local anesthetic agent, 1-cyclohexylamino-2-propanol benzoate hydrochloride, occurring as a white, bitter powder with a slight aromatic odor, which is soluble in water, ethanol, and chloroform, but not in ether. Used for infiltration and topical anesthesia. Adverse reactions may include nausea, vomiting, euphoria, restlessness, vertigo, anxiety, disorientation, vasodilation, hypotension, bradycardia, hypersensitivity, shock, respiratory failure, and death. A variety of other disorders may be associated. Trademark: Cyclaine.

hexylresorcinol (hek″sil-re-zor′sĭ-nol) an antiseptic and anthelmintic agent, 4-hexyl-1,3-dihydroxybenzene, occurring as white to yellowish crystals with a faint odor and an astringent, numbing taste, which is freely soluble in alcohol, methanol, glycerol, ether, chloroform, benzene, and vegetable oils, and slightly soluble in water. It is irritating to the oral mucosa and respiratory tract and to the skin; its solution in alcohol has vesicant properties. Trademarks: Caprokol and Sucrets.

Hey's saw [William *Hey*, English surgeon, 1736–1819] see under SAW.

Hf hafnium.

Hg 1. mercury (L. *hydrargyrum*). 2. hemoglobin.

HHS Department of Health and Human Services; see under DEPARTMENT.

hiatus (hi-a′tus) [L.] a general anatomical term for a gap, cleft, or opening. **h. of canal for greater petrosal nerve,** an opening in the petrous part of the temporal bone in the floor of the middle cranial fossa that transmits the greater petrosal nerve and a branch of the middle meningeal artery. Called also *h. canalis facialis, h. canalis nervi petrosi majoris* [NA], *h. of facial canal, h. of fallopian canal, h. fallopii, false h. of fallopian canal, h. for greater superficial petrosal nerve, Ferrein's foramen,* and *superficial petrosal fissure*. **h. of canal for lesser petrosal nerve,** the small, laterally placed opening on the anterior surface of the pyramid of the temporal bone that transmits the lesser petrosal nerve. Called also *h. canalis nervi petrosi minoris* [NA]. **h. cana′lis facia′lis, h. cana′lis ner′vi petro′si majo′ris** [NA], h. of canal for greater petrosal nerve. **h. cana′lis ner′vi petro′si mino′ris** [NA], h. of canal for lesser petrosal nerve. **ethmoidal h., h. ethmoida′lis,** semilunar h. **h. of facial canal, h. of fallopian canal, h. fallo′pii, false h. of fallopian canal, h. for greater superficial petrosal nerve,** h. of canal for greater petrosal nerve. **maxillary h., h. maxilla′ris** [NA], **h. of maxillary sinus,** a very irregular opening on the medial surface of the maxillary sinus, in the articulated skull, being largely filled by parts of several adjoining bones. Called also *maxillary foramen*. **semilunar h., h. semiluna′ris** [NA], the deep semilunar groove anterior and inferior to the bulla of the ethmoid bone; the anterior ethmoidal air cells, the maxillary sinus, and sometimes the frontonasal duct drain through it via the ethmoid infundibulum. Called also *ethmoidal h.* and *h. ethmoidalis*. **subarcuate h.,** subarcuate fossa of temporal bone; see under FOSSA.

HIBAC Health Insurance Benefits Advisory Council; see under COUNCIL.

hibernation (hi″ber-na′shun) [L. *hiberna* winter] the dormant state in which certain animal species pass the winter. **artificial h.,** a state of reduced metabolism, muscle relaxation, and a twilight sleep resembling narcosis, produced pharmacodynamically by controlled inhibition of the sympathetic nervous system and reducing the level of the homeostatic reactions of the organism.

Hibernyl trademark for *pholcodine*.

hiccough (hik′up) hiccup.

hiccup (hik′up) an involuntary spasmodic contraction of the diaphragm, causing a beginning inspiration which is suddenly checked by closure of the glottis, causing the characteristic sound. Spelled also *hiccough*.

hidro- [Gr. *hidrōs* sweat] a combining form denoting relation to sweat or to a sweat gland.

hidrocystoma (hid″dro-sis-to′mah) [*hidro-* + *cystoma*] a retention cyst of a sweat gland, causing obstruction of the duct, occurring as a discrete, deeply seated, noninflammatory vesicle, about 1 to 5 mm in diameter. It occurs most commonly on the face in middle-aged women exposed to excessive heat and humidity. Called also *Robinson's disease.*

hidropoiesis (hid″ro-poi-e′sis) [hidro- + Gr. *poiesis* formation] the formation and secretion of sweat.

hiemalis (hi″ĕ-ma′lis) pertaining to or occurring in winter.

Higashi, Ototaka see Chédiak-Higashi SYNDROME.

Highmore, antrum of [Nathaniel *Highmore*, English surgeon, 1613–1685] maxillary SINUS.

hila (hi′lah) [L.] plural of *hilum.*

hili (hi′li) [L.] plural of *hilus.*

Hill, Archibald Vivian [born 1886] an English biochemist, noted for his work on heat loss in muscle contraction; co-winner, with Otto Fritz Meyerhof, of the Nobel prize for medicine and physiology in 1922, for his discovery relating to heat production in muscle.

Hill's stopping [Asa *Hill*, American dentist, 1815–1874] see under STOPPING.

hillock (hil′ok) a small prominence or elevation. **axon h.,** implantation CONE.

Hilton's law, muscle [John *Hilton*, English surgeon, 1804–1878] see under LAW, and see aryepiglottic MUSCLE.

hilum (hi′lum), pl. *hi′la* [L.] hilus.

hilus (hi′lus), pl. *hi′li* [L. "a small thing"] a general anatomical term for a depression or pit at that part of an organ where the nerve or vessel enters. Called also *hilum.* **h. of lymph node, h. lymphoglan′dulae, h. no′di lymphat′ici** [NA], the indentation on the lymph node where the arteries enter and the veins and afferent lymphatic vessels leave.

HIMA Health Industry Manufacturers Association.

hindgut (hind′gut) the part of the primitive gut, caudal to the midgut, which evolves from the tail fold of the splanchnopleure, and specializes into a part of the small intestine and all of the colon and rectum. A pit at its extremity (proctodeum) develops into the rectum.

hinge (hinj) a device that connects two structures together, allowing free or limited movement on its axis. See also hinge STRESS-BREAKER. **Ancorvis h.,** trademark for a *hinge stress-breaker* for removable dentures. **h. area,** hinge AREA. **Gerber h.,** a hinge stress-breaker for partial dentures.

hinge-bow (hinj′bo) adjustable axis FACE-BOW.

Hippocrates of Cos [late 5th century B.C.] the famous Greek physician who is generally regarded as the "Father of Medicine." Many of the writings of Hippocrates and his school have survived — the so-called *Corpus Hippocraticum,* but it is not certain which were written by Hippocrates himself; these writings are usually characterized by the stress laid on treatment and prognosis. The collection of writings of Hippocrates contains references to the teeth and their diseases, including comments on formation of the teeth, relation of the teeth to speaking, erosion and decay of the teeth, toothache and extraction (only loose teeth should be extracted), dental instruments, mouthwashes, dentifrices, relations between malformation of the skull and palate and irregularities of the teeth, scurvy, necrosis of the jaw, jaw fractures, role of atmospheric conditions in diseases of the teeth, dental and gingival symptoms of systemic diseases, and ulcers due to sharp or broken teeth. An oath which appears in the body of work attributed to Hippocrates and his school, and known as the Hippocratic oath, has been the ethical guide of the medical profession since those days. It is as follows:

I swear by Apollo the physician, by Æsculapius, Hygeia, and Panacea, and I take to witness all the gods, all the goddesses, to keep according to my ability and my judgment the following Oath: To consider dear to me as my parents him who taught me this art; to live in common with him and if necessary to share my goods with him; to look upon his children as my own brothers, to teach them this art if they so desire without fee or written promise; to impart to my sons and the sons of the master who taught me and the disciples who have enrolled themselves and have agreed to the rules of the profession, but to these alone, the precepts and the instruction. I will prescribe regimen for the good of my patients according to my ability and my judgment and never do harm to anyone. To please no one will I prescribe a deadly drug, nor give advice which may cause his death. Nor will I give a woman a pessary to procure abortion. But I will

preserve the purity of my life and my art. I will not cut for stone, even for patients in whom the disease is manifest; I will leave this operation for practitioners [specialists in this art]. In every house where I come I will enter only for the good of my patients, keeping myself far from all intentional ill-doing and all seduction, and especially from the pleasures of love with women or with men, be they free or slaves. All that may come to my knowledge in the exercise of my profession or outside my profession or in daily commerce with men, which ought not to be spread abroad, I will keep secret and will never reveal. If I keep this oath faithfully, may I enjoy my life and practice my art, respected by all men and in all times; but if I swerve from it or violate it, may the reverse be my lot.

hippocratic (hip″po-krat′ik) pertaining to or described by Hippocrates of Cos, or pertaining to the school of medicine founded by him.

hippocratism (hip-pok′rah-tizm) the system of medicine attributed to Hippocrates and his school, based on imitating the processes of nature, and emphasizing treatment and prognosis.

Hirschfeld's canal [I. *Hirschfeld,* American dentist] interdental CANAL.

Hirschfeld's file, silver point see under FILE and POINT.

Hirschfeld-Dunlop file see Hirschfeld FILE.

hirsutism [her′sut-izm] abnormal hairiness, especially in women.

His histidine.

His, duct of [Wilhelm *His,* German anatomist and embryologist, 1831–1904] thyroglossal DUCT.

His' line, plane see under LINE and PLANE.

Hiserpia trademark for *reserpine.*

Hislosine trademark for *carbinoxamine maleate* (see under CARBINOXAMINE).

hist- see HISTO-.

Histabromamine trademark for *bromodiphenhydramine hydrochloride* (see under BROMODIPHENHYDRAMINE).

Histacuran trademark for *climizole.*

Histadyl trademark for *methapyrilene hydrochloride* (see under METHAPYRILENE).

histaminase [E.C.1.4.3.6] (his-tam′ĭ-nās) an oxidoreductase that catalyzes oxidation of primary monoamines and diamines, including histamine. It is present in various tissues, particularly the kidneys and the intestinal mucosa. Used in the treatment of allergic diseases and intestinal intoxication. Called also *diamine oxidase.*

histamine (his′tah-mēn, his′tah-min) an amine, beta-imidazolylethylamine, formed by decarboxylation of histidine, found in many tissues. One fraction, bound to heparin, occurs in mast cells and basophils, where it cannot be metabolized or exert effect while in the bound state. It is released by antigen-antibody complexes when the mast cells are degranulated. The second fraction is found in the mast cells of the gastric mucosa, where it plays a role in gastric secretion. The third fraction is found in the hypothalamus from where it is released by reserpine, thereby playing a role in blood pressure regulation. Therapeutically, histamine is of little importance, except as a diagnostic aid and in experimental studies; endogenous histamine plays a role in allergy, anaphylaxis, and gastric hypersecretion. **h. antagonist, h. blocking agent,** histamine INHIBITOR. **h. receptor,** histamine RECEPTOR.

histidine (his′ti-din) a heterocyclic, naturally occurring, neutral amino acid, 2-amino-3-(5-imidazolyl)-propionic acid, which is essential for the growth of infants and for nitrogen equilibrium in adults. Histidine is obtained from many proteins by the action of sulfuric acid and water. It is also found in the saliva. The decarboxylation of histidine results in the formation of histamine. Abbreviated *His.* See also amino ACID.

histio- [Gr. *histion,* dim. of *histos* web, tissue] a combining form denoting relationship to tissue. See also words beginning HISTO-.

histiocyte (his′ti-o-sit″) [Gr. *histion,* dim. of *histos* web, woven thing, tissue + *kytos* hollow vessel] a large phagocytic stellate or fusiform cell of the reticuloendothelial system, which serves as the scavenger cell of the body, primarily concerned with ingesting and digesting dead cells, foreign bodies, and other debris. Histiocytes generally occupy a fixed position near small blood vessels in connective tissue and, upon demand, as in inflammation, migrate by ameboid movement to the site of infection. They are usually present in small numbers in the dental pulp but, in the presence of an inflammatory process, their population is increased, either by migration from other tissues or by differentiation of mesenchymal cells in the capillary bed. Called also *macrophage.*

histiocytosis (his″te-o-si-to′sis) a condition marked by the abnormal appearance of histiocytes in the blood. **lipid h.,** Niemann-Pick DISEASE. **h. X,** a condition in which histiocytes phagocytize normal circulating cholesterol. The term embraces Letterer-Siwe disease, Hand-Schüller-Christian disease, and eosinophilic granuloma. Called also *nonlipid reticuloendotheliosis.*

HISTLINE History of Medicine Online; an acronym for a data base containing references to articles, monographs, symposia, and other publications dealing with the history of medicine and related subjects. It is the source of *Bibliography of the History of Medicine,* published by the National Library of Medicine.

histo-, hist- [Gr. *histos* web, woven thing; tissue] a combining form denoting relationship to tissue. See also words beginning *histio-.*

histochemistry (his″to-kem′is-tre) [*histo- + chemistry*] that branch of histology which deals with the application to histological preparations of methods of physical and chemical analysis that permit identification of chemical substances in their normal sites in tissues. Chemical methods permit identification of lipids by their uptake of certain fat-soluble dyes, the staining of carbohydrates by means of a reagent that produces a colored compound with the products of their oxidation, the demonstration of deoxyribonucleoprotein by staining of a special aldehyde made available by mild hydrolysis, and the localization of enzymes. Physical methods consist of the identification of nucleoproteins by taking advantage of absorption of ultraviolet light at specific wavelengths (ultraviolet spectrophotometry), absorption of x-rays of selected wavelengths by calcium and other elements (historadiography), emission of x-rays of specific wavelengths by elements bombarded by an electron beam (electron microprobe analysis), and emission of ionizing particles from unstable isotopes incorporated in tissue components (radioautography).

histoclastic (his″to-klas′tik) [*histo- + Gr. klastos* broken] breaking down tissue; said of certain cells.

histocompatibility (his″to-kom-pat″ĭ-bil′ĭ-te) [*histo- + compatibility*] the quality of being histocompatible. **major h. complex,** in mammals, a region of the chromosome that determines the major transplantation antigens and has a major role in graft rejection, controls immune responses to various types of antigen, and determines the susceptibility to the development of immunologically mediated diseases. Abbreviated *MHC.* See *major h. complex (of man)* and *major h. complex (of mouse),* and see also histocompatibility antigens, under ANTIGEN. **major h. complex (of man),** the major genetic histocompatibility system in man, which controls over 50 human leukocyte antigens (HLA). The antigens, which are glycoproteins, are determined by alleles within the locus of chromosome 6 (see illustration) and are involved in controlling the formation of some complement components and in graft rejection and are associated with the pathogenesis of such diverse disorders as ankylosing spondylitis, gluten-sensitive enteropathy, and multiple sclerosis. A comparable system is found in the mouse, which determines the H-2 antigens. Called also *HLA* or *HL-A complex, HLA* or *HL-A system,* and *human MHC.* **major h. complex (of mouse),** the major genetic histocompatibility immunogenetic system in the mouse, which determines the H-2 antigens (comparable to the human leukocyte antigens). The antigens are controlled by the arrangement of alleles within the locus of the chromosome 17 (see illustration), covering the length of DNA

MHC Man (HLA)

6th chromosome:

Loci	HLA-D	HLA-B	HLA-C	HLA-A
Antigen	LD	SD	SD	SD

Nomenclature of HLA

NEW	OLD	ORIGINAL
HLA-A	SD1	1st locus
HLA-B	SD2	2nd locus
HLA-C	SD3	3rd locus
HLA-D	LD1	—
HLA-DR		

Schematic representation of the human major histocompatibility complex (MHC), illustrating chromosomal loci (HLA) and their gene products and the lymphocyte detectable (LD) and serologically detectable (SD) antigens. (From J. A. Bellanti: Immunology II. Philadelphia, W. B. Saunders Co., 1978.)

Mouse MHC (H-2)

17th chromosome (9th linkage group):

Regions	K	I	Ss-Slp	G	D
Subregions		I-A I-B I-C			
Loci	H-2K	Ir-1A Ir-1B Ir-1C I-E I-J	Ss	H-2G	H-2D
Antigen	SD	LD-1			SD
Function or product		Immune response genes (genetic control of immune response)	Suppressor function	Serum substance and C4	H-2 antigen on RBC

Schematic representation of the mouse MHC (H-2), depicting regions, subregions, loci, antigens, and their gene functions and products. (From J. A. Bellanti: Immunology II. Philadelphia, W. B. Saunders Co., 1978.)

equivalent to 0.5 recombination unit; tissues grafted between animals having different arrangements will undergo rejection. The H-2 locus serves as a genetic and tissue typing marker and genes within the locus control the immune responses of the animal. Two loci, H-2K and H-2D determine about 50 antigenic specificities. The H-2 antigen has a molecular weight of 28,000 to 32,000 daltons and is found in all tissues except sperm. Called also *H-2 complex, H-2 system,* and *mouse MHC.*

histocompatible (his″to-kom-pat′ĭ-b′l) capable of being accepted and remaining functional; said of that relationship between the genotypes of donor and host in which a graft will not be rejected.

histodifferentiation (his″to-dif″er-en″she-a′shun) [*histo- + differentiation*] the acquisition of histologic characteristics during development.

histogenesis (his″to-jen′ĕ-sis) [*histo- + Gr. genesis* production] the formation or development of tissues from undifferentiated cells of the germ layers of the embryo. See also table at TISSUE.

histoincompatibility (his″to-in″kom-pat″ĭ-bil′ĭ-te) [*histo- + incompatibility*] the condition of not being accepted or remaining functional; said of that relationship between genotypes of donor and host in which a graft generally will be rejected.

histologist (his-tol′o-jist) one who specializes in histology.

histology (his-tol′o-je) [*histo- + -logy*] that branch of anatomy which deals with the study of the composition and function of minute structures of tissue. Called also *microscopical anatomy* and *minute anatomy.* See also CYTOLOGY, MORPHOLOGY, and TISSUE. **pathological h.,** histopathology.

histone (his′tōn) a group of simple proteins having an open unfolded structure. Histones are soluble in water but insoluble in dilute ammonia, and can be heat-coagulated only with difficulty. Histones are characterized by a very high content of basic amino acids. Many are poisonous and contain large amounts of phosphorus. Blood treated with histones is altered so that it does not coagulate readily. They have been found in the urine in leukemia and febrile conditions. Histones forming complexes with nucleic acids are known as *nucleohistones.* They are thought to be important in the molecular organization of DNA in the nucleus and its junctions.

histopathology (his″to-pah-thol′o-je) [*histo- + pathology*] the study of composition and function of tissues under pathological conditions. Called also *pathological histology.* See also cellular PATHOLOGY.

Histoplasma (his″to-plaz′mah) a genus of deuteromycetous fungi (Fungi Imperfecti). **H. capsula′tum,** a species occurring as a small oval cell, 1 to 5 μ in diameter, at 37°C and as mycelium with conidia at 25° C, which is the cause of histoplasmosis. Its teleomorph state is *Ajellomyces capsulatus,* an ascomycete.

histoplasmosis (his″to-plaz-mo′sis) an infectious systemic disease caused by the fungus *Histoplasma capsulatum.* In the mild or subclinical form, it is manifested by pneumonia, malaise, weight loss, and lymph node involvement. In the disseminated chronic form, the symptoms may include anemia, lymph node enlargement, fever, hepatosplenomegaly, pulmonary involvement, ulceration of the pharynx, anus, genitalia, nose, and mouth, and erythema nodosum. Vegetative or ulcerative lesions covered by a nonspecific, indurated gray membrane of the buccal mucosa, gingiva, tongue, palate, and lips are the principal oral manifestations. Called also *Darling's disease*.

history (his'to-re) 1. a systematic record of past events relating to a particular people, country, period, persons, etc. 2. a continuous systematic record of past events, usually written in chronological order. See also RECORD[1]. **dental h.,** a record containing complete information on all aspects of the patient's oral health, his or her general health conditions, and care received in the past. **family h.,** information on the clinical status and history of members of the patient's immediate family. Abbreviated *F.H.* **medical h.,** the records of past diseases and events that may affect the health of the patient and are of interest to his physician.

histotome (his'to-tōm) [*histo-* + Gr. *tomē* a cut] microtome.

histotomy (his-tot'o-me) [*histo-* + Gr. *tomnein* to cut] microtomy.

histotoxic (his"to-tok'sik) [*histo-* + Gr. *toxikon* poison] poisonous to tissues.

Histril trademark for *diphenylpyraline*.

Histyn trademark for *diphenylpyraline*.

hives (hīvz) urticaria.

HLA, HL-A human leukocyte antigen; see major histocompatibility complex (of man), under HISTOCOMPATIBILITY.

H & M Special trademark for an *amalgam alloy* (see under AMALGAM).

HMC 1. major histocompatibility complex; see under HISTOCOMPATIBILITY. 2. hypertelorism-microtia-clefting SYNDROME.

HMO health maintenance ORGANIZATION.

HMSS Hospital Management Systems Society.

h𝜈 photon ENERGY.

HN2 mechlorethamine.

H₂O water.

²H₂O heavy WATER.

H₂O₂ hydrogen PEROXIDE.

Ho holmium.

hoarseness (hōrs'nes) a rough quality of voice; trachyphonia.

Hobbs, Lucy B. the first woman dentist in the United States, who graduated from the Ohio College of Dental Surgery in 1866.

Hodge see DENTINOGENESIS imperfecta (Capdepont-Hodge syndrome).

Hodgkin, Alan Lloyd [born 1914] an English physiologist; cowinner, with John Carew Eccles and Andrew Fielding Huxley, of the Nobel prize for medicine and physiology in 1963, for discoveries concerning the ionic mechanisms involved in excitation and inhibition in the peripheral and central portions of the nerve cell membrane.

Hodgkin, W. E. see Rapp-Hodgkin ectodermal DYSPLASIA.

Hodgkin's disease (granuloma, syndrome) [Thomas *Hodgkin*, English physician, 1798–1866] see under DISEASE.

Hodostin trademark for *neostigmine methyl sulfate* (see under NEOSTIGMINE).

hoe (ho) a cutting dental instrument having its cutting edge at a right angle to the axis of its blade and no constriction at the junction of its shank and blade; used for breaking down tooth structure undermined by caries, smoothing cavity walls, and sharpening line and point angles. See also *surgical h.* and hoe SCALER. See illustration. **h. scaler,** hoe SCALER. **surgical h.,** a surgical instrument with a flattened, fish-tail–shaped blade with a pronounced convexity in its terminal portion. The cutting edge is beveled with rounded edges and projects beyond the long axis of the handle to preserve the effectiveness of the instrument when the blade is reduced by sharpening. It is generally used for detaching the pocket wall after gingivectomy incision, but it is also useful for smoothing root surfaces in periodontal surgical procedures. See illustration.

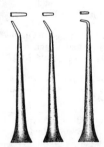

Hoes. (From V. R. Park and J. R. Ashman: A Textbook for Dental Assistants. 2nd ed. Philadelphia, W. B. Saunders Co., 1975.)

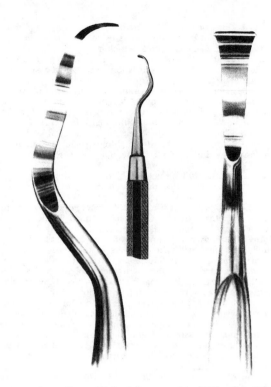

Surgical hoe. (From F. A. Carranza, Jr.: Glickman's Clinical Periodontology. 5th ed. Philadelphia, W. B. Saunders Co., 1979.)

Hoffman, Ernst [German neurologist, born 1868] see infantile muscular ATROPHY (Werdnig-Hoffman syndrome).

Hofmann's bacillus [Georg von *Hofmann-Wellendof*, Austrian bacteriologist] *Corynebacterium pseudodiphthericum;* see under CORYNEBACTERIUM.

holandric (hol-an'drik) [Gr. *holos* entire + *aner* man] inherited exclusively through the male. See holandric INHERITANCE.

holder (hōld'er) 1. a device for keeping something in place or position. 2. a person who possesses or holds something. **certificate h.,** subscriber (3). **exposure h., film h.,** cassette. **foil h.,** an instrument used for retaining a foil pellet in place while it is being condensed in a cavity or to retain a bulk of gold while additions are made. Called also *foil assistant*. **Gardner's needle h.,** a needle holder with a groove in the beak to hold and direct the suture needle. **matrix h.,** matrix RETAINER. **needle h.,** a forceps used to hold the needle in passing a suture; a suture forceps. Called also *acutenaculum*. **policy h.,** under a group insurance purchase plan, the employer, labor union, or trustee to whom the group contract is issued (third party). In a plan providing for individual or family enrollment, the person to whom the contract is issued (first party or beneficiary). **rubber dam h.,** a device, usually a metal clip, for holding a rubber dam in place.

hole (hōl) an aperture, opening, or cavity in or through something. **pour h.,** an aperture in investment or other mold material leading to the prosthesis space into which prosthetic material is poured.

holism (hōl'izm) [Gr. *holos* whole] the conception of man as a functioning whole.

holistic (ho-lis'tik) considering man as a functioning whole, or relating to the conception of man as a functioning whole.

Hollenback condenser [George M. *Hollenback*] pneumatic CONDENSER.

holmium (hol'me-um) [L. *Holmia* Stockholm] a rare earth, occurring as a crystalline solid with a metallic luster, which reacts slowly with water, and is soluble in dilute acids. Symbol, Ho; atomic number, 67; atomic weight, 164.9304; valence, 3; specific gravity, 8.803; melting point, 1470°C; group IIIB of the periodic table. It has one natural isotope, ¹⁶⁵Ho, and several artificial radioactive ones, 150–164 and 166–170. Used in electronic technology and electrochemistry.

holo- [Gr. *holos* entire] a combining form meaning entire, or denoting relationship to the whole.

Holocaine trademark for *phenacaine hydrochloride* (see under PHENACAINE).

holocrine (hol'o-krīn) [*holo-* + Gr. *krinein* to separate] wholly secretory; pertaining to secretion through disintegration of the whole glandular cell; as in a holocrine gland. Cf. MEROCRINE.

holodontography (hol″o-don-tog′rah-fe) the use of holography in dentistry; see HOLOGRAPHY.

hologram (hol-o′gram″) [*holo-* + Gr. *gramma* that which is produced] a three-dimensional record on a photographic plate, film, or slide obtained by holography, upon which the interference pattern produced by the reinforcement or cancellation of two different intersecting wave fronts is recorded. By changing position, the viewer may observe objects blocked out by foreground objects, thus allowing three-dimensional observation. See illustration.

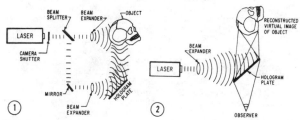

Fig. 1. Exposing the hologram.
Fig. 2. Viewing the hologram.

1, Exposing the hologram. *2,* Viewing the hologram. (From J. M. Young and B. R. Altschuller: Laser holography in dentistry. J. Prosthet. Dent., *38*(2):217, 1977.)

holography (hol-og′rah-fe) [*holo-* + Gr. *graphein* to write] the technique of recording reflected light waves from an object, especially by using a laser, to produce a three-dimensional image on a photographic plate, film, or slide (see HOLOGRAM). The method allows observation of details not available through light photography, such as minute movements or contouring of the examined object, part, or organ. See illustration. See also INTERFEROMETRY and LASER. **laser h.,** see HOLOGRAPHY and laser INTERFEROMETRY. **real-time h.,** holography which permits the observation and recording of dimensional changes as they occur.

Holopon trademark for *methscopolamine bromide* (see under METHSCOPOLAMINE).

holoprosencephaly (hol″o-pros″en-sef′ah-le) a congenital abnormality characterized by failure of cleavage of the prosencephalon with faulty midline facial development; cyclopia, cleft lip and palate, low-set ears, ocular defects, hypertelorism, and other anomalies may be associated.

Holt, M. see frontometaphyseal DYSPLASIA (Gorlin-Holt syndrome).

Holtermüller-Wiedemann syndrome [K. *Holtermüller,* German physician; Hans Rudolf *Wiedemann,* German physician] cloverleaf SKULL.

Holz phlegmon see under PHLEGMON.

Holzknecht unit [Guido *Holzknecht,* radiologist in Russia, 1872–1931] see under UNIT.

Homapin trademark for *homatropine methylbromide* (see under HOMATROPINE).

homatropine (ho-mat′ro-pēn) a poisonous alkaloid, *endo-α-*hydroxybenzeneacetic acid 8-methyl-8-azabicyclo[3,2,1]oct-3-yl ester. It is obtained by the condensation of tropine and mandelic acid, occurring in D-, L-, and DL-forms. Used as an anticholinergic drug. Called also *tropine mandelate.* **h. hydrobromide,** the hydrobromide salt of homatropine, occurring as a white, photosensitive, crystalline powder or white crystals that are soluble in water, ethanol, and chloroform, but not in ether. It is a poisonous antimuscarinic agent, used chiefly in ophthalmological therapy. **h. methylbromide,** the methylbromide salt of homatropine, occurring as a white, odorless, photosensitive powder that is soluble in water and ethanol, but not in ether and acetone. It is a poisonous, semisynthetic, quaternary ammonium antimuscarinic substance, used chiefly in gastrointestinal disorders and as a mydriatic agent. Trademarks: Esopin, Homapin, Mesopin, Novatropine.

home (hōm) a place of residence. **nursing h.,** an institution primarily engaged in providing nursing care, rehabilitation services, and other forms of health care to injured, disabled, or sick inpatients and elderly residents. See also extended care FACILITY.

homeo-, homeo-, homoio- [Gr. *homoios* like, resembling, unchanging] a combining form denoting sameness, similarity, or a constant unchanging state.

homeopathy (ho″me-op′ah-the) [*homeo-* + Gr. *pathos* disease] a

system of therapeutics founded by Samuel Hahnemann (1755–1843), in which diseases are treated by drugs which are capable of producing in healthy persons symptoms like those of the disease to be treated, the drug being administered in minute doses.

homeostasis (ho″me-o-sta′sis) [*homeo-* + Gr. *stasis* standing] maintenance of a narrow range in the internal environment through the operation of different functional systems of the body in harmony with each other. It often involves a negative feedback, as in control mechanisms for carbon dioxide, one of which involves increased carbon dioxide in the blood triggering increased pulmonary ventilation, which in turn causes a decrease in the carbon dioxide concentration of the blood. **immunologic h.,** the normal state of the adult animal in which it produces antibodies or develops cell-mediated immunity to foreign antigens but not to its own antigens.

homo- [Gr. *homos* same] 1. a combining form meaning the same. 2. a prefix in chemical nomenclature indicating the addition of one CH_2 group to the main compound.

homoarterenol hydrochloride (ho″mo-ar″te-re′nol) NORDEFRIN hydrochloride.

homocodeine (ho″mo-ko′dēn) pholcodine.

homocytotropic (ho″mo-si″to-trop′ik) [*homo-* + Gr. *kytos* hollow vessel   *tropos* a turning] having an affinity for cells of the same species.

homocytotropin (ho″mo-si″to-trop′in) a cytotropic antibody derived from the same species; see cytotropic ANTIBODY.

homodont (ho′mo-dont) [*homo-* + Gr. *odous* tooth] having teeth which are morphologically of the same type. Cf. HETERODONT.

homodromous (ho-mod′ro-mus) [*homo-* + Gr. *dromos* running] moving or acting in the same direction.

homogenate (ho-moj′ē-nāt) material subjected to homogenization, as tissue that is finely shredded and mixed.

homogeneity (ho″mo-je-ne′ĭ-te) the state or quality of being homogeneous.

homogeneous (ho″mo-je′ne-us) [*homo-* + Gr. *genos* kind] consisting of or composed of similar elements or ingredients; of a uniform quality throughout.

homogenesis (ho″mo-jen′ē-sis) [*homo-* + Gr. *genesis* production] the reproduction by the same process in each generation. Cf. HETEROGENESIS.

homogenization (ho-moj″ē-ni-za′shun) the act or process of rendering homogeneous.

homograft (ho′mo-graft) [*homo-* + *graft*] homologous GRAFT.

homolateral (ho″mo-lat′er-al) [*homo-* + L. *latus* side] situated on or pertaining to the same side. Called also *ipsilateral.* Cf. CONTRALATERAL.

homologous (ho-mol′o-gus) [Gr. *homologos* agreeing, correspondent] 1. corresponding in structure, position, origin, etc., as *(a)* the feathers of a bird and the scales of a fish, *(b)* antigen and its specific antibody, *(c)* allelic chromosomes. 2. allogeneic.

homoplant (ho′mo-plant) homologous GRAFT.

homoplasty (ho′mo-plas″te) [*homo-* + Gr. *plassein* to shape] transplantation of tissues or organs from an individual of the same species or from a member of another inbred strain.

homopolymer (ho″mo-pol′ĭ-mer) [Gr. *homos* same + *polymer*] a polymer containing the same repeating unit. **chlorethene h.,** POLYVINYL chloride. **ethene h.,** polyethylene. **tetrafluorethene h.,** polytetrafluoroethylene.

homopolysaccharide (ho″mo-pol″e-sak′ah-rīd) a polysaccharide made up of only one type of recurring monomeric (monosaccharide) units, as in starch, which contains only D-glucose units. Homopolysaccharides containing glucose, e.g., starch and glycogen, are called *glucans;* those containing mannose units are *mannans.*

homozygosity (ho″mo-zi-gos′ĭ-te) [*homo-* + *zygosity*] the state of possessing an identical pair of alleles at a given locus or loci. Cf. HETEROZYGOSITY.

homozygote (ho″mo-zi′gōt) [*homo-* + *zygote*] an individual having a pair of identical alleles at a given locus or loci on a pair of homologous chromosomes. See also COMPOUND (4). Cf. HETEROZYGOTE.

homozygous (ho″mo-zi′gus) having an identical pair of alleles at a given locus or loci. Cf. HETEROZYGOUS.

hood (hood) a flexible covering. **tooth h.,** dental OPERCULUM.

Hooft's syndrome [C. *Hooft*] familial HYPOLIPIDEMIA.

hook (hook) a curved or angular piece or metal or other rigid material for catching, pulling, elevating, or exerting traction on something. **elastic h.,** molar h. **embrasure h.,** a device used as a support for a unit of a removable prosthesis, forming a hook that extends into the embrasure above the contact area between two adjacent teeth to engage the buccal or labial angles of each tooth so as to resist movement in a cervical direction. Called also *incisal h.* **incisal h.,** embrassure h. **intermaxillary h.,** one bent into the arch wire of an orthodontic appliance, such as a Begg appliance. **molar h.,** one attached on the lingual or buccal aspects of the molar bands for engaging elastics on an orthodontic appliance. Called also *elastic h.* **sliding h.,** a movable attachment used on an orthodontic wire.

Hooke's law [Robert *Hooke,* English physician, 1635–1703] see under LAW.

hook-up (hook′up) the method of arranging circuits, appliances, and electrodes for a particular purpose or method.

Hoorweg's law see under LAW.

HOP high oxygen PRESSURE.

Hor. decub. abbreviation for L. *ho′ra decu′bitus,* at bedtime.

Hor. interm. abbreviation for L. *ho′ris interme′diis,* at the intermediate hours.

hormion (hor′me-on) [Gr. *hormos* a wreath] a craniometric landmark, being the median anterior point of the spheno-occipital suture.

hormone (hor′mōn) [Gr. *hormaein* to set in motion] originally, a substance secreted directly into the bloodstream by a gland, which produces a biological or physiological effect in some unrelated organ or tissue. The scope of the term has been expanded to also include substances of similar activity produced synthetically and substances secreted by organs other than the classic endocrine glands. **adrenal cortex h.,** a steroid hormone synthesized by the adrenal cortex from cholesterol, those with 21 carbons in the ring being corticosteroids and those with 19 carbons adrenal androgens. Adrenal cortex hormones are divided into those that promote gluconeogenesis (glucocorticoids), including cortisol and corticosterone, and those that act on the distal tubules of the kidneys to enhance the reabsorption of sodium ions from the tubular fluid into the plasma (mineralocorticoids); glucocorticoids are of greater importance in dental therapeutics. Small amounts of progesterone and estrogens are also found in hormonal secretions of the adrenal cortex, but they are not considered as adrenocorticosteroids. Called also *adrenocortical h., adrenal cortex steroid, adrenocorticosteroid, corticoid,* and *corticosteroid.* **adrenal medulla h's,** the hormonally active catecholamines, epinephrine and norepinephrine. **adrenocortical h.,** adrenal cortex h. **adrenocorticotropic h.,** a protein hormone of the anterior pituitary gland, representing a straight chain polypeptide containing 39 amino acids. It is believed to be secreted by the chromophobe cells. Its functions include regulation of the production and secretion of glucocorticoids by the fascicular and reticular zones of the adrenal cortex. Administration of adrenocorticotropic hormone produces increases in the secretion of glucocorticoids and 17-ketosteroids. Large doses produce hypertrophy of the adrenal cortex, hyperglycemia, negative nitrogen balance, redistribution of fat in the face and trunk, hypercholesterolemia, ketonemia, eosinopenia, and retention of sodium and chloride ions. Used therapeutically to stimulate production of glucocorticoids in conditions which indicate cortisone or cortisol therapy. Called also *ACTH, adrenocorticotropin,* and *corticotropin.* **androgenic h.,** androgen. **antidiuretic h. (ADH),** vasopressin. **estrogenic h.,** estrogen. **follicle stimulating h.,** a gonadotropic hormone of the anterior pituitary which stimulates the growth and maturation of the ovarian follicles and prepares them for ovulation, and increases spermatogenesis in the testes. Abbreviated *FSH.* **gonadotropic h.,** a hormone having a stimulating effect on the gonads. It may be produced by the anterior pituitary gland, and includes follicle stimulating hormone, prolactin, and luteinizing hormone (see specific hormones). The placenta also produces one called *chorionic gonadotropin,* which sustains the corpus luteum. Called also *gonadotropin.* **growth h.,** somatotropic h. **growth h. release inhibiting factor (GH-RIF),** somatostatin. **interstitial cell stimulating h.,** luteinizing h. **lactogenic h.,** prolactin. **luteinizing h.,** a gonadotropic hormone of the anterior pituitary gland, which controls ripening of ovarian follicles and secretion of estrogen in the female, and stimulation of the interstitial cells of the testis and production of androgens in the male. Abbreviated *LH.* Called also *interstitial cell stimulating h. (ICSH).* **melanocyte stimulating h.,** a factor in the intermediate lobe of the pituitary, representing a straight polypeptide chain similar to that of adrenocorticotropin, which influences pigment granules in cold-blooded vertebrates in changing the coloring of their skin. The role of this hormone in humans is not known. Abbreviated *MSH.* Called also *intermedin* and *melanotropin.* **parathyroid**

h., a polypeptide hormone of the parathyroid gland which affects calcium and phosphate metabolism and influences the development of bones and teeth. A small amount of vitamin D is necessary for its activity. It increases the renal tubular secretion of phosphate and bone resorption by osteocytes and osteoclasts, as well as calcium absorption by the small intestine so that the blood calcium level is increased. Insufficient secretion of parathyroid hormone causes hypoparathyroidism and excessive secretion produces hyperparathyroidism. Neuromuscular irritability is inversely related to the plasma ionic calcium level. Side effects may include hypercalcemia and nervous system depression. Abbreviated *PTH.* Called also *parathormone.* **progestational h.,** progestin. **sex h.,** any hormone that influences the sex organs and functions of the body. Female sex hormones include estrogens and progestins and male sex hormones include androgens. **somatotropic h.,** a hormone produced by the anterior pituitary gland, probably by the acidophils. It is an anabolic polypeptide which stimulates growth, delays amino acid catabolism and accelerates their incorporation into proteins, induces positive nitrogen balance associated with an increase in tissue nitrogen and a decrease in urea nitrogen, antagonizes the action of insulin, increases blood sugar, increases muscle glycogen, and stimulates fat mobilization from body fat deposits. Secretion of somatotropic hormone is controlled by a hypothalamic secretion, somatotropin releasing factor. Used in the treatment of growth retardation before epiphyseal closure. Called also *growth h. (GH)* and *somatotropin.* **steroid h.,** a hormonally active steroid compound. See *adrenal cortex h.* and *sex h.* See also STEROID. **thyroid h.,** any hormone produced by the thyroid gland; see TRIIODOTHYRONINE and THYROXINE. **thyroid stimulating h.,** thyrotropic h. **thyrotropic h.,** a glycoprotein hormone presumably produced by the basophils of the anterior pituitary gland. Its principal function is to regulate the production and release of thyroid hormone by the thyroid gland. Its production and release are regulated by the level of thyroxine in the blood and a neurohumoral factor in the hypothalamus, as well as hypothalamic thyrotropic hormone releasing factor. Called also *thyrotropin, thyroid stimulating h. (TSH),* and *thyrotropin.*

horn (horn) [L. *cornu*] 1. one of the paired processes that arise from the upper part of the head in some animals. 2. a pointed projection or excrescence on the body. See also CORNU. **cicatricial h.,** a hard, dry outgrowth from a cicatrix, commonly scaly and very rarely osseous. **cutaneous h.,** a horny excrescence of the skin, due to excessive keratinization, occurring most commonly on the face and scalp. Called also *cornu cutaneum.* **greater h. of hyoid bone,** a bony projection extending dorsally from the lateral border of the hyoid bone, to which it is connected by a cartilaginous synchondrosis; it ossifies during middle life. The thyrohyoid ligament is attached to a tubercle at its tip; the hyoglossus and constrictor pharyngis muscles attach to the cranial surface, near its lateral border; the digastricus and stylohyoideus muscles insert near the junction with the body; and the thyrohyoid membrane and the thyrohyoideus attach to its lateral border. Called also *lateral h. of hyoid bone, greater cornu of hyoid bone, cornu majus ossis hyoidei* [NA], and *thyrohyal.* **inferior h. of thyroid cartilage,** one of the symmetrical, short and thick caudal extensions projecting from the lower corners of the laminae of the thyroid cartilage, terminating with a small oval articular facet for articulation with the cricoid cartilage. Called also *cornu inferius cartilaginis thyroideae* [NA]. **lateral h. of hyoid bone,** greater h. of hyoid bone. **lesser h. of hyoid bone,** a small, conical eminence projecting upward on either side of the hyoid bone at the angle of junction between the body and the greater horns. It is connected to the body by a synchondrosis of fibrous tissue which may ossify during middle life. The styloid ligament is attached at its apex and the chondroglossus muscle originates at its medial side. Called also *superior h. of hyoid bone, ceratohyal, lesser cornu of hyoid bone,* and *cornu minus ossis hyoidei* [NA]. **mucosal h.,** a horny excrescence of the mucous membrane, such as of the lip, due to excessive keratinization. **h. of pulp,** an extension of the pulp into an accentuation of the roof of the pulp chamber directly uner a cusp or a developmental lobe of the tooth. **superior h. of hyoid bone,** lesser h. of hyoid bone. **superior h. of thyroid cartilage,** one of the two symmetrical, long and narrow cranialward extensions projecting from the upper corners of the laminae of the thyroid cartilage, ending with conical extremities for attachment of the lateral thyrohyoid ligament. Called also *cornu superius cartilaginis thyroideae* [NA]. **h's of thyroid cartilage,** one of the two symmetrical pairs of horns projecting from the laminae of the thyroid cartilage. See *inferior h. of thyroid cartilage* and *superior h. of thyroid cartilage.* Called also *cornua cartilaginis thyroideae.*

Horner's muscle [William Edmonds *Horner*, American anatomist, 1793–1853] lacrimal part of orbicular muscle of eye; see under PART.

Horner's syndrome [Johann Friedrich *Horner*, Swiss ophthalmologist, 1831–1886] Bernard-Horner SYNDROME. See also paratrigeminal SYNDROME (incomplete Horner's syndrome).

Horner's teeth see under TOOTH.

Horsley's wax [Sir Victor Alexander Haden *Horsley*, English surgeon, 1857–1916] see under WAX.

Hortega cell [Pio del Rio *Hortega*, Spanish histologist in Buenos Aires, 1882–1945] microgliocyte.

Horton's headache, neuralgia [Bayard Taylor *Horton*, American physician, born 1895] cluster HEADACHE.

hospice (hos′pis) a facility which provides palliative and supportive care for terminally ill patients and their families, either directly or on a consulting basis.

hospital (hos′pit-'l) [L. *hospitalium*, from *hospes* host, guest] an institution for the treatment of the sick. "An institution suitably located, constructed, organized, managed, and personneled, to supply, scientifically, economically, efficiently, and unhindered, all or any recognized part of the complex requirements for the prevention, diagnosis, and treatment of physical, mental, and the medical aspect of the social ills; with functioning facilities for training new workers in the many special professional, technical and economic fields essential to the discharge of its proper functions; and with adequate contacts with physicians, other hospitals, medical schools and all accredited health agencies engaged in the better health program." — Council on Medical Education. **affiliated h.,** one that is affiliated with some health program. **closed h.,** one in which only members of the staff are permitted to treat patients. **h. dentistry,** hospital DENTISTRY. **investor-owned h.,** proprietary h. **proprietary h.,** a privately owned hospital operated for profit. Called also *investor-owned h.* **teaching h.,** one that provides undergraduate or graduate medical or dental education or internship or residency and is affiliated with a medical or dental school. Hospitals which train auxiliary medical or dental personnel are not considered as teaching hospitals. **voluntary nonprofit h.,** one operated under the sponsorship of a community, religious order, or other nonprofit agency.

hospitalization (hos″pit'l-i-za′shun) 1. the confinement of a patient in a hospital for at least an overnight stay, or the period of such confinement. 2. insurance that provides coverage for all or some of a patient's hospital costs. See INSURANCE.

host (hōst) [L. *hospes*] 1. an animal or plant that harbors or nourishes another organism (parasite). 2. the recipient of an organ or other tissue transplanted from another organism (the donor). **h. site,** host SITE.

hot (hot) 1. characterized by high temperature. 2. dangerously radioactive.

Hotchkiss' operation [Lucius Wales *Hotchkiss*, American surgeon, 1860–1926] see under OPERATION.

Houghton's law LAW of fatigue.

housing (how′zing) 1. a shelter, dwelling, or lodging. 2. anything that covers or protects. **protective h.,** tube h. **tube h.,** a part of the x-ray generator which encloses the x-ray tube and prevents leakage of radiation outside the generator. Called also *protective h.* See also *tube h., diagnostic* and *tube h., therapeutic.* **tube h., diagnostic,** a housing that encloses the x-ray tube of a generator used for diagnostic purposes; present safety standards require that the leakage of radiation should be less than 1 R per hour at a distance of 1 m from the tube target when the tube is operating at its maximum continuous rate current for the maximum rated voltage. **tube h., therapeutic,** a housing that encloses the x-ray tube of a generator used for therapeutic purposes; present safety standards require that the leakage of radiation should be less than 1 R per minute at any point on the surface of the housing when the tube is operating at its maximum continuous rate current for the maximum rated voltage.

Houssay, Bernardo Alberto [1887–1971] an Argentinean endocrinologist; co-winner, with Carl F. Cori and Gerty Theresa Cori, of the Nobel Prize for medicine and physiology in 1947, for discovery of the part played by the hormone of the anterior pituitary lobe in the metabolism of sugar.

Houwer, A. W. M. see Sjögren's SYNDROME (Gougerot-Houwer-Sjögren syndrome).

Howard's method [Benjamin Douglas *Howard*, American physician, 1840–1900] see artificial RESPIRATION.

Howe's color scale see under SCALE.

Howe's solution [P. *Howe*] ammoniacal silver nitrate SOLUTION.

Howell body [W. H. *Howell*] Howell-Jolly BODY.

Howell-Jolly body [W. H. *Howell*; Justin *Jolly*, French histologist, 1870–1953] see under BODY.

Howmedica III trademark for a nickel-chromium base-metal crown and bridge alloy that is used with fused porcelain veneers.

Howship's lacuna [John *Howship*, English surgeon, 1781–1841] resorption LACUNA.

Hozay, Jean see van Bogaert-Hozay SYNDROME.

HP house PHYSICIAN.

HPI history of present illness.

Hruska attachment (unit) see under ATTACHMENT.

HS Haynes stellite; see HS21 ALLOY and HS31 ALLOY.

h.s. abbreviation for L. *ho′ra som′ni*, at bedtime.

HSA health systems agency.

5-HT 5-hydroxytryptamine.

Huët, G. J. see Pelger-Huët ANOMALY and pseudo-Pelger-Huët ANOMALY.

Hueter, Karl [German surgeon, 1838–1882] see Vogt's POINT (Vogt-Hueter point).

Hueter's maneuver see under MANEUVER.

Hu-Friedy elevator see under ELEVATOR.

Hughlings Jackson's syndrome [John *Hughlings Jackson*, English neurologist, 1834–1911] Jackson-MacKenzie SYNDROME.

Huguier's canal [Pierre Charles *Huguier*, French surgeon, 1804–1873] CANALICULUS of chorda tympani.

Hullihen, Simon P. [1810–1857] an American dentist, considered to be the "father" of oral surgery, who made special contributions to surgical therapy of harelip and cleft palate and removal of carcinoma of the mouth and jaws with the reconstruction of the jaws and lips.

Humby knife see under KNIFE.

humectant (hu-mek′tant) [L. *humectus*, from *humectare* to be moist] 1. moistening. 2. a moistening or diluent substance.

humidity (hu-mid′ĭ-te) [L. *humiditas*] the degree of moisture, especially of that in the air.

humor (hu′mor), pl. *humors, humo′res* [L. "a liquid"] a fluid or semifluid substance; used in anatomical nomenclature to designate certain fluids in the body. See also HUMORALISM and humoral THEORY. **aqueous h., h. aquo′sus** [NA], the fluid occupying the anterior and posterior chambers of the eye.

humoral (hu′mor-al) pertaining to the humors of the body. See also humoral THEORY.

humoralism (hu′mor-al-izm″) the doctrine that all diseases arise from some change of the humors of the body. See humoral THEORY.

Humorsol trademark for *demecarium bromide* (see under DEMECARIUM).

Hünermann, Carl see Conradi-Hünermann SYNDROME.

hunger (hung′ger) a craving, as for food. **oxygen h.,** see ANOXIA and HYPOXIA.

Hunt, William E. [American physician] see Tolosa-Hunt SYNDROME.

Hunt's neuralgia, syndrome [James Ramsay *Hunt*, American neurologist, 1872–1937] see geniculate NEURALGIA and see under SYNDROME.

Hunter, John [1728–1793] a Scottish anatomist and surgeon who made many outstanding contributions to the study of medicine and dental histology, pathology, and embryology. His *Natural History of the Human Teeth*, published in 1771, and his *Practical Treatise on the Diseases of the Teeth*, published in 1778, are considered as landmarks in the history of dentistry. Hunter attempted to establish a nomenclature of the teeth; to describe the physiology of mastication; established the need for removing diseased dental pulp; named the incisor, cuspid, bicuspid, and molar teeth; and devised orthodontic appliances.

Hunter's glossitis [William *Hunter*, English physician, 1861–1937] see under GLOSSITIS.

Hunter-Hurler syndrome [Charles *Hunter*; Gertrud *Hurler*, Austrian pediatrician] see under SYNDROME.

Hunter-Schreger bands [Bernhard Gottlieb *Schreger*, German anatomist, 1766–1825] lines of Schreger; see under LINE.

Hurler, Gertrud [Austrian pediatrician] see Hunter-Hurler SYNDROME.

Hurricane gel see under GEL.

Hurricane topical solution see under SOLUTION.

Hürthle cells [Karl *Hürthle*, German histologist, born 1860] see under CELL.

Huschke's canal, foramen of [Emil *Huschke*, German anatomist, 1797–1858] see under CANAL and FORAMEN.

Hutchinson's freckle, teeth, triad [Sir Jonathan *Hutchinson*, English physician, 1828–1913] see under FRECKLE, TOOTH, and TRIAD.

Hutchinson-Gilford syndrome [Sir J. *Hutchinson;* Hastings *Gilford*, British physician, 1861–1941] see under SYNDROME.

Huxley, Andrew Fielding [born 1917] an English physiologist; co-winner, with John Carew Eccles and Alan Lloyd Hodgkin, of the Nobel prize for medicine and physiology in 1963, for discoveries concerning the ionic mechanisms involved in excitation and inhibition in peripheral and central parts of the nerve cell membrane.

Huxley's plane see under PLANE.

HVJ hemagglutinating virus of Japan; see parainfluenza virus type 1, under VIRUS.

HVL half-value LAYER.

hyal- see HYALO-.

hyalin (hi′ah-lin) [Gr. *hyalos* glass] a translucent substance, one of the products of amyloid degeneration.

hyaline (hi′ah-lin) [Gr. *hyalos* glass] glassy and transparent, or nearly so.

hyalinization (hi″ah-lin″ĭ-za′shun) conversion to a substance resembling glass.

hyalinosis (hi″ah-lin-o′sis) hyaline DEGENERATION. **h. cu′tis et muco′sae,** Urbach-Wiethe SYNDROME.

hyalo-, hyal- [Gr. *hyalos* glass] a combining form denoting resemblance to glass.

Hyalococcus (hi″ah-lo-kok′us) [*hyalo-* + *kokkos* berry] *Klebsiella.* **H. pneumo′niae,** *Klebsiella pneumoniae;* see under KLEBSIELLA.

hyalogen (hi-al′o-jen) [*hyalo-* + Gr. *gennan* to produce] an albuminous substance occurring in cartilage and other tissues, and converted to hyalin.

hyalomere (hi′ah-lo-mēr′) [*hyalo-* + Gr. *meros* part] a zone of smooth or finely fibrillar pale blue cytoplasm surrounding the central granular portion of a blood platelet in dry smears stained with a Romanovskii's stain. See also GRANULOMERE.

hyaloplasm (hi′ah-lo-plazm″) [*hyalo-* + Gr. *plasma* anything formed] 1. an amorphous, fluid, finely granular substance of the cytoplasm of cells in which cellular components form a colloidal suspension. Called also *amorphous cell matrix, cell sap, cytolymph, enchylema, interfilar mass, interfilar substance, interfibrillar substance of Flemming, paramitome,* and *paraplasm.* 2. axoplasm.

hyaloserositis (hi″ah-lo-se″ro-si′tis) [*hyalo-* + *serum* + *-itis*] inflammation of serous membranes marked by hyalinization of the serous exudate into a pearly investment of the organs concerned.

hyalosome (hi-al′o-sōm) [*hyalo-* + Gr. *sōma* body] a structure resembling the nucleolus of a cell, but staining only slightly.

hyaluronidase [E.C.3.2.1.36; 3.2.1.37] (hi″ah-lu-ron′ĭ-dās) an enzyme, hyaluronate glycanohydrolase, that catalyzes the hydrolysis of hyaluronic acid. It is present in leeches, snake and spider venom, testes, and malignant tissues, and is produced by a number of bacteria noted for their invasive properties, such as pneumococcus, certain strains of staphylococci, streptococci, and gas gangrene bacilli. By hydrolyzing hyaluronic acid, which is a mucopolysaccharide consisting of acetylglucosamine and glucuronic acid acting as a cementing substance of the tissue, hyaluronidase facilitates penetration of venoms into tissues and invasion of bacteria. Decomposition by hyaluronidase of hyaluronic acid occurs by making it no longer precipitable with acetic acid, depolymerization with coincident decrease of its viscosity, and liberation of reducing sugars. It is sometimes added to local anesthetic solutions. Hyaluronidase is antagonized by an enzyme present in normal blood plasma, called *anti-invasin I.* Called also *diffusion factor, Duran-Reynals factor, spreading factor, hyaluronoglucuronidase, invasin,* and *mucinase.* See also INVASIVENESS.

hyaluronoglucuronidase (hi″ah-lu-ron″o-glu″ku-ron′ĭ-dās) hyaluronidase.

Hyasorb trademark for *penicillin G potassium* (see under PENICILLIN).

hybridoma (hi″brĭ-do′mah) two fused lymphocytes forming hybrid cells that synthesize hybrid molecules with many possible associations between heavy and light chains of immunoglobulins from each parent cell.

Hyclorate trademark for *clofibrate.*

hydantoin (hi-dan′to-in) a crystalline base, 2,4-imidazolidinedione, that is soluble in water, ether, and alcohol. Hydantoin derivatives are used in the treatment of epilepsy. See also fetal hydantoin SYNDROME and PHENYTOIN.

Hydeltrasol trademark for *prednisolone sodium phosphate* (see under PREDNISOLONE).

Hydol trademark for *hydroflumethiazide.*

hydr- see HYDRO-.

hydracid (hi-dras′id) a binary acid (see under ACID).

hydralazine (hi-dral′ah-zēn) an antihypertensive agent, 1-hydrazinophthalazine, which decreases arterial blood pressure and increases heart rate, stroke volume, and cardiac output. Used therapeutically as the hydrochloride salt, which occurs as a white to off-white, odorless, crystalline powder that is soluble in water and ethanol and very slightly soluble in ether. Anorexia, headache, cardiac arrhythmia, vertigo, nausea, sweating, nasal congestion, paresthesia, edema, tremor, and muscle cramps are the most common side reactions. Drug fever, urticaria, skin rash, polyneuritis, gastrointestinal hemorrhage, anemia, polycythemia, acute rheumatoid state, and a lupus erythematosus–like condition may occur. Trademark: Apresoline.

Hydramycin trademark for *doxycycline hyclate* (see under DOXYCYCLINE).

hydranencephaly (hi″dran-en-sef′ah-le) complete or almost complete absence of the cerebral hemispheres, the space being filled with cerebrospinal fluid.

hydrargyri (hi-drar′ji-ri) genitive of *hydrargyrum* (mercury).

hydrargyrism (hi-drar′ji-rizm) chronic mercury poisoning. See MERCURY.

hydrargyrum (hi-drar′ji-rum), gen. *hydrar′gyri* [L. "liquid silver"] mercury.

hydrarthrosis (hi″drar-thro′sis) [*hydr-* + Gr. *arthron* joint + *-osis*] the presence of watery fluid in the cavity of a joint.

hydratase (hi′drah-tās) hydro-lyase. **aconitate h.** [E.C.4.2.1.3], a hydro-lyase that catalyzes the conversion of citric acid to *cis*-aconitic acid and isocitric acid in oxidative carbohydrate metabolism (Krebs cycle). Called also *aconitase.* **fumarate h.** [E.C.4.2.1.2], a hydro-lyase that catalyzes the conversion of fumaric acid to malic acid. Active in the oxidative metabolism of carbohydrates (Krebs cycle). Called also *fumarase.* **2-phosphoglycerate h., phosphopyruvate h.,** enolase.

hydrate (hi′drāt) [L. *hydras*] a compound whose molecule combines with a molecule(s) of water (known as *water of crystallization*) to form a loose chemical combination which, when allowed to evaporate slowly, produces well-defined crystals, as in dental plaster that is formed by combining calcium sulfate with water, $(CaSO_4)_2 \cdot H_2O$. Hydrates are further classified according to the number of water molecules contained in the compound, as monohydrates (whose crystals contain one water molecule), dihydrates (two molecules of water), trihydrates (three molecules of water), etc. Called also *hydrated compound.* See also anhydrous COMPOUND. **ammonium h.,** AMMONIUM hydroxide. **ferric h.,** ferric HYDROXIDE.

hydrated (hi′drāt-ed) [L. *hydratus*] combined with water; forming a hydrate or a hydroxide.

hydration (hi-dra′shun) combination with water sometimes, but not always, resulting in the production of hydrates.

hydraulics (hi-draw′liks) [*hydr-* + Gr. *aulos* pipe] the branch of physics and engineering dealing with liquids in motion and the mechanisms and laws governing their movement. See also HYDRODYNAMICS.

hydrazide (hi′drah-zīd) an acyl hydrazine, such as R • CO • NH • NH₂. **isonicotinic acid h.,** isoniazid.

hydrazine (hi′drah-zin) a compound, H_2NNH_2, occurring as a colorless, fuming, hygroscopic liquid, which is miscible with water and alcohol. Used in the production of antibacterial and antihypertensive drugs, antioxidants, and various chemical products. Called also *anhydrous h.* and *diamine.* **anhydrous h.,** hydrazine.

Hydrea trademark for *hydroxyurea.*

hydremia (hi-dre′me-ah) [*hydr-* + Gr. *haima* blood + *-ia*] excess of water in the blood.

Hydrenox trademark for *hydroflumethiazide.*

Hydrex trademark for *calcium hydroxide cement* (see under CEMENT).

hydric (hi′drik) pertaining to or combined with hydrogen; containing replaceable hydrogen.

Hydril trademark for *hydrochlorothiazide.*

hydro-, hydr- [Gr. *hydōr* water] 1. a combining form denoting relationship to water or to hydrogen. 2. a combining form denoting presence of fluid in an organ indicated by the word stem to which it is affixed, as in hydrarthrosis.

hydroa (hid-ro′ah) a vesicular eruption attended with intense itching and burning, occurring on surfaces of the body exposed to sunlight. **h. aestiva′le,** a recurrent vesicular eruption occurring most commonly in prepubertal boys during the spring and summer months, and affecting only the parts of the body exposed to sunlight, including the face and dorsum of the hands. The vesicles and bullae, which appear shortly after exposure to sunlight, may become umbilicated and covered with crust, and may be followed by varioliform scarring. Sometimes the bullae show a central depression, like a vaccinia vesicle, which is converted into a thick black crust that, after separation, reveals a variola-like scar; hence, the synonym *hydroa vacciniforme*. Called also *recurrent summer eruption*. **h. puero′rum,** an eruption that may affect any part of the skin, including the face, usually occurring during the first year of life, and usually preceded by and associated with itching and burning sensation. Red vesicles frequently coalesce to form bullae. Each attack lasts about two weeks. Spontaneous recovery occurs at puberty. **h. vaccinifor′me,** h. aestivale.

hydrobromide (hi″dro-bro′mīd) a salt of an organic base and hydrobromic acid. Called also *hydrogen bromide*.

Hydrocal trademark for Class I *dental stone* (see under STONE).

hydrocarbon (hi″dro-kar′bon) a large group of organic compounds containing only carbon and hydrogen, which are derived chiefly from petroleum, coal tar, and vegetable sources. Hydrocarbons are divided into alicyclic, aliphatic, and aromatic, according to the arrangement of the atoms and the chemical properties of the compounds. **alicyclic h.,** one having a cyclic structure and aliphatic properties. **aliphatic h′s,** straight-chain hydrocarbons consisting chiefly of carbon atoms in chains, including paraffins (alkanes), olefins, acetyls, and acyclic terpenes. **aromatic h′s,** a major group of unsaturated cyclic hydrocarbons containing one or more closed chains with six carbons and three double bonds in their structure (benzene rings). Most are derived from petroleum and coal tar, and are characterized by a strong typical odor. Aromatic hydrocarbons have a wide chemical application because of their high reactivity and chemical versatility; the most important ones include benzene, toluene, naphthalene, anthracene, and phenanthrene. **carcinogenic h.,** a condensed nuclear aromatic hydrocarbon that tends to cause cancer. **cyclic h.,** one of the series of hydrocarbons having the general formula C_nH_{2n}, the carbon atoms being thought of as having a closed ring structure. **halogenated h.,** a hydrocarbon in which one or more of the hydrogen atoms has been replaced by fluorine, chlorine, bromine, or iodine. **saturated h.,** a hydrocarbon in which all four valencies for the carbon atoms are satisfied; one that has the maximum number of hydrogen atoms for a given carbon structure, such as methane, ethane, propane, cyclopropane, and the butanes. **unsaturated h.,** a hydrocarbon in which one or more double or triple bonds exist between the carbon atoms; an alicyclic or aliphatic hydrocarbon that has less than the maximum number of hydrogen atoms for a given carbon structure, such as ethylene, acetylene, propylene, cyclobenzene, and the butenes.

Hydro-Cast trademark for a *denture reliner* (see under RELINER).

hydrocephalus (hi-dro-sef′ah-lus) [*hydro-* + Gr. *kephalē* head] an abnormal accumulation of fluid in the cranial vault, causing enlargement of the head and brain atrophy.

hydrochlorothiazide (hi″dro-klo″ro-thi′ah-zīd) a benzothiadiazine diuretic, 6-chloro-3,4-dihydro-2*H*-1,2,4-benzothiadiazine-7-sulfonamide 1,1-dioxide, occurring as a white, odorless, crystalline powder that is soluble in sodium hydroxide solutions, dimethylformamide, and methanol, slightly soluble in water, and insoluble in ether, chloroform, benzene, and mineral acids. Used in the treatment of hypertension, usually as an adjunct to other hypotensive drugs. Also used in the treatment of edema, liver cirrhosis, congestive heart failure, and other diseases. Adverse effects may include gastrointestinal, neurological, allergic, respiratory, and other disorders, including leukopenia, agranulocytosis, thrombocytopenia, aplastic anemia, purpura, hyperglycemia, glycosuria, and other conditions occurring in benzothiadiazine therapy. Called also *chlorosulthiadil*. Trademarks: Bremil, Cidrex, Dichlorosal, Diclotride, Esidrex, Hydril, HydroDIURIL, Hydrosoluric, Hypothiazide, Urodiazin.

Hydrocodin trademark for *dihydrocodeine*.

hydrocodone (hi″dro-ko′dōn) a semisynthetic opium alkaloid, 4,5α-epoxy-3-methoxy-17-methylmorphinan-6-one, occurring as prisms that are soluble in ethanol and dilute acids, but not in water. It is an addictive analgesic and antitussive agent. Called also *dihydrocodeinone*. Trademarks: Bekadid, Dicodid. **h. bitartrate,** a bitartrate salt of hydrocodone, occurring as a fine white crystalline powder or solids that are soluble in water, slightly soluble in ethanol, and insoluble in ether and chloroform. It is an addictive analgesic and antitussive agent. Called also *dihydrocodeinone bitartrate* and *dihydrocodeinone tartrate*. Trademarks: Calmodid, Codinovo, Dicodrine, Duodin, Norgan.

hydrocolloid (hi″dro-kol′loid) [*hydro-* + Gr. *kollōdēs* glutinous] a colloid system in which water is the dispersion medium. **h. conditioner,** hydrocolloid CONDITIONER. **h. impression material,** see impression material, irreversible hydrocolloid and impression material, reversible hydrocolloid, under MATERIAL. **irreversible h.,** a hydrocolloid which can be converted by chemical reaction from the sol to the gel condition, but cannot be reverted to a sol by any simple means. **reversible h.,** a hydrocolloid which can be reverted from the gel to the sol condition by increase in temperature, brought about by physical changes to form gel lattices. **h. syringe,** hydrocolloid SYRINGE.

hydrocortisone (hi″dro-kor′tĭ-zōn) a glucocorticoid, 11β,17α-21-trihydroxy-4-pregnene-3,20-dione, occurring as a white, odorless, bitter, crystalline powder that is readily soluble in ethanol and acetone, and slightly soluble in water, ether, and chloroform. Conversely, through a feedback mechanism, it controls ACTH secretion. Hydrocortisone is involved in protein, lipid, and carbohydrate metabolism and in immune and inflammatory responses of the body. Used in the treatment of adrenocortical insufficiency and as an anti-inflammatory and antiallergic agent. In dentistry, used in the treatment of sensitive dentin, pulpal reactions to surgery, oral ulcers associated with skin diseases, temporomandibular joint lesions, and in tissue transplantation. Side reactions may include euphoria, mental depression, psychoses, hypertension, anorexia, peptic ulcer, susceptibility to infection, abnormal fat distribution, moon face, edema, potassium loss, alkalosis, and osteoporosis. Called also *cortisol* and *17-hydroxycorticosterone*. Trademarks: Cremesone, Cort-Dome, Cortifoam, Epicort, Hydrocortone. **h. acetate,** the acetate ester of hydrocortisone, occurring as a white, odorless, crystalline powder that is slightly soluble in ethanol and chloroform and insoluble in water. Used in ointments and suspensions for intra-articular and topical administration. Called also *cortisol acetate*. Trademarks: Hydrocortistat, Litraderm. **h. 21-(dihydrogen phosphate),** h. phosphate. **h. 21-(disodium phosphate),** h. sodium phosphate. **h. phosphate,** a dihydrogen phosphate derivative of hydrocortisone; used for injections. Called also *hydrocortisone . 21-(dihydrogen phosphate)*. Trademark: Cortiphate. **h. sodium phosphate,** the disodium salt of hydrocortisone phosphate, occurring as a white to yellowish, odorless, bitter powder that is readily soluble in water, slightly soluble in ethanol, and insoluble in chloroform and ether. Used for intravenous, intramuscular, intrasynovial, and intralesional injections. Called also *hydrocortisone 21-(disodium phosphate)*. Trademark: Actocortin. **h. sodium succinate,** a salt of hydrocortisone, occurring as a white, odorless, hygroscopic powder that is soluble in water and ethanol, slightly soluble in acetone, and insoluble in chloroform. Used for injections. Trademarks: Corlan, Intracort, Nordicort, Solu-Cortef.

Hydrocortistat trademark for *hydrocortisone acetate* (see under HYDROCORTISONE).

Hydrocortone trademark for *hydrocortisone*.

hydrodiffusion (hi″dro-di-fu′zhun) diffusion in an aqueous medium.

HydroDiuril trademark for *hydrochlorothiazide*.

hydrodynamics (hi″dro-di-nam′iks) that branch of the science of mechanics which treats of the movement of fluids and of solids contained in fluids. See also HYDRAULICS.

hydroflumethiazide (hi″dro-floo″me-thi′ah-zīd) a benzothiadiazine diuretic, 3,4-dihydro-6-(trifluoromethyl)-2*H*-1,2,4-benzothiadiazine-7-sulfonamide 1,1-dioxide, occurring as a white to creamy, odorless, crystalline powder that is soluble in acetone and ethanol and very slightly soluble in water. Used chiefly in the treatment of edema in congestive heart failure, liver cirrhosis, and in mild forms of hypertension. Adverse reactions may include gastrointestinal, neurological, allergic, respiratory, and other disorders, including leukopenia, agranulocytosis, thrombocytopenia, aplastic anemia, purpura, hyperglycemia, glycosuria, and other conditions occurring during benzothiadiazine therapy. Called also *dihydromethiazide* and *methforylthiazidine*. Trademarks: Bristab, Diucardin, Hydol, Hydrenox, Rodiuran, Saluron.

hydrogen (hi′dro-jen) [*hydro-* + Gr. *gennan* to produce] the lightest and most abundant element in nature, occurring as an odorless, colorless, tasteless gas that becomes explosively volatile when mixed with oxygen, chlorine, or air. Symbol, H; atomic number, 1; atomic weight, 1.0079; density, 0.08988 gm/l; valence, 1; group IA of the periodic table. It occurs as ¹H (protium), ²H (deuterium), and ³H (tritium). Hydrogen is nontoxic, but may act as a simple asphyxiant. With oxygen, it forms water. **h. bond,** hydrogen BOND. **h. bridge,** hydrogen BRIDGE. **h.**

bromide, hydrobromide. **h. cyanide,** hydrocyanic ACID. **h. fluoride,** hydrogen FLUORIDE. **h. halide,** hydrogen HALIDE. **heavy h.,** deuterium. **h. iodide,** a strong, irritant, colorless gas, HI, that is soluble in water. Used in the production of hydriodic acid. Called also *anhydrous hydriodic acid.* **h. ion concentration,** hydrogen ion CONCENTRATION. **h. peroxide,** hydrogen PEROXIDE. **h. sulfate,** sulfuric ACID.

hydrogenase [E.C.1.11 and 1.12] (hi″dro-jen-ās) a subclass of oxidoreductases, the enzymes of which catalyze the reduction of various substances by means of molecular hydrogen. **fumaric h.,** succinate DEHYDROGENASE.

hydrogenation (hi″dro-jě-na′shun) causing to combine with hydrogen; saturation of aliphatic unsaturated compounds with hydrogen; cracking higher hydrocarbons to gasoline by hydrogen.

Hydro-Jel Alginate see under ALGINATE.

hydrolase [E.C.3] (hi′dro-lās) any of a major class of enzymes involved in catalysis of hydrolytic reactions, and including digestive enzymes. See also ENZYME classification. **acetylcholine h.,** acetylcholinesterase. **dipeptidyl-peptide h.,** proteinase. **peptide h.** [E.C.3.4], any of a group of enzymes that catalyze protein hydrolysis by attacking peptide bonds, thus producing protein degradation. Peptide hydrolases are divided into peptidases and proteinases. Peptidases [E.C.4.11 to 4.15] are those enzymes that catalyze hydrolysis of single amino acids from the N-terminus of peptide chains, hydrolysis of residues from the C-terminus, and split off dipeptide units from either the N- or C-terminus. Proteinases [E.C.3.4.21 to 3.4.24] consist of a large number of hydrolases which attack protein substrates at internal peptide bonds. Called also *peptidohydrolase, protease* and *proteolytic enzyme.* **phosphoric monoester h.,** phosphatase.

Hydrolose trademark for *methylcellulose.*

hydro-lyase [E.C.4.2.1] (hi″dro-li′ās) a subsubclass of carbon-oxygen lyases, the enzymes of which cleave the C–O bond; the reaction being associated with the elimination of water. Called also *hydratase.* **carbonate h.,** carbonate DEHYDRATASE.

hydrolysis (hi-drol′ĭ-sis), pl. *hydrol′yses* [hydro- + Gr. *lysis* dissolution] the splitting of a compound by the addition of water, the hydroxyl group being incorporated in one fragment, and the hydrogen atom in the other.

Hydromedin trademark for *ethacrinic acid* (see under ACID).

hydromorphone (hi″dro-mor′fōn) a semisynthetic opium alkaloid, 4,5α-epoxy-3-hydroxy-17-methymorphinan-6-one, occurring as a fine, white, odorless, crystalline powder that is affected by light and is soluble in ethanol and chloroform and slightly soluble in water. It is an addicting analgesic. Called also *dihydromorphinone.* Trademarks: Dimorphone, Novolaudon. **h. hydrochloride,** a hydrochloride salt of hydromorphone that is soluble in water, sparingly soluble in ethanol, and insoluble in ether. It is an addicting analgesic, being a morphine derivative, that is stronger and more toxic than the parent compound. Used chiefly in postoperative pain, myocardial infarction, and cancer. Trademarks: Dilaudid, Laudicon, Hymorphan.

Hydromox trademark for *quinethazone.*

Hydron trademark for a hydrophilic *acrylic resin* (see under RESIN).

Hydronol trademark for *isosorbide.*

hydroparotitis (hi″dro-par″o-ti′tis) distention of the parotid gland with watery fluid.

hydropericardium (hi″dro-per″ĭ-kar′de-um) [hydro- + *pericardium*] abnormal accumulation of fluid in the pericardial cavity. Called also *pericardial edema.*

hydrophilia (hi-dro-fil′e-ah) [hydro- + Gr. *philein* to love +-*ia*] the property of readily absorbing water or moisture.

hydrophilic (hi″dro-fil′ik) readily absorbing water or moisture; hygroscopic.

hydrophobia (hi″dro-fo′be-ah) [hydro- + Gr. *phobein* to be affrighted by + -*ia*] rabies.

hydrophobic (hi″dro-fo′bik) 1. pertaining to or affected by hydrophobia (rabies). 2. not readily absorbing water, or being adversely affected by water.

hydrophthalmos (hi″drof-thal′mos) [hydro- + Gr. *ophthalmos* eye] distention of the eyeball by a watery effusion.

hydrops (hi′drops) [L.; Gr. *hydor* water] the presence of abnormal fluids in the tissues or in a body cavity. Called also *dropsy.* See also EDEMA. **endolymphatic h.,** Ménière's DISEASE. **h. feta'lis,** ERYTHROBLASTOSIS fetalis.

hydroquinone (hi″dro-kwi-nōn) a demelanizing agent, *p*-dihydroxybenzene, occurring as fine, white needles that dissolve in water, alcohol, chloroform, and ether, and darken on

exposure to air. Used in the treatment of freckling and other conditions characterized by hyperpigmentation. Believed to inhibit the enzyme tyrosinase, thus preventing the conversion of tyrosine to dihydroxyphenylalanine, and the synthesis of melanin. Also used as a reducer and developer of photographic and x-ray plates. Ingestion may cause tinnitus, nausea, vomiting, tachypnea, cyanosis, convulsions, delirium, collapse, and death. Side effects may include a burning sensation, rash, irritation, and allergic reactions. Called also *1,4-benzenediol* and *tecguinol.* See also developing SOLUTION.

hydrorrhea (hi″dro-re′ah) [hydro- + Gr. *rhoia* flow] a copious watery discharge.

Hydrosaluric trademark for *hydrochlorothiazide.*

hydrosol (hi′dro-sol) [hydro- + *sol*] a colloidal suspension (sol) in which the dispersion medium is water, as in gel.

hydrothorax (hi″dro-tho′raks) [hydro- + *thorax*] an abnormal collection of fluids in the pleural cavity. Called also *pleural edema.* **chylous h.,** chylothorax.

Hydroton trademark for *chlorthalidone.*

Hydrotricine trademark for *tyrothricin.*

hydroxide (hi-drok′sīd) 1. an inorganic compound in which a hydroxyl radical (OH) or a hydroxide ion (OH^-) combines with other radicals or atoms. 2. in the older literature, an inorganic base consisting of a metal in compound form with a hydroxyl (OH) radical. **ammonium h.,** AMMONIUM hydroxide. **ferric h.,** a compound, $Fe(OH)_3$, occurring as a brown substance soluble in water, alcohol, acids, and ether. Used in dextran-iron complex as a source of iron, and in various pharmaceutical preparations. Formerly used as an antidote in arsenic poisoning. Also used as a black pigment in ceramic restorations. Called also *iron h., ferric hydrate, iron hydrate,* and *iron oxide.* **iron h.,** ferric h. **potassium h.,** POTASSIUM hydroxide.

hydroxocobalamin (hi-drok″so-ko-bal′ah-min) hydroxycobalamin.

hydroxy- a chemical prefix indicating presence of the hydroxyl (OH) group.

***p*-hydroxyacetanilide** (hi-drok″se-as″ě-tan′ĭ-lĭd) acetaminophen.

hydroxyamphetamine (hi-drok″se-am-fet′ah-mēn) a sympathomimetic, *p*-(2-aminopropyl)phenol, occurring as white crystals that are soluble in water, ethanol, chloroform, and ethyl acetate. Used as a nasal decongestant, as a mydratic, in controlling blood pressure in spinal anesthesia, in providing relief in heart block, in preventing syncope in certain diseases, and in the treatment of orthostatic hypotension. Side reactions may include nausea, vomiting, gastrointestinal irritation, blood pressure elevation, arrhythmia, substernal pain, headache, and sweating. Dental patients receiving the drug may exhibit excessive nervousness. Trademarks: Paredrine, Pulsoton. **h. hydrobromide,** the hydrobromide salt of hydroxyamphetamine, occurring as a white, crystalline powder that is readily soluble in water and ethanol, slightly soluble in chloroform, and almost insoluble in ether. **h. hydrochloride,** the hydrochloride salt of hydroxyamphetamine, occurring as crystals that are soluble in water and ethanol, but not in ether.

hydroxyapatite (hi-drok″se-ap′ah-tīt) a calcium phosphate compound, $Ca_{10}(PO_4)_6(OH)_2$, which is an apatite derivative and one of the two mineral constituents of bones and teeth (the other is $CaCO_3$). In the teeth, it is the principal mineral component of the hard tissue, forming crystals that are the integral parts of the tooth structure. In the tooth, it is soluble in acids of soft drinks and in carbohydrate fermentation products, but its OH ion is readily exchanged for the F ion from fluorides, resulting in a fluoroapatite not susceptible to acid decay. See also FLUORIDATION and FLUORIDE.

2-hydroxybenzamide (hi-drok″se-benz-am′ĭd) salicylamide.

***p*-hydroxybenzylpenicillin** (hi-drok″se-ben″zil-pen′ĭ-sil′in) penicillin X.

hydroxycarbamide (hi-drok″se-kar-bam′ĭd) hydroxyurea.

25-hydroxycholecalciferol (hi-drok″se-ko″lě-kal-sif′ě-rol) a vitamin D_3 metabolite, 9,10-secocholesta-5,7,10(19)-triene-3β, 25-diol, formed in the liver by side-chain hydroxylation of carbon-25. It is an intermediate in the formation of 1α,25-dihydroxycholecalciferol, which is the biologically active form of vitamin D_3, and is involved in the absorption of calcium from the intestinal tract and the resorption of phosphate in the renal tubule. Abbreviated 25-*HCC.*

hydroxycobalamine (hi-drok″se-ko-bal′ah-mēn) vitamin B_{12a}.

11-hydroxycorticosteroid (hi-drok″se-kor′ti-ko-ste′roid) a C_{11} glucocorticoid produced by the zona fasciculata of the adrenal cortex, which responds to adrenocorticotropic hormone, and is involved in protein, lipid, and carbohydrate metabolism. See also GLUCOCORTICOID and STEROID.

17-hydroxycorticosteroid (hi-drok″se-kor″ti-ko-ste′roid) a C_{17} glucocorticoid produced by the zona fasciculata of the adrenal cortex, which responds to adrenocorticotropic hormone stimulation, and is involved in protein, lipid, and carbohydrate metabolism. See also GLUCOCORTICOID and STEROID.

17-hydroxycorticosterone (hi-drok″se-kor″tĭ-ko′stĕ-rōn) hydrocortisone.

2-hydroxydiphenyl (hi-drok″se-di-fen′il) orthophenylphenol.

hydroxyl (hi-drok′sil) the univalent CH group which combines with other groups of an organic compound; its H being replaceable by positive elements and the entire radical by halogens.

Hydroxyline trademark for a *cavity liner* (see under LINER), consisting of calcium hydroxide in a resin solution.

hydroxylysine (hi″drok-sil′ĭ-sin) a basic, naturally occurring nonessential amino acid found in collagen and structural proteins, 2,6-diamino-5-hydroxy-hexanoic acid. Abbreviated *Hyl.*

o-hydroxyphenylmercuric chloride (hi-drok″se-fen″il-mer-ku″rik) a toxic antiseptic agent, occurring as a white or pinkish, fine crystalline powder or solid that is readily soluble in hot water, alcohol, and hot benzene and sparingly in chloroform. Used especially in soaps. It is a constituent of mercocresols. Called also *chloromercuriphenol* and *o-(chloromercuri)phenol.*

hydroxyproline (hi-drok″se-pro′lēn) a heterocyclic, naturally occurring, nonessential amino acid, 4-hydroxy-2-pyrrolidinecarboxylic acid, produced by hydrolysis of collagen and elastin. Abbreviated *Hypo.* See also amino ACID and PROLINE.

8-hydroxyquinoline (hi-drok″se-kwin′o-lēn) a fungistatic disinfectant of moderate toxicity, occurring as white crystals or powder that darkens when exposed to light. It is soluble in alcohol, acetone, chloroform, benzene, and mineral acids, but not in water and ether. Called also *oxine, oxychinolin, oxyquinoline,* and *8-quinolinol.* **8-h. sulfate,** the sulfate salt of 8-hydroxyquinoline, occurring as a yellow, crystalline powder with a slight odor and a burning taste, which is soluble in water and glycerol, slightly soluble in alcohol, and insoluble in ether. Used as an antiperspirant, deodorant, and antiseptic drug. Included in some ointments, nasal sprays, gargles, eyewashes, and foot powders. Called also *oxine sulfate, oxyquinoline sulfate,* and *8-quinolinol sulfate.*

5-hydroxytryptamine (hi-drok″se-trip′tah-mēn) a substance, 3-(β-aminoethyl)-5-hydroxyindole, first found as a vasoconstrictor factor in the serum of coagulated blood (hence the synonyms *serotonin* and *vasotonin*) and, later, as a gut-stimulating factor in the gastric mucosa and other tissues. It has been found to be widely distributed in animal and plant tissues. 5-Hydroxytryptamine is believed to serve as a transmitter substance released by neurons in the brain, being a target for various centrally active drugs. Pharmacologically, it stimulates or inhibits smooth muscles and nerves. Effects are variable, including stimulation of afferent nerves of the respiratory system; vasoconstriction or vasodilation; depending on the dose, the resting tonus and the vascular bed; production of positive inotropic and chronotropic effects on the heart; and stimulation of intestinal motility. Blood pressure responds to the administration of 5-hydroxytryptamine by an initial repressor phase, followed by a pressor phase and, finally, a prolonged depressor phase. In mammals, it is synthesized from dietary tryptophan, which is first hydroxylated to 5-hydroxytrophan and then decarboxylated to 5-hydroxytryptamine. It has primary application in physiological and pharmacological studies. Abbreviated *5-HT.* Called also *enteramine* and *thrombocytin.*

hydroxyurea (hi-drok″se-u-re′ah) a substituted urea compound, $CH_4N_2O_2$, occurring as a white, odorless, tasteless, photosensitive powder that is soluble in water and hot ethanol. It acts on the enzyme ribonucleoside diphosphate reductase and interferes with the synthesis of DNA, thereby suppressing cell division of rapidly proliferating cells, especially those in the bone marrow. Used in the treatment of chronic granulocytic leukemia, melanoma, and other cancers. Adverse reactions may include stomatitis, oral ulcers, alopecia, skin rash, predisposition to infection, fetal abnormalities, nausea, vomiting, diarrhea, headache, vertigo, hallucinations, convulsions, pruritus, elevated blood urea nitrogen, hyperuricemia, nephrolithiasis, and bone marrow depression with leukopenia, megaloblastic anemia, and, less commonly, thrombocytopenia. Called also *hydroxycarbamide.* Trademarks: Hydrea, Litalir.

hydroxyzine (hi-drok′sĭ-zēn) a compound, 2-[2-[4-[(4-chlorophenyl)phenylmethyl]-1-piperazinyl]ethoxy]ethanol. Its salts are antianxiety drugs with mild antihistaminic, antiemetic, and anticholinergic properties. **h. dihydrochloride,** h. hydrochloride. **h. hydrochloride,** a dihydrochloride salt of hydroxyzine, occurring as a white, odorless powder that is readily soluble in chloroform and water, slightly soluble in acetone, and insoluble in ether. Used in the treatment of anxiety conditions, irritability, tension, confusion, certain allergic diseases, and alcoholism. In dentistry, the drug is used to allay apprehension

before dental procedures and in pre- and postoperative medication. Adverse reactions include drowsiness, xerostomia, and involuntary motor activity, including tremor. Its use is contraindicated in pregnancy and hypersensitivity. Called also *h. dihydrochloride.* Trademarks: Alamon, Atarax. **h. pamoate,** a pamoate derivative of hydroxyzine, having pharmacological properties, uses, and adverse reactions similar to those of the hydrochloride salt. Trademark: Vistaril.

Hygeia [Gr. *Hygieia*] one of two sisters, the other being Panacea, who were daughters of Æsculapius, the mythical god of healing, and who assisted in the rites at the early temples of healing.

hygiene (hi′jēn) [Gr. *hygieia* health] 1. the science of health and its preservation. 2. a condition or practice conductive to the preservation of health, as by cleanliness. **dental h., oral h. food h.,** measures necessary for ensuring the safety, wholesomeness, and soundness of food at all stages from its growth, production, or manufacture until its final consumption. **mouth h., oral h. oral h.,** the personal maintenance of cleanliness and hygiene of the teeth and oral structures by toothbrushing, tissue stimulation, gum massage, hydrotherapy, and other procedures recommended by the dentist or dental hygienist for the preservation of dental and oral health. Called also *dental h.* and *mouth h.* See also oral hygiene INDEX. **Oral H. Instruction,** see under INSTRUCTION.

hygienist (hi-je′nist, hi′je-en″ist) a specialist in hygiene. **dental h.,** a dental auxiliary who has completed at least a two-year program in an accredited school or dental college and who has been licensed by a state's board of dental examiners to practice dental prophylaxis. Upon completing the educational and licensing requirements, dental hygienists receive the title Registered Dental Hygienist (RDH). Some schools offer, in addition, bachelor's and master's degree programs to dental hygienists. They work under the direction and supervision of a dentist and their functions include scaling and polishing the teeth, dental radiography, and teaching oral hygiene. In some states they are permitted to apply fluoride solution to the teeth. Formerly called *dental nurse.* See also dental AUXILIARY. **Registered Dental H. (RDH),** see *dental h.*

Hygratyl trademark for *dihydrotachysterol.*

hygro- [Gr. *hygros* moist] a combining form meaning moist or denoting relationship to moisture.

hygroma (hi-gro′mah), pl. *hygro′mata* [hygro- + -oma] a fluid-distended sac, cyst, or bursa. **cystic h.,** cavernous LYMPHANGIOMA.

hygroscopic (hi″gro-skop′ik) 1. taking up and retaining moisture readily; hydrophilic. 2. pertaining to chemical compounds which take up water on exposure to atmospheric conditions. Compounds taking up sufficient water to finally dissolve are said to be deliquescent.

Hygroton trademark for *chlorthalidone.*

Hykinone trademark for *menadione sodium bisulfite* (see under MENADIONE).

Hyl hydroxylysine.

Hymorphan trademark for *hydromorphone hydrochloride* (see under HYDROMORPHONE).

Hynes pharyngoplasty see under PHARYNGOPLASTY.

hyo- [Gr. *hyoeides* shaped like the letter U] a combining form meaning U-shaped, or hyoid.

hyobasioglossus (hi″o-ba″se-o-glos′us) the basal part of the hyoglossus muscle.

hyoepiglottic (hi″o-ep″ĭ-glot′ik) pertaining to the hyoid bone and the epiglottis.

hyoglossal (hi″o-glos′al) [hyo- + Gr. *glōssa* tongue] pertaining to the hyoid bone and the tongue.

hyoglossus (hi″o-glos′us) hyoglossal MUSCLE.

hyoid (hi′oid) [Gr. *hyoeides* U-shaped] 1. shaped like the Greek letter upsilon (ʋ). 2. pertaining to the hyoid bone.

Hyosan trademark for *dichlorophen.*

hyoscine (hi′o-sin, hi′o-sēn) scopolamine. **h. methyl bromide,** METHSCOPOLAMINE bromide.

hyoscyamine (hi″o-si′ah-mēn) an alkaloid usually obtained from *Hyoscyamus* and other solanaceous plants, [3(S)-endo]-α-(hydroxymethyl)-benzeneacetic acid 8-methyl-8-azabicyclo [3,2,1] oct-3-yl ester. It is a white crystalline powder that deteriorates when exposed to air, and is soluble in water, benzene, alcohol, chloroform, and dilute acids. The levorotatory isomer of the racemic mixture is known as *atropine.* It is an antimuscarinic agent used chiefly as the hydrobromide and sultate salts, its properties being similar to that of atropine. Therapeutically, hyoscyamine is used mainly as an antispasmodic.

Hyoscyamus (hi″o-si′ah-mus) [L.; Gr. *hys* swine + *kyamos* bean] a genus of solanaceous plants, yielding some medically important alkaloids, including hyoscyamine.

hyothyroid (hi″o-thi′roid) pertaining to the hyoid bone and the thyroid cartilage; thyrohyoid.

Hyp hydroproline.

hypalgesia (hi″pal-je′ze-ah) [hypo- + Gr. *algēsis* pain] diminished capacity to perceive pain. Called also *hypalgia* and *hypoalgesia*. See also ANALGESIA. **unilateral h.,** hemihypalgesia.

hypalgia (hi-pal′je-ah) hypalgesia.

Hypaque trademark for *diatrizoate sodium* (see under DIATRIZOATE).

hyper- [Gr. *hyper* above] a prefix signifying above, beyond, or excessive. See also words beginning SUPER-.

hyperacidity (hi″per-ah-sid′ĭ-te) excessive acidity; superacidity.

hyperactive (hi″per-ak′tiv) hyperkinetic.

hyperactivity (hi″per-ak-tiv′ĭ-te) hyperkinesia.

hyperacusis (hi″per-ah-ku′sis) [hyper- + Gr. *akousis* hearing] abnormal acuteness of the sense of hearing, or a painful sensitiveness to sounds. Called also *acoustic* or *auditory hyperesthesia*.

hyperacute (hi″per-ah-kūt) extremely acute; superacute.

hyperalgesia (hi″per-al-je′ze-ah) [hyper- + Gr. *algēsis* pain] excessive sensitivity to pain. Called also *hyperalgia*. See also HYPERESTHESIA and PAIN (1). Cf. ANALGESIA and ANESTHESIA.

hyperalgia (hi-per-al′je-ah) [hyper- + Gr. *algos* pain] hyperalgesia.

hyperalimentation (hi″per-al″ĭ-men-ta′shun) the administration or consumption of nutrients beyond normal requirements. Called also *superalimentation*. **continuous pump/tube enteric h.,** enteral h. **enteral h.,** introduction of a complete liquid diet through a small feeding tube passed transnasally into the stomach and distal to the pylorus in patients with gastrointestinal dysfunction. Called also *continuous pump/tube enteric h.* and *enteral therapy*. See also parenteral FEEDING. **parenteral h.,** parenteral infusion of nutrients, such as glucose, proteins, lipids, electrolytes, vitamins, and other substances in the restoration of negative nitrogen balance and deficiencies of nutrients in patients with gastrointestinal dysfunction. The nutrients are usually instilled intravenously, sometimes into the subclavian artery, and infrequently under the skin. Called also *parenteral hyperalimentation therapy* and *total parenteral nutrition (TPN)*. See also parenteral FEEDING.

hyperbaric (hi″per-bār′ik) [hyper- + Gr. *baros* weight] characterized by greater than normal pressure or weight; applied to gases under greater than atmospheric pressure, as hyperbaric oxygen, or to a solution of greater specific gravity than another taken as a standard of reference. See also hyperbaric MEDICINE.

hyperbarism (hi″per-bar′izm) exposure to environmental pressure that exceeds the pressure within body tissues, fluids and cavities, usually that of 1 atmosphere at sea level.

hyperbetalipoproteinemia (hi″per-ba″tah-lip″o-pro″te-in-e′me-ah) [hyper- + β-lipoprotein + Gr. *haima* blood + -ia] the presence in the blood of excessive amounts of β-lipoprotein. See hyperlipoproteinemia II. **familial h.,** hyperlipoproteinemia II.

hyperbilirubinemia (hi″per-bil″ĭ-roo″bĭ-ne′me-ah) an excess of bilirubin in the blood, indicating excessive red cell destruction, faulty uptake of bilirubin by the liver, reduced hepatic conjugation of bilirubin, reduced excretion of conjugated bilirubin, and other forms of defective pigment metabolism. Jaundice and green discoloration of the teeth are the principal cutaneous and oral symptoms, respectively.

hyperbrachycephalic (hi″per-brak″e-sĕ-fal′ik) pertaining to or characterized by extreme brachycephaly. See hyperbrachycephalic SKULL.

hyperbrachycephaly (hi″per-brak″e-sef′ah-le) a condition characterized by a short broad skull. See hyperbrachycephalic SKULL.

hypercalcemia (hi″per-kal-se′me-ah) an excess of calcium in the blood caused by excessive gastrointestinal calcium absorption, excessive bone resorption, decreased osteogenesis, excessive calcium binding in serum, or decreased calcium excretion by the kidneys. It may be associated with hyperparathyroidism, hypervitaminosis D, Burnett's syndrome, osteoporosis, multiple myeloma, sarcoidosis, and neoplasms. **idiopathic h. of infancy,** elfin facies SYNDROME.

hypercalcinuria (hi″per-kal″sĭ-nu′re-ah) an excess of calcium in the urine, usually caused by an increase in the amount of calcium filtered by the renal glomeruli or by a decrease in the amount reabsorbed by the renal tubules. It is usually seen associated with hyperparathyroidism, hyperthyroidism, Cush-

ing's syndrome (1), renal rickets, osteomalacia, starvation and insufficient dietary phosphate intake, osteoporosis, osteitis fibrosa generalisata, bone neoplasms, hypervitaminosis D, and sarcoidosis. Called also *hypercalciuria*.

hypercalciuria (hi″per-kal″sĭ-u′re-ah) hypercalcinuria.

hypercapnia (hi″per-kap′ne-ah) [hyper- + Gr. *kapnos* smoke + -ia] abnormally high amount of carbon dioxide in the blood. Cf. ACAPNIA and HYPOCAPNIA.

hypercementosis (hi″per-se″men-to′sis) a regressive change of teeth characterized by excessive development of secondary cementum on the surface of the teeth, which may occur on any part of the root, but the apical two-thirds are most commonly affected. The principal causes include accelerated elongation of a tooth, inflammation, tooth repair, and osteitis deformans; some cases are idiopathic. In young individuals, tooth eruption may be delayed, leading to curvature of the roots and ankylosis between the bone and root surface. Excessive amounts of secondary or cellular cementum (osteocementum) is the principal histological feature. Restricted hypercementosis may result in spurs. Called also *cementosis*, *cementum hyperplasia*, and *cementum hypertrophy*.

hyperchloremia (hi″per-klo-re′me-ah) excess of chloride in the blood.

hypercholesterolemia (hi″per-ko-les″ter-ol-e′me-ah) [hyper- + *cholesterol* + Gr. *haima* blood + -ia]. An excess of cholesterol in the blood, believed to lead to arteriosclerosis. **essential familial h., familial h.,** hyperlipoproteinemia II.

hyperchondroplasia (hi″per-kon″dro-pla′se-ah) [hyper- + Gr. *chondros* cartilage + *plassein* to form] excessive development of cartilage. See Marfan's SYNDROME.

hyperchylomicronemia (hi″per-ki″lo-mi″kro-ne′me-ah) [hyper- + *chylomicron* + Gr. *haima* blood + -ia] the presence in the blood of excessive amounts of chylomicrons, resulting in blood turbidity. It occurs after meals, at the time when ingested fats are transported from the intestine to the liver, muscles, and adipose tissue. Persistent hyperchylomicronemia may indicate hyperlipoproteinemia or diabetic acidosis. See also alimentary LIPEMIA. **familial h.,** hyperlipoproteinemia I.

hyperdolichocephalic (hi″per-dol″ĭ-ko-sĕ-fal′ik) [hyper- + *dolicho-* + Gr. *kephalē* head] characterized by or pertaining to an extremely elongated narrow head. See hyperdolichocephalic SKULL.

hyperdontia (hi″per-don′she-ah) an anomaly characterized by the presence of an excessive number of teeth.

hyperemia (hi″per-e′me-ah) [hyper- + Gr. *haima* blood + -ia] an abnormal increase in the amount of blood in the vessels of a part, leading to engorgement. **active h., arterial h.,** hyperemia due to relaxation of the arterioles. **collateral h.,** increased flow of blood through collateral vessels when the flow through the main artery is arrested. **dental pulp h.,** excessive accumulation of blood in the dental pulp resulting in vascular congestion and forcing out some of the interstitial fluid to make way for the blood, which may be due to an increased arterial flow (active h.) or to diminished venous flow (passive h.). It may occur as a result of such factors as bacterial invasion of the pulp through carious dentin; exposure of the dentin to saliva over long periods of time; thermal shock, especially when inadequately cooled high-speed burs or polishing devices are used; prolonged contact of the dentin with burs during cavity preparation; thermal conduction of hot or cold food through extensive restorations; excessive dehydration of dentin with alcohol, chloroform, or air blasts; trauma as in disturbed occlusal relationship, traumatic injuries, galvanic shock due to the use of dissimilar metals in restorations; contact with a freshly placed amalgam filling or occlusion with a gold restoration; and irritation of exposed dentin, e.g., by acids or drugs, such as arsenic trioxide or silver nitrate. The condition is ordinarily painless but exposure to sweet and sour foods may cause sharp pain, especially if it is due to cervical caries or abrasion. Called also *pulp h.* **passive h., venous h.,** hyperemia due to obstructed outflow of blood from a part. **pulp h.,** dental pulp h.

hyperesthesia (hi″per-es-the′ze-ah) [hyper- + Gr. *aisthēsis* sensation + -ia] abnormally increased sensitiveness of the skin or of an organ of special sense. See also HYPERALGESIA and PAIN (1). Cf. ANALGESIA and ANESTHESIA. **acoustic h., auditory h.,** hyperacusis. **cerebral h.,** that which is due to a cerebral lesion. **gustatory h.,** hypergeusesthesia. **oneiric h.,** increase of sensitiveness or of pain during sleep and dreams. **unilateral h.,** hemihyperesthesia.

hypereuryprosopic (hi″per-u″re-pro-sop′ik) pertaining to or characterized by a very low and wide face. See hypereuryprosopic SKULL.

hyperextension (hi″per-ek-sten′shun) [hyper- + *extension*] the act or process of extension, whereby the parts go through an arc extending their angle, but go beyond the straight line.

hyperfunction (hi"per-funk'shun) excessive activity of an organ or system; superfunction.

hypergeusesthesia (hi"per-gūs"es-the'ze-ah) [hyper- + Gr. *geusis* taste + *aisthēsis* perception + -*ia*] excessive or abnormal acuteness of the sense of taste. Called also *gustatory hyperesthesia.*

hyperglobulinemia (hi"per-glob"u-lin-e'me-ah) [hyper- + *globulin* + Gr. *haima* blood + -*ia*] excessively high globulin content of the blood. **idiopathic h.,** Waldenström's SYNDROME.

hyperglycemia (hi"per-gli-se'me-ah) [hyper- + Gr. *glykys* sweet + *haima* blood + -*ia*] abnormally increased content of sugar in the blood; the concentration of a glucose level above 90 mg/100 ml of blood. Hyperglycemia is considered as one of the principal symptoms of diabetes mellitus and other disorders of the islands of Langerhans. See also renal threshold for glucose, under THRESHOLD.

hyperglyceridemia (hi"per-glis"er-ĭ-de'me-ah) [hyper- + *glyceride* + Gr. *haima* blood + -*ia*] a condition characterized by the presence of excessive amounts of blood glycerides, usually triglycerides.

Hyperhidrit trademark for *urea peroxide* (see under UREA).

hyperhidrosis (hi"per-hi-dro'sis) [hyper- + Gr. *hidrōsis* sweating] excessive perspiration. **gustatory h.,** excessive sweating associated with eating, usually occurring in the preauricular region of the face and forehead.

hyperinsulinism (hi"per-in'su-lin-izm) excessive secretion of insulin by the islands of Langerhans, resulting in hypoglycemia. See also hypoglycemic SHOCK.

hyperkalemia (hi"per-kah-le'me-ah) [hyper- + L. *kalium* potassium + Gr. *haima* blood + -*ia*] abnormally high potassium concentration in the blood, usually associated with cardiac and neuromuscular complications. Electrocardiographic changes (elevated T waves and depressed P waves, and intraventricular block), flaccid paralysis, and cardiac standstill are the most common complications of severe intoxication. It is most often due to faulty renal potassium excretion, deficiency of adrenal steroids, the use of aldosterone antagonists, or the administration of other agents inhibiting sodium-potassium exchange by the renal tubules. It may also be produced by excessive rapid intravenous administration of potassium. Oral potassium rarely produces excessive blood concentrations unless renal function is impaired. Called also *hyperpotassemia* and *kalemia.*

hyperkeratosis (hi"per-ker"ah-to'sis) [hyper- + Gr. *keras* horn + -*osis*] 1. hypertrophy or thickening of the stratum corneum of the skin, or any disease characterized by thickened stratum corneum. 2. hypertrophy of the cornea. **h. complex,** oral LEUKOPLAKIA. **h. excen'trica,** Mibelli's DISEASE. **focal palmoplantar and marginal gingival h.,** a syndrome, transmitted as an autosomal dominant trait, characterized by focal hyperkeratosis of the palms and soles, being particularly prominent over the weight bearing areas, heels, toe pads, and metatarsal heads; hyperhidrosis of the hyperkeratotic areas; and marginal hyperkeratosis involving the labial and lingual portions of the attached gingiva. Lesions of the palms and soles appear around the time of puberty in most patients; those of the gingiva appear during early childhood and increase in severity with age. **h. lin'guae,** black TONGUE. **oral h.,** hypertrophy of the stratum corneae of the oral epithelium. See oral LEUKOPLAKIA. **h. palma'ris et planta'ris,** a hereditary, congenital skin disease characterized by thickening of the stratum corneum of the skin of the palms and soles, usually associated with other hereditary conditions. Called also *keratosis palmaris et plantaris.* **h. sim'plex,** oral LEUKOPLAKIA.

hyperkinesia (hi"per-ki-ne'ze-ah) [hyper- + Gr. *kinēsis* motion + -*ia*] abnormally increased motor function or activity; excessive movement; hyperactivity.

hyperleptoprosopic (hi"per-lep"to-pro-so'pik) [hyper- + *lepto-* + Gr. *prosōpon* face] pertaining to or characterized by a very high and narrow face. See hyperleptoprosopic SKULL.

hyperlipemia (hi"per-li-pe'me-ah) [hyper- + Gr. *lipos* fat + *haima* blood + -*ia*] a condition characterized by the presence in the blood of excessive amounts of lipids. See also LIPEMIA. **carbohydrate-induced h., essential h.,** hyperlipoproteinemia III. **essential h.,** hyperlipoproteinemia III. **familial fat-induced h., idiopathic h.,** hyperlipoproteinemia I. **mixed h.,** hyperlipoproteinemia V. **postalimentary h.,** elevated lipid level in the blood following a meal, characterized by the turbidity of plasma, due to the presence of chylomicrons. **retention h.,** hyperlipoproteinemia I.

hyperlipoproteinemia (hi"per-lip"o-pro"te-in-e'me-ah) an excess of lipoproteins in the blood, due to a disorder of lipoprotein metabolism, and occurring as an acquired or familial condition. **h. I.,** a familial form, probably transmitted as a recessive trait, believed to be caused by faulty removal of chylomicrons and other triglyceride-rich lipoproteins from the blood due to lipopro-

tein lipase deficiency, and characterized by persistent hyperchylomicronemia that usually disappears after a few days of a fat-free-diet. Both α- and β-lipoproteins are low in the blood. It usually becomes apparent during infancy and childhood and is manifested by persistent blood turbidity, xanthomas, hepatosplenomegaly, abdominal pain, lipemia retinalis, and the presence of foam cells in the bone marrow, spleen, and liver. Oral manifestations may include xanthomas of the mucous membrane. Called also *Bürger-Grütz syndrome, familial fat-induced hyperlipemia, familial hyperchylomicronemia, idiopathic hyperlipemia,* and *retention hyperlipemia.* **h. II,** a hereditary form, transmitted as a dominant trait, characterized by the presence in the blood of high concentrations of β-lipoproteins and by hypercholesterolemia in association with normal levels of blood triglycerides. Complications include lipid deposits in the skin, tendons, eyes, and vascular endothelium; xanthomatosis; arteriosclerosis, especially of the coronary vessels, leading to myocardial infarction and cardiac failure; and hyperuricemia. Called also *essential familial hypercholesterolemia, familial hyperbetalipoproteinemia, familial hypercholesterolemia, familial hypercholesterolemic xanthomatosis, familial xanthoma* and *xanthoma tuberosum multiplex.* **h. III,** a hereditary form of hyperlipoproteinemia, transmitted as a dominant trait, characterized by increased amounts of β- and pre-β-lipoproteins in the blood and carbohydrate-induced hyperglyceridemia in patients on normal diets. Xanthomatosis and arteriosclerosis leading to myocardial infarction are often associated. Called also *carbohydrate-induced hyperlipemia* and *essential hyperlipemia.* **h. IV,** a hereditary form, transmitted as a dominant trait, characterized by increased amounts of pre-β-lipoproteins in the blood and slight hyperglyceridemia in patients on normal diets. **h. V,** a hereditary form of hyperlipoproteinemia characterized by hyperchylomicronemia associated with hyperprebetalipoproteinemia in the presence of normal or low α- and β-lipoproteins in the blood, observed in patients on normal diets. The condition is believed to be induced by both fats and carbohydrates. Symptoms are similar to those in hyperlipoproteinemia I; they include persistent blood turbidity, xanthomas, hepatomegaly, splenomegaly, abdominal pain, and lipemia retinalis. Oral manifestations include xanthomas of the oral mucosa, especially of the palate. Called also *mixed hyperlipemia.*

hypermagnesemia (hi"per-mag"ne-se'me-ah) [hyper- + *magnesium* + Gr. *haima* blood + -*ia*] an abnormally large magnesium content in the blood plasma, usually in excess of 4 mEq per liter. See MAGNESIUM.

hypermetria (hi"per-me'tre-ah) [hyper- + Gr. *metron* measure] see DYSMETRIA.

hypermineralization (hi"per-min"er-al-i-za'shun) the presence of excessive mineral elements in the tissues or body.

hypermobility (hi"per-mo-bil'ĭ-te) [hyper- + *mobility*] excessive mobility of an organ, usually a joint. **temporomandibular joint h.,** excessive mobility of the temporomandibular joint, usually caused by partial dislocation of the head of the condyle from the glenoid fossa of the temporal bone.

hypermorph (hi'per-morf) [hyper- + Gr. *morphē* form] 1. a person who is tall but of low sitting height, with bony and narrow arms and legs, slender body, narrow nose, lips, shoulders, and thorax. 2. an allele that is excessively productive.

hypermotility (hi"per-mo-til'ĭ-te) excessive or abnormally increased motility.

hypermyotonia (hi"per-mi"o-to'ne-ah) [hyper- + Gr. *mys* muscle + *tonos* tension + -*ia*] excessive muscle tonus.

hypermyotrophy (hi"per-mi-ot'ro-fe) [hyper- + Gr. *mys* muscle + *trophē* nourishment] excessive development of the muscular tissue.

hypernatremia (hi"per-nah-tre'me-ah) [hyper- + L. *natrium* sodium + Gr. *haima* blood + -*ia*] an excessive amount of sodium in the blood.

hypernitremia (hi"per-ni-tre'me-ah) [hyper- + *nitrogen* + Gr. *haima* blood + -*ia*] excessive nitrogen in the blood.

hypernormal (hi"per-nor'mal) [hyper- + *normal*] in excess of what is normal.

Hyperol trademark for *urea peroxide* (see under UREA).

hyperostosis (hi"per-os-to'sis) [hyper- + Gr. *osteon* bone + -*osis*] hypertrophy of bone. **h. cortic'alis defor'mans juveni'lis,** an autosomal recessive disorder characterized by multiple fractures beginning early in life, with bowing of all extremities. Roentgen examination reveals thickening of frontal, parietal, and occipital bones with deepened diploic spaces; osteoporosis; and signs of healing and healed fractures with bowing and angulation of long bones and widening of the medullary cavities of unfractured bones. Serum alkaline phosphatase is elevated, but it drops to normal levels when healing takes place. Called also *Bakwin-Eiger syndrome, chronic idiopathic hyperphosphatasia, congenital chronic idiopathic hyperphosphatasemia, juvenile Paget's disease,* and *osteoclasia desmalis familiaris.* **h. cortica'lis generalisa'ta,** an autosomal recessive disorder characterized by thickening and osteosclerosis of the base of the skull, calvaria, mandible, clavicles, and ribs, and hyperplasia of the diaphyseal cortex, often associated with elevated blood alkaline phosphatase. The onset is at puberty. Stenosis of the cranial foramina may produce facial paralysis, and the thickening of the base of the skull may cause optic atrophy and hearing disorders. Called also *chronic hyperphosphatasemia* and *van Buchem's syndrome.* **infantile cortical h.,** cortical hyperostoses, transmitted as an autosomal dominant trait, affecting infants under six months of age. It involves several bones at the same time, usually the mandible and, less frequently, the clavicle, tibia, ulna, femur, ribs, humerus, and fibula, and is usually associated with bilateral swelling of the affected tissue, hyperirritability, fever, and roentgenographic signs of neo-osteogenesis. Unilateral or bilateral thickening and sclerosis of the cortex of various bones are usually present on the roentgenogram. Puffy jaws and cheeks give the face a characteristic appearance. Dysphagia, pleurisy, leukocytosis, high sedimentation rate, and excess of blood alkaline phosphatase are the common symptoms. The ocular signs may include edema around the orbits, proptosis, and conjunctivitis. Asymmetric deformity of the mandible, usually in the angle and ramus area, associated with severe malocclusion are sometimes present. Called also *Caffey's syndrome, Caffey-Silverman syndrome,* and *Caffey-Smyth disease.*

hyperparathyroidism (hi"per-par″ah-thi'roid-izm) a rare disease occurring most commonly in adult women, in which hyperactivity of the parathyroid glands produces excessive amounts of parathyroid hormone resulting in hypercalcemia and hypercalciuria. Weakness, constipation, vomiting, nausea, anorexia, muscular hypotonicity, and conjunctival calcification are the most common symptoms. Pancreatitis, nephrocalcinosis, and osteitis fibrosa cystica generalisata are frequently associated. Giant cell tumors or pseudocysts of the jaws, osteoporotic changes in the cranium and jaws due to calcium and phosphorus disturbances, bone resorption, drifting of the teeth leading to malocclusion, and spacing of the teeth may be the early symptoms. The characteristic radiologic signs are general radiolucency of the bones, especially of the mandible, and a "ground-glass" appearance of the bone, with a partial loss of the lamina dura around the teeth. Small cystic areas in the calvarium and sharply defined radiolucencies in the maxilla or mandible suggesting eosinophilic granuloma or multiple myeloma are common. The most common histologic feature is an osteoclastic resorption of the trabeculae of the spongiosa and along the blood vessels of the cortex. See also Recklinghausen's DISEASE (2). **primary h.,** hyperparathyroidism usually caused by adenoma of the parathyroid glands and, less commonly, primary hyperplasia or carcinoma. **secondary h.,** hyperparathyroidism in which excessive production of parathyroid hormone is caused by chronic renal insufficiency or calcium-wasting diseases, such as metastatic carcinoma, multiple myeloma, rickets, and osteomalacia.

hyperphonia (hi"per-fo'ne-ah) [*hyper-* + Gr. *phōnē* voice + *-ia*] excessively energetic phonation, as in stuttering. Called also *superenergetic phonation.*

hyperphosphatasemia (hi"per-fos″fah-tas-e'me-ah) the presence in the blood of an excessive amount of phosphatase. **chronic h.,** HYPEROSTOSIS corticalis generalisata. **congenital chronic idiopathic h.,** HYPEROSTOSIS corticalis deformans juvenilis.

hyperphosphatasia (hi"per-fos″fah-ta'ze-ah) abnormally increased phosphatase level in the body. **chronic idiopathic h.,** HYPEROSTOSIS corticalis deformans juvenilis.

hyperphosphatemia (hi"per-fos″fah-te'me-ah) an excessive amount of phosphates in the blood, usually observed in osteolytic bone lesions, some bone neoplasms, diabetic acidosis, nephritis, osteoporosis, hypervitaminosis D, menopause and gonadal insufficiency, acromegaly, and preadolescent growth.

hyperpituitarism (hi"per-pī-tu'ī-tah-rism) any condition due to hypersecretion of any of the hormones of the pituitary gland, especially a condition associated with excessive production of growth hormone by an acidophil adenoma. See also ACROMEGALY, GIGANTISM, and Cushing's SYNDROME (1).

hyperplasia (hi"per-pla'ze-ah) [*hyper-* + Gr. *plasis* formation] the abnormal multiplication or increase in the number of cells in normal arrangement in a tissue, brought about by increased mitotic activity. It is considered to be a self-limiting process and is not etiologically related to neoplasia. Hyperplastic tissue sometimes regresses after removal of the source of irritation but in some cases of focal or diffuse proliferation of oral tissue, there is no regression after removal of the irritant. Cf. HYPERTROPHY and NEOPLASIA. **cementum h.,** hypercementosis. **chronic perforating pulp h.,** tooth resorption, internal; see under RESORPTION. **condylar h.,** usually unilateral enlargement of the condyle, probably caused by inflammatory processes, resulting in slowly progressive elongation of the face with deviation of the chin away from the affected side. Malocclusion is usually present, and pain may be associated. **Dilantin h.,** Dilantin GINGIVITIS. **h. fascia'lis progressi'va,** progressive myositis ossificans; see under MYOSITIS. **fibrous h. of gingiva,** FIBROMATOSIS gingivae. **fibrous inflammatory h.,** development of masses of collagenized, fibrous, connective tissue along the borders of ill-fitting dentures, usually in the mucolabial or mucobuccal fold areas in which the denture flange fits, and also in other areas where chronic irritation exists, such as in the gingival and buccal areas and angle of the mouth. A lesion may present a pedunculated sessile, hyperkeratinized, ulcerated, hard or soft mass, sometimes associated with secondary inflammation, typically made up of stratified squamous epithelium, usually of normal thickness or slightly acanthotic. The connective tissue is composed of coarse bundles of collagen fibers, sometimes separated by fibroblastic nuclei; small vascular channels; inflammatory cells; and occasionally areas of dystrophic calcification, metaplastic ossification, or myxomatous degeneration. Hyperkeratosis and parakeratosis are seldom present; vascularity is sparse. Called also *denture injury tumor, epulis fissuratum,* and *redundant tissue.* **focal epithelial h.,** 1. Hyperplasia of the mucous membrane of the lips, tongue, and, less commonly, the buccal mucosa, floor of the mouth, and palate, presenting soft, painless, round to oval, sessile papules about 1 to 4 mm in diameter, which sometimes become confluent. The surface of the papules is usually soft, but it may become rough, having the same color as the surrounding mucosa. Histologically, lesions show acanthosis, papillomatosis, and parakeratosis, with inflated surface cells and mitotic figures. The condition usually occurs in children and young adults and has familial predilection, lasting for several months, sometimes years, before running its course. A viral etiology is suspected but virological tests are usually negative. 2. Heck's DISEASE. **giant follicular h.,** giant follicle LYMPHOMA. **gingival h.,** noninflammatory enlargement of the gingivae produced by factors other than local irritation. It is not common, and is most often associated with phenytoin (Dilantin) therapy. See also gingival ENLARGEMENT. **inflammatory fibrous h.,** the enlargement and overgrowth of tissues found in the mucobuccal and/or labial fold, produced by dentures that no longer exhibit an anatomical relationship to the alveolar ridges. **inflammatory papillary h.,** papillary h. **papillary h.,** inflammatory hyperplasia of the mucosa of the hard palate usually observed in edentulous patients with ill-fitting dentures and, rarely, in patients with a full complement of teeth. A typical lesion is composed of numerous papillary projections of less than 1 mm in diameter that tend to coalesce and form a plaquelike area, and is usually restricted to the vault of the hard palate, but it may spread to the lingual slope or the alveolar ridge or, less frequently, over the crest of the ridge of the buccal aspect. Histologically, the tissue shows numerous small vertical projections made up of stratified squamous ep'thelium and a central core of connective tissue. It is not considered to be neoplastic but sometimes it may be found to contain foci of pseudoepitheliomatous hyperplasia. Usually, the hyperplasia tends to regress after removal of the denture. Called also *inflammatory papillary h., multiple papillomas of the palate,* and *papillomatosis.* **primary pseudoepitheliomatous h.,** a nonmalignant hyperplastic lesion that closely resembles well-differentiated epidermoid carcinoma, occurring most often on the skin and sometimes on the oral mucosa, especially the lips. It typically begins as a small papule that rapidly develops into a firm, hemispherical nodule about 1–2 cm in diameter, with a depressed central core consisting of a proliferating epithelial peg covered by a layer of keratin, from the bottom of which islands of epithelium spread out. Most lesions undergo spontaneous regression. Called also *keratoacanthoma, tumor-like molluscum sebaceum, multiple primary selfhealing squamous epithelioma,* and *tumor-like keratosis.* **pseudocarcinomatous h.,** pseudoepitheliomatous h. **pseudoepitheliomatous h.,** nonmalignant epithelial hyperplasia closely resembling squamous cell carcinoma, usually occurring in a variety of lesions, particularly in granulomatous processes, such as granuloma inguinale, blastomycosis, at the edges of chronic ulcers, and overlying granular cell myoblastoma. Called also *pseudocarcinomatous h.* **pulp h.,** hyperplastic PULPITIS. **unilateral h.,** hemihyperplasia.

hyperploid (hi'per-ploid) [*hyper-* + *-ploid*] 1. having one or more added chromosomes or chromosome segments in the complement, as in Down's syndrome. 2. an individual or cell having one or more chromosomes or chromosome segments in the complement.

hyperploidy (hi"per-ploi'de) [*hyper-* + *ploidy*] the state or condition of being hyperploid.

hyperpnea (hi"per-ne'ah) [*hyper-* + Gr. *pnoia* breath] an increase in the depth and rate of the respiration, often with a rate of pulmonary ventilation great enough to cause over-respiration; polypnea. Cf. HYPOPNEA.

hyperpotassemia (hi"per-pot"ah-se'me-ah) hyperkalemia.

hyperprognathous (hi"per-prog'nah-thus, hi"per-prog-na'thus) [*hyper-* + Gr. *pro* before + *gnathos* jaw] pertaining to or characterized by severe protrusion of the jaw, or prognathism. See hyperprognathous SKULL.

hyperptyalism (hi"per-ti"al-izm) [*hyper-* + Gr. *ptyalon* spittle] excessive flow of saliva. Called also *hypersalivation, ptyalism, ptyalorrhea,* and *sialorrhea.*

hypersalivation (hi"per-sal"i-va'shun) excessive flow of saliva. Called also *hyperptyalism, ptyalism, ptyalorrhea,* and *sialorrhea.*

hypersensitivity (hi"per-sen'si-tiv"i-te) a state of altered reactivity in which the body reacts with an exaggerated response to a foreign agent. Hypersensitivity reactions are pathologic processes induced by immune responses and may be classified as immediate or delayed (although the time required for the two reactions may be similar). The immediate form includes *type I,* typified by atopic hypersensitivity and anaphylaxis due to antigen reacting with antibody or mediator cells such as basophils; *type II,* in which injury is produced by antibody against antigens on tissues (e.g., nephrotoxic nephritis); and *type III,* in which injury is produced by antigen-antibody complexes (e.g., Arthus reaction) and complexes formed by slight antigen excess (e.g., serum sickness). The delayed form includes *type IV,* in which the hypersensitivity reactions are lymphocyte-mediated (e.g., contact dermatitis). See also ALLERGY. **contact h.,** a type IV hypersensitivity reaction of the skin produced by contact with a chemical substance having the properties of an antigen or hapten, which occurs as a result of the interaction of sensitized lymphocytes with the contactant, either directly or after complexing with tissue components. It includes contact dermatitis. **delayed h.,** a type IV hypersensitivity reaction mediated by T-lymphocytes to a specific antigen. Skin test reactions of this type have a slow onset and reach maximum intensity in about 24 hours. It is involved in the graft rejection, autoimmune disease, and contact dermatitis, as well as in antimicrobial immunity. **drug h.,** drug REACTION. **immediate h.,** hypersensitivity reactions, including types I, II, and III, which are mediated by antibody. The most rapid hypersensitivity reaction is type I and is termed *anaphylaxis.* It is characterized by a rapid response after the challenge and it can be either systemic (generalized) or localized (cutaneous), associated with immune mechanisms which may be operative, but most have a mediation pathway involving the release of active substances from mediator cells. The primary effect of these mediators is interaction with target cells, producing a functional alteration, e.g., contraction of smooth muscle, increase of vascular permeability, or increased secretion. Types II and III reactions may occur over a protracted period. **pulp h.,** hypersensitive PULPALGIA. **tooth h.,** see hypersensitive PULPALGIA and hypersensitive TOOTH.

hypersplenism (hi"per-splen'izm) any hematological disorder resulting from the destruction of blood cells by apparently increased splenic activity.

Hyperstat trademark for *diazoxide.*

hypersusceptibility (hi"per-su-sep"ti-bil'i-te) a condition of abnormally increased susceptibility to foreign agents, such as poisons, infective agents, or agents which in the normal individual are entirely innocuous; specifically, an extreme reactivity of the body to the second injection of an anaphylactogenic substance. See ANAPHYLAXIS.

hypertaurodontism (hi"per-taw"ro-don'tizm) [*hyper-* + *taurodontism*] form of taurodontism in which the roots of a tooth do not branch at all.

hypertelorism (hi-per-te'lo-rizm) [*hyper-* + Gr. *telouros* distant] abnormally increased distance between two organs, or parts, such as the eyes.

hypertension (hi"per-ten'shun) [*hyper-* + *tension*] abnormally

high tension, especially of the blood against the arterial walls; various criteria for its threshold are used, a common one being that in which the resting systolic pressure is greater than 160 mm Hg and the diastolic pressure is over 90 mm Hg. **ocular h.,** excessively high pressure of the aqueous humor of the eye. **portal h.,** increase in blood pressure within the portal vein above the normal pressure of 5 to 10 mm Hg; it is due to obstruction of the portal vein, and is a frequent complication of liver cirrhosis.

hyperthermia (hi"per-ther'me-ah) [*hyper-* + Gr. *therme* heat + *-ia*] fever; abnormally high body temperature. See FEVER. **malignant h.,** a rapid rise of body temperature associated with muscular rigidity, respiratory and metabolic acidosis, transient hyperkalemia, myoglobinuria, and increased blood enzymes, especially creatine phosphokinase, which may result in death. It may be precipitated by inhalation anesthesia and muscle relaxants, and occurs usually during the first anesthetic experience, but it has been also reported in patients with previously uncomplicated anesthesia.

hyperthyroidism (hi"per-thi'roid-izm) a condition resulting from excessive production of thyroid hormones, usually associated with diffuse hyperplasia and hypertrophy of the thyroid gland or toxic adenoma. Symptoms include increased metabolic rate, rapid heart rate, hyperactivity, emotional instability, flushing, peculiar facies, and intolerance to heat. Exophthalmic goiter is frequently associated. Hyperthyroid mothers tend to give birth to children with congenital hyperthyroidism. Oral manifestations may include alveolar atrophy in advanced cases, and, in children, shedding of the deciduous teeth earlier than normal and accelerated eruption of the permanent teeth. See also GOITER and Plummer's DISEASE.

Hypertonalum trademark for *diazoxide.*

hypertonia (hi"per-to'ne-ah) [*hyper-* + Gr. *tonus* tone] a condition of increased tone of the skeletal muscles.

hypertonic (hi"per-ton'ik) [*hyper-* + Gr. *tonos* tone] 1. pertaining to hypertonia. 2. pertaining to a hypertonic solution; sometimes used alone to denote such a solution.

hypertonicity (hi"per-to-nis'i-te) 1. the state or quality of being hypertonic; usually applied to a solution. 2. having a greater total concentration of ions in the blood plasma.

hypertrichosis (hi"per-trik-o'sis) [*hyper-* + Gr. *thrix* hair + *-osis*] a condition characterized by excessive growth of hair.

hypertrophic (hi"per-trof'ik) pertaining to or marked by hypertrophy.

hypertrophy (hi-per'tro-fe) [*hyper-* + Gr. *trophe* nutrition] the abnormal enlargement or overgrowth of an organ or a part brought about by enlargement of the existing cells. Cf. HYPERPLASIA and NEOPLASIA. **cementum h.,** hypercementosis. **functional h.,** hypertrophy of an organ or part due to its increased activity. See also *physiologic h.* **hemangiectatic h.,** Klippel-Trenaunay-Weber SYNDROME. **hemifacial h.,** abnormal unilateral hypertrophy of facial and oral structures. It is usually congenital and may occur alone but is most frequently found in combination with unilateral hypertrophy of other structures and co-occurring with various congenital defects. Enlargement of one side of the palate, maxilla, mandible, lips, uvula, and tongue are the principal manifestations. Enlargement of the permanent teeth on the affected side, except for the third molars, with ipsilateral premature eruption and sheeding of teeth may also occur. Called also *unilateral facial h., facial hemihypertrophy,* and *Friedreich's disease.* **physiologic h.,** temporary increase in the size of an organ or part due to its physiologic activity. See also *functional h.* **simple familial cranial h.,** Klippel-Feldstein SYNDROME. **unilateral h.,** hemihypertrophy. **unilateral facial h.,** hemifacial h.

hypertropia (hi"per-tro'pe-ah) [*hyper-* + Gr. *tropein* to turn] upward deviation of the visual axis of the eye when fusion is a possibility.

hyperuricacidemia (hi"per-u"rik-as"i-de'me-ah) hyperuricemia.

hyperuricemia (hi"per-u"ri-se'me-ah) excess of uric acid in the blood, as in gout and Lesch-Nyhan syndrome. Called also *hyperuricacidemia.*

hyperventilation (hi"per-ven"ti-la'shun) an increase in alveolar ventilation in excess of that required to maintain normal arterial blood oxygen and carbon dioxide pressures, resulting in the lowering of arterial carbon dioxide tension (hypocapnia) with a rise of arterial hydrogen ion concentration (respiratory alkalosis), with little change in the arterial oxygen pressure. It is a common emergency in the dental office, often being a manifestation of acute anxiety.

hypervitaminosis (hi″per-vi′tah-mĭ-no′sis) vitamin intoxication; a condition due to the intake of excessive amounts of vitamins. For specific vitamin intoxications, see the vitamin involved.

hypervolemia (hi″per-vo-le′me-ah) [hyper- + volume + Gr. haima blood + -ia] abnormal increase in the volume of the circulating blood plasma.

hypnalgia (hip-nal′je-ah) [hypno- + Gr. algos pain + -ia] pain occuring during sleep.

hypno- [Gr. hypnos sleep] a combining form denoting relationship to sleep.

hypnoanesthesia (hip″no-an″es-the′ze-ah) induction of the anesthetic state by hypnosis.

hypnosis (hip-no′sis) an artificially induced passive state in which there is increased amenability and responsiveness to the suggestions and commands of the hypnotist. In hypnosis, a drowsy phase is followed by a light or deep sleep, depending on the cooperation of the subject. Although this sleep seems normal, a part of the subject's mind remains aware of the outside world and of the hypnotist's wishes. In certain cases, when the use of anesthetics is not advisable, hypnosis has been used during dental treatment, setting of fractures, and other surgical procedures, usually in addition to analgesics. Called also *hypnotism*.

hypnotic (hip-not′ik) [Gr. hypnotikos] 1. inducing sleep. 2. pertaining to or of the nature of hypnotism. 3. any drug that depresses the activity of the central nervous system, reducing cortical excitability and producing sleep. In small doses, some hypnotics may produce relaxation without inducing sleep, thus acting as sedatives. Because of their common quality of allaying anxiety, hypnotics and sedatives are often jointly referred to as antianxiety drugs (formerly called minor tranquilizers). They are used to induce sleep in insomnia, as an adjunct in psychiatric therapy, and in preanesthetic medication. In dentistry, they may be used the night before a contemplated surgical operation to promote sleep. Some ultrashort-acting hypnotics are also used in general anesthesia.

hypnotism (hip′no-tizm) 1. the method or practice of inducing hypnosis. 2. hypnosis.

hypnotist (hip′no-tist) one who induces hypnosis.

hypo (hi′po) 1. a popular designation for a hypodermic inoculation or syringe. 2. a contraction of sodium thiosulfate, used as a photographic fixing agent.

hypo- [Gr. hypo under] a prefix signifying beneath, under, or deficient. In chemistry, it denotes that the principal element in the compound is combined in its lowest state of valence. See also words beginning SUB-.

hypoacusis (hi″po-ah-ku′sis) [hypo- + Gr. akousis hearing] a slightly diminished auditory sensitivity, with hearing threshold levels above the normal limit so that the impairment is measureable in decibels. See also DEAFNESS. Cf. DYSACUSIS (1).

hypoadrenalism (hi″po-ah-dre′nal-izm) abnormally diminished activity of the adrenal cortex. Called also *adrenal insufficiency*.

hypoalgesia (hi″po-al-je′ze-ah) hypalgesia.

hypobaric (hi″po-bar′ik) [hypo- + Gr. baros weight] characterized by less than normal pressure or weight; applied to gases under less than atmospheric pressure or to a solution of lower specific gravity than another taken as a standard of reference. See also hypobaric SOLUTION.

hypobarism (hi″po-bar′izm) the condition resulting from exposure to ambient gas pressure or atmospheric pressures that are below those within body tissues, fluids, cavities.

Hypo-Cal trademark for a cavity liner (see under LINER), consisting of an aqueous suspension of calcium hydroxide.

Hypo-Cal powder see under POWDER.

hypocalcemia (hi″po-kal-se′me-ah) calcium deficiency in the blood caused by inadequate gastrointestinal calcium absorption, inadequate bone resorption, excessive formation of bone, or excessive calcium excretion by the kidneys. It is relatively uncommon in man but may be observed in association with hypoparathyroidism, pseudohypoparathyroidism, osteomalacia, and rickets. Experimental calcium deficiency usually produces tetany, blood coagulation disorders, generalized paralysis, capillary disorders, internal hemorrhage, gastric ulcers, and cataracts. **constitutional chronic h.,** pseudohypoparathyroidism.

hypocalcification (hi″po-kal″sĭ-fĭ-ka′shun) [hypo- + calcification] insufficient calcification. **enamel h.,** a form of amelogenesis imperfecta believed to be transmitted as an autosomal dominant or recessive trait, due to faulty mineralization of enamel.

It is characterized by a normal appearance of the tooth crown at eruption, which shortly thereafter assumes a white chalky (white enamel, opaque enamel) appearance and gradually undergoes brown discoloration. The affected teeth are soft and rough. Called also *enamel hypomaturation* and *enamel hypomineralization*. **enamel and dentin h.,** faulty development of the dental enamel and dentin, which is different from amelogenesis imperfecta and dentinogenesis imperfecta, resulting from failure of crystallization processes, characterized by softness of the tooth substance.

hypocalcipexy (hi″po-kal″sĭ-pek″se) deficient calcium fixation.

hypocalciuria (hi″po-kal″se-u′re-ah) an abnormally diminished amount of calcium in the urine, usually caused by a decrease in the volume of calcium filtered by the renal glomeruli or an increase in the volume of calcium reabsorbed by the renal tubules. It may be caused by insufficient dietary calcium intake, excessive phosphate intake, pregnancy, lactation, rickets, osteomalacia, vitamin D deficiency, acromegaly, steatorrhea, hyperparathyroidism, or hypothyroidism.

hypocapnia (hi″po-kap′ne-ah) [hypo- + Gr. kapnos smoke + -ia] abnormally low content of carbon dioxide in the blood, usually produced by pulmonary hyperventilation. Cf. ACAPNIA and HYPERCAPNIA.

hypochloremia (hi″po-klo-re′me-ah) an abnormally diminished level of chloride in the blood.

hypochlorite (hi″po-klo′rīt) a compound containing the radical ClO. See also CALCIUM hypochlorite and SODIUM hypochlorite.

hypochondria (hi″po-kon′dre-ah) 1. plural of hypochondrium. 2. hypochondriasis.

hypochondriac (hi″po-kon′dre-ak) 1. pertaining to the hypochondrium or to hypochondriasis. 2. a person affected with hypochondriasis.

hypochondriasis (hi″po-kon-dri′ah-sis) [so called because the hypochondrium, and especially the spleen, was supposed to be the seat of this disorder] morbid anxiety about one's health.

hypochondrium (hi′po-kon′dre-um), pl. hypochon′dria [hypo- + Gr. chondros cartilage] the upper lateral region of the abdomen, about the costal cartilages, on either side of the epigastric region.

hypochromatism (hi″po-kro′mah-tizm) [hypo- + chromatin] abnormally deficient pigmentation; especially deficiency of the chromatin in a cell nucleus. Called also *hypochromia*.

hypochromia (hi″po-kro′me-ah) [hypo- + Gr. chrōma color + -ia] 1. abnormal decrease in the hemoglobin content of the erythrocytes. 2. hypochromatism.

hypochromic (hi″po-kro′mik) pertaining to or marked by hypochromia or hypochromatism.

hypocomplementemic (hi″po-kom″plĕ-men-te′mik) denoting or involving lowered levels of complement in the blood.

hypocondylar (hi″po-kon′dĭ-lar) below a condyle.

hypocone (hi′po-kōn) [hypo- + Gr. kōnos cone] the distolingual cusp of a maxillary molar tooth. See also METACONE, PARACONE, and PROTOCONE.

hypoconid (hi″po-ko′nid) [hypo- + Gr. kōnos cone + -id] the distobuccal cusp of a mandibular molar tooth. See also METACONID, PARACONID, and PROTOCONID.

hypoconulid (hi″po-kon′u-lid) the fifth, or distal, cusp of a mandibular molar tooth; usually found on the mandibular first molar. See also HYPOCONID, METACONID, PARACONID, and PROTOCONID.

hypocrine (hi′po-krin) due to endocrine hypofunction.

hypocythemia (hi″po-si-the′me-ah) [hypo- + Gr. kytos cell + haima blood + -ia] a deficiency in the number of erythrocytes in the blood. **progressive h.,** aplastic ANEMIA.

hypoderm (hi′po-derm) [hypo- + Gr. derma skin] subcutaneous FASCIA.

hypodermic (hi″po-der′mik) [hypo- + Gr. derma skin] 1. applied or administered beneath the skin. 2. hypodermic injection.

hypodontia (hi″po-don′she-ah) [hypo- + Gr. odous tooth + -ia] partial absence of the teeth. A relatively common congenital condition characterized by absence of one or more teeth because of absence of their anlage, which is seldom associated with other anomalies. Called also *partial anodontia*. See also ANODONTIA and OLIGODONTIA.

hypoesthesia (hi″po-es-the′ze-ah) [hypo- + Gr. aisthēsis sensation + -ia] abnormally decreased sensitivity of the skin or of a special sense.

hypofibrinogenemia (hi″po-fi-brin′o-jĕ-ne′me-ah) abnormally low fibrinogen content of the blood. See also AFIBRINOGENEMIA.

hypogammaglobulinemia (hi″po-gam″ah-glob″u-lĭ-ne′me-ah) [hypo- + gamma globulin + Gr. haima blood + -ia] an immunological condition characterized by deficiency of immunoglobulins (gamma globulins). See also AGAMMAGLOBULINEMIA. **acquired h.,** that occurring after early childhood, characterized by deficiency of all immunoglobulins with resulting predisposition to infection, but without associated thymus abnormalities. It may occur in both sexes at any age but those in the 30–50 age group are the most susceptible. **congenital h.**, sex-linked recessive AGAMMAGLOBULINEMIA. **sex-linked recessive h.**, sex-linked recessive AGAMMAGLOBULINEMIA. **transient h.**, physiologic hypogammaglobulinemia occurring in normal infants at about three months of age and lasting to 18 months of age or more.

hypogeusesthesia (hi″po-gus′es-the′ze-ah) [*hypo-* + Gr. *geusis* taste + *aisthēsis* perception + *-ia*] abnormally diminished acuteness of the sense of taste. Called also *hypogeusia.*

hypogeusia (hi″po-gu′ze-ah) hypogeusesthesia.

hypoglobulinemia (hi″po-glob″u-li-ne′me-ah) [*hypo-* + *globulin* + Gr. *haima* blood + *-ia*] a deficiency of immunoglobulins (gamma globulins). See AGAMMAGLOBULINEMIA and HYPOGAMMAGLOBULINEMIA. **congenital h.**, a sex-linked deficiency of immunoglobulins. See sex-linked recessive AGAMMAGLOBULINEMIA. **physiologic h.**, a temporary form of hypogamma-globulinemia occurring in normal infants at about three months of age. When prolonged to 18 months of age or more, it is called *transient hypogammaglobulinemia.*

hypoglossal (hi″po-glos′al) [*hypo-* + Gr. *glōssa* tongue] situated or occurring underneath the tongue.

hypoglycemia (hi″po-gli-se′me-ah) [*hypo-* + Gr. *glykys* sweet + *haima* blood + *-ia*] a condition characterized by diminishing of glucose concentration in the blood to less than 50 mg per 100 ml. It is a symptom of a variety of diseases, including starvation, liver diseases, hypofunction of the adrenal cortex, poisoning, excessive production of insulin by the islands of Langerhans, or excessive administration of insulin or sulfonylureas. Clinical signs are varied: an inadequate supply of glucose to the nervous system may produce confusion, hallucinations, hyperactivity, convulsions, and coma; excessive production of epinephrine usually results in tachycardia, sweating, pallor, and hypertension; hunger is a common sign, and eating carbohydrate usually terminates hypoglycemic states. The condition may also occur as a result of excessive doses of insulin. See also hypoglycemic SHOCK.

hypoglycemic (hi″po-gli-se′mik) 1. pertaining to, characterized by, or producing hypoglycemia. 2. an agent that produces hypoglycemia.

hypohydration (hi″po-hi-dra′shun) dehydration.

hypokalemia (hi″po-ka-le′me-ah) [*hypo-* + L. *kalium* potassium + Gr. *haima* blood + *-ia*] abnormally low potassium level of the blood.

hypokinesia (hi″po-ki-ne′ze-ah) [*hypo-* + Gr. *kinesis* motion + *-ia*] abnormally decreased motor activity or function.

hypolarynx (hi″po-lar′inks) the infraglottic compartment of the larynx from the true vocal cords to the first tracheal ring.

hypolethal (hi″po-le′thal) not sufficient to cause death.

hypolipemia (hi″po-li-pe′me-ah) any condition characterized by abnormally decreased blood fats; hypolipidemia. **familial h.**, a familial syndrome combining clinical and biochemical abnormalities. The clinical features include growth retardation beginning during the second year of life, erythematosquamous skin lesions on the face and limbs, abnormalities of the hair, nails, and teeth, and occasionally tapetoretinal degeneration. The biochemical findings include decreased blood lipids, depressed blood ATP and phospholipids, increased tubular phosphate reabsorption, abnormal tryptophan metabolism with indoluria and aminoaciduria, and faulty glycolysis. Called also *h. S and Hooft's syndrome.* **h. S,** familial h.

hypolipidemia (hi″po-lip″ĭ-de′me-ah) a condition characterized by an abnormally decreased amount of blood fats; hypolipemia.

hypomagnesemia (hi″po-mag″ne-se′me-ah) [*hypo-* + *magnesium* + Gr. *haima* blood + *-ia*] an abnormally low magnesium content of the blood plasma. See MAGNESIUM.

hypomaturation (hi″po-mat″u-ra′shun) [*hypo-* + *maturation*] inability to reach full maturity; incomplete maturation.

hypometria (hi″po-me′tre-ah) [*hypo-* + Gr. *metron* measure] see DYSMETRIA.

hypomicron (hi″po-mi′kron) submicron.

hypomineralization (hi″po-min″er-al-i-za′shun) [*hypo-* + *mineralization*] insufficient mineralization. **enamel h.**, enamel HYPOCALCIFICATION.

hyponatremia (hi″po-nah-tre′me-ah) [*hypo-* + L. *natrium* sodium + Gr. *haima* blood + *-ia*] deficiency of sodium in the blood.

hyponychium (hi″po-nik′e-um) [*hypo-* + Gr. *onyx* nail] [NA] the thickened epidermis underneath the free distal end of the nail.

hypoparathyroidism (hi″po-par″ah-thi′roid-izm) a metabolic disease produced by defective action or removal of the parathyroid glands, characterized by high serum phosphate and low serum calcium, tetany, short stature, round face, numbness and tin-

gling in the fingers and toes, malformed nails sometimes infected with *Candida,* laryngeal stridor, dyspnea, cyanosis, tonic muscle contraction, dry and coarse skin, thin patchy head hair and scant axillary and pubic hair, and calcification in the basal ganglia. Principal oral manifestations include delayed dentition, tooth retention, enamel defects, dentinal dysplasia, incomplete root formation, and narrowing of the apical foramina. See also PSEUDOHYPOPARATHYROIDISM and DiGeorge's DISEASE. **idiopathic h.**, a rare form of obscure etiology, which may be congenital, sometimes with familial incidence, or may appear sporadically in children and adolescents. **postoperative h.**, a form produced by inadvertent removal or injury of the parathyroid gland, usually during thyroid surgery, characterized by a wide range of symptoms, from temporary tingling in the fingers and toes, following a minor injury, to frank tetany and other symptoms.

hypopharyngoscopy (hi″po-far″in-gos′ko-pe) [*hypopharynx* + Gr. *skopein* to view] instrumental examination of the hypopharynx.

hypopharynx (hi″po-far′inks) that division of the pharynx which lies below the upper edge of the epiglottis and opens into the larynx and esophagus.

hypophonia (hi″po-fo′ne-ah) [*hypo-* + Gr. *phōnē* voice + *-ia*] defective speech due to lack of phonation and resulting in whispering. Called also *subenergetic phonation.*

hypophosphatasia (hi″po-fos″fah-ta′ze-ah) a hereditary metabolic disease, transmitted as an autosomal recessive trait, characterized by blood alkaline phosphatase deficiency, urinary excretion of ethanolamine phosphate, and hypercalcemia. The serum alkaline phosphatase level is relative to the severity of symptoms — in severe cases the disease is diagnosed at birth and death ensues shortly; in milder cases, the symptoms may go unrecognized until adulthood. Failure of calcification of the calvarium, dyspnea, cyanosis, vomiting, constipation, renal calcinosis, movement disorders, failure to thrive, beading of the costochondral junctions, and rachitic bone changes, including bowing, are the most common symptoms. Spontaneous, or after slight trauma, loss of primary teeth is usually the first symptom. Other oral manifestations include absence of cementum, with resulting lack of attachment of the teeth to bone by the periodontal ligament, loose teeth, hypererupted teeth, wide pulp chambers, and areas of hypocalcification. See also HYPOPHOSPHATEMIA, ODONTOHYPOPHOSPHATASIA, and vitamin d–resistant RICKETS.

hypophosphatemia (hi″po-fos-fah-te′me-ah) an abnormally decreased level of phosphate in the blood, which may be observed in hyperparathyroidism, rickets, osteomalacia, hyperinsulinism, pregnancy, some bone diseases, hypervitaminosis D, lactation, and Addison's disease. See also HYPOPHOSPHATASIA.

hypophysis (hi-pof′ĭ-sis) [*hypo-* + Gr. *phyein* to grow] [NA] pituitary GLAND. **h. cer′ebri,** pituitary GLAND.

hypopituitarism (hi″po-pi-tu′ĭ-tah-rizm) a condition characterized by pituitary insufficiency. For hypopituitarism in children, see pituitary DWARFISM; in adults, see Sheehan's SYNDROME and Simmonds' SYNDROME.

hypoplasia (hi″po-pla-ze-ah) [*hypo-* + Gr. *plasis* formation + *-ia*] failure of an organ to achieve full adult size because of incomplete development. **condylar h.**, incomplete development of the mandibular condyle, which may be congenital or due to perinatal or postnatal trauma, radiation injury, infection, inflammation, or other factors. It usually produces faulty temporomandibular articulation, facial asymmetry, and malocclusion. Complications are usually more severe in the unilateral form than in the bilateral. **enamel h.**, a form of amelogenesis imperfecta characterized by incomplete formation of the dental enamel, which may be transmitted as an X-linked or autosomal dominant trait, or it may be associated with vitamin A, C, or D deficiency, measles, chickenpox, scarlet fever, congenital syphilis (Hutchinson's teeth), prematurity, birth injuries, Rh incompatibility, trauma, local infection, or Morquio's disease. It may exhibit only small grooves, pits, and fissures on the enamel surface in mild cases; deep horizontal rows of pits in severe cases; or absence of enamel in extreme cases (enamel aplasia), associated with yellow, reddish, or brown discoloration of the teeth. Called also *hypoplastic e.* and *enamel agenesia.* See also mottled ENAMEL, enamel HYPOCALCIFICATION, and Turner's TOOTH. **granulocytic h.**, agranulocytosis. **Turner's h.**, Turner's tooth. **unilateral h.**, hemihypoplasia.

hypopnea (hi″po-ne′ah) [*hypo-* + Gr. *pnoia* breath] a decrease in the depth and rate of the respiration, often with a rate of pulmonary ventilation sufficiently decreased to cause under-respiration. Cf. HYPERPNEA.

hypoproteinemia (hi″po-pro″ti-ne′me-ah) abnormal decrease in the amount of protein in the blood, sometimes resulting in edema and fluid accumulation in serous cavities.

hypoprothrombinemia (hi″po-pro-throm″bin-e′me-ah) a blood coagulation disorder characterized by prolonged plasma prothrombin time. Prothrombin deficiency, as well as deficiency of other coagulation factors having influence on prothrombin utilization, such as factors V, VII, and X, and of vitamin K are believed to be the cause. A bleeding tendency similar to that seen in mild hemophilia occurs; spontaneous bleeding is rare but hemorrhage may occur after trauma and surgery, including tooth extraction and tonsillectomy. Salicylates, propylthiouracil, and vitamin A are suspected as having hypoprothrombinemic effect. See also PARAHEMOPHILIA. **congenital h.,** parahemophilia.

hypoptyalism (hi″pop-ti′al-izm) [*hypo-* + Gr. *ptyalon* spittle] decreased secretion of saliva. Called also *hyposalivation* and *hyposialosis.*

hyposalivation (hi″po-sal″i-va′shun) hypoptyalism.

hyposialosis (hi″po-si″ah-lo′sis) [*hypo-* + *sialosis*] hypoptyalism.

hyposulfite (hi″po-sul′fit) a compound containing the radical S₂O₄. **h. of gold and sodium,** GOLD sodium thiosulfate. **sodium h.,** SODIUM thiosulfate.

hypotelorism (hi″po-tel′o-rizm) [*hypo-* + Gr. *tēlouros* distant] 1. abnormally decreased distance between two organs or parts. 2. ocular h. **ocular h., orbital h.,** abnormally decreased distance between the eyes.

hypotension (hi″po-ten′shun) [*hypo-* + *tension*] abnormally low blood pressure. **controlled h.,** induced h. **induced h.,** lowered blood pressure produced with hypotensive drugs to assist hemostasis and reduce blood loss in certain types of surgery. Called also *controlled h.* See also hypotensive ANESTHESIA.

hypotensive (hi″po-ten′siv) 1. characterized by or causing diminished tension or pressure, or abnormally low blood pressure. 2. an agent that causes the lowering of blood pressure. See also *antihypertensive.* 3. a person with hypotension.

hypothalamus (hi″po-thal′ah-mus) [NA] the portion of the diencephalon which forms the floor and part of the lateral wall of the third ventricle. It is made up of collections of neurons known as *hypothalamic nuclei* and bundles of axons or fiber tracts which connect it with other structures. Fibers of the pituitary stalk originate in the supraoptic, paraventricular, and tuberal nuclei and terminate in the posterior pituitary gland. The hypothalamus is involved in various functions, including the regulation of the release of pituitary hormones, heart rate, appetite, rage, mating behavior, blood sugar, and vasopressin and oxytocin production and secretion.

hypothermia (hi″po-ther′me-ah) [*hypo-* + Gr. *thermē* heat + *-ia*] low temperature; especially a state of low core body temperature below the normal 98.6°F (37°C). Hypothermia may occur naturally, e.g., if a person falls asleep or unconscious while exposed to extreme cold, or it may be induced artificially for surgical purposes, such as to reduce body metabolism and slow the heart during cardiovascular surgery.

hypothesis (hi-poth′e-sis) [Gr. *hypotithenai;* from *hypo-* + *tithenai* to put more at] a supposition that appears to explain a group of phenomena; a proposition or theory assumed to be true and offered for discussion. **lattice h.,** a theory of the nature of the antigen-antibody reaction which postulates reaction between multivalent antigen and divalent antibody to give an antigen-antibody complex of a lattice-like structure. For example, the formation of a precipitate consists of antigen molecules linked to antibody molecules to form a visible complex. **linear h.,** an assumption that a dose-effect curve derived from data in the high dose and high dose–rate ranges may be extrapolated through the low dose and low dose–rate range to zero. **Lyon h.,** all X chromosomes in a cell in excess of one are inactivated (in the form of sex chromatin) on a random basis in all mammalian cells at an early stage of embryogenesis. In effect, then, the normal human female is a mosaic for heterozygous X-linked genes, since the paternal X chromosome is inactivated in some cells and the maternal one in the remainder. Hence, females heterozygous for an X-linked disorder often exhibit some stigmata for the condition. **sliding-filament h.,** the stretching of individual muscle fibers raises the number of tension-developing bridges that can be formed between the sliding

contractile protein elements (actin and myosin) and thus augments the force of the next muscle contraction. **threshold h.,** the hypothesis that no radiation injury occurs below a dose level of irradiation. **unitarian h.,** the theory that antibody is a single species of modified serum globulin regardless of the overt consequences of its reaction with homologous antigen, e.g., agglutination, precipitation, complement fixation, etc.

Hypothiazide trademark for *hydrochlorothiazide.*

hypothyroidism (hi″po-thi′roid-izm) a condition resulting from an inability of the thyroid gland to produce sufficient hormone. **congenital h.,** cretinism. **primary h.,** diminished production of thyroid hormone due to a primary lesion in the thyroid gland. **secondary h.,** diminished production of thyroid hormone due to decreased production of thyrotropin by the pituitary gland.

hypotonia (hi″po-to′ne-ah) [*hypo-* + Gr. *tonos* tone + *-ia*] a condition characterized by abnormally diminished tone, tension, or activity. See also muscle SPLINTING. **unilateral h.,** hemihypotonia.

hypotonic (hi-po-ton′ik) [*hypo-* + Gr. *tonos* tone] 1. pertaining to hypotonia. 2. pertaining to a hypotonic solution; sometimes used alone to denote such a solution.

hypotonicity (hi″po-to-nis′ĭ-te) 1. the state or quality of being hypotonic. 2. a condition of a muscle characterized by decreased tonus; hypotonia.

hypotrichosis (hi″po-tri-ko′sis) [*hypo-* + Gr. *thrix* hair + *-osis*] presence of less than the normal amount of hair. See also ALOPECIA.

hypotrophy (hi-pot′ro-fe) [*hypo-* + Gr. *trophē* nutrition] 1. trophic deficiency; degeneration of vital functions. Called also *abionergy* and *abiotrophy.* 2. bacterial nutrition in which the organism is nourished by its host's nutrition.

Hypovase trademark for *prazosin hydrochloride* (see under PRAZOSIN).

hypovitaminosis (hi″po-vi″tah-min-o′sis) a condition resulting from deficiency of one or more vitamins. For specific vitamin deficiencies, see the vitamin involved.

hypoxanthine (hi″po-zan′thēn) a product of nucleic acid breakdown, 6-oxypurine, being an intermediate product of uric acid synthesis, formed from adenylic acid and itself a precursor of xanthine. It occurs as a white to creamy powder that is readily soluble in dilute acids and alkalies and slightly soluble in boiling water. **h. riboside,** inosine.

hypoxemia (hi″pok-se′me-ah) [*hypo-* + *oxygen* + Gr. *haima* blood + *-ia*] deficient oxygen content of the blood. See also ANOXEMIA, ANOXIA and HYPOXIA.

hypoxia (hi-pok′se-ah) [*hypo-* + *oxygen* + *-ia*] decreased oxygen content or tension; decreased oxygen content in the tissue. See also ANOXIA.

hypsi- [Gr. *hypsi* high] a combining form meaning high.

hypsicephalic (hip″se-sĕ-fal′ik) [*hypsi-* + Gr. *kephalē* head] pertaining to or characterized by a high vaulted skull. See hypsicephalic SKULL.

hypsicephaly (hip″se-sef′ah-le) a condition characterized by a high cranial vault. See hypsicephalic SKULL and OXYCEPHALY.

hypsiloid (hip′sĭ-loid) [Gr. *hypsiloeidēs* in the shape of an Υ] shaped like the Greek letter Υ, capital upsilon. See also HYOID and UPSILOID.

hypsistaphylia (hip″si-stah-fil′e-ah) [*hypsi-* + Gr. *staphylē* uvula + *-ia*] a condition characterized by an unusually high-arched, narrow palate. See also hypsistaphyline SKULL.

hypsistaphyline (hip″si-staf′ĭ-lin) [*hypsi-* + Gr. *staphylē,* a bunch of grapes, uvula] characterized by a palate with a high arch, or pertaining to hypsistaphylia. See hypsistaphyline SKULL.

hypsistenocephalic (hip″se-sten″o-sĕ-fal′ik) [*hypsi-* + Gr. *stenos* narrow + *kephalē* head] See hypsistenocephalic SKULL.

hypsistenocephaly (hip″se-sten″o-sĕ-fal′e) [*hypsi-* + Gr. *stenos* narrow + *kephalē* head] a condition characterized by a skull with a high, curved vertex, prominent cheek bones, and prognathic jaws.

hypso- [Gr. *hypsos* height] a combining form denoting relationship to height.

hypsocephalous (hip″so-sef′ah-lus) [*hypso-* + Gr. *kephalē* head] having a high vertex. See also hysicepahlic SKULL.

hypsodont (hip′so-dont) [*hypso-* + Gr. *odous* tooth] an individual having teeth with abnormally high crowns. Cf. BRACHYDONT.

hysteresis (his″tĕ-re′sis) [Gr. *hysterēsis* a lagging behind] a lagging or retardation of an effect.

Hytakerol trademark for *dihydrotachysterol.*

Hytrast trademark for a suspension of two organic iodides; used as a water-insoluble contrast medium in radiography, including sialography.

Hz hertz.

I iodine.

¹²⁵I IODINE-125.

¹³¹I IODINE-131.

i isochromosome; see CHROMOSOME nomenclature.

Ia see Ia ANTIGEN.

-ia a word termination indicating state or condition.

IADR International Association for Dental Research; an association established in 1920 to promote the advancement of the research in all branches of dental science and to contribute directly to the development of oral health service.

IAG International Academy of Gnathology (see under ACADEMY).

IAO International Association for Orthodontics (see under ASSOCIATION).

IAOM International Association of Oral Myology (see under ASSOCIATION).

-iasis a word termination denoting a process or condition resulting thereon, particularly a morbid condition. See -SIS.

iatric (i-at'rik) [Gr. *iatrikos*] pertaining to medicine or to a physician.

iatro- [Gr. *iatros* physician] a combining form denoting relationship to medicine or to a physician.

iatrogenesis (i″at-ro-jen′ĕ-sis) [*iatro-* + Gr. *genesis* production] the creation of an abnormal state or condition in a patient, occurring as a result of inadvertent or erroneous treatment by a physician, surgeon, or dentist. See also IATROGENIC.

iatrogenic (i″at-ro-jen′ik) [*iatro-* + Gr. *gennan* to produce] resulting from the activity of physician, dentist, or other health professional.] Originally applied to disorders induced in the patient by autosuggestion based on the physician's examination, manner, or discussion, the term is now applied to any adverse condition in a patient occurring as the result of treatment by a physician or surgeon and, by extension, a dentist.

Ibn Rushd see AVERROES.

Ibn Sinā see AVICENNA.

Ibn Zuhr see AVENZOAR.

ibuprofen (i-bu′pro-fen) an analgesic, antipyretic, and antiinflammatory agent, 2-(4-isobutylphenyl)propionic acid, occurring as a white crystalline powder or a colorless solid with a slight characteristic odor and taste, which is very slightly soluble in water and readily soluble in organic solvents. Used in the treatment of rheumatoid arthritis, osteoarthritis, and other painful conditions. Gastrointestinal disorders are the principal side reactions. Trademarks: Emodin, Motrin.

IC inspiratory CAPACITY.

-ic in chemical nomenclature, a suffix indicating a higher valence, as compared with *-ous*, as in fer*rous* (valence 2) and fer*ric* (valence 3). Also, a suffix indicating acids, such as those of the binary and ternary groups.

ICDA International Classification of Diseases, Adapted; see under CLASSIFICATION.

ice (īs) a solid or frozen form of water; usually the common low-density form melting at 0°C at 1 atmosphere. **dry i.,** carbon dioxide SNOW.

ICF intermediate care FACILITY.

ichthammol (ik′tham-ol) an irritant and topical antiseptic, ammonium ichthosulfonate, obtained by sulfation and ammoniation of a distillate from bituminous schists, and containing nitrogenous bases, acids, unsaturated hydrocarbons, and thiophene derivatives. It occurs as a yellow to brownish-black, viscous liquid with a specific odor, which is miscible with water, glycerol, propylene glycol, fats, oils, and lanolin. Called also *bituminol* and *sulfonated bitumen*. Trademarks: Ictiol, Lithol, Perichthol.

ichthyo- [Gr. *ichthys* fish] a combining form denoting relationship to fish or to a fishlike appearance.

ichthyosis (ik″the-o′sis) [*ichthyo-* + *-osis*] a skin disease characterized by abnormal keratinization, giving it a dry, rough, scaly appearance. Called also *fish-skin disease* and *xeroderma*.

icosahedral (i-ko′sah-he′dral) pertaining to an icosahedron.

icosahedron (i-ko′sah-he′dron) a solid figure having 20 faces.

ICRP International Commission on Radiological Protection.

ICRU International Commission on Radiation Units and Measurements.

ICSH interstitial cell stimulating hormone; see luteinizing HORMONE.

ictal (ik′tal) [L. *ictus* stroke] pertaining to, characterized by, or caused by a stroke or an acute epileptic seizure.

icterus (ik′ter-us) [L., Gr. *ikteros*] jaundice. **i. gra′vis neonato′rum,** ERYTHROBLASTOSIS fetalis.

Ictiol trademark for *ichthammol*.

ictus (ik′tus) [L. "stroke"] a seizure, stroke, blow, or sudden attack. See also SEIZURE. **i. laryn′gis,** Charcot's VERTIGO.

ICTV International Committee for the Taxonomy of Viruses.

ICU intensive care UNIT.

ID 1. intradermal. 2. inside DIAMETER.

I.D. infective DOSE.

I.D.₅₀ median infective dose; that amount of pathogenic microorganisms which will produce infection in 50 percent of the test subjects.

Id 1. infradentale. 2. interdentale.

Id. abbreviation for L. *i′dem*, the same.

-id [Gr. *eidos* form, shape] a word termination meaning having the shape of, or resembling.

-ide a suffix signifying a binary compound of a nonmetallic element, such as a chloride or a sulfide.

identification (i-den″ti-fi-ka-shun) the act or process of establishing the unique characteristics of something. **dental i.,** unique identification of a person through the characteristics of his teeth or dental work, such as identification of a corpse by matching his dentures or dentition with an existing dental chart and records. See also forensic DENTISTRY and INQUEST. **medicolegal i.,** the use of modern medical methods in the application of law and justice, as in determining the type of weapon used through the characteristics of the gunshot wound or establishing the proof of rape through the characteristics of semen stains. See also forensic MEDICINE.

identity (i-den′ti-te) the aggregate of characteristics by which an individual is recognized by himself and others.

Idexur trademark for *idoxuridine*.

IdI INTERDENTALE inferius.

idio- [Gr. *idios* own, peculiar] a combining form denoting relationship to the self or to one's own, or to something separate and distinct.

idiocy (id′e-o-se) severe mental deficiency. **amaurotic familial i.,** Tay-Sachs DISEASE. **mongoloid i.,** Down's SYNDROME.

idioglossia (id″e-o-glos′e-ah) [*idio-* + Gr. *glōssa* tongue + *-ia*] imperfect articulation with utterance of meaningless vocal sounds.

idiopathic (id″e-o-path′ik) of the nature of an idiopathy; self-originated; of unknown causation; essential.

idiopathy (id″e-op′ah-the) [*idio-* + Gr. *pathos* disease] a morbid state of spontaneous origin.

idiosyncrasy (id″e-o-sin′krah-se) [*idio-* + Gr. *synkrasis* mixture] 1. a habit or quality of body or mind peculiar to any individual. 2. an abnormal susceptibility to some drug, protein, or other agent which is peculiar to the individual. **drug i.,** drug REACTION. **food i.,** food INTOLERANCE.

idiotype (id′e-o-tīp) 1. genotype. 2. a genetic specificity associated with a single or with very few individuals due to unique antigenic determinants associated with a variable portion of the Fab fragments of immunoglobulins; seen primarily in patients with mononuclear gammopathies.

IDL Index to Dental Literature; see under INDEX.

Ido-K trademark for *menadione sodium bisulfite* (see under MENADIONE).

Idomethine trademark for *indomethacin*.

idoxuridine (i″doks-ur′i-dēn) a thymidine antimetabolite, 2′-deoxy-5-iodouridine, occurring as a white, photosensitive, odorless, crystalline powder that is soluble in sodium hydroxide solutions, slightly soluble in water, hydrochloric acid solutions, acetone, methanol, ethanol, dioxane, and ethyl acetate, and insoluble in ether and chloroform. Formerly considered an antineoplastic drug, it is now used chiefly as an antiviral agent in the treatment of herpes simplex infection of the eye. Ocular application may cause epithelial edema, corneal stippling, inflammation, itching, and photophobia. Abbreviated *IDU, IDUR,* and *IUDR.* Trademarks: Dendrid, Herplex, Idexur, Iduridin, Stoxil.

IdS INTERDENTALE superius.

IDU, IDUR idoxuridine.

Iduridin trademark for *idoxuridine*.

IER immunoelectrophoresis.

IF initiating FACTOR.

Ig immunoglobulin.

IgA IMMUNOGLOBULIN A. secretory IgA, see IMMUNOGLOBULIN A.

IgA1, IgA2 allotypic subclasses of immunoglobulin A (IgA).

IgD IMMUNOGLOBULIN D.

IgD1, IgD2 allotypic subclasses of immunoglobulin D (IgD).

IgE IMMUNOGLOBULIN E.

IgE1 a subclass of immunoglobulin E (IgE).

IgG IMMUNOGLOBULIN G.

IgG1, IgG2, IgG3, IgG4 subclasses of immunoglobin G (IgG).

IgM IMMUNOGLOBULIN M.

IgM1 a subclass of immunoglobin M (IgM).

IgND IMMUNOGLOBULIN E.

Ihring, von see VON IHRING.

Ii INCISION inferius.

Ikaklomine trademark for *clomiphene citrate* (see under CLOMI-PHENE).

Ile isoleucine.

ileitis (il″e-i′tis) [*ileum* + *-itis*] inflammation of the ileum. **regional i., terminal i.,** Crohn's DISEASE.

ileum (il′e-um) [L.] [NA] the terminal part of the small intestine which empties into the large intestine.

ileus (il′e-us) [L.; Gr. *eileos*, from *eilein* to roll up] obstruction of the intestine.

illness (il′ness) a condition marked by pronounced deviation from the normal healthy state; sickness. **acute i.,** acute DISEASE. **chronic i.,** chronic DISEASE. **disabling i.,** an illness causing any degree of interference with the ability of an individual to carry out his ordinary activities. Called also *incapacitating i.* **incapacitating i.,** disabling i. **radiation i.,** radiation SICKNESS. **terminal i.,** illness from which there is no hope of recovery. Called also *terminal disease.*

illumination (ĭ-lu″mĭ-na′shun) [L. *illuminatio*] the lighting up of a part, cavity, organ, or object for inspection.

illuminator (ĭ-lu″mĭ-na′tor) the source of light for viewing an object, as one for viewing a radiograph. **Abbe's i.,** Abbe's CONDENSER.

illusion (ĭ-lu′zhun) [L. *illusio*] a false interpretation of a sensory impression.

Ilosone trademark for *erythromycin estolate* (see under ERYTHROMYCIN).

Ilotycin trademark for *erythromycin.*

IM 1. Index Medicus; see under INDEX. 2. intramuscularly (by intramuscular injection).

image (im′ij) [L. *imago*] a likeness or representation of physical objects, persons, animals, or other things. See also ROENTGENOGRAM and RADIOGRAPH. **i. amplification,** image-tube INTENSIFICATION. **invisible i.,** latent i. **latent i.,** an invisible image created upon a radiosensitive or photosensitive emulsion on the photographic film through the passage of x-rays or rays in the visible spectrum, which is rendered visible by the subsequent chemical developing process. Called also *invisible i.* **manifest i.,** the visible image on the developed film. Called also *visible i.* See also film PROCESSING and x-ray FILM. **radiographic i.,** an image of a structure or tissue produced by the passage of x-rays. It is at first latent, but is rendered visible through the use of a fluorescent screen or subsequent chemical developing process of the exposed film. Called also *x-ray i.* See also RADIOGRAPH. **radioisotope i.,** a quasipictorial representation of the distribution of radioactive materials in the body. **visible i.,** manifest i. **x-ray i.,** radiographic i.

imbalance (im-bal′ans) the state or condition of lack of equilibrium between opposing forces, weight, amount, and the like. **occlusal i.,** imperfect relationship between the upper and lower teeth during closure or functional jaw movements. See MALOCCLUSION.

imbecility (im″be-sil′ĭ-te) [L. *imbecillitas*] a former category of mental retardation comprising mentally retarded persons of the second lowest order. See mental RETARDATION. **phenylpyruvic i.,** phenylketonuria.

imbibition (im″bĭ-bish′um) [L. *imbibere* to drink] absorption or soaking up of a liquid by a solid or gel.

imbricated (im′brĭ-kāt″ed) [L. *imbricatus*; *imbrex* tile] overlapping like tiles or shingles.

ImD₅₀ immunizing DOSE.

Imerslund-Gräsbeck syndrome [Olga *Imerslund*; Ralph *Gräsbeck*, Finnish physician] see under SYNDROME.

Imferon trademark for dextran *iron complex* (see under COMPLEX).

imide (im′īd) 1. a compound containing the bivalent group,

R
  ＼NH, in which R is an acyl radical. 2. a compound from acid
R／

anhydrides in which O is replaced by NH.

imido- a prefix denoting the presence in a compound of the

                    R
                     ＼
bivalent group   NH, where R is an acid radical.
                     ／
                    R

imidole (im′ĭ-dol) pyrrole.

imine (im′in) an organic compound having a carbon-to-nitrogen double bond, R—CH. See also imino acids, under ACID.

‖
NH

imino- a prefix used to denote the presence of the NH group attached to one or two carbon atoms, as =C:NH.

imipramine (īmip′rah-mēn) an antidepressant agent, 10,11-dihydro-*N*,*N*-dimethyl-5*H*-dibenz [*b*,*f*] azepine-5-propanamine. Used therapeutically as the hydrochloride salt, which occurs as a white, odorless, crystalline powder that is soluble in water, ethanol, and acetone, but not in ether and benzene. It may cause fetal abnormalities, hypotension, seizures, tremor, diplopia, hallucinations, agitation, confusion, and agranulocytosis. Most side reactions occur in patients over 65 years of age. Trademarks: Dimipressin, Imiprin, Tofranil.

Imiprin trademark for *imipramine hydrochloride* (see under IMIPRAMINE).

immature (im″ah-tūr′) [L. *in* not + *maturus* mature] not fully developed.

immediate (ĭ-me′de-it) [L. *in* not + *mediatus* mediate] direct; with nothing intervening; occurring without delay.

immersion (ĭ-mer′shun) [L. *immersio*] 1. the placing or plunging of a body into a liquid. 2. the use of the microscope with the object and object glass both covered with a liquid.

immiscible (ĭ-mis′ĭ-b'l) not susceptible of being mixed.

immobility (im″mo-bil′ĭ-te) the state or condition of being immovable.

immobilization (im-mo″bil-ĭ-za′shun) the act of rendering immovable. See ANKYLOSIS. **tooth i.,** a fixing or splinting technique to stabilize loose teeth.

immobilize (im-mo′bil-īz) [L. *in* not + *mobilis* movable] to render incapable of being moved, as by a cast or splint.

immunity (ĭ-mu′nĭ-te) [L. *immunitas*] 1. the condition of being immune; security against a particular disease; nonsusceptibility to the invasive or pathogenic effects of foreign microorganisms or to the toxic effect of antigenic substances. Called also *functional* or *protective i.* See also *active i., nonspecific i.,* and *passive i.* 2. heightened responsiveness to antigenic challenge that leads to more rapid binding or elimination of antigen than in the nonimmune state; it includes both humoral and cell-mediated immunity. 3. the capacity to distinguish foreign material from self, and to neutralize, eliminate, or metabolize that which is foreign by the physiologic mechanisms of the immune response. See also immune SYSTEM. **acquired i.,** specific immunity attributable to the presence of antibody in response to antigenic stimulation or the introduction of preformed antibody or specifically sensitized lymphoid cells. See *active i.* and *passive i.* **active i.,** acquired immunity attributable to the presence of antibody or of immune lymphoid cells formed in response to antigenic stimulation. It involves active host participation after exposure to immunogen, either naturally through a subclinical or clinical infectious disease or by vaccination, having an onset after a latent period. Humoral and cell-mediated immunity are the chief components of the process. The duration of active immunity may be long-lived and dependent on the persistence of lymphocytes capable of recognizing the specific antigen. Called also *actual i.* **actual i.,** active i. **adoptive i.,** permanent specific immunity produced by the administration of immunologically competent and committed cells from a previously sensitized donor to a previously unsensitized individual. **antibacterial i.,** immunity against the action of bacteria or against their products, i.e., the ability to resist infection by bacteria. **antiblastic i.,** immunity due to forces antagonistic to the growth and multiplication of the microorganism in the body of the host organism, or *in vitro*. **antitoxic i.,** immunity against toxins, attributable to the presence of specific antitoxins in the immune individual. **antiviral i.,** immunity against viruses. **artificial i.,** acquired (active or passive) immunity produced by deliberate exposure to an antigen, such as in vaccination or by transfer of humoral or cellular factors of immunity. Cf. *natural i.* **bacteriolytic i.,** antibacterial immunity usually attributable to humoral factors but that may also be due to cellular immune factors. **cell-mediated i., cellular i.,** immunity mediated by specifically sensitized lymphocytes that differentiate under the influence of the thymus (T-lymphocytes). The effector arm is carried out directly by the sensitized lymphocytes or by specifically-released cell products formed upon interaction of immunogen with sensitized lymphocytes; the products, called *lymphokines*, include migration inhibitory factor, cytotoxin, interferon, macrophage activating factors, ˙nd several others, and are believed to be the effector molecules of cellular immunity. It is responsible for resistance to infection caused by certain types of bacteria, fungi, and viruses, certain forms of resistance to cancer, delay˙d hypersensitivity reactions, certain autoimmune diseases, and allogenic graft rejection. Abbreviated *CMI.* See accompanying illustration and see illustration at LYMPHOCYTE. **cellular theory of i.,** Metchnikoff's THEORY. **charitable i.,** in malpractice, a doctrine in use in some states that nonprofit or charitable hospitals and other health facilities are not subject to suit for malpractice under certain conditions. **community i.,** herd i. **congenital i.,** the immunity which an individual possesses at birth, including that passively acquired by transplacental passage from the mother. **cross i.,** immunity produced by inoculation with an agent (e.g., bacterium, fungus, or virus) that is effective against organisms different from, but closely related to, the agent inducing the immunity. It is usually due to the presence of identical or similar determinants in the species involved. **familial i.,** genetic i. **functional i.,** immunity (1). **genetic i.,** immunity determined by the genetic constitution of the individual. Called also *familial i., inherent i., inherited i., and innate i.* **governmental i.,** a doctrine that, subject to certain qualifications, the government cannot be sued for the negligent acts of its officers, agents, or employees, as in malpractice suits, unless it consents to such a suit. **herd i.,** the resistance of a group to a disease because of the immunity of a large proportion of the members and the consequent lessening of the likelihood of an affected individual coming into contact with a susceptible individual. Called also *community i.* **humoral i.,** immunity mediated by factors found in the noncellular elements of the blood such as antibody; the biologic amplification system consisting of the complement system, which, under some conditions, leads to the inactivation and removal of infective agents and, under other conditions, results in tissue damage; and the kallikrein system which produces vasoactive peptides (kinins) that increase capillary permeability. Certain proteins involved in blood coagulation may also act to amplify the immune response during the interaction of antigen .with antibody. See accompanying illustration and see illustration at LYMPHOCYTE. **infection i.,** active immunity by reason of an existing or past infection by the same or antigenically related microorganism. **inherent i., inherited i., innate i.,** genetic i. **intrauterine i., natural,** passive immunity acquired by the fetus as a consequence of the passage of maternal IgG antibodies from the immune mother through the placenta into the fetal circulation. Called also *placental i.* See also *natural i.* **local i.,** immunity manifested predominantly in a restricted anatomical region or type of tissue; antibodies of the class termed secretory or exocrine IgA account for many manifestations of local immunity. **maturation i.,** increase in resistance to disease that comes with development of cells involved in the immune response. **mixed i.,** passive immunity succeeded by active immunity as a consequence of serovaccination, e.g., administration of tetanus toxoid together with antitoxin if the immune status of the patient is in doubt. **native i.,** a nonimmunologic resistance of an individual to harmful agents, due to a genetic endowment that provides for the capacity to prevent access into the body of the harmful agent or to neutralize and eliminate it from the body. **natural i.,** the capacity of the normal (not specifically immunized) individual to respond immunologically; immunity inherited or acquired passively *in utero* or through the maternal milk, or acquired actively by clinical or subclinical infection. See also *intrauterine i.* Cf. *artificial i.* **nonspecific i.,** a sum of immune responses to foreign potentially harmful macromolecules, microorganisms, or metazoa, which does not involve the recognition of a specific antigen or a specific response against such an antigen, but consists of chemical and physical barriers to infection, phagocytosis, inflammatory response, and the action of various substances, such as lysozyme and interferon. **opsonic i.,** immunity due to the presence of opsonins. **passive i.,** acquired immunity produced by the administration of preformed antibody or specifically sensitized lymphoid cells or their products from an actively immunized host. No host participation is involved in the production of the immune factors, and the onset is immediate. The duration of this type of immunity is transitory. **phagocytic i.,** immunity attributable to the activity of phagocytes in the engulfment and destruction of pathogenic agents. **placental i.,** intrauterine i. **postoncolytic i.,** immunity to tumor development following regression of a previously existing tumor. Blocking factors or antigens shedding from the tumor often mask an underlying immunity, which becomes manifest after reduction in the tumor burden. **protective i.,** immunity (1). **residual i.,** immunity which remains for varying periods after the complete disappearance of the infection or toxemia. **specific i.,** an immune response concerned with the recognition of the foreignness of the specific antigens (a foreign macromolecule, microorganism, or metazoon) and its disposal.

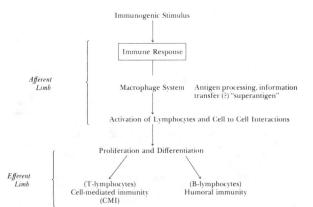

Effector mechanisms that mediate specific immunologic responses. (From J. A. Bellanti: Immunology II. Philadelphia, W. B. Saunders Co., 1978.)

It is a discriminatory process consisting of (*a*) specificity, whereby antigens originating from different species, individuals, and organs (species, individual, and organ specificity) are distinguished and differentiated; (*b*) heterogeneity, whereby cell types and products are induced to interaction with a diversity of responses commensurate with the variety of cell types, giving rise to specific antibodies; and (*c*) memory, whereby there is an augmentation of the specific response through proliferation and differentiation of cells upon subsequent exposure to an immunogen. **toxin-antitoxin i.,** an active antitoxic immunity produced by injecting a nearly neutral mixture of diphtheria toxin and antitoxin.

immunization (im″u-ni-za′shun) the process of rendering a subject immune, or of becoming immune. **active i.,** the synthesis of an immune response to an antigen by the cells of the host. Called also *isopathic i.* **collateral i.,** inoculation with an organism other than the one causing an existing infection. **isopathic i.,** active i. **occult i.,** immunization produced in some unknown, spontaneous way.

immuno- [L. *immunitas* exemption from public service or burden] a combining form relating to immunity.

immunoassay (im″u-no-as′sa) the quantitation of humoral or cellular immune factors. It may be performed *in vivo*, as in the measurement of a response to a graded challenge to a microorganism, a toxin, or a tumor; or *in vitro*, e.g., the determination of the ability of an antigen to react with antibody.

immunobiology (im″u-no-bi-ol-′o-je) that branch of biology dealing with immunologic effect. It encompasses a broad area that includes simple immune responses in lower forms of life and the responses of higher forms of life to infectious disease, growth and development, antigen recognition phenomena, hypersensitivity, heredity, aging, cancer, and transplantation.

immunochemistry (im″u-no-kem′is-tre) that branch of biological science concerned with the chemical basis of immune phenomena and their interactions.

immunocompetence (im″u-no-kom′pē-tens) the ability or capacity to develop an immune response (i.e., antibody production and/or cell-mediated immunity) following exposure to antigen. Called also *immunologic competence.*

immunocyte (im″u-no-sīt′) a lymphocyte capable of responding to a specific antigen stimulus and differentiating either along a pathway leading to the production of antibody or to the induction of cell-mediated events such as delayed hypersensitivity.

immunodeficiency (im″u-no-de-fish′en-se) an absence or reduction of the capacity to respond to antigen stimuli due to a defect in the cells responsible for the immune response, which may involve T-lymphocytes and/or B-lymphocytes or macrophages. It may be hereditary or be acquired as a result of disease or treatment with immunosuppressive drugs.

immunoelectrophoresis (ī-mu″no-e-lek″tro-fo-re′sis) a method whereby mixtures of antigens are identified after they have been separated on the basis of their electrophoretic mobilities by electrophoresis in agar, cellulose acetate, or another supporting medium. Antiserum is then added, usually in a trough parallel to the line of migration and permitted to diffuse toward the separated antigens. **counter i.,** a sensitive precipitation technique in which antigen and antibody migrate in opposing directions toward each other in an electric field due to their electric mobilities. This results in a concentration of the reagents at their line of interaction and the formation of a precipitate. The technique is used, for example, to detect hepatitis antigen in human serum. **rocket i.,** electrophoresis of a mixture of antigens or a single antigen into a layer of agar containing antiserum. Cone-shaped areas of precipitate are produced by each antigen-antibody system in the antibody layer. See also Lawrell TECHNIQUE. **two-dimensional i.,** a technique whereby separation of a mixture of antigens is accomplished in one direction on the basis of their electrophoretic mobilities in an electrical field and then electrophoresed in a second dimension into a layer containing antiserum. The resultant precipitin arcs permit an effective resolution of the antigenic components.

immunofiltration (im″u-no-fil-tra′shun) the extraction of antibodies in pure form by subjection of serum to insoluble specific antigen, the antigen then being removed from the antibody by treatment with soluble carriers. Called also *electrosyneresis*.

immunofluorescence (im″u-no-floo″o-res′ens) a technique employing antigens or antibodies that have been labeled with a fluorescent dye and which increases the sensitivity of the detection of their interaction. Fluorescein isocyanate or isothiocyanate bound onto antigens or serum antibodies, which give off a yellow green fluorescence, are the common fluorescent dyes used. The procedure may be used to detect the presence of antigen or antibody in tissues or as the basis of a very sensitive quantitative assay for either antigen or antibody. Called also *fluorescent antibody method* or *technique*.

immunogen (im′u-no-jen) [*immuno-* + Gr. *gennan* to produce] any substance capable of eliciting an immune response, including substances which, when introduced into the body, stimulate humoral or cell-mediated immunity, or those which stimulate protective immunity. Immunogens are generally substances which are genetically foreign to the host but, on occasion, body constituents may be recognized as foreign substances and elicit an immune response. Effective immunogens have a molecular weight greater than 10,000 but smaller molecules, such as insulin (5,000) and glucagon (4,600) may under certain conditions function as immunogens. Proteins are usually good immunogens and complex carbohydrates are also effective. Most lipids and nucleic acids behave as haptens. See also ANTIGEN.

immunogenetics (im″u-no-jĕ-net′iks) [*immuno-* + *genetics*] the field of immunology and genetics concerned with all processes involved in immune responses that may have a genetic basis, including all the factors that control the immunologic responsiveness of the host to foreign elements, as well as the transmission of antigenic specificities from generation to generation. In the past, the term was restricted to genetic markers on immunoglobulin polypeptide chains.

immunogenicity (im″u-no-jĕ-nis′ĭ-te) the property of a substance (immunogen) which endows it with the capacity to provoke for a particular species or strain a specific immune response, consisting of either the elaboration of antibody, the development of cell-mediated immunity, or both. See also ANTIGENICITY.

immunoglobulin (im″u-no-glob′u-lin) a serum protein with antibody properties. It is composed of four polypeptide chains held together by disulfide bonds; two similar light chains, each of about 214 amino acid residues; and two similar heavy chains of 450 to 550 amino acid residues. Each chain has an N-terminal amino acid and a C-terminal amino acid. Intrachain disulfide bonds create compact *domains* of folded amino acids — two for each light chain and four or five for each heavy chain. The sequence of the amino acids on the domain at the N-terminal end is *variable* and accounts for the antibody specificity of the antibody molecule; the sequence of amino acids for the remaining domains is relatively *constant* from molecule to molecule within a class. There are five classes of immunoglobulins (abbreviated *Ig* or designated by the Greek letter γ), identified by antigenic determinants on the heavy chains as IgG, IgM, IgA, IgE, and IgD. Subclasses of IgG, IgA, IgM, and of the light chains have been identified by antigenic determinants on the polypeptide chains. Mild reduction of the interchain disulfide bonds can dissociate the molecule into four polypeptide chains. Digestion with papain can split the antibody into three units, two of which have antigen-binding activity. Abnormal immunoglobulins (paraproteins) include myeloma protein and Bence Jones protein. Diseases associated with immunoglobulin disorders include heavy chain disease, light chain disease, macroglobulinemia, agammaglobulinemia, and multiple myeloma. Called also *gamma globulin* (γ-*globulin*), *immune globulin*, *immune protein*, and *immunoprotein*. See illustration and table. **i. domain,** immunoglobulin DOMAIN. **i. A (IgA),** an immunoglobulin present in small amounts (representing 5 to 10 percent of serum immunoglobulins), but constituting the major immunoglobulin class in external secretions, mainly saliva, tears, colostrum, and gastrointestinal and respiratory fluids. Serum IgA exists in monomer form, and has two allotypic classes: IgA1 and IgA2 (γ₁A and γ₂A globulins, respectively). Secretory (exocrine) IgA exists chiefly as a dimer of IgA (SC) complexed to a J chain and to another chain called a *secretory piece* or *component*. Its principal function appears to be related to immunity against infections of the respiratory and intestinal tracts. Secretory IgA is called also *secretory IgA, secretory IgA globulin*, and *secretory γA globulin*. Called also *γA globulin, globulin A, IgA globulin*, and *protein A*. **i. D (IgD),** an immuno-

SOME PHYSICAL AND BIOLOGIC PROPERTIES OF HUMAN IMMUNOGLOBULIN CLASSES

CLASS	MEAN SERUM CONCENTRATION (mg/100 ml)	MOLECULAR WEIGHT	$S_{20.w}$	MEAN SURVIVAL T/2 (days)	BIOLOGIC FUNCTION	HEAVY CHAIN DESIGNATION	NO. OF SUBCLASSES
IgG or γG	1240	150,000	7	23	1. Fix complement 2. Cross placenta 3. Heterocytotropic antibody	γ	4
IgA or γA	280	170,000	7, 10, 14	6	1. Secretory antibody 2. Properdin pathway	α	2
IgM or γM	120	890,000	19	5	1. Fix complement 2. Efficient agglutination	μ	1
IgD or γD	3	150,000	7	2.8	1. Lymphocyte surface receptor	δ	2
IgE or γE	.03	196,000	8	1.5	1. Reaginic antibody 2. Homocytotropic antibody	ε	1

(From J. A. Bellanti: Immunology II. Philadelphia, W. B. Saunders Co., 1978.)

MOLECULAR STRUCTURE OF IMMUNOGLOBULINS
THE FIVE CLASSES

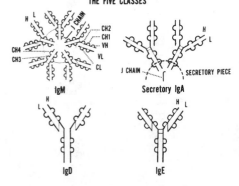

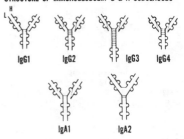

STRUCTURE OF IMMUNOGLOBULIN G & A SUBCLASSES

Schematic representation of the basic four polypeptide chain, monomeric unit structure of immunoglobulin molecules. (From Dorland's Illustrated Medical Dictionary. 26th ed. Philadelphia, W. B. Saunders Co., 1981.)

globulin class present in serum in very small quantities. The effector functions of IgD are unknown but its presence on the surface of B lymphocytes suggests that it may play a receptor role. It has two subclasses: IgD1 and IgD2 (γ_1D and γ_2D globulins, respectively). Called also *γD globulin, globulin D, and protein D.* **i. E (IgE),** an immunoglobulin class found in normal serum in very small amounts. It is a glycoprotein, and has reaginic activity, including the ability to fix cells, particularly mast cells, and to provoke release of histamine, slow-reacting substances, and other agents. Its level may be elevated in some types of asthma, eczema, and parasitic disease. It has a single subclass: IgE1 (γ_1E globulin). Called also *globulin E, IgND,* and *protein E.* **exocrine i.,** see *i. A.* **i. G (IgG),** a major immunoglobulin class found in human serum, which is important in immunity against many diseases and is involved in hypersensitivities. It has four subclasses: IgG1, IgG2, IgG3, and IgG4 (γ_1G, γ_2G, γ_3G, and $_4$G globulins, respectively). Called also *γG globulin, globulin G,* and *protein G.* **i. M (IgM),** an immuno-globulin class consisting of five monomer units. It is involved in the early immune response, being detectable by the third day, peaking by the fifth or sixth day, and rapidly diminishing thereafter. IgM plays a role in the internal invasion of bacteria through its cytolytic and agglutinating properties. It has a single subclass: IgM1 (γ_1M globulin) Called also *M globulin, globulin M, macroglobulin,* and *protein M.* **secretory i., secretory i. A (IgA),** see *i. A.* **serum i. A,** see *i. A.*

immunoglobulinopathy (im″u-no-glob″u-lin-op′ah-the) gammopathy.

immunohematology (im″u-no-hem″ah-tol′o-je) the branch of hematology concerned with immune properties and mechanisms, as when dealing with blood groups.

immunologic, immunological (im″u-no-loj′ik, im″u-no-loj′e-kal) pertaining to immunology.

immunologist (im″u-nol′o-jist) one who is an expert or specializes in immunology.

immunology (im″u-nol′o-je) that branch of biomedical science concerned with the study of all aspects of the immune response, including immunopathology and the immune mechanisms that endow the animal with the capacity to recognize materials as foreign to itself and to produce antibodies and sensitized lymphocytes that lead to the ability of the host to neutralize, eliminate, or metabolize them with or without injury to its own tissues. See also IMMUNOPATHOLOGY.

immunopathology (im″u-no-pah-thol′o-je) that branch of immunology concerned with the study of immune responses associated with disease. The reactions may be due to immune specificities directed to the patient's own tissues (*autoimmune disease*) or to antibodies or lymphocytes reacting with foreign antigens, and may involve the activation of complement and the release of mediators that lead to inflammation.

immunopotentiation (im″u-no-po-ten″she-a′shun) the augmentation of the host's nonspecific or specific immune responses. The augmentation may be induced by various biologically active substances, including adjuvants, such as Freund's adjuvant and alum. An intense immune response to substances such as mycobacteria may result in nonspecific activation of effector cells, such as macrophages, with a resultant nonspecific immunity.

immunoprecipitation (im″u-no-pre-sip″ĭ-ta′shun) precipitation due to the formation of complexes of antigen reacting with specific antibody.

immunoprophylaxis (im″u-no-pro″fi-lak′sis) the prevention of disease by the use of vaccines, or other agents, which provide the host with an immune mechanism to resist invasion by a microorganism or cancer or to neutralize a toxic substance.

immunoprotein (im″u-no-pro′te-in) immunoglobulin.

immunoreaction (ĭ-mu″no-re-ak′shun) the reaction of an antigen with antibody or a specific lymphocyte, which may result in recognized or unrecognized manifestations.

immunoselection (im″u-no-se-lek′shun) the selection from an array of lymphocytes with a variety of specificities, of those lymphocytes with receptors complementary to determinants of an antigen. The interaction of antigen with receptors on the lymphocyte may induce a proliferative response with the generation of antibody effector lymphocytes and memory cells.

immunosorbent (im″u-no-sor′bent) an insoluble support for antigen or antibody used to adsorb homologous antibodies or antigens, respectively, from a mixture; the antibodies or antigens so removed may then be eluted in pure form. See also absorption METHOD.

immunosuppressant (im″u-no-su-presh′ant) immunosuppressive.

immunosuppression (im″u-no-su-presh′un) the prevention or diminution of expression of immune response through the use of agents such as radiation, antimetabolites, cytotoxic agents, and anti-inflammatory drugs. Most commonly used in preventing graft rejection. Certain therapeutic procedures may also result in the generation of suppressor cells that are cytotoxic and cause a reduction in immune responses. Called also *immune suppression.*

immunosuppressive (im″u-no-su-pres′iv) 1. pertaining to or inducing immunosuppression. 2. immunosuppressive AGENT.

immunotherapy (ĭ-mu″no-ther′ah-pe) therapy of diseases through the use of active or passive specific immunization or nonspecifically, as in immunopotentiation.

IMP individual Medicaid PRACTITIONER.

IMPA incisal mandibular plane ANGLE.

impact (im′pakt) [L. *impactus*] a sudden and forcible collision. **i. force, i. load,** impact FORCE. **i. strength,** impact STRENGTH.

impaction (im-pak′shun) [L. *impactio*] the condition of being firmly lodged or wedged. **dental i.,** the condition in which a tooth is blocked by a physical barrier, usually other teeth, so that its eruption is prevented. See also impacted TOOTH. **distoangular i.,** prevention of eruption of a tooth that lies obliquely in the bone, the crown pointing distally toward the ramus. **food i.,** forceful wedging of food into the periodontium by occlusal forces, which may occur interproximally or in relation to the vestibular or oral tooth surfaces. It is a common cause of gingival and periodontal diseases. See also plunger CUSP. **food i., lateral,** impaction of food interproximally through the act of lateral pressure of lips, cheeks, and tongue, occurring most likely when the gingival embrasure is enlarged by tissue destruction in periodontal diseases or by recession. **horizontal i.,** inability of a tooth that lies in a horizontal position to erupt. **mesioangular i.,** prevention of eruption of a tooth that lies obliquely in the bone, the crown pointing in a mesial direction, usually in contact with the distal surface of the root or crown of another tooth. **vertical i.,** prevention of eruption of a tooth that lies in its normal vertical position by the lack of space for eruption.

impalpable (im-pal′pah-b'l) [L. *in* not + *palpare* to feel] impossible or too small or fine to be detected by touch.

impar (im′par) [L. "unequal"] a general anatomical term meaning unpaired; having no fellow; azygous.

impedance (im-pēd′ans) the opposition to the flow of an alternating current, which is the vector sum of ohmic resistance plus additional resistance, if any, due to induction, to capacity, or to both. Symbol Z. See also impedance ANGLE.

Imperacin trademark for *oxytetracycline hydrochloride* (see under OXYTETRACYCLINE).

imperfection (im″per-fek′shun) the quality of not being perfect or being defective. **lattice i.,** LATTICE imperfection.

imperforate (im-per′fo-rāt) [L. *imperforatus*] not open; lacking a normal opening. See also words beginning ATRETO-.

impermeable (im-per′me-ah-b'l) [L. *in* not + *per* through + *meare* to move] not permitting passage, as of fluid.

impervious (im-per′ve-us) [L. *impervius*] impenetrable; not affording a passage.

impetiginization (im″pe-tij″ĭ-ni-za′shun) the development of impetigo on an area previously affected with some other skin disease.

impetigo (im″pĕ-ti′go) [L.] a streptococcal infection of the skin characterized by fragile, grouped, pinhead-sized vesicles or pustules that become confluent and rupture early, forming rapidly enlarging and spreading erosions with bright yellow crusts that are attached in the center and have elevated margins. **i. pityroi′des, i. sic′ca,** PITYRIASIS alba.

impingement (im-pinj′ment) 1. encroachment or infringement. 2. an area of traumatization of the periodontal ligament caused by an occlusal force on a tooth that produces laterally directed stress. 3. an area of overcompaction, displacement, or compression of a tissue by a unit of a partial denture.

implant[1] (im-plant′) to insert or graft an object or material, such as an alloplastic or radioactive material, a drug capsule, or tissue, into the body of the recipient.

implant[2] (im′plant) 1. an object or material, such as an alloplastic or radioactive material or tissue, partially or totally inserted or grafted into the body for prosthetic, therapeutic, diagnostic, or experimental purposes. See also INSERT and GRAFT. 2. dental i. i. **abutment,** implant ABUTMENT. **alloplastic i.,** an implant made of an alloplastic synthetic material, such as inert metals, ceramics, or plastics. **i. anchor,** endosteal implant ANCHOR. **arthroplastic i.,** an implant for the arthroplastic reconstruction of a joint, such as a cast chrome alloy prosthesis for the glenoid fossa. **blade i.,** a thin wedge-shaped endosseous implant which derives its retention from its anteroposterior width rather than its depth, having a post protruding through the mucoperiosteum to provide abutment for a denture. **i. button,** intramucosal INSERT. **i. cast,** implant CAST. **CM i.,** endosseous i., CM. **dental i.,** a prosthetic device of alloplastic material implanted into the oral tissues beneath the mucosal or periosteal layer to provide support and retention to a partial or full denture. Some authorities restrict the use of the term *implant* to only those devices which have at least one part emerging into the oral cavity through the mucous layer. Endosseous, subperiosteal, mucosal, transosseous, and endodontic implants are the most commonly used dental implants. **endodontic i.,** a metallic implant extending through the root canal of a tooth into the periapical bone structure, to serve as lengthening of the root of a pulpless tooth. **i. denture,** implant DENTURE. **endodontic endosseous i.,** endodontic PIN. **endosseous i.,** a dental implant, usually of metal or, less commonly, of ceramic or polymeric material, consisting of a blade, screw, pin, or vent, which is inserted into the jaw bone through the alveolar or basal bone, either directly or through the root canal and the apex of a tooth, with a post protruding through the mucoperiosteum into the oral cavity to serve as an abutment for dentures or orthodontic appliances, or to serve in fracture fixation. Called also *endosteal i.* See illustration. **endosseous i., ceramic,** one constructed of silicate or porcelain. **endosseous i., CM** [Fr. *crête manche*], a narrow-diameter screw implant for thin ridges. Called also *CM i.* **endosseous i., endodontic,** endodontic PIN. **endosseous i., helicoid,** a two-piece endosseous implant consisting of a helical steel spring (female part) that is inserted into bone, and another part (male part) that may be placed postoperatively and serves as the abutment. **endosseous i., needle,** a thin pin usually implanted into the bone in groups of three in a tripodal form. Called also *pin endosseous i.* **endosseous i., pin,** endosseous i., needle. **endosseous i., spiral,** a hollow or solid corkscrew-type of endosseous implant. **endosseous vent i.,** vent plant, endosseous; see under PLANT. **endosteal i.,** endosseous i. **fabricated i.,** one designed and produced to meet special requirements. **i. framework,** implant SUBSTRUCTURE. **helicoid endosseous i.,** endosseous i., helicoid. **i. infrastructure,** implant SUBSTRUCTURE. **intraosseous i.,** a bone fixation tube used to obtain a canal traversed by a metal tube serving as a denture support. **intra-**

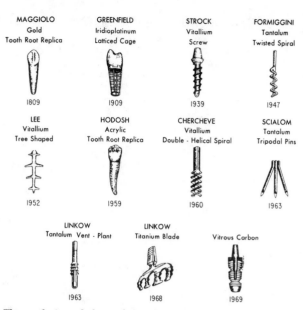

MAGGIOLO	GREENFIELD	STROCK	FORMIGGINI
Gold	Iridioplatinum	Vitallium	Tantalum
Tooth Root Replica	Latticed Cage	Screw	Twisted Spiral
1809	1909	1939	1947
LEE	HODOSH	CHERCHEVE	SCIALOM
Vitallium	Acrylic	Vitallium	Tantalum
Tree Shaped	Tooth Root Replica	Double - Helical Spiral	Tripodal Pins
1952	1959	1960	1963

LINKOW	LINKOW	
Tantalum Vent - Plant	Titanium Blade	Vitrous Carbon
1963	1968	1969

The evolution of the endosseous implant showing the many variations in design and materials from the early attempts up to the more recent. (From R. B. Steiner and R. D. Thompson: Oral Surgery and Anesthesia. Philadelphia, W. B. Saunders Co., 1977.)

periosteal i., a frame, usually made of a chrome-cobalt alloy, fabricated to conform to the shape of the bone, implanted beneath the outer or fibrous layer of the periosteum and resting firmly on the bone, with a post protruding into the oral cavity to serve as an abutment for dentures. Used most commonly for upper fixed bridges and in the treatment of cleft palate. See also implant DENTURE and subperiosteal IMPLANT. **magnetic i.,** denture MAGNET. **i. mesostructure,** implant MESOSTRUCTURE. **i. model,** implant CAST. **monostructure i.,** a series of splinted copings, each over an implant abutment or a natural prepared tooth, being an intermediate superstructure which serves to engage a denture. **mucosal i.,** intramucosal INSERT. **i. neck,** implant POST. **needle endosseous i.,** endosseous i., needle. **oral i.,** any device implanted into oral hard or soft tissue for prosthetic, therapeutic, or diagnostic purposes. See also *dental i.* **pin endosseous i.,** endosseous i., needle. **polymer tooth i.,** a resin replica of the extracted tooth inserted into the socket immediately after the extraction. **i. post,** implant POST. **prosthetic i.,** a prosthetic device implanted either totally or partially into the tissue. **i. restoration,** implant DENTURE. **i. screw,** implant SCREW. **self-tapping i.,** one that cuts its own path into the bone. See also vent plant, endosseous, under PLANT. **spiral endosseous i.,** endosseous i., spiral. **stock i.,** a prefabricated implant, usually endosseous, that is available in standard sizes and forms. **i. structure, intermediate,** implant structure, intermediate; see under STRUCTURE. **subdermal i.,** one shaped like a collar button, which is invaginated into the epithelium. **subperiosteal i.,** a dental implant, consisting of a metal frame, usually made of a chrome-cobalt alloy, implanted under the periosteum and resting on the bone, with a post protruding into the oral cavity, being firmly bound by the mucoperiosteum. Used most commonly as an abutment for upper fixed bridges and in the treatment of cleft palate. See also *intraperiosteal i.,* implant DENTURE, implant SUBSTRUCTURE and subperiosteal implant one-phase TECHNIQUE. **subperiosteal i., anterior,** a subperiosteal implant in the anterior part of an edentulous mandible, with or without posterior subperiosteal extensions, which supplies abutments in the two cuspid regions. **subperiosteal i., complete,** a subperiosteal implant used for an entire edentulous jaw. **subperiosteal i. one-phase technique,** subperiosteal implant one-phase TECHNIQUE. **subperiosteal i., unilateral,** one that is used in one quadrant only, usually serving as an abutment for a free-end denture base. **subperiosteal i., universal,** a complete subperiosteal implant in a semiedentulous jaw, being similar to that for a completely edentulous jaw with the peripheral struts circumventing the natural teeth. **i. substructure,** implant SUBSTRUCTURE. **i. substructure interspace,** implant substructure INTERSPACE. **i. superstructure,** implant SUPERSTRUCTURE. **i. superstructure, temporary,** implant surgical SPLINT. **i. superstructure neck,** implant POST. **transosseous i., transosteal i.,** a dental implant consisting of a bolt passed vertically through the mandible, usually in the region of the canine or first premolar teeth, fixed in placed with a nut, with a post protruding from the top end of the bolt into the oral cavity to provide attachment to a denture, sometimes fitting over a pontic cemented to the post. **two-piece i.,** an endosseous or subperiosteal implant, having the substructure implanted as the first stage of operation, and a separate threaded abutment screwed into it some time after the implantation as the second stage. **universal subperiosteal i.,** subperiosteal i., universal. **vent i., endosseous,** vent plant, endosseous; see under PLANT.

implantation (im″plan-ta′shun) [L. *in* into + *plantare* to set] 1. the insertion of an organ or tissue, such as a tooth, skin, or tendon, in a new site in the body. 2. attachment of the blastocyst to the epithelial lining of the uterus, its penetration through the epithelium, and its embedding in the compact layer of the endometrium occurring about six days after fertilization of the oocyte. 3. the insertion or grafting into the body of biological living, inert, or radioactive material.

implantodontics (im″plan-to-don′tiks) the branch of dentistry dealing with the implantation of artificial devices and materials into the oral hard and soft tissues for prosthetic, therapeutic, or diagnostic purposes; dental implantology.

implantodontist (im″plan-to-don′tist) 1. a dentist who specializes in the practice of implantodontics. 2. IMPLANTOLOGIST.

implantodontology (im-plan″to-don-tol′o-je) IMPLANTOLOGY.

implantologist (im″plan-tol′o-jist) a dentist who specializes in dental implantology. Called also *implantodontist.*

implantology (im″plan-tol′o-je) the study and practice of implantation of artificial devices and materials into the oral hard tissues. Called also *implantodontics* and *implantodontology.*

impressio (im-pres′se-o), pl. *impressio′nes* [L.] an indentation, or concavity; impression. Used in anatomical nomenclature as a general term for such a structure. **i. trigem′ini os′sis tempora′lis** [NA], trigeminal impression of temporal bone; see under IMPRESSION.

impression (im-presh′un) [L. *impressio*] 1. a slight indentation or depression. See *impressio.* 2. a negative copy or the impressed reverse of the surface of any object. 3. an effect produced upon the mind, body, or senses by some external factors. 4. dental i. **anatomic i.,** an impression of the form of a dental arch or portion thereof that records the structures in a passive or unstrained form, making possible a static relationship of a prosthesis produced from such an impression. **basilar i.,** platybasia. **bridge i.,** an impression made for the purpose of constructing or assembling a fixed restoration, fixed partial denture, or bridge. **cleft palate i.,** an impression of the upper jaw made in patients with cleft palate, to be used in the prosthetic repair of the defect. **closed mouth i.,** a dental impression made while the mouth is closed and with the patient's muscular activity molding the borders. **complete denture i.,** 1. one made of the entire edentulous arch of the maxilla or mandible, for the purpose of construction of a complete denture. 2. a negative registration of the entire denture-bearing stabilizing area of the maxilla or mandible. 3. a negative registration of the entire denture foundation and border seal areas of the edentulous mouth. **composite i.,** sectional i. **i. compound,** impression COMPOUND. **correctable i.,** one that may be altered by removing from or adding impression material to its surface or borders. **corrective i.,** a secondary impression made with a mix of impression plaster, zinc oxide–eugenol pastes, or hydrocolloids, placed in a tray produced by the primary impression method, a final impression being obtained with plaster that is spread over the compound, a thin layer of which reproduces the fine detail of the denture area. **dental i.,** an imprint or negative likeness of the teeth and/or edentulous areas, made in plastic material which becomes hardened or set while in contact with the tissue. It is later filled with plaster of Paris or artificial stone to produce a facsimile of the oral structures present. Impressions may be made of the full complement of teeth, of areas where some teeth have been removed, or in a mouth from which all teeth have been extracted. They are classified according to material of which they are made, such as *reversible* and *irreversible hydrocolloid impression, modeling plastic impression, plaster impression, wax impression, silicone impression,* or *Thiokol rubber impression,* etc. **digastric i.,** digastric FOSSA (1). **direct i.,** a technique for making an impression directly from the tissue, as in fabricating gold restorations, such as inlays, where wax is placed into the cavity prepared in the tooth and is subsequently carved in situ to resemble the missing tooth (wax pattern). The pattern is then removed from the tooth and a gold casting is made from it. Called also *direct technique.* Cf. *indirect i.* **direct bone i.,** an impression of denuded bone used in the construction of denture implants. **elastic i.,** one made of an elastic impression material that will allow registration of under-

cut areas by springing over projecting areas and then returning to its original position. **final i.,** secondary i. **fluid wax i.,** wax i., fluid. **functional i.,** an impression of the supporting structures in their functional form, as that of the functional ridge made with the use of a specially molded tray and/or type of impression material that displaces soft and flabby tissue. It is thus made of firm tissues which are not displaced and are therefore considered as being capable of giving support to a denture base. See also functional RIDGE. **hydrocolloid i. (reversible and irreversible),** see *dental i.* **indirect i.,** a technique for making an impression, whereby an impression is first obtained of the tooth and the prepared cavity, and then the impression is removed from the mouth and filled with stone in order to produce a cast of the tooth and the prepared cavity. The stone model (die) is then removed from the impression and the wax pattern is formed on the die, the gold casting being fabricated from the pattern. Called also *indirect technique.* Cf. *direct i.* **lower i.,** mandibular i. **mandibular i.,** an impression of the mandibular jaw and related tissues and dental structures. Called also *lower i.* **i. material,** impression MATERIAL. **maxillary i.,** an impression of the maxillary jaw and related tissues and dental structures. Called also *upper i.* **mercaptan i.,** one made with mercaptan (polysulfide); see impression material, polysulfide, under MATERIAL. **modeling plastic i.,** an impression made in modeling plastic. See *dental i.* **partial denture i.,** a negative copy of the partially edentulous dental arch or its section made for the purpose of constructing a partial denture. **pickup i.,** a dental impression made after the superstructure frame has been inserted in place on the abutments and the oral tissue has healed following implantation. **pickup i., subperiosteal,** subperiosteal pickup i. **plaster i.,** an impression made in dental plaster. See *dental i.* **i. plaster,** impression PLASTER. **preliminary i.,** primary i. **prepared cavity i.,** a negative likeness of a prepared cavity, made with the use of impression materials. **presurgical i.,** an overextended impression of the intact mandible, which serves for the formation of a surgical cast tray for the implantation. **primary i.,** an impression of an edentulous mouth made with a Type II impression compound (tray compound), softened by heat, placed on an impression tray, and pressed against the tissue before it hardens. The primary impression usually lacks fine details of the tissue and is often used as a tray on which other types of impression materials (Type I) are used to line its surface to be placed against the tissue for the reproduction of fine details on the secondary impression. Called also *preliminary i.* and *snap i.* See also *wash i.* **secondary i.,** an impression made by lining with an impression material, such as plaster, zinc oxide–eugenol pastes, or hydrocolloids, in a tray produced by the primary impression method for the reproduction of fine details of an edentulous mouth. Called also *final i.* See also *corrective i.* **sectional i.,** a dental impression made in sections or two or more parts. Called also *composite i.* **silicone i.,** an impression made in silicone. See *dental i.* **snap i.,** primary i. **subperiosteal pickup i.,** an impression of the oral mucosa and the superstructure following subperiosteal implantation, after the surgical wound has healed and the superstructure has been placed over the abutments. **surgical bone i.,** an impression of the bone selected as a support for an subperiosteal implant substructure, made after lifting the mucoperiosteum and exposing the bone proper. **Thiokol rubber i.,** an impression made in Thiokol rubber impression materials. See *dental i.* **trigeminal i. of temporal bone,** the shallow impression in the floor of the middle cranial fossa on the petrous part of the temporal bone, lodging the semilunar ganglion of the trigeminal nerve. Called also *fossa of gasserian ganglion* and *impressio trigemini ossis temporalis* [NA]. **upper i.,** maxillary i. **wash i.,** a technique whereby rough outlines of dental or oral structures on a preliminary impression are lined with a layer of a similar or dissimilar light body impression material to be reintroduced into the mouth for the reproduction of fine details of the teeth and oral structures on the secondary impression. Called also *wash method* and *wash technique.* **wax i.,** an impression made in wax. See *dental i.* **i. wax,** impression WAX. **wax i., fluid,** one made by brushing wax in the liquid state on structures of which the impression is made. **welded inlay i.,** a dental impression produced by incremental welding of the impression compound by heat and impression into an inmobilized matrix.

impressiones (im-pres″e-o′nēz) [L.] plural of *impressio.*

impulse (im′puls) 1. a sudden pushing force. 2. a sudden uncontrollable determination to act. 3. nerve i. 4. the burst of radiation generated during a half cycle of alternating current. **nerve i., neural i.,** the electrochemical process propagated along nerve fibers and their synapses.

In 1. indium. **2.** inion.

in inch.

in- **1.** [L. *in* in, into] a prefix signifying in, within, or into. **2.** [L. *in* not] a negative or privative prefix. **3.** an intensive prefix.

in² square INCH.

in³ cubic INCH.

Inacid trademark for *indomethacin.*

inaction (in-ak'shun) [*in*-(2) + L. *actio* act] imperfect response to a normal stimulus.

inactivate (in-ak'tĭ-vāt) to render inactive; to destroy the activity of.

inactivation (in-ak"tĭ-va'shun) interruption or arrest of any activity.

inadequacy (in-ad'ĕ-kwah-se) [*in*-(2) + L. *adaequare* to make equal] the quality or state of not being able to perform fully; incompetence; insufficiency. **velopharyngeal i.,** faulty velopharyngeal closure with resulting passage of air and sound into the nasopharyngeal and nasal cavities and hypernasal quality of speech.

Inamycin trademark for *novobiocin.*

inanimate (in-an'ĭ-māt) [*in*-(2) + L. *animatus* alive] **1.** without life. **2.** lacking in animation.

inanition (in"ah-nish'un) [L. *inanis* empty] a condition characterized by marked weakness, extreme weight loss, and a decrease in metabolism resulting from prolonged and severe insufficiency of food.

Inapsine trademark for *droperidol.*

inarticulate (in"ar-tik'u-lāt) [*in*-(2) + L. *articulatus* joined] not having joints; disjointed; not uttered like articulate speech.

in articulo mortis (in ar-tik'u-lo mor'tis) [L.] at the very point of death.

inassimilable (in"ah-sim'ĭ-lah-b'l) [*in*-(2) + *assimilable*] not susceptible of being utilized as nutriment.

inborn (in'born) formed or implanted during intrauterine life.

inbreeding (in'brēd-ing) the mating of closely related individuals, or individuals having closely similar genetic constitutions. See also CONSANGUINITY.

incandescent (in"kan-des'ent) [L. *incandescens* glowing] glowing with light and heat; emitting light on being heated. See also thermionic EMISSION.

incarceration (in-kar"ser-a'shun) [*in*-(1) + L. *carcer* prison] unnatural retention or confinement of a part, as may occur in hernia.

incarnative (in-kar'nah-tiv) [L. *incarnare* to invest in flesh] **1.** promoting the formation of granulations. **2.** an agent that promotes granulations.

incasement (in'kās'ment) the act of surrounding or state of being enclosed, as with a case.

incertae sedis (in-ser'te se'dis) [L.] of uncertain or doubtful affiliation or position; said of taxa.

inch (inch) a unit of length, being one-twelfth of a foot, or one-thirty-sixth of a yard, or equivalent to 2.54 centimeters. Abbreviated *in.* See also *Tables of Weights and Measures* at WEIGHT. **cubic i.,** a unit of measure, being equal to a cube each side of which measures 1 inch. It is equal to 16.387 cubic centimeters; 57.75 cubic inches equal 1 quart. Abbreviated *cu in* or *in³.* See also *Tables of Weights and Measures* at WEIGHT. **square i.,** a unit of measure, being equal to a square both sides of which measure 1 inch. It is equivalent to 6.451 square centimeters. Abbreviated *sq in* or *in².* See also *Tables of Weights and Measures* at WEIGHT.

incidence (in'sĭ-dens) [L. *incidere,* from *in* + *cedere,* to occur] an expression of the rate at which a certain event occurs, as the number of new cases of a specific disease occurring during a certain period. See also PREVALENCE. **angle of incidence,** ANGLE of incidence.

incident (in'sĭ-dent) [L. *incidens* falling upon] falling or striking upon, as incident radiation.

incineration (in-sin"ĕ-ra'shun) [*in*-(1) + L. *cineres* ashes] the act or process of burning to ashes; cremation.

incipient (in-sip'e-ent) beginning to exist; coming into existence.

incisal (in-si'zal) **1.** cutting. **2.** pertaining to the cutting edges of incisor and cuspid teeth.

incision (in-sizh'un) [L. *incidere,* from *in* into + *caedere* to cut] **1.** a cut, or a wound produced by cutting with a sharp instrument. **2.** the act of cutting. **3.** the biting and tearing of food into manageable pieces, involving the incisor and canine teeth. **4.** an odontologic landmark; see *i. inferius* and *i. superius.* **angular i.,** in oral surgery, a marginal incision combined with an oblique incision running from the gingival crevice to the buccal or labial sulcus, the oblique incision being placed mesial to the marginal incision so that the operative field remains under direct vision. Used in flap operations on the facial aspects of the alveolus in both the maxillae and mandible. **crucial i.,** a cross-shaped incision. **external bevel i.,** an incision that reduces the thickness of gingiva from the outside, as in gingivectomy or gingivoplasty. **Fergusson's i.,** an incision for excision of the upper jaw; it runs along the junction of the nose with the cheek, around the ala of the nose to the median line, and descends to bisect the upper lip. Called also *Weber-Fergusson* and *Fergusson's operation.* **i. infe'rius,** an odontologic landmark, being the tip of the crown of the most anterior mandibular central incisor. Abbreviated *Ii.* **inner bevel i., internal bevel i.,** inverse bevel i. **inverse bevel i., inverted bevel i.,** incision that reduces the thickness of the gingivae from the inside. Called also *inner bevel i., internal bevel i.,* and *reverse bevel i.* **marginal i.,** in oral surgery, the incision made in the marginal gingiva and used in areas where the dental arch is concave or straight, i.e., the entire premolar and molar areas and palatally and lingually in the incisor region. **preauricular i.,** one anterior to the external ear that permits access to the temporomandibular joint and/or the zygomatic arch and/or the articular eminence. **relief i., relieving i.,** one made to relieve tension in tissue. **reverse bevel i.,** inverse bevel i. **Risdon i.,** incision of the soft tissues in the area beneath the angle of the mandible that permits access to the lateral surface of the mandibular ramus, subcondylar neck, and condylar area. **i. supe'rius,** an odontologic landmark, being the tip of the crown of the most anterior maxillary central incisor. Abbreviated *Is.* **trapezoid i.,** in oral surgery, a marginal incision combined with two terminal oblique incisions; used in the anterior regions of the maxillae and mandible when large areas of bone have to be exposed, such as in cyst operations and apicoectomies. **Weber-Fergusson i.,** Fergusson i. **Wilde's i.,** exposure of the mastoid process by an incision behind the auricle, the bone being opened if necessary; done for mastoid abscess.

incisive (in-si'siv) [L. *incisivus*] **1.** having the power or quality of cutting. **2.** pertaining to the incisor teeth.

incisivus (in-si'siv-us [L.] **1.** incisive. **2.** incisive MUSCLE. **i. la'bii inferio'ris,** incisive muscle of lower lip; see under MUSCLE. **i. la'bii superio'ris,** incisive muscle of upper lip; see under MUSCLE.

incisolabial (in-si"zo-la'be-al) denoting the incisal and labial surfaces of an anterior tooth.

incisolingual (in-si"zo-ling'gwal) denoting the incisal and lingual surfaces of an anterior tooth.

incisoproximal (in-si"zo-prok'sĭ-mal) denoting the incisal and proximal surfaces of an anterior tooth.

incisor (in-si'zer) [L. *incidere* to cut into] **1.** adapted for cutting. **2.** incisor TOOTH. **hawk-bill i.,** shovel-shaped i. **Hutchinson's i's,** Hutchinson's teeth; see under TOOTH. **central i.,** incisor tooth, first; see under TOOTH. **lateral i.,** incisor tooth, second; see under TOOTH. **medial i.,** incisor tooth, first; see under TOOTH. **second i.,** incisor tooth, second; see under TOOTH. **shovel-shaped i.,** an incisor tooth with very prominent lingual marginal ridges bordering a concave lingual surface. Called also *hawk-bill i.* **winged i.,** a rotation deformity of a maxillary incisor in which the distal edge of the tooth protrudes labially.

incisura (in-si-su'rah), pl. *incisu'rae* [L.] a cut, notch, or incision. A general anatomical term for an indention or depression, chiefly on the edge of a bone or other structure. Called also *incisure.* See also NOTCH. **i. ethmoida'lis os'sis fronta'lis** [NA], ethmoidal notch of frontal bone; see under NOTCH. **i. fronta'lis** [NA], frontal INCISURE. **i. interarytenoi'dea laryn'gis** [NA], interarytenoid NOTCH. **i. jugula'ris os'sis occipita'lis** [NA], jugular notch of occipital bone; see under NOTCH. **i. jugula'ris os'sis tempora'lis** [NA], jugular notch of temporal bone; see under NOTCH. **i. lacrima'lis maxil'lae** [NA], lacrimal notch of maxilla; see under NOTCH. **i. mandib'ulae** [NA], sigmoid notch of mandible; see under NOTCH. **i. mastoi'dea os'sis tempora'lis** [NA], mastoid NOTCH. **i. nasa'lis maxil'lae** [NA], nasal notch of maxilla; see under NOTCH. **i. parieta'lis os'sis tempora'lis** [NA], parietal notch of temporal bone; see under NOTCH. **i. Rivi'ni,** tympanic NOTCH. **i. sphenopalati'na os'sis palati'ni** [NA], sphenopalatine notch of palatine bone; see under NOTCH. **i. supraorbita'lis** [NA], supraorbital INCISURE. **i. thyroi'dea infe'rior** [NA], thyroid notch, inferior; see under NOTCH. **i. thyroi'dea supe'rior** [NA], thyroid notch, superior; see under NOTCH. **i. tympan'ica** [NA], tympanic NOTCH.

incisurae (in"si-su're) [L.] plural of *incisura.*

incisure (in-si'zhŭr) [L. *incisura*] a cut, notch, or incision. Called also *incisura.* **digastric i. of temporal bone,** mastoid NOTCH. **ethmoidal i. of frontal bone,** ethmoidal notch of frontal bone;

see under NOTCH. **frontal i.,** a notch located in the supraorbital margin of the frontal bone medial to the supraorbital notch or foramen, for transmission of branches of the supraorbital nerve and vessels. It is frequently converted into a foramen (frontal foramen) by a bridge of osseous tissue. Called also *frontal incisure, frontal notch,* and *incisura frontalis* [NA]. **Henle's palatine i.,** sphenopalatine notch of palatine bone; see under NOTCH. **inferior maxillary i.,** lacrimal margin of maxilla; see under MARGIN. **interarytenoid i.,** interarytenoid NOTCH. **jugular i. of temporal bone,** jugular notch of temporal bone; see under NOTCH. **lacrimal i. of maxilla,** lacrimal notch of maxilla; see under NOTCH. **i. of mandible,** sigmoid notch of mandible; see under NOTCH. **mastoid i. of temporal bone,** mastoid NOTCH. **maxillary i., inferior,** lacrimal margin of maxilla; see under MARGIN. **nasal i. of frontal bone,** nasal margin of frontal bone; see under MARGIN. **nasal i. of maxilla,** nasal notch of maxilla; see under NOTCH. **palatine i.,** pterygoid FISSURE. **palatine i. of Henle,** sphenopalatine notch of palatine bone; see under NOTCH. **parietal i. of temporal bone,** parietal notch of temporal bone; see under NOTCH. **pterygoid i.,** pterygoid FISSURE. **semilunar i. of mandible,** sigmoid notch of mandible; see under NOTCH. **Rivinus' i.,** tympanic NOTCH. **sigmoid i. of mandible,** sigmoid notch of mandible; see under NOTCH. **sphenopalatine i. of palatine bone,** sphenopalatine notch of palatine bone; see under NOTCH. **supraorbital i.,** a notch in the lateral two-thirds of the supraorbital margin of the frontal bone, for transmission of the supraorbital nerve and vessels to the forehead. It may be bridged by fibrous tissue, which is sometimes ossified, forming a bony aperture (*supraorbital foramen*). Called also *incisura supraorbitalis* [NA], *supraorbital notch,* and *supraorbital sulcus.* **thyroid i., inferior,** thyroid notch, inferior; see under NOTCH. **thyroid i., superior,** thyroid notch, superior; see under NOTCH.

incitant (in-sīt'ant) an inciting or causative agent, as one that causes infectious diseases or induces an allergic reaction.

inclinatio (in″klĭ-na'she-o), pl. *inclinatio'nes* [L.] inclination.

inclination (in″klĭ-na'shun) [L. *inclinatio* a leaning] 1. a deviation from the horizontal or vertical slant; a sloping or leaning. 2. deviation of the long axis of a tooth from the perpendicular line, as the *mesial inclination* of the incisors or the *lingual* or *inward inclination* of a molar. 3. deviation of a portion of the surface of a tooth from the general plane of that surface. 4. in describing the angles with the surface of a tooth at which the walls of a cavity may be cut, or of the relation of the opposing walls to each other, as *outward inclination, inward inclination,* etc. 5. inclination of enamel rods from a line perpendicular to the surface of a tooth. **axial i.,** the alignment of a tooth in a vertical plane in relation to its basal bone structure. **condylar i., lateral,** the direction of the lateral condyle path. **condylar guidance i., condylar guide i.,** the angle of inclination of the condylar guidance to an accepted horizontal plane. **lateral condylar i.,** the direction of the lateral condyle path. **lingual i.,** deviation of a tooth from the vertical, in the direction of the tongue.

inclinationes (in″kli-na″she-o'nēz) [L.] plural of *inclinatio.*

incline (in'klīn) 1. an inclined surface; a slope. 2. to deviate from the vertical or horizontal slant. **guiding i's,** the planes and occlusal ridges that determine the path of the supporting cusp during normal lateral and protrusive working excursions. They include the bucco-occlusal inclines (lingual inclines of the buccal cusps) of the maxillary posterior teeth, the lingual inclines of the maxillary anterior teeth, and the linguo-occlusal inclines (buccal inclines of the lingual cusp) of the mandibular posterior teeth. See also GUIDANCE.

inclusion (in-kloo'zhun) [L. *inclusio*] 1. the act of enclosing or condition of being enclosed. 2. anything that is enclosed; often used alone to refer to cell inclusion. **cell i.,** a usually lifeless, often temporary, constituent of the cytoplasm of a cell, such as an accumulation of proteins, fats, carbohydrates, pigments, secretory granules, crystals, or other insoluble materials. **dental i.,** 1. a tooth so surrounded with bony material that it is unable to erupt. 2. a cyst of oral soft tissue or bone.

incoagulability (in″ko-ag″u-lah-bil'ĭ-te) the state of being incapable of coagulation.

incoherent (in″ko-hēr'ent) [*in*-(2) + L. *cohaerere* to cling together] without proper sequence; disordered; denoting an inability to think or articulate one's thoughts clearly.

incompatibility (in″kom-pat″ĭ-bil'ĭ-te) the quality of being incompatible, as blood of ABO and Rh types. **blood i.,** see incompatible BLOOD. **chemical i.,** the quality of not being miscible with another given substance without a chemical change. **physiologic i.,** the quality of not being administrable with another given remedy due to their antagonistic pharmacologic effects. **therapeutic i.,** opposition in therapeutic effect between two or more remedies.

incompatible (in″kom-pat'ĭ-b'l) [L. *incompatibilis*] not suitable for combination, simultaneous administration, or transplantation from one individual to another; mutually repellent.

incompetence (in-kom'pĕ-tens) [*in*-(2) + L. *competens* sufficient] 1. physical or mental inadequacy or insufficiency. 2. the legal status of a person determined by the court to be unable to manage his own affairs. **palatal i.,** the inability of an apparently anatomically normal soft palate to function as the palatopharyngeal sphincter valve.

incompetency (in-kom'pe-ten″se) incompetence. **palatal i.,** the inability of a defective soft palate to effect a functional palatopharyngeal sphincter valve.

incompressible (in″kom-pres'ĭ-b'l) not susceptible of being squeezed together.

incontinence (in-kon'tĭ-nens) [L. *incontinentia*] the inability to refrain from yielding to desires or urges, such as the urge to defecate (*fecal i.*) or urinate (*urinary i.*). cf. CONTINENCE. **bladder i.,** urinary i. **fecal i.,** inability to voluntarily control the anal sphincter, associated with involuntary defecation and flatus. Called also *rectal i.* **rectal i.,** fecal i. **urinary i.,** inability to voluntarily control sphincter muscles of the bladder and urethra, associated with episodes of involuntary urination. Called also *bladder i.*

incontinentia (in-kon″tĭ-nen'she-ah) [L.] incontinence. **Naegeli's i. pigmen'ti,** Naegeli's SYNDROME. **i. pigmen'ti,** Bloch-Sulzberger SYNDROME. **i. pigmen'ti of Asboe-Hansen,** Asboe-Hansen's DISEASE.

incoordination (in″ko-or″dĭ-na'shun) [*in*-(2) + *coordination*] lack of the normal adjustment of muscular motion; failure of organs to work harmoniously.

Incortin trademark for *cortisone acetate* (see under CORTISONE).

increment (in'kre-ment) [L. *incrementum*] growth, increase, augmentation; the amount by which a given quantity or value is increased.

incretory (in'kre-to-re) pertaining to internal secretion; endocrine.

incubation (in″ku-ba'shun) [L. *incubatio*] the induction of development, as (*a*) the development of an infectious disease from the entrance of the pathogen to the appearance of clinical symptoms (see also incubation PERIOD and cf. DECUBATION); (*b*) the development of disease-producing microorganisms in an intermediate or in the ultimate host; or (*c*) the development of microorganisms or other cells in appropriate media.

incubator (in'ku-ba-tor) 1. an apparatus for maintaining a constant and suitable temperature for the development of eggs, cultures of microorganisms, or other living cells. 2. an apparatus for maintaining a premature infant in an environment of proper temperature and humidity.

incurvation (in″ker-va'shun) [L. *incurvare* to bend in] a condition of being bent in.

IND investigational new DRUG.

in d. abbreviation for L. *in di'es*, daily.

Indema trademark for *phenindione.*

indemnification (in-dĕm-nĭ-fi-ka-shun) protecting or insuring against possible damage, hurt, loss, etc. **i. schedule,** see ALLOWANCE.

indemnity (in-dem'nĭ-te) 1. protection or security against damage or loss. 2. compensation for damages or loss sustained. 3. protection from liabilities or penalties incurred by one's actions. See also schedule of allowances, under ALLOWANCE. **aggregate i.,** the maximum dollar amount payable for any disability, period of disability, or covered service under an insurance policy. **i. allowance,** indemnity ALLOWANCE. **i. benefit,** indemnity PROGRAM. **i. plan,** indemnity PROGRAM.

indentation (in″den-ta'shun) [L. *indentatio*] 1. a condition of being notched. 2. a notch, pit, or depression. 3. the act or process of indenting. 4. a depression in the surface of material being tested, made in determining its relative hardness; see HARDNESS test.

indenter (in-den'ter) a device for making indentations or depressions. **Brinell i.,** Brinell hardness indenter POINT. **Knoop i.,** Knoop hardness indenter POINT. **i. point,** hardness indenter POINT. **Rockwell i.,** Rockwell hardness indenter POINT. **Vickers i.,** Vickers hardness indenter POINT.

index (in'deks), pl. *indexes, in'dices* [L.] 1. something that serves as an indicator. 2. the forefinger, or the second digit of the hand. 3. a core or mold used in dentistry to record or maintain the relative position of a tooth or teeth to one another and/or to a cast; a guide, usually of plaster of Paris, used to reposition teeth or casts or parts in order to reproduce their original position. 4.

an expression of the ratio of one dimension to another, determined by multiplying the smaller value by 100 and dividing by the larger value. See also EQUATION and QUOTIENT. **ACH i.,** an index for nutritional condition of children based on measurements of arm girth, chest depth, and hip width. **alveolar i.,** gnathic i. **antibacterial i.,** in competitive inhibition, the minimal value of the ratio of inhibitor to metabolite just sufficient to prevent the growth of the organism. **auricular i.,** the relation of the width to the height of the ear. **auriculoparietal i.,** the ratio of the breadth of the skull between the auricular points to its greatest breadth. **auriculovertical i.,** the ratio of the height of the skull above the auricular point to its greatest height (vertex). **Ayala's i.,** Ayala's QUOTIENT. **Broders' i.,** an index of malignancy based on the fact that the more undifferentiated the cell of a tumor, the more malignant is the tumor. Grade 1 contains one fourth undifferentiated cells; Grade 2, one half undifferentiated cells; Grade 3, three fourths undifferentiated cells; Grade 4, all cells undifferentiated. Called also *Broders' classification.* **calcium i.,** the relative amount of calcium in the blood compared with that in a 1:6000 solution of calcium oxide. **calculus i.,** see *oral hygiene i.* **calculus i., simplified (CI-S),** see *oral hygiene i., simplified.* **calculus surface i.,** an index for short-term studies of calculus accumulation. The four mandibular incisors are graded for presence (1) or absence (0) of calculus on each of four surfaces (lingual, facial, mesial, and distal). The total number of surfaces with calculus is the index, 16 being the maximum possible score. **catalase i.,** a number representing the proportion between the amount (in gm) of hydrogen peroxide decomposed by 1 ml of blood, as compared with the erythrocyte count of the same blood. **I.-Catalogue,** Index-Catalogue of the Library of the Surgeon General's Office, published from 1880 to 1950; replaced by Current List of Medical Literature published to 1959; replaced by Index Medicus. **centromeric i.,** the ratio of the length of the shorter arm of a mitotic chromosome to the total length of the chromosome. **cephalic i.,** a numerical expression of the ratio of various proportions of the skull in a living person. The formula:

$$\frac{\text{maximum cranial breadth} \times 100}{\text{maximum cranial length}}$$

is used in classifying skulls as dolichocephalic, ultradolichocephalic, hyperdolichocephalic, mesocephalic, brachycephalic, hyperbrachycephalic, and ultrabrachycephalic. The formula:

$$\frac{\text{basion-bregma height} \times 100}{\text{maximum cranial length}}$$

may be used for classifying skulls as seen in profile, according to the height of their cranial vaults, as chamecephalic, orthocephalic, and hypsicephalic. The formula:

$$\frac{\text{basion-bregma height} \times 100}{\text{maximum cranial breadth}}$$

permits classification of skulls, as seen in an anterior view, according to the height of their cranial vaults, as tapeinocephalic, metriocephalic, and acrocephalic. The equivalent of *cephalic index* in a dry skull is *cranial index.* See also CEPHALOMETRY and entries under SKULL. **cephalo-orbital i.,** a numerical expression of the cranial capacity, obtained by the following formula:

$$\frac{\text{cranial capacity} \times 100}{\text{capacity of two orbits}} = \text{cephalo-orbital index}$$

cephalorhachidian i., cerebrospinal i. **cerebral i.,** the ratio of the greatest transverse to the greatest anteroposterior diameter of the cranial cavity. Called also *endocranial i.* **cerebrospinal i.,** cephalorhachidian index; a number obtained by the following formula:

$$\frac{\text{final cerebrospinal pressure} \times \text{vol. CSF withdrawn}}{\text{initial cerebrospinal pressure}}$$

chemotherapeutic i., therapeutic i. **color i.,** an expression of the relative amount of hemoglobin contained in the erythrocyte compared with that of a normal individual of the patient's age and sex; divide the percentage of hemoglobin by the percentage of erythrocytes. **Colour I.,** a publication of the Society of Dyers and Colourists and the American Association of Textile Chemists and Colorists containing a list of dyes and dye inter-

mediates. **cranial i.,** one used in craniometry in measuring and classifying dry skulls according to their length/breath proportions. See *cephalic i.* **Cumulated I. Medicus,** an annual publication of the National Library of Medicine, comprising 12 monthly issues of the *I. Medicus.* Abbreviated *CIM.* **cytophagic i.,** the relative phagocytic power of leukocytes from a different source used as a standard. **debris i.,** see *oral hygiene i.* **debris i., simplified (DI-S),** see *oral hygiene i., simplified.* **degenerative i.,** 1. an index indicating the accumulation of granules in the cytoplasm. 2. an index reflecting the increased number of neutrophilic leukocytes with narrow, deeply staining nuclei in the peripheral blood. **dental i.,** a craniometric index obtained by the following formula:

$$\frac{\text{dental length} \times 100}{\text{basinasal length}}$$

Called also *Flower's i.* **I. to Dental Literature,** a quarterly bibliography sponsored jointly by the National Library of Medicine and the American Dental Association from the MEDLARS data base. Abbreviated *IDL.* **Dunning-Leach i.,** gingival-bone COUNT. **effective temperature i.,** an index indicating the warmth due to air temperature, air movement, and humidity. **endemic i.,** the percentage of persons in any locality affected with an endemic disease. **endocranial i.,** cerebral i. **facial i.,** a numerical expression of the ratio of various proportions of the face, obtained by the following formula:

$$\frac{\text{facial height} \times 100}{\text{zygomatic breadth}}$$

Using the facial index, the skull may be classified as hypereuryprosopic, euryprosopic, mesoprosopic, leptoprosopic, and hyperleptoprosopic. See also *morphologic face i.* and *physiognomic upper face i.* **Flower's i.,** dental i. **generation i.,** the number that shows the rate of increase from generation to generation; in the binary division of bacteria, if all survive the rate will be 2; if some die, the rate will be less. **gingival i. (GI),** an index for assessing the quality, severity, and quantity of gingival disease. The circumference of the gingival margin is divided into the vestibular, oral, mesial, and distal margins, and the following score is used: 0 = normal gingiva; 1 = mild inflammation; 2 = moderate inflammation; 3 = severe inflammation. The scores for each tooth are totaled and divided by 4 to determine the gingival index for the tooth. Totaling all the indices and dividing by the number of the teeth in the mouth provides the gingival index for the individual. **gingival-bone i., gingival-bone count i.,** gingival-bone COUNT. **gingival periodontal i.,** an index for measuring gingival and periodontal health, using the gingival status, periodontal status, and irritation index as parameters, and dividing the mandible and maxilla into one anterior and two posterior segments. The gingival status: 0 = firm and tightly adapted tissue; 1 = slight inflammation; 2 = inflammation encircles one or more teeth; 3 = marked inflammation with ulceration, hemorrhage, and other changes. The area with the highest score is the gingival score for the entire segment; the gingival status is obtained by dividing the total score by the number of segments. The periodontal status (assessed with a periodontal probe): 0 = the probe does not extend apical to the cementoenamel junction; 4 = up to 3 mm apical to the cementoenamel junction; 5 = 3–6 mm apical to the cementoenamel junction; 6 = 6 mm of more apical to the cementoenamel junction. The area with the highest score is the periodontal score; the status is determined by dividing the total score by the number of segments. The irritation index: 0 = no materia alba or calculus; 1 = slight amount of materia alba or calculus, no more than 2 mm from the gingival margin; 2 = materia alba covers up to one-half of the crown or gross supragingival calculus; 3 = materia alba or supragingival calculus covers more than one-half of the crown. The area with the highest score for the entire segment and the irritation index is obtained by dividing the total score by the number of segments. **gingival recession i.,** a modification of the PMA index, used for assessing gingival recession, rather than the condition of the attached gingiva. Abnormalities of the gingival papilla (P) and marginal gingiva (M) in relation to each tooth are recorded, plus gingival recession (R) if the root is exposed. The index expressed in percentage is obtained by dividing the number of affected teeth by the total number of teeth present and multiplying by 100. Similar determination can be made for papillary and marginal gingival diseases. **gnathic i.,** the degree of prominence of the upper jaw, expressed as a percentage of the distance from basion to nasion. Called also *alveolar i.* See also total profile ANGLE. **Greene-Vermillion i.,** oral hygiene i., simplified. **height i., height-length i., height-breadth i.,** the relation of the cranial height to the cranial length. See also *vertical i.* **hematopneic i.,** a figure denoting the intensity of blood oxygenation. **Hench-Aldrich i.,** Hench-Aldrich TEST. **hemolytic i.,** a numerical expression of the erythrocyte destruction rate; the average of a 4-day quantitation of fecal urobilinogen (in mg) multiplied by 100 is divided by the hemoglobin (in gm/100 ml) multiplied by total blood volume divided by 100. **hemophagocytic i.,** the relative phagocytic power of leukocytes in the presence of serum. Called also *opsonocytophagic i.* **irritation i.,** see *gingival periodontal i.* **Krebs leukocyte i.,** the number obtained by dividing the percentage of neutrophils by the percentage of lymphocytes. **length-breadth i.,** the breadth of the skull or head expressed as a percentage of its length. **maxilloalveolar i.,** the distance between the two most lateral points on the external surface of the upper alveolar margin, usually opposite the middle of the second permanent molar teeth, divided by the maxilloalveolar length. **I. Medicus,** a bibliography of the principal biomedical literature of the world produced by the MEDLINE system from the MEDLARS data base and published monthly and cumulated annually. Abbreviated *IM.* **mitotic i.,** an expression of the number of mitoses found in a stated number of cells. **Mohs i.,** Mohs hardness number; see under HARDNESS. **monocyte-leukocyte i.,** the number obtained by dividing the number of lymphocytes by the number of monocytes. **morphologic face i.,** a craniometric index obtained by the following formula:

$$\frac{\text{basion-nasion distance} \times 100}{\text{bizygomatic breadth}}$$

opsonic i., a measure of opsonic activity, usually of an antiserum, determined by the ratio of the number of microorganisms phagocytized by normal leukocytes in the presence of the antiserum of an individual to the number phagocytized in serum from a normal individual. See also OPSONIN. **opsonocytophagic i.,** hemophagocytic i. **oral hygiene i.,** a quantitative index for estimating the status of oral hygiene in population groups. The index is composed of the combined *debris index* and *calculus index,* each index based on 12 numerical determinations representing the amount of debris or calculus on the buccal and lingual surfaces of each of three segments of each dental arch: (1) the segment distal to the right cuspid; (2) the segment distal to the left cuspid; and (3) the segment mesial to the right and left first bicuspid. The individual indexes are derived from scores based on the fraction of tooth surface area covered by debris or calculus. Abbreviated *OHI.* Called also *oral hygiene score.* **oral hygiene i., simplified (OHI-S),** an index for determining oral hygiene, using a combination of the *debris index* and the *calculus index.* In the debris index (DI-S) the teeth scored are the vestibular surface of the first fully erupted molar in the right and left maxilla, the vestibular surface of the maxillary right central incisor, and the lingual surface of the first fully erupted molar on the right and left sides of the mandible. 0 = no debris or stain present: 1 = soft debris covering less than one-third on the tooth and the presence of extrinsic stains; 2 = soft debris covering more than one-third, but less than two-thirds, of the tooth surface; 3 = soft debris covering more than two-thirds of the tooth surface. The calculus index (CI-S): 0 = no calculus present; 1 = supragingival calculus on less than one-third of tooth surface; 2 = supragingival calculus covering more than one-third, but less than two-thirds, of the tooth surface; 3 = supragingival calculus covering more than two-thirds of tooth surface. Teeth scored are the same as in the debris index. The indices are calculated by totaling the scores and dividing by 6. Called also *Greene-Vermillion i.* **palatal i.,** palatine i. **palatal height i.,** a numerical expression of the arching of the palate, obtained by the following formula:

$$\frac{\text{palatal height} \times 100}{\text{palatal breadth}} = \text{palatal height index}$$

Using this index, the palate may be classified as chamestaphyline, orthostaphyline, and hypsistaphyline. **palatine i., palatomaxillary i.,** a numerical expression of the ratio of various proportions of the palate, obtained by the following formula:

$$\frac{\text{palatal breadth} \times 100}{\text{palatal length}} = \text{palatine index}$$

Using the palatine index, the palate may be classified as leptostaphyline and brachystaphyline. **periodontal i.,** a quantitative index for scoring gingival and periodontal disease, where 0 = negative finding, 1 = mild gingivitis, 2 = gingivitis, 4 = an early notchlike resorption of the alveolar crest on the radio-

graph, 6 = gingivitis with pocket formation, 8 = advanced destruction with loss of masticatory function.

$$\text{Periodontal index} = \frac{\text{sum of individual scores}}{\text{number of teeth present}}$$

According to the periodontal index, the value for individuals with clinically normal gingivae is from 0 to 0.2; for those with a clinical diagnosis of gingivitis, from 0.3 to 0.9, for those with severe gingivitis with incipient destructive disease, from 0.7 to 1.9; for those with established destructive disease, from 1.6 to 5.0; and for those with severe terminal destructive disease, from about 3.8 to 8.0. Abbreviated *PI.* Called also *periodontal score and Ramfjord i.* **periodontal disease i.,** a quantitative index of the periodontal health of individuals, small groups, and large populations. It is determined on the basis of the examination of six teeth: right first molar, left central incisor, and left first premolar in the maxillary arch; left first molar, right central incisor, and left first premolar in the mandibular arch. Gingivitis is scored on a scale of 0 to 3 on the basis of the extent of inflammation. When the gingival pocket extends below the cementoenamel junction, but not more than a distance of 3 mm, the tooth is given a score of 4. When the pocket extends 3 to 6 mm, the score is 5, and when it extends more than 6 mm, the score is 6. Abbreviated *PDI.* Called also *Russell i., periodontal disease rate,* and *periodontal disease score.* See also *oral hygiene i.* **phagocytic i.,** 1. the average number of bacteria ingested per leukocyte of a patient's blood. 2. the proportion in the blood of multinuclear neutrophil leukocytes with nuclei having three or more lobes. **physiognomic upper face i.,** an anthropometric index based on the following formula:

$$\frac{\text{nasion-stomion distance} \times 100}{\text{bizygomatic breadth}}$$

Pirquet's i. (of nutritional status), multiply the weight in grams by 10, divide the product by the sitting height in centimeters and extract the cube root of this quotient. A result lower than 0.945 indicates faulty nutrition. See also PELIDISI. **plaque i. (PI),** 1. an index for assessing plaque with the use of a dye-containing rinse or wafer and the following score (all teeth are scored except third molars): 0 = no plaque; 1 = separate flecks of plaque at the cervical margin; 2 = a thin continuous band of plaque, up to 1 mm, at the cervical margin; 3 = a band of plaque wider than 1 mm, but covering less than one-third of the crown; 4 = plaque covering at least one-third, but no more than two-thirds, of the crown; 5 = plaque covering two-thirds or more of the crown. The index is determined by dividing the total score by the number of examined teeth. 2. the circumference of the gingival margin is divided into the vestibular, oral, mesial, and distal areas. The following score is used: 0 = no plaque in the gingival area; 1 = a thin film adhering to the marginal gingival and adjacent area of the tooth; 2 = moderate accumulation of soft deposits within the gingival pocket on the marginal gingiva and/or adjacent tooth surface; 3 = abundance of soft matter within the gingival pocket and/or on the gingival margin and adjacent tooth surface. The index is obtained by totaling all the indices and dividing by the number of teeth in the mouth. **PMA i.,** the index used to record the prevalence and severity of gingivitis. The gingiva mesial to each tooth on the vestibular surface is divided into the interdental papilla (P), the marginal gingiva (M), and the attached gingiva (A). Each unit is scored as to presence (1) or absence (0) of inflammation. P, M, and A values are totaled separately, added together, and expressed in one figure (the PMA index). The index is computed from findings in the maxillary and mandibular incisors, canines, and premolars, which have been found to represent 82 to 85 percent of the gingival inflammation in the entire mouth. Called also *Schour-Massler i.* See also *gingival recession i.* **ponderal i.,** an index of body mass determined by dividing the height in inches by the cube root of the weight in pounds. **Pont i.,** the relation of the width of the four incisors to the width between the first premolars and the width between the first molars. **prothrombin i.,** the time of clotting of control plasma, divided by the time of clotting of the patient's blood. **Quarterly Cumulative I. Medicus,** a former publication of the American Medical Association, in which was indexed the principal medical literature of the world; replaced by Cumulated I. Medicus. Abbreviated *QCIM.* **Ramfjord i.,** periodontal i. **refraction i., i. of refraction,** refractive i. **refractive i.,** the refractive power of a medium compared with that of air, which is assumed to be 1. Symbol n or n_{D}. See also interference MICROSCOPE and phase MICROSCOPE. **refractive i., absolute,** an expression of the ratio of the velocity of light in air to its velocity in a specific substance. **refractive i., relative,** an expression of the ratio of the absolute refractive indexes of two different optically dense substances. **retention i.,** an index for assessing retentive factors on the tooth surface adjacent to the marginal gingiva. The circumference of the marginal gingiva is divided into the vestibular, oral, mesial, and distal areas, and the following scores are used: 0 = no caries, calculus, or imperfect margin of dental restoration; 1 = supragingival cavity, calculus, or imperfect margin of dental restoration; 2 = subgingival cavity, calculus, or imperfect margin of dental restoration; 3 = large cavity, abundance of calculus, or grossly insufficient marginal fit of dental restoration. The scores for each tooth are totaled and divided by 4 to determine the retention index for a tooth; totaling all the indices and dividing by the number of the teeth in the mouth provides the retention index for the individual. **Russell i.,** periodontal disease i. **salivary Lactobacillus i.,** the count of lactobacilli per 1 ml of saliva, used in the past as an index of cariogenic activity. **salivary urea i.,** Hench-Aldrich TEST. **saturation i.,** a number indicating the hemoglobin content of an individual's red blood cells as compared with the normal, obtained by dividing the percentage of hemoglobin by the percentage by volume of the cells. **Schour-Massler i. PMA i. sedimentation i.,** the logarithm of the number of millimeters of sedimentation of erythrocytes that would have occurred in 100 minutes at the maximum rate of sedimentation observed at 10-minute intervals over a 2 to 2½-hour period. **simplified calculus i. (CI-S),** see *oral hygiene i., simplified.* **simplified debris i. (DI-S),** see *oral hygiene i., simplified.* **simplified oral hygiene i. (OHI-S),** see *oral hygiene i., simplified.* **therapeutic i.,** an index derived from animal experiments and calculated as the ratio of the lethal dose (or toxic dose) in 50 per cent of those so treated to the effective dose (or therapeutic dose) in 50 per cent of the companion population. It is a population statistic calculated by probit plot; most frequently it is DL_{50}/ED_{50}. Called also *chemotherapeutic i.* **vertical i.,** an anthropometric index obtained by the following formula:

$$\frac{\text{height of skull} \times 100}{\text{length of skull}}$$

vital i., the ratio of births to deaths within a given time in a population. Called also *birth-death ratio.* **volume i.,** the index indicating the size of an erythrocyte as compared with the normal. It is the quotient obtained by dividing the volume of erythrocytes (expressed in percentage of the normal) by the number of erythrocytes (expressed in percentage of the normal). **zygomaticoauricular i.,** the ratio between the zygomatic and auricular diameters of the skull.

indication (in″dĭ-ka′shun) [L. *indicatio*] 1. anything serving to point out something. 2. sign or circumstance which points to or shows the cause, pathology, treatment, or issue of an attack of disease; that which points out; that which serves as a guide or warning.

indicator (in′dĭ-ka″ter) [L.] in chemistry, a substance which, when added to another substance, shows its chemical characteristics, such as acidity or alkalinity, by changing its own physical properties, such as color, or when used in a titration, to indicate the point at which the reaction is complete.

indigency (in′dĭ-jen″se) poverty; inability to support oneself. **medical i.,** a condition whereby a person is unable, through his own resources, to provide himself and his dependents with adequate medical care, without depriving himself and his dependents of basic necessities.

indigestible (in″dĭ-jes′tĭ-b′l) [*in*-(2) + *digestible*] not susceptible of being digested.

indigestion (in″dĭ-jes′chun) lack or failure of digestion; commonly used to denote vague abdominal discomfort after meals.

Indiloy trademark for a *high copper alloy* (see under ALLOY), also containing a small amount of indium.

indirect (in″dĭ-rekt′) [L. *indirectus*] 1. not straight or immediate; circuitous. 2. acting through an intermediary agent.

indiscriminate (in″dis-krim′ĭ-nāt) [*in*-(2) + *discrimen* distinction] affecting various parts without distinction.

indisposition (in″dis-po-zish′un) the condition of being slightly ill; a slight illness.

indium (in′de-um) [from the brilliant indigo line in its spectrum] a metallic element. Symbol, In; atomic number, 49; atomic weight, 114.82; melting point, 156.61°C; specific gravity, 7.31;

valences, 1, 2, 3; group IIIA of the periodic table. It occurs as two natural isotopes (113 and 115) and several artificial radioactive ones (107–112, 114, 116–124). Indium is a very soft, silvery white, ductile, malleable metal, which gives a high-pitched "cry" when bent. It is unaffected by air and water and resistant to alkalies, but attacked by mineral acids. Used in low-melting alloys. Indium is relatively nontoxic on contact and when administered orally, but very toxic when given intravenously or subcutaneously.

individual (in″dĭ-vij′u-al) 1. of or relating to one person. 2. a single human being or organism, as distinguished from a group. 3. single; separate. **eligible i.,** beneficiary.

Indocid trademark for *indomethacin.*

Indoklon trademark for *flurothyl.*

indole (in′dōl) a compound, 2,3-benzopyrrole, occurring as white to yellowish leaflets, turning red on exposure to light or air, and having an unpleasant odor in high concentrations, but changing to pleasant in solution. Indole is obtained from coal tar and indigo, and produced by the decomposition of tryptophan in the intestine, being responsible in part for the peculiar odor of the feces. It is also found in cultures of *Vibrio cholerae* and other bacteria; a color test for its production is used in classifying enteric bacteria. In cases of intestinal obstruction, indole accumulates in the intestine and is found in large quantities in the urine in conjugated form. Used in the production of perfumes, drugs, and flavoring agents.

indolent (in′do-lent) [*in*-(2) + L. *dolens* painful] causing little pain, as an indolent tumor; slow growing, as an indolent lesion.

Indomed trademark for *indomethacin.*

indomethacin (in″do-meth′ah-sin) a synthetic nonaddicting analgesic, antipyretic, and anti-inflammatory drug, 1-(*p*-chlorobenzoyl)-5-methoxy-2-methylindole-3-acetic acid, occurring as a pale yellow to yellow tan, odorless, slightly bitter, crystalline powder that is sensitive to light and is soluble in chloroform, ether, and ethanol, but not in water. Used in the treatment of rheumatoid arthritis, ankylosing spondylitis, osteoarthritis, and gouty arthritis. Its side reactions are sometimes severe and may include gastrointestinal lesions, such as ulcers, hemorrhage, pain, colitis, gastritis, nausea, vomiting, and epigastric distress; ocular disorders, including blurring of vision and corneal and retinal lesions; hepatotoxicity; hematologic complications, such as aplastic anemia, hemolytic anemia, agranulocytosis, leukopenia, thrombocytopenic purpura, and hemorrhagic disorders; hypersensitivity; neurological and mental disorders; deafness; coma; ulcerative stomatitis; epistaxis; hypoglycemia; and glycosuria. Trademarks: Comfortid, Idomethine, Inacid, Indocid, Indomed, Mezolin.

inducer (in-dūs′er) 1. something that causes an event or process to occur. 2. an appliance used for electric induction. 3. a substance that induces protein synthesis. By combining with repressor, it inactivates the inhibiting effect of repressor on operator genes that forestalls messenger RNA transcription, thereby activating protein synthesis. See also REPRESSOR.

induction (in-duk′shun) [L. *inductio*] 1. the act or process of inducing or causing to occur. 2. the appearance of an electric current or of magnetic properties in a body because of the presence of another electric current or magnetic field nearby. 3. the production of an electromotive force by a changing magnetic or electrical field.

inductor (in-duk′ter) tissue elaborating a chemical substance which acts to determine the growth and differentiation of embryonic parts.

induration (in″du-ra′shun) [L. *induratio*] 1. the quality of being hard; the process of hardening. See also SCLEROSIS. 2. an abnormally hard spot or place.

-ine suffix indicating an alkaloid, an organic base, or a halogen.

inert (in-ert′) having little or no chemical action.

inertia (in-er′she-ah) [L.] inactivity, inability to move spontaneously.

in extremis (in-ekstre′mis) [L. "at the end"] at the point of death.

Inf. abbreviation for L. *infun′de*, pour in.

infancy (in′fan-se) the early period of life; see INFANT.

infant (in′fant) [L. *infans,* from *in* not + *fans* speaking] young child; considered to designate the human young from birth or from the termination of the newborn period (the first four weeks of life) to the time of assumption of erect posture (12 to 14 months); it is regarded by some to extend to the end of the first 24 months of life. **battered i.,** battered CHILD. **floppy i.,** a condition of infants characterized by difficulty in holding the head up, sluggish movements, and flaccid paralysis. **newborn i.,** the human young during the first two to four weeks after birth.

infantile (in'fan-tīl) [L. *infantilis*] pertaining to an infant or to infancy.

infantilism (in-fan'tĭ-lĭzm) condition in which the characters of childhood persist in adult life. Cf. PROGERIA. **Herter's i.,** celiac DISEASE. **intestinal i.,** celiac DISEASE. **pancreatic i.,** Andersen's SYNDROME.

infarct (in'farkt) [L. *infarctus*] localized area of ischemic necrosis caused by occlusion of the arterial blood supply or venous drainage; most infarcts are a complication of embolic occlusion of arteries. Called also *infarction*. **anemic i.,** white i. **bland i.,** one whose necrotic tissue is not infected by pathogenic bacteria. **bone i.,** a necrotic area of bone caused by the interruption of the arterial blood supply. **hemorrhagic i.,** 1. red i. 2. one caused by an obstruction of the arterial blood supply, where collateral circulation developed as a response to the incident caused extravasation of large amounts of hemoglobin into spongy tissue, thus giving it a hemorrhagic appearance. **hemorrhagic i., transient,** white i. **pale i.,** white i. **red i.,** local tissue necrosis due to obstruction of a venous blood outlet followed by hemorrhagic extravasation of blood into the surrounding tissue, thus giving it a red appearance. Called also *hemorrhagic i.* **septic i.,** one in which there is infection of the necrotic tissue by pathogenic organisms, which are usually present in the tissue prior to the injury. **white i.,** local necrosis caused by interruption of the arterial supply. Initially, the development of collateral circulation to the injured area may produce seepage of blood into the necrotic area, giving it a hemorrhagic appearance. In solid tissues, the released hemoglobin will soon diffuse out or be converted into hemosiderin and, within 24 to 48 hours, the tissue will assume a pale appearance; the spongy tissue will remain hemorrhagic for long periods of time. Called also *anemic i., pale i.,* and *transient hemorrhagic i.*

infarction (in-fark'shun) [L. *infarcire* to stuff in] 1. an infarct. 2. formation of an infarct. **myocardial i.,** development of coagulation necrosis in the heart tissue due to ischemia resulting from obstruction of the coronary artery by a thrombus or arteriosclerosis. See also coronary OCCLUSION. **pulmonary i.,** localized necrosis of lung tissue caused by obstruction of the arterial blood flow, most often due to pulmonary embolism. Clinical signs vary from nonexistent to chest pain, dyspnea, hemoptysis, and tachycardia. See also pulmonary EMBOLISM.

infection (in-fek'shun) 1. invasion of the body by pathogenic microorganisms and the reaction of the tissue to their presence; often applied to the presence of microorganisms within the tissues, whether or not this results in detectable pathologic effects. 2. a general term applied to invasion of the body by bacteria, protozoa, helminths, and viruses; an infectious disease. Cf. INFESTATION. **aerial i.,** airborne i. **airborne i.,** infection by inhalation of organisms suspended in air. Called also *aerial i.* **apical i.,** one situated at the apex of the root of a tooth as a consequence of an infection in the root canal. **contact i.,** direct i. **cross i.,** one transmitted between individuals infected with different pathogenic microorganisms. **direct i.,** one produced by direct contact with another person. Called also *contact i.* **droplet i.,** one due to inhalation of respiratory pathogens suspended on liquid particles exhaled by someone already infected. **dustborne i.,** infection by pathogens which have become affixed to particles of dust. **ectogenous i., exogenous i. endogenous i.,** one due to reactivation of organisms already present in the body in a dormant focus. **exogenous i.,** one due to organisms not normally present in the body but which have gained entrance from the outside. Called also *ectogenous i.* **focal i.,** one in which pathogenic microorganisms exist in circumscribed areas, from where they or their toxins spread through the blood stream or lymphatic channels to distant sites. Systemic diseases suspected of being caused by oral foci of infection include rheumatoid arthritis, valvular heart diseases, subacute bacterial endocarditis, and various gastrointestinal, ocular, cutaneous, and renal diseases. See also FOCUS of infection. **generalized salivary gland virus i.,** cytomegalic inclusion DISEASE. **herd i.,** an infection of any large group (human or animal). **inapparent i.,** subclinical i. **indirect i.,** infection transmitted by water, food, or other indirect means. **latent i.,** a phase of an established infection in which the pathogenic microorganisms became dormant and symptoms of disease are no longer apparent, as in latent syphilis. **mass i.,** one produced by a large number of pathogenic microorganisms. **metastatic i.,** pyemia. **mixed i.,** one due to different microorganisms. **phytogenic i.,** one due to plant organisms. **pyogenic i.,** one due to pus-producing microorganisms, such as *Staphylococcus aureus, Streptococcus pyogenes,* and a variety of other bacteria, fungi, and viruses. **secondary i.,** one that follows an infection with another pathogenic microorganism. **silent i.,** subclinical i. **subclinical i.,** one in which there are no detectable clinical symptoms. Called also *inapparent i.* and

silent i. **Vincent's i.,** acute necrotizing GINGIVITIS. **water-borne i.,** an exogenous infection caused by pathogenic microorganisms which are transmitted through water. **zoogenic i.,** one due to animal organisms, such as protozoa or helminths.

infectiosity (in-fek"she-os'ĭ-te) the degree of infectiousness of microorganisms.

infectious (in-fek'shus) caused by or being capable of producing a disease that may be transmitted; infective.

infectiousness (in-fek'shus-nes) the state or quality of being infectious.

infective (in-fek'tiv) [L. *infectivus*] capable of producing infection; infectious.

inferior (in-fe're-or) [L. "lower"; neut. *inferus*] lower; situated below, or directed downward. An anatomical term used in reference to the lower surface of an organ or other structure, or to the lower of two (or more) similar structures.

inferolateral (in"fer-o-lat'er-al) [L. *inferus* lower + lateral] situated below and to one side.

inferomedian (in"fer-o-me'de-an) [L. *inferus* low + median] situated in the middle of the underside.

inferoposterior (in"fer-o-pos-tēr'e-or) [L. *inferus* low + *posterior*] situated below and behind.

infertile (in'fer-til) not fertile; exhibiting infertility.

infestation (in-fes-ta'shun) parasitic attack or subsistence on the skin or its appendages, as by insects, mites, or ticks; sometimes used to denote parasitic invasion of the tissues or organs, as by helminths. Cf. INFECTION.

infiltrate (in-fil'trāt) 1. to penetrate the interstices of a tissue or substance. 2. material deposited by infiltration.

infiltration (in"fil-tra'shun) [*in-*(1) + *filtration*] a form of degeneration in which there is diffusion or accumulation in the tissue of substances not normal to it. **adipose i.,** fatty i. **calcareous i.,** a deposit of lime and magnesium salts in the tissues. **calcium i.,** a deposit of calcium salts within the tissues of the body. See also CALCIFICATION. **cellular i.,** the migration and accumulation of cells within the tissues. **fatty i.,** the accumulation of fat within normal cells, occurring as a result of flooding of the cells by excessive circulating levels of lipids. Called also *adipose i.* See also fatty DEGENERATION. **inflammatory i.,** that formed by inflammatory exudation penetrating the interstices of a tissue. **serous i.,** an abnormal accumulation of lymph in a tissue.

infirm (in-firm') [L. *infirmis,* from *in* not + *firmus* strong] 1. weak and feeble, as from disease or old age. 2. one who is weak and feeble.

infirmary (in-fir'mah-re) [L. *infirmarium*] a short-term inpatient and outpatient medical care facility, usually established by organizations or institutions for their personnel, such as one at a university or a military establishment.

inflammation (in"flah-ma'shun) [L. *inflammatio,* from *inflammare* to set on fire] a tissue response to injury by agents such as heat, cold, radiant energy, electricity, chemical agents, mechanical trauma, or bacterial or other infection. It is a protective reaction which serves to destroy, dilute, and wall off (sequester) both the injurious agent and injured tissue, the degree of response being determined by the severity of the injurious stimulus and the reactive capability of the host. Histologically, the reaction involves dilatation of blood vessels with increased permeability and blood flow, exudation of fluids, including plasma proteins, and leukocytic migration into the inflammatory focus. Clinical signs have classically been characterized as localized heat (calor), redness (rubor), swelling (edema), pain (dolor), loss of function (functio laesa), and usually, the appearance of pus. The process may be localized or it may be accompanied by systemic changes, including fever, loss of appetite, listlessness, and debility. The febrile reaction is caused by endogenous pyrogens, lipoproteins from the cell membrane of leukocytes, and exogenous pyrogens, such as bacterial endotoxins, acting upon the temperature control centers of the brain, particularly the hypothalamus. The swelling and redness are largely due to escape of fluid into the perivascular tissue (exudation and transudation). Inflammatory involvement of specific organs or tissues is designated by the suffix *-itis,* as in *tonsillitis.* **acute i.,** that of sudden onset, having the classical signs (see under *inflammation),* associated with vascular congestion and proteinous exudation containing neutrophils, macrophages, and some lymphocytes (*exudative i.*). **adhesive i.,** that which promotes the adhesion of contiguous surfaces. **atrophic i.,** that which results in atrophy and may lead to a deformity. Called also *fibroid i.* **catarrhal i.,** inflammation of any mucus-secreting mucosa, which is associated with excessive elaboration of mucin and copious discharge of mucus and epithelial debris, such as seen in the common cold. **chronic i.,** an inflammatory reaction occurring as a result of repeated or persistent injuries, characterized by a sustained reaction with slow progress, and marked chiefly by the formation of new connective tissue and a proliferative (fibroblastic), rather than an exudative response; usually resulting in permanent tissue damage. **diffuse i.,** that which spreads over a large area, being both interstitial and parenchymatous. **disseminated i.,** that which has a number of distinct foci. **exudative i.,** an inflammatory reaction associated with proteinous exudation containing neutrophils, macrophages, and some lymphocytes. See also *acute i.* **fibrinous i.,** that associated with exudation of coagulated fibrin. **fibroid i.,** atrophic i. **focal i.,** that confined to a single focus or a few limited spots or foci. **granulomatous i.,** that accompanied by the formation of a granuloma or granulomas. See GRANULOMA. **hyperplastic i.,** that which leads to the formation of new connective tissue fibers. **hypertrophic i.,** that marked by increase in size of the elements of the affected tissue. **interstitial i.,** that affecting chiefly the stroma of an organ. **membranous i.,** pseudomembranous i. **metastatic i.,** that which spreads to distant parts by the conveyance of infectious material through the circulatory system. **necrotic i.,** that accompanied by necrosis or death of cells in the affected tissues and organs. See also NECROSIS. **obliterative i.,** that which results in the narrowing of a lumen of a tubular organ, resulting in obstruction. **pseudomembranous i.,** an acute inflammatory reaction, usually to a necrotizing toxin, such as the diphtheria exotoxin, characterized by the formation on a mucosal surface of a false membrane (pseudomembrane) made up of precipitated fibrin, necrotic epithelium, and inflammatory white cells. The toxin causes necrosis of the epithelial surface, resulting in desquamation. The outpouring of fibrinosuppurative exudate traps the necrotic and cellular debris, producing a dirty gray-white, rubbery membrane which layers the inflamed eroded surface, most commonly in the pharynx, larynx, and respiratory passages. Called also *membranous i.* **purulent i.,** suppurative i. **serous i.,** that associated with the production of serous exudate. **subacute i.,** a condition being an intergrade between acute and chronic inflammation, and having some elements of the exudative vascular response modified by proliferation of fibroblasts and infiltration of eosinophils and the mononuclear inflammatory cells of the chronic reaction. **suppurative i.,** that associated with the production of pus. Called also *purulent i.* **ulcerative i.,** that in which there is ulceration of the affected tissue.

inflation (in-fla′shun) [L. *in* into + *flare* to blow] 1. distention with air, gas, or a fluid. 2. the act or process of distending with air or with a gas.

influenza (in″flu-en′zah) [Ital.] an acute viral infection involving the respiratory tract, caused by a number of serologically distinct strains of influenza virus, designated A (with many subgroups), B, and C. It occurs in isolated cases, in epidemics, or in pandemics striking many continents simultaneously or in sequence, and is marked by inflammation of the nasal mucosa, pharynx, and conjunctiva, and by headache and severe, often generalized myalgia. Involvement of the myocardium and of the central nervous system occur infrequently. A necrotizing bronchitis and interstitial pneumonia are prominent features of severe influenza and account for the susceptibility of patients to secondary bacterial pneumonia due to *Diplococcus pneumoniae, Haemophilus influenzae,* and *Staphylococcus aureus.* The incubation period is one to three days and the disease ordinarily lasts for three to ten days. Popularly called *flu.*

Influenzavirus (in″flu-en″zah-vi′rus) a genus of orthomyxoviruses, causing influenza in man and other animals. **I. type A,** a virus associated with human, porcine, equine, and avian influenza. According to the WHO system for the designation of surface glycoprotein antigens, there are four hemagglutinins of the human subtype (H0, H1, H2, H3), one of the swine subtype (Hsw1), two of the equine subtype (Heq1, Heq2), and eight of the avian subtype (Hav1–Hav8); antigenic categories and neuraminidase being classified into two human (N1, N2), two equine (Heq1, Heq2), and four avian (Hav1–Hav4) forms. The human subtype causes influenza and sometimes pneumonia in man, occasionally associated with encephalitis and other complications. The porcine subtype causes influenza and pneumonia in swine, usually in association with *Haemophilus influenzae suis,* also causing human influenza. The equine subtype causes respiratory disease in horses, also producing experimen-

tal infection in human volunteers. The avian subtype (called also *fowl plague virus*) causes diseases in fowl, varying in severity from a mild respiratory disorder to a fatal condition. **I. type B,** a type causing influenza and sometimes pneumonia in man. **I. type C,** a type which probably causes an influenza-like disease in man.

influenzavirus (in″flu-en″zah-vi′rus) any virus of the genus *Influenzavirus.* Written also *influenza virus.*

infra- [L. *infra* beneath] a prefix meaning situated, formed, or occurring beneath the element indicated in the word stem to which it is affixed. See also words beginning HYPO- and SUB-.

infrabulge (in′frah-bulj) the surface of a tooth gingival to the height of contour, or sloping cervically; the surface of the crown of a tooth cervical to the clasp guideline (see survey LINE [3]) or surveyed height of contour, being the retention area of a tooth. Cf. *suprabulge.*

infraclusion (in″frah-kloo′zhun) malocclusion in which a tooth has failed to erupt fully and reach the line of occlusion and is out of contact with the opposing tooth. Called also *infraversion.*

infraconstrictor (in″frah-kon-strik′tor) the inferior constrictor muscle of the pharynx.

infraction (in-frak′shun) [*in*-(1) + L. *fractio* break] an incomplete fracture. See under FRACTURE.

infradentale (in″frah-den-ta′le) an osteometric landmark, being the tip of the alveolar process between the mandibular central incisors. Abbreviated *Id.* See illustration at CEPHALOMETRY.

infraglenoid (in″frah-gle′noid) below the fossa of the glenoid cavity; subglenoid.

infrahyoid (in″fra-hi′oid) below the hyoid bone; subhyoid.

inframandibular (in″frah-man-dib′u-lar) beneath the mandible or the lower jaw; submandibular.

inframarginal (in″frah-mar′ji-nal) below the margin or border; submarginal.

inframaxillary (in″frah-mak′si-lār″e) beneath the upper jaw or maxilla; submaxillary.

infraorbital (in″frah-or′bi-tal) situated beneath or on the floor of the orbit; suborbital.

infrared (in-frah-red′) denoting thermal radiation between the red waves and the radio waves. Called also *ultrared.* See infrared rays, under RAY.

infrasonic (in″frah-son′ik) below the frequency range of the waves normally perceived as sound by the human ear; subsonic.

infrastructure (in″frah-struk′chur) substructure (2). **implant i.,** implant SUBSTRUCTURE.

infratemporal (in″frah-tem′po-ral) below the temporal fossa.

infratonsillar (in″frah-ton′si-lar) [*infra-* + *tonsillar*] below the tonsil.

infraversion (in″frah-ver′zhun) [*infra-* + L. *version* a turning] infraclusion.

infundibula (in″fun-dib′u-lah) [L.] plural of *infundibulum.*

infundibular (in″fun-dib′u-lar) pertaining to or of the nature of an infundibulum.

infundibuliform (in″fun-dib′u-li-form″) [*infundibulum* + L. *forma* form] shaped like a funnel.

infundibulum (in″fun-dib′u-lum), pl. *infundib′ula* [L. "funnel"] 1. any funnel-shaped or cone-shaped passage or part, used in anatomical nomenclature for such a structure. 2. pituitary STALK. **ethmoidal i. of cavity of nose,** a passage connecting the cavity of the nose with the anterior ethmoidal cells and the frontal sinus. Called also *i. ethmoidale cavi nasi* [NA], *i. nasi,* and *i. of nose.* **ethmoidal i. of ethmoid bone,** a variable sinuous passage extending from the middle nasal meatus through the ethmoidal labyrinth, communicating with the anterior ethmoidal cells and often with the frontal sinus. Called also *i. ethmoidale ossis ethmoidalis* [NA], *i. nasi,* and *i. of nose.* **i. ethmoida′le ca′vi na′si** [NA], ethmoidal i. of cavity of nose. **i. ethmoida′le os′sis ethmoida′lis** [NA], ethmoidal i. of ethmoid bone. **i. hypothal′ami** [NA], **i. of hypothalamus,** pituitary STALK. **i. of nose, i. na′si,** 1. ethmoidal i. of cavity of nose. 2. ethmoidal i. of ethmoid bone.

infusion (in-fu′zhun) 1. [L. *infusio,* from *in* into + *fundere* to pour] the act or process of steeping a substance or drug in water, without boiling, to extract those ingredients which are soluble. 2. [L. *infusum*] the solution of preparation produced by such a process. 3. the process of introducing by gravity a fluid other than blood, as a saline solution, into a vein or other parts. Cf. INJECTION (1), INSTILLATION, and INSUFFLATION.

ingate (in′gāt) sprue (2).

ingestion (in-jes′chun) the act of taking in solid foods, medicines, etc., by mouth. See also DIGESTION.

Ingrassia's apophysis, process, wing [Giovanni Filippo *Ingras-*

sia, Italian anatomist, 1510–1580; the first to describe the tooth germ] see great wing of the sphenoid bone and small wing of sphenoid bone, under WING.

ingravescent (in″grah-ves′ent) [L. *in* upon + *gravesci* to grow heavy] gradually increasing in severity.

ingrowth (in′grōth) an inward growth; something that grows inward or into.

INH isonicotinic acid hydrazide; see ISONIAZID.

inhalant (in-ha′lant) a substance that is or may be taken into the body by way of the nose and trachea, or through the respiratory system. **ammonia i.,** SPIRIT of ammonia, aromatic.

inhalation (in″hah-la′shun) [L. *inhalatio*] 1. the drawing of air or other substances into the lungs. 2. a substance to be inhaled as a vapor.

inhaler (in-ha′ler) an apparatus for administering vapor or aero-solized remedies by inhalation. **Allis′ i.,** an apparatus for administering ether by the drop method.

inherent (in-her′ent) [L. *inhaerens* sticking fast] belonging by nature and not as a result of change or circumstance; intrinsic; innate.

inheritance (in-her′ĭ-tans) [L. *heredito* inherit] 1. the acquisition of characteristics or qualities by transmission from parent to offspring. See also GENETICS and HEREDITY. 2. that which is transmitted from parent to offspring. 3. the act or process of inheriting. **alternative i.,** inheritance in which the traits are inherited from one parent. **autosomal dominant i.,** autosomal dominant CHARACTER. **autosomal recessive i.,** autosomal recessive CHARACTER. **dominant i.,** see autosomal dominant CHARACTER and X-linked dominant CHARACTER. **holandric i.,** sex-linked inheritance, whereby a trait caused by a Y-linked gene is transmitted by an affected male to all his sons but to none of his daughters. See also sex-linked CHARACTER. **mendelian i.,** Mendel's LAW. **monofactorial i.,** inheritance of traits from a single gene. **multifactorial i.,** polygenic i. **polygenic i., quantitative i.,** inheritance of quantitative characters, such as skin color, height, and intelligence in humans, which is dependent on the cumulative action of several or many different genes (polygenes), each of which produces a slight effect on the total condition. Called also *multifactorial i.* **recessive i.,** see autosomal recessive CHARACTER and X-linked recessive CHARACTER. **sex-linked i.,** sex-linked CHARACTER. **X-linked dominant i.,** X-linked dominant CHARACTER. **X-linked recessive i.,** X-linked recessive CHARACTER.

inhibition (in″hĭ-bish′un) [L. *inhibere* to restrain, from *in* + *habere* to have] arrest or restraint of a process. **enzyme i.,** prevention of the normal enzyme catalytic reaction from materializing, usually through the use of a chemical substance (enzyme inhibitor). **enzyme i., competitive,** inhibition of the normal substrate-enzyme combination in which the substrate and the enzyme inhibitor compete for the same locus on the enzyme. **reciprocal i.,** the inhibition of one group of muscles on excitation of their antagonists, a phenomenon resulting from reciprocal innervation.

inhibitor (in-hib′ĭ-tor) 1. any substance that interferes with a chemical reaction, growth, or other biological activity. See also RETARDER. 2. a chemical substance that acts to inhibit, or hold in check, the action of a tissue organizer or the growth of microorganisms. 3. a mechanical device for controlling mouth breathing. **aldosterone i.,** any substance that inhibits the action of aldosterone; see aldosterone inhibitor DIURETIC. **antidiuretic hormone i.,** antidiuretic hormone inhibitor DIURETIC. **calculus i.,** see *plaque and calculus i.* **carbonic anhydrase i.,** a substance blocking the action of carbonic anhydrase (carbonate dehydratase); see carbonic anhydrase inhibitor DIURETIC. **cholesterol i.,** a chemical substance that suppresses the production of cholesterol by the body or decreases the level of cholesterol in the blood. **cholinesterase i.,** a chemical substance that neutralizes cholinesterase, thereby preventing acetylcholinesterase from terminating the transmitter action of acetylcholine at the junctions of the cholinergic nerve endings with their effector organs or postsynaptic sites. They cause acetylcholine to accumulate at cholinoceptive sites and thus are potentially capable of producing effects similar to those of continuous stimulation of cholinergic fibers throughout the central and peripheral nervous system. Pharmacologically, they are used as cholinomimetic agents and also as insecticides and nerve gases. Clinical use of cholinesterase inhibitors produces excessive salivation. Called also *anticholinesterase, anticholinesterase agent,* and *anticholinesterase drug.* **coagulation i.,** anticoagulant. **competitive i.,** antimetabolite. **enzyme i.,** a substance that can combine with an enzyme or with enzyme-substrate complex in such a manner as to prevent the normal catalytic reaction. **fibrinolytic i.,** an agent that inhibits the action of

fibrinolytic anticoagulants; see anticoagulant ANTAGONIST. **folic acid i.,** folic acid ANALOGUE. **H₁ i., H₁ receptor i.,** a competitive histamine antagonist which blocks histamine mediation at the H₁ receptor. Principal H₁ inhibitors include diphenhydramine, pyrilamine, chlorpheniramine, chlorcyclizine, promethazine, and various ethanolamines, ethylenediamines, alkylamines, piperazines, and phenothiazines. They inhibit the effect of histamine on capillary permeability and vascular bronchial and other types of smooth muscle, also having local anesthetic properties. Specifically, they suppress itching due to histamine, inhibit the stimulant action of histamine on adrenal chromaffin cells, counteract histamine-evoked salivary and other exocrine secretions, control gastric acid secretion (only when H₂ is also administered), diminish edema in anaphylaxis, both stimulate and depress the central nervous system, counter motion sickness, have anticholinergic activity on the autonomic nervous system, and cause transient hypotension. Therapeutically H₁ inhibitors are used in allergy and motion sickness. Called also *H₁ antagonist* and *H₁ blocking agent.* **H₂ i., H₂ receptor i.,** a competitive histamine antagonist which blocks histamine mediation at the H₂ receptor. Principal H₂ inhibitors are burimamide and metiamide. Inhibition of histamine-stimulated gastric secretion is their principal pharmacologic property. Together with H₁ inhibitors, they influence vasoconstriction. Used chiefly in the treatment of peptic ulcer, Zollinger-Ellison syndrome, and other conditions characterized by excessive gastric secretion. Called also *H₂ antagonist* and *H₂ blocking agent.* **histamine i.,** an agent that counteracts physiologic effects of histamine either by blocking its mediation at the H₁ or H₂ receptors (see *H₁ i.* and *H₂ i.*) or by inhibiting its release from mast cells. Called also *antihistaminic, histamine antagonist,* and *histamine blocking agent.* **monoamine oxidase i.,** any substance that has the ability to block oxidative deamination of monoamines. By blocking monoamine (amine) oxidase, the inhibitors enhance the activity of catecholamines which, otherwise, would have been neutralized by the enzyme, thus acting as sympathomimetics. They elevate the mood of depressed persons, influence sleep patterns, lower blood pressure, and provide relief in angina pectoris. Both hypotension and hypertension, agitation, hallucinations, hyperreflexia, hyperpyrexia, convulsions, brain lesions, liver disorders, cardiovascular complications, excessive central stimulation, tremor, insomnia, hyperhidrosis, agitation, and other disorders are among the adverse reactions. Phenelzine and tranylcypromine are two prototypes of monoamine oxidase inhibitors. **plaque and calculus i.,** a chemical preventive agent which inhibits plaque formation or its attachment to the tooth, destroys or removes the plaque before it calcifies, or alters the chemistry of the plaque as to prevent calcification and, thus, reduces calculus formation. Some inhibitors are incorporated in toothpastes, mouthwashes, chewing gum, and lozenges. **purine i.,** purine ANALOGUE. **pyrimidine i.,** pyrimidine ANALOGUE.

iniac (in′e-ak) pertaining to the inion.

iniad (in′e-ad) toward the inion.

iniencephaly (in″e-en-sef′ah-le) [Gr. *inion* occiput + *enkephalos* brain] a congenital abnormality characterized by malformation of the nape of the neck and of the brain, associated with enlargement of the foramen magnum, and absence of the laminal and spinal processes or the cervical, dorsal, and sometimes lumbar vertebrae; the brain and much of the spinal cord occupy a single cavity.

inio- [Gr. *inion* occiput] a combining form denoting relationship to the occiput.

inion (in′e-on) [Gr. "back of the head"] the tip of the external occipital protuberance (see under PROTUBERANCE). Abbreviated *In.* See also illustration at CEPHALOMETRY.

iniopagus (in″e-op′ah-gus) [*inion* + Gr. *pagos* thing fixed] conjoined symmetrical twins fused at the occiput.

iniops (in′e-ops) [*inion* + Gr. *ōps* eye] double-faced monster with the posterior face incomplete.

initial (in-nish′al) [L. *initialis,* from *initium* beginning] pertaining to the beginning or to the earliest stage of a process or activity.

initiator (ĭ-nish′e-āt″or) 1. something or someone who originates, sets going, or begins some process or action. 2. a chemical agent added to a resin to initiate polymerization.

injectio (in-jek′she-o), pl. *injectio′nes* [*in*-(1) + L. *jacere* to throw] injection.

injection (in-jek′shun) [L. *injectio*] 1. the act of forcibly introducing a liquid into a part, as into the subcutaneous tissues, the vascular tree, or an organ. Cf. INFUSION (3), INSTILLATION, and INSUFFLATION. 2. a substance so forced or administered. Officially, in pharmacy, a solution of a medicament suitable for injection. **hypodermic i.,** subcutaneous i. **jet i.,** injection of a substance in solution through the intact skin by a very fine jet of the solution under high pressure. **i. molding,** injection MOLDING. **parenchymatous i.,** one made into the substance of an organ. **subcutaneous i.,** an injection made into the subcutaneous tissue. Called also *hypodermic i.*

injector (in-jek'tor) a device or instrument for making injections.

injury (in'ju-re) [L. *injuria,* from *in* not + *jus* right] harm or hurt; a wound or maim; usually applied to damage inflicted to the body by an external force. **cotton roll i.,** an iatrogenic injury produced when the dry cotton roll is roughly removed from the mouth and the mucosa adhering to it is torn. **denture i.,** an injury resulting from wearing of artificial dentures. Most common denture injuries include traumatic ulcer, inflammation, hyperplasia, and allergic conditons. **electric i.,** tissue injury or sudden death, depending on the amount of current and its pathways, produced by the passage of an electric current through the body. The electric current injures the tissue by the transformation of electrical energy into heat, causing burns, or by interruption of neural conduction, such as respiratory impulses from the medulla or cardiac rhythm. See also electric BURN. **factitial i.,** accidentally self-induced injury. **iatrogenic i.,** injury resulting from the activity of physicians, dentists, or other health professionals. See IATROGENESIS and IATROGENIC. **radiation i.,** any local or systemic tissue damage caused by exposure to ionizing radiations. Cutaneous changes usually include erythema a few days after exposure, followed by depigmentation, ulcers, necrosis, atrophy, hyperpigmentation, telangiectasis, keratosis, alopecia, and sometimes, neoplasms. Oral lesions include redness of the mucosa, followed by edema, ecchymoses, and fibrous pseudomembranes of the oral mucosa. The tongue may become covered by opalescent plaques that develop into yellowish pseudomembranes. Gingival hemorrhage, loosening of teeth, bone necrosis, osteomyelitis of the jaws, presence of small red dots on the orifices of the excretory ducts of the minor salivary glands of the palate, atrophy, and xerostomia may be associated. See also radiation SICKNESS and RADIOSENSITIVITY, and see table at IRRADIATION.

inlay (in'la) in dentistry, a restoration made outside of a tooth to correspond with the form of a prepared cavity and then cemented into the tooth. See also ONLAY (2). **i. II B,** trademark for a medium hard *dental casting gold alloy* (see under GOLD). **American Gold "M" i. medium,** trademark for a medium hard *dental casting gold alloy* (see under GOLD). **American Gold "M-H" i.,** trademark for a medium hard *dental casting gold alloy* (see under GOLD). **Baker i.,** trademark for a *dental casting gold alloy* (see under GOLD). **Baker i. extra hard,** trademark for an extra hard *dental casting gold alloy* (see under GOLD). **Baker i. hard,** trademark for a hard *dental casting gold alloy* (see under GOLD). **i. burnout,** wax BURNOUT. **cast i.,** gold i. **i. casting wax,** dental inlay casting WAX. **Crown K i.,** trademark for a soft *dental casting gold alloy* (see under GOLD). **epithelial i.,** a method of securing epithelialization of an unhealed deep wound. A mold of the wound cavity is taken and covered with a graft of epidermis, the whole being inserted into the wound cavity, and the edges then approximated with sutures. The mold is removed after 10 days, leaving the cavity completely epithelialized. Called also *Esser operation.* See also epithelial ONLAY. **i. furnace,** inlay FURNACE. **gold i.,** an inlay made of a dental casting gold alloy (see under GOLD). Called also *cast i.* **Goldsmith I i.,** trademark for a soft *dental casting gold alloy* (see under GOLD). **Jelenko special i.,** trademark for a soft *dental casting gold alloy* (see under GOLD). **Leff light i.,** trademark for a soft *dental casting gold alloy* (see under GOLD). **Libra II i. and crown,** see under LIBRA. **Mowrey B i.,** trademark for a medium hard *dental casting gold alloy* (see under GOLD). **i. pattern wax,** dental inlay casting WAX. **porcelain i.,** one made of porcelain. **Sterngold i., Sterngold Bridgette i.,** trademark for a hard *dental casting gold alloy* (see under GOLD). **Veribest 22 Kt i.,** trademark for a soft *dental casting gold alloy* (see under GOLD).

I.N.N. International Nonproprietary Names; the nonproprietary designation recommended by the World Health Organization for any pharmaceutical preparation. Such names are selected according to general principles set forth by the World Health Organization, and lists are published periodically in the *WHO Chronicle.*

innate (in'nāt) [*in*-(1) + L. *nasci* to be born] inborn; congenital.

innervation (in'er-va'shun) [L. *in* into + *nervus* nerve] the distribution or supply of nerves to a part. **double i.,** innervation of a structure by two kinds of nerve fibers, e.g., sympathetic and parasympathetic. **reciprocal i.,** the innervation of muscles around the joints, where the motor centers are so connected in pairs that when one is excited, the center of the corresponding antagonist is inhibited. See also Sherrington's LAW (2).

innidiation (ĭ-nid″e-a'shun) [*in*-(1) + L. *nidus* nest] the development of cells in a part to which they have been carried by metastasis.

innocent (in'o-sent) [L. *innocens,* from *in* not + *nocere* to harm] harmless; benign not malignant; not tending of its nature to a fatal issue.

innocuous (ĭ-nok'u-us) harmless.

innominate (ĭ-nom'ĭ-nāt) [L. *innominatus* nameless, from *in* not + *nomen* name] not having a name; nameless. The term has been applied to certain structures better identified by their descriptive names, as the innominate (petrous) canaliculus or innominate (brachiocephalic) artery.

Innovar trademark for an intravenous basal anesthetic mixture of fentanyl citrate (a narcotic analgesic) and droperidol (a neuroleptic); used in premedication for anesthesia and as an adjunct for induction and maintenance of anesthesia. Its use is contraindicated in infants and in patients with a history of myasthenia gravis and asthma.

innoxious (ĭ-nok'shus) [*in*-(2) + L. *noxius* harmful] not injurious, not hurtful.

ino- [Gr. *is, inos* fiber] a combining form denoting relationship to a fiber, or fibrous material.

inoblast (in'o-blast) [*ino*- + Gr. *blastos* germ] any connective tissue cell in the formative stage.

inochondritis (in″o-kon-dri'tis) [*ino*- + Gr. *chondros* cartilage + *-itis*] inflammation of a fibrocartilage.

inoculation (ĭ-nok″u-la'shun) [L. *inoculatio,* from *in* into + *oculus* bud] in the strict sense, the introduction of viable microorganisms into a host. The term has been generalized to include the introduction into the host of nonviable vaccines, antigens, or other substances.

inophragma (in″o-frag'mah) [*ino*- + Gr. *phragmos* a fencing in] a segment of the sarcomere consisting of the Z and M bands. Called also *ground membrane.*

Inophylline trade name for a preparation of *aminophylline.*

inorganic (in″or-gan'ik) [*in*-(2) + *organic*] 1. having no organs. 2. pertaining to substances not of organic origin. 3. pertaining to compounds that do not contain carbon; see inorganic COMPOUND.

inosinate (in-o'sĭ-nāt) a salt of inosinic acid.

inosine (in'o-sin) a nucleoside, $C_{10}H_{12}O_5N_4$, resulting from the cleavage of inosinic acid; it is a compound of hypoxanthine and ribose. Inosine is an intermediate in animal purine metabolism. Called also *hypoxanthine riboside.*

inositol (in-o'sĭ-tol, in-os'ĭ-tol) an isomer of glucose, hexahydroxycyclohexane, occurring as nonhygroscopic crystals with a sweet taste, which are soluble in water and alcohol, but not in most organic solvents. Because it was found to promote the growth of certain yeasts, and later to be of importance in animal nutrition, it was classified as a member of the vitamin B complex, but its presence in large amounts in animal tissues and the unavailability of a coenzyme of which inositol is a constituent seem to rule out the possibility that it is a true vitamin. Human deficiency has not been recorded and its need in human nutrition has not been established. Previously used in the treatment of lipid metabolism disorders and scurvy, but it has not been shown to be therapeutically effective. Inositol is excreted in large amounts in diabetes mellitus. Its derivative, *myo*-inositol, was found to be essential for the growth of some malignant cells in vitro. Found chiefly in muscles, viscera, and various plants. Experimental deficiency may cause alopecia, retarded growth, and lactation disorders. Called also *meat sugar* and *mouse antialopecia factor.*

inpatient (in'pa-shent) 1. a patient who is hospitalized for at least overnight and is provided with room, board, and continuous general medical and nursing service. 2. pertaining to medical services in a hospital to a patient admitted for at least an overnight stay. Cf. OUTPATIENT. **hospital i.,** see *inpatient* (1).

input (in'put) 1. that which is put in. 2. the power or energy supplied to a machine. 3. in computer technology, information or data transferred or to be transferred from an external source into the internal storage of the computer. Cf. OUTPUT.

inquest (in'kwest) [*in*-(1) L. *in* into + *quaerere* to seek] legal inquiry into the conditions surrounding violent or unexplained death, before the coroner or medical examiner and usually a jury, sometimes also involving dental identification. See also CORONER, dental IDENTIFICATION, and medical EXAMINER.

insalivation (in"sal-ĭ-va'shun) [*in*-(1) + *saliva*] the moistening of food with saliva during mastication.

inscriptio (in-skrip'she-o), pl. *inscriptio'nes* [L., from *in* upon + *scribere* to write] inscription. **i. tendin'ea,** tendinous INSCRIPTION.

inscription (in-skrip'shun) [L. *inscriptio*] 1. a mark, or line. 2. that part of a prescription which contains the names and amounts of the ingredients. See PRESCRIPTION. **tendinous i.,** a fibrous band that crosses the belly of a muscle and more or less completely divides it into two parts. Called also *inscriptio tendinea, intersectio tendinea,* and *tendinous intersection.*

inscriptiones (in-skrip"she-o'nēz) [L.] plural of *inscriptio.*

insecticide (in-sek'tĭ-sīd) [L. *insectum* insect + *caedere* to kill] 1. selectively destructive to insects. 2. any substance selectively poisonous to insects.

insenescence (in"se-nes'ens) the process of growing old.

insensible (in-sen'sĭ-b'l) [*in*-(2) L. + *sensibilis* appreciable] 1. not appreciable by or perceptible to the senses. 2. devoid of consciousness or of sensibility.

insert (in'sert) 1. to put in, introduce, or implant something into something else. 2. something that is implanted. See also IMPLANT. **intramucosal i.,** a nonreactive metal stud, consisting of a base, cervix, and head, attached to a prosthesis that is inserted into a small pocket of oral mucosa through a hole in the mucosa made immediately prior to fitting the denture; most commonly used for added retention of full upper dentures. Called also *mucosal i.* and *implant button.* **mucosal i.,** intramucosal i.

insertion (in-ser'shun) [L. *insertio,* from *in* into + *serere* to join] 1. the site of attachment of an organ or part, as the site of attachment of the distal portion of the muscle to a supporting structure, such as a bone. Cf. ORIGIN. 2. the process of placing a filling or inlay in a dental cavity or part to be restored. 3. the placing of a dental prosthesis in the mouth. See also PATH of insertion. 4. a type of translocation in which a broken part of a chromosome is inserted into a nonhomologous chromosome. Abbreviated *ins.* See also TRANSLOCATION.

insidious (in-sid'e-us) [L. *insidiosus* deceitful, treacherous] coming on in a stealthy manner; of gradual and subtle development.

in situ (in si'tu) [L.] in the natural or normal place without invasion of neighboring tissues.

insoluble (in-sol'u-b'l) [*in*-(2) + L. *solvere* to dissolve] not susceptible of being dissolved.

insomnia (in-som'ne-ah) [*in*-(2) + L. *somnus* sleep + *-ia*] inability to sleep; abnormal wakefulness.

inspection (in-spek'shun) [L. *inspectio, inspicere* to behold] examination by the eye.

inspiration (in"spĭ-ra'shun) [L. *inspirare,* from *in* in + *spirare* to breathe] the act or process of drawing air into the lungs.

inspissation (in"spis-sa'shun) [L. *inspissatio*] the act or process of thickening by means of evaporation.

installation (in'stah-la'shun) 1. the act or process of placing something in position for service or use. 2. a system of machinery or other apparatus. **multiple-tube i.,** a radiologic facility in which there is more than one x-ray source in the same room or in adjacent rooms, being sufficiently close to each other as to pose a potential radiation hazard from their combined workload, thereby requiring special protection.

instep (in'step) the dorsal part of the arch of the foot. See TARSUS (1).

instillation (in"stil-la'shun) [L. *instillare* to put in little by little] the act or process of pouring or administering a liquid very gradually, drop by drop. Cf. INFUSION (3), INJECTION (1), and INSUFFLATION.

institute (in'stĭ-toot) an organization established to further or promote a cause or to enforce certain standards. **American National Standards I.,** the national clearing house for standards. The American National Standards Committee MD156 for Dental Materials and Devices is one of its arms. Abbreviated ANSI. Formerly called *American Standards Association.* **American I. of Oral Biology,** a professional organization open to all members of the dental profession who are interested in emphasizing the oral biologic basis for the practice of dentistry. Abbreviated *AIOB.* **National I. of Occupational Safety and Health,** an agency of the United States government having the responsibility of enforcing all mandatory industrial safety and health standards, including those for dental laboratories. Abbreviated *NIOSH.* **Research I.,** see American Dental Association in Appendix.

instruction (in-struk'shun) 1. the giving of directions or commands. 2. the act or practice of furnishing with knowledge or teaching; training; education. **Oral Hygiene I.,** a program whereby dental patients are instructed in methods of oral

health and plaque control through proper brushing techniques, recommended nutrition, and other aspects of oral hygiene. Abbreviated OHI. Called also *Oral Therapy Control Program* and *Plaque Control Program.*

instrument (in'stroo-ment) [L., from *in* + *struere* to build] a device, apparatus, or appliance for the performance of a delicate operation or procedure. See *dental i.* **beam guiding i.,** an instrument used during radiography to facilitate correct alignment of the central ray. **carving i.,** carver. **condensing i.,** condenser (3). **cone-socket i.,** an instrument in which the shank and blade (or nib) are separate from the handle and the shank is threaded to be screwed into it. **cutting i.,** any instrument used for cutting. In dentistry, a wide variety of handcutting and rotary engine-driven instruments, such as burs, wheels, disks, and points, are used for cutting hard and soft tissues in the mouth, for removing deposits from the teeth, and for finishing restorations. See also *handcutting i.* **dental i.,** any instrument used in the practice of dentistry. See DENTISTRY and see specific specialties, such as ENDODONTICS, ORTHODONTICS, PERIODONTICS, etc. **diamond rotary i.,** a rotary cutting instrument in which metal surfaces are impregnated with bits of industrial diamonds; used with high-speed handpieces for cutting hard tissue, usually in the washed field techniques. Called also *diamond stone.* See illustration. See also DIAMOND (1), diamond

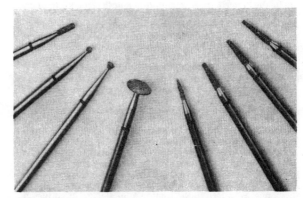

Assorted diamond stones. (From H. O. Torres and A. Ehrlich: Modern Dental Assisting. 2nd ed. Philadelphia, W. B. Saunders Co., 1980; courtesy of Dent-tal Ez.)

BUR, and diamond DISK. **double-ended i.,** one supplied with blades (or nibs) on both ends. **endodontic i.,** see ENDODONTICS and root canal THERAPY. **Kirkland i's,** a set of curets for gingivectomy, especially adapted for removing diseased tissues following the gingivectomy incision and cleansing the root surfaces. They also provide accessibility to all tooth surfaces for the removal of deposits and smoothing the roots. See also Kirkland KNIFE. **i. grasp,** instrument GRASP. **handcutting i.,** any instrument that is held in hand and used for cutting. In dentistry, a variety of hand-operated instruments, including chisels, hatchets, hoes, angle formers, gingival margin trimmers, spoons, excavators, scalers, files, and knives. See DENTISTRY. **long-handled i.,** an instrument made of one piece of metal. **occlusal adjustment i's,** see occlusal ADJUSTMENT. **orthodontic i.,** see ORTHODONTICS. **paralleling i.,** parallelometer. **periodontal i.,** one of several instruments designed for specific purposes in periodontal diagnosis and therapy. Called also periodontal *armamentarium* and *periodontal instrumentarium.* See PERIODONTICS. **root canal i., root canal therapy i.,** see root canal THERAPY. **rotary i.,** any cutting instrument driven by power derived from the dental engine or air pressure, such as burs, disks, and wheels. Those operating at 500 to 6,000 rpm are referred to as conventional, regular, or slow instruments; those rotating at 6,000 to 60,000 rpm are known as medium high-speed instruments; and those which are driven at speeds of 60,000 to 300,000 rpm are called ultra–high-speed instruments. See also HANDPIECE.

instrumental (in"stroo-men'tal) pertaining to or performed by instruments.

instrumentarium (in"stroo-men-ta're-um) the instruments or equipment required for any particular operation or purpose; the physical adjuncts with which a physician or dentist combats disease. See also ARMAMENTARIUM. **endodontic i.,** endontic instruments; see ENDODONTICS and root canal THERAPY. **periodontal i.,** periodontal instruments; see PERIODONTICS.

instrumentation (in″stroo-men-ta′shun) the use of instruments; work performed with instruments.

insuccation (in″su-ka′shun) [L. *insuccare* to soak in, from *in* into + *succus* juice] the thorough soaking of a drug before preparing an extract from it.

insufficiency (in″su-fish′en-se) [L. insufficientia, from *in* not + *sufficiens* sufficient] the quality or state of being insufficient or inadequate to the performance of the allotted duty; incompetence; inadequacy. See also DEFICIENCY and INCOMPETENCE. **adrenal i.,** hypoadrenalism. **muscular i.,** the inability of a muscle to do its normal work by a normal contraction. **palatal i.,** the inability of the soft palate to perform its normal function, where the palatopharyngeal sphincter is incomplete. **velopharyngeal i.,** inability to achieve velopharyngeal closure, due to muscular dysfunction, deficiency of the soft palate or superior constrictor muscle, cleft palate, or other disorders, often resulting in defective speech.

insufflation (in″sŭ-fla′shun) [*in*-(1) + L. *sufflatio* a blowing up] the act or process of blowing a vapor, gas, air, or powder into a body cavity or any empty space. Cf. INFUSION (3), INJECTION (1), and INSTILLATION. **endotracheal i.,** introduction of air into the trachea through a tube passed into the larynx; employed to inflate the lungs in surgery. **mouth-to-mouth i.,** mouth-to-mouth respiration; see artificial RESPIRATION.

insulation (in″su-la′shun) [L. *insulare* to make an island of] 1. the act or process of preventing transfer of energy, such as electricity, heat, or sound, by means of surrounding an object with a shield made of material that is a poor conductor of a specific type of energy. 2. material used as a shield to prevent transfer of energy.

insulin (in′su-lin) [L. *insula* island + -*in* ending indicating a chemical compound] a hormone produced by the β-cells of the islands of Langerhans, composed of two polypeptide chains (proinsulin) containing 21 and 30 amino acids, respectively, joined at two points by disulfide bridges (cysteine). Insulin secretion is regulated by the blood sugar level; the increase of glucose increases the insulin content. Its principal function consists of carbohydrate metabolism regulation. Specifically, it decreases the blood sugar content, increases glucose oxidation, increases muscle glycogen, decreases gluconeogenesis, and decreases ketogenesis. A preparation of the active principle of the pancreas is used in the treatment of diabetes mellitus and sometimes in other conditions. It is inactivated when taken orally, by proteolytic enzymes and acids. Excessive amounts may produce shock. See also DIABETES mellitus and hypoglycemic SHOCK.

Insulon trademark for *mephenytoin.*

insurance (in-shur′ans) the contractual relationship which exists when one party, for a consideration, agrees to reimburse another for loss to a person or thing caused by designated contingencies. The first party is the *insurer* (see CARRIER); the second, the *insured* (see BENEFICIARY); the contract, the *insurance policy;* the consideration, the *premium;* the person or thing, the *risk;* and the contingency, the *hazard* or peril. Insurance may be offered on a profit or nonprofit basis, to groups or individuals. **accident and health i.,** insurance under which benefits are payable in case of disease, accidental injury, or, in some cases, accidental death. **i. administrative agent,** carrier (5). **all risk i.,** a method of insuring whereby coverage is provided against all perils, except those specifically excluded by the contractual conditions. **catastrophic health i.,** major medical POLICY. **certificate of i.,** CERTIFICATE of insurance. **contributory i.,** contributory PLAN. **dental i.,** health insurance which provides coverage in diseases and injuries of the oral and dental systems. **disability income i.,** a form of health insurance that provides periodic payments to replace income when the insured is unable to work as a result of injury or disease. See also workmen's COMPENSATION. **dread disease i.** specified disease i. **employer's liability i.,** insurance against common-law liability of an employer for accidents to employees. See also workmen's COMPENSATION. **first dollar i.,** insurance against the entire loss covered by the policy, without a deductible clause. **group i.,** a policy protecting a specific minimum number of persons, usually of the same employer. **guaranteed renewable i.,** an insurance policy that is renewable at the option of the insured until a stated time, such as the seventieth birthday of the insured. Called also *noncancelable i.* **health i.,** insurance against loss by disease or accidental bodily injury, usually covering the medical costs of treating disease or injury and, in some instances, other losses, such as

loss of present or future earnings. Health insurance may be either individual or group. **health i. for aged and disabled,** the social insurance program authorized by title XVIII of the Social Security Act. See MEDICARE. **health i., individual,** health insurance providing coverage for individuals (and usually their dependents) rather than a group. **health i., supplemental,** health insurance which covers medical expenses not covered by health insurance already held by the insured. **liability i.,** a contract to have an insurer indemnify or pay for any liability or loss in return for the payment of premiums by the insured. **malpractice liability i.,** insurance against alleged professional negligence resulting from improper discharge of professional duties or failure to meet the standards of care. See also MALPRACTICE. **malpractice i., sponsored,** a malpractice insurance plan which involves an agreement by a professional society to sponsor a particular insurer's malpractice insurance coverage, and cooperate with the insurer in the administration of the coverage. **national health i.,** the organization of finances and the distribution of funds to providers for health care of the population. See also national health SERVICE. **no-fault i.,** insurance whereby liability is determined solely as a result of an accident, without an effort to determine the responsibility for the accident. In most instances, awards are determined in advance upon the type and severity of the accident, without awards for pain or suffering. **noncancellable i.,** guaranteed renewable i. **noncontributory i.,** insurance in which the employer pays all the premium; so-called because the employee does not contribute to the cost of the insurance. **self i.,** setting aside of funds by an individual or organization to meet medical or dental care expenses. Written also *self-insurance.* **specified disease i.,** an insurance which provides benefits, usually in large amounts or with high maximums, toward the expense of the treatment of specified disease(s) named in the policy. Called also *dread disease i.* **Supplementary Medical I.,** Part B of Medicare. See MEDICARE.

insured (in-shurd′) beneficiary.

insurer (in-shur′er) carrier (5). **nonprofit i.,** not-for-profit CARRIER. **primary i.,** primary **payer.**

intake (in-tak′) the substances, or the quantities thereof, taken in and utilized by the body. **caloric i.,** the food ingested or otherwise taken into the body.

Intal trademark for *cromolyn sodium* (see under CROMOLYN).

integument (in-teg′u-ment) [L. *integumentum*] a covering or investment; the skin. **common i.,** the covering of the body, or skin, including its various layers and appendages. Called also *integumentum commune* [NA]. See also SKIN.

integumentum (in-teg″u-men′tum) [L. *in* on + *tegere* to cover] integument. **i. commu′ne** [NA], common INTEGUMENT.

in tela (in te′lah) [L.] in tissue; relating especially to stained histological preparations.

intensification (in-ten″si-fi-ka′shun) [L. *intensus* intense + *facere* to make] the act or process of making something more intense or stronger. **image i.,** intensification of the radiographic image, as through the use of the intensifying screen. **image-tube i.,** the use of electronic image amplification by means of an electron-image or electron multiplier tube, capable of producing apparent intensification of the order of 500 to 1,500 times. Called also *image amplification.* **screen i.,** see intensifying SCREEN.

intensimeter (in″ten-sim′ĕ-ter) a device for measuring the intensity of x-rays, based on the variation of electric resistance of a selenium cell under influence of radiation at different intensities.

intensionometer (in′ten″se-o-nom′ĕ-ter) an inometric instrument for measuring the intensity of x-rays. Two series of plates, separated by an air gap that serves as the dielectric, are connected to opposite terminals in a closed chamber. An electric circuit is completed when the air becomes ionized by the x-rays, and the difference in electric potential is registered by deflection of a galvanometer needle.

intensity (in-ten′sĭ-te) [L. *intensus* intense, from *in* on + *tendere* to stretch] the strength or force of an activity. **i. of electric field,** the force exerted on a unit charge in an electric field. **radiant i.,** radiation i. **radiation i.,** the energy or the number of photons or particles of any radiation incident upon a unit area or flowing through a unit of solid material per unit of time. Called also *radiant i.* See also neutron FLUX. **i. of radioactivity,** see *radiation i.* and neutron FLUX.

intensive (in-ten′siv) [L. *intensus,* from *in* on + *tendere* to stretch] of great force or intensity.

inter- [L. *inter* between] a prefix meaning situated, formed, or occurring between elements indicated by the word stem to which it is affixed. See also INTRA-.

interaction (in′ter-ak′shun) reciprocal action or influence. **antigen-antibody i.,** antigen-antibody REACTION. **drug i.,** a response elicited by two or more drugs acting simultaneously.

interalveolar (in″ter-al-ve′o-lar) between alveoli.

intercalate (in-ter′kah-lāt) [L. *intercalatus*] to insert between.

intercellular (in″ter-sel′u-lar) situated between the cells of any cellular structure.

intercondylar (in″ter-kon′dĭ-lar) situated between two condyles.

intercricothyrotomy (in″ter-kri″ko-thi-rot′o-me) [*inter-* + *cricothyroid* + Gr. *tomē* a cutting] incision of the larynx through the cricothyroid membrane; inferior laryngotomy. Called also *conotomy.* See also superior TRACHEOTOMY.

intercuspal (in″ter-kus-p′l) between cusps.

intercuspation (in″ter-kus-pa′shun) the fitting together of cusps of opposing teeth in occlusion. The cusp-to-fossa relationship of the upper and lower posterior teeth to each other. Called also *interdigitation.*

intercusping (in″ter-kusp′ing) the occlusion of the cusps of the teeth of one jaw with the depression in the teeth of the other jaw.

interdent (in″ter-dent) a double-ended knife designed for removing interdental tissue during periodontal surgery.

interdental (in″ter-den′tal) [*inter-* + L. *dens* tooth] situated between the proximal surfaces of adjacent teeth of the same arch or between any two teeth in the same arch. See also INTEROCCLUSAL and INTERPROXIMAL.

interdentale (in″ter-den-ta′le) a craniometric landmark located between the right and left central incisors, in the midline on the tip of the alveolar septum. Abbreviated *Id.* Called also *point Id.* See illustration at CEPHALOMETRY. **i. inferius,** the midline point between the right and left lower central incisors. Abbreviated *IdI.* Called also *point IdI.* **i. superius,** the midline point between the right and left upper central incisors. Abbreviated *IdS.* Called also *point IdS.*

interdentium (in″ter-den′she-um) interproximal SPACE.

interdigitation (in″ter-dij″ĭ-ta-shun) [*inter-* + L. *digitus* digit] 1. an interlocking of parts by finger-like processes. 2. any one of a set of finger-like processes. 3. intercuspation.

interface (in′ter-fās) 1. a surface serving as a common boundary or space. 2. the area of contact between the walls of a cavity preparation of a tooth and a restoration. 3. in chemistry, the area of contact between two immiscible phases of a dispersion, including: solid/solid (alloys), liquid/liquid (water and oil), solid/gas (smoke and air), solid/liquid (clay and water), and liquid/gas (water and air). 4. in computer technology, a common boundary between automatic data-processing systems or parts of a single system.

interfacial (in″ter-fa′shal) pertaining to an interface.

interference (in″ter-fer′ens) [*inter-* + probably L. *fero, ferre* to bring, to carry, or *ferio, ferire* to strike, to knock] 1. opposition or hampering of an action or procedure. 2. the process in which two or more light, sound, or electromagnetic waves of the same frequency combine to reinforce or cancel each other, the amplitude of the resulting wave being equal to the sum of the amplitudes of the combining waves. 3. an interplay of two intrinsic pacemakers in the heart, one or the other dominating the rhythm. 4. any premature contact point along the occlusal surface of the teeth that prevents maximum contact, function, and proper alignment in full occlusion. See also occlusal contact, deflective, under CONTACT. **cuspal i's,** occlusal contact, deflective; see under CONTACT. **occlusal i's,** occlusal contacts hampering or hindering smooth, gliding, harmonious jaw movements with the teeth maintaining contact.

interferometer (in″ter-fer-om′ĕ-ter) an instrument for measuring lengths or movements by means of the phenomena caused by the interference of two rays of light or sound.

interferometry (in″ter-fer-om′ĕ-tre) a form of holography that permits recording responses of an object to the phenomena caused by interference of two rays of light or sound (acoustic interferometry), thus permitting the measurement of minute movements. In dentistry, it is used chiefly to study the effect of stress on various structures, such as dentures. **laser i.,** that in which a laser light beam is used. See also HOLOGRAPHY.

interferon (in″ter-fēr′on) a class of small soluble proteins produced and released by cells invaded by a virus, which induce in noninfected cells the formation of an antiviral protein that inhibits viral multiplication; although not virus-specific, interferons are more effective in animal cells of the same species that produced them. Interferon production may also be induced by certain bacteria, rickettsiae, etc., and by specifically sensitized lymphocytes following interaction with specific antigen or antigen-antibody complex. The latter form, known as *Type II* or *immune interferon,* is capable of affecting antibody production and cell-mediated immunity. **immune i.,** see *interferon.*

interfibrillar (in″ter-fi′bril-ar) [*inter* + L. *fibrilla* small fiber] between or among fibrils.

interfrontal (in″ter-fron′tal) between the halves of the frontal bone.

interfurca (in″ter-fur′kah), pl. *interfur′cae* [*inter-* + L. *furca* fork] the area lying between and at the base of divided tooth roots.

interfurcae (in″ter-fur′se) [L.] plural of *interfurca.*

intergemmal (in′ter-jem′al) [*inter-* + L. *gemma* bud] between buds, such as taste buds.

interglobular (in″ter-glob′u-lar) [*inter-* + L. *globulus* globule] between or among globules, as of the dentin.

intergonial (in″ter-go′ne-al) between the tips of the two angles of the mandible.

intergrade (in′ter-grād) [*inter-* + L. *gradus* a step] a step or stage between two other stages.

interior (in-tēr′e-or) [L. "inner"; neut. of *interius*] 1. situated inside; inward. 2. an inner part of cavity.

interkinesis (in″ter-ki-ne′sis) [*inter-* + Gr. *kinēsis* motion] a short resting phase sometimes occurring between the first and second division in meiosis, characterized by the presence of two chromatids which tend to diverge due to a lack of attraction. Formerly called *resting phase.*

interlabial (in″ter-la′be-al) [*inter-* + L. *labium* lip] between the lips, or between any two labia.

interlobar (in″ter-lo′bar) [*inter-* + L. *lobus* lobe] between lobes.

interlobular (in″ter-lob′u-lar) [*inter-* + L. *lobulus* lobule] between lobules.

interlock (in′ter-lok′) 1. to engage or interlace one with another. 2. a device which controls access to an area of radiation hazard, either by locking the area to the outside personnel or by removing the hazard before the personnel enter the area.

intermaxilla (in″ter-mak′sil′ah) intermaxillary BONE.

intermaxillary (in″ter-mak′sĭ-lār″e) situated between the maxillae or jaws.

intermediate (in″ter-me′de-āt) [*inter-* + L. *medius* middle] 1. placed between; intervening; resembling, in part, each of two extremes. 2. a substance formed in a chemical process that is essential to the formation of the end product of the process.

intermedin (in″ter-me′din) melanocyte stimulating HORMONE.

intermission (in″ter-mish′un) [L. *intermissio,* from *inter* between + *mittere* to send] an interval; a period of temporary cessation, as between two occurrences or paroxysms.

intermittent (in″ter-mit′ent) [L. *intermittens,* from *inter* between + *mittere* to send] occurring at separated intervals; having periods of activity.

intermural (in-ter-mu′ral) [*inter-* + L. *murus* wall] interparietal; situated between the walls of an organ or organs.

intermuscular (in″ter-mus′ku-lar) [*inter-* + L. *muscularis* muscular] situated between muscles.

intern (in′tern) [Fr. *interne*] 1. an advanced student undergoing on the job training, especially a graduate of a medical or dental school serving and residing in a hospital preparatory to being licensed to practice medicine or dentistry. See also INTERNSHIP. Cf. RESIDENT. 2. to confine within certain geographical or physical boundaries.

internal (in-ter′nal) [L. *internus*] situated or occurring within or on the inside; many anatomical structures formerly called internal are now termed *medial.*

internarial (in″ter-na′re-al) [*inter-* + L. *nares* nostrils] situated between the nostrils.

internasal (in″ter-na′zal) situated between the nasal bones.

International System of Units see SI.

internist (in-ter′nist) a physician who specializes in internal medicine.

internship (in′tern-ship) a period of on the job training, usually in a hospital, which is part of a larger educational program. In medicine, dentistry, podiatry, and some other health professions it consists of a one year program of graduate medical education. See also INTERN (1). Cf. RESIDENCY.

internus (in-ter′nus) [L.] internal; an anatomical term denoting something situated nearer to the center of an organ or a cavity.

interocclusal (in″ter-o-kloo′zal) situated between the occlusal surfaces of cusps of opposing teeth of the mandibular and maxillary arches. See also INTERDENTAL and INTERPROXIMAL.

interoceptor (in″ter-o-sep′tor) any of the specialized nerve endings that are concerned with perceiving and relaying to the central nervous system of visceral stimuli, such as hunger, visceral pain, or thirst. See also RECEPTOR (6).

interoinferiorly (in″ter-o-in-fēr′e-or′le) inwardly and in a downward position or direction.

interorbital (in″ter-or′bĭ-tal) [*inter-* + L. *orbita* orbit] situated between the orbits.

interosseous (in″ter-os′e-us) [*inter-* + L. *os* bone] between bones.

interpalpebral (in″ter-pal′pĕ-bral) [*inter-* + L. *palpebra* eyelid] between the eyelids.

interparietal (in″ter-pah-ri′ĕ-tal) [*inter-* + L. *paries* wall] 1. intermural; situated between the walls of an organ or organs. 2. situated between the parietal bones. See interparietal BONE.

interparoxysmal (in″ter-par″ok-siz′mal) occurring between paroxysms.

interphase (in′ter-fāz) the interval between two successive cell divisions, during which the chromosomes are not individually distinguishable and the normal physiological processes proceed. Formerly called *resting phase.*

interpolar (in″ter-po′lar) [*inter-* + L. *polus* pole] situated between two poles.

interpolation (in-ter″po-la′shun) 1. surgical implantation of tissue. 2. the determination of intermediate values in a series on the basis of observed values.

interposition (in″ter-po-zish′un) the act of placing between.

interproximal (in″ter-prok′sī-mal) between adjoining surfaces, as the space between adjacent teeth. See also INTERDENTAL and INTEROCCLUSAL.

interradicular (in″ter-rah-dik′u-lar) between the roots of multirooted teeth.

intersectio (in″ter-sek′she-o), pl. *intersectio′nes* [L., from *inter* between + *secare* to cut] intersection. **i. tendin′ea,** tendinous INSCRIPTION.

intersection (in″ter-sek′shun) [L. *intersectio*] a site at which one structure cuts across another; a general term denoting a cutting across, or between. Called also *intersectio.* **tendinous i.,** tendinous INSCRIPTION.

intersectiones (in″ter-sek″she-o′nēz) [L.] plural of *intersectio.*

interseptal (in″ter-sep′tal) between septa.

interspace (in′ter-spās) a space between two similar structures. **implant substructure i.,** any of the spaces between the primary and secondary struts of the implant substructure that allows infiltration of tissue in an implant denture.

interstice (in-ter′stis) [L. *interstitium*] a small interval, space, or gap in a tissue or structure.

interstitial (in″ter-stish′al) [L. *interstitialis,* from *inter* between + *sistere* to set], pertaining to or situated in the interstices of a tissue.

intertrigo (in″ter-tri′go) [*inter-* + L. *terere* to rub] a chafe or chafed patch of the skin which occurs especially on opposed surfaces; also the erythema or eczema that may result from a chafe of the skin. **i. labia′lis,** angular STOMATITIS.

interval (in′ter-val) [*inter-* + L. *vallum* rampart] the space or gap between two objects or parts; the lapse of time between two occurrences. **P-R i.,** see ELECTROCARDIOGRAPHY.

intestine (in-tes′tin) [L. *intestinus* inward, internal; Gr. *enteron*] the lower portion of the digestive system, being a tubular structure extending from the pyloric opening of the stomach to the anus. Called also *bowel, gut,* and *intestinum.* See also terms beginning ENTERO-. **large i.,** a tubular structure with a caliber that is generally larger than that of the small intestine. It is about 5 feet in length, its upper end connecting with the small intestine at the ileocecal junction and the other end joining the anus. It receives the digested food from the small intestine and evacuates it out of the body through peristaltic action, absorbing along the way most of the water content of the waste material and some nutrients which have been liberated by the intestinal bacteria, such as vitamins and certain sugars. Called also *intestinum crassum* [NA]. **small i.,** a tough membranous tubular structure in which most digestive activity takes place. It is about 18 feet in length, its upper end connecting with the stomach and the other end emptying into the large intestine at the ileocecal junction. Through its rhythmic contractions, the peristaltic waves, the intestine macerates its contents as a part of the digestive function and propels the digested food into the large intestine. Water, electrolytes, and nutrients are absorbed into the system in the small intestine. Called also *intestinum tenue* [NA].

intestinum (in″tes-ti′num), pl. *intesti′na* [L., from *intestinus* inward, internal] intestine. **i. cras′sum** [NA], large INTESTINE. **i. ten′ue** [NA], small INTESTINE.

intima (in′tĭ-mah) [L.] 1. something innermost. 2. TUNICA intima.

Intocostrin trademark for *tubocurarine chloride* (see under TUBOCURARINE).

intolerance (in-tol′er-ans) [*in-*(2) L. + *tolerare* to bear] inability to withstand or consume. **food i.,** a variety of gastrointestinal disorders attributed in whole or in part to nonallergic mechan-

isms incited by specific foods or properties of foods. Called also *food idiosyncrasy.* Cf. gastrointestinal ALLERGY.

intoxication (in-tok″sī-ka′shun) [L. *in* intensive + Gr. *toxicon* poison] 1. poisoning; the state of being poisoned. 2. the condition produced by excessive use of an alcohol, especially ethanol. **serum i.,** serum SICKNESS.

intra- [L. *intra* within] a prefix meaning situated, formed, or occurring within the element indicated by the word stem to which it is affixed. See also INTER-.

intra-arterial (in″trah-ar-te′re-al) within an artery.

intra-articular (in″trah-ar-tik′u-lar) within a joint.

intrabuccal (in″trah-buk′al) within the mouth or within the cheek.

intracapsular (in″trah-kap′su-lar) within a capsule.

intracartilaginous (in″trah-kar′tĭ-laj′ĭ-nus) within a cartilage; endochondral.

intracavitary (in″trah-kav′ī-tār″e) [*intra-* + *cavitary*] within a cavity.

intracellular (in″trah-sel′u-lar) [*intra-* + *cellular*] within a cell.

intracerebellar (in″trah-ser″ĕ-bel′ar) [*intra-* + *cerebellum*] within the cerebellum.

intracerebral (in″trah-ser″ĕ-bral) [*intra-* + *cerebrum*] within the cerebrum.

intracoronal (in″trah-ko-ro′nal) within the crown of a tooth.

intracorporeal (in″trah-kor-po′re-al) [*intra-* + *corporeal*] within the body.

intracorpuscular (in″trah-kor-pus′ku-lar) [*intra-* + *corpuscular*] within a corpuscle.

Intracort trademark for *hydrocortisone sodium succinate* (see under HYDROCORTISONE).

intracranial (in″trah-kra′ne-al) [*intra-* + *cranial*] within the cranium.

intractable (in-trak′tah-b'l) resistant to cure, relief, or control.

intracutaneous (in″trah-ku-ta′ne-us) [*intra-* + *cutaneous*] within the skin.

intracystic (in″trah-sis′tik) within a cyst.

intradermal (in″trah-der′mal) [*intra-* + *dermal*] within the dermis.

intrafistular (in″trah-fis′tu-lar) within a fistula.

intragalvanization (in″trah-gal″van-i-za′shun) the galvanization of the inner surface of an organ or structure.

intraglandular (in″trah-glan′du-lar) [*intra-* + *glandular*] within a gland.

intrahyoid (in″trah-hi′oid) within the hyoid bone.

intralaryngeal (in″trah-lah-rin′je-al) [*intra-* + *laryngeal*] within the larynx.

intraligamentous (in″trah-lig″ah-men′tus) within a ligament.

intralingual (in″trah-ling′gwal) [*intra-* + *lingual*] within the tongue.

intralobar (in″trah-lo′bar) [*intra-* + *lobar*] within a lobe.

intralobular (in″trah-lob′u-lar) [*intra-* + *lobular*] within a lobule.

intramastoiditis (in″trah-mas″toi-di′tis) inflammation of the mastoid antrum and the cells of the mastoid process.

intramural (in″trah-mu′ral) [*intra-* + L. *murus* wall] 1. within the walls, boundaries, or enclosing units. 2. within the wall of an organ; intraparietal.

intramuscular (in″trah-mus′ku-lar) [*intra-* + *muscular*] within or into the substance of a muscle, as in intramuscular injection.

intranarial (in″trah-na′re-al) within the nostrils.

intranasal (in″trah-na′zal) [*intra-* + *nasal*] within the nose.

intranatal (in″trah-na′tal) occurring during birth.

intraoperative (in″trah-op′er-ah′tiv) occurring during the course of a surgical operation.

intraoral (in″trah-o′ral) [*intra-* + *oral*] within or into the mouth.

intraorbital (in″trah-or′bī-tal) [*intra-* + *orbit*] within the orbit.

intraosseous (in″trah-os′e-us) [*intra-* + *osseous*] within a bone.

intraparietal (in″trah-pah-ri′ĕ-tal) [*intra-* + *parietal*] within the wall of an organ; intramural.

intrastitial (in″trah-stish′al) within the cells or fibers of a tissue.

intravasation (in-trav″ah-za′shun) the entrance of foreign material into a blood vessel.

intravascular (in″trah-vas′ku-lar) [*intra-* + *vascular*] within or into a vessel or vessels.

intravenation (in″trah-ve-na′shun) the entrance or injection of foreign matter into a vein.

intravenous (in″trah-ve′nus) [*intra-* + *venous*] within or into a vein, as in intravenous injection.

intraversion (in″trah-ver′zhun) in orthodontics, malocclusion in which the teeth or other maxillary structures are too near the median plane. Called also *introversion.* Cf. EXTRAVERSION.

intravital (in″trah-vi′tal) occurring during life.

intra vitam (in′trah vi′tam) [L.] during life.

intrinsic (in-trin′sik) [L. *intrinsecus* situated on the inside] 1.

inherent; necessary; essential. 2. situated wholly within, or on the inside.

intro- [L. *intro* within] a prefix meaning into or within.

introflexion (in″tro-flek′shun) [*intro-* + L. *flexio* bending] a bending inward.

intromission (in″tro-mish′un) [*intro-* + L. *mittere* to send] the insertion of one part or instrument into another.

Intropin trademark for *dopamine*.

introversion (in″tro-ver′shun) [*intro-* + L. *versio* a turning] 1. the turning outside in, more or less completely, of an organ. 2. introversion.

intrusion (in-troo′zhun) in orthodontic therapy, a technique of depressing a tooth back into the occlusal plane or an effort to prevent its eruption or elongation during the correction of an excessive overbite. Called also *tooth depression*. Cf. EXTRUSION (3).

intubation (in″tu-ba′shun) [*in*-(1) + L. *tuba* tube] the insertion of a tube, especially the introduction of a tube into the larynx through the glottis, through which anesthetic gases are administered. Also performed in diphtheria and edema of the glottis to allow air to pass into the lungs. **endotracheal i.,** insertion of a tube through the trachea to assure a clear airway and prevent entrance of foreign material into the tracheobronchial tree. **nasal i.,** insertion of a tube into the respiratory or gastrointestinal tract through the nose. **oral i.,** insertion of a tube into the respiratory or gastrointestinal tract through the mouth.

intumescentia (in″tu-mě-sen′she-ah) pl. *intumescen′tiae* [L. "enlargement, swelling"] a general anatomical term for an enlargement or swelling. **i. tympan′ica,** an enlargement on the tympanic branch of the glossopharyngeal nerve. Called also *Valentin's ganglion*.

intumescentiae (in″tu-mě-sen′she-e) [L.] plural of *intumescentia*.

intussusception (in″tus-sus-sep′shun) [L. *intus* within + *suscipere* to receive] a receiving within; prolapse of one part into another, such as one part of the intestine into the lumen of an immediately adjoining part. See also *invagination*.

inunction (in-ung′shun) [L. *in* into + *unguere* to anoint] 1. the act of anointing or of applying an ointment with friction. 2. an ointment made with lanolin as a menstrum; inunctum.

inunctum (in-ungk′tum) [L.] inunction (2).

in utero (in u′ter-o) [L.] within the uterus; said of fetal conditions.

Inv 1. Inv group antigen (see Km ANTIGEN) 2. see Inv FACTOR.

inv inversion (2). See also CHROMOSOME nomenclature.

invagination (in-vaj′ĭ-na′shun) [L. *invaginatio*, from *in* within + *vagina* sheath] the infolding of one part within another. See also *intussusception*.

invalid (in′vah-lid) [L. *invalidus*, from *in* not + *validus* strong] 1. not well and strong. 2. one who is unable to carry out his accustomed work; one who is disabled by illness or infirmity.

invasin (in-va′zin) hyaluronidase.

invasion (in-va′zhun) [L. *invasio*, from *in* into + *vadere* to go] 1. the attack or onset of a disease. 2. the simple harmless entrance of bacteria into the body or their deposition in the tissues, as distinguished from infection. 3. the infiltration and active destruction of surrounding tissue, a characteristic of malignant neoplasms. **furca i.,** a condition in which a bifurcation or trifurcation becomes denuded in periodontal disease. The mandibular first molars tend to be affected most commonly and the maxillary premolars remain the least affected; the number of furcations affected increasing with age. Tooth mobility, sensitivity to temperature changes, and pain are common, but the affected teeth may be symptom-free. The condition may be classified as Class I — an incipient lesion in the furca; Class II — variable degrees of bone destruction in the furca, but not extending through the furcation to another tooth surface; and Class III — bone resorption extending through the interfurca. Called also *denuded furca*, *denuded furcation*, and *furca involvement*.

invasiveness (in-va′siv-nes) 1. the ability of a microorganism to enter the body and to spread more or less widely throughout the tissues; the organism may or may not cause an infection or disease. 2. the ability to infiltrate and actively destroy surrounding tissue, said of malignant neoplasms.

Inversine trademark for *mecamylamine*.

inversion (in-ver′zhun) [L. *inversio*, from *in* into + *vertere* to turn] 1. a turning inward, inside out, upside down, or other reversal of the normal relation of a part. 2. a structural chromosome aberration, consisting of the inverted reunion of the middle segment after breakage of a chromosome at two points, resulting in a change in sequence of genes or nucleotides. Abbreviated *inv*. See also CHROMOSOME aberration.

invertase (in-ver′tās) β-FRUCTOFURANOSIDASE.

invertebrate (in-ver′tě-brāt) 1. any animal lacking a spinal column; a nonvertebrate animal. 2. having no spinal column.

invertin (in-ver′tin) β-FRUCTOFURANOSIDASE.

invest (in′vest) to surround, envelop, or embed in an investment material or tissue.

investing (in-vest′ing) 1. the act or process of covering or enveloping wholly or in part an object, such as a denture, tooth, wax form, crown, etc., with a refractory investment material before curing, soldering, or casting. 2. the covering or enveloping of a tissue or part by another tissue, such as a fascia. See also OBDUCENT. **i. the pattern,** surrounding the wax pattern with an investment material, such as a mix of a plaster, for low temperature casting, or a mix consisting of dental stone, a refractory, and a silica, for high temperature casting. Upon hardening, the investment forms a mold into which casting materials are poured. **vacuum i.,** subjecting the water-investment mixture to a vacuum during the investing procedure, in order to remove air bubbles from the mixture.

investment (in-vest′ment) 1. any tissue, such as fascia, that envelops or covers other tissues or parts. 2. a material applied as a soft paste to a pattern that, upon hardening, will form a mold for casting. In restorative and prosthetic dentistry, a material applied around a wax pattern which is a reproduction of a missing tooth structure, a part of a denture, or appliance, which will harden to form a mold into which materials, such as molten metal or alloy, porcelain, or resin, are poured in the fabrication of dental restorations, dentures, or appliances outside the oral cavity. Plaster of Paris (β-hemihydrate of gypsum) is the usual investment for materials hardening at low temperatures. Refractory investments, such as silica-bonded or phosphate-bonded materials, are used for casting molten metals or alloys or for baking porcelain restorations. The refractory investments usually consist of a powdered refractory, binder, and modifier. A crystalline silica, mostly quartz and cristobalite, is the most commonly used refractory, boric acid and sodium and other chlorides being used as modifiers, and the α-hemihydrate of gypsum (see dental STONE) is the usual binder. Called also *cast i*. **cast i.,** investment (2). **i. cast,** refractory CAST. **casting i.,** material from which the mold is made in fabrication of gold or cobalt-chromium castings. **cristobalite i.,** a dental investment in which cristobalite represents the silica component. **dental i.,** a mixture of the α-hemihydrate of gypsum and silica, used to form molds for the casting of dental restorations in metals and alloys; the α-hemihydrate being used because of its strength and hardness and the silica to produce an expansion of the mold following elimination of the wax pattern by burnout, when the investment is heated above the temperature at which the gypsum dihydrate reverts to the hemihydrate. Investments for casting dental gold alloys are classified into three types: *Type I*, used for the casting of inlays or crowns and when the alloy casting shrinkage compensation is accomplished chiefly by thermal expansion of the investment; *Type II*, used for the casting of inlays, the major mode of compensation being by the hygroscopic expansion of the investment; and *Type III*, used in the construction of partial dentures with gold alloys. See illustration at MOLD. **quartz i.,** a dental investment in which quartz represents the silica component. **refractory i.,** see *investment*.

inv ins inverted insertion. See INSERTION (4), and see also CHROMOSOME nomenclature.

in vitro (in vi′tro) [L.] within a glass; observable in a test tube.

in vivo (in vi′vo) [L.] within the living body.

involucra (in″vo-lu′krah) [L.] plural of *involucrum*.

involucrum (in″vo-lu′krum), pl. *involu′cra* [L. *in* into + *volvere* to wrap] a covering or sheath, such as contains the sequestrum of a necrosed bone.

involution (in″vo-lu′shun) [L. *involutio*, from *in* into + *volvere* to roll] 1. a rolling or turning inward over a rim. 2. a retrograde change, the reverse of evolution; applied especially to a lessening of the size of a tissue.

involvement (in-volv′ment) including something or someone in an activity. **furca i.,** furca INVASION.

iodate (i′o-dāt) any salt of iodic acid; a compound containing the radical IO₃.

iodemia (i″o-de′me-ah) [*iodine* + Gr. *haima* blood + *-ia*] the presence of iodides in the blood.

iodide (i′o-dīd) any binary compound of iodine; a compound of iodine with an element or radical. Iodide inhibits the release of thyroid hormone from the thyroid gland.

iodine (i′o-dīn, i′o-din) [Gr. *ioeides* violet-like, from the color of its vapor] a halogen occurring as bluish black scales or plates with a metallic luster and a characteristic odor and sharp taste and a violet corrosive vapor. Symbol, I; atomic number, 53; atomic weight, 126.9045; valences, 1, 3, 5, 7; group VIIA of the periodic table. It occurs in nature as ^{127}I, but isotopes range from 117 to 139. Radioactive tracer isotopes are 124, 125, 128, and 132, ^{131}I being most commonly used. Iodine is soluble in alcohol, carbon disulfide, ether, chloroform, and other organic solvents, but not in water. The body normally contains 20 to 30 mg of iodine, 50 percent in the muscles, 20 percent in the thyroid gland, 10 percent in the skin, and 6 percent in the bones. It is essential in thyroid hormones and deficiency may cause goiter. In iodine-poor areas, particularly inland and at high altitudes, iodine is added to the drinking water and table salt. Iodine is used in the treatment of hyperthyroidism, as a topical antiseptic, and as an antidote in alkaloid poisoning, and its salts are used in contrast media. Radioactive iodine is used in the diagnosis and treatment of thyroid diseases. In dentistry iodine is used in tincture, applied topically to the mucous membranes as an antiseptic and in disclosing solutions. For daily requirements of iodine, see table at NUTRITION. Ingestion of iodine tincture, especially of more than 30 ml, causes poisoning, which is characterized by brown staining of the oral mucosa (*i. stomatitis*), vomiting of blue vomitus, abdominal pain, gastroenteritis, diarrhea sometimes with bloody stools, edema of the glottis, aspiration pneumonia, dehydration, shock, and death. Toxic reactions are due to the corrosive action of the drug. When ingested, it combines with foodstuffs in the digestive system and the element reaches the blood stream in the form of iodides, with little iodine being absorbed from the intestinal tract. Gastric lavage with a starch solution and sodium thiosulfate solution or protein are used in the treatment of iodine poisoning. Called also *iodism*. See also iodine MUMPS. **i. disclosing solution**, iodine disclosing AGENT. **i. mumps**, iodine MUMPS. **i.-125**, ^{125}I, a radioactive isotope of iodine, having a half-life of 60 days and emitting both beta and gamma rays. Used in the diagnosis and treatment of both benign and malignant disease of the thyroid gland and in scintiscanning of such organs as the lung, liver, kidney, and other parts of the body. **i.-131**, ^{131}I, a radioactive isotope of iodine, having a half-life of 8.04 days and emitting both beta and gamma rays. Used in the diagnosis and treatment of both benign and malignant disease of the thyroid gland and in scintiscanning of such organs as the lung, liver, kidney, and other parts of the body. **povidone-i.**, povidone-iodine. **protein-bound i.**, iodine bound to proteins in the body serum, determination of which constitutes a test of thyroid function. **radioactive i.**, any of the radioactive isotopes of iodine, including ^{124}I, ^{125}I, ^{128}I, ^{131}I, and ^{132}I: ^{131}I and ^{125}I are the most commonly used as tracers and in radiotherapy. Called also *radioiodine*. **i. solution**, a transparent, reddish brown liquid, with the odor of iodine, consisting of iodine and sodium iodide in purified water, each 100 ml of which contains 1.8–2.2 gm iodine and 2.1–2.6 gm sodium iodide. Used as a topical anti-infective agent. **i. solution, compound**, i. solution, strong. **i. solution, strong**, a transparent, deep brown liquid, with the odor of iodine, consisting of iodine and potassium iodide in purified water, each 100 ml of which contains 4.5–5.5 gm iodine and 9.5–10.5 gm potassium iodide. Used as a source of iodine. Called also *compound i. solution* and *Lugol's solution*. **i. stomatitis**, see *iodine*. **i. tincture**, a preparation of iodine and sodium iodide in diluted alcohol, each 100 ml of which contains 1.8–2.2 gm iodine and 2.1–2.6 gm sodium iodide. Used as a topical antiseptic. **i. tincture, strong**, an alcoholic solution of iodine and potassium iodide, each 100 of which contains 6.8–7.8 gm iodine and 4.7–5.5 gm potassium iodide; used as an irritant and antiseptic agent.

iodism (i′o-dizm) iodine poisoning; see IODINE.

Iodochlorol trademark for *chloriodized oil* (see under OIL).

iodoform (i-o′do-form) [*iodine* + *formyl*] a compound with local analgesic, antiseptic, and irritant properties, CHI$_3$. It occurs as a greenish yellow powder or crystals with a strong penetrating odor that are slightly soluble in water or alcohol, but are soluble in olive oil, ether, chloroform, and glycerol, and decomposes at high temperature yielding iodine. Used in antiseptic dusting powder for open wounds. In dentistry, it is impregnated into gauze and ointments for use as dressings in extraction sockets; formerly used in root canal and periodontal treatment. Called also *triiodomethane*.

Iodopaque trademark for *acetrizoate sodium* (see under ACETRIZOATE).

iodophor (i-o′do-for) [*iodine* + Gr. *phoros* bearing] a combination or complex iodine with a solubilizing agent or carrier that liberates free iodine in solution, nonionic surface-active agents sometimes being employed as carriers. Povidone-iodine is the most common iodophor used in dentistry.

Iodosol trademark for *thymol iodide* (see under THYMOL).

Iodothymol trademark for *thymol iodide* (see under THYMOL).

Iodotope trademark for *radioactive sodium iodide* (see under SODIUM).

Ioduril trademark for *sodium iodide* (see under SODIUM).

ion (i′on) [Gr. *iōn* going] an electrically charged atom or molecule. If positively charged, it is called a *cation*; if negatively charged, it is called an *anion*. **hydrogen i.**, the nucleus of the hydrogen atom or a hydrogen atom that has lost its electron; it bears a positive charge equivalent to the negative charge of the electron and is called a proton. Symbol H$^+$. **hydrogen i. concentration**, hydrogen ion CONCENTRATION; see also *pH*.

ionization (i″on-i-za′shun) 1. the act or process of removing one or more electrons from atoms or molecules, thereby creating ions, usually resulting from very high temperatures, electrical discharges, or irradiation. See also ionizing RADIATION. 2. electrolytic dissociation or breaking up of a molecule into two or more negatively and positively charged components (ions); usually when a polar compound is dissolved in water. **avalanche i.**, the multiplicative process in which a single charged particle, accelerated by a strong electric field, produces additional charged particles through collision with neutral gas molecules. Called also *Townsend i.* **i. chamber**, ionization CHAMBER. **primary i.**, 1. in the collision theory, the ionization produced by the primary particles (e.g., photons or electrons). 2. in counter tubes, the total ionization produced by incident radiation without gas amplification. **root canal i.**, ELECTROSTERILIZATION. **secondary i.**, particles, usually electrons, ejected by recoil when a primary ionizing particle passes through matter, each secondary particle constituting a delta ray. **Townsend i.**, avalanche i.

ionizer (i″o-ni′zer) electrolyzer.

ionomer (i-on′o-mer) a polymer having covalent bonds between the constituents of the long-chain molecules, and ionic bonds between the chains. **glass i. cement**, glass ionomer CEMENT. **i. resin**, ionomer RESIN.

ionometry (i″o-nom′e-tre) an instrument for the measurement of the intensity or quantity of radiation from an ionizing radiation source.

iontophoresis (i-on″to-fo-re′sis) the introduction by means of electric current of ions of soluble salts into the tissue, usually for therapeutic purposes. The method is based on the principle of electrolysis, whereby a salt, such as NaCl, placed in solution will undergo ionization (NaCl $\rightleftharpoons$ Na$^+$ + Cl$^-$). The introduction of a positive electrode (anode) and a negative electrode (cathode) into the solution, and passing of direct current through the solution will result in concentration of chlorine ions (Cl$^-$) at the positive pole and sodium ions (Na$^+$) at the negative pole. When used in dentistry, one electrode is attached to the tooth and the other is held in the hand. Previously, in endodontics, the cathode was introduced in the root canal and an iodide-iodine solution or a zinc iodide-iodine solution was used as the electrolyte; now, the anode is used in the canal. Called also *electrolytic medication, electromedication,* and *ionic medication*. **root canal i.**, ELECTROSTERILIZATION.

iophendylate (i″o-fen′di-lāt) a contrast medium, ethyl 10-(*p*-iodophenyl)undecylate occurring as a viscous liquid that is insoluble in water, but soluble in alcohol, benzene, and other organic solvents, and darkens when exposed to air. Used in radiography, including sialography and myelography. Emulsified iophendylate adheres to the mucous membranes and is miscible with tissue fluids. Trademarks: Ethiodan, Myodil, Neurotrast, Pantopaque.

iota (i-o′ta) [Gr. *iōta* letter I, *ι*] 1. the ninth letter of the Greek alphabet. 2. a very small quantity of anything.

iotacism (i-o′ah-sizm) excessive use of the sound of the Greek letter iota (English *e*, as in be) in speaking.

iothalamate (i″o-thal′ah-māt) a salt of iothalamic acid; used as a radiopaque medium.

IPA individual practice ASSOCIATION.

IPPB intermittent positive pressure BREATHING.

iproniazid (i″pro-ni′ah-zid) a monoamine oxidase inhibitor, 4-pyridinecarboxylic acid 2-(1-methylethyl)hydrazide, occurring as a crystalline substance that is soluble in water and ethanol. Used as an antidepressant agent. Also used in the treatment of tuberculosis. Trademarks: Euphozid, Marsilid.

ipsilateral (ip″si-lat′er-al) [L. *ipse* self + *latus* side] situated on, pertaining to, or affecting the same side, as opposed to contralateral; homolateral.

Ipsilon trademark for *aminocaproic acid* (see under ACID).

Ipsoclip attachment (unit) see under ATTACHMENT.

Ir iridium.

Iradicav acidulated phosphate fluoride solution see under SOLUTION.

Ircon trademark for a preparation of *ferrous fumarate* (see under FUMARATE).

Irene trademark for *desipramine hydrochloride* (see under DESIPRAMINE).

Irgasan DP 300 trademark for *triclosan*.

irides (ir'ĭ-dēz) [L.; Gr.] plural of *iris*.

iridium (i-rid'e-um, ĭ-rid'e-um) [L.; Gr. *iris* rainbow, from the tinge of its salts] a metallic element. Symbol, Ir; atomic number, 77; atomic weight, 192.22; melting point, 2443°C; Brinell hardness number, 218; valences, 1, 2, 3, 4, 6; group VIII of the periodic table. It has two naturally occurring isotopes (191, 193) and several artificial radioactive ones (182–190, 191, 192, 194–198). Iridium is a silvery white metal that is the hardest and most corrosion resistant of all known elements, being insoluble in acid and only slowly soluble in aqua regia and in fused alkalies.

Iridocin trademark for *ethionamide*.

Iridoviridae (ir"ĭ-do-vi'rĭ-de) [L. *iridescere* to gleam like a rainbow + *virus*] a family of icosahedral enveloped viruses with a single linear molecule of double-stranded DNA, which replicate in the cell cytoplasm. The diameter of the virion is 130 nm and the number of capsomers in the virion is 1500. The family consists of the single genus, *Iridovirus*, and several unclassified viruses.

Iridovirus (ir"ĭ-do'vi-rus) a genus of viruses of the family Iridoviridae, isolated originally from insects, but recently, also found in vertebrates. Called also *iridescent virus*.

Iris (i'ris) a genus of perennial herbs, the roots of which yield orris.

iris (i'ris), pl. *ir'ides* [Gr. "rainbow," "halo"] the circular pigmented membrane behind the cornea, perforated by the pupil, which widens or narrows, allowing transmission of light through the lens.

iritis (i-ri'tis) [*iris* + *-itis*] inflammation of the iris.

Irium trademark for *sodium lauryl sulfate* (see under SODIUM).

Iromon trademark for a preparation of *ferrous gluconate* (see under GLUCONATE).

iron (i'ern) [L. *ferrum*] a metallic element. Symbol, Fe; atomic number, 26; atomic weight, 55.847; melting point, 1536°C; Brinell hardness number, 60; valences, 2, 3 and 1, 4, 6; group VIII of the periodic table. It has three naturally occurring isotopes (54, 57, 58) and several artificial radioactive ones (52, 53, 55, 59–61). Iron occurs as a silvery grayish, ductile, malleable, magnetic metal that is oxidized in moist air and is attacked by acids. When alloyed with carbon manganese, chromium, nickel, and other elements, it forms steels. It is distributed in the animal body in both ionic (inorganic) and nonionic (organic) forms, chiefly in the cells of the liver, spleen, and bone marrow. Of the 3.5 gm of iron content in the human body, 70 percent is found in hemoglobin, myoglobin, and enzymes, and 30 percent in hemosiderin and ferritin. Iron-containing enzymes are those involved in electron transfer, including cytochrome oxidase, succinic dehydrogenase, and xanthine oxidase. Iron is absorbed through the alimentary canal and, in its ferrous form, passes into the blood where it is bound to transferrin. The excess is oxidized to the ferric state and combines with apoferritin to form ferritin, which is excreted from the body. The chief function of iron is the transportation of oxygen to the tissues in hemoglobin and cellular oxidation processes via the cytochrome system. There being no reserve of iron in the body, it must be taken daily. Depletion of iron leads to iron deficiency anemia (see under ANEMIA). Various ferrous salts are used in the treatment of anemia, but the absorption of all ferric salts is poor. Side effects to intramuscular administration include pain at the injection site, skin discoloration, inflammatory response, inguinal lymphadenopathy, and abdominal pain. Ingestion of an excessive amount of an iron salt can be fatal. Symptoms are usually present 30 minutes after intake of the iron salt, gastrointestinal disorders being the most common findings. Nausea, vomiting, pallor, lassitude, drowsiness, hematemesis, diarrhea with green and tarry stools, cardiovascular collapse, and shock are the most common symptoms. Death may occur within 6 hours, but sometimes there may be a period of transient improvement that is followed by death within 12 to 48 hours. Hemorrhagic gastroenteritis and liver injury are usually found at autopsy. Iron poisoning is very rare in adults. Prolonged intake of therapeutic doses may produce constipation, nausea, epigastric pain, diarrhea, melena, and rickets due to interference with phosphorus absorption. For daily requirements of iron, see table at NUTRITION. See also terms beginning FERR-, FERRIC-, FERRO-, and SIDERO-. **α-i.,** the body-centered cubic magnetic form of iron existing up to 768°C (1414°F). **available i.,** that portion of iron in the food which can be separated from the total iron content by digestive processes, the ferrous form being more absorbable than the ferric form. **β-i.,** the nonmagnetic form of iron existing between 768 and 910°C (1414 and 1670°F). **i. carbonate,** ferrous CARBONATE. **cast i.,** an eutectic iron-carbon alloy containing 2 to 6.67 percent carbon, which may exist in the form of graphite or a carbide. It is more brittle than steel, and is used in the cast rather than the wrought condition. Called also *cast i.* See also carbon STEEL. **i. chloride,** 1. ferrous CHLORIDE. 2. ferric CHLORIDE. **Δ-i.,** a body-centered form of iron existing over the temperature range of 1390 to 1534°C (2534 to 2793°F). Called also *Δ-ferrite.* **i. dichloride,** ferrous CHLORIDE. **elemental i., reduced i. γ-i.,** the face-centered cubic form of iron existing in the temperature range of 910 to 1390°C (1670 to 2536°F). **i. gluconate,** ferrous GLUCONATE. **i. hydrate, i. hydroxide,** ferric HYDROXIDE. **i. lactate,** ferrous LACTATE. **liquid i.,** iron liquefied by heating to above 1534°C (2793°F) at 1 atm. **metallic i., reduced i. i. oxide,** ferric HYDROXIDE. **i. protochloride,** *ferrous* CHLORIDE. **i. protosulfate,** ferrous SULFATE. **radioactive i.,** any radioactive iron isotope, including ^{52}Fe, ^{53}Fe, ^{55}Fe, ^{59}Fe, ^{60}Fe, and ^{61}Fe; ^{55}Fe (half-life 4 years) and ^{59}Fe (half-life 47 days) are the most commonly used in hematological studies. Called also *radioiron.* **reduced i.,** finely powdered metallic iron, with particles ranging in size from 2 to 6 μm, obtained by precipitation with hydrogen from a solution of a soluble iron salt; used in the form of oral preparations or for enrichment of bread and cereals for the treatment of iron deficiency conditions. Called also *elemental i.* and *metallic i.* **i. sorbitex,** a complex of iron, sorbitol, and citric acid stabilized with dextrin. Used parenterally in the treatment of iron deficiency. Called also *glucitol iron complex.* Trademark: Jectofer. **i. sulfate,** ferrous SULFATE.

iron-dextran (i'ern-dek'stran) see dextran iron COMPLEX.

Ironate trademark for a preparation of *ferrous sulfate* (see under SULFATE).

ironing (i'er-ning) spatulation (2).

Irosul (i'ro-sul) trademark for a preparation of *ferrous sulfate* (see under SULFATE).

Irox trademark for a preparation of *ferrous gluconate* (see under GLUCONATE).

irradiation (ir-ra"de-a'shun) [L., from *in* into + *radiare* to emit rays] the act or process of exposing an object to radiant energy. **interstitial i.,** therapeutic irradiation by the insertion into tissues of radioactive materials, such as radiogold, radon, or radium, through the use of hollow seeds or capsules. See also radium NEEDLE, radiogold SEED, and radon SEED. **orthovoltage i.,** low-voltage x-irradiation in the range of 150 to 250 kilovolts, used in teletherapy. Formerly used extensively in oral cancer but, because of its relatively more harmful effect on the bone than the soft tissue, it is now used infrequently. **specific area i.,** irradiation of a specific area of the body. Called also *specific area radiation.* **whole-body i.,** exposure of the entire body to external ionizing radiations. Called also *whole-body exposure.* See table. See also radiation SICKNESS and RADIOSENSITIVITY.

LEVELS OF WHOLE-BODY EXPOSURE TO RADIATION

Dose in Rads	Probable Effect
10 to 50	No obvious effect except, probably, minor blood changes
50 to 100	Vomiting and nausea for about one day in 5 to 10% of exposed personnel. Fatigue, but no serious disability. Transient reduction in lymphocytes and neutrophils.
100 to 200	Vomiting and nausea for about one day, followed by other symptoms of radiation sickness in about 25 to 50% of personnel. No deaths anticipated. A reduction of approximately 50% in lymphocytes and neutrophils will occur.

Table continued on following page

LEVELS OF WHOLE-BODY
EXPOSURE TO RADIATION (Continued)

Dose in Rads	Probable Effect
200 to 350	Vomiting and nausea in nearly all personnel on first day, followed by other symptoms of radiation sickness, e.g., loss of appetite, diarrhea, minor hemorrhage. About 20% die within 2 to 6 weeks after exposure; survivors convalesce for about 3 months, although many have a second wave of symptoms at about 3 weeks. Up to 75% reduction in all circulating blood elements.
350 to 550	Vomiting and nausea in most personnel on first day, followed by other symptoms of radiation sickness, e.g., fever, hemorrhage, diarrhea, emaciation. About 50% die within one month; survivors convalesce for about 6 months.
550 to 750	Vomiting and nausea (or at least nausea) in all personnel within 4 hours after exposure, followed by severe symptoms of radiation sickness, as above. Up to 100% die; few survivors convalesce for about 6 months.
1000	Vomiting and nausea in all personnel within 1 to 2 hours. All die within days.
5000	Incapacitation almost immediately (minutes to hours). All personnel will die within one week.

(From S. Warren: The Pathology of Ionizing Radiation. 1961. Courtesy of Charles C Thomas, Publisher, Springfield, Illinois.)

irreversible (ir″re-ver′si-b'l) incapable of being reversed.

irrigation (ir″ĭ-ga′shun) [L. *irrigatio*, from *in* into + *rigare* to carry water] washing by a stream of water or other fluid. See also LAVAGE. **endodontic i.**, irrigation of the pulp canal during root canal therapy. See also endodontic irrigating SYRINGE. **oral i.**, the washing of the teeth and oral structures with an oral irrigator.

irrigator (ir′ĭ-ga″tor) [L. "waterer"] a device for performing irrigation. **oral i.**, a device for washing of the teeth and oral structures by a stream of water that may be cold or warm, steady or pulsating. In one type, the pressure is created by a built-in pump using water from a reservoir, an adjustable dial regulating the water pressure. The other type is attached to a water faucet. It is an oral hygiene aid, recommended for use in conjunction with toothbrushing, to remove food debris. It is designed to retard the accumulation of plaque and calculus and to reduce gingival inflammation and pocket depth, as well as increase gingival keratinization. When used incorrectly, it may injure the gingival tissue.

irritability (ir″ĭ-tah-bil′ĭ-te) [L. *irritabilitas*, from *irritare* to tease] 1. the quality of being responsive to a stimulus. 2. excessive responsiveness to slight stimuli.

irritant (ir′ĭ-tant) [L. *irritans*] 1. giving rise to irritation. 2. an agent which acts locally on the skin and mucous membranes causing hyperemia, inflammation and, in severe cases, vesication. Irritants producing only hyperemia are known as *rubefacients*, and those causing blisters (vesicles) are known as *vesicants*. Some irritants, when taken internally, exert emetic or cathartic action. 3. a painful stimulus.

irritation (ir″ĭ-ta′shun) [L. *irritatio*] 1. the act of stimulating. 2. a state of excessive excitation and undue sensitivity. 3. the act of producing excessive excitation.

Is INCISION superius.

ischemia (is-ke′me-ah) [Gr. *ischein* to suppress + *haima* blood + *-ia*] loss of blood supply to a tissue due to mechanical obstruction, which may result in cell death and coagulation necrosis. **cardiac i.**, heart i., myocardial i., ischemic heart DISEASE.

ischo- [Gr. *ischein* to suppress] a combining form meaning suppressed, or denoting relationship to suppression.

Ishikawa, H. [Japanese physician] see Puretić-Ishikawa SYNDROME.

Isicaine trademark **for** *lidocaine*.

island (i′land) a cluster of cells or an isolated piece of tissue. See also ISLET. **i's of Langerhans**, islands of irregular structure in the pancreas composed of cells smaller than the surrounding cells, representing the endocrine portion of the pancreas. They produce glucagon, hyperglycemic factor, probably by means of the α-cells, and insulin, a hypoglycemic factor, by means of the β-cells. Called also *islets of Langerhans*. See also DIABETES mellitus.

islet (i′let) a cluster of cells or an isolated piece of tissue. See also ISLAND. **i's of Langerhans**, islands of Langerhans; see under ISLAND.

-ism [Gr. *-izō* + *-mos*] a word termination meaning state, condition, or fact of being, or the process or result of an action.

Ismelin trademark **for** *guanethidine sulfate* (see under GUANETHIDINE).

ISO International Standards Organization (see under ORGANIZATION).

iso- [Gr. *isos* equal] a prefix or combining form meaning equal, alike, or the same.

ISO/TC106 see COMMITTEE TC106.

isoadrenaline hydrochloride (i″so-ah-dren′ah-lin) NORDEFRIN hydrochloride.

isoagglutination (i″so-ah-gloo′tĭ-na-shun) agglutination of erythrocytes of individuals of the same species but different blood groups. See also HEMAGGLUTINATION.

isoagglutinin (i″so-ah-gloo′tĭ-nin) [iso- + *agglutinin*] an isoantibody that causes agglutination of erythrocytes of individuals of the same species but with different blood groups. Called also *isohemagglutinin*.

isoallele (i″so-ah-lēl′) an allelic gene which is considered as being normal but can be distinguished from another allele by its differing phenotypic expression when in combination with a dominant mutant allele.

isoalloxazine (i″so-ah-lok′sah-zēn) an isomer of alloxazine from which riboflavin and other flavins are derived.

isoamyl (i″so-am′il) an amyl isomer (see AMYL). **i. nitrite**, amyl NITRITE.

isoanaphylaxis (i″so-an″ah-fi-lak′sis) anaphylaxis produced by the administration of serum from the same species, as in man by the administration of human serum.

isoantibody (i″so-an′tĭ-bod″e) an antibody produced by one individual that reacts with antigens (isoantigens) of another individual of the same species. Called also *alloantibody*.

isoantigen (i″so-an′tĭ-jen) allogeneic ANTIGEN.

isobamate (i″so-bam′āt) carisoprodol.

isobar (i′so-bar) [iso- + Gr. *baros* weight] 1. a line on a map or chart depicting the boundaries of an area of constant pressure. 2. one of two or more different elements of the same atomic mass but of different atomic numbers; the sum of their nucleons is the same but there are more protons in one than in the others.

Isobide trademark **for** *isosorbide*.

isobutyl (i″so-bu′til) an isomeric form of butyl $(CH_3)_2 CHCH_2-$ or i-C_4H_9-.

Isocaine trademark **for** *mepivacaine hydrochloride* (see under MEPIVACAINE).

isocarboxazid (i″so-kar-bok′sah-zid) a monoamine oxidase inhibitor, 5-methyl-3-isoxazolecarboxylic acid 2-benzylhydrazide, occurring as a white, crystalline powder with a slight characteristic odor, which is soluble in ethanol and chloroform and slightly soluble in water. Used in the treatment of certain types of mental depression. Its adverse reactions are similar to those of other monoamine oxidase inhibitors. Trademark: Marplan.

Isochinol trademark **for** *dimethisoquin hydrochloride* (see under DIMETHISOQUIN).

isochromosome (i″so-kro′mo-sōm) a structural chromosome aberration, consisting of the presence of a median centromere and two identical arms, formed by the transverse, rather than the normal longitudinal splitting of a replicating chromosome. Abbreviated *i*. See also CHROMOSOME aberration.

Isocillin trademark **for** *penicillin V potassium* (see under PENICILLIN).

isocytotoxin (i″so-si″to-tok′sin) a cytotoxin that is toxic for homologous cells of the same species.

Isodin trademark **for** *oxazepam*.

Isodine trademark **for** *povidone-iodine*.

isoeffect (i″so-e-fekt′) an effect midway between two reference points.

isoelectric (i″so-e-lek′trik) having no variation in electric potential.

iso-elixir (i″so-e-lik″ser) iso-ELIXIR.

isoenzyme (i″so-en′zīm) a multiple form of a protein catalyst which may exist in a single species, the various forms differing chemically, physically, and/or immunologically, but catalyzing the same reaction. For example, lactate dehydrogenase may exist in several forms arising from different tetramer combinations of two subunits. In principle, the term is restricted to those multiple forms which arise from genetically determined differences in primary structure, and not to those derived by modification of the same primary sequence. In practice, it is used as an operational term in dealing with enzyme proteins with the same catalytic activities, but separable by suitable methods, such as electrophoresis. Called also *isozyme*.

isoetharine (i″so-eth′ah-rēn) a sympathomimetic drug with predominantly β-adrenergic activity, 3,4-dihydroxy-α-[1-(isopropylamino)propyl]benzyl alcohol. Used chiefly as a bronchodilator. Tachycardia, arrhythmia, nausea, vertigo, and headache are the principal side effects. Trademarks: Dilabron, Neoisuprel.

isoflurane (i″so-floo′rān) an anesthetic,1-chloro-2,2,2,-trifluoroethyl difluoromethyl ether, occurring as a clear colorless liquid with a slight odor, which is miscible with fats and oils. Trademark: *Forane*.

isogeneic (i″so-jĕ-ne′ik) [*iso-* + Gr. *genos* kind] syngeneic.

isogenous (i-soj′ĕ-nus) developed or originating from the same cell.

Isoglaucon trademark for *clonidine hydrochloride* (see under CLONIDINE).

isograft (i′so-graft″) isologous GRAFT.

isohemagglutination (i″so-hem″ah-gloo″tĭ-na′shun) agglutination of erythrocytes caused by a hemagglutinin from another individual of the same species but with a different blood group. Called also *isoagglutination*.

isohemagglutinin (i″so-hem″ah-gloo′tĭ-nin) [*iso-* + *hemagglutinin*] an isoantibody that causes hemagglutination in individuals of the same species but with different blood groups. Called also *isoagglutinin*.

isohemolysis (i″so-he-mol′ĭ-sis) hemolysis of the blood corpuscles of an animal by the lysins in serum from another animal of the same species.

isoimmunization (i″so-im″u-ni-za′shun) development of antibodies against an antigen derived from a genetically dissimilar individual of the same species. See also ISOANTIGEN.

isolateral (i″so-lat′er-al) [*iso-* + L. *latus* side] having sides that are equal or identical; equilateral.

isoleucine (i″so-lu′sin) an aliphatic, naturally occurring, amino acid that is essential for growth in humans, 2-amino-3-methylvaleric acid. Isoleucine is also found in the saliva. Abbreviated *Ile*. See also amino ACID.

isologous (i-sol′o-gus) characterized by the identical genotype.

isomer (i′so-mer) [*iso-* + Gr. *meros* part] 1. one of the two or more distinct compounds of the same molecular formula, each molecule possessing an identical number of atoms of each element, but in different arrangement. See ISOMERISM. 2. one of two or more nuclides with the same numbers of neutrons and protons in their nuclei, but with different energies. *cis-*i., one in which the hydrogen atoms attached to two atoms with double bonds are substituted adjacently on the same side of the molecule. Cf. *trans-*i. +i., dextrorotatory i. −i., levorotatory i. *d-*i., *dextro-*i., dextrorotatory i. **dextrorotatory i.**, one which, when in solution, has the property of rotating the plane of polarized light to the right or clockwise; its chemical properties being otherwise identical with those of a levorotatory isomer of the same compound. Also written +*i.*, d-*i.*, and dextro-*i*. *l-*i., *levo-*i., levorotatory i. **levorotatory i.**, one which, when in solution, has the property of rotating the plane of polarized light to the left or counterclockwise, its chemical properties being otherwise identical with those of a dextrorotatory isomer of the same compound. Also written −*i.*, l-*i.*, and levo-*i*. *m-*i., *meta-*i., one having the substitution in a derivative of a benzene ring of two atoms separated by an intervening carbon atom or 1,3-position in the ring. *o-*i., *ortho-*i., one having the substitution in a derivative of a benzene ring of two atoms linked to neighboring carbon atoms or 1,2-position in the ring. *p-*i., *para-*i., one having the substitution in a derivative of a benzene ring of two atoms linked to opposite carbon atoms or 1,4-position in the ring. *trans-*i., one in which the hydrogen atoms attached to two carbon atoms with double bonds are substituted in the opposite location to the carbon axis. Cf. cis-*i*.

isomerase [E.C.5] (i-som′er-ās) any of a major class of enzymes involved in catalyzing geometric or stereoisometric changes within a molecule. See also ENZYME classification. *cis-trans-*i. [E.C.5.2], a subclass of isomerases, the enzymes of which catalyze geometric or stereoisometric changes within a molecule by rearranging the geometry of groups attached to carbon-carbon double bonds.

isomeric (i″so-mer′ik) pertaining to or exhibiting isomerism.

Isomerine trademark for *dexchlorpheniramine maleate* (see under DEXCHLORPHENIRAMINE).

isomerism (i-som′ĕ-rizm) [*iso-* + Gr. *meros* part] the possession by two or more distinct compounds of the same molecular formula, each molecule possessing an identical number of atoms of each element, but in different arrangement. Isomerism is divided into two broad classifications: *structural isomerism* and *stereoisomerism* (spatial or stereochemical isomerism). **chain i.**, structural isomerism in which the compounds differ in regard to the linkage in the basic chain of carbon atoms. Called also *nuclear i. cis-*i., see *cis-*ISOMER. **functional group i.**, structural isomerism dependent upon the presence of different functional groups, such a compound being of distinct chemical types, e.g., ethyl alcohol, C_2H_5OH, and dimethyl ether, CH_3OCH_3. **geometric i.**, stereoisomerism usually described as being dependent upon some form of restricted rotation, enabling the component parts of the molecule to occupy a different spatial position. Thus, *cis-* and *trans-*dichloroethylene are said to be geometric isomers, the isomerism resulting from the lack of freedom of rotation about the double bond. In the case of *cis-* and *trans-*decalin, however, the rigidity of the fused ring structure is responsible for the isomerism. *meta-*i., see *meta-*ISOMER. **nuclear i.**, chain i. **optical i.**, a type of stereoisomerism in which an appreciable number of molecules exhibit any of the following effects on polarized light: the isomers (*a*) rotate the plane of polarization: to the *same* degree in *opposite* directions (enantiomorphism), (*b*) rotate the plane of polarization to a *different* degree in either the same direction or in opposite directions, or (*c*) have no effect on the plane because of so-called internal compensation (diastereoisomerism). *ortho-*i., see *ortho-*ISOMER. *para-*i., see *para-*ISOMER. **position i.**, structural isomerism in which the position occupied by an atom or group differs with reference to the same fundamental carbon chain, e.g., *n*-propyl chloride, $CH_3CH_2CH_2Cl$, and isopropyl chloride, $CH_3CHClCH_3$. Called also *substitution i*. **spatial i., stereochemical i.**, stereoisomerism. **structural i.**, the possession by two or more compounds of the same molecular formula but of different structural formulas, the linkages of the atoms being different, in contrast with stereoisomerism, in which the structural arrangements of the atoms are the same. **substitution i.**, position i. *trans-*i., see *trans-*ISOMER.

isomerization (i-som″er-i-za′shun) the process whereby any isomer, whether structural or stereochemical, is converted into another, usually requiring special conditions of temperature, pressure, or catalysts.

isometric (i″so-met′rik) [*iso-* + Gr. *metron* measure] 1. maintaining, or pertaining to, the same measure of length; of equal dimensions. 2. not isotonic.

isometry (i-som′ĕ-tre) [*iso-* + Gr. *metron* measure] equality of dimensions. See bisecting angle TECHNIQUE (for Cieszynski's rule of isometry).

Isonal trademark for *mephobarbital*.

isoniazid (i″so-ni′ah-zid) a compound, 4-pyridinecarboxylic acid, occurring as a colorless or white, odorless crystalline solid or powder that is soluble in water and alcohol and slightly soluble in ether and chloroform. It is the most potent of known bacteriostatic drugs used in the treatment of tuberculosis. In patients in whom the process of acetylation is slow, the drug may cause restlessness, insomnia, muscle twitching, hyperreflexia, paresthesia, convulsions, neurological disorders, and various other disorders. Called also *isonicotinic acid hydrazide* (INH). Trademarks: Niconyl, Nydrazid.

isonipecaine (i″so-nip′ĕ-kān) meperidine.

Isophen trademark for *methamphetamine hydrochloride* (see under METHAMPHETAMINE).

Isophrin trademark for *phenylephrine hydrochloride* (see under PHENYLEPHRINE).

isopropanol (i″so-pro′pah-nol) isopropyl ALCOHOL.

isopropyl (i″so-pro′pil) an isomeric form of propyl, $(CH_3)_2$— or i-C_3H_7—. **i. alcohol**, isopropyl ALCOHOL.

isopropylarterenol (i″so-pro″pil-ar″te-re′nol) isoproterenol.

isopropylnorepinephrine (i″so-pro″pil-nor″ep-ĭ-nef′rin) isoproterenol.

isoproterenol (i″so-pro″te-re′nol) a catecholamine, 3,4-dihydroxy-α-[(isopropylamino)methyl]benzyl alcohol. Used therapeutically as the hydrochloride salt, which occurs as a white crystalline powder with a bitter taste, and is soluble in water and alcohol, but not in organic solvents. Isoproterenol is a powerful sympathomimetic drug acting on the β-receptors, and its pharmacological effects include lowering of peripheral vascular resistance, especially in skeletal muscles and in renal and mesenteric vascular beds; raising cardiac output; relaxation of smooth muscles, particularly of the gastrointestinal system and bronchi; release of free amino acids; increase of blood sugar level; and stimulation of insulin secretion. Used as a bronchodilator and cardiac stimulant. Side effects may include arrhythmia, myocardial necrosis, headache, tremor, anginal pain, vertigo, nausea, sweating, and sometimes, cardiac reactions. Called also *isopropylnorepinephrine* and *isopropylarterenol*. Trademarks: Aleudrin, Aludrine, Isorenin, Isuprel, Isupren, Neodrenal.

Isorbid trademark for *isosorbide dinitrate* (see under ISOSORBIDE).

Isorenin trademark for *isoproterenol*.

isosmotic (i″sos-mot′ik) having the same osmotic pressure.

isosorbide (i″so-sor′bĭd) an osmotic diuretic, 1,4:3,6-dianhydro-D-glucitol. Trademarks: Hydronol, Isobide. **i. dinitrate**, the dinitrate salt of isosorbide. In the undiluted form, occurring as white, odorless, crystalline rosettes that are soluble in acetone and chloroform and sparingly soluble in ethanol and water; in diluted form, it is a white, odorless powder. It is a peripheral organonitrate vasodilator, used in the treatment of angina pectoris. Headache and paradoxical anginal pain are the chief side effects. Vertigo, orthostatic hypotension, and mild gastrointestinal disorders may occur. Called also *dinitrosorbide*. Trademarks: Cardis, Isorbid, Maycor, Sorbitrate, Sorquad, Vasorbate.

isotactic (i″so-tak′tik) pertaining to a chemical compound in which the radicals are always in the same position, as in a polymer. Cf. ATACTIC and SYNDIOTACTIC.

isotherm (i′so-therm) [*iso-* + Gr. *thermē* heat] a line on a map or chart depicting the boundaries of an area in which the temperature is the same. Called also *isothermal line*.

isothermal (i″so-ther′mal) [*iso-* + Gr. *thermē* heat] isothermic; having the same temperature.

isothermic (i″so-ther′mik) isothermal; having the same temperature.

isothermognosis (i″so-ther″mo-no′sis) [*iso-* + Gr. *thermē* heat + *gnōsis* recognition] a sense perception disorder in which pain, cold, and heat stimuli are all perceived as heat.

isotone (i′so-tōn) one of two or more different nuclides having the same number of neutrons but a different number of protons in their nuclei.

isotonia (i″so-to′ne-ah) [*iso-* + Gr. *tonos* tone] 1. a condition of equal tone, tension, or activity. 2. equality of osmotic pressure between two elements of a solution or between two different solutions.

isotonic (i″so-ton′ik) [*iso-* + Gr. *tonos* tone] 1. pertaining to isotonia. 2. pertaining to an isotonic solution. Sometimes used alone to denote such a solution.

isotope (i′so-tōp) [*iso-* + Gr. *topos* place] one of two or more atoms with the same atomic number but different atomic weights, having the same number of nuclear protons but different numbers of neutrons. Isotopes have very nearly the same chemical properties, but somewhat different physical properties. See also NUCLIDE. **radioactive i.**, radioisotope. **stable i.**, a nonradioactive isotope that does not transmute into another element. **tracer i.**, radioactive TRACER.

isotransplantation (i″so-trans″plan-ta′shun) [*iso-* + *transplantation*] the transplantation of an isogeneic graft.

isoxsuprine hydrochloride (i-sok′su-prēn) a sympathomimetic drug, 4-hydroxy-α-[1-[(1-methyl-2-phenoxyethyl)amino]ethyl]-benzenemethanol hydrochloride, occurring as a white, odorless, bitter, crystalline powder that is slightly soluble in water and ethanol. Used as a vasodilator in vascular disorders of the brain, peripheral vessels, and skeletal muscles. Also used in threatened abortion and dysmenorrhea. Nausea, vomiting, vertigo, weakness, cardiac arrhythmias, hypotension, and skin rashes are its principal side effects. Trademarks: Dilavase, Duvadilan, Vasodilan, Vasoplex, Vadosilan, Vasotran.

isozyme (i′so-zīm) isoenzyme.

Isphamycin trademark for *chlortetracycline hydrochloride* (see under CHLORTETRACYCLINE).

isthmi (is′mi) [Gr.] plural of isthmus.

isthmic (is′mik) pertaining to an isthmus.

isthmus (is′mus), pl. *isth′mi* [Gr. *isthmos*] a narrow connection between two bodies or parts. **anterior i. of fauces, i. of fauces. i. of fauces, i. fau′cium** [NA], a constricted aperture located between the dorsal end of the oral cavity and the pharynx, bounded by the soft palate, dorsum of the tongue, and the palatoglossal arch. Called also *anterior i. of fauces*. See also FAUCES.

Isuprel trademark for *isoproterenol*.

Isupren trademark for *isoproterenol*.

itch (ich) a skin disorder characterized by an unpleasant sensation that provokes the desire to scratch the skin. Called also PRURITUS. **barber's i.**, 1. TINEA barbae. 2. SYCOSIS barbae (1). **Boeck's i.**, Norwegian i. Norwegian SCABIES.

itching (ich′ing) a cutaneous or mucous sensation that provokes the desire to scratch or rub. See PRURITUS.

iter (i′ter) [L.] a way or tubular passage. **i. den′tium**, the area through which a permanent tooth makes its appearance.

-ites [Gr. *-itēs*, a masculine termination agreeing with *hydrōps* dropsy (understood) — as in tympanites] a word termination indicating dropsy of a part denoted by the stem to which it is affixed.

-itides plural form of *-itis*.

-itis, pl. *it′ides* [*-itis*, a feminine adjectival termination agreeing with Gr. *nosos* (understood) — e.g., neuritis = Gr. *hē neuritis nosos*, the disease of the nerves, which soon becomes the inflammatory disease] a word termination denoting inflammation of the part indicated by the word stem to which it is attached.

IU international UNIT.

IUB International Union of Biochemistry.

IUDR idoxuridine.

IV intravenously (by intravenous injection).

ivory (i′vo-re) [L. *ebur*, *eburneus*] 1. the bonelike substance (modified dentin) of the tusks of elephants or of such large mammals as the walrus. 2. dentin.

Ivory clamp see under CLAMP.

Ivoseal trademark for a *denture reliner* (see under RELINER), believed to be prepared from ethyl alcohol plasticizers, and acrylic resins.

IVT intravenous TRANSFUSION.

Ivy loop wiring [Robert Henry *Ivy*, English-born American plastic and maxillofacial surgeon] see under WIRING.

Ivy method see bleeding TIME.

J

J joule.

J-9 trademark for a hard *dental casting gold alloy* (see under GOLD).

J-13 trademark for an extra hard *dental casting gold alloy* (see under GOLD).

jacket (jak′et) an enveloping structure or garment, especially a covering for the trunk or for the upper part of the body. See also jacket CROWN. **porcelain j.**, a jacket crown made of porcelain.

jackscrew (jak′skroo) 1. a jack consisting of a screw steadied by a threaded support and carrying a plate or other part bearing the load. 2. a threaded device used in orthodontic appliances for the separation or approximation of teeth or jaw segments. See also jackscrew APPLIANCE and orthodontic SCREW. See illustration.

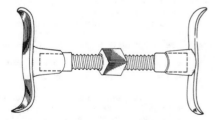

Jackscrew. (From T. M. Graber: Orthodontics — Principles and Practice. 3rd ed. Philadelphia, W. B. Saunders Co., 1972.)

j. appliance, jackscrew APPLIANCE. **j. regainer-maintainer,** jackscrew REGAINER-MAINTAINER.

Jackson appliance (crib) [Victor Hugo *Jackson,* American dentist, 1850–1929] see under APPLIANCE.

Jackson's epilepsy (seizures), law, syndrome [John Hughlings *Jackson,* English neurologist, 1834–1911] see under EPILEPSY and LAW, and see Jackson-MacKenzie SYNDROME.

Jackson's safety triangle [Chevalier *Jackson,* American laryngologist, 1865–1958] see under TRIANGLE.

Jackson-MacKenzie syndrome [J. H. *Jackson;* Sir Stephen *MacKenzie,* London physician, 1844–1909] see under SYNDROME.

jacksonian (jak″so-ne′an) named after John Hughlings *Jackson,* as jacksonian seizures (see Jackson's EPILEPSY).

Jacob, François [born 1920] a French biologist; co-winner, with André Michael Lwoff and Jacques Lucien Monod, of the Nobel prize for medicine and physiology in 1965, for discoveries concerning the genetic control of enzymes and virus synthesis.

Jacob's disease [O. *Jacob*] see under DISEASE.

Jacob's syndrome [Eugene C. *Jacobs,* American physician, born 1905] oculo-orogenital SYNDROME.

Jacobi's disease [E. *Jacobi*] POIKILODERMA atrophicans vasculare.

Jacobson's canal, cartilage, nerve, organ, plexus, sulcus [Ludwig Levin *Jacobson,* Danish anatomist, 1783–1843] see tympanic CANALICULUS, vomeronasal CARTILAGE, tympanic NERVE, vomeronasal ORGAN, tympanic PLEXUS, SULCUS promontorii cavi tympani, and tympanic sulcus of temporal bone, under SULCUS.

Jacod's syndrome, triad, [Maurice *Jacod,* French neurologist] retrosphenoidal space SYNDROME.

Jacquart's angle see ophryospinal ANGLE.

Jadassohn-Lewandowski syndrome [Josef *Jadassohn,* German dermatologist in Bern, 1863–1936] PACHYONYCHIA congenita.

Jadassohn-Tièche nevus [J. *Jadassohn;* Max *Tièche*] blue NEVUS.

Jadelot's line (furrow) [Jean François Nicolas *Jadelot,* French physician, 1791–1830] see under LINE.

Jaffe-Lichtenstein syndrome [Henry L. *Jaffe;* Louis *Lichtenstein*] see under SYNDROME.

Janar trademark for fluoride preparations used in dental caries prevention; see under RINSE.

Jansen's syndrome [W. Murk *Jansen,* Dutch physician, 1867–1935] metaphyseal DYSOSTOSIS.

Jaquette scaler see under SCALER.

Jarcho-Levin syndrome [S. *Jarcho,* American physician; P. M. *Levin,* American physician] see under SYNDROME.

jaundice (jawn-dis) [Fr. *jaunisse,* from *jaune* yellow] a condition associated with the presence in the blood of excessive amounts of bilirubin causing pigmentation of all of the organs in the body, especially the skin and sclera. Called also *icterus.* **acholuric familial j.,** hereditary SPHEROCYTOSIS. **acquired hemolytic j.,** acquired hemolytic anemia characterized by a low erythrocyte count, jaundice, spherocytosis, and splenomegaly, probably due to the presence of abnormal hemolysins. Called also *Abrami's disease, Hayem-Widal syndrome,* and *icterohemolytic anemia.* **catarrhal j.,** infectious HEPATITIS. **epidemic j.,** infectious HEPATITIS. **homologous serum j.,** homologous serum HEPATITIS.

jaw (jaw) either of two bony structures in most vertebrates that border the mouth and bear teeth. **abnormally large j.,** prognathism. **big j.,** actinomycosis. **bird-beak j.,** the condition produced by protrusion of the upper jaw. Called also *parrot j.* **j. brace,** mouth PROP. **cleft j.,** CLEFT jaw. **crackling j.,** noise (crepitation) in the normal or diseased temporomandibular joint associated with jaw movement. **Hapsburg j.,** mandibular prognathism usually associated with a thick overdeveloped lower lip (*Hapsburg lip*), as seen in members of the Hapsburg family. **Heidelberg j.,** a fossilized human mandible of the early Middle Pleistocene age found in 1907 near Heidelberg, Germany. **lower j.,** mandible. **lumpy j.,** actinomycosis. **parrot j.,** bird-beak j. **phossy j.,** phosphorus NECROSIS. **pipe j.,** a painful condition of the jaws caused by carrying a tobacco pipe in the mouth. **upper j.,** maxilla. **wide j.,** eurygnathism.

JCAH Joint Commission on Accreditation of Hospitals; see under COMMISSION.

JDE Journal of Dental Education.

Jectofer trademark for IRON sorbitex (see under IRON).

Jeghers, Harald Joseph [American physician, born 1904] see Peutz-Jeghers SYNDROME.

jejunum (je-joo′num) [L. "empty"] that portion of the small intestine which extends from the duodenum to the ileum.

Jelcone trademark for a *silicone impression material* (see under MATERIAL).

Jeleko No. 7 trademark for an extra hard *dental casting gold alloy* (see under GOLD).

Jelenko Durocast trademark for a hard *dental casting gold alloy* (see under GOLD).

Jelenko Modulay trademark for a *dental casting gold alloy* (see under GOLD).

Jelenko special inlay see under INLAY.

Jelenko super wire see under WIRE.

Jelenko surveyor see under SURVEYOR.

Jellin trademark for fluocinolone acetonide (see under FLUOCINOLONE).

jelly (jel′e) [L. *gelatina*] a soft substance which is coherent, tremulous, and more or less translucent; generally, a colloidal semisolid mass. **mineral j.,** petrolatum. **paraffin j.,** petrolatum. **petroleum j.,** petrolatum. **white petroleum j.,** white PETROLATUM.

Jel-Span trademark for a nickel-chromium base-metal crown and bridge alloy, also containing some beryllium. Inhalation of dust during melting, milling, or grinding may cause beryllium poisoning.

Jeltrate trademark for an *irreversible hydrocolloid impression material* (see under MATERIAL).

Jenkins' porcelain [N. S. *Jenkins,* American dentist in Paris and Dresden, 1840–1919] see under PORCELAIN.

Jenner, Edward [1749–1823] an English physician who conducted the first controlled experiment that led to the process of producing immunity to smallpox by inoculation (vaccination) with coxpox (vaccinia) vaccine.

Johnson, Frank Chambliss [American pediatrician, 1894–1934] see Stevens-Johnson SYNDROME.

Johnson's method see root canal filling method, Johnson's, under METHOD.

Johnson twin wire appliance [Joseph E. *Johnson,* American orthodontist] see under APPLIANCE.

joint (joint) [L. *junctio* a connection, joining] 1. the place of union between two or more bones. See also *articulatio* and *junctura.* 2. the place where two parts of a structure are united or joined. **Ackermann bar j.,** a multiple sleeve joint of a bar attachment in a dental prosthesis. Called also *Ackermann bar.* **amphidiarthrodial j.,** cartilaginous j. **arthrodial j.,** a synovial joint in which the opposed surfaces are flat or only slightly curved. See also *plane j.* **axial rotation j.,** a type of Steiger's joint in a dental prosthesis that allows some up and down play. **ball-and-socket j.,** spheroidal j. **bar j.,** an element in a bar attachment that allows movement between the two components in a dental prosthesis. **bar j., single sleeve,** the joint element of a bar attachment, consisting of a wrought wire bar and an open-sided sleeve built into the impression surface that fits over the bar when the denture is inserted. It allows some side-to-side and rotary movement around the wire, while resisting lateral movements. **biaxial j.,** a joint permitting movement in two of the assumed three mutually perpendicular axes, or having two degrees of freedom. See also biaxial MOVEMENT. **bilocular j.,** one in which the synovial cavity is divided into two compartments by an interarticular cartilage, as the temporomandibular joint. **bleeders' j.,** hemorrhage into a joint in persons suffering from blood coagulation disorders, such as hemophilia. Called also *hemophilic j.* **Budin's j.,** a band of cartilage seen at birth between the squamous and the two condylar portions of the occipital bone. **butt j.,** a joint formed by two structures joining each other end-to-end without overlapping. In dental restoration, a joint formed between the abutment and the restoration, where the restoration rests on the shoulder of a prepared tooth. **cartilaginous j.,** one in which two bones are connected by a mass of cartilage which acts as their growth center, such as a synchondrosis and symphysis. Called also *amphidiarthrodial j., slightly movable j., amphiarthrosis,* and *junctura cartilaginea* [NA]. **composite j., compound j.,** a type of synovial joint in which more than two bones are involved. Called also *articulatio composita* [NA], *composite articulation,* and *compound articulation.* **condylar j., condyloid j.,** one in which an ovoid head of one bone moves in an elliptical activity of another, permitting all movements except axial rotation. Called also *articulatio condylaris* [NA]. **diarthrodial j.,** synovial j. **Dolder bar j.,** Dolder bar joint ATTACHMENT. **false j.,** pseudoarthrosis. **fibrocartilaginous j.,** symphysis. **fibrous j.,** one in which two or more bones are connected by fibrous tissue; it includes suture, syndesmosis, and gomphosis. Called also *immovable j., synarthrodial j., junctura fibrosa* [NA], and *synarthrosis.* **freely movable j.,** synovial j. **ginglymoid j.,** ginglymus. **gliding j.,** plane

j. **hemophilic j.,** bleeders' j. **hinge j.,** ginglymus. **immovable j.,** fibrous j. **ligamentous j.,** syndesmosis. **mandibular j.,** temporomandibular j. **mixed j.,** one combining features of different types of joints. **multiaxial j.,** spheroidal j. **multiple sleeve j.,** a joint of a bar attachment, consisting of several short sleeves that may be bent to follow the vertical contours, as well as the curvature of the ridge in a dental prosthesis. **pivot j.,** rotary j. **plane j.,** a type of synovial joint in which the opposed surfaces are flat or only slightly curved. Called also *gliding j., articulatio plana* [NA], and *gliding articulation.* **polyaxial j.,** spheroidal j. **rotary j.,** a uniaxial joint in which one bone pivots within a bony or an osseoligamentous ring. Called also *pivot j., articulatio trochoidea* [NA], *pivot articulation,* and *trochoidal articulation.* **rotation j.,** a type of Steiger's joint in a dental prosthesis that does not allow vertical movements. **saddle j.,** a joint having two saddle-shaped surfaces at right angles to each other. Called also *sellar j., articulatio sellaris* [NA], and *saddle articulation.* **sellar j.,** saddle j. **simple j.,** one in which only two bones articulate. Called also *articulatio simplex* [NA] and *simple articulation.* **slightly movable j.,** cartilaginous j. **socket j. of tooth,** gomphosis. **solder j.,** the union produced by soldering two pieces of metal. **spheroidal j.,** a type of synovial joint in which a spheroidal surface of one bone ("ball") moves within a concavity ("socket") on the other bone. Called also *ball-and-socket j., multiaxial j., polyaxial j., articulatio spheroidea* [NA], *ball-and-socket articulation,* and *spheroidal articulation.* **Steiger's j.,** a flexible major connector that joins two parts of a removable denture, allowing a limited amount of play between the parts, thus serving as a stress-breaker. It consists of the female part, which is a vertical sleeve attached to the removable crown or a clasp-retained part of a denture, and the male unit, which is a flattened rod attached to the denture saddle, fitting within the sleeve of the female part. Retention is provided by a screw which passes through the female part and into the male part. One type, the *axial rotation joint,* has a longitudinal opening which allows the screw to move up and down along the sleeve; the other type, the *rotation joint,* has a round hole that does not allow any vertical play. Called also *Steiger's attachment* and *Steiger's connector.* **synarthrodial j.,** fibrous j. **synovial j.,** one in which a fibrous capsule connects two bones, providing a space between the two bones, which is lined with a synovial membrane, thus allowing free movement of the joint. Called also *diarthrodial j., freely movable j., through j., diarthrosis,* and *junctura synovialis* [NA]. **temporomandibular j.,** one of the two joints between the cranium and the mandible, formed by the head of the condyle of the mandible resting in the mandibular fossa of the squamous part of the temporal bone. It is enclosed in the articular capsule and its surface is lined with fibrocartilage, rather than hyaline cartilage. A disk between the condyle and mandibular fossa divides the articular space into the inferior and superior synovial cavities. The auriculotemporal and masseteric branches of the mandibular nerve innervate the joint, and the superficial branch of the external carotid artery provides the blood supply. The joint is unique in that it allows both hinge and gliding movement, thus being a ginglymoarthrodial joint, the lower part doing the hinge movement and the upper the gliding. The action of the joint is coupled with that of its fellow of the opposite side and consists of opening and closing the jaws, protrusion and retrusion of the mandible, and lateral movement of the mandible. In the opening and closing movements, the disk slides anteriorly on the articular tubercle and the condyle moves in a hingelike motion while the mandible rotates on its axis near the center of the ramus. Opening of the jaws is associated with gliding of the condyle forward; during protrusion the disk glides forward; and lateral movement is accompanied by the disk gliding forward while its fellow of the opposite side remains in place. The movements of the joints are accomplished through the action of the lateral pterygoid, digastric, mylohyoid, geniohyoid, masseter, and temporal muscles, and the temporomandibular, stylomandibular, and sphenomandibular ligaments. Called also *mandibular j., articulatio mandibularis, articulatio temporomandibularis* [NA], *craniomandibular articulation, mandibular articulation, maxillary articulation, temporomandibular articulation,* and *temporomaxillary articulation.* See also temporomandibular dysfunction SYNDROME. See illustration. **temporomandibular j., lower,** synovial cavity, inferior, of temporomandibular joint; see under CAVITY. **temporomandibular j. syndrome,** see under SYNDROME. **temporomandibular j., upper,** synovial cavity, superior, of temporomandibular joint; see under CAVITY. **through j.,** synovial j. **tinner's j.,** a joint formed by foil being folded together in a manner similar to that of sheet metal, as when making a platinum matrix for porcelain paste. **uniaxial j.,** one permitting movement in only one of the assumed three mutually perpendicular axes, or having only one degree of freedom. **unilocular j.,** a synovial joint having only one cavity.

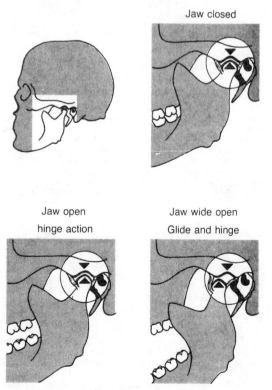

Jaw closed

Jaw open
hinge action

Jaw wide open
Glide and hinge

Hinge and glide action of the temporomandibular joint. (From H. O. Torres and A. Ehrlich: Modern Dental Assisting. 2nd ed. Philadelphia, W. B. Saunders Co., 1980.)

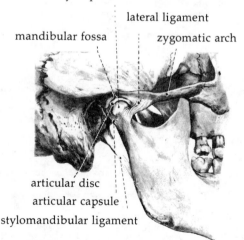

condylar process of mandible

lateral ligament

mandibular fossa   zygomatic arch

articular disc
articular capsule
stylomandibular ligament

The temporomandibular joint with part of the capsule removed. (From J. Langman and M. W. Woerdeman: Atlas of Medical Anatomy. Philadelphia, W. B. Saunders Co., 1978.)

Jolly, Justin [French histologist, 1870–1953] see Howell-Jolly BODY.

Jones, Henry Bence see BENCE JONES.

Jones' disease [William A. *Jones*] cherubism.

Jones' nasal splint [John *Jones,* American surgeon, 1729–1791] see under SPLINT.

Jordan's anomaly see under ANOMALY.

Joseph's clamp see under CLAMP.

Joseph's saw see under SAW.

Joule, James Prescott [English physicist, 1818–1889] see JOULE.

joule (jool) [named after J. P. *Joule*] originally, the energy expended by a current of 1 ampere flowing for 1 second through a resistance of 1 ohm. In SI, a unit of potential, kinetic, mechanical, electrical, magnetic, or thermal energy required to displace the point of application of the force of 1 newton by a distance of 1 meter in the direction of the force. Symbol *J.* See also SI.

J/s symbol for *joule per second;* see WATT.

Ju jugale.

juga (joo′gah) plural of *jugum.*

jugal (joo′gal) [L. *jugalis, jugum* yoke] 1. connecting like a yoke. 2. pertaining to the cheek or cheek bone (zygomatic bone).

jugale (joo-ga′le) a craniometric point at the angle formed by the masseteric and maxillary edges of the malar bone. Abbreviated *Ju.* Called also *jugal point.* See illustration at CEPHALOMETRY.

jugate (joo′gāt) 1. locked together. 2. marked by ridges.

jugular (jug′u-lar) [L. *jugularis,* from *jugulum* neck] pertaining to the neck, or to a jugular vein.

jugum (joo′gum), pl. *ju′ga* [L. "a yoke"] a general term for a depression or ridge connecting two structures. **ju′ga alveola′ria mandib′ulae** [NA], depressions on the anterior surface of the alveolar process of the mandible, between the ridges caused by the roots of the incisor teeth. **ju′ga alveola′ria maxil′lae** [NA], depressions on the anterior surface of the alveolar process of the maxilla, between the ridges caused by the roots of the incisor teeth. **ju′ga cerebra′lia os′sium cra′nii,** cerebral ridges of cranial bones; see under RIDGE. **j. sphenoida′le** [NA], the portion of the body of the sphenoid bone that connects the lesser wings.

juice (jōōs′) [L. *jus* broth] any fluid derived from animal or plant tissue or bodily secretion. Called also *succus.* **cancer j.,** a milky juice obtained from cancerous tissue, and containing cancer cells. **gastric j.,** the liquid secretion of the glands of the stomach. Called also *succus gastricus.*

jumping (jump′ing) 1. to spring into the air; to leap. 2. to pass over intervening steps, to advance rapidly from one level to another, or to change abruptly from one point to another. **j. the bite,** correction of cross-bite. See also Kingsley APPLIANCE.

junction (junk′shun) [L. *junctum* to join] a point or line of meeting or of coming together. See also JOINT and JUNCTURA. **amelodentinal j.,** dentinoenamel j. **cementodentinal j.,** dentinocemental j. **cementoenamel j.,** the line at which the cementum covering the root of a tooth and the enamel of the tooth meet, designated anatomically as the *cervical line.* **dentinocemental j.,** the line of fusion between the dentin and the cementum. Called also *cementodentinal j.* **dentinoenamel j.,** the plane of meeting between the dentin and enamel on the crown of a tooth, which is generally sigmoid in shape, being uneven and scalloped. Pointed or spindle-shaped processes of dentin,sometimes penetrate the junction and enter the enamel; some dentinal tubules penetrate into the enamel and end blindly. Called also *amelodentinal j.* **dentogingival j.,** the zone of meeting of the cementum and the gingiva, consisting of the epithelial attachment and the gingival fibers. **dermoepidermal j.,** the plane of meeting between the dermis and epidermis. **intermediate j.,** ZONULA adherens. **interneuronal j.,** synapse. **mucogingival j.,** a sharp scalloped, generally indistinct, line running parallel with the free margin, which separates the gingival tissue from that of the oral mucosa; seen under the microscope. Called also *mucogingival line.* **myoneural j.,** the point of junction of a nerve fiber with the muscle which it innervates. **osseous j.,** the union or junction between two or more bones. Called also *junctura ossium.* See ARTICULATION, JOINT, and JUNCTURA. **synaptic j.,** synapse. **tight j.,** ZONULA occludens.

junctura (junk-tu′rah), pl. *junctu′rae* [L. "a joining"] a general term used in anatomical nomenclature to designate the site of union between two structures. See also JOINT and JUNCTION. **j. cartilagin′ea** [NA], cartilaginous JOINT. **j. fibro′sa** [NA], fibrous JOINT. **j. os′sium,** osseous JUNCTION. **j. synovia′lis** [NA], synovial JOINT.

juncturae (junk-tu′re) [L.] plural of *junctura.*

Jürgens, Rudolf [1898–1961] see Willebrand-Jürgens SYNDROME.

jurisprudence (joor″is-proo′dens) [L. *juris prudentia* knowledge of law] the scientific study or application of the principles of law and justice. **dental j.,** the application of the principles of law as they relate to the practice of dentistry, to the obligations of the practitioner to his patient, and to the relations of dentists to each other and to society in general. This term and *forensic dentistry* are sometimes used as synonyms, but some authorities consider the first as a branch of law and the second as a branch of dentistry. See also *medical j.* and forensic DENTISTRY. **medical j.,** the application of the principles of law as they relate to the practice of medicine, to the obligations of the practitioner to his patient, and to the relations of physicians to each other and to society in general. This term and *forensic medicine* are sometimes used as synonyms, but some authorities consider the first as a branch of law and the second as a branch of medicine. See also *dental j.* and forensic MEDICINE.

Justi resin cement see under CEMENT.

juvenile (joo′vĕ-nil, joo′vĕ-nīl) 1. pertaining to youth or childhood; young or immature. 2. a youth or child; a young animal. 3. a cell or organism intermediate between the immature form and mature form.

juxta- [L. *juxta* near] a combining form meaning near, in the vicinity.

juxta-articular (juks″tah-ar-tik′u-lar) [*juxta-* + L. *articulus* joint] situated near a joint or in the region of a joint.

juxtaposition (juks″tah-po-zish′un) [*juxta-* + L. *positio* place] apposition.

K

K 1. kelvin. 2. kerma. 3. potassium (L. *kalium*). 4. electrostatic CAPACITY. 5. Kell FACTOR. 6. equilibrium CONSTANT.

°K degree on the Kelvin scale; see absolute TEMPERATURE.

k KILO-.

Ka kathode; see CATHODE.

Kadon primer see under PRIMER.

Kafocin trademark for *cephaloglycin.*

Kahler's disease [Otto *Kahler,* Austrian physician, 1849–1893] multiple MYELOMA.

Kahn's test [Herbert *Kahn*] see under TEST.

kaino- [Gr. *kainos* new, fresh] see CENO-(1).

Kaiser see Kirkland-Kaiser PACK.

kala-azar (kah′lah ah-zar′) [Hindi "black fever"] visceral LEISHMANIASIS.

kalemia (kah-le′me-ah) [L. *kalium* potassium + Gr. *haima* blood + *-ia*] the presence of potassium in the blood; see HYPERKALEMIA.

kali (ka′li, kah′le) [Ger.] POTASSIUM carbonate.

kalium (ka′le-um) [L.] potassium.

kaliuresis (ka″le-u-re′sis) [L. *kalium* potassium + Gr. *ouresis* a making water] the excretion of potassium in the urine.

kaliuretic (ka″le-u-ret′ik) 1. pertaining to, characterized by, or promoting kaliuresis. 2. an agent that promotes kaliuresis.

kallidin (kal′lĭ-din) a plasma kinin produced by glandular kallikreins acting on the plasma γ_2-globulin. It is a polypeptide made of ten amino acids (decapeptide), having the following sequence: H-Ly-Arg-Pro-Pro-Gly-Phe-Ser-Pro-Phe-Arg-OH. Pharmacologically, it causes vasodilatation, increases capillary permeability, produces edema, evokes pain, and contracts or relaxes various extravascular smooth muscles. See also plasma kinins, under KININ.

kallikrein (kal″lĭ-kre′in) any of a group of proteolytic enzymes present in the pancreas, saliva, lymph, urine, and blood plasma, which by acting on γ_2-globulin, liberate bradykinin and kallidin; plasma kallikrein produces bradykinin and exocrine kallikrein produces kallidin. See also plasma kinins, under KININ.

Kalymin trademark for *pyridostigmine bromide* (see under PYRIDOSTIGMINE).

Kamycin trademark for *kanamycin sulfate* (see under KANAMYCIN).

Kanacedin trademark for *kanamycin sulfate* (see under KANAMYCIN).

Kanacin trademark for *kanamycin sulfate* (see under KANAMYCIN).

kanamycin (kan″ah-mi′sin) an aminoglycoside antibiotic which acts on the bacterial ribosome. It is elaborated by *Streptomyces kanamyceticus* and occurs as a white, odorless, crystalline powder that is soluble in water, but not in organic solvents. It comprises three components; A (usually designated as kanamycin), B, and C. It is active against gram-negative bacteria, including *Klebsiella, Aerobacter, Enterobacter, Brucella, Neisseria, Haemophilus, Shigella, Salmonella, Escherichia coli, Serratia marcescens*, and strains of *Proteus*, as well as gram-positive bacteria, including *Staphylococcus aureus* and *S. epidermis*. Used in the treatment of septicemia, urinary tract infections, bacterial endocarditis, peritonitis, and pneumonia. Side effects include auditory, visual, and renal disorders, headache, pruritus, rash, drug fever, and vomiting. **k. sulfate**, the sulfate salt of kanamycin, having actions and uses similar to those of the parent drug. Trademarks: Cantrex, Kamycin, Kanacedin, Kanacin, Kantrex.

Kanone trademark for *menadione*.

Kantrex trademark for *kanamycin sulfate* (see under KANAMYCIN).

kaolin (ka'o-lin) a native aluminum silicate, powdered and freed from gritty particles by elutriation, occurring as a soft white or yellowish white powder with a claylike taste, used as an absorbent and demulcent. It is also used in dental porcelain to add strength to the molded tooth prior to firing and toughness and opacity to the fused porcelain and as a sunscreen for protecting the lips from ultraviolet rays. Called also *argilla, bolus alba,* and *China clay*.

Kaplan, Eugene 1. see familial nonspherocytic ANEMIA (Zueler-Kaplan syndrome). 2. thalassemia–hemoglobin C disease (Zueler-Kaplan syndrome).

Kaposi's sarcoma (angiomatosis), varicelliform eruption (dermatitis) [Moritz *Kaposi*-Kohn, Austrian dermatologist, 1837–1902] see under SARCOMA and ERUPTION.

Kaposi-Spiegler sarcomatosis [M. *Kaposi*-Kohn; Eduard *Spiegler*, Vienna dermatologist, 1860–1908] benign LYMPHADENOMATOSIS.

Kappadione trademark for *menadiol sodium diphosphate* (see under MENADIOL).

Kappaxin trademark for *menadione*.

Kari rinse see under RINSE.

Karidium liquid, phosphate fluoride topical gel, phosphate fluoride topical solution, tablets see under GEL, LIQUID, SOLUTION, and TABLETS.

Karion trademark for *sorbitol*.

Karolyi effect [M. *Karolyi*, Hungarian dentist, 19th and 20th centuries] bruxism.

karyo- [Gr. *karyon* nucleus, nut] a combining form denoting relationship to a nucleus. See also words beginning CARYO-.

karyogamy (kar″e-og'ah-me) [*karyo-* + Gr. *gamos* marriage] cell conjugation followed by union of nuclei.

karyogenesis (kar″e-o-jen'ĕ-sis) [*karyo-* + Gr. *genesis* production] the development of the nucleus of a cell.

karyokinesis (kar″e-o-ki-ne'sis) [*karyo-* + Gr. *kinesis* motion] the division of the cell nucleus in cell division.

karyoklasis (kar″e-ok'lah-sis) [*karyo-* + Gr. *klasis* breaking] the breaking down of the cell nucleus or nuclear membrane.

karyology (kar″e-ol'o-je) [*karyo-* + *-logy*] the branch of cytology which deals with the cell nucleus.

karyolymph (kar″e-o-limf″) [*karyo-* + *lymph*] the liquid ground substance of the cell nucleus in which the chromatin material and nucleolus are suspended. Called also *nuclear sap*.

karyolysis (kar″e-ol'ĭ-sis) [*karyo-* + Gr. *lysis* dissolution] the dissolution of the cell nucleus with a gradual loss of the chromatin. See also NECROSIS.

karyoplasm (ka're-o-plazm″) [*karyo-* + Gr. *plasma* plasm] the semifluid form of the protoplasmic fluid in the cell nucleus. See NUCLEOPLASM.

karyopyknosis (kar″e-o-pik-no'sis) [*karyo-* + *pyknōsis*] pyknosis.

karyorrhexis (kar″e-o-rek'sis) [*karyo-* + Gr. *rhēxis* breaking] rupture of the cell nucleus in which the chromatin disintegrates into formless granules which are extruded from the cell. See also NECROSIS.

karyosome (kar'e-o-sōm″) [*karyo-* + Gr. *sōma* body] irregular clumps of chromatin (heterochromatin) dispersed in the nuclei of cells that are not in division. Called also *chromatin nucleolus, chromatin particle, chromocenter, false nucleolus,* and *nucleinic nucleolus*.

karyotype (kar'e-o-tīp) [*karyo-* + *type*] the full chromosome set; by extension, the photomicrograph of chromosomes arranged according to the Denver nomenclature. See CHROMOSOME nomenclature, Denver, and see illustration at CHROMOSOME.

kat katal.

kat-, kata- [Gr. *kata* down] a prefix signifying down, against. See also words beginning CATA-.

katal (kat'al) the unit of enzymic activity, being the amount of activity that converts 1 mole of substrate per second. Logarithmic multiples of this unit may be expressed by adding prefixes, such as micro-, nano-, or pico-. Abbreviated *kat*. See also enzyme UNIT.

Katonil trademark for *chlormerodrin*.

Kaufmann see Abderhalden-Fanconi SYNDROME (Abderhalden-Kaufmann-Lignac syndrome).

Kavitan trademark for *menadione sodium bisulfite* (see under MENADIONE).

Kavit-G trademark for *menadione*.

Kayvisyn trademark for *vitamin K₅ hydrochloride* (see under VITAMIN).

Kazanjian's forceps, operation, splint, T bar [Varaztad Hovhannes *Kazanjian*, Armenian-born American plastic and maxillofacial surgeon, born 1879] see under FORCEPS, OPERATION, SPLINT, and BAR.

KBG KBG SYNDROME.

kc kilocycle.

Keegan's operation [Denis Francis *Keegan*, English surgeon, 1840–1920] see under OPERATION.

Kefglycin trademark for *cephaloglycin*.

Keflex trademark for *cephalexin*.

Keflin trademark for *cephalothin sodium* (see under CEPHALOTHIN).

Keflodin trademark for *cephaloridine*.

Kelene trademark for *ethyl chloride* (see under CHLORIDE).

Kell antigen (factor), blood groups [named after the person in whom antibodies to the Kell antigen were first discovered] see under ANTIGEN and BLOOD GROUP.

Kelly, Adam Brown [1865–1941] see Plummer-Vinson SYNDROME (Paterson and Brown Kelly syndrome, Paterson-Kelly syndrome, Paterson-Kelly webs).

Kelly hemostat see under HEMOSTAT.

Kelly's operation [Joseph Dominic *Kelly*, American surgeon, born 1888] arytenoidopexy.

keloid (ke'loid) [Gr. *kēlē* tumor + *eidos* form] a sharply elevated, irregularly-shaped, progressively enlarging scar due to the formation of excessive amounts of collagen in the corium during connective tissue repair. **Addison's k.**, morphea. **k. of gums**, FIBROMATOSIS gingivae.

kelvin (kel'vin) [named after Lord *Kelvin*] the SI unit of thermodynamic temperature equal to 1/273.15 of the absolute temperature of the triple point of water. Abbreviated *K*. See also absolute TEMPERATURE, Kelvin SCALE, and SI.

Kelvin scale, thermometer [Lord William Thomson *Kelvin*, British physicist, 1824–1907] see under SCALE and THERMOMETER. See also KELVIN.

Kemadrin trademark for *procyclidine hydrochloride* (see under PROCYCLIDINE).

Kempe, C. H. [American physician] see battered CHILD (Caffey-Kempe syndrome).

Kenacort trademark for *triamcinolone*.

Kenalog trademark for *triamcinolone acetonide* (see under TRIAMCINOLONE).

Kendall, Edward Calvin [1886–1972] an American chemist; co-winner, with P. S. Hench and T. Reichstein, of the Nobel prize for medicine and physiology in 1950, for discoveries concerning the adrenal cortex hormones.

Kennedy bar 1. see under BAR. 2. continuous CLASP.

Kennedy classification [Edward *Kennedy*] see under CLASSIFICATION.

keno- [Gr. *kenos* empty] see CENO-(2).

Kent zinc cement see under CEMENT.

kerasin (ker'ah-sin) a cerebroside containing lignoceric acid; it yields on hydrolysis galactose, sphingosine, and lignoceric acid. It is obtained from brain tissue.

keratan sulfate (ker'ah-tan) an acid mucopolysaccharide made up of repeating disaccharide units of N-acetylglucosamine, galactose, and galactose 6-sulfate *Keratan sulfate I* is found in the cornea and *keratan sulfate II* in skeletal tissue, the two keratans differing in the nature of the amino sugar present. Abbreviated KS.

keratenite (ker-at'ĕ-nīt) the natural anhydrous form of calcium sulfate.

keratin (ker'ah-tin) a fibrous protein found chiefly in the epidermis, hair, and nails, and in wool, which is produced by keratinocytes, consisting of folded, probably in a helical fashion, peptide chains with −S−S cross-linkages between adjacent chains. Keratin is insoluble in dilute alkalies, strong acids, organic solvents, and water, thus giving the skin its protective qualities and nails and hair their tough flexible characteristics. **hard k.**, keratin found in the hair and nails, forming a more or less compact homogeneous mass. **soft k.,** keratin found in the epidermis, which sloughs continuously in fine loose scales and becomes structurally integrated with the shrunken, non-nucleated dead cells, thus forming a tough elastic horny upper layer of the skin.

keratinization (ker″ah-tin″i-za′shun) the process of impregnating the stratum corneum of the epidermis with keratin, so that it is structurally integrated with the shrunken, non-nucleated dead cells, thus forming a tough elastic horny upper layer of the skin. Called also *cornification.*

keratinocyte (ke-rat′ĭ-no-sīt) the epidermal cell which synthesizes keratin; constituting 95 percent of the epidermal cells and, with the melanocytes, forming the binary cell system of the epidermis. In its various successive stages it is known as basal cell, prickle cell, and granular cell. Called also *malphighian cell.*

keratitis (ker″ah-ti′tis) [kerato- + -itis] inflammation of the cornea.

kerato- [Gr. keras horn, cornea] a combining form denoting relationship to the horny tissue, or to the cornea. See also words beginning CERATO-.

keratoacanthoma (ker″ah-to-ak″an-tho′mah) [kerato- + acanthoma] primary pseudoepitheliomatus HYPERPLASIA.

keratoconjunctivitis (ker″ah-to-kon-junk″tĭ-vi′tis) inflammation of the cornea and conjunctiva. **k. sic′ca,** Sjögren's SYNDROME.

keratoconus (ker″ah-to-ko′nus) [kerato- + Gr. kōnos cone] a conical protrusion of the cornea.

keratocyst (ker″ah-to-sist) [kerato- + cyst] an odontogenic cyst lined with keratinized epithelium. See also CYST.

keratogenesis (ker″ah-to-jen′ĕ-sis) [kerato- + Gr. genesis production] the formation of horny tissue or material.

keratohyalin (ker″ah-to-hi′ah-lin) a substance found in granules in the granular layer of the epidermis, the origin and chemistry of which is unclear, but which may be involved in the process of keratinization. Spelled also *keratohyaline.* See also keratohyalin granules, under GRANULE.

keratohyaline (ker″ah-to-hi′ah-lĭn) 1. both horny and hyaline. 2. pertaining to keratohyalin or to the keratohyalin granules of the granular layer of the epidermis. 3. keratohyalin.

keratoid (ker′ah-toid) [kerato- + Gr. eidos form] resembling horn or corneal tissue.

keratolysis (ker″ah-tol′ĭ-sis) [kerato- + Gr. lysis dissolution] a cutaneous condition characterized by dissolution and peeling of the horny layer of the epidermis. **k. bullo′sa heredita′ria,** EPIDERMOLYSIS bullosa. **k. neonato′rum,** Ritter's DISEASE.

keratolytic (ker″ah-to-lit′ik) 1. pertaining to, characterized by, or producing keratolysis. 2. an agent (caustic) that induces desquamation of horny tissue by loosening cornified epithelium and causing it to swell and soften. Used in the treatment of some dermatophytoses, warts, corns, and acneiform and eczematous skin diseases. Called also *desquamating agent.*

keratoma (ker″ah-to′mah), pl. *keratomas, kerato′mata* [kerato- + -oma] a horny or keratoid tumor. See KERATOSIS. **k. excen′tricum,** Mibelli's DISEASE. **senile k.,** actinic KERATOSIS.

keratomata (ker″ah-to′mah-tah) plural of *keratoma.*

keratomycosis (ker″ah-to-mi-ko′sis) [kerato- + Gr. mykēs fungus + -osis] fungous disease of the cornea. **k. lin′guae,** black TONGUE.

keratosis (ker″ah-to′-sis), pl. *kerato′ses* [kerato- + -osis] 1. any horny growth, such as a wart or callosity. 2. any condition attended ⎣ y horny growths. **actinic k.,** a sharply outlined, red or skin-colored, flat or elevated, verrucous or keratotic growth, which may develop into a cutaneous horn, and may give rise to a squamous cell carcinoma; it usually affects the middle-aged or elderly, especially those of fair complexion, and is caused by excessive exposure to sun. Called also *solar k.,* and formerly *senile k.* and *senile keratoma.* **focal (oral) k.,** oral LEUKOPLAKIA. **k. follicula′ris,** a skin disease, usually beginning during childhood as discrete flesh-colored keratotic papules, which become crust-covered and, by coalescence, produce papillomatous, vegetating, tumor-like growths on the head, neck, back, chest, and groin; ulcerations and secondary infection may occur, causing an offensive odor. The oral lesions appear as minute, whitish papules which feel rough upon palpation, and are usually found on the gingivae, tongue, buccal mucosa, and hard and soft palates; other mucosal surfaces, such as the vulva, larynx, and pharynx, may be involved. It appears to be inherited as an irregular autosomal dominant trait, although isolated cases are common. Called also *k. vegetans, Darier's disease, dyskeratosis follicularis vegetans,* and *White's disease.* **k. follicula′ris serpigino′sa,** perforating ELASTOSIS. **inverted follicular k.,** Helwig's DISEASE. **k. labia′lis, k. lin′guae,** oral LEUKOPLAKIA. **k. ni′gricans,** ACANTHOSIS nigricans. **nonspecific (oral) k.,** oral LEUKOPLAKIA. **k. palma′ris et planta′ris,**

HYPERKERATOSIS palmaris et plantaris. **k. pharyn′gea,** a condition characterized by projection of numerous white horny masses from the tonsils and from the orifices of the lymph follicles in the wall of the pharynx. **senile k., solar k.,** actinic k. **tumor-like k.,** primary pseudoepitheliomatous HYPERPLASIA. **k. veg′etans, k. follicularis.**

Kerckring's ossicle [Theodorus Kerckring, Dutch anatomist, 1640–1693] see under OSSICLE.

kerma (ker′mah) [kinetic energy released in material] a unit of quantity that represents the kinetic energy transferred to charged particles by the uncharged particles per unit mass of the irradiated medium. Abbreviated *K.*

kernel (ker′nel) that part of an atom left after removal of the valence electrons.

kerosene, kerosine (ker′o-sēn) a hydrocarbon, chiefly of the methane series, being a distillation product of petroleum, occurring as a pale yellow or clear, mobile, oily liquid with a characteristic odor. Used as a fuel, as a reagent, and in insecticides. Owing to its defatting action, contact with the skin may cause irritation leading to infection; inhalation may cause headache, drowsiness, and coma; and ingestion may result in vomiting and diarrhea. Called also *coal oil* and *paraffin.*

Kerr equalizing paste see under PASTE.

Kerr Luralite a trademark for a hard *zinc oxide–eugenol impression paste* (see under PASTE).

Kerr Permplastic trademark for a *polysulfide impression material* (see under MATERIAL).

Kerr sealer see under SEALER.

Kerr Speraloy trademark for an *amalgam alloy* (see under AMALGAM).

Kerr Spher-A-Caps trademark for preproportioned *dental amalgam* (see under AMALGAM) in disposable capsules, containing 49.82 to 50.18 percent mercury.

Kerr Topical Flura-Gel see under GEL.

Kerr Traycon trademark for a *silicone impression material* (see under MATERIAL).

Kesling appliance, spring [Harold D. Kesling, American orthodontist, born 1901] see under APPLIANCE and SPRING.

Kessodrate trademark for *chloral hydrate* (see under CHLORAL).

Ketajet trademark for *ketamine hydrochloride* (see under KETAMINE).

Ketalar trademark for *ketamine hydrochloride* (see under KETAMINE).

ketamine hydrochloride (ket′ah-mēn) a rapid-acting general anesthetic, 2-(o-chlorophenyl)-2-(methylamino)-cyclohexanone hydrochloride, occurring as a white crystalline powder with a characteristic odor, which is soluble in water, methanol, ethanol, and chloroform. It produces deep analgesia, normal pharyngeal-laryngeal reflexes, normal or slightly enhanced muscle tone, cardiovascular and respiratory stimulation, and, occasionally, minimal respiratory depression. Used as the sole anesthetic for diagnostic and surgical procedures, for the induction of anesthesia prior to the administration of other anesthetics, and as a supplement for agents such as nitrous oxide. Temporary increase of the pulse rate and blood pressure and psychological reactions ranging from pleasant dream-like states to hallucinations and delirium are the principal side reactions. Trademarks: Ketajet, Ketalar, Ketanest, Vetalar.

Ketanest trademark for *ketamine hydrochloride* (see under KETAMINE).

keto- a chemical prefix indicating the presence of the keto or carbonyl group, : C : O.

ketoacidosis (ke″to-ah″sĭ-do′-sis) acidosis accompanied by the accumulation of ketone bodies (ketosis) in the body tissues and fluids, as in diabetic acidosis.

ketogenesis (ke″to-jen′ĕ-sis) [ketone + Gr. genesis production] the production of ketone bodies.

ketone (ke′tōn) a class of organic compounds having a functional

$$\overset{\text{O}}{\underset{\|}{}}$$

group—C—which is attached to two carbon atoms, and having a name ending in –one, propanone (acetone) being a typical ketone. **k. body,** ketone BODY. **dimethyl k.,** acetone.

β-ketopropane (ba″tah-ke″to-pro′pān) acetone.

ketose (ke′tōs) a carbohydrate containing a ketone group.

ketosis (ke-to′sis) a condition characterized by an abnormally elevated concentration of ketone bodies in body tissues and fluids, characterized by a specific odor detectable in the breath, and considered to be one of the principal symptoms of diabetes mellitus.

17-ketosteroid (ke-to′ste-roid) a group of steroids produced by the zona fasciculata and zona reticularis of the adrenal cortex and, in smaller amounts, by the testes, which are characterized by the presence of a ketone group on C_{17} (see STEROID). 17-Ketosteroids are present in the urine of normal human adults and, in excessive amounts, in adrenal neoplasms. Principal 17-ketosteroids include progesterone and dehydroepiandrosterone.

keV kiloelectron VOLT.

key (ke) an instrument for opening a lock, or a device for making or breaking an electric circuit; by extension, any tool for revealing specific information. **dental k.,** an instrument formerly used for tooth extraction, believed to have been developed early in 18th century, consisting of a handle, stock, convex rest, claw, and claw hinge. Later models included various modifications; for example, some types had projections from the shaft to the site opposite to the attachment of the claw and others had the claw in the form of a semicircle. **torquing k.,** an orthodontic instrument used to facilitate the engaging of rectangular arch wires into the edgewise brackets.

keyway (ke'wa) the slot into which the male portion of a precision attachment fits.

kg kilogram.

kg-cal kilocalorie; see large CALORIE.

kg/cm² kilogram per square centimeter. See also mechanical STRESS.

kg-m kilogram-meter.

kg × m/s² a symbol for acceleration of the mass of 1 kilogram the distance of 1 meter per second squared. See NEWTON.

KHN Knoop hardness number; see under HARDNESS.

Kidd antigen (factor), blood groups [named after the mother of the child in whom Kidd antigen was first discovered] see under ANTIGEN and BLOOD GROUP.

kidney (kid'ne) [L. *ren;* Gr. *nephros*] either of the two organs in the lumbar region that filter the blood, excreting the end-products of body metabolism in the form of urine, and regulating the concentrations of hydrogen, sodium, potassium, phosphate, and other ions in the extracellular fluid. Called also *ren.* See also terms beginning RENO- and NEPHRO-. **artificial k.,** extracorporeal DIALYSIS. **middle k.,** mesonephros. **permanent k.,** metanephros.

Kiel graft see under GRAFT.

Kienböck unit [Robert *Kienböck,* American radiologist, 1871–1953] see under UNIT.

kieselguhr (ke'zel-goor) a type of diatomaceous earth, used as a filler in dental materials, such as hydrocolloid impression materials, and as a mild abrasive and polishing agent.

Kiesselbach's area (space) [Wilhelm *Kiesselbach,* German physician, 1839–1902] see under AREA.

kil (kil) a white, sticky, soapy clay from the Black Sea region; when sterilized, used as an ointment base.

Killax trademark for *tetraethyl pyrophosphate* (see under PYROPHOSPHATE).

killer (kil'er) someone or something that destroys life or neutralizes or does away with active qualities of anything. **k. cell,** killer CELL. **pain k.,** popular name for *analgesic* (3).

Killian's operation [Gustav *Killian,* German surgeon, born 1891] see under OPERATION.

killing (kil'ing) deprivation of life. **mercy k.,** euthanasia (2).

kilo- [Fr., from Gr. *chilioi* thousand] in the metric system, a combining form denoting a quantity 1000 (10^3) times the unit designated by the root with which it is combined. Abbreviated *k.* See also metric SYSTEM and *Tables of Weights and Measures* at WEIGHT.

kilocalorie (kil″o-kal'o-re) [*kilo-* + *calorie*] large CALORIE.

kilocycle (kil″o-si'k'l) [*kilo-* + *cycle*] a unit of 1000 (10^3) cycles, e.g., 1000 cycles per second; applied to the frequency of electromagnetic waves. Abbreviated *kc.*

kilogram (kil'o-gram) [*kilo-* + *gram*] the standard unit of mass (weight) in the metric system or in SI, which is based on the weight of 1 liter of pure water at 4°C (the temperature of the maximum density of water) at sea level. A block of platinum and iridium kept by the International Bureau of Weights and Measures in Paris is used as a standard weight for 1 kilogram. It contains 1,000 grams and 1,000,000 milligrams, and is equivalent to 2.204623 pounds avoirdupois weight and to 2.679229 pounds apothecaries weight. Abbreviated *kg.* See also SI and *Tables of Weights and Measures* at WEIGHT.

kilogram-meter (kil″o-gram-me'ter) a unit of work, representing the energy required to raise 1 kilogram of weight 1 meter vertically against gravitational force at sea level, being equiva-

lent to about 7.2 foot-pounds and equal to 1000 gram-meters. Abbreviated *kg-m.*

kiloliter (kil'o-le″ter) [*kilo-* + *liter*] a unit of volume in the metric system, being 1000 (10^3) liters, or the equivalent of 264.18 U.S. gallons. Abbreviated *kl.* See also *Tables of Weights and Measures* at WEIGHT.

kilomegacycle (kil″o-meg′ah-si″k'l) [*kilo-* + *megacycle*] a unit of 1000 (10^3) megacycles or 1,000,000,000 (10^9) cycles per second; applied to the frequency of electromagnetic waves. Abbreviated *kMc.*

kilometer (kil'o-me″ter) [*kilo-* + *meter*] a unit of length in the metric system, being 1000 (10^3) meters, or the equivalent of 3280.83 feet, 1093.6121 yards, or about five-eighths of a mile. Abbreviated *km.*

kilonem (kil'o-nem) [*kilo-* + *nem*] a unit of nutritive value, being the equivalent of 667 calories. See also NEM.

kilounit (kil″o-u'nit) a quantity equivalent to 1000 (10^3) units.

kilovolt (kil″o-vōlt) [*kilo-* + *volt*] a unit of electrical pressure or electromotive force, being 1,000 (10^3) volts. In radiology, the electromotive force responsible for the penetrating ability of x-rays. Abbreviated *kv.*

kilovoltage (kil″o-vōl'tij) electromotive force measures in kilovolts. In radiology, the potential difference between the anode and cathode of an x-ray tube. See also MEGA-, ORTHO-, and SUPERVOLTAGE. **constant potential k.,** in radiology, the potential of a constant voltage generator, in constant potential kilovolts. Abbreviated *kvcp.* **effective k.,** equivalent k. **equivalent k.,** in radiology, the kilovoltage of monoenergetic radiation having the same half-value layer as the heterogeneous beam produced by a peak kilovoltage in question. Called also *effective k.* **k. peak,** kilovolt PEAK.

kilowatt (kil″o-wot) a unit of electric power, being 1,000 (10^3) watts.

kilowatt-hour (kil'o-wot-aw'er) a unit of electric energy equal to that expended by 1 kilowatt in 1 hour. Abbreviated *kw-hr.*

kilurane (kil'u-rān) a unit of radioactivity, being 1000 (10^3) uranium units.

kinase (ki'nās) 1. a phosphotransferase [E.C.2.7.1 to 2.7.5] or a pyrophosphotransferase [E.C.2.7.6] that catalyzes the transfer of a high-energy group of a donor, usually adenosine triphosphate. 2. any hydrolase [E.C.3.4] that activates zymogen, variously named according to its source as enterokinase, staphylokinase, and so on. **hexo-k.,** hexokinase. **phosphoenolpyruvate k.,** pyruvate k. **phosphoglycerate k.** [E.C.2.7.2.3], a phosphotransferase with a carboxyl group as acceptor, which, in carbohydrate metabolism, converts 1,3-diphosphoglyceric acid to 3-phosphoglyceric acid in the presence of ADP. **pyruvate k.** [E.C.2.7.1.40], a phosphotransferase that occurs in all tissues of the body. It catalyzes the transfer of a phosphate group from ATP to pyruvate to form ADP and phosphoenolpyruvate, and also phosphorylates hydroxylamine and fluoride in the presence of carbon dioxide. Called also *phosphoenolypyruvate k. phosphoenolypyruvate-ADP transphosphatase,* and *phosphoenol transphosphorylase.*

kindred (kin'dred) an extended family group.

kine- see KINESIO-.

kinesio-, kine- [Gr. *kinēsis* movement] a combining form denoting relationship to movement. See also words beginning CINE- and CINESIO-.

kinesiology (ki-ne″se-ol'o-je) [*kinesio-* + *-logy*] the study of movement as it relates to physiological processes, physical principles, and anatomy of the body. See also MOVEMENT.

kinetic (ki-net'ik) [Gr. *kinētikos*] pertaining to or producing motion.

kinetics (ki-net'iks, ki-net'iks) [Gr. *kinētikos* of or for putting in motion] the branch of dynamics that pertains to the turnover, or rate of change, of a specific factor (e.g., erythrocytes — erythrokinetics, leukocytes — leukokinetics, or iron — ferrokinetics), commonly expressed as units of amount per unit time. **chemical k.,** the rates of chemical reactions and the actual steps involved in converting reactants to products.

kineto- [Gr. *kinētos* movable] a combining form meaning movable.

kinetochore (ki-ne'to-kōr) [*kineto-* + Gr. *chora* space] centromere.

King's operation arytenoidopexy.

kingdom (king'dum) [Anglo-Saxon *cyningdom*] traditionally, one of the three categories into which natural objects are usually classified: the *animal kingdom,* including all animals; the *plant kingdom,* including all plants; and the *mineral kingdom,* including all objects and substances without life. A fourth kingdom, the *Protista,* includes all single-celled organisms. Currently, one of the two categories of forms of life: the Procaryotae, including two divisions, the *Bacteria* and *Cyanobac-*

teria (blue-green algae), which is characterized by cells lacking true nuclei (prokaryotic cells); and the Eucaryotae, including higher plants and animals, fungi, protozoa, and most algae, which is characterized by cells having true nuclei (eukaryotic cells). See also TAXONOMY.

Kingsley, Norman William [1829–1913] an American dentist, considered to be the "father" of modern orthodontics. He designed a cleft-palate obturator and interdental splint. See Kingsley PLATE and Kingsley SPLINT.

kinin (ki′nin) any of a large group of vasodilator polypeptides, found widely distributed in nature, which have pharmacological properties resembling those of bradykinin (see *plasma k.*), and containing the same nonapeptide fragment. **hornet k.,** a kinin which, together with histamine, 5-hydroxytryptamine, and acetylcholine, forms the dolorogenic component of hornet venom. **plasma k.,** either of two kinins, bradykinin and kallidin, originally observed in the urine as hypotensive factors and later found to occur also in the saliva, blood plasma, and other tissues. Bradykinin is made up of nine amino acids (nonapeptide) and kallidin of ten (decapeptide). They are cleaved from kininogens in plasma γ_2-globulin with the participation of a group of proteolytic enzymes (kallikreins) present in the plasma, lymph, urine, saliva, pancreatic, and exocrine secretions; plasma kallikreins liberating bradykinin and glandular kallikreins liberating kallidin. Pharmacologically, they cause vasodilatation, increase capillary permeability, produce edema, evoke pain, and contract or relax various extravascular smooth muscles. **wasp k.,** a kinin which, together with histamine and 5-hydroxytryptamine, forms the dolorogenic component of wasp venom.

kininogen (ki′nin-o-jen″) an α_2-globulin of plasma that is a precursor of the kinins.

Kinnier Wilson's disease [Samuel Alexander *Kinnier Wilson,* English neurologist, 1878–1936] hepatolenticular DEGENERATION.

kinnogenase (ki″no-jen′ās) kallikrein.

kino- [Gr. *kinein* to move] a combining form denoting relationship to motion.

kinosophere (ki′no-sfēr) [*kino-* + Gr. *sphaira* sphere] aster.

Kipca trademark for *menadiol sodium diphosphate* (see under MENADIOL).

Kirkland instruments, knife, periodontal pack see under INSTRUMENT, KNIFE, and PACK.

Kirkland-Kaiser pack see under PACK.

Kirschner wire [Martin *Kirschner,* German surgeon, 1879–1942] see under WIRE.

kit (kit) a set or collection of instruments, parts, or supplies designed and assembled to serve a specific purpose. **Messerann k.,** a trademark for a kit used to remove broken instruments and sections of silver points from root canals. It consists of a hollow trepan bur, which is used to create a space around the broken fragment, and an extractor, which grasps and extricates fragments from the canal.

Kitasato, Shibasaburo [1852–1931] a Japanese bacteriologist who, with Emil Adolph von Behring, first described antitoxins.

kiting (kīt′ing) increasing the quantity of a drug ordered by a prescription by illegal practices, such as adding zeros to the number shown on the prescription.

K-Jet trademark for *phytonadione.*

kl kiloliter.

Klebs-Loeffler bacillus [T.A.E. *Klebs*] *Corynebacterium diphtheriae;* see under CORYNEBACTERIUM.

Klebsiella (kleb″se-el′ah) [named after T. A. E. *Klebs*] a genus of gram-negative, facultatively anaerobic bacteria of the family Enterobacteriaceae, made up of nonmotile, encapsulated rods, about 0.3 to 1.5 by 0.6 to 6.0 μm in size, found singly, in pairs, or in short chains. The organisms ferment glucose with the production of acid and gas; most strains produce 2,3-butanediol as an end product of glucose fermentation, and lactic, formic, and acetic acids are fermented in small amounts. Some strains are resistant to standard doses of penicillin, but may be sensitive to higher doses. They are variably sensitive to ampicillin, cephalosporins, streptomycin, tetracyclines, neomycin, polymyxin B, sulfonamides, and nitrofurantoin. Resistant strains occur with increasing frequency. Called also *Hyalococcus.* **K. friedländeri,** *K. pneumoniae.* **K. ozae′nae,** a species associated with ozena and atrophic diseases of the upper respiratory tract. Called also *Bacillus mucosus ozaenae, B. ozaenae,* and *Bacterium ozaenae.* **K. pneumon′iae,** a species subdivided into several biotypes, and occurring as a thick type (adhering to guinea pig and other animal red cells) and a thin type (adhering to cells treated with tannic acid). The species is widely distributed in nature, and is found in soil, water, and grain. The organisms also inhabit the intestines of man and animals, and occur in association with various diseases, such as urinary tract infections. *K. pneumoniae* is the etiologic agent of a type of pneumonia (Friedländer's) and other infectious diseases of the human respiratory tract. Called also *K. friedländeri, Bacillus pneumoniae, Bacterium pneumoniae crouposae, Friedländer's bacillus, Hyalococcus pneumoniae,* and *pneumobacillus.* **K. rhinoscleroma′tis,** a species isolated from patients with rhinoscleroma. Called also *Bacterium rhinoscleromatis.*

Kleeblattschädel cloverleaf SKULL.

Klein-Waardenburg syndrome [D. *Klein;* P. Johannes *Waardenburg*] see under SYNDROME.

Kleinschmidt's syndrome, [Hans *Kleinschmidt,* German physician, 1885–1977] see under SYNDROME.

Klemidox trademark for *climizole.*

Klestadt's cyst [Walter D. *Klestadt,* American physician, born 1883] nasoalveolar CYST.

Klinefelter's syndrome [Harry Fitch *Klinefelter,* Jr., American physician, born 1912] see under SYNDROME.

Klinomycin trademark for *minocycline.*

Klippel-Feil syndrome [Maurice *Klippel,* French neurologist, 1858–1942; André *Feil,* French neurologist, born 1884] see under SYNDROME.

Klippel-Feldstein syndrome [M. *Klippel;* E. *Feldstein,* French physician] see under SYNDROME.

Klippel-Trenaunay-Weber syndrome [M. *Klippel;* P. *Trenaunay;* Frederick Parkes *Weber,* British physician, 1863–1962] see under SYNDROME.

Kloropercha N-Ø trademark for a preparation of *chloropercha.*

Klottone trademark for *menadione.*

Km Km FACTOR.

km kilometer.

K-Mart see under DENTIFRICE.

kMc kilomegacycle.

Knapp No. 2 trademark for medium hard *dental casting gold alloy* (see under GOLD).

knee (ne) 1. the site of articulation between the thigh and leg. Called also *genu* [NA]. 2. any structure bent like the knee. **k. of aquaeduc′tus fallo′pii,** GENICULUM of facial canal.

Kniest's disease (syndrome) [W. *Kniest*] see under DISEASE.

knife (nīf) 1. a cutting instrument. 2. an instrument used to remove or smooth the rough margin of a metallic restoration, such as gold foil, or tissue in a surgical procedure. See illustration. **Blair k.,** one with a long sharp blade used to cut skin

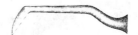

Knife used for gold foil and amalgam restorations. (From H. O. Torres and A. Ehrlich: Modern Dental Assisting. 2nd ed. Philadelphia, W. B. Saunders Co., 1980; courtesy of S. S. White Div. of Pennwalt Corp.)

grafts. **Buck k.,** a periodontal knife with pear-shaped cutting points, used for interdental incision during gingivectomy. **button k.,** a small knife used for the cutting of cartilage. **carving k.,** carver. **cautery k.,** one connected to an electric battery, so that the tissues may be seared while being cut, in order to prevent bleeding. **electric k., endotherm k.,** a knife-shaped electrode or steel needle which cuts by causing dissolution of tissue when activated by a high-frequency current. **finishing k.,** a small knife with a finely tempered blade; used in trimming and finishing edges of fillings and in carving wax cores preparatory to casting. **gold k.,** a knife, usually contra-angled, used to trim direct filling gold. **Goldman-Fox k.,** any of a group of knives designed for incision and contouring of gingival tissues in periodontal surgery. **Humby k.,** one with a roller attached, used for cutting skin grafts of varying thickness; the distance between the roller and the knife blade can be varied by means of a calibration device. **interdental k.,** a periodontal knife designed for interdental tissue removal in periodontal surgery. **Kirkland k.,** a periodontal knife which consists of a thin, flattened blade attached to the handle by an angulated shank, the outer edge being elliptical and the inner straight; used for primary gingivectomy. See illustration. See also gingival LANCET and Kirkland instruments, under INSTRUMENT. **Merrifield k.,** a periodontal knife with a long, narrow, triangular blade; used in gingivectomy. **Monahan-Lewis k.,** a periodontal knife with

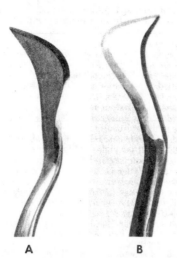

A   **B**

Kirkland Gingivectomy Knife. *A*, 15K; *B*, 16K. (From F. A. Carranza, Jr.: Glickman's Clinical Periodontology. 5th ed. Philadelphia, W. B. Saunders Co., 1979.)

detachable blades. **Orban k.,** a periodontal knife having a spear-shaped blade attached to the handle by an offset shank to provide accessibility to interproximal areas. The blade has two cutting edges, formed by the junction of the rounded outer surface and the flat inner surface, and tapers to a sharp point. **periodontal k.,** a surgical knife used for gingivectomy and other periodontal surgery. It is usually a double-ended instrument, having paired scaler-shaped blades attached to an angulated shank. The entire periphery of the blade is a cutting edge, formed by the junction of the outer and inner surfaces. The tip of the blade is extended to provide access to proximal surfaces. See also INTERDENT. **plaster k.,** a knife for cutting and trimming plaster models. **surgical k.,** see LANCET and SCALPEL.

knitting (nit′ing) the physiological process of repair of a fractured bone.

knob (nob) a bulbous mass or protuberance. **terminal k's,** synaptic terminals; see under TERMINAL.

Knollide trademark for *potassium iodide* (see under POTASSIUM).

Knoop hardness indenter point, hardness number, hardness scale, hardness test see under POINT and HARDNESS.

knot (not) 1. an intertwining of the ends or parts of one or more threads, sutures, or strips of cloth so they cannot be separated easily. Knots have been used in the rotation of teeth. 2. in anatomy, any knoblike swelling or protuberance, as a node. **Ahern's k.,** enamel k. **enamel k.,** an area of epithelial cell concentration in the stellate reticulum of a developing tooth. It is a temporary structure present during the cap stage of odontogenesis, disappearing before enamel formation begins. Called also *Ahern's knot*. **Hensen's k.,** primitive k., Hensen's NODE.

Koch's bacillus [Robert *Koch*, German bacteriologist, 1843–1910; he discovered the phenomenon of delayed hypersensitivity to tuberculosis (cell-mediated immunity), and was winner of the Nobel prize for medicine in 1905] *Mycobacterium tuberculosis;* see under MYCOBACTERIUM.

Kocher's operation [Emil Theodor *Kocher*, Swiss surgeon, 1841–1917; he was the first to perform thyroidectomy, and was winner of the Nobel prize for medicine in 1909] see under OPERATION.

Koeber's saw see under SAW.

koilo- [Gr. *koilos* hollow] a combining form denoting hollow or concave.

koino- [Gr. *koinos* shared in common] see CENO-(3).

Kollidon trademark for *povidone*.

Kölliker's column, membrana eboris of [Rudolf Albert von *Kölliker*, Swiss anatomist and histologist, 1817–1905] see under COLUMN, and see DENTIN.

Kombetin trademark for *strophanthin*.

Konakion trademark for a phytonadione preparation.

Koplik's spots [Henry *Koplik*, New York pediatrician, 1858–1927] see under SPOT.

Korff's fibers see under FIBER.

Kornberg, Arthur [born 1918] an American physician and biochemist; co-winner, with Severo Ochoa, of the Nobel prize for medicine and physiology in 1959, for work in the discovery of enzymes for producing nucleic acids artificially.

Kornzweig, Abraham L. see ACANTHOCYTOSIS (Bassen-Kornzweig syndrome).

Körte-Ballance operation [Werner *Körte*, Berlin surgeon, 1853–1937; Sir Charles Alfred *Ballance*, British surgeon, 1856–1936] see under OPERATION.

Kotogen trademark for *menadione sodium bisulfite* (see under MENADIONE).

Kozhenikov's epilepsy [Aleksei Iakovlevich *Kozhenikov*, Russian physician, 1853–1902] see under EPILEPSY.

KR key-ridge.

Kr krypton.

Krause, Fedor [German surgeon, 1857–1937] see Hartley-Krause OPERATION.

Krause's bulbs (corpuscles, end-bulbs), line, membrane, transverse suture of [Wilhelm Johann Friedrich *Krause*, German anatomist, 1833–1910] see under BULB; and see Z BAND and infraorbital SUTURE.

Krause's posterior jugular process of occipital bone see paramastoid PROCESS.

Krebs cycle [Sir Hans Adolf *Krebs*, German biochemist in England, born 1900; co-winner, with Fritz A. Lipmann, of the Nobel prize for medicine and physiology in 1953, for the discovery of the Krebs cycle] see under CYCLE.

Krebs' leukocyte index [Carl *Krebs*, Danish pathologist, born 1892] see under INDEX.

Kresantin trademark for *metacresyl acetate* (see under METACRESYL).

Krex impression corrective trademark for a soft *zinc oxide-eugenol impression paste* (see under PASTE).

Krimer's operation see under OPERATION.

Krisovski's sign see under SIGN.

Krogh, August [1874–1949] a Danish physiologist noted for his research on the capillaries; winner of the Nobel prize for medicine and physiology in 1920.

Krönlein's operation [Rudolf Ulrich *Krönlein*, Swiss surgeon, 1847–1910] see under OPERATION.

krypto- [Gr. *kryptos* hidden] for words beginning thus, see those beginning CRYPTO-.

krypton (krip′ton) [Gr. *kryptos* hidden] a gaseous element. Symbol, Kr; atomic number, 36; atomic weight, 83.80; density, 3.733 gm/l; valence, 0; group 0 of the periodic table. It occurs as six stable isotopes (78, 80, 82, 83, 84, 86) and several artificial radioactive ones (74–77, 79, 81, 85, 87–95, 97). Kyrpton is a noble, nontoxic, noncombustible, colorless, and odorless gas, slightly soluble in water, which combines with fluorine at liquid nitrogen temperature. Used in high-speed photography, lasers, and electric bulbs. **k.-85,** ^{85}**Kr,** a radioactive isotope of krypton, having a half-life of 10.3 years and emitting beta rays with a small component of gamma rays; used as an activator of phosphorus in self-luminous markers and in medical research, particularly in tracing blood flow.

KS KERATAN sulfate.

Ku 1. Peltz factor (see Kell GROUP). 2. kurchatovium (see ELEMENT 104).

Kühne's spindle, terminal plates [Wilhelm Friedrich *Kühne*, German physiologist, 1837–1900] see neuromuscular SPINDLE, and see under PLATE.

Kulenkampff-Tarnow syndrome [C. *Kulenkampff*] see under SYNDROME.

Küntscher nail [Gerhard *Küntscher*, German surgeon, born 1902] see under NAIL.

Kupffer's cell [Karl Wilhelm von *Kupffer*, German anatomist, 1829–1902] see under CELL.

Kurchatov, Igor Vasilevich [Russian nuclear physicist, 1903–1960] see KURCHATOVIUM.

kurchatovium [named after Igor Vasilevich *Kurchatov*] a proposed name for *element 104* (see under ELEMENT).

Kurloff see KURLOV.

Kurlov's (Kurloff's) body [Mikkail Georgevich *Kurlov*, Russian physician, born 1859] see under BODY.

Kurth, Heinrich [1860–1901] a German bacteriologist.

Kurthia (kur′the-ah) [named after H. *Kurth*] a genus of generally nonpathogenic bacteria of the family Corynebacteriaceae, occurring as gram-positive, non–acid-fast, strictly aerobic rods, about 0.8 by 2.0 to 8.0 μm in size. They have been isolated from human feces in mild cases of food poisoning and under normal conditions, from the intestinal contents of chickens, and from manure, stagnant fresh water, and milk.

Küstner, Heinz [German physician, born 1876] see Prausnitz-Küstner REACTION and REAGIN (1) (Prausnitz-Küstner antibody).

Küttner's ganglion (hauptganglion of) see under GANGLION.

Küttner's tumor [H. *Küttner*] submandibular chronic sclerosing SIALADENITIS.

kv kilovolt.

kvcp constant potential KILOVOLTAGE.

kvp kilovolt PEAK.

kwashiorkor (kwash-e-or'kor) [local name in Gold Coast, Africa, "displaced child"] a syndrome of protein deficiency in children who have been weaned and maintained on an adequate or almost adequate caloric intake on a diet of cereals, such as manioc, which are poor in proteins, occurring chiefly in tropical and subtropical regions. Symptoms include protruding abdomen, edema, growth retardation, fatty liver, hepatomegaly, sparsity of hair, dyspigmentation of hair with streaks or gray and red, dyspigmentation of the skin, dermatitis desquamativa, jaundice, diarrhea, apathy, irritability, anorexia, muscle weakness, tremor, macrocytic, microcytic, or normocytic anemia, hemoglobin deficiency, hypocholesterolemia, hypoalbuminemia, ketonuria, potassium deficiency, enlargement of the lacrimal glands, and oral symptoms, including enlargement of the parotid and submandibular glands, sialadenosis, deficient salivation or sialorrhea, and changes in amylase concentrations of the saliva.

kw-hr kilowatt-hour.

kyphosis (ki-fo'sis) [Gr. *kyphōsis* humpback] abnormal backward curvature of the spine; hunchback. cf. LORDOSIS and SCOLIOSIS.

L

L 1. libra (pound, balance). 2. liter. 3. lethal (fatal). 4. left; usually stamped on paired instruments to differentiate left-handed instruments from the right-handed ones. 5. lambda (2).

L. 1. Latin. 2. length. 3. lumbar. 4. coefficient of induction.

L₀ a symbol for *limes nul*, i.e., a toxin-antitoxin mixture which is completely neutralized and therefore will not kill an animal.

L+ a symbol for *limes tod*, i.e., a toxin-antitoxin mixture which contains one fatal dose in excess and which will kill the experimental animal.

L- 1. a prefix signifying levorotatory. 2. a chemical prefix (small capital) which specifies that the substance corresponds in configuration to the standard substance, i.e., belongs to the same configurational family. In carbohydrate nomenclature, L refers to the *highest numbered* asymmetric carbon atom. In amino acid nomenclature, under rules adopted in 1947, L refers to the configurational family to which the lowest numbered asymmetric carbon atom, i.e., the 2-carbon atom or α-carbon atom, belongs. Opposite of D-.

l 1. liter. 2. azimuthal quantum NUMBER.

l 1. a prefix signifying levorotatory. 2. a prefix used with one of the additional symbols (+) or (−), especially in amino acid nomenclature in the literature from 1923 until approximately 1947, with reference to the configurational family to which the 2-carbon atom or α-carbon atom of the amino acid belongs, the actual direction of the rotation in a specified solvent being indicated by the plus or minus sign, as in, $l(+)$alanine; opposed to $d(−)$- or $a(+)$-, as in $d(−)$alanine or $d)+)$cystine. Opposite of *d*-.

Λ the capital of the Greek letter lambda.

λ the eleventh letter of the Greek alphabet. Symbol for *decay constant*. See LAMBDA.

La 1. lambda. 2. lanthanum.

Labarraque's solution [Antoine Germain *Labarraque*, French chemist, 1777–1850] see SODIUM hypochlorite.

label (la'b'l) something that identifies; an identifying mark, tag, etc. **radioactive l.,** a radioactive atom, usually one that does not interfere with the chemistry of the substance studied or the normal functions of the body, attached to a molecule; used for metabolic studies; a radioactive isotope introduced into tissue to identify the role of the normal element in metabolism.

labia (la'be-ah) [L.] plural of *labium*.

labial (la'be-al) [L. *labialis*] 1. pertaining to a lip, or labium. 2. toward the lips. In dental anatomy, the term is used to refer to the vestibular (or facial) surface of the incisors and canines that faces the lips. Cf. BUCCAL. See illustration at SURFACE.

labialism (la'be-ah-lizm") defective speech, with use of labial sounds.

labially (la'be-al-e) toward the lips.

labio- [L. *labium* lip] a combining form denoting relationship to a lip, especially to the lips of the mouth. See also terms beginning CHEILO-.

labioalveolar (la"be-o-al-ve'o-lar) 1. pertaining to the lip and dental alveoli. 2. pertaining to the labial side of the dental alveolus.

labioaxiogingival (la"be-o-ak"se-o-jin'jĭ-val) pertaining to or formed by the labial, axial, and gingival walls of a tooth cavity preparation. Called also *axiolabiogingival*.

labiocervical (la"be-o-ser'vĭ-kal) 1. pertaining to the labial surface of the neck of an anterior tooth. 2. labiogingival.

labiochorea (la"be-o-ko-re'ah) [*labio-* + *chorea*] a choreic stiffening of the lips in speech, with stammering. Called also *labiochoreic stuttering*.

labioclination (la"be-o-kli-na'shun) deviation of an anterior tooth from the vertical, in the direction of the lips.

labiodental (la"be-o-den'tal) 1. pertaining to the lips and teeth. 2. a speech sound produced by the contact of the lips with the teeth, such as *f* and *v*.

labiogingival (la"be-o-jin'jĭ-val) pertaining to or formed by the labial and gingival walls of a tooth cavity. Called also *labiocervical*.

labioglossolaryngeal (la"be-o-glos"o-lah-rin'je-al) pertaining to the lips, tongue, and larynx.

labioglossopharyngeal (la"be-o-glos"o-fah-rin'je-al) pertaining to the lips, tongue, and pharynx.

labiograph (la'be-o-graf") [*labio-* + Gr. *graphein* to record] an instrument for recording the motion of the lips.

labioincisal (la"be-o-in-si'zal) pertaining to or formed by the labial and incisal surfaces of a tooth.

labiolingual (la"be-o-ling'gwal) 1. pertaining to the lips and the tongue. 2. pertaining to the labial and lingual surfaces of an anterior tooth.

labiology (la"be-ol'o-je) the study of the movements of the lips.

labiomental (la"be-o-men'tal) [*labio-* + L. *mentum* chin] pertaining to the lip and chin.

labiomycosis (la"be-o-mi-ko'sis) [*labio-* + Gr. *mykēs* fungus] any disease of the lips caused by a fungus, such as thrush.

labionasal (la"be-o-na'zal) pertaining to the lip and nose.

labiopalatine (la"be-o-pal'ah-tin) pertaining to the lip and palate.

labioplacement (la"be-o-plās'ment) displacement of a tooth toward the lip.

labioplasty (la'be-o-plas"te) cheiloplasty.

labioproximal (la"be-o-prok'sĭ-mal) of or pertaining to both the proximal and labial surfaces of a tooth. Called also *proximolabial*.

labiotenaculum (la"be-o-te-nak'u-lum) [*labio-* + *tenaculum*] an instrument or device for holding the lip.

labioversion (la"be-o-ver'zhun) displacement of a tooth labially from the line of occlusion.

labium (la'be-um), pl. *la'bia* [L.] lip; one of the two fleshy margins of the mouth. See also LIP. **l. infe'rius o'ris** [NA], lower lip. See LIP (2). **l. mandibula're,** lower lip. See LIP (2). **l. maxilla're,** upper lip. See LIP (2). **l. o'ris** [NA], LIP (2). **l. supe'rius o'ris** [NA], upper lip. See LIP (2). **l. voca'le,** a projection at each side of the rima glottidis.

laboratory (lab'o-rah-to"re) [L. *laboratorium*] a facility intended and equipped for performing experimental work or investigative procedures, for the preparation of drugs or chemicals, or to serve as a workshop for analytical work or for the design and preparation of special purpose appliances. **dental l.,** a facility equipped for the fabrication of appliances and fixed or removable dental prostheses prescribed by a dentist, which operates under the direction of a dental technician. It may be a part of the dental office or a separate facility. Some dental laboratories are commercial enterprises providing services to dentists.

labrale (lah-bra'le) an anthropometric landmark situated in the midsagittal plane on the vermilion border of the lip **l. infe'rius,** the lowermost point, in the midsagittal plane, on the vermilion border of the lower lip. Abbreviated *Li*. Called also *point Li*. **l. supe'rius,** the uppermost point, in the midsagittal plane, on the vermilion border of the upper lip. Abbreviated *Ls*. Called also *point Ls*. See illustration at CEPHALOMETRY.

labrum (la'brum) [L.] a general anatomical term for an edge, brim, or lip.

labyrinth (lab'ĭ-rinth) [Gr. *labyrinthos*] 1. an intricate combination of passages in which it is difficult to find one's way. 2. any system of intercommunicating cavities or canals, especially that constituting the internal ear. Called also *labyrinthus*. 3.

internal EAR. **4.** an intricate entrance into a darkroom that prevents light from the outside shining into the room while the personnel enters or leaves the room. **5.** a system of entrances into a high-voltage therapy room that prevents x-rays from escaping to the outside of the room. **ethmoid l.,** either of the paired lateral masses of the ethmoid bone, consisting of thin-walled cellular cavities, the ethmoidal cells, interposed between two vertical plates of bone. The lateral plate forms part of the orbit and the medial plate forms part of the nasal cavity. The superior surface is made up of half-broken cells which are completed by the edges of the ethmoidal notch of the frontal bone. The lateral surface has irregular cellular cavities which are closed by the sphenoidal conchae and orbital processes of the palatine bones; the smooth surface forms the orbital lamina, which covers the posterior ethmoidal cells and forms part of the wall of the orbit. The thin, rough lamella of the medial surface forms part of the lateral wall of the nasal cavity. Called also *labyrinthus ethmoidalis* [NA], *lateral mass of ethmoid bone,* and *massa lateralis ossis ethmoidalis.*

labyrinthectomy (lab″ĭ-rin-thek′to-me) [*labyrinth* + Gr. *ektomē* excision] excision of the labyrinth.

labyrinthi (lab″ĭ-rin′thi) [L.] plural of *labyrinthus.*

labyrinthine (lab″ĭ-rin′thīn) pertaining to a labyrinth.

labyrinthitis (lab″ĭ-rin-thi′tis) [*labyrinth* + *-itis*] inflammation of the labyrinth (internal EAR).

labyrinthotomy (lab″ĭ-rin-thot′o-me) [*labyrinth* + Gr. *temnein* to cut] surgical incision into the labyrinth (internal EAR).

labyrhinthus (lab″ĭ-rin′thus), pl. *labyrin′thi* [L.; Gr. *labyrinthos*] a general anatomical term for a system of intercommunicating cavities or canals. Called also *labyrinth.* **l. ethmoida′lis** [NA], ethmoid LABYRINTH.

lac (lak), pl. *lac′ta,* gen. *lac′tis* [L.] **1.** milk. **2.** any milklike medicinal preparation. **3.** shellac. **garnet l., gum l.,** shellac. **stick-l.,** see SHELLAC.

laceration (las″er-a′shun) [L. *laceratio*] **1.** the act of tearing. **2.** a wound produced by tearing.

Lacolin trademark for *sodium lactate* (see under SODIUM).

lacrima (lak′rĭ-mah) [L.] tear (1).

lacrimal (lak′rĭ-mal) [L. *lacrimalis,* from *lacrima* tear] pertaining to the tears.

lacrimation (lak″rĭ-ma′shun) [L. *lacrimatio*] the secretion and discharge of tears. **gustatory l.,** paroxysmal unilateral lacrimation during the act of eating or drinking, appearing after facial palsy, which may be caused by misdirected nerve fiber regeneration. Ageusia and facial tic are often associated. Called also *paroxysmal l., Bogorad's syndrome,* and *crocodile tears.* See also gustolacrimal REFLEX. **paroxysmal l.,** gustatory l.

lacta (lak′tah) [L.] plural of *lac.*

lactacidemia (lak-tas″ĭ-de′me-ah) [*lactic acid* + Gr. *haima* blood + *-ia*] the presence in the blood of excessive amounts of lactic acid.

lactaciduria (lak-tas″ĭ-du′re-ah) [*lactic acid* + Gr. *ouron* urine + *-ia*] the presence in the urine of lactic acid.

lactalbumin (lak″tal-bu′min) albumin found in milk, consisting of about 12 percent of the whey. Called also *milk albumin.*

β-lactamase I (ba″tah-lak′tah-māz) penicillinase.

β-lactamase II (ba″tah-lak′tah-māz) cephalosporinase.

lactase (lak′tās) β-GALACTOSIDASE.

lactate (lak′tāt) a salt of lactic acid, containing the radical CH_3–CHOH · COO–. Sometimes the terms *lactate* and *lactic acid* are used interchangeably. **ferrous l.,** a compound, $Fe(C_6H_{10}O_6)$, occurring as greenish-white crystals with a specific odor that darken when exposed to air and are readily soluble in water and alkali, but not in alcohol. Used in the treatment of iron deficiency anemia. Called also *iron lactate.* See also IRON. **iron l.,** ferrous l.

lactic (lak′tik) pertaining to milk or to lactic acid.

lactin (lak′tin) lactose.

Lactinex a mixture of viable cultures of *Lactobacillus acidophilus* and *L. bulgaricus;* used in the treatment of herpes labialis, certain gastrointestinal disorders, and acne.

lactis (lak′tis) [L.] genitive of *lac.*

lactivorous (lak-tiv′o-rus) [L. *lac* milk + *vorare* to devour] feeding or subsisting on milk.

lacto- [L. *lac, lactis* milk] a combining form denoting relationship to milk.

Lactobacillaceae (lak″to-bas″il-la′se-e) [*Lactobacillus* + *-aceae*] a family of nonsporulating bacteria, occurring as gram-positive, nonmotile (rare strains are motile), anaerobic to facultative, straight or curved rods, usually found singly or in chains. It consists of the genus *Lactobacillus.* Formerly called *Lactobacteriaceae.*

lactobacilli (lak″to-bah-sil′li) plural of *lactobacillus.*

Lactobacillus (lak″to-bah-sil′us) [*lacto-* + *bacillus*] a genus of bacteria of the family Lactobacillaceae, occurring as gram-positive (becoming gram-negative with age and increased acidity), nonsporulating rods, which vary from long and slender to short coccobacilli. The members are saccharoclastic organisms; their metabolism is fermentative, at least half of the end-product being lactic acid. They are characteristically aciduric, having an optimal pH of about 5.5 to 5.8 or less, and growing at 5.0 or less. The species are divided into the homofermentative group, producing only lactic acid, and the heterofermentative, producing lactic acid and other end-products of fermentation. Lactobacilli are nonpathogenic generally but may be associated with pathologic conditions, such as febrile diseases and endocarditis. They occur in fermenting animal and plant products where carbohydrates are available, being found in the mouth, vagina, and intestinal tracts of warm-blooded animals; also found in dairy products, water, sewage, beer, wine, fruits, pickled vegetables, and sourdough and mash. In the oral cavity and saliva, they tend to occur in greater concentrations in the presence of dental caries than in caries-free mouths; complete restoration of carious lesions diminishes the oral flora of lactobacilli. The role in dental caries is not yet understood. **L. bre′vis,** a heterofermentative species isolated from the oral cavities, intestinal tract, and feces of humans and rats, and from milk, kefir, cheese, sauerkraut, spoiled tomato products, sourdough, silage, and manure, and producing, in addition to lactic acid, carbon dioxide, acetic acid, ethanol, and mannitol. They occur as straight, short rods, about 0.7 to 1.0 by 2.0 to 4.0 μm in size, with rounded ends, and are found singly or in short chains. **L. buch′neri,** a heterofermentative species producing, in addition to lactic acid, carbon dioxide, acetic acid, ethanol, and mannitol; it is similar to *L. brevis.* **L. bulgar′icus,** a homofermentative species that produces a fermented product known as *Bulgarian* or *bulgaricus milk.* **L. ca′sei,** a homofermentative species isolated from milk, cheese, and other dairy products. **L cellobio′sus,** a heterofermentative species found in the human mouth, which produces in addition to lactic acid, carbon dioxide, acetic acid, ethanol, and mannitol. It occurs as nonmotile and nonflagellated rods, 0.5 to 1.0 by 3.0 to 5.0 μm or more in size. **L. curva′tus,** a homofermentative species isolated from manure, milk, and silage, and from patients with endocarditis. **L. delbruec′kii,** a homofermentative species isolated from potato and vegetable mashes. **L. fermen′tum, L. ga′yoni,** a heterofermentative species, occurring as nonmotile rods of variable size (0.5 to 1.0 by 3.0 μm or more), sometimes found in pairs or in chains. The species has been isolated from the mouth and feces of humans and rats, turkey cecum, yeast, milk products, sourdough, fermenting plants, wine, manure, and silage. Also called *L. longus, Bacterium gayoni,* and *Lactobacterium longum.* **L. helvet′icus,** a homofermentative species isolated from sour milk and cheeses. **L. jensen′ii,** a homofermentative species isolated from the human vagina. **L. lac′tis,** a homofermentative species that acidifies and coagulates milk. **L. leichman′nii,** a homofermentative species isolated from yeast and grain mash. **L. lon′gus,** *L. fermentum.* **L. saliva′rius,** a homofermentative species producing mainly L(+)-lactic acid and small amounts of D(–)-lactic acid. It occurs as rods, about 0.6 to 0.9 by 1.5 to 5.0 μm in size, with rounded ends, found singly, in pairs, and in chains. They are nonmotile, nonflagellated, gram-positive organisms, which have been isolated from the human mouth, mouth and intestinal tract of the hamster, and intestinal tract of poultry.

lactobacillus (lak″to-bah-sil′us), pl. *lactobacilli.* Any microorganism of the genus *Lactobacillus.* **heterofermentative l.,** any strain of *Lactobacillus* that produces lactic acid and also another end-product of fermentation, including *L. brevis, L. buchneri, L. cellobiosus, L. coprophilus, L. desidiosus, L. fructinorans, L. heterohiochii, L. hilgardii, L. trichodes,* and *L. viridescans.* **homofermentative l.,** any strain of *Lactobacillus* that produces only lactic acid as the end-product of fermentation, which includes: a group producing D(–)-lactic acid — *L. delbrueckii, L. leichmannii, L. bulgaricus, L. jensenii, L. lactis;* a group producing DL-lactic acid — *L. acidophilus, L. helveticus;* a group producing mainly L(+)-lactic acid and small amounts of D(–)-lactic acid — *L. salivarius;* a group producing DL-lactic acid (ribose fermented) — *L. casei, L. xylosus;* a group producing DL-lactic acid (ribose fermented) — *L. casei, L. curvatus, L. plantarum;* a group producing DL-lactic acid (ribose fermentation equivocal — *L. laryngiformis;* and a group producing D(–)-lactic acid (ribose not fermented) — *L. coryniformis, L. homohiochii.*

Lactobacteriaceae (lak″to-bak″te-re-a′se-e) former name for Lactobacillaceae.

Lactobacterium (lak″to-bak″te′re-um) former name for *Lactobacillus*. **L. lon′gus,** *Lactobacillus fermentum;* see under LACTOBACILLUS.

lactoflavin (lak′to-fla″vin) [*lacto-* + L. *flavus* yellow] riboflavin.

lactogen (lak′to-jen) any substance that enhances lactation, the principal one being prolactin.

lactone (lak′tōn) 1. an aromatic liquid, $C_{10}H_8O_4$, prepared by distillation from lactic acid. 2. tablets containing lactic acid bacteria; used in preparing buttermilk. 3. a cyclic organic compound in which the chain is closed by ester formation between a carboxyl and a hydroxyl group in the same molecule. **macrocytic l.,** a lactone containing 12 or more carbon atoms in the primary ring. See also MACROLIDE.

lactose (lak′tōs) [L. *saccharum lactis*] a disaccharide present in milk, 4-O-β-D-galactopyranosyl-D-glucose, which, on hydrolysis with acids and certain enzymes (lactases), yields glucose and galactose. It is synthesized in the mammary glands of mammals from glucose in the blood and obtained commercially from milk whey. Lactose may not be tolerated in certain persons after weaning, owing to reduced lactase activity. Used in infant foods and special diets, as an osmotic laxative and diuretic, as a tablet and capsule diluent, in baking mixtures, to produce lactic acid fermentation, in ensilage and food products, as a chromatographic absorbent, and in culture media. Called also *lactin* and *milk sugar.*

lacuna (lah-ku′nah), pl. *lacu′nae* [L.] 1. a small pit or hollow cavity; used in anatomical nomenclature to designate such a compartment within or between other body structures. 2. a defect or gap. See also LAKE. **absorption l.,** resorption l. **blood l.,** a space, lake, or vacuole in the syncytiotrophoblastic layer of the blastocyst, which collects blood from the uterine vessels rupturing during the embryonic development and merges with other lacunae to form a communicating network or labyrinth, thus giving the trophoblast its spongy texture. It becomes the intervillous space of the placenta. Called also *trophoblastic lacuna.* **l. of bone,** a lenticular cavity in the bone matrix, which contains an osteocyte. **cartilage l.,** a cavity in the matrix of cartilage, which contains the cells. Normally, there is a single cell in each lacuna, but during the division, two, four, or eight cells may be found in a single lacuna. Called also *cartilage nidus.* **Howship's l.,** see resorption l. **l. pharyn′gis,** a depression at the pharyngeal end of the auditory tube. **resorption l.,** a pit or concavity found in bones undergoing resorption, frequently containing osteoclasts. Similar lacunae also may be found in eroding surfaces of cementum, in which cementoclasts may or may not be located. Called also *absorption l.* and *Howship's l.* **trophoblastic l.,** blood l.

lacunae (lah-ku′ne) [L.] plural of *lacuna.*

LADD lacrimoauriculodentodigital SYNDROME.

Laevosan trademark for *fructose.*

lag (lag) the period of time elapsing between the application of a stimulus and the resulting reaction. **screen l.,** persistence on the intensifying screen of glow after the cessation of irradiation, usually due to some imperfection in the screen. Called also *afterglow.*

Lagrange's scissors [Pierre Félix *Lagrange,* French ophthalmologist, 1857–1928] see under SCISSORS.

lake (lāk) [L. *lacus*] 1. to undergo separation of hemoglobin from the erythrocytes; a phenomenon sometimes occurring in the blood. 2. a circumscribed collection of fluid in a hollow or depressed area. See also LACUNA.

Laki-Lóránd defect, factor [Koloman (Kálmán) *Laki,* Hungarian-born American biochemist, born 1909; Lászlo *Lóránd,* Hungarian-born American biochemist] see FACTOR XIII.

laliatry (lah-li′ah-tre) [Gr. *lalia* talking + *iatria* therapy] the study and treatment of disorders of speech. Called also *logopedics.*

lallation (lah-la′shun) a speech defect in which *l* is pronounced instead of *r,* or in which an *l* sound is mispronounced.

lalo- [Gr. *lalein* to babble, speak] a combining form denoting relationship to speech, or babbling. See also terms beginning LOGO-.

lalopathology (lal″o-pah-thol′o-je) [*lalo-* + *pathology*] the branch of medicine which deals with disorders of speech.

lalopathy (lah-lop′ah-the) [*lalo-* + Gr. *pathos* illness] logopathy.

laloplegia (lal″o-ple′je-ah) [*lalo-* + Gr. *plēgē* stroke] logoplegia.

lalorrhea (lal″o-re′ah) [*lalo-* + Gr. *rhoia* flow] logorrhea.

lambda (lam′dah) [Gr. letter *lambda* λ, Λ] 1. the eleventh letter of the Greek alphabet. 2. the craniometric point at the site of the posterior fontanelle where the lambdoid and sagittal sutures meet; used as a cephalometric landmark. Abbreviated *L* or *La.* See illustration at CEPHALOMETRY. 3. decay CONSTANT.

lambdacism, lambdacismus (lam′dah-sizm; lam-dah-siz′mus)

[Gr. *lambdakismos*] 1. the substitution of *l* for *r* in speaking. 2. inability to utter correctly the sound of *l.*

lambdoid (lam′doid) [Gr. *lambda* + *eidos* form] shaped like the Greek letter Λ or λ, as in lambdoid suture.

lambert (lam′bert) [named after J. H. *Lambert*] a unit of brightness, being the brightness of a perfect diffuser emitting 1 lumen per square centimeter. The unit generally used is one-thousandth of this and is called a *millilambert.* When the area chosen is 1 square foot the unit is called *foot lambert.* **foot l.,** see *lambert.*

Lambert's cosine law [Johann Heinrich *Lambert,* German physicist and mathematician, 1728–1777] see under LAW. See also LAMBERT.

Lamblia (lam′ble-ah) [named after Vilem Dušan *Lambl,* Czech physician, 1824–1895] *Giardia.*

lamella (lah-mel′ah), pl. *lamel′lae* [L., dim. of *lamina*] 1. a thin leaf or plate, as of bone. See also LAMINA. 2. a medicated disk or wafer prepared from gelatin, glycerin, and distilled water, and containing a small quantity of an alkaloid, to be inserted under the eyelid. **annulate lamellae,** cytoplasmic organelles consisting of parallel arrays of cisternae exhibiting small annuli or circular fenestrae at very regular intervals along their length. **articular l.,** the layer of bone to which an articular cartilage is attached. **cementum l.,** a layer of cementum deposited directly over the older less vital cementum. See also resting LINE (2). **circumferential l., external,** circumferential l., outer. **circumferential l., inner,** circumferential l., internal, one of the osseous lamellae deposited around the marrow cavity and situated in close proximity to the endosteum. Called also *endosteal l.* **circumferential l., outer,** one of the osseous lamellae that surround the outer surface of the bone and situated in close proximity to the periosteum. Called also *external circumferential l., periosteal l.,* and *peripheral l.* **l. of compact bone,** osseous l. **concentric l.,** haversian l. **enamel lamellae,** imperfectly calcified areas of enamel located generally in the cervical enamel but also found in the interdigitating surface of the premolars and molars. They are foliaceous structures visible only under the microscope, which may extend from the surface to the dentinoenamel junctions and beyond. There are three principal types. Type I, a developmental type caused by faulty mineralization, characterized by lamellae that reach the dentinoenamel junctions. Type II, also a developmental type, characterized by crevices and cracks extending into the dentin, which contain exogenous cellular elements and other components, and packed with nonmineralized materials. These two types are considered to be variants of *lamellae verae.* Type III, a posteruptive type. Called also *l. spuriae.* **endosteal l.,** circumferential l., inner. **ground l.,** interstitial l. **haversian l.,** one of the bony lamellae forming rings about the haversian canal. Called also *concentric l.* **intermediate l.,** interstitial l. **interstitial l.,** an irregular osseous lamella situated in the interstitial spaces between the haversian systems. Called also *ground l.* and *intermediate l.* **osseous l.,** a thin layer of calcified interstitial substance of compact bone, about 3 to 7 μ in thickness, which shows variations in density of the compact bone in cross sections. Called also *l. of compact bone.* **periosteal l., peripheral l.,** circumferential l., outer. **punctate l.,** a lamella of stained decalcified bone in which collagenous fibers run across in a section. **lamel′lae spu′riae,** enamel lamellae. **striated l.,** a lamella of stained decalcified bone in which collagenous fibers run longitudinally in a section. **lamellae ve′rae,** developmental enamel lamellae, including Types I and II lamellae; see *enamel l.* **type I l.,** see *enamel l.* **type II l.,** see *enamel l.* **type III l.,** see *enamel l.*

lamellae (lah-mel′e) plural of *lamella.*

lamellar (lah-mel′ar) pertaining to or resembling lamellae.

lamelliform (lah-mel′ĭ-form) [*lamella* + L. *forma* form] resembling or having the appearance of a lamella.

lamina (lam′ĭ-nah), pl. *lam′inae* [L.] a thin flat plate, or layer; used in anatomical nomenclature as a general term to indicate such a structure, or a layer of a composite structure. Called also *layer.* See also LAMELLA. **alar l., l. ala′ris,** alar PLATE. **basal l.,** 1. a mucopolysaccharide layer on which the basal surfaces of epithelial cells that face connective tissues rest. It is in the form of a sheet that follows the contours of cell surfaces, being about 400 to 700 Å wide, which is separated from the cell surface by a light area. Under high magnification it appears as a weblike mass of delicate filaments. Originally, the basal lamina was believed to be derived from the connective tissue, but now considered to be a product of the epithelial cells. 2. basal PLATE (1). **buccal l., buccogingival l.,** vestibular l. **l. cartilag′inis**

cricoideae [NA], l. of cricoid cartilage. l. **cartilag′inis thy-roi′deae** [NA], l. of thyroid cartilage. **cribriform l. of ethmoid bone,** cribriform plate of ethmoid bone; see under PLATE. l. **cribro′sa os′sis ethmoida′lis** [NA], cribriform plate of ethmoid bone; see under PLATE. **l. of cricoid cartilage,** a quadrate, deep lamina which forms the posterior part of the cricoid cartilage. Internally, a ridge on the midline of its dorsal surface attaches fibers of the esophagus; externally, the surface provides a depression for the cricoarytenoideus posterior muscle. Called also *lamina cartilaginis cricoideae* [NA]. **l. den′sa,** the part of the basal lamina of the epithelial attachment of Gottlieb that is adjacent to the enamel. **dental l.,** a horizontal band which projects perpendicularly from the vestibular lamina and extends into the substance of the primitive gum, assuming a horseshoe-like shape to conform with the dental arches. It arises during the seventh week of embryonic growth during the lamina-bud stage of odontogenesis, originating in the epithelial lining of the stomodeal ectoderm, and continuing to function until all the primordia for the permanent teeth have been produced at about four years of age. Following the formation of the successional lamina, the dental lamina undergoes retrogressive changes. The vestigial remains may cause abnormalities, including enamel accretions, epithelial pearls, odontogenic cysts, or supernumerary teeth. Called also *l. dentalis* and *dentogingival l.* See also *successional l.* and tooth BUD. **dental l., lateral,** a lateral band of cells believed to be functionally and structurally similar to the parent dental lamina, which connects the developing tooth germ to the dental lamina. Concavities in the lateral lamina formed by the invading mesenchyma are known as the *enamel niches.* Called also *lateral enamel strand.* **l. denta′lis,** dentogingival l., dental l. **descending l. of sphenoid bone,** pterygoid PROCESS. **l. du′ra,** bundle BONE. **elastic l., external,** elastic membrane, external; see under MEMBRANE. **elastic l., internal,** elastic membrane, internal; see under MEMBRANE. **external l.,** glycocalyx. **external l. of cranial bones,** the outer compact layer of bone of the flat bones of the head. Called also *outer l. of cranial bones, outer plate of cranial bones,* and *outer table of bones of skull.* **external l. of pterygoid process,** pterygoid plate, lateral; see under PLATE. **horizontal l. of ethmoid bone,** cribriform plate of ethmoid bone; see under PLATE. **l. horizonta′lis os′sis palati′ni** [NA], horizontal plate of palatine bone; see under PLATE. **inferior l. of sphenoid bone,** pterygoid PROCESS. **l. inter′na os′sium cra′nii** [NA], internal l. of cranial bone. **internal l. of cranial bone,** the inner plate of the cranial bone; the inner compact layer of bone of the flat bones of the skull. Called also *l. interna ossium cranii* [NA], *inner plate of cranial bone,* and *inner table of bone of skull.* **internal l. of pterygoid process,** pterygoid plate, medial; see under PLATE. **labial l.,** vestibular l. **lateral l. of pterygoid process,** l. latera′lis proces′sus pterygoi′dei [NA], pterygoid plate, lateral; see under PLATE. **l. lu′cida,** the part of the basal lamina of the epithelial attachment of Gottlieb to which the hemidesmosomes are attached. **medial l. of pterygoid process,** l. media′lis proces′sus pterygoi′dei [NA], pterygoid plate, medial; see under PLATE. **orbital l.,** l. orbita′lis os′sis ethmoida′lis [NA], a thin, oblong plate forming the lateral surface of the labyrinth of the ethmoid bone, which covers the middle and posterior ethmoidal cells and forms part of the medial wall of the orbit. It articulates with the orbital plate of the frontal bone, maxilla, orbital process of the palatine bones, lacrimal bone, and sphenoid bone. Called also *l. papyracea, orbital plate of ethmoid bone, os planum,* and *paper plate.* **outer l. of cranial bones,** external l. of cranial bones. **palatine l. of maxilla,** palatine process of maxilla; see under PROCESS. **l. papyra′cea,** orbital l. **perpendicular l. of ethmoid bone,** perpendicular plate of ethmoid bone; see under PLATE. **l. perpendicula′ris os′sis ethmoida′lis** [NA], perpendicular plate of ethmoid bone; see under PLATE. **l. perpendicula′ris os′sis palati′ni** [NA], perpendicular plate of palatine bone; see under PLATE. **l. pretrachea′lis fas′ciae cervica′lis** [NA], cervical visceral FASCIA. **l. prevertebra′lis fas′ciae cervica′lis** [NA], prevertebral FASCIA. **l. profun′da fas′ciae tempora′lis** [NA], the deep or inner layer of the lower part of the temporal fascia. **l. pro′pria muco′sae** [NA], the connective tissue coat of a mucous membrane just deep to the epithelium and basement membrane. Called also *membrana propria* and *proper mucous membrane.* **rudimentary l.,** the dental lamina undergoing retrogressive changes following the formation of the successional lamina. **successional l.,** a continuation of the dental lamina, situated lingually to the developing deciduous teeth, which gives rise to the epithelial germs that differentiate into the permanent teeth. **l. superfi-**

cia′lis fas′ciae tempora′lis [NA], the superficial or outer layer of the lower part of the temporal fascia. **supraglandular elastic l.,** a layer of elastic fibers that separates the submucosa from the lamina propria in the soft palate. **l. of thyroid cartilage, l. cartilag′inis thyroi′dea,** one of the symmetrical right and left cartilaginous plates which form the thyroid cartilage. Called also *lamina cartilaginis thyroideae* [NA]. **vestibular l.,** a germinal band that forms during the seventh week of embryonic growth, during the lamina-bud stage of tooth development. It arises together with the dental lamina (the two being virtually indistinguishable at first) from the epithelial lining of the stomodeal ectoderm. Later, it invades the connective tissue and forms the epithelial wall that separates the connective tissue of the lip from that of the gingivae, thus giving shape to the mandible and maxilla. Its central cells divide into the outer epithelial sheet which forms the vestibular mucosa and the inner sheet which forms the gingival mucosa; the cleft between the sheets forming the vestibule of the mouth. Called also *buccal l., buccogingival l., labial l.,* and *lip furrow band.*

laminae (lam′ĭ-ne) [L.] plural of *lamina.*

laminagram (lam′ĭ-nah-gram) a roentgenogram of a selected layer of the body made by body-section roentgenography.

laminagraph (lam′ĭ-nah-graf) an x-ray generator for making roentgenograms of a layer of tissue at a selected depth.

laminagraphy (lam″ĭ-nag′rah-fe) [L. *lamina* + Gr. *graphein* to write] a body section radiographic technique accomplished by moving the x-ray source and film in parallel planes and at a predetermined angle to the film surface. See also TOMOGRAPHY.

laminar (lam′ĭ-nar) [L. *laminaris*] made up of, or arranged in, laminae or layers.

laminated (lam′ĭ-nāt″ed) made up of thin layers of laminae; stratified.

lamp (lamp) an apparatus for furnishing light or heat. **annealing l.,** an alcohol lamp for heating and purifying gold foil to be used for filling tooth cavities. **mercury vapor l.,** a lamp in which the arc is struck in mercury and is enclosed in a quartz burner; used in light therapy. **mouth l.,** a lamp used for intraoral lighting in areas of the mouth where illumination from the dental operating light is insufficient; usually a part of the dental unit. **quartz l.,** a mercury vacuum lamp made of melted quartz glass embedded in a running water-bath, used as a source of ultraviolet rays. **ultraviolet l.,** one which produces ultraviolet rays.

lamprophonia (lam″pro-fo′ne-ah) [Gr. *lampros* clear + *phōnē* voice + *-ia*] clearness of voice.

Lamy, Maurice see Maroteaux-Lamy SYNDROME.

lanatoside (lah-nat′o-sīd) any of a group of cardiac glycosides obtained by extraction of the wet leaves of *Digitalis lanata.* The group consists of *lanatoside A* ($C_{49}H_{76}O_{19}$; digilanide A, Adigal), *lanatoside B* ($C_{49}H_{76}O_{20}$; digilanide B), *lanatoside C* ($C_{49}H_{76}O_{20}$; digilanide D, Allocor, Ceglunat, Cedilanid, Celadigal), and *lanatoside D* ($C_{49}H_{76}O_{21}$). Used in the treatment of congestive heart failure and atrial fibrillation.

Lanatoxin trademark for *digitoxin.*

lance (lans) [L. *lancea*] 1. lancet. 2. to cut or incise with a lancet.

lancet (lan′set) [L. *lancea* lance] a small pointed and two-edged surgical knife. See also KNIFE. **abscess l.,** a wide-bladed lancet with one convex and one concave edge. **gingival l., gum l.,** a knife for incising the gingivae. See also Kirkland KNIFE. **laryngeal l.,** a delicate knife for operations within the larynx; it is operated through a cannula. **spring l.,** one having a blade held by a spring mechanism.

lancinating (lan′sĭ-nāt″ing) [L. *lancinas*] tearing, darting, or sharply cutting, as lancinating pain.

Landeker-Steinberg light see under LIGHT.

landmark (land′mark) a readily recognizable skeletal or soft tissue structure used as a point of reference in establishing the location of another structure or in determining certain measurements. See also entries under POINT and illustrations at CEPHALOMETRY. **bilateral l.,** any of the symmetrically situated somatometric or cephalometric landmarks on various body structures. Called also *bilateral point.* **bony l.,** an area or spot on a bone, which serves as a landmark for osteometric measurements. Called also *bony point.* **cephalometric l′s,** see illustration at CEPHALOMETRY. **chromosome l′s,** constant and distinct morphological features that are important aids in identifying a chromosome, such as centromeres, telomeres, or some well-defined bands. See also chromosome BAND, chromosome BANDING, and CHROMOSOME nomenclature. **craniometric l′s,** see illustration at CEPHALOMETRY. **midsagittal l.,** a somatometric landmark situated on the median or midsagittal plane. Called also *midsagittal point.* **soft tissue l.,** an area or point on a soft tissue, which serves as a landmark for somatometric measurements. Called also *soft tissue point.*

Landomycin trademark for *oleandomycin*.

Landouzy-Déjérine dystrophy (atrophy) [Louis Théophile Joseph *Landouzy*, French physician, 1845–1917; Joseph Jules *Déjérine*, French physician, 1849–1917] see under DYSTROPHY.

Landsteiner's nomenclature (classification) of blood groups [Karl *Landsteiner*, Austrian physician in the United States, 1868–1940; winner of the Nobel prize for medicine and physiology in 1930, for discovery of human blood groups] see Landsteiner's nomenclature (classification) of blood groups and ABO blood groups, under BLOOD GROUP.

Lane plates [Sir William Arbuthnot *Lane*, English surgeon, 1856–1943] see under PLATE.

Lang crown, bridge, and inlay trademark for a *zinc phosphate cement* (see under CEMENT).

Lange's syndrome [Cornelia de *Lange*, Dutch pediatrician, 1871–1950] de Lange's SYNDROME.

Langenbeck see VON LANGENBECK.

Langer-Giedion syndrome [L. O. *Langer*; A. *Giedion*] see trichorhinophalangeal DYSPLASIA (2).

Langerhans, islands (islets) of [Paul *Langerhans*, German pathologist, 1847–1888] see under ISLAND.

Langhans' layer [Theodor *Langhans*, German pathologist, 1839–1915] cytotrophoblast.

Langley's ganglion [John Newport *Langley*, English physiologist, 1852–1925] see under GANGLION.

Languepin, Anne see Fèvre-Languepin SYNDROME.

Lanimerck trademark for *deslanoside*.

lanolin (lan′o-lin) [L. *lana* wool + *oleum* oil] a purified fatlike substance from the wool of sheep. It is a waxy substance made up of various aliphatic, steroid and triterpenoid high-molecular-weight alcohols, fatty acids, and 25 to 30 percent water, occurring as a yellowish, tenacious semisolid mass with a slight odor. Lanolin is insoluble in water, but readily mixes with it and is soluble in alcohol, benzene, chloroform, ether, carbon disulfide, acetone, and ether. Used as an ointment base. Called also *wool fat*. **anhydrous l.**, lanolin that contains not more than 0.25 percent water; used as an adsorbent ointment base.

Lanoxin trademark for *digoxin*.

lanthanum (lan′thah-num) [Gr. *lanthanein* to be concealed] the most reactive of the rare earths, occurring as a silvery white, malleable, ductile metal, which is soft enough to be cut with a knife. Symbol, La; atomic number, 57; atomic weight, 138.9055; valence, 3; specific gravity, 6.18; melting point, 920°C; group IIIB of the periodic table. It occurs in two stable isotopes, 138 and 139; ^{138}La is radioactive and has a half-life of 1.12×10^{11} years. Radioactive isotopes include 125–137 and 140–144. Lanthanum oxidizes rapidly when exposed to air, is attacked by water, and is soluble in acids. Used in electronic and space technologies and in biology, as a specific antagonist of calcium. See also rare EARTH. **l. group, l. series,** rare EARTH.

Lanvis trademark for *thioguanine*.

lapis (la′pis, lap′is) [L.] stone. **aerosus l.**, calamine (2). **l. calamina′ris,** calamine (2). **l. imperia′lis, l. inferna′lis, l. luna′ris,** SILVER nitrate.

lard (lard) [L. *lardum*] the purified internal fat of the abdomen of the hog.

Largon trademark for *propiomazine hydrochloride* (see under PROPIOMAZINE).

Larixin trademark for *cephalexin*.

Larocin trademark for *amoxicillin*.

Larodopa trademark for *levodopa*.

Larsen's syndrome [Loren J. *Larsen*, American physician, born 1914] see under SYNDROME.

Larsson, Tage see Sjögren-Larsson SYNDROME.

laryngalgia (lar″in-gal′je-ah) [*larynx* + Gr. *algos* pain + *-ia*] pain in the larynx.

laryngeal (lah-rin′je-al) of or pertaining to the larynx.

laryngectomy (lar″in-jek′to-me) [*larynx* + Gr. *ektomē* excision] excision of the larynx.

laryngendoscope (lar″in-jen′do-skōp) [*laryngo-* + Gr. *endon* within + *skopein* to examine] an instrument for viewing the interior of the larynx.

laryngismus (lar″in-jiz′mus) [L.; Gr. *laryngismos* a whooping] spasm of the larynx. **l. strid′ulus,** a condition marked by sudden laryngeal spasm, with a crowing inspiration and the development of cyanosis. It occurs in laryngeal inflammations and as an independent disease, especially in connection with rickets. Called also *Millar's asthma, spasmodic croup,* and *Wichmann's asthma.* See also STRIDOR.

laryngitis (lar″in-ji′tis) inflammation of the larynx, a condition attended with dryness and soreness of the throat, hoarseness, cough, and dysphagia. Called also *angina laryngea.* See also acute CORYZA. **acute catarrhal l.**, a form characterized by aphonia or hoarseness, pain and dryness of the throat, dyspnea, a wheezy cough, and fever. **atrophic l.**, a severe form of chronic catarrhal laryngitis associated with atrophic changes. **chronic catarrhal l.**, that occurring as a sequela of acute catarrhal laryngitis, or, less frequently, due to recurring inflammation, characterized by atrophy of the glands of the mucous membrane. See also *atrophic l.* and *l. sicca.* **croupous l.**, that occurring chiefly in infants or small children, characterized by a resonant barking cough, hoarseness, and stridor. Infection, allergy, foreign body, or neoplasms may be the cause. Laryngeal diphtheria was once a common cause but is now relatively rare. **diphtheric l.**, diphtheric CROUP. **Haemophilus influenzae B l.**, Kleinschmidt's SYNDROME. **membranous l.**, that attended with the formation of a false membrane. See also membranous CROUP. **phlegmonous l.**, a usually fatal complication of erysipelas, smallpox, and other pathologic conditions, attended with submucous suppuration and edema. **l. sic′ca**, chronic laryngitis in which the usual secretions are gluelike; it often accompanies atrophic rhinitis. **subglottic l.**, inflammation of the under surface of the vocal cords. **syphilitic l.**, chronic laryngitis due to syphilitic involvement of the larynx. **ventricular l., l. ventricularis,** congenital dilatation or herniation of the sacculus or appendix of the laryngeal ventricle. **vestibular l.**, viral laryngitis in which edema forms a ring outlining the vestibule of the larynx.

laryngo- [Gr. *larynx* larynx] a combining form denoting relationship to the larynx.

laryngocele (lah-ring′go-sēl) [*laryngo-* + Gr. *kēlē* hernia] a congenital anomalous air sac communicating with the cavity of the larynx, which may become manifest as an enlargement seen as a tumor-like lesion on the outside of the neck; the enlargement is increased by intralaryngeal pressure, as from coughing.

laryngocentesis (lah-ring″go-sen-te′sis) [*laryngo-* + Gr. *kentēsis* puncture] surgical puncture of the larynx.

laryngofissure (lah-ring″go-fish′ūr) the operation of opening the larynx by a median incision through the thyroid cartilage with the formation of a wide window; done for the removal of cancer of the larynx. Called also *median laryngotomy.*

laryngography (lar″ing-gog′rah-fe) [*laryngo-* + Gr. *graphein* to write] 1. a description of the larynx. 2. roentgenography of the larynx with use of a contrast medium.

laryngology (lar″ing-gol′o-je) [*laryngo-* + *-logy*] that branch of medicine which deals with the throat, pharynx, larynx, and tracheobronchial tree and their diseases.

laryngomalacia (lah-ring″go-mah-la′she-ah) [*laryngo-* + Gr. *malakia* softness] flaccidity of the epiglottis and aryepiglottic folds.

laryngopathy (lar″ing-gop′ah-the) [*laryngo-* + Gr. *pathos* disease] any disease of the larynx.

laryngopharyngeal (lah-ring″go-fah-rin′je-al) pertaining to the larynx and pharynx.

laryngopharynx (lah-ring″go-fah′rinks) [*laryngo-* + *pharynx*] the portion of the pharynx which lies below the upper edge of the epiglottis and opens into the larynx and esophagus. Called also *laryngeal pharynx, laryngopharyngeal cavity, pars laryngea pharyngis* [NA], and *pharyngolaryngeal cavity.*

laryngoplasty (lah-ring′go-plas″te) [*laryngo-* + Gr. *plassein* to mold] plastic surgery of the larynx.

laryngoplegia (lar″ing-go-ple′je-ah) [*laryngo-* + Gr. *plēgē* stroke + *-ia*] paralysis of the larynx.

laryngoptosis (lah-ring″go-to′sis) [*laryngo-* + Gr. *ptōsis* fall] an abnormally low position of the larynx which may be congenital or acquired, or dropping of the larynx occurring as an aging process.

laryngopyocele (lah-ring″go-pi′o-sēl) a suppurative form of laryngocele.

laryngorrhagia (lar″ing-go-ra′je-ah) [*laryngo-* + Gr. *rhēgnynai* to break*] hemorrhage from the larynx.

laryngorrhaphy (lar″ing-gor′ah-fe) [*laryngo-* + Gr. *rhaphē* suture] the operation of suturing the larynx.

laryngoscopy (lar″ing-gos′ko-pe) [*laryngo-* + Gr. *skopein* to examine] examination of the interior of the larynx.

laryngospasm (lah-ring′go-spazm) [*laryngo-* + Gr. *spasmos* spasm] spasmodic closure of the larynx.

laryngostat (lah-ring′go-stat) a device for holding a source of radioactive material within the larynx.

laryngostenosis (lah-ring″go-ste-no′sis) [*laryngo-* + Gr. *stenōsis* contracture] a narrowing or stenosis of the larynx.

laryngostomy (lar″ing-gos′to-me) [*laryngo-* + Gr. *stomoun* to provide with an opening] surgical incision into the larynx.

laryngostroboscope (lar″ing-go-strōb′o-skōp) [*laryngo-* + Gr. *strophos* whirl + *skopein* to examine] an apparatus for observing the intralaryngeal phenomena of phonation.

laryngotome (lah-ring′go-tōm) an instrument used in laryngotomy.

laryngotomy (lar″ing-got′o-me) [*laryngo-* + Gr. *tomē* a cutting] surgical incision of the larynx. **complete l.,** the longitudinal slitting of the entire larynx. **inferior l.,** intercricothyrotomy. **intercricothyroid l.,** superior TRACHEOTOMY. **median l.,** laryngofissure. **superior l., subhyoid l., thyrohyoid l.,** incision of the larynx through the thyrohyoid membrane.

laryngotracheal (lah-ring″go-tra′ke-al) pertaining to the larynx and trachea.

laryngotracheotomy (lah-ring″go-tra″ke-ot′o-me) incision of the larynx and trachea.

laryngoxerosis (lah-ring″go-ze-ro′sis) [*laryngo-* + Gr. *xērōsis* a drying up] dryness of the larynx.

larynx (lar′inks) [Gr. "the upper part of the windpipe"] [NA] a structure that connects the pharynx with the trachea, forming a triangular box which is flat and triangular dorsally, bounded ventrally by vertical ridges, and narrow and cylindrical caudally. It is situated at the top of the trachea and below the root of the tongue and the hyoid bone, and is composed of cartilages held together by muscles and ligaments. The larynx serves as a sphincter which guards the entrance to the trachea; the epiglottis, a flap at the base of the tongue, shuts off the larynx as it is lifted up during deglutition and so prevents entry of food and liquids into the air passages. It also serves as the organ of voice, housing two vocal cords which extend from the back to the front wall of the larynx. The larynx is formed by nine cartilages —the thyroid (which forms the Adam's apple), cricoid, epiglottis, two arytenoid, two corniculate, and two cuneiform cartilages. Before puberty, the larynx in males and females differs little in size, but after puberty, its size increases substantially in males, while increasing only slightly in females. **artificial l.,** an electromechanical device which, when activated by the motions of the neck in speech, simulates laryngeal activity and thus enables a laryngectomized person to converse.

laser (la′zer) [*L*ight *A*mplification by *S*timulated *E*mission of *R*adiation] a device which amplifies electromagnetic energy at various optical frequencies in an extremely intense, small, and nearly nondivergent beam of bright light of a single color. Capable of mobilizing intense heat and power when focused at close range, it is used as a tool in surgical procedures, in diagnosis, and in physiological research studies. Its forerunner was the maser, and it was originally called *optical maser.* See also HOLOGRAPHY. **l. interferometry,** laser INTERFEROMETRY. **l. holography,** see HOLOGRAPHY and laser INTERFEROMETRY.

Lasix trademark for *furosemide.*

Lassar's pastes see ZINC oxide.

lassitude (las′ĭ-tūd) [L. *lassitudo* weariness] weakness; exhaustion.

latency (la′ten-se) the state of seeming inactivity, as that occurring between the instant of stimulation and the beginning of response. See also latent PERIOD.

latent (la′tent) [L. *latens* hidden] not manifest; concealed; hidden.

laterad (lat′er-ad) toward a side or a lateral aspect.

lateral (lat′er-al) [L. *lateralis*] on the side; farther from the median plane.

lateralis (lat″er-a′lis) [L.] lateral; a general term used in anatomical nomenclature to denote a structure situated farther from the midplane of the body.

laterality (lat″er-al′ĭ-te) a relationship to one side, such as a tendency, in voluntary motor acts, to use preferentially the organs (hand, foot, ear, eye) of the same side.

latero- [L. *latus* side] a combining form denoting relationship to the side.

laterodetrusion (lat″er-o-de-tru′zhun) the direction in which the condyle moves outwardly and downwardly in the side shift preparatory to swallowing a large bolus of food.

laterodeviation (lat″er-o-de″ve-a′shun) deviation to one side.

lateroflexion (lat″er-o-flek′shun) flexion to one side.

laterognathism (lat″ter-o-nah′thizm) asymmetry of the mandible due to an irregular growth of the mandible, fractures, tumors, or bone diseases, as well as soft tissue disorders, such as hypertrophy or atrophy of some tissues.

lateroposition (lat″er-o-po-zish′un) displacement to one side.

lateroprotrusive (lat″er-o-pro-tru′siv) pertaining to the direction of jaw movement that has both sideward and forward components.

lateroretrusive (lat″er-o-re-tru′siv) pertaining to the direction of a cusp or condyle movement that has both lateral and backward components.

laterotrusion (lat″er-o-tru′zhun) the outward thrust of the rotating condyle or the condyle on the bolus side during mastication. **procurrent l.,** one in which the working side condyle is rotated as it is thrust laterally.

latex (la′tex) [L. "fluid"] a viscid, milky juice secreted by certain species of shrubs and trees, in which minute globules of natural rubber are suspended in a watery serum. Natural rubber latex is obtained from the tree *Hevea braziliensis.* Coagulation of latex is prevented by protective colloids, but can be induced by addition of acetic or formic acid. See also RUBBER.

lathe (lāth) a mechanical device for working metals, wood, and other materials, which holds the material and rotates it about a horizontal axis against a cutting tool. **dental laboratory l.,** an electrically driven lathe which rotates burs, stones, brushes, and wheels, held by metal chucks in order to polish appliances. The chucks are attached to shafts which protrude from the left and right sides of the lathe, so that either side may be used.

latissimus (lah-tis′ĭ-mus) [L.] widest; used in anatomical nomenclature as a term denoting a broad structure, as a muscle.

latitude (lat′ĭ-tūd) in photography, the ability of an emulsion on a photographic plate to record the brightness of various objects in their true proportion to one another. **film exposure l.,** the range between the minimum and maximum radiation exposure which yields radiographic images, the latitude varying directly with kilovoltage and inversely with the contrast. **object l.,** the range between the minimum and maximum object densities recorded on a radiograph.

lattice (lat′is) a structure of strips arranged to form a diagonal pattern of intersecting narrow strips. **Brevais l., crystal l.,** space l. **cubic l.,** a space lattice in which all edges are the same length and all angles between faces are 90°. **hexagonal l.,** a space lattice having two edges equal and two angles equal. **l. imperfection,** an abnormal arrangement or displacement of atoms in the space lattice of a crystalline structure, such as point defects or dislocations. **orthorhombic l.,** a space lattice in which all edges are unequal, but the interfacial angles are all 90°. **space l.,** a pattern formed by the spatial distribution of atoms or radicals in a crystal, with atoms maintaining their relative position, or interatomic distance, to one another. The lattice may have a cubic, hexagonal, orthorhombic, or other geometric form. Most crystalline materials used in dentistry tend to form a cubic type of lattice. Called also *Brevais l.* and *crystal l.* See illustration.

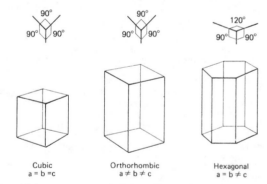

Cubic
a = b =c

Orthorhombic
a ≠ b ≠ c

Hexagonal
a = b ≠ c

Three of the seven general classes of crystal systems. (From J. I. Routh, D. P. Eyman, and D. J. Burton: Essentials of General, Organic and Biochemistry. 3rd ed. Philadelphia, W. B. Saunders Co., 1977.)

latus (la′tus) [L.] 1. broad, wide. 2. an anatomical term denoting the side or flank.

laudanum (law′dah-num) OPIUM tincture.

Laudicon trademark for *morphone hydrochloride* (see under MORPHONE).

laughter (laf′ter) a series of spasmodic and partly involuntary expirations with inarticulate vocalization, normally indicative of merriment, often a hysteric manifestation or a reflex result of tickling.

Laumonier's ganglion [Jean Baptiste Philippe Nicolas Réné *Laumonier,* French surgeon, 1749–1818] 1. carotid GANGLION; 2. carotid ganglion, inferior; see under GANGLION.

Lauren's operation see under OPERATION.

Lauritzen electroscope dosimeter PENCIL.

Lauromicina trademark for *erythromycin estolate* (see under ERYTHROMYCIN).

lavage (lah-vahzh′) [Fr.] the washing out of an organ. See also IRRIGATION.

laveur (lah-vur′) [Fr.] an instrument for performing lavage or irrigation.

law (law) a uniform or constant fact or principle. **all or none l.,** the principle whereby stimulation of a nerve or muscle fiber will cause an action potential to travel over the entire fiber or not at all, and function, once initiated, becomes independent of the intensity of the stimulus. Stimulation of any single atrial or ventricular fiber of the heart will cause an action potential to travel over the entire atrial or ventricular muscle mass, because of the syncytial nature of the heart muscle, but in all other muscles and nerves, the principle is limited to individual fibers; i.e., stimulation of a fiber causes an action potential to travel over the entire single fiber, or not to travel at all. Called also *all or none, all or none effect, all or nothing principle,* and *Bowditch's law.* **Ångström's l.,** the wavelengths of the light absorbed by a substance are the same as those given off by it when luminous. **Aran's l.,** fractures of the base of the skull (except those by contrecoup) resulting from injuries to the vault, the fractures extending by radiation along the line of shortest circle. **Arndt-Schulz l.,** weak stimuli increase physiologic activity and very strong stimuli inhibit or abolish activity. **l's of articulation,** a set of rules to be followed in arranging teeth to produce a balanced articulation. **Avogadro's l.,** equal volumes of all perfect gases at the same temperature and pressure contain the same number of molecules, or, in the case of monatomic gases, of atoms. **Barfurth's l.,** the axis of the tissue in a regenerating structure is at first perpendicular to the cut. **Bell's l., Bell-Magendie l.,** the anterior roots of the spinal nerves are motor roots, and the posterior are sensory. **Behring's l.,** an old term for an example of passive immunization with antiserum, in which the blood and serum of an immunized person, when transferred to another subject, will render the latter immune. Called also *von Behring's l.* **Bergonié-Tribondeau l.,** the sensitivity of cells to radiation varies directly with the reproductive capacity of the cells and inversely with their degree of differentiation. **Bowditch's l.,** 1. all or none l. 2. nerves cannot be tired out by stimulation. **Boyle's l.,** The volume occupied by a gas at constant temperature is inversely proportional to the pressure. **Bunsen-Roscoe l.,** the photochemical effect produced is equal to the product of the intensity of the illumination and the duration of exposure. **Charles' l.,** when the amount and the pressure of a gas remain constant, the volume is directly proportional to the absolute temperature. Called also *Gay-Lussac's l.* **Colles' l., Colles-Baumès l.,** a child that is affected with congenital syphilis, its mother showing no sign of the disease, will not infect its mother. **Collin's l.,** in infants and children, if after removal of a neoplasm, metastasis or recurrence does not occur for a period equivalent to the age of the patient plus nine months, the possibility of such occurrence is slight. **l. of conservation of energy,** energy can neither be created nor destroyed and therefore the total amount of energy in the universe remains constant. See also *first l. of thermodynamics.* **l. of conservation of mass,** matter can neither be created nor destroyed, and therefore the total amount of mass in the universe remains constant. **l. of constant energy consumption,** Rubner's l. (1). **l. of constant growth quotient,** Rubner's l. (2). **l. of constant proportions,** l. of definite proportions. **l. of contrary innervation,** Meltzer's l. of contrary innervation. **Coulomb's electromagnetic l.,** the force between two similar magnetic poles varies inversely as the square of the distance between them. **Coulomb's electrostatic l.,** the force between two electric charges varies: (*a*) inversely as the squares of their distance apart; (*b*) directly as the product of their electric charges. **Coutard's l.,** in radiotherapy, the point of origin of a mucous membrane tumor is the last site to heal following irradiation. **Curie's l.,** all substances may be rendered radioactive by the influence of the emanations of radium and substances thus influenced hold their radioactivity longer when enclosed in some material through which the emanations cannot pass. **Dalton's l.,** the total pressure of a mixture of gases that are not in chemical combination is equal to the sum of the pressures of the individual gases. See also *Henry's l.* **l. of definite proportions,** when two or more elements combine, they always combine in a fixed, or definite, proportion by weight. Called also *l. of constant proportions* and *Proust's l.* See also *l. of multiple proportions.* **displacement l.,** Wien's displacement l. **Draper's l.,** only the rays that are absorbed by a photochemical substance will produce a chemical change in it. **Dulong and Petit l.,** elementary atoms or molecules have an equal atomic heat capacity, although certain elements of low atomic weight and high melting point obey the law only at high temperatures. **Edinger's l.,** a gradual increase in the function of the neuron causes at first increased growth, but if irregular and excessive, then it leads to atrophy and degeneration. **Einstein-Starck l. (of photochemical equivalence),** according to the quantum theory,

quanta of light are absorbed at random during irradiation; the absorption of one quantum of light by a molecule (or atom) produces only one activated molecule (or atom). **l. of excitation,** above threshold, increased electrical stimulation of a motor nerve causes a graded contractile response until a maximum response is achieved. **l. of facilitation,** when an impulse has passed once through a certain set of neurons to the exclusion of others, it will tend to take the same course on a future occasion, and each time it traverses this path the resistance in the path will be smaller. See also FACILITATION. **Fajans' l.,** the product left after the emission of alpha rays has a valence less than that of the parent radioactive substance; the product left after the emission of beta rays has a valence greater by one than that of the parent radioactive substance. **Fajans-Soddy l.,** when an alpha particle is expelled from a radioactive substance, the product is two places lower in the periodic table. A beta ray change (expulsion of an electron) produces a rise of one place. **Faraday's l.,** *I.* in electrolysis, the amount of an ion liberated in any given time is proportional to the strength of the current. *II.* 1 faraday (96.489 coulombs) liberates 1 gm equivalent of an ion by electrolysis. **l. of fatigue,** when the same muscle or group of muscles is kept in constant action until fatigue sets in, the total work done, multiplied by the rate of work, is constant. Called also *Houghton's l.* **Fechner's l.,** the intensity of a sensation produced by a varying stimulus is proportional to the logarithm of that stimulus. Called also *Weber-Fechner's principle.* **first l. of thermodynamics,** see *l's of thermodynamics.* **Gay-Lussac's l.,** Charles' l. **Gerhardt-Semon l.,** peripheral and central lesions affecting the recurrent laryngeal nerve cause the vocal cord to assume a position between abduction and adduction, the paralysis of the parts being incomplete. **Gompertz's l.,** there is a quantitative relation between the probability of death from a given disease and age. **Good Samaritan l.,** a law enacted in some states which absolves physicians or dentists rendering aid in an emergency situation from malpractice liability for alleged damages, unless there is evidence of willful wrongdoing. Called also *Good Samaritan legislation.* **Graham's l.,** the rate of diffusion of a gas is inversely proportional to the square root of its density. **l. of gravitation,** all bodies attract each other with a force that is proportional to their masses and inversely proportional to the square of their distance apart. Called also *Newton's l.* **Grotthus' l.,** only those rays of ultraviolet light that are absorbed produce a chemical reaction. **Guldberg and Waage l.,** the velocity of a chemical reaction is proportional to the active masses of the reacting substances. Called also *mass l.* and *l. of mass action.* **Hanau's l's of articulation,** a set of physical laws that must be observed in the formation of the occlusal surfaces of natural dentition or dentures, to assure establishment or production of balanced articulation. See Thieleman's PRINCIPLE. **Hardy-Weinberg l.,** in population genetics, a law concerned with the relation between gene frequencies and genotype frequencies within populations. It states that the proportions of the three genotypes determined by two alleles (*A* and *a*) occurring with a frequency of *p* and *q*, respectively, in a randomly mating population will remain constant from one generation to the next: $AA = p^2, Aa = 2pq, aa = q^2$. Mutation, selection, migration, and genetic drift can disturb this equilibrium. Called also *Hardy-Weinberg equilibrium, Hardy-Weinberg formula,* and *Hardy-Weinberg ratio.* **Henry's l.,** a slightly soluble gas that dissolves in a definite mass of liquid at a given temperature, and does not unite chemically with the solvent, is very nearly directly proportional to the partial pressure of that gas. See also *Dalton's l.* **Hilton's l.,** a nerve trunk which supplies the muscles of any given joint also supplies the muscles which move the joint and the skin over the insertion of such muscles. **Hooke's l.,** within the elastic limit of any body the ratio of the stress to the strain produced is constant. See also ELASTICITY. **Hoorweg's l.,** for a given voltage there is a minimal duration of stimulus necessary to cause an action potential. **Houghton's l.,** l. of fatigue. **l. of independent assortment,** the members of gene pairs segregate independently during meiosis. See also *Mendel's l.,* and LINKAGE (2). **l. of inverse square,** the intensity of radiation is inversely proportional to the square of the distance between the point of source and the irradiated surface. **isodynamic l.,** in the production of heat in the body the different foodstuffs are interchangeable in accordance with their heat-producing values. **Jackson's l.,** after a convulsion, simple neurological functions are recovered before more complex ones. **Lambert's cosine l.,** the intensity of radiation on an absorbing surface varies as the cosine of the angle of incidence for parallel rays. **Lossen's l.,** Lossen's RULE. **malthusian l.,** the hypothesis that population tends to outrun the means available to sustain it. **mass l., l. of mass action,** Guldberg and Waage l. **Meltzer's l. of contrary innervation,** all living functions are continually controlled by two opposing forces; augmentation or action on the one hand, and inhibition on the other. **Mendel's l., mendelian l.,** in the inheritance of certain traits or characters, the offspring are not intermediate in character between the parents but inherit from one or the other parent in this respect. For example, if a pea plant with the factor tallness (TT) is mated with one with the factor shortness (SS) then some of the offspring will inherit TT, some TS, and some SS in the ratio: TT, 2TS, SS. The TT's are homozygous (pure) tall, the SS's are homozygous short, and the TS's are heterozygous. Which parent the TS ones resemble will depend on whether T or S is dominant. The TT's mated with TT's breed pure as do the SS's with SS's. The TS's mated with TS's again produce TT's, TS's and SS's in the same rato as above. TS's mated with TT's or SS's give the same combinations but in a different ratio. Today, Mendel's law is usually expressed as the *law of independent assortment* and the *law of segregation.* Called also *mendelian inheritance.* **Mendeleev's l.,** periodic l., **Metchnikoff's l., Mechnikov's l.,** whenever the body is attacked by bacteria, the polymorphonuclear leukocytes and the large mononuclear leukocytes quickly become protective phagocytes. **Meyer's l.,** the internal structure of fully developed normal bone represents the lines of greatest pressure or traction and affords the greatest possible resistance with the least possible amount of material. **Müller's l.,** l. of specific irritability. **l. of multiple proportions,** if an element unites with another element in more than one proportion by weight to form two or more compounds, these proportions by weight bear a ratio to one another that may be expressed in small whole numbers. See also *l. of definite proportions.* **Nernst's l.,** the current required to stimulate muscle action varies as the square root of its frequency. **Newland's l.,** a forerunner of the periodic law, in which the chemical elements, arranged in order of their atomic weights, showed a repetition of properties in octaves. **Newton's l., l. of gravitation. Newton's l. of motion I,** every body continues in its state of rest or of uniform motion in a straight line except insofar as it may be compelled to change that state by the action of some outside force. **Newton's l. of motion II,** change of motion is proportional to force applied and takes place in the direction of the line of action of the force. **Newton's l. of motion III,** to every action there is always an equal and opposite reaction. **Nysten's l.,** rigor mortis affects first the muscles of mastication, next those of the face and neck, then those of the upper trunk and arms, and last of all those of the legs and feet. **Ohm's l.,** the strength of an electric current varies directly as the electromotive force, and inversely as the resistance. **Pascal's l.,** pressure applied to a liquid at any point is transmitted equally in all directions. See also PASCAL. **periodic l.,** if the chemical elements are arranged in the sequence of their atomic numbers, they fall into distinctive periods of 2, 8, 8, 18, 18, and 32 elements. Called also *Mendeleev's l.* See also ELEMENT (2). **Pfeiffer's l.,** an old term for an example of passive transfer of antibody in serum, in which the blood serum of an animal immunized against a disease will, when introduced into the body of another (susceptible) animal, protect the recipient by destroying the bacteria causing that disease. **Poiseuille's l.,** the volume flow in a tube is (a) directly proportional to the pressure drop along the length of the tube and to the fourth power of the radius of the tube, and (b) is inversely proportional to the length of the tube and to the viscosity of the fluid. See also VISCOSITY. **Prévost's l.,** in a lateral cerebral lesion the head is turned toward the side involved, **Proust's l.,** l. of definite proportions. **Raoult's l.,** molar weights of nonvolatile nonelectrolytes when dissolved in a definite weight of a given solvent under the same conditions lower the solvent's freezing point, elevate its boiling point, and reduce its vapor pressure equally for all such solutes. **l. of reciprocal proportions,** two chemical elements that unite with a third element do so in proportions that are multiples of those in which they unite with each other. Called also *Walton's l.* **reciprocity l.,** the time required for a given radiographic exposure is inversely proportional to the milliamperage employed. **l. of referred pain,** referred pain only arises from irritation of nerves which are sensitive to those stimuli that produce pain when applied to the surface of the body. **l. of refreshment,** the refreshment of a laboring muscle depends on the rate of supply of arterial blood and the number of open capillaries. **l. of relativity,** simultaneous and successive sensations modify each other. **Ritter's l.,** both the opening and closing of an electric current produce

stimulation in a nerve. **Rubner's l.,** 1. (*law of constant energy consumption*) the rapidity of growth is proportional to the intensity of the metabolic process. 2. (*law of constant growth quotient*) the same fractional part of the entire energy is utilized for growth; this fractional part is called the *growth quotient.* **Schroeder van der Kolk's l.,** the sensory fibers of a mixed nerve are distributed to the parts moved by muscles innervated by the motor fibers of that nerve. Called also *van der Kolk's l.* **second l. of thermodynamics,** see *l's of thermodynamics.* **l. of segregation,** in each generation the ratio of (a) pure dominants, (b) dominants giving descendants in the proportion of three dominants to one recessive, and (c) pure recessives is 1:2:1. This ratio follows from the fact that the two alleles of a ·gene cannot be a part of a single gamete, but must segregate to different gametes. See also *Mendel's l.* and MEIOSIS. **Semon's l., Semon-Rosenbach l.,** in progressive organic diseases of the motor laryngeal nerves, the abductors of the vocal cords (posterior cricoarytenoids) are the first, and occasionally the only, muscles affected. **Sherrington's l.,** 1. every posterior spinal nerve root supplies a definite region of the overlying skin, although fibers from adjacent spinal segments may also supply such a region to a lesser extent. 2. when a muscle receives a nerve impulse to contract, its antagonist simultaneously receives an impulse to relax. See reciprocal INNERVATION. **l. of specific irritability,** every sensory nerve reacts to one form of stimulus and gives rise to one form of sensation only, though if under abnormal conditions it be excited by other forms of stimuli, the sensation evoked will be the same. Called also *Müller's l.* **Stokes' l.,** a muscle situated above an inflamed membrane is often affected with paralysis. **Teevan's l.,** fractures of bones occur in the line of extension and not in the line of compression. **l's of thermodynamics,** *zeroth law:* two systems in thermal equilibrium with a third system are in thermal equilibrium with each other. *First law:* energy is conserved in any process; i.e., the energy gained (or lost) by a system is exactly equal to the energy lost (or gained) by the surroundings. See also *l. of conservation of energy. Second law:* there is always an increase in entropy in any naturally occurring (spontaneous) process. *Third law:* absolute zero is unattainable. **third l. of thermodynamics,** see *l's of thermodynamics.* **L. of Twelve Tables,** Roman laws (c. 450 B.C.) listing heavy fines for anyone causing "the tooth of another man to fall." **van der Kolk's l.,** Schroeder van der Kolk's l. **Virchow's l.,** the cell elements of tumors are derived from normal and preexisting tissue cells. **von Behring's l.,** Behring's l. **Waller's l., wallerian l.,** if the sensory fibers of the root of a spinal nerve be divided on the central side of the ganglion, the fibers of the peripheral side of the cut do not degenerate; while those that remain connected with the cord degenerate. **Walton's l., l. of reciprocal proportions. Wien's displacement l.,** in radiation therapy, the wavelength of maximum intensity becomes shorter as the temperature of the body increases. Called also *displacement l.* **Wolff's l.,** a bone, normal or abnormal, develops the structure most suited to resist forces acting upon it. **zeroth l. of thermodynamics,** see *l's of thermodynamics.*

Lawrence, Ernest Orlando [1901–1958] an American physicist; builder of the first cyclotron for the production of high-energy particles, and winner of the Nobel prize for physics in 1939. See also LAWRENCIUM.

Lawrence's syndrome [R. D. *Lawrence*] lipoatrophic DIABETES.

lawrencium (law-ren'se-um) [named after E. O. *Lawrence*] an artificial radioactive element of the actinide series produced by bombarding californium with boron ions. Symbol, Lr (formerly Lw); atomic number, 103; atomic mass number, 157; valence, 3(?). Several isotopes are known to exist (255–260). Originally discovered as the isotope ^{257}Lr, whose number has been changed to 258, having a half life of 4.2 sec and emitting alpha rays.

laxative (lak'sah-tiv) [L. *laxativus*] 1. aperient; mildly cathartic. 2. a chemical substance that facilitates the passage and elimination of feces; see CATHARTIC.

Laxin trademark for *phenolphthalein.*

layer (la'er) a sheetlike mass of substance of nearly uniform thickness, several of which may be superimposed, one above another. Called also *lamina* and *stratum.* **adamantine l.,** dental ENAMEL. **ameloblastic l.,** the inner layer of cells of the enamel organ, created by its invagination, which forms the enamel prism. **basal l., basal l. of epidermis,** the innermost layer of the malpighian layer of the epidermis, bordering on the corium, consisting mostly of the keratinocytes which give rise to all other cells of the stratified epidermis, and some melanocytes. Called also *stratum basale epidermidis* [NA], and *stratum cylindricum epidermidis* [NA alternative]. Sometimes called also *germinative l.* or *germinative layer of epidermis.* **basement l.,** basement MEMBRANE. **Beilby's l.,** see metallographic

POLISHING. **blastodermic l.,** germ l. **boundary l.,** glycocalyx. **cambium l.,** the internal layer of the periosteum. See PERIOSTEUM. **cell-rich l.,** a layer of the dental pulp situated between the pulp core and Weil's basal layer, which is richly supplied with cellular elements, including reticular fibers, mesenchymal cells, fibroblasts, and macrophages, and contains blood vessels and nerves. Called also *cell-rich zone*. **cementogenic l.,** a layer of cementoblasts in which cementum is produced. **clear l., clear l. of epidermis,** the clear, translucent layer of the epidermis, located between the granular and horny layers, and consisting of closely packed, flattened cells in which the nuclei are indistinct or absent. This layer is usually present only in especially thick epidermis, such as that of the palms and soles. Called also *stratum lucidum epidermidis* [NA]. **Dobie's l.** Z BAND. **enamel l., inner,** the inner, concave wall of the enamel organ. **enamel l., outer,** the outer, convex wall of the enamel organ. **ependymal l.,** the innermost layer of the wall of the neural tube, which appears during the fourth week of embryonic development and lines the neurocoele. It differentiates regionally into the roof plate and floor plate and its cells persist as an epithelial lining for the cavities of the central nervous system. **germ l.,** one of the three embryonic layers (ectoderm, mesoderm, and endoderm) evolved from the blastula through the process of gastrulation, which give raise to specific tissues and organs of the body. Called also *blastodermic l.* **germinative l., germinative l. of epidermis,** 1. malpighian l. 2. basal l. **granular l., granular l. of epidermis,** the layer of the epidermis located just above the prickle-cell layer; in the palms and soles, it is separated from the horny layer by the clear layer. It consists mostly of rhomboidal and flattened keratinocytes containing a dense collection of darkly staining, irregularly-shaped keratohyaline granules. This layer is three to five cells deep in the thick epidermis of the palms and soles, but is thinner in other body areas, or may be absent. Called also *stratum granulosum epidermidis* [NA]. **granular l. of Tomes,** a layer of imperfectly calcified dentin made of small interglobular spaces immediately beneath the dentinocemental junction in the root of a tooth. Called also *Tomes' granular l.* **half-value l.,** the thickness of a given substance which, introduced in the path of a given beam of rays, will reduce its intensity to one half of the initial value. Abbreviated *HVL.* Called also *half-value thickness.* See also homogeneity COEFFICIENT. **horny l., horny l. of epidermis,** the outermost layer of the epidermis, consisting of stratified layers of dead keratinocytes, which provide the protective shield against external noxious agents. Called also *stratum corneum epidermidis* [NA]. **investing l. of cervical fascia,** the part of the cervical fascia which sheathes the superficial infrahyoid muscles and invests the structures of the neck. Called also *investing cervical fascia.* **Langhans' l.,** cytotrophoblast. **malpighian l.,** the deepest layer of the epidermis and the mucous membrane, whose cells are actively engaged in mitosis. It is comprised of the basal and prickle-cell layers, and is responsible for initiation of the keratinization process. Called also *germinative l., germinative l. of epidermis, stratum dentatum epidermidis,* and *stratum germinativum epidermidis* [Malpighii]. **mantle l.,** a layer of the neural tube situated between the ependymal and marginal layers. It appears during the fourth week of embryonic development and contains the bulk of the cell mass (perikaryon) of the neurons, differentiating into the gray substance of the central nervous system. **marginal l.,** the narrow, practically cell-free outermost layer of the wall of the neural tube, made up of a fibrous sheath, which appears during the fourth week of embryonic development and differentiates into the white substance of the central nervous system. **mucous l.,** malpighian l. **odontoblastic l.,** the epithelioid odontoblastic zone, one to five layers thick, which forms the outer surface of the dental pulp adjacent to the dentin, resting on the zone of Weil. Its function consists of producing and maintaining the dentin. See also ODONTOBLAST. **Ollier's l., osteogenetic l.,** the innermost layer of the periosteum. **passivating l.,** a thin layer of chromic oxide (Cr_2O_3) formed on the surface of stainless steel, which provides a barrier against corrosion and tarnish. Called also *passivating film.* See also stainless STEEL. **peptidoglycan l.,** in the bacterial cell, a single, bag-shaped macromolecule, or network, entirely surrounding the cytoplasmic elements of the cell, composed of glycan strands cross-linked by short peptides. See also cell WALL and PEPTIDOGLYCAN. **polish l.,** see metallographic POLISHING. **prickle-cell l.,** the spinous layer of the malpighian layer of the epidermis, located between the granular and basal layers, and consisting mostly of keratinocytes which appear to be joined to each other by numerous short cytoplasmic processes or prickles (prickle cells). Called also *spinous l., spinous l. of epidermis,* and *stratum spinosum epidermidis* [NA]. **second half-value l.,** the additional thickness of material needed to reduce the beam from one half to one

fourth of its original exposure rate. **spinous l., spinous l. of epidermis,** prickle-cell l. **subendothelial l.,** the middle, fibrous layer of the tunica intima of typical blood vessels, located between the endothelium and internal elastic membrane. **submantle l.,** a layer of interglobular dentin usually situated just below the cover (mantle) dentin. **submucous l.,** submucous MEMBRANE. **submucous l. of pharynx,** submucous membrane of pharynx; see under MEMBRANE. **subodontoblastic l.,** Weil's basal l. **subpapillary l.,** the layer of the corium immediately underlying the layer containing the dermal papillae. **subserous l.,** subserous FASCIA. **Tomes' granular l.,** granular l. of Tomes. **trophic l.,** entoderm. **vegetative l.,** entoderm. **vertical l. of ethmoid bone,** perpendicular plate of ethmoid bone; see under PLATE. **Weil's basal l.,** a clear, relatively cell-free layer, located just inside the odontoblastic layer and overlying the cell-rich zone of the dental pulp, which is visible during the inactive phase of dentinogenesis. It is made up of delicate fibrils embedded in the ground substance. In dentinogenesis, the fibrils are incorporated into the matrix. The few cellular elements include mesenchymal cells, fibroblasts, macrophages, and cytoplasmic extensions of odontoblasts. The tissue is innervated by some unmyelinated nerve fibers and supplied by a capillary network. Called also *subodontoblastic l., cell-free zone, cell-poor zone,* and *Weil's basal zone.*

Lazarus complex [named after *Lazarus,* a brother of Mary and Martha whom Jesus raised from the dead] see under COMPLEX.

lb pound.

lb/in² pounds per square inch (psi). See also mechanical STRESS.

LCM lymphocytic choriomeningitis (virus); see under VIRUS.

LD 1. lethal DOSE. 2. linguodistal (see DISTOLINGUAL).

LD₅₀ 1. median lethal DOSE: 2. median infective DOSE.

LD₅₀|₃₀ a dose which is lethal for 50 percent of the test subjects within 30 days subsequent to exposure. See also lethal dose, median, under DOSE.

LDG lingual developmental GROOVE.

LDL low-density lipoprotein; see β-LIPOPROTEIN.

LDS Licentiate in Dental Surgery.

LE lupus erythematosus; see also LE CELL.

Leach see gingival-bone COUNT (Dunning-Leach index).

lead[1] (lĕd) any of the conductors connected to the electrocardiograph. Also any of the records made by the electrocardiograph, varying with the part of the body from which the current is led off.

lead[2] (led) [L. *plumbum*] a heavy metal. Symbol, Pb; atomic number, 82; atomic weight, 207.2; specific gravity, 11.35; melting point, 327.4°C; valences, 2, 4; group IVB of the periodic table. It is a soft, grayish blue, ductile metal, soluble in nitric acid and insoluble in water (but dissolving slowly in water containing weak acid solution), and resistant to corrosion. Lead is a poor conductor of electricity and a good sound and vibration absorber, being relatively impenetrable to ionizing radiation. It is toxic and may be absorbed through the gastrointestinal and respiratory tracts; only about 8 to 12 percent of orally ingested lead is absorbed into the tissue. In the soft tissue, lead is found chiefly in the kidneys, followed by the liver, with only small amounts accumulating in the brain. Over a period of time, it is redistributed in bones, teeth, and hair. On x-ray examination, lead forms rings of increased density in the ossification centers of the epiphyses. It penetrates the placental barrier, causing abnormalities in animals, but teratogenesis in humans has not been established. Used in radiation protection; formerly used as an astringent. Lead poisoning is caused by massive ingestion of lead salts (acute form), or cumulative retention of small amounts of inhaled lead vapor or dust or through drinking of water pumped through lead pipes (chronic form). Symptoms are similar in both forms, including stippling of the erythrocytes and inhibition of hemoglobin synthesis, resulting in hypochromic anemia; abdominal colic (lead colic), associated with nausea, vomiting, and constipation, degeneration of the cortical and ganglionic neurons, associated with diffuse edema of the gray and white matter, often followed by depression, psychotic changes, and coma; peripheral nerve lesions, usually myelin degeneration and neuritis, chiefly of the motor nerves, resulting in foot-drop and wrist-drop; and radiographic density of the epiphyseal ends of bones in children. Oral manifestations include a thin blue-black line (lead line) in the marginal gingivae; the pigmentation is often diffuse and may involve other areas of the oral cavity. Excessive salivation, a metallic taste, and salivary gland swelling may occur. Lead projectiles embedded in the skin or muscle may also cause poisoning. Called also *plumbism* and *saturnism*. **l. dioxide,** a compound, PbO₂, occurring as brown, hexagonal crystals, which are soluble in glacial acetic acid but insoluble in water and alcohol. It is a highly toxic compound that presents a fire hazard in contact with organic material. Used in various industrial processes and as a curing or oxidizing agent for polysulfide rubber. Called also *l. oxide brown, l. peroxide,* and *l. superoxide*. **l. oxide brown, l. peroxide, l. superoxide,** l. dioxide.

leaf (lēf) an organ, usually green, of vascular plants, which is attached to the plant by a stem. **Digitalis l.,** see DIGITALIS.

leaflet (lēf′let) a structure resembling a small leaf, especially a cusp of a heart valve.

leakage (lēk′ij) 1. the escape of fluid from a vessel or other container. See also MICROLEAKAGE. 2. the escape of radiation through the protective shielding of an x-ray machine.

leash (lēsh) a bundle of cordlike structures, as nerves, blood vessels, fibers, and the like.

LeChâtelier's principle [Henry Louis *LeChâtelier,* French chemist, 1850–1936] see under PRINCIPLE.

lecithin (les′ĭ-thin) [Gr. *lekithos* egg yolk] a phospholipid originally isolated from egg yolk, being an ester of phosphatidic acid and choline, consisting of esters of glycerol with two molecules of long-chain aliphatic acids and one of phosphoric acid, the latter being esterified with the alcohol group of cholines. It is a hygroscopic, white, paraffin-like substance, which is soluble in alcohol and organic solvents, but is insoluble in water, although it can be dispersed in a colloidal state. Lecithins comprise the bulk of the total lipids of animal and plant cells, and are found in the nerve tissue, especially in the white and gray matter, blood plasma, erythrocytes, liver, muscles, intestines, and other tissues, being involved in transporting fats from one tissue to another and serving as essential components of the protoplasm of all body cells. Lecithins are also believed to be involved in blood coagulation, sodium and potassium transport, amino acid metabolism, and other vital functions. Those in which the oleic acid on the central carbon atom has been removed by hydrolysis are known as *lysolecithin;* those which form complexes with proteins are known as *lecithoproteins.* Lecithins may be obtained from soybean, and are used as lipotropic agents, digestible surfactants,and emulsifiers. Called also *choline phosphoglyceride, phosphatidyl choline,* and *phosphatidylcholine.*

lecithoprotein (les″ĭ-tho-pro′te-in) [*lecithin* + *protein*] a conjugated protein which contains lecithin as the prosthetic group.

Le Dentu's suture [Jean François Auguste *Le Dentu,* French surgeon, 1841–1926] see under SUTURE.

Ledercillin-VK trademark for *penicillin V potassium* (see under PENICILLIN).

Ledermycin trademark for *demeclocycline.*

ledge (lej) 1. a relatively narrow, shelflike, horizontal projection in a structure. 2. a plateau-like bone margin caused by resorption of a thickened bony plate. **crown l.,** a shoulder, usually at the junction of the gingival and middle third of the lingual surface of a tooth, prepared on an abutment tooth to give support to a denture, such as a full or three-quarter crown restoration. Called also *shoulder.*

ledging (lej′ing) the creation of a ledge or shelf, as one created in the wall of the root canal during endodontic instrumentation.

Lee denture [J. H. *Lee*] see under DENTURE.

Leeuwenhoek, Antonij van [1632–1723] a Dutch microscopist and naturalist whose pioneer work contributed to the development of modern microscopy. His many discoveries include the red blood cells, the capillary circulation of the blood, and the tubular structure of the dentin, and he is believed to have been the first to observe bacteria under the microscope.

Lefèvre, Paul see Papillon-LeFèvre SYNDROME.

Leff trademark for a *dental casting gold alloy* (see under GOLD).

Leff "C" trademark for a hard *dental casting gold alloy* (see under GOLD).

Leff hard trademark for an extra hard *dental casting gold alloy* (see under GOLD).

Leff light inlay see under INLAY.

Leff medium soft trademark for a medium hard *dental casting gold alloy* (see under GOLD).

Le Fort's fracture, suture see under FRACTURE and SUTURE.

leg (leg) the lower limb, especially the part from the knee to the foot. Called also *crus* [NA].

Legal's disease [Emmo *Legal,* German physician, 1859–1922] CEPHALALGIA pharyngotympanica.

Legential trademark for *sodium gentisate.*

Legionella (le″jun-el′ah) a genus of bacteria of the family Legion-

ellaceae, occurring as rod-shaped (0.3 to 0.4 by 2.0 to 3.0 μm in size) or filamentous, gram-negative, fastidious organisms, which have a narrow optimal pH and temperature ranges and will not grow anaerobically. They do not reduce nitrates, use carbohydrates, degrade urea, and appear to possess decarboxylases for lysine and ornithine or an arginine dihydrolase. **L. pneumoph′ila,** a species that is the causative agent of legionnaires' disease and Pontiac fever; it occurs in several different immunologic groups.

Legionellaceae (le″jun-el-la′se-e) [*Legionella* + *-aceae*] a family of bacteria that consists of the genus *Legionella.*

legislation (lej″is-la′shun) 1. the making of laws. 2. a law(s). **Good Samaritan l.,** Good Samaritan LAW.

Leichtenstern, Otto [German physician, 1845–1900] see Strümpell-Leichtenstern ENCEPHALITIS.

Leiner's dermatitis [Karl *Leiner,* Austrian physician, 1871–1930] see under DERMATITIS.

leio- [Gr. *leios* smooth] a combining form meaning smooth.

leiomyoma (li″o-mi-o′mah) [*leio-* + Gr. *mys* muscle + *-oma*] a benign tumor derived from smooth muscle, which may arise anywhere in the body but occurs most commonly in the uterus. Oral leiomyoma, which is rare, affects most commonly the posterior part of the tongue, with the soft palate, floor of the mouth, and buccal mucosa being less frequently involved. Typically, it is a well-defined but unencapsulated, slow-growing, firm, painless, usually superficial, but often pedunculated mass. Histologically, it is made up of interlacing bundles of smooth muscle fibers interspersed by connective tissue; some are composed of vascular tissue with disorganized smooth muscle layers — they may be derived from the smooth muscle of blood vessels. **malignant l.,** leiomyosarcoma.

leiomyosarcoma (li″o-mi″o-sar-ko′mah) [*leio-* + Gr. *mys* muscle + *sarcoma*] a very rare, malignant form of leiomyoma, in the uterus or retroperitoneal region, from where it may metastasize through the lymphatic system to other organs. It is grossly similar to leiomyoma, except that it may be larger and softer and have a tendency to necrosis and hemorrhage. Histologically, it is also similar to leiomyoma, except for the presence of anaplasia and mitoses.

Leishmania (lēsh-ma′ne-ah) [named after Sir William B. *Leishman*] a genus of protozoa of the subphylum Mastigophora, found chiefly in the reticuloendothelial cells of the skin or viscera of vertebrates. The organisms have two stages in their life cycle, a leptomonad stage, spent in the intestine of an insect host, and a leishmanial form, developing in the vertebrate host. The leptomonad stage is elongate and possesses a free flagellum, and the leishmanial stage is round or oval and has no free flagellum.

leishmaniasis (lēsh″mah-ni′ah-sis) any infection caused by the protozoan parasite *Leishmania.* **cutaneous l.,** a sandfly-borne infection caused by *Leishmania tropica,* seen most commonly in countries of the Middle East, Mediterranean littoral, Africa, and South America. It first appears, after an incubation period ranging from several weeks to several months, in the form of papules on the exposed skin, followed by ulceration and scabs. Called also *tropical l., Aleppo boil, Alibert's disease, Baghdad boil, Biskra button, Borovskii's disease, Chiclero ulcer, Delhi boil, Kandahar sore, Lahore sore,* and *oriental boil.* **mucocutaneous l., naso-oral l., nasopharyngeal l.,** a chronic, probably sandfly-borne, disease seen most commonly in Central and South America, caused by infection with *Leishmania braziliensis,* a microorganism virtually indistinguishable from *L. tropica.* Lesions are similar to those seen in the cutaneous form, except that the mucous membranes of the pharynx, larynx, nose, oral cavity, and other organs are involved, as well as the skin. Called also *bouba braziliana, espundia, forest yaws,* and *uta.* **tropical l.,** cutaneous l. **visceral l.,** a chronic disease caused by infection with *Leishmania donovani,* which occurs mainly in India, Brazil, northern China, southern Russia, and western Africa. It involves primarily the reticuloendothelial system, and is characterized by hepatosplenomegaly, lymphadenopathy, fever, weakness, and weight loss. Called also *black fever, febrile tropical splenomegaly, kala-azar,* and *ponos.*

Lejeune's syndrome [Jérôme *Lejeune*] crying cat SYNDROME.

Le Mayeur, Jean Pierre [1761–1806] a French-born American dentist who influenced the development of dental practice in the United States.

Lemli, Luc see Smith-Lemli-Opitz SYNDROME.

lemmoma (lem′o-mah) neurilemmoma.

lemnisci (lem-nis′si) plural of *lemniscus.*

lemniscus (lem-nis′kus), pl. *lemnis′ci* [L.; Gr. *lēmniskos* fillet] a ribbon or band; a general anatomical term for such a structure, especially in the central nervous system.

Lemoflur trademark for a *sodium fluoride* preparation (see under FLUORIDE).

lemoran (le′mo-ran) levorphanol.

length (length) an expression of the longest dimension of an object, or of the measurement between the two ends. In measuring the human body, *length* and *height* are sometimes used interchangeably. See also INCH, METER, and *Tables of Weights and Measures* at WEIGHT, and see entries at INDEX. **anterior arch l., arch l. arch l.,** the height of the dental arch measured from the line connecting the first premolars to the most labial point on the anterior arch, along the midline or midsagittal plane, usually to the point between the maxillary central incisors. Called also *anterior arch l.* **basialveolar l.,** the distance from the basion to the lower end of the intermaxillary suture. **basinasal l.,** the distance form basion to nasion. **bond l.,** the distance between bonded atoms in a molecule. **cranial l.,** the distance from the glabella to the opisthocranium. **l. of cranial base,** the distance from basion to nasion, and on the roentgenogram from nasion to Bolton point. **l. of crown (buccal),** measurement of the crown of posterior teeth, from the crest of buccal cusp or cusps, to the crest of curvature at the cementoenamel junction. See table of *Measurement of the Permanent Teeth of Man* at TOOTH. **l. of crown (labial),** measurement of the crown of anterior teeth, from the curvature at the cementoenamel junction, to the incisal edge. See table *Measurement of the Permanent Teeth of Man* at TOOTH. **crown-heel l.,** an expression of the measurement from the crown of the head to the sole in embryos, fetuses, and infants; the equivalent of *standing height* in older individuals. **dental l.,** an expression of the distance between the mesial surface of the first premolar and the distal surface of the third molar of the upper jaw. See tooth MEASUREMENT. **equilibrium l.,** the length of unattached (cut free from bony attachments), relaxed muscle at which tension at rest is minimal, essentially zero. **gauge l.,** original length, or length used as a standard or to compare with, as in the determination of percentage elongation in calculating ductility of materials. **Hensen's l.,** M BAND. **l. of mandible,** a projected length of the mandible measured from pogonion to a vertical plane tangential to the most posterior points of the condyles and right angles to the plane of the lower border of the mandible. **maxilloalveolar l.,** the distance from the prosthion to the midpoint of the tangent to the posterior margin of the tuberosity of the maxilla. **l. of palate,** the distance from the orale to the staphylion. **resting l.,** the length of muscle at which the contraction tension is minimal. **l. of root,** measurement of the root from the apex, to the crest of curvature at crown cervix. See table *Measurement of the Permanent Teeth of Man* at TOOTH. **span l.,** the length of the beam between two supports. **l. of stay,** the length of an inpatient's stay in a hospital or other health facility, usually measured as an average number of days spent in a facility per admission or discharge. Abbreviated *LOS.* **wave l.,** wavelength.

lenitive (len-ĭ-tiv) [L. *lenire* to soothe] demulcent.

lens (lenz) [L. "lentil"] 1. a piece of glass or other transparent substance, so shaped as to converge or scatter the rays of light. 2. the transparent biconvex body of the eye, constituting part of its refractive mechanism; the crystalline lens. **achromatic l.,** one corrected for chromatic aberration. **aplanatic l.,** one that serves to correct spherical aberration. **apochromatic l.,** one corrected for chromatic and spherical aberration. **biconcave l.,** one that has both surfaces concave. Called also *concavoconcave l.* **biconvex l.,** one that has both surfaces convex. **bicylindrical l.,** one that has both surfaces cylindrical. **bispherical l.,** one that is spherical on both sides. **compound l.,** one made up of two or more segments. **concave l.,** a lens with one or both (biconvex) surfaces curved like a section of the interior of a hollow sphere; it disperses the rays of light. **concavoconcave l.,** biconcave l. **concavoconvex l.,** one that has one concave surface and one convex surface. Called also *periscopic l.* **converging l., convex l.,** a lens curved like a section of the exterior of a hollow sphere; it brings light to a focus. **convexoconcave l.,** one that has one convex and one concave surface. **crossed l.,** one with front and back surfaces of different curvatures. **crystalline l.,** lens (2). **dispersing l.,** one that disperses the rays of light. Called also *minus l.* **minus l.,** dispersing l. **immersion l.,** immersion OBJECTIVE. **planoconcave l.,** a lens with one plane and one concave side. **planoconvex l.,** a lens with one plane and one convex side. **periscopic l.,** concavoconvex l. **spherical l.,** one that is a segment of a sphere.

lentigines (len-tij′ĭ-nēz) [L.] plural of *lentigo.*

lentigo (len-ti′go), pl. *lentig′ines* [L. "freckle"] a round or oval, flat, brown, pigmented spot on the skin due to increased deposition of melanin and associated with an increased number of melanocytes in the skin. Cf. FRECKLE.

Lentin trademark for *carbachol.*

Lentivirinae (len″tĭ-vi′rĭ-ne) a subfamily of retroviruses, having virions 60 to 90 nm in diameter with 30 to 40 nm cores, and surface projections that are 10 nm long. The RNA genome is composed of subunits and assumes a coiled configuration in the virion. Maturation takes place by budding through the plasma membrane, followed by condensation of the cores and morphological transition to single-walled particles. Lentiviruses cause disease in sheep. Called also *Maedi virus, progressive interstitial pneumonia virus, progressive pneumonia virus,* and *Visna virus.*

Lentivirus (len″tĭ-vi′rus) any virus of the subfamily Lentivirinae.

lentula (len′chu-lah, len-too′lah) lentulo.

lentulo (len′chu-lo, len-too′lah) an engine-driven, flexible stainless steel wire spiral rotating endodontic instrument used in a handpiece to place cement into the prepared root canal in root canal therapy. Called also *lentula, lentula carrier, lentulo paste carrier,* and *paste carrier.* See illustration at root canal THERAPY.

Lenz-Majewski dwarfism (syndrome) [W. D. *Lenz;* F. *Majewski*] see under DWARFISM.

Leonides [2nd and 3rd centuries A.D.] a Greek surgeon who flourished in Rome, and whose writings are cited by Aëtius.

leontiasis (le″on-ti′ah-sis) [Gr. *leōn* lion] the leontine facies (*facies leontina*) of lepromatous leprosy, due to nodular invasion of the subcutaneous tissue of the face, giving it a vaguely leontine appearance. **l. os′sea, l. os′sium,** hypertrophy of the bony structures of the face and jaws, especially evident in the paranasal areas, giving the head a leonine appearance. Called also *megalocephaly.*

Leostesin trademark for *lidocaine.*

lepido- a combining form meaning flake or scale.

Leporipoxvirus (lē-por′ĭ-poks-vi′rus) a genus of poxviruses, causing poxlike diseases in rabbits, hares, and squirrels.

lepra (lep′rah) [Gr. "the leprosy, which makes the skin scaly"] leprosy; (prior to the mid 19th century) psoriasis. The term is now largely obsolete.

leproma (lep-ro′mah) [*lepra* + *-oma*] a tumor-like granulomatous nodule, the characteristic lesion of leprosy.

leprosy (lep′ro-se) [Gr. *lepros* scaly, scabby, rough] a chronic, infectious, disfiguring disease caused by *Mycobacterium leprae,* characterized by granulomatous lesions (lepromas) in the skin, mucous membranes, and peripheral nervous system. It is only slightly contagious and is quite rare in the cooler zones of the world. Two principal or polar types are recognized: lepromatous and tuberculoid. The lesion is usually made up of epithelioid cells and lymphocytes in fibrous stroma. Vacuolated macrophages (lepra cells) are present throughout. Called also *elephantiasis graecorum, Hansen's disease,* and *lepra.* **lepromatous l.,** that polar type of leprosy marked by the development of lepromas and invariably by the presence of *Mycobacterium lepra* in abundance from the onset. The lesions present as symmetric, brown-red, granular nodules diffusely distributed over the body; they have a tendency to break down and ulcerate. The face, ears, brows, and perioral and nasal areas are characteristically involved, sometimes leading to the development of facies leonina and destruction of a part of the eyebrows. In advanced cases, there may be perforation of the nasal septum and development of saddle nose. Nodular infiltration may produce macrocheilia, progressing through scarring to microstomia. Gingival and tongue lesions, gingival hyperplasia with loosening of the teeth, perforation of the palate, loss of the uvula, and scarring of the vocal cords may occur. Facial bone changes, known as *Møller-Christenson's syndrome,* consisting of atrophy of the anterior nasal spine, defects of the pyriform aperture, and atrophy of the maxillary anterior alveolar process may develop. It is the only form that may regularly serve as a source of infection to others, until treatment is begun. Called also *nodular l.* **macular l., maculocutaneous l., neural l.,** tuberculoid l. **nodular l.,** lepromatous l. **tuberculoid l.,** that polar type of leprosy in which, due to high-cell mediated resistance to the infection, *Mycobacterium lepra* are few or lacking by ordinary methods of examination, and nerve damage occurs very early, so that all skin lesions are denervated from the start, often with dissociation of sensation. Affected patients are rarely a source of infection to others. Called also *macular l., maculocutaneous l.,* and *neural l.*

lepto- [Gr. *leptos* slender] a combining form meaning slender, thin, or delicate.

leptocephalic (lep″to-sĕ-fal′ik) pertaining to or characterized by a tall, narrow skull. Called also *leptocephalous*. See also DOLI-CHOCEPHALIC and OXYCEPHALIC.

leptocephalous (lep″to-sef′ah-lus) leptocephalic.

leptocephaly (lep″to-sef′ah-le) [*lepto-* + Gr. *kephalē* head] a condition characterized by tallness and narrowness of the skull. See DOLICHOCEPHALY and OXYCEPHALY.

leptocyte (lep′to-sīt) [*lepto-* + Gr. *kytos* cell] target CELL.

leptodontous (lep″to-don′tus) [*lepto-* + Gr. *odous* tooth] having slender teeth.

leptoprosope (lep-top′ro-sōp) a person exhibiting leptoprosopia.

leptoprosopia (lep″to-pro-so′pe-ah) [*lepto-* + Gr. *prosopon* face + *-ia*] a condition characterized by narrowness of the face, with slender features, round, open orbits, long nose, narrow nostrils, and small mouth. See also leptoprosopic SKULL.

leptoprosopic (lep″to-pro-so′pik) characterized by a narrow face or pertaining to leptoprosopia.

Leptospira (lep″to-spi′rah) [*lepto-* + Gr. *speira* coil] a genus of flexuous, helical bacteria of the family Spirochetaceae, order Spirochaetales, made up of finely coiled cells (0.1 μm in diameter and 6 to 20 μm or more in length), with one or both ends hooked. The organisms are motile by means of axial filaments (aristyle), and are aerobic, using atmospheric oxygen. Some strains are pathogenic and cause infectious jaundice and various febrile conditions in man, human diseases being frequently derived from infected animal reservoirs. **L. icteroi′des,** *L. interrogans.* **L. inter′rogans,** a species containing all the serotypes of the genus, which comprise all pathogenic and saprophytic strains with no known hosts. Called also *L. icteroides, Spirochaeta biflexa, S. icterogenes, S. icterohaemorrhagiae, S. interrogans,* and *S. nodosa.*

leptostaphyline (lep″to-staf′ĭ-lĭn) [*lepto-* + Gr. *staphylē* bunch of grapes, uvula] pertaining to or characterized by a narrow palate. See leptostaphyline SKULL.

leptotene (lep′to-tēn) [*lepto-* + Gr. *tainia* ribbon] the first stage of the first division of meiosis, characterized by the appearance of the chromosomes as thin uncoiled threads.

Leptotrichia (lep″to-trik′e-ah) [*lepto-* + Gr. *thrix* hair] a genus of gram-negative, anaerobic, rod-shaped bacteria of the family Bacteroidaceae. Formerly called *Leptothrix.* **L. aerog′enes,** *Eubacterium saburreum;* see under EUBACTERIUM. **L. bucca′lis,** a species isolated from the human oral cavity, frequently from precarious, transitional, and carious plaques, occurring as anaerobic, unbranching, nonmotile, nonsporulating rods (about 1.0 to 1.5 by 5.0 to 15.0 μm in size), with one or both ends rounded or pointed. In older cultures, filaments may be up to 200 μm long and cells may assume coccoid shapes or present bullous swellings as they undergo lysis. Initially, the organisms are gram-positive but may become gram-negative in older cultures. Fructose, glucose, maltose, mannose, and sucrose are fermented with production of acid but no gas; cellobiose, salicin, and trehalose are usually fermented; galactose, lactose, raffinose, and starch may be fermented. An initial pH of 7.2 to 7.4 is required for optimum growth. Called also *Fusobacterium fusiforme* and *Leptothrix buccalis.*

leptotrichosis (lep″to-trī-ko′sis) infection with microorganisms of the genus *Leptotrichia.*

Leptothrix (lep′to-thriks) [*lepto-* + Gr. *thrix* hair] former name for *Leptotrichia.* **L. bucca′lis,** *Leptotrichia buccalis;* see under LEPTOTRICHIA.

leptothrix (lep′to-thriks) any microorganism of the genus *Leptothrix* (*Leptotrichia*).

Lergefin trademark for carbinoxamine maleate (see under CAR-BINOXAMINE).

Lergigan trademark for promethazine.

Leritine trademark for anileridine.

Leroy's syndrome [L. G. *Leroy*] see under SYNDROME.

Lesch-Nyhan syndrome [Michael *Lesch,* American physician, born 1939; William L. *Nyhan,* Jr., American physician, born 1926] see under SYNDROME.

lesion (le′zhun) [L. *laesio, laedere* to hurt] any pathological or traumatic disorder of tissue or loss of function of a part. **benign lymphoepithelial l.,** Mikulicz's DISEASE. **central giant cell l.,** central giant cell GRANULOMA. **Ghon's l.,** primary l. **gross l.,** one that is visible to the naked eye. **histologic l.,** microscopic l. **lymphoepithelial l., benign,** Mikulicz's DISEASE. **microscopic l.,** a minute lesion that is visible only under the microscope. Called also *histologic l.* **molecular l.,** a minute lesion that is not visible even under the microscope. **organic l.,** structural l. **peripheral l.,** one of a nerve ending. **peripheral giant cell l.,** giant cell EPULIS. **precancerous l.,** a nonmalignant lesion that may lead

to the development of cancer. **primary l.,** the original and characteristic lesion of a disease. **primary l., calcified,** Ghon's FOCUS. **primary (tuberculous) l.,** the initial tuberculous lesion usually located in the lungs, and less commonly in the intestine, tonsil, skin, or any mucous membrane, including the oral mucosa, from where it spreads out to lymph nodes. Called also *Ghon's l.* and *Ghon's tubercle.* **structural l.,** one that produces organic changes in a tissue. Called also *organic l.* **systemic l.,** one involving a system or a group of organs with a common function. **total l.,** one involving the whole of an organ or the diameter of a conducting tract. **trophic l.,** one manifested by a disturbance in the nutrition of a part.

Lesser's triangle see under TRIANGLE.

LET [*linear energy transfer*] the amount of energy transferred per unit path length, considering the mass, charge, and velocity. **high LET,** radiation characteristic of particles with a high mass, e.g., x-rays and gamma rays. **low LET,** radiation characteristic of particles with a low mass, e.g., protons and alpha particles.

lethal (le′thal) [L. *lethalis,* from *lethum* death] deadly; fatal.

lethargy (leth′ar-je) [Gr. *lēthargia* drowsiness] a condition of drowsiness.

Letterer's reticulosis [Erich *Letterer,* German physician, born 1895] Letterer-Siwe DISEASE.

Letterer-Siwe disease [E. *Letterer;* Sture August *Siwe,* German physician, born 1897] see under DISEASE.

Leu leucine.

leucine (lu′sin) an aliphatic, naturally occurring amino acid, 2-aminoisocaproic acid, that is essential for growth of infants and for certain nitrogen metabolic processes in human adults. It is also found in the saliva. Abbreviated *Leu.*

leucite (loo′sīt) a whitish or grayish mineral, potassium aluminum silicate, $KAlSi_2O_6$, found in alkali vulcanic rocks. Also produced during the melting of porcelain paste by fused feldspar.

leuco- [Gr. *leukos* white] a combining form meaning white; see also words beginning LEUKO-.

leucocidin (lu″ko-si′din) leukocidin.

Leucocristine trademark for *vincristine.*

Leucogen trademark for *asparaginase.*

Leucoline trademark for *quinoline.*

Leuconostoc (lu″ko-nos′tok) a genus of bacteria of the family Streptococcaceae, which are gram-positive, nonsporogenic, nonmotile, and nonpathogenic to man and animals, and are found on fruits, in milk and dairy products, and in wine.

leucovorin (lu″ko-vo′rin) citrovorum FACTOR.

leukemia (lu-ke′me-ah) [Gr. *leukos* white + *haima* blood + *-ia*] a malignant, frequently fatal disease of the blood-forming organs, characterized by proliferation of immature leukocytes and their infiltration in the bone marrow, lymph nodes, liver, spleen, and other tissues. The etiology is unknown but chronic exposure to radiations and to some drugs and chemicals and infection with some viruses are known to have leukemogenic effects. Chromosomal defects found consistently in leukemic patients also suggest a possible genetic factor. Leukemia is classified clinically on the basis of (1) duration and character of the disease — *acute* or *chronic;* (2) the type of cell involved — *myeloid* (*myelogenous*), *lymphoid* (*lymphogenous*), or *monocytic;* (3) increase or nonincrease in the number of abnormal cells in the blood — *leukemic* or *aleukemic* (subleukemic). **acute l.** a form of leukemia occurring most commonly in children and young adults, characterized by a sudden onset followed by anemia, weakness, fever, thrombocytopenia, leukemic infiltrations, pallor, weakness, lassitude, lymph node enlargement, petechiae, ecchymoses, hepatosplenomegaly, and susceptibility to infection. Oral and respiratory infections are common. Oral manifestations may include pallor of the mucous membranes, gingival hemorrhage, fungiform papillae on the tongue, petechiae and ecchymoses, persistent bleeding after tooth extraction, gingival swelling, loose teeth, ulceration of the oral mucosa and tonsils, and xerostomia. **aleukemic l., aleukocythemic l.** that in which the leukocyte count is either normal or below normal. Called also *subleukemic l.* **chronic l.,** a form of leukemia occurring most commonly in adult and elderly patients, characterized by an insidious onset and discrete initial symptoms, such as a mild leukocytosis or a few enlarged lymph nodes, which may be present for months or years without being detected. Anorexia, weight loss, weakness, anemia, thrombocytopenia, and hepatosplenomegaly usually follow. Oral manifestations may include gingivitis, gingival hyperplasia, gingival hemorrhage, prolonged bleeding after tooth extraction, petechiae, ecchymoses, purpuric lesions, ulceration, loose teeth, enlargement of the salivary glands and tonsils, xerostomia, and destruction of the alveolar bone. It may include the myelocytic, lymphocytic, and monocytic types. **lymphogenous l.,** lymphoid l. **lymphoid l.,** that associated with hyperplasia and overactivity of the lymphoid tissue, in which the leukocytes are lymphocytes or lymphoblasts. Called also *lymphogenous l.* **megakaryocytic l.**, hemorrhagic THROMBOCYTHEMIA. **monocytic l.**, that in which the predominating leukocytes are identified as monocytes. **myeloblastic l.**, that in which myeloblasts predominate. **myelocytic l.**, **myelogenous l.**, **myeloid granulocytic l.**, that arising from myeloid tissue in which the granular, polymorphonuclear leukocytes and their precursors predominate. **subleukemic l.**, aleukemic l.

leukemic (lu-ke′mik) pertaining to or affected with leukemia.

leukemoid (lu-ke′moid) [*leukemia* + Gr. *eidos* form] resembling leukemia; characterized by blood and sometimes clinical findings resembling true leukemia.

Leukeran trademark for *chlorambucil.*

Leukerin trademark for *mercaptopurine.*

leukexosis (lu″kek-so′sis) an aggregation of dead leukocytes in one of the channels of the body.

leuko- [Gr. *leukos* white] a combining form meaning white, or denoting relationship to a white blood cell, or leukocyte, or to the white matter of the brain.

leukoblast (lu′ko-blast) [*leuko-* + Gr. *blastos* germ] an immature granulocyte.

leukocidin (lu″ko-si′din) [*leukocyte* + L. *caedere* to kill] a substance produced by some pathogenic bacteria, which is toxic to polymorphonuclear leukocytes, killing the cell with or without lysis. Written also *leucocidin.* **Neisser-Wechsberg l.**, a leukocidin produced by staphylococci, which destroys rabbit but not human leukocytes; it is identical with α-staphylolysin. **Panton-Valentine (P-V) l.**, a substance produced by staphylococci, which inhibits phagocytosis by human heterophils, being active on both human and rabbit polymorphonuclear leukocytes.

leukocyte (lu′ko-sīt) [*leuko-* + Gr. *kytos* cell] a white cell or white blood cell. Leukocytes are produced in the bone marrow (granulocytes) and the lymph nodes (agranulocytes) and are transported to different parts of the body where they participate in reparative and defense processes. They pass through the capillary walls and, using their power of ameboid movement, move in the direction of inflammation, governed by chemical substances released by injured tissue (chemotaxis) and protect the body by transporting antibodies and by engulfing and destroying invading microorganisms (phagocytosis). During their development leukocytes are known as *myeloblasts, myelocytes, lymphoblasts, lymphocytes, metamyelocytes, basophils, eosinophils, granulocytes, monocytes,* and *neutrophils.* Called also *white corpuscle.* See also table of *Reference Values in Hematology* in Appendix. **acidophilic l.**, eosinophil. **l. aggregation,** concentration of white blood cells at an inflammatory focus. **basophilic l.**, basophil (2). **l. count,** determination of the number of leukocytes in a measured volume of blood. An increased leukocyte count is *leukocytosis;* a reduced count is *leukopenia.* Called also *white cell count.* See table of *Reference Values in Hematology* in Appendix. **l. count, differential,** a leukocyte count indicating counts for individual leukocytes. See table of *Reference Values in Hematology* in Appendix. **eosinophilic l.**, eosinophil. **granular l.**, granulocyte. **irritation l.**, Türk CELL. **juvenile l.**, metamyelocyte. **lymphoid l.**, agranulocyte. **mast l.**, basophil (2). **l. migration,** the passage of leukocytes through the vascular wall; diapedesis. **neutrophilic l.**, neutrophil (1). **nongranular l.**, agranulocyte. **polymorphonuclear l.**, **polynuclear l.**, neutrophil (2). **Türk irritation l.**, Türk CELL.

leukocytosis (lu″ko-si-to′sis) an increase in the number of leukocytes in the blood, usually seen in various diseases, such as hemorrhage, infection, and inflammatory conditions. See also LEUKOCYTE count. **eosinophilic l.**, see EOSINOPHILIA (2). **lymphocytic l.**, an increase in the total white cell count with a predominance in the number of lymphocytes, usually occurring in chronic inflammatory diseases, such as tuberculosis, syphilis, malaria, and whooping cough, and in Hodgkin's disease. **neutrophilic l.**, that characterized by an increase in the number of neutrophils in the blood, occurring in diseases caused by pyogenic microorganisms, acute massive hemorrhage, malignant neoplasms, gout, nephritis, and diseases with necrotic changes, such as myocardial infarction.

leukoderma (lu″ko-der′mah) [*leuko-* + Gr. *derma* skin] an acquired type of localized loss of melanin pigmentation of the skin.

leukodystrophy (lu″ko-dis′tro-fe) [*leuko-* + *dystrophy*] any dystrophic disorder of the white matter of the brain. **metachromatic l.**, a familial disease characterized by metachromasia in the myelin sheath and lipid deposits in the nerve cells. In children, the syndrome is marked by loss of motor activity with spastic seizures and atactic signs, blindness, oculomotor disorders, and death within two years. In adults, the course is slower and is marked chiefly by schizophreniform symptoms; patients may

survive up to 20 years. A juvenile form has also been described. Called also *familial progressive cerebral sclerosis, Greenfield's disease, Scholz's syndrome, sulfatide lipidosis,* and *van Bogaert-Nyssen-Peiffer syndrome.*

leukoedema (lu″ko-e-de′mah) [*leuko-* + *edema*] a disorder of the buccal mucosa which resembles early leukoplakia, characterized by the presence of a filmy opalescence of the mucosa in the early stages to a whitish-gray cast with a coarsely wrinkled surface in the later stages, associated with intracellular edema of the spinous or malpighian layer.

leukokeratosis (lu″ko-ker′ah-to′sis) [*leuko-* + *keratosis*] oral LEUKOPLAKIA. **congenital l.**, white sponge NEVUS.

leukopenia (lu″ko-pe′ne-ah) [*leukocyte* + Gr. *penia* poverty] abnormal reduction in the number of leukocytes in the blood, usually below 5,000 per cu mm, due to various diseases, such as bacterial, protozoal, or viral infections, allergic conditions, debilitated states, bone marrow disorders caused by ionizing radiations or various drugs and chemicals, various hematopoietic disorders, and other conditions of diverse etiology. Called also *aleukocytosis.* **idiopathic l.**, **malignant l.**, **pernicious l.**, agranulocytosis.

leukoplakia (lu″ko-pla′ke-ah) [*leuko-* + Gr. *plax* plate + *-ia*] 1. a white patch on the mucous membrane which will not rub off. See also CARCINOMA in situ. **l. bucca′lis**, the presence of white thickened patches on the mucous membrane of the cheeks. See *oral l.* **l. lingua′lis**, the presence of white thickened patches on the mucous membrane of the tongue. See *oral l.* **oral l.**, a condition marked by white, thick patches on the oral mucosa produced by hyperkeratosis of the epithelium. It is a benign lesion that provides favorable conditions for the development of epidermoid carcinoma. Histologically, it presents a thickening of the stratified squamous epithelium with hyperkeratosis, hyperplasia, inflammatory infiltration, and degeneration of epithelial cells. The term leukoplakia is commonly used to designate only the precancerous keratosis, but sometimes it is also used for any condition characterized by oral white patches that cannot be readily rubbed or stripped off, excluding conditions normally associated with leukoplakia-like lesions, such as lichen planus, burns, syphilis, etc. The etiology is unknown, but alcohol, irritation, vitamin deficiencies, infections, endocrine disorders, and, chiefly, tobacco are considered as contributing factors. Called also *focal (oral) keratosis, hyperkeratosis complex, hyperkeratosis simplex, intraepithelial carcinoma, keratosis labialis, keratosis linguae, leukokeratosis, nonspecific (oral) keratosis, oral hyperkeratosis, pachyderma oralis, psoriasis buccalis,* and *psoriasis linguae.* See also STOMATITIS nicotina. **speckled l.**, see ERYTHROPLASIA of Queyrat.

leukopoiesis (lu″ko-poi-e′sis) [*leukocyte* + Gr. *poiein* to make] the formation and development of leukocytes.

leukotaxine (lu″ko-tak′sin) a crystalline nitrogenous polypeptide that appears when tissue is injured, which can be recovered from inflammatory exudates, and that promotes leukocytosis and increases capillary permeability and diapedesis of leukocytes.

leukotaxis (lu″ko-tak′sis) [*leukocyte* + Gr. *taxis* arrangement] the cytotaxis of leukocytes; the tendency of leukocytes to collect in regions of injury and inflammation.

leukovirus (lu″ko-vi′rus) Oncovirinae.

Leunase trademark for *asparaginase.*

Levadone trademark for the *l*-form of *methadone hydrochloride* (see under METHADONE).

levallorphan tartrate (lev″al-lor′fan) a narcotic antagonist, 17-allylmorphinan-3-ol, occurring as a white, odorless, crystalline powder that is soluble in water and ethanol, but not in chloroform and ether. It is a partial agonist of the nalorphine type, which competes with morphine-like compounds for opioid receptor sites, also producing autonomic, endocrine, analgesic, and respiratory depressant effects similar to those caused by morphine. Used in the treatment of respiratory depression induced by opioid narcotics, but not barbiturates, anesthetics, or nonnarcotic agents. Adverse reactions may include dysphoria, miosis, lethargy, vertigo, drowsiness, gastric disorders, sweating, pallor, nausea, sense of heaviness of the limbs and, in high doses, hallucinations, dreams, disorientation, and feeling of unreality. Lorfan.

levarterenol (lev″ar-tēr′ē-nol) the levorotatory isomer of norepinephrine, *l*-β-(3,4-dihydroxyphenyl)-α-aminoethanol. **l. bitartrate,** a salt of levarterenol, *l*-β-(3,4-dihydroxyphenyl)-α-aminoethanol bitartrate, occurring as a white or grayish, odorless, crystalline powder that darkens on exposure to light and air and is soluble in water and ethanol, but not in chloroform and ether. It is a sympathomimetic drug with pharmacological and toxic properties similar to those of norepinephrine. Used chiefly for support of blood pressure in fluid replacement therapy in shock and hypertensive states. Also used in local anesthesia. Adverse reactions may include respiratory difficulty, slow and forceful heart beat, headache, and anxiety. Hypertension, photophobia, retrosternal pain, pallor, sweating, vomiting, necrosis at the site of injection, cardiac arrhythmias, shock, and intestinal necrosis are some of its principal side effects. Called also *noradrenaline acid tartrate*. Trademark: Levophed.

levator (le-va′tor), pl. *levato′res* [L. *levare* to raise] 1. [NA] a muscle for elevating an organ or structure into which it is inserted. 2. a surgical instrument used to raise depressed osseous fragments in fractures of the skull and other bones. **l. an′guli o′ris,** levator muscle of angle of mouth; see under MUSCLE. **l. glan′dulae thyroi′deae,** levator muscle of thyroid gland; see under MUSCLE. **l. la′bii superio′ris,** levator muscle of upper lip; see under MUSCLE. **l. la′bii superio′ris alae′que na′si,** levator muscle of upper lip and ala of nose; see under MUSCLE. **l. men′ti,** mentalis MUSCLE. **l. pala′ti,** levator veli palatini MUSCLE. **l. pal′pebrae superio′ris,** levator muscle of upper eyelid; see under MUSCLE. **l. ve′li palati′ni,** levator veli palatini MUSCLE.

levatores (lev″ah-to′rēz) [L.] plural of *levator*.

level (lev′el) 1. relative position, rank, or concentration. 2. a cerebrospinal center for combining or integrating impulses; the first level is spinal, the second is brainstem, the third is cortical. 3. in orthodontics, to reduce the curve of Spee by intrusion and/or extrusion of the teeth in an arch.

lever (le′ver, lev′er) a bar or a rigid device used to lift, dislodge, or move an object by placing one end underneath or in contact with the object and bringing pressure to bear upon the other end.

leverage (lev′er-ij) power gained by the use of the lever, as in certain instruments, such as forceps, pliers, etc., or in surgical and orthodontic appliances. **denture l.,** stabilization of a denture, without transmitting tipping stresses or torque to abutment teeth.

Levin, P. M. [American physician] see Jarcho-Levin SYNDROME.

levo- [L. *laevus* left] 1. a combining form denoting relationship to the left. 2. a chemical prefix indicating levorotatory.

levocompound (le″vo-kom′pound) levorotatory ISOMER.

levodopa (le″vo-do′pah) a centrally acting muscle relaxant, 3-hydroxy-L-tyrosine, occurring as a white, crystalline powder that darkens on exposure to air and humidity and dissolves in water, ethanol, and chloroform. Used in the treatment of parkinsonism, in which it abolishes sialorrhea, dysphagia, speech difficulties, and postural instability. Adverse reactions often include gastrointestinal disorders, such as nausea, anorexia, vomiting, epigastric pain, flatulence, and some instances of peptic ulcer and gastrointestinal hemorrhage; involuntary movements usually starting with the tongue and face and progressing to the arms, hands, and trunk; cardiovascular disorders, such as hypotension, tachycardia, and atrial fibrillation; neurological disorders, including nervousness, anxiety, insomnia, tremor, hallucinations, delusions, delirium, and psychotic episodes; and easy sexual arousal and loss of sexual inhibitions. Orodental complications usually consist of xerostomia, acceleration of carious processes, forceful tongue protrusions, biting movements, clenching, damage to the teeth and supporting structures, inability to retain dentures, and inflammatory lesions. Called also L-*dopa*. Trademarks: Bendopa, Biodopa, Dopal, Dopar, Dopasol, Larodopa, Veldopa.

Levo-Dromoran trademark for *levorphanol tartrate* (see under LEVORPHANOL).

levomeprazine (le″vo-mep′rah-zēn) methotrimeprazine.

Levomycetin trademark for *chloramphenicol.*

levonordefrin (le″vo-nor-def′rin) the *l*-form of nordefrin, *l*-1-(3,4-dihydroxyphenyl)-2-aminopropanol, occurring as a white to buff, odorless, crystalline powder that is freely soluble in aqueous solutions of mineral acids, slightly soluble in acetone, chloroform, ethanol, and ether, and insoluble in water. It is a sympathomimetic drug used as a vasoconstrictor in local anesthetic solutions and as a nasal decongestant. Trademark: Neo-Cobefrin.

Levophed trademark for *levarterenol bitartrate* (see under LEVARTERENOL).

Levoprome trademark for *methotrimeprazine.*

Levorenine trademark for *epinephrine.*

levorotatory (le″vo-ro′tah-to-re) [*levo-* + L. *rotare* to turn] turning to the left, pertaining to the property of chemical compounds, when in solution, of rotating the plane of polarized light to the left or counterclockwise. The prefixes *l-* and L- and the symbol − are used in organic chemistry to distinguish levorotatory from dextrorotatory isomers.

levorphan (lev′or-fan) LEVORPHANOL tartrate..

levorphanol tartrate (le-vor′fah-nol) the *l*-form of 3-hydroxy-*N*-methylmorphinan, occurring as a white, odorless, crystalline powder that is soluble in water and ethanol, but not in chloroform or ether. It is a semisynthetic opium alkaloid, being an addicting analgesic used in severe or moderate pain. Called also *lemoran* and *levorphan:* Trademark: Levo-Dromoran.

Levothyl trademark for the *l*-form of *methadone hydrochloride* (see under METHADONE).

Levugen trademark for *fructose.*

levulose (lev′u-lōs) fructose.

Lévy, Robert see Creyx-Lévy SYNDROME.

Lewandowski's tuberculid [Felix *Lewandowski*, Hamburg dermatologist, 1879–1921] see under TUBERCULID. See also PACHYONYCHIA congenita (Jadassohn-Lewandowski syndrome).

Lewis see Monahan-Lewis KNIFE.

Lewis antigen (factor), blood groups [named after the person in whom antibodies to the Le^a Lewis antigen were first discovered] see under ANTIGEN and BLOOD GROUP.

Lewis concept, theory [Gilbert Newton *Lewis*, American chemist, 1875–1946] see under CONCEPT and THEORY.

Leyden's paralysis [Ernst Victor von *Leyden*, German physician, 1832–1910] see under PARALYSIS.

Leydig's cell [Franz von *Leydig*, German anatomist, 1821–1908] see under CELL.

LFD lateral facial dysplasia. See first and second brachial arch SYNDROME.

LH luteinizing HORMONE.

Lhermitte-Cornil-Quesnel syndrome [Jean *Lhermitte*, French neurologist, 1877–1959; Lucien *Cornil*, French neurologist] see under SYNDROME.

Li 1. lithium. 2. LABRALE inferius.

liability (li″ah-bil′ĭ-te) [Fr. *lier* to bind] a responsibility, debt, or obligation under existing laws. **common law l.,** the responsibility for injuries or damages imposed upon a party, because of his actions, by that part of the law based upon custom and usage as established by the courts, as distinguished from liability under statutes passed by a legislative body, which is known as statutory law. **joint l.,** in health insurance, an arrangement whereby participating doctors sign contracts with the insurer and assume liability for fulfilling the commitments in the subscribers' contracts.

Lib. abbreviation for L. *li′bra*, a pound.

libra (li′brah) [L.] 1. pound. 2. balance.

Libra II inlay and crown trademark for a medium hard *dental casting gold alloy* (see under GOLD).

Libra III crown and bridge trademark for a hard *dental casting gold alloy* (see under GOLD).

Libra IV extra hard trademark for an extra hard *dental casting gold alloy* (see under GOLD).

Libritabs trademark for *chlordiazepoxide.*

Librium trademark for *chlordiazepoxide hydrochloride* (see under CHLORDIAZEPOXIDE).

license (li′sens) [L. *licere* to be permitted] a permit granted by a government agency to a person to engage in a given profession or occupation.

licensure (li′sen-shur) the process by which a government agency grants permission to persons to engage in a given profession or occupation by certifying that those licensed have attained the minimal degree of competency necessary to ensure that the public health, safety, and welfare will be reasonably well protected. See also ACCREDITATION and CERTIFICATION.

licentiate (li-sen′she-āt) [L. *licentia* license] one holding a license granted by an agency of government entitling him to engage in a given profession or occupation.

lichen (li′ken) [Gr. *leichēn* a tree-moss] 1. any of the many thallophytic plants consisting of a symbiotic combination of an alga and a fungus. 2. any of a wide range of skin diseases characterized by the presence of small, firm papules set close together. **l. al′bus,** l. sclerosus et atrophicus. **l. nit′idus,** a slowly progressive skin eruption consisting of small, glistening, flesh-colored to reddish-yellow papules or macules that occur in groups (without coalescing) on various parts of the body, with a special predilection for the genital area, elbows, axillae, palms of the hands, abdomen, and, occasionally, the oral mucosa and tongue. The typical lesion is located beneath the epidermis and is composed of hosts of lymphocytes, histiocytes, and giant cells. Called also *Pinkus' disease*. **l. pila'ris,** a condition in which there is a horn or spine in the center of each hair follicle. Called also *l. spinulosus*. **l. pla'nus,** a usually chronic or subacute, inflammatory skin disease, occurring most often in adults. It is marked by multiple, small, crimson to purple, topped, angular or polygonal papules; the plane apex of each being usually flat or depressed and covered with a horny film. Oral lesions usually accompany cutaneous lesions and, sometimes, occur alone; the buccal mucosa, lips, gingivae, floor of the mouth, and palate are affected in a descending order of frequency. Typically, oral lesions consist of radiating white or gray, velvety, threadlike lines arranged in a reticular pattern, at the intersection of which there may be minute, white, elevated dots or streaks (*Wickham's striae*). The lesions may coalesce and form bluish white, angular plaques or papules with radiating striae at the periphery. A burning sensation of the affected areas is a common symptom. Drug sensitivity and emotional factors are suspected as contributing causes, but the etiology is unknown. Called also *l. psoriasis* and *l. ruber planus*. See also Atabrine STOMATITIS. **l. psori'asis, l. ru'ber pla'nus,** l. planus. **l. sclero'sus et atroph'icus,** a chronic atrophic skin disease characterized by irregular, firm, flat-topped papules the color of ivory or mother-of-pearl, with erythematous halos surrounding the white spots. Individual papules are round or oval, and have a shining smooth surface, and contain dark, comedo-like plugs or minute depressions caused by former plugs. In advanced stages, coalescing papules may form large lesions and atrophy may occur. Bullae, hemorrhage, hyperpigmentation, and exfoliation may also occur. Leukoplakia-like white plaques may involve the oral mucosa. It occurs predominantly in women, the upper chest, back, and anogenital area being the common sites. Called also *l. albus, chronic atrophic lichenoid dermatitis, Hallopeau's disease, von Zumbusch's disease, white spot disease,* and *Zumbusch's disease*. **l. spinulo'sus,** l. pilaris.

lichenification (li″ken-ĭ-fĭ-ka′shun) thickening of the skin, with exaggeration of its normal markings and furrows, such as seen in persistent scratching.

Lichtenstein, Louis see Jaffe-Lichtenstein SYNDROME.

licorice (lik′o-ris) glycyrrhiza.

lid (lid) an eyelid.

Liddel and Sherrington reflex [Edward George Tandy *Liddel*, British physiologist, born 1895; Sir Charles Scott *Sherrington*, English physiologist, 1857–1952] stretch REFLEX.

lidocaine (li′do-kān) a topical anesthetic, 2-diethyl-amino-2′6′-aceto-xylidide, occurring as a white or yellowish crystalline powder with a characteristic odor, which is very soluble in alcohol and chloroform, readily soluble in benzene, ether, and oils, and insoluble in water. Also used as an antiarrhythmic agent. Called also *lignocaine*. Trademarks: Duncaine, Isicaine, Leostesin, Lidothesin, Xylocaine, Zylestesin. **l. hydrochloride,** the hydrochloride salt of lidocaine, occurring as a bitter, odorless, white crystalline powder that is very soluble in water and alcohol, readily soluble in chloroform, and insoluble in ether. It is a potent local anesthetic, used in all types of local anesthesia, alone or in combination with epinephrine and other substances. Also a component of local anesthetic solutions (see under SOLUTION). Nausea, vomiting, muscular twitching, chills, drowsiness, unresponsiveness, and depression are the principal side effects. It is partially detoxified in the liver. Trademarks: Alphacaine, Codescaine, Octacaine, Xylocaine. See also table at ANESTHETIC.

Lidothesin trademark for *lidocaine*.

lie (li) presentation (2).

lien (li′en) [L.] [NA] spleen.

Liéou, Young Choen see Barré-Liéou SYNDROME.

life (līf) [L. *vita*; Gr. *bios* or *zōe*] 1. the aggregate of vital phenomena; a certain peculiar stimulated condition of organized matter; that obscure principle whereby organized beings are peculiarly endowed with certain powers and functions not associated with inorganic matter. 2. the duration of an earthly existence. See also EMBRYOLOGY, ONTOGENY, and PHYLOGENY. **average l.,** mean l. **half-l.,** half-life. **mean l.,** the average of the lives of all individual atoms of a radioactive substance. Called also *average l.* **radioactive l.,** the theoretical time required for a radioactive substance to lose all of its activity by decay. See also DECAY and HALF-LIFE. **shelf l.,** the length of time a chemical substance may be stored without deterioration.

ligament (lig′ah-ment) [L. *ligamentum*] 1. a band of connective tissue that serves to connect and strengthen joints and support the visceral organs. Ligaments are tough and flexible but not extensible; they are made up of parallel bundles interlaced with bundles of collagen fibers. Most are white and shiny, but ligaments which connect the laminae of the vertebrae and the ligamentum nuchae in lower animals are yellow. Called also

ligamentum. 2. a double layer of peritoneum extending from one visceral organ to another. 3. cordlike remnants of fetal tubular structures that are nonfunctional after birth. **accessory l.,** any ligament that strengthens or supports another. **accessory l. of Henle, lateral,** temporomandibular l. **accessory l. of Henle, medial,** sphenomandibular l. **alar l's,** two strong bands that pass from the posterolateral part of the tip of the dens of the axis upward and laterally to the condyles of the occipital bone; they limit rotation of the head. Called also *ligamenta alaria* [NA]. **alveolodental l.,** periodontal l. **annular l's, tracheal,** tracheal annular l's. **anterior petrosphenoid l.,** sphenopetrosal SYNCHONDROSIS. **apical dental l., apical odontoid l.,** a cord of tissue extending from the tip of the dens of the axis of the occipital bone. Called also *ligamentum apicis dentis axis* [NA] and *ligamentum apicis dentis epistrophei.* **arytenoepiglottic l., aryepiglottic** FOLD. **l's of auricle, l's of auricle of external ear,** the three ligaments, anterior, superior, and posterior, that help attach the auricle to the side of the head. Called also *l's of Valsalva* and *ligamenta auricularia.* **Berry's l.,** thyrohyoid l. **canthal l.,** 1. palpebral l., lateral. 2. palpebral raphe, lateral; see under RAPHE. **capsular l.,** joint CAPSULE. **cemental l.,** circular dental l., periodontal l. **ceratocricoid l., anterior,** a fibrous band that extends from the anterior surface of the tip of the inferior cornu of the thyroid cartilage forward and downward and is attached to the side of the arch of the cricoid cartilage. Called also *ligamentum ceratocricoideum anterius.* **ceratocricoid l's, lateral,** fibrous bands that extend downward and back from the tip of the inferior cornu of the thyroid cartilage and are attached to the lower, lateral, outer surface of the lamina of the cricoid cartilage. Called also *ligamenta ceratocricoidea lateralia.* **ceratocricoid l's, posterior,** fibrous bands that extend from the posterior surface of the inferior cornu of the thyroid cartilage near its tip upward, backward, and medially, and are attached to the superior lateral margin of the lamina of the cricoid cartilage. Called also *ligamenta ceratocricoidea posteriora.* **cricoarytenoid l., posterior,** the ligament extending from the lamina of the cricoid cartilage to the medial surface of the base and muscular process of the arytenoid cartilage. Called also *triquetral l., ligamentum cricoarytenoideum posterius* [NA], and *posterior cricoarytenoid cartilage.* **cricopharyngeal l., cricosantorinian l.,** a ligament extending from the cricoid lamina to the midline of the pharynx. Called also *ligamentum cricopharyngeum* [NA]. **cricothyroarytenoid l.,** elastic cone of larynx; see under CONE. **cricothyroid l.,** a flat ligament extending from the inferior thyroid notch down to arcus of the cricoid cartilage, forming the anterior part of the elastic cone of the larynx. Called also *ligamentum cricothyroideum* [NA] and *ligamentum cricothyreoideum medium.* **cricotracheal l.,** an extrinsic ligament of the larynx; it connects the cricoid cartilage with the first ring of the trachea. Called also *ligamentum cricotracheale* [NA]. **dental l., apical,** apical dental l. **dentoalveolar l.,** periodontal l. **external l. of temporomandibular articulation, external l. of mandibular articulation,** temporomandibular l. **extrinsic l's of larynx,** l's of larynx, extrinsic. **Ferrein's l.,** vocal cord, true; see under CORD. **gingivodental l.,** periodontal l. **glenoid l. of mandibular fossa,** a ring of fibrocartilage connected with the rim of the mandibular fossa. **hammock l.,** a fibrous structure developing from the dental sac. It is part of the periodontal ligament below the growing end of the root of the tooth. Called also *suspensory l.* **l. of Henle, lateral accessory,** temporomandibular l. **l. of Henle, medial accessory,** sphenomandibular l. **hyoepiglottic l.,** a triangular elastic ligamentous band which attaches the caudal part of the anterior surface of the epiglottis to the cranial border of the body of the hyoid bone. Called also *ligamentum hypoepiglotticum* [NA]. **hyothyroid l., hyothyroid l., lateral,** thyrohyoid l. **hyothyroid l., middle,** thyrohyoid l., middle. **interarticular l.,** any ligament situated within the capsule of a joint. **intermaxillary l.,** pterygomandibular RAPHE. **intrinsic l's of larynx,** l's of larynx, intrinsic. **l's of larynx, extrinsic,** ligaments which connect the thyroid cartilage and epiglottis with the hyoid bone, and the cricoid cartilage with the trachea. **l's of larynx, intrinsic,** ligaments which connect laryngeal cartilages to each other. **lateral accessory l. of Henle,** temporomandibular l. **lateral hyothyroid l., lateral thyrohyoid l.,** thyrohyoid l. **lateral maxillary l., lateral l. of temporomandibular articulation,** temporomandibular l. **lateral l. of temporomandibular articulation,** temporomandibular l. **lateral l. of temporomandibular joint,** temporomandibular l. **maxillary l., lateral,** temporomandibular l. **maxillary l., middle,** sphenomandibular l. **middle hyothyroid l.,** thyrohyoid l., middle. **middle maxillary l.**, sphenomandibular l. **middle pharyngeal l.**, RAPHE of pharynx. **middle thyrohyoid l.**, thyrohyoid l., middle. **palpebral l., lateral**, a ligament that anchors the lateral end of the superior and inferior tarsal plates to the margin of the orbit. Called also *canthal l.* and *ligamentum palpebrale laterale* [NA]. **palpebral l., medial**, a short fibrous band that connects the medial ends of the tarsi to the bones of the orbit, an anterior bundle passing in front of the lacrimal sac and being attached to the frontal process of the maxilla, and a posterior bundle passing behind the lacrimal sac and being attached to the posterior crest of the lacrimal bone. Called also *ligamentum palpebrale mediale* [NA], *tendo oculi*, and *tendo palpebrarum*. **periodontal l.**, the fibrous connective tissue that surrounds the root of a tooth and separates it from the alveolar bone. The ligament extends from the base of the gingival mucosa to the fundus of the bony socket, and its main function consists of holding the tooth in its socket. It is also involved in tooth development, transport of metabolic substances to the dental tissue, and passage of blood vessels, nerves, and lymphatics to the tooth. The ligament is made up of fibrous elements, collagen fibers being the chief component, which are organized into bundles; and principal fibers arranged along the length of the root, which serve in anchoring the tooth to its alveolus. In addition to collagen fibers, the ligament contains the reticular fibers, which are usually associated with the vascular channels; elastic fibers, which are usually located with the afferent blood vessels; oxytalan fibers, which follow the collagen fibers and are inserted into either the cementum or the bone; and Shapey's fibers, which are a part of the principal fibers. Functionally, the periodontal fibers are classified as the gingival fibers, which attach to the cementum and to the gingiva and support the vestibular and oral gingivae; transseptal fibers, which attach to the cementum, connecting it with the cementum of the adjoining teeth, supporting the interproximal gingivae and securing the adjacent teeth; alveolar crest fibers, which attach to the cementum and to the alveolar crest and anchor the tooth to the alveolus and oppose lateral stresses; horizontal fibers, which attach to the cementum and to the occlusal third of the alveolus and resist lateral pressures; oblique fibers, which attach to the cementum and to two-thirds of the alveolus, and sustain occlusal stresses and suspend and anchor the tooth in its socket; apical fibers, which attach to the cementum and to the alveolar fundus and prevent the tooth from vestibulo-oral tipping; and interradicular fibers, which attach to the cementum and the crest of the interradicular septum and resist tipping and torque. Called also *alveolodental l.*, *cemental l.*, *circular dental l.*, *dentoalveolar l.*, *gingivodental l.*, *alveolar periosteum*, *alveolodental membrane*, *dental periosteum*, *desmodont*, *peridental membrane*, *periodontal membrane*, and *periosteum alveolare*. See also PERIODONTIUM. **petrosphenoid l.**, 1. sphenopetrosal SYNCHONDROSIS. 2. sphenooccipital SYNCHONDROSIS (1). **petrosphenoid l., anterior**, sphenopetrosal SYNCHONDROSIS. **pharyngeal l., pharyngeal l., middle**, RAPHE of pharynx. **pterygomandibular l., pterygomaxillary l.**, pterygomandibular RAPHE. **pterygospinal l., pterygospinous l.**, a fibrous band of the pterygoid fascia that extends from the upper part of the superior border of the lateral pterygoid plate to the spine of the sphenoid bone. The ligament sometimes ossifies, creating the pterygospinous foramen. Called also *ligamentum pterygospinale* [NA] and *ligamentum pterygospinosum*. **Rauber's tubopharyngeal l.**, salpingopharyngeal FOLD. **salpingopharyngeal l.**, salpingopharyngeal FOLD. **Sappey's l.**, the thicker posterior part of the capsule of the temporomandibular joint. **sphenomandibular l.**, a thin but strong aponeurotic band formed by the pterygoid fascia, which extends from the angular spine of the sphenoid bone downward medial to the temporomandibular articulation and attaches to the lingula of the mandible. Called also *medial accessory l. of Henle*, *middle maxillary l.*, and *ligamentum sphenomandibulare* [NA]. **stylohyoid l.**, a fibrous aponeurotic cord that attaches to the tip of the styloid process of the temporal bone and the lesser cornu of the hyoid bone, and sometimes is partially ossified. Called also *ligamentum stylohyoideum* [NA]. **stylomandibular l., stylomaxillary l., stylomylohyoid l.**, a strong aponeurotic band extending from the suprahyoid fascia, between the deep surface of the parotid and the posterior belly of the digastric muscle, which is attached superiorly to the tip of the styloid process of the temporal bone and inferiorly to the angle and posterior margin of the ramus of the mandible. Called also *ligamentum stylomandibulare* [NA]. **suspensory l.**, hammock l. **sutural l.**, a

layer of fibrous membrane between the opposed bones of a suture or immovable joint. **synovial l.**, a large synovial fold. **temporomandibular l.**, a thick, fibrous band made up of two short, narrow fasciculi; it reinforces the lateral wall of the articular capsule and attaches superiorly to the lateral border of the articular tubercle of the postglenoid process, and inferiorly to the posterior and lateral border of the neck of the condyle of the mandible. It covers the postglenoid process and is covered by the parotid gland and by the integument. Called also *external l. of mandibular articulation*, *external l. of temporomandibular articulation*, *lateral accessory l. of Henle*, *lateral maxillary l.*, *lateral l. of temporomandibular articulation*, *lateral l. of temporomandibular joint*, and *ligamentum laterale articulationis temporomandibularis* [NA]. **thyroepiglottic l.**, a fibrous band that attaches the petiolus of the epiglottis to the thyroid cartilage just below the superior notch. Called also *ligamentum thyreoepiglotticum* and *ligamentum thyroepiglotticum* [NA]. **thyrohyoid l., thyrohyoid. l., lateral**, an extrinsic ligament, consisting of a round elastic cord formed by the posterior border of the thyrohyoid membrane; it extends from the tip of the superior horn of the thyroid cartilage upward to the tip of the greater horn of the hyoid bone. It sometimes contains triticeal cartilaginous nodules which are occasionally ossified. Called also *Berry's l.*, *hyothyroid l.*, *lateral hyothyroid l.*, *ligamentum hyothyreoideum*, and *ligamentum thyrohyoideum* [NA]. **thyrohyoid l., middle, thyrohyoid l., median**, an extrinsic ligament of the larynx, formed by the thick middle part of the thyrohyoid membrane, which attaches its upper end to the body of the hyoid bone and its lower end to the superior incisure of the thyroid cartilage. Called also *middle hyothyroid l.*, *ligamentum hyothyreoideum medianum*, and *ligamentum thyrohyoideum medianum* [NA]. **tracheal annular l's**, circular horizontal ligaments that join the tracheal cartilages together. Called also *ligamenta annularia trachealia* and *ligamenta anularia trachealia* [NA]. **triquetral l.**, cricoarytenoid l., posterior. **tubopharyngeal l. of Rauber**, salpingopharyngeal FOLD. **l's of Valsalva**, l's of auricle. **ventricular l. of larynx**, vestibular l. **vestibular l.**, the membrane that extends from the thyroid cartilage in front to the anterolateral surface of the arytenoid cartilage behind; it lies within the vestibular fold, above the vocal ligament. Called also *ventricular l. of larynx*, *glandular crest of larynx*, *ligamentum ventriculare*, and *ligamentum vestibulare* [NA]. **vocal l.**, one of two strong bands of yellow elastic tissue, which extends from the angle of the thyroid cartilage ventrally, to the vocal process of the arytenoid cartilage dorsally. It is within the vocal fold, below the vestibular ligament. Called also *ligamentum vocale* [NA].

ligamenta (lig″ah-men′tah) [L.] plural of *ligamentum*.
ligamentum (lig″ah-men′tum), pl. *ligamen′ta* [L.] ligament. **ligamen′ta ala′ria** [NA], alar ligaments; see under LIGAMENT. **ligamen′ta annula′ria trachea′lia**, tracheal annular ligaments; see under LIGAMENT. **ligamen′ta anula′ria trachea′lia** [NA], tracheal annular ligaments; see under LIGAMENT. **l. a′picis den′tis ax′is** [NA], l. a′picis den′tis epistro′phei, apical dental LIGAMENT. **ligamen′ta auricula′ria** [NA], ligaments of auricle; see under LIGAMENT. **l. ceratocri′deum ante′rius**, ceratocricoid ligament, anterior; see under LIGAMENT. **ligamen′ta ceratocricoi′dea latera′lia**, ceratocricoid ligaments, lateral; see under LIGAMENT. **ligamen′ta ceratocricoi′dea posterio′ra**, ceratocricoid ligaments, posterior; see under LIGAMENT. **l. cricoarytenoi′deum poste′rius** [NA], cricqarytenoid ligament, posterior; see under LIGAMENT. **l. cricopharyn′geum** [NA], cricopharyngeal LIGAMENT. **l. cricothyroi′deum** [NA], l. cricothyreoi′deum me′dium, cricothyroid LIGAMENT. **l. cricotrachea′le** [NA], cricotracheal LIGAMENT. **l. hyoepiglot′ticum** [NA], hyoepiglottic LIGAMENT. **l. hyothyreoi′deum latera′le**, thyrohyoid LIGAMENT. **l. hyothyreoi′deum media′num**, thyrohyoid ligament, middle; see under LIGAMENT. **l. latera′le articulatio′nis temporomandibula′ris** [NA], temporomandibular LIGAMENT. **l. palpebra′le latera′le** [NA], palpebral ligament, lateral; see under LIGAMENT. **l. palpebra′le media′le** [NA], palpebral ligament, medial; see under LIGAMENT. **l. pterygospina′le** [NA], l. pterygospino′sum, pterygospinal LIGAMENT. **l. sphenomandibula′re** [NA], sphenomandibular LIGAMENT. **l. stylohyoi′deum** [NA], stylohyoid LIGAMENT. **l. stylomandibula′re** [NA], stylomandibular LIGAMENT. **l. temporomandibula′re**, temporomandibular LIGAMENT. **l. thyreoepiglot′ticum, l. thyreoepiglot′ticum**, thyroepiglottic LIGAMENT. **l. thyrohyoi′deum** [NA], l. thyrohyoi′deum latera′le, thyrohyoid LIGAMENT. **l. thyrohyoi′deum media′num** [NA], thyrohyoid ligament, middle; see under LIGAMENT. **l. ventricula′re**, vestibular LIGAMENT. **l. vestibula′re** [NA], vestibular LIGAMENT. **l. voca′le** [NA], vocal LIGAMENT.

ligand (li′gand, lig′and) [L. *ligare* to tie or bind] a group of ions or atoms (coordinating atoms) around a central metal ion (central atom) in a coordination compound bound by covalent bonds with the central ion, as oxygen is bound to the central ion atoms of hemoglobin. The term is also used to indicate any ion or molecule that reacts to form a complex with another molecule, frequently a macromolecule. See also CHELATE. **bidentate l.,** a chelate which bonds to a metal ion through two sites, such as ethylenediamine. **monodentate l.,** a ligand which bonds through one lone pair of electrons. **polydentate l.,** chelate.

ligase [E.C.6] (li′gās, lig′ās) any of a major class of enzymes that catalyze the linking together of two molecules with the breaking of a pyrophosphate bond of ATP or a similar triphosphate. Called also *synthetase.* See also ENZYME classification. **acid–amino acid l.,** pepetide SYNTHETASE. **acid-ammonia l.,** amide SYNTHETASE. **acid-thiol l.** [E.C.6.2.1], a subclass of ligases, the enzymes of which synthesize acyl-CoA derivatives. **carbon–nitrogen l.** [E.C.6.3.3], a subclass of ligases, the enzymes of which catalyze the formation of C−N bonds. See CYCLO-LIGASE.

ligate (li′gāt) to tie or bind with a ligature.

ligation (li-ga′shun) 1. the application of a ligature. 2. teeth l. **interdental l.,** a suturing technique used to join facial and lingual flaps. See illustration. **sling l.,** sling SUTURE. **surgical l.,**

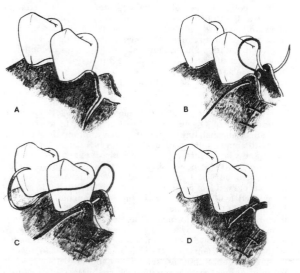

Interdental ligation. *A,* Facial and lingual flaps to be sutured. *B,* The vertical incision is closed by simple, interrupted sutures; the needle is inserted through the facial aspect of the facial papilla and through the lingual papilla from its inner side. *C,* The needle is reversed through the same interdental space. *D,* A tie is made on the facial side. (From F. A. Carranza: Glickman's Clinical Periodontology. 5th ed., Philadelphia, W. B. Saunders Co., 1979.)

1. a technique used in the past to expose an unerupted tooth, in which a metal ligature was placed around the cervix, the free ends being fixed to a fine metal chain, which in turn was fixed to an orthodontic appliance for the purpose of placing traction on the unerupted tooth and causing its eruption. 2. ligation of a blood vessel by tying it in controlling hemorrhage or of a secretory duct in preventing escape of fluids. **teeth l.,** the binding together of teeth with wire, thread, or other material for their stabilization and immobilization as a method of tooth movement in orthodontic therapy or following traumatic injury.

ligature (lig′ah-chūr) [L. *ligatura*] 1. any substance such as catgut, cotton, silk, or wire, used to tie a vessel or strangulate a part. See also SUTURE. 2. ligature WIRE. **grass-line l.,** one made of fibers of a grass-cloth plant (ramie), which shrinks upon becoming wet with saliva and, thus, effects a limited amount of tooth movement. **interlacing l., interlocking l.,** a continuous suture in which the loops interlock. **lateral l.,** one so applied as to check, but not to interrupt, the distal blood flow. **occluding l.,** one that occludes the blood supply to distal tissue. **soluble l.,** one of prepared animal membrane which is subsequently absorbed, the time of absorption depending upon the method of preparation and the size of the ligature. **steel l.,** one of steel filaments used to bind teeth together to secure their stabilization and immobilization or to reduce minor tooth movement. **thread-elastic l.,** an elastic thread used for various forms of orthodontic

therapy, such as assisting in eruption of impacted teeth, closing spaces, and rotating teeth.

light (līt) the electromagnetic radiation having a velocity of about 3×10^{10} cm (186,284 miles) per second, and the vibrations in space being at right angles to the direction of transmission. Frequently construed as limited to the range of wavelength between 3900 and 7700 angstroms, which provides the stimulus for the subjective sensation of sight, but sometimes considered as including part of the ultraviolet and infrared ranges as well. **actinic l.,** light rays capable of producing chemical effects. **axial l., central l.,** light whose rays are parallel to each other and to the optic axis. **coherent l.,** light of a single frequency that travels in intense, nearly perfect, parallel rays without appreciable divergence. **cold l.,** a light transmitted through a quartz or plastic structure to dissipate the heat. The lamp may be applied directly to the skin and is used for transillumination of the tissues for diagnostic purposes. **diffused l.,** that which has been scattered by reflection and refraction. **infrared l.,** infrared rays; see under RAY. **Landeker-Steinberg l.,** a light that emits a spectrum similar to that of the sun except that the ultraviolet waves are eliminated; used therapeutically. **monochromatic l.,** one of the colors of the spectrum into which light is divided by a prism. **neon l.,** a light that contains no ultraviolet and no infrared rays. **oblique l.,** the light that falls obliquely on a surface. **operating l.,** a lamp for illuminating the operating area. In a dental unit, it is usually a spotlight mounted on an extension arm. **polarized l.,** light the vibrations of which are made over one plane or in circles or ellipses. **reflected l.,** light whose rays have been turned back from an illuminated surface. **refracted l.,** light whose rays have been bent out of their original course by passing through a transparent membrane. **safe l.,** light used in dark rooms in which photographic and x-ray film is developed. It is usually a yellow or red-orange light from which those rays in the spectrum to which films are sensitive have been screened out by special filters. Written also *safelight.* **transmitted l.,** light the rays of which have passed through an object. **ultraviolet l.,** ultraviolet rays; see under RAY. **white l.,** that produced by a mixture of all wavelengths of electromagnetic energy perceptible as light.

Lightwood's syndrome [Reginald *Lightwood*] Lightwood-Albright SYNDROME.

Lightwood-Albright syndrome [Reginald *Lightwood;* Fuller *Albright,* born 1900] see under SYNDROME.

Lignac's disease [G. O. E. *Lignac*] Abderhalden-Fanconi SYNDROME.

Lignac-Fanconi disease [G. O. E. *Lignac;* Guido *Fanconi,* Swiss biochemist, born 1832] Abderhalden-Fanconi SYNDROME.

ligneous (lig′ne-us) [L. *lignum* wood] woody; having a wooden feeling.

lignocaine (lig′no-kān) lidocaine.

limb (lim) 1. one of the paired appendages of the body used in locomotion or grasping; in man, an arm or a leg. 2. a structure or part resembling an arm or leg.

limbi (lim′bi) [L.] plural of *limbus.*

limbic (lim′bik) pertaining to a limbus or margin; forming a border around.

limbus (lim′bus), pl. *lim′bi* [L.] an outer edge, border, or margin; a general anatomical term for such a structure. See also BORDER, LIP, and MARGIN. **alveolar l. of mandible, l. alveola′ris mandib′ulae,** alveolar arch of mandible; see under ARCH. **alveolar l. of maxilla, l. alveola′ris maxil′lae,** alveolar arch of maxilla; see under ARCH. **l. foram′inis ova′lis,** the border of the oval foramen. Called also *crista dividens.*

lime (līm) 1. CALCIUM oxide. 2. the fruit of *Citrus acida,* the juice of which contains ascorbic acid; it has antiscorbutic properties. **burnt l.,** CALCIUM oxide. **hydrated l.,** CALCIUM hydroxide. **slaked l.,** CALCIUM hydroxide. **unslaked l.,** CALCIUM oxide.

limen (li′men), pl. *lim′ina* [L.], 1. threshold, as of a stimulus. 2. a general anatomical term for the beginning point, boundary, or threshold of a structure. **l. na′si** [NA], threshold of the nose; a ridge marking the boundary between the nasal cavity proper and the vestibule.

limina (lim′ĭ-nah) [L.] plural of *limen.*

liminal (lim′ĭ-nal) [L. *limen* threshold] pertaining to limen; barely perceptible.

liminometer (lim″ĭ-nom′ĕ-ter) [*limen* + Gr. *metron* measure] an instrument for measuring the strength of stimulus applied over a tendon and determining the reflex threshold.

limit (lim′it) [L. *limes* boundary], a boundary, as one that confines. **age l.,** in insurance, the definition of the lower and upper age limits, as those specified in a dental plan contract for eligibility of children and adults. **assimilation l.,** the amount of carbohydrate that an organism can metabolize without causing glycosuria. Called also *saturation limit.* **elastic l.,** the extent elastc material may be deformed without impairing its ability to return to its original dimensions. There are minor differences between the elastic and proportional limits. See also Hooke's LAW. **l. on liability,** in insurance, a limit on dollar coverage contained in an insurance policy, such as a limit on the amounts payable for an individual claim in malpractice insurance. **proportional l.,** the limit measured as the deviation from linearity in the stress-strain curve of a continuously increased loaded specimen. There are minor differences between the elastic and proportional limits. When the amount of stress exceeds the proportional limit, permanent deformation of the material under stress occurs. See also DEFORMATION (2). **saturation l.,** assimilation l. **solubility l.,** see point DEFECT. **time l's,** in insurance, the periods of time within which a notice of claim must be filed.

limitation (lim-i-ta′shun) 1. the setting or establishing of limits or boundaries, thereby limiting or restricting something as to extent, amount, continuance, procedure, etc. 2. exclusion (3).

Linc alloy see under ALLOY.

Lincocin trademark for *lincomycin.*

Lincomix trademark for *lincomycin.*

lincomycin (lin″ko-mi′sin) a broad-spectrum antibiotic produced by *Streptomyces lincolnensis,* methyl 6,8-dideoxy-6-(1-methyl-4 - propyl - 2 - pyrrolidinecarboxamido) - 1 - thio - D - erythro - D - galacto-octapyranoside. Used therapeutically as the hydrochloride salt, which occurs as a white, odorless, bitter, crystalline powder that is freely soluble in water, methanol, and ethanol, slightly soluble in acetone, and insoluble in nonpolar organic solvents. It suppresses protein metabolism by binding bacterial ribosomes, being active against various gram-positive organisms, chiefly staphylococci, streptococci, clostridia, and corynebacteria. Oral administration may cause diarrhea, glossitis, stomatitis, vomiting, pruritus, skin rash, urticaria, vaginitis, and potentially fatal colitis. Neutropenia, leukopenia, and thrombopenia may follow parenteral administration. Less common adverse reactions may include hypersensitivity, angioedema, anaphylaxis, photosensitization, and cardiac arrest. Intestinal yeast overgrowth may occur. Trademarks: Albiotic, Collimycin, Frademicina, Lincocin, Lincomix, Myvicin.

Lind, James [1716–1794] a British naval surgeon and founder of naval hygiene, whose controlled study on scurvy resulted in lime juice being issued to British sailors during long ocean voyages; thus virtually eradicating scurvy under these circumstances.

Lindemann bur see under BUR.

line (lin) [L. *linea*] 1. a stripe, streak, mark, or narrow ridge. Called also *linea.* See also BAND. 2. in anthropometry, an imaginary line connecting different anatomical landmarks. See also AXIS and PLANE. **absorption l.,** one of the dark lines of the spectrum due to absorption of light by the substance (usually an incandescent gas or vapor) through which the light has passed. Cf. absorption BAND. **accretion l.,** incremental l. **alveolar l.,** a term sometimes used for upper facial height. See under HEIGHT. Called also *alveolonasal l., alveolar point–nasal point l., alveolar point–nasion l., nasal point–alveolar point l.,* and *nasion–alveolar point l.* **alveolar point–basion l.,** alveolobasilar l. **alveolar point–nasal point l., alveolar point–nasion l.,** alveolar l. **alveolobasilar l.,** a line from the basion to the upper alveolar point. Called also *alveolar point–basion l.* and *basion–alveolar point l.* **alveolonasal l.,** alveolar l. **Amberg's l.,** a line dividing into two halves the angle formed by the anterior border of the mastoid process and the temporal line; it indicates the most easily accessible part of the lateral sinus for a mastoid operation. Called also *lateral sinus l.* **Amici's l.,** Z BAND. **l. angle,** line ANGLE. **ANS-Opis l.,** His′ l. (1). **aplastic l.,** a cement line formed by a smooth layer of basophilic material. Called also *limiting l.* See also *cement l.* **aplastic resorption l.,** a cement line formed by a layer of basophilic material with an eroded and irregular surface, which is characteristic of bone undergoing resorption. See also *cement l.* **arcuate l. of occipital bone, external superior,** nuchal l., superior. **arcuate l. of occipital bone, highest,** nuchal l., highest. **arcuate l. of occipital bone, inferior,** nuchal l., inferior. **arcuate l. of occipital bone, superior,** nuchal l., superior. **arcuate l. of occipital bone, supreme,** nuchal l., highest. **auricular point–bregma l.,** auriculobregmatic l. **auric-**

ulobregmatic l., a line from the auricular point to the bregma (Po-Br). Called also *auricular point–bregma l., bregma–auricular point l.,* and *Broca's point–bregma l.* **basinasal l.,** Huxley's plane when viewed on edge; see under PLANE. Called also *basion–nasion l., nasion–basion l.,* and *nasobasilar l.* **basiobregmatic l.,** one from the basion to the bregma. Called also *basion-bregma l.* and *bregma-basion l.* **basion–alveolar point l.,** alveolobasilar l. **basion–bregma l.,** basiobregmatic l. **basion–nasion l.,** basinasal l. **biauricular l.,** a line passing over the vertex from one porion to the other. **bismuth l.,** a thin blue-black line in the marginal gingiva around the teeth, sometimes confined to the gingival papilla, observed in bismuth poisoning. See also *gingival l.* (2), BISMUTH, bismuth PIGMENTATION, and gingival STOMATITIS. **blood l.,** a line of direct descent through several generations. **blue l.,** lead l. **bregma–auricular point l.,** auriculobregmatic l. **bregma–basion l.,** basiobregmatic l. **Bridgett's l.,** one drawn on the premastoid lamina after a simple mastoid operation to show the course of the facial canal in order to prevent injury of the facial nerve in performing a radical mastoid operation. **Broca's point–bregma l.,** auriculobregmatic l. **Burton's l.,** lead l. **calcification l.,** incremental l. **Camper's l.,** Camper's PLANE. **canthomeatal l.,** the line joining the lateral canthus of the eye and superior border of the external auditory meatus. **cell l.,** a group of animal cells derived from a primary culture at the time of the first subculture; it is considered to be an *established cell line* when it demonstrates the potential for indefinite subculture in vitro. **cement l., cementing l.,** a layer of a refractile, dark-staining material around groups of lamellae, visible under the microscope as a thin line in cross sections of a bone. See also *aplastic l., aplastic resorption l., resting l.,* and *reversal l.* **cervical l.,** an anatomical landmark determining the junction of the enamel- and cementum-covered portions of a tooth (cementoenamel junction); the dividing line between the crown and the root portions of a tooth. **Clapton's l.,** copper l. **contour l.,** l. of Owen. **copper l., Corrigan's l.,** a greenish, reddish, or purplish line on the gingivae symptomatic of poisoning with copper salts. Called also *Clapton's l.* and *Corrigan's sign.* See also *gingival l.* (2). See also COPPER. **cruciate l.,** cruciate EMINENCE. **curved l. of occipital bone, highest,** nuchal l., highest. **curved l. of occipital bone, inferior,** nuchal l., inferior. **curved l. of occipital bone, superior,** nuchal l., superior. **curved l. of occipital bone, supreme,** nuchal l., highest. **Daubenton's l.,** Daubenton's PLANE. **l. defect,** dislocation (2). **demarcation l.,** a line formed in the secondary dentin by dentinal tubules displaced by shifting of the cell bodies of the odontoblasts due to crowding or some strong stimulus, indicating the change in cell orientation. **De Salle's l.,** nasal l. **developmental l's,** developmental grooves; see under GROOVE. **dislocation l.,** a plane of atoms that is discontinuous in the space lattice in a crystalline structure. See also DISLOCATION (2). **Dobie's l.,** Z BAND. **l. of draw,** the direction or plane of withdrawal or seating of a removable or cast restoration. **dynamic l's,** lines on the face, e.g., laugh lines and frown lines, which develop as a result of repetitious right-angle pull on the skin by the muscles of expression; they are considered a sign of aging. **l's of Ebner,** delicate lines indicating periods of rest between daily increments of dentin, which are visible on ground sections of a tooth, particularly on slightly acid-etched sections. Called also *imbrication l's of Ebner, incremental l's of Ebner,* and *von Ebner's l's.* **ectental l.,** the line of junction between the ectoderm and entoderm. **embryonic l.,** the primitive tract in the center of the germinal area. **established cell l.,** see *cell l.* **facial l.,** a line connecting the nasion with the pogonion, gnathion, or menton. Called also *nasion–pogonion l.* and *pogonion–nasion l.* **finish l.,** in cavity preparation, a minimal line of demarcation of the wall of the preparation at the cavosurface angle. **Frankfort Horizontal l.,** Frankfort Horizontal PLANE. **frown l.,** see *dynamic l's.* **fulcrum l.,** an axis that extends from one abutment tooth to another, about which a partial denture can rotate during function. **fulcrum l., retentive,** an imaginary line connecting the retentive points of clasp arms on retaining teeth adjacent to mucosa-borne denture bases, around which a denture tends to rotate when subjected to such forces as the pull of sticky foods. **fulcrum l., stabilizing,** an imaginary line connecting occlusal rests around which the denture will rotate under masticatory forces. **genal l.,** one of Jadelot's lines, extending from the nasal line near the mouth toward the malar bone. **gingival l.,** 1. a line determined by the level to which the gingiva extends on a tooth; although it tends to follow the curvature of the cervical line, the two rarely coincide. Called also *gum l.* 2. any linear discoloration on the gingiva, such as that seen in lead poisoning (*lead l.*), bismuth poisoning (*bismuth l.*), or copper poisoning (*copper l.*). **glabella–inion l.,** Schwalbe's l. **glabella–lambda l.,** Hamy's l. **glabella–pogonion l.,** Topinard's l. **Gl-In line,** Schwalbe's l.

Gl-La l., Hamy's l. **Gottinger's l.,** one along the upper border of the zygomatic arch. **Granger l.,** a curved line seen in roentgenograms of the skull, indicating the position of the optic groove. **grid l's,** shadows on a radiograph caused by the grid. See GRID (3). **Gubler's l.,** a line connecting the apparent orgins of the roots of the fifth cranial nerve. **guide l.,** guideline. **gum l.,** gingival l. (1). **guide l.,** guideline. **Hamy's l.,** Hamy's plane when viewed on edge; see under PLANE. Called also *glabella–lambda l.* and *Gl–La l.* **His' l.,** 1. His' plane when viewed on edge; see under PLANE. Called also *ANS-Opis l.* 2. Martin's l. **imbrication l's of cementum,** incremental l's of cementum. **imbrication l's of Ebner,** l's of Ebner. **imbrication l's of Pickerill,** lines formed by ends of rod bundles which overlie one another and are arranged in scalariform fashion on the surface of the crown of a tooth, seen on longitudinal sections of a tooth together with the incremental lines, but forming areas not completely contained in the enamel. Called also *Pickerill's imbrication l's.* See also *incremental l.* **incremental l.,** one of the lines showing the successive layers deposited in a tissue. In the enamel, they are brown striations visible under transmitted light and colorless in reflected light. They may be observed under the microscope in longitudinal sections as oblique lines running inward from the surface and toward the root and in cross sections as rings similar to those in a tree trunk. Dry dentin often shows a series of somewhat parallel lines caused by imperfectly calcified dentin arranged in layers. Called also *accretion l., calcification l., l. of Retzius, ring of Retzius, stria of Retzius,* and *zone of Retzius.* See also *l's of Ebner, imbrication l's of Pickerill,* and *neonatal l.* **incremental l's of cementum,** very fine dark lines, present in longitudinal sections of a tooth, which follow the contour of the root and border with wider light bands, revealing the cyclic activity of cementogenesis. Called also *imbrication l's of cementum.* **incremental l's of Ebner,** l's of Ebner. **isoeffect l's,** in radiotherapy, lines on a rectangular graph representing doses of radiation having tumoricidal effects and those having complicating necrotic effects in normal tissues. **isothermal l.,** isotherm. **Jadelot's l.,** one of the lines of the face in young children, the genal, labial, nasal, and oculozygomatic lines, described as being indicative of specific types of diseases. Called also *Jadelot's furrow.* **K l's, L l's, M l's, N l's, O l's, P l's,** groups of lines in an x-ray spectrum, determined by the stability level to which the replacement electron "drops"; the K lines come from the level nearest the nucleus of the atom and have the shortest wavelength. **Krause's l.,** Z BAND. **L l's,** see *K l's.* **labial l.,** one of Jadelot's lines, extending laterally from the angle of the mouth; said to indicate disease of the lungs. **lambda–nasion l.,** Virchow's l. **lateral sinus l.,** Amberg's l. **laugh l.,** see *dynamic l's.* **lead l.,** a thin blue-black line in the marginal gingivae, presumably due to precipitation of lead sulfide in the tissue, observed in lead poisoning. Called also *blue l., Burton's l.,* and *Burton's sign.* See also *gingival l.* (2), and see LEAD²' and lead STOMATITIS. **limiting l.,** aplastic l. **lip l.,** a line of the level to which the margin of either lip extends on the teeth. **lip l., high,** the greatest height to which the maxillary lip is raised. **lip l., low,** the lowest position of the lower lip during the act of smiling or voluntary retraction. **liquidus l.,** liquidus. **load l.,** an imaginary line joining any two positive supports of a denture, the fulcrum line being always a load line, but the load line not always being a fulcrum line. **M l.,** M BAND. **M l's,** see *K l's.* **magnetic l's of force,** lines indicating direction of force in a magnetic field. **Martin's l.,** Martin's plane when viewed on edge; see under PLANE. Called also *His' l.* and *nasion–inion l.* See illustration at CEPHALOMETRY. **median l.,** 1. the median plane when viewed on edge; see under PLANE. 2. median l. of face. **median l., anterior,** an imaginary vertical line on the anterior surface of the body, dividing the surface equally into right and left sides. Called also *linea mediana anterior* [NA]. **median l., posterior,** an imaginary vertical line on the posterior surface of the body dividing the surface equally into right and left sides. Called also *linea mediana posterior* [NA]. **median l. of face,** an imaginary vertical line drawn through the center of the face, passing between the central incisors, dividing both the mandibular and maxillary dental arches into right and left sides. **mesenteric l.,** a plaque of brown or black dots which may coalesce to form a thin, dark line on the enamel at the cervical margin of a tooth; its presence is often associated with a relative freedom from dental caries. **Morgan's l.,** a secondary crease in the lower eyelids in atopic dermatitis. Called also *Dennie's sign.* **mucogingival l.,** mucogingival JUNCTION. **mylohyoid l. of mandible,** a ridge on the internal surface of the body of the mandible, running from the base of the symphysis to the ascending ramus behind the last molar tooth. It gives attachment to the mylohyoid muscle and superior constrictor of the pharynx. Called also *internal oblique l. of mandible, internal*

oblique ridge, linea mylohyoidea mandibulae [NA], *linea obliqua mandibulae interna,* and *mylohyoid ridge.* **N l's,** see *K l's.* **nasal l.,** one of Jadelot's lines, extending from the ala nasi in a semicircle around the mouth. Called also *De Salle's l.* **nasal point–alveolar point l.,** nasion–alveolar point l. **nasion–basion l.,** basinasal l. **nasion–inion l.,** Martin's l. **nasion–lambda l.,** Virchow's l. **nasion–pogonion l.,** facial l. **nasobasilar l.,** basinasal l. **nasolabial l.,** one from the ala nasi to the angle of the mouth. **neonatal l.,** a line seen on longitudinal sections of a tooth, showing a demarcation between the structures present at birth and those deposited postnatally. In cross sections, the lines are seen as rings (neonatal rings), and their variations indicate adaptational changes in tooth formation. The shock at birth is registered in the enamel as an exaggerated incremental line; in the dentin, an exaggerated line of Owen is formed during the perinatal adjustment of the infant to its new environment. **nuchal l., highest,** a sometimes indistinct line on the outer surface of the occipital bone, arching upward from the external occipital protuberance and running toward the lateral angle, giving attachment to the epicranial aponeurosis. Called also *highest arcuate l. of occipital bone, highest curved l. of occipital bone, highest semicircular l. of occipital bone, supreme arcuate l. of occipital bone, supreme nuchal l., supreme curved l. of occipital bone, supreme semicircular l. of occipital bone,* and *linea nuchae suprema* [NA]. **nuchal l., inferior,** a faintly marked line and the lowest of the three nuchal lines found on the outer surface of the occipital bone, extending laterally from the middle of the external occipital crest to the jugular process, giving attachment to the nuchal ligament. Called also *inferior arcuate l. of occipital bone, inferior curved l. of occipital bone,* and *linea nuchae inferior* [NA]. **nuchal l., median, nuchal l., middle,** a sometimes indistinct ridge on the outer surface of the occipital bone, running from the foramen magnum to the external occipital protuberance, giving attachment to the ligamentum nuchae. Called also *middle nuchal l., crista occipitalis externa* [NA], *external occipital crest,* and *linea nuchae mediana.* **nuchal l., superior,** a curved line on the outer surface of the occipital bone, extending from the external occipital protuberance toward the lateral angle, and giving attachment medially to the trapezius muscle and laterally to the sternocleidomastoid muscle. Called also *superior arcuate l. of occipital bone, external superior arcuate l. of occipital bone, superior curved l. of occipital bone, superior semicircular l. of occipital bone,* and *linea nuchae superior* [NA]. **nuchal l., supreme,** nuchal l., highest. **O l's,** see *K l's.* **oblique l., external,** a ridge of osseous structure on the body of the mandible extending from the anterolateral border to the mandibular ramus, passing downward and forward, after covering the buccocervical portion of the third molar, and ending by blending into the body of the mandible, lateral to the molar teeth. **oblique l. of mandible,** a ridge on the external surface of the body of the mandible, extending posteriorly from each mental tubercle, which is continuous with the anterior border of the ascending ramus on either side. It gives attachment to the depressor labii inferioris and depressor anguli oris muscles. Called also *linea obliqua mandibulae* [NA]. **oblique l. of mandible, internal,** mylohyoid l. of mandible. **oblique l. of thyroid cartilage,** a line on the external surface of the lamina of the thyroid cartilage, extending between the two thyroid tubercles. Called also *linea obliqua cartilaginis thyroideae* [NA]. **l. of occlusion,** the alignment of the occluding surfaces of the teeth in a horizontal plane. **oculozygomatic l.,** one of Jadelot's lines, extending outward from the medial canthus toward the zygoma; said to be a sign of some disorder of the nervous system. **l. of Owen,** one of the sweeping bands seen on longitudinal section which outline the growth of the coronal or radicular dentin. The bands represent a lag of several days between the calcification phases, each lasting about four days, and (16 μ of new dentin deposited as incremental bands that originate at the incisal edge or cusp tips of a tooth and expand apically (rootward) and centrally (pulpward). Called also *contour l.* See also *neonatal l.* **P l's,** see *K l's.* **Pickerill's imbrication l's,** imbrication l's of Pickerill. **pogonion–glabella l.,** Topinard's l. **pogonion–nasion l.,** facial l. **Poirier's l.,** a line from the nasofrontal angle to a point just above the lambda. **precentral l.,** a line on the head, extending from a point midway between the inion and the glabella downward and forward. **primitive l.,** primitive STREAK. **profile l.,** Camper's PLANE. **recessional l.,** one of the lines or markings on the teeth due to recession, in the formative period of the teeth, of the soft tissue which gives place to the dentin. **Reid's base l.,** a line from the infraorbital ridge to the external auditory meatus and the middle line of the occiput. **resorption l.,** an intense blue line which separates the resorptive from reparative processes of the cementum, being the boundary where cementoclasts disappear and cementoblasts reappear. **resting l.,** 1. a cement line formed by a layer of basophilic material which separates old from newly formed bone. See also *cement l.* 2. a line between new cementum deposited over a layer of the older less vital cementum. See also cementum LAMELLA. **retentive fulcrum l.,** an imaginary line connecting the retentive points of clasp arms, around which the denture tends to rotate when subjected to forces, such as the pull of sticky foods. **l. of Retzius,** incremental l. **reversal l.,** a cement line formed by a layer of basophilic material and having a surface with a scalloped appearance, which is characteristic of apposition of bone adjacent to the aplastic resorption lines. See also *cement l.* **l's of Schreger,** the dark and light lines visible under reflected light in a ground section of a tooth, which terminate at the dentinoenamel junctions coinciding with the enamel prism curvatures. The dark bands are known as *diazones* and the light ones as *parazones.* Called also *Hunter-Schreger bands, Schreger's bands, Schreger's striae,* and *zones of Schreger.* **Schwalbe's l.,** Schwalbe's plane when viewed on edge; see under PLANE. Called also *glabella–inion l.* and *Gl–In l.* **segmental l's,** developmental grooves; see under GROOVE. **semicircular l. of frontal bone,** temporal l. of frontal bone. **semicircular l. of occipital bone, highest,** nuchal l., highest. **semicircular l. of occipital bone, superior,** nuchal l., superior. **semicircular l. of occipital bone, supreme,** nuchal l., highest. **semicircular l. of parietal bone, inferior,** temporal l., inferior. **semicircular l. of parietal bone, superior,** temporal l., superior. **simian l.,** simian CREASE. **solidus l.,** solidus. **sternomastoid l.,** one from the heads of the sternomastoid to the mastoid process. **supraorbital l.,** one across the forehead, just above the root of the external angular process of the frontal bone. **survey l.,** 1. the line indicating the height of a tooth after the cast has been positioned according to the chosen path of insertion. 2. a line produced on a cast of a tooth by a surveyor scriber, marking the greatest height of contour in relation to the chosen path of insertion of the restoration. 3. a line drawn on a tooth or teeth by means of a surveyor for the purpose of determining the position of the various parts of a clasp or clasps. Called also *clasp guideline.* See also dental SURVEYOR. **sylvian l.,** a line on the head extending from the external angular process of the frontal bone to a point three-fourths of an inch below the most prominent point of the parietal bone. It coincides with the direction of the fissure of Sylvius. **temporal l. of frontal bone,** a ridge extending upward and backward from the zygomatic process of the frontal bone, dividing into superior and inferior parts that are continuous with corresponding lines on the parietal bone, and giving attachment to the temporal fascia. Called also *semicircular l. of frontal bone, crista temporalis, external frontal crest, linea temporalis ossis frontalis* [NA], *and temporal crest of frontal bone.* **temporal l., inferior, temporal l. of parietal bone, inferior,** a curved line on the external surface of the parietal bone, marking the limit of attachment of the temporal muscle. Called also *inferior semicircular l. of parietal bone, inferior semicircular ridge of parietal bone,* and *linea temporalis inferior ossis parietalis* [NA]. **temporal l., superior, temporal l. of parietal bone, superior,** a curved line on the external surface of the parietal bone, above and parallel to the inferior temporal line, giving attachment to the temporal fascia. Called also *superior semicircular l. of parietal bone, linea temporalis superior ossis parietalis* [NA], and *superior semicircular ridge of parietal bone.* **Thompson's l.,** a red line observed on the gingivae in pulmonary tuberculosis. **thyroid red l.,** an erythematous line produced by irritation of the skin on front of the neck and upper part of the chest in patients with hyperthyroidism. **Topinard's l.,** one from the glabella to the pogonion. Called also *glabella–pogonion l.* and *pogonion–glabella l.* **vibrating l.,** an imaginary line across the palate which separates its movable portion, the hard palate, from its immovable portion, the soft palate. **Virchow's l.,** one from the nasion to the lambda. Called also *lambda–nasion l.* and *nasion–lambda l.* **von Ebner's l's,** l's of Ebner. **von Ihring's l.,** von Ihring's plane when viewed on edge; see under PLANE. **Wagner's l.,** a thin whitish line at the junction of the epiphysis and diaphysis of a bone, formed by preliminary calcification. **white l. of pharynx,** RAPHE of pharynx. **Z l.,** Z BAND.

linea (lin′e-ah), pl. *lin′eae* [L.] a stripe, streak, mark, or narrow ridge; used in anatomical nomenclature as a general term to designate a streak or narrow ridge on the surface of some structure. Called also *line.* **l. media′na ante′rior** [NA], median line, anterior; see under LINE. **l. media′na poste′rior** [NA], median line, posterior; see under LINE. **l. mylohoi′dea mandib′ulae** [NA], mylohyoid line of mandible; see under LINE. **l. nu′chae infe′rior** [NA], inferior nuchal LINE. **l. nu′chae media′na,** median nuchal LINE. **l. nu′chae supe′rior** [NA], superior nuchal LINE. **l. nu′chae supre′ma** [NA], highest nuchal LINE. **l. obli′qua cartilag′inis thyroi′deae** [NA], oblique line of thyroid cartilage; see under LINE. **obli′qua mandib′ulae** [NA], oblique line of mandible; see under LINE. **l. obli′qua mandib′ulae inter′na,** mylohyoid line of mandible; see under LINE. **l. tempora′lis infe′rior os′sis parieta′lis** [NA], temporal line, inferior; see uner LINE. **l. tempora′lis os′sis fronta′lis** [NA], temporal line of frontal bone; see under LINE. **l. tempora′lis supe′rior os′sis parieta′lis** [NA], temporal line, superior; see under LINE.

lineae (lin′e-e) [L.] plural of *linea.*

lineage (lin′e-ij) [L. *linea* line] descent traced down from or back to a common ancestor. **cell l.,** the developmental history of cells as traced from the first division of the original cell or cells.

linear (lin′e-ar) [L. *linearis*] pertaining to or presenting a line; pertaining to one dimension.

liner (lin′er) material applied to the inside of the walls of a cavity or container, for protection or insulation of the surface. See also RELINER. **cavity l.,** a cavity lining agent used for the protection of the pulp from irritation and to neutralize the free acid of zinc phosphate and silicate cements. It is usually applied to a shallow prepared cavity or, sometimes, over a cavity base and, on evaporation of the solvent, it forms a thin residual film. Cavity liners are aqueous or volatile organic liquid suspensions or dispersions of zinc phosphate or calcium hydroxide, methylcellulose and natural or synthetic resin being often used as the dispersing or suspending medium. See also cavity PRIMER. Available under various trademarks. **cushion l.,** resilient l. **Handi-l.,** HANDI-LINER. **resilient l., soft l.,** a material applied to the tissue side of a denture to provide a soft lining to the parts of a denture coming in contact with soft tissue and to cushion its contact with the tissues. Resins, such as acrylic and silicone resins, that have been rendered elastomeric by plasticizers, are generally used as resilient liners. Called also *cushion l.* See also tissue CONDITIONER. **Speed l.,** trademark for a temporary denture base reliner.

Lingraine trademark for *ergotamine tartrate* (see under ERGOTAMINE).

Lingran trademark for *ergotamine tartrate* (see under ERGOTAMINE).

lingua (ling′gwah), pl. *lin′guae* [L. "tongue"] [NA] 1. the movable, muscular organ in the mouth and in the pharynx, subserving the functions of taste, mastication, articulation, and deglutition. See TONGUE. 2. any organ or structure having a shape similar to that of the tongue. **l. fraena′ta,** ankyloglossia. **l. geograph′ica,** benign migratory GLOSSITIS. **l. ni′gra,** black TONGUE. **l. plica′ta,** fissured TONGUE. **l. villo′sa ni′gra,** black TONGUE.

linguae (ling′gwe) [L.] plural of *lingua.*

lingual (ling′gwal) [L. *lingualis*] pertaining to or toward the tongue; glossal. In dental anatomy, the term is used to refer to the surface of a tooth directed toward the tongue (or oral cavity) and opposite the vestibular (or facial) surface. Used synonymously with *oral.* See illustration at SURFACE.

linguale (ling-gwa′le) the point at the upper end of the symphysis of the lower jaw on its lingual surface.

lingualis (ling-gwa′lis), pl. *lingua′les* [L.] relating to the tongue.

lingually (ling′gwal-le) toward the tongue.

lingula (ling′gu-lah), pl. *lin′gulae* [L., dim. of *lingua*] a general anatomical term for a small tonguelike structure. **l. of mandible, l. mandib′ulae** [NA], a sharp spine on the lateral surface of the ramus of the mandible, on the bony ridge surrounding the mandibular foramen, which gives attachment to the sphenomandibular ligament. Called also *mandibular spine.* **l. of sphenoid, sphenoidal l., l. sphenoida′lis** [NA], a slender ridge of bone on the lateral margin of the carotid sulcus, projecting backward between the body and great wing of the sphenoid bone. Called also *anterior petrosal process.*

lingulae (ling′gu-le) [L.] plural of *lingula.*

lingular (ling′gu-lar) pertaining to a lingula.

linguo- [L. *lingua* tongue] a combining form denoting relationship to the tongue. See also words beginning GLOSSO-.

linguoaxial (ling″gwo-ak′se-al) pertaining to the lingual and axial walls of a cavity preparation of a tooth.

linguoaxiogingival (ling″gwo-ak″se-o-jin′ji̇-val) pertaining to or formed by the lingual, axial, and gingival walls of a tooth cavity preparation. Called also *axiolinguocervical* and *axiolinguogingival.*

linguocervical (ling″gwo-ser′vĭ-kal) 1. **pertaining** to the lingual surface of the neck of a tooth; cervicolingual. 2. linguogingival.

linguoclusion (ling″gwo-kloo′zhun) an occlusion in which the dental arch or groups of teeth are lingual to normal; lingual occlusion.

linguodental (ling″gwo-den′tal) 1. **pertaining** to the tongue and teeth. 2. a speech sound produced with the aid of the tongue and teeth, as *th*.

linguodistal (ling″gwo-dis′tal) distolingual. Abbreviated *LD*.

linguogingival (ling″gwo-jin′jĭ-val) **pertaining** to the tongue and gingiva; pertaining to or formed by the lingual and gingival walls of a cavity preparation of a tooth.

linguoincisal (ling″gwo-in-si′zal) **pertaining** to or formed by the lingual and incisal surfaces of a tooth.

linguomesial (ling″gwo-me′ze-al) **pertaining** to or formed by the lingual and mesial surfaces of a tooth, or the lingual and mesial walls of a cavity preparation of a tooth.

linguo-occlusal (ling″gwo-o-kloo′zal) **pertaining** to or formed by the lingual and occlusal surfaces of a tooth.

linguopapillitis (ling″gwo-pap″ĭ-li′tis) inflammation or ulceration of the papillae of the edges of the tongue.

linguoplacement (ling″gwo-plās′ment) lingual PLACEMENT.

linguoplate (ling″gwo-plāt) lingual PLATE.

linguoproximal (ling″gwo-prok′sĭ-mal) of or pertaining to both the proximal and lingual surfaces of a tooth. Called also *proximolingual*.

linguopulpal (ling″gwo-pul′pal) **pertaining** to or formed by the lingual and pulpal walls of a tooth cavity.

linguoversion (ling″gwo-ver′zhun) **displacement** of a tooth lingually from the line of occlusion.

liniment (lin′ĭ-ment) [L. *linimentum, linere* to smear] an oily liquid preparation to be used on the skin. **camphor l.,** a preparation of camphor and cottonseed oils; used as a local irritant to the skin. **camphor and soap l.,** a preparation of green soap, camphor, rosemary oil, ethanol, and distilled water; used as a local irritant to the skin. **chloroform l.,** a preparation of chloroform with camphor and soap liniment; used as a local irritant to the skin. **medicinal soft soap l.,** green soap TINCTURE.

linimentum (lin″ĭ-men′tum) [L.] liniment. **s. sapo′nis mol′lis,** green soap TINCTURE.

lining (lin′ing) 1. material used for covering or investing, especially the inner surface of something. 2. the act or process of covering or investing, especially the inner surface of something. 3. cavity l. **cavity l.,** an inner coating, as of varnish or other protective substance, to cover a cavity wall — usually a resinous film-forming agent dissolved in a volatile solvent, or a suspension of calcium hydroxide in a solution of a synthetic resin. The lining seals the dentinal tubules and protects the pulp before the restoration is inserted.

link (lingk) anything connecting one thing to another. **siloxane l.,** a link in a straight-chain compound (siloxane) so arranged that each silicon atom is linked with four oxygen atoms. See also silicone polymers, under POLYMER.

linkage (lingk′ij) 1. the connection between different atoms in a chemical compound. 2. **the association of two genes** having loci close together on the same chromosome or the same nucleic acid molecule, which are transmitted together, thus being an exception to Mendel's law of independent assortment. See also ASSOCIATION (3) and SYNTENY.

Liomycin trademark for *doxycycline hyclate* (see under DOXYCYCLINE).

lip (lip) [L. *labium*] 1. any margin or marginal portion of an organ or part. 2. one of two fleshy margins of the mouth, situated beneath the nose, above the chin, and bounded on both sides by the cheeks, which are connected to each other by thin folds (labial commissures) at the corners of the mouth. The upper lip borders onto the nose, and is separated from the cheeks by the nasolabial sulci which start at each side of the wings of the nose, from where they diverge at about a 90 degree angle, passing downward at some distance from the corners of the mouth. A vertical groove, the philtrum, connects the nose with the upper lip. The lower lip is not separated from the cheeks early in life but, later in life, it is separated by furrows (labiomarginal sulci), passing in posteriorly convex arches close to the corners of the mouth. The labiomental groove divides the lower lip from the chin. The surface of the lips is entirely bound by epithelium; that which covers the external surface is considered to be epidermis because it is keratinized. The integument contains sweat glands, sebaceous glands, and hairs, which are more prominent in males than females. The inner surface is covered by nonkeratinized epithelium and the lamina propria. The tissue contains labial vessels, nerves, areolar tissue, fat, and mixed labial glands that form an almost continuous layer. The border of the lips is also covered by nonkeratinized epitheli-

um. Translucency of the stratum lucidum, showing capillaries and papillae beneath the surface, gives the characteristic red color to the vermilion border. A slight protrusion in the vermilion zone of the upper lip, just below the philtrum, is called the tubercle of the upper lip. Each lip is connected in the midline to the corresponding gingiva by a fold of mucous membrane (labial frenum). The orbicularis oris muscle provides the musculature of the lips. Called also *labium oris* [NA]. See also terms beginning CHEILO- and LABIO-. **cleft l.,** CLEFT lip. **double l.,** redundancy of the submucous tissue and mucous membrane of the lip on either side of the median line. **Hapsburg l.,** a thick overdeveloped lower lip usually associated with mandibular prognathism (*Hapsburg jaw*), as seen in members of the Hapsburg family. **inferior l., lower l.,** the fleshy margin of the inferior border of the mouth. See LIP (2). Called also *inferior l., labium inferius oris* [NA], and *labium mandibulare*. **l. plumper,** lip PLUMPER. **superior l., upper l.,** the fleshy upper margin of the superior border of the mouth. See LIP (2). Called also *superior l., labium maxillare,* and *labium superius oris* [NA].

lipase (lip′ās, li′pās) [Gr. *lipos* fat + *-ase*] 1. a group of widely occurring enzymes that catalyze the hydrolysis of lipids, found in milk, saliva, adipose tissue, the pancreas, stomach, and other tissues. See also lipid METABOLISM. 2. triacylglycerol l. **triacylglycerol l.** [E.C.3.1.1.3], a carboxylic ester hydrolase that catalyzes the hydrolysis of fats, being a component of pancreatic juice and acting only on an ester-water interface, the outer ester links being preferentially hydrolyzed. Called also *triglyceride l., steapsin,* and *tributyrase*. **triglyceride l.,** triacylglycerol l.

Lipavlon trademark for *clofibrate*.

lipemia (li-pe′me-ah) [lipo- + Gr. *haima* blood + *-ia*] the presence in the blood of excessive amounts of fats. See also HYPERLIPEMIA. **alimentary l.,** increase in the blood of fats (chylomicrons) following a meal, associated with increased blood turbidity. See also HYPERCHYLOMICRONEMIA. **l. retina′lis,** a pale cast to the retina, usually associated with a marked increase in light reflex of the retinal vessels; a symptom of hyperlipemia.

lipid (lip′id) any of a group of organic substances which are insoluble in water, but are soluble in alcohol, ether, chloroform, and other nonpolar solvents. All lipids derive their properties from the hydrocarbon nature of a major portion of their structure. Lipids serve as structural components of membranes, as a source of energy, as a protective coating on the surface of some organisms, and as cell-surface components concerned with cell recognition, species specificity, and tissue immunity. They are also involved in calcification of the cartilage. In the U.S.A., the term embraces fatty acids, glycerol-containing compounds (neutral fats and phosphoglycerides), fats which do not contain glycerol (sphingolipids, aliphatic alcohols and waxes, terpenes, and steroids), lipoproteins, proteolipids, phosphatidopeptides, lipoamino acids, lipopolysaccharides, and some vitamins. In Great Britain, the term is restricted to compounds which, on hydrolysis, yield alcohol or a sugar, a base, and a fatty acid, and does not include neutral fats, fatty acids, or sterols. There are also numerous other classifications of lipids. Called also *lipoid*. **blood l.,** any fat or lipid present in the blood. The lipids of the blood are constantly changing in concentration as lipids are added by absorption from the intestine, by synthesis, and by removal from fat depots, being the highest immediately after meals. Average values for young adults are:

	mg/100 ml
Total lipids	510
Triglycerides	150
Phospholipids	200
Total cholesterol	160

The triglycerides, phospholipids, and cholesterol in the plasma are combined with protein as lipoprotein complexes, which are bound to the α- and β-globulin fractions of the plasma proteins and are transported in this form. A small amount of nonesterified fatty acids is present in the blood and is bound to the albumin fraction of the plasma for transportation. **complex l's,** saponifiable lipids having fatty acids as components, including acylglycerols, phosphoglycerides, sphingolipids, and waxes. On alkaline hydrolysis, they yield soaps (salts of fatty acids). **compound l's,** lipids which, in addition to an alcohol and fatty acids, contain some other chemical group. The two subdivisions are phospholipids (lecithins, cephalins, phosphoinositides, plasmalogens, phosphatidic acids, and spingomyelins); and glycolipids (cerebrosides and gangliosides), characterized by their content of phosphoric acid and carbohydrate, respectively. Lipoproteins are also sometimes included in this group, although they are usually classified as conjugated proteins. **l. metabolism,** the process by which lipids (fats) are absorbed and used by the body. Dietary fats entering the intestine are mostly neutral fats (triglycerides) with small amounts of phospholipids, cholesterol, and cholesterol esters. They are emulsified in the intestine by bile salts, mainly ionized sodium salts, breaking the fat globules into small sizes so that the digestive enzymes can act on their surfaces, being assisted in the fragmentation by movements of the small intestine. Digestion is accomplished by water-soluble enzymes, lipases, present in the pancreatic juice and the epithelial cells of the small intestine, breaking down triglycerides into glycerol and fatty acids or into monoglycerides and fatty acids. From the intestine, fats are absorbed into the lymph. After passing through the intestinal epithelium, lipids are resynthesized into new molecules of triglycerides, which aggregate and enter the lymph nodes as minute dispersed droplets, the chylomicrons. Most cholesterol and phospholipids also enter the chylomicrons and are together transported up the thoracic duct and emptied into the venous circulation. Some short-chain fatty acids are absorbed directly into the blood from the intestine. Most chylomicrons are removed from the circulating blood as they pass through the capillaries of adipose tissue and are hydrolyzed into fatty acids and glycerol by lipoprotein lipase, to be stored in the fat cells. Once in the cells, fatty acids are resynthesized into triglycerides, to be split again into fatty acids and glycerol when they are needed for energy. They are transported to mitochondria by an enzyme-catalyzed process that employs carnitine as a carrier substance and, once in the mitochondria, the fatty acids are split away from the carnitine to be oxidized. Large amounts of triglycerides appear in the liver during starvation, in diabetes mellitus, and in other conditions in which fats are used extensively for energy. In addition to triglycerides, the liver also contains phospholipids and cholesterol, where they are synthesized. About 40 to 45 percent of energy is derived from lipids in the American diet. See also LIPOLYSIS. **nonsaponifiable l.,** see *simple l's.* **saponifiable l.,** see *complex l's.* **simple l's,** according to one classification, nonsaponifiable lipids that do not contain fatty acids, including terpenes, steroids, and prostaglandins. According to another classification, lipids containing only fatty acids and some type of alcoholic compound, including fats and waxes.

lipidosis (lip″ĭ-do′sis) any disorder of lipid metabolism; lipoidosis. **cerebroside l.,** Gaucher's DISEASE. **ganglioside l.,** Tay-Sachs DISEASE. **glycolipid l.,** Fabry's DISEASE. **sphingomyelin l.,** Niemann-Pick DISEASE. **sulfatide l.,** metachromatic LEUKODYSTROPHY.

Lipiodol trademark for *iodized oil* (see under OIL).

Lipmann, Fritz Albert [born 1899] a German-born biochemist in the United States; co-winner, with Sir Hans Adolf Krebs, of the Nobel prize for medicine and physiology in 1953, for the discovery of coenzyme A and its importance in intermediary metabolism. See also phosphogluconate PATHWAY (Warburg-Dickens-Lipmann pathway).

lipo- [Gr. *lipos* fat] a combining form denoting relationship to fat.

lipoatrophy (li″po-at′ro-fe) [lipo- + *atrophy*] atrophy of the fatty tissue, especially the subcutaneous fat depot.

lipoblast (lip′o-blast) [lipo- + Gr. *blastos* germ] a young cell of the connective tissue which develops into a fat cell.

lipochondrodystrophy (lip″o-kon″dro-dis′tro-fe) [lipo- + Gr. *chondros* cartilage + *dystrophy*] Hunter-Hurler SYNDROME.

lipocyte (lip′o-sīt) [lipo- + *-cyte*] fat CELL.

lipogenesis (lip″o-jen′ĕ-sis) [lipo- + *genesis*] the formation of fat; the transformation of nonfat materials into body fat. See LIPID metabolism.

lipogranulomatosis (lip″o-gran″u-lo-mah-to′sis) a disorder of lipid metabolism in which yellow nodules of lipid matter are deposited in the skin and mucosae, giving rise to granulomatosis. **disseminated l., Farber's l.,** Farber's SYNDROME.

lipoid (lip′oid) [lipo- + Gr. *eidos* form] 1. fatlike; resembling fat. 2. lipid.

lipoidosis (lip″oi-do′sis) any disorder of lipid metabolism; lipoidosis. **hereditary dystrophic l.,** Fabry's DISEASE.

lipolysis (li-pol′ĭ-sis) [lipo- + Gr. *lysis* dissolution] 1. the hydrolysis or splitting up of fats or fatty tissue. Called also *adipolysis.* 2.

the hydrolysis of triglycerides to free fatty acids, as shown in the equation:

$$\text{triglycerides} \xrightarrow[\text{lipase}]{\text{activated}} \text{glycerol + fatty acids}$$

The process is enhanced by hormones, such as epinephrine, which stimulate the production of cyclic-3′,5′-AMP and depressed by prostaglandins, which decrease the production of cyclic-3′,5′-AMP.

lipoma (lip-o′mah) [lipo- + *-oma*] a fatty tumor; a tumor made up of fat cells. Typically, a benign tumor presenting a poorly delimited, thinly encapsulated, soft, multilobular mass made up of mature fat cells exhibiting various amounts of collagen strands. It may be located anywhere in the body, but is found most commonly in the subcutaneous regions containing abundant amounts of fat. It is a rare oral tumor, but those located in the mouth may be found on the tongue, floor of the mouth, buccal mucosa, gingiva, and mucobuccal and labial folds. **malignant l.,** liposarcoma.

lipomatosis (lip″o-mah-to′sis) an abnormal, localized, or tumorlike accumulation of fat in the tissues.

lipopenia (lip″o-pe′ne-ah) [lipo- + Gr. *penia* poverty] deficiency of lipids in the body.

lipoprotein (lip″o-pro′te-in) [lipo- + *protein*] a conjugated protein in which lipids are the prosthetic group. Lipoproteins are found chiefly in the blood serum (*soluble l's*) and in nerve tissue and subcellular cell components (*insoluble l's*); their molecular weight is about 200,000 to 5,000,000, and their lipid content varies from 5 to 97 percent. Function of lipoproteins is related mainly to the transport of lipids. By association with proteins (which are soluble), lipids (which are insoluble) may be transported in the blood serum in the form of lipoproteins. Lipoproteins may be separated from other proteins on the basis of their solubility, electrophoretic mobility, and ultracentrifugation. Fractionation in cold EtOH/H₂O yields two fractions which may be identified with α₁- and β-lipoproteins; zone electrophoresis yields three fractions: the α₁, α₂, and β; and ultracentrifugation separates lipoproteins on the basis of their relative densities (molecular weight being inversely proportional to the density) measured in Svedberg flotation units (Sf). See also HYPERLIPOPROTEINEMIA. **α-l.,** a high-density plasma lipoprotein which contains more protein (45–55 percent) and less lipids than other lipoproteins, has electrophoretic mobility in the α-range, floats between densities 1.063 and 1.21 gm per ml in the ultracentrifuge, participates in the transport of most phospholipids, and is synthesized in the intestine. Called also *high-density l.* (HDL). See also Tangier DISEASE. **β-l.,** a low-density plasma lipoprotein which contains 25 percent protein and 75 percent lipid, has electrophoretic mobility in the β-range, floats between densities 1.006 and 1.063 gm per ml in the ultracentrifuge, participates in the transport of cholesterol, and is synthesized in the liver. Called also *low-density l.* (LDL). **high-density l.,** α-l. **insoluble l.,** the lipoprotein fraction that is insoluble in water, usually occurring in nerve tissue and subcellular cell components. **low-density l.,** β-l. **prebeta-l.,** a very low-density lipoprotein which contains about 10 percent protein, 55 percent triglyceride, 20 percent phospholipid, and 15 percent cholesterol, floats between densities 0.95 and 1.006 gm per ml in the ultracentrifuge, and participates in the transport of triglycerides. Called also *very low-density l.* (VLDL). **soluble l.,** the water-soluble fraction of lipoprotein, usually occurring in the blood serum. **very low-density l.,** prebeta-l.

lipoproteinosis (lip″o-pro″te-in-o′sis) [lipoprotein + *-osis*] a condition characterized by abnormal deposits of lipoproteins. **Urbach's l.,** Urbach-Wiethe SYNDROME.

liposarcoma (lip″o-sar-ko′mah) [lipo- + *sarcoma*] a malignant lipoma; it is an uncommon tumor, occurring most frequently in elderly persons, in the peritoneal and mediastinal fat.

lipotropic (lip″o-trop′ik) having an affinity for fats or oils, and thus acting on fat metabolism by hastening the removal of or decreasing the deposit of fat in the body.

lipping (lip′ing) 1. a wedge-shaped shadow in the roentgenogram of chondrosarcoma between the cortex and the elevated periosteum. 2. the development of a bony overgrowth, as in osteoarthritis or on the jaw as a result of peripheral buttressing bone formation.

Lipschütz bodies [Benjamin *Lipschütz*, Austrian physician, 1878–1931] see under BODY.

Liq. liquor.

liquefacient (lik″wĕ-fa′shent) [L. *liquefaciens*] 1. having the quality to convert a solid material into a liquid; producing liquefaction. 2. an agent capable of producing liquefaction.

liquefaction (lik″wĕ-fak′shun) [L. *liquefactio; liquere* to flow + *facere* to make] 1. the conversion of a solid material into a liquid form; dissolution. 2. colliquative NECROSIS. **gas l.,** the conversion of gas into a liquid form, brought about by cooling and compression, resulting in a decrease of the average kinetic energy of the molecules sufficiently to allow intermolecular forces of attraction to pull the molecules together. Called also *condensation.*

liquid (lik′wid) [L. *liquidus, liquere* to flow] 1. a fluid; a substance that flows readily in its natural state. 2. a state of matter intermediate between a solid and a gas, having no fixed shape, but occupying the entire space afforded within the walls of their container. Liquids have a definite volume, their density being lower than that of solids and being nearly incompressible. See also LIQUIDUS. **Fluorident l.,** trademark for an aqueous fluoride solution, 100 ml of which contain 2 gm sodium fluoride and 0.34 gm hydrogen fluoride, which is acidulated with 0.98 gm phosphoric acid; used in dental caries control. **Fluoritab l.,** trademark for a solution, four drops (0.17 ml) of which contain 2.21 mg sodium fluoride, being equivalent to 1 mg fluoride ion; used in dental caries prevention. **Karidium l.,** trademark for a solution, eight drops (0.5 ml) of which contain 2.21 mg sodium fluoride, being equivalent to 1 mg fluoride ion and 10 mg sodium chloride; used in dental caries prevention. **Nebs analgesic l.,** trademark for an analgesic solution, 5 ml of which contain 120 mg acetaminophen and various amounts of glycerol, propylene glycol, alcohol elixir, and coloring, flavoring, and preservative substances. **Pulpdent l.,** trademark for a *cavity liner* (see under LINER), consisting of an aqueous suspension of calcium hydroxide in methylcellulose. **Topicale l.,** trademark for an anesthetic solution for topical application, containing 18 percent benzocaine, 0.1 percent benzalkonium chloride, and various amounts of flavoring agents dissolved in a water-soluble polyethylene glycol base.

Liquidomonas (lik″wid-o-mo′nas) *Pseudomonas.* **L. fluores′cens,** *Pseudomonas fluorescens;* see under PSEUDOMONAS.

Liquidovibrio cholerae (lik″wid-o-vib′re-o kol′er-e) *Vibrio cholerae;* see under VIBRIO.

liquidus (lik′wĭ-dus) a temperature/concentration curve of a solution on the phase diagram (see under DIAGRAM), indicating its liquid phase. Called also *liquidus curve* and *liquidus line.* Cf. SOLIDUS.

Liquiphene trademark for *phenylmercuric acetate* (see under ACETATE).

liquor (lik′er; li′kwor), pl. *liquors, liquo′res* [L.] 1. a liquid, especially an aqueous solution, or a solution obtained by distillation. 2. a general anatomical term for certain fluids of the body. See also FLUID, LIQUID, and SOLUTION. **l. cerebrospina′lis** [NA], cerebrospinal FLUID.

liquores (li-kwo′rēz) [L.] plural of *liquor.*

liquorice (lik′er-is) glycyrrhiza.

liquorrhea (li″kwo-re′ah) [*liquor* + Gr. *rhoia* flow] an excessive discharge of any body fluid.

Liranol trademark for *promazine.*

lisp (lisp) 1. a speech defect consisting of pronouncing *s* and *z* like or nearly like *th* sounds. 2. defective production of the sibilant sounds caused by improper tongue placement or by abnormality of the articulatory mechanism. **dental l.,** production of the sibilant sounds with the tongue close to or touching the upper front teeth. **lateral l.,** production of the sibilant sounds with the tongue raised so that the breath is emitted laterally over or around the sides of the tongue. **lingual protrusion l.,** production of the sibilant sounds with the tongue between the teeth.

lisping (lisp′ing) see LISP.

lissencephaly (lis″sen-sef′ah-le) [Gr. *lissos* smooth + *enkephalos* brain] agyria.

Lister's dressing [Baron Joseph *Lister*, English surgeon, 1827–1912; his publication in 1867 of the principles of antiseptic surgery made "clean" operations a reality, and catalyzed the development of modern surgery] see under DRESSING.

Listerella (lis″ter-el′ah) *Listeria.* **L. hepatolyt′ica,** *Listeria monocytogenes;* see under LISTERIA.

Listeria (lis-ter′e-ah) [named after Joseph *Lister*] a genus of small, coccoid, gram-positive, nonsporulating, aerobic to microaerophilic, rod-shaped bacteria of uncertain affiliation, which are parasites of poikilothermic and warm-blooded animals, including man. **L. monocytog′enes,** a pathogenic species, occurring as small coccoid rods (about 0.4 to 0.5 by 0.5 to 2.0 μm in size), with rounded ends, slightly curved in some

cultures, found singly and in V-shaped or parallel pairs. In lower animals, infection causes septicemic or encephalomyelitic disease in sporadic or epizootic form. In man, it produces an upper respiratory disease, with angina, lymphadenitis, and conjunctivitis, or a septicemic disease which may be transmitted transplacentally in pregnant women, or it may assume an encephalitic form. Human disease is often associated with a monocytosis. The organisms are sensitive to tetracycline, chloramphenicol, erythromycin, ampicillin, neomycin, and other antibiotics, being less sensitive to penicillin and sulfonamides, and resistant to polymyxin B. Called also *Bacterium monocytogenes, B. monocytogenes hominis, Corynebacterium infantisepticum, C. parvulum, Erysipelothrix monocytogenes,* and *Listerella hepatolytica.*

Listerine see under DENTIFRICE.

Liston's forceps, operation [Robert *Liston*, Scottish surgeon in London, 1794–1847] see under FORCEPS and OPERATION.

Litalir trademark for *hydroxyurea.*

liter (le′ter) the standard unit of volume in SI or in the metric system, which is based on the space occupied by 1 kilogram of pure water at 4°C (the temperature at which a given volume of water weighs the most at sea level; 1 liter contains 1000 cubic centimeters or milliliters and is equivalent to 1.0567 liquid quarts. Abbreviated *l.* Written *litre* in Great Britain. See also *Tables of Weights and Measures* at WEIGHT.

lithiasis (lĭ-thi′ah-sis) [*litho-* + *-iasis*] a condition characterized by the formation of calculi and concretions. **salivary l.,** sialolithiasis.

lithium (lith′e-um) [Gr. *lithos* stone] the lightest and least reactive of the alkali metals and the lightest solid element, occurring as a very soft silvery metal that yellows on exposure to moist air. Symbol, Li; atomic number, 3; atomic weight, 6.941; valence, 1; specific gravity, 0.534; melting point, 180.54°C; group IA of the periodic table. Natural isotopes include ^{7}Li and ^{6}Li; artificial radioactive isotopes include ^{5}Li, ^{8}Li, and ^{9}Li, all being unstable with a half-life of less than 1 sec. When introduced into a biological system, lithium mimics sodium and is, thus, useful in the study of membrane potential. Used in the treatment of neurological disorders and thyrotoxicosis. Also used as a fluxing agent for dental porcelain. Poisoning is caused by chronic or excessive intake of lithium or its salts. Chronic poisoning may be marked by polydipsia; polyuria; kidney lesions, sometimes associated with nephrogenic diabetes insipidus; hematological changes, including increased leukocyte count and aplasia anemia; allergic reactions, such as vasculitis and dermatitis; and ECG and EEG changes. Acute poisoning may be characterized by vomiting, diarrhea, ataxia, convulsions, nausea, abdominal pain, mental confusion, hyperreflexia, dysarthria, arrhythmia, hypotension, albuminuria, coma, and death. There is no specific antidote for lithium poisoning; therapy is largely supportive.

litho- [Gr. *lithos* stone] a combining form denoting relationship to stone or to a calculus.

Lithol trademark for *ichthammol.*

lithotroph (lith′o-trōf) [*litho-* + Gr. *trophē* nutrition] chemolithotroph; see chemolithotrophic CELL.

Liticon trademark for *pentazocine.*

Litocon trademark for *pentazocine.*

Litraderm trademark for *hydrocortisone acetate* (see under HYDROCORTISONE).

litre (le′ter) [Fr.] liter (in Great Britain).

Little's area [James Laurence *Little*, American physician, 1836–1885] Kiesselbach's AREA.

livedo (lĭ-ve′do) [L.] a discolored spot or patch on the skin, commonly due to passive congestion. **l. telangiectat′ica,** permanent mottling of the skin due to an anomaly of the capillaries of the skin.

liver (liv′er) [L. *jecur;* Gr. *hēpar*] 1. a large gland of dark-red color situated in the upper part of the abdomen on the right side, which is essential to life. Its domed upper surface fits closely against and is adherent to the inferior surface of the right diaphragmatic dome, and it has a double blood supply from the hepatic artery and the portal vein. It comprises thousands of minute lobules (lobuli hepatis), the functional units of the liver. Its manifold functions include the storage and filtration of blood, secretion of bile, excretion of bilirubin and other substances formed elsewhere in the body, and numerous metabolic functions, including the conversion of sugars into glycogen, which it stores. Called also *hepar* [NA]. 2. the same gland of certain animals sometimes used as food or from which pharmaceutical products are prepared. See also terms beginning HEPAT- and HEPATO-. **l. starch**, glycogen.

Liviatin trademark for *doxycycline*.

livid (liv′id) [L. *lividus* lead-colored] discolored, as from the effects of contusion or congestion; black and blue.

lividity (lĭ-vid′ĭ-te) [L. *lividitas*] the quality of being livid; discoloration, as of dependent parts, by the gravitation of the blood. **postmorten l.**, LIVOR mortis.

livor (li′vor), pl. *livo′res* [L.] discoloration; livedo. **l. mor′tis**, discoloration appearing on dependent parts of the body after death, as a result of stagnation of the blood due to cessation of circulation. Called also *postmortem l.*

Lizars′ operation [John *Lizars*, Edinburgh surgeon, 1787(c.)–1860] see under OPERATION.

LLF Laki-Lóránd factor; see FACTOR XIII.

load (lōd) the quantity of a measurable entity borne by an object or organism, such as the work (work load) required of an individual, or the body content, as of water, salt, or heat, especially as it varies from normal. **dynamic l.**, dynamic STRESS. **impact l.**, impact FORCE. **occlusal l.**, the total force exerted on the teeth through the occlusal surfaces during mastication, consisting of the vertical and lateral forces. See also occlusal FORCE. **patient l.**, a number of patients treated within a specified period of time. **static l.**, static STRESS.

loading (lōd′ing) 1. in insurance, the amount added to the expected or coverage amounts payable to the insured needed to meet anticipated liabilities for expenses, contingencies, profits, or special situations. Generally, loading costs in group health insurance range from 5 to 25 percent, and in individual health insurance up to 40 or 60 percent. 2. administration of sufficient quantities of a substance to test the subject's ability to metabolize it.

lobar (lo′ber) pertaining to, or affecting a lobe.

lobate (lo′bāt) [L. *lobatus*] provided with lobes, or disposed in lobes.

lobe (lōb) [L. *lobus*; Gr. *lobos*] 1. a more or less well-defined portion of any organ; especially of the brain and glands. Lobes are demarcated by fissures, sulci, and connective tissue, and by their shape. See also LOBUS. 2. a part of a tooth formed by any one of the separate points of the beginning of calcification. **anterior l. of hypophysis, anterior l. of pituitary gland**, pituitary gland, anterior; see under GLAND. **frontal l.**, the anterior portion of the cerebral hemisphere which, for the most part, consists of an associative area and contains centers for the sense of smell and for speech. Called also *lobus frontalis* [NA]. **neural l.**, PARS nervosa hypophyseos. **occipital l.**, the posterior portion of the cerebral hemisphere, extending from the posterior pole to the parieto-occipital fissure on the medial surface, but continuous with the parietal lobe on the lateral surface. Called also *lobus occipitalis* [NA]. **olfactory l.**, the olfactory apparatus on the lower surface of the frontal lobe. Called also *lobus olfactorius*. **parietal l.**, the upper central lobe of the cerebral hemisphere, joining the temporal lobe below, the frontal lobe in front, and the occipital lobe on the side. Called also *lobus parietalis* [NA]. **pyramidal l. of thyroid gland**, an occasional third lobe of the thyroid gland which extends upward from the isthmus, continuous with the thyroglossal duct, to the hyoid bone; it is the remains of the thyroid stalk of the fetus. Called also *lobus pyramidalis glandulae thyroideae* [NA]. **temporal l.**, the lower lateral lobe of the cerebral hemisphere, having an auditory area and the center for memory. Called also *lobus temporalis* [NA]. **l. of thyroid gland**, either of the lobes (right or left) of the thyroid gland, closely applied to either side of the trachea, cricoid cartilage, and thyroid cartilage. Called also *lobus glandulae thyroideae* [NA].

lobectomy (lo-bek′to-me) [*lobe* + Gr. *ektomē* excision] excision of a lobe, as of the thyroid gland or the submandibular gland.

lobeline (lob′ĕ-lin) a compound, 2-[6-(2-hydroxy-2-phenylethyl)-1-methyl-2-piperidinyl]-1-phenylethanone, obtained from the herb and seeds of *Lobelia inflata*. The term is commonly used to designate a mixture of all *Lobelia inflata* alkaloids; sometimes used as a synonym for α-l. **α-l., alpha-l.**, the L-form of lobeline, occurring as colorless crystals that are soluble in hot ethanol, chloroform, benzene, ether, and, slightly, water. Used as a respiratory stimulant and in treating symptoms of tobacco withdrawal. Called also *inflatine*. **l. hydrochloride**, the hydrochloride salt of lobeline, occurring as a white, bitter, granular powder that is soluble in water, ethanol, and chloroform. Used in the treatment of tobacco withdrawal symptoms, and has been used as a respiratory stimulant. Trademarks: Lobron, Zoolobelin.

lobi (lo′bi) [L.] plural of *lobus*.

Lobron trademark for *lobeline hydrochloride* (see under LOBELINE).

Lobstein's syndrome [Johann Friedrich Georg Christian Martin *Lobstein* Strasbourg surgeon, 1777–1835] see under SYNDROME.

lobule (lob′ul) [L. *lobulus*] a small lobe. See also LOBULUS. **l's of thyroid gland**, irregular areas on the surface of the thyroid gland produced by entrance into the gland of fibrous trabeculae from the sheath. Called also *lobuli glandulae thyroideae* [NA].

lobuli (lob′u-li) [L.] plural of *lobulus*.

lobulus (lob′u-lus), pl. *lob′uli* [L., dim. of *lobus*] a small lobe; used in anatomical nomenclature as a general term to designate a small lobe or one of the primary divisions of a lobe. Called also *lobule*. **lob′uli glan′dulae thyroi′deae** [NA], lobules of thyroid gland; see under LOBULE.

lobus (lo′bus), pl. *lo′bi* [L.] lobe; used in anatomical nomenclature as a general term to designate a more or less well-defined portion of any organ. See also LOBE. **l. ante′rior hypophys′eos** [NA], pituitary gland, anterior; see under GLAND. **l. fronta′lis** [NA], frontal LOBE. **l. glan′dulae thyroi′deae** [NA], LOBE of thyroid gland. **l. occipita′lis** [NA], occipital LOBE. **l. olfacto′rius**, olfactory LOBE. **l. parieta′lis** [NA], parietal LOBE. **l. poste′rior hypophys′eos** [NA], pituitary gland, posterior; see under GLAND. **l. pyramida′lis glan′dulae thyroi′deae** [NA], pyramidal lobe of thyroid gland; see under LOBE. **l. tempora′lis** [NA], temporal LOBE.

Locacorten trademark for *flumethasone 21-pivalate* (see under FLUMETHASONE).

local (lo′k′l) [L. *localis*] restricted to or pertaining to one spot or part; not general.

localization (lo″kah-li-za′shun) 1. the determination of the site or place of any process or lesion. 2. restriction to a circumscribed or limited area. 3. the making of a radiograph for the purpose of identifying a site in relation to surrounding tissues. **selected l.**, the tendency of microorganisms to infect a specific variety of tissue.

localized (lo′kah-lizd) restricted to a limited region or to one or more spots; not general.

Localyn trademark for *fluocinolone acetonide* (see under FLUOCINOLONE).

locater (lo-ka′ter) locator.

locator (lo′ka-tor) an instrument, device, or apparatus by which the location of an object is determined. **abutment l.**, a thin resin base made on a diagnostic cast in which holes have been cut to predetermine the locations of the cuspid and molar teeth on a subperiosteal implant. **Berman-Moorhead l.**, an instrument for locating metallic fragments embedded in body tissues. **electroacoustic l.**, an apparatus that amplifies into an audible click the contact of a probe with a solid object; used in locating foreign objects within the body.

Loc. dol. abbreviation for L. *lo′co dolen′ti*, to the painful spot.

loci (lo′si) [L.] plural of *locus*.

lockjaw (lok′jaw) 1. tetanus. 2. trismus.

lockpin (lok′pin) lock PIN.

locomotion (lo″ko-mo′shun) [L. *locus* place + *movere* to move] moving from one place to another.

locomotor (lo″ko-mo′tor) pertaining to locomotion, or to organs and systems of the body involved in locomotion.

Locorten trademark for *flumethasone 21-pivalate* (see under FLUMETHASONE).

locular (lok′u-lar) pertaining to a loculus.

loculi (lok′u-li) [L.] plural of *loculus*.

loculus (lok′u-lus), pl. *loc′uli* [L.] a small space or cavity.

locus (lo′kus), pl. *lo′ci* [L. place] 1. place; a general anatomical term for a site in the body. 2. the position of a gene on a chromosome, different forms of genes (alleles) being found at the same position on homologous chromosomes. **complex l.**, one within which mutation and recombination can occur at more than one site. **l. mino′ris resisten′tiae**, a site of lessened resistance; an area, structure, or organ offering little resistance to invasion by microorganisms and/or their toxins.

Lodosin trademark for *carbidopa*.

Lodosyn trademark for *carbidopa*.

Loefflerella (lef″ler-el′ah) former name for a genus of bacteria, now assigned to the genus *Pseudomonas*. **L. mal′lei**, *Pseudomonas mallei*; see under PSEUDOMONAS. **L. pseudomal′lei**, *Pseudomonas pseudomallei*; see under PSEUDOMONAS.

Logan bow see under BOW.

logasthenia (log″as-the′ne-ah) [*logo-* + *asthenia*] a disorder of that faculty of the mind which deals with the comprehension of speech. See also ASTHENIA.

logo- [Gr. *logos* word] a combining form denoting relationship to words or speech. See also terms beginning LALO-.

logoclonia (log″o-klon′e-ah) [logo- + Gr. *klonos* tumult + -*ia*] spasmodic repetition of the end syllables of words.

logopathy (log-op′ah-the) [logo- + Gr. *pathos* illness] a disorder of speech. Called also *lalopathy*.

logopedics (log″o-pe′diks) laliatry.

logoplegia (log″o-ple′je-ah) [logo- + Gr. *plēgē* stroke] paralysis of the organs of speech. Called also *laloplegia*.

logorrhea (log″o-re′ah) [logo- + Gr. *rhoia* flow] excessive or abnormal volubility. Called also *lalorrhea*.

logospasm (log′o-spazm) [logo- + spasm] the spasmodic utterance of words.

-logy [Gr. *logos* word, reason] a word termination meaning the science or study of, or a treatise on, the subject designated by the stem to which it is affixed.

Londomycin trademark for *methacycline*.

longissimus (lon-jis′ĭ-mus [L.] longest; a general term denoting a long structure, as a muscle. **l. cap′itis**, longissimus muscle of head; see under MUSCLE.

longitudinal (lon″jĭ-tu′dĭ-nal) [L. *longitudinalis*] lengthwise; parallel to the long axis of the body or an organ.

longitudinalis (lon″jĭ-tu″dĭ-na′lis) [L.] longitudinal. **l. infe′rior lin′guae**, longitudinal muscle of tongue, inferior; see under MUSCLE. **l. supe′rior lin′guae**, longitudinal muscle of tongue, superior; see under MUSCLE.

longus (long′gus) [L.] long; a general term denoting a long structure, as a muscle.

loop (lōop) a sharp turn or twist in a cordlike structure. Called also ANSA. **cervical l.**, a structure consisting of the outer and inner enamel epithelium, being the basalmost area of the enamel organ that forms a narrow rim for its concavity. It evolves into Hertwig's epithelial sheath, which determines the number, the size, and the shape of roots of the teeth. **Henle's l.**, a U-shaped turn in a portion of the renal tubule with a descending limb from the proximal convoluted tubule and an ascending limb to the distal convoluted tubule. **l. of hypoglossal nerve**, ANSA cervicalis. **T l.**, a loop on an arch wire in an orthodontic appliance resembling the letter T. **vertical l.**, a U-shaped bend in the arch wire, which aids in the opening and closing of spaces in the arch.

lophodont (lof′o-dont) having molar teeth with crested occlusal ridges.

Lóránd, László [Hungarian-born American biochemist] see FACTOR XIII (Laki-Lóránd factor).

lordosis (lor-do′sis) [Gr. *lŏrdosis*] abnormal inward curvature of the spine. Cf. SCOLIOSIS and KYPHOSIS.

Lorenz, Heister [1683–1758] a German surgeon who was the first to produce removable dental prostheses fashioned of ivory or hippotamus tusks.

Lorfan trademark for *levallorphan tartrate* (see under LEVALLORPHAN).

Loridine trademark for *cephaloridine*.

Lortat-Jacob's disease [Denise *Lortat-Jacob*] benign mucosal PEMPHIGOID.

LOS LENGTH of stay.

Losantin trademark for *calcium hypochlorite* (see under CALCIUM).

loss (los) 1. the inadvertent failure to retain something in such a way that it cannot be immediately recovered. 2. the state of being deprived of something. 3. in insurance, any diminution in quantity, quality, or value of property, resulting from the occurrence of some peril or hazard, which serves as the basis for a claim under the terms of an insurance policy. **hearing l.**, deafness.

Lossen's rule (law) [Herman Friedrich *Lossen*, German surgeon, 1842–1909] see under RULE.

Loticort trademark for *fluorometholone*.

Lotrimin trademark for *clotrimazole*.

Lotusate trademark for *talbutal*.

Louis-Bar's syndrome [Denis *Louis-Bar*, French physician] ATAXIA teleangiectasia.

Low, George Carmichael [English physician, 1872–1952] see Castellani-Low SYMPTOM.

Löwenberg's forceps [Benjamin Benno *Löwenberg*, otologist in Vienna and Paris, born 1836] see under FORCEPS.

Lowry's syndrome [R. B. *Lowry*] see under SYNDROME. See also Coffin-Lowry SYNDROME.

lozenge (loz′enj) [Fr.] a sweetened medicated tablet or a troche. **Flura-Loz l.**, trademark for lozenges containing 2.21 mg sodium fluoride (equivalent to 1 mg of fluoride ion), a dye, flavoring agents, and excipients; used in dental caries prevention.

Lozi-Tabs tablets see under TABLET.

LP-2 trademark for a *polysulfide impression material* (see under MATERIAL).

LPN licensed practical NURSE.

Lr lawrencium.

Ls LABRALE superius.

LSD, LSD-25 lysergic acid diethylamide; see under ACID.

LT lymphotoxin.

Lu lutetium.

Lubarsch's syndrome [Otto *Lubarsch*, German pathologist, 1860–1933] see under SYNDROME.

lubricant (loo′brĭ-kant) an oily liquid applied to moving parts of a mechanism in order to reduce friction, heat, or wear, or to surfaces in close contact to prevent them from adhering to one another. **die l.**, a substance that prevents a wax pattern from adhering to the die and allows it to be separated without sticking.

Luc, Henry [French laryngologist, 1855–1925] see Caldwell-Luc OPERATION.

Lucent trademark for a *silicophosphate cement* (see under CEMENT).

Lucibacterium (lu″sĭ-bak-te′re-um) a genus of gram-negative, facultatively anerobic bacteria of the family Vibrionaceae; found in sea water and on the surfaces of dead marine animals.

Lucite trademark for a thermoplastic acrylic resin of the methyl methacrylate type, occurring as a clear, transparent plastic, used in lacquers, coatings, adhesives, and modifiers for other resins. Also used in restorative dentistry. See also methyl METHACRYLATE.

Ludwig's angina [Wilhelm Friedrich von *Ludwig*, German surgeon, 1790–1865] see under ANGINA.

lues (lu′ēz) [L. "a plague"] syphilis.

lug (lug) 1. a projecting part that supports something. 2. the part of a dental casting that projects. **occlusal l.**, occlusal REST. **retention l.**, a piece of metal soldered either to an orthodontic band or to an artificial crown to create greater undercut for retention of a prosthesis.

Lugol's solution [Jean Guillaume Auguste *Lugol*, French physician, 1786–1851] strong iodine solution; see under IODINE.

Lumbrical trademark for *piperazine*.

lumen (lu′men), pl. *lu′mina* [L. "light"] 1. the cavity or channel within a tube or tubular organ. 2. the SI unit of light flux; it is the flux emitted in a unit solid angle by a uniform point source of 1 candela. See also CANDELA and LUX.

lumina (lu′min-ah) [L.] plural of *lumen*.

Luminal trademark for *phenobarbital*.

luminescence (lu″mĭ-nes′ens) emission of light produced by the action of biological or chemical processes or by radiation, or any other cause except high temperature (which produces incandescence). See also FLOURESCENCE and PHOSPHORESCENCE.

Lumirelax trademark for *methocarbamol*.

lumisterol (loo′brĭ-ste′rol) a compound, $9\beta, 10\alpha$ - ergosta - 5, 7, 22-trien-3β-ol, prepared by ultraviolet irradiation of ergosterol. See also VITAMIN D$_1$.

Lundquist, G. R. [1894–1972] an American periodontologist and dental educator.

lung (lung) [L. *pulmo*; Gr. *pneumōn, pleumōn*] the organ of respiration, being one of the two symmetrically located spongy structures in the lateral cavities of the chest, which serve to remove waste carbon dioxide from the blood and to replenish the blood with oxygen to be used by tissues for metabolic processes. **artificial l.**, oxygenator. **collapsed l.**, see ATELECTASIS and PNEUMOTHORAX.

Lunorium trademark for a *cobalt-chrome alloy* (see under ALLOY).

lunula (lu′nu-lah), pl. *lu′nulae* [L., dim. of *luna* moon] a general anatomical term for a small crescentic or moonshaped area.

lunulae (lu′nu-le) [L.] plural of *lunula*.

lupiform (lu′pĭ-form) [*lupus* + L. *forma* form] 1. resembling lupus. 2. resembling a wen.

lupoid (lu′poid) 1. pertaining to lupus vulgaris. 2. a variant of sarcoidosis marked by small papular lesions.

Lupolen trademark for *polyethylene*.

lupus (lu′pus) [L. "wolf" or "pike"] a nonspecific term originally used to designate various types of tuberculosis of the skin, later extended to mean any skin condition characterized by chronic destructive lesions with ulceration, hypertrophy, and degeneration. Alone, the term now may mean any specific form, such as *lupus vulgaris, lupus tuberculosus, or disseminated lupus erythematosus*. **l. erythemato′sus**, an autoimmune collagen disease, usually chronic but sometimes acute, which is characterized by erythematous scaling patches of various configurations and sizes which cause scarring and atrophy, and by the presence of LE cells. **l. erythemato′osus, acute disseminated,** disseminated lupus erythematosus occurring most commonly in middle-aged women, which is characterized by severity of symptoms, and associated with physical deterioration often leading to death. **l. erythemato′sus, chronic discoid,** a mucocutaneous form occurring chiefly in adults, most commonly in females. It begins with the appearance of small erythematous scaling lesions of the skin, chiefly on the cheeks, neck, and exposed parts of the chest and arms. The lesions, which are usually well-defined and have sharp margins, become covered with a gray adherent scale that extends slowly into the follicles, giving it the "carpet tack" appearance. Atrophy, alopecia, telangiectasia, marginal hyperpigmentation, and central depigmentation, scarring, and photosensitivity are usually associated. The pathologic picture includes hyperkeratosis with keratotic plugs, atrophy of the stratum malpighii, liquefactive degeneration of the basal cells, perivascular, chiefly lymphocytic, infiltrate, and basophilic degeneration of collagen. Oral lesions, which are present in some cases, include erythematous papules or plaques and ulcers covered with membranes and red atrophic lesions surrounded by white keratotic borders, which are found most commonly on the vermilion border of the lip or the buccal mucosa. Scale formation on the labial lesions, atrophy of the lingual papillae, and lesions of the palate may occur, with a tendency to develop hemorrhage, edema, or squamous cell carcinoma. **l. erythematosus, disseminated,** l. erythematosus, systemic. **l. erythemato′sus, systemic,** a form characterized by mucocutaneous lesions and a wide variety of systemic symptoms due to involvement of the connective tissue of the vascular system, skin, mucous membranes, and serous and synovial membranes. Prodromal symptoms include fatigue, arthralgia, weakness, low-grade fever, and thoracic and abdominal pain, followed by polyarthritis, pleurisy, pericarditis, peritonitis, perihepatitis, perisplenitis, remittent fever, leukopenia, hematuria, albuminuria, hypertension, edema, renal insufficiency, and mucocutaneous lesions. A positive LE test is the principal diagnostic feature. Roughly symmetric ("butterfly") erythematous patches of the face, which coalesce and spread over to the cheeks and across the bridge of the nose, and hands, presenting itching, elevated red macules covered by gray membranes, with pigmented borders and, sometimes, depigmented central areas are the chief skin lesions. Oral lesions, which are sometimes present, include well-defined, elevated white plaques with a periphery often surrounded by telangiectasis, and associated with erosion, ulcers, and scarring; the buccal mucosa is most often affected, but the lips, palate, and tongue also may be affected. Called also *disseminated l. erythematosus.* **l. hypertroph′icus,** see *l. vulgaris.* **l. maculo′sus,** see *l. vulgaris.* **l. papillo′sus,** see *l. vulgaris.* **l. per′nio,** sarcoidosis. **l. pla′nus,** see *l. vulgaris.* **l. psoriasifor′mis,** see *l. vulgaris.* **l. vulga′ris,** a persistent form of primary tuberculous disease of the skin, affecting most commonly the face, characterized by small, soft, reddish, yellowish, or reddish-brown nodules in the corium, which may be flat or slightly elevated and may or may not be covered with scales. In severe cases, the cartilage of the nose and ears may be destroyed. The mucosa of the mouth, pharynx, and nose may be involved; a typical lesion is usually an ulcer, which sometimes heals spontaneously but frequently forms a flaccid lesion with ill-defined borders, made up of confluences of several ulcers. Intraoral adhesions, especially of the soft palate and lips with resulting microstomia, may occur. Depending on the form and nature of the lesions, the condition may be called *lupus hypertrophicus, maculosus, papillosus, planus,* and *psoriasiformis.* Called also *tuberculosis cutis luposa.* See also oral TUBERCULOSIS.

Luride drops, topical gel, topical solution see under DROP, TABLET, GEL, and SOLUTION.

Luscha's cartilage, laryngeal cartilage, tonsil [Hubert von *Luscha,* German anatomist, 1820–1875] see sesamoid cartilage of vocal ligament, under CARTILAGE, and see pharyngeal TONSIL.

Lustraloy trademark for an *amalgam alloy* (see under AMALGAM).

lute (loot) [L. *lutum* mud] luting AGENT.

lutecium (lu-te′she-um) lutetium.

lutetium (lu-te′she-um) [*Lutetia* ancient name for Paris] a rare earth, occuring as a silvery white, ductile metal, which reacts slowly with water and is soluble in acids. Symbol, Lu; atomic number, 71; atomic weight, 174.97; valence, 3; melting point, 16.52°C; group IIIB of the periodic table. It occurs as two natural isotopes; ^{175}Lu and ^{176}Lu; the latter being radioactive with a half-life of 2.2×10^{10} years and emitting beta rays. Artificial radioactive isotopes include 155, 156, 167–174, and 177–180. Used in nuclear technology. Written also *lutecium.*

Lutheran antigen (factor), blood groups [named after the person in whose blood the first antigen was discovered] see under ANTIGEN and BLOOD GROUP.

Lutz's disease [Alfredo *Lutz*] South American BLASTOMYCOSIS.

Lutz-Miescher disease [Wilhelm *Lutz,* Swiss dermatologist, 1888–1958; Guido *Miescher,* 1877–1961] perforating ELASTOSIS.

Lutz-Splendore-de Almeida disease [A. *Lutz;* A. *Splendore;* Floriano Paulo *de Almeida,* Brazilian physician] South American BLASTOMYCOSIS.

lux (luks) [L. "light"] the SI unit of illumination, being 1 lumen per square meter. Called also *meter candle.*

luxatio (luk-sa′she-o) [L.] dislocation. **l. imper′fecta,** a sprain.

luxation (luk-sa′shun) [L. *luxatio*] 1. dislocation. 2. partial or complete detachment of a tooth from its socket. **temporomandibular l.,** temporomandibular joint DISLOCATION. **habitual temporomandibular joint l.,** temporomandibular joint dislocation, recurrent; see under DISLOCATION.

Luxene trademark for a heat-cured denture base acrylic resin.

LVN licensed vocational nurse; see licensed practical NURSE.

Lw formerly, lawrencium; now Lr.

Lwoff, André Michael [born 1902] a French microbiologist and virologist; co-winner, with François Jacob and Jacques Lucien Monod, of the Nobel prize for medicine and physiology in 1965, for discoveries concerning the genetic control of enzymes and virus synthesis.

lyase [E.C.4] (li′as) any of a major class of enzymes that catalyze the removal of chemical groups without hydrolysis or oxidation, by cleaving C—C, C—O, C—N, and other bonds. Two substrates are involved in the unidirectional reaction. When acting on the single substrate, a molecule is eliminated leaving an unsaturated residue. See also ENZYME classification. **aldehyde l.** [E.C.4.1.2.], a subsubclass of lyases, including enzymes that act on carbon-carbon bonds and catalyze the reversal of an aldol condensation with the formation of an aldehyde. In carbohydrate metabolism, aldehyde lyases catalyze the conversion of fructose-1,6-diphosphate to glyceraldehyde-3-phosphate and dihydroxy acetone phosphate. Called also *aldolase.* **argininosuccinate l.** [E.C.4.3.2.1], an amidine-lyase that catalyzes the conversion of argininosuccinic acid to fumaric acid and arginine in the formation of urea in protein metabolism. Called also *arginine succinase* and *arginosuccinase.* **carbon-carbon l.** [E.C.4.1], a subclass of lyases, including enzymes that catalyze the removal of chemical groups by cleaving the C—C bonds. **carbon-nitrogen l.** [E.C.4.3], a subclass of lyases, including enzymes that catalyze the removal of chemical groups by cleaving the C—N bond; the reaction being associated with the elimination of ammonia and the formation of a double bond. **carbon-oxygen l.** [E.C.4.2], a subclass of lyases, including enzymes that catalyze the removal of chemical groups by cleaving the C—O bond, leading to the production of unsaturated substances with the formation of water. **carbon-sulfur l.** [E.C.4.4], a subclass of lyases, including enzymes that catalyze the removal of chemical groups by cleaving the C—S bond, with the elimination of H_2S or substituted H_2S. **phosphorus-oxygen l.** [E.C.4.6], a subclass of lyases, including enzymes that catalyze the removal of chemical groups by cleaving the P—O bond.

Lydol trademark for *meperidine hydrochloride* (see under MEPERIDINE).

lye (li) POTASSIUM hydroxide.

Lyell's syndrome [Aian *Lyell*] toxic epidermal NECROLYSIS.

Lyman rays see under RAY.

lymph (limf) [L. *lympha* water] a transparent, yellowish, watery liquid of alkaline reaction contained within the lymphatic system. It serves as a vehicle for excess fluid in the interstitial spaces and for substances leaked out of the blood capillaries, allowing them to be reabsorbed by the lymph capillaries or through the thoracic duct; for foreign antigens to be carried from the site of invasion through the filtering system of lymph nodes; for blood proteins to be transported from the liver to the blood stream; and for fats to be absorbed from the intestines into the system. The protein content of lymph from the peripheral vessels is about 1 percent; from the liver about 5 percent; and from the thoracic duct, about 2–4 percent. The lymph from the thoracic duct also has about 5–15 percent fat content, giving it a milky appearance (chyle). In addition, lymph contains most diffusible substances found in the blood, including glucose, urea, creatinine, amino acids, blood cells, and other blood components. The circulation of lymph is accomplished by the contraction of muscles surrounding the lymphatic vessels, thus propelling it through a series of non-return valves (lymph pump). Called also *lympha* [NA] and *lymphatic fluid.* **aplastic l., corpuscular l.,** lymph that contains an excess of leukocytes and does not tend to become organized. **croupous l.,** inflammatory lymph that tends to the formation of a false membrane.

euplastic l., fibrinous l., that which tends to coagulate and become organized. **inflammatory l.**, the lymph produced by inflammation, as in a wound. **intercellular l.**, lymph occupying the intercellular spaces of tissues. **intravascular l.**, the lymph of the lymph vessels. **plastic l.**, inflammatory lymph that has a tendency to become organized. **l. pump**, lymph PUMP. **tissue l.**, lymph derived from the tissues and not from the blood.

lymph- see LYMPHO-

lympha (lim′fah) [L. "water"] [NA] lymph.

lymphaden (lim′fah-den) [lymph- + Gr. adēn gland] lymph NODE.

lymphadenectasis (lim-fad″ĕ-nek′tah-sis) [lymph- + Gr. adēn gland + ektasis distention] enlargement of a lymph node.

lymphadenectomy (lim-fad″ĕ-nek′to-me) [lymph- + Gr. adēn gland + ektomē excision] excision of a lymph node or nodes.

lymphadenhypertrophy (lim-fad″en-hi-per′tro-fe) [lymph- + Gr. adēn gland + hypertrophy] hypertrophy of a lymph node.

lymphadenitis (lim-fad″ĕ-ni′tis) [lymph- + Gr. adēn gland + -itis] inflammation of the lymph nodes. **caseous l.**, lymphadenitis associated with tuberculosis of some other part, but showing tubercle bacilli in the lymphatics. Called also paratuberculous l. **nonbacterial regional l.**, cat-scratch DISEASE. **paratuberculous l.**, caseous l. **regional l.**, cat-scratch DISEASE. **tuberculoid l.**, inflammation of the lymph nodes similar to that seen in tuberculous lymphadenitis; it may be caused by such disorders as sarcoidosis, regional enteritis, leprosy, syphilis, and certain fungal infections. **tuberculous l.**, tuberculosis of the lymph nodes, involving most often the cervical and mediastinal nodes, due to lymphatic spread from a primary pulmonary infection or to hematogenous dissemination. Affected nodes may suppurate, with formation of draining sinuses. See also SCROFULA. **tuberculous cervical l.**, scrofula.

lymphadeno- [lymph- + Gr. adēn gland] a combining form denoting relationship to a lymph node or nodes.

lymphadenocele (lim-fad′ĕ-no-sēl″) [lymph- + adenocele] a cyst of a lymph node. Called also adenolymphocele.

lymphadenocyst (lim-fad′ĕ-no-sist″) [lymph- + Gr. adēn gland + cyst] a degenerated lymph node caused by occlusion of its incoming lymph vessels. By dilatation of the lymph sinuses it becomes a fine-meshed network.

lymphadenogram (lim-fad′ĕ-no-gram′) a roentgenogram of the lymph nodes.

lymphadenography (lim-fad″ĕ-nog′rah-fe) [lymph- + Gr. adēn gland + graphein to write] roentgenographic visualization of the lymph nodes, following injection of radiopaque material into a lymphatic vessel.

lymphadenoid (lim-fad″ĕ-noid) [lymph- Gr. adēn gland + eidos form] resembling the tissue of lymph nodes; lymphadenoid tissue. See under TISSUE.

lymphadenoleukopoiesis (lim-fad″ĕ-no-lu″ko-poi-e′sis) the production of leukocytes by the lymphadenoid tissue.

lymphadenoma (lim″fad-ĕ-no′mah) a benign tumor of lymphadenoid tissue. **multiple l.**, Hodgkin's DISEASE. **sebaceous l.**, an extremely rare benign tumor of the salivary glands, believed to represent hyperplasia of heterotopic sebaceous glands, found almost exclusively in the middle-aged and elderly. The lesion is firm, encapsulated, cystic, yellow gray in color. Sebum is often found in ducts and sebaceous glands making up a typical tumor.

lymphadenomatosis (lim-fad″ĕ-no-mah-to′sis) a condition marked by the presence of multiple lymphomas. **benign l.**, a rare benign recurrent tumor of the lymphoreticular tissue, which presents a pink to red violet papule or nodule, usually occurring on the face, ear lobes, nipples, and scrotum. Pathologically, it is characterized by a thin epidermis and dense infiltrates in the midcutis or masses consisting of mature lymphocytes and reticulum cells. Called also Bäfverstedt's syndrome, Kaposi-Spiegler sarcomatosis, lymphadenosis cutis benigna, multiple sarcoid, and sarcomatosis cutis.

lymphadenopathy (lim-fad″ĕ-nop′ah-the) [lymph- + Gr. adēn gland + pathos disease] disease of the lymph nodes.

lymphadenosis (lim-fad″ĕ-no′sis) [lymph- + Gr. adēn gland + -osis] hypertrophy or proliferation of lymphoid tissue. **acute l.**, infectious MONONUCLEOSIS. **l. cu′tis benig′na**, benign LYMPHADENOMATOSIS.

lymphadenotomy (lim-fad″ĕ-not′o-me) incision of a lymph node.

lymphadenovarix (lim-fad″ĕ-no-va′riks) enlargement of the lymph nodes from the pressure of dilated lymph vessels.

lymphagogue (lim′fah-gog) an agent that promotes the production of lymph.

lymphangiectasis (lim-fan″je-ek′tah-sis) [lymph- + Gr. angeion vessel + ektasis distention] dilatation of the lymphatic vessels.

lymphangiectomy (lim-fan″je-ek′to-me) [lymph- + Gr. angeion vessel + ektomē excision] excision of one or more lymphatic vessels.

lymphangio- [lymph- + Gr. angeion vessel] a combining form denoting relationship to a lymphatic vessel or vessels.

lymphangiogram (lim-fan′je-o-gram″) a roentgenogram of the lymphatic vessels.

lymphangiography (lim-fan″je-og′rah-fe) [lymph- + Gr. angeion vessel + graphein to write] roentgenography of the lymphatic vessels following the injection of a contrast medium.

lymphangioma (lim-fan″je-o′mah) a benign tumor composed of lymph spaces and channels, which is the counterpart in the lymphatic system of hemangioma of blood vessels. It is typically present at birth, usually as a small growth that may be missed. Two types have been differentiated: capillary lymphangioma and cavernous lymphoangioma. **capillary l.**, a lymphangioma made up of small lymphatic channels, occurring in the head and neck region, and in the axilla, rarely found in other sites. Called also simple l. **cavernous l.**, a lymphangioma composed of cavernous lymphatic spaces, considered as an analogue of angioma cavernosum, occurring most often in the neck and axilla. It is the most common type of oral lymphangioma, usually found on the tongue, but may also occur on the palate and buccal mucosa. A superficial oral lesion may appear as a papillary growth of the same color and texture as the mucosa; a deep lesion exhibits diffuse nodules and masses, also of the same color and texture as the mucosa, often resulting in macroglossia or macrocheilia. Typically, it is made up of a soft, spongelike, red-pink mass, containing dilated cystic spaces filled with lymph, lined by endothelial cells, and separated by scant stroma, containing aggregates of lymphocytes, lymphatic tissue, and islands of fat or muscle. The lesion is well-defined and nonencapsulated with finger-like projections extending in all directions. Called also cystic hygroma. **simple l.**, capillary l.

lymphangioplasty (lim-fan′je-o-plas″te) [lymph- + Gr. angeion vessel + plassein to form] surgical restoration or correction of lymphatic vessels.

lymphangiotomy (lim-fan″je-ot′o-me) [lymphangio- + Gr. temnein to cut] incision into a lymphatic vessel.

lymphangitis (lim″fan-ji′tis) [lymphangio- + -itis] inflammation of a lymphatic vessel or vessels.

lymphatic (lim-fat′ik) [L. lymphaticus] pertaining to or containing lymph, as in the lymphatic system or a lymphatic vessel; by extension, the term is sometimes used alone to designate a lymphatic vessel. **afferent l.**, lymphatic vessel, afferent; see under VESSEL. **efferent l.**, lymphatic vessel, efferent; see under VESSEL.

lymphedema (lim″fe-de′mah) [lymph- + edema] edema due to accumulation of excessive amounts of lymph, which is secondary to obstruction of the lymphatic system in conditions such as cancer, elephantiasis, or abnormalities of the lymphatic structures. Called also lymphatic edema.

lympho-, lymph- [L. lympha water] a combining form denoting relationship to lymph.

lymphoblast (lim″fo-blast) [lympho- + Gr. blastos germ] a lymphocyte in its germinative stage; a developing lymphocyte.

lymphoblastoma (lim″fo-blas-to′mah) [lymphoblast + -oma] a neoplasm of the lymphoid tissue, made up of lymphoblasts. It is a malignant tumor that may arise in a single lymph node or in groups of nodes, sometimes leading to lymphatic leukemia. Called also lymphoblastic lymphoma. **macrofollicular l.**, giant follicle LYMPHOMA.

lymphoblastosis (lim″fo-blas-to′sis) excess of lymphoblasts in the blood. **acute benign l.**, infectious MONONUCLEOSIS.

lymphocyte (lim′fo-sīt) [lympho- + Gr. kytos hollow vessel] a spherical cell of the lymphoid cell series, 7 μ to 20 μ in diameter, which has a large, round nucleus that tends to be indented when viewed under the electron microscope and scanty cytoplasm that is usually transparent and does not show basophilic staining but may contain azurophilic granules, and generally lacks a well-developed endoplasmic reticulum. They are motile cells and some may exhibit phagocytosis. These cells are the principal cells involved in the specificity and the generation of cell-mediated and humoral immunity. See illustration at IMMUNITY. See also table of Reference Values in Hematology in Appendix. **active l's**, see B-l's. **B-l's, bursa-equivalent l's**, small lymphocytes derived from stem cells which differentiate in the bursa of Fabricius in birds and in the mammalian bursal equivalent tissue. The location of the bursal equivalent tissue is not known but gut-associated lymphoid tissue (GALT), fetal liver, and bone marrow are considered as the primary sites of origin of B-lymphocytes. Under stimulation, by an antigen, macrophage processed antigen, or mitogens, they may transform into large, active blast cells (active lymphocytes or large pyroninophyllic cells), which may become antibody-producing plasma cells. Following stimulation, an alternate pathway of differentiation leads to the production of memory cells which upon re-encountering with specific immunogen, have the capacity to proliferate and differentiate into cell lines responsible for humoral immunity. In lymph nodes and in the spleen, B-lymphocytes proliferate in the germinal centers found in the cortical areas where they form lymphoid follicles. They are principally involved in antibody-mediated humoral immunity, however, recent observations have shown that they may also produce lymphokines, such as migration inhibitory factor. Called also *B-cells* and *thymus-independent l's*. **l. count,** table of *Reference Values in Hematology* in Appendix. **l. helper,** helper CELL. **large l.,** one with a diameter of 12 μ or more. **long-lived l.,** a small lymphocyte which may survive for months, even years, without dividing. These cells are believed to be T-lymphocytes, and are also believed to be memory cells for specific antigens and to play an important role in immune surveillance. **medium l.,** one with a diameter ranging from 8 μ to 12 μ, one with a diameter of 8 μ or less. **T-l's, thymus-dependent l's,** lymphocytes derived from or dependent on the thymus, for the acquisition of properties involved in cell-mediated immune reactions, such as graft-versus-host reaction, delayed hypersensitivity, and tumor rejection. They are incapable of differentiating into plasma cells but give rise to cells capable of producing factors that trigger cell-mediated reactions leading to inflammation and to cell-mediated events, including migration inhibitory factor, substances chemotactic for mononuclear and granulocytic cells, a cytotoxic factor capable of injuring various cell types, interferon, and several other factors. Some factors are released upon interaction of sensitized lymphocytes with antigens; others may remain cell-bound, all leading to the destruction of foreign target cells or to the damage of host cells. Following stimulation, an alternate pathway of differentiation leads to the production of memory cells which, upon re-encountering with specific immunogens, have the capacity to proliferate and differentiate into cell lines responsible for cell-mediated immunity. Called also *T-cells*. See also LYMPHOKINE. **thymus-independent l's,** B-l's.

lymphocytoma (lim″fo-si-to′mah) [*lymphocyte* + *-oma*] a neoplasm of the lymphoid tissue, made up of adult lymphocytes. It is a malignant tumor that may arise in single lymph nodes or in groups of nodes, sometimes leading to lymphatic leukemia. Called also *lymphocytic lymphoma.*

lymphocytopenia (lim″fo-si″to-pe′ne-ah) reduction in the number of lymphocytes in the blood. See also leukocyte count, differential, under COUNT.

lymphocytosis (lim″fo-si-to′sis) excess of lymphocytes in the blood or in any effusion. See also leukocyte count, differential, under COUNT.

lymphoepithelioma (lim″fo-ep″i-the″le-o′mah) a transitional cell carcinoma associated with massive lymphoid infiltrate within the fibrous stroma. **nasopharyngeal l.,** a tumor variously considered to be reticulum cell sarcoma or anaplastic carcinoma with lymphocytic infiltration; it originates in the nasopharynx and metastasizes to the cervical lymph nodes. It is a common cause of Garcin's syndrome. Called also *Schmincke's tumor.*

lymphoglandula (lim″fo-glan′du-lah), pl. *lymphoglan′dulae* [*lympho-* + L. *glandula* gland] lymph NODE. **lymphoglan′dulae auricula′res posterio′res,** auricular lymph nodes, posterior; see under NODE. **lymphoglan′dulae cervica′les profun′dae,** cervical lymph nodes, deep; see under NODE. **lymphoglan′dulae cervica′les superficia′les,** cervical lymph nodes, superficial; see under NODE. **lymphoglan′dulae facia′les profun′dae,** buccal lymph nodes; see under node. **lymphoglan′dulae lingua′les,** lingual lymph nodes; see under NODE. **lymphoglan′dulae occipita′les,** occipital lymph nodes; see under NODE. **lymphoglan′dulae paroti′deae,** parotid lymph nodes; see under NODE. **lymphoglan′dulae submandibula′res,** submandibular lymph nodes; see under NODE.

lymphogranuloma (lim″fo-gran″u-lo′mah) 1. any disease characterized by granulomatous lesions. 2. Hodgkin's DISEASE. **l. inguina′le, l. trop′icum, l. venereum. l. vene′reum,** a disease occurring in a venereal and a nonvenereal form, most frequently in tropical climates, and caused by *Chlamydia.* In cases transmitted by sexual intercourse, the initial lesion at the site of entry progresses to lymphadenitis, discharging sinuses, elephantiasis in males, and rectal stricture in females. The disease may be also transmitted by genito-oral contact; the initial oral lesion at the site of entry progresses to lymphadenitis, inflammation of adjacent tissues, obliteration of the lymphatic vessels, discharging sinuses, and hyperplastic cicatrization. In the nonvenereal form, an oculoglandular syndrome may develop.

Oral manifestations in systemic forms are rare but when they occur, they may include ulcerative and vegetative lesions of the pharynx and tongue. Called also *l. inguinale, l. tropicum, benign inguinal lymphogranulomatosis, climatic bubo, Durand-Nicolas Favre disease, fifth venereal disease, Frei's bubo, Frei's disease, lymphomatosis inguinalis suppurativa subacuta, lymphopathia venereum, Nicolas-Favre disease, poradenitis nostras,* and *tropical bubo.*

lymphogranulomatosis (lim″fo-gran″u-lo-mah-to′sis) a condition characterized by the presence of multiple lymphogranulomas. **l. benig′na,** sarcoidosis. **benign inguinal l.,** LYMPHOGRANULOMA venereum. **l. malig′na, malignant l.,** Hodgkin's DISEASE.

lymphoid (lim′foid) [*lymph-* + Gr. *eidos* form] resembling or pertaining to lymph or tissue of the lymphatic system.

lymphokine (lim′fo-kīn) a general term for soluble mediators released by sensitized lymhocytes on contact with antigen and believed to play a role in macrophage activation, lymphocyte transformation, and reactions associated with cell-mediated immunity. Lymphokines are also released by the action of mitogens, such as phytohemagglutinin and concanavalin A, upon normal lymphocytes.

lymphokinesis (lim″fo-ki-ne′sis) [*lympho-* + Gr. *kinēsis* movement] 1. the movement of the endolymph in the semicircular canals. 2. the circulation of lymph in the body.

lymphoma (lim-fo′mah) a primary, usually malignant, tumor of the lymph nodes derived from the basic cells of the lymphoid tissue, the lymphocytes, lymphoblasts, reticulum cells, and plasma cells; **a** general term used for any neoplastic disease of the lymphoid tissue, including lymphocytoma, lymphosarcoma, lymphoblastoma, giant follicle lymphoma, reticulum cell sarcoma, Hodgkin's disease, plasmacytoma, and Burkitt's lymphoma. Called also *malignant l.* **African l.,** Burkitt's l. **Burkitt's l.,** a unique form of lymphoma, usually of the retroperitoneal and jaw areas, which also may involve the kidneys, liver, ovaries, adrenal glands, thyroid gland, testes, and gastrointestinal tract. It is usually found in areas of the world up to 1500 meters above sea level where the temperature never falls below 12° C and the annual rain fall is at least 60 cm, principally in Central Africa, New Guinea, and Colombia. Viruses, especially the Epstein-Barr virus, are the suspected pathogens. The jaw tumor usually originates in the alveolar process, growing rapidly and producing gross deformity and displacement and exfoliation of the teeth. It usually extends through the periosteum and invades surrounding soft tissue, but the skin remains normal. Typically, it presents a soft, grayish, fleshy mass composed of cells lying intermediate between immature lymphocytes and reticulum cells, with a spattering of large phagocytic histiocytic cells, the so-called "starry-sky" effect. Called also *African l.* and *Burkitt's tumor.* **follicular l.,** giant follicle l. **giant follicle l.,** a lymphoma characterized by the combined proliferation of lymphoblasts and reticulum cells within lymphoid follicles, resulting in an increase in the number and size of germinal follicles. The course is initially benign but there is often malignant transformation. It may occur at any age but middle-aged individuals are most commonly affected, beginning insidiously with painless enlargement of superficial lymph nodes, followed by splenomegaly, fever, debility, weight loss, and anemia. Oral manifestations are rare but tumor masses may be found on the palate, tonsils, and nasopharynx. Called also *follicular l.,* Brill-Symmers disease, giant follicular hyperplasia, and *macrofollicular lymphoblastoma.* **lymphoblastic l.,** lymphoblastoma. **lymphocytic l.,** lymphocytoma. **malignant l.,** lymphoma. **multiple l's,** lymphomatosis.

lymphomatoid (lim-fo′mah-toid) resembling lymphoma.

lymphomatosis (lim″fo-mah-to′sis) a condition characterized by the presence of multiple lymphomas. **l. inguina′lis suppurati′va subacu′ta,** LYMPHOGRANULOMA venereum.

lymphomatous (lim-fo′mah-tus) pertaining to or of the nature of lymphoma.

lymphonodi (lim″fo-no′di) [L.] plural of *lymphonodus.*

lymphonodus (lim″fo-no′dus), pl. *lymphono′di* [*lympho-* + L. *nodus* knot] lymph NODE.

lymphopathia (lim″fo-path′e-ah) any disease of the lymphatic system. **l. vene′reum,** LYMPHOGRANULOMA venereum.

lymphopathy (lim-fop′ah-the) [*lympho-* + Gr. *pathos* disease] any disease of the lymphatic system.

lymphopenia (lim-fo-pe′ne-ah) [*lymphocyte* + Gr. *penia* poverty] deficiency of lymphocytes in the circulating blood. It may be related to thymic hypoplasia and is associated with agammaglobulinemia. See also ALYMPHOCYTOSIS, and see leukocyte count, differential, under COUNT.

lymphosarcoma (lim″fo-sar-ko′mah) [*lympho-* + *sarcoma*] a common type of malignant lymphoma that may originate at any site, and is composed of lymphocytes or lymphoblasts. It is derived from lymphoid tissue and enlarges by progressive expansile, invasive, contiguous growth, and may metastasize by the lymphatic route. Typically, it presents a grayish to pink, soft tumor often showing areas of necrosis. The palate, gingiva, buccal mucosa, mandible, floor of the mouth, and tonsils are the principal sites of oral tumors. Swelling is the initial symptom, and is usually followed by rapid growth of the lesion, bone destruction, and loosening of the teeth. Eventually, the tumor becomes large, fungating, necrotic, and foul-smelling. **reticulum cell l.**, reticulum cell SARCOMA. **sclerosing l.**, a form occurring mainly in childhood, in which the tumor has a fine collagenous stroma and the lymphocytes are arranged in serried rows between the fibers, often giving the tumor a distinctive whorled pattern.

lymphotoxin (lim″fo-tok′sin) a mediator liberated from specifically sensitized lymphocytes by antigen or by nonspecific stimulants, such as phytohemagglutinin, which appears to be associated with target-cell injury and inhibits the capacity of cells to divide. It has a molecular weight of 80,000 to 150,000, is heat stable, and resists RNase, DNase, and trypsin but is destroyed by chymotrypsin. Its biological role is unknown, but it is possible that it destroys cells directly. Abbreviated *LT*.

lyo- [Gr. *lyein* to dissolve] a combining form meaning dissolved.

Lyogen trademark for *fluphenazine hydrochloride* (see under FLUPHENAZINE).

Lyon hypothesis [Mary L. *Lyon*, British geneticist] see under HYPOTHESIS.

lyonization (li″on-ĭ-za′shun) the process or state of being inactivated; said of X chromosomes. See Lyon HYPOTHESIS.

lyophilic (li″o-fil′ik) [*lyo-* Gr. *philein* to love] having an affinity for or attracting liquids; pertaining to a colloid system in which the disperse phase (analogous to the solute) is a liquid and attracts the continuous phase (analogue to the solvent). See also COLLOID and HYDROPHILIC.

lyophobic (li″o-fo′bik) [*lyo-* + Gr. *phobein* to fear] repelling liquids; pertaining to a colloid system in which the disperse phase (equivalent to the solute) has no attraction for the continuous phase (equivalent to the solvent). See also COLLOID and HYDROPHOBIC.

lyophylization (li-of″ĭ-li-za′shun) the creation of a stable preparation of a biological substance, such as blood plasma, by rapid freezing and dehydration of the frozen product under high vacuum.

lyophilizer (li-of″ĭ-li-zer) an appliance used in lyophilization; a freeze drier.

lyosol (li′o-sol) a sol in which the dispersion medium is a liquid.

lyosorption (li″o-sorp′shun) the adhesion of a liquid to a solid; as the adsorption of a solvent film on suspended particles.

Lyovac trademark for *dactinomycin*.

Lys lysine.

Lysalgo trademark for *mefenamic acid* (see under ACID).

lysate (li′sāt) 1. the material formed by the lysis of cells. 2. a medicinal preparation obtained from an animal organ by means of artificial digestion.

lysergide (li′ser-jīd) *lysergic acid diethylamide* (see under ACID).

lysin (li′sin) [Gr. *lyein* to dissolve] an antibody which has the power of causing dissolution of cells, including hemolysin, bacteriolysin, cytolysin, etc., which usually involves activation and participation of the complement sequence. **α-l.**, α-STAPHYLOLYSIN. **β-l.**, β-STAPHYLOLYSIN. **γ-l.**, γ-STAPHYLOLYSIN. **δ-l.**, δ-STAPHYLOLYSIN.

lysine (li′sin) a basic, naturally occurring amino acid, 2,6-diaminohexanoic acid, which is essential for the growth of human infants and for certain nitrogen metabolic processes in adults. It is generally abundant in animal proteins but not in cereal proteins. Leucine is also found in the saliva. Used as a food enrichment of wheat-based foods. Abbreviated *Lys*. See also amino ACID.

lysis (li′sis) [Gr. "dissolution; a loosing, setting free, releasing"] 1. the destruction of cells, as in hemolysis, bacteriolysis, etc. 2. decomposition of a chemical agent.

lyso- [Gr. *lysis* dissolution] a combining form, indicating lysis or dissolution.

Lysodren trademark for *mitotane*.

lysolecithin (li″so-les′ĭ-thin) a lecithin from which the oleic acid on the central carbon atoms has been removed by hydrolysis, as by an enzyme in cobra venom or that of some insects and spiders. Injection of lysolecithin causes hemolysis.

lysosome (li′so-sōm) [*lyso-* + Gr. *sōma* body] one type of minute body seen with phase or electron microscopy in many kinds of cells, containing various soluble hydrolytic enzymes (hydrolases) that exhibit an optimum pH in the acid range. Its membrane is a lipoprotein that prevents the enzymes from escaping into the cytoplasm, and also prevents the substrate from entering the cell. It is normally involved in the process of localized intracellular digestion of substances ingested and contained within a phagosome. Injury to a lysosome is followed by the uncontained release into the cell of the enzymes, which may damage the cell and give rise to inflammation and result in the pathologic aspects of certain diseases, such as autoimmune disease and wasting, as in muscular dystrophy. One of the main functions suggested for lysosomes is to help clear tissues of dead cells, as in phagocytosis and pinocytosis when they are believed to be involved in hydrolysis of phagocytosed material. See also PHAGOSOME.

lysozyme [E.C.3.2.1.17] (li′so-zīm) [Gr. *lysis* dissolution + *zymē* leaven] a hydrolase that catalyzes the hydrolysis of 1,4-β-linkages between *N*-acetylmuramic acid and 2-acetamido-2-deoxy-D-glucose residues in a mucopolysaccharide or mucopeptide and dissolves the cell-wall substance of certain bacteria. It is effective in lysing *Micrococcus lysodeikticus* and, to a lesser extent, *Escherichia coli* and *Salmonella typhosa*. Found in egg white, tears, saliva, and various body fluids, where it acts as an antibacterial agent. Called also *muramidase* and *mucopeptide glycohydrolase*.

lyssa (lis′ah) [Gr. "frenzy"; "*the worm* under the tongue of dogs, removed because of the belief that it caused rabies"] 1. rabies. 2. lingual SEPTUM.

Lyssavirus (lis′ah-vi′rus) a genus of rhabdoviruses, comprising several viruses, three of which are assoociated with human infection: rabies, Kontonkan, and Duvenhage viruses.

lyssavirus (lis″ah-vi′rus) any virus of the genus *Lyssavirus*.

lysso- [Gr. *lyssa* frenzy] a combining form denoting relationship to rabies.

lytic (lit′ik) [Gr. *lytikos* dissolving] 1. pertaining to lysis or to a lysin. 2. producing lysis. 3. a word termination denoting lysis of a substance or dissolution of something indicated by the stem to which it is affixed.

M

M 1. mega-. 2. meter. 3. minim. 4. molarity. 5. molar (solution); the expression M/10, M/100, etc., denotes the strength of a solution in comparison with the molar, as tenth molar, hundredth molar, etc.

M. abbreviation for L. *macera're*, macerate; *manipulus*, handful; *mil*, *mil'le*, thousand; *mis'ce*, mix; *mistu'ra*, mixture.

3-M see 3-M SYNDROME.

m 1. meter. 2. milli-. 3. molality. 4. magnetic quantum NUMBER.

μ the twelfth letter of the Greek alphabet. See MU. Symbol for *micron*, *micro-*, and *dipole moment*.

m- meta-.

m$_s$ spin quantum NUMBER.

ma milliampere.

MAC 1. maximum allowable cost; see under PROGRAM. 2. maximum allowable concentration; usually pertaining to concentrations of noxious substances in the environment.

Mac. abbreviation for L. *macera're*, macerate.

Macalister, ethmoidal process of, ethmoidal spine of see sphenoidal CREST.

McArdle's disease [B. *McArdle*] GLYCOGENOSIS V.

McCall curet see under CURET.

McCall's epithelial solvent [J. O. *McCall*] see under SOLVENT.

McCall's festoon see under FESTOON.

McCall scaler see under SCALER.

McCollum tube see under TUBE.

McCullum attachment see under ATTACHMENT.

McCune-Albright syndrome [D. *McCune*; Fuller *Albright*, Boston physician, born 1900] Albright's SYNDROME (1).

McDonough's syndrome [Kenneth B. *McDonough*, American physician, 1902–1974] see under SYNDROME.

maceration (mas″er-a′shun) [L. *maceratio*] the softening of a solid by soaking; abnormal softening of tissue by repeated trauma or inappropriate soaking with dressings wet with saline or draining fluids.

McEwen's point see under POINT.

Macewen's triangle [Sir William *Macewen*, Scottish surgeon, 1848–1924] suprameatal TRIANGLE.

Machacek see Bloom's SYNDROME (Bloom-Torre-Machacek syndrome).

machine (mah-shen′) [L. *machina*] a contrivance or apparatus for the production, conversion, or transmission of energy, so that it may be used for productive purposes. **casting m.**, a mechanical device for casting molten metals and alloys in prosthetic and restorative dentistry. In one type, the molten metal is forced into the mold under air pressure; in the vacuum type, the metal is drawn into the mold under reduced air pressure; and in the centrifugal type, the alloy is fused in a crucible separate from the ring and thrown into the mold under centrifugal force. **heart-lung m.**, a combination blood pump (artificial heart) and blood oxygenator (artificial lung) used in open-heart surgery. **Taggart's m.**, **Taggart's compressed-gas casting m.**, a casting machine operated by the use of a combination of compressed nitrous oxide and natural gas to heat gold preparatory to forcing it into a mold. **x-ray m.**, x-ray GENERATOR.

MacKenzie's syndrome [Sir Stephen *MacKenzie*, London physician, 1844–1909] see Jackson-MacKenzie SYNDROME.

Macleans see under DENTIFRICE.

McLeod phenotype [named after the person in whom the McLeon phenotype was first discovered] see under PHENOTYPE and see Kell blood groups, under BLOOD GROUP.

Macodyn trademark for *oxytetracycline hydrochloride* (see under OXYTETRACYCLINE).

macro- [Gr. *makros* large, or long] a combining form meaning large, or of abnormal size or length. See also words beginning MEGA- and MEGALO-.

macroanalysis (mak″ro-ah-nal′ĭ-sis) chemical analysis using 0.1 to 0.2 gm of the substance under study.

macrocephalia (mak″ro-se-fa′le-ah) macrocephaly.

macrocephaly (mak″ro-sef′ah-le) [*macro-* + Gr. *kephalē* head] a condition characterized by excessive size of the head. Called also *macrocephalia*. See also HYDROCEPHALUS.

macrocheilia (mak″ro-ki′le-ah) [*macro-* + Gr. *cheilos* lip + *-ia*] excessive size of the lips. Called also *macrolabia*. See also PACHYCHEILIA.

macrocheilitis (mak″ro-ki′li-tis) [*macro-* + *cheilitis*] inflammation and swelling of the lips. **essential granulomatous m.**, CHEILITIS granulomatosa.

macrochemistry (mak″ro-kem′is-tre) [*macro-* + *chemistry*] chemistry in which the reactions may be seen with the naked eye.

macrocrania (mak″ro-kra′ne-ah) abnormal increase in the size of the skull, the facial area being disproportionately small in comparison.

macrocyclic (mak″ro-sik′lik) pertaining to a chemical compound having a ring of more than seven carbon atoms.

macrocyte (mak″ro-sīt) [*macro-* + *-cyte*] an abnormally large erythrocyte, i.e., one larger than 9 μ in diameter, such as is seen in macrocytic anemia. See also MEGALOCYTE.

macrocytic (mak″ro-sit′ik) pertaining to or of the nature of a macrocyte.

macrocythemia (mak″ro-si-the′me-ah) [*macrocyte* + Gr. *haima* blood + *-ia*] a condition in which the erythrocytes are larger than normal. See macrocytic ANEMIA.

macrodont (mak′ro-dont) having large teeth; characterized by macrodontia. Called also *megadont*.

macrodontia (mak″ro-don′she-ah) [*macro-* + Gr. *odous* tooth + *-ia*] a developmental disorder characterized by increase in size of the teeth. Called also *macrodontism, megadontia,* and *megalodontia*. **relative generalized m.**, a condition in which teeth of normal size give the appearance of being abnormally large in proportion to abnormally small jaws. **single tooth m.**, macrodontia involving only a single tooth. A variant of this condition may be seen in facial hemihypertrophy, in which the teeth of the involved side are larger than those on the unaffected side. **true generalized m.**, a form of macrodontia in which all the teeth are larger than normal.

macrodontic (mak″ro-don′tik) pertaining to or affected by macrodontia.

macrodontism (mak″ro-don′tizm) macrodontia.

macrogenia (mak″ro-jen′e-ah) [*macro-* + Gr. *genys* jaw] enlargement of the jaw, especially the chin, which may involve only the osseous or soft-tissue components or both the bony and soft tissues.

macrogingivae (mak″ro-jin-ji′ve) [*macro-* + *gingivae*] FIBROMATOSIS gingivae.

macroglia (mak-rog′le-ah) astrocytes and oligodendrocytes considered together; originally, used synonymously with astroglia.

macroglobulin (mak″ro-glob′u-lin) IMMUNOGLOBULIN M. **γ-m.**, IMMUNOGLOBULIN M (IgM).

macroglobulinemia (mak″ro-glob″u-lĭ-ne′me-ah) [*macroglobulin* + Gr. *haima* blood + *-ia*] a condition characterized by increase in macroglobulins in the blood. **primary m.**, Waldenström's m. **Waldenström's m.**, a condition characterized by the presence in the blood of abnormally large amounts of macroglobulin (IgM), associated with deficiency of IgG globulin resulting in the increased susceptibility to infection. Symptoms include weakness, lethargy, mucosal bleeding, hepatomegaly, lymphadenopathy, and sometimes Raynaud's syndrome, congestive heart failure, mental disorders, fundal abnormalities, and disorders of visual acuity. Oral manifestations consist of spontaneous gingival bleeding, often with continuous oozing of blood; bleeding ulcers on the tongue, palate, buccal mucosa, or gingivae; and focal, painful hyperemia. Prolonged bleeding after tooth extraction is common. Salivary gland involvement with xerostomia may occur. Hematologic changes include increased sedimentation rate, autohemagglutination, rouleau formation, coagulation disorders, peripheral vascular occlusion, and serum hyperviscosity. Poorly-defined cell infiltrations may be found in the bone marrow, lymph nodes, spleen, and liver. The total serum protein is usually increased. Sharp peaks in the β and γ region are found on paper electrophoresis. Ultracentrifugation shows high molecular weight proteins of 15S or more in concentrations greater than 5 percent. Called also *macroglobulinemia syndrome* and *primary macroglobulinemia*.

macroglossia (mak″ro-glos′e-ah) [*macro-* + Gr. *glōssa* tongue + *-ia*] presence of an excessively large tongue, which may be congenital or may develop as a result of a tumor or edema due to obstruction of lymphatic vessels, or it may occur in association with hyperpituitarism or acromegaly. It also may be associated with malocclusion, because of pressure of the tongue on the teeth, sometimes also resulting in crenation or scalloping of the lateral borders of the tongue. Called also *megaglossia* and *megaloglossia*. See also PACHYGLOSSIA. **unilateral m.**, hemimacroglossia.

macrognathia (mak″ro-na′the-ah) [*macro-* + Gr. *gnathos* + *-ia*] a condition characterized by abnormally large jaws. **mandibular m.**, development of an abnormally large mandible. See also PROGNATHISM. **maxillary m.**, development of an abnormally large maxilla. See also PROGNATHISM and maxillary PROTRUSION.

Macrogol trademark for *polyethylene glycol* (see under GLYCOL).

macrogyria (mak″ro-ji′re-ah) [*macro-* + Gr. *gyros* ring + *-ia*] a reduction in the number of sulci of the cerebrum, sometimes with increase in the brain substance, resulting in excessive size of the gyri. Called also *pachygyria*.

macrolabia (mak″ro-la′be-ah) [*macro-* + L. *labium* lip + *-ia*] macrocheilia.

macrolide (mak′ro-līd) any of a group of antibiotic macrocytic lactones containing 12 or more carbon atoms in the primary ring. The group includes amphotericin B, erythromycin, nystatin, and rifampin, which are official in the United States. Oleandomycin, spiramycin, and troleandomycin are unofficial macrolides, and are classified as erythromycin-type macrolides.

macromolecule (mak″ro-mol′ē-kul) [*macro-* + L. *molecula* little mass] a very large molecule constructed from many smaller organic building-block molecules (monomers), linked together by repetitive formation of covalent bonds, and constructed into polymeric chain structures. The macromolecules of animal cells fall into three main classes: polysaccharides, proteins, and nucleic acids.

macrophage (mak′ro-fāj) [*macro-* + Gr. *phagein* to eat] a large, stellate or fusiform leukocyte, about 15 to 80 μ in diameter, believed by some authorities to derive from lymphocytes and by others from monocytes. They have irregular contours and blunt pseudopodia, and their motility is similar to that of monocytes. The nucleus is small and near the nucleus there is a centrosome closely associated with the Golgi apparatus; the mitochondria are short and usually congregate around the centrosome. Many macrophages are fixed along the bundles of collagen fibers — these are known as fixed *macrophages* or *histiocytes*. When stimulated by inflammation, they detach from the fibers and become motile — these are known as free *macrophages*. Macrophages phagocytize by extending pseudopodia around foreign particles and taking them into the cytoplasm in vacuoles. They are scavenger cells and, in addition to foreign substances, remove from the tissue dead cells, extravasated erythrocytes, and other debris. The macrophages of the connective tissue are called *clasmatocytes, rhagiocrine cells,* and *resting wandering cells;* those along the blood vessels are called *adventitial cells*. **armed m.**, one that has acquired a specific mediator released from sensitized T-lymphocytes and has the ability to specifically kill target cells.

macrophthalmia (mak″rof-thal′me-ah) [*macro-* + Gr. *ophthalmos* eye + *-ia*] abnormal enlargement of the eyeball.

macropolycyte (mak″ro-pol′e-sīt) [*macro-* + *polycyte*] a hypersegmented, unusually large neutrophil, about 16 to 25 μ, having six to ten lobes. Macropolycytes are usually observed in the circulating blood in pathological conditions, such as folic acid deficiency and pernicious anemia. Called also *giant neutrophil*. See also POLYCYTE and PROPOLYCYTE.

macroprosopia (mak″ro-pro-so′pe-ah) [*macro-* + Gr. *prosōpon* face + *-ia*] excessive size of the face.

macrorhinia (mak″ro-rin′e-ah) [*macro-* + Gr. *rhis* nose + *-ia*] excessive size of the nose.

macroscopic (mak″ro-skop′ik) [*macro-* + Gr. *skopein* to examine] visible to the naked eye without the microscope.

macroscopy (mah-kros′ko-pe) [*macro-* + Gr. *skopein* to examine] examination with the naked eye without the microscope.

macrosis (mah-kro′sis) [*macro-* + *-osis*] increase in size.

macrostomia (mak″ro-sto′me-ah) [*macro-* + Gr. *stoma* mouth + *-ia*] an abnormally large mouth sometimes associated with lateral facial cleft.

macrotome (mak′ro-tōm) [*macro-* + Gr. *tomē* cut] an apparatus for cutting large sections of tissue for anatomical study.

macrotooth (mak′ro-tōōth) an excessively large tooth.

McShirley electromallet [R. C. *McShirley*] electromallet CONDENSER.

macula (mak′u-lah), pl. *mac′ulae* [L.] 1. a stain or spot; used in anatomical nomenclature as a general term to designate an area distinguishable by color or otherwise from its surroundings. 2. macule. **m. adher′ens,** desmosome.

maculae (mak′u-le) [L.] plural of *macula.*

macular (mak′u-lar) pertaining to or characterized by the presence of macules.

maculate (mak′u-lāt) [L. *maculatus* spotted] spotted or blotched.

maculation (mak″u-la′shun) [L. *macula* spot] the condition of being spotted; the formation of spots or macules.

macule (mak′ūl) 1. a circumscribed spot not raised above the level of the skin, which is not palpable, such as a freckle. 2. macula.

MAD methylandrostendiol; see METHANDRIOL.

madefaction (mad″ĕ-fak′shun) [L. *madefacere* to moisten] an old term for the act or process of moistening.

madidans (mad′ĭ-dans) an old term for moist or wet.

Madribol trademark for *sulfadimethoxine.*

mafenide (maf′en-īd) a sulfonamide, α-amino-*p*-toluenesulfonamide, occurring as a white, crystalline powder that is soluble in water. It acts against some strains of both grampositive and gram-negative bacteria, being particularly effective against *Pseudomonas aeruginosa* and anaerobic organisms. Used chiefly in antibacterial therapy of superficial wounds, including burns. Systemic hyperchloremic acidosis, hyperventilation, pain at the site of application, hypersensitivity, agranulocytosis, and fungal superinfection are some potential side reactions. Trademarks: Marfanil, Sulfamylon.

Mag. abbreviation for L. *mag′nus,* large.

magaldrate (mag′al-drāt) an antacid, tetrakis(hydroxymagnesium) decahydroxydialuminate dihydrate, occurring as a white, odorless, crystalline powder that is soluble in mineral acid solutions, but not in water and ethanol. Called also *aluminum magnesium hydroxide* and *magnesium aluminate hydrate.* Trademark: Riopan.

Magan trademark for *magnesium salicylate* (see under SALICYLATE).

Magcal trademark for a *magnesium oxide* preparation (see under MAGNESIUM).

Magendie, François [French physiologist, 1783–1855] see Bell's LAW (Bell-Magendie law).

magistery (maj′is-ter′e) [L. *magisterium; magister* master] 1. a precipitate. 2. any subtle or masterly preparation.

magistral (maj′is-tral) [L. *magister* master] 1. pertaining to a master. 2. pertaining to a medicine that is prepared in accordance with a physician's prescription; see magistral DRUG.

Magitot's disease [Emile *Magitot,* French dentist, 1833–1896] periodontoclasia.

Maglite trademark for a *magnesium oxide* preparation (see under MAGNESIUM).

Magnan's movement [Valentin Jacques Joseph *Magnan,* French physician, 1835–1916] see under MOVEMENT.

magnesia (mag-ne′zhe-ah) MAGNESIUM oxide. **m. mag′ma,** MILK of magnesia. **calcined m.,** MAGNESIUM oxide. **milk of m.,** MILK of magnesia. **m. us′ta,** MAGNESIUM oxide.

magnesium (mag-ne′ze-um) [*Magnesia,* a district in Thessaly, a region in ancient Greece] an alkaline metal. Symbol, Mg; atomic number, 12; atomic weight, 24.305; valence, 2; specific

gravity, 1.738; melting point, 648°C; group IIA of the periodic table. Magnesium has three natural isotopes, 24, 25, and 26. It is a silvery metal, soluble in acids, but not in water and, in the powdered state, ignites at 650°C, being the lightest of all structural metals. Magnesium is essential to life and an average adult has about 20 to 28 gm in the body (about 50 percent in bone, 45 percent as an intracellular cation, and 5 percent in the extracellular fluid). It is believed to be bound loosely to enamel, carious enamel having less magnesium than healthy. Legumes, whole grain, seafoods, and nuts are the principal sources of magnesium. Along with calcium, it acts to control neuromuscular transmission, sometimes synergistically, and at other times antagonistically. It is also a prosthetic ion for essential enzymes, including those involved in the phosphorylation of glucose in its anaerobic metabolism and its oxidative decarboxylation, in fatty acid degradation, in the activation of amino acids in the formation of cyclic AMP, in the synthesis of proteins, and in the synthesis and degradation of DNA. Magnesium salts are used as a cathartic, antacid, and CNS depressant in the treatment of seizures, pregnancy toxemias, and hypomagnesemia. Magnesium deficiency is associated with conditions such as chronic diarrhea, steatorrhea, alcoholism, prolonged intravenous feeding with magnesium-deficient solutions, diabetes mellitus, pancreatitis, postdiuretic electrolyte imbalance, renal tubular lesions, hyperaldosteronism, hypokalemia, and other diseases associated with hypocalcemia and hypokalemia. Symptoms may include neuromuscular dysfunction, tetany, hyperirritability, psychotic behavior, tachycardia, hypertension, electrolyte disorders, nephrocalcinosis, and other changes in the skeletal and cardiac muscle. Liver and kidney disorders, neuromuscular disturbances, and dental enamel hypoplasia may be produced in experimental animals by magnesium deficient diets. For daily requirements of magnesium, see table at NUTRITION. Magnesium poisoning is caused by elevated magnesium concentrations due to intake of large amounts of magnesium salts, such as magnesium-containing antacids or cathartics, in the presence of renal insufficiency. Symptoms may include ECG changes, sedation, confusion and, with plasma concentrations in excess of 4 mEq per liter, decrease of the deep-tendon reflexes, respiratory paralysis, and, in very high magnesium concentrations, heart block. **m. aluminate hydrate,** magaldrate. **m. carbonate hydroxide,** an antacid and cathartic, $(MgCO_3)_4 \cdot Mg(OH)_2 \cdot 5H_2O$, occurring as an odorless, white, amorphous solid that is insoluble in water or alcohol and is incompatible with acids. It is used also in dentifrices, particularly tooth powders to facilitate the pouring of the powder. It does not affect the pH of the saliva and is not absorbable from the oral and gastrointestinal mucous membranes to produce central nervous system depressant action. **m. hydrate,** m. hydroxide. **m. hydroxide,** a compound, $Mg(OH)_2$, occurring as amorphous powder that is soluble in dilute acids, but not in water, produced by hydration of magnesium oxide. A suspension of 7.0 to 8.5 percent magnesium hydroxide in water is known as *milk of magnesia* (see under MILK). Called also *m. hydrate.* **m. mesotrisilicate,** m. trisilicate. **m. oxide,** a gastric antacid, MgO, occurring as a white, fine powder that is slightly soluble in water and is readily soluble in acids, but not in ethanol. On combining with water, it forms magnesium hydroxide. It is used also in dentifrices to facilitate flowing. Called also *magnesia, calcined magnesia* and *magnesia usta.* Trademarks: Magcal, Maglite. **m. salicylate,** magnesium SALICYLATE. **m. silicate, hydrous,** talc. **m. sulfate,** a compound, $MgSO_4$; the heptahydrate, $(MgSO_4 \cdot 7H_2O)$, occurs in nature as the mineral epsomite, which forms efflorescent crystals or powder with a bitter saline taste. It dissolves in water and, at a slower rate, glycerol and alcohol. Used as a cathartic. Also used in solution for soaking inflamed areas to reduce swelling. Called also *bitter salts* and *Epsom salts.* **m. trisilicate,** a compound of magnesium oxide and silicon dioxide, $Mg_2O_8Si_3$. In hydrated form, it is a fine, white, odorless, tasteless powder that is insoluble in water and ethanol, but decomposes in mineral acids with the liberation of silicic acid. Used as an antacid and adsorbent. Called also *m. mesotrisilicate.* Trademark: Trisomin.

magnet (mag′net) [L. *magnes;* Gr. *magnēs* magnet] a body capable of attracting magnetizable substances, such as iron or steel, and producing a magnetic field external to itself. **denture m.,** a magnet used for additional retention of dentures, usually a small cylinder, measuring 6.35 × 3.55 × 2.54 mm (0.24 × 0.14 × 0.10 inches), and made of a nonreactogenic platinum-cobalt alloy, one end of the cylinder having a negative polarity and the other a positive polarity. One magnet is implanted into the mandible under the periosteum (mandibular magnet) and the other is attached to the denture, its poles being opposite of those in the mandible. Called also *magnetic implant*.

magnetism (mag′nĕ-tizm) magnetic attraction or repulsion.

magnification (mag″nĭ-fĭ-ka′shun) [L. *magnificatio*, from *magnus* great + *facere* to make] 1. apparent increase in size, as with the use of a lens. 2. making something greater in actual size. 3. the ratio of apparent (image) size to real size.

maim (mām) 1. to disable by a wound; to dismember by violence. 2. a dismemberment or disablement effected by violence.

main (măn) [Fr.] hand. **m. en griffe,** clawhand.

maintainer (măn-tān′er) something that keeps or maintains in another thing existence or continuancy. **band and bar space m.,** one in which a bar bridging the edentulous area to be maintained is soldered to two orthodontic bands fitted onto the teeth on both sides of the space. **band and crib space m.,** a cantilever space maintainer in which a crib, attached to an orthodontic band on the abutment tooth, extends across the edentulous space and presses against the tooth on the other side of the space. **broken stress space m.,** one in which the bar bridging the edentulous area to be maintained is fitted with a stress breaker, such as a ball-and-socket joint, to allow vertical movement of the supporting teeth and, to a lesser degree, adjustive labial or lingual movement. **cantilever space m.,** one in which the arm or crib bridging the edentulous space to be maintained is supported by only one abutment tooth, being attached to a crown or orthodontic band in a cantilever fashion. **crown and bar space m.,** one in which a bar bridging the edentulous space to be maintained is soldered to two steel crowns on both sides of the space. **crown and crib space m.,** a cantilever space maintainer in which a crib, attached to a stainless steel crown, projects across the edentulous space and presses against the tooth on the other side of the space. **fixed-removable space m.,** one equipped with a locking attachment which allows the dentist, but not the patient, to remove the appliance. **fixed space m.,** one soldered to a steel crown or orthodontic band and can not be removed. **Gerber space m.,** a cantilever space maintainer equipped with spring-loaded arms to provide the desired degree of pressure against another tooth. By applying constant pressure, the device pushes back the tooth across the edentulous area, thus serving as a space regainer. See illustra-

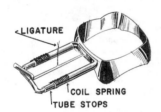

Gerber space maintainer. (From T. M. Graber: Orthodontics — Principles and Practice. 3rd ed. Philadelphia, W. B. Saunders Co., 1972; courtesy Unitek Corp.)

tion. **Mayne space m.,** a cantilever space maintainer, in which the arm is bent around the space for the unerupted tooth and is placed against a tooth on the other side of the space to prevent it from crowding the space; thus providing room for the erupting tooth. See illustration. **removable space m.,** any space maintainer that may be removed by the patient. **space m.,** 1. an orthodontic appliance, fixed or removable, used for maintaining the space created by a prematurely lost tooth or the space to be filled by a tooth still to be erupted. See also space REGAINER and space RETAINER. 2. separator.

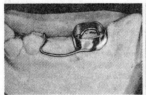 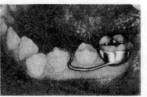

Mayne space maintainer. (From T. M. Graber: Orthodontics — Principles and Practice. 3rd ed. Philadelphia, W. B. Saunders Co., 1972; courtesy W. R. Mayne.)

maintenance (măn′tĕ-nans) the act or process of keeping something in an existing state. **preventive health m.,** the periodic assessment of the health and fitness of an individual for the early detection of abnormalities so as to institute prompt preventive treatment of correctable conditions, for monitoring and preventive maintenance to postpone disability and death for uncorrectable diseases, and health education and counseling for the nondiseased.

Majewski's syndrome [F. *Majewski*] see under SYNDROME. See also Lenz-Majewski DWARFISM.

majoon (mah-joon′) ganja.

makro- for words thus beginning, see those beginning MACRO-.

mal (mahl) [Fr.; L. *malum* ill] illness; sickness; disease.

mal- [L. *malus* bad] a combining form denoting false, evil, or bad.

mala (ma′lah) [L.] [NA alternative] bucca.

malabsorption (mal″ab-sorp′shun) faulty absorption of nutrients by the intestine.

malacia (mah-la′she-ah) [Gr. *malakia*] 1. the morbid softening of a part or tissue. Also used with combining forms to denote specific conditions, such as osteomalacia. 2. craving for spiced foods.

malacic (mah-la′sik) marked by malacia or abnormal softness.

malaco- [Gr. *malakos* soft] a combining form denoting a condition of abnormal softness.

malacoma (mal″ah-ko′mah) [*malaco-* + *-oma*] an abnormally soft spot or part.

malacoplakia (mal″ah-ko-pla′ke-ah) [*malaco-* + Gr. *plax* plaque] the formation of soft patches on the mucous membrane.

malacotic (mal″ah-kot′ik) soft; inclined to malacia; said of teeth.

malactic (mah-lak′tik) 1. softening; emollient. 2. an agent which softens; emollient.

maladie (mal″ah-de′) [Fr.] a disease.

malady (mal′ah-de) [Fr. *maladie*] a disease or illness.

malagma (mah-lag′mah) [Gr.] an emollient or cataplasm.

malaise (mal-āz′) [Fr.] a feeling of indisposition; ill-being.

malalignment (mal″ah-līn′ment) displacement out of line, especially displacement of the teeth from their normal relation to the line of the dental arch. See MALOCCLUSION.

malar (ma′lar) [L. *mala* cheek] pertaining to the cheek or cheek bone.

malare (ma-la′re) the midpoint of the intersection between the projection of the coronoid process and the lower contour of the malar bone.

malaria (mah-la′re-ah) [It. "bad air"] an infectious febrile disease caused by protozoa of the genus *Plasmodium,* transmitted by the bites of infected mosquitoes of the genus *Anopheles.* It is characterized by attacks of chills, fever, and sweating, occurring at intervals which depend on the time required for development of a new generation of parasites in the body. After recovery from the acute attack, the disease has a tendency to become chronic, with occasional relapse.

Malassez's rest (epithelial rest of) [Louis Charles *Malassez,* French physiologist, 1842–1909] see under REST.

Malassezia (mal″ah-se′ze-ah) [named after Louis Charles *Malassez*] a genus of deuteromycetous fungi (Fungi Imperfecti), most members of which occur as unicellular organisms with budding cells and reproduce by blastospores cut off from the mother cell by the developing cross-wall. Several species are common members of the normal skin flora. Called also *Pityrosporon* and *Pityrosporum.* **M. fur′fur,** a species that is a customary resident of normal skin, but is capable of causing disease (pityriasis versicolor). Called also *Pityrosporum furfur* and *P. orbiculare.* **M. ova′le,** a lipid-dependent species that is abundant in sebaceous areas, such as the skin of the face and scalp, which is capable of causing a type of pityriasis versicolor, particularly the actinic or follicular form. Called also *Pityrosporum ovale.*

malassimilation (mal″ah-sim″ĭ-la′shun) [*mal-* + L. *assimilatio* a rendering like] imperfect, faulty, or disordered assimilation.

malathion (mal″ah-thi′on) an organophosphorus compound, *O,O*-dimethyl-*S*-(1,2-dicarboxyethyl)dithiophosphate, occurring as a brown to yellow liquid with a characteristic odor, which is slightly soluble in water and is miscible with several organic solvents. It decomposes when pH is below 5 or above 7. Malathion is an anticholinesterase agent used as an insecticide, having a relatively low toxicity for warm-blooded animals. Its residues disappear in a few days to 2 weeks after application. Ingestion of 60 gm is estimated as being fatal to humans. Called also *mercaptothion* and *phosphothion.*

maleate (ma′le-āt) a salt of maleic acid containing the radical —OCO·CH : CH·COO—.

maleruption (mal″e-rup′shun) faulty eruption of a tooth, so that it is out of its normal position.

malformation (mal″for-ma′shun) [L. *malus* evil + *formatio* a forming] defective or abnormal formation; a deformity. See also

ABNORMALITY, ANOMALY, and DEFORMITY. **Rieger's m.,** see Rieger's SYNDROME.

malfunction (mal-funk′shun) dysfunction.

Malgaigne's fossa, Malgaigne's triangle [Joseph François *Malgaigne*, French surgeon, 1806–1865] superior carotid TRIANGLE.

Malherbe's epithelioma [A. *Malherbe*] benign calcifying EPITHELIOMA.

malignancy (mah-lig′nan-se) [L. *malignare* to act maliciously] 1. a tendency to progress in virulence; the quality of being malignant. 2. a malignant tumor.

malignant (mah-lig′nant) [L. *malignans* acting maliciously] tending to be progressively worse and to result in death. Having the properties of anaplasia, invasion, and metastasis; said of tumors.

malingering (mah-ling′ger-ing) the willful, deliberate, and fraudulent feigning or exaggeration of the symptoms of illness or injury, done for the purpose of a consciously desired end. Called also *pathomimia*.

malinterdigitation (mal″in-ter-dij″ĭ-ta′shun) failure of interdigitation of parts which are normally so related.

malleability (mal″ĕ-ah-bil′ĭ-te) 1. the quality of a material of being able to be shaped by hammering or by pressure exerted by rollers. See also DUCTILITY. 2. the ability of material to withstand permanent deformation under compressive stress.

malleable (mal′e-ah-b'l) [L. *malleare* to hammer] capable of being beaten out into thin sheets by blows from a hammer or pressure from a roller; said of metals.

Malleomyces (mal″e-o-mi′sēz) [L. *malleus* glanders + Gr. *mykēs* fungus] a former genus of gram-negative, aerobic bacilli, the species of which have been now assigned to the genus *Pseudomonas*. **M. mal′lei,** *Pseudomonas mallei;* see under PSEUDOMONAS. **M. pseudomal′lei,** *Pseudomonas pseudomallei;* see under PSEUDOMONAS.

mallet (mal′et) a hammer-like tool with a head commonly of wood, plastic, or some other relatively soft material, used for driving another tool that has a plastic or wooden handle, or to strike a surface so as not to leave a mark. See also HAMMER. **automatic m.,** mechanical CONDENSER. **Bonwill m.,** a mechanical condenser driven by an electromagnetic engine.

malleus (mal′e-us) [L. "hammer"] 1. [NA] the largest of the auditory ossicles, and the one attached to the tympanic membrane; its club-shaped head articulates with the incus. Called also *hammer* and *plectrum*. 2. glanders.

malnutrition (mal″nu-trish′un) any disorder of nutrition that may result in poor health. Malnutrition may be due to consumption of insufficient amounts of food (undernutrition), consumption of excessive amounts of food (overnutrition), or consumption of an unbalanced variety of food so that the ratio of nutrients to one another is not in proper proportion for their efficient utilization by the body. See table of *Recommended Daily Dietary Allowances* in Appendix.

malocclusion (mal″o-kloo′zhun) such malposition and contact of the maxillary and mandibular teeth as to interfere with the

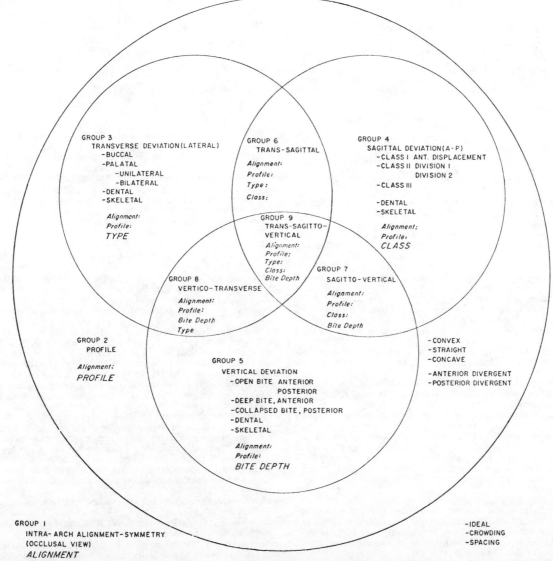

Modified Venn diagram for classification of malocclusion. (From J. L. Ackermann and W. R. Proffitt: The characteristics of malocclusion: a modern approach to classification and diagnosis. Am. J. Orthodont, 56:443–454, 1969.)

highest efficiency during the excursive movements of the jaw that are essential for mastication. Originally classified by Angle into four major groups, depending on the anteroposterior jaw relationship as indicated by interdigitation of the first molar teeth, but Class IV is no longer used (see table). See illustration.

ANGLE'S CLASSIFICATION OF MALOCCLUSION

Class I (Neutroclusion). Normal anteroposterior relationship of the jaws, as indicated by correct interdigitation of maxillary and mandibular molars, but with crowding and rotation of teeth elsewhere, i.e., a dental dysplasia or an arch length deficiency.

Class II (Distoclusion). The lower dental arch is posterior to the upper in one or both lateral segments; the lower first molar is distal to the upper first molar.

    Division 1. Bilaterally distal with narrow maxillary arch and protruding upper incisors.

      Subdivision. Unilaterally distal with other characteristics the same.

    Division 2. Bilaterally distal with normal or square-shaped maxillary arch, retruded maxillary central incisors, labially malposed maxillary lateral incisors, and an excessive overbite.

      Subdivision. Unilaterally distal with other characteristics the same.

Class III (Mesioclusion). The lower arch is anterior to the upper in one or both lateral segments; lower first molar is mesial to upper first molar.

    Division. Mandibular incisors are usually in anterior crossbite.

      Subdivision. Unilaterally mesial, with other characteristics the same.

Class IV. The occlusal relations of the dental arches present the peculiar condition of being in distal occlusion upon one lateral half, and in mesial occlusion upon the other half of the mouth.

Ackerman-Proffitt classification, a method of classifying malocclusion on the basis of its unique and overlapping morphological characteristics, using a modified Venn diagram to divide the condition into nine groups. Since the degrees of alignment of symmetry are common to all dentitions, this is represented as the outer envelope of the diagram (Group 1); the profile is affected in several forms of malocclusion, hence it becomes a major set within the diagram subset (Group 2); deviations in three planes of space, lateral (transverse), anteroposterior, and vertical, are represented by Groups 3 to 9, which include the overlapping or interlocking subsets, all within the profile or Group 2 set. See illustration. **closed-bite m.,** closed BITE. **deflective m.,** that in which all the teeth cannot be closed while the condyles are held in their rearmost position. To gain occlusal contacts, the jaw must be moved anteriorly, laterally, or anterolaterally, as the deflectors demand in their guidance. **openbite m.,** open BITE.

Malonal trademark for *barbital.*

malonyl (mal′o-nil) the divalent radical, OCCH₂CO.

malonylurea (mal″o-nil-u-re′ah) barbituric ACID.

Malpighi, Marcello [1628–1694] an Italian anatomist. See MALPIGHIAN.

malpighian (mal-pig′i-an) named after or described by Marcello *Malpighi,* as malpighian cell and malpighian layer. (see under CELL and LAYER).

malposition (mal″po-zish′un) [mal- + L. *positio* placement] abnormal or anomalous position. **jaw m.,** any abnormal position of the lower jaw. See MALOCCLUSION.

malpractice (mal-prak′tis) [mal- + practice] professional negligence resulting from improper discharge of professional duties or failure to meet the standard of care, which results in harm to a client or patient. See also malpractice liability INSURANCE and NEGLIGENCE. **medical m.,** professional negligence in the administration of and failure to meet the established standards in the administration of therapy, diagnosis, or any other form of medical care.

malpraxis (mal-prak′sis) malpractice.

malt (mawlt) [L. *maltum*] grain, for the most part barley, which has been soaked, made to germinate, and then dried; it contains dextrin, maltose, and diastase. It is nutritive and digestant, aiding in the digestion of starchy foods. **m. sugar,** maltose.

maltase (mawl′tās) α-GLUCOSIDASE.

Malthus, Rev. Thomas [1766–1834] an English economist. See MALTHUSIAN.

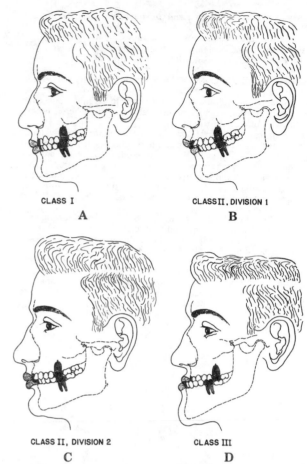

Angle's Classification of Malocclusion. *A,* Class 1: mesiodistal first molar relationship normal; tooth irregularities elsewhere. *B,* **Class II, Division 1:** lower first molar distal to upper first molar. Mandibular retrusion usually reflected in patient profile. *C,* **Class II, Division 2:** lower first molar distal to upper first molar. Deep overbite often reflected in patient profile. *D,* **Class III malocclusion:** lower first molar mesial to upper first molar. Mandibular prognathism usually reflected in patient profile. (From T. M. Graber: Orthodontics — Principles and Practice. 3rd ed. **Philadelphia, W. B. Saunders Co., 1972.)**

malthusian (mal-thoo′se-an) named after Rev. Thomas *Malthus,* as malthusian law (see under LAW).

maltobiose (mawl″to-bi′ōs) maltose.

maltodextrin (mawl″to-dek′strin) a dextrin convertible into maltose.

maltose (mawl′tōs) a disaccharide, 4-*O*-α-D-glucopyranosyl-D-glucopyranose, present in germinating grains, which is also formed in the animal body by the action of enzymes on starch in the process of digestion. Commercially, it is made by the partial hydrolysis of starch by acid in the manufacture of corn syrup. On hydrolysis, it forms two molecules of glucose. Maltose is a white crystalline substance, about one-third as sweet as sucrose, which is soluble in water and, slightly, in alcohol. It is present in small amounts in many carbohydrate foods, due to partial breakdown of starch during cooking, and is also a component of beer and ale, being responsible for their caloric content. Used as a nutrient and sweetener, as a parenteral supplement for sugar for diabetics, in culture media, in the manufacture of drugs, as a fermentable intermediate in brewing, and as a stabilizer for polysulfides. Called also *maltobiose* and *malt sugar.*

malturned (mal-ternd′) turned abnormally; said of teeth twisted on their central axes.

malum (ma′lum) [L.] disease. **m. rus′ti,** Rust's DISEASE. **m. suboccipita′le,** Rust's DISEASE.

malunion (mal-un′yon) union of the fragments of a fractured bone in a faulty position. See faulty UNION, NONUNION, and vicious UNION.

mamelon (mam′ĕ-lon) [Fr. "nipple"] 1. one of the three rounded protuberances on the incisal edges of newly erupted incisor teeth. 2. the nipplelike elevation in the umbilicus.

Mamiesan trademark for *dicyclomine hydrochloride* (see under DICYCLOMINE).

mamilla (mah-mil'ah), pl. *mamil'lae* [L., dim. of *mamma* a breast] nipple (1).

mamillae (mah-mil'le) [L.] plural of *mamilla*.

man (man) 1. an adult male member of the human race. 2. a human being; an individual, *Homo sapiens*, at the highest level of animal development.

management (man'ij-ment) 1. the act, manner, or practice of managing, directing, handling, or controlling a business, organization, etc. 2. the person(s) responsible for management; executives collectively. **Training in Expanded Auxiliary M.,** see TEAM.

Mandelamine trademark for *methenamine mandelate* (see under METHENAMINE).

mandible (man'dĭ-b'l) [L. *mandibula*] the horseshoe-shaped bone forming the lower jaw and serving as the bony framework for the floor of the mouth and providing support of the lower teeth. It presents a horizontal portion, and two vertical portions, the rami, which articulate with the skull at the temporomandibular joint. The mandible is ossified in the membrane covering the outer surface of Meckel's cartilage, and develops in two halves from a single center which appears at about the sixth week of fetal life. At birth the two parts of the bone are joined by a fibrous symphysis which ossifies during the first year of life. Called also *inferior maxillary bone, lower jaw, lower jaw bone, lower maxilla, mandibula* [NA], and *submaxilla*. Cf. MAXILLA. See illustration. **disappearing m.,** a very rare condition characterized by osteolysis and resorption of the mandible. **protruding m.,** prognathism. **retrognathic m.,** mandibular RETROGNATHIA. **retruded m.,** mandibular RETROGNATHIA. **short m.,** brachygnathia.

mandibula (man-dib'u-lah), pl. *mandib'ulae* [L.] [NA] mandible.

mandibulae (man-dib'u-le) plural of *mandibula*.

mandibular (man-dib'u-lar) pertaining to the mandible.

mandibulectomy (man-dib"-lik'to-me) surgical removal of the mandible. **unilateral m.,** hemimandibulectomy.

mandibulofacial (man-dib"u-lo-fa'shal) pertaining to the mandible and face.

mandibulopharyngeal (man-dib"u-lo-fah-rin'je-al) pertaining to the mandible and the pharynx.

Mandoz trademark for *methenamine mandelate* (see under METHENAMINE).

mandrel (man'drĕl) 1. a shaft which holds a rotating device, such as a grinding wheel, sandpaper disk, circular saw, or headstock of a lathe. 2. a shaft in a handpiece that holds a disk, stone, or cup used for grinding or polishing. Written also *mandril*. **disk m.,** one having a slip-on or a split head to hold a polishing disk, allowing it to be rotated forward or backward in the handpiece. Called also *Moore's m.* **endosseous implant needle m.,** a device into which needle implants fit and which, after being engaged into the contra-angle handpiece, is used to drive the needles into the bone. **Moore's m.,** disk m. **Morgan's m.,** a disk mandrel with a split head, for holding polishing disks with metal cores by frictional contact. **snap-on m.,** one with a split end for holding rubber polishing cups.

mandril (man'dril) mandrel.

maneuver (mah-noo'ver) any dextrous proceeding. **Heimlich m.,** a technique for removing foreign matter from the trachea of a choking victim, also recommended as a preliminary step in the emergency treatment of accident victims in need of artificial ventilation, carried out to clear material that may prevent adequate ventilation of the lungs before administering mouth-to-mouth respiration. In the dental chair, the patient is left in the chair while the rescuer sits astride him and the second rescuer turns the head to the side and prepares to evacuate the ejected material. Placing both hands, one on top of the other, between the xiphoid process and the umbilicus, the rescuer suddenly presses inward and upward, thus forcing the diaphragm upward, compressing the lungs and expelling the obstruction. In the standing position, the rescuer stands behind the victim and wraps his arms around the waist, allowing the victim's head, arms, and upper torso to hang forward. A fist is made with one hand and held with the other. The fist is then placed against the victim's abdomen at a point slightly above the umbilicus and below the rib cage. The fist is then pressed suddenly into the victim's abdomen with a forceful upward thrust. In the supine position, the victim is placed on his back with the head turned to one side. The rescuer kneels astride the victim's hips and places both hands on his abdomen, one hand upon the other. The heel of the lower hand is placed slightly above the umbilicus and below the rib cage. Pressure is applied to the victim's abdomen with a forceful upward thrust. The maneuver may be repeated if necessary. See also RESUSCITATION. **Hueter's m.,** downward and forward pressure on the patient's tongue by the left forefinger during intubation.

Manexin trademark for *mannitol hexanitrate* (see under MANNITOL).

manganese (man'gah-nĕs) [L. *manganum, manganesium*] a metallic element. Symbol, Mn; atomic number, 25; atomic weight, 54.938; melting point, 1245°C; Mohs hardness index, 5; valences, 2, 3, 4, 6, 7; group VIIB of the periodic table. It occurs as one stable isotope, 55, and several artificial radioactive ones, 49–54 and 56–58. In a pure form, manganese is a grayish white, lustrous, brittle metal that resembles iron, which reacts with

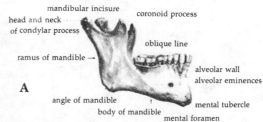

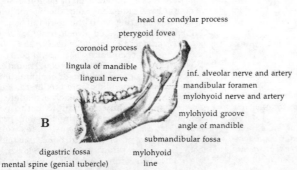

A, The mandible seen from the right side. *B*, Medial view of the right half of the mandible. (From J. Langman and M. W. Woerdeman: Atlas of Medical Anatomy. Philadelphia, W. B. Saunders Co., 1978.)

water and dissolves in mineral acids. It occurs in trace amounts (about 10 to 20 mg) in tissues, the highest concentration being in the liver, muscles, and bones. It is generally elevated in the saliva of children in endemic dental caries areas. Manganese serves as an activator of liver arginase, thus being essential in the formation of urea, and other enzymes, including mitochondrial respiratory enzymes and cholinesterase. Plant foods, including tea, are the principal sources of manganese. Manganese deficiency is rare, but may cause production of excessive amounts of ammonium compounds in the body and bone lesions. Inhalation of dust and fumes may cause parkinsonism-like disorders, including spastic gait, emotional disorders, paralysis, and weakness. Manganese-substituted austenitic stainless steels are used in dentistry.

manganic (man-gan′ik) pertaining to manganese as a trivalent element.

manganous (man′gah-nus) pertaining to manganese as a divalent element.

manganum (man′gah-num) [L.] manganese.

manifestation (man′ĭ-fĕ-sta′shun) the occurrence of events that are readily perceived, as changes occurring on the skin or tongue, in the eyes, etc., in certain diseases.

manipulation (mah-nip″u-la′shun) [L. *manipulare* to handle] skillful or dextrous treatment by the hand; performance of a function or operation through the use of the hand or hands. **conjoined m.**, manipulation with both hands.

manipulator (mah-nip″u-la′tor) [L. *manipulare* to handle] a device or instrument for handling objects without the necessity of touching them. **amalgam m.**, an instrument for shaping and carving amalgam restorations.

Mann, Ludwig [German neurologist, 1866–1936] see Wernicke-Mann HEMIPLEGIA.

manna (man′ah) dried exudation of the plant *Fraxinus ornus*, which grows in the Mediterranean Basin and Asia Minor. Used as a cathartic. **m. sugar**, mannitol.

mannite (man′īt) mannitol.

mannitol (man′ĭ-tol) a sugar alcohol, HOCH₄(CHOH)₄CH₂OH, widely distributed in plants and fungi, and obtained from manna and seaweeds. It occurs as an odorless, sweetish, white, crystalline powder that is soluble in water and alkaline solutions, slightly soluble in ethanol and pyridine, and insoluble in ether. Used chiefly as an osmotic diuretic. Also used as a diagnostic agent in kidney function tests and to reduce intraocular pressure and cerebrospinal fluid in surgery. Called also *manna sugar, mannite,* and D-*mannitol.* Trademark: *Osmitrol.* **m. hexanitrate**, a compound formed by the nitration of mannitol, occurring as long needles that are unstable and will explode on percussion. It is soluble in ethanol and ether, but not in water. It is a vasodilator most commonly used in the prevention of angina pectoris. Nausea, vomiting, headache, and hypotension may occur during therapy. Called also *m. nitrate* and *nitromannite.* Trademarks: Manexin, Maxitate, Nitranitol. **m. nitrate**, m. hexanitrate.

manometer (mah-nom′ĕ-ter) [Gr. *manos* thin + *metron* measure] an instrument for measuring the pressure or tension of liquids or gases. See also SPHYGMOMANOMETER.

manpower (man′pow-er) the body of persons available to perform a certain task or function; personnel. **health m.**, collectively, all persons working to provide health services whether as individual practitioners or employees of health institutions and programs; whether or not professionally trained; and whether or not subject to public regulation.

Man. pr. abbreviation for L. *ma′ne pri′mo,* early in the morning.

mantle (man′t′l) [L. *mantellum* cloak] an enveloping cover or layer. **glycoprotein m.**, glycocalyx.

manual (man′u-al) [L. *manualis,* from *manus* hand] pertaining to, performed by, or operated by the hand or hands.

manubria (mah-nu′bre-ah) [L.] plural of *manubrium.*

manubrium (mah-nu′bre-um), pl. *manu′bria* [L.] a general anatomical term for a handlelike structure or part.

manudynamometer (man″u-di″nah-mom′ĕ-ter) [L. *manus* hand + Gr. *dynamis* force + *metron* measure] an apparatus for measuring the force of the thrust of an instrument.

manus (ma′nus), pl. *ma′nus* [L.] [NA] the hand. **m. ca′va**, a hand deformed by a deep hollowing of the palm. **m. exten′sa**, backward deviation of the hand. Called also *m. superextensa.* **m. flex′a**, forward deviation of the hand. **m. pla′na**, flattening of the arch formed normally by the proximal row of the carpal bones. Called also *flat hand.* **m. superexten′sa**, m. extensa. **m. val′ga**,

clubhand marked by deflection of the hand toward the radial side. **m. va′ra**, clubhand marked by deflection of the hand to the ulnar side.

MAO monoamine oxidase; see amine OXIDASE.

MAP Medical Audit Program; see under PROGRAM.

map (map′) a two-dimensional graphic representation of arrangement in space. **genetic m.**, a graphic representation of the linear arrangement of genes on a chromosome.

Mapharsen trademark for *oxophenarsine.*

mapping (map′ing) delineation or representation of anything. **chromosome m.**, the locating of the relative position of genes on a chromosome.

mar marker chromosome; see genetic MARKER. See also CHROMOSOME nomenclature.

Marboran trademark for *methisazone.*

Marchand's cell [Felix Jacob *Marchand,* German pathologist, 1846–1923] adventitial CELL.

Marchesani-Weill syndrome [Oswald *Marchesani,* 1900–1952; G. *Weill*] Marchesani's SYNDROME.

Marchiafava's hemolytic anemia [Ettore *Marchiafava,* Italian physician, 1847–1935] Marchiafava-Micheli SYNDROME.

Marchiafava-Micheli syndrome [E. *Marchiafava;* F. *Micheli,* Italian physician] see under SYNDROME.

Marcus Gunn's phenomenon, syndrome [Robert *Marcus Gunn,* English ophthalmologist 1850–1909] Gunn's SYNDROME.

Marden-Walker syndrome [P. M. *Marden;* W. A. *Walker*] see under SYNDROME.

Marevan trademark for *warfarin sodium* (see under WARFARIN).

Marfan's syndrome [Bernard Jean Antonin *Marfan,* French physician, 1858–1942] see under SYNDROME.

Marfanil trademark for *mafenide.*

margin (mar′jin) an edge or border. See also BORDER and MARGO. **alveolar m.**, alveolar ARCH. **alveolar m. of mandible**, alveolar arch of mandible; see under ARCH. **alveolar m. of maxilla**, alveolar arch of maxilla; see under ARCH. **anterior m. of parietal bone**, frontal m. of parietal bone. **cavosurface m.**, the area formed by the cavity wall and the external tooth surface. **coronal m. of frontal bone**, coronal m. of frontal bone. **coronal m. of parietal bone**, frontal m. of parietal bone. **free gingival m.**, **free gum m.**, marginal GINGIVA. **frontal m. of great wing of sphenoid bone**, a roughened area on the great wing of the sphenoid bone where it articulates with the frontal bone; it is situated at the upper lateral margin of the orbital surface of the great wing where this meets the cerebral and temporal surfaces. Called also *parietofrontal m. of great wing of sphenoid bone, margo frontalis alae magnae,* and *margo frontalis alae majoris* [NA]. **frontal m. of parietal bone**, the edge of the parietal bone that articulates with the frontal bone along the coronal suture. Called also *anterior m. of parietal bone, coronal m. of parietal bone, frontal border of parietal bone,* and *margo frontalis ossis parietalis* [NA]. **gingival m., gum m.**, marginal GINGIVA. **incisal m.**, the crest of the biting edge of an incisor tooth. **inconsistent m.**, periodontal defect in marginal bone; see under DEFECT. **infraorbital m. of maxilla**, the short rounded edge of the maxilla where the orbital surface becomes continuous with the anterior surface. Called also *infraorbital border of maxilla, infraorbital ridge of maxilla,* and *margo infraorbitalis maxillae* [NA]. **infraorbital m. of orbit**, the inferior edge of the entrance of the orbit, formed by the infraorbital process of the zygomatic bone and the infraorbital margin of the maxilla. Called also *infraorbital border of orbit* and *margo infraorbitalis orbitae* [NA]. **lacrimal m. of maxilla**, the posterior border of the frontal process of the maxilla where it articulates with the lacrimal bone. Called also *lacrimal border of maxilla, inferior maxillary incisure,* and *margo lacrimalis maxillae* [NA]. **lambdoid m. of occipital bone**, the edge of the occipital bone extending from the lateral angle to the superior angle, articulating with the parietal bone to help form the lambdoid suture. Called also *parietal m. of occipital bone* and *margo lambdoideus squamae occipitalis* [NA]. **lambdoid m. of parietal bone**, occipital m. of parietal bone. **malar m.**, zygomatic m. of great wing of sphenoid bone. **mamillary m.**, mastoid m. of occipital bone. **mastoid m. of occipital bone**, the edge of the occipital bone extending from the lateral angles to the inferior angle; the posterior half of each articulates with the mastoid portion and the anterior half with the petrous part of the temporal bone that bears the mastoid process. Called also *mamillary m.* and *margo mastoideus squamae occipitalis* [NA]. **mastoid m. of parietal bone**, mastoid angle of parietal bone; see under ANGLE. **nasal m.**, the lower, free margin of the ala nasi and septum nasi that surrounds the external naris. Called also *margo nasi.* **nasal m. of frontal bone**, the articular surface, on each nasal part of the frontal bone, which articulates with the nasal bones and with the frontal process of the maxilla. Called also *margo nasalis ossis frontalis* [NA], *nasal border of frontal bone,* and *nasal incisure of frontal bone.* **occipital m. of parietal bone,** the edge of the parietal bone that articulates with the occipital bone at the lambdoid suture. Called also *lambdoid m. of parietal bone, margo occipitalis ossis parietalis* [NA], and *occipital border of parietal bone.* **occipital m. of temporal bone,** the border of the petrous part of the temporal bone that articulates with the occipital bone along the occipitomastoid suture. Called also *margo occipitalis ossis temporalis* [NA], and *occipital border of temporal bone.* **parietal m. of frontal bone,** the posterior border of the frontal bone, semicircular in shape, which articulates with the parietal bone. Called also *coronal m. of frontal bone, margo parietalis ossis frontalis* [NA], and *parietal border of frontal bone.* **parietal m. of great wing of sphenoid bone,** the superior extremity of the squamous margin of the great wing of the sphenoid bone. Called also *angulus parietalis ossis sphenoidalis, margo parietalis alae majoris* [NA], and *parietal angle of sphenoid bone.* **parietal m. of occipital bone,** lambdoid m. of occipital bone. **parietal m. of parietal bone,** sagittal m. of parietal bone. **parietal m. of temporal bone, parietal m. of temporal squama,** the superior border of the squamous part of the temporal bone where it articulates with the parietal bone. Called also *parietal m. of temporal squama, margo parietalis ossis temporalis* [NA], *margo parietalis squamae temporalis,* and *parietal border of temporal bone.* **parietofrontal m. of great wing of sphenoid bone,** frontal m. of great wing of sphenoid bone. **sagittal m. of parietal bone,** the edge of the parietal bone that articulates with the other parietal bone along the sagittal suture. Called also *parietal m. of parietal bone, m. of parietal bone,* and *margo sagittalis ossis parietalis* [NA]. **sphenoidal m. of parietal bone,** sphenoid angle of parietal bone; see under ANGLE. **sphenoidal m. of temporal bone, sphenoidal m. of temporal squama,** the anterior border of the temporal bone, articulating with the great wing of the sphenoid bone. Called also *margo sphenoidalis ossis temporalis* [NA], *margo sphenoidalis squamae temporalis, sphenoidal border of temporal bone,* and *sphenoidal border of temporal squama.* **sphenotemporal m. of parietal bone,** squamous m. of parietal bone. **squamous m. of great wing of sphenoid bone,** the border of the great wing of the sphenoid bone that articulates with the squama of the temporal bone; its superior extremity is known as the *parietal margin of great wing of the sphenoid bone.* Called also *margo squamosus alae majoris* [NA] and *margo squamosus alae magnae.* **squamous m. of parietal bone,** the inferior edge of the parietal bone, which articulates with the sphenoid and temporal bones along the squamous suture. Called also *sphenotemporal m. of parietal bone, temporal m. of parietal bone, margo squamosus ossis parietalis* [NA], and *squamous border of parietal bone.* **superior m. of parietal bone,** sagittal m. of parietal bone. **supraorbital m. of frontal bone,** the anteroinferior edge of the frontal bone, bending down laterally to the zygomatic bone and medially to the frontal process of the maxilla; it marks the junction between the squama and the orbital part of the frontal bone. Called also *margo supraorbitalis ossis frontalis* [NA], *orbital crest, supraorbital arch of frontal bone,* and *supraorbital rim of frontal bone.* **supraorbital m. of orbit,** the superior edge of the entrance to the orbit, formed by the supraorbital margin of the frontal bone. Called also *margo supraorbitalis orbitae* [NA] and *supraorbital rim of orbit.* **temporal m. of parietal bone,** squamous m. of parietal bone. **temporal m. of zygomatic bone,** the posterior superior margin of the zygomatic bone, forming a curve similar to the letter S. It is continuous with the zygomatic arch and serves as attachment for the temporal fascia. Its posterior inferior border provides attachment for the masseter muscle. Called also *margo temporalis ossis zygomatici* and *temporal border of zygomatic bone.* **m. of tongue, m. of tongue, lateral,** the lateral border of the body of the tongue. Called also *margo lateralis linguae* and *margo linguae* [NA]. **zygomatic m. of great wing of sphenoid bone,** the border on the great wing of the sphenoid bone that separates the temporal and orbital surfaces and articulates with the zygomatic bone. Called also *malar m., jugular crest of great wing of sphenoid bone, malar crest of great wing of sphenoid bone, margo zygomaticus alae magnae, margo zygomaticus alae majoris* [NA], and *zygomatic crest of great wing of sphenoid bone.*

marginal (mar′jĭ-nal) [L. *marginalis,* from *margo* margin] pertaining to a margin or border.

margines (mar′jĭ-nēz) [L.] plural of *margo.*

margo (mar′go), pl. *mar′gines* [L.] an edge or border; used in anatomical nomenclature as a general term to designate the edge of a structure. Called also *border* and *margin.* See also LIMBUS. **m. alveola′ris,** alveolar ARCH. **m. fronta′lis a′lae**

majo′ris [NA], **m. fronta′lis a′lae mag′nae,** frontal margin of great wing of sphenoid bone; see under MARGIN. **m. fronta′lis os′sis parieta′lis** [NA], frontal margin of parietal bone; see under MARGIN. **m. infraorbita′lis maxil′lae** [NA], infraorbital margin of maxilla; see under MARGIN. **m. infraorbita′lis or′bitae** [NA], infraorbital margin of orbit; see under MARGIN. **m. lacrima′lis maxil′lae** [NA], lacrimal margin of maxilla; see under MARGIN. **m. lambdoi′deus squa′mae occipita′lis** [NA], lambdoid margin of occipital bone; see under MARGIN. **m. latera′lis lin′guae, m. lin′guae** [NA], MARGIN of tongue. **m. mastoi′deus squa′mae occipita′lis** [NA], mastoid margin of occipital bone; see under MARGIN. **m. nasa′lis os′sis fronta′lis** [NA], nasal margin of frontal bone; see under MARGIN. **m. na′si,** nasal MARGIN. **m. occipita′lis os′sis parieta′lis** [NA], occipital margin of parietal bone; see under MARGIN. **m. occipita′lis os′sis tempora′**[NA], occipital margin of temporal bone; see under MARGIN. **m. parieta′lis a′lae majo′ris,** [NA], parietal margin of great wing of sphenoid bone; see under MARGIN. **m. parieta′lis os′sis fronta′lis** [NA], parietal margin of frontal bone; see under MARGIN. **m. parieta′lis os′sis tempora′lis** [NA], **m. parieta′lis squa′mae tempora′lis,** parietal margin of temporal bone; see under MARGIN. **m. sagitta′lis os′sis parieta′lis** [NA], sagittal margin of parietal bone; see under MARGIN. **m. sphenoida′lis os′sis tempora′lis** [NA], **m. sphenoida′lis squa′mae tempora′lis,** sphenoidal margin of temporal bone; see under MARGIN. **m. squamo′sus a′lae majo′ris** [NA], **m. squamo′sus a′lae mag′nae,** squamous margin of great wing of sphenoid bone; see under MARGIN. **m. squamo′sus os′sis parieta′lis** [NA], squamous margin of parietal bone; see under MARGIN. **m. supraorbita′lis or′bitae** [NA], supraorbital margin of orbit; see under MARGIN. **m. supraorbita′lis os′sis fronta′lis** [NA], supraorbital margin of frontal bone; see under MARGIN. **m. tempora′lis os′sis zygomat′ici,** temporal margin of zygomatic bone; see under MARGIN. **m. zygomat′icus a′lae majo′ris** [NA], **m. zygomat′icus a′lae mag′nae,** zygomatic margin of great wing of sphenoid bone; see under MARGIN.

Maridex trademark for *dexamethasone.*

Marie-Sainton syndrome [Pierre *Marie,* French physician, 1853–1940; Raymond *Sainton*] cleidocranial DYSPLASIA. See also Bekhterev-Strümpell-Marie SYNDROME and Brissaud-Marie SYNDROME.

mariguana (mar″ĭ-hwah′nah) marihuana.

marihuana (mar″ĭ-hwah′nah) [Portuguese] A crude cannabinoid preparation of the leaves and flowering tops of the plant *Cannabis sativa,* usually employed in cigarettes and inhaled as smoke for its euphoric properties. Sometimes written *mariguana* and *marijuana.* See also CANNABINOID.

marijuana (mar″ĭ-hwah′nah) marihuana.

mark (mark) a blemish; a spot, usually pigmented, on the surface of the skin or mucous membrane. **lightning m.,** a burn mark on the skin characterized by an arborizing pattern, due to an injury of high intensity electric current. See also electric BURN. **portwine m.,** NEVUS flammeus. **static m's,** marks on a radiograph in the form of the branching of tree limbs, smudges, or black spots, due to discharges of static electricity on the film surface. **witness m's,** subperiosteal, small hemispherical depressions prepared in the bone surface instead of abutment grooves as a guide for seating the abutment posts of the implant.

marker (mark′er) something used for marking or identifying objects; an identifying characteristic or feature. **AM m.,** an allotypic determinant found only on the heavy chain of IgA. **genetic m.,** any genetically controlled phenotypic difference or trait that may be used in genetic studies. **periodontal pocket m.,** a set of instruments shaped like cotton pliers. One tip is sharp and bent at a right angle, and the other is blunt and slightly bowed to conform to the tooth contour when it is inserted into the pocket. The blades are joined to the shank with a goose-neck bend to improve accessibility to different tooth surfaces. To mark a pocket, the blunt tip is aligned in the long axis of the tooth and inserted to the bottom of the pocket. The ends are pressed together, creating an external bleeding point which corresponds to the bottom of the pocket. Multiple markings are used to trace the course of pockets on individual surfaces of a tooth. **Richey condyle m.,** trademark for a compass-like instrument for locating the axis in the use of a dental articulator.

marking (mark′ing) a conspicuous line or spot visible on a surface. **carbon m.,** a marking made on the occlusal surface when the mandibular teeth are brought in contact with the maxillary teeth in the centric path of closure, or when the mandible is carried through its excursive movements with mandibular and maxillary teeth in contact; performed to detect occlusal interferences.

marmoreal (mar-mo're-al) resembling marble, as bone in osteopetrosis.

Marochetti's blister see under BLISTER.

Maroteaux-Lamy syndrome [Pierre *Maroteaux;* Maurice *Lamy*] see under SYNDROME.

Marplan trademark for *isocarboxazid.*

marrow (mar'o) 1. the soft material that fills the cavities of the bones. See *bone m.* 2. any substance resembling bone marrow. See also MEDULLA. **bone m.,** a loosely knit gelatinous to semifluid tissue rich in fat, which is partially compartmentalized in cavities of the bones by trabeculae protruding into the cavity. It is made up of a meshwork of connective tissue containing branching fibers, the meshes being filled with marrow cells consisting variously of fat cells, large nucleated cells or myelocytes, and giant cells or megakaryocytes. Called also *medulla ossium.* See *red m.* and *yellow m.* **depressed m.,** bone marrow exhibiting decreased hematopoietic activity. **fat m.,** yellow m. **hematopoietic m.,** red m. **red m., red bone m.,** bone marrow whose principal function is hematopoiesis, which is found in adults, chiefly in the cavities of the vertebrae, ribs, sternum, pelvis, scapulae, skull, and proximal ends of the humerus and femur, and contains mainly hematopoietic cells. It is supplied by a rich vascular system, consisting chiefly of central arteries which send out branches that terminate in capillary beds within the bone or the periphery of the marrow space; some capillaries reenter the marrow and form large venous sinuses that often intercommunicate with each other. Its cellular composition consists of neutrophils, eosinophils, basophils, mast cells, erythrocytes, lymphocytes, plasma cells, monocytes, and megakaryocytes. Biopsy of the red marrow may also contain nonhematopoietic cells, such as reticulum cells, osteoblasts, osteoclasts, and Schwann cells. Called also *hematopoietic m.* and *medulla ossium rubra* [NA]. **yellow m., yellow bone m.,** bone marrow in which fat cells predominate, which is not involved in hematopoiesis, and is found ordinarily in the large cavities of long bones. Under some abnormal conditions, such as in certain types of anemias, it may be replaced by the red marrow. Called also *fat m.* and *medulla ossium flava* [NA].

Marshall's syndrome [D. *Marshall*] see under SYNDROME.

Marshall Hall facies, method of [*Marshall Hall,* English physician, 1790–1887] see under FACIES, and see artificial RESPIRATION.

Marsilid trademark for *iproniazid.*

Marsin trademark for *phenmetrazine hydrochloride* (see under PHENMETRAZINE).

marsupialization (mar-su"pe-al-i-za'shun) [L. *marsupium* pouch] the creation of a pouch; applied especially to surgical exteriorization of a cyst by resection of the anterior wall and stretching the edges over the external incision where they are sutured, thereby establishing an open pouch of what was formerly an enclosed cyst. In treating an oral cyst, the cyst lumen is open to the oral environment to provide a small window which is maintained with a short segment of nylon, a plastic tube, or a rubber dam wick. The cyst usually collapses in several weeks or months and eventually shrinks or disappears entirely. Called also *cyst fenestration.* See also cyst EXTIRPATION and Partach's OPERATION.

martensite (mar'ten-zīt) a supersaturated, body-centered tetragonal solid solution of carbon and iron.

Martialis, Marcus Valerius [A.D. 43(?)–104(?)] a Roman epigrammatist born in Spain, who provides the earliest record of artificial teeth made of bone or ivory. Martialis' works mention Cascellius and his curing of tooth diseases and tooth extraction.

Martin's line, plane see under LINE and PLANE.

Martin-Albright syndrome [Eric *Martin;* Fuller *Albright,* Boston physician, born 1900] pseudohypoparathyroidism.

Martin de Gimard's syndrome [*Martin* Jules Louis Alexander *de Gimard,* born 1858] de Gimard's SYNDROME.

Martricin trademark for *tyrothricin.*

Marzine trademark for *cyclizine.*

MAS, mas milliampere-second.

masarium (mah-sa're-um) former name for *technetium.*

maser (ma'zer) [microwave amplification by stimulated emission of radiation] a device which amplifies microwave energy into an extremely intense, small, and nearly nondivergent beam of monochromatic radiation in the microwave region with all

waves in phase. It was the forerunner of the laser. **optical m.,** laser.

mask (mask) [Fr. *masque*] 1. to cover or conceal, as the masking of the nature of a disorder by the presence of unrelated signs, symptoms, organisms, etc. 2. in audiometry, to obscure or diminish a sound by the presence of another sound of different frequency. 3. an appliance for shading, protecting, or medicating the face. 4. in dentistry, to camouflage metal parts of a prosthesis by covering with opaque material. **full-face m.,** a device used in anesthesia to confine the gas to be delivered through the mask into the respiratory tract through the nose or mouth. **meter m.,** an oxygen-breathing mask designed to provide fixed percentage admixture of air and oxygen. **rubber dam m.,** rubber dam PAD. **Stent m.,** a plastic resinous material which sets into a very hard substance; used in surgery for making molds shaped to keep grafts in place. See also STENT (2). **Wanscher's m.,** a mask for ether anesthesia. **Yankauer's m.,** a mask used in ether anesthesia.

masking (mask'ing) 1. the act of covering, concealing, or disguising. See MASK. 2. an opaque covering to camouflage the metal parts of a dental prosthesis.

mass (mas) [L. *massa*] 1. a lump or body made up of cohering particles. See also MASSA. 2. a cohesive mixture suitable for being made up into pills. 3. that characteristic of matter which gives it inertia. The mass of a hypothetical atom of atomic weight 1.000 (dalton) is 1.648×10^{-24} gm, and the mass of any other atom may be found by multiplying this number by the atomic weight of the atom. The standard unit of mass in SI or in the metric system is the kilogram; in the avoirdupois and apothecaries' weights it is the pound. **atomic m.,** the mass of a neutral atom of a nuclide, usually expressed in atomic mass units *(amu);* being $^1/_{12}$ the mass of the carbon-12 isotope. **electron m.,** atomic mass of the electron, estimated as being approximately 0.00055 amu. **inner cell m.,** see BLASTOCYST. **interfilar m.,** hyaloplasm (1). **intermediate cell m.,** nephrotome. **lateral m. of ethmoid bone,** ethmoid LABYRINTH. **neutron m.,** atomic mass of the neutron, being estimated as approximately 1.00894 amu. **outer cell m.,** see BLASTOCYST. **proton m.,** atomic mass of the proton, estimated as being approximately 1.00758 amu. **Stent m.,** a plastic resinous material which sets into a very hard substance; used in surgery for making molds shaped to keep grafts in place. See also STENT (2).

massa (mas'ah), pl. *mas'sae* [L.] a unified lump, or mass of material; a general anatomical term for an accumulation of cells or cohesive tissue. Called also *mass.* **m. latera'lis os'sis ethmoida'lis,** ethmoid LABYRINTH.

massae (mas'se) [L.] plural of *massa.*

massage (mah-sahzh') [Fr.; Gr. *massein* to knead] the systematic stroking, rubbing, or kneading of the body. **cardiac m.,** rhythmic compression of the heart by pressure applied manually over the sternum (closed or external method) or directly to the heart through an opening in the chest wall (open or internal method), which is done to empty the ventricles in an effort to circulate the blood, and also to stimulate the heart so that it will resume its pumping action. Called also *heart m.* See also cardiopulmonary RESUSCITATION. **gingival m., gum m.,** the systematic application of frictional rubbing and stroking to the gingiva for cleansing purposes and for improving tissue tone, circulation, and keratinization of the gingival tissue. Called also *gingival stimulation* and *ulotripsis.* **heart m.,** cardiac m.

Massel see PMA INDEX (Schour-Massel index).

masseter (mas-se'ter) [Gr. *masētēr* chewer] masseter MUSCLE.

Massler see PMA INDEX (Schour-Massler index).

mast- see MASTO-.

Mastadenovirus (mas-tad"ĕ-no-vi'rus) a genus of adenoviruses isolated from mammalian hosts.

Masterone trademark for *dromostanolone propionate* (see under DROMOSTANOLONE).

mastic (mas'tik) [L. *mastiche;* Gr. *mastiche*] a concrete resinous exudation from the mastic tree, *Pistacia lentiscus,* indigenous to the Mediterranean region composed chiefly of mastinic and masticonic acids. It occurs as pale yellow or greenish-yellow, globular, elongated or tear-shaped substance with a slightly balsamic odor and terebene taste, which is soluble in ethanol, chloroform, and ether, partially soluble in oil turpentine, and insoluble in water. Widely used in Greece as a characteristically flavored chewing gum base. In dentistry, used chiefly as a component of some cavity varnishes. Called also *mastix* and *pistachia galls.* Trademark: Mastisol.

mastication (mas"tĭ-ka'shun) [L. *masticare* to chew] the process of chewing food in preparation for swallowing and digestion, consisting of incision, crushing and diminishing the size of large particles, and milling or trituration of the food preparatory to deglutition. See also masticating CYCLE, masticatory FORCE, masticatory movements, under MOVEMENT, and muscles of mastication, under MUSCLE. **bilateral m.,** chewing of food simultaneously on both sides of the mouth, with multidirectional, alternating bilateral masticatory movements. **unilateral m.,** chewing of food on one side of the mouth, occurring in persons eating soft nonabrasive foods and in conditions where normal occlusal patterns are disturbed by dental and periodontal irregularities or diseases, being a result of adaptation to occlusal interferences.

masticatory (mas'tĭ-kah-to"re) 1. subserving or pertaining to mastication. 2. a remedy to be chewed but not swallowed.

Mastigophora (mas"tĭ-gof'o-rah) [Gr. *mastix* whip + *phorein* to bear] a subphylum of protozoa comprising those having one or more flagella throughout the life cycle and a simple centrally located nucleus. Most are free-living, but many are parasitic in both invertebrates and vertebrates, including man. Genera parasitic to man include *Chilomastix, Trichomonas, Giardia, Trypanosoma,* and *Leishmania.* Called also *Flagellata.*

Mastisol trademark for *mastic.*

mastix (mas'tiks) mastic.

masto-, mast- [Gr. *mastos* breast] a combining form denoting relationship to the breast or to the mastoid process.

mastocyte (mas'to-sīt) [Ger. *Mast* fattening feed + *-cyte*] a connective tissue cell whose specific physiologic function remains unknown; capable of elaborating basophilic, metachromatic cytoplasmic granules which contain histamine, heparin, and, in certain species (e.g., rat and mouse), serotonin. Called also *mast cell.*

mastodynia (mas"to-din'e-ah) [*masto-* + Gr. *odynē* pain] pain in the breast.

mastoid (mas'toid) [Gr. *mastos* breast + *eidos* form] 1. pertaining to or having a conical shape similar to a nipple or a breast. 2. pertaining to the mastoid process or bone.

mastoidale (mas"toi-da'le) the lowest point on the mastoid process.

mastoidalgia (mas"toi-dal'je-ah) [*mastoid* + *-algia*] pain in the mastoid region.

mastoidectomy (mas"toi-dek'to-me) [*mastoid* + Gr. *ektomē* excision] excision of the mastoid cells or the mastoid process of the temporal bone.

mastoideum (mas-toi'de-um) mastoid BONE.

mastoiditis (mas"toi-di'tis) inflammation of the mastoid antrum. **Bezold's m.,** mastoiditis associated with escape of pus into the digastric groove and the head of the sternocleidomastoid muscle.

mastoidotomy (mas"toi-dot'o-me) [*mastoid* + Gr. *temnein* to cut] surgical incision of the mastoid process or bone.

masto-occipital (mas"to-ok-sip'ĭ-tal) pertaining to the mastoid bone or process and the occipital bone.

mastoparietal (mas"to-pah-ri'ĕ-tal) pertaining to the mastoid bone or process and the parietal bone.

masurium (mah-su-re'um) former name for *technetium.*

mat (mat) 1. a protective material or pad placed under an object or a protective covering of a floor. 2. maternal origin; see CHROMOSOME nomenclature. **m. foil,** mat FOIL. **m. gold,** mat GOLD.

matching (mach'ing) comparison for the purpose of selecting objects having similar or identical characteristics. **blood m.,** BLOOD matching. **cross m.,** determination of the compatibility of the blood, without necessarily determining its exact type, by placing the erythrocytes of the donor in the recipient's serum and, conversely, the erythrocytes of the recipient in the donor's serum. Absence of agglutination indicates compatibility. Written also *crossmatching.* **donor-recipient m.,** 1. in organ transplantation, the determination of the histocompatibility of a donor's tissue with that of the recipient. 2. in transfusion of red blood cells, the determination and comparison for compatibility of the groups and types of antigens on the red cell surface. See table.

mater (ma'ter) [L.] mother. **dura m.** [L. "hard mother"], the outermost, toughest, and most fibrous of the three membranes (meninges) enveloping the brain and spinal cord. Called also *pachymeninx.* **pia m.,** [L. "tender mother"] the innermost of the three membranes (meninges), composed of loose connective tissue, which envelops the brain and spinal cord and supports their blood vessels.

materia (mah-te're-ah), pl. *mate'riae* [L.] matter, or substance. **m. al'ba,** a whitish or cream-colored cheesy mass deposited around the necks of the teeth, composed of food debris, mucin, and dead epithelial cells, which serves as a medium for the growth of microorganisms and as a factor in the development of marginal gingivitis. It is usually deposited on neglected dental plaque and indicates poor oral hygiene. Calcified materia alba forms *dental calculus.* **m. den'tica,** that branch of study which deals with medicinal substances used in the practice of dentistry. **m. med'ica,** that branch of medical study which deals with drugs, their sources, preparations, and uses; pharmacology.

materiae (mah-te're-e) [L.] plural of *materia.*

material (mah-te're-al) substance or element from which a concept may be formulated, or an object constructed. **acceptable m.,** any dental material which has been evaluated under the provisions of the acceptance program of the Council of Dental Materials and Devices of the American Dental Association, based on evidence of safety and usefulness established by biological, laboratory, and/or clinical evaluations. Products found both useful and safe are listed in the *Guide to Dental Materials and Devices* and are awarded the Seal of Acceptance, which may be used in advertising, in brochures, and on packages. Called also *acceptable product.* **agar impression m.,** impression m., reversible hydrocolloid. **alginate impression m.,** impression m., irreversible hydrocolloid. **baseplate m.,** any dental material used in the construction of a baseplate, including silver, gold, aluminum, platinum, alloys, and plastics. **blockout m.,** any material used for blockout or to eliminate undercuts on master casts prior to duplication, usually a mixture of wax and clay, hard inlay wax, or a mixture of baseplate wax, adhesive wax, gutta-percha, kaolin, and coloring matter. See also BLOCKOUT and blockout WAX. **cast m.,** CAST material. **coating m.,** a substance, usually a porous, nonmetallic, biologically acceptable substance, such as a carbon, polymer, or ceramic substance, applied over the surface of a metallic implant, so that tissues may proliferate into its substance. **colloid impression m.,** see *impression m., irreversible hydrocolloid* and *impression m., reversible hydrocolloid.* **composite m.,** a three-dimensional combination of at least two chemically different materials with a distinct interface separating the components. **dental m.,** any material used in dental practice, particularly a material used in the production of dental bases, restorations, impressions, or prostheses. The most commonly used dental materials include metal alloys, acrylic resins, cements, porce-

PRINCIPLES OF DONOR-RECIPIENT MATCHING

PRINCIPLE	METHOD USED FOR TESTING
1. No transplantation across ABO incompatibility	Hemagglutination
2. No transplantation in presence of positive cross-match	Lymphocytotoxicity, leukagglutination
3. Attempt to obtain best HLA match from ABO-compatible potential donors	Lymphocytotoxicity
4. Attempt to obtain transplant from donor inducing least mixed lymphocyte response from ABO-compatible, satisfactorily matched, potential donors	Mixed lymphocyte culture reactivity

(From J. A. Bellanti: Immunology II. Philadelphia, W. B. Saunders Co., 1978.)

LINEAR COEFFICIENTS OF THERMAL EXPANSION AND THERMAL CONDUCTIVITY FOR SOME IMPORTANT DENTAL MATERIALS

Material	Linear Coefficient of Thermal Expansion	Coefficient of Thermal Conductivity
	cm./cm.·°C.	cal.·cm./sec.·°C.·cm.²
Dental polymers		
Inlay wax	$\alpha = 350 \times 10^{-6}$	$k = 0.00009$
Impression compound	250	
Silicone rubber	200	
Polysulfide rubber	150	0.0004
Polymethyl methacrylate	81	0.0005
Dental metals		
Amalgam	25	0.055
Co-Cr	18–22	0.165
Gold inlay	14–16	0.80
Gold foil	14–15	0.70
Stainless steel	11	
Dental ceramics		
Tooth (across crown)	11	0.0003–0.002
Silicate cement	8	0.0005
Porcelain	4	

(From E. H. Greener, J. K. Harcourt, and E. P. Lautenschlager: Materials Science in Dentistry. Elmsford, New York, Pergamon Press; adapted from Skinner and Phillips [1967] and Peyton et al. [1971].)

lain, shellac, waxes, vulcanite, polyvinyls, and silicones. See tables. **duplicating m.,** duplicating COMPOUND. **elastic impression m.,** impression m., elastic. **elastomeric impression m.,** impression m., elastomeric. **m. fatigue,** material FATIGUE. **filling m.,** any material used for filling dental cavities or the root canal, including gold, amalgam, dental cements, gutta-percha, zinc oxide–eugenol, chloropercha, and other substances. **m. hardness,** see table at HARDNESS. **hydrocolloid impression m.,** see *impression m., irreversible hydrocolloid* and *impression m., reversible hydrocolloid.* **impression m.,** any material used for making impressions of the teeth and oral structures for the purpose of producing artificial teeth and dentures. They include substances such as plasters, which harden and become rigid in the mouth by a chemical reaction; thermoplastic materials, which are softened by exposure to heat before use and harden once removed from the mouth; and elastic materials, which remain flexible after removal from the mouth. Impression materials include dental plasters, metallic oxide pastes, impression compounds (Types I and II), reversible and irreversible colloids (agar and alginate impression materials), silicone base materials, and duplicating materials. **impression m., alginate,**

APPROXIMATE ROOM TEMPERATURE PROPERTIES OF SOME MATERIALS OF DENTAL INTEREST

Material	Elastic Modulus (E)	Proportional Limit	Ultimate Tensile Strength	Elongation in Tension	Compressive Strength	Elongation in Compression
	kg./cm.²	kg./cm.²	kg./cm.²	%	kg./cm.²	%
Pure gold	9.1×10^5	210	1340	45	1340	45
Casting gold (hard)	9.1×10^5	4900	7000	2	7000	2
316 stainless steel, annealed	20.4×10^5	2450	5600	50	5600	50
Cast Co-Cr	21.1×10^5	4200	7000	3		
Dental amalgam	2.1×10^5	560	560	0	3500	1
Silicate cement	2.1×10^5		(Poor)	0	1750	0
Plaster of Paris						
$\frac{W}{P} = 0.45$			(Poor)	0	126	0
$\frac{W}{P} = 0.55$			(Poor)	0	91	0
Dental stone						
$\frac{W}{P} = 0.30$			(Poor)	0	245	0
Polymethyl methacrylate	3.5×10^4	280	560	2	770	3
Enamel	4.8×10^5	700	700	0	2700	0
Dentin	1.4×10^5	420	420	0	2500	1

*$\frac{W}{P}$ = water to powder ratio.

(From E. H. Greener, J. K. Harcourt, and E. P. Lautenschlager: Materials Science in Dentistry. Elmsford, New York, Pergamon Press, 1972.)

impression m., irreversible hydrocolloid. **impression m., elastic,** a material which will produce an impression that would be sufficiently elastic to be withdrawn from the mouth over sharp undercuts and return to its original shape without distortion, while retaining an accurate impression of a tooth. Rubber, reversible and irreversible hydrocolloids, and silicone base materials are the principal elastic materials. Cf. *impression m., inelastic.* **impression m., elastomeric,** an elastic impression material which is soft and rubber-like, technically known as an elastomer. Elastomeric materials include polysulfide, silicone, and polyether prepolymer base materials. Called also *rubber impression m.* **impression m., heavy body,** see *impression m., polysulfide,* and *impression m., silicone.* **impression m., inelastic,** an impression material, such as plaster, that hardens into a rigid solid upon setting. Used chiefly for making impressions for full dentures where there are no undercuts that would prevent removal of the impression without distortion or fracture. Impressions made of inelastic material are sometimes fractured intentionally to remove the pieces which then may be reassembled. Cf. *impression m., elastic.* **impression m., irreversible hydrocolloid,** an elastic impression material that changes from a sol to a gel but not from a gel to a sol. Main constituents are a soluble alginate, a reactor, such as calcium sulfate (dihydrate, hemihydrate, or anhydrite), and a retarder, such as trisodium phosphate. Also included are potassium titanium fluoride, which gives the material a stonelike surface and acts as an accelerator for the setting of gypsum components; zinc oxide; and diatomaceous earth, which serves as a filler. Some types contain triethanol amine alginate and carbonates substituting for phosphate. Such materials may be classified as fast setting (gelation time of 1–2 min) and normal setting (2–4 min). Upon mixing with water, the three components start to dissolve, the retarder tying up the reactor briefly to allow the placing of the material in the mouth on an impression tray. Gelation occurs by chemical reaction whereby the sol hardens to an elastic gel, the temperature not being a factor in the reaction. Used chiefly in partial and complete prosthodontics, orthodontics, and less frequently, study casts and fixed bridge prosthodontics. Called also *alginate impression m.* Trademarks: Algident, Coe Alginate, Hydro-Jel A, Jeltrate, Opotow Jelset, Palginex 75, Plastodent Elastic Impression Powder, UniJel. **impression m., light body,** see *impression m., polysulfide,* and *impression m., silicone.* **impression m., plaster,** impression PLASTER. **impression m., polyether,** an elastomeric material used chiefly in fixed partial prosthodontics and for quadrant inlay and crown impressions. Both the polyether base and the aromatic sulfonate ester reactor are available as pastes, which are mixed before being used for making impressions on a tray. The material also contains a colloidal silica as a filler and a plasticizer, such as glycolether phthalate. A body modifier or thinner is used to reduce stiffness of the material. Called also *polyether rubber.* **impression m., polysulfide,** an elastomeric material used chiefly in fixed partial prosthodontics and for quadrant inlay and crown impressions. Also used as a wash or secondary impression material for complete dentures and as a stabilizing liner for occlusion rims. Impressions are made by mixing the polysulfide base (prepolymer base) and a peroxide (usually lead peroxide) until the contrasting colors of the two components are completely blended. Various fillers, plasticizers, coloring pigments, and deodorizers are also included in the material, such as sulfur, zinc oxide, zinc sulfide, silica, titanium dioxide, calcium carbonate, and organic amines. The addition of lead peroxide causes both lengthening of the polymer chain and oxidation of terminal −SH groups and crosslinking by oxidation of pendant −SH groups. Three types are used: *Class 1,* a heavy body type, with high viscosity, used most commonly with a custom-made tray; *Class 2,* a regular body type, with medium viscosity, used generally with a custom-made tray; and *Class 3,* a light body type, with low viscosity, used most commonly with a syringe. Trademarks: Coe Flex, Kerr Permaplastic, LP-2, Mieradent 70, Omniflex, ProFlex, Sta-Tic. **impression m., regular body,** see *impression m., polysulfide,* and *impression m., silicone.* **impression m., reversible hydrocolloid,** an elastic impression material that can change from a sol to a gel and back to a sol. Agar is its principal constituent, having a gelation temperature of about 37°C (99°F) and a liquefaction temperature of 60 to 70°C (108 to 126°F). Other components include water, borates, sulfates, hard wax, thixotropic materials; some materials also contain fillers added for viscosity, strength, and rigidity, such as diatomaceous earth, clay, silica, rubber, and other substances. Thymol and glycerin are sometimes added as a bactericide and plasticizer, respectively. Pigments and flavoring agents are usually added. The addition of hydrochloric acid decreases the rigidity of the gel. The material is placed in an impression tray in the sol condition and impressed against the tissue, cold water circulating through tubes on the outside of the tray while it is held in place. When the material has gelled, the tray is removed and the impression is prepared for the pouring of the dental stone. Called also *agar impression m.* Trademarks: Deelastic, Rubberloid, Surgident. **impression m., rubber,** impression m., elastomeric. **impression m., silicone,** an elastomeric material used chiefly in fixed partial prosthodontics and for quadrant inlay and crown impressions. Also used as the wash or secondary impression material for complete dentures. The base material is a silicone liquid which, upon mixing with silica powder, produces a paste. Polymerization is carried out by the use of a catalyst (tin octoate) and a reactor (alkyl silicate). Four types are used: *Class 1,* a heavy body type, with high viscosity, used chiefly with custom-made trays; *Class 2,* a regular body type with a medium viscosity, also used with custom-made trays; *Class 3,* a light body material with a low viscosity, used mainly with a syringe; and *putty silicone,* a doughlike material used with trays. The addition of a diluting agent to a heavy body material will allow it to be used with a syringe. See also SILICONE. Trademarks: Citricon, Elasticon, Flexicon, Jelcone, Kerr Traycon, SIR, Xantopren. **impression m., thermoplastic,** an impression material which is soft at higher temperatures but hardens in the oral environment. **impression m., wash,** Type I impression material used to line the surface of a tray produced by the primary impression method, for the reproduction of fine details of structures of an edentulous mouth through the secondary impression method. **inelastic impression m.,** impression m., inelastic. **investment m.,** investment. **polyether impression m.,** impression m., polyether. **polysulfide impression m.,** impression m., polysulfide. **provisionally acceptable m.,** a dental material which, on the basis of biological, laboratory, and/or clinical evaluations, has been established as lacking sufficient evidence to justify classification as "acceptable," but for which there is reasonable evidence of safety and usefulness, including clinical feasibility. Materials classified as "provisionally acceptable" are listed in the *Guide to Dental Materials and Devices,* published by the Council on Dental Materials and Devices of the American Dental Association, but the Council may authorize the use of a suitable statement to define specifically the area of usefulness in this category. Provisionally acceptable materials are reviewed annually for up to 3 years. Called also *provisionally acceptable product.* **refractory m.,** refractory (3). **restorative m.,** any material used in dental restorations which, according to G. V. Black's criteria, should be adaptable to cavity walls, be indestructible by oral fluids, should not alter its shape or volume after insertion, have adequate strength and hardness, have the degree of resistance to attrition that is comparable to that of tooth structure, have a harmonious and stable color, be nonirritating, have low thermal conductivity, and be easy to manipulate. No present restoration material encompasses all of these ideal characteristics. Gold and alloys, porcelain, amalgams, resins, and cements are the principal restorative materials. **rubber impression m.,** impression m., elastomeric. **m's science,** materials SCIENCE. **silicone impression m.,** impression m., silicone. **temporary m.,** a dental material used in temporary restorations, usually a composite resin, unfilled resin, silicate cement, silicophosphate cement, polycarboxylate cement, zinc phosphate cement, low-fusing metal, zinc oxide–eugenol cement, and gutta-percha. **tissue-equivalent m.,** see tissue EQUIVALENT. **unacceptable m.,** a dental material which, in the judgment of the Council on Dental Materials and Devices of the American Dental Association, is dangerous to the health of the user, or is obsolete, markedly inferior, or useless. Called also *unacceptable product.* **wash impression m.,** impression m., wash.

matrices (ma'tri-sēz) [L.] plural of *matrix.*

matrix (ma'triks), pl. *ma'trices* [L.] 1. a seat of a tissue or organ. 2. the groundwork on which anything is cast, or that basic material from which a thing develops. 3. a mold or a form for casting. 4. basic material which binds together the material in an agglomerated mass. 5. a plastic or metal strip used to support and shape a plastic restorative material. See also matrix RETAINER. 6. a piece of gold or platinum foil fitted against the sides and bottom of a cavity, used as a mold in which porcelain for an inlay is baked. 7. an intergranular substance which serves as a cementing material for other particles, such as phosphate compounds serving as a cementing material for zinc oxide particles. **amalgam m.,** a metal strip, usually of stainless steel or other material not reacting with mercury, about 0.0015 to 0.002 inch thick, adapted to a prepared cavity to supply the missing wall, thereby confining and contouring the plastic amalgam mass during condensation. **amorphous cell m.,** hyaloplasm (1). **m. band,** matrix BAND. **bone m.,** the intercellular material representing the bulk of the bone,

made up of collagen fibril bundles and ground substance. Embedded in the matrix are the lacunae in which osteocytes are found and the canaliculi through which canaliculi communicate with each other and form a syncytium-like network. Its inorganic component consists chiefly of submicroscopic crystals of an apatite of calcium and phosphate and of citrate and carbonate ions. The apatite crystals, which are deposited in the form of slender needles 200 to 400 Å in length by 15 to 30 Å in thickness, are located within the substance of the collagen fibers. Bone matrix also serves as a storage depot for magnesium and sodium. Called also ground *substance of bone.* **cartilage m.,** a component of cartilage in which chondrocytes are embedded. It is made up of the ground substance consisting of chondromucoprotein, a copolymer of mucoprotein, chondroitin-4-sulfate (chondroitin sulfate A) and chondroitin-6-sulfate (chondroitin sulfate C), and fine collagen fibrils. **celluloid m.,** a strip of celluloid used to compress, contain, and contour resin or cement restorative materials. **custom m.,** one that is precontoured, fitted, and stabilized in order to provide for restoration of physiologic contours and contact. **dentin m.,** the intercellular material of dentin, made up of organic and inorganic matter; its inorganic component represents 25 percent of the total volume and 80 percent of the total weight. It is a form of connective tissue, both its formed and unformed constituents being of ectomesenchymal origin; the formed elements are collagenous and the unformed part (ground substance) is made up chiefly of mucopolysaccharides, being closely related to the chondroitin sulfate of the cartilage. During its early development, the matrix is organic in nature, but later it becomes mineralized by calcium phosphate. The collagen fibrils of the matrix are 3 μ in diameter and show bands at regular intervals. **direct porcelain m.,** a platinum-foil matrix adapted directly to the tooth preparation for the direct technique. **functional m.,** the contiguous and motivating soft tissue organs and tissues in the growth of the craniofacial complex. **m. holder,** matrix RETAINER. **plastic m.,** a matrix of resin or plastic for use with cold-curing resin or cement. **platinum m.,** one of wrought platinum foil, usually 0.001 inch or less in thickness, adapted to a die of a preparation for a fired porcelain restoration. It serves as a vehicle to carry and maintain the application of porcelain when it is placed in a furnace for firing. **resin m.,** in a composite resin, the resin component which forms a matrix for the filler material. The most commonly used resin is a compound derived from an epoxy resin and a methacrylate resin, where the reaction sites (oxirane group) of the epoxy molecule were replaced by methacrylate groups, the hybrid molecule being polymerized through the methacrylate group. The compound is sometimes classified as a thermosetting methacrylate resin. See also DIMETHACRYLATE. **m. retainer,** matrix RETAINER. **T-band m.,** a metal band cut with a T-shaped projection at one end, the lugs being bent over to engage the band as it encircles the tooth.

Matromycin trademark for *oleandomycin.*

matter (mat'er) 1. anything that possesses mass and occupies space, existing in three states, solid, liquid, or gas, depending on the temperature and pressure. 2. pus. **gray m.,** gray SUBSTANCE. **white m.,** white SUBSTANCE.

Matulane trademark for *procarbazine hydrochloride* (see under PROCARBAZINE).

maturate (mat'u-rāt) 1. to mature. 2. to suppurate.

maturation (mat"u-ra'shun) [L. *maturatio; maturus* ripe] the stage or process of becoming mature.

mature (mah-chur') [L. *maturus*] 1. to come to maturity, or ripen. 2. fully developed; ripe.

maturity (mah-chur'ĭ-te, mah-tur'ĭ-te) 1. the period of attainment of maximal development. 2. the state or quality of being fully grown, or mature. 3. in the firing of dental porcelain, the last stage whereby the porcelain undergoes vitrification. True color and translucency of the porcelain and sheen on its surface are the signs of maturity of fired porcelain. See also high biscuit FIRING, maturing TEMPERATURE, and VITRIFICATION.

Matut. abbreviation for L. *matuti'nus,* in the morning.

Mauthner's membrane, sheath [Ludwig *Mauthner,* Austrian ophthalmologist, 1840–1894] axolemma.

Maxidex trademark for *dexamethasone.*

maxilla (mak-sil'ah), pl. *maxil'lae* [L.] [NA] an irregularly shaped bone that with its fellow forms a major part of the bony framework of the facial skeleton and assists in forming the roof of the mouth, the floor of the orbit, and the sides of the nasal cavity, and bears the upper teeth. It consists of the body of the maxilla and the zygomatic, nasal, palatine, and alveolar processes. The anterior (facial) surface presents inferiorly a series of

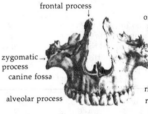

lacrimal notch
ant. lacrimal crest
frontal process
orbital surface
infraorbital groove
openings of
alveolar canals
zygomatic process
maxillary tuberosity
nasal notch
infraorbital foramen
palatine process
ridges caused by
roots of teeth
alveolar process
canine fossa

A

frontal process
nasolacrimal groove
contact area with
nasal bone
ethmoidal crest
nasal surface
nasal notch
ant. nasal spine
contact area with
ethmoid bone
ethmoidal air cells
invading maxilla
maxillary hiatus
greater palatine groove
incisive canal
palatine process

B

frontal process
orbital surface
infraorbital margin
contact area for
zygomatic bone
infraorbital foramen
nasal notch
ant. surface
ridges caused by
roots of teeth
zygomatic
process
canine fossa
alveolar process
intermaxillary suture

C

A, Right maxilla (lateral aspect). *B*, Right maxilla (medial aspect). *C*, Maxillae (frontal aspect). (From J. Langman and M. W. Woerdeman: Atlas of Medical Anatomy. Philadelphia, W. B. Saunders Co., 1978.)

eminences which correspond to the roots of the teeth, and is separated superiorly from the orbital aspect by the infraorbital ridge, medially by the nasal notch, and posteriorly by the zygomatic process. The posterior (infratemporal) surface articulates with the palatine bone and is bounded by the posterior edge of the zygomatic process. The superior (orbital) surface forms part of the floor of the orbit and is bounded by the lacrimal notch and the inferior orbital fissure. The medial (nasal) surface forms an opening to the maxillary sinus. Its superior border has some broken air cells which are closed by the ethmoid and lacrimal bones. It ossifies from one center in the maxilla proper and one in the premaxilla. The suture between the two portions of the maxilla persists into adult life. Called also *superior maxillary bone, supermaxilla, supramaxilla, upper jaw,* and *upper jaw bone.* Cf. MANDIBLE. See illustration and also see illustration at MANDIBLE. **lower m.,** mandible.

maxillae (mak-sĭl′e) [L.] plural of *maxilla.*

maxillary (mak′sĭ-ler″e) [L. *maxillaris*] pertaining to the maxilla.

maxillectomy (mak″sĭ-lek′to-me) [*maxilla* + Gr. *ektomē* excision] excision of the maxilla. **partial m.,** hemimaxillectomy.

maxillitis (mak″sĭ-li′tis [*maxilla* + *-itis*] inflammation of the maxilla.

maxillodental (mak′sĭl″o-den′tal) pertaining to or affecting the maxillae and the teeth.

maxillofacial (mak-sĭl″o-fa′shal) pertaining to the maxillae and the face.

maxillofrontale (mak″sĭl-o-fron-ta′le) the craniometric point where the prolongation of the anterior crest crosses the maxillofrontal suture. Abbreviated *Mf.* See illustration at CEPHALOMETRY.

maxillojugal (mak-sĭl″o-ju′gal) pertaining to the maxilla and the zygoma.

maxillolabial (mak-sĭl″o-la′be-al) pertaining to the maxilla and the lip.

maxillomandibular (mak-sĭl″o-man-dib′u-lar) pertaining to the maxilla and the mandible.

maxillopalatine (mak-sĭl″o-pal′ah-tīn) pertaining to the maxilla and the palate or palatine bone.

maxillopharyngeal (mak-sĭl″o-fah-rin′je-al) pertaining to the maxilla and the pharynx.

maxillotomy (mak″sĭ-lot′o-me) surgical sectioning of the maxilla which allows movement of all or a part of the maxilla into the desired position. Called also *maxillary osteotomy.*

maxima (mak′sĭ-mah) [L.] plural of *maximum.*

maximal (mak′sĭ-mal) the greatest possible; the reverse of minimal.

Maximed trademark for *protriptyline hydrochloride* (see under PROTRIPTYLINE).

maximum (mak′sĭ-mum), pl. *max′ima* [L. "greatest"] 1. the greatest, highest, or largest number, quantity, or degree attainable. 2. the acme of a process, such as a disease. **annual policy m.,** maximum annual BENEFIT.

Maxipen trademark for *phenethicillin.*

Maxitate trademark for *mannitol hexanitrate* (see under MANNITOL).

Maxiton trademark for *dextroamphetamine sulfate* (see under DEXTROAMPHETAMINE).

maxwell (maks′wel) [named after James Clerk *Maxwell*] the unit of magnetic flux, replaced in SI by the weber.

Maxwell, James Clerk [1831–1878] a British physicist. See MAXWELL.

May-Hegglin anomaly (syndrome) [Richard *May;* Robert *Hegglin*] see under ANOMALY.

Maycor trademark for *isosorbide dinitrate* (see under ISOSORBIDE).

mayer (ma′er) [named after J. R. von *Mayer*] a unit of heat capacity; it is the capacity of a body that is warmed 1°C by 1 joule. Abbreviated *my.*

Mayer, Julius Robert von [1814–1878] a German physicist. See MAYER.

Mayne muscle control appliance, space maintainer [W. R. *Mayne,* American orthodontist] see under APPLIANCE and MAINTAINER.

M.B. abbreviation for L. *Medici′nae Baccalau′reus,* Bachelor of Medicine.

m.b. abbreviation for L. *mis′ce be′ne,* mix well.

MBC maximum breathing CAPACITY.

MBDG mesiobuccal developmental GROOVE.

MC Master of Surgery (L. *Magis′ter Chirur′giae*); Medical Corps.

Mc 1. megacurie. 2. megacycle. 3. see MAC.

mc millicurie.

μc microcurie.

MCA multiple congenital anomaly.

mcg microgram.

MCH mean corpuscular hemoglobin; an expression of the average hemoglobin content of a single cell in micrograms, obtained by multiplying the hemoglobin in grams by 10 and dividing by the number of red cells (in millions).

mch millicurie-hour.

MCHC mean corpuscular hemoglobin concentration; an expression of the average hemoglobin concentration in percent, obtained by multiplying the hemoglobin in grams by 100 and dividing by the hematocrit determination.

mc-hr millicurie-hour.

μC hr microcurie-hour.

mCi millicurie.

μCi microcurie.

mcoul millicoulomb.

μcoul microcoulomb.

MCV 1. mean corpuscular volume; an expression of the average volume of individual erythrocytes in cubic microns, obtained by multiplying the hematocrit determination by 10 and dividing by the number of erythrocytes (in millions). 2. mean clinical value; a number obtained by assigning a numerical value to the response as noted in a number of patients receiving a specific treatment, adding these numbers, and dividing by the number of patients treated.

MD Doctor of Medicine (see under DOCTOR).

Md mendelevium.

MD156 see American National Standards Committee MD156 for Dental Materials and Devices, under COMMITTEE.

Me 1. methyl. 2. menton.

meal (mēl) 1. a portion of food or foods taken at some particular and usually stated or fixed time. 2. a coarsely ground substance, prepared from various grains. **bismuth m.,** one containing an opaque bismuth preparation; used in radiography. **opaque m.,** a light meal, sometimes a glass of buttermilk, which contains some substance opaque to x-rays, so that the outline of the intestinal tract can be determined during radiography.

mean (mēn) an average; a numerical value intermediate between two extremes. In statistical methods, the abscissa of the center of gravity of the variables or of the frequency polygon. **arithmetical m.,** the arithmetical average. **geometrical m.,** the antilogarithm of the arithmetical mean of the logarithm of a series of values.

measles (me′zelz) an acute, viral disease of children, usually transmitted by direct contact. The incubation period is 10–12 days; in the prodromal stage small red spots (*Koplik's spots*) appear on the buccal and pharyngeal mucosa, in association with mild fever, conjunctivitis, coryza, and cough; and in the third stage a maculopapular rash erupts over the neck and face and descends to the body, arms, and legs, and the fever is high. Neutropenia is common. Koplik's spots usually increase in number and coalesce to form small patches. Complications may include bronchopneumonia, otitis media, sinusitis, laryngitis, and encephalomyelitis. Inflammation, congestion, swelling, and ulceration of the gingiva, palate, and throat may also occur. Called also *rubeola*. See also measles VIRUS. **German m.,** rubella.

measure (mezh′er) [L. *mensurare*] 1. to determine the extent of quantity of a substance. 2. a specific extent or quantity of a substance. 3. a graduated scale by which the dimensions or mass of an object or substance may be determined. See also SI.

measurement (mezh′er-ment) [L. *mensuratio*] the act or process of determining the size or dimensions of an object. **tooth m.,** determination of the dimensions of a tooth, usually with the use of the Boley gauge: *length of crown* (labial), from the curvature at the cementoenamel junction, to the incisal edge, in anterior teeth; *length of crown* (buccal), from the crest of buccal cusp or cusps, to the crest of curvature at the cementoenamel junction, in posterior teeth; *length of root*, from the apex of the root, to the crest of curvature at crown cervix; *mesiodistal diameter of crown*, from the crest of curvature on the mesial surface, to the crest of curvature on the distal surface; *mesiodistal diameter of crown at the cervix*, from the junction of crown and root on the mesial surface, to the junction of crown and root on the distal surface; *labiolingual diameter of crown*, from the crest of curvature on the labial surface, to the crest of curvature on the lingual surface, in anterior teeth; *labiolingual diameter of crown at the cervix*, from the junction of crown and root on the labial surface, to the junction of crown and root on the lingual surface, in anterior teeth; *curvature of cementoenamel junction on the mesial*, from the crest of curvature at the cementoenamel junction, labial and lingual surfaces, to the crest of curvature at the cementoenamel junction on the mesial surface, in anterior teeth; *curvature of cementoenamel junction on the distal*, from the crest of curvature at the cementoenamel junction on the labial and lingual surfaces, to the crest of curvature at the cementoenamel junction on the distal surface, in anterior teeth; *buccolingual diameter of crown*, from the crest of curvature on the buccal surface, to the crest of curvature on the lingual surface, in posterior teeth; *buccolingual diameter of crown at the cervix*, from the junction of crown and root on the buccal surface, to the junction of crown and root on the lingual surface, in posterior teeth; *curvature of cementoenamel junction on the mesial*, from the crest of curvature at the cementoenamel junction on the mesial surface, to the crest of curvature of cementoenamel junction, buccal and lingual surface, in posterior teeth; *curvature of cementoenamel junction on the distal*, from the crest of curvature of cementoenamel junction on the distal surface, to the crest of curvature at the cementoenamel junction on the buccal and lingual surfaces, in posterior teeth. See also table of *Tooth measurements* at TOOTH.

meat (mēt) any edible flesh, especially that of mammals. **m. sugar,** inositol.

meatus (me-a′tus), pl. *mea′tus* [L. "a way, path, course"] an opening; in anatomical nomenclature used as a general term to designate an opening or some passageway in the body. **m. acus′ticus exter′nus** [NA], external acoustic m. **m. acus′ticus exter′nus cartilagin′eus** [NA], cartilaginous external acoustic m. **m. acus′ticus exter′nus os′seus** [NA], bony external acoustic m. **m. acus′ticus inter′nus** [NA], internal acoustic m. **m. acus′ticus inter′nus os′seus** [NA], bony internal acoustic m. **m. audito′rius exter′nus,** external acoustic m. **m. audito′rius exter′nus cartilagin′eus,** cartilaginous external acoustic m. **m. audito′rius exter′nus os′seus,** bony external acoustic m. **m. audito′rius inter′nus,** internal acoustic m. **m. audito′rius inter′nus os′seus,** bony internal acoustic m. **bony common nasal m.,** the space on either side of the nasal septum bounded by the bones of the cranium. Called also *m. nasi communis osseus* [NA]. **bony external acoustic m., bony external auditory m.,** the opening in the external surface of the temporal bone, posterior to the condyle of the mandible and anterior to the mastoid air cells. Called also *m. acusticus externus osseus* [NA] and *m. auditorius externus osseus.* **bony inferior nasal m.,** the opening in the cranium overhung by the inferior nasal concha. Called also *m. nasi inferior osseus* [NA]. **bony internal acoustic m., bony internal auditory m.,** the opening on the posterior surface of the petrous part of the temporal bone through which the facial, intermediate, and vestibulocochlear nerves, and the labyrinthine artery pass. Called also *meatus acusticus internus osseus* [NA] and *m. auditorius internus osseus.* **bony middle nasal m.,** the opening in the cranium overhung by the middle bony nasal concha. Called also *m. nasi medius osseus* [NA]. **bony nasopharyngeal m.,** the opening in the cranium between the posterior edges of the middle and inferior bony nasal conchae and the choanae. Called also *m. nasopharyngeus osseus* [NA]. **bony superior nasal m.,** a channel-like opening in the cranium inferior to the superior bony nasal concha. Called also *m. nasi superior osseus* [NA]. **cartilaginous external acoustic m., cartilaginous external auditory m.,** the cartilaginous part of the external acoustic meatus, found lateral to the bony part. Called also *m. acusticus externus cartilagineus* [NA] and *m. auditorius externus cartilagineus.* **common nasal m.,** the anterior space on either side of the nasal septum into which the three nasal meatuses open. Called also *m. nasi communis.* **m. con′chae ethmoturbina′lis mino′ris** superior nasal m. **m. con′chae maxilloturbina′lis,** **m. con′chae turbina′lis majo′ris** [NA], inferior nasal m. **external acoustic m., external auditory m.,** the narrow passage of the external ear leading to the tympanic membrane. Called also *m. acusticus externus* [NA] and *m. auditorius externus.* **inferior nasal m.,** the space beneath the inferior nasal concha, into which the nasolacrimal duct opens. Called also *m. conchae maxilloturbinalis, m. conchae turbinalis majoris,* and *m. nasi inferior* [NA]. **internal acoustic m., internal auditory m.,** the passage in the petrous part of the temporal bone, through which the facial, intermediate, and vestibulocochlear nerves and the labyrinthine artery pass. Called also *m. acusticus internus* [NA] and *m. auditorius internus.* **middle nasal m.,** the space beneath the middle nasal concha, with which the anterior ethmoidal cells of the labyrinth and frontal and maxillary sinuses communicate. Called also *m. nasi medius* [NA]. **m. na′si commu′nis,** common nasal m. **m. na′si commu′nis os′seus** [NA], bony common nasal m. **m. na′si infe′rior** [NA], inferior nasal m. **m. na′si infe′rior os′seus** [NA], bony inferior nasal m. **m. na′si me′dius** [NA], middle nasal m. **m. na′si me′dius os′seus** [NA] bony middle nasal m. **m. na′si supe′rior** [NA], superior nasal m. **m. na′si supe′rior os′seus** [NA], bony superior nasal m. **nasopharyngeal m., m. nasopharyn′geus** [NA], the part of the nasal cavity coinciding with the bony nasopharyngeal cavity. Called also *posterior nasal sulcus.* **m. nasopharyn′geus os′seus** [NA], bony nasopharyngeal m. **superior nasal m.,** the narrow cavity below the superior nasal concha, with which the posterior ethmoidal cells communicate. Called also *m. conchae ethmoturbinalis minoris, m. nasi superior* [NA], and *ethmoid fissure.*

Mebaral trademark for *mephobarbital.*

mecamylamine (mek″ah-mil′ah-mēn) a nondepolarizing ganglionic blocking agent, N,2,3,3-tetramethylbicyclo [2.2.1] heptan-2-amine, used therapeutically as the hydrochloride salt, which occurs as a white, odorless, crystalline powder that is soluble in water and chloroform, slightly soluble in benzene, and insoluble in ether. Used in the treatment of hypertension. Orthostatic hypotension, blurring of vision, xerostomia, diarrhea followed by constipation, paralytic ileus, nausea, vomiting, urinary retention, fatigue, and impotence are some of the side reactions. Tremor, delusions, and hallucinations may occur. Trademarks: Inversine, Mekamine, Mevasine, Reveramine.

mechanic (me-kan′ik) a person who is skillful in the building or operation of machinery, tools, or equipment; a craftsman or artisan. **dental m.,** denturist.

mechanism (mek′ah-nizm) [Gr. *mēchanē* machine] 1. a machine or machine-like structure. 2. the manner of combination of parts which subserve a common function. **extrinsic m.,** extrinsic SYSTEM. **intrinsic m.,** intrinsic SYSTEM.

mechanoreceptor (mek″ah-no-re-sep′tor) a sensory receptor (see receptor [6]) that is excited by mechanical pressure or deformations, such as those responding to sound, touch, and muscular contraction. Called also *pressure receptor.*

mechlorethamine (me″klor-eth′ah-mēn) the first nitrogen mustard developed, 2′,2′-dichloro-*N*-methyldiethylamine, occurring as a mobile liquid with a faint odor, which is slightly soluble in water and miscible with organic solvents and oils. It is a poison with vesicant and necrotizing properties. Called also *nitrogen mustard* and *HN2*. Trademark: Stickstofflost. **m. hydrochloride**, the hydrochloride salt of mechlorethamine, occurring as a white, hygroscopic, crystalline powder that is soluble in water and ethanol. It was the first nitrogen tried clinically as an antineoplastic agent. Used as a cytotoxic drug in the treatment of Hodgkin's disease and lymphomas. Also used in mycosis fungoides and rheumatoid arthritis. Adverse reactions may include nausea, vomiting, bone marrow depression with leukopenia and thrombocytopenia, bleeding tendency, skin eruptions, predisposition to infection, menstrual disorders, hyperuricemia, alopecia, metallic taste, headache, drowsiness, fetal abnormalities, induration and sloughing of the skin and mucous membranes, and thrombophlebitis. Trademarks: Cloramin, Dichloren, Mustargen, Mustine.

Mechnikov, Ilia Ilich see METCHNIKOFF.

Mecholyl trademark for *methacholine*.

Meciclin trademark for *demeclocycline hydrochloride* (see under DEMECLOCYCLINE).

Meckel's cartilage (rod), plane [Johann Friedrich *Meckel* (the younger), German anatomist, 1781–1833] see under CARTILAGE and PLANE.

Meckel's ganglion [Johann Friedrich *Meckel* (the elder), German anatomist, 1714–1774] pterygopalatine GANGLION.

meckelectomy (mek″el-ek′to-me) [*Meckel's* ganglion + Gr. *ektomē* excision] surgical removal of Meckel's lesser (submandibular) ganglion.

mecocephalic (me″ko-sĕ-fal′ik) [Gr. *mēkos* length + Gr. *kephalē* head] dolichocephalic.

mecrylate (mĕ-kri′lāt) a cyanoacrylate compound, 2-cyano-2-propanoic acid methyl ester, produced when formaldehyde is condensed with the corresponding alkyl cyanoacetates. It is an adhesive substance originally developed as a commercial bonding agent. Used as a tissue adhesive and as a pit and fissure sealant. Trademarks: AD/here, Coapt, Eastman Kodak 910.

MED 1. minimal effective DOSE. 2. minimal erythema DOSE.

Medawar, Peter B. [born 1915] an English biologist; co-winner, with Sir Frank Macfarlane Burnet, of the Nobel prize for medicine and physiology in 1960, for the theoretical solution to the problem of transplanting tissues and organs from one animal to another.

Medex (med′eks) [Fr. *médicin extension* extension of the physician] a physician assistant program developed specifically for former military medical corpsmen with independent duty experience, generally consisting of three months of university training and twelve months of preceptorship.

media (me′de-ah) [L.] 1. plural of *medium* 2. TUNICA media.

mediad (me′de-ad) [L. *medium* middle + *ad* toward] toward a median line or plane.

medial (me′de-al) [L. *medialis*] 1. pertaining to the middle; closer to the median plane or the midline of the body or a structure; median or mesial. Many anatomical structures formerly called internal are now termed medial. 2. pertaining to the middle layer.

Medialan trademark for *sodium lauroyl sarcosinate* (see under SODIUM).

medialis (me″de-a′lis) medial; a general anatomical term denoting a structure situated nearer to the median plane or the midline of a body or structure.

median (me′de-an) [L. *medianus*] situated in the median plane or in the midline of a body or structure; medial or mesial.

medianus (me″de-a′nus) [L.] median, or situated in the middle; a general anatomical term denoting structures lying in the median plane, that is, the plane dividing the body into right and left halves.

mediastina (me″de-as-ti′nah) [L.] plural of *mediastinum*.

mediastinum (me″de-as-ti′num), pl. *mediasti′na* [L.] 1. a median septum or partition. 2. [NA] the mass of tissues and organs separating the two lungs. It contains the heart and its large vessels, trachea, esophagus, thymus, lymph nodes, and other structures and tissues.

mediator (me′de-a″tor) an object or structure by which something is mediated, such as (1) a structure of the nervous system that transmits impulses eliciting a specific response; (2) a chemical substance (see transmitter SUBSTANCE) that induces activity in tissues, such as nerve or muscle; or (3) a substance released

from cells as the result of the interacton of antigen with antibody, e.g., allergen with antibody on a mast cell, or by the action of antigen with a sensitized lymphocyte, e.g., release of lymphokines.

Medicaid (med′ĭ-kād) a federally-aided but state-operated and administered program providing medical benefits to certain low-income persons in need of health and medical care, which was authorized by title XIX of the Social Security Act. The program provides benefits to persons who are normally qualified to receive welfare cash payments, including the poor, aged, blind, disabled, and members of families with dependent children where one parent is absent, incapacitated, or unemployed. Under certain circumstances, states may provide Medicaid coverage for children under the age of 21 who are not categorically related. Subject to broad federal guidelines, states determine the benefits covered, program eligibility, rates of payments for providers, and methods of administration of the program. Called also *Medical Assistance Program*. **M. Management Information System**, a computerized claim reporting system used by Medicaid in some states.

medical (med′ĭ-kal) pertaining to medicine. **major m.**, major medical POLICY.

medicament (med′ĭ-kah-ment) [L. *medicamentum*] any medicinal substance or a remedy used in the treatment of disease.

medicamentous (med″ĭ-kah-men′tus) pertaining to, used in, or caused by drugs or a remedy or remedies used in the treatment of disease.

Medicare (med′ĭ-kār) a nationwide health insurance program for persons aged 65 and over, for persons eligible for social security disability payments, and for persons with kidney disease requiring kidney transplantation or dialysis, which was enacted as title XVIII — Health Insurance for the Aged — of the Social Security Act. It is available without regard to income, and is financed by money from payroll taxes and premiums from beneficiaries. The program has two parts: *Part A* provides hospital insurance available to all qualified beneficiaries under the Medicare criteria; *Part B* provides medical insurance coverage for services, such as physician's services, outpatient services, and home health care. Participation under Part B is voluntary and beneficiaries pay monthly premiums. Part B is called also *Supplementary Medical Insurance (SMI)* and *medigap policy*. No dental services are provided under the program.

medicated (med′ĭ-kāt″ed) imbued with a medical substance.

medication (med″ĭ-ka′shun) [L. *medicatio*] 1. the process or act of impregnation with a medicine. 2. the administration of remedies in the treatment of disease. See also DRUG. **conservative m.**, treatment aimed to build up the vital powers of the patient. **electrolytic m.**, iontophoresis. **ionic m.**, iontophoresis. **maintenance m.**, administration of a drug or drugs in dosage sufficient to maintain at the desired level the influence of a drug achieved by earlier administration. See maintenance DOSE. **preanesthetic m.**, **preoperative m.**, premedication. **root canal electrolytic m.**, **root canal ionic m.**, see ELECTROSTERILIZATION. **sublingual m.**, the administration of medicine by placing it beneath the tongue.

medicinal (me-dis′ĭ-nal) [L. *medicinalis*] 1. having healing qualities. 2. pertaining to a medicine or to healing.

medicine (med′ĭ-sin) [L. *medicina*] 1. the art and science of the diagnosis and treatment of disease and the maintenance of health. 2. any drug or remedy. **clinical m.**, the study of disease by direct examination of the living patient. **community m.**, that branch of medicine which is concerned with the study of health and disease in populations; see *preventive m.*, community health CARE, primary CARE, and public HEALTH. See also community DENTISTRY. **comparative m.**, the study of phenomena basic to the diseases of all species. **compound m.**, a medicinal preparation containing a mixture of several drugs. **defensive m.**, the practice of medicine based on safeguards against potential malpractice suits, whereby a physician, in order to protect himself, may elect to order more diagnostic tests than the condition would indicate; to refuse to perform any risky therapeutic procedure, even when such a procedure is clinically desirable; to rely heavily on consultants, regardless of costs to the patient; or to undertake any protective measure in an effort to minimize the hazard of a malpractice suit. **environmental m.**, that branch of medicine which considers the effects of the environment on man, including rapid population growth, changes and extremes in temperature, alterations in atmospheric pressure, water and air pollution, radiation, travel, etc. See also ECOLOGY and ENVIRONMENT. **experimental m.**, the study of disease based on experimentation in animals. See also human EXPERIMENTATION. **family m.**, the medical specialty concerned with the planning and provision of the comprehensive primary health care of a family, whether involving only one member, several members, or all members of the family. Called also *family practice*. See also family PHYSICIAN and general PRACTICE. **forensic m.,** that branch of medicine dealing with the application of medical knowledge to the purposes of law. This term and jurisprudence are sometimes used as synonyms, but some authorities consider the first as a branch of medicine and the second as a branch of law. Called also *legal m.* See also medical EXAMINER, medical JURISPRUDENCE, and medicolegal IDENTIFICATION. **geriatric m.,** geriatrics. **group m.,** group PRACTICE. **hyperbaric m.,** the treatment of diseases in an environment of higher than atmospheric pressure through the use of a special pressure chamber. **internal m.,** that branch of medicine dealing especially with the delivery of health care in disorders of the internal structures of the human body. See also INTERNIST. **legal m.,** forensic m. **magistral m.,** magistral DRUG. **mental m.,** psychiatry. **nuclear m.,** that branch of medicine concerned with the use of radioactive isotopes in the diagnosis and treatment of diseases. **official m.,** official DRUG. **officinal m.,** officinal DRUG. **oral m.,** 1. a branch of dentistry dealing with the relationship between oral and systemic diseases, including the oral manifestations of systemic diseases. 2. dentistry. **patent m.,** a drug or remedy protected by a trademark, available without prescription. **preclinical m.,** 1. medical practice devoted to keeping the well well and preventing or postponing the development of clinical conditions in the near sick; preventive medicine. 2. the first two years of the usual curriculum in a medical school. **preventive m.,** the branch of medicine which aims at the prevention of disease; preclinical medicine. **proprietary m.,** proprietary DRUG. **psychosomatic m.,** a system of medicine which aims at discovering the exact nature of the relationship of the emotions and bodily function, affirming the principle that the mind and body are one; the simultaneous application of physiologic and psychologic techniques in the study and treatment of illness. **social m.,** phases of preventive medicine and the care of the sick which concern the community as a whole or large groups of persons rather than the individual. **space m.,** the branch of medicine concerned with conditions to be encountered by man in space. **tropical m.,** that branch of medicine concerned with diseases occurring chiefly in tropical and subtropical climates.

medico- [L. *medicina* medicine] a combining form denoting relationship to medicine.

medicodental (med″ĭ-ko-den′tal) pertaining to both medicine and dentistry.

medicolegal (med″ĭ-ko-le′gal) pertaining to medicine and law. See forensic MEDICINE and medical JURISPRUDENCE.

medifrontal (me″dĭ-fron′tal) median and frontal; pertaining to the middle of the forehead.

MEDIHC Military Experience Directed Into Health Careers; a cooperative program of the Department of Health, Education, and Welfare and the Department of Defense to help individuals, trained in health skills while in the armed services, to utilize those skills after returning to civilian life.

Medin, Karl Oskar [Swedish physician, 1847–1928] see POLIOMYELITIS (Heine-Medin disease).

medioccipital (me″de-ok-sip′ĭ-tal) midoccipital.

mediolateral (me″de-o-lat′er-al) pertaining to the middle and to one side.

medionecrosis (me″de-o-ne-kro′sis) [*medio-* + *necrosis*] necrosis of the tunica media of a blood vessel. Called also *medial necrosis*.

medio-occipital (me″de-o-ok-sip′ĭ-tal) midoccipital.

medisect (me′dĭ-sekt) [L. *medius* middle + *secare* to cut] to divide or dissect medially.

medium (me′de-um), pl. *mediums* or *me′dia* [L. "middle"] 1. means. 2. a substance which transmits impulses. 3. culture m. **clearing m.,** a substance used for rendering histologic specimens transparent. **contrast m.,** radiopaque m. **culture m.,** a substance, or a combination of various substances, used for the propagation or growth of microorganisms or tissue cells. **dispersion m., disperse m., dispersive m.,** continuous PHASE. **nutrient m.,** a culture medium to which certain nutrient materials have been added. **radiopaque m.,** a substance that may be injected into a cavity or region to increase its density in x-ray examination and thereby aid in diagnosis. Called also *contrast m.* **separating m.,** in dentistry, a substance applied to the investment surface of a denture flask to protect the resin from the surfaces in the mold space to avoid incorporation of water into the resin from the gypsum, thereby preventing crazing of the denture, and keeping the dissolved polymer and free monomer from soaking into the mold surface, and making separation of the investing material from the resin possible. Water-soluble alginates and water-insoluble alginates (treated with alkali earth metals) are

most commonly used as separating media. Formerly, a thin sheet of tin foil burnished over the mold surface (tin foil substitute) was used to separate the gypsum from the resin. Called also *separating agent*.

medius (me′de-us) [L.] in the middle; an anatomical term used in reference to a structure lying between two other structures that are anterior and posterior, superior and inferior, or internal and external in position.

MEDLARS *MED*ical *L*iterature *A*nalysis and *R*etrieval *S*ystem; a registered acronym for a computerized biomedical information storage and retrieval system of the National Library of Medicine, which contains a bibliographic data base consisting of more than 5,000,000 journal articles published since 1965. Materials in the system are published in *Index Medicus, Index to Dental Literature*, and other bibliographies, and are accessible to direct computer on-line searching through MEDLINE.

MEDLINE *MED*LARS on *Line;* an acronym for an on-line computer system used to gain direct access to bibliographic data in the MEDLARS data base.

Medopren trademark for *methyldopa*.

Medrate trademark for *methylprednisolone*.

Medrol trademark for *methylprednisolone*.

medulla (me-dul′lah) [L.] the middle, inmost part; used in anatomical nomenclature to designate the inmost portion of an organ or structure. Called also *marrow*. **adrenal m.,** the inner part of the adrenal gland, which synthesizes, stores, and secretes the hormonally active catecholamines epinephrine and norepinephrine. It is surrounded by the adrenal cortex, and is composed of networks of cords of polyhedral chromaffin cells that secrete hormones. Called also *m. glandulae suprarenalis* [NA]. **m. glan′dulae suprarena′lis** [NA], adrenal m. **m. of lymph node, m. no′di lymphat′ici** [NA], the central part of a lymph node, comprising cords and sinuses. Called also *substantia medullaris lymphoglandulae*. **m. oblonga′ta** [NA], a part of the brain stem that is continuous above with the pons and below with the spinal cord, lying anterior to the cerebellum. It contains ascending and descending nerve tracts that assist in the control of the right side of the body by the left cerebral hemisphere and the left side by the right hemisphere. It also assists in dealing with vital functions, such as respiration, circulation, and special senses. **m. os′sium,** bone MARROW. **m. os′sium fla′va** [NA], yellow MARROW. **m. os′sium ru′bra** [NA], red MARROW. **m. spina′lis** [NA], spinal CORD.

medullae (mĕ-dul′e) [L.] plural of *medulla*.

medullary (med′u-lār″e) [L. *medullaris*] pertaining to the medulla or marrow.

medullated (med′u-lāt″ed) possessing a medulla or myelin sheath; myelinated. Said of a nerve fiber.

medullation (med″u-la′shun) the formation of a medulla or marrow, especially the formation of the medullary sheath around a nerve fiber.

mega- [Gr. *megas* big, great] 1. a combining form designating great size. See also words beginning MACRO- and MEGALO-. 2. in the metric system, a combining form denoting a quantity one million (10^6) times the unit designated by the root with which it is combined. Abbreviated *M*. See also metric SYSTEM.

megacurie (meg″ah-ku′re) [*mega-* + *curie*] a unit of radioactivity, being one million (10^6) curies. Abbreviated *Mc*.

megacycle (meg′ah-si″k'l) [*mega-* + *cycle*] a unit of one million (10^6) cycles e.g., 1,000,000 cycles per second; applied to the frequency of electromagnetic waves. Abbreviated *Mc*.

megadont (meg′ah-dont) [*mega-* + Gr. *odous* tooth] macrodont.

megadontia (meg″ah-don′she-ah) macrodontia.

megadyne (meg′ah-dīn″) [*mega-* + *dyne*] one million (10^6) dynes.

megaglossia (meg″ah-glos′e-ah) [*mega-* + Gr. *glōssa* tongue + *ia*] macroglossia.

megakaryoblast (meg″ah-kar′e-o-blast) [*mega-* + Gr. *karyon* nucleus + *blastos* germ] an immature megakaryocyte, about 15 to 50 μ in diameter, having nongranular, basophilic cytoplasm and a large oval or kidney-shaped nucleus with numerous nucleoli. When the cell enlarges and reaches 20 to 80 μ in diameter, and the cytoplasmic granulation begins to appear, the cell is known as a *promegakaryocyte*.

megakaryocyte (meg″ah-kar′e-o-sīt) [*mega-* + Gr. *karyon* nucleus + *kytos* hollow vessel] the giant cell, ranging in size from 35 to 160 μ in diameter, which gives rise to blood platelets. In adults, megakaryocytes are found chiefly in the bone marrow, and also in the lungs and spleen; in the fetus, they occur successively in the liver, spleen, and bone marrow. They have irregularly lobed ring nuclei that stain brilliant blue with Wright stain; the cytoplasm is light blue and is packed, except for the periphery, with azurophilic granules. Each megakaryocyte has several, sometimes as many as 23, mature nuclei with dense chromatin and no nucleoli. Megakaryocytes derive from megakaryoblasts and develop into promegakaryocytes before maturation.

megalo- [Gr. *megas, megalē* big, great] a combining form designating great size. See also words beginning MACRO- and MEGA-.

megaloblast (meg′ah-lo-blast) [*megalo-* + Gr. *blastos* germ] an erythroblast that is larger than the normoblast and has a nucleus containing chromatin having the appearance of a fine meshwork. The stages of development of megaloblasts are similar to those of normal erythrocytes and, during their development, the cells are known as *promegaloblasts, basophilic megaloblasts, polychromatic megaloblasts,* and *orthochromatic megaloblasts.* See also ERYTHROPOIESIS and megaloblastic ANEMIA.

megalocephaly (meg″ah-lo-sef′ah-le) [*megalo-* + Gr. *kephalē* head] 1. any condition characterized by a head that is unusually large in proportion to the body. 2. LEONTIASIS ossea.

megalocyte (meg′ah-lo-sīt) [*megalo-* + Gr. *kytos* hollow vessel] an extremely large erythrocyte, i.e., one measuring 12 to 25 μ in diameter. See also MACROCYTE.

megalodontia (meg″ah-lo-don′she-ah) [*megalo-* + Gr. *odous* tooth + *-ia*] macrodontia.

megaloglossia (meg″ah-lo-glos′e-ah) [*megalo-* + Gr. *glōssa* tongue + *-ia*] macroglossia.

megaloscope (meg′ah-lo-skōp″) [*megalo-* + Gr. *skopein* to examine] a large magnifying lens; a magnifying speculum or mirror.

-megaly [Gr. *megaleios* magnificent, *megalē* great] a word termination meaning enlargement of a structure.

Megamycine trademark for *methacycline.*

megaprosopous (meg″ah-pros′o-pus) [*mega-* + Gr. *prosōpon* face] having a large face.

Megasphaera (meg′ah-sfe′rah) a genus of gram-negative, anaerobic bacteria of the family Veillonellaceae, occurring as relatively large coccoid cells (2 μm or more in diameter), which have been isolated from the gastrointestinal tract of animals.

megaunit (meg′ah-u″nit) [*mega-* + *unit*] a quantity one million (10^6) times that of a standard unit.

megavolt (meg′ah-vōlt) [*mega-* + *volt*] a unit of electricity, being a million (10^6) volts.

megavoltage (meg″ah-vōl′tij) a very high voltage. In ionizing radiation therapy, voltage greater than 2 megavolts. cf. SUPERVOLTAGE.

Méglin's point [J. A. *Méglin,* French physician, 1756–1824] see under POINT.

megohm (meg′ōm) [*mega-* + *ohm*] one million (10^6) ohms.

Meibom, Heinrich [1638–1700] a German anatomist. See MEIBOMIAN.

meibomian (mi-bo′me-an) named after or described by Heinrich *Meibom,* as meibomian foramen (see FORAMEN cecum of tongue).

meio- [Gr. *meiōn* smaller] a combining form denoting decrease in size or number. See also terms beginning MIO-.

meiosis (mi-o′sis) [Gr. *meiōsis* diminution] a special type of cell division by which gametes are produced, occurring in maturation of sex cells and by means of which each daughter nucleus receives half the number of chromosomes characteristic of the somatic cells of the species. Meiosis differs from mitosis in that in mitosis each daughter cell is identical to the parent cell. Meiosis is divided into two divisions. FIRST DIVISION: Prophase I has five stages: 1. *Leptotene* — the chromosomes appear as thin threads for the first time (the DNA has already duplicated).

Meiosis (only two of the 23 human chromosome pairs are shown, the chromosomes from one parent in black, from the other parent in outline). FIRST MEIOTIC DIVISION: *A, leptotene* — first appearance of chromosomes as thin threads; *B, zygotene* — pairing (synapsis) of chromosomes; *C, pachytene* — chromosomal thickening and shortening, the individual chromatids becoming visible; *D, diplotene* — longitudinal separation of chromatids, the centromere remaining intact and a chiasma being formed (NOTE: prophase includes *A* to *D* plus diakinesis [not shown]); *E, metaphase* — movement of chromosomes into the equatorial plane; *F, anaphase* — separation of pairs, one member going to each pole; *G, telophase* — cell division, each of the two daughter cells being haploid. SECOND MEIOTIC DIVISION: *prophase* (not shown) — chromosomes being visible; *H, metaphase* — movement of chromosomes into equatorial plane; *I, anaphase* — division of centromeres, the chromatids going to opposite poles; *J, telophase* — cell division, each daughter cell being diploid. (From J. S. Thompson and M. W. Thompson: Genetics in Medicine. 2nd ed. Philadelphia, W. B. Saunders Co., 1973.)

2. *Zygotene* — the homologous chromosomes pair up (synapsis). 3. *Pachytene* — the chromosomes coil tightly and thicken; they stain darker than before. 4. *Diplotene* — the two components of each bivalent chromosome begin longitudinal separation; the two chromatids remain together and the halves of each bivalent chromosome are in contact through the chiasmata; there is an exchange of materials between the chromatids. 5. *Diakinesis* — the chromosomes coil tighter and stain deeper than before. *Prometaphase:* the nuclear membrane is disrupted; the spindles are organized; the spindles mediate the orientation of centromeres. *Metaphase I:* the nuclear membrane disappears; the chromosomes move to the equatorial plate. *Anaphase I:* the two members of the homologous pairs of chromosomes move to opposite poles. *Telophase I:* the chromosomes are regrouped at the cell poles, each pole receiving one-half of the original chromosome number. *Interkinesis:* the interphase between the first and second division of meiosis, which may be absent under some conditions. SECOND DIVISION: *Prophase II:* this stage occurs only in situations where there is no interkinesis; it consists of contraction of chromosomes by coiling. *Metaphase II:* organization of spindles; the centromeres line up on the equators of the second division spindles. *Anaphase II:* sister centromeres and chromatids separate at the poles. *Telophase II:* the nuclei are reconstituted and cell membranes form between the four nuclei, producing four cells which develop into gametes in males, whereas in females three of the four abort as polar nuclei. See illustration. Cf. MITOSIS. **m. I.,** first division of meiosis. **m. II,** second division of meiosis.

meiotic (mi-ot′ik) pertaining to, characteristic of, or characterized by meiosis.

Meissner's oval corpuscles, touch corpuscles, tactile corpuscles [Georg *Meissner*, German physiologist, 1829–1905] tactile corpuscles; see under CORPUSCLE.

Mejchar, B. see Edlan-Mejchar OPERATION.

Mekamine trademark for *mecamylamine.*

melanin (mel′ah-nin) [Gr. *melas* black] an endogenous, nonhemoglobin-derived, brown-black pigment synthesized from tyrosine in melanocytes. Tyrosinase catalyzes the oxidation of tyrosine to dihydroxyphenylalanine (dopa), and dopa is polymerized and then coupled with protein to produce melanin. The pigment is normally found in the basal malpighian layer of the epidermis and mucous membrane of the gingivae and remainder of the oral cavity. Melanin is also found in pigmented nevi (moles) and their malignant counterpart, melanocarcinoma.

melanizer (mel′ah-ni″zer) melanizing AGENT.

melano- [Gr. *melas* black] a combining form meaning black, or denoting relation to melanin.

melanoameloblastoma (mel″ah-no-ah-mel″o-blas-to′mah) [Gr. *melas* black + Old Fr. *amel* enamel + Gr. *blastos* germ + -*oma*] a benign tumor of the jaw, usually of the anterior maxilla, most frequently observed in infants under the age of six months. It presents a rapidly growing nonulcerated dark lesion, resulting in displacement of the tooth buds and distortion of the jaw. Histologically, it consists of basophilic epithelial cells surrounded by hyalinized stroma, with melanin pigment being present in the cells. It is believed not to be odontogenic in nature but to be of neuroectodermal origin. Called also *benign pigmented neuroectodermal tumor of infancy, melanotic ameloblastoma, melanotic progonoma, pigmented ameloblastoma, pigmented anlage tumor,* and *retinal anlage tumor.*

melanoblast (mel′ah-no-blast″, mĕ-lan′o-blast) [*melano-* + Gr. *blastos* germ] a cell originating from the neural crest that differentiates into a melanocyte.

melanocarcinoma (mel″ah-no-kar″sĭ-no′mah) [*melano-* + *carcinoma*] malignant MELANOMA.

melanocyte (me-lan′o-sīt) the cell responsible for the synthesis of melanin, which is stellate in form with long protoplasmic processes extending into the basal cells and the malpighian layer of the epidermis, while the cell proper generally remains at the dermoepithelial junction. The nucleus has a round to oval shape; ovoid nuclei are oriented parallel with the dermoepidermal junction and round ones are at right angles to the junction. Minute brown to black melanin granules (melanosomes) are generally present in the melanocytes in the nonwhite population, but are seldom observed in members of the white race. Melanocytes are more prominent in the lining of the papillary gingiva than other parts of the oral mucosa in whites; in nonwhites, they occur in most regions of the gingiva and the oral mucosa.

melanocytoma (mel″ah-no-si-to′mah) [*melanocyte* + -*oma*] a tumor made up of melanocytes. **dermal m.,** blue NEVUS.

melanoderm (mel′ah-no-derm) [*melano-* + Gr. *derma* skin] a person belonging to one of the black races.

melanoderma (mel″ah-no-der′mah) [*melano-* + Gr. *derma* skin]

abnormally increased amount of melanin in the skin, either due to an increase in the production of melanin by the melanocytes normally present or to an increase in the number of melanocytes, with production of hyperpigmented skin. **senile m.,** pigmentation of the skin in the aged.

melanofibroma (mel″ah-no-fi-bro′mah) [*melano-* + *fibroma*] blue NEVUS.

melanogenesis (mel″ah-no-jen′ĕ-sis) the production of melanin. See also melanizing AGENT.

melanoglossia (mel″ah-no-glos′e-ah) [*melano-* + Gr. *glōssa* tongue + -*ia*] black TONGUE.

melanoid (mel′ah-noid) [*melano-* + Gr. *eidos* form] 1. resembling melanin; of dark color. 2. a material resembling melanin.

melanoleukoderma (mel″ah-no-lu″ko-der′mah) [*melano-* + Gr. *leukos* white + *derma* skin] a mottled appearance of the skin, as in chronic arsenic poisoning. See ARSENIC.

melanoma (mel″ah-no′mah) [*melano-* + -*oma*] a tumor made up of melanin-pigmented cells. The term is commonly used to refer to *malignant melanoma.* **benign mesenchymal m.,** blue NEVUS. **malignant m.,** a black-brown malignant neoplasm of the melanin-producing cells, which is one of the most deadly human neoplasms; most tend to enlarge and to metastasize early. It is usually surrounded by erythema, and may be associated with satellite lesions. Histologically, it extends from the dermoepidermal junction into the dermis, and is characterized by mitosis, anaplasia, inflammatory infiltrates, and multinucleated bizarre giant tumor cells. Involvement of the oral cavity is relatively uncommon; when found in the mouth they are usually located on the maxillary alveolar ridge and palate. Called also *melanoma, black cancer, melanocarcinoma,* and *melanosarcoma.*

melanophore (mel″ah-no-fōr″) [*melano-* + Gr. *phoros* bearing] a cell that transports melanin granules from melanocytes to peripheral cells, such as epidermal cells and phagocytes. See also CHROMATOPHORE.

melanoplakia (mel″ah-no-pla′ke-ah) [*melano-* + Gr. *plax* plate + -*ia*] presence of pigmented patches on the oral mucosa.

melanosarcoma (mel″ah-no-sar-ko′mah) [*melano-* + *sarcoma*] malignant MELANOMA.

melanosis (mel″ah-no′sis) [*melano-* + -*osis*] a condition characterized by abnormal pigmentation. **Dubreuilh's m.,** Hutchinson's FRECKLE. **extrasacral dermal m., oculocutaneous m.,** Ota's NEVUS. **jute-spinner's m.,** a condition marked by brown, to violet-brown, or bronze-pigmented macules and patches on the forehead, neck, and face, occasionally involving other areas of the skin unprotected by clothing, such as the hands and forearms. It was a common occupational disease in Germany during World War I. Photosensitization following exposure to tar, jute, and aniline-containing chemicals is suspected as the causative factor. It is considered to be identical with *reticulated pigmented poikiloderma.* Called also *Riehl's m.* and *tar m.* **Ordóñez' m.,** a condition marked by generalized melanoderma, especially of exposed parts of the body, melanosis of the mucous membranes of the mouth, eyes, and vulva, brown pigmentation of the nails, and dark discoloration of viscera; observed in malnourished persons living at high altitudes. Pituitary disorders are suspected as contributing factors. **precancerous m.,** Hutchinson's FRECKLE. **Riehl's m.,** tar m., jute-spinner's m.

melanosome (mel′ah-no-sōm) any of the granules within the melanocytes that contain the pigment melanin.

melanotrichia (mel″ah-no-trik′e-ah) [*melano-* + Gr. *thrix* hair + -*ia*] hyperpigmentation of the hair. Called also *melanotrichosis.* **m. lin′guae,** black TONGUE.

melanotrichosis (mel″ah-no-trī-ko′sis) [*melano-* + Gr. *thrix* hair + -*osis*] melanotrichia. **m. lin′guae,** black TONGUE.

melanotropin (mel″ah-no-trop′in) melanocyte stimulating HORMONE.

melarsoprol (mel-ar′so-prōl) an antiprotozoal drug, 2-[4-[(4,6-diamino-1,3,5-triazin-2-yl)amino]phenyl]-1,3,2-dithiarsolane-4-methanol, occurring as a creamy or grayish, bitter powder with a slight odor, which is slowly soluble in propylene glycol and insoluble in water, ethanol, and ether. Used chiefly in the treatment of trypanosomiasis. Trademark: Arsobal.

melasma (mĕ-laz′mah) [Gr. *melas* black] a disease characterized by dark pigmentation of the skin. Called also *chloasma.* **suprarenal m.,** Addison's DISEASE.

Meleril trademark for *thioridazine.*

melfalan (mel′fah-lan) melphalan.

meli- [Gr. *meli* honey] a combining form meaning sweet, or denoting a relationship to honey. See also words beginning GLUCO-.

melibiase (mel″ĭ-bi′ās) α-GALACTOSIDASE.

melioidosis (me″le-oi-do′sis) [Gr. *melis* a distemper of asses + *eidos* resemblance] an infectious bacterial disease of rodents, transmissible to man, caused by *Pseudomonas pseudomallei*, and occurring in tropical climates, particularly in Southeast Asia. In man, it may assume three general forms: an acute septicemia with diarrhea; a subacute typhoidal form with pulmonary symptoms and local abscess formation; and a chronic form, which may localize in any tissue as small caseous nodules. It was formerly believed that mortality was 95 percent or more, but recent studies indicate that the infection is more common and milder than originally suspected.

melitis (me-li′tis) [Gr. *melon* cheek + *-itis*] inflammation of the cheek.

Melitoxin trademark for *dicumarol*.

Melkersson-Rosenthal syndrome [E. *Melkersson*, Swedish physician; Curt *Rosenthal*, German physician] see under SYNDROME.

Mellaril trademark for *thioridazine*.

Melnick-Needles syndrome [John Charles *Melnick*, American physician, born 1928; Carl F. *Needles*, American physician] see under SYNDROME.

meloschisis (me-los′ki-sis) [Gr. *melon* cheek + *schisis*] a facial cleft. See oblique facial CLEFT.

Melotte's metal [George W. *Melotte*, American dentist, 1835–1915] see under METAL.

melphalan (mel′fah-lan) a nitrogen mustard, 4-[bis(2-chloroethyl)amino]-L-phenylalanine, occurring as an off-white to buff powder with a faint odor, which is soluble in dilute mineral acids, slightly soluble in ethanol and methanol, and insoluble in water, ether, and chloroform. It is a cytotoxic drug, used in the treatment of plasma-cell myeloma, Burkitt's tumor of the jaw, lymphocytic leukemia, osteosarcoma, melanoma, reticulum-cell sarcoma, and other neoplasms. Adverse reactions may include nausea, vomiting, aphthous ulcers, hemorrhagic tendency, azotemia, predisposition to infection, bone marrow depression with anemia, thrombocytopenia, and neutropenia. Called also *alanine nitrogen mustard, melfalan,* L-*phenylalanine mustard* and L-*sarcolysine*. Trademarks: Alkeran, Sarcocloria.

Melsedin trademark for *methaqualone hydrochloride* (see under METHAQUALONE).

melting (melt′ing) to become liquid or liquefied; the transformation of a solid into a liquid by means of heat; fusion. See also melting POINT.

Meltrol trademark for *phenformin hydrochloride* (see under PHENFORMIN).

Meltzer's law of contrary innervation [Samuel James *Meltzer*, American physiologist, 1851–1920] see under LAW.

member (mem′ber) [L. *membrum*] 1. a part of the body distinct from the rest in function and position. 2. a limb. 3. a person belonging to a group or organization, as one who participates in a dental plan and is eligible for benefits under that plan. See BENEFICIARY.

membra (mem′bra) [L.] plural of *membrum*.

membrana (mem-brah′nah), pl. *membra′nae* [L.] thin skin; a term used in anatomy to designate a thin layer of tissue which covers a surface or divides a space or organ. See also MEMBRANE. **m. adamanti′na** primary CUTICLE. **m. ebo′ris** of Kölliker, dentin. **m. elas′tica laryn′gis**, fibroelastic membrane of larynx; see under MEMBRANE. **membra′nae decid′uae** [NA], decidua. **m. elas′tica laryn′gis, m. fibroelas′tica laryn′gis** [NA], fibroelastic membrane of larynx; see under MEMBRANE. **m. fibro′sa cap′sulae articula′ris** [NA], fibrous membrane of articular cavity; see under MEMBRANE. **m. germinati′va**, blastoderm. **m. hyothyroi′dea**, thyrohyoid MEMBRANE. **m. muco′sa na′si**, mucous membrane, nasal; see under MEMBRANE. **m. pituito′sa**, mucous membrane, nasal; see under MEMBRANE. **m. prefor-ma′ta**, a term used in the past to denote a thick, limiting line of dentin first appearing between ameloblasts and odontoblasts in dentinogenesis. **m. pro′pria**, LAMINA propria mucosae. **m. quadrangula′ris** [NA], quadrangular MEMBRANE. **m. sero′sa**, serous MEMBRANE. **m. synovia′lis cap′sulae articula′ris** [NA], synovial membrane of articular capsule; see under MEMBRANE. **m. thyreohyoi′dea, m. thyrohyoi′dea** [NA], thyrohyoid MEMBRANE. **m. tym′pani** [NA], tympanic MEMBRANE.

membranaceous (mem″brah-na′shus) [L. *membranaceus*] of the nature of a membrane.

membranae (mem-bra′ne) [L.] plural of *membrana*.

membranate (mem′brah-nāt) having the character of a membrane.

membrane (mem′brān) [L. *membrana*] a thin layer of tissue which covers a surface or divides a space or organ. See also MEMBRANA. **accidental m.**, false m. **adamantine m.**, primary CUTICLE. **adventitious m.**, a membrane not normal to the part. **alveolodental m.**, periodontal LIGAMENT. **basement m.**, the delicate layer of extracellular condensation of mucopolysaccharides and proteins forming a membrane separating epithelium from connective tissue of most organs, including those of oral and perioral structures, underlying immediately the basal lamina. Its thickness varies from about 0.02 mm in the nasal cavity and respiratory tract to an almost imperceptible thinness in the gastrointestinal system, and being quite thick in the nasopharynx and very thin in the sublingual sulcus. The thickness of the basement membrane of blood vessels in the dental pulp increases with age. Called also *subepithelial m.* and *basement layer*. **Bichat's m.**, Henle's fenestrated m. **Brunn's m.**, the epithelium of the olfactory region of the nose. **buccopharyngeal m.**, pharyngobasilar FASCIA. **cell m.**, plasma m. **chromatic m.**, a continuous layer of chromatin substance situated on the internal surface of a nuclear membrane. **cloacal m.**, the thin, temporary barrier formed by fusion of the ectoderm and entoderm at the caudal end of the primitive streak during the third week of embryonic development; it separates the hindgut from the exterior. It breaks down at the end of the eighth week of development, forming external openings for the gastrointestinal and genitourinary tracts. **complex m.**, a membrane made up of several layers differing in structure. **cricothyroid m., cricovocal m.**, elastic cone of larynx; see under CONE. **croupous m., diphtheritic m.**, false m. **cytoplasmic m.**, plasma m. **dentinoenamel m.**, a continuous thin membrane laid down by ameloblasts adjoining the basement membrane separating them from the dentin in an early developing tooth. **dialyzing m.**, a type of a semipermeable membrane that will permit the crystalloids suspended in solution to pass through but not the colloids. **elastic m.**, a variety of membrane composed largely of elastic fibers. **elastic m., external**, a thin elastic membrane forming a boundary between the tunica media and the tunica adventitia. Called also *elastica externa* and *external elastic lamina*. **elastic m., internal**, an elastic membrane forming a boundary between the tunica intima and tunica media, particularly noticeable in arteries of median caliber. Called also *elastica interna* and *internal elastic lamina*. **elastic m. of larynx**, fibroelastic m. of larynx. **enamel m.**, 1. enamel CUTICLE. 2. the inner layer of cells within the enamel organ of the tooth germ in the fetus. Called also *Hannover's intermediate m.* **endoneural m.**, neurilemma. **erythrocyte m.**, erythrocyte STROMA. **exocoelomic m.**, Heuser's m. **false m.**, a dirty gray-white, rubbery membrane, usually of the pharynx, larynx, or respiratory passages, produced by an acute inflammatory response, usually to a necrotizing toxin, such as the diphtheria exotoxin, which causes necrosis and desquamation of the epithelial layer, resulting in the outpouring of fibrinosuppurative exudate which traps the necrotic and cellular debris, forming layers of pseudomembranes on the inflamed eroded surfaces. The layers adhere closely to the underlying necrotic ulcerated areas and are difficult to remove and leave bleeding surfaces if stripped forcibly. Called also *accidental m., croupous m., diphtheritic m.,* and *pseudomembrane*. **fenestrated m.**, one of the multiply perforated elastic sheets of the tunica intima and tunica media of arteries. **fetal m's**, auxiliary embryonic structures that develop from the zygote, not all considered as being membranous in the histological and anatomical sense, which are concerned with the protection, nutrition, respiration, and excretion of the embryo and fetus. They include the yolk sac, amnion, chorion, allantois, placenta, and umbilical cord. The placenta and fetal membranes separate from the fetus at birth and are discarded as the afterbirth. See illustration. **fibroelastic m. of larynx**, a broad sheath of fibroelastic tissue beneath the mucous coat of the larynx. Its upper (cranial) portion extends between the arytenoid cartilage and the epiglottis and forms the quadrangular membrane; the lower (caudal) portion forms with its fellow of the opposite side the *conus elasticus*. Called also *elastic m. of larynx, membrana elastica laryngis,* and *membrana fibroelastica laryngis* [NA]. **fibrous m. of articular cavity**, the outer of two layers of the articular capsule of a synovial joint. Called also *membrana fibrosa capsulae articularis* [NA] and *stratum fibrosum capsulae articularis*. **germinal m.**, blastoderm. **ground m.**, inophragma. **Hannover's intermediate m.**, enamel m. (2). **Henle's elastic m.**, a fenestrated layer between the outer and middle tunics of certain arteries. **Henle's fenestrated m.**, a subendothelial fibroelastic fenestrated layer in the tunica intima of an artery. Called also *Bichat's m.* **Heuser's m.**, a delicate sac of mesoblastic tissue that develops as a lining of the blastocyst cavity during the second week of embryonic development. Called also

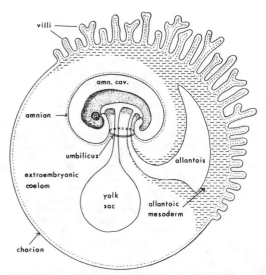

Amnion, chorion, and other embryonic membranes surrounding
the embryo of a placental mammal; *amn. cav.* = amniotic cavity.
(From B. I. Balinsky: Introduction to Embryology. 4th ed. Philadelphia, W. B. Saunders Co., 1975.)

exocoelomic m. **hyoglossal m.**, the part of the oral mucosa
which connects the tongue with the hyoid bone. **hyothyroid m.**,
thyrohyoid m. **intersutural m.**, the pericranium lying between
the cranial sutures. **ivory m.**, dentin. **Krause's m.**, Z BAND.
laryngeal m., mucous m., laryngeal. **limiting m.**, 1. any membrane which constitutes the border of some tissue or structure.
2. viral ENVELOPE. **Mauthner's m.**, axolemma. **medullary m.**,
endosteum. **mucous m.**, the lining of tubular and hollow structures, consisting of the covering of the free surface, the epithelial layer, and beneath it the lamina propria, which is composed
of the basement membrane and the papillary, reticular, and
muscular layers. In the oral cavity the muscular layer is absent
and in the soft palate it is replaced by the elastic lamina. Called
also *mucosa* and *tunica mucosa* [NA]. **mucous m., lingual,**
mucous m. of tongue. **mucous m., laryngeal, mucous m. of**
larynx, the mucous coat, with associated glands and cilia, of
the larynx. The part lining the anterior surface of the epiglottis
and the upper half of its posterior surface, the aryepiglottic
folds, and the vocal cords are covered with stratified squamous
epithelium. In the adult, ciliated epithelium usually begins at
the base of the epiglottis and extends down the larynx; the cilia
beat toward the mouth, thus propelling foreign particles, bacteria, and mucus from the lungs toward the exterior of the body.
Called also *laryngeal m., laryngeal mucosa,* and *tunica mucosa laryngis* [NA]. **mucous m., masticatory,** the oral mucous
membrane covering the parts of the mouth involved in the
masticatory activity, including the gingivae, hard palate, and
dorsum of the tongue. Called also *masticatory mucosa.* **mucous**
m. of mouth, mucous m., oral. **mucous m., nasal, mucous m. of**
nose, the mucous membrane lining the nasal cavity, consisting
of connective tissue and epithelium made up of pseudostratified
ciliated columnar epithelium with goblet cells. The columnar
cells interspersed among the goblet cells are provided with
cytoplasmic projections (cilia), which propel the secretions of
the goblet cells and other cells toward the postnasal choanae
through their beating movements. It is divided into an olfactory
region and a respiratory region (see under REGION). Called also
*schneiderian m., membrana mucosa nasi, membrana pituito-
sa, nasal mucosa,* and *tunica mucosa nasi* [NA]. **mucous m.,**
oral, the mucous membrane lining the oral cavity. Its epithelium is of the stratified squamous type, being keratinized in areas
exposed to abrasive forces and nonkeratinized in protected
areas. Nuclei of the superficial cells tend to shrink and degenerate, and the somewhat flattened bodies of these cells are shed in
large quantities and are found in the saliva. Keratohyalin may
be found in some superficial cells and glycogen is sometimes
located in the middle and superficial layers. The posterior oral
mucosa contains lymphocytes which migrate across the epithelium. The entire membrane is well supplied with blood vessels,
lymphatic and nerve endings, the nerve endings belonging to
the sensory branches of the trigeminal nerve. The lamina
propria contains a wide assortment of salivary glands. Called
also *mucous m. of mouth, oral mucosa,* and *tunica mucosa oris*
[NA]. **mucous m., palatal, mucous m. of palate,** the mucosal

lining of the palate. That of the hard palate consists of keratinized stratified squamous epithelium and a lamina propria
whose superior border extends into the epithelium, forming tall
and slender papillae; palatal glands are found in the connective
tissue of the posterolateral region and pellets of fat are contained in the anterolateral region. The lining of the soft palate
consists of nonkeratinized stratified squamous epithelium and
a compact lamina propria; the submucous membrane, which
contains palatal glands, is separated from the lamina propria by
a layer of elastic fibers, the supraglandular elastic lamina.
Called also *palatal mucosa.* **mucous m., pharyngeal, mucous m.**
of pharynx, the mucous lining of the pharynx. The lower
section of the pharynx and a part of its nasal region are lined
with stratified squamous epithelium. Toward the fornix, the
epithelium becomes stratified columnar, ciliated with many
goblet cells. On the lateral side of the nasal region the ciliated
epithelium continues downward beyond the aperture of the
eustachian tube. Stratified squamous epithelium may replace
the ciliated epithelium with age. The mucosa is provided with a
thick, dense, elastic layer and a loose submucous layer that is
well developed only in the lateral part of the nasal region and in
areas where the pharynx joins the esophagus; in all other parts,
the mucosa is adjacent to the muscular wall. The lamina
propria consists of a dense connective tissue network. Papillae
occur in areas covered with stratified squamous epithelium and
are absent in areas lined with pseudostratified ciliated columnar epithelium. Mucous glands are present in the mucosa lined
with stratified squamous epithelium and mixed glands are
located in regions covered with ciliated epithelium. Called also
pharyngeal mucosa and *tunica mucosa pharyngis* [NA].
mucous m., proper, LAMINA propria mucosae. **mucous m., sub-**
lingual, the mucous covering of the sublingual sulcus. It is a
thin relatively transparent membrane surfaced by a thin layer
of nonkeratinized stratified squamous epithelium that shows
through the rich vascular bed beneath the mucosa, hence its
red color. The deep layers of tissue are often diffuse and contain
sublingual glands and fat cells. The connective tissue papillae
are broad and shallow. Called also *sublingual mucosa.* **mucous**
m. of tongue, the mucous covering of the tongue, having a
structure similar to that of other parts of the oral cavity. The
covering of the ventral surface is relatively thin and has nonkeratinized epithelium. The dorsal mucosa is tougher and bears
the lingual papillae. Its epithelium has variable thickness,
being much thicker around the papillae than elsewhere. The
lamina propria of the dorsal mucosa consists of an irregularly
arranged dense fibrous connective tissue which serves as the
epimysium around the muscles, the epineurium around the
nerves, the adventitia around the blood vessels, and the parenchyma and the excretory units around the salivary glands.
Called also *lingual mucous m., lingual mucosa,* and *tunica
mucosa linguae* [NA]. **mucous m., vestibular,** the mucous
lining of the oral vestibule, consisting of nonkeratinized stratified squamous epithelium, the underlying lamina propria, and
elastic fibers. The seromucous labial glands are contained in
the lamina propria. Called also *vestibular mucosa.* **Nasmyth's**
m., primary CUTICLE. **nuclear m.**, the condensed double layer of
lipids and proteins that encloses the nucleoplasm, separating it
from the cytoplasm, and comprising an inner and an outer
membrane closely opposed. Called also *nuclear envelope.* **ob-**
turator m. of larynx, thyrohyoid m. **oronasal m.**, an epithelial
plate separating the mouth cavity from the olfactory pit, which
thins and ruptures during the seventh week of embryonic
development. **peridontal m.**, periodontal LIGAMENT. **peridental**
m., periodontal m., periodontal LIGAMENT. **plasma m.**, the extremely thin membrane that envelops a cell. It is thought to be
made up of a phospholipid layer with structural proteins and
enzymatically active proteins interspersed in the membrane,
having a hydrophobic zone and being traversed by protein
"studs" believed to be permeases involved in active transport of
small substrates, such as amino acids and carbohydrates, to the
cell interior. Under the electron microscope the membrane is
seen as a trilaminar structure, all three layers of which constitute jointly the *unit membrane.* It forms an uninterrupted
boundary for the cell, functioning as though it has ultramicroscopic pores, the size of which determines the size of the
molecules that can pass through the membrane. The membrane demonstrates selective permeability, with factors such as
electric charge, lipid solubility, and water content determining
whether a substance will pass through the membrane through
osmotic processes. In most prokaryotic cells and in plant cells, a
rigid cell wall lies exterior to the plasma membrane, the two

structures being joined together by internal hydrostatic pressure. In bacteria, invaginations of the membrane form internal organelles known as *mesosomes.* Called also *cell m., cytoplasmic m.,* and *plasmalemma.* See illustration at BACTERIUM. **pseudoserous m.,** a membrane resembling serous membrane, but differing from it in structure. **pyogenic m.,** a membrane which produces pus. **pyophylactic m.,** a fibrinous membrane lining a pus cavity and tending to prevent reabsorption of injurious materials. **quadrangular m.,** the upper part of the fibroelastic membrane of the larynx. Called also *membrana quadrangularis* [NA]. **red cell m.,** erythrocyte STROMA. **schneiderian m.,** mucous m., nasal. **Schwann's m.,** neurilemma. **semipermeable m.,** a membrane that allows free passage to one substance but not to others, such as allowing a solvent to pass through but preventing solutes from diffusing. See also OSMOSIS. **serous m.,** a loose layer of connective tissue covered by a layer of mesothelium, lining the serous cavities, such as those of the pleura, peritoneum, and pericardium. Called also *membrana serosa, serous tunic,* and *tunica serosa* [NA]. **subepithelial m.,** basement m. **subimplant m.,** a fibrous connective tissue layer between the inner surface of the subperiosteal implant framework and the bone surface, formed by the regenerating periosteum, which bears the vertical and lateral stresses applied against the abutments. **submucous m.,** a layer of loose connective tissue situated between a mucous membrane and subjacent tissues. In the oral cavity, it is found only in the soft palate. Called also *submucosa, submucous layer,* and *tela submucosa* [NA]. **submucous m. of pharynx,** the submucosa underlying the mucous membrane of the pharynx. Called also *submucosa of pharynx, submucous layer of pharynx,* and *tela submucosa pharyngis* [NA]. **synaptic m.,** the layer separating the neuroplasm of an axon from that of the body of the nerve cell with which it makes synapsis. **synovial m. of articular capsule,** the inner of the two layers of the joint capsule of a synovial joint, composed of loose connective tissue and having a free smooth surface that lines the joint cavity and secretes a lubricating fluid. Called also *membrana synovialis capsulae articularis* [NA] and *stratum synoviale capsulae articularis.* **tarsal m.,** orbital SEPTUM. **tendinous m.,** aponeurosis. **thyrohyoid m.,** a broad fibroelastic sheet attached to the cranial border of the thyroid cartilage and to the front of its superior cornu, and to the dorsal surface of the hyoid bone and its greater cornua. Its middle part is known as the *middle thyrohyoid ligament.* Called also *hyothyroid m., obturator m. of larynx, membrana hyothyroidea, membrana thyreohyoidea,* and *membrana thyrohyoidea* [NA]. **tympanic m.,** the obliquely placed, thin membranous partition between the external acoustic meatus and the middle ear. Called also *eardrum* and *membrana tympani* [NA]. **unit m.,** see plasma m. **Z m.,** Z BAND.

membranoid (men'brah-noid) [*membrane* + Gr. *eidos* form] resembling a membrane.

membranous (mem'brah-nus) [L. *membranosus*] pertaining to or of the nature of a membrane.

membrum (mem'brum), pl. *mem'bra* [L.] a limb, or member, of the body; used as a general anatomical term to designate one of the limbs.

memory (mem'o-re) [L. *memoria*] 1. that mental faculty by which sensations, impressions, and ideas are recalled. 2. the capacity of a computer to store information subject to recall. 3. relaxation (3). 4. storage (2). **elastic m.,** the property of a material, such as wax, enabling it, after being warmed, bent, and coiled, to return to its original form on rewarming. **immunologic m.,** the capacity of the immune system to respond more rapidly and strongly to subsequent antigenic challenge than to the first exposure, whereby the memory cells (B- and T-lymphocytes) store information on the antigen during the primary response so that they will respond to the same antigen more vigorously during the secondary response.

menadiol sodium diphosphate (men"ah-di'ol) a vitamin of the K group, 2-methyl-1,4-naphthalenediol diphosphoric acid ester tetrasodium salt, occurring as a white to pinkish, hygroscopic powder with a characteristic odor and a salty taste, which is soluble in water, but not in ethanol, methanol, ether, and acetone. It is synthesized from menadione, and is converted to menadione in the body. Used for correcting vitamin K deficiency and its attendant deficiency of prothrombin and related clotting factors with resulting hemorrhagic disorders. When indicated, used prior to dental surgical procedures. Called also *menadione diphosphate tetrasodium salt.* Trademarks: Kappadione, Kipca, Procoagulo, Synka-Vit, Synkavite.

menadione (men"ah-di'on) a vitamin of the K group, 2-methyl-1,4-naphthalenedione, having pharmacological properties similar to other substances in the group. It occurs as a bright yellow, crystalline powder with a faintly acrid odor, which decomposes on exposure to sunlight, and is soluble in ethanol, benzene, and vegetable oil, sparingly soluble in chloroform and carbon tetrachloride, and insoluble in water. Used in correcting vitamin K deficiency and its attendant deficiency of prothrombin and related clotting factors. When indicated, used prior to dental surgical operations. Menadione powder is irritating to the mucous membranes and skin and its solution in alcohol has vesicant properties. Excessive doses may cause hyperprothrombinemia and a tendency toward thrombosis. Called also *vitamin K_3* and *vitamin $K_{2(0)}$.* Trademarks: Aquinone, Kanone, Kappaxin, Kativ-G, Klottone, Thyloquinone. **m. diphosphate tetrasodium salt,** MENADIOL sodium diphosphate. **m. sodium bisulfite,** the sodium bisulfite of menadione, converted in the body to menadione, occurring as a white, crystalline, hygroscopic powder that is very soluble in water, slightly soluble in ethanol, and insoluble in ether and benzene. Its pharmacological and toxicological properties are similar to those of the parent compound. Trademarks: Hemodal, Hykinone, Ido-K, Kavitan, Kotogen.

menaquinone (me"nah-kwi-nōn', me"nah-kwin'ōn) vitamin K_2.

Mende's syndrome [Irmgard *Mende,* German physician] see under SYNDROME.

Mendel's law [Gregor Johann *Mendel,* Austrian monk and naturalist, 1822–1884] under LAW.

Mendeleev's periodic law, periodic table [Dimitri Ivanovich *Mendeleev,* Russian chemist, 1834–1907] see periodic LAW, and see ELEMENT (2). See also MENDELEVIUM.

mendelevium (men"dě-le've-um) [named after D. I. *Mendeleev*] a synthetic radioactive element of the actinide series. Symbol, Md (formerly Mv); atomic number, 101; valences, 2, 3. The isotope ^{256}Md (half-life 1.5 hr) was first produced by bombarding einsteinium-253 with helium ions. The heaviest and most stable isotope is ^{258}Md (half-life 60 days).

mendelian (men-del'e-an) named after G. J. *Mendel,* as mendelian law (see Mendel's LAW).

Menhydrinate trademark for *dimenhydrinate.*

Ménière's disease (syndrome) [Prosper *Ménière,* French physician, 1799–1862] under DISEASE.

meningeal (mě-nin'je-al) pertaining to the meninges.

meninges (mě-nin'jēz) [Gr., pl. of *mēninx* membrane] the three membranes that envelop the brain and the spinal cord; the dura mater, pia mater, and arachnoid.

meningitis (men"in-ji'tis) [Gr. *mēninx* membrane + *-itis*] any inflammatory disease of the meninges. **mumps m.,** an aseptic meningitis secondary to mumps. **torula m.,** European BLASTOMYCOSIS.

meningo- [Gr. *mēninx* membrane] combining form denoting relationship to the meninges.

meningocele (mě-ning'go-sēl) [*meningo-* + Gr. *kēlē* hernia] hernial protrusion of the meninges through a defect in the skull or vertebral column.

meningococcemia (mě-ning"go-kok-se'me-ah) [*meningococcus* + Gr. *haima* blood + *-ia*] the presence of meningococci (*Neisseria meningitidis*) in the blood.

meningococci (mě-ning"go-kok'si) plural of *meningococcus.*

meningococcidal (mě-ning"go-kok-si'dal) [*meningococcus* + L. *caedere* to kill] destroying meningococci (*Neisseria meningitidis*).

meningococcosis (mě-ning"go-kok-ko'sis) infection caused by meningococci (*Neisseria meningitidis*).

meningococcus (mě-ning"go-kok'us), pl. *meningococ'ci* [*meningo-* + Gr. *kokkos* berry] *Neisseria meningitidis;* see under NEISSERIA.

meningoencephalocele (mě-ning"go-en-sef'ah-lo-sēl") [*meningo-* + Gr. *enkephalos* brain + *kēlē* hernia] protrusion of the meninges and other brain substance through a cranium bifidum or a traumatic opening in the cranium. See also ENCEPHALOCELE.

meningomyelocele (mě-ning"go-mi'ě-lo-sēl") [*meningo-* + Gr. *myelos* + *kēlē* hernia] hernial protrusion of the meninges through a defect in the vertebrae.

meninx (me'ninks), pl. *menin'ges* [Gr. *mēninx* membrane] a membrane, especially one of the three membranes that envelop the brain and the spinal cord. See MENINGES.

meniscectomy (men"ĭ-sek'to-me) [*meniscus* + Gr. *ektomē* excision] the excision of an intra-articular disk or meniscus, as of the temporomandibular joint.

menisci (men-is'si) [L.] plural of *meniscus.*

meniscus (mě-nis'kus), pl. *menis'ci* [L.; Gr. *mēniskos* crescent] 1. a crescent-shaped structure appearing at the surface of a liquid column, as in a pipet or buret, made concave or convex by the influence of capillarity. 2. any crescent-shaped structure. See also DISCUS and DISK. **articular m., m. articula′ris** [NA], interarticular DISK. **m. of sternoclavicular joint,** interarticular disk of sternoclavicular joint; see under DISK. **m. of temporomandibular joint,** interarticular disk of temporomandibular joint; see under DISK.

Menkes' syndrome [John H. *Menkes*, Austrian-born American physician, born 1928] see under SYNDROME.

meno- [Gr. *mēn* month; *mēniaia* the menses] a combining form denoting relationship to the menses.

menogingivitis (men″o-jin″ji-vi′tis) [*meno-* + *gingivitis*] gingivitis occurring in conjunction with the menstrual cycle. See also menstruation GINGIVITIS. **periodic transitory m.,** gingivitis characterized by discomfort, sensitiveness, and redness and congestion of the gingiva with bleeding under the normal stress of mastication, occurring just prior to menstruation, in amenorrhea, after hysterectomy, before and after ectopic pregnancy, and during and after menopause. See also menstruation GINGIVITIS.

menopause (men′o-pawz) [*meno-* + Gr. *pausis* cessation] cessation of menstruation in the human female, signaling the end of reproductive capability. Menopause may be associated with thinning of the oral epithelium, a burning sensation of the tongue, or dryness of the mouth, sometimes without associated diminution of saliva.

menorrhagia (men″o-ra′je-ah) [*meno-* + Gr. *rhēgnynai* to burst forth] excessive uterine bleeding occurring at the regular intervals of menstruation, the period of flow being of greater than usual duration.

menses (men′sez) [L., pl. of *mensis* month] the monthly flow of blood from the female genital tract; see MENSTRUATION.

menstruation (men″stroo-a′shun) the cyclic, physiologic uterine bleeding which normally recurs, usually at approximately four-week intervals, in the absence of pregnancy.

menstruum (men′stroo-um) [L. *menstruus* menstruous; it was long believed that the menstrual fluid had a peculiar solvent quality] a solvent medium.

mental (men′tal) 1. [L. *mens* mind] pertaining to the mind. 2. [L. *mentum* chin] pertaining to the chin. See also GENIAL.

mentalis (men-ta′lis) relating to the chin.

menthol (men′thol) A compound, 5-methyl-2-(1-methylethyl)-cyclohexanol, occurring as needle-like crystals, fused masses, or crystalline powder, with a peppermint taste and odor, prepared from peppermint and other mint oils or by hydrogenation of thymol. It is soluble in ethanol, chloroform, ether, hexane, glacial acetic acid, mineral oil, fixed and volatile oils, and, slightly, water. Used chiefly as a flavoring agent. Also used in counterirritant throat lozenges, inhalers for nasal congestion, headache, and neuralgia, and in mentholated cigarettes. In dentistry, used in some zinc oxide–eugenol cements. Called also *peppermint camphor.*

mento- [L. *mentum* chin] a combining form denoting relationship to the chin. See also words beginning GENIO-.

mentolabial (men″to-la′be-al) [*mento-* + L. *labium* lip] pertaining to the chin and lip.

menton (men′ton) a cranial osteometric landmark, being the lowest point of the mandibular symphysis on the lateral jaw projection as seen on x-ray films. Abbreviated *Me.* Called also point *Me.* See illustration at CEPHALOMETRY.

mentum (men′tum) [L.] the chin.

mepasin (mep′ah-sin) mepazine.

mepazine (mep′ah-zēn) a phenothiazine tranquilizer, 10[(1-methyl-3-piperidinyl)methyl]10*H*-phenothiazine, used therapeutically as either the hydrochloride monohydrate or acetate salt. The hydrochloride salt occurs as photosensitive crystals with a slightly bitter taste, which are soluble in ethanol and chloroform, slightly soluble in water, and insoluble in ether and benzene. The acetate salt occurs as a white crystalline powder with an acetic acid odor, which turns pink on exposure to light and air. Used especially in the treatment of mental disorders, nausea, vomiting, hiccups, and acute porphyria, and in controlling apprehension and anxiety in surgical patients. Side effects are similar to those associated with chlorpromazine, with bone marrow depression, agranulocytosis, seizures, and failure to respond to pressor agents being the principal ones. It is contraindicated with narcotics, barbiturates, and alcohol. Called also *mepasin, MPMP,* and *pecazine.* Trademarks: Nothiazine, Pacatal.

mepenzolate bromide (mē-pen′zo-lāt) an antimuscarinic drug, 3-hydroxyl-1,1-dimethylpiperidinium bromide benzilate, occurring as a white or creamy powder that is soluble in water, methanol, and ethanol, slightly soluble in chloroform, and insoluble in ether. Used chiefly in the treatment of gastrointestinal disorders. Xerostomia, blurring of vision, and other dis-

orders may occur during therapy. Trademarks: Cantil, Cantril, Trancolon.

Mepergan trademark for an analgesic preparation containing meperidine hydrochloride and promethazine hydrochloride.

meperidine (mē-peri′i-dēn) a nonopioid narcotic analgesic, 1-methyl-4-phenyl-4-piperidin carboxylic acid ethyl ester. Used similarly to morphine. Called also *isonipecaine* and *pethidine.* **m. hydrochloride,** the hydrochloride salt of meperidine, occurring as a white, odorless, crystalline powder that is soluble in water, ethanol, and sparingly in ether. It has pharmacological properties similar to those of morphine, with analgesia and sedation being its chief effects. Used similarly to morphine in controlling severe pain, preoperative and postoperative medication, and for obstetric analgesia. Adverse reactions may include vertigo, nausea, vomiting, sweating, euphoria, weakness, headache, agitation, tremor, hallucinations, disorientation, and various gastrointestinal, genitourinary, and cardiovascular disorders. Respiratory depression with arrest, cardiovascular shock, and cardiac arrest may occur. Abuse may lead to habituation and addiction. Trademarks: Algil, Demerol, Dolantin, Dolenal, Dolvanol, Mephedine, Lydol, Pantalgine, Spasmodolin, Spasmomedal.

Mephedine trademark for *meperidine hydrochloride* (see under MEPERIDINE).

mephenesin (mē-fen′ĕ-sin) a skeletal muscle relaxant, 3-(2-methylphenoxy)-1,2-propanediol, occurring as a white, bitter, crystalline powder with a numbing effect on the tongue, that is soluble in ethanol, propylene glycol, chloroform, water, and ether. Trademarks: Atensin, Mepherol, Relaxar, Relaxil, Spasmolyn.

mephentermine (mē-fen′ter-mēn) a sympathomimetic amine, N-, α,α-trimethylphenethylamine, occurring as a liquid with a typical fishy amine odor, which is soluble in ethanol and ether, but not in water. It has some cardiovascular activity and central nervous system stimulant effects; when given systemically, it elevates blood pressure and stimulates the heart and, when given topically, causes vasoconstriction. Used chiefly as a nasal decongestant. Side effects may include cardiac arrhythmia, tachycardia, precordial pain, respiratory disorders, weakness, vertigo, tremor, and anxiety. Excessive doses may produce hypertensive crises. Trademarks: Vialin, Wyamine. **m. sulfate,** the sulfate salt of mephentermine, occurring as a white, odorless crystalline powder or crystals that are soluble in water and ethanol but not in chloroform. Its pharmacological and toxicological properties are similar to those of the parent compound. Used to support blood pressure in spinal anesthesia and in treatment with ganglionic blocking agents or in postural hypotension. Also used as a nasal decongestant. Trademarks: Mephine, Wyamine.

mephenytoin (mē-fen′i-to-in) an anticonvulsant, 5-ethyl-3-methyl-5-phenyl-2,4-imidazolidinedione, occurring as a white crystalline powder that is readily soluble in chloroform, ethanol, and alkali hydroxide solution and slightly soluble in ether and water. Used in the treatment of epilepsy. Side effects may include leukopenia, neutropenia, agranulocytosis, thrombocytopenia, pancytopenia, eosinophilia, monocytosis, leukocytosis, anemias, severe skin lesions, Stevens-Johnson syndrome, ataxia, diplopia, fatigue, choreiform movements, tremor, jaundice, and polyarthropathy. Trademarks: Insulon, Mesantoin, Phenantoin.

Mepherol trademark for *mephenesin.*

Mephine trademark for *mephentermine sulfate* (see under MEPHENTERMINE).

mephobarbital (mef″o-bar′bi-tal) A long-lasting barbiturate derivative, 5-ethyl-1-methyl-5-phenyl-2,4,6-(1*H*,3*H*,5*H*)-pyrimidinetrione, occurring as a white, odorless, bitter, crystalline powder that is readily soluble in chloroform and alkali hydroxide and carbonate solutions and slightly soluble in ethanol, ether, and water. Used as a hypnotic and sedative, and as an anticonvulsive agent in the treatment of epilepsy. Abuse may lead to potentially fatal acute or chronic intoxication and to habituation or addiction. Trademarks: Isonal, Mebaral, Prominal.

Mepiben trademark for *diphenylpyraline.*

mepivacaine (mē-piv′ah-kān) a local anesthetic, 1-methyl-2′6′-pipecoloxylidide. **m. hydrochloride,** the hydrochloride salt of mepivacaine, occurring as white, odorless crystals that are readily soluble in water and methanol, slightly soluble in chloroform, and insoluble in ether. Used in infiltration, nerve block, and epidural anesthesia. Also used in dental procedures of short duration without vasoconstrictors. Nausea, vomiting, muscular twitching, chills, drowsiness, and depression are the principal side reactions. Trademarks: Arestocaine, Carbocaine, Isocaine, Scandicain.

meprobamate (mĕ-pro′bah-măt, mep″ro-bam′ăt) a minor tranquilizer, 2-methyl-2-propyl-1,3-propanediol dicarbamate, occurring as a white powder with a characteristic odor and a bitter taste, which is readily soluble in alcohol and acetone and slightly soluble in water and ether. Used in insomnia, anxiety, and tension. Prolonged use may lead to habituation. Trademarks: Equanil, Miltown. **isopropyl m.** carisoprodol.

mepyramine (mĕ-pir′ah-mēn) pyrilamine.

mEq, meq milliequivalent.

mer (mer) [Gr. *meros* part] monomeric repeat unit of a polymer.

meractinomycin (mer-ak″tĭ-no-mi′sin) dactinomycin.

meralluride (mer-al′lu-rīd) a mercurial diuretic consisting of a mixture of *N* - [[3 - (hydroxymercuri) - 2 - methoxypropyl] - carbamoyl]-succinamic acid and theophylline in molecular proportions. Used therapeutically as the sodium salt, which occurs as a white to yellowish powder that is soluble in glacial acetic acid, alkali hydroxide solutions, and hot water, in the treatment of edematous diseases, congestive heart failure, the nephrotic syndrome, glomerulonephrosis, and ascites. Adverse reactions include acute stomatitis and other complications occurring during mercurial diuretic therapy (see under DIURETIC). Trademarks: Dilurgen, Mercardan, Mercuhydrin, Mercuretin.

merbromin (mer-bro′min) the disodium salt of 2′7′-dibromo-4′-(hydroxymercuric) fluorescein, derived from dibromofluorescein and mercuric acetate, occurring as odorless, iridescent, green scales or granules that are soluble in water, giving a deep red solution, but not in organic solvents. It is a very toxic substance which, in solutions and tinctures, is used as a disclosing agent for dental plaque and as a topical antiseptic for surgical preparation of the skin. Called also *DOMF* and *solution No. 220.* Trademarks: Chromargyre, Flavurol, Mercurochrome, Mercurochrome-220 soluble, Mercurophage, Planochrome.

Mercaleukin trademark for *mercaptopurine.*

mercaptan (mer-kap′tan) [L. *mercurium captans* seizing or combining with mercury] sulfhydryl. **polyfunctional m.,** POLYSULFIDE polymer.

mercapto- prefix indicating the presence of the sulfhydryl group, SH, in a chemical compound.

mercaptomerin sodium (mer″kap-tom′er-in) a mercurial diuretic, [3 - [[(3-carboxy-2,2,3-trimethylcyclopentyl)carbonyl]amino] - 2 - methoxypropyl] (mercaptoacetato-*S*) mercury disodium salt, occurring as a white, hygroscopic powder or solid with a honeycomb structure, which is freely soluble in water and ethanol and slightly soluble in chloroform and ether. Used in the treatment of edematous diseases, congestive heart failure, nephrotic syndrome, glomerulonephrosis, and ascites. Adverse reactions include acute stomatitis and other complications associated with mercurial diuretic therapy (see under DIURETIC). Trademarks: Diucardyn, Thiomerin.

mercaptopurine, 6-mercaptopurine (mer-kap″to-pu′rēn) an antimetabolite purine analogue either of adenine (6-aminopurine) or hypoxanthine (6-hydroxypurine), 1,7-dihydro-6*H*-purine-6-thione monohydrate. It occurs as an odorless, yellow, crystalline powder that is soluble in hot ethanol and dilute alkali solutions, slightly soluble in diluted sulfuric acid, and insoluble in water, acetone, and ether. Its biological effect is due not to the base itself, but to its riboside formed by the cell, the cell thus performing a "lethal synthesis" by producing a substance which interferes with metabolic processes. In its action mercaptopurine interferes with the conversion of inosinic acid into adenylic and guanylic acid and inhibits biosynthesis of purine by feedback inhibition, i.e., the excess concentration of the false metabolite which inhibits an early stage of biosynthesis. Used in the treatment of cancer, chiefly certain types of leukemia, as an immunosuppressive agent in tissue transplantation, and in therapy of ulcerative colitis. Bone marrow depression with thrombocytopenia, leukopenia, and anemia; predisposition to infection and hemorrhage; gastrointestinal disorders, including ulceration, nausea, vomiting, and diarrhea; and oral disorders, including stomatitis and mucosal ulcers, are the principal side reactions. Called also *6MP* and *6-purinethiol.* Trademarks: Leukerin, Mercaleukin, Purinethol.

mercaptothion (mer-kap″to-thi′on) malathion.

Mercardan trademark for *meralluride.*

Mercazole trademark for *methimazole.*

Mercloran trademark for *chlormerodrin.*

mercocresols (mer″ko-kre′solz) an antiseptic preparation containing *o*-hydroxyphenylmercuric chloride and a tricresol with an amyl group substitution, forming a tincture for external use. Used in the treatment of minor superficial wounds and infections and as a prophylactic disinfectant for surgical preparation of the intact skin, teeth, or rubber dam. In dilution, also used for topical application to mucous membranes and for irrigation of body cavities and deep infected wounds. See also MERCRESIN.

Mercoral trademark for *chlormerodrin.*

Mercresin trademark of an antiseptic and disinfectant preparation containing 0.2 percent mercocresols in a mixture of acetone, 10 percent ethyl alcohol, and 50 percent water and coloring matter.

Mercuhydrin trademark for *meralluride.*

Mercuretin trademark for *meralluride.*

mercurial (mer-ku′re-al) [L. *mercurialis*] 1. pertaining to mercury. 2. a mercury preparation.

mercurialism (mer-ku′re-al-izm) chronic mercury poisoning. See MERCURY.

mercurialized (mer-ku′re-al-īzd) treated with mercury; containing mercury.

mercuric (mer-ku′rik) pertaining to mercury as a bivalent element; a mercury compound containing the Hg atom. **m. oxide, yellow,** see under OXIDE.

Mercurochrome (mer-ku′-ro-krōm) trademark for *merbromin.* **M.-220 soluble,** trademark for *merbromin.*

Mercurophage trademark for *merbromin.*

mercurothiolate (mer-ku″ro-thi′o-lăt) thimerosal.

mercurous (mer′ku-rus) pertaining to mercury as a monovalent element; a compound of monovalent mercury.

mercury (mer′ku-re) [L. *mercurius hydrargyrum*] a heavy metal. Symbol, Hg; atomic number, 80; atomic weight, 200.59; specific gravity, 13.546; valences, 1, 2; melting point, −38.87°C; group IIB of the periodic table. Natural mercury isotopes include 196, 198–202, and 204; other isotopes range in mass number 189–206. It occurs as a silvery, heavy, mobile liquid metal, soluble in sulfuric and nitric acid, but insoluble in water, hydrochloric acid, alcohol, and ether. Solid mercury is a white, ductile, soft metal. Mercury and its salts have been used therapeutically as purgatives, as alternatives in chronic inflammation, and as antisyphilitics, intestinal antiseptics, disinfectants, and astringents. In dentistry, mercury preparations are used for the treatment of minor oral infections and for disinfection of the oral field prior to injections and in endodontic procedures. Also used in dental amalgams. Called also *liquid silver* and *quicksilver.* Acute mercury poisoning, most commonly due to ingestion of mercury bichloride, is characterized by immediate abdominal pain and vomiting, followed by inflammation and edema of the gastric mucosa, associated with necrosis and focal or massive confluent ulcers. Renal changes include acute necrosis and calcium deposits. Severe, necrotizing ulcerative colitis may result. The subacute or chronic form (mercurialism) is characterized chiefly by neurological and oral changes. Myelin degeneration of the peripheral nerves and central nervous system are the principal neurological changes. Oral symptoms consist of increased salivation, metallic taste, enlarged and painful tongue, swollen and hyperemic gingivae, ulcers of the gingivae, palate, and tongue, loosening of teeth and sometimes exfoliation, and pigmentation of the mucosa, characterized by grayish blue lines in the margins of the gingivae. An ashen gray skin pigmentation may be present. Mercury may also produce allergy and acrodynia. Toxic reactions from absorption of mercury from dental amalgam may occur. Mercury poisoning is called also *hydrargyrism.* **m. acetate,** mercuric ACETATE. **m. alloy,** amalgam. **m. amide chloride,** ammoniated m. **ammoniated m.,** a compound, HgNH$_2$Cl, occurring as a white odorless powder or pulverulent solids that darken when exposed to light and are soluble in warm hydrochloric, nitric, and acetic acids and ammonia, but not in water. Used chiefly in ointments for the treatment of bacterial and fungal infections and parasite infestations. Side reactions may include hypersensitivity and mercury poisoning. Ancient names given by alchemists include *sal sapientiae* and *alembroth.* Called also *amminomercuric chloride, mercury amide chloride,* and *white precipitate.* **m. bichloride,** mercuric CHLORIDE. **dental m.,** pure mercury used in dental amalgams. The purity of mercury can be determined by the appearance of its surface, whereby mercury containing less than 0.001 percent copper, zinc, tin, lead, bismuth, cadmium, arsenic, antimony, and other contaminants has a glossy, mirror-like surface. Also, because of the wetting properties of contaminants, impure mercury cannot be completely poured out of a glass container. Gold and silver in the amounts of up to 0.1 percent do not alter the appearance of the surface, but their presence in mercury can be determined by volatilizing mercury; the presence of a residue indicates contamination. Trademarks: Argentum, Crown, Moyco, ProMercury, Spectropure. **m. dispenser,** mercury DISPENSER. **m. perchloride,** mercuric CHLORIDE.

mereprine (mer'ĕ-prēn) doxylamine.

Merezine trademark for preparations of *cyclizine.*

Merfamin trademark for *thimerosal.*

meridian (mĕ-rid'e-an) [L. *meridianus*] an imaginary line forming a great circle on the surface of a spherical body, passing through opposite poles.

meridiani (mĕ-rid"e-a'ni) [L.] plural of *meridianus.*

meridianus (mĕ-rid"e-a'nus), pl. *meridia'ni* [L. from *medius* middle + *dies* day] meridian.

Merismopedia gonorrhoeae (me"ris-mo-po'de-ah gon"o-re'e) *Neisseria gonorrhoeae;* see under NEISSERIA.

Merkel's cells [Friedrich Sigmund *Merkel*, German anatomist, 1845–1919] see under CELL.

Merkel's corpuscles (disks) [Friedrich Sigmund *Merkel*, German anatomist, 1845–1919] see under CORPUSCLE.

Merkel's muscle [Karl Ludwig *Merkel*, German anatomist, 1812–1876] ceratocricoid MUSCLE.

Merkel-Ranvier cells [F. S. *Merkel;* Louis Antoine *Ranvier*, French pathologist, 1835–1922] Merkel's cells; see under CELL.

mero- [Gr. *meros* part] a combining form meaning part.

merocrine (mer'o-krĭn) [*mero-* + Gr. *krinein* to separate] partly secreting; as in a merocrine gland. Cf. HOLOCRINE.

meromyosin (mer"o-mi'o-sin) *myosin.*

Merrifield knife see under KNIFE.

Mershon arch see under ARCH.

Mersolite trademark for *phenylmercuric acetate* (see under ACETATE).

Merten, D. F. see Singleton-Merten SYNDROME.

Merthiolate trademark for *thimerosal.*

Mertorgan trademark for *thimerosal.*

Merzonin trademark for *thimerosal.*

mesad (me'sad) [Gr. *mesos* middle] toward the median line or plane, mesiad.

mesal (me'sal) mesial.

Mesantoin trademark for *mephenytoin.*

mescaline (mes'kah-lēn) a psychogenic agent, 3,4,5-tri-methoxybenzenethanamine, which is the principal alkaloid of peyote, the dried flowering tops of the cactus *Lophophora williamsii*, occurring as a crystalline substance that is soluble in water, ethanol, chloroform, and benzene, but not in ether. Used chiefly in experimental studies; in humans, it produces hallucinations, sympathomimetic autonomic effects, hyperreflexia, tremors, and various psychotic changes. Used by certain American Indians for religious purposes.

mesencephalon (mes"en-sef'ah-lon) [*meso-* + Gr. *enkephalos* brain] midbrain.

mesenchyma (mĕ-seng'kĭ-mah) [*meso-* + Gr. *enchyma* infusion] the meshwork of embryonic connective tissue of mesodermal and, to a lesser extent, ectodermal origin, from which are formed the connective tissue, and also the blood and lymphatic vessels. The mesenchyma originating from the neural crest (*ectomesenchyme*) forms the visceral arches and the anterior portion of the trabeculae cranii; that originating from the endoderm (*endomesenchyme* or *endomesoderm*) gives rise to the branchial arch cartilages, dermal bones, dentin, adrenal medulla, and pigment cells. It is made up of stellate cells, the protoplasmic processes of which meet those of adjacent cells, forming a cellular network. A jelly-like ground substance fills the intercellular spaces. By the end of the second month, the fibrous elements become prominent and the presence of fibroblasts is noted. Called also *mesenchyme.*

mesenchyme (mes'eng-kīm) mesenchyma.

Mesentol trademark for *ethosuximide.*

MeSH (mesh) Medical Subject Headings; acronym for a thesaurus published by the National Library of Medicine, which is used for the computerized medical information system on line (MEDLINE), and a number of printed biomedical bibliographies, including *Index Medicus* and *Index to Dental Literature.*

mesiad (me'ze-ad) toward the middle; mesad.

mesial (me'ze-al) toward or situated in the middle, median, nearer the middle line of the body or nearer the center of the dental arch.

mesially (me'ze-al"e) toward the median line.

mesien (me'ze-en) pertaining to the mesion.

mesio- [Gr. *mesos* middle] a combining form indicating relationship to the middle; specifically, the mesial surface of a tooth or the mesial wall of a tooth cavity. See also words beginning MESO-.

---

mesioaxial (me"ze-o-ak'se-al) pertaining to or formed by the mesial and axial walls of a tooth cavity preparation. Called also *axiomesial.*

mesioaxiogingival (me"ze-o-ak"se-o-jin'jĭ-val) pertaining to or formed by the mesial, axial, and gingival walls of a tooth cavity preparation. Called also *axiomesiocervical* and *axiomesiogingival.*

mesioaxioincisal (me"ze-o-ak"se-o-in-si'zal) pertaining to or formed by the mesial, axial, and incisal walls of a tooth cavity preparation. Called also *axiomesioincisal.*

mesiobuccal (me"ze-o-buk'kal) pertaining to or formed by the mesial and buccal surfaces of a tooth, or the mesial and buccal walls of a cavity preparation of a tooth. Called also *buccomesial.*

mesiobucco-occlusal (me"ze-o-buk"ko-ŏ-kloo'zal) pertaining to or formed by the mesial, buccal, and occlusal surfaces of a tooth.

mesiobuccopulpal (me"ze-o-buk"ko-pul'pal) pertaining to or formed by the mesial, buccal, and pulpal walls of a tooth cavity.

mesiocervical (me"ze-o-ser'vĭ-kal) 1. pertaining to the mesial surface of the neck of a tooth. 2. mesiogingival.

mesioclination (me"ze-o-kli-na'shun) deviation of a tooth from the vertical, in the direction of the tooth next mesial (anterior) to it in the dental arch.

mesioclusion (me"se-o-kloo'zhun) malocclusion in which the mandibular arch is in an anterior position in relation to the maxillary arch (prognathism). Generally considered as identical with Class III in Angle's classification of malocclusion (see MALOCCLUSION). Called also *anterior,* or *protrusive, occlusion* and *anteroclusion.* **bilateral m.,** that occurring on both sides. **unilateral m.,** that occurring only on one side.

mesiodens (me'ze-o-denz), pl. *mesioden'tes* [*mesio-* + Gr. *dens* tooth] the most common supernumerary tooth, appearing singly or in pairs as a small tooth with a cone-shaped crown and a short root, between the maxillary central incisors; they may be erupted, impacted, or even inverted.

mesiodentes (me"ze-o-den'tēz) [L.] plural of *mesiodens.*

mesiodistal (me"ze-o-dis'tal) pertaining to the mesial and distal surfaces of a tooth.

mesiogingival (me"ze-o-jin'jĭ-val) pertaining to or formed by the mesial and gingival walls of a tooth cavity, called also *mesiocervical.*

mesiognathic (me"ze-o-nath'ik) malposition of one or both jaws ahead of the frontal plane or forehead.

mesioincisodistal (me"ze-o-in-si"zo-dis'tal) pertaining to the mesial, incisal, and distal surfaces of an anterior tooth.

mesiolabial (me"ze-o-la'be-al) pertaining to or formed by the mesial and labial surfaces of a tooth, or the mesial and labial walls of a cavity preparation of a tooth.

mesiolabioincisal (me"ze-o-la"be-o-in-si'zal) pertaining to or formed by the mesial, labial, and incisal surfaces of a tooth.

mesiolingual (me"ze-o-ling'gwal) pertaining to or formed by the lingual and mesial surfaces of a tooth, or the lingual and mesial walls of a tooth cavity preparation. Called also *linguomesial.*

mesiolinguoincisal (me"ze-o-ling"gwo-in-si'zal) pertaining to or formed by the mesial, lingual, and incisal surfaces of a tooth.

mesiolinguo-occlusal (me"ze-o-ling"gwo-ŏ-kloo'zal) pertaining to or formed by the mesial, lingual, and occlusal surfaces of a tooth.

mesiolinguopulpal (me"ze-o-ling"gwo-pul'pal) pertaining to or formed by the mesial, lingual, and pulpal walls of a cavity preparation of a tooth.

mesion (me'se-on) [Gr. *mesos* middle] the plane that divides the body into right and left symmetric halves. Called also *meson.*

mesio-occlusal (me"ze-o-ŏ-kloo'zal) pertaining to or formed by the mesial and occlusal surfaces of a tooth, or the mesial and occlusal walls of a tooth cavity.

mesio-occlusion (me"ze-o-ŏ-kloo'zhun) mesioclusion.

mesio-occlusodistal (me"ze-o-ŏ-kloo"so-dis'tal) pertaining to the mesial, occlusal, and distal surfaces of a posterior tooth.

mesiopulpal (me"ze-o-pul'pal) pertaining to or formed by the mesial and pulpal walls of a cavity preparation of a tooth.

mesiopulpolabial (me"ze-o-pul"po-la'be-al) pertaining to or formed by the mesial, pulpal, and labial walls of a cavity preparation of a tooth.

mesiopulpolingual (me"ze-o-pul"po-ling'gwal) pertaining to or formed by the mesial, pulpal, and lingual walls of a cavity preparation of a tooth.

mesioversion (me"ze-o-ver'zhun) deviation of a tooth from the vertical, in the direction of the tooth next mesial (anterior) to it in the dental arch.

meso- [Gr. *mesos* middle] 1. a prefix signifying middle. See also words beginning MESIO-. 2. a chemical prefix signifying inactive or without effect on polarized light.

mesocephalic (mes″o-sĕ-fal′ik) [*meso-* + Gr. *kephalē* head] characterized by or pertaining to a skull having an average breadth-length index. See mesocephalic SKULL.

mesocranic (mes″o-kra′nik) having a cranial index between 75.0 and 79.9.

mesoderm (mes′o-derm) [*meso-* + Gr. *derma* skin] the middle of the three primary germ layers of the embryo, lying between the ectoderm and the entoderm. From it are derived the connective tissue, bone, cartilage, muscles, blood, blood vessels, lymphatics, lymphoid organs, notochord, pleura, pericardium, peritoneum, kidneys, and gonads. See also GASTRULATION and germ LAYER. **lateral m., lateral plate m.,** the part of the embryonic mesoderm that, in conjunction with the ectoderm and entoderm, forms the periphery of the embryonic disk. The embryonic coelom develops within it. **somatic m.,** the part of the lateral mesoderm next to the ectoderm, being the outer of the two layers into which the mesoderm divides. The somatic mesoderm and the ectoderm are known collectively as the *somatopleure*. **peraxial, m.,** the mesoderm on each side of the notochord and neural tube, which gives rise to the paired somites. **splanchnic m.,** mesoderm that lies next to the entoderm; being the inner of the two layers of the embryonic mesoderm. The splanchnic mesoderm and the entoderm are known collectively as the *splanchnopleure*.

mesodont (mes′o-dont) [*meso-* + Gr. *odous* tooth] having a dental index between 42 and 44.

mesodontic (mes″o-don′tik) having medium-sized teeth.

mesodontism (mes′o-don′tizm) the state of having medium-sized teeth, or a dental index between 42 and 44.

mesoglia (mĕ-sog′le-ah) microglia.

mesognathic (mes″og-na′thik) mesognathous.

mesognathous (mĕ-sog′nah-thus) [*meso-* + Gr. *gnathos* jaw] pertaining to or characterized by moderate protrusion of the jaw. Called also *mesognathic*. See mesognathic SKULL.

mesomelic (mes″o-mel′ik) [*meso-* + Gr. *melus* limb] pertaining to or affecting the midportion of the limb.

mesomorph (mes′o-morf) [*mesoderm* + Gr. *morphē* form) an individual having a type of body build in which tissues derived from the mesoderm predominate. There is relative preponderance of muscle, bone, and connective tissue, usually with heavy, hard physique of rectangular outline. This somatotype is classified between the ectomorph and the endomorph.

meson (mes′on, me′zon) [Gr. *mesos* middle] 1. mesion. 2. a subatomic, short-lived particle of a mass less than that of a proton but more than that of an electron, carrying either a positive or a negative electric charge. Called also *mesotron*. π **m.,** a positively or negatively charged particle with a mass 285 times that of an electron, having a mean life of 2×10^{-8} sec, and decaying into μ meson. Abbreviated π m. **μm.,** a positively or negatively charged particle with a mass 215 times that of an electron. Abbreviated μm.

mesonasal (mes″o-na′zal) situated in the middle of the nose.

mesonephroi (mes″o-nef′roi) [Gr.] plural of *mesonephros*.

mesonephros (mes″o-nef′ros), pl. *mesoneph′roi* [*meso-* + Gr. *nephros* kidney] the embryonic kidney that precedes the permanent kidney (metanephros) and serves in the embryo as a temporary excretory organ overlapping the initial activity of the kidney. It originates in the fourth and fifth weeks by developing from the nephrogenic cord, and consists of the renal units, collecting duct, and urinary duct; its long tube in the lower part of the body running parallel with the spinal axis and joining at right angles a row of twisting tubes. It undergoes regression during the early fetal period as the permanent kidney develops. Called also *corpus Wolffi*, *middle kidney*, and *wolffian body*.

mesophragma (mes″o--frag′mah) [*meso-* ∝ Gr. *phragmos* a fencing in] M BAND.

mesophryon (me-sof′re-on) [*meso-* + Gr. *ophrys* eyebrow] the glabella or its central point.

Mesopin trademark for *homatropine methylbromide* (see under HOMATROPINE).

mesoprosopic (mes″o-pro-sop′ik) [*meso-* + Gr. *prosōpon* face] pertaining to or characterized by a face of moderate width and height. See mesoprosopic SKULL.

mesorrhine (mes′o-rin) [*meso-* + Gr. *rhis* nose] having a nasal index between 48 and 53.

mesoseme (mes′o-sēm) [*meso-* + Gr. *sēma* sign] having an orbital index between 83 and 89.

mesosome (mes′o-sōm) [*meso-* + Gr. *sōma* body] an invagination of the plasma membrane of a bacterial cell, forming an internal organelle. Mesosomes may assume vesicular, lamellar, or tubular forms, and more than one type may be found in a single cell. Their function has not been fully established, but they have been linked with replication and apportionment of DNA to daughter cells during cell division and have been considered as septum initiators during cell division. See also illustration at BACTERIUM.

mesostaphyline (mes″o-staf′ĭ-lĭn) [*meso-* + Gr. *staphylē* a bunch of grapes, uvula] pertaining to or characterized by a palate with a moderate width. See mesostaphyline SKULL.

mesostructure (mes′o-struk′chur) a middle or intermediate structure. **m. bar,** mesostructure BAR. **implant m.,** that part of an endosseous implant which is located between the internally threaded vent plants and the superstructure. It is attached to the implant with screws, and contains a system of internal threads which allows the superstructure to be screwed into it. **integral intraoral bilateral posterior m.,** mesostructure BAR.

mesotaurodontism (mes″o-taw″ro-don′tizm) [*meso-* + *taurodontism*] a form of taurodontism in which roots branch only in the middle.

mesotendineum (mes″o-ten-din′e-um) the delicate connective tissue sheath attaching a tendon to its fibrous sheath. Called also *mesotendon* and *mesotenon*.

mesotendon (mes″o-ten′don) mesotendineum.

mesotenon (mes″o-ten′on) mesotendineum.

mesothelioma (mes″o-the″le-o′mah) a tumor derived from the mesothelial tissue.

mesothelium (mes″o-the′le-um) [*meso-* + *epithelium*] [NA] the surface layer of the mesoderm, which is bound to the coelom and lines the body cavity of the embryo. In the adult, it forms the simple squamous-cell layer of the epithelium which covers the surface of all true serous membranes.

mesotron (mes′o-tron) meson (2).

messenger (mes′en-jer) one who or that which bears or transmits a message or performs an errand. **second m.,** ADENOSINE 3′5′-cyclic phosphate. **m. RNA,** see RNA.

Mestinon trademark for *pyridostigmine bromide* (see under PYRIDOSTIGMINE).

Mesulfa trademark for *sulfamerazine*.

mesuranic (mes″u-ran′ik) [*meso-* + Gr *ouranos* palate of the mouth] having a maxilloalveolar index between 110.0 and 114.9.

Met methionine.

met (met) a unit of measurement of heat production by the body; the metabolic heat produced by a resting-sitting subject, being 50 kilocalories per 1 m²/hr.

meta- [Gr. *meta* after, beyond, over] 1. a prefix indicating change, transformation, exchange, after, or next. 2. in organic chemistry, a prefix in structural isomerism indicating the substitution in a derivative of a benzene ring of two atoms separated by an intervening carbon atom or 1,3-position in the ring. See meta-ISOMER. 3. in inorganic chemistry, a less hydrated acid or salt. 4. a polymeric compound.

metabasis (me-tab′ah-sis) [*meta-* + Gr. *bainein* to go] 1. a change in the manifestations or course of a disease. 2. metastasis, or change in the site of a morbid process from one region of the body to another.

metabiosis (met″ah-bi-o′sis) [*meta-* + Gr. *biosis* way of life] the dependence of one organism upon another for its existence.

metabolic (met″ah-bol′ik) pertaining to or of the nature of metabolism.

metabolimeter (met″ah-bo-lim′ĕ-ter) an apparatus for measuring basal metabolism.

metabolism (me-tab′o-lizm) [Gr. *metaballein* to turn about, change, alter] the sum of all the physical and chemical processes by which living substance is produced and maintained, and also the transformation by which energy is made available for the use of the organism. See also ANABOLISM, CARBOHYDRATE metabolism, CATABOLISM, LIPID metabolism, and PROTEIN metabolism. **basal m.,** the minimal energy expended for the maintenance of respiration, glandular activity, and other vegetative functions of the body. The basal metabolic rate (BMR) is measured under basal conditions, whereby the subject has not eaten for at least 12 hours; after a night of restful sleep; without performing strenuous exercise, the subject remaining at complete rest in a reclining position for at least 30 minutes prior to the test; after insuring that the subject is free of any physical or psychic stress; at the temperature of the air in the range of 68 to 80°F. BMR is determined by calculating from the quantity of oxygen used the quantity of heat liberated in the body, according to the following steps: O_2 consumed in 1 hour; calories liberated per liter of O_2 burned; calories liberated per hour; body surface area in m^2; calories per m^2 per hour; excess calories above normal. BMR equals 1800 C/day and 1200 C/day for a standard 70 kg male and a 50 kg female, respectively. **carbohydrate m.,** CARBOHYDRATE metabolism. **energy m.,** the metabolic processes by which energy is released. **inborn error of m.,** a genetically determined biochemical disorder in which a specific enzyme defect produces a metabolic block that may have pathologic consequences at birth (e.g., phenylketonuria) or in later life (e.g., diabetes mellitus). Called also *enzymopathy.* **intermediary m.,** chemical reactions occurring in the cell in which various interrelated multienzyme systems participate, exchanging both matter and energy between the cell and its environment. Its functions include: obtaining chemical energy from fuel molecules or from absorbed sunlight; conversion of exogenous nutrients into the building blocks, or precursors, of macromolecular cell components; assembling such building blocks into proteins, nucleic acids, lipids, and other components; and formation and degradation of biomolecules in specialized functions of cells. **lipid m.,** LIPID metabolism. **protein m.,** PROTEIN metabolism.

metabolite (me-tab′o-līt) any substance produced by metabolic processes, or an intermediate product of metabolism. **m. antagonist,** antimetabolite.

metabutoxycaine hydrochloride (met″ah-bu-tok′sĕ-kān) a local anesthetic of short duration, 2-(dimethylamino)ethyl-3-amino-2-butoxybenzoate hydrochloride, occurring as a white crystalline solid that is very soluble in water and alcohol, slightly soluble in acetone and chloroform, and very slightly soluble in ether. Used for infiltration and nerve block anesthesia in dental procedures.

metacentric (met″ah-sen′trik) [*meta-* + Gr. *kentron;* L. *centrum* center] having the center or centromere near the middle. See metacentric CHROMOSOME.

metachromasia (met″ah-kro-ma′ze-ah) [*meta-* + Gr. *chrōma* color] 1. a condition in which tissues do not stain true with a given stain. 2. staining in which the same stain colors different tissues in different tints. 3. the change of color produced by staining.

metachromatic (met″ah-kro-mat′ik) [*meta-* + Gr. *chrōmatikos* relating to color] staining differently with the same dye, said of tissues in which different elements take on different colors when a certain dye is applied. By extension, said of dyes by which different tissues are stained differently.

metachronous (me-tak′ro-nus) [*meta-* + Gr. *chronos* time] occurring at different times.

metacone (met′ah-kōn) [*meta-* + Gr. *kōnos* cone] the distobuccal cusp of a maxillary molar tooth. See also HYPOCONE, PARACONE, PROTOCONID, and TRIGONE (2).

metaconid (met″ah-kon′id) [*meta-* + Gr. *kōnos* cone + *-id*] the mesiolingual cusp of a mandibular molar tooth. See also HYPOCONID, PARACONID, PROTOCONID, and TRIGONID.

metaconule (met″ah-kon′ūl) the small intermediate cusp between the metacone and the protocone of the upper molar teeth of mammals, sometimes also present in man.

metacortandracin (met″ah-kor-tan′drah-sin) prednisone.

metacortandralone (met″ah-kor-tan′drah-lōn) prednisolone.

metacresol (met″ah-kre′sol) metacresyl. **m. acetate** METACRESYL acetate.

metacresyl (met″ah-kre′sil) one of the three isometric forms of cresol, and the most strongly antiseptic of the group. Written also *m*-cresyl. Called also *metacresol.* **m. acetate,** a strong bactericidal and fungicidal drug, $CH_3C_6H_4OCOCH_3$, occurring

as a colorless oily liquid with a characteristic phenolic odor, which is insoluble in water or glycerol and miscible with alcohol, ether, and other organic solvents. Used in root canal therapy. Called also *acetylmetacresol,* m-*cresyl acetate, meta-cresol acetate, metacresylic acid, 3-methylphenol,* and m-*tolyl acetate.* Trademarks: Cresantin, Kresantin.

Metadorm trademark for *methaqualone hydrochloride* (see under METHAQUALONE).

Metahydrin trademark for *trichlormethiazide.*

metainfective (met″ah-in-fek′tiv) occurring after an infection; usually applied to a febrile state occurring during convalescence from an infectious disease.

metal (met′l) [L. *metallum;* Gr. *metallon*] 1. any element that tends to form positive ions in solution and whose oxides form hydroxides rather than acids with water. Physically, most metals are characterized by heat and electric conductivity, fusibility, hardness, luster, ductility, and suitability to be formed and machined. Structurally, metals differ from non-metals by their lattice structure. Metals represent about three-quarters of all elements. See also metallic SOLID and periodic table at ELEMENT. 2. in dentistry, a term sometimes used to mean alloy. **alkali m.,** a group of metals, which includes lithium, sodium, potassium, rubidium, cesium, and francium, belonging to group IA of the periodic table. Except for francium, members of this group are characterized by their silvery appearance, fusibility, and melting points that become lower with increasing atomic weight. Most react violently with water and are strongly electropositive; their basicity increases with atomic weight. None of the alkali metals is found in nature because of their very high reactivity. **alkaline earth m.,** a group of metals, including calcium, barium, strontium, and radium, belonging to group IIA of the periodic table. They are grayish white, extrudable, malleable, and easily oxidized in air. Their melting and boiling points are higher than those of alkali metals. **alloy-forming m.,** see table at ALLOY. **m. annealing,** metal ANNEALING. **Babbitt's m.,** an alloy of tin, copper, and antimony; a very low melting metal used for dies. **base m., basic m.,** any metal whose compounds with oxygen are not decomposable by heat alone, retaining oxygen at high temperatures, including zinc, aluminum, tin, iron, and lead. **cast m.,** a metal which, after melting, is poured into a mold where it solidifies to a desired shape, or is extruded to form pipes and rods. When worked in the cold state by drawing, rolling, or hammering, it becomes wrought metal. **cliche m.,** a fusible alloy containing tin, lead, antimony, and bismuth; no longer used. **counterdie m.,** any hard, fusible alloy suitable for counterdies. **d'Arcet's m.,** an alloy of lead, bismuth, and tin; a fusible metal formerly used for dies. **m. deformation,** see DEFORMATION (2). **earth m.,** any metal of group III of the periodic table. **fusible m.,** an alloy that melts at a relatively low temperature, as at or around the boiling point of water. Bismuth, lead, and tin are usually the principal components. **heavy m.,** any metal with a density above 4. Heavy metals vary in chemical, biological, and physical characteristics, but most form stable complexes with a number of ligands, sulfur, and nitrogen. Their principal biologic effect is exerted through combination with sulfhydryl groups. Most exert a toxic effect on rapidly proliferating tissues, such as the bone marrow, or on microorganisms. Most heavy metals are no longer used therapeutically; their present importance lies in their occupational and environmental toxicity. Arsenic, an-

COMPOSITION LIMITS OF HIGH STRENGTH PRECIOUS METAL WIRES USED IN DENTISTRY

TYPE No.	GOLD (%)	PLATINUM (%)	PALLADIUM (%)	SILVER (%)	COPPER (%)	NICKEL (%)	ZINC (%)
1	25–30	40–50	25–30	...	...	...	...
2	54–60	14–18	1– 8	7–11	11–14	0–1	0–2
3	45–50	8–12	20–25	5– 8	7–12	...	0–1
4	62–64	7–13	0– 6	9–16	7–14	0–2	0–1
5	64–70	2– 7	0– 5	9–15	12–18	0–2	0–1
6	56–63	0– 5	0– 5	14–25	11–18	0–3	0–1
7	10–28	0–25	20–37	6–30	14–21	0–2	0–2
8	...	0– 1	42–44	38–41	16–17	0–1	...

Fractional percentages of iridium, indium, and rhodium have not been included. (From Walter S. Crowell, **"Gold Alloys in Dentistry,"** *Metals Handbook:* Properties and Selection of Metals, Vol. 1, 8th ed., Lyman, T. **(ed.). American Society for Metals, 1961, pg. 1188.)**

timony, bismuth, silver, gold, mercury, and lead are the principal heavy metals of biological and toxicological importance. **implant m.,** any inert metal used for implants; silver, tantalum, ticonium, and vitallium being most commonly used. **light m.,** a metal with a density below 4. **Melotte's m.,** a soft fusible alloy consisting of bismuth, lead, and tin; used for dies and counterdies. **noble m.,** a metal that reacts only to a limited extent with other metals and does not readily oxidize when exposed to humid air or water or is readily attacked by common acids. Gold and silver are the most commonly used noble metals in dentistry; platinum, palladium, iridium, rhodium, ruthenium, and osmium are also included in this group. Called also *precious m.* See also inert ELEMENT. **precious m.,** noble m. **rare m.,** a nonspecific term usually denoting the less common metallic elements, including barium, calcium, strontium, beryllium, bismuth, cadmium, cobalt, gallium, germanium, hafnium, indium, lithium, boron, silicon, manganese, molybdenum, rhenium, selenium, tantalum, niobium, tellurium, thallium, thorium, titanium, tungsten, uranium, vanadium, zirconium, and the rare earths. **rare earth m.,** rare EARTH. **m. sol,** metal SOL. **white m.,** 1. any of a group of alloys having a relatively low melting point, and usually containing tin, lead, or antimony as the principal component. 2. any metal which, when not oxidized, is characterized by a white lustrous color, including silver, nickel, tin, aluminum, and zinc. **wrought m.,** a metal that is first cast and then worked in the cold state into a desired shape by drawing, rolling, or hammering, being more resistant to fractures and more flexible than cast metal. Used in orthodontic wires, springs, and some instruments.

metal-ceramics (met″l-sĕ-ram′iks) see metal-ceramic RESTORATION.

metalizing (met‴l-īz′ing) making something metallic, as when treating the surface of impression material with metals so that it will conduct electricity before electroplating. The process consists of burnishing a metalizing agent, such as bronzing powder suspended in oil of almonds, suspensions of silver powder, and powdered graphite, on the surface of the impression with a brush.

metallic (mĕ-tal′ik) 1. pertaining to, consisting of, or of the nature of metal, as in luster, resonance, hardness, or appearance. 2. made of metal.

metalloid (met″l-oid) [*metal* + Gr. *eidos* form] 1. any element that behaves like a metal under certain conditions, but does not ionize positively when in solution, such as carbon, silica, or boron. 2. a group of chemical substances which have properties intermediate between metals and nonmetals. Metalloids generally have a medium degree of electronegativity and their oxides form neither strong acids nor strong bases. Some authorities consider carbon, germanium, silicon, arsenic, antimony, selenium, and tellurium as metalloid substances, some of which are classifed as nonmetals by others. Sometimes called incorrectly nonmetal. 3. resembling a metal.

metallophilic (me-tal″o-fil′ik) [*metal* + Gr. *philein* to love] having an affinity for metal-containing stains.

metalloprotein (me-tal″o-pro′te-in) a conjugated protein in which the prosthetic group is a metal. Principal metalloproteins are enzymes such as tyrosinase, arginase, and xanthine oxidase.

metalloproteinase [E.C.3.4.24] (me-tal″o-pro′te-in-ās″) a subsubclass of peptide hydrolases, the enzymes of which utilize a metal ion in the catalytic mechanism.

metalloscopy (met″l-os′ko-pe) [*metal* + Gr. *skopein* to examine] observation on the effects of applying metal to the body.

metallum (met′ah-lum) [L.] metal. **m. paradox′um,** tellurium. **m. problema′tum,** tellurium.

metallurgy (met″l-er′je) [*metal* + Gr. *ergon* work] the science, art, or technology dealing with the processes involved in the separation of metals from their ores, the technique of making or compounding the alloys, the techniques of working or heat-treating of metals, and the mining of metals. **physical m.,** the science dealing with the study of the physical properties and internal structure of metals and alloys.

Metamine trademark for *trolnitrate phosphate* (see under TROLNITRATE).

metamorphosis (met″ah-mor′fō-sis) [*meta-* + Gr. *morphōsis* a shaping, bringing into shape] change of shape or structure, particularly a transition from one developmental stage to another. **fatty m.,** any normal or pathologic transformation of fat, including fatty infiltration and fatty degeneration. **tissue m.,** any change in tissues, either normal or pathologic.

metamyelocyte (met″ah-mi-el′o-sīt) [*meta-* + *myelocyte*] an immature myelocyte in an advanced stage of development, following the promyelocyte stage, characterized by the presence of granules that fill the cytoplasm, except for the centrosome, and a horseshoe- or sausage-shaped nucleus. Called also *juvenile cell, form, leukocyte,* or *neutrophil,* and *young form.* See MYELOCYTE.

Metandren trademark for *methyltestosterone.*

metanephrine (met″ah-nef′rin) a naturally occurring biodegradation product of epinephrine found in the urine and in certain tissues, 4-hydroxy-3-methoxy-α-(methylaminomethyl)benzenemethanol.

metanephroi (met″ah-nef′roi) [Gr.] plural of *metanephros.*

metanephros (met″ah-nef′ros), pl. *metaneph′roi* [*meta-* + Gr. *nephros* kidney] the permanent kidney made up of an aggregate of tubules which drain into a common duct. Its drainage ducts (ureter, pelvis, calices, and straight tubules) derive from the ureteric bud of the mesonephric duct, and its secretory unit (Bowman's capsule, convolute tubules, and Henle's loop) derive from the nephrogenic cord.

metaphase (met′ah-fāz) [*meta-* + *phase*] the second stage of cell division (mitosis or meiosis), during which the contracted chromosomes, each consisting of two chromatids, are arranged in the equatorial plane of the spindle prior to separation. See MEIOSIS and MITOSIS.

Metaphen trademark for *nitromersol.*

metaphosphate (met″ah-fos′fāt) a salt or ester of metaphosphoric acid.

metaphosphoric (met″ah-fos-for′ik) pertaining to metaphosphoric acid.

Metaphyllin trademark for *aminophylline.*

metaphysis (me-taf′ĭ-sis), pl. *metaph′yses* [*meta-* + Gr. *phyein* to grow] a wide part on the shaft of the long bone at the junction of the epiphysis and the diaphysis. During development it serves as the zone of cartilage proliferation and contains the growth zone. In the adult it is continuous with the epiphysis.

metaplasia (met″ah-pla′ze-ah) [*meta-* + Gr. *plassein* to form] a reversible change in which one adult cell type (epithelial or mesenchymal) is replaced by another adult cell type. Cf. ANAPLASIA and DYSPLASIA (2). **adaptive m.,** adaptive substitution of cells more sensitive to stress by other cell types better able to withstand the adverse environment, as seen in squamous metaplasia. **atypical m.,** dysplasia. **epithelial m.,** that occurring in epithelium exposed to protracted mechanical trauma, chronic irritation in prolonged inflammation, or prolonged vitamin A deficiency. The most common type is the replacement of columnar cells by stratified squamous epithelium. **mesenchymal m.,** that in which primitive mesenchymal cells differentiate into any other form of mesenchymal cell. Under certain circumstances, cells are transformed into more highly differentiated forms, such as osteoblasts, fat cells, macrophages, or histiocytes. **m. of pulp,** transformation of the usual types of cells normally found in the pulp tissue into entirely different types. **retrograde m.,** retroplasia. **squamous m.,** replacement of the normal secretory columnar epithelium by nonfunctioning stratified squamous epithelium, occurring in organs such as the respiratory tract in response to chronic irritation by various conditions, including habitual cigarette smoking or chronic infection; or in the salivary glands, pancreas, and other secretory organs due to conditions such as calculi; or in the bronchi in vitamin A deficiency.

Metaprel trademark for *metaproterenol sulfate* (see under METAPROTERENOL).

metaprotein (met′ah-pro′te-in) [*meta-* + *protein*] a protein derivative produced by hydrolysis.

metaproterenol sulfate (met″ah-pro-ter′ĕ-nol) a beta-adrenergic agonist with bronchodilator and cardiovascular actions, 5-[1-hydroxy-2-[(1-methylethyl)amino]ethyl]-1,3-benzenediol sulfate, occurring as a white to off-white, odorless, bitter, photosensitive powder that oxidizes on exposure to air and is soluble in water and ethanol. Used chiefly in the treatment of bronchial asthma. Side effects may include tachycardia, arrhythmia, precordial pain, headache, vertigo, excessive sweating, and anxiety. Trademarks: Alotec, Alupent, Metaprel, Novasmasol.

metaraminol bitartrate (met″ah-ram′ĭ-nol) a sympathomimetic with vasoconstrictor and cardiac actions, α-(1-aminoethyl)-3-hydroxybenzenemethanol bitartrate, occurring as a white, odorless, crystalline powder that is soluble in ethanol and water, but not in ether and chloroform. Used to elevate blood pressure in anesthesia and acute hypotension. Overdoses may cause hypertensive crises, tachyarrhythmias, pallor, precordial pain, weakness, vertigo, tremor, respiratory-distress, and anxiety. Trademarks: Aramine, Metaril, Pressonex, Pressorol.

Metaril trademark for *metaraminol bitartrate* (see under METARAMINOL).

metarteriole (met″ar-te″re-ōl) a precapillary.

Metastab trademark for *methylprednisolone*.

metastasis (me-tas′tah-sis) [*meta*- + Gr. *stasis* stand] the transfer of disease from one organ to another not directly connected with it. It may be due either to the transfer of pathogenic microorganisms or to transfer of cells, as in malignant tumors. The capacity to metastasize is a characteristic of all malignant tumors; they usually metastasize through the blood vessels, lymphatic channels, and direct transplantation. **biochemical m.**, the transportation from the point of production and the deposition in previously normal tissues of abnormal or pathologically produced biochemical substances which bring about immunological or other changes in the tissues. **calcareous m.**, the formation of bone salts in soft tissues, such as the kidneys, in osteomalacia. **direct m.**, that in the direction of the blood or lymph stream. **implantation m.**, that brought about by transfer of tumor cells by fluid and their implantation in a distal location. **paradoxical m.**, retrograde m., that taking place in a direction opposite to that of the blood or lymph stream. **transplantation m.**, that from one tissue to another.

Meta-Synephrine trademark for *phenylephrine hydrochloride* (see under PHENYLEPHRINE).

metathalamus (met″ah-thal′ah-mus) a part of the diencephalon.

Metaxan trademark for *methantheline bromide* (see under METHANTHELINE).

Metazon trademark for *phenylephrine hydrochloride* (see under PHENYLEPHRINE).

Metchnikoff's law, theory [Elie (Ilia, Ilich) *Metchnikoff* (Mechnikov), Russian zoologist in Paris, 1845–1916; discoverer of phagocytes and phagocytosis, and co-winner, with Paul Ehrlich, of the Nobel prize for medicine and physiology in 1908] see under LAW and THEORY.

Meteorex trademark for *simethicone*.

meter (me′ter) [Gr. *metron* measure; Fr. *mètre*] 1. the standard unit of length in the metric system or in SI. It was originally based on one ten-millionth of the distance from the equator to the North Pole, now established by the Eleventh General Conference of Weight and Measures as the 1,650,763.73 wavelengths of the orange-red line of krypton 86, which is the equivalent to 39.37 inches. Its standard is established as the length of a bar of an alloy of platinum and iridium preserved in a vault at the International Bureau of Weights and Measures, near Paris. Abbreviated *m*. Written *metre* in Great Britain. See also SI and Tables of Weights and Measures at WEIGHT. 2. an apparatus devised to measure the quantity of anything passing through it, such as gas, liquid, amperes, etc. **m. candle**, lux. **condenser roentgen-m.**, a boxlike dosimeter consisting of an electroscope, a device for charging the electroscope with its attached electrode, and a lamp to illuminate the scale reading in roentgenograms. The ionization chamber is situated in the receptacle at one end of the box. The passage of x-rays causes a loss in potential of the electrometer according to the degree of ionization in the chamber, the scale marker indicating the number of roentgens. The measurements are made at specific intervals, usually for 1 minute each time, exposing the chamber to radiations at specified distances from the x-ray tube. Called also *r-m*. and *roentgen-m*. **dosage m., dose m.**, dosimeter. **integrating radiation m.**, an instrument consisting in principle of an ionization chamber feeding responses to an integrating system, for the determination of the total accumulated radiation exposure. **r-m.**, condenser roentgen-m. **radiation m.**, dosimeter. **rate m.**, a radiation detector whose output is proportional to instantaneous radiation intensity (rate of radioactive emissions). **roentgen-m.**, condenser roentgen-m. **venturi m.**, venturimeter.

-meter [Gr. *metron* measure] a word termination designating relationship to measurement, or denoting especially an instrument used in measuring.

Meterazine trademark for *prochlorperazine*.

meth (meth) a popular name for *methamphetamine*.

methacholine (meth″ah-ko′lēn) an acetylcholine-like cholinomimetic agent, acetyl-β-methylcholine, which has predominantly muscarinic and some nicotinic actions. It stimulates the salivary, sweat, and other exocrine secretions; dilates most blood vessels, while constricting some veins; decreases the heart rate in high doses, sometimes causing conduction block; stimulates gastrointestinal secretions, increasing peristalsis and defecation; increases gastric secretions; stimulates autonomic ganglia; and stimulates the skeletal neuromuscular junctions, sometimes also causing fasciculation and twitching. Used chiefly as a vasodilator in the treatment of Raynaud's disease, phlebitis, frostbite, scleroderma, and other vascular diseases. Trademark: Mecholyl. **m. bromide**, the bromide salt of methacholine, occurring as a hygroscopic, white crystalline powder

with an alkaline slight odor, which is soluble in water and ethanol, but not in ether and benzene. Its pharmacological properties are similar to those of the parent compound. Trademark: Amechol. **m. chloride**, the chloride salt of methacholine, occurring as a deliquescent, odorless, white, crystalline powder or white or colorless crystalline solids that are soluble in water, chloroform, and ethanol. Its pharmacological properties are similar to those of the parent compound.

Methacolimycin trademark for *colistimethate sodium* (see under COLISTIMETHATE).

methacrylate (meth-ak′rĭ-lāt″) an ester of methacrylic acid. **bisphenol A glycidyl m.**, a phenol-methacrylate polymer, 2-methy-(1-methylethylidene)bis(4, 1-phenyleneoxy-(2-hydroxy-3,1-propanedylo)-2-propanoic acid ester. Used as a pit and fissure sealant. Originally, an amine-benzoyl peroxide mixture was used as the catalyst. The benzoin methyl ester catalyst is currently used to make the polymerization induction sensitive to ultraviolet light. The sealant is applied directly to the enamel and is converted to a hard, glasslike solid when exposed to ultraviolet rays. Called also *Bis-BMA*. Trademarks: Nuva-Seal, Epoxylite 9075. **methyl m.**, a methyl ester of methacrylic acid, being a clear, transparent liquid at room temperature. Its melting point, $-54.4°F$ ($-48°C$); boiling point, $213.4°F$ ($100.8°C$); density, 0.945 gm/cm^3 at $68°F$ ($20°C$); and heat polymerization, 12.0 kg-cal/molecule. Methyl methacrylate has a high vapor pressure, and it is an organic solvent. Ultraviolet light, heat, and catalysts can be used to initiate polymerization. Twenty-one percent shrinkage occurs during polymerization of the pure monomer. By itself, polymerized methyl methacrylate monomer becomes polymethyl methacrylate. In dental practice, the liquid monomer is usually mixed with the polymer in the powdered form which, by swelling, forms a dough, which is then packed into the mold where the monomer is polymerized. Written also *methylmethacrylate*. **polymethyl m.**, an acrylic resin that is a polymethyl ester of methacrylic acid, produced by polymerization of methyl methacrylate. Benzoyl peroxide is the most commonly used catalyst. It is a transparent solid with a Knoop hardness number of 18 to 20, tensile strength of approximately $8,500$ lbs in^2 (600 kg/cm^2), specific gravity of 1.19, and modulus of elasticity of approximately $35,000$ lbs/in^2 ($24,000$ kg/cm^2). Polymethyl methacrylate is resistant to discoloration and aging processes. It softens at $260°F$ ($125°C$), and can be molded as a thermoplastic material. Depolymerization takes place between the melting point and $400°F$ ($200°C$) and about 90 percent of the material polymerizes to the monomeric form. The resin takes up water by imbibition and the polar carboxyl group can form hydrogen bridges with the water. It is soluble in organic solvents, including chloroform and acetone. That used in prosthodontics is usually pigmented to simulate the natural tissue. In dental use, on mixing the polymerized resin in powder form with the monomer, a plastic dough is formed, which is packed into the denture mold and polymerization of the added monomer is induced by heating. The resin is completely translucent to x-rays and a powdered bismuth glass is sometimes added to provide radiopacity. Shrinkage during polymerization and susceptibility to some antiseptic solutions are the major disadvantages of polymethyl methacrylate in dental prosthetics. The term is sometimes used synonymously with *acrylic resin* (see under RESIN). Abbreviated *PMMA*. Written also *polymethylmethacrylate*. See also polymethyl methacrylate CEMENT. **thermosetting m. resin**, see under RESIN.

methacycline (meth″ah-si′klen) a semisynthetic tetracycline antibiotic, 4 - dimethylamin - 1,4,4a,5,5a,6,11,12a - octahydro-3,5,10,12,12a-pentahydroxy - 6 - methylene-1,11-dioxo-2-naphthacenecarboxamide. Used orally as the hydrochloride salt, which occurs as a yellow to dark yellow, odorless, bitter, crystalline powder that is readily soluble in water, slightly soluble in alcohol, and insoluble in ether and chloroform. Its antimicrobial properties and toxicity are similar to those of other tetracyclines. Trademarks: Londomycin, Megamycine, Metilenbiotic, Optimycin, Pindex, Rondomycin.

methadone hydrochloride (meth′ah-don) a synthetic, nonopioid, narcotic analgesic and sedative, 6-dimethylamino-4,4-diphenyl-3-heptanone hydrochloride, occurring as a white, odorless, crystalline powder or colorless crystalline solids that are soluble in water, ethanol, and chloroform, but not in ether and in ether and glycerol. It is similar in action to morphine, and is used chiefly for the relief of pain. Also used for the suppression of the narcotic abstinence syndrome in withdrawal therapy for narcotic dependence. It also has antitussive properties. Adverse reactions may include vertigo, nausea, vomiting, sweating, euphoria, weakness, headache, agitation, tremor, hallucinations, disorientation, and various gastrointestinal, genitourinary, and cardiovascular disorders. Abuse may lead to habituation and addiction. Trademarks for the *dl*-form: Adanon, Algidon, Algolysin, Amidon, Butalgin, Depridol, Dolophine, Fenadone, Heptadon, Phenadone, Physeptone; for the *l*-form: Levadone, Levothyl, Polamidon.

Methaform trademark for *chlorobutanol.*

methamphetamine (meth″am-fet′ah-men) an amphetamine derivative, *d-N*,α-dimethylphenethylamine, occurring as a clear, colorless, slowly volatile mobile liquid, which is a vasoconstrictor with actions similar to those of the parent compound. Like amphetamine, repetitive use of methamphetamine or its derivatives leads to drug dependence of the amphetamine type. Called also *desoxyephedrine* and, popularly, *meth.* Trademark: Norodin. See also AMPHETAMINE. **m. hydrochloride,** the hydrochloride salt of methamphetamine, which occurs as an odorless, white crystalline powder or solids that are soluble in water, ethanol, and chloroform and slightly soluble in ether. It is a sympathomimetic drug with a strong central nervous system stimulant action, used in the treatment of narcolepsy, parkinsonism, epilepsy, hyperkinetic children, and orthostatic hypotension, and as an appetite depressant. Dental patients receiving methamphetamine exhibit excessive nervousness. Side reactions may include insomnia, restlessness, hyperactivity, euphoria, dysphoria, headache, tremor, hypertension, tachycardia, arrhythmia, xerostomia, nausea, diarrhea, urticaria, skin rash, impotence, hypersensitivity, and other disorders. Trademarks: Adipex, Amphedroxyn, Desfedrin, Dexephrin, Dexoval, Isophen, Methedrine, Pervitin, Syndrox.

methanal (meth′ah-nal) formaldehyde.

methandienone (meth″an-di″ĕ-nōn) methandrostenolone.

Methandiol trademark for *methandriol.*

methandriol (meth-an′dre-ol) an anabolic steroid with androgenic properties, 17α-methyl-5-androstene-3β,17β-diol. Called also *methylandrostendiol (MAD).* Trademarks: Methandiol, Metidione, Neutrosteron, Notandron, Stenediol.

methandrostenolone (meth-an″dro-sten′o-lōn) a steroid hormone with strong anabolic and weak androgenic properties, 17β-hydroxy-17-methylandrosta-1,4-dien-3-one, occurring as an odorless, white, crystalline powder or white crystals that are freely soluble in ethanol, chloroform, and glacial acetic acid, slightly soluble in ether, and insoluble in water. Used chiefly to promote nitrogen anabolism and weight gain in debilitating diseases and following infections, burns, injuries, and surgery. Also used to relieve pain in some types of osteoporosis and arthritis. Side effects may include virilization, acne, sodium retention with edema, and cholestatic edema. By potentiating prothrombopenic anticoagulants, it may also enhance the development of hemorrhage in patients on anticoagulant therapy. Called also *methandienone.* Trademarks: Danabol, Dianabol, Nabolin, Nerobol, Stenolon.

methane (meth′ān) a hydrocarbon, CH$_4$, occurring as a colorless, odorless, flammable gas, produced by decomposition of organic matter, being the first member of the paraffin hydrocarbon series. It is a major component of coal and natural gas, which, although nonpoisonous, may cause asphyxia and, when mixed with oxygen or air, may become explosive. Hydrocarbons of the methane series include ethane, propane, butane, pentane, hexane, heptane, octane, nonane, and decane. Called also *marsh gas* and *methyl hydride.*

Methanide trademark for *methantheline bromide* (see under METHANTHELINE).

methanol (meth′ah-nol) methyl ALCOHOL

methantheline bromide (mĕ-thăn′the-lēn) a synthetic quaternary ammonium compound, diethyl(2-hydroxyethyl)methylammonium bromide xanthene-9-carboxylate, occurring as a white or nearly white odorless powder with a bitter taste, which is soluble in water, alcohol, and chloroform. It has antimuscarinic properties and blocks the response of smooth muscle, heart, and secretory cells to exogenous as well as endogenous acetylcholine; in larger doses, it exerts anticholinergic action on autonomic ganglia and skeletal muscles, producing pupillary dilation, xerostomia, decreased sweating, moderate tachycardia, decreased gastric contraction, delayed emptying of the stomach, and decreased gastric secretion. Used chiefly in the treatment of duodenal ulcer, hyperhidrosis, sialorrhea, and various gastrointestinal disorders. In dentistry, used mainly to control the flow of saliva during dental procedures. Side effects may

include xerostomia, blurred vision, mydriasis, feeling of epigastric fullness, heartburn, difficulty in urination, decreased libido, and constipation. Restlessness, euphoria, fatigue, psychotic episodes, skin rashes, and exfoliative dermatitis sometimes occur. Trademarks: Avagal, Banthine, Metaxan, Methanide, Methanthine, Vagantin.

Methanthine trademark for *methantheline bromide* (see under METHANTHELINE).

methapyrilene hydrochloride (meth″ah-pir′ĭ-lēn) an antihistaminic drug, 2-[[2(dimethylamino)ethyl]-2-thenylamino]pyridine monohydrochloride, occurring as a white crystalline powder with a faint odor, which dissolves in water, alcohol, and chloroform, and is insoluble in ether and benzene. It blocks histamine mediation at the H$_1$ receptor, and also has mild sedative and local anesthetic properties. Used in the treatment of allergic diseases; also used in proprietary sleep medications. Trademarks: Dormin, Histadyl, Restryl, Sleepwell, Thenylene, Thenylpyramine.

methaqualone (mĕ-thah′kwah-lōn) a nonbarbiturate hypnotic and sedative, 2-methyl-3-*c*-tolyl-4(3*H*)-quinazolinone, occurring as a bitter, odorless, white, crystalline powder that is soluble in ethanol, chloroform, hydrochloric acid solutions, ether, and, slightly, water. Adverse reactions may include headache, drowsiness, nausea, fatigue, vertigo, xerostomia, epigastric discomfort, emesis, restlessness, tachycardia, anorexia, diarrhea, urticaria, exanthema, paresthesia, and aplastic anemia. The drug is potentially addictive. Called also *metolquizolone, MTQ,* and *ortonal.* Trademarks: Cateudyl, Citexal, Dormigen, Noctilene, Quaalude, Somnafac. **m. hydrochloride,** the hydrochloride salt of methaqualone, occurring as a white, odorless, crystalline powder that is freely soluble in chloroform and acetone, sparingly soluble in water and ethanol, and very slightly soluble in ether and benzene. Its pharmacological and toxicological properties are those of the parent compound. Trademarks: Melsedin, Metadorm, Optimil, Revonal, Sedaquin, Sleepinal.

metharbital (me-thăr′bĭ-tal) an *N*-methylated derivative of barbital, 5,5-diethyl-1-methyl-2,4,6(1*H*,3*H*,5*H*)-pyrimidinetrione, occurring as a white, crystalline powder with an aromatic odor that is soluble in ether, ethanol, and water. Used as an anticonvulsant in the treatment of some types of epilepsy. Side effects may include gastric distress, drowsiness, irritability, skin rashes, and vertigo. Trademark: Gemonil.

methdilazine hydrochloride (meth-di′lah-zēn) an antihistaminic drug which blocks histamine at the H$_1$ receptor, 10-[(1-methyl-3-pyrrolidylmethyl)methyl] phenothiazine monohydrochloride. It occurs as a light tan crystalline powder with a bitter numbing taste, which is stable in the crystalline form, but not in solution when exposed to light, and is freely soluble in water, alcohol, chloroform, and hot isopropyl alcohol. Used in the treatment of allergic diseases. It is contraindicated in newborn infants, and in various conditions, including asthma, glaucoma, peptic ulcer, prostatic hypertrophy, and in conjunction with other phenothiazines and antihistaminics. Side effects may include vertigo, dryness of the mouth and mucous membranes, gastrointestinal disorders, and skin rash. Trademarks: Dilosyn, Disyncran, Tacaryl.

Methedrine trademark for *methamphetamine hydrochloride* (see under METHAMPHETAMINE).

methemoglobin (met-he′mo-glo′bin) a compound formed from hemoglobin by oxidation of the ferrous to the ferric state with essentially ionic bonds; it does not combine with oxygen.

methemoglobinemia (met″he-mo-glo″bĭ-ne′me-ah) [*methemoglobin* + Gr. *haima* blood + *-ia*] the presence of methemoglobin in the blood, resulting in inability of hemoglobin to combine efficiently with oxygen with secondary cyanosis. It may be drug-induced or be due to a defect in the enzyme NADH methemoglobin reductase (an autosomal recessive trait) or to an abnormality in hemoglobin M (an autosomal dominant trait).

methenamine (meth″en-am′in) an anti-infective agent, hexamethylenetetramine, occurring as an odorless, white, crystalline powder or colorless crystals that are soluble in water, ethanol, chloroform, and, slightly, ether. Used in the treatment of urinary tract infections. Nearly 30 percent of the drug is converted to formaldehyde in the stomach, unless it is administered in enteric-coated capsules. Hematuria, frequent urination, diarrhea, skin rashes, bladder irritation, and other disorders may occur during therapy. Called also *hexamine.* Trademarks: Aminoform, Cystamin. **m. mandelate,** a compound formed by mixing methenamine and mandelic acid in water or ethanol, occurring as a white, odorless, sour, crystalline powder that is soluble in water, ethanol, chloroform, and ether. Its pharmacological and toxicological properties are similar to those of methenamine, except that mandelic acid is excreted into the urine with the use of methenamine mandelate. Trademarks: Cedulamin, Mandelamine, Mandoz, Uronamin.

methflorylthiazidine (meth-flor″il-thi-az′ĭ-dēn) hydroflumethiazide.

Methicil trademark for *methylthiouracil.*

methicillin (meth′ĭ-sil′in) a broad-spectrum, highly penicillinase-resistant, semisynthetic penicillin, 6-(2,6-dimethoxybenzamido)-3,3-dimethyl - 7 - oxo-5-thia-1-azabicyclo[3,2,0]heptane-2-carboxylic acid. Used therapeutically as the monosodium salt, which occurs as a white, odorless, fine crystalline powder that is soluble in water, methanol, and pyridine, slightly soluble in propyl and amyl alcohols, chloroform, and ethylene chloride, and insoluble in benzene, acetone, and ether. It is less potent than penicillin G against hemolytic streptococci, pneumococci, and *Treponema,* but more potent against staphylococci. The drug is destroyed in the stomach and is well absorbed intramuscularly. Toxic reactions, particularly hypersensitivity, are typical of other penicillins; hemolytic anemia and other anemias may occur. Called also 2,6-*dimethoxyphenylpenicillin* and *dimethoxyphenyl penicillin.* Trademarks: Azapen, Belfacillin, Celbenin, Staphcillin.

methimazole (meth-im′ah-zol) a thyroid antagonist, 1-methylimidazole-2-thiol, occurring as white or buff, crystalline powder with a faint characteristic odor, which is soluble in water, ethanol, chloroform, and ether. Used in the treatment of hyperthyroidism and in the preparation of hyperthyroid patients for surgery. Agranulocytosis is the most serious adverse reaction; sore throat, purpuric rash, headache, pain and stiffness in the joints, paresthesia, nausea, and loss or depigmentation of the hair may occur. Called also *thiamizole.* Trademarks: Basolan, Danantizol, Favistan, Frentirol, Mercazole, Strumazol.

methionine (me-thi′o-nin) a sulfur-containing, naturally occurring amino acid, 2-amino-4-methylmercaptobutyric acid, which is essential for the growth of infants and certain nitrogen metabolic processes in adults. Methionine is also found in trace amounts in the saliva. Used as a dietary supplement and lipotropic agent. Abbreviated *Met.* See also amino ACID.

methisazone (me-this′ah-zōn) an antiviral drug, 2-(1,2-dihydro-1-methyl-2-oxo-3H-indol-3-ylidene)hydrazinecarbothioamide. It is believed to interfere with the synthesis of a protein required for assembly and morphogenesis of viruses, without affecting replication of viral DNA and RNA. Used in the treatment of smallpox, eczema vaccinatum, and vaccinia gangrenosa. Side effects may include vomiting, nausea, and reversible amnesia. Called also 3-*thiosemicarbazone.* Trademarks: Marboran, Viruzona.

methocarbamol (meth″o-kar′bah-mol) a centrally acting muscle relaxant, 3-(o-methoxyphenoxy)-1,2-propanediol-1-carbamate, occurring as an odorless, white powder with a slight characteristic odor that is soluble in water, ethanol, and chloroform, but not in benzene. Used in muscle spasms, paralysis agitans, cerebral palsy, multiple sclerosis, cerebrovascular accidents, and orthopedic procedures. Side effects may include vertigo, drowsiness, headache, fever, skin rashes, urticaria, gastrointestinal discomfort, flushing, muscular incoordination, hypotension, bradycardia, and metallic taste. Sloughing and thrombophlebitis may occur after injections. Trademarks: Lumirelax, Myolaxene, Neuraxin, Relestrid, Robaxin, Tresortil.

Methocel trademark for *methylcellulose.*

Methocillin-S trademark for *cloxacillin.*

method (meth′ud) [Gr. *methodos*] the manner of performing any act or operation. See also TECHNIQUE and TEST. **absorption m.,** the separate and selective removal of agglutinins from specific immune sera by the addition of homologous particulate antigen(s) (e.g., bacterial cells or red blood cells) to the immune sera, or by the passage of specific immune sera through columns containing antigen of an insoluble support (immunosorbent) with which the homologous antibody combines and is thereby removed from the serum. The method may also be applied to precipitating soluble antigens; precipitation of nondesirable antibodies from antiserum with appropriate antigens may result in improved specificity toward antigens. **Altmann-Gersh m.,** the freeze drying method of preparing tissue for histologic study. **Arthur's m.,** arthurizing. **banding m.,** chromosome BANDING. **Bass' m.,** see TOOTHBRUSHING. **Buist's m.,** see artificial RESPIRATION. **Callahan's m.,** 1. root canal filling m., Callahan's. 2. a method of tracing and opening up root canals by applying 50 percent sulfuric acid solution at the root orifice and working it into the canal by means of a broach; remnants of pulp tissue are thus destroyed and removed and the dentinal walls enlarged. **C-banding m.,** C-BANDING. **Caspersson's m.,** a cytogenetic method which demonstrates a distinctive bandlike

fluorescence pattern in chromosomes after quinacrine staining. Plants were originally used, but Caspersson pioneered the human work as well. The method is considered as the pioneer work in chromosome banding. Called also *Caspersson's technique.* See also chromosome BANDING and Q bands, under BAND. **Charters' m.,** see TOOTHBRUSHING. **chloropercha m.,** root canal filling m., chloropercha. **chromosome alkali denaturation and re-association m.,** C-BANDING. **Delphi m.,** a method whereby weighting or index factors are assigned to parameters that are not readily quantifiable, on the basis of a consensus or majority opinion of a group of unprejudiced experts. **diffusion m.,** root canal filling m., Johnson's. **Duke m.,** see bleeding TIME. **Eve's m.,** see artificial RESPIRATION. **Feulgen m.,** histological staining with Feulgen stain. See also F-BANDING. **fluorescent antibody m.,** immunofluorescence. **Fones' m.,** Fones' method of TOOTHBRUSHING. **Giemsa m.,** G-BANDING. **Howard's m.,** see artificial RESPIRATION. **Ivy m.,** see bleeding TIME. **Johnson's m.,** root canal filling m., Johnson's. **Kazanjian's suspension m.,** Kazanjian's OPERATION (2). **Laborde's m.,** the making of rhythmical traction movements on the tongue with the use of Laborde's forceps in order to stimulate the respiratory center in asphyxiation. **lateral condensation m.,** root canal filling m., lateral condensation. **m. of Marshall Hall,** see artificial RESPIRATION. **mouth-to-mouth m.,** see artificial RESPIRATION. **multiple cone m.,** root canal filling m., lateral condensation. **m. of postural respiration,** m. of prone respiration, see artificial RESPIRATION. **Purmann's m.,** extirpation of the aneurysmal sac in aneurysm. **"ready m.,"** m. of Marshall Hall; see artificial RESPIRATION. **retrofilling m.,** see RETROFILLING. **reverse filling m.,** see RETROFILLING. **Romanovskii's (Romanovsky's, Romanowsky's) m.,** Romanovskii's STAIN. **root canal filling m., Callahan's,** a root canal therapy method, whereby the canal is first dried and then flooded with a rosin in chloroform solution, followed by placement of a gutta-percha cone to or near the end of the canal and pumping it up and down into the canal while it is maneuvered apically, as it dissolves in the solution. Additional gutta-percha cones are packed with root canal pluggers, should any space remain in the coronal portion of the root canal. Called also *Callahan's m.* **root canal filling m., chloropercha,** a method of filling a root canal with gutta-percha cones dissolved in a chloroform-rosin solution, as in Callahan's and Johnson's methods of root canal filling. Called also *chloropercha m.* **root canal filling m., diffusion** root canal filling m., Johnson's. **root canal filling m., Johnson's,** a modification of Callahan's method, in which the canal is initially flooded with alcohol, thus allowing the chloroform component of the chloroform-rosin solution to diffuse. Alcohol being present deeply in the dentin facilitates rosin dissolved in the chloroform to be carried into dentin through the mechanism of diffusion. Called also *diffusion m., diffusion root canal filling m.,* and *Johnson's m.* **root canal filling m., lateral condensation,** a method of filling a root canal in which the main portion of the canal is filled with a well-fitting primary gutta-percha cone or silver point in conjunction with sealer cement or paste and the remaining canal space is packed with auxiliary gutta-percha cones. Spreaders and pluggers are used to force gutta-percha into the canal laterally and sometimes vertically. Called also *lateral condensation m., multiple cone m.,* and *multiple cone root canal filling m.* **root canal filling m., multiple cone,** root canal filling m. lateral condensation. **root canal filling m., retrograde,** retrograde FILLING. **root canal filling m., sectional,** a method of filling a root canal in which gutta-percha cones are cut into 2 to 3 mm sections and, after lubricating the canal with a substance such as eucalyptol, the cut sections are carried on the heated end of an apex plugger and packed in the canal individually until it is filled. Called also *sectional m., segmentation m.,* and *segmentation root canal filling m.* **root canal filling m., segmentation,** root canal filling m., sectional. **root canal filling m., silver point (cone),** a method of filling a root canal in which a prefitted silver point is sealed into the apical portion of the root canal. Irregularities in the canal that are not sealed with the point are obliterated with gutta-percha by lateral condensation or segmentation. Called also *silver point (cone) m.* **root canal filling m., single cone,** a method of filling a root canal with a single, well-fitting gutta-percha cone or silver point in conjunction with a sealer cement or paste. Called also *single cone m.* **root canal filling m., vertical condensation,** a method of filling a root canal by alternately heating and vertically condensing gutta-percha until the apical third of the canal is filled. The coronal portion of the canal is then filled with warmed 2 to 4 mm sections of gutta-percha cones. Called also *vertical condensation m.* **root-end filling m.,** see RETROFILLING. **Schafer's m.,** see artificial RESPIRATION. **sectional m., segmentation m.,** root canal filling m., sectional. **silver point (cone) m.,** root canal filling m., silver point (cone). **Silvester's m.,** see artificial RESPIRATION. **single cone m.,** root canal filling m., single cone. **split-cast m.,** 1. a method for placing indexed casts on an articulator to facilitate their removal and replacement on the instrument. 2. a method for checking the ability of an articulator to receive or be adjusted to a maxillomandibular relation record. Called also *split cast mount.* **Stillman's m.,** Stillman's method of TOOTHBRUSHING. **Taggard's m.,** disappearing CORE. **vertical condensation m.,** root canal filling m., vertical condensation. **wash m.,** wash IMPRESSION.

Methodist 1. an ancient sect or school which based the practice of medicine on a few simple rules and theories. This school, influenced by Asclepiades, was founded (c. 50 B.C.) by Themison of Laodicea. The Methodists believed that disease is caused either by a narrowing of the internal pores of the body (*status strictus*) or by their excessive relaxation (*status laxus*). Such extreme simplification of the nature of disease is discernible as late as 18th century, for example, in the so-called *brunonian system* (John Brown, 1735–1788). 2. a believer in or practitioner of the Methodist theory of medicine.

methohexital sodium (meth″o-hek′sĭ-tal) an ultrashort-acting barbiturate, α-DL-1-methyl-5-allyl-5-(l-methyl-pentynyl)barbituric acid sodium salt, occurring as a white to cream-colored crystalline powder with a bitter taste that is soluble in water. Used as an intravenous anesthetic and in preanesthetic medication. Muscle twitching, tremor, hiccups, spasmodic coughing, laryngospasm, respiratory stridor, hypotension, thrombophlebitis, headache, skin rash, nausea, and vomiting are the principal adverse reactions. Contraindicated in porphyria and hypersensitivity to barbiturates. The drug is addictive and subject to regulations of the Controlled Substances Act. Trademark: Brevital.

Methoplain trademark for *methyldopa.*

methotrexate (meth″o-trek′sāt) a folic acid analogue, L-(+)-N-[p - [[2,4 - diamino - 6 - pteridinyl)methyl]methylamino]benzoyl]glutamic acid, occurring as an orange-brown, crystalline powder that is soluble in dilute solutions of alkali hydroxides and carbonates, slightly soluble in dilute hydrochloric acid, and insoluble in water, ethanol, chloroform, and ether. Used in the treatment of lymphocytic leukemia, choriocarcinoma, osteogenic sarcoma of the lungs, oropharynx, breast, and testes, and other cancers. Also used in mycosis fungoides, psoriasis, and psoriatic arthritis, and as an immunosuppressive agent in tissue transplantation. Adverse reactions may include ulcerative stomatitis, hemorrhagic tendency, predisposition to infection, alopecia, fetal abnormalities, hepatotoxicity, diarrhea, intestinal perforation, and depression of the bone marrow with leukopenia, thrombocytopenia, and anemia. Called also *amethopterin, 4-amino-10-methylfolic acid,* and *methylaminopterin.*

methotrimeprazine (meth″o-tri-mep′rah-zēn) a nonaddicting analgesic with sedative properties, 2-methoxy-N,N,β-trimethyl-10H-phenothiazine-10-propanamine, occurring as a white, odorless, crystalline powder that is unstable on exposure to light and is soluble in chloroform, ether, and boiling alcohol, sparingly soluble in methanol and cold ethanol, and insoluble in water. Used in severe pain, in preanesthetic medication to allay apprehension, and in other types of analgesia in which respiratory depression is to be avoided. Orthostatic hypotension, vertigo, disorientation, amnesia, slurred speech, blurred vision, nausea, vomiting, xerostomia, nasal congestion, pain at the site of injection, and chills are the principal side reactions. Leukopenia, agranulocytosis, and jaundice may occur. Called also *levomeprazine.* Trademarks: Levoprome, Neozine, Nirvan, Tisercin.

methoxamine hydrochloride (mĕ-thok′sah-mēn) a directly acting sympathomimetic amine with a pressor action and moderate β-adrenergic receptor blocking properties, α-(1-aminoethyl)-2,5-dimethoxybenzenemethanol hydrochloride. It occurs as an odorless, crystalline powder or white crystalline plates that are soluble in ethanol and water, but not in chloroform and ether. Used in the treatment of hypotension and to support blood pressure during anesthesia. Also used to induce reflex bradycardia in the treatment of paroxysmal atrial tachycardia and in cardiac arrhythmias. Sometimes used as a nasal decongestant. Adverse reactions may include pilomotor erection, tingling of

the extremities, and excessive urination. Large doses may cause hypertensive crises. Called also *2,5-dimethoxynorephedrine hydrochloride.* Trademarks: Pressomin, Vasoxyl.

methoxsalen (me-thok′sah-len) a compound, 6-hydroxy-7-methyl-5-benzofuranacrylic acid δ-lactone, occurring as white to cream-colored, odorless, fluffy needles that are soluble in acetone, acetic acid, boiling alcohol, and some alkalies, but not in water. Used to promote repigmentation in vitiligo and to increase skin tolerance to sunlight. In the presence of ultraviolet light, methoxsalen thickens the stratum corneum, induces an inflammatory reaction in the skin, and increases the amount of melanin in the skin. Usually applied topically. Oral administration increases its effectiveness, but also may cause gastrointestinal and neurological reactions. Overexposure to ultraviolet rays may produce severe sunburn. Contraindicated in liver diseases and photosensitivity.

methoxyflurane (me-thok″sĕ-floo′rān) a potent inhalation anesthetic, 2,2-dichloro-1,1-difluoroethyl, occurring as a clear, mobile, nonexplosive, nonflammable liquid with a fruity odor, which is slightly soluble in water and is miscible with olive oil, chloroform, ethyl alcohol, acetone, and benzene. Used in dentistry for brief exodontic procedures to prolonged dental operations up to 4 hours. In smaller doses, it produces light anesthesia with muscle relaxation and analgesia. Sometimes used in conjunction with nitrous oxide. Adverse reactions may include hypotension, depression of respiration, and kidney disorders. The drug is contraindicated in conjunction with epinephrine, tetracyclines, and gentamicin, and in patients with a history of liver disease. Trademark: Penthrane.

methoxyphenamine hydrochloride (mĕ-thok″se-fen′ah-mēn) a directly acting sympathomimetic with β-adrenergic stimulant properties without stimulating the heart, o-methoxy-N,α-dimethylphenethylamine hydrochloride, occurring as a white, crystalline powder that is freely soluble in water, ethanol, and chloroform and slightly soluble in ether. Used as a bronchodilator agent in the treatment of bronchial asthma. It is also a weak antihistaminic agent acting on the H_1 receptors; used in the treatment of hay fever, urticaria, and other allergic diseases. Side effects may include xerostomia, drowsiness, and wakefulness. Trademarks: Orthoxine, Ortodrinex, Proamsa.

methscopolamine (meth″sko-pol′ah-mēn) a semisynthetic quaternary ammonium derivative of scopolamine, N-methylscopolammonium, which has antimuscarinic properties. Used chiefly in the treatment of peptic ulcer, diarrhea, and intestinal hypermotility. Also used in the treatment of sialorrhea and hyperhidrosis. Its side effects are similar to those of atropine. **m. bromide,** the bromide salt of methscopolamine, occurring as an odorless, white, crystalline powder or white crystals that are freely soluble in water, slightly soluble in ethanol, and insoluble in acetone and chloroform. Its pharmacological and toxicological properties are similar to those of the parent compound. Called also *hyoscine methyl bromide* and *scopolamine methylbromide.* Trademarks: Diopal, Holopon, Pamine. **m. nitrate,** the nitrate salt of methscopolamine, occurring as an odorless, tasteless, white, crystalline powder that is freely soluble in water and ethanol. Its pharmacological and toxicological properties are similar to those of the parent compound. Called also *scopolamine methylnitrate.* Trademark: Skopyl.

methsuximide (meth-suk′sĭ-mĭd) an antiepileptic agent, 1,3-dimethyl-3-phenyl-2,5-pyrrolidinedione, occurring as a white to grayish, odorless, crystalline powder that is soluble in hot water, ethanol, ether, and chloroform. Side effects may include nausea, vomiting, anorexia, weight loss, diarrhea, constipation, abdominal pain, eosinophilia, leukopenia, monocytosis, pancytopenia, insomnia, drowsiness, ataxia, irritability, headache, visual disorders, hiccups, and periorbital edema and hyperemia. Trademarks: Celontin, Petinutin.

methyclothiazide (meth″ĭ-klo-thi′ah-zīd) a thiazide (benzothiadiazine) diuretic agent with antihypertensive properties, 6-chloro-3 - (chloromethyl) - 3,4 - dihydro - 2 - methyl-2H-1,2,4-benzothiadiazine - 7 - sulfonamide 1,1-dioxide, occurring as an odorless, tasteless, white, crystalline powder that is freely soluble in acetone and pyridine, slightly soluble in methanol and ethanol, and very slightly soluble in benzene, chloroform, and isopropanol. Adverse reactions may include anorexia, gastritis, irritation, nausea, vomiting, abdominal discomfort, vertigo, paresthesias, headache, leukopenia, purpura, skin rashes, photosensitivity, necrotizing angiitis, anaphylaxis, agranulocytosis, thrombocytopenia, aplastic anemia, orthostatic hypotension, fever, muscle spasms, hyperglycemia, glycosuria, hematuria, and blurred vision. Trademarks: Aquatensen, Duretic, Enduron, Naturon.

methyl (meth′il) [Gr. *methy* wine + *hylē* wood] the chemical group or radical CH_3—. Sometimes abbreviated *Me.* **m. acetate,**

an ester, $CH_2CO_2CH_3$, occurring as a colorless, volatile liquid with a fragrant odor, which is miscible in water and organic solvents. Used as a solvent. It may cause irritation of the skin and mucous membranes and, in high concentration, inhalation of fumes may produce narcosis. **m. aldehyde,** formaldehyde. **m. ethylene,** propylene. **m. glycol,** propylene GLYCOL. **m. hydride,** methane. **m. methacrylate,** methyl METHACRYLATE. **m. salicylate,** methyl SALICYLATE.

methylamine (meth'il-am'in) a compound, CH_3NH_2, occurring as a colorless gas with a strong ammoniacal odor; used in the production of drugs, insecticides, fungicides, surface active agents, and in various chemical processes. Called also *aminomethane* and *monomethylamine.*

methylaminopterin (meth"il-am"ĭ-nop'ter-in) methotrexate.

methylandrostendiol (meth"il-an"dro-sten'de-ol) methandriol.

methylbenzene (meth"il-ben'zēn) toluene.

methylbenzethonium chloride (meth"il-ben"zĕ-tho'ne-um) a general purpose local anti-infective agent, N,N-dimethyl-N-[2-[2-[methyl - 4 - (1,1,3,3 - tetramethylbutyl)phenoxy] ethoxy]ethyl]-benzenemethanaminium chloride, occurring as odorless, colorless bitter crystals that are soluble in water, alcohol, chloroform, and hot benzene. Trademark: Diaparene.

methylbutyrase (meth"il-bu'tĭ-rās) carboxylesterase.

methylcatechol (meth"il-kat'ĕ-kol) guaiacol.

methylcellulose (meth"il-sel'u-lōs) a methyl ester of cellulose, occurring as odorless, tasteless, nonpoisonous granules that are soluble in cold water and insoluble in hot water, ether, chloroform, and alcohol. In water, methylcellulose swells to a viscous, colloidal solution. Used as food additive and thickening agent for cosmetics and drugs. Also employed in the preparation of gels which serve as vehicles for drugs, such as fluoride gels. Sometimes used as a laxative. Trademarks: Bogolax, Cellumeth, Cethylose, Cethytin, Collothyl, Cologel, Hydrolose, Methocel, Nicel, Syncelose, Tylose. See also CARBOXYMETHYLCELLULOSE. **hydroxypropyl m.,** the propylene glycol ether of methylcellulose, in which both hydroxypropyl and methyl groups are attached to the anhydriglucose rings of cellulose by ether linkages; used as a suspending agent for drugs.

methyldopa (meth"il-do'pah) a dopamine derivative, L-3-(3,4-dihydroxyphenyl)-2-methylalanine, occurring as a white to yellowish white, odorless, and tasteless powder that is soluble in dilute hydrochloric acid, water and slightly in alcohol. It has adrenergic neuron blocking properties, and its mechanism of action is believed to consist of inducing the release of norepinephrine and an interference with its release in response to stimuli. The metabolites of methyldopa are believed to displace norepinephrine from the storage sites and to act as false transmitters in adrenergic mediation. Having independent hypotensive properties, probably through a peripheral and central vasodepressor action, methyldopa is used chiefly in the treatment of hypertension. In dentistry, it is used chiefly as a vasoconstrictor agent in local anesthesia, in gingival retraction, and to control postoperative bleeding. Somnolence, occasional orthostatic hypotension, vertigo, nausea, headache, impotence, diarrhea, stuffy nose, and bradycardia are the most common side effects. Trademarks: Aldomet, Aldometil, Dopamet, Medopren, Methoplain, Presinol.

methylene (meth"il-ēn) the bivalent hydrocarbon radical, CH_2. **m. blue,** methylene BLUE. **m. oxide,** formaldehyde.

methylhexabital (meth"il-heks-ab'ĭ-tal) hexobarbital.

N-methylhydrazine (meth"il-hi'drah-zēn) PROCARBAZINE hydrochloride.

methylmethacrylate (meth"il-meth-ak'rĭ-lāt) methyl METHACRYLATE.

Methylococcus (meth"il-o-kok'kus) [*methyl* + Gr. *kokkos* berry] a genus of gram-negative, aerobic cocci of the family Methylomonadaceae.

Methylomonadaceae (meth"il-o-mo"nah-da"se-e) [*Methylomonas* + *-aceae*] a family of gram-negative, aerobic bacteria, occurring as rods or cocci. Their metabolism is respiratory, using molecular oxygen as a terminal electron acceptor. Methane and methanol are their only known sources of carbon and energy. It consists of the genera *Methylomonas* and *Methylococcus.*

Methylomonas (meth"il-o-mo'nas) [*methyl* + Gr. *monas* unit] a genus of gram-negative, aerobic rods of the family Methylomonadaceae.

methylmorphine (meth"il-mor'fēn) codeine. **m. phosphate,** CODEINE phosphate.

methylparaben (meth"il-par'ah-ben) an antiseptic substance, 4-hydroxybenzoic acid methyl ester, occurring as a white crystalline powder or colorless crystalline solids with a faint odor and a slightly burning taste, which are soluble in water, ethanol, ether, acetone, glycerol, oils, fats and slightly in benzene and carbon tetrachloride. Used chiefly as a preservative for thera-

peutic and other preparations containing vegetable or animal fats and oils that are susceptible to decomposition, such as antibiotic and corticosteroid preparations. Allergic reactions are the principal side effects. Trademarks: Methyl Parasept, Nipagin M, Tegosept M.

Methyl Parasept trademark for *methylparaben.*

methylphenidate (meth"il-fen'ĭ-dāt) an antidepressant agent, α-phenyl-2-piperidineacetic acid methyl ester, occurring as a crystalline substance that is soluble in ethanol, ethyl acetate, and ether, but not in water. Adverse effects may include drowsiness, xerostomia, tremor, fatigue, weakness, blurred vision, constipation, urinary retention, edema, tachycardia, and orthostatic hypotension. Anemias and other hematopoietic changes may occur with large doses. Trademarks: Centedrin, Phenidylate, Ritalin. **m. hydrochloride,** the hydrochloride salt of methylphenidate, occurring as an odorless, white, crystalline powder that is freely soluble in water, methanol, and ethanol and slightly soluble in chloroform and acetone. Its pharmacological and toxicological properties are similar to those of the parent compound.

3-methylphenol (meth"il-fen'ol) METACRESYL acetate.

methylprednisolone (meth"il-pred'nĭ-so-lōn) a synthetic glucocorticoid that is a 6α-methyl derivative of progesterone, 11β,17,21-trihydroxy - 6 - α-methylpregna-1,4-diene-3,20-dione, occurring as an odorless white, crystalline powder that is slightly soluble in ethanol, methanol, acetone, chloroform, and ether, and is insoluble in water. Used in the treatment of adrenocortical insufficiency and as an anti-inflammatory and antiallergic agent. In dentistry, used in sensitive dentin, postoperative pulpal reactions, oral ulcer, arthritic temporomandibular disorders, and in tissue transplantation. Adverse reactions are similar to those of other glucocorticoids, but sodium and water retention is less severe than with the use of prednisolone. Trademarks: Medrate, Medrol, Metastab, Promacortine, Urbasol. **m. acetate,** the acetate salt of methylprednisolone, occurring as a white, odorless, crystalline powder that is soluble in dioxane, sparingly soluble in acetone, ethanol, chloroform, and methanol, slightly soluble in ether, and insoluble in water. Used in ointments and sterile suspensions for intramuscular, intra-articular, and intralesional injections, and for topical application. Trademarks: Depo-Medrate, Depo-Medrol, Depo-Medrone. **m. sodium succinate,** a salt of methylprednisolone, occuring as a white, odorless, hygroscopic solid that is soluble in water and ethanol, slightly soluble in acetone, and insoluble in chloroform. Used for intramuscular, intra-articular, intravenous, and intralesional injections. Trademarks: Solu-Medrol, Urbason-Solubile.

methylpromazine (meth"il-pro'mah-zēn) trimeprazine.

Methylpyrimal trademark for *sulfamerazine.*

methylrosaniline chloride (meth"il-ro-zan'ĭ-lēn) gentian VIOLET.

methyltestosterone (meth"il-tes-tos'ter-ōn) a testicular hormone, 17β-hydroxy - 17 - methylandrost - 4 - en - 3 - one, occurring as a slightly hygroscopic, photosensitive, odorless, crystalline powder or creamy white crystals that are soluble in ethanol, methanol, ether, and other organic solvents, but not in water. Used chiefly in substitutional therapy of testicular insufficiency, such as that occurring in climacteric syndrome and hypogonadism, impotence, and other endocrine disorders. Also used in treating such conditions as osteoporosis, Addison's disease, pituitary insufficiency, and malnutrition. Adverse effects may include hirsutism, hoarseness, precocious puberty, epiphyseal closure, increased libido in both males and females, priapism, weight gain, edema, hypercalcemia, hypersensitivity, and skin rashes. Trademarks: Androsan, Metandren, Synadrotabs, Testoviron.

methyltheobromine (meth"il-the"o-bro'mēn) caffeine.

methylthiouracil (meth"il-thi"o-u'rah-sil) a propylthiouracil analogue, 2,3-dihydro - 6 - methyl - 2 - thioxo-4(1H)pyrimidinone, occurring as bitter, odorless, white, crystalline powder that is freely soluble in ammonia and alkali hydroxide solutions, slightly soluble in ethanol, chloroform, and ether, and very slightly soluble in water. It is a thyroid antagonist, used chiefly in the preparation of hyperthyroid patients for surgery and in the treatment of hyperthyroidism. Side effects may include granulocytopenia, leukopenia, drug fever, arthralgia, and dermatitis. Abbreviated *MTU.* Trademarks: Alkiron, Antibason, Besecil, Methicil, Muracil, Thyreostat I.

methyltransferase [E.C.2.1.1.] (meth"il-trans'fer-ās) a subclass of transferases, including enzymes that catalyze transmethylation, e.g., the transfer of methyl groups from methionine (Sadenosylmethionine) to nicotinamide to form *N*-methyl-nicotinamide, to guanidinoacetic acid to form creatine, or in the formation of methylated bases of nucleic acids. Called also *transmethylase.*

5-methyluracil (meth″i-u′rah-sil) thymine.

methylxanthine (meth″il-zan′thēn) a methyl derivative of xanthine, such as caffeine, theobromine, and theophylline.

methyprylon (meth″ĭ-pri′lon) a hypnotic, 3,3-diethyl-5-methyl-2,4-piperidinedione, occurring as a white, crystalline powder with a slight characteristic odor, which is soluble in water, ethanol, chloroform, ether, and benzene. Used in insomnia. Adverse effects may include morning drowsiness, vertigo, diarrhea, esophagitis, nausea, vomiting, headache, paradoxical excitement, skin rashes, and isolated causes of thrombocytopenia and neutropenia. Abuse may lead to addiction or habituation. Trademarks: Dimerin, Noctan, Noludar.

methysergide (meth″ĭ-ser′jĭd) a methylated ergot preparation (+)-9,10-didehydro-*N*-1-(hydroxymethyl)propyl-1,6-dimethyl-ergoline-8-β-carboxamide. Used as potent serotonin antagonist in the prophylaxis of vascular (migraine) headache. Nausea, abdominal cramps, vertigo, restlessness, insomnia, drowsiness, confusion, epigastric pain, vomiting, diarrhea (or constipation), myalgia, arthralgia, paresthesias, skin rashes, hypotension, edema, weight gain, tachycardia, neutropenia, and eosinophilia may occur. Also available as the maleate salt. Trademark: Sansert.

Methyton trademark for *phytonadione.*

Meticortelone trademark for *prednisolone sodium succinate* (see under PREDNISOLONE).

Meticorten trademark for *prednisone.*

Metidione trademark for *methandriol.*

Metilar trademark for *paramethasone.*

Metilenbiotic trademark for *methacycline.*

Metol trademark for a film developer, *N*-methyl-*p*-aminophenyl sulfate, $CH_3NHC_6H_4OH\cdot H_2SO_4$. See also developing SOLUTION and film PROCESSING.

metolazone (mĕ-tōl′ah-zōn) an osmotic diuretic agent with antihypertensive properties, 7-chloro-1,2,3,4-tetrahydro-2-methyl-4-oxo-3-o-tolyl-6-quinazolinesulfonamide, occurring as a light-sensitive, colorless, odorless, tasteless, crystalline powder that is insoluble in water and ethanol. It inhibits sodium reabsorption in the proximal convoluted tubules. Adverse effects may include sodium depletion, hypokalemia, increase in extracellular fluid volume, and hypersensitivity. Trademark: Zaroxolyn.

metolquizolone (me″tol-kwi′zo-lōn) methaqualone.

metopic (me-top′ik) pertaining to the forehead; frontal.

Metopirone trademark for *metyrapone.*

metopism (met′o-pizm) the persistence of the frontal suture. See metopic SUTURE.

metopo- [Gr. *metōpon* forehead] a combining form denoting relationship to the forehead. See also words beginning FRONTO-.

metopodynia (met″o-po-din′e-ah) [*metopo-* + Gr. *odynē* pain] frontal headache.

metopopagus (met″o-pop′ah-gus) [*metopo-* + Gr. *pagos* thing fixed] a craniopagus in which the fusion is in the region of the forehead.

metre (me′ter) meter (in Great Britain)

metric (met′rik) [Gr. *metron* measure] pertaining to the meter or to the metric system (see under SYSTEM). See also DECIMAL and *Tables of Weights and Measures* at WEIGHT.

metriocephalic (met″re-o-sĕ-fal′ik) [Gr. *metrios* moderate + *kephalē* head] pertaining to or characterized by a skull with an average height of the cranial vault. See metriocephalic SKULL.

Metromycin trademark for *oleandomycin.*

metronidazole (me″tro-ni′dah-zōl) an antiprotozoal agent, 2-methyl-5-nitroimidazole-1-ethanol; occurring as cream-colored, odorless crystals or crystalline powder. Used in the treatment of amebiasis and lambliasis. Also used in the treatment of acute necrotizing ulcerative gingivitis. In large doses, it may cause headache, nausea, dry mouth, stomatitis, vomiting, diarrhea, confusion, ataxia, dizziness, paresthesia, and rash.

Metroprione trademark for *metyrapone.*

metrostasis (me-tros′tah-sis) [Gr. *metron* measure + *stasis* a setting] a state in which the length of a muscle fiber is relatively fixed, and at which length it contracts and relaxes.

-metry [Gr. *metrein* to measure] a word termination meaning the act of measuring, or the measurement of, the object measured being indicated by the word stem to which it is affixed.

M. et sig. abbreviation for L. *mis′ce et sig′na,* mix and write a label.

Metycaine trademark for *piperocaine hydrochloride* (see under PIPEROCAINE).

metyrapone (mĕ-ter′ah-pōn) a compound, 2-methyl-1,2-di-3-pyridyl-1-propanone, occurring as a white to amber, photosensitive, crystalline powder with a characteristic odor, which is soluble in methanol and chloroform. It blocks the enzymatic activity leading to the synthesis of cortisol and corticosterone, while stimulating ACTH secretion and inducing an increase in the urinary 17-hydroxycorticosteroid excretion. Used as a diagnostic agent in pituitary function tests. Adverse effects may include thrombophlebitis, anorexia, nausea, abdominal discomfort, diarrhea, vertigo, headache, and sedation. Trademarks: Metopirone, Metroprione.

Mev, MeV million electron volts; see electron VOLT.

Mevasine trademark for *mecamylamine.*

Mexatol trademark for *phenylephrine hydrochloride* (see under PHENYLEPHRINE).

Mexocine trademark for *demeclocycline hydrochloride* (see under DEMECLOCYCLINE).

Meyenburg-Altherr-Uehlinger syndrome, [H. *Meyenburg,* Swiss pathologist; Franz *Altherr,* Swiss physician; E. *Uehlinger,* Swiss pathologist] chronic atrophic POLYCHONDRITIS.

Meyer's disease [Hans Wilhelm *Meyer,* Danish physician, 1824–1895] see under DISEASE.

Meyer's law see under LAW.

Meyer, organ of [George Hermann von *Meyer,* anatomist in Zürich, 1815–1892] see under ORGAN.

Meyerhof, Otto Fritz [1884–1951] a German physiologist, noted for his work on the metabolism of muscles; co-winner, with Archibald Vivian Hill, of the Nobel prize for medicine and physiology in 1922. See Embden-Meyerhof PATHWAY.

Meyer-Schwinckerath and Weyers syndrome [Gerd *Meyer-Schwinckerath;* Helmut *Weyers,* German physician] oculo-dento-osseous DYSPLASIA.

Mezolin trademark for *indomethacin.*

Mf maxillofrontale.

μf microfarad.

MFP monofluorophosphate; see SODIUM monofluorophosphate.

MF-Y gold see under GOLD.

Mg magnesium.

mg milligram.

μg microgram.

MHC major histocompatibility complex; see under HISTOCOMPATIBILITY.

MHN Mohs hardness number; see under HARDNESS.

mho (mo) [*ohm* spelled backwards] siemens.

MHS multiphasic health SCREENING.

MIB Medical Impairment Bureau; see under BUREAU.

Mibelli's disease [Vittorio *Mibelli,* Italian dermatologist, 1860–1910] see under DISEASE.

micelle (mi-sel′) 1. a unit of living matter, visible or invisible, made up of one or more molecules, and having the power of growth and division. Called also *gemma.* 2. a supermolecular colloid particle, most often a packet of chain molecules in parallel arrangement.

Micheli, F. [Italian physician] see Marchiafava-Micheli SYNDROME and THALASSEMIA minor (Rietti-Greppi-Micheli syndrome).

Micofur trademark for *nifuroxime.*

Micoserina trademark for *cycloserine.*

micr- see MICRO-.

micra (mi′krah) [Gr.] plural of *micron.*

Micro II trademark for a *high copper alloy* (see under ALLOY).

micro-, micr- [Gr. *mikros* small] 1. a combining form designating small size. 2. in the metric system, a combining form denoting one-millionth (10^{-6}) of the unit designated by the root with which it is combined. Symbol μ. See also metric SYSTEM and *Tables of Weights and Measures* at WEIGHT.

microabscess (mi″kro-ab′ses) [*micro-* + *abscess*] a very small or minute abscess.

microanalysis (mi″kro-ah-nal′ĭ-sis) [*micro-* + *analysis*] the analysis of minute quantities of material.

microanatomy (mi″kro-ah-nat′o-me) [*micro-* + *anatomy*] microscopic anatomy; histology.

microangiopathy (mi″kro-an″je-op′ah-the) [*micro-* + Gr. *angeion* vessel + *pathos* disease] disease of the small blood vessels.

Microbacterium (mi″kro-bak-te′re-um) a genus *incertae sedis* presently incorporated into the family Corynebacteriaceae, made up of small diphtheroid, rod-shaped bacteria with rounded ends, which are gram-positive and nonmotile; they are found in dairy products and characterized by relatively high resistance to heat.

microbe (mi′krōb) [*micro-* + Gr. *bios* life] a general term for a minute living organism, applied especially to those minute forms of life capable of causing disease in animals, and including bacteria and blue green algae (prokaryotes), protozoa (eukaryotic protists), and fungi (karyotic organisms).

microbial (mi-kro′be-al) of or pertaining to or caused by microbes.

microbicidal (mi-kro″bĭ-si′dal) [*microbe* + L. *caedere* to kill] destructive to microbes.

microbicide (mi-kro′bĭ-sid) [*microbe* + L. *caedere* to kill] an agent that destroys microbes.

microbioassay (mi″kro-bi″o-as′a) determination of the active power of a nutrient or other factor by noting its effect on the growth of a microorganism, as compared with the effect of a standard preparation.

microbiologist (mi″kro-bi-ol′o-jist) one who is an expert in microbiology.

microbiology (mi″kro-bi-ol′o-je) [*micro-* + Gr. *bios* life + *-logy*] the science which deals with the study of microorganisms, including bacteria, fungi, viruses, and protozoa.

microbiota (mi″kro-bi-o′tah) the microscopic living organisms of a region; the combined microflora and microfauna of a region. See also ZOOGLEA. **dental m.**, an adherent microbial mass found on the tooth surface and in the gingival crevice, together with sloughed tissue cells and exudates bound in a semipermeable slime.

microblepharia (mi″kro-blĕ-fa′re-ah) [*micro-* + Gr. *blepharon* eyelid + *-ia*] a condition characterized by abnormal shortness of the vertical dimension of the eyelids.

microblepharon (mi″kro-blef′ah-ron) an abnormally small eyelid.

Microbond 2000 trademark for a nickel-chromium base-metal crown and bridge alloy, also containing beryllium. Inhalation of dust during melting, milling, or grinding may cause beryllium poisoning.

Microbond NP trademark for a nickel-chromium base-metal crown and bridge alloy.

microbrenner (mi″kro-bren′er) [*micro-* + Ger. *Brenner* burner] a needle-pointed electric cautery.

microburet (mi″kro-bu-ret′) a buret with a capacity of the order of 0.1 to 10 ml, with graduated intervals of 0.001 to 0.02 ml.

microcalorie (mi″kro-kal′o-re) the heat required to raise the temperature of 1 ml distilled water from 0 to 1°C. See also CALORIE.

microcentrum (mi″kro-sen′trum) [*micro-* + *centrum*] centrosome.

microcephaly (mi″kro-sef′ah-le) [*micro-* + Gr. *kephalē* head] abnormal smallness of the head.

microcheilia (mi″kro-ki′le-ah) [*micro-* + Gr. *cheilos* lip] abnormal smallness of the lips.

microchemistry (mi″kro-kem′is-tre) [*micro-* + *chemistry*] 1. quantitative and qualitative reactions performed with minute amounts (a few milligrams or milliliters) of substances studied, using miniature apparatus. 2. chemical studies performed with the use of the microscope, such as chemical reactions performed on a microscopic slide with minute quantities of substances studied.

microcirculation (mi″kro-ser″ku-la′shun) circulation of the blood through a system of fine vessels of about 100 microns or less in diameter.

Micrococcaceae (mi″kro-kok-ka′se-e) [*Micrococcus* + *-aceae*] a family of gram-positive, aerobic or facultatively anaerobic, motile or nonmotile coccoid bacteria, some members of which are pathogenic to man. It includes the genera *Micrococcus and Staphylococcus.*

micrococci (mi″kro-kok′si) plural of *micrococcus.*

Micrococcus (mi″kro-kok′us) [*micro-* + Gr. *kokkos* berry] a genus of gram-positive bacteria of the family Micrococcaceae, occurring as aerobic, nonmotile, spherical coccoid cells, 0.5 to 3.5 μm in diameter, found in pairs and dividing in more than one plane to form irregular clusters, tetrads, or cubical pockets. **M. au′reus,** *Staphylococcus aureus;* see under STAPHYLOCOCCUS. **M. aerog′enes,** *Peptococcus aerogenes;* see under PEPTOCOCCUS. **M. anaero′bius,** *Peptococcus anaerobius;* see under PEPTOCOCCUS. **M. asaccharolyt′icus,** *Peptococcus asaccharolyticus;* see under PEPTOCOCCUS. **M. cit′reus,** *Staphylococcus aureus;* see under STAPHYLOCOCCUS. **M. epider′midis,** *Staphylococcus epidermidis;* see under STAPHYLOCOCCUS. **M. foe′tidus,** *Peptostreptococcus anaerobius;* see under PEPTOSTREPTOCOCCUS. **M. gazog′enes,** *Veillonella alcalescens;* see under VEILLONELLA. **M. gonococ′cus, M. gonorrhoe′ae,** *Neisseria gonorrhoeae;* see under NEISSERIA. **M. hy′icus,** *Staphylococcus epidermidis;* see under STAPHYLOCOCCUS. **M. intracellula′ris,** *Neisseria meningitidis;* see under NEISSERIA. **M. lactilyt′icus,** *Veillonella alcalescens;* see under VEILLONELLA. **M. lu′teus, M. lysodeik′ticus,** a nonpathogenic species found in dust and water and on the skin of various animals, including man. Called also *Sarcona lutea, Staphylococcus afermentans,* and *Staphylococcus flavocyaneus.* **M. meliten′sis,** *Brucella*

melitensis; see under BRUCELLA. **M. meningi′tidis,** *Neisseria meningitidis;* see under NEISSERIA. **M. pneumo′niae,** *Streptococcus pneumoniae;* see under STREPTOCOCCUS. **M. pyocya′neus,** *Pseudomonas aeruginosa;* see under PSEUDOMONAS. **M. pyog′enes, M. pyog′enes var. au′reus,** *Staphylococcus aureus;* see under STAPHYLOCOCCUS. **M. ro′seus,** a nonpathogenic species isolated from dust, water, and salt-containing foods. Called also *Staphylococcus roseus.* **M. scarlati′nae,** *Streptococcus pyogenes;* see under STREPTOCOCCUS. **M. variabi′lis,** *Peptococcus anaerobius;* see under PEPTOCOCCUS. **M. va′rians,** a nonpathogenic species found in milk, dairy products, animal carcasses, dust, and soil. Called also *Staphylococcus lactis.* **M. violagabriel′lae,** *Staphylococcus epidermidis;* see under STAPHYLOCOCCUS.

micrococcus (mi″kro-kok′us) 1. an organism of the genus *Micrococcus.* 2. a spherical microorganism of extremely small size.

microcolony (mi′kro-kol′o-ne) a microscopical colony of bacteria.

microcomputer (mi″kro-kom-pu′ter) a smaller version of a computer, usually consisting of a microprocessing unit assembled on a printed circuit board with memory and auxiliary circuits. See also MINICOMPUTER.

microcoulomb (mi″kro-koo′lom) [*micro-* + *coulomb*] a unit of quantity of electric current, being one-millionth (10^{-6}) of a coulomb. Abbreviated μ*coul.*

microcrania (mi″kro-kra′ne-ah) [*micro-* + L. *cranium;* Gr. *kranion* skull + *-ia*] abnormal smallness of the skull, the cranial cavity being reduced in all diameters, and the facial area being disproportionately large in comparison.

microcurie (mi″kro-ku′re) a unit of radioactivity, being one-millionth (10^{-6}) curie, or the quantity of radioactive material in which the number of nuclear disintegrations is 3.7×10^4 per second. Abbreviated μ*c* or μ*Ci.*

microcurie-hour (mi′kro-ku″re-owr′) a unit of exposure equivalent to that obtained by exposure for 1 hour to radioactive material disintegrating at the rate of 3.7×10^4 atoms per second. Abbreviated μ*C hr.*

microcyst (mi′kro-sist) [*micro-* + *cyst*] a very small cyst.

microcyte (mi′kro-sīt) [*micro-* + Gr. *kytos* hollow vessel] an abnormally small erythrocyte, i.e., one 6 μ or less in diameter, such as seen in microcytic anemia.

microcythemia (mi″kro-si-the′me-ah) [*microcyte* + Gr. *haima* blood + *-ia*] a condition in which the erythrocytes are smaller than normal. See microcytic ANEMIA.

microcytic (mi″kro-sit′ik) pertaining to or of the nature of a microcyte.

microdermatome (mi″kro-der′mah-tōm) an instrument for cutting very thin skin sections.

microdetermination (mi″kro-de-ter″mĭ-na′shun) a chemical method in which minute quantities of the substance to be examined are used.

microdissection (mi″kro-di-sek′shun) dissection of tissue or cells under the microscope.

microdont (mi′kro-dont) [*micro-* + Gr. *odous* tooth] having an abnormally small tooth or teeth.

microdontia (mi″kro-don′she-ah) [*micro-* + Gr. *odous* tooth + *-ia*] a developmental disorder characterized by abnormal smallness of the teeth. **relative generalized m.,** a condition in which teeth of normal size give the appearance of being abnormally small in proportion to abnormally large jaws. **single tooth m.,** that involving only a single tooth, most frequently the maxillary lateral incisor and the third molar. **true generalized m.,** a form in which all the teeth are smaller than normal.

microdose (mi′kro-dōs) [*micro-* + Gr. *dosis* a giving] a very small dose.

microelectrophoresis (mi″kro-e-lek″tro-fo-re′sis) electrophoresis in which migrating particles are observed by light microscopy; submicroscopic particles, such as viruses, are made visible by aggregation or are absorbed onto carriers, such as collodion particles or finely ground glass.

microembolus (mi″kro-em′bo-lus), pl. *microem′boli* [*micro-* + *embolus*] an embolus of microscopic size.

microfarad (mi″kro-far′ad) a unit of electrical capacity, being one-millionth (10^{-6}) of a farad. Abbreviated μ*f.*

microfauna (mi″kro-faw′nah) the animal life, visible only under the microscope, which is present in or characteristic of a special location.

microfiche (mi′kro-fēsh) [*micro-* + Gr. *fiche* small card] a sheet of microfilm containing a number of separate images.

microfilament (mi″kro-fil′ah-ment) [*micro-* + *filament*] any of the filaments about 60 Å in diameter found in the cytoplasmic ground substance.

microfilaria (mi″kro-fi-la′re-ah) [*micro-* + L. *filum* thread] the prelarval stage of Filarioidea in the blood of man and in the tissue of the vector. This term is sometimes incorrectly used as a genus name.

microfilm (mi′kro-film) 1. a film, usually 16- or 35-mm, bearing miniaturized photographs of printed or documentary material, such as books or journals. Generally used in libraries to preserve valuable or older materials or save storage space for bulky books and documents. 2. a film on which microcopies are made. 3. to produce a microfilm.

microflora (mi″kro-flo′rah) the plant life, visible only under the microscope, which is present in or characteristic of a special location.

microgamma (mi″kro-gam′mah) picogram.

microgenesis (mi″kro-jen′ĕ-sis) [*micro-* + *genesis*] development of an abnormally small part.

microgenia (mi″kro-jen′e-ah) [*micro-* + Gr. *genys* jaw] underdevelopment of the mental symphysis of the mandible, resulting in a very small chin; a similar appearance is caused by malocclusion with excessive prominence of the alveolar structures.

microglia (mi-krog′le-ah) [*micro-* + *neuroglia*] the tissue made up of microgliocytes. Called also *mesoglia*.

microgliocyte (mi-krog′le-o-sīt) [*microglia* + *cyte*] a small neuroglial cell, said to be of mesodermal origin, which has a small round to oblong or angular nucleus and two or more branching processes. It is found in both the gray and white substance and its function consists of phagocytizing injured and dead cells in the nervous system. Called also *gitter cell* and *Hortega cell*. Collectively, such cells are called *microglia*. See illustration at NERVE.

microglobulin (mi″kro-glob′u-lin) [*micro-* + *globulin*] γL-GLOBULIN.

microglossia (mi″kro-glos′e-ah) [*micro-* + Gr. *glōssa* tongue + *-ia*] presence of an undersized or rudimentary tongue.

micrognathia (mi″kro-na′the-ah) [*micro-* + Gr. *gnathos* jaw + *-ia*] a congenital or acquired condition characterized by abnormal smallness of the jaw. See also BRACHYGNATHIA and RETROGNATHIA. Cf. PROGNATHISM. **mandibular m.**, abnormal smallness of the mandible associated with recession of the chin; micromandible. **maxillary m.**, abnormal smallness of the maxilla associated with retraction of the middle third of the face; micromaxilla.

microgram (mi′kro-gram) [*micro-* + *gram*] a unit of mass (weight) in the metric system, being one-millionth (10^{-6}) of a gram or one-thousandth (10^{-3}) of a milligram. Abbreviated μg or mcg. Symbol γ.

micrograph (mi′kro-graf) 1. an instrument for recording extremely small movements. It acts by making a greatly magnified record of the minute motions on a photographic film. One type is a ballistocardiograph. 2. photomicrograph.

micrography (mi-krog′rah-fe) [*micro-* + Gr. *graphein* to write] 1. an account of microscopic objects. 2. examination with the microscope.

microhm (mi′krōm) [*micro-* + *ohm*] one-millionth part of an ohm.

microincineration (mi″kro-in-sin″er-a′shun) the incineration of minute specimens of tissue or other substance for identification from the ash of the elements composing it.

microinjector (mi″kro-in-jek′tor) an instrument for injecting minute amounts of fluids or drugs.

microleakage (mi″kro-lēk′ij) the seepage of microorganisms, fluids, and debris along the interface between a restoration or cement (and the walls of a cavity preparation). Such leakage can progress through the dentin at the floor of the cavity preparation, and into the pulp. See illustration.

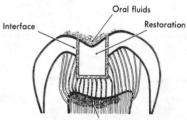

Oral fluids

Interface

Restoration

Penetration into pulp

Schematic diagram of the microleakage phenomenon. In this case the penetration of possible irritants from the oral cavity has extended along the entire tooth-restoration interface, through the dentin, and into the pulp. (From R. W. Phillips: Skinner's Science of Dental Materials. 7th ed. Philadelphia, W. B. Saunders Co., 1973; modified from M. Massler: Adhesive Restorative Materials. Spencer, Ind., Owens Litho Service, 1961.)

microlesion (mi″kro-le′zhun) [*micro-* + *lesion*] a minute lesion.

microline (mi′kro-līn) potassium FELDSPAR.

microliter (mi′kro-le″ter) [*micro-* + *liter*] a unit of volume in the metric system, being one-millionth (10^{-6}) of a liter or one-thousandth (10^{-3}) of a milliliter (cubic centimeter). It is equivalent to 0.01623108 minims. Abbreviated μl.

microlith (mi′kro-lith) [*micro-* + Gr. *lithos* stone] a minute concretion or calculus.

micromandible (mi″kro-man′di-b'l) [*micro-* + *mandible*] extreme smallness of the mandible; mandibular micrognathia.

micromanipulator (mi″kro-mah-nip′u-la″tor) an attachment to a microscope for manipulating tiny instruments used in examination and dissection of minute objects under the microscope.

micromanometer (mi″kro-man-om′ĕ-ter) [*micro-* + *manometer*] an apparatus for indicating gas or vapor pressure from a very small sample, as of blood, fluid, etc.

micromaxilla (mi″kro-mak-sil′ah) [*micro-* + *maxilla*] extreme smallness of the maxilla; maxillary micrognathia.

micromelia (mi″kro-me′le-ah) [*micro-* + Gr. *melos* limb + *-ia*] a condition characterized by abnormal shortness of the extremities.

micrometer[1] (mi-krom′ĕ-ter) [*micro-* + Gr. *metron* measure] an instrument for measuring objects seen through the microscope.

micrometer[2] (mi′kro-me″ter) micron (1).

micromethod (mi″kro-meth′od) any technique involving use of exceedingly small quantities of material.

micrometry (mi-krom′ĕ-tre) [*micro-* + *-metry*] the measurement of microscopic objects.

micromicro- a prefix used in naming units of measurement to indicate one-millionth of one-millionth (10^{-12}) of the unit designated by the root with which it is combined. Now supplanted by the prefix *pico-*.

micromicrocurie (mi″kro-mi″kro-ku′re) picocurie.

micromicrogram (mi″kro-mi′kro-gram) [*micro-* + *microgram*] a former name for *picogram*. Abbreviated μμg.

micromicron (mi″kro-mi′kron) a unit of linear measure in the metric system, being 10^{-6} micron, 10^{-9} millimeter, or 10^{-12} meter. Abbreviated μμ.

micromilligram (mi″kro-mil′ĭ-gram) [*micro-* + *milligram*] a unit of mass (weight) in the metric system, being one-millionth (10^{-6}) of a milligram. Abbreviated μmg.

micromillimeter (mi″kro-mil′ĭ-me″ter) [*micro-* + *millimeter*] a unit of length in the metric system, being one-millionth (10^{-6}) of a millimeter, and equivalent to the nanometer and the millimicron. Abbreviated μmm.

micromole (mi″kro-mol) one-millionth (10^{-6}) of a mole. Abbreviated μmole.

micromolecular (mi″kro-mo-lek′u-lar) pertaining to or composed of small molecules.

micron (mi′kron), pl. *microns*, *mi′cra* [Gr. *mikros* small] 1. a unit of length in the metric system, being one-thousandth (10^{-3}) of a millimeter and one-millionth (10^{-6}) of a meter; it is equivalent to 0.000039 inch. Abbreviated μ. See *Tables of Weights and Measures* at WEIGHT. Called also *micrometer* (μm). 2. a microscopic colloid particle varying in size from 10^{-3} to 10^{-5} cm.

microneedle (mi″kro-ne′d'l) a fine glass needle for use in microsurgery.

micronize (mi′kro-nīz) [Gr. *micron* a small thing] to reduce to a fine powder; to reduce to particles of a micron in diameter.

micronucleus (mi″kro-nu′kle-us) [*micro-* + *nucleus*] 1. a small nucleus. 2. nucleolus.

micronutrient (mi″kro-nu′tre-ent) any essential dietary element required only in small quantities, e.g., trace elements.

microorganism (mi″kro-or′gan-izm) [*micro-* + *organism*] a minute living organism, usually microscopic. Those of medical interest include bacteria, viruses, fungi, algae, and protozoa. **aerobic m.**, see AEROBE. **anaerobic m.**, see ANAEROBE.

microparasite (mi″kro-par′ah-sīt) a parasitic microorganism.

microphone (mi′kro-fōn) [*micro-* + Gr. *phōnē* voice] a device for converting an acoustic signal into an electric signal for purpose of amplification or transmission.

microphonia (mi″kro-fo′ne-ah) [*micro-* + Gr. *phōnē* voice + *-ia*] weakness of the voice.

microphthalmia (mi″krof-thal′me-ah) [*micro-* + Gr. *ophthalmos* eye + *-ia*] abnormal smallness of the eyes.

micropipet (mi″kro-pi-pet′) a pipet for handling small quantities of liquids (up to 1 ml).

microprecipitation (mi″kro-pre-sip″ĭ-ta′shun) precipitation with a minute amount (1/2 to 1 drop or less) of reagent observed under a microscope.

microprobe (mi′kro-prōb) a minute probe, as one used in microsurgery. **laser m.**, a laser beam utilized to vaporize a minute area of tissue, as in a biopsy specimen, which is then subjected to emission spectrography.

microradiography (mi″kro-ra″de-og′rah-fe) [*micro-* + *radiography*] a process by which a radiograph of a small or very thin object is produced on fine-grained photographic film under conditions which permit subsequent microscopic examination or enlargement of the radiograph at linear magnifications of up to several hundred and with the resolution approaching the resolving power of the photographic emulsion (about 1000 lines per millimeter).

microreaction (mi″kro-re-ak′shun) a qualitative chemical reaction performed with minute reagents under the microscope.

microrhinia (mi″kro-rin′e-ah) [*micro-* + Gr. *rhis* nose] abnormal smallness of the nose.

microroentgen (mi″kro-rent′gen) [*micro-* + *-roentgen*] one-millionth of a roentgen. Abbreviated μR.

microscope (mi′kro-skōp) [*micro-* + Gr. *skopein* to view] 1. an instrument used to obtain an enlarged image of small objects and reveal details of structure not otherwise distinguishable. See also EYEPIECE, LENS, and OBJECTIVE. 2. optical m. **binocular m.**, one which has two eyepieces, making possible simultaneous viewing with both eyes. **centrifuge m.**, one built into a high-speed centrifuge, by which a magnified image of a specimen undergoing centrifugation may be produced. **comparison m.**, one which permits simultaneous viewing of parts of images of two separate specimens, involving two microscopes bridged together with a comparison eyepiece, or one microscope with two body tubes and lens systems. **compound m.**, one that consists of two lens systems, one above the other, in which the image formed by the system nearer the object (objective) is further magnified by the system nearer the eye (eyepiece). **darkfield m.**, one with a central stop in the condenser, permitting diversion of the light rays and illumination of the object from the side, so that the details appear light against a dark background. **electron m.**, one in which the light source is replaced by electrons emitted by a tungsten filament, their effective wavelength being determined by the voltage by which they are accelerated; shaped magnetic or electronic fields take the place of glass lenses, and a fluorescent screen replaces the human eye for direct viewing or for photography. **fluorescence m.**, one used for the examination of specimens stained with fluorochromes or fluorochrome complexes, e.g., a fluorescein-labeled antibody, which fluoresces in ultraviolet rays. The image seen is due to emission from the specimen that has absorbed the primary exciting light and re-emitted light of longer wavelength and lower energy, which is filtered to ensure that only the desired secondary emission from the specimen will contribute to the image. **infrared m.**, one in which radiation of 800 mμ or longer wavelength is used as the image-forming energy. **interference m.**, one for observing the same kind of refractile detail in specimens as does the phase microscope but using two separate beams of light that are recombined with each other in the image plane, one focused through the specimen and the other, a comparison beam, through a neutral area. It allows direct quantitative measurement of retardation and of the related quantities of refraction index and, consequently, the thickness of the specimen. See also *phase m.* **ion m.**, an electron microscope modified to use ions (e.g., of lithium) instead of electrons. **light m.**, one in which the specimen is viewed under visible light. The light comes through a numerical aperture which is a measure of the size or angle of the cone of light delivered by the illuminating condenser lens to the object plane and of the cone of light emerging from the object that is collected by the objective lens. Light coming through the fine details of the object is diffracted into directions different from that of its original propagation, the wider the angle at which the light is diffracted, the finer the detail. The resolving power of a light microscope is relative to the number of the numerical aperture, its theoretical limit being approximately 0.25 μ. The probe size to be associated with the light is about that of its wavelength, or about 0.5 μ. Called also *optical m.* **measuring micrometer m.**, an instrument for measuring small objects or distances to 0.001 mm, consisting of a specimen stage and a stand supporting the lens system and micrometer. The lens is equipped with a cross hair which is focused on a point on one side of the specimen and a reading is taken on the micrometer gauge. **opaque m.**, one with vertical illumination or with the condenser built around the objective for viewing opaque specimens. **operating m.**, one designed for use in delicate surgical procedures. **optical m.**, light m. **phase m.**, **phase-contrast m.**, one which alters the phase relationships of the light passing through and that passing around the object, the contrast permitting visualization of the object without staining or other special preparation. It converts small differences in the refrac-

tive index, which cannot be appreciated by the eye, into differences in intensity that can be seen. See also *interference m.* **polarizing m.**, one for the histological examination at the molecular level, based on the principle that, when a ray of plane polarized light strikes tissues or cells that are crystalline or fibrous, it acts as if it were split into two rays polarized in planes perpendicular to one another, the two rays having different velocities. Objects with high degree of molecular orientation have different refractive indexes depending upon the plane of vibration of the ray of polarized light with respect to the orientation of the molecules. It contains a polarizer, analyzer, and means for measurement of the alteration of the polarized light by the specimen. **reflecting m.**, one in which mirrors are used instead of lenses. **simple m.**, one consisting of a single lens; a magnifying glass. **stereoscopic m.**, a binocular biobjective microscope, or a binocular mono-objective microscope modified to give a three-dimensional view of the specimen. **ultraviolet m.**, one which uses ultraviolet light, with the aid of quartz as the reflecting lenses, instead of visible light. **x-ray m.**, one in which a beam of x-rays is used instead of light, the image usually being reproduced on film.

microscopic (mi″kro-skop′ik) of very small size; visible only under the microscope.

microscopy (mi-kros′ko-pe) [*micro-* + Gr. *skopein* to view] examination under or observation by means of the microscope. **immunofluorescent m.**, identification by means of a fluorescent microscope of antigens exposed to homologous antibodies labeled with a fluorescent tracer.

microsection (mi″kro-sek′shun) a very thin section for examination under the microscope. Sections for the light microscope are 5 to 10 μ; those for the electron microscope are 50 to 100 μ (5 to 10 nm).

microsecond (mi′kro-sek″und) one-millionth (10^{-6}) of a second. Abbreviated μsec.

microslide (mi′kro-slīd) the slide on which objects for microscopical examination are mounted.

microsome (mi′kro-sōm) [*micro-* + Gr. *sōma* body] a minute particle of a cell rich in nucleic acids, being a vesicular fragment of the endoplasmic reticulum.

microsomia (mi″kro-so′me-ah) [*micro-* + Gr. *sōma* body + *-ia*] smallness of the body. **hemifacial m.**, first and second branchial arch SYNDROME.

microspectrophotometry (mi″kro-spek″tro-fo-tom′ĕ-tre) a histochemical method combining microscopy with spectrophotometry.

microspectroscope (mi″kro-spek′tro-skōp) [*micro-* + *spectroscope*] a spectroscope to be used in connection with a microscope for the examination of the spectra of microscopic objects.

microsphygmia (mi-kro-sfig′me-ah) [*micro-* + Gr. *sphygmos* pulse + *-ia*] a pulse that is difficult to perceive by the finger.

Microspira (mi″kro-spi′rah) [*micro-* + Gr. *speira* coil] a former name for small, spiral microorganisms now assigned to the genus *Vibrio*. **M. alben′sis**, *Vibrio cholerae* (biotype *albensis*); see under VIBRIO. **M. dun′bari**, *Vibrio cholerae* (biotype *albensis*); see under VIBRIO. **M. fink′leri**, *Vibrio cholerae* (biotype *proteus*); see under VIBRIO. **M. pro′tea**, *Vibrio cholerae* (biotype *proteus*); see under VIBRIO.

Microspironema (mi″kro-spi″ro-ne′mah) [*micro-* + Gr. *speira* coil + *nēma* thread] *Treponema*. **M. pal′lidum**, *Treponema pallidum*; see under TREPONEMA.

Microsporon (mi-kros′po-ron) a genus name no longer used in bacteriological taxonomy. **M. diphtherit′icum**, *Corynebacterium diphtheriae*; see under CORYNEBACTERIUM.

Microsporum (mi-kros′po-rum) [*micro-* + Gr. *sporos* seed] a genus of dermatophytes which cause various forms of tinea, including tinea corporis, tinea capitis, and tinea barbae.

microstat (mi′kro-stat) the stage and finder of a microscope.

microstomia (mi″kro-sto′me-ah) [*micro-* + Gr. *stoma* mouth + *-ia*] abnormal smallness of the mouth.

microsurgery (mi′kro-ser″jer-e) dissection of minute structures under the microscope by means of instruments held in the hand, as in microsurgery of the larynx.

microsyringe (mi″kro-ser′inj) a syringe fitted with a screw-thread micrometer head for the accurate control of minute measurements.

microthrombi (mi″kro-throm′bi) [L.] plural of *microthrombus*.

microthrombus (mi″kro-throm′bus), pl. *microthrom′bi* [*micro-* + *thrombus*] a small thrombus located in a capillary or other small blood vessel.

microtia (mi-kro′she-ah) [*micro-* + Gr. *ous* ear + *-ia*] a developmental abnormality characterized by hypoplasia or aplasia of the pinna of the ear, associated with a blind or absent external auditory meatus.

Microtin trademark for *cephalothin sodium* (see under CEPHALO-THIN)

microtome (mi'kro-tōm) [*micro-* + Gr. *tomē* a cut] an instrument for cutting very thin slices of tissue for microscopical study. See also ULTRAMICROTOME.

microtomy (mi-krot'o-me) [*micro-* + Gr. *tomnein* to cut] the cutting into thin sections. Called also *histotomy*.

microtonometer (mi"kro-to-nom'ĕ-ter) a small tonometer for measuring the oxygen and carbon dioxide tension in the blood.

microtrauma (mi"kro-traw'mah) a slight trauma or lesion; a microscopic lesion.

microtubule (mi"kro-tu'būl) a cylindrical hollow-appearing structure in the cytoplasmic ground substance of many motile cells, especially erythrocytes; microtubules, which increase in number during mitosis, are found in the mitotic spindle.

microunit (mi'kro-u"nit) one-millionth (10⁻⁶) of a standard unit. Abbreviated μU.

microvilli (mi"kro-vil'i) [L.] plural of *microvillus*.

microvillus (mi"kro-vil'us), pl. *microvil'li* [L. "a tuft of hair"] one of the minute cylindrical processes on the free surface of a cell. See brush BORDER.

microviscosimeter (mi"kro-vis"ko-sim'ĕ-ter) an instrument for measuring the viscosity in minute quantities of materials.

microvolt (mi'kro-volt) [*micro* + *volt*] one-millionth of a volt. Abbreviated μv.

microwatt (mi'kro-wat) [*micro-* + *watt*] one-millionth of a watt. Abbreviated μw.

microwave (mi'kro-wāv) [*micro-* + *wave*] an electromagnetic wave of very high frequency and of short wavelength, considered by some authorities as ranging between 1 millimeter and 1 meter, or between 1 centimeter and 1 meter. Called also *ultrashort wave*.

microzoon (mi"kro-zo'on) [*micro-* + Gr. *zōon* animal] a microscopic animal organism.

micrurgy (mi'krur-je) [*micro* + Gr. *ergon* work] a micromanipulative method in the field of a microscope. See also MICROMANIPULATOR.

midbody (mid'bod-e) 1. a body or a mass of granules developed in the equatorial region of the spindle during the anaphase of mitosis. 2. the middle region of the trunk.

midbrain (mid'brān) a short, narrow, constricted portion of the brain stem, just below the thalamus, which connects the pons and the cerebellum with the forebrain. Among its structures, it contains the center for visual reflexes, the nucleus of the mesencephalic root of the trigeminal nerve, the nucleus of the trochlear nerve, and the nucleus of the oculomotor nerve. Called also *mesencephalon*.

midfrontal (mid-fron'tal) pertaining to the middle of the forehead.

midgut (mid'gut) the intermediate region of the primitive gut between the foregut and hindgut, opening into the yolk sac, which exists for a brief period during the fourth week of embryonic life, before constriction of the yolk stalk and detachment from the gut at the end of the fifth week. It gives rise to the distal part of the duodenum, jejunum, ileum, cecum, appendix, ascending colon, and right half of the transverse colon.

midoccipital (mid"ok-sip'ĭ-tal) pertaining to or located in the middle of the occiput. Called also *medioccipital* and *midiooccipital*.

midplane (mid'plān) the median plane of a bilateral structure.

midsection (mid-sek'shun) a cut through the middle of any organ or part.

Mielucin trademark for *busulfan*.

Mieradent 70 trademark for a *polysulfide impression material* (see under MATERIAL).

Miescher's cheilitis, disease, elastoma, and syndrome [Guido *Miescher*, Swiss dermatologist, 1877–1961] see CHEILITIS granulomatosa and perforating ELASTOSIS, and see under SYNDROME.

MIF migration inhibitory FACTOR.

migraine (mi'grān, me'grān) [Fr., from Gr. *hemikrania* an affection of half of the head] a pain syndrome characterized by periodic headache of varied degree of severity, lasting from a few minutes to several days, often associated with nausea, vomiting, flushing, gastrointestinal disorders, vertigo, and photophobia. The headache is usually unilateral at the beginning but may spread to other parts of the head. Attacks may be preceded by various prodromal symptoms (preheadache), such

as scotoma, visual field defects, and visual disorders. The pain is usually throbbing and aching, and may involve the temporal, frontal, retro-orbital, and, less commonly, the parietal, occipital, and suboccipital areas. Painful contractions of the neck and head muscles may occur. Called also *blind headache, hemicrania, migrainous neuralgia,* and *sick headache.* See also vascular HEADACHE. **cervical m.,** 1. Barré-Liéou SYNDROME. 2. Bärtschi-Rochain's SYNDROME. **hemiplegic m., ophthalmoplegic h.,** migraine associated with hemiplegia that may persist after the headache. Called also *hemiplegic headache* and *ophthalmoplegic headache.*

migration (mi-gra'shun) [L. *migratio*] the act or process of moving or wandering from one point to another, usually some point foreign to the normal location. **leukocyte m.,** LEUKOCYTE migration. **physiologic mesial m.,** a gradual process of movement of the teeth mesially, as they wear their proximal contact areas and become flattened. **tooth m., pathologic,** drifting of the teeth due to destruction of tooth-supporting structures by periodontal disease or failure to replace missing teeth. The teeth may move in any direction; mobility and rotation of the involved teeth are usually associated. Migration occurs most frequently in the anterior region, but posterior teeth may also migrate. Pathologic migration in the occlusal or incisal direction is termed *extrusion* or *elongation.* Called also *abnormal tooth mobility* and *pathologic tooth wandering.* See also pathologic tooth MOBILITY, and tooth MOVEMENT. **tooth m., physiologic,** change of position of the teeth during their growth and development. It may be a passive process in which the tooth itself remains in position while the surrounding tissue migrates (preeruptive translocation), or it may be an active process in which the tooth itself changes position. One form of active migration consists of an occlusal movement as a result of natural wearing of the tooth surface, and the other is the mesial drift occurring as a consequence of natural approximal wearing of tooth surfaces. Called also *physiologic drift.*

Mikulicz's aphthae, cells, disease, syndrome [Johann (Jan) von *Mikulicz*-Radecki, surgeon in Berlin, 1850–1905] see PERIADENITIS mucosa necrotica and see under CELL, DISEASE, and SYNDROME.

Mikulicz-Radecki see MIKULICZ.

milia (mil'e-ah) [L.] plural of *milium*.

miliaria (mil"e-a're-ah) [L. *milium* millet] a syndrome of cutaneous changes associated with sweat retention and extravasation occurring at different levels in the skin.

miliary (mil'e-a-re) [L. *miliaris* like a millet seed] 1. resembling a millet seed. 2. characterized by the formation of lesions resembling millet seeds, as in miliary tuberculosis.

milieu (me-lyuh') [Fr.] surroundings; environment.

milium (mil'e-um), pl. *mil'ia* [L. "millet seed"] a small whitish nodule in the skin, especially of the face. Milia are spheroidal masses of lamellated keratin lying just under the epidermis, often associated with vellus hair follicles. Called also *whitehead.*

milk (milk) [L. *lac*] 1. a white fluid secreted by the mammary gland, forming the natural food for young mammals. 2. the milk produced by cows, goats, sheep, and certain other domestic animals that is used for human consumption, either in the natural state or processed into dairy products, such as butter, cheese, or yogurt. **m. albumin,** lactalbumin. **m. of magnesia,** a 7.0 to 8.5 percent aqueous suspension of magnesium hydroxide, occurring as an opaque, white, viscous suspension which settles out on standing, with small quantities of citric acid and flavoring agents added. Used as a cathartic and antacid. Also used as an alkaline mouthwash. It is insoluble in the saliva and, thus, is not absorbed through the oral mucosa. It may be used topically as a protective to irritated mucosa, especially in the presence of mild xerostomia. It is claimed to have neutralizing effects on oral acidity, preventing dental caries; this last property is questioned. Called also *magnesia magma.* **m. sugar,** lactose.

mill (mil) a machine or device for working materials into a desired form, or performing other mechanical operations. **colloid m.,** a device designed to mechanically disintegrate by grinding of a substance into fine particles of colloidal size, or to reduce the size of particles.

Millar's asthma [John *Millar*, British physician, 1733–1805] LARYNGISMUS stridulus.

Millard's syndrome [Auguste L. J. *Millard*, French physician, 1830–1915] Millard-Gubler SYNDROME.

Millard-Gubler syndrome [A. L. J. *Millard*; Adolphe Marie *Gubler*, French physician, 1821–1879] see under SYNDROME.

Miller Apexo elevator see under ELEVATOR.

Miller's collutory see under COLLUTORY.

Miller's elevator see under ELEVATOR.

Miller's theory [Willoughby Dayton *Miller*, American dentist and oral pathologist 1853–1907, who spent most of his professional life in Germany. His discovery that gangrenous pulp may serve as a center of infection to other parts is considered as a landmark in the development of modern endodontics. He is considered to be a founder of the theory on the bacterial origin of dental caries.] acidogenic THEORY.

milli- [L. *mille* thousand] in the metric system, a combining form denoting one-thousandth (10^{-3}) of the unit designated by the root with which it is combined. Symbol *m*. See also metric SYSTEM and *Tables of Weights and Measures* at WEIGHT.

milliammeter (mil″e-am′ĕ-ter) an ammeter which registers a current in milliamperes.

milliampere (mil″e-am′pēr) [*milli-* + *ampere*] one-thousandth of an ampere. Abbreviated *ma*.

milliampere-minute (mil″e-am″pēr-min′ut) a unit of electrical quantity equivalent to that delivered by 1 milliampere in 1 minute.

milliampere-second (mil″e-am″per-sek′und) a unit of electrical quantity equivalent to that delivered by 1 milliampere in 1 second. In roentgenography, it determines the quantity and intensity of x-ray production. Abbreviated *mas*.

millicoulomb (mil″ĭ-koo′lom) a unit of quantity of current, being one-thousandth (10^{-3}) of a coulomb. Abbreviated *mcoul*.

millicurie (mil′ĭ-ku′re) a unit of radioactivity, being one-thousandth (10^{-3}) curie, or the quantity of radioactive material in which the number of nuclear disintegrations is 3.7×10^7 per second. Abbreviated *mc* or *mCi*.

millicurie-hour (mil′ĭ-ku′re-owr″) a unit of dose equivalent to that obtained by exposure for 1 hour to radioactive material disintegrating at the rate of 3.7×10^7 atoms per second. Abbreviated *mch* or *mc-hr*.

milliequivalent (mil″ĭ-e-kwiv′ah-lent) the number of grams of solute contained in 1 milliliter (cubic centimeter) of a normal solution. Abbreviated *mEq* or *meq*.

milligram (mil′ĭ-gram) [*milli-* + *gram*] a unit of mass (weight) in the metric system, being one-thousandth (10^{-3}) of a gram and equivalent to 0.015432 grains. One-thousandth of a milligram is a microgram. Abbreviated *mg*.

millilambert (mil″ĭ-lam′bert) one-thousandth of a lambert.

milliliter (mil′ĭ-le″ter) [*milli-* + *liter*] a unit of volume of fluid in the metric system, being one-thousandth (10^{-3}) of a liter and consisting of 1000 microliters. It corresponds to 1 cubic centimeter and is equivalent to 16.231 minims. Abbreviated *ml*.

millimeter (mil″ĭ-me′ter) [*milli-* + *meter*] a unit of length in the metric system, being one-thousandth (10^{-3}) of a meter and one-tenth (10^{-1}) of a centimeter. It is equivalent to about 0.03937 inch. Abbreviated *mm*. **cubic m.**, a unit of volume in the metric system, being a cube each side of which measures 1 millimeter; 1000 cubic millimeters are equivalent to 1 cubic centimeter. Abbreviated mm^3. **square m.**, a unit in the metric system used for measuring minute areas, being a square both sides of which measure 1 millimeter; 100 square millimeters are equivalent to 1 square centimeter. Abbreviated mm^2.

millimicro- a prefix used in naming units of measurement to indicate one-thousandth of one-millionth (10^{-9}) of the unit designated by the root with which it is combined. Now supplanted by the prefix *nano-*.

millimicrocurie (mil″ĭ-mi″kro-ku′re) former name for *nanocurie*. Abbreviated *mμc*.

millimicrogram (mil″ĭ-mi′kro-gram) [*milli-* + *microgram*] a former name for *nanogram*. Abbreviated *mμg*.

millimicroliter (mil″ĭ-mi″kro-le′ter) [*milli-* + *microliter*] a former name for *nanoliter*.

millimicron (mil″ĭ-mi′kron) [*milli-* + *micron*] a unit of length in the metric system, being one-thousandth (10^{-3}) of a micron, and equivalent to the nanometer and the micromillimeter. Abbreviated *mμ*. Called also *millimu*.

millimole (mil′ĭ-mōl) one-thousandth (10^{-3}) of a mole. Abbreviated *mM*.

millimu (mil′ĭ-mu) [*milli-* + *mu* (Gr. letter μ)] millimicron.

milling-in (mil′ing-in) correcting or perfecting occlusal disharmonies of natural or artificial teeth by the use of abrasives between their occluding surfaces while the dentures are rubbed together in the mouth or on the articulator. See also GRINDING-IN and selective GRINDING.

millinormal (mil′ĭ-nor′mal) having a concentration one-thousandth of normal; said of solutions. Abbreviated *mN*.

millirad (mil′ĭ-rad) [*milli-* + *rad*] a unit of absorbed radiation, being one-thousandth (10^{-3}) rad. Abbreviated *mrad*.

milliroentgen (mil′ĭ-rent′gen) a unit of dose equal to one-thousandth (10^{-3}) roentgen. Abbreviated *mR* or *mr*.

millisecond (mil′ĭ-sek′ond) [*milli-* + *second*] a unit of time, being one-thousandth (10^{-3}) second. Abbreviated *msec*.

milliunit (mil′ĭ-u″nit) [*milli-* + *unit*] one-thousandth (10^{-3}) of a standard unit. Abbreviated *mU*.

millivolt (mil′ĭ-vōlt) one-thousandth of a volt. Abbreviated *mv*.

Milontin trademark for *phensuximide*.

Milton's disease, urticaria [John Laws *Milton*, London dermatologist, 1820–1898] Quincke's EDEMA.

Miltown trademark for *meprobamate*.

mimesis (mi-me′sis) [Gr. *mimēsis* imitation] the simulation of one disease or bodily process by another.

mimetic (mi-met′ik) [Gr. *mimētikos*] 1. marked by simulation of another bodily process or disease. Called also *mimic*. 2. a word termination indicating simulation of a function, process, etc., designated by the root to which it is affixed, as *sympathomimetic*.

mimic (mim′ik) mimetic (1).

min. abbreviation for L. *min′imum*, a minim.

mind (mīnd) [L. *mens*; Gr. *psyche*] the faculty, or function of the brain, by which an individual becomes aware of his surroundings and of their distribution in space and time, and by which he experiences feeling, emotions, and desires, and is able to attend, to remember, to reason, and to decide.

mineral (min′er-al) [L. *minerale*] a nonorganic homogeneous solid substance, usually a constituent of the earth's crust. **m. jelly,** petrolatum. **m. white,** gypsum.

mineralization (min″er-al-i-za′shun) the addition of mineral matter to the body with resulting hardening of the tissue. See also CALCIFICATION.

mineralocorticoid (min″er-al-o-kor′tĭ-koid) any of a group of adrenal cortex hormones produced in the zona glomerulosa, which are affected little by adrenocorticotropic hormone. Their chief function is to maintain the water-electrolyte balance, chiefly through the mechanism of reabsorption of sodium by the renal tubules and also through their influence on the distribution of sodium, potassium, water, and hydrogen ions between the cellular and extracellular fluids. Principal mineralocorticoids include aldosterone, deoxycorticosterone, and dehydroepiandrosterone.

minicomputer (min″ĭ-kom-pu′ter) a small computer, usually a parallel binary system with 8-, 12-, 16-, 18-, 24-, or 32-bit word length incorporating semiconductor or magnetic core memory offering from 4K words to 64K words of storage and a cycle time of 0.2 to 8 microsecond or less. See also MICROCOMPUTER.

minim (min′im) [L. *minimum*] a unit of capacity (liquid or wine measure) that has been accepted as being equal to a drop. It is the equivalent of 0.0166 fluid drams, 0.00013 pints, 0.00376 cubic inches, or 0.06161 cubic centimeters or milliliters. See also *Tables of Weights and Measures* at WEIGHT.

minima (min′ĭ-mah) [L.] plural of *minimum*.

minimal (min′ĭ-mal) [L. *minimus* least] smallest or least; the smallest possible; the reverse of maximal.

Minimax 178 trademark for an *amalgam alloy* (see under AMALGAM).

minimum (min′ĭ-mum), pl. *min′ima* [L. "smallest"] the least; the smallest or lowest number, quantity, or degree attainable.

Minipress trademark for *prazosin hydrochloride* (see under PRAZOSIN).

Minkowski-Chauffard syndrome [Oskar *Minkowski*, German physician, 1858–1931] hereditary SPHEROCYTOSIS.

Minocin trademark for *minocycline*.

minocycline (mi-no-si′klēn) a semisynthetic tetracycline antibiotic, 4,7 - bis(dimethylamino) - 1,4,4a,5,5a,6,11,12a - octahydro - 3,10,12,12a - tetrahydroxy - 1,11 - dioxo - 2 - naphthacenecarboxamide. Administered orally and intravenously as the hydrochloride salt, occurring as a yellow, odorless, slightly hygroscopic, crystalline powder that darkens on exposure to strong light and moisture and dissolves in water, alcohol, alkali hydroxide, and carbonate solutions, but not in chloroform and ether. Used to eliminate meningococci from the nasopharynx. It has toxic properties similar to those of other tetracyclines. Trademarks: Klinomycin, Minocin, Vectrin.

mio- [Gr. *meiōn* smaller] a combining form denoting less. See also terms beginning MEIO-.

miosis (mi′o-sis) [Gr. *meiōsis* diminution] 1. contraction of the pupil. 2. a diminution of symptoms of disease.

Miracryl Clear trademark for a heat-cured denture base acrylic resin.

Mirchamp's sign see under SIGN.

Miromorfalil trademark for *nalorphine hydrochloride* (see under NALORPHINE).

Mirontin trademark for *phensuximide*.

mirror (mir′or) [Fr. *miroir*] a polished surface that reflects light to yield images of objects in front of it. **concave m.,** one with a concave reflecting surface. **convex m.,** one with a convex reflecting surface. **dental m.,** mouth m. **frontal m., head m.,** a circular mirror strapped to the head of the examiner, used to reflect light into a cavity, especially in connection with nasal, pharyngeal, and laryngeal examinations and to some extent in surgery of these organs. **mouth m.,** a small mirror, magnifying or nonmagnifying, used to reflect the operating field in the oral cavity, to retract the tissue and tongue, and to protect the tissue from injury during operation. The mirror may be mounted either on the front or the reverse side of the handle. Called also *dental m.* See illustration. **plane m.,** one with a flat reflecting surface.

Sterilizable mouth mirror. (From H. O. Torres and A. Ehrlich: Modern Dental Assisting. 2nd ed. Philadelphia, W. B. Saunders Co., 1980; courtesy of S. S. White Div. of Pennwalt Corp.)

misce (mis′e) [L.] mix.
miscible (mis′ĭ-b′l) susceptible of being mixed.
mist. abbreviation for L. *mistu′ra,* a mixture.
mistura (mis-tu′rah) [L.] mixture.
Misulban trademark for *busulfan.*
Mithracin trademark for *mithramycin.*
mithramycin (mith″rah-mi′sin) an antibiotic isolated from cultures of several strains of *Streptomyces,* occurring as a yellow solid that is soluble in alcohols, acetone, ethyl acetate, water, and chloroform and slightly soluble in ether and benzene. It is a cytotoxic drug that inhibits the synthesis of RNA and acts on plasma calcium concentration. Used in the treatment of cancer, especially disseminated testicular carcinoma. Also used in the treatment of severe hypercalcemia and hypercalciuria, particularly in cases of parathyroid carcinoma. It is a very toxic drug acting on the bone marrow, liver, and kidneys, producing hematological disorders, including thrombocytopenia and hemorrhagic diathesis. Gastrointestinal, cutaneous, and neurological disorders may also occur. Called also *aurelic acid, aureolic acid,* and *mitramycin.* Trademark: Mithracin.
mitigate (mit′ĭ-gāt) [L. *mitigare* to soften] to moderate; to render milder.
mitis (mi′tis) [L.] mild; moderate.
mito- [Gr. *mitos* thread] a combining form meaning threadlike, or denoting relationship to a thread.
mitochondria (mi″to-kon′dre-ah, mit″o-kon′dre-ah), pl. *mitochon′drion* [mito- + Gr. *chondrion* granule] small spherical to rod-shaped components (organelles) suspended in the cytoplasm of cells and enclosed in a double membrane, the inner one having infoldings called *cristae,* and the outer layer forming a smooth boundary. The foldings of the inner membrane contain the enzymes involved in the formation of adenosine triphosphate (ATP) by the process of oxidative phosphorylation. The liquid within the inner compartment contains protein, neutral fat, phospholipids, nucleic acids, and the enzymes of the fatty acid and Krebs cycles and the respiratory pathway. The nucleic acids are RNA and very small amounts of DNA. The principal function of mitochondria consists of the production of energy resulting from the oxidation of foodstuff. Called also *chondriosomes.*
mitochondrion (mi″to-kon′dre-on) singular of *mitochondria.*
mitogen (mi′to-jen) a substance that induces mitosis.
mitogenesis (mi″to-jen′ĕ-sis) [mito- + Gr. *genesis* production] the production, or causation, of mitosis.
mitoses (mi-to′sez) plural of *mitosis.*
mitoquinone (mi″to-kwĭ-nōn) ubiquinone.
Mitosan trademark for *busulfan.*
mitosis (mi-to′sis), pl. *mito′ses* [mito- + -osis] a method of indirect division of a cell, consisting of a complex of various processes, by means of which the two daughter nuclei normally receive identical complements of the number of chromosomes characteristic of the somatic cells of the species. Mitosis, the process by which the body grows and replaces cells, is divided into four phases. 1. *Prophase:* formation of paired chromosomes; disappearance of nuclear membrane; appearance of the achromatic spindle; formation of polar bodies. 2. *Metaphase:* arrangement of chromosomes in the equatorial plane of the central spindle to form the monaster. Chromosomes separate into exactly similar halves. 3. *Anaphase:* the two groups of daughter chromosomes separate and move along the fibers of the central spindle, each toward one of the asters, forming the diaster. 4. *Telophase:* the

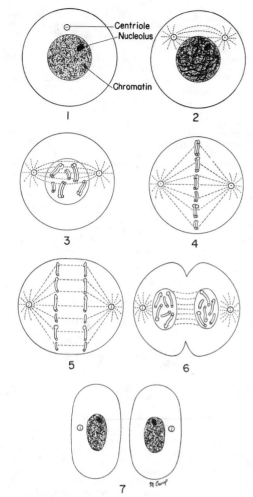

Mitosis shown as occurring in a cell of a hypothetical animal with a diploid chromosome number of 6 (haploid number 3); one pair of chromosomes is short, one pair is long and hooked, and one pair is long and knobbed. *1,* Resting stage. *2,* Early prophase: centriole divided and chromosomes appearing. *3,* Later prophase: centrioles at poles, chromosomes shortened and visibly doubled. *4,* Metaphase: chromosomes arranged on equator of spindle. *5,* Anaphase: chromosomes migrating toward poles. *6,* Telophase: nuclear membranes formed; chromosomes elongating; cytoplasmic divisions beginning. *7,* Daughter cells: resting phase. (From C. A. Villee, W. F. Walker, and R. D. Barnes: General Zoology. 5th ed. Philadelphia, W. B. Saunders Co., 1978.)

daughter chromosomes resolve themselves into a reticulum and the daughter nuclei are formed; the cytoplasm divides, forming two complete daughter cells. See illustration. Cf. *meiosis.* **heterotypic m.,** mitosis in which the halves of bivalent chromosomes move away from each other toward the poles, as occurs in the first, or reductional, division of meiosis. **homeotypic m.,** the ordinary type of cell division in mitosis, as occurs also in the second, or equational, division of meiosis. **multicentric m.,** pluripolar m. **pathologic m.,** atypical, asymmetrical mitosis indicative of malignancy. **pluripolar m.,** cell division that results in the formation of more than two daughter cells.
mitotane (mi′to-tān) an antineoplastic, 1-chloro-2-[2,2-dichloro-1-(4-chlorophenyl)ethyl]benzene, occurring as a white, tasteless, crystalline powder with an aromatic odor, which is soluble in ethanol, ether, hexane, oils, and fats, but not in water. Side effects include bone marrow depression with leukopenia, thrombocytopenia, and various other disorders. Called also *o,p′-DDD.* Trademark: Lysoderm.
mitotic (mi-tot′ik) pertaining to mitosis.
mitral (mi′tral) 1. shaped like a miter. 2. pertaining to the mitral valve of the heart.
mitramycin (mit′rah-mi′sin) mithramycin.
mix (miks) 1. to put substances, things, and the like together into one mass, collection, or assemblage. 2. an act or instance of mixing. 3. a mixture. **water m. of cement,** one that has an

insufficient amount of powder in proportion to liquid, producing a cement with inadequate strength and resistance to solubility of oral fluids.

mixer (mik′ser) 1. a receptacle for diluting a drop of blood preparatory to counting the corpuscles. 2. any device for mixing gases, liquids, or solids. **amalgam m.**, triturator.

mixing (miks′ing) the putting together of substances, elements, or other things, into one mass, collection, or assemblage, generally with thorough blending of the constituents. **vacuum m.**, a method for mixing a material, such as plaster of Paris or investing or impression materials, in a vacuum, in order to avoid trapping air in the material.

mixture (miks′chur) [L. *mixtura, mistura*] a combination of different ingredients, as a fluid resulting from combining a fluid with other fluids, or with solids, or a suspension of a solid in a liquid. See also MISTURA. **racemic m.**, racemate. **eutectic m.**, eutectic ALLOY.

Miyagawa, Yoneji [born 1885] a Japanese bacteriologist.

Miyagawanella (mi″yah-ga″wah-nel′ah) [named after Y. *Miyagawa*] a former genus of microorganisms, the species of which (and the diseases associated with them) are now assigned to the genus *Chlamydia* as follows: *M. lymphogranulomato′sis* (*lymphogranuloma venereum*) and *M. bronchopneumoniae* (mouse pneumonitis) are assigned to *Chlamydia trachomatis*. The species *M. bo′vis* (calf enteritis), *M. fe′lis* (feline pneumonitis), *M. illi′nii* (pneumonitis), *M. louisia′nae* (Louisiana pneumonitis), *M. opos′sumi* (opossum encephalitis), *M. ornitho′sis* (ornithosis), *M. o′vis* (enzootic abortion of ewes), *M. pe′coris* (sporadic bovine encephalomyelitis), *M. pneumo′niae* (human pneumonitis), and *M. psitta′ci* (psittacosis) are assigned to the single species *Chlamydia psittaci*.

MKS meter-kilogram-second system; a system of measurements in which the units, e.g., the newton, are based on the meter as the unit of length, the kilogram as the unit of mass, and the second as the unit of time.

ml milliliter.

μl microliter.

ML-2 filter see under FILTER.

MLA Medical Library Association.

MLD 1. median lethal DOSE. 2. minimum lethal DOSE.

MLG mesiolingual GROOVE.

MLR mixed lymphocyte REACTION.

MLNS mucocutaneous lymph node SYNDROME.

MLT median lethal TIME.

mM millimole.

mm millimeter.

mm² square MILLIMETER.

mm³ cubic MILLIMETER.

mμ millimicron.

μm micrometer²; see MICRON (2).

μ m μ MESON.

μμ micromicron.

mμc millimicrocurie; see NANOCURIE.

μμC micromicrocurie; see PICOCURIE.

mμg millimicrogram; see NANOGRAM.

μmg micromilligram.

μμg micromicrogram; see PICOGRAM.

MMIS Medicaid Management Information System; see under MEDICAID.

MMM see 3-M SYNDROME.

μmm micromillimeter.

μmole micromole.

mmpp millimeters partial pressure (partial pressure expressed in millimeters of mercury).

Mn manganese.

mN millinormal.

MN/m² meganewtons per square meter. See also mechanical STRESS.

mnemonic (ne-mon′ik) [Gr. *mnēmonikos* pertaining to memory] pertaining to, characterized by, or promoting recollection, or memory.

MO mesial and occlusal.

Mo molybdenum.

mobility (mo-bil′ĭ-te) [L. *mobilitas*] the state or condition of being mobile, or having freedom of motion. **tooth m.**, horizontal and, to a lesser degree, axial movement of a tooth in response to various forces, with return of the tooth to its original position, once the pressure is removed. See also elastic RECOIL, periodontal PULSE, and tooth MIGRATION. **tooth m., abnormal,** tooth m., pathologic. **tooth m., normal,** tooth m., physiologic. **tooth m., pathologic,** excessive tooth mobility, usually brought about by the loss of alveolar bone and periodontal ligament, which may occur as a result of trauma from occlusion, periodontal inflammatory and degenerative changes, and hormonal changes, such as those associated with pregnancy and with the use of hormonal contraceptives. Called also *abnormal tooth m.* See

also pathologic tooth MIGRATION. **tooth m., physiologic,** horizontal and, to a lesser degree, axial movement of a tooth in response to normal forces, as in occlusion. It occurs in two stages: the initial or intrasocket stage, in which the tooth moves within the confines of the periodontal ligament, associated with viscoelastic distortion of the ligament and redistribution of periodontal fluids, interbundle content, and fibers; and the second stage, which occurs gradually and entails elastic deformation of the alveolar bone in response to increased horizontal forces. The tooth itself is also deformed by the impact of a force applied to the crown, but not to a clinically significant degree. The mobility varies during a 24-hour period, being highest upon arising in the morning. Called also *normal tooth m.*

mobilization (mo″bĭ-li-za′shun) the process of making a fixed or ankylosed part movable.

mobilometer (mo″bil-om′ĕ-ter) 1. an instrument for measuring the consistency of liquids. 2. a mechanical or electronic device for measuring tooth mobility. Called also *periodontometer.*

Möbius′ syndrome [Paul Julius *Möbius*, German neurologist, 1853–1907] congenital facial DIPLEGIA.

mock-up (mok′up) a full-sized model of an apparatus or other equipment constructed out of substitute materials, used in instruction or for study and improvement of design.

MOD mesial, occlusal, and distal.

mode (mōd) in statistics, the value or item in a variations curve which shows the maximum frequency of occurrence.

model (mod′′l) 1. something that represents or simulates something else; a replica. 2. a reasonable facsimile of the body or any of its parts, such as dental arches or facial structures, usually made of durable material colored to simulate the tissue represented. Some elaborate models may contain removable parts to show anatomical interrelationships between different structures and parts. Used for demonstration and teaching purposes. 3. dental CAST. **animal m.**, any condition found in an animal that is of value in studying a biological phenomenon, e.g., a pathological mechanism of an animal disorder useful in studying human disease. **chemical m.**, a structural model showing atomic configuration of a compound or molecule. **implant m.**, implant CAST. **liquid drop m.**, a model in which the atomic nucleus is imagined to behave in the manner of a drop of liquid. **study m.**, diagnostic CAST. **m. trimmer,** model TRIMMER. **Watson-Crick m.**, double HELIX.

moderator (mod′er-a-tor) 1. anything keeping something within reasonable or proper limits. 2. in nuclear physics, a substance, such as graphite or beryllium, used to cut down the flux of subatomic particles or radiation by absorption of the same.

Modern Tenacin trademark for a dental *zinc phosphate cement* (see under CEMENT).

modification (mod″ĭ-fi-ka′shun) the process or result of changing the form or characteristics of an object or substance. **racemic m.**, racemate.

modifier (mod′ĭ-fi-er) something that alters or changes; in the plural, modifying factors (polygenes). **body m.**, a substance, usually a liquid, that modifies the body or viscosity of other substances, such as varnishes or rubber cements. See THINNER. **glass m.**, a substance, such as potassium, sodium, and calcium oxides, capable of interrupting the integrity of the silicon network, acting as fluxes in lowering the softening temperature of glass by reducing the amount of cross-linking between the oxygen and glass formers.

modioliform (mo″de-o′lĭ-form) shaped like the hub of a wheel.

modiolus (mo-di′o-lus) [L. "nave," "hub"] 1. [NA] the central pillar or columella of the cochlea. 2. a point near the corner of the mouth where several muscles of facial expression converge.

Moditen trademark for *fluphenazine hydrochloride* (see under FLUPHENAZINE).

Mod. praesc. abbreviation for L. *mo′do praescrip′tio,* in the way directed.

modulus (moj′u-lus, mod′ju-lus) 1. a coefficient pertaining to a physical property. 2. that number by which the logarithms in one system are multiplied to yield the logarithms in another. 3. the quantity by which two given quantities can be divided to yield the same remainders. **bulk m.**, see *m. of elasticity.* **elastic m.**, m. of elasticity. **m. of elasticity,** any of several coefficients of elasticity of a body, expressing the ratio between a stress or force per unit area which acts to deform the body and the corresponding fractional deformation caused by the stress; the stress required to produce unit strain, which may be a change in length (*Young′s m.*); or a twist or shear (*m. of rigidity* or *m. of torsion*); or a change of volume (*bulk m.*), expressed in dynes/cm². It is usually indicative of the stiffness of a material — the higher the modulus of elasticity, the more rigid the material. Called also *elastic m.* and *coefficient of elasticity.* See also *mechanical strain* and mechanical STRESS. **m. of resilience,** the energy required to stress a given volume of material in one direction from zero up to the proportional limit of the material, measured by the ability of the material to withstand the momentary effect of an impact load while stresses remain within the proportional limit. It is determined by dividing the square of the proportional limit by twice the modulus of elasticity. **m. of rigidity,** see *m. of elasticity.* **m. of rupture,** flexure STRENGTH. **shear m.,** a value comparable to the modulus of elasticity, based on a shear stress instead of a tension stress. **m. of torsion,** see *m. of elasticity.* **Young's m.,** see *m. of elasticity.*

Moebius see MÖBIUS.

Moeller see MÖLLER.

Moens, E. see De Barsy-Moens-Dierckx SYNDROME.

mogi- [Gr. *mogis* with difficulty] a combining form meaning difficult, or with difficulty.

mogilalia (moj-e-la′le-ah) [*mogi-* + Gr. *lalia* chatter] difficulty in speech; stuttering.

mogiphonia (moj-e-fo′ne-ah) [*mogi-* + Gr. *phōnē* voice] difficulty in making vocal sounds.

Mohr's syndrome [O. L. *Mohr,* Norwegian physician] oral-facial-digital SYNDROME (2).

Mohs hardness number (index), hardness scale, hardness test [Friedrich *Mohs*] see under HARDNESS.

moiety (moi′ĕ-te) [Fr. *moitié,* from L. *medietas, medius* middle] any equal part; a half.

mol mole (3).

molality (mo-lal′ĭ-te) the number of moles of solute per 1 kilogram (1000 gm) of solution. Symbol, *m.* See also molal SOLUTION and MOLARITY.

molar (mo′lar) [L. *molaris* to do with grinding] 1. molar TOOTH. 2. pertaining to molecules in bulk or moles per volume, as in molecular solution. See also molar SOLUTION. **anchor m.,** a molar tooth on which a band is fitted to serve as anchorage for an orthodontic appliance. **m. band,** molar BAND. **first m.,** molar tooth, first; see under TOOTH. **fourth m.,** distomolar. **m. hook,** molar HOOK. **impacted m.,** a molar tooth that is prevented from erupting, or from taking its place in normal occlusion. **Moon's m's,** Moon's TEETH. **mulberry m.,** a malformed first molar characterized by dwarfing of the cusps and hypertrophy of the enamel surrounding the cusp, with agglomeration of masses of globules, giving it the appearance of a mulberry; seen in congenital syphilis and certain other diseases. Called also *mulberry tooth.* **second m.,** molar tooth second; see under TOOTH. **sixth-year m.,** the first permanent molar, so called because it usually erupts at the age of six years, immediately posterior to the last molar of the deciduous dentition. See *molar tooth, first,* under TOOTH. **supernumerary m.,** paramolar. **third m.,** molar tooth, third; see under TOOTH. **twelfth-year m.,** the second permanent molar, so called because it usually erupts at the age of 12 years. See *molar tooth, second,* under TOOTH.

molariform (mo-lar′ĭ-form) [*molar* + L. *forma* form] shaped like a molar; showing molar-like characteristics.

molarity (mol-ar′ĭ-te) the number of moles of solute per 1 liter (1000 ml) of solution. Symbol, *M.* See also MOLALITY and molar SOLUTION.

mold (mōld) 1. any one of a large group of parasitic and saprophytic fungi which cause mold or moldiness; also, the desposits or growth produced by such fungi. 2. a device or form for giving a

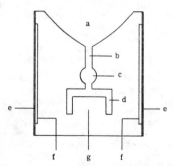

Diagrammatic representation of an inlay casting mold: *a,* crucible; *b,* ingate or sprue; *c,* reservoir; *d,* inlay mold; *e,* casting ring; *f,* asbestos liner; *g,* investment. (From R. W. Phillips: Skinner's Science of Dental Materials. 7th ed. Philadelphia, W. B. Saunders Co., 1973.)

desired shape to a liquid or plastic substance. 3. an object formed in a mold; also the shape of a molded object, as the shape of an artificial tooth. See illustration. **mother matrix m.,** a negative form, usually in sections, used for making positive casts.

molding (mōld′ing) the act or process of shaping, or fashioning of an object; giving shape to an object. **border m.,** the shaping of an impression material by the manipulation or action of the tissues adjacent to the borders of an impression. Called also *tissue m.* and *muscle trimming.* **compression m.,** a method of molding in which compression is used to pack the material in and to express its excess from the mold. In molding of dentures, the teeth are embedded in the investing medium of the lower half of the denture flask, after the baseplate is positioned, and once the investing material has hardened, it is coated with a soap solution to prevent the stone or plaster mixture in the upper half from adhering to that in the lower half. Two methods of pouring the material may be used: The *one-pour technique* (single-pour technique) whereby the material is poured into the flask in a single stage, and the *two-pour technique* (double-pour technique, or capping) whereby the investment material is poured into the upper half, leaving the occlusal and incisal surfaces of the teeth exposed. When the initial pour has set, the surface is saturated with water to prevent moisture from being drawn from it by the second pour. A second mix of material is used to complete the fill of the upper half of the flask. After the investing material has set in the top half, the flask is heated to soften the wax and the two halves are separated, the teeth remaining in the upper half. See illustration at FLASK. **injection m.,** the act or process of forcing a plastic material, such as a softened resin, into the mold space under pressure. See illustration at FLASK. **tissue m.,** border m.

mole (mōl) [L. *moles* a shapeless mass] 1. a circumscribed new growth of the skin of congenital origin, presenting a small elevated flat or pedunculated, often pigmented lesion; a nevus. 2. a fleshy mass or tumor of the uterus. 3. the SI unit of amount of a substance, being that quantity of a substance (in a system) containing as many elementary entities (atoms, ions, molecules, or radicals) as there are carbon atoms in 12 gm of carbon-12, or that amount of a chemical compound whose mass in grams is equivalent to its formula mass (see GRAM-MOLECULE and GRAM MOLECULAR WEIGHT). A mole is considered to be equal to 6.023×10^{23} (Avogadro's number) elementary entities. Abbreviated *mol.* See also SI. **pigmented m.,** pigmented cellular NEVUS.

molecular (mo-lek′u-lar) of, pertaining to, or composed of molecules.

molecule (mol′ĕ-kul) [L. *molecula* little mass] an aggregation of atoms; a chemical combination of two or more atoms that form a specific chemical substance. **carrier m.,** a molecule, usually a protein, which transports other substances across the cell membrane. In facilitated diffusion, it combines with substances, thus making them lipid-soluble, rotates within the membrane, or assists substances to pass through membrane pores. After passing to the other side of the membrane, the carrier breaks away from the ligand and moves back to pick up another molecule of substance to be carried through the membrane. Called also *carrier protein, porter, translocase,* and *transport system.* See also DIFFUSION and facilitated DIFFUSION. **diatomic m.,** one composed of two atoms. **hexatomic m.,** one containing six atoms. **homonuclear m.,** one composed of atoms of the same element. **monatomic m.,** one composed of a single atom. **nonpolar m.,** one formed by combinations of atoms held together by nonpolar bonds, in which the electrical potential is symmetrically distributed. **octahedral m.,** one in which six atoms are distributed around a central atom. **polar m.,** one formed by combinations of atoms held together by polar bonds, in which the electrical potential is not symmetrically distributed. **square planar m.,** one in which the bonded atoms are located at the corners of a square with the central atom located in the center of the square. **tetrahedral m.,** one in which four atoms are bonded to a central atom. **tetratomic m.,** one containing four atoms. **triangular m.,** one in which three atoms are bonded to a central atom. Called also *trigonal m.* **triatomic m.,** one composed of three atoms. **trigonal m.,** triangular m. **trigonal bipyramidal m.,** one in which five atoms are located around the central atom.

Moll's gland [Jacob Antonius *Moll,* Dutch ophthalmologist, 1832–1914] ciliary GLAND.

Möller's disease, glossitis [Julius Otto Ludwig *Möller,* 1819–1887] see infantile SCURVY, and see under GLOSSITIS.

Möller-Barlow disease [J. O. L. *Möller;* Sir Thomas *Barlow,* British physician, 1845–1945] infantile SCURVY.

Møller-Christenson's syndrome [Peter Vilhelm *Møller-Christenson,* Danish professor of medical history and osteologist, born 1903] see under SYNDROME.

Mollicutes (mol-lĭ-ku'tēz) [L. *mollis* soft + *cutis* skin] a class of prokaryotic microorganisms (kingdom Procaryotae), comprising the smallest of the living organisms. The Mollicutes is considered to be unrelated to the bacteria because of their unusual physical structure, i.e., they lack a true cell wall. They occur as pleomorphic, coccoid, or filamentous cells with a tendency to produce myceloid structures, which are bounded by a single triple-layered pliable membrane (hence the name). It consists of the order Mycoplasmatales.

molluscum (mo-lus'kum) [L. *molluscus* soft] 1. one of a group of skin diseases marked by the presence of soft, rounded growths. 2. m. contagio'sum. **m. contagio'sum,** an infectious disease of the skin, which may also involve any part of the body, including the oral mucosa and lips. The lesions form pinhead- to pea-sized pearly, white umbilicate nodules with proliferation and hyperplasia of the epidermal cells. Oral lesions tend to be globular in shape at first and become later umbilicate, their most common location being the dorsal surface of the tongue and, less commonly, the lips. **m. seba'ceum,** primary pseudoepitheliomatous HYPERPLASIA.

Molt elevator see under ELEVATOR.

molugram (mol'u-gram) gram-molecule.

Mol wt molecular WEIGHT.

molybdenum (mo-lib'dĕ-num) [Gr. *molybdos* lead] a metallic element. Symbol, Mo; atomic number, 42; atomic weight, 95.94; melting point, 2617°C; specific gravity, 10.22; valence, 3; group VI of the periodic table. It occurs in seven natural isotopes: 92, 94–98, and 100; artificial radioactive isotopes include 88–91, 93, 99, and 101–105. Molybdenum is found in nature only in a bound form. It occurs as a gray metal or black powder, soluble in hot concentrated sulfuric and nitric acids, but not in water, sulfuric acid, and other solvents. It is a necessary trace element in plant nutrition; in animals, it is a component of xanthine oxidase, aldehyde oxidase, nitrate reductase, and hydrogenase, being absorbed in the intestine and excreted mainly with the urine, with little tissue retention except in the bones, liver, and kidneys. It is believed to have some cariostatic effects in children. Generally, molybdenum is considered to be relatively nontoxic, but excessive amounts may cause anemia, decreased copper retention, and skeletal and muscular lesions in sheep, cattle, and rats.

moment (mo'ment) 1. an indefinitely short period of time; an instant. 2. the present or any other particular instant. 3. in statistics, the mean or expected value of the product formed by multiplying together a set of one or more variates or variables, each to a specific power. 4. a tendency to produce motion. 5. m. of force. **m. arm,** moment ARM. **bending m.,** a measure of the bending effort at any point in a beam, measured in units of force times distance. **bending m., maximum,** the highest bending moment in a beam under any specific loading conditions, being a limiting factor in the capacity of a beam. **dipole m.,** in a dipole, the distance in centimeters between the charges multiplied by the quantity of charge in electrostatic units. Symbol, μ. **m. of force,** the effectiveness of a force to produce rotation about an axis, measured by the product of the force and the perpendicular distance from the line of action of the force to the axis. Called also *m. of torque.* **m. of inertia,** a measure of the effectiveness of a mass in rotation. In the rotation of a rigid body not only the body's mass but the distribution of the mass about the axis of rotation determines the change in the angular velocity resulting from the action of a given torque for a given time. **m. of torque,** m. of force.

momentum (mo-men'tum) [L.] the quantity of motion measured by the product of mass and velocity.

mon- see MONO-.

monad (mon'ad) [Gr. *monas* a unit] 1. a single-celled protozoon or a single-celled coccus. 2. a univalent radical or element. 3. in meiosis, one member of a tetrad.

Monahan-Lewis knife see under KNIFE.

monamide (mon-am'īd) a compound having only one amide group ($CONH_2$).

monamine (mon-am'in) a compound having only one amine (HN_2) group.

monangle (mon'ang-g'l) having only one angle; Black's term for a dental instrument having only one angulation in the shank connecting the handle, or shaft, with the working portion of the instrument, known as the blade, or nib.

monangled (mon'ang-g'ld) monoangled.

monarthric (mon-ar'thrik) pertaining to or affecting a single joint; monarticular.

monarticular (mon"ar-tik'u-lar) monarthritic.

monatomic (mon"ah-tom'ik) [*mono-* + Gr. *atomos* indivisible] 1. pertaining to a molecule consisting of a single atom (monatomic molecule). 2. pertaining to an atom or atomic group having one free valency.

Mondonesi's reflex [Filippo *Mondonesi,* Italian physician] bulbomimic REFLEX.

Monge's disease [Carlos *Monge,* Peruvian physician, born 1884] see under DISEASE.

mongolism (mon'go-lizm) [*Mongol,* a member of one of the chief ethnological divisions of Asiatic peoples] 1. Down's SYNDROME; so called because of facial characteristics typical of this condition. 2. see Turner-mongolism POLYSYNDROME.

mongoloid (mon'go-loid) [see *mongolism*] 1. pertaining to or resembling the Mongols. 2. pertaining to or characteristic of mongolism (see Down's SYNDROME), as mongoloid slant of the palpebral fissures, whereby the outer rims slant upward.

Monilia (mo-nil'e-ah) former name for *Candida.*

monilial (mo-nil'e-al) pertaining to or caused by *Monilia* (see CANDIDA).

moniliasis (mon-ĭ-li'ah-sis) candidiasis. **oral m.,** thrush.

moniliosis (mo-nil"e-o'sis) candidiasis.

monitor (mon'ĭ-tor) [L. "one who reminds"] 1. to check constantly on a state or condition of a patient under anesthesia, undergoing surgery, or in an intensive care unit, by employing the senses of touch, sight, hearing, or smell or by means of devices which operate chemically, physically, or electronically to measure the adequacy of various physiological functions. 2. an apparatus used to observe or record such physiological signs. 3. to check periodically or continuously on the amount of ionizing radiation or radioactivity present in a given location. **central station m.,** in an intensive care unit, a system whereby the information on the respiratory rate, pulse rate, electrocardiogram, blood pressure, temperature, and other vital signs of a patient or several patients is remotely displayed at the central station for continuous monitoring. Some systems also provide for closed circuit television and computer analysis of some selected data such as the electroencephalogram and electrocardiogram.

monitoring (mon'ĭ-tor"ing) observing, checking, or recording periodically or continuously. **area m.,** in radiology, routine monitoring of the level of radiation in any particular area. **personnel m.,** in radiology, monitoring of individuals exposed to radiation sources for possible contamination, including examination of clothing, body excretions and secretions, breath, etc.

mono-, mon- [Gr. *monos* single] a combining form denoting one or single; limited to one part; in chemistry, combined with one atom. See also words beginning UNI-.

monoangled (mon'o-ang'g'ld) having one angle or bend; monangled.

monobasic (mon"o-ba'sik) [*mono-* + Gr. *basis* base] having but one base; unibasal; applied to an acid having only one replaceable atom of hydrogen and therefore yielding only one series of salts, as HCl.

monobenzone (mon"o-ben'zōn) a compound, *p*-(benzyl)phenol, occurring as white, odorless, almost tasteless, crystalline powder that is soluble in alcohol and acetone, but not in water. It inhibits the enzyme tyrosinase, thus preventing the conversion of tyrosine to dihydroxyphenylalanine, a precursor of melanin, and the synthesis of melanin. Used as a depigmenting agent in severe freckling and other conditions characterized by hyperpigmentation. Dermatitis, erythema, and eczema are the most common side reactions.

monoblast (mon'o-blast) [*mono-* + Gr. *blastos* germ] the cell which is the precursor of the mature monocyte. It is usually more than 14 μ in diameter and nonmotile, and has basophilic or grayish cytoplasm, fine stringy chromatin, and one or two large nucleoli.

monoblock (mon'o-blok) functional ACTIVATOR. **Andresen m.,** functional ACTIVATOR. **m. appliance,** functional ACTIVATOR.

monochloroethane (mon"o-klo-ro-eth'ăn) ethyl CHLORIDE.

monochromatic (mon"o-kro-mat'ik) [*mono-* + Gr. *chrōma* color] 1. existing in or having only one color. 2. pertaining to or characterized by perception of a single color band in the spectrum. 3. staining with only one dye at a time. 4. pertaining to or located within a single wavelength in the spectrum, as the monochromatic radiation.

monoclinic (mon"o-klin'ik) [*mono-* + Gr. *klinein* to incline] pertaining to crystals in which the vertical axis is inclined to one lateral axis, but is at right angles to the other.

Monocortin trademark for *paramethasone acetate* (see under PARAMETHASONE).

Monocortin S trademark for *paramethasone disodium phosphate* (see under PARAMETHASONE).

monocyclic (mon"o-si'klik) 1. pertaining to one cycle. 2. in chemistry, having a molecular structure containing only one ring.

monocyte (mon′o-sīt) [*mono-* + Gr. *kytos* hollow vessel] an agranulocyte representing about 3 to 8 percent of the leukocyte count in the blood. Typical monocytes are about 9 to 12 μm in diameter and resemble large monocytes. They have cytoplasm that is opaque, grayish blue in appearance, and filled with fine reddish-blue granules; large nuclei that may have two or more concentric rows of small neutral vacuoles; fine, skeinlike, or lacy chromatin; and protoplasm with a foamy, ground glass–like appearance. Motility of monocytes is characterized by waving and sliding motion of the cell. Monocytes are believed to derive from a specific stem cell (monoblast) and during their development they are known as *promonocytes*. **m. count,** see table of *Reference Values in Hematology* in Appendix. **young m.,** promonocyte.

monocytopenia (mon″o-si″to-pe′ne-ah) [*monocyte* + Gr. *penia* poverty] a decrease in the number of monocytes in the blood. See also table of *Reference Values in Hematology* in Appendix.

monocytosis (mon″o-si-to′sis) an increase in the number of monocytes in the blood. See also LEUKOCYTE count, differential, and see table of *References Values in Hematology* in Appendix.

Monod, Jacques Lucien [born 1910] a French biochemist; cowinner, with François Jacob and André Michael Lwoff, of the Nobel prize for medicine and physiology in 1965, for discoveries concerning the genetic control of enzymes and virus synthesis.

monodentate (mon″o-den′tāt) 1. having one tooth or a toothlike structure. 2. monodentate LIGAND.

monoethanolamine (mon″o-eth″ah-nol′ah-mēn) ethanolamine.

monoethylamine (mon″o-eth″il-am′in) ethylamine.

monogenesis (mon′o-jen′ĕ-sis) [*mono-* + Gr. *genesis* production] 1. the production of only male or female offspring. 2. the theory that all things develop from a single cell. See also ORTHOGENESIS.

monoglyceride (mon″o-glis′er-īd) [*mono-* + *glyceride*] a glyceride in which a single hydroxyl group of glycerol is esterified with a fatty acid.

monograph (mon′o-graf) 1. a publication dealing with a particular subject or field appearing in the form of a book, as opposed to a publication appearing periodically (a periodical, or serial). 2. a treatise on a particular subject. **drug m.,** a rule, established by the Food and Drug Administration, which prescribes for drugs (or classes of drugs) the kinds and amounts of ingredients they may contain, the conditions for which they may be used therapeutically, and directions for use, including warnings and other information which their labels must bear. It also states conditions under which they may be marketed as safe and effective drugs.

monohydrate (mon″o-hi′drāt) [*mono-* + Gr. *hydōr* water] a hydrate containing one molecule of water for every molecule of other substance in the compound, as in sodium carbonate, $Na_2CO_3 \cdot H_2O$.

monohydric (mon″o-hi-drik) containing only one hydroxyl group.

Mono-Kay trademark for *phytonadione*.

monomaxillary (mon″o-mak′sī-ler″e) affecting or pertaining to one jaw.

monomer (mon′o-mer) [Gr. *monos* single + *meros* part] a single molecule; usually a simple molecule, or mer, of a relatively low-molecular-weight which, during the process of polymerization, combines with similar molecules to form a large molecule or polymer.

monomeric (mon″o-mer′ik) [*mono-* + Gr. *meros* part] pertaining to, made of, or affecting a single segment, as distinguished from dimeric, polymeric, etc. In genetics, determined by a gene or genes at a single locus either in the heterozygous or homozygous state.

monomethylamine (mon′o-meth′il-am′in) methylamine.

monomolecular (mon″o-mo-lek′u-lar) unimolecular.

mononuclear (mon″o-nu′kle-ar) [*mono-* + *nucleus*] 1. pertaining to a single nucleus; having but one nucleus; mononucleate; uninucleated. 2. a cell having a single nucleus, especially a monocyte of the blood or tissues.

mononucleate (mon″o-nu′kle-āt) [*mono-* + *nucleus*] having but one nucleus; uninucleated.

mononucleosis (mon″o-nu″kle-o′sis) the presence of an abnormally large number of mononuclear leukocytes (monocytes) in the blood. **infectious m.,** an acute infectious disease, probably of viral etiology; most cases are associated with the Epstein-Barr virus. It occurs predominantly in children and young adults, and is characterized by pharyngitis, tonsillitis, lymphadenitis, splenomegaly, high concentration of heterophil antibodies

against sheep erythrocytes, and absolute lymphocytosis with the presence of abnormal but mature lymphocytes. Manifestations include irregular fever, malaise, headache, sore throat, enlarged tonsils and pharyngeal lymphoid tissue, diphtheroid pseudomembranes, peritonsillar edema, stomatitis, gingivitis, and less commonly, petechiae of the palate and ulcers of the oral mucosa. Called also *acute benign lymphoblastosis, acute infectious adenitis, acute lymphadenosis, glandular fever, monocytic angina, Filatov's disease,* and *Pfeiffer's disease.* See also Epstein-Barr VIRUS.

mononucleotide (mon″o-nu′kle-o-tīd) see NUCLEOTIDE.

monopathy (mo-nop′ah-the) [*mono-* + Gr. *pathos* disease] a disease affecting a single part.

monophasic (mon″o-fa′zik) [*mono-* + Gr. *phasis* phase] occurring in a single phase or stage. Cf. DIPHASIC and TRIPHASIC.

monophosphatase (mon″o-fos′fah-tās) see PHOSPHATASE.

monophosphate (mon″o-fos′fāt) a compound having one phosphate group, usually phosphoric acid in ester linkage to a hydroxyl group in the compound. **adenosine m.,** adenylic ACID. **uridine m. (UMP),** uridylic ACID.

monophyodont (mon″o-fi′o-dont) [*mono-* + Gr. *phyein* to grow + *odous* tooth] having only one set of teeth, all being permanent.

monosaccharide (mon″o-sak′ah-rīd) a class of carbohydrates that includes the simplest carbohydrates. They are derivatives of straight-chain polyhydric alcohols, having the same general formula $(CH_2O)_n$, and occur as colorless, water-soluble, crystalline substances with a sweet taste. Monosaccharides are classified according to the number of carbon atoms in the chain into diose $(C_2H_4O_2)$, triose $(C_3H_6O_3)$, tetrose $(C_4H_8O_4)$, pentose $(C_5H_{10}O_5)$, hexose $(C_6H_{12}O_6)$, and heptose $(C_7H_{14}O_7)$. Those containing an aldehyde group are termed *aldoses;* those with a ketone group are *ketoses.* Called also *simple sugar.*

monosilane (mon″o-si′lān) silane.

monosome (mon′o-sōm) 1. the unpaired sex chromosome. See also RIBOSOME. 2. the single chromosome present in monosomy.

monosomy (mon′o-so″me) [*mono-* + Gr. *sōma* body] aneuploidy; the absence of one chromosome of one pair in an otherwise diploid cell. **9p m.,** deletion of the short arm of chromosome 9, associated with somatic and mental retardation, trigonocephaly, craniostenosis, high forehead, pointed eyebrows, protruding eyes, oblique palpebral fissures, epicanthus, short nose with a long and flat saddle, nostrils with forward openings, long upper lip that overhangs the lower lip, aplastic philtrum, small mouth, receding chin, malformed ears, short and sometimes webbed neck, elongated thorax with wide-spaced nipples, and a variety of genital, cardiovascular, hand, and other abnormalities. Called also *chromosome 9p monosomy syndrome.* **12p m.,** chromosome 12p, partial deletion SYNDROME. **partial 12p m.,** chromosome 12p, partial deletion SYNDROME.

monostotic (mon″os-tot′ik) [*mono-* + Gr. *osteon* bone] pertaining to or affecting a single bone.

monotropic (mon″o-trop′ik) [*mono-* + Gr. *tropos* a turning] affecting only one particular species of bacterium or one variety of tissue. See also POLYTROPIC.

monovalence (mon″o-va′lens) the state or condition of being monovalent.

monovalent (mon″o-va′lent) 1. univalent. 2. denoting an antibody capable of combining with only one antigenic species, or an antigen capable of combining with only one antibody species.

monoxide (mon-ok′sīd) 1. an oxide containing but one atom of oxygen. 2. CARBON monoxide. **dinitrogen m.,** nitrous OXIDE.

monoxychlorosene (mon-ok″se-klor′o-sēn) oxychlorosene.

Monson curve [W. G. *Monson,* American dentist] see under CURVE. See also reverse CURVE (anti-Monson curve).

monster (mon′ster) [L. *monstrum*] a fetus or infant with such pronounced developmental anomalies as to be grotesque and usually nonviable. Called also *teras.*

Montague's plane see under PLANE.

Moon's tooth (molar) [Henry *Moon,* English oral surgeon, 19th century] see under TOOTH.

Moore's mandrel disk MANDREL.

Moorehead's retractor [Frederick Brown *Moorehead,* American dentist] see under RETRACTOR.

Moorhead see Berman-Moorhead LOCATOR.

Mor. sol. abbreviation for L. *mo′re sol′ito,* in the usual way.

Morax, Victor [1866–1935] a French physician.

Moraxella (mo″rak-sel-ah) [named after Victor *Morax*] a genus of gram-negative bacteria of the family Neisseriaceae, occurring as short plump rods, often approaching the coccoid shape, which are parasitic on the mucous membranes. They are nonsporogenous, aerobic organisms, about 1.0 to 1.5 by 1.5 to 2.5 μm in size, usually found in pairs and short chains, characterized by an inability to form acid from glucose. They are highly sensitive to penicillin. Formerly called *Diplobacillus*. **M. bo′vis**, a species causing keratoconjunctivitis in cattle. Called also *Haemophilus bovis*. **M. lacuna′ta**, a species suspected of causing conjunctivitis in man; formerly reported frequently, now rarely. Called also *Bacillus lacunatus* and *Diplobacillus moraxaxenfeld*. **M. nonliquefa′ciens**, a species of uncertain pathogenicity, found in the human upper respiratory tract, patricularly in the nose. **M. osloen′sis**, a species of uncertain pathogenicity, found in the human upper respiratory tract. **M. phenylpyru′vica, m. polymor′pha**, a species isolated in various pathological conditions.

Morbicid trademark for a solution of *formaldehyde*.

morbid (mor′bid) [L. *morbidus* sick] pertaining to or affected with disease; diseased.

morbidity (mor-bid′ĭ-te) 1. the condition of being diseased or morbid. 2. the rate of sickness; the ratio of sick to well persons in a community.

Morbillivirus (mor-bil′ĭ-vi′rus) a genus of paramyxoviruses, comprising several viruses, one of which, measles virus, is pathogenic to man.

morbillivirus (mor-bil′ĭ-vi′rus) any virus of the genus *Morbillivirus*.

morbus (mor′bus) [L.] disease. **m. ang′licus, m. ang′lorum**, rickets. **m. maculo′sus hemorrag′icus**, thrombocytopenic purpura, idiopathic; see under PURPURA.

Morgagni's glandular foramen, ventricle [Giovanni Battista *Morgagni*, Italian anatomist and pathologist, 1682–1771; he was a professor at Padua, and the founder of pathological anatomy, whose clinicopathological reports were published in 1761 under the title *De sedibus et causis morborum* ("The Seats and Causes of Disease") See FORAMEN cecum of tongue and VENTRICLE of larynx.

Morgan, Thomas Hunt [1866–1945] an American biologist; winner of the Nobel prize for medicine and physiology in 1933, for discoveries concerning the hereditary function of the chromosomes.

Morgan's line see under LINE.

Morgan's mandrel see under MANDREL.

Morganella (mor″gah-nel′ah) [named after Harry de Reimer *Morgan*] a proposed generic name for bacteria now included under the genus *Proteus*. **M. morga′nii**, *Proteus morganii*; see under PROTEUS.

morgue (morg) [Fr.] a place where dead bodies may be temporarily kept, for identification or until claimed for burial.

moribund (mor′ĭ-bund) [L. *moribundus*] about to die; in a dying state.

Moronal trademark for *nystatin*.

-morph [Gr. *morphē* form] a word termination denoting relationship to form or shape.

morphea (mor-fe′ah) [Gr. *morphē* form] a disease of the skin, sometimes also involving the oral mucosa, marked by pinkish patches, lines, or bands, bordered by a purplish halo. Individual lesions are firm, well-defined, and slightly elevated or depressed, beginning as red or purple areas of various sizes and, as they expand, their centers become whitish or yellowish, while the borders remain purple. They may undergo involution, followed by atrophy and scarring. The mucosa of the cheeks, palate, and tongue may be involved, and the periodontal ligament may be widened. Called also *Addison's keloid, circumscribed scleroderma*, and *localized scleroderma*.

morphine (mor′fēn) [L. *morphina, morphinum*] the principal and most active of the opium alkaloids, 7,8-didehydro-4,5-epoxy-17-methylmorphinan-3,6-diol, occurring as colorless crystals that have a bitter taste and an alkaline reaction and are slightly soluble in water, alcohol, and ether. Morphine is an addicting narcotic which produces analgesia without loss of consciousness. Its effects include EEG changes similar to those in natural sleep, constriction of the pupil, respiratory depression; decreased hydrochloric acid secretion in the stomach, diminished pancreatic and biliary secretion, depressed peristaltic waves in the colon with resulting constipation, increased ureteral tone and contractions, and dilatation of cutaneous blood vessels. Mental clouding and euphoria are usually associated; dysphoria sometimes displaces euphoria. Morphine is used chiefly to relieve pain, as a sedative, and in the treatment of sleeplessness, cough, dyspnea, and diarrhea. In high doses, it is used to induce anesthesia. Abuse leads to habituation and addiction. See also OPIOID. **m. antagonist**, see narcotic ANTAGONIST. **m. hydrochloride**, the hydrochloride salt of morphine, $C_{17}H_{19}NO_3HCl + 3H_2O$, which occurs in the trihydrate form as white flakes or crystalline powder with bitter taste. Used as a narcotic and analgesic in some countries, but rarely in the United States. **m. sulfate**, the sulfate salt of morphine, which occurs in the pentahydrate form as a fine crystalline solid or powder that is soluble in water and alcohol, but insoluble in

chloroform and ether. Used in dental surgery to lessen pain, to promote sleep, and to facilitate anesthesia. Similarly to morphine, it produces analgesia without loss of consciousness or dulling of the tactile sense to a significant degree. It is incompatible with alkalies, tannic acid, iodic acid, potassium permanganate, borax, chlorates, ferric chloride, lead acetate, magnesia, spirit nitrous ether, mercury bichloride, and gold salts. Adverse reactions may include vomiting, constipation, respiratory depression, and other symptoms.

morpho- [Gr. *morphē* form] a combining form denoting relationship to form.

morphodifferentiation (mor″fo-dif″er-en″she-a′shun) the arrangement of formative cells in the development of tissues or organs, which leads to production of the ultimate shape of the structure.

morphodone hydrochloride (mor′fo-dōn) PHENADOXONE hydrochloride.

morphogenesis (mor″fo-jen′ĕ-sis) [morpho- + Gr. *gennan* to produce] the development and evolution of form.

morphology (mor-fol′o-je) [morpho- + *-logy*] the science of the forms and structure of organized beings.

morphometry (mor-fom′ĕ-tre) [morpho- + Gr. *metron* measure] the measurement of the body. See also ANTHROPOMETRY.

morphoplasm (mor′fo-plazm) [morpho- + Gr. *plasma* anything formed] a substance of the cellular reticulum.

morphosis (mor-fo′sis) [Gr. *morphōsis* a shaping, bringing into shape] the process of formation of a part or organ.

-morphous [Gr. *morphē* shape, form] a word termination indicating the manner of shape or form.

Morquio's disease (syndrome) [Louis *Morquio*, Urugauyan physician, 1867–1935] see under DISEASE.

Morquio-Ullrich syndrome [L. *Morquio*; Otto *Ullrich*, German physician, 1894–1957] Morquio's DISEASE.

mors (morz) [L.] death.

morsal (mor′sal) [L. *morsus* bite] taking part in mastication; said of teeth. Also applied to the masticating surfaces of a bicuspid or molar.

morsicatio (mor-sic′at-io) [L.] biting. **m. bucca′rum**, cheek BITING.

morsus (mor′sus) [L.] bite; sting. **m. huma′nus**, a bite by a human being.

mortal (mor′tal) [L. *mortalis*] 1. subject to death, or destined to die. 2. fatal; causing or terminating in death.

mortality (mor-tal′ĭ-te) 1. the state or condition of being subject to death. 2. in life insurance, the ratio of deaths that take place to expected deaths. 3. death RATE. **actual m.**, the number of deaths in 1,000,000 insured lives, over a period of 100 years. **annual actual m.**, the number of deaths per 100 insured lives. **tabular m.**, the expected death rate per 1000 insured persons as shown in the mortality table.

mortar (mor′tar) [L. *mortarium*] a bell-shaped or urn-shaped vessel of glass, iron, porcelain, or other material, in which drugs are beaten, crushed, or ground with a pestle.

Morton's plane see under PLANE.

morula (mor′u-lah) [L. *morus* mulberry] a cluster of blastomeres which develops by mitotic division from the zygote during the third day after fertilization, forming a mulberry-like structure which, in turn, is transformed into a larger hollow structure (blastocyst) with a central cavity (blastocoele) during the first week of embryonic development. Called also *embryonic sphere, segmentation sphere, vitelline sphere*, and *yolk sphere*. See illustration at CLEAVAGE.

Moryl trademark for *carbachol*.

mosaic (mo-za′ik) [Gr. *mouseion*; L. *opus mosicum, opus musivum*] 1. a pattern made of numerous small pieces fitted together. 2. an individual or tissue with at least two cell lines differing in genotype or karyotype, derived from a single zygote. Cf. CHIMERA.

mosaicism (mo-sa′ĭ-sizm) the presence in an individual of two or more cell lines that are karyotypically or genotypically distinct and are derived from a single zygote. **trisomy 8 m.**, TRISOMY 8. **trisomy 9 m.**, TRISOMY 9 mosaicism.

Mosatil trademark for *calcium disodium edetate* (see under CALCIUM).

Mosetig-Moorhof wax [Albert von *Mosetig-Moorhof*, German surgeon, 1838–1907] see under WAX.

moss (mos) 1. any plant or species of the cryptogamic class Musci. 2. any material obtained from the cryptogamic class Musci. **Irish m.**, carrageenan.

Moss, Melvin L. [American dentist, born 1921] see Gorlin-Chaudhry-Moss SYNDROME.

Mosse's syndrome (polycythemia) [Max *Mosse*, German physician, born 1873] see under SYNDROME.

motile (mo'til) capable of spontaneous or voluntary movement.

motility (mo-til'ĭ-te) the ability to move spontaneously. **gliding m.,** a continuous and regular movement across solid substrates by certain prokaryotic cells having no detectable locomotor organelles.

motion (mo'shun) [L. *motio*] the act or process of changing position in space of a body. See also MOVEMENT and Newton's laws of motion, under LAW. **molecular m.,** a state of constant rapid motion of both solute and solvent molecules in a solution. **Newton's laws of m.,** see under LAW. **plane m.,** the combined motions of translation and rotation of a rigid body in which all parts move in parallel planes.

motoneuron (mo″to-nu'ron) a peripheral neuron that conveys motor impulses to peripheral organs, such as muscles. Called also *motor nerve* and *motor neuron.* **alpha m.,** large neurons in the anterior portion of the spinal cord that give rise to large alpha fibers which innervate skeletal muscle fibers. **gamma m.,** a small neuron of the anterior portion of the spinal cord that gives rise to the gamma (fusimotor) fibers which innervate intrafusal fibers of the muscle spindle. **heteronymous m.,** one supplying fibers other than the one from which the afferent impulses originate. **homonymous m.,** one supplying the muscle from which the afferent impulses originate. **lower m.,** a neuron consisting of an anterior horn cell in the central nervous system whose axon passes to a peripheral muscle or organ to cause movement or secretion. Called also *lower motor neuron.* **upper m.,** a neuron of the central portion of the descending (motor) tract, whose cell body is situated in the motor cortex and whose axon synapses with anterior horn cells. Called also *upper motor neuron.*

motor (mo'tor) [L.] 1. any device that transforms energy into motive force. 2. a muscle, nerve, or center that effects or produces movement. 3. producing or subserving motion. **induction m.,** a motor in which a series of electromagnets is used around a rotor to produce a rotating magnetic field, thus causing the rotor to spin around. **m. nerve, m. neuron,** motoneuron.

Motrin trademark for *ibuprofen.*

mottling (mot'ling) a condition of covering with spots or blotches, as in mottled enamel.

moulage (moo-lahzh') [Fr. "molding"] the making of molds or models of wax or plaster, as of a structure or a lesion; also such a mold or model.

mount (mownt) 1. to fix on or in a support. 2. a support, backing, setting, or the like, on which something may be fixed. 3. to prepare specimens and slides for study. **split cast m.,** split cast MOUNTING. **x-ray m.,** a windowed, stiff material on which radiographs may be arranged in an order corresponding with the chart of the teeth.

mountant (mownt'ant) a medium, such as a natural resin, polymer, or glycerol, in which objects are embedded for study, especially with the microscope. Called also *mounting medium.*

mounting (mownt'ing) 1. the preparation of specimens and slides for study. The chief media used in mounting large specimens are alcohol and glycerin jelly; for microscopic objects on slide, Canada balsam and glycerin. 2. attachment, in the laboratory, of the maxillary and/or mandibular cast to an articulator. **split cast m.,** 1. a dental cast with key grooves on its base, mounted on the articulator for the purpose of easy removal and accurate replacement. Split mounting metal plates may be used instead of grooves in casts. Called also *split cast mount.* 2. split cast METHOD.

mouse (mows) 1. a small rodent belonging to the genus *Mus*, frequently used as an experimental animal. 2. a small weight, or movable structure. **nude m., nu nu m.,** a mouse with congenital absence of the thymus, associated with a marked deficiency of T-lymphocytes and with hairlessness.

mouth (mowth) [L. *os*] an opening or aperture; specifically, the anterior opening to the digestive tube. See oral CAVITY. See also terms beginning ORO- and STOMATO-. **Ceylon sore m.,** tropical SPRUE. **denture sore m.,** denture STOMATITIS. **dry m.,** xerostomia. **m. flora,** the microorganisms normally residing in the oral cavity. See table. **glass-blowers' m.,** swelling of the parotid gland in glass-blowers. See also parotid gland PNEUMOTOCELE. **m. inflammation,** stomatitis. **m. prop,** mouth PROP. **putrid sore m.** acute necrotizing GINGIVITIS. **m. rehabilitation,** oral REHABILITATION. **sore m.,** stomatodynia. **m. stick,** mouthstick. **supernumerary m.,** a congenital abnormality characterized by the presence of an accessory oral opening. **tapir m.,** a condition, often observed in patients with Landouzy-Déjérine dystrophy, marked by thick, separated lips that cannot be pursed, due to weakness and atrophy of the orbicular oris muscle, giving the face a tapir-like appearance. **trench m.,** acute necrotizing GINGIVITIS; so called because it occurred in troops in the trenches during World War I. **m. wash,** mouthwash. **white m.,** thrush.

APPROXIMATE PROPORTIONAL DISTRIBUTION OF PROMINENT BACTERIA ON VARIOUS ORAL SURFACES AND IN SALIVA*

	Gingival Crevice	Coronal Plaque	Tongue Dorsum	Buccal Mucosa	Saliva
Streptococcus salivarius	<0.5	<0.5	20	11	20
S. mitis	8	15	8	60	20
S. sanguis	8	15	4	11	8
S. mutans	?	0–50	<1	<1	<1
Enterococci	0–10	<0.1	<0.01	<0.1	<0.1
Gram + filaments,† including *Actinomyces, Nocardia, Rothia, Corynebacterium, Bacterionema, Leptotrichia* and others	35	42	20	?	15
Lactobacilli	<1	<0.005	<0.1	<0.1	<1
Veillonella species	10	2	12	1	10
Neisseria species	<0.5	<0.5	<0.5	<0.5	<1
Bacteroides oralis	5	5	4	?	?
B. melaninogenicus	6	<1	<1	<1	<1
Vibrio sputorum	5	1	<0.5	<0.5	?
Spirochetes (*Treponema, Borrelia* species)	2	<0.1	<0.1	<0.1	<0.1
Fusobacterium	3	4	1	?	<1
Hemophilus species	+	?	+	+	5

*Data are expressed as a percent of the total flora cultivable on anaerobically incubated blood agar.

†The oral distribution of individual species in this group has not been determined.

(From J. H. Shaw, E. A. Sweeney, C. C. Cappuccino, and S. M. Meller: Textbook of Oral Biology. Philadelphia, W. B. Saunders Co., 1978.)

mouthrinse (mowth'rins) a solution, usually medicated, used for cleansing or treating diseases of the oral mucosa; mouthwash. See also RINSE. **Fluorigard m.,** trademark for a solution containing 0.05 percent sodium fluoride, 15 percent glycerin, 5 percent alcohol, and various amounts of detergents, preservatives, sweetening agents, and dyes; used in dental caries prevention. **Point-Two m.,** trademark for an aqueous solution containing 0.2 percent sodium fluoride, 15 percent glycerin, 5 percent alcohol, and various amounts of surface-active agents and preservative, coloring, and flavoring agents; used in dental caries control.

mouthstick (mowth-stik) a device held in the mouth by a handicapped person which allows the person to perform certain basic functions without the use of the hands. The devices include simple mouth-held sticks which permit only the most rudimentary activities, prostheses with grasping devices which are operated by use of the jaws, battery-operated telescopic wands, electronic microswitch hand-mouth devices, and a variety of other mouth-held prostheses. Called also *bite stick, mouthstick appliance,* and *mouthstick prosthesis.*

mouthwash (mowth'wosh) a solution, usually medicated, used for cleansing the mouth or treating diseases of the oral mucosa; mouthrinse. **antibacterial m.,** one used to remove or destroy oral bacteria, and usually containing quarternary ammonium compounds, phenolic derivatives, and other antibacterial agents as active substances. **astringent m.,** one used for flocculating and precipitating proteinaceous material in the mouth so that it can be removed by flushing. Zinc chloride, zinc acetate, and aluminum potassium sulfate are the most commonly used active substances. **buffered m.,** any mouthwash whose acidity has been lowered by a buffer. **concentrated m.,** any mouthwash that should be diluted before being used. **cosmetic m.,** one used chiefly for cosmetic purposes and cleansing of the mouth and teeth. It usually contains water, alcohol, and flavoring and coloring agents. Essential oils, such as oil of cinnamon or peppermint, surface active agents for solubilization of the essential oils and for cleansing, and various flavoring substances are the principal components. **deodorizing m.,** one used to deodorize the breath, containing antibacterial agents and deodorants. **therapeutic m.,** one used to relieve infection, prevent dental caries, or mitigate other pathological conditions of the mouth, teeth, or throat.

Mouton, Claude [18th century] a French dentist whose work, *Essai d'odontotechnique,* is considered to be the first book on mechanical dentistry. He also invented a method of applying artificial teeth fixed to adjoining natural teeth by springs and clasps.

movement (moov'ment) the act of moving; motion. See also terms beginning CINE-, KINE-, and KINESIO-. **active m.,** a voluntary movement produced by muscular activity, as opposed to passive movement. **ameboid m.,** the most primitive form of locomotion by a living organism, such as amebae, and cells, such as leukocytes, based on a mechanism whereby the flow of intracellular fluids produces pseudopodia, and moves them along the body against the resistance of the liquid medium, or gliding the organism in the desired direction. **angular m.,** a movement which changes the angle between the bones, as in flexion, extension, abduction, and adduction. **associated m.,** a movement of parts which act together. **associated m., contralateral,** a movement on the paralyzed side in hemiplegia, associated with active movement of the corresponding part on the unaffected side. **automatic m.,** a movement produced by automatic processes, such as one originated by defense or reflex mechanisms or the autonomic nervous system, as opposed to one produced by willful processes under the control of the central nervous system. **Bennett m.,** the lateral shift of the mandibular condyles and articular disks in the direction of the working bite as the lower jaw swings in preparation for mastication. Called also *Bennett shift, lateral shift of mandible,* and *side shift of mandible.* See also Bennett ANGLE. **biaxial m.,** movement around two axes at right angles to each other, such as movement of the saddle joint. See also biaxial JOINT. **bodily m.,** TRANSLATION (2). **bodily m. (of tooth),** movement of the crown and root apex at the same rate and direction, thus maintaining the same axial inclination. See also *tipping m. (of tooth).* **border m.,** any extreme compass of mandibular movement limited by bone, ligaments, or soft tissues; usually applied to horizontal mandibular movements. **border m., posterior,** a movement of the mandible in its most posterior relation, occurring in the vertical plane from the level of occlusal contact to the level of maximal opening of the jaws. **border tissue m.,** the action of the muscles and other structures adjacent to the

borders of a denture. **brownian m., brownian-Zsigmondy m., brunonian m.,** the rapid, random, vibratory motion of particles in a colloidal solution, caused by bombardment of the particles by the molecules of the dispersion medium, the velocity of movement varying inversely with the size of particles and depending on the viscosity of the medium. **buccal m.,** movement in the buccal direction, as of teeth in orthodontic therapy. **choreic, choreiform m's,** irregular, jerky movements of muscles or groups of muscles. **cutting m.,** a masticatory movement, such as movement of incisors and canines to bite off a piece of food. **distal m.,** tooth movement in the distal direction. **dystonic m.,** a large slow, amplified athetoid movement. **empty m.,** tooth contact during swallowing or without anything between the teeth. See also empty SWALLOWING. **envelope of border m's,** see under ENVELOPE. **excessive m.,** hyperkinesia. **excursive m.,** excursion. **forced m.,** a movement caused by an injury to a motor center or a conducting path. **gliding m.,** a translatory movement in which one surface glides over another, without any angular or rotary movements, being the simplest kind of motion of a joint. In the temporomandibular joint, it is the second phase of mouth opening, involving both the lower and upper compartments of the joint, and consisting of a gliding of the condyle and miniscus forward and downward along the articular elimence. This occurs alone during protrusion and lateral movements of the mandible, and in combination with the hinge movement during wide opening of the mouth. Called also *gliding action.* See illustration at temporomandibular JOINT. **grinding m.,** a masticatory movement, such as the movement of the molars and premolars to comminute a piece of food. **hinge m.,** a movement rotational around a single axis or hinge, such as a movement of the temporomandibular joint during the first phase of mouth opening, in which only the lower compartment of the joint is used, with the condyle rotating around a point on the undersurface of the meniscus and the mandible dropping downward and backward. Called also *hinge action.* See illustration at temporomandibular JOINT. **hinge m., terminal,** a border movement of the mandible in its most retruded position from which opening and lateral movements can be performed comfortably. See also centric RELATION. **index m.,** a movement of the cephalic part of a body about the fixed caudal part. **intermediary m., intermediate m.,** mandibular movements between the extremes of mandibular excursions. See also EXCURSION. **jaw m.,** mandibular m. **labial m.,** movement in the labial direction, as of teeth in orthodontic therapy. **lateral m.,** any movement to one side of an established position. **lingual m.,** movement in the lingual direction, as of teeth in orthodontic therapy. **Magnan's m.,** forward and backward movement of the tongue when it is drawn out, observed in dementia paralytica. Called also *trombone tremor of tongue.* **mandibular m.,** any movement of which the mandible is capable. Called also *jaw m.* See *gliding m.* and *hinge m.* **mandibular m., free,** any movement of the mandible without interference. **mandibular m., functional,** any movement of the mandible which occurs in the performance of some function, as mastication, swallowing, articulation of vocal sounds, yawning, facial expression, or any other normal action. See also *masticatory m.,* EXCURSION, POSITION, and RELATION. **mandibular m., opening,** opening m. **mandibular m., perverted,** any nonfunctional or unintended mandibular movement, as in unusual facial expression or holding an object between the teeth, which sometimes results in malocclusion. **masticatory m's,** those movements of the mandible occurring in the mastication of food, which include cutting and grinding movements. They may be initiated consciously but are essentially governed by automatic rhythms which vary from person to person but are quite stable in an individual. The process consists of excursion of the mandible during chewing, opening, closing, protruding, lateral and lateral protrusive movements that are governed by the size and consistency of food bolus, the patient's pain threshold, the anatomic structure and functioning of the temporomandibular joints, the masticatory muscles, the restraining ligaments, the presence of disease, and other factors. **mesial m.,** mesial DRIFT. **opening m., opening mandibular m.,** a mandibular movement occurring during jaw separation. **opening m., posterior,** the opening movement of the mandible about the terminal hinge axis. **orthodontic tooth m.,** corrective movement of a tooth or teeth, sometimes through the bone without causing the root to be resorbed or damaged, with the use of orthodontic techniques and appliances. **passive m.,** any movement of the body effected by a force entirely outside of the organism. **pendulum m's,** in tooth extraction, rocking movements in the faciolingual plane. **protrusive m.,** forward movement of the mandible associated with forward and downward sliding of the articular disks of the temporomandibular joint. See also PROTRUSION and protrusive jaw RELATION. **retrusive m.,** backward movement of the mandible associated with backward and upward movement of the articular disks of the temporomandibular joints. **rotational m.,** 1. a movement around an axis. See also *hinge m.* 2. in tooth extraction, movement designed to rotate a tooth around its longitudinal axis. **spontaneous m.,** one originated within the organism. **synkinetic m.,** any minor, unconscious movement that accompanies major voluntary movements, such as the facial contortions in severe exertion. **tipping m. (of tooth),** movement of a tooth in any direction, while its apex remains in almost the original position. See also *bodily m. (of tooth).* **tooth m.,** displacement of a tooth from its normal position in a dental arch, occurring either by bodily or tipping movement. It results from excessive tongue pressure, lack of equilibrium between the lingual and labial pressure, faulty tooth-supporting structures, malocclusion, failure to replace missing teeth, a purposeful orthodontic procedure, and other factors. Specific forms include labial, lingual, and distal movements. See also pathologic tooth MIGRATION. **translatory m.,** motion of a body at any instant when all points within the body are moving at the same velocity and in the same direction. See also *gliding m.* **uniaxial m.,** hinge m.

Mowrey No. 1 wire see under WIRE.

Mowrey No. 8 trademark for an extra hard *dental casting gold alloy* (see under GOLD).

Mowrey 12% wire see under WIRE.

Mowrey 120 trademark for a hard *dental casting gold alloy* (see under GOLD).

Mowrey 695 trademark for an *amalgam alloy* (see under AMALGAM).

Mowrey B inlay see under INLAY.

Mowrey S-1 trademark for a soft *dental casting gold alloy* (see under GOLD).

Mowrey S-3 trademark for a hard *dental casting gold alloy* (see under GOLD).

moxa (mok'sah) a cone of dried leaves, usually of *Artemisia moxa* (wormwood), used in moxibustion.

moxibustion (mok"sĭ-bus-chun) [*moxa* + (com)*bustion*] an ancient Chinese method of therapy, eventually adopted in Japan and other countries, consisting of placing ignited cones of dried leaves of *Artemisia moxa* (wormwood) on different spots of the human body, for the production of counterirritation. It is believed by its practitioners to restore the equilibrium of the bodily functions, and is used for a wide variety of morbid conditions.

Moyco trademark for *dental mercury* (see under MERCURY).

MP mesial PIT.

mp melting POINT.

6MP mercaptopurine.

MPD maximum permissible DOSE.

MPMP mepazine.

MQ cement see under CEMENT.

MR mental RETARDATION.

mR milliroentgen.

mr milliroentgen.

μR microroentgen.

mrad millirad.

mRNA messenger RNA.

m/s meter per second; the unit of velocity in SI.

m/s² meter per second squared; the unit of acceleration in SI.

msec millisecond.

μsec microsecond.

MSH melanocyte stimulating HORMONE.

MTQ methaqualone.

MTU methylthiouracil.

MTV mammary tumor virus of mice; see under VIRUS.

mU milliunit.

mu (mu) μ, the twelfth letter of the Greek alphabet. It is used as a symbol for the prefix *micro-* and for *micron.*

μU microunit.

MUC maximum urinary concentration; see under SOLUTION.

mucicarmine (mu"sĭ-kar'min) a stain containing carmine, aluminum chloride, and distilled water, which is specific for mucin.

muciferous (mu-sif'er-us) [*mucus* + L. *ferre* to bear] secreting mucus.

muciform (mu'sĭ-form) [*mucus* + L. *forma* form] resembling mucus.

mucigen (mu'sĭ-jen) [*mucus* + Gr. *gennan* to produce] the substance produced by the endoplasmic reticulum and refined by the Golgi apparatus, which is the intracellular forerunner of mucus. It stains pink with mucicarmine.

mucigenous (mu-sij'ĕ-nus) producing mucus.

mucigogue (mu'sĭ-gog) [*mucus* + Gr. *agōgos* leading] 1. stimulating the secretion of mucus. 2. an agent that stimulates the secretion of mucus.

mucilage (mu'sĭ-lij) [L. *mucilago*] 1. an artificial viscid paste of gum or dextrin used in pharmacy as a vehicle or excipient, or in therapy as a demulcent. 2. a naturally formed viscid principle of a plant, consisting of a gum dissolved in the juices of the plant. See also ACACIA and TRAGACANTH.

mucin (mu'sin) [L. *mucus*] a glycoprotein or mucoprotein, depending on the classification used, occurring in mucus, gastric and intestinal juices, saliva, and other secretions. Salivary mucin, because of its slippery properties, facilitates the propulsion of the food bolus into and through the gastrointestinal tract.

mucinase (mu'sĭ-nās) hyaluronidase.

mucinogen (mu-sin'o-jen) [*mucin* + Gr. *gennan* to produce] a precursor of mucin.

mucinoid (mu'sĭ-noid) [*mucin* + *-oid*] 1. resembling mucin. Called also *mucoid.* 2. myxoid (1).

mucinolytic (mu"sĭ-no-lit'ik) [*mucin* + Gr. *lysis* dissolution] dissolving or splitting of mucin.

mucinosis (mu"si-no'sis) a condition characterized by abnormal deposits of mucopolysaccharides (mucins) in the skin. **cutaneous focal m.,** a condition characterized by the presence of nodules or dome-shaped elevations on the skin of the face, trunk, and extremities. Histologically, the lesions are characterized by a mucinous accumulation interspersed with spindle-shaped fibroblasts. **oral focal m.,** a solitary lesion of the oral cavity with a predilection for the mucosa attached to the bone, but sometimes also involving the buccal mucosa and tongue. It usually appears as a rounded elevation resembling a fibroma, which is of the same color as the surrounding mucosa and is asymptomatic, with the exception of slight tenderness. The presence of myxomatous connective tissue surrounded by a relatively dense but normal collagenous fibrous connective tissue is the principal histologic feature.

mucinous (mu'sĭ-nus) resembling or marked by the formation of mucin.

muciparous (mu-sip'ah-rus) [*mucus* + L. *parere* to produce] producing or secreting mucin, as in a mucous gland.

mucitis (mu-si'tis) inflammation of the mucous membrane.

muco- [L. *mucus*] a combining form denoting relationship to mucus or the mucous membranes.

mucocele (mu'ko-sēl) [*mucus* + Gr. *kēlē* tumor] a cavity dilated with accumulated mucous extravasation; mucous retention cyst. **maxillary sinus m.,** maxillary sinus retention CYST.

mucoid (mu'koid) [*mucin* + *-oid*] 1. a conjugated protein identified with glycoproteins (or mucoproteins, depending on the classification used), containing as a conjugated group mucopolysaccharides with multiple units of acetyl galactosamine sulfate and glucuronic or iduronic acids in glycosidal linkage. Mucoid is found in the cartilage (chondromucoid), egg white (ovomucoid), bone (osseomucoid), tendons (tendomucoid), etc. They are soluble in water and are resistant to denaturation. 2. mucinoid (1). 3. myxoid (1).

mucolytic (mu"ko-lit'ik) 1. destroying or dissolving mucus. 2. an agent that destroys or dissolves mucus.

mucomembranous (mu"ko-mem'brah-nus) pertaining to or composed of mucous membrane.

mucopeptide (mu"ko-pep'tīd) peptidoglycan. **m. glycohydrolase,** lysozyme.

mucoperiosteal (mu"ko-per"e-os'te-al) consisting of mucous membrane and periosteum.

mucoperiosteum (mu"ko-per"e-os'te-um) periosteum having a mucous surface.

mucopolysaccharide (mu"ko-pol"e-sak'ah-rīd) a group of heteropolysaccharides, usually containing two types of alternating monosaccharide units of which at least one has an acidic group, either a carboxyl or sulfuric group. When occurring as complexes with specific proteins, they are known as *mucins* or *mucoproteins.* Hyaluronic acid, chondroitin 4-sulfate, dermatan sulfate, keratan sulfate, and heparin are the principal mucopolysaccharides. Called also *acid m.* and *glycosaminoglucuronoglycan.* **acid m.,** mucopolysaccharide.

mucopolysaccharidosis (mu"ko-pol"e-sak'ah-rid-o-sis) a disorder characterized by faulty polysaccharide metabolism. **m. I,** Hurler's syndrome; see Hunter-Hurler SYNDROME. **m. II,** Hunter's syndrome; see Hunter-Hurler SYNDROME. **m. III,** Sanfilippo's SYNDROME. **m. IV,** Morquio's DISEASE. **m. V,** Scheie's SYNDROME. **m. VI,** Maroteaux-Lamy SYNDROME (1).

mucoprotein (mu″ko-pro′te-in) [muco- + protein] a conjugated protein containing a protein and a carbohydrate, chiefly hexosamine, occurring as a jelly-like, sticky, or slippery substance, providing lubrication and, in some instances, functioning as flexible intercellular cement. According to some authorities, compounds containing more than 4 percent carbohydrates are classified as mucoproteins, whereas those having less than 4 percent are glycoproteins. Other classifications identify mucins, mucoids, chondroproteins, and various plasma proteins containing hexoses or other carbohydrates as either mucoproteins or glycoproteins. α_1-m., orosomucoid.

Mucor (mu′kor) [L.] a genus of true fungi of the class Zygomycetes, the members of which form delicate, white tubular filaments. The fungi are ordinarily nonpathogenic saprophytes and are often found as mold on bread. It is a cause of mucormycosis, but only in the presence of severe predisposing factors, such as diabetes mellitus.

mucormycosis (mu″kor-mi-ko′sis) an infection usually caused by fungi of the genera *Absidia, Mucor,* and *Rhizopus.* It is relatively rare, but may be associated with debilitating conditions, such as cancer and diabetes mellitus. The superficial infection may involve the external ear, fingernails, and skin. The visceral infection may involve the lungs, gastrointestinal tract, and head and neck. The nasal cavity is believed to be a portal of entry, from where the infection may extend to the paranasal sinuses, pharynx, palate, orbit, and brain. A typical lesion may present a mass of necrotic tissue in the maxilla. The fungi often penetrate blood vessel walls and produce thromboses.

mucosa (mu-ko′sah) [L. "mucus"] see mucous MEMBRANE. **alveolar m.,** a thin, soft, and fragile part of the oral mucosa, being the mucosal alveolar lining which is continuous with the mucous membrane of the cheek, lips, and floor of the mouth. **hypermobile m.,** excessive mobility of the oral mucosa, most commonly occurring in the anterior segment of the maxillary arch and, less commonly, on any part of the arch, usually brought about by atrophy of the alveolar bone which leaves a pendulous mass of mucosal tissue unsupported by bone. **laryngeal m.,** mucous membrane, laryngeal; see under MEMBRANE. **lingual m.,** mucous membrane of tongue; see under MEMBRANE. **masticatory m.,** mucous membrane, masticatory; see under MEMBRANE. **nasal m.,** mucous membrane, nasal; see under MEMBRANE. **oral m.,** mucous membrane, oral; see under MEMBRANE. **palatal m.,** mucous membrane, palatal; see under MEMBRANE. **pharyngeal m.,** mucous membrane, pharyngeal; see under MEMBRANE. **sublingual m.,** mucous membrane, sublingual; see under MEMBRANE. **vestibular m.,** mucous membrane, vestibular; see under MEMBRANE.

mucosal (mu-ko′sal) pertaining to the mucous membrane.

mucositis (mu″ko-si′tis) inflammation of a mucous membrane. **m. necrot′icans agranulocyt′ica,** agranulocytosis.

mucosocutaneous (mu-ko″so-ku-ta′ne-us) pertaining to a mucous membrane and the skin.

mucostatic (mu″ko-stat′ik) 1. arresting the secretion of mucus. 2. denoting the normal relaxed condition of the tissues of the mucosa of the jaws.

mucous (mu′kus) [L. mucosus] pertaining to or resembling mucus; also, secreting mucus.

mucoviscidosis (mu″ko-vis″ĭ-do′sis) a disease of the exocrine glands, occurring chiefly in children but also in adults; so called because of the abnormally viscous mucoid secretions associated with the condition. It is transmitted as a recessive trait, and is characterized by obstruction of the pancreatic ducts, chronic pulmonary disorders, high levels of sodium chloride and potassium in the sweat, and susceptibility to infection. Complications include dilatation and eosinophilic concretions in the pancreatic duct and degeneration and fibrosis of the pancreas; bronchial obstruction; pulmonary insufficiency, pulmonary abscesses, atelectasis, cor pulmonale, hypertension, pneumothorax, hemoptysis, asphyxia, emphysema, anoxia, and carbon monoxide retention; abdominal distention, diarrhea, foul-smelling stools, meconium ileus, malnutrition, exorbitant appetite, and duodenal ulcer; liver cirrhosis; short stature; delayed puberty; clubbing of the fingers; and diabetes mellitus. Oral features include hypertrophy of the submandibular glands, dilated salivary ducts, eosinophilic concretions in the salivary ducts, and somewhat elevated levels of sodium chloride, urea, and uric acid in the saliva. Called also *cystic fibrosis of pancreas.*

mucro (mu′kro), pl. *mucro′nes* [L. "a sharp point"] the pointed end of a part or organ.

mucronate (mu′kro-nat) [L. *mucro* a sharp point] having a spine-like tip or end.

mucus (mu′kus) [L.] a slippery, viscid liquid which lubricates and

protects mucous membranes from noxious elements, composed chiefly of mucin, a protein-carbohydrate complex, water, inorganic salts, desquamated cells, and leukocytes. It is produced by gastric, intestinal, salivary, and other mucous glands; the palatine, posterior lingual, and sublingual glands are the principal salivary glands involved in its secretion. Mucus is soluble in water but not in alcohol, ether, or other organic solvents. See also MYXOID.

mud (mud) moist or wet earth. **dentin m.,** ground dentin accumulating in the bottom of the root canal during its shaping.

muffle (muf′'l) part of a furnace, usually removable or replaceable, in which material may be placed for processing, without exposing it to the direct action of the fire. See also porcelain FURNACE.

Mühlemann appliance propulsor.

Mulder, angle of [Johannes *Mulder,* Dutch anatomist, 1769–1810] see under ANGLE.

mulibrey *mu*scles, *li*ver, *br*ain, and *ey*e; see mulibrey NANISM.

muller (mul′er) a kind of pestle, flat at the bottom, used for grinding drugs upon a slab of similar material.

Muller, W. see Geiger-Muller COUNTER.

Müller's ganglion superior ganglion of glossopharyngeal nerve; see under GANGLION.

Müller's law see LAW of specific irritability.

mulling (mul′ing) the final step of mixing dental amalgam, consisting of the kneading of the triturated mass to complete the amalgamation.

Mult-Form Dual Purpose Impression Paste see under PASTE.

multi- [L. *multus* many, much] a combining form meaning many or much. See also terms beginning POLY- and PLURI-.

multiarticular (mul″te-ar-tik′u-lar) pertaining to or affecting several joints.

multicellular (mul″tĭ-sel′u-lar) [multi- + L. *cellula* cell] 1. composed of many cells. 2. containing many hollow spaces or compartments.

multicentric (mul″ti-sen′trik) [multi- + center] having many centers or points of origin.

multicontaminated (mul″ti-kon-tam′ĭ-nāt″ed) contaminated by several different species or types of microorganisms.

multicuspid (mul″ti-kus′pid) [multi- + cuspid] having many cusps, such as a tooth with many cusps. Called also *multicuspidate.*

multicuspidate (mul″ti-kus′pĭ-dāt) multicuspid.

multidentate (mul″ti-den′tāt) [multi- + L. *dens* tooth] having many teeth or toothlike processes.

multifactorial (mul″tĭ-fak-to′re-al) pertaining to or due to many factors.

multifamilial (mul″tĭ-fah-mil′e-al) affecting several successive generations of a family.

multifid (mul′tĭ-fid) [multi- + L. *fidere* to split] cleft or divided into many parts.

multifocal (mul″tĭ-fo′kal) arising from or pertaining to many foci.

multiform (mul′tĭ-form) [multi- + L. *forma* form] having many forms; polymorphic.

multiglandular (mul″tĭ-glan′du-lar) pertaining to, derived from, or affecting several glands; pluriglandular.

multi-infection (mul″tĭ-in-fek′shun) infection with several varieties of organisms.

multilobar (mul″tĭ-lo′bar) having numerous lobes.

multilobular (mul″tĭ-lob′u-lar) [multi- + L. *lobulus* lobule] having many lobules.

multilocular (mul″tĭ-lok′u-lar) [multi- + L. *loculus* cell] having many cells or compartments, as a multilocular cyst.

multinucleate (mul″tĭ-nu′kle-āt) [multi- + *nucleus*] having several nuclei.

multiple (mul′tĭ-p'l) [L. *multiplex*] manifold; occurring in or affecting various parts of the body at once.

multipolar (mul″tĭ-po′lar) [multi- + L. *polus* pole] having more than two poles or processes.

multirooted (mul″tĭ-root′ed) having many roots; said of molar teeth.

multiterminal (mul″tĭ-ter′mĭ-nal) having several sets of terminals so that several electrodes may be used.

multivalent (mul″tĭ-va′lent) [multi- + L. *valere* to have value] 1. having the power of combining with three or more univalent atoms. 2. active against several strains of an organism.

Mummery, pink tooth of see internal tooth RESORPTION.

mummification (mum″ĭ-fi-ka′shun) conversion into a state resembling that of a mummy; dry GANGRENE. **pulp m.,** a method used in the past in treating the dental pulp by removing the coronal portion of devitalized pulp (usually with arsenic trioxide) and preserving the remaining pulp, usually with paraformaldehyde. See also mummified PULP.

mumps (mumps) any condition characterized by enlargement of the parotid gland; specifically, an acute contagious viral infection usually occurring in children, marked by unilateral or bilateral inflammation and swelling of the parotid glands, sometimes associated with involvement of the submandibular and submaxillary glands. After an incubation period of two to three weeks, it is manifested by chills, fever, headache, swelling in the parotid area, and difficulty in mastication and swallowing. Complications may include involvement of the testes, ovaries, pancreas, mammary glands, prostate, epididymis, and heart. Orchitis, occasionally resulting in sterility, is a relatively common serious complication in adult males. Called also *angina parotidea* and *epidemic parotitis*. See also mumps VIRUS. **chemical m.**, iodine m. **iodine m.**, bilateral swelling of the salivary glands, which sometimes accompanies the administration of iodine or iodine compounds. Called also *chemical m.* See also IODINE. **metastatic m.**, mumps associated with involvement of other glands or organs. **nutritional m.**, chronic, asymptomatic, bilateral enlargement of the parotid and/or submaxillary glands, occurring endemically in populations suffering from malnutrition. **single m.**, that which affects only one of the parotid glands. **surgical m.**, acute postoperative PAROTITIS.

Münchmeyer's syndrome [Ernst *Münchmeyer*, German physician, 1846–1880] progressive myositis ossificans; see under MYOSITIS.

Munsell, Hazel E. [American nutritionist, born 1891] see Sherman-Munsell unit of vitamin A, under UNIT.

Muracil trademark for *methylthiouracil*.

mural (mu′ral) [L. *muralis*, from *murus* wall] pertaining to, associated with, or resembling a wall, as of a vessel or cavity.

muramidase (mu-ram′ĭ-dās) lysozyme.

murein (mu′rān), mu′rēn) peptidoglycan.

muriform (mu′rĭ-form) resembling a wall, particularly a brick or stone wall; said of organisms having both longitudinal and transverse septa.

Murk Jansen's syndrome [W. *Murk Jansen*, Dutch physician, 1867–1935] metaphyseal DYSOSTOSIS.

murmur (mur′mur) [L.] an auscultatory sound, particularly a periodic sound of short duration of cardiac or vascular origin, observed in normal or abnormal conditions.

muscarine (mus′kah-rin) an alkaloid, tetrahydro-4β-hydroxy-$N,N,N,5\alpha$-tetramethyl-2α-furanmethanaminium, of the toadstool *Amanita muscaria*, also found in decaying fish. It is a very poisonous substance of little or no therapeutic value, which acts on the muscarinic receptors in the postganglionic parasympathetic impulses. Intake of toxic doses may cause sialorrhea, lacrimation, diaphoresis, nausea, vomiting, diarrhea, miosis, bradycardia, circulatory shock, and death.

muscarinic 1. pertaining to muscarine. 2. muscarinic DRUG.

muscle (mus′l) [L. *musculus*] an organ made up of a reddish, fleshy tissue, representing about 40 percent of total body weight, whose contractions provide motor power for the animal body. Three types of muscles are recognized: striated muscle, which is responsible for locomotion, movement of the limbs and head, mastication, maintenance of posture, facial expression, and other forms of voluntary motor activity; smooth muscle, which invests the hollow organs and blood vessels and is responsible for the peristaltic function of the digestive organs and tonus of the visceral organs and blood vessels; and a specialized muscle of the heart (myocardium), which is responsible for pumping blood through the body. Called also *musculus* [NA]. See also terms beginning *myo-*. **Aeby's m.**, depressor m. of lower lip. **agonistic m.**, a muscle opposed in action by another muscle, its antagonist. **Albinus' m.**, risorius m. **antagonistic m.**, a muscle that acts in opposition to the action of another muscle, its agonist. Called also *antagonist*. **antigravity m.**, a skeletal muscle which is responsible for maintaining normal posture, and assists the body in resisting the constant pull of gravity. **articular m.**, a muscle that is attached at one end to the membrane of a synovial joint. Called also *musculus articularis* [NA]. **aryepiglottic m., aryepiglotticus m.**, an inconstant fascicle of the oblique arytenoid muscle which arises from the apex of the arytenoid cartilage, continues around the lateral margin of the cartilage into the aryepiglottic fold, and inserts into the lateral margin of the epiglottis. Called also *Hilton's m., aryepiglotticus* and *musculus aryepiglotticus* [NA]. **arytenoid m., arytenoideus m.**, an intrinsic muscle of the larynx, consisting of

an oblique part (*arytenoid m., oblique*), and a transverse part (*arytenoid m., transverse*). Called also *arytenoideus* and *musculus arytenoideus*. **arytenoid m., oblique, arytenoideus obliquus m.**, the oblique part of the arytenoid muscle, consisting of two fasciculi, each connecting the base of one arytenoid cartilage with the apex of the other, and forming an X. It is innervated by the recurrent laryngeal nerve. Its function consists of approximating the arytenoid cartilages and closing the inlet of the larynx. Fibers continuing from the oblique arytenoid muscle around the lateral margin of the cartilage and into the aryepiglottic fold form the aryepiglottic muscle. Called also *arytenoideus obliquus* and *musculus arytenoideus obliquus* [NA]. **arytenoid m., transverse, arytenoideus transversus m.**, the transverse part of the arytenoid muscle which transversely connects the two opposite arytenoid cartilages. The recurrent laryngeal nerve provides innervation. Its function consists of approximating the arytenoid cartilages. Called also *arytenoideus transversus* and *musculus arytenoideus transversus* [NA]. **auricular m., anterior**, a thin, delicate facial muscle that arises from the anterior part of the superficial temporal fascia and inserts into the cartilage of the helix of the ear. It is innervated by the facial nerve. Its function consists of drawing the auricle forward. Called also *musculus attrahens aurem* and *musculus auricularis anterior* [NA]. **auricular m., posterior**, a thin facial muscle consisting of two or three fasciculi, which arises from the mastoid process and inserts into the cartilage of the ear. It is innervated by the facial nerve. Its function consists of drawing the auricle backward. Called also *musculus auricularis posterior* [NA] and *musculus retrahens aurem*. **auricular m., superior**, a thin, fan-shaped facial muscle that arises from the temporal area of the epicranial aponeurosis and inserts into a tendon to the cartilage of the ear. It is innervated by the facial nerve. Its function consists of raising the auricle. Called also *musculus attolens aurem* and *musculus auricularis superior* [NA]. **bipennate m., bipenniform m.**, a muscle in which the fasciculi converge like the plumes of feathers to both sides of a tendon. Called also *musculus bipennatus* [NA]. **buccinator m.**, a facial muscle, presenting a thin and wide square muscular plate, which occupies the space between the maxilla and the mandible of the cheek and forms the lateral wall of the oral cavity, and is covered by the buccopharyngeal fascia and the buccal fat pad. The parotid duct perforates it opposite to the upper second molar tooth. It arises from the buccinator ridge of the mandible and the alveolar process of the maxilla. The pterygomandibular raphe provides a tendinous inscription between the buccinator and constrictor of the pharynx muscles. It inserts into the orbicular muscle at the corner of the mouth. Innervation is provided by the buccal branch of the facial muscle. It retracts the angle of the mouth and compresses the cheek, keeping it taut during opening and closing of the mouth. Called also *cheek m., buccinator*, and *musculus buccinator* [NA]. **buccopharyngeal m.**, the part of the constrictor pharyngis superior muscle arising from the pterygomandibular raphe. Called also *musculus buccopharyngeus* and *pars buccopharyngea musculi constrictoris pharyngis superioris* [NA]. **ceratocricoid m., ceratocricoideus m.**, a muscular fasciculus arising from the cricoid cartilage and inserting on the inferior horn of the thyroid cartilage. Called also *Merkel's m., ceratocricoideus*, and *musculus ceratocricoideus* [NA]. **ceratopharyngeal m., ceratopharyngeus m.**, the part of the constrictor pharyngis medius muscle arising from the greater horn of the hyoid bone. Called also *ceratopharyngeus, musculus ceratopharyngeus*, and *pars ceratopharyngea musculi constrictoris pharyngis medii* [NA]. **cheek m.**, buccinator m. **canine m.**, levator m. of angle of mouth. **cardiac m.**, myocardium. **chin m.**, mental m. **chondroglossus m.**, an extrinsic muscle of the tongue, sometimes considered as a part of the hyoglossus muscle. It is about 2 cm long and originates at the medial side and base of the lesser cornu of the hyoid bone and inserts into the substance of the tongue. Its function consists of depressing and retracting the tongue. The hypoglossal nerve provides innervation. Called also *chondroglossus* and *musculus chondroglossus* [NA]. **chondropharyngeal m., chondropharyngeus m.**, the portion of the constrictor pharyngis medius muscle arising from the lesser cornu of the hyoid bone. Called also *chondropharyngeus, musculus chondropharyngeus*, and *pars chondropharyngea musculi constrictoris pharyngis medii* [NA]. **compressor m. of naris**, transverse part of nasal muscle; see under PART. **constrictor pharyngis inferior m.**, the largest of the three constrictor muscles of the pharynx that arises from the sides of the cricoid cartilage and the thyroid cartilage, and also from the oblique line on the side of the lamina of the thyroid cartilage, and after passing dorsalward and medialward, inserts with its fellow of the opposite side into the fibrous raphe in the posterior median line of the pharynx. It is innervated by the vagus and the external branch of the superior laryngeal nerve. Its function consists of constricting the pharynx in deglutition. Called also *inferior constrictor m. of pharynx, constrictor pharyngis inferior,* and *musculus constrictor pharyngis inferior* [NA]. **constrictor pharyngis medius m.,** a fan-shaped muscle of the pharynx that is somewhat smaller than the inferior and larger than the superior constrictor, arising from the cornua of the hyoid and stylohyoid ligament, and inserting into the posterior median fibrous raphe of the posterior wall of the pharynx. The pharyngeal plexus of the vagus nerve provides innervation. Its function consists of constricting the pharynx in swallowing. Called also *middle constrictor m. of pharynx, constrictor pharyngis medius,* and *musculus constrictor pharyngis medius* [NA]. **constrictor pharyngis superior m.,** a thin, pale, quadrilateral muscle of the pharynx, which is the smallest of the three constrictors of the pharynx; it arises from the medial pterygoid plate, pterygomandibular raphe, mylohyoid line of the mandible, mucous membrane of the floor of the mouth, and by a few fibers from the side of the tongue, and inserts into the median raphe of the posterior wall of the pharynx, and, by its uppermost fibers, into the

pharyngeal tubercle. The vagal nerve, through the pharyngeal plexus, provides innervation. It constricts the pharynx in swallowing. Called also *superior constrictor m. of pharynx, constrictor pharyngis superior,* and *musculus constrictor pharyngis superior* [NA]. **m. contraction,** see under CONTRACTION. **corrugator supercilii m.,** a slender, pyramidal facial muscle situated at the medial end of the eyebrow, under the frontal belly of the occipitofrontal muscle and the orbicular muscle of the eye. It arises from the medial end of the superciliary arch and inserts into the skin of the eyebrow. The temporal branch of the facial nerve innervates the muscle. Its function consists of drawing the skin of the forehead medially downward above the nose, producing the vertical wrinkles of the forehead characteristic of a frown. Called also *corrugator supercilii* and *musculus corrugator supercilii* [NA]. **cricoarytenoid m., lateral, cricoarytenoideus lateralis m.,** an intrinsic muscle of the larynx that arises from the cranial border of the arch of the cricoid cartilage and inserts into the front of the

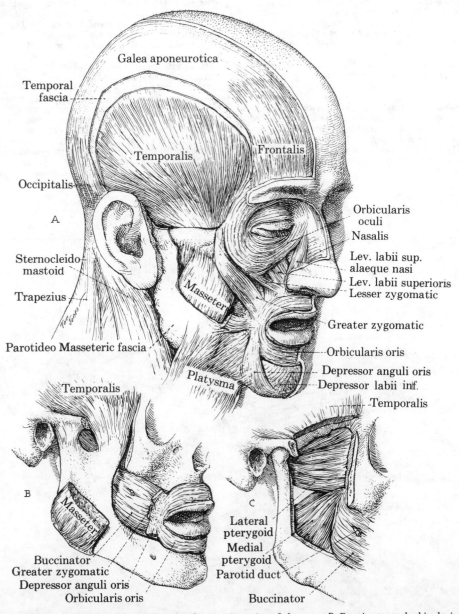

Muscles of the head and face. *A,* Muscles of face and scalp, showing insertion of platysma. *B,* Buccinator and orbicularis oris. *C,* Pterygoid muscles. (From Dorland's Illustrated Medical Dictionary. 26th ed. Philadelphia, W. B. Saunders Co., 1981; adapted from Jones and Shepard.)

muscular process of the arytenoid cartilage. The recurrent laryngeal nerve provides innervation. Its function consists of closing the glottis. Called also *cricoarytenoideus lateralis* and *musculus cricoarytenoideus lateralis* [NA]. **cricoarytenoid m., posterior, cricoarytenoideus posterior m.,** an intrinsic muscle of the larynx that arises from the back of the cricoid cartilage and inserts into the back of the muscular process of the arytenoid cartilage. The recurrent laryngeal nerve provides innervation. Its function consists of separating the vocal cords and opening the glottis. Called also *cricoarytenoideus posterior* and *musculus cricoarytenoideus posterior* [NA]. **cricopharyngeal m., cricopharyngeus m.,** the portion of the constrictor pharyngis inferior muscle arising from the cricoid cartilage. Called also *cricopharyngeus, musculus cricopharyngeus,* and *pars cricopharyngea musculi constrictoris pharyngis inferioris* [NA]. **cricothyroid m., cricothyroideus m.,** an intrinsic triangular muscle of the larynx that arises from the front and side of the cricoid cartilage and inserts into the lamina of the thyroid cartilage. Its fibers form two groups, the pars obliqua, which slants backward to the anterior border of the inferior horn, and the pars recta, which runs to the thyroid cartilage. The external branch of the superior laryngeal nerve provides innervation. The action of the muscle produces tension and elongation of the vocal folds. Called also *cricothyroideus* and *musculus cricothyroideus* [NA]. **cross striated m.,** striated m. **cutaneous m.,** a striated muscle that inserts into the skin. Called also *musculus cutaneus* [NA]. **depressor m. of angle of mouth,** a facial muscle arising from the oblique line of the mandible, being continuous at its origin with the platysma, and whose fibers form a triangle by converging toward the corner of the mouth, into which it is inserted by a single slender fasciculus, together with the orbicular muscle of the mouth and the risorius muscle. The facial nerve provides innervation. It pulls down the corner of the mouth. Called also *triangular m., depressor anguli oris, musculus depressor anguli oris* [NA], *musculus triangularis,* and *triangularis.* **depressor m. of lower lip,** a small, square facial muscle that arises from the

anterior portion of the lower border of the mandible and inserts into the integument of the lower lip. At the origin, its fibers are continuous with the platysma. The lateroinferior part is covered by the depressor of the angle of the mouth. The facial nerve provides innervation. It pulls the lower lip down and a little laterally in the expression of irony. Called also *Aeby's m., quadrate m. of lower lip, square m. of lower lip, depressor labii inferioris, musculus depressor labii inferioris* [NA], *musculus quadratus labii inferioris,* and *musculus quadratus menti.* **depressor m. of nasal septum,** a facial muscle of the nose situated between the mucosa and muscles of the lip; it arises from the incisive fossa of the maxilla and inserts into the nasal septum and ala of the nose. It draws the ala of the nose downward and constricts the opening of the naris. Called also *depressor septi nasi, musculus depressor alae nasi* and *musculus depressor septi nasi* [NA]. **depressor m., superciliary,** a part of the orbicularis oris muscle which is inserted into the eyebrow and is responsible for drawing it downward. Called also *depressor supercilii* and *musculus depressor supercilii* [NA]. **digastric m.,** a suprahyoid muscle consisting of two bellies united by an intermediate tendon, which is situated between the mastoid process and the mental symphysis. The smaller anterior belly arises from the inner side of the lower border of the mandible near the symphysis and the larger posterior belly from the mastoid notch of the temporal bone. The intermediate tendon, which unites the two bellies, perforates the stylohyoid muscle and fastens to fibers of the cervical fascia; these fibers form a loop around the tendon and are attached to the greater cornu of the hyoid bone, thus forming a pulley. It raises the hyoid bone and assists in opening the jaws. The anterior belly is innervated by the mylohyoid branch of the trigeminal nerve and the posterior belly by the digastric branch of the facial nerve. Called also *musculus digastricus* [NA]. **dilator m. of nose,** alar part of nasal muscle; see under PART. **m. of ear,** 1. auricular m., anterior. 2. auricular m., posterior. **emergency m.,** a muscle which is not ordinarily required in acts performed with moderate force, but is called upon to assist the prime movers in acts requiring great force. **epicranial m.,** the muscular covering of the top of the skull; the skull muscles. Called also *musculus epicranius* [NA]. See *occipitofrontal m.* and *temporoparietal m.* **m's of expression,** facial m's. **extra-**

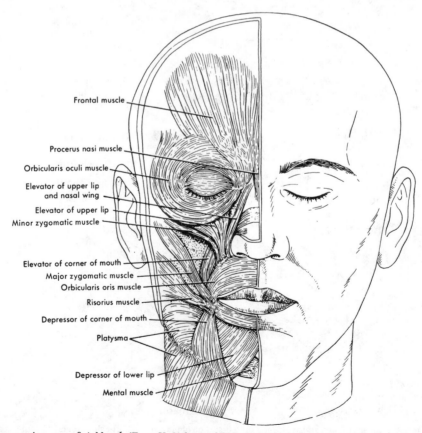

Frontal muscle

Procerus nasi muscle

Orbicularis oculi muscle

Elevator of upper lip
and nasal wing

Elevator of upper lip

Minor zygomatic muscle

Elevator of corner of mouth

Major zygomatic muscle

Orbicularis oris muscle

Risorius muscle

Depressor of corner of mouth

Platysma

Depressor of lower lip

Mental muscle

Muscles of facial expression, superficial layer. (From H. Sicher and E. L. DuBrul: Oral Anatomy. 7th ed., St. Louis, The C. V. Mosby Co., 1980; modified and redrawn from H. Sicher and J. Tandler: Anatomie für Zahnärzte. Vienna and Berlin, Springer, 1928.)

ocular m's, the six voluntary muscles that move the eyeball, including the superior, inferior, middle, and lateral recti, and the superior and inferior oblique muscles. Called also *musculi bulbi* [NA]. **extrinsic m.,** a muscle that does not arise in the same part in which it is inserted. **extrinsic m. of tongue,** m. of tongue, extrinsic. **m's of eyelid,** a group of facial muscles responsible for opening and closing the eyelids and for moving the eyebrows, thus producing the wrinkles of the forehead. They include the orbicular muscles of the eyes, levator muscles of the upper eyelids, and corrugator supercilii muscles. **facial m's, m's of facial expression,** a group of cutaneous muscles of the facial structures, which includes the muscles of the scalp, ear, eyelids, nose, and mouth, and the platysma. They generally arise from the fascia or bones of the face and insert into the skin. Embryologically, facial muscles derive from the second branchial, or hyoid arch. The facial nerve innervates all muscles in this group. Called also *m's of expression*. **fixation m., fixator m.,** one of the muscles that serves to hold a part of the body in a fixed or steady position. **flaccid m.,** hypotonic m. **frontal m.,** frontal belly of occipitofrontal muscle; see under BELLY. **fusiform m.,** a spindle-shaped muscle in which the fibers are approximately parallel to the long axis of the muscle but converge upon a tendon at either end. Called also *musculus fusiformis* [NA]. **genioglossus m., geniohyoglossus m.,** one of the paired extrinsic muscles of the tongue that arises from the mental tubercle or spine of the inner surface of the mandible. At their origin the right and left muscles blend together, but a short distance away, they separate. The anterior fibers insert into the tip of the tongue, the posterior reach its base, and the remaining ones fan out, inserting near the free dorsal surface. It protrudes and depresses the tongue. The hypoglossal nerve provides innervation. Called also *genioglossus, geniohyoglossus, musculus genioglossus* [NA], and *musculus geniohyoglossus*. **geniohyoid m.,** a thin suprahyoid muscle that arises above the anterior end of the mylohyoid line from the inner surface of the mandible and inserts into the anterior surface of the hyoid bone. It pulls the hyoid bone upward and forward or exerts a downward and backward pull on the mandible. A branch of the first cervical nerve, through the hypoglossal nerve, provides innervation. Called also *geniohyoideus* and *musculus geniohyoideus* [NA]. **glossopalatine m.,** palatoglossus m. **glossopharyngeal m.,** the part of the constrictor pharyngis superior muscle arising from the side of the root of the tongue. Called also *glossopharyngeus, musculus glossopharyngeus,* and *pars glossopharyngea musculi constrictoris pharyngis superioris* [NA]. **greater zygomatic m.,** zygomatic m., greater. **grinning m.,** risorius m. **heart m.,** myocardium. **Hilton's m.,** aryepiglottic m. **Horner's m.,** lacrimal part of orbicular muscle of eye; see under PART. **hyoglossal m.,** an extrinsic muscle of the tongue that arises from the upper border of the greater horn of the hyoid bone and parts of its body and inserts at the side of the tongue. It is a thin muscular plate with delicate fibers running straight upward into the tongue. Its function consists of depression and retraction of the tongue. The hypoglossal nerve provides innervation. The lingual artery runs deep to it. Called also *hyoglossus* and *musculus hyoglossus* [NA]. **m's of hyoid bone,** infrahyoid m's and suprahyoid m's. **hypertonic m.,** a muscle exhibiting increased passive resistance to stretching. In dentistry, the condition may accompany malocclusion or temporomandibular joint dysfunction. Hypertonicity and hyperreflexia of the trunk and limb musculature result from lesions of the pyramidal tract. Called also *spastic m.* **hypotonic m.,** a muscle exhibiting diminished passive resistance to stretching. Called also *flaccid m.* **incisive m. of lower lip,** a small facial muscle that arises from the mandible at the height of the canine eminence near the origin of the mental muscle and close to the alveolar border and runs toward the corner of the mouth, intermingling with other facial muscles. Its function is not well defined. It is innervated by the buccal branch of the facial nerve. Called also *incisivus labii inferioris* and *musculus incisivus labii inferioris*. **incisive m. of upper lip,** a small facial muscle that arises from the alveolar eminence of the canine near the alveolar crest and, after passing over the fornix of the upper vestibule, forms the lateral band of the orbicular muscle of the mouth, running toward the corner of the mouth. Its function is not well defined. It is innervated by the buccal branch of the facial nerve. Called also *incisivus labii superioris* and *musculus incisivus labii superioris*. **inferior constrictor m. of pharynx,** constrictor pharyngis inferior m. **inferior longitudinal m. of tongue,** longitudinal m. of tongue, inferior. **infrahyoid m's,** a group of muscles of the neck that extend between the hyoid bone above and the sternum, clavicle, and scapula below, and include the sternohyoid, sternothyrohyoid, thyrohoid, and omohyoid muscles. They participate in deglutition by depressing the larynx and the hyoid bone after

they have been drawn up with the pharynx, and in respiration by tensing the lower cervical fascia during the act of inspiration. Called also *ribbon m's* and *musculi infrahyoidei* [NA]. **intrinsic m.,** a muscle whose origin and insertion are both in the same part. **intrinsic m. of tongue,** m. of tongue, intrinsic. **involuntary m's,** smooth m. **laryngeal m's,** muscles of the larynx, especially the intrinsic muscles confined in the larynx, which open and close the glottis and regulate the degree of tension of the vocal folds. They include the cricothyroideus, cricoarytenoideus posterior and lateralis, arytenoideus, thyroarytenoideus, and vocalis muscles. **lesser zygomatic m.,** zygomatic m., lesser. **levator m. of angle of mouth,** a facial muscle presenting a deep muscular layer in the upper lip, which arises from the canine fossa of the maxilla and inserts into the orbicular muscle of the mouth and the skin at the angle of the mouth. It is innervated by the facial nerve. Its function consists of raising the angle of the mouth and pulling it medially. Called also *canine m., caninus, levator anguli oris, musculus levator anguli oris,* and *musculus levator anguli oris* [NA]. **levator menti m.,** mental m. **levator palati m.,** levator veli palatini m. **levator m. of thyroid gland,** an inconstant muscle arising on the isthmus or pyramid of the thyroid gland and inserting into the body of the hyoid bone. Called also *levator glandulae thyroideae* and *musculus levator glandulae thyroideae* [NA]. **levator m. of upper eyelid,** a muscle lying within the orbit, which arises from the orbital plate of the lesser wing of the sphenoid bone and inserts into the upper eyelid. It elevates the upper eyelid when contracted and permits it to close when relaxed. Innervation is provided by the oculomotor nerve. Called also *levator palpebrae superioris* and *musculus levator palpebrae superioris* [NA]. **levator m. of upper lip,** a muscle of facial expression arising along a broad line from the lower margin of the orbit immediately above the infraorbital foramen, with some fibers being attached to the maxilla and others to the zygomatic bone. The fibers pass the nasolabial sulcus and insert into the upper lip near the vermilion zone, some fibers being interlaced with those of the orbicular muscle of the mouth. Its functions consist of elevating the upper lip and moving it forward and dilating the nostril; together with the levator muscle of upper lip and ala of nose and the lesser zygomatic muscle, it participates in forming the nasolabial furrow. Innervation is provided by the buccal branches of the facial nerve. Called also *quadrate m. of upper lip, square m. of upper lip, levator labii superioris, musculus levator labii superioris* [NA], *musculus quadratus labii superioris,* and *quadratus labii superioris*. Formerly called *caput infraorbitale musculi quadrati labii superioris, infraorbital head of levator muscle of upper lip,* and *infraorbital head of quadratus labii superioris muscle* because it was once considered to be one of three heads of the levator muscle of the upper lip. **levator muscle of upper lip and ala of nose,** a muscle of facial expression arising from the upper part of the frontal process of the maxilla, which divides into two sections: one section inserts into the greater alar cartilage of the skin and the other extends into the lip where it joins the levator of the upper lip. Its functions consist of elevating the upper lip and corner of the mouth and dilating the nostril; together with the lesser zygomatic muscle and the levator muscle of upper lip, it participates in forming the nasolabial furrow. Innervation is provided by the buccal branches of the facial nerve. Called also *levator labii superioris alaeque nasi,* and *musculus levator labii superioris alaeque nasi* [NA]. Formerly called *angular head of levator muscle of upper lip, angular head of quadratus labii superioris muscle, caput angulare musculi quadrati labii superioris,* and *nasal head of levator labii superioris alaeque nasi muscle,* because it was once considered to be one of three heads of the levator muscle of the upper lip. **levator veli palatini m.,** a muscle of the palate situated lateral to the choanae and deep to the torus tubarius, which arises at the apex of the petrous portion of the temporal bone and cartilaginous part of the auditory tube and inserts into the aponeurosis of the soft palate. It is innervated by the pharyngeal plexus of the vagus nerve. It raises the soft palate. Called also *levator palati, levator veli palatini, musculus levator palati, musculus levator veli palatini* [NA], *petrosalpingostaphylinus,* and *petrostaphylinus*. **longissimus capitis m.,** longissimus m. of head. **longissimus m. of head,** a muscle that arises from the transverse processes of four or five upper thoracic vertebrae and inserts into the mastoid process of the temporal bone. It is innervated by the cervical nerve. Its function consists of rotating the head. Called also *longissimus capitis m., longissimus capitis,* and *musculus longissimus capitis* [NA]. **longitudinal**

m. of tongue, inferior, an intrinsic muscle, forming a narrow band, present on the inferior surface of the tongue beneath the mucosa. It arises under the surface at the base of the tongue and inserts at its tip, some fibers blending with the fibers of the styloglossus muscle and others being connected with the body of the hyoid bone. Its function consists of changing the shape of the tongue in mastication and deglutition. Called also *longitudinalis inferior linguae* and *musculus longitudinalis inferior linguae* [NA]. **longitudinal m. of tongue, superior,** an intrinsic muscle of the tongue, presenting a thin plaque immediately under the mucosa of the dorsum of the tongue, which arises from the submucosa and the septum of the tongue and inserts at the margins of the tongue. Its function consists of changing the shape of the tongue in mastication and deglutition. Called also *longitudinalis superior linguae* and *musculus longitudinalis superior linguae* [NA]. **major zygomatic m.,** zygomatic m., major. **masseter m.,** a quadrilateral superficial muscle of mastication that is partially divided into superficial and deep portions (*pars superficialis* and *pars profunda*). The larger superficial portion arises from the lower border of the zygomatic bone by a fibrous aponeurosis and inserts into the angle and the lower border of the ramus of the mandible. The smaller deep portion arises from the lower border and medial surface of the zygomatic arch and inserts into the upper half of the ramus and lateral surface of the coronoid process of the mandible. It elevates the mandible. Innervation is provided by the masseteric nerve from the mandibular division of the trigeminal nerve. Called also *masseter* and *musculus masseter* [NA]. **m's of mastication,** a group of muscles responsible for the movement of the jaws during the process of mastication. They include the masseter, temporal, and medial and lateral pterygoid muscles. All are innervated by the mandibular division of the trigeminal nerve. **mental m., mentalis m.,** a small conical facial muscle that arises from the incisive fossa of the mandible, inserts into the integument of the chin, and is innervated by the facial nerve. Its function consists of assisting in raising and protruding the lower lip and wrinkling the skin of the chin. Called also *chin m.,* *levator menti m.,* *levator menti,* *musculus levator menti,* and *musculus mentalis* [NA]. **Merkel's m.,** ceratocricoid m. **middle constrictor m. of pharynx,** constrictor pharyngis medius m. **minor zygomatic m.,** zygomatic m., lesser. **m's of mouth,** a group of facial muscles responsible for closing and opening of the mouth and for generation of wrinkles and furrows around the mouth in facial expression. They include the levator muscle of the angle of the mouth, levator muscle of the upper lip, zygomatic muscle, risorius muscle, depressor muscle of the lower lip, depressor muscle of the angle of the lip, mental muscle, transverse muscle of the chin, orbicular muscle of the mouth, and buccinator muscle. **multipenniform m.,** a muscle in which the fasciculi converge like the plumes of feathers toward several tendons. Called also *musculus multipennatus.* **multiunit smooth m.,** see *smooth m.* **mylohyoid m.,** a suprahyoid flat and triangular muscle that, with its fellow of the opposite side, forms the floor of the mouth. It arises along the mylohyoid line of the mandible, the posterior fibers originating from the region of the alveolus of the lower third molar, and inserts into the hyoid bone and median raphe. It participates in the acts of mastication, deglutition, sucking, and blowing by raising the hyoid bone and tongue. The mylohyoid nerve from the inferior alveolar branch of the mandibular division of the trigeminal nerve provides innervation. Called also *diaphragm of mouth, diaphragma oris, musculus mylohyoideus* [NA], *mylohyoideus,* and *oral diaphragm.* **mylopharyngeal m.,** the part of the constrictor pharyngis superior muscle arising from the mylohyoid ridge of the mandible. Called also *musculus mylopharyngeus, mylopharyngeus,* and *pars mylopharyngea musculi constrictoris pharyngis superioris* [NA]. **nasal m.,** a facial muscle consisting of a transverse part, which arises from the maxilla and passes over the lower part of the bridge of the nose to join the nasal muscle of the opposite side, and an alar part, which is attached to the greater alar cartilage on one end and to the integument at the point of the nose at the other end. It is innervated by the buccal branch of the facial nerve. Its function consists of dilating the nasal opening and widening and flattening the nose. Called also *musculus nasalis* [NA]. **nasolabial m.,** a small facial muscle that forms the medial band of the orbicular muscle of the mouth and connects the upper lip to the septum of the nose. It is innervated by the buccal branch of the facial nerve. Called also *musculus nasolabialis.* **nonstriated m.,** smooth m. **m's of nose,** a group of facial muscles

responsible for dilating and constricting the nares during respiratory processes and producing transverse wrinkles over the bridge of the nose. They include the procerus muscle, nasal muscle, and depressor muscle of the nasal septum. All are innervated by the buccal branches of the facial nerve. **occipital m.,** occipital belly of occipitofrontal muscle; see under BELLY. **occipitofrontal m.,** the muscular covering of the scalp and a part of the epicranial muscle, which extends from the occipital bone to the eyebrows and is made up of the occipital and frontal bellies, joined together by the epicranial aponeurosis, and the temporoparietal muscle. Called also *musculus occipitofrontalis* [NA]. **omohyoid m.,** a long, narrow, two-bellied infrahyoid muscle. The inferior belly runs obliquely upward and forward, crossing the posterior triangle of the neck, and unites with the superior belly by a central tendon. The superior belly runs upward and forward to the inferior border of the hyoid bone. It arises from the cranial border of the scapula and inserts into the caudal border of the hyoid bone, and draws the hyoid bone caudalward. Branches of the cervical loop (*ansa cervicalis*), containing fibers of the second and third and possibly first cervical nerves provide innervation. Called also *musculus omohyoideus* [NA] and *omohyoideus.* **orbicular m.,** a muscle that encircles a body opening, such as the eye or the mouth. Called also *musculus orbicularis* [NA] and *orbicularis.* **orbicular m., of eye,** an oval facial muscle which arises from the nasal part of the frontal bone and the medial palpebral ligament and surrounds the eyelid. It consists of the palpebral part, which arises from the medial palpebral ligament and is inserted into the lateral palpebral raphe; the lacrimal part, which arises from the orbital surface of the lacrimal bone and is inserted into the tarsal cartilage; and the orbital part, which blends with the frontal belly of the occipitofrontal and corrugator muscles. Fibers inserted into the eyebrow and responsible for its drawing downward are known as the *superciliary depressor muscle.* It is innervated by the temporal and zygomatic branches of the facial nerve. Its function consists of opening and closing the eyelids. Called also *musculus orbicularis oculi* [NA], *musculus orbicularis palpebrarum, sphincter of eye,* and *sphincter of eyelid.* **orbicular m. of mouth,** a facial muscle which occupies the entire width of the lips and consists of numerous fibers running in different directions and interlacing with each other, some deriving from other facial muscles. In a strict sense it represents a functional, but not anatomical, unit. Fibers of the orbicular muscle arise from and insert into different facial structures. Their function consists of serving as a sphincter muscle which closes and protrudes the mouth and keeps food on the occlusal surfaces of the teeth in the region of the lips. It is innervated by buccal branches of the facial nerve. Called also *musculus orbicularis oris* [NA], *orbicularis ortis,* and *sphincter oris.* **orbital m.,** a muscle of the orbital area, which arises from the orbital periosteum and inserts into the fascia of the inferior orbital fissure. It is innervated by the sympathetic fibers. Its function consists of protruding the eye. Called also *musculus orbitalis* [NA] and *orbitalis.* **palatoglossus m.,** an extrinsic muscle of the tongue, which arises under the surface of the soft palate and inserts at the side of the tongue, and helps in elevating the tongue and constricting the fauces. It is innervated by the pharyngeal plexus of the vagus nerve. Called also *glossopalatine m., glossopalatinus, musculus glossopalatinus, musculus palatoglossus* [NA], and *palatoglossus.* **palatopharyngeal m.,** a fleshy muscle of the palate that, together with the mucosa covering it, forms the palatopharyngeal arch. It arises from the soft palate, where it divides into two fasciculi. The posterior fasciculus lies in contact with the mucous membrane and joins with its fellow of the opposite side. The thicker anterior fasciculus lies in the soft palate and joins in the middle line with its fellow of the opposite side. It is inserted with the stylopharyngeal muscle into the posterior border of the thyroid cartilage. The pharyngeal plexus of the vagus nerve provides innervation. It aids in deglutition. Called also *pharyngopalatine m., musculus palatopharyngeus* [NA], *musculus pharyngopalatinus, palatopharyngeus,* and *pharyngopalatinus.* **penniform m.,** a muscle in which the fasciculi converge, like the plumes of a feather, to one side of the tendon and run the entire length of the muscle. Called also *musculus unipennatus* [NA] and *unipennate muscle.* **pharyngopalatine m.,** palatopharyngeal m. **platysma m.,** platysma. **procerus m.,** a slender pyramidal muscle of the nose, which arises from the fascia covering the nasal bone and upper part of the lateral nasal cartilage, inserts into the skin between the eyebrows, and is innervated by the buccal branch of the facial nerve. Its function consists of drawing the medial angles of the eyebrows down and producing transverse wrinkles across the root of the nose in facial expression. Called also *musculus procerus* [NA] and *procerus.* **m.**

protein, muscle PROTEIN. **pterygoid m., external,** pterygoid m., lateral. **pterygoid m., internal,** pterygoid m., medial. **pterygoid m., lateral,** a short, conical muscle of mastication that arises with two heads: the upper head originates on the lateral surface of the great wing of the sphenoid bone and the infratemporal crest; the lower head originates on the lateral surface of the lateral pterygoid plate. It inserts into a depression in the anterior part of the neck of the condyle of the mandible and the temporomandibular joint capsule. Its function consists of opening the jaws, protruding the mandible, and moving the mandible from side to side. The lateral pterygoid nerve from the mandibular division of the trigeminal nerve provides innervation. Called also *external pterygoid muscle, musculus pterygoideus externus, musculus pterygoideus lateralis* [NA], *pterygoideus externus,* and *pterygoideus lateralis.* **pterygoid m., medial,** a thick square muscle of mastication that occupies the medial side of the ramus of the mandible, which arises from the lateral pterygoid plate and the grooved surface of the pyramidal process of the palatine bone. It inserts into a triangular area on the medial surface of the ramus and angle of the mandible. Its function consists of elevation of the mandible. The medial pterygoid nerve from the mandibular division of the trigeminal nerve provides innervation. Called also *internal pterygoid m., musculus pterygoideus internus, musculus pterygoideus medialis* [NA], *pterygoideus internus,* and *pterygoideus medialis.* **pterygopharyngeal m.,** the part of the constrictor pharyngis superioris muscle arising from the caudal part and hamulus of the medial pterygoid plate. Called also *musculus pterygopharyngeus, pars pterygopharyngea musculi constrictoris pharyngis superioris* [NA], and *pterygopharyngeus.* **quadrate m. of lower lip,** depressor m. of lower lip. **quadrate m. of upper lip,** levator m. of upper lip. **radiated m.,** a muscle in which the fasciculi converge to a narrow tendinous point. **rectus capitis anterior m.,** a muscle of the neck that arises from the atlas and inserts into the basilar process of the occipital bone. It is innervated by the first and second cervical nerves. Its function consists of flexing and supporting the head. Called also *musculus rectus capitis anterior* [NA], and *rectus capitis anterior.* **rectus capitis lateralis m.,** a muscle at the side of the neck that arises from the atlas and inserts into the jugular process of the occipital bone. It is innervated by the first and second nerves. Its function consists of flexing and supporting the head. Called also *musculus rectus capitis lateralis* [NA] and *rectus capitis lateralis.* **rectus capitis posterior major m.,** a muscle of the neck that arises from the axis and inserts into the occipital bone. It is innervated by the suboccipital nerve. Its action consists of extending the head. Called also *musculus rectus capitis posterior major* [NA] and *rectus capitis posterior major.* **rectus capitis posterior minor m.,** a muscle of the neck that arises from the atlas and inserts into the occipital bone. The suboccipital nerve provides innervation. Its function consists of extending the head. Called also *musculus rectus capitis posterior minor* [NA] and *rectus capitis posterior minor.* **m. relaxant,** muscle RELAXANT. **ribbon m's,** infrahyoid m's. **Riolan's m.,** palpebral part of orbicular muscle of eye; see under PART. **risorius m.,** a triangular facial muscle that arises from the fascia of the masseter muscle and inserts into the skin at the angle of the mouth. It is innervated by the buccal branch of the facial nerve. Its function consists of pulling the corner of the mouth laterally in grinning expression. Called also *Albinus' m., grinning m., smiling m., musculus risorius* [NA], and *risorius.* **salpingopharyngeal m.,** a muscle of the pharynx that arises from the auditory tube near its orifice and inserts in the posterior part of the palatopharyngeal muscle. The pharyngeal plexus of the vagus nerve provides innervation. Its function consists of raising the nasopharynx in deglutition. Called also *musculus salpingopharyngeus* [NA] and *salpingopharyngeus.* **m's of scalp,** the muscular covering of the skull; the epicranial muscles. See *occipitofrontal m.* and *temporoparietal m.* **skeletal m's,** striated muscles attached to bones and typically cross at least one joint. Called also *musculi skeleti* [NA]. See *striated m.* **smiling m.,** risorius m. **smooth m.,** a type of muscle without transverse striations, having spindle-shaped fibers, each with a single rod-shaped nucleus. It is sometimes divided into *multiunit smooth muscle* and *visceral smooth muscle* (also known as *unitary smooth muscle*). The multiunit type is found in blood vessels and in the iris, and is composed of discrete smooth muscle fibers about 100 to 200 microns in length and 10 microns in diameter; this type contracts only when stimulated by a nerve. The visceral type is found in most visceral organs of the body and is composed of smooth muscle fibers that are crowded together; when one fiber is stimulated, the impulse is conducted to the surrounding fibers by ephaptic conduction. Smooth muscle is innervated by nerves from the

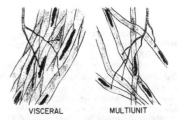

VISCERAL   MULTIUNIT

Visceral and smooth muscle. (From A. C. Guyton: Textbook of Medical Physiology. 6th ed. Philadelphia, W. B. Saunders Co., 1981.)

autonomic nervous system, composed mainly of unmyelinated fibers, and is subject to autonomic nerve impulses, rather than the voluntary control of the striated muscles. Called also *involuntary m., nonstriated m.,* and *unstriated m.* See illustration. **somatic m.,** striated m. **m. spasm,** see SPASM (1). **spastic m.,** hypertonic m. **sphincter m.,** sphincter. **spinalis capitis m.,** a muscle of the neck that arises from the cervical vertebrae and inserts into the occipital bone. It is innervated by the spinal nerves. Its function consists of extending the head. Called also *musculus spinalis capitis* [NA]. **splenius capitis m.,** a muscle which rotates the head, arising from the back of the neck and spinal vertebrae and inserting into the occipital bone. It is innervated by the middle and lower cervical nerves. Called also *musculus splenius capitis* [NA]. **square m. of lower lip,** depressor m. of lower lip. **square m. of upper lip,** levator m. of upper lip. **sternocleidomastoid m.,** a muscle of the neck that rotates the head. One of its heads arises from the sternum and the other from the clavicle, inserting into the superior nuchal line of the occipital bone. The accessory nerve and the cervical plexus provide innervation. Called also *musculus sternocleidomastoideus* [NA], *sternomastoid muscle,* and *sternocleidomastoideus.* **sternohyoid m.,** a thin infrahyoid muscle that arises from a line extending from the lateral part of the inner surface of the sternum and inserts by a short tendon into the inferior border of the hyoid bone. The right and left muscles separate widely at the origin but merge in the middle of their course and lie side by side. Its function consists of drawing the hyoid bone inferiorly. The ansa cervicalis from the first, second, and third cervical nerves provides innervation. Called also *musculus sternohyoideus* [NA] and *sternohyoideus.* **sternomastoid m.,** sternocleidomastoid m. **sternothyroid m.,** a muscle of the neck that arises from the sternum and inserts into the thyroid cartilage. It is innervated by the ansa cervicalis. Its function consists of depressing the thyroid cartilage. Called also *musculus sternothyroideus* [NA] and *sternothyroideus.* **strap m's,** muscles of the anterior neck, particularly those of the thyroid cartilage and hyoid bone. **striated m.,** a muscle characterized by cross striations. Striated muscles are responsible for voluntary movements of the body and are generally attached to the skeletal structures by tendons (in which case they are called *skeletal muscles*). Some striated muscles, such as those of facial expression, are attached to the skin and other nonskeletal structures. A striated muscle is made up of bundles of fibers, or fasciculi, and covered by a thin layer of connective tissue (epimysium). Connective tissue septa (endomysium) divides the fasciculi. Each fasciculus contains a number of parallel fibers which consist of several thousand myofibrils which, in turn, are formed by parallel bundles of myofilaments arranged into sarcomeres, the contractile units of the muscle. Actin and myosin filaments are the structural components of the myofilaments. Called also *cross striated m., somatic m., striped m.,* and *voluntary m.* **styloglossus m.,** an extrinsic muscle of the tongue that arises from the styloid process and inserts at the margin of the tongue. Its function consists of raising and retracting the tongue. The hypoglossal nerve provides innervation. Called also *musculus styloglossus* [NA] and *styloglossus.* **stylohyoid m.,** a slender suprahyoid muscle that arises from the styloid process and inserts into the hyoid bone. A tendon of the digastric muscle perforates it near insertion. It draws the hyoid bone and the tongue upward. A branch of the facial nerve provides innervation. Called also *musculus stylohyoideus* [NA] and *stylohyoideus.* **stylopharyngeal m.,** a long, slender muscle of the pharynx that arises from the styloid process. After passing downward, some of its fibers merge with those of the constrictor muscles and others join the palatopharyngeal muscle and insert into the posterior border of the thyroid cartilage. Innervation is provided by the glossopharyngeal nerve. Its function consists of raising and dilating the pharynx in swallowing. Called also *musculus stylopharyngeus* [NA] and *stylopharyngeus*. **superior constrictor m. of pharynx,** constrictor pharyngis superior m. **superior longitudinal m. of tongue,** longitudinal m. of tongue, superior. **suprahyoid m's,** a group of muscles that attach the hyoid bone to the skull and are located between the skull and the mandible and the hyoid bone, including the digastric, geniohyoid, mylohyoid, and stylohyoid muscles. Their function consists of elevating the hyoid bone and, with it, the larynx or depressing the mandible. Called also *musculi suprahyoidei* [NA]. **synergic m., synergistic m.,** one of the muscles that assists another in performing an action. Called also *synergist*. **temporal m.,** a fan-shaped muscle of mastication which covers the temporal area; it arises in a wide field on the lateral surface of the skull from the temporal fossa and the deep surface of the temporal fascia. Fibers converge downward toward a tendon which inserts into the medial surface, apex, and anterior border of the coronoid process, and the anterior border of the ramus of the mandible near the molar tooth. It elevates and retracts the mandible. The deep temporal nerves from the mandibular division of the trigeminal nerve provide innervation. Called also *musculus temporalis* [NA] and *temporalis*. **temporoparietal m.,** a thin, flat and broad sheet of muscular tissue spreading over the temporal fascia; it arises from the temporal fascia anterior to the ear and inserts into the lateral border of the epicranial aponeurosis. Its functions include tightening the scalp, drawing back the skin of the temples, wrinkling the forehead, and widening the eyes in the production of facial expressions. It is innervated by the temporal branch of the facial nerve. Called also *musculus temporoparietalis* [NA]. **tensor palati m.,** tensor veli palatini m. **tensor veli palatini m.,** a thin muscle of the palate that arises from the scaphoid fossa at the base of the medial pterygoid plate, from the spine of the sphenoid, and from the lateral wall of the auditory tube, and inserts into the palatine aponeurosis and into the surface behind the transverse ridge of the horizontal part of the palatine bone. It is innervated by the mandibular division of the trigeminal nerve. Its function consists of tensing the soft palate and opening the auditory tube. Called also *tensor palati m., musculus tensor palati, musculus tensor veli palatini* [NA], *tensor palati,* and *tensor veli palatini*. **thyroarytenoid m., thyroarytenoideus m.,** a broad thin intrinsic muscle of the larynx that arises from the caudal half of the angle of the thyroid cartilage and from the middle cricothyroid ligament and inserts into the base and anterior surface of the arytenoid cartilage. Its medial fibers form the vocal muscle and are inserted into the vocal process of the arytenoid cartilage. The recurrent laryngeal nerve provides innervation. Its function consists of shortening and relaxing the vocal folds and narrowing the rima of the glottis. Called also *musculus thyroarytenoideus* [NA] and *thyroarytenoideus*. **thyroepiglottic m., thyroepiglotticus m.,** a muscle composed of fibers of the thyroarytenoid muscle which are prolonged into the aryepiglottic fold and continue to the margin of the epiglottis. It arises from the lamina of the thyroid cartilage and inserts into the epiglottis. The recurrent laryngeal nerve provides innervation. Its function consists of closing the inlet to the larynx. Called also *musculus thyroepiglotticus* [NA] and *thyroepiglotticus*. **thyrohyoid m.,** a small, square infrathyroid muscle that arises from the oblique line of the thyroid cartilage and inserts into the lateral part of the body and the medial part of the greater horn of the hyoid bone. It draws the hyoid bone inferiorly and draws the thyroid cartilage superiorly in raising and changing the form of the larynx. Fibers from the first and probably second cervical nerves provide innervation. Called also *musculus thyrohyoideus* [NA] and *thyrohyoideus*. **thyropharyngeal m.,** the part of the constrictor pharyngis inferior muscle arising from the thyroid cartilage. Called also *musculus thyropharyngeus, pars thyropharyngea musculi constrictoris pharyngis inferioris* [NA], and *thyropharyngeus*. **m. of tongue, extrinsic,** any of a group of five muscles of the tongue which have their origin outside the tongue, including the genioglossus, hyoglossus, chondroglossus, styloglossus, and palatoglossus muscles. **m. of tongue, intrinsic,** any of a group of muscles which are contained entirely within the tongue, including the inferior and superior longitudinal, transverse, and vertical muscles of the tongue. **m.**

tonus, muscle TONUS. **m. of tragus,** a short, flattened vertical band on the lateral surface of the tragus, innervated by the auriculotemporal and posterior auricular nerves. Called also *musculus tragicus* [NA]. **transverse m. of chin,** a small facial muscle occurring only in 50 percent of the population; it is formed by superficial fibers of the depressor muscle of the angle of the mouth which turn back and cross to the opposite side. Called also *musculus transversus menti* [NA]. **transverse m. of nape,** a thin muscle present in about 25 percent of the population, arising from the external occipital protuberance or from the superior nuchal line and inserts with the posterior auricular muscle or joins the posterior edge of the sternocleidomastoid muscle. It may be either superficial or deep to the trapezius. Called also *musculus occipitalis minor, musculus transversus nuchae* [NA], and *occipitalis minor*. **transverse m. of tongue,** an intrinsic muscle that arises from the fibrous septum of the tongue and inserts into the submucous fibrous tissue at the dorsum and margins of the tongue. It is innervated by the hypoglossal nerve. Its function consists of changing the shape of the tongue in mastication and deglutition. Called also *musculus transversus linguae* [NA] and *transversus linguae*. **triangular m.,** depressor m. of angle of mouth. **m. trimming,** border MOLDING. **unipennate m.,** penniform m. **unitary smooth m.,** see *smooth m.* **unstriated m.,** smooth m. **m. of uvula,** a muscle that arises from the posterior nasal spine of the palatine bone and aponeurosis of the soft palate and inserts into the uvula. The pharyngeal plexus of the vagus nerve provides innervation. Its function consists of raising the uvula. Called also *musculus uvulae* [NA]. **ventricularis m.,** fibers of the thyroarytenoid muscle which run into the vestibular fold at the side of the epiglottis. Called also *musculus ventricularis* and *ventricularis*. **vertical m. of tongue,** an intrinsic muscle of the tongue that arises from the dorsal fascia of the tongue and inserts at the sides and base of the tongue. It is innervated by the hypoglossal nerve. Its function consists of changing the shape of the tongue in mastication and deglutition. Called also *musculus verticalis linguae* [NA] and *verticalis linguae*. **visceral smooth m.,** see *smooth m.* **vocal m., vocalis m.,** a band of medial fibers of the thyroarytenoid muscle that arises from the thyroid cartilage and inserts into the vocal process of the arytenoid cartilage. It is innervated by the recurrent laryngeal nerve. Its function consists of shortening the vocal folds. Called also *musculus vocalis* [NA] and *vocalis*. **voluntary m.,** striated m. **zygomatic m.,** zygomatic m., greater. **zygomatic m., greater,** one of the principal muscles of facial expression situated in the middle face, which arises from the frontal process of the zygomatic bone, its flat band running downward and forward to the corner of the mouth, where it may be divided by the canine muscle into superficial and deep parts. It is generally inserted at the level of the corner of the mouth but some fibers may extend into the mucous membrane of the lower lip. A buccal branch of the facial nerve provides innervation. It pulls the corner of the mouth upward and laterally in laughing. Called also *zygomatic m., zygomaticus major m., musculus zygomaticus, musculus zygomaticus major* [NA], *zygomaticus,* and *zygomaticus major*. **zygomatic m., lesser, zygomatic m., minor,** a muscle of facial expression, which is the weakest and most variable of the superficial muscles of the upper lip. It arises from the malar surface of the zygomatic bone behind the zygomaticomaxillary suture and inserts into the upper lip near the midline somewhat below or at the side of the ala of the nose. In some instances, its fibers may be replaced by those of the orbicular muscle of the eye; sometimes the lesser zygomatic muscle is missing completely. Its functions consist of elevating the upper lip and dilating and nostril; together with the levator muscle of upper lip and the levator muscle of upper lip and ala of nose; it participates in forming the nasolabial furrow. Called also *zygomaticus minor m.* and *musculus zygomaticus minor* [NA]. Formerly called *caput zygomaticum musculi quadrati labii superioris, zygomatic head of levator muscle of upper lip,* and *zygomatic head of quadratus labii superioris muscle* because it was once considered to be one of three heads of the levator muscle of the upper lip. **zygomaticus major m.,** zygomatic m., greater. **zygomaticus minor m.,** zygomatic m., lesser.

muscular (mus′ku-lar) [L. *muscularis*] 1. pertaining to or composing muscle. 2. having a well-developed musculature.

muscularis (mus″ku-la′ris) [L.] 1. muscular; pertaining to muscles. 2. pertaining to the tunica muscularis.

musculature (mus′ku-lah-chur) the muscular apparatus of the body or a part.

musculi (mus′ku-li) [L.] plural of *musculus*.

musculo- [L. *musculus* muscle] a combining form denoting a relationship to a muscle.

musculocutaneous (mus″ku-lo-ku-ta′ne-us) pertaining to the muscles and skin.

musculoskeletal (mus″ku-lo-skel′ĕ-tal) pertaining to or comprising the skeleton and the muscles, as musculoskeletal system.

musculotendinous (mus″ku-lo-ten′dī-nus) pertaining to muscles and tendons.

musculotonic (mus″ku-lo-ton′ik) pertaining to muscular contractility.

musculotropic (mus″ku-lo-trop′ik) having a special affinity for or exerting its principal effect upon muscle tissue.

musculus (mus′ku-lus), pl. *mus′culi* [L., dim. of *mus* mouse, because of a fancied resemblance to a mouse of a muscle moving under the skin] [NA] an organ that has the power to contract. See also MUSCLE. **m. articula′ris** [NA], articular MUSCLE. **m. aryepiglot′ticus** [NA], aryepiglottic MUSCLE. **m. arytenoi′deus**, arytenoid MUSCLE. **m. arytenoi′deus obli′quus** [NA], arytenoid muscle, oblique; see under MUSCLE. **m. arytenoi′deus transver′sus** [NA], arytenoid muscle, transverse; see under MUSCLE. **m. attol′lens au′rem**, auricular muscle, superior; see under MUSCLE. **m. attra′hens au′rem**, auricular muscle, anterior; see under MUSCLE. **m. auricula′ris ante′rior** [NA], auricular muscle, anterior; see under MUSCLE. **m. auricula′ris poste′rior** [NA], auricular muscle, posterior; see under MUSCLE. **m. auricula′ris supe′rior** [NA], auricular muscle, superior; see under MUSCLE. **m. bipenna′tus** [NA], bipennate MUSCLE. **m. buccina′tor** [NA], buccinator MUSCLE. **m. buccopharyn′geus**, buccopharyngeal MUSCLE. **mus′culi bul′bi** [NA], extraocular muscles; see under MUSCLE. **m. cani′nus**, levator muscle of angle of mouth; see under MUSCLE. **m. ceratocricoi′deus** [NA], ceratocricoid MUSCLE. **m. ceratopharyn′geus**, ceratopharyngeal MUSCLE. **m. chondroglos′sus** [NA], chondroglossus MUSCLE. **m. chondropharyn′geus**, chondropharyngeal MUSCLE. **m. compres′sor na′ris**, transverse part of nasal muscle; see under PART. **m. constric′tor pharyn′gis infe′rior** [NA], constrictor pharyngis inferior MUSCLE. **m. constric′tor pharyn′gis medius** [NA], constrictor pharyngis medius MUSCLE. **m. constric′tor pharyn′gis supe′rior** [NA], constrictor pharyngis superior MUSCLE. **m. corruga′tor supercil′ii** [NA], corrugator supercilii MUSCLE. **m. cricoarytenoi′deus latera′lis** [NA], cricoarytenoid muscle, lateral; see under MUSCLE. **m. cricoarytenoi′deus poste′rior** [NA], cricoarytenoid muscle, posterior; see under MUSCLE. **m. cricopharyn′geus**, cricopharyngeal MUSCLE. **m. cricothyroi′deus** [NA], cricothyroid MUSCLE. **m. cuta′neus** [NA], cutaneous MUSCLE. **m. depres′sor a′lae na′si**, depressor muscle of nasal septum; see under MUSCLE. **m. depres′sor an′guli o′ris** [NA], depressor muscle of angle of mouth; see under MUSCLE. **m. depres′sor la′bii inferio′ris** [NA], depressor muscle of lower lip; see under MUSCLE. **m. depres′sor sep′ti na′si** [NA], depressor muscle of nasal septum; see under MUSCLE. **m. depres′sor supercil′ii** [NA], depressor muscle, superciliary; see under MUSCLE. **m. digas′tricus** [NA], digastric MUSCLE. **m. dila′tor na′ris**, **m. dilata′tor na′ris**, alar part of nasal muscle; see under PART. **m. epicra′nius** [NA], epicranial MUSCLE. **m. fronta′lis**, frontal belly of occipitofrontal muscle; see under BELLY. **m. fusifor′mis** [NA], fusiform MUSCLE. **m. genioglos′sus** [NA], **m. geniohyoglos′sus**, genioglossus MUSCLE. **m. geniohyoi′deus** [NA], geniohyoid MUSCLE. **m. glossopalati′nus**, palatoglossus MUSCLE. **m. glossopharyn′geus**, glossopharyngeal MUSCLE. **m. hyoglos′sus** [NA], hyoglossal MUSCLE. **m. incisi′vus la′bii inferio′ris**, incisive muscle of lower lip; see under MUSCLE. **m. incisi′vus la′bii superio′ris**, incisive muscle of upper lip; see under MUSCLE. **mus′culi infrahyoi′dei** [NA], infrahyoid muscles; see under MUSCLE. **m. leva′tor an′guli o′ris** [NA], levator muscle of angle of mouth; see under MUSCLE. **m. leva′tor glan′dulae thyroi′deae** [NA], levator muscle of thyroid gland; see under MUSCLE. **m. leva′tor la′bii superio′ris**, levator muscle of upper lip; see under MUSCLE. **m. leva′tor la′bii superio′ris alae′que na′si** [NA], levator muscle of upper lip and ala of nose; see under MUSCLE. **m. leva′tor men′ti**, mental MUSCLE. **m. leva′tor pala′ti**, levator veli palatine MUSCLE. **m. leva′tor pal′pebrae superio′ris** [NA], levator muscle of upper eyelid; see under MUSCLE. **m. leva′tor ve′li palati′ni** [NA], levator veli palatini MUSCLE. **m. longis′simus cap′itis** [NA], longissimus muscle of head; see under MUSCLE. **m. longitudina′lis infe′rior lin′guae** [NA], longitudinal muscle of tongue, inferior; see under MUSCLE. **m. longitudina′lis supe′rior lin′guae** [NA], longitudinal muscle of tongue, superior; see under MUSCLE. **m. masse′ter** [NA], masseter MUSCLE. **m. menta′lis** [NA], mentalis MUSCLE. **m. multipenna′tus**, multipenniform MUSCLE. **m. mylohyoi′deus** [NA], mylohyoid MUSCLE. **m. mylopharyn′geus**, mylopharyngeal MUSCLE. **m. nasa′lis** [NA], nasal MUSCLE. **m. nasolabia′lis**, nasolabial MUSCLE. **m. occipita′lis**, occipital belly of occipitofrontal muscle; see under BELLY. **m. occipita′lis mi′nor**, transverse muscle of nape; see under MUSCLE. **m. occipitofronta′lis** [NA], occipitofrontal MUSCLE. **m. omohyoi′deus** [NA], omohyoid MUSCLE. **m. orbicula′ris** [NA], orbicular MUSCLE. **m. orbicula′ris oc′uli** [NA], **m. orbicula′ris palpebra′rum**, orbic-

ular muscle of eye; see under MUSCLE. **m. orbicula′ris o′ris** [NA], orbicular muscle of mouth; see under MUSCLE. **m. orbita′lis** [NA], orbital MUSCLE. **m. palatoglos′sus** [NA], palatoglossus MUSCLE. **m. palatopharyn′geus** [NA], palatopharyngeal MUSCLE. **m. pharyngopalati′nus**, palatopharyngeal MUSCLE. **m. proce′rus** [NA], procerus MUSCLE. **m. pterygoi′deus exter′nus**, pterygoid muscle, lateral; see under MUSCLE. **m. pterygoi′deus inter′nus**, pterygoid muscle, medial; see under MUSCLE. **m. pterygoi′deus latera′lis** [NA], pterygoid muscle, lateral; see under MUSCLE. **m. pterygoi′deus media′lis** [NA], pterygoid muscle, medial; see under MUSCLE. **m. pterygopharyn′geus**, pterygopharyngeal MUSCLE. **m. quadra′tus la′bii inferio′ris**, depressor muscle of lower lip; see under MUSCLE. **m. quadra′tus la′bii superio′ris**, levator muscle of upper lip; see under MUSCLE. **m. quadra′tus men′ti**, depressor muscle of lower lip; see under MUSCLE. **m. rec′tus cap′itis ante′rior** [NA], rectus capitis anterior MUSCLE. **m. rec′tus cap′itis latera′lis** [NA], rectus capitis lateralis MUSCLE. **m. rec′tus cap′itis poste′rior ma′jor** [NA], rectus capitis posterior MUSCLE. **m. rec′tus cap′itis poste′rior mi′nor** [NA], rectus capitis posterior minor MUSCLE. **m. retra′hens au′rem**, auricular muscle, posterior; see under MUSCLE. **m. riso′rius** [NA], risorius MUSCLE. **m. salpingopharyn′geus** [NA], salpingopharyngeal MUSCLE. **mus′culi skel′eti** [NA], skeletal MUSCLE. **m. sphinc′ter** [NA], sphincter. **m. spina′lis cap′itis** [NA], spinalis capitis MUSCLE. **m. sple′nius cap′itis** [NA], splenius capitis MUSCLE. **m. sternocleidomastoi′deus** [NA], sternocleidomastoid MUSCLE. **m. sternohyoi′deus** [NA], sternohyoid MUSCLE. **m. sternothyroi′deus**, [NA], sternothyroid MUSCLE. **m. styloglos′sus** [NA], styloglossus MUSCLE. **m. stylohyoi′deus** [NA], stylohyoid MUSCLE. **m. stylopharyn′geus** [NA], stylopharyngeal MUSCLE. **mus′culi suprahyoi′dei** [NA], suprahyoid muscles; see under MUSCLE. **m. tempora′lis** [NA], temporal MUSCLE. **m. temporoparieta′lis** [NA], temporoparietal MUSCLE. **m. ten′sor pala′ti**, tensor veli palatini MUSCLE. **m. ten′sor tar′si**, lacrimal part of orbicular muscle of eye; see under PART. **m. ten′sor ve′li palati′ni** [NA], tensor veli palatini MUSCLE. **m. thyroarytenoi′deus** [NA], thyroarytenoid MUSCLE. **m. thyroepiglot′ticus** [NA], thyroepiglottic MUSCLE. **m. thyrohyoi′deus** [NA], thyrohyoid MUSCLE. **m. thyropharyn′geus**, thyropharyngeal MUSCLE. **m. trag′icus** [NA], MUSCLE of tragus. **m. transver′sus lin′guae** [NA], transverse muscle of tongue; see under MUSCLE. **m. transver′sus men′ti** [NA], transverse muscle of chin; see under MUSCLE. **m. transver′sus nu′chae** [NA], transverse muscle of nape; see under MUSCLE. **m. triangula′ris**, depressor muscle of angle of mouth; see under MUSCLE. **m. unipenna′tus** [NA], penniform MUSCLE. **m. u′vulae** [NA], MUSCLE of uvula. **m. ventricula′ris**, ventricularis MUSCLE. **m. vertica′lis lin′guae** [NA], vertical muscle of tongue; see under MUSCLE. **m. voca′lis** [NA], vocal MUSCLE. **m. zygomat′icus**, zygomatic muscle, greater; see under MUSCLE. **m. zygomat′icus ma′jor** [NA], zygomatic muscle, greater; see under MUSCLE. **m. zygomat′icus mi′nor** [NA], zygomatic muscle, lesser; see under MUSCLE.

mushbite (mush′bīt) a procedure used in the past for making simultaneously an impression of both upper and lower teeth and/or associated structures by having the subject bite on a mass of plastic material placed between the jaws. Written also *mush bite*.

Musitano, Carlo [1635–1714] an Italian priest and physician, originator of a theory that dental caries is caused by minute organisms or worms developing from insect eggs introduced into the oral cavity with food.

mustard (mus′tard) [L. *sinapis*] 1. a plant of the genus *Brassica*. 2. the ripe seeds of *Brassica nigra* (black mustard) and *B. alba* (white mustard). When mustard seeds are crushed and moistened, volatile oils are liberated; these oils give mustard its counterirritant, stimulant, and revulsant properties. **alanine nitrogen m.**, melphalan. **nitrogen m.**, 1. any of a group of chemical substances homologous with dichlorodiethyl sulfide (mustard gas) and having the bis-(2-chloroethyl) group, to which various other groups, such as amino acids, substituted phenyl groups, and pyrimidine bases, may be attached. Nitrogen mustards are alkylating agents used in the treatment of neoplastic diseases, such as Hodgkin's disease and lymphomas. A wide variety of adverse reactions may occur, including vomiting, nausea, leukopenia, thrombocytopenia, susceptibility to infection, hemorrhagic diathesis, maculopapular eruptions, herpes zoster, menstrual irregularities, fetal abnormalities, subcutaneous indurations, and thrombophlebitis. 2. mechlorethamine. L-**phenylalanine m.**, melphalan. **quinacrine m.**, QUIN-

ACRINE mustard. **uracil m.,** a nitrogen mustard, 5-[bis(2-chloroethyl)amino]-2,4-(1*H*,3*H*)-pyrimidinedione, occurring as an off-white, odorless, crystalline powder that is slightly soluble in water, acetone, and ethanol and insoluble in chloroform. It is a cytotoxic drug, having some antimetabolite properties, used in the treatment of lymphocytic leukemia, Hodgkin's disease, and other lymphomas, primary macroglobulinemia, and certain other neoplasms. Adverse reactions may include nausea, vomiting, diarrhea, pruritus, dermatitis, irritability, depression, amenorrhea, oligospermia, susceptibility to infection, hyperuricemia, kidney disorders, and bone marrow depression with hematological disorders. Called also *demethyldopan, desmethyldopan,* and *uramustine.*

Mustargen trademark for *mechlorethamine hydrochloride* (see under MECHLORETHAMINE).

Mustine trademark for *mechlorethamine hydrochloride* (see under MECHLORETHAMINE).

Mutabase trademark for *diazoxide.*

mutagen (mu′tah-jen) [*mut*ation + *gen*esis] any chemical or physical agent that induces mutation.

mutarotation (mu″tah-ro-ta′shun) a special type of tautomerism involving either (*a*) the transformation of one optical isomer into another, or (*b*) the transformation of one structural isomer into another (both possessing asymmetric centers and optical activity). With each type the rotatory power of a freshly prepared solution of the compound will change, under a variety of conditions, until an equilibrium value is set up which (unlike in racemization) will not be zero.

mutation (mu-ta′shun) [L. *mutatio,* from *mutare* to change] 1. a change in form, quality, or some other characteristic. 2. a permanent heritable change in the genetic material; usually restricted to change in a single gene (*point m.*), but sometimes is used for any structural chromosomal change. Mutation includes a loss, gain, or exchange of genetic material. See also DELETION (2), TRANSDUCTION, and TRANSLOCATION. **genomic m.,** a mutation in which there is a change in the number of complete chromosomes; if the result is a whole multiple of the haploid set of the chromosomes, it is a *ploidic mutation.* **induced m.,** a genetic mutation caused by external factors which are experimentally or accidentally produced. See also TRANSDUCTION. **missense m.,** a mutation in which changes in a codon produce a single amino acid substitution in a polypeptide chain. **natural m.,** a genetic mutation occurring without the intervention of any known external factors. **nonsense m.,** a mutation in which insertion or deletion of a single base alters a codon for a particular amino acid, so that a sequence of amino acids is altered and a polypeptide is lacking in biological activity. **ploidic m.,** see *genomic m.* **point m.,** mutation involving a single gene, which is not associated with changes in other parts of the chromosome. It involves the substitution of one base for another within a triplet, which may result in changes in the codon, so that codes for different amino acids are altered, leading to changed polypeptide chains, such as those in abnormal hemoglobins. **somatic m.,** a genetic mutation occurring in a somatic cell, providing the basis for a mosaic condition.

muton (mu′ton) [*mut*ation + Gr. *-on* neuter ending] the smallest unit of alterable material in a gene, being a unit of DNA (a nucleotide) which, when altered, gives rise to mutation.

M.V. abbreviation for L. *Med′icus Veterinar′ius,* veterinary physician.

Mv formerly, mendelevium; now Md.

mv. millivolt.

μv microvolt.

μw microwatt.

my mayer.

my- See MYO-.

Myacyne trademark for *neomycin.*

myalgia (mi-al′je-ah) [*my-* + *algia*] pain in the muscle or muscles.

Myambutol trademark for *ethambutol.*

myasthenia (mi″as-the′ne-ah) [*my-* + Gr. *astheneia* weakness] a disease characterized by muscular weakness. **m. gra′vis,** a disorder occurring in both sexes at any age, but affecting most commonly middle-aged women. It is presumably caused by faulty synaptic transmission at the myoneural junction, in which abnormal fatigability and paralysis are produced by muscular activity or administration of cholinesterase antagonists. The voluntary muscles of the face, larynx, and throat are affected initially, but other muscles also become involved. Difficulty in mastication and swallowing toward the end of a meal, ptosis, diplopia, slurred speech and weak voice after prolonged talking, inability to close the mouth, weakness of the leg muscles after a walk, dyspnea, hyperventilation, and repetitive movements are the principal signs. Myocarditis, thymic tumors and hyperplasia, and ocular changes are frequently associated. Death usually occurs within two years. Called also *asthenic bulbar paralysis, bulbospinal paralysis,* and *Erb-Goldflam syndrome.*

Myasul trademark for *sulfamethoxypyridazine.*

myc- see MYCO-.

mycelium (mi-se′le-um), pl. *myce′lia* [*myc-* + Gr. *hēlos* nail] the mass of threadlike processes (hyphae) constituting the fungal thallus.

mycet- see MYCO-.

Mycifradin trademark for *neomycin.*

myco-, myc-, mycet- [Gr. *mykēs* fungus] a combining form denoting relationship to a fungus.

Mycobacteriaceae (mi″ko-bak-te″re-a′se-e) [*Mycobacterium* + *-aceae*] a family of bacteria of the order Actinomycetales, consisting of the genus *Mycobacterium.* Called also *Proactinomycetaceae.*

Mycobacterium (mi″ko-bak-te′re-um) [*myco-* + *baktērion* small rod] a genus of bacteria of the family Mycobacteriaceae, order Actinomycetales, occurring as aerobic, acid-alcohol fast, grampositive, nonmotile organisms without endospores, conidia, or capsules. They are slightly curved or straight rods, about 0.2 to 0.6 by 1.0 to 10.0 μm in size; filamentous or mycelium-like forms may occur, but may be modified by even a slight disturbance, causing the organisms to assume coccoid or rod shapes. The genus includes obligate parasites, saprophytes, and intermediate forms. **M. absces′sus,** *M. chelonei.* **M. africa′num,** a species isolated from sputum of a tuberculous patient in Senegal, causing human tuberculosis in tropical Africa. **M. a′vidum,** *Propionibacterium avidum;* see under PROPIONIBACTERIUM. **M. a′vium,** a species which produces tuberculosis in domestic fowl and other birds, believed to be also pathogenic to man. Called also *M. tuberculosis avium, M. tuberculosis var. avium, M. tuberculosis typus avium, M. tuberculosis typus gallinaceus,* and *Bacillus tuberculosis.* **M. bal′nei,** *M. marinum.* **M. borstelen′se,** *M. chelonei.* **M. bo′vis,** a species isolated originally from tubercles in cattle, which causes tuberculosis in man and other primates, domestic and wild ruminants, carnivores, including dogs and cats, and some birds. In man, most commonly children, the infection is usually acquired by infected milk, producing a hilar pulmonary infection, or a tracheobronchial lymphatic or mesenteric infection with a tendency to generalization. *M. bovis* is also pathogenic to rabbits, guinea pigs, and other experimental animals. The antigenic properties of tuberculin produced from *M. bovis* and *M. tuberculosis* have identical actions. Called also *M. tuberculosis* var. *bovis* and *M. tuberculosis typus bovinus.* **M. chelon′ei,** a species that produces synovial lesions and gluteal abscesses, also found in human sputum. Experimental infection causes gross lesions in various organs. Called also *M. abscessus* and *M. borstelense.* **M. diphthe′riae,** *Corynebacterium diphtheriae;* see under CORYNEBACTERIUM. **M. e′qui,** *Corynebacterium equi;* see under CORYNEBACTERIUM. **M. fla′vum** var. *tortuo′sum, Eubacterium tortuosum;* see under EUBACTERIUM. **M. gas′tri,** a nonpathogenic species isolated from human gastric lavage and sputum, also found in soil. **M. gordo′nae,** a nonpathogenic species found in human sputum and gastric lavage. **M. influen′zae,** *Haemophilus influenzae;* see under HAEMOPHILUS. **M. intracellula′re,** a species occurring as transiently filamentous rods that become coccobacillary; found in human pulmonary secretions associated with tuberculosis-like lung disease and in surgical specimens in such cases. Called also *Nocardia intracellularis.* **M. joh′nei,** *M. paratuberculosis.* **M. kansas′ii,** the etiologic agent of a tuberculosis-like disease in man, frequently isolated from pulmonary secretions or tubercles in man. Colonies grown in dark are nonpigmented; those cultivated in light or when exposed to light when colonies are young, become brilliant yellow. Called also *M. luciflavum, group I photochromogen,* and *yellow bacillus.* **M. lep′rae,** a noncultivable species isolated from human leprosy tissue. It is an obligate intracellular parasite in man, confined largely to the skin, testes, and peripheral nerves, and occurs as rods with parallel sides and rounded ends, about 0.3 to 0.5 by 1.0 to 8.0 μm in size. Its growth can be inhibited by diaminodiphenyl sulfone, isoniazid, paraminosalicylic acid, and cycloserine. Called also *Bacillus leprae, Hansen's bacillus,* and *leprosy bacillus.* **M. lepraemu′rium,** a noncultivable species causing an endemic disease (rat, or murine, leprosy) in wild rats, characterized by lesions of the skin and lymph nodes with alopecia, induration, and ulceration. Written also *M. leprae murium* and called also *rat* *leprosy bacillus.* **M. lep′rae mu′rium,** *M. lepraemurium.* **M. limo′sum,** *Eubacterium limosum;* see under EUBACTERIUM. **M. lucifla′vum,** *M. kansasii.* **M. lympho′philum,** *Propionibacterium lymphophilum;* see under PROPIONIBACTERIUM. **M. mari′num,** a species, isolated originally from diseased fish and from aquariums, occurring in man in skin lesions resulting from abrasions occurring in swimming pools, sometimes causing granuloma. Called also *M. balnei.* **M. paratuberculo′sis,** a species isolated from the intestinal mucosa of cattle suffering from chronic diarrhea. Called also *M. johnei* and *Johne's bacillus.* **M. peregrin′um,** a species, various strains of which have been isolated from bronchial aspirations in a child, nasal exudate in a cow, sputum in man, and from soil. **M. pseudodiphtherit′icum,** *Corynebacterium pseudodiphtheriticum;* see under CORYNEBACTERIUM. **M. scrofula′ceum,** a species found in human secretions, particularly pus from suppurating cervical lymphadenitis in children. Also occurring in human sputum and gastric lavage, sometimes in association with pulmonary diseases, and occasionally found in soil. **M. ter′rae,** a nonpathogenic species isolated from human sputum and gastric lavage. **M. trivia′le,** a nonpathogenic species isolated from human sputum. **M. tuberculo′sis,** a species causing tuberculosis, most commonly pulmonary, in man and other primates, and in dogs and other animals, being also pathogenic to experimental animals, such as guinea pigs and hamsters but relatively nonpathogenic for rabbits, cats, goats, fowl, and bovines. Low-virulence strains have been isolated in urogenital tuberculosis, scrofuloderma, and lupus erythematosus. The organism occurs as straight or slightly curved rods, singly or, occasionally, in threads, about 0.3 to 0.6 by 1.0 to 4.0 μm in size. Some strains are sensitive to streptomycin, para-aminosalicylic acid, isoniazid, and other drugs, but the organisms may mutate and develop resistance to any of these drugs. Called also *Bacillus tuberculosis, Bacterium tuberculosis, M. tuberculosis* var. *hominis, M. tuberculosis typus humanus,* and *tubercle bacillus.* **M. tuberculo′sis a′vium, M. tuberculo′sis** var. **a′vium,** *M. avium.* **M. tuberculo′sis ty′pus a′vium,** *M. avium.* **M. tuberculo′sis ty′pus bovi′nus,** *M. bovis.* **M. tuberculo′sis ty′pus gallina′ceus,** *M. avium.* **M. tuberculo′sis ty′pus huma′nus,** *M. tuberculosis.* **M. tuberculo′sis** var. **bo′vis,** *M. bovis.* **M. tuberculosis** var. **hom′inis,** *M. tuberculosis.* **M. tuberculo′sis o′vis,** *Corynebacterium pseudotuberculosis;* see under CORYNEBACTERIUM. **M. ul′cerans,** a species isolated from human ulcerative skin lesions. **M. xeno′pi,** a species isolated from skin granulomas of the toad *Xenopus laevis.* In man, sometimes isolated from chronic pulmonary diseases and, more frequently, from secretions associated with genitourinary diseases. **M. xero′sis,** *Corynebacterium xerosis;* see under CORYNEBACTERIUM.

Mycoderma (mi″ko-der′mah) *Acetobacter.*

mycology (mi-kol′o-je) [*myco-* + *-logy*] the science and study of fungi.

Mycoplasma (mi″ko-plaz′mah) [*myco-* + Gr. *plasma* anything formed] a genus of prokaryotic, gram-negative, mostly facultatively, anaerobic microorganisms of the family Mycoplasmataceae, order Mycoplasmatales. The members lack a true cell wall and are bounded by a single triple-layered membrane, about 7.5 to 10 nm in thickness, and occur as pleomorphic cells, from spherical to ovoid, 125 to 250 nm in diameter, to slender branched filaments up to 150 μm in diameter. All species require cholesterol or other sterols for growth, most using either glucose or arginine. They are resistant to penicillin G, methicillin, and nafcillin and variably susceptible to erythromycin and other antibiotics. Mycoplasmas are weakly pathogenic and cause disease only as secondary invaders, but a few are frankly pathogenic. Many are common inhabitants of the genitourinary tract and of the oral cavity, generally found in the saliva, tooth scrapings, and carious material. Called also *Asterococcus* and *Schizoplasm.* Formerly called *pleuropneumonia-like organisms* (*PPLO*). **M. alkales′cens,** a species isolated from the nasal cavity of cattle. **M. bovirhi′nis,** a species found in the nose and upper respiratory tract of cattle. **M. ca′nis,** a species isolated from the upper respiratory tract, throat, and genital tract of dogs. **M. cy′nos,** a species isolated from the upper respiratory tract, conjunctivae, and genital tract of a dog. **M. feliminu′tum,** a small-colony species originally isolated from the oral cavity of a cat. **M. fe′lis,** a nonpathogenic species commonly found in the oral and nasal cavities, conjunctivae, and genital tract of cats. **M. fermen′tans,** a species isolated from the human oropharynx and urogenital tract, sometimes occurring in association with gynecological diseases and rheumatoid arthritis. Called also *Asterococcus fermentans* and *Schizoplasma fermentans.* **M. hom′inis,** a species isolated from the urogenital tract and, less commonly, from the oropharynx of man and nonhuman primates. It is a potentially pathogenic species, ranging in length

from 2 to 5 up to 30 μm, suspected of causing pharyngitis and respiratory diseases in man. Called also *Asterococcus hominis* and *Schizoplasma hominis.* **M. hyorhi′nis,** a species isolated from the nasal cavity of swine, suspected of being an etiologic agent of swine pneumonia and other diseases. **M. hyosyn′oviae,** a species isolated from synovial fluid, nasal secretions, and tonsils of swine. **M. maculo′sum,** a species isolated from the upper respiratory tract, throat, and genitourinary tract of dogs. **M. mycoi′des,** a species causing pleuropneumonia and other diseases in ruminants, occurring as two subspecies. Called also *M. peripneumoniae* and *Bovimyces pleuropneumoniae.* **M. neurolyt′icum,** a species inhabiting the upper respiratory tract of healthy and diseased mice. **M. ora′le,** a species inhabiting the oropharynx of man and nonhuman primates, subdivided into three biochemically and serologically distinct strains. It is a facultative anaerobe, about 8 to 10 μm in length, which is resistant to erythromycin. Called also *M. pharyngis* and *Schizoplasma orale.* **M. ovipneumo′niae,** a species isolated from the nose, trachea, lungs, and paranasal sinuses of lambs; associated with pneumonia. **M. peripneumo′niae,** *M. mycoides.* **M. pharyn′gis,** *M. orale.* **M. pneumo′niae,** a species occurring as filaments, 2 to 5 μm in length, being the etiologic agent of cold-hemagglutin–associated primary atypical pneumonia in man and various respiratory complications. Called also *Eaton agent* and *Schizoplasma pneumoniae.* **M. prima′tum,** a nonpathogenic species that has been isolated from the oral cavity and urogenital tract of monkeys. **M. pulmo′nis,** a species that is commonly found in the respiratory tract, including the nares and oropharynx, of mice and rats. **M. saliva′rium,** a species that has been isolated from the oropharynx of man and nonhuman primates. The organisms are nonpathogenic, facultative anaerobes, occurring in four strains as short, almost bacillary filaments, about 0.6 to 1.0 μm in length, which are highly resistant to erythromycin. Called also *Asterococcus salivarius* and *Schizoplasma salivarium.* **M. spu′mans,** a species isolated from the upper respiratory tract, throat, and genitourinary tract of dogs.

mycoplasma (mi″ko-plaz′mah), pl. *mycoplas′mas, mycoplas′-mata.* Any microorganism of the genus *Mycoplasma.*

mycoplasmal (mi″ko-plaz′mal) of, pertaining to, or caused by mycoplasmas.

Mycoplasmataceae (mi″ko-plaz″mah-ta′se-e) [*Mycoplasma* + *-aceae*] a family of prokaryotic microorganisms of the order Mycoplasmatales, class Mollicutes, which requires cholesterol or other sterols for growth. It consists of the genus *Mycoplasma.*

Mycoplasmatales (mi″ko-plaz″mah-ta′lēz) an order of prokaryotic microorganisms of the class Mollicutes, which consists of two families, the Mycoplasmataceae, characterized by a requirement for cholesterol or other sterols, and the Acholeplasmataceae, which do not require sterols.

mycoplasmosis (mi″ko-plaz-mo′sis) infection with mycoplasmas.

mycosis (mi-ko′sis) [*myco-* + *-osis*] any disease caused by infection with a fungus.

Mycosporin trademark for *clotrimazole.*

mycostasis (mi-kos′tah-sis, mi″ko-sta′sis) [*myco-* + Gr. *stasis* a stopping] inhibition of the growth of fungi; fungistasis.

mycostat (mi′ko-stat) an agent that inhibits the growth of fungi.

Mycostatin trademark for *nystatin.*

mycotic (mi-kot′ik) pertaining to or caused by fungi; fungal.

mycotoxin (mi″ko-tok′sin) a fungal toxin.

mycteric (mik-ter′ik) [Gr. *myktēr* nostril] pertaining to the nasal cavities.

mycteroxerosis (mik-ter-o-ze-ro′sis) [Gr. *myktēr* nostril + *xeros* dry] dryness of the nostril.

Mydplegic trademark for *cyclopentolate hydrochloride* (see under CYCLOPENTOLATE).

Mydriatine trademark for *phenylpropanolamine hydrochloride* (see under PHENYLPROPANOLAMINE).

Mydrilate trademark for *cyclopentolate hydrochloride* (see under CYCLOPENTOLATE).

myelin (mi′ĕ-lin) [Gr. *myelos* marrow] a lipoidal substance forming a sheath around certain nerve fibers. See myelin SHEATH.

myelinated (mi′ĕ-li-nāt″ed) possessing a myelin sheath; medullated. Said of a nerve fiber.

myelitis (mi″ĕ-li′tis) [Gr. *myelos* marrow + *-itis*] 1. inflammation of the bone marrow. 2. inflammation of the spinal cord.

myelo-, myel- [Gr. *myelos* marrow] a combining form denoting relationship to the spinal cord, bone marrow, or myelin sheath.

myeloblast (mi'ĕ-lo-blast) [*myelo-* + Gr. *blastos* germ] an immature cell of the bone marrow, varying in size from 10 to 20 μ, which is not normally found in the circulating blood. Myeloblasts develop into myelocytes and granulocytes and, in some pathological conditions, lymphocytes. It has a large oval or round nucleus and two to five nucleoli. In certain conditions, such as leukemia, nuclei may have indentations suggesting lobulations; these myeloblasts are known as *Rieder cells*. Myeloblasts resembling plasma cells but retaining the nuclear pattern of myeloblasts are known as *Türk cells*. In certain pathological conditions *Auer bodies* may be found in the cytoplasm of myeloblasts.

myeloblastemia (mi"ĕ-lo-blas-te'me-ah) [*myeloblast* + Gr. *haima* blood + *-ia*] the presence of myeloblasts in the circulating blood.

myeloblastosis (mi"ĕ-lo-blas-to'sis) [*myeloblast* + *-osis*] the presence of an excess of myeloblasts in the circulating blood.

myelocyte (mi'e-lo-sīt) [*myelo-* + Gr. *kytos* hollow vessel] an immature cell in the bone marrow, which represents the developmental stage of the leukocyte following the myeloblast and in turn is followed by the granulocyte. An early myelocyte is known as a *promyelocyte*, and is characterized by fewer than 10 granules in the cytoplasm and by lack of indentation of the nucleus. In the next stage of development, the cell is known as a *metamyelocyte* and the cell body is filled with granules, except for the centrosome. The cell then undergoes mitosis and its nucleus shows the initial stages of polymorphism, assuming the shape of a horseshoe or sausage, and divides into two lobes. Mitochondria are still present but difficult to detect because of the numerous granules; the nucleoli are no longer visible. Those with heterophilic granules develop into heterophils (*neutrophils* in man); those with eosinophilic granules into eosinophils; and those with basophilic granules, into basophils. The average time of maturation of a myeloblast into a mature granulocyte is about 3 to 4 days. **m. count**, see table of *Reference Values in Hematology* in Appendix.

myelocythemia (mi"ĕ-lo-si-the'me-ah) [*myelocyte* + Gr. *haima* blood + *-ia*] an excess in the number of myelocytes in the blood. See also leukocyte count, differential, under COUNT.

myelocytosis (mi"ĕ-lo-si-to'sis) the presence of an excessive number of myelocytes in the blood; myelosis.

myelography (mi"ĕ-log'rah-fe) [*myelo-* + Gr. *graphein* to write] roentgenographic examination of the spinal cord and subarachnoid space, usually after injection of a contrast medium into the subarachnoid space.

Myeloleukon trademark for *busulfan*.

myeloma (mi"ĕ-lo'mah) [*myelo-* + *-oma*] 1. a tumor composed of cells of the type normally found in the bone marrow. 2. any medullary tumor. **endothelial m.**, Ewing's SARCOMA. **multiple m.**, a fatal neoplastic disease of middle or later age, characterized by abnormal proliferation of plasma cells derived from reticulum cells in the bone marrow; abnormal serum and urinary proteins, chiefly urinary excretion of Bence Jones protein (a thermosensitive protein of low-molecular weight), associated with immune disorders; and abnormal deposits of amyloid. In a typical lesion containing an aggregate of plasma cells and deposits of amyloid, cells vary in size and shape and are arranged in sheets with very little connective stroma. Symptoms include pain, spontaneous fractures, anemia, nephritis, and neurological disorders. Oral tumors, usually of the mandible, and less commonly of the maxilla, are accompanied by pain, swelling, numbness, and mobility of the teeth. Gingival enlargement or epulides are typical extraosseous lesions. Called also *Kahler's disease* and *myelosis*. **plasma cell m.**, a general term for a group of neoplastic conditions, including plasmacytoma, multiple myeloma, diffuse myelomatosis, and plasma cell leukemia, having in common abnormal plasma cell proliferation. All disorders in this group are characterized by one or more of the following features: abnormal infiltration or accumulations of plasma cells, usually in bone, deposits of amyloid, and serum or urinary paraproteins. **plasma cell m., solitary**, a controversial lesion histologically similar to multiple myeloma, considered by some to be an early form of multiple myeloma, and by others as a separate, unrelated entity. It may occur in the jaws and, less frequently, in the soft tissue of the nose, pharynx, and mouth. The presenting symptoms are similar to those seen in multiple myeloma, with pain, spontaneous fractures, and swelling being the principal ones. Called also *solitary plasmacytoma*.

myelopathy (mi"ĕ-lop'ah-the) [*myelo-* + Gr. *pathos* disease] 1. any disease of the spinal cord. 2. any disease of the bone marrow.

Myelosan trademark for *busulfan*.

myelosis (mi'e-lo'sis) 1. the proliferation of bone marrow tissue; myelocytosis. 2. multiple tumors of the spinal cord. 3. multiple MYELOMA. **aplastic infantile funicular m.**, Fanconi's ANEMIA.

myiasis (mi'yah-sis) [Gr. *myia* fly + *-iasis*] infestation of the body by fly maggots. **oral m.**, infestation of the mouth tissue by fly larvae, which lay their eggs in dental sockets or in necrotic tissue of the mouth; it occurs most commonly in India and Pakistan. **traumatic m.**, infestation of wounds or ulcers with fly larvae.

Mylaxen trademark for *hexafluorenium bromide* (see under HEXAFLUORENIUM).

Mylepsin trademark for *primidone*.

Myleran trademark for *busulfan*.

mylo- [Gr. *myle* a mill, in pl. *mylai* molar teeth] a combining form denoting relationship to molar teeth or to the posterior portion of the lower jaw.

Mylocon trademark for *simethicone*.

mylohyoid (mi-lo-hi'oid) [*mylo-* + *hyoid*] pertaining to the molar teeth, or to the posterior portion of the mandible, and the hyoid bone.

mylohyoideus (mi"lo-hi-o-id'e-us) mylohyoid MUSCLE.

mylopharyngeus (mi'lo-far-in'je-us) mylopharyngeal MUSCLE.

Mylosul trademark for *sulfamethoxypyridazine*.

Mynol cement see under CEMENT.

myo-, my- [Gr. *mys* muscle] a combining form denoting relationship to muscle.

myoblast (mi'o-blast) [*myo-* + Gr. *blastos* germ] an embryonic muscle cell which differentiates into a muscle fiber.

myoblastoma (mi"o-blas-to'mah) [*myoblast* + *-oma*] a benign tumor typically presenting as a well-defined, spherical, grayish to yellow-tan nodule about 0.5 to 2.0 cm in diameter, which has a normal, sometimes slightly hyperkeratotic cover. It may occur in any part, but is most commonly located in the tongue, and is composed of strands and fascicles of large cells showing granular, eosinophilic cytoplasm, sometimes related to striated muscle fibers or peripheral myelinated nerves. Some authorities suggest that it is probably not derived from striated muscle, as the name implies. Myoblastoma is quite similar to congenital epulis but it is believed that they are two separate entities. Called also *granular cell m.*, *Abrikossoff's tumor*, *Abrikossov's tumor*, and *myoblastic myoma*. **granular cell m.**, myoblastoma. **malignant granular cell m.**, alveolar soft part SARCOMA.

myocarditis (mi"o-kar-di'tis) [*myocardium* + *-itis*] inflammation of the muscular wall of the heart. See also CARDITIS.

myocardium (mi"o-kar'de-um) [*myo-* + Gr. *kardia* heart] [NA] the middle and muscular layer of the heart wall, having a striated appearance similar to voluntary muscle. In contrast to other muscles, the myocardial fibers intertwine and produce a continuous branching network, so that the impulse is allowed to pass through the entire muscle without disruptions, hence the all-or-none action in myocardial contraction. Called also *cardiac muscle* and *heart muscle*.

Myochrisine (mi"o-kri'sin) trademark for a preparation of *gold sodium thiomalate* (see under GOLD).

myoclonus (mi-ok'lo-nus) [*myo-* + Gr. *klonos* turmoil] rapid contractions of an entire muscle, a portion of a muscle, or a group of muscles, occurring in one or several parts of the body. **facial m.**, a condition characterized by frequent shocklike myoclonic contractions of the facial muscles, usually beginning at the orbicularis oculi as fine intermittent twitchings, and spreading slowly to muscles of the lower part of the face, affecting most commonly the retractors of the angle of the mouth. The spasms are usually hemifacial and affect middle-aged and elderly women; they usually last a few seconds and are often precipitated by fatigue and tension. Facial contracture and lip closure and pursing may occur in prolonged cases, and the sense of taste may be lost over the anterior portion of the tongue. The etiology is unknown but irritation of the nerve and lesions of the geniculate ganglion have been suggested as possible causes. Called also *clonic facial spasm* and *hemifacial spasm*. **palatal m.**, a relatively rare, usually bilateral, condition in which the palatal muscles undergo continuous up-and-down contractions, sometimes accompanied by an objective clicking in the ear, produced by the eustachian tube snapping open and shut, and ipsilateral synchronous clonic movements of the muscles of the face, tongue, pharynx, and diaphragm. Called also *palatal nystagmus*.

Myocrisin (mi"o-kri'sin) trademark for a preparation of *gold sodium thiomalate* (see under GOLD).

myocyte (mio'sīt) [*myo* + *-cyte*] a muscle cell. **Anichkov's m.**, a cell found in Aschoff's bodies in the heart in rheumatic fever, considered by some as an altered fibroblast and by others as an altered myocyte. It is a large differentiated mesenchymal, occasionally multinucleate cell, with the nuclear chromatin aggregated into the center forming a slender wavy ribbon with fine leglike projections (hence, the synonym *caterpillar cell*). Called also *Anichkov's cell*.

Myodil trademark for *iophendylate*.

myodystrophia (mi″o-dis-tro′fe-ah) muscular DYSTROPHY. **m. congen′ita**, Guérin-Stern SYNDROME.

myofibril (mi″o-fi′bril) [*myo-* + L. *fibra* fiber] a thin fibril of the skeletal muscle cell, consisting of parallel bundles of myofilaments arranged in the contractile units (sarcomeres), and crossed by light and dark bands which give the muscle its characteristic striations. Called also *sarcostyle*. See illustration at MUSCLE.

myofilament (mi″o-fil′ah-ment) [*myo-* + *filament*] any of the numerous elongated polymerized protein molecules that make up a myofibril, and which are responsible for muscle contraction. Each myofibril has about 1500 myosin filaments (see A BAND), and about 3000 actin filaments (see I BAND). See illustration at MUSCLE.

myofunctional (mi″o-funk′shun-al) 1. pertaining to muscular function. 2. pertaining to the use of muscles as an adjunct in orthodontic therapy.

myoglobin (mi″o-glo′bin) [*myo-* + *globin*] a conjugated protein composed of one molecule of heme and having a molecular weight of about 17,000. It binds oxygen, thus providing a labile reserve of oxygen to muscle cells during peak or intermittent muscular activity. Called also *muscle hemoglobin*.

myognathus (mi-og′nah-thus) [*myo-* + Gr. *gnathos* jaw] a developmental abnormality characterized by the presence of a supernumerary lower jaw attached to the normally placed mandible.

myography (mi-og′rah-fe) [*myo-* + Gr. *graphein* to write] recording of muscular contraction.

myo-inositol (mi″o-in-o′sĭ-tol, mi″in-os′ĭ-tol) see INOSITOL.

Myolaxene trademark for *methocarbamol*.

myolipoma (mi″o-li-po′mah) [*myo-* + Gr. *lipos* fat + *-oma*] myoma (leiomyoma) containing fatty or lipomatous elements.

myologia (mi″o-lo′je-ah) myology; in NA terminology, *myologia* encompasses the nomenclature relating to the muscles and to the bursae and synovial sheaths.

myology (mi-ol′o-je) [*myo-* + Gr. *logos* treatise] the study of muscles, and the body of knowledge relating thereto.

myolysis (mi-ol′ĭ-sis) [*myo-* + Gr. *lysis* dissolution] degeneration or disintegration of muscle tissue.

myoma (mi-o′mah), pl. *myomas*, *myo′mata* [*myo-* + *-oma*] any tumor made up of muscular tissue, including leiomyoma, leiomyosarcoma, rhabdomyoma, rhabdomyosarcoma, and myoblastoma. **myoblastic m.,** myoblastoma. **m. striatocellula′re,** rhabdomyoma.

myomata (mi-o′mah-tah) [L.] plural of *myoma*.

myomere (mi′o-mēr) [*myo-* + Gr. *meros* part] myotome (2).

Myo-Monitor trademark for a device used for determination of Myo-Monitor centric. It is a solid-state electronic instrument delivering small amounts of DC current through electrodes placed over the coronoid notch of the ramus of the mandible. The instrument is designed to simulate all muscles involved in mandibular movements and it positions the mandible in Myo-Monitor centric.

myopathy (mi-op′ah-the) [*myo-* + Gr. *pathos* suffering] a disease of a muscle or muscles.

myopia (mi-o′pe-ah) [Gr. *myein* to shut + *ōps* eye + *-ia*] an error of refraction, in which the rays of light entering the eye are brought to a focus in front of the retina, as a result of the eyeball being too long. Called also *nearsightedness*.

myosin (mi′o-sin) [Gr. *mys* muscle] a contractile protein, forming a heavy molecule with a molecular weight of about 460,000, which is made up of two heavy chains wound around each other and folded at the end into a globular structure to form a head, and four light chains forming a tail. The amino acid sequence has not been established, but 1800 amino acid residues have been found in myosin treated with urea or guanine solutions. Myosin attacks glutamic-pyruvic transaminase, inosine triphosphate, and cytidine triphosphate and hydrolyzes the terminal phosphate group of adenosine triphosphate. This last activity is stimulated by calcium and inhibited by magnesium ions. Myosin filaments form the A bands of striated muscle and participate in its contraction by sliding along the actin filaments, thus reducing the length of the sarcomere. Called also *meromycin*. See also A BAND, ACTIN, ACTOMYOSIN, and ratchet THEORY. **m. B.,** actomyosin.

myositis (mi″o-si′tis) [Gr. *myos* of muscle + *-itis*] inflammation of a voluntary muscle. See also DERMATOMYOSITIS. **generalized m. ossif′icans, interstitial ossifying m.,** progressive m. ossificans. **m. ossif′icans circumscrip′ta,** traumatic m. ossificans. **progressive m. ossif′icans,** an uncommon, probably hereditary, disease of children and adolescents, characterized by myositis followed by ossification and replacement of striated muscles, tendons, ligaments, and aponeuroses of the major joints, as well as other organs; the muscle cells are gradually replaced by collagenous tissue which is later converted into cartilage and bone. Any skeletal muscle may undergo ossifying changes, but the tongue, larynx, and diaphragm seem to be unaffected. The masseter muscle is often involved, leading to fixation of the jaws. Called also *generalized m. ossificans, interstitial ossifying m., exostosis luxurians, fibrositis ossificans, hyperplasia fascialis progressiva*, and *Münchmeyer's syndrome*. **traumatic m. ossif′icans,** a condition characterized by the deposit of fibrous tissue and bone at the site of traumatic muscle injury, occurring usually in young males exposed to heavy physical strain. The lesion, initially a hemorrhage, undergoes formation of granulation tissue and fibrous scarring, followed by formation of cartilage and endochondral ossification. In some cases, calcification may occur and be followed by ossification. The masseter and temporal muscle may undergo ossification following a traumatic injury, leading to difficulty in opening the mouth. Called also *m. ossificans circumscripta* and *ossifying hematoma*.

myotasis (mi-ot′ah-sis) [*myo-* + Gr. *tasis* stretching] stretching of muscle.

myotatic (mi″o-tat′ik) [*myo-* + Gr. *teinein* to stretch] performed or induced by stretching or extending a muscle.

myotome (mi′o-tōm) [*myo-* + Gr. *tomē* a cut] 1. an instrument for performing myotomy. 2. the muscle plate of a somite that develops into voluntary muscle. Called also *myomere*. 3. a group of muscles innervated by a single spinal segment.

myotomy (mi-ot′o-me) [*myo-* + Gr. *tomē* a cutting] the cutting of a muscle or muscle tissue.

myotonia (mi″o-to′ne-ah) [*myo-* + Gr. *tonos* tension] increased muscular irritability and contractility with decreased power of relaxation; tonic spasm of muscle. See also PARAMYOTONIA. **acquired m., m. acquis′ita,** increased muscular rigidity and spasm when movements are initiated and a decrease in the degree of relaxation even when the muscle is at rest, associated with normal mechanical and electrical excitability of the motor nerves but with abnormally heightened mechanical and electrical excitability. Facial muscles may be involved. It usually develops in adults after trauma, acute infection, or intoxication. Called also *Talma's disease*. **atrophic m.,** myotonic DYSTROPHY. **m. congen′ita, congenital m.,** a rare disease, inherited as an autosomal dominant trait, usually beginning during childhood, characterized by myotonia and hypertrophy of the voluntary muscles, with inability to relax the muscles immediately after forceful contraction. Ptosis, difficulty in turning the eyes to the side, and inability to open the eyes rapidly are the ocular symptoms. The muscles are large, the muscles of the thighs, forearms, and shoulder being especially affected, giving the patient a "herculean" appearance. The muscles of the neck and the masseter muscles of the face are usually involved, and the muscles of the tongue, although not hypertrophied, are affected. Sudden movement, such as sneezing, may produce a prolonged spasm of the muscles of the tongue, face, larynx, and chest. Called also *hereditary m., ataxia muscularis, congenital muscular dystrophy*, and *Thomsen's disease*. **m. congen′ita intermit′tens,** congenital PARAMYOTONIA. **hereditary m.,** m. congenita.

myotonic (mi″o-ton′ik) 1. pertaining to or characterized by myotonia. 2. pertaining to the tonic function of muscle.

myotonus (mi-ot′o-nus) [*myo-* + Gr. *tonos* tone] the normal slight contraction of a muscle.

myria- [Gr. *myrios* numberless] a combining form meaning a great number.

Myricin (mir′ĭ-sin) [L. *myrica* myrtle] 1. a crystalline principle, $C_{30}H_{61}C_{16}H_{31}O_2$, from beeswax. 2. an astringent and antiluetic preparation from wax myrtle, *Myrica cerifera*.

Myristica (mi-ris′tĭ-kah) [L.; Gr. *myrizein* to anoint] a genus of trees of tropical countries, *M. fragrans*, the nutmeg tree, it is the source of myristica.

myristica (mi-ris′tĭ-kah) the dried ripe seed of *Myristica fragrans* deprived of its seed coat and arillode and with or within a coating of lime, the source of myristica oil. Used in flavoring foods and pharmaceutical preparations. Ingestion of large quantities causes stupor, drowsiness, and death. Called also *nutmeg* and *nux moschata*.

myrmecia (mer-me′she-ah) [Gr. *myrmēx* ant + *-ia*] a wart resembling somewhat an anthill.

myrtiform (mur′tĭ-form) [L. *myrtiformis; myrtus* myrtle + *forma* shape] shaped like a leaf or berry of the myrtle.

Mysoline trademark for *primidone*.

mysticomimetic (mis'ti-ko-mi-met'ik) mysticomimetic AGENT.

Myvicin trademark for *lincomycin*.

myxadenitis (miks"ad-ĕ-ni'tis) [*myxo-* + Gr. *adēn* gland + *-itis*] inflammation of a mucous gland. **m. labia'lis,** CHEILITIS glandularis apostematosa.

myxedema (mik"sĕ-de'mah) [*myxo-* + Gr. *oidema* swelling] a condition usually observed in adults, resulting from diminished ability to produce hormones by the thyroid gland, most often caused by atrophy of the gland, characterized by a lowered metabolic rate. Symptoms include weakness, lethargy, slow speech, edema of the face and eyelids, sensation of cold, cold clammy skin, decreased sweating, dry and coarse skin, pallor, coarse hair, cardiac enlargement, faulty memory, constipation, and weight gain. A thick protruding tongue appears to be the only constant oral manifestation. Called also *adult cretinism*. **congenital m., infantile m.,** cretinism. **juvenile m.,** a disease of older children and adolescents caused by deficiency of thyroid hormone secondary to insufficiency or lack of the thyroid gland, in which the genitalia are usually normal but puberty is delayed and the growth is retarded and is characterized by a disproportionately long trunk. It may be present at birth but early development is undisturbed. Other symptoms may include areas of ossification, epiphyseal dysgenesis, hypometabolism, and hypercholesteremia. Generally, symptoms are less severe than in cretinism but more severe than in adult myxedema. Delayed tooth eruption and enlarged protruding tongue possibly leading to malocclusion are the principal oral symptoms.

myxo- [Gr. *myxa* mucus] a combining form denoting relationship to mucus, or slime.

myxofibroma (mik"so-fi-bro'mah) a fibroma containing myxomatous tissue. **odontogenic m.,** odontogenic MYXOMA.

myxoid (mik'soid) [*myxo-* + *-oid*] 1. resembling mucus. 2. mucinoid (1).

myxoma (mik-so'mah), pl. *myxomas, myxo'mata* [*myxo-* + *-oma*] a benign soft tissue tumor made up of fibrous tissue resembling primitive mesenchyme, occurring predominantly in the subcutaneous spaces in contact with the muscular aponeuroses and fascia. Other locations that may be involved include bones, the retroperitoneal area, and the genitourinary tract. True oral myxomas are rare; those found in the oral cavity usually represent fibrous tumors that have undergone myxomatous degeneration. **odontogenic m.,** a benign central tumor of the jaws, derived from the mesenchymal part of the tooth germ, either the dental papilla, follicle, or periodontal ligament, which usually grows slowly and does not metastasize, but may infiltrate adjacent tissues. It is made up of spindle-shaped and stellate cells, some with intermeshed fibrillar processes, and intercellular mucoid substance. Tiny capillaries and occasional collagen strands may be found in the tissue. Called also *odontogenic myxofibroma*.

myxosarcoma (mik"so-sar-ko'mah) a sarcoma containing myxomatous tissue.

N

N. 1. nitrogen. 2. newton. 3. a symbolic reference for the number of neutrons in an atomic nucleus. 4. normal or normality (see normal SOLUTION). 5. nasion.

n. 1. normal; neutron; nano-(2): 2. symbol for *refractive index* (see under INDEX). 3. symbol for *principal quantum number* (see under NUMBER).

n$_D$ symbol for *refractive index* (see under INDEX).

2 N symbol for *double-normal;* see under SOLUTION.

N2 trademark for therapeutic root canal sealer containing paraformaldehyde, corticosteroids, and lead tetroxide added to increase radiopacity and hardness of the material.

NA Nomina Anatomica; the official anatomical terminology approved by the Sixth International Congress of Anatomists at Paris in 1955, with later emendations. See also *The Language of Medicine and Dentistry — An Introductory Note*, page ix.

Na 1. chemical symbol for *sodium* (L. *natrium*). 2. nasion.

Nabolin trademark for *methandrostenolone*.

NACA processor trademark for a medium capacity automatic film processor.

NAD 1. nicotinamide-adenine DINUCLEOTIDE. 2. no appreciable disease.

NADL National Association of Dental Laboratories.

NADP nicotinamide-adenine dinucleotide phosphate; see under DINUCLEOTIDE.

Naegeli's syndrome (incontinentia pigmenti) [Oskar *Naegeli*, Swiss dermatologist, 1871–1938] see under SYNDROME.

nafcillin (naf-sil'in) a semisynthetic penicillin, 6-(2-ethoxy-1-naphthamido)-3,3-dimethyl-7-oxo-4-thia-1-azabicyclo[3,2,0] heptane-2-carboxylic acid, which is a broad-spectrum penicillinase-resistant antibiotic. Used as the sodium salt, occurring as a white to yellowish powder with a slight characteristic odor, which dissolves in water, chloroform, and alcohol. Used in the treatment of penicillinase-producing gram-positive bacteria, particularly staphylococci. Also effective against streptococci, pneumococci, *Treponema*, and other bacteria. Its toxicity is similar to that of other penicillins. Trademarks: Naftopen, Unipen.

NaFpak powder see under POWDER.

NaFrinse acidulated solution, rinse see under SOLUTION and RINSE.

Naftopen trademark for *nafcillin*.

Nageotte, Jean [French pathologist, 1866–1948] see Babinski-Nageotte SYNDROME.

Nager's acrofacial dysostosis [F. R. *Nager*] DYSOSTOSIS mandibularis.

Nager-de Reynier syndrome [F. R. *Nager; J. P. de Reynier*] DYSOSTOSIS mandibularis.

nail [nāl] [L. *unguis;* Gr. *onyx*] 1. the horny plate on the dorsal surface of a finger or toe, made up of hard keratin. 2. a rod of metal, bone, or other material, used for fixation of the ends of the fragments of fractured bones. **fracture n.,** a metal nail (usually of stainless steel or other inert metal) used to fasten together the fragments of a broken bone. **Küntscher n.,** a tubular metal nail for the intramedullary fixation of fractures.

nailing (nāl'ing) the operation of fixing or fastening of a fractured bone with a nail. **intramedullary n., marrow n., medullary n.,** the fixation of a fractured long bone by insertion of a steel nail into the marrow cavity of the bone. Called also *intramedullary fixation* and *medullary fixation*.

Nalline trademark for *nalorphine*.

nalorphine (nal'or-fēn) a narcotic antagonist, 7,8-didehydro-4,5-epoxy-17-(2-propylmorphinan-3,6-diol, occurring as a white crystalline powder that is soluble in water, ether, ethanol, acetone and dilute alkali. It is the prototype for partial agonists of the nalorphine type, competing with morphine-like drugs for opioid receptor sites, and also producing autonomic, endocrine, analgesic, and respiratory depressant effects similar to those of morphine. Nalorphine does not produce symptoms of abstinence when given alone, but can cause severe withdrawal symptoms in addicts and in nonaddicts who have received narcotics. Used to alleviate postoperative pain; as a specific antidote in acute narcotic poisoning, inhibiting the action of morphine, methadone, meperidine, and other narcotic drugs; and in the diagnosis of narcotic addiction. Called also *allorphine, N-allylnormorphine,* and *antorphine*. Trademarks: Anarcon, Nalline, Norfin. **n. hydrochloride,** the hydrochloride salt of nalorphine, occurring as a white, odorless, crystalline powder that darkens on exposure to air and light and is soluble in water, ethanol, and alkali hydroxide solution, but not in ether and chloroform. Its pharmacological properties are similar to those of the parent compound. Trademark: Miromorfalil.

naloxone (nal-oks'ōn) a pure narcotic antagonist that competes with morphine-like compounds for opioid receptor sites, 17-allyl-4,5α-epoxy-3,14-dihydroxymorphinan-6-one, occurring as chloroform-soluble crystals. Used in the treatment of depression produced by narcotics, and in restoring a normal level of alertness following the use of narcotics, as in ambulatory dental practice. Trademark: Narcon. **n. hydrochloride,** the hydrochloride salt of naloxone, occurring as an off-white, odorless, bitter powder that is affected by moisture and light and is soluble in water, slightly soluble in ethanol, and insoluble in ether and chloroform. Its pharmacological properties are similar to those of the parent compound.

name (nām) a word(s) used to designate a person, place, or thing, distinguishing it from another. **established n.,** DRUG established name. **generic n.,** DRUG generic name. **systematic n.,** in chemical nomenclature, a name of a substance based on the systematic chemical structure of a compound. **trivial n.,** in chemical nomenclature, any name of a substance that is not based on the systematic structure of a compound; it may be an abbreviation or any name given for convenience. **United States Adopted N.,** see USAN.

NANB nonA-nonB; see Au ANTIGEN.

Nance's leeway space see under SPACE.

nandrolone (nan'dro-lōn) a synthetic androgenic steroid, 17β-hydroxyestr-4-en-3-one, occurring as a crystalline substance that is soluble in ethanol, ether, and chloroform. Used chiefly in the treatment of chronic wasting diseases and conditions characterized by negative nitrogen balance. Called also *19-nortestosterone.*

nanism (na'nizm) [L. *nanus* dwarf] underdevelopment of body; dwarfism. **Hanhart's n.,** hereditary proportionate dwarfism associated with adiposogenital dystrophy, transmitted as a simple recessive trait, and occurring in closely inbred groups. Growth retardation is usually observed between the ages of one and a half to six years, after a normal infancy and early childhood. Heavy deposits of adipose tissue on the breast and abdomen, underdevelopment of secondary sex characteristics, typical facies, and diminished or absent libido are the principal features. Occasionally, brachycephaly and mental retardation are seen. Called also *Hanhart's syndrome.* **mulibrey n.,** a hereditary syndrome, transmitted as an autosomal recessive trait, combining abnormalities of the *mu*scles, *li*ver, *br*ain, and *ey*e (hence the name *mulibrey*). It is characterized by progressive growth failure of prenatal onset, triangular face with hydrocephaloid skull, thinness, muscular hypotonia, a peculiar voice due to venous congestion caused by pericardial constriction, and pigment dispersion and yellowish dots in the fundi of the eye. Two-thirds of the affected patients have cutaneous nevi flammei and one-third have cystic fibrous dysplasia of the tibia. **symptomatic n.,** that in which there is defective dentition, ossification, and sexual development.

nano- [Gr. *nanos;* L. *nanus* dwarf] 1. a combining form denoting small size. 2. in the metric system, a combining form denoting one-billionth (10⁻⁹) of the unit designated by the root with which it combined. Abbreviated *n.* Formerly called *millimicro-.* See also metric SYSTEM and *Tables of Weights and Measures* at WEIGHT.

nanocephaly (na"no-sef'ah-le) [*nano-* + Gr. *kephalē* head] abnormal smallness of the head.

nanocurie (na"no-ku're) a unit of radioactivity, being one-billionth (10⁻⁹) of a curie, or the quantity of radioactive material in which the number of nuclear disintegrations is 3.7×10, or 37, per second. Abbreviated *nc* or *nCi.* Formerly called *millimicrocurie* ($m\mu c$).

nanogram (na'no-gram) [*nano-* + *gram*] a unit of mass (weight) in the metric system, being one-billionth (10⁻⁹) of a gram. Abbreviated *ng.* Formerly called *millimicrogram.*

nanoid (na'noid) [*nano-* + Gr. *eidos* form] dwarfish; resembling a dwarf.

nanoliter (na"no-le'ter) [*nano-* + *liter*] a unit of volume in the metric system, being one-billionth (10⁻⁹) of a liter. Abbreviated *nl.* Formerly called *millimicroliter.*

nanometer (na"no-me'ter) [*nano-* + *meter*] a unit of length in the metric system, being one-billionth (10⁻⁹) of a meter and equivalent to the micromillimeter and the millimicron. Abbreviated *nm.*

nanosecond (na"no-sek'ond) [*nano-* + *second*] a unit of time, being one-billionth (10⁻⁹) of a second. Abbreviated *ns* or *nsec.*

nanounit (na"no-u'nit) [*nano-* + *unit*] one-billionth (10⁻⁹) of a standard unit. Abbreviated *nU.*

nanus (na'nus) [L.; Gr. *nanos*] a dwarf.

NAP nasion, point A, pogonion; see ANGLE of convexity.

napex (na'peks) the region of the scalp just below the occipital protuberance.

naphazoline (naf-az'o-lēn) a directly acting sympathomimetic, 2-(1-naphtylmethyl)-2-imidazoline. Used as the hydrochloride salt, which occurs as a- white, odorless, bitter, crystalline powder that is readily soluble in water and ethanol, slightly soluble in chloroform, and insoluble in ether. Used as a local vasoconstrictor, chiefly for relief of nasal congestion. Hypertension, bradycardia, sweating, excessive sedation, and occasional coma in children are the principal side reactions. Trademarks: Coldan, Niazol, Privine, Sanorin, Vasocon.

naphthalene (naf'thah-lēn) [L. *naphthalinum*] an aromatic hydrocarbon, $C_{10}H_8$, occurring as monoclinic primastic plates, white scales, or balls, being the most abundant constituent of coal tar. It volatilizes at room temperature and is soluble in hot water, alcohol, ether, chloroform, benzene, and other organic solvents. Used as a moth repellent and fungicide and in the synthesis of various products. Formerly used in the treatment of typhoid fever. Ingestion or absorption of large quantities may cause nausea, vomiting, headache, hematuria, hemolytic ane-

mia, fever, liver necrosis, convulsions, and coma. Called also *naphthalin.*

naphthalin (naf'thah-lin) naphthalene.

Naprosine trademark for *naproxen.*

naproxen (nah-proks'en) an anti-inflammatory, analgesic, and antipyretic agent, (+)-6-methoxy-α-methyl-2-naphthaleneacetic acid. It may cause gastrointestinal bleeding. Trademarks: Naprosine, Proxen.

napsylate (nap'sĭ-lāt) a naphthalene substituted by a sulfonate group. See PROPOXYPHENE napsylate.

Napsylgesic trademark for *propoxyphene napsylate* (see under PROPOXYPHENE).

Narcan trademark for *naloxone hydrochloride* (see under NALOXONE).

narco- [Gr. *narkē* numbness] a combining form denoting relationship to stupor or to a stuporous state.

narcoma (nar-ko'mah) stupor or coma produced by narcotics.

Narcon trademark for *naloxone.*

narcosis (nar-ko'sis) [Gr. *narkōsis* a benumbing] a condition characterized by stupor or insensibility.

narcotic (nar-kot'ik) [Gr. *narkotikos* benumbing, deadening] 1. pertaining to or producing narcosis. 2. any drug which dulls senses and reduces pain, whose extended use may produce drug dependence, including heroin, morphine, meperidine, and methadone. According to the Comprehensive Drug Abuse Prevention Act, a narcotic is any drug, whether produced directly or indirectly by extraction from substances of vegetable origin, or independently by means of chemical synthesis, or by combination of extraction and chemical synthesis: opium, coca leaves, and opiates; a compound, manufacture, salt, derivative or preparation of opium, coca leaves, or opiates; and a substance (and any compound, manufacture, salt, derivative, or preparation thereof) which is chemically identical with any of the substances referred to above. Called also *narcotic drug.* See also narcotic ANALGESIC. **n. antagonist,** narcotic ANTAGONIST.

Narcotile trademark for *ethyl chloride* (see under CHLORIDE).

Nardil trademark for *phenelzine sulfate* (see under PHENELZINE).

nares (na'rēz) [L.] [NA] plural of *naris;* the external orifices of the nose. Called also *nostrils.* **posterior n.,** choana (2).

Nargesic tablets see under TABLET.

Naridan trademark for *oxyphencyclimine hydrochloride* (see under OXYPHENCYCLIMINE).

naris (na'ris), pl. *na'res* [L.] one of the openings of the nose. Called also *nostril.*

Narphen trademark for *phenazocine hydrobromide* (see under PHENAZOCINE).

nasal (na'zal) [L. *nasalis*] pertaining to the nose.

nasalis (na-za'lis) [L.] nasal.

nasality the quality of speech sounds when the nasal cavity is used as a resonator.

nascent (nas'ent, na'sent) [L. *nascens*] 1. just born; just coming into existence. 2. just liberated from a chemical combination.

NASDAD National Association of Seventh-Day Adventist Dentists (see under ASSOCIATION).

nasioiniac (na"ze-o-in'e-ak) pertaining to the nasion and inion.

nasion (na'ze-on) [L. *nasus* nose] an anthropometric landmark locating the point where the intranasal and nasofrontal sutures meet; it corresponds roughly to the depression at the root of the nose just below the level of the eyebrows. Abbreviated *N* or *Na.* Called also *nasal point* and *point Na.* See illustration at CEPHALOMETRY.

nasitis (na-zi'tis) inflammation of the nose; rhinitis.

Nasmil trademark for *cromolyn sodium* (see under CROMOLYN).

Nasmyth's membrane [Alexander *Nasmyth,* Scottish surgeon in London, died 1847] enamel CUTICLE.

naso- [L. *nasus* nose] a combining form denoting relationship to the nose. See also terms beginning RHINO-.

nasoantral (na"zo-an'tral) pertaining to the nose and the maxillary antrum.

nasoantritis (na"zo-an-tri'tis) inflammation of the nose and the maxillary antrum.

nasobronchial (na"zo-brong'ke-al) pertaining to the nasal cavities and the bronchi.

nasociliary (na"zo-sil'e-a"re) pertaining to the eyes, brow, and root of the nose, as the nasociliary nerve.

nasofrontal (na"zo-frun'tal) pertaining to the nasal and frontal bones.

nasograph (na'zo-graf) an instrument for measuring the nose.

nasolabial (na"zo-la'be-al) [*naso-* + L. *labium* lip] pertaining to the nose and lip.

nasolacrimal (na″zo-lak′ri-mal) pertaining to the nose and lacrimal apparatus.

nasomanometer (na″zo-mah-nom′ĕ-ter) a manometer for measuring intranasal pressure.

naso-oral (na″zo-o′ral) pertaining to the nose and mouth.

nasopalatine (na″zo-pal′ah-tīn) pertaining to the nose and palate.

nasopharyngeal (na″zo-fah-rin′je-al) pertaining to the nasopharynx; rhinopharyngeal.

nasopharyngitis (na″zo-far″in-ji′tis) inflammation of the nasopharynx; pharyngorhinitis.

nasopharyngoscope (na″zo-fah-rin′go-skōp) a lighted, telescopic endoscope for use in examination of the nasopharynx and the pharyngeal end of the auditory tube.

nasopharynx (na″zo-far′inks) [naso- + pharynx] the part of the pharynx above the level of the soft palate, communicating with the posterior nares and the auditory tube. Similarly to the soft palate and its appendages, the nasopharynx is lined by nonkeratinized stratified squamous epithelium which rests on a well developed lamina propria. No submucosa is present. In swallowing, the nasopharynx is closed off by the uvula during the passage of food from the mouth to the esophagus. Called also *epipharynx, nasal pharynx, pars nasalis pharyngis* [NA], and *pharyngonasal cavity.*

nasorostral (na″zo-ros′tral) pertaining to the rostrum of the nose.

nasoscope (na′zo-skōp) [naso- + Gr. *skopein* to examine] a lighted instrument for the examination of the nasal cavity.

nasoseptal (na″zo-sep′tal) pertaining to the nasal septum.

nasoseptitis (na″zo-sep-ti′tis) inflammation of the nasal septum.

nasospinale (na″zo-spi-na′le) an anthropometric landmark situated at the base of the anterior nasal spine, at the point at which a horizontal line tangential to the lower margins of the nasal aperture is intersected by the midsagittal plane. Abbreviated *Ns.* Called also *point Ns.* See illustration at CEPHALOMETRY.

nasoturbinal (na″zo-tur′bĭ-nal) pertaining to the nose and turbinate bone.

Nastenon trademark for *oxymetholone.*

nasus (na′sus) [L.] [NA] nose. **n. exter′nus** [NA], external nose.

Natacillin trademark for *hetacillin potassium* (see under HETACILLIN).

natal (na′tal) [L. *natus* birth] pertaining to birth.

National Formulary see under FORMULARY.

native (na′tiv) [L. *nativus*] normal to a location; uncombined with other elements or unaltered from its natural state.

Natrionex trademark for *acetazolamide.*

natrium (na′tre-um) gen. *na′trii* [L.] sodium.

natriuresis (na″tre-u-re′sis) [L. *natrium* sodium + Gr. *ourēsis* a making water] the excretion of abnormal amounts of sodium in the urine.

natriuretic (na″tre-u-ret′ik) 1. pertaining to natriuresis. 2. an agent that promotes excretion of large amounts of sodium in the urine. See also DIURETIC.

Natulan trademark for *procarbazine hydrochloride* (see under PROCARBAZINE).

natural (nat′u-ral) [L. *naturalis,* from *natura* nature] existing or occurring in nature or under natural conditions; neither artificial nor pathologic.

Natural Coe-Lor trademark for a heat-cured denture base acrylic resin.

Naturon trademark for *methyclothiazide.*

naturopath (na′chur-o-path″) a practitioner of naturopathy. A person who has received a degree of Doctor of Naturopathy (N.D.) from an approved school of naturopathy and who has been licensed to practice naturopathy; licensing laws vary from state to state.

naturopathy (na″chur-op′ah-the) a drugless system of therapy, making use of physical forces such as air, light, water, heat, massage, etc.

nausea (naw′se-ah) [L.; Gr. *nausia* seasickness] an unpleasant sensation, vaguely referred to the epigastrium and abdomen, and often culminating in vomiting.

Nautazine trademark for *cyclizine.*

Navane trademark for *thiothixene hydrochloride* (see under THIOTHIXENE).

navel (na′vel) 1. a cicatricial depression in the middle of the abdomen, marking the point of attachment of the umbilical cord. Called also *umbilicus* [NA]. 2. any structure similar to the navel. **enamel n.,** in the cap stage of odontogenesis, a slight indentation in the outer dental epithelium of a developing tooth,

in the end of the enamel cord. It is a temporary structure which disappears before enamel formation begins.

navicular (nah-vik′u-lar) [L. *navicula* boat] boat-shaped; scaphoid.

N.B. abbreviation for L. *no′ta be′ne,* note well.

Nb niobium.

NBME National Board of Medical Examiners; see under BOARD.

nc nanocurie.

NCHSR National Center for Health Services Research.

nCi nanocurie.

N/cm² newtons per square centimeter.

NCRP National Council for Radiation Protection and Measurements; see under COUNCIL.

ND Doctor of Naturopathy (see NATUROPATH).

Nd neodymium.

NDA 1. National Dental Association. 2. new drug application (see under APPLICATION).

Ne neon.

Neamine trademark for *neomycin A.*

nearsightedness (nēr-sīt′ed-nes) myopia.

Neazina trademark for *sulfamethazine.*

Neazolin trademark for *sulfisoxazole.*

Nebs analgesic liquid, tablets see under LIQUID and TABLET.

necessity (ně-ses′ĭ-te) something necessary or indispensable. **pharmaceutic n., pharmaceutical n.,** a substance that itself has no therapeutic value, but is necessary for the production or preparation of pharmaceutical preparations, including excipient, filtering, enteric coating, flavoring, coloring, diluting, emulsifying, and suspending agents, and ointment bases. Called also *pharmaceutic* or *pharmaceutical aid.*

neck (nek) 1. the portion of the body connecting the head and trunk (called also *collum* [NA]); the lower front portion of the neck is called the *cervix* and the back is called the *nucha.* 2. any constricted, necklike portion of the body connecting two structures or organs. See also terms beginning CERVICO-. **bull n.,** massive swelling of the neck, as in malignant diphtheria. **bur n.,** the narrowing part of the bur which connects the shank with the head. See BUR. **n. of condyle, n. of condyloid process of mandible,** n. of mandible. **implant n., implant superstructure n.,** implant POST. **n. of mandible,** the constricted portion of the mandible below the articular part, being flattened in front and having a concavity on its medial surface (*pterygoid fossa*), and a smooth semicircular notch (*sigmoid notch*), which forms the upper border of the ramus. Called also *n. of condyle, n. of condyloid process of mandible, collum mandibulae* [NA], and *collum processus condyloidei mandibulae.* **n. of tooth,** the constricted part of the tooth at the junction of the crown and root or roots. Called also *cervix dentis* and *collum dentis* [NA]. **wry n.,** torticollis.

necrectomy (nek-rek′to-me) [necro- + Gr. *ektomē* excision] the excision of necrotic tissue.

necro- [Gr. *nekros* dead body; dead] a combining form denoting relationship to death or to a dead body, cells, or tissue.

necrobiosis (nek″ro-bi-o′sis) [necro- + Gr. *biosis* life] the physiologic degeneration and death of cells or tissue followed by replacement, such as the constant degeneration and replacement of cells of the epidermis or blood. Called also *bionecrosis.* See also GANGRENE and NECROSIS.

necrocytosis (nek″ro-si-to′sis) [necro- + Gr. *kytos* cell + -osis] cell DEATH. See also NECROSIS.

necrogenic (nek″ro-jen′ik) [necro- + Gr. *gennan* to produce] productive of necrosis or death.

necrogenous (ně-kroj′ě-nus) [necro- + Gr. *gennan* to produce] originating from dead matter.

necrology (ně-krol′o-je) [necro- + -logy] the statistics or records of deaths.

necrolysis (ně-krol′ĭ-sis) [necro- + Gr. *lysis* dissolution] separation or exfoliation of tissue due to necrosis. **toxic epidermal n.,** an exfoliative skin disease in which erythema rapidly spreads over the entire body, followed by the formation of large flaccid bullae and later by skin that appears scalded and separates from the body in sheets, much as in a second degree burn. Staphylococci of phage group two (in infants) and a toxic reaction to various drugs (in adults) are the usual causes. Called *Lyell's syndrome* and *scalded skin syndrome.*

necronectomy (nek″ro-nek′to-me) [necro- + Gr. *ektomē* excision] the excision of necrotic tissue.

necropsy (nek′rop-se) [Gr. *nekros* dead + *opsis* view] examination of a body after death; autopsy.

necroses (ně-kro′sēz) [Gr.] plural of *necrosis.*

necrosis (ne-kro′sis), pl. *necro′ses* [Gr. *nekrōs* death + -osis] death of tissue, especially as individual cells or groups of cells in localized areas, brought about by the degradative action of enzymes on the lethally injured cells. The process begins when cell injury triggers the activation and release of lysosomal enzymes in the injured cells which cause their disintegration (*autolysis*). Injury also produces an inflammatory reaction associated with migration of polymorphonuclear leukocytes to the focus of injury, the malignant cells contributing their lysosomal enzymes to the degradation of injured cells (*heterolysis*). Also involved in the process are changes in cell nuclei, consisting of shrinkage (*pyknosis*), fragmentation (*karyorrhexis*), and, ultimately, destruction (*karyolysis*). Cell death is followed by progressive proteolysis and digestion of the carcass (*colliquative n.*) and immediate removal of liquefied debris, or coagulation and temporary mummification of the carcass (*coagulation n.*) for later removal. See also cell DEATH, GANGRENE, and NECROBIOSIS. **avascular n.,** that due to deficient blood supply. See also *coagulation n.* **caseous n., caseation n.,** cheesy n. **cheesy n.,** necrosis, most commonly occurring in tuberculosis, characterized by conversion of tissue into a granular, eosinophilic mass of amorphous fat and proteins, with total loss of cell detail, giving it the appearance of cottage cheese. Cheesy necrosis of the dental pulp is one of the causes of its death. Called also *caseous n.* and *caseation n.* See also necrotic PULP. **coagulation n., coagulative n.,** necrosis in which dead cells are converted to an acidophilic opaque mass, usually with loss of the nucleus but with the preservation of its basic shape to permit recognition of cell boundaries, whereby cell debris is temporarily mummified; occurring most commonly when the tissue loses its blood supply. Called also *dry n.* and *ischemic n.* **colliquative n.,** necrosis in which dead cells are digested and liquefied through the action of protein-splitting enzymes into the leukocyte-containing proteinaceous fluid which is a part of pus. This type is encountered most commonly in focal bacterial lesions, being one of the principal causes of dental pulp death. The enzymes are believed to originate from leukocytes and bacteria, including staphylococci, streptococci, and *Escherichia coli.* Called also *liquefaction n., liquefactive n.,* and *moist n.* See also necrotic PULP. **dry n.,** that in which the necrotic tissue becomes dry. See *coagulation n.* **embolic n.,** coagulation necrosis of an infarct following embolism. **epiphyseal ischemic n.,** osteochondrosis. **exanthematous n.,** an acute necrotizing process involving the gingivae, jaw bones, and contiguous soft tissues, which primarily affects children; it resembles gangrenous stomatitis, except that there is a slight odor, tendency to be self-limited, low mortality rate, and normal leukocyte count. **fat n.,** necrosis of fatty tissue, in which the neutral fats in the cells are split into fatty acids and glycerol. **focal n.,** the presence of small foci of necrosis. **gangrenous n.,** gangrene. **gangrenous pulp n.,** necrosis of the pulp tissue due to ischemia with superimposed bacterial infection, representing an advanced stage of untreated pulpitis. Called also *pulp gangrene.* See also necrotic PULP. **gummatous n.,** see GUMMA. **intrauterine facial n.,** first and second branchial arch SYNDROME. **ischemic n.,** coagulation n. **liquefaction n., liquefactive n.,** colliquative n. **medial n.,** medionecrosis. **moist n.,** that in which the dead tissue becomes wet and soft. See *colliquative n.* **mummification n.,** dry GANGRENE. **phosphorus n.,** necrosis of the jaw, sometimes associated with deposition of new subperiosteal bone, occurring in workers exposed to yellow phosphorus fumes. It is now very rare. Called also *phosphonecrosis* and *phossy jaw.* See also PHOSPHORUS. **n. progre′diens,** progressive sloughing. **pulp n.,** necrotic PULP. **radiation n.,** necrosis at the site of radiation injury. **radium n.,** necrosis of the jaw bone in workers in radium plants. **septic n.,** that resulting from bacterial infection. **simple n.,** degeneration of the protoplasm and nucleus of the cells without changes in the appearance of the tissue. **superficial n.,** that which affects only the outer layers of a bone. **total n.,** that which affects all parts of a bone.

necrotic (ně-krot′ik) pertaining to or characterized by necrosis.

necrotizing (nek′ro-tīz″ing) causing necrosis.

necrotomy (ne-krot′o-me) [Gr. *nekros* death + *tomē* a cutting] 1. dissection (1). 2. the excision of a sequestrum. **osteoplastic n.,** removal of a sequestrum from a bone after first lifting a flap of the bone, which is replaced after the operation.

need (nēd) 1. a requirement. 2. a lack of something wanted. 3. destitution or poverty. **accrued n's, accumulated n's,** the amount of treatment needed by an individual or group at any given time. In dental plans, the term usually refers to conditions at the time of enrollment. Called also *backlog.* **certificate of n.,** CERTIFICATE of need.

needle (ne′d′l) [L. *acus*] 1. a slender, sharp instrument, usually made of steel, with an eye for thread, used for sewing or suturing. 2. a sharp, pointed indicator on a dial. 3. any sharp, slender object. See also terms beginning ACU-. **aneurysm n.,** one with a handle, used in ligating blood vessels. **aspirating n.,** a long hollow needle for removing fluid from a cavity. **atraumatic**

n., swaged n. Deschamps' n., one with the eye near the point, and a long handle attached; used in ligating deep-seated arteries. **exploring n.,** a long, grooved, eyeless needle so constructed that it may puncture an abscess, tumor, or any tissue containing fluid and allow a few drops to flow through the groove. **Gillmore n.,** an instrument, available as either a ¼- or 1-lb needle, used for the penetration test in determining the setting time of a material such as plaster of Paris. See illustration. See

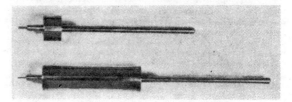

Set of Gillmore needles. (From R.W. Phillips: Skinner's Science of Dental Materials. 7th ed. Philadelphia, W. B. Saunders Co., 1973.)

also setting TIME. **Hagedorn's n.,** one of several suture needles which are flat from side to side, and have a straight cutting edge near the point and a large eye. **harelip n.,** a needle (or pin) introduced through the edges of the wound in harelip operation, a figure-of-8 suture being applied over the needle. Called also *harelip pin.* **n. holder,** needle HOLDER. **hypodermic n.,** a slender, hollow needle attached to the barrel of a hypodermic syringe. **ligature n.,** a slender needle with a long handle and an eye in its curved end, used for passing a ligature underneath an artery. **noncutting n.,** a suture needle designed to inflict the least possible trauma. **nontarnish n.,** one resistant to tarnishing during the sterilization processes. **radioactive n.,** in radiation therapy, a sealed source of radioactive material inserted into the region of a tumor. **radium n.,** a hollow, straight needle containing radium in its cavity, used in intracavitary and interstitial treatment of lesions in regions such as the maxillary sinuses, lips, floor of the mouth, buccal mucosa, and the tongue. **Reverdin n.,** a suture needle having an eye which can be opened and closed by means of a slide. **Silverman n.,** an instrument for taking tissue specimens, consisting of an outer cannula, an obturator, and an inner split needle with longitudinal grooves in which the tissue is retained when the needle and cannula are withdrawn. **stop n.,** one with a shoulder that prevents it from being inserted beyond a certain distance. **surgical n.,** suture n. **suture n.,** a usually curved needle for suturing tissues. Called also *surgical n.* See illustration.

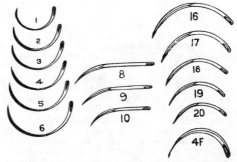

Suture needles. (From H. O. Torres and A. Ehrlich: Modern Dental Assisting. 2nd ed. Philadelphia, W. B. Saunders Co., 1980; courtesy of Hu-Friedy Mfg. Co., Inc.)

swaged n., one permanently attached to the suture material. Called also *atraumatic n.* **Vicat's n.,** a needle used in the penetration test in determining the setting time of materials, such as plaster or stone. See also setting TIME.

Needles, Carl F. [American physician] see Melnick-Needles SYNDROME.

needy (ne′de) one who is in a state of want; poor; destitute. **categorically n.,** persons who are eligible to receive public assistance. Under Medicaid, persons who are blind, aged, disabled, or are members of families with children under 18 (or 21, if in school) where one parent is absent, incapacitated, or unemployed are considered as being categorically needy, providing that they also meet specified income and resources requirements established by individual states. **medically n.,** under the Medicaid program, persons who possess sufficient resources to pay their basic living expenses but are unable to pay their medical expenses.

NEFA nonesterified fatty acids; see under ACID.

negative (neg′ah-tiv) [L. *negativus*] 1. contradictory of or denying something; opposite to *positive.* 2. a mathematical quantity that has a minus or less than zero value. Symbol −. 3. indicating a lack or absence. 4. a reverse impression or mold. 5. the plate of a voltaic or electrolytic cell that is at the lower potential. 6. in photography, a plate or film whose image is inverted, where light areas appear dark and shadows light. Used to produce positive photographs by transilluminating the negative onto a photosensitive surface.

neglect (ně-glekt′) to fail or to be remiss or careless in performing one's task.

negligence (neg′li-jens) the state or fact of being neglectful, or being indifferent or careless; failure to exercise the proper or reasonable care that a prudent person would be expected to exercise, as when failing to protect the patient from undue damage or injury during the performance of a diagnostic or therapeutic procedure. See also MALPRACTICE. **contributory n.,** failure on the part of the patient to follow the doctor's instructions.

Negri, Silvio see SILVIO NEGRI.

Neill-Dingwall syndrome [Catherine A. *Neill,* American physician, born 1921; Mary M. *Dingwall*] Cockayne's SYNDROME.

Neisser, Albert Ludwig Siegmund [1855–1916] a German physician.

Neisser-Wechsberg leukocidin [Max *Neisser,* German physician, 1869–1938; Friedrick *Wechsberg,* German physician] see under LEUKOCIDIN.

Neisseria (nīs-se′re-ah) [named after A. L. S. *Neisser*] a genus of gram-negative bacteria of the family Neisseriaceae, occurring as cocci, singly or in pairs with adjacent sides flattened, about 0.6 to 1.0 μm in diameter; tetrads occur sometimes. The members are aerobic or facultatively anaerobic, nonendosporogenous, and nonmotile organisms, sometimes having capsules and fimbriae, which produce catalase and cytochrome oxidase. They are parasitic on mammalian mucous membranes, including those of the oral cavity; some species are pathogenic. In the oral cavity, they have been found on the lips, tongue, and cheeks, and in plaque and the saliva; mean proportions were less than 1 percent of the cultivable flora. Most species are sensitive to penicillin, streptomycin, tetracyclines, the macrolide group of polymyxin B sulfate, and related drugs. **N. fla′va,** *N. subflava.* **N. flaves′cens,** a rare species isolated from the cerebrospinal fluid in patients with meningitis and from the blood in patients with septicemia. **N. gonorrhoe′ae,** a species which causes gonorrhea and other infections in man, found in purulent discharges, blood, conjunctiva, joints, petechiae in the skin, and cerebrospinal fluid. In most cases, it is susceptible to penicillin. Called also *Diplococcus gonorrhoeae, gonococcus, Gonococcus neisseri, Merismopedia gonorrhoeae, Micrococcus gonococcus,* and *M. gonorrhoeae.* **N. haemoly′sans,** *Gemella haemolysans;* see under GEMELLA. **N. meningi′tidis,** a species causing epidemic cerebrospinal fever, found in the cerebrospinal fluid, nasopharynx, blood, conjunctiva, joints, discharge in venereal diseases, and petechiae in skin; also found in the nasopharynx of normal persons. Called also *N. weichselbaumii, meningococcus, Micrococcus intracellularis,* and *M. meningitidis.* **N. muco′sa,** a potentially pathogenic species isolated from the human rhinopharynx. Called also *Diplococcus mucosus.* **N. perfla′va,** *N. subflava.* **N. sic′sa,** a species isolated from the nasopharynx, saliva, and sputum in man. Called also *Diplococcus siccus.* **N. subfla′va,** a species isolated from the human nasopharynx and, less commonly, from the cerebrospinal fluid in cases of meningitis. Called also *N. flava* and *N. perflava.* **N. weichselbau′mii,** *N. meningitidis.*

Neisseriaceae (nis-se″re-a′se-e) [*Neisseria* + *-aceae*] a family of spheroid bacteria, occurring in pairs or in masses with adjacent sides flattened, or as rods in pairs or short chains. The members are aerobic, nonflagellated, and gram-negative organisms, some being parasitic, some saprophytic, and others pathogenic. The family includes the genera *Acinetobacter, Branhamella, Moraxella,* and *Neisseria.*

nem (nem) [acronym for Ger. *Nahrungs Einheit Milch* "nutritional unit milk"] a unit of nutrition equivalent to the nutritive value of 1 gm of breast milk.

Nematoda (nem″ah-to′dah) [Gr. *něma* thread + *eidos* form] a class of tapered cylindrical helminths, the roundworms, characterized by longitudinally oriented muscles and by a triradiate esophagus.

nematode (nem′ah-tōd) any individual belonging to the class Nematoda.

nematodiasis (nem″ah-to-di′ah-sis) infection by nematodes.

Nembutal trademark for *pentobarbital.*

neo- [Gr. *neos* new] a combining form meaning new or strange.

Neo-Atromid trademark for *clofibrate.*

Neobar trademark for *barium sulfate* (see under BARIUM).

Neocid trademark for *chlorophenothane.*

Neo-Cobefrin trademark for *levonordefrin.*

Neo-Devomit trademark for *cyclizine.*

Neodrenal trademark for *isoproterenol.*

Neodrol trademark for *stanolone.*

neodymium (ne″o-dim′e-um) [Gr. *neos* new + *didymos* twin, so named because it was considered to be an "inseparable twin of lanthanum"] a rare earth, occurring as a soft, malleable, yellowish metal. Symbol, Nd; atomic number, 60; atomic weight, 144.24; specific gravity, 6.80; melting point, 1021°C; valence, 3; group IIIB of the periodic table. It has seven naturally occurring isotopes: 142–146, 148, and 150; 144 is radioactive with a half-life of 2.4×10^{15} years and emits alpha rays. Artificial radioactive isotopes include 138–141, 147, 149, and 151. Neodymium tarnishes on exposure to air and liberates hydrogen from water, being soluble in dilute acids. Its salts may be irritating to the skin and eyes. Used in electronic and space technologies.

Neo-Erycinum trademark for *erythromycin estolate* (see under ERYTHROMYCIN).

neohippocratism (ne″o-hip-pok′rah-tizm) a school of medicine (and by implication dentistry) which tends toward a humanistic view of disease focused on the individual patient and scientific observation by the physician, representing a return to the hippocratic theory and practice, with emphasis on observational and bedside medicine.

Neohydrin trademark for *chlormerodrin.*

Neoisuprel trademark for *isoetharine.*

Neolate trademark for *neomycin.*

Neo-Mercazole trademark for *carbimazole.*

Neo-Metantyl trademark for *propantheline bromide* (see under PROPANTHELINE).

Neomin trademark for *neomycin.*

neomycin (ne′o-mi″sin) an aminoglycoside antibiotic which acts on the bacterial ribosome and is elaborated by *Streptomyces fradiae,* occurring as a white to yellowish powder or cryodesiccated, odorless, hygroscopic solid that is soluble in water, slightly soluble in alcohol, and insoluble in acetone, chloroform, and ether. It comprises three components; neomycins A, B, and C. Neomycin is active against a wide sprectrum of gram-positive and gram-negative bacteria (except *Pseudomonas*) and against acid-fast bacilli and actinomycetes. Used in the treatment of burns, wounds, ulcers, furunculosis, dermatoses, otitis, and various infections. Parenteral administration may cause hypersensitization and nephrotoxic and neurotoxic complications, including lesions of the eighth cranial nerve with auditory disorders. Trademarks: Fradiomycin, Myacyne, Mycifradin, Neolate, Neomine, Nivemycin, Vonamycin. **n. A,** one of the three components of the neomycin complex, $C_{12}H_{26}N_4O_6$. Trademark: Neamine. **n. B.,** one of the three components of the neomycin complex, $C_{23}H_{46}N_6O_{13}$. Trademarks: Actilin, Enterfram, Framycetin, Soframycin. **n. C,** one of the three components of the neomycin complex, $C_{23}H_{46}O_{13}$. **n. sulfate,** the sulfate salt of neomycin, having a potency of not less than 180 mcg of the base activity per milligram.

neon (ne′on) [Gr. *neos* new] a rare gaseous element. Symbol, Ne; atomic number, 10; atomic weight, 20.179; specific gravity, 0.6964; group 0 of the periodic table. It occurs as three stable isotopes, 20–22, and five short-lived artificial radioactive ones, 17–19, 23, and 24. Neon is a colorless, odorless, tasteless, nontoxic, inert gas, which does not form compounds, but ionizes in electric discharge tubes. Used in electronic and electrical technologies and in gaseous filters for antifog devices.

neonatal (ne″o-na′tal) [*neo-* + L. *natus* born] pertaining to the period immediately after birth.

neoplasia (ne″o-pla′ze-ah) [*neo-* + Gr. *plassein* to form] formation of a neoplasm, or an abnormal mass of tissue, the growth of which exceeds and is uncoordinated with that of the normal tissues and persists in the same excessive manner after cessation of the stimuli which evoke the change. Cf. HYPERPLASIA and HYPERTROPHY. **radiation n.,** formation of a neoplasm at the site of radiation injury.

neoplasm (ne′o-plazm) [*neo-* + Gr. *plasma* formation] a new growth comprising an abnormal mass of tissue, the growth of which exceeds and is uncoordinated with that of the normal tissues and persists in the same excessive manner after cessation of the stimuli which evoke the change. The mass is purposeless and virtually autonomous, but depends on the host for nutrition, respiration, and vascular supply. Neoplasms may be benign or malignant. See also CANCER and TUMOR. **benign n.,** benign TUMOR. **malignant n.,** malignant TUMOR.

neoplastic (ne″o-plas′tik) pertaining to or like a neoplasm.

Neorickettsia (ne″o-rĭ-ket′se-ah) a genus of bacteria of the tribe Ehrlichieae, family Rickettsiaceae, occurring as small, gram-negative, nonmotile, coccoid, often pleomorphic organisms, found in the reticular cells of lymphoid tissues of dogs and other canines and in certain flukes. They are not known to be pathogenic for man.

neostigmine (ne″o-stig′mēn) a quaternary ammonium compound with cholinomimetic properties, 3-[[(dimethylamino)carbonyl]oxy]-*N,N,N*-trimethylbenzenaminium, which acts as an anticholinesterase agent on the esteratic site to form the inactive dimethylcarbamoyl enzyme. Its principal sites of action are the bowel, urinary bladder, and skeletal muscles; to a lesser degree, it acts on the pupils, heart, blood pressure, and secretory organs. Used chiefly in the form of its bromide and methyl sulfate salts, in the treatment of postanesthetic disorders, such as bladder atony and intestinal paresis, and in therapy of myasthenia gravis. Also used as an antidote in curare poisoning and in therapy of myotonia congenita, glaucoma, and esotropia. Side effects may include nausea, vomiting, diarrhea, abdominal cramps, excessive salivation, increased bronchial secretions, bronchoconstriction, excessive sweating, miosis, muscle cramps, fasciculation and muscle twitching, and weakness. Called also *synstigmin.* Trademarks: Eustigmin, Philostigmin, Proserine, Prostigmin. **n. bromide,** the bromide salt of neostigmine, occurring as a white, odorless, bitter, crystalline powder that is soluble in water and ethanol, but not in ether. Called also *synstigmin bromide.* **n. methyl sulfate,** a methyl sulfate derivative of neostigmine, occurring as a white, odorless, bitter, crystalline powder that is soluble in water and ethanol. Trademarks: Hodostin, Normastigmin, Stiglyn, Stigmosan.

Neo-Synephrine trademark for *phenylephrine hydrochloride* (see under PHENYLEPHRINE).

Neo-Thyreostat trademark for *carbimazole.*

neotype (ne′o-tīp) a strain of bacteria that replaces a type culture which no longer exists, and that agrees with the original description of the taxon and is acceptable by international agreement. See also indicator STRAIN.

Neozine trademark for *methotrimeprazine.*

nepheline (nef′ĕ-lin) a feldspathoid mineral, NaAlSiO₄, essentially made up of sodium aluminum silicate. **n. syenite,** a mixture containing approximately 50 percent sodium feldspar, 25 percent potassium feldspar, and 25 percent nepheline. Used as a substitute for potassium feldspar in dental porcelain; said to possess an extended maturing range.

nephr- see NEPHRO-.

Nephril trademark for *polythiazide.*

nephritides (nĕ-frit′ĭ-dez) plural of *nephritis.*

nephritis (nĕ-fri′tis), pl. *nephriti′des* [Gr. *nephros* kidney + *-itis*] inflammation of the kidney; a focal or diffuse proliferative or destructive process which may involve the glomerulus, tubule, or interstitial tissue. Cf. NEPHROSIS.

nephro-, nephr- [Gr. *nephros* kidney] a combining form denoting relationship to the kidney.

nephrocalcinosis (nef″ro-kal″sĭ-no′sis) [*nephro-* + *calcium* + *-osis*] a condition characterized by precipitation of calcium phosphate in the tubules of the kidney, with resultant renal insufficiency. **n. infan′tum,** Lightwood-Albright SYNDROME.

Nephron benzocaine ointment see under OINTMENT.

nephropathy (nef′rop′ah-the) [*nephro-* + Gr. *pathos* disease] disease of the kidneys. **evolutive tubular n.,** Lightwood-Albright SYNDROME.

nephrosclerosis (nef″ro-skle-ro′sis) [*nephro-* + Gr. *sklērōsis* hardening] hardening of the kidney due to renovascular disorders.

nephroses (ne-fro′sēz) plural of *nephrosis.*

nephrosis (ne-fro′sis), pl. *nephro′ses* [*nephro-* + *-osis*] any disease of the kidney, especially any disease of the kidneys characterized by degenerative lesions of the renal tubules — as opposed to nephritis — and marked by edema, albuminuria, and decreased serum albumin (*nephrotic syndrome*).

nephrotome (nef′ro-tōm) [*nephro-* + Gr. *tomē* a cutting] a short plate of cells extending ventrolaterally from a somite, being the segmented divisions of the mesoderm that connect the mesoderm somite with the lateral plates of the unsegmented mesoderm. Its tubule merges with that of the caudally adjacent tubule in forming a segmental duct (pronephric duct). The serially arranged nephrotome plates serve in the development of the kidneys and their ducts, by first giving rise to the pronephroi, mesonephroi, and metanephroi. Called also *intermediate cell mass* and *middle plate.*

neptunium (nep-tu′ne-um) [named after the planet *Neptune*] a radioactive element in the actinide (transuranium) series. Symbol, Np; atomic number, 93; atomic weight, 237.0482; valences, 3, 4, 5, 6; specific gravity, 20.25. The first neptunium isotope was 239, obtained by bombarding uranium with high-speed deuterons. ²³⁷Np is the most stable isotope, having a half-life of 2.14×10^6 years and emitting alpha rays; it is obtained in gram quantities as a by-product in the production of plutonium.

Nernst's law see under LAW.

Nerobol trademark for *methandrostenolone.*

nerve (nerv) [L. *nervus;* Gr. *neuron*] 1. a cordlike structure, visible to the naked eye, comprising a collection of nerve fibers which convey impulses between a part of the central nervous system and some other body region. It consists of a connective tissue sheath (epineurium) enclosing bundles (funiculi or fasciculi) of nerve fibers, each bundle being surrounded by its own sheath of connective tissue (perineurium), the inner surface of which is formed by a membrane of flattened mesothelial cells; very small nerves consist of only one funiculus derived from the parent nerve. Within each such bundle, the individual microscopic nerve fibers are surrounded by interstitial connective tissue (endoneurium). An individual nerve fiber (an axon with its covering sheath) consists of formed elements in a matrix of protoplasm (axoplasm), the entire structure being enclosed in a thin membrane (axolemma). Each nerve fiber is enclosed by a cellular sheath (neurilemma), from which it may or may not be separated by a lipid layer (myelin sheath) derived from neurilemmal cells. Called also *nervus* [NA]. See illustrations. See also terms beginning NEURO-. 2. popular name for *dental pulp.*

abducent n., a cranial nerve that supplies the lateral rectus muscle of the eye, which arises in the pons, emerging from the brain in the furrow between the inferior border of the pons and the medulla oblongata, and enters the orbit through the superior orbital fissure. It communicates with the carotid and cavernous plexuses and with the trigeminal nerve. Called also *cranial n. VI, sixth cranial n., nervus abducens* [NA], and *nervus cranialis VI.* **accessory n., accessory n., spinal,** a mixed motor and parasympathetic cranial nerve that arises by cranial roots from the side of the medulla oblongata, and by spinal roots from the side of the cervical segment of the spinal cord. The roots unite and the nerve thus formed divides into an internal branch (from the cranial roots) and an external branch (from the spinal roots). The internal branch indistinguishably joins the vagus nerve in the jugular foramen and supplies the muscles of the pharynx, soft palate, and larynx; the external branch supplies the sternocleidomastoid and trapezius muscles. Called also *cranial n. XI, eleventh cranial n., n. of Willis, nervus accessorius* [NA], and *nervus cranialis XI.* **acoustic n.,** vestibulocochlear n. **afferent n.,** any nerve that conveys impulses from peripheral organs to the central nervous system, such as a sensory nerve. Called also *centripetal n., esodic n.,* and *afferent neuron.* **alveolar n., anterior superior,** alveolar branches of infraorbital nerve, anterior superior; see under BRANCH. **alveolar n., inferior,** a branch of the mandibular division of the trigeminal nerve. It is a mixed motor and sensory nerve that descends with the inferior alveolar artery, first passing between the two pterygoid muscles, then winding around the lower border of the lateral pterygoid muscle, and, finally, entering into the mandibular canal through the mandibular foramen. Just before entering the foramen, it gives off the mylohyoid nerve and, further along, divides into several additional branches, including the inferior dental, mental, inferior gingival, and incisive nerves. Called also *inferior dental n.* and *nervus alveolaris inferior* [NA]. **alveolar n., middle superior,** alveolar branch of infraorbital nerve, middle superior; see under BRANCH. **alveolar n., posterior superior,** alveolar branches of maxillary nerve, posterior superior; see under BRANCH. **alveolar n's, superior,** dental branches arising from the maxillary and infraorbital nerves. Called also *nervi alveolares superiores* [NA]. See *alveolar branches of infraorbital nerve* and *alveolar branches of maxillary nerve,* under BRANCH. **alveolar n., superior posterior,** alveolar branches of maxillary nerve, posterior superior; see under BRANCH. **Arnold's n.,** auricular branch of vagus nerve; see under BRANCH. **articular n.,** a peripheral nerve that supplies a joint and its associated strictures. Called also *nervus articularis* [NA]. **auditory n.,** vestibulocochlear n. **auricular n's, anterior,** sensory branches of the auriculotemporal nerve that innervate the skin of the anterosuperior part of the external ear. Called also *nervi auriculares anteriores* [NA]. **auricular n., great,** a general sensory nerve originating from the cervical plexus; it sends branches to the skin over the parotid gland and mastoid process, and both surfaces of the auricle. Called also *nervus auricularis magnus* [NA]. **auricular n., posterior,** a sensory branch of the facial nerve, running behind the ear and supplying the auricularis posterior and intrinsic muscles of the auricle and the occipitofrontal muscle. Called also *nervus auricularis posterior* [NA]. **auriculotemporal n.,** a sensory branch of the mandibular division of the trigeminal nerve, which usually arises by two roots that encircle the middle meningeal artery,

runs posteriorly along the medial side of the neck of the mandible, turns up under the parotid gland, and passes over the root of the zygomatic arch. It divides into several branches, including branches communicating with the facial nerve and otic ganglion, anterior auricular branches, branches to the external acoustic meatus, articular branches, parotid branches, and superficial temporal branches. Called also *nervus auriculotemporalis* [NA]. **autonomic n.,** a nerve in the autonomic nervous system; see autonomic nervous SYSTEM. **Bock's n.,** pharyngeal branch of the pterygopalatine ganglion; see under BRANCH. **buccal n., buccinator n.,** a sensory branch of the mandibular division of the trigeminal nerve which arises on the anterolateral part of the mandibular nerve and passes between the two heads of the

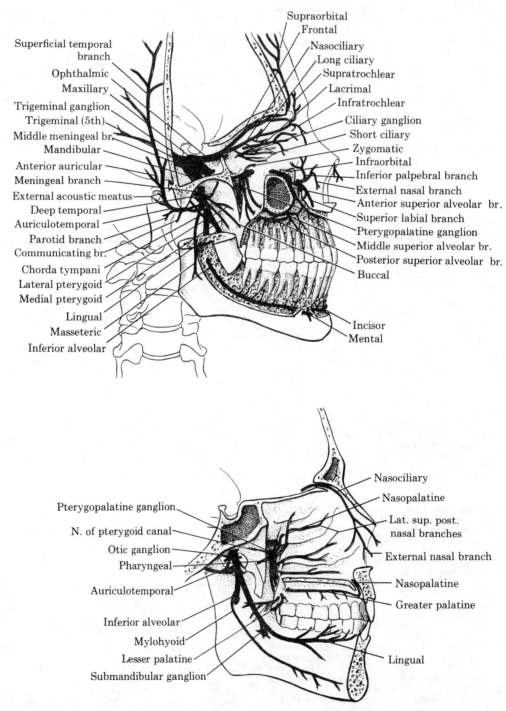

Deep nerves shown in relation to bones of face. (From Dorland's Illustrated Medical Dictionary. 26th ed. Philadelphia, W. B. Saunders Co., 1981.)

lateral pterygoid muscle to emerge from under the anterior border of the masseter muscle. On the surface of the buccal muscle, it divides into branches that form a plexus with branches of the facial nerve, and innervate almost the entire mucosa of the cheek except for its posterosuperior area, and the oral mucosa, including the adjacent gingivae. Called also *nervus buccalis* [NA] and *nervus buccinatorius*. **caroticotympanic n's,** two sympathetic branches originating in the carotid plexus which form the tympanic plexus together with the tympanic nerve and innervate the tympanic region. Called also *nervi caroticotympanici* [NA]. **carotid n's, external,** sympathetic nerve fibers, arising from the superior cervical ganglion and running along the external carotid artery; they form the external carotid plexus and innervate cranial blood vessels and glands. Called also *nervi carotici externi* [NA]. **carotid n., internal,** a sympathetic nerve, originating in the superior cervical ganglion, which forms the internal carotid plexus and innervates the cranial blood vessels and glands. Called also *nervus caroticus internus* [NA]. **carotid sinus n.,** BRANCH of glossopharyngeal nerve to carotid sinus. **centrifugal n.,** efferent n. **centripetal n.,** afferent n. **cerebral n's,** cranial n's. **cervical n's,** the eight pairs of nerves that arise from the cervical

segments of the spinal cord; the ventral branches of the upper four nerves form the cervical plexus. Called also *nervi cervicales* [NA]. **chorda tympani n.,** a mixed sensory and parasympathetic nerve that arises from the facial nerve via the intermediate nerve, passes through the canaliculus of the chorda tympani, crosses the tympanic cavity, and emerges from the skull on the medial surface of the spine of the sphenoid bone to be joined by a communication from the otic ganglion and, further on, to unite with the lingual nerve between the lateral pterygoid muscles. Special afferent fibers for taste, which supply the anterior two-thirds of the tongue and are distributed with branches of the lingual nerve, represent the major part of the chorda tympani. It also contains preganglionic parasympathetic fibers from the intermediate nerve, which are responsible for the secretory motor activity of the submandibular, sublingual, and lingual glands. Called also *chorda tympani* [NA]. **ciliary n's, long,** two or three branches of the nasociliary nerve that contain sensory fibers supplying the internal parts of

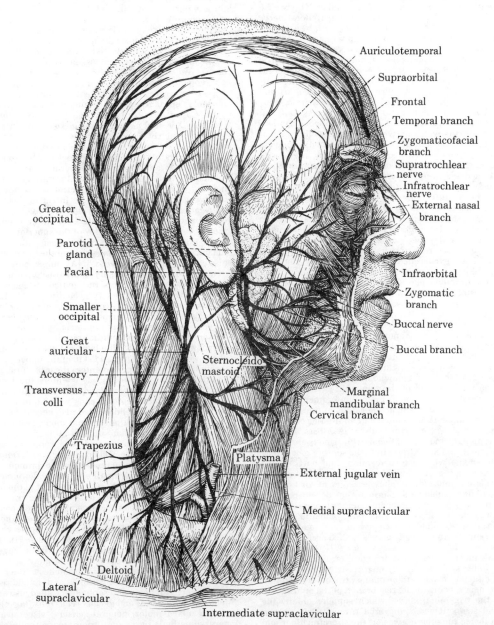

Superficial nerves and muscles of head and neck. Portions of the parotid gland and platysma muscle are shown cut away. (From Dorland's Illustrated Medical Dictionary. 26th ed. Philadelphia, W. B. Saunders Co., 1981; adapted from Jones and Shepard.)

the eyeball. Called also *nervi ciliares longi* [NA]. **ciliary n's, short,** mixed parasympathetic, sympathetic, and general sensory nerves that arise from the ciliary ganglion and innervate the smooth muscle and tunics of the eye. Called also *nervi ciliares breves* [NA]. **cochlear n.,** the nerve of hearing, being the part of the vestibulocochlear nerve that consists of sensory fibers arising from the bipolar cells of the spiral ganglion and supplying the cochlea. Called also *nervus cochleae, pars cochlearis nervi octavi* [NA], and *pars cochlearis nervi vestibulocochlearis.* **cranial n's,** the twelve pairs of nerves that are attached to the base of brain and leave the cranial cavity through the foramina in the skull. Called also *cerebral n's, nervi cerebrales,* and *nervi craniales* [NA]. **cranial n's, I (first cranial n's),** olfactory n's. **cranial n., II (second cranial n.),** optic n. **cranial n., III (third cranial n.),** oculomotor n. **cranial n., IV (fourth cranial n.),** trochlear n. **cranial n., V (fifth cranial n.),** trigeminal n. **cranial n., VI (sixth cranial n.),** abducent n. **cranial n., VII (seventh cranial n.),** facial n. **cranial n., VIII (eighth cranial n.),** vestibulocochlear n. **cranial n., IX (ninth cranial n.),** glossopharyngeal n. **cranial n., X (tenth cranial n.),** vagus n. **cranial n., XI (eleventh cranial n.),** accessory n. **cranial n., XII (twelfth cranial n.),** hypoglossal n. **cutaneous n.,** any peripheral nerve that supplies the skin. Called also *nervus cutaneus* [NA]. **dental n., inferior,** alveolar n., inferior. **depressor n.,** 1. a nerve that depresses or lessens the activity of an organ. 2. an inhibitory nerve whose stimulation depresses motor activity. **digastric n.,** digastric branch of facial nerve; see under BRANCH. **efferent n.,** any nerve that conveys impulses from the central nervous system to peripheral organs. Called also *centrifugal n.* and *efferent neuron.* **eighth cranial n.,** vestibulocochlear n. **eleventh cranial n.,** accessory n. **n. of equilibrium,** vestibular n. **esodic n.,** afferent n. **ethmoidal n's, anterior,** branches containing sensory filaments which derive from the nasociliary nerve as it passes through the anterior ethmoidal foramen, supplying the mucosa of the upper and anterior nasal septum, lateral wall of the nasal cavity, and the skin of the lower bridge and tip of the nose. Called also *anterior ethmoidal branches of nasociliary nerve, nervi ethmoidales anteriores,* and *rami anteriores nervorum nasociliarium.* **ethmoidal n., posterior,** a branch of the nasociliary nerve that contains sensory fibers which leave the orbit through the posterior ethmoidal foramen to supply the posterior ethmoidal and sphenoidal sinuses. Called also *nervus ethmoidalis posterior* [NA]. **exciter n.,** one that conveys impulses resulting in excitation and increased functional activity. **excitoreflex n.,** a visceral nerve that produces reflex action. **n. of external acoustic meatus,** a sensory branch of the auriculotemporal nerve that supplies the skin lining the external acoustic meatus and sends a filament to the tympanic membrane. Called also *nervus meatus acustici externi* [NA] and *nervus meatus auditorii externi.* **facial n.,** a cranial nerve that originates at the inferior border of the pons by two roots, one sensory and one motor; from there it passes into the acoustic meatus and into the facial canals. Within the tympanic cavity it makes a U-shaped turn to form the geniculum. The roots fuse at the geniculum and become swollen by the presence of the geniculate ganglion. From the geniculum it runs posteriorly in the wall of the tympanic cavity and dips toward the stylomastoid foramen. From the foramen it enters the parotid gland and divides near the ramus of the mandible into a superior temporofacial branch and an inferior cervicofacial branch, both of which further subdivide. Fibers from the motor root supply the muscles of facial expression in the scalp, external ear, face, and neck; those from the sensory root supply the anterior tongue with taste perception, and parts of the acoustic meatus, soft palate, and pharynx with sensation. The parasympathetic component supplies secretory motor fibers to the submandibular, sublingual, lacrimal, nasal, and palatine glands. Branches include the stapedius and posterior auricular nerves, parotid plexus, digastric, temporal, zygomatic, buccal, lingual, marginal mandibular and cervical rami, and a communicating ramus with tympanic plexus. Called also *cranial n. VII, seventh cranial n., nervus cranialis VII, and nervus facialis* [NA]. **facial n., temporal,** temporal branches of facial nerve; see under BRANCH. **fifth cranial n.,** trigeminal n. **first cranial n's,** olfactory n's. **fourth cranial n.,** trochlear n. **frontal n.,** a sensory nerve, being the largest branch of the ophthalmic division of the trigeminal nerve, which supplies chiefly the forehead and scalp. It enters the orbit through the superior fissure, and inside the orbit it gives off the supratrochlear and supraorbital nerves and a branch to the frontal sinus. Called

also *nervus frontalis* [NA]. **ganglionated n.,** any nerve having a ganglionic connection; a sympathetic nerve. **glossopharyngeal n.,** a mixed cranial nerve, consisting of visceral and somatic sensory fibers and general visceral efferent motor fibers that innervate the tongue, pharynx, parotid glands, and tonsils. It originates by several roots on the lateral side of the upper part of the medulla oblongata, from where it passes through the jugular foramen and, once outside the skull, runs anteriorly between the internal jugular vein and the internal carotid artery to divide into several branches. The part in the jugular foramen has two enlargements, the superior and inferior ganglia. Branches include the tympanic and carotid sinus nerves, and the pharyngeal, tonsillar, stylopharyngeal, and lingual branches. The nerve to the stylopharyngeus muscle is motor; the lingual branch conducts taste from the posterior one-third of the tongue. It communicates with the vagus nerve, facial nerve, and superior cervical sympathetic ganglion. Called also *cranial nerve IX, ninth cranial nerve, nervus cranialis IX,* and *nervus glossopharyngeus* [NA]. **n. of hearing,** cochlear n. **Hering's n.,** BRANCH of glossopharyngeal nerve to carotid sinus. **hypoglossal n.,** the motor nerve of the tongue. It is a cranial nerve that originates by several rootlets from the medulla oblongata in the ventrolateral sulcus between the olive and the pyramid. Its rootlets form two separate bundles that enter the dura mater and pass through the hypoglossal canal, where the rootlets unite. It then runs beneath the internal carotid artery and internal jugular vein downward and forward; loops around the occipital artery near the angle of the mandible, and curves toward the skull above the hyoid bone to innervate the styloglossus, hyoglossus, and genioglossus muscles and intrinsic muscles of the tongue. It communicates with the vagus nerve, pharyngeal plexus, and sympathetic, lingual, and spinal nerves, and gives off meningeal, thyrohyoid, geniohyoid, and muscular branches, and the superior ramus of the ansa cervicalis. Called also *cranial n. XII, twelfth cranial n., nervus cranialis XII,* and *nervus hypoglossus* [NA]. **infraorbital n.,** a sensory branch of the maxillary division of the trigeminal nerve that enters the orbit through the inferior orbital fissure and passes through the infraorbital groove, infraorbital canal, and infraorbital foramen to give off several branches, including the middle and anterior superior alveolar, inferior palpebral, internal and external nasal, and superior labial branches. Called also *nervus infraorbitalis* [NA]. **infratrochlear n.,** a branch that contains sensory fibers which are given off by the nasociliary nerve just before it enters the anterior ethmoidal foramen; it runs beneath the pulley of the superior oblique muscle, supplying the skin of the root of the upper bridge of the nose and the lower eyelid, the conjunctiva, and the lacrimal duct. Called also *nervus infratrochlearis* [NA]. **intermediate n., intermediary n.,** the smaller sensory and parasympathetic root of the facial nerve that connects the geniculate ganglion with the brain. Called also *nervus intermedius* [NA]. **Jacobson's n.,** tympanic n. **jugular n.,** a communicating branch between the superior cervical ganglion and the vagus and glossopharyngeal nerves. Called also *nervus jugularis* [NA]. **lacrimal n.,** a small sensory branch of the ophthalmic division of the trigeminal nerve, which innervates the lacrimal gland, conjunctiva, lateral commissure of the eye, and skin of the upper eyelid. It passes through the dura mater and enters the orbit through the superior orbital fissure. In the orbit, it enters the lacrimal gland, giving off filaments to the gland and the conjunctiva and, after piercing the orbital septum, ends with filaments of the facial nerve in the upper eyelid. Called also *nervus lacrimalis* [NA]. **laryngeal n., inferior,** the terminal motor branch of the recurrent laryngeal nerve that supplies all intrinsic muscles of the larynx, except the cricothyroid, and communicates with the internal laryngeal nerve. Called also *nervus laryngeus inferior* [NA]. **laryngeal n., recurrent,** a mixed branch of the vagus nerve containing parasympathetic, visceral afferent, and motor fibers. It arises on the right side in the root of the neck near the subclavian artery and on the left side in the cranial part of the thorax on the left side of the arch of the aorta, passing upward behind the common carotid artery and between the trachea and the esophagus toward the larynx, to provide nerve supply to all its muscles, except the cricothyroid muscle. Its branches include the inferior laryngeal nerve to the laryngeal muscles, pharyngeal branches to the constrictor pharyngis inferior muscle, sensory and secretory motor branches to the mucous membrane of the larynx and vocal folds, and, in addition, branches to the heart, trachea, and esophagus. Called also *nervus laryngeus recurrens* [NA] and *nervus recurrens.* **laryngeal n., superior,** a mixed motor, general sensory, visceral afferent, and parasympathetic nerve that originates in the inferior ganglion of the vagus nerve. It passes deep to the internal carotid artery and along the pharynx to the superior cornu of the thyroid cartilage and divides into external and internal branches. The external branch supplies the inferior constrictor muscle of the pharynx and cricothyroid muscle; the internal branch supplies the mucous membrane of the back of the tongue and larynx. It communicates with the superior cervical sympathetic ganglion, pharyngeal plexus, and the superior sympathetic cardiac and recurrent nerves. Called also *nervus laryngeus superior* [NA]. **lingual n.,** a branch of the mandibular division of the trigeminal nerve. It is a sensory nerve that descends to the tongue, first between the medial pterygoid muscle and the mandible, then under the mucous membrane of the floor of the mouth to the side of the tongue, supplying innervation to the anterior two-thirds of the tongue and floor of the mouth. Its branches include the sublingual nerve, a lingual branch, a branch to the isthmus of the fauces, and branches communicating with the hypoglossal nerve and chorda tympani. Called also *nervus lingualis* [NA]. **mandibular n., mandibular division of trigeminal n.,** the largest of the three divisions of the trigeminal nerve. It is a mixed nerve, containing the entire motor portion of the trigeminal nerve and sensory fibers. The sensory root derives from the inferior angle of the trigeminal ganglion and the motor root represents the entire motor root of the trigeminal ganglion. It enters the infratemporal fossa through the foramen ovale to give off several branches. The sensory branches supply the mucous membrane and skin of the temporal region, external auricular meatus, cheek, lower lip, lower part of the face, tongue, and mastoid air cells; the mandible, including its teeth and gingivae; the temporomandibular articulation; and parts of the dura mater and cranium. The motor branches supply the masticatory muscles, mylohyoid, anterior belly of the digastric muscle, tensor veli palatini, and tensor tympanic muscles. Branches include the meningeal branch and medial pterygoid, masseteric, deep temporal, lateral pterygoid, buccal, auriculotemporal, lingual, and inferior alveolar nerves. Called also *inferior maxillary n.* and *nervus mandibularis* [NA]. **masseteric n.,** a mixed motor and sensory branch of the mandibular division of the trigeminal nerve that passes above the pterygoideus lateralis muscle to the mandibular notch, innervates the masseter muscle, and gives off a filament to the temporomandibular articulation. Called also *nervus massetericus* [NA]. **masticator n.,** motor root of trigeminal nerve; see under ROOT. **maxillary n., maxillary division of trigeminal n.,** one of the three divisions of the trigeminal nerve. It is a sensory nerve originating from the trigeminal ganglion, leaving the cranial cavity through the foramen rotundum, then crossing the pterygopalatine fossa, and entering the orbit through the inferior orbital fissure. In the posterior part of the orbit it becomes the

infraorbital nerve. It supplies the skin of the middle part of the face, nasal cavity, lower eyelid, side of the nose, and upper lip, and the mucous membrane of the nasopharynx, maxillary sinus, soft palate, tonsil, maxillary gingivae, and teeth. Its branches include the middle meningeal, zygomatic, and pterygopalatine nerves and posterior superior alveolar, middle superior alveolar, anterior superior alveolar, inferior palpebral, infraorbital, nasopalatine, and lateral nasal branches. Called also *nervus maxillaris* [NA]. **maxillary n., inferior,** mandibular n. **medullated n.,** myelinated n. **meningeal n., middle,** a sensory branch of the maxillary nerve arising near its origin from the trigeminal ganglion in the middle cranial fossa. It accompanies the middle meningeal artery through the foramen spinosum and supplies the dura mater. Called also *dural branch of maxillary nerve, middle meningeal branch of maxillary nerve, nervus meningeus medius,* and *ramus meningeus medius nervi maxillaris* [NA]. **mental n.,** a sensory branch of the inferior alveolar nerve which emerges through the mental foramen and divides into three filaments, one supplying the skin of the chin and two others innervating the skin and mucous membrane of the lower lip. All three branches communicate with branches of the facial nerve. Called also *nervus mentalis* [NA]. **mixed n.,** any peripheral nerve that contains both motor and sensory fibers and is capable of transmitting impulses to and from the central nervous system at once. **motor n.,** motoneuron. **motor n. of tongue,** hypoglossal n. **myelinated n.,** a nerve, especially a peripheral nerve, whose fibers (axons) are encased in a myelin sheath, which in turn may be enclosed by a neurilemma. Called also *medullated n.* Cf. *unmyelinated n.* **mylohyoid n.,** a motor branch that leaves the inferior alveolar nerve just before it enters the mandibular foramen, and continues in the groove of the ramus of the mandible to supply the mylohyoid muscle and the anterior belly of the digastric muscle. Called also *nervus mylohyoideus* [NA]. **nasal n.,** nasociliary n. **nasociliary n.,** a sensory nerve, being a branch of the ophthalmic division of the trigeminal nerve, which passes through the orbit by entering it between the two heads of the rectus lateralis muscle and leaving through the anterior ethmoidal foramen as the anterior ethmoidal nerve. It then enters the cranial cavity above the cribriform plate of the ethmoid bone and reaches the nasal cavity through the nasal fissure. It gives off branches that supply the nose, eye, lacrimal sac, and ethmoidal and frontal sinuses. Its branches include a branch communicating with the ciliary ganglion, the long ciliary nerves, the intratrochlear nerve, the ethmoidal branches, and the internal and external nasal branches. Called also *nasal n.* and *nervus nasociliaris* [NA]. **nasopalatine n.,** a parasympathetic and sensory branch of the pterygopalatine ganglion, which passes through the sphenopalatine foramen, down the nasal septum, and through the incisive foramen to supply the septum and anterior part of the hard palate. It communicates with its fellow of the opposite side and the greater palatine nerve. Called also *Scarpa's n.* and *nervus nasopalatinus* [NA]. **ninth cranial n.,** glossopharyngeal n. **nonmedullated n.,** unmyelinated n. **occipital n., greater,** a general sensory and motor branch of the second cervical nerve that supplies the semispinalis capitis muscle and skin of the back of the scalp. Called also *nervus occipitalis major* [NA]. **occipital n., least,** occipital n., third. **occipital n., lesser,** a general sensory branch of the second and third cervical nerves that supplies the side of the scalp and the cranial surface of the auricle. Called also *nervus occipitalis minor* [NA]. **occipital n., third,** a general sensory branch of the third cervical nerve that supplies the skin of the upper part of the back of the neck and head. Called also *least occipital n.* and *nervus occipitalis tertius* [NA]. **oculomotor n.,** a nerve that supplies the levator muscle of the upper eyelid and all extrinsic eye muscles, except for the lateral rectus and superior oblique muscles. It is a motor nerve that carries some parasympathetic fibers to eye structures and is believed to contain proprioceptive fibers. It originates in the brain stem medial to the cerebral peduncles and emerges through the superior orbital fissure; its superior division sending branches to the rectus superior and levator palpebrae muscles, and its inferior division sending branches to the rectus medialis, rectus inferior, and obliquus inferior muscles, and providing the motor root of the ciliary ganglion. It communicates with the ophthalmic division of the trigeminal nerve and the postganglionic fibers of the superior cervical ganglion. Called also *cranial n. III, third cranial n., nervus cranialis III,* and *nervus oculomotorius* [NA]. **olfactory n's,** the nerves of smell, consisting of about 20 bundles of

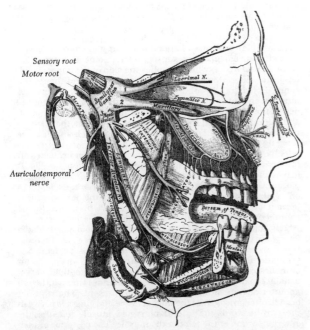

Sensory root
Motor root

Auriculotemporal
nerve

Distribution of the maxillary and mandibular nerves. (From H. Gray: Gray's Anatomy. 29th ed. C. M. Goss [ed.], Philadelphia, Lea & Febiger, 1973.)

unmyelinated fibers, a lateral group deriving from the olfactory mucosa of the concha, and a medial group from the septum. The fibers form a plexiform network in the mucous membrane of the superior nasal concha and the opposite part of the nasal septum and pass through the foramina of the cribriform plate of the ethmoid bone to the olfactory bulb. Called also *cranial n's I, first cranial n's, n's of smell, nervi craniales I,* and *nervi olfactorii* [NA]. **ophthalmic n., ophthalmic division of trigeminal n.,** one of the three divisions of the trigeminal nerve, originating at the trigeminal ganglion and supplying sensory fibers to the eye, lacrimal gland and sac, nasal mucosa and frontal sinus, external nose, upper eyelid, forehead, and scalp. Its branches include the tentorial branch and the lacrimal, frontal, and nasociliary nerves. Called also *nervus ophthalmicus* [NA]. **optic n.,** the nerve of sight; from the retina it passes out of the orbit through the optic canal, some of its fibers crossing over to the opposite side in the optic chiasm. Crossed and uncrossed fibers continue as the optic tract, over the surface of the cerebral peduncle to the third ventricle, where the tract divides into two roots. Called also *cranial n. II, second cranial n., nervus cranialis II,* and *nervus opticus* [NA]. **orbital n.,** zygomatic n. **pain n.,** any sensory nerve that conducts pain stimuli. **palatine n., anterior,** palatine n., greater. **palatine n., greater,** a nerve consisting of parasympathetic, sympathetic, and sensory fibers, which originates in the pterygopalatine ganglion, passes through the pterygopalatine canal, and emerges on the hard palate through the greater palatine foramen. It divides into several branches, including the posterior inferior nasal branches and the lesser palatine nerve, which supply the palate, gingivae, and parts of the soft palate, some branches reaching as far as the incisor teeth. It communicates with the nasopalatine nerve. Called also *anterior palatine n., descending branch of pterygopalatine ganglion, descending branch of sphenopalatine ganglion, nervus palatinus anterior,* and *nervus palatinus major* [NA]. **palatine n's, lesser, palatine n's, medial, palatine n's, middle, palatine n's, posterior,** parasympathetic, sympathetic, and sensory branches originating in the pterygopalatine ganglion, which emerge through the lesser palatine foramen to supply the soft palate, uvula, and tonsil. Together with tonsillar branches of the glossopharyngeal nerve, they form a plexus around the tonsil. Called also *nervi palatini minores* [NA], *nervi palatini posteriores,* and *nervus palatinus medius*. **parasympathetic n.,** a nerve in the parasympathetic nervous system. **parotid n.,** parotid branches of auriculotemporal nerve; see under BRANCH. **peripheral n.,** any nerve situated outside the brain and the spinal cord (the central nervous system). See peripheral nervous SYSTEM. **petrosal n., deep,** a nerve containing postganglionic fibers from the superior cervical sympathetic ganglion, which pass through the pterygopalatine ganglion and supply the lacrimal, nasal, and palatine glands. Called also *nervus petrosus profundus* [NA]. **petrosal n., greater, petrosal n., greater superficial,** a mixed sensory and parasympathetic nerve that originates in the geniculate ganglion, passes through a hiatus in the canal for the greater petrosal nerve into the middle cranial fossa, runs beneath the dura mater and the trigeminal ganglion on the anterior surface of the petrous part of the temporal bone, and joins the deep petrosal nerve to form the nerve of the pterygoid canal. Its parasympathetic fibers from the intermediate nerve forms a root of the pterygopalatine ganglion, and its sensory fibers from the peripheral processes of the geniculate ganglion supply the soft palate through the lesser palatine nerve, sending filaments to the auditory tube. It also reaches the lacrimal, nasal, and palatine glands and the nasopharynx through the pterygopalatine ganglion. Called also *nervus petrosus major* [NA] and *nervus petrosus superficialis major*. **petrosal n., lesser,** a nerve given off by the tympanic plexus that carries parasympathetic fibers from the tympanic nerve to the otic ganglion, serving as its parasympathetic root. It emerges from the tympanic cavity through the canal for the lesser petrosal nerve and passes within the cranium to the sphenopetrosal fissure, or the foramen ovale, or a foramen nearby before joining the otic ganglion. Called also *middle superficial petrosal n., nervus petrosus minor* [NA], *nervus petrosus superficialis minor,* and *parasympathetic root of otic ganglion*. **petrosal n., middle superficial,** petrosal n., lesser. **pneumogastric n.,** vagus n. **pressor n.,** any nerve whose stimulation results in increased vascular tension. **n. of pterygoid canal,** a mixed sympathetic and parasympathetic nerve, arising in the foramen lacerum by the union of the greater petrosal and deep petrosal nerves, and enters the pterygoid canal, where it is joined by the ascending sphenoidal branch from the otic ganglion and gives off branches to the mucous membrane of the sphenoidal sinus; as it leaves the anterior opening of the canal, it joins the pterygopalatine ganglion. Called also *vidian n., facial root, nervus canalis pterygoidei* [NA], and *radix facialis*. **pterygoid n., external,** pterygoid n., lateral. **pterygoid n., internal,** pterygoid n., medial. **pterygoid n., lateral,** a motor branch of the mandibular division of the trigeminal nerve that often arises with the buccal nerve and innervates the deep surface of the lateral pterygoid muscle. Called also *external pterygoid n., nervus pterygoideus externus,* and *nervus pterygoideus lateralis* [NA]. **pterygoid n., medial,** a motor branch of the mandibular division of the trigeminal nerve that passes through the otic ganglion without interruption, and sends out two slender branches: one to the tensor veli palatini muscle, which enters the muscle near its origin, and the other to the tensor tympani. Terminally, it supplies the medial pterygoid muscle. Called also *internal pterygoid n., nervus pterygoideus internus, nervus pterygoideus medialis* [NA]. **pterygopalatine n's,** two short trunks that derive from the maxillary division of the trigeminal nerve, uniting it with the pterygopalatine ganglion and dividing into the orbital, posterior inferior nasal, posterior superior nasal, and pharyngeal branches, and the lesser palatine nerves. The trunks consist chiefly of trigeminal somatic afferent fibers. Called also *sphenopalatine n's, nervi pterygopalatini* [NA], and *nervi sphenopalatini*. **recurrent laryngeal n.,** laryngeal n., recurrent. **Scarpa's n.,** nasopalatine n. **second cranial n.,** optic n. **secretory n.,** any efferent nerve whose stimulation increases secretory activity of a gland. **sensory n.,** an afferent nerve that conveys impulses from peripheral organs to the central nervous system. Called also *sensory neuron*. **seventh cranial n.,** facial n. **·n. of sight,** optic n. **sinus n.,** BRANCH of glossopharyngeal nerve to carotid sinus. **sixth cranial n.,** abducent n. **n's of smell,** olfactory n's. **somatic n.,** any nerve that innervates the skeletal muscles and somatic tissues. **sphenopalatine n's,** pterygopalatine n's. **spinal n's,** the 31 pairs of nerves that arise from the spinal cord and pass out between the vertebrae. They consist of fibers conveying somatic and visceral, afferent and efferent impulses. The somatic afferent fibers convey sensation for pain, temperature, and touch from the skin, and proprioception and deep pain from muscles and joints; the visceral afferent fibers convey reflex impulses which do not reach consciousness; and the somatic efferent fibers convey motor stimuli to the skeletal muscles. Called also *nervi spinales* [NA]. **spinal accessory n.,** accessory n. **stapedial n., stapedius n.,** a motor nerve originating from the facial nerve and supplying the stapedius muscle. Called also *nervus stapedius* [NA]. **stylohyoid n.,** stylohyoid branch of facial nerve; see under BRANCH. **stylopharyngeal n.,** stylopharyngeal branch of glossopharyngeal nerve; see under BRANCH. **sublingual n.,** a parasympathetic and general sensory branch of the lingual nerve that supplies the sublingual glands and the mucous membrane of the floor of the mouth overlying the glands. Called also *nervus sublingualis* [NA]. **submaxillary n's,** glandular branches of submandibular ganglion; see under BRANCH. **supraorbital n.,** a sensory nerve, being a continuation of the frontal nerve, which supplies the skin of the upper eyelid, forehead, anterior scalp, and mucous membrane of the frontal sinus. It leaves the orbit through the supraorbital notch or foramen and gives off filaments to the upper eyelid and continues to the forehead, where it divides into the medial (frontal) and lateral branches; the medial branch supplies the scalp in front of the parietal bone, and the lateral branch supplies the scalp up to the lambdoid suture. Called also *nervus supraorbitalis* [NA]. **supratrochlear n.,** a sensory nerve that branches off the frontal nerve and supplies the forehead and upper eyelid. It leaves the orbit at the medial end of the supraorbital margin, passing above the pulley of the obliquus superior muscle, gives off a filament which communicates with the infratrochlear branch of the nasociliary nerve, gives off filaments to the conjunctiva and the upper eyelid, and divides into branches which supply the skin of the lower and mesial parts of the forehead. Called also *nervus supratrochlearis* [NA]. **sympathetic n.,** a nerve in the sympathetic nervous system. See sympathetic nervous SYSTEM. **temporal n's, deep,** motor branches of the mandibular division of the trigeminal nerve, usually consisting of an anterior and posterior ramus, although an intermediate branch may also be present. The anterior branch often arises from the buccal nerve and emerges between the two heads of the lateral pterygoid muscle to enter the anterior portion of the temporalis muscle. The posterior branch (and the intermediate, if present) pass close to the bone of the temporal fossa and enter the deep surface of the muscle. Called also *nervi temporales profundi* [NA] [*anterior et posterior*].

temporal facial n., temporal branches of facial nerve; see under BRANCH. temporomalar n., zygomatic n. n. of tensor tympani, a motor nerve originating in the mandibular division of the trigeminal nerve through the otic ganglion that innervates the tensor tympani muscle. Called also *nervus tensoris tympani* [NA]. n. of tensor veli palatini, a motor branch of the mandibular division of the trigeminal nerve through the nerve of the medial pterygoid muscle and the otic ganglion; it innervates the tensor veli palatini muscle. Called also *nervus tensoris veli palatini* [NA]. tenth cranial n., vagus n. tentorial n., tentorial branch of ophthalmic nerve; see under BRANCH. terminal n's, nerve filaments, collectively termed the terminal nerve, originating in the cerebral hemisphere in the region of the olfactory trigone and passing through the cribriform plate of the ethmoid bone to the nasal mucosa. Their bundles join the olfactory bundles and the vomeronasal nerves and, in the nasal cavity, they communicate with the medial nasal branch of the anterior ethmoidal branch of the ophthalmic division of the trigeminal nerve. Their fibers are unmyelinated and have ganglion cells along their course. Called also *nervi terminales* [NA]. third cranial n., oculomotor n. tonsillar n's, tonsillar branches of glossopharyngeal nerve; see under BRANCH. trifacial n., trigeminal n. trigeminal n., the largest of the cranial nerves, being the principal sensory nerve of the face, mouth, teeth, and nasal cavity, and the motor nerve of the muscles of mastication. It arises from the trigeminal nuclei in the mesencephalon, pons, and spinal cord, emerging on the lateral surface of the pons, from where it passes to the apex of the petrous portion of the temporal bone. Here the sensory root expands into the trigeminal ganglion which gives off three major divisions of the trigeminal nerve (hence the name *trigeminal*): the ophthalmic, maxillary, and mandibular nerves. Called also *cranial n. V, fifth cranial n., trifacial n., nervus cranialis V,* and *nervus trigeminus* [NA]. See illustration. trochlear n., the smallest of the cranial nerves that supplies the superior oblique muscle. It originates in the midbrain and its fibers decussate across the median plane, emerging into the orbit through the superior orbital fissure. It is a motor nerve, and it communicates with the sympathetic nerves and with the ophthalmic division of the trigeminal nerve. Called also *cranial n. IV; fourth cranial n., nervus cranialis IV,* and *nervus trochlearis* [NA]. twelfth cranial n., hypoglossal n. tympanic n., a mixed general sensory and parasympathetic branch of the glossopharyneal nerve. It arises from the inferior ganglion of the glossopharyngeal nerve and runs to the tympanic cavity where it assists in forming the tympanic plexus. It supplies the mucous membrane of the tympanic cavity, mastoid air cells, auditory tube and, through the otic ganglion, the parotid gland. Called also *Jacobson's n.* and *nervus tympanicus* [NA]. unmyelinated n., a nerve whose fibers (axons) are not encased in a myelin sheath, and which may or may not be enclosed by a neurilemma. Unmyelinated

nerves are generally smaller than myelinated ones and make up the trunks and branches of the autonomic nervous system. Called also *nonmedullated n.* Cf. *myelinated n.* vagus n., a mixed cranial nerve, having somatic and visceral afferent and general and special visceral efferent fibers that originate by eight or ten rootlets on the lateral side of the medulla oblongata and wander through the neck, thorax, and abdomen (hence the name *vagus*). After leaving the medulla, the rootlets form a flat cord and pass beneath the cerebellum to the jugular foramen to leave the cranial cavity. In the foramen, it presents the superior ganglion and the inferior ganglion just after leaving the foramen. It supplies sensory fibers to the ear, tongue, pharynx, and larynx; motor fibers to the pharynx, larynx, and esophagus; and parasympathetic fibers to the heart and thoracic and abdominal viscera. Its branches innervating the head and neck include the superior and recurrent laryngeal nerves and the meningeal, auricular, and pharyngeal branches. It communicates with the accessory, glossopharyngeal, facial, jugular, accessory, hypoglossal, and accessory nerves. Called also *cranial n. X, pneumogastric n., tenth cranial n., nervus cranialis X,* and *nervus vagus* [NA]. vascular n., a nerve branch that supplies the wall of a blood vessel. Called also *nervus vascularis* [NA]. vasoconstrictor n., a vasomotor nerve whose stimulation results in contraction of the blood vessels. vasodilator n., a vasomotor nerve whose stimulation results in dilation of the blood vessels. vasomotor n., one supplying motor innervation to the blood vessels; its stimulation results in vasoconstriction or vasodilatation. vasosensory n., one supplying sensory innervation to the blood vessels. vestibular n., the nerve of equilibrium, being the part of the vestibulocochlear nerve arising from bipolar cells in the vestibular ganglion and dividing peripherally and into a superior and an inferior part, with receptors in the semicircular canal, utricle, and saccule. Called also *n. of equilibrium, nervus vestibuli, pars vestibularis nervi octavi* [NA], and *pars vestibularis nervi vestibulocochlearis.* vestibulocochlear n., a sensory cranial nerve that supplies the organs of hearing and equilibrium. It has two separate roots (cochlear and vestibular), emerging between the pons and the medulla oblongata behind the facial nerve and entering the internal acoustic meatus together with the facial nerve. It consists of two distinct sets of fibers: the cochlear nerve (nerve of hearing) that derives its fibers from the cochlear root and supplies the hearing receptors, and the vestibular nerve (nerve of equilibrium) that derives its fibers from the vestibular root and supplies the equilibrium receptors. Centrally, the two sets of fibers are united into a single trunk. Called also *acoustic n., auditory n., cranial n. VIII, eighth cranial n., nervus acusticus, nervus cranialis*

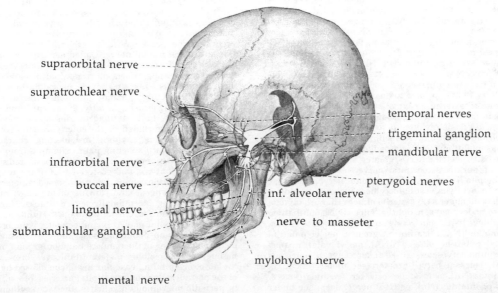

The trigeminal nerve with its branches. (From J. Langman and M. W. Woerdeman: Atlas of Medical Anatomy. Philadelphia, W. B. Saunders Co., 1978.)

VIII, and *nervus vestibulocochlearis* [NA]. **vidian n.**, n. of pterygoid canal. **n. of Willis**, accessory n. **zygomatic n.**, a sensory branch of the maxillary division of the trigeminal nerve that arises in the pterygopalatine fossa and enters the orbit through the inferior orbital fissure. It supplies the skin of the temples and adjacent parts of the face through the zygomaticofacial and zygomaticotemporal branches, and communicates with the lacrimal nerve. Called also *orbital n.*, *temporomalar n.*, and *nervus zygomaticus* [NA]. **zygomaticofacial n.**, zygomaticofacial branch of zygomatic nerve; see under BRANCH. **zygomaticotemporal n.**, zygomaticotemporal branch of zygomatic nerve, see under BRANCH.

nervi (ner'vi) [L.] plural of *nervus*.

nervone (ner'vōn) a cerebroside, $C_{48}H_{91}O_8N$, isolated from nerve tissue.

nervus (ner'vus), pl. **ner'vi** [L.] a nerve. **n. abdu'cens** [NA], abducent NERVE. **n. accesso'rius** [NA], accessory NERVE. **n. acus'ticus**, vestibulocochlear NERVE. **n. alveola'ris infe'rior** [NA], alveolar nerve, inferior; see under NERVE. **ner'vi alveola'res superio'res** [NA], alveolar nerves, superior; see under NERVE. **n. articula'ris** [NA], articular nerve; see under NERVE. **ner'vi auricula'res anterio'res** [NA], auricular nerves, anterior; see under NERVE. **n. auricula'ris mag'nus** [NA], auricular nerve, great; see under NERVE. **n. auricula'ris poste'rior** [NA], auricular nerve, posterior; see under NERVE. **n. auriculotempora'lis** [NA], auriculotemporal NERVE. **n. bucca'lis** [NA], **n. buccinato'rius**, buccal NERVE. **n. cana'lis pterygoi'dei** [NA], NERVE of pterygoid canal. **ner'vi carot'ici exter'ni** [NA], carotid nerves, external; see under NERVE. **ner'vi caroticotympan'ici** [NA], caroticotympanic nerves; see under NERVE. **n. carot'icus inter'nus** [NA], carotid nerve, internal; see under NERVE. **ner'vi cerebra'les**, cranial nerves; see under NERVE. **ner'vi cervica'les** [NA], cervical nerves; see under NERVE. **ner'vi cilia'res bre'ves** [NA], ciliary nerves, short; see under NERVE. **ner'vi cilia'res lon'gi** [NA], ciliary nerves, long; see under NERVE. **n. coch'leae**, cochlear NERVE. **ner'vi crania'les** [NA], cranial nerves; see under NERVE. **ner'vi crania'les I**, olfactory nerve's; see under NERVE. **n. crania'lis II**, optic NERVE. **n. crania'lis III**, oculomotor NERVE. **n. crania'lis IV**, trochlear NERVE. **n. crania'lis V**, trigeminal NERVE. **n. crania'lis VI**, abducent NERVE. **n. crania'lis VII**, facial NERVE. **n. crania'lis VIII**, vestibulocochlear NERVE. **n. crania'lis IX**, glossopharyngeal NERVE. **n. crania'lis X**, vagus NERVE. **n. crania'lis XI**, accessory NERVE. **n. crania'lis XII**, hypoglossal NERVE. **n. cuta'neus** [NA], cutaneous NERVE. **nervi ethmoida'les anterio'res**, ethmoidal nerves anterior; see under NERVE. **n. ethmoida'lis poste'rior** [NA], ethmoidal nerve, posterior; see under NERVE. **n. facia'lis** [NA], facial NERVE. **n. fronta'lis** [NA], frontal NERVE. **n. glossopharyn'geus** [NA], glossopharyngeal NERVE. **n. hypoglos'sus** [NA], hypoglossal NERVE. **n. infraorbita'lis** [NA], infraorbital NERVE. **n. infratrochlea'ris** [NA], infratrochlear NERVE. **n. interme'dius** [NA], intermediate NERVE. **n. jugula'ris** [NA], jugular NERVE. **n. lacrima'lis** [NA], lacrimal NERVE. **n. laryn'geus infe'rior** [NA], laryngeal nerve, inferior; see under NERVE. **n. laryn'geus recur'rens** [NA], laryngeal nerve, recurrent; see under NERVE. **n. laryn'geus supe'rior** [NA], laryngeal nerve, superior; see under NERVE. **n. lingua'lis** [NA], lingual NERVE. **n. mandibula'ris** [NA], mandibular NERVE. **n. masseter'icus** [NA], masseteric NERVE. **n. masticato'rius**, motor root of trigeminal nerve; see under ROOT. **n. maxilla'ris** [NA], maxillary NERVE. **n. mea'tus acus'tici exter'ni** [NA], **n. mea'tus audito'rii exter'ni**, NERVE of external acoustic meatus. **n. menin'geus me'dius**, meningeal nerve, middle; see under NERVE. **n. menta'lis** [NA], mental NERVE. **n. mylohyoi'deus** [NA], mylohyoid NERVE. **n. nasocilia'ris** [NA], nasociliary NERVE. **n. nasopalati'nus** [NA], nasopalatine NERVE. **n. occipita'lis ma'jor** [NA], occipital nerve, greater; see under NERVE. **n. occipita'lis mi'nor** [NA], occipital nerve, lesser; see under NERVE. **n. occipita'lis ter'tius** [NA], occipital nerve, third; see under NERVE. **n. octa'vus**, vestibulocochlear NERVE. **n. oculomoto'rius** [NA], oculomotor NERVE. **ner'vi olfacto'rii** [NA], olfactory nerves; see under NERVE. **n. ophthal'micus** [NA], ophthalmic NERVE. **n. op'ticus** [NA], optic NERVE. **n. palati'nus ante'rior, n. palati'nus ma'jor** [NA], palatine n., greater. **ner'vi palati'ni me'dii, ner'vi palati'ni mino'res** [NA], **ner'vi palati'ni posterio'res**, palatine nerves, lesser; see under NERVE. **n. petro'sus ma'jor** [NA], petrosal nerve, greater; see under NERVE. **n. petro'sus mi'nor** [NA], petrosal nerve, lesser; see under NERVE. **n. petro'sus profun'dus** [NA], petrosal nerve, deep; see under NERVE. **n. petro'sus superficia'lis ma'jor**, petrosal nerve, greater; see under NERVE. **n. petro'sus superficia'lis mi'nor**, petrosal nerve, lesser; see under NERVE. **n. pterygoi'deus**

exter'nus, pterygoid nerve, lateral; see under NERVE. **n. pterygoi'deus inter'nus**, pterygoid nerve, medial; see under NERVE. **n. pterygoi'deus latera'lis** [NA], pterygoid nerve, lateral; see under NERVE. **n. pterygoi'deus media'lis** [NA], pterygoid nerve, medial; see under NERVE. **ner'vi pterygopalati'ni**, pterygopalatine nerves; see under NERVE. **n. recur'rens**, laryngeal nerve, recurrent; see under NERVE. **ner'vi sphenopalati'ni**, pterygopalatine nerves; see under NERVE. **ner'vi spina'les** [NA], spinal nerves; see under NERVE. **n. spino'sus**, meningeal branch of mandibular nerve; see under BRANCH. **n. stape'dius** [NA], stapedial NERVE. **n. sublingua'lis** [NA], sublingual NERVE. **n. supraorbita'lis** [NA], supraorbital NERVE. **n. supratrochlea'ris** [NA], supratrochlear NERVE. **ner'vi tempora'les profun'di** [NA] [**anterior et posterior**], temporal nerves, deep; see under NERVE. **n. tenso'ris tym'pani** [NA], NERVE of tensor tympani. **n. tenso'ris ve'li palati'ni** [NA], NERVE of tensor veli palatini. **n. tento'rii**, tentorial branch of ophthalmic nerve; see under BRANCH. **ner'vi termina'les** [NA], terminal nerves; see under NERVE. **n. trigem'inus** [NA], trigeminal NERVE. **n. trochlea'ris** [NA], trochlear NERVE. **n. tympan'icus** [NA], tympanic NERVE. **n. va'gus** [NA], vagus NERVE. **n. vascula'ris** [NA], vascular NERVE. **n. vestib'uli**, vestibular NERVE. **n. vestibulocochlea'ris** [NA], vestibulocochlear NERVE. **n. zygomat'icus** [NA], zygomatic NERVE.

Nesacaine trademark for *chloroprocaine hydrochloride* (see under CHLOROPROCAINE).

NESO Northeastern Society of Orthodontists.

Nesontil trademark for *oxazepam*.

Nespan trademark for *tybamate*.

net (net) a meshlike structure of interlocking fibers or strands. See also NETWORK.

Nethalide trademark for *pronethalol*.

nettle-rash (net''l-rash) urticaria.

network (net'work) a meshlike structure of interlocking fibers or strands. See also NET. **National Health Professions Placement N.**, a nationwide program aimed at improving access to and the availability of health care throughout the United States, particularly in underserved areas. Abbreviated *NHPPN*.

Neubauer's artery [Ernst *Neubauer*, German anatomist, 1742–1777] thyroid artery, lowest; see under ARTERY.

Neuber's operation see under OPERATION.

Neumann's aphthosis disease [Isidor Elder von Heilward *Neumann*, Austrian dermatologist, 1837–1906] see PEMPHIGUS vegetans and Stevens-Johnson SYNDROME.

Neumann's cells, sheath of [Ernst *Neumann*, German pathologist, 1834–1918] see under CELL and SHEATH.

neur- see NEURO-.

neurad (nu'rad) toward a neural axis or aspect.

neural (nu'ral) [L. *neuralis*; Gr. *neuron* nerve] pertaining to a nerve or to the nerves.

neuralgia (nu-ral'je-ah) [*neur-* + *-algia*] pain which extends along the course of one or more nerves, characterized by recurrence of spasmodic attacks of sharp pain, and usually caused by inflammatory diseases or injury. See also CAUSALGIA and PAIN. **Arnold's n.**, recurrent laryngeal n. **atypical facial n.**, atypical facial PAIN. **auriculotemporal n.**, recurrent laryngeal n. **ciliary n.**, a unilateral nasociliary nerve disorder, characterized by paroxysmal congestion of the anterior segment of the eye, rhinorrhea, and neuralgia at the inner angle of the eye at the side of the frontal nerve. Called also *supraorbital n.* and *Charlin's syndrome*. **cranial n.**, neuralgia along the course of a cranial nerve. **epileptiform n.**, trigeminal n. **n. facia'lis ve'ra**, geniculate n. **geniculate n.**, severe neuralgia in herpes zoster viral infection of the geniculate ganglion. Called also *n. facialis vera*, *Hunt's n.*, *otic n.*, *Ramsay Hunt's n.*, and *geniculate otalgia*. See also Hunt's SYNDROME. **glossopharyngeal n.**, a rare condition occurring chiefly in the elderly, which may be precipitated by swallowing, yawning, or coughing, characterized by paroxysms of sharp shooting pain extending from the trigger zone in the posterior pharynx or tonsillar fossa, and spreading to the ear, nasopharynx, and posterior part of the tongue. Occasional severe attacks may be interspersed among numerous mild attacks. Syncope and slowing of the heart rate may be associated during exceptionally severe attacks. **Harris' n.**, histamine n., Horton's n., cluster HEADACHE. **Hunt's n.**, geniculate n. **mandibular joint n.**, vertex and occipital pain, otalgia, glossodynia, and pain about the nose and eyes, associated with disturbed function of the temporomandibular joint. **migrainous n.**, migraine. **nasociliary n.**, pain in the eyes, brow, and root of the nose. **occipital n.**, vascular headache caused by distention of the postauricular and/or occipital arteries. **otic n.**, geniculate n. **periodic migrainous n.**, cluster HEADACHE. **Ramsay Hunt's n.**, geniculate n. **recurrent laryngeal n.**, neuralgia of the recurrent laryngeal nerve. Called also *Arnold's n.*, *auriculotemporal n.*, and *superior laryngeal n.* **Sluder's n.**, sphenopalatine n.

sphenopalatine n., neuralgia of the lower half of the face, affecting most often menopausal women, and usually occurring unilaterally in the maxilla, teeth, ear, mastoid, around the eyes, at the base of the nose, and beneath the zygoma. The occipital area, neck, shoulder, axilla, breast, arms, and hands may be involved. The pain is recurrent and persists from a few minutes to several days. Contrary to trigeminal neuralgia, it cannot be produced by external stimulation but some cases appear to be associated with tooth extraction. There may be nasal congestion, rhinorrhea, ocular hyperemia, excessive lacrimation, and paresthesia of the skin over the lower half of the face. Vasoconstriction of the vessels supplying the nasal mucosa has been suggested as the etiologic factor; other evidence indicates that the condition is due to vasodilatation of the internal maxillary artery, especially the portion supplying the sphenopalatine ganglion. Called also *Sluder's n., pterygopalatine syndrome,* and *Sluder's headache.* See also *vidian n.* **superior laryngeal n.,** recurrent laryngeal n. **supraorbital n.,** ciliary n. **temporomandibular n.,** temporomandibular dysfunction SYNDROME. **n. traumat'ica,** bruxism. **trifacial n.,** trigeminal n. **trigeminal n.,** unilateral, paroxysmal, stabbing pain of high intensity in the area supplied by the second or third division of the trigeminal nerve, usually occurring during middle life, and of unknown etiology. Attacks are sudden and pain may persist a few seconds to several minutes and then disappear as promptly as they arise; they may be associated with spasmodic contraction of the facial muscles, hence the synonym *tic douloureux.* Sometimes it may be precipitated by touching a "trigger zone" located on the vermilion border of the lips, nasal alae, cheeks, and around the eyes. Called also *epileptiform n., tortua facies, trifacial n., Fothergill's disease* and *prosopalgia.* **trigeminal nonsympathetic n.,** sudden trigeminal neuralgia associated with Bernard-Horner syndrome and a vasomotor disorder in the area supplied by the trigeminal nerve. Called also *Bonnet's syndrome.* **vidian n.,** irritation or inflammation of the vidian nerve associated with attacks of neuralgic pain in the nose, face, eye, ear, head, neck, and shoulder, which are usually unilateral, often nocturnal, and may be associated with subjective symptoms of nasal sinusitis. Called also *Vail's syndrome.*

neurasthenia (nu"ras-the'ne-ah) [*neur-* + Gr. *astheneia* debility] a neurosis marked chiefly by chronic abnormal fatigability, lack of energy, feelings of inadequacy, moderate depression, inability to concentrate, loss of appetite, insomnia.

Neuraxin trademark for *methocarbamol.*

neurectomy (nu-rek'to-me) [*neur-* + Gr. *ektomē* excision] the excision of a part of a nerve.

neurectopia (nu"rek-to'pe-ah) [*neur-* + Gr. *ektopos* out of place + *-ia*] displacement of a nerve or abnormal situation of a nerve.

neurexeresis (nur"ek-ser'ĕ-sis) [*neur-* + Gr. *exairein* to extract] the operation of tearing out (avulsion) of a nerve.

neurilemma (nu"rĭ-lem'mah) [*neur-* + Gr. *eilēma* a sheath] the thin membrane spirally enwrapping the myelin layers of a myelinated nerve fiber or the axon of an unmyelinated nerve fiber. It is made up of attenuated nucleated cells, there being one cell for each internodal segment between nodes of Ranvier. Called also *endoneural membrane, neurolemma, Schwann's membrane,* and *sheath of Schwann.* See illustration at NERVE.

neurilemmoma (nu"rĭ-lĕ-mo'mah) [*neur-* + Gr. *eilēma* a sheath + *-oma*] a common benign tumor of the neurilemma, which is typically a slow-growing encapsulated nodule, most commonly located about the neck and head and in various other organs. Oral and paraoral locations include the maxillary sinus, floor of the mouth, tongue, palate, lips, salivary glands, and retropharyngeal, nasopharyngeal, and retrotonsillar areas. Some cases have been reported as central lesions of bones, including the mandible. It is composed of elongated or spindle-shaped nuclei aligned in the shape of pallisades, with intracellular fibers arranged between the rows of nuclei; some are made up of a disorderly arrangement of cells and fibers with areas of edema fluid and microcysts. Small hyaline structures may be present. Called also *lemmona, neurinoma, perineural fibroblastoma,* and *schwannoma.* **malignant n.,** malignant SCHWANNOMA.

neurinofibrolipomatosis (nu"rĭ-no-fi"bro-lip"o-mah-to'sis) Recklinghausen's DISEASE (1).

neurinoma (nu"rĭ-no'mah) [*neur-* + *-oma*] neurilemmoma. **ameloblastic n.,** a tumor combining the characteristics of ameloblastoma and neurilemmoma. Most authorities believe that this is a co-occurrence of two separate tumors.

neurinomatosis (nu"ri-no"mah-to'sis) development of numerous neurinomas (see NEURILEMMOMA). **n. centra'lis et periph'erica,** Reckinghausen's DISEASE (1).

neuritic (nu-rit'ik) pertaining to or affected with neuritis.

neuritis (nu-ri'tis) [*neur-* + *-itis*] inflammation of a nerve. See also NEUROPATHY. **disseminated n.,** polyneuritis. **multiple n.,** polyneuritis.

neuro-, neur- [Gr. *neuron* nerve] a combining form denoting relationship to a nerve or nerves, or to the nervous system.

neuroadventitia (nu"ro-ad"ven-tish'e-ah) adventitia formed by nerve fibers. **perivascular n.,** a sheath for an artery formed by nerve fibers, sometimes found in the dental pulp and seldom if ever encountered in other tissues of the body.

neuroanatomy (nu"ro-ah-nat'o-me) [*neuro-* + *anatomy*] that branch of science which is concerned with the anatomy of the nervous system.

neuroblast (nu'ro-blast) [*neuro-* + Gr. *blastos* germ] any embryonic cell which develops into a nerve cell or neuron; an immature nerve cell.

neuroblastoma (nu"ro-blas-to'mah) [*neuroblast* + *-oma*] a highly malignant tumor of the nervous system, composed chiefly of neuroblasts, which may be located in the adrenal glands, in the sympathetic chain, as well as in the bladder and other visceral organs, and the lips, nose, and jaws. Typically, it is a lobular, soft lesion weighing between 80 to 150 gm, presenting as a grayish mass with areas of hemorrhage and necrosis and, sometimes, foci of calcification. Histologically, it is composed of small and dark lymphocyte-like cells frequently arranged in masses without any pattern; rosettes may be found in some tumors. **olfactory n.,** a rare, invasive, destructive tumor, believed to originate from the olfactory apparatus, found most frequently in the nasal cavity and nasopharynx. It typically appears as a painful swelling made up of densely packed masses of small darkly staining cells with poorly defined eosinophilic cytoplasm and regular round vesicular nuclei. Called also *esthesioneuroblastoma* and *esthesioneuroepithelioma.*

neurocoele (nu'ro-sēl) [*neuro-* + Gr. *koilon* hollow] the neural canal; the cavity or lumen of the embryonic neurocranium.

neurocranium (nu"ro-kra'ne-um) [*neuro-* + Gr. *kranion* cranium] in skull development, the part of the cranium which encloses the brain. The components of the membranous neurocranium include the frontal, parietal, and interparietal bones, occipital and squamous portions of the temporal bone, and nasal and lacrimal bones. The components of the cartilaginous neurocranium include the supraoccipital and orbitosphenoid bones, temporal wing, and otic capsule.

neurodendrite (nu"ro-den'drit) [*neuro-* + Gr. *dendron* tree] dendrite.

neurodendron (nu"ro-den'dron) [*neuro-* + Gr. *dendron* tree] dendrite.

neuroepithelium (nu"ro-ep"ĭ-the'le-um) [*neuro-* + *epithelium*] 1. simple columnar epithelium made up of cells specialized to serve as sensory cells for the reception of external stimuli, as the sensory cells of the cochlea, vestibule, nasal mucosa, and tongue. 2. the epithelium of the ectoderm, from which the cerebrospinal axis is developed.

neurofibril (nu"ro-fi'bril) one of the delicate threads running in every direction through the cytoplasm of the body of a nerve cell and extending into the axon and the dendrites of the cell.

neurofibroma (nu"ro-fi-bro'mah) [*neuro-* + *fibroma*] a tumor derived from the nerve fiber fasciculus. **multiple n.,** see Recklinghausen's DISEASE (1).

neurofibromatosis (nu"ro-fi"bro-mah-to'sis) Recklinghausen's DISEASE (1).

neurofibrosarcoma (nu"ro-fi"bro-sar-ko'mah) [*neuro-* + *fibrosarcoma*] malignant SCHWANNOMA.

neurogenic (nu"ro-jen'ik) [*neuro-* + Gr. *gennan* to produce] 1. forming nervous tissue, or stimulating nervous energy. 2. originating in the nervous system.

neuroglia (nu-rog'le-ah) [*neuro-* + Gr. *glia* glue] the supporting structure of nervous tissue, consisting of a fine web of tissue made up of modified ectodermal elements, in which are enclosed peculiar branched cells, the neuroglial cells. The neuroglial cells are of three types: the astrocytes, oligodendrocytes, and microgliocytes. Astrocytes and oligodendrocytes appear to play a role in myelin formation, transport of material to neurons, and maintenance of the ionic environment of neurons. Called also *blind web* and *glia.* See illustration at NERVE.

Neurohr spring-lock attachment [F. G. *Neurohr,* American dentist] see under ATTACHMENT.

Neurohr-Williams shoe (rest shoe) [F. G. *Neurohr*] see under SHOE.

neurohumor (nu"ro-hu'mor) transmitter SUBSTANCE.

neurohypophysis (nu"ro-hi-pof'ĭ-sis) [*neuro-* + *hypophysis*] [NA alternative] pituitary gland, posterior; see under GLAND.

neurolemma (nu″ro-lem′mah) [*neuro-* + Gr. *eilēma* sheath] neurilemma.

neuroleptanalgesia (nu″ro-lep″tan-al-je′ze-ah) [*neuro-* + Gr. *leptos* slender + *an* neg. + *algēsis* pain + *-ia*] a state of quiescence, altered awareness, and analgesia produced by the administration of a combination of a narcotic analgesic and a neuroleptic agent.

neuroleptanesthesia (nu″ro-lep″tan-es-the′ze-ah) [*neuro-* + Gr. *leptos* slender + *an* neg. + *aisthēsis* sensation] a state of neuroleptanalgesia and unconsciousness, produced by the combined administration of a narcotic analgesic and a neuroleptic agent, together with the inhalation of nitrous oxide and oxygen.

neuroleptic (nu″ro-lep′tik) 1. antipsychotic. 2. antipsychotic DRUG.

neurology (nu-rol′o-je) that branch of medical science which deals with the nervous system, both normal and in disease.

neuroma (nu-ro′mah) [*neuro-* + *-oma*] a tumor made up of nerve cells and nerve fibers. **amputation n.,** a lesion most commonly occurring at the end of an amputated limb but also found in the oral cavity, which is not a true neoplasm but an attempt to repair a damaged or sectioned nerve. In the oral cavity, it presents hyperplasia of nerve fibers and their supportive structures, showing a small, slow-growing nodule or swelling of the mucous membrane or, less frequently, a central bone lesion, and is typically located on the alveolar ridge in edentulous areas near the mental foramen, or on the lips or tongue. It is usually composed of a mass of irregular, often interlacing neurofibrils and Schwann cells in a connective tissue stroma. Called also *post-traumatic n.* and *traumatic n.* **multiple mucosal n's,** a dominantly inherited syndrome of mucosal neuromas, usually present early in life and involving the lips, tongue, conjunctiva, larynx, and nostril. It is associated with medullary thyroid carcinoma; pheochromocytoma; secondary hyperparathyroidism; blubbery lips; eversion of the upper eyelids; Scheuermann's disease, slipped femoral epiphyses; medullated corneal nerves; and gastrointestinal disorders, such as intestinal ganglioneuromatosis and diarrhea, and failure of axon flare following intracutaneous injection of histamine. Called also *syndrome of multiple mucosal neuromas.* **post-traumatic n.,** amputation n. **traumatic n.,** amputation n.

neuromuscular (nu″ro-mus′ku-lar) pertaining to muscles and nerves.

neuron (nu′ron) [Gr. "nerve"] a conducting cell of the nervous system, typically consisting of a cell body (perikaryon) with its surrounding cytoplasm, organelles, and inclusion bodies; a large and vesicular nucleus containing a prominent nucleolus with a sex element being clearly visible; several short radiating processes (dendrites); and one long process (axon), which terminates in twiglike branches (telodendrons) and sometimes has branches (collaterals) projecting along its course. The axon together with its covering or sheath forms the nerve fiber. The cytoplasm contains mitochondria and a Golgi apparatus. There is apparently no mitotic division of neurons. The specialized structures include neurofibrils and Nissl granules. Pigment granules may be found in some neurons. Called also *nerve cell.* See illustration at NERVE. **afferent n.,** afferent NERVE. **bipolar n.,** one having two axons arising from opposite poles. **central n.,** one located within the central nervous system. **efferent n.,** efferent NERVE. **motor n.,** motoneuron. **motor n., lower,** lower MOTONEURON. **motor n., upper,** upper MOTONEURON. **multipolar n.,** one having several axons. **postganglionic n.,** one that originates in the autonomic ganglia, whose fibers continue beyond the ganglion to peripheral organs and blood vessels. See also gray rami communicantes, under RAMUS. **postsynaptic n.,** one that conveys impulses away from a synapse. See also SYNAPSE. **preganglionic n's,** neurons whose cell bodies are located in the central nervous system and whose fibers (preganglionic fibers) terminate in the autonomic ganglia. See also white rami communicantes, under RAMUS. **presynaptic n.,** one that conveys impulses toward a synapse. **sensory n.,** sensory NERVE. **unipolar n.,** one having only one axon.

neuronal (nu′ro-nal) pertaining to a neuron or neurons.

neuronevus (nu″ro-ne′vus) [*neuro-* + *nevus*] intradermal NEVUS. **blue n.,** blue NEVUS.

neuropathic (nu″ro-path′ik) pertaining to or characterized by neuropathy.

neuropathy (nu-rop′ah-the) [*neuro-* + *-pathy*] any condition characterized by pathological changes in the peripheral nervous system. The term is also sometimes used to distinguish noninflammatory conditions of the peripheral nervous system from inflammatory lesions (see NEURITIS).

neurorrhaphy (nu-ror′ah-fe) [*neuro-* + Gr. *rhaphē* stitch] the suturing of a cut nerve; nerve suture.

Neurosin trademark for *calcium glycerophosphate* (see under CALCIUM).

neuroses (nu-ro′sēz) plural of *neurosis.*

neurosis (nu-ro′sis), pl. *neuro′ses* [*neur-* + *-osis*] an emotional disorder due to unresolved conflicts, anxiety being its chief characteristic. Called also *psychoneurosis.* Cf. PSYCHOSIS. **occlusal habit n.,** bruxism.

neuroskeleton (nu″ro-skel′e-ton) endoskeleton.

neurotomy (nu-rot′o-me) [*neuro* + Gr. *temnein* to cut] 1. the surgical cutting of a nerve. 2. the dissection or anatomy of the nerves. **retrogasserian n.,** retrogasserian RHIZOTOMY.

neurotoxin (nu″ro-tok′sin) a substance that is poisonous or destructive to nerve tissue, especially an exotoxin which is characterized by a marked affinity for nerve tissue. **tetanus n.,** tetanospasmin.

Neurotrast trademark for *iophendylate.*

neurotrophy (nu-rot′ro-fe) [*neuro-* + Gr. *trophē* nutrition] supply through the nervous system of influences necessary for the maintenance of tissue.

neutral (nu′tral) [L. *neutralis, neuter* neither] 1. not engaged or aligned on either side; in the middle of two extremes. 2. not electrically charged. 3. in chemistry, neither basic nor acid; having a pH of 7.

neutralization (nu′trah-li-za′shun) 1. the rendering of something neutral; the inactivation of extreme or harmful qualities of something. 2. the rendering of a solution neutral by adding a base to an acid solution or an acid to an alkaline or basic solution, until it achieves a pH of 7.

Neutrapen trademark for *penicillinase.*

neutrino (nu-tre′no) a hypothetical elementary particle with no charge and small mass, 6×10^{-30} gm, emitted with an electron in radioactive or other changes, such as beta decay.

neutroclusion (nu″tro-kloo′zhun) malocclusion characterized by irregularities of individual teeth, but with normal mesiodistal or normal anteroposterior relation of the mandibular to the maxillary arch. Generally regarded as identical with Class I in Angle's classification of malocclusion (see MALOCCLUSION). **complex n.,** that involving facial features. **simple n.,** that not involving facial features.

neutron (nu′tron) an electrically neutral or uncharged particle of matter existing along with protons in atoms of all elements except for the mass 1 isotope of hydrogen. Its mass is about 1.67 $\times 10^{-27}$ kg. A free neutron is unstable and decays with a half-life of about 13 minutes into an electron, proton, and neutrino. Abbreviated *n.* **epithermal n.,** one having an energy level of a few hundredths electron volt to 100 electron volts. **fast n.,** one having an energy level exceeding 10^5 electron volts. **intermediate n.,** one having an energy level of 100 to 100,000 electron volts. **slow n.,** 1. thermal n. 2. one having an energy level up to 100 electron volts. **thermal n.,** one having an energy level of about 0.025 electron volt. Called also *slow n.*

neutropenia (nu″tro-pe′ne-ah) [*neutrophil* + Gr. *penia* poverty] a decrease in the number of neutrophilic leukocytes in the blood. See also AGRANULOCYTOSIS. **chronic hypoplastic n.,** neutropenia characterized by granulocytic hypoplasia of the bone marrow, recurrent infections, splenomegaly, and lesions of the skin and oral mucosa. Recurrent ulcerations of the gingivae, lips, and buccal mucosa, dental abscesses, gingivitis, severe reactions to dental extraction, and canker sores are the principal oral lesions. **cyclic n.,** periodic AGRANULOCYTOSIS. **congenital n.,** a congenital absence of neutrophils, inherited as an autosomal recessive trait, associated with a lowered resistance to bacterial infections, principally severe otitis media and skin infections. Serum gamma globulin is normally elevated and bone marrow granulopoiesis is depressed. Oral complications may include blister-like lesions filled with clear, nonpurulent fluid, found on the oral mucosa, lips, and tongue, which recur at regular intervals of four to six weeks, often associated with fetid gingivitis, necrotic changes, and pharyngitis. Called also *Felty's syndrome* and *infantile genetic agranulocytosis.* **malignant n.,** agranulocytosis. **periodic n.,** periodic AGRANULOCYTOSIS. **primary splenic n.,** a syndrome consisting of splenomegaly and neutropenia. Myeloid hyperplasia of the bone marrow, leukopenia, granulocytopenia, lymphadenopathy, anemia, weight loss, weakness, fatigue, and skin pigmentation are the usual features. Oral changes consist chiefly of recurrent ulcer of the oral mucosa, presenting a clean, punched-out lesion about 2 mm in diameter. When associated with rheumatoid arthritis, the disorder is known as *Felty's syndrome.*

neutrophil (nu′tro-fil) [L. *neuter* neither + Gr. *philein* to love] 1. any cell, structure, or histologic element readily stainable by neutral dyes. 2. a granulocyte occurring as a spherical cell, about 7 to 9 μ in diameter, having a nucleus with three to five irregularly oval to angular lobes connected by slender chromatin threads, and cytoplasm containing fine inconspicuous granules. Stained cells show deep purplish-blue nuclei and coarse chromatin network and pink cytoplasm with pink to violet-pink granules. Granules fill most of the cell, except for a small clear area in the center which contains diplosomes. The peripheral layer of the cytoplasm forms pseudopodia. Blood smears of human females show appendages about 1.5 μ in diameter, which are attached to the nucleus by a chromatin thread, believed to be XX chromosomes. Neutrophils arise in the bone marrow from stem cells and, after a series of divisions, undergo maturation as myeloblast, promyelocyte, metamyelocyte, band cell, and mature neutrophil. With maturation, there is a sequential appearance of the primary (azurophilic) and secondary (specific) granules; the primary granules are electron-dense structures about 0.4 μ in diameter, appearing early in maturation and being similar to lysosomes, the secondary granules are about 0.3 μ in diameter and are less dense. After about 12 hours in the blood, neutrophils enter the tissues where they complete their life span in a few days. They are the first to appear at the site of inflammation and participate in the breakdown and ingestion of foreign materials and the killing of microorganisms, believed to be under the control of cellular and humoral factors. Called also *polymorphonuclear n., neutrophilic cell* or *granulocyte,* and *neutrophilic, polymorphonuclear,* or *polynuclear leukocyte.* See also table of *Reference Values in Hematology* in Appendix. **n. count,** see table of *Reference Values in Hematology* in Appendix. **filamented n.,** one having two or more lobes connected by a filament of chromatin. **giant n.,** macropolycyte. **juvenile n.,** metamyelocyte. **nonfilamented n.,** one whose lobes are connected by thick strands of chromatin. **polymorphonuclear n.,** neutrophil (2). **rod n., stab n.,** one whose nucleus is not divided into segments.

neutrophilia (nu″tro-fil′e-ah) increase in the number of neutrophils in the blood; it is the most common form of leukocytosis and may result from various diseases, including acute infections, intoxications, hemorrhage, and malignant neoplasms. See also LEUKOCYTE count and table of *Reference Values in Hematology* in Appendix.

Neutrosteron trademark for *methandriol.*

nevi (ne′vi) [L.] plural of *nevus.*

nevoid (ne′void) resembling a nevus.

nevus (ne′vus), pl. *ne′vi* [L. *naevus*] a circumscribed new growth of the skin of congenital origin, presenting a small elevated flat or pedunculated, often pigmented lesion. Called also *birthmark* and *mole.* **blue n.,** a sharply defined, round or oval, slightly elevated, hard, blue to blue-black benign melanocytic tumor. Individual nevi vary in size from 2 to 15 mm, and are found most commonly on the face, forearms, hands, and buttocks, and occasionally may be located in the oral cavity. Histologically, it consists of mixtures of melanocytes, fibrillar cells, collagenous fibrous tissue, and nerve-like cells. Spindle-shaped, bipolar, dendritic cells grouped in the lower two-thirds of the cutis are the principal pathological feature. Called also *Jadassohn-Tièche n., benign mesenchymal melanoma, blue neuronevus, chromatophoroma, dermal melanocytoma,* and *melanofibroma.* **Cannon's n.,** white sponge n. **compound n.,** a lesion composed of an intradermal nevus and an overlying junctional nevus. **dermoepidermal n.,** 1. Hutchinson's FRECKLE. 2. junctional n. **n. flam′meus,** a capillary hemangioma usually present at birth, and occurring most commonly on the face and neck, and less frequently on the trunk and extremities. Crying, coughing, or exposure to cold may produce changes in the color of the lesion. Called also *port-wine mark* and *port-wine stain.* See also capillary HEMANGIOMA. **n. flam′meus, post-traumatic,** a nevus flammeus of the part of the face supplied by the trigeminal nerve, associated with ipsilateral weakness and hyperesthesia of the arm and leg. It occurs following a head injury, and is probably caused by damage of the spinal cord and the cervical autonomic nerves resulting in vasomotor disorders. Called also *Fegeler's syndrome.* **n. follicula′ris,** cystic adenoid EPITHELIOMA. **n. fuscoceru′leum ophthalmomaxilla′ris,** Ota's n. **n. hypertroph′icus,** Klippel-Trenaunay-Weber SYNDROME. **intradermal n.,** a pigmented cellular nevus located in the dermis, sometimes also found in the oral mucosa. Called also *neuronevus.* **Jadassohn-Tièche n.,** blue n. **junctional n.,** a pigmented cellular nevus which involves the junction of the dermis and epidermis, sometimes also located in the oral mucosa. Called also *dermoepidermal n.* and *marginal n.* **marginal n.,** junctional n. **melanophoric n.,** Naegeli's SYNDROME. **oral epithelial n.,** white sponge n. **Ota's n.,** a pigmented nevus of the eyelids, nose, zygomatic and frontal regions, ear lobes, retroauricular region, and anterior portion of the scalp, usually noted at birth or during the first decade. Commonly, the lesions are unilateral, macular or slightly raised, and tan-brown, slate blue, black, or purple. Ipsilateral hyperpigmentation of the cornea, conjunctiva, sclera, uvea, optic papilla, optic nerve, and orbit is fre-

quently associated. There also may be pigmentation of the external auditory canal, oral mucosa, gingivae, pharynx, hard palate, nasal mucosa, and leptomeninges. Females, usually of the Oriental and dark-skinned races, are most often affected. Called also *aberrant mongolian spot, extrasacral dermal melanosis, nevus fuscoceruleus ophthalmomaxillaris,* and *oculocutaneous melanosis.* **pigmented cellular n.,** a superficial pigmented mole of the skin and mucous membrane, present in varying numbers on almost everybody, which is composed of melanocytes, the pigment-producing cells; the color of lesions varies, depending on the amount of melanin, from flesh color to brown or black. Pigmented nevi, usually of the intradermal or junctional type, may also appear on the oral mucosa, most commonly on the gingiva, lips, and palate. Called also *pigmented mole.* **n. pigmento′sus systemat′icus,** Bloch-Sulzberger SYNDROME. **tardive n.,** Hutchinson's FRECKLE. **vascular n.,** ANGIOMA cavernosum. **white sponge n.,** a condition, transmitted as an autosomal dominant trait, characterized by spongy white lesions of the oral and nasal mucosae, in which thickened spongy folded mucosa covers the nasal septum, conchae, cheeks, tongue, palate, gums, and floor of the mouth. The lesions, which are asymptomatic, may be found in newborn infants, increasing in severity until adolescence. Called also *Cannon's n., oral epithelial n., congenital leukokeratosis, familial white folded dysplasia,* and *white folded gingivostomatitis.*

New Concept see under DENTIFRICE.

Newlands' law [John Alexander Raina *Newlands,* British chemist, 1838–1898] see under LAW.

newton (nu′ton) [named for Sir Isaac *Newton*] the SI unit of force, being equal to the force required to give a mass of 1 kilogram an acceleration of 1 meter per second squared, calculated: force = mass × acceleration, or $1 N = 1 kg × m/s^2$. Abbreviated N. See also SI.

Newton's law of motion [Sir Isaac *Newton,* English mathematician, physicist, and astronomer, 1643–1727] see under LAW. See NEWTON and NEWTONIAN.

newtonian (nu′to′ne-an) named after Sir Isaac *Newton,* as newtonian aberration (see under ABERRATION).

Ney articulator, surveyor see under ARTICULATOR and SURVEYOR.

Ney gold color elastic trademark for a low noble metal dental wrought gold wire alloy.

Ney-Oro A-A trademark for a soft *dental casting gold alloy* (see under GOLD).

Ney-Oro B-2 trademark for an extra hard *dental casting gold alloy* (see under GOLD).

Ney-Oro elastic no. 4 trademark for a high noble metal dental wrought gold wire alloy.

NF National FORMULARY.

ng nanogram.

NHI 1. National Health Insurance. 2. National Health Institute.

NHMRC National Health and Medical Research Council.

NHPPN National Health Professions Placement Network (see under NETWORK).

NHSC National Health Service Corps; see under CORPS.

Ni nickel.

niacin (ni′ah-sin) nicotinic ACID.

niacinamide (ni″ah-sin′ah-mīd) nicotinamide.

NIAID National Institute of Allergy and Infectious Diseases.

nialamide (ni-al′ah-mīd) a monoamine oxidase inhibitor, 2-[2-(benzylcarbamoyl)-ethyl]hydrazide, occurring as bitter crystals that are soluble in solutions of acidic solvents and slightly soluble in water. Used as an antidepressive agent. Adverse reactions are similar to those of other monoamine oxidase inhibitors. Trademarks: Espril, Niamid, Niaquitil, Nyazid.

NIAMD National Institute of Arthritis and Metabolic Diseases.

Niamid trademark for *nialamide.*

Niaquitil trademark for *nialamide.*

Niazol trademark for *naphazoline.*

nib (nib) in dentistry, the working part of a condenser, connected to the handle by the shank, which comes into contact with restorative material within a prepared cavity, its end, the face, being smooth or serrated. The nib corresponds to the blade in an excavating or cutting instrument. Called also *condenser point.*

niccolum (nik′o-lum) [L.] nickel.

Nicel trademark for *methylcellulose.*

niche (nich) 1. a recess in a wall or the like. 2. a defect in an otherwise even surface, especially a depression or recess in the wall of a hollow organ. **enamel n.,** either of two depressions between the lateral dental lamina and the developing tooth germ, one pointing distally (distal enamel n.) and the other mesially (mesial enamel n.).

NICHHD National Institute of Child Health and Human Development.

nickel (nik′′l) [L. *niccolum;* Ger. *Nickel* Satan or "Old Nick"] a metallic element. Symbol, Ni; atomic number, 28; atomic weight, 58.71; specific gravity, 8.908; melting point, 1455°C; valences, 2, 3; group VIII of the periodic table. It occurs as five naturally occurring isotopes, 58, 60–62, and 64, and several artificial radioactive ones, 56, 57, 59, 63, and 65–67. Nickel is a lustrous, white, hard, ferromagnetic metal that is slowly attacked by dilute hydrochloric and sulfuric acids and readily attacked by nitric acid, but not by alkali hydroxides. It is a trace element which takes the place of cobalt in aiding the synthesis of hemoglobin in the bone marrow and participates in the metabolism of fatty acids or their esters by serving as a catalyst in hydrogenation. It also combines with porphyrins to form *meta*-porphyrin. Used as a component in stainless steels and nickel-chromium wires for the production of orthodontic arch wires and springs. Contact may cause dermatitis and ingestion usually produces vomiting, nausea, and diarrhea. **n.-chromium alloy,** nickel-chromium ALLOY. **cobalt-chromium-n. alloy,** cobalt-chromium-nickel ALLOY.

Nicolas-Favre disease [Joseph *Nicolas,* French physician, born 1869; Maurice *Favre,* French physician, 1876–1954] LYMPHOGRANULOMA venereum.

Niconyl trademark for *isoniazid.*

Nicorine trademark for *nikethamide.*

Nicot's herb [Jean *Nicot* de Villemain, 1530–1600, who is said to have introduced tobacco in France] *Nicotiana.*

Nicotiana (nik′′o-she′a-nah) [named after Jean *Nicot* de Villemain] a genus of solaceous annual plants, native to tropical and subtropical America, from which tobacco is derived. Called also *Nicot's herb.*

nicotinamide (nik′′o-tin′ah-mīd) the amide of nicotinic acid, which is a component of the vitamin B complex, pyridine-3-carboxylic acid amide. It occurs as water-soluble crystals. In tissue, it is derived from nicotinic acid, and as the functional component of codehydrogenase I and II, it plays an essential role in electron transport in respiratory reactions. Therapeutically, nicotinamide is used in the treatment and prevention of pellagra. Called also *niacinamide, nicotinic acid amide, vitamin B₃,* and *vitamin PP.* See also PELLAGRA.

nicotine (nik′o-tēn) [L. *nicotiana* tobacco] a poisonous alkaloid from tobacco leaves, 1-methyl-2-(3-pyridyl)pyrrolidine, occurring as a yellowish, oily, hygroscopic liquid that turns brown on exposure to air or light, and is miscible in water and soluble in alcohol, chloroform, ether, and oils. Nicotine is a ganglionic stimulant with unpredictable effects, which may increase the heart rate by excitation of sympathetic or paralysis of parasympathetic cardiac ganglia, or it can slow the rate by paralysis of sympathetic or stimulation of parasympathetic cardiac ganglia. It stimulates the peripheral nerves, followed by depression. Small doses stimulate the autonomic ganglia, but with large doses, initial stimulation is followed by blockade. Small doses evoke the discharge of catecholamines, but large doses prevent their release. Small doses stimulate the central nervous system, but large doses may cause tremors and convulsions. Nicotine also stimulates sensory receptors, causes vomiting, exerts an antidiuretic action, and causes initial stimulation of salivary and bronchial secretions, followed by inhibition. Nicotine is absorbed from the oral, gastrointestinal, and respiratory mucosa and through the skin, most of it being metabolized in the liver and some in the lungs and kidneys. It is excreted in the urine, acidity of the urine enhancing the rate of excretion. Used as an antiparasitic insecticidal and as an antitetanic drug. Nicotine poisoning is usually caused by ingestion of nicotine-containing insecticide sprays or tobacco products, most commonly by children. Acute poisoning is usually characterized by nausea, salivation, abdominal pain, vomiting, diarrhea, cold sweat, headache, dizziness, hearing and visual disorders, confusion, weakness, prostration, hypotension, breathing difficulty, collapse, convulsions, and death.

nicotinic (nik-o-tin′ik) 1. pertaining to nicotine. 2. nicotinic DRUG.

nidi (ni′di) [L.] plural *nidus.*

NIDR National Institute of Dental Research.

nidus (ni′dus), pl. *ni′di* [L. "nest"] 1. the point of origin or focus. 2. nucleus (2). **cartilage n.,** cartilage LACUNA

Nielsen's syndrome [Herman *Nielsen,* Danish physician] see under SYNDROME.

Niemann-Pick disease [Albert *Niemann,* German pediatrician, 1880–1921; Ludwig *Pick,* German physician, born 1868] see under DISEASE.

Nifos T trademark for *tetraethyl pyrophosphate* (see under PYROPHOSPHATE).

Nifulidone trademark for *furazolidone.*

nifuroxime (ni′′fur-ok′sēm) a topical antibacterial and antiprotozoal agent, 5-nitro-2-furancarboxaldehyde oxime, occurring as pale yellow or greenish crystals that darken on exposure to light and are soluble in water, methyl alcohol, and ethyl alcohol. Trademark: MICOFUR.

night-grinding (nīt-grīnd′ing) bruxism.

nightshade (nīt′shād) a plant of the genus *Solanum.* **deadly n.,** belladonna (1).

NIGMS National Institute of General Medical Sciences.

nigricans (ni′gri-kans) [L.] black or blackish.

nigrities (ni-grish′e-ēz) [L.] blackness. **n. lin′guae,** black TONGUE.

NIH National Institutes of Health.

nikethamide (ni-keth′ah-mīd) a weak analeptic, N,N-diethyl-3-pyridinecarboxamide, occurring as a clear to pale yellow, slightly viscous liquid that crystallizes on exposure to cold, with a faintly bitter taste and a faint warm aftertaste, which is miscible with water, ethanol, and ether. Used as a respiratory stimulant, mainly in treating anesthetic overdosage, asphyxia of the newborn, cardiac decompensation, shock, respiratory depression, acute alcoholic intoxication, and poisoning with carbon monoxide and various hypnotic and narcotic substances. Also used in the treatment of pellagra. Overdosage may cause convulsions and fatal respiratory paralysis. Called also *nicotinic acid diethylamide.* Trademarks: Anacardone, Carbamidal, Cardamine, Cardiamid, Cormed, Cormid, Eucoran, Nicorine, Salvacard, Stimulin.

Nikolsky's (Nikolskii's) sign [Petr Vasilyevich (Vasilevich) *Nikolsky,* Russian dermatologist, 1858–1940] see under SIGN.

Nilevar trademark for *norethandrolone.*

NIMH National Institute of Mental Health.

NINDB National Institute of Neurological Diseases and Blindness.

niobium (ni-o′be-um) [named after *Niobe,* daughter of Tantalus, a character in Greek mythology] a metallic element. Symbol, Nb; atomic number, 41; atomic weight, 92.9064; valences, 2, 3, 4, 5, being usually pentavalent; melting point, 2468°C; group VB of the periodic table. ⁹³Nb is the natural isotope; artificial radioactive isotopes include 88–92 and 94–101. Niobium is a steel-gray, lustrous, ductile, malleable metal that is resistant to oxygen and halogens at room temperature and is attacked by hot nitric, hydrochloric, sulfuric, and phosphoric acids. It is unaffected by aqua regia at room temperature, but attacked by alkalies at all temperatures. Used in steel alloys and in nuclear technology. Called also *columbium.*

Nionate trademark for a preparation of *ferrous gluconate* preparation (see under GLUCONATE).

NIOSH National Institute of Occupational Safety and Health (see under INSTITUTE).

Nipagin A trademark for *ethylparaben.*

Nipagin M trademark for *methylparaben.*

Nipasol trademark for *propylparaben.*

Nipecotan trademark for *anileridine.*

niperyt (ni′per-it) PENTAERYTHRITOL tetranitrate.

Nipodal trademark for *prochlorperazine.*

nippers (nip′erz) a strong hinged pliers with cutting beaks. **bone n.,** rongeur. **plate n., wire n.,** nippers for cutting metal plate or wire.

nipple (nip′′l) 1. the pigmented projection of the anterior surface of the mammary gland, surrounded by the areola; it gives outlet to milk from the breast. Called also *mammary papilla, mamilla, papilla mammae* [NA], *staphylion,* and *thelium.* 2. an artificial nipple made of rubber or other elastic nontoxic material, through which an infant sucks milk or other liquid from a bottle. Improperly designed nipples are believed to cause faulty tooth development that may lead to malocclusion.

Niranium trademark for a high-fusing chromium-cobalt casting alloy.

Nirvan trademark for *methotrimeprazine.*

Nisentel trademark for *alphaprodine hydrochloride* (see under ALPHAPRODINE).

Nisentil trademark for *alphaprodine hydrochloride* (see under ALPHAPRODINE).

Nisotin trademark for *ethionamide.*

Nissl bodies (granules, substance) [Franz *Nissl,* neurologist in Heidelberg, 1860–1919] see under BODY.

Nitranitol trademark for *mannitol hexanitrate* (see under MANNITOL).

Nitranol trademark for mannitol hexanitrate (see under MANNI-TOL).

nitrate (ni'trāt) [L. *nitratum*] a salt of nitric acid, containing the radical —NO₃. Nitrates are the principal form of nitrogen available to higher plants from the soil and are assimilated into the form of ammonia by being first reduced to nitrites and subsequently to ammonia. Nitrates are used in food preservation, particularly sausages, and are sometimes suspected as being the cause of methemoglobinemia. **phenylmercuric n., basic,** a mixture of phenylmercuric nitrate (C₆H₅HgNO₃) and phenylmercuric hydroxide (C₆H₅HgOH), occurring as a white, crystalline powder that is affected by light, and is slightly soluble in water, ethanol, and glycerol, becoming increasingly soluble in the presence of nitric acid or alkali hydroxides. It is a basic salt, being unstable and decomposing into the basic compounds on contact with water; its Hg component is 62.75 to 63.50 percent. Used chiefly as a topical antibacterial agent for the prevention and therapy of superficial abrasions, wounds, and infections. Sometimes used to disinfect dental instruments, but its effectiveness is believed to be limited. Trademark: Merphenyl.

nitration (nī-tra'shun) the introduction of a nitro group (—NO₂) into a chemical compound.

nitrazepam (ni-trah'ze-pam) an anticonvulsant and hypnotic drug, 1,3-dihydro-7-nitro-5-phenyl-2*H*-1,4-benzodiazepin-2-one, occurring as a crystalline substance that is soluble in ethanol, acetone, chloroform, and ethyl acetate, but not in water, ether, and benzene. Trademarks: Benzalin, Eunoctin, Nitrepax, Pelson, Sonnolin.

nitremia (ni-tre'me-ah) azotemia.

nitric (ni'trik) pertaining to or containing nitrogen, applied especially to compounds containing nitrogen with a higher valence than that contained in the nitrous compounds. See also nitric ACID.

nitride (ni'trīd) a binary compound of nitrogen with a metal.

nitrite (ni'trīt) any salt of nitrous acid or a compound containing the radical —NO₂. Nitrites are antagonists of norepinephrine, acetylcholine, histamine, and similar agents and act as smooth muscle relaxants, particularly of the blood vessels. Pharmacologically, they are general vasodilators and are used chiefly in therapy of angina pectoris. They are denitrated by the glutathione–organic nitrate reductase system of the liver. Headache is the most common complication of nitrite therapy; dizziness, weakness, nausea, and hypotension being sometimes associated. Alcohol exacerbates the severity of symptoms. Acute poisoning may include nausea, vomiting, abdominal cramps, headache, confusion, delirium, brachycardia, brachypnea, convulsions, methemoglobinemia, shock, and death. Chronic exposure may produce headache, hallucinations, and mucocutaneous eruptions. Poisoning usually occurs in industrial workers. See also NITROGLYCERIN. **amyl n.,** a mixture of isomers containing C₅H₁₁NO₂; chiefly isoamyl nitrite, (CH₃)₂CHCH₂CH₂ONO. It is a flammable yellowish liquid, with a peculiar, ethereal, fruity odor, which is volatile at low temperature. It is inhaled as a vapor to relieve the symptoms of angina pectoris and in the treatment of cyanide poisoning. **isoamyl n.,** see *amyl n.*

nitritocobalamin (ni"tri-to"ko-bal'ah-min) a member of the vitamin B₁₂ group in which the cyanide group is replaced by a nitrite group. Called also *nitrocobalamin* and *vitamin B₁₂c*. See VITAMIN B₁₂.

nitro (ni'tro) a colloquial name for *nitroglycerin.*

nitro- a chemical prefix indicating presence of the group —NO₂ or

$$-N\overset{\displaystyle O}{\underset{\displaystyle O}{\big\Vert}}$$

Nitro-Bid trademark for *nitroglycerin.*

nitrocobalamin (ni"tro-ko-bal'ah-min) nitritocobalamin.

Nitrofural trademark for *nitrofurazone.*

nitrofurantoin (ni"tro-fu-ran'to-in) an antibacterial agent, N-(5-nitro-2-furfurylidene)-1-aminohydantoin, occurring as a yellow, odorless powder or crystals with a bitter aftertaste, which are soluble in water, alcohol, and dimethylformamide. It is effective against *Escherichia coli, Klebsiella, Proteus, Pseudomonas, Aerobacter, Staphylococcus, Streptococcus, Pneumococcus, Clostridium,* and *Bacillus subtilis.* Used chiefly in the treatment of urinary infections. Side effects include nausea, vomiting, diarrhea, impotency, hypersensitivity, headache, vertigo, malaise, nystagmus, and neurological complications. Trademarks: Furadantin, Furantoin, Orafuran.

nitrofurazone (ni"tro-fu'rah-zōn) a broad-spectrum antibacterial agent derived from furan, 5-nitro-2-furaldehyde semicarba-zone, occurring as a yellow, odorless, almost tasteless crystalline powder with a bitter aftertaste, which darkens on exposure to light, and is slightly soluble in water, alcohol, and propylene glycol, readily soluble in polyethylene glycol mixtures, and insoluble in chloroform and ether. Used topically in the treatment of infections of the skin and mucous membranes. Trademarks: Aldomycin, Chemofuran, Furacin, Furesol, Nitrofural, Vabrocid.

nitrogen (ni'tro-jen) [Gr. *nitron;* L. *nitrum* native soda + Gr. *gennan* to produce] a gaseous element. Symbol, N; atomic number, 7; atomic weight, 14.0067; specific gravity, 0.9673; valences, 1, 2, 3, 4, 5; group VA of the periodic table. ¹⁴N and ¹⁵N are the natural isotopes; artificial isotopes include five short-lived isotopes, 12, 13, and 16–18. It is an odorless, tasteless, diatomic gas constituting about four-fifths of common air. Chemically, nitrogen is almost inert, but forms by combination of nitric acid and ammonia. Nitrogen is a component of proteins — the average protein of the diet contains about 16 percent nitrogen. When metabolized, about 90 percent of the protein nitrogen is excreted in the urine in the form of urea, uric acid, creatinine, and other products. The total quantity of protein metabolized by the body is estimated by the amount of nitrogen excreted in the urine (see nitrogen BALANCE). Nitrogen is soluble in the blood and body fluids and when released as bubbles of gas by reduction of atmospheric pressure causes reduction of atmospheric pressure in divers and painful articular symptoms (see decompression SICKNESS). Although not a toxic substance, it is a simple asphyxiant. Called also *azote.* See also terms beginning AZO-. **n. balance,** nitrogen BALANCE. **n. cycle,** nitrogen CYCLE. **n. dioxide,** a poisonous substance, NO₂, occurring as a red to red-brown gas or yellow liquid. It is found in automotive exhaust fumes and is thus considered a major pollutant. Used in various industrial processes and as an oxidant in the production of oxidized cellulose. Inhalation, even of a short duration, may cause pneumonia, pulmonary edema, and death. **n. fixation,** nitrogen FIXATION. **n. mustard,** nitrogen MUSTARD.

nitroglycerin (ni-tro-glis'er-in) a low-molecular-weight organic nitrate, glyceryl trinitrate, occurring as a pale yellow, viscous liquid that is readily soluble in ether and alcohol and slightly soluble in water. It is highly explosive and sensitive to shock and heat, and it is used in the production of dynamite. Therapeutically, it is a general vasodilator used chiefly in angina pectoris and, as an ointment, in topical therapy of Raynaud's disease and trophic ulcers. Also used to dilate peripheral arteries in differentiating organic occlusion by palpation or angiography. Nitroglycerin is rapidly denitrated by the glutathione–organic nitrate reductase system of the liver. Headache is the most common complication of nitroglycerin therapy; dizziness, weakness, nausea, and hypotension may be associated. Alcohol exacerbates the severity of symptoms. Acute poisoning may include nausea, vomiting, abdominal cramps, headache, confusion, delirium, brachycardia, brachypnea, convulsions, methemoglobulinemia, shock, and death. Chronic exposure may produce headache, hallucinations, and mucocutaneous eruptions. Poisoning usually occurs in industrial workers. Called also *nitro, trinitroglycerin,* and *trinitroglycerol.* Trademarks: Nitro-Bid, Nitrol, Nitrostat.

Nitrol trademark for *nitroglycerin.*

nitromannite (ni'tro-man'īt) MANNITOL hexanitrate.

nitromersol (ni"tro-mer'sol) an organic mercurial antiseptic, 5-methyl-2-nitro-7-oxa-8-mercurabicyclo(4,2,0)octa-1,3,5,-triene, occurring as a yellow, odorless, tasteless powder or granules. Used as a disinfectant for instruments and as a topical antiseptic in the treatment of cutaneous and mucosal infections, including those of the oral cavity, such as acute necrotizing ulcerative gingivitis. Trademark: Metaphen.

nitron (ni'tron) the name suggested for the molecular weight of a radium emanation.

nitroso- a chemical prefix indicating the presence of the group —N:O.

nitrosourea (ni-tro"so-u-re'ah) a urea compound which is substituted with one or two nitroso groups. Some nitrosourea compounds, such as carmustine and streptozotocin, exhibit cytotoxic properties and are used as antineoplastic agents.

Nitrostat trademark for *nitroglycerin.*

nitrous (ni'trus) pertaining to a compound containing nitrogen in its lowest valency. See also nitrous ACID.

Nivelona trademark for *diphemanil methylsulfate* (see under DIPHEMANIL).

Nivemycin trademark for *neomycin*.

Nivitin trademark for *sorbitol*.

Nivocillin trademark for *doxycycline hyclate* (see under DOXY-CYCLINE).

NK Nomenklatur Kommission; a committee of the Anatomical Society of Germany which has given supplementary names to the terminology of anatomy.

nl nanoliter.

NLM National Library of Medicine.

NLN National League for Nursing.

nm nanometer.

N/m² a symbol for pressure exerted by 1 newton over an area of 1 m². See PASCAL. See also mechanical STRESS.

N × m a symbol for newton by meter; see JOULE.

NMA National Malaria Association; National Medical Association.

NMRI Naval Medical Research Institute.

NMSS National Multiple Sclerosis Society.

nn. abbreviation for L. *ner'vi*, nerves.

NND New and Nonofficial Drugs (see under DRUG).

No nobelium.

No. abbreviation for L. *nu'mero*, to the number of.

Noack's acrocephalosyndactyly [M. *Noack*] Pfeiffer's SYN-DROME.

Nobel, Alfred Bernard [1833–1896] a Swedish chemist and engineer; inventor of dynamite. Nobel established the Nobel prize whereby awards are usually given annually for outstanding achievements in chemistry, physics, medicine and physiology, literature, and in the interest of world peace. First presented in 1901. An award for achievement in economics has since been added.

nobelium (no-be'le-um) [named after A. B. *Nobel*] a synthetic radioactive element. Symbol, No; atomic number, 102; valences, 2, 3. Its longest-lived known isotope is ²⁵⁹No; because all nobelium isotopes are very short-lived its chemical properties have not yet been determined.

Nobil Ceram trademark for a nickel-chromium base-metal crown and bridge alloy, also containing some beryllium. Inhalation of dust during melting, milling, or grinding may cause beryllium poisoning.

Nobillium alloy see under ALLOY.

noble (no'b'l) in chemistry, pertaining to an element that does not combine with or reacts only to a limited extent with other elements, such as noble gases or noble metals.

Noble 1 trademark for a soft *dental casting gold alloy* (see under GOLD).

Noble 2 trademark for a medium hard *dental casting gold alloy* (see under GOLD).

Noble 3 trademark for a hard *dental casting gold alloy* (see under GOLD).

Noble 4, Noble 18, Noble 19 trademarks for an extra hard *dental casting gold alloy* (see under GOLD).

Nocard, Edmond Isidore Etienne [1850–1903] [French veterinarian, 1850–1903] Preisz-Nocard bacillus; see *Corynebacterium pseudotuberculosis*, under CORYNEBACTERIUM.

Nocardia (no-kar'de-ah) [named after E. I. E. *Nocard*] a genus of bacteria of the family Nocardiaceae, order Actinomycetales, separable into more than 40 species and three morphological groups according to the degree of mycelial development: extensive, limited, and very limited. Some species are pathogenic, several inhabit the oral cavity, and the remainder are saprophytic. Individual species may or may not be acid-fast, and all are aerobic, fragment into bacillary or coccoid forms, and produce chains of spores by simple fragmentation of hyphal branches. Called also *Proactinomyces*. **N. asteroi'des,** a species causing infection of the lungs in man, from where it spreads to other parts of the body. It also has been isolated from soil. Called also *Actinomyces asteroides, A. eppingeri, Cladothrix asteroides, Procactinomyces asteroides, Streptothrix asteroides,* and *S. eppingerii*. **N. brasilien'sis,** a species isolated from various human lesions and from soil, and causing pulmonary infection in man; it occurs most commonly in tropical zones. Called also *Actinomyces brasiliensis, Discomyces brasiliensis,* and *Streptothrix brasiliensis*. **N. dentocario'sus,** *Rothia dentocariosa;* see under ROTHIA. **N. intracellula'ris,** *Mycobacterium intracellulare;* see under MYCOBACTERIUM. **N. israe'li,** *Actinomyces israelii;* see under ACTINOMYCES. **N. lu'tea,** a species isolated from the lacrimal gland in actinomycosis. Called also *Actinomyces luteus*. **N. mu'ris rat'ti,** *Streptobacillus moniliformis;* see under STREPTOBACILLUS. **N. sali'vae,** *Rothia dentocariosa;* see under ROTHIA.

Nocardiaceae (no-kar''de-a'se-e) [*Nocardia* + *-aceae*] a family of gram-positive, acid-fast to partially acid-fast, nonmotile, obligate aerobic bacteria of the order Actinomycetales, and including the genus *Nocardia*.

nocardial (no-kar'de-al) pertaining to or caused by *Nocardia*.

nocardiasis (no''kar-di'ah-sis) nocardiosis.

nocardiosis (no-kar-de-o'sis) infection with microorganisms of the genus *Nocardia;* nocardiasis.

noci- [L. *nocere* to injure] a combining form denoting relation to injury or to a noxious or deleterious agent or influence.

nociceptor (no''se-sep'tor) a sensory receptor that detects damage in the tissues or pain, whether due to physical or chemical modalities. Also called *nociceptive receptor*.

nociperception (no''se-per-sep'shun) the perception of injurious stimuli.

Noct. abbreviation for L. *noc'te*, at night.

Noctan trademark for *methyprylon*.

Noctec trademark for *chloral hydrate* (see under CHLORAL).

Noctilene trademark for *methaqualone*.

node (nōd) [L. *nodus* knot] a swelling or protuberance. See also NODULE and NODUS. **auricular anterior n's,** auricular lymph n's, anterior. **auricular lymph n's, anterior,** one to three nodes anterior to the tragus, receiving the afferent vessels draining the lateral surface of the auricula and the scalp of the temporal region. Their efferent vessels drain into the superior deep cervical nodes. Called also *auricular anterior n's, preauricular lymph n's, superficial parotid lymph n's, extraparotid lymph glands, nodi lymphatici parotidei superficiales,* and *nodi lymphatici preauriculares*. **auricular lymph n's, posterior,** two small nodes on the insertion of the sternocleidomastoid muscle; receiving the afferent vessels draining the posterior part of the external acoustic meatus, the upper part of the cranial surface of the pinna, and the posterior part of the temporoparietal region. Their efferent vessels drain into the superior deep cervical nodes. Called also *auricular posterior n's, retroauricular lymph n's, lymphoglandulae auriculares posteriores,* and *nodi lymphatici retroauriculares* [NA]. **auricular posterior n's,** auricular lymph n's, posterior. **buccal lymph n's,** a variable number of lymph nodes lying on a line between the angle of the mandible and the angle of the mouth, receiving the afferent vessels draining the temporal and infratemporal fossae and the nasopharynx. Their efferent vessels drain into the superior deep cervical nodes. Called also *deep facial lymph n's, internal maxillary lymph n's, lymphoglandulae faciales profundae,* and *nodi lymphatici buccales* [NA]. **cervical n's,** cervical lymph n's. **cervical n., superficial lateral,** one of the cervical lymph nodes situated on the surface of the sternocleidomastoid muscle, near the parotid gland at the site where the external jugular vein emerges from the gland. Its afferent vessels drain the parotid region and the auricula. Called also *nodus lymphaticus cervicalis superficialis lateralis* [NA]. **cervical lymph n's,** nodes which receive the afferent vessels from the neck, including the submandibular, submental, superior cervical, anterior cervical, and deep cervical lymph nodes. Called also *cervical n's* and *lymph n's of neck*. See illustration. **cervical lymph n's, anterior,** a group of lymph nodes ventral to the larynx and trachea. They consist of superficial vessels on the anterior jugular vein, and deep vessels on the middle cricothyroid ligament as well as ventral to the trachea, which drain the lower larynx, thyroid gland, and cranial part of the trachea. Their efferent vessels from the anterior cervical lymph nodes drain into the superior deep cervical nodes. **cervical lymph n's, deep,** a group of numerous large lymph nodes that form a chain along the internal jugular vein, extending from the base of the skull to the root of the neck, lying near the pharynx, esophagus, and trachea, consisting of the *superior deep cervical nodes* and *inferior deep cervical nodes*. Called also *lymphoglandulae cervicales profundae* and *nodi lymphatici cervicales profundae* [NA]. **cervical lymph n's, inferior deep,** nodes extending beyond the posterior margin of the sternocleidomastoid muscle into the supraclavicular triangle, along the subclavian vein and the brachial plexus; they receive the afferent vessels draining the back of the scalp and neck, the superficial pectoral region, the arms, and sometimes, the liver. Their efferent vessels of the inferior and superior deep cervical lymph nodes unite to form the jugular trunk which joins the subclavian vein and the thoracic duct. **cervical lymph n's, superficial,** nodes along the external jugular vein as it emerges from the parotid gland, being superficial to the sternocleidomastoid muscle; they receive afferent vessels from the auricula and parotid region. Their efferent vessels drain into the superior deep cervical nodes. Called also *lymphoglandulae cervicales superficiales* and *nodi lymphatici cervicales superficiales* [NA]. **cervical lymph n's, superior deep,** nodes under the sternocleidomastoid muscle, along the internal jugular vein and the accessory nerve, which receive afferent vessels draining the occipital part of the scalp, auricula, back of the neck, and parts of the tongue, larynx, thyroid gland, trachea, nasopharynx, nasal cavity, palate, and esophagus. They also receive efferent vessels from various lymph nodes of the head and neck. Their efferent vessels of the inferior and superior deep cervical lymph nodes unite to form the jugular trunk, which joins the subclavian vein and the thoracic duct. **delphian n.,** a lymph node encased in the fascia in the midline, just anterior to the thyroid isthmus, so called because it is exposed first at surgery and, if diseased, is indicative of disease in the thyroid gland, but not of a specific disease process. **facial lymph n's,** a group of lymph nodes, including the mandibular, infraorbital, and maxillary nodes, which receive the afferent vessels draining the eyelids, conjunctiva, and skin and mucous membrane of the nose and cheeks. Their efferent vessels drain into the submandibular nodes. Called also *facial n's.* **facial lymph n's, deep,** buccal lymph n's. **facial n's,** facial lymph n's. **Hensen's n.,** a thickening at the cranial end of the primitive streak. Called also *primitive n., Hensen's knot,* and *primitive knot.* **infraorbital n's,** infraorbital lymph n's. **infraorbital lymph n's,** facial nodes which receive the afferent vessels from the infraorbital region, their efferent vessels draining into the submandibular nodes. Called also *infraorbital n's* and *maxillary lymph n's.* **jugulodigastric n.,** Küttner's GANGLION. **lingual lymph n's,** two or three small nodes on the lymphatic vessels of the tongue, situated on the hyoglossus and under the genioglossus muscles. Called also *lymphoglandulae linguales* and *nodi lymphatici linguales* [NA]. **lymph n.,** any of the small, oval or bean-shaped organs, ranging in size from 1 to 25 mm in diameter, which are situated intermittently along the course of lymphatic vessels and act as filters for substances carried with the lymph and are a site for the formation of lymphocytes. A node consists of an outer cortical and an inner medullary part made up of a reticular framework containing masses of densely packed lymphocytes in various stages of development. The lymph enters a node through the afferent lymphatic vessels and flows through the outer capsule into the subcapsular sinuses, from where it passes through the medullary sinuses and out through the hilus and into the efferent vessels. No particulate matter or large molecules can be absorbed from the lymphatic vessels into the blood vessels, hence all foreign substances, including bacteria, must pass through the lymph nodes where they are filtered out and phagocytized by the lymphocytes. Called also *ganglion lymphaticus, globate gland, lymphaden, lymph gland, lymphoglandula, lymphonodus,* and *nodus lymphaticus* [NA]. **lymph n's, preauricular,** auricular lymph n's, anterior. **lymph n's of head,** lymph nodes which receive the lymph from the lymphatic vessels of the head, including the occipital, posterior and anterior auricular, parotid, deep facial, lingual, and retropharyngeal lymph nodes. See illustration. **lymph n's of neck,** cervical lymph n's. **mandibular lymph n's,** the facial lymph nodes situated near the angle of the mandible on its outer

surface. Their afferent vessels drain the lymph from the eyelids, conjunctiva, and skin and mucosa of the nose and cheeks, and their efferent vessels drain into the submandibular nodes. Called also *nodi lymphatici mandibulares* [NA]. **maxillary lymph n's,** infraorbital lymph n's. **maxillary lymph n's, internal,** buccal lymph n's. **occipital lymph n's,** one to three small lymph nodes situated in the back of the head, near the occipital insertion of the semispinalis capitis muscle. Their afferent vessels drain the occipital region of the scalp, and their efferent vessels drain into the cervical nodes. Called also *lymphoglandulae occipitales* and *nodi lymphatici occipitales* [NA]. **paratracheal lymph n's,** a group of small inferior deep cervical nodes, situated alongside the recurrent nerve of the trachea and esophagus. **parotid lymph n's,** lymph nodes consisting of nodes embedded in the substance of the parotid gland and the subparotid nodes situated on the lateral wall of the pharynx. Their afferent vessels drain the root of the nose, eyelids, frontotemporal region, external acoustic meatus, tympanic cavity, posterior palate, and floor of the nasal cavity; their efferent vessels drain into the superior deep cervical nodes. The subparotid nodes receive afferent vessels from the nasal part of the pharynx and the posterior portion of the nasal cavities; their efferent vessels also drain into the superior deep cervical nodes. Called also *lymphoglandulae parotideae* and *nodi lymphatici parotidei.* **parotid lymph n's, deep,** subparotid lymph n's. **parotid lymph n's, superficial, preauricular lymph n's,** auricular lymph n's, anterior. **Parrot's n.,** Parrot's SIGN. **prelaryngeal n.,** a lymph node anterior to the larynx that helps drain the thyroid gland. **pretracheal n.,** a lymph node of the anterior cervical region that helps drain the thyroid gland. **primitive n.,** Hensen's n. **n. of Ranvier,** an interruption or notch in the myelin sheath of a peripheral nerve, found more or less regularly every 1 to 2 mm. See illustration at NERVE. **retroauricular lymph n's,** auricular lymph n's, posterior. **retropharyngeal lymph n's,** one to three nodes deep in the neck in the buccopharyngeal fascia, behind the upper part of the pharynx. Their afferent vessels drain the nose, nasal part of the pharynx, and auditory tubes; their efferent vessels drain into the deep cervical nodes. Called also *nodi lymphatici retropharyngei* [NA]. **Rosenmüller's n.,** palpebral part of lacrimal gland; see under PART. **Stahr's n.,** a submandibular lymph node situated on the facial artery as it turns over the mandible. Called also *Stahr's gland.* **subdigastric n's,** tonsillar lymph n's. **submandibular lymph n's,** three to six nodes in the submandibular triangle, under the mandible and on the surface of the submandibular gland. Their afferent vessels drain the facial and submental nodes and the cheeks, nose, upper lip, lateral portion of the lower lip, gingivae, and anterior portion of the tongue; their efferent vessels drain into the superior deep cervical nodes. Called also *lymphoglandulae submandibulares* and *nodi lymphatici submandibulares* [NA].

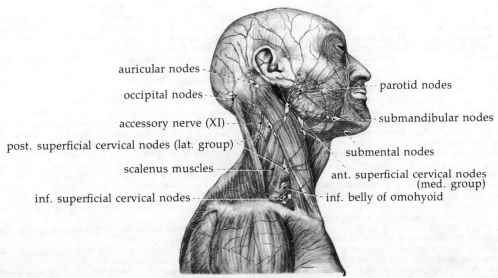

auricular nodes --

occipital nodes --

accessory nerve (XI) --

post. superficial cervical nodes (lat. group) -

scalenus muscles --

inf. superficial cervical nodes --

-- parotid nodes

-- submandibular nodes

-- submental nodes

-- ant. superficial cervical nodes (med. group)

-- inf. belly of omohyoid

Superficial lymph nodes of the head and neck. (From J. Langman and M. W. Woerdeman: Atlas of Medical Anatomy. Philadelphia, W. B. Saunders Co., 1978.)

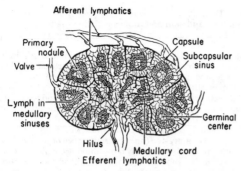

Afferent lymphatics

Primary nodule

Valve

Capsule

Subcapsular sinus

Lymph in medullary sinuses

Germinal center

Hilus

Medullary cord

Efferent lymphatics

Functional diagram of a lymph node. (From A. C. Guyton: Textbook of Medical Physiology. 6th ed. Philadelphia, W. B. Saunders Co., 1981; redrawn from Ham: Histology. J. B. Lippincott Co., 1971.)

submental lymph n's, cervical nodes situated between the anterior portions of the digastric muscle. Their afferent vessels drain the floor of the mouth, apex of the tongue, and central part of the lower lip; their efferent vessels drain into the submandibular and deep cervical nodes. Called also *suprahyoid lymph n's* and *nodi lymphatici submentales* [NA]. **subparotid lymph n's,** parotid lymph nodes situated on the lateral wall of the pharynx, at the inferior part of the parotid gland. Their afferent vessels drain the nasal part of the pharynx and the posterior part of the nasal cavity; their efferent vessels, together with other efferent vessels of the parotid nodes, drain into the superior deep cervical nodes. Called also *deep parotid lymph n's* and *subparotid lymph glands.* **suprahyoid lymph n's,** submental lymph n's. **tonsillar lymph n's,** a pair of superior deep cervical nodes lying just below the posterior belly of the digastric muscle, which usually become swollen and may be palpated in inflammation of the pharynx and tonsils. Called also *subdigastric n's.* **prelaryngeal n.,** a lymph node anterior to the larynx that helps drain the thyroid gland.

nodi (no'di) [L.] plural of *nodus.*

nodose (no'dōs) [L. *nodosus*] characterized by the presence of nodes or projections on the surface.

nodosity (no-dos'ĭ-te) [L. *nodositas*] 1. the quality of being nodose. 2. a node.

No-Doz trademark for a preparation of *caffeine.*

nodular (nod'u-lar) 1. having the appearance of a node. 2. marked with nodules.

nodulation (nod"u-la'shun) the presence or development of nodules.

nodule (nod'ul) [L. *nodulus* little knot] a small, circumscribed, solid, elevated lesion of the skin more than 5 mm in diameter, such as a pigmented nevus. **Bohn's n's,** inclusion cysts along the buccal and lingual aspects of the dental ridges and on the palate away from the raphe, found in newborn infants; considered to be remnants of mucous-gland tissue trapped during fetal development. Called also *Bohn's pearls.* **enamel n.,** enameloma. **lingual thyroid n.,** a nodule in or near the base of the tongue, near the foramen cecum, usually about 2 to 3 cm in diameter, containing a follicle of thyroid tissue, indicating incomplete descent of the thyroid gland during the embryonic development. **lymph n., lymphatic n.,** 1. lymph NODE. 2. one of the collections of lymphoid elements scattered in the submucous tissues of the respiratory tract, intestine, and genitourinary tract, being particularly well developed in structures such as tonsils, where they guard the entrances of the gastrointestinal and respiratory tracts, and in Peyer's patches in the gastrointestinal system. They are poorly developed in the fetus or in germ-free animals but develop rapidly following exposure to antigens. Phagocytic as well as lymphoid elements are found in the nodules, which are thus capable of reacting in specific and nonspecific immunity. The nodules synthesize IgA and IgE and, contiguous with external structures, elaborate a secretory form of antibody that is effective against pathogens in the external environment. Called also *nodulus lymphaticus* and *nodus lymphaticus* [NA]. **pulp n.,** denticle (2). **secondary n's,** germinal CENTER.

noduli (nod'u-li) [L.] plural of *nodulus.*

nodulous (nod'u-lus) nodose.

nodulus (nod'u-lus), pl. *nod'uli* [L., dim. of *nodus*] a small knot or node; used in anatomical nomenclature as a general term to designate a comparatively minute collection of tissue. See also NODE, NODULE, and NODUS. **n. lymphat'icus,** 1. lymph NODULE. 2. lymph FOLLICLE. **nod'uli lymphat'ici laryn'gei,** laryngeal lymphatic follicles; see under FOLLICLE.

nodus (no'dus), pl. *no'di* [L.] a knot, a node; used in anatomical nomenclature as a general term to designate a small mass of tissue. See also NODE, NODULE, and NODULUS. **n. jugulodigas'tricus,** Küttner's GANGLION. **n. lymphat'icus** [NA], lymph NODE. **no'di lymphat'ici bucca'les** [NA], buccal lymph nodes; see under NODE. **no'di lymphat'ici cervica'les profun'dae** [NA], cervical lymph nodes, deep; see under NODE. **no'di lymphat'ici cervica'les superficia'les** [NA], cervical lymph nodes, superficial; see under NODE. **n. lymphat'icus jugulodigas'tricus** [NA], Küttner's GANGLION. **n. lymphat'icus juguloomohyoi'deus** [NA], one of the deep cervical lymph nodes lying on the internal jugular vein just above the tendon of the omohyoid muscle. **no'di lymphat'ici lingua'les** [NA], lingual lymph nodes; see under NODE. **no'di lymphat'ici mandibula'res** [NA], mandibular lymph nodes; see under NODE. **no'di lymphat'ici occipita'les** [NA], occipital lymph nodes; see under NODE. **no'di lymphat'ici paroti'dei,** parotid lymph nodes; see under NODE. **no'di lymphatici paroti'dei superficia'les,** auricular lymph nodes, anterior; see under NODE. **no'di lymphat'ici preauricula'res,** auricular lymph nodes, anterior; see under NODE. **no'di lymphat'ici retroauricula'res,** auricular lymph nodes, posterior; see under NODE. **no'di lymphat'ici retropharyn'gei** [NA], retropharyngeal lymph nodes; see under NODE. **no'di lymphat'ici submandibula'res** [NA], submandibular lymph nodes; see under NODE. **no'di lymphat'ici submenta'les** [NA], submental lymph nodes; see under NODES.

no-fault (no'fawlt) see no-fault INSURANCE.

Noludar trademark for *methyprylon.*

noma (no'mah) [Gr. *nomē* spreading] a severe gangrenous disease of the oral and facial tissues, occurring essentially in children recovering from infectious diseases, but it has also been reported in debilitated adults, such as concentration camp inmates. An early symptom is a small vesicle or ulcer on the buccal or gingival mucosa, which rapidly becomes necrotic and spreads to the surrounding tissues of the jaws, lips, and cheeks, presenting a fetid, dark, gangrenous mass surrounded by indurated tissue with a waxlike shine; the tongue and palate sometimes may be involved. Pain, fever, and general malaise are associated. Complications may include toxemia and pneumonia. *Borrelia vincentii* and immune mechanisms have been suggested as possible, causative agents. Called also *cancrum oris, corrosive ulcer, gangrenous stomatitis,* and *stomatonecrosis.*

nomen (no'men), pl. *no'mina* [L.] name. **n. du'bium,** the name of an organism representing an unidentifiable taxon. **n. nu'dum,** the name of an organism without a definition, description, or indication of the taxon to which it is intended to apply.

nomenclature (no'men-kla"chur) [L. *nomen* name + *calare* to call] terminology; especially a classified system of names. **ADA Uniform Code on Dental Procedures and N.,** see under CODE. **Chicago n.,** see CHROMOSOME nomenclature. **chromosome n.,** CHROMOSOME nomenclature. **dental n.,** a system of terminologies in all branches of dentistry and related fields, as organized and classified by official professional bodies which were assigned to and given the authority to systematize dental terminology. Called also *dentonomy* and *odontonomy.* **Denver n.,** see CHROMOSOME nomenclature. **Landsteiner's n. of blood groups,** see under BLOOD GROUP. **Paris n.,** see CHROMOSOME nomenclature. **Wiener's n.,** see Rh blood groups, under BLOOD GROUP.

nomina (no'mi-nah) [L.] plural of *nomen.*

Nomina Anatomica (no'mi-nah an-ah-tom'ĭ-kah) [L. "anatomical names"] the official body of anatomical nomenclature, applied specifically to that revised by the International Anatomical Nomenclature Committee appointed by the Fifth International Congress of Anatomists held at Oxford in 1950, and approved by the Sixth, Seventh, Eighth, Ninth, and Tenth Congresses of Anatomists held in Paris, 1955, New York, 1960, Wiesbaden, 1965, Leningrad, 1970, and Tokyo, 1975. The abbreviation NA is used to identify official anatomical terms. See also *The Language of Medicine and Dentistry — An Introductory Note,* page xi.

nomo- [Gr. *nomos* law] a combining form denoting relationship to usage or law.

non- 1. [L. *non* not] a combining form meaning not. 2. [L. *nonus* ninth] a prefix meaning ninth.

nonadherent (non"ad-he'rent) not adherent to or connected with adjacent structures.

nonan (no'nan) [L. *nonus* ninth] recurring every ninth day, or at intervals of eight days.

nonane (no'năn) a nine-carbon straight chain hydrocarbon of the methane series, C_9H_{20}, occurring as a colorless, volatile liquid. Used in organic synthesis, in the production of biodegradable detergents, and in other chemical processes. Inhalation of fumes may cause narcosis.

nonapeptide (non″ah-pep'tīd) [non-(2) + peptide] a polypeptide containing nine amino acids.

nondisjunction (non″dis-junk'shun) failure of paired chromosomes or sister chromatids to disjoin at anaphase, either in a mitotic division or in the first or second meiotic division. See also CHROMOSOME aberration.

nonmetal (non-met'al) 1. a chemical substance which does not display the chemical and physical characteristics of a metal. A nonmetal consists of a group of electronegative elements that are generally polyvalent and exist in nature in various stages of oxidation, including halogens, phosphorus, sulfur, boron, carbon, silicon, oxygen, hydrogen, nitrogen, and the noble gases. Called also *nonmetallic element*. 2. any substance that is not a metal, e.g., a plastic, wax, or petroleum. 3. incorrectly, metalloid.

nonocclusion (non″o-kloo'zhun) open BITE.

nonpenetrant (non-pen'ĕ-trant) [non-(1) + L. penetrare to enter into] pertaining to a genotype which is not phenotypically expressed.

non rep., non repetat. abbreviation for L. non repeta'tur, do not repeat (placed on prescriptions that are not to be refilled).

nonunion (non-ūn'yun) failure of the ends of a fractured bone to unite; faulty union. See also MALUNION.

Noonan's syndrome [J. A. *Noonan*] see under SYNDROME.

noradrenaline (nor″ah-dren'ah-lin) norepinephrine. **n. acid tartrate**, LEVARTERENOL bitartrate.

Norbide trademark for *boron carbide* (see under BORON).

Nord appliance (plate) see under APPLIANCE.

nordefrin hydrochloride (nor-def'rin) a long-acting vasoconstrictor, dl-α-(1-aminoethyl)-3,4-dihydroxyphenyl) alcohol hydrochloride, occurring as a white crystalline solid that is soluble in water and alcohol, but not in water. Used chiefly in local anesthetic solutions, as a local nasal decongestant, and sometimes in the treatment of hypotension. Called also *homoarterenol hydrochloride* and *isoadrenaline hydrochloride*. Trademarks: Corbadrin, Corbasil, Cobefrin, Lirotil. See also LEVONORDEFRIN.

Nordicort trademark for *hydrocortisone sodium succinate* (see under HYDROCORTISONE).

Norephedrane trademark for *amphetamine*.

norepinephrine (nor″ep-ĭ-nef'rin) a catecholamine, 4-(2-amino-1-hydroxyethyl)-1,2-benzenediol. It is a chemical mediator liberated by postganglionic adrenergic nerves, having pharmacological and chemical properties similar to those of epinephrine. It differs from epinephrine in that it lacks the methyl substitution in the amino group. Of several isomers, the l-form (see LEVARTERENOL) is the most active; this form is used mainly in the form of its bitartrate salt. Pharmacologically, norepinephrine is a sympathomimetic and vasopressor agent that acts chiefly on the α-receptors; increases blood pressure and peripheral resistance of blood vessels, also reducing blood flow to the kidneys, brain, liver, and muscles; increases stroke volume of the heart; alters EEG; increases blood sugar; and increases the respiratory volume. Called also *arterenol* and *noradrenaline*.

norethandrolone (nor″eth-an'dro-lōn) a synthetic androgen with anabolic properties, 17-hydroxy-19-norpregn-4-en-3-one, occurring as a crystalline substance that is soluble in ethanol, benzene, ether,. and ethyl acetate, but not in water. Trademarks: Nilevar, Solevar.

norethindrone (nor-eth'in-drōn) a progestational hormone 17-hydroxy-19-nor-17α-pregn-4-en-20-yn-3-one, occurring as an odorless, white, crystalline powder that is soluble in chloroform and dioxane, slightly soluble in ether, and insoluble in water. Used in the treatment of various gynecological disorders and as a component of some oral contraceptives. Adverse reactions may include ulcerative stomatitis, nausea, vomiting, diarrhea, weight gain, fatigability, hirsutism, and skin pigmentation. Trademarks: Norluten, Primolut N.

Norfin trademark for *nalorphine*.

Norgan trademark for *hydrocodone bitartrate* (see under HYDROCODONE).

Norglycin trademark for *tolazamide*.

Norit trademark for *activated charcoal* (see under CHARCOAL).

Norluten trademark for *norethindrone*.

norm (norm) [L. norma rule] a standard; a fixed rule. **medical care n's**, numerical or statistical measures of a usual observed performance in the delivery of medical care, against which the quality of medical services is compared.

norma (nor'mah) [L.] 1. a norm; a standard. 2. an outline es-

tablished to define the aspects of the cranium. **n. ante'rior**, n. frontalis. **n. basila'ris**, the outline of the inferior aspect of the skull. Called also *n. inferior*. **n. facia'lis**, n. frontalis. **n. fronta'lis**, the outline of the skull viewed toward the face. Called also *n. anterior* and *n. facialis*. See illustration at SKULL. **n. infe'rior**, n. basilaris. **n. latera'lis**, the outline of the skull viewed from the side. Called also *n. temporalis*. See illustration at SKULL. **n. occipitalis**, n. poste'rior, the outline of the skull viewed from behind. **n. sagitta'lis**, the outline of a sagittal section through the skull. **n. supe'rior**, n. verticalis. **n. tempora'lis**, n. lateralis. **n. ventra'lis**, the outline of the inferior aspect of the skull. **n. vertica'lis**, the outline of the skull viewed from above. Called also *n. superior*.

normal (nor'mal) [L. norma rule] 1. agreeing with the regular and established type. 2. in chemistry, (a) denoting a solution containing in each 1000 ml 1 gm equivalent weight of the active substance; (b) denoting aliphatic hydrocarbons in which no carbon atom is combined with more than two other carbon atoms; (c) denoting salts formed from acids and bases in such a way that no acidic hydrogen of the acid remains nor any of the basic hydroxyl of the base. 3. in bacteriology, not immunized or otherwise bacteriologically treated.

normality (nor-mal'ĭ-te) 1. the state of being normal. 2. the number of gram-equivalent weights of solute per 1 liter (1000 ml) of solution. The equivalent in grams is that quantity of the active reagents which brings into reaction 1 gram of hydrogen. Designated N.

Normastigmin trademark for *neostigmine methyl sulfate* (see under NEOSTIGMINE).

Normet trademark for *clofibrate*.

normo- [L. norma rule] a combining form meaning conforming to the rule; normal or usual.

normoblast (nor'mo-blast) [normo- + Gr. blastos germ] an immature erythrocyte in its late stage of development, characterized by the presence of hemoglobin and a cell nucleus. **acidophilic n.**, orthochromatic n. **basophilic n.**, an early normoblast similar to a pronormoblast, except for the disappearance of the nucleoli and the basophilic characteristic of the cytoplasm, whose chromatin presents a granular coarse material and the nuclear material assumes a wheel-spoke arrangement. Called also *basophilic erythroblast*, *early erythroblast*, and *rubricyte*. **orthochromatic n.**, an immature erythrocyte following the polychromatic stage in erythropoiesis, characterized by its almost full complement of hemoglobin, in which the basophilic spongioplasm is not readily demonstrable and the nucleus undergoes pyknotic degeneration. Called also *acidophilic n*. **polychromatic n.**, an immature erythrocyte following the basophilic stage in erythropoiesis, characterized by the beginning of elaboration of hemoglobin, decreasing basophilia, disappearance of nucleoli, and decrease in the size of the nucleus. The cell may contain a few pink spots near the nucleus indicating the presence of hemoglobin. Called also *late erythroblast*, *polychromatic erythroblast*, and *polychromatocyte*.

normocyte (nor'mo-sīt) [normo- + Gr. kytos hollow vessel] an erythrocyte that is normal in size, shape, hemoglobin content, such as seen in normocytic anemia.

normocytic (nor″mo-sit'ik) pertaining to or of the nature of a normocyte.

Norodin trademark for *methamphetamine*.

Norpramin trademark for *desipramine hydrochloride* (see under DESIPRAMINE).

nostrum (nos'trum) [L. "our own"] a patent or quack remedy.

norsulfazole (nor-sul'fah-zōl) sulfathiazole.

19-nortestosterone (nor″tes-tos'tĕ-rōn) nandrolone.

Nothiazine trademark for *mepazine*.

Northrop, John Howard [born 1891] an American chemist; cowinner, with James Batcheller Sumner and Wendell Meredith Stanley, of the Nobel prize for chemistry in 1946, for pioneering work in crystallizing proteins.

Nortrilen trademark for *nortriptyline hydrochloride* (see under NORTRIPTYLINE).

nortriptyline hydrochloride (nor-trip'tĭ-lēn) an antidepressant agent, 3-(10,11-dihydro-5H-dibenzo[a,d]cyclohepten-5-ylidine)-N-methyl-1-propanamine hydrochloride, occurring as a white powder with a characteristic odor, which is soluble in water and chloroform, slightly soluble in methanol, and insoluble in ether, benzene, and other organic solvents. It interferes with the transport, release, and storage of catecholamines and acts as a histamine, serotonin, and acetylcholine inhibitor. Side effects may include xerostomia, drowsiness, confusion, tremor, seizures, orthostatic hypotension, tachycardia, and heart block. Excitement and agitation may also occur. Trademarks: Acetexa, Nortrilen, Norzepine, Sensival.

Norzepine trademark for *nortriptyline hydrochloride* (see under NORTRIPTYLINE).

nose (nōz) [L. *nasus*; Gr. *rhis*] the specialized structure of the face that serves as an organ of the sense of smell and as part of the respiratory apparatus by providing for the intake of air and by warming and filtering breathed air. Sometimes used to mean *external nose*. Called also *nasus* [NA]. See also nasal CAVITY, paranasal SINUSES, and terms beginning NASO- and RHINO-. **brandy n.,** ACNE rosacea. **external n.,** the part of the nose that protrudes on the face. It is made up of an osteocartilaginous framework, and is covered externally by muscles and skin, and lined internally by mucous membrane. Its most distal part is known as the *apex*. Two orifices below, which are separated from each other by a median septum, the *anterior nares*, serve for the intake of air. The stiff hairs in the nares, the *vibrissae*, arrest foreign subtances carried with inspired air. The union of the two lateral surfaces forms the *dorsum;* its upper part supported by the nasal bones known as the *bridge*. The flaring cartilaginous expansions forming the outer side of each nostril are known as the *alae nasi*. Called also *nasus externus* [NA] and *promontorium faciei*. **saddle n., saddle-back n., swayback n.,** a nose with a sunken bridge, such as seen in congenital syphilis.

noso- [Gr. *nosos* disease] a combining form denoting relationship to disease. See also words beginning PATHO-.

nosogenic (nos″o-jen′ik) pathogenic.

nosography (no-sog′rah-fe) [*noso-* + Gr. *graphein* to write] a written account or description of diseases.

nosology (no-sol′o-je) [*noso-* + *-logy*] the science of the classification of diseases.

nostril (nos′tril) one of the external orifices of the nose. Called also *naris*.

Notandron trademark for *methandriol*.

notatin (no′ta-tin) glucose OXIDASE.

notation (no-ta′shun) 1. a critical or explanatory note; annotation. 2. a set or system of marks or symbols to identify something. **Palmer n.,** a method in which lower case letters are used to identify teeth on a dental chart (1). See dental CHART.

notch (noch) an indentation or depression, especially one on the edge of a bone or other organ. See also INCISURA. **buccal n.,** the notch in the flange of a denture that accommodates the buccal frenum. **ethmoidal n. of frontal bone,** a space which separates the two orbital plates of the frontal bone, in which the cribriform plate of the ethmoid bone is lodged. Called also *ethmoidal incisure of frontal bone* and *incisura ethmoidalis ossis frontalis* [NA]. **frontal n.,** frontal INCISURE. **interarytenoid n.,** the posterior portion of the aditus laryngis between the two arytenoid cartilages. Called also *incisura interarytenoidea laryngis* [NA] and *interarytenoid incisure.* **interclavicular n. of occipital bone,** jugular n. of occipital bone. **interclavicular n. of temporal bone,** jugular n. of temporal bone. **jugular n. of occipital bone,** a notch on the anterior surface of the jugular process of the occipital bone, forming the posterior wall of the jugular foramen. It may be divided into two by a bony spicule, the intrajugular process. Called also *interclavicular n. of occipital bone* and *incisura jugularis ossis occipitalis* [NA]. **jugular n. of temporal bone,** a prominent depression on the inferior surface of the petrous part of the temporal bone, forming the anterior and lateral walls of the jugular foramen. It lodges the superior bulb of the internal jugular vein in its lateral part and the glossopharyngeal, vagus, and accessory nerves in its medial part. Called also *interclavicular n. of temporal bone, incisura jugularis ossis temporalis* [NA], and *jugular incisure of temporal bone.* **labial n.,** the notch in the labial flange of an upper or lower denture that accommodates the labial frenum. **lacrimal n. of maxilla,** an indentation on the posterior border of the frontal process of the maxilla that lodges the lacrimal sac. Called also *incisura lacrimalis maxillae* [NA] and *lacrimal incisure of maxilla.* **mandibular n.,** sigmoid n. of mandible. **mastoid n.,** a deep groove on the medial surface of the mastoid process of the temporal bone that gives attachment to the posterior belly of the digastric muscle. Called also *digastric fossa, digastric groove, digastric incisure of temporal bone, incisura mastoidea ossis temporalis* [NA], and *mastoid incisure of temporal bone.* **nasal n. of maxilla,** the large notch in the anterior border of the maxilla that forms the lateral and inferior margins of the anterior nasal aperture. Called also

incisura nasalis maxillae [NA] and *nasal incisure of maxilla.* **palatine n.,** pterygoid FISSURE. **palatine n. of palatine bone,** sphenopalatine n. of palatine bone. **parietal n. of temporal bone,** the notch found on the upper margin of the temporal bone where the squamous and parietomastoid sutures meet. Called also *incisura parietalis ossis temporalis* [NA], *parietal incisure of temporal bone,* and *parietosphenoid fissure.* **parotid n.,** the notch between the ramus of the mandible and the mastoid process of the temporal bone. **pterygoid n.,** pterygoid FISSURE. **rivinian n., Rivinus' n.,** tympanic n. **sigmoid n. of mandible,** a smooth, semicircular notch on the upper edge of the ramus of the mandible, forming a sharp upper border of the ramus between the condyle and the coronoid process. Called also *mandibular n., incisura mandibulae* [NA], *incisure of mandible, semilunar incisure of mandible,* and *sigmoid incisure of mandible.* **sphenopalatine n. of palatine bone,** an incisure situated on the posterior border of the palatine bone, between the orbital and sphenoidal processes; it is converted into the sphenopalatine foramen by the undersurface of the sphenoid bone. Called also *palatine n. of palatine bone, incisura sphenopalatina ossis palatini* [NA], *palatine incisure of Henle,* and *sphenopalatine incisure of palatine bone.* **supraorbital n.,** supraorbital INCISURE. **thyroid n., inferior,** a notch at the lower part of the anterior border of the thyroid cartilage. Called also *incisura thyroidea inferior* [NA] and *inferior thyroid incisure.* **thyroid n., superior,** a deep V-shaped notch which separates the laminae of the thyroid cartilage at their upper junction, just above the laryngeal prominence. Called also *incisura thyroidea superior* [NA] and *superior thyroid incisure.* **trigeminal n.,** a notch in the superior border of the petrosal portion of the temporal bone, near the apex, for transmission of the trigeminal nerve. **tympanic n.,** a defect in the upper portion of the tympanic part of the temporal bone, between the greater and lesser tympanic spines, which is filled in by the pars flaccida of the tympanic membrane. Called also *rivinian n., Rivinus' n., incisura Rivini, incisura tympanica* [NA], *rivinian foramen,* and *Rivinus' foramen.*

notifiable (no′tī-fī″ah-b'l) denoting that which should be made known; said of diseases that are required to be made known to a proper public health agency.

noto- [Gr. *nōton* back] a combining form denoting relationship to the back.

notochord (no′to-kord) [*noto-* + Gr. *chordē* cord] the rod-shaped cord made up of large cells with thick membranes and abundant cytoplasm, which derives from Hensen's node (*primitive knot*) and grows cranially between the ectoderm and entoderm during the third week of embryonic development, dividing the primitive axis of the body in the presomite embryo. The migrating notochord cells (*notochordal process*) move in the direction of the prochordal plate until reaching the blastopore, where the outpocketing of the blastopore in the process is followed by the formation of the notochordal canal which, in turn, provides temporary communication at the site of the primitive pit between the cavities of the yolk sac and amnion. The vertebral column and the caudal part of the base of the skull develop around the cells of the notochord. Called also *chorda dorsalis, head process,* and *notochordal plate.*

Notoral trademark for *penicillin G potassium* (see under PENICILLIN).

not-self (not′self) an expression used to denote antigenic constituents foreign to the organism; see SELF.

A4Novamidon trademark for *aminopyrine.*

Novamin trademark for *dimenhydrinate.*

Novasmasol trademark for *metaproterenol sulfate* (see under METAPROTERENOL).

Novatropine trademark for *homatropine methylbromide* (see under HOMATROPINE).

Novecyl trademark for *salicylamide.*

Novicodin trademark for *dihydrocodeine.*

novobiocin (no″vo-bi′o-sin) an antibiotic produced by cultures of *Streptomyces spheroides, S. niveus,* and other species, N-[7-[[3-O-(aminocarbonyl)-5,5-di-C-methyl-4,0-methyl-α-L-lyxopyranosyl]oxy]-4-hydroxy-8-methyl-2-oxo-2H-1-benzopyran-3-yl]-4-hydroxy-3-(3-methyl-2-butenyl)benzamide, occurring as a pale yellow crystalline substance that is soluble in acetone, ethyl acetate, amyl acetate, lower alcohols, pyridine, and alkaline aqueous solutions. It is active against grampositive bacteria, such as *Staphylococcus aureus,* being only moderately active against gram-negative bacteria. Strains of staphylococci develop resistance to novobiocin. Side effects may include leukopenia, anemia, pancytopenia, agranulocytosis, thrombocytopenia, nausea, vomiting, diarrhea, abdominal pain, intestinal hemorrhage, vertigo, drowsiness, arthritis, conjunctivitis, alopecia, pneumonia, jaundice, hyperbilirubinemia, and myocarditis. Called also *crystallinic acid.* Trademarks: Albamycin, Biotexin, Cardelmycin, Inamycin, Spheromycin, Vulcamycin. **n. calcium,** the calcium salt dihydrate of novobiocin, occurring as a white, odorless, crystalline powder that is soluble in water, ethanol, ether, and chloroform. It is a semisynthetic form of novobiocin, having pharmacological and toxicological properties similar to those of the parent compound. **n. sodium,** the monosodium salt of novobiocin, occurring as a white, hygroscopic, odorless, crystalline powder that is soluble in water, ethanol, glycerol, and propylene glycol. It is a semisynthetic form of novobiocin, having pharmacological and toxicological properties similar to those of the parent compound.

Novocain, Novocaine trademarks for *procaine hydrochloride* (see under PROCAINE).

Novocamid trademark for *procainamide hydrochloride* (see under PROCAINAMIDE).

Novocell trademark for *oxidized cellulose* (see under CELLULOSE).

Novocillin trademark for *penicillin G sodium* (see under PENICILLIN).

Novodox trademark for *doxycycline hyclate* (see under DOXYCYCLINE).

Novolaudon trademark for *hydromorphone.*

Novol-benzocaine solution see under SOLUTION.

Novomycetin trademark for *chloramphenicol.*

Novotrone trademark for *sulfoxone sodium* (see under SULFOXONE).

Novoxapin trademark for *doxepin hydrochloride* (see under *doxepin*).

Novy's bacillus [Frederick George *Novy,* American bacteriologist, 1864–1957] *Clostridium novyi;* see under CLOSTRIDIUM.

noxa (nok′sah), pl. *nox′ae* [L. "harm"] an injurious, harmful agent, act, or influence.

Noxaben trademark for *dicloxacillin sodium* (see under DICLOXACILLIN).

Noxal trademark for *disulfiram.*

noxious (nok′shus) [L. *noxius*] harmful; not wholesome.

NP new patient.

Np neptunium.

Ns nasospinale.

ns nanosecond.

NSD nominal single DOSE.

nsec nanosecond.

NSNA National Student Nurses' Association.

nsq not sufficient quantity.

NSS normal saline SOLUTION.

nU nanounit.

nucha (nu′kah) [L.] [NA] the nape, scruff, or back of the neck. See also CERVIX and NECK.

nuchal (nu′kal) pertaining to the nucha, or back of the neck.

Nuchar trademark for *activated charcoal* (see under CHARCOAL).

Nuck's glands [Anton *Nuck,* Dutch anatomist, 1650–1742] lingual glands, anterior; see under GLAND.

nuclear (nu′kle-ar) pertaining to a nucleus.

nucleated (nu′kle-āt″ed) [L. *nucleatus*] having a nucleus or nuclei.

nucleation (nu″kle-a′shun) the act or process of forming a nucleus. **heterogeneous n.,** in the process of crystallization, the formation of nuclei around atoms coming in contact with surfaces or particles in the melt which they can wet, whereby the surface energy is reduced and a nucleus formed. Heterogeneous nucleation can occur without supercooling of the liquid. See also solidification NUCLEUS. **homogenous n.,** in the process of crystallization, the formation of nuclei around clusters of atoms (embryos) which aggregate in a supercooled liquid, without the presence of foreign particles. See also solidification NUCLEUS.

nucleocapsid (nu″kle-o-kap′sid) in viral structure, a unit of the viral nucleic acid with its protective protein coat, the capsid.

nucleofugal (nu″kle-of′u-gal) [*nucleus* + L. *fugere* to flee] moving away from a nucleus.

nucleohistone (nu″kle-o-his′tōn) a nucleoprotein composed of a histone–DNA complex. According to some hypotheses, histones surround individual double-stranded DNA helices, form bridges between adjacent coils, and block some areas of the DNA molecule, thereby permitting only parts of the DNA base sequences to act as templates for the formation of messenger RNA and thus controlling protein biosynthesis.

nucleoid (nu′kle-oid) 1. resembling a nucleus. 2. a nucleus-like body sometimes seen in the center of an erythrocyte. 3. the nuclear region of a bacterium, which is not limited by a membrane. See BACTERIUM and prokaryotic CELL.

nucleolar (nu-kle′o-lar) pertaining to a nucleolus.

nucleoli (nu-kle′o-li) [L.] plural of *nucleolus.*

nucleoloid (nu′kle-o-loid) resembling a nucleolus.

nucleolonema (nu″kle-o″lo-ne′mah) [*nucleolus* + Gr. *nēma* thread] one of several coarse strands formed by a finely granular substance that surrounds the pars amorpha in the nucleolus. Called also *nucleoloneme.*

nucleoloneme (nu″kle-o′lo-nēm) nucleolonema.

nucleolus (nu-kle′o-lus), pl. *nucle′oli* [L., dim. of *nucleus*] a rounded, refractile, vacuole-like achromatin body placed eccentrically in the cell nucleus; most somatic cells contain from one to four nucleoli. Its size varies, being large in rapidly growing embryonic cells and in cells active in protein synthesis and smaller in other cells. It contains RNA and stains with basic dyes. It is composed of a dense central area, the pars amorpha, surrounded by coarse strands, the nucleolonema. In some instances, it is compacted into a dense homogeneous mass. Nucleoli are formed during mitosis and are associated with specific regions of chromosomes. Called also *micronucleus* and *plasmosome.* **chromatin n., false n., nucleinic n.,** karyosome.

nucleon (nu′kle-on) a constituent of an atomic nucleus; a proton or neutron.

nucleoplasm (nu′kle-o-plazm″) [*nucleus* + Gr. *plasma* something formed] the protoplasmic fluid or semifluid of the cell nucleus. It is a slightly chromophilic ground substance, which contains chiefly proteins, RNA, and enzymes, and which fills the space in the cell nucleus around the chromosomes, nucleoli, and granules. In its colloidal state, it is sometimes referred to as *karyolymph* and in its semifluid state as *karyoplasm* but, generally, the three terms are considered synonymous. See also CYTOPLASM.

nucleoprotamine (nu″kle-o-pro-tam′in) a complex of protamine and a nucleic acid.

nucleoprotein (nu″kle-o-pro′te-in) [*nucleic acid* + *protein*] a conjugated protein consisting of a complex of nucleic acids or polynucleotides and proteins, subdivided into *ribonucleoprotein* and *deoxyribonucleoprotein,* depending on whether the nucleic acid is primarily of the ribose (RNA) or deoxyribose (DNA) type, and *nucleohistone* or *nucleoprotamine.*

nucleoside (nu′kle-o-sīd″) a compound obtained during partial decomposition (hydrolysis) of nucleic acids, and consisting of a sugar and a nitrogenous base. It is formed when a purine or pyrimidine base is combined with β-D-ribose or β-2-deoxy-D-ribose. Specific nucleosides include adenosine, cytidine, guanosine, and uridine. See also NUCLEOTIDE.

nucleotide (nu′kle-o-tīd″) one of the building blocks of nucleic acids, formed by a phosphoric acid attached to a hydroxyl group of the pentose sugar in the nucleoside by an ester linkage. All nucleotides include D-ribose in their structure and are designated as acids because of the ionizable hydrogen of the phosphate group. Adenylic and uridylic acids and adenosine triphosphate are typical nucleotides. See also NUCLEOSIDE. **adenine n.,** adenylic ACID. **adenosine n.,** adenylic ACID. **diphosphopyridine n. (DPN),** nicotinamide-adenine DINUCLEOTIDE. **triphosphopyridine n. (TPN),** nicotinamide-adenine dinucleotide phosphate; see under DINUCLEOTIDE.

nucleotidyl (nu″kle-o-tīd′il) a nucleotide residue.

nucleotidyltransferase [E.C.2.7.7] (nu″kle-o-tīd″il-trans′fer-ās) a subclass of transferases, including enzymes that catalyze the transfer of a nucleotidyl residue from nucleoside phosphates to polymer forms. **DNA n.** [E.C.2.7.7.7], a transferase that transfers phosphorus-containing groups. It catalyzes the formation of DNA from deoxyribonucleoside triphosphates, with single-stranded DNA serving as a template. Called also *DNA polymerase.* **RNA n.** [E.C.2.7.7.6], a transferase that transfers phosphorus-containing groups. It catalyzes the formation of RNA from the four nucleoside triphosphates (which contain the bases adenine, guanine, cytosine, and uracil), with single-stranded DNA serving as a template. Called al *RNA polymerase.*

nucleus (nu′kle-us), pl. *nu′clei* [L., dim. of *nux* nut] 1. cell n. 2. [NA] a group of nerve cells located within the central nervous system and bearing a direct relationship to the fibers of a particular nerve. Called also *nidus.* 3. in organic chemistry, the combination of atoms forming the central element or basic framework of the molecule. **n. amyg′dalae,** amygdaloid BODY. **n. of atom, atomic n.,** the small, positively charged core of an atom. It is about $\frac{1}{10,000}$ the diameter of the atom, or about 10^{-13} cm, but contains nearly all the atom's mass. All nuclei contain both protons and neutrons, except the nucleus of ordinary hydrogen, which consists of a single proton. **caudate n., n. cauda′tum** [NA], an elongated, arched gray mass closely related to the lateral ventricle throughout its entire extent. The caudate nucleus and putamen form a functional unit of the corpus striatum. **cell n.,** a spheroid body within a cell bounded on the outside by the limiting or nuclear membrane which separates it from the cytoplasm. It contains DNA, RNA, proteins, and lipids. The DNA occurs in combined form with histones and other proteins to form chromatin, which is present in interchangeable states of condensation and dispersion. In dividing cells chromatin becomes condensed into elongated structures, the chromosomes, which are present in cells of all species. In cells not in division, chromatin forms irregular clumps known as chromatin particles or karyosomes. Also contained in the nucleus are round, refractile achromatin bodies (nucleoli) placed eccentrically. Cell nuclei divide by mitosis or meiosis, the latter resulting in the production of gametes or meiospores. **crystal n.,** n. of crystallization, solidification n. **cyclopentane n.,** cyclopentane RING. **cyclopenta-perhydrophenanthrene n.,** cyclopenta-perhydrophenanthrene RING. **n. descenden′tis ner′vi trigem′ini,** n. of mesencephalic tract of trigeminal nerve. **heterocyclic n.,** the basic ring structure of a heterocyclic compound (see under COMPOUND). **lenticular n.,** lentiform n. **lentiform n., n. lentifor′mis** [NA], the part of the corpus striatum comprising the putamen and globus pallidus; it lies just lateral to the internal capsule. Called also *lenticular n.* **masticatory n., n. masticato′rius,** motor n. of trigeminal nerve. **n. of mesencephalic tract of trigeminal nerve,** strands of cells in the lateral part of the central gray matter of the rostral part of the fourth ventricle in the mesencephalon. It is the only central nervous system site of primary sensory neurons, its cells resembling dorsal root ganglion cells. The peripheral processes of its cells, which form the mesencephalic tract, carry proprioceptive impulses; the central processes have widespread cerebellar and brain stem connections, including the motor nucleus of the trigeminal nerve. Called also *nucleus descendentis nervi trigemini* and *nucleus tractus mesencephalicus nervi trigemini* [NA]. **motor n. of trigeminal nerve, n. moto′rius ner′vi trigem′ini** [NA], the nucleus of origin of the motor fibers of the trigeminal nerve which innervate the muscles of mastication and the tensor tympani and tensor veli palatini muscles. It is located in the dorsolateral part of the pons, just medial to the main sensory nucleus and the entering sensory root. Called also *masticatory n.* and *n. masticatorius.* **n. ner′vi oculomoto′rii** [NA], n. of oculomotor nerve. **n. ner′vi trochlea′ris** [NA], n. of trochlear nerve. **nu′clei ner′vi trigem′ini** [NA], nuclei of trigeminal nerve. **n. of oculomotor nerve,** the origin of fibers of the oculomotor nerve, situated in the tegmentum of the midbrain immediately ventral to the central gray matter. Called also *n. nervi oculomotorii* [NA]. **perhydrocyclopentanophenanthrene n.,** cyclopentaperhydrophenanthrene RING. **phenanthrene n.,** phenanthrene RING. **poisoning of nuclei,** POISONING of nuclei. **principal sensory n. of trigeminal nerve,** the nucleus of termination of afferent fibers of the trigeminal nerve, carrying impulses for sensation, touch, and pressure, located in the dorsolateral part of the middle of the pons, just lateral to the entering trigeminal root fibers. Called also *n. sensorius principalis nervi trigemini* [NA], *n. sensorius superior nervi trigemini,* and *superior sensory n. of trigeminal nerve.* **n. senso′rius infe′rior ner′vi trigem′ini,** n. of spinal tract of trigeminal nerve. **n. senso′rius principa′lis ner′vi trigem′ini** [NA], n. senso′rius supe′rior ner′vi trigem′ini, principal sensory n. of trigeminal nerve. **sensory n.,** the nucleus of termination of the afferent (sensory) fibers of a peripheral nerve. **solidification n.,** in the process of crystallization, a nucleus that develops in a supercooled liquid from a cluster of atoms (embryo) that has reached the critical radius, the volume-free energy balancing the surface-free energy, and, in turn, gives rise to dendrites. It is the first element of a developing crystal having the space lattice. Called also *crystal n.* and *n. of crystallization.* See also heterogeneous and homogeneous NUCLEATION. **spinal n. of trigeminal nerve,** n. of spinal tract of trigeminal nerve. **n. of spinal tract of trigeminal nerve,** a column of cells which lies along the medial aspect of the spinal tract, extending from the level of entry of the trigeminal nerve in the pons to the second cervical segment of the spinal cord, where it is continuous with the posterior gray column. It has several cytoarchitectonic subdivisions and the fibers of the spinal tract end in it. Called also *spinal n. of trigeminal nerve, n. sensorius inferior nervi trigemini,* and *n. tractus spinalis nervi trigemini* [NA]. **sterol n.,** cyclopentaperhydrophenanthrene RING. **superior sensory n. of trigeminal**

nerve, principal sensory n. of trigeminal nerve. **n. trac′tus mesencephal′icus ner′vi trigem′ini** [NA], n. of mesencephalic tract of trigeminal nerve. **n. trac′tus spina′lis ner′vi trigem′ini** [NA], n. of spinal tract of trigeminal nerve. **nuclei of trigeminal nerve,** the nuclear complex of the trigeminal nerve, located chiefly in the pons and medulla oblongata, but also in the mesencephalon and upper cervical cord. See motor n. of trigeminal nerve, n. of mesencephalic tract of trigeminal nerve, principal sensory n. of trigeminal nerve, and n. of spinal tract of trigeminal nerve. Called also nuclei nervi trigemini [NA]. **n. of trochlear nerve,** a group of cells in the ventral part of the gray matter on the dorsal surface of the medial longitudinal fasciculus in the lower part of the midbrain. Called also nucleus nervi trochlearis [NA].

nuclide (nu′klĭd) a general term applicable to all atomic forms of the elements, comprising all their isotopic forms. The nuclear constitution of a nuclide is specified by the number of protons, Z; number of neutrons, N; and energy content. Or by the atomic number, Z; mass number A (= N + Z) and atomic mass. The term is often used erroneously as a synonym for *isotope;* isotopes are the various forms of a single element and all have the same atomic number and number of protons, whereas nuclides comprise all the isotopic forms of all the elements. **radioactive n.,** radionuclide.

Nufluor chewable tablets, gel see under TABLET and GEL.

NUG necrotizing ulcerative gingivitis; see acute necrotizing GINGIVITIS.

Nuhn's glands [Anton *Nuhn,* German anatomist, 1814–1880] lingual glands, anterior; see under GLAND. See also Blandin-Nuhn CYST.

nullipara (nŭ-lip′ah-rah) [L. *nullus* none + *parere* to bring forth, to bear] a woman who has never borne a viable child; also written *para 0.*

number (num′ber) a symbol, as a figure or word, expressive of a certain value or of a specified quantity determined by count. **acid n.,** the number of milligrams of potassium hydroxide necessary to neutralize the free fatty acids in 1 gram of fat, it represents a measure of the amount of free fatty acids in the fat. **ADA procedure n's,** see *ADA Uniform Code on Dental Procedures and Nomenclature;* see under CODE. **atomic n.,** the number of protons in the nucleus; the electrical charge of these protons determining the number and arrangement of the outer electrons of the atom, thereby establishing the chemical and physical properties of the element. Abbreviated *at no.* Symbol Z. See also ELEMENT (2). **Avogadro's n.,** the number of particles, real or imaginary, of the type specified by the chemical formula of certain substances in 1 mole of the substance; the value currently assigned to the number is 6.023×10^{23}. Called also *Avogadro's constant.* **azimuthal quantum n.,** quantum n., azimuthal. **Brinell n., Brinell hardness n.,** see under HARDNESS. **coordination n.,** the number of ligands in the primary coordination sphere; the valence number of the central atom of addition compounds indicating the number of molecules or atoms linked to that atom. **diploid chromosome n.,** see DIPLOID. **E.C. n.,** see ENZYME classification. **group n.,** in insurance, the master contract policy number which identifies a specific health insurance plan. **hardness n.,** HARDNESS number. **IMP n.,** a nine digit identification number provided by Medicaid in some states for the individual Medicaid practitioner. **Knoop n., Knoop hardness n.,** see under HARDNESS. **magnetic quantum n.,** quantum n., magnetic. **mass n.,** the whole number nearest to the atomic weight of an element or isotope, being the number of nucleons (protons and neutrons) in the nucleus of an atom. Symbol A. **Mohs n., Mohs hardness n.,** see under HARDNESS. **oxidation n.,** the numerical charge of the ions of an element. **polar n.,** the number of valences (positive or negative) possessed by an atom in a compound. Called also *valence n.* **principal quantum n.,** quantum n., principal. **quantum n.,** 1. the number which indicates the energy level of the electron orbit or the number of quanta. See also Bohr ATOM and orbital THEORY. 2. quantum n., principal. **quantum n., azimuthal,** that which is relative to the shapes of the orbitals, being given the principal quantum numbers −1 (0, 1, 2, 3, etc.). Orbitals with values of 0, 1, 2, and 3 are commonly referred as s, p, d, and f orbitals. Symbol *l.* **quantum n., magnetic,** that which is related to the orientation of a given orbital in the magnetic field, being given values of 2l + m for each azimuthal quantum number. Symbol *m.* **quantum n., principal,** the number which corresponds to the energy level of electrons in an atom and their relative position in relation to the nucleus. Quantum number 1 is assigned to the electron having the lowest energy level which is located in the orbit closest to the nucleus (K orbit) and each following orbit is assigned the consecutive number. Symbol *n.* See also electron ORBIT. **quantum n., spin,** the quantum number related to the spin of the electron in an atom, having values of $+\frac{1}{2}$ and $-\frac{1}{2}$ for each magnetic quantum number (m) value. Each orbital can contain two electrons with opposing spins, where the spin quantum number values must have the opposite. Symbol m_s. **Rockwell n., Rockwell hardness n.**, see under HARDNESS. **scleroscope n.**, a number indicative of the hardness of tested material, determined by the scleroscope test (see under TEST). **spin quantum n.**, quantum n., spin. **valence n.**, polar n. **Vickers n., Vickers hardness n.**, see under HARDNESS.

numbness (num′nes) lack of the sense of touch.

nummiform (num′ĭ-form) [L. *nummus* coin + *forma* form] shaped like a small coin.

nummular (num′u-lar) [L. *nummularis*] 1. of the size or shape of a coin. 2. made up of coinlike disks. 3. piled like coins, in a rouleau.

Numorphan trademark for *oxymorphone hydrochloride* (see under OXYMORPHONE).

Nupercaine trademark for *dibucaine hydrochloride* (see under DIBUCAINE).

Nuran trademark for *cyproheptadine hydrochloride* (see under CYPROHEPTADINE).

nurse (ners) 1. a person who is especially prepared in the scientific basis of nursing and who meets certain prescribed standards of education and clinical competence. 2. to provide services that are essential to or helpful in the promotion, maintenance, and restoration of health and well-being. See also NURSING. **n. anesthetist,** a clinical nurse specialist with special training in anesthesiology, who assists the anesthesiologist and administers anesthesia under his supervision. **charge n.,** one who is in charge of a patient care unit of a hospital or other health care institution. Called also *head n.* **circulating n.,** an operating room nurse whose responsibility includes preparation and keeping in readiness and obtaining equipment, materials, and instruments needed for the surgical procedure, without directly assisting the surgeon. See also *scrub n.* **n. clinician,** a registered nurse, referred to as a *nurse clinician* or as a *nurse practitioner*, who has well-developed competencies in utilizing a broad range of cues. These cues are used for prescribing and implementing both direct and indirect nursing care and for articulating nursing therapies with other planned therapies. Nurse clinicians demonstrate expertise in nursing practice and insure ongoing development of expertise through clinical experience and continuing education. Generally minimal preparation for this role is the baccalaureate degree. See also *occupational health n. clinician* and *occupational health n. coordinator.* **clinical n. specialist,** a registered nurse with a high degree of knowledge, skill, and competence in a specialized area of nursing. These skills are made directly available through the provision of nursing care to clients and indirectly available through guidance and planning of care with other nursing personnel. Clinical nurse specialists hold a master's degree in nursing, preferably with an emphasis in clinical nursing. Called also *n. specialist.* **community health n.,** public health n. **dental n.,** 1. a dental auxiliary trained to provide dental care for school children. Called also *New Zealand dental nurse* because the program originated in New Zealand. 2. formerly, dental HYGIENIST. **general duty n.,** a registered nurse who sees to the general nursing care of patients in a hospital or other health care institution. **graduate n.,** a graduate of a school of nursing, often used to designate one who has not been registered or licensed to practice. Formerly called *trained n.* **head n.,** charge n. **hospital n.,** one employed by a hospital. **industrial n.,** occupational health n. **licensed practical n.,** a graduate of a school of practical nursing whose qualifications have been examined by a state board of nursing and who has been legally authorized to practice as a licensed practical or vocational nurse (LPN or LVN), under the supervision of a physician or a registered nurse. **licensed vocational n.,** see *licensed practical n.* **New Zealand dental n.,** dental n. (1). **occupational health n.,** a registered nurse employed by business, industry, or an organization for the purpose of conserving, protecting, or restoring the health of workers; prevention of disease and injury of employed workers at and through their place of employment; making first-level diagnoses; and assessment of physical and emotional needs. In addition, this nurse provides total patient care in conjunction with the physician. Called also *industrial n.* **occupational health n. clinician,** a nurse clinician who performs all the functions of the occupational health nurse. This nurse has also had specialized preparation through education in a clinical area and is expected to demonstrate a high degree of skill in the application of basic knowlege in both physical and behavioral sciences, i.e., physical examination, mental health counseling, etc. **occupational health n. consultant,** an occupational health nurse who is responsible for in-plant health services, for occu-

pational health needs of workers, and who is involved in human relations activities. The nurse consultant plans, develops, and implements educational and other activities for other occupational health nurses, acts in an advisory capacity to employers, management, labor, and other interested bodies, and works with community agencies and professional organizations in occupational health programs. **occupational health n. coordinator,** an occupational health nurse clinician who develops, implements, evaluates, supervises, and coordinates the delivery of health care services to employees. **office n.,** a registered nurse employed in a physician's office to assist in health care delivery. **operating room n.,** a clinical nurse specialist with special training in surgery, who assists the surgeon in the operating room. See also *circulating n.* and *scrub n.* **pediatric n.,** a clinical nurse specialist with special training in pediatrics, who delivers nursing care to sick and/or well children. **practical n.,** a person who has had practical experience in nursing care but who is not a graduate of any kind of nursing school; not to be confused with a *licensed practical nurse.* **n. practitioner,** see *n. clinician.* **private n., private duty n.,** one who attends an individual patient, usually on a fee-for-service basis, and who may specialize in a special class of diseases. Called also *special n.* **psychiatric n.,** a clinical nurse specialist with special training in psychiatry, who cares for mentally ill patients. **public health n.,** an especially prepared registered nurse employed in a community agency to safeguard the health of persons in the community, giving care to the sick in their homes, promoting health and well-being by teaching families how to keep well, and assisting in programs for the prevention of disease. Called also *community health n.* See also *visiting n.* **registered n.,** a graduate nurse who has been legally authorized (registered) to practice after examination by a state board of nurse examiners or similar governmental agency, and who is legally entitled to use the designation RN. **school n.,** an especially prepared registered nurse employed in a school system or public health agency to assist in safeguarding the health of students and to teach health practices. **scrub n.,** an operating room nurse who assists other members of the operating team and works directly with the surgeon at the side of the patient, and whose duties consist of providing and arranging the sterile instruments, drapes, and supplies necessary for the operation and handing them to the surgeon as needed. See also *circulating n.* **special n.,** 1. private n. 2. a nurse who specializes in a particular class of cases. **n. specialist,** a clinical n. specialist. **student n.,** former name for NURSING student. **trained n.,** former name for *graduate n.* **visiting n.,** an especially prepared registered nurse employed by a private or nongovernmental institution to safeguard the health of persons in an organization or a preselected group, giving care to the sick in their homes, promoting health and well-being, and teaching families how to keep well, and assisting in programs for the prevention of diseases. See also *public health n.*

nursing (ners′ing) the provision of services that are essential to or helpful in the promotion, maintenance, and restoration of health and well-being or in the prevention of illness, as of infants, of the sick and injured, or of others for any reason unable to provide such services for themselves. Specific types of nursing functions are sometimes designated according to the age of the patients being cared for (e.g., pediatric or geriatric nursing), or their particular health problems (e.g., gynecologic, medical, obstetrical, orthopedic, psychiatric, surgical, or urological nursing, or the like), or the setting in which the services are provided (e.g., office, school, community health, or occupational health nursing). See also NURSE. **n. facility,** nursing FACILITY. **n. home,** nursing HOME. **n. student,** a person enrolled in a basic program of nursing education. Formerly called *student nurse.*

nut (nut) [L. *nux*; Gr. *karyon*] a seed element, as of various trees, usually enclosed in a coating of variable hardness.

nutgall (nut′gawl) an excrescence growing on oak trees, produced by insect eggs and larvae embedded in the plant tissues. It is a source of gallic and tannic acids. Called also *gall.*

nutmeg (nut′meg) myristica.

nutrient (nu′tre-ent) [L. *nutriens*] 1. a substance or ingredient that affects nutritive or metabolic processes of the body. 2. pertaining to or providing nutrition; feeding; nourishing.

nutrition (nu-trish′un) [L. *nutritio*] 1. the sum of the processes involved in taking in nutriments and their assimilation and utilization, including physiological processes dealing with ingestion, digestion, absorption, transport, and utilization of nu-

FOOD AND NUTRITION BOARD, NATIONAL ACADEMY OF SCIENCES — NATIONAL RESEARCH COUNCIL
RECOMMENDED DAILY DIETARY ALLOWANCES[a], REVISED 1980
Designed for the maintenance of good nutrition of practically all healthy people in the U.S.A.

	Age (years)	Weight (kg)	Weight (lb)	Height (cm)	Height (in)	Protein (g)	Vitamin A (μg RE)[b]	Vitamin D (μg)[c]	Vitamin E (mg α-TE)[d]
Infants	0.0–0.5	6	13	60	24	kg × 2.2	420	10	3
	0.5–1.0	9	20	71	28	kg × 2.0	400	10	4
Children	1–3	13	29	90	35	23	400	10	5
	4–6	20	44	112	44	30	500	10	6
	7–10	28	62	132	52	34	700	10	7
Males	11–14	45	99	157	62	45	1000	10	8
	15–18	66	145	176	69	56	1000	10	10
	19–22	70	154	177	70	56	1000	7.5	10
	23–50	70	154	178	70	56	1000	5	10
	51+	70	154	178	70	56	1000	5	10
Females	11–14	46	101	157	62	46	800	10	8
	15–18	55	120	163	64	46	800	10	8
	19–22	55	120	163	64	44	800	7.5	8
	23–50	55	120	163	64	44	800	5	8
	51+	55	120	163	64	44	800	5	8
Pregnant						+30	+200	+5	+2
Lactating						+20	+400	+5	+3

[a]The allowances are intended to provide for individual variations among most normal persons as they live in the United States under usual environmental stresses. Diets should be based on a variety of common foods in order to provide other nutrients for which human requirements have been less well defined. See individual entries for detailed discussion of allowances and of nutrients not tabulated.

[b]Retinol equivalents. 1 retinol equivalent = 1 μg retinol or 6 μg β carotene.

[c]As cholecalciferol. 10 μg cholecalciferol = 200 IU of vitamin D.

[d]α-tocopherol equivalents. 1 mg d-α tocopherol = α-TE.

[e]1 NE (niacin equivalent) is equal to 1 mg of niacin or 60 mg of dietary tryptophan.

trients and excretion of waste products. See also DIET and MALNUTRITION. See table. 2. nutriment. **parenteral n.,** parenteral FEEDING. **total parenteral n. (TPN),** parenteral HYPERALIMENTATION.

Nuva-Lite trademark for a bisphenol A glycidyl methacrylate pit and fissure sealant polymerized by ultraviolet light.

Nuva-Seal trademark for *bisphenol A glycidyl methacrylate* (see under METHACRYLATE).

Nuva-System tooth conditioner see under CONDITIONER.

nux (nuks) [L.] nut. **n. moscha′ta,** myristica.

Nyazid trademark for *nialamide.*

nycto- [Gr. *nyx* night] a combining form denoting relationship to night.

nyctohemeral (nik″to-hem′er-al) [nycto- + Gr. *hēmera* day] pertaining to phenomena regularly recurring during the night and day. See under RHYTHM.

nycturia (nik-tu′re-ah) [nycto- + Gr. *ouron* urine + -ia] abnormally frequent urination during the night.

NYD not yet diagnosed.

Nydrazid trademark for *isoniazid.*

Nygaard-Otsby frame see under FRAME.

Nyhan, William L., Jr. [American physician, born 1926] see Lesch-Nyhan SYNDROME and Sakati-Nyhan-Tisdale SYNDROME.

nylidrin hydrochloride (nil′ĭ-drin) a sympathomimetic amine, 4-hydroxy-α-[1-[(1-methyl-3-phenylpropyl)amino]ethyl]benzenemethanol hydrochloride, occurring as a white, tasteless, odorless, crystalline powder that is soluble in water and ethanol and slightly soluble in ether and chloroform. It decreases blood pressure in hypertensive subjects, but increases pressure in hypotensive patients, having little effect in normotensive persons. It has also vasodilator effects, particularly on the skeletal muscles. Used chiefly in the treatment of vasospastic diseases of extremities. Side effects include nervousness and cardiac ar-

rhythmias. Trademarks: Arlidin, Befedon, Dilatal, Opino, Rydrin.

nylon (ni′lon) a plastic fiber in which fiber-forming substances are long-chain synthetic polyamide having recurring polyamide groups (−CONH−) as an integral part of the polymer chain. It can be extruded when molten into fibers, sheets, or objects of various shapes, toughness, strength, and electricity, which are resistant to moisture and microbial degradation. Used in the production of synthetic fibers for various textile and domestic purposes, and as nonabsorbable suture material in surgical procedures.

Nyssen, René see metachromatic LEUKODYSTROPHY (von Bogaert-Nyssen-Peiffer syndrome).

nystagmus (nis-tag′mus) [Gr. *nystagmos* drowsiness, from *nystazein* to nod] an involuntary rapid movement of the eyeball. **palatal n.,** palatal MYOCLONUS.

Nystan trademark for *nystatin.*

nystatin (nis′tah-tin) an antifungal macrolide antibiotic, $C_{47}H_{75}NO_{17}$, elaborated by *Streptomyces noursei, S. aureus,* and other species, occurring as a yellow to light tan, hygroscopic powder with a cereal-like odor, which is affected by exposure to light, air, and humidity, is slightly soluble in water, ethyl alcohol, methyl alcohol, *n*-propyl alcohol, and *n*-butyl alcohol, and is insoluble in organic solvents. It causes potassium leakage through the cell membrane, being effective against several types of yeasts and molds, but is used mostly in the treatment of candidiasis. Occasionally, it may cause nausea, vomiting, and diarrhea. Also applied topically to the tissue surface prior to denture insertion. Trademarks: Candio-Hermal, Diastatin, Fungicidin, Moronal, Mycostatin, Nystavescent.

Nystavescent trademark for *nystatin.*

Nysten's law [Pierre Hubert *Nysten,* French pediatrician, 1771–1818] see under LAW.

nystigmin (ni-stig′min) neostigmine.

FOOD AND NUTRITION BOARD, NATIONAL ACADEMY OF SCIENCES — NATIONAL RESEARCH COUNCIL
RECOMMENDED DAILY DIETARY ALLOWANCES, REVISED 1980 *(Continued)*
Designed for the maintenance of good nutrition of practically all healthy people in the U.S.A.

Water-Soluble Vitamins							Minerals					
Vitamin C (mg)	Thiamin (mg)	Riboflavin (mg)	Niacin (mg NE)[e]	Vitamin B-6 (mg)	Folacin[f] (μg)	Vitamin B-12 (μg)	Calcium (mg)	Phosphorus (mg)	Magnesium (mg)	Iron (mg)	Zinc (mg)	Iodine (μg)
35	0.3	0.4	6	0.3	30	0.5[g]	360	240	50	10	3	40
35	0.5	0.6	8	0.6	45	1.5	540	360	70	15	5	50
45	0.7	0.8	9	0.9	100	2.0	800	800	150	15	10	70
45	0.9	1.0	11	1.3	200	2.5	800	800	200	10	10	90
45	1.2	1.4	16	1.6	300	3.0	800	800	250	10	10	120
50	1.4	1.6	18	1.8	400	3.0	1200	1200	350	18	15	150
60	1.4	1.7	18	2.0	400	3.0	1200	1200	400	18	15	150
60	1.5	1.7	19	2.2	400	3.0	800	800	350	10	15	150
60	1.4	1.6	18	2.2	400	3.0	800	800	350	10	15	150
60	1.2	1.4	16	2.2	400	3.0	800	800	350	10	15	150
50	1.1	1.3	15	1.8	400	3.0	1200	1200	300	18	15	150
60	1.1	1.3	14	2.0	400	3.0	1200	1200	300	18	15	150
60	1.1	1.3	14	2.0	400	3.0	800	800	300	18	15	150
60	1.0	1.2	13	2.0	400	3.0	800	800	300	18	15	150
60	1.0	1.2	13	2.0	400	3.0	800	800	300	10	15	150
+20	+0.4	+0.3	+2	+0.6	+400	+1.0	+400	+400	+150	h	+5	+25
+40	+0.5	+0.5	+5	+0.5	+100	+1.0	+400	+400	+150	h	+10	+50

[f] The folacin allowances refer to dietary sources as determined by *Lactobacillus casei* assay after treatment with enzymes (conjugates) to make polyglutamyl forms of the vitamin available to the test organism.

[g] The recommended dietary allowance for vitamin B-12 in infants is based on average concentration of the vitamin in human milk. The allowances after weaning are based on energy intake (as recommended by the American Academy of Pediatrics) and consideration of other factors, such as intestinal absorption.

[h] The increased requirement during pregnancy cannot be met by the iron content of habitual American diets nor by the existing iron stores of many women; therefore the use of 30–60 mg of supplemental iron is recommended. Iron needs during lactation are not substantially different from those of nonpregnant women, but continued supplementation of the mother for 2–3 months after parturition is advisable in order to replenish stores depleted by pregnancy.

O

O 1. oxygen. 2. pint (L. *octarius*). 3. orale. 4. see BLOOD GROUP O.

o. 1. abbreviation for L. *oc'ulus*, eye; *octa'rius*, pint. 2. opening.

o- chemical abbreviation for ORTHO.

¹⁸O heavy OXYGEN.

O₂ diatomic OXYGEN.

O₃ ozone.

Ω the capital of the Greek letter omega. Symbol for *ohm*.

Ω⁻¹ a symbol for *ohm⁻¹*; see SIEMENS.

ω the twenty-fourth and last letter of the Greek alphabet. See OMEGA.

OAB see ABO blood groups, under BLOOD GROUP.

OASHDI Old-Age, Survivors, Disability and Health Insurance; see under PROGRAM.

oasis (o-a'sis), pl. *oa'ses* [Gr. "a fertile islet in a desert"] an island or spot of healthy tissue in a diseased area.

oath (ōth) a solemn declaration or affirmation. **o. of Hippocrates, hippocratic o.,** see HIPPOCRATES.

OAV oculoauriculovertebral SYNDROME.

OB obstetrics.

ob- [L. *ob* against] a prefix signifying against, in front of, towards.

obducent (ob-du'sent) [L. *obducere* to draw over, to cover] serving as a cover, covering. See also INVESTING.

obduction (ob-duk'shun) [L. *obductio*] a medicolegal autopsy.

Obedrex trademark for *fenfluramine hydrochloride* (see under FENFLURAMINE).

obelion (o-be'le-on) [Gr. dim. of *obelos* a spit] a point on the sagittal suture where it is crossed by a line which connects the parietal foramina.

Obepar trademark for *phendimetrazine tartrate* (see under PHENDIMETRAZINE).

Obesedrin trademark for *dextroamphetamine sulfate* (see under DEXTROAMPHETAMINE).

obesity (o-bēs'ĭ-te) [L. *obesitas*] an increase in body weight beyond the limitation of skeletal and physical requirement, as the result of an excessive accumulation of fat in the body. Called also *adiposis*.

obfuscation (ob"fus-ka'shun) [L. *obfuscatio* a darkening] the act or process of rendering or becoming obscure; a darkening.

ObG, ObGyn obstetrics and gynecology.

object (ob'jekt) something that is visible or tangible.

objective (ob-jek'tiv) [L. *objectivus*] 1. a lens or combination of lenses in a microscope or telescope that is nearest to the object under examination. 2. a result for whose achievement an effort is made. 3. perceptible to the external senses. 4. pertaining to those symptoms and manifestations which may be observed by a person other than the patient in contradistinction to the subjective signs, which are apparent only to the patient. **achromatic o.,** a microscope objective in which the chromatic aberration is corrected for light of two wavelengths and the spherical aberration is corrected for that of one wavelength. **apochromatic o.,** a microscope objective in which the chromatic aberration is corrected for light of three wavelengths and the spherical aberration is corrected for that of two. **dry o.,** a microscope objective designed to be used without a liquid between its tip and the cover glass over the specimen. **fluorite o.,** a microscope objective in which some of the lenses are made from fluorite instead of glass. **immersion o.,** a microscope objective designed to have its tip and the cover glass over the specimen connected by a liquid instead of by air. The liquid may be water (water immersion) or a specially prepared oil (oil immersion). Called also *immersion lens.* **semiapochromatic o.,** a microscope objective in which the correction of chromatic and spherical aberrations is between those of the achromatic and apochromatic objectives.

obligate (ob'lĭ-gāt) [L. *obligatus*] essential; necessary; compulsory; not facultative; limited to a single life condition; able to survive only in a particular environment or to assume only a particular role, as an obligate anaerobe.

oblique (ŏ-blēk', ŏ-blīk) [L. *obliquus*] slanting; inclined; between a horizontal and a perpendicular direction.

obliquity (ob-lik'wĭ-te) the state of being oblique, or slanting.

obliquus (ob-li'kwus) [L.] oblique.

obliteration (ob-lit″er-a'shun) [L. *obliteratio*] the act or process of completely blotting out, or erasing, or entirely removing, whether by disease, surgical procedure, degeneration, or any other means.

oblongata (ob″long-ga'tah, ob'long-gah'tah) [L., a feminine adjective; literally, "made oblong"] oblong; frequently used alone to mean the *medulla oblongata.*

Obramycin trademark for *tobramycin.*

O'Brien's akinesia [Cecil Starling *O'Brien,* American ophthalmologist, born 1889] see under AKINESIA.

obstruction (ob-struk'shun) [L. *obstructio*] the act, process, or state of being blocked or clogged.

obtund (ob-tund') [L. *obtundere*] to render dull or blunt; to render less acute.

obtundent (ob-tun'dent) [L. *obtundens*] 1. having the power to dull sensibility or to soothe pain. 2. a soothing or partially anesthetic medicine.

obturate (ob″tu-rāt) to close or occlude.

obturation (ob″tu-ra'shun) [L. *obturatio* stopping up] the act or process of closing or occluding. **canal o.,** the final stage of root canal therapy, which is done after extirpation of the pulp and disinfection and preparation of the canal, consisting of filling the entire root canal completely and densely with a nonirritating hermetic sealing agent. **retrograde o.,** retrograde FILL-ING.

obturator (ob'tu-ra″tor) [L.] 1. any structure, natural or artificial, which closes an opening. 2. a prosthesis used to close an acquired or congenital opening in the palate (cleft palate). See also artificial PALATE. 3. speech-aid PROSTHESIS. **Case's velum o.,** a device of soft rubber posteriorly combined with hard vulcanite, used to replace the anterior part of a defective palate.

occipital (ok-sip'ĭ-tal) [L. *occipitalis*] pertaining to the occiput.

occipitalis (ok-sip″ĭ-ta'lis) [L.] occipital muscle; see occipital belly of occipitofrontal muscle, under BELLY. **o. mi′nor,** transverse muscle of nape; see under MUSCLE.

occipitalization (ok-sip″ĭ-tal-i-za'shun) synostosis of the atlas with the occipital bone. **o. of atlas,** platybasia.

occipito- [L. *occipitalis* occipital] a combining form denoting relationship to the occiput or to the occipital bone.

occipitoatloid (ok-sip″ĭ-to-at'loid) pertaining to the occipital bone and the atlas.

occipitoaxoid (ok-sip′ĭ-to-ak'soid) pertaining to the occipital bone and the axis.

occipitobasilar (ok-sip″ĭ-to-bas'ĭ-ler) pertaining to the occiput and the base of the skull.

occipitocalcarine (ok'sip″ĭ-to-kal'kar-ĭn) both occipital and calcarine.

occipitocervical (ok-sip″ĭ-to-ser′vĭ-kal) pertaining to the occiput and the neck.

occipitofacial (ok-sip″ĭ-to-fa'shal) pertaining to the occiput and the face.

occipitofrontal (ok-sip″ĭ-to-fron'tal) pertaining to the occiput and the forehead.

occipitomastoid (ok-sip″ĭ-to-mas'toid) pertaining to the occipital bone and the mastoid process.

occipitomental (ok-sip″ĭ-to-men'tal) pertaining to the occiput and the chin.

occipitoparietal (ok-sip″ĭ-to-pah-ri′e-tal) pertaining to the occipital and parietal bones or lobes of the brain.

occiput (ok'sĭ-put) [L.] [NA] the back of the head. Called also *o. cranii* and *o. of cranium.*

occipitotemporal (ok-sip″ĭ-to-tem'po-ral) pertaining to the occipital and temporal bones.

occipitothalamic (ok-sip″ĭ-to-thaň-lam'ik) pertaining to the occipital lobe and the thalamus.

occlude (ŏ-klood') 1. to close, shut, or stop up. 2. to bring the mandibular teeth into contact with the maxillary teeth.

occluder (ŏ-klood'er) a form of dental articulator.

occlusal (ŏ-kloo'zal) 1. pertaining to occlusion. 2. pertaining to the contacting surfaces of opposing teeth or of opposing occlusion rims, or to the masticating surfaces of the premolar and molar teeth.

occlusion (ŏ-kloo'zhun) [L. *occlusio*] 1. the act or process of closure or of being closed or shut off. 2. the trapping of a material, either gas or liquid, within cavities of a solid. 3. the relationship between all the components of the masticatory system in normal function, dysfunction, and parafunction, including the morphological and functional features of contacting surfaces of opposing teeth and restorations, occlusal trauma and dysfunction, neuromuscular physiology, the temporomandibular joint and muscle function, swallowing and mastication, psychophysiological status, and the diagnosis, prevention, and treatment of functional disorders of the masticatory system. See also MALOCCLUSION and BITE. 4. momentary complete closure of some area in the vocal tract, causing stoppage of the breath and accumulation of pressure. **abnormal o.,** malocclusion. **acentric o.,** a condition in which the habitual voluntary closure pattern of the mandible does not coincide with centric relation, producing primary premature tooth contacts in the centric path of closure. Called also *eccentric o.* **adjusted o.,** in dental restoration, increase or decrease of occlusal contacts in an effort to attain a balanced or functional occlusion between the opposing structures. **o. analysis,** occlusal ANALYSIS. **anatomic o.,** that in which the arrangement of natural teeth in the same and opposing arch is defined by dental and/or skeletal landmarks rather than functional criteria. **anterior o.,** mesioclusion. **attritional o.,** that in which each tooth wears occlusally and proximally as it erupts. According to P. R. Begg, occlusion may be considered as normal, although differing from ideal, when teeth become worn, attrition serving as a corrective factor in adjusting the size and shape of teeth, determined by evolutional, physiological, adaptive, environmental, or nutritional factors, for their physiological needs. See also active ERUPTION and continuous ERUPTION. **balanced o.,** that in which the occlusal contact of the teeth on the working side of the jaw is accompanied by the harmonious contact of the teeth on the opposite (balancing) side. The occlusion of artificial teeth may be *mechanically balanced,* as on an articulator, without reference to physiologic considerations, or *physiologically balanced,* functioning in harmony with the temporomandibular joint and the neuromuscular system. Called also *balanced bite* and *occlusal balance.* **buccal o.,** the position of a posterior tooth when it is outside (buccal to) the line of occlusion. **centric o.,** that in the vertical and horizontal position of the mandible in which the cusps of the mandibular and maxillary teeth interdigitate maximally. Ideally, the lingual cusps of the maxillary bicuspids make contact with the marginal ridges of the mandibular bicuspids and the marginal ridges of the second bicuspid and first molar. The mesial lingual cusps of the maxillary molar occlude in the central fossae of the mandibular molars, while the distal cusps of the maxillary molars occlude on the marginal ridges of the mandibular molars. Similarly, the supporting cusps of the mandibular teeth occlude on the marginal ridges and fossae of the maxillary molars and bicuspids. Abbreviated CO. Called also *intercuspal position, acquired centric, habitual centric, intercuspal position,* and *tooth-to-tooth position.* See also centric POSITION and centric RELATION. **centric o., handheld,** that obtained by hand coupling the casts of a pair of molars that allow their main stamp cusps to be seated mutually in the central fossae of their opposite numbers. **centric relation o.,** that when the jaws are in centric relation. **convenience o.,** the assumed position of maximum intercuspation when there is occlusal interference in the centric path of closure, being anterior, lateral, anterolateral, etc., to the true centric occlusion. Called also *convenience jaw relation.* **coronary o.,** obstruction of the coronary artery, usually caused by closure of its lumen by cholesterol deposits in arteriosclerosis, thrombosis, or other causes, but rarely by embolism. It is often associated with myocardial infarction with resulting coagulation necrosis in the heart muscle due to local ischemia from an interrupted blood supply, and presenting painful pressure in the chest, occasionally radiating to the arms, throat, and back, a state of shock, profuse perspiration, and anxiety. Sudden death is common. Incidents of vomiting and nausea may be erroneously interpreted as signs of acute indigestion. Commonly called *heart attack.* See also coronary ARTERIOSCLEROSIS, coronary ΤHROMBOSIS, and myocardial INFARCTION. **crossbite o.,** that in which the lower teeth overlap the upper teeth. See also CROSSBITE. **cuspid protected o.,** complete cuspid guidance provided in dental restorations to protect the occlusion and to prevent occlusal dysfunctions. **distal o.,** the position of the lower tooth when it is distal to its opposite number in the maxilla. Called also *postnormal o.* **eccentric o.,** acentric o. **edge-to-edge o., end-to-end o.,** that in which the anterior maxillary and mandibular teeth meet along their incisal edges when the mandible is in centric position. Called also *edge-to-edge bite* and *end-to-end bite.* **functional o.,** such contact of the maxillary and mandibular teeth as will provide the highest efficiency in the centric position and during all excursive movements of the jaw that are essential to mastication, without producing trauma. **gliding o.,** relation between the opposing teeth when they are in motion. See ARTICULATION. **habitual o.,** the consistent relationships of the teeth in the maxilla to those of the mandible when the teeth in both jaws are brought into maximum contact, such relationships varying from individual to individual; the ideal habitual occlusion is centric occlusion, but it is seldom attained without dental intervention. See also *ideal o., normal o.,* and HABIT. **hyperfunctional o.,** traumatic o. **ideal o.,** perfect interdigitation of the upper and lower teeth, associated with neuromuscular harmony in the masticatory system; stable jaw relationship when the teeth make contact in centric relation; centric occlusion slightly in front of centric relation; the distance between centric relation and centric occlusion of about 0.1 to 0.2 mm in the temporomandibular joints and about 0.5 mm at the level of the teeth; an unrestricted glide with maintained occlusal contacts between centric relation and centric occlusion; complete freedom for smooth gliding occlusal contact movements in the various excursions both from centric occlusion and centric relation; and the occlusal guidance in various excursions on the working rather than on the balancing side. **labial o.,** the position of an anterior tooth when it is outside (labial to) the line of occlusion. **lateral o.,** that of the teeth when the lower jaw is moved to the right or left of centric position. **lingual o.,** malocclusion in which the tooth is lingual to the line of the normal dental arch. Called also *linguoclusion.* **locked o.,** an occlusal relationship in which lateral and protrusive mandibular movements are limited. **malfunctional o.,** malocclusion. **mechanically balanced o.,** see *balanced o.* **mesial o.,** the position of the lower tooth when it is mesial to its opposite number in the maxilla. Called also *prenormal o.* **milled-in o.,** see *milled-in path,* under PATH. **neutral o.,** normal o. **normal o.,** the contact of the upper and lower teeth in centric relation, taking into consideration adaptive changes of the masticatory system in the absence of recognizable pathologic manifestations, or where temporomandibular joint-muscle-pain dysfunction and centrally induced disturbance are effectively controlled. Called also *neutral o.* See also *physiologic o.* **pathogenic o.,** an occlusal relationship that is capable of producing pathologic changes in the supporting tissues. See also *traumatic o.* **physiologic o.,** that which is in harmony with the functioning of the temporomandibular joint and the neuromuscular system, occlusal stresses being distributed normally on the teeth and their supporting structures. See also *normal o.* **physiologically balanced o.,** see *balanced o.* **posterior o.,** distocclusion. **postnormal o.,** distal o. **prenormal o.,** mesial o. **protrusive o.,** mesioclusion. **retrusive o.,** distocclusion. **spherical form of o.,** an arrangement of teeth that places their occlusal surfaces on the surface of an imaginary sphere, about 8 inches in diameter, with its center above the level of the teeth. See also Monson CURVE. **terminal o.,** the relationship of opposing occlusal surfaces that provides the maximum natural or planned contact and/or intercuspation. **traumatic o.,** progressive injury to the supporting structure of the teeth as a result of occlusal dysfunction, which may or may not include periodontal pocket formation or modify the progress or severity of periodontal disease. Malocclusion, faulty oral habits, temporomandibular joint dysharmony, loss of teeth, loss of periodontal support, dental caries, faulty dental restorations and appliances, faulty orthodontic therapy, and displacement of teeth are some of the principal predisposing factors. Called also *periodontal traumatism.* See also *traumatogenic o.,* BRUXISM, MALOCCLUSION, oral HABIT, and occlusal TRAUMA. **traumatic o., primary,** abnormal occlusal stress acting upon basically normal periodontal structures. **traumatic o., secondary,** abnormal occlusal stress acting upon weakened periodontal structures; the effect of occlusal forces which may not be abnormal but are excessive for weakened periodontal structures. **traumatogenic o.,** abnormal occlusion capable of producing injury to the teeth, residual ridges, and periodontal structures. See *traumatic o.* **working o.,** the contact made between the teeth on the side toward which the mandible is moved. Called also *working bite relation.*

occlusive (o-kloo′siv) pertaining to or affecting occlusion.

occlusocervical (o-kloo″so-ser′vĭ-kal) pertaining to the occlusal surface and neck of a tooth.

occlusometer (ok″loo-som′ĕ-ter) gnathodynamometer.

occlusorehabilitation (o-kloo″zo-re″hah-bil″ĭ-ta′shun) occlusal REHABILITATION.

occult (ŏ-kult′) [L. *occultus*] obscure; concealed from observation; difficult to understand.

occupancy (ok′u-pan-se) 1. the act of occupying or the state of being occupied. 2. the period of time during which a unit quantity of a substance, administered in a specified way, is present in, or occupies, a part of the body before it is excreted or broken down. **hospital o.,** the percent of hospital beds occupied during a given period.

Oceanomonas (o″she-an″o-mo′nas) a proposed name for a genus of bacteria now assigned to the genus *Vibrio.* **O. alginolyt′ica, O. enterit′idis,** *Vibrio parahaemolyticus;* see under VIBRIO.

ocher (o′ker) any of the colored earthy powders consisting of hydrated ferric oxides, sand, clay, and other substances. **chrome o.,** chromic OXIDE.

Ochoa, Severo [born 1905] an American physician and biochemist; co-winner, with Arthur Kornberg, of the Nobel prize for medicine and physiology in 1959, for work in the discovery of enzymes for producing nucleic acids artificially.

octa- [L. *octō;* Gr. *okto* eight] a combining form meaning eight. See also OCTO-.

Octacaine trademark for *lidocaine hydrochloride* (see under LIDOCAINE).

octadecanoate (ok″tah-dek″ah-no′āt) systematic name for stearate, denoting that it has 18 (L. *octa* eight + *deca* ten) carbon atoms in a straight chain.

octamethyl pyrophosphoramide (ok″tah-meth″il-pir″o-fos-for′ah-mīd) a highly toxic cholinesterase inhibitor, bis[bisdimethylaminophosphorous] anhydride, occurring as a viscous liquid that is miscible with water and soluble with most organic solvents. Used chiefly as an insecticide. Abbreviated OMPA. Trademarks: Pestox III, Schradan.

octan (ok′tan) [L. *octō* eight] recurring every eighth day, or at intervals of seven days.

octane (ok′tān) an eight-carbon straight chain hydrocarbon of the methane series, C_8H_{18}, obtained from petroleum, occurring as an oily colorless, volatile liquid. Used as an organic solvent and in various chemical processes. It may be narcotic in high concentrations.

octapeptide (ok″tah-pep′tīd) [*octa-* + *peptide*] a polypeptide containing eight amino acids.

Octatensine trademark for *guanethidine.*

octo- [L. *octō* eight] a combining form denoting eight. See also OCTA-.

octoate (ok′to-āt) a salt of octanoic (caprylic) acid. Called also *caprylate.* **stannous o., tin o.,** a tin salt of octanoic (caprylic) acid; used as a catalyst in the polymerization of silicone. Called also *stannous caprylate* and *tin caprylate.*

ocular (ok′u-lar) [L. *ocularis; oculus* eye] pertaining to the eye.

oculi (ok′u-li) [L.] plural of *oculus.*

oculo- [L. *oculus* eye] a combining form denoting relationship to the eye.

oculofacial (ok″u-lo-fa′she-al) pertaining to the eyes and the face.

oculomandibulodyscephaly (ok″ku-lo-man-dib″u-lo-dis-sef′ah-le) Hallermann-Streiff SYNDROME.

oculomotor (ok″u-lo-mo′tor) [*oculo-* + L. *motor* mover] pertaining to movements of the eye, as the oculomotor muscle.

oculonasal (ok″u-lo-na′zal) pertaining to the eye and the nose.

oculus (ok′u-lus), pl. *oc′uli* [L.] [NA] the eye.

o.d. abbreviation for L. *om′ne di′e,* once a day.

odaxesmus (o″dak-sez′mus) [Gr. *odaxēsmos* an itching] the biting of the tongue or cheek in an epileptic seizure. See also entries under BITING.

ODD oculodentodigital dysplasia; see oculodento-osseous DYSPLASIA.

odontalgia (o-don-tal′je-ah) [*odonto-* + *-algia*] pain in a tooth or in the teeth; toothache; odontodynia. **phantom o.,** pain in the area from which a tooth has been removed. Called also *ghost pain.*

odontalgic (o-don-tal′jik) pertaining to or characterized by odontalgia or toothache.

odontectomy (o″don-tek′to-me) [*odonto-* + Gr. *ektomē* excision] excision or removal of a tooth. See tooth EXTRACTION.

odontexesis (o″don-teks′e-sis) [*odonto-* + Gr. *xesis* scraping] a term used in the past to denote the scaling of teeth. See also APOXESIS.

odontic (o-don′tik) [Gr. *odous* tooth] pertaining to a tooth; dental.

odontinoid (o-don″tĭ-noid) [Gr. *odous* tooth + *eidos* form] resembling a tooth; toothlike.

odonto- [Gr. *odous* tooth] a combining form denoting relationship to a tooth or to the teeth. See also DENTO-.

odontoameloblastoma (o-don″to-am′ĕ-lo-blas-to′mah) ameloblastic ODONTOMA.

odontoblast (o-don′to-blast) [*odonto-* + Gr. *blastos* germ] one of the connective tissue cells forming the odontoblastic layer of the dental pulp and responsible for depositing dentin. A mature cell resembles an osteoblast, its height reflecting the shape of the nucleus. The tall cells are usually found in the coronal pulp and the cuboidal in the root portion. The nuclei, which usually contain one or more nucleoli, tend to be more oval in taller cells in the coronal portion than those in the root. The nuclear membrane, about 50 Å in thickness, is double-walled; its inner wall contains numerous annuli or pores, with granules about 150 Å in diameter. The cell membrane is about 100 Å in width. The cytoplasmic organelles include diplosomes, Golgi apparatus, mitochondria, and cytoplasmic granules. Terminal bars are found on the dentinal surface, and processes projecting into the dentinal tubules extend from the cell surface. Called also *dentin cell* and *fibrilloblast*.

odontobothrion (o-don″to-both′re-on) [*odonto-* + Gr. *bothrion* a small trench] dental ALVEOLUS.

odontobothritis (o-don″to-both-ri′tis) [*odontobothrium* + *-itis*] alveolitis.

odontobothrium (o-don″to-both-re′um) [*odonto-* + Gr. *bothrion* little] dental ALVEOLUS.

odontochirurgical (o-don″to-ki-rur′jĭ-kal) [*odonto-* + L. *chirurgia* surgery] a term formerly used to denote relationship to dental surgery.

odontoclamis (o-don″to-kla′mis) [*odonto-* + Gr. *klamys* cloak] dental OPERCULUM.

odontoclasia (o-don″to-kla′ze-ah) [*odonto-* + Gr. *klasis* a breaking + *-ia*] external tooth RESORPTION.

odontoclast (o-don′to-klast″) [*odonto-* + Gr. *klasis* a breaking] a cell, cytomorphologically similar to the osteoclast, which is involved in tooth resorption; the cavities thus produced by resorption are known as *resorption lacunae*.

odontoclastoma (o-don″to-klast-o′mah) [*odontoclast* + *-oma*] internal tooth RESORPTION.

odontodynia (o-don″to-din′ĕ-ah) [*odonto-* + Gr. *odynē* pain] pain in a tooth or in the teeth; toothache; odontalgia.

odontodysplasia (o-don′to-dis-pla′se-ah) [*odonto-* + *dysplasia*] a localized arrested tooth development, which appears to involve most commonly the anterior teeth, usually on one side of the midline, most often the maxillary central and lateral incisors. Roentgenographically, the teeth have a ghostlike appearance. Calcification and bits of prismatic enamel may be found in the pulp, and the enamel is thin and absent in part. Called also *ghost teeth* and *odontogenic dysplasia*.

odontogen (o-don′to-jen) [*odonto-* + Gr. *gennan* to produce] the substance which develops into the dentin of the teeth.

odontogenesis (o-don″to-jen′ĕ-sis) [*odonto-* + Gr. *genesis* production] development and formation of the teeth. The process is divided into the incipient stage (see lamina-bud STAGE); the proliferative stage (see cap STAGE); the morphodifferentiation and histodifferentiation stage (see bell STAGE); the apposition and calcification stage (see APPOSITION [3]); and tooth eruption (see under ERUPTION). See illustration. **o. imperfec′ta,** DENTINOGENESIS imperfecta.

odontogenic (o-don″to-jen′ik) 1. forming teeth. 2. arising in tissues which give origin to the teeth.

odontogenous (o″don-toj′ĕ-nus) arising or originating in the teeth, or a dental condition.

odontogram (o-don′to-gram) [*odonto-* + Gr. *gramma* mark, record] the tracing made by an odontograph.

odontograph (o-don′to-graf) [*odonto-* + Gr. *graphein* to write] an instrument for recording the unevenness of the surface of tooth enamel.

odontography (o″don-tog′rah-fe) [*odonto-* + Gr. *graphein* to write] 1. a description of the teeth. 2. the use of the odontograph. Called also *dentography*.

odontohypophosphatasia (o-don″to-hi″po-fos″fah-ta′ze-ah) hypophosphatasia associated with dental symptoms, including hy-

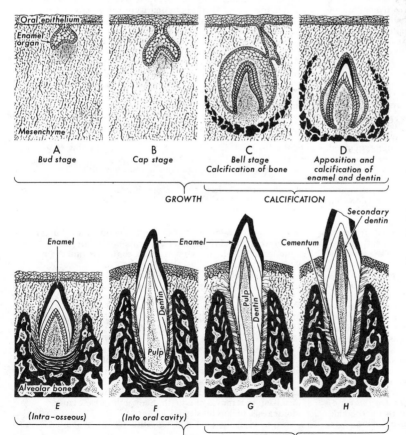

A — Bud stage
B — Cap stage
C — Bell stage / Calcification of bone
D — Apposition and calcification of enamel and dentin

GROWTH   CALCIFICATION

Oral epithelium
Enamel organ
Mesenchyme

Enamel
Enamel
Secondary dentin
Cementum
Dentin
Pulp
Alveolar bone

E (Intra-osseous)
F (Into oral cavity)
G
H

ERUPTION   ATTRITION

Diagram of life cycle of a human deciduous incisor. The normal resorption of the root is not indicated. Enamel and bone are drawn in black. (From W. Bloom and D. W. Fawcett: A Textbook of Histology. 10th ed. Philadelphia, W. B. Saunders Co., 1975; redrawn and modified from Schour and Massler.)

pocementogenesis, premature exfoliation of the anterior teeth, presence of shell teeth, loss of alveolar bone usually limited to the anterior teeth, and absence of severe gingival inflammation. See also HYPOPHOSPHATASIA.

odontoiatria (o-don″to-e-at′re-ah) [odonto- + Gr. iatreia treatment] treatment of diseases of the teeth; dentistry.

odontoid (o-don′toid) [odonto- + Gr. eidos form] resembling a tooth; toothlike. Called also dentoid.

odontolith (o-don′to-lith) [odonto- + Gr. lithos stone] dental CALCULUS.

odontolithiasis (o-don″to-lĭ-thi′ah-sis) a condition marked by the presence of dental calculus.

odontologist (o″don-tol′o-jist) a dentist.

odontology (o″don-tol′o-je) [odonto- + -logy] the sum of knowledge regarding the teeth. See DENTISTRY.

odontolysis (o-don-tol′ĭ-sis) [odonto- + Gr. lysis dissolution] the resorption of dental tissue. See tooth RESORPTION.

odontoma (o-don-to′mah) [odonto- + -oma] 1. any tumor of odontogenic origin. 2. a mixed tumor of odontogenic origin, in which both the epithelial and mesenchymal cells exhibit complete differentiation, resulting in the formation of tooth structures. See composite o. **o. adamanti′num,** ameloblastic o. **ameloblastic o.,** a rare, slow-growing, mixed tumor of odontogenic origin, which combines the characteristics of composite odontoma and ameloblastoma, and occurs more commonly on the mandible than on the maxilla. It may contain columnar, squamous, and epithelial cells, together with ameloblasts, enamel, dentin, osteodentin, stellate reticulum-like tissue, dental papilla, and other tissues and cells, both in a relatively undifferentiated and highly differentiated form. Called also o. adamantinum, adamanto-odontoma, and odontoameloblastoma. **complex composite o.,** see composite o. **composite o.,** an odontogenic tumor of the jaws, most commonly of the molar region, composed of both the ectodermal and mesodermal components of the tooth apparatus. A type that consists of calcified dental tissue exhibiting complete differentiation, resulting in the formation of enamel and dentin that bear resemblance to normal tooth structures, is known as compound composite odontoma; a type in which calcified dental tissue presents a disorganized mass bearing no similarity to normal tooth structure is known as complex composite odontoma. **compound composite o.,** see composite o. **coronal o., coronary o.,** one associated with the crown of a tooth, or one formed at the time when the crown of the tooth was developing. **cystic o.,** one in which there is a cystic structure associated with the tumor. **dilated o.,** DENS in dente. **embryoplastic o.,** a soft odontoma formed in the period that precedes the formation of the dental tissues. **fibrous o.,** one containing fibrous elements. **gestant o.,** DENS in dente. **mixed o.,** an odontogenic neoplasm containing different elements of the tooth structure. **radicular o.,** one associated with the root of a tooth, or one formed at the time when the root of the tooth was developing. **soft mixed o.,** ameloblastic FIBROMA.

Odontomyces viscosus (o-don″to-mi′sēz vis-ko′sus) Actinomyces viscosus; see under ACTINOMYCES.

odontonomy (o″don-ton′o-me) [odonto- + Gr. onoma name] dental NOMENCLATURE.

odontopathy (o′don-top′ah-the) [odonto- + Gr. pathos illness] any disease of the teeth.

odontoperiosteum (o-don″to-per″e-os′te-um) periodontium.

odontophobia (o-don″to-fo′be-ah) [odonto- + phobia] morbid fear associated with the teeth, as that aroused by the sight of teeth, or abnormal dread of dental operations.

odontoprisis (o-don″to-pri′sis) [odonto- + Gr. prisis sawing] bruxism.

odontoradiograph (o-don″to-ra′de-o-graf) a roentgenograph of a tooth or of the teeth.

odontoschism (o-don′to-skizm) [odonto- + Gr. schisma cleft] a fissure of a tooth.

odontoscopy (o″don-tos′ko-pe) the taking of dental impressions.

odontoseisis (o-don″to-si′sis) [odonto- + Gr. seisis a shaking] looseness of the teeth.

odontosis (o″don-to′sis) [Gr. odous tooth] the formation or eruption of the teeth.

odontotheca (o-don″to-the′kah) [odonto- + Gr. thēkē case] dental SAC.

odontotomy (o″don-tot′o-me) [odonto- + Gr. tomē a cutting] the cutting into a tooth, especially incision into an occlusal groove. **prophylactic o.,** in preventing dental caries developing in pits and fissures, a cut into enamel to include all pits and fissures, followed by restoration with silver amalgam. A modification of the method consists of grinding to eliminate pits and fissures and polishing the adjacent tooth structure into depressions that will allow efficient self-cleansing.

odontotripsis (o-don″to-trip′sis) [odonto- + Gr. tripsis rubbing] wearing away of the teeth. See also ABRASION (2) and WEAR.

odor (o′dor) [L.] a volatile emanation that is perceived by the sense of smell.

-odynia [Gr. odynē pain] a word ending meaning pain.

odyno- [Gr. odynē pain] a combining form meaning pain.

odynophagia (od″ĭ-no-fa′je-ah) [odyno- + Gr. phagein to eat] pain on deglutition; painful swallowing.

Odysseus Ulysses.

Oersted, Hans Christian [1777–1851] a Danish physicist.

oersted (er′sted) [named after H. C. Oersted] the unit of magnetizing force. Symbol H.

oesophagus (ĕ-sof′ah-gus) [Gr. oisophagos] esophagus.

OFD see oral-facial-digital SYNDROME (1 and 2).

official (o-fish′al) [L. officialis, officium duty] in pharmacology, pertaining to an official drug (see under DRUG).

officinal (o-fis′ĭ-nal) [L. officinalis; from officina shop] kept in stock in pharmacies; see under DRUG.

off-line (of′līn) operating independently of the main computer.

offspring (of′spring) progeny or descendants. First generation offspring are designated on genetic charts as F_1, the second generation as F_2, etc. See also GENERATION, PROGENY, and SIBLING.

-ogen [Gr. gennan to produce] a suffix denoting a precursor.

ogive (o′jīv) an S-shaped curve; a term used in biometry.

OH hydroxyl.

Ohara's disease [Shoichiro Ohara, Japanese physician] see under DISEASE.

OHI 1. Oral Hygiene INSTRUCTION. 2. oral hygiene INDEX.

OHI-S oral hygiene index, simplified; see under INDEX.

Ohl elevator see under ELEVATOR.

ohm (ōm) [named after George S. Ohm] the SI unit of electric resistance, being that resistance through which a difference potential of 1 volt will produce a current of 1 ampere. Symbol Ω. See also SI. **international o., legal o.,** the resistance to a constant current by a column of mercury at 0°C, 14.4521 grams in mass, of constant cross-sectional area and 106.300 centimeters in length. **reciprocal o.,** siemens.

Ohm's law [George S. Ohm, German physicist, 1787–1854] see under LAW. See also OHM.

ohmmammeter (om′am-mĕ″ter) an ohmmeter and ammeter combined.

ohmmeter (om′mĕ-ter) an instrument for measuring electric resistance in ohms.

-oic in chemical nomenclature, a name ending indicating an acid.

-oid [Gr. eidos form, shape] a word termination signifying resemblance to the thing specified by the stem to which it is affixed.

Oidal trademark for salicylamide.

oil (oil) [L. oleum] an unctuous, combustible substance which is easily liquefiable on warming, and is soluble in ether, but not in water. **allspice o.,** o. of pimenta. **almond o.,** the fixed oil obtained by expression from the kernels of varieties of Prunus amygdalus, occurring as a clear, pale straw-colored or colorless, odorless, oily liquid with a bland taste, which is miscible with ether, chloroform, benzene, and hexane, and slightly soluble in ethanol. It does not congeal until cooled to −20°C. Used as an emollient and flavoring agent. Called also expressed almond o., sweet almond o., and oleum amygdalae expressum. **almond o., bitter,** the volatile oil obtained from kernels of Prunus amygdalus deprived of fixed oil, or from other kernels containing amygdalin, such as apricots, cherries, plums, and peaches, occurring as a colorless to yellow, refractive liquid with a characteristic odor and the taste of benzaldehyde. Slightly soluble in water and miscible with ethanol, ether, and oils. It is a highly toxic substance containing hydrogen cyanide. Used as a flavoring agent after deprivation of hydrogen cyanide. Formerly used as a topical antipruritic. Called also volatile bitter almond o. **almond o., expressed,** almond o. **almond o., sweet,** almond o. **anise o.,** the volatile oil obtained from the dried, ripe fruit of Pimpinella anisum or of Illicium verum, occurring as a colorless or pale yellow oily liquid with the odor of anise, which is slightly soluble in water and alcohol. Used chiefly as a flavoring agent, and has been used as a carminative and expectorant. **arachis o.,** peanut o. **o. of betula,** methyl SALICYLATE. **bitter almond o.,** almond o., bitter. **caraway o.,** the volatile oil distilled from the dried ripe fruit of Carum carvi, occurring as a colorless or pale yellow liquid that darkens with age, and is soluble in ethanol, but not in water. Used as a flavoring agent. Called also oleum cari. **cassia o.,** the volatile oil distilled from the leaves and twigs of the Chinese cinnamon (Cinnamomum cassia). See cinnamon o. **castor o.,** the fixed oil from the seeds of *Ricinus communis,* and consisting chiefly of the glycerides of ricinoleic and isoricinoleic acids. It is a pale yellowish to colorless, transparent, viscid liquid with a faint odor and a bland taste followed by a nauseating aftertaste, which is soluble in ethanol and miscible with dehydrated ethanol, glacial acetic acid, chloroform, and ether. Used in the manufacture of various chemical products, such as embalming fluid, synthetic resins and fibers, and lubricants. Also used as an emollient and cathartic. Called also *o. of palma Christi, ricinus o.* and *tangatangan o.* **cedro o.,** lemon o. **China o.,** BALSAM of Peru. **chloriodized o.,** a chlorinated and iodinated peanut oil, containing about 7.5 percent chlorine and about 27 percent iodine. Used as a water-insoluble contrast medium in radiography, including sialography. It may cause adverse reactions when retained in the salivary glands. Trademark: Iodochlorol. **cinnamon o.,** the volatile oil distilled from the leaves and twigs of cinnamon. Two forms exist: one produced from Ceylon cinnamon *(Cinnamomum zeylanicum),* the other from Chinese cinnamon *(Cinnamomum cassia);* the latter, also known as cassia oil, is the official one. It occurs as a yellowish or brownish liquid which darkens with time and on exposure to the air, with the characteristic odor and taste of cinnamon. Used in dentistry chiefly as a flavoring agent. Formerly used as a weak antiseptic. **clove o.,** the volatile oil distilled from the dried flower buds of *Eugenia caryophillus,* occurring as a colorless or pale yellow liquid with the characteristic taste and odor of cloves, which darkens and thickens on exposure to air. It is slightly soluble in water and freely soluble in ethanol. Phenol eugenol is its chief constituent. Used chiefly as an analgesic to alleviate toothache. Clove oil mixed with zinc oxide into a paste is used as a cavity base. It may be used to reduce ammoniacal silver nitrate. When clove oil comes in contact with the mucous membranes burns may occur. Its active ingredient, eugenol, when mixed with zinc oxide, forms zinc oxide–eugenol cement (see under CEMENT). **coal o.,** kerosene. **coconut o.,** the fixed oil obtained by expression or extraction from the kernels of seeds of ·*Cocos nucifera* (coconut), occurring as a white, semisolid, lardlike fat that is soluble in ethanol, ether, chloroform, and carbon disulfide, but not in water. It is a digestible fat containing glycerides of lauric, capric, myristic, palmitic, and oleic acids, as well as cholesterol. Used in the production of oleomargarine, hydrogenated shortenings, synthetic cocoa butter, soaps, cosmetics, emulsions, detergents, drugs, fatty alcohols, and methyl esters. Also used as an ointment base. Called also *copra o.* **cod liver o.,** the partially destearinated fixed oil obtained by expression from fresh livers of the fish *Gadus morrhua* and other species of cod, occurring as a pale yellow, thin, oily liquid with a bland, slightly fishy odor and taste, which is soluble in chloroform, ether, carbon disulfide, and ethyl acetate, but not in water. Used as a source of vitamins A and D. Trademarks: Gaduol, Tunol. **copra o.,** coconut o. **coriander o.,** the volatile oil distilled from the dried ripe fruits of *Coriandrum sativum,* occurring as a colorless or yellowish liquid with an aromatic odor and a spicy taste, which is soluble in ethanol, ether, and chloroform. Used chiefly as a flavoring agent. **corn o.,** the refined fixed oil obtained from the embryo of *Zea mays* (corn), occurring as a clear, light yellow, oily liquid with a faint characteristic taste and odor, which is miscible with ether, chloroform, benzene, and hexane and is slightly soluble in ethanol. Used as a solvent and vehicle for injections, in the production of soaps, and as an edible cholesterol-free cooking oil. Called also *maize o.* **cottonseed o.,** the fixed refined oil from the seeds of *Gossypium hirsutum* and other species of the same genus, occurring as a pale yellow, oily, odorless liquid with a bland taste, which is miscible with ether, chloroform, hexane, and carbon disfulfide, and is slightly soluble in ethanol. Used in zinc oxide–eugenol preparations, as a solvent and vehicle for injections, and in the production of soaps, lubricants, and cosmetics. Also used as a source of polyunsaturated, cholesterol-free fatty acids in the preparation of cooking oils, oleomargarine, and lard substitutes. Sometimes used as a laxative. **distilled o.,** volatile o. **drying o.,** a fixed oil that thickens and hardens on exposure to air, especially when spread out in a thin layer. **earth-nut o.,** peanut o. **essential o.,** volatile o. **ethereal o.,** 1. a compound of ether with heavy oil of wine. 2. volatile o. **ethiodized o.,** an ethyl ester of iodinated fatty acid of poppyseed oil, containing about 37 percent bound iodine. Used as a water-insoluble contrast medium in radiography, including sialography. Trademark: Ethiodol. **eucalyptus o.,** the volatile oil distilled from fresh leaves of *Eucalyptus globulus* and other species of the same genus, occurring as a colorless or pale

yellow liquid with a characteristic aromatic odor and a spicy cooling taste, which is miscible with ethanol, but insoluble in water. It has antiseptic and expectorant properties. Used in the treatment of chronic bronchitis and also used as a flavoring agent. Formerly used to treat the root canal in preparation for filling. In endodontics, used as a solvent for gutta-percha for root canal filling and in the liquid portion of certain root canal sealers. It may cause burns of mucous membranes on contact. **expressed o.,** fixed o. **expressed almond o.,** almond o. **fatty o.,** fixed o. **fixed o.,** a fatty substance of vegetable and animal organisms, which does not evaporate on warming. Fatty oils contain esters (usually glycerol esters) of fatty acids. Called also *expressed o.* and *fatty o.* **flaxseed o.,** linseed o. **gaultheria o.,** methyl SALICYLATE. **o. green,** chromic OXIDE. **groundnut o.,** peanut o. **halibut liver o.,** the fixed oil obtained from livers of the fish *Hippoglossus hippoglossus* (halibut), occurring as a pale yellow liquid with a slightly fishy odor and taste, which is soluble in ethanol, ether, chloroform, and carbon disulfide, but not in water. Used as a source of vitamins A and D. **heavy o.,** an oily product obtained by the action of sulfuric acid on alcohol. **iodized o.,** a combination of vegetable oils and iodine, containing about 38 to 42 percent combined iodine. It is a thick, viscous, oily liquid that decomposes and darkens when exposed to air and light. Used as a water-insoluble contrast medium in radiography, including sialography. Adverse reactions may occur when it is retained in the salivary glands. Trademark: Lipiodol. **juniper o., juniperberry o.,** the volatile oil distilled from the dried ripe fruit of *Juniperus communis,* occurring as a pale greenish yellow liquid with the odor and taste of juniper berries, which is soluble in ethanol, miscible with carbon disulfide, benzene, chloroform, and amyl alcohol, and insoluble in water. Used as a flavoring agent, as a diuretic agent, and in the preservation of catgut sutures. **lavender o., lavender flowers o.,** the volatile oil distilled from the fresh flowering tops of *Lavendula officinalis,* occurring as a colorless or yellow liquid that is miscible with dehydrated ethanol and carbon disulfide and slightly soluble in water. Linalool, linalyl acetate, geraniol, pinene, limonene, and cineol are its principal components. Used as an aromatic, carminative, and flavoring agent. **lemon o.,** the volatile oil expressed from fresh peel of *Citrus limonum* (lemon), occurring as a pale yellow or greenish yellow liquid that is miscible with carbon disfulfide and glacial acetic acid, soluble in ethanol, and slightly soluble in water. Limonene, terpinene, phellandrene, and pinene are its principal components. Used as a flavoring agent. Called also *cedro o.* **light mineral o.,** **light white mineral o.,** mineral o., light. **linseed o.,** a drying oil obtained from the dried ripe seed of *Linum usitatissimum* (linseed), occurring as a yellowish liquid with a peculiar odor and bland taste, which gradually thickens and darkens on exposure to air. It is slightly soluble in ethanol, and is miscible with chloroform, ether, petroleum ether, carbon disulfide, and oil turpentine. Glycerides of linolenic, oleic, stearic, palmitic, and myristic acids are its principal components. It has been used as a laxative. Used in liniments, pastes, medicinal soft soap, and saponated cresol solutions. Called also *flaxseed o.* and *raw linseed o.* **maize o.,** corn o. **mineral o., light, mineral o., light white,** a mixture of liquid hydrocarbons obtained from petroleum, occurring as a colorless, transparent, odorless, tasteless, oily liquid that is miscible with fixed oils (but not with castor oil), soluble in volatile oils, and insoluble in water and ethanol. Used to cleanse dry and inflamed skin. Also used in heat sterilization of dental instruments. Heated to 150°C (300°F), it will destroy vegetative microorganisms in 15 minutes; at 125°C (260°F), all the organisms will be destroyed in 20 to 30 minutes. No longer used as a vehicle for nose and throat medications because of the hazard of lipoid pneumonia. Called also *light liquid paraffin, light liquid petrolatum,* and *light white mineral o.* See also STERILIZATION. **o. of mustard,** the oil derived from the seeds of species of *Brassica.* Volatile mustard oil is from the seeds of black mustard (see ALLYL isothiocyanate). Expressed mustard oil is obtained from the seeds of black or white mustard and occurs as a straw-colored, brownish yellow, or greenish brown liquid that is miscible with chloroform and ether, slightly soluble in ethanol, and insoluble in water. Used in the manufacture of oleomargarine, soaps, lubricants, and edible oils. **myristica o.,** the volatile oil from the dried kernels of the ripe seed of *Myristica fragrans* (nutmeg). Used as a flavoring agent. Called also *nutmeg o.* **nut o.,** peanut o. **nutmeg o.,** myristica o. **olive o.,** the fixed oil obtained from the ripe fruit of *Olea europeae,* occurring as a pale yellow or light greenish oily liquid with a characteristic slight odor and taste, which is miscible with carbon disulfide, chloroform, and ether and is slightly soluble in ethanol. It is the principal source of dietary fats in some areas, such as the Mediterranean countries, and is used in the preparation of cerates, ointments, liniments, and plasters and as an emollient, laxative, and cholagogue. Also used in the preparation of zinc oxide cements in packs for retarding the setting of cements. Called also *sweet o*. **o. of orange,** the volatile oil obtained from the fresh peel of the ripe fruit of *Citrus sinensis* (orange), occurring as a yellow or orange liquid with a characteristic taste and odor of orange peels, which is miscible with ethanol, carbon disulfide, and glacial acetic acid. Used mainly as a flavoring agent and for the removal of zinc oxide–eugenol cements. Called also *sweet orange o*. **o. of palma Christi,** castor o. **peanut o.,** the refined fixed oil from seed kernels of one or more of the cultivated varieties of *Arachis hypogaea*, occurring as a colorless or pale yellow, oily liquid with a characteristic nutty odor and a bland taste. It is a cholesterol-free edible oil, frequently used as an adulterant for olive oil. Also used as a solvent in preparing oil solutions for injections and for preparing liniments, ointments, plasters, and soaps. Called also *arachis o., earth-nut o., groundnut o.,* and *nut o*. **peppermint o.,** a volatile oil distilled from the fresh flowering plant *Mentha piperita*, occurring as a colorless or pale yellow liquid with the penetrating odor of peppermint and a pungent cooling taste, which is soluble in ethanol and slightly soluble in alcohol. It is the chief constituent of menthol. Used chiefly as a flavoring agent; formerly used as a carminative, antiseptic, and local anesthetic agent. **pimenta o., o. of pimento,** a volatile oil distilled from the fruit of *Pimenta officinalis* (allspice), occurring as a colorless, yellow, or reddish liquid with the odor and taste of allspice. Used as a carminative, stimulant, and flavoring agent. Called also *allspice o*. **raw linseed o.,** linseed o. **ricinus o.,** castor o. **o. of rose,** the volatile oil from fresh flowers of *Rosa gallica, R. damascena,* and other species of roses, occurring as a colorless or pale yellow, viscous liquid with a fragant odor, which is soluble in fatty oils and chloroform and slightly soluble in water and ethanol. Used as a flavoring agent for lozenges and ointments and a perfuming agent. Called also *attar of roses*. **safflower o.,** a drying oil from the seeds of the safflower, *Carthomus tinctorius*, occurring as a straw-colored liquid. It is an edible, cholesterol-free oil used in the production of drugs, dietetic foods, hydrogenated shortening, alkyl resins, paints, and other products. **spearmint o.,** the volatile oil distilled from the fresh overground parts of *Mentha spicata (M. viridis)* or *Mentha cardiaca*, occurring as a colorless, yellow, or greenish yellow liquid with the characteristic odor and taste of spearmint, which is soluble in ethanol and, slightly, in water. Used chiefly as a flavoring agent; has been used as a carminative. **sweet o.,** olive o. **sweet almond o.,** almond o. **sweet birch o.,** methyl SALICYLATE. **sweet orange o.,** o. of orange. **tangatangan o.,** castor o. **teaberry o.,** methyl SALICYLATE. **theobroma o.,** the fat from the roasted seed of *Theobroma cacao*, occurring as a yellowish, white solid with a faint, agreeable odor and a bland or chocolate-like taste, depending on the method of extraction, which is soluble in boiling alcohol, ether, and chloroform, slightly soluble in cold alcohol, and insoluble in water. It consists of glycerides of stearic, palmitic, oleic, lauric, and lower fatty acids, and melts at between 30 and 35°C. Used in dentistry as a protector against dehydration of soft tissues and to temporarily protect silicate cements from moisture during setting or to protect them from dehydrating after they are set. Also used in suppositories, ointments, and emollients. Called also *cacao butter* and *cocoa butter*. **thyme o.,** the volatile oil distilled from the flowering plant of *Thymus vulgaris*, occurring as a colorless to reddish-brown liquid with a pleasant odor of thymol and a sharp taste, which is soluble in ethanol and, slightly, in water. Used as a flavoring agent for drugs; has been used as a rubefacient, expectorant, counterirritant, antiseptic, and carminative agent. **turpentine o.,** the volatile oil distilled from the oleoresin obtained from *Pinus palustris* and other species of *Pinus* (pine), occurring as a colorless liquid with a disagreeable odor and taste, which is soluble in ethanol, insoluble in water, and miscible with benzene, chloroform, ether, carbon disulfide, and oils. Used chiefly as a solvent for oils, resins, and varnishes. Also used as a rubefacient and counterirritant. Exposure to its vapors may cause headache, vertigo, nausea, and eye irritation. Ingestion may cause bladder irritation and severe poisoning. Called also *spirit of turpentine*. **turpentine o., rectified,** turpentine oil treated with sodium hydroxide and distillation to remove its disagreeable odor and taste, otherwise having the same properties as turpentine oil. **o. of vitriol,** sulfuric ACID. **volatile o.,** an oil which evaporates readily. The volatile oils occur in aromatic plants, hence their characteristic odor. Called also *distilled o., essential o.,* and *ethereal o*. **volatile bitter almond o.,** almond o., bitter. **white mineral o.,** mineral o. **o. of wintergreen,** methyl SALICYLATE.

ointment (oint′ment) [L. *unguentum*] a semisolid preparation for external application to the body, and usually containing a medicinal substance. Ointments are applied to the skin or mucous membranes by inunction and should be of such composition that they soften, but not necessarily melt, when applied. Called also *salve, unction,* and *unguent*. **absorption o.,** one with a water-absorbing base. **o. base,** a vehicle for medicinal substances intended for external application to the body, selected for their compatibility with the skin or mucous membrane, stability, pliability, nonirritating and nonsensitizing properties, inertness, ability to absorb water or other liquids, and ability to release incorporated medications into the skin or mucous membrane. Ointment bases may be classified as oleaginous bases (including vegetable oils, animal fats, or mineral oils), absorption bases (characterized by water-absorbing properties), emulsion bases (including water-in-oil and oil-in-water emulsions), and water-soluble bases. **emulsion o.,** one with a base that is an emulsion, either an oil-in-water or water-in-oil. **Nephron benzocaine o.,** trademark for a benzocaine preparation used in dental anesthesia for topical application, 100 mg of which contains 18 gm of benzocaine and various amounts of flavoring agents in a polyethylene glycol base. **oleaginous o.,** one with an oily ointment base. **simple o.,** 1. white o. 2. yellow o. **Topical o.,** trademark for an anesthetic ointment for topical application, containing 18 percent benzocaine, 0.1 percent benzalkonium chloride, and various amounts of flavoring agents dissolved in a water-soluble polyethylene glycol base. **water-soluble o.,** one with a water-soluble base. **white o.,** an oleaginous ointment consisting of 95 percent white petrolatum and 5 percent white wax. Used as an emollient or vehicle for other ointments. Called also *simple o*. **yellow o.,** an oleaginous ointment consisting of 95 percent petrolatum and 5 percent yellow wax. Used as an emollient or vehicle for other ointments. Called also *simple o*.

Oktadin trademark for *guanethidine*.

Okuniewski see Sterling-Okuniewski SIGN.

-ol in chemical nomenclature, a name ending indicating an alcohol or phenol.

olea (o′le-ah) [L.] plural of *oleum*.

oleaginous (o″le-aj′ĭ-nus) [L. *oleaginus*] oily; greasy; unctuous.

Oleandocetine trademark for *troleandomycin*.

oleandomycin (o″le-an′do-mi″sin) a broad-spectrum macrolide antibiotic, $C_{35}H_{61}NO_{12}$, elaborated by *Streptomyces antibioticus*, occurring as a white amorphous powder that is readily soluble in acids, methanol, ethanol, butanol, and acetone, moderately soluble in water, and insoluble in hexane, ether, and carbon tetrachloride. It has properties similar to those of erythromycin, but is less effective and more toxic. Oleandomycin is effective against gram-positive cocci, including staphylococci, streptococci, and pneumococci, and against strains of gram-negative bacteria, including *Haemophilus, Mycoplasma, Neisseria, Clostridium, Treponema, Fusobacterium, Borrelia vincenti,* and *Corynebacterium*. Trademarks: Amimycin, Landomycin, Matromycin, Romicil.

olefin (o′le-fin) [*oleo-* + L. *facere* to make] an unsaturated hydrocarbon with a general formula C_nH_{2n}, having one or more double bonds, thus being chemically reactive. See also ALKENE.

olein (o′le-in) triolein.

oleo- [L. *oleum* oil] a combining form denoting relationship to oil.

oleoinfusion (o′le-o-in-fu′zhun) [*oleo-* + *infusion*] a preparation made by infusing a drug in oil.

oleoresin (o″le-o-rez′in) 1. a semisolid mixture of the resin and the essential oil of plants, such as pines and other plants, from which they are derived, having a pungent taste and a peculiar odor. Sometimes called *balsam*. 2. a compound prepared by exhausting a drug by percolation with a volatile solvent, such as acetone, alcohol, or ether, and evaporating the solvent.

oleosus (o″le-o′sus) [L.] oily; greasy; accompanied by an oily secretion.

oleovitamin (o″le-o-vi′tah-min) a fish liver oil preparation containing vitamin A or vitamins A and D; used as dietary supplements. **o. D$_2$,** VITAMIN D$_2$. **o. D$_3$,** VITAMIN D$_3$.

oleum (o′le-um) pl. o′lea [L.] 1. oil. 2. sulfuric acid, fuming; see under ACID. **o. amyg′dalae expres′sum,** almond OIL. **o. ca′ri,** caraway OIL.

olfaction (ol-fak′shun) [L. *olfacere* to smell] smelling; the sense of smell.

olfactory (ol-fak′to-re) [L. *olfacere* to smell] pertaining to the sense of smell.

oligemia (ol″ĭ-ge′me-ah) [*oligo-* + Gr. *haima* blood + *-ia*] a condition in which there is a decreased volume of the blood. See also ANEMIA, OLIGOCHROMEMIA and OLIGOCYTHEMIA.

oligo- [Gr. *oligos* little] a combining form meaning few, little, or scanty.

oligochromemia (ol″ĭ-go-kro-me′me-ah) [*oligo-* + Gr. *chrōma* color + *haima* blood + *-ia*] a condition in which there is a decreased volume of hemoglobin in the blood. See also ANEMIA, OLIGEMIA, and OLIGOCYTHEMIA.

oligocythemia (ol″ĭ-go-si-the′me-ah) [*oligo-* + *-cyte* + Gr. *haima* blood + *-ia*] deficiency of the red cell elements in the blood. Called also *oligocytosis*. See also ANEMIA, ERYTHROCYTE count, OLIGEMIA, and OLIGOCHROMEMIA. See also table of *Reference Values in Hematology* in Appendix.

oligocytosis (ol″ĭ-go-si-to′sis) oligocythemia.

oligodendrocyte (ol″ĭ-go-den′dro-sīt) [*oligo-* + Gr. *dendron* tree + *kytos* a hollow vessel] a neuroglial cell of ectodermal origin, having a round to oval nucleus but no nucleoli, which is rich in chromatin, and has several slender, long processes. They are found in the central nervous system near smaller blood vessels, as satellites to some large nerve cells, or between the fibers of the white substance, and are believed to be involved in the formation and preservation of the myelin sheath. Collectively, such cells are called *oligodendroglia*.

oligodendroglia (ol″ĭ-go-den-drog′le-ah) [*oligo-* + Gr. *dendron* tree + *neuroglia*] the tissue composed of oligodendrocytes.

oligodontia (ol″ĭ-go-don′she-ah) [*oligo-* Gr. *odous* tooth *-ia*] absence of many teeth, usually associated with small size of the existing teeth and other anomalies. See also ANODONTIA, HYPODONTIA, and PSEUDOANODONTIA.

oligodynamic (ol′ĭ-go-di-nam′ik) [*oligo-* + Gr. *dynamis* power] active in minute quantities, said of the effect of heavy metal ions on the living cell.

oligophrenia (ol″ĭ-go-fre′ne-ah) [*oligo-* + Gr. *phrēn* mind + *-ia*] former name for defective mental development. See mental RETARDATION. **phenylpyruvic o.,** phenylketonuria.

oliguria (ol″ĭ-gu′re-ah) [*oligo-* + Gr. *ouron* urine + *-ia*] a condition characterized by a diminished output of urine.

Ollier's layer [Léopold Louis Xavier Edouard *Ollier*, French surgeon, 1830–1900] see under LAYER.

ololiqui (o″lo-lik′e) a hallucinogenic principle from the seeds of the morning glory, *Rivea corymbosa*.

Ol. oliv. abbreviation for L. *o′leum oli′vae*, olive oil.

Olsen stiffness tester see under TESTER.

o.m. abbreviation for L. *om′ni ma′ne*, every morning.

-oma [Gr. *ōma*, perhaps adapted from *onkōma* a swelling] a word termination meaning tumor, swelling, or neoplasm of the part indicated by the stem to which it is attached. Hence, *osteoma* (*osteo-* + *-oma*) is a tumor of a bone.

Omca trademark for *fluphenazine hydrochloride* (see under FLUPHENAZINE).

omega (o-meg′ah) ω,Ω, the twenty-fourth and last letter of the Greek alphabet.

Omn. bih. abbreviation for L. *om′ni biho′ra*, every two hours.

Omn. hor. abbreviation for L. *om′ni ho′ra*, every hour.

Omniflex trademark for a *polysulfide impression material* (see under MATERIAL).

Omn. noct. abbreviation for L. *om′ni noc′te*, every night.

Omnopon Pantopon.

omohyoid (o″mo-hi′oid) [Gr. *ōmos* shoulder + *hyoid*] pertaining to the shoulder and the hyoid bone.

omohyoideus (o″mo-hi-oi′de-us) omohyoid MUSCLE.

OMPA OCTAMETHYL pyrophosphoramide.

omphalo- [Gr. *omphalos* the navel] a combining form denoting relationship to the umbilicus.

omphalocele (om′fah-lo-sēl″) [*omphalo-* + Gr. *kēlē* hernia] congenital protrusion of the intestine through an abdominal wall defect at the umbilicus.

ON onlay.

o.n. abbreviation for L. *om′ni noc′te*, each night.

onco- [Gr. *onkos* mass, bulk] a combining form denoting relationship to a neoplasm, tumor, swelling, or mass.

oncocytoma (ong″ko-si-to′mah) [*oncocyte* + *-oma*] oxyphil ADENOMA.

oncogenesis (ong″ko-jen′ĕ-sis) [*onco-* + Gr. *genesis* production, generation] the production or generation of neoplasms.

oncogenic (ong″ko-jen′ik) giving rise to neoplasms or causing oncogenesis, as oncogenic or tumor producing viruses. Called also *cancerigenic*.

oncogenicity (ong″ko-jĕ-nis′ĭ-te) the quality or property of being able to cause neoplasm formation.

oncology (ong-kol′o-je) [*onco-* + *-logy*] the sum of knowledge or study of tumors or neoplasms. Formerly called *cancerology*.

oncolysis (ong-kol′ĭ-sis) [*onco-* + Gr. *lysis* dissolution] the lysis or destruction of tumor cells.

oncolytic (ong″ko-lit′ik) pertaining to or characterized by oncolysis.

oncornavirus (ong″kor″nah-vi′rus) [*onco-* + *RNA* + *virus*] Oncovirinae.

oncosis (ong-ko′sis) a condition characterized by the development of tumors or neoplasms.

oncotic (ong-kot′ik) pertaining to, caused by, or marked by, swelling.

Oncovin trademark for *vincristine sulfate* (see under VINCRISTINE).

Oncovirinae (ong″ko-vi′rĭ-ne) a subfamily of retroviruses, having virions that are approximately spherical, about 80 to 120 nm in diameter, their envelope projecting with knobs and spikes, and containing an icosahedral core shell within which there is a ribonucleoprotein structure. Oncoviruses cause tumors in avian, mammalian, reptilian, and piscine hosts. Called also *leukovirus* and *oncornavirus*. **type A O.,** viral particles which are precursor forms of oncoviruses, represented in thin sections of infected cells as complete or incomplete ringlike nucleoids enclosed in shell membranes. **type B O.,** viral particles which, in thin sections of infected cells, have dense eccentric nucleoids within inner shells that themselves are contained in unit membrane envelopes covered with spikes. This group of oncoviruses causes mainly mammary tumors, e.g., mouse mammary carcinoma; a related virus may be associated with human mammary cancer. **type C O.,** viral particles which, in thin sections of infected cells, have central spherical nucleoids contained in unit membrane envelopes. All leukemia and sarcoma viruses belong to this type.

oncovirus (ong″ko-vi′rus) [*onco-* + *virus*] any virus of the subfamily Oncovirinae.

-one [Gr. *ōnē*, a feminine partronymic suffix] in chemistry, a suffix used in forming the name of a compound from that of a parent compound, or from a root representing the occurrence of the compound, or from a root representing a characteristic property of the compound, such as *acetone* from *acetic acid*, *hydrazone* from *hydrazine*, *coumarone* from *courmarin*, *histone* from Gr. *histion*, animal tissue, *peptone* from Gr. *pepsis* digestion, and so on.

One-Iron trademark for a preparation of *ferrous fumarate* (see under FUMARATE).

onlay (on′la) 1. something that rests over something else; overlay. 2. a cast metal restoration which onlays or overlays cusps, thereby lending strength to the restored tooth. See overlay DENTURE, and see also INLAY. 3. a graft applied or laid on the surface of an organ or structure. Abbreviated *ON*. **cast gold o.,** the gold casting containing an intracoronal design, also covering the cusps of the restored tooth. **epithelial o.,** an epithelial graft the edges of which are not completely approximated to the edges of the wound, thus permitting new epithelium to grow out around the margin. See also epithelial INLAY.

on-line (on′līn) operating as part of or directly connected with the main computer.

ontogenic (on″to-jen′ik) pertaining to ontogeny.

ontogeny (on-toj′ĕ-ne) [Gr. *on* existing ┼ *gennan* to produce] the development of the individual organism, from sexual repro-

ONTOGENY

Prenatal life	*Ovum.* Fertilization to end of first week. *Embryo.* Second to eighth week, inclusive. *Fetus.* Third to tenth lunar month, inclusive.	

Birth

Postnatal life	*Newborn.* Neonatal period; birth to end of second week. *Infancy.* Third week until assumption of erect posture at end of first year.	
	Childhood.	*Early.* Milk-tooth period; second to sixth year, inclusive. *Middle.* Permanent-tooth period; 7 to 9 or 10 years, inclusive. *Later.* Prepuberal period; from 9 or 10 years to 12–15 years in females and to 13–16 years in males.

Puberty

Adolescence. The six years following puberty.

Adult. Prime and transition. Between 20 and 60 years.
Old age and senescence. From 60 years on.

Death

(From L. B. Arey: Developmental Anatomy. 7th ed. Philadelphia, W. B. Saunders Co., 1974.)

duction to death. See also EMBRYOLOGY, LIFE, and PHYLOGENY. See table.

oo- / operation 563

oo- [Gr. *ōon* egg] a combining form denoting relationship to an egg or ovum. See also words beginning ovo-.

oocyte (o'o-sīt) [*oo-* + *-cyte*] a developing egg cell in the ovary. It derives during the third month of fetal life from the oogonium, which differentiates into the *primary oocyte*, having reached prophase of the first meiotic division at birth, but remains in the suspended state (dictyotene) until sexual maturation is reached. The *secondary oocyte* is derived from the primary oocyte shortly before ovulation by the first and second meiotic divisions, but it is arrested at metaphase or anaphase up to the time of fertilization. If fertilized, the secondary oocyte divides into an ootid and the second polar body; otherwise it perishes. See also OOGENESIS.

oogenesis (o″o-jen′ĕ-sis) [*oo-* + Gr. *genesis* production] the formation of the ovum. The process begins with the development of the oogonium (primordial germ cell) in the follicular tissue of the fetal ovary. By the third month of fetal life, the oogonium begins to differentiate into the primary oocyte which, at birth has reached the prophase of the first meiotic division but remains in the suspended state (dictyotene) until sexual maturation is reached. With puberty, the first meiotic division resumes and the follicles begin to mature. By telophase, each daughter cell receives 23 chromosomes, giving rise to one functional gamete and three (sometimes two) abortive polar bodies. The second meiotic division takes place in the secondary oocyte but is arrested at metaphase or anaphase up to the time of fertilization. Cell division is completed after fertilization, usually after the oocyte has already descended into the uterus. Cf. SPERMATOGENESIS.

oogonium (o″o-go′ne-um) [*oo-* + Gr. *gonē* generation] the primordial germ cell of the ovary that develops in the follicular tissue of the fetal ovary, and begins to differentiate by mitosis and meiosis by the third month of fetal life into the primary oocyte. See also OOGENESIS.

ootid (o′o-tid) a ripe ovum; one of four cells derived from the two consecutive divisions of the primary oocyte. See also OOCYTE and OOGENESIS.

Op opisthocranion.

opacifier (o-pas″ĭ-fi′er) a substance that renders a translucent or transparent object opaque. Metallic oxides, particularly zirconium oxide, are the most common opacifiers used in dental porcelain. Called also *opaquing agent*.

opacity (o-pas′ĭ-te) [L. *opacitas*] 1. the state or quality of being impenetrable to rays or light. 2. An opaque area.

opalescence (o″pah-les′enz) the quality or state of being opalescent. **fixation o.,** a temporary cloudiness of a radiograph sometimes occurring in freshly made fixer which soon disappears after washing and drying, which is believed to be caused by the reaction of gelatin to high concentrations of sodium thiosulfate in a fresh fixer; it may also occur when ammonium thiosulfate is used as a clearing agent.

opalescent (o″pah-les′ent) showing a milky iridescence, like an opal.

opalgia (o-pal′je-ah) [Gr. *ops* face + *-algia*] facial NEURALGIA.

Opalski's syndrome [Adam *Opalski*, Polish physician, 1879–1963] see under SYNDROME.

opaque (o-pāk′) [Lat. *opacus*] impervious to light rays, or by extension to roentgen rays or other electromagnetic vibrations; neither transparent nor translucent.

OPD outpatient department; see OUTPATIENT, ambulatory CARE, and ambulatory hospital CARE.

open (o′pen) 1. exposed, uncovered, as an open wound. 2. interrupted, as an open circuit, so that the electric current is interrupted. 3. not closed or obstructed.

opener (o′pe-ner) a device used for opening something that is closed. **dynamic bite o.,** trismus STENT.

opening (o′pen-ing) 1. an aperture, orifice, or open space. See also OSTIUM. 2. the act or process of becoming open or creating an opening. **access o.,** root canal ACCESS. **anterior o. of orbital cavity,** orbital APERTURE. **external o. of aqueduct of cochlea,** external aperture of canaliculus of cochlea; see under APERTURE. **o. for lesser superficial petrosal nerve,** superior aperture of tympanic canaliculus; see under APERTURE. **midpalatal o., midpalatal suture o.,** separation of the palatine bones at the midpalatal suture, brought about by the action of an orthodontic appliance. See also maxillary EXPANSION. **nasal o. of facial skeleton,** piriform APERTURE. **orbital o.,** orbital APERTURE. **piriform o.,** piriform APERTURE. **o. for smaller superficial petrosal nerve,** superior aperture of tympanic canaliculus; see under APERTURE. **o. of sphenoidal sinus,** APERTURE of sphenoid sinus. **superior o. of tympanic canal,** superior aperture of tympanic canaliculus; see under APERTURE. **o. for tympanic branch of**

glossopharyngeal nerve, inferior aperture of tympanic canaliculus; see under APERTURE. **vertical o.,** vertical DIMENSION.

operable (o′per-ah-b'l) subject to being operated upon with a reasonable degree of success; appropriate for surgical removal.

operation (op″er-a′shun) [L. *operatio*] 1. any act performed with instruments or by the hands of a surgeon; a surgical procedure. 2. any effect produced by an agent employed in therapy. **Abbé-Eastlander o.,** the transfer of a full-thickness flap from one lip to fill a defect in the other lip, using an arterial pedicle to ensure survival of the graft. **Anderson's o.,** longitudinal splitting of a tendon followed by sliding along of the cut surface to produce lengthening of the tendon. **Anel's o.,** dilatation of the lacrimal duct with a probe, followed by an astringent injection. **Baum's o.,** one formerly used for the stretching of the facial nerve by an incision below the ear. **Billroth's o.,** 1. excision of the tongue by making a transverse incision below the symphysis of the jaw and joining it by two incisions, one on each side, parallel to the body of the mandible, with preliminary ligation of the lingual arteries. 2. partial resection of the stomach. 3. pyloroplasty with anterior gastroenterostomy. **Blaskovics' o.,** for epicanthus, resection of a semilunar piece of skin from an epicanthal fold nearer to the side of the nose than the canthus, followed by closure with black silk sutures. **Bose's o.,** a method of tracheotomy. **Brewer's o.,** closure of wounds of arteries by application of a special rubber plaster. **Brophy's o.,** one for cleft palate (with or without cleft lip), consisting of the forcible approximation of the freshened palate margins, which are held in position by special sutures supported by lead plates. **Burckhardt's o.,** a method of incision formerly used to drain a retropharyngeal abscess from the outside of the neck. **Caldwell-Luc o.,** 1. the operation of opening into the maxillary sinus by way of an incision into the supradental fossa opposite the premolar teeth, usually done to remove tooth roots or abnormal tissue from the sinus. 2. in compound zygomaticomaxillary fractures, the packing of the maxillary sinus by approaching the atrium through the canine fossa of the maxilla above the tooth apices, thus allowing the reduction of displaced fragments of the zygoma by upward and outward pressure. Fragments that may herniate into the maxillary sinus are elevated into position and held by packing the sinus with selvage gauze permeated with petrolatum. An antrostomy is performed beneath the inferior turbinate bone, and the end of the packing is brought out into the nasal cavity or through a mucosal incision. **Carnochan's o.,** one used in the past to remove Meckel's ganglion and a part of the fifth cranial nerve in the treatment of neuralgia; incision is made below the orbit, and the ganglion is reached by trephination through the maxillary antrum. **Carpue's o.,** Indian RHINOPLASTY. **Carter's o.,** reconstruction of the bridge of the nose by transplanting a piece of bone from the rib. **Cheever's o.,** complete tonsillectomy through the neck, no longer performed. **Chiene's o.,** exposure of the retropharyngeal space by lateral cervical incision along the posterior border of the sternocleidomastoid muscle; no longer performed. **Coakley's o.,** one used in the past in diseases of the frontal sinus by incising through the cheek, removing the anterior wall, and curetting away the mucous membrane. **Commando's o.,** one for management of oral cancer, consisting of resection of the primary lesion and the regional lymphatic nodes. **Denonvilliers' o.,** plastic correction of a defective ala nasi by transferring a triangular flap from the adjacent side of the nose. **Edlan-Mejchar o.,** a vestibular extension operation which produces vestibular deepening in patients without periodontal pockets, but with little or no gingiva remaining around the mandibular anterior teeth. **Esser o.,** epithelial INLAY. **exploratory o.,** surgical incision into an area of the body for the purpose of inspection and palpation of organs and tissues to determine the cause of unexplained symptoms. **Fergusson's o.,** Fergusson's INCISION. **flap o.,** any operation involving the raising of a full-thickness mucoperiosteal flap of tissue. In periodontology, an operation to secure greater access to granulation tissue and osseous defects, consisting of detachment of the gingivae, the alveolar mucosa, and/or a portion of the palatal mucosa. In oral and maxillofacial surgery, an operation to expose the overlying bone and then remove it in the surgical extraction of a tooth. **Gillies' o.,** a technique for reducing fractures of the zygoma and the zygomatic arch through an incision in the temporal region above the hairline. **Grant's o.,** excision of tumors of the lip by removing a square block of tissue containing the tumor, and then making an oblique incision extending down and out from each angle of the wound.

The triangular flaps thus formed are drawn toward the center and sutured. **Hartley-Krause o.,** excision of the gasserian ganglion and its roots to relieve facial neruralgia; no longer performed. **Heath's o.,** division of the ascending rami of the mandible with a saw for ankylosis, performed within the oral cavity; now rarely performed. **Hotchkiss' o.,** in epithelioma of the cheek, surgical removal of the lateral half of the mandible and part of the maxilla, followed by plastic restoration of tissue by means of a flap drawn up from the side of the neck. **Indian o.,** Indian RHINOPLASTY. **Italian o.,** tagliacotian RHINOPLASTY. **Kazanjian's o.,** 1. a technique of surgical extension of the buccal vestibular sulcus of edentulous ridges to increase their height and to improve denture retention. 2. in compound zygomaticomaxillary fractures, the use of extraskeletal fixation for support of the fractured zygomatic compound. A small hole is drilled through the infraorbital rim, and a stainless steel wire is inserted with both ends brought out through the wound, where they are twisted together into a loop or hook. Rubber band traction between the suspension wire and an outrigger on a head cap provides support for the zygomatic fragments. Called also *Kazanjian's suspension method.* **Keegan's o.,** a modification of the Indian rhinoplasty for reconstructing the nose, the flap being taken mainly from one side of the forehead. **Kelly's o.,** arytenoidopexy. **Killian's o.,** excision of the anterior wall of the frontal sinus, removal of the diseased tissue, and formation of a permanent communication with the nose. **King's o.,** arytenoidopexy. **Kocher's o.,** 1. thyroidectomy performed by one median incision and two lateral ones, the latter being carried upward almost to the angle of the jaw. 2. excision of the tongue through an incision extending from the symphysis of the jaw to the hyoid bone and thence to the mastoid process. **Körte-Ballance o.,** anastomosis of the facial and hypoglossal nerves. **Krimer's o.,** uranoplasty in which mucoperiosteal flaps from each side of the palatal cleft are sutured together at the median line. **Krönlein's o.,** 1. resection of the outer wall of the orbit for the removal of an orbital tumor without excising the eye. 2. exposure of the third branch of the trigeminal nerve for facial neuralgia; no longer performed. **Lauren's o.,** a plastic operation for closure of a cicatricial opening following mastoid operation. **Liston's o.,** one for the excision of the upper jaw. **Lizars' o.,** excision of the upper jaw by a curved incision extending from the angle of the mouth to the malar bone. **Neuber's o.,** filling a bone cavity with skin flaps taken from the sides of the wound. **Partsch's o.,** a technique for marsupialization of dental cysts; see MARSUPIALIZATION. **Regnoli's o.,** excision of the tongue through a median opening below the lower jaw, reaching from the chin to the hyoid bone. **Reverdin's o.,** a method for taking an epidermic graft and transplanting it to a defect. **Ridell's o.,** excision of the anterior and inferior walls of the frontal sinus for chronic inflammation. **Schede's o.,** excision of the necrosed part of a bone, all dead bone and diseased tissue being scraped away, and the cavity permitted to fill with blood clot, the latter being kept moist and aseptic with a cover of gauze and rubber tissue, and eventually becoming organized. **Schönbein's o.,** staphyloplasty in which a flap of mucous membrane from the posterior wall of the pharynx is stitched to the velum palati, shutting off the nose from the mouth. **Sédillot's o.,** 1. a method of staphylorrhaphy. 2. a flap operation for restoring the upper lip. **Serre's o.,** one for correction of skin contractures that distort the angle of the mouth, involving switching of a skin and subcutaneous tissue flap from one lip to another. **Sistrunk's o.,** a surgical procedure for removal of thyroglossal cysts and sinuses. **Sluder's o.,** removal of the tonsil along with its capsule. **Sorrin o.,** a flap technique in the treatment of periodontal abscesses, whereby a semilunar incision is made in the attached gingiva below the lesion, and the flap is raised to provide an access to the abscess for curettage. **Stein's o.,** one for reconstruction of the lower lip with flaps taken from the upper lip. **tagliacotian o.,** tagliacotian RHINOPLASTY. **Textor's o.,** removal of thin, split-thickness skin grafts by means of a razor, skin-graft cutting knife, or dermatome. **Thiersch's o.,** removal of skin grafts by means of a razor. **Toti's o.,** dacryocystorhinostomy. **Whitehead's o.,** removal of the tongue with scissors, the operation being performed within the mouth.

operative (op′er-ah-tiv, op′rah-tiv, op′ĕ-ra″tiv) [L. *operativus*] 1. pertaining to an operation. 2. effective; not inert.

operator (op′er-a-tor) 1. one who performs an operation. 2. operator GENE.

operatory (op″ĕ-rah-to′re) a working space, as an area or room equipped with a dental chair and appropriate equipment in which the dentist provides dental treatment for his patients. Called also *treatment area.*

opercula (o-per′ku-lah) [L.] plural of *operculum.*

opercular (o-per′ku-lar) pertaining to an operculum.

operculectomy (o-per″ku-lek′to-me) the surgical removal of a mucosal flap partially or completely covering an unerupted tooth.

operculitis (o-per″ku-li′tis) pericoronitis.

operculum (o-per′ku-lum), pl. *oper′cula* [L.] a lid or covering structure. **dental o.,** the hood of gingival tissue overlying the crown of an erupting tooth. Called also *odontoclamis* and *tooth hood.*

operon (op′ĕ-ron) [L. *opera* exertion + Gr. *-on* neuter ending] a segment of a chromosome consisting of an operator gene and the closely linked structural gene or genes whose action it controls; the operon codes for single messenger RNA molecules and acts as a unit of genetic transcription and genetic regulation.

ophryon (of′re-on) [Gr. *ophrys* eyebrow + *-on* neuter ending] a craniometric landmark located at the middle point of the transverse supraorbital line. Called also *supranasal point.*

Ophthaline trademark for *proparacaine hydrochloride* (see under PROPARACAINE).

ophthalm- see OPHTHALMO-.

ophthalmia (of-thal′me-ah) [Gr., *ophthalmos* eye + *-ia*] severe inflammation of the eye, or its deep structures.

ophthalmo-, ophthalm- [Gr. *ophthalmos* eye] a combining form denoting relationship to the eye.

ophthalmologist (of′thal-mol′o-jist) a physician who specializes in the diagnosis and medical and surgical treatment of diseases and defects of the eye and related structures.

ophthalmology (of″thal-mol′o-je) [*ophthalmo-* + *-logy*] that branch of medicine dealing with the eye, its anatomy, physiology, pathology, and related subjects.

ophthalmoplegia (of-thal″mo-ple′je-ah) [*ophthalmo-* + Gr. *plēgē* stroke + *-ia*] paralysis of the ocular muscles. **painful o.,** Tolosa-Hunt SYNDROME. **sympathetic o.,** Bernard-Horner SYNDROME.

ophthalmorhinostomatohygrosis (of-thal″mo-ri″no-sto″mah-to-hi′gro-sis) Creyx-Lévy SYNDROME.

Ophthetic trademark for *proparacaine hydrochloride* (see under PROPARACAINE).

opiate (o′pe-āt) 1. an opium alkaloid. Principal opiates include morphine, codeine, thebaine, and paraverine. 2. a term sometimes used to refer to a narcotic analgesic; opioid.

Opino trademark for *nylidrin hydrochloride* (see under NYLIDRIN).

Opinsul trademark for *sulfamethoxypyridazine.*

opioid (o′pī-oid) [*opium* + Gr. *eidos* form, shape] 1. opium-like. 2. narcotic ANALGESIC. **o. antagonist,** narcotic ANTAGONIST. **o. receptor,** opioid RECEPTOR.

Opis for opisthion.

opisthiobasial (o-pis″the-o-ba′se-al) pertaining to or connecting opisthion and basion; it is the plane of the foramen magnum of the skull.

opisthion (o-pis′the-on) [Gr. *opisthios* rear, posterior] the midpoint of the posterior border of the foramen magnum. Abbreviated *Opis* or *Ops.* See also BASION. See illustration at CEPHALOMETRY.

opisthionasial (o-pis″the-o-na′ze-al) pertaining to or connecting the opisthion and nasion.

opistho- [Gr. *opisthen* behind, at the back] a combining form meaning backward and/or denoting relationship to the back.

opisthocranion (o-pis″tho-kra′ne-on) [*opistho-* + Gr. *kranion* the upper part of the head] a craniometric landmark determined instrumentally to indicate the posterior end of the maximum cranial length measured along the midline of the glabella. Abbreviated *Op.* See also maximum occipital POINT and illustration at CEPHALOMETRY.

opisthogenia (o-pis″tho-je′ne-ah) defective development of the jaws following ankylosis of the jaw.

opisthognathism (o″pis-thog′nah-thizm) the condition of having receding jaws.

opisthotonos (o″pis-thot′o-nos) [*opistho-* + Gr. *tonos* tension] a form of spasm in which the head and the heels are bent backward, associated with convex dorsal arching of the back, occurring most commonly in tetanus and in shock therapy, sometimes so violently as to cause compression fractures of the vertebrae.

Opitz's syndrome, trigonocephaly syndrome [John M. *Opitz,* American physician, born 1935] see under SYNDROME. See also Herrmann-Opitz SYNDROME, Herrmann-Pallister-Opitz SYNDROME, and Smith-Lemli-Opitz SYNDROME.

Opitz-Frias syndrome [J. M. *Opitz;* J. L. *Frias*] G SYNDROME.

opium (o′pe-um) [L.; Gr. *opion*] the air-dried exudate from incised unripe capsules of *Papaver somniferum* or its variety, *album,* yielding some 20 alkaloids: morphine (about 9.5 percent by weight), codeine, thebaine, and papaverine, being the most important clinically, because of their narcotic and analgesic effects. Therapeutically, opium is used chiefly as a narcotic analgesic, sedative expectorant, and antidiarrheal agent. Crude opium is largely used in the production of morphine, codeine, and other opium alkaloids. Because it is highly addictive, the production of opium is restricted, and the cultivation of the plants from which it is obtained is prohibited by most nations under an international agreement. Called also *crude o.* and *gum o.* **camphorated o. tincture,** paregoric. **crude o.,** opium. **denarcotized o., o. deodora'tum, deodorized o.,** powdered opium from which the odor and certain nauseating constituents have been removed by treatment with purified petroleum benzin. Used as a narcotic and antidiarrheal agent. **granulated o.,** opium reduced to a coarse powder produced by drying crude opium at not above 70° C and adjusted with lactose or other inert diluent to contain 10–10.5% anhydrous morphine. Used chiefly for preparing tincture of opium. It is a narcotic analgesic; abuse leads to addiction. **gum o.,** opium. **powdered o., o. pulvera'tum,** opium dried at a temperature not exceeding 70° C, reduced to a very fine powder, and adjusted with lactose or other inert diluent to contain 10 to 10.5 percent of anhydrous morphine. Used as a narcotic analgesic. See also PAREGORIC. **o. tincture,** a preparation, obtained by percolation of granulated opium and concentration of the product, each 100 ml of which yields 0.95 to 1.05 gm. of anhydrous morphine; used as an antiperistaltic. Called also *laudanum.*

Opotow Jelset trademark for an *irreversible hydrocolloid impression material* (see under MATERIAL).

Ops opisthion.

opsonin (op-so'nin) [Gr. *opsonein* to buy victuals] 1. an antibody that renders bacteria and other cells susceptible to phagocytosis. 2. a nonantibody substance, which may be derived from the C3 or C4 component of complement, capable of rendering bacteria susceptible to phagocytosis. The basic proteins, protamine, globulin, and lysozyme have been shown to be opsonins. Two proteins, one a β-globulin and the other an α_1-globulin, are opsonic without the aid of complement and are not basic proteins. These are called *phagocytosis promoting factor (PPF).*

opsonization (op"so-ni-za'shun) the rendering of bacteria and other antigenic or nonantigenic elements subject to phagocytosis by coating them with opsonins.

Optaloy trademark for an *amalgam alloy* (see under AMALGAM).

Optaloy II trademark for a *high copper alloy* (see under ALLOY).

optician (op-tish"an) a person who is expert in the science, craft, and art of optics as applied to the translation, filling, and adapting of ophthalmic prescriptions, products, and accessories. The licensing of dispensing opticians varies from state to state.

optimal (op'ti-mal) the best; the most favorable.

Optimil trademark for *methaqualone hydrochloride* (see under METHAQUALONE).

Optimycin trademark for *methacycline.*

option (op'shun) the power or freedom of choosing from among various alternatives. **dual o.,** an option, provided by federal legislation, which requires employers to give their employees the choice to enroll in a local health maintenance organization rather than in a conventional employer-sponsored health program. Called also *dual choice.* **high o.,** in health insurance, one of two or more levels of insurance which may be chosen by the subscriber, whereby the benefits covered are essentially the same except that the high option provides lower deductibles and other cost-sharing requirements and more generous time or quantity limits than the low option, the premium for the high option being higher. **low o.,** in health insurance, levels of insurance which may be chosen by the subscriber, whereby the benefits covered are essentially the same but the low option provides higher deductibles and other cost-sharing requirements and less generous time or quantity limits than the high option, the premium for the low option being lower.

opto- [Gr. *optos* seen] a combining form meaning visible, or denoting relationship to vision or sight.

optometrist (op-tom'e-trist) a practitioner of optometry, who is a graduate of an approved school with a program leading to a Doctor of Optometry degree (DO), and who is licensed by a state board or committee of optometry to examine and test the eyes and to treat visual defects by prescribing and adapting corrective lenses and other optical aids, and by establishing programs of exercises.

optometry (op'tom'e-tre) measurement of the powers of vision and the adaptation of prisms or lenses for the aid thereof, utilizing any means other than drugs.

OR operating room.

Or orbitale.

ora[1] (o'rah), pl. *or'ae* [L.] an edge or margin.

ora[2] (o'rah) [L.] plural of *os,* mouth.

Orabase oral protective paste see under PASTE.

Oracillin trademark for *penicillin V.*

α-Oracillin trademark for *phenethicillin.*

Oracil-VK trademark for *penicillin V potassium* (see under PENICILLIN).

orad (o'rad) [L. *os, oris* mouth + *-ad* toward] toward the mouth.

Oradexon trademark for *dexamethasone.*

Oradian trademark for *chlorpropamide.*

orae (o're) [L.] plural of *ora,* edge.

Orafuran trademark for *nitrofurantoin.*

oral (o'ral) [L. *oralis*] pertaining to the mouth or toward the oral cavity. In dental anatomy, the term is used to refer to the surface of a tooth directed toward the oral cavity (or tongue) and opposite the vestibular (or facial) surface. Used synonymously with *lingual.* See illustration at SURFACE.

Oral-B see under TOOTHBRUSH.

orale (o-ra'le) a craniometric landmark being the point in the midline of the maxillary suture just lingual to the central incisors in the alveolar process. Abbreviation O. See illustration at CEPHALOMETRY.

oralogy (o-ral'o-je) [L. *oralis* pertaining to the mouth + *-logy*] stomatology.

Oramid trademark for *salicylamide.*

Orasone trademark for *prednisone.*

Ora Tone trademark for a heat-cured denture base acrylic resin.

orb (orb) [L. *orbis* circle, disk] a sphere; the eyeball.

Orban file, knife [B. *Orban,* American periodontologist] see under FILE and KNIFE.

orbicular (or-bik'u-lar) [L. *orbicularis*] round, circular, or spherical.

orbicularis (or-bik"u-la'ris) [L.] 1. orbicular. 2. orbicular MUSCLE. **o. oc'uli,** orbicular muscle of eye; see under MUSCLE. **o. o'ris,** orbicular muscle of mouth; see under MUSCLE.

orbiculi (or-bik'u-li) [L.] plural of *orbiculus.*

orbiculus (or-bik'u-lus), pl. *orbic'uli* [L., dim. of *orbis* orb, circle] a structure shaped like a small circle, or disk.

Orbinamon trademark for *thiothixene.*

orbit (or'bit) [L. *orbita*] 1. the conical bony cavity which houses the eyeball and its associated muscles, vessels, and nerves. It is situated on the anterior aspect of the skull and its entrance is bounded by the frontal, zygomatic, and maxillary bones, with the frontal bone providing the upper boundary. The roof is formed by the orbital plate of the frontal bone; a small triangular area close to the apex is formed by a part of the lesser wing of the sphenoid bone that is perforated by the optic canal. The lateral wall is made up by the orbital surface of the greater wing of the sphenoid bone and by the frontal process of the zygomatic bone. The zygomatic, maxillary, and palatine bones form the floor. The medial wall is formed by the maxilla, lacrimal bone, ethmoid bone, and sphenoid bone. The ridges surrounding the orbital opening protect the eye. Called also *eye socket, orbita* [NA] and *orbital cavity.* 2. a curved path traced by a satellite about a celestial body. 3. to move or travel in an orbital or elliptical path. **electron o.,** in the orbital theory, the path of electrons moving around the nucleus of an atom, generally corresponding to the orbital shell, in which the electrons are assumed to oscillate at certain levels in relation to the nucleus. The orbits are commonly designated with letters K, L, M, and N, each letter representing a special distance from the nucleus, and corresponding to different energy levels of electrons; the K orbit is the closest to the nucleus and has the lowest energy level and is thus designated with the atomic number 1. Called also *nuclear o.* See also Bohr ATOM, orbital THEORY, and quantum NUMBER. **nuclear o.,** see *electron o.* and electron ORBITAL. **terminal functional o.,** the phase of the masticating cycle between the closing and opening cycles of the mandible, in which the opposing teeth are in occlusal contact.

orbita (or'bi-tah), pl. *or'bitae* [L. "mark of a wheel"] [NA] orbit (1).

orbitae (or'bi-te) [L.] plural of *orbita.*

orbital (or'bi-tal) [L. *orbitalis*] 1. pertaining to the orbit. 2. electron o. **electron o.,** in the orbital theory, a three-dimensional wave that has a cloudlike structure and indefinite boundaries, but occupies in an atom a position relative to the nucleus (nuclear orbit) and has a specific energy level which is relative to its position in relation to the nucleus. The orbital levels and the movement of electrons are expressed by wave functions and quantum numbers. See also Bohr ATOM, electron ORBIT, and quantum NUMBER. **molecular o.,** an electron cloud associated with more than one nucleus. **s, p, d, and f, o's,** see quantum number, azimuthal, under NUMBER.

orbitale (or"bi-ta'le) an anthropometric landmark, being the lowest point on the inferior margin of the orbit. Abbreviated *Or*. Called also *point Or*. See illustration at CEPHALOMETRY.

orbitalis (or″bĭ-ta′lis) [L.] 1. pertaining to the orbit. 2. orbital MUSCLE.

orbito- [L. *orbita* "mark of a wheel"] a combining form denoting relationship to an orbit.

orbitonasal (or″bĭ-to-na′zal) pertaining to the orbit and the nose.

orbitosphenoid (or″bĭ-to-sfe′noid) [orbito- + sphenoid] a part of the presphenoid consisting of the small wings. Called also *orbitosphenoidal bone*.

orbitostat (or′bĭ-to-stat) an instrument for measuring the axis of the orbit.

orbitotemporal (or″bĭ-to-tem′po-ral) pertaining to the orbit and temporal regions or bone.

orbitotomy (or″bĭ-tot′o-me) [orbito- + Gr. *tomnein* to cut] incision or opening into the orbit through the orbital margin.

Orbivirus (or″bĭ-vi′rus) [L. *orbis* a circular object + *virus*] a genus of reoviruses, occurring as nonenveloped icosahedral particles about 50 to 60 nm in diameter, having double-stranded RNA that is found in 10 pieces. The genus includes a number of arthropod-borne viruses, some strains being pathogenic to vertebrates.

orbivirus (or″bĭ-vi′rus) any virus of the genus *Orbivirus*.

orchitis (or-ki′tis) inflammation of a testis. **mumps o., o. parotid′ea**, orchitis associated with mumps.

order (or′der) [L. *ordo* a line, row, or series] a taxonomic category subordinate to a class and superior to a family.

ordinate (or′dĭ-nāt) one of the lines used as a base of reference in graphs; see ABSCISSA.

Ordóñez melanosis [J. Hernando *Ordóñez*, Columbian physician] see under MELANOSIS.

Oreton-F trademark for *testosterone*.

organ (or′gan) [L. *organum*; Gr. *organnon*] a somewhat independent part of the body arranged according to a characteristic structural plan, and performing a special function or functions. It is composed of various tissues, one of which is primary in function. A collection of organs united for the express purpose of executing a specific function or group of functions in the body is known as a *system*. See also ORGANON and ORGANUM. **cement o.**, a name used in the past for the embryonic tissue that develops into the cement layer of the tooth. **Chievitz's o.**, an embryonic outgrowth behind the parotid gland which may merge into the latter or may disappear. **effector o.**, an organ, such as a muscle or gland, which secretes or contracts in direct response to nerve impulses. Called also *effector*. **enamel o.**, a circumscribed, knoblike mass of ectodermal cells arising from the dental lamina. During the cap stage of odontogenesis, it assumes a caplike shape, becoming a double-walled sac during the third month of fetal development, which is composed of an outer, convex wall (outer enamel layer) and an inner, concave wall (inner enamel layer). Between the two is a filling of looser ectodermal cells which transforms into a stellate reticulum. The enamel organ first produces the enamel and then encases the crown portion of the future tooth, molding its shape and depositing enamel there. Later, it elongates and models the root portion of the dental papilla, which organizes in response to its influences. See also tooth BUD. **end o.**, end-organ. **Golgi tendon o.**, a mechanoreceptor found in the tendons, usually near the junction with the muscle, consisting of a capsule which contains enlarged tendon fasciculi. The nerve fibers, having lost their myelin sheath on entering the capsule, subdivide and enter between the tendon fibers. The organ is activated by any increase in pressure exerted by contraction or stretch of the muscle, thus being responsible for lengthening reaction. Called also *neurotendinous o., neurotendinous spindle*, and *tendon spindle*. **gustatory o.**, the organ concerned with the perception of taste, consisting chiefly of the taste buds. Called also *o. of taste, organon gustus*, and *organum gustus* [NA]. **o. of hearing and equilibrium**, vestibulocochlear o. **Jacobson's o.**, vomeronasal o. **lymphatic o.**, a collective term used in anatomical nomenclature to denote any organ concerned with collecting, transporting, and filtering of lymph, and which is made up of lymphoid or adenoid tissue, including the lymph nodes, lymphatic vessels, tonsils, spleen, and thymus. See also lymphatic SYSTEM. **o.'s of mastication**, masticatory SYSTEM. **Meyer's o.**, an area of circumvallate papillae on either side of the posterior part of the tongue. **neurotendinous o.**, Golgi tendon o. **olfactory o.**, the specialized structures subserving the function of the sense of smell, including the olfactory region of the nasal mucosa containing the bipolar cells or origin of the olfactory nerves, and the olfactory glands. Called also *o. of smell, organon olfactus*, and *organum olfactus* [NA]. **sense o., sensory o.**, an organ that receives stimuli which give rise to sensations, i.e., an organ which translates certain forms of energy into nerve impulses that are perceived as special sensations. Sense organs are characterized by highly specialized neuroreceptors and relationships, and include the visual, vestibulocochlear, olfactory, and gustatory organs. Called also *o. of special sense, organon sensuum*, and *organum sensuum*. **o. of smell**, olfactory o. **o. of special sense**, sense o. **target o.**, one that is affected by a particular hormone. **terminal o.**, one situated at either end of a reflex arc. **o. of taste**, gustatory o. **vestibulocochlear o.**, a collective term in anatomical nomenclature applied to those structures outside the central nervous system concerned with balance and hearing, and comprising the internal, middle, and external ear. Called also *o. of hearing and equilibrium, organon auditus, organum oticum, organum stato-acousticum*, and *organum vestibulocochleare* [NA]. **o. of vision, visual o.**, a collective term in anatomical nomenclature applied to those structures outside the central nervous system concerned with vision, and comprising the eye and the accessory organs of the eye. Called also *organon visus* and *organum visus* [NA]. See also EYE. **vomeronasal o.**, a short rudimentary canal just above the vomeronasal cartilage, opening in the side of the nasal septum and passing from there blindly upward and backward. Called also *Jacobson's o., organon vomeronasale*, and *organum vomeronasale* [NA].

organa (or′gah-nah) plural of *organum* [L.] and *organon* [Gr.].

organelle (or″gan-el′) [L. *organella*] 1. a specific particle of membrane-bound substance present in practically all cells, such as nuclei, centrioles, mitochondria, Golgi complexes, endoplasmic reticulum, lysosomes, microbodies, microtubules, and possibly filaments. Organelles are organized units of living substance having important specific functions in cell metabolism. Together with inclusions, they form a colloidal suspension in the hyaloplasm.

organic (or-gan′ik [L. *organicus*; Gr. *organikos*] 1. pertaining to an organ or the organs. 2. having an organized structure. 3. arising from an organism. 4. pertaining to substances derived from living organisms. 5. pertaining to chemical substances that contain carbon, with the exception of oxides of carbon and carbonates. See organic COMPOUND. 6. pertaining to or cultivated by the use of animal or vegetable fertilizers, rather than synthetic chemicals.

organism (or′gah-nizm) any individual living thing, whether animal or plant. **aerobic o.**, aerobe. **anaerobic o.**, anaerobe. **autotrophic o.**, autotrophic CELL. **chemolithotrophic o.**, chemolithotrophic CELL. **chemo-organotrophic o.**, chemo-organotrophic CELL. **chemotrophic o.**, chemotrophic CELL. **heterotrophic o.**, heterotrophic CELL. **photolithotrophic o.**, photolithotrophic CELL. **photo-organotrophic o.**, photo-organotrophic CELL. **phototrophic o.**, phototrophic CELL. **pleuropneumonia-like o.** (PPLO), former name for *Mycoplasma*.

organization (or″gah-ni-za′shun) 1. the process of organizing or of becoming organized. 2. the replacement of blood clots by fibrous tissue. See HEMOSTASIS. 3. any organized body, group, or structure. **health maintenance o.**, an organized system of health care which provides a comprehensive health maintenance and treatment service for an enrolled group of persons through a prepaid aggregate fixed sum or capitation arrangement. Included are ambulatory physician care, outpatient preventive service, inpatient hospital and physician care, and emergency service. Abbreviated *HMO*. **International Standards O.**, an international, nongovernmental organization whose objective is the development of international standards. The American National Standards Institute is the American Representative to the organization. A committee, TC106 — Dentistry, is responsible for the standardization of terminology, test methods, and specifications for dental materials, instruments, appliances, and equipment. Abbreviated *ISO*. **mutual benefit o.**, a fraternal or social organization or corporation established for the relief of its members from specified perils or costs, such as the costs of illness. **Professional Standards Review O.** a federally sponsored program charged with comprehensive and ongoing review of services provided under the Medicare, Medicaid, and Maternal and Child Health programs, and administered by the Bureau of Quality Assurance. The program is staffed with local physicians, osteopaths, and other professionals whose duties consist of establishing the criteria, norms, and standards for diagnosis and treatment of diseases encountered in the local PSRO jurisdiction, and review of services which are inconsistent with the established norms. This established peer review process is used to determine for purposes of reimbursement under these programs whether services are: medically necessary; provided in accordance with professional criteria, norms, and standards; and, in the case of institutional services, rendered in an appropriate setting. Abbreviated *PSRO.* See also peer REVIEW. **O. of Teachers of Oral Diagnosis,** a professional association of dentists who are involved in teaching oral diagnosis, having as its objective the advancement and promotion of the study of oral diagnosis and medicine. Abbreviated *OTOD.* **World Health O.,** an international agency associated with the United Nations and based in Geneva. It was established in 1948 to help improve the health of the world population by preventing and controlling communicable diseases through various programs. Abbreviated *WHO.*

organo- [Gr. *organon* organ] 1. a combining form denoting relationship to an organ. 2. a combining form denoting relationship to an organic chemical compound.

organoid (or'gah-noid) [*organ* + Gr. *eidos* form] 1. resembling an organ. 2. a structure which resembles an organ.

organometallic (or"gah-no-mě-tal'ik) 1. pertaining to the carbon-metal linkage. 2. pertaining to any compound in which a metal is attached directly to a carbon.

organon (or'gah-non), pl. *or'gana* [Gr.] organ. **o. audi'tus,** vestibulocochlear ORGAN. **o. gus'tus,** gustatory ORGAN. **o. olfac'tus,** olfactory ORGAN. **o. sen'suum,** sense ORGAN. **o. vi'sus,** ORGAN of vision. **o. vomeronasa'le,** vomeronasal ORGAN.

organophosphate (or"gah-no-fos'făt) Any organic compound containing phosphorus. Organophosphates include: (1) phospholipids, or phosphatides, which are found in nature in the form of lecithins, certain proteins, and nucleic acids; (2) esters of phosphinic acids which are used mainly as plasticizers, insecticides, flame retardants, and resin modifiers; (3) pyrophosphates which serve as the basis for cholinesterase inhibitors and are used as insecticides; and (4) phosphoric esters of glycerol, glycol, and sorbitol. Called also *organophosphorus compound.*

organotrophic (or"gah-no-trof'ik) chemo-organotrophic; see chemo-organotrophic CELL.

organotropic (or"gah-no-trop'ik) pertaining to or characterized by organotropism.

organotropism (or-gah-not'ro-pizm) [*organo-* + Gr. *tropē* a turning] the special affinity of chemical compounds or of pathogenic agents for particular tissues or organs of the body.

organum (or'gah-num), pl. *or'gana* [L.] organ. **o. gus'tus** [NA], gustatory ORGAN. **o. olfac'tus** [NA], olfactory ORGAN. **or'gana uropoët'ica** [NA], urinary SYSTEM. **o. o'ticum, o. statoacousti'cum, o. vestibulocochlea're** [NA], vestibulocochlear ORGAN. **o. vi'sus** [NA], ORGAN of vision. **o. sen'suum** [NA], sense ORGAN. **o. vomeronasa'le** [NA], vomeronasal ORGAN.

Oribasius [325–403] a famous physician and medical writer who became physician to the Emperor Julian. His *magnum opus* was an encyclopedia of medicine in 70 volumes, of which only 17 survive; these are invaluable, for they contain extracts from the works of many important physicians of antiquity (e.g., Dioscorides, Galen, Antyllus).

orifice (or'ĭ-fis) [L. *orificium*] an opening into a cavity in the body. Called also *opening, orificium,* and *ostium.* **o. of the mouth,** the longitudinal opening of the mouth, between the lips, which provides the entrance to the oral cavity. Called also *oral fissure* and *rima oris* [NA].

orificia (or"ĭ-fish'e-ah) [L.] plural of *orificium.*

orificial (or"ĭ-fish'al) pertaining to an orifice.

orificium (or"ĭ-fish'e-um), pl. *orific'ia* [L.] an opening into a cavity in the body. Called also *opening, orifice,* and *ostium.*

origin (or'ĭ-jin) [L. *origo* beginning] 1. a source or beginning. 2. the site from which a muscle arises and is attached to a supporting structure, such as a bone. See also INSERTION.

Orinase trademark for *tolbutamide.*

Oriodide trademark for radioactive sodium iodide (see under soDIUM).

Orlon trademark for an acrylic resin obtained by polymerization of acrylonitrile, which is resistant to mineral acids, common solvents, weak alkalies, and other substances. Called also *fiber A* and *polyacrylonitrile.*

Orn ornithine.

ornithine (or'nĭ-thin) a naturally occurring, nonessential amino acid, 2,5-diaminovaleric acid, which is obtained from arginine. On decomposition, it gives rise to putrescine. Ornithine is an intermediate in urea biosynthesis. Used as an anticholesteremic agent. Abbreviated *Orn.* See also amino ACID. **o. carbamoyltransferase,** ornithine CARBAMOYLTRANSFERASE. **o. transcarboxylase,** ornithine CARBAMOYLTRANSFERASE.

oro- 1. [L. *os, oris* mouth] a combining form denoting relationship to the mouth. 2. [Gr. *oros* the watery part of the blood (serum), or whey]; see ORRHO-.

orofacial (o"ro-fa'shal) pertaining to the mouth and face.

orolingual (o"ro-ling'gwal) [*oro-*(1) + L. *lingua* tongue] pertaining to the mouth and tongue.

oromaxillary (o"ro-mak'sĭ-ler"e) [*oro-*(1) + *maxilla*] pertaining to the tongue and maxilla or maxillary region.

oronasal (o"ro-na'zal) [*oro-*(1) + L. *nasus* nose] pertaining to the mouth and nose.

Oronol trademark for *aurothioglucose.*

oropharynx (o"ro-far'inks) [*oro-*(1) + *pharynx*] that part of the pharynx which lies between the soft palate and the upper edge of the epiglottis. Called also *oral pharynx, pars oralis pharyngis* [NA], *pharyngo-oral cavity,* and *vestibule of pharynx.*

orosomucoid (o"ro-so-mu'koid) [*oro-*(2) + *mucoid*] a mucoid rich in galactose, mannose, glucosamine, fucose, and sialic acid. Orosomucoid is soluble in various acids, and has a pH of 8.6 and a molecular weight of about 41,000. Its blood content usually increases in inflammatory diseases and decreases in lipoid nephrosis, returning to the normal levels after symptoms have subsided. Called also *acid glycoprotein* and α_1-mucoprotein.

orrho- [Gr. *orrhos* serum] a combining form denoting relationship to serum.

orris (or'is) the root of species of *Iris;* used in dentifrices, perfumes, and other preparations.

ortho- [Gr. *orthos* straight] 1. a prefix meaning straight, normal, correct, etc. 2. in organic chemistry, a prefix in structural isomerism indicating the substitution in a derivative of a benzene ring of two atoms in neighboring positions. Abbreviated *o-.* See *ortho-*ISOMER. Usually written in italics and disregarded in alphabetization. Also, a prefix indicating a highly hydrated acid or salt.

orthocephalic (or"tho-sě-fal'ik) [*ortho-* + Gr. *kephalē* head] pertaining to or characterized by a skull of an average height-length index. Called also *orthocephalous.* See orthocephalic SKULL.

orthocephalous (or"tho-sef'ah-lus) orthocephalic.

orthocheilia (or"tho-ke'le-ah) a condition characterized by straight lips.

orthochromatic (or"tho-kro-mat'ik) [*ortho-* + Gr. *chrōma* color] normally colored or stained.

orthochromophil (or"tho-kro'mo-fil) [*ortho-* + Gr. *chrōma* color + *philein* to love] staining normally with neutral stain. See also orthochromatic NORMOBLAST.

orthoclase (or'tho-klās, or'tho-klāz) potassium FELDSPAR.

orthodentin (or"tho-den'tin) [*ortho-* + *dentin*] straight-tubed dentin, as seen in the teeth of mammals.

orthodontia (or"tho-don'she-ah) orthodontics. **surgical o.,** surgical ORTHODONTICS.

orthodontic (or"tho-don'tik) pertaining to orthodontics.

orthodontics (or"tho-don'tiks) [*ortho-* + Gr. *odous* tooth] that branch of dentistry concerned with the supervision, guidance, and correction of the growing or mature dentofacial structures, including those conditions that require movement of teeth or correction of malrelationships and malformations of their related structures and the adjustment of relationships between and among teeth and facial bones by the application of forces and/or the stimulation and redirection of functional forces within the craniofacial complex. Major responsibilities of orthodontic practice include the diagnosis, prevention, interception, and comprehensive treatment of all forms of malocclusion of the teeth and associated alterations in their surrounding structures; the design, application, and control of functional and corrective appliances; and the guidance of the dentition and its supporting structures to attain and maintain optimum occlusal relations in physiologic and esthetic harmony among facial and cranial structures. Various instruments are used for producing, fitting, and removing orthodontic appliances. The most commonly used instruments include band pushers, seaters, and adapters; wire, ligature, and pin cutters; band removers; files; mallets; mirrors; explorers; scissors; Boley gauge and calipers; scalers; cementation instruments; welding and soldering instruments; and a variety of pliers. Called also *dentofacial orthopedics, orthodontia,* and *orthodontology.* **corrective o.,** that phase of orthodontics concerned with the correction of malocclusion with proper appliances and prevention of its sequelae. **interceptive o.,** that phase of orthodontics concerned with intercepting and correcting conditions which might result in severe cases of malocclusion. **preventive o., prophylactic o.,** that phase of orthodontics concerned with preservation of the integrity of proper occlusion through the use of orthodontic procedures and devices, such as space maintainers. **surgical o.,** orthodontic therapy involving surgical procedures or orthognathic surgery, including resections and ostectomies, cosmetic surgery, and the surgical uncovering of impacted teeth, and positioning and transpositioning of teeth. Called also *surgical orthodontia.*

orthodontist (or″tho-don′tist) a dentist who specialized in orthodontics.

orthodontology (or″tho-don-tol′o-je) orthodontics.

orthogenesis (or″tho-jen′ĕ-sis) [ortho- + Gr. *genesis* production] 1. progressive evolution in a given direction, as opposed to several directions. 2. the theory that the course of evolution is fixed and predetermined. See also MONOGENESIS (2).

orthognathia (or″thog-nath′e-ah) [ortho- + Gr. *gnathos* jaw] the branch of oral medicine dealing with the cause and treatment of malposition of the bones of the jaw.

orthognathic (or″thog-na′thik) 1. pertaining to orthognathia. 2. orthognathous.

orthognathous (or-thog′nah-thus) [ortho- + Gr. *gnathos* jaw] pertaining to or characterized by minimal protrusion of the mandible or minimal prognathism. Called also *orthognathic.* See orthognathous SKULL.

Orthomyxoviridae (or″tho-mik″so-vi′rĭ-de) [ortho- + *myxa* mucus + *virus*] a family of viruses with pleomorphic, spherical, or filamentous virions 80 to 120 nm in diameter, and helical nucleocapsids 6 to 90 nm in diameter contained in a protein shell with an outer lipid envelope studded with projections of hemagglutinin and neuraminidase. The genome consists of single-stranded RNA in several segments, which is transcribed to complementary mRNA by polymerase. It comprises a single genus, *Influenzavirus,* which includes the pathogenic agents of influenza.

orthomyxovirus (or″tho-mik″so-vi′rus) any virus of the family Orthomyxoviridae.

Orthopantomograph trademark for a panoramic x-ray machine. See PANTOMOGRAPHY.

orthopedic (or″tho-pe′dik) [ortho- + Gr. *pais* child] pertaining to the correction of deformities; pertaining to orthopedics.

orthopedics (or″tho-pe′diks) [ortho- + Gr. *pais* child] that branch of surgery which is specially concerned with the preservation and restoration of the function of the skeletal system, its articulations and associated structures. **Crozat dental o.,** 1. gnathologic o. 2. see Crozat APPLIANCE. **dentofacial o.,** orthodontics. **functional jaw o.,** an orthodontic principle approach proposed by Haupl and advanced by Schwarz, for the use of muscle force to effect changes in jaw position and tooth alignment with a removable appliance, such as the Andresen, Frankel, Nord, Schwarz, or Bimler appliance. See also active PLATE. **gnathologic o.,** an orthodontic specialty based on the use of the Crozat appliance to encourage and guide the growth of the bony structure itself so that there will be room for all the teeth in their proper places, resulting in arch development. Called also *Crozat dental o.* **oral o.,** a concept in dentistry concerned with postural relationships of the jaws, both normal and abnormal; analysis of the harmful effects of improper relationship of the mandible and the maxilla on dental and other related structures; the diagnosis and correction of such malrelationship; and the treatment and/or prevention of disturbances resulting therefrom.

orthophenylphenol (or″tho-fen′il-fe′nol) a phenol derivative occurring as nearly white or light buff crystals that are soluble in alcohol and sodium hydroxide solutions, but not in water. Used in various topical germicidal and fungicidal preparations. Called also *2-hydroxydiphenyl, orthoxenol,* and *o-phenylphenol.* Trademark: Dowicide 1.

orthophosphate (or″tho-fos′fāt) a salt of orthophosphoric acid; a compound of the type M_3PO_4. **calcium o.,** CALCIUM phosphate, basic. **calcium o.,** CALCIUM phosphate, tribasic. **dicalcium o.,** CALCIUM phosphate, dibasic. **disodium o.,** sodium PHOSPHATE, dibasic. **tricalcium o.,** CALCIUM phosphate, tribasic.

orthopnea (or″thop-ne′ah) [ortho- + Gr. *phoia* breath] difficult breathing except in an upright position.

Orthopoxvirus (or″tho-poks-vi′rus) [ortho- + *pox* + *virus*] a genus of brick-shaped poxviruses, whose virions measure 218×270 nm and are surrounded by outer envelopes containing threads about 9 nm wide. These poxviruses parasitize various vertebrates, including the rabbit, monkey, cow, buffalo, camel, mouse, and raccoon, and, two types, vaccinia and variola viruses, are involved in human infections.

Orthoreovirus (or″tho-re″o-vi′rus) a genus of reoviruses, occurring as particles about 70 nm in diameter, enclosing nucleoids 35 nm across. Their virions have a molecular weight of $127 \times$

10^6 to 131×10^6 and their core has a constant molecular weight of 52×10^6. There are 20 capsomers in the periphery, 127 being the total number of capsomers in the virion. Some strains have been isolated in cases of diarrhea, a variety of respiratory, gastrointestinal, and neurological diseases, exanthema, hepatitis, and febrile conditions, but their etiologic role in these conditions has not been established. Called also *echovirus 10* and *hepatoencephalomyelitis virus.*

orthosilicate (or″tho-sil′ĭ-kāt) a salt of silic acid containing the radical $\equiv SiO_4$. **ethyl o.,** a silicate used as a cross-linking agent in the vulcanization of silicone rubber. Called also *tetraethyoxysilane.*

orthostaphyline (or″tho-staf′ĭ-lin) [ortho- + Gr. *staphylē* a bunch of grapes, uvula] pertaining to or characterized by a palate of moderate height. See orthostaphyline SKULL.

orthosurgical (or″tho-ser′jĭ-kal) pertaining to surgical orthodontics.

orthotopic (or″tho-top′ik) [ortho- + Gr. *topos* place] occurring at the normal place or upon the proper part of the body.

orthovoltage (or″tho-vol′tij) in roentgenotherapy, voltage in the range of 30 to 400 kilovolts or 30,000 to 400,000 (10^3) volts. See also MEGAVOLTAGE and SUPERVOLTAGE.

orthoxenol (or″tho-zen′ol) orthophenylphenol.

Orthoxine trademark for *methoxyphenamine hydrochloride* (see under METHOXYPHENAMINE).

Orticalm trademark for *reserpine.*

Ortin trademark for *trolnitrate phosphate* (see under TROLNITRATE).

Ortizon trademark for *urea peroxide* (see under UREA).

Ortner's syndrome [Norbert *Ortner,* Austrian physician] see under SYNDROME.

Ortodrinex trademark for *methoxyphenamine hydrochloride* (see under METHOXYPHENAMINE).

Orton's enamel cleaver [Charles H. *Orton,* American dentist, 20th century] see under CLEAVER.

ortonal (or′ton′al) methaqualone.

Os osmium.

os[1] (os), gen. *o′ris,* pl. *o′ra* [L. "an opening, or mouth"] any orifice of the body; [NA] the mouth.

os[2] (os), gen. *os′sis,* pl. *os′sa* [L.] bone; used in anatomical nomenclature as a general term which is combined with an appropriate adjective to designate a specific type of bony structure. See BONE. **o. pneumat′icum** [NA], pneumatic BONE. **o. basila′re,** a term applied to the sphenoid and occipital bones. **os′sa cra′nii** [NA], cranial bones; see under BONE. **o. epitympan′icum,** a bone of very early fetal life which becomes the posterior portion of the squama that aids in forming the mastoid cells. **o. ethmoida′le** [NA], ethmoid BONE. **os′sa fa′ciei** [NA], facial bones; see under BONE. **o. fronta′le** [NA], frontal BONE. **o. hyoi′deum** [NA], hyoid BONE. **o. in′cae,** interparietal BONE. **o. incisi′vum** [NA], incisive BONE. **o. interparieta′le** [NA], interparietal BONE. **o. lacrima′le,** lacrimal BONE. **o. mastoi′deum,** mastoid BONE. **o. nasa′le** [NA], nasal BONE. **o. occipita′le** [NA], occipital BONE. **o. palati′num** [NA], palatine BONE. **o. parieta′le** [NA], parietal BONE. **o. pla′num** [NA], 1. flat BONE. 2. orbital LAMINA. **o. sphenoida′le** [NA], sphenoid BONE. **os′sa sutura′tum** [NA], wormian bones; see under BONE. **o. tempora′le** [NA], temporal BONE. **os′sa Wor′mi,** wormian bones; see under BONE. **o. zygomat′icum** [NA], zygomatic BONE.

oscedo (os-se′do) [L.] the act of yawning.

oscillation (os″ĭ-la′shun) [L. *oscillare* to swing] a backward and forward motion, like a pendulum. Also vibration, fluctuation, or variation.

oscillator (os′ĭ-la″tor) an apparatus for producing oscillations; an electric circuit designed to generate alternating current at a particular frequency.

-ose a suffix indicating a sugar or higher saccharide.

OSHA Occupational Safety and Health Administration (see under ADMINISTRATION).

-osis a word termination denoting a process, often a disease or morbid process, or sometimes conveying the meaning of abnormal increase. See also -SIS.

Osler's disease [Sir William *Osler,* Canadian-born physician and medical educator, 1849–1919; he was successively professor of medicine at McGill University, the University of Pennsylvania, Johns Hopkins University, and the University of Oxford] POLYCYTHEMIA vera. See also hereditary hemorrhagic TELANGIECTASIA (Rendu-Weber-Osler syndrome).

Osmitrol trademark for MANNITOL.

osmium (oz′me-um) [Gr. *osmē* odor, so named because of the odor of the vapor, OsO_4, produced by oxidation of the element] a metallic element. Symbol, Os; atomic number, 76; atomic weight, 190.2; valences 2, 3, 4, 6, 8; specific gravity, 22.5; melting point, 3000°C; group VIII of the periodic table. It occurs in seven natural isotopes (184, 186–190, 192) and several artificial radioactive ones (181–183, 185, 191, 193–195). Osmium is a white metal of the platinum group that is attacked by fused alkalies and is insoluble in acids and aqua regia. On heating in air, it gives off poisonous fumes of osmium trioxide. Used in some alloys and in various industrial processes. **o. tetroxide,** a compound, OsO₄, occurring as colorless or slightly yellow crystals or crystalline granules with a pungent odor. Used as a fixative in preparing histologic specimens. It is an irritant that may cause injuries to the eyes, mucous membranes, skin, and respiratory tract. Called also *osmic acid.*

osmo- 1. [Gr. *osmē* smell] a combining form denoting relationship to smell or odors. 2. [Gr. *ōsmos* impulse] a combining form denoting relationship to an impulse, or to osmosis.

osmosis (oz-mo'sis, os-mo'sis) [Gr. *ōsmos* impulsion] the passage of a solvent from the area of low concentration of solute to an area of high concentration of solute, across a semipermeable membrane that allows free passage of the solvent but not the solute. See illustration. See also DIFFUSION (1) and osmotic PRESSURE.

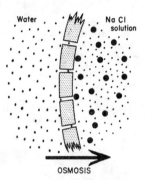

OSMOSIS

Osmosis at a cell membrane when a sodium chloride solution is placed on one side of the membrane and water on the other side. (From A. C. Guyton: Textbook of Medical Physiology. 6th ed. Philadelphia, W. B. Saunders Co., 1981.)

osmotic (os-mot'ik) pertaining to or of the nature of osmosis.

Osnervan trademark for *procyclidine hydrochloride* (see under PROCYCLIDINE).

ossa (os'ah) [L.] plural of *os.*

Ossalin trademark for a preparation of *sodium fluoride* (see under FLUORIDE).

osseomucoid (os″e-o-mu'koid) [L. *os,* bone + *mucoid*] a mucoid in the bone tissue, containing as a prosthetic group chondroitin sulfates with multiple units of acetyl galactosamine sulfate and glucuronic or iduronic acid in glycosidal linkage.

osseous (os'e-us) [L. *osseus*] of the nature or quality of bone; bony.

ossicle (os'sĭ-k'l) [L. *ossiculum*] a small bone. **Bertin's e.,** sphenoidal CONCHA. **Kerckring's o.,** a small bone of early life which becomes the basilar process of the occipital bone. **Riolan's o.,** one of the small bones occasionally seen in sutures between the bones of the skull, usually between the mastoid portion of the temporal bone and the occipital bone. Called also *Riolan's bone.* See also wormian bones, under BONE. **sphenoturbinal o.,** sphenoidal CONCHA.

ossiferous (ŏ-sif'er-us) [L. *os* bone + *ferre* to bear] producing bone.

ossific (ŏ-sif'ik) [L. *os* bone + *facere* to make] forming or becoming bone.

ossification (os″ĭ-fĭ-ka'shun) [L. *ossificatio*] the formation of bone or of a bony substance; the conversion of fibrous tissue or of cartilage into bone or bony substance. **cartilaginous o., endochondral o., intracartilaginous o. intracartilaginous o.,** ossification which takes place in cartilage, occurring chiefly in long bones, progressing from the center toward the extremity of the bone. It begins in centers of ossification with cartilage cells enlarging and forming rows. Deposition of calcareous material is associated with separation of cells from each other by longitudinal columns of calcified matrix, which subsequently become bridged by transverse bars that isolate the cells and cause them to atrophy, thus forming spaces which become primary areolae. Simultaneously, osteoblasts on the contact surface of the perichondrium form a thin layer of bony tissue between the cartilage and the perichondrium by the intramembranous mode of ossification. Perichondrium thus transformed in the process to periosteum consists of blood vessels and osteoblasts and

osteoclasts. In the second stage, the membrane bone is perforated by the osteogenic layer of the periosteum and the action of osteoclasts causes fusion of primary areolae into secondary areolae or medullary spaces. Called also *cartilaginous o.* and *endochondral o.* **intramembranous o.,** ossification which takes place in a membrane, rather than cartilage, occurring in the development of some bones, including the roof and sides of the skull. The membrane preceding the bone is made up of connective tissue composed of fibers and granular cells of the matrix, which eventually form the periosteum, with the osteoblasts being present in the periphery. Early in the process, there is the development of a network of spicules which contain at their growing points osteogenic fibers and granular cells and radiate from the centers of ossification toward the periphery. Deposition of calcareous granules is associated with darkening of the membrane; fusing of granules results in the membrane becoming transparent. Ossification of osteogenic fibers is associated with embedding of osteoblasts in the lacunae and continuous deposition of new layers of bone under the periosteum. **perichondral o., periosteal o.,** subperiosteal o. **subperiosteal o.,** ossification in which a process similar to that in intramembranous ossification produces a thin layer of bone between the perichondrium and cartilage, which takes place simultaneously with intracartilaginous ossification. The action of osteoblasts cause the development of bone by apposition on the contact surface of the perichondrium and its subsequent transformation to the periosteum. Called also *perichondral o.* and *periosteal o.*

ossifluence (ŏ-sif'lu-ens) softening of bony tissue.

ossiform (os'ĭ-form) [L. *os* bone + *forma* shape] resembling bone.

ossifying (os'ĭ-fi″ing) changing or developing into bone.

Ossin trademark for a preparation of *sodium fluoride* (see under FLUORIDE).

osteal (os'te-al) bony; osseous.

ostealgia (os″te-al'je-ah) [osteo- + -algia] pain in a bone or bones.

ostearthrotomy (os″te-ar-throt'o-me) [osteo- + Gr. *arthron* joint + *temnein* to cut] excision of an articular end of a bone.

ostectomy (os-tek'to-me) [osteo- + Gr. *ektomē* excision] the excision of a bone or a portion of a bone.

osteitis (os″te-i'tis) [osteo- + -itis] inflammation of the bone in which the cortex is predominantly involved. **alveolar o.,** dry SOCKET. **condensing o.,** chronic focal sclerosing OSTEOMYELITIS. **o. defor'mans,** a disease of obscure etiology, usually affecting adults over 40 years of age. It is characterized by extensive localized remodeling of one or several bones, including the sacrum, spine, especially the maxilla, and, less frequently, the skull, pelvis, femur, and tibia. The principal pathological findings are bone thickening, spontaneous fractures, areas of osteomalacia and sclerosis, bone resorption, osteoblastic bone deposition, presence of nonlamellar bone, mosaic areas, extensive vascularity, disorganization of the cortex, bone hypertrophy, and bowing of the tibiae and femora. When the jaws are involved the affected bone exhibits progressive enlargement, the palate becomes flattened, the alveolar ridges become widened, the teeth become loose and migrate, producing spacing, and edentulous patients experience difficulty in wearing their appliances because of expansion of the jaw. When associated with angioid streaks, it is known as *Terry's syndrome.* Called also *multiple osteomalacia* and *Paget's disease.* **o. fibro'sa cys'tica,** 1. Jaffe-Lichtenstein SYNDROME. 2. Recklinghausen's DISEASE (2). **o. fibro'sa cys'tica dissemina'ta, o. fibro'sa dissemina'ta,** Albright's SYNDROME (1). **o. fibro'sa generalisa'ta,** Recklinghausen's DISEASE (2). **radiation o.,** pathologic changes in bone following exposure to ionizing radiations. **renal o. fibro'sa generalisa'ta,** renal RICKETS. **syphilitic o. of newborn,** Parrot's DISEASE (1).

Ostensin trademark for *trimethidinium methosulfate* (see under TRIMETHIDINIUM).

osteo- [Gr. *osteon* bone] a combining form denoting relationship to a bone or to bones.

osteoarthritis (os″te-o-ar-thri'tis) [osteo- + Gr. *arthron* joint + -itis] a degenerative disease of the joints, characterized by degeneration of the articular cartilage and hypertrophy of bone at the articular margins, accompanied chiefly by pain which may be relieved by rest, clicking and snapping of the joint, stiffness, and, less commonly, subluxation. It affects chiefly weight-bearing joints of elderly persons. Systemic symptoms are usually absent. The temporomandibular joint may be involved, usually as a consequence of trauma or loss of teeth associated with disturbed balance of the joint. Ankylosis is rare. Loss of elasticity of the tissues, surface erosions, horizontal fissures which may separate the cartilage from the underlying bone, vertical cracks which may extend through the cartilage into the subchondral bone, degeneration of the cartilage, calcification, ossification, and exostoses are the principal histological features. Called also *chronic senescent arthritis* and *hypertrophic arthritis*.

osteoarthropathy (os″te-o-ar-throp′ah-the) [*osteo-* + Gr. *arthron* joint + *pathos* disease] any disease of the joints and bones.

osteoarticular (os″te-o-ar-tik′u-lar) pertaining to or affecting bones and joints.

osteoblast (os′te-o-blast″) [*osteo-* + Gr. *blastos* germ] a bone cell which arises from a fibroblast and forms an osteogenic layer adjacent to the growing bone (osteoblastic layer). An active cell has an irregularly cuboid shape and is about 15 to 25 μ in diameter. Its cytoplasmic components consist of mitochondria and Golgi apparatus; a concentration of structures, varying in size from 0.3 to 6.0 μ, may be observed in the cytoplasm. The nucleus is large and spherical in shape and contains a prominent nucleolus. Inactive cells have cuboidal or squamous shapes and little or no cytoplasmic granules. Osteoblasts are involved in bone growth and their function is believed to be one of matrix production and mineralization. Called also *Gegenbaur's cell* and *skeletogenous cell*.

osteoblastic (os″te-o-blas′tik) pertaining to or of the nature of osteoblasts.

osteoblastoma (os″te-o-blas-to′mah) [*osteoblast* + *-oma*] a benign, rather vascular tumor of bone characterized by the formation of osteoid tissue and primitive bone. Called also *giant osteoid osteoma*.

osteocartilaginous (os″te-o-kar″ti-laj′i-nus) pertaining to or composed of bone and cartilage.

osteocementum (os″te-o-se-men′tum) [*osteo-* + *cementum*] a hard bonelike secondary cementum, typically arranged in concentric layers around the root and frequently showing numerous resting lines, such as occurring in hypercementosis.

osteochondral (os″te-o-kon′dral) pertaining to bone and cartilage.

osteochondritis (os″te-o-kon-dri′tis) [*osteo-* + Gr. *chondros* cartilage + *-itis*] inflammation of both bone and cartilage. **o. subepiphysa′ria,** metaphyseal DYSOSTOSIS. **syphilitic o.,** Parrot's DISEASE (1).

osteochondrodystrophia (os″te-o-kon″dro-dis-tro′fe-ah) [*osteo-* + *chondro-* + *dystrophia*] Morquio's DISEASE. **o. defor′mans,** Morquio's DISEASE.

osteochondrodystrophy (os″te-o-kon″dro-dis-tro′fe) Morquio's DISEASE. **hereditary o.,** Morquio's DISEASE.

osteochondroma (os″te-o-kon-dro′mah) [*osteo-* + Gr. *chondros* cartilage + *-oma*] osteoma blended with chondroma; a benign tumor consisting of projecting adult bone capped by cartilage.

osteochondromatosis (os″te-o-kon″dro-mah-to′sis) the presence of multiple osteochondromas.

osteochondropathy (os″te-o-kon-drop′ah-the) [*osteo-* + Gr. *chondros* cartilage + *pathos* disease] any disease of both bone and cartilage.

osteochondrosis (os″te-o-kon-dro′sis) a disease of growth or ossification centers in children, which begins as a degeneration or necrosis followed by regeneration or recalcification. Called also *epiphyseal ischemic necrosis*.

osteoclasia (os″te-o-kla′ze-ah) [*osteo-* + Gr. *klasis* a breaking + *-ia*] the absorption and destruction of bone tissue. See also bone RESORPTION. **o. desma′lis familia′ris,** HYPEROSTOSIS corticalis deformans juvenilis.

osteoclasis (os-te-ok′lah-sis) [*osteo-* + Gr. *klasis* a breaking] the surgical fracture or refracture of bone.

osteoclast (os′te-o-klast″) [*osteo-* + Gr. *klan* to break] 1. a large bone cell, usually found in the periosteum in resorption lacunae, but also in other parts of the bone, which contain as many as 50 nuclei. In younger osteoclasts, the nuclei tend to be ovoid and their membranes have smooth surfaces, and in older ones, the membranes are folded and the chromatin material is denser; in the last stage of development, the nuclei may appear pyknotic. The cell surface continuous to the bone surface usually has a brush border. The functions of the osteoclast include destruction and resorption of bone. Upon cessation of bone destruction, osteoclasts disappear. They are prominent in the areas of resorption when the germ of the permanent teeth begins to develop and the pressure causes resorption of the bony

partition between the two teeth, then of the root, and finally of a part of the enamel of the deciduous teeth. 2. an instrument for use in the surgical fracture or refracture of bone.

osteoclastic (os″te-o-klas′tik) pertaining to or of the nature of an osteoclast; destructive to bone.

osteoclastoma (os″te-o-klasto′mah) giant cell EPULIS.

osteocranium (os″te-o-kra′ne-um) [*osteo-* + Gr. *kranion* cranium] the fetal cranium during its stage of ossification.

osteocyte (os′te-o-sīt″) an osteoblast that has become embedded in the lacuna of the bone matrix. It is a biconvex cell, ranging in diameter from 10 to more than 30 μ, having an eccentric nucleus, and containing mitochondria and Golgi apparatus in the organelles and basophilic granular incisions in the cytoplasm. Thin cytoplasmic projections reach out through apertures in the cell wall and through canaliculi in the matrix, some of which communicate with their fellows from adjacent cells and form a syncytium-like network, while others project toward the blood vessels and the periosteum. Called also *bone cell, bone corpuscle,* and *osseous cell.*

osteodentin (os″te-o-den′tin) [*osteo-* + *dentin*] dentin that resembles bone; seen in the teeth of certain fish and pathologically in other lower species, and in man, being produced by rapid formation of secondary dentin, with entrapment of cells.

osteodentinoma (os″te-o-den-ti-no′mah) an odontoma composed of bone and dentin.

osteodynia (os″te-o-di′ne-ah) [*osteo-* + Gr. *odynē* pain] pain in a bone.

osteodysplasty (os″te-o-dis-plas′te) [*osteo-* + *dys-* + Gr. *plassein* to form] abnormal bone development. See Melnick-Needles SYNDROME.

osteodystrophia (os″te-o-dis-tro′fe-ah) osteodystrophy. **o. fibro′sa,** Albright's SYNDROME (1). **o. generalisa′ta,** Recklinghausen's DISEASE (2).

osteodystrophy (os″te-o-dis′tro-fe) [*osteo-* + *dystrophy*] defective formation of bone. Called also *osteodystrophia*.

osteoepiphysis (os″te-o-ĕ-pif′ĭ-sis) any bony epiphysis.

osteofibroma (os″te-o-fi-bro′mah) [*osteo-* + *fibroma*] a tumor containing both osseous and fibrous elements.

osteofibrosis (os″te-o-fi-bro′sis) a condition characterized by the presence of fibrous lesions of the bone. **o. defor′mans juveni′lis,** Jaffe-Lichtenstein SYNDROME.

osteofluorosis (os″te-o-floo″o-ro′sis) skeletal changes, usually consisting of osteomalacia and osteosclerosis, caused by the chronic intake of excessive quantities of fluorides.

osteogen (os′te-o-jen″) [*osteo-* + Gr. *gennan* to produce] the basic bone making element of osteogenic fibers, making up the inner layer of the periosteum, from which bone is formed.

osteogenesis (os″te-o-jen′ĕ-sis) [*osteo-* + Gr. *gennan* to produce] the formation of bone; the development of the bones. Called also *osteosis*. **o. imperfec′ta,** abnormal brittleness of the bones, often associated with dentinogenesis imperfecta. Called also *brittle bones* and *fragilitas ossium*. See also Blegvad-Haxthausen SYNDROME, Lobstein's SYNDROME, van der Hoeve's SYNDROME, and Vrolik's SYNDROME. **o. imperfec′ta congen′ita,** Vrolik's SYNDROME. **c. imperfec′ta tar′da,** Lobstein's SYNDROME.

osteogenic (os″te-o-jen′ik) [*osteo-* + Gr. *gennan* to produce] pertaining to osteogenesis; derived from or composed of any tissue involved in the growth or repair of bone.

osteoid (os′te-oid) [*osteo-* + Gr. *eidos* form] 1. resembling bone. 2. the organic matrix of bone; young bone which has not undergone calcification. Called also *prebone*.

osteologia (os″te-o-lo′je-ah) in NA terminology it encompasses the nomenclature relating to the bones; osteology.

osteologist (os″te-ol′o-jist) a specialist in osteology.

osteology (os″te-ol′o-je) [*osteo-* + Gr. *logos* treatise] the scientific study of the bones; applied also to the body of knowledge relating to the bones. Called also *osteologia* [NA].

osteolysis (os″te-ol′ĭ-sis) [*osteo-* + Gr. *lysis* dissolution] disintegration of bone, believed to consist of softening and liquefaction of the organic matrix followed by a leaching out of the inorganic components; loss of the inorganic components caused by disturbances in the normal equilibrium is followed by the reversion of the organic components to connective tissue.

osteoma (os″te-o′mah) [*osteo-* + *-oma*] an uncommon benign tumor composed of bone tissue; it is usually a solitary lesion but multiple tumors also occur. It is rarely located in the jaws; when oral and paraoral structures are involved, the mandibular condyle, angle of the inferior border of the mandible, lateral surface of the mandible, palate, and paranasal sinuses are the most frequent sites. Osteoma of periosteal origin presents a hard, spherical, nodular, painless, slow-growing lesion on the surface of the bone, which may produce asymmetry of the jaw or occlude a sinus. Osteoma of endosteal origin (*endosteal o.*) is a central lesion separated from the surrounding bone by a fibrous capsule. **endosteal o.**, see *osteoma*. **giant osteoid o.**, osteoblastoma. **osteoid o.**, a benign tumor of bone, most commonly affecting young persons, made up of fibrous tissue containing osteoid or calcified, poorly formed spicules of bone. It presents a discrete, reddish-brown nodule usually arising within the cortical bone, surrounded by a zone of delicate porous bone, and about this zone, dense sclerotic bone. The jaws are seldom involved.

osteomalacia (os″te-o-mah-la′she-ah) [osteo- + Gr. *malakia* softening] a deficiency disease of adult age, characterized by disorders of mineralization and softening of the bones due to lack of vitamin D and calcium and phosphate deficiency. Called also *adult rickets*. **multiple o.**, OSTEITIS deformans.

osteomatosis (os″te-o-mah-to-sis) formation of multiple osteomas. **hereditary polyposis and o.**, Gardner's SYNDROME.

osteometric (os″te-o-met′rik) pertaining to osteometry.

osteometry (os″te-om′ĕ-tre) [osteo- + Gr. *metron* measure] the measurement of the dimensions and proportions of bones in a dry skeleton. See also ANTHROPOMETRY and CRANIOMETRY.

osteomyelitis (os″te-o-mi″ĕ-li′tis) [osteo- + Gr. *myelos* marrow + *-itis*] inflammation of bone beginning in the bone marrow and extending to involve the periosteum. After pus in the medullary cavity and beneath the periosteum interrupts the blood supply, the calcified tissue becomes the seat of infection, and gradually becomes necrotic. **acute intramedullary o.**, acute suppurative o. of jaw. **acute subperiosteal o.**, an acute form characterized by an accumulation of exudate beneath the periosteum. Formation of periapical abscesses and escape of pus along the surface of bone, producing periodontal abscesses and separation of the periosteum from the cortex usually occurs, associated with draining of pus through multiple intraoral and extraoral sinuses, severe swelling, pain, and labial anesthesia or paresthesia. **acute suppurative o. of jaw**, an acute condition of either jaw that may follow periapical dental infection, characterized by spreading of infection throughout the medullary spaces, causing necrosis of the bone. Teeth may become loosened and tender to percussion, and pus is discharged through multiple sinuses. Called also *acute intramedullary o.* **bloodborne o.**, hematogenous o. **chronic diffuse sclerosing o.**, osteomyelitis that may affect all bones at any age. Oral lesions occur most commonly in edentulous elderly individuals, usually in the mandible. It has usually a mild course, with occasional acute episodes, associated with suppuration, and sometimes external draining fistulae. Vague pain and a bad taste in the mouth are occasionally the only symptoms. The lesion shows dense, irregular trabeculae of bone — some bordered by active layers of osteoblasts. Focal areas of osteoclastic activity sometimes occur. Polymorphonuclear leukocytes and plasma cells may be present in lesions undergoing an acute phase. **chronic focal sclerosing o.**, osteomyelitis occurring most often in children and young adults, which may involve the jaws, usually adjacent to a mandibular first molar with a large carious lesion. It represents a high tissue reaction to a mild bacterial infection entering through a carious lesion. Histologically, it is characterized by a dense mass of bony trabeculae with little interstitial marrow tissue. Called also *condensing osteitis*. **chronic intramedullary o.**, chronic suppurative o. of jaw. **chronic subperiosteal o.**, a protracted inflammatory disease, which may also involve the jaws, usually occurring after the acute phase of an infection subsides or as a result of interruption of the blood supply to the bone following a prolonged dysplasia. **chronic suppurative o. of jaw**, a chronic condition of either jaw that may develop after the acute phase subsides, characterized by the presence of multiple intraoral and extraoral discharging sinuses, sometimes thickening of the bone producing facial asymmetry, and periodic acute exacerbations. The infection is localized but bacteria in the dead bone are inaccessible to body defense, thus the chronic course. Called also *chronic intramedullary o.* **Garré's o.**, nonsuppurative sclerosing osteomyelitis marked by increased density and gradual development of a spindle-shaped sclerotic thickening of the cortex. The long bones are most commonly affected, but involvement of the mandible may also occur, marked by a hard, nontender mass of bone overlying the affected jaw. Staphylococci, streptococci, and mixed organisms appear to be the pathogens most commonly associated with the disease. Called also *sclerosing nonsuppurative o.*, *o. sicca*, and *idiopathic cortical sclerosis*. **hematogenous o.**, pyogenic osteomyelitis in which pathogenic bacteria enter the bone through the hematogenous route. Called also *bloodborne o.* **o. of jaw in newborn infants**, acute osteomyelitis, usually of the maxilla, believed to be a result of small abrasions caused at the time of delivery by inserting the fingers into the mouth of an infant to aid delivery or to clean mucus from the mouth. Involvement of the mandible is usually rare; it may be produced by fractures of the mandible. **pyogenic o.**, osteomyelitis caused by any of the pyogenic bacteria. **radiation o.**, osteomyelitis following exposure to large doses of ionizing radiations, followed by bacterial invasion. The jaws may be affected because of the possibility of contamination through the teeth or through a breach in the oral mucosa. Pathological fracture is a frequent complication. **Salmonella o.**, typhoid o. **sclerosing nonsuppurative o.**, **o. sic′ca**, Garré's o. **syphilitic o.**, a chronic, now relatively rare, inflammatory disease of the bone, including the jaws, seen in tertiary syphilis. It may produce granulomatous and necrotizing lesions resulting in decalcification, partial destruction, and sclerosis of the tissue. **tuberculous o.**, osteomyelitis caused by tubercle bacilli, involving the epiphyses of the long bones, vertebrae, and phalanges. The onset is usually insidious, characterized at first by swelling. Involvement of the jaws is usually secondary to pulmonary tuberculosis and is produced through the hematogenous route; some cases of periapical tuberculoma may result in extension of infection into the jaw bones. The lesion in the jaws shows necrosis associated with sequestration and draining sinuses similar to that seen when other bones are affected. Gingival involvement may occur. See also oral TUBERCULOSIS. **typhoid o.**, osteomyelitis occurring as a late complication of typhoid or paratyphoid fever, usually involving the vertebrae, ribs, long bones, and occasionally the jaws. Called also *Salmonella o.*

osteon (os′te-on) [osteo- + Gr. *on* neuter ending] the basic unit of structure of compact bone, comprising a haversian canal and its concentrically arranged lamellae, of which there may be 4 to 20, each 3 to 7 μ thick, in a single (haversian) system; such units are directed mainly in the long axis of the bone.

osteonecrosis (os″te-o-ne-kro′sis) [osteo- + Gr. *nekrosis* death] necrosis of bone. **radiation o.**, osteoradionecrosis.

osteopath (os′te-o-path) a practitioner of osteopathy; Doctor of Osteopathy (DO).

osteopathia (os″te-o-path′e-ah); any disease of a bone; osteopathy. **o. acidot′ica pseudorachit′ica**, Fanconi-Albertini-Zellweger SYNDROME. **o. fibro′sa generalisa′ta**, Recklinghausen's DISEASE (2).

osteopathology (os″te-o-pah-thol′o-je) pathology or disease of bone; also the field of study of diseases of bone.

osteopathy (os″te-op′ah-the) [osteo- + Gr. *pathos* disease] 1. any disease of a bone; osteopathia. 2. a system of therapy founded by Andrew Taylor Still and based on the theory that the body is capable of making its own remedies against diseases and other toxic conditions when it is in normal structural relationship and has favorable environmental conditions and adequate nutrition. It utilizes generally accepted physical, medicinal, and surgical methods of diagnosis and therapy, while placing chief emphasis on the importance of normal body mechanics and manipulative methods of detecting and correcting faulty structure. **disseminated condensing o.**, Albers-Schönberg's DISEASE. **hunger o.**, disturbances of the skeletal system observed in famine areas, characterized by a reduction in the amount of normally calcified bone, and attributed to dietary deficiencies and associated hormonal dysfunctions.

osteopenia (os″te-o-pe′ne-ah) [osteo- Gr. *penia* poverty] reduced bone mass due to a decrease in the rate of osteoid synthesis to a level insufficient to compensate normal bone lysis.

osteoperiosteal (os″te-o-per″ĭ-os′te-al) pertaining to bone and its periosteum.

osteoperiostitis (os″te-o-per″ĭ-os-ti′tis) inflammation of a bone and its periosteum. **alveolodental o.**, periodontitis.

osteopetrosis (os″te-o-pe-tro′sis) [osteo- + Gr. *petra* stone + *-osis*] a disease characterized by bone condensation. See Albers-Schönberg's DISEASE.

osteophyma (os″te-o-fi′mah) [osteo- + Gr. *phyma* growth] a tumor or outgrowth of a bone.

osteophyte (os′te-o-fit″) [osteo- + Gr. *phyton* plant] a bony excrescence or outgrowth.

osteophytosis (os″te-o-fi-to′sis) formation of osteophytes.

osteoplaque (os′te-o-plak) a layer of bone.

osteoplasty (os′te-o-plas″te) [osteo- + Gr. *plassein* to form] plastic surgery of the bones; reshaping or remodeling of bone.

osteoporosis (os″te-o-po-ro′sis) [osteo- + Gr. *poros* passage + *-osis*] an acquired systemic disorder that may affect any bone, including the jaws, characterized by abnormal rarefaction of the involved bone. It is believed to stem from failure of the osteoblasts to lay down bone matrix. Studies suggest that inadequate formation of proteinaceous matrix may be due to excessive catabolic activity of glucocorticoids, and to a negative calcium balance. Thinning of the cortical bone, resorption of cancellous bone spicules, enlargement of the medullary cavity, and bone loss are the characteristic features. Absence of the teeth without a prosthetic replacement; immobilization over long periods following fractures, paralysis, or other conditions; interference with the blood supply; use of steroid hormones; postmenopausal and gonadal disorders; metabolic disorders, such as hyperthyroidism and diabetes mellitus; and vitamin C deficiency are among the etiologic factors. **o. of disuse,** atrophy of bone tissue due to lack of re-formation of laminae in the absence of stimuli necessary for their replacement in new stress lines. See also disuse ATROPHY. **fetal o.,** Vrolik's SYNDROME.

osteoradionecrosis (os"te-o-ra"de-o-ne-kro'sis) necrosis of bone following irradiation, characterized by a chronic painful infection and necrosis followed by sequestration. It may involve the mandible and, less frequently, the maxilla. Called also *radiation osteonecrosis.*

osteorrhagia (os"te-o-ra'je-ah) [*osteo-* + Gr. *rhēgnynai* to burst out] hemorrhage from the bone tissue.

osteorrhaphy (os"te-or'ah-fe) [*osteo-* + Gr. *rhaphē* suture] the suturing or wiring of bones.

osteosarcoma (os"te-o-sar-ko'mah) [*osteo-* + *sarcoma*] osteogenic SARCOMA.

osteosclerosis (os"te-o-skle-ro'sis) [*osteo-* + Gr. *sklērosis* hardening] the hardening or abnormal denseness of bone. See also EBURNATION. **o. congen'ita dif'fusa,** Albers-Schönberg's DISEASE. **congenital o.,** achondroplasia.

osteosis (os"te-o'sis) [Gr. *osteon* bone + *-osis*] 1. any morbid process of bone. 2. osteogenesis.

osteosynovitis (os"te-o-sin"o-vi'tis) synovitis together with osteitis of the neighboring bones.

osteosynthesis (os"te-o-sin'thĕ-sis) [*osteo-* + *synthesis*] surgical fastening of the ends of a fractured bone by sutures, rings, plates, or other mechanical means.

osteothrombophlebitis (os"te-o-throm"bo-fle-bi'tis) inflammation extended through intact bone by a progressive thrombophlebitis of small venules, such as sometimes occurs in the mastoid bone.

osteothrombosis (os"te-o-throm-bo'sis) thrombosis of the veins of a bone.

osteotome (os'te-o-tōm") [*osteo-* + Gr. *tomē* a cut] a chisel-like instrument for cutting bone.

osteotomoclasis (os"te-o-to-mok'lah-sis) [*osteo-* + Gr. *tomos* section + *klasis* breaking] correction of curvature of bone by partial division with the osteotome, followed by forcible fracture.

osteotomy (os"te-ot'o-me) [*osteo-* + Gr. *temnein* to cut] the cutting of a bone. **blind o.,** closed o. **block o.,** that in which a section of bone is removed. **C-form o.,** a form of mandibular osteotomy used for correcting retrognathism. See illustration. **closed o.,**

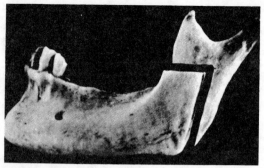

Inverted L-form osteotomy. (From B. Levine and D. S. Topazian: The intraoral inverted-L double oblique osteotomy of the mandibular ramus: a new technique for correction of mandibular prognathism. J. Oral Surg., 34(1):522, 1976.)

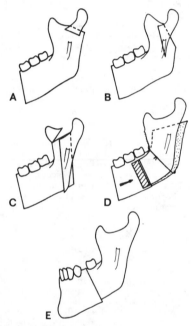

Common techniques for the correction of mandibular prognathism. *A,* Osteotomy in the condylar neck. *B,* Subcondylar oblique osteotomy. *C,* Vertical osteotomy of the ramus. *D,* Sagittal splitting of the ramus. *E,* Osteotomy of the body. (From D. E. Waite: Textbook of Practical Oral Surgery. 2nd ed. Philadelphia, Lea & Febiger, 1978.)

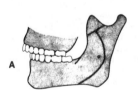 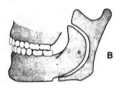

A, Outline of bony cut for C-form osteotomy with coronoidectomy. *B,* C-form osteotomy advancement of mandible without coronoidectomy (different case). (From D. E. Waite: Textbook of Practical Oral Surgery. 2nd ed. Philadelphia, Lea & Febiger, 1978.)

that performed without directly visualizing the bone, as by passing a Gigli saw behind the back of the condyle through small skin or mucosal incisions and cutting through the bone. Called also *blind osteotomy.* **o. of condylar neck,** that of the condylar neck of the mandible for correction of prognathism, which may be performed blindly or through an extraoral approach. See illustration. **cuneiform o.,** the removal of a wedge of bone. **cup-and-ball o.,** that in which the distal fragment is pointed and the proximal fragment is recessed. **hinge o.,** curvilinear cutting of a bone. **L-form o., inverted,** a type of mandibular osteotomy used for correcting retrognathism. See illustration. **linear o.,** the sawing or linear cutting of a bone. **mandibular o.,** that of the mandible in correction of its defects. See illustration. **maxillary o.,** maxillotomy. **open o.,** that performed under direct vision. **perforation o.,** that performed through intact overlying mucosa by means of a bur. **sagittal**

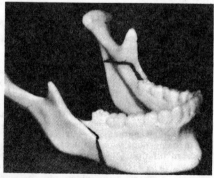

Sagittal split osteotomy. Bony incision (cut) outlined on model. (From D. E. Waite: Textbook of Practical Oral Surgery. 2nd ed. Philadelphia, Lea & Febiger, 1978.)

split o., surgical sagittal splitting of the ramus of the mandible in correction of prognathism. See illustration. **segmental alveolar o.,** that in which the bone is cut horizontally apical to the apices of teeth to facilitate repositioning of tooth-bone segments. **subcondylar oblique o.,** in prognathism, a technique in which the line of osteotomy begins in the sigmoid notch midway between the coronoid process and the condylar neck and proceeds diagonally downward to the posterior border of the vertical ramus of the mandible. See illustration. **vertical o. of ramus of mandible,** in prognathism, that in which the line of resection proceeds vertically from the deepest aspect of the sigmoid notch to the lower border of the mandible in the angle area, the mandibular foramen remaining in the anterior side of the line and the small proximal fragment together with the condyle being moved laterally. See illustration.

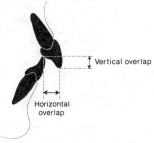

Vertical overlap

Horizontal overlap

(Modified from T. M. Graber: Orthodontics — Principles and Practice. 3rd ed. Philadelphia, W. B. Saunders Co., 1972.)

osteotribe, osteotrite (os′te-o-trīb″, os′te-o-trīt″) [osteo- + Gr. tribein to rub] an instrument for rasping bone.
osteotrophy (os″te-ot′ro-fe) [osteo- + Gr. trophē nutrition] nutrition of bone.
osteotylus (os″te-ot′ĭ-lus) [osteo- + Gr. tylos callus] the callus enclosing the end of a broken bone.
ostia (os′te-ah) [L.] plural of ostium.
ostial (os′te-al) pertaining to an ostium.
ostium (os′te-um), pl. os′tia [L.] an opening; used in anatomical nomenclature as a general term to designate an opening into a tubular organ, or between two cavities within the body. Called also opening, orifice, and orificium. **o. cardi′acum** [NA], the orifice between the stomach and the esophagus and the upper (cardiac) part of the stomach. Called also cardia. **pharyngeal o. of auditory tube, o. pharyn′geum tu′bae auditi′vae** [NA], an opening to the auditory tube on the lateral wall of the nasopharynx.
Ostranorm trademark for dihydroergotamine mesylate (see under DIHYDROERGOTAMINE).
Ostrocilline trademark for penicillin V benzathine (see under PENICILLIN).
ot- see OTO-.
Ota's nevus [M. T. Ota, Japanese physician] see under NEVUS.
otagra (o-tag′rah) otalgia.
otalgia (o-tal′je-ah) [Gr. ōtalgia] pain in the ear; earache. Called also otagra. **o. denta′lis,** reflex pain in the ear due to dental disease. **geniculate o.,** geniculate NEURALGIA. **reflex o.,** otalgia dependent upon some lesion of the buccal cavity or nasopharynx.
OTC over-the-counter (drug); see under DRUG.
otitis (o-ti′tis) [ot- + -itis] inflammation of the ear. **o. me′dia,** inflammation of the middle ear, or typanum, most often occurring in infants and young children, which frequently follows or accompanies an upper respiratory infection. The principal symptoms of the acute form are earache, hearing loss, fever, and a feeling of fullness and pressure in the ear. As the infection progresses pressure builds up behind the tympanic membrane and may cause perforation or rupture of it; this is followed by drainage of exudate into the external acoustic meatus. The chronic condition is almost always associated with perforation of the tympanic membrane. This form may complicate an upper respiratory disease or be associated with mastoiditis. Frequent symptoms are drainage from the ear, ringing in the ear, and hearing loss. Called also tympanitis.
oto-, ot- [Gr. ous, ōtos ear] a combining term denoting relationship to the ear.
otoantritis (o″to-an-tri′tis) otitis involving the attic of the tympanum and the mastoid antrum.
otoblennorrhea (o″to-blen″o-re′ah) [oto- + Gr. blenna mucus + rhoia flow] mucous discharge from the ear.
otocephalus (o″to-sef′ah-lus) [oto- + Gr. kephalē head] a monster lacking the lower jaw and having ears united below the face.

otocranium (o″to-kra′ne-um) [oto- + Gr. kranion skull] 1. the chamber of the petrous bone that lodges the internal ear. 2. the auditory portion of the cranium. Called also petromastoid.
OTOD Organization of Teachers of Oral Diagnosis (see under ORGANIZATION).
otogenous (o-toj′ĕ-nus) [oto- + Gr. gennan to produce] originating within the ear.
otolaryngology (o″to-lar″in-gol′o-je) that branch of medicine which treats the diseases of the ear, nose, and throat.
otologist (o-tol′o-jist) a physician who specializes in otology.
otology (o-tol′o-je) [oto- + -logy] that branch of medicine which deals with the ear.
otomastoiditis (o″to-mas″toid-i′tis) mastoiditis associated with otitis.
otopharyngeal (o″to-fah-rin′je-al) pertaining to the ear and pharynx.
otoplasty (o′to-plas″te) [oto- + Gr. plassein] surgical reconstruction of the ear; plastic surgery of the ear.
otopyorrhea (o″to-pi″o-re′ah) [oto- + Gr. pyon pus + rhein to flow] a copious purulent discharge from the ear.
otopyosis (o″to-pi-o′sis) [oto- + Gr. pyon pus + -osis] a suppurative disease of the ear.
otorhinolaryngology (o″to-ri″no-lar″in-gol′o-je) [oto- + Gr. rhis nose + larynx + -logy] that branch of medicine that treats the ear, nose, pharynx, and larynx.
otorhinology (o″to-ri-nol′o-je) [oto- + Gr. rhis nose + -logy] that branch of medicine which treats diseases of the nose and ear.
otorrhagia (o″to-ra′je-ah) [oto- + Gr. rhēgnynai to burst forth] hemorrhage from the ear.
otorrhea (o″to-re′ah) [oto- + Gr. rhoia to flow] a discharge from the ear.
ototomy (o-tot′o-me) [oto- + Gr. tomē a cutting] the dissection of or anatomy of the ear.
Otsby see Nygaard-Otsby FRAME.
ouabain (wah-ba′in) a poisonous cardiac glycoside from Strophanthus gratus, Acokanthera ouabaio, and other plants, 3-[(6-deoxy-α-L-mannopyranosyl)oxy]-1,5,11α,14,19-pentahydroxycard-20-(22)-enolide. It occurs as a photosensitive, white, odorless, crystalline powder or crystals that are soluble in water and ethanol. Used in the treatment of congestive heart failure. Called also acocantherin, gratus strophanthin, and G-strophanthin. Trademark: Strovidal.
oulectomy (oo-lek′to-me) ulectomy.
oulitis (oo-li′tis) ulitis.
ounce (ouns) [L. uncia] a unit of weight in both the avoirdupois and apothecaries' weights. The avoirdupois ounce is one-sixteenth of a pound or 437.5 grains, or 28.3495 grams. The apothecaries' ounce is one-twelfth pound, or 480 grains, or 31.103 grams. Symbol ℥. Abbreviated oz. See also Tables of Weights and Measures at WEIGHT. **fluid o.,** a unit of capacity (liquid or wine measure) in the apothecaries' system, which is equivalent to 480 minims, 8 fluid drams, 0.0625 pints, or 29.5729 cubic centimeters. Abbreviated fl oz. Written also fluidounce. **troy o.,** an ounce consisting of 480 grains, 20 pennyweights, 0.083 pounds, and 31.103 grams.
ourari (oo-rar′e) curare.
-ous a chemical suffix indicating a lower valence, as compared with -ic, as in ferrous (valence 2) and ferric (valence 3).
outline (out′līn) the line by which a figure or object is defined; a contour. **basal seat o.,** an outline on the mucous membrane or on a cast of the entire area that is to be covered by a denture. See also basal SEAT.
outpatient (out′pa-shent) 1. a patient who comes to the hospital, clinic, or dispensary for diagnosis and/or treatment but does not occupy a bed. 2. pertaining to medical services rendered in a hospital without admitting the patient; ambulatory. See also ambulatory CARE and ambulatory hospital CARE. Cf. INPATIENT. **hospital o. care,** ambulatory hospital CARE. **o. care,** 1. ambulatory CARE. 2. ambulatory hospital CARE.
outpocketing (out-pok′et-ing) evagination.
output (out′put) 1. the quantity produced in a given time. 2. the act of turning out. 3. the current, voltage, power, or signal produced by an electrical or electronic system. 4. Information transferred from the memory bank of a computer to a secondary or external storage or to an on-line device. Cf. INPUT. **cardiac o.,** see circulation RATE.
oval (o′val) [L. ovalis] egg-shaped; having the outline of an egg.
ovalbumin (o″val-bu′min) [L. ovum egg + albumin] an albumin in the whites of eggs. Called also egg albumin.
ovalocyte (o′vah-lo-sīt) an oval erythrocyte found in various forms of anemia, as well as in normal individuals.

ovalocytosis (o-val″o-si-to′sis) the presence in the blood of abnormally large numbers of ovalocytes, as in elliptocytosis.

ovarium (o-va′re-um), pl. *ova′ria* [L.] [NA] ovary.

ovary (o′vah-re) [L.] the female gonad; one of the two sexual glands, one on each side of the pelvic cavity, in which ova are formed and from where they descend into the uterine cavity through the fallopian tubes. Called also *ovarium* [NA].

OVD occlusal vertical dimension; see vertical dimension, contact, under DIMENSION.

oven (uv′en) a heated chamber or enclosed compartment. **dry heat o.,** a dry heat sterilizer, consisting of a box in which an electric unit raises the air temperature to more than 160° C (320° F). See also dry heat STERILIZATION.

overbite (o′ver-bīt) vertical OVERLAP (1). **deep o.,** closed BITE. **horizontal o.,** horizontal OVERLAP.

overclosure (o″ver-klo′sur) the loss of occlusal vertical dimension. **reduced interarch distance o.,** loss of occlusal or contact vertical dimension.

overdenture (o′ver-den′chur) overlay DENTURE.

overdosage (o′ver-do′sij) administration of a drug or another agent in amounts that are greater than the standard or prescribed dosage.

overeruption (o″ver-e-rup′shun) supraclusion.

overgrafting (o″ver-graft′ing) the application of a second graft over a previously healed graft from which the epithelium has been removed, as a means of reinforcing split thickness grafts.

overgrowth (o′ver-grōth) excessive growth of a part, due either to increase in size of the constituent cells (hypertrophy) or to an increase in their number (hyperplasia).

overhang (o′ver-hang) 1. something that juts over and extends beyond the main structure, hanging over something below. 2. the extension over the margins of a tooth cavity of an excessive amount of filling material.

overjet (o′ver-jet) horizontal OVERLAP.

overjut (o′ver-jut) horizontal OVERLAP.

overlap (o′ver-lap) 1. to cover and extend beyond a certain point. 2. anything that lies or extends over and partially covers something. **horizontal o.,** that condition in which the incisal or buccal cusp ridges of the maxillary teeth extend labially or buccally to the incisal margins and ridges of the mandibular teeth when the jaws are in habitual occlusion. Called also *horizontal overbite, overjet,* and *overjut.* See illustration. **vertical o.,** 1. that condition in which the incisal ridges of the maxillary anterior teeth extend below the incisal ridges of the mandibular anterior teeth when the jaws are in centric occlusion. Called also *overbite.* See illustration. 2. the distance that the teeth lap over their antagonists. 3. the relationship of the maxillary incisors to the mandibular incisors when the incisal edges pass each other in centric occlusion. **vertical o., deep,** closed BITE.

overlay (o′ver-la) 1. a covering over an already existing structure; onlay. 2. overlay DENTURE.

overnutrition (o′ver-nu-trish′un) malnutrition due to the consumption of excessive amounts of food. See table at NUTRITION.

overriding (o″ver-rīd′ing) the slipping of either part of a fractured bone past the other.

ovi- see OVO-.

ovo-, ovi- [L. *ovum* egg] a combining form denoting relationship to an egg, or to ova. See also words beginning OO-.

ovoid (o′void) [*ovo-* + Gr. *eidos* form] shaped like an egg.

ovomucoid (o′vo-mu′koid) [*ovo-* + *mucoid*] a heat-stable mucoid in egg white, which represents about 10 percent of its protein content.

Owen, line of [Sir Richard *Owen,* English anatomist and paleontologist, 1804–1892] see under LINE.

Owren's syndrome [Paul A. *Owren*] 1. hemolytic CRISIS. 2. parahemophilia.

oxacillin (oks″ah-sil′in) a broad-spectrum semisynthetic penicillin, 3,3-dimethyl - 6 - (5-methyl-3-phenyl - 4 - isoxozolecarboxamido)-7-oxo-4-thia-1-azabicyclo[3,2,0]heptane-2-carboxylic acid, occurring as an odorless, fine, crystalline powder that is readily soluble in water, methanol, and dimethylsulfoxide, slightly soluble in ethanol, chloroform, pyridine, and methyl acetate, and insoluble in ethyl acetate, ether, benzene, and ethylene chloride. Generally used as the sodium salt in the treatment of infections due to penicillinase-producing gram-positive bacteria, particularly staphylococcal infections. Its pharmacological and toxic properties are similar to those of other penicillins, but may also cause nausea, vomiting, diarrhea, fever, eosinophilia, hairy tongue, and rarely candidiasis. Trademarks: Bactocill, Bristopen, Cryptocillin, Prostaphlin.

Oxacycline trademark for *oxytetracycline.*

oxalate (ok′sah-lāt) a salt of oxalic acid.

Oxalid trademark for *oxyphenbutazone.*

Oxamycin trademark for *cycloserine.*

oxandrolone (ok-san′dro-lōn) an androgenic steroid, 17β-hydroxy-17-methyl-2-oxa-5α-androstan-3-one, occurring as a white, odorless, photosensitive, crystalline powder that is soluble in chloroform, sparingly soluble in ethanol and acetone, and insoluble in water. Used in the treatment of wasting disease in children, conditions characterized by negative nitrogen balance, retarded growth, and osteoporosis. It may cause leukopenia, liver lesions, cholestatic jaundice, virilization, and other disorders. Trademarks: Anavar, Provitar, Vasorome.

oxazepam (oks-az′e-pam) a mild sedative, 7-chloro-1,3-dihydro-3-hydroxy-5-phenyl-2*H*-1,4-benzodiazepin-2-one, occurring as a creamy white to yellowish, odorless, bitter powder that is slightly soluble in ethanol, chloroform, and ether and insoluble in water. Used to control anxiety, tension, agitation, and symptoms associated with alcoholic intoxication. Adverse reactions may include transient drowsiness, vertigo, headache, syncope, skin rashes, lethargy, edema, slurred speech, tremor, altered libido, leukopenia, and jaundice. Trademarks: Adumbran, Bonare, Enidrel, Isodin, Nesontil, Propax, Rondar, Serax, Serenid, Seresta, Sobril.

oxhydrase (oks-hi′drās) oxidase. **amino acid o.,** amino acid OXIDASE.

oxidant (ok′si-dant) 1. the electron acceptor in an oxidation-reduction reaction. 2. a substance that releases free oxygen, thus being destructive to anaerobic bacteria. Hydrogen and metallic peroxides are the principal oxidants used in dental practice.

oxidase (ok′si-dās) an oxidoreductase that catalyzes an oxidation reaction involving molecular oxygen or where O_2 is an acceptor. Called also *oxhydrase.* **adrenalin o.,** amino o. **amino o.** [E.C.1.4.3.4], an oxidoreductase that acts on the CH−NH_2 group of donors with oxygen as acceptor. It is widely distributed in animal tissue, its function consisting of breaking of biologically active amines. Tryptamine derivatives, chiefly catecholamines and histamine, are the principal substrates. Called also *adrenal o., monoamine o. (MAO), tyramine o.,* and *tyraminase.* **amino acid o.,** an oxidoreductase that acts on the CH−NH_2 group of donors. It is a flavoprotein that catalyzes the splitting off of the amino group (NH_2) of an amino acid to form an imino acid which is hydrolyzed to a keto acid and ammonia. Called also *amino acid oxhydrase.* See also DEAMINATION. **D-amino acid o.** [E.C.1.4.3.3], an oxidoreductase (a flavoprotein) that catalyzes oxidation of D-amino acids. **diamine o.,** histaminase. **glucose o.** [E.C.1.1.3.4], an oxidoreductase that is a toxic flavoprotein derived from *Penicillium notatum,* which catalyzes the oxidation of glucose to gluconic acid. Called also *aeroglucose dehydrogenase, notatin, penatin,* and *penicillin B.* **L-amino acid o.** [E.C.1.4.3.2], an oxidoreductase that catalyzes the oxidation of L-amino acids. Certain examples also catalyze the oxidation of 2-hydroxy acids. It is a flavoprotein found in the liver and kidneys; also occurring in snake venom. **monoamine o.,** amino o. **pyruvate o., pyruvic o.** [E.C.1.2.3.3], an oxidoreductase with oxygen as an acceptor, which is involved in oxidative metabolism of carbohydrates where pyruvic acid forms acetyl CoA, and in turn transfers the acetyl group to oxaloacetic acid to make the citric acid in the Krebs cycle. **tyramine o.**

oxidation (ok″si-da′shun) originally, a term meaning combining of oxygen with another substance. Now defined as the process occurring when an element loses electrons or increases in valence number thereby losing negative charges and becoming more electropositive. See also OXIDATION-REDUCTION.

oxidation-reduction (ok″si-da′shun-re-duk′shun) a chemical reaction whereby electrons are removed (oxidation) from atoms of the substance being oxidized and transferred to atoms being reduced (reduction). The total number of valence increases must equal the total number of valence decreases, or the total electrons lost must equal the total electrons gained. Called also *redox.* See also chemical EQUATION.

oxide (ok′sīd) [L. *oxidum*] any compound of oxygen with an element or radical. **arsenous o.,** ARSENIC trioxide. **chrome o.,** see chromic o. **chromic o.,** a compound, Cr_2O_3, occurring as light to dark green, fine, hexagonal, hard crystals that are slightly soluble in acids and alkalies but not in water, alcohol, and acetone. Used as an abrasive and pigment material, in the production of alloys, and in various chemical and industrial processes. It can also form on the surface of iron-chromium alloy (stainless steel) as a tough, transparent oxide layer (passivating layer) that provides a barrier against further oxidation and protects the steel from corrosion and tarnishing. Called also *chrome o., anadonis green, chrome green, chrome ocher, green cinnabar, green oxide of chromium, green rouge, leaf green, oil green,* and *ultramarine green.* **ethyl o.,** ethyl ETHER. **ethylene o.,** oxide ETHYLENE. **ferric o.,** a substance Fe_2O_3, appearing in nature as the mineral hematite or maghemite, its color and appearance depending upon the size and shape of its particles and the amount of combined water it contains. Used as a pigment and as a fine polishing agent for metals. Also used as a sunscreen in protecting the lips from the effects of ultraviolet rays. In dentistry, it is used for polishing metal restorations. Available in the form of sticks for application on a rag wheel or felt cone to attain a high gloss after the preliminary polishing with pumice and tripoli. Called also *jeweler's rouge* and *ferric sesquioxide.* **green o. of chromium,** chromic o. **iron o.,** ferric HYDROXIDE. **mercuric o.,** a yellow to orange-yellow, heavy, odorless powder, HgO, that decomposes and becomes discolored on exposure to light, is soluble in diluted hydrochloric or nitric acids, but not in water and alcohol. Used chiefly in ointments for topical antiseptic therapy. Called also *yellow precipitate.* **methylene o.,** formaldehyde. **nitrous o.,** a colorless asphyxiant gas, N_2O, with a slight sweetish taste and a pleasant odor. In oral surgery, used in psychosedation, the pain control depending on the concomitant use of local anesthesia, the nitrous oxide acting chiefly as a sedative to allay apprehension, whereby the patient experiences total loss of pain sensibility, but not consciousness. Also used as an inhalation anesthetic agent, either as a nitrous oxide–oxygen mixture alone or with narcotic premedication, or with halothane, vinyl ether, methoxyfluorane, or thiopental used as adjuncts. Its muscle relaxant properties are enhanced by the use of neuromuscular blocking agents. Called also *dinitrogen monoxide, factitious air, hyponitrous acid anhydride,* and *laughing gas.* **stannic o.,** a compound, SnO_2, occurring as a white or slightly grayish powder, found in nature as the mineral cassiterite, or produced through a reaction between tin and concentrated nitric acid at high temperatures. Used as a polishing agent for glass, metals, and, especially, to produce a high polish on metallic dental restorations. Called also *tin o., white tin o., flowers of tin, putty powder, stannic anhydride, tin ash,* and *tin dioxide.* **sulfurous o.,** SULFUR dioxide. **tin o.,** stannic o. **titanic o.,** TITANIUM dioxide. **white tin o.,** stannic o.

oxidoreductase [E.C.1] (ok″sĭ-do-re-duk′tās) any of a major class of enzymes involved in catalyzing oxidation-reduction reactions in cells. See also ENZYME classification. **transaminating o.,** aminotransferase.

oximeter (ok-sim′ĕ-ter) an instrument for measuring oxygen saturation of the blood, usually by measuring the arterial oxygen saturation by colorimetric changes in the arterial circulation of the earlobe.

oximinotransferase [E.C.2.6.3.1] (ok-sim″ĭ-no-trans′fer-ās) a transferase that catalyzes the transfer of oxime from pyruvate-oxime to form pyruvate and acetoxime. Called also *transoximinase.*

oxine (oks′ēn) 8-hydroxyquinoline. **o. sulfate,** 8-HYDROXYQUINOLINE sulfate.

Oxirane trademark for *ethylene oxide* (see under ETHYLENE).

oxirane (ok′sĭ-rān) the oxygen atom of the epoxide ring,

$$-\underset{|}{C}-\underset{|}{C}-$$
$$\diagdown O \diagup$$

oxole (oks′ōl) furan.

oxomethane (ok′so-meth′ān) formaldehyde.

oxophenarsine (ok″so-phen-ar′sēn) an antitrypanosomal agent, 2-amino-4-arsenosophenol hydrochloride, occurring as a white or whitish powder that is soluble in water and ethanol. Sometimes also used in the treatment of acute necrotizing ulcerative gingivitis. Trademark: Mapharsen.

oxosilane (oks″o-sil′ān) siloxane.

oxprenolol hydrochloride (oks-pren′o-lol) a coronary vasodilator, 1-[(1-methylethyl)amino] - 3 - [2-(2-propenyloxy)phenoxy]-2-propanol. Trademark: Trasicor.

oxtriphylline (oks-trif′ĭ-lēn) a central nervous system stimulant, choline theophyllinate, occurring as a white, crystalline powder with an amine-like odor, which is soluble in water and ethanol and slightly in chloroform. Used in the treatment of respiratory obstructive disorders. Side effects may include gastric distress, cardiac arrhythmias, and central nervous system stimulation. Called also *theophylline cholinate.* Trademark: Choledyl.

oxy- [Gr. *oxys* keen] a combining form meaning (*a*) sharp, quick,

or sour, or (*b*) denoting the presence of oxygen in a compound.

oxy-acid (ok″sī-as′id) see ternary acids, under ACID.

Oxybiocycline trademark for *oxytetracycline hydrochloride* (see under OXYTETRACYCLINE).

Oxybiotic trademark for *oxytetracycline hydrochloride* (see under OXYTETRACYCLINE).

Oxycel trademark for *oxidized cellulose* (see under CELLULOSE).

oxycephaly (ok″se-sef′ah-le) [*oxy-* + Gr. *kephalē* head] a condition characterized by a high vertical index of the skull (hypsicephaly and acrocephaly), in which the head assumes an ovid shape, its top being narrow and pointed. Called also *steeple head, steeple skull, tower head, tower skull,* and *turricephaly.* See also ACROCEPHALY, HYPSICEPHALY, hypsistenocephalic SKULL, and LEPTOCEPHALY.

oxychinolin (oks″sĕ-chin′o-lin) 8-hydroxyquinoline.

oxychlorosene (ok″sĕ-klor′o-sēn) a buffered organic hypochlorous acid derivative, $C_{20}H_{35}ClO_4S$, with surfactant and antiseptic properties. Used in surgical antisepsis and as a local irrigant in neoplasm surgery to destroy detached viable cells to prevent metastases. Called also *monoxychlorosene.* Trademark: Clorpactin.

oxycodone (ok″sĕ-ko′dōn) a semisynthetic opium alkaloid, 4,5α-epoxy-14-hydroxy-3-methoxy-17-methylmorphinan-6-one, occurring as long rods that are soluble in ethanol and chloroform, but not in water and ether. It is an addicting analgesic used similarly to morphine. Trademarks: Dihydrone, Percodan. **o. hydrochloride,** the hydrochloride salt of oxycodone, occurring as an odorless, white, crystalline powder with a bitter saline taste, which is soluble in water and ethanol. It is an addicting analgesic and antitussive agent used similarly to codeine. Trademark: Dinarkon, Eubine, Eucodal, Oxycon, Tecodin, Thecodine.

Oxycon trademark for *oxycodone hydrochloride* (see under OXYCODONE).

oxygen (ok′sī-jen) [Gr. *oxys* sour + *gennan* to produce] a gaseous element. Symbol, O; atomic number, 8; atomic weight, 15.9994; specific gravity, 1.10535; valence, 2; group VIA of the periodic table. It occurs as the diatomic gas, O_2, and as ozone, O_3. Its natural isotopes include 16, 17, and 18 (*heavy o.*); artificial radioactive isotopes include 13–15, 19, and 20. It is the most abundant element of the earth's crust, constituting about 20 percent by weight of the atmospheric air and being essential to life. Oxygen is a colorless, odorless, and tasteless gas, soluble in water and alcohol, and liquefiable at −218°C, when it becomes a slightly bluish liquid. With hydrogen, it forms water and, with carbon and hydrogen, it is the chemical basis for organic compounds. Oxygen forms numerous covalently-bonded compounds, including oxides of nonmetals; organic compounds, such as alcohols, aldehydes, and carboxylic acids; and common acids and their salts. Animals and lower plants take up oxygen from the atmosphere and return it as carbon dioxide and higher (green) plants assimilate carbon dioxide in the presence of sunlight and evolve free oxygen through the process of photosynthesis; nearly all free oxygen in the atmosphere having been formed by photosynthesis. In animals, the inspired oxygen is carried to the lungs where, in the alveoli, it is combined with hemoglobin to be transported with the bloodstream to peripheral tissues to participate in oxidative energy metabolism. Oxygen inhalation therapy is used in oxygen deficiency conditions due to injuries, diseases, faulty metabolic processes, or lack of oxygen in the atmosphere. Untoward effects may include pulmonary atelectasis when filling the alveoli with oxygen produces airway obstruction with subsequent alveolar collapse; oxygen apnea caused by depression of responsivity to carbon dioxide by the respiratory centers; retrolental fibroplasia caused by exposure of premature infants to high concentration of oxygen; and oxygen poisoning when breathing 80 percent oxygen for more than 12 hours, characterized by irritation of the respiratory tract, decreased vital capacity, coughing, nasal stuffiness, sore throat, substernal discomfort, tracheobronchitis, pulmonary congestion, and atelectasis. Breathing of pure oxygen at an increased pressure does not appear to produce poisoning. Oxygen is not combustible, but supports combustion of other substances, thereby presenting an explosion hazard. **o. deficiency,** see ANOXIA and HYPOXIA. **diatomic o.,** a molecule consisting of two oxygen atoms, O_2; the naturally-occurring form of oxygen. **heavy o.,** an oxygen isotope of atomic weight 18, ^{18}O, occurring in proportions 8 parts to 10,000 of ordinary oxygen. Used as a tracer in biomedical experiments. **o. lack,** see ANOXIA and HYPOXIA. **molecular o.,** oxygen, O_2, whose atoms are joined in pairs, as in the atmosphere. **monatomic o.,** an oxygen molecule consisting of a single atom. **o. saturation,** oxygen SATURATION. **triatomic o.,** ozone.

oxygenator (ok″si-jĕ-na′tor) a device which mechanically oxygenates venous blood extracorporeally. Called also *artificial lung.* See also extracorporeal CIRCULATION.

oxyhemoglobin (ok″se-he″mo-glo′bin) a compound formed from combination of hemoglobin with oxygen, used for transporting oxygen from the lungs to the tissue.

oxyhydrase (ok″si-hi′drās) oxidase.

Oxylone trademark for *fluorometholone.*

oxymetazoline hydrochloride (ok″sĕ-met-az′o-lēn) a sympathomimetic agent with vasoconstrictor properties, 6-*tert*-butyl-3-2-imidazolin-2-ylmethyl)-2,4-dimethylphenol monohydrochloride, occurring as a white, odorless, crystalline powder that is soluble in water and ethanol, but not in benzene, chloroform, and ether. Used topically in the treatment of nasopharyngitis, sinusitis, hay fever, otitis media, and aerotitis media. Side effects may include sneezing and burning and stinging at the site of application. Trademark: Afrin.

oxymetholone (ok″sĕ-meth′olŏn) an androgenic steroid with anabolic properties, 17β-hydroxy-2-(hydroxymethylene)-17-methyl-5α-androstan-3-one, occurring as a white to creamy, odorless, crystalline powder or crystals that are soluble in chloroform and dioxane, slightly soluble in ether and ethanol, and insoluble in water. Used in the treatment of conditions in which there are a negative nitrogen balance and osteoporosis and to promote weight gain in debilitating diseases. It is also used in therapy of aplastic anemia. Side effects may include nausea, vomiting, anorexia, glossopyra, changes in libido, acne, decreased gonadotropin secretion, virilization, gynecomastia, sodium retention with edema, and hemorrhagic diathesis. Called also *anasterone.* Trademarks: Adroyd, Anadrol, Nastenon, Protanabol, Synasteron.

oxymethylene (ok″sĕ-meth′ĭ-lēn) formaldehyde.

oxymorphone hydrochloride (ok″sĕ-mor′fōn) a semisynthetic opium alkaloid, 4,5α-epoxy-3,14-dihydroxy-17-methylmorphinan-6-one hydrochloride, occurring as a white powder or crystalline solids that darken on exposure to light and are soluble in water and sparingly in ethanol and ether. It is an addictive analgesic used in the treatment of pain similarly to morphine. Called also *dihydrohydroxymorphinone.* Trademark: Numorphan.

Oxymycin trademark for *oxytetracycline.*

oxynervon (ok″se-ner′vŏn) a cerebroside containing a hydroxy derivative of nervonic acid.

oxyphenbutazone (ok″sĕ-fen-bu′tah-zōn) a phenylbutazone derivative with analgesic, antipyretic, and anti-inflammatory properties, 4-butyl-1-(4-hydroxyphenyl)-2-phenyl-3,5-pyrazolidinedione. It occurs as a white to yellowish, odorless, crystalline powder that is soluble in ethanol, ether, and acetone and very slightly soluble in water. Used in the treatment of gout, rheumatoid arthritis, rheumatoid spondylitis, osteoarthritis, psoriatic arthritis, thrombophlebitis, and certain other inflammatory and painful conditions. Water retention, skin rash, nausea, vertigo, stomatitis, hepatitis, hypertension, psychotic disorders, leukopenia, agranulocytosis, thrombocytopenia, visual disorders, lethargy, constipation, diarrhea, anemia, hemorrhagic complications, fever, and cardiac arrhythmias are the potential side reactions. Trademarks: Crovaril, Flogoril, Oxalid, Tanderil, Visubutina.

oxyphencyclimine hydrochloride (ok″sĕ-fen-si′klĭ-mēn) an atropine-like antimuscarinic agent (1,4,5,6-tetrahydro-1-methyl-2-pyrimidyl)methyl-α-phenylcyclohexaneglycolate monohydrochloride, occurring as a white, odorless, bitter, crystalline powder that is soluble in water, slightly soluble in ethanol, chloroform, and methylene chloride, and insoluble in ether. It decreases the secretion of gastric juice in large doses and decreases gastric motility without affecting gastric secre-

tion in lower doses. Used chiefly in the treatment of peptic ulcer. Side effects are similar to those of atropine. Trademarks: Antulcus, Daricon, Naridan, Setrol.

oxyphenonium bromide (ok″sĕ-fe-no′ne-um) a quaternary ammonium antimuscarinic agent which decreases gastric secretion and motility, 2-[(cyclohexylhydroxyphenylacetyl)oxy]-*N,N*-diethyl-*N*-methylethanaminium bromide, occurring as a white, crystalline powder that is soluble in water and ethanol, but not in ether and acetone. Used mainly in the treatment of peptic ulcer. Side effects may include xerostomia, blurred vision, mydriasis, epigastric discomfort, heartburn, impotence, difficult urination, constipation, and skin rashes. Trademarks: Antrenyl, Spasmophen.

oxyphilic (ok″se-fil′ik) [*oxy-* + Gr. *philein* to love] stainable with an acid dye.

oxyquinoline (ok″se-kwin′o-lēn) 8-hydroxyquinoline. **o. sulfate,** 8-HYDROXYQUINOLINE sulfate.

oxytalan (oks-it′ah-lan) a connective tissue fiber found typically in the periodontal ligament of man and other animals, including monkeys. It is stained with aldehyde fuchsin after oxidation. On electron microscopic examination, fibrillar and amorphous components are revealed.

Oxytetracid trademark for *oxytetracycline.*

oxytetracycline (ok″sĕ-tet″rah-si′klēn) a natural tetracycline antibiotic elaborated by cultures of *Streptomyces rimosus,* 4-(dimethylamino) - 1,4,4a,5,5a,6,11,12a-octahydro-3,5,6,10,12,12a - hexahydroxy - 6 - methyl - 1,11 - dioxo - 2 - naphthacenecarboxamide. It occurs as a pale yellow to tan, odorless, crystalline powder that darkens on exposure to sunlight, deteriorates in solutions of pH below 2, and is readily soluble in dilute hydrochloric acid and slightly soluble in water and alcohol. Therapeutic uses and toxicity of oxytetracycline are similar to those of other tetracyclines. Trademarks: Berkmycen, Biostat, Oxacycline, Oxymycin, Oxytetracid, Ryomycin, Terramycin, Tetramel. **o. calcium,** a calcium salt of oxytetracycline, occurring as a yellow to brownish, tasteless, odorless, crystalline powder that discolors on the exposure to light, oxidizes on exposure to air, is soluble in dilute acids, and is insoluble in water. Used in oral suspensions. **o. hydrochloride,** the hydrochloride salt of oxytetracycline, occurring as a yellow, odorless, slightly bitter, hygroscopic, crystalline powder that darkens on exposure to sunlight, air, and heat. It is soluble in water, ethanol, and methanol, slightly soluble in dehydrated ethanol, and insoluble in chloroform and ether. Used orally and parenterally. Trademarks: Bio-Mycin, Geomycin, Imperacin, Macodyn, Oxybiocycline, Oxybiotic.

oxytocin (ok″se-to′sin) an octapeptide hormone believed to be formed in the neuronal cells of the hypothalamic nuclei, from where it migrates along the axons and is stored in the nerve cell endings in the posterior pituitary gland. It stimulates contraction of the uterine muscle and is used to induce labor.

Oz see Oz FACTOR.

oz ounce.

ozena (o-ze′nah) [Gr. *ozaina* a fetid polypus in the nose] a condition of the nose, of varying etiology, associated with an offensive-smelling discharge. **o. laryn′gis,** a condition of the larynx associated with a foul-smelling discharge, usually related to atrophic rhinitis.

ozocerite (o-zo′kĕ-rīt) a mineral wax occurring as a yellowish-brown to green or black, greasy, waxy mixture of hydrocarbons. It is soluble in petroleum, benzene, turpentine, ether, carbon disulfide, slightly soluble in ethanol, and insoluble in water. Its specific gravity is 0.85 to 0.95 and has a melting point of 55 to 110°C. Used in ointments, cosmetics, dental waxes, and various industrial processes. Called also *fossil wax.* Spelled also *ozokerite.*

ozokerite (o-zo′kĕ-rīt) ozocerite. **purified o.,** ceresin.

ozone (o′zōn) [Gr. *ozē* stench] triatomic oxygen, O_3, occurring as a bluish explosive gas, produced in the atmosphere by electric discharge and by electrolysis of alkaline perchlorate solutions. Used as a disinfectant, by virtue of its oxidizing properties, in water and sewage purification, in bleaching, and in various chemical processes. High concentrations are irritating to the respiratory tract, eye, and mucous membranes.

P

P phosphorus.

P. abbreviation for *position*, *presbyopia*, L. *prox'imum* (near), L. *pon'dere* (by weight), L. *pugil'lus* (handful), *pulse*, and *pupil*.

P$_i$ inorganic PHOSPHATE.

P$_1$, P-one symbol for parental GENERATION.

p. 1. symbol for short arm of a chromosome; see under ARM. See also CHROMOSOME nomenclaure. 2. pico-.

p- chemical abbreviation for *para-*.

PA 1. physician ASSISTANT. 2. posteroanterior PROJECTION.

P-A posteroanterior PROJECTION.

Pa 1. protactinium. 2. pascal.

PABA *p*-aminobenzoic ACID.

PAC an analgesic mixture containing phenacetin, aspirin, and caffeine.

Pacatal trademark for *mepazine*.

Pacchioni, Antonio [1665–1726] an Italian antomist. See PAC-CHIONIAN.

pacchionian (pak″e-o-ne′an) named after or described by Antonio *Pacchioni*, as pacchionian bodies (see arachnoidal granulations, under GRANULATION) and pacchionian depressions (see granular foveolae, under FOVEOLA).

pacemaker (pas′mak-er) an object or substance that influences the rate at which a certain phenomenon occurs; often used alone to indicate the natural cardiac pacemaker or an artificial cardiac pacemaker. In biochemistry, a substance whose rate of reaction sets the pace for a series of interrelated reactions. **artificial p.,** cardiac p., artificial. **cardiac p.,** the group of cells rhythmically initiating the heart beat, characterized physiologically by a slow loss of membrane potential during diastole. **cardiac p., artificial,** a device designed to stimulate, by electrical impulses, contraction of the heart muscle at a certain rate; used particularly in heart block or in the absence of normal function of the sinoatrial node. It may be connected from the outside or implanted within the body. Electrical and electronic devices, such as those used in a dental office, including motorized dental chairs, pulp testers, electrosurgical equipment, ultrasonic scaling devices, etc., may adversely affect the operation of certain types of pacemakers. Called also *artificial p.* and, popularly, *pacemaker*.

Pacemaker Fluorinse, Nafeen solution, Nafeen tablets, topical fluoride gel, topical fluoride solution see under GEL, RINSE, SOLUTION, and TABLET.

pachy- [Gr. *pachys* thick, clotted] a combining form meaning thick.

pachyblepharon (pak″e-blef′ah-ron) [*pachy-* + Gr. *blepharon* eyelid] a thickening of the eyelid, chiefly near the border.

pachycephalia, pachycephaly (pak″e-sē-fa′le-ah; pak″e-sef′ah-le) [*pachy-* + Gr. *kephalē* head] abnormal thickness of the bones of the skull.

pachycheilia (pak″e-ki′le-ah) [*pachy-* + Gr. *cheilos* lip + *-ia*] thickness of the lips. See also MACROCHEILIA.

pachyderma (pak″e-der′mah) [*pachy-* + Gr. *derma* skin] abnormal thickening of the skin. **p. circumscrip′ta, p. laryn′gis,** localized warty epithelial thickenings of the vocal cords. **p. ora′lis,** oral LEUKOPLAKIA. **p. verruco′sa,** a condition characterized by papillomatous growths on the vocal cords.

pachyglossia (pak″e-glos′e-ah) [*pachy-* + Gr. *glōssa* tongue + *-ia*] abnormal thickness of the tongue. See also MACROGLOSSIA.

pachygnathous (pah-kig′nah-thus) [*pachy-* + Gr. *gnathos* jaw] having a large jaw. See also MACROGNATHIA.

pachygyria (pak″e-ji′re-ah) [*pachy-* + Gr. *gyros* ring + *-ia*] see MACROGYRIA, and see agyria-pachygyria SYNDROME.

pachymeninx (pak″e-me′ninks) [*pachy-* + Gr. *mēninx* membrane] dura MATER.

pachymucosa (pak″e-mu-ko′sah) [*pachy-* + *mucosa*] abnormal thickening of the mucosa. **p. al′ba,** leukoplakia with thickening of the mucous membrane.

pachynsis (pah-kin′sis) [Gr.] a thickening, especially an abnormal thickening.

pachyonychia (pak″e-o-nik′e-ah) [*pachy-* + Gr. *onyx* nail + *-ia*] thickening of the nails. **p. congen′ita,** congenital thickening of the nails, transmitted as an autosomal dominant trait, which may be associated with hyperhidrosis, hyperkeratosis palmaris et plantaris, hair abnormalities, follicular keratosis, dyskeratosis of the cornea, steatocystoma multiplex, and bullae. Oral manifestations include focal or generalized, white, opaque thickening of the mucosa, involving the buccal mucosa, tongue, or lips; natal teeth; and, sometimes, perlèche. Called also *Jadassohn-Lewandowski syndrome* and *polykeratosis congenita*.

pachytene (pak′-e-tēn) [*pachy-* + Gr. *tainia* ribbon] the third stage of the first division in meiosis, characterized by coiling and thickening of chromosomes, associated with their staining darker than in the earlier stages.

pacifier (pas′ĭ-fi-er) exerciser (2).

Pacini's corpuscles [Filippo *Pacini*, Italian anatomist, 1812–1883] lamellar corpuscles; see under CORPUSCLE.

Pacinia (pah-sin′e-ah) a proposed genus name for bacteria now assigned to the genus *Vibrio*. **P. chol′erae-asiat′icae,** *Vibrio cholerae;* see under VIBRIO. **P. fink′leri,** *Vibrio cholerae* (biotype *proteus*); see under VIBRIO. **P. loef′fleri,** *Corynebacterium diphtheriae;* see under CORYNEBACTERIUM. **P. metschnikovi,** *Vibrio cholerae* (biotype *proteus*); see under VIBRIO. **P. neis′seri,** *Corynebacterium xerosis;* see under CORYNEBACTERIUM.

pacinian (pah-sin′e-an) named after or described by Filippo *Pacini,* as pacinian corpuscles (see lamellar corpuscles, under CORPUSCLE).

Pacinol trademark for *fluphenazine*.

Pacinox trademark for *capuride*.

Pacitane trademark for *trihexylphenidyl hydrochloride* (see under TRIHEXYLPHENIDYL).

pack (pak) 1. treatment by wrapping a patient in blankets, sheets, or towels, wet or dry; also, the blankets, sheets, or towels used for this purpose. 2. a dressing inserted firmly into a wound or body cavity, as the nose, principally for stopping hemorrhage. See also COMPRESS and TAMPON. **Coe-P.,** trademark for a periodontal pack consisting of a mixture of metallic oxides, lorothidol, nonionizing carboxylic acids, and chlorothymol. **cyanoacrylate p.,** *N*-butyl cyanoacrylate applied as a periodontal dressing either in drops or as a spray, which solidifies in 5 to 10 seconds, moisture, heat, and pressure acting as catalysts for polymerization. **eugenol p.,** a periodontal pack containing eugenol. Typically, it is a mixture of a powder (usually containing zinc oxide, rosin, asbestos fibers, and zinc acetate), and a liquid, containing eugenol and olive or peanut oil. **Kirkland-Kaiser p.,** trademark for a periodontal pack prepared from a powder (consisting of zinc oxide, powdered rosin, and tannic acid flakes) and a liquid, consisting of one part peanut oil and two parts eugenol. **Kirkland periodontal p.,** trademark for a periodontal dressing. In the powder form, 100 gm of the preparation contain 40 gm zinc oxide, 40 gm rosin, and 20 gm tannic acid. In the liquid form, 100 ml contain 46.5 ml eugenol, 46.5 mg peanut oil, and 7.5 gm rosin. **periodontal p.,** a surgical dressing applied over the surgical wound in periodontal operations to provide a matrix for the regeneration of tissue and enhance healing processes. Called also *periodontal cement* and *periodontal dressing*. Trademarks: Coe-Pack, Kirkland-Kaiser p., Kirkland periodontal p. **periodontal noneugenol p.,** one in which some other substance is substituted for eugenol, such as a mixture of powder containing zinc oxide, powdered rosin, and zinc bacitracin, and an ointment containing hydrogenated fat. **pressure p.,** one made of folded sterile gauze and pressed against the wound. **throat p.,** a moistened gauze pack used as a posterior pharyngeal seal, especially around a noncuffed endotracheal tube; also used to prevent materials from being displaced into the pharynx. **wax p.,** a periodontal pack, consisting of a mixture of cocoa butter and paraffin, cut into strips and applied after gingivectomy.

packer (pak′er) an instrument for introducing a dressing into body cavities, such as the nose.

packet (pak′it) a small bundle, parcel, or package. **film p.,** a small, light-proof, moisture resistant, sealed envelope containing photographic or x-ray film.

packing (pak′ing) 1. the act of filling a wound or cavity with dressing material. 2. the substance used for filling a cavity. 3. denture p. **denture p.,** the act of filling and compressing a denture base material into a mold in a flask.

Pacs trademark for preproportioned *dental amalgam* (see under AMALGAM) in disposable capsules, containing 47.01 to 49.52 percent mercury.

pad (pad) cushionlike mass of soft material. See also CUSHION. **buccal fat p.,** an encapsulated mass of fat in the cheek, separated from the subcutaneous fascia by a fascial cleft and situated between the masseter and the external surface of the buccinator muscles. It is especially prominent in infants and is said to assist in the act of sucking, hence the synonyms *sucking pad* or *suctorial pad*. Called also *masticatory fat p.* *adipose body of cheek, corpus adiposum buccae* [NA], *fatty ball of Bichat,* and *sucking cushion*. **gum p's,** edentulous segments of the maxilla and the mandible that correspond to the underlying primary teeth. **masticatory fat p.,** buccal fat p. **occlusal p.,** a pad which covers the occlusal surface of a tooth. **Passavant's p.,** Passavant's BAR. **retrodiscal p.,** retroarticular CUSHION. **retromolar p.,** a mass of tissue, frequently pear-shaped, which is located at the distal termination of the mandibular residual ridge, made up of the retromolar papilla and the retromolar glandular prominence. Called also *pear-shaped area.* **rubber dam p.,** the absorbent piece of mannelette or gauze, which is placed between the rubber dam and the face to protect the face from contact with the rubber and with the clips of the dam holder. Called also *rubber dam mask.* **sucking p., suctorial p.,** buccal fat p.

PAF platelet-activating FACTOR.

Paget abscess, disease, juvenile disease [Sir James *Paget,* English surgeon, 1814–1899] see under ABSCESS, and see OSTEITIS deformans and HYPEROSTOSIS corticalis deformans juvenilis.

pain (pān) [L. *poena, dolor;* Gr. *odynē, algos*] 1. a physical condition which may range from a mild sensation of discomfort to excruciating agony. It is a manifestation and alerting process of injury by an external agent, or the presence of damaging processes in the body, which also serves to localize the affected area and as a protective mechanism, initiating a reflex action allowing an organ or part to be removed from the source of injury. See also CAUSALGIA, HYPERALGESIA, HYPERESTHESIA, and NEURALGIA. 2. mental anguish or stress. **aching p.,** deep pain with varying degree of severity, which is not felt on the surface of the body. **atypical facial p.,** a painful syndrome characterized by dull aching or throbbing, rather than paroxysms of pain, such as seen in trigeminal, glossopharyngeal, or postherpetic neuralgia, occurring in areas supplied by various nerve groups, including the fifth and ninth cranial nerves and the second and third cervical nerves. Attacks last from a few days to several months and seem to occur following dental work or sinus manipulation, but examination of the teeth, nose, sinuses, ears, and temporomandibular joints seldom reveals any abnormalities. A psychogenic etiology has been suggested. Called also *atypical facial neuralgia* and *facial causalgia.* **boring p.,** pain with a sensation as of being pierced with a sharp instrument. Called also *torebrating p.* **chest p.,** pain in the chest region, often indicating the presence of diseases of the heart, respiratory system, or esophagus. **deep p.,** dull, aching, or boring pain of deep organs, which tends to radiate. **epicritic p.,** sharp and localized cutaneous pain that is rapidly transmitted to the brain by A (δ) nerve fibers. **ghost p.,** phantom ODONTALGIA. **heterotopic p.,** referred p. **intractable p.,** pain which is not amenable to relief by treating its source. **p. killer,** analgesic (3). **lancinating p.,** a sharp, darting pain. **pricking p.,** pain which may be produced by pricking the skin with a needle, cutting it with a knife, or diffuse but strong irritation of large areas of the skin. **pulpal p.,** pulpalgia. **referred p.,** pain in a part other than that in which the cause that produced it is situated, as pain in the temporomandibular region in tooth diseases. Called also *heterotropic p.* See also dental HEADACHE and LAW of referred pain. **root p.,** pain caused by disease of the sensory nerve roots, occurring in the cutaneous areas supplied by the affected roots. **tooth p.,** see ODONTALGIA and TOOTHACHE. **torebrating p.,** boring p. **unilateral p.,** hemialgesia. **wandering p.,** a pain which repeatedly changes its location. Called also *dolor vagus.*

pair (pār) a combination of two related, similar, or identical entities or objects. **ion p.,** a pair of ions formed when an atom loses an electron to another, each atom becoming an ion.

pairing (pār'ing) 1. the act or process of joining into pairs. 2. the process of selecting a compatible donor and host, usually by typing or matching in transplantation and immunology. 3. joining of homologous chromosomes in pairs in meiosis. See also SYNAPSIS.

Pakoral-Xu trademark for a large-capacity automatic film processor.

palata (pal-ah'tah) [L.] plural of *palatum.*

palatal (pal'ah-tal) pertaining to the palate; sometimes used to designate the lingual surface of a maxillary tooth.

palate (pal'at) [L. *palatum*] the partition which serves as the roof of the oral cavity and the floor of the nasal cavity, consisting anteriorly of the hard palate and posteriorly of the soft palate. Called also *floor of nasal cavity, palatum* [NA], *roof of mouth, roof of oral cavity,* and *uraniscus.* See also terms beginning PALATO- and URANO-. See illustration. **artificial p.,** a prosthetic device used to close a cleft palate, an obturator. **bony p., bony hard p.,** the bony framework of the hard palate consisting of the palatine process of the maxilla and the horizontal part of the palatine bone. Called also *palatum durum osseum* and *palatum osseum* [NA]. See also *hard p.* **brachystaphyline p.,** see

Bones of the palate. (From J. Langman and M. W. Woerdeman: Atlas of Medical Anatomy. Philadelphia, W. B. Saunders Co., 1978.)

brachystaphyline SKULL. **chamestaphyline p.,** see chamestaphyline SKULL. **cleft p.,** CLEFT palate. **gothic p.,** an unusually high and pointed hard palate. Called also *palatum ogivale.* **hard p.,** the anterior, rigid portion of the palate, bounded anteriorly and laterally by the alveolar arches and the gingivae and joined posteriorly with the soft palate. Its bony framework (*bony p.*) is formed by the palatine process of the maxilla and the horizontal part of the palatine bone. A raphe running along the median line from the palatine papilla divides the palate into two lateral halves, which in turn are subdivided into the anterior, or fatty, zones and the posterior, or glandular, zones, which are separated by a convex line connecting the mesial halves of the two first molars; fat lobules are packed into the spaces of the anterior zone and glands occupy the spaces in the posterior zone. A dense structure covers the hard palate. Strands of connective tissue attach the lamina propria of the mucosa to the periosteum. The anterior part on both sides of the raphe is covered by a pale pink corrugated mucosa, having irregular transverse rugae, and the posterior parts are covered by smooth, thin, and somewhat deeper red, stratified epithelium. Called also *palatum durum* [NA]. Cf. *soft p.* **high p., high-arched p.,** see hypsistaphyline SKULL. **hypsistaphyline p.,** see hypsistaphyline SKULL. **leptostaphyline p.,** see leptostaphyline SKULL. **low p., low-arched p.,** see chamestaphyline SKULL. **mesostaphyline p.,** see mesostaphyline SKULL. **orthostaphyline p.,** see orthostaphyline SKULL. **pendulous p.,** palatine UVULA. **pipe-smokers' p.,** STOMATITIS nicotina. **premaxillary p.,** primary p. **primary p.,** that portion of the palate contributed by the median nasal process. Called also *premaxillary p.* **secondary p.,** the palate proper, formed by fusion of the lateral palatine processes. **short p.,** see brachystaphyline SKULL. **smoker's p.,** STOMATITIS nicotina. **soft p.,** the posterior part of the palate made up of a thick fold of mucous membrane which encloses a system of muscles, an aponeurosis, blood vessels, nerves, lymphoid tissue, and mucous glands. It is suspended anteriorly from the hard palate, its sides blending with the pharynx, and its posterior portion forming the uvula. In its relaxed position, the soft palate is continuous with the roof of the mouth. During the process of deglutition or sucking, it becomes elevated, thus separating the nasal cavity and nasopharynx from the posterior part of the oral cavity and the oral portion of the pharynx. It is covered by a thin, loosely textured mucosa that shows through the rich vascularization beneath, thus giving the soft palate a red color with a yellowish hue. The epithelium is nonkeratinized, having a lamina propria and submucosa which are less compact than those of the hard palate. The palatine glands are located in the submucosa. Its musculature consists of the uvular, levator and tensor palati, glossopalatine, and palatopharyngeal muscles. The vibrating line separates the mobile from the immobile parts of the palate. The palatine arteries provide the blood supply. Called also *palatum molle* [NA], *velum palati,* and *velum palatinum.* Cf. *hard p.* **wide p.,** see brachystaphyline SKULL.

Palatex 51 trademark for a self-cured denture base acrylic resin.

palatine (pal'ah-tīn) [L. *palatinus*] pertaining to the palate.

palatitis (pal″ah-ti'tis) [*palate + -itis*] inflammation of the palate. **p. nicoti'na,** STOMATITIS nicotina.

palato- [L. *palatum* palate] a combining form denoting relationship to the palate; sometimes used instead of *linguo-* in terms referring to the lingual surface of maxillary teeth. See also terms beginning URANISCO- and URANO-.

palatoglossal (pal″ah-to-glos′al) pertaining to the palate and tongue.

palatoglossus (pal″ah-to-glos′us) palatoglossus MUSCLE.

palatognathous (pal″ah-tog′nah-thus) [*palate* + Gr. *gnathos* jaw] having a cleft palate.

palatogram (pal′ah-to-gram″) a graphic representation of the area of the palate contacted by the tongue.

palatograph (pal′ah-to-graf) an instrument used in palatography.

palatography (pal″ah-tog′rah-fe) [*palate* + Gr. *graphein* to write] the recording of the movements of the palate in speech.

palatomaxillary (pal″ah-to-mak″sĭ-ler′e) pertaining to the palate and the maxilla.

palatomyography (pal″ah-to-mi-og′rah-fe) [*palate* + Gr. *mys* muscle + *graphein* to write] the recording of muscular movements of the palate.

palatonasal (pal″ah-to-na′zal) [*palato-* + *nasal*] pertaining to the palate and the nose.

palatopagus (pal″ah-top′ah-gus) [*palato-* + Gr. *pagos* that which is firmly set] congenital oral TERATOMA.

palatopharyngeal (pal″ah-to-fah-rin′je-al) [*palato-* + *pharyngeal*] pertaining to the palate and the pharynx.

palatopharyngeus (pal″ah-to-fah-rin-je′us) palatopharyngeal MUSCLE.

palatoplasty (pal′ah-to-plas″te) [*palate* + Gr. *plassein* to form] plastic reconstruction of the palate. Called also *uraniscoplasty* and *uranoplasty*. See also URANOSTAPHYLOPLASTY.

palatoplegia (pal″ah-to-ple′je-ah) [*palato-* + Gr. *plēgē* stroke] paralysis of the palate. Called also *uranoplegia*.

palatoproximal (pal″ah-to-prok′sĭ-mal) pertaining to the palatal (lingual) and proximal surfaces of the maxillary teeth.

palatorrhaphy (pal″ah-tor′ah-fe) [*palato-* + Gr. *raphē*) to close by sewing] surgical correction of cleft palate, the cleft involving the soft palate and the soft tissues over the hard palate. Called also *uraniscorrhaphy* and *uranorrhapy*. See also URANOSTAPHYLORRHAPHY.

palatoschisis (pal″a-tos′kĭ-sis) [*palato-* + Gr. *schisis* cleft] CLEFT palate.

palatum (pal-ah′tum), pl. *pala′ta* [L.] [NA] palate. **p. du′rum** [NA], hard PALATE. **p. du′rum os′seum,** bony PALATE. **p. fis′sum,** CLEFT palate. **p. mol′le** [NA], soft PALATE. **p. ogiva′le,** gothic PALATE. **p. os′seum** [NA], bony PALATE.

paleo- [Gr. *palaios* old] a combining form meaning old.

Palginex 75 trademark for a fast-setting irreversible hydrocolloid impression material (see under MATERIAL).

pali-, palin- [Gr. *palin* backward, again] a combining form meaning again, often denoting pathologic repetition.

palin see PALI-.

palinesthesia (pal″in-es-the′ze-ah) [*palin-* + Gr. *aisthēsis* sensation] the rapid termination of the anesthetic state and the restoration to consciousness of a person under general anesthesia; it may be induced by the injection of weak hydrochloric acid; now discontinued because of ineffectiveness and potential harmfulness of the method.

palladium (pah-la′de-um) [named after the asteroid *Pallas*, discovered about the same time as the element], a metallic element. Symbol, Pd; atomic number, 46; atomic weight, 106.4; specific gravity, 12.0; melting point 1554°C; Brinell hardness number, 46; valences 2, 3, 4; group VIII of the periodic table. It occurs in six natural isotopes (102, 104–106, 108, 110) and several artificial radioactive ones (98–101, 103, 107, 109, 111–115). Palladium is a silvery white, ductile metal which absorbs up to 800 times its volume of hydrogen and is attacked by hot concentrated nitric and boiling sulfuric acids; it is soluble in aqua regia and fused alkalies; and is insoluble in organic acids. Used in gold, silver, and copper alloys in dentistry and in various industrial processes. **silver-p. alloy,** see under ALLOY.

pallesthesia (pal″es-the′ze-ah) [Gr. *pallein* to shake + *aisthēsis* perception] sensibility to vibrations; the peculiar vibrating sensation felt when a vibrating tuning-fork is placed against a subcutaneous bony prominence of the body. Called also *bone sensibility*.

palliate (pal′e-āt) to reduce the severity of; to relieve.

palliative (pal′e-a″tiv) [L. *palliatus* cloaked] 1. affording relief, but no cure. 2. an alleviating medicine.

Pallister, P. D. see Hermann-Pallister-Opitz SYNDROME.

pallium (pal′e-um) [L. "cloak"] [NA] cerebral CORTEX.

pallor (pal′or) [L.] paleness; absence of skin coloration.

palm (palm) [L. *palma*] 1. the hollow of the hand. 2. any of a family of tropical and subtropical trees and shrubs having a stem and a crown of large pinnate or fan-shaped leaves.

Palmer notation see dental CHART (1).

palmitin (pal′mĭ-tin) tripalmitin.

palpable (pal′pah-b'l) perceptible by touch or palpation.

palpation (pal-pa′shun) [L. *palpatio*] the act of feeling with the hand; the application of the fingers with light pressure to the surface of the body for the purpose of determining the consistence of the parts beneath in physical diagnosis.

palpebra (pal′pĕ-brah), pl. *pal′pebrae* [L.] [NA] eyelid; either of the two movable folds (upper and lower) that protect the anterior surface of the eye. **p. infe′rior** [NA], lower EYELID. **p. supe′rior** [NA], UPPER EYELID.

palpebrae (pal′pĕ-bre) [L.] plural of *palpebra*.

palpebral (pal′pĕ-bral) [L. *palpebralis*] pertaining to the eyelids.

palpitation (pal′pī-ta′shun) [L. *palpitatio*] unduly rapid action of the heart. See ARRHYTHMIA.

palsy (pawl′ze) paralysis. **Bell's p.,** peripheral, usually unilateral, paralysis of the facial nerve, with a mild onset consisting of pain and swelling behind the ear and pain and stiffness of the neck, followed within a few hours by exacerbation of pain, excessive lacrimation, vertigo, fever, tinnitus, impaired hearing, distorted speech, and paralysis. In severe cases, the affected side of the face becomes immobile, the labiofacial fold is erased, the mouth is drawn toward the unaffected side, the forehead cannot be wrinkled, the upper eyelid cannot be closed, whistling becomes impossible, and the sense of taste becomes distorted. Spontaneous recovery occurs in most cases within two weeks. Adults are most commonly affected, especially after an exposure to draft or cold, although cold in itself is not considered to be the etiologic factor. Called also *refrigeration p., facial paralysis,* and *seventh nerve paralysis.* **pseudobulbar p.,** amyotrophic lateral SCLEROSIS. **refrigeration p.,** Bell's p. **shaking p.,** parkinsonism. **spastic bulbar p.,** pseudobulbar PARALYSIS.

Paludrine trademark for *proguanil hydrochloride* (see under PROGUANIL).

2-PAM chloride PRALIDOXIME chloride.

Pamine trademark for *methscopolamine bromide* (see under METHSCOPOLAMINE).

pamplegia (pam-ple′je-ah) total paralysis.

pan- [Gr. *pan* all] a prefix signifying all.

Panacea [Gr. *Panakeia*] one of two sisters, the other being Hygeia, who were daughters of Æsculapius, the mythical god of healing; they assisted in the rites at the temples of healing and fed the sacred snakes.

panacea (pan″ah-se′ah) [Gr. *panakeia*] 1. a universal remedy. 2. an ancient name for a healing herb or its juice.

panarteritis (pan″ar-te-ri′tis) [*pan-* + *arteritis*] any diffuse inflammatory disease of the arterial system. **p. nodo′sa,** PERIARTERITIS nodosa.

panarthritis (pan″ar-thri′tis) [*pan-* + *arthritis*] any diffuse inflammatory disease of all the joints.

panatrophy (pan-at′ro-fe) [*pan-* + *atrophy*] diffuse atrophy; general atrophy.

pancarditis (pan″kar-di′tis) [*pan-* + *carditis*] inflammation of all three layers of the heart, involving the endocardium, myocardium, and pericardium.

panchondritis (pan-kon-dri′tis) chronic atrophic POLYCHONDRITIS.

panchromatic (pan″kro-mat′ik) sensitive to all colors; applied to photographic emulsions.

pancreas (pan′kre-as), pl. *pancre′ata* [*pan-* + Gr. *kreas* flesh] a large, elongated racemose gland situated transversely behind the stomach, between the spleen and the duodenum, composed of both endocrine and exocrine tissue. The endocrine part, consisting of the islands of Langerhans, is responsible for producing and secreting directly into the blood stream the hormone insulin, which plays a major role in carbohydrate metabolism, and glucagon, which has an effect opposite to insulin. The exocrine part produces and secretes into the duodenum pancreatic juice, which contains enzymes essential to the digestion of proteins.

pancreata (pan-kre′ah-tah) [Gr.] plural of *pancreas*.

pancreatitis (pan″kre-ah-ti′tis) inflammation of the pancreas; it is caused most often by alcoholism or biliary tract diseases, and is less commonly associated with hyperlipemia, hyperparathyroidism, abdominal trauma, vasculitis, or uremia.

pancuronium bromide (pan-ku-ro′ne-um) a nondepolarizing neuromuscular blocking agent, 1,1′-[3α,17β-bis(acetyloxy)-5α-androstane-2β, 16β -diyl]bis[1-methylpiperidinium]dibromide, occurring as a white, hygroscopic, photosensitive powder that is soluble in water, ethanol, and chloroform. Used in the treatment of cardiovascular diseases, bronchial asthma, and other conditions in which muscle relaxation is needed. Also used to produce muscle relaxation in anesthesia, to relax laryngeal muscles in endotracheal intubation, and in electroshock therapy. Side effects may include slight hypertension, increased heart rate, excessive salivation, and skin rashes. Trademark: Pavulon.

pancytopenia (pan″si-to-pe′ne-ah) [pan- + cyto- + Gr. *penia* poverty] deficiency of all three formed elements of the blood, the erythrocytes, leukocytes, and blood platelets. See also aplastic ANEMIA. **congenital p.,** Fanconi's ANEMIA.

panel (pan″l) a body of persons gathered to conduct a public discussion, serve as advisers, or the like. **closed p.,** in a prepayment insurance plan, a group of doctors sharing office facilities who provide stipulated services to an eligible group for a set premium. The beneficiary is limited in selecting the doctor to the panel members only; the doctor is obliged to accept any beneficiary as his patient. **open p.,** in health insurance, a plan in which any licensed doctor may elect to participate, the beneficiary has choice from among all licensed doctors, and the doctor may accept or refuse any beneficiary. **screening p.,** either of two types of fact-finding bodies used in malpractice disputes: one type is a physicians' defense panel which seeks to develop the best possible defense for the physician who faces a malpractice claim, and the other is a joint physician-lawyer panel whose purpose is to look at the facts of the case for the physician and the plaintiff and decide on its merits.

Panelipse trademark for a method of panoramic radiography. See PANTOMOGRAPHY.

panesthesia (pan″es-the′ze-ah) [pan- + Gr. *aisthēsis* perception] the sum of the sensations experienced.

Panmycin trademark for *tetracycline.*

panmyelophthisis (pan-mi″ĕ-lof′thi-sis) [pan- + Gr. *myelos* marrow + *phthisis* wasting] aplasia of the bone marrow. See aplastic ANEMIA.

panniculus (pah-nik′u-lus), pl. *pannic′uli* [L., dim. of *pannus* cloth] a layer of membrane. **p. adipo′sus** [NA], a layer of fatty tissue under the skin. Called also *subcutaneous fatty tissue.* See also subcutaneous FASCIA.

Panoral trademark for a method of panoramic radiography. See PANTOMOGRAPHY.

Panorex trademark for a radiographic system that uses two axes of rotation to obtain a panoramic radiograph of the dental arches and their associated structures. See also PANTOMOGRAPHY.

Panparnit trademark for *caramiphen hydrochloride* (see under CARAMIPHEN).

pansinusitis (pan″si-nu-si′tis) inflammation involving all the paranasal sinuses.

pant- see PANTO-.

Pantheline trademark for *propantheline bromide* (see under PROPANTHELINE).

panto-, pant- [Gr. *pas, pantos* all] a combining form meaning all, the whole.

Pantocaine trademark for *tetracaine hydrochloride* (see under TETRACAINE).

pantograph (pan′to-graf) [panto- + Gr. *graphein* to write] 1. an instrument for copying a plane figure to any desired scale. 2. a pair of face-bows fixed to both jaws by means of clutches, designed to inscribe centrically related points and arcs leading to them on segments of planes related to the three craniofacial planes. The maxillary planes are attached to the maxillary bow, and the inscribing styluses are attached to the mandibular bow. See illustration at FACE-BOW.

Pantomatic trademark for an automatic film developer used in dentistry for developing x-ray film.

Pantomicina trademark for *erythromycin stearate* (see under ERYTHROMYCIN).

pantomography (pan″to-mog′rah-fe) a method of tomography for visualization of body curved surfaces at any depth. In dentistry, it may be used for roentgenography of the maxillary and mandibular dental arches and their associated structures. Called also *panoramic radiography.*

Pantopaque trademark for *iophendylate.*

Pantopon trademark for a preparation containing the hydrochlorides of the opium alkaloids, exhibiting the pharmacological properties of morphine, codeine, papaverine, and other opium alkaloids. It occurs as a water-soluble, yellowish gray, crystalline powder. Used as a narcotic analgesic and antitussive agent. Abuse may lead to addiction. Called also *Omnopon* and *Papaveretum.*

panus (pa′nus) [L. "swelling"] a lymph gland inflamed but not suppurating.

papain [E.C.3.4.22.2] (pah-pa′in, pah-pi′in) an SH-proteinase derived from the latex of the papaw, *Carica papaya,* which catalyzes the hydrolysis of proteins and polypeptides to amino acids. It cleaves preferentially arginine, lysine, and phenylalanine, hydrolyzing native immunoglobulins. In surgery, it has been used as a protein decongestant, as a topical application in the treatment of sloughing and infected wounds, and to prevent postoperative adhesions. Also used in blood grouping serology to treat red cells for the purpose of enhancing their agglutination activity with incomplete antibodies. Called also *papainase.*

papainase (pah-pa′in-ās, pah-pi′in-ās) papain.

Papanicolaou's classification, test (smear) [George Nicolas *Papanicolaou,* Greek physician and histologist in the U.S., 1883–1962] see under TEST.

Papaver (pah-pav′er) a genus of plants comprising the poppies. *P. somniferum,* a pink to purplish pink and purple species, and its variety *album,* a silvery-white species, are the source of opium. The unripe capsules when scarified yield a white latex which upon drying is known as *crude opium,* containing some 20 alkaloids, including morphine, codeine, and thebaine. Because opium is highly addictive, the cultivation of the plants from which it is obtained is prohibited by most nations under an international agreement.

Papaveretum Pantopon.

papaverine (pah-pav′er-in) an opium alkaloid that is also produced synthetically, 1-[(3,4-dimethoxyphenyl)methyl]-6,7-dimethoxyisoquinoline. It occurs as a white or a white crystalline powder that is soluble in ether, chloroform, hot benzene, aniline, glacial acetic acid, and acetone, but not in water. Unlike other opium alkaloids, it has no analgesic effect but is a powerful relaxant of smooth muscle and is a cerebral vasodilator.

paper (pa′per) a material chiefly obtained from wood pulp, rags, or other fibrous substances, used for writing, printing, etc. Also, a sheet(s) of such material. **articulating p.,** paper strips, coated with ink- or dye-containing wax, used for the marking or locating of occlusal interferences or deflective or interceptive occlusal contacts.

papilla (pah-pil′lah), pl. *papil′lae* [L.] a small, nipple-shaped projection or elevation. **arcuate papillae of tongue,** fungiform papillae. **calciform papillae,** vallate papillae. **capitate papillae, circumvallate papillae,** vallate papillae. **papil′lae con′icae** [NA], **conical papillae,** sparsely scattered large elevations on the tongue surface, often considered as a modified type of filiform papillae. **papil′lae, co′rii** [NA], p. of corium. **papillae of corium,** conical extensions of the collagen fibers, the capillary blood vessels, and sometimes the nerves of the corium into corresponding spaces among the downward- or inward-projecting rete ridges on the undersurface of the epidermis. On the forehead and ear they are lacking; on the face, neck, and pubes the relations are reversed and "rete pegs" extend inward or downward into spaces among a network of dermal ridges. Called also *papillae corii* [NA], *dermal papillae,* and *skin papillae.* **corolliform papillae of tongue,** filiform papillae. **dental p., p. den′tis** [NA], a small mass of condensed mesenchymal tissue in the enamel organ, which differentiates into dentin and dental pulp. The innermost layer consists of a cell-free zone of reticular fibers which constitute the basement membrane. Numerous relatively undifferentiated cells are found elsewhere, mostly the stellate or fusiform cells with numerous protoplasmic processes which intercommunicate. The intercellular space consists of a network of argyrophilic fibrils and ground substances. **dermal papillae,** papillae of corium. **filiform papillae, papil′lae filifor′mes** [NA], numerous minute, threadlike projections arranged in rows parallel with the two rows of vallate papillae over the anterior two-thirds of the dorsal surface of the tongue, except at the apex of the organ, where they are directed transversely. They are about 2.5 mm long and consist of a core of loose fibrous connective tissue capped by keratinized stratified squamous epithelium. Elastic fibers give them firmness and elasticity. The larger and longer filiform papillae are sometimes termed *conical papillae.* Called also *corolliform papillae of tongue, simple papillae of tongue, papillae simplices, small papillae of tongue, villous papillae of tongue,* and *lingual villi.* **papil′lae folia′tae** [NA], foliate papillae. **foliate papillae,** parallel projections, inconstant in number, near the posterior border of the tongue, in front of the anterior pillars of the fauces, which bear taste buds and excretory ducts from von Ebner's glands. At birth, they appear as well-developed mucosal ridges but undergo progressive atrophic changes, and in adult life present rudimentary, foldlike elevations. Called also *papillae foliatae* [NA], *columns of folds of tongue,* and *taste ridges.* **fungiform papillae, papil′lae fungifor′mes** [NA], numerous, large, red, knoblike projections found on the dorsal surface of the tongue, chiefly at the sides and apex, which bear taste buds. They are about 1.9 mm in length, and are narrow at their attachment but broad at their free ends. Called also *arcuate papillae of tongue, medial papillae of tongue,* and *obtuse papillae of tongue.* **gingival p.,** a cone-shaped pad of the interdental gingival tissue between two contiguous teeth, consisting of a central core of densely collagenous connective tissue covered by stratified squamous epithelium. It is tapered toward the interproximal contact area and the mesial and distal surfaces are slightly concave, as viewed from the labial, buccal, and lingual aspects. On the vestibular and oral sides the papilla tends to be high, filling the embrasures of the dental arch, but between these areas, the edges of the papilla tend to be depressed. Its lateral borders and tips are formed by a continuation of the marginal gingiva from the adjacent teeth. Called also *interdental p.* and *interproximal p.* See also *retromolar p.* and *interdental* GINGIVA. **gustatory p.,** a papilla which bears taste buds. See *lingual papillae.* **p. inci-si'va** [NA], incisive p. **incisive p.,** an oval projection situated on the palate just anterior to the palantine raphe and immediately posterior to the central incisors, overlying the oral orifice of the nasopalatine ducts. It is lined with a smooth epithelial tissue containing keratinized cells similar to those in other parts of the hard palate. Called also *palatine p.* and *papillar incisiva* [NA]. **interdental p., interproximal p.,** gingival p. **lingual papillae, papil'lae lingua'les** [NA], projections of the corium found on the dorsal surface of the tongue, giving the tongue its characteristic roughness, including the vallate, fungiform, filiform, foliate, conical, and simple papillae. Called also *gustatory p.* **p. mam'mae** [NA], mammary p., nipple (1). **medial papillae of tongue,** fungiform papillae. **obtuse papillae of tongue,** fungiform papillae. **palatine p.,** incisive p. **parotid p., p. paroti'dea** [NA], the small papilla marking the orifice of the parotid duct in the mucous membrane of the cheek. **retrocuspid p.,** a circumscribed round or oval dome-shaped sessile nodule found on the lingual aspect of the mandibular canines near the mucogingival junction. It results from frictional irritation during mastication and phonation and has normal histological and anatomical features that regress with age and require no treatment. **retromolar p.,** a small papilla made up of gingival tissue, which is located at the foot of the mandibular ramus and is attached to the most inferior part of the anterior border of the ramus. Together with the retromolar glandular prominence, it forms the retromolar pad. See also *gingival p.* **simple papillae of tongue, papillae sim'plices,** 1. papillae found over the entire surface of the tongue, consisting of microscopic projections, each containing a capillary loop. 2. filiform papillae. **skin papillae,** papillae of corium. **small papillae of tongue,** filiform papillae. **sublingual p.,** sublingual CARUNCLE. **papil'lae valla'tae** [NA], vallate papillae. **vallate papillae,** eight to twelve large papillae which arise in the bottoms of shallow, walled troughs or depressions on the dorsal surface of the tongue, and are arranged in the form of a V in front of the sulcus terminalis. Each is a cone, the broader end of which projects above the surface of the tongue, being about 1 to 2 mm wide. Their walls are studded with smaller secondary papillae and taste buds are present in large numbers on the walls of the papillae and of the depressions. Secretions from von Ebner's glands discharge into the deepest parts of the troughs. Called also *calciform papillae, capitate papillae, circumvallate papillae,* and *papillae vallatae* [NA]. **villous papillae of tongue,** filiform papillae.

papillae (pah-pil'e) [L.] plural of *papilla.*

papillary (pap'ĭ-ler″e) pertaining to or resembling a papilla, or nipple.

papillate (pap'ĭ-lāt) marked by papilla-like or nipple-like projections.

papillectomy (pap″ĭ-lek'to-me) [*papilla* + Gr. *ektomē* excision] excision of a papilla.

papilledema (pap″il-ĕ-de'mah) [*papilla* + *edema*] edema of the optic papilla.

papillitis (pap″ĭ-li'tis) [*papilla* + *-itis*] inflammation of a papilla. **chronic lingual p.,** Möller's GLOSSITIS.

papilloma (pap″ĭ-lo'mah) [*papilla* + *-oma*] a benign wartlike tumor originating from surface epithelium. An oral papilloma usually presents as a well-circumscribed pedunculated lesion, most commonly of the gingivae, palate, lips, tongue, and buccal mucosa with a corrugated surface resembling a cauliflower, varying in size from a few millimeters to several centimeters. Histologically, it consists of long, thin, finger-like projections extending above the surface of the mucosa, made up of a stratified squamous epithelium and containing central connective tissue cores. Nonkeratinized papillomas are generally soft; those covered with keratin may be firm. The term is often used in connection with any elevated soft tissue growth. Some authorities identify verruca vulgaris with oral papilloma because of their histopathological similarities, although the characteristic vacuolated cells and inclusions present in skin lesions are absent in oral papillomas. **multiple p's of palate,** papillary HYPERPLASIA. **Riga's p.,** Riga-Fede DISEASE.

papillomatosis (pap″ĭ-lo″mah-to'sis) 1. the development of multiple papillomas. 2. papillary HYPERPLASIA.

Papillomavirus (pap″ĭ-lo″mah-vi'rus) [*papillo-* + *-oma* + *virus*] a genus of papovaviruses, which may be arthropod-borne. The diameter of the virion is 50 to 55 nm and the molecular weight of the DNA is 5×10^6 dl. Papillomaviruses are host-specific and cause papillomatous tumors.

papillomavirus (pap″ĭ-lo″mah-vi'rus) any virus of the genus *Papillomavirus.*

Papillon-Léage and Psaume syndrome [Papillon-Léage, French dentist; J. *Psaume,* French dentist] oral-facial-digital SYNDROME (1).

Papillon-Lefèvre syndrome [M. M. *Papillon;* Paul *Lefèvre*] see under SYNDROME.

Papovaviridae (pap″o-vah-vi'rĭ-de) [*papilloma, polyoma,* and *vacuolating agent* + *virus* + *-idae*] a family of naked icosahedral viruses containing a single molecule of double-stranded cyclic DNA which replicates in the host cell nucleus. The diameter of the virion is 45 to 55 nm and the number of capsomers in the virion is 72. Most papovaviruses produce benign tumors that may undergo malignant degeneration. It consists of the genera *Papillomavirus* and *Polyomavirus.*

papovavirus (pap″o-vah-vi'rus) any virus of the family Papovaviridae.

papular (pap'u-lar) [L. *papularis*] consisting of or characterized by the presence of papules.

papule (pap'ul) [L. *papula*] a circumscribed, solid elevated lesion up to 5 mm in diameter, which may be palpable, such as an acne pimple. **dry p.,** the papule of chancre. **prurigo p.,** a dome-shaped papule with a small transient vesicle on top, followed by crusting or lichenification, which is characteristic of prurigo. **split p's,** fissured papular syphilides sometimes seen at the corners of the mouth.

papulosis (pap-u-lo'sis) any condition marked by the presence of multiple papules.

papyraceous (pap″ĭ-ra'shus) [L. *papyraceus*] like paper; chartaceous.

para (par'ah) [L. *parere* to bring forth, to bear] a woman who has produced a viable child regardless of whether or not the child was living at birth. Called *para-1* (also written *para I, 1-para*) or *primipara* after one pregnancy, *para-2* (also written *para II, 2-para*) or *secundipara* after two pregnancies, *para-3* (also written *para III, 3-para*) or *tripara* after three pregnancies, etc. A woman who has never produced a viable child is called *para 0* or *nullipara.* See also PUERPERA.

para- [Gr. *para* beyond] 1. a prefix meaning beside, beyond, accessory to, apart from, against, etc. 2. in organic chemistry, a prefix in structural isomerism indicating the substitution in a derivative of a benzene ring of two atoms linked to opposite carbon atoms in the ring. Abbreviated *p-.* See *para-isomer.* Usually written in italics and disregarded in alphabetization.

para-acetphenetidin (par″ah-as″et-fe-net'ĭ-dēn) phenacetin.

para-agglutinin (par″ah-ah-gloo″tĭ-nin) partial AGGLUTININ.

paracentesis (par″ah-sen-te'sis) [*para-* + Gr. *kentēsis* puncture] surgical puncture of a cavity for the aspiration of fluid.

paracentral (par″ah-sen'tral) near the center.

paracetaldehyde (par-as″et-al'de-hĭd) paraldehyde.

paracetamol (par-as″et-am'ol) acetaminophen.

parachlorophenol (par″ah-klo″ro-fe'nol) a highly toxic compound, 4-chloro-1-hydroxybenzene, occurring as a white or transparent crystalline solid, sometimes with a yellowish or pinkish hue, with a penetrating, unpleasant odor, which is soluble in water, benzene, and ether. It is absorbed through the skin, and intake, inhalation, or contact may produce severe irritation to the exposed tissues. Used in dentistry as a topical anti-infective agent for treatment of infected root canal and periapical infections and is incorporated into various drugs thus used. Also used in the synthesis of drugs and dyes and as a denaturant agent for alcohol. Called also p-*chlorophenol* and *paramonochlorophenol.* **camphorated p.,** a compound produced by combining parachlorophenol with camphor, 100 gm of which contain 35 gm parachlorophenol and 65 gm camphor. Used in the treatment of infected root canal and periapical infections. **liquefied p.,** a liquid preparation, 100 gm of which contain 98 gm parachlorophenol and 2 gm glycerol. Used in root canal therapy and in the treatment of para-apical infection.

Paracoccidioides brasiliensis (par″ah-kok-sid″e-oi-dēz brah-sil″e-en'sis) a species of deuteromycetous fungi (Fungi Imperfecti), which is a multiple-budding yeastlike fungus at 37°C and a mycelium at 25°C. It is the etiologic agent of South American blastomycosis.

paracoccidioidomycosis (par″ah-kok-sid″e-oi″do-mi-ko'sis) South American BLASTOMYCOSIS.

Paracodin trademark for *dihydrocodeine*.

paracone (par′ah-kōn) [*para*-(1) + Gr. *kōnos* cone] the mesiobuccal cusp of a maxillary molar tooth of mammals, which normally occludes between the paraconid and hypoconid of the respective lower molar. See also HYPOCONE, METACONE, PROTOCONE, and TRIGONE (2).

paraconid (par′ah-ko′nid) [*para*-(1) + Gr. *kōnos* cone + *-id*] the mesiobuccal cusp of a mandibular molar tooth. See also HYPOCONID, METACONID, PROTOCONID, and TRIGONID.

paradental (par″ah-den′tal) 1. having some connection with or relation to dentistry. 2. periodontal.

paradentitis (par″ah-den-ti′tis) periodontitis.

paradentium (par″ah-den′she-um) periodontium (1).

paradentosis (par″ah-den-to′sis) periodontosis.

paraffin (par′ah-fin) [L. *parum* little + *affinis* akin] 1. a class of aliphatic hydrocarbons C_nH_{2n+2}, having straight chains consisting chiefly of carbon atoms, and varying with increasing molecular weight from gases (methane) to waxy solids. See also ALKANE. 2. kerosene. 3. paraffin WAX. 4. paraffin COMPOUND (see open CHAIN). **hard p.,** paraffin WAX. **p. jelly,** petrolatum. **light liquid p.,** light mineral OIL. **liquid p.,** mineral OIL. **white soft p.,** white PETROLATUM. **yellow soft p.,** petrolatum.

Paraflex trademark for *chlorzoxazone*.

parafunction (par″ah-funk″shun) 1. disordered or perverted function. 2. bruxism.

Paragit trademark for *trihexyphenidyl hydrochloride* (see under TRIHEXYPHENIDYL).

parahemophilia (par″ah-he″mo-fil′e-ah) a congenital disorder of blood coagulation, transmitted as an autosomal recessive trait, in which deficiency of prothrombin (coagulation factor V) results in a hemophilia-like syndrome, with epistaxis, susceptibility to bruising, and hemorrhage after tooth extraction. In severe cases, hemorrhage into the gastrointestinal tract and central nervous system, hematomas, and spontaneous gingival bleeding may be observed. Called also *p. A, Ac-globulin deficiency, congenital hypoprothrombinemia, hemophiloid state A, labile factor deficiency, Owren's syndrome, parahemophilia syndrome,* and *proaccelerin deficiency.* See also HYPOPROTHROMBINEMIA. **p. A,** parahemophilia.

parakeratosis (par″ah-ker″ah-to′sis) abnormal thickening of the stratum corneum (horny layer), with retention of nuclei or nuclear fragments. It is seen normally in the true mucous membrane of the mouth and vagina. **p. annula′ris,** Mibelli's DISEASE. **p. centrifuga′ta atro′phicans,** Mibelli's DISEASE.

paraldehyde (par-al′de-hīd) a hypnotic and sedative agent, 2,4,6-trimethyl-1,3,5-trioxane, occurring as a transparent, colorless liquid with a specific disagreeable taste and a pungent odor, which is poorly soluble in water and is miscible with ethanol, chloroform, ether, and volatile oils. It may be irritating to the throat and lungs. Called also *paracetaldehyde*.

paralgesia (par″al-je′se-ah) [*para*-(1) + Gr. *algesis* sense of pain + *-ia*] an abnormally painful sensation; a painful paresthesia.

parallax (par′ah-laks) [Gr. "in turn"] an apparent displacement of an object as seen from two different points. In radiography, parallax may cause unsharpness of an x-ray image when a film is wet and the emulsions are swollen.

parallelometer (par″ah-lel-om′ĕ-ter) [*parallel* + Gr. *metron* measure] an instrument for determining the exact parallel relationships of lines, surfaces, and structures in dental prostheses and casts. Some instruments are equipped with a drill attachment for parallel pin insertion. Called also *paralleling instrument*. Trademark: Paramax II. See also dental SURVEYOR. See illustration.

paralysis (pah-ral′ĭ-sis), pl. *paralyses* [*para*-(1) + Gr. *lyein* to loosen] loss or impairment of motor function in a part due to lesions of the neural or muscular mechanism; also, by analogy, impairment of sensory function (*sensory p.*). See also PALSY. **p. ag′itans,** see PARKINSONISM. **ascending p.,** spinal paralysis that progresses cephalad. **association p.,** bulbar p. **asthenic bulbar p.,** MYASTHENIA gravis. **bilateral p.,** paralysis affecting both sides of the body; diplegia. **brachiofacial p.,** paralysis affecting the face and an arm. **bulbar p., bulbar p., progressive,** paralysis due to changes in the motor centers of the medulla oblongata; a chronic, usually fatal disease, most commonly affecting persons over 50 years of age but also occurring in the course of amyotrophic lateral sclerosis, syringobulbia, and multiple sclerosis. It is marked by progressive paralysis and atrophy of the muscles of the lips, tongue, mouth, pharynx, and larynx, and is due to degeneration of the nerve nuclei of the floor of the fourth ventricle. Called also *association p., Duchenne's p., glossolabiolaryngeal p., labial p., labioglossolaryngeal p.,* and *labioglossopharyngeal p.* **bulbar p., spastic,** pseudobulbar p. **bulbospinal p.,** MYASTHENIA gravis. **central p.,** any paralysis due to a lesion of the brain or spinal cord. **Céstan's p.,** Céstan-Chenais SYNDROME. **congenital abducens-facial p., congenital facial p., congenital oculofacial p.,** congenital facial DIPLEGIA. **cruciate p.,** paralysis affecting one side of the face and the opposite side of the body. **divers' p.,** paralysis occurring as a result of too rapid reduction of pressure on deep-sea divers. See also decompression SICKNESS. **Duchenne's p.,** bulbar p. **facial p.,** 1. weakening or paralysis of the facial nerve, as in Bell's palsy. Called also *facioplegia* and *prosopoplegia*. 2. Bell's PALSY. **general p.,** DEMENTIA paralytica. **glossolabiolaryngeal p.,** bulbar p. **Gubler's p.,** Millard-Gubler SYNDROME. **hypoglossal p.,** paralysis due to a lesion of the hypoglossal nucleus of the hypoglossal nerve at any point. **immune p., immnological p.,** the absence of immune response to a specific antigen, usually induced by very large doses of antigen. See immunologic TOLERANCE. **Indian bow p.,** paralysis of the thyroarytenoid muscles. **infantile p.,** poliomyelitis. **labial p., labioglossolaryngeal p., labioglossopharyngeal p.,** bulbar p. **laryngeal p.,** paralysis of one of the laryngeal muscles. **Leyden's p.,** partial or complete oculomotor paralysis and contralateral hemiplegia due to lesions of the nucleus of the third cranial nerve and its ventral fibers crossing the midbrain and the pyramidal tract. Called also *hemiplegia alternans superior peduncularis* and *hemiplegia oculomotorica*. **lingual p.,** paralysis of the tongue. **local p.,** paralysis of one muscle or of a group of muscles. **masticatory p.,** paralysis of the muscles of mastication. **medullary tegmental p.,** Babinski-Nageotte SYNDROME. **mimetic p.,** paralysis of muscles of facial expression. **motor p.,** paralysis of voluntary muscles, resulting in their loss of the power of contraction. **palatopharyngeal p.,** Tapia's SYNDROME. **parotitic p.,** paralysis accompanying mumps. **Parrot's p.,** Parrot's DISEASE (1). **phonetic p.,** paralysis of the muscles of speech. **pressure p.,** paralysis, generally temporary, caused by pressure on a nerve trunk. **progressive bulbar p.,** bulbar p. **progressive hemifacial p.,** facial HEMIATROPHY. **pseudobulbar p.,** spastic weakness of the muscles innervated by the cranial nerves, i.e., the muscles of the face, pharynx, and tongue, due to bilateral lesions of the corticospinal tract; it is often accompanied by uncontrolled weeping or laughing. Called also *supranuclear p.* and *spastic bulbar palsy*. **pseudohypertrophic muscular p.,** Duchenne's DYSTROPHY. **sensory p.,** impairment of sensory function. **seventh nerve p.,** Bell's PALSY. **supranuclear p.,** pseudobulbar p. **trigeminal p.,** paralysis due to a lesion of the trigeminal nerve, marked by sensory loss in the face and weakness of the muscles of mastication. **unilateral p.,** hemiplegia. **uveoparotitic p.,** Heerfordt's SYNDROME.

paralytic (par″ah-lit′ik) [Gr. *paralytikos*] 1. affected with or pertaining to paralysis. 2. a person affected with paralysis.

paramagnetic (par″ah-mag-net′ik) 1. pertaining to or having the property of being attracted by a magnet, and of assuming a position parallel to that of a magnetic force. 2. pertaining to a substance that has magnetic properties stronger than those of air; i.e., a magnetic permeability over 1. See also DIAMAGNETIC.

paramastoid (par″ah-mas′toid) situated near the mastoid process.

Paramax II trademark for a parallelometer equipped with a drill attachment for parallel pin insertion. See illustration at PARALLELOMETER.

paramedian (par″ah-me′de-an) [*para*-(1) + L. *medianus* median] situated near the midline or midplane. Called also *paramesial*.

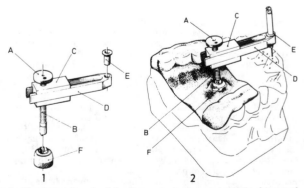

1. The several parts of the Paramax instrument. (*A*) Locking and height-adjustment wheel, with markings. (*B*) Pivot pin. (*C*) Guide block. (*D*) Bar. (*E*) Bur bushing. (*F*) Ball joint with the support. 2. Paramax instrument mounted on the baseplate. (From P. Goransson and A. Parmlid: A paralleling instrument, Paramax II, and the Kodex drills. J. Prosthet. Dent., 34(1):31, 1975.)

paramedical (par″ah-med′ĭ-kal) having some connection with or relation to the science or practice of medicine; adjunctive to the practice of medicine in the maintenance or restoration of health and normal functioning.

paramesial (par″ah-me′se-al) [*para-*(1) + Gr. *mesos* middle] paramedian.

parameter (pah-ram′ĕ-ter) [Gr. *parametrein* to measure one thing by another] 1. one of the independent variables in a set of parametric equations. A variable whose measure is indicative of a quantity or function that cannot itself be precisely determined by direct methods, e.g., blood pressure and pulse rate are parameters of cardiovascular function. 2. a variable entering into the mathematical form of any distribution such that the possible value of the variable corresponds to different distribution.

paramethasone (par″ah-meth′ah-sōn) a synthetic glucocorticoid derived from 16α-methylpregnenolone, 6α-fluoro-11β,17,21-trihydroxy-16α-methylpregna-1,4-diene-2,30-dione. Used in the treatment of adrenocortical insufficiency and as an anti-inflammatory and anti-allergic agent. In dentistry, used to treat sensitive dentin, postoperative pulpal reactions, oral ulcers in skin diseases, and arthritic temporomandibular lesions, and in tissue transplantation. Its side reactions are those common to all glucocorticoids. Trademarks: Cortiden, Flumethone, Haldrate, Metilar, Paramezone. **p. acetate**, the acetate salt of paramethasone, occurring as a fluffy, odorless, white, crystalline powder that deteriorates on exposure to light and is soluble in ethanol, acetone, chloroform, ether, and methanol, but not in water. Administered orally. Trademarks: Haldrone, Monocortin, Sintecort. **p. disodium phosphate**, a soluble disodium phosphate derivative of paramethasone. Trademarks: Monocortin S, Solu-Dilar.

Paramezone trademark for *paramethasone*.

paramitome (par″ah-mi′tōm) [*para-*(1) + Gr. *mitos* thread] hyaloplasm (1).

paramolar (par″ah-mo′lar) [*para-*(1) + *molar*] a supernumerary molar, usually a small and rudimentary tooth, most commonly found in the maxilla, situated buccally or lingually to one of the molars or interproximally between the first or second and third molars. Called also *accessory buccal cusp, paramolar tubercle,* and *supernumerary molar.*

paramonochlorophenol (par″ah-mo-no-klor″o-fe′nol) parachlorophenol.

paramorphine (par″ah-mor′fēn) thebaine.

paramyosin (par″ah-mi′o-sin) tropomyosin A.

paramyotonia (par″ah-mi″o-to-ne′ah) [*para-*(1) + Gr. *mys* muscle + *tonos* tension + *-ia*] a myotonia-like condition characterized by tonic spasms of muscle, without muscle wasting. **congenital p.**, a hereditary disease, transmitted as a dominant trait, present from infancy, in which myotonia of the pharyngeal, orofacial, and distal muscles is precipitated by exposure to cold. Facial grimacing, closing of the eyelids, and clenching of the hands may be produced by brief exposures; longer exposures result in severe flaccid weakness of the extremities with abolition of deep reflexes. Called also *Eulenburg's disease* and *myotonia congenita intermittens.*

Paramyxoviridae (par″ah-mik″so-vi′rĭ-de) a family of viruses with pleomorphic, spherical virions 100 to 200 nm in diameter, occasionally larger. The virion is made up of a rigid, helical nucleocapsid in a lipid-containing envelope with surface projections, the envelope being acquired by budding through the cell membrane. The genome is linear single-stranded (−)RNA which is transcribed into complementary mRNA by polymerase. It comprises three genera: *Pneumovirus* (includes respiratory syncytial virus), *Paramyxovirus* (includes mumps and parainfluenza viruses), and *Morbillivirus* (includes measles virus).

Paramyxovirus (par″ah-mik″so-vi′rus) a genus of paramyxoviruses consisting of several viruses, of which mumps and parainfluenza viruses are pathogenic to man.

paramyxovirus (par″ah-mik″so-vi′rus) any virus of the family Paramyxoviridae or of the genus *Paramyxovirus.*

parangi (pah-ran′je) Ceylonese name for yaws.

paraoperative (par″ah-op′er-a″tiv) pertaining to the accessories essential to operative surgery, such as care of instruments and gloves, sterilization, etc.

paraoral (par″ah-o′ral) 1. situated near or around the mouth. 2. administered by some other route than the mouth, said of medication.

paraplasm (par″ah-plazm) [*para-*(1) + Gr. *plasma* something formed] 1. hyaloplasm (1). 2. an abnormal growth.

paraplegia (par″ah-pie′je-ah) [*para-*(1) + Gr. *plēgē* stroke + *-ia*] paralysis of the legs and lower part of the body. **unilateral p.**, hemiparaplegia.

paraplegic (par″ah-plej′ik) 1. pertaining to or of the nature of paraplegia. 2. a person with paraplegia.

Parapoxvirus (par″ah-poks-vi′rus) a genus of poxviruses, which are 220 to 300 nm long. It includes orf, paravaccinia, and bovine papular stomatitis viruses, which may cause infection in man.

paraprotein (par″ah-pro′te-in, par″ah-pro′tēn) [*para-*(1) + *protein*] originally, a term used to denote an abnormal serum protein of restricted electrophoretic mobility, seen in the electrophoretogram as a narrow band or spike, such as myeloma proteins and Bence Jones protein. By common usage, the term is now applied to a monoclonal serum immunoglobulin that represents the protein synthesized by a single clone of lymphoid cells.

paraproteinemia (par″ah-pro″te-in-e′me-ah) any of a group of diseases characterized by the presence in the blood of paraproteins. Principal paraproteinemias include heavy chain disease, multiple myeloma, Waldenström's macroglobulinemia, malignant lymphoma, amyloidosis, and Hodgkin's disease. Called also *plasma cell dyscrasia.*

parapsis (par-ap′sis) [*para-*(1) + Gr. *hapsis* touch] perversion of the sense of touch.

pararhizoclasia (par″ah-ri″zo-kla′ze-ah) [*para-*(1) + Gr. *rhiza* root + *klasis* destruction + *-ia*] Inflammatory destruction of the deep layers of the alveolar process and the periodontal ligament around the root of a tooth. See also *perirhizoclasia.*

pararhotacism (par″ah-ro′tah-sizm) [*para-*(1) + Gr. *rho* the Greek letter *r*] imperfect pronunciation of the sound of the letter *r.*

pararthria (par-ar′thre-ah) [*para-*(1) + Gr. *arthron* articulation] disordered or imperfect utterance of speech.

parasigmatism (par″ah-sig′mah-tizm) [*para-*(1) + Gr. *sigma* the Greek letter *s*] imperfect pronunciation of *s* and *z* sounds.

parasinoidal (par″ah-si-noi′dal) situated along the course of a sinus.

parasite (par″ah-sīt) [*para-*(1) + Gr. *sitos* food] 1. a plant or animal which lives upon or within another living organism at whose expense it obtains some advantage. 2. the less completely developed, smaller of conjoined twins, which is attached to the autosite. **accidental p.**, an organism parasitizing an animal other than the usual host. Called also *incidental p.* **celozoic p.**, one which lives in a body cavity of the host. **cytozoic p.**, one which lives in body cells of the host. **eurytrophic p.**, an ectoparasite which can feed on various hosts. **facultative p.**, an organism which may be parasitic upon another but which is capable of independent existence. **hematozoic p.**, a parasite which lives in the blood of the host. **incidental p.**, accidental p. **intermittent p.**, one which lives in its host only at times, being free living during the interval. Called also *occasional p.* **karyozoic p.**, one which lives in cell nuclei. **malarial p.**, *Plasmodium.* **obligatory p.**, one which cannot live apart from its host. **occasional p.**, intermittent p. **periodic p.**, one that resides in its hosts for short periods. **permanent p.**, one which lives in its host from early life until maturity or death. **specific p.**, one normal to its current host. **spurious p.**, an organism which is parasitic on hosts other than man, but which may pass through the human body without causing harm. **stenotrophic p.**, an ectoparasite which can feed on one host only. **temporary p.**, one which lives free of its host during part of its life cycle. Called also *transient p.* **teratoid p.**, a fetal parasite which appears as a tumor-like mass. **transient p.**, temporary p.

parasitemia (par″ah-si-te′me-ah) the presence of parasites in the blood.

parasitic (par″ah-sit′ik) [Gr. *parasitikos*] pertaining to, of the nature of, or caused by a parasite.

parasiticidal (par″ah-sit″ĭ-si′dal) destructive to parasites.

parasiticide (par″ah-sit′ĭ-sīd) [L. *parasitus* a parasite + *caedere* to kill] 1. destructive to parasites. 2. an agent that is destructive to parasites.

parasitism (par″ah-si″tizm) 1. symbiosis in which one population (or individual) adversely affects the other, but cannot live without it. 2. infection or infestation with parasites.

parasitization (par″ah-sit″ĭ-za′shun) infection or infestation with parasites.

parasitologist (par″ah-si-tol′o-jist) an expert in parasitology.

parasitology (par″ah-si-tol′o-je) [Gr. *parasitos* parasite + *-logy*] the study of parasites and parasitism.

parasitosis (par″ah-si-to′sis) [Gr. *parasitos* parasite + *-osis*] a condition caused by infection or infestation with parasites.

paraspasm (par′ah-spazm) a spasm of the corresponding muscles on both sides of the body. Called also *paraspasmus.*

paraspasmus (par″ah-spaz′mus) paraspasm. **p. facia′le**, a painless motor disturbance affecting both sides of the face.

paraspecific (par″ah-spe-sif′ik) having curative properties in addition to the specific one.

Paraspen trademark for *acetaminophen*.

parasympathetic (par″ah-sim″pah-thet′ik) [*para*-(1) + *sympathetic*] 1. of or pertaining to the division of the nervous system that, together with the sympathetic division, forms the autonomic nervous system. See parasympathetic SYSTEM. 2. the craniosacral portion of the autonomic nervous system.

parasympatholytic (par″ah-sim″pah-tho-lit-ik) [*parasympathetic* + Gr. *lytikos* dissolving] 1. dissolving or interrupting impulses of the parasympathetic nervous system. 2. a drug or substance blocking impulses of the parasympathetic nervous system. The term applies to blocking of impulses mediated at both nicotinic and muscarinic receptors but it is sometimes used as a synonym for antimuscarinic drugs (see under DRUG).

parasympathomimetic (par″ah-sim″pah-tho-mi-met′ik) [*parasympathetic* + Gr. *mimetikos* imitative] 1. producing effects resembling those of stimulation of the parasympathetic nervous system. 2. parasympathomimetic DRUG.

parathion (par″ah-thi′on) an agricultural insecticide that is very toxic to warm-blooded animals, *O,O*-diethyl *O-p*-nitrophenyl phosphorothiate. Acute poisoning may cause anorexia, nausea, vomiting, diarrhea, excessive salivation, pupillary constriction, bronchial constriction, muscle twitching, convulsions, coma, and death.

parathormone (par″ah-thor′mōn) parathyroid HORMONE.

parathyroid (par″ah-thi′roid) [*para*-(1) + *thyroid*] 1. parathyroid GLAND. 2. situated beside or near the thyroid gland.

paratope (par′ah-tōp) the combining site on an antigen molecule that corresponds and reacts with the epitope of the antigen. See also antigenic DETERMINANT.

parazone (par′ah-zōn) one of the light bands, alternating with dark bands (diazones) that form the lines of Schreger, seen under reflected light in a ground section of a tooth. It is believed that it is an area in which the enamel prisms have been cut in longitudinal section.

Par-Cast trademark for an extra hard *dental casting gold alloy* (see under GOLD).

Paré, Ambroise [French surgeon, 1510–1590] the most celebrated surgeon of the Renaissance, who reformed the treatment of gunshot wounds by abolishing cauterization with boiling oil. He also practiced ligation of arteries after amputation, and reintroduced podalic version into obstetrics. His famous aphorism, *Je le pensay, et Dieu le guarit* ("I dressed him and God healed him"), first appeared in 1585, in the fourth edition of his collected works. He is credited with the introduction of artificial eyes, teeth, hands, and legs. Among his works are extensive writings on dentistry, including descriptions of tooth extraction and reimplantation. Paré is credited with being the first to close perforations of the palate by means of an obturator.

Paredrine trademark for *hydroxyamphetamine*.

paregoric (par″ē-gor′ik) [Gr. *paregorikos* consoling] a preparation of powdered opium, anise oil, benzoic acid, camphor, diluted alcohol, and glycerin, each 100 ml of which yields 35 to 45 mg anhydrous morphine. Used as an antiperistaltic, especially in the treatment of diarrhea. Formerly called *camphorated opium tincture*.

parenchyma (pah-reng′kĭ-mah) [Gr. "anything poured in beside"] a functional element of an organ, as distinguished from its framework, or stroma.

parent (par′ent) 1. a father or a mother. See also PEDIGREE. 2. any organism that produces or generates another. 3. a radionuclide that upon radioactive decay or disintegration yields a specific nuclide (decay product or daughter), either directly or as a later member of a radioactive series. See also PRODUCT.

parenteral (pah-ren′ter-al) [*para*-(1) + Gr. *enteron* intestine] not through the alimentary canal but rather by injection through some other route, as subcutaneous, intramuscular, intraorbital, intracapsular, intraspinal, intrasternal, intravenous, etc.

Parenzyme trademark for a trypsin preparation.

paresis (pah-re′sis, par′ĕ-sis) [Gr. "relaxation"] a slight form of paralysis or partial loss of muscular power. **general p.,** DEMENTIA paralytica. **unilateral p.,** hemiparesis.

paresthesia (par″es-the′ze-ah) [*para*-(1) + Gr. *aisthēsis* perception] an abnormal sensation, such as burning, prickling, tingling, numbness, formication, etc. **postoperative p.,** numbness, burning, or prickling after surgery, as numbness of the lip, sometimes with drooping of the lip and drooling of saliva, following oral surgery and due to injury of the mental or mandibular nerve. **unilateral p.,** hemiparesthesia.

pargyline (par′gĭ-lēn) a monoamine oxidase inhibitor with vasodilator effects, *N*-methyl-*N*-2-propynylbenzylamine. Administered as the hydrochloride salt, which occurs as white, crystalline powder with a slight characteristic odor, and is soluble in water, ethanol, and chloroform and slightly soluble in acetone and benzene. Used in the treatment of hypertensive crises. Adverse reactions may include tachycardia, nausea, vomiting, restlessness, tremor, muscle twitching, dyspnea, cyanosis, mydriasis, and shock. Overdosage may change the effect from hypotensive to hypertensive. Trademarks: Eudatin, Eutonyl, Supirdyl.

Parham band [F. W. *Parham*, American surgeon, 1885–1927] see under BAND.

paries (pa′re-ez), pl. *pari′etes* [L.] a wall; a general anatomical term for the wall of an organ or body cavity. See also *floor, roof,* and *wall*. **p. carot′icus ca′vi tym′pani** [NA], the anterior wall of the tympanic cavity, related to the carotid canal, in which is lodged the internal carotid artery. **p. infe′rior or′bitae** [NA], FLOOR of orbit. **p. jugula′ris ca′vi tym′pani** [NA], the floor of the tympanic cavity that is in intimate relation with the jugular fossa, which lodges the bulb of the internal jugular vein. **p. labyrin′thicus ca′vi tym′pani** [NA], the medial wall of the tympanic cavity. **p. latera′lis or′bitae** [NA], lateral wall of orbit; see under WALL. **p. mastoi′deus ca′vi tym′pani** [NA], the posterior wall of the tympanic cavity, related to the mastoid portion of the temporal bone. **p. media′lis or′bitae** [NA], medial wall of orbit; see under WALL. **p. membrana′ceus ca′vi tym′pani** [NA], the outer, or lateral, wall of the tympanic cavity, formed mainly by the tympanic membrane. **p. membrana′ceus tra′cheae** [NA], the posterior part of the wall of the trachea where the cartilaginous rings are deficient. **p. supe′rior or′bitae** [NA], ROOF of orbit. **p. tegmenta′lis ca′vi tym′pani** [NA], the roof of the tympanic cavity, related to part of the petrous portion of the temporal bone. See also TEGMEN tympani.

parietal (pah-ri′ĕ-tal) [L. *parietalis*] 1. pertaining to the walls of a cavity. 2. pertaining to or located near the parietal bone, as the parietal lobe.

parietes (pah-ri′ĕ-tēz) [L.] plural of *paries*.

parieto- [L. *paries* wall] a combining form denoting relationship to a wall.

parietofrontal (pah-ri″ĕ-to-fron′tal) [*parieto*- + *frontal*] pertaining to the parietal and frontal bones, gyri, or fissures.

parieto-occipital (par-ri″ĕ-to-ok-sip′ĭ-tal) [*parieto*- + *occipital*] pertaining to the parietal and occipital bones or lobes.

parietosphenoid (pah-ri″ĕ-to-sfe′noid) [*parieto*- + *sphenoid*] pertaining to the parietal and sphenoid bones.

parietosquamosal (pah-ri″ĕ-to-skwah-mo′sal) [*parieto*- + *squamosal*] pertaining to the parietal bone and the squamous portion of the temporal bone.

parietotemporal (pah-ri″ĕ-to-tem′po-ral) [*parieto*- + *temporal*] pertaining to the parietal and temporal bones or lobes.

Paris nomenclature see CHROMOSOME nomenclature, Paris.

Parkemed trademark for *mefenamic acid* (see under ACID).

Parkes Weber's syndrome [Frederick *Parkes Weber*, British physician, 1863–1962] Klippel-Trenaunay-Weber SYNDROME.

Parkinsan trademark for *trihexyphenidyl hydrochloride* (see under TRIHEXYPHENIDYL).

Parkinson's disease, facies [James *Parkinson*, English physician, 1755–1824] see PARKINSONISM, and see under FACIES.

parkinsonism (par′kin-sun-izm″) a chronic disorder of the central nervous system characterized by masklike facies (Parkinson's facies) with a wide-eyed, unblinking expression, sialorrhea, and greasy skin; dysarthria; stooped posture; cogwheel rigidity; slowness of movement; alternating tremor; and abnormal gait. Involuntary tremor usually begins in one hand and gradually spreads to both arms and legs; it may disappear momentarily on voluntary movements or during sleep. Pathologically, degenerative and necrotizing lesions are usually found in the basal ganglia and cerebral cortex. Four principal varieties of disease are most commonly recognized: Parkinson's disease (paralysis agitans), which normally occurs during the sixth decade; encephalic parkinsonism, which follows encephalitis and is observed in both children and adults; arteriosclerotic muscular rigidity, which is a disease of old age; and drug-induced parkinsonism, which may be present at any age. Called also *shaking palsy*. **drug-induced p.,** see *parkinsonism*. **encephalic p.,** see *parkinsonism*. **unilateral p.,** hemiparkinsonism.

Parnate trademark for *tranylcypromine*.

Parnite trademark for *tranylcypromine*.

Parodyne trademark for *antipyrine*.

parotid (pah-rot′id) [*para*-(1) + Gr. *ous* ear] situated or occurring near the ear. See also parotid GLAND.

parotidosis (pah-rot-id′o-sis) [*parotid* + -*osis*] a disorder of the parotid gland. See also SIALADENOSIS. **diabetic p.,** a disorder of the parotid glands characterized by usually bilateral and retromandibular enlargement, observed in diabetic patients.

parotitis (par″o-ti′tis) inflammation of the parotid gland. See also SIALADENITIS. **acute postoperative p.,** acute inflammation of the parotid gland, believed to be caused by a retrograde infection following surgery, especially abdominal operations. *Staphylococcus aureus, S. pyogenes, Streptococcus viridans,* and, less frequently, pneumococci and coli bacteria are the principal pathogens. General debilitation, dehydration, and decreased salivary secretion are the precipitating factors. It is accompanied by pain, swelling in the parotid area, reddening of the overlying skin, edema, trismus, and severe headache. Called also *retrograde sialadenitis* and *surgical mumps.* **collagen p.,** collagen *sialadenitis.* **epidemic p.,** mumps. **p. phlegmono'sa,** parotitis associated with suppuration. **recurrent p.,** chronic recurrent, usually unilateral, pyogenic parotitis seen in children and adults, characterized by hyposialosis, enlargement in the parotid area, and purulent saliva.

paroxysm (par'ok-sizm) [Gr. *paroxysmos*] 1. a fit, seizure, or wave of pain or convulsion. 2. a sudden recurrence, usually periodic, or intensification of symptoms.

paroxysmal (par'ok-siz'mal) recurring in paroxysms.

Parpanit trademark for *caramiphen hydrochloride* (see under CARAMIPHEN).

Parrot's disease (paralysis, pseudoparalysis), scars (cicatrices, rhagades), sign (nodes) [Jules Marie *Parrot,* French physician, 1839–1883] see ACHONDROPLASIA, and see under SCAR and SIGN.

Parry-Romberg syndrome [Caleb Hillier *Parry,* English physician, 1755–1822; Moritz Heinrich *Romberg,* German physician, 1795–1873] facial HEMIATROPHY.

pars (parz), pl. *par'tes* [L.] a division or part; used in anatomical nomenclature to designate a particular portion of a larger area, organ, or structure. **p. ala'ris mus'culi nasa'lis** [NA], alar part of nasal muscle; see under PART. **p. alveola'ris mandib'ulae** [NA], alveolar part of mandible; see under PART. **p. amor'pha,** the dense, spherical granular body forming the central area of the nucleolus, surrounded by coarse strands, the nucleolonema. **p. basila'ris os'sis occipita'lis** [NA], basilar PART. **p. buccopharyn'gea mus'culi constricto'ris pharyn'gis superio'ris,** buccopharyngeal MUSCLE. **p. cartilagin'ea sep'ti na'si** [NA], cartilaginous part of nasal septum; see under PART. **p. cephal'ica syste'matis sympath'ici,** cephalic part of sympathetic nervous system; see under PART. **p. ceratopharyn'gea mus'culi constricto'ris pharyn'gis me'dii** [NA], ceratopharyngeal MUSCLE. **p. cervica'lis syste'matis sympath'ici,** cervical part of sympathetic nervous system; see under PART. **p. chondropharyn'gea mus'culi constricto'ris pharyn'gis me'dii** [NA], chondropharyngeal MUSCLE. **p. cochlea'ris ner'vi octa'vi** [NA], **p. cochlea'ris ner'vi vestibulocochlea'ris,** cochlear NERVE. **p. corpo'ris adipa'ta,** fatty zone of hard palate; see under ZONE. **par'tes corpo'ris huma'ni** [NA], the category in anatomical nomenclature embracing the names of the various parts of the human body. **p. corpo'ris glandulo'sa,** glandular zone of hard palate; see under ZONE. **p. corpo'ris ra'phe,** raphe ZONE. **p. cricopharyn'gea mus'culi constricto'ris pharyn'gis inferio'ris** [NA], cricopharyngeal MUSCLE. **p. dista'lis lo'bi anterio'ris hypophys'eos** [NA], the main body of the anterior pituitary gland. **p. glossopharyn'gea mus'culi constricto'ris pharyn'gis superio'ris** [NA], glossopharyngeal MUSCLE. **p. horizonta'lis os'sis palati'ni,** horizontal plate of palatine bone; see under PLATE. **p. infundibula'ris lo'bi anterio'ris hypophys'eos** [NA], the upward extension of the anterior pituitary gland, which forms a thin cloak of cells on the anterior surface of the pituitary stalk. Called also *p. tuberalis lobi anterioris hypophyseos.* **p. intercartilagin'ea ri'mae glot'tidis** [NA], RIMA glottidis cartilaginea. **p. interme'dia lo'bi anterio'res hypophys'eos** [NA] an ill-defined region between the pars distalis of the anterior lobe of the pituitary gland and the posterior lobe. Assigned in some systems of nomenclature as a component of the anterior lobe and in others as part of the posterior lobe. See also pituitary GLAND. **p. intermembrana'cea ri'mae glot'tidis** [NA], RIMA glottidis membranacea. **p. labia'lis mus'culi orbicula'ris o'ris** [NA], labial part of orbicular muscle of mouth; see under PART. **p. lacrima'lis mus'culi orbicula'ris oc'uli** [NA], lacrimal part of orbicular muscle of eye; see under PART. **p. laryn'gea pharyn'gis** [NA], laryngopharynx. **p. latera'lis os'sis occipita'lis** [NA], lateral part of occipital bone; see under PART. **p. margina'lis mus'culi orbicula'ris o'ris** [NA], marginal part of orbicular muscle of mouth; see under PART. **p. mastoi'dea os'sis tempora'lis,** mastoid BONE. **p. membrana'cea sep'ti na'si** [NA], membranous septum of nose; see under SEPTUM. **p. mo'bilis sep'ti na'si** [NA], mobile septum of nose; see under SEPTUM. **p. mus'culi constricto'ris pharyn'gis superio'ris,** buccopharyngeal MUSCLE. **p. mylopharyn'gea mus'culi constricto'ris pharyn'gis superio'ris** [NA], mylopharyngeal MUSCLE. **p. nasa'lis os'sis fronta'lis** [NA], nasal process of frontal bone; see under PROCESS. **p. nasa'lis pharyn'gis** [NA], nasopharynx. **p. nervo'sa hypophys'eos,** the main body of the posterior pituitary

gland. Called also *infundibular process* and *neural lobe.* **p. obli'qua mus'culi cricothyroi'dei** [NA], oblique part of cricothyroid muscle; see under PART. **p. ora'lis pharyn'gis** [NA], oropharynx. **p. orbita'lis mus'culi orbicula'ris oc'uli** [NA], orbital part of orbicular muscle of eye; see under PART. **p. orbita'lis os'sis fronta'lis** [NA], orbital plate of frontal bone; see under PLATE. **p. os'sea sep'ti na'si** [NA], bony part of nasal septum; see under PART. **p. palpebra'lis glan'dulae lacrima'lis** [NA], palpebral part of lacrimal gland; see under PART. **p. palpebra'lis mus'culi orbicula'ris oc'uli** [NA], palpebral part of orbicular muscle of eye; see under PART. **p. parasympath'ica syste'matis nervo'si autonom'ici** [NA], parasympathetic nervous SYSTEM. **p. perpendicula'ris os'sis palati'ni,** perpendicular plate of palatine bone; see under PLATE. **p. petro'sa os'sis tempora'lis** [NA], petrous BONE. **p. profun'da glan'dulae parot'idis** [NA], deep part of parotid gland; see under PART. **p. profun'da mus'culi masse'teris,** [NA], deep part of masseter muscle; see under PART. **p. pterygopharyn'gea mus'culi constricto'ris pharyn'gis superio'ris** [NA], pterygopharyngeal MUSCLE. **p. squamo'sa os'sis tempora'lis** [NA], temporal SQUAMA. **p. superficia'lis mus'culi masse'teris** [NA], superficial part of masseter muscle; see under PART. **p. sympath'ica syste'matis nervo'si autonom'ici** [NA], sympathetic nervous SYSTEM. **p. thyropharyn'gea mus'culi constricto'ris pharyn'gis inferio'ris** [NA], thyropharyngeal MUSCLE. **p. transver'sa mus'culi nasa'lis** [NA], transverse part of nasal muscle; see under PART. **p. tubera'lis lo'bi anterio'ris hypophyseo's,** p. infundibularis lobi anterioris hypophyseos. **p. tympan'ica os'sis tempora'lis** [NA], tympanic BONE. **p. vestibula'ris ner'vi octa'vi** [NA], **p. vestibula'ris ner'vi vestibulocochlea'ris,** vestibular NERVE.

part (part) [L. *pars,* a portion, piece] a general anatomical term used to designate a part or portion of a structure or organ. Called also *pars.* **alar p. of nasal muscle,** the part of the nasal muscle that arises from the maxilla below the nose and inserts into the greater alar cartilage. Its function consists of widening the opening of the nares. Called also *dilator muscle of nose, dilator naris, musculus dilatator naris, musculus dilator naris,* and *pars alaris musculi nasalis* [NA]. **alveolar p. of mandible,** the alveolar process of the mandible, consisting of the superior body of the mandible, which surrounds and supports the teeth. Called also *pars alveolaris mandibulae* [NA]. See also alveolar PROCESS. **basilar p., basilar p. of occipital bone,** the thick, roughly quadrilateral plate of the occipital bone. It extends anteriorly from the foramen magnum and, in young persons, is joined to the sphenoid bone by cartilage. In the early twenties the cartilaginous plate becomes ossified and the basilar part of the occipital bone and the sphenoid bone form a continuous plate. The posterior concave edge forms the anterior rim of the occipital foramen. On the inferior surface, about 1 cm anterior to the foramen magnum, a small elevation, the pharyngeal tubercle, provides attachment to the pharyngeal raphe. The upper surface is slightly depressed and ascends anteriorly, and is a part of the basal slope, the clivus, which supports the medulla oblongata and the pons. The lateral borders are joined with the temporal bone by the petro-occipital fissure. The shallow furrow along the lateral border on the upper surface contains a venous sinus, the inferior petrosal sinus. The longus capitis and rectus capitis muscles are attached on either side of the midline, and immediately anterior to the foramen magnum, the anterior atlanto-occipital membrane is attached. Called also *basilar process, occipital process of occipital bone,* and *pars basilaris ossis occipitalis* [NA]. **bony p. of nasal septum,** that part of the nasal septum composed posterosuperiorly of the perpendicular plate of the ethmoid bone and posteroinferiorly of the vomer. Called also *pars ossea septi nasi* [NA]. **cartilaginous p. of nasal septum,** the plate of cartilage forming the anterior part of the nasal septum. Called also *cartilaginous nasal septum, pars cartilaginea septi nasi* [NA], and *septum cartilagineum nasi.* **cephalic p. of sympathetic nervous system,** the part of the sympathetic nervous system that derives from the superior cervical ganglion, consisting of the internal carotid nerve and branches that accompany the vertebral artery and branches of the external carotid artery. It supplies various structures of the head, including the sweat glands, muscles of the scalp, facial arteries, and the salivary glands. Called also *pars cephalica systematis sympathici.* **cervical p. of sympathetic nervous system,** the cervical portion of the sympathetic trunk, consisting of the superior, middle, and inferior ganglia. Called also *pars cervicalis systematis sympathici.* **condylar p. of occipital bone,** lateral p. of occipital bone. **cranial p. of accessory nerve,**

internal branch of accessory nerve; see under BRANCH. **cranio-sacral p. of autonomic nervous system,** parasympathetic nervous SYSTEM. **deep p. of masseter muscle,** the portion of the masseter muscle arising from the lower border and medial surface of the zygomatic arch and inserting into the upper half of the ramus and lateral surface of the coronoid process of the mandible. Called also *pars profunda musculi masseteris* [NA]. **deep p. of parotid gland,** that part of the parotid gland located deep to the facial nerve. Called also *pars profunda glandulae parotidis* [NA]. **exoccipital p. of occipital bone,** lateral p. of occipital bone. **horizontal p. of palatine bone,** horizontal plate of palatine bone; see under PLATE. **jugular p. of occipital bone,** lateral p. of occipital bone. **labial p. of orbicular muscle of mouth,** the part of the orbicular muscle of the mouth whose fibers are restricted to the lips. Called also *pars labialis musculi orbicularis oris* [NA]. **lacrimal p. of orbicular muscle of eye,** a small part of the orbicular muscle of the eye, about 12 mm in length and 6 mm in breadth, arising from the posterior lacrimal ridge of the lacrimal bone, passing behind the medial palpebral ligament and the lacrimal sac, and dividing into upper and lower segments which are inserted into the upper and lower tarsal cartilages. Called also *Horner's muscle, musculus tensor tarsi, pars lacrimalis musculi orbicularis oris* [NA], and *tensor tarsi.* **lateral p. of occipital bone,** one of the two parts of the occipital bone at the lateral edges of the foramen magnum. They are flat bones which are somewhat thinner in their posterior aspects than their anterior portions. They articulate with the atlas through the occipital condyles which project on their anterior surfaces. Short perforations at the base of each condyle (hypoglossal canals) provide an exit for the hypoglossal nerve and an entry for the meningeal branch of the ascending pharyngeal artery. A depression on the posterior aspect of the condyle (condyloid fossa) is the point of contact with the atlas. A canal through the floor of the fossa (condyloid canal) provides a passage for the veins which connect the intracranial and extracranial veins (condylar emissaria). A quadrilateral bony plate (jugular process) is located on the lateroposterior part of the condyle, and is excavated by a small projection (jugular notch), which, together with the opposing notch on the temporal bone, forms the borders of the jugular foramen. The jugular process is surrounded by the sigmoid sulcus. The superior surface of the lateral part forms the jugular groove, which overlays the hypoglossal canal, and is crossed by a groove for the glossopharyngeal, vagus, and accessory nerves. Called also *condylar p. of occipital bone, exoccipital p. of occipital bone, jugular p. of occipital bone,* and *pars lateralis ossis occipitalis* [NA]. **mamillary p. of temporal bone,** mastoid BONE. **marginal p. of orbicular muscle of mouth,** the part of the orbicular muscle of the mouth, whose fibers blend with those of adjacent muscles. Called also *pars marginalis musculi orbicularis oris* [NA]. **membranous p. of nasal septum,** membranous septum of nose; see under SEPTUM. **oblique p. of cricothyroid muscle,** the fibers of the cricothyroid muscle that are inserted into the inferior horn, caudal margin, and inner surface of the thyroid cartilage. Called also *pars obliqua musculi cricothyroidei* [NA]. **occipital p. of occipital bone,** occipital SQUAMA. **orbital p. of lacrimal gland,** the main and superior part of the lacrimal gland, connected loosely to the periosteum of the orbit and resting on a fascial sheet extending between the superior and lateral rectus muscles. Called also *glandulae lacrimalis superior.* **orbital p. of orbicular muscle of eye,** a thick, reddish portion of the orbicular muscle of the eye that arises from the medial palpebral ligament and the medial margin of the orbit and surrounds it and the palpebral part of the muscle, inserting laterally in the cheek. Called also *pars orbitalis musculi orbicularis oculi* [NA]. **palpebral p. of lacrimal gland,** the part of the lacrimal gland that projects laterally into the upper eyelid. Called also *glandula lacrimalis inferior, palpebral process, pars palpebralis glandulae lacrimalis* [NA], *Rosenmüller's gland,* and *Rosenmüller's node.* **palpebral p. of orbicular muscle of eye,** a thin, pale portion of the orbicular muscle of the eye that arises from the bifurcation of the medial palpebral ligament. Its fibers interdigitate laterally to form the lateral palpebral raphe. Called also *palpebralis musculi orbicularis oculi* [NA] and *Riolan's muscle.* **parasympathetic p. of autonomic nervous system,** parasympathetic nervous SYSTEM. **perpendicular p. of palatine bone,** perpendicular plate of palatine bone; see under PLATE. **squamous p. of occipital bone,** occipital SQUAMA. **squamous p. of temporal bone,** temporal SQUAMA. **superficial p. of masseter muscle,** the part of the masseter muscle that arises from the lower border of the zygomatic bone by a fibrous aponeurosis and

inserts into the angle of the lower border of the ramus of the mandible. Called also *pars superficialis musculi masseteris* [NA]. **transverse p. of nasal muscle,** the part of the nasal muscle that arises from the canine eminence of the maxilla and joins by common aponeurosis its fellow of the opposite side. It depresses the nasal cartilage and helps dilate the nasal aperture. ·Called also *compressor muscle of naris, compressor naris, musculus compressor naris,* and *pars transversa musculi nasalis* [NA].

Parterol trademark for *dihydrotachysterol.*

partes (par'tēz) [L.] plural of *pars.*

participant (par-tis'i-pant) 1. one who has a part or share, as with others. 2. beneficiary.

particle (par'tĭ-k'l) [L. *particula,* dim. of *partus* part] a tiny mass of material. **alpha p., α-p.,** 1. a positively-charged heavy particle, consisting of a nucleus of the helium isotope made up of two protons and two neutrons, which is ejected from some types of atoms of radioactive materials at speeds ranging from 9,000 to 20,000 miles per second. Streams of alpha particles form intensely ionizing radiations that may be stopped by a sheet of paper and are thus less dangerous than the two other radioactive emissions, beta particles and gamma rays. Those which do not collide with other matter, eventually collect two free electrons and become atoms of helium. Called also *alpha ray.* Streams of alpha particles are called *alpha radiation.* 2. glycogen granules (see under GRANULE) occurring in groups. **beta p., β-p.,** 1. a high-speed electron emitted from a nucleus of radioactive materials during radioactive decay, having a single electrical charge and a mass equal to approximately $\frac{1}{1837}$ that of a proton. A negatively charged beta particle is identical to an electron; a positively charged particle is known as a *positron.* They travel in straight paths at speeds greater than alpha particles and are capable of penetrating tissues up to about 1 cm in thickness but are stopped by a thin sheet of metal. Streams of beta particles *(beta radiation)* may cause skin burns. Called also *beta ray.* 2. isolated glycogen granules (see under GRANULE). **chromatin p.,** karyosome. **crystalline p's,** particles observable under a light microscope in a variety of cells, believed by some to be proteins, usually iron-containing bodies probably derived from hemoglobin. They are found mainly in association with organelles: nucleus, endoplasmic reticulum, mitochondria, Golgi apparatus, lysosomes, and inclusions, as well as in a free state in the cytoplasm. Called also *crystalline bodies.* **Dane p.,** a viral particle 40 to 42 nm in diameter having a 27-nm core, which is probably the infective virion of the hepatitis B virus (see under VIRUS). **elementary p.,** a subatomic particle, such as the electron, proton, neutron, positron, meson, neutrino, and the like. **fat p.,** lipid GRANULE. **high-velocity p's,** nuclear particles, such as electrons, protons, and deuterons, given high speeds in an accelerator. **indirectly ionizing p's,** uncharged particles which can liberate directly ionizing particles or can initiate a nuclear transformation. **lipid p.,** lipid GRANULE. **viral p.,** virion.

Partsch's operation see under OPERATION.

part. vic. abbreviaton for L. *parti'tis vi'cibus,* in divided does.

party (par'te) 1. a group of persons with common purposes or opinions who participate in some activity. 2. one of the litigants (a person or a group) in a legal proceeding. 3. one who signs a legal document. **first p.,** beneficiary. **second p.,** in health insurance, an organization that provides benefits, such as a commercial insurance company, Medicare or Medicaid, or Blue Cross. See CARRIER (5). **third p.,** in health insurance, the agency that pays for services provided by the carrier to the beneficiary. See third party PAYER.

parulis (pah-roo'lis) [*para*-(1) + Gr. *oulon* gum] an elevated nodule at the site of a fistula draining a chronic periapical abscess, occurring most commonly in pulpally involved deciduous teeth. Called also *gumboil* (also written *gum boil*).

parvo- [L. *parvus* small] a combining form meaning small.

Parvoviridae (par'vo-vi'rĭ-de) [*parvo-* + *virus* + *-idae*] a family of small, naked, icosahedral viruses which replicate in the host cell nucleus, having virions about 18 to 26 nm in diameter and 32 capsomers in the virion. The genome is single-stranded DNA. The family consists of the genera *Parvovirus* and *Densovirus* (a virus of invertebrates) and the adenoassociated virus group.

Parvovirus (par'vo-vi'rus) a genus of parvoviruses, having virions 19 to 24 nm in diameter, icosahedral symmetry, and 32 capsomers in the virion. Parvoviruses are not pathogenic to man, but infect various animals, including rats, cattle, dogs, pigs, mink, cats, mice, and geese.

parvovirus (par'vo-vi'rus) any virus of the family Parvoviridae or of the genus *Parvovirus.*

Pa × s pascals per second; see dynamic VISCOSITY and POISE.

PAS 1. para-aminosalicylic acid; see aminosalicylic ACID. 2. Professional Activity Study; see under STUDY.

PASA para-aminosalicylic acid; see aminosalicylic ACID.

Pasara trademark for *calcium aminosalicylate* (see under AMINO-SALICYLATE).

pascal (pas'kahl) [named after Blaise *Pascal*] the SI unit of pressure, being equal to the pressure exerted by 1 newton evenly distributed over an area of 1 m². Abbreviated *Pa*. See also SI.

Pascal's law [Blaise *Pascal*, French scientist, 1623–1662] see under LAW.

Passavant's bar (cushion, pad, ridge) [Philip Gustav *Passavant*, German surgeon, 1815–1893] see under BAR.

passer (pas'er) one who or that which transfers or conveys something from one place to another. **foil p.**, a pointed or forked instrument used to carry pellets of gold foil through an annealing flame or from the annealing tray to the prepared cavity for compaction. Called also *foil carrier*.

passivate (pas'ĭ-vāt) to render the surface of a metal less reactive chemically.

passive (pas'iv) [L. *passivus*] neither spontaneous or active; not produced by active efforts.

passivity (pas-siv'ĭ-te) in dentistry, the condition of rest assumed by the teeth, surrounding tissue, and denture when a removable partial denture is in place but not under masticatory pressure.

Passow's syndrome [A. *Passow*] see under SYNDROME.

paste (pāst) [L. *pasta*] a semisolid preparation, generally for external use, of a fatty base, a viscous or mucilaginous base, or a mixture of starch and petrolatum. **Abbot's p.**, a paste made of arsenic trioxide, morphine, and creosote; formerly used to devitalize the dental pulp. **base p.**, a paste containing substances, such as polysulfide, silicone, or polyether, which upon mixing with an appropriate reactor, will form a polymer. See also impression MATERIAL. **Caulk impression p.**, trademark for a hard zinc oxide–eugenol impression paste. **Coe-Pak p.**, trademark for two types of antiseptic and astringent preparations. *Paste 1* contains 45 percent zinc oxide, 32 percent magnesium oxide, 11 percent peanut oil, 6 percent mineral oil, 3 percent rosin, and other components and is bacteriostatic in small quantities. *Paste 2* contains 53 percent polymerized rosin, 30 percent coconut fatty acid, 4 percent ethyl cellulose and lanolin, 3 percent Peru balsam, 3 percent chloroethymol, and other formulating agents. **denture p.**, a mechanical denture cleanser, consisting of an abrasive powder combined with a dilute acid, used for brushing dentures. **denture adherent p.**, see denture ADHESIVE. **filler p.**, a paste used for filling the root canal system, as opposed to the use of solid filling materials, such as silver or gutta-percha cones and sealer cements. **Kerr equalizing p.**, trademark for a hard *zinc oxide–eugenol impression paste*. **Lassar's p's**, see ZINC oxide. **metallic oxide p.**, a paste containing metallic oxides, usually zinc oxide, commonly used as an impression material or to be placed over oral tissues after extraction or periodontal surgery to aid in retention of medicines and to promote healing. Most metallic pastes are produced by mixing zinc oxide and eugenol and allowing them to set. Noneugenol pastes exclude eugenol to avoid soft tissue irritation and use instead aliphatic carboxylic acids. **Multi-Form dual purpose impression p.**, trademark for a soft *zinc oxide–eugenol impression paste*. **noneugenol p.**, see *metallic oxide p.* **Orabase oral protective p.**, trademark for a protective ointment, 100 gm of which contains 16.75 gm sodium carboxymethylcellulose, 16.75 gm pectin, 16.75 gm gelatin, and an ointment base consisting of 5.0 gm polyethylene resin and 95.0 gm mineral oil. Used as a protective coating or as a vehicle for substances applied topically to the moist surfaces of the mucous membrane of the oral cavity and gingivae. **pressure-indicating p.**, a soft mixture used to disclose areas of contact or pressure in dentures. **pumice p.**, a paste made of ground pumice mixed with water or an antiseptic solution; used as a dental abrasive and polishing agent. See PUMICE. **tooth p.**, see DENTIFRICE. **Wachs p.**, a zinc oxide–eugenol root canal sealer. **zinc oxide p's**, see ZINC oxide. **zinc oxide–eugenol p.**, a metallic oxide paste produced by commercially prepared pastes of zinc oxide and eugenol. Upon setting, the mixture forms a paste consisting mainly of unreacted zinc oxide embedded in a matrix of zinc eugenolate crystals with excess eugenol probably absorbed by the zinc oxide and zinc eugenolate. The exact formulation of the ingredients is unknown but it is believed to consist of 85 percent zinc oxide and 15 percent rosin and a liquid to consist of 60 percent oil of cloves, 35 percent Canada balsam and 5 percent balsam of Peru. The paste is used as an impression material for edentulous mouths and as a reline impression material for dentures. Also placed over oral tissues after extractions and periodontal surgery to aid in retention of medicines and to promote healing. **zinc oxide–eugenol impression p.**, ZOE

impression p., a paste consisting mainly of zinc oxide, eugenol, and rosin with various additives, such as oil of cloves, Canada balsam, balsam of Peru, gum silica filler, lanolin, and other substances incorporated as needed, which upon mixing sets into a hard mass, being essentially a matrix of zinc eugenolate crystals in which unreacted zinc oxide is embedded. Some formulations substitute eugenol for the higher aliphatic carboxylic acids. Zinc salts, such as zinc acetate, are the principal accelerators. Used chiefly as corrective washes, veneer impressions, temporary liners or stabilizers in dentures and occlusion rims, for recording jaw relations, and for cementing gnathological clutches. Trademarks: Caulk Impression P., Coe-Flo, Kerr Equalizing P., Kerr Luralite, Krex P., Plastopaste, Superpaste.

Pasteur, Louis [1822–1895] a French chemist and bacteriologist, whose research led to the development of the germ theory of disease upon which the science of microbiology is based. Pasteur coined the term "vaccine" in honor of Edward Jenner's contribution toward the development of cowpox (vaccinia) vaccine, and he was responsible for the development of the technique of vaccination by attenuated and killed microorganisms.

Pasteurella (pas"te-rel-ah) [named after Louis *Pasteur*] a genus of gram-negative, facultatively anaerobic bacteria of uncertain affiliation, occurring as nonmotile ovoid or rod-shaped cells, about 1.4 by 0.4 μm in size, found singly or in pairs or short chains, which are parasitic in mammals, including man, and birds. The members are catalase positive, frequently oxidase positive, and gelatinase negative. **P. chol'erae-gallina'rum**, *P. multocida*. **P. coag'ulans**, *Bacteroides coagulans;* see under BACTEROIDES. **P. haemolyt'ica**, a species found in enzootic pneumonia of sheep and in septicemia of lambs. **P. multo'cida**, a species occurring as coccobacilli or short rods in cultures from diseased tissues or as pleomorphic forms from healthy animals, with longer bacillary forms and occasional short filaments. Found in a wide variety of pathological conditions in animals, including ruminants, cats, dogs, fowl, and swine; pathological conditions include hemorrhagic septicemia of ruminants, respiratory diseases, turkey cholera, etc. Human pasteurellosis most commonly takes the form of a wound infection, frequently following an animal bite or scratch, with localized swelling, abscesses, bronchiectasis, pneumonia, meningitis, and septicemia being the common symptoms. The organisms are sensitive to penicillin. Called also *P. cholerae-gallinarum, P. septica, Bacillus polaris septicus, Bacterium bipolare multocidum,* and *B. multocidum.* **P. novi'cida**, *Francisella novicida;* see under FRANCISELLA. **P. parahaemolyt'ica**, *Vibrio parahaemolyticus;* see under VIBRIO. **P. pes'tis**, *Yersinia pestis;* see under YERSINIA. **P. pneumotro'pica**, a species occurring as rods, about 1.2 by 0.5 μm in size, with occasional longer forms, sometimes found in the human respiratory tract and in infections caused by dog bites. It is a cause of enzootic diseases of mice, rabbits, and other laboratory animals, resulting in abscesses and respiratory diseases, and is frequently present in the nasal cavity of laboratory animals. **P. pseudotuberculo'sis**, *Yersinia pseudotuberculosis;* see under YERSINIA. **P. sep'tica**, *P. multocida.* **P. tularen'sis**, *Francisella tularensis;* see FRANCISELLA. **P. ure'ae**, a species occurring as rod-shaped or pleomorphic cells, found in the nasal cavity of healthy persons, sometimes causing ozena and other infections.

pasteurellosis (pas"ter-ĕ-lo'sis) infection with microorganisms of the genus *Pasteurella.*

pasteurization (pas"ter-i-za'shun) [Louis *Pasteur*] the process of heating milk or other liquids to a moderate temperature for a definite time, often to 60°C for 30 minutes. This exposure kills most species of pathogenic bacteria and considerably delays other bacterial development.

pat paternal origin. See also CHROMOSOME nomenclature.

Patau's syndrome [Klaus *Patau*] see under SYNDROME.

patch (pach) [L. *pittacium;* Gr. *pittakion*] an area differing from the rest of the surface, in either color or texture, or both; the aggregation of several isolated or confluent lesions. **mucous p.**, a flat, rounded, grayish white, slightly raised erosion covered by a soggy membrane with an erythematous halo, occurring most often on the oral mucosa, and sometimes on the anal and genital mucosa, in secondary syphilis. It contains vast numbers of treponemata and therefore is highly infectious. **Peyer's p.**, an oval elevated area of lymphoid tissue on the mucosa of the small intestine. **smokers' p's**, STOMATITIS nicotina.

patency (pa'ten-se) [L. *patens* open] the condition of being wide open.

patent (pa'tent) [L. *patens*] 1. open, unobstructed, or not closed. 2. apparent; evident.

Paterson and Brown Kelly syndrome [Donald Rose PATERSON, Welsh laryngologist, 1863–1939; Adam *Brown Kelly,* 1865–1941] Plummer-Vinson SYNDROME.

Paterson-Kelly syndrome, webs [D. R. Paterson; A. B. *Kelly*] Plummer-Vinson SYNDROME.

path (path) 1. a particular course that is followed, or a route that is ordinarily traversed. 2. a set of nerve fibers along which a nervous impulse may move. **centric p. of closure,** the path traversed by the mandible during closure when its associated neuromuscular mechanisms are in a balanced state of tonus, usually resulting in a hinge movement of the mandible during closure. **condyle p.,** the course followed by the mandibular condyle during the various movements of the mandible. **condyle p., lateral,** the path of the condyle in the glenoid fossa when lateral movements of the mandible are made. **condyle p., protrusive,** the path of the condyle when the mandible is moved forward from its centric position. **generated occlusal p.,** occlusal p., generated. **idling p.,** the path that a stamp cusp travels when the bolus is being treated on the other side of the mouth. See also *working p.* **incisor p.,** the course followed by the incisal edges of the lower anterior teeth in movement of the mandible from the position of normal occlusion to that of edge-to-edge contact with opposing incisors. **p. of insertion,** that direction or path of the removable partial denture that permits the proper relation of the prosthesis to the hard and soft tissues on insertion, on removal, in function, and at rest. Called also *p. of removal.* **ionization p.,** the trail of ion pairs produced by ionizing radiation in its passage through matter. Called also *ionization track.* **lateral condyle p.,** condyle p., lateral. **mean free p.,** in nuclear physics, the average distance a particle travels between collisions. **occlusal p.,** the course followed by the occlusal surfaces of the lower teeth in movements of the mandible. **milled-in p.,** 1. the contour carved by various mandibular movements into the occluding surface of an occlusion rim by teeth or studs placed in the opposing occlusion rim. The curves or contour may be carved into wax, modeling plastic, or plaster of Paris. Called also *milled-in curve* and *milled-in occlusion.* 2. gliding movements of occlusion rims which are composed of materials, including abrasives. **occlusal p., generated,** a registration of the paths of movement of the occlusal surfaces of mandibular teeth on a plastic or abrasive surface attached to the maxillary arch. **p. of placement,** a seldom used term referring to the direction in which a restoration moves from the point of initial contact of its rigid parts with the supporting teeth to the terminal resting position, with rests seated and the denture base in contact with the tissue. See also *p. of insertion.* **p. of removal,** see *p. of insertion.* **working p.,** the path that the stamp cusps make when working on the bolus, deflecting it at first in the direction of the cusps and, after the fibrous contents have been reduced to the point of being ready for swallowing, traveling along with the working grooves. See also *idling p.*

pathfinder (path'find-er) root canal PROBE.

patho- [Gr. *pathos* disease] a combining form denoting relationship to disease. See also words beginning NOSO-.

pathoanatomy (path"o-ah-nat'o-me) morbid ANATOMY.

Pathocil trademark for *dicloxacillin sodium* (see under DICLOXACILLIN).

pathodontia (path"o-don'she-ah) dental PATHOLOGY.

pathogen (path"o-jen) [*patho-* + Gr. *gennan* to produce] any disease-producing microorganism or material.

pathogenesis (path"o-jen'ĕ-sis) [*patho-* + *genesis*] the development of morbid conditions or of disease. See also ETIOLOGY.

pathogenic (path-o-jen'ik) giving origin to disease or to morbid conditions. Called also *nosogenic.*

pathogenicity (path"o-jĕ-nis'ĭ-te) the quality of producing or the ability to produce pathologic changes or disease.

pathognomonic (path"og-no-mon'ik) [*patho-* + Gr. *gnōmonikos* fit to give judgment] specifically distinctive or characteristic of a disease or pathologic condition; a sign or symptom on which a diagnosis can be made.

pathognomy (path-og'no-me) [*patho-* + Gr. *gnōmē* a means of knowing] the science of signs and symptoms of disease.

pathologic (path"o-loj'ik) indicative of or caused by a morbid condition.

pathologist (pah-thol'o-jist) an expert in pathology.

pathology (pah-thol'o-je) [*patho-* + *-logy*] that branch of medicine which treats the essential nature of disease, especially of the structural and functional changes in cells, tissues, and organs of the body which cause or are caused by disease. **cellular p.,** that which regards the cells as starting points of the phenomena of disease and that every cell descends from some preexisting cell. See also cell THEORY and HISTOPATHOLOGY. **comparative p.,** that which institutes comparison between various diseases of the human body and those of the lower animals. **clinical p.,** pathology applied to the solution of clinical problems, especially the use of laboratory methods in clinical diagnosis. **dental p.,** the branch of pathology which treats dental changes in disease. Called also *pathodontia.* See also *oral p.* **experimental p.,** the study of artificially induced disease processes. **general p.,** that which takes cognizance of pathologic conditions which may occur in various diseases and in different organs. **geographical p.,** pathology in its geographic and climatic relations. **internal p.,** medical p. **medical p.,** that which relates to morbid processes which are not accessible to operative intervention. Called also *internal p.* **oral p.,** the branch of pathology which treats the structural and functional changes in cells, tissues, and organs of the body that cause or are caused by disease. See also *dental p.* **speech p.,** the study and treatment of functional and organic speech defects and disorders. **surgical p.,** the pathology of disease processes which are surgically accessible for diagnosis or treatment. See also BIOPSY.

pathomimia (path"o-mim'e-ah) malingering. **p. muco'sae o'ris,** cheek BITING.

patho-occlusion (path"o-o-kloo'zhun) a former name for pathologic occlusion. See MALOCCLUSION.

pathosis (pah-tho'sis) [*patho-* + *-osis*] a pathological or morbid condition; a disease.

pathway (path'wa) a path or course, especially a course followed in the attainment of a specific end. In neurology, the nerve structures through which a sensory impression is conducted to the cerebral cortex, or through which an impulse passes from the brain to the skeletal musculature or other organ. **activation p.,** see *complement activation p.* **alternative p.,** see *complement activation p., alternative.* **classical p.,** see *complement activation p., classical.* **complement activation p., alternative,** a pathway of complement activation that is not fully understood. It is initiated by agents, such as bacterial endotoxins, zymosan, and inulin, which bypass the C1, C4, C2 steps of the complement sequence, probably in the absence of specific antibody, and may also be activated by myeloma IgA and IgG.

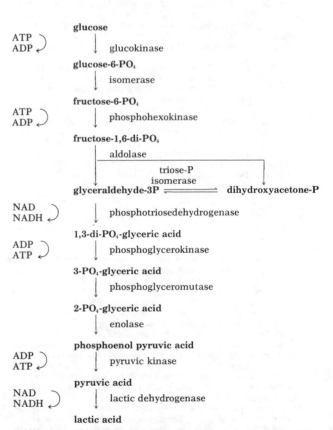

Embden-Meyerhof Pathway. (Adapted from J. I. Routh, D. P. Eyman, and D. J. Burton: Essentials of General, Organic and Biochemistry. 3rd ed. Philadelphia, W. B. Saunders Co., 1977.)

The critical function of the pathway is the generation of C3 convertase, which activates the C3 molecule. At least four factors are involved in the activation of the alternative pathway: *factor B* (C3 proactivator, C3PA), which is activated by factor $\bar{D}$; *factor $\bar{D}$* (C3 proactivator convertase, C3PA convertase), which cleaves factor B into two fragments; *initiating factor* (IF), believed to initiate the reaction that generates the formation of an active convertase, C3b,$\bar{B}$, which can form new C3b molecules from C3 or act as a convertase for C5; and *properdin,* which exerts a stabilizing effect on C5 convertase (C3b,$\bar{B}$) and produces a stable C5 convertase (C3b$\bar{B}$P). With cleavage of C5 to C5b + C5a, the pathway continues in a fashion similar to that of the classical pathway. Called also *properdin p.* See also COMPLEMENT. **complement activation p., classical,** a pathway of complement activation that is triggered by the interaction of IgM or IgG with specific antigen. The interaction results in a conformational change on the Fc fragment of the immunoglobulin molecule. The mechanism is illustrated by the hemolytic action of complement (C) on the red blood cell (E) surface after it has been sensitized with antibody (A). The nine complement components or groups (C1 through C9) are divided into three units: recognition unit, C1; activation unit, C4, C2, C3; and membrane unit, C5, C6, C7, C8, C9. The sequence proceeds as follows:

$$EA + C \xrightarrow[Ca^{++}]{} EA\overline{C1} \ (C1 \text{ esterase activity activates C4 and C2})$$

$$EA\overline{C1} + C4 + C2 \rightarrow EA\overline{C1,4b,2a} \ (C3 \text{ convertase}) + C4a + C2b$$

$$EA\overline{C1,4b,2a,3b} + C5 + C6 + C7 \rightarrow EAC1,4b,2a,3b,5b,6,7 + C5a$$

$$EA\overline{1 \rightarrow 7} + C8 + C9 \ EA1 \rightarrow 9 - \text{lysis}$$

The structural damage resulting in lysis is first seen slowly with C8 but C9 accelerates the process. Depressions can be seen on the red cell surface at the site of lysis. See also COMPLEMENT. **Embden-Meyerhof p.,** a pathway of oxidative metabolism of carbohydrates; the anaerobic pathway of glycolysis from glucose to lactate. See illustration. See also Krebs CYCLE. **infection p.,** a pathway along which infection may spread, such as tissue spaces which provide natural pathways along which dental infection spreads to produce cellulitis. See also tissue spaces, under SPACE. **pentose p.,** phosphogluconate p. **phosphogluconate p.,** an alternate pathway of carbohydrate oxidation, in which glucose-6-phosphate is oxidized, through a series of reactions, to glyceraldehyde-3-phosphate and fructose-6-phosphate. The primary purpose of the pathway in most cells is to generate reducing power in the cytoplasm in the form of NADPH. The pentoses that are formed, especially ribose, are used in the synthesis of nucleic acids, whereas the glyceral-

dehyde and fructose phosphates enter the Embden-Meyerhof pathway. Called also *pentose p., Warburg-Dickens-Lipman p., hexose monophosphate shunt, oxidative shunt,* and *pentose shunt.* See illustration. **properdin p.,** complement activation p., alternative. **Warburg-Dickens-Lipman p.,** phosphogluconate p.

-pathy [Gr. *pathos* disease] a work termination denoting a morbid condition or disease.

patient (pa'shent) [L. *patiens*] a person who is ill or who is undergoing treatment. In dental practice, an individual who has established a professional and legally binding relationship with a dentist for the delivery of dental health care, after the dentist has accepted the person as the patient. See also ACCEPTANCE. **emergency p.,** an acutely ill or injured person who requires immediate care and special diagnostic and therapeutic services. **hospital p.,** a person who has been admitted to a hospital for treatment or diagnosis. See also INPATIENT and OUTPATIENT.

pattern (pat'ern) a form or model designed as a guide for imitation or copying. **investing the p.,** INVESTING the pattern. **occlusal p.,** the form or design of the occluding surfaces of a tooth or teeth; these forms may be based on natural or modified anatomic or nonanatomic concepts of teeth. **trabecular p.,** the trabecular arrangement of the alveolar bone in relation to the marrow spaces. **wax p.,** a pattern made from a casting wax, being a reproduction of a missing tooth structure or a dental appliance, from which the outline of the mold is made for the casting of a restoration or an appliance. In the casting of an inlay or crown, the cavity is prepared in the tooth and the pattern is carved, either directly in the tooth or on the die which is a reproduction of the tooth and the prepared cavity. See also direct IMPRESSION and indirect IMPRESSION. **wear p.,** the topographic distribution of tooth wear due to masticatory activity and oral habits.

Paul's test [Gustav *Paul,* Austrian physician, 1859–1935] see under TEST.

Pautrier, Lucien M. [French dermatologist, 1876–1959] see median rhomboid GLOSSITIS (Brocq-Pautrier glossitis or syndrome).

Paveril trademark for *dimoxyline.*

Pavlov's reflex [Ivan Petrovich *Pavlov,* Russian physiologist, 1849–1936; winner of the Nobel prize for medicine and physiology in 1904] conditioned REFLEX.

Pavulon trademark for *pancuronium bromide* (see under PANCURONIUM.)

payer (pa'er) one who pays. **primary p.,** an insurer who is obligated to pay prior to any liability of other, secondary insurers. Under law, Medicare is a primary payer with respect to Medicaid to persons eligible under both programs. Called also *primary insurer.* See also coordination of benefits CLAUSE.

The Phosphogluconate Pathway

Phosphogluconate pathway. (From J. I. Routh, D. P. Eyman, and D. J. Burton: Essentials of General, Organic and Biochemistry. 3rd ed. Philadelphia, W. B. Saunders Co., 1977.)

third party p., the agency that pays for services provided by the carrier (second party) to the beneficiary (first party) under a specific reimbursement formula.

payment (pa'ment) a monetary compensation; that which is paid. **claim p.,** payment made directly either to the insured as a reimbursement for an expenditure covered under terms of the insurance plan or to the dentist for services rendered under the contract. **progress p.,** in health insurance, interim payment by the purchaser to the carrier for use as an operating fund. **third party p.,** see third party PAYER.

Pb lead.

PBZ trademark for *tripelennamine.*

P.C. abbreviation for *pon'dus civi'le,* avoirdupois weight (see under WEIGHT).

pc picocurie.

p.c. abbreviation for L. *post ci'bum,* after meals.

PCA passive cutaneous ANAPHYLAXIS.

pcf pounds per cubic feet; see specific WEIGHT.

pCi picocurie.

Pcs preconscious.

PCV packed-cell VOLUME.

Pd palladium.

PDI periodontal disease INDEX.

PDR Physicians' Desk Reference; see under REFERENCE.

Peak see under DENTIFRICE.

peak (pēk) the top or upper limit of a graphic tracing or of any variable. **kilovolt p.,** the maximum electrical pressure or electromotive force, or the peak of the voltage curve. In radiology, maximum electrical energy used in an x-ray exposure. Abbreviated *kvp.*

Peale, Charles W. [1741–1827] an American dentist who was the first to make porcelain teeth. He also developed a process for incorporating platinum in porcelain.

pearl (perl) 1. a small calcareous concretion from various species of mollusks. 2. a small medicated granule. **p. ash,** POTASSIUM carbonate. **Bohn's p's,** Bohn's nodules; see under NODULE. **enamel p.,** enameloma. **epidermal p's,** rounded concentric masses of epithelial cells found in certain papillomas and epitheliomas. Called also *epithelial p's* and *pearly bodies.* **epithelial p's,** 1. epidermic p's. 2. Serres' GLAND. **Epstein's p's,** multiple, firm, white, or grayish white inclusion cysts on the palatal or alveolar mucosa of newborn infants, found along the midpalatine raphe, considered to be remnants of epithelial tissue trapped along the raphe during fetal development. They are small keratin-containing lesions lined by stratified squamous epithelium, which are usually shed within a few weeks of life. Called also *Epstein's disease.* **P. Drops,** see under DENTIFRICE.

pearlite (per'līt) the two-phase mixture of ferrite and cementite which is formed from the decomposition of austenite at 0.8 percent carbon content (eutectoid composition); so named because of the characteristic mother-of-pearl appearance of the microstructure. See also SPHEROIDITE.

pecazine (pe'kah-zēn) mepazine.

Pecquet, duct of [Jean *Pecquet,* French anatomist, 1622–1674] thoracic DUCT.

pectin (pek'tin) a polysaccharide in the cell walls of all plants, in which it functions as an intercellular cementing substance. It consists of a mixture of methyl esterified galacturonan, galactan, and araban (molecular weight 20,000 to 400,000), and occurs as a white, coarse, odorless powder with a mucilaginous taste, which is soluble in water. Used as a food preservative and protectant. **p. sugar,** arabinose.

pedes (pe'dēz) [L.] plural of *pes.*

pedia- [Gr. *pais, paidos* child] a combining form denoting relationship to a child. See also PEDO-(1).

Pediamycin trademark for *erythromycin ethylsuccinate* (see under ERYTHROMYCIN).

pediatrics (pe"de-at'riks) [*pedia-* + Gr. *iatrikē* surgery, medicine] that branch of medicine which treats of the child and its development and care and of the diseases of children and their treatment.

pedicle (ped'ĭ-k'l) [L. *pediculus,* dim. of *pes* foot] 1. any slender stalk; a peduncle. 2. the constricted portion of a nonsessile tumor which serves as a stem to connect it to the body. 3. a slender tubed stalk connecting a graft to the body. See also pedicle FLAP.

pedigree (ped'ĭ-gre) [L. *pedis* foot + *de* of + *grūs* crane] a list for tracing ancestry, used in human genetics in the analysis of mendelian inheritance. See also CHARACTER and INHERITANCE, and see illustration.

□	Male	■ ●	Heterozygotes for autosomal recessive
○	Female	⊙	Carrier of X –linked recessive
□—○	Mating	⬚	Death
	Parents and Children 1 boy 1girl (in order of birth)	↓	Abortion or stillbirth sex unspecified
△○	Dizygotic twins	↗■	Propositus
△	Monozygotic twins		Method of identifying persons in a pedigree
◇	Sex unspecified		Here the propositus is Child 2 in Generation II
◢ ③	Number of children of sex indicated		
■ ●	Affected individuals	□—○	Consanguineous marriage

Symbols commonly used in pedigree charts. (From J. S. Thompson and M. W. Thompson: Genetics in Medicine. 3rd ed. Philadelphia, W. B. Saunders Co., 1980.)

Pediococcus (pe"de-o-kok'us) [Gr. *pedium* a plane surface + L. *coccus* berry] a genus of gram-positive, nonmotile, nonsporogenic, coccoid bacteria of the family Streptococcaceae, found in fermenting plant material, especially in spoiled beer, and rarely in milk and dairy products. **P. hom'ari,** *Aerococcus viridans;* see under AEROCOCCUS.

pedo- 1. [Gr. *pais, paidos* child] a combining form denoting relationship to a child. See also PEDIA-. 2. [L. *pes, pedis* foot] a combining form denoting relationship to the foot.

pedodontia (pe"do-don"she-ah) pedodontics.

pedodontics (pe"do-don'tiks) [*pedo-*(1) + Gr. *odous* tooth] the division of dentistry concerned with the diagnosis and treatment of conditions of the teeth and mouth in children, including restoring and maintaining the primary, mixed, and permanent dentition; applying preventive measures for dental caries and periodontal disease; preventing, intercepting, and correcting occlusal problems; and training the child to accept dental care. Called also *dentistry for children, pediatric dentistry,* and *pedodontia.*

pedodontist (pe"do-don'tist) a dentist who specializes in pedodontics.

peduncle (pe-dung'k'l) [L. *pedunculus*] a narrow structure which connects a smaller part to a main body; a stalk; a stem. See also PEDUNCULUS.

pedunculated (pĕ-dung'ku-lāt"ed) having a peduncle; opposed to sessile, or attached on a broad base.

pedunculus (pe-dung'ku-lus) [L.] peduncle; an anatomical term for collections of nerve fibers coursing between different areas in the central nervous system.

peer (pēr) a person who is equal to another in rank, ability, education, experience, or qualifications. **p. review,** peer REVIEW.

Peeso pliers [F. A. *Peeso,* American dentist, 1858–1928] see under PLIERS.

PEG polyethylene GLYCOL.

peg (peg) a projecting structure. **epithelial p.,** a basal cell occasionally growing down into the connective tissue and forming a finger-like peg, which is separated by conical masses of loose connective tissue, the papillae. **rete p's,** the invaginations of the epidermis into the dermis at the dermatoepidermal junction; the invaginations of the epithelium into the adjacent connective tissue.

Peganone trademark for *ethotoin.*

Peiffer, Jurgen see metachromatic LEUKODYSTROPHY (van Bogaert-Nyssen-Peiffer syndrome).

pelentan. (pĕ-len'tan) ETHYL biscoumacetate.

Pelger-Huët anomaly [Karel *Pelger,* Dutch physician, 1885–1931; G. J. *Huët*] see under ANOMALY; see also pseudo-Pelger-Huët ANOMALY.

pelidisi (pel"ĭ-de'se) [a term coined from L. *pondus decies linearis divisus sidentis (altitudo)* meaning weight ten line divided sitting height] the unit of Pirquet's index for determining the nutritive condition of children. It is obtained by dividing the cube root of 10 times the weight (in grams) by the sitting height (in centimeters). A pelidisi of 94 or less indicates undernutrition; of 95 to 100, good nutrition, and of 101 or above, overnutrition.

pelidnoma (pel″id-no′mah) [Gr. *pelidnōma* a livid spot] a discolored spot or patch on the skin.

pellagra (pel-lag′rah, pel-la′grah) [It. *pelle* skin + *agra* rough] a syndrome caused by nicotinic acid deficiency, characterized by dermatitis, diarrhea, and dementia. Dermatitis occurs symmetrically in any region, but most commonly in areas of exposure to sunlight. Initial redness and thickening of the skin are followed by hyperkeratosis and scaling, vascularization, inflammation, edema, and, eventually, desquamation. Areas of depigmentation and increased pigmentation may occur; subcutaneous fibrosis and scarring may be found in chronic cases; and mucous membranes also may become involved. Diarrhea is presumed to be due to atrophy of the columnar epithelium of the gastrointestinal tract mucosa, followed by submucosal inflammation, which may lead to ulceration. Dementia is usually based upon degeneration of the ganglion cells of the brain, associated with degeneration of the tracts of the spinal cord. Microcytic anemia is sometimes associated. Oral changes consist of burning sensation of the tongue, which becomes swollen and pressed against the teeth, causing indentations; its tip and lateral margins become red. A fiery red color and pain of the oral mucosa, giving the mouth a sensation as though it had been scalded, characterize advanced stages. Tenderness and ulcers, usually beginning at the interdental gingival papillae, and spreading to other parts of the mouth, are usually present. See also *oculo-orogenital* SYNDROME.

pellet (pel′et) 1. a small rounded mass of material. 2. a small pill or granule, such as a small mass of steroid hormone, to be implanted under the skin to provide for its slow absorption. **cotton p.,** a rolled ball of cotton about ⅛ to ⅜ inch in diameter, used for the topical application of medicinal preparations. Larger spheres of cotton are referred to as *balls*; those of smaller size are known as *pledgets*. **foil p.,** FOIL pellet. **foil p., gold foil p.,** a loosely rolled piece of gold foil; used as a direct filling material in dental restoration. See also gold FOIL.

pellicle (pel′i-k'l) [L. *pellicula*] 1. a delicate cuticle or film. 2. a thin layer or film on the surface of a liquid. **acquired p.,** an acellular, bacteria-free film which is deposited on the teeth after eruption. Microscopically, it is made up of three layers: the subsurface layer, which is basically dendritic in appearance and fills the pores or demineralized areas of enamel; the surface layer, which is normally less than 1 μ in thickness; and the suprasurface layer, which is up to 10 μ in thickness, and is located under plaque and in areas not accessible to brushing. The subsurface and surface layers are believed to be formed by salivary glycoproteins and the suprasurface layer by salivary glycoproteins, as well as by bacterial debris and dead epithelial cells. When removed from the teeth, the pellicle reappears within 20 minutes. Called also *acquired cuticle*. **brown p.,** a brownish gray to black film formed over a period of time on the surface of the teeth, resulting from poor hygiene and brushing habits. See also PLAQUE.

pellicular, pelliculous (pel-lik′u-lar; pel-lik′u-lus) characterized by or pertaining to a pellicle.

pellucid (pel-lu′sid) [L. *pellucidus*, from *per* through + *lucere* to shine] translucent.

pelo- [Gr. *pelos* mud] a combining form denoting relationship to mud.

Pelson trademark for *nitrazepam.*

Peltz antigen (factor) [named after the person in whom Peltz antigen (Ku antigen) was first discovered] see Ku ANTIGEN, and see Kell blood groups, under BLOOD GROUP.

pelvis (pel′vis), pl. *pel′ves* [L.; Gr. *pyelos* an oblong trough] 1. [NA] the lower portion of the trunk of the body, bounded anteriorly and laterally by the two hip bones and posteriorly by the sacrum and coccyx. 2. renal p. **renal p., p. rena′lis** [NA], the expansion from the upper end of the ureter into which the calices open.

Pemal trademark for *ethosuximide.*

pemphigoid (pem′fi-goid) [Gr. *pemphix* blister + *eidos* form] 1. resembling pemphigus. 2. a chronic, generalized, bullous skin eruption characterized by bullae beneath the intact epidermis in the absence of acantholysis. 3. bullous p. **benign mucosal p.,** a chronic bullous disease of elderly persons, involving primarily the conjunctival and oral mucous membranes, with scarring. Associated lesions of the face, neck, scalp, legs, and genitalia are seen in about half of the cases. Entropion with secondary blindness, and synechiae of the palpebral and bulbar conjunctivae are common. The bullae of the oral mucosa, most commonly affecting the gingivae and edentulous ridges, develop from vesicles about 3 to 6 mm in diameter, which rupture and coalesce, leaving shallow ulcers, and, eventually, mild scarring. Histologically, the lesions are similar to those seen in erythema multiforme, with subepithelial bullae and late fibrosis. Called also *cicatricial pemphigoid, Lortat-Jacob's disease,*

and *mucosynechial dermatitis.* **bullous p.,** a chronic, generalized, bullous skin eruption, suspected of having an autoimmune etiology, usually occurring in elderly patients, with or without oral lesions. The lesions resemble those seen in pemphigus vulgaris, with erythematous patches and large, tense, nongrouped bullae beneath the epidermis in the absence of acantholysis. Pruritus is common but the general health is seldom affected and the eruption disappears within a few months, sometimes, years. Oral lesions, when present, consist of small vesicles similar to those seen in erythema multiforme bullosum. Called also *benign pemphigus.* **cicatricial p.,** benign mucosal p.

pemphigus (pem′fi-gus) [Gr. *pemphix* blister] 1. any of a group of acute or chronic diseases of unknown etiology, occurring in several phases and sometimes accompanied by constitutional symptoms. They are characterized by the presence of bullae developing in cycles or in continuous succession on the skin and mucous membranes, acantholysis, and intracellular antiepithelial antibodies. **benign p.,** bullous PEMPHIGOID. **chronic malignant p.,** p. vulgaris. **p. erythemato′sus,** an eruption of bullous crusted lesions, usually on the face and chest. On the face, they may occur in the "butterfly" distribution similar to that seen in seborrheic dermatitis and lupus erythematosus. Histologically, it is classified with the permphigus group because of the presence of acantholysis. Pemphigus vulgaris usually develops. Oral lesions are rare, but when present they usually appear with the development of pemphigus vulgaris. The course is slow and remissions are common. Called also *seborrheic p.* and *Senear-Usher syndrome.* **p. folia′ceus,** a chronic form of symmetrical pemphigus in adults, in which flaccid bullae characterize the early phases and generalized exfoliation predominates in the later stages. The bullae are slightly elevated and rupture readily, discharging malodorous fluid, revealing a reddish or purplish moist surface beneath. The lesions spread slowly and symmetrically and, within a few months, the entire body may be covered with exfoliative lesions. The hair and nails are commonly lost. Nikolsky's sign and acantholysis are always present. Oral lesions are rare. Called also *Cazenave's disease.* **p. papilla′ris,** p. vegetans. **seborrheic p.,** p. erythematosus. **p. veg′etans,** a variant of pemphigus vulgaris in which many of the bullous lesions are replaced by malodorous, verrucoid hypertrophic vegetative masses, which are usually found on the skin and not on the mucous membranes, except for the vermilion border of the lips. The initial stages are similar to those in pemphigus vulgaris but the denuded ulcerative areas become hypertrophied and are characterized by the presence of vegetative granulation tissue. The lesions may further become dry and verrucous. Secondary bacterial infection is always present. Called also *p. papillaris, condylomatosis pemphigoides maligna, erythema bullosum vegetans,* and *Neumann's disease.* See also DERMATITIS vegetans. **p. vulga′ris,** a rare relapsing form of pemphigus, most often affecting adults of Jewish extraction. The oral and vaginal mucosae are the first sites involved, from where lesions spread to other parts. Lesions are initially tense, later, flaccid bullae of various sizes, which rupture, leaving denuded erosion ulcers; they appear without prodromal symptoms or may be preceded by slight itching or burning, and are usually painful. Symptoms include Nikolsky's sign (separation of the epidermis upon drawing the finger over the surface of apparently normal skin), general malaise, leukocytosis, eosinophilia, increased sedimentation rate (in advanced cases), anemia, and lowered serum protein levels. Secondary bacterial infection of the bullae and ulcers produces a characteristic odor, and leads to septicemia; death is common in untreated cases. Histologically, lesions show disruption of the intercellular connections of the epidermis (acantholysis). The acantholytic cells have rounded, sharply defined, deeply stained cytoplasm and round, swollen, and hyperchromic nuclei. Called also *chronic malignant p.*

Pen-A trademark for *ampicillin.*

Pen A/N trademark for *ampicillin sodium* (see under AMPICILLIN).

penatin (pen′ah-tin) glucose OXIDASE.

pencil (pen′sil) something shaped or used like a pencil. **dosimeter p.,** DOSIMETER pencil.

penetrability (pen″ĕ-trah-bil′ĭ-te) the ability of a beam of x-rays to penetrate matter, the degree of penetrability being determined by kilovoltage and filtration.

penetrance (pen′ĕ-trans) [L. *penetrare* to enter into] the ability of a genotype to be expressed in a phenotype, determined as a percentage; when less than 100 percent penetrance occurs, **the**

condition is known as *reduced penetrance*. When an individual who has a genotype which characteristically produces an abnormal phenotype but who is phenotypically normal, the trait is said to be *nonpenetrant*, or 0 percent. See also EXPRESSIVITY. **complete p.**, penetrance in which all the homozygous recessive traits show one phenotype, in which all the homozygous dominants show another phenotype, and in which all the heterozygotes are alike. **reduced p.**, see *penetrance*.

penetrant (pen′ĕ-trant) [L. *penetrare* to enter into] pertaining to penetrance, i.e., pertaining to a genotype which is phenotypically expressed.

penetration (pen″ĕ-tra′shun) [L. *penetratio*] 1. the act of piercing or entering deeply. 2. the act of piercing or entering a substance or tissue by x-rays. See also HARDNESS (3).

penetrometer (pen″ĕ-trom′ĕ-ter) an apparatus for measuring the penetrating power and intensity of x-rays, consisting of increments of an absorber through which a radiographic exposure is made on film, to permit determination of the amounts of radiation reaching the film by measuring film density. Called also *step-wedge*.

-penia [Gr. *penia* poverty, need] a word termination indicating an abnormal reduction in number of the element denoted by the root to which it is affixed, as leukopenia.

penicillin (pen″ĭ-sil′in) any of a family of natural or semisynthetic antibiotics obtained from cultures of the fungus *Penicillium*. The parent compound of penicillins is (2S-*cis*)-4-thia-1-azabicyclo[3,2,0]heptane-carboxylic acid; all being derivatives of penicillanic acid. They were the first antimicrobial substances isolated from cultures of fungi, thus originating the era of antibiotics. Penicillins have a broad spectrum of activity, inhibiting bacterial cell formation, being effective against strains of both gram-positive and gram-negative bacteria. In low concentrations, they are bacteriostatic; in high concentrations, they are bactericidal. Some bacteria develop resistance to penicillins and elaborate a penicillin-destroying enzyme, penicillinase. Penicillins are used in the treatment of infections due to gram-positive bacteria, chiefly staphylococcal, streptococcal, pneumococcal, and clostridial infections, and in diseases caused by gram-negative bacteria, particularly *Treponema* and *Meningococcus* infections. Also used in infections due to *Escherichia coli*, and in diphtheria, anthrax, Vincent's infection, actinomycosis, leptospirosis, rheumatic fever, and other infectious diseases. Their toxicity is relatively low, but allergic reactions, including anaphylaxis, may occur. Penicillin therapy often alters the bacterial and fungal flora. Blood coagulation disorders due to the suppression of enteric bacteria which synthesize vitamin K may also occur. Very high doses are neurotoxic. Topical application may cause dermatitis. Penicillins numbered with Roman numerals are alphabetized according to the Roman numeral. **allylmercapto-p.**, p. O. **American p.**, p. G sodium. **p. amido-β-lactamhydrolase**, see PENICILLINASE. **D-α-aminobenzyl p.**, ampicillin. **p. AT**, p. O. **p. B**, glucose OXIDASE. **benzathine G p.**, p. G benzathine. **benzathine p., V**, p. V benzathine. **benzethacil diamine p.**, p. G benzathine. **benzyl p.**, p. G. **biosynthetic p's**, semisynthetic p's. **p. BT**, a natural penicillin. Called also *butylmercaptomethylpenicillin* and *butylthiomethylpenicillin*. **butylmercaptomethyl p.**, p. BT. **butylthiomethyl p.**, p. BT. **calcium p. V**, p. V calcium. **3-o-chlorophenyl-5-methyl-4-isoxazolyl p.**, cloxacillin. **p. dihydro F.**, dihydropenicillin. **2,6-dimethoxyphenyl-p.**, methicillin. **dimethoxyphenyl p. sodium**, methicillin. **disodium carboxybenzyl-p.**, carbenicillin. **p. F.**, a natural penicillin, 2-pentenylpenicillin, which is less stable than penicillin G. Called also *p. I*. **p. G**, a natural penicillin, 3,3-dimethyl-7-oxo-6[(phenylacetyl)aminoi]-4-thia-1-azabicyclo[3,2,0] heptane-2-carboxylic acid. Used therapeutically in various salts; considered as a prototype for all penicillins. Called also *p. II* and *benzylpenicillin*. **p. G benzathine**, a semisynthetic penicillin consisting of penicillin G compounded with *N,N′*-dibenzylethylenediamine, occurring as an odorless white crystalline powder that is soluble in benzene, acetone, formamide, and alcohol and is slightly soluble in water. Its low water-solubility allows it to be released slowly when administered intramuscularly. Antibacterial and toxic properties are similar to those of other penicillins. Used chiefly in the treatment of infections due to penicillinase-producing bacteria. Called also *benzethacil diamine penicillin*. Trademarks: Beacillin, Bicillin, Cillenta, Tardocillin. **p. G hydrabamine**, a semisynthetic penicillin, *N,N′*-bis(dehydroabietyl)-ethylenediamine dipenicillin G. Trademark: Compocillin. **p. G potassium**, the monopotassium salt of penicillin G, occurring as odorless, colorless crystals or white crystalline powder, which is moderately hygroscopic and decomposes on prolonged exposure to heat and is soluble in water, dextrose solution, glycerol, and alcohols. It is a semisynthetic penicillin which is resistant to penicillinase and is, thus, used in the treatment of infections due to penicillinase-producing bacteria. Its pharmacological properties and toxicity are similar to those of other penicillins. Used chiefly in patients on sodium restricted diets. Prolonged use may lead to potassium intoxication. Called also *benzylpenicillin potassium* and *potassium benzylpenicillinate*. Trademarks: Eskacillin, Hyasorb, Notoral, Pentid. **p. G procaine**, a semisynthetic penicillin consisting of penicillin G compounded with 2-(diethylamino)ethyl-*p*-aminobenzoate, occurring as white crystals or white microcrystalline powder, which is practically odorless and dissolves in alcohol and chloroform and is slightly soluble in water. Its low solubility in water allows it to be absorbed very slowly when administered intramuscularly. Pharmacological properties and toxicity are similar to those of other penicillins. Called also *benzylpenicillin procaine* and *procaine benzylpenicillinate*. Trademarks: Afsillin, Aquacillin, Avloprocil, Crysticillin, Dorsalin, Premocillin. **p. G sodium**, the monosodium salt of penicillin G, occurring as colorless or white crystals or as a white or yellowish crystalline powder, which is odorless, decomposes on exposure to heat, and is soluble in water, isotonic sodium chloride or glucose solutions, alcohol, glycerol, and other alcohols. It is a semisynthetic penicillin which is resistant to penicillinase and is, thus, used in the treatment of infections due to penicillinase-producing bacteria. Its pharmacological properties and toxicity are similar to those of other penicillins. Massive doses or prolonged use may result in sodium intoxication with expanded extracellular spaces and edema. Called also *American p.*, *benzylpenicillin sodium*, and *sodium benzylpenicillinate*. Trademarks: Novocillin, Veticillin. **hydrabamine p. G**, p. G hydrabamine. **hydrabamine phenoxymethyl p., hydrabamine p. V**, p. V hydrabamine. **p. I**, p. F. **p. II**, p. G. **p. III**, p. X. **p. IV**, p. K. **p. K**, a natural penicillin, *n*-heptylpenicillin, being less stable than penicillin G, but having the same pharmacological properties. Called also *p. IV*. **p. MV**, phenethicillin. **p. N**, a broad-spectrum, penicillinase-resistant, water-soluble antibiotic elaborated by the fungi *Cephalosporium*, *Paecilomyces persicimus*, and *Penicillium chrysogenum*, 6-(D-5-amino-5-carboxyvaleramido)-3,3-dimethyl-7-oxo-4-thia-1-azabicyclo[3,2,0] heptane-2-carboxylic acid. It is active against both gram-positive and gram-negative microorganisms, including *Sarcina lutea*, *Proteus vulgaris*, *Salmonella typhimurium*, and *Streptococcus pneumoniae*. Called also *adicillin* and *cephalosporin N*. Trademark: Synnematin B. **natural p's**, penicillins obtained from unmodified cultures of the mold *Penicillium*; they include penicillin BT, F, G, K, O, and X, and dihydropenicillin F. See also *semisynthetic p*. **p. O**, a natural penicillin, 3,3-dimethyl-7-oxo-6[[(2-propenylthio)acetyl]amino]-4-thia-1-azabicyclo[3,2,0]-heptane-2-carboxylic acid. Called also *p. AT*, *allylmercaptopenicillin*, and *allylmercaptopenicillinic acid*. **p. O potassium**, the potassium salt of penicillin O. **p. 152**, phenethicillin. **phenoxymethyl p.**, phenethicillin. **potassium p. G**, p. G potassium. **potassium p. O**, p. O potassium. **p. potassium phenoxymethyl, potassium p. V**, p. V potassium. **procaine p. G**, p. G procaine. **semisynthetic p's**, penicillins produced from cultures of the mold *Penicillium*, to which various substances other than culture media components, such as acids, amines, or amides, have been added. They are often more acid-stable and more penicillinase-resistant than natural penicillins. Principal semisynthetic penicillins include ampicillin, carbenicillin, cloxacillin sodium, dicloxacillin sodium, methicillin sodium, nafcillin sodium, oxacillin sodium, penicillin G salts, penicillin V and its salts, phenethicillin potassium, hetacillin potassium, floxacillin, carbenicillin, and amoxicillin. Called also *biosynthetic p's*. See also *natural p*. **sodium p. G**, p. G sodium. **p. V**, a broad-spectrum, semisynthetic penicillin, 3,3-dimethyl-7-oxo-6-(phenoxyacetyl) amino]-4-thia-1-azabicyclo[3,2,0] heptane-2-carboxylic acid, prepared from cultures of the mold *Penicillium* in the presence of 2-phenoxyethanol with an autolysate of yeast as the source of nitrogen. Penicillin V occurs as a white, odorless, crystalline powder that is soluble in alcohol and acetone, slightly soluble in water, and insoluble in fixed oils. It is active in the D-form; the DL-form being less active and the L-form being inactive. Its pharmacological and toxic properties are similar to those of other penicillins, but it is less potent than penicillin G. Allergic reactions are less common with oral administration than with the intramuscular injection. Called also *phenoxymethylenepenicillic acid* and *phenoxymethylpenicillin*. Trademarks: Fenacilin, Oracillin, Pen-Oral, Phenopenicillin. **p. V benzathine**, a semisynthetic penicillin consisting of penicillin V compounded with *N,*

N'-dibenzylethylenediamine. It occurs as a white, tasteless, crystalline powder with a characteristic odor, being less soluble than the parent compound. Used similarly to penicillin V. Called also **p. V DBED**. Trademarks: Bicillin V, Ostrocilline. **p. V calcium,** a calcium salt of penicillin V. Trademarks: Bantogen, Calcipen V, Septocillin. Stabilin V, Uticillin VK. **p. V DBED,** p. V benzathine. **p. V hydrabamine,** a semisynthetic penicillin consisting of penicillin V compounded with N,N'-bis[(1,2,3,4,4a,9,10,10a-octahydro-7-isopropyl-1,4a-dimethyl-1-phenanthryl)methyl]ethylenediamine. It occurs as a white powder with a characteristic odor, which is very slightly soluble in water, alcohol, and ether, and freely soluble in chloroform. It is somewhat less potent but otherwise similar in action and toxicity to penicillin V. Because of its low solubility in water, it is less susceptible to hydrolysis by gastric juice. Called also *hydrabamine phenoxymethyl penicillin.* Trademarks: Abbocillin-V, Compocillin-V. **p. V potassium,** the monopotassium salt of penicillin V, occurring as a white, odorless powder that is very soluble in water, slightly soluble in acetone, and slightly soluble in alcohol, and insoluble in acetone. Its pharmacological and toxic properties are similar to those of the parent compound. Because of its solubility, it is believed to enter the blood faster than other penicillins. Called also *p. potassium phenoxymethyl.* Trademarks: Arcacil, Beromycin, Calciopen K, Compocillin VK, Fenoxypen, Isocillin, Ledercillin-VK, Oracil-VK, Pfizerpen VK, Robicillin VK. **p. X,** a natural penicillin, *p*-hydroxybenzylpenicillin, being somewhat less active than penicillin G. Called also *p. III.*

penicillinase [E.C.3.5.2.6] (pen″ĭ-sil′ĭ-nās) a hydrolase that acts on carbon-nitrogen bonds, other than peptide bonds, which inactivates penicillins. It is produced by certain bacteria and converts penicillin into inactive penicilloic acid by liberation of a second carboxyl group, thus rendering antibiotics inactive and causing the bacteria to become resistant to penicillin. A purified preparation from cultures of *Bacillus cereus* is used in the treatment of reactions to penicillin. Called also *β-lactamase I.* and *penicillin amido-β-lactamhydrolase.* Trademark: Neutrapen.

penicillin-fast (pen″ĭ-sil′in-fast) resistant to the action of penicillin; said of certain strains of bacteria.

penicilliosis (pen″ĭ-sil″e-o′sis) infection with the fungus *Penicillium,* usually a pulmonary infection.

Penicillium (pen″ĭ-sil′e-um) [L. *penicillum* brush] a genus of deuteromycetous fungi (Fungi Imperfecti) that develop fruiting organisms resembling a broom or the bones of the hand and fingers. Some species are the source of antibiotics, including penicillin. A few species rarely produce opportunistic infections in man.

penis (pe′nis) [L.] the male organ of copulation and urination.

Penitracin trademark for *bacitracin.*

penniform (pen′ĭ-form) [L. *penna* feather + *forma* form] shaped like a feather; having the appearance of a feather.

Penny antigen (factor) [named after the person in whom antibodies to the Penny factor (Kp^a antigen) were first discovered] see Kp^a ANTIGEN, and see Kell blood groups, under BLOOD GROUP.

pennyweight (pen′e-wāt) a unit of weight in the troy system, being equivalent to 24 grains, 0.05 ounces, or 1.555 grams. Abbreviated *pwt* or *dwt.* See also *Tables of Weights and Measures* at WEIGHT.

Pen-Oral trademark for *penicillin V.*

Penplenum trademark for *hetacillin.*

Penrose drain [Charles Bingham *Penrose,* American physician, 1862–1925] see under DRAIN.

Pen-Sint trademark for *dicloxacillin.*

pent-, penta- [Gr. *pente* five] 1. a combining form meaning five. 2. in chemical nomenclature, generally used in connection with molecules made up of five similar parts; the number of each type of monodentate ligand in a coordination compound. The number of chelate or complicated ligands is indicated with the prefix *pentakis-.*

pentabasic (pen″tah-ba′sik) having five replaceable atoms of hydrogen in the molecule.

pentachlorin (pen″tah-klo′rin) chlorophenothane.

pentaerythritol (pen″tah-ĕ-rith′rĭ-tol) an alcohol prepared by treating acetaldehyde with formaldehyde in an aqueous solution of calcium hydroxide, 2,2-bis(hydroxymethyl)-1,3-propanediol. It occurs as a white, crystalline powder that is readily esterified by organic acids and is soluble in water, slightly soluble in ethanol, and insoluble in benzene, carbon tetrachloride, ether, and other solvents. Used in the production of resins, rosins, varnishes, drugs, plasticizers, insecticides, and other chemical processes. Called also *pentaerythrityl.* **p. tetranitrate,** the nitric acid ester of pentaerythritol, occurring as a white to ivory powder with a faint mild odor, which is soluble in acetone, slightly soluble in ethanol and ether, and insoluble

in water. It is a cardiovascular drug that slowly releases nitrite ions, thus acting as a coronary vasodilator. Used in the prevention of angina pectoris. Side effects may include headache and nausea. Undiluted pentaerythritol tetranitrate can be exploded by percussion or by heat. Called also *niperyt, pentaerythrityl tetranitrate (PTEN),* and *penthrit.*

pentaerythrityl (pen″tah-e-rith′ri-til) pentaerythritol. **p. tetranitrate,** PENTAERYTHRITOL pentanitrate.

pentakis- in chemical nomenclature, a prefex indicating the presence of five similar chelate or complicated ligands in a coordination compound. See also prefix PENT-(2).

Pentalgine trademark for *meperidine hydrochloride* (see under MEPERIDINE).

pentamer (pen′tah-mer) [*penta-* + Gr. *meros* part] 1. a chemical compound (polymer) having a combination of five simpler molecules (monomers). 2. a capsomer having five structural subunits.

pentane (pen′tān) n-pentane; a five-carbon straight-chain hydrocarbon of the methane series, C_5H_{12}, obtained by distillation of petroleum, and occurring as a clear, colorless, flammable liquid. Pentane may produce anesthesia in high concentrations when inhaled, ingested, or injected.

pentazocine (pen-taz′o-sēn) a synthetic nonopiate analgesic, 1,2,3,4,5,6-hexahydro-6,11-dimethyl-3-(3-methyl-2-butenyl)-2,6-methano-3-benzazocin-8-ol, occurring as a white to tan, odorless, slightly bitter, crystalline powder that is soluble in chloroform, ethanol, acetone, ether, and acidic solutions, sparingly soluble in benzene and ethyl acetate, and insoluble in water. It exerts a morphine-like action without precipitating withdrawal symptoms at high doses, but suppresses withdrawal at low doses of morphine. Used to alleviate moderate to severe pain. Nausea, vomiting, diarrhea, constipation, abdominal distress, vertigo, sedation, euphoria, headache, dreams, insomnia, syncope, visual blurring, hallucinations, skin rash, urticaria, facial edema, hypotension, tachycardia, and, rarely, respiratory depression and urinary retention are the principal adverse reactions. Trademarks: Fortalgesic, Fortalin, Fortral, Litocon, Liticon, Sosigon, Talwin. **p. hydrochloride,** the hydrochloride salt of pentazocine, occurring as a white crystalline powder that is soluble in ethanol, chloroform, and water, slightly soluble in acetone, and insoluble in ether and benzene. Its pharmacological properties are similar to those of the parent compound. **p. lactate,** a sterile injectable solution prepared from pentazocine base, lactic acid, and sodium hydroxide in a buffered solution.

2-pentenylpenicillin (pen″tĕ-nil-pen″ĭ-sil′in) penicillin F.

Penthrane trademark for *methoxyflurane.*

penthrit (pen′thrit) PENTAERYTHRITOL tetranitrate.

Pentid trademark for PENICILLIN G potassium.

pentobarbital (pen″to-bar′bĭ-tal) a short-acting, hypnotic and sedative barbiturate, 5-ethyl-5-(1-methylbutyl)barbituric acid, occurring as a white, odorless powder that is very soluble in alcohol, chloroform, and ether, and very slightly soluble in water. It is used for sedation in mild anxiety states and tension, insomnia, hypertension, and coronary, gastrointestinal, convulsive, and psychoneurotic disorders. Also used in preoperative medication and in allaying apprehension before dental interventions. Indications, contraindications, and side-effects are similar to those of other barbiturates. It is an addictive drug subject to the regulation of the Controlled Substances Act. Called also *pentobarbitone.* Trademark: Nembutal. **p. sodium,** the monosodium salt of pentobarbital, occurring as a white, odorless, slightly bitter white powder that is very soluble in water, freely soluble in alcohol, and insoluble in ether. Its indications, contraindications, and adverse effects are similar to those of the parent compound, but its action is shorter. Like the parent compound, it is an addictive drug subject to the regulation of the Controlled Substances Act. Called also *pentobarbitone sodium.*

pentobarbitone (pen″to-bar′bĭ-tōn) British form of *pentobarbital.* **p. sodium,** PENTOBARBITAL sodium.

pentolinium tartrate (pen″to-lin′e-um) nondepolarizing ganglionic blocking agent, 1,1′-pentamethylnebis (1-methylpyrrolidinium hydrogen tartrate), occurring as a nonhygroscopic solid with an acid taste, which is freely soluble in water, slightly soluble in ethanol, and insoluble in ether and chloroform. Used in the treatment of malignant hypertension. Orthostatic hypotension, blurring of vision, xerostomia, urinary retention, fatigue, impotence, and other complications of ganglionic blocking agent therapy are the side reactions. Trademark: Ansolysen.

pentosan (pen'to-san) any member of a group of pentose polysaccharides having the composition $(C_5H_8O_4)_n$, which are found in various foods and juices. It yields pentose on hydrolysis.

pentose (pen'tōs) a monosaccharide containing five carbon atoms in a molecule, $C_5H_{10}O_5$. **p. pathway, p. shunt,** phosphogluconate PATHWAY.

pentosyl (pen'to-sil) a radical of pentose.

pentosyltransferase [E.C.2.4.2] (pen"to-sil-trans'fer-ās) a subsubclass of glycosyltransferases, including enzymes that catalyze the transfer of a pentosyl group, as from uridine to orthophosphate to form uracil. Called also *transpentosylase.*

Pentothal trademark for *thiopenthal sodium* (see under THIOPENTHAL).

pentyl (pen'til) amyl.

penumbra (pĕ-num'brah), pl. *penum'brae* [L. *pene* almost + *umbra* shadow] marginal unsharpness or blurring surrounding the true shadow on a radiographic image due to the slightly different angles of x-rays that are projected onto the examined object and the film from various points on the target. Cf. UMBRA. **transmission p.,** the region of free space irradiated by photons which have traversed only part of the thickness of the collimator, i.e., the part of the collimator at its lower edge.

penumbrae (pĕ-num'bre) [L.] plural of *penumbra.*

Pen-Vee trademark for *penicillin V.*

peppermint (pep'er-mint) the dried leaves and flowering tops of *Mentha piperita* L. (Labiatae), having carminative, gastric stimulant, and counter-irritant properties. **p. camphor,** menthol.

pepsin [E.C.3.4.23.1] (pep'sin) [Gr. *pepsis* digestion] an acid proteinase secreted by the gastric glands as pepsinogen. It has no digestive activity at first, becoming activated after secretion in the gastric juice by coming in contact with previously formed pepsin in the presence of hydrochloric acid. Pepsin catalyzes the hydrolysis of food proteins to amino acids, having active proteolytic properties in a highly acid medium (pH 2.0–3.0) and becoming rapidly deactivated in an alkaline medium. It cleaves preferentially phenylalanine and leucine, although other bonds may be also split. Crude preparations from swine and beef stomachs have been used as a digestive aid. Called also *p. A.* **p. A,** pepsin. **p. B.** [E.C.3.4.23.2] a form of pepsin that catalyzes the hydrolysis of gelatin. **p. C** [E.C.3.4.23.3], a form of pepsin that is active with hemoglobin as a substrate.

pepsinogen (pep-sin'o-jen) [*pepsin* + Gr. *gennan* to produce] an inactive precursor of pepsin secreted by the gastric glands, which is activated in the gastric juice by coming in contact with previously formed pepsin in the presence of hydrochloric acid.

Pepsodent see under DENTIFRICE.

peptidase [E.C.4.11 to 4.15] (pep'tĭ-dās) [*peptide* + *-ase*] a group of peptide hydrolases which free the N-terminal or C-terminal amino acids from peptide chains in degradation of proteins. Called also *exopeptidase.* See also peptide HYDROLASE.

peptide (pep'tīd) [Gr. *pepton,* neuter of *peptos,* cooked, digested + *-ide*] a compound of low molecular weight, yielding two or more amino acids on hydrolysis. Peptides are the constituent parts of proteins. They are formed by loss of water from the NH_2 and COOH groups of adjacent amino acids, and are distinguished as di-, tri-, tetra-(etc.) peptides, depending on the number of amino acids in the molecule. See also POLYPEPTIDE. **p. bond,** peptide BOND. **p. C,** see PROINSULIN. **p. hydrolase,** peptide HYDROLASE. **p. peptidohydrolase,** proteinase. **p. synthetase,** peptide SYNTHETASE.

peptidoglycan (pep"tĭ-do-gli'kan) a heteropolymer consisting of a backbone of a polysaccharide containing alternating units of N-acetylglucosamine and muramic acid. In bacterial cells, it is a bag-shaped macromolecule that surrounds the cytoplasmic element of the cell, being composed of glycan strands crosslinked by short peptides. The glycan strand consists of repeating units of β-1,4-N-acetylgucosamine-β-1,4-N-acetylmuramic acid. The N-terminus of the peptide subunit is bound through the carboxyl group of muramic acid. The peptide subunits of adjacent glycans are often joined directly through the unbound amino group of diamino-pimelic acid or lysine and the C-terminal of D-alanine, or indirectly through an interpeptide bridge. Called also *glycosaminopeptide, murein,* and *mucopeptide.* See also cell WALL and peptidoglycan LAYER.

peptidohydrolase (pep"tĭ-do-hi'dro-lās) peptide HYDROLASE. **peptide p.,** proteinase.

Peptococcaceae (pep"to-kok-ka'se-e) [*Peptococcus* + *-aceae*] a family of gram-positive coccoid bacteria, consisting of the genera *Peptococcus, Peptostreptococcus, Ruminococcus,* and *Sarcina.*

Peptococcus (pep"to-kok'us) [Gr. *pepton* digestion + L. *coccus* berry] a genus of gram-positive bacteria of the family Peptococcaceae, occurring as cocci, singly, in pairs or tetrads, or as irregular masses of spherical cells, 0.5 to 1.0 or, exceptionally, 1.6 μm in diameter. They are nonmotile, nonsporogenous, penicillin-sensitive organisms, which have been isolated in humans from the skin and intestinal, respiratory, and female urogenital tracts, and from appendicitis, cystitis, pleurisy, gingivitis, postpartum septicemia, and tonsillitis; also isolated from sheep lymphadenitis and tidal mud. Their pathogenicity is uncertain. **P. aerog'enes,** a species isolated from cases of puerperal fever, and from the female genital tract, tonsils, and nose. Called also *Micrococcus aerogenes* and *Staphylococcus aerogenes.* **P. anaero'bius,** a species isolated from the human appendix, female genital tract, draining paranasal sinuses, from cases of cystitis, and from tidal mud. Called also *P. glycinophilus, P. variabilis, Diplococcus glycinophilus, D. magnus anaerobius, Micrococcus anaerobius, M. variabilis,* and *Staphylococcus anaerobius.* **P. asaccharolyt'icus,** a species isolated from the human large intestine, oral cavity, pleura, uterus, and vagina. Called also *Micrococcus asaccharolyticus* and *Staphylococcus asaccharolyticus.* **P. constella'tus,** a species isolated from the human tonsils, appendix, nose, throat, gingiva, and, occasionally, from the skin and vagina and from cases of purulent pleurisy. Called also *Diplococcus constellatus.* **P. glycinoph'ilus, P. variabi'lis,** *P. anaerobius.*

peptone (pep'tōn) [Gr. *pepton,* neuter of *peptos* cooked, digested + *-one*] a secondary derived protein, being a partially hydrolyzed protein that is lower in molecular weight than a proteose. On hydrolysis, peptones yield peptides and amino acids, and are readily soluble in water and coagulable by heat. Collectively known as *polypeptides.*

peptostreptococcus (pep"to-strep"to-kok'us) a genus of gram-positive bacteria of the family Peptococcaceae, occurring as anaerobic, nonsporogenous, nonmotile, nonflagellated, spherical to ovoid cells, about 0.7 to 1.0, occasionally, 0.3 to 0.5 μm in diameter, found in pairs or in chains. The members are potentially pathogenic and penicillin-sensitive. They have been isolated from the female genital tract under normal and pathological conditions; the blood in puerperal fever; the respiratory and intestinal tract under normal conditions; the oral cavity and in dental plaque; and in cases of septic wounds and appendicitis. **P. anaero'bius,** a species averaging 0.8 μm in diameter, arranged in chains, which has been isolated in man from cases of gangrene, infected wounds, puerperal fever, appendicitis, pleurisy, paranasal sinusitis, and osteomyelitis, and from the intestinal tract, oral cavity, and genital secretions. Called also *Micrococcus foetidus, Streptococcus anaerobius, S. foetidus,* and *S. putridus.* **P. lanceola'tus,** a species having large ovoid cells, 1.2 to 1.4 μm in diameter, with pointed ends, occurring in short chains and in pairs, which has been isolated in man from cases of diarrhea, dental infection, vulvovaginitis, and abscesses. Called also *Streptococcus lanceolatus.* **P. mi'cros,** a species having small spheroid cells, 0.3 to 0.5 μm in diameter, occurring in long chains or in pairs, which has been isolated in man from cases of pleurisy, puerperal septicemia, appendicitis, actinomycosis, cerebral abscesses, and dental abscesses. Called also *Streptococcus anaerobius micros* and *S. micros.* **P. par'vulus,** a species of small spherical cells, about 0.3 to 0.4 μm in diameter, occurring in short chains and sometimes in pairs, which has been isolated from the human respiratory tract and oral cavity. Called also *Streptococcus parvulus.* **P. produc'tus,** a species of spherical cells, about 0.7 to 1.2 μm diameter, occurring in chains of 6 to 20 cells, which has been isolated in man from cases of gangrene and pelvic abscesses and from the blood and urine. Called also *Streptococcus productus.*

per- [L. *per* through] 1. a combining form meaning throughout, thoroughly, or completely. 2. in chemistry, a prefix denoting a compound containing an element in its highest state of oxidation, as perchloric acid. 3. in chemistry, presence of a peroxy group, $-O-O-$, as perchromic acid.

Perazyl trademark for *chlorcyclizine.*

Percaine trademark for *dibucaine hydrochloride* (see under DIBUCAINE)

Percapyl trademark for *chlormerodrin.*

percent (per-sent') [*per-* + L. *centum* one hundred] one one-hundredth part; 1/100. Written also *per cent.* Symbol %. **atomic p.,** ATOMIC percent. **p. volume in volume,** the number of milliliters of an active constituent in 100 ml of solution. Symbol *v/v.* **weight p.,** the ratio of the weight of the components to the total weight of the whole multiplied by 100. **p. weight in volume,** the number of grams of an active constituent in 100 ml of solution. Symbol *w/v.* **p. weight in weight,** the number of grams of an active constituent in 100 gm of solution. Symbol *w/w.*

per cent (per sent') percent.

percentage (per-sen'tij) a rate or portion per hundred. Called also *percent*. Symbol %. **p. elongation**, elongation (2).

percentile (per-sen'tīl, per-sen'til) 1. of, pertaining to, or used in percentage. 2. one of 100 equal parts of a series divided in order of their measurable magnitude.

perception (per-sep'shun) [L. *perceptio* a gathering together] the conscious awareness of a sensory stimulus.

perchlorate (per-klo'rāt) any salt of perchloric acid containing the radical ClO_4^-.

perchloride (per-klo'rīd) a chloride that contains more chlorine than the corresponding normal chloride; an organic compound in which all the hydrogen atoms are substituted by chlorine. **mercury p.**, mercuric CHLORIDE.

perchlormethane (per'klor-meth'ān) CARBON tetrachloride.

Percodan trademark for *oxycodone*.

Percogesic tablets see under TABLET.

percolation (per'ko-la'shun) [L. *percolatio*] the extraction of the soluble parts of a drug by causing a liquid solvent to flow slowly through it.

percussion (per-kush'un) [L. *percussio*] listening to the sounds produced by striking a part with short, sharp blows; used as an aid in diagnosing the condition of underlying parts.

per cutem (per ku'tem) [L.] through the skin.

Peredrine trademark for *hydroxyamphetamine hydrobromide* (see under HYDROXYAMPHETAMINE).

perennial (pe-ren'i-al) [L. *perennis*, from *per* through + *annus* year] 1. perpetual, everlasting. 2. lasting or continuing through the year.

Perfex repair resin see under RESIN.

perfluoroethylene (per-floo'or-o-eth'ĭ-lēn) tetrafluoroethylene.

perforation (per'fo-ra'shun) [L. *perforare* to pierce through] 1. the act or process of piercing or penetrating through a surface or layer. 2. accidental opening through a wall or tissue. 3. an opening made in a wall or tissue. **Bezold's p.**, perforation of the inner surface of the mastoid bone. **mechanical p.**, an artificial opening made by piercing or cutting through a surface or layer. **pathologic p.**, an opening or hole produced in a tissue surface or structure by a pathologic process, as may occur in internal resorption of a tooth. **tooth p.**, an opening or hole through a wall of a tooth.

Perhydrol-Urea trademark for *urea peroxide* (see under UREA).

peri- [Gr. *peri* around] a prefix meaning around.

Periactin trademark for *cyproheptadine hydrochloride* (see under CYPROHEPTADINE).

periadenitis (per'e-ad"ĕ-ni'tis) [*peri-* + Gr. *adēn* gland + *-itis*] inflammation of the tissue around a gland. **p. muco'sa necrot'ica recur'rens**, a recurrent disease of the mucous membranes of unknown etiology, generally considered to be a severe form of recurrent aphthous stomatitis. It is characterized by the development of deep crateriform ulcers with inflamed borders which leave scars after healing, thus differing from herpes simplex and ordinary recurrent aphthous stomatitis in which there is no scarring. The mucosa of the lips, cheeks, tongue, palate, and anterior tonsillar pillars are most commonly involved, and the pharynx, larynx, and genitalia also are affected sometimes. The gingivae are seldom if ever involved. The recurrent episodes of disease are spaced over a period of several years. Called also *chronic necrotic stomatitis*, *Mikulicz's aphthae*, *recurring scarring aphthae*, and *Sutton's disease*.

periangiitis (per'e-an"je-i'tis) [*peri-* + Gr. *angeion* vessel + *-itis*] inflammation of the tissue surrounding a blood or lymph vessel.

periapex (per'e-a'peks) the tissue which surrounds the root apex of a tooth (the periodontal ligament and alveolar bone).

periapical (per'e-ap'ĭ-kal) [*peri-* + L. *apex* tip] situated at or surrounding the apex of a tooth.

periarteritis (per'e-ar"tĕ-ri'tis) [*peri-* + Gr. *arteria* artery + *-itis*] inflammation involving the external coat of an artery and its surrounding tissue. **p. nodo'sa**, an inflammatory vascular disease, identified with the collagen diseases, involving small and medium-sized arteries and, sometimes, veins. It is characterized by the development of nodules on the affected vessels, involving any system, but the gastrointestinal tract, kidneys, and lungs are affected most frequently. Microscopically, lesions are initially characterized by mucoid degeneration and acute fibrinoid necrosis of the arterial walls, followed by leukocyte infiltration, cellular exudation, fibroblastic proliferation, formation of granulation tissue, and inflammatory infiltration. It may have many causes but the allergic theory is most widely accepted. Called also *necrotizing angiitis*, *panarteritis nodosa*, and *polyarteritis nodosa*.

periarticular (per'e-ar-tik'u-lar) [*peri-* + L. *articulus* joint], around a joint.

pericarditis (per'i-kar-di'tis) [*pericardium* + *-itis*] inflammation of the pericardium.

pericardium (peri"ĭ-kar'de-um) [*peri-* + Gr. *kardia* heart] the fibroserous sac which encloses the heart and the roots of the great vessels.

pericellular (per'ĭ-sel'u-lar) [*peri-* + L. *cellula* cell] surrounding a cell.

pericemental (per'ĭ-se-men'tal) pertaining to the pericementum or periodontal ligament.

pericementitis (per'ĭ-se-men-ti'tis) [*pericementum* + *-itis*] inflammation of the pericementum (periodontal ligament). See PERIODONTITIS. **apical p.**, apical ABSCESS. **chronic suppurative p.**, marginal PERIODONTITIS. **rarefying p. fibrosa** periodontosis.

pericementoclasia (per'ĭ-se-men"to-kla'ze-ah) [*pericementum* + Gr. *klasis* breaking] a term used in the past to denote disintegration of the periodontal ligament (pericementum) and alveolar bone without loss of the overlying gingival tissue, resulting in pocket formation. See also PERIODONTITIS.

pericementum (per'ĭ-se-men'tum) [*peri-* + L. *caementum* cement] periodontal LIGAMENT.

pericentral (per'ĭ-sen'tral) surrounding a center.

pericephalic (per'ĭ-sĕ-fal'ik) surrounding the head.

perichondritis (per'ĭ-kon-dri'tis) inflammation of the perichondrium. **chondrolytic p.**, **diffuse p.**, chronic atrophic POLYCHONDRITIS.

perichondrium (per'ĭ-kon'dre-um) [*peri-* + Gr. *chondros* cartilage] a dense fibrous connective tissue which encloses cartilage, except for parts exposed to the synovial fluid in joints, and merges with the cartilage on one side and the adjacent connective tissue on the other. During embryonic life, the cells on the chondrogenic layer differentiate into chondrocytes and secrete matrix, thus building new layers on the surface of cartilage in the process of appositional growth.

Perichthol trademark for *ichthammol*.

pericline (per'i-klīn) sodium FELDSPAR.

pericoronal (per'ĭ-kor'o-nal) around the crown of a tooth.

pericoronitis (per'ĭ-kor"o-ni'tis) [*peri-* + L. *corona* crown + *-itis*] inflammation of the gingiva surrounding the crown of a tooth. It occurs most frequently around partially erupted or impacted third molars, the space between the crown and the tooth and the overlying gingival flap being a favorable area for food debris and bacterial growth. The affected flap is usually infected, red, swollen, suppurating, and tender with pain radiating to the ear, throat, and floor of the mouth. A foul taste and inability to close the jaws are the common symptoms. The lesion may become localized and form a pericoronal abscess or it may spread posterior to the base of the tongue and make swallowing difficult. Lymphadenitis, peritonsilar abscess, cellulitis, and Ludwig's angina are possible complications. Called also *operculitis*.

pericranial (per'ĭ-kra'ne-al) pertaining to the pericranium.

pericranitis (per'ĭ-kra-ni'tis) inflammation of the external periosteum of the skull.

pericranium (per'ĭ-kra'ne-um) [*peri-* + Gr. *kranion* cranium] the external periosteum of the skull.

pericystic (per'ĭ-sis'tik) situated about a cyst.

pericyte (per'ĭ-sīt) [*peri-* + *-cyte*] one of the peculiar elongated cells with the power of contraction, found spirally wrapped about capillaries outside the basement membrane. Called also *p. of Zimmerman* and *Rouget cell*. **p. of Zimmerman**, pericyte.

peridens (per'ĭ-dens) [*peri-* + L. *dens* tooth] a supernumerary tooth appearing elsewhere than the midline of the dental arch.

peridental (per'ĭ-dent'tal) periodontal (1).

periderm (per'ĭ-derm) [*peri-* + Gr. *derma* skin] 1. the superficial flattened outer layer of the embryonic epidermis, made up of large squamoid cells, which appears within the second week of the second month of the embryonic development. In the human embryo, it is loosened by the hair which grows beneath it, and generally disappears before birth. Called also *epitrichium*. 2. the cuticle (eponychium and hyponychium), the only part of the periderm which persists after birth.

peridontium (per'ĭ-don'she-um) periodontium.

peridontoclasia (per'ĭ-don"to-kla'se-ah) periodontoclasia.

Peridres trademark for a periodontal dressing. In the powder form, 100 gm contains 49 mg rosin, 46 mg zinc oxide, 3 gm tannic acid, and 2 gm kaolin. In the liquid form, each 100 ml contain 98 ml eugenol, 2 ml thymol, and coloring agents.

perifascicular (per'ĭ-fah-sik'u-lar) surrounding or around a fasciculus of nerve or muscle fibers.

perifocal (per″ĭ-fo′kal) around or surrounding a focus, such as a focus of infection.

perifolliculitis (per″ĭ-fo-lik-u-li′tis) [peri- + folliculitis] inflammation around the hair follicle, which may involve the face and lips. Necrosis of the surrounding tissue and leukocytic liquefaction, associated with abscess formation, pain, and fever may develop. See also deep FOLLICULITIS.

periglandular (per″ĭ-glan′du-lar) surrounding a gland or glands.

periglossitis (per″ĭ-glŏ-si′tis) inflammation of the tissue around the tongue.

periglottic (per″ĭ-glot′ik) situated around the tongue.

periglottis (per″ĭ-glot′is) [peri- + Gr. glotta tongue] the mucous membrane of the tongue.

peri-implantoclasia (per″e-im-plan″to-kla′se-ah) [peri- + implant + Gr. klasis breaking] a pathological tissue reaction surrounding implanted foreign material, characterized by local inflammation. **exfoliative p.,** a condition in which degenerative changes surrounding an implant cause its exfoliation, exposing deeply-implanted structures. **necrotic ulcerative p.,** necrotic complications of ulcerative peri-implantoclasia, associated with hyperplasia, hyperemia, edema, sloughing, and a bleeding tendency, usually due to an oral infection combined with food impaction and salivary calculi. **resorption p.,** a condition in which the supporting bone structure beneath an implant is undergoing resorption, usually due to excessive masticatory pressure with resulting atrophy, excessive increase of the vertical dimension, or insufficient metal coverage of the supporting bone structures. **traumatic p.,** degenerative inflammatory changes surrounding an implant, due to trauma resulting from displacement or distortion, fractures, or excessive forces exerted on the implant. **ulcerative p.,** ulcerative changes around a subperiosteal implant, with hyperplasia, hyperemia, edema, and pain, sometimes resulting in abscesses, due to oral infections, loose screws, surgical infection, galvanic action of dissimilar metals, and other causes. **ulcerative p., necrotic,** necrotic ulcerative p.

perikaryon (per″ĭ-kar′e-on) [peri- + Gr. karyon nucleus] the cell body as distinguished from the nucleus and the processes; applied particularly to neurons.

perikymata (per″ĭ-ki′mah-tah) [pl., peri- + Gr. kyma wave] the numerous small transverse ridges on the surface of the enamel of permanent teeth, representing overlapping prism groups. With continued abrasion, the surface of the enamel becomes eroded and the perikymata become obliterated.

perilaryngeal (per″ĭ-lah-rin′je-al) situated around the larynx.

perilaryngitis (per″ĭ-lar″in-ji′tis) inflammation of the tissues around the larynx.

periligamentous (per″ĭ-lig″ah-men′tus) situated around a ligament.

perilobar (per″ĭ-lo′bar) surrounding or around a lobe.

perilymph (per″ĭ-limf) [peri- + L. lymph] the fluid contained within the space separating the membranous from the osseous labyrinth of the ear; it is separate from the endolymph. Called also perilympha [NA].

perilympha (per″ĭ-lim′fah) [NA] perilymph.

perilymphadenitis (per″ĭ-lim″fad-ĕ-ni′tis) inflammation of the tissues around the lymph nodes.

perilymphangitis (per″ĭ-lim″fan-ji′-tis) inflammation of the tissues around the lymphatic vessels.

perilymphatic (per″ĭ-lim-fat′ik) 1. pertaining to the perilymph. 2. pertaining to the tissues around a lymphatic node or vessel; around a lymphatic node or vessel.

perimeter (pĕ-rim′ĕ-ter) [peri- + Gr. metron measure] 1. the circumference, border, or outer boundary of a two-dimensional object. 2. an instrument for determining the extent of the peripheral visual field of a curved surface. **dental p.,** an instrument for measuring the circumference of a tooth.

perimyositis (per″ĭ-mi″o-si′tis) inflammation of the connective tissue around muscles.

perimysium (per″ĭ-mis′e-um) [peri- + Gr. mys muscle] [NA] a collagenous septum surrounding fascicles of skeletal muscles. Called also p. internum. **p. exter′num,** epimysium. **p. inter′num,** perimysium.

perinatal (per″ĭ-na′tal) [peri- + L. natus born] pertaining to or occurring in the period shortly before and after birth; in medical statistics, generally considered to begin with completion of 28 weeks of gestation and variously defined as ending one to four weeks after birth.

perineural (per″ĭ-nu-ral) [peri- + neural] surrounding a nerve or nerves.

perineurium (per″ĭ-nu′re-um) [peri- + Gr. neuron nerve] a sheath of dense connective tissue surrounding each bundle (fasciculus) of nerve fibers.

Perio-Aid trademark for an interdental tip, being a holder for the end of a toothpick used for cleansing interdental spaces.

period (pe′re-od) [peri- + Gr. hodos way] an interval or division of time; the time for the regular recurrence of a phenomenon. **benefit p.,** the period of time for which payments for benefits covered by an insurance policy are available. The availability of certain benefits may be limited over a specified time period, e.g., one dental examination during a one-year period. The benefit period is usually defined by a set unit of time, such as a year (benefit, contract, or policy year), but it may be also tied to a spell of illness. Deductible and annual maximum amounts are calculated from various specified dates during the calendar year, but some policies calculate deductible and annual maximum amounts from the first of January. Called also policy p. **enrollment p.,** a period during which an individual may enroll for insurance or health maintenance organization benefits. There are two kinds of enrollment periods for supplementary medical insurance of Medicare, the initial enrollment period (the seven months beginning three months before and ending three months after the month a person first becomes eligible, usually by turning 65); and the general enrollment period (the first three months of each year). Most contributory group insurance has an annual enrollment period when members of the group may elect to begin contributing and become covered. **fibrillogenic p.,** the period during osteogenesis, cementogenesis, or dentinogenesis in which the appropriate cells engage in fibril production for formation of matrix. **grace p.,** in insurance, a specified time, after a plan's premium payment is due, in which the protection of the plan continues subject to actual receipt of the premium within that time. **incubation p.,** the interval of time required for development; the period of time between the moment of entrance of the infecting organism into the body and the first symptoms of the consequent disease, or between the moment of entrance into a vector and the time at which the vector is capable of transmitting the disease. **inductive p.,** latent p. (2). **latent p.,** 1. a seemingly inactive period, as that between exposure of tissue to an injurious agent and the manifestation of response, or that between the instant of stimulation and the beginning of response. 2. the period in either the primary or the secondary immune response extending from the introduction of an antigen into an immunocompetent animal to the appearance of detectable specific antibodies or of sensitized lymphocytes in the serum, during which the immunogen is recognized as foreign and processed and antibody formation is initiated. Called also inductive p., and inductive phase. **policy p.,** benefit p. **silent p.,** 1. an interval in the course of a disease in which the symptoms become very mild or disappear for a time. 2. in electromyography, a momentary pause in tracings associated with reflex stimulation. **waiting p.,** in health insurance, the period of time between enrollment in a plan and the date when an insured person is entitled to receive benefits.

periodic (pe″re-od′ik) [Gr. periodikos] recurring at regular intervals. **p. table,** see table at ELEMENT.

periodicity (pe″re-o-dis′ĭ-te) recurrence at regular intervals of time. See also CHRONOBIOLOGY, CYCLE, and RHYTHM.

periodontal (per″e-o-don′tal) [peri- + Gr. odous tooth] 1. pertaining to or occurring around a tooth; peridental. 2. pertaining to the periodontal ligament or periodontium.

periodontalgia (per″e-o-don-tal′je-ah) pain arising in the periodontal ligament, usually as a result of infective or traumatic inflammation.

periodontia (per″e-o-don′she-ah) 1. plural of periodontium. 2. periodontics.

periodontics (per″e-o-don′tiks) [peri- + Gr. odous tooth] that branch of dentistry that deals with the diagnosis, prevention, and treatment of periodontal diseases. In current terminology, the term periodontics is used usually in a more restrictive sense than the term periodontology, which comprises the scientific study of the structures and function of the periodontium in both health and disease. But, sometimes, these terms are used interchangeably. Called also periodontia. **preventive p.,** a program for the preservation of the natural dentition by preventing the onset, progress, and recurrence of gingivitis and periodontal disease, involving the cooperative effort of the dentist, his ancillary personnel, and the patient. See also interceptive restorative DENTISTRY, oral PROPHYLAXIS, preventive DENTISTRY, and TOOTHBRUSHING.

periodontist (per″e-o-don′tist) a dentist who specializes in periodontics.

periodontitis (per″e-o-don-ti′tis) [periodontium + -itis] 1. an inflammatory disease of the periodontium, or the supporting tissues of the teeth, or a gingival inflammatory lesion extending into the adjacent bone, which, when left untreated, may lead to loss of bone and periodontal extension. Called also *alveolodental osteoperiostitis* and *cementoperiostitis*. 2. marginal p. **apical p., apical chronic p.,** apical GRANULOMA. **chronic apical p.,** apical GRANULOMA. **p. complex,** see PERIODONTOSIS. **marginal p.,** an inflammatory periodontal disease which begins as a simple marginal gingivitis and is caused by calculus, impacted food debris, materia alba, or irritation by fillings. Minute ulcerations of the crevicular epithelium are the initial symptom. If left untreated, the inflammation will migrate along the tooth toward the apex, producing periodontal pockets and destruction of the periodontal and alveolar structures (periodontoclasia and alveoloclasia), causing the teeth to become loose. Swelling, edema, hyperemia, and bleeding of the gingivae, detachment of the tissue from the tooth structure, and recession of soft tissue, expulsion of suppurative material on pressure from periodontal pockets (hence the synonym *pyorrhea*), and halitosis are the principal symptoms. The condition is observed most frequently among adult and elderly patients, but it also occurs in children. Called also *p. simplex, primary p., simple p., alveolodental periostitis, chronic suppurative pericementitis, Fauchard's disease, gingivitis expulsiva, pyorrhea, pyorrhea alveolaris, Riggs' disease,* and *schmutz pyorrhea.* **prepubertal p.,** loss of bone around multiple teeth in children sometimes observed in periodic agranulocytosis. **primary p.,** marginal p. **secondary p.,** see PERIODONTOSIS. **simple p., p. sim′plex,** marginal p. **suppurative apical p.,** apical abscess, chronic; see under ABSCESS.

periodontium (per″e-o-don′she-um), pl. *periodon′tia* [*peri-* + Gr. *odous* tooth] the tissues that invest or help to invest and support the teeth, including the periodontal ligament, gingivae, cementum, and alveolar and supporting bone. In NA terminology, the term periodontium is restricted to the periodontal ligament. Called also *alveolar periosteum, odontoperiosteum, paradentium,* and *peridontium.*

periodontoclasia (per″e-o-don″to-kla′se-ah) [*periodontium* + Gr. *klasis* breaking] destruction of the periodontal structures. See marginal PERIODONTITIS. Called also *Magitot's disease* and *peridontoclasia.*

periodontology (per″e-o-don-tol′o-je) [*peri-* + Gr. *odous* tooth + *-logy*] that branch of dentistry that deals with the scientific study of the structures and function of the periodontium in both health and disease. In current terminology, the term *periodontology* is used usually in a broader sense than the term *periodontics,* which is restricted to the diagnosis, prevention, and treatment of periodontal diseases. But, sometimes, these terms are used interchangeably.

periodontometer (per″e-o-don-tom′ĕ-ter) mobilometer (2).

periodontosis (per″e-o-don-to′sis) [*periodontium* + *-osis*] a chronic degenerative periodontal disease characterized by early migration and loosening of teeth in the absence of inflammation, followed by destruction of the periodontal tissue and loss of the teeth. The initial symptoms include desmolysis of the periodontal fibers and, probably, cessation of cementogenesis, associated with alveolar resorption, edema, and capillary proliferation of the epithelial attachment along the root which, when left untreated, advance to gingival inflammation, pocket formation, trauma from occlusion, and bone loss. This last stage is sometimes referred to as *periodontal syndrome, secondary periodontitis,* and *periodontitis complex.* The existence of this disease is not accepted by many authorities. Called also *alveolar atrophy* and *rarefying pericementitis fibrosa.*

perioral (per″e-o′ral) [*peri-* + L. *os* mouth] situated or occurring around the mouth.

periorbita (per″e-or′bĭ-tah) [*peri-* + L. *orbita* orbit] the periosteal covering of the bones forming the orbit.

periorbital (per″e-or′bĭ-tal) situated around the orbit.

periorbititis (per″e-or′bĭ-ti′tis) inflammation of the periorbita.

periosteal (per″e-os′te-al) pertaining to the periosteum.

periosteomyelitis (per″e-os″te-o-mi″ĕ-li′tis) [*peri-* + Gr. *osteon* bone + *myelos* marrow + *-itis*] inflammation of the entire bone, including the periosteum and marrow.

periosteorrhaphy (per″e-os″te-or′ah-fe) [*periosteum* + Gr. *rhaphē* suture] the suturing together of the margins of severed periosteum.

periosteotome (per″e-os′te-o-tōm) [*periosteum* + Gr. *tomē* a cutting] an instrument for cutting the periosteum or for separating the periosteum from the bone. In oral surgery, an instrument designed to fit under the free gingiva, which is used prior to the

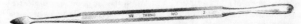

Periosteotome. (From H. O. Torres and A. Ehrlich: Modern Dental Assisting. 2nd ed. Philadelphia, W. B. Saunders Co., 1980; courtesy of S. S. White, Div. of Pennwalt Corp.)

placement of the surgical forceps in tooth extraction to loosen the gingival cuff from the root. Called also *periosteal elevator* and *subperiosteal e.* See illustration.

periosteotomy (per″e-os″te-ot′o-me) [*periosteum* + Gr. *tomē* a cutting] surgical incision or slitting of the periosteum.

periosteum (per″e-os′te-um) [*peri-* + Gr. *osteon* bone] [NA] a specialized connective tissue which covers all bones of the body, except the cartilaginous extremities, and is incorporated with tendons or ligaments when they are attached to the bone. It consists of two closely united layers, the external layer made up chiefly of collagenous tissue and a few fat cells, and the deep one composed of elastic fibers arranged into layers of dense membranous networks. A network of fine lymphatic vessels and nerves may be present. Early in life the periosteum is thick and richly supplied with blood vessels and unites with the epiphyseal cartilage, separated from the bone by a layer of soft tissue containing osteoblasts. In older persons it becomes thinner and less vascular and the osteoblasts are converted into the epithelioid layer. **alveolar p., p. alveola′re,** periodontal LIGAMENT. **dental p.,** periodontal LIGAMENT.

periostitis (per″e-os-ti′tis) [*periosteum* + *-itis*] inflammation of the bone in which the periosteum is predominantly involved. **alveolodental p.,** marginal PERIODONTITIS. **p. hyperplas′tica,** progressive diaphyseal DYSPLASIA. **suppurative p.,** periostitis characterized by diffuse suppuration, resulting in necrosis.

periostosteitis (per″e-os-tos″te-i′tis) inflammation involving both bone and its tissue covering (periosteum).

peripheral (pĕ-rif′ĕ-ral) 1. pertaining to, in the direction of, or situated at or near the periphery. 2. a device that can be used in conjunction with a computer without being its integral part.

periphery (pĕ-rif′er-e) [Gr. *periphereia,* from *peri-* around + *pherein* to bear] the external or outward part of a surface. **denture p.,** denture BORDER.

periphlebitis (per″ĭ-fle-bi′tis) [*peri-* + Gr. *phleps* vein + *-itis*] inflammation of the tissues around a vein, or of the external coat of a vein.

periradicular (per″ĭ-rah-dik′u-lar) around or surrounding a root, especially the root of a tooth.

perirhizoclasia (per″ĭ-ri″zo-kla′se-ah) [*peri-* + Gr. *rhiza* root + *klasis* destruction + *-ia*] inflammatory destruction of tissues immediately arround the root of a tooth, i.e., pericementum, cementum, and the superficial layers of the alveolar process. See also PARARHIZOCLASIA.

perisinusitis (per″ĭ-si″nu-si′tis) inflammation of the tissues around a sinus.

Periston trademark for *povidone.*

peritectic (per″ĭ-tek′tik) pertaining to the phase intermediate between a solid and a liquid in the melting of a solid. See also peritectic ALLOY.

perithelium (per″ĭ-the′le-um) [*peri-* + Gr. *thēlē* nipple] the layer of connective tissue surrounding the capillaries and smaller vessels. Called also *pericapillary cells.*

Peritol trademark for *cyproheptadine hydrochloride* (see under CYPROHEPTADINE).

peritoneum (per″ĭ-to-ne′um) [L.; Gr. *peritonaion,* from *per* around + *teinein* to stretch] [NA] the serous membrane lining the abdominal and pelvic walls.

peritonitis (per″ĭ-to-ni′tis) inflammation of the peritoneum due to either bacterial invasion or chemical irritation. The sterile type may be caused by bleeding into the peritoneal cavity, escape of bile from a perforated biliary system, pancreatic enzymes, surgically introduced foreign matter, such as talcum powder, and other chemical agents. The bacterial form may occur secondary to such primary disorders as ruptured peptic ulcer, appendicitis, cholecystitis, diverticulitis, or strangulated bowel. Abdominal pain and tenderness, constipation, vomiting, and fever are the most common symptoms.

peritonsillar (per″ĭ-ton′sĭ-lar) situated around a tonsil.

peritonsillitis (per″ĭ-ton′sĭ-li′tis) inflammation of the peritonsillar tissues.

perlèche (per-lesh) [Fr.] single or multiple fissures and cracks at the corners of the mouth that may be caused by a primary or superimposed infection with microorganisms, such as *Candida albicans,* staphylococci, and streptococci; poor hygiene; drooling; overclosure of the jaws in edentulous patients and in patients with ill-fitting dentures; riboflavin deficiency (see ARIBOFLAVINOSIS) in which it may be the first sign, or other causes. It may be unilateral or bilateral, and begins as areas of pallor at the angles of the mouth, with a feeling of dryness and a burning sensation, followed by maceration and fissuring radiating from the oral commissures. The fissures become deep and covered by a dry yellow crust that can be removed without causing bleeding. In advanced stages, the lesions, which may be painful, may spread to the lips and cheeks and become red and shiny due to desquamation of the epithelium. Called also *angular cheilosis, angulus infectiosus,* and *migrating cheilitis.*

Perma-Bond trademark for a nickel-chromium base-metal crown and bridge alloy, also containing beryllium. Inhalation of dust during melting, milling, or grinding may cause beryllium poisoning.

Permastril trademark for *dromostanolone.*

permeability (per″me-ah-bil′ĭ-te) the property or state of being permeable. See also OSMOSIS. **capillary p.,** passage of substances across the capillary wall, accomplished by diffusion of lipid-soluble substances and gases directly through the membrane and water-soluble substances and larger molecules through pores which are 80 to 90 Å in diameter, about 25 times larger than the water molecule. **magnetic p.,** a property of materials modifying the action of magnetic poles placed therein and modifying the magnetic induction resulting when the material is subjected to a magnetic field or magnetizing force. Magnetic permeability of a substance is determined as the ratio of the magnetic induction in the substance to the magnetizing field to which it is subjected.

permeable (per′me-ah-b′l) [L. *per* through + *meare* to pass] not impassable; pervious; that may be traversed.

permease (per′me-ās) a stereospecific membrane transport system. The term was introduced to emphasize the resemblance of these systems in bacteria to enzymes, with respect to kinetics of function and control of formation, but it does not imply either that permeases are enzymes or that they differ from the membrane transport systems of cells other than bacteria.

permeation (per″me-a′shun) the act of spreading or penetrating a substance, tissue, or organ. See also permeation ANESTHESIA.

pero- [Gr. *pēros* maimed] a combining form meaning maimed or deformed.

Peronine trademark for *benzylmorphine hydrochloride* (see under BENZYLMORPHINE).

peroral (per-o′ral) [L. *per* through + *os, oris* the mouth] performed through or administered through the mouth.

per os (per os) [L.] by mouth; oral administration.

peroxidase [E.C.1.11.1.7] (pe-rok′si-dās) an oxidoreductase that acts on hydrogen peroxide as acceptor. It is one of a group of hemoproteins which catalyze the oxidation of some organic substrates in the presence of hydrogen peroxide. Peroxidases occur widely in plants (e.g., horseradish); there is weak peroxidase activity in the kidney and leukocytes of animals, which may explain the peroxidative activity of pus. Substrates which have been reported, in addition to peroxides, include phenols, reduced glutathione, ferrocytochrome C, and NADH.

peroxide (pe-rok′sīd) any compound which contains the bivalent O-O group, one of the oxygen atoms being bound loosely in the molecule and thus being released readily. Peroxides are generally strong oxidizing agents and present a fire risk when in contact with combustible materials. Called also *superoxide.* **benzoyl p.,** BENZOYL peroxide. **benzoyl p., dibenzoyl p.,** BENZOYL peroxide. **carbamide p.,** UREA peroxide. **dibenzoyl p.,** BENZOYL peroxide. **hydrogen p.,** an oxygen-liberating agent, H_2O_2, occurring as a colorless, bitter liquid that is unstable and breaks down readily to form molecular oxygen and water. A 1.5 to 3.0 percent aqueous solution is effective as an oral wound cleanser, its foaming action also dislodging debris from fissures and crevices. It is believed to be effective against some infections caused by anaerobic bacteria, such as acute necrotizing gingivitis. Hydrogen peroxide is a caustic substance and continued use in mouthwashes may lead to the development of hypertrophy of filiform papillae of the tongue. A 30 percent aqueous solution is a strong oxidizing agent used for the bleaching of vital and pulpless teeth. It may cause irritation and injuries of the oral soft tissue. When stored in a warm place, it may explode spontaneously. Trademark: Superoxol. **lead p.,** LEAD peroxide. **urea p., urea hydrogen p.,** UREA peroxide.

Perphenan trademark for *perphenazine.*

perphenazine (per-fen′ah-zēn) a tranquilizing agent, 4-[3-(2-chlorophenathiazin-10-yl)propyl]-1-pierazineethanol, occurring as a white to creamy, odorless, bitter powder that is soluble in ethanol, chloroform, and acetone, sparingly soluble in ether, and insoluble in water. Used in the management of psychotic disorders and apprehension prior to surgery. Side effects may include drowsiness, parkinsonian-like syndrome, dystonia, dyskinesia, torticollis, ticks, restlessness, hyperreflexia, seizures,

postural hypotension, bradycardia, agranulocytosis, eosinophilia, leukopenia, hemolytic anemia, thrombocytopenic purpura, pancythopenia, and hypersensitivity. Trademarks: Decentan, Fentazin, Perphenan, Trilafon, Trilifan.

per primam; per primam intentionem (per pri′mam in-ten″she-o′nem) [L.] by first intention; see primary UNION.

per rectum (per rek′tum) [L.] by way of the rectum.

per saltum (per sal′tum) [L.] by·a leap or bound; denoting a sudden evolutionary development without intermediate stages.

Persantine trademark for *dipyridamole.*

Persitol trademark for *triethylenemelamine.*

per secundam; per secundam intentionem (per se-kun′dam in-ten″she-o′nem) [L.] by second intention; see secondary UNION.

personality (per″su-nal′ĭ-te) that which constitutes, distinguishes, and characterizes a person as an entity over a period of time; the total reaction of a person to his environment. **split p.,** a popular and erroneous name for schizophrenia.

personnel (per″son-nel′) a group of persons usually employed in the same organization, business, or service. **allied health p.,** specially trained and licensed (when necessary) health workers other than physicians, dentists, podiatrists, and nurses. Called also *paramedical p.* **ancillary p.,** in health care delivery, members of a team, other than physicians and dentists. In dentistry, persons employed by a dentist, such as secretaries, receptionists, bookeepers, or other clerical workers, but excluding dental assistants, dental hygienists, and laboratory assistants. Usually referred to as *ancillary.* See also dental AUXILIARY. **auxiliary dental p.,** see dental AUXILIARY. **paramedical p.,** allied health p.

pertechnetate (per-tek′nĕ-tāt) a salt of pertechnetic acid. See also TECHNECIUM. **sodium p.,** a sodium salt of pertechnetic acid; used in scintigraphy and other scanning techniques, particularly of the brain, salivary glands, tissue grafts, and bones.

Pertik's diverticulum [Otto *Pertik,* Hungarian physician, 1852–1913] see under DIVERTICULUM.

Pertofrane trademark for *desipramine hydrochloride* (see under DESIPRAMINE).

pertussis (per-tus′is) [L. *per-* intensive + *tussis* cough] whooping COUGH.

Pervitin trademark for *methamphetamine hydrochloride* (see under METHAMPHETAMINE).

pes (pes), pl. *pe′des,* gen. *pe′dis* [L.] [NA] the foot. Used also to designate a footlike part.

Pestisella pestis (pes″ti-sel′ah pes′tis) *Yersinia pestis;* see under YERSINIA.

Pestivirus (pes″ti-vi′rus) a genus of togaviruses, having a virion 40 nm in diameter, which cause diseases in swine and lambs.

pestivirus any virus of the genus *Pestivirus.*

pestle (pes′l) [L. *pestillum*] an implement for pounding drugs in a mortar.

pestology (pes-tol′o-je) the branch of science concerned with pests.

Pestox III trademark for *octamethyl pyrophosphoramide* (see under OCTAMETHYL).

-petal [L. *petere* to seek] a word termination meaning directed or moving toward the point of reference being indicated by the word stem to which it is affixed, as centripetal (toward the center), corticipetal (toward the cortex), etc.

petechia (pe-te′ke-ah), pl. *pete′chiae* [L.] a pinpoint, nonraised, round, purplish red spot caused by intradermal or submucous hemorrhage. Cf. ECCHYMOSIS.

petechiae (pe-te′ke-e) [L.] plural of *petechia.*

petechial (pe-te′ke-al) characterized by or of the nature of petechiae.

Peter of Abano [1250 to c. 1316] physician, philosopher, astrologer; an outstanding professor in the University of Padua whose opinions caused him to be tried for heresy during the Inquisition. His works include the *Consiliator differentiarum* (an attempt to reconcile Arabian and Greek medicine) and *De venenis* (a book on poisons). He was also known as *Pietro d'Abano* and *Petrus Apponus.*

Peters' anomaly [A. *Peters*] see under ANOMALY.

Petges-Cléjat syndrome [G. *Petges,* French dermatologist; C. *Cléjat,* French dermatologist] poikilodermatomyositis.

pethidine (peth′ĭ-dēn) meperidine.

Petidon trademark for *trimethadione.*

Petinimid trademark for *ethosuximide.*

Petinutin trademark for *methsuximide.*

petiole (pet′e-ōl) [L. *petiolus*] a stem, stalk, or pedicle. **epiglottic p.,** the pointed lower end of the epiglottic cartilage, which is attached to the back of the thyroid cartilage. Called also *cushion of epiglottis* and *petiolus epiglottidis* [NA].

petiolus (pĕ-ti′o-lus) [L., dim. of *pes* foot] petiole; a stem, stalk, or pedicle. **p. epiglot′tidis** [NA], epiglottic PETIOLE.

Petit, Alexis Therése [French physicist, 1791–1820] see Dulong and Petit LAW.

Petnidan trademark for *ethosuximide*.

Petrassi, G. see Fanconi-Petrassi SYNDROME.

Petri dish [Julius Richard *Petri*, German bacteriologist, 1852–1921] see under DISH.

petrifaction (pet″rĭ-fak-shun) [L. *petra* stone + *facere* to make] conversion into a stonelike substance.

petrolate (pet′ro-lāt) petrolatum.

petrolatum (pet″ro-la′tum) [L.] a purified mixture of semisolid hydrocarbons, chiefly in the methane series, being a colloidal system of nonstraight-chain solid hydrocarbons. It occurs as a yellowish to light amber, semisolid, odorless, and tasteless mass that is transparent in thin masses, being insoluble in water, almost insoluble in alcohol, but freely soluble in benzene, carbon disulfide, chloroform, and turpentine oil. Used as an ointment base; also used as a protective dressing and soothing application to the skin and mucous membranes, and as an emollient and lubricating agent. Called also *amber p., yellow p., mineral jelly, petroleum jelly, paraffin jelly, petrolate,* and *yellow soft paraffin.* Trademark: Vaseline. **amber p.,** petrolatum. **heavy liquid p.,** mineral OIL. **light liquid p.,** light mineral OIL. **liquid p., p. liqui′dum,** mineral OIL. **white p.,** a wholly or nearly decolorized form of petrolatum which, in thin layers, is completely transparent even at 0°C, having all the other properties and uses of petrolatum. Called also *white petroleum jelly* and *white soft paraffin.* **yellow p.,** petrolatum.

petroleum (pĕ-tro′le-um) [L. *petra* stone + *oleum* oil], a complex mixture of paraffinic, cycloparaffinic (naphthenic), and aromatic hydrocarbons, also containing some sulfur, nitrogen, and oxygen compounds, which is said to have originated from decomposing plant and animal sources about 10 to 20 million years ago. It is a flammable, viscous, dark-brown, oily liquid from which gasoline, kerosene, and other products are obtained by distillation. **p. jelly,** petrolatum.

petromastoid (pet″ro-mas′toid) 1. pertaining to the petrous portion of the temporal bone and its mastoid process. 2. otocranium (2).

petro-occipital (pet″ro-ok-sip′ĭ-tal) pertaining to the petrous portion of the temporal bone and to the occipital bone.

petropharyngeus (pet″ro-fah-rin′je-us) an occasional muscle arising from the lower surface of the petrous portion of the temporal bone and inserted into the pharynx.

petrosal (pĕ-tro′sal) [L. *petrosus* rocky] pertaining to the petrous portion of the temporal bone.

petrosalpingostaphylinus (pet″ro-sal-ping″go-staf″ĭ-li′nus) [Gr.; L. *petra* stone + *salpinx* tube + *staphylē* uvula] levator veli palatini MUSCLE.

petrosectomy (pet″ro-sek′to-me) [Gr.; L. *petra* stone + *ektomē* excision] excision of the cells of the apex of the petrous portion of the temporal bone.

petrositis (pet″ro-si′tis) [Gr.; L. *petra* stone + *-itis* inflammation] inflammation of the petrous portion of the temporal bone.

petrosphenoid (pet″ro-sfe′noid) pertaining to the sphenoid bone and the petrous portion of the temporal bone.

petrosquamosal (pet″ro-skwah-mo′sal) pertaining to the petrous and squamous portions of the temporal bone.

petrostaphylinus (pet″ro-staf″ĭ-li′nus) levator veli palatini MUSCLE.

petrous (pet′rus) [L. *petrosus* rocky] 1. resembling a rock; hard; stony. 2. pertaining to the petrous portion of the temporal bone.

Petrus Apponus see PETER OF ABANO.

Peutz-Jeghers syndrome [J. L. A. *Peutz,* Dutch physician; Harold Joseph *Jeghers;* American physician, born 1904] see under SYNDROME.

pexic (pek′sik) [Gr. *pēxis* fixation, putting together] having the ability of fixing substances.

pexis (pek′sis) [Gr. *pēxis*] 1. the fixation of matter. 2. surgical fixation, usually by suturing.

-pexy [Gr. *pēxis* fixing, putting together] a word termination meaning fixation.

Peyer's patch [Johann Conrad *Peyer,* Swiss anatomist, 1653–1712] see under PATCH.

peyote (pa-o′te) 1. a Mexican cactus of the genus *Lophophora,* especially *L. williamsii.* 2. mescaline.

Pfaff, Philip a dentist to Frederick the Great of Prussia. He was the first to use plaster models for prostheses.

pFc′ noncovalently bonded dimer of the C-terminal immunoglobulin of the Fc fragment that may be produced after pepsin digestion of IgG.

Pfeiffer's disease [Emil *Pfeiffer,* German physician, 1846–1921] infectious MONONUCLEOSIS.

Pfeiffer's law, phenomenon [Richard Friedrich Johann *Pfeiffer,* German bacteriologist, 1858–1945; in 1894, with Bordet, he elucidated the action of complement and antibody in cell lysis] see under LAW and PHENOMENON.

Pfeiffer's syndrome (acrocephalosyndactyly) [R. A. *Pfeiffer*] see under SYNDROME.

Pfeifferella mallei (pfi″fer-el′ah mal′e-i) *Pseudomonas mallei;* see under PSEUDOMONAS.

Pfizer-E film coated tablets see under TABLET.

Pfizerpen VK trademark for *penicillin V potassium* (see under PENICILLIN).

PG prostaglandin.

Pg pogonion.

pg picogram.

PGA 1. see PROSTAGLANDIN. 2. pteroylglutamic acid; see folic ACID.

PGB see PROSTAGLANDIN.

PGE see PROSTAGLANDIN.

PGF see PROSTAGLANDIN.

pH the symbol of hydrogen ion (H⁻) concentration, expressed in numbers corresponding to the acidity or alkalinity of an aqueous solution, originally defined as the negative logarithm (base 10) of the concentration of hydrogen ions (equivalent per liter). The range extends from 14 ("pure" base) to 0 ("pure" acid), pH 7 being neutral; or from about 1 for 0.1 N hydrochloride to about 13 for 0.1 N sodium hydroxide, pH of less than 7 indicating acidity and pH of more than 7 indicating alkalinity.

phage (fāj) bacteriophage.

-phagia, -phagy [Gr. *phagein* to eat] a word termination denoting a perversion of appetite, such as geophagia, or relationship to eating or swallowing, such as aerophagy.

phago- [Gr. *phagein* to eat] a combining form denoting relationship to ingesting or engulfing.

phagocyte (fag′o-sīt) [*phago-* + *-cyte*] a cell having a capacity to ingest microorganisms or other foreign matter, e.g., a leukocyte.

phagocytin (fag′o-si′tin) a substance contained in neutrophils, which destroys phagocytized bacteria.

phagocytosis (fag′o-si-to′sis) [*phago-* + Gr. *kytos* a hollow vessel] an immune process involving a complex biochemical mechanism, in which potentially harmful foreign macromolecules, microorganisms, metazoa, or particles are engulfed by phagocytes. Stages of the process involve the recognition of particle to be ingested, movement toward the particle (chemotaxis), attachment, ingestion, digestion, and elimination of the ingested material. During the attachment phase, the contact is established through the surface properties of the particle, e.g., hydrophobicity and surface tension, or involving the participation of receptors on the plasma membrane of the phagocyte. Most unencapsulated bacteria are rapidly destroyed, but encapsulated strains, such as pneumococcus, are taken up poorly and not destroyed rapidly. The presence of some serum proteins, e.g., complement or antibodies (opsonins) enhance the attachment of the coated bacteria. During ingestion, the phagocyte, through the process of endocytosis, takes up the particle into the cytoplasm and encloses it within a vacuole (phagosome). Actin- and myosin-like proteins appear to participate in ingestion through the formation of microfilaments. Phagosomes fuse with lysosomes and the lysosomes release their enzymes within the phagolysosome wherein digestion takes place. The remaining residual body is expelled by the process of exocytosis. Cf. *pinocytosis.* **p. promoting factor (PPF),** see OPSONIN (2).

phagolysosome (fag″o-li′so-sōm) [*phago-* + *lysosome*] a cell formed by fusion of a phagosome with a lysosome during the process of phagocytosis. See PHAGOCYTOSIS.

phagosome (fag′o-sōm) [*phago-* + Gr. *sōma* body] an intracellular vesicle in a phagocytic cell formed by the process of endocytosis, in which the plasma membrane in contact with a foreign body invaginates and becomes pinched off within the cytoplasm. See also PHAGOCYTOSIS.

-phagy see -PHAGIA.

phanero- [Gr. *phaneros* visible] a combining form meaning visible or apparent.

phanerogenic (fan″er-o-jen′ik) [*phanero-* + Gr. *gennan* to produce] having a known cause. Cf. CRYPTOGENIC.

phantasticant (fan-ta′stĭ-kant) 1. psychedelic. 2. psychedelic AGENT.

phantom (fan′tom) [Gr. *phantasma* an appearance] 1. an image or impression not evoked by actual stimuli. 2. A model of the body or of a specific part thereof. 3. a device that simulates the conditions encountered when radiation or radioactive material is deposited in vivo and permits a quantitative estimation of its effects. **heterogeneous p.,** a phantom simulating the heterogeneity of the human body. **homogeneous p.,** a phantom made of one material only.

phar., pharm. pharmacy; pharmaceutical; pharmacopeia.

PharmB 1. abbreviation for L. *Pharmaciae Baccalaureus.* 2. Bachelor of Pharmacy. See PHARMACIST.

PharC pharmaceutical chemist.

PharD Doctor of Pharmacy.

PharG Graduate in Pharmacy.

PharM Master of Pharmacy.

pharmaceutic (fahr″mah-su′tik) [Gr. *pharmakeutikos*] pertaining to pharmacy or to drugs.

pharmaceutical (fahr″mah-su′tĭ-kal) 1. pertaining to pharmacy or to drugs; pharmaceutic. 2. a medicinal drug.

pharmaceutics (fahr″mah-su′tiks) 1. pharmacy (1). 2. pharmaceutical preparations.

pharmaceutist (fahr″mah-su′tist) a pharmacist.

pharmacist (far′mah-sist) a person who is a graduate of an approved school of pharmacy and is licensed to prepare and sell or dispense drugs and compounds and to make up prescriptions. Called also *apothecary* and *druggist.*

pharmaco- [Gr. *pharmakon* medicine] a combining form denoting relationship to a drug or medicine.

pharmacochemistry (fahr″mah-ko-kem′is-tre) pharmaceutical CHEMISTRY.

pharmacodiagnosis (fahr″mah-ko-di″ag-no′sis) the employment of drugs in the diagnosis of disease.

pharmacodynamic (fahr″mah-ko-di-nam′ik) [*pharmaco-* + Gr. *dynamis* power] pertaining to the effects of medicine or drugs.

pharmacodynamics (fahr″mah-ko-di-nam′iks) the study of the action of drugs on living systems.

pharmacoendocrinology (fahr″mah-ko-en″do-kri-nol′o-je) the study of the influence of drugs on the activity of the endocrine system.

pharmacogenetics (fahr″mah-ko-jĕ-net′iks) the response of biochemical genetics to the action of drugs, and their genetically controlled variations.

pharmacognosy (fahr″mah-kog′no-se) [*pharmaco-* + Gr. *gnōsis* knowledge] that branch of pharmacology which deals with the biological, biochemical, and economic features of natural drugs and their constituents.

pharmacokinetics (fahr″mah-ko-ki-net′iks) the study of the action of a drug in the body over a period of time, including the process of absorption, distribution, localization in tissue, biotransformation, and excretion.

pharmacologic (fahr″mah-ko-loj′ik) pertaining to pharmacology or to the properties of and reactions to drugs.

pharmacologist (fahr″mah-kol′o-jist) one who makes a study of the action of drugs.

pharmacology (fahr″mah-kol′o-je) the science which deals with the study of the action of drugs on living systems.

pharmacometrics (fahr″mah-ko-met′riks) [*pharmaco-* + Gr. *metron* measure] the comparative evaluation of drug activity, distinguished from bioassay in that substances with different chemical constitutions are compared.

pharmacopedia, pharmacopedics (fahr″mah-ko-pe′de-ah, fahr″mah-ko-pe′diks) [*pharmaco-* + Gr. *paideia* instruction] the science which deals with the properties and preparation of drugs.

pharmacopeia (fahr″mah-ko-pe′ah) [*pharmaco-* + Gr. *poiein* to make] an authoritative treatise on drugs and their preparations; a book containing a list of products used in medicine, with descriptions, chemical tests for determining identity and purity, and formulas for certain mixtures of these substances. It also generally contains a statement of average dosage. Written also *pharmacopoeia.* See USP. **United States P.,** see USP.

pharmacopeial (fahr″mah-ko-pe′al) pertaining to or recognized by a pharmacopeia.

pharmacophore (fahr″mah-ko-for″) [*pharmaco-* + Gr. *phoros* bearing] the group of atoms in a drug molecule which is responsible for the action of the compound.

pharmacopoeia (fahr-mah-ko-pe′ah) pharmacopeia.

pharmacoradiography (fahr″mah-ko-ra″de-o-og′rah-fe) pharmacoroentgenography.

pharmacoroentgenography (fahr″mah-ko-rent″gen-og′rah-fe) roentgenographic examination of a body organ under the influence of a drug which best facilitates such examination.

pharmacotherapeutics (fahr″mah-ko-ther″ah-pu′tiks) the study of the uses of drugs in the treatment of disease.

pharmacotherapy (fahr″mah-ko-ther′ah-pe) the treatment of disease by drugs.

pharmacy (fahr′mah-se) [Gr. *pharmakon* medicine] 1. the art of preparing, compounding, and dispensing medicines. 2. a place fo the preparation, compounding, and dispensing of drugs and medicinal supplies; a drugstore or apothecary's shop. **chemical p.,** pharmaceutical CHEMISTRY.

pharyngalgia (far″in-gal′je-ah) [*pharyngo-* + *-algia*] pain in the pharynx; pharyngodynia.

pharyngeal (fah-rin′je-al) [L. *pharyngeus*] pertaining to the pharynx.

pharyngectomy (far″in-jek′to-me) [*pharyngo-* + Gr. *ektomē* excision] excision of the pharynx.

pharyngemphraxis (far″in-jem-frak′sis) [*pharyngo-* + Gr. *emphraxis* stoppage] obstruction of the pharynx.

pharyngeus (far-in′je-us) [L.] pharyngeal.

pharyngismus (far″in-jiz′mus) muscular spasm of the pharynx.

pharyngitic (far″in-jit′ik) affected with or of the nature of pharyngitis.

pharyngitis (far″in-ji′tis) [*pharyngo-* + *-itis*] inflammation of the pharynx. **acute p.,** inflammation with pain in the throat, especially on swallowing, dryness, followed by moisture of the pharynx, congestion of the mucous membrane, and fever. Called also *catarrhal p.* and *angina catarrhalis.* See also CORYZA. **aphthous p.,** herpangina. **atrophic p.,** a chronic pharyngitis which leads to wasting of the submucous tissue accompanied by dryness and thickened secretions. **catarrhal p.,** acute p. **chronic p.,** that which results from repeated acute attacks or is due to tuberculosis or syphilis; it is attended with excessive secretion, and in the severe ulcerated forms by pain and dysphagia. **croupous p.,** membranous p. **diphtheric p.,** pharyngeal DIPHTHERIA. **follicular p.,** sore throat with enlargement of the pharyngeal glands. Called also *glandular p.* **gangrenous p.,** that characterized by gangrenous patches. **glandular p.,** follicular p. **gonococcal p.,** that due to infection with *Neisseria gonorrhoeae,* transmitted through oral or orogenital contact with a person having gonorrheal infection. The throat may show diffuse erythema and edema, with or without small punctate pustules in the tonsillar area and uvula. In some instances, the condition is asymptomatic, the presence of infection being demonstrated only through throat cultures. See also GONORRHEA. **granular p.,** chronic pharyngitis in which the mucous membrane becomes granular. **p. herpet′ica,** membranous or aphthous sore throat; a form of acute pharyngitis characterized by the formation of vesicles, which give place to excoriations. Called also *benign croupous angina.* **hypertrophic p.,** a chronic form which leads to thickening of the submucous tissues. **p. kerato′sa,** pharyngomycosis. **membranous p.,** that with a fibrous exudate leading to the formation of a false membrane. Called also *croupous p.* **phlegmonous p.,** acute parenchymatous tonsillitis attended with the formation of abscesses. **p. sic′ca,** an atrophic pharyngitis in which the throat becomes dry. **p. ulcero′sa,** the formation of ulcers covered by yellow, membrane-like deposits in the pharynx, with fever, pain, and prostration. Called also *angina nosocomii.* **vesicular p., p. vesicula′ris,** herpangina.

pharyngo- [Gr. *pharynx* pharynx] a combining form denoting relationship to the pharynx.

pharyngoamygdalitis (fah-ring″go-ah-mig″dah-li′tis) pharyngitis associated with tonsillitis.

pharyngocele (fah-ring′go-sēl) [*pharyngo-* + Gr. *kēlē* hernia] hernial protrusion of a part of the pharynx; a hernial pouch or other cystic deformity of the pharynx.

pharyngodynia (fah-ring″go-din′e-ah) [*pharyngo-* + Gr. *odynē* pain] pain in the pharynx; pharyngalgia.

pharyngoepiglottic (fah-ring″go-ep″ĭ-glot′ik) pertaining to the pharynx and epiglottis.

pharyngoesophageal (fah-ring″go-e-sof″ah-je″al) pertaining to the pharynx and esophagus.

pharyngoglossus (fah-ring″go-glos′us) the muscular fibers from the superior constrictor of the pharynx to the tongue.

pharyngolaryngeal (fah-ring″go-lah-rin′je-al) pertaining to the pharynx and the larynx.

pharyngolaryngitis (fah-ring″go-lar″in-ji′tis) [*pharyngo-* + *larynx* + *-itis*] pharyngitis associated with laryngitis.

pharyngolith (fah-ring′go-lith) [*pharyngo-* + Gr. *lithos* stone] a concretion in the pharynx.

pharyngolysis (far″ing-gol′ĭ-sis) [*pharyngo-* + Gr. *lysis* dissolution] paralysis of the pharynx.

pharyngomaxillary (fah-ring″go-mak′sĭ-ler″e) pertaining to the pharynx and the maxillae.

pharyngomycosis (fah-ring″go-mi-ko′sis) [*pharyngo-* + *mycosis*] any fungal disease of the pharynx. Called also *pharyngitis keratosa.*

pharyngonasal (fah-ring″go-na′sal) pertaining to the pharynx and the nose.

pharyngo-oral (fah-ring″go-o′ral) pertaining to the pharynx and mouth.

pharyngopalatine (fah-ring″go-pal′ah-tīn) pertaining to the pharynx and the palate.

pharyngopalatinus (fah-ring″go-pal′ah-tīn′us) palatopharyngeal MUSCLE.

pharyngopathy (far″ing-gop′ah-the) [*pharyngo-* + Gr. *pathos* disease] disease of the pharynx.

pharyngoperistole (fah-ring″go-pĕ-ris′to-le) [*pharyngo-* + Gr. *peristolē* contracture] narrowing of the pharynx.

pharyngoplasty (fah-ring″go-plas′te) [*pharyngo-* + Gr. *plassein* to form] plastic surgery of the pharynx. **Hynes p.**, a technique of pharyngoplasty accomplished by muscle transposition.

pharyngoplegia (far″ing-go-ple′je-ah) [*pharyngo-* + Gr. *plēgē* stroke] paralysis of the pharynx.

pharyngorhinitis (fah-ring″go-ri-ni′tis) [*pharyngo-* + *rhinitis*] inflammation of the nasopharynx; nasopharyngitis.

pharyngorhinoscopy (fah-ring″go-ri-nos′ko-pe) [*pharyngo-* + *rhino-* + Gr. *skopein* to examine] examination of the rhinopharynx with a rhinoscope.

pharyngorrhagia (far″ing-go-ra′je-ah) [*pharyngo-* + Gr. *rhēgnynai* to break forth] hemorrhage from the pharynx.

pharyngorrhea (far″ing-go-re′ah) [*pharyngo-* + Gr. *rhoia* flow] a discharge of mucus from the pharynx.

pharyngosalpingitis (fah-ring″go-sal″pin-ji′tis) inflammation of the pharynx and the auditory tube.

pharyngoscope (fah-ring′go-skōp) [*pharyngo-* + Gr. *skopein* to examine] an instrument for examination of the pharynx.

pharyngoscopy (far″ing-gos′ko-pe) [*pharyngo-* + Gr. *skopein* to examine] direct visual examination of the pharynx.

pharyngospasm (fah-ring′go-spazm) [*pharyngo-* + Gr. *spasmos* spasm] spasm of the pharynx.

pharyngostenosis (fah-ring″go-ste-no′sis) [*pharyngo-* + Gr. *stenosis* narrowing] narrowing or stenosis of the lumen of the pharynx.

pharyngostoma (fah″ring-gos′to-mah) [*pharyngo-* + Gr. *stoma* mouth] the opening formed by pharyngostomy.

pharyngostomy (fah″ring-gos′to-me) [*pharyngo-* + Gr. *stomoun* to provide an opening, or mouth] the surgical creation of an artificial opening into the pharynx.

pharyngotherapy (fah-ring″go-ther′ah-pe) the treatment of pharyngeal disorders, especially the irrigation of the nasopharynx in infectious diseases.

pharyngotome (fah-ring′go-tōm) a cutting instrument used in pharyngeal surgery.

pharyngotomy (far″ing-got′o-me) [*pharyngo-* + Gr. *tomē* a cutting] surgical incision of the pharynx.

pharyngotonsillitis (fah-ring″go-ton″sĭ-li′tis) pharyngitis associated with tonsillitis.

pharyngoxerosis (fah-ring″go-ze-ro′sis) [*pharyngo-* + Gr. *xērōsis* dryness] dryness of the pharynx.

pharynx (far′inks) [Gr. "the throat"] [NA] a part of the digestive tube made up of mucous, fibrous, and muscular coats, which forms a sac between the mouth and nares and the esophagus. It is continuous below with the esophagus and it communicates above with the larynx, mouth, nasal passages, and auditory tubes. The part above the level of the soft palate is the *nasopharynx*, communicating with the posterior nares and the auditory tube. The lower portion consists of the *oropharynx*, which lies between the soft palate and the upper edge of the epiglottis, and the *laryngopharynx*, which lies below the upper edge of the epiglottis and opens into the larynx and esophagus. It is separated from the mouth by the soft palate and the uvula, which hangs from the top of the back of the mouth, above the root of the tongue. In swallowing, the uvula lifts up, closing the nasopharynx as food passes from the mouth to the esophagus; at the same time, the pharynx is drawn upward and dilated to receive food, and after the bolus is received, the muscles relax and it descends to allow food to be conveyed into the esophagus. Pharyngeal muscles include the constrictor inferior, medius, and superior, and the stylopharyngeus, salpingopharyngeus, and palatopharyngeus muscles. **laryngeal p.**, laryngopharynx. **nasal p.**, nasopharynx. **oral p.**, oropharynx.

phase (fāz) [Gr. *phasis* an appearance] 1. the view that a thing presents to the eye. 2. any one of the varying aspects or stages through which a disease or process may pass. 3. any physically or chemically distinct, homogenous, and mechanically separable part of a system, e.g., the ice and steam phases of water. 4. the fraction of a whole period of an oscillatory motion which has elapsed since the motion last passed through its null position in a positive direction. 5. a stage in solidification processes. **α-p.**, α-solid SOLUTION. **β-p.**, β-solid SOLUTION. **continuous p.**, that portion of a colloid system in which the disperse phase (the

analogue of the solute in solution) is dispersed; it is analogous to the solvent in a solution. Called also *dispersion, disperse,* or *dispersive medium.* **p. diagram,** phase DIAGRAM. **discontinuous p.,** disperse p. **disperse p.,** the internal or discontinuous portion of a colloid system; it is analogous to the solute in a solution. Called also *discontinuous p.* and *internal p.* **functional p. (of tooth eruption),** see eruptive STAGE (2). **γ-p.,** a solid phase of an alloy entering an amalgam system. In dental amalgam, it is the solid phase of the silver-tin alloy, Ag_3Sn, which forms the core for the amalgam when mixed with mercury. Two phases are formed during the process of mixing (trituration): the γ_1-phase which crystallizes as a body-centered cubic structure with the formula Ag_2Hg_3, and the γ_2-phase which has a hexagonal space lattice, with the formula $Sn_{7-8}Hg$. The $\gamma_1 + \gamma_2$ phases form a matrix around the original particles, thereby inducing hardening. Trituration abrades off the surface of the alloy particles to permit the mercury to react. **inductive p.,** latent PERIOD (2). **internal p.,** disperse p. **prefunctional p. (of tooth eruption),** see eruptive STAGE (2). **resting p.,** former term for INTERPHASE or INTERKINESIS. **synaptic p.,** zygotene.

Phasealloy trademark for a *high copper alloy* (see under ALLOY).

PHC premolar aplasia, hyperhidrosis, canities prematura; see Böök's SYNDROME.

Phe phenylalanine.

Phebuzine trademark for *phenylbutazone.*

Phemerol trademark for *benzethonium chloride* (see under BENZETHONIUM).

phen- in chemical nomenclature, a prefix derived from *phenol,* indicating a benzene derivative.

phenacaine hydrochloride (fen′ah-kān) a local anesthetic, *N,N′*-bis(*p*-ethoxyphenyl)acetamidine hydrochloride, occurring as odorless, bitter, white crystals that are soluble in alcohol, boiling water, and chloroform. Used topically in ophthalmology. Also used in dental preparations, such as root canal dressings. Trademarks: Holocaine, Tanicaine.

phenacemide (fĕ-nas′ĕ-mīd) an anticonvulsant, *N*-(aminocarbonyl)benzeneacetamide, occurring as a white, odorless, crystalline powder that is slightly soluble in ethanol, acetone, chloroform, and ether and is insoluble in water. Used in severe forms of epilepsy. Adverse effects may include gastrointestinal disorders, anorexia, weight loss, headache, drowsiness, insomnia, vertigo, paresthesias, mental changes, blood dyscrasias, and nephritis. Called also *phenylacetylurea.* Trademark: Phenurone.

phenacetin (fĕ-nas′ĕ-tin) an analgesic and antipyretic drug with minor anti-inflammatory properties, *N*-(4-ethoxyphenyl)-acetamide, occurring as a white, odorless, slightly bitter, crystalline powder or scales that are soluble in water, ethanol, ether, chloroform, and boiling water. Used in the treatment of mild pain of the musculoskeletal system, and included in various proprietary analgesic preparations. Excessive use may cause renal damage. Called also *acetophenetidin, acetphenetidin, para-acetphenetidin, p-acetophenetide, p-ethoxyacetanilide.*

phenacetylurea (fĕ-nas′ĕ-til-u-re′ah) phenacemide.

Phenadone trademark for the *dl*-form of *methadone hydrochloride* (see under METHADONE).

phenadoxone hydrochloride (fen″ah-dok′sōn) a narcotic analgesic, 6-morpholino-4,4-diphenyl-3-heptanone hydrochloride, occurring as a crystalline substance that is soluble in water, methanol, ethanol, and chloroform, slightly soluble in acetone, and insoluble in ethyl acetate, acetate, and benzene. Abuse may lead to addiction. Called also *heptazone hydrochloride,* and *morphodone hydrochloride.* Trademarks: Heptalgin, Heptalin, Supralgin.

phenanthrene (fe-nan′thrēn) a tricyclic aromatic hydrocarbon, $C_{14}H_{10}$, derived from coal tar, occurring as colorless shining crystals that are soluble in alcohol, ether, benzene, carbon disulfide, and acetic acid, but are insoluble in water. Used in the production of drugs, dyestuffs, and other substances and in biochemical research. Contact may cause photosensitization of the skin. It is suspected of having carcinogenic properties. **p. ring,** phenanthrene RING.

Phenantoin trademark for *mephenytoin.*

Phenaphen trademark for an analgesic preparation containing aspirin, phenacetin, phenobarbital, and hyoscyamine sulfate.

phenazacillin (fen″ah-zah-sil′in) hetacillin.

Phenazine trademark for *phendimetrazine tartrate* (see under PHENDIMETRAZINE).

phenazocine (fĕ-naz′o-sēn) a nonopiate, addicting analgesic, 1,2,3,4,5,6-hexahydro-6,11-dimethyl-3-(2-phenethyl)-2,6-methano-benzazocin-8-ol. Called also *phenethylazocaine* and *phenobenzorphan*. **p. hydrobromide,** the hydrobromide salt of phenazocine, occurring as a white powder that is soluble in ethanol, water, and acetone, but not in ether and carbon tetrachloride. Used in pre- and postoperative medication and in controlling painful conditions. Nausea, vomiting, constipation, and, less commonly, respiratory depression, hypotension, bradycardia, tachycardia, vertigo, and pruritus are potential side reactions. Trademarks: Narphen, Prinadol, Xenagol.

phenazone (fen′ah-zōn) antipyrine.

phencyclidine (fen-si′klī-dēn) an anesthetic, 1-(1-phenylcyclohexy)piperidine. Used therapeutically in the form of the hydrochloride salt, which occurs as a white to creamy white, odorless, bitter, crystalline powder or granules, that are freely soluble in water, alcohol, and chloroform, and sparingly soluble in dilute hydrochloric acid. Used to produce general and, more commonly, basal anesthesia. Restlessness, disorientation, tremor, euphoria, hypersalivation, anxiety, convulsions, hyperpnea, respiratory and cardiac arrest, emesis, hypothermia, shock, and death are the potential side effects. Trademark: Sernyl and Sernylan.

Phendextro trademark for *dexchlorpheniramine maleate* (see under DEXCHLORPHENIRAMINE).

(phendimetrazine tartrate (fen″di-met′rah-zēn) an indirectly acting sympathomimetic agent with predominantly central nervous stimulant actions, (+)3,4-dimethyl-2-phenylmorpholine tartrate, occurring as a white, odorless, bitter, crystalline powder that is soluble in methanol and ethanol. Used as an appetite depressant. Side effects may include insomnia, irritability, vertigo, headache, glossitis, xerostomia, headache, tachycardia, cardiac arrhythmias, hypertension, abdominal discomfort, nausea, constipation, urinary disorders, and cystitis. Trademarks: Adophen, Bacarate, Obepar, Phenazine, Reducto, Statobex.

phene (fēn) see CHARACTER (3).

Phenedrine trademark for *amphetamine.*

phenelzine sulfate (fen′el-zēn) a monoamine oxidase inhibitor, (2-phenethyl)hydrazine, occurring as a white to yellowish powder with a specific odor, which is soluble in water and insoluble in organic solvents. Used in the treatment of mental depression. Adverse reactions are similar to those of other monoamine oxidase inhibitors. Trademarks: Nardil, Phenodyn.

Phenergan (fen′er-gan) trademark for *promethazine.*

phenethicillin (fĕ-neth″ī-sil′in) a semisynthetic penicillin, 3,3-dimethyl-7-oxo-6-[(1-oxo-2-phenoxypropyl)amino]-4-thia-1-azabicyclo[3,2,0]heptane-2-carboxylic acid. Used therapeutically in the form of the potassium salt, occurring as colorless, moderately hygroscopic crystals that are freely soluble in water, in the treatment of infections caused by penicillinase-producing bacteria, particularly staphylococcal infections. Its actions and toxicity are similar to those of other penicillins. Called also *penicillin MV, penicillin-152,* and *phenoxymethyl penicillin.* Trademarks: Alfacillin, Alpen, Feneticilline, Maxipen, α-Oracillin, Synapen, Syncillin.

phenethylazocine (fen-eth″il-az′o-sēn) phenazocine.

phenformin hydrochloride (fen-for′min) an oral hypoglycemic, N-(2-phenylethyl)-imidodicarbonimidic diamide monohydrochloride, occurring as a white, odorless, bitter, crystalline powder that is soluble in water and ethanol, but not in chloroform and ether. It increases the clearance of insulin into muscle and thus promotes muscle glucose uptake. Used in the treatment of diabetes mellitus. Also used to lower blood cholesterol and triglyceride levels in myocardial infarction. Adverse effects may include metallic taste, anorexia, nausea, vomiting, lactic acidosis, and ethanol intolerance. Weight loss, asthenia, and ketonuria may occur. Trademarks: Dipar, Meltrol.

Phenidylate trademark for *methylphenidate.*

phenindamine (fĕ-nin′dah-mēn) a weak antihistaminic drug that blocks histamine medication at the H₁ receptor, 2,3,4,9-tetrahydro-2-methyl-9-phenyl-1H-indeno[2,1-c]pyridine. Used therapeutically in the form of the tartrate salt, occurring as a white powder with a faint odor, which is soluble in water and alcohol, but not in chloroform, ether, and benzene. Used in the treatment of allergic diseases. Side effects may include nervousness, nausea, arrhythmia, vomiting, and insomnia. Trademark: Thephorin.

phenindione (fen-in′di-ōn) an oral prothrombopenic anticoagulant, 2-phenyl-1,3-indandione, occurring as white, crystalline powder with a slight odor, which is soluble in chloroform, methanol, and alkali hydroxide solutions, but not in water. Used in the treatment and prevention of thromboembolic diseases. Headache, fever, malaise, rash, pyrexia, leukopenia, erythematous lesions, renal lesions, albuminuria, diarrhea, hepatitis, agranulocytosis, and hypersensitivity are some of the potential side reactions. Spontaneous gingival bleeding and hemorrhagic complications in surgical patients may occur. Trademarks: Athrombon, Danilone, Hedulin, Indema, Thrombasal.

pheniprazine (fen-ip′rah-zēn) an antihypertensive agent, (1-methyl-2-phenylethyl)hydrazine.

phenmetrazine hydrochloride (fen-met′rah-zēn) a sympathomimetic agent with central actions, 3-methyl-2-phenylmorpholine hydrochloride, occurring as a white, crystalline powder that is soluble in water, ethanol, and chloroform. Used as an appetite depressant. It is potentially addictive. Trademarks: Marsin, Preludin.

phenobarbital (fe″no-bar′bĭ-tal) a long-acting barbiturate, hypnotic, and sedative, 5-phenyl-5-ethylbarbituric acid. It occurs as white, odorless crystals or white crystalline powder, which may exhibit polymorphism, and is soluble in water, alcohol, chloroform, and ether. Used in the treatment of epilepsy, psychoneurotic states, hypertension, gastrointestinal disorders, and coronary disease. Also used in preoperative and postoperative medication. It is an addictive drug. Adverse reactions may include skin rash and eruptions of the oral mucosa. Generally, indications and contraindications are those of other barbiturates. Called also *phenobarbitone* and *phenylethylmalonylurea.* Trademarks: Gardinal, Luminal. **p. sodium,** the sodium salt of phenobarbital, occurring as white, bitter, odorless, hygroscopic, flaky crystals or crystalline granules or powder, which is very soluble in water, readily soluble in alcohol, and insoluble in ether and chloroform. On exposure to air, it decomposes rapidly with the formation of free phenobarbital. Its uses, indications, contraindications, and side reactions are the same as those of phenobarbital and other barbiturates. Called also *soluble p.* and *phenobarbitone sodium.* **soluble p.,** p. sodium.

phenobarbitone (fe″no-bar′bĭ-tōn) British name for phenobarbital. **p. sodium,** phenobarbital SODIUM.

phenobenzorphan (fe″no-benz′or-fan) phenazocine.

Phenodyn trademark for *phenelzine sulfate* (see under PHENELZINE).

phenol (fe′nol) 1. a highly toxic and caustic substance, $C_6H_5 \cdot OH$, obtained by the distillation of coal tar, occurring as colorless to light pink needles or a crystalline mass with a characteristic odor, which darkens on exposure to light, and is soluble in water, ethanol, glycerol, chloroform, ether, and oils. In the solid state, used to cauterize and whiten the skin and mucous membranes. It is liquefied by the addition of 10 percent water. Used as a germicidal, antipruritic, local anesthetic, and radiopaque agent; now largely replaced by less toxic substances. Also used to cauterize small wounds and bites. In dentistry, used chiefly for sterilization and disinfection and in the preparation of mouthwashes. Phenol produces a flammable vapor and may cause severe chemical burns of the skin and mucous membranes. Called also *carbolic acid, phenylic acid,* and *phenylic alcohol.* 2. any organic compound containing one or more hydroxyl groups attached to an aromatic or carbon ring.

phenolphthalein (fe″nol-thal′ē-in) an irritant cathartic agent, 3,3-bis(4-hydroxyphenyl)-1-(3H)-isobenzofuranone, occurring as a white to yellowish, odorless, crystalline powder that is soluble in ethanol and ether, but not in water. It is a component of several proprietary laxatives. Also used as an indicator in titration for mineral and organic acids, most alkalis, some alkaloids, and other substances in biochemical analysis. Trademark: Laxin.

phenomenon (fe-nom′ĕ-non), pl. *phenom′ena* [Gr. *phainomenon* thing seen] any sign or objective symptom; any observable occurrence or fact. See also REACTION, SIGN, SYMPTOM, and TEST. **Arthus p.,** Arthus REACTION. **Bell's p.,** an outward and upward movement of the eyes during attempted closure of the eyelids, occurring in some forms of facial paralysis. **blanching p.,** development of a white zone when the skin of a normal person is gently stroked with a broad flat instrument or is gently stretched, caused by direct vasoconstriction of the superficial blood vessels of the skin. **Bordet-Gengou p.,** complement FIXATION. **Danysz's p.,** toxin in carefully calibrated amounts will be neutralized by antitoxin when mixed all at once, but when the same amount of toxin is added in divided portions there is a decrease of the neutralizing influence of the antitoxin. **dental p.,** thermal and tactile sensations in the gingiva with toothache, produced by repeated foradic stimulation of hyperesthetic lines in the body. **Gunn's p.,** Gunn's SYNDROME. **Koch p.,** increased specific reactivity to antigens of the tubercle bacillus during the course of tuberculous disease. It was observed by Koch on rechallenge of already infected guinea pigs with tubercle bacilli, and represents a cellular hypersensitivity response analogous to the tuberculin reaction. **LE p.,** see LE CELL. **Marcus Gunn's p.,** Gunn's SYNDROME. **Pfeiffer's p.,** cholera vibrios, introduced into the peritoneal cavity of a guinea pig that has been immunized against cholera, lose their motility and disintegrate. The disintegration can be followed under the microscope by removing a portion of the peritoneal contents from time to time. The same result is observed if a bacteriolytic serum (against cholera) is introduced along with the bacteria into the peritoneal cavity of a normal guinea pig. **prezone p., prozone p.,** prozone. **Shwartzman p., Shwartzman-Sanarelli p.,** a nonimmunologic inflammatory reaction resulting in hemorrhage and necrosis of certain organs after injection of endotoxin into animals presensitized 6 to 48 hours earlier by a primary injection of endotoxin. **sickling p.,** the appearance of sickle-shaped erythrocytes in the blood due to the presence of sickle cell hemoglobin which is insoluble and causes the formation of tactoids (doubly-refracting rodlike particles) when oxygen tension and pH of the blood are reduced. The phenomenon is the principal symptom of sickle cell anemia. **Simonsen p.,** splenomegaly induced in animals due to a graft-versus-host reaction. Simonsen first reported the response in young chickens by injecting 18-day-old embryos intravenously with adult fowl leukocytes. **Theobald Smith's p.,** guinea pigs which have been used for standardizing diphtheria antitoxin and have thus been injected with a small dose of blood serum become highly susceptible to the serum and may die very promptly if given a rather large second dose of the same serum a few weeks later. See ANAPHYLAXIS. **Tyndall p.,** a path of light through a heterogeneous medium is made visible by the solid particles, as a beam of light passed through a colloidal solution is made visible by the reflection of light from the moving colloidal particles, or a sunbeam in air due to suspended particles. Called also *Tyndall effect.*

Phenopenicillin trademark for *penicillin V.*

phenothiazine (fe″no-thi′ah-zēn) a compound, thiodiphenylamine, occurring as yellow, rhombic leaflets or diamond-shaped plates that are readily soluble in benzene, ether, and hot acetic acid and are slightly soluble in alcohol and mineral oil. Used chiefly as an insecticide, anthelmintic, and urinary antiseptic drug. Side effects may include agranulocytosis, toxic hepatitis, hemolytic anemia, tachycardia, and abdominal cramps. Derivatives of phenothiazine have a wide variety of pharmacological properties, including gangliolytic, adrenolytic, antifibrillatory, antiedema, antipyretic, antishock, anticonvulsant, and antiemetic properties. They also enhance the activity of analgesic and sedative and hypnotic drugs. Chlorpromazine is the prototype of the phenodiazines.

phenotype (fe′no-tīp) [Gr. *phainein* to show + *typos* type] the observable expression of the constitution, including the physical, biochemical, and physiological nature of an individual, as determined by hereditary factors (the genotype) and environmental influences. See also TRAIT (2). **K⁰ p.,** a very rare phenotype, the possessors of which appear to lack all detectable Kell antigens. K⁰ individuals are K-k-KP (a−b−) Js(a−b−), but some have a rare antibody (called *anti-Ku* or *anti-K5*), which reacts with every Kell phenotype except K⁰. See Kell blood groups, under BLOOD GROUP. **McLeod p.,** a phenotype in the Kell blood groups (see under BLOOD GROUP), being probably a genetic defect in a gene unrelated to the Kell locus, but whose action or product is required for the expression of Kell antigens.

phenoxy- in chemical nomenclature, a prefix indicating the presence of the group OC₆H₅, composed of phenyl and an atom of oxygen.

phenoxybenzamine (fe-nok″se-ben′zah-mēn) a haloalkylamine preparation, N-(2-chloroethyl)-N-(1-methyl-2-phenoxyethyl)-benzylamine, occurring as a white, crystalline, odorless powder that is soluble in water, alcohol, and chloroform, but not in ether. It is an α-adrenergic blocking drug, used as the hydrochloride salt in the treatment of Raynaud's disease, acrocyanosis, frostbite, phlebitis, thrombophlebitis, diabetic gangrene, causalgia, skin ulcers, malignant hypertension, vascular collapse, and vasospastic diseases. Side effects may include drowsiness, postural hypotension, stuffy nose, gastric irritation, vomiting, convulsions, and shock. The drug combines irreversibly with the smooth muscle adrenergic receptors and its action may last for several days. Trademarks: Dibenyline, Dibenzyline.

phenoxymethylpenicillin (fe-nok″se-meth″il-pen″i-sil′in) penicillin V.

phenoxypropanediol (fe-nok″se-pro-pan″e-di′ōl) one of the first substances used as a centrally acting muscle relaxant, 3-phenoxy-1,2-propanediol. Trademark: Antodyne.

phensuximide (fen-suk′sī-mīd) an anticonvulsant drug, 1-methyl-3-phenyl-2,5-pyrrolidinedione, occurring as a white, odorless, crystalline powder that is soluble in ethanol and slightly souble in water and chloroform. Used in the treatment of some types of epilepsy. Side effects may include nausea, vomiting, anorexia, weakness, drowsiness, ataxia, lethargy, pruritus, skin rashes, erythema multiforme, hematuria, granulocytopenia, leukopenia, and pancytopenia. Trademarks: Milontin, Mirontin, Succitimal.

phentermine (fen′ter-mēn) sympathomimetic agent with weak cardiovascular and central actions, α,α-dimethylbenzene-ethanamine, occurring as a colorless, mobile, oily liquid with an amine-like odor, that is soluble in chloroform, ether, ethanol, dilute acids and, slightly, water. Used as an appetite depressant. It is potentially addictive. **p. hydrochloride,** the hydrochloric salt of phentermine, occurring as a white, odorless, crystalline powder that is soluble in water, chloroform, and ethanol, slightly soluble in acetone and benzene, and insoluble in ether. Its properties are similar to those of the parent compound. Trademarks: Fastin, Wilpo.

phentolamine (fen-tol′ah-mēn) an adrenergic blocking agent, 2-[N-(m-hydroxyphenyl)-p-toluidinomethyl]imidazole, occurring as a white or slightly grayish, crystalline, odorless powder that is soluble in water and alcohol and slightly soluble in chloroform and ether. Used in the form of the hydrochloride and mesylate salts as a diagnostic aid in pheochromocytoma, in the treatment of hypertension, and in the prevention of skin necrosis from extravasation of norepinephrine. Formerly used in the treatment of Raynaud's disease, arterial spasms, and arterial occlusion. Flushing, tachycardia, orthostatic hypotension, cardiac arrhythmias, stuffy nose, gastrointestinal disorders, and physical weakness are the most common complications. Trademark: Regitine.

Phenurone trademark for *phenacemide.*

phenyl (fen′il, fe′nil) a univalent radical, C₆H₅.

phenylalanine (fen″il-al′ah-nin) an aromatic, naturally occurring amino acid that is essential for certain nitrogen metabolic processes in humans, 2-amino-3-phenylpropionic acid. It is also found in the saliva. Abbreviated *Phe.* See also amino ACID.

phenylbutazone (fen″il-bu′tah-zōn) an aminopyrine antipyretic, analgesic, and anti-inflammatory agent with mild uricosuric effects, 4-butyl-1,2-diphenyl-3,5-pyrazolidinedione, occurring as a white, crystalline powder that is soluble in ethanol, acetone, and ether, and slightly soluble in water. Used in the treatment of gout, rheumatoid arthritis, rheumatoid spondylitis, osteoarthritis, psoriatic arthritis, and thrombophlebitis. Side effects may include agranulocytosis, nausea, edema, reactivation of peptic ulcer, water retention, skin rash, epigastric distress, vertigo, stomatitis, hepatitis, hypertension, psychotic disorders, leukopenia, thrombocytopenia, central nervous system stimulation, anemia, lethargy, constipation, diarrhea, hemorrhagic disorders, fever, and cardiac arrhythmias. Trademarks: Antadol, Butadion, Fenibutol, Buzon, Fenibutol, Phebuzine, Reudox.

phenylephrine hydrochloride (fen″il-ef-rin) a sympathomimetic drug, l-1-(m-hydroxyphenyl)-2-methylaminoethanol hydrochloride, occurring as a white, bitter, odorless, crystalline solid that is soluble in water and ethanol. It has strong α-adrenergic and weak β-adrenergic properties, activating blood pressure through arteriolar constriction. Used in the treatment of paroxysmal atrial tachycardia, as a local vasoconstrictor in solutions of local anesthetics, as a mydriatic, nasal decongestant, and pressor agent in hypotensive states. It has a potential value in reducing blood loss in oral surgery. Hypotensive crises, cardiac arrhythmias, pallor, respiratory distress, weakness, and anginal pain in cardiac patients are the principal adverse reactions. Trademarks: Adrianol, Isophrin, Meta-Synephrine, Metazon. Mexatol, Neo-Synephrine.

phenylethylene (fen″il-eth′i-lēn) styrene.

phenylethylmalonylurea (fen′il-meth″il-mal′o-nil-u-re′ah) phenobarbital.

phenylketonuria (fen″il-ke″to-nu′re-ah) an inborn error of me-. tabolism, transmitted as an autosomal recessive trait, attributable to a deficiency of or a defect in phenylalanine hydrolase, the enzyme that catalyzes the conversion of phenylalanine to tyrosine, resulting in accumulation of phenylalanine and its metabolic products in the body fluids. It results in mental retardation, neurologic manifestations (e.g., hyperkinesia, epilepsy, and microcephaly), light pigmentation, eczema, and a mousy odor, unless treated with diets low in phenylalanine. Affected patients, who are usually blond and blue-eyed, may suffer poor coordination, tremor, dystonia, and athetoid movements. Their head circumference averages nearly 2 cm less than normal. Prominent maxillae, wide interdental spaces, and enamel hypoplasia may occur. Two types of the disease have been recognized: the usual variant, in which patients tolerate higher levels of phenylalanine in the diet, and a transient variant, in which tolerance increases during infancy and early childhood. Abbreviated *PKU*. Called also *Følling's disease, phenylpyruvic imbecility, phenylpyruvic oligophrenia,* and *phenyluria*. See also PKU SCREENING.

phenylmercuric (fen″il-mer-ku′rik) denoting a compound containing the radical C_6H_5Hg-, some of which have bacteriostatic and bactericidal properties. **p. acetate,** phenylmercuric ACETATE. **p. nitrate** phenylmercuric NITRATE.

phenylpropanolamine hydrochloride (fen″il-pro″pah-nol′am-in) an indirectly acting sympathomimetic agent with strong adrenergic and weak central stimulant effects, α-(1-aminoethyl)benzenemethanol hydrochloride. It occurs as a white, photosensitive, crystalline powder with a slight aromatic odor, which is soluble in water and ethanol, but not in ether. Used chiefly as a nasal decongestant in hay fever and bronchodilator in bronchial asthma. Side effects may include restlessness, insomnia, headache, nausea, cardiac arrhythmia, and hypertension. Trademarks: Mydriatine, Propadrine.

phenylpropylmethylamine hydrochloride (fen″il-pro″pil-meth″il-am′ēn) a sympathomimetic with vasoconstrictor actions, *N,β*-dimethylphenethylamine hydrochloride, occurring as a volatile liquid that is freely soluble in ethanol, ether, and benzene, but not in water. Used as a nasal decongestant. Elevated blood pressure and excessive nervousness may occur. Trademark: Vonedrine.

phenyluria (fen″il-u′re-ah) [*phenyl-* + *-uria*] presence of phenyl in the urine. See PHENYLKETONURIA.

phenytoin (fen′ī-to-in) an anticonvulsant and cardiac depressant, 5,5-diphenyl-2,4-imidazolidinedion, occurring as a white, odorless powder that is soluble in hot ethanol, slightly soluble in cold ethanol, ether, and chloroform, and insoluble in water. Used in the treatment of epilepsy and as an antiarrhythmic. Side reactions may include nystagmus, diplopia, mydriasis, vertigo, confusion, slurring of speech, ataxia, tremor, nausea, vomiting, constipation, scarlatiniform and morbilliform skin rashes, exfoliative or purpuric dermatitis, lupus erythematosus, Stevens-Johnson syndrome, thrombocytopenia, leukopenia, agranulocytosis, granulocytopenia, pancytopenia, susceptibility to infection, liver damage, hirsutism, and gingival hyperplasia. Called also *diphenylhydantoin*. Trademark: Dilantin. See also Dilantin GINGIVITIS and fetal hydantoin SYNDROME. **p. sodium, p. soluble,** the sodium salt of phenytoin, occurring as a white, odorless, hygroscopic powder that is soluble in water and ethanol, but insoluble in ether and chloroform, which on exposure to air absorbs carbon dioxide with the liberation of phenytoin. Trademarks: Danten, Dihydan Soluble, Diphentoin, Diphenylan Eptin, Solantoin.

phial (fi′al) [Gr. *phiale*] a small bottle; vial.

Philadelphia chromosome see under CHROMOSOME.

Philinos of Cos [c. 250 B.C.] a Greek physician who was a pupil of Herophilus, and is believed to have been one of the founders of the Empiric school of medicine.

philosophy (fĭ-los′o-fe) 1. the critical study of the basic principles and concepts in a field of knowledge. 2. a system or doctrine. **Begg's p.,** Begg's THEORY. **Crozat p.,** a philosophy based on the use of the Crozat appliance to encourage and guide the growth of the bony structure so that there will be room for all the teeth in their proper places, resulting in arch development. See Crozat APPLIANCE and gnathologic ORTHOPEDICS.

Philostigmin trademark for *neostigmine.*

philtrum (fil′trum) [Gr. *philtron* love potion] [NA] the vertical depression or groove in the median portion of the upper lip, just below the nasal septum.

Philumenus [2nd century A.D.] a Greek physician of the Eclectic school whose works are quoted by Oribasius and Aëtius.

pHisoHex trademark for *hexachlorophene.*

Phix trademark for *phenylmercuric acetate* (see under ACETATE).

phleb- see PHLEBO-.

phlebectasia (fleb″ek-ta′ze-ah) [*phleb-* + Gr. *ektasis* dilatation + *-ia*] a dilatation of a vein or veins; varicosity. **p. laryn′gis,** dilatation of the veins of the larynx, especially those of the vocal cords.

phlebectomy (fle-bek′to-me) [*phleb-* + Gr. *ektomē* excision] excision of a vein, or a part of a vein.

phlebectopia (fleb″ek-to′pe-ah) [*phleb-* + Gr. *ektopos* out of place + *-ia*] abnormal displacement of a vein.

phlebitis (fle′bi-tis) [*phleb-* + *-itis*] inflammation of a vein or veins. See also THROMBOPHLEBITIS. **sinus p.,** inflammation of venous sinuses.

phlebo-, phleb- [Gr. *phleps, phlebos* vein] a combining form denoting relationship to a vein or veins. See also terms beginning VENO-.

phleboclysis (fle-bok′lĭ-sis) [*phlebo-* + Gr. *klysis* injection] injection of fluid into a vein. **drip p., slow p.,** slow or drop-by-drop instillation of a fluid into a vein.

phlebogenous (fle-boj′ĕ-nus) [*phlebo-* + Gr. *gennan* to produce] originating in a vein.

phlebography (fle-bog′rah-fe) [*phlebo-* + Gr. *graphein* to write] 1. roentgenography of a vein or veins by use of contrast medium. Called also *venography*. 2. the graphic tracing of the venous pulse. 3. a description of the veins.

phlebolith (fleb′o-lith) [*phlebo-* + Gr. *lithos* stone] a calculus or concretion in a vein.

phlebolithiasis (fleb″o-lĭ-thi′ah-sis) [*phlebo-* + *lithiasis*] a condition characterized by the presence of phleboliths.

phlebology (flĕ-bol′o-je) [*phlebo-* + *-logy*] the study of the veins and their diseases.

phlebomanometer (fleb″o-mah-nom′ĕ-ter) an instrument for the direct measurement of venous blood pressure.

phlebophlebostomy (fleb″o-flĕ-bos′to-me) [*phlebo-* + Gr. *phleps* vein + *stomoun* to provide with an opening, or mouth] surgical vein to vein anastomosis.

phleboplasty (fleb′o-plas″te) [*phlebo-* + Gr. *plassein* to form] plastic repair of a vein.

phleborrhagia (fleb″o-ra′je-ah) [*phlebo-* + Gr. *rhēgnynai* to burst forth] copious hemorrhage from a vein; venous hemorrhage.

phleborrhaphy (flĕ-bor′ah-fe) [*phlebo-* + Gr. *rhaphē* suture] the suturing of a vein; venesuture, venisuture.

phleborrhexis (fleb″o-rek′sis) [*phlebo-* + Gr. *rhēxis* rupture] rupture of a vein.

phlebosclerosis (fleb″o-skle-ro′sis) [*phlebo-* + Gr. *sklērōsis* hardening] fibrous thickening and hardening of the wall of the veins.

phlebostenosis (fleb″o-stĕ-no′sis) [*phlebo-* + Gr. *stenōsis* narrowing] stenosis or constriction of a vein.

phlebothrombosis (fleb″o-throm-bo′sis) [*phlebo-* + *thrombosis*] presence of a thrombus in a vein, without inflammation. Phlebothrombosis associated with inflammation is called *thrombophlebitis*.

phlebotome (fleb′o-tōm) a knife or lancet used in phlebotomy.

phlebotomy (flĕ-bot′o-me) [*phlebo-* + Gr. *tomē* a cutting] incision of a vein; venesection.

phlegm (flem) [Gr. *phlegma*] a ropy, viscid, mucous secretion, such as that produced by the mucosa of the respiratory passages and discharged through the mouth.

phlegmon (fleg′mon) [Gr. *phlegmatikos*] inflammation of connective tissue. See CELLULITIS (2). **Dupuytren's p.,** suppurative phlegmon in the anterolateral portion of the neck on one side. See also facial and cervical CELLULITIS. **Escat's p.,** a juxtatonsillar, odontogenic, periosteal abscess. **facial and cervical p.,** facial and cervical CELLULITIS. **p. of floor of mouth,** Ludwig's ANGINA. **Holz p.,** a chronic cellulitis of the floor of the mouth and neck. **ligneous p.,** phlegmon of the neck, characterized by induration of the subcutaneous connective tissue with little suppuration, fever, or pain, and running a chronic course. Called also *Reclus' disease* and *woody p*. See also facial and cervical CELLULITIS. **woody p.,** ligneous p.

phlegmonous (fleg′mon-us) pertaining to or attended by phlegmon; see CELLULITIS (2).

phlogistic (flo-jis′tik) [Gr. *phlogistos*] inflammatory.

phlogo- [Gr. *phlox, phlogos* flame] a combining form denoting relation to inflammation.

phlogogenic (flo″go-jen′ik) [*phlogo-* + Gr. *gennan* to produce] causing inflammation.

phobia (fo′be-ah) [Gr. *phobos* fear] any persistent abnormal fear or dread. Used as a word termination designating abnormal or morbid fear of, or aversion to the subject indicated by the stem to which it is affixed, as *odontophobia*.

pholcodine (fol′ko-dēn) a narcotic analgesic, 7,8-didehydro-4,5α-epoxy-17-methyl-3-(2-morpholinoethoxy)morphinan-6α-ol, occurring as a crystalline, bitter substance that is freely soluble in ethanol, chloroform, and benzene and slightly soluble in water and ether. Used as an antitussive agent. Called also *homocodeine,* and *β-morpholinylethylmorphine*. Trademarks: Glycodine, Hibernyl, Pectolin, Prodromine.

phon (fōn) [Gr. *phōnē* voice] a unit of the subjective loudness of a sound.

phon- see PHONO-.

phonal (fo'nal) pertaining to the voice.

phonasthenia (fo"nas-the'ne-ah) [phon- + asthenia] weakness of the voice; difficult phonation from fatigue.

phonation (fo-na'shun) the utterance of vocal sounds by means of vocal cord vibrations. **subenergetic p.,** hypophonia. **superenergetic p.,** hyperphonia.

phoneme (fo'nēm) [Gr. phōnēma a sound made, a thing spoken] a group of closely related speech sounds, all of which have the same distinctive acoustic characteristics in spite of their differences, being basic units of spoken language. Often called *speech sound.*

phonetics (fo-net'iks) the science of vocal sounds.

phono-, phon- [Gr. phōnē voice] a combining form denoting relationship to sound or voice.

phonoautograph (fo-no-aw'to-graf) [phon- + Gr. autos self + graphein to write] an apparatus which registers vibrations of the air caused by the voice.

-phore (fōr) [Gr. phoros bearing] a word termination signifying a carrier of an element designated by the stem to which it is affixed, as a melanophore.

-phoresis (fo-re'sis) [Gr. phorēsis a being borne] a word termination indicating transmission, as electrophoresis, etc.

Phos-Flur chewable tablets, oral rinse supplement, see under TABLET and RINSE.

phosphatase [E.C.3.1.3.] (fos'fah-tās") [phosphate + -ase] a subclass of hydrolases, including enzymes that catalyze the hydrolysis of esters of orthophosphoric acid. Called also *glycerophosphatase, phosphomonoesterase,* and *phosphoric monoester hydrolase.* **acid p.** [E.C.3.1.3.2], a hydrolase active in an acid medium, having optimal activity of pH 6 for the enzymes in mammalian erythrocytes and yeasts; pH 5 for enzymes in the prostate, epithelium, spleen, kidneys, blood plasma, pancreas, liver, and rice bran; and pH 3 to 4 for enzymes of other types. Some acid phosphatase also occurs in the ground substance of the dental pulp along the collagen fibers. It catalyzes the hydrolysis of an orthophosphoric ester and phosphorylation. Called also *acid phosphomonoesterase.* **alkaline p.** [E.C.3.1.3.1], a hydrolase active in an alkaline medium (optimal activity at about pH 9.3). It catalyzes the hydrolysis of an orthophosphoric monoester by the cleavage of the phosphate group from an organic ester linkage, also being involved in the catalysis of transphosphorylation. Alkaline phosphatase is found chiefly in the blood serum, leukocytes, bone, kidneys, spleen, lungs, adrenal cortex, seminiferous tubules, and mammary glands; large amounts are found in pulpal odontoblasts, particularly during active calcification, but also when the pulp undergoes an inflammatory state. Called also *alkaline phosphomonoesterase.*

phosphate (fos'fāt) [L. phosphas] a salt of phosphoric acid containing the radical PO_4, being the principal mineral component of the skeleton. Phosphates are essential in the metabolism of fats and carbohydrates, in energy transfer, and in the maintenance of the hydrogen ion concentration through the phosphate buffering system. They are a bound form of phosphorus present in all animal or plant cells, about 80 percent being found in the skeletal system and teeth. High phosphate intake may decrease the body calcium level; deficiency may produce dental changes similar to those seen in rickets. Phosphates introduced into the body fluids have little pharmacological effect; those introduced into the gastrointestinal system are rapidly excreted and, in large amounts, produce a cathartic action. Ingestion of very large amounts of phosphates may produce poisoning associated with lowering of the pH of the urine and reduction of the concentration of Ca^{2+} and symptoms of hypocalcemia. Dietary phosphate supplements have been reported to have cariostatic effects. See also HYPOPHOSPHATASIA, HYPOPHOSPHATEMIA, PHOSPHORUS, and vitamin D–resistant RICKETS. **acid p.,** a phosphate in which only one or two of the three hydrogen atoms are taken up or replaced. **acid calcium p.,** CALCIUM phosphate, monobasic. **adenosine p.,** ADENOSINE phosphate. **alkaline p.,** a phosphate of an alkaline metal, as sodium or potassium. **bone p.,** CALCIUM phosphate. **calcium p.,** CALCIUM phosphate. **calcium monohydrogen p., dibasic calcium p.,** CALCIUM phosphate, dibasic. **dibasic sodium p.,** a phosphate compound, HNa_2PO_4, occurring in either anhydrous or hydrated form. Used in dyeing and in the production of enamels, ceramics, and detergents. Also tested as a potential cariostatic agent. In anhydrous form, it may cause irritation of the skin and mucous membranes. Abbreviated DSP. Called also *disodium orthophosphate.* **dicalcium p.,** CALCIUM phosphate, dibasic. **organic p.,** organophosphate. **precipitated calcium p.,** CALCIUM phosphate, tribasic. **primary calcium p.,** CALCIUM phosphate, monobasic. **secondary calcium p.,** CALCIUM phosphate, dibasic. **tertiary calcium p., tricalcium p.,** CALCIUM phosphate, tribasic.

phosphate-fluoride (fos'fāt-floo'o-rīd) a substance containing both a phosphate and a fluoride, such as a fluoride solution acidulated with orthophosphoric acid.

phosphatide (fos'fah-tīd) phospholipid. **glycerol p.,** phospholipid.

phosphatidylcholine (fos-fat"ĭ-dil-ko'lēn) lecithin.

phosphatidylethanolamine (fos-fat"ĭ-dil-eth"ah-nol-ah'mēn) cephalin.

phosphatidylinositide (fos-fat"ĭ-dil-in-o'sĭ-tīd) a group of compounds obtained from the crude cephalin fractions of tissues, sometimes classified as cephalins, mainly on the basis of solubility. They contain residues of inositol and phosphatide, occurring in a variety of tissues and especially concentrated in the brain. Called also *phosphoinositide.*

phosphatidylserine (fos-fat"ĭ-dil-se'rēn) cephalin.

phosphocreatine (fos"fo-kre'ah-tin) CREATINE phosphate.

6-phosphofructokinase [E.C.2.7.1.11] (fos"fo-fruk"to-ki'nās) a phosphotransferase that, in the presence of ATP and ADP, catalyzes the conversion of fructose-6-phosphate to fructose-1,6-diphosphate in the oxidative metabolism of carbohydrates. Called also *phosphohexokinase.*

phosphoglucomutase [E.C.2.7.5.1] (fos"fo-gloo"ko-mu'tās) a phosphotransferase that catalyzes the conversion of glucose-6-phosphate to glucose-1-phosphate in the process of glycogenesis. The enzyme requires glucose 1,6-diphosphate as an essential cofactor. The human enzyme exhibits multiple molecular forms (isoenzymes), which are controlled by three separate genetic loci. Called also *glucose phosphomutase.*

phosphoglyceride (fos"fo-glis'er-īd) phospholipid. **choline p.,** lecithin.

phosphohexokinase (fos"fo-hek'-so-ki'nās) 6-PHOSPHOFRUCTO-KINASE.

phosphohydrolase (fos"fo-hi'dro-lās) phosphatase. **pyrophosphate p.,** inorganic PYROPHOSPHATASE.

phosphoinositide (fos"fo-in-o'sĭ-tīd) phosphatidylinositide.

Phospholine trademark for *echothiophate iodide* (see under ECHOTHIOPHATE).

phospholipid (fos"fo-lip'id) a class of lipids containing one or more fatty acid molecules and one phosphoric acid radical and, usually, a nitrogenous base, found in all animal and vegetable cells, chiefly cell membranes. The liver and, to a lesser extent, the intestine are the primary sites of phospholipid synthesis. Functions of phospholipids include transporting fatty acids through the intestinal mucosa into the lymph; blood coagulation, whereby thromboplastin is composed mainly of one of the cephalins; insulation of nerves, sphingomyelin being a component of the myelin sheath; metabolism, in which phospholipids serve as donor of phosphate radicals; and forming the structural elements of cell membranes. The major types of phospholipids are cephalins, lecithins, and sphingomyelins. Called also *glycerol phosphatide, phosphatide,* and *phosphoglyceride.* **platelet p.,** platelet factor 3; see under FACTOR.

phosphomonoesterase (fos"fo-mon"o-es'ter-ās) phosphatase. **acid p.,** acid PHOSPHATASE. **alkaline p.,** alkaline PHOSPHATASE.

phosphomutase [E.C.2.7.5] (fos"fo-mu'tās) a phosphotransferase with regeneration of donors, which catalyzes intermolecular transfer of phosphoryl groups. **glucose p.,** phosphoglucomutase.

phosphonate (fos'fo-nāt) a carbon-phosphate compound. Such compounds may be related to inorganic pyrophosphates in structure but possess stable $P-C-P$ bonds instead of $P-O-P$ bonds; they are stable to both enzymatic and chemical hydrolysis.

phosphonecrosis (fos"fo-ne-kro'sis) phosphorus NECROSIS.

phosphoprotein (fos"fo-pro'te-in) a conjugated protein, such as casein and vitellin, in which phosphoric acid is esterified with a hydroxyamino acid.

phosphor (fos'for) a substance capable of emitting light when exposed to light and other radiations. See also PHOSPHORESCENCE.

phosphorate (fos'for-āt) an organic compound containing the radical P_2O_4.

phosphorescence (fos"fo-res'ens) the emission of radiation by a substance as a result of previous absorption of radiation of high or greater energy (shorter wavelength), which may continue for a considerable time after cessation of the ionizing radiation. See also FLUORESCENCE and LUMINESCENCE.

phosphorescent (fos"fo-res'ent) pertaining to or exhibiting phosphorescence; phosphorus.

phosphoric (fos'fo-rik) pertaining to or containing pentavalent phosphorus, as in phosphoric acid.

phosphorism (fos'fo-rizm) phosphorus poisoning. See PHOSPHO-RUS.

phosphorous (fos'for-us, fos-for'us) 1. phosphorescent. 2. containing trivalent phosphorus, as in phosphorous acid.

phosphoruria (fos"for-u're-ah) [*phosphorus* + Gr. *ouron* urine + *-ia*] the presence of free phosphorus in the urine.

phosphorus (fos'fo-rus) [Gr. *phōs* light + *phorein* to carry] a nonmetallic element, occurring in nature in phosphate rock or apatite. Symbol, P; atomic number, 15; atomic weight, 30.974; valences, 1, 3, 4, 5; group VA of the periodic table. ^{31}P is the naturally occurring phosphorus isotope; artificial isotopes include 28–30 and 32–34. Phosphorus is a crystalline, waxlike, transparent solid that ignites spontaneously in air at 30°C (86°F); dissolves in carbon disulfide, but not in water and alcohol; and exhibits phosphorescence at room temperature. It exists in three allotropic forms: white, black, and red. Phosphorus is present in bones and teeth and in all plant and animal cells, being about one-half the concentration of calcium, the skeleton containing more than 80 percent of the body's phosphorus. All phosphorus in the body is in the bound form, occurring as phosphates. Milk and cheese are the chief sources of dietary phosphorus, meat and vegetables being also good sources. Phosphorus has been used in the treatment of rickets and other bone diseases and nervous system diseases. Inorganic phosphorus is highly toxic. Phosphorus poisoning, due to ingestion or inhalation of large doses of free phosphorus, may cause gastrointestinal and liver diseases, skin eruptions, oliguria, circulatory collapse, fatty changes of the peripheral nerves and central nervous system, coma, and death. External contact may result in severe burns. Chronic poisoning may have an effect similar to that of a single toxic dose or may be manifested primarily as a focal necrotizing process in the bones of the face, particularly the maxilla and mandible (see phosphorus NECROSIS), sometimes associated with spontaneous fractures. Weight loss and anemia are the chief presenting symptoms of chronic poisoning. For daily requirements of phosphorus, see table at NUTRITION. **p.-32**, ^{32}**P**, radioactive p. **amorphous p.**, red p. **black p.**, phosphorus occurring as black, stable crystals, which are relatively nontoxic. **ordinary p.**, white p. **organic p. compound**, organophosphate. **radioactive p.**, any radioactive phosphorus isotope. The most commonly used in medicine is ^{32}P, which has a half-life of 14.3 days and emits beta rays; used chiefly in hematology, particularly in the treatment of polycythemia vera and bone marrow examination, including red cell volume determination. Called also *radiophosphorus*. **red p.**, phosphorus occurring as a red to violet powder, which is relatively nontoxic unless it contains white phosphorus as an impurity. Called also *amorphous p.* **regular p.**, white p. **white p.**, phosphorus occurring as white or yellowish transparent crystals which darken on exposure to light and are exceedingly poisonous. Called also *ordinary p., regular p.,* and *yellow p.* **yellow p.**, white p.

phosphoryl (fos'for-il) the trivalent radical ≡P:O.

phosphorylase [E.C.2.4.1.1] (fos-for'ĭ-lās) a hexosyltransferase that, in the presence of inorganic phosphate, catalyzes reversibly the phosphorylic cleavage of the α-1,4-linkage of glycogen to yield glucose-1-phosphate. It occurs in plants and various animal tissues. In the liver, phosphorylase is involved in the conversion of glycogen to free glucose; its activity is stimulated by glucagon. Called also *amylophosphorylase* and *polyphosphorylase.* **citrulline p.**, ornithine CARBAMOYLTRANSFERASE.

phosphorylation (fos"for-ĭ-la'shun) the process of enzymatically introducing the trivalent PO₄ group into an organic molecule. **oxidative p.**, the formation of high-energy phosphate bonds by phosphorylation of ADP to ATP, during which electrons are transferred from the substrate to oxygen; it occurs in mitochondria. See also PHOTOPHOSPHORYLATION. **photosynthetic p.**, photophosphorylation.

phosphothion (fos"fo-thi'on) malathion.

phosphotransferase [E.C.2.7.1 to 2.7.5] (fos"fo-trans'fer-ās) a sub-subclass of transferases, including enzymes that catalyze the transfer of a phosphorus-containing group, subdivided according to the acceptor group, which may be an alcohol group [E.C.2.7.1], a carboxyl group [E.C.2.7.2], a nitrogenous group [E.C.2.7.3], or a phosphate group [E.C.2.7.4]. Called also *transphosphatase.* See also KINASE (1).

phot- See PHOTO-.

photic (fo'tik) pertaining to light.

photo-, phot- [Gr. *phōs, phōtos* light] a combining form denoting relationship to light.

Photobacterium (fo"to-bak-te're-um) [*photo-* + Gr. *baktērion* small rod] a genus of gram-negative, facultatively anaerobic bacteria of the family Vibrionaceae, made up of motile or nonmotile, asporogenous, coccoid or occasionally rod-shaped cells, 1.0 to 2.5 μm in length and 0.4 to 1.0 μm in width. They are found in sea water, in the alimentary tracts of some fishes, and on the luminous organs of some fishes and cephalopods. **P. dun'bari, Vibrio chol'erae** (biotype *albensis);* see under VIBRIO.

photochemical (fo"to-kem'e-kal) pertaining to the chemical properties of light; chemically reactive in the presence of light or other radiation.

photochemistry (fo-to-kem'is-tre) [*photo-* + *chemistry*] the branch of chemistry which deals with the chemical properties or effects of light rays or other radiation; actinochemistry.

photochromogen (fo"to-kro'mo-jen) [*photo-* + Gr. *chrōma* color + *gennan* to produce] a microorganism whose pigmentation develops as a result of exposure to light, specifically *Mycobacterium kansasii* (pathogenic for man), which is yellow-orange if grown in the light, and almost colorless if grown in the dark. **group I p.**, *Mycobacterium kansasii;* see under MYCOBACTERIUM.

photodermatitis (fo"to-der"mah-ti'tis) dermatitis due to overexposure to sunlight.

photoelectron (fo"to-e-lek'tron) [*photo-* + *electron*] an electron ejected from the orbit of an atom that has collided with short wavelength radiation, such as x-rays, with resulting transfer of energy from the photon to the electron; it is a source of secondary radiations of x-rays. See also photoelectric EMISSION.

photofluorography (fo"to-floo"or-og'rah-fe) the photographic recording of fluoroscopic images on small films, using a fast lens; used in mass roentgenography. Called also *fluorography* and *fluororoentgenography,* and sometimes *abreugraphy* (see ABREU).

photography (fo-tog'rah-fe) the process of making images on a sensitized material by exposure to light or other radiant energy.

photolithotroph (fo"to-lith'o-trof) [*photo-* + Gr. *lithos* stone + *trophē* nutrition] photolithotrophic CELL.

photomeson (fo"to-mes'on) a meson, usually a pi meson, ejected from the nucleus by an impinging photon.

photometer (fo-tom'ĕ-ter) [*photo-* + Gr. *metron* measure] a device for measuring the intensity of light.

photomicrograph (fo"to-mi'kro-graf) [*photo-* + Gr. *mikros* small + *graphein* to record] the photograph of a minute object as seen under the light microscope, produced by ordinary photographic methods. Called also *micrograph.*

photomicrography (fo"to-mi-krog'rah-fe) the production of a photomicrograph.

photomicroscope (fo"to-mi'kro-skōp) [*photo-* + Gr. *mikros* small + *skopein* to examine] a camera and a microscope combined for making a photomicrograph.

photomicroscopy (fo"to-mi-kros'ko-pe) photography of enlarged pictures of minute objects with the photomicroscope.

photomultiplier (fo"to-mul"tĭ-pli'er) photomultiplier TUBE.

photon (fo'ton) the carrier of a quantum of electromagnetic energy, which has no mass or electric charge, but has an effective momentum. See also QUANTUM. **Compton p.**, a high-energy photon which, after colliding with an atom, displaces an orbital electron (recoil electron) out of the atom, thus causing ionization. During the collision, it gives some of its energy to the electron and becomes displaced from its course, sometimes striking other electrons in the orbit. See also Compton EFFECT.

photo-organotroph (fo"to-or"gah-no-trof) photo-organotrophic CELL.

photopharmacology (fo"to-far"mah-kol'o-je) [*photo-* + *pharmacology*] the study of the effects of light and other radiations on drugs and on their pharmacological action.

photophobia (fo"to-fo'be-ah) [*photo-* + Gr. *phobein* to be affrighted by] abnormal intolerance to light.

photophore (fo'to-fōr) [*photo-* + Gr. *phoros* bearing] a light-bearing instrument for examination of the nose and larynx.

photophosphorylation (fo"to-fos"for-ĭ-la'shun) light reaction in which ATP is formed, occurring in chloroplasts during photosynthesis; it is analogous to mitochondrial oxidative phosphorylation.

$$ADP + P_i \xrightarrow{\text{light energy}} ATP$$

Called also *photosynthetic phosphorylation.*

photoptarmosis (fo"to-tar-mo'sis) [*photo-* + Gr. *ptarmos* sneezing + *-osis*] sneezing caused by the influence of light.

photoradiometer (fo″to-ra″de-om′ĕ-ter) an apparatus for measuring the quantity of roentgen rays penetrating any given surface.

photoreaction (fo″to-re-ak′shun) a chemical reaction produced by the influence of light; a photochemical reaction.

photoreception (fo″to-re-sep′shun) [*photo-* + L. *receptio,* from *recipere* to receive] the process of detecting radiant energy, usually of the wavelengths between 3900 and 7700 Å, being the range of visible light.

photoscan (fo′to-skan) a two-dimensional representation (map) of the gamma rays emitted by a radioisotope, revealing its varying concentration in a body tissue, differing from a scintiscan only in that the printout mechanism is a light source exposing a photographic film.

photosensitive (fo″to-sen′sĭ-tiv) 1. sensitive to light, as emulsion of the photographic film. 2. exhibiting an abnormally heightened reaction to sunlight. See also PHOTODERMATITIS.

photosensitization (fo″to-sen″sĭ-ti-za′shun) the development of abnormally heightened reactivity of the skin to sunlight.

Photospirillum dunbari (fo″to-spi-ril′um dun′bar-i) *Vibrio cholerae* (biotype *albensis);* see under VIBRIO.

photostable (fo″to-sta″b′l) [*photo-* + L. *stabilis* stable] resistant to light; unchanged by the influence of light.

photosynthesis (fo″to-sin′thĕ-sis [*photo-* + Gr. *synthĕsis* to put together] the basic chemical process of synthesizing complex organic material, in which molecular oxygen and carbohydrates are produced from carbon dioxide and water and the action of light in the presence of chlorophyll, which may be represented as follows:

$$6\ CO_2 + H_2O \xrightarrow[\text{chlorophyll}]{\text{sunlight}} C_6H_{12}O_6\ (\text{carbohydrate}) + 6\ O_2.$$

The process is initiated by the absorption of light by chlorphyll, which produces an excited-state molecule in which several electrons are raised from their normal energy level to a higher level in the double bond structure of chlorophyll. These electrons flow from chlorophyll and ultimately to an iron-containing protein, ferredoxin, and bring about the reduction of NADP to form NADPH, which is used in the CO_2 fixation reaction of photosynthesis. Some of the electrons flow through flavin pigment to plastoquinone, then to cytochrome pigments, and back to chlorophyll and their normal energy level. During the cycle some of the energy is given up by coupling in the reaction of ADP with inorganic phosphate (P_i) to form ATP, which is used in the CO_2 fixation reaction of photosynthesis. The electrons used in the formation of NADPH and ATP are replenished by a reaction in which the OH ions of water form oxygen and donate electrons to chlorophyll through a cytochrome chain. See also PHOTOPHOSPHORYLATION.

phototimer (fo″to-ti′mer) a timing device used in photography and radiography to give a desired exposure. In radiography, it is a special device mounted beneath the Bucky-Potter diaphragm and the cassette tray, which consists of a fluorescent screen that, upon being irradiated with x-rays, gives off a glow that activates the photoelectric cell. The electricity generated in the cell flows to the condenser until it reaches sufficient current to permit discharge; the discharge initiates a series of events that leads to the opening of a relay and termination of the x-ray exposure. See also TIMER.

phototroph (fo″to-trof) [*photo-* + Gr. *trophē* nutrition] phototrophic CELL.

phrenosin (fren′o-sin) a cerebroside, *N*-[1-[β-D-galactopyraminosyloxy)methyl] - 2 - hydroxy - 3 - heptadecenyl] - 2 - hydroxytetracosanamide, obtained from brain and other nerve tissues. On hydrolysis it yields galactose, sphingosine, and phrenosinic acid. Called also *cerebron.*

phthalate (thal′āt) a salt of phthalic acid containing the radical $C_6H_4(COO)_2$=.

phthalylsulfathiazole (thal″il-sul″fah-thi′ah-zōl) a sulfonamide, 4′-(2-thiazolysulfamoyl)phthalanilic acid, occurring as a white or yellowish, bitter, odorless, crystalline powder that darkens on exposure to light and is soluble in alkali hydroxide solutions, slightly soluble in ether and alcohol, and insoluble in water and chloroform. Used in antibacterial therapy. Skin rash, low-grade fever, malaise, headache, anorexia, and anuria are some of the potential side effects. Trademarks: Entexidin, Sulfathalidine, Teleudron.

Phycomycetes (fi″ko-mi-se′tēz) [Gr. *phykos* seaweed + *mykēs* fungus] a former class of fungi, which has been divided into several other divisions, some of which are no longer considered fungi. The true fungi of this group have been placed in the class Zygomycetes, which contains genera of medical importance.

phyla (fi′lah) plural of *phylum.*

phylloquinone (fil′o-kwin′ōn) phytonadione.

phylogenic (fi″lo-jen′ik) pertaining to phylogeny.

phylogeny (fi-loj′ĕ-ne) [Gr. *phylon* tribe + *genesis* generation] the complete developmental history of a race or group of animals. See also EMBRYOLOGY and LIFE. Cf. ONTOGENY.

phylum (fi′lum), pl. *phy′la* [L.; Gr. *phylon* race] a primary or main division of the animal or of the vegetable kingdom, grouping organisms which are assumed to have a common ancestry.

Physeptone trademark for the *dl*-form of *methadone hydrochloride* (see under METHADONE).

physical (fiz′ĭ-kal) [Gr. *physikos*] pertaining to the body, to material things, or to physics.

physician (fĭ-zish′un) an authorized practitioner of medicine, as one graduated from a college of medicine or osteopathy and licensed by the appropriate board. See also DOCTOR and PRACTITIONER. **admitting p.,** the physician responsible for admission of a patient to a hospital or other inpatient health facility. **p. assistant,** physician ASSISTANT. **attending p.,** the physician who is responsible for the care given a patient in a hospital or other health program. **family p.,** a personal physician, oriented to the whole patient, who practices both scientific and humanistic medicine. Family physicians may provide care for only one member of the family, but more often do so for several or all members, regardless of age. Usually they provide medical care in more than one of the traditional specialty fields of medicine, and coordinate the care obtained by referral to or consultation with other physicians and allied health personnel. Some specialize and become subject to specialty board examination. They assume responsibility for the patients' comprehensive and continuing health care. Called *family practitioner.* See also general PRACTITIONER. **personal p.,** the physician who assumes responsibility for the comprehensive medical care of an individual on a continuing basis. See also *family p.* **primary care p.,** a physician who is an expert in primary health care, who may be a specialist in any of several specialties. **resident p.,** a graduate and licensed physician resident in a hospital. See also RESIDENT.

physics (fiz′iks) [Gr. *physis* nature] the science that deals with natural laws and phenomena, but especially with matter and energy in terms of motion and force.

physio- [Gr. *physis* nature] a combining form denoting relationship to nature, as in *physiology,* or denoting physical, as in *physiotherapy.*

physiologic (fiz″e-o-loj′ik) normal; not pathologic; characteristic of or conforming to the normal functioning or state of the body or a tissue or organ; physiological.

physiological (fiz″e-o-loj′ĭ-kal) pertaining to physiology; physiologic.

physiology (fiz″e-ol′o-je) [*physio-* + *-logy*] 1. the science which treats of the functions of the living organism and its parts, and of the physical and chemical factors and processes involved. 2. the basic processes underlying the functioning of a species or class of organisms, or any of its parts or processes. **comparative p.,** the study of organ functions in various types of animals in an effort to discern similarities and differences in physiology among members of the entire animal kingdom or a subdivision thereof. **dental p.,** the study of the function and functional form of the teeth and supporting tissues. **general p.,** the science of the mechanisms involved in the diverse functions occurring in all living species. **morbid p., pathologic p.,** the study of altered, disturbed, and abnormal functions or of function of diseased tissues; physiopathology.

physiopathology (fiz″e-o-pah-thol′o-je) [*physio-* + *pathology*] the science of functions in disease, or as modified by disease; morbid or pathologic physiology.

physiotherapy (fiz″e-o-ther′ah-pe) physical THERAPY.

physique (fĭ-zēk′) bodily structure, organization, and development. Called also *body type* and *habitus.*

physo- [Gr. *physa* air] a combining form denoting relationship to air or gas.

physocele (fi′so-sēl) [*physo-* + Gr. *kēlē* tumor] 1. a tumor filled with gas. 2. a hernial sac filled with gas.

physostigmine (fi″so-stig′mēn) an alkaloid of *Physostigma venenosum,* (3a*S-cis*)-1,2,3,3,α,8,8α-hexahydro-1,3α,8-trimethylpyrrolo[2,3-*b*]indole-5-ol methylcarbonate (ester), which is the oldest of the anticholinesterases. It occurs as a white crystalline powder that turns red on exposure to air, and is soluble in water, alcohol, benzene, chloroform, and oils. Used therapeutically as the sulfate, salicylate, or sulfite salts, chiefly in ophthalmology. Also used to stimulate the intestines and urinary bladder.

phyto- [Gr. *phyton* plant] a combining form denoting relationship to a plant or plants.

phytomenadione (fi″to-men″ah-di′ōn) phytonadione.

phytonadione (fi″to-nah-di″ōn) a vitamin, 2-methyl-1,4-naphthoquinone, occurring as a clear, yellow, viscous, odorless liquid that decomposes on exposure to sunlight and is soluble in ethanol, benzene chloroform, ether, and vegetable oil, but not in water. It is the only natural form of vitamin K which is found in plants, such as alfalfa. Used for correcting vitamin K deficiency and its attendant deficiency of prothrombin and related clotting factors with resulting hemorrhagic disorders. When indicated, used prior to dental surgical procedures. Called also *phytomenadione, phylloquinone,* and *vitamin K₁*. Trademarks: Aquamephyton, K-Jet, Konakion, Methyton, Mono-Kay.

phytotoxin (fi″to-tok′sin) [*phyto- + toxin*] an exotoxin produced by certain species of higher plants. Phytotoxins are resistant to proteolytic digestion, and are effective when taken by mouth. In the broadest sense a phytotoxin is any toxic substance of plant origin.

PI 1. periodontal INDEX. 2. plaque INDEX.

pia (pi′ah) [L.] tender; soft. **p. ma′ter,** pia MATER.

piastrinemia (pi-as″tri-ne′me-ah) [It. *piastre* coin + Gr. *haima* blood + *-ia*] thrombocythemia.

pica (pi′kah) [L.] compulsive craving for unnatural articles of food, such as clay or dirt (geophagia), flaked paint, starch, plaster, etc., most frequently observed in patients suffering from iron-deficiency anemia. The eating of paint may result in lead poisoning (see LEAD) and the eating of abrasive articles often causes wearing out of dentures and tooth abrasion. Treatment of anemia with iron usually eliminates the craving.

pick (pik) any pointed or other sharp device for removing objects from areas that are difficult to access. **apical p.,** apical ELEVATOR. **crane p.,** an elevator for the removal of root fragments of mandibular molar teeth fractured during extraction. Its sharp pointed end may be placed in a small hole drilled in the buccal aspect of a retained root or portion of an impacted crown, with the buccal shelf of the bone serving as a fulcrum for lifting the tooth upward. **root p.,** apical ELEVATOR. **tooth p.,** toothpick.

Pick, Ludwig [German physician, born 1868] see Niemann-Pick DISEASE.

Pickerill's imbrication lines see under LINE.

pickler (pik′ler) a device used for pickling (metallic surfaces) after casting. Called also *acid treating unit.* See illustration.

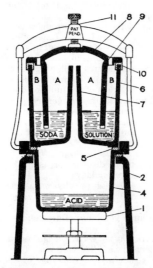

Hanau acid treating unit: (1) Electric heating assembly with pilot light; (2) base supporting the unit; (4) acid pot; (5) acid gasket; (6) soda water pot; (7) fume escape tower; (8) bell, fume trap; (9) vent holes; (10) rubber gasket; (11) yoke with locking screw. (From V. R. Park, J. R. Ashman, and G. J. Shelly: A Textbook for Dental Assistants. 2nd ed. Philadelphia, W. B. Saunders Co., 1975; courtesy of the Hanau Engineering Co., Inc.)

pickling (pik′ling) 1. the process of cleansing newly cast metallic surfaces and removal of oxides and other impurities from metal objects by immersion in an acid solution (see pickling SOLUTION), usually containing sulfuric, hydrochloric, or phosphoric acid; the rate of cleansing varying inversely with the concentration and temperature of solution. 2. a method of food preservation with the use of organic acid (usually acetic acid), sugar, salt, and spices.

pico- [It. *pico* small] in the metric system, a combining form denoting one-trillionth (10⁻¹²) of the unit designated by the root with which it is cominbed. Symbol *p*. Formerly called *micromicro-*. See also metric SYSTEM.

picocurie (pi′ko-ku′re) [*pico- + curie*] a unit of radioactivity, being one-trillionth (10⁻¹²) of a curie, or that quantity of radioactive material in which the number of nuclear disintegrations is 3.7 × 10⁻², or 0.037 per second. Abbreviated *pc* or *pCi*. Formerly called *micromicrocurie* (μμC).

picogram (pi′ko-gram) [*pico- + gram*] a unit of mass (weight) in the metric system, being one-trillionth (10⁻¹²) of a gram. Abbreviated *pg*. Formerly called *microgamma* and *micromicrogram*.

picopicogram (pi″ko-pi′ko-gram [*pico- + picogram*] a unit of mass (weight) in the metric system, being one-trillionth (10⁻¹²) of a picogram, or one-septillionth (10⁻²⁴) of a gram, or the equivalent of 1 avogram. Abbreviated *ppg*.

Picornaviridae (pi-kor″nah-vi′ri-de) [*pico- + RNA + virus + -idae*] a family of naked icosahedral viruses that contain linear single-stranded RNA and replicate in the cell cytoplasm. The diameter of the virion is 20 to 30 nm and there are 32 capsomers in the virion. The RNA is infectious and acts as a messenger for translation, its molecular weight is 2.5 × 10⁶ to 3.0 × 10⁶. A mature virion contains four major polypeptides resulting in posttranslational cleavage of a single precursor. According to one classification, the family consists of the genera *Enterovirus* and *Rhinovirus*. In some classifications, the family also includes the tentative genus *Aphthovirus*. The family formerly included the genus *Calcivirus*.

picornavirus (pi-kor″nah-vi′rus) any virus of the family Picornaviridae.

picounit (pik″o-u′nit) [*pico- + unit*] a quantity one-trillionth (10⁻¹²) of a standard unit.

picrate (pik′rāt) a salt of picric acid.

picro- [Gr. *pikros* bitter] a combining form meaning bitter.

picrotoxin (pik″ro-tok′sin) an active principle, C₃₀H₃₄O₁₃, obtained from the seed (*cocculus indicus*) of *Anamita cocculus*, occurring as flexible, shining, odorless, bitter, photosensitive, prismatic crystals that are soluble in water, boiling alcohol, dilute acids and alkalies, and sparingly soluble in ether and chloroform. It is a powerful central nervous system stimulant, used as an antidote in acute barbiturate poisoning. Called also *cocculin*.

piece (pēs) a part or portion. **end-p.,** END-PIECE. **eye p.,** eyepiece. **Fab p.,** Fab. **Fc p.,** Fc. **Fd p.,** Fd. **secretory p.,** a glycopeptide component of secretory immunoglobuin A. Called also *secretory component, T component,* and *transport component*.

pier (pēr) intermediate ABUTMENT.

Pierre Robin's syndrome [*Pierre Robin,* French physician, 1867–1950] Robin's ANOMALAD.

Pietrantoni's syndrome [L. *Pietrantoni,* Italian physician] see under SYNDROME.

pigment (pig′ment) [L. *pigmentum* paint] 1. any dye or paint; a paintlike medicinal preparation to be applied to the skin. 2. any normal or abnormal coloring matter of the body.

pigmentation (pig″men-ta′shun) the deposition of coloring matter; the coloration or discoloration of a part by a pigment. **amalgam p.,** see ARGYRIA. **bismuth p.,** pigmentation of the oral mucosa, especially of the gingivae and cheeks, sometimes also involving the lips, ventral surface of the tongue, and any localized area of inflammation of the oral mucosa. A thin blue-black line (*bismuth line*) of the marginal gingivae, sometimes confined to the gingival papilla, may be present. The pigment represents precipitated granules of bismuth sulfide produced by the action of hydrogen sulfide on bismuth in the tissue. See also BISMUTH and bismuth STOMATITIS.

pigmented (pig′ment-ed) containing or impregnated with pigment.

pilar, pilary (pi′lar; pil′a-re) [L. *pilaris*] pertaining to the hair.

pill (pil) [L. *pilula*] a small globular or oval medicated mass to be swallowed; a tablet. **sleeping p.,** 1. any pill containing a sleep-inducing substance; a soporific. 2. a popular name for a barbiturate-containing pill.

pillar (pil′ar) [L. *pila*] a supporting column, usually occurring in pairs; used in anatomical nomenclature for such a structure. See also COLUMN and COLUMNA. **p. of fauces, anterior,** palatoglossal ARCH. **p. of fauces, posterior,** palatopharyngeal ARCH.

p. of soft palate, 1. palatopharyngeal ARCH. 2. palatoglossal ARCH.

pilo- [L. *pilus* hair] combining form denoting relationship to hair.

pilocarpine (pi″lo-kar′pēn) an alkaloid obtained from *Pilocarpus jaborandi* or *P. microphyllus,* (3S-*cis*)-3-ethyldihydro-4-[(1-methyl-1H-imidazol-5-yl)methyl]-2(3H)-furanone, occurring as colorless or yellow, hygroscopic crystals that are soluble in water, alcohol, and chloroform and slightly soluble in ether. It is a cholinomimetic drug that stimulates autonomic effector cells and acts on cholinergic postganglionic nerve impulses. Used chiefly in ophthalmology and in the treatment of conditions characterized by deficient salivary secretion.

pilonidal (pi″lo-ni′dal) [*pilo-* + Gr. *nidus* nest] having hair for a nidus. See pilonidal CYST.

piminodine esylate (pi-min′o-dēn) an addictive analgesic, 1-(3-enilinopropyl)-4-phenylisonipecotate monoethanesulfonate, occurring as a colorless, slightly bitter, crystalline solid that is soluble in alcohol and chloroform and slightly soluble in water and ether. Trademark: Alvodine.

pimple (pim′p'l) a papule or pustule

pin (pin) 1. a long slender metal rod for the fixation of the ends of fractured bones. See also FIXATION. 2. a peg or dowel by means of which an artificial crown is fixed to the root of a tooth. **cemented p.,** a threaded pin that is inserted into a dentinal channel and cemented with zinc phosphate cement in place; used in pin-supported restorations. **channel shoulder p. (CSP),** see channel shoulder pin TECHNIQUE. **endodontic p.,** an endosseous implant consisting of a straight or threaded pin inserted into the bony tissue of the jaw through the root canal and apex of a tooth. Called also *endodontic endosseous implant.* See also DOWEL. **friction p., friction-retained p.,** a metal pin of larger diameter than its accommodating hole drilled in dentin, and having a spiral channel threaded into it. It is retained in the tooth structure by friction alone; used in pin-supported restorations. **harelip p.,** harelip NEEDLE. **incisal guide p.,** a metal rod attached to the upper member of an articulator, touching the incisal guide table, which maintains the established vertical separation of the upper and lower arms of the articulator. **lock p.,** a soft metal pin used to attach an arch wire to an orthodontic bracket. Written also *lockpin.* **retention p.,** the frictional grip of small metal projections extending from a metal casting into the dentin. **Roger-Anderson p.,** one formerly used in extra-oral fixation of mandibular fractures and prognathism. **screw p.,** one threaded so that it may be screwed into a dentinal channel. **self-threading p.,** a pin screwed into a hole of smaller diameter prepared in the dentin. **sprue p.,** sprue FORMER. **Steinmann p.,** a metal rod for the internal fixation of fractures. See nail EXTENSION. **TMS (thread mate system) p.,** a threaded pin that is screwed into the dentinal post hole; used in pin-supported restorations.

Pinaud's triangle hypoglossohyoid TRIANGLE.

Pin-Dalbo attachment see under ATTACHMENT.

Pindborg's tumor [Jens Jørgen *Pindborg,* Danish oral pathologist, born 1921] see calcifying epithelial odontogenic TUMOR.

Pindex trademark for *methacycline.*

pineal (pin′e-al) [L. *pinealis; pinea* pine cone] 1. shaped like a pine cone. 2. pertaining to the pineal gland.

ping-ponging (ping pong′ing) the practice of unnecessarily passing a patient from one doctor to another.

Pinkus' disease [Felix *Pinkus,* German dermatologist, born 1868] LICHEN nitidus.

pinlay (pen′la) a gold inlay which is retained by means of one or more pins placed within the tooth structure.

pinledge (pin′lej) a flat floor or shoulder prepared within the tooth structure, into which pin holes are drilled to accommodate pins in a pin retained cast restoration.

pinna (pin′ah) [L. "wing"] the projecting, shell-like part of the external ear lying outside of the head; the flap of the ear. Called also *auricle* and *auricula* [NA].

pinocytosis (pi″no-si-to′sis) [Gr. *pinein* to drink + *kytos* cell + *-osis*] the imbibition of liquids by cells, especially the phenomenon in which minute incuppings or invaginations are formed in the cell membrane, which close and then pinch off to form free fluid-filled vesicles (pinocytosis vesicles). Cf. PHAGOCYTOSIS.

pinosome (pi′no-sōm) [Gr. *pinein* to drink + *sōma* body] pinocytotic VESICLE.

pint (pint) [L. *octarius*] a unit of capacity (liquid or dry), being one-half of a quart or one-eighth of a gallon. Symbol O. Abbreviated *pt.* See also *Tables of Weights and Measures* at WEIGHT. **British imperial p.,** one-half of the British imperial quart, being equivalent to 4 gills (34.678 cubic inches), or 568.26 cubic centimeters. **U.S. p.,** one-half of U.S. quart, being equivalent to 4 gills (28.875 cubic inches), or 0.473 liter.

pinta (pēn′tah) [Sp. "painted"] a form of treponematosis, being a

chronic dyschromic dermatosis endemic in certain parts of tropical America, and characterized by the presence on the skin of spots, which may be white, coffee colored, blue, red, or violet. It is caused by *Treponema carateum* (the Wassermann reaction is usually positive), and is believed to be transmitted usually by direct person-to-person contact.

pio- [Gr. *piōn* fat] a combining form denoting relationship to fat. See also words beginning LIPO-.

pion (pi′on) a nuclear particle with mass intermediate between an electron and a proton.

Pipanol trademark for *trihexyphenidyl hydrochloride* (see under TRIHEXYPHENIDYL).

piperazine (pi-per′ah-zēn) an anthelmintic agent, hexahydropyrazine, occurring as white lumps or flakes with an ammoniacal odor, which are soluble in water and ethanol, but not in ether. Side effects may include vertigo, urticaria, visual disorders, ataxia, and hypotonia. Trademark: Lumbrical.

piperocaine hydrochloride (pi′per-o-kān) a local anesthetic, 3-(2-methylpiperidino)propyl benzoate hydrochloride, occurring as an odorless white powder or small crystals that are soluble in water, alcohol, and chloroform, but not in ether. Trademark: Metycaine.

pipet (pi-pet′) pipette.

pipette (pi-pet′) [Fr.] 1. a glass or transparent plastic tube used in measuring or transferring small quantities of liquid or gas. Also written *pipet.* 2. to dispense fluid or gas by means of a pipette.

piranhalysis (pi″ran-hal′ĭ-sis) fragmentation of pinocytotic vesicles by repeated collisions with lysosomes that subdivide them into smaller pieces.

Piridazol trademark for *sulfapyridine.*

piriform (pir′ĭ-form) [L. *pirum* a pear + *forma* form] pear-shaped. Written also *pyriform.*

Piriton trademark for *chlorpheniramine maleate* (see under CHLORPHENIRAMINE).

Pirmazin trademark for *sulfamethazine.*

Pirogoff's triangle [Nikolai Ivannovich *Pirogoff* (Pirogov), Russian surgeon, 1810–1881] hypoglossohyoid TRIANGLE.

Pirogov see PIROGOFF.

Pirquet's index see under INDEX.

pit (pit) 1. a hollow fovea or indentation. 2. a pockmark. 3. a small, steep-sided depression or fault in the dental enamel, usually at the junction of two or more grooves, found commonly in the occlusal surfaces of bicuspids and molars, at the ends of facial grooves in molars, and occasionally in lingual surfaces of incisors. Considered as belonging to Class I cavities of Black's classification of dental caries (see dental caries classification, under CARIES). See also FISSURE (2). 4. to indent, or to become and remain for a few minutes indented by pressure. **anal p.,** proctodeum. **basilar p.,** a depression in the crown of an incisor tooth above its neck. **p. caries,** pit CARIES. **central p.,** a minute depression at the point of intersection of developmental grooves on the central aspect of the occlusal surfaces of the molar teeth, being a potential site for dental caries. Abbreviated CP. See illustration at GROOVE. **commissural lip p.,** a congenital malformation of the lips, probably genetically transmitted, characterized by unilateral or bilateral depressions at the corners of the mouth on the vermilion surface, sometimes associated with fistulae from which fluid may be expressed. **distal p.,** a minute depression located at the point of intersection of developmental grooves on the distal aspect of the occlusal surface of bicuspid and molar teeth, being a potential site of dental caries. Abbreviated DP. See illustration at GROOVE. **lip p.,** a congenital, probably genetically transmitted, circular depression or a transverse slit about 0.5 to 2.5 cm in depth, forming a blind fistula, usually occurring symmetrically on the vermilion border of either lip, but more commonly on the lower lip. If often exudes viscid saliva on pressure. **mesial p.,** a minute depression at the point of intersection of developmental grooves on the mesial aspect of the occlusal surface of a bicuspid or mandibular molar tooth, being a potential site for dental caries. Abbreviated MP. See illustration at GROOVE. **nasal p.,** the primordium of the nasal cavity. Nasal pits appear as paired shallow depressions in the nasal placodes or ectoderm of the rostral part of the head which overhangs the mouth region. By the fifth week they become limited by U-shaped elevations with their limbs directed toward the oral cavity, the lateral limb forming the nasolateral prominence or process and the median limb forming the nasomedial prominence or process. Called also *olfactory p.* **oblong p. of arytenoid cartilage,** a depression on the anterolateral surface of the arytenoid cartilage, separated from the triangular pit above by the arcuate crest. Called also *fovea oblongata cartilaginis arytenoideae* [NA] and *oblong fovea of arytenoid cartilage*. **olfactory p.**, nasal p. **pterygoid p.**, pterygoid fossa of mandible; see under FOSSA. **p. sealant**, see pit and fissure SEALANT. **stomodeal p.**, stomodeum. **triangular p. of arytenoid cartilage**, a depression on the anterolateral surface of the arytenoid cartilage, separated from the oblong pit below by the arcuate crest. Called also *fovea triangularis cartilaginis arytenoideae* [NA].

pitch (pich) [L. *pix*] 1. a dark, lustrous, more or less viscous residue from the distillation of tar and other substances. 2. a natural asphalt of various kinds. 3. the quality of sound dependent on the frequency of vibration of the waves producing it. **Burgundy p.**, an aromatic, oily resin from Norway spruce, European silver fir, and other types of pine trees. It is characterized by extreme tackiness and is soluble in acetone and alcohol. Used in plasters, surgical tapes, and impression compounds.

pituitary (pĭ-tu-'ĭ-tār''e) 1. pertaining to the pituitary gland. 2. pituitary GLAND. 3. a pharmaceutical preparation of the pituitary gland of animals.

pityriasis (pit''ĭ-ri'ah-sis) [Gr. *pityron* bran + -*iasis*] any disease of the skin or mucous membrane characterized by the formation of branny scales. **p. al'ba**, a common skin disorder of the face and neck in children and adolescents, which consists of one or many unevenly round or oval, hypopigmented, sometimes slightly reddened, finely scaling macules 1 to 4 cm in diameter. If untreated, it usually persists from one to several years, and often recurs. Called also *erythema streptogenes*, *impetigo pityroides*, and *impetigo sicca*. **p. lin'guae**, benign migratory GLOSSITIS. **p. macula'ta et circina'ta**, p. rosea. **p. ro'sea**, an acute, self-limited, inflammatory disease of the skin. It is characterized by oval or circinate macules distributed symmetrically over the trunk and extremities, the individual lesions of which are usually yellowish, pinkish, or reddish, and vary in size from 0.5 to 5.0 cm.; a single large plaque precedes the general eruption by about one to two weeks. The eruption disappears normally after four to eight weeks and recurrences are rare. It may be associated with oral lesions, which occur simultaneously or subsequently to skin lesions, and are present during the most severe phase of disease and clear with the skin lesions. The buccal mucosa is affected most commonly but the tongue and palate may also be involved. Initially, the oral lesions appear as erythematous macules with or without central areas of grayish desquamation; they may be single or multiple, are irregular in shape, occasionally show a raised border, and vary in size from a few millimeters to 1 or 2 cm in diameter. Called also *herpes tonsurans maculosus*, *pityriasis maculata et circinata*, and *squamous roseola*. **p. versic'olor**, a common chronic, noninflammatory and usually symptomless disorder, characterized only by the occurrence of multiple macular patches of all sizes and shapes, varying from whitish in pigmented skin to fawn-colored or brown in pale skin; seen most frequently in hot, humid tropical regions, and caused by *Malassezia furfur*. Called also tinea *versicolor*.

pityroid (pit''ĭ-roid) [Gr. *pityron* bran + *eidos* form] furfuraceous, branny.

Pityrosporon (pit''ĭ-ros'po-ron) *Malassezia*.

Pityrosporum (pit''ĭ-ros'po-rum) *Malassezia*. **P. fur'fur**, *Malassezia furfur*; see under MALASSEZIA. **P. orbicula're**, *Malassezia furfur*; see under MALASSEZIA.

pivot (piv'ot) 1. that on which something turns. 2. a pin or short shaft on the end of which something rests and turns. 3. the point of rotation for a removable partial denture. **occlusal p.**, an elevation contrived on the occlusal surface, usually in the molar region, designed to act as a fulcrum and to induce sagittal mandibular rotation. **occlusal p., adjustable**, an occlusal pivot which may be adjusted vertically by means of a screw or other means.

PKU phenylketonuria.

placebo (plah-se'bo) [L. "I will please"] an inactive substance or preparation given to satisfy the patient's symbolic need for drug therapy, and used in controlled studies to determine the efficacy of medicinal substances. Also, a procedure with no intrinsic therapeutic value, performed for such purposes.

placement (plās'ment) position or arrangement, as of the teeth. **lingual p.**, displacement of a tooth toward the tongue. Called also *linguoplacement*.

placenta (plah-sen'tah), pl. *placentas*, *placen'tae* [L. "a flat cake"] an organ characteristic of true mammals during pregnancy, joining mother and offspring, providing endocrine secretion and selective exchange of soluble, but not particulate, blood-borne substances through an apposition of uterine and trophoblastic vascularized parts.

placentatation (plas''en-ta'shun) a series of events associated with the development and functioning of a placenta, including implantation of the blastocyst in the uterus, differentiation of the uterine lining into a specialized decidual membrane, development of a placenta, and the fetal-maternal relations during pregnancy.

Placidyl trademark for *ethchlorvynol*.

placode (plak'ŏd) [Gr. *plax* plate + *eidos* form] a platelike structure, especially a thickened plate of ectoderm in the early embryo, from which a sense organ develops.

plagiocephaly (pla''je-o-sef'ah-le) [Gr. *plagios* oblique + *kephalē* head] a malformation characterized by the skull appearing larger on one side than the other, being skewed to one side due to premature union of the sutures on one half of the skull and compensatory development of the other half.

plague (plāg) [L. *plaga, pestis;* Gr. *plēgē* stroke] an acute febrile, infectious disease with high fatality rate, caused by *Pasteurella pestis*. **Pohvant Valley p.**, tularemia.

plan (plan) a procedure or design for carrying out an action. See also INSURANCE. **Blue Cross p.**, any of more than 70 nonprofit, tax-exempt health service prepayment organizations providing coverage for health care and related services, all of which voluntarily belong to the Blue Cross Association (see under ASSOCIATION). Originally, the plans were largely associated with hospitals but their association with the American Hospital Association ended in 1972 and, at present, they are community services organizations with governing bodies with membership including a majority of public representatives. They often have a cooperative arrangement with Blue Shield plans and coverage for both plans is frequently sold jointly. Most plans are regulated by state insurance commissioners under special enabling legislation. Unlike most private companies, they usually provide service rather than indemnity benefits, and often pay hospitals on the basis of reasonable costs rather than charges. See also *Blue Shield p.* **Blue Shield p.**, any of numerous nonprofit, tax-exempt plans established to provide coverage for physicians' services, all of which voluntarily belong to the Association of Blue Shield Plans (see under ASSOCIATION). The plans often have a cooperative arrangement with Blue Cross plans and coverage for both plans is frequently sold jointly. Most plans are regulated by state insurance commissioners under special enabling legislation. They provide coverage to groups and private business and, in addition, to government sponsored programs, including Medicare (Part B), Medicaid, and CHAMPUS. See also *Blue Cross p.* **budget payment p.**, divided payment p. **communitywide p.**, a plan under which a contract for prepaid health or dental benefits is made available to any group in the community at established premium rates. **comprehensive coverage p.**, a prepaid insurance plan in which all necessary dental services are covered, usually offered by commercial insurance firms. It provides stated cash allowances for selected procedures, plus usually about 70 percent coinsurance for the basic dental care and about 50 percent for orthodontic or periodontal treatment. **contributory p.**, a group insurance plan in which at least a part of the premium is paid by the employee, the remainder being paid by the employer or union. Called also *contributory insurance*. **Delta Dental P's**, a prepaid dental care program arranged for groups of consumers, which are sponsored, endorsed, and organized by state dental associations and administered for the societies by local insurance companies. Under most of these plans, payments are made to the participating dentists on the basis of usual, customary, and reasonable fees. Sometimes called *blue tooth* because of their similarity to the Blue Shield prepaid medical care plan. **dental p.**, an insurance policy offering a prepaid dental care program. **dental service p.**, a plan which either provides dental services to the insured or makes provisions for dental care and pays the dentist for services rendered. Called also *service p.* **divided payment p.**, a payment plan whereby patients are allowed to remit on a regular basis, usually each month, an agreed upon sum until the entire amount due is received. Called also *budget payment p., installment payment p.,* and *postpayment p.* **fee-for-service p.**, a health insurance plan providing for payment to the doctor for each service rendered rather than on the basis of salary or capitation fee. **group purchase p.**, a health insurance plan which is available for purchase by groups of persons, usually employees of a firm, members of a union, or members of a fraternal organization. **incentive p.**, **incentive copayment p.**, incentive PROGRAM. **indemnity p.**, indemnity PROGRAM. **installment payment p.**, divided payment p. **noncontributory p.**, a group insurance plan in which the entire premium is paid by the employer or union. See also *employer-sponsored p.* Cf. *contributory p.* **package p.**, major insurance policies obtained in a single package or through a single insurance company. **post-payment p.**, divided payment p. **prepaid dental p.**, a program that finances the cost of dental care in advance of receipt of service; it may be offered by a prepayment organization, such as a Blue Shield plan, a primary insurance company, or a dental service corporation, such as Delta Dental Plans. Called also *prepaid dental program.* **reduced fee p.**, a health insurance program in which the fees established for some or all services are lower than those usually charged for services in the community. In some industrial plants, employers make lower fees possible by partially subsidizing the cost of providing care (e.g., furnishing rent-free facilities and paying costs of utilities). In welfare plans with limited funds, doctors may accept lower fees than they usually charge. **service p.**, dental service p. **treatment p.**, an initial tentative outline of therapeutic measures to be undertaken in accordance with diagnostic data and indications.

Planck's constant, theory [Max Karl Ernst Ludwig *Planck,* German physicist, 1858–1947] see under CONSTANT, and see quantum THEORY.

plane (plān) [L. *planus*] 1. a flat or level surface defined by three points. In craniometry and cephalometry, sometimes used interchangeably with line because when viewed from the side (lateral projection), as in an x-ray, it appears as a line. Called also *planum.* See also AXIS and LINE, and see illustration at CEPHALOMETRY. 2. a specified level. 3. to rub away or abrade. See PLANING. 4. a superficial incision in the wall of a cavity or between tissue layers. **acanthion–bony external auditory meatus p.**, Camper's p. **Aeby's p.**, Huxley's p. **alveolar point–**

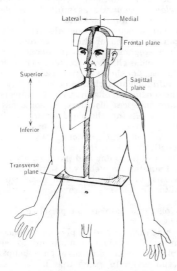

Planes of the body (Davenport). Anterior view, in the anatomical position, with standard planes of reference shown by cleavages. (From Dorland's Illustrated Medical Dictionary. 26th ed. Philadelphia, W. B. Saunders Co., 1981.)

auricular point p., Meckel's p. **ANS–Op p.**, anterior nasal spine–opisthion p., His' p. **auricular point–alveolar point p.**, Meckel's p. **auriculo-orbital p.**, Frankfort Horizontal p. **axial p.**, one parallel with the long axis of a structure. **axiolabiolingual p.**, one parallel with the long axis of an anterior tooth and passing through its labial and lingual surfaces. **axiomesiodistal p.**, one parallel with the long axis of a tooth and passing through its mesial and distal surfaces. **Baer's p.**, one passing through the upper border of the zygomatic arches. **Ba–Na p.**, Huxley's p. **base p.**, an imaginary plane upon which is estimated the retention of an artificial denture. **basion–nasion p.**, Huxley's p. **basion–opisthion p.**, Daubenton's p. **bite p.**, 1. biteplane. 2. occlusal p. **Blumenbach's p.**, a plane determined by the base of a skull from which the lower jaw has been removed. **Bolton p.**, **Bolton–nasion p.**, one passing at a right angle to the median plane, and determined in profile by the line connecting the nasion and postcondylare. Called also *nasion–postcondylare p.* and *postcondylare–nasion p.* **Broca's p.**, one passing from the tip of the interalveolar septum between the upper central incisors to the lowermost point of the occipital condyle. Called also *French p.* **buccolingual p.**, one passing through the buccal and lingual surfaces of a posterior tooth. **Camper's p.**, one

passing from the acanthion to the center of the bony external auditory meatus. See illustration at CEPHALOMETRY. Called also *acanthion–bony external auditory meatus p., Camper's line,* and *prolife line.* **coronal p.**, frontal p. **cusp p.**, the small imaginary plane in which two buccal cusp tips and the highest lingual cusp are located. **Daubenton's p.**, one passing through the opisthion and the lower edges of the orbits. Called also *basion–opisthion p., opisthion–basion p., opisthion–orbitale p.,* and *Daubenton's line.* **external auditory meatus–orbitale p.**, von Ihring's p. **eye–ear p.**, Frankfort Horizontal p. **facial p.**, any of several planes passing through craniometric or cephalometric landmarks of the face. **Frankfort Horizontal p.**, a horizontal plane represented in profile by a line between the lowest point on the margin of the orbit to the highest point on the margin of the auditory meatus, adopted at the 13th General Congress of German Anthropologists (the "Frankfort Agreement"), Frankfurt-am-Main, 1882, and finally by the International Agreement for the Unification of Craniometric and Cephalometric Measurements, Monaco, 1906. Sometimes referred to as *Frankfort Horizontal* and *Frankfort Horizontal line.* Abbreviated *FH.* Called also *auriculo-orbital p.* and *eye–ear p.* **French p.**, Broca's p. **frontal p.**, any plane passing longitudinally through the body from side to side, at right angles to the median plane, and dividing the body into front and back parts. So called because such a plane roughly parallels the frontal suture of the skull. Called also *coronal plane* because one of these planes passes through the coronal suture. **glabella–inion p.**, Schwalbe's p. **glabella–lambda p.**, Hamy's p. **guide p.**, **guiding p.**, 1. any plane that guides movement. 2. a part of an orthodontic appliance that causes a change in the occlusal relation of the maxillary and mandibular teeth and permits their movement to a normal position. 3. two or more vertically parallel surfaces of abutment teeth, so shaped as to direct the path of placement and removal of a partial denture. **Hamy's p.**, one passing from the glabella to the lambda. Called also *glabella–lambda p.* and *lambda–glabella p.* **His' p.**, one passing from the anterior nasal spine to the opisthion. **horizontal p.**, 1. any plane passing through a body, at right angles to both the median and the frontal plane, and dividing the body into upper and lower parts. Called also *transverse p.* 2. a plane passing through a tooth at right angles to its long axis. **Huxley's p.**, one passing from basion to nasion. Called also *Aeby's p., Ba–Na p., basion–nasion p.,* and *Na–Ba p.* See also basicranial AXIS. **inion–glabella p.**, Schwalbe's p. **inion–nasion p.**, Martin's p. **labiolingual p.**, one passing through the labial and lingual surfaces of an anterior tooth. **lambda–glabella p.**, Hamy's p. **Martin's p.**, one passing from the nasion to the inion. Called also *inion–nasion p.* and *nasion–inion p.* **mean foundation p.**, the mean of the various irregularities in form and inclination of the basal seat (denture-supporting tissues). The ideal condition for denture stability exists when the mean foundation plane is most nearly at right angles to the direction of force. **Meckel's p.**, one passing through the auricular and alveolar points. Called also *alveolar point–auricular point p.* and *auricular point–alveolar point p.* **median p.**, the imaginary plane passing longitudinally through the middle of the body from front to back and dividing it into right and left halves. Called also *midsagittal p.* See also *saggital p.* **median–raphe p.**, the median plane of the head. **mesiodistal p.**, one passing through the mesial and distal surfaces of a tooth. **midsaggittal p.**, median p. **Montague's p.**, one passing from nasion to porion. Called also *nasion–porion p., Na–Po p., Po–Na p.* and *porion–nasion p.* **Morton's p.**, one passing through the most projecting points of the parietal and occipital protuberances. **p. motion**, plane MOTION. **Na–Ba p.**, Huxley's p. **Na–Po p.**, Montague's p. **nasion–basion p.**, Huxley's p. **nasion–inion p.**, Martin's p. **nasion–porion p.**, Montague's p. **nasion–postcondylare p.**, Bolton p. **nuchal p.**, the rough and irregular surface of the occipital squama located between the foramen magnum and the superior nuchal line. Called also *planum nuchale.* **occipital p.**, the surface of the occipital squama above the highest nuchal line that is covered by the occipital muscle. Called also *planum occipitale.* **occlusal p., p. of occlusion**, the hypothetical horizontal plane formed by the contacting surfaces of the upper and lower teeth when the jaws are closed. Called also *bite p.* **Op–ANS p.**, His' p. **opisthion–anterior nasal spine p.**, His' p. **opisthion–basion p.**, Daubenton's p. **opisthion–orbitale p.**, Daubenton's p. **orbital p.**, one passing through the two orbital points and perpendicular to the Frankfort Horizontal plane. Called also *planum orbitale.* **orbitale–bony external auditory meatus p.**, von Ihring's p. **orbitale–opisthion p.**, Daubenton's p. **parasagittal p.**, sagittal p. **princi-**

pal p., in radiology, the plane which contains the central ray of a radiation beam. **Po–Na p., porion–nasion p.,** Montague's p. **postcondylare–nasion p.,** Bolton's p. **p. of reference,** one that is used as a base of comparison when several measurements are taken. **sagittal p.,** any vertical plane that passes through the body parallel to the median plane (or to the sagittal suture) and divides the body into left and right parts. Called also *parasagittal p.* See also *median p.* **Schwalbe's p.,** one from the glabella to the inion. Called also *glabella–inion p.* and *inion–glabella p.* **semicircular p. of frontal bone,** temporal surface of frontal bone; see under SURFACE. **semicircular p. of parietal bone,** temporal p. **semicircular p. of squama temporalis,** temporal surface of temporal squama; see under SURFACE. **slip p.,** a plane along which a dislocation moves in the space lattice of a crystalline structure. When the slip planes occur in groups, the metal surface becomes irregular and causes a diffuse reflection of the light, when viewed through a metallurgical microscope. See illustration at SLIP. **p. of superimposition,** a plane, accepted as reasonably stable during growth, upon which successive tracings are superimposed at various stages of growth; most often S–N is chosen, with S registered. **temporal p.,** the depressed area on the side of the skull below the inferior temporal line. Called also *planum temporale* and *semicircular plane of parietal bone.* **tooth p.,** any hypothetical plane passing through a tooth. **transverse p.,** horizontal p. **vertical p.,** any plane of the body perpendicular to the horizontal plane and dividing the body into left and right, or front and back portions, as the sagittal and frontal planes. **von Ihring's p.,** one from the orbitale to the center of the bony external auditory meatus. Called also *external auditory meatus–orbitale p.* and *orbitale–bony external auditory meatus p.*

planigraphy (plah'nig'rah-fe) a body section radiographic technique accomplished by motion of the x-ray source and film along planes parallel to each other and to the film surface. See also TOMOGRAPHY.

planimeter (pla-nim'ĕ-ter) [L. *planus* plane + Gr. *metron* measure] an instrument for measuring the area of surfaces.

planing (plān'ing) the plastic surgery procedure of abrading disfigured skin to promote reepithelization with minimal scarring. It may be done by means of sandpaper, emery paper, low- or high-speed wire brushes, etc. (surgical planing, dermabrasion), or by application of caustic substances such as phenol or trichloracetic acid (chemical planing, chemabrasion). **root p.,** smoothing the roughened root surface of a tooth after subgingival scaling or curettage.

Planochrome trademark for *merbromin.*

plant (plant) 1. any member of the vegetable group of living organisms. 2. equipment or apparatus for a particular mechanical process. 3. to insert or set firmly in the ground or some other body. Also, that which is inserted or set firmly in the ground or some other body. See also IMPLANT¹ and IMPLANT². **vent p., endosseous,** a self-tapping screw-type implant with a large vent inside the screw.

planum (pla'num), pl. *pla'na* [L.] a flat surface, determined by the position of three points in space. Called also *plane.* Used in anatomical nomenclature to designate a more or less flat surface of a bone or other structure. **p. nucha'le,** nuchal PLANE. **p. occipita'le,** occipital PLANE. **p. orbita'le,** orbital PLANE. **p. tempora'le,** temporal PLANE.

plaque (plak) [Fr.] 1. any patch or flat area. 2. a blood platelet. 3. dental p. **attachment p.,** hemidesmosome. **bacterial p.,** dental p. **p. and calculus inhibitor,** plaque and calculus INHIBITOR. **p. control,** plaque CONTROL. **P. Control Program,** Oral Hygiene Instruction; see under INSTRUCTION. **dental p.,** a soft, thin film of food debris, mucin, and dead epithelial cells deposited on the teeth, providing the medium for the growth of various microorganisms, principally, *Lactobacillus acidophilus* and other lactobacilli, streptococci, micrococci, and other cocci, *Cladothrix placoides, Leptothrix buccalis,* actinomycetes, and *Neisseria.* In the first few days, plaque appears as a dense meshwork of cocci with occasional rod forms, almost to the exclusion of other microorganisms; as the plaque matures, filaments and threads increase gradually, while cocci decrease. The main inorganic components are calcium and phosphorus with small amounts of magnesium, potassium, and sodium. The organic matrix consists of polysaccharides, proteins, carbohydrates, lipids, and other components. Plaque plays an etiologic role in the development of dental caries and periodontal and gingival diseases and provides the base for the development of materia alba, and calcified plaque forms dental calculus. Called also *bacterial p.* and *microbial p.* See also brown PELLICLE. **p. index,** plaque

INDEX. **p. inhibitor,** plaque and calculus INHIBITOR. **microbial p.,** dental p.

Plasdone trademark for *povidone.*

plasm (plazm) plasma; formative substance. **germ p.,** the reproductive and hereditary substance of individuals that is passed on from the germ cell in which an individual originates in direct continuity to the germ cells of succeeding generations.

plasma (plaz'mah) [Gr. "anything formed or molded"] 1. blood p. 2. cytoplasm or protoplasm. 3. a mixture of starch and glycerol, used as an ointment base. **blood p.,** the fluid portion of the blood, which serves as a vehicle for the formed elements, nutrients carried to the tissue, wastes carried away from the tissues, and various chemical substances of the body, such as proteins, salts, and hormones carried to their destinations. Plasma is composed of water (90 percent); proteins, mainly fibrinogen, globulins, and albumin; salts (0.9 percent), chiefly sodium, potassium, calcium, magnesium, iron, and copper; sugar (0.9 percent); various trace elements; and other substances necessary to sustain life. Transfusion of blood plasma is used in various complications of blood loss, such as shock, to replace lost blood volume and to restore deficient coagulation factors. Blood plasma from which fibrinogen has been separated, is known as blood serum (see under SERUM). Fresh frozen plasma has coagulation factors; stored plasma lacks labile coagulation factors. See also table of *Reference Values for Blood, Plasma, and Serum* in appendix. **p. kinin,** plasma KININ. **p. membrane,** plasma MEMBRANE.

plasmacyte (plaz'mah-sīt) [*plasma* + *-cyte*]. plasma CELL.

plasmacytoma (plaz″mah-si-to'mah) [*plasmacyte* + *-oma*] a neoplasm composed of plasma cells. The most common form is *multiple myeloma,* occurring as multiple neoplasms in the bone; a less common form is *solitary plasma cell myeloma,* occurring as a single focus in a bone. Also relatively uncommon is primary plasmacytoma of the soft tissue, which usually originates in the lymphoid tissue in and about the nasopharynx and oropharynx, and is chiefly characterized by enlargement. It is made up of masses or sheets of typical adult plasma cells and, sometimes, multinucleated plasma cells. Most cases are associated with the production of abnormal globulins resulting in a variety of immunological disorders; in some cases, there is spilling of plasma cells into the blood stream, producing leukemia. See also plasma cell MYELOMA. **extramedullary p.,** a soft-tissue plasma cell tumor, histologically similar to multiple myeloma, usually found on the gingiva, palate, floor of the mouth, tongue, tonsils, pillar and nasal cavity, nasopharynx, and paranasal sinuses, as well as in some visceral organs. It presents a sessile or polypoid reddish mass which becomes lobulated. **solitary p.,** plasma cell myeloma, solitary; see under MYELOMA.

plasmacytosis (plaz″mah-si-to'sis) the presence of excess plasma cells in the blood.

plasmalemma (plaz″mah-lem'ah) 1. plasma MEMBRANE. 2. a thin peripheral layer of the ectoplasm in a fertilized egg.

plasmalogen (plaz-mal'o-jen) a group of phospholipids similar to the lecithin-cephalin group, except that the fatty acid residue in the α position is replaced by a vinyl ether in the ether linkage to glycerol. In most tissues, plasmalogens are characterized by a large content of highly unsaturated fatty acids. They are present in blood platelets, liberating higher fatty aldehydes on hydrolysis, and may be related to the specialized function of platelets in blood coagulation.

plasmin [3.4.21.7] (plaz'min) a serine proteinase, formed from a plasma protein plasminogen. It cleaves selectively arginine and lysine, digesting fibrin threads and other clotting factors, such as fibrinogen, factor V, factor VIII, prothrombin, and factor XII, thus causing lysis of blood clot. Conversion of plasminogen to plasmin occurs through the action of an activator urokinase produced in the body and by a streptococcal enzyme streptokinase. Plasmin dissolves blood clot and allows clearing extraneous blood from tissues, sometimes opening clotted vessels. Excessive production of plasmin leads to hypocoagulability of the blood. Called also *fibrinase* and *fibrinolysin.* See also FIBRINOLYSIS.

plasminogen (plaz-min'o-jen) a plasma protein containing a euglobulin which, when activated by an enzyme, such as urokinase or streptokinase, forms plasmin. Called also *profibrinolysin.* See also FIBRINOLYSIS.

plasmo- [Gr. *plasma*] a combining form denoting relationship to plasma, or to the substance of a cell.

plasmocytosis (plaz″mo-si-to'sis) the presence of excess plasma cells in the blood; plasmacytosis. **gingival p.,** plasma cell GINGIVITIS.

plasmodia (plaz-mo'de-ah) plural of *plasmodium.*

Plasmodium (plaz'mo-de'um) a genus of protozoa of the subphylum Sporozoa, parasitic in the red blood cells of lizards, birds and mammals, including man; the malarial parasite. **P. fal-cip'arum**, the species which causes falciparum malaria in man. **P. mala'riae**, the species which causes quartan malaria in man. **P. vi'vax**, the species causing vivax malaria.

plasmodium (plaz-mo'de-um), pl. *plasmo'dia* [*plasmo-* + Gr. *eidos* form] 1. a parasite of the genus *Plasmodium*. 2. a multinucleate continuous mass of protoplasm.

plasmolemma (plaz"mo-lem'ah) plasma MEMBRANE.

Plasmosan trademark for *povidone*.

plasmosome (plaz'mo-sōm) [*plasmo-* + Gr. *sōma* body] 1. nucleolus. 2. [pl.] mitochondria.

plasmozyme (plaz'mo-zīm) [*plasmo-* + Gr. *zymē* yeast] prothrombin.

-plast [Gr. *plastos* formed] a word termination denoting any primitive living cell.

plaster (plas'ter) [L. *emplastrum*] 1. any semisolid, viscous preparation, sometimes medicated, which may be spread over the skin to provide protection, to serve as a counterirritant, or used for other purposes. 2. dental p. 3. p. of Paris. **adhesive p.**, former name for adhesive TAPE. **adhesive p., sterile**, adhesive tape, sterile; see under TAPE. **dental p.**, a semisolid paste that hardens to form a stonelike solid. It is produced from gypsum (CaSO$_4$ · 2H$_2$O), which on heating gives up part of its water and forms a fine white powder. When mixed with water, two molecules of the dehydrated gypsum combine with one molecule of water, producing gypsum hemihydrate, (CaSO$_4$)$_2$ · H$_2$O, and forming a paste which sets rapidly to re-form hard crystalline gypsum, expanding slightly as it hardens. The material produced by heating at atmospheric pressure is known as β-hemihydrate, and that produced by heating in an autoclave under steam pressure is known as α-hemihydrate. According to ADA specifications, dental plasters are classified into four types: *Type I*, a β-hemihydrate, or plaster of Paris, occurring as a white, chalky solid, which is easily breakable (see *impression p.*). *Type II*, a β-hemihydrate, occurring as a white, chalky solid, whose strength varies with specific needs (see *model p.*). *Types III* and *IV*, both of which are α-hemihydrates, occurring as a tough, stonelike solid; the former has a dry compressive strength of 500 to 700 kg/cm^2 (7100–9900 psi), and the latter a dry compressive strength of 800 kg/cm^2 (11,400 psi) and a very low setting expansion (see dental STONE). See table. **p. headcap**, plaster HEADCAP. **impression p.**, Type I dental plaster (of ADA specifications; see *dental p.*) with a relatively low strength to allow

ADA CLASSIFICATION FOR DENTAL GYPSUM PRODUCTS

	ADA Specifications	Traditional Terminology
Type I	Plaster, impression	Impression plaster
Type II	Plaster, model	Model or lab plaster
Types III and IV	Dental stone	Class I stone or Hydrocal; Class II stone; Densite, or improved stone

(Modified from R. W. Phillips: Elements of Dental Materials. Philadelphia, W. B. Saunders Co., 1977.)

easy breaking of the impression in the mouth without injury to the adjacent tissues. It is a white chalky solid, sometimes colored to distinguish it from the cast material, composed of the β-hemihydrate of gypsum, or plaster of Paris (see GYPSUM hemihydrate), which is modified by flavoring agents, gums, and various chemical additives which alter its setting time and handling properties. Potato starch or other starches are sometimes added to reduce the strength of the plaster. Used for making impressions for complete dentures, impressions of labial sections for immediate denture, transfer of copings in crowns and bridges, and recording jaw relations and also as "wash" liners for final impressions. See also impression MATERIAL. **lab p.**, model p. **model p.**, Type II dental plaster (of ADA specifications; see *dental p.*) used to produce dental models. It is a chalky white solid, sometimes colored to simulate tissues, which is generally harder than the impression plaster, its hardness varying according to the need. It is composed of the β-hemihydrate of gypsum (see GYPSUM hemihydrate). Called also *lab p.* **p. of Paris**, the β-hemihydrate of gypsum (see GYPSUM hemihydrate), which, when mixed with water, forms a

paste that sets rapidly to re-form hard crystalline gypsum, expanding slightly as it hardens. Plaster of Paris is used in making casts and bandages to support or immobilize body parts. Modifiers are added to plaster of Paris to produce impression plaster.

plastic (plas'tik) [L. *plasticus*; Gr. *plastikos*] 1. tending to build up tissues or to restore a lost part. 2. conformable; capable of being molded. 3. a permanently deformable material; an organic material which has been shaped by plastic deformation, usually formed in a softened condition and then made to harden. 4. synthetic p. **modeling p.**, impression COMPOUND. **synthetic p.**, a synthetically produced nonmetallic, pliable compound, usually derived from organic compounds, which can be molded into a desirable form and then hardened. Synthetic plastics are fibrous, rubber-like, or resinous or hard, rigid substances made up of polymers of high molecular weight, the molecular morphology determining whether they are fibers, rubber-like products, or resins. Sometimes called *synthetic*.

plasticity (plas-tis'ĭ-te) 1. the quality of being plastic or moldable, usually applying to a semisolid substance. 2. the ability of early embryonic cells to alter in conformity with the immediate environment.

plasticizer (plas'tĭ-si"zer) an organic compound added to a polymer to improve its flow, reduce brittleness, and lower the softening point, usually accomplished through increasing the solubility of the monomer in the total mixture and by dispersing the interchain attractive forces. The action of a plasticizer is the partial neutralization of the secondary bonds or intermolecular forces which normally prevent the resin molecules from slipping past one another when the material is stressed. Plasticizing of a resin can also be accomplished by copolymerization with a suitable comonomer. Most commonly used plasticizers are nonvolatile organic liquids with low-melting points, such as phtalate, adipate, and sebacate esters, including ethylene glycol and its derivatives, trioresyl phosphate, castor oil, and the like. Used sparingly in dental resins.

plastics (plas'tiks) 1. plastic materials. See PLASTIC (3). 2. plastic SURGERY.

Plastodent elastic impression powder see under POWDER.

Plastopaste trademark for a soft *zinc oxide–eugenol impression paste* (see under PASTE).

plastoquinone (plas"to-kwin'ōn) a quinone occurring in chloroplasts, which is involved in the transport of electrons during photosynthesis.

plasty (plas'te) [Gr. *plassein* to form, mold, shape] the surgical repair and reconstruction of a defective part; plastic surgery. Also used as a word termination meaning the shaping or the surgical formation of, or pertaining to plastic surgery. **W-p.**, a technique of plastic surgery used mainly in the repair of straight scars that require the redistribution of tension. It consists of excising a series of consecutive small triangular areas of tissue on each side of the wound or scar, and imbricating the resultant flaps. **Z-p.**, a plastic operation for the relaxation of contractures, in which a Z-shaped incision is made, the middle bar of the Z being over the contracted scar, and the triangular flaps rotated so that their apices cross the line of contracture.

plate (plāt) [Gr. *platē*] 1. a flat structure or layer. 2. dental p.; sometimes, by extension, incorrectly used to designate a complete denture. **active p.**, active plate APPLIANCE. **alar p.**, either of the pair of longitudinal zones of the embryonic neural tube dorsal to the sulcus limitans, from which are developed the dorsal gray columns of the spinal cord and the sensory centers of the brain. Called also *dorsolateral p., wing p., alar lamina,* and *lamina alaris*. **bandelette p.**, an orthodontic appliance used to "straighten" teeth by tying them to metal plates with brass or silver wire threaded through two small holes for each tooth. The appliance is believed to have been developed by Pierre Fauchard. **basal p.**, 1. either of the pair of longitudinal zones of the embryonic neural tube ventral to the sulcus limitans, from which are developed the ventral gray columns of the spinal cord and the motor centers of the brain. Called also *ventrolateral p.,* and *basal lamina*. 2. the fused parachordal cartilages, precursors of the occipital bone. 3. the portion of the basal decidua that becomes an integral part of the placenta. **base p.**, baseplate. **basic p.**, the principal part of the active plate appliance, consisting of an acrylic plate which carries all working parts of the appliance, serves as an anchorage, and becomes an active part of the appliance itself. See also active plate APPLIANCE. **bite p.**, a simple type of removable orthodontic appliance which makes use of adhesion to the palate to provide part of the anchorage needed for the desired tooth movement; used to stimulate eruption of the posterior teeth and to decrease the amount of anterior overbite. It is generally made of acrylic resin with appurtances attached as needed. If the anterior teeth are spaced excessively, a labial wire may be used for retraction; a variety of clasps may be added around the molar teeth. Some models may have divided plastic plates, the separate parts being movable to facilitate the desired tooth movement. Written also *biteplate*. See also Hawley RETAINER and occlusal STENT. See illustration. **bone p.,** a metal bar with perforations for the

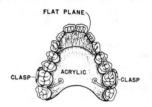

Maxillary bite plate. (From T. M. Graber: Orthodontics — Principles and Practice. 3rd ed. Philadelphia, W. B. Saunders Co., 1972.)

insertion of screws, used to immobilize fractured segments. **clinoid p.,** the portion of the sphenoid bone behind the sella turcica. **Coffin p., Coffin split p.,** an orthodontic appliance used in the past to expand the upper teeth and, more recently, in cleft palate therapy for segmental expansion. It consists of a vulcanite plate to fit the palatal or lingual and sometimes the occlusal surfaces of the teeth and into which a screw has been vulcanized. The appliance is joined anteroposteriorly at the median line and the two halves exert a lateral pressure controlled by adjustment of the screw or spring wire. Called also *Coffin appliance*. See also *expansion p.* **cortical p.,** the dense outer portion of the alveolar process overlying the spongiosa, being a continuation of the bony plate, which is located on the vestibular and oral aspects of the mandible and maxilla, it meets the cribriform plate at the crest of the alveolus, and consists of a compact bone composed of haversian systems; circumferential lamellae, whose thickness varies, being thinner near the median line and becoming thicker along the dental arches, until it reaches its maximum width in the molar area; and interstitial spaces (remnants of haversian and circumferential lamellae). Numerous Volkmann's canals, which tend to be more numerous in the maxilla but larger in the mandible, provide entry for the blood vessels, lymphatics, and nerves. **p. of cranial bone, inner,** internal lamina of cranial bones; see under LAMINA. **p. of cranial bone, outer,** external lamina of cranial bone; see under LAMINA. **cribriform p. of alveolar process,** a thick bony plate of the alveolar process which lines the tooth sockets (alveoli), being supported by trabacular bone and fibers of the periodontal ligament inserting into it. It is perforated by numerous Volkmann's canals for the passage of nerves and lymphatic and blood vessels supplying the periodontal ligament. Its endosteal lamellae are arranged in layers conforming to the shape of the adjacent marrow spaces and other lamellae belong to the haversian systems or their remains. The outer, or periosteal, lamellae, which face the periodontal ligament, are those with which the principal collagen-fiber bundles, as Sharpey's fibers are inserted. It is composed of bundle bone, which contains large amounts of more calcified cementing substance than the surrounding bones and thus more resistant to x-rays, appearing on dental radiographs as a thin radiopaque line (hence the synonym *lamina dura*). Called also *alveolar bone proper*. See also bundle BONE. **cribriform p. of ethmoid bone,** the horizontal plate of the ethmoid bone forming the roof of the nasal cavity. The posterior border of a triangular process projecting from the middle of the plate into the cranial fossa (crista galli) serves as attachment for the falx cerebri, and two small projections on the anterior border fit into depressions of the frontal bone, forming the foramen cecum. Perforations on the sides of the crista galli (olfactory foramina) offer passage for the olfactory nerves. On either side of the crista galli at the anterior part of the plate there is a small fissure occupied by a process of the dura mater. A notch or foramen lateral to the fissure transmits the anterior ethmoidal vessels and nerves. Called also *cribriform lamina of ethmoid bone, cribrum, horizontal lamina of*

ethmoid bone, and *lamina cribrosa ossis ethmoidalis* [NA]. **deck p.,** roof p. **dental p.,** a plate of acrylic resin, metal, or other material, which is fitted to the shape of the mouth and serves to support artificial teeth. **die p.,** a plate of metal containing dies for forming the cusps in shell crowns. **dorsal p.,** roof p. **dorsolateral p.,** alar p. **end p.,** a flattened discoid expansion at the neuromuscular junction, where a myelinated motor nerve fiber joins a skeletal muscle fiber. It contains a receptor which combines with acetylcholine, thus allowing the impulse to pass through the junction, and another which combines with acetylcholinesterase, which inactivates acetylcholine, thus controlling the transmission of impulses across the junction. Called also *motor p.* **equatorial p.,** the platelike collection of chromosomes at the equator of the spindle in karyokinesis. **ethmovomerine p.,** the central part of the ethmoid bone in the fetus. **expansion p.,** a bite plate bisected and the halves connected by the expansion screw. The turning of the screw expands the plate and applies force against the teeth to be moved. Called also *split p.* See also orthodontic SCREW. See illustration. **floor p.,** the unpaired ventral longitudinal zone of the neural tube, forming its floor. Called also *ventral p.* **frontal p.,** a fetal plate of cartilage between the sides of the ethmoid cartilage and the sphenoid bone. **frontonasal p.,** the fetal plate from which the

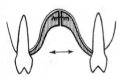

Schematic cross section of expansion plate inserted in narrow upper jaw. (From A. M. Schwarz and M. Gratzinger: Removable Orthodontic Appliances. Philadelphia, W. B. Saunders Co., 1968.)

external nose is developed. **growth p.,** the area between the epiphysis and diaphysis of long bones, within which growth in length occurs. **Hawley bite p.,** a bite plate used with a Hawley retainer. **horizontal p. of palatine bone,** the horizontal part of the palatine bone, forming the posterior part of the hard palate. Its smooth superior (nasal) surface forms the back part of the floor of the nasal cavity and its rough inferior (palatine) surface forms the hard palate. The serrated anterior border articulates with the palatine process of the maxilla, and the posterior concave border attaches the soft palate. The medial serrated border articulates with its fellow of the opposite side; its superior edge forms a ridge which, together with the one of the opposite side, forms the nasal crest and articulates with the vomer. Called also *horizontal part of palatine bone, lamina horizontalis ossis palatini* [NA], and *pars horizontalis ossis palatini*. **jumping-the-bite p.,** Kingsley APPLIANCE. **Kingsley p.,** Kingsley APPLIANCE. **Kühne's terminal p's,** the motor end plates of nerves in the muscle spindles. **Lane p's,** steel plates with holes for screws, used in fixing the fragments of a fractured bone. **lingual p.,** a major partial denture connector formed as a lingual bar extended to cover the cingula of the lower anterior teeth. When used on the maxillary arch it is often referred to as a *palatal plate*. Called also *lingual apron, lingual shield, lingual strap,* and *linguoplate*. See also continuous CLASP. **middle p.,** nephrotome. **motor p.,** end p. **muscle p.,** myotome (2). **neural p.,** a thickened area of the ectoderm, dorsal to the notochord, which develops during the third week of embryonic life, being at first flat and thin but thickening and becoming stratified rapidly. By the time somites begin to appear, it folds into a neural groove to become the neural tube from which the brain and spinal cord develop. **Nord p., Nord expansion p.,** Nord APPLIANCE. **notochordal p.,** notochord. **oral p.,** pharyngobasilar FASCIA. **orbital p. of ethmoid bone,** orbital LAMINA. **orbital p. of frontal bone,** the horizontal part of the frontal bone that forms the greater part of the roof of the orbit and the floor of the anterior cranial fossa; it is separated from its fellow of the opposite side by the ethmoidal notch. Called also *pars orbitalis ossis frontalis* [NA]. **outer p. of cranial bones,** external lamina of cranial bones, see under LAMINA. **palatal p.,** see lingual p. **palate p.,** that part of the palatine bone which forms a lateral half of the roof of the mouth. **paper p.,** orbital LAMINA. **parietal p.,** a thin lamina of the ethmoid bone that forms part of the nasal septum. **perpendicular p. of ethmoid bone,** a thin lamina which descends from the inferior surface of the cribriform plate and forms a part of the nasal septum. Its anterior border articulates with the spine of the frontal bone and the crest of the nasal bones and its posterior border articulates with the sphenoid crest and with the vomer. Its somewhat thicker inferior border serves for attachment of the septal cartilage of the nose. Many foramina leading from the cribriform plate lodge olfactory nerve filaments. Called also *lamina perpendicularis ossis ethmoidalis* [NA], *perpendicular lamina of ethmoid bone, perpendicular layer of ethmoid bone,* and *vertical layer of ethmoid bone.* **perpendicular p. of palatine bone,** the flat, oblong, thin, vertical bony plate that extends superiorly on either side from the palatine bone. Its inferior or nasal surface forms part of the inferior meatus of the nose; somewhat higher is the conchal crest and a depression above forms the middle meatus. The rough maxillary surface articulates with the maxilla. Its smooth posterosuperior portion forms part of the pterygopalatine fossa, and its smooth anterior portion forms part of the wall of the maxillary sinus. A groove on the posterior part of the maxillary surface forms the pterygopalatine canal for transmission of the palatine vessels and nerve. The thin anterior border forms the maxillary process which fits into the maxillary sinus. A groove in the posterior border articulates with the medial pterygoid plate of the sphenoid bone. Called also *vertical p. of palatine bone, lamina perpendicularis ossis palatini, pars perpendicularis ossis palatini* [NA], and *perpendicular part of palatine bone.* **pharyngeal p.,** pharyngobasilar FASCIA. **prechordal p.,** prochordal p. **prochordal p.,** a thickened plate in the cranial end of the embryo, formed by the endodermal cells near the edge of the germinal disk, cephalad to the notochord, which combines with the ectoderm to develop into the buccopharyngeal membrane. Called also *prechordal p.* **pterygoid p., external,** pterygoid p., lateral. **pterygoid p., internal,** pterygoid p., medial. **pterygoid p., lateral,** either of a pair of bony plates projecting downward from the roots of the great wings of the sphenoid bone. Its lateral surface forms part of the medial wall of the infratemporal fossa, and gives attachment to the lateral pterygoid muscle. Its medial surface forms part of the pterygoid fossa and gives attachment to the medial pterygoid muscle. Called also *external pterygoid p., external lamina of pterygoid process, lamina lateralis processus pterygoidei* [NA], and *lateral lamina of pterygoid process.* **pterygoid p., medial,** either of a pair of bony plates projecting downward from the roots of the great wings of the sphenoid bone, forming the lateral boundary of the ipsilateral posterior aperture of the nasal cavity (choana) and the most posterior part of the lateral wall of the nasal cavity. The lateral surface forms part of the pterygoid fossa and the medial surface forms the lateral boundary of the choana. A projection on the inferior surface is known as the *vaginal process* and a prominence between the posterior edge of the process and the medial border of the scaphoid fossa is named the *pterygoid tubercle.* The posterior edge of the plate serves as attachment for the pharyngeal aponeurosis and the constrictor pharyngis muscles attach to its inferor third. An angular process (*processus tubarius*) projecting from the posterior edge of the plate supports the auditory tube. Called also *internal pterygoid p., internal lamina of pterygoid process, lamina medialis processus pterygoidei* [NA], and *medial lamina of pterygoid process.* **roof p.,** the longitudinal zone of the neural tube forming its roof. Called also *deck p.,* and *dorsal p.* **Sherman p.,** a chrome-cobalt alloy or stainless steel bone plate that can be affixed to a fracture site with screws; frequently used in open reduction of mandibular fractures. **split p.,** expansion p. **spring p.,** a dental plate held in place by the elasticity of the material which abuts against natural teeth. **ventral p.,** floor p. **ventrolateral p.,** basal p. (1). **vertical p. of palatine b.,** perpendicular p. of palatine bone. **wing p.,** alar p.

plateau (plah-to′) 1. an elevated and level area. 2. the range of Geiger-Müller counter tube potential for which the counting rate is essentially independent of voltage. **Geiger p.,** the voltage range over which only small changes in counting rate occur. See also Geiger-Müller COUNTER.

platelet (plāt′let) 1. any small plate or platelike structure. 2. blood p. **p. adhesiveness,** viscidity of the blood platelet surface to exposed collagen in areas of vascular injury, occurring in the presence of the free amino groups of collagen, considered to be one of the principal mechanisms of hemostasis. After adhering to collagen, platelets degranulate and release ADP, which results in further aggregation of platelets and building up of the platelet mass. In vitro, blood platelets adhere to glass, but the mechanism is not yet fully understood. **p. aggregation,** aggregation of blood platelets at the site of a vascular injury in the initial stages of hemostasis, precipitated by agitation and collision between individual platelets. See illustration. **blood p.,** a colorless, biconcave, round disk varying in size from 2 to 5 μm in diameter, the average being 3 μ, while some may reach 25 to 50 μ, especially during blood regeneration. Some platelets may have bizzare forms, such as the shape of a dumbbell, cigar, or Indian club. Platelets originate from megakaryocytes in the

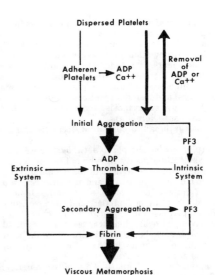

Adenosine diphosphate (ADP) appears to provide a common basis for the action of a variety of substances known to induce platelet aggregation. The action of ADP requires Ca^{++}, fibrinogen and one other protein cofactor. Removal of ADP or Ca^{++} results in dispersion of platelets. (From B. S. Leavell and O. A. Thorup, Jr.: *Fundamentals of Clinical Hematology.* 4th ed. Philadelphia, W. B. Saunders Co., 1976.)

bone marrow, and are known as *megakaryoblasts* and *promegakaryocytes* during their development. Cells consist of a membrane surrounding the cytoplasmic reticulum, Golgi apparatus, endoplasmic reticulum, well-defined granules of high density, granules with clear interiors, small mitochondria, and microvesicles and tubuli. When stained by Romanovskii's method, platelets show a purple granular portion occupying the central part (granulomere) and a smooth pale portion (hyalomere). Blood platelets have three principal properties: adhesiveness, aggregation, and agglutination. Their major functions include hemostasis, blood coagulation, antibody transport, phagocytosis, and storage and transport of chemical substances, such as serotonin, epinephrine, and histamine. Biochemically, platelets require a constant supply of ATP; use glucose as the principal source of energy; contain all of the enzymes of the glycolytic pathway and citric acid cycle; have at least 15 different proteins, most of which are found in the blood plasma; and are associated with coagulation factors II, V, VIII, IX, X, XI, XII, and XIII. Called also *blood disk* and *thrombocyte.* See also table of *Reference Values in Hematology* in Appendix. **blood p. count,** determination of the number of circulating blood platelets in a measured volume of blood, usually a cubic millimeter. See table of *Reference Values in Hematology* in Appendix. **p. cofactor I,** FACTOR VIII. **p. cofactor II,** FACTOR IX. **p. count,** blood p. count. **p. factor,** platelet FACTOR.

plating (plāt′ing) 1. the act of applying bacterial culture media to glass plates; the cultivation of bacteria on plates. 2. a thin coating of gold, silver, or similar material. 3. the application of plates to fractured bones for the purpose of holding the fragments in place. **gold p.,** 1. the application of a thin layer of gold on another metal by the process of electrolysis. 2. the adaptation of a layer of gold on the surface of copper, brass, or other metal by burnishing it with a rapidly revolving gold-wire brush.

platinic (plah-tin′ik) pertaining to a compound containing quadrivalent platinum.

Platinore trademark for a high-fusing chromium-cobalt casting alloy.

platinous (plat′ĭ-nus) pertaining to a compound containing divalent platinum.

platinum (plat′ĭ-num) [L.] a noble metal. Symbol, Pt; atomic number, 78; atomic weight, 195.09; specific gravity, 21.37; melting point, 1769°C; Brinnell hardness number, 97; valences, 2, 4; group VIII of the periodic table. It has six natural isotopes: 190, 191, 194–196, 198; 190 and 191 are radioactive (half-life 6.9 × 10^{11} and 10^{15} years, respectively). Artificial radioactive isotopes include 173–189, 191, 193, and 199–201. Platinum occurs as a silver-gray, lustrous, malleable and ductile metal, insoluble in mineral and organic acid, but soluble in aqua regia and attacked by fused alkalies. It also occurs as a black powder (platinum black) and as a spongy substance (spongy platinum), both having a strong affinity for oxygen and acting as oxidizing and catalytic agents. It is added to some gold alloys to reduce the ductility and increase the strength and hardness of dental appliances. Inhalation of dust of platinum salts may cause irritation to oral and respiratory mucosa associated with sneezing, coughing, apnea, cyanosis, and rhinorrhea. Contact with the skin may cause dermatitis.

platy- [Gr. *platys* broad] a combining form meaning broad or flat.

platybasia (plat″e-ba′se-ah) [*platy-* + Gr. *basis* base (of the skull) + *-ia*] a skull abnormality in which the cervical vertebrae appear to have pushed the floor of the occipital bone upward. Called also *basilar impression*, and *occipitalization of atlas.*

platycelous (plat″e-se′lus) [*platy-* + Gr. *koilos* hollow] having vertebrae flat in front, or cephalad, and concave caudad.

platycephalic (plat″e-sĕ-fal′ik) [*platy-* + Gr. *kephalē* head] wide-headed; having a breadth-height index of less than 70.

platycephaly (plat″e-sef′ah-le) an abnormally wide head.

platycrania (plat″e-kra′ne-ah) [*platy-* + Gr. *kranion* skull + *-ia*] a flattened condition of the skull.

platyglossal (plat″e-glos′al) [*platy-* + Gr. *glossa* tongue] having a broad, flat tongue.

platyhelminth (plat″e-hel′minth) one of the Platyhelminthes.

Platyhelminthes (plat″e-hel-min′thēz) [*platy-* + Gr. *helmins* worm] a phylum of acoelomate, dorsoventrally flattened, bilaterally symmetrical animals, commonly known as flatworms, and including the classes Turbellaria, Trematoda, and Cestoidea.

platyrrhine (plat′e-rīn) [*platy-* + Gr. *rhis* nose] having a broad nose; having a nasal index exceeding 53.

platysma (plah-tiz′mah) [Gr.] [NA] a broad and flat facial muscle that covers most of the lateral and anterior regions of the neck. It arises from the fascia of the cervical region and some of its fibers insert into the mandible below the oblique line, others insert into the subcutaneous tissue and skin of the lower face, while still others may reach the orbicular muscle of the eye and the greater zygomatic muscle. It acts to wrinkle the skin of the neck, to draw down the lower lip and corner of the mouth, and to open the mouth. The cervical branch of the facial nerve provides innervation. Called also *platysma muscle.*

platystaphyline (plat″e-staf′ĭ-līn) [*platy-* + Gr. *staphylē* palate] having a broad, flat palate.

platytrope (plat′e-trōp) [*platy-* + Gr. *tropein* to turn] either of two symmetrical parts on opposite sides of the body; a lateral homologue.

Plaut's angina, ulcer [Hugo Carl *Plaut*, German physician, 1858–1928] see necrotizing ulcerative GINGIVOSTOMATITIS and necrotizing ulcerative GINGIVITIS.

Plaut-Vincent stomatitis [H. C. *Plaut*; Henri *Vincent*, French physician, 1862–1950] acute necrotizing GINGIVITIS.

Pleasants' disease [John E. *Pleasants*, American dentist] see under DISEASE.

Pleasure curve reverse CURVE.

plectrum (plek′trum) [L., from Gr. *plektron* anything to strike with] 1. palatine UVULA. 2. malleus (1). 3. styloid process of temporal bone; see under PROCESS.

pledget (plej′et) 1. a small compress or tuft, as of wool or lint. 2. a small spherical mass of rolled cotton less than 1/8 inch in diameter, commonly used for the topical application of medicinal substances. Larger balls are known as *cotton pellets.*

-plegia [Gr. *plēgē* a blow, stroke] a word termination meaning paralysis, or stroke.

pleiotropy (pli-ot′ro-pe) [Gr. *pleiōn* more + *tropē* a turning] 1. the quality of having affinity for several different types of tissue, representing derivatives of the different primary germ layers. 2. production by a single gene of multiple effects in a phenotype.

pleo- [Gr. *pleōn* more] a combining form meaning more.

pleomorphic (ple″o-mor′fik) [*pleo-* + Gr. *morphē* form] occurring in various distinct forms).

pleomorphism (ple″o-mor′fizm) the assumption of various distinct forms by a single organism or species; also the property of crystallizing in two or more forms.

Plesiomonas (ple″se-o-mo′nas) [Gr. *plesios* neighbor + *monas* unit] a genus of gram-negative, facultatively anaerobic bacteria of the family Vibrionaceae, occurring as motile (by polar flagella), lophotrichous cells, 3.0 μm in length and 0.8 to 1.0 μm in width. Their metabolism is both respiratory and fermentative, with acid, but not gas, being produced during carbohydrate

breakdown. **P. shigelloi′des**, a species isolated from the feces of man and monkeys and from the lymph nodes of canines and fowl, which is a cause of human gastroenteritis.

plesiotherapy (ple″se-o-ther′ah-pe) [Gr. *plesios* near + *therapeia* cure] radiotherapy in which the source of radiation is at a short distance from the tissue being treated, usually no further than 1 to 2 cm from the irradiated area. It may be applied externally as well as internally. See also external RADIOTHERAPY and internal RADIOTHERAPY. Cf. TELETHERAPY.

plethora (pleth′o-rah) [L.; Gr. *plēthōrē* fullness, satiety] a general term denoting a red florid complexion, or specifically, an excessive amount of blood.

pleura (ploor′ah), pl. *pleur′ae* [Gr. "rib," "side"] the serous membrane investing the lungs and lining the thoracic cavity, completely enclosing a potential space known as the *pleural cavity.*

pleurae (ploor′e) [L.] plural of *pleura.*

pleurisy (ploor′ĭ-se) [Gr. *pleuritis*] inflammation of the pleura, with exudation into its cavity and upon its surface.

pleuropneumonia-like organism (ploor″o-nu-mo′nĭ-ah-lĭk or′gah-nizm) former name for a microorganism of the genus *Mycoplasma;* abbreviated *PPLO.*

Plexiglas trademark for thermoplastic polymers of the methyl methacrylate type.

plexus (plek′sus), pl. *plex′us, plexuses* [L. "braid"] a network or tangle; a general anatomical term for a network of lymphatic vessels, nerves, or veins. **p. articula′ris,** a small venous plexus near the outer aspect of the temporomandibular joint. **p. auricula′ris poste′rior,** a sympathetic nerve plexus on the posterior auricular artery. **autonomic p's, p. autonom′ici** [NA], extensive networks of nerve fibers and cell bodies associated with the autonomic nervous system. Called also *p. sympathici.* **basilar p., p. basila′ris** [NA], a venous plexus of the dura mater situated over the basilar part of the occipital bone and the posterior portion of the body of the sphenoid, extending from the cavernous sinus to the foramen magnum, and communicating with other dural sinuses. Called also *basilar sinus.* **p. carot′icus commu′nis** [NA], carotid p., common. **p. carot′icus exter′nus** [NA], carotid p., external. **p. carot′icus inter′nus** [NA], **carotid p.,** carotid p., internal. **carotid p., common,** a nerve plexus on the common carotid artery, formed by branches of the internal and external carotid plexuses and the cervical sympathetic ganglia, and supplying sympathetic fibers to the head and neck via branches accompanying the cranial blood vessels. Called also *p. caroticus communis* [NA]. **carotid p., external,** a nerve plexus located around the external carotid artery, formed by the external carotid nerves from the superior cervical ganglion, and supplying sympathetic fibers which accompany branches of the external carotid artery. Called also *p. caroticus externus* [NA]. **carotid p., internal,** a nerve plexus on the internal carotid artery, formed by the internal carotid nerve, which supplies sympathetic fibers to the branches of the internal carotid artery, to the tympanic plexus, to the nerves in the cavernous sinus, and, directly or indirectly, to certain cranial parasympathetic ganglia through which they pass. Called also *carotid p.* and *p. caroticus internus* [NA]. **cavernous p., p. caverno′sus,** a plexus of sympathetic nerve fibers related to the cavernous sinus of the dura mater. **cavernous p's of conchae, p. caverno′si concha′rum,** numerous venous plexuses in the thick membrane of the nasal conchae. **dental p., inferior, p. denta′lis infe′rior** [NA], a plexus of nerve fibers from the inferior alveolar nerve, situated around the roots of the lower teeth. **dental p., superior, p. denta′lis supe′rior** [NA], a plexus of fibers from the superior alveolar nerve, situated around the roots of the upper teeth. Called also *Bochdalek's ganglion.* **facial p., p. of facial artery,** a nerve plexus along the facial artery. Called also *p. maxillaris externus.* **infraorbital p.,** a nerve plexus situated deep to the levator muscle of the upper lip, formed by superior labial branches of the infraorbital nerve and branches of the facial nerve. **intermediate p.,** a continuous anastomosing network of the principal fiber bundles of the periodontal ligament between the tooth and bone. **intracavernous p.,** a network of venous channels connecting the two cavernous sinuses across both the roof and floor of the pituitary fossa. **Jacobson's p.,** tympanic p. **jugular p., p. jugula′ris,** a plexus of lymphatic vessels along the internal jugular vein. **laryngeal p.,** a nerve plexus on the outer surface of the inferior constrictor of the pharynx; it is an offshoot of the pharyngeal plexus and is made up of fibers from the sympathetic and external laryngeal nerves. **lingual p., p. lingua′lis,** a nerve plexus accompanying the lingual artery. **lymphatic p., p. lymphat′icus** [NA], an interconnecting network of lymphatic vessels, being most abundant in the mucous membranes of the respiratory and digestive system. The salivary glands have deep perilobular plexuses. **p. maxilla′ris exter′nus,** facial p. **p. maxilla′ris inter′nus,** a nerve plexus accompanying the maxillary artery. **p. menin'geus,** a nerve plexus accompanying the middle meningeal artery. **nasopalatine p.,** a nerve plexus near the incisor foramen. **nerve p., nervous p.,** a plexus made up of intermingled nerve fibers. **occipital p., p. occipita'lis,** a nerve plexus accompanying the occipital artery. **ophthalmic p., p. ophthal'micus,** a nerve plexus accompanying the ophthalmic artery. **parotid p. of facial nerve, p. paroti'deus ner'vi facia'lis** [NA], a plexus formed by anastomosis of the terminal branches of the temporal, zygomatic, buccal, marginal mandibular, and cervical rami of the facial nerve, arising in the parotid gland. **periarterial p., p. periarteria'lis** [NA], a network of autonomic and sensory nerve fibers in the adventitia of an artery, some of which are following the course of the artery to reach and innervate other structures and some of which innervate the artery itself. **pharyngeal p.,** a venous plexus posterolateral to the pharynx, formed by the pharyngeal veins, communicating with the pterygoid venous plexus, and draining into the internal jugular vein. Called also *p. pharyngeus* [NA]. **pharyngeal p. of vagus nerve,** a plexus formed chiefly by fibers from branches of the vagus nerves, but also containing fibers from the glossopharyngeal nerves and sympathetic trunks, and supplying motor, general sensory, and sympathetic innervation to the muscle and mucosa of the pharynx and soft palate, except for the tensor veli palatini muscle. Called also *p. pharyngeus nervi vagi* [NA]. **p. pharyn'geus** [NA], pharyngeal p. **p. pharyn'geus ascen'dens,** a nerve plexus accompanying the ascending pharyngeal artery. **p. pharyn'geus ner'vi va'gi** [NA], pharyngeal p. of vagus nerve. **pseudocavernous p.,** a network of blood vessels in the bilaminar region of the temporomandibular joint. With forward movement of the mandible, the blood vessels become filled with blood, helping to fill the space formed by the excursion of the mandible, and as the mandible moves back, they empty. **pterygoid p., p. pterygoi'deus** [NA], an extensive network of veins corresponding to the second and third parts of the maxillary vein, situated on the lateral surface of the medial pterygoid muscle and on both surfaces of the lateral pterygoid muscle, and draining into the facial vein. It communicates with the cavernous sinus and with the facial vein through the deep facial and angular veins. Its tributaries include the inferior alveolar, middle meningeal, deep temporal, masseteric, buccal, posterior superior alveolar, pharyngeal, descending palatine, and infraorbital veins and the vein of the pterygoid canal. Its tributaries anastomose with the inferior ophthalmic and ethmoidal veins and may communicate with the superior sagittal sinus. **p. of Raschkow,** a delicate plexus of nerve fibers beneath the odontoblasts in the dental papilla during the formation of dentin. **Stensen's p.,** the venous network around the parotid duct. **subclavian p., p. subcla'vius** [NA], a sympathetic nerve plexus on the subclavian artery, arising from the cervicothoracic ganglion, contributing to the branches of the subclavian artery. **p. sympath'ici,** autonomic *p's.* **p. tempora'lis superficia'lis,** a plexus of nerve fibers accompanying the superficial temporal artery. **thyroid p., inferior,** a nerve plexus accompanying the inferior thyroid artery and supplying fibers to the larynx, pharynx, and thyroid region. Called also *p. thyroi'deus infe'rior.* **thyroid p., superior,** a nerve plexus accompanying the superior thyroid artery to the larynx, pharynx, and thyroid region. Called also *p. thyroi'deus supe'rior.* **thyroid p., unpaired,** a venous plexus investing the surface of the thyroid gland. Called also *p. thyroideus impar* [NA]. **p. thyroi'deus im'par** [NA], thyroid p., unpaired. **p. thyroi'deus infe'rior,** thyroid p., inferior. **p. thyroi'deus supe'rior,** thyroid p., superior. **tonsillar p.,** a plexus around the tonsil, formed by communications between the middle and posterior palatine nerves and the tonsillar branches of the glossopharyngeal nerve; fibers are supplied to the tonsil, soft palate, and region of the fauces. **Trolard's p.,** venous p. of hypoglossal canal. **tympanic p., p. tympan'icus** [NA], a plexus on the promontory of the middle ear formed by the tympanic and caroticotympanic nerves. It gives off the lesser petrosal nerve, a continuation of the tympanic nerve, which terminates in the otic ganglion as its parasympathetic root, and sensory branches, which innervate the mucous membrane of the tympanic cavity, auditory tube, and the mastoid air cells. It communicates with the greater petrosal nerve through a branch. Called also *Jacobson's p.* **vascular p., p. vasculo'sus** [NA], a network of intercommunicating blood vessels. **p. veno'sus** [NA], venous p. **p. veno'sus cana'lis hypoglos'si** [NA], venous p. of hypoglossal canal. **p. veno'sus carot'icus inter'nus** [NA], venous p., internal carotid. **p. veno'sus foram'inis ova'lis** [NA], venous p. of foramen ovale. **p. veno'sus suboccipita'lis** [NA], venous p., suboccipital. **venous p.,** a network of intercommunicating veins. Called also *p. venosus* [NA]. **venous p., internal carotid,** a venous plexus around the petrosal portion of the internal carotid artery,

through which the cavernous sinus communicates with the internal jugular vein. Called also *p. venosus caroticus internus* [NA]. **venous p., suboccipital,** that part of the external vertebral plexus which lies on and in the suboccipital triangle, receives the occipital vein of the scalp, and drains into the vertebral vein. Called also *p. venosus suboccipitalis* [NA]. **venous p. of foramen ovale,** a venous plexus that connects the cavernous sinus through the foramen ovale with the pterygoid plexus and the pharyngeal plexus. Called also *rete foraminis ovalis.* Called also *p. venosus foraminis ovalis* [NA]. **venous p. of hypoglossal canal,** a venous plexus surrounding the hypoglossal nerve in its canal, and connecting the occipital sinus with the vertebral vein and with the longitudinal vertebral venous sinuses. Called also *Trolard's p., p. venosus canalis hypoglossi* [NA], and *rete canalis hypoglossi.*

-plexy [Gr. *plēxis* a stroke] a word termination meaning a stroke, or seizure.

plica (pli'kah), pl. *pli'cae* [L.] a fold. Used in anatomical nomenclature to designate a ridge or fold. See also FOLD. **p. aryepiglot'tica** [NA], aryepiglottic FOLD. **epiglottic p.,** a fold of mucous membrane between the tongue and the epiglottis. **p. fimbria'ta** [NA], fimbriated FOLD. **p. glossoepiglot'tica,** glossoepiglottic FOLD. **p. glossoepiglot'tica latera'lis,** glossoepiglottic fold, lateral; see under FOLD. **p. glossoepiglot'tica media'na,** glossoepiglottic fold, median; see under FOLD. **p. lacrima'lis** [NA], **p. lacrima'lis Has'neri,** lacrimal FOLD. **p. muco'sa,** a mucous fold; a fold of mucous membrane. **p. ner'vi laryn'gei,** FOLD of laryngeal nerve. **pli'cae palati'nae transver'sae,** palatine folds; see under FOLD. **p. palpebronasa'lis** [NA], epicanthus. **p. salpingopalati'na** [NA], salpingopalatine FOLD. **p. salpingopharyn'gea** [NA], salpingopharyngeal FOLD. **p. semiluna'ris** [NA], semilunar FOLD. **p. sero'sa,** a fold of serous membrane; a serosal fold. **p. sublingua'lis** [NA], sublingual FOLD. **p. triangula'ris** [NA], triangular FOLD. **p. ventricula'ris, p. vestibula'ris** [NA], vestibular FOLD. **p. voca'lis** [NA], vocal cord, true; see under CORD.

plicadentin (pli"kah-den'tin) [*plica + dentin*] a modification of the dentin in which the fibers diverge in many lines from the central pulp cavity of the tooth, as the teeth of reptiles and certain fish.

plicae (pli'se) [L.] plural of *plica.*

plicate (pli'kāt) [L. *plicatus*] plaited or folded.

plication (pli-ka'shun) the taking of tucks in any structure to shorten it, or in the walls of a hollow viscus; a folding.

pliers (pli'erz) small tong-jawed pincers for bending metals or holding small objects; also used in dental work. **Allen's root p.,** an instrument for removing fragments of bone broken off from tooth roots or from the alveolar process in extraction of teeth. **band p.,** stretching p. **band-removing p.,** band REMOVER. **band soldering p.,** light pliers with a locking device for the long beaks over a lap joint while soldering. **clasp bending p.,** one with one round nose and one concave, used chiefly for bending and shaping wire and clasps. **contouring p.,** heavy pliers with one nose convex and the other concave, used for contouring of banding metal. **cotton p.,** delicate pliers with long flattened jaws, used for holding or applying cotton or paper points. See illustration. **cusp forming p.,** strong pliers used in forming cusps in metal crowns. **cutting p.,** any strong pliers equipped with a sharp edge for cutting wire, metal plate, etc. **eagle's beak p.,** one with noses resembling an eagle's beak, used for bending wire or metal plate. **flat nose p.,** one with two flat noses. **foil p., foil carrying p.,** one with delicate jaws for carrying or folding gold, tin, or platinum foil. See illustration. **ligature tying p.,** one used for tying ligatures; a needle-holder used for tying ligatures. See illustration. **matrix p.,** one with long, curved jaws, one having a slot near the end and the other a projection to fit; used for placing and removing a matrix between two teeth. **ortho-**

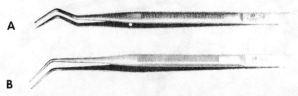

A, Cotton pliers. *B,* Foil pliers. (From H. O. Torres and A. Ehrlich: Modern Dental Assisting. 2nd ed. Philadelphia, W. B. Saunders Co., 1980.)

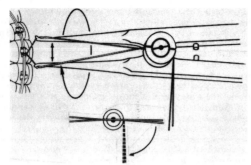

Ligature-typing pliers. (From T. O. Torres and A. Ehrlich: Modern Dental Assisting. 2nd ed. Philadelphia, W. B. Saunders Co., 1980.)

dontic p., any of various pliers used in the preparation, fitting, and removal of orthodontic appliances. See illustration. **Peeso p.,** one designed for contouring bands and other parts of crowns and artificial dentures. **round p.,** one with round noses. **serrated p.,** one in which the jaws are serrated to insure a better grasp. **silver-point p.,** a type of pliers or forceps used to remove silver points extending into the pulp chamber, which can be locking or nonlocking. Narrow hemostats are often substituted for silver point pliers. **smooth p.,** one with smooth jaws. **soldering p.,** light pliers with long flattened jaws shaped to a point, used for soldering, particularly transporting pieces of solder to a desired point. **Steiglitz p.,** a type of silver-point pliers. **stretching p.,** one whose jaws are designed as a hammer and anvil, with the handles sufficiently long to develop a high leverage ratio;

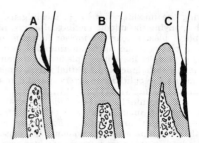

Different types of periodontal pockets. *A*, Gingival pocket. There is no destruction of the supporting periodontal tissues. *B*, Suprabony pocket. The base of the pocket is coronal to the level of the underlying bone. Bone loss is horizontal. *C*, Intrabony pocket. The base of the pocket is apical to the level of the adjacent bone. Bone loss is vertical. (From F. A. Carranza, Jr.: Glickman's Clinical Periodontology. 5th ed. Philadelphia, W. B. Saunders Co., 1979.)

used to enlarge metal bands or to thin the contact area of matrix bands. Called also *band pliers*.

Pliny the Elder (Gaius Plinius Secundus) [A.D. 23–79] a Roman naturalist and encyclopedist whose writings contain comments on the teeth and their diseases, such as that in the human teeth there exists a poisonous substance having the effect of dimming the brightness of a mirror when the teeth are presented uncovered before it; scratching painful gums with the tooth of a man who has suffered violent death has curative effects; touching a tooth with a piece of wood from a tree that has been struck by lightning will cure toothache; the ashes of stag's horn rubbed over loose and aching teeth will make them firm and soothe the pain; the ashes of the head of a hare offer a good dentifrice; mouth odors may be eliminated with ashes of mice mixed with honey; washing the mouth with the blood of a tortoise three times a year will protect against toothache.

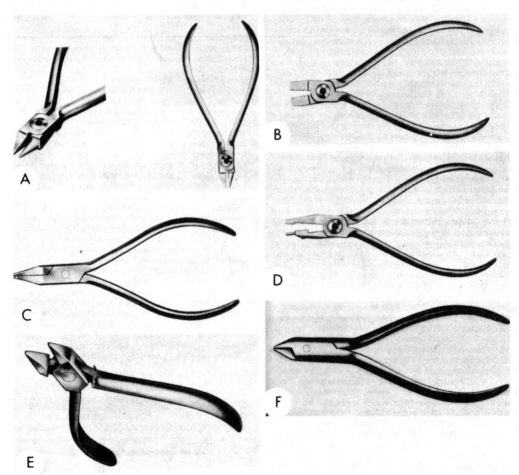

Orthodontic pliers. *A*, Wire-bending pliers (Angle), two views. *B*, Lingual arch–forming pliers. *C*, Loop pliers (Tweed). *D*, Loop-forming pliers. *E*, Clasp-bending pliers (Universal-Adams). *F*, Clasp-adjusting pliers (Aderer type). (From H. O. Torres and A. Ehrlich: Modern Dental Assisting. 2nd ed. Philadelphia, W. B. Saunders Co., 1980; courtesy of Rocky Mountain Dental Products, Denver, Colorado.)

-ploid [Gr. *-ploos* a fold, as in *diploos* + *eidos* form] a word termination denoting (in adjectives) the condition in regard to degree of multiplication of chromosome sets in the karyotype, or (in nouns) an individual or cell having chromosome sets of the particular degree of multiplication in the karyotype indicated by the root to which it is attached, as aneuploid, polyploid, etc.

ploidy (ploi'de) [Gr. *-ploos* a fold, as in *diploos*, + *eidos* form] the status of the number of chromosome sets per cell; used also as a word termination denoting the condition in regard to the degree of multiplication of chromosome sets, as *aneuploidy, diploidy, haploidy,* etc.

plosive (plo'siv) a speech sound produced by suddenly releasing air pressure, such as *p, d,* and *t.*

plug (plug) a substance or mass which obstructs an opening. **Dittrich's p.,** a yellowish or gray caseous mass consisting of debris, fats, and bacteria, found in the sputum of patients with bronchial diseases. **mucous p.,** a plug formed by secretion of mucous glands, such as the salivary glands, thought to be incompletely mineralized calculi.

plugger (plug'er) a metal instrument designed to pack and condense restorative material within a prepared cavity. See CONDENSER (3). **amalgam p.,** amalgam CONDENSER. **automatic p.,** mechanical CONDENSER. **back-action p.,** back-action CONDENSER. **endodontic p.,** root canal filling CONDENSER. **foil p.,** gold CONDENSER. **foot p.,** foot CONDENSER. **gold p.,** gold CONDENSER. **Ladamore p.,** a type of a long-tipped root canal filling condenser. **Luks p.,** a type of a fine-tipped root canal filling condenser having a single curve to its working tip. **reverse p.,** back-action CONDENSER. **root canal p.,** root canal filling CONDENSER.

pluglet (plug'let) a compressed tablet for use in pressure anesthesia of the dental pulp. Called also *billet.*

plumbism (plum'bizm) lead poisoning. See LEAD.

plumbum (plum'bum) [L.] lead.

Plummer's adenoma, disease [Henry Stanley *Plummer,* American physician, 1874–1937] see under ADENOMA and DISEASE.

Plummer-Vinson syndrome [H. S. *Plummer;* Porter Paisley *Vinson,* American surgeon, 1890–1959] see under SYNDROME.

plumper (plum'per) [*plump,* well rounded or filled out] lip p. **lip p.,** an acrylic cushion attached to a denture. See lip habit APPLIANCE and Mayne muscle control APPLIANCE.

Plurazol trademark for *sulfapyridine.*

pluri- [L. *plus* more] a combining form meaning several or more. See also terms beginning POLY- and MULTI-.

pluricytopenia (ploor″ĭ-si′to-pe′ne-ah) [*pluri-* + *cytopenia*] deficiency of several cellular elements of the blood.

pluriglandular (ploor″ĭ-glan′du-lar) [*pluri-* + *glandular*] pertaining to, derived from, or affecting several glands; multiglandular.

pluriorificial (ploor″e-or′ĭ-fish′al) [*pluri-* + L. *orificium* orifice] pertaining to or affecting several orifices of the body.

Pluronic F68 trademark for poloxamer 188.

Pluronic F88 trademark for poloxamer 238.

Pluronic F108 trademark for poloxamer 338.

Pluronic F127 trademark for poloxamer 407.

plutonium (ploo-to′ne-um) [named after the planet *Pluto*] a transuranium element of the actinide series, first produced as the isotope 238 by bombarding uranium with deuterons. Symbol, Pu; atomic number, 94; atomic weight, 239.11; valences, 3, 4, 5, 6. The most stable plutonium isotopes are 242 and 244; there are numerous unstable ones (232–246). ^{239}Pu (half-life 24,360 years) is of major importance because of its fissionable properties by both high- and low-energy neutrons. Plutonium is a highly toxic bone-seeking poison used as a source in thermoelectric generators and in nuclear weapons.

Pm *promethium.*

π m π MESON.

PMA 1. see PMA INDEX. 2. Pharmaceutical Manufacturers Association (see under ASSOCIATION). 3. phenylmercuric ACETATE.

PMAS phenylmercuric ACETATE.

PMIS PSRO Management Information System; see under SYSTEM.

PMMA polymethyl METHACRYLATE.

PMP patient medication PROFILE.

-pnea [Gr. *pnoia* breath] a word termination denoting relationship to breathing.

pneo- [Gr. *pnein* to breathe] a combining form denoting relationship to the breath or to breathing.

pneuma- see PNEUMATO-.

pneumatic (nu-mat′ik) [L. *pneumaticus;* Gr. *pneumatikos*] of or pertaining to air or respiration.

Pneumatist 1. a school or sect of ancient medicine, founded by Athenaeus of Attalia, and based on the action and constitution of the *pneuma,* or vital air, which passed from the lungs into the heart and arteries and was then disseminated throughout the body. Among other members of this school were Agathinus of Sparta, Archigenes of Apamea, Aretaeus of Cappadocia, and Antyllus. 2. a believer in or practitioner of the Pneumatist theory of medicine.

pneumato-, pneuma- [Gr. *pneuma, pneumatos* air] a combining form denoting relationship to air or gas, or to respiration.

pneumatocele (nu-mat′o-sēl) [*pneumato-* + Gr. *kēlē* hernia] 1. hernial protrusion of lung tissue. 2. an air-containing cyst of the lung. 3. a tumor or sac containing gas. **p. cra′nii, extracranial p.,** a gaseous tumor beneath the scalp after a fracture of the skull that communicates with the paranasal sinuses. **intracranial p.,** pneumatocephalus. **parotid gland p.,** enlargement of the parotid glands due to forcing air into the parotid ducts. See also glass-blowers' MOUTH.

pneumatosis (nu″mah-to′sis) [*pneumato-* + *-osis*] the presence of air or gas in an abnormal situation in the body.

pneumo-, pneumono- [Gr. *pneumōn* lung] a combining form denoting relationship to the lungs. *Pneumo-* is also used as a combining form to denote relationship to air or to the breath.

pneumobacillus (nu″mo-bah-sil′us) *Klebsiella pneumoniae;* see under KLEBSIELLA.

pneumocephalus (nu″mo-sef′ah-lus) [*pneuma-* Gr. *kephalē* head] the presence of air in the intracranial cavity. Called also *intracranial pneumatocele.*

pneumoencephalography (nu″mo-en-sef′ah-log′rah-fe) [*pneuma-* + *encephalography*] roentgenographic visualization of the fluid-containing structures of the brain following the introduction into the spinal canal of air, oxygen, or helium.

pneumogram (nu″mo-gram″) [*pneumo-* + Gr. *gramma* mark] 1. the tracing or graphic record of respiratory movements. 2. a roentgenogram made after the injection of air into a cavity or part. Called also *aerogram.*

pneumography (nu-mog′rah-fe) 1. [*pneumo-* + Gr. *graphein* to write] an anatomical description of the lungs or graphic recording of the respiratory movement. 2. [*pneuma-* + Gr. *graphein* to write] roentgenographic visualization of a part after introducing air, oxygen, helium, or other inert gas.

pneumonia (nu-mo′ne-ah) [Gr. *pneumōnia*] inflammation of the lungs. **bronchial p., catarrhal p., lobular p.,** bronchopneumonia.

pneumono- see PNEUMO-.

pneumothorax (nu″mo-tho′raks) [*pneumo-* + Gr. *thōrax* thorax] collapse of a portion of the lung or the entire lung due to an accumulation of air or gas in the pleural cavity; it may occur spontaneously, or it may follow trauma to, and perforation of the chest wall, or be performed surgically for diagnostic or therapeutic purposes. See also ATELECTASIS.

Pneumovirus (nu″mo-vi′rus) [*pneumo-* + *virus*] a genus of paramyxoviruses, which includes the respiratory syncytial virus of humans and bovines and the pneumonia virus of mice.

pneumovirus (nu″mo-vi′rus) any virus of the genus *Pneumovirus.*

PNHA Physicians National Housestaff Association.

PNS posterior nasal SPINE (2).

PO phosphate.

P.O. abbreviation for L. *per os,* by mouth; orally.

Po 1. polonium. 2. porion.

Po₂ symbol for oxygen partial pressure (tension); also written Po_2, pO_2, pO_2.

pock (pok) a pustule, especially one of the lesions of smallpox.

pocket (pok′et) a saclike space or cavity. **absolute p.,** a term used in the past for a periodontal pocket that occurs in periodontal diseases and is associated with a diseased gingiva and deepening of the crevice, due to destruction of the periodontal tissue. **complex p.,** a spiral-type periodontal pocket that originates on

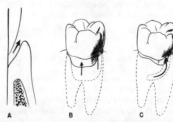

Classification of periodontal pockets according to involved tooth surfaces. *A,* Simple pocket. *B,* Compound pocket. *C,* Complex pocket. (From F. A. Carranza: Glickman's Clinical Periodontology. 5th ed. Philadelphia, W. B. Saunders Co., 1979.)

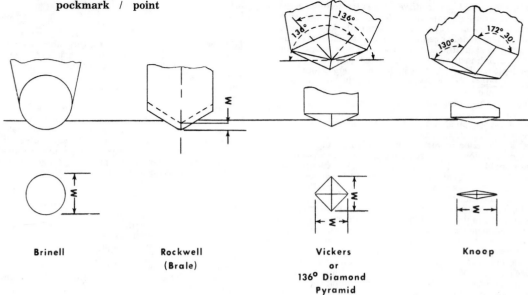

Brinell   Rockwell   Vickers   Knoop
                 (Brale)   or
                                         136° Diamond
                                            Pyramid

Diagrammatic representation of various hardness indenter points impressed into a surface. In each of the tests the dimensions of the indentation that are measured in order to determine the hardness are designated by "M." *Brinell test* — a steel ball is used. The hardness is calculated from the diameter of the indentation. *Rockwell* — a conical diamond indenter point is shown, but the same principle would apply if the steel ball indenter were used. The dotted line represents the penetration of the indenter point upon application of the minor load, and the solid line indicates the penetration under the major load. *Vickers* or 136° diamond pyramid — a pyramidal point of a diamond is used. Hardness is determined from the average length of the diagonals. *Knoop* — the rhomboidal pyramid of a diamond is used. Hardness is determined from the length of the long axis of the indentation. (From R. W. Phillips: Skinner's Science of Dental Materials. 7th ed. Philadelphia, W. B. Saunders Co., 1973.)

one tooth surface and twists around the tooth to involve one or more additional surfaces. The only communication with the gingival margin is at the surface where the pocket originates. See illustration. **compound p.,** a periodontal pocket involving more than one tooth surface and communicating with the marginal gingiva along each of the affected surfaces. See illustration. **gingival p.,** a clinically patent gingival pouch that develops as a result of pathological conditions, such as inflammation, food impaction, calculus, irritation, and other conditions, leading to separation of the gingival epithelium from the surface of the teeth. See illustration. See also *periodontal p.* **infrabony p., intra-alveolar p.,** intrabony p. **intrabony p.,** a periodontal pocket associated with intrabony defects. Called also *infrabony p., intra-alveolar p.,* and *subcrestal p.* See illustration. **periodontal p.,** a gingival sulcus deepened into the periodontal ligament apically to the original level of the resorbed alveolar crest. See illustrations. **Rathke's p.,** Rathke's POUCH. **relative p.,** a gingival pocket formed by gingival enlargement without destruction of the underlying periodontal tissues. The crevice is deepened because of the increased bulk of the gingiva. Called also *pseudopocket.* **Seessel's p.,** Seessel's POUCH. **simple p.,** a periodontal pocket involving only one tooth surface. See illustration. **subcrestal p.,** intrabony p. **suprabony p., supracrestal p.,** a periodontal pocket in which the bottom is coronal to the underlying bone. See illustration.

pockmark (pok'mark) a depressed scar left by a pustule, especially one left by a lesion of smallpox.

POE proof of eligibility; see CERTIFICATE of eligibility.

Pog pogonion.

pogonion (po-go'ne-on) [Gr., dim. of *pōgōn* beard] a craniometric landmark, being the most anterior point in the contour of the chin in the sagittal plane. Abbreviated *Pg* or *Pog.* Called also *mental point* and *point Pog.* See illustration at CEPHALOMETRY.

-poiesis [Gr. *poiein* to make] a word termination meaning formation.

poikilo- [Gr. *poikilos* varied] a combining form meaning varied or irregular.

poikilocyte (poi'ki-lo-sīt) [*poikilo-* + Gr. *kytos* hollow vessel] an erythrocyte showing abnormal variation in shape.

poikilocytosis (poi"ki-lo-si-to'sis) [*poikilocyte* + *-osis*] a condition characterized by the presence in the blood of poikilocytes.

poikiloderma (poi"ki-lo-der-mah) [*poikilo-* + Gr. *derma* skin] a condition characterized by a mottled appearance of the skin, due to atrophic and pigmentary changes. Called also *mottled skin.* **p. atroph'icans vascula're,** poikiloderma which resembles radiodermatitis clinically, characterized by extensive telangiec-

tasia, pigmentation, and atrophy of the skin and oral mucosa. Initially, red patches appear on various parts of the body, and enlarge gradually, eventually occupying large areas. Individual lesions range in color from red to brown and consist of telangiectases, minute petechial hemorrhages, pigmented areas, and lichenoid papules covered by scales. Called also *Jacobi's disease.* **p. congenita'le,** Rothmund-Thomson SYNDROME. **reticulated pigmented p.,** poikiloderma of the face and neck, affecting most often menopausal women, characterized by an irregular reticulated network of symmetrical patches of pigmented and atrophic macular lesions, which are reddish brown and covered by small scales. It progresses from initial erythema, to edema and pruritus, to pigmentation around the hair follicles, to dryness of the skin, to desquamation, and occasionally, to follicular keratosis. This disorder is considered to be identical with *jute-spinner's melanosis.* Called also *Civatte's disease.*

poikilodermatomyositis (poi"ki-lo-der"mah-to-mi"o-si'tis) poikiloderma characterized by extensive telangiectasia and pigmentation of the skin and mucous membranes and by atrophy of the muscles and myositis. Called also *Petges-Cléjat syndrome.*

point (point) [L. *punctum*] 1. a small area or spot; the sharp end of an object. See also PUNCTUM. 2. to approach the surface, like the pus of an abscess, at a definite spot or place. 3. a tapered, pointed endodontic instrument used for exploring the depth of the root canal in root canal therapy (see under THERAPY). Called also *root canal p.* See *absorbent p.* and *silver p.* 4. mounted p. 5. an anthropometric landmark from which measurements are made. See also LANDMARK and illustrations at CEPHALOMETRY. 6. a measure of weight or precious stones, being equal to 0.01 metric carats. **p. A,** subspinale. **abrasive p.,** a mounted point having a diamond surface or made of carborundum. **p. of an abscess,** the place at which the pus comes nearest to the surface. **absorbent p.,** a cone of variable width and taper, most commonly composed of paper or a paper product, used in drying or maintaining a liquid disinfectant in the root canal of a tooth. Called also *paper p.* **acupuncture p.,** specific exterior body locations into which needles are inserted in acupuncture. **alveolar p.,** the center of the anterior margin of the alveolar arch. **p. angle,** point ANGLE. **p. ANS,** nasal spine, anterior (2); see under SPINE. **p. Ar,** articulare. **auricular p.,** Broca's p. **p. B,** supramentale. **p. Ba, p. ba,** basion. **Barker's p.,** a point 1¼ inches above and 1¼ inches behind the middle external auditory meatus, used to apply the trephine in abscess of the temporosphenoid lobe. **p. bb,** Bolton p. **bilateral p.,** bilateral LANDMARK. **p. Bo,** Bolton p. **boiling p.,** the temperature at which a liquid will boil, being the temperature at which the vapor pressure of a material equals the pressure exerted by the surrounding atmosphere. At sea level, the boiling point for water is 100°C or 212°F. **boiling p., normal,** the temperature at which a liquid boils, the vapor pressure of a substance being 1 atmosphere. **Bolton p.,** a craniometric landmark located at the top of the convex curvature of the retrocondylar fossa, posterior to the condyle and between it and the basal surface of the occipital bone. Abbreviated *B, bb, Bo,* and *BP.* Called also *point bb* and *point Bo.* See illustration at CEPHALOMETRY. **bony p., bony** LANDMARK. **bony end–p.,** an area or point on a bone, which serves as a landmark for osteometric measurements. **Brinell hardness indenter p., Brinell indenter p.,** a ball of hardened steel used for determining the Brinell number in testing materials for hardness. Called also *Brinell indenter.* See illustration. See also under HARDNESS. **Broadbent registration p.,** the midpoint of the perpendicular from the center of the sella turcica to the Bolton plane. Abbreviated *R.* Called also *point R.* **Broca's p.,** an osteometric landmark, being the center of the opening of the external auditory meatus. Called also *auricular p.* **carborundum p.,** an abrasive mounted point made of carborundum. **p. Cd, condylar p.,** condylion. **central-bearing p.,** the contact point of a central-bearing prosthodontic device. See also central-bearing DEVICE. **p. centric,** point CENTRIC. **cold rigor p.,** that point of low temperature at which the activity of a cell ceases. **condenser p.,** nib. **contact p.,** contact AREA (2). **convenience p.,** a small depression at the edge of the floor of the prepared cavity, placed there to retain the first piece of direct filling gold during the process of compaction. See direct filling gold COMPACTION. **craniometric p.,** any of various points of reference assumed for use in craniometry. **critical p.,** the temperature at or above which a gas cannot be liquefied by pressure alone. **p. defect,** point DEFECT. **diamond p.,** an abrasive mounted point having its surface impregnated with diamond chips. **p. douloureux,** painful p. **p. of election,** that point at which any particular surgical operation is done by preference. **end p.,** in titration, the highest dilution of a substance that produces a reaction with a given volume of another substance. **equivalence p.,** in titration, the point at which the number of gram equivalent weights of the two reactants is exactly the same. **eye p.,** eyepoint. **freezing p.,** the temperature at which a liquid begins to freeze, especially the temperature at which a liquid and solid are in a state of equilibrium; that of pure water at sea level (1 atm) is 0°C, or 32°F. Cf. *melting p.* **gingival p.,** the point on the sagittal surface of the incisor of the sectioned oriented cast near the gingival line and midway between the labial and lingual surfaces of the tooth. **p. Gl,** glabella (2). **p. Gn,** gnathion. **p. Go,** gonion. **gutta-percha p.,** gutta-percha CONE. **hardness indenter p.,** a point made of a hard material used for hardness tests. Called also *indenter p.* See illustration. See also HARDNESS number. **hinge-axis p.,** a reference point on the skin corresponding with the terminal mandibular (hinge) axis of the mandible. **Hirschfeld's silver p.,** a calibrated silver rod used to record the depth of periodontal pockets on radiographs. See also periodontal PROBE. **p. Id,** interdentale. **p. IdI,** INTERDENTALE inferius. **p. IdS,** INTERDENTALE superius. **p. Ii,** INCISION inferius. **immunodominant p.,** the portion of the antigenic determinant (see under DETERMINANT) most critical to establishing specificity. **indenter p.,** hardness indenter p. **p. Is,** INCISION superius. **isoelectric p.,** the point of electric neutrality; the pH value at which a dipolar ion of a charged molecule does not migrate in an electric field in a solution. **isoionic p.,** the pH value of a solution at which a specific ion (usually a protein) contains as many negative charges as positive charges. **jugal p.,** jugale. **jugomaxillary p.,** a craniometric landmark, being the point at the anteroinferior angle of the zygomatic bone. **Knoop hardness indenter p., Knoop indenter p.,** an indenter having a diamond head ground to an elongated pyramidal form with a ratio of diagonals of 7.11 to 1, used for determining the Knoop number in testing materials for hardness. Called also *Knoop indenter.* See illustration. See also under HARDNESS. **p. KR,** key RIDGE. **lacrimal p's,** outlets of the lacrimal canaliculi. Called also *puncta lacrimalia.* **leak p.,** renal threshold for glucose; see under THRESHOLD. **p. Li,** LABRALE inferius. **p. Ls,** LABRALE superius. **McEwen's p.,** a point above the inner canthus of the eye, which is tender in acute frontal sinusitis. **maximum occipital p.,** a craniometric landmark, being the point on the occipital bone farthest from the glabella. See also OPISTHOCRANION. **p. Me,** menton. **median mandibular p.,** a craniometric landmark, being the point on the anteroposterior center of the mandibular ridge in the median sagittal plane, at the site of former mandibular symphysis. **Méglin's p.,** a point where the greater palatine nerve emerges from the great palatine foramen. **melting p.,** the temperature at which a solid begins to liquify; that of pure water at sea level (1 atm) is 0°C, or 32°F. Abbreviated *mp.* Cf. *freezing p.* **mental p.,** pogonion. **metopic p.,** glabella (2). **mid-**

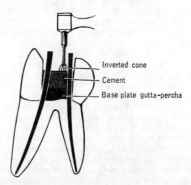

Mounted diamond points. (From V. R. Park and J. R. Ashman: A Textbook for Dental Assistants. 2nd ed. Philadelphia, W. B. Saunders Co., 1975.)

sagittal p., midsagittal LANDMARK. **motor p.,** 1. the point at which a motor nerve enters the muscle. 2. any point on the skin over a muscle at which the application of galvanic stimulation will cause contraction of a corresponding muscle. **mounted p.,** an abrasive or polishing instrument mounted in straight or contra-angle handpieces, having either a diamond or carborundum surface for abrasive purposes or being made of wood and used with pumice for polishing purposes. Called also *rotary mounted p.* See illustration. **p. Na, nasal p.,** nasion. **p. Ns,** nasospinale. **occipital p.,** a craniometric landmark, being the most posterior point on the occipital bone. **p. Or,** orbitale. **ossification p.,** CENTER of ossification. **painful p.,** one of the tender points along the course of certain nerves in neuralgia. Called also *p. douloureux* and *Valleix's p.* **paper p.,** absorbent p. **p. PNS,** nasal spine, posterior (2); see under SPINE. **p. Po,** porion. **p. Pog,** pogonion. **pour p.,** the temperature at which a liquid just begins to flow. **p. Pr,** prosthion. **preauricular p.,** an anthropometric landmark, being a point on the posterior root of the zygomatic arch just in front of the auricular point. **pressure p.,** 1. a point of extreme sensibility to pressure. 2. one of various locations on the body at which digital pressure may be applied for the control of hemorrhage. **pressure-arresting p.,** a point at which pressure arrests spasm. **pressure-exciting p.,** a point at which pressure produces spasm. **p. Ptm,** pterygomaxillary FISSURE (2). **p. R,** Broadbent registration p. **retromandibular tender p.,** a point behind the superior extremity of the mandible below the lobule of the ear and in front of the mastoid process of the temporal bone. Pressure on this point elicits extreme pain in meningitis. **Rockwell hardness indenter p., Rockwell indenter p.,** a conical diamond indenter or a ball of hardened steel, used for determining the Rockwell number in testing materials for hardness. Called also *Rockwell indenter.* See illustration. **root canal p.,** point (3). **rotary mounted p.,** mounted p. **p. S,** sella (3). **p. Sa,** a craniometric landmark, being the most anterior point of the anterior contour of the sella turcica. Abbreviated *Sa.* **p. SE,** sphenoethmoidal SUTURE (2). **p. Si,** a craniometric landmark, being the most inferior point on the lower contour of the sella turcica. Abbreviated *Si.* **silver p.,** a tapered and elongated silver plug which is cemented into the root canal in endodontic therapy as a root canal filling. Called also *silver cone.* See illustration. **p. Sn,** subnasale. **p. SO,** spheno-occipital SYNCHONDROSIS (2). **soft tissue p.,** soft tissue LANDMARK. **p. S. Or,** supraorbitale. **p. Sp,** a craniometric landmark, being the most posterior point on the posterior contour of the sella turcica. Abbreviated *Sp.* **p. Sph,** sphenoidale. **spinal p.,** subnasal p. **p. St,** stomion. **starting p.,** convenience p. **subnasal p.,** the central point of the root of the anterior nasal spine. Called also *spinal p.* **subtemporal p.,** a craniometric landmark, being the point where the sphenotemporal suture and infratemporal crest inter-

Inverted cone
Cement
Base plate gutta-percha

Silver point (cone). (From R. P. Sommer, R. D. Ostrander, and M. C. Crowley: Clinical Endodontics. 3rd ed. Philadelphia, W. B. Saunders Co., 1966.)

sect. **supra-auricular p.,** a craniometric landmark, being the point at the root of the zygomatic process of the temporal bone, directly above the auricular point. **supranasal p.,** ophryon. **supraorbital p.,** a tender spot just above the supraorbital notch in neuralgia. **sylvian p.,** a point on the surface of the skull 29 to 32 mm behind the external angular process of the frontal bone. **thermal death p.,** the degree of heat required to kill a given microorganism in a stated length of time. **p. Tr,** tragion. **Valleix's p.,** painful p. **Vickers hardness indenter p., Vickers indenter p.,** an indenter having a diamond head ground to a pyramidal form, used for determining the Vickers number in testing materials for hardness. Called also *Vickers indenter.* See illustration. See also under HARDNESS. **vital p.,** a point in the medulla oblongata, at the respiratory center, puncture of which causes immediate death. **Vogt's p., Vogt-Hueter p.,** a point of the intersection of a horizontal line, two finger-breadths above the zygoma, with a vertical line a thumb-breadth behind the ascending sphenofrontal process, used for trephination in traumatic meningeal hemorrhage. **white p.,** an abrasive mounted point of quartz, used for sharpening instruments and for polishing porcelain and metallic castings. **wood p.,** a mounted point, used with pumice for polishing. **p. Z,** a craniometric landmark, being a point formed by a line perpendicular to the nasion-menton line through the anterior nasal spine. **p. Zy,** zygion.

pointer (point'er) a contusion at a bony eminence.

pointing (point'ing) 1. making something to have a sharp or tapered end. 2. in occlusal adjustment, the restoration of cusp point contours.

Poirier's gland, line [Paul *Poirier*, French surgeon, 1853–1907] see under GLAND and LINE.

poise (poiz) [named after J. M. *Poiseville*] the unit of dynamic viscosity of a liquid, being the number of grams per centimeter per second. The commonly used unit is the *centipoise*, or one-hundredth of a poise.

Poiseuille's law [Jean Leonard Marie *Poiseuille*, French physiologist, 1799–1869] see under LAW.

poison (poi'zn) [L. *potio* draft; *toxicum*; Gr. *toxikon*] any substance which, when ingested, inhaled, or absorbed, or when applied to, injected into, or developed within the body, in relatively small amounts, by its chemical action may cause damage to structure or disturbance of function.

poisoning (poi'zun-ing) the morbid condition produced by a poison. For specific types of poisoning, see the toxic agent, as LEAD, MERCURY, etc. **blood p.,** septicemia. **food p.,** harmful effects following ingestion of food contaminated with pathogenic bacteria, toxic fungal or bacterial products, and chemical substances, or the presence in food of allergens. Vomiting, diarrhea, enteritis, and prostration are the most common clinical manifestations. **milk p.,** milk alkali SYNDROME. **p. of nuclei,** formation of deposits on the nuclei of crystallization by foreign substances, such as sodium chloride, so that further crystallization is retarded. See also gypsum RETARDER.

Polamidon trademark for the *l*-form of *methadone hydrochloride* (see under METHADONE).

Polaramine trademark for DEXCHLORPHENIRAMINE MALEATE (see under DEXCHLORPHENIRAMINE).

polarity (po-lar'ĭ-te) 1. the fact or condition of having poles. 2. the exhibition of opposite effects at the two extremities. 3. the presence of an axial gradient and exhibition by a nerve of both anelectrotonus and catelectrotonus. 4. the orientation of intracellular structures to the tissue as a whole.

polarization (po-lar"ĭ-za'shun) the production or condition of polarity. **angle of p.,** ANGLE of polarization.

Polaronil trademark for *chlorpheniramine maleate* (see under CHLORPHENIRAMINE).

Policort trademark for *dexamethasone.*

policy (pol'ĭ-se) 1. a course of action adopted and pursued by an organization or government. 2. insurance p. **annual p. maximum,** maximum annual BENEFIT. **catastrophe p.,** major medical p. **claims incurred p.,** a form of malpractice insurance under which the insured is covered for any claim arising from an incident which occurred or is alleged to have occurred during the policy period, regardless of when the claim is made. **claims made p.,** a form of malpractice insurance in which the insured is covered for any claim made, rather than an injury occurring, while the policy is in force. **extra cash p.,** an insurance policy which pays cash benefits to hospitalized individuals in fixed amounts unrelated to the individual's medical expenses or income, the policy usually being sold separately from other health insurance. **p. holder,** policy HOLDER. **insurance p.,** the document embodying the insurance contract. **major medical p.,** health insurance designed to offset catastrophic or extraordinary medical expenses. Generally, such policies do not provide first dollar coverage, but do provide benefit payments of 75 to 80 percent of all types of medical expenses above a certain base amount paid by the insured. Some policies have limited coverage of dental procedures, such as injury to sound natural teeth, extraction of impacted teeth which require hospitalization, some periodontal surgery, such as gingivectomy, transplantation, osteoplasty, and treatment of temporomandibular joint dysfunction. Called also *catastrophe p., catastrophic health insurance,* and *major medical service.* Sometimes called *major medical.* **master p.,** in insurance, a document that states the complete terms of the contract which covers a group of persons. Individuals covered under the group policy are issued certificates of insurance as evidence of their coverage. **maximum p. benefit,** maximum annual BENEFIT. **medigap p.,** Part B of Medicare. See MEDICARE. **supplemental health insurance p.,** Part B of Medicare. See MEDICARE. **trolley car p.,** a facetious name for an insurance policy which makes it almost impossible to collect payments; so-called because it is as though all benefits are excluded, except those for being hit by a trolley car. **p. year,** see benefit PERIOD.

policyholder (pol"ĭ-se-hol'der) policy HOLDER.

polio (po'le-o) poliomyelitis.

polio- [Gr. *polios* gray] a combining form denoting relationship to the gray matter of the nervous system.

poliomyelitis (po"le-o-mi"ĕ-li'tis) [*polio-* + Gr. *myelos* marrow + *-itis*] an acute disease caused by polioviruses, involving various parts of the central nervous system, including the cranial nerves, cerebral cortex, posterior column of the spinal cord, and especially the anterior horns and motor nuclei of the brain stem. Clinical manifestations may range from no apparent illness to flaccid paralysis and respiratory failure due to destruction of the respiratory center of the brain. There may be subsequent atrophy of groups of muscles, resulting in contractures and deformity. Involvement of the nuclei of cerebral nerves may cause masticatory paralysis with resulting mandibular movement disorders and temporomandibular disturbances. Polioviruses are often present in the oral cavity and carious teeth and exposed pulp may be portals of entry for the viruses. The disease is now largely controlled by vaccines. Called also *infantile paralysis, Heine-Medin disease,* and *polio.*

poliovirus (po"le-o-vi'rus) [*poliomyelitis* + *virus*] a picornavirus of the genus *Enterovirus,* which causes poliomyelitis. Infection prior to vaccination was generally universal, occurring as an inapparent disease of the upper respiratory tract and the gastrointestinal system, sometimes also invading the central nervous system with resulting paralysis of the nerves of the anterior horns of the spinal cord. The virus usually enters the body orally, and initially multiplies in the oropharyngeal and intestinal mucosa, the tonsils and Peyer's patches being involved in early infection. From the primary site, the virus enters the lymph nodes and blood, sometimes without progressing any further, but in some cases, it replicates in the viscera, producing viremia and invading the central nervous system. Polioviruses occur in three serotypes: type 1 being responsible for about 85 percent of paralytic poliomyelitis, type 2 for 5 percent, and type 3 for 10 percent. Called also *Heine-Medin disease virus* and *poliomyelitis virus.* Written also *polio virus.*

Poliseptil trademark for *sulfathiazole.*

polish (pol'ish) 1. to produce a smooth, glossy surface, especially by rubbing or friction, or by the application of a substance, such as wax. 2. a smooth and glossy surface produced by rubbing or friction or by the application of a substance, such as wax. 3. a polishing agent.

polisher-stimulator (pol'ish-er-stim"u-la'tor) a slender interdental tip made of plastic. Abbreviated *P/S.*

polishing (pol'ish-ing) 1. the creation of a smooth and glossy surface finish by rubbing or buffing, as of a denture. 2. material obtained by abrasion of a solid, such as that produced by the milling of rice; rice polishings are a rich source of vitamin B. **p. brush,** polishing BRUSH. **electro-p.,** electropolishing. **metallographic p.,** the production of a smooth, mirror-like, scratch-free surface on a metal without the use of a film (as by waxing), accomplished by the use of extremely fine abrasives. The process involved is believed to consist of the removal with the polishing agent of materials from the surface, molecule by molecule, and filling in fine scratches and irregularities by the powdered particulates being removed from the surface. The microcrystalline layer on the surface thus produced is known as the *polish layer* or *Beilby layer.*

pollen (pol'en) the mass of microspores (male fertilizing elements) of flowering plants. Many pollens, especially the airborne pollens, are allergens.

pollution (po-lu'shun) [L. *pollutio*] the act or process of rendering something impure or dirty. **air p., atmospheric p.,** the rendering of the atmosphere impure by discharging into the air foreign material in concentrations which are harmful to man and his environment. The term is sometimes used only in connection with man-made pollution and excludes the pollutants of natural origin, such as pollen, products of volcanic activity or of the decay of rocks and organic matter, and dusts from outside the earth's atmosphere.

polonium (po-lo′ne-um) [L. *Polonia* Poland] a very rare natural element of the actinide series. Symbol, Po; atomic number, 84; atomic weight, 210; melting point, 254°C; specific gravity, 9.4; valences, 4, occasionally 2 and 6; group VIA of the periodic table. Isotopes range from 193 to 218; all are radioactive. Polonium is a radioactive poison, occurring as a bismuth-like metal that dissolves by concentrated sulfuric and nitric acids and aqua regia, and by dilute hydrochloric acid. Formerly called *radium F.*

poloxamer (pol-oks′ah-mer) a class of polymers consisting of polyethylene glycols and polypropylene glycols; α-hydro-ω-hydroxypoly(oxyethylene)poly(oxypropylene)poly(oxyethylene)-block copolymers. The molecular weight of *p. 188* is 8350; *p. 238*, 10,800; *p. 407*, 12,500, and *p. 338*, 14,000. Poloxamers are surface-active substances occurring as odorless, tasteless, water-soluble, white, opaque flakes; used in dentifrices and mouthwashes. Believed to be nontoxic in standard concentrations. Trademarks: Pluronic 188, 238, 407, and 338.

poly- [Gr. *polys* many] a combining form meaning many or much. See also terms beginning MULTI- and PLURI-.

polyacrylonitrile (pol″e-ak″rĭ-lo-ni′tril) Orlon.

polyadenitis (pol″e-ad″ĕ-ni′tis) [*poly-* + Gr. *adēn* gland + *-itis*] inflammation of several or many glands.

polyadenoma (pol″ĕ-ad″ĕ-no′mah) adenoma of many glands.

polyadenopathy (pol″e-ad″ĕ-nop′ah-the) any disease affecting several glands.

polyalcohol (pol″e-al′ko-hol) polyhydric ALCOHOL.

polyarteritis (pol″e-ar′tĕ-ri′tis) [*poly-* + Gr. *artēria* artery + *-itis*] inflammation involving multiple arteries. **p. nodo′sa,** PERIARTERITIS nodosa. **rhinogenic p.,** Wegener's GRANULOMATOSIS.

polyarthritis (pol″e-ar-thri′tis) [*poly-* + Gr. *arthron* joint + *-itis*] an inflammation of several joints together. **ankylosing p.,** Bekhterev-Strümpell-Marie SYNDROME. **p. rheumat′ica acu′ta,** rheumatic FEVER.

polyblast (pol′e-blast) [*poly-* + Gr. *blastos* germ] originally, a name for the mononuclear exudate cells in inflamed tissues, believed to arise from the wandering cells of the tissue and from hypertrophied nongranular leukocytes which have left the blood stream. As now used, it is a synonym for *macrophage.*

polyblennia (pol″e-blen′e-ah) [*poly-* + Gr. *blenna* mucus + *-ia*] the secretion of excessive quantity of mucus.

polycarbonate (pol″e-kar′bon-āt) see polycarbonate RESIN.

polycarboxylate (pol″e-kar-bok′sĭ-lāt) a salt of polycarboxylic acid. **p. cement,** polycarboxylate CEMENT.

polychondritis (pol″e-kon-dri′tis) [*poly-* + *chondritis*] inflammation involving many cartilages. **chronic atrophic p., relapsing p.,** a disease of the articular and nonarticular cartilage, suspected of being hereditary, frequently affecting the nose, throat, and ears. A wide variety of symptoms may include recurrent nasal inflammation, tenderness of the nasal septum, rhinorrhea, epistaxis, and saddle nose; middle and inner ear lesions, deafness, tinnitus, and red swollen ears; and recurrent laryngeal inflammation, dyspnea, obstruction of the airways, cough, and hoarseness. Fever, malaise, and arthralgia may occur. Ocular symptoms may include conjunctivitis and iritis. The erythrocyte sedimentation rate is elevated. Called also *chondrolytic perichondritis, diffuse perichondritis, generalized chondromalacia,* and *Meyenburg-Altherr-Uehlinger syndrome.*

polychromatic (pol″e-kro-mat′ik) [*poly-* + Gr. *chrōma* color] exhibiting many colors.

polychromatocyte (pol″e-kro-mat′o-sīt) [*poly-* + Gr. *chrōma* color + *kytos* cell] 1. a cell that is stainable with various stains or colors. 2. polychromatic NORMOBLAST.

polychromatophil (pol″e-kro-mat′o-fil) [*poly-* + Gr. *chrōma* color + *philein* to love] having affinity for various stains; stainable with different kinds of stains or colors.

Polycycline trademark for *tetracycline* (1).

polycyte (pol′e-sīt) [*poly-* + Gr. *kytos* hollow vessel] a hypersegmented neutrophil of normal size. See also MACROPOLYCYTE and PROPOLYCYTE.

polycythemia (pol″e-si-the′me-ah) [*poly-* + Gr. *kytos* cell + *haima* blood + *-ia*] an abnormally large number of erythrocytes in the circulating blood, ranging from 7 to 12 million cells per cubic millimeter. See also ERYTHROCYTE count. **absolute p.,** an increase in the total red cell mass. **Mosse's p.,** Mosse's SYNDROME. **myelopathic p.,** p. vera. **relative p.,** relatively excessive concentration of erythrocytes in the circulating blood resulting from

loss of the fluid portion of the blood; it may occur as an acute transient condition or it may be chronic. **p. ru′bra,** p. vera. **secondary p.,** erythrocytosis. **splenomegalic p.,** p. vera. **transient p.,** relative polycythemia of brief duration. **p. ve′ra,** absolute polycythemia occurring most commonly in middle-aged males, with splenomegaly and cyanosis being the most constant symptoms. Headache, gas pains, and belching are the typical presenting symptoms. It is characterized by flushing, itching of the skin after a bath, ecchymoses, neuralgia, thickening of the phalanges, dyspnea, vertigo, lassitude, weakness, tinnitus, and dyspepsia. Other symptoms may include transitory blindness, mesenteric thrombosis, gangrene, and hemorrhage from various organs. Oral manifestations include purplish red coloration of the mucosa, especially of the tongue and gingivae and swelling and bleeding from the gingivae, and ecchymoses, hematomas, and submucosal petechiae are common. Recurrent infection may occur. The erythrocyte count and hemoglobin level are grossly elevated with the erythrocyte count reaching sometimes 10,000,000 cells per cmm. Leukocytosis, increased number of blood platelets, and bone marrow hyperplasia are other hematological features. When associated with liver cirrhosis, it is known as *Mosse's syndrome.* Called also *myelopathic p., p. rubra, splenomegalic p., erythremia, Osler's disease, Vaquez's disease,* and *Vaquez-Osler disease.*

polydentate (pol″e-den′tāt) 1. characterized by or having several teeth or toothlike structures. 2. a polydentate ligand; a chelate.

polydipsia (pol″e-dip′se-ah) [*poly-* + Gr. *dipsa* thirst + *-ia*] excessive thirst.

polydysplasia (pol″e-dis-pla′ze-ah) [*poly-* + *dysplasia*] faulty development in several types of tissues or several organs or systems; multiple dysplasia.

polyether (pol″e-e′ther) a polymer in which the repeating unit contains the —(CH₂—CHR—O—)ₙ group. It is cured by the reaction between aziridine rings, the main chain being probably a copolymer of ethylene oxide and tetrahydrofuran. Cross-linking is brought about by an aromatic sulfonate ester. It forms a rigid elastomeric substance. **p. impression material,** impression material, polyether; see under MATERIAL. **p. rubber,** impression material, polyether; see under MATERIAL.

polyethylene (pol″e-eth′ĭ-lēn) a product of polymerization of liquid ethylene at high temperatures, occurring as a tough, plastic solid with milky transparency that can be molded into sheets or objects of various shapes and sizes. It is resistant to water, nonoxidizing acids and alkalies, alcohols, ethers, and ketones. Polyethylene is not resistant to heat and its products are highly flammable. Used in the production of laboratory tubings, bags, prostheses, and various other products. Called also *ethene homopolymer.* Trademarks: Agilene, Alathon, Alkathene, Lupolen, Polythene. **p. glycol,** polyethylene GLYCOL.

Poly-G trademark for *polyethylene glycol* (see under GLYCOL).

polygene (pol′e-jēn) [*poly-* + *gene*] a group of nonallelic genes which individually have little effect but act cumulatively in exerting a phenotypic effect. Called also *cumulative genes* and *quantitative genes.* See also multifactorial genes, under GENE.

polyglucose (pol″e-gloo′kōs) a polysaccharide composed only of glucose moieties.

Polyglycol E trademark for *polyethylene glycol* (see under GLYCOL).

polygnathus (po-lig′nah-thus) [*poly-* + Gr. *gnathos* jaw] a double monster with the autosite and the parasite united at the jaws.

polyhedral (pol″e-he′dral) [*poly-* + Gr. *hedra* seat, base] having many faces or sides.

polyhydric (pol″e-hi′drik) containing more than two hydroxyl groups.

cis-1,4-**polyisoprene** (pol″e-i′so-prēn) the principal chemical component of rubber. See RUBBER (1).

polykeratosis (pol″e-ker″ah-to′sis) [*poly-* + *keratosis*] keratosis involving several organs. **p. congen′ita,** PACHYONYCHIA congenita.

polymer (pol′ĭ-mer) [Gr. *polys* many + *meros* part] a chemical compound consisting of a large organic molecule (macromolecule) built up by repetition of smaller, simpler monomeric units (mers), sometimes occurring as a simple chain and, other times, as branched or interconnected chains forming three-dimensional networks. The most desired qualities of polymeric materials being the ability to be molded into complex shapes, while in a softened condition, and hardness, resistance to abrasion, and chemical inertness, after hardening by polymerization. In dentistry, they are used for a variety of purposes, as impression materials, dental waxes, denture base materials, restoration materials, and cements. See also dental MATERIAL, dental WAXES, and degree of POLYMERIZATION. **addition p.,** see addition POLYMERIZATION. **block p.,** block COPOLYMER. **chlorethylene p.,** POLYVINYL chloride. **chloroethylene p.,** POLYVINYL chloride. **condensation p.,** a compound formed by the repeated reaction of smaller molecules (monomers) involving at the same time the elimination of water or other simple compounds (e.g., nylon). See also condensation POLYMERIZATION. **cross-linked p.,** one in which individual strands are connected through a process of cross-linking, the cross-linkage forming bridges between the linear macromolecules to form a three-dimensional network that alters the strength, solubility, and water sorption of the substance:

$$\cdots -M-M-M-Y-M-M-M-Y- \cdots$$
$$|$$
$$Y$$
$$|$$
$$\cdots -M-Y-M-M-M-Y- \cdots$$

graft p., graft COPOLYMER. **polysulfide p.,** POLYSULFIDE polymer. **random p.,** random COPOLYMER. **silicone p's,** SILICONE polymers. **tetrafluoroethylene p.,** polytetrafluoroethylene. **thermoplastic p.,** one that softens and flows when heated and can be remelted many times without change. See also thermoplastic RESIN. **thermosetting p.,** one that, when heated to its melting point, undergoes a permanent change and is set to a solid which cannot be remelted. See also thermosetting RESIN.

polymerase (pol'im'er-ās) any enzyme that catalyzes polymerization. See LIGASE. **DNA p.,** DNA NUCLEOTIDYLTRANSFERASE. **RNA p.,** RNA NUCLEOTIDYLTRANSFERASE.

polymeric (pol"ĭ-mer'ik) [*poly-* + Gr. *meros* part] 1. pertaining to, made of, or affecting several segments, as distinguished from monomeric, dimeric, etc. 2. exhibiting the characteristics of a polymer.

polymerization (pol"ĭ-mer"ĭ-za'shun) a chemical process in which, through a series of reactions, a macromolecule, or polymer, is formed from large numbers of single molecules known as monomers; a reaction whereby a large number of low-molecular-weight molecules (mers) of one or more species form a single large molecule of high molecular weight. The four stages of polymerization include: induction or initiation, when the molecules of the initiator become energized or activated and start to transfer their energy to the monomer molecules; propagation, when monomers join to form chains; termination, when the chain reactions are terminated by either direct coupling or by exchange of a hydrogen atom from one growing chain to another; and chain transfer, when the active state is transferred from an activated radical to an inactive molecule, and a new nucleus for further growth is created. See also CURING. **addition p.,** polymerization in which succeeding monomers are added to the molecule to increase the size of the polymer, the macromolecules being formed from smaller units, or monomers, without change in composition, since the monomer and polymer have the same empirical formulas. The process proceeds without the formation of byproducts. **condensation p.,** a chemical reaction in which the joining of the mers to form polymers is accompanied by the formation of byproducts, such as water, ammonia, or hydrochloric acid. See also condensation RESIN. **degree of p.,** the number of repeat mer units in a chain, calculated according to the following formula:

$$DP = \frac{\text{average MW}}{\text{mer weight}}$$

Polymers, such as man-made plastics, natural rubbers, wool, and cellulose have a degree of polymerization in the range of 500 to 1500. The average degree of polymerization is calculated by dividing the total number of structural units by the total number of molecules. Abbreviated *DP*. **p. shrinkage,** polymerization SHRINKAGE.

polymethacrylate (pol"e-meth-ak'rĭ-lāt") a methacrylate polymer (see METHACRYLATE).

polymethyl (pol"e-meth'il) a chemical substance having two or more CH₃ (methyl) groups. **p. methacrylate,** polymethyl METHACRYLATE.

polymethylmethacrylate (pol"e-meth"il-meth-ah-krī-lāt") see polymethyl METHACRYLATE.

polymorphic (pol"e-mor'fik) [*poly-* + Gr. *morphē* form] having many forms; multiform.

polymorphism (pol"e-mor'fizm) [*poly-* + Gr. *morphē* form] the state or quality of occurring in several different forms. **chromo-**

somal p., the occurrence of one or several chromosomes in two or more structural forms, including the presence, absence, or minor variations of certain chromosomal segments, not necessarily with associated physical abnormality. See also MONOSOMY and TRISOMY. **genetic p.,** the occurrence in a population of two or more genetically determined phenotypes in such proportions that the rarest of them cannot be maintained by mutation alone.

polymyalgia (pol"e-mi-al'je-ah) myalgia affecting several muscles.

polymyositis (pol"e-mi"o-si'tis) [*poly-* + Gr. *mys* muscle + *itis*] inflammation of several muscles; multiple myositis.

polymyxin (pol"e-mik'sin) an antibiotic complex isolated from cultures of *Bacillus polymyxa*. **p. B,** a mixture of polymyxins B₁ and B₂, which is chemically identical with colistin, except for the substitution of a residue of D-phenylalanine for that of D-leucine. Used therapeutically in the form of the sulfate salt, occurring as a white to buff, odorless powder or with a faint odor, which is soluble in water and slightly soluble in alcohol. It is a cationic detergent with a molecular weight of about 1000, which affects the permeability of the cell membrane. Its antibacterial activity is limited to gram-negative bacteria. Side effects include vertigo, weakness, paresthesias of the mouth and face, facial flushing, incoordination, ataxia, dysarthria, dyssynergia, renal damage, dyspnea, slurred speech, blurred vision, areflexia, myasthenia, diplopia, ptosis, dysphagia, and blood disorders. Suprainfection with gram-positive organisms may occur. Trademark: Aerosporin. **p. E,** COLISTIN sulfate.

polyneuralgia (pol"e-nu-ral'je-ah) [*poly-* + *neuralgia*] neuralgia affecting several nerves.

polyneuritis (pol"e-nu-ri'tis) [*poly-* + Gr. *neuron* + *-itis*] inflammation of several nerves; multiple neuritis. **acute infectious p.,** Guillain-Barré SYNDROME.

polynucleotide (pol"e-nu'kle-o-tīd) a polymer of mononucleotides formed by a sequence of nucleotides (of DNA or RNA), in which the 3' position of the sugar of one nucleotide is linked through a phosphate group with the 5' position of the sugar of the adjacent nucleotide.

polyodontia (pol"e-o-don'she-ah) [*poly-* + Gr. *odous* tooth + *-ia*] the presence of supernumerary teeth.

polyol (pol'e-ol) polyhydric ALCOHOL.

Polyomavirus (pol"e-o-mah-vi'rus) [*poly-* + *-oma* + *virus*] a genus of oncogenic papovaviruses, in which the diameter of the virion is about 45 nm and the molecular weight of the DNA is 3×10^6. Tumors caused by the virus may undergo malignant degeneration. Under some conditions, viral particles containing reduced amounts of DNA (defective viruses) may be produced. Hybrids between adenoviruses and polyoma viruses have been produced in the laboratory.

polyoncosis (pol"e-ong-ko'sis) a condition characterized by the development of multiple tumors.

polyostotic (pol"e-os-tot'ik) [*poly-* + Gr. *osteon* bone] pertaining to or affecting several bones.

polyp (pol'ip) [Gr. *polypous* a morbid excrescence] a morbid excrescence, or protruding growth, from mucous membrane; classically applied to a growth of the mucous membrane of the nose, the term is now applied to such protrusions from any mucous membrane. **choanal p.,** a nasal polyp that arises from the maxillary sinus and projects anteriorly into the nasopharynx. **gum p.,** a small pedunculated growth on the gingiva. **p. of larynx,** a smooth, rounded, sessile or pedunculated nodule, usually occurring on the true vocal cords, which may become ulcerated as a result of the trauma inflicted by the opposing vocal cords. **nasal p.,** a focal accumulation of edema fluid in the mucosa of the nose, with hyperplasia of the associated submucosal connective tissue. **pulp p.,** hyperplastic PULPITIS.

polypapilloma tropicum (pol"e-pap"ĭ-lo'mah trōp'ĭ-kum) [*poly-* + *papilloma*] yaws.

polypeptide (pol"e-pep'tīd) [*poly-* + *peptide*] a structural unit of proteins which, on hydrolysis, yields more than two amino acids; distinguished as tripeptides, tetrapeptides, etc., according to the number of amino acids contained. See also PEPTIDE and PEPTONE. **p. chain,** polypeptide CHAIN.

polyphagia (pol"e-fa'je-ah) [*poly-* + Gr. *phagein* to eat] excessive or voracious eating.

polypharmacy (pol"e-fahr'mah-se) [*poly-* + Gr. *pharmakon* drug] 1. simultaneous administration of several drugs in combination or separately. 2. the administration of excessive medication.

polyphase (pol'e-fāz) [*poly-* + *phase*] having several phases.

polyphasic (pol"e-fa'zik) having or existing in many phases; having unlike particles in the disperse phase.

polyphosphorylase (pol"e-fos-for'ĭ-lās) phosphorylase.

polyphyodont (pol"e-fi'o-dont) [*poly-* + Gr. *phyein* to produce + *odous* tooth] developing several sets of teeth successively throughout life.

polypi (pol'ĭ-pi) [L.] plural of *polypus*.

polyplegia (pol"e-ple'je-ah) [*poly-* + Gr. *plēgē* stroke + *-ia*] simultaneous paralysis of several muscles.

polyploid (pol'e-ploid) [*poly-* + *-ploid*] 1. having more than two full sets of homologous chromosomes; there may be three (triploid), four (tetraploid), five (pentaploid), etc. 2. an individual or cell having more than two full sets of homologous chromosomes.

polyploidy (pol'e-ploi"de) [*poly-* + *ploidy*] the state of being polyploid.

polypnea (pol"ip-ne'ah) [*poly-* + Gr. *pnoia* respiration] a condition in which the rate of respiration is increased; hyperpnea; panting.

polyposis (pol"e-po'sis) the presence of multiple polyps. **familial p.,** a hereditary condition, transmitted as an autosomal dominant trait, characterized by the presence of multiple adenomatous polypi of the intestine, usually the colon, which may undergo malignant degeneration. When associated with mucocutaneous pigmentation, it is known as *Peutz-Jeghers syndrome;* when associated with cysts of the skin, osteomas, fatty tumors of the mesentery, follicular odontomas, and dentigerous cysts, it is known as *Gardner's syndrome.* **hereditary p. and osteomatosis,** Gardner's SYNDROME. **melanoplakia-small intestinal p.,** Peutz-Jeghers SYNDROME.

polypotome (po-lip'o-tōm) [*polyp* + Gr. *tomē* a cutting] a cutting instrument for removing polyps.

polypotrite (po-lip'o-trīt) [*polyp* + L. *terere* to crush] instrument for crushing polyps.

polypus (pol'ĭ-pus), pl. *pol'ypi* [L.; Gr. *polypous*] a polyp.

polyradiculoneuritis (pol"e-rah-dik"u-lo-nu-ri'tis) [*poly-* + L. *radix* root + Gr. *neuron* nerve + *-itis*] Guillain-Barré SYNDROME.

polyribosome (pol"e-ri'bo-sōm) a complex made up of ribosomal subunits assembled among themselves by the filaments of messenger RNA containing the genetic information; they play a role in the synthesis of peptides. Called also *ergosome* and *polysome.*

polyrrhea (pol"e-re'ah) [*poly-* + Gr. *rhoia* flow] a copious fluid discharge.

polysaccharide (pol"e-sak'ah-rīd) a class of high-molecular-weight carbohydrates which, on hydrolysis, yield chiefly monosaccharides or related products, most commonly glucose and, to a lesser extent, mannose, galactose, xylose, arabinose, and glucuronic, galacturonic, and mannuric acids, also containing glucosamine, galactosamine, and sialic and uronic acids. Some polysaccharides are linear polymers, others are branched, all being linked by glycosidic bonds. Polysaccharides differ from simple sugars by being insoluble in water and lacking a sweet taste. When dissolved, they form colloidal solutions due to their large molecules. Most have a terminal monomer present as a reducing sugar. Some polysaccharides are formed from pentoses and hexoses and many are mixed. Those composed of repeating glucose units are known as *glucans* and those made up of mannose units are *mannans.* Starch, glycogen, dextrin, and cellulose are principal polysaccharides. See also HETEROPOLYSACCHARIDE, HOMOPOLYSACCHARIDE, and MUCOPOLYSACCHARIDE. **bacterial p.,** one found in bacteria, especially in bacterial capsules. **immune p.,** one which can function as a specific antigen. **mixed p.,** heteropolysaccharide. **soluble p.,** one which dissolves in water. **specific p.,** a soluble polysaccharide found in microorganisms which in high dilution precipitate specifically the antisera of the corresponding organisms. **storage p's,** those polysaccharides, of which starch is the most abundant in plants and glycogen in animals, usually deposited as granules in the cytoplasm of cells, to be used for metabolic purposes and for energy. **structural p's,** those that serve as structural elements in cell walls and coats, intercellular spaces, and connective tissue and give shape, elasticity, or rigidity to plant and animal tissues, also providing protection and support to unicellular organisms.

polyserositis (pol"e-se-ro-si'tis) general inflammation of serous membranes with serous effusion.

polysialia (pol"e-si-a'le-ah) [*poly-* + Gr. *sialon* saliva + *-ia*] ptyalism.

polysiloxane (pol'ĕ-si'lok-sān) a polymer of silicone dioxide; see SILOXANE. **dimethyl p.,** simethicone.

polysinusectomy (pol"e-si"nu-sek'to-me) excision of the diseased membrane of several of the paranasal sinuses.

polysinusitis (pol"e-si-nu-si'tis) [*poly-* + *sinusitis*] inflammation of several sinuses at once.

polysome (pol'e-sōm) polyribosome.

polysomy (pol'e-so'me) [*poly-* + *chromosome*] an excess of a particular chromosome, resulting from meiotic chromosomal disjunction. The chromosome may be duplicated three (trisomy), four (tetrasomy), or more times.

polysorbate (pol"e-sor'bāt) a generic name for esters of sorbitol and its anhydrides condensed with polymers of ethylene oxide, which are surfactant agents used as emulsifiers and dispersing agents for drugs designed for internal use: *p. 20,* $C_{58}H_{114}O_{26}$, is polyoxyethylene 20 sorbitan monolaurate; *p. 40,* $C_{62}H_{122}O_{26}$, is polyoxyethylene 20 sorbitan monopalmitate; *p. 60,* $C_{64}H_{126}O_{26}$, is polyethylene 20 sorbitan monostearate; *p. 65,* $C_{100}H_{194}O_{28}$, is polyethylene 20 sorbitan tristearate; *p. 80,* $C_{64}H_{124}O_{26}$, is polyethylene 20 sorbitan monooleate; *p. 85,* $C_{100}H_{188}O_{28}$, is polyethylene 20 sorbitan trioleate.

polystyrene (pol"e-sti'rĕn) a thermoplastic synthetic resin produced by the polymerization of styrene (vinyl benzene). It occurs as a transparent, hard solid with a high strength and impact resistance, which is resistant to organic acids, alkalies, and alcohols, but is attacked by organic solvents. Unmodified polystyrene yellows when exposed to light. It can be copolymerized with various resins. Used in the construction of denture bases. Called also *polyvinyl benzene.* Trademarks: Dylene, Trycite.

polysulfide (pol"e-sul'fīd) a binary sulfur compound containing more sulfur than is required by the normal valency of the metal, as in sodium sulfide, Na_2S. **p. accelerator, p. catalyst, p. coreactant,** polysulfide ACCELERATOR. **p. polymer,** a synthetic rubber, having the structural formula:

$$\left[\begin{array}{c} -(CH_2)_x S - S - \\ \parallel \quad \parallel \\ S \quad S \end{array} \right]$$

It occurs as a solid or liquid obtained by the reaction of sodium polysulfide with organic dichlorides, occurring as a resilient, hard substance, some formulations having a strong odor. Used in dentistry as a base for polysulfide impression materials (see under MATERIAL). Called also *polyfunctional mercaptan, polysulfide rubber,* and *thiorubber.* Trademark: Thiokol.

polysyndrome (pol'e-sin'drom) a condition combining the characteristics of several syndromes. **Turner-mongolism p.,** a syndrome combining the characteristics of both Turner's syndrome and Down's syndrome. Its principal features include growth and mental retardation, shieldlike chest, poorly developed breasts, absent body hair, brachycephaly, short neck with folding, low hairline, oblique palpebral fissures, squat nose, scrotal or normal tongue, high or cleft palate, short hands and feet, frequent cubitus valgus, hypoplastic or peniform clitoris, and the XO/G + karyotype, mosaic for XO in most instances.

polytetrafluoroethylene (pol"e-tet"rah-floo"or-o-eth'ĭ-lēn) a tough, nonflammable, chemically inert plastic, obtained by homopolymerization of tetrafluoroethylene, and composed of very long chains of linked CF_2 units. It does not dissolve in any known substance, but deteriorates with age and on prolonged contact with fluorine, hot plasticizers, and polymeric waxes. Used in the production of tubing and sheets for chemical laboratories, surgical implants, nonsticking cooking dishes, insulators, and various other products. Called also *tetrafluoroethene homopolymer* and *tetrafluoroethylene polymer.* Trademarks: Fluoroflex, Teflon.

Polythene trademark for *polyethylene.*

polythiazide (pol"e-thi'ah-zīd) a benzothiadiazine diuretic with antihypertensive properties, 6-chloro-3,4-dihydro-2-methyl-3-[[(2,2,2-trifluoroethyl)thio]methyl]-2 *H*-1,2,4-benzothiadiazine-7-sulfonamide 1,1-dioxide. It occurs as a white, crystalline powder with a characteristic odor, which is soluble in methanol, acetone, and dimethylformamide, but not in water and chloroform. Side effects are those of the benzothiadiazine diuretics. Trademarks: Drenusil, Nephril, Renese.

polytropic (pol"e-trop'ik) [*poly-* + Gr. *tropos* a turning] affecting many kinds of bacteria or many varieties of tissues. See also MONOTROPIC.

polyunsaturated (pol"e-un-sach'ĕ-rāt-ed) having many unsaturated bonds and tending to be liquid at room temperature; said of fats and oils.

polyurethane (pol"e-u're-thān) a class of thermoplastic polymers produced by condensation of a polyisocyanate and a hydroxyl-containing material such as a polyol or drying oil. Polyurethanes are characterized by the presence of the methane group, $-NH \cdot CO \cdot O-$, many containing urethane or a free isocyanate group. They are produced as fibers, coatings, moldable resins, elastomers, and foams, and have high elastic modules, good electrical resistance, high moisture resistance, and crystalline structure. Some are used as pit and fissure sealants, having a rubbery consistency and providing protection for limited periods. Most also contain fluorides and are used as short-term sealants and long-term fluoridation vehicles. Elmex Protector and Epoxylite 9070 are the principle polyurethane pit and fissure sealants.

polyuria (pol"e-u're-ah) [poly- + Gr. *ouron* urine + -ia] excretion of an abnormally large volume of urine in a given period.

polyvalent (po-liv'ah-lent) having more than one valency.

Polyvidone trademark for *povidone.*

polyvinyl (pol"e-vi'nil) a compound having a number of vinyl units, $CH_2:CH-$, in a polymerized form. **p. acetate,** a product of polymerization of vinyl acetate, occurring as a colorless, odorless, tasteless, nontoxic, transparent thermoplastic solid, which is resistant to weathering and ultraviolet rays, but has a relatively low softening point (35–40 C). It is insoluble in water, gasoline, oils, and fats, but soluble in low-molecular-weight alcohols, esters, benzene, and chlorinated hydrocarbons. Used in the production of denture bases and maxillofacial prostheses. Abbreviated *PVAc.* **p. benzene,** polystyrene. **p. chloride,** a product of polymerization of vinyl chloride, which is a thermoplastic polymer occurring as a tasteless, odorless, nontoxic white powder or colorless granules. It is resistant to weathering and moisture, but darkens when exposed to ultraviolet rays, thus requiring stabilizers to prevent discoloration, and is combustible but self-extinguishing. Polyvinyl chloride resists most acids, fats, oils, and fungi. With the use of plasticizers, it may be compounded into flexible and rigid forms, and may be processed by molding or extrusion. Used in producing denture bases and maxillofacial prostheses. Abbreviated *PVC.* Called also *chloroethene, chlorethylene polymer,* and *homopolymer.* Trademarks: Breon, Geon, Velcic, Vinacort, Vybak.

polyvinylpyrrolidone (pol"e-vi"nil-pir-rol'ĭ-dōn) povidone. **p.-iodine,** povidone-iodine.

Pompe's syndrome [J. C. *Pompe*] GLYCOGENOSIS II.

POMR problem oriented medical RECORD.

Ponderax trademark for *fenfluramine hydrochloride* (see under FENFLURAMINE).

Pondimin trademark for *fenfluramine hydrochloride* (see under FENFLURAMINE).

ponos (po'nos) visceral LEISHMANIASIS.

pons (ponz), pl. *pon'tes,* gen. *pon'tis* [L. "bridge"] 1. any slip of tissue connecting two parts of an organ. Called also BRIDGE. 2. [NA] that part of the central nervous system lying between the medulla oblongata and the mesencephalon, ventral to the cerebellum, and contains the nuclei of the fifth, sixth, seventh, and eighth cranial nerves. See also brain STEM.

Ponstan trademark for *mefenamic acid* (see under ACID).

Ponstel trademark for *mefenamic acid* (see under ACID).

Pontal trademark for *mefenamic acid* (see under ACID).

pontes (pon'tēz) plural of *pons.*

pontic (pon'tik) [L. *pons, pontis* bridge] an artificial tooth on a fixed partial denture, which replaces the lost natural tooth, restores its function, and usually occupies the space previously occupied by the natural crown.

Pont index see under INDEX.

Pontocaine trademark for *tetracaine hydrochloride* (see under TETRACAINE).

pool (pōol) 1. any grouping of interests, organizations, funds, etc., for common advantage of the participants. 2. any facility or resource shared by members of a particular group of people. **insurance p.,** an organization of insurers or reinsurers through which particular types of risks are shared or pooled. The risk of high loss by any particular insurance company is transferred to the group as a whole (the insurance pool) with premiums, losses, and expenses shared in agreed amounts. **recirculating p.,** lymphocytes found in the circulating blood, which traverse a circumscribed pathway from lymph nodes through lymphatic channels to the blood, through the postcapillary venules, and back to the lymphatic system. The passage occurs through a process in which the endothelial cells invaginate and allow lymphocytes to pass directly through. The pool consists primarily of T-lymphocytes that are characterized by their long life spans and are believed to function as memory cells. See also postcapillary VENULE.

poradenitis (pōr"ad-ĕ-ni'tis) [Gr. *poros* pore + *adēn* gland + -itis] a disease of the lymph nodes of the ileum characterized by small abscesses. **p. nos'tras,** LYMPHOGRANULOMA venereum.

porcelain (por'sĕ-lin) 1. a white, translucent, dense ceramic material produced by fusing under high temperature of a mixture of feldspar, kaolin, quartz, whiting, and other substances. It has a high impact strength, is impermeable to liquids and gases, and is resistant to chemicals except hydrofluoric acid and hot caustic solutions. Specific gravity is 2.4; Mohs hardness number 6–7; and compression strength 100,000 psi. Used in cooking utensils, laboratory ware, corrosion-resistant equipment, electrical resistors, and other products. See table. 2. dental p. **aluminous p.,** dental porcelain in which the quartz is replaced by alumina (Al_2O_3). Aluminous porcelain is generally stronger than the quartz type, alumina crystals tending to prevent the development of cracks in porcelain jackets. **Ames plastic p.,** trademark for a *silicate cement* (see under CEMENT). **p. cement,** former name for *silicate cement* (see under CEMENT). **p. cervical contact and single bake techniques,** see under TECHNIQUE. **p. cervical ditching technique,** see under TECHNIQUE. **dental p.,** a type of porcelain used in dental restorations, either jacket crowns or inlays, artificial teeth, or metal-ceramic crowns. It is essentially a mixture of particles of feldspar and quartz, the feldspar melting first and providing a glass matrix for the quartz. Dental porcelain is produced by mixing ceramic powder (a mixture of quartz, kaolin, pigments, opacifiers, a suitable flux, and other substances) with distilled water. The resulting paste is applied to the matrix made from an impression of the prepared tooth, the surface of which is covered by a thin platinum sheet, using various methods of condensation, such as vibration, pressure, spatulation, whipping, brush application, and gravitation techniques, all of which are designed to cause the particles to settle and become closely packed, while the excess water is displaced to the surface from where it is blotted out. The ceramic paste is then placed in the furnace and fired; firing under vacuum reduces the porosity of the porcelain. After the first firing, the surface of porcelain restorations is rough and porous and requires additional firing to the glaze stage (vitrification) to allow it to become smooth and translucent. When a lower fusion point is desired, substances such as sodium or potassium carbonate and borax or boric acid are added to the powder. Nepheline syenite (a mixture of potash and sodium feldspar and nephelite) is sometimes substituted for feldspar; alumina may replace silica, particularly when pins are used in the restoration; some types of glass may be used as a constituent of porcelain; and lithia and potassium silicate are sometimes used as fluxing agents. The terms *dental ceramic* and *dental porcelain* are sometimes used synonymously. **p. firing,** see FIRING (2). **p. furnace,** porcelain FURNACE. **high-fusing p., high temperature maturing p.,** a type of dental porcelain which has a fusing temperature of 1300 to 1370°C (2360–2500°F); generally used in the fabrication of artificial teeth by commercial manufacturers and rarely in dental laboratories. **Jenkins' p.,** a durable low-fusing porcelain of stable color; used especially for inlays. **low-fusing p., low temperature maturing p.,** a type of dental porcelain which has a fusing temperature of 870 to 1065°C (1600–1950°F). It is the porcelain of choice for making restorations and dentures in dental laboratories. Technically, classified as glass, rather than as a porcelain. **medium-fusing p., medium temperature maturing p.,** a type of dental porcelain which has a fusing temperature of 1090 to 1260°C (2000–2300°F); a porcelain of choice for making restorations and dentures in dental laboratories. Technically, classified as glass, rather than as a porcelain. **opaque p.,** nontranslucent dental porcelain, generally used as an initial layer to mask the color of the tooth dentin or the color of the metal if it is to be fused to a cavity for a metal-ceramic restoration. The opaque layer is normally covered with other porcelains to simulate the color and translucency of tooth structures. Metallic oxides, such as zirconium oxide, are used as the opaquing agents. **S. S. White new filling p.,** trademark for a *silicate cement* (see under CEMENT). **synthetic p.,** silicate CEMENT.

PORCELAIN

	Feldspar	Kaolin	Quartz	Whiting	Pigments and Opacifiers
Industrial porcelain dinnerware	27	45	27.5	0.5	—
Denture teeth body	70–90	1–10	1–18	—	1–3

(From William P. Lee: Ceramics. New York, Reinhold Publishing Company, 1961.)

porcelaneous (por″sĕ-la′ne-us) pertaining to or resembling porcelain.

pore (por) [L. *porus;* Gr. *poros*] a small opening. Called also *porus*. **capillary p.,** a minute opening through the capillary wall, about 80 to 90 Å in diameter, which allows certain molecules and water-soluble substances to pass through. See also capillary PERMEABILITY. **external acoustic p.,** the outer end of the external acoustic meatus. Called also *porus acusticus externus* [NA]. **external osseous acoustic p.,** the outer end of the bony external acoustic meatus, in the tympanic portion of the temporal bone. Called also *porus acusticus externus osseus* [NA]. **gustatory p.,** the small opening of the taste bud onto the surface of the tongue, through which the peripheral end of the taste cell protrudes and forms the gustatory hair. Called also *taste p.* and *porus gustatorius* [NA]. **internal acoustic p.,** the opening in the internal acoustic meatus. Called also *porus acusticus internus* [NA]. **internal osseous acoustic p.,** the opening into the internal acoustic meatus, found on the posteromedial portion of the internal surface of the petrous part of the temporal bone. Called also *porus acusticus internus osseus* [NA]. **membrane p.,** a minute opening in the cell membrane, about 8 Å in diameter, which allows transport of substances across the cell membrane between the intracellular and extracellular fluids. See also DIFFUSION. **sweat p.,** the opening in the duct of the sweat gland on the surface of the skin. Called also *porus sudoriferus* [NA]. **taste p.,** gustatory p.

porion (po′re-on) [Gr. *poros* pore + *-on* neuter ending] a craniometric landmark, being the most lateral point on the roof of the bony external auditory meatus, vertically over the middle of the meatus. Abbreviated *Po.* Called also *point Po.* See illustration at CEPHALOMETRY. **cartilaginous p.,** a landmark used in living persons in cephalometry, located at the point where the superior margin of the cartilaginous external auditory meatus is in contact with the ear-rod of the cephalostat.

porokeratosis (po″ro-ker″ah-to′sis) [Gr. *poros* pore + *keratosis*] Mibelli's DISEASE. **p. centrifuga′ta atro′phicans,** Mibelli's DISEASE.

porosity (po-ros′ĭ-te) 1. the condition of having minute openings or pores. 2. a pore. **back pressure p.,** the occurrence of pores in a dental casting due to failure to completely eliminate gases from the mold, with resulting back pressure that prevents the molten alloy from entirely filling the mold. **occluded gas p.,** porosity of a metal due to heating it in the oxidizing part of the flame. **shrink-spot p.,** areas of porosity in cast metal developing as it solidifies from its molten state, due to shrinking without additional metal being allowed to flow into the mold. **solidification p.,** porosity developing as the result of faulty spruing or heating of either the metal or the investment.

porous (po′rus) possessing pores or minute interstices, thus being permeable to liquids or gases.

porphin (por′fin) a heterocyclic structure of four linked pyrrole rings, linked by methylene (—CH═) bridges, in the center of which may be a metal. The porphin ring is a structural part of many compounds in plants and animals, including hemoglobin, myoglobin, and chlorophyll.

porphyria (por-fe′re-ah, por-fi′re-ah) a disturbance of porphyrin metabolism, characterized by the abnormal accumulation of ferroprotoporphyrin in the erythrocyte precursors in the bone marrow or in the liver, and by the presence of porphyrins in the urine and feces. **acquired p.,** porphyria characterized by abnormal porphyrin pigmentation at some part of the body, abnormal deposits of ferroporphyrins, and the presence of porphyrins in the urine and feces, resulting from liver neoplasms, intoxication by hexachlorobenze fungicides, or other causes. **acute intermittent p.,** hepatic porphyria transmitted as an autosomal dominant trait, characterized by abdominal pain and sensory and motor neurologic manifestations. **combined p.,** mixed p. **p. congen′ita, congenital erythropoietic p.,** erythropoietic p. **p. cuta′nea tar′da,** hepatic porphyria, transmitted as an autosomal dominant trait, characterized by cutaneous photosensitization and accumulation of porphyrin in the liver. **erythropoietic p.,** an inborn error of metabolism, suspected of being transmitted as an autosomal recessive trait, characterized by abnormal deposits of ferroporphyrin in the red cell precursors in the bone marrow. It is marked by cutaneous changes, including the formation of vesicles and bullae and photosensitivity, which may be absent during the neonatal period, but becomes apparent during the first years of life; porphyrinuria; and red to brownish discoloration of the deciduous and permanent teeth, yielding a red fluorescence under the fluorescent microscope. Skin eruptions appear chiefly on the face, back of the hands, and other exposed parts of the body, and rupture, leaving depressed, pigmented scars. The serous fluid usually exhibits red fluorescence. Called also *p. congenita, congenital erythropoietic p., photosensitive p.,* and *Gunther's syndrome.* **hepatic**

p., p. hepat′ica, a group of inborn errors of metabolism characterized by abnormal deposits of porphyrins in the liver, including *acute intermittent p., p. cutanea tarda,* and *mixed p.* **mixed p.,** hepatic porphyria, transmitted as an autosomal dominant trait, characterized by cutaneous photosensitization, abdominal symptoms, motor and sensory neurologic disorders, and hepatic accumulation of porphyrins. Called also *combined p.* **photosensitive p.,** erythropoietic p.

porphyrin (por′fi-rin) any of a group of cyclic compounds based on the porphin ring. They are normal pigments of the body found in hemoglobin, myoglobin, and cytochrome complexes with iron (iron porphyrins). See also PORPHYRIA. **iron p.,** a chelate complex of porphyrin (protoporphyrin) with iron. See PROTOPORPHYRIN.

porphyrinuria (por″fi-ri-nu′re-ah) [*porphyrin* + Gr. *ouron* urine + *-ia*] the presence in the urine of porphyrins in excessive amounts, giving it a red to brown color; the characteristic sign of porphyria.

port (port) 1. an aperture in a surface. 2. an aperture in the protective tube housing of an x-ray generator, through which the useful radiation beam emerges from the head of the machine.

porta (por′tah), pl. *por′tae* [L.] and entrance or portal; used in anatomical nomenclature to designate an opening, especially the site of entrance to an organ of the blood vessels and other structures supplying or draining it.

portal (por′tal) 1. an entrance or gateway. Called also *porta.* 2. pertaining to a porta, or entrance.

portepolisher (port-pol′ish-er) a cleansing and polishing hand instrument constructed to hold a wooden point, to be used in a dental engine for applying polishing paste and burnishing teeth. Written also *porte-polisher.* See illustration. **contra-angle p.,** a portepolisher angulated at 60° for use in the posterior part of the mouth.

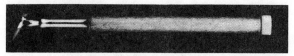

Portepolisher. (From F. A. Carranza, Jr.: Glickman's Clinical Periodontology. 5th ed. Philadelphia, W. B. Saunders Co., 1979.)

porte-polisher (port-pol′ish-er) portepolisher.

porter (por′ter) one who or that which carries or transports something. See carrier MOLECULE.

portio (por′she-o), pl. *portio′nes* [L.] a part or division, a general anatomical term for a portion of an organ or structure. **p. ma′jor ner′vi trigem′ini,** sensory root of trigeminal nerve; see under ROOT. **p. mi′nor ner′vi trigem′ini,** motor root of trigeminal nerve; see under ROOT.

portiones (por″she-o′nēz) [L.] plural of *portio.*

Portsmouth syndrome see under SYNDROME.

porus (po′rus), pl. *po′ri* [L.; Gr. *poros* passage] a pore; a small cavity or opening; used in anatomical nomenclature as a general term to designate certain openings in the body. **p. acus′ticus exter′nus** [NA], external acoustic PORE. **p. acus′ticus exter′nus os′seus** [NA], external osseous acoustic PORE. **p. acus′ticus inter′nus** [NA], internal acoustic PORE. **p. acus′ticus inter′nus os′seus** [NA], internal osseous acoustic PORE. **p. gustato′rius** [NA], gustatory PORE. **p. sudorif′erus** [NA], sweat PORE.

-posia [Gr. *posis* drinking + *-ia*] a word termination denoting relationship to drinking, or to intake of fluids.

position (po-zish-un) [L. *positio*] 1. a situation of an object or part relative to a point of reference. See also RELATION. 2. a bodily posture or attitude assumed by the patient to achieve comfort in certain conditions, or the particular disposition of the body and extremities to facilitate the performance of certain diagnostic or therapeutic procedures. 3. the situation of the fetus in the pelvis. Cf. PRESENTATION (2). **anatomical p.,** the position of the human body, standing erect, with the palms of the hands turned forward; used as the position of reference in description of the site or direction of various structures or parts as established in official anatomical nomenclature. **anteroposterior p., A-P p.,** anteroposterior PROJECTION. **backward p.,** occlusal retrusive p. **Caldwell p.,** a roentgenographic position with the forehead and nose against the x-ray plate, giving a posteroanterior projection for demonstration of the frontal sinuses and the anterior ethmoidal cells. **centric p.**, the rest position of the mandible, as it is influenced by the muscle tone, while the patient remains standing or is sitting with his jaw open, from which the teeth will come into centric occlusion, when the jaw is closed. Called also *muscular p.* See also centric OCCLUSION and centric. RELATION. **condylar hinge p.**, hinge p., condylar. **contact p., retruded**, centric RELATION. **distoangular p.**, in tooth impaction, the tilting of the crown of an unerupted tooth in the distal direction. **dorsal p.**, the posture of a person lying on his back. Called also *supine p.* See also *horizontal p.* **eccentric p.**, eccentric RELATION. **Fowler's p.**, the position in which the head of the patient's bed is raised 18 to 20 inches above the level; the knees are also elevated. **Fuchs' p.**, a roentgenographic position which gives an oblique view of the zygomatic arch projected free of superimposed structures. **hinge p.**, the position of the condyle in the temporomandibular joint from which an opening by hinge movement is possible beyond the amplitude of rest position. **hinge p., condylar**, the position of the condyles in the glenoid fossa at which hinge axis movement is possible. **hinge p., mandibular**, a position of the mandible that allows the condyles movements on the hinge axis during the opening or closing of the jaws. **hinge p., terminal**, centric RELATION. **horizontal p.**, 1. the position assumed by a person lying on his back (*dorsal p.*) with limbs extended. 2. in tooth impaction, the horizontal position of an unerupted tooth. **intercuspal p.**, centric OCCLUSION. **jaw-to-jaw p.**, centric RELATION. **lateral p.**, 1. lateral RELATION. 2. in radiography, a position distant from the medial plane or midline of the body or structure. **lateral decubitus p.**, one in which the patient rests on the side during the radiographic examination, usually of the chest or abdomen. **lateral occlusal p.**, lateral RELATION. **ligamentous p.**, centric RELATION. **mandibular hinge p.**, hinge p., mandibular. **mandibular rest p.**, rest p., mandibular. **median occlusal p.**, median RELATION. **mesio-angular p.**, in tooth impaction, the tilting of the crown of an unerupted tooth in the mesial direction. **most retruded p.**, centric RELATION. **muscular p.**, centric p. **occlusal p.**, a functional position of the jaws when the mandible is closed, in which contact between some, or all, upper and lower teeth occurs, which may or may not coincide with centric occlusion. Called also *occlusal relation.* **occlusal p., lateral**, lateral RELATION. **occlusal p., median**, median RELATION. **occlusal p., protrusive**, jaw relation, protrusive; see under RELATION. **occlusal retrusive p.**, occlusal position in which the mandible is retruded from its median position. Called also *backward p.* **physiologic rest p.**, rest p. **posterior border p.**, the most posterior position of the mandible at any specific vertical relation to the maxilla. Called also *posterior border jaw relation.* **P-A p.**, **posteroanterior p.**, posteroanterior PROJECTION. **postural resting p.**, rest p. **protrusive occlusal p.**, jaw relation, protrusive; see under RELATION. **respiratory rest p.**, rest p., respiratory. **rest p.**, the position of the mandible when its muscles are at rest and the body is in the upright standing or sitting position, the eyes being focused toward the horizon; the lips are slightly touching and the distance between the upper and lower teeth has the free-way space of about 2 to 5 mm. Abbreviated *PRP.* Called also *physiologic rest p., postural rest p., rest relation*, and *rest jaw relation.* **rest p., electromyographic**, rest position with minimal muscle activity as determined electromyographically. **rest p., physiologic**, rest p. **rest p., respiratory**, the position of the mandible and its associated soft tissue structures at the completion of the expiratory phase of the respiratory cycle. **resting p., postural**, rest p. **retruded p., retruded contact p.**, centric RELATION. **Rose's p.**, one intended to prevent aspiration or swallowing of blood, as from an injured lip: the patient on his back with head hanging over the end of the table in full extension so as to enable the patient to bleed over the margins of the inverted upper incisors. **supine p.**, dorsal p. **screw p., screw-post. terminal hinge p.**, centric RELATION. **tooth p.**, the position of a tooth in the dental arch in relation to the bone in alveolar process, its adjacent teeth, and the opposing teeth. See also centric OCCLUSION. **tooth-to-tooth p.**, centric OCCLUSION. **Trendelenburg's p.**, one in which the patient is supine on the table or bed, the head of which is tilted downward 30 to 40 degrees, and the table or bed angulated beneath the knees. **vertical p.**, in tooth impaction, vertical situation of an unerupted tooth.

positioner (po-zish'un-er) a resilient elastoplastic removable orthodontic appliance fitting over the occlusal surfaces of the teeth, designed to obtain limited tooth movement and stabilization, usually at the end of therapy to obtain final tooth position during finishing.

positive (poz'ĭ-tiv) [L. *positivus*] having a value greater than zero; indicating existence or presence of a condition, organism, etc., as chromatin positive or Wassermann positive; characterized by affirmation or cooperation. Sometimes indicated by the symbol +.

positron (poz'ĭ-tron) an elementary particle with the mass of an electron but charged positively. It is emitted in some radioactive disintegrations and is formed in pair production by the interaction of high-energy gamma rays with matter. Called also *antielectron, beta-plus*, and *positive electron.* Symbol β^+.

posology (po-sol'o-je) [Gr. *posos* how much + *-ology*] the science of dosage, or a system of dosage.

Pospischill-Feyrter aphthoid (disease) see under APHTHOID.

post (pōst) 1. a piece of wood, metal, or other material firmly secured in an upright position, usually to support something. 2. an elongated metallic projection fitted within the prepared root canal, serving to retain a crown restoration; a dowel. **abutment p.**, 1. implant ABUTMENT. 2. implant p. **implant p.**, a constricted part on that portion of the subperiosteal or intraperiosteal implant which protrudes into the oral cavity and serves as an abutment for a denture. Called also *abutment p., implant neck*, and *implant superstructure neck.* **P. W. (Pullen-Warner) split p.**, trademark for a device used for locking parts of a sectional denture through the application of frictional resistance. It is a metal post split longitudinally, consisting of two half-round sections of wire, the flat surfaces being face-to-face, surrounded by a stainless steel tube.

post- [L. *post* after] a prefix signifying after or behind, in time or place.

postalbumin (post"al-bu'min) α_1-FETOPROTEIN.

postameloblast (post"ah-mel'o-blast") a cellular structure of the reduced enamel epithelium; an ameloblast in the postsecretory stage of enamel formation.

postanesthetic (post"an-es-thet'ik) after anesthesia.

postaurale (post"aw-ra'le) an anthropometric landmark, the most posterior point on the helix of the ear.

postbuccal (post-buk'al) situated behind the buccal region.

postcibal (post-si'bal) [*post-*   L. *cibum* food] occurring after ingestion of food; postprandial.

post cibum (post si'bum) [L.] after meals.

postcondensation (post-kon"den-sa'shun) completion of compaction, of the surface of a direct filling gold restoration after the gold has been positioned in place, usually with the aid of a condenser with a large face and fine serrations. Called also *aftercondensation.*

postcondylar (post-kon'dĭ-lar) behind the condyle.

postcondylare (post"kon-dĭ-lar'e) the highest point of the curvature behind the occipital condyle.

postcranial (post-kra'ne-al) situated posterior or inferior to the cranium or skull.

posthole (pōst'hōl) a hole prepared within the root canal space, which accommodates a post or dowel in a dental restoration.

postembryonic (post"em-bre-on'ik) [*post-* + Gr. *embryon* embryo] occurring after the embryonic stage.

posteriad (pos-tēr'e-ad) toward the posterior surface of the body.

posterior (pos-tēr'e-or) [L. "behind"; neut. *posterius*] situated in back of, or in the back part of, or affecting the back part of an organ; used in reference to the back or dorsal surface of the body.

postero- [L. *posterus* behind] a combining form denoting relationship to the posterior part.

posteroanterior (pos"ter-o-an-tēr'e-or) from back to front, or from the posterior to the anterior surface. In roentgenology, denoting direction of the beam from the x-ray source to the beam exit surface.

posterooclusion (pos"ter-o-kloo'zhun) distoclusion.

posteroexternal (pos"ter-o-eks-ter'nal) situated on the outer side of a posterior aspect.

posteroinferior (pos"ter-o-in-fēr'e-or) situated on a posterior and inferior aspect.

posterointernal (pos"ter-o-in-ter'nal) situated within and toward the back.

posterolateral (pos"ter-o-lat'er-al) situated behind and at one side.

posteromedial (pos"ter-o-me'de-al) situated toward the middle of the back.

posteromedian (pos"ter-o-me'de-an) situated on the midline of the back.

posteroparietal (pos"ter-o-pah-ri'ĕ-tal) situated at the back of the parietal bone.

posterosuperior (pos"ter-o-su-pēr'e-or) situated behind and above.

posterotemporal (pos"ter-o-tem'po-ral) situated at the back of the temporal bone.

posterula (pos-ter'u-lah) [L.] the space between the nasal conchae and the posterior nares.

postethmoid (post-eth'moid) behind the ethmoid bone.

postexed (pos-tekst') bent backward.

postextraction (post"eks-trak'shun) after extraction; occurring after extraction.

postfebrile (post-feb'ril) occurring after or as the result of a fever.

postganglionic (post"gang-gle-on'ik) situated posterior or distal to a ganglion; said especially of autonomic nerve fibers so located.

postglenoid (post-gle'noid) situated behind the glenoid fossa.

postgrippal (post-grip'al) occurring after influenza.

posthemorrhagic (post-hem"o-raj'ik) occurring after or as the result of hemorrhage.

posthumous (pos'tu-mus) [L. *postumus* coming after] occurring after death; born after the father's death.

posthyoid (post-hi'oid) situated or occurring behind the hyoid bone.

posthypnotic (post"hip-not'ik) succeeding the hypnotic state.

posthypophysis (post"hi-pof'ĭ-sis) pituitary gland, posterior; see under GLAND.

postmastoid (post-mas'toid) situated behind the mastoid process of the temporal bone.

post mortem (post mor'tem) [L.] after death.

postmortem (post-mor'tem) [L.] occurring or performed after death; pertaining to the period after death.

postnares (post-na'rēs) the posterior nares.

postnarial (post-na're-al) pertaining to the posterior nares.

postnasal (post-na'zal) [post- + L. *nasus* nose] situated or occurring behind the nose.

postnatal (post-na'tal) [post- + L. *natalis* natal] occurring after birth, with reference to the newborn. Cf. POSTPARTUM.

postoperative (post-op'er-a"tiv) occurring after operation; after surgery.

postoral (post-o'ral) [post- + L. *os* mouth] behind the mouth.

postorbital (post-or'bĭ-tal) behind the orbit.

postpalatine (post-pal'ah-tīn) behind the palate, or behind the palatine bone.

post partum (post par'tum) [L.] after childbirth, or after delivery.

postpartum (post-par'tum) occurring after childbirth or after delivery, with reference to the mother. Cf. POSTNATAL.

postpharyngeal (post-fah-rin'je-al) situated or occurring behind the pharynx.

postprandial (post-pran'de-al) [post- + *prandial*] occurring after a meal; postcibal.

postradiation (post"ra-de-a'shun) following exposure to radiation.

postresection (post"re-sek'shun) a condition that has become evident after a surgical procedure has been accomplished.

postscreening (post-skrēn'ing) in dental health delivery, the examination by designated dentists, usually on a sample basis, to determine if services have been rendered adequately and in accordance with prescribed administrative procedures. See also quality CONTROL and SCREENING (4). Cf. PRESCREENING.

postsphenoid (post-sfe'noid) [post- + *sphenoid*] the part of the sphenoid bone posterior to the tuberculum sellae; it develops separately and unites with the anterior portion (presphenoid) between the seventh and eighth months of fetal life. Called also *postsphenoidal bone.*

postsynaptic (post"sĭ-nap'tik) situated distal to the synaptic cleft, as the postsynaptic neuron.

post-traumatic (post"traw-mat'ik) occurring after injury.

postulate (pos'tu-lāt) [L. *postulatum* demanded] anything assumed or taken for granted.

postural (pos'chu-ral) pertaining to posture or position.

posture (pos'chur) [L. *postura*] attitude of the body; carriage; the position of the limbs and other parts of the body as a whole. See also POSITION.

POT postoperative TREATMENT.

potash (pot'ash) 1. POTASSIUM carbonate. 2. POTASSIUM hydroxide. **p. aluminosilicate,** potassium FELDSPAR. **caustic p.,** POTASSIUM hydroxide. **p. feldspar,** potassium FELDSPAR.

potassa (po-tas'ah) POTASSIUM hydroxide.

potassemia (pot"ah-se'me-ah) [*potassium* + Gr. *haima* blood + *-ia*] the presence of an abnormally large amount of potassium in the blood; hyperkalemia.

potassium (po-tas'e-um) [Engl. *potash;* L. *kalium;* Arab. *qali*] a metallic element of the alkali group. Symbol, K; atomic number, 19; atomic weight, 39.102; specific gravity, 0.89; group IA of the periodic table. Natural isotopes include 39, 40,

and 41, K⁴⁰ being radioactive. Potassium is a soft, silvery-white metal that becomes brittle at low temperatures and is soluble in liquid ammonia, aniline, mercury, and sodium. It has valence 1 and rapidly oxidizes and reacts violently with water. Its function in the body consists of maintenance of water balance and osmotic pressure, acid-base balance, and neuromuscular irritability, whereby K is the chief cation of intracellular fluids, and Na is the chief cation and Cl the chief anion of extracellular fluid. Legumes, whole grain, fruits, and vegetables are its principal dietary sources. For recommended daily requirements, see table at NUTRITION. See also HYPERPOTASSEMIA. **p. alum,** see ALUM (1). **p. aluminosilicate,** potassium FELDSPAR. **p. benzylpenicillinate,** PENICILLIN G. potassium. **p. bromide,** a compound, KBr, occurring as white cubical crystals or as a granular powder, which is readily soluble in water and alcohol. Used as a restrainer in developing solution for x-ray film. Formerly used as a sedative and anticonvulsant. Large doses may produce central nervous system depression and mental deterioration. Prolonged exposure may cause skin eruption. See also developing SOLUTION. **exsiccated p. alum,** exsiccated ALUM. **p. carbonate,** a hygroscopic, odorless, white, crystalline or granular powder, K_2CO_3, that is soluble in water, but not in alcohol, forming a strongly alkaline aqueous solution. Used in various chemical, industrial, and pharmaceutical processes. It is a strong irritant and is caustic on contact. Called also *kali, pearl ash, potash,* and *salt of tartar.* **p. chlorate,** a highly explosive compound, $KClO_3$, occurring as white granules or powder, soluble in water. It is an oxygen-liberating substance, formerly used as a topical anti-infective in the treatment of diseases of the skin and mucous membranes, including necrotizing ulcerative gingivitis and in the treatment of thyroid diseases. It is irritating to the digestive system and kidneys and may cause hemolysis and methemoglobinemia. **p. feldspar,** potassium FELDSPAR. **p. hydrate,** p. hydroxide. **p. hydroxide,** a compound, KOH, occurring as white, deliquescent pieces, lumps, pellets, or flakes with a crystalline fracture that absorb water and carbon dioxide from the air and are soluble in water, ethanol, glycerol, and, slightly, ether. Potassium hydroxide is an extremely corrosive substance, the ingestion of which causes severe burns to the mouth, throat, and digestive system, resulting in collapse and death; if not immediately fatal, stricture of the esophagus will result. It is very irritating on contact or inhalation. Used as a caustic and in the production of various substances, such as soaps and drugs. Called also *p. hydrate, caustic potash, lye, potash,* and *potassa.* **p. iodide,** a compound, KI, occurring as colorless or white, cubical crystals, white granules, or powder, which is slightly deliquescent in moist air and liberates in small quantities iodine and iodate and is soluble in water, alcohol, and glycerol. Used as an expectorant, in the treatment of thyroidism, and as a component of iodine tincture. Trademark: Knollide. **p. permanganate,** a water-soluble compound, $KMnO_4$, occurring as dark purple or bronzelike crystals that are sweet with astringent aftertaste. It is an oxygen-liberating compound used extensively in the past as a topical anti-infective preparation in the treatment of fungal and bacterial diseases of the skin and mucous membranes, including acute necrotizing ulcerative colitis. Also used as a topical oxidizing agent in treating snake bite and ivy poisoning. Dilute solutions may cause mild irritation and concentrated solutions may be caustic. **p. silicate,** a compound with variable composition, having a formula $K_2Si_2O_5$ to $K_2Si_3O_7$, occurring as colorless or yellowish, translucent to transparent, hygroscopic glasslike pieces that are soluble in water only at high temperatures and under pressure. Used as a fluxing agent in dental porcelain. Also used in the manufacture of glass and refractory material and in various industrial processes. **p. sulfate,** a compound, K_2SO_4, occurring as colorless or white, odorless, hard crystals with a bitter, saline taste that are soluble in water but insoluble in alcohol. It has been used as a cathartic, but it has a strong irritant action on the stomach. Used as an accelerator to shorten the setting time of dental plaster, dental stone, and plaster of Paris, and to reduce their setting expansion. Called also *sal polychrestum* and *tartarus vitriolatus.*

potential (po-ten'shal) [L. *potentia* power] 1. stored up energy ready for action. 2. electron tension or electromotive force, as measured by the capacity of producing electric effects in bodies of a different state of electrization. 3. the force necessary to separate one electron from an atom, resulting in the formation of an ion pair. **action p.,** the electrical mechanism of transmission of impulses, brought about by a stimulus that produces an abrupt increase in the permeability of the membrane to sodium and potassium resulting in a transient discharge of the membrane potential and depolarization of the cell. See also *membrane p.* and sodium PUMP. **cell p.,** electromotive FORCE. **p. difference,** voltage. **electrical p.,** potential of separated electric charges to perform work when flowing through a system. It is the basis of most physiological functions. The difference in potential between two points is measured in volts. See VOLTAGE. **ionization p.,** the potential necessary to separate one electron from an atom, resulting in the formation of an ion pair. **ionization p., primary,** in collision theory, the ionization produced by the primary particles as contrasted with the total ionization which includes secondary ionization. **membrane p.,** the electrical potential which exists on the two sides of a membrane or across the wall of a cell. It results from an unequal distribution of cations and anions across the membrane or plasmalemma.

potentiation (po-ten"she-a'shun) the synergistic action of two substances, such as drugs, being greater than the sum of the effects of each used alone.

Potter see Bucky's DIAPHRAGM (Bucky-Potter diaphragm).

Potter's disease (syndrome), facies [E. I. *Potter,* American physician] see under DISEASE and FACIES.

Potts' elevator see under ELEVATOR.

pouch (powch) a pocket or saclike formation. See also SPACE. **branchial p's,** endodermal outpocketings of the pharyngeal portion of the foregut, which arise in succession in five pairs toward the end of the fourth week of embryonic development. Each develops a dorsal and ventral wing and expands, pushing aside the mesenchyme and coming in contact with the ectoderm of the corresponding groove; together with the groove, it forms a closing plate that may rupture and complete the gill slit condition observed in lower vertebrates. In higher vertebrates, the first pouch differentiates into the auditory tube and the tympanic cavity of the middle ear; the second becomes the fossa and covering epithelium of the palatine tonsil; and the third, fourth, and fifth give rise to the thymus, parathyroid glands, and some pharyngeal structures. Called also *pharyngeal p's.* See table at branchial ARCHES. **craniobuccal p., craniopharyngeal p.,** Rathke's p. **neurobuccal p.,** Rathke's p. **pharyngeal p's,** branchial p's. **Rathke's p.,** a diverticulum from the embryonic buccal cavity, from which the anterior lobe of the pituitary gland is developed. The lumen of Rathke's pouch persists in adults as a small colloid-filled cyst and clefts at the juncture of the pars distalis and the neurohypophysis. Called also *craniobuccal p., craniopharyngeal p., neurobuccal p.,* and *Rathke's pocket.* **Seessel's p.,** a transient outpouching of the embryonic pharynx rostrad of the pharyngeal membrane and caudal to Rathke's pouch. Called also *Seessel's pocket.* **temporal p., superficial,** temporal space, superficial; see under SPACE.

pound (pownd) [L. *pondus* weight; *libra* pound] a unit of mass (weight) in both the avoirdupois and apothecaries' weights. The avoirdupois pound contains 16 ounces, or 7000 grains, and is equivalent to 453.592 grams. The apothecaries' pound contains 12 ounces, or 5760 grains, and is equivalent to 373.242 grams. Abbreviated *lb.* See also *Tables of Weights and Measures* at WEIGHT. **troy p.,** one containing 5760 grains, 240 pennyweights, or 12 ounces.

pour (por) the flowing of a liquid from one container into another. **double-p. technique, single-p. technique,** see compression MOLDING.

povidone (po'vĭ-dōn) a synthetic polymer, poly[1-(2-oxo-1-pyrrolidinyl)ethylene], occurring as a white to creamy white, odorless powder. It consists principally of linear 1-vinyl-2-pyrrolidone groups, produced as a series of products having mean molecular weights ranging from about 10,000 to about 700,000. Used as dispersing and suspending agent, and has been used as plasma volume expander. Called also *polyvidone* and *polyvinylpyrrolidone (PVP).* Trademarks: Bolinan, Killidon, Periston, Plasdone, Plasmosan, Vinisil, Haemodyn (in solution).

povidone-iodine (po'vĭ-dōn i'o-dīn) an iodophor, being a complex of iodine and povidone, occurring as a fine brown powder that is readily soluble in water and alcohol, forming a stable compound that liberates iodine on contact with reducing substances and biological materials. It provides about 10 percent available iodine. Used as a topical antiseptic agent in a solution containing about 1 percent available iodine. Also used in surgical scrubs. Abbreviated *PVP-I.* Called also *iodine-polyvinylpyrrolidone complex.* Trademarks: Betadine, Disadine, Isodine, Proviodine.

powder (pow'der) [L. *pulvis*] a substance made up of an aggrega-

tion of small particles obtained by the grinding or trituration of a solid drug. **Co-Re-Ga denture adhesive p.,** trademark for a *denture adhesive* (see under ADHESIVE), 100 gm of which contains 94.6 to 98.86 gm gum karaya, 0.5 to 4.76 gm water soluble ethylene oxide, 240 mg calcium silicate, and 400 mg flavoring agents. **denture p.,** a mechanical denture cleanser consisting of an abrasive powder, such as calcium phosphate, used for brushing dentures. **denture adherent p.,** see denture ADHESIVE. **dusting p.,** an inert and insoluble fine powder used as a protective and absorbent to cover and protect epithelial surfaces, ulcers, and wounds, to prevent friction, to protect tissues from outside irritants, and to absorb moisture. Also used for dusting surgeons' rubber gloves. **Hypo-Cal p.,** trademark for a powder containing calcium hydroxide and barium sulfate in a 4:1 ratio. **NaFpak p.,** trademark for a sodium fluoride powder, also containing coloring and sweetening agents. The powder is available in 2 or 3 gm packages which, when dissolved in 1000 or 1500 ml of water, will produce a 0.2 percent aqueous solution used as a mouthrinse for dental caries control. **Plastodent elastic impression p.,** trademark for an *irreversible hydrocolloid impression material* (see under MATERIAL). **putty p.,** stannic OXIDE. **Pycopay tooth p.,** trademark for a dentifrice containing a mixture of pancreatic enzymes and a mixture of abrasive powder, chiefly sodium chloride and sodium bicarbonate. Used to retard calculus formation. **talcum p.,** talc. **tooth p.,** dentifrice.

power (pow'er) [L. *posse* to have power] 1. capability; potency; the ability to act. 2. the rate at which work is accomplished. 3. a measure of magnification, as of a microscope. 4. electric p. **stopping p.,** a measure of the effect of a substance upon the kinetic energy of a charged particle passing through it. **throwing p.,** the ionic penetration of the electric field in a concave structure, as during electroplating an impression for a full crown.

pox (poks) 1. any eruptive or pustular disease, especially of viral origin. 2. former name for SYPHILIS. **cow p.,** cowpox.

Poxviridae (poks"vi'rĭ-de) [*pox* + *virus* + *-idae*] a family of brick-shaped viruses that are the largest of the animal viruses, being 200 to 300 nm in diameter, which contain double-stranded DNA and replicate in the cytoplasm, and whose virions have complex morphology with dense central portions surrounded by envelopes. The family consists of six genera: *Orthopoxvirus, Parapoxvirus, Capripoxvirus, Avipoxvirus, Leporipoxvirus,* and *Entomopoxvirus,* and several unclassified viruses. All of the genera, except *Entomopoxvirus,* infect vertebrates.

poxvirus (poks-vi'rus) any virus of the family Poxviridae.

PPF phagocytosis promoting factor; see OPSONIN (2).

ppg picopicogram.

PPLO pleuropneumonia-like organism; see MYCOPLASMA.

ppm parts per million.

PR prosthion.

Pr praseodymium.

practice (prak'tis) [Gr. *praktikē*] the utilization of one's knowledge in a particular profession, as the exercise of one's knowledge in the practical recognition, prevention, and treatment of diseases. **p. administration,** practice ADMINISTRATION. **contract p.,** the treatment of the members of a specified group for a lump sum, or at so much per member. See also INSURANCE. **dental p., general,** dental practice whereby a dentist does not limit his practice to a single specialty and engages in several areas of dentistry which are within the scope and range of his training and ability. **family p.,** family MEDICINE. **general p.,** the provision of comprehensive health care as a continuing responsibility regardless of age or sex of the patient or of the condition that may temporarily require the services of a specialist. See also *dental p., general,* and family MEDICINE. **group p.,** the practice of medicine or dentistry by a group of physicians or dentists, usually representing various specialties. Called also *group medicine.* **individual p.,** solo p. **office p.,** the elements of medical, dental, or other professional practice that take place in the practitioner's office. **prepaid group p.,** one involving a group of three or more practitioners providing services in return for a fixed periodic prepayment made in advance of the use of service. **private p.,** a practice of medicine or dentistry in which the practitioner and his practice are independent of any external policy control. It usually requires that the practitioner be self-employed, except when he is salaried by a partnership in which he is a partner with similar practitioners. **solo p.,** the practice of medicine or dentistry by a single physician or dentist, assisted by only auxiliary personnel. Called also *individual p.* Cf. *group p.*

practitioner (prak-tish'un-er) one who has complied with the requirements and who is engaged in the practice of medicine, such as an appropriately licensed medical physician, an appropriately licensed dentist, an osteopathic physician with an unlimited license, and an appropriately licensed podiatrist. **dental p.,** a dentist who engages in the clinical practice of dentistry. **family p.,** family PHYSICIAN. **general p.,** a physician oriented to the whole patient, who provides medical care in more than one of the traditional specialty fields of medicine, and who coordinates the care obtained by referral to or consultation with medical specialists and allied health personnel. Abbreviated *GP.* See also family PHYSICIAN and general PRACTICE. **individual Medicaid p.,** one who has accepted patients whose fees are paid by the Medicaid program. Abbreviated *IMP.* **nurse p.,** see NURSE clinician.

practolol (prak'to-lol) an isoproterenol derivative, 4'-[2-hydroxy-3-(isopropylamino)propoxy] acetanilide. It is a cardioselective β-adrenergic blocking agent used in heart diseases. Trademarks: Dalzic, Eraldin.

Prader-Willi syndrome [A. *Prader;* H. *Willi*] see under SYNDROME.

prae- for words beginning thus, see those beginning PRE-.

pralidoxime chloride (pral"ĭ-doks'ēm) a cholinesterase reactivator, compound, 2-[(hydroxyimino)methyl]-1-methylpyridinium chloride, occurring as a white to yellowish, crystalline powder that is soluble in water and methanol, slightly soluble in ethanol, and insoluble in acetone. Used as an anticholinesterase antidote in organophosphate poisoning. By attaching the quaternary portion of the molecule to the anionic site of the cholinesterase molecule, it brings the oxime into proximity of the poisoned esteratic site. Rapid injection may cause vertigo, tachycardia, nausea, headache, weakness, nausea, and blurred vision. Called also 2-*PAM chloride.* Trademark: Protopam.

pramocaine hydrochloride (pram'o-kān) pramoxine hydrochloride.

pramoxine hydrochloride (pram-ok'sēn) a surface anesthetic, 4-[3-(4-butoxyphenoxy)propyl]morpholine hydrochloride, occurring as a white, crystalline powder with a numbing taste and a slight aromatic odor, which is soluble in water, chloroform, and ethanol and slightly soluble in ether. Used to treat superficial lesions, itching, and dermatoses, and in certain intubation procedures. Called also *pramocaine hydrochloride.* Trademark: Tronothane.

prandial (pran'de-al) [L. *prandium* breakfast] pertaining to a meal.

Prantal trademark for *diphemanil methylsulfate* (see under DIPHEMANIL).

praseodymium (pra"ze-o-dim'e-um, pra"se-o-dim'e-um) [Gr. *prasios* green + *didymos* twin] a rare earth, occurring as a yellowish metal. Symbol, Pr; atomic number, 59; atomic weight, 140.9077; melting point, 930° C; specific gravity, 6.78–6.81; valences, 3, 4; group IIIB of the periodic table; ^{141}Pr is the only natural isotope; artificial radioactive isotopes include 134–140 and 142–149. It tarnishes readily on exposure to air, ignites to oxide, liberates hydrogen from water, and is soluble in dilute acids. Used in various industrial processes.

P. rat. aetat. abbreviation for L. *pro ratio'ne aeta'tis,* in proportion to age.

Prausnitz-Küstner antibody, reaction [Carl Willy *Prausnitz,* German physician, born 1876; Heinz *Küstner,* German physician, born 1876] see REAGIN (1) and see under REACTION.

Pravocaine trademark for *propoxycaine hydrochloride* (see under PROPOXYCAINE).

prazosin hydrochloride (prah'zo-sin) an antihypertensive agent, 1 - (4 - amino,6,7 - dimethoxy - 2 - quinazolinyl) - 4 - (2 - furanylcarbonyl)-piperazine hydrochloride. Trademarks: *Hypovase, Minipress, Sinetens.*

pre- [L. *prae* before] a prefix signifying before, in time or place.

prealbumin (pre'al-bu'min) a serum protein consisting of four equal chains, which has the molecular weight of 50,000 to 62,000 and an electrophoretic mobility faster than albumin. **thyroxine-binding p.,** a prealbumin with the molecular weight of 54,000, which serves as a thyroxine carrier in the blood plasma.

preameloblast (pre"ah-mel'o-blast") enamel epithelium, inner; see under EPITHELIUM.

preanesthesia (pre"an-es-the'se-ah) preliminary anesthesia; light anesthesia or narcosis induced by medication as a preliminary to administration of a general anesthetic.

preaurale (pre'aw-ra'le) a cephalometric landmark, the point at which a straight line from the postaurale, perpendicular to the long axis of the auricle, meets the base of the auricle.

preauricular (pre"aw-rik'u-lar) [*pre-* + *auricular*] situated in front of an auricle or the ear.

preauthorization (pre-aw'thor-ĭ-za'shun) prior AUTHORIZATION.

prebase (pre'bās) that part of the dorsum of the tongue lying in front of the base.

prebone (pre'bon) osteoid (2).

precancer (pre'kan-ser) a condition which tends eventually to become malignant.

precancerosis (pre"kan-ser-o'sis) a nonmalignant condition that is likely to become malignant; a condition of early cancer. **Bowen's p.,** CARCINOMA in situ.

precancerous (pre-kan'ser-us) pertaining to a pathologic process that tends to become malignant.

precapillary (pre-kap'ĭ-ler"e) a vessel lacking complete coats, intermediate between an arteriole and a true capillary. Called also *metarteriole.*

precementum (pre"se-men'tum) cementoid.

precertification (pre"ser-tĭ-fĭ-ka'shun) prior AUTHORIZATION.

precipitate (pre-sip'ĭ-tat) 1. [L. *praecipitatum*] the deposit of an insoluble substance in a solution. 2. [L. *praecipitare* to cast down] the act or process of depositing an insoluble substance in a solution. 3. occurring with undue rapidity. 4. in immunology, the insoluble product of interaction between soluble macromolecular antigen and the homologous antibody (e.g., the visible antigen-antibody complex formed as a consequence of the reaction of pneumococcus capsular polysaccharide in solution with specific antiserum). See also IMMUNOPRECIPITATION. **white p.,** ammoniated MERCURY. **yellow p.,** mercuric oxide, yellow; see under OXIDE.

precipitation (pre-sip"ĭ-ta-shun) [L. *praecipitatio*] the act or process of producing a precipitate; the deposition of an insoluble substance in a solution. **group p.,** precipitation by a precipitin in an antiserum of an antigen common to a group of closely related microorganisms. **p. hardening,** precipitation HARDENING.

precipitin (pre-sip'ĭ-tin) an antibody which reacts with soluble antigen to form a precipitate. See also precipitin TEST.

precocious (pre-ko'shus) premature development or occurrence.

Precortal trademark for *prednisone.*

Precortancyl trademark for *prednisolone.*

precritical (pre-krit'ĭ-kal) previous to the occurrence of the crisis.

precursor (pre'ker-sor) [L. *praecursor* a forerunner] 1. something that precedes. 2. in clinical medicine, a sign or symptom that heralds another. 3. in biological processes, a substance from which another, usually more active or mature substance is formed. 4. in biochemistry, an intermediate compound or molecular complex present in a living organism which, when activated, is converted to a specific functional substance. For example, ergosterol, which is activated by ultraviolet rays to vitamin D, or prothrombin, which is activated to thrombin. Three systems for naming precursors are used: the prefix *pro-* (as in prothrombin), the use of the suffix *-ogen* (as in trypsinogen), and the use of the prefix *pre-;* the latter has failed to gain wide acceptance.

predeciduous (pre"de-sid'u-us) [*pre-* + L. *deciduus,* from *decidere* to fall off] see predeciduous teeth, under TOOTH.

predental (pre-den'tal) preceding and preparing for the regular dental course of study, as predental education.

predentin (pre-den'tin) [*pre-* + *dentin*] the soft fibrillar substance composing the primitive dentin and forming the narrow band of dentinal matrix immediately external to the layer of odontoblasts, in the inner layer of the circumpulpar dentin. Called also *dentinoid.*

predetermination (pre"de-ter"mĭ-na'shun) the settling or deciding in advance. **p. of benefits,** prior AUTHORIZATION.

predisposing (pre"dis-pōz'ing) conferring a tendency to disease.

predisposition (pre"dis-po-zish'un) [*pre-* + L. *disponere* to dispose] susceptibility to certain conditions.

Prednelan trademark for *prednisolone.*

Prednesol trademark for *prednisolone sodium phosphate* (see under PREDNISOLONE).

prednisolone (pred'nĭ-so"lōn) a glucocorticoid, 11β,17,21-trihydroxypregna-1,4-diene-3,20-dione, occurring as a white, odorless, crystalline powder that is soluble in ethanol, chloroform, acetone, and very slightly soluble in water. Used in the treatment of adrenocortical insufficiency and as an anti-inflammatory and antiallergic agent. In dentistry, used in the treatment of sensitive dentin, pulpal reactions to surgery, oral ulcers, and rheumatoid temporomandibular disorders, and in tissue transplantation. Side reactions may include euphoria, mental depression, psychoses, hypertension, anorexia, peptic ulcer, susceptibility to infection, abnormal fat distribution, moon face, edema, potassium loss, alkalosis, and osteoporosis. Trademarks: Cortalone, Delta-Cortef, Delta-Stab Deltacortril, Dicortol, Meticortelone, Precortancyl, Prednelan. **p. acetate,** an ester of prednisolone, occurring as an odorless, white, crystalline powder, soluble in ethanol, slightly soluble in chloroform and acetone, and insoluble in water. Used in sterile suspension for topical application or intramuscular, intra-articular, or intralesional injections. Trademarks: Deltacortenolo, Meticortelone, Pricortin. **p. 21-(disodium phosphate),** p. sodium phosphate. **methyl-p.,** methylprednisolone. **p. phosphate sodium,** p. sodium phosphate. **p. 21-(hydrogen succinate),** p. succinate. **p. 21-succinate sodium,** p. sodium succinate. **p. sodium phosphate,** the disodium phosphate salt of prednisolone, occurring as a white to yellowish, odorless, slightly hygroscopic powder or granules, readily soluble in water and methanol, slightly soluble in ethanol and chloroform, and very slightly soluble in acetone. Used for topical application and for intra-articular, intravenous, or intralesional injections. Called also *p. 21-(disodium phosphate)* and *p. phosphate sodium.* Trademarks: Hydeltrasol, Prednesol, Solucort. **p. sodium succinate,** a soluble salt of prednisolone, used for intravenous, intramuscular, intra-articular, and intralesional injections. Called also *p. 21-succinate sodium.* **p. succinate,** an ester of prednisolone, occurring as an odorless, creamy white powder that is freely soluble in ethanol and acetone and slightly soluble in water. Called also *p. 21-(hydrogen succinate).*

prednisone (pred'ni-son) a synthetic glucocorticoid derived from cortisone, 17,21-dihydroxypregna-1,4-dione-3,11,20-trione, but having some mineralocorticoid activity. It occurs as a white, odorless, crystalline powder that is slightly soluble in water, ethanol, chloroform, and methanol. Used in the treatment of adrenocortical insufficiency and as an anti-inflammatory and anti-allergic agent. Also used in the treatment of cancer. In dentistry, used in the treatment of sensitive dentin, pulpal reactions to surgery, oral ulcers in skin diseases, arthritic temporomandibular joint disorders, and in tissue transplantation. Side reactions include euphoria, mental depression, psychoses, hypertension, anorexia, peptic ulcer, susceptibility to infection, abnormal fat distribution, moon face, edema, potassium loss, alkalosis, and osteoporosis. Called also Δ-¹cortisone, delta-E, deltacortisone, Δ¹-dehydrocortisone, and *metacortandracin.* Trademarks: Bicortone, Decortin, Deltasone, Delta Prenovis, Deltisone, Deltra, Encorton, Meticorten, Orasone, Ultracorten.

preepiglottic (pre″ep-ĭ-glot'ik) situated or occurring in front of the epiglottis.

preeruptive (pre″e-rup'tiv) preceding an eruption.

Prefaxil trademark for *tolazoline hydrochloride* (see under TOLAZOLINE).

prefrontal (pre-fron'tal) 1. situated in the anterior part of the frontal lobe or region. 2. the central part of the ethmoid bone.

preganglionic (pre″gang-gle-on'ik) situated anterior or proximal to a ganglion; said especially of autonomic nerve fibers so located.

pregnancy (preg'nan-se) [L. *praegnans* with child] the condition of having a developing embryo or fetus in the body. In humans, duration of pregnancy is about 266 days after conception or fertilization of the ovum. Pregnancy is roughly divided in three trimesters of about three calendar months each or, more precisely, into the embryonic period lasting from the fertilization through the first eight weeks of pregnancy, and the fetal period during the remainder of pregnancy. During the first period the conceptus is known as the *embryo* and during the second period it is referred to as the *fetus.* See also GESTATION. **p. gingivitis,** pregnancy GINGIVITIS. **p. tumor,** pregnancy GINGIVITIS.

pregnane (preg'nān) a class of steroid compounds having a two-carbon side chain at C-17. See also STEROID.

preheadache (pre-hed'ak) a group of symptoms which may precede the onset of migraine, including scintillating scotomas, visual field defects, such as hemianopsia, and hemiplegia. See also MIGRAINE.

prehension (pre-hen'shun) [L. *prehensio*] the act of seizing or grasping, as with the teeth or hand.

prehyoid (pre-hi'oid) in front of the hyoid bone.

prehypophyseal (pre″hi-po-fiz'e-al) pertaining to or derived from the anterior lobe of the pituitary gland.

prehypophysis (pre″hi-pof'ĭ-sis) pituitary gland, anterior; see under GLAND.

preictal (pre-ik'tal) [*pre-* + L. *ictus* stroke] occurring before a stroke or an attack, as before an acute epileptic attack.

preimmunization (pre-im″u-ni-za'shun) artificial immunization in very young infants.

Preisz-Nocard bacillus [Hugo *Preisz,* Hungarian bacteriologist, 1860–1940; Edmond Isidore Étienne *Nocard,* French veterinarian, 1850–1903] *Corynebacterium pseudotuberculosis;* see under CORYNEBACTERIUM.

prelacrimal (pre-lak'rĭ-mal) in front of the lacrimal sac.

prelaryngeal (pre″lah-rin'je-al) in front of the larynx.

Preludin trademark for *phenmetrazine hydrochloride* (see under PHENMETRAZINE).

premature (pre-mah-tūr') [L. *prematurus* early ripe] 1. occurring before the proper time, as in premature contact. 2. premature INFANT.

prematurity (pre″mah-tu'rĭ-te) 1. an event or happening occurring earlier than expected. 2. the condition of an infant born after a gestation period of less than 37 weeks. 3. a condition of tooth contacts which diverts the mandible from a normal path of closure. See also premature CONTACT. **occlusal p.,** premature CONTACT.

premaxilla (pre″mak-sil'ah) a separate bone element derived from the median nasal process in the embryo, which in humans later fuses with the maxilla. Called also *premaxillary bone.* See also incisive BONE.

premaxillary (pre-mak'sĭ-ler″e) 1. situated in front of the maxilla. 2. pertaining to the premaxilla.

premedical (pre-med'ĭ-kal) preceding and preparing for the regular medical course of study, as premedical education.

premedication (pre″med-ĭ-ka'shun) preliminary medication before anesthesia to allay apprehension of the patient, to provide a basal state of depression in preparation for anesthesia, to protect against undesirable reflexes, and to dry secretions in the respiratory tract, its principal objective being to provide a patient who is comfortably sedated, free from apprehension, and able to cooperate in the preliminary preparations for anesthesia. Called also *preanesthetic medication* and *preoperative medication.* **dental p.,** medication used to produce psychic sedation prior to dental treatment. Called also *dental pretreatment sedation* and *dental psychosedation.*

premenstrual (pre-men'stroo-al) occurring before menstruation.

premium (pre'me-um) 1. in insurance, the amount or consideration paid by an insured person or policy holder (or on his behalf) by an insurer or third party for insurance coverage under an insurance policy, usually paid in periodic amounts. **deposit p.,** in health insurance, a dollar amount, per beneficiary per contract year, deposited with the carrier usually at the beginning of a program, ordinarily based on the estimated cost, and used as an operating fund from which charges for services are paid. **earned p.,** that portion of a policy's premium payment for which the protection of the policy has already been given. **fixed p.,** in dental plans, a specified amount charged for insurance which is not changed by such factors as size of family or initial year versus maintenance year of dental care coverage. Called also *set p.* **scaled p.,** in dental plans, used loosely to describe a premium that will vary, as in an adjustment of individual premium in accordance with size of the family unit, or establishment of one premium for coverage during the initial year under a dental plan with a lower premium for subsequent (maintenance) years of coverage. **set p.,** fixed p. **unearned p.,** that part of the premium applicable to the unexpired part of the policy period.

Premocillin trademark for *penicillin G procaine* (see under PENICILLIN).

premolar (pre-mo'lar) [*pre-* + L. *molaris* molar] 1. any of the eight permanent teeth in man that replace the molars of the deciduous dentition. In zoology, those teeth which succeed the deciduous molars regardless of the number to be succeeded. See premolar teeth, under TOOTH. 2. situated in front of the molar teeth. **first p.,** premolar tooth, first; see under TOOTH. **second p.,** premolar tooth, second; see under TOOTH. **two-pointed p.,** a bicuspid tooth. See premolar teeth, under TOOTH.

premonitory (pre-mon'ĭ-to-re) [L. *premonitorius*] serving as a warning, as a premonitory symptom.

premorbid (pre-mor'bid) occurring before the development of disease.

premunition (pre″mu-nish'un) an immunity induced by a nonprogressive parasitic infection in a host, which permits the host to resist a further infection as long as the initial parasitic relationship persists; elimination of the parasite results in the loss of the immunity.

prenares (pre-na'rēz) the nostrils or nares.

prenasale (pre″na-sa'le) a cephalometric landmark being the most projecting point, in the median plane, at the tip of the nose.

prenatal (pre-na'tal) [*pre-* + L. *natalis* natal] existing or occurring before birth, with reference to the fetus.

preneoplastic (pre″ne-o-plas'tik) before the development or existence of a tumor.

preoperative (pre-op'er-a″tiv) preceding an operation; before surgery.

preoral (pre-o'ral) [*pre-* + L. *os* mouth] situated in front of the mouth.

prepalatal (pre-pal'ah-tal) situated in front of the palate.

preparation (prep"ah-ra'shun [L. *praeparatio*] 1. the act or process of making ready. 2. a medicine or drug made ready for use. 3. an anatomical or pathological specimen made ready and preserved for study. **access p.**, endodontic CAVITY. **biomechanical p.**, the procedures involved in exposing, enlarging, cleansing, and shaping the pulp chamber and root canal of a tooth by mechanical means. **cavity p.**, a procedure for establishing in a tooth the biochemically acceptable form necessary to receive and retain a restoration, accomplished with the use of rotary and handcutting instruments. Elements of cavity preparation include the resistance form, retention form, convenience form, removal of carious tissue, finish of the cavity wall, and cavity toilet. See also cavity LINING, cavity TOILET, and prepared CAVITY. **depo-p.**, see under D. **p. GK-101**, a carious dentin softener consisting of a solution of sodium hypochlorite, sodium chloride, and sodium hydroxide. **medicinal p.**, drug. **mouth p.**, all the procedures necessary to prepare the mouth to receive, support, and retain a denture. **slice p.**, a cavity preparation for Class II restoration, whereby the proximal portion is formed by removing a slice of the proximal convexity of the tooth to achieve cleansable margins and a line of draw and a tapered keyway of two keyed grooves or channels are formed in the proximal surface to provide retention form.

prepayment (pre-pa'ment) 1. payment in advance; payment for services to be received. See also prepaid dental PLAN and prepaid group PRACTICE. 2. sometimes used to mean INSURANCE.

prepolymer (pre-pol'ĭ-mer) a substance which upon reacting with a catalyst will form a polymer.

preprandial (pre-pran'de-al) [*pre-* + *prandial*] before meals.

prepubertal (pre-pu'ber-tal) occurring before puberty.

presby- [Gr. *presbys* old] a combining form meaning old or denoting relationship to old age.

prescreening (pre-skrēn'ing) in dental health delivery, the review by designated dentists of patients' examination records as a prerequisite of the authorization of some or all types of treatment. See also quality CONTROL and SCREENING, (4). Cf. POSTSCREENING.

prescription (pre-skrip'shun) [L. *praescriptio*] a written direction for the preparation and administration of a remedy. A prescription consists of the heading or *superscription* – that is, the symbol ℞ or the word Recipe, meaning "take"; the *inscription*, which contains the names and quantities of the ingredients; the *subscription*, or directions for compounding; and the *signature*, usually introduced by the sign S, for *signa* "mark," which gives the directions for the patient which are to be marked on the receptacle. **p. drug**, prescription DRUG.

presenility (pre"sĕ-nil'ĭ-te) premature old age.

presenium (pre-se'ne-um) the period immediately preceding old age.

presentation (prez'en-ta'shun) 1. the bringing forth; the introduction. 2. the relationship of the long axis of the fetus to that of the mother. Called also *lie*. Cf. POSITION (3). **case p.**, a consultation between the doctor and patient in which the doctor presents his diagnostic findings and recommendations for treatment.

preservative (pre-zer'vah-tiv) 1. something that keeps something else in existence and safe from harm of injury. 2. a substance or preparation added to a product for the purpose of destroying or inhibiting the multiplication of microorganisms. **film p.**, a chemical substance, such as sodium sulfite, which preserves a photographic or x-ray film by preventing its oxidation. **food p.**, a substance used to preserve foods from spoiling and to prolong its freshness.

Presinol trademark for *methyldopa*.

prespermatid (pre-sper'mah-tid) secondary SPERMATOCYTE.

presphenoid (pre-sfe'noid) [*pre-* + *sphenoid*] the part of the sphenoid bone anterior to the tuberculum sellae; it develops separately and unites with the posterior portion (*postsphenoid*) between the seventh and eighth months of fetal life. Called also *presphenoidal bone*.

Pressomatic attachment (unit) see under ATTACHMENT.

Pressomin trademark for *methoxamine hydrochloride* (see under METHOXAMINE).

Pressonex trademark for *metaraminol bitartrate* (see under METARAMINOL).

pressor (pres'or) tending to increase blood pressure.

pressoreceptor (pres"o-re-sep'tor) a neuroreceptor sensitive to pressure changes, such as in the walls of the aortic arch and carotid sinus which are responsive to arterial blood pressure changes.

Pressorol trademark for *metaraminol bitartrate* (see under METARAMINAL).

pressure (presh'ur) [L. *pressura*] stress or strain, whether by compression, pull, thrust, or shear. See also TENSION and TONUS. **after p.**, a sense of pressure which lasts for a short period after removal of the actual pressure. **arterial p.**, see *blood p.* **atmospheric p.**, the pressure exerted by the atmosphere at sea level, being 14.6974 psi or 1.0333 kg/cm²; see ATMOSPHERE (3). **back p.**, 1. pressure produced by a gas or liquid under compression. See also back pressure POROSITY. 2. the pressure caused by damming back of the blood in a heart chamber and its tributaries due to an obstructive heart valve or failing myocardium. **basal blood p.**, see *blood p.* **biting p.**, occlusal p. **blood p.**, the pressure of the blood against the walls of the blood vessels. In clinical practice, the term applies usually to arterial pressure measured at the upper arm, usually by means of a sphygmomanometer. Maximum pressure occurs near the end of the contraction phase of the heart beat and is termed *systolic* pressure; minimum pressure occurs during the relaxation or dilation phase and is termed *diastolic* pressure. *Mean blood pressure* is the diastolic pressure plus one-third the *pulse pressure*, which is the difference between the systolic and the diastolic pressure; *basal blood pressure* is the pressure during a quiet or basal condition. The highest pressure occurs in the aorta, averaging approximately 100 mm Hg, falling progressively throughout the systemic circulation, until it reaches approximately 0 mm Hg at the right atrium. Under normal conditions, systolic pressure is about 120 mm Hg, and diastolic about 80 mm Hg, depending on cardiac output and the diameter and elasticity of the walls of the arteries. The volume and viscosity of the blood, age of the individual, body position and other factors, such as size and fit of the cuff of the sphygmomanometer, also influence the reading. **brain p.**, the capillary venous pressure in the brain. **capillary p.**, the blood pressure in the capillaries. **cerebrospinal p.**, the pressure of the cerebrospinal fluid, normally 100–150 mm Hg. **colloid osmotic p.**, oncotic p. **diastolic p.**, see *blood p.* **high oxygen p.**, oxygen pressure in excess of 1 atmosphere. Abbreviated HOP. Called also *hyperbaric oxygen p.* **hydrostatic p.**, pressure exerted by a fluid on a surface. **hyperbaric oxygen p.**, high oxygen p. **maximum blood p.**, see *blood p.* **mean blood p.**, see *blood p.* **minimum p.**, see *blood p.* **negative p.**, a pressure of less than that of the atmosphere, or 14.69 psi or 1 atm at sea level. **occlusal p.**, pressure exerted on the occlusal surfaces of the teeth when the jaws are brought into apposition. Called also *biting p.* **oncotic p.**, osmotic pressure exerted by colloids. Called also *colloid osmotic p.* **osmotic p.**, the pressure necessary to prevent the flow of a solvent across a semipermeable membrane, depending on the relative concentration of solute in solution on either side of the membrane. Hence, to prevent the flow from the side where the solution is less dense to where it is denser, the concentration of solute must be equalized. **osmotic p., effective**, that part of the total osmotic pressure of a solution which governs the tendency of its solvent to pass through a semipermeable bounding membrane or across another boundary. **partial p.**, the pressure exerted by each of the constituents of a mixture of gases. **positive p.**, pressure greater than that of the atmosphere, or 14.69 psi or 1 atm at sea level. **pulse p.**, see *blood p.* **SI unit of p.**, pascal. **systolic p.**, see *blood p.* **tongue p.**, pressure exerted by the tongue against the teeth, considered to be a contributory factor in malocclusion. **vapor p.**, the pressure (usually expressed in milliliters of mercury) at which a liquid and its vapor are in equilibrium at a definite temperature. Once the vapor pressure reaches the atmospheric pressure (14.69 psi or 1 atm at sea level), the liquid boils. **venous p.**, the blood pressure in a vein.

presynaptic (pre"sĭ-nap'tik) situated proximal to the synaptic cleft, or before crossing the synaptic cleft, as the presynaptic neuron.

pretragal (pre-tra'g'l) [*pre-* + *tragal*] situated in front of the tragus.

pretreatment (pre-trēt'ment) prior AUTHORIZATION.

prevalence (prev'ah-lens) the total number of cases of a disease in existence at a certain time in a designated area. See also INCIDENCE.

prevention (pre"ven-shun) [L. *praeventiio* anticipating] 1. hindering, thwarting, or obstructing something from happening. 2. warding off illness; prophylaxis. **primary p.**, **secondary p.**, **tertiary p.**, see preventive DENTISTRY.

preventive (pre-ven'tiv) serving to avert the occurrence of.

Prévost's law [Jean Louis *Prévost*, Swiss physician, 1838–1927] see under LAW.

prezone (pre'zōn) prozone.

Price's rule [W. A. *Price*, American dentist] see bisecting angle TECHNIQUE.

Pricortin trademark for *prednisolone acetate* (see under PREDNISOLONE).

prilocaine hydrochloride (pril′o-kăn) an anesthetic, 2-propylamino-*o*-propionotoluidide hydrochloride, occurring as a white, odorless crystalline powder with an initially acid and then bitter taste, which is readily soluble in water and alcohol, slightly soluble in chloroform, very slightly soluble in acetone, and insoluble in ether. Used for local and regional nerve block anesthesia. In dentistry, used in local anesthetic solutions with or without epinephrine for dental infiltration and mandibular nerve block. Methemoglobinemia and drowsiness are the principal adverse effects. Trademarks: Citanest, Xylonest.

Primaclone trademark for *primidone*.

Primamycin trademark for *hamycin*.

primaquine phosphate (pri′mah-kwin) an antimalarial agent, *N*¹-(6-methoxy-8-quinolinyl)-1,4-pentanediamine, occurring as an orange colored, odorless, bitter, crystalline powder that is soluble in water, but not in chloroform and ether. It is tolerated in therapeutic doses by Caucasians; large doses are not well tolerated by those blacks and other individuals whose erythrocytes are deficient in glucose-6-phosphate dehydrogenase. Adverse effects may include abdominal cramps, epigastric distress, anemia, methemoglobinemia, leukocytosis, leukopenia, and other disorders.

primary (pri′mer-e, pri′mah-re) [L. *primarius* principal; *primus* first] principal; first in order.

Primates (pri-ma′tēz) [L. *primus* first] the highest order of mammals, including man, apes, monkeys, and lemurs.

primed (prīmd) immunologically activated by initial exposure to antigen; capable of recognition and enhanced response upon further exposure to the same antigen. See also primary immune REACTION and secondary immune REACTION.

primer (pri′mer) a substance which prepares for or facilitates the action of another. **Bonfil p.**, trademark for a cavity primer to be used with a restorative resin, containing an unsaturated acid, such as methacrylic acid, an acid amide, such as acrylamide, and a polymerizable solvent, such as liquid methyl methacrylate monomer. **Bowen's cavity p.**, a coupling agent capable of copolymerizing with a dental material, thus enhancing bonding of the material to tooth surface. Chemically, it is an alcoholic solution of the addition-reaction product of *N*-phenylglycine and glycidyl methacrylate. Called also *surface-active comonomer*. **cavity p.**, a substance which enhances adaptation of resin filling materials to cavity walls by inducing wetting between the resinous material and the treated dentin and enamel surfaces. Some cavity primers contain acrylics or composite resins. See also cavity LINER. **Kadon p.**, trademark for a cavity primer to be used with a resin restorative material, containing an unsaturated acid, such as methacrylic acid, an acid amide, such as acrylamide, and a polymerizable solvent, such as liquid methyl methacrylate monomer. **polyurethane p.**, a cavity primer based on polyurethanes, frequently used in conjunction with amalgam. **Sevriton cavity seal p.**, trademark for a cavity primer for an acrylic resin, consisting of phosphoric acid ester glycerol dimethacrylate, methacrylic acid, methyl methacrylate, and probably a trace of methacrylic anhydride.

primidone (pri′mĭ-dōn) an anticonvulsant drug, 5-ethyldihydro-5-phenyl-4,6(1*H*,5*H*)-pyrimidinedione, occurring as a white, odorless, slightly bitter crystalline powder that is slightly soluble in water, ethanol, and organic solvents. Used alone or in combination with other drugs in the treatment of epilepsy. Side reactions may include ataxia, vertigo, nausea, anorexia, vomiting, fatigue, irritability, emotional disorders, diplopia, nystagmus, skin rash and, rarely, megaloblastic anemia. Gingival pain may occur. Called also *2-desoxyphenobarbital*. Trademarks: Mylepsin, Mysoline, Primacolone, Sertan.

primigravida (pri″mĭ-grav′ĭ-dah) [L. *prima* first + *gravida* pregnant] a woman pregnant for the first time; also written *gravida I*.

priming (prīm′ing) 1. the act or process of making ready or preparing. 2. the escape into the condenser of a liquid being distilled. **complement p.**, complement activation PATHWAY.

primipara (pri-mip′ah-rah), pl. *primap′arae* [L. *prima* first + *parere* to produce] a woman who has had one pregnancy which resulted in a viable child; also written *para-1*, *para-I*, and *1-para*.

primitive (prim′ĭ-tiv) [L. *primitivus*] first in point of time; existing in a simple form, or showing little evolution.

Primolut N trademark for *norethindrone*.

primordia (prī-mor′de-ah) [L.] plural of *primordium*.

primordial (pri-mor′de-al) [L. *primordialis*] original or primitive; of the simplest and most undeveloped character.

primordium (pri-mor′de-um), pl. *primor′dia* [L. "the beginning"] the earliest or primary stage in the development of an organ or structure; an anlage, rudiment, or germ. **tooth p.**, tooth *bud*.

Prinadol trademark for *phenazocine hydrobromide* (see under PHENAZOCINE).

principle (prin′sĭ-p'l) [L. *principium*] 1. a law of conduct. 2. a chemical component. 3. a substance on which certain of the properties of a drug depend. **all or nothing p.**, all or none LAW. **antipernicious anemia p.**, cyanocobalamin. **p. of ethics**, CODE of ethics. **Le Châtelier's p.**, a system at chemical equilibrium will react to an applied stress so as to remove that stress. **pressor p.**, vasopressin. **Thielemann's p.**, the balanced occlusion is equal to the product of condylar guidance and incisal guidance divided by the product of the cusp angle, curve of Spee, and the plane of occlusion determined according to the following formula:

$$\text{balanced occlusion} = \frac{CG \cdot IG}{PO \cdot CH \cdot CS}$$

where *CG* = condylar guidance, *IG* = incisal guidance, *PO* = plane of occlusion, *CH* = cusp height, and *CS* = curve of Spee. Orthodontic or prosthetic treatment may alter these factors, except for condylar guidance. Called also *Hanau's quint* and *Thielemann's formula*. **Weber-Fechner p.**, Fechner's LAW.

Priscoline trademark for *tolazoline hydrochloride* (see under TOLAZOLINE).

Prisilidene trademark for alphaprodine hydrochloride (see under ALPHAPRODINE).

prism (prizm) [Gr. prisma] 1. a solid with a triangular or polygonal cross section. 2. a transparent body having two plane faces that are not parallel, used to deviate rays of light. **adamantine p's, enamel p's. enamel p's**, the structural units of the tooth enamel, consisting of parallel rods or prisms composed mainly of hydroxyapatite crystals and organic substance and held together with a cement substance, each enveloped in a sheath that stains differently than the prism (see enamel SHEATH). The average diameter of a prism is 4 μ, being narrower at its origin at the dentinoenamel junction, and increasing in width toward the external surface. Externally, the prisms are marked by regular striations, which are believed to represent cyclic deposition of enamel matrix. Called also *adamantine p's, enamel columns, enamel rods*, and *prismata adamantina* [NA].

prisma (priz′mah), pl. *pris′mata* [Gr.] prism. **pris′mata adaman′tina**, enamel prisms; see under PRISM.

prismata (priz′mah-tah) [L.] plural of *prisma*.

prismatic (priz-mat′ik) shaped like a prism; produced by a prism.

prismoid (priz′moid) resembling a prism.

Pristacin trademark for *cetylpyridinium chloride* (see under CETYLPYRIDINIUM).

private (pri′vit) pertaining to or affecting a particular person or group. See private antigens, under ANTIGEN.

Privenal trademark for *hexobarbital sodium* (see under HEXOBARBITAL).

privilege (priv″ĕ-lij) a special advantage, right, benefit, immunity, or exemption enjoyed by or granted to a person, group, etc. **conversion p.**, in group health insurance, the right of the insured to change his or her insurance to another form, without medical examination, upon termination of the policy in force, usually upon termination of employment or other source of membership in the group. **staff p.**, the privilege, granted by a hospital or other inpatient health facility, to a physician, dentist, or other practicing health professional to join the hospital's staff and hospitalize private patients in the hospital.

Privine trademark for *naphazoline*.

p.r.n. abbreviation for L. *pro re nata*, as required.

Pro proline.

pro- [L., Gr. *pro* before] 1. a prefix signifying before or in front of. 2. a prefix denoting a precursor.

proaccelerin (pro″ak-sel′er′in) FACTOR V.

Pro-Actidil trademark for *triprolidine*.

Proactinomyces (pro″ak-tĭ-no-mi′sēz) *Nocardia*. **P. asteroi′des**, *Nocardia asteroides*; see under NOCARDIA. **P. israe′li**, *Actinomyces israelii*; see under ACTINOMYCES. **P. mu′ris**, *Streptobacillus moniliformis*; see under STREPTOBACILLUS.

Proactinomycetaceae (pro″ak-tĭ-no-mi″sē-ta′se-e) Mycobacteriaceae.

proactivator (pro-ak′tĭ-va″tor) the inactive precursor form of an activator, or a factor that requires a chemical change, usually by an enzyme, to become an activator. For example, a substance present in plasma (*plasminogen p.*) that is adsorbed onto fibrin during clotting and which, when activated, will convert plasminogen to plasmin; or factor B (C3 proactivator) which is involved in activation of the alternate pathway of complement. **C3 p.**, FACTOR B. **C3 p. convertase**, factor D̄.

ProAlloy trademark for an *amalgam alloy* (see under AMALGAM).

Proasma trademark for *methoxyphenamine hydrochloride* (see under METHOXYPHENAMINE).

proband (pro′band) [Ger.; from L. *probare* to prove] propositus.

Pro-Banthine trademark for *propantheline bromide* (see under PROPANTHELINE).

probe (prōb) [L. *proba; probare* to test] a slender instrument designed for introduction into a wound, cavity, or sinus tract for purposes of exploration. **Anel's p.,** a delicate probe for the lacrimal puncta and canals. **blood flow p.,** an implanted cuff that fits around a surgically exposed artery or vein to detect blood flow. **blunt p.,** one in which the blade has a blunt end. **Bowman's p.,** one of a set of probes for use in the nasal ducts. **Brackett's p.,** a delicate and flexible probe of silver wire for exploring dental fistulas. **calibrated p.,** a periodontal probe calibrated in millimeters. **cross p.,** a fine periodontal probe used for the diagnosis and examination of calculus on the root surface in the periodontal or gingival pocket. **drum p.,** one with an attachment which emits a sound when it comes in contact with a foreign body. **electric p.,** one which on contact with a foreign body completes an electric circuit, thereby producing sound. **eyed p.,** one with a slit near one end through which a ligature or tape may be drawn. **Fox-Williams p.,** a relatively thick periodontal probe graduated at 1, 2, 3, 5, 7, 8, 9, and 10 mm, used for determining the depths of periodontal pockets. **Glickman's periodontal p.,** a periodontal probe having the

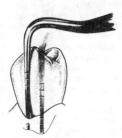

Glickman Periodontal Probe #26G. (From F. A. Carranza, Jr.: Glickman's Clinical Periodontology. 5th ed. Philadelphia, W. B. Saunders Co., 1979.)

calibrated blade offset from the shank at a 90° angle. See illustration. **lacrimal p.,** one designed for use in the lacrimal passages. **Marquis p.,** trademark for a thin periodontal probe with a rounded tip and graduations in 3-mm units, alternately colored chrome and black; used for determining the depths of periodontal pockets. **Michigan p.,** trademark for a thin periodontal probe marked at 3-, 6-, and 8-mm. **periodontal p., pocket p.,** one graduated in millimeters, used to measure the depth and determine the outline of a periodontal pocket and the condition of the crevicular epithelium. **root canal p.,** a slender, flexible, and smooth or edged metal, hand-operated endodontic instrument, usually made of soft iron wire; used for tracing the course of and exploring root canals. Called also *pathfinder, pathfinder broach,* and *smooth broach.* See illustration at root canal THERAPY. **scissors p.,** a long, delicate pair of scissors that can be used as a probe. **Williams' periodontal p.,** a periodontal probe having a tapered rodlike blade at a 45° angle to the shank and handle, used to measure retractable gingival tissue and to locate the base of periodontal pockets.

Probecid trademark for *probenecid.*

Proben trademark for *probenecid.*

probenecid (pro-ben′ĕ-sid) a uricosuric agent, 4-[(ipropylamino)sulfonyl]benzoic acid, occurring as a white, odorless, crystalline powder that is soluble is alkali solutions, ethanol, chloroform, and acetone, but not in water and dilute acids. It inhibits the tubular reabsorption of urate and increases urinary excretion of uric acid, thus decreasing serum uric acid levels. It also decreases urinary levels of aminosalicylic acid, aminoketosteroids, and sodium iodomethamate. By blocking renal tubular secretion of penicillins and other antibiotics, probenecid enhances their action, therefore it is used as an adjunct in antibiotic therapy. Adverse reactions include occasional gingivitis, anorexia, nausea, vomiting, excessive urination, vertigo, anemia, nephrotic syndrome, liver necrosis, and aplastic anemia. Trademarks: Benemid, Probecid, Proben.

procainamide hydrochloride (pro-kan′ah--mīd) a cardiac depressant, 4-amino-N-[2-(diethylamino)ethyl]benzamide monohydrochloride, occurring as a white to tan, odorless, crystalline powder that is soluble in water and ethanol, slightly soluble in chloroform, and very slightly soluble in benzene and ether. Used as an antiarrhythmic and antifibrillatory drug. Anorexia, nausea, vomiting, flushing, diarrhea, weakness, neuroses with

hallucinations, fever, muscle and joint pain, malaise, pruritus, angioedema, urticaria, and other hyposensitivity reactions may occur. Lupus erythematosus–like reactions and potentially fatal complications, such as agranulocytosis, hypotension with shock, coronary insufficiency, and cardiac rhythm disorders, may also occur. Called also *procaine amide hydrochloride.* Trademarks: Novocamid, Procardyl, Pronestyl.

procaine (pro′kān) a local anesthetic, 2-diethylaminoethyl-*p*-aminobenzoate. **p. amide hydrochloride,** PROCAINAMIDE hydrochloride. **p. benzylpenicillinate,** PENICILLIN G procaine. **p. esterase,** carboxylesterase. **p. hydrochloride,** the hydrochloride salt of procaine, occurring as white, odorless crystals or crystalline powder that is soluble in water and alcohol, slightly soluble in chloroform, and insoluble in ether. Used in infiltration, nerve block, epidural block, spinal block, and intravenous anesthesia. Procaine hydrochloride also has antispasmodic, antipruritic, and antiarrhythmic properties. In dentistry, frequently used in a solution also containing butetheamine, tetracaine, propoxycaine, and a vasoconstrictor agent, such as epinephrine, phenylephrine, levarterenol, or levonordefrin. Its adverse effects are similar to those of other local anesthetics. Trademarks: Ethocaine, Novocain, Novocaine, Syncaine. **p. penicillin G,** PENICILLIN G procaine.

procallus (pro-kal′us) [*pro-* + *callus*] provisional CALLUS.

procarbazine (pro-kar′bah-zēn) a substituted hydrazine compound, N-isopropyl-α-(2-methylhydrazino)-*p*-toluamide monohydrochloride, occurring as a white to yellowish, bitter, crystalline powder with a slight odor, which is soluble in water, methanol, and ethanol, and is slightly soluble in chloroform, benzene, ether, and acetone. It is a cytotoxic drug believed to inhibit DNA, RNA, and protein synthesis, having also weak monoamine oxidase inhibitor properties. Used in the treatment of Hodgkin's disease and other neoplastic diseases. Principal side reactions include bone marrow depression with leukopenia and thrombocytopenia, nausea, and vomiting. Hypertension, cough, anorexia, xerostomia, dysphagia, stomatitis, predisposition to infection, paresthesia, hemorrhagic tendency, and a variety of gastrointestinal, neurological, and dermatological complications may occur. Called also *N-methylhydrazine.* Trademarks: Matulane, Natulan.

Procardyl trademark for *procainamide hydrochloride* (see under PROCAINAMIDE).

Procaryotae (pro-kar′e-o′te) [*pro-* + Gr. *karyon* nucleus] a kingdom of microorganisms made up of single prokaryotic cells or simple associations of prokaryotic cells, and comprises two divisions: the Cyanobacteria, which includes the blue-green algae (see under ALGAE), and the Bacteria, which includes all prokaryotic organisms that are not blue-green algae (see BACTERIUM). Sometimes, prokaryotic organisms that lack a true cell wall are considered unrelated to the Bacteria and are placed in a separate class — the Mollicutes. Cf. EUCARYOTAE.

procaryote (pro-kar′e-ōt) prokaryote.

procaryotic (pro″kar-e-ot′ik) prokaryotic.

procedure (pro-se′dur) [L. *procedere,* from *pro* forward + *cedere* move] a series of steps by which a desired result is accomplished. See also METHOD. **push-back p.,** push-back TECHNIQUE.

procerus (pro-se′rus) [L.] 1. long, slender. 2. procerus MUSCLE.

process (pros′es) [L. *processus*] 1. a prominence or projection, as of bone. See also PROCESSUS. 2. a series of operations leading to the achievement of a specific result; used also as a verb to designate subjection to such a series of operations designed to produce desired changes in the original material, or achieve other result. **aliform p. of sphenoid bone,** small wing of sphenoid bone; see under WING. **alveolar p.,** the superior process of the mandibular and the inferior process of the maxillary bones, which is excavated into eight deep cavities on each side to receive and support the teeth. It consists of the cribriform plate (alveolar bone proper), which provides the bony lining for the alveolus, being a thick bony layer perforated by openings for nerves and blood and lymphatic vessels supplying the periodontal ligament; the cortical plate, which is a continuation of the bony plate of the maxillary and mandibular bones; and spongy bone, which also continues from the cancellous bone of the maxilla and mandible. Two tables of compact bone and an intervening diploë of spongy bone are produced during the developmental stage, the outer table forming the cortical plate, the inner plate producing the cribriform plate, and the trabeculae making up the spongy bone. The roots of the teeth are separated from those of neighboring teeth by spongy bone, forming interdental septa. Called also *processus alveolaris.* See also *alveolar p. of maxilla* and alveolar part of maxilla, under PART. **alveolar p., supporting,** the part of the alveolar process consisting of cancellous trabeculae and the facial and lingual plates of compact bone. **alveolar p. of mandible,** alveolar part of mandible; see under PART. **alveolar p. of maxilla,** the thick parabolically curved ridge that projects downward and forms the free lower border of the maxilla; it is in front of and lateral to the palatine process and it bears the teeth. When the maxillae are articulated with each other, the alveolar processes together form the alveolar arch. It extends from the base of the tuberosity posterior to the last molar to the median line anteriorly, where it articulates with its fellow of the opposite side, and merges with the palatine process medially and with the zygomatic process laterally. The process has a facial and a lingual surface with ridges corresponding to the surfaces of the roots of the teeth invested. The bone is made up of the labiobuccal and lingual plates of very dense but thin cortical tissue separated by interdental septa of cancellous bone. The buccinator muscle arises from the outer surface. Called also *dental p.* and *processus alveolaris maxillae* [NA]. See also *alveolar p.* under PART. **angular p. of frontal bone, external,** zygomatic p. of frontal bone. **basilar p.,** basilar PART. **p. of Blumenbach,** uncinate p. of ethmoid bone. **p. of cartilage of nasal septum posterior,** a narrow flat strip of cartilage that extends backward and upward along the groove on the upper margin of the vomer and below the perpendicular plate of the ethmoid bone, from the septal cartilage nearly to the sphenoid bone. Called also *posterior sphenoidal p., processus posterior sphenoidalis* [NA], and *processus sphenoidalis septi cartilaginei.* **Civinini's p. of external pterygoid plate,** pterygospinous p. **clinoid p., anterior,** a bony process formed by the medial end of the posterior border of the small wing of the sphenoid bone. Called also *processus clinoideus anterior* [NA]. **clinoid p., middle,** one of two small eminences on the internal surface of the intracranial surface of the body of the sphenoid bone, situated on either side of the anterior part of the pituitary fossa. Called also *middle petrosal p.* and *processus clinoideus medius* [NA]. **clinoid p., posterior,** one of the two tubercles on the superior angle of either side of the dorsum sellae of the body of the sphenoid bone, giving attachment to the tentorium of the cerebellum. Called also *posterior superior petrosal p.* and *processus clinoideus posterior* [NA]. **condyloid p.,** mandibular CONDYLE. **coronoid p. of mandible,** the anterior part of the upper end of the ramus of the mandible, presenting a thin, triangular bony projection that is somewhat roughened anterior to the tip to give attachment to a part of the temporal muscle. Called also *temporal p. of mandible, corone, coronoid,* and *processus coronoideus mandibular* [NA]. **dental p.,** alveolar p. of maxilla. **ensiform p. of sphenoid bone,** small wing of sphenoid bone; see under WING. **epiphyseal p.,** epiphysis. **ethmoidal p. of inferior nasal concha,** a bony projection above and behind the maxillary process of the inferior nasal concha. Called also *processus ethmoidalis conchae nasalis inferioris* [NA]. **ethmoidal p. of Macalister,** sphenoidal CREST. **frontal p., external,** nasal spine of frontal bone; see under SPINE. **frontal p. of maxilla,** a large, strong, irregular bony process that projects from the upper and anterior part of the body of the maxilla. Laterally, it is a part of the continuation of the infraorbital margin; anteriorly, it articulates with the nasal bone, and superiorly, with the frontal bone. Its medial surface is directed toward the nasal cavity. The smooth lateral surface gives attachment to the levator labii superioris alaeque nasi and the orbicularis oculi muscles and the medial palpebral ligament. Its lateral surface closes the anterior ethmoidal cells. Inferior to this is the ethmoidal crest which articulates with the middle nasal concha, forming the upper limit of the atrium of the middle meatus; its anterior part forms the agger nasi. The lateral margin forms the anterior lacrimal crest and at its junction with the orbital surface is the lacrimal tubercle. Called also *nasal p. of maxilla* and *processus frontalis maxillae* [NA]. **frontal p. of zygomatic bone,** a thick, serrated, upward projecting triangular process of the zygomatic bone lying behind the malar surface and between the orbital and temporal surfaces. Its anterior edge is smooth and forms part of the orbit; its superior edge articulates with the frontal bone; its posterior serrated edge articulates with the great wing of the sphenoid bone and the orbital surface of the maxilla. At the junction with the sphenoid and maxillary bones, the process forms the anterior boundary of the orbital fissure. Called also *frontosphenoidal p. of zygomatic bone, processus frontalis ossis zygomatici* [NA] and *processus frontosphenoidalis ossis zygomatici.* **frontonasal p.,** the median elevation between the medial limb

of U-shaped elevations or processes that develop during the fifth week of embryonic life and surround the nasal pit, their limbs being directed toward the oral cavity. It develops into the forehead and the bridge of the nose. Called also *frontonasal elevation prominence.* **frontosphenoidal p. of zygomatic bone,** frontal p. of zygomatic bone. **greater p. of ethmoid bone,** hamate p. of ethmoid bone, uncinate p. of ethmoid bone. **hamular p. of lacrimal bone,** lacrimal HAMULUS. **hamular p. of sphenoid bone,** pterygoid HAMULUS. **head p.,** notochord. **infundibular p.,** PARS nervosa hypophyseos. **Ingrassia's p.,** small wing of sphenoid bone; see under WING. **intrajugular p. of occipital bone,** a bony spicule projecting laterally above the hypoglossal canal, which divides the jugular notch of the occipital bone into a lateral and medial part. Called also *middle jugular p. of occipital bone* and *processus intrajugularis ossis occipitalis* [NA]. **intrajugular p. of temporal bone,** a small ridge on the petrous part of the temporal bone that separates the jugular notch into a medial and a lateral part, corresponding to similar parts of the jugular notch of the facing temporal bone. Called also *processus intrajugularis ossis temporalis* [NA]. **jugular p., jugular p. of occipital bone,** an irregular process extending laterally from the posterior part of the condyle of the occipital bone, which forms the posterior boundary of the jugular foramen. From the lateral aspect, it forms a quadrilateral or triangular area, joining the jugular area of the temporal bone. The junction is made up of a plate of cartilage which ossifies after the age of 25 years. Its rough inferior surface gives attachment to the rectus capitis lateralis muscle and the lateral atlanto-occipital ligament, and also gives rise to a downward projection, the paramastoid process. Called also *jugular spine* and *processus jugularis ossis occipitalis* [NA]. **jugular p. of occipital bone of Krause, posterior,** paramastoid p. of occipital bone. **jugular p. of occipital bone, middle,** intrajugular p. **Krause's posterior jugular process of occipital bone,** paramastoid p. **lacrimal p.,** lacrimal p. of inferior nasal concha. **lacrimal p. of inferior nasal concha,** a process on the inferior nasal concha that articulates with the lacrimal bone. Called also *lacrimal p., nasal p. of inferior turbinate bone* and *processus lacrimalis conchae nasalis inferioris* [NA]. **lateral nasal p.,** nasolateral p. **Macalister's ethmoidal p.,** sphenoidal CREST. **malar p.,** zygomatic p. of maxilla. **mamillary p. of temporal bone,** mastoid p. **mandibular p.,** one of the processes formed by bifurcation of the first branchial arch in the embryo, which unites ventrally with its fellow to form the lower jaw. **marginal p. of malar bone,** marginal tubercle of zygomatic bone; see under TUBERCLE. **mastoid p.,** a conical process projecting forward and downward from the external surface of the temporal bone just posterior to the external acoustic meatus; it gives attachment to the sternocleidomastoideus, splenius capitis, and longissimus capitis muscles. A deep groove on its medial side (mastoid notch) gives attachment to the digastricus muscle, and medial to this, the occipital groove lodges the occipital artery. Called also *mamillary p. of temporal bone* and *processus mastoideus ossis temporalis* [NA]. **maxillary p.,** one of the processes formed by bifurcation of the first branchial arch in the embryo, which joins with the ipsilateral median nasal process in the formation of the upper jaw. **maxillary p. of inferior nasal concha,** a bony process descending from the ethmoid process of the inferior nasal concha. Called also *processus maxillaris conchae nasalis inferioris* [NA]. **maxillary p. of zygomatic bone,** a rough, triangular process of the zygomatic bone which articulates with the maxilla. **mental p.,** mental PROTUBERANCE. **muscular p. of arytenoid cartilage,** the lateral and posterior lower angular projection of the arytenoid cartilage, to which the cricoarytenoid muscles are attached. Called also *processus muscularis cartilaginis arytenoideae* [NA]. **nasal p. of frontal bone,** the small, irregularly shaped process that projects downward from the medial part of the squama of the frontal bone to articulate with the nasal bones and the frontal process of the maxillary bones. Called also *pars nasalis ossis frontalis* [NA], *prefrontal bone, prefrontal bone of von Bardeleben,* and *von Bardeleben's prefrontal bone.* **nasal p. of inferior turbinate bone,** lacrimal p. of inferior nasal concha. **nasal p., lateral,** one of the two limbs of the horseshoe-shaped elevation, bounding a nasal pit in the embryo, which participates in formation of the side and wing of the nose. **nasal p. of maxilla,** frontal p. of maxilla. **nasal p., median,** one of the two limbs of the horseshoe-shaped elevation bounding a nasal pit in the embryo, which participates with the ipsilateral maxillary process in forming half of the upper jaw. **nasolateral p.,** the lateral limb of U-shaped elevations that develop during the fifth week of embryonic life and surround the nasal pit, their limbs being directed toward the oral cavity. It develops into the sides of the wings of the nose. Called also *lateral nasal p., nasolateral elevation,* and *nasolateral prominence.* **notochordal p.,** a midline cord of cells migrating from the area of Hensen's node (primitive knot) of the primitive streak in the direction of the prochordal plate. It develops into the notochord. **occipital p. of occipital bone,** basilar PART. **p. of odontoblast, odontoblastic p.,** a slender protoplasmic process in a dentinal tubule, which is a cytoplasmic extension of the cell body. Odontoblastic processes extend from the dentinoenamel junction and cementodentinal junction to the cell bodies of odontoblasts in the dental pulp. Some form the enamel spindles and extend through the amelodentinal junction into the enamel. In the peripheral dentin or mantle dentin, they tend to bifurcate, some subdividing to form a protoplasmic arborization which joins with the collaterals from the adjacent processes. Called also *dentinal fiber.* **orbital p. of palatine bone,** a bony process projecting superiorly and laterally from the uppermost part of the vertical plate of the palatine bone, to which it is connected by a constricted neck. Its superior or orbital surface forms a part of the floor of the orbit; its lateral surface forms a part of the inferior orbital fissure; its anterior or maxillary surface articulates with the maxilla; its posterior or sphenoidal surface presents the opening of the air cell usually communicating with the sphenoidal sinus; its medial or ethmoidal surface articulates with the labyrinth of the ethmoid bone. Called also *processus orbitalis ossis palatini* [NA]. **palatine p. of maxilla,** a horizontal bony plate arching medially from the nasal surface, which forms the floor of the nose and the roof of the mouth. With its fellow of the opposite side, it forms three-fourths of the hard palate. Its concave, rough inferior surface contains pits for the palatine glands and is perforated by numerous foramina for passage of blood vessels and nerves. A groove (or canal) near the last molar transmits the greater palatine vessels and nerve. In the midline behind the incisor teeth is the incisive foramen opening into the incisive canal, or the foramen of Stensen, transmitting the branches of the septal artery and the nasopalatine nerve. Two additional canals, the foramina of Scarpa, may also be present for transmission of the nasopalatine nerves. Young skulls may show a delicate suture extending from the incisive foramen to the interval between the lateral incisor and the canine tooth; anterior to it is the premaxilla. Its posterior thin edge joins the palatine bone at the point of the greater palatine foramen. The anterior portion is progressively thicker and is continuous with the alveolar process surrounding the roots of the anterior teeth. Called also *palatine lamina of maxilla* and *processus palatinus maxillae* [NA]. **palatine p., lateral,** a shelflike projection developing from each maxillary process region of the upper jaw in the embryo, later fusing with each other and with the nasal septum to form the palate. Called also *palatine shelf.* **palatine p., median,** a shelflike projection developing from each median nasal process in the embryo, which participates with its fellow in forming the premaxillary portion of the upper jaw. Called also *palatine shelf.* **palpebral p.,** palpebral part of lacrimal gland; see under PART. **paracondyloid p. of occipital bone,** paramastoid p. **paramastoid p., paramastoid p. of occipital bone, paroccipital p. of occipital bone,** a process projecting downward from the inferior surface of the jugular process of the occipital bone, which sometimes reaches the transverse process of the atlas. Called also *Krause's posterior jugular p. of occipital bone, paracondyloid p. of occipital bone, posterior jugular p. of occipital bone of Krause,* and *processus paramastoideus ossis occipitalis* [NA]. **petrosal p.,** one of the two sharp bony projections inferior to the notches for the passage of the abducent nerve, situated on either side of the dorsum sellae on the superior surface of the body of the sphenoid bone, which articulates with the apex of the petrous part of the temporal bone, and forms the median boundary of the foramen lacerum. **petrosal p., anterior,** sphenoidal LINGULA. **petrosal p., middle,** clinoid p., middle. **petrosal p., posterior superior,** clinoid p., posterior. **pterygoid p.,** one of the two bony processes which project perpendicularly from the point of junction of the great wings and body of the sphenoid bone, each consisting of a lateral and medial plate. The plates are separated by a cleft (pterygoid fissure) the margins of which articulate with the pyramidal process of the palatine bone. The line of fusion of the two plates is marked by the pterygopalatine groove. A V-shaped fossa (pterygoid fossa) situated between the two plates diverging posteriorly, contains the pterygoideus medialis and tensor veli palatini muscles. A small depression superior to this fossa (scaphoid fossa) gives origin to the tensor veli palatini muscle. Called also *descending lamina of sphenoid bone, inferior lamina of sphenoid bone, processus pterygoideus ossis sphenoidalis* [NA], *pterygoid bone,* and *trapezoid bone of Henle.* **pterygospinous p.,** a small spine on the posterior edge of the lateral pterygoid plate of the sphenoid bone, giving attachment to the pterygospinous ligament. Called also *Civinini's process of external pterygoid plate, Civinini's spine, processus pterygospinosus* [NA], and

processus pterygospinosus Civinini. **pyramidal p. of palatine bone,** a strong bony process which projects laterally from the junction of the horizontal and vertical plates of the palatine bone and fits into the interval between the inferior extremity of the pterygoid plates, helping to form the pterygoid fossa. Its rough posterior surface articulates with the pterygoid plates; the pterygoideus medialis muscle attaches to its grooved intermediate area. The rough anterior part of the lateral surface articulates with the maxilla. A triangular area between the tuberosity of the maxilla and the pterygoid plate forms the infratemporal fossa. The lesser palatine foramina at the base of the pyramidal process transmit the lesser palatine nerves. Called also *processus pyramidalis ossis palatini* [NA] and *pyramidal tuberosity of palatine bone.* **retromandibular p. of parotid gland,** an irregularly wedge-shaped portion of the parotid gland passing medially behind the ramus of the mandible almost to the wall of the pharynx. Called also *processus retromandibularis glandulae parotidis.* **small p. of Soemmering,** marginal tubercle of zygomatic bone; see under TUBERCLE. **sphenoidal p. of palatine bone,** a small, thin, bony process that projects upward and medially from the posterior part of the superior margin of the perpendicular plate of the palatine bone. Its superior surface articulates with the pterygoid process and the sphenoidal concha. It reaches the ala of the vomer and presents a groove that forms the pharyngeal canal. The rough portion of the lateral surface articulates with the pterygoid plate and the smooth portion forms a part of the pterygopalatine fossa, with the anterior border forming a part of the sphenopalatine notch. The posterior border articulates with the pterygoid plate. The concave medial surface forms a part of the lateral wall of the nasal cavity. Called also *processus sphenoidalis ossis palatini* [NA]. **sphenoidal p., posterior,** p. of cartilage of nasal septum, posterior. **spinous p.,** any slender, pointed projection; a spine. **styloid p. of temporal bone,** a long spine projecting downward from the inferior surface of the temporal bone just anterior to the stylomastoid foramen, giving attachment to three muscles and two ligaments. Called also *plectrum* and *processus styloideus ossis temporalis* [NA]. **temporal p. of mandible,** coronoid p. of mandible. **temporal p. of zygomatic bone,** the posterior, long, narrow, and serrated process of the zygomatic bone that articulates with the zygomatic process of the temporal bone. Called also *processus temporalis ossis zygomatici* [NA]. **Tomes' p.,** a finger-like projection of the ameloblast, occurring during the secretory phase of the cell during amelogenesis, which extends from the point of separation of the adjacent cell membrane to the distal free surface. **uncinate p. of ethmoid bone,** a curved bony plate that extends inferiorly and posteriorly from the anterior part of the labyrinth of the ethmoid bone, and forms part of the medial wall of the maxillary sinus and articulates with the ethmoid process of the inferior nasal concha. Called also *p. of Blumenbach, greater p. of ethmoid bone, hamate p. of ethmoid bone, hamulus of ethmoid bone, processus uncinatus ossis ethmoidalis* [NA]. **uncinate p. of lacrimal bone,** lacrimal HAMULUS. **vaginal p. of sphenoid bone,** a projecting small plate on the inferior surface of the body of the sphenoid bone on either side, running medially from the medial pterygoid plate to articulate with the wing of the vomer and with the sphenoid process of the palatine bone. Called also *processus vaginalis ossis sphenoidalis* [NA]. **vocal p.,** the process of the arytenoid cartilage to which the vocal ligament is attached. Called also *processus vocalis* [NA]. **xiphoid p. of sphenoid bone,** small wing of sphenoid bone; see under WING. **zygomatic p. of frontal bone,** a thick, strong process of the frontal bone, situated at the lateral end of the supraorbital margin and articulating with the zygomatic bone, and from which the temporal line starts. Called also *external angular p. of frontal bone* and *processus zygomaticus ossis frontalis* [NA]. **zygomatic p. of maxilla,** a roughly triangular eminence that articulates with the zygomatic bone and marks the separation of the anterior, infratemporal, and orbital surfaces of the body of the maxilla. Its lower border is situated directly over the first molar tooth. Called also *malar p., zygomatico-orbital p. of maxilla,* and *processus zygomaticus maxillae* [NA]. **zygomatic p. of temporal bone,** a long, strong, arched bony process projecting from the lower portion of the squama of the temporal bone, passing forward from just above the entrance of the external acoustic meatus to join the zygomatic bone and thus forming the zygomatic arch. Its anterior end articulates with the zygomatic bone, and the posterior end arises from the squama by the anterior and posterior roots. Its convex lateral surface gives attachment to the masseter muscle, while the short and thick inferior border attaches some of its fibers. Its thin and sharp superior border gives attachment to the temporal fascia. Called also *processus zygomaticus ossis temporalis* [NA] and *zygoma*. **zygomatico-orbital p. of maxilla,** zygomatic p. of maxilla.

processing (pros'es-ing) a series of operations, events, or steps leading to the achievement of a specific goal. **film p.,** a series of steps leading to the conversion of the latent image on the exposed photographic or x-ray film into the manifest image by reducing the exposed silver salts to metallic silver grains, thus rendering them black and giving shape to the image. The steps include development, consisting of immersion of the exposed film in the developing solution, where the reduction of silver salts occurs, followed by immersion in the water bath and acid bath. The exposed film is immersed in the fixing solution, where the film surface is hardened and the manifest image is fixed. The last stage consists of washing, rinsing, and drying the film. See also film DEVELOPMENT and film FIXATION. **film p., automatic,** film processing through the use of a device which mechanically transports the film through a series of solutions under controlled conditions.

processor (pros'es-or) one who handles or processes something. **claim p.,** an employee of an organization responsible for payment of benefits who processes routine claims.

processus (pro-ses'sus) [L.] a prominence or projection; used in anatomical nomenclature as a general term to designate such a mass projecting from a larger structure. See also PROCESS. **p. ala'ris os'sis ethmoida'lis,** frontal HAMULUS. **p. alveo'laris,** alveolar PROCESS. **p. alveola'ris max'illae** [NA], alveolar process of maxilla; see under PROCESS. **p. clinoi'deus ante'rior** [NA], anterior clinoid PROCESS. **p. clinoi'deus me'dius** [NA], middle clinoid PROCESS. **p. clinoi'deus poste'rior** [NA], posterior clinoid PROCESS. **p. condyla'ris mandib'ulae** [NA], mandibular CONDYLE. **p. coronoi'deus mandib'ulae** [NA], coronoid process of mandible; see under PROCESS. **p. ethmoida'lis con'chae nasa'lis inferio'ris** [NA], ethmoidal process of inferior nasal concha; see under PROCESS. **p. fronta'lis maxil'lae** [NA], frontal process of maxilla; see under PROCESS. **p. fronta'lis os'sis zygomat'ici** [NA], frontal process of zygomatic bone; see under PROCESS. **p. frontosphenoida'lis os'sis zygomat'ici,** frontal process of zygomatic bone; see under PROCESS. **p. intrajugula'ris os'sis occipita'lis** [NA], intrajugular process of occipital bone; see under PROCESS. **p. intrajugula'ris os'sis tempora'lis** [NA], intrajugular process of temporal bone; see under PROCESS. **p. jugula'ris os'sis occipita'lis** [NA], jugular PROCESS. **p. lacrima'lis con'chae nasa'lis inferio'ris** [NA], lacrimal process of inferior nasal concha; see under PROCESS. **p. margina'lis os'sis zygomat'ici,** marginal tubercle of zygomatic bone; see under TUBERCLE. **p. mastoi'deus os'sis tempora'lis** [NA], mastoid PROCESS. **p. maxilla'ris con'chae nasa'lis inferio'ris** [NA], maxillary process of inferior nasal concha; see under PROCESS. **p. muscula'ris cartilag'inis arytenoi'deae** [NA], muscular process of arytenoid cartilage; see under PROCESS. **p. orbita'lis os'sis palati'ni** [NA], orbital process of palatine bone; see under PROCESS. **p. palati'nus maxil'lae** [NA], palatine process of maxilla; see under PROCESS. **p. paramastoi'deus os'sis occipita'lis** [NA], paramastoid PROCESS. **p. poste'rior sphenoida'lis** [NA], PROCESS of cartilage of nasal septum, posterior. **p. pterygoi'deus os'sis sphenoida'lis** [NA], pterygoid PROCESS. **p. pterygospino'sus** [NA], **p. pterygospino'sus Civinini,** pterygospinous PROCESS. **p. pyramida'lis os'sis palati'ni** [NA], pyramidal process of palatine bone; see under PROCESS. **p. retromandibula'ris glan'dulae parot'tidis,** retromandibular process of parotid gland; see under PROCESS. **p. sphenoida'lis os'sis palati'ni** [NA], sphenoidal process of palatine bone; see under PROCESS. **p. sphenoida'lis sep'ti cartilagin'ei,** process of cartilage of nasal septum, posterior; see under PROCESS. **p. styloi'deus os'sis tempora'lis** [NA], styloid process of temporal bone; see under PROCESS. **p. tempora'lis os'sis zygomat'ici** [NA], temporal process of zygomatic bone; see under PROCESS. **p. tuba'rius,** an angular process projecting dorsally from the middle of the posterior edge of the medial pterygoid plate of the sphenoid bone; it supports the pharyngeal end of the auditory tube. **p. uncina'tus os'sis ethmoida'lis** [NA], uncinate process of ethmoid bone; see under PROCESS. **p. vagina'lis os'sis sphenoida'lis** [NA], vaginal process of sphenoid bone; see under PROCESS. **p. voca'lis** [NA], vocal PROCESS. **p. zygomat'icus maxil'lae** [NA], zygomatic process of maxilla; see under PROCESS. **p. zygomat'icus os'sis fronta'lis** [NA], zygomatic process of frontal bone; see under PROCESS. **p. zygomat'icus os'sis tempora'lis** [NA], zygomatic process of temporal bone; see under PROCESS.

procheilia (pro-kel'e-ah) protruding lips.

procheilon (pro-ki'lon) [*pro-* + Gr. *cheilon* lip] TUBERCLE of upper lip.

prochlorpemazine (pro″klor-pem'ah-zēn) prochlorperazine.

prochlorperazine (pro″klor-per'ah-zēn) an antiemetic and tranquilizer, 2-chloro-10-[3 - (4-methyl-1-piperazinyl) propyl]-10*H*-phenothiazine, occurring as a clear, pale yellow, viscous liquid that is sensitive to light, and is soluble in ethanol, chloroform, and ether and slightly soluble in water. Adverse reactions may include restlessness, dystonia, pseudoparkinsonism, dyskinesia, and contact dermatitis; children with infections and dehydration ·are particularly susceptible. Agranulocytosis may occur. Called also *chlormeprazine* and *prochlorpemazine.* Trademarks: Capazine, Meterazine, Nipodal. **p. dimaleate,** the dimaleate salt of prochlorperazine, having properties similar to those of the parent drug. Trademarks: Compazine, Emetiral, Stemetil.

Procoagulo trademark for *menadiol sodium diphosphate* (see under MENADIOL).

Procomat trademark for a small-capacity automatic film processing unit.

proconvertin (pro″kon-ver'tin) FACTOR VII.

proconvertin-convertin (pro″kon-ver'tin-kon-ver'tin) FACTOR VII.

ProcoSol sealer see under SEALER.

proctodeum (prok″to-de'um) [Gr. *proktos* anus + *hodaios* pertaining to a way] an invagination in the ectoderm under the root of the tail adjacent to the primitive hindgut of the embryo at the point where later the anus is formed. Called also *anal pit.*

procumbency (pro-kum'ben-se) excessive labioaxial inclination of the incisors.

procumbent (pro-kum'bent) lying on the face; prone.

procyclidine hydrochloride (pro-si'kli-dēn) a skeletal muscle relaxant with weak antimuscarinic and antispasmodic actions, α-cyclohexyl-α-phenyl-1-pyrrolidinepropanol hydrochloride. It occurs as a white, crystalline powder with a characteristic odor, which is soluble in water, ethanol, and chloroform and slightly soluble in ether. Used chiefly as an antiparkinsonism drug. Adverse reactions may include blurred vision, tachycardia, dry skin, xerostomia, headache, irritability, sedation, constipation, weakness, insomnia, vomiting, tinnitus, and suppurative parotitis. Trademarks: Kemadrin, Osnervan.

Procyclomin trademark for *dicyclomine hydrochloride* (see under DICYCLOMINE).

Procytox trademark for *cyclophosphane.*

Prodixamon trademark for *propantheline bromide* (see under PROPANTHELINE).

prodromal (pro-dro'mal) premonitory; indicating the onset of a disease or morbid state.

prodrome (pro'drōm) [L. *prodromus;* Gr. *prodromos* forerunning] a forerunner of disease; a premonitory sign or symptom of a disease.

prodromic (pro-dro'mik) prodromal.

Prodromine trademark for *pholcodine.*

product (prod'ukt) something brought into existence. **acceptable p.,** acceptable MATERIAL. **biological p.,** biological (2). **decay p.,** a nuclide, whether stable or radioactive, formed by the radioactive decay of another nuclide (parent). Called also *daughter.* **provisionally acceptable p.,** provisionally acceptable MATERIAL. **unacceptable p.,** unacceptable MATERIAL.

production (pro-duk'shun) the act or process of producing something; output. **pair p.,** an absorption process for x-rays and gamma rays in which the incident photon is annhilated in the vicinity of the nucleus of the absorbing atom with subsequent production of an electron and positron pair, occurring only when the incident photon energies exceed 1.02 MeV.

Pro-Entra trademark for *triprolidine.*

proerythroblast (pro″ĕ-rith'ro-blast) pronormoblast.

Profemin trademark for *furosemide.*

Proffit, William R. [American dentist] see Ackerman-Proffit classification, under MALOCCLUSION.

profibrinolysin (pro″fi-bri-no-li'sin) see plasminogen.

profile (pro'fil) an outline of the shape or form of an object, such as the face from the lateral view; the sagittal outline form of the face. By extension, a graph representing quantitatively a set of characteristics subjected to tests. See also CEPHALOMETRY, face FORM, FACIES, and NORMA. **facial p.,** the sagittal outline form of the face. See also face FORM. **patient drug p.,** patient medication p. **patient medication p.,** a record or a set of records containing information on the types of medications dispensed to the patient. Abbreviated *PMP.* Called also *patient drug p.*

proflavine (pro-fla'vin) an acridine dye, 3,6-diaminoacridinium. The dihydrate occurs as an orange to brownish red powder that dissolves in water and slightly soluble in ether, chloroform, and petrolatum. When diluted, the solution becomes fluorescent. It is a topical antiseptic which is active in vitro against certain oral bacteria and yeasts. Called also *diaminoacridine.*

ProFlex trademark for a *polysulfide impression material* (see under MATERIAL).

Profundol trademark for *talbutal*.

profundometer (pro"fun-dom'ĕ-ter) an apparatus for locating a foreign body by the fluoroscope by obtaining three lines of sight which intersect at the foreign body.

profundus (pro-fun'dus) [L.] deep; an anatomical term denoting a structure situated deeper than another from the surface of the body.

progenia (pro-je'ne-ah) [*pro-* + L. *gena* chin] prognathism.

progeny (proj'ĕ-ne) [L. *progignere* to bring forth] offspring or descendants.

progeria (pro-je're-ah) [*pro-* + Gr. *gēras* old age + *-ia*] premature development of characteristics suggesting old age, such as graying of hair, wrinkling of skin, etc. See also GERODERMA and Hutchinson-Gilford SYNDROME. Cf. INFANTILISM. **p. adulto'rum,** Werner's SYNDROME.

progesterone (pro-jes'te-rōn) a steroid substance, pregna-4-ene-3,20-dione, containing a 21 carbon atom ring, unsaturated at the 4 position, and substituted at the 3 and 20 carbon with oxygen (see STEROID for nomenclature). It is the prototype for endogenous progestins, synthesized by the animal ovaries and also produced synthetically. It occurs as a white, odorless, crystalline powder that is soluble in ethanol, acetone, and dioxane, sparingly soluble in vegetable oils, and insoluble in water. Its biochemical and pharmacological actions, toxicity, and uses are similar to those of all progestins.

progestin (pro-jes'tin) [*pro-* + L. *gestatio*, from *gestare* to bear] a female sex hormone secreted by the ovaries during the second half of the menstrual cycle. Its chief function is the promotion of secretory changes in the endometrium in its preparation for implantation of the fertilized ovum, acting only on the uterus that has already been sensitized by estrogens. Progestins are used in the treatment of functional uterine bleeding, premenstrual tension, dysmenorrhea, endometriosis, threatened and habitual abortion, and some uterine cancers; in suppression of postpartum lactation; as oral contraceptives; and in ovarian function tests. Adverse reactions may include nausea and vomiting similar to those seen in pregnancy, diarrhea edema, weight gain, fatigability, hirsutism, urticaria, vulvar pruritus, a tendency to galactorrhea and vaginal candidiasis, hyperpigmentation, headache, and hypertension. Some progestins exhibit both estrogenic and androgenic activity and may cause masculinization, especially of the female fetus. Women receiving progestins may exhibit oral changes similar to those observed in pregnancy, including gingival inflammation, hyperemia, swelling, loss of tissue tone, tenderness, ulcerations, and bleeding. Chemically, all progestins are steroids, being structurally similar to progesterone which is their prototype. In addition to natural progestins, there are numerous synthetic substances with pharmacologically similar properties.

Proglicem trademark for *diazoxide*.

proglossis (pro-glos'is) [Gr. *proglōssis*] the tip or apex of the tongue.

prognathia (pro-na'the-ah) [*pro-* + Gr. *gnathos* jaw + *-ia*] prognathism. **p. inferior,** prognathism. **maxillary p.,** maxillary PROTRUSION. **p. superior,** maxillary PROTRUSION.

prognathism (prog'nah-thizm) [*pro-* + Gr. *gnathos* jaw + *-ism*] a condition marked by abnormal protrusion of the mandible. Called also *abnormally large jaw, caput progeneum, exognathia, progenia,* and *prognathia.* See also Hapsburg JAW, mandibular MACROGNATHIA, and prognathous SKULL. Cf. BRACHYGNATHIA, MICROGNATHIA, and RETROGNATHIA. **relative p.,** that in which the mandible is normal, while the maxilla is hypoplastic.

prognathic (prog-na'thik) prognathous.

prognathous (prog'nah-thus, prog-na'thus) [*pro-* + Gr. *gnathos* jaw] pertaining to or characterized by protrusion of the lower jaw or prognathism; having projecting jaws; having a gnathic index above 103, the teeth being in mesiocclusion.

prognathometer (prog"nah-thom'ĕ-ter) [*prognathous* + Gr. *metron* measure] an instrument or device used for measuring the degree of facial prognathism.

prognosis (prog-no'sis) [Gr. *prognōsis* foreknowledge] a forecast as to the probable result of an attack of disease; the prospect as to recovery from a disease as indicated by the nature and symptoms of the case. **dental p.,** an evaluation of the results to be achieved from a dental treatment. **denture p.,** an opinion or judgment given in advance to treatment of the prospects for success in the construction of dentures and for their usefulness.

progonoma (pro"go-no'mah) [*pro-* + *gonos* sperm + *-oma*] a tumor due to misplacement of tissue as the result of fetal atavism to a stage which does not occur in the life history of the species, but which does occur in ancestral forms of the species. **melanotic p.,** melanoameloblastoma.

program (pro'gram) 1. a plan or schedule to be followed. 2. a set of instructions written in computer language that directs the computer in accomplishing its task. **Civilian Health and Medical P. of Uniformed Services,** see CHAMPUS. **Civilian Health and Medical P. of Veterans Administration,** see CHAMPVA. **dental assisting p.,** a program at a college level, usually a one year course that fulfills the educational requirements for dental assisting approved by the Commission on Accreditation of Dental and Auxiliary Educational Programs. Upon completing the program, graduates become eligible for certification examination. See also dental ASSISTANT, and see *Accredited Dental Assisting Programs* in the Appendix. **Federal Employees Health Benefits P.,** an employer-sponsored contributory group health insurance program for federal employees, contracted with several nongovernmental providers, such as the Blue Cross and Blue Shield plans, the Aetna Life Insurance Company, and other insurance companies. Abbreviated *FEHBP.* **Hospital Insurance P,** a compulsory portion of Medicare which automatically enrolls all persons aged 65 or over, entitled to benefits under Old-Age, Survivors, Disability and Health Insurance or railroad retirement, disabled persons under 65 who have been eligible for disability for over two years, and insured workers and their dependents requiring renal dialysis or kidney transplantation. It covers, after various cost-sharing requirements are met, inpatient hospital care and care in skilled nursing facilities and home health agencies. **incentive p., incentive copayment p.,** in dental health insurance, a program that encourages dental care through offering an incentive for regular (usually annual) visits to a dentist. A program paying 70 percent of the cost of dental treatment during the first year, for example, may increase the benefit to 80 percent during the second year if the subscriber visits the dentist each year as stipulated in the program. Conversely, there may be a corresponding percentage reduction in the copayment if the covered individual fails to visit the dentist in a given year, but never below the initial copayment level. Called also *incentive plan* and *incentive copayment plan.* **indemnity p.,** in health insurance, a program that provides specific cash reimbursement for specified covered services, which may be made either to the enrollee or on assignment to the doctor. Called also *scheduled p., indemnity benefit,* and *indemnity plan.* **maximum allowable cost p.,** a federal program which limits reimbursement for prescription drugs under the Medicare and Medicaid programs, and Public Health Service projects to the lowest cost at which the drug is generally available, plus a reasonable dispensing fee, the acquisition cost, or the providers' usual and customary charge to the general public for the drug. Abbreviated *MAC.* **Medical Assistance P.,** Medicaid. **Medical Audit P.,** an extension of the Professional Activity Study (see under STUDY), which produces quarterly reports developed by hospital departments that are used in conducting a comprehensive medical audit and a retrospective utilization review. Abbreviated *MAP.* **Old-Age, Survivors, Disability and Health Insurance P.,** a program administered by the Social Security Administration which provides monthly cash benefits to retired and disabled workers and their dependents and to survivors of insured workers; also providing health insurance benefits for persons 65 years of age or older and for the disabled under the age of 65. Abbreviated *OASHDI.* **Oral Therapy Control P.,** Oral Hygiene Instruction; see under INSTRUCTION. **Plaque Control P.,** Oral Hygiene Instruction; see under INSTRUCTION. **prepaid dental p.,** prepaid dental PLAN. **Quality Assurance P. for Medical Care in Hospital,** a program developed by the American Hospital Association for use by hospital administrations and medical staffs in the development of a hospital program to assure the quality of the care given. Abbreviated *QAP.* **regional medical p's,** originally, programs which were federally sponsored, regionally coordinated arrangements among medical schools, research institutions, and hospitals for research and training and for demonstration of patient care in the fields of heart disease, cancer, stroke, and other major diseases. They were established within defined geographic areas composed of part or parts of one or more states, and consisted of one or more medical centers, research centers, and diagnostic and treatment stations. Some parts of the program were discontinued and efforts have been directed toward regionalization of patient care services. **scheduled p.,** indemnity p.

proguanil hydrochloride (pro-gwan'il) CHLOROGUANIDE hydrochloride.

proinsulin (pro-in'su-lin) a precursor of insulin. It is a long, single-chain polypeptide, molecular weight of 8,000 to 10,000, produced by the β-cells of the islands of Langerhans and converted to active insulin by forming disulfide crosslinks at the chain and by the splitting off of an inactive peptide portion (called *peptide C*) by cellular enzymes.

projection (pro-jek′shun) [*pro-* + L. *jacere* to throw] 1. a throwing forward, especially the act of referring impressions made on the sense organs to their proper source, so as to locate correctly the objects producing them. 2. the act of extending or jutting out or a part that juts out. 3. in radiology, the position of a part of the body in relation to the x-ray film and the x-ray beam. **anteroposterior p., A-P p.,** in radiography, placing the film at the posterior position, with x-rays passing from the anterior to the posterior aspect of the radiographed part. Abbreviated *A-P.* Called also *anteroposterior position.* **base film p.,** see *submentovertex p.* **bregma-mentum p.,** in radiography, examination of the temporomandibular joint and the mandible, whereby the film is placed beneath the chin, with the rays directed downward through the junction of the coronal and sagittal sutures (bregma) to the chin (mentum). **Caldwell p.,** a projection used in producing a posteroanterior oblique radiograph of the skull, including the frontal and anterior ethmoid sinuses, made with a central ray entering the back of the head 23° above the canthomesial line. **enamel p.,** enamel SPUR. **extradental p.,** a projection in which the radiographic film is placed between the teeth and the tissue of the cheek or lip. **isometric p.,** the projection of a x-ray beam that produces an image of the same dimensions as the object being examined. **lateral jaw p., lateral oblique p. of mandible,** a radiographic examination in which the film is placed adjacent to the ramus or the body of the mandible, with the rays directed obliquely upward from the opposite side and the central beam directed at the examined part. The vertical angulation is such as to cast the image of the mandible superior and/or anterior to the examined area. **lateral sinus p.,** a radiographic examination in which two views (one of the body and one of the ramus of the mandible) are used for visualization. **lateral skull p.,** a radiographic examination in which the film is placed parallel to the sagittal plane of the head with the rays directed at right angles to the plane of the film and sagittal plane, whereby the entire skull is shown on the radiograph. **low p.,** in radiography, a view of the mastoid process with the central ray oriented 15° caudad and 15° toward the face, the sagittal plane of the skull parallel with the cassette. **mental p.,** a radiographic examination in which the film is placed beneath the chin with the radiation directed through the long axis of the mandibular central incisors while the mouth is open; used in the examination of the mental process. **orthoradial p.,** a projection in which the central ray is perpendicular to the tangent to the dental arch. **P-A p.,** posteroanterior p. **posteroanterior p.,** in oral radiography, a projection in which the film is placed anteriorly to the examined part, with x-rays passing from the posterior to the anterior aspect along the canthomeatal line. Abbreviated *P-A.* Called also *P-A p.* and *posteroanterior position.* **roentgenographic p.,** one in which the body is in such a position that the part to be x-rayed will be at a desired angle and distance in relation to the radiographic plate. Called also *roentgenographic view.* **submentovertex p.,** a projection in skull radiography in which the central beam enters under the chin at right angles to the canthomeatal line. Called also *base film p.* **Towne p.,** a projection in skull radiography in which the central ray enters the frontal bone at 30° to the canthomeatal line. **Towne p., reverse,** in radiography, a projection in a posteroanterior orientation where the head is tilted forward so that the canthomeatal line forms a 30° angle with the horizontal line. **Waters p.,** a projection in skull radiography in which the central beam is projected through the chin 37° below the canthomeatal line; used chiefly for an anteroposterior view of the maxillary sinuses.

prokaryote (pro-kar′e-ōt) an organism made up of prokaryotic cells, i.e., cells without true nuclei. Bacteria, blue-green algae, and mycoplasmas are prokaryotes. See PROCARYOTAE. Written also *procaryote.* Cf. EUKARYOTE.

prokaryotic (pro″kar-e-ot′ik) [*pro-* + Gr. *karyon* nucleus] pertaining to prokaryotic cells or prokaryotic organisms (prokaryotes). Written also *procaryotic.* Cf. EUKARYOTIC.

prolabium (pro-la′be-um) [*pro-* + L. *labium* lip] the prominent median part of the upper lip.

prolactin (pro-lak′tin) a gonadotropic hormone produced by the anterior lobe of the pituitary gland, which stimulates and sustains lactation in postpartum mammals. Called also *lactogen* and *lactogenic hormone.*

prolamin (pro-lam′in) any of the simple proteins obtained from cereals, which yield only α-amino acids on hydrolysis, and are soluble in diluted (70–80 percent) alcohol but are insoluble in water and absolute alcohol. Zein in corn and glutenin in wheat are typical prolamins. Called also *alcohol-soluble protein.*

prolapse (pro-laps′) [L. *prolapsus;* from *pro* before + *labi* to fall] the falling down or sagging of an organ or part.

proliferation (pro-lif″ē-ra′shun) [L. *proles* offspring + *ferre* to bear] 1. an excessively rapid spread. 2. the reproduction or multiplication of similar forms, such as cells.

proline (pro′lēn, pro′lin) a naturally occurring, nonessential, heterocyclic amino acid (imino acid), 2-pyrrolidinecarboxylic acid, which is present in all proteins. Abbreviated *Pro.* See also amino ACID and HYDROXYPROLINE. **p. carboxypeptidase,** proline CARBOXYPEPTIDASE.

Prolixin trademark for *fluphenazine hydrochloride* (see under FLUPHENAZINE).

Promacortine trademark for *methylprednisolone.*

Promantina trademark for *promethazine.*

promazine (pro′mah-zēn) a tranquilizer, *N,N*-dimethyl-10*H*-phenothiazine-10-propanamine. Used therapeutically as the hydrochloride salt, which occurs as a white or yellowish, odorless, hygroscopic crystalline powder that becomes discolored and oxidized on exposure to air, and is soluble in water, chloroform, ethanol, and methanol. Used in the treatment of mental disorders, nausea, and vomiting, and for the relief of tension and apprehension in surgical patients. Adverse reactions are similar to those of chlorpromazine. Trademarks: Ampazine, Esparin, Liranol, Promwill, Sinophenin, Tomil.

promegakaryocyte (pro-meg″ah-kar″e-o-sīt) [*pro-* + *megakaryocyte*] a megakaryocyte in the stage of development following the megakaryoblast. It is a cell about 20 to 80 μ, having cytoplasmic granulation, and exhibiting multiple nuclear divisions without cell division. The cell eventually develops several, sometimes as many as 23, mature nuclei with dense chromatin and no nucleoli and becomes a megakaryocyte.

promegaloblast (pro-meg′ah-lo-blast″) an early megaloblast, about 19 to 27 μ in diameter, in which there are three to five nucleoli and the cytoplasm is usually basophilic. The nuclear chromatin is distributed uniformly without clumping.

ProMercury trademark for *dental mercury* (see under MERCURY).

promethazine (pro-meth′ah-zēn) a strong antihistaminic of prolonged action that acts on the H₁ receptor, 10-(2-dimethylaminopropyl)-phenothiazine. Used therapeutically as the hydrochloride salt, occurring as a white to yellowish, odorless crystalline powder that is slowly oxidized, especially in the presence of humidity, and changes to blue when exposed to air. It is soluble in water, hot dehydrated alcohol, and chloroform. Used in the treatment of allergy and anaphylaxis, in surgical sedation, in the prevention of nausea and vomiting associated with anesthesia, as an adjunct with analgesics in controlling postoperative pain, in the treatment of motion sickness, and as an antitussive agent. Dryness of the mouth, blurring of vision, and mild hypotension are its chief side effects. Overdosage may result in hyperexcitability, nightmares, convulsions, and coma. Trademarks: Atosil, Diprazin, Dorme, Fargan, Fenazil, Provigan, Lergigan, Phenergan, Promantina, Prothazin, Remsed.

prometaphase (pro-met′ah-fāz) the phase of mitosis which generally begins with the disintegration of the nuclear membrane. When this has occurred, a more fluid zone is noted in the center of the cell in which the chromosomes move freely and in apparent disorder, making their way toward the equator. In meiosis, the phase is characterized by disruption of the nuclear membrane and organization of spindles.

promethium (pro-me′the-um) [named after *Prometheus,* a character in Greek mythology] a radioactive rare earth of the lanthanide series. Symbol, Pm; atomic number, 61; atomic weight, 145; melting point, 1168°C; specific gravity, 7.22; valence, 3. All known promethium isotopes are radioactive and have mass numbers 140–154; ¹⁴⁵Pm has a half-life of 18 years and ¹⁴⁷Pm of 2.62 years. Promethium is a radioactive poison occurring as a silvery white metal. Used as a β-ray source for thickness gauges and in luminescent paint for watch dials and in various nuclear technologies.

Prominal trademark for *mephobarbital.*

prominence (prom′i-nens) [L. *prominentia*] a protrusion or projection. See also PROMINENTIA. **frontonasal p.,** frontonasal PROCESS. **laryngeal p.,** a subcutaneous projection on the front of the neck, formed by the laryngeal cartilage at the line of fusion of the laminae, being most distinct at its cranial part and more pronounced in males than in females. Called also *Adam's apple, prominentia laryngea* [NA], and *thyroid eminence.* **nasolateral p.,** nasolateral PROCESS. **retromolar glandular p.,** an aggregation of buccal and retromolar glands immediately behind the retromolar papilla, together forming the retromolar pad.

prominentia (prom″i-nen′she-ah), pl. *prominen′tiae* [L.] a protrusion or projection. Used in anatomical nomenclature. See also PROMINENCE. **p. laryngea** [NA] laryngeal PROMINENCE.

promonocyte (pro-mon′o-sīt) [*pro-* + *monocyte*] a cell intermediate in the development between the monoblast and monocyte. It has most of the characteristics of the mature monocyte, including its size and motility, but has more numerous mitochondria, a nucleus that is moderately indented, and fewer red bodies. Called also *young monocyte.*

promontoria (prom″on-to′re-ah) [L.] plural of *promontorium.*

promontorium (prom″on-to′re-um), pl. *promonto′ria* [L.] promontory; a projecting eminence or process. **p. faci′ei**, external NOSE. **p. tym′pani** [NA], PROMONTORY of tympanic cavity.

promontory (prom′on-to″re) [L. *promontorium*] a projecting eminence or process. See also EMINENCE, PROCESS, and PROMONTORIUM. **p. of tympanic cavity**, the prominence on the medial wall of the tympanic cavity, formed by the first turn of the cochlea. Called also *promontorium tympani* [NA].

promoter (pro-mo′ter) a substance in a catalyst which increases the rate of activity of the latter.

Promwill trademark for *promazine.*

promyelocyte (pro-mi′e-lo-sīt) [*pro-* + *myelocyte*] a myelocyte in its earliest stage of development, having cytoplasm with fewer than 10 granules and a nucleus without indentations. It develops into a metamyelocyte.

pronasion (pro-na′ze-on) the most prominent point on the tip of the nose when the head is placed in the eye-ear (horizontal) plane.

prone (prōn) [L. *pronus* inclined forward] lying face downward.

pronephroi (pro-nef′roi) [Gr.] plural of *pronephros.*

pronephros (pro-nef′ros), pl. *pronephroi* [*pro-* + Gr. *nephros* kidney] the primordial kidney; an excretory structure or its rudiments developing in the embryo before the mesonephros. Its duct is later used by the mesonephros, which arises caudal to it. Nonfunctional in man, it consists of several pairs of rudimentary pronephric tubules arising from the nephrogenic cord; the pronephroi appear in human embryos during the fourth week of development and undergo retrogressive changes soon thereafter.

Pronestyl trademark for *procainamide hydrochloride* (see under PROCAINAMIDE).

pronethalol (pro-neth′ah-lol) an isoproterenol derivative, α-[(isopropylamino)methyl]2-naphthalenemethanol; used as a β-adrenergic blocking drug. Trademarks: Alderin, Nethalide.

prong (prong) a conical projection, such as a conical root of a tooth.

pronormoblast (pro-nor′mo-blast) an early precursor of an erythrocyte, appearing as a round or oval cell about 12 μ to 19 μ in size, with a large nucleus and a thin rim of basophilic cytoplasm. Nucleoli are present but may not be prominent. Called also *lymphoid hemoblast* and *proerythroblast.* See also ERYTHROCYTE and ERYTHROPOIESIS.

Prontosil trademark for an orange-red, crystalline dye, *p*-[(2,4-diaminophenyl)azo]-benzenesulfonamide, the hydrochloride salt of which was the forerunner of the sulfonamide drugs.

pronucleus (pro-nu′kle-us) [*pro-* + *nucleus*] the precursor of a nucleus. **female p.**, the haploid nucleus of the fully mature ovum which loses its nuclear envelope and liberates its chromosomes to meet in synapsis with those similarly derived from the male pronucleus, thus forming the zygote. See also FERTILIZATION. **male p.**, the nuclear material in the head of a spermatozoon after it has penetrated the ovum and acquired a pronuclear membrane in forming the zygote. See also FERTILIZATION.

proof (proōf) evidence establishing truthfulness of a claim. **p. of eligibility (POE)**, CERTIFICATE of eligibility. **p. of loss**, in health insurance, verification of services rendered by the submission of claim forms that may be accompanied by radiographs, study models, and/or diagnostic material that justify the need for the service.

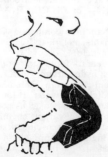

Mouth prop. (From H. O. Torres and A. Ehrlich: Modern Dental Assisting. 2nd ed. Philadelphia, W. B. Saunders Co., 1980; courtesy of Hu-Friedy Mfg. Co., Inc.)

prop (prop) anything used to serve as a support or to shore something up. **mouth p.**, a device inserted between the jaws to maintain an open position of the mandible. Called also *jaw brace.* See illustration.

Propacil trademark for *propylthiouracil.*

Propadrine trademark for *phenylpropanolamine hydrochloride* (see under PHENYLPROPANOLAMINE).

propane (pro′pān) a hydrocarbon of the methane series, C_3H_8, occurring as a colorless, flammable gas with a specific odor. Used as a fuel and a refrigerant and in chemical synthesis. Inhalation may cause narcosis. Called also *diamethylmethane.*

propantheline bromide (pro-pan′the-lēn) a quaternary ammonium compound with antimuscarinic properties, (2-hydroxyethyl)diidopropylmethylammonium bromide xanthene-9-carboxylate, occurring as white, bitter, odorless crystals that are soluble in water, ethanol, and chloroform, but not in ether and benzene. Used in the treatment of peptic ulcer through suppression of gastric secretion and decrease of gastric motility. Also used as an antisialogogue. Side reactions may include xerostomia, blurred vision, mydriasis, heartburn, decreased libido, constipation, restlessness, euphoria, fatigue, psychotic episodes, skin rash, and dermatitis. Trademarks: Neo-Metantyl, Pantheline, Pro-Banthine, Prodixamon.

proparacaine hydrochloride (pro-par′ah-kān) a topical anesthetic, 3-amino-4-propoxybenzoic acid 2-(diethylamine)ethyl ester monohydrochloride, occurring as a white to buff, odorless, crystalline powder that discolors on exposure to air and is soluble in water, ethanol, and methanol, but not in ether and benzene. Used chiefly in ophthalmology. Called also Alcaine, Ophthaline, Ophthetic.

Propax trademark for *oxazepam.*

2-propenal (pro-pe′nal) acrolein.

propene (pro′pēn) propylene.

2-propenenitrile (pro″pēn-ni′tril) acrylonitrile.

properdin (pro′per-din) a relatively heat-labile, normal serum protein that participates in the alternative pathway of complement activation. It migrates as a β-globulin in its inactive form and as a γ-globulin when active. Its role appears to be in the formation of a stable C_5 convertase. **p. pathway**, complement activation pathway, alternative; see under PATHWAY.

prophase (pro′fāz) the first stage in cell reduplication. In mitosis, the stage during which the chromosomes become visible (because of supercoiling of DNA), the cell nucleus starts to lose its identity, and the centrioles begin to migrate. In meiosis, the prophase of the first division consists of five stages: leptotene, zygotene, pachytene, diplotene, and diakinesis. In the second meiotic division, prophase resembles that in mitotic division. See MEIOSIS and MITOSIS.

prophylactic (pro″fĭ-lak′tik) [Gr. *prophylaktikos*] 1. tending to ward off disease; pertaining to prophylaxis. 2. an agent that tends to ward off disease.

prophylaxis (pro″fĭ-lak′sis) [Gr. *prophylassein* to keep guard before] the prevention of disease; preventive treatment. **causal p.**, removal of the cause of a disease. **collective p.**, the protection of the community from infection. **dental p.**, oral p. **drug p.**, the use of drugs in the prevention of infection. **individual p.**, the prevention of infection in an individual. **oral p.**, in a narrow sense, cleansing the teeth in the dental office, including removal of plaque, materia alba, calculus, and stains from the exposed and unexposed surfaces of the teeth by scaling and polishing of the teeth as a preventive measure for the control of local irritational factors. A comprehensive oral prophylaxis program involves using a disclosing solution or wafer in plaque detection; removing of supra- or subgingival plaque and calculus; cleansing and polishing of the teeth; applying topical caries-preventing agents; checking of restorations and prostheses and correcting overhanging margins and proximal contours of restorations; cleansing removable prostheses; and checking for signs and symptoms of food impaction. Called also *prophylactic dentistry* and *dental prophylaxis.* See also preventive PERIODONTICS.

Propionibacteriaceae (pro″pe-on″ĭ-bak-te″re-a′se-e) [*Propionibacterium* + *-aceae*] a family of coryneform bacteria, occurring as gram-positive, non–spore-forming, anaerobic to aerotolerant, pleomorphic, branching or regular rods or filaments whose major metabolic products include carbon dioxide, propionic and acetic acids, or mixtures of organic acids, including butyric, formic, lactic, and other monocarboxylic acids. It includes the genera *Eubacterium* and *Propionibacterium.*

Propionibacterium (pro″pe-on″ĭ-bak-te′re-um) [*pro-* + Gr. *pion* fat + *baktērion* little rod] a genus of bacteria of the family Propionibacteriaceae, occurring as anaerobic to aerotolerant, gram-positive, non–spore-forming, nonmotile, pleomorphic rods, which may be diphtheroid or club-shaped with one end rounded and the other end tapered or pointed and stained less intensely. They are found in dairy products, human skin, and human and animal intestines. Some species are suspected of being pathogenic. **P. ac′nes,** a species isolated from normal human skin, human intestines, and from wounds, blood, pus, and soft tissue abscesses, which are pathogenic for some experimental animals. Called also *Actinobacterium liquefaciens, Bacillus acnes, B. anaerobius diphtheroides, B. hepatodystrophicus, B. parvus liquefaciens, Corynebacterium acnes, C. anaerobium, C. parvus,* and *C. parvum infectiosum.* **P. a′vidum,** a species isolated from the blood, pus, infected wounds, brain, feces, and submaxillary and other types of abscesses in man. Called also *Bacteroides avidus, Corynebacterium avidum,* and *Mycobacterium avidum.* **P. granulo′sum,** a species isolated from the intestinal tract and from abscess materials in man. Called also *Corynebacterium granulosum* and *C. pyogenes bovis.* **P. lympho′philum,** a species isolated from urinary tract infections and from lymph nodes in Hodgkin's disease in man. Called also *Bacillus lymphophilus, Corynebacterium lymphophilum,* and *Mycobacterium lymphophilum.*

propiomazine (pro″pe-o-ma′zēn) a hypnotic and sedative, 1-[10-(2-dimethylaminopropyl)-phenothiazin-2-yl]-1-propanone, occurring as a yellow, odorless powder that is soluble in water and alcohol, but not in benzene. The hydrochloride salt is used to allay apprehension and restlessness before and during surgery. It enhances the effect of central nervous system depressants. Adverse reactions may include drowsiness, xerostomia, moderate hypertension, and, rarely, tachycardia and hypotension. Trademark: Largon.

propionate (pro-pi′o-nāt) a salt or ester of propionic acid. Sodium propionate is used in the treatment of dermatomycoses, and calcium propionates are used as mold inhibitors in bread.

propionyloxybutane (pro-pi″o-nil-ok″sē-bu′tān) propoxyphene.

propolycyte (pro-pol′e-sit) [*pro-* + *polycyte*] a hypersegmented promyelocyte having a complex nucleus, which is of a normal size. See also MACROPOLYCYTE and POLYCYTE.

propositus (pro-poz′ĭ-tus), pl. *propos′iti* [L. *proponere* to put on view] in genetic studies, the first member of a family to draw attention to a given trait. Called also *index case* and *proband.* See also PEDIGREE.

Propox trademark for *propoxyphene hydrochloride* (see under PROPOXYPHENE).

propoxycaine hydrochloride (pro-pok′sē-kān) a powerful local anesthetic, 2-diethylaminoethyl-4-amino-2-propoxybenzoate hydrochloride, occurring as white, odorless crystals that are sensitive to light, and are soluble in water, slightly soluble in alcohol and chloroform, and insoluble in acetone and ether. Used in infiltration and nerve block anesthesia, alone or in combination with other anesthetics. It is allergenic and causes adverse reactions common to other local anesthetics. Trademarks: Blocain, Provocaine, Ravocaine.

Propoxychel trademark for *propoxyphene hydrochloride* (see under PROPOXYPHENE).

propoxyphene (pro-pok′se-fēn) a compound, (*S*)-α-[2-(dimethylamino) - 1 - methylethyl] - α - phenylbenzeneethanol propanoate. Its salts and isomers are used as analgesics. Called also *dextropropoxyphene, propionyloxybutane,* and *d-propoxyphene.* **d-p.,** propoxyphene. **p. hydrochloride,** the α-d-hydrochloride salt of propoxyphene, occurring as a white, odorless, bitter, crystalline powder that is soluble in water, ethanol, chloroform, and acetone, but not in water. It is an analgesic drug, used in mild to moderate pain. The *l*-form has anti-inflammatory and antipyretic properties, but the *d*-form does not. Ingestion of excessive amounts may cause toxic psychoses and convulsions. Other adverse reactions may include sedation, vertigo, nausea, vomiting, constipation, abdominal pain, skin rash, headache, lassitude, euphoria, and visual disorders. Physical and psychological dependence may develop. Trademarks: Algafan, Antalvic, Darvon, Depromic, Dolene, Erantin, Femadol, Propox, Propoxychel. **p. napsylate,** the α-d-napsylate monohydrate salt of propoxyphene, occurring as a white, odorless, bitter, crystalline powder that is soluble in methanol, ethanol, chloroform, and acetone, and slightly soluble in water. Used in larger doses than the hydrochloride salt as an analgesic drug in mild to moderate pain. Adverse reactions are similar to those of the hydrochloride salt. Trademarks: Darvon-N, Doloxene, Napsylgesic.

propranolol (pro-pran′o-lol) an isoproterenol derivative, 1-(isopropylamino)-3-(1-naphthyloxy)-2-propanol, occurring as a white or off-white, odorless powder with a bitter taste, which is soluble in water and alcohol, slightly soluble in chloroform, and insoluble in ether. It is a β-adrenergic blocking agent, used normally in the form of the hydrochloride salt as an antiarrhythmic drug. Nausea, vomiting, diarrhea, constipation, dizziness, depression, lassitude, asthenia, paresthesia, visual disorders, erythematous rash, fever, sore throat, orthostatic hypotension, and syncope are the most common side effects; occasionally, hallucinations and hypoglycemia may occur. Trademark: Avlocardyl.

proprietary (pro-pri′ĕ-ter′e) a proprietary medicine or drug; "any chemical, drug, or similar preparation used in the treatment of diseases, if such article is protected against free competition as to name, product, composition, or process of manufacture by secrecy, patent, trademark, or copyright, or by any other means."

proprioceptive (pro″pre-o-sep′tiv) receiving stimuli within the tissues of the body, as within muscles and tendons.

proprioception (pro″pre-o-sep′shun) a sense providing knowledge of the position of those parts and regions of the body containing skeletal muscles, bones, and joints.

proprioceptor (pro″pre-o-sep′tor) any of the specialized nerve endings that are concerned with the position of the body. The labyrinth and receptors for movement are not usually considered proprioceptors, which are for position rather than movement. Although the otolith is in part a static receptor, it is mainly a dynamic one.

proptosis (prop-to′sis) [Gr. *proptōsis* a fall forward] a forward displacement; a projecting, as of the eyeballs in exophthalmos.

propulsor (pro-pul′sor) an orthodontic appliance similar in principle to the activator, but also having a tissue-borne part, so that the retrusive forces on the maxillary anterior segment are transmitted directly to the alveolar bone. The appliance engages the basal bone to eliminate functional retrusion, and to take advantage of favorable growth that may occur in the mandible as the maxillary arch is being held by the retrusive force or the orofacial muscles. Called also *Mühlemann appliance.* See also functional jaw ORTHOPEDICS. See illustration.

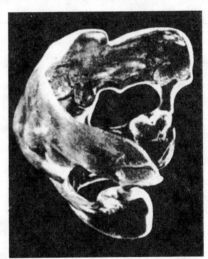

Propulsor. (From T. M. Graber: Orthodontics — Principles and Practice. 3rd ed. Philadelphia, W. B. Saunders Co., 1972; courtesy of R. Hotz.)

Propycil trademark for *propylthiouracil.*

propyl (pro′pil) a radical of the three-carbon hydrocarbon of the methane series, C_3H_7— or $CH_3CH_2CH_2$—. See also ISOPROPYL.

***n*-propylamine** (pro″pil-am′in) a compound, $CH_3CH_2CH_2NH_2$; occurring as a flammable, colorless liquid; used as an intermediate laboratory reagent.

Propyl Chemosept trademark for *propylparaben.*

propylene (prop′ĭ-len) a hydrocarbon, C_3H_6, occurring as a colorless gas obtained from petroleum, which is soluble in alcohol and ether, but only slightly soluble in water. It has anesthetic properties and, in polymerized form, is used as polypropylene plastic. Also used in the production of various chemicals. Propylene is a simple asphyxiant, causing unconsciousness in high concentrations. Because it is highly inflammable, it presents explosion and fire risks. Called also *methyl ethylene* and *propene.* **p. glycol,** propylene GLYCOL.

propylhexedrine (pro″pil-hek′sē-drēn) a sympathomimetic amine with no central excitatory properties, N,α-dimethyl-cyclohexaneethanamine, occurring as a clear, colorless, volatile liquid with a characteristic amine-like odor, which absorbs carbon dioxide from the air and is slightly soluble in water and miscible with ethanol, chloroform, and ether. Used chiefly as a vasoconstrictor and nasal decongestant. Trademark: Benzedrex.

propylparaben (pro″pil-par′ah-ben) an antifungal agent, 4-hydroxybenzoic acid propyl ester, occurring as a white powder or colorless crystalline solids without odor or with a faint odor, which is soluble in ethanol, ether, and hot water, and slightly soluble in cold water. Used chiefly as a preservative for therapeutic and other preparations containing vegetable or animal fats and oils that are susceptible to decomposition, such as antibiotic and corticosteroid preparations. Allergic reactions are the principal side effect. Trademarks: Chemocide PK, Nipasol, Propyl Chemosept, Propyl Parasept, Solbrol P.

Propyl Parasept trademark for *propylparaben*.

propylthiouracil (pro″pil-thi″o-u′rah-sil) a thyroid antagonist, 2,3-dihydro-6-propyl-2-thioxo-4(1*H*)pyrimidinone, occurring as bitter, starchy, white, crystalline powder that is freely soluble in ammonia and alkali hydroxide solutions and slightly soluble in water, ethanol, chloroform, and ether. Used chiefly in the preparation of hyperthyroid patients for surgery and in the treatment of hyperthyroidism. Side effects may include granulocytopenia, leukopenia, drug fever, arthralgia, dermatitis, and compensatory hyperplasia of the thyroid gland. Trademarks: Propacil, Propycil, Propyl-Thyracil, Prothyran, Thyreostat II.

Propyl-Thyracil trademark for *propylthiouracil*.

prorating (pro-rāt′ing) 1. making arrangements on a basis of proportional distribution; dividing or distributing proportionately. 2. prorating CLAUSE.

proscillaridin A (pro-sil-ar′ĭ-din) a cardiac glycoside, 3β-[(6-deoxy-α-L-mannopyranosyl)oxyl]-14-hydroxybufa-4,20,22-trienolide.

prosection (pro-sek′shun) a carefully programmed dissection for demonstration of anatomic structures.

prosencephalon (pros″en-sef′ah-lon) [Gr. *prosō* before + *enkephalon* brain] forebrain.

Proserine trademark for *neostigmine*.

proso- [Gr. *proso* forward] a prefix meaning forward or anterior.

prosody (pros′o-de) [Gr. *prosodos* a solemn procession] the variation in stress, pitch, and rhythm of speech by which different shades of meaning are conveyed.

prosopalgia (pros″o-pal′je-ah) [*prosopo-* + Gr. *algos* pain] trigeminal NEURALGIA.

prosopantritis (pros″o-pan-tri′tis) [*prosopo-* + Gr. *antron* cavity + *-itis*] inflammation of the frontal sinuses.

prosopectasia (pros″o-pek-ta′ze-ah) [*prosopo-* + Gr. *ektasis* expansion + *-ia*] oversize of the face.

prosopo- [Gr. *prosōpon* face] a combining form denoting relationship to the face.

prosopoanoschisis (pros″o-po-ah-nos′kĭ-sis) [*prosopo-* + Gr. *ana* up + *schisis* cleft] facial cleft, oblique; see under CLEFT.

prosopodysmorphia (pros″o-po-dis-mor′fe-ah) [*prosopo-* + *dys-* + Gr. *morphē* form + *-ia*] facial HEMIATROPHY.

prosoponeuralgia (pros″o-po-nu-ral′je-ah) [*prosopo-* + *neuralgia*] neuralgia of the face.

prosopoplegia (pros″o-po-ple′je-ah) [*prosopo-* + Gr. *plēgē* stroke] facial PARALYSIS.

prosoposchisis (pros″o-pos′kĭ-sis) [*prosopo-* + Gr. *schisis* cleft] congenital fissure or cleft of the face.

prosopospasm (pros′o-po-spazm) [*prosopo-* + *spasm*] spasm of the muscles of the face.

prostaglandin (pros″tah-glan′din) a group of autacoid substances which are C_{20} unsaturated fatty acids, designated according to the constituent groups on the five-membered ring as E,A,B, and F. The main classes are further subdivided according to the number of double bonds in the side chains, indicated by the subscript 1, 2, or 3, reflecting the fatty acid precursor. Prostaglandins are found in almost every tissue and body fluid, their production being influenced by a variety of stimuli involving most biological activities. The major biological function of prostaglandins is either activation or inhibition of adenylate cyclase in cells, and their biosynthesis is one of the mechanisms of the pharmacological actions of certain drugs, as of anti-inflammatory drugs, such as aspriin. They influence bone metabolism, and their administration stimulates bone resorption *in vitro*. Administration of prostaglandins also increases blood calcium levels. Complement-mediated immune cytotoxicity against bone cells (leading to bone resorption) is believed to be mediated by prostaglandins. It appears that gingival tissue produces factors stimulating prostaglandin synthesis, thus contributing to the alveolar bone loss accompanying periodontal disease.

Prostaphlin, Prostaphlin-A trademarks for *oxacillin*.

prostata (pros′tah-tah) [L.] [NA] prostate.

prostate (pros′tāt) [Gr. *prostates* one who stands before] a gland of the male reproductive system, which surrounds the neck of the bladder and the urethra. It produces part of the seminal fluid which accounts for the fluid state of semen. Called also *prostata* [NA] and *prostatic gland*.

prostheses (pros-the′sēz) [Gr.] plural of *prosthesis*.

prosthesis (pros-the′sis), pl. *prosthe′ses* [Gr. "a putting to"] an artificial substitution for a missing organ or tissue, used for functional or cosmetic reasons, or both. **cleft palate p.**, a prosthetic device, such as an obturator, used to correct cleft palate. See also artificial PALATE and OBTURATOR (2). **complete dental p.**, **complete denture p.**, complete DENTURE. **definitive p.**, one to be used over an extended period of time; a permanent prosthesis. **dental p.**, a replacement for one or more of the teeth or other oral structure, ranging from a single tooth to a complete denture. See also BRIDGE and DENTURE. **dental p., complete**, complete DENTURE. **cranial p.**, a prosthetic device used for correcting defects of the skull. **expansion p.**, one used to expand the lateral segment of the maxilla in bilateral or unilateral cleft of the palate and alveolar processes. See also EXPANSION. **expansion p., fixed**, an expansion prosthesis that remains in position for the duration of the treatment. **expansion p., removable**, an expansion prosthesis that may be removed from the mouth during the course of treatment. **feeding p.**, a prosthesis worn by a young infant with a cleft palate to increase sucking power and to eliminate the escape of food through the nose. **fixed p.**, a dental prosthesis firmly attached to natural teeth, roots, or implants, usually by a cementing agent; normally not capable of removal by the patient and only with difficulty by the dentist. **fixed p., fixed bridge p.**, partial denture, fixed; see under DENTURE. **mandibular guide-plane p.**, one with an extension designed to direct a resected mandible into an occlusal contact relationship with the maxilla. **maxillofacial p.**, a prosthetic replacement for those regions in the maxilla, mandible, and face that are missing or defective because of surgical intervention, trauma, pathology, or developmental malformations. See also maxillofacial PROSTHETICS. **mouthstick p.**, mouthstick. **overlay p.**, overlay DENTURE. **partial denture p.**, partial denture, removable; see under DENTURE. **permanent p.**, see *definitive p.* **postsurgical p.**, an artificial replacement of a missing part or parts after a surgical operation. **provisional p.**, an interim prosthesis designed for use for varying periods of time. **speech-aid p.**, a device designed to obturate an unrepaired cleft of the hard or soft palate and to perform as a substitute for the structures used for normal speech. Called also *obturator* and *speech bulb*. **superimposed p.**, the overlay of artificial teeth on the surfaces of natural teeth to improve occlusion, arch form, and esthetics. **surgical p.**, a prosthetic device used to assist in a surgical procedure and placed at the time of surgery. **swing-lock p.**, swing-lock DENTURE. **telescopic p.**, overlay DENTURE. **temporary p.**, one which is used temporarily until a permanent device is applied. **therapeutic p.**, a device used for transporting and retaining a therapeutic agent, such as a radium carrier. Called also *therapeutic appliance*.

prosthetic (pros-thet′ik) serving as a substitute; pertaining to or involving prostheses.

prosthetics (pros-thet′iks) the science and art dealing with design, fabrication, fitting, and servicing prostheses. **complete denture p.**, the restoration of an edentulous mouth; the replacement of the natural teeth and their associated structures by artificial substitutes. Called also *full denture p.* See also complete DENTURE. **dental p.**, denture p., prosthodontics. **facial p.**, maxillofacial p. **full denture p.**, complete denture p. **maxillofacial p.**, that branch of prosthodontics which is concerned with anatomic, functional, and cosmetic reconstruction by means of synthetic substitutes of those regions of the maxilla, mandible, and face that have been damaged, absent, or malformed due to illness, injury, congenital defects, or surgical intervention. Called also *facial p.* and *maxillofacial prosthodontics*. See also maxillofacial PROSTHESIS.

prosthetist (pros′thĕ-tist) [Gr. *prosthetes* one who adds] a person skilled in prosthetics and practicing its application; prosthodontist. See also DENTURIST.

prosthion (pros′the-on) [Gr. *prosthios* the foremost + *-on* neuter ending] a craniometric landmark located at the point of the maxillary alveolar process that projects most anteriorly in the midline of the maxilla; used for measuring upper facial height and in determining the gnathic index. Abbreviated *Pr*. Called also *point Pr*. See illustration at CEPHALOMETRY.

prosthodontia (pros″tho-don″she-ah) prosthodontics.

prosthodontics (pros″tho-don′tiks) [*prosthesis* + Gr. *odous* tooth] that branch of dentistry pertaining to the restoration and maintenance of oral functions, comfort, appearance, and health of the patient by the replacement of missing teeth and contiguous tissues with artificial substitutes. Called also *dental prosthetics, denture prosthetics, prosthetic dentistry,* and *prosthodontia.* See also BRIDGE, DENTURE, DENTURISM, PROSTHESIS, and RESTORATION. **American Board of P.,** see under BOARD. **complete p.,** that branch of prosthodontics which is concerned with the design and application of complete dentures. **crown and bridge p.,** that branch of prosthodontics dealing with the complete restoration of a single tooth, or the replacement of one or more teeth by a fixed partial denture. See also partial denture, fixed, under DENTURE. **fixed p., fixed bridge p.,** that branch of prosthodontics concerned with replacement and/or restoration of teeth by nonremovable prostheses and with the design, production, and fitting of fixed partial dentures. See also partial denture, fixed, under DENTURE. **maxillofacial p.,** maxillofacial PROSTHETICS. **partial p.,** that branch of prosthodontics concerned with replacement and/or restoration of only a part of the maxillary or mandibular arches, with either fixed or removable prostheses. See also partial denture, fixed and partial denture, removable, under DENTURE. **removable p.,** that branch of prosthodontics concerned with restoration of missing teeth and associated structures by prostheses that can be removed and replaced when indicated. See also removable DENTURE. **removable partial p.,** that branch of prosthodontics dealing with the design, production, and application of removable partial dentures. See also partial denture, removable, under DENTURE.

prosthodontist (pros″tho-don′tist) a dentist who specializes in prosthodontics. Sometimes called *prosthetist.*

Prostigmin trademark for *neostigmine.*

prostration (pros-tra′shun) [L. *prostratio*] a condition of loss of strength; extreme exhaustion.

prot- see PROTO-.

protactinium (pro″tak-tin′e-um) [Gr. *protos* first] a radioactive element of the actinide series. Symbol, Pa; atomic number, 91; atomic weight, 231.0359; melting point, 1600°C; specific gravity, 15.37; valences, 4, 5. All known protactinium isotopes are radioactive, the longest-lived isotope being ^{231}Pa, which decays by alpha emission and has a half-life of about 33,000 years. The first isotope discovered was ^{234}Pa with a half-life of 1.175 min. Protactinium is a radioactive poison, occurring as a shiny malleable metallic mass that easily tarnishes on exposure to air. Called also *brevium, protoactinium,* and *uranium X (UX).*

protaminase (pro-tam′ i-nās) carboxypeptidase B.

protamine (pro′tah-min) any of a group of simple proteins, occurring in the spermatozoa of fish. The molecular weight of protamines is about 5,000; thus they are the smallest known proteins. They are strongly basic in reaction and soluble in water, dilute acids, and ammonia. They precipitate other proteins. Protamine occurring with nucleic acids is known as *nucleoprotamine.* **p. sulfate,** a purified mixture of simple proteins from the sperm or testes of certain types of fish, occurring as a fine, white, hygroscopic, crystalline powder that is sparingly soluble in water. It is an anticoagulant antagonist which neutralizes heparin; used in the treatment of hemorrhagic complications of heparin therapy.

Protanabol trademark for *oxymetholone.*

protean (pro′te-an) [Gr. *Proteus* a many-formed deity] 1. assuming different shapes; changeable in form. 2. a primary derived protein that is insoluble in water, obtained by treatment of original protein with water, heat, or acids, or by its exposure to a mechanical factor, such as agitation. Fibrin obtained from fibrinogen is an example of a protean.

protease (pro′te-ās) [*protein* + *-ase*] peptide HYDROLASE.

Protect see under DENTIFRICE.

protection (pro-tek′shun) 1. the act of keeping from or defending against harm, injury, or attack. 2. one who or that which provides defense against harm or injury. 3. coverage (2).

protective (pro-tek′tiv) [L. *protegere* to cover over] 1. affording defense or immunity. 2. an agent that affords defense against a deleterious influence, such as a substance applied to the skin or mucous membrane to avoid contact with possible irritants. Protectives are usually insoluble and chemically inert substances, such as dusting powders or materials that form an adherent, continuous, flexible, or semirigid coat when applied to tissues to be protected. Demulcents and emollients are also considered as protectives. See also ABSORBENT and SCREEN. **mechanical p.,** one forming either a flexible or semirigid coating, used to provide occlusive protection from external environment, to provide mechanical support to injured tissues, and to serve as a vehicle for active substances. Collodions and plasters are the principal mechanical protectives.

protein (pro′te-in, pro′tēn) [Gr. *protos* first] any of a group of some 3000 different complex organic nitrogenous compounds containing carbon, hydrogen, oxygen, and sulfur; phosphorus, iodine, and iron being found in some specialized proteins. Protein is the principal constituent of the cell protoplasm, and is made by plant cells by the process starting with photosynthesis, through synthetic processes from carbon dioxide, water, nitrates, sulfates, and phosphates. Animals can synthesize only a limited amount of proteins from inorganic sources and are mainly dependent on plants or other animals for their source of proteins. Proteins are used in the body for growth of new tissue, for maintenance of existing tissues, and as a source of energy. When used for energy, they are broken down by oxidation to form simple substances, such as water, carbon dioxide, sulfates, phosphates, and nitrogen compounds, which are excreted. Protein molecular weight varies from 6000 to 50,000,000. Proteins are essentially combinations of α-amino acids in peptide linkages. See also amino ACID, nitrogen CYCLE, and PEPTIDE. See illustration. **p. A,** 1. IMMUNOGLOBULIN A (IgA). 2.

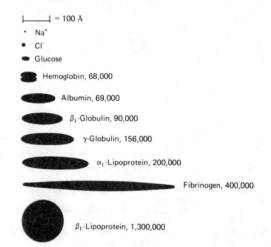

| | = 100 Å

· Na⁺

● Cl⁻

◖ Glucose

▬ Hemoglobin, 68,000

⬬ Albumin, 69,000

⬬ β₁-Globulin, 90,000

⬬ γ-Globulin, 156,000

⬬ α₁-Lipoprotein, 200,000

▬ Fibrinogen, 400,000

● β₁-Lipoprotein, 1,300,000

Relative dimensions of various protein molecules. (From J. I. Routh, D. P. Eyman, and D. J. Burton: Essentials of General, Organic, and Biochemistry. 3rd ed. Philadelphia, W. B. Saunders Co., 1977; after J. L. Oncley: Conference on the Preservation of the Cellular and Protein Components of Blood, published by the American Red Cross, Washington, D.C.)

AGGLUTINOGEN A. 3. a protein found in extracts of *Staphylococcus aureus,* which reacts serologically with various human sera. Called also *staphylococcal p. A.* **alcohol-soluble p.,** prolamin. **Bence Jones p.,** a heat-sensitive protein found in the urine of patients with paraproteinemias, especially multiple myeloma, and in trace amounts under normal conditions, which is believed to occur as the result of production of abnormally large numbers of light chains without the corresponding number of heavy chains. It is an abnormal immunoglobulin (paraprotein) having a sedimentation constant of 2 to 4S, molecular weight of 23,000 or 46,000, and electrophoretic mobility of β- and γ-globulin. Bence Jones protein is considered to be a protein fragment, consisting solely of L chains, either single or joined together by a disulfide bond. It is classified as either type κ or λ, similar to heavy chains. See also Bence Jones PROTEINURIA. **blood p.,** a protein found in the blood, including albumin, globulin, fibrinogen, and globin. See also *plasma p.* and *serum p.* **carrier p.,** 1. a protein which, when coupled to a hapten, renders the hapten capable of eliciting an immune response. 2. carrier MOLECULE. **coagulated p.,** an insoluble form which certain proteins assume when denatured by heat, alcohol, or other agents. **conjugated p's,** proteins which are combined in nature with nonprotein substances, in which the protein molecule is united to a nonprotein molecule, the prosthetic group, other than salts. They include: phosphoprotein, nucleoprotein, glycoprotein, chromoprotein, lipoprotein, and metalloprotein. **contractile p.,** a muscle protein involved in the contractile process. Principal contractile proteins include actin, myosin, tropomyosin, and troponin. **C-reactive p.,** a serum globulin that forms a precipitate with the somatic C-polysaccharide of the pneumococcus (hence its name), and is a sensitive indicator of the existence and severity of inflammation of infectious or noninfectious origin. Called also *acute phase globulin.* Abbreviated CRP. **defense p.,** protective p. **denatured p.,** derived p's, primary. **derived p's,** derivatives of the protein molecule formed by the action of heat, acids, alkalies, water, enzymes, alcohol, radiant energy, or mechanical shock. **derived p's, primary,** protein derivatives produced by denaturation of native proteins, including proteans, metaproteins, and coagulated proteins. Called also *denatured p's.* See also DENATURATION. **derived p's, secondary,** proteins formed during the progressive hydrolysis of proteins, their molecular weight depending on the extent of the hydrolytic cleavage of the original protein. Secondary derived proteins include peptoses, peptones, and peptides. **fast chain p's,** fast CHAINS; see under CHAIN. α_1-**fetospecific serum p.,** α_1-fetoprotein. **p. D,** IMMUNOGLOBULIN D (IgD). **p. E,** IMMUNOGLOBULIN E (IgE). **fibrous p.,** one of the two broad classes of proteins, the proteins of which are insoluble in water or dilute salt solutions, and consist of elongated polypeptide chains arranged in a parallel fashion along a single axis, each helically coiled along its length, to yield long fibers or sheets. X-ray diffraction shows the presence of amorphous regions in which the chains are distributed randomly, interspersed with "crystalline" regions in which the adjacent chains are arranged with the same regularity as found in true crystals. They are the basic structural elements of the connective tissue, keratin and collagen being the main proteins of the principal fibrous proteins. Cf. *globular p.* **p. G,** IMMUNOGLOBULIN G (IgG). **globular p.,** one of the two broad classes of proteins, the members of which consist of tightly folded polypeptide chains, forming compact spherical or globular shapes, which are easily soluble and readily diffusible. Most globular proteins have a mobile or dynamic function, forming enzymes, antibodies, and hormones, and having a transport function, such as serum albumin and hemoglobin. Cf. *fibrous p.* **heavy chain p's,** heavy chains; see under CHAIN. **immune p.,** immunoglobulin. **iron-binding p.,** transferrin. **light chain p's,** light chains; see under CHAIN. **p. M,** IMMUNOGLOBULIN M (IgM). **p. metabolism,** the process by which proteins are absorbed and used by the body. The process begins with mastication when meat and other protein-bearing foods are broken down into small fragments and thus made susceptible to enzymatic digestion, but the digestive processes begin in the stomach when proteins are attacked by a gastric enzyme (pepsin), which first digests collagen, the constituent of intercellular connective tissue of meat, and then splits other proteins into proteoses, peptones, and large peptides through breaking (hydrolysis) of the peptide linkages between the amino acids. Pepsin digestion occurs in an acidic environment, being most active at pH 2. Upon leaving the stomach, products of partial digestion by pepsin are attacked by the pancreatic enzymes trypsin, chymotrypsin, and carboxypeptidase, further breaking proteins into small polypeptides, dipeptides, and some amino acids. Epithelial peptidases of the small intestine (amino polypeptidase and dipeptidases) hydrolyze the remaining peptide linkages, breaking the peptides into amino acids, which are then transported across the intestinal epithelium to be carried by the blood to various organs to serve in tissue reconstruction. **muscle p.,** the protein component of the muscle. See *contractile p.* **myeloma p.,** a paraprotein found in various forms of myeloma, having an abnormal number of light or heavy chains, or a number of disulfide bonds between the chains. **native p.,** unchanged animal or vegetable protein, especially as it occurs in foods. **oligomeric p's,** proteins made up of several chains, such as hemoglobin which consists of four polypeptide chains. **plasma p.,** a protein found in the blood plasma, including globulin, albumin, and fibrinogen, Originally, 50 percent ammonium sulfate was used to precipitate globulin and 100 percent for albumin; later methods include ultracentrifugation, electrophoresis, and immunological techniques. The movement of protein molecules in the ultracentrifuge is related to their net mass, as determined in terms of Svedberg units (see under UNIT). Three major fractions are thus identified: fraction A = 4S — molecular weight, 70,000; fraction G = 7S —molecular weight, 160,000; and fraction M = 19S — molecular weight, 1,000,000. Fraction A consists mostly of albumin, fraction G of γ-globulin, and fraction M of macroglobulins. Five components may be identified electrophoretically: albumin α_1 and α_2, γ-globulin, and fibrinogen. See also *serum p.,* FIBRINOGEN, plasma ALBUMIN, and plasma GLOBULIN. **primary derived p's,** derived p's, primary. **protective p.,** a protein formed within the body and serving as a protection against disease. Principal protective proteins include antibodies (complexes with foreign proteins), complement (complexes with antigen-antibody sys-

tems), fibrinogen (precursor of fibrin in blood coagulation), and thrombin (component of blood clotting mechanism). Called also *defense p.* **p. 4S,** a plasma protein fraction having the sedimentation coefficient 4×10^{-13}, consisting chiefly of plasma albumin and representing protein with the smallest molecules (MW = 70,000) of the blood protein group. Protein 4S corresponds to fraction A. **secondary derived p's,** derived p's, secondary. **serum p.,** a protein found in the blood serum. Major classes of serum proteins include globulin and albumin. Properties of serum proteins are similar to those of plasma proteins, except for fibrinogen which is separated during the preparation of blood serum. See *plasma p.,* serum ALBUMIN, and serum GLOBULIN. **silver p.,** SILVER protein. **simple p's,** naturally occurring proteins which yield only α-amino acids and their derivatives on hydrolysis. They include: albumin, globulin, glutein, prolamine, albuminoids, histone, and protamine. Called also *unconjugated p's.* **slow chain p.,** slow CHAIN. **spike p's,** glycoproteins that project from the viral envelope. **staphylococcal p. A,** p. A (3). **storage p.,** any protein stored in various substances and tissues of the body, such as those stored in egg white (ovalbumin) and milk (casein), or involved in iron storage in the spleen (ferritin). **transport p.,** a protein capable of binding and transporting specific types of molecules. Principal transport proteins include hemoglobin (transport of oxygen in vertebrates), hemocyanin (transport of oxygen in invertebrates), myoglobin (transport of oxygen in muscle), serum albumin (transport of fatty acids), and ceruloplasmin. **unconjugated p.,** simple p.

proteinase [E.C.3.4.21 to 3.4.24] (pro′te-in-ās″) [*protein* + -*ase*] a group of peptide hydrolases which catalyze protein hydrolysis by attacking internal peptide bonds. Called also *p. peptidohydrolase, dipeptidyl-peptide hydrolase,* and *endopeptidase.* See also peptide HYDROLASE. **acid p.** [E.C.3.4.23], an enzyme which catalyzes the hydrolysis of protein, and having a pH optimum in the acid region. **serine p.** [E.C.3.4.21], an enzyme which catalyzes the hydrolysis of proteins, having histidine and serine in the active center involved in the catalytic processes. **SH-p.** [E.C.3.4.22], an enzyme which catalyzes protein hydrolysis, having cysteine in the active center and involved in the catalytic processes.

proteinochromogen (pro″te-in-o-kro′mo-jen) former name for *tryptophan;* so called because it gave a red color with bromine.

proteinosis (pro″te-in-o′sis) [*protein* + -*osis*] a condition characterized by abnormal accumulation of proteins in the tissues. **lipoid p.,** Urbach-Wiethe SYNDROME.

proteinuria (pro″te-in-u′re-ah) [*protein* + Gr. *ouron* urine + -*ia*] the presence in the urine of excessive amounts of blood proteins. See also ALBUMINURIA. **Bence Jones p.,** the presence of Bence Jones protein in the urine, usually but not exclusively, observed in multiple myeloma. It is commonly associated with reduction of serum immunoglobulins, pulmonary infections, osteolytic lesions, painful fractures, and renal insufficiency due to intratubular deposits of light chain proteins, with consequent atrophy. Called also *Bence Jones albuminuria* and *light chain disease.*

proteoglycan (pro″te-o-gli′kan) a glycoprotein having a very high content of carbohydrate. Called also *chondromucoprotein.*

proteolysis (pro″te-ol′ĭ-sis) [*protein* + Gr. *lysis* dissolution] the hydrolysis of proteins into proteoses, peptones, and other products by means of enzymes. See also Proteolysis-chelation THEORY.

proteolytic (pro″te-o-lit′ik) 1. pertaining to, characterized by, or promoting proteolysis. 2. pertaining to a proteolytic enzyme. See peptide HYDROLASE.

proteose (pro′te-ōs) [*protein* + -*ose*] a secondary derived protein, constituting the highest molecular weight group and thus being the least hydrolyzed state of the original protein. Proteoses are generally more readily soluble in water than the original protein and are noncoagulable by heat.

Proteus (pro′te-us) [Gr. *Prōteus* a many-formed deity] a genus of gram-negative, unencapsulated, nonsporogenous, facultatively anaerobic bacteria of the family Enterobacteriaceae, made up of straight or slightly curved rods, 1.0 to 2.5 μm in length and 0.4 to 0.6 μm in breadth, frequently occurring in end-to-end pairs and short chains. Ovoid forms are common, and long, curved, filamentous cells predominate in swarming cultures, the swarming phenomenon being the consequence of active motility by peritrichous flagella. The organisms occur alone or in association with other organisms in various pathological conditions of the eye and ear, in cases of pleurisy, peritonitis, abscesses, cystitis, pyelonephritis, urinary tract infections, and various hospital-acquired infections; in infections of the digestive tract, such as infant diarrhea; and in certain types of food poisoning. They are also found in feces, often increasing in number during or immediately after attacks of diarrhea caused by other organisms, and are common in soil and water containing decaying matter of animal origin and present in large numbers in sewage, being associated with putrefaction. Many strains are drug-resistant. **P. enter'icus,** *P. rettgeri.* **P. incon'stans,** a species found in human feces and urine, which may be associated with gastroenteritis and urinary tract infection. It is sensitive to kanamycin and gentamicin but resistant to most other antibiotics. Called also *P. stuartii, Bacillus inconstans, Providencia alcalifaciens, P. inconstans,* and *P. stuartii.* **P. mirab'ilis,** a species found in pathologic material of human origin, and in feces, sewage, soil, and decomposing matter, especially of animal origin. **P. morga'nii,** a species most frequently found in human feces, often associated with summer diarrhea of infants. It is sensitive to nitrofurantoin and tetracyclines. Called also *Morganella morganii* and *Salmonella morgani.* **P. rettge'ri,** a species associated with epidemic gastroenteritis and other human conditions, and also isolated from feces in fowl. Called also *P. entericus, Bacterium rettgeri,* and *Shigella rettgeri.* **P. stuar'tii,** *P. inconstans.* **P. vulga'ris,** a species often occurring as a secondary invader in a variety of localized suppurative pathologic processes in man, and found in feces, sewage, soil, pathologic material, and decomposing matter, particularly of animal origin. It occurs as several serotypes: the X strains agglutinate in antiserum to certain of the rickettsia, X-19 strains in antisera to the typhus group, and X-K in antisera to the tsutsugamushi group, in the Weil-Felix reaction, used for diagnostic purposes.

Prothazin trademark for *promethazine.*

Prothromadin trademark for *warfarin sodium* (see under WARFARIN).

prothrombin (pro-throm'bin) [*pro-* Gr. *thrombos* clot + *in* chemical suffix] a blood protein that in the process of coagulation is converted to thrombin by an extrinsic or intrinsic prothrombin activator. It is an α_2-globulin, having a molecular weight of 68,700, and is present in normal plasma in a concentration of about 15 mg/100 ml, being an unstable protein that readily breaks up into smaller compounds (thrombin) with a molecular weight of 33,700. Prothrombin is formed continually by the liver, vitamin K being necessary for its production. The rate of formation of thrombin is almost directly proportional to the quantity of prothrombin activator available, which in turn is approximately proportional to the degree of trauma to the vessel or to the blood. Prothrombin deficiency results in hypoprothrombinemia and parahemophilia. Called also *factor II, factor XA, plasmozyme, serozyme,* and *thrombogen.* See also blood COAGULATION and Quick's TEST. **p. accelerator,** FACTOR V. **p. activator,** a factor that converts prothrombin to thrombin in blood coagulation. In the extrinsic mechanism, its formation begins with blood coming in contact with injured tissue and consists of three steps: the injured tissue releases a proteolytic enzyme (factor III tissue factor, tissue thromboplastin) and tissue phospholipids; the enzyme complexes with factor VII and the resulting complex, in the presence of phospholipids, acts on factor X to form activated factor X; the activated factor X complexes with tissue phospholipids and with factor V to form prothrombin activator. In the intrinsic mechanism, trauma of the blood itself starts a five-step process: the contact of collagen in the vascular wall with factor XII causes it to be converted into a proteolytic enzyme, activated factor XII, while the damaged blood causes blood platelets to release platelet phospholipids, platelet factor 3; activated factor XII causes factor XI to become activated; activated factor XI in turn activates factor IX; activated factor IX, together with factor VIII and platelet factor 3, activates factor X; activated factor X complexes with the phospholipids and factor V to form prothrombin activator. Called also *complete thromboplastin.* See also blood COAGULATION. **p. deficiency,** hypoprothrombinemia. **p. deficiency, congenital,** parahemophilia. **p. F,** vitamin K.

prothrombinase [E.C.3.4.21.6] (pro-throm'bin-ās) a serine proteinase which is a precursor that, in the presence of an extrinsic or intrinsic prothrombin factor, forms thrombin. Called also *factor XA.* See also PROTHROMBIN activator.

Prothyran trademark for *propylthiouracil.*

protium (pro'te-um) ordinary or light hydrogen; symbol H¹. See HYDROGEN.

proto-, prot- [Gr. *protos* first] a combining form meaning first.

protoactinium (pro"to-ak-tin'e-um) protactinium.

protocone (pro'to-kōn) [*proto-* + Gr. *kōnos* cone] the principal mesiolingual cusp of the upper molar of man and certain mammals, such as the opossum and dog. See also HYPOCONID, METACONID, PARACONID, and TRIGONE (2).

protoconid (pro"to-ko'nid) [*proto-* + Gr. *kōnos* cone + *-id*] the mesiobuccal cusp of the lower molars of primitive mammals and in man, being greatly modified in many higher mammals and completely disappearing in some. See also HYPOCONID, METACONID, PARACONID, and TRIGONID.

proton (pro'ton) [Gr. *prōtos* first + *-on* neuter ending] 1. a positively charged fundamental particle of the atom, which has a mass approximately that of the nucleus of the hydrogen atom, or 1.67×10^{-27} kg (about 1840 times that of the electron), and the positive charge of 1.6×10^{-19} coulomb. Protons are constituents of all nuclei. The atomic number (Z) of an atom is equal to the number of protons in its nucleus. 2. the primitive rudiment of a part; a primordium or anlage.

Protopam trademark for *pralidoxime chloride* (see under PRALIDOXIME).

protopathic (pro"to-path'ik) [*proto-* + Gr. *pathos* disease] pertaining to protopathic sensibility, the ability of the receptors in the viscera to perceive pain. Such pain is often poorly localized, of low intensity, and poorly defined.

protoplasia (pro-to-pla'se-ah) primary formation of tissue.

protoplasm (pro'to-plazm) [*proto-* + Gr. *plasma* plasm] the only known form of matter in which life is manifested. It is a viscid, translucent polyphasic colloid with water as the continuous phase, which makes up the essential material of all plant and animal cells. It is composed mainly of proteins, lipids, carbohydrates, and inorganic salts. The protoplasm surrounding the nucleus is known as the *cytoplasm* and that composing the nucleus as the *nucleoplasm.* **superior p.,** endoplasmic RETICULUM.

protoplast (pro'to-plast) [*proto-* + Gr. *plastos* formed] 1. the type or model of some organic being. 2. a bacterial or plant cell deprived of its rigid wall, but with its plasma membrane still intact; the cell is dependent for its integrity on an isotonic or hypertonic medium.

protoporphyrin (pro"to-por'fi-rin) a porphyrin having four methyl groups, two vinyl groups, and two propionic acid groups, which forms quadrilaterate chelate complexes with metal ions, such as iron, magnesium, zinc, nickel, cobalt, and copper. Chelate complexes of protoporphyrin with iron in the ferrous state are called *heme*; with iron in the ferric state, are called *hematin.*

prototropy (pro-tot'ro-pe) [*proton* + Gr. *tropē* a turning] the more usual type of tautomerism, which is the result of a mobile hydrogen ion. Cf. ANIONOTROPY.

prototype (pro"to-tīp) [*proto-* + Gr. *typos* type] the original type or form after which other types or forms are developed.

protoveratrine (pro"to-ver'ah-trēn) a name applied to alkaloids (protoveratrines A and B) isolated from *Veratrum album* and *V. viride.* Formerly used in the treatment of hypertension.

Protozoa (pro"to-zo'ah) a phylum comprising the simplest organisms of the animal kingdom, consisting of unicellular organisms that range in size from submicroscopic to macroscopic; most are free-living, but some lead commensalistic, mutualistic, or parasitic existences. Protozoa are usually divided into four subphyla: Sarcodina (amebae), having pseudopodia during most of the life cycle; Mastigophora (flagellates), having one or more flagella during most of the life cycle; Ciliophora (ciliates and suctorians), having cilia during some stage of development; and Sporozoa, having no locomotor organs in the adult stages and reproducing by sporulation.

protozoa (pro"to-zo'ah) plural of *protozoon.*

protozoacide (pro"to-zo-'ah-sīd) destructive to protozoa; an agent destructive to protozoa.

protozoal (pro"to-zo'al) pertaining to or caused by protozoa.

protozoology (pro"to-zo-ol'o-je) the study of protozoa.

protozoon (pro"to-zo'on), pl. *protozo'a* [*proto-* + Gr. *zōon* animal] a primitive animal organism consisting of a single cell; any individual organism belonging to the Protozoa.

protraction (pro-trak'shun) [L. *protrahere* to drag forth from a place] 1. drawing out or lengthening. 2. extension or protrusion. 3. mandibular p. 4. a condition in which the teeth or other maxillary or mandibular structures are situated anterior to their normal position. **mandibular p.,** 1. the protrusive movement of the mandible initiated by the lateral and medial pterygoid muscles acting simultaneously. Cf. mandibular RETRACTION. 2. a facial anomaly in which the gnathion lies anterior to the orbital plane. See also PROGNATHISM. **maxillary p.,** facial anomaly in which the subnasion is anterior to the orbital plane.

protractor (pro-trak'tor) [*pro-* + L. *trahere* to draw] an instrument for extracting bits of bone, bullets, or other foreign material from wounds.

protriptyline hydrochloride (pro-trip'tĭ-lēn) an antidepressant agent with anticholinergic properties, *N*-methyl-5*H*-dibenze-[*a,d*]cycloheptene-5-propylamine hydrochloride, occurring as a white to yellowish, odorless, bitter, crystalline powder that is soluble in water, methanol, chloroform, and ethanol but not in ether. Adverse reactions may include aggravation of anxiety, tachycardia, postural hypotension, paradoxical hypertension, headache, cardiac arrhythmia, nausea, vomiting, intracranial hemorrhage, and xerostomia. Trademarks: Concordin, Maximed, Triptil.

protrusion (pro-troo'zhun) [L. *protrudo* to thrust forward] the state of being thrust forward or laterally, as in masticatory movements of the mandible. See also PROGNATHISM and mandibular PROTRACTION. **bimaxillary p.,** the projection of both the maxilla and the mandible beyond normal limits in relation to the cranial base. **bimaxillary dentoalveolar p.,** the positioning of the entire dentition forward with respect to the facial profile. **double p.,** a definite labioversion of the maxillary and mandibular anterior teeth. **forward p.,** protrusion of the mandible forward from the centric position. See also PROGNATHISM and mandibular PROTRACTION. **jaw p.,** 1. see PROGNATHISM. 2. see mandibular PROTRACTION. **lateral p.,** a protrusion of the mandible to the side from the centric position. **mandibular p.,** 1. see PROGNATHISM. 2. see mandibular PROTRACTION. **maxillary p.,** abnormal protrusion of the maxillae, usually resulting from maxillary macrognathia, maxillary alveolar protrusion, or the position of the upper front teeth. Called also *maxillary prognathia* and *superior prognathia*. **maxillary alveolar p.,** the protrusion of the alveolar processes of the maxillae.

protuberance (pro-tu'ber-ans) [pro- + L. *tuber* bulge] a bulge, projecting part, or prominence; an apophysis, process, or swelling; a general anatomical term for such structures. Called also *protuberantia*. **p. of chin,** mental p. **external occipital p.,** a prominence situated halfway between the summit of the outer surface of the squama of the occipital bone and the foramen magnum; it gives attachment to the ligamentum nuchae. Called also *external occipital spine, inion,* and *protuberantia occipitalis externa* [NA]. **internal occipital p.,** a bony projection at the intersection of the four divisions of the cruciate eminence, on the internal surface of the squama of the occipital bone. Called also *internal occipital spine* and *protuberantia occipitalis interna* [NA]. **mental p., mental p., external,** a triangular prominence on the anterior external surface of the body of the mandible, formed by splitting of the ridge of the symphysis menti, with the mental tubercle at its base. Called also *p. of chin, external mental spine, external mental tubercle, mental process,* and *protuberantia mentalis* [NA].

protuberantia (pro-tu"ber-an'she-ah) [L.] protuberance; a bulge, projecting part, or prominence; a general anatomical term for such structures. Called also *protuberance*. **p. menta'lis** [NA], mental PROTUBERANCE. **p. occipita'lis exter'na** [NA], external occipital PROTUBERANCE. **p. occipita'lis exter'na** [NA], internal occipital PROTUBERANCE.

proud (prowd) characterized by exuberant granulation tissue. See proud FLESH.

Proust's law [Louis Joseph *Proust,* French chemist, 1755–1826], LAW of definite proportions.

Providencia (pro"vĭ-den'se-ah) a generic name proposed for *Proteus inconstans*. **P. alcalifa'ciens, P. incon'stans, P. stuar'tii,** *Proteus inconstans;* see under PROTEUS.

provider (pro-vīd'er) one who or that which furnishes or supplies something or makes something available, such as medical care. **p. of health care, direct,** an individual who is a direct provider of health care (including a physician, dentist, nurse, podiatrist, or physician assistant) in that the individual's primary current activity is the provision of health care to individuals or the administration of facilities or institutions (including hospitals, long-term care facilities, outpatient facilities, and health maintenance organizations) in which such care is provided and, when required by state law, the individual has received professional training in the provision of such care or in such administration and is licensed or certified for such provision or administration. **p. of health care, indirect,** an individual who holds a fiduciary position with, or has a fiduciary interest in, any entities engaged in the provision of health care or such research or instruction or in producing drugs or such other articles; receives, either directly or through his spouse, more than one-tenth of his gross annual income from any one or combination of any phase of health care delivery; is a member of the immediate family of an individual engaged in health care delivery; or is engaged in issuing any policy or contract of individual or group health insurance or hospital or medical service benefits. **individual p.,** an individual who is engaged in health care delivery, including a physician, dentist, nurse, podiatrist, or physician assistant engaged in direct provision of

health care, administration of health care facilities, or related activities. See *direct p. of health care* and *indirect p. of health care.* **institutional p.,** an institution which receives cost-related reimbursement for health care delivery, such as a hospital, skilled nursing facility, home health agency, or certain providers of outpatient physical therapy services.

Provigan trademark for *promethazine*.

Proviodine trademark for *povidone-iodine*.

provirus (pro-vi'rus) the genome of an animal virus integrated (by crossing over) into the chromosome of the host cell, and thus replicated in all of its daughter cells.

provision (pro-vizh-un) 1. the act of supplying or providing something. 2. something provided. 3. a clause in a legal document or agreement, providing a stipulation or qualification. **comparability p.,** in Medicare, a provision that the reasonable charge for a service may not be higher than charges payable for comparable services insured under comparable circumstances by a carrier for its non-Medicare beneficiaries. See also usual, customary, and reasonable fees, under FEE. **grandfather p.,** grandfather CLAUSE.

provisional (pro-vizh'un-al) formed or performed for temporary purposes; temporary.

provitamin (pro-vi'tah-min) a precursor of a vitamin; a substance from which the animal organism can form vitamin. **p. A.** carotene.

Provitar trademark for *oxandrolone*.

provocative (pro-vok'ah-tiv) stimulating the appearance of a sign, reflex, reaction, or therapeutic effect.

Prower defect, factor see FACTOR X.

Proxabrush trademark for an interproximal toothbrush available as small tapered or cylindrical nylon brushes fitting into a handle.

Proxen trademark for *naproxen*.

proximad (prok'sĭ-mad) toward the proximal end or in a proximal direction.

proximal (prok'sĭ-mal) [L. *proximus* next] nearest to any point of reference, as the surface of a tooth which is adjacent to the tooth under consideration. Opposed to *distal*.

proximate (prok'sĭ-mat) [L. *proximatus* drawn near] immediate or nearest.

proximobuccal (prok"sĭ-mo-buk"l) pertaining to both the proximal and buccal surfaces of a tooth.

proximolabial (prok"sĭ-mo-la'be-al) labioproximal.

proximolingual (prok"sĭ-mo-ling'gwal) linguoproximal.

proximo-occlusal (prok"sĭ-mo-ok-loo'zal) pertaining to both the proximal and occlusal surfaces of a tooth.

prozone (pro'zōn) the phenomenon exhibited by some sera, which give effective agglutination reactions when diluted but do not visibly react with antigen particles when undiluted or only slightly diluted. It is not simply due to antibody excess, but often involves a special class of antibodies, blocking or incomplete antibodies, which react with the corresponding particulate antigen in an anomalous manner. The bound antibody not only fails to elicit agglutination, but actively inhibits it. Called also *agglutinoid reaction, prezone, prezone phenomenon,* and *prozone phenomenon*.

PRP physiologic rest position or postural rest position; see rest POSITION.

Pruralgan trademark for *dimethisoquin hydrochloride*.

prurigo (proo-ri'go) [L. "the itch"] a group of skin diseases of unknown etiology, characterized by itching. The typical lesion is the prurigo papule, a dome-shaped eruption with a small transient vesicle on top, followed by crusting or lichenification. **Besnier's p.,** atopic DERMATITIS.

pruritus (proo-ri'tus) [L. from *prurire* to itch] 1. itching. 2. any condition characterized by itching.

P/S polisher-stimulator.

ps per second.

Psaume, J. [French dentist] see oral-facial-digital SYNDROME (1) (Papillon-Léage and Psaume syndrome).

pseud- see PSEUDO-.

pseudarthrosis (su"dar-thro'sis) [pseud- + Gr. *arthrōsis* joint] false joint; an inadequate union of a fractured bone due to failure to form a normal callus, whereby a dense fibrous tissue remains as the end stage of the repair process. Called also *pseudoarthrosis*.

pseudo-, pseud- [Gr. *pseudēs* false] a combining form signifying false or spurious.

pseudoanaphylaxis (su"do-an"ah-fi-lak'sis) acute shock, similar to that in anaphylaxis, which is not caused by an immunological reaction but is associated with the liberation of large amounts of histamine and other mediators, due to the administration of certain substances, such as bee or snake venom, india ink, or acetic acid. Called also *anaphylactoid reaction.*

pseudoanodontia (su″do-an″o-don′she-ah) [*pseudo-* + *anodontia*] a condition characterized by the presence of multiple unerupted permanent teeth. See also *anodontia* and *oligodontia.*

pseudoarthrosis (su″do-ar-thro′sis) pseudarthrosis.

Pseudobacterium (su″do-bak-te′re-um) a proposed generic name that includes various strains of bacteria assigned to different genera. **P. aerofa′ciens,** Eubacterium aerofaciens; see under Eubacterium. **P. cadav′eris,** *Eubacterium budayi;* see under Eubacterium. **P. capillo′sum,** *Bacteroides capillosus;* see under Bacteroides. **P. coag′ulans,** *Bacteroides coagulans;* see under Bacteroides. **P. cylindroi′des,** *Eubacterium cylindroides;* see under Eubacterium. **P. frag′ilis,** *Bacteroides fragilis;* see under Bacteroides. **P. freun′dii,** *Fusobacterium mortiferum;* see under Fusobacterium. **P. furco′sum,** *Bacteroides furcosus;* see under Bacteroides. **P. inaequa′lis, P. incommu′nis,** *Bacteroides fragilis;* see under Bacteroides. **P. len′tum,** *Eubacterium lentum;* see under Eubacterium. **P. mortif′erum, P. necrot′icum,** *Fusobacterium mortiferum;* see under Fusobacterium. **P. putre′dinis,** *Bacteroides putredinis;* see under Bacteroides. **P. recta′le,** *Eubacterium rectale;* see under Eubacterium. **P. ser′pens,** *Bacteroides serpens;* see under Bacteroides. **P. unca′tum,** *Bacteroides fragilis;* see under Bacteroides. **P. ventrio′sum,** *Eubacterium ventriosum;* see under Eubacterium.

pseudobacterium (su″do-bak-te′re-um) [*pseudo-* + Gr. *baktērion* small rod] a cell that resembles a bacterium.

pseudocartilage (su″do-kar′tĭ-lij) chondroid tissue.

pseudocholinesterase (su″do-ko″lin-es′ter-ās) cholinesterase (1).

pseudocrypt (su′do-kript) a folding of tissue that gives an appearance of a crypt, such as those seen on the ceiling of the nasopharynx, forming the pharyngeal tonsils.

pseudocyst (su′do-sist) [*pseudo-* + *cyst*] an abnormal or dilated space resembling a cyst, which is not lined with epithelium. See also cyst.

pseudodiphtheria (su″do-dif-the′re-ah) a condition similar to diphtheria, in which there is the development of false membrane not due to *Corynebacterium diphtheriae.* Called also *false diphtheria.* See also membranous croup. **Epstein's p.,** the development of pseudomembranes on the soft palate in young infants.

pseudofolliculitis (sud″o-fo-lik″u-li′tis) [*pseudo-* + *folliculitis*] a condition resembling folliculitis. **p. bar′bae,** a condition, seen predominantly in Negroes who shave, usually in the submandibular region, characterized by erythematous papules and, less commonly, pustules, containing ingrown hairs whose tips can easily be freed up. The hairs show a confused pattern, growing in all directions; some hairs emerge from curved follicles, and reenter the skin and grow downward. It is called incorrectly *sycosis barbae.*

pseudoglobulin (su″do-glob′u-lin) [*pseudo-* + *globulin*] a class of globulins which are soluble in water. Cf. euglobulin.

pseudohemophilia (su″do-he″mo-fil′e-ah) [*pseudo-* + *hemophilia*] a condition similar to hemophilia, characterized by a bleeding tendency in the presence of normal platelet count, normal clotting time, normal serum fibrinogen, and normal prothrombin time. Epistaxis and cutaneous hemorrhages, occurring either spontaneously or after minor injury, are the principal features. Oral manifestations include gingival bleeding without cause or after a minor irritation, such as brushing, and prolonged severe hemorrhage after tooth extraction. **p. B,** Willebrand-Jürgens syndrome.

pseudohermaphroditism (su″do-her-maf′ro-dit-izm) a condition in which the gonads are of one sex but one or more contradictions exist in the morphologic criteria of sex.

pseudohypoparathyroidism (su″do-hi″po-par″ah-thi′roid-izm) a familial disorder, probably transmitted as an X-linked dominant trait, in which, in spite of apparently normal production of parathyroid hormone, there are symptoms of idiopathic hypoparathyroidism: tetanic and epileptiform convulsions; short stature, round face, and thick skull; cataract; nail fragility; brachymetatarsia and brachymetacarpia; ectopic bone formation; and prolonged Q-T interval. Hypocalcemia and hyperphosphatemia are also present. Histologically, the parathyroid glands are normal or hyperplastic. Oral manifestations include delayed dentition, hypoplasia of the enamel, amelogenesis imperfecta, tooth resorption, exostoses of the mandible, and pulp stones. Called also *constitutional chronic hypocalcemia, hy-*

poparathyroid cretinism, and *Martin-Albright syndrome.* See also pseudopseudohypoparathyroidism.

pseudomembrane (su″do-mem′brăn) false membrane.

Pseudomonadaceae (su″do-mo″nah-da″se-e) [*Pseudomonas* + *-aceae*] a family of gram-negative saprophytic or phytopathogenic, aerobic, rod-shaped bacteria found chiefly in soil and water; some species are also found in animals, including man. It includes the genera *Gluconobacter, Pseudomonas, Xanthomonas,* and *Zoogloea.*

Pseudomonas (su″do-mo′nas) [*pseudo-* + Gr. *monas* unit] a genus of gram-negative bacteria of the family Pseudomonadaceae, made up of single, straight or curved rods, about 0.5 to 1.0 μm in width and 1.5 to 4.0 μm in length, which are motile by polar flagella. The organisms are strict aerobes, except for species which depend on denitrification for anaerobic respiration; their metabolism is respiratory; and they are catalase positive. The genus comprises several hundred species, including a large number of species incertae sedis; most are saprophytic, found in soil, water, and decomposing matter, some being phytopathogenic. Several species are pathogenic for animals, including man. Called also *Liquidomonas.* **P. aerugino′sa,** a species made up of gram-negative, unencapsulated, nonsporogenous rods, 1.5 to 3.0 μm in length and 0.5 μm in breadth, frequently united in pairs and short chains, each having a single polar flagellum by which it is actively motile. They stain readily with aniline dyes. The polysaccharide of the cell wall has endotoxic activity, and a number of extracellular toxic factors are produced, including a lethal glycolipoprotein slime, a leucocidin, and a heat-labile protein exotoxin. Originally considered nonpathogenic saprophytes, these bacteria are now believed to be involved in a number of pathologic processes, and have been isolated from blue or blue-green stains sometimes appearing on surgical dressings, and from urinary tract infections, burns, infected wounds, meningitis, bacteremia, middle ear infections, endocarditis, pneumonia, and water-borne diarrheal diseases. They are occasionally pathogenic to plants. The organisms are drug-resistant, usually showing multiple resistance to three or more antibiotics. Called also *P. pyocyanea, Bacillus aeruginosa, B. pyocyaneus, Bacterium aerugineum, B. aeruginosum, B. pyocyaneum,* and *Micrococcus pyocyaneus.* **P. cepa′cia,** a species found chiefly in soil and rotten onions; some strains have been isolated from cases of human urinary tract infection. Called also *P. multivorans.* **P. enteri′tis,** *Vibrio parahaemolyticus;* see under Vibrio. **P. fluores′cens,** a species found in soil and water, and associated with spoilage of eggs, cured meats, fish, and milk, and sometimes associated with pathological conditions in man. Called also *Bacillus fluorescens, Bacterium fluorescens,* and *Liquidomonas fluorescens.* **P. mal′lei,** a species occurring as small, gram-negative, aerobic rods, straight or slightly curved, usually with rounded ends, and often of irregular contour, ranging in size from 2.0 to 5.0 μm in length and 0.5 to 1.0 μm in breadth. They stain with aqueous aniline dyes, but not readily. In pus they are sometimes found in the leukocytes but more often are extracellular. The organisms are pathogenic chiefly for horses, causing glanders, but man and other animals, such as cats, dogs, goats, sheep, swine, and cattle, may also be infected. The mucous membrane of the nose, especially when abraded, and the conjunctiva, are suspected as the principal points of entry. Called also *Acinetobacter mallei, Actinobacillus mallei, Bacillus mallei, glanders bacillus, Loefferella mallei, Malleomyces mallei,* and *Pfeifferella mallei.* **P. multiv′orans,** *P. cepacia.* **P. pseudomal′lei,** a causative agent of melioidosis, occurring as short, motile rods, about 0.8 by 1.5 μm in size, singly or in short chains, which liquify gelatin and ferment some carbohydrates. It is suspected of producing two thermolabile exotoxins, one lethal and necrotizing and the other lethal only. The species has been isolated from soil and water in tropical regions. Called also *Bacterium whitmori, Bacillus pseudomallei, Loefflerella pseudomallei, Malleomyces pseudomallei,* and *Whitmore's bacillus.* **P. pyocya′nea,** *P. aeruginosa.*

pseudoparalysis (su″do-pah-ral′ĭ-sis) false paralysis; apparent loss of muscular power without true paralysis, marked by defective coordination of movement or by repression of movement on account of pain. **Parrot's p.,** Parrot's disease (1). **syphilitic p.,** Parrot's disease (1).

pseudopocket (su″do-pok′et) a false pocket; especially a pocket formed by enlarged gingivae without apical migration of the junctional epithelium; see relative pocket.

pseudopodia (su″do-po′de-ah) plural of *pseudopodium.*

pseudopodium (su″do-po′de-um), pl. *pseudopo′dia* [*pseudo-* + Gr. *pous* foot] a temporary protrusion of the cytoplasm of an ameboid cell, serving for purposes of locomotion or to engulf food.

pseudopseudohypoparathyroidism   (su″do-su″do-hi″po-par″ah-thi'roid-izm) a syndrome, probably transmitted as an X-linked dominant trait, in which certain features characteristic of pseudohypoparathyroidism are present (round face, short stature, brachymetatarsia, brachymetacarpia, and ectopic bone formation), but in which blood calcium and phosphate levels are normal. Delayed dentition is the most frequent dental complication. Called also *Albright's syndrome*.

pseudoptyalism (su"do-ti'al-izm) accumulation and dribbling of saliva due to dysphagia.

pseudoxanthoma elasticum (su"do-zan-tho'mah e-las'tĭ-kum) a skin disease characterized by the presence of coalescing soft, chamois-yellow to orange, pinhead- to pea-sized papules, which give rise to patches of plaques of various sizes. The flexural folds of the skin become lax or stretched. Oral lesions may occur, usually in the form of ivory to yellow papules on the inner surface of the lips and gingivolabial sulcus. Cardiovascular involvement usually includes degenerative arterial changes and gastrointestinal hemorrhage. Angioid streaks are sometimes associated. It is familial in many cases, probably transmitted as a recessive trait with partial sex limitation to the female. Called also *Darier's disease*.

psi pounds per square inch (lb/in²). See also mechanical STRESS.

psilosis (si-lo'sis) [Gr. *psilōsis* a stripping bare] tropical SPRUE.

psoriasis (so-ri'ah-sis) [Gr. *psōriasis*] a chronic, recurrent papulosquamous disease of the skin, characterized by the presence of reddish-brown papules or plaques, covered by distinctive silvery gray scales. **p. bucca'lis**, 1. oral LEUKOPLAKIA. 2. a probably psoriatic disease of the mouth, characterized by yellow-brown plaques with areas of bluish-gray thickening of the mucous membrane of the cheek. **p. lin'guae**, 1. oral LEUKOPLAKIA. 2. a probably psoriatic disease of the mouth, characterized by yellow-brown plaques with areas of bluish-gray thickening of the tongue.

PSRO Professional Standards Review Organization; see under ORGANIZATION. See also PSRO Management Information System, under SYSTEM.

psych- see PSYCHO-.

psyche (si'ke) [Gr. *psyche* the organ of thought and judgment] the human faculty for thought, judgement, and emotion; the mental life, including both conscious and unconscious processes.

psychiatrist (si-ki'ah-trist) a physician who specializes in psychiatry.

psychiatry (si-ki'ah-tre) [*psych-* + Gr. *iatreia* healing] the branch of medicine which deals with the study, treatment, and prevention of mental illness. Called also *mental medicine*. Cf. PSYCHOLOGY.

psycho-, psych-, [Gr. *psyche* the organ of thought and judgment] a combining form denoting relationship to the psyche, or to the mind.

psychoactive (si"ko-ak'tiv) acting on or influencing mood. See psychoactive AGENT.

psychodelic (si"kĕ-del'ik) [*psycho-* + Gr. *delos* manifest, evident] 1. pertaining to or characterized by changes in psychic processes (i.e., perception, thought, feeling, mood, and behavior) without necessarily being associated with significant changes in metabolic, sensorimotor, and autonomic processes. Called also *phantasicant*. 2. psychodelic AGENT.

psychodysleptic (si"ko-dis-lep'tik) [*psycho-* Gr. *dys* bad + *lepsis* a taking hold] 1. capable of producing abnormalities of mental function or of being mind-disturbing. 2. psychotoxic AGENT.

psychogenic (si"ko-jen'ik) 1. having an emotional or psychologic origin. 2. psychoactive AGENT.

psychologist (si-kol'o-jist) a qualified specialist in psychology.

psychology (si-kol'o-je) [*psycho-* + *-logy*] that branch of science which deals with the mind and mental processes. Cf. PSYCHIATRY.

psychoneuroses (si"ko-nu-ro'sēz) [Gr.] plural of *psychoneurosis*.

psychoneurosis (si"ko-nu-ro'sis), pl. *psychoneuro'ses* [*psycho-* + Gr. *neuron* nerve + *-osis*] neurosis.

psychopharmacology (si"ko-fahr"mah-kol'o-je) [*psycho-* + Gr. *pharmakon* medicine + *-logy*] the science dealing with drugs used to alter the mental state and behavior.

psychosedation (si"ko-se-da'shun) a procedure whereby the patient is rendered free from fear and apprehension through the administration of a psychosedative agent. Sometimes used in dental procedures with the application of nitrous oxide. See also relative ANALGESIA. **dental p.**, dental PREMEDICATION.

psychosedative (si"ko-sed'ah-tiv) an agent that allays apprehension by its action on subcortical centers, while producing minimal motor and sensory impairment because of its limited effect on the cerebral cortex. Nitrous oxide is the most commonly used psychosedative agent.

psychoses (si-ko'sēz) [Gr.] plural of *psychosis*.

psychosis (si-ko'sis), pl. *psycho'ses* [*psych-* + *-osis*] 1. any major mental disorder of organic and/or emotional origin characterized by derangement of the personality and loss of contact with reality, often with delusions, hallucinations, or illusions. Cf. NEUROSIS. 2. an old name for any mental disorder.

psychosomatic (si"ko-so-mat'ik) [*psycho-* + Gr. *sōma* body] pertaining to the mind-body relationship; having bodily symptoms of psychic, emotional, or mental origin; commonly used to refer to a group of disorders thought to be caused in part or in whole by emotional disturbances but presenting as physiologic derangements.

psychotherapeutic (si"ko-ther"ah-pu'tik) 1. pertaining to treatment of abnormalities of mental function. 2. pertaining to agents used in the treatment of disorders of mental function; a psychotherapeutic AGENT.

psychotogenic (si-kot"o-jen'ik) 1. producing a state of psychosis. 2. psychotomimetic AGENT.

psychotomimetic (si-kot"o-mi-met'ik) [*psychosis* + Gr. *mimetikos* imitative] 1. pertaining to, characterized by, or producing manifestations resembling those of a psychosis. 2. psychotomimetic AGENT.

psychotoxic (si"ko-tok'sik) 1. causing abnormalities of mental function. 2. psychotoxic AGENT.

psychotropic (si"ko-tro'pik) [*psycho-* + Gr. *trope* a turning] exerting an effect upon the mind; capable of modifying mental activity; usually applied to drugs that affect the mental state. See also psychoactive AGENT.

Pt platinum.

pt pint.

PTA plasma thromboplastin antecedent; see FACTOR XI. **PTA deficiency,** see FACTOR XI.

PTC plasma thromboplastin component; see FACTOR IX.

PTEN PENTAERYTHRITOL tetranitrate.

pter a symbol for an end of the short arm of a chromosome. See also chromosome ARM and CHROMOSOME nomenclature.

pteridine (ter'ĭ-dēn) a compound, pyrazino[2,3-*d*]pyrimidine, occurring as water-soluble yellow plates. A combination of *p*-aminobenzoic acid and pteridine forms pteroid acid which, in turn, in combination with glutamic acid, forms folic acid.

pterion (te're-on) [Gr. *pteron* wing] a point at the junction of the frontal, parietal, temporal, and great wing of the sphenoid bone; about 3 cm behind the external angular process of the orbit.

pterygium (tĕ-rij'e-um) [Gr. *pterygion* wing] 1. any winglike structure. 2. an abnormal triangular fold of membrane in the interpalpebral fissure. **popliteal p. syndrome,** Fèvre-Languepin SYNDROME. **p. universa'lis,** Guérin-Stern SYNDROME.

pterygoid (ter'ĭ-goid) [Gr. *pterygōdes* like a wing] shaped like a wing.

pterygoideus (ter"ĭ-goi'de-us) [L., from Gr. *pterygōdes*] 1. pterygoid; shaped like a wing. 2. musculus pterygoideus. See pterygoid muscle, medial and pterygoid muscle, lateral, under MUSCLE. **p. exter'nus,** pterygoid muscle, lateral; see under MUSCLE. **p. inter'nus,** pterygoid muscle, medial; see under MUSCLE. **p. latera'lis,** pterygoid muscle, lateral; see under MUSCLE. **p. media'lis,** pterygoid muscle, medial; see under MUSCLE.

pterygomandibular (ter"ĭ-go-man-dib'u-lar) pertaining to the pterygoid process and the mandible.

pterygomaxillary (ter"ĭ-go-mak'sĭ-ler'e) pertaining to a pterygoid process and the maxilla.

pterygopalatine (ter"ĭ-go-pal'ah-tin) pertaining to a pterygoid process and to the palatine bone.

pterygopharyngeus (ter"ĭ-go-far-in'je-us) pterygopharyngeal MUSCLE.

PTH parathyroid HORMONE.

Ptm pterygomaxillary FISSURE (2).

ptosis (to'sis) [Gr. "fall"] prolapse or drooping of an organ or part, such as the eyelid. See also BLEPHAROPTOSIS.

-ptosis [Gr. *ptōsis* fall] a word termination indicating downward displacement.

ptyalagogue (ti-al'ah-gog) [*ptyalo-* + Gr. *agōgos* leading] an agent that promotes the flow of saliva; sialagogue.

ptyalase (ti'ah-lās) [*ptyalin* + *-ase*] salivary AMYLASE.

ptyalectasis (ti"ah-lek'tah-sis) [*ptyalo-* + Gr. *ektasis* distention] 1. operative dilatation of a salivary duct. 2. dilatation of one of the ducts of the salivary glands.

ptyalin (ti'ah-lin) [Gr. *ptyalon* spittle] salivary α-AMYLASE.

ptyalism (ti'ah-lizm) [Gr. *ptyalismos*] excessive flow of saliva. Called also *hyperptyalism, hypersalivation, polysialia, ptyalorrhea, sialism, sialismus,* and *sialorrhea*.

ptyalize (ti′ah-līz) to increase or stimulate the secretion of saliva.

ptyalo- [Gr. *ptyalon* spittle] a combining form denoting relationship to the saliva. See also terms beginning SIALO-.

ptyalocele (ti-al′o-sēl) [*ptyalo-* + Gr. *kēlē* tumor] a cystic tumor containing saliva. **sublingual p.,** ranula.

ptyalogenic (ti″ah-lo-jen′ik) [*ptyalo-* + Gr. *gennan* to produce] formed from or by the action of saliva.

ptyalography (ti″ah-log′rah-fe) [*ptyalo-* + Gr. *graphein* to write] roentgen examination of the salivary ducts or glands; sialography.

ptyalolithiasis (ti″ah-lo-li-thi′ah-sis) [*ptyalo-* + Gr. *lithos* stone] sialolithiasis.

ptyalolithotomy (ti″ah-lo-li-thot′o-me) [*ptyalo-* + Gr. *tomē* a cutting] surgical removal of salivary calculi; sialolithotomy.

ptyalorrhea (ti″ah-lo-re′ah) [*ptyalo-* + Gr. *rhoia* flow] excessive flow of saliva. Called also *hyperptyalism, hypersalivation, ptyalism,* and *sialorrhea.*

Pu plutonium.

puberty (pu′ber-te) [L. *pubertas*] the age of observable sexual maturation; it is typically 13 to 16 years of age for boys and 12 to 14 years of age for girls. **precocious p.,** early sexual maturity, usually caused by pathological processes.

public (pub′lik) pertaining to of or affecting the people as a whole, as in public health. See also public antigens, under ANTIGEN.

Puente's disease CHEILITIS glandularis apostematosa.

puerpera (pu-er′per-ah) [L. *puer* child + *parere* to bring forth, to bear] a woman who has just given birth to a child. See also PARA.

puerperium (pu″er-pe′re-um) [L.] the period of confinement after childbirth.

pulp (pulp) [L. *pulpa* flesh] 1. any soft, juicy animal or vegetable tissue. 2. dental p. **coronal p.,** that part of the dental pulp contained in the pulp chamber or the crown portion of the pulp cavity. Called also *pulpa coronale* [NA]. **dead p., p. death,** necrotic p. **dental p.,** a richly vascularized and innervated connective tissue of mesodermal origin, contained in the central cavity of a tooth and delimited by the dentin, and having formative, nutritive, sensory, and protective functions. The portion housed in the tooth chamber proper is known as *coronal pulp*; that within the root as *radicular pulp.* Its size and shape change, being larger early in life and decreasing thereafter. It receives the blood vessels, lymphatics, and nerves through the apical ·canal at the tip of the root. In a transverse section, it consists of a peripheral cellular layer, odontoblastic layer, cell-free fibrous layer, zone of Weil, and cell-rich zone. The remaining portion consists of the pulp proper. The cellular components include fibrocytes, mesenchymal cells, and histiocytes. The pulp may undergo regressive changes, including fatty degeneration, fibrosis, atrophy, cystic disorders, metaplasia, and calcific regression. Called also *endodontium* and *pulpa dentis* [NA], and is popularly referred to as *the nerve.* See also ENDODONTICS. **devitalized p.,** necrotic p. **enamel p.,** stellate RETICULUM. **exposed p.,** a condition in which the dental pulp becomes exposed to the external environment and is thus susceptible to bacterial invasion. It is usually caused by pathological changes in the hard tissues of the tooth, including carious lesions or tooth resorption; trauma, such as fracture of the crown of the tooth; mechanical factors, as through penetration of sound dentin during tooth preparation; and various dental procedures. **p. gangrene,** gangrenous pulp NECROSIS. **hyperactive p., hypersensitive p.,** hypersensitive PULPALGIA. **p. mummification,** pulp MUMMIFICATION. **mummified p.,** the dry, shriveled dental pulp seen in dry gangrene. **p. necrosis,** necrotic p. **necrotic p., nonvital p.,** death of the dental pulp with or without bacterial invasion, occurring in pulp which has been deprived of its blood and nerve supply. Absence of living tissue may be evidenced by pulp insensitivity to stimulation by electricity, heat, cold, or trauma. Cheesy necrosis and colliquative necrosis are the two most common forms. Called also *dead p., devitalized p.,* and *p. necrosis.* See also gangrenous pulp NECROSIS. **p. proper,** the central mass of the dental pulp, containing most of the cellular elements, as well as large blood, lymph, and nerve structures located in a framework of fibrils and ground substance. Cells are mainly fibroblasts; mesenchymal cells are few and always confined to the capillary bed. Defense cells, such as histiocytes, plasma cells, lymphocytes, polyblasts, and eosinophils, are also scarce under normal conditions and, when protection is needed, their population is increased, either by migration from other tissues or by differentiation of mesenchymal cells. Called also *pulp core.* **putrescent p.,**

a necrotic pulp which has been invaded by putrefactive microorganisms and is characterized by a particularly foul odor. **radicular p.,** that part of the dental pulp contained in the root canal of a tooth. Called also *pulpa radicularis* [NA]. **p. stone,** denticle. **transitional p.,** see transitional pulp STAGE. **vital p.,** dental pulp characterized by vascularity and sensation; one that is not necrotic. See also pulp vitality tests, under TEST.

pulpa (pul′pah), pl. *pul′pae* [L. "flesh"] pulp. **p. coron′ale** [NA], coronal PULP. **p. den′tis** [NA], dental PULP. **p. radicula′ris** [NA], radicular PULP.

pulpal (pul′pal) pertaining to the pulp.

pulpalgia (pul-pal′je-ah) pain in the dental pulp. **acute p.,** pulpalgia having a rapid onset; it may be referred to as *incipient* (such as a mild discomfort after anesthesia), *moderate* (a discomfort usually recurring over several days but may be well tolerated by the patient), or *advanced* or *severe* (a severe pain usually caused by a closed pulp chamber with retention of fluids in the cavity). **advanced acute p.,** see *acute p.* **chronic p.,** vague pain in the pulp of a tooth that has decayed over a long period of time, usually showing hypersensitivity to temperature changes or touch; it is often associated with discomfort in adjacent teeth in the arch. **hyperactive p.,** hypersensitive p. **hypersensitive p.,** pulpalgia characterized by short, sharp shooting pain precipitated by temperature changes, sweet or sour foods, touch, or other factors, commonly occurring after the placement of new restorations, root planing, or periodontal surgery. Called also *hyperactive p., hyperactive pulp, hypersensitive pulp,* and *pulp hypersensitivity.* See also hypersensitive TOOTH. **incipient acute p.,** see *acute p.* **moderate acute p.,** see *acute p.* **severe acute p.,** see *acute p.*

Pulpdent cavity liner see under LINER.

Pulpdent liquid see under LIQUID.

Pulpdent pulp capping agent see under AGENT.

pulpectomy (pul-pek′to-me) [*pulp* + Gr. *ektomē* excision] complete extirpation of the dental pulp. See also root canal THERAPY.

pulpitis (pul-pi′tis), pl. *pulpit′ides* [*pulp* + *-itis*] inflammation of the dental pulp, usually due to bacterial infection in dental caries, tooth fracture, or other conditions causing exposure of the pulp to bacterial invasion. Chemical irritants, thermal factors, as in dental restoration with the use of material transmitting heat or cold to the pulp, hyperemic changes, and other factors may also cause pulpitis. **acute p.,** pulpitis having a short and relatively severe course, occurring usually in a tooth with a large carious lesion or a restoration with a defective margin, associated with recurrent caries. It is believed to follow pulp hyperemia, and is marked by severe pain produced by heat or cold, which characteristically continues even after the thermal stimulus has been removed; pain is more severe in closed types of acute pulpitis, because of lack of escape of inflammatory exudate. Small pus-containing abscesses (see pulp ABSCESS), arising from breakdown of leukocytes and bacteria, may occur in the early stages. Vascular dilatation, hyperemia, edema, presence of polymorphonuclear leukocytes in vascular channels, and collection of leukocytes beneath surfaces of carious lesions are the principal histologic features. **anachoretic p.,** that caused by bacteria circulating in the blood stream, which settle at sites of pulpal inflammation resulting from a chemical or mechanical injury. **p. aper′ta,** open p. **chronic p.,** pulpitis, occurring in both a closed and an open form, characterized by a protracted course and relatively mild symptoms. Contrary to acute pulpitis, there is only a mild, dull ache and à mild reactivity to thermal stimuli. It is characterized by inflammatory exudate, infiltration of the tissue by mononuclear cells, chiefly lymphocytes and plasma cells, prominent capillaries, fibroblastic activity, and necrosis. **p. clau′sa,** closed p. **closed p.,** that characterized by the absence of a direct communication between the dental pulp and the oral environment. Called also *p. clausa.* **generalized p.,** that which involves the entire dental pulp. **hyperplastic p., hyperplastic p., chronic,** a chronic productive type of pulpitis, usually occurring in teeth with large carious lesions, and most often affecting children and young adults. It is characterized by proliferation of the dental pulp tissue, filling the cavity with a pedunculated or sessile, pinkish-red, fleshy mass. The hyperplastic tissue is basically granulation tissue made up of connective tissue fibers interspersed with small capillaries. Inflammatory cell infiltration, usually plasma cells and lymphocytes, sometimes admixed with polymorphonuclear leukocytes is a common histologic feature. Called also *hypertrophic p., hyperplastic pulposis, pulp hyperplasia,* and *pulp polyp.* **hypertrophic p.,** hyperplastic p. **irreversible p.,** severe pulpitis with a minimal probability of recovery, which may be acute, subacute, or chronic, and partial or total. The affected pulp may be infected or sterile. An exudate is always present and pain is usually present when the exudate is confined to the root canal, being moderate to severe (depending on the degree of inflammation), sharp or dull, or referred, throbbing, or constant. If the exudate is vented, pain may be alleviated. Some types of irreversible pulpitis are characterized by spasmodic episodes of pain; in others prolonged pain occurs, especially after sudden changes of temperature, and continues even after the stimulus is removed. Change of posture may also be a cause of episodes of pain in some cases. **open p.,** that characterized by the presence of a direct communication between the dental pulp and the oral environment. Called also *p. aperta.* **partial p.,** that in which inflammatory processes involve only a part of the dental pulp. **reversible p.,** pulpitis characterized by a sharp, hypersensitive response to thermal changes, especially cold, with pain subsiding immediately after the stimulus is removed; it is usually asymptomatic unless provoked by an external stimulus. It is caused most commonly by defective restorations or restorative procedures, or dental caries; sweet foods contacting dentin or rubbing areas of cervical erosion, abrasion, or fracture of the crown of a tooth exposing vital dentin may also be a cause. Reparative processes usually occur after the causative agent is removed, but if the cause is not removed, degenerative processes will lead to irreversible pulpitis. **suppurative p.,** that usually caused by extension of a carious process into the dental pulp. **total p.,** that in which inflammatory processes involve the entire dental pulp. **ulcerative p.,** a form of chronic pulpitis characterized by deposition of collagen about the inflamed area, resembling granulation tissue, seen on the exposed surface of the pulp.

pulpless (pulp′les) without pulp.

pulpoma (pul″po-mah) tooth resorption, internal; see under RESORPTION.

pulposis (pul-po′sis) any disease of the dental pulp. **hyperplastic p.,** hyperplastic PULPITIS.

pulpotomy (pul-pot′o-me) [*pulp* + Gr. *tomē* a cutting] partial excision of the dental pulp. The operation is usually performed in the treatment of pulpitis, and all pathologically changed pulp tissue is removed for the purpose of preserving its remaining normal radicular portion. Called also *pulp amputation.*

pulse (puls) [L. *pulsus* stroke] 1. the rhythmic expansion of an artery produced by the rise and fall in blood pressure with the diastolic and systolic phases of heart contraction, being a shock wave that travels along the fibers of the arteries. Normal pulse rate at birth is about 130 beats per minute, decreasing to 50 to 90 beats in adults. Changes in the regularity and rate of the pulse rate usually indicate exertion, physical or mental stress, or an illness. It is usually felt just inside the wrist below the thumb by placing two or three fingers lightly upon the radial artery, the thumb never being used because its own pulse is likely to be confused with the one being taken. The instrument for registering the movements, form, and force of the arterial pulse is known as a *sphygmograph.* Called also *arterial p.* See also terms beginning with SPHYGMO-. 2. a brief surge, as of current or voltage. **abrupt p.,** one which strikes the finger rapidly. **allorhythmic p.,** one marked by irregularities in rhythm. **arterial p.,** pulse (1). **carotid p.,** the pulse in the carotid artery, above the clavicle and below the angle of the mandible; used in timing the phases of the cardiac cycle. **dropped-beat p.,** intermittent p. **frequent p.,** one which is faster in rate than normal, being more than 90 beats per minute. Called also *quick p.* **infrequent p.,** one which is slower in rate than normal, being less than 50 beats per minute. **intermittent p.,** one in which beats are dropped. Called also *dropped-beat p.* **irregular p.,** one in which the beats occur at irregular intervals. **jerky p.,** one in which the artery is suddenly and markedly distended. Called also *sharp p.* **periodontal p.,** the return of the teeth to their original position after forces applied against them, as in mastication, are removed, consisting of a pulsating movement associated with the normal pulsation of the periodontal vessels which occurs in synchrony with the cardiac cycle. **p. pressure,** see blood PRESSURE. **quick p.,** 1. one which strikes the finger smartly and leaves it quickly. Called also *short p.* 2. frequent p. **radial p.,** the pulse felt over the radial artery, on the thumb side of the inner wrist; most commonly used for reading the pulse rate. **sharp p.,** jerky p. **short p.,** quick p. (1). **venous p.,** the pulsation in a vein, usually observed at the right jugular vein just above the sternoclavicular joint.

Pulsoton trademark for *hydroxyamphetamine.*

pulsus (pul′sus), pl. *pul′sus* [L.] pulse.

pulv. abbreviation for L. *pul′vis,* powder.

pumice (pum′is) a substance of vulcanic origin, found chiefly in the Lipari Islands and in the Greek archipelagos, and occurring as a light, hard rough porous gray substance or powder. It consists mainly of silicates of aluminum, potassium, and sodium, being insoluble in water or acids. Pumice is ground in various grits (flour of pumice) and mixed with water or an

antiseptic solution to be used as an abrasive paste (pumice paste) in dentistry. It is generally used as the first polishing agent for metal dentures and orthodontic appliances, followed by tripoli and rouge. **flour of p.,** see *pumice.*

pump (pump) an apparatus or mechanism drawing or propelling fluids or gases. **lymph p.,** a mechanism for propelling lymph through the lymphatic system. Compression of lymphatic vessels by their smooth muscle pushes the lymph through a series of one-way valves in the veseels. Additional propulsion is by contraction of skeletal muscles surrounding many of the vessels and pulsations of adjacent arteries. **sodium p.,** active transport of intracellular sodium across the cell membrane in the system of maintenance of intracellular and extracellular sodium-potassium balance. The process is based on the transport of intracellular sodium across the cell membrane against the greater extracellular concentration by a carrier (believed to be a lipoprotein) which, after releasing sodium at the outer surface of the membrane, binds the extracellular potassium to be transported against the greater intracellular concentration. Energy is supplied by MgATP reacting with lipoprotein which acts as ATPase in breaking the potassium carrier complex into inorganic P, Mg, and ADP. The sodium pump is involved in maintaining membrane potential and transmitting impulses by nerves and muscles, preventing cell swelling by excessive intracellular sodium concentration, glandular secretion, and other functions of the body. See also active TRANSPORT (2).

punch (punch) an instrument or a tool for perforating, indenting, or cutting out holes. **Ainsworth p.,** a lightweight rubber dam punch. **pin p.,** one for perforating a metal backing to receive the pins for fastening artificial teeth. **plate p.,** one for cutting out parts of a dental plate. **rubber dam p.,** a hand instrument for punching holes in a rubber dam in order to permit the passage of the dam over the crowns of the teeth. It has a platform with graduated holes and a sharpened stylus to cut the holes in the rubber dam. **S. S. White p.,** trademark for a rubber dam punch.

punched-out (puncht′owt) having the appearance of substance or tissue having been removed with a punch.

puncta (punk′tah) [L.] plural of *punctum.*

punctate (punk′tāt) 1. [L. *punctum* point] resembling or marked with points or dots. 2. the fluid obtained by an exploratory puncture.

punctiform (punk′ti-form) [L. *punctum* point + *forma* form] like a point; located in a point.

punctum (punk′tum), pl. *punc′ta* [L.] an extremely small spot, or point; used in anatomical nomenclature as a general term to designate an extremely small area, or point or projection. See also POINT. **punc′ta lacrima′lia,** lacrimal points; see under POINT.

puncture (punk′tur) [L. *punctura*] 1. the act of piercing or penetrating with a pointed object or instrument. 2. a wound so made. **apical p.,** dental TREPHINATION. **dental p.,** dental TREPHINATION.

puppet (pup′et) an artificial figure representing a human being or an animal, manipulated by rods, hand, or wires. **happy p., p. child,** happy-puppet SYNDROME.

Pur purple; see color coding table at root canal THERAPY.

Purecal trademark for *precipitated calcium carbonate* (see under CALCIUM).

Puretić's syndrome [B. *Puretić,* Yugoslav physician] Puretić-Ishikawa SYNDROME.

Puretić-Ishikawa syndrome [B. *Puretić;* H. *Ishikawa,* Japanese physician] see under SYNDROME.

purine (pu′rēn) [L. *purum* pure + *urine*] a colorless crystalline heterocyclic compound, which is not found free in nature, but is variously substituted to produce a group of compounds known as *purines* or *purine bases* (purine bodies), of which uric acid is a metabolic end product. The purines formed by the hydrolysis of nucleosides in the tissue undergo catabolic changes, the nucleosides adenosine, inosine, guanosine, and xanthosine being split into ribose plus adenine, hypoxanthine (6-oxypurine), guanine, and xanthine (2,6-dioxypurine), respectively. See also nitrogenous BASE. **p. antagonist, p. inhibitor,** purine ANALOGUE. **methyl p's,** alkaloids formed from purines by substituting methyl groups, usually in positions 1, 3, 7. The principal ones are caffeine, theobromine, and theophylline.

6-purinethiol (pu″ri-neth′i-ol) mercaptopurine.

Purinethol trademark for *mercaptopurine.*

Purmann's method [Matthaeus Gottfried *Purmann,* German surgeon, 1648–1711; he was the first to use sealing wax for taking impressions] see under METHOD.

purpura (pur'pu-rah) [L. "purple"; Gr. *porphyra* a mollusk from which a purple dye was obtained] a condition characterized by the presence of confluent petechiae or ecchymoses over any part of the the body, caused by escape of blood from capillaries into the skin or mucous membranes. **allergic nonthrombocytopenic p., anaphylactoid p.,** Schönlein-Henoch SYNDROME. **athrombocytopenic p.,** Glanzmann's SYNDROME. **athrombopenic p., essential** Schönlein-Henoch SYNDROME. **p. ful'minans,** a rare form of nonthrombocytopenic purpura of unclear etiology, characterized by large areas of gangrene and hemorrhage of the skin, associated with chills, fever, shock, coma, and death. It appears suddenly in children and young adults convalescing from a variety of infectious diseases, such as streptococcal pharyngitis, scarlet fever, chickenpox, meningococcemia, and rubella. There is intravascular coagulation and stasis and deficiency of blood coagulation factors V and VIII. **gangrenous p.,** de Gimard's SYNDROME. **p. hemorrha'gica,** thrombocytopenic p. **p. hyperglobuline'mica,** Waldenström's SYNDROME. **p. infectio'sa acu'ta,** Schönlein-Henoch SYNDROME. **infectious p.,** thrombocytopenic or nonthrombocytopenic purpura associated with various infectious diseases, such as Rocky Mountain spotted fever, typhus, meningococcemia, bacterial endocarditis, chickenpox, smallpox, scarlet fever, measles, tuberculosis, infectious mononucleosis, and infectious hepatitis. The course is relatively mild and is similar to that seen in idiopathic thrombocytopenic purpura. **p. necrot'isans,** de Gimard's SYNDROME. **p. rheumat'ica, Schönlein-Henoch p.,** Schönlein-Henoch SYNDROME. **thrombocytopathic p.,** Glanzmann's SYNDROME. **thrombocytopenic p.,** purpura associated with thrombocytopenia. Called also *p. hemorrhagica.* See *idiopathic thrombocytopenic p.* and *symptomatic thrombocytopenic p.* **thrombocytopenic p., idiopathic, thrombocytopenic p., primary,** thrombocytopenic purpura occurring in acute, chronic, and recurrent forms. The acute form most commonly affects children, and is characterized by a sudden onset of purpura and ecchymoses of the skin and mucous membranes, internal bleeding, and recovery in a few weeks or months. The chronic form is characterized by an insidious onset, a long history of a tendency to bruise or abnormal menstrual bleeding, frequent remissions, and, sometimes, enlarged spleen. The recurrent form is similar to the chronic form, but differs in having a normal platelet count between relapses. Thrombocytopenia, sometimes associated with platelet levels of only a few thousand per cubic millimeter of blood, the presence of giant platelets, prolonged bleeding time, and positive tourniquet test are the most common features. Gingival bleeding, sometimes in absence of skin lesions, petechiae of the oral mucosa, and occasional ecchymoses are the principal oral symptoms. Called also *Werlhof's p., essential thrombocytopenia, morbus maculosus hemorrhagicus,* and *Werlhof's disease.* **thrombocytopenic p., symptomatic,** thrombocytopenic purpura associated with deficiency of blood platelets which complicates various diseases, such as smallpox, measles, rubella, systemic lupus erythematosus, and infectious mononucleosis, or is precipitated by hypersensitivity to certain drugs, such as apronalide, quinine, digitoxin, quinidine, chlorothiazide, chlorpropramide, meprobamate, phenylbutazone, sulfonamides, and some antihistaminics. It is accompanied by internal bleeding, presence of petechiae and ecchymoses on the skin and mucous membranes, and severe decrease in the blood platelet count. Oral symptoms include gingival bleeding and ecchymoses and petechiae of the mucosa. The immunologic mechanism of lysis of blood platelets is believed to be the cause; antibodies are suspected to cause platelet lysis by fixation of complement, which is specifically antidrug, rather than antiplatelet. **p. variolo'sa,** an old term for hemorrhagic VARIOLA. **Werlhof's p.,** *thrombocytopenic p.,* idopathic.
purulent (pu'roo-lent) [L. *purulentus*] consisting of or containing pus; associated with the formation of or caused by pus.
pus (pus), pl. *pu'ra,* gen. *pu'ris* [L.] a thick fluid composed of large numbers of viable and necrotic polymorphonuclear leukocytes and necrotic tissue debris that is partially liquefied by proteases, peptidases, and lipases liberated from dead leukocytes, usually resulting from the presence of pyogenic bacteria in inflammatory processes, or by injury produced by chemical agents, such as turpentine or silver nitrate. Called also *matter, purulent exudate,* and *suppurative exudate.*
pusher (poosh'er) one who or that which presses on or against something with force in order to move it. **band p.,** an orthodontic instrument designed to apply pressure against an orthodontic band when adapting it to a tooth. See illustrations.

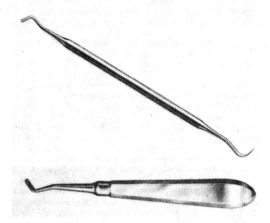

Band pushers. (From H. O. Torres and A. Ehrlich: Modern Dental Assisting. 2nd ed. Philadelphia, W. B. Saunders Co., 1980.)

pustule (pus'tul) [L. *pustula*] a circumscribed, elevated lesion of the skin of less than 5 mm in diameter, which contains pus. **malignant p.,** anthrax.
pustulosis (pus"tu-lo'sis) a condition marked by an outbreak of pustules. **p. herpet'ica infan'tum,** Kaposi's varicelliform ERUPTION.
putamen (pu-ta'men) [L. "shell"] [NA] the larger and more lateral part of the lentiform nucleus.
putrefy (pu'tre-fi) to decompose, with the production of foulsmelling compounds; a term applied especially to the decomposition of proteins and other organic matter.
putrescence (pu-tres'ens) partial or complete rottenness.
putty (put'e) a pliable, sticky material. **p. powder** stannic OXIDE. **silicone p.,** see impression material, silicone, under MATERIAL.
PVAc POLYVINYL acetate.
PVC POLYVINYL chloride.
PVD postural vertical DIMENSION.
PVP polyvinylpyrrolidone; see POVIDONE.
PVP-I povidone-iodine.
pwt pennyweight.
pycno- PYKNO-.
Pycopay see under DENTIFRICE.
pyel- see PYELO-.
pyelitis (pi"ē-li'tis) [*pyel-* + *-itis*] inflammation of the pelvis of the kidney.
pyelo-, pyel- [Gr. *pyelos* pelvis] a combining form denoting relationship to the pelvis of the kidney.
pyelonephritis (pi"ē-lc-nē-fri'tis) [*pyelo-* + Gr. *nephros* kidney + *-itis*] inflammation of the kidney and its pelvis, beginning in the interstitium and rapidly extending to involve the tubules, glomeruli, and blood vessels, due to bacterial infection. It is more common in females than in males. Symptoms include fever, chills, lumbar pain, painful urination with increased frequency, and tenderness in the costovertebral angle.
pyemia (pi-e'me-ah) [Gr. *pyon* pus + *haima* blood + *-ia*] a general septicemia in which secondary foci of suppuration occur and multiple abscesses are formed. Called also *metastatic infection.* **cryptogenic p.,** that in which the source of infection is unknown.
pykno- [Gr. *pyknos* thick, frequent] combining form meaning thick, compact, or frequent. Sometimes written *pycno-.*
pyknocyte (pik'no-sīt) [*pykno-* + *-cyte*] a distorted contracted erythrocyte.
pyknodysostosis (pik"no-dis"os-to'sis) [*pykno-* + *dysostosis*] Maroteaux-Lamy SYNDROME (2).
Pyknolepsinum trademark for *ethosuximide.*
pyknosis (pik-no'sis) [Gr. *pyknōsis* condensation] a thickening; especially degeneration of a cell in which the nucleus shrinks in size and the chromatin condenses to a solid, structureless mass. Called also *karyopyknosis.* See also NECROSIS.
Pyle's disease, syndrome [Edwin *Pyle*, American physician, born 1891] metaphyseal DYSPLASIA.
pyo- [Gr. *pyon* pus] a combining form denoting relationship to pus.
pyoderma (pi"o-der'mah) [*pyo-* + Gr. *derma* skin] any purulent skin disease. Called also *pyodermatitis.* **p. veg'etans, p. verruco'sum,** DERMATITIS vegetans.

pyodermatitis (pi″o-der″mah-ti′tis) an old name for pyoderma. **p. veg′etans,** DERMATITIS vegetans.

pyogenesis (pi″o-jen′ĕ-sis) [*pyo-* + Gr. *genesis* production] the formation of pus.

pyogenic (pi″o-jen′ik) producing pus.

pyogenous (pi-oj′ĕ-nus) caused by pus.

Pyopen trademark for *carbenicillin disodium* (see under CARBENICILLIN).

pyoptysis (pi-op′tı-sis) [*pyo-* + Gr. *ptysis* spitting] spitting of purulent matter.

pyorrhea (pi″o-re′ah) [*pyo-* + Gr. *rhoia* flow] a discharge of pus. 2. marginal PERIODONTITIS. **p. alveola′ris,** marginal PERIODONTITIS. **schmutz p.,** marginal PERIODONTITIS.

pyorrheal (pi″o-re′al) pertaining to or characterized by pyorrhea.

pyostomatitis (pi″o-sto″mah-ti′tis) [*pyo-* + *stomatitis*] a suppurative inflammation of the mouth. **p. veg′etans,** inflammation of the mouth beginning with minute flat miliary abscesses of uniform size, tending to conglomerate and becoming proliferative, soft, red, folded, and verrucose. The primary lesions appear as multiple small pustules with a yellowish tip and a reddened base, spreading within a few weeks to involve the entire oral cavity. As the lesions become chronic, the buccal mucosa proliferates to form folds, and the miliary abscesses are found on the summits of the rugae and in the deep invaginations. Mild pain is usually present. Microscopically, there is pronounced hyperkeratosis and acanthosis with broadening and elongation of the rete pegs. Connective tissue presents a granulomatous inflammatory process with unruptured miliary abscesses, associated with degeneration of the epithelium and focal areas of surface necrosis.

PYP pyrophosphate. **Techne-Scan PYP,** trademark for *stannous pyrophosphate* (see under PYROPHOSPHATE).

Pyradone trademark for *aminopyrine*.

pyramid (pir′ah-mid) [Gr. *pyramis*] a pointed or cone-shaped structure or part; a general anatomical term for such a structure. Called also *pyramis*. **petrous p.,** petrous BONE.

pyramidal (pī-ram′ĭ-dal) [L. *pyramidalis*] pertaining to, or shaped like a pyramid.

pyramides (pi-ram′ĭ-dēz) [Gr.] plural of *pyramis*.

Pyramidon trademark for *aminipyrine*.

pyramis (pir′ah-mis), pl. *pyram′ides* [Gr.] pyramid; a general anatomical term for any pointed or cone-shaped structure or part. **p. os′sis tempora′lis,** petrous BONE.

Pyranisamine (pi″rah-nis′ah-mēn) trademark for *pyrilamine*.

pyrazinamide (pi″rah-zin′ah-mīd) an antimicrobial agent, pyrazinecarboxamide, occurring as a white, odorless, crystalline powder that is soluble in water, chloroform, and ether and slightly soluble in ethanol. Used chiefly in the treatment of tuberculosis. Adverse effects may include fever, anorexia, liver lesions, malaise, retention of uric acid, arthralgia, and vomiting. Called also *pyrazinoic acid amide*. Trademarks: Aldinamide, Tebrazid.

pyrethrin (pi-rēth′rin) an active insecticidal substance, pyrithrin I or II, occurring in the flowers of perennial herbs of the genus *Chrysanthemum (Pyrethrum)*. Pyrethrins are relatively nontoxic to mammals, but exposure to excessive amounts may cause hypersensitivity, dermatitis, nausea, vomiting, tinnitus, headache, and various central nervous system disorders.

pyreto- [Gr. *pyteros* fever] a combining form denoting relationship to fever.

Pyrex glass see under GLASS.

pyrexia (pi-rek′se-ah) [Gr. *pyressein* to be feverish] abnormal elevation of body temperature; fever.

Pyriamid trademark for *sulfapyridine*.

Pyribenzamine trademark for *tripelennamine*.

pyridine (pir′ĭ-dēn) a heterocyclic compound, C_5H_5N, occurring as a yellowish or colorless, flammable liquid with a nauseating odor and sharp taste, which is found in coal tar, bone oil, tobacco smoke, and various organic matters. Used as a solvent, in chemical techniques, and in the manufacturing of drugs, vitamins, fungicides, and other products. Exposure may cause mental depression, skin and mucous membrane irritation, gastrointestinal disorders, and kidney and liver diseases.

pyridostigmine bromide (pir′ĭ-do-stig′mēn) a cholinomimetic (quaternary ammonium anticholinesterase) agent,3-[[(dimethylamino)carbonyl]oxy]-1-methylpyridinium bromide, occurring as a white, hygroscopic, crystalline powder with an agreeable characteristic odor. It is soluble in water, ethanol, and chloroform, slightly soluble in solvent hexane, and insoluble in ether. Used chiefly in the treatment of myasthenia gravis. Trademarks: Kalymin, Mestinon, Regonol.

pyridoxal (pir′ĭ-dok′sal) a water-soluble compound of the vitamin

B complex, 3-hydroxy-5-(hydroxymethyl)-2-methyl-4-pyridinecarboxaldehyde, occurring as crystals that are soluble in water and ethanol. It is one of the three forms of vitamin B_6 (the other two are pyridoxamine and pyridoxine), having metabolic and pharmacological properties identical to those of pyridoxine. For daily requirements of the forms of vitamin B_6, see table at NUTRITION. **p. phosphate,** a coenzyme of amino acid metabolism, 2-methyl-3-hydroxy-4-formyl-5-pyridylmethylphosphoric acid. See PYRIDOXINE phosphate.

pyridoxamine (pir′ĭ-dok′sah-min) a water-soluble compound of the vitamin B complex, 4-(amino-methyl)-5-hydroxy-6-methyl-3-pyridinemethanol, being one of the three forms of vitamin B_6 (the other two are pyridoxine and pyridoxal). Used clinically as the dihydrochloride salt, occurring as a crystalline powder that is soluble in water and ethanol. Its pharmacological and metabolic activities are those of pyridoxine. For daily requirements of the forms of vitamin B_6, see table at NUTRITION.

pyridoxine (pir′ĭ-dok′sēn) a water-soluble vitamin of the B complex, 3-hydroxy-6-methyl-3,4-pyrimidinedimethanol, being one of the three forms of vitamin B_6 (the other two are pyridoxal and pyridoxamine). It is found in yeasts, rice polishings, cereals, egg yolk and, in moderate amounts, in the liver, kidneys, muscles, and fish. Used clinically as the hydrochloride salt, which occurs as a white crystalline powder or colorless or white crystals that are soluble in water, ethanol, and propylene glycol, sparingly soluble in acetone, and insoluble in ether and chloroform. In the body, pyridoxine is converted to pyridoxal phosphate, which serves as a coenzyme for amino acid metabolism, including decarboxylation, transamination, and racemization. It is also concerned with fatty acid metabolism erythropoiesis, biosynthesis of hemoglobin, other metabolic processes, and the active transport of amino acids and metallic ions across cell membranes. Used therapeutically in pyridoxine deficiency. The symptoms of pyridoxine deficiency are believed to be epileptiform convulsions, failure to grow, anemia, skin lesions, neuritis, and various lesions of the nervous system. Symptoms of deficiency, especially neuritis, may be produced by pyridoxine antagonists. Oral manifestations may include perlèche, glossitis, edema of the tongue, glossodynia, atrophy of the lingual papillae, especially on the tip, and a purplish cast of the tongue. For daily requirements of forms of vitamin B_6, see table at NUTRITION.

pyriform (pir′ĭ-form) piriform.

pyrilamine (pi-ril′ah-mēn) an antihistaminic agent with low sedative effects that acts on the H_1 histamine receptor, 2-[(2-dimethylaminoethyl)-*p*-methoxybenzyl)amino]pyridine. Used therapeutically in the form of the maleate salt, occurring as white, crystalline powder with a faint odor that is soluble in water, alcohol, and chloroform, and very slightly soluble in ether and benzene. Also used in various antitussive preparations. Called also *mepyramine*. Trademarks: Antallergan, Anthisan, Pyranisamine.

pyrimidine (pi-rim′ĭ-dēn) an organic compound, which is the fundamental form of the pyrimidine bases, some being constituents of nucleic acids. See also nitrogenous base and pyrimidine bases, under BASE. **p. antagonist, p. inhibitor,** pyrimidine ANALOGUE.

pyrimidinetrione (pi-rim′ĭ-din-tri′ōn) barbituric ACID.

Pyrisept trademark for *cetylpyridinium chloride* (see under CETYLPYRIDINIUM).

pyro- [Gr. *pyr* fire] a combining form meaning fire or heat or, in chemistry, produced by heating.

pyrocatechol (pi-ro-kat′ĕ-kol) [*pyro-* + *catechu* rubiaceous plant *Ourouparia gambir*] a crystallizable substance obtained from catechu, 1,2-dihydroxybenzene. Formerly used as external antiseptic. It may cause eczematous dermatitis. Pyrocatechol forms the aromatic portion of catecholamines. Called also *catechol*.

pyrogen (pi′ro-jen) [*pyro-* + *gennan* to produce] a chemical substance, such as a protein, a breakdown product of protein, a mucopolysaccharide, or any other substance capable of increasing body temperature. See also CALOR and FEVER. **bacterial p.,** endotoxin. **distilled water p.,** a filtrable thermostable product of bacterial activity that accumulates in distilled water and tends to cause severe chills when the water is injected into the body. **endogenous p.,** a pyrogen originating within the body, believed to be a lipoprotein derived from cell membranes of phagocytized neutrophils and monocytes, which acts upon the central nervous system, especially the temperature-regulating center in the hypothalamus that controls the production and dissipation of body heat. It is believed to be produced as a result of phagocytosis caused by invading foreign organisms and by the action of exogenous pyrogens on the leukocytes and, possibly, the blood plasma, thus acting as an intermediate agent in producing fever by exogenous pyrogens, such as bacterial endotoxins. Called also *leukocytic p.* **exogenous p.,** a pyrogen originating from the outside of the body, as from invading toxic foreign organisms, or being injected into the tissue. It is believed to act on the leukocytes and, possibly, the blood plasma, thus causing the release of endogenous pyrogens which, in turn, act on the temperature-regulating center of the hypothalamus in producing fever. **leukocytic p.,** endogenous p.

pyroglobulin (pi″ro-glob′u-lin) [*pyro-* + *globulin*] a globulin which precipitates out from serum at 56°C and redissolves when the serum is cooled. Pyroglobulins are found most commonly in multiple myeloma.

pyrometer (pi-rom′ĕ-ter) [*pyro-* + Gr. *metron* measure] an instrument for measuring the intensity of heat, especially for temperatures which cannot be measured with a mercury thermometer. See also porcelain FURNACE.

Pyronil trademark for *pyrrobutamine.*

pyrophosphatase [E.C.3.6.1] (pi″ro-fos′fah-tās) a group of hydrolases that act on acid anhydrides; they catalyze the hydrolysis of central pyrophosphate linkages. **ATP p.** [E.C.1.6.1.8], a hydrolase acting on acid anhydrides, which catalyzes the splitting of adenosine triphosphate to AMP and pyrophosphate. Called also *ATPase.* **inorganic p.** [E.C.3.6.1.1], a type of pyrophosphatase occurring in a wide variety of tissues, which catalyzes the hydrolysis of pyrophosphate to two orthophosphates. Called also *pyrophosphate phosphohydrolase.*

pyrophosphate (pi″ro-fos′fāt) a salt of pyrophosphoric acid. **calcium p.,** CALCIUM pyrophosphate. **ditin p.,** *stannous p.* **p. phosphohydrolase,** inorganic PYROPHOSPHATASE. **stannous p.,** $Sn_2P_2O_7$, occurring as white, free-flowing crystals that are insoluble in water, but soluble in concentrated acid and alkali. Used as a diagnostic aid in radioactive bone scanning and as an ingredient in certain dentifrices. Called also *ditin p., diphosphoric acid tin salt,* and *ditin diphosphate.* Trademark: Techne-Scan PYP. **tetraethyl p.,** a cholinesterase inhibitor,

diphosphoric acid tetraethyl ester, occurring as a dark amber to colorless liquid that is miscible with water, but not with petroleum oils. Used as an insecticide. It is very poisonous to insects and warm-blooded animals. Abbreviated *TEPP.* Sometimes written *tetraethylpyrophosphate.* Trademarks: Bladan, Killax, Nifos T, Tetron.

pyrophosphokinase (pi″ro-fos fo-ki′nās) pyrophosphotransferase.

pyrophosphotransferase [E.C.2.7.6] (pi″ro-fos′fo-trans′fer-ās) a sub-subclass of transferases, the enzymes of which catalyze the transfer of pyrophosphate, as from ATP to thiamine to form AMP and thiamine pyrophosphate. Called also *diphosphotransferase* and *pyrophosphokinase.* See also KINASE (1).

Pyroplast trademark for a dimethacrylate resin; used for a veneer on metal crowns or as a jacket for a prepared tooth.

pyrrobutamine (pir″ro′bu′tah-mēn) an antihistaminic drug with low sedative effects that blocks histamine mediation at the H_1 receptor, 1-[4-(*p*-chlorophenyl)-3-phenyl-2-butenyl] pyrrolidine. Used in the form of the phosphate salt in the treatment of allergic diseases. It occurs as a white crystalline powder with a faint odor, which is readily soluble in water, slightly soluble in alcohol, and insoluble in ether and chloroform. Trademark: Pyronil.

Pyrrocycline-N trademark for *rolitetracycline nitrate* (see under rolitetracycline).

pyrrole (pir′ōl) a compound, C_4H_5N, occurring as a colorless liquid (when freshly distilled) with chloroform-like odor, which darkens and readily polymerizes by the action of light. It is soluble in alcohol, ether, and acids, but insoluble in water and dilute alkalies. Used in the production of pharmaceuticals. Pyrrole is moderately toxic on ingestion or inhalation of its fumes. Called also *azole, divinylenimine,* and *imidole.*

pyruvate (pi″roo-vāt) a salt or ester of pyruvic acid,

$$CH_3-\overset{\overset{\displaystyle O}{\|}}{C}-\overset{\overset{\displaystyle O}{\|}}{C}-O^-.$$

In biochemistry, the term is used interchangeably with pyruvic acid, even though pyruvate technically refers to the negatively charged ion; the reason being that at cellular pH most of the pyruvic acid is in the form of the anion. **p. kinase,** pyruvate KINASE.

pyuria (pi-u′re-ah) [Gr. *pyon* pus + *ouron* urine + *-ia*] the presence of pus in the urine.

Q

Q. electric quantity.

q symbol for the long arm of a chromosome. See also chromosome ARM and CHROMOSOME nomenclature.

q.2h. abbreviation for L. *qua′que secun′da ho′ra,* every two hours.

q.3h. abbreviation for L. *qua′que ter′tia ho′ra,* every three hours.

q.4h. abbreviation for L. *qua′que quar′ta ho′ra,* every four hours.

QAP Quality Assurance Program for Medical Care in Hospital; see under PROGRAM.

QCIM Quarterly Cumulative Index Medicus; see under INDEX.

q.d. abbreviation for L. *qua′que di′e,* every day.

QF quality FACTOR.

q.h. abbreviation for L. *qua′que ho′ra,* every hour.

q.i.d. abbreviation for L. *qua′ter in di′e,* four times a day.

q.l. abbreviation for L. *quan′tum li′bet,* as much as desired.

q.n.s. quantity not sufficient.

q.p. abbreviation for L. *quan′tum pla′ceat,* as much as desired.

q.q.h. abbreviation for L. *qua′que quar′ta ho′ra,* every four hours.

Qq.hor. abbreviation for L. *qua′que ho′ra,* every hour.

QRS see ELECTROCARDIOGRAPHY.

q.s. abbreviation for L. *quan′tum sa′tis,* sufficient quantity.

q.suff. abbreviation for L. *quan′tum suf′ficit,* as much as suffices.

qt quart.

qter symbol for an end of the long arm of a chromosome. See also chromosome ARM and CHROMOSOME nomenclature.

Quaalude trademark for *methaqualone.*

quack (kwak) one who fraudulently misrepresents his qualifications or ability in the diagnosis and treatment of diseases or the effects to be achieved by the treatment he offers. See also CHARLATAN.

quackery (kwak′er-e) the fraudulent misrepresentation of one's ability and experience in the diagnosis and treatment of disease or of the effects to be achieved by the treatment offered. Called also *empiricism.*

quadrangle (kwod′rang-g'l) [L. *quadratus* squared + *angulus* angle] 1. a figure having four angles, or sides. 2. Black's term for a dental instrument having four angulations in the shank connecting the handle, or shaft, with the working portion of the instrument, the blade or nib.

quadrangular (kwod-rang′gu-lar) [*quadri-* + L. *angulus* angle] having four angles.

quadrant (kwod′rant) [L. *quadrans* quarter] 1. one quarter of a circle; that portion of the circumference of a circle that subtends an angle of 90 degrees. 2. any one of four corresponding parts or quarters. 3. each of four sections or quarters of dentition, determined by an imaginary midline, dividing each dental arch into two halves. The four quarters are the maxillary right and left and the mandibular left and right quadrants. In the primary dentition each quadrant contains the central incisor, lateral incisor, canine, first molar, and second molar. In the permanent dentition each quadrant contains the central incisor, lateral incisor, canine, first premolar, second premolar, first molar, second molar, and third molar. See illustration and see additional illustrations at dental CHART.

Maxillary right | Maxillary left

Anterior

Posterior

Posterior

Posterior

Posterior

Anterior

Mandibular right | Mandibular left

Occlusal views of the dental arches divided into quadrants. Also indicated are the anterior and posterior teeth. (From H. O. Torres and A. Ehrlich: Modern Dental Assisting. 2nd ed. Philadelphia, W. B. Saunders Co., 1980.)

quadrat (kwod'rat) [L. *quadratus* squared] a rectangular, usually square plot used in ecological studies.

quadrate (kwod'rāt) [L. *quadratus* squared] square or squared; four-sided.

quadratus (kwod-ra'tus) [L.] 1. squared; four-sided. 2. musculus quadratus. See depressor muscle of lower lip and levator muscle of upper lip, under MUSCLE. **q. la'bii inferio'ris**, depressor muscle of lower lip; see under MUSCLE. **q. la'bii superio'ris**, levator muscle of upper lip; see under MUSCLE. **q. men'ti**, depressor muscle of lower lip; see under MUSCLE.

quadri- [L. *quadratus* squared] a combining form denoting four, or fourfold.

quadribasic (kwod″rĭ-ba'sik) having four replaceable atoms of hydrogen.

quadricuspid (kwod″rĭ-kus'pid) [*quadri-* + L. *cuspis* point] 1. having four cusps; said of a tooth, or of a semilunar (aortic or pulmonary) heart valve with four cusps. 2. a tooth with four cusps.

quadrigeminal (kwod″rĭ-jem'ĭ-nal) [L. *quadrigeminus*] fourfold, or in four parts; forming a group of four.

quadrilateral (kwod″rĭ-lat'er-al) [*quadri-* + L. *latus* side] 1. having four sides. 2. a four-sided figure, or postulate.

quadrilocular (kwod″rĭ-lok'u-lar) [*quadri-* + L. *loculus* a small space] having four cells, cavities, or chambers.

quadrisection (kwod″rĭ-sek'shun) [*quadri-* + L. *sectio* cut] division into four parts.

quadrivalent (kwod″rĭ-va'lent) [*quadri-* + L. *valere* to be worth] having a chemical valence or combining power of four.

quadrupl. abbreviation for L. *quadruplica'to*, four times as much.

Qualimet trademark for a nickel-chromium base-metal crown and bridge alloy.

qualitative, qualitive (kwol'ĭ-ta″tiv, kwol'ĭ-tiv) [L. *qualitativus*] pertaining to quality.

quality (kwol'ĭ-te) [L. *qualitas*] 1. a characteristic, property, or attribute; a feature. 2. in radiology, the ability of a particular form or type of ionizing radiation to penetrate matter.

quanta (kwon'tah) [L.] plural of *quantum*.

quantimeter (kwon-tim'ĕ-ter) [*quantum* + L. *metrom* measure] an apparatus for measuring the quantity of x-rays generated by a tube.

quantum (kwon'tum), pl. *quan'ta* [L. "as much as"] a unit of energy. See quantum THEORY. See also PHOTON. **q. number**, quantum NUMBER.

quarantine (kwor'an-tēn) [It. *quarantina*] isolation of persons or animals suspected of having been exposed to a communicable disease in order to prevent the infection from spreading.

quart (kwort) [L. *quartus* fourth] a unit of capacity (liquid or solid), being one-fourth of a gallon and consisting of 2 pints. Abbreviated **qt**. See also *Tables of Weights and Measures* at WEIGHT. **British imperial q.**, one-fourth of the British imperial gallon, being equivalent to 2 pints (69.355 cubic inches), or 1.136 liters. **U.S. q.**, one-fourth of the U.S. gallon, being equivalent to 2 pints (57.75 cubic inches), or 0.946 liters.

quartz (kwarts) a crystalline form of silicon dioxide. Quartz is a component of dental porcelain which forms a refractory skeleton about which the other materials in the porcelain (kaolin and feldspar) may fuse and flow. It helps the crown hold its form during firing, as its fusion temperature is very high, but does undergo some dissolution in the liquid portion of the porcelain. The coefficient of thermal expansion of the undissolved quartz may form a component of the over-all coefficient of expansion of the porcelain. Quartz is also used as a component of dental investments. **fused q.**, amorphous silica showing no inversion at any temperature below its fusion point.

quasi- [L. *quasi* as if, as though] a prefix signifying almost, seemingly, or resembling.

Quat., quat. abbreviation for L. *quat'tuor,* four.

quater in die (kwah'ter in de'a) [L.] four times a day. Abbreviated *q.i.d.*

quaternary (kwah'ter-ner″e, kwah-ter'nah-re) [L. *quaternarius*, from *quattuor* four] 1. fourth in order. 2. containing four elements or groups.

Quatrachlor trademark for *benzethonium chloride* (see under BENZETHONIUM).

Quatrefage's angle [Jean Louis Armand de *Quatrefage* de Bréau, French naturalist, 1810–1892] parietal ANGLE.

Quatrex trademark for *tetracycline hydrochloride* (see under TETRACYCLINE).

quench (kwench) 1. to satisfy or allay thirst. 2. to cool suddenly by plunging into a liquid, as in tempering steel.

Quesnel see Lhermitte-Cornil-Quesnel SYNDROME.

Queyrat's erythroplasia [Auguste *Queyrat*, French dermatologist, born 1872] see under ERYTHROPLASIA.

quicklime (kwik'līm) CALCIUM oxide.

Quick's test [Armand J. *Quick*, American physician, born 1894] see under TEST.

quicksilver (kwik-sil'ver) mercury.

quinacrine (kwin'ah-krin) an acridine derivative, 6-chloro-9-[[4-(diethylamino)-1-methylbutyl]-amino-2-methoxyadine]. **q. bands**, see under BAND. **q. hydrochloride**, the dihydrochloride salt of quinacrine, occurring as a bright yellow crystalline powder. It has been used as an anthelmintic in the treatment of intestinal large tapeworms, but has mostly been replaced by less toxic agents. Formerly used as an antimalarial. It is used for staining chromosomes (see Q bands, under BAND). Its use may be associated with transient psychosis and oral lesions similar to those seen in lichen planus (see Atabrine STOMATITIS). Trademark: Atabrine. **q. mustard**, 2-methoxy-6-chloro-9-[4-bis(beta-chloroethyl)amino-1-methylbutylamino]acridine. A nitrogen mustard analogue of quinacrine used primarily as a stain in chromosome banding. See also Q-BANDING.

quinalbarbitone (kwin″al-bar'bĭ-tōn) secobarbital. **q. sodium**, SECOBARBITAL sodium.

Quincke's edema (disease) [Heinrich Irenaeus *Quincke*, physician in Kiel, 1842–1922] see under EDEMA.

quinethazone (kwin-eth'ah-zōn) a quinazoline diuretic agent with antihypertensive properties, 7-chloro-2-ethyl-1,2,3,4-tetrahydro-4-oxo-6-quinazolinesulfonamide, occurring as a white to yellowish, bitter, odorless, crystalline powder that is soluble in polyethylene glycol, propylene glycol, ethanol, alkali hydroxide and carbamate solutions, slightly soluble in pyridine, and very slightly soluble in water. It has pharmacological and toxicological properties similar to those of thiazide diuretics. Trademarks: Aquamox, Hydromox.

quinidine (kwin'ĭ-dēn) a dextrorotatory isomer of quinine, 6-methoxy-α-(5-vinyl-2-quinuclidinyl)-4-quinolinemethanol, obtained from *Cinchona* and other plants. It occurs as colorless, lustrous crystals that are efflorescent on exposure to air and are soluble in chloroform, alcohol, and ether, and very slightly in water. Pharmacologically, it is similar to quinine, being somewhat less toxic. Quinidine depresses skeletal and cardiac muscles and increases the duration of the effective refractory period, decreases excitability, and slows the rate of conduction of the wave of excitation. Used in the treatment of arrhythmias. Called also *β-quinine*.

quinine (kwi′nīn, kwin′in, kwin′en) the major alkaloid from the bark of the plant *Cinchoma officinalis*, occurring as a white, amorphous, odorless powder or crystals with a bitter taste, which is soluble in alcohol, ether, chloroform, carbon disulfide, oils, glycerol, alkalies, and acids, and slightly soluble in water. It has analgesic, anesthetic, local irritant, cardiac depressant, and moderate antipyretic properties. Quinine also destroys unicellular organisms, including certain bacteria, trypanosomes, infusoria, yeasts, plasmodia, spermatozoa, and salt-water amebae. Other pharmacological properties include sensory nerve stimulation followed by paralysis in larger doses, edema, pain, and fibrosis; gastric pain, nausea, and vomiting following oral administration of large doses; pain, sterile abscesses, thrombosis, and sclerosis after injection; curariform effect on the muscle; and inhibition of gastric secretion. Quinine is absorbed chiefly through the small intestine and metabolized by the liver, but some is excreted unchanged in the urine. Used chiefly in the treatment of malaria.

quinoid (kwin′oid) containing the chromatophoric group:

quinoline (kwin′o-lēn) a poisonous, aromatic compound derived from coal tar or produced by heating aniline with glycerol and nitrobenzene in the presence of sulfuric acid. It occurs as a colorless, hygroscopic liquid with a penetrating odor, which darkens with age and is soluble in water, alcohol, ether, and

carbon disulfide. Used in the treatment of malaria, as a preservative for anatomical specimens, as a solvent for resins, and in the production of various drugs, such as niacin. Called also *chonoleine* and *chinoline*. Trademark: Leucoline.

quinone (kwi-nōn′, kwin′ōn) a compound, 2,5-cyclohexadiene-1,4-dione, occurring as yellow crystals with an irritating odor, solube in ether and alcohol, being only slightly soluble in hot water. It is a highly toxic substance, which may cause necrotic lesions, erythema, dermatitis, and discoloration. Used as an oxidizing agent. Called also *benzoquinone*. See also UBIQUINONE.

Quinq. abbreviation for L. *quin′que*, five.

quinquecuspid (kwin″kwĕ-kus′pid) [L. *quinque* five + *cuspis* point] 1. having five cusps. 2. a tooth with five cusps.

quinquetubercular (kwin″kwĕ-tu-ber′ku-lar) having five tubercles or cusps.

quinsy (kwin′ze) [Gr. *kynanche* sore throat] peritonsillar ABSCESS. **lingual q.,** suppurative inflammation of the lingual tonsil.

quint (kwint) a combination of five of a kind. **Hanau's q.,** Thielemann's PRINCIPLE.

quint. abbreviation for L. *quin′tus*, fifth.

quintan (kwin′tan) [L. *quintanus* of the fifth] recurring every fifth day.

Quotane trademark for *dimethisoquin hydrochloride* (see under DIMETHISOQUIN).

quotient (kwo′shent) a number obtained as the result of division. See also EQUATION and INDEX. **growth q.,** that portion of the entire food energy which is utilized for the purpose of growth. See also Rubner's LAW (2). **Ayala's q.,** a quotient in examination of the cerebrospinal pressure, obtained by dividing the pressure after removal of 10 ml of cerebrospinal fluid by 10. Normal values are 5.5 to 6.5. A value under 5 indicates a small reservoir, as in subarachnoid block; over 7 means a large reservoir, as may be encountered in serous meningitis or hydrocephalus. Called also *Ayala's equation* and *Ayala's index*.

q.v. abbreviation for L. *quan′tum vis*, as much as you please, and for *quod vi′de*, which see.

R

R 1. roentgen. 2. Rankine or Réamur (see under SCALE). 3. organic RADICAL (in chemical formulas). 4. rough COLONY. 5. Broadbent registration POINT. 6. right; usually stamped on paired instruments to differentiate right-handed instruments from left-handed ones.

R. abbreviation for L. *remo′tum*, far.

r 1. formerly, roentgen; now R. 2. ring CHROMOSOME; see also CHROMOSOME nomenclature.

℞ symbol for L. *rec′ipe*, take. See PRESCRIPTION.

Ra radium.

rabbetting (rab′et-ing) impaction of the denticulated broken surfaces of a fractured bone.

Rabenhorst syndrome cardioacrofascial SYNDROME.

rabid (rab′id) [L. *rabidus*] affected with rabies.

rabies (ra′bēz) [L. *rabere* to rage] an acute infectious disease of the central nervous system, usually fatal in mammals ranging from bats to cattle, caused by an RNA virus. Human infection results from the bite of a rabid animal, such as a bat, wolf, dog, cat, mongoose, or other animal. The incubation period in man is from one to three months, being shorter after bites near the brain and after those farther away. The earliest symptoms are numbness and tingling around the site of infection; soon generalized hyperexcitability occurs, followed by fever, paralysis of the muscles of deglutition and glottal spasm at first provoked by drinking of fluids or by the sight of fluids, and maniacal behavior. Convulsions, tetany, and respiratory paralysis are the terminal events. Called also *hydrophobia* and *lyssa*.

racemase [E.C.5.1.1] (ra′se-mās) a subclass of isomerases which catalyze racemization.

racemate (ra′sĕ-māt) an equimolecular mixture of two enantiomorphic isomers, being optically inactive in solution because of the presence of the same number of dextro- and levorotatory molecules. In the solid state, it may have the properties of a loosely bound molecular compound. Called also *raceme, racemic form, racemic mixture,* and *racemic modification*.

raceme (ra-sēm′) [L. *racemus* a bunch of grapes] racemate.

racemic (ra-se′mik) made up of two enantiomorphic isomers and therefore optically inactive.

racemization (ra″sĕ-mi-za″shun) the transformation of one-half of the molecules of an optically active compound into molecules which possess exactly the opposite (mirror-image) configura-

tion, with complete loss of rotatory power because of the statistical balance between equal numbers of dextro- and levorotatory molecules. Cf. MUTAROTATION.

racemose (ras′ĕ-mōs) [L. *racemus* a bunch of grapes] resembling a bunch of grapes on its stalk; staphyline.

racephedrine (ra-sef′e-drin) the *dl*-form of ephedrine (see EPHEDRINE). **r. hydrochloride,** the *dl*-form of ephedrine hydrochloride (see EPHEDRINE hydrochloride).

rachianesthesia (ra″ke-an″es-the′ze-ah) anesthesia produced by the injection of the anesthetic into the spinal canal; spinal anesthesia.

Racine's syndrome [W. *Racine*] see under SYNDROME.

rad (rad) [acronym for *r*adiation *a*bsorbed *d*ose] a unit of measurement of the absorbed dose of ionizing radiation. It corresponds to an energy transfer of 100 ergs per gram of any absorbing material (including tissue). Cf. GRAY.

radectomy (ra-dek′to-me) [L. *radix* root + Gr. *ektomē* excision] resection of the root of a tooth, in whole or in part.

radial (ra′de-al) [L. *radialis*] 1. pertaining to the radius. 2. radiating; spreading outward from a common center.

radiant (ra de-ant) [L. *radians*] 1. diverging from a common center. 2. a radioactive substance.

radiatio (ra-de-a′she-o), pl. *radiatio′nes* [L.] a radiating structure; used in anatomical nomenclature to designate a collection of nerve fibers connecting different portions of the brain. See also RADIATION.

radiation (ra-de-a′shun) [L. *radiatio*] 1. divergence from a common center. 2. a radiating structure made up of divergent elements, as one of the fiber tracts of the brain. Called also radiatio. 3. The act or process of radiating, as pain radiating from one part of the body to another. 4. the act or process of transfer of energy in the form of waves or particles from one place to another without a material carrier. 5. a ray. 6. radiant energy or beam. See also IRRADIATION, radiation INJURY, and radiation SICKNESS. **actinic r.,** radiation beyond the violet end of the spectrum that produces chemical effects. In roentgenography, actinic rays produce photochemical effects, such as the production of a latent image in a film emulsion by visible light or x-rays. Called also *actinic rays* and *chemical rays*. **alpha r., α-r.,** streams of alpha particles; see alpha PARTICLE. **annihilation r.,** photons produced when an electron and positron unite and cease to exist; the annihilation of a positron-electron pair results in two photons, each of 0.51 Mev energy. **background r.,** in a given area, the sum total of radiations arising from radioactive materials located in the vicinity, cosmic rays, radioactive materials present in the building, and all other radiations that are not emitted by the x-ray generator or any other radiation-generating devices directly applicable to the technique used. Called also *natural r.* **beta r., β-r.,** streams of beta particles; see beta PARTICLE. **braking r.,** bremsstrahlung. **r. build-up,** radiation BUILD-UP. **central r.,** central RAY. **characteristic r.,** radiation emitted when an electron is ejected from an atom due to bombardment by an outside electron of a certain energy. Electrons ejected from the K, L, M, N, and O orbits of an atom give rise to the K, L, M, N, and O radiations (or rays), respectively. Vacancies on orbits from which electrons have been ejected are filled immediately by electrons from adjacent lower energy shells, whereby ejection of an electron from the K shell results in filling the vacancy with an electron from the L shell, thus giving rise to the characteristic radiation of the K electron. Characteristic radiations of the commonly used contrast agents, such as iodine or barium, are used for diagnostic purposes, whereby selecting an appropriate energy diagnostic x-ray maximum absorption of x-rays by the iodine or barium contrast media can be achieved, thus deriving the highest possible contrast between the contrast medium and surrounding tissue, e.g., 70 KVP x-rays being maximally absorbed by iodinated contrast material. Called also *discrete r.* and *characteristic ray.* See also *homogeneous r.* **corpuscular r.,** particle r. **cosmic r.,** cosmic rays; see under RAY. **discrete r.,** characteristic r. **electromagnetic r.** radiation transferred by means of oscillatory variation in electric and magnetic fields, which includes radio waves, microwaves, infrared waves, visible light, ultraviolet rays, x-rays, and gamma rays. See table. See also electro-

APPROXIMATE WAVELENGTH RANGE OF ELECTROMAGNETIC WAVES

Radiations	Wavelengths in Å Units
Radio waves	10^{14} to 10^{11}
Hertzian waves	10^{10} to 10^{9}
Short electric waves	10^{8}
Infrared rays	10^{7} to 10^{5}
Visible light rays	10^{4}
Ultraviolet light rays	10^{3}
X-rays	10^{2} to 10^{-1}
Gamma rays	10^{-2}
Cosmic rays	10^{-4}

magnetic waves, under WAVE. **fluorescent r.,** energy emitted as an electromagnetic photon, sometimes within the visible spectrum, after irradiation of a tissue or another structure with x-rays or ultraviolet rays, the wavelength of fluorescent rays being longer than that of the energy absorbed. Called also *fluorescent rays.* See also FLUORESCENCE and secondary rays, under RAY. **gamma r., γ-r.,** see gamma rays; see under RAY. **hard r.,** radiation of higher effective energies and shorter wavelengths. Called also *hard rays.* See also HARDNESS (3). Cf. *soft r.* **heterogeneous r.,** radiation consisting of a beam of particles of various energies, or having different frequencies, or containing different types of particles. See also *white r.* and BREMSSTRAHLUNG. **homogeneous r.,** radiation consisting of an extremely narrow band of frequencies or a beam of monoenergetic particles of a single type. Called also *homogeneous beam.* See also *characteristic r.* and *monochromatic r.* **infrared r.,** infrared rays; see under RAY. **internal r.,** interstitial r. **interstitial r.,** radiation emitted by sources, such as radium or radon, inserted directly into the tissue. Called also *internal r.* **ionizing r.,** any radiation capable of displacing electrons from atoms or molecules, thereby producing ions. Ionizing radiations include alpha rays, beta rays, gamma rays, cosmic rays, and x-rays, and short wave ultraviolet light. **irritative r.,** radiation with ultraviolet rays to the point of erythema. **K r.,** see *characteristic r.* **L r.,** see characteristic r. **leakage r.,** radiation which escapes through the protective shielding of an x-ray generator. **M r.,** see *characteristic r.* **monochromatic r.,** electromagnetic radiation of a single wavelength or in which all photons have the same energy. Called also *monochromatic beam* and *monochromatic rays.* See also *homogeneous r.* **monoenergetic r.,** radiation of a given type, as of alpha, beta, or gamma rays, in which all particles or photons originate with and have the same energy. **N r.,** see *characteristic r.* **natural r.,** background r. **O r.,** see

characteristic r. **particle r.,** radiation other than x-rays and gamma rays, such as alpha-, beta-, proton-, neutron-, positron-, and deuteron-radiations, consisting of particles of definite mass and charge, generated through spontaneous decay of natural and artificial radioactive materials or generated artificially by accelerating neutrons or electrons propelled by a cyclotron or betatron. Called also *corpuscular r.* **photochemical r.,** any radiation capable of producing chemical changes. **primary r.,** radiation coming directly from the target of the anode of an x-ray tube, or radiation given off directly from a radioactive substance. Called also *direct ray, primary beam,* and *primary ray.* See also useful BEAM. **remnant r.,** part of the primary radiation that emerges from irradiated tissues and consists of unabsorbed primary and secondary rays generated in the tissue; it is that ionizing radiation which produces the radiographic image. Called also *remnant rays.* **scattered r.,** scattered rays; see under RAY. **secondary r.,** secondary rays; see under RAY. **secondary scattered r.,** scattered rays; see under RAY. **soft r.,** roentgen rays of long wavelength and little penetrating power. Called also *soft rays.* See also grenz rays, under RAY. Cf. *hard r.* **specific area r.,** specific area IRRADIATION. **stem r.,** x-rays given off from parts of the anode other than the target, particularly from the target support. **stray r.,** radiation other than that in the useful beam, including leakage radiation, scattered radiation, and secondary radiation. Called also *stray rays.* **thermal r.,** electromagnetic radiation emitted from the fireball produced by a nuclear explosion. **ultraviolet r.,** ultraviolet rays; see under RAY. **useful r.,** useful BEAM. **white r.,** a spectral distribution of x-rays ranging from very low energy photons to those produced by the peak kilovoltage applied across an x-ray tube; it connotes a similarity of the intensity/energy curve from an x-ray tube to the continuous optical spectrum obtained from white light. See also *heterogeneous r.* and BREMSSTRAHLUNG. **x-ray r.,** see x-rays, under RAY.

radical (rad'ĭ-kal) [L. *radicalis*] 1. directed to the cause; going to the root or source of a pathological process, such as radical surgery. 2. a group of atoms that behaves in a chemical reaction as a single atom. **acid r.,** 1. the electronegative element which combines with hydrogen to form an acid. 2. all of the acid except the hydroxyl group. **alcohol r.,** all of the alcohol molecule except the hydrogen atom of the −OH group; an alkoxy radical. **free r.,** a molecular fragment having one or more unpaired electrons, being highly reactive and short-lived with a half-life of 10^{-5} sec in an aqueous solution or less. It is conventionally indicated by a dot, as in Cl • or (C_2H_5) •.

radices (rad'ĭ-sēz) [L.] plural of *radix.*

radiciform (ra-dis'ĭ-form) [L. *radix* root + *forma* shape] shaped like a root, especially like the root of a tooth.

radicle (rad'ĭ-k'l) [L. *radicula*] a minute root; a minute branch of a blood vessel or nerve.

radicula (rah-dik'u-lah) [L.] radicle.

radicular (rah-dik'u-lar) pertaining to a root or a radicle.

radiculum (rah-dik'u-lum) [L. *radicula*] a small root; radicle. **r. appendicifor'me,** accessory ROOT.

radiectomy (ra″de-ek'to-me) [L. *radix* root + Gr. *ektomē* excision] excision of the root of a tooth; excision of one or the roots of a multirooted tooth.

radii (ra'de-i) [L.] plural of *radius.*

radio- [L. *radius* ray] a combining form denoting relationship to radiation.

radioactive (ra″de-o-ak'tiv) having the property of radioactivity.

radioactivity (ra″de-o-ak-tiv'ĭ-te) emission of radiant energy from an unstable atomic nucleus during decay of certain materials, accompanied by ejection of alpha and beta particles and gamma rays. **artificial r., induced r.,** that produced by bombarding an element with high velocity particles, as the radioactivity of synthetic radionuclides. **natural r.,** that of naturally occurring radioisotopes.

radioautography (ra″de-o-aw-tog'rah-fe) autoradiography.

radiobiology (ra″de-o-bi-ol'o-je) that branch of science concerned with the study of the principles, mechanisms, and effects of ionizing radiation on living matter.

radiocalcium (ra″de-o-kal'se-um) radioactive CALCIUM.

radiocarbon (ra″de-o-kar'bon) radioactive CARBON.

radiochemistry (ra″de-o-kem'is-tre) that branch of science concerned with the study of the chemical properties and reactions of radioactive materials.

radiocobalt (ra″de-o-ko'bawlt) radioactive COBALT.

radiode (ra'de-ōd) an instrument for the therapeutic application of a radioactive source.

radiodermatitis (ra″de-o-der′mah-ti′tis) [radio- + dermatitis] dermatitis caused by exposure to ionizing radiations; actinodermatitis.

radiodiagnosis (ra″de-o-di″ag-no′sis) diagnosis by means of x-rays and roentgenography.

radiodontics (ra″de-o-don′tiks) dental RADIOLOGY.

radiodontist (ra″de-o-don′tist) dental RADIOLOGIST.

radioecology (ra″de-o-e-kol′o-je) that branch of science concerned with the study of the effects of radiations on the living matter in the natural environment.

radioelement (ra″de-o-el′ĕ-ment) any chemical element having radioactive properties.

radiogen (ra′de-o-jen) any substance emitting radiation.

radiogenesis (ra″de-o-jen′ĕ-sis) the production of rays or radioactivity; actinogenesis.

radiogenic (ra″de-o-jen′ik) [radio- + Gr. gennan to produce] produced by irradiation.

radiogold (ra′de-o-gold) radioactive GOLD.

radiogram (ra′de-o-gram″) radiograph.

radiograph (ra′de-o-graf″) the film produced by radiography. Called also radiogram. See also IMAGE and ROENTGENOGRAM. **bite-wing r.,** a type of dental radiograph that reveals the crowns, necks, the coronal thirds of the roots of both the upper and lower teeth and the dental arches, produced on dental x-ray film that has a central protruding tab or wing on which the teeth close to hold the film in position (bite-wing film). **composite r.,** an image produced by superimposing two or more radiographs, as in superimposing a radiograph of bony tissue, whose exposed border has been cut away, on a radiograph of soft tissues. **extraoral r.,** a radiograph of the teeth and facial bones made by placing the film against the side of the head or face and projecting x-rays from a position opposite to the side of the head and face. **follow-up r.,** one made during or after therapy to allow the follow-up of the progress of disease and to ascertain the effectiveness of therapy. **interproximal r.,** an intraoral radiograph for depicting interproximal features of the teeth and the interdental bone crests, made on a film positioned by bite-wing tabs on which the teeth are closed. **intra-oral r.,** one produced on a film placed intraorally. **occlusal r.,** an intraoral radiograph made with the film held between the occluded teeth. **panoramic r.,** an extraoral body-section radiograph on which an entire maxilla, or both the maxilla and the mandible, are depicted on a single film. See PANTOMOGRAPHY. **periapical r.,** a radiograph made by the intraoral placement of film for disclosing the apices of the teeth and their contiguous tissues.

radiographic (ra″de-o-graf′ik) pertaining to or produced by radiography.

radiography (ra″de-og′rah-fe) [radio- + Gr. graphein to write] the making of a record (radiograph) of internal structures of the body by passage of x-rays or gamma rays through the body to act on specially sensitized film. See also FLUOROSCOPY, ROENTGENOGRAPHY, X-RAY GENERATOR, and x-ray TUBE. **body section r.,** tomography. **electron r.,** radiography in which an x-ray generator is used but, instead of the conventional x-ray film, the latent image is generated by an electrostatic method using a special imaging chamber. **mass r.,** radiographic examination of large groups of the population. **panoramic r.,** pantomography. **selective r.,** radiographic examination of groups of the population, selected on some special common basis. **serial r.,** the taking of several exposures of a selected area at arbitrary intervals. **spot film r.,** the making of localized instantaneous radiographs of a small anatomic area obtained (a) by rapid exposure during fluoroscopy to provide a permanent record of a transiently observed abnormality, or (b) by limitation of radiation passing through the area to improve definition and detail of the image produced. **stereoscopic r.,** stereoradiography.

radioimmunity (ra″de-o-ĭ-mu′nĭ-te) a condition of decreased sensitivity to radiation sometimes produced by repeated irradiation.

radioimmunoassay (ra″de-o-im″u-no-as′a) an assay for the determination of antigen or antibody concentration by using a radioactive-labeled substance that reacts with the substance under test. Abbreviated RIA. **liquid-phase r.,** radioimmunoassay carried out in solution. Called also soluble-phase r. **solid phase r.,** radioimmunoassay on a supporting matrix to which the antigen (ligand) or antibody is adsorbed or covalently linked. **soluble-phase r.,** liquid-phase r.

radioimmunoelectrophoresis (ra″de-o-im″u-no-e-lek″tro-fo-re′sis) immunoelectrophoresis in which precipitates are identified by adding the corresponding radioactive-labeled antigen or antibody and subjecting it to autoradiography.

radioiodine (ra″de-o-i′o-dīn) radioactive IODINE.

radioiron (ra″de-o-i′ern) radioactive IRON.

radioisotope (ra″de-o-i′so-tōp) an isotope that transmutes into another element with emission of corpuscular or electromagnetic radiations. Such isotopes occur naturally or may be produced by bombardment of a common chemical element with high velocity particles. Called also radioactive isotope. See table.

TABLE OF COMMON RADIOISOTOPES

Element	Isotope	Half-Life	Element	Isotope	Half-Life
Arsenic	As^{76}	26.7 hr.	Plutonium	*Pu^{239}	24.3×10^3 yr.
Bromine	Br^{82}	36 hr.		Pu^{241}	13 yr.
Calcium	Ca^{41}	1×10^5 yr.		Pu^{242}	3.8×10^5 yr.
	Ca^{45}	180 days	Potassium	*K^{40}	1×10^9 yr.
	Ca^{47}	4.7 days	Radium	*Ra^{226}	16.2×10^2 yr.
Carbon	*C^{14}	5.6×10^3 yr.	Radon	*Rn^{222}	3.82 days
Chlorine	Cl^{136}	3×10^5 yr.	Silver	Ag^{110}	24 sec.
Cobalt	Co^{58}	71 days		Ag^{111}	7.5 days
Copper	Cu^{64}	12.8 hr.	Sodium	Na^{22}	2.6 yr.
Gold	Au^{198}	2.69 days		Na^{24}	15 hr.
Hydrogen	*H^3	12.3 yr.	Strontium	Sr^{85}	64 days
Iodine	I^{129}	1×10^7 yr.		Sr^{89}	51 days
	I^{131}	8.05 days		Sr^{90}	28 yr.
Iron	Fe^{55}	2.9 yr.	Sulfur	S^{35}	87 days
	Fe^{59}	45 days	Thorium	Th^{228}	1.91 yr.
Lead	Pb^{202}	1×10^5 yr.		*Th^{232}	1.4×10^{10} days
	*Pb^{210}	19.4 yr.	Tin	Sn^{113}	119 days
Mercury	Hg^{197}	65 hr.	Uranium	U^{233}	1.6×10^5 yr.
	Hg^{203}	47 days		*U^{234}	2.5×10^5 yr.
Molybdenum	Mo^{99}	67 hr.		*U^{235}	7.1×10^8 yr.
Nickel	Ni^{59}	8×10^4 yr.		*U^{238}	4.5×10^9 yr.
	Ni^{63}	125 yr.	Zinc	Zn^{65}	245 days
Phosphorus	P^{32}	14.2 days			

*Naturally occurring radioactive isotopes. (Modified from G. W. Shafer, M. K. Hine, and B. M. Levy: A Textbook of Oral Pathology. 3rd ed. Philadelphia, W. B. Saunders Co., 1974.)

radiolesion (ra″de-o-le′zhun) a lesion caused by radiation injury (see under INJURY).

radiologic, radiological (ra″de-o-log′ik, ra″de-o-loj′ĭ-kal) pertaining to radiology.

radiologist (ra″de-ol′o-jist) a physician who has been licensed to practice in radiology after successfully fulfilling the requirements for the degree of Doctor of Medicine, completing a 1-year internship and a 3-year residency, and passing medical specialty board examinations. See also ROENTGENOLOGIST. Cf. radiologic TECHNOLOGIST. **dental r.**, a dentist who specializes in the interpretation of radiographic findings. Called also *radiodontist.*

radiology (ra″de-ol′o-je) the science dealing with the study and application of radiations and radioactive substances, especially in the treatment and diagnosis of disease. See also ROENTGENOLOGY. **dental r.**, the branch of radiology dealing primarily with the orofacial structures. Called also *oral r.* and *radiodontics.* **oral r.**, dental r. **therapeutic r.**, radiotherapy.

radiolucency (ra″de-o-lu′sen-se) the property of being radiolucent.

radiolucent (ra-de-o-lu′sent) [*radio-* + L. *lucere* to shine] pertaining to substances and materials that permit the passage of radiant energy, such as x-rays. Radiolucent substances, such as adipose tissues, gas, and air, appear on the exposed film as dark areas. See also RADIOTRANSPARENCY.

radiometer (ra″de-om′ĕ-ter) an instrument for measuring radiant energy. Called also *roentgenometer.* See also METER. **pastille r.**, a radiation meter consisting of a color index by means of which the color changes in the pastilles, before and after irradiation, may be estimated. **photographic r.**, a radiation meter that uses strips of photographic paper which, after exposure to radiation and development, are compared with a half-tone color index.

radiomicrometer (ra″de-o-mi-krom′ĕ-ter) [*radio-* + Gr. *mikros* small + *metron* measure] a radiation meter for detecting minute changes of radiant energy.

radiomimetic (rad″de-o-mi-met′ik) [*radio-* + Gr. *mimetikos* imitative] 1. exerting effects similar to those of ionizing radiation. 2. an agent capable of exerting effects similar to those of ionizing radiation, said of alkylating agents (see under AGENT).

radionecrosis (ra″de-o-ne-kro′sis) necrotic changes in tissue or ulceration due to radiant energy. See also radiation INJURY.

radionuclide (ra″de-o-nu′klīd) a nuclide which has an unstable nucleus and emits radiation. Called also *radioactive nuclide.* See RADIOISOTOPE.

radiopacity (ra″de-o-pās′ĭ-te) the property of being radiopaque.

radiopaque (ra″de-o-pāk) [*radio-* + L. *opacus* dark, obscure] pertaining to substances and materials that do not permit the passage of radiant energy, such as x-rays. Radiopaque substances, such as bones and other calcium-containing tissues, appear on the exposed film as light or white areas.

radioparent (ra″de-o-par′ent) permitting the passage of radiation.

radiophosphorus (ra″de-o-fos′fo-rus) radioactive PHOSPHORUS.

radiophysics (ra″de-o-fiz′iks) the physics of radiology.

radioresistance (ra″de-o-re-zis′tans) resistance, as of a tissue or cell, to irradiation.

radiosensitive (ra″de-o-sen′si-tiv) sensitive to radiant energy, as x-ray or other radiation, said of tissue, skin, or tumors.

radiosensitivity (ra″de-o-sen″sĭ-tiv′ĭ-te) sensitivity of tissues to radiations. See table. See also radiation INJURY, radiation SICKNESS, and whole-body IRRADIATION.

radiotelemetry (ra″de-o-tel-em′ĕ-tre) the determination or measurement of various factors, the specific data being transmitted by radio waves from the object of measurement to the recording apparatus.

radiotherapy (ra″de-o-ther′ah-pe) [*radio-* + Gr. *therapeia* cure] the treatment of diseases by ionizing radiation. Called also *radiation therapy* and *therapeutic radiology.* See also ROENTGENOTHERAPY. **external r.**, that in which the source of radiation and the radioactive particles are external to the tissue being treated. See also PLESIOTHERAPY and TELETHERAPY. **internal r.**, plesiotherapy in which the source of radiation is placed within the body, either within the tissues (*interstitial*) or in a body cavity (*intracavitary*) through the use of radiation needles or radon or radiogold seeds. **interstitial r.**, that administered with the radioactive element contained in devices (e.g., needles or wire) inserted directly into the tissue. **intracavitary r.**, that in which the radioactive element is introduced into a natural body cavity.

RADIOSENSITIVITY OF SPECIALIZED CELLS AND THEIR TUMORS

Radio-sensitivity	Normal Cells	Tumors
High	Lymphoid, hematopoietic (marrow), germ cells, intestinal epithelium, ovarian follicular cells	Leukemia—lymphoma, seminoma, dysgerminoma, granulosa cell carcinoma
Fairly high	Epidermal epithelium, adnexal structures (hair follicles, sebaceous glands), oropharyngeal stratified epithelium, urinary bladder epithelium, esophageal epithelium, gastric gland epithelium, ureteral epithelium	Squamous cell carcinoma of skin, oropharyngeal, esophageal, cervical and bladder epithelium, adenocarcinoma of gastric epithelium
Medium	Connective tissue, glia, endothelium, growing cartilage or bone	Endothelio- and angiosarcomas, astrocytomas, the vasculature and connective tissue elements of all tumors
Fairly low	Mature cartilage or bone cells, mucous or serous gland epithelium, pulmonary epithelium, renal epithelium, hepatic epithelium, pancreatic epithelium, pituitary epithelium, thyroid epithelium, adrenal epithelium, nasopharyngeal nonstratified epithelium	Liposarcoma, chondrosarcoma, osteogenic sarcoma, adenocarcinoma of: breast epithelium hepatic epithelium renal epithelium pancreatic epithelium thyroid epithelium adrenal gland epithelium colon epithelium, squamous cell cancer of the lung
Low	Muscle cells, ganglion cells	Rhabdomyosarcoma, leiomyosarcoma, ganglioneuroma

(From S. L. Robbins and R. S. Cotran: Pathologic Basis of Disease. 2nd ed. Philadelphia, W. B. Saunders Co., 1979; adapted from R. Rubin and G. W. Casarett: Clinical Radiation Pathology, Philadelphia, W. B. Saunders Co., 1968.)

radiotomy (ra"de-ot'o-me) [radio- + Gr. *tomē* a cutting] a body section radiographic technique. See TOMOGRAPHY.

radiotransparency (ra"de-o-trans-par'en-se) the quality of being pervious to x-rays or other forms of radiation. See also RADIOLUCENT.

radisectomy (ra"dĭ-sek'to-me) root AMPUTATION.

radium (ra'de-um) [so called from its radiant quality] a rare radioactive element in the uranium decay series. Symbol, *Ra*; atomic weight 226; atomic number 88; half-life 1622 years. It is found mainly in pitchblende and undergoes spontaneous disintegration with formation of a gas called *radon* (half-life 3.85 days). In this process radium emits alpha particles. Radon (alpha emitter) on deposit in solid form disintegrates into a series of decay products: radium A (half-life 3 min), radium B (half-life 26.7 min), and radium C (half-life 19.5 min). The beta particles and gamma radiations used in clinical therapy originate from radium B and C. With radium in a sealed container and the same number of atoms of each decay product disintegrating per second, radium and its decay products are in equilibrium. In this state the formation of beta particles and gamma rays reaches its maximum. In clinical gamma-ray therapy, shielding off of the beta particles can be accomplished by a metallic container, e.g., of gold or platinum. A glass wall container permits irradiation with beta particles as well as gamma rays. **r. emanation,** radon. **r. F,** polonium.

radius (ra'de-us), pl. *ra'dii* [L. "spoke" (of a wheel)] 1. a straight line from the center to the limit of a circle; the semidiameter of a circle. 2. the bone on the outer or thumb side of the forearm. **r. fix'us,** a straight line from the hormion to the inion.

radix (ra'diks), pl. *rad'ices* [L.] the lowermost part, or a structure by which something is firmly attached. See also ROOT. **r. clin'ica** [NA], clinical ROOT. **r. den'tis** [NA], the portion of a tooth embedded in the dental alveolus. See ROOT of tooth. **r. descen'dens [mesencephalica] ner'vi trigem'ini,** mesencephalic tract of trigeminal nerve; see under TRACT. **r. facia'lis** [NA], NERVE of pterygoid canal. **r. in rad'ice,** DENS in dente. **rad'ices crania'les ner'vi accesso'rii** [NA], cranial roots of accessory nerve; see under ROOT. **r. lin'guae** [NA], ROOT of tongue. **r. lon'ga gan'glii cilia'ris,** communicating branch of nasociliary ganglion with nasociliary nerve; see under BRANCH. **r. moto'ria ner'vi trigem'ini** [NA], motor root of trigeminal nerve; see under ROOT. **r. na'si** [NA], ROOT of nose. **r. ner'vi facia'lis,** ROOT of facial nerve. **r. senso'ria ner'vi trigem'ini** [NA], sensory root of trigeminal nerve; see under ROOT. **rad'ices spina'les ner'vi accesso'rii** [NA], spinal roots of accessory nerve; see under ROOT. **r. supe'rior an'sae cervica'lis** [NA], superior root of ansa cervicalis; see under ROOT. **r. sympath'ica gan'glii submaxilla'ris,** sympathetic root of submandibular ganglion; see under ROOT.

radon (ra'don) a heavy, colorless, gaseous, radioactive element. Symbol Rn; atomic weight 222; atomic number, 86. It is obtained by the breaking up of radium, and is used in radiotherapy. Called also *radium emanation (RE).* Cf. RADIUM. ^{219}Rn is a radioactive isotope of the actinium radioactive series; ^{220}Rn is a radioactive isotope of the thorium radioactive series.

Raeder's syndrome [J. G. *Raeder*] paratrigeminal SYNDROME.

Rafluor topical gel, topical solution see under GEL and SOLUTION.

raising (rāz'ing) the act or process of elevating or lifting. **r. bite,** increase of the vertical height of the teeth, usually by means of prosthetic restoration.

rale (rahl) [Fr. *râle* rattle] an abnormal respiratory sound resembling a rattle in auscultation. Depending on the presence of fluid in the air passages, rales are distinguished as *moist* or *dry,* both usually indicating some type of pathological condition.

Ramfjord index [Sigurd P. *Ramfjord,* American dentist] periodontal INDEX.

rami (ra'mi) [L.] plural of *ramus.*

Ramibacterium (ra"mĭ-bak-te're-um) [L. *ramus* branch + Gr. *baktērion* little rod] a former genus name for bacteria made up of nonsporulating, anaerobic, gram-positive microorganisms found in the intestinal tract and sometimes associated with purulent infections. Its species have now been assigned to other genera. **R. alactolyt'icum, R. den'tium,** *Eubacterium alactolyticum;* see under EUBACTERIUM.

ramification (ram"ĭ-fi-ka'shun) [*ramus* + L. *facere* to make] 1. the act or process of branching, or distribution in branches. 2. a branch or set of branches. 3. the manner of branching. **apical r.,** the branching of the apical foramen of a tooth near its apex to form two or more ramifications. **apical r.,** root canal, accessory; see under CANAL.

ramify (ram"ĭ-fi) [*ramus* + L. *facere* to make] 1. to branch; to diverge in various directions. 2. to transverse in branches. 3. the manner of branching.

ramollissement (rah"mol-es-maw') [Fr.] softening.

Ramón y Cajal, Santiago [1852–1934] a Spanish histologist; co-winner, with Camillo Golgi, of the Nobel prize for medicine and physiology in 1906, in recognition of their work on the structure of the nervous system.

ramose (ra'mos) [L. *ramus* branch] branching; having many branches.

rampant (ram'pant) violent in action; progressing or prevailing without restraint.

rampart (ram'part) a broad elevation or mound encircling something. **maxillary r.,** a ridge or mound of epithelial cells seen in that portion of the jaw of the embryo which is to become the alveolar border.

Ramphenol trademark for a preparation, 100 mg of which contain 35 gm parachlorophenol and 65 gm camphor; used in root canal therapy and in periapical infection.

Ramsay Hunt's neuralgia, syndrome [James *Ramsay Hunt,* American neurologist, 1872–1937] see geniculate NEURALGIA and Hunt's SYNDROME.

Ramsden's eyepiece [Jesse *Ramsden,* English instrument maker and optician, 1735–1800] see under EYEPIECE.

ramuli (ram'u-li) [L.] plural of *ramulus.*

ramulus (ram'u-lus), pl. *ram'uli* [L., dim. of *ramus*] a small branch or terminal division.

ramus (ra'mus), pl. *ra'mi* [L.] a branch; used in anatomical nomenclature as a general term to designate a smaller structure given off by a larger one, or into which the larger structure divides. **ra'mi alveola'res superio'res anterio'res ner'vi infraorbita'lis** [NA], alveolar branches of infraorbital nerve, anterior superior; see under BRANCH. **r. alveola'ris supe'rior me'dius ner'vi infraorbita'lis** [NA], alveolar branch of infraorbital nerve, middle superior; see under BRANCH. **ra'mi alveola'res superio'res posterio'res ner'vi maxilla'ris** [NA], alveolar branches of maxillary nerve, posterior superior; see under BRANCH. **r. anastomot'icus,** anastomotic BRANCH. See communicating BRANCH. **r. anastomot'icus arte'riae menin'geae me'diae cum arte'ria lacrima'li** [NA], anastomotic branch of middle meningeal artery with lacrimal artery; see under BRANCH. **r. anastomot'icus gan'glii o'tici cum chor'da tym'pani,** communicating branch of otic ganglion with chorda tympani; see under BRANCH. **r. anastomot'icus gan'glii o'tici cum ner'vo auriculotempora'li,** communicating branch of otic ganglion with auriculotemporal nerve; see under BRANCH. **r. anastomot'icus gan'glii o'tici cum ra'mo menin'geo ner'vi mandibula'ris,** communicating branch of otic ganglion with meningeal branch of mandibular nerve; see under BRANCH. **r. anastomot'icus ner'vi facia'lis cum ner'vo glossopharyn'geo,** communicating branch of facial nerve with glossopharyngeal nerve; see under BRANCH. **r. anastomot'icus ner'vi facia'lis cum plex'u tympan'ico,** communicating branch of facial nerve with tympanic plexus; see under BRANCH. **r. anastomot'icus ner'vi glossopharyn'gei cum ra'mo auricula'ri ner'vi va'gi,** communicating branch of glossopharyngeal nerve with auricular branch of vagus nerve; see under BRANCH. **r. anastomot'icus ner'vi lacrima'lis cum ner'vo zygomat'ico,** communicating branch of lacrimal nerve with zygomatic nerve; see under BRANCH. **r. anastomot'icus ner'vi laryn'gei superio'ris cum ner'vo laryn'geo inferio're,** communicating branch of superior laryngeal nerve with inferior laryngeal nerve; see under BRANCH. **ra'mi anastomot'ici ner'vi lingua'lis cum ner'vo hypoglos'so,** communicating branches of lingual nerve with hypoglossal nerve; see under BRANCH. **r. anastomot'icus ner'vi va'gi cum ner'vo glossopharyn'geo,** communicating branch of vagus nerve with glossopharyngeal nerve; see under BRANCH. **ra'mi anastomot'ici ner'vi auriculotempora'lis cum ner'vo facia'li,** communicating branches of auriculotemporal nerve with facial nerve; see under BRANCH. **r. ante'rior arte'riae thyroi'deae superio'ris** [NA], anterior branch of superior thyroid artery; see under BRANCH. **r. ante'rior ner'vi auricula'ris mag'ni** [NA], anterior branch of great auricular nerve; see under BRANCH. **ra'mi anterio'res nervo'rum nasocilia'rum,** ethmoidal nerves, anterior; see under NERVE. **ra'mi auricula'res anterio'res arte'riae tempora'lis superficia'lis** [NA], anterior auricular branches of superficial temporal artery; see under BRANCH. **r. auricula'ris arte'riae auricula'ris posterio'ris** [NA], auricular branch of posterior auricular artery; see under BRANCH. **r. auricula'ris arte'riae occipita'lis** [NA], auricular branch of occipital artery; see under BRANCH. **r. auricula'ris ner'vi va'gi** [NA], auricular branch of vagus nerve; see under BRANCH. **ra'mi bucca'les ner'vi facia'lis** [NA], buccal branches of facial nerve; see under BRANCH. **r. caroticotympan'icus arte'riae carot'idis inter'nae,** caroticotympanic branch of internal carotid artery; see under BRANCH. **r. col′li ner′vi facia′lis** [NA], cervical branch of facial nerve; see under BRANCH. **r. commu′nicans** [NA], communicating BRANCH. **ra′mi communican′tes al′bae,** communicating branches, white; see under BRANCH. **r. commu′nicans gan′glion cili′are,** communicating branch of ciliary ganglion of nasociliary nerve; see under BRANCH. **r. commu′nicans gan′glii o′tici cum ner′vo auriculo-tempora′li** [NA], communicating branch of otic ganglion with auriculotemporal nerve; see under BRANCH. **r. commu′nicans gan′glii o′tici cum ra′mo menin′geo ner′vi mandibula′ris** [NA], communicating branch of otic ganglion with meningeal branch of mandibular nerve; see under BRANCH. **r. commu′nicans gan′glii cilia′ris cum ner′vo nasocilia′ri** [NA], communicating branch of ciliary ganglion with nasociliary nerve; see under BRANCH. **ra′mi communican′tes gan′glii submandibula′ris cum ner′vo linguali** [NA], communicating branches of submandibular ganglion with lingual nerve; see under BRANCH. **ra′mi communican′tes gan′glii submaxilla′ris cum ner′vo lingua′li,** communicating branches of submandibular ganglion with lingual nerve; see under BRANCH. **r. commu′nicans gan′glii o′tici cum chor′da tym′pani** [NA], communicating branch of otic ganglion with chorda tympani; see under BRANCH. **ra′mi communican′tes, gray,** communicating branches, gray; see under BRANCH. **ra′mi communican′tes ner′vi auriculotempora′lis cum ner′vo facia′li** [NA], communicating branches of auriculo-temporal nerve with facial nerve; see under BRANCH. **r. commu′nicans ner′vi facia′lis cum ner′vo glossopharyn′geo** [NA], communicating branch of facial nerve with glossopharyngeal nerve; see under BRANCH. **r. commu′nicans ner′vi facia′lis cum plex′u tympan′ico** [NA], communicating branch of facial nerve with tympanic plexus; see under BRANCH. **r. commu′nicans ner′vi glossopharyn′gei cum ra′mo auricula′ri ner′vi va′gi** [NA], communicating branch of glossopharyngeal nerve with auricular branch of vagus nerve; see under BRANCH. **r. commu′nicans ner′vi lacrima′lis cum ner′vo zygomat′ico** [NA], communicating branch of lacrimal nerve with zygomatic nerve; see under BRANCH. **r. commu′nicans ner′vi laryn′gei inferio′ris cum ra′mo laryn′geo inter′no** [NA], communicating branch of inferior laryngeal nerve with internal laryngeal branch; see under BRANCH. **r. commu′nicans ner′vi laryn′gei recurren′tis cum ra′mo laryn′geo inter′no,** communicating branch of inferior laryngeal nerve with internal laryngeal branch; see under BRANCH. **r. commu′nicans ner′vi laryn′gei superio′ris cum ner′vo laryn′geo inferio′re** [NA], communicating branch of superior laryngeal nerve with inferior laryngeal nerve; see under BRANCH. **r. commu′nicans ner′vi lingua′lis cum chor′da tym′pani** [NA], communicating branch of lingual nerve with chorda tympani; see under BRANCH. **ra′mi communican′tes ner′vi lingua′lis cum ner′vo hypoglos′so** [NA], communicating branches of lingual nerve with hypoglossal nerve; see under BRANCH. **r. commu′nicans ner′vi nasocilia′ris cum ganglio′ne cilia′ri** [NA], communicating branch of nasociliary ganglion with nasociliary nerve; see under BRANCH. **r. commu′nicans ner′vi va′gi cum ner′vo glossopharyn′geo** [NA], communicating branch of vagus nerve with glossopharyngeal nerve; see under BRANCH. **ra′mi communican′tes nervo′rum spina′lium** [NA], communicating branches of spinal nerves; see under BRANCH. **ra′mi communican′tes, white,** communicating branches, white; see under BRANCH. **r. cricothyroi′deus arte′riae thyroi′deae superio′ris** [NA], cricothyroid branch of superior thyroid artery; see under BRANCH. **ra′mi denta′les arte′riae aιveola′ris inferio′ris** [NA], dental branches of inferior alveolar artery; see under BRANCH. **ra′mi denta′les arte′riae alveola′ris superio′ris posterio′ris** [NA], dental branches of posterior superior alveolar artery; see under BRANCH. **ra′mi denta′les arteria′rum alveola′rium superio′rum anterio′rum** [NA], dental branches of anterior superior alveolar arteries; see under BRANCH. **ra′mi denta′les inferio′res plex′us denta′lis inferio′ris** [NA], dental branches of inferior dental plexus; see under BRANCH. **ra′mi denta′les superio′res plex′us denta′lis superio′ris** [NA], dental branches of superior dental plexus, superior; see under BRANCH. **r. descen′dens arte′riae occipita′lis,** descending branch of occipital artery; see under BRANCH. **r. digas′tricus ner′vi facia′lis** [NA], digastric branch of facial nerve; see under BRANCH. **ra′mi dorsa′les lin′guae arte′riae lingua′lis** [NA], dorsal lingual branches of lingual artery, see under BRANCH. **ra′mi esopha′gei arte′riae thyroi′deae inferio′ris** [NA], esophageal branches of inferior thyroid artery; see under BRANCH. **r. exter′nus ner′vi accesso′rii** [NA], external branch of accessory nerve; see under BRANCH. **r. exter′nus ner′vi laryn′gei superio′ris** [NA], external branch of superior laryngeal nerve; see under BRANCH. **r. fronta′lis arte′riae tempora′lis superficia′lis** [NA], frontal branch of superficial temporal artery; see under BRANCH. **ra′mi gingiva′les inferio′res plex′us denta′lis inferio′ris** [NA], gingival branches of inferior

dental plexus, inferior; see under BRANCH. **ra′mi gingiva′les superio′res plex′us denta′lis superio′ris** [NA], gingival branches of superior dental plexus, superior; see under BRANCH. **ra′mi glandula′res arte′riae facia′lis** [NA], **ra′mi glandula′res arte′riae maxilla′ris exter′nae,** glandular branches of facial artery; see under BRANCH. **ra′mi glandula′res gan′glii submandibula′ris** [NA], glandular branches of submandibular ganglion; see under BRANCH. **gray ra′mi communican′tes,** communicating branches, gray; see under BRANCH. **r. hyoi′deus arte′riae lingua′lis,** suprahyoid branch of lingual artery; see under BRANCH. **r. hyoi′deus arte′riae thyroi′deae superio′ris,** infrahyoid branch of superior thyroid artery; see under BRANCH. **r. infrahyoi′deus arte′riae thyroi′deae superio′ris** [NA], infrahyoid branch of superior thyroid artery; see under BRANCH. **ra′mi intergangliona′res** [NA], interganglionic branches; see under BRANCH. **r. inter′nus ner′vi accesso′rii** [NA], internal branch of accessory nerve; see under BRANCH. **r. inter′nus ner′vi laryn′gei superio′ris** [NA], internal branch of superior laryngeal nerve; see under BRANCH. **ra′mi isth′mi fau′cium ner′vi lingua′lis** [NA], branches from lingual nerve to isthmus of fauces; see under BRANCH. **r. of jaw, r. of mandible. ra′mi labia′les superio′res ner′vi infraorbita′lis** [NA], labial branches of infraorbital nerve, superior; see under BRANCH. **ra′mi laryngopharyn′gei gan′glii cervica′lis superio′ris** [NA], laryngopharyngeal branches of superior cervical ganglion; see under BRANCH. **r. latera′lis ner′vi supraorbita′lis** [NA], lateral branch of supraorbital nerve; see under BRANCH. **r. lingua′lis ner′vi facia′lis** [NA], lingual branch of facial nerve; see under BRANCH. **ra′mi lingua′les ner′vi glossopharyn′gei** [NA], lingual branches of glossopharyngeal nerve; see under BRANCH. **ra′mi lingua′les ner′vi hypoglos′si** [NA], lingual branches of hypoglossal nerve; see under BRANCH. **ra′mi lingua′les ner′vi lingua′lis** [NA], lingual branches of lingual nerve; see under BRANCH. **r. of mandible, r. mandib′ulae** [NA], a quadrilateral process projecting upward and backward from the posterior part of the body of mandible, and ending on the other end at the temporomandibular joint in a saddle-like indentation (sigmoid notch) between the coronoid and condylar processes. The principal landmark on the lateral surface is an oblique ridge which attaches the masseter muscle. Landmarks on the medial aspect include the mandibular foramen which gives entrance to the alveolar vessels and communicates with the mandibular canal; the lingula mandibulae, a ridge on the margin of the foramen which attaches the sphenomandibular ligament; the mylohyoid groove which accommodates the mylohyoid vessels and nerves; and a rough surface posterior to the groove which attaches the pterygoideus medialis muscle. Piercing the ramus is the mandibular canal running under the alveoli and opening to the exterior near the bicuspid teeth through the mental foramen. The parotid gland rests against the posterior border. The inferior border joins the posterior border at the angle of the mandible. Called also **r. of jaw. r. margina′lis mandib′ulae ner′vi facia′lis** [NA], marginal mandibular branch of facial nerve; see under BRANCH. **ra′mi mastoi′dei arte′riae auricularis posterio′ris** [NA], mastoid branches of posterior auricular artery; see under BRANCH. **r. mastoi′deus arte′riae occipita′lis** [NA], mastoid branch of occipital artery; see under BRANCH. **r. media′lis ner′vi supraorbita′lis** [NA], medial branch of supraorbital nerve; see under BRANCH. **r. membra′nae tym′pani ner′vi auriculotempora′lis** [NA], branch to tympanic membrane of auriculotemporal nerve; see under BRANCH. **r. menin′geus accesso′rius arte′riae menin′geae me′diae** [NA], accessory meningeal branch of middle meningeal artery; see under BRANCH. **r. menin′geus arte′riae occipita′lis** [NA], meningeal branch of occipital artery; see under BRANCH. **r. menin′geus [me′dius] ner′vi maxilla′ris** [NA], meningeal nerve, middle; see under NERVE. **r. menin′geus ner′vi mandibula′ris** [NA], meningeal branch of mandibular nerve; see under BRANCH. **r. menin′geus ner′vi va′gi** [NA], meningeal branch of vagus nerve; see under BRANCH. **ra′mi menta′les ner′vi menta′lis** [NA], mental branches of mental nerve; see under BRANCH. **ra′mi muscula′res** [NA], muscular branches; see under BRANCH. **r. mus′culi stylopharyn′gei ner′vi glossopharyn′gei** [NA], stylopharyngeal branch of glossopharyngeal nerve; see under BRANCH. **r. mylohyoi′deus arte′riae alveola′ris inferio′ris** [NA], mylohyoid branch of inferior alveolar artery; see under BRANCH. **ra′mi nasa′les anterio′res ner′vi ethmoida′lis anterio′ris,** nasal branches of anterior ethmoidal nerve; see under BRANCH. **r. nasa′lis exter′nus ner′vi ethmoida′lis anterio′ris** [NA], nasal branch of anterior ethmoidal nerve, external; see under

BRANCH. ra'mi nasa'les exter'ni ner'vi infraorbita'lis [NA], nasal branches of infraorbital nerve, external; see under BRANCH. ra'mi nasa'les inter'ni ner'vi ethmoida'lis anterio'ris [NA], nasal branches of anterior ethmoidal nerve, internal; see under BRANCH. ra'mi nasa'les inter'ni ner'vi infraorbita'les [NA], nasal branches of infraorbital nerve, internal; see under BRANCH. ra'mi nasa'les latera'les ner'vi ethmoida'lis anterio'ris [NA], nasal branches of anterior ethmoidal nerve, lateral; see under BRANCH. ra'mi nasa'les media'les ner'vi ethmoida'lis anterio'ris [NA], nasal branches of anterior ethmoidal nerve, medial; see under BRANCH. ra'mi nasa'les ner'vi ethmoida'lis anterio'ris [NA], nasal branches of anterior ethmoidal nerve; see under BRANCH. ra'mi nasa'les posterio'res inferio'res [latera'les] gan'glii pterygopalati'ni [NA], nasal branches of pterygopalatine ganglion, inferior posterior, lateral; see under BRANCH. ra'mi nasa'les posterio'res inferio'res [latera'les] gan'glii sphenopalati'ni, nasal branches of pterygopalatine ganglion, inferior [lateral] posterior; see under BRANCH. ra'mi nasa'les posterio'res media'les gan'glii pterygopalati'ni [NA], ra'mi nasa'les posterio'res superio'res media'les gan'glii sphenopalati'ni, nasal branches of pterygopalatine ganglion, superior [medial] posterior; see under BRANCH. ra'mi nasa'les posterio'res superio'res [latera'les] gan'glii pterygopalati'ni [NA], ra'mi nasa'les posterio'res superio'res [latera'les] gan'glii sphenopalati'ni, nasal branches of pterygopalatine ganglion, superior [lateral] posterior; see under BRANCH. r. occipita'lis arte'riae auricula'ris posterio'ris [NA], occipital branch of posterior auricular artery; see under BRANCH. ra'mi occipita'les arte'riae occipita'lis [NA], occipital branches of occipital artery; see under BRANCH. r. occipita'lis ner'vi auricula'ris posterio'ris [NA], occipital branch of posterior auricular nerve; see under BRANCH. ra'mi orbita'les gan'glii pterygopalati'ni [NA], orbital branches of pterygopalatine ganglion; see under BRANCH. ra'mi palpebra'les inferio'res ner'vi infraorbita'lis [NA], palpebral branches of infraorbital nerve, inferior; see under BRANCH. ra'mi palpebra'les ner'vi infratrochlea'ris [NA], palpebral branches of infratrochlear nerve; see under BRANCH. r. parieta'lis arte'riae tempora'lis superficia'lis [NA], parietal branch of superficial temporal artery; see under BRANCH. ra'mi paroti'dei arte'riae tempora'lis superficia'lis [NA], parotid branches of superficial temporal artery; see under BRANCH. ra'mi paroti'dei ner'vi auriculotempora'lis [NA], parotid branches of auriculotemporal nerve; see under BRANCH. ra'mi paroti'dei ve'nae facia'lis [NA], parotid branches of facial vein; see under BRANCH. r. petro'sus arte'riae menin'geae me'diae [NA], petrosal branch of middle meningeal artery; see under BRANCH. r. petro'sus superficia'lis arte'riae menin'geae me'diae, petrosal branch of middle meningeal artery; see under BRANCH. ra'mi pharyn'gei arte'riae pharyn'geae ascenden'tis [NA], pharyngeal branches of ascending pharyngeal artery; see under BRANCH. r. pharyn'geus gan'glii pterygopalati'ni [NA], pharyngeal branch of pterygopalatine ganglion; see under BRANCH. ra'mi pharyn'gei ner'vi glossopharyn'gei [NA], pharyngeal branches of glossopharyngeal nerve; see under BRANCH. ra'mi pharyn'gei ner'vi va'gi [NA], pharyngeal branches of vagus nerve; see under BRANCH. r. poste'rior arte'riae thyroi'deae superio'ris [NA], posterior branch of superior thyroid artery; see under BRANCH. r. poste'rior ner'vi auricula'ris mag'ni [NA], posterior branch of great auricular nerve; see under BRANCH. postganglionic rami, communicating branches, gray; see under BRANCH. preganglionic ra'mi, communicating branches, white; see under BRANCH. ra'mi pterygoi'dei arte'riae maxilla'ris [NA], ra'mi pterygoi'dei arte'riae maxilla'ris inter'nae, pterygoid branches of maxillary artery; see under BRANCH. r. si'nus carot'ici ner'vi glossopharyn'gei [NA], branch of glossopharyngeal nerve to carotid sinus; see under BRANCH. ra'mi sternocleidomastoi'dei arte'riae occipita'lis [NA], sternocleidomastoid branches of occipital artery; see under BRANCH. r. sternocleidomastoi'deus arte'riae thyroi'deae superio'ris [NA], sternocleidomastoid branch of superior thyroid artery; see under BRANCH. r. stylohyoi'deus ner'vi facia'lis [NA], stylohyoid branch of facial nerve; see under BRANCH. r. stylopharyn'geus ner'vi glossopharyn'gei, stylopharyngeal branch of glossopharyngeal nerve; see under BRANCH. ra'mi submaxilla'res gan'glii submaxilla'ris, glandular branches of submandibular ganglion; see under BRANCH. r. superficia'lis arte'riae transver'sae col'li [NA], cervical artery, superficial; see under ARTERY. r. supe'rior ner'vi oculomoto'rii [NA], superior branch of oculomotor nerve; see under BRANCH. r. suprahyoi'deus arte'riae linga'lis [NA], suprahyoid branch of lingual artery; see under BRANCH. r.

sympath'icus ad gan'glion submandibula're [NA], see sympathetic root of submandibular ganglion, under ROOT. ra'mi tempora'les ner'vi facia'lis [NA], temporal branches of facial nerve; see under BRANCH. ra'mi tempora'les superficia'les ner'vi auriculotempora'lis [NA], temporal branches of auriculotemporal nerve, superficial; see under BRANCH. r. tento'rii ner'vi ophthal'mici [NA], tentorial branch of ophthalmic nerve; see under BRANCH. r. thyreohyoi'deus ner'vi hypoglos'si, r. thyreohyoi'deus an'sae cervica'lis, thyrohyoid branch of ansa cervicalis; see under BRANCH. r. thyrohyoi'deus an'sae cervica'lis [NA], thyrohyoid branch of ansa cervicalis; see under BRANCH. r. tonsilla'ris arte'riae facia'lis [NA], r. tonsilla'ris arte'riae maxilla'ris exter'ni, tonsillar branch of facial artery; see under BRANCH. ra'mi tonsilla'res ner'vi glossopharyn'gei [NA], tonsillar branches of glossopharyngeal nerve; see under BRANCH. ra'mi trachea'les arte'riae thyroi'deae inferio'ris [NA], tracheal branches of inferior thyroid artery; see under BRANCH. white ra'mi communican'tes, communicating branches, white; see under BRANCH. ra'mi zygomat'ici ner'vi facia'lis [NA], zygomatic branches of facial nerve; see under BRANCH. r. zygomaticofacia'lis ner'vi zygomat'ici [NA], zygomaticofacial branch of zygomatic nerve; see under BRANCH. r. zygomaticotempora'lis ner'vi zygomat'ici [NA], zygomaticotemporal branch of zygomatic nerve; see under BRANCH.

Ranephrine trademark for a vasoconstrictor preparation, being a 1:500 aqueous solution of racemic epinephrine with 1 percent benzyl alcohol serving as a preservative.

range (rānj) 1. the difference between the upper and lower limits of a variable or of a series of values. 2. the portion of the earth in which a given species is found. **melting r.**, a temperature range at which a given substance, such as an alloy, will melt, having the lower and upper limits, the substance being both molten and solid within the range. See also phase DIAGRAM.

ranine (ra'nīn) [L. *raninus*, from *rana* frog] pertaining to a frog, or a ranula, or the lower surface of the tongue, or the sublingual (ranine) artery.

Ranke's angle [Hans Randolph *Ranke*, Dutch anatomist, 1849–1887] see under ANGLE.

Rankine scale, thermometer [William J. M. *Rankine*, Scottish physicist, died 1872] see under SCALE and THERMOMETER.

ranula (ran'u-lah) [L. dim of *rana* frog] a form of rention cyst of the floor of the mouth, usually due to obstruction of the ducts of the submaxillary or sublingual glands, presenting a slowly enlarging painless deep burrowing mucocele of one side of the mouth. Called also *sublingual cyst* and *sublingual ptyalocele*. See also mucous retention CYST.

Ranvier, node of [Louis Antoine *Ranvier*, French pathologist, 1835–1922] see under NODE. See also Merkel cells (Merkel-Ranvier cells), under CELL.

Raoult's law [François Marie *Raoult*, French chemist, 1830–1901] see under LAW.

Rapacodin trademark for DIHYDROCODEINE.

raphe (ra'fē) [Gr. *rhaphē*] a seam; a general anatomical term for the line of union of two symmetrical parts of an organ or structure. See also SEAM and SUTURE. **longitudinal r. of tongue**, median sulcus of tongue; see under SULCUS. **palatine r.**, **r. pala'ti** [NA], a narrow whitish streak in the midline of the palate, extending from the incisive papilla to the tip of the uvula; it may present as a ridge in front and as a groove posteriorly. Called also *cutaneous suture of palate* and *longitudinal ridge of hard palate*. See also median palatine SUTURE. **palpebral r., lateral, r. palpebra'lis latera'lis** [NA], a thin horizontal band of connective tissue extending from the margin of the frontosphenoidal process of the zygomatic bone, from where it passes to the lateral commissure of the eyelids, and splits into two parts which are attached to corresponding margins of the eyelids. Called also *canthal ligament*. **r. of pharynx, r. pharyn'gis** [NA], a more or less distinct band of connective tissue extending downward from the base of the skull along the posterior wall of the pharynx in the median plane, and giving attachment to the constrictor muscle of the pharynx. Called also *middle pharyngeal ligament, pharyngeal ligament*, and *white line of pharynx*. **pterygomandibular r., r. pterygomandibula'ris** [NA], a tendinous inscription between the buccinator and superior constrictor of the pharynx muscles. It attaches to the pterygoid hamulus and the posterior end of the mylohyoid line of the mandible. The buccal fat pad separates it from the mandible and the mucous membrane provides the covering for the lateral surface. Called also *intermaxillary ligament, pterygomandibular ligament*, and *pterygomaxillary ligament*.

Rapicidin trademark for *tyrocidine hydrochloride* (see under TYROCIDINE).

Rapp-Hodgkin ectodermal dysplasia [R. S. *Rapp*; W. E. *Hodgkin*] see under DYSPLASIA.

raptus (rap'tus) [L.] a sudden, violent attack.

rarefaction (ra″ĕ-fak′shun) [L. *rarefactio*] the condition of being or becoming less dense, diminution in density and weight, but not in volume.

Raschkow, plexus of see under PLEXUS.

rash (rash) a temporary eruption of the skin. **drug r.,** DERMATITIS medicamentosa. **nettle r.,** urticaria. **wandering r.,** benign migratory GLOSSITIS.

rasion (ra′zhun) [L. *rasio*] the grating of drugs with a file.

rasp (rasp) 1. to scrape or abrade with a rough instrument. 2. a coarse file. **bone r.,** bone FILE. **R-type r.,** rat-tail FILE.

raspatory (ras′pah-to-re) [L. *raspatorium*] a file or rasp for surgical use; a xyster.

Rastinon trademark for *tolbutamide*.

rasura (rah-su′rah) [L.] scrapings of filings.

rat (rat) a small omnivorous rodent of the genus *Rattus* and related genera of the family Muridae. Albino mutants of *R. norvegicus* (Norway, sewer, or wharf rat) are used as laboratory animals. Rats are vectors of various human diseases.

rate (rāt) an expression of the speed or frequency with which a certain event or circumstance occurs in relation to a certain period of time, a specific population, or some other fixed standard. **absorbed dose r.,** dose r. (2). **basal metabolism r. (BMR),** see basal METABOLISM. **birth r.,** an expression of the number of births occurring in one year. **case r.,** morbidity r. **case fatality r.,** the number of deaths caused by a specific disease, expressed as a percentage of or otherwise related to the total number of cases of disease. **circulation r.,** an expression of the amount of blood pumped per minute by the heart through the body. **critical cooling r.,** in steel, the minimum cooling rate which allows the transformation of austenite to martensite, rather than to ferrite plus carbide. **death r.,** the ratio of the total number of deaths in a specified area to the population, generally figured in terms of the number of deaths per 1,000, 10,000, or 100,000 of population. Called also *mortality r.* **DEF r.,** an expression of dental caries experience in deciduous teeth. The DEF rate is calculated by adding the number of decayed primary teeth requiring filling (D), decayed primary teeth requiring extraction (E), and primary teeth successfully filled (F). Missing primary teeth are not included in the calculation. **DMF r.,** an expression of the condition of the teeth based on the number of teeth that are decayed, missing, or indicated for removal and of those filled or bearing restorations. The rate is calculated by adding the number of carious permanent teeth requiring filling (D), the carious permanent teeth requiring extraction (*Mr*), the permanent teeth previously extracted because of caries (*Mp*), and the filled permanent teeth (F). The number of DMF teeth per child of a specific age or age group is calculated by using the following formula:

$$\frac{D \text{ teeth} + Mr \text{ teeth} + Mp \text{ teeth} + F \text{ teeth}}{\text{number of children examined}} = DMF$$

dose r., 1. the amount of any agent, such as a drug, administered per unit of time. 2. in radiology, the dose of ionizing radiation measured in rads, absorbed per unit of time, usually expressed in rads per second. Called also *absorbed dose r.* and *exposure r.* 3. exposure r. **erythrocyte sedimentation r.,** see under ERYTHROCYTE. **exposure r.,** 1. an exposure to ionizing radiation, usually expressed in roentgens per minute. Called also *dose r.* 2. dose r. (2). **fatality r.,** the number of deaths, caused by a specific circumstance or disease, expressed as the absolute or relative number of deaths among the individuals encountering the circumstance or having the disease. Called also *lethality r.* **growth r.,** an expression of the increase in size of an organic object per unit time, calculations usually being made as to both the absolute and the relative increment. **heart r.,** the number of contractions of the ventricles of the heart per unit of time (usually a minute). It usually corresponds to the pulse rate, but pathologically some of the contractions of the left ventricle may be so weak that they fail to produce peripheral pulse waves, so that the rate of the pulse at the wrist is less than that of the heart. See also PULSE (1). **lethality r.,** fatality r. **morbidity r.,** the number of cases of a given disease occurring during a specified period per 1,000, 10,000 or 100,000 of population. Called also *case r.* and *sickness r.* **mortality r.,** death r. **occupancy r.,** a measure of inpatient health facility use, determined by dividing available bed days by patient days. **output exposure r.,** in radiology, the exposure to radiation at a specified point per unit of time, usually expressed in roentgens per minute. **periodontal disease r.,** periodontal disease INDEX. **pulse r.,** the rate of pulsation noted in a peripheral artery per minute. See PULSE (1). See also *heart r.* **reaction r.,** the velocity with which a reactant or reactants undergo chemical change. **respiration r.,** an expression of the number of sequences of inspiration and expiration, occurring per minute. **sickness r.,** morbidity r. **spring r.,** SPRING rate.

Rathke's pouch (pocket), trabeculae [Martin Heinrich *Rathke*, German anatomist, 1793–1860] see under POUCH, and see TRABECULAE cranii.

rating (rāt′ing) classification; relative standing; grading. **insurance r., community,** the distribution of insurance premiums based upon the past and probable distribution of illness and expense for a large group of persons. **insurance r., experience,** the determination of insurance premiums based on the past and probable future distribution of illness and expenses for an individual or a small group of individuals seeking insurance. **insurance r., retrospective,** a procedure that adjusts the final premium, normally after the expiration of the policy, in accordance with the actual experience of the insured during the term of the policy for which the premium is paid.

ratio (ra′she-o) [L.] an expression of the quantity of one substance, factor, or entity in relation to that of another; the relationship between two quantities expressed as the quotient of one divided by the other. **alloy-mercury r.,** in a dental amalgam, the parts by weight of alloy to be combined with the proper amount of mercury. With the small-grained alloys, the ratios of 50 to 51 percent mercury is common, with some alloys being as little as 48 to 49 percent. The use of low mercury-alloy ratios is known as the *Eames technique* or the *minimal mercury technique.* **birth-death r.,** vital INDEX. **grid r.,** in radiology, the ratio of the height of the lead strips to the width of the interspacing of a grid, having direct effect on the contrast and density of the image and on the scatter-ray absorption. **Hardy-Weinberg r.,** Hardy-Weinberg LAW. **holdaway r.,** a means of expressing the relationship of the pogonion and the lower incisor to the nasion-basion plane; used in roentgenographic cephalometric diagnosis. **tissue-air r.,** in radiology, the ratio of the absorbed dose at a given point in a phantom to the absorbed dose which would be measured at the same point in free air within a volume of the phantom material just sufficient to provide the maximum electronic buildup at the point of measurement. Abbreviated *TAR.* **water-powder r., W/P r.,** the proportions of water and gypsum hemihydrate in the preparation of dental plaster, plaster of Paris, or dental stone. In mixing dental stone, 30 ml of water per 100 gm of powder, the proportion of water to powder (the W/P ratio) is 30/100 or 0.30; if 28 ml of water are mixed with 100 gm of water, the W/P ratio is 0.28.

rational (rash′un-al) [L. *rationalis* reasonable] accordant with reason; based upon reasoning and not upon simple experience.

rationale (rash″un-al′) [L.] a rational exposition of principles; the logical basis of a procedure.

Rauber, tubopharyngeal ligament of [August Antinous *Rauber*, German anatomist, 1841–1917] salpingopharyngeal FOLD.

Rautenberg antigen (factor) [named after the person in whom antibodies to the Rautenberg factor (Kp^b antigen) were first discovered] see Kp^b ANTIGEN, and see Kell blood groups, under BLOOD GROUP.

Rauwolfia (raw-wol′fe-ah) a genus of tropical trees and shrubs indigenous to Asia, now growing also in other parts of the world, including over 100 species, and providing various alkaloids of medical interest including reserpine. Many species have been used as sources of other medicines. **R. serpenti′na,** a species containing various alkaloids, of which reserpine is the most important therapeutically.

rauwolfia (raw-wol′fe-ah) a preparation of the dried rhizome and sometimes the aerial stem of *Rauwolfia.* **r. serpenti′na,** a dried preparation of the rhizome and sometimes the aerial stem of *Rauwolfia serpentina*, containing all the alkaloids of the plant, including no less than 0.15 percent reserpine-rescinnamine group alkaloids. It is an adrenergic neuron blocking agent with hypotensive and sedative effects. See also RESERPINE.

Ravocaine trademark for *propoxycaine hydrochloride* (see under PROPOXYCAINE).

ray (ra) [L. *radius* spoke] 1. a more or less distinct portion of radiant energy, proceeding in a specific direction from the source. See also RADIATION. 2. one of the individual elements at the distal end of the limb of an early embryo, foretelling development of the metacarpal or metatarsal bones and the phalanges. **actinic r's,** actinic RADIATION. **alpha r., α-r.,** alpha PARTICLE. **anode r's,** positive r's. **Becquerel r's,** former name for rays emitted from uranium and other radioactive substances, and now known as alpha, beta, and gamma rays. **beta r., β-r.,** beta PARTICLE. **border r's, borderline r's, Bucky's r's,** grenz r's. **cathode r's,** a stream of electrons emitted by the cathode, or negative electrode, as in a vacuum tube or by thermionic emission in an x-ray tube. See also electron STREAM. **central r.,** the part of the primary radiation that leaves the port at right angles to the long axis of the x-ray tube and is the portion of the useful beam directed to the center of the film or structure to be radiographed. Called also *central beam* and *central radiation.* **characteristic r.,** characteristic RADIATION. **chemical r's,** actinic RADIATION. **cosmic r's,** radiation of many sorts but mostly atomic nuclei (protons) with very high energy, originating outside the earth's atmosphere. Called also *cosmic radiation.* **delta r's, δ-r's,** secondary ionizing particles, usually electrons, ejected by recoil when a primary ionizing particle passes through matter. See also secondary IONIZATION. **direct r.,** primary RADIATION. **fluorescent r's,** fluorescent RADIATION. **gamma r's, γ-r's,** uncharged electromagnetic radiations from the nuclei of isotopes during a nuclear reaction. They consist of high energy photons, have no mass and no electric charge, and travel with the speed of light; they have extremely short wavelength and high frequencies; they ionize matter by the ejection of high speed electrons from the absorbing material; and they have high tissue penetration capacity and may destroy tissue and cause burns. Called also *gamma radiation.* **glass r's,** the rays formed in an x-ray tube by the cathode rays striking the glass wall of the tube, so called to distinguish them from the x-rays originating at the anticathode. **Goldstein's r's,** rays formed when x-rays pass through some transparent medium. Called also *s r's.* **grenz r's,** very soft x-rays having a long wavelength (about 2 Å), lying between the x-rays and ultraviolet rays, which are generated at low kilovoltage, between 5 and 15 kvp. Called also *border r's, borderline r's, Bucky's r's,* and *infra-roentgen r's.* See also *intermediate r's* and soft RADIATION. **hard r's,** hard RADIATION. **incident r.,** see REFLECTION (4). **indirect r's,** rays formed at the surface of the glass of the cathode-ray tube. **infrared r's,** radiations lying just beyond the red end of the spectrum; their wavelengths range between 7700 and 500,000 Å. Called also *infrared light* and *infrared radiation.* **infra-roentgen r's,** grenz r's. **intermediate r's,** rays in the wavelengths between ultraviolet rays and x-rays. See also *grenz r's.* **K r.,** see characteristic RADIATION. **L r.,** see characteristic RADIATION. **luminous r's,** the visible rays of the spectrum. **Lyman r's,** electromagnetic vibrations of wavelength between 600 and 12,300 Å. **M r.,** see characteristic RADIATION. **monochromatic r's,** monochromatic RADIATION. **N r.,** see characteristic RADIATION. **necrobiotic r's,** short ultraviolet rays which kill living cells. **O r.,** see characteristic RADIATION. **paracathodic r's,** rays formed by the impaction of cathode rays against a body (anticathode) in their path. See also *x-r's.* **parallel r's,** rays which travel paths that are parallel or nearly parallel. They are rays originating from a source at an infinite distance, or may be primary stronger x-rays which strike the object and film at increased target-film distance and travel in paths more nearly parallel to each other. Divergent rays may be made parallel by means of a convex lens or a concave mirror. They are used chiefly in teleroentgenography. **positive r's,** a stream of positively charged particles traveling at high speed from the anode under the influence of an applied voltage. Called also *anode r's.* **primary r.,** primary RADIATION. **reflected r.,** see REFLECTION (4). **remnant r's,** remnant RADIATION. **roentgen r's, x-r's.** **s r's,** Goldstein's r's. **Sagnac r's,** secondary beta rays formed when gamma rays are reflected from a metal surface. **scattered r's,** rays from the primary beam that have been deflected during their passage through tissues or substances, whose energy may or may not have been attenuated with associated change in their wavelength. Called also *secondary scattered r's, scattered radiation,* and *secondary scattered radiation.* See also *secondary r's,* BACKSCATTER, and SCATTERING. **secondary r's,** 1. rays emitted during the interaction of primary radiation with substances or tissues. 2. any rays that have been generated in substances or tissues exposed to primary radiation, or primary radiation that has been deviated with or without change of energy (scattered radiation), including fluorescent radiation. Called also *secondary radiation.* **secondary scattered r's,** scattered r's. **soft r's,** soft RADIATION. **stray r's,** stray RADIATION. **ultraviolet r's,** rays or radiation between the violet rays and the x-rays with wavelengths between 1800 and 3900 Å, having strong actinic and chemical properties. Called also *ultraviolet light* and *ultraviolet radiation.* **useful r's,** useful BEAM. **x-r's,** electromagnetic radiation of extranuclear origin, with a wavelength of less than 5 Å, which are produced when electrons moving at high velocity impinge on various substances, especially the heavy metals. They are generated by

passing a high voltage current through a Collidge tube, and can penetrate most substances in varying degree. They are able to affect a photographic plate, and are used for revealing the presence and position of fractures or foreign bodies or of radiopaque substances purposely introduced. Because of their ability to cause certain substances to fluoresce, it is possible to determine the size, shape, and movements of various organs through the use of fluoroscopy. They strongly ionize and destroy tissue and, because of this property, are used in treating various pathological conditions, such as cancer. Called also *roentgen r's* and *x-radiation.* See also x-ray GENERATOR; x-ray tube, hot cathode, under TUBE; and characteristic RADIATION. **x-r's, supervoltage,** x-rays produced by voltages ranging from 250 kvp to 3 Mev.

Raymond-Céstan syndrome [Fulgence *Raymond,* French neurologist, 1844–1910; Etienne Jacques Marie *Céstan,* French physician, 1872–1932] see under SYNDROME.

Rb rubidium.

RBC red blood cell (see ERYTHROCYTE); red blood (cell) count (see erythrocyte COUNT).

RBE relative biological EFFECTIVENESS.

rcp reciprocal TRANSLOCATION. See also CHROMOSOME nomenclature.

RC-Prep trademark for a preparation of a calcium-chelating agent used in endodontic therapy. It consists of 15 percent EDTA and 10 percent urea peroxide in a water-soluble base. It facilitates instrumentation in root canal therapy by its lubrication of the root canal and by its chelating action on the dentin. It also reacts with sodium hypochlorite irrigating solution to cause a slow release of oxygen bubbles, thus producing a foaming action which assists in dislodging debris on the walls of the root canal.

RCT random controlled TRIAL.

rd rutherford.

RDA dental assistant, registered; see under ASSISTANT.

RDH Registered Dental Hygienist; see dental HYGIENIST.

RE 1. radium emanation; see RADON. 2. reticuloendothelial SYSTEM.

Re rhenium.

re- [L.] a prefix signifying back, again, contrary, and the like.

reabsorption (re″ab-sorp′shun) 1. the act or process of absorbing again, as the selective absorption by the kidneys of substances (glucose, proteins, sodium, etc.) already secreted into the renal tubules, and their return to the circulating blood. 2. resorption.

reactance (re-ak′tans) the weakening of an alternating electric current caused by passage through a coil of wire.

reaction (re-ak′shun) [*re-* + L. *agere* to act] 1. opposite action, or counteraction; the response to a specific stimulus. 2. the phenomena caused by the action of chemical agents; a chemical process in which one substance is transformed into another substance or substances. See also PHENOMENON, REAGENT, and TEST. **adverse r.,** an undesired reaction, usually harmful to the body, elicited by side effects of a drug or another agent administered for therapeutic purposes in a standard dose and form. Called also *side r.* **agglutinoid r.,** prozone. **allergic r.,** a reaction characterized by altered local or general reactivity of the animal body to an antigenic substance, often accompanied by physiological disturbances and tissue damage. **allograft r.,** the rejection of an allogenic graft that occurs in a normal host after an immune response has been mounted. Called also *homograft r.* See also graft REJECTION. **anaphylactoid r.,** pseudoanaphylaxis. **antigen-antibody r.,** an immune process usually divided into three categories: (1) primary antigen-antibody reaction consisting of the initial binding of antigen with two or more available antigen-binding sites on any given antibody molecule, during which no visible manifestation occurs; (2) secondary reaction, usually with visible manifestations, including precipitation, agglutination, complement-dependent reactions, neutralization, and cytotropic effects; and (3) tertiary reaction, being biologic expressions of the antigen-antibody interactions sometimes serving as a protective mechanism but at other times leading to disease through immunologic injury. The initial reaction is a specific one between the antigenic determinant and antibody reactive group, which is stabilized by certain nonspecific forces. Called also *antigen-antibody interaction.* **Arthus r.,** localized anaphylaxis, characterized by the development of an inflammatory lesion, classically an ulcer, marked by edema, hemorrhage, and necrosis, which occurs within hours after interdermal injection of an antigen to which the animal already has precipitating antibody. It is generally considered an immediate hypersensitivity, or is classed as a type III reaction. Arthus reactions usually occur in antibody excess. In the presence of antigen excess soluble complexes are usually formed. Antigen-antibody complexes formed in the presence of complement adhere to the vascular epithelium and are encircled by fibrin, blood platelets, and polymorphonuclear neutrophils. Plugging of the vessels is followed by exudation into surrounding tissues of fluid laden with neutrophils. Type III reaction refers to numerous hypersensitivity states in which antigen-antibody complexes initiate the lesion, including serum sickness and glomerulonephritis. The reaction is considered as being peculiar to rabbits, but other animals, including man, may develop similar reactions under certain conditions. For generalized anaphylactic phenomena, see generalized ANAPHYLAXIS. Called also *Arthus phenomenon*. **bimolecular r.,** a chemical reaction involving two molecules in forming the transitional state. **Bordet-Gengou r.,** complement FIXATION. **delayed r.,** a reaction, such as an allergic reaction, occurring hours to days after exposure to an inducer. The term is usually used to refer to lymphokine-mediated responses but delayed reaction may also be associated with antibody-mediated reaction. Called also *delayed response*. **drug r.,** an adverse reaction to the systemic or topical administration of drugs. Based on the time of onset, drug reactions may be classified as: *immediate*, mediated primarily by the IgE reaginic antibodies, occurring within minutes of drug administration, and may be characterized by urticaria, hypotension, and shock (when life-threatening, termed anaphylactic or anaphylactoid); *accelerated*, occurring 1 to 72 hours after drug administration, and almost always manifested by urticaria, with morbilliform eruption and laryngeal edema sometimes being associated; *late*, beginning three days after drug administration, thought to be mediated by soluble antigen-antibody complexes in which the antibodies are primarily IgG and IgM, and presenting various forms of skin eruption, serum sickness, and drug fever; and *unusually late*, occurring more than three days after drug administration, usually triggered by various mechanisms, such as IgG cytolytic reactions, antigen-antibody complexes, and other immune reactions, and manifested chiefly by hemolytic anemia, thrombocytopenia, granulocytopenia, erythema multiforme–like eruption, acute renal insufficiency, lupus-like syndrome, and cholestatic jaundice. Cutaneous manifestations of drug reaction may include contact dermatitis, urticaria, angioedema, erythematous eruption, erythema multiforme–like eruptions, erythema nodosum, purpura, exfoliative dermatitis, fixed drug eruption photosensitivity, phototoxicity, and photoallergy. Called also *drug allergy, drug hypersensitivity, drug idiosyncrasy*, and *drug sensitivity*. **equation r., r. equation,** chemical EQUATION. **eutectic r.,** a reaction taking place during the solidification and melting of a eutectic alloy, expressed as follows: liquid $\rightleftharpoons$ α-solid solution + β-solid solution. See also *peritectic r.* **eutectoid r.,** in steel, the decomposition, upon cooling below the eutectoid temperature, of austenite (a single phase) to pearlite (two phases). **first-order r.,** one in which the reaction rate is proportional to the first power of the concentration of a reactant. **fright r.,** involuntary contraction of extraocular and facial muscles of animals during states of fright and anger. **graft-vs-host r.,** the immunological reaction of a graft rich in immunologically competent cells against the genetically non-identical tissues of the recipient. The graft is not rejected because of the recipient's immunological immaturity (as in the newborn) or its genetic make-up (as in F_1 hybrid disease), or because it has been treated with whole-body irradiation or immunosuppression. The grafted elements, on the other hand, become sensitized to the tissues of the host and react against them. Tissues especially rich in immunologically competent cells capable of inducing a graft-vs-host reaction include the spleen, lymph nodes, thoracic duct lymph, and to a lesser degree the bone marrow and peripheral blood. See also graft REJECTION. **hemagglutination-inhibition r.,** the inhibition of agglutination of red cells. If agglutination is caused by hemagglutinating viruses, inhibition is accomplished by antiviral antibodies. If agglutination is the result of antibodies to antigens of or adsorbed to the surfaces of red cells, inhibition may be due to antigens or haptens that react with reactive sites on the antibody and prevent its access to the antigen or red cell. **heterophil antibody r.,** a reaction produced by antibody against a heterophil antigen. **homograft r.,** allograft r. **hypersensitivity r.,** see HYPERSENSITIVITY. **r. of identity,** in the two-dimensional double diffusion test (Ouchterlony test), wells filled with antigen solution opposed by one filled with antiserum form lines of precipitate which fuse and form a continuous line if the antigens in the two solutions are identical. If the line of precipitation is continuous but has a spurlike projection, the antigens are only partially identical but share antigenic determinants (*r. of partial identity*). If two intersecting lines are formed, the antigens are different (*r. of nonidentity*). **immediate r.,** an antibody-mediated reaction, such as an allergic reaction, occurring usually within minutes after exposure to an antigen.

Called also *immediate response*. **immune r.,** immune RESPONSE. **light r.,** the reaction involving the conversion of light energy into chemical energy, especially during photosynthesis. **mixed lymphocyte r. (MLR),** a reaction initiated by mixing lymphocytes from genetically dissimilar individuals, which causes a stimulation in DNA synthesis in both cell populations (two-way MLR). If one of the cell populations is inactivated, e.g., by x-irradiation, the unirradiated population becomes activated (one-way MLR). **monomolecular r.,** unimolecular r. **neutral r.,** a reaction that is neither acid nor basic, i.e., a pH of 7. **neutralization r.,** a reversible reaction between an acid and a metallic hydroxide or base in which water and a salt are formed and both the acid and the base are neutralized. **r. of nonidentity,** see *r. of identity*. **nuclear r.,** a reaction involving a change in an atomic nucleus, such as fission or fusion, as distinct from a chemical reaction, which is limited to changes in the electron structure surrounding the nucleus. See also nuclear FISSION and nuclear FUSION. **oxidation-reduction r.,** see OXIDATION-REDUCTION. **r. of partial identity,** see *r. of identity*. **patch r.,** patch TEST. **peritectic r.,** a reaction taking place during the solidification of a peritectic alloy, expressed as follows: liquid + β-solid solution $\rightarrow$ α-solid solution. See also *eutectic r.* **photochemical r.,** photoreaction. **PK r.,** Prausnitz-Küstner r. **Prausnitz-Küstner r.,** a skin reaction for the detection and assay of human reagin (IgE). The intradermal inoculation of a non-atopic individual with serum containing reaginic antibody results in fixation of the reaginic antibody to the epidermal mast cells and diffusion of the other immunoglobulins away from the site of injection. Injection of specific antigen into the site of reagin attachment 48 hours later results in the immediate appearance of a wheal-and-flare response that can be graded in intensity. The danger of transferring serum hepatitis has precluded the use of this test clinically. It was also used to determine the donor's sensitivity to various antigens. Abbreviated *PK r*. Called also *passive transfer test*. **Quellung r.,** a swelling of the polysaccharide capsule of pneumococci or other microorganisms, due to the interaction with specific anticapsular antibodies. **reversible r.,** a chemical reaction which is in a state of equilibrium and can occur in either direction, from left to right and from right to left; a reaction in which the product reacts to re-form the reactants. Double arrows indicate a reversible reaction. $A + B \rightleftharpoons C + D$. See also chemical EQUILIBRIUM. **second-order r.,** one in which the reaction time is proportional to the concentration of each of two reactants or to the second power of the concentration of one reactant. **side r.,** adverse r. **solid state r.,** a reaction taking place between substances in their solid state, such as one occurring during the formation of some alloys (gold, platinum, or palladium alloys), whereby on heating to a temperature below the lower limit of the melting range and allowing the two components of the alloy to cool down slowly, the atoms of one metal diffuse and penetrate into the lattice of the other, forming a superlattice. The gold-copper system is an example of an alloy formed through the solid state reaction. **third-order r.,** one in which the reaction time is proportional to the concentration of each of three reactants, or proportional to the concentration of one of two reactants and to the second power of the concentration of the other, or proportional to the third power of the concentration of a single reactant. **T-lymphocyte–antigen r.,** a three-stage immunological reaction. The *primary* stage consists of binding of antigen or processed antigen with an antigen receptor on the surface of a sensitized T-lymphocyte. The *secondary* (morphologic or biochemical) phase is made up of the *in vitro* manifestations of cell-mediated immunity that presumably result from the membrane perturbations established after the primary interaction and are detected indirectly through morphologic or biochemical events. The changes may be detected by the observation of blast cell transformation with subsequent mitosis and chemical uptake of radioactive precursors into DNA or RNA. The *tertiary* phase is the biologic expression of earlier events and consists of the generation of helper or suppressor T-lymphocytes for T-T and T-B interactions; the generation of cytotoxic T-lymphocytes; the generation of T-lymphocytes that elaborate the effector molecules (mediators) of cell-mediated immunity; and the generation of memory T-lymphocytes. **transfusion r.,** immune and nonimmune complications occurring during or after transfusion of whole blood or blood products. Nonimmune reactions usually include infection secondary to transfusion of contaminated blood (hepatitis) and cardiac failure due to the rapid transfusion. The immune reactions result from the passive transfer or active formation of antibodies to foreign alloantigens of red cells, white cells, platelets, or gamma globulin; less commonly, immune complications may also result from the passive transfusion of allergic antibodies that can initiate hypersensitivity phenomena in the recipient (e.g., reagin-mediated urticaria). **trimolecular r.,** a chemical reaction involving three molecules in forming the transitional state. **unimolecular r.,** a chemical reaction involving only one molecule in forming the transitional state. Called also *monomolecular r.* **wheal-flare r.,** a cutaneous sensitivity reaction to skin injury or antigen, due to production of histamine, and characterized by edematous elevation and erythematous flare. It may occur in generalized anaphylactic reactions or after the administration of antigen into the skin as a diagnostic procedure. See also triple RESPONSE. **zero-order r.,** one in which the reaction time is independent of the concentration of reactant or reactants.

reactivator (re-ak′tĭ-va″tor) an agent that makes something active again or restores effectiveness or the ability to function. **cholinesterase r's,** chemical substances which neutralize anticholinesterase substances, thereby allowing cholinesterase to be reactivated and to destroy acetylcholine after it has completed its function as a transmitter of cholinergic impulses and, thus, stabilizing the cholinergic activity of the autonomic nervous system. Their function is believed to consist principally of displacing dialkylphosphate groups from organic phosphate cholinesterase inhibitors and dimethylcarbamoyl groups from physostigmine or neostigmine. Used chiefly in the treatment of poisoning by anticholinesterases.

reactor (re-ak′tor) 1. one who or that which reacts. 2. a container or vat in which chemical substances are undergoing a reaction. 3. a chemical substance bringing about a chemical reaction, such as one causing conversion of a sol to a gel or one initiating polymerization. See also CATALYST.

Reactrol trademark for *climizole.*

reagent (re-a′jent) [*re-* + L. *agere* to act] a substance employed to produce a specific chemical reaction. See also REACTION.

reagin (re′ah-jin) 1. antibody of the IgE immunoglobulin class which attaches to mast cells and basophils, and which interacts with its antigen to induce the release of histamine and other vasoactive amines. It is a cytotropic antibody, present in the serum of naturally hypersensitive individuals and can confer specific immediate hypersensitivity to nonreactive individuals. Called also *Prausnitz-Küstner (PK) antibody* and *reaginic antibody.* 2. a complement-fixing antibody interacting with cardiolipin in the Wassermann test for syphilis.

reamer (re′mer) an endodontic instrument for enlarging root canals, consisting of a triangular shaft twisted into a loosely spiraled serrated instrument. See also root canal FILE, and see illustration at root canal THERAPY. **A-type r.,** an engine-driven reamer with a long, tapered, pyramid-shaped head, which is square in cross-section, with four straight side-cutting blades with a groove between the edges, connected to the shank by a short narrow neck. **B-1 r.,** an engine-driven reamer having an elongated, flame-shaped head set on a long noncutting shaft for mounting in a contra-angle handpiece; used in root canal preparation. **B-2 r.,** an engine-driven reamer operated with a special handpiece, having a cylindrical working head with two cutting edges forming a spiral. **D-type r.,** an engine-driven reamer having a short, tapered, flattened pyramid-shaped head, which is square in cross-section, with four straight cutting blades separated by grooves, connected to the shank by a short, heavy neck. **G-type r.,** Gates-Glidden DRILL. **K-type r.,** a hand-operated or engine-driven tapered and pointed reamer having a spiral cutting edge, sometimes serrated, which is used to enlarge root canals by a rotary cutting action. It is produced from a carbon or stainless steel triangular blank made from stainless or carbon steel wire, twisted so as to produce a series of spirals into the operating head; it has 0.80 to 0.28 cutting flutes per millimeter of operating head. It is quite similar to a root canal file, except for the number of cutting flutes. The identification symbol is an equilateral triangle. Called also *Kerr r.* **Kerr r.,** a trademark for a K-type reamer. **Ko-type r.,** an engine-driven reamer having an elongated and tapering head with slightly spiraling side cutting blades that are somewhat similar to those of a fissure bur without crosscuts; used with either a straight or a contra-angle handpiece as an orifice enlarger in root canal therapy. **M-type r.,** an engine-driven reamer having a spherical head with six to eight cutting blades, connected to the shank by a long and slightly flexible neck; used with either a straight or a contra-angle handpiece as an orifice-widener in root canal therapy. **O-type r.,** an engine-driven reamer having an elongat-

ed head with side-cutting spiraling blades with a wide rake angle, connected to the shank by a short sturdy neck, used in root canal therapy. **P-type r.,** Peeso DRILL. **quarter-turn r.,** an engine-driven reamer operated with a special endodontic handpiece, being a tapered and pointed, straight instrument, quadrangular in cross section, and having four straight side-cutting edges; used to enlarge or widen the root canal by cutting its axial walls. **T-type r.,** an engine-driven reamer having an elongated and slightly tapering head with 12 to 16 straight side-cutting blades separated by grooves; used with either a straight or a contra-angle handpiece as an orifice widener in root canal therapy.

reasonable skill, care, and judgment the responsibility of the dentist and auxiliary, to possess and use that reasonable degree of knowledge and skill that is ordinarily possessed by dentists or auxiliaries practicing in the same community.

reattachment (re″ah-tach′ment) 1. joining together parts that have been separated. 2. the recementing of a dental crown or other prosthesis. 3. reembedding of new periodontal ligament fibers into new cementum and the attachment of gingival epithelium to tooth surface previously denuded by disease. Called also *new attachment.*

rebase (re-bās′) the process of refitting a denture by means of the replacement of the denture base material without changing the occlusal relations of the teeth.

rebasing (re-bās′ing) the replacement of a denture base with the use of the teeth from the old denture. In rebasing, an impression of the soft tissue is made, using the existing denture as an impression tray; a stone cast is constructed in the corrected denture; the denture and cast are mounted, while the correct vertical and horizontal relationships between the cast and the denture teeth are maintained; the teeth are indexed in position; the teeth are removed from the old denture base; the teeth are reassembled in the index of the mounting device in their original relationship to the cast; and the new denture is constructed. The term is sometimes confused with *denture relining.*

recall (rĕ-kal′) 1. to call back; summon to return. 2. in dental practice, regularly scheduled appointments for periodic examination, treatment, or preventive care. **preventive r.,** regularly scheduled appointments for preventive periodic dental care.

receptaculum (re″sep-tak′u-lum), pl. *receptac′ula* [L.] a receptacle or container; that which serves for receiving or containing something. **r. chy′li,** CISTERNA chyli.

receptor (re-sep′tor) 1. a specific chemical grouping on the surface of the plasma or nuclear membrane that can combine with hormones or drugs so that they may affect the cell. 2. a specific chemical grouping on the surface of an immunologically competent cell with the capability of combining specifically with antigen. 3. a chemical group on the surface of the protoplasmic, colloidal molecule that fixes drugs or poisons and thereby renders them effective. 4. a hypothetical group in a cell that has the power of combining with and thus anchoring a haptophore group of a toxin or other substance. 5. one of the lateral chains of a cell that combines with foreign substances. Receptors for antigens may remain attached to T lymphocytes or may be cast off into the blood plasma by plasma cells (mature B lymphocytes). In either case, they retain their combining power and so function as antibodies. See also Ehrlich's side-chain THEORY. 6. a sensory nerve terminal that receives stimuli and relays them to the central nervous system. Called also *sensory r.* See also *electromagnetic r.,* CHEMORECEPTOR, EXTERORECEPTOR, INTERORECEPTOR, MECHANORECEPTOR, NOCICEPTOR, and THERMORECEPTOR. **acetylcholine r.,** cholinergic r. **adrenergic r.,** a drug receptor on an effector organ innervated by postganglionic adrenergic fibers of the sympathetic nervous system, which is stimulated by norepinephrine, epinephrine, and various adrenergic drugs, and blocked by adrenergic-blocking or adrenolytic drugs. Called also *adrenoceptor* and *adrenoreceptor.* **α-adrenergic r.,** an adrenergic receptor that is stimulated mainly by norepinephrine and, to a lesser extent, by epinephrine, having both excitatory and inhibitory effects on the effector organs. Responses to stimulation include: constriction and dilatation of the arterioles of the heart, skin, mucous membranes, skeletal muscles, brain, lungs, and abdominal viscera; constriction of the salivary glands; contraction of the iris, gastric sphincter, muscles of the bladder, uterus, pilomotor muscles, and splenic capsule; control of intestinal motility; and pancreatic, sweat gland, and salivary secretions. **β-adrenergic r.,** an adrenergic receptor that is stimulated by epinephrine and, to a lesser degree, by norepinephrine, having both excitatory and inhibitory effects on the effector organs. Responses to stimulation include: relaxation of the bronchial, ciliary, and certain bladder muscles; increased contractility, conduction velocity, and rate of the heart; constriction and dilatation of the arterioles of the heart, skeletal muscles, lungs, and abdominal viscera; decreased motility and tonus of the stomach and intestines; uterine contraction, contraction and relaxation of the splenic capsule; glycolysis and gluconeogenesis in the liver; increased secretion by the β-cells of the islands of Langerhans; lipolysis; secretion of amylase by the salivary glands; and synthesis of melatonin by the pineal gland. **cholinergic r.,** a molecular structure on the effector cells through which acetylcholine acts on organs controlled by the autonomic nervous system. The effect of acetylcholine on the exocrine glands, smooth muscle, and heart may be blocked by atropine and that on the autonomic ganglia and the voluntary junction by tubocurarine; since muscarine exerts the former action and nicotine the latter, the corresponding receptors are termed muscarinic (M) and nicotinic (N) receptors. Stimulation of cholinergic receptors produces: iris contraction; decreased contractility rate of the heart; increased conduction velocity at the cardiac atria; decreased conduction velocity at the His-Purkinje system of the heart; decreased contractility at the cardiac ventricles; dilatation of the arterioles of the heart, skin, mucous membranes, brain, lungs, abdominal viscera, and salivary glands; contraction of smooth muscles of the bronchi; stimulation of the bronchial glands; increased motility and tonus of the stomach and intestines; relaxation of gastric and intestinal sphincters; stimulation of gastric and intestinal secretions; contraction of the gallbladder and urinary bladder; relaxation of the sphincter of the bladder; increased motility and tonus of the ureters; erection of the penis; increased secretion of epinephrine and norepinephrine by the adrenal medulla; increased glycogen secretion; increased secretion of potassium and water by the salivary glands; and increased secretion by the lacrimal, nasopharyngeal, and sweat glands, and the pancreas. **contact r.,** a sense organ which responds to stimuli from objects in contact with the body. **contiguous r.,** a receptor which must be in direct contact with the stimulant, such as touch and taste receptors. **distance r.,** a sense organ which responds to stimuli from objects remote from the body, as a receptor for the stimuli of hearing, vision, or smell. **dominant r.,** a type of drug receptor. **drug r.,** a cellular chemical structure, usually of a cell membrane, but also found in other cellular elements, such as a protein or a lipoprotein, or an extracellular substance, such as cholinesterase, which is receptive to or has a chemical affinity for a specific drug. The effect of the drug is believed to cause a transmitter substance first to bind with the receptor, resulting in changes in the molecular structure of the receptor compound, and bringing about changes in cell membrane permeability to ions and ionic changes altering the membrane potential; thus, eliciting action potentials (as in smooth muscle), or causing electrotonic effects on cells (as in glandular cells) to produce a response. Another suspected mechanism consists of the activation of enzyme in the cell membrane, the enzyme in turn promoting chemical reaction in the cell. Called also *receptive substance.* See also occupation THEORY. **electromagnetic r.,** a receptor which detects light on the retina of the eye. **exteroceptive r.,** exteroceptor. **gustatory r.,** a chemoreceptor for the sense of taste; a taste bud. **H₁ r.,** see *histamine r.* **H₂ r.,** see *histamine r.* **histamine r.,** a chemical structure believed to be similar to a drug receptor, which mediates the activity of histamine, and is found on cell membrane of smooth muscle, particularly of the bronchi and blood vessels. Two types are recognized: H₁ and H₂ receptors. H₁ is blocked by pyralamine and other classic histamine antagonists, and is involved in histamine-induced bronchoconstriction, vasoconstriction, and vasodilation, although the hypotensive effects of histamine are not completely abolished by H₁, unless H₂ is also administered. H₂ is blocked by buramamide and metiamide, and is involved in histamine stimulation of gastric-acid secretion. H₁ receptors in capillaries are suspected of being also involved in the production of the histamine wheal. See also H₁ INHIBITOR and H₂ INHIBITOR. **hormone r.,** a specific molecular structure on cells with which endogenous substances, such as hormones, react or to which they bind. **interoceptive r.,** interoceptor. **M r., muscarinic r.,** see *cholinergic r.* **N r., nicotinic r.,** see *cholinergic r.* **nociceptive r.,** nociceptor. **olfactory r.,** a chemoreceptor for the sense of smell; the olfactory organ. **opioid r.,** a membrane-bound proteolipid with a mass of about 60,000 daltons, believed to be a receptor site for morphine-like drugs; the opioid drug receptor. **pain r.,** a nociceptor for the sense of pain. **pressure r.,** mechanoreceptor. **proprioceptive r.,** proprioceptor. **sensory r.,** receptor (6). **temperature r.,** thermoreceptor. **r. of the third order,** a former term for a receptor which possesses two combining groups only, a haptophore group for combining with the foreign toxin, and a complementophile group which combines with the complement that carries the zymotoxic element; this group included the lysins.

recess (re′ses) [L. *recessus*] a cavity, indentation, or a hollow space. Called also *recessus.* See also CAVITY and FOSSA. **pharyngeal r.,** a wide, slitlike lateral extension in the wall of the nasopharynx, cranial and dorsal to the pharyngeal orifice of the auditory tube. Called also *r. of Rosenmüller, recessus pharyngeus* [NA], *recessus pharyngeus Rosenmülleri, Rosenmüller's cavity,* and *Rosenmüller's fossa.* **piriform r.,** piriform SINUS. **r. of Rosenmüller,** pharyngeal r. **sphenoethmoidal r.,** the most superior and posterior part of the nasal cavity above the superior nasal concha, formed by the angle of junction of the sphenoid and ethmoid bones, into which the sphenoidal sinus opens. Called also *recessus sphenoethmoidalis* [NA].

recession (re-sesh′un) [L. *recedere* to draw back or away] the act or process of drawing away of a tissue or part from its normal position. **bone r.,** apical regression associated with pathologic changes of the periodontal ligament, resulting from bone resorption with decreased support for a tooth. **gingival r.,** the drawing back of the gingivae from the necks of the teeth with subsequent exposure of the root surfaces, beginning as a thin break in the free gingiva adjacent to the center of the tooth. Abnormal or excessive exposure of the root surface is known as *pathologic recession,* the distinction between normal and abnormal being of degree. Called also *gingival atrophy.* See also passive ERUPTION and gingival recession INDEX. **gingival r. index,** see gingival recession INDEX. **pathologic r.,** see *gingival r.*

recessive (re-ses′iv) 1. tending to recede; not exerting a ruling or controlling influence. 2. in genetics, pertaining to a recessive characteristic. See autosomal recessive CHARACTER and X-linked recessive CHARACTER.

recessus (re-ses′sus), pl. *reces′sus* [L.] a recess; a small cavity, indentation, or a hollow space; an anatomical term for such a space. See also CAVITY and FOSSA. **r. epitympan′icus** [NA], attic. **r. pharyn′geus** [NA], **r. pharyn′geus Rosenmül′leri,** pharyngeal RECESS. **r. pirifor′mis** [NA], piriform SINUS. **r. sphenoethmoida′lis** [NA], sphenoethmoidal RECESS.

recipe (res′ĭ-pe) 1. [L.] take; used at the head of a prescription, and usually indicated by the symbol ℞. See PRESCRIPTION. 2. a formula for the preparation of a specific combination of ingredients.

recipient (rĕ-sip′e-ent) one who receives, as blood in transfusion, or a tissue or organ graft. **universal r.,** a person thought to be able to receive blood of any "type" without agglutination of the donor cells.

reciprocation (re-sip′ro-ka′shun) [L. *reciprocare* to move backward and forward] 1. to give and receive in exchange; the complementary interaction of two distinct entities. 2. the means by which one part of a removable partial denture framework is made to counter the effect created by another part of the framework. **active r.,** the means by which one part of a restoration is made to counter the effects created by another. **passive r.,** reciprocation in a clasp unit achieved by the use of a rigid part of the clasp, located on or above the height of contour line or on a guiding plane and opposite to the retentive arm, performed in the presence of a similar action by another component of the removable partial denture located across the arch.

reciprocity (res′ĭ-pros′ĭ-te) 1. a mutual or cooperative exchange or relationship. 2. in licensure of health manpower, the recognition by one state of the licenses of another state when the latter extends the same recognition to licenses of the former state. See also ENDORSEMENT (3).

Recklinghausen's disease [Friedrich Daniel von *Recklinghausen,* German pathologist, 1833–1910] see under DISEASE.

Recklinghausen-Applebaum disease [F. D. von *Recklinghausen*] hemochromatosis.

Reclus' disease, [Paul *Reclus,* French surgeon, 1847–1914] ligneous PHLEGMON.

recoil (re-koil′) the act or process of drawing or springing back. **elastic r.,** a spring-like recoil, being the first phase of return of the teeth to their original position after forces applied against them, as in mastication, are removed.

recombinant (re-kom′bĭ-nant) a new cell or individual that results from genetic recombination.

recombination (re″kom-bĭ-na′shun) 1. the reunion of formerly united but separated elements. 2. the formation of a new combination of linked genes by crossing over.

recon (re′kon) [*rec*ombination + Gr. *-on* neuter ending] the smallest unit of genetic material in a gene (corresponding to a single nucleotide), which is exchangeable but not divisible by genetic recombination between homologous linkage structures of chromosomes.

record¹ (rek'ord) 1. information committed to, and preserved in, writing. 2. a permanent register of anything. 3. in a dental office, a written document pertaining to any professional or business activity. Records are generally classified as patient records (acquaintance forms, case histories, dental charts, records of treatment and prescriptions, radiographs, insurance forms and correspondence, study casts, financial records, recall records, and laboratory work authorizations) and business records (unpaid bills, expense records, payroll records, business correspondence, canceled checks and bank statements, income and expense records, financial statements, and income tax records). **centric interocclusal r.**, interocclusal r., centric. **centric maxillomandibular r.**, maxillomandibular r., centric. **centric occluding relation r.**, occluding centric relation r. **chew-in r., functional**, 1. a record of the natural chewing movements of the mandible made on the occlusion rim by the teeth or scribing studs. 2. a record of movements of the mandible made on the occluding surface of the opposing occlusion rim by the teeth or scribing studs and produced by simulated chewing movements. 3. a record of lateral and protrusive movements of the mandible made on the occlusal surface of the occlusion rim by the teeth or scribing studs on an opposing rim; produced during simulated movements of bruxism. **3-D r.**, three-dimensional r. **dental r.**, dental CHART. **eccentric interocclusal r.**, interocclusal r., eccentric. **eccentric maxillomandibular r.**, maxillomandibular r., eccentric. **face-bow r.**, a record made with a face-bow of the position of the hinge axis and/or the condyles, used to orient the maxillary and/or mandibular casts to the opening and closing axis of the articulator. **functional chew-in r.**, chew-in r., functional. **insurance summary r.**, a chronological organizational record for keeping track of insurance claims in process. **interocclusal r.**, a record of the positional relation of the opposing teeth or jaws to each other. It is made on the occlusal surfaces of occlusion rims or the teeth in a plastic material that hardens, such as plaster of Paris, wax, or zinc oxide–eugenol paste. **interocclusal r., centric**, a record of the centric jaw position (relation). **interocclusal r., eccentric**, a record of a jaw relation other than the centric relation. **interocclusal r., lateral**, a record of a lateral eccentric jaw position. Called also *lateral checkbite*. **interocclusal r., protrusive**, one of a protruded eccentric jaw relation. **jaw relation r.**, a registration of any positional relationship of the mandible in reference to the maxillae; these records may be of any of the many vertical, horizontal, or orientation relations. **jaw relation r., terminal**, terminal jaw relation r. **lateral check-bite interocclusal r.**, interocclusal r., lateral. **lateral interocclusal r.**, interocclusal r., lateral. **maxillomandibular r.**, a record of the relation of the mandible to the maxillae. Called also *maxillomandibular registration*. **maxillomandibular r., centric**, a record of the relation of the mandible to the maxillae when the mandible is in centric position. **maxillomandibular r., eccentric**, a record of the relation of the mandible to the maxillae when the mandible is in any position other than centric. **medical r.**, a written account of a patient's illnesses and the medical procedures applied. **occluding centric relation r.**, one of centric relation made at the established occlusal vertical dimension. Called also *centric occluding relation r.* **problem oriented medical r.**, a system of organizing a patient's health information in terms of specific problems, with each problem being assigned a number and treatment being referenced to the number of the problem involved. The concept is also applicable to dental records. Abbreviated *POMR*. **profile r.**, a record showing the sagittal outline form or profile of the face. See also facial PROFILE. **protrusive r.**, a record of the forward position of the mandible with reference to the maxillae. **protrusive interocclusal r.**, interocclusal r., protrusive. **r. rim**, occlusion RIM. **terminal jaw relation r.**, a record of the relationship of the mandible to the maxilla made at the vertical relation of occlusion and at the centric position. **three-dimensional r.**, a maxillomandibular interocclusal record. Called also *3-D r.*

record² (re'kord) to set down or register in a permanent form, such as a registration obtained with a face-bow.

recovery (rě-kov'er-e) 1. the act of getting back or regaining something. 2. in annealing a cold-worked metal, the stage when internal stresses begin to disappear, before any changes in the microstructure can be observed. See metal ANNEALING.

recrudescence (re″kroo-des'ens) [L. *recrudescere* to become sore again] the recurrence of symptoms after a temporary abate-

ment. The chief distinction between a recrudescence and a relapse is the time interval, a recrudescence occurring after some days or weeks, a relapse after some weeks or months.

recruitment (re-kroot'ment) 1. an increase in the number of individual nerve fibers discharging as the intensity of a stimulus increases. 2. activation of progressively more motor units in a muscle to increase the force of contraction. Called also *spatial summation*. 3. a gradual increase of a reflex to a maximum following a prolonged stimulus of unaltered intensity.

recrystallization (re-kris″tah-lī-za'shun) the act or process of reestablishing a normal crystalline structure. In annealing a cold-worked metal, the stage when distorted grains are replaced by new strain-free grains with a regular crystalline structure. See metal ANNEALING. **r. temperature**, recrystallization TEMPERATURE.

Rect. abbreviation for L. *rectifica'tus*, rectified.

rectification (rek″tǐ-fǐ-ka'shun) [L. *rectificatio*] 1. the act or process of making something straight or correct. 2. the redistillation of a liquid to purify it. 3. restriction of the flow of electric current to only one direction, thereby converting alternating current to direct current. See also SELF-RECTIFICATION. **full-wave r.**, rectification of the entire wave of alternating current to direct current by means of valve tubes or a mechanical device. **half-wave r.**, rectification of one-half the sine wave of alternating current by means of valve tubes or a mechanical device. In an x-ray generator, half-wave rectification allows only half the current impulses to produce x-rays, current flowing in the opposite direction being blocked.

rectifier (rek'tǐ-fī″er) 1. a device used for converting an alternating current to a direct current. 2. a device used for preventing or limiting the flow of current in the opposite direction. **full-wave r.**, an apparatus for rectifying the entire wave of an alternating current in an x-ray generator. **half-wave r.**, an apparatus for rectifying half of the sine wave in an x-ray generator. **thermionic r.**, a rectifier consisting of a valve in which the electrons are supplied by a heated electrode.

rectum (rek'tum) [L. "straight"] [NA] the distal portion of the large intestine.

rectus (rek'tus) [L.] 1. straight; a general term denoting a straight structure. 2. rectus MUSCLE. **r. cap'itis ante'rior**, rectus capitis anterior MUSCLE. **r. cap'itis latera'lis**, rectus capitis lateralis MUSCLE. **r. cap'itis poste'rior ma'jor** [NA], rectus capitis posterior major MUSCLE. **r. cap'itis poste'rior mi'nor** [NA], rectus capitis posterior minor MUSCLE.

recumbent (re-kum'bent) lying down.

recuperation (re-ku″per-a'shun) [L. *recuperatio*] the recovery of health and strength.

recurrence (re-kur'ens) [*re-* + L. *currere* to return] occurring again; the return of symptoms after a remission.

recurrent (re-kur'ent) [L. *recurrens* returning] 1. running back, or toward the source. 2. returning after intermissions.

recurvation (re″kur-va'shun) [L. *recurvatio*] a backward bending or curvature.

Red see color coding table at root canal THERAPY.

red (red) [L. *rubrum*] 1. one of the primary colors produced by the longest waves of the visible spectrum. 2. a red dye or stain.

Redig. in pulv. abbreviation for L. *rediga'tur in pul'verem*, let it be reduced to powder.

Red. in pulv. abbreviation for L. *reduc'tus in pul'verem*, reduced to powder.

redintegration (red-in″tě-gra'shun) [L. *redintegratio*] the restoration or repair of a lost or damaged part.

redislocation (re″dis-lo-ka'shun) dislocation recurring after reduction.

redox (red'oks) mutual reduction and oxidation; see OXIDATION-REDUCTION.

redressement (re-dres-maw') [Fr.] 1. a second or repeated dressing. 2. correction of a deformity.

reductase (re-duk'tās) dehydrogenase. **acceptor r.**, dehydrogenase. **aldehyde r.**, alcohol DEHYDROGENASE. **fumarate r.**, succinate DEHYDROGENASE.

reduction (re-duk'shun) [L. *reductio*] 1. the bringing of something to a smaller size, number, or amount. 2. in chemistry, originally the term meant taking away of oxygen from a substance, but it is now defined as the process occurring when an element gains electrons or decreases in valence, thereby becoming more electronegative. See also OXIDATION-REDUCTION. 3. the correction of a fracture, dislocation, or hernia. **closed r.**, the repositioning of fractured bones without making a surgical opening to the fracture site. In cases of fractures of the mandible or maxilla, accomplished by inter- or intramaxillary fixation. **open r.**, the repositioning of fractured bones by making a surgical opening to the fracture site, allowing direct visualization of the fracture and permitting stabilization by transosseous wires or bone plates.

Reducto trademark for *phendimetrazine tartrate* (see under PHENDIMETRAZINE).

redundant (re-dun'dant) more than necessary; superfluous.

reef (rēf) an infolding or tuck of tissue, as a tuck made in plication.

Reese's dysplasia (syndrome) [Algeron Beverly *Reese*, American ophthalmologist, born 1906] see under DYSPLASIA.

Reese-Blodi syndrome [A. B. *Reese*; Frederick C. *Blodi*, American physician, born 1917] Reese's DYSPLASIA.

reference (ref'er-ens) 1. the act or process of directing the attention or thoughts to something. 2. something for which a name or designation stands. 3. a direction of a source for assistance or information. **Physician's Desk R.**, an annual compendium of information concerning drugs (chiefly the prescription drugs) and diagnostic products, which is published for the use of physicians, dentists, and other health professionals. Abbreviated *PDR*.

referral (rĕ-fer'al) the practice of sending a patient to another practitioner or to another program for services or consultation which the referring practitioner is not prepared or qualified to provide. Referral for services involves a delegation of responsibility for patient care to another practitioner or program, and the referring practitioner may or may not follow up to ensure that services are received.

reflected (re-flekt'ed) turned or bent back; mirrored.

reflection (re-flek'shun) [L. *reflexio*] 1. a turning or bending back; a bending back upon its course. 2. an image produced by reflection. 3. the elevation or folding back of the mucoperiosteum to expose the underlying bone. 4. the turning back of a ray of light, sound, heat, or other ray when it strikes against a surface that it does not penetrate. The ray before reflection is known as the *incident ray*, after reflection, it is the *reflected ray*.

reflector (re-flek'tor) a device for reflecting light or sound. **dental r.**, a mouth mirror used to reflect light rays upon the field of action during a dental operation or examination.

reflex (re'fleks) [L. *reflexus*] 1. an immediate involuntary response of the body to a stimulus received by a receptor or a sense organ. 2. reflected. 3. a reflected image of an object. **allied r's**, reflexes in which two afferent stimuli use the same common pathway or produce effects on two synergistic muscles. **antagonistic r's**, those which oppose each other and are unable simultaneously to travel the final common pathway. **attitudinal r's**, those having to do with body position, e.g., tonic-labyrinthine reflexes, the position of the head influencing the tone of the limb muscles. **audito-oculogyric r.**, a turning of both eyes in the direction of a sudden sound. **autonomic r.**, a response of smooth muscle, glands, and conducting tissue and contractility of the heart, which alters the functional state of the innervated organ. For example, the aortic and carotid sinus reflexes mediate sympathetic vasomotor stimulation affecting heart rate and contractility. **axon r.**, a reflex resulting from a stimulus applied to one branch of a nerve which sets up an impulse that moves centrally to the point of division of the nerve where it is reflected down the other branch to the effector organ. **bulbomimic r.**, in coma from cerebrovascular injury, pressure on the eyeball causes contraction of the facial muscles on the side opposite to the lesion; in coma from systemic diseases, e.g., diabetes or uremia, the reflex occurs on both sides. Called also *facial r.* and *Mondonesi's r.* **carotid sinus r.**, pressure on or in the carotid artery at the level of its bifurcation, owing to external pressure or uncomfortable head position, causes reflex slowing of the heart rate, vasodilation, and hypotension. See also carotid sinus SYNDROME. **chain r.**, a series or cascade of reflexes, each serving as a stimulus to the next one. **chin r.**, stroking of the chin causes closing of the mouth. **concealed r.**, one elicited by a stimulus but concealed by a more dominant reflex elicited by the same stimulus. **conditional r.**, conditioned r. **conditioned r.**, one that does not occur naturally but that may be passively developed by regular association of some physiological function with an unrelated outside event, such as ringing of a bell or flashing of a light. Soon the physiological function starts whenever the outside event occurs (Pavlov, 1911). Called also *conditional r.* and *Pavlov's r.* **convulsive r.**, one in which several muscles contract without coordination. Both agonists and antagonists may contract simultaneously, as in strychnine poisoning. **coordinated r.**, one in which several muscles react so as to produce an orderly and useful movement. **corneomandibular r.**, movement of the lower jaw toward the side opposite the eye whose cornea is lightly touched, the mouth being open. Called also *corneopterygoid r.* **corneomental r.**, unilateral wrinkling of the muscles of the chin when pressure is applied to the cornea. **corneopterygoid r.**, corneomandibular r. **delayed r.**, a conditioned reflex whose efferent portion occurs some time after the stimulus provoking it has been received. **esophagosalivary r.**, Roger's

r. facial r., bulbomimic r. **faucial r.**, reflex vomiting caused by irritation of the fauces. **flexor r.**, flexion r., one initiated by a noxious stimulus, such as stepping on a sharp object, which causes an organ to withdraw from the source of painful stimulation, thus protecting it from injury. During mastication, an encounter of teeth or other tissue with a hard object similarly causes the jaw to open. It is a polysynaptic reflex involved in contraction of flexor muscles with a simultaneous inhibition of extensor muscles that takes precedence over other reflexes. Called also *nociceptive r.* and *withdrawal r.* **gag r.**, pharyngeal r. **gustolacrimal r.**, an anomalous reflex by which food taken into the mouth tends to stimulate the secretion not only of saliva but to a lesser extent also of tears. See gustatory LACRIMATION. **inverse stretch r.**, stretch r., inverse. **jaw r.**, jaw jerk r., closure of the mouth caused by a downward blow on the lower jaw while it hangs passively open; it is seen only rarely in health, but it is very noticeable in lesions of the corticospinal tract. Called also *mandibular r.* See also *stretch r.* **Liddel and Sherrington r.**, stretch r. **lip r.**, a reflex pouting of the lips in sleeping babies which occurs on tapping near the angle of the mouth. **mandibular r.**, jaw r. **Mondonesi's r.**, bulbomimic r. **motor r.**, one brought about by stimulation upon the periphery of the motor mechanism; for example, a stretch reflex elicited by deformation of a tendon. **myotatic r.**, stretch r. **nasolabial r.**, sudden retroversion of the head, stretching of the back, retroversion of the arms at the shoulder, extension and pronation of the forearms, and extension and adduction of the legs, elicited by a slight vertical sweeping motion touching the tip of the nose. It frequently occurs in healthy infants, and disappears around the fifth month of life. **nasomental r.**, contraction of the mentalis muscle on tapping the side of the nose. **nociceptive r.**, flexor r. **nostril r.**, reduction of the size of the opening of the naris, said to occur on the affected side in pulmonary disease. **nursing r.**, sucking r. **oculopharyngeal r.**, rapid deglutition together with spontaneous closing of the eyes when a very cold substance reaches the pharynx. **palatal r.**, palatine r., stimulation of the palate causing swallowing elevation of the soft palate. Called also *swallowing r.* **pathologic r.**, any reflex occurring as a result of a pathologic condition. **Pavlov's r.**, conditioned r. **pharyngeal r.**, contraction of the constrictor muscles of the pharynx and gagging elicited by touching the back of the pharynx. Called also *gag r.* **phasic r.**, an active and coordinated movement occurring as a response to stimulation. It is in contrast to a postural reflex. **postural r.**, one involved in the maintenance of posture. It is in contrast to a phasic reflex. Called also *static r.* **proprioceptive r.**, one that is initiated by stimulation of proprioceptors, e.g., the carotid sinus reflex. **psychogalvanic r.**, decreased electric resistance of the body as a result of emotional agitation. **Roger's r.**, profuse salivation on irritation or distension of the lower esophagus. It occurs acutely after swallowing an excessively large bolus that cannot easily enter the stomach, and is also associated with carcinoma. Called also *esophagosalivary r.* **rooting r.**, a reflex of the newborn in which stimulation of the cheek or the lip causes the infant to turn his mouth and face to the stimulus and the lips to purse ready for sucking. **spinal r.**, any reflex arc whose afferent and efferent arms make functional contact in the spinal cord. **static r.**, postural r. **stretch r.**, reflex contraction of a muscle in response to passive longitudinal stretching; the muscle spindle being the receptor. This type of reflex is active during reflex and voluntary contraction of both flexor and extensor muscles. The jaw jerk is a stretch reflex in which contraction of the temporal and masseter muscles is activated by downward percussion of the chin or by tapping the lower incisors or the tendon of the masseter muscle. Called also *Liddel and Sherrington r.* and *myotatic r.* **stretch r., inverse**, one which, upon severe stretching of a muscle, causes it to relax, the Golgi tendon organ being the receptor for the stimulus. **sucking r.**, a sucking movement of the mouth elicited by the touching of an object to an infant's lips. Called also *nursing r.* **swallowing r.**, palatal r. **withdrawal r.**, flexor r.

reflux (re'fluks) [re- + L. *fluxus* flow] backward or return flow or regurgitation.

Refobacin trademark for *gentamicin sulfate* (see under GENTAMICIN).

refract (rĕ-frakt') [L. *refringere* to break apart] 1. to cause to deviate. 2. to ascertain errors of ocular refraction.

refraction (re-frak'shun) 1. the act or process of refracting; specifically, the determination of refractive errors of the eye. 2. the deviation of light in passing obliquely from one medium to another of different density, occurring at the surface of junction between the two media. See also refractive INDEX, and phase MICROSCOPE.

refractory (re-frak'to-re) [L. *refractorius*] 1. not readily yielding to treatment. 2. capable of withstanding extremely high temperatures. 3. any material that has low thermal conductivity and is capable of withstanding extremely high temperatures. Crystalline silicates, such as quartz and cristobalite, are examples of refractory materials. See INVESTMENT. **r. investment,** see INVESTMENT.

regainer (re-gān'er) 1. a device that recovers or restores something previously lost. 2. space r. **coil spring space r.,** a cantilever space regainer, in which a tooth on one side of the space to be expanded is fitted with an orthodontic tube equipped with horizontal tubes on the buccal and lingual sides. The U-crib with coil springs is fitted into the tubes, its other end pressing against the other tooth across the space, with the resultant reciprocal force tipping the teeth away from the space. See illustration. **space r.,** a space maintainer that pushes back teeth

Regalloy trademark for a high-fusing chromium-cobalt casting alloy.

Regelan trademark for *clofibrate.*

regeneration (re-jen''er-a'shun) [re- + L. *generare* to produce, bring to life] the growth and differentiation of new cells and intercellular substance to form new tissue or parts. In the oral tissue, it consists of fibroplasia, endothelial proliferation and deposition of interstitial ground substance and collagen, and the maturation of connective tissue. It takes place by growth from the same type of tissue as that which has been destroyed, or from its precursor. In the periodontal structures, regeneration is a continuous physiological process, gingival epithelium being replaced by epithelium and the underlying connective tissue and periodontal ligament deriving from connective tissue. Bone and cementum are replaced by connective tissues, not the existing bone or cementum.

regimen (rej'i-men) [L. "guidance"] a strictly regulated scheme of diet, exercise, or other activity designed to achieve certain ends.

regio (re'je-o), pl. *regio'nes* [L. "a space enclosed by lines"] a plane area or section with either definite or approximate boundaries, usually on the surface of the body. See also AREA and

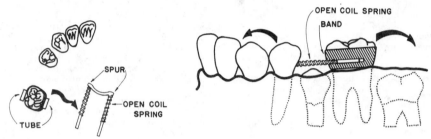

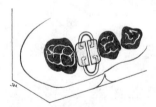

Cantilever coil spring space regainer. (From T. M. Graber: Orthodontics — Principles and Practice. 3rd ed. Philadelphia, W. B. Saunders Co., 1972; courtesy H. P. Hitchcock.)

that have crowded the edentulous area. See also Graber space MAINTAINER, space MAINTAINER, and space RETAINER. **split acrylic spring space r.,** a space regainer consisting of a spring made of a 0.032-inch stainless wire soldered to form an ellipse. The ellipse is compressed into the edentulous space to be increased, between the teeth and embedded into acrylic resin. The acrylic mass is split, thus releasing the spring action of the wire which then begins to push against the teeth. See illustration.

Split acrylic spring space regainer. (From T. M. Graber: Orthodontics — Principles and Practice. 3rd ed. Philadelphia, W. B. Saunders Co., 1972.)

regainer-maintainer (re-gān'er-mān-tān'er) an orthodontic appliance combining the characteristics of a space regainer and a maintainer. **jackscrew r.m.,** an adjustable orthodontic appliance in which the arm bridging the edentulous space, soldered to the orthodontic bands fitted over the two teeth on both sides of the space, is equipped with a jackscrew, thus allowing precise regulation of the pressure applied to the teeth. See illustration.

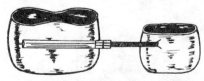

Jackscrew regainer-maintainer. (From T. M. Graber: Orthodontics — Principles and Practice. 3rd ed. Philadelphia, W. B. Saunders Co., 1972.)

REGION. **r. auricula'ris,** auricular REGION. **r. bucca'lis** [NA], buccal REGION. **regio'nes cap'itis** [NA], the various anatomical regions of the head, including the frontal, parietal, occipital, temporal, and infratemporal regions. **regio'nes col'li** [NA], the various anatomical regions of the neck, including the anterior, sternocleidomastoid, lateral, and posterior regions. **r. col'li ante'rior** [NA], anterior region of neck; see under REGION. **r. col'li latera'lis** [NA], posterior region of neck (2); see under REGION. **r. col'li poste'rior** [NA], posterior region of neck (1); see under REGION. **regio'nes cor'poris** [NA], **regio'nes cor'poris huma'ni,** regions of the body; the various anatomical areas, or subdivisions, demarcated on the surface of the human body for the purpose of topographical description. **regio'nes faci'ei** [NA], facial REGIONS; see under REGION. **r. fronta'lis** [NA], frontal REGION. **r. hyoi'dea,** hyoid REGION. **r. infraorbita'lis** [NA], infraorbital REGION. **r. infratempora'lis** [NA], infratemporal REGION. **r. labia'lis infe'rior,** labial region, inferior; see under REGION. **r. labia'lis supe'rior,** labial region, superior; see under REGION. **r. laryn'gea,** laryngeal REGION. **r. mastoi'dea,** mastoid REGION. **r. menta'lis** [NA], mental REGION. **r. nasa'lis** [NA], nasal REGION. **r. nu'chae,** nuchal REGION. **r. occipita'lis** [NA], occipital REGION. **r. olfacto'ria** [NA], olfactory REGION. **r. ora'lis** [NA], oral REGION. **r. orbita'lis** [NA], orbital REGION. **r. palpebra'lis infe'rior,** palpebral region, inferior; see under REGION. **r. palpebra'lis supe'rior,** palpebral region, superior; see under REGION. **r. parieta'lis** [NA], parietal REGION. **r. parotideomasseter'ica** [NA], parotideomasseteric REGION. **r. respirato'ria** [NA], respiratory REGION. **r. sternocleidomastoi'dea** [NA], sternocleidomastoid REGION. **r. subhyoi'dea,** subhyoid REGION. **r. submandibula're,** **r. submaxilla'ris,** submandibular TRIANGLE. **r. submenta'lis,** submental REGION. **r. supraorbita'lis,** supraorbital REGION. **r. tempora'lis** [NA], temporal REGION. **r. thyroi'dea,** thyroid REGION. **r. zygomati'ca** [NA], zygomatic REGION.

region (re'jun) [L. *regio*] a plane area or section with either definite or approximate boundaries. See also AREA and REGIO. **anterior r. of neck, anteromedial r. of neck,** the region of the neck situated on its anterior aspect. Called also *regio colli anterior* [NA]. **auricular r.,** the region of the head on either side, about the ear. Called also *regio auricularis.* **basilar r.,** the base of the skull. **bilaminar r.,** the region of the temporomandibular joint that contains the pseudocavernous plexus, an extensive network of blood vessels. In the superior layer there are numerous elastic fibers which take the form of fenestrated membranes. In the inferior layer, the elastic fibers are absent, while collagen components, blood, and lymph channels are numerous; this layer participates in the formation of the lining of the inferior synovial cavity, sometimes becoming ruffled to form villi which project into the synovial cavity. **buccal r.,** the region of the cheek; a facial region situated at the side of the oral cavity. Called also *regio buccalis* [NA]. **chromosome r.,** any region of a chromosomal arm lying between two adjacent landmarks. In each arm, the region closest to the centromere is identified as No. 1, and other regions numbered consecutively toward the telomeric ends. See also chromosome BAND, and see Chicago nomenclature and Paris nomenclature, under CHROMOSOME. **constant r.,** constant DOMAIN. **facial r's,** the areas into which the face is divided, including the *buccal* (side of oral cavity), *infraorbital* (below the eye), *mental* (chin), *nasal* (nose), *oral* (lips), *orbital* (eye), *parotideomasseter* (angle of the jaw), and *zygomatic* (cheek bone). Called also *regiones faciei* [NA]. **frontal r.,** the region of the head overlying the frontal bone; the forehead. Called also *regio frontalis* [NA]. **hyoid r.,** the part of the anterior region of the neck about the hyoid bone. Called also *regio hyoidea*. **immunoglobulin r.,** immunoglobulin DOMAIN. **infraorbital r.,** a facial region situated beneath the eye, adjacent to the nasal region. Called also *regio infraorbitalis* [NA]. **infratemporal r.,** the region of the head on either side, about the infratemporal fossa. Called also *regio infratemporalis* [NA]. **labial r., inferior,** the facial region about the lower lip. Called also *regio labialis inferior*. **labial r., superior,** the facial region about the upper lip. Called also *regio labialis superior*. **laryngeal r.,** the part of the anterior region of the neck overlying the larynx. Called also *regio laryngea*. **mastoid r.,** the region of the head on either side, about the mastoid process of the temporal bone. Called also *regio mastoidea*. **mental r.,** the region of the face about the chin. Called also *regio mentalis* [NA]. **mylohyoid r.,** the region on the lingual surface of the mandible to which the mylohyoid muscle is attached. **r. of nape,** nuchal r. **nasal r.,** the facial region about the nose. Called also *regio nasalis* [NA]. **nuchal r.,** the part of the posterior region of the neck adjoining the posterior region of the neck. Called also *r. of nape* and *regio nuchae*. **occipital r.,** the region of the head overlying the occipital bone. Called also *regio occipitalis* [NA]. **ocular r.,** orbital r. **olfactory r.,** the superior region of the nasal cavity, the mucosa of which contains most of the receptors for the sense of smell. It occupies the covering of the superior nasal concha and the opposite septum, and is confined to the area of the fossa which is walled off by the ethmoid bone. Called also *regio olfactoria* [NA]. **oral r.,** the region of the face about the mouth. Called also *regio oralis* [NA]. **orbital r.,** a part of the facial region about the eye. Called also *ocular r.* and *regio orbitalis* [NA]. **palpebral r., inferior,** the facial region about the lower eyelid. Called also *regio palpebralis inferior*. **palpebral r., superior,** the facial region about the upper eyelids. Called also *regio palpebralis superior*. **parietal r.,** the region of the head on either side, about the parietal bone. Called also *regio parietalis* [NA]. **parotideomasseteric r.,** the facial region on either side, about the parotid gland and the masseter muscle. Called also *regio parotideomasseterica* [NA]. **posterior r. of neck,** 1. the region of the neck between the occipital region above and the regions of the back below. Called also *regio colli posterior* [NA]. 2. the region of the neck lateral to the sternocleidomastoid region. Called also *regio colli lateralis* [NA] and *trigonum colli laterale*. **proportional r.,** in radiology, the range of operating voltage for the counter tube or ionization chamber in which the gas amplification is greater than 1 and is independent of the primary ionization; the range in which the pulse size is proportional to the number of ions produced as a result of the initial ionizing event. **pterygomaxillary r.,** the region of the face, about the zygoma and the prominence of the lower jaw. **respiratory r.,** the part of the nasal cavity below the olfactory region. Called also *regio respiratoria* [NA]. **sternocleidomastoid r.,** the region of the neck overlying the sternocleidomastoid muscle. Called also *regio sternocleidomastoidea* [NA]. **subhyoid r.,** the part of the anterior region of the neck below the hyoid bone. Called also *regio subhyoidea*. **submandibular r., submaxillary r.,** submandibular TRIANGLE. **submental r.,** the part of the anterior region of the neck beneath the chin. Called also *regio submentalis*. **supraorbital r.,** the region of the head immediately above the orbit. Called also *regio supraorbitalis*. **temporal r.,** the region of the head on either side, about the temporal bone. Called also *regio temporalis* [NA]. **thyroid r.,** the part of the anterior region of the neck about the thyroid gland. Called also *regio thyroidea*. **variable r.,** variable DOMAIN. **vestibular r.,** the lowest and the movable portion of the nose; it is lined with stratified epithelium and possesses hairs and sebaceous glands. **zygomatic r.,** the facial region on either side, about the zygomatic bone. Called also *regio zygomatica* [NA].

regional (re'jun-al) pertaining to, limited to, or affecting a certain region or regions.

regiones (re"je-o'nēz) [L.] plural of *regio*.

registrant (rej'is-trant) a nurse who is listed on the books of a registry as available for duty.

registrar (rej'is-trar) 1. an official keeper of records. 2. in British hospitals, a resident specialist who acts as assistant to the chief or attending specialist.

registration (re"ji-stra'shun) 1. the act of recording. 2. certification. 3. in dentistry, the making of a record of the jaw relations, present or of those desired, in order to transfer them to an articulator to facilitate proper construction of a dental prosthesis. **functional occlusal r.,** a dynamic registration of opposite dentition. **maxillomandibular r.,** maxillomandibular RECORD. **tissue r.,** the accurate recording of the shape of tissues by means of impression material.

registry (rej'is-tre) 1. an office where a nurse may have her or his name listed as being available for duty. 2. a central agency for the collection of pathologic material and related clinical, laboratory, x-ray, and other data in a specific field of pathology, so organized that the data can be properly processed and made available for study.

Regitine trademark for *phentoalamine*.

Regnoli's operation see under OPERATION.

Regonol trademark for *pyridostigmine bromide* (see under PYRIDOSTIGMINE).

regression (re-gre'shun) [L. *regressio* a return] 1. a return to a form or earlier state; returning to former unhealthy or inferior condition; retrogression; reversion. 2. a subsidence of symptoms or of a disease process. **calcific r. of pulp,** see pulp CALCIFICATION. **focal calcific r. of pulp,** denticle (2). **calcific r. of pulp, focal,** DENTICLE (2).

regurgitation (re-gur"ji-ta'shun) [re- + L. *gurgitare* to flow] a backward flowing, as of undigested food, or the backward flowing of blood into the heart, or between the chambers of the heart when a valve is incompetent. See also VOMITING.

rehabilitation (re"hah-bil"ĭ-ta'shun) 1. the restoration of normal form and function after injury or illness. 2. the restoration of an ill or injured patient to self-sufficiency or in gainful employment at his highest attainable skill in the shortest possible time, using combined medical, social, and vocational measures. **mouth r.,** oral r. **occlusal r.,** treatment methods for the restoration of the dentition to its optimum functional state, entailing adjustment of occlusal tooth surfaces through selective grinding, orthodontic alignment of teeth, prosthetic restoration, surgical correction of diseased parts, and other dental procedures, aimed at restoring normal masticatory function, proper esthetic appearance of the teeth and facial expression, improved phonetics, and preservation of the teeth and the periodontal ligament. Called also *occlusorehabilitation*. **oral r.,** correction, treatment, and improvement of the dentition through procedures that may range from a single amalgam restoration to complete mouth reconstruction by means of extensive crown and bridgework. Called also *mouth r*.

rehydration (re"hi-dra'shun) the restoration of water or of fluid content of a body or a substance which has become dehydrated.

Reichert's canal, cartilages [Karl Bogislaus *Reichert*, German anatomist, 1811–1883] see Hensen's CANAL, and see under CARTILAGE.

Reichert's syndrome [Frederick Leet *Reichert*, American physician, born 1894] see under SYNDROME.

Reichstein, Tadeus [born 1897] a Polish-born chemist in Switzerland; co-winner, with Philip S. Hench and Edward Calvin Kendall, of the Nobel prize for medicine and physiology in 1950, for their discoveries concerning the adrenal cortical hormones.

Reid's base line [Robert William *Reid*, Scottish anatomist, 1851–1939] see under LINE.

Reilly, William Anthony see Alder's ANOMALY (Alder-Reilly anomaly).

reimbursement (re"im-bers'ment) payment for expense, damage, or loss incurred; refund; repayment; compensation. **cost-based r., cost-related r.,** a method of payment for health care programs by third parties, typically Blue Cross plans or government agencies, whereby the amount of payment is based on the costs to the provider of delivering the service.

reimplantation (re"im-plan-ta'shun) replacement of an organ or other structure, such as a tooth (with vital or nonvital pulp), in the site from which it was previously lost or removed, either accidentally or intentionally. Called also *replantation*. See also

TRANSPLANTATION. **intentional r., intentional tooth r.,** 1. reimplantation of a tooth into the same alveolus after its removal for endodontic treatment outside the mouth. 2. reimplantation of a tooth after its accidental avulsion.

reinfection (re″in-fek′shun) a second infection by the same pathogenic agent.

reinforcement (re″in-fors′ment) the increasing of force or strength.

Reinke's edema [Friedrich *Reinke*] see under EDEMA.

reinstatement (re″in-stāt′ment) 1. the act of putting back or establishing again, as in a former position or state. 2. in insurance, the resumption of a policy which has lapsed.

reinsurance (re-in′shur-ans) a protection of insurance companies against excessive losses by purchasing insurance with other companies that assume a portion of the liability.

reintubation (re″in-tu-ba′shun) intubation performed a second time.

Reiter's disease [Hans *Reiter*, German physician, born 1881] see under DISEASE.

rejection (re-jek′shun) 1. the act or process of refusing to accept; throwing away; discarding. 2. graft r. **first set r.,** rejection of a graft that has been planted for the first time onto a previously unprimed host. See *graft r.* **graft r.,** the process by which the immune system of the host recognizes antigenic differences, becomes sensitized against, and attempts to eliminate the donor graft. With the exception of autografts and isografts, some degree of rejection occurs with every transplant. In *primary (first-set) rejection,* the host encounters the histocompatibility antigens on the surface of the cells of the graft for the first time, followed by sensitization. Sensitized lymphocytes then encounter the specific antigens of the graft, and initiate immune injury. In *hyperacute rejection,* there is an immediate response because of preformed antibody, associated with fibrin deposition, platelet aggregation, neutrophil infiltration, and graft failure. In *acute rejection,* the response occurs after about the sixth day and proceeds rapidly to graft failure, characterized by intermediate pain, swelling, and sloughing. Acute rejection occurs most often in heterologous grafting where the tissue is transplanted from a donor of a phylogenetically different species, and is less common in homologous grafting where tissue is transplanted from a donor who is of the same species as the host but is genetically dissimilar. Immunologically-determined rejection practically never occurs in isologous grafting where tissue is transplanted between genetically identical individuals, as between identical twins, or between individuals differing only at a single genetic region, and in autologous grafting performed within the same individual. See also GRAFT. **second set r.,** rejection of a graft by a host who has already rejected tissue from the same donor or tissue carrying similar histocompatibility antigen as the rejected graft.

Rela trademark for *carisoprodol.*

relapse (re-laps′) [L. *relapsus*] the return of symptoms some weeks or months after abatement. Cf. RECRUDESCENCE.

relation (re-la′shun) [L. *relatio* a carrying back] the condition or state of one object or entity when considered in connection with another. See also POSITION (1). **acentric r.,** eccentric r. **buccolingual r.,** the position of a tooth or space in the dental arch in relation to the tongue and the cheek. **centric r., centric jaw r.,** the position of the mandible obtained principally by operator guidance so that the condyles are in the rearmost uppermost position in the fossae of the temporomandibular joint. In this position hinge axis type movements can be made for up to about 25 mm. Centric relation is the most stable frame of reference for transferring jaw relations to the articulator and is a position reached by some individuals in swallowing and bruxism. An interference to stable jaw closure in centric relation is a common cause of temporomandibular dysfunction syndrome. Abbreviated *CR.* Called also *median retruded r.; jaw-to-jaw, ligamentous most retruded, muscular, retruded, retruded contact,* and *terminal hinge position; retruded centric;* and *true centric.* See also centric POSITION, retrusive EXCURSION, and hinge movement, terminal, under MOVEMENT. **convenience jaw r.,** convenience OCCLUSION. **cusp-fossa r.,** in centric occlusion, the relation between a stamp cusp and its fossa so that the cross and oblique grooves of the fossa form arcs about the condylar axes. The cusp is thus allowed to leave its fossa by either of these grooves and return to its three contact points

without sliding. **dynamic r.,** relations existing between two objects or entities when one or both of them are moving or constantly changing, as the relations between the mandible and the maxillae. **eccentric r., eccentric jaw r.,** any relation of the mandible to the maxilla other than the centric relation. Called also *acentric r.* and *eccentric position.* **eccentric jaw r., acquired,** an eccentric relation of the mandible to the maxilla that is assumed in order to bring the teeth into centric occlusion. **intermaxillary r., jaw r. jaw r.,** any relation of the mandible to the maxilla, variously designated as *centric, eccentric, median, occlusal, protrusive,* and so on. Called also *intermaxillary r.* and *maxillomandibular r.* **jaw r., centric,** centric r. **jaw r., convenience,** convenience OCCLUSION. **jaw r., eccentric,** eccentric r. **jaw r., median,** median r. **jaw r., median retruded,** centric r. **jaw r., posterior border,** posterior border POSITION. **jaw r., protrusive,** an occlusal position in which the mandible is protruded. Called also *protrusive occlusal position.* See also PROGNATHISM and protrusive EXCURSION. **jaw r., surgical,** the establishment and recording of the vertical dimension and centric relation between the surgically exposed bone surface and the opposite jaw at the time of the surgical bone impression. **jaw-to-jaw r.,** the muscular and temporomandibular joint positioning of the mandible in relation to the maxillae with regard to tooth positioning, or intercuspation. **jaw r., unstrained,** that maintained when a state of balanced tonus exists among all the muscles involved, being achieved without undue or unnatural force and causing no distortion of the tissue of the temporomandibular joints. **lateral r., lateral occlusal r.,** the relation of the mandible to the maxilla when the lower jaw is in a position to either side of centric relation. Called also *lateral position* and *lateral occlusal position.* See also lateral EXCURSION. **maxillomandibular r.,** jaw r. **median r., median jaw r., median occlusal r.,** the relation between the maxilla and the mandible when the lower jaw is in the median sagittal plane, without being displaced to either side. Under ideal conditions, median and centric relations should coincide. Called also *median occlusal position.* **median retruded jaw r.,** centric r. **occluding r.,** the jaw relation at which the opposing teeth occlude. **occlusal r.,** occlusal POSITION. **occlusal r., lateral,** lateral r. **occlusal r., median,** median r. **posterior border jaw r.,** posterior border POSITION. **protrusive jaw r.,** jaw r., protrusive. **rest r., rest jaw r.,** rest POSITION. **retruded jaw r., median,** centric r. **ridge r.,** the positional relation of the mandibular ridge to the maxillary ridge. **static r.,** one existing between two objects or entities that are not in motion. **unstrained jaw r.,** jaw r., unstrained. **working bite r.,** working OCCLUSION.

relationship (re-la′shun-ship″) a connection, association, or involvement. See also RELATION. **buccolingual r.,** the position of a space or tooth in relation to the tongue and the cheek.

relaxant (re-lak′sant) [L. *relaxare* to loosen] 1. lessening or reducing tension. 2. an agent that lessens tension. 3. muscle r. **centrally acting muscle r.,** see *muscle r.* **muscle r.,** a drug that aids in reducing muscle tension. Included in the group of muscle relaxants are drugs which interrupt afferent reflex pathways, as by local anesthesia, sometimes used to relieve localized muscle spasms; drugs which block neuromuscular transmission (*neuromuscular blocking agents*), which are further subdivided into those which act on the motor end-plate membrane of the myoneural junction (*competitive, stabilizing,* or *curariform agents*), thus inhibiting the response of the junction to acetylcholine, and those which completely depolarize the muscle fibers (*depolarizing agents*); and the *centrally acting agents,* which include drugs used in the treatment of Parkinson's disease and related syndromes, and drugs acting centrally to depress the degree of selectivity of neural systems in controlling muscle tone, used in the treatment of muscle spasm, tetanus, and certain orthopedic disorders. **skeletal muscle r.,** see *muscle r.*

Relaxar trademark for *mephenesin.*

relaxation (re″lak-sa′shun) 1. a lessening of tension. 2. a phenomenon whereby internal stresses and strains in a material are removed after its return to a normal shape following deformation and resumption of atoms to their normal position in the space lattice; a change in shape and contour of the solid due to the rearrangement in its atomic or molecular position, occurring as a relief to stresses and strains through the process of diffusion. Called also *memory.* See DIFFUSION (2).

Relaxil trademark for *mephenesin.*

release (re-lēs′) 1. liberate; to set free. 2. to allow to be done or known. 3. the relinquishment of a right, claim, etc., to another; also, the document in which such relinquishment is acknowledged. **r. of information,** in health insurance, a form signed by the patient giving the physician or dentist permission to release whatever information is necessary to the processing of his insurance claim.

Relestrid trademark for *methocarbamol*.

relief (re-lēf') [L. *relevatio*] 1. the mitigation or removal of pain or distress. 2. the projection of a figure, part, or structure above the ground on which it is formed. 3. the reduction or elimination of undesirable pressure or force from a specific area under a denture base. See also relief AREA, relief CHAMBER, and relief SPACE. 4. a thin lining of adhesive or hard baseplate wax in the master cast beneath lingual bar connectors or bar portions of the lingual plates, areas where major connectors will contact thin tissue, and beneath framework extension onto bridge areas for attachment of resin bases, which correspond accurately to the tissue topography. See also BLOCKOUT. **r. area,** relief AREA. **r. chamber,** relief CHAMBER. **gingival r.,** relief given to removable partial denture units at all gingival crossings to avoid impingement.

reline (re-līn') 1. to replace or put in a new lining or liner, material applied to the inside of a cavity or container. 2. to resurface the denture side of a denture with new base material to make it fit more accurately. See also RELINER and RELINING.

reliner (re-līn'er) material used in the process of relining. **denture r.,** a material, usually a self-curing resin, applied and cured against the old denture base, which provides a soft cushion to a denture. Available under numerous trademarks. **Just Treatment r.,** trademark for a *denture reliner*, prepared by mixing polyethyl methacrylate powder with a liquid containing ethyl alcohol.

relining (re-līn'ing) the replacement of a lining or liner. **denture r.,** resurfacing the tissue side of a denture in order to compensate for changes in the soft tissue occurring during the wearing of the denture and to achieve an accurate fit. See also denture RELINER and REBASING.

rem (rem) [acronym for *r*oentgen *e*quivalent *m*an] the quality of any ionizing radiation that produces biological effects in man equivalent to 1 rad of x-rays. **man-r., person-r.,** the product of the average individual dose in a population multiplied by the number of individuals in the population.

Remak, fibers of [Robert *Remak*, German neurologist, 1815–1865] gray fibers; see under FIBER.

remedial (re-me'de-al) [L. *remedialis*] curative, acting as a remedy.

remedy (rem'ě-de) [L. *remedium*] anything that cures, palliates, or prevents disease; see DRUG, MEDICINE, and THERAPEUTIC.

remineralization (re-min″er-al-i-za'shun) the restoration of mineral elements, as to the human body.

remission (re-mish'un) [L. *remissio*] a diminution or cessation of symptoms of a disease; also the period during which such diminution occurs.

remittence (re-mit'ens) temporary abatement, without actual cessation, of symptoms of a disease.

remittent (re-mit'ent) [L. *remittere* to send back] having periods of abatement and of exacerbation.

remnant (rem'nant) something remaining; a residue; a vestige. **enamel organ r.,** primary CUTICLE.

remodeling (re-mod″l-ing) 1. reconstruction; changing of shape; reshaping. 2. the arrangement of components. **temporomandibular joint r., adaptive,** a slow remodeling of the articular surfaces of the temporomandibular joint to enable it to adapt to changing occlusal forces. **temporomandibular joint r., peripheral,** an adaptive form of remodeling, in which there is addition of bone to the articular surface of the condyle of the mandible, and also at the neck of the condyle, occurring most often on the anterior condylar margin, sometimes producing lipping of the joint margins. **temporomandibular joint r., progressive,** an adaptive form of remodeling, in which there is addition of bone to the articular surface of the condyle of the mandible, which brings it closer to the joint cavity. **temporomandibular joint r., regressive,** an adaptive form of remodeling, in which changes occur on the articular eminence of the temporal bone and the posterior aspect of the articular surface of the condyle of the mandible, leading to a loss of convexity or flattening of the joint.

remover (re-moo'ver) an agent or device used to move something from its place or position. **band r.,** an orthodontic instrument designed for removing orthodontic bands from the teeth. Called also *band-removing pliers*. See illustrations. **crown r.,** an instrument for removing artificial crowns from the teeth. Most commonly it is a hooked bar that is applied to the cervical margin of the retainer; the weight against the handle provides the lever action which dislodges the crown.

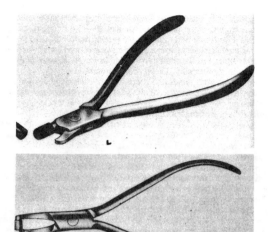

Band removers. (From H. O. Torres and A. Ehrlich: Modern Dental Assisting. 2nd ed. Philadelphia, W. B. Saunders Co., 1980.)

Remsed trademark for *promethazine*.

ren (ren), pl. *re'nes*, gen. *re'nis* [L.] kidney.

renal (re'nal) [L. *renalis*] pertaining to the kidney.

renaturation (re-na″chur-a'shun) restoration of native properties to proteins after their denaturation; believed to consist of refolding polypeptide chains to their original state and return of amino acid residues to their original position in the chains.

Rendu-Weber-Osler syndrome [Henry Jules Louis Marie *Rendu*, French physician, 1844–1902; Frederick Parkes *Weber*, British physician, 1863–1962; Sir William *Osler*, Canadian-born physician and medical educator, 1849–1919] hereditary hemorrhagic TELANGIECTASIA.

renes (re'nēz) [L.] plural of *ren*.

Renese trademark for *polythiazide*.

renewal (re-nu'al) 1. the act of beginning, or making new again; restoring; replenishing. 2. in insurance, an acceptance of a premium for a new policy term.

reniform (ren'i-form) [*ren* + L. *forma* form] shaped like a kidney.

reno- [Gr. *ren* kidney] a combining form denoting relationship to the kidneys.

REO respiratory enteric orphan (virus); see REOVIRIDAE.

Reomax trademark for *ethacrinic acid* (see under ACID).

Reoviridae (re″o-vi'ri-de) [respiratory and enteric orphan + *virus* + *-idae*] a family of arboviruses with naked virions having double icosahedral capsids, and a genome of 10 segments of double-stranded RNA, which replicate in the cell cytoplasm. The diameter of the virion is 70–75 nm and the number of capsomers in the virion is 32 to 92. Reoviruses have been isolated from feces and respiratory secretions of healthy and diseased individuals, the throat being their common habitat, but there is little evidence that they are related to any pathologic condition. The family consists of three genera: *Orthoreovirus, Orbivirus,* and *Rotavirus*. Several additional types have been provisionally assigned to this family.

reovirus (re″o-vi'rus) any virus of the family Reoviridae.

reoxidation (re-ok″si-da'shun) the act of taking up oxygen again, as by hemoglobin in the blood.

Rep. abbreviation for L. *repeta'tur*, let it be repeated.

rep (rep) [acronym for *r*oentgen *e*quivalent *p*hysical] an absolute unit of absorbed dose of any ionizing radiation with a magnitude of 93 ergs per gram. It has been superseded by *rad*.

repair (re-pār') 1. to restore something to good or workable condition. 2. the physical or mechanical restoration of damaged or diseased tissues by the growth of healthy new cells or by surgical apposition. 3. in dentistry, rejoining of broken parts of either the base or the framework, or the replacement of deteriorated or lost segments of the partial denture. **tooth r., histologic,** a reparative process in a tooth consisting of reduction or limitation of inflammatory infiltrate; elaboration of secondary cementum on previously resorbed root surfaces; and regeneration of previously resorbed alveolar bone or collagen fill-in of bony defects. **tooth r., periapical,** the repair of the apical periodontium. **tooth r., radiographic,** repair of the tooth tissue determined on the basis of follow-up radiographs.

repetatur (re″pe-ta′tur) [L.] let it be repeated.

replant (re-plant′) to restore a structure to its original site, as to reinsert a tooth into the alveolar socket from which it has been displaced.

replantation (re″plan-ta′shun) reimplantation.

replenisher (re-plen′ish-er) an agent that restores what has been lost, used up, or is lacking.

repletion (re-ple′shun) [L. *repletio*] the condition of being full.

replication (re″pli-ka′shun) 1. a turning back of a part so as to form a duplication. 2. repetition of an experiment to ensure accuracy. 3. the process of duplicating or reproducing DNA strands. The process occurs when the hydrogen bonds between the bases break, and the strands replicate as they unwind, each strand acting as a model or template for the formation of a new complementary chain. See also DNA, TEMPLATE, TRANSCRIPTION, and TRANSLATION. **conservative r.,** replication of DNA in which the original molecule remains intact and a completely new one is formed. **dispersive r.,** nonconservative r. **nonconservative r.,** replication of DNA in which parental nucleotide bases are distributed in both strands of each daughter molecule. Called also *dispersive r.* **semiconservative r.,** replication of DNA in which the strands separate longitudinally so that each daughter molecule has one new and one parental strand.

replicator (rep″li-ka′tor) a device which duplicates or reproduces something. **gnathic r.,** an apparatus for registering and reproducing functional jaw motions.

reposition (re″po-zish′un) [L. *repositio*] replacement in the normal position.

repositioning (re″po-zish′un-ing) the replacement of a structure or part to its normal site. **jaw r.,** the changing of any relative position of the mandible to the maxillae, usually by altering the occlusion of the natural or artificial teeth. **muscle r.,** surgical replacement of a muscle attachment into a more acceptable functional position.

repository (re-poz′i-to-re) 1. a place where something is stored. 2. an injection, usually intramuscular, of a long-acting drug, which is slowly absorbed and is, therefore, prolonged in its action.

repressor (re-pres′or) [L. "restrainer"] 1. that which restrains or inhibits. 2. a substance coded for by a regulator gene which acts through the cytoplasm to repress the synthesis of specific proteins or groups of related proteins by binding to their corresponding operator genes, thus forestalling messenger RNA transcription. See also COREPRESSOR and INDUCER.

repulsion (re-pul′shun) [*re-* + L. *pellere* to drive] 1. the act of driving apart or away; the force which tends to drive two bodies apart. 2. the occurrence on opposite chromosomes in a double heterozygote of two mutant alleles. Cf. COUPLING.

Rescue Squad see under GEL.

research (re-serch′, re′serch) 1. to study or investigate thoroughly and carefully. 2. the study of laws, theories, and hypotheses through a systematic examination of pertinent facts and their interpretation. **clinical r.,** human EXPERIMENTATION.

resection (re-sek′shun) [L. *resectio*] excision of a portion of an organ or other structure. **bone r.,** ostectomy. **interdental r.,** interdental DENUDATION. **root r., root end r.,** apicoectomy.

Reserpex trademark for *reserpine*.

reserpine (res′er-pēn, re-ser′pin) an alkaloid from the rhizomes of various species of *Rauwolfia*, especially *R. serpentina*, 11,17α-dimethoxy-18β-[(3,4,5-trimethoxybenzoyl) oxy]-3β, 20-α-yohimban-16β-carboxylic acid methyl ester. It occurs as a white, pale buff, or yellowish, odorless powder that darkens on exposure to light, and is soluble in alcohol, chloroform, and acetic acid, is slightly soluble in benzene, and is insoluble in water. It is an adrenergic neuron blocking agent that depletes catecholamine-containing granules of the postganglionic sympathetic neurons. Reserpine is also a sedative that depletes serotonin and catecholamines in the brain, but its central action is not fully understood. Used in the treatment of hypertension; formerly used in psychoses. In dentistry, used chiefly as a vasoconstrictor in local anesthesia, in gingival retraction, and in controlling postoperative bleeding. Stuffy nose, nausea, bradycardia, salivation, weight gain, diarrhea, suicidal tendencies, gastric hypersecretion, and hypotension are the most common side effects. Trademarks: Alserin, Austrapine, Crysto-

serpine, Hiserpia, Orticalm, Reserpoid, Reserpex, Rivasin, Sandril, Serpasol, Serpiloid, Serpine.

Reserpoid trademark for *reserpine*.

reserve (re-zerv′) something kept in store for future use. **alkali r., alkaline r.,** the amount of conjugate base components of the blood buffers; since bicarbonate is the most important of these conjugate bases, the term *blood bicarbonate* is often used to mean alkali reserve. **cardiac r.,** the potential ability of the heart to perform a wide range of work beyond that required under basal conditions.

reservoir (rez′er-vwar) 1. a place where something is collected or accumulated. 2. in anatomy, a structure serving as a storage space for fluid. See CISTERNA. 3. an alternate host or passive carrier of a pathogenic organism. 4. in a mold, a dilated space in the ingate, formed by a piece of wax attached to the sprue former, serving as a storage space for molten metal in preventing localized shrinkage porosity. When the molten metal flows into the mold, the fused metal in the reservoir is the last to solidify so that any voids in the mold caused by shrinkage are filled from the reservoir. See also illustration at MOLD.

res gestae [L. "part of the action"] a statement made spontaneously at the time of an alleged negligent act.

reshaping (re-shāp′ing) a restoration or change of shape, as of a crown, bridge, or denture. **surgical r.,** 1. plastic SURGERY. 2. in periodontics, gingivoplasty, osteoplasty, and ostectomy.

residency (rez′i-den-se) a period of one to seven years of on the job training, usually in a hospital, which may be either a part of a formal educational program or be undertaken separately after completion of the formal program, normally required toward the fulfillment of requirements for credentialing in medicine, dentistry, and other health professions. See also RESIDENT. Cf. INTERNSHIP.

resident (rez′i-dent) a graduate and licensed physician or dentist receiving training in a specialty in a hospital. See also RESIDENCY and resident PHYSICIAN. Cf. INTERN (1).

residua (re-zid′u-ah) [L.] plural of *residuum*.

residual (re-zid′u-al) [L. *residuus*] remaining or left behind; pertaining to a residue.

residue (rez′i-du) [L. *residuum*, from *re* back + *sidere* to sit] a remainder; remnant; that which remains after the removal of other substances.

residuum (re-zid′u-um), pl. *resid′ua* [L.] a residue.

resilience (re-zil′e-ens) [L. *resilire* to leap back] 1. the property of being able to return to the original form after distortion, as by bending, compressing, or stretching. 2. the ability to recover readily from an illness. 3. resiliency (2).

resiliency (re-zil′yen-se) 1. resilience. 2. the capacity of a material, such as orthodontic wire, for the elastic storage of energy when it is stressed, as by elastic deformation; being the combined effect of stiffness and working range and not being related to size or form of stressed material.

resin (rez′in) [L. *resina*] a mixture of carboxylic acids, essential oils, and terpenes, occurring as exudations on various trees and shrubs. Resins are highly combustible and electrically nonconductive semisolids or amorphous solids that are insoluble in water, while some are soluble in ethanol and others in carbon tetrachloride, ether, and volatile oils. Most are soft and sticky, but harden after exposure to cold. Rosin and balsam are some commonly occurring natural resins. Used in varnishes, adhesives, and other products. Resins are also produced synthetically. **acrylic r.,** one of the thermoplastic polymers or copolymers of acrylic acid; methacrylic acid, their esters, or acrylonitrile, being derivatives of ethylene and containing a vinyl group in their structural formula. The monomers of acrylic resins are colorless liquids readily polymerized in the presence of light, heat, or catalysts, such as benzoyl peroxide. They have low specific gravity, shock resistance, and stability to weathering and various chemical substances, and are soluble in aromatic and chlorinated hydrocarbons, esters, and ketones. Addition of acrylic anhydride, acrylamide, or glycol esters converts acrylic resins into thermosetting resins. In powder form, they may be injection- and compression-molded or, in dough form, may be molded in gypsum molds. *Methyl methacrylate* and *polymethyl methacrylate* are the most commonly used acrylic resins in dentistry. Called also *acrylic.* The term is sometimes used synonymously with *polymethyl methacrylate* (see under METHACRYLATE). **activated r.,** self-curing r. **alkyd r.,** a polyester polymer with cross-links. **autopolymer r.,** self-curing r. **r. benjamin,** benzoin (1). **r. benzoin,** benzoin (1). **r. cement,** resin CEMENT. **cold-curing r.,** self-curing r. **composite r.,** a synthetic resin, usually acrylic based, to which a high percentage (about 75 to 80 percent) of an inert filler has been added — glass beads or rods, borosilicate glass powder, and natural silica being the most commonly used fillers. Binding of the filler to the resin is produced by priming the filler particles with a coupling agent, such as silanes. Used chiefly in dental restorative procedures. Called also *filled r*. See also *unfilled r*. and composite MATERIAL. **condensation r.,** one formed through the process of condensation polymerization. Polymers whose repeating units are joined by functional groups, such as amide, urethane, ester, or sulfide linkages, even without the formation of a byproduct, are also classified as condensation resins. **copolymer r.,** a synthetic resin which is the product of polymerization of two or more monomers or polymers. **r. crazing,** resin CRAZING. **crown and bridge r.,** a resin used in the construction of crown and dental bridges, including vinyl-acrylic resin, acrylic resins, and composite resins, especially those processed under dry heat in a vacuum. **cyanoacrylate r.,** a resin based on alkyl 2-cyanoacrylates prepared by pyrolizing poly(alkyl)-2-cyanoacrylates, produced when formaldehyde is condensed with the corresponding alkyl cyanoacetates. Used experimentally in surgical sutures and for periodontal dressings. Also used in various industrial products. **dammar r.,** dammar. **dental r.,** any of a wide variety of synthetic resins used in dentistry, including those used as elastomeric impression materials, in the restoration of missing teeth or missing tooth structures, in denture bases, and in dentures, polymethyl methacrylate being the one used most commonly. **denture base r.,** any resin used for the construction of a denture base, including heat-curing and self-curing acrylic resins and vinyl-acrylic combinations. **direct filling r.,** a resin or a composite, usually an acrylic, that is inserted directly into the prepared cavity and allowed to polymerize at mouth temperature. It is a self-curing resin available as a powder polymer and a liquid monomer, the powder particles being somewhat smaller than those of the denture base resin. Various hues of powder are available to match different shades of teeth. Two types are used: a composite resin (one containing a high concentration of filling materials) and an unfilled resin (one having no or only small amounts of filling materials). At least three methods of applying the resin are in general use: the pressure technique (see pressure FILLING), the nonpressure (bead) technique (see bead technique FILLING), and a combination pressure and nonpressure technique (see flow technique FILLING). **epoxy r.,** a thermosetting resin based on the reactivity of the epoxide group (an organic compound containing a reactive group produced by the union of an oxygen atom and other atoms, usually carbon). Epoxy resins have the ability to polymerize by both addition and condensation and form a tight cross-linked polymer network, being characterized by toughness, adhesibility, chemical resistance, dielectric properties, and dimensional stability. Polybasic acids, boron trifluoride, anhydrides, and, chiefly, polyfunctional amines are the cross-linking agents. Epoxy resins may be cured at room temperature and adhere to metals, wood, and glass. Several modified types are used as denture base material, but problems of color stability, water sorption, and tissue irritation still remain to be solved. Called also *epoxy*. **filled r.,** composite r. **r. filler,** resin FILLER. **heat-curing r.,** any resin that can be polymerized by the use of heat. **ionomer r.,** a copolymer of ethylene and a vinyl monomer with an acid group, such as methacrylic acid. Ionomer resins are cross-linked polymers in which the linkages are ionic as well as covalent bonds. Ionomer resins are transparent, tough, resilient, and thermoplastic solids with high resistance to abrasion and cracking, and cannot be dissolved completely in common solvents. Used in mercury flasks, break-resistant bottles, and other products. **kauri r.,** a hard resin from the bark of the kauri tree, sometimes found in a fossil form. It is soluble in alcohols and ketones but not in water. Used in varnishes and as a component of impression compounds. **r. matrix,** resin MATRIX. **natural r.,** see *resin*. **Perfex repair r.,** a trademark for a self-curing *repair resin*. **polycarbonate r.,** a polyester of carbonic acid in which the carbonate is repeated in the linear chain, produced by the polymeric condensation of bisphenols with a phosgene or its derivatives. It is a thermoplastic material having physical properties similar to those of polymethyl methacrylate. Studied for use in denture bases and as a direct filling resin. **polyurethane r.,** see POLYURETHANE. **quick-cure r.,** self-curing r. **repair r.,** any resin used to repair an acrylic denture that has been fractured in service. Self-curing resins are usually preferred because the use of heat-curing tends to warp the denture during processing. **restorative r.,** a synthetic resin used in restorative dentistry, self-curing acrylic-based resin, e.g., dimethacrylate, composite (filled) or unfilled, being used most commonly. **self-curing r.,** any resin which can be polymerized by the addition of an activator and a catalyst without the use of external heat. Called also *activated r.*, *autopolymer r.*, *cold-curing r.*, and *quick-cure r*. **synthetic r.,** a man-made high polymer produced by a chemical reaction between two or more substances in the presence of a catalyst or heat, including synthetic rubbers, siloxanes, and silicones. **thermoplastic r.,** a resin, usually a linear polymer, which can be made to soften and take a new shape by the application of heat and pressure. Thermoplastic resins are fusible, and are usually soluble in organic solvents. **thermoset r., thermosetting r.,** a resin, usually a three-dimensional, cross-linked polymer which can be molded to final shape during polymerization but, once the reaction has taken place, the product is stable to heat and cannot be made to flow under pressure or to melt. Some thermosetting resins may be made more pliable by the addition of plasticizers. They are generally insoluble and infusible. **thermosetting methacrylate r.,** a compound derived from an epoxy resin and a methacrylate resin, where the reaction sites (oxirane group) of the epoxy molecule were replaced by methacrylate groups, the hybrid molecule being polymerized through the methacrylate group. Used as a resin matrix in composite resins. **ultraviolet light-cured r.,** a resin, such as an acrylic-based resin, that polymerizes under the influence of ultraviolet rays, rather than a chemical activator. An ultraviolet light-sensitive chemical, such as benzoin methyl ether, is substituted for the conventional peroxide initiator. When used as a direct filling resin, the polymer-monomer mixture with an ultraviolet light-sensitive initiator is inserted into the prepared cavity and an ultraviolet light gun is used to initiate polymerization. **unfilled r.,** a resin, such as polymethyl methacrylate, that does not contain or contains very small amounts of inert filler materials. See also *composite r*. **vinyl r's,** resins produced by the polymerization of ethylene monomers. See VINYL acetate and VINYL chloride. **yellow r.,** rosin.

resina (re-zi′nah) [L.] resin.

resinoid (rez′ĭ-noid) 1. resembling a resin. 2. a substance resembling a resin.

resinous (rez′ĭ-nus) [L. *resinosus*] of the nature of a resin; pertaining to a resin.

res ipsa loquitur [L. "the facts speak for themselves"] in malpractice, a legal doctrine or presumption that, when an injury occurs to a plaintiff through a situation under the sole and exclusive control of the defendant and where such injury would not normally occur if the one in control had used due care, then it is presumed the defendant is negligent. Applies, for example, in the case of a surgeon who leaves a sponge in the abdomen.

resistance (re-zis′tans) [L. *resistentia*] 1. the act or capacity of opposing or withstanding something. 2. the opposition by a conductor to the passage of an electric current. 3. the natural ability of a normal organism to remain unaffected by noxious agents in its environment, such as poisons, toxins, irritants, and pathogenic microorganisms. Resistance is for the most part a genetic endowment of an entire species with respect to a particular agent. If the resistance is absolute, all members of the species are insusceptible to a specific agent. If the resistance is relative, racial and individual differences become manifest within the species, one race or member being more resistant than another. See also IMMUNITY. **abrasion r.,** resistance of a substance or material to abrasion and wear, hardness being generally indicative of the resistance capacity, with some exceptions, such as rubber, which, although soft, is very resistant to abrasion. **r. to fluid flow,** viscosity. **hemolytic r.,** see osmotic FRAGILITY. **peripheral r.,** the resistance to the passage of the blood through the small vessels, especially the arterioles. **solubility r.,** the ability to resist by a substance the dissolving action of a liquid, as when a dental material resists the action of saliva. **vital r.,** the natural resistance of an individual to the untoward effects of infections, diseases in general, fatigue, overwork, and the like.

resite (res′īt) an insoluble, infusible compound formed by further reaction of resole under heat.

resol (res′ōl) a single-stage synthetic resin produced from a phenol and an aldehyde.

resole (res′ōl) a relatively low-molecular-weight condensation polymer of alcohol formed by interaction of phenol and formaldehyde; it is thermoplastic and soluble in alcohol. See also BAKELITE.

resolution (rez′o-lu′shun) [L. *resolutum*, from *resolvere* to unbind] 1. the subsidence of a pathologic state, as the subsidence of an inflammation, or the softening and disappearance of a swelling. 2. the perception as separate of two adjacent objects or points. In microscopy, it is the minimal distance at which two adjacent objects can be distinguished as separate. The resolving power of an instrument depends on the wavelength of the radiation used and the numerical aperture of the system; it is expressed in microns distance or lines per millimeter. See also image DEFINITION.

resonance (rez′o-nans) [L. *resonantia*] 1. the prolongation and intensification of sound produced by the transmission of its vibrations to a cavity, especially a sound elicited by percussion. Decrease of resonance is called *dullness*; absence of resonance, *flatness.* 2. a vocal sound as heard in auscultation.

resorcin (rĕ-zor′sin) resorcinol.

resorcinol (re-zor′si-nol) a phenol derivative, 1,3-benzenediol, occurring as white needles or powder with a faint characteristic odor and a sweetish taste and a bitter aftertaste, which becomes pinkish on exposure to light and air and dissolves in water, alcohol, glycerol, and ether, and is slightly soluble in chloroform. Used as a topical antibacterial and antifungal agent and as a local irritant. Called also *resorcin.*

resorcinolphthalein (re-zo″sĭ-nol-thal′ĕ-in) fluorescein.

resorption (re-sorp′shun) [L. *resorbere* to swallow again] the act or process of resorbing; assimilation of substances or structures previously produced by the body; reabsorption. **bone r.,** resorption of calcified bone tissue, the mechanism of which is believed to involve demineralization due to reversal of the cation exchange and lacunar resorption by osteoclasts, resulting in bone destruction. Increased oxygen tension and accelerated synthesis of citric acid with its local accumulation are believed to be involved in the process. **cementum r.,** resorption occurring, in descending order of frequency, in the apical third of the root, in the middle, or in the gingival portion. It may be due to systemic or local causes, with occlusal trauma, orthodontic manipulation, pressure from malaligned erupting teeth, cysts and tumors, and other lesions being the principal causes, or it may occur without an apparent cause (idiopathic r.). Microscopically, a focus of resorption appears as baylike concavities in the root surface, multinucleated giant cells and large mononuclear macrophages being found adjacent to cementum undergoing resorption. Sites of resorption may coalesce to form large areas of destruction. The process may extend into the dentin or pulp, but is usually painless. **central r.,** tooth r., internal. **external r.,** see *tooth r., external.* **extracanalicular r.,** tooth r., external. **frontal r.,** resorption of the lamina dura of the alveolar bone adjacent to the periodontal ligament. **idiopathic r.,** resorption of calcified tissue without apparent cause. **internal r.,** see *tooth r., internal.* **intracanalicular r.,** tooth r., internal. **lacunar bone r.,** destruction of bone due to the action of osteoclasts, which begins as decalcification of the mineral salts caused by a decrease of hydrogen ion concentration, and followed by proteolytic reaction of the matrix, resulting in the liberation of calcium salts, destruction of inorganic and organic bone components, and phagocytosis of the organic matrix after the inorganic salts have been removed. **osteoclastic r.,** bone resorption due to the activity of osteoclasts and characterized by the formation of Howship's lacunae on its surface. **physiologic bone r.,** physiologic bone ATROPHY. **pressure r.,** bone or tooth resorption precipitated by excessive mechanical or occlusive force. **pressure bone r.,** bone resorption due to sustained pressure. **rear r.,** osteoclastic resorption of the supporting bone of the alveolar process from the bone marrow spaces, producing thinning and fragmentation of the bone. **root r.,** resorption in which cementum and/or dentin is lost from the root of a tooth, due to cementoclastic or osteoclastic activity in conditions such as trauma of occlusion or neoplasms. **senile bone r.,** physiologic bone ATROPHY. **tooth r.,** resorption of calcified dental tissue, involving demineralization due to reversal of the cation exchange and lacunar resorption by osteoclasts. A hypothesis has been proposed that the condition is triggered by increased oxygen tension and accelerated synthesis of citric acid. Called also *odontolysis.* See also resorption LACUNA. **tooth r., external,** resorption of calcified dental tissue, beginning on the external surface, usually at the apex or the lateral surface of the root, as a result of a tissue reaction in the periodontal or pericoronal tissue, increasing in severity with age. Principal causative factors in resorption include periapical inflammation, tooth reimplantation, tumors and cysts, excessive mechanical or occlusive forces, and impaction of teeth. Spontaneous resorption sometimes may occur in endocrine disorders. The lesion begins on the surface of the root, extending to the cementum, dentin, and eventually into the root canal. Irregular infractious defects, lined by numerous osteoclasts, Howship's lacunae, and granulation tissue are the principal histologic features. External resorption which ramifies into the dentin is sometimes called *internal resorption.* Called also *extracanalicular r.* **tooth r., internal,** an unusual form of tooth resorption beginning centrally in a tooth, and apparently initiated by a peculiar inflammatory hyperplasia of the pulp. It is usually symptomless in the early stages. A pink hued area on the crown showing the hyperplastic vascular pulp tissue filling the resorbed area is the most prominent sign. Histologically, the condition presents a variable degree of resorption of the inner or pulpal surface of the dentin and proliferation of the pulp tissue filling the defect. The term *odontoclastoma* applies to a lacunar variety showing osteoclasts or odontoclasts. External resorption which ramifies into the dentin is sometimes called *internal resorption.* Called also *central r., intracanalicular r., chronic perforating pulp hyperplasia, endodontoma, internal pulp granuloma, Mummery's pink tooth, pink spot disease, pink tooth, pink tooth of Mummery,* and *pulpoma.* **undermining r.,** bone resorption in which pressure produces a cell-free zone in the compressed periodontal ligament. **unerupted tooth r.,** external resorption of unerupted teeth.

respiration (res′pĭ-ra′shun) [L. *respiratio*] the absorption of oxygen and elimination of carbon dioxide from the atmosphere and the cells of the body, respectively. The process consists of pulmonary ventilation, including the inflow (inspiration) of the air and outflow (expiration) of carbon dioxide; diffusion of oxygen from the pulmonary alveoli to the blood and of carbon dioxide from the blood to the alveoli; transport of oxygen to, and of carbon dioxide from, the body cells; and regulation of respiratory activity through humoral and neurological mechanisms. A widely dispersed group of neurons in the reticular substance of the medulla oblongata and pons, the respiratory center, is responsible for regulating the respiratory rate and pulmonary ventilation so that the blood oxygen content remains almost static during strenuous exercise or other types of respiratory stress. This is accomplished by changes of carbon dioxide and hydrogen ion concentration acting upon the respiratory center and changes in oxygen concentration affecting the peripheral chemoreceptors which, in turn, influence the respiratory center. In normal adults the respiratory rate is about 17 breaths per minute. See also BREATHING and VENTILATION (2). **artificial r.,** respiration which is maintained by artificial means. Among the various methods of artificial respiration are the following: *Buist's method* is employed in asphyxiation of the newborn and consists of holding the infant alternately on the stomach and back. *Eve's method:* " . . . the victim is laid face downward on a stretcher and is well wrapped with blankets. His wrists and ankles are lashed to the handles. Then he is hoisted on a trestle or sling and rocking is begun. The first tilt should be head down and steep (50 degrees) and should produce full expiration by the weight of the abdominal contents pressing on the diaphragm. It will also force aortic blood through the coronaries and empty the stomach and lungs of water. Then full inspiration is produced by tilting the foot end down to 50 degrees. The rocking is done a dozen times a minute through an angle of 45 degrees each way." (J.A.M.A.) *Method of Marshall Hall:* Put the body prone, gently press on the back, then removing the back pressure, turn the body on its side and press a little more, repeating this formula 16 times every minute. It is also known as the *method of prone* or *postural respiration,* or "ready method." *Howard's method:* Place the body supine, with a cushion under the back, so that the head is lower than the abdomen: the arms are held over the head, forcible pressure is made with both hands inward and upward, over the lower ribs, about 16 times per minute. *Mouth-to-mouth method:* The rescuer applies his mouth directly to the mouth of the patient and regularly inflates the patient's lungs with his own expired air. *Schafer's method:* Patient prone with forehead on one of his arms: straddle across patient with knees on either side of his hips, and press with both hands firmly upon the back over the lower ribs; then raise your body slowly at the same time relaxing the pressure with your hands. Repeat this forward and backward movement about every five seconds. *Silvester's method:* Patient supine: the arms are pulled firmly over the head to raise the ribs, and kept there until air ceases to enter the chest. The arms are brought down to the chest, and are pressed against it for a second or so after air ceases to escape. Repeat 16 times per minute. See illustration. See also RESPIRATOR and see cardiopulmonary RESUSCITATION. **cell r.,** the process in the living cell by which organic substances are oxidized and chemical energy is released. **Cheyne-Stokes r.,** a regularly oscillating respiratory pattern with recurring apneic and hyperpneic periods, seen in some types of brain injury. **external r.,** the exchange of carbon dioxide and oxygen by diffusion between the external environment and the bloodstream. See also *respiration.* **internal r.,** the exchange of oxygen and carbon dioxide between the bloodstream and the cells of the body. Called also *tissue r.* **mouth-to-mouth r.**, see *artificial r.* **r. rate**, respiration RATE. **stridulous r.**, a high-pitched sound occurring during respiration, due to adduction of the vocal cords. **stertorous r.**, snoring. **tissue r.**, internal r.

respirator (res′pĭ-ra″tor) an apparatus to qualify the air that is breathed through it, or a mechanical device for giving artificial respiration or to assist in pulmonary ventilation in respiratory failure. Called also *ventilator.* See also artificial RESPIRATION.

respiratory (re-spi′rah-to″re) pertaining to respiration.

respirometer (res″pĭ-rom′ĕ-ter) an instrument for determining the character of the respiratory movements.

respondeat superior [L. "let the master answer"] in malpractice, a form of vicarious liability, whereby an employer is held liable for the wrongful acts of an employee even though the employer's conduct is without fault.

response (re-spons′) [L. *respondere* to answer, reply] an action or movement due to the application of a stimulus. **anamnestic r.**, secondary immune r. **autoimmune r.**, the immune response in which antibodies or immune lymphoid cells are produced against the body's own tissues. This may or may not be responsible for signs and symptoms of disease. **booster r.**, secondary immune r. **delayed r.**, delayed REACTION. **immediate r.**, immediate REACTION. **immune r.**, specifically altered reactivity of the animal body following exposure to antigen, manifested by antibody production, cell-mediated immunity, or immunological tolerance. Called also *immune reaction.* See *primary immune r.* and *secondary immune r.* **memory r.**, secondary immune r. **primary immune r.**, the specific response to a single dose of a foreign substance (antigen) introduced into an immunocompetent animal, causing specific antibodies to appear in the serum or the induction of sensitized lymphocytes. The process consists of (1) the latent period (see under PERIOD [2]) extending from the introduction of the antigen to the time when specific antibodies or sensitized lymphocytes begin to appear in the serum; (2) the logarithmic phase when the antibody concentration increases logarithmically; (3) the transitory plateau or steady state; and (4) the decline phase when the rate of antibody catabolism is greater than that of its production. See also *secondary immune r.* **recall r.**, secondary immune r. **second set r.**, secondary immune r. **secondary immune r.**, rapid reappearance of specific antibodies or increase in titer in the serum following the administration of an antigen to immunocompetent animals that have been previously primed with a single dose of the same antigen (*primary immune r.*). The resultant

response leads to higher titers, longer persistence of antibody with greater avidity for antigens. This response serves as the principle for giving booster doses of vaccines. Called also *anamnestic r., booster r., memory r., recall r.,* and *second set r.* See also HYPERSENSITIVITY. **triple r. (of Lewis)**, a reaction of the skin to stroking with a blunt instrument: first an erythematous line develops at the site of stroking, owing to the release of histamine or a histamine-like substance, then a flare develops around the red line, and lastly a wheal is formed as a result of local edema. This sequence of responses also follows the cutaneous injection of histamine, which suggests that local injury results in the release of histamine-like substances. A similar response is induced when allergen is administered to allergic patients in cutaneous test reactions. See also *wheal-flare r.*

rest (rest) 1. repose or inactivity, especially after exertion. 2. a fragment of embryonic tissue that has been retained within the adult organism. Called also *embryonic r., epithelial r.,* and *fetal r.* 3. that part of a removable partial denture which rests on the abutment tooth, usually in a prepared seat, and thus prevents movement of the denture toward the soft tissue and assists in providing occlusal support. **r. area**, rest AREA. **auxiliary r.**, a denture rest that is not used as a component part of a primary direct retainer. **auxiliary implant r.**, in a subperiosteal implant, a small metal protrusion through the mucosa connected to the labial or buccal and lingual (peripheral) frame to furnish additional support for the superstructure of an implant denture between the abutments. **auxiliary occlusal r.**, a rest used in indirect retainers for removable partial dentures, being located on the occlusal surface as far away from the distal extension as possible. **bed r.**, confinement of a patient to bed. **cingulum r.**, lingual r. **continuous bar r.**, continuous CLASP. **embryonic r.**, **epithelial r.**, rest (2). **epithelial r's of Malassez**, Malassez's r's. **fetal r.**, rest (2). **finger r.**, a part of a dental instrument or device in which the fingers of the working hand are allowed to rest on the teeth or adjacent tissues. **incisal r.**, a metallic part or extension of a removable partial denture which rests on the prepared incisal edge of an anterior abutment tooth. **internal r.**, a rigid metallic extension of a fixed or removable partial denture which contacts an intracoronal preparation in a cast restoration of a tooth. **intracoronal r.**, indirect RETAINER. **lingual r.**, a metallic part or extension of a removable partial denture which rests on the prepared lingual surface of an

---

Place one hand under the patient's chin and the other on top of his head. Lift up on the chin and push down on the top of the head to tilt the head backwards.

While holding the jaw forward pinch the nostrils closed with the other hand to prevent leakage of air through the nose.

Blowing into the lungs causes the chest to expand. When the chest has expanded adequately remove your mouth from the patient's so that he can exhale.

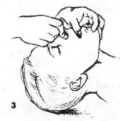

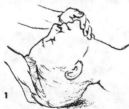

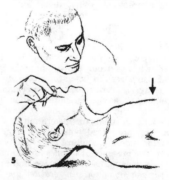

Put the thumb of the hand under the jaw into the patient's mouth; grasp the jaw and pull it forward.

Take a deep breath; place your mouth tightly over the patient's and blow forcefully into his lungs.

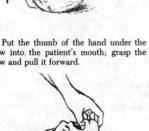

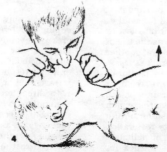

Repeat this sequence of maneuvers every 3 to 4 seconds until other means of ventilation are available.

If you cannot open his mouth blow through his nose. In infants cover both mouth and nose with your mouth. Blow gently into a child's mouth, and in infants use only small puffs from your cheeks.

Technique of artificial respiration by mouth-to-mouth method (Nealon). (From Dorland's Illustrated Medical Dictionary. 26th ed. Philadelphia, W. B. Saunders Co., 1981.)

anterior abutment tooth, and thus provides support or indirect retention. Called also *cingulum r.* **Malassez's r.,** the remaining cells of root sheath in the periodontal ligament, which persist, sometimes forming an epithelial network, and on occasion develop into a dental cyst. Called also *epithelial r. of Malassez.* **occlusal r.,** a rest placed on the occlusal surface of a posterior tooth for transmitting occlusal stresses parallel to its long axis and holding the clasp in its predetermined position, being a component of removable partial dentures. Called also *occlusal lug* and *occlusal stop.* **precision r.,** a prefabricated, rigid, metallic extension of a fixed or removable partial denture, consisting of two closely fitted interlocking parts, the insert of which fits into a box-type rest or keyway (female) portion of the attachment in the cast restoration of a tooth. **recessed r.,** a rigid extension of a partial denture which contacts a definite seat prepared in the surface of a tooth. **root r.,** an endodontically treated root, covered by a low, dome-shaped coping, used as a vertical rest under the denture base of a removable denture. **semiprecision r.,** a denture rest, sometimes supplemented by a spring-loaded plunger or clip, which fits into an abutment of a tooth into an especially deepened seat in an abutment to provide added retention. See illustration at semiprecision ATTACHMENT. **surface r.,** a rigid extension of a partial denture which contacts the unaltered extracoronal surface of a tooth.

restbite (rest'bīt) the relation of the teeth when the jaw is at rest.

restenosis (re″stě-no′sis) recurrent stenosis.

restiform (res′tĭ-form) [L. *restis* rope + *forma* form] shaped like a rope.

restitution (res″tĭ-tu′shun) [L. *restitutio*] an active process of restoration.

Re-Stor trademark for a temporary *denture reliner* (see under RE-LINER).

restoration (res″to-ra′shun) [L. *restaurare* to review, rebuild] 1. the act of renewing, rebuilding, or reconstruction. 2. the return to a previous state or condition, as of health. 3. prosthetic r. 4. the process of replacing by artificial means a missing, damaged, or diseased tooth or teeth or any part thereof. See also restorative DENTISTRY. 5. the act of re-forming the contours of parts of teeth destroyed by lesions or injury, thereby restoring their functional properties. **alloy r.,** a dental restoration made of an alloy. Abbreviated *AR.* **buccal r.,** the replacement, usually with silver alloy, gold, or acrylic resin, of the buccal portion of a posterior tooth lost through caries or injury. **cusp r.,** restoration of the summit of a cusp or the incisal edge of a tooth with restorative material for functional or cosmetic reasons. Called also *capping, shoeing cusp, tipping,* and *tipping of cusp.* **direct gold r.,** a dental restoration in which gold is compacted directly into a prepared cavity. **distal extension r.,** partial denture, distal extension; see under DENTURE. **facial r.,** the replacement, usually with silver alloy, gold, or acrylic resin, of the facial portion of a posterior tooth lost through caries or injury. **implant r.,** implant DENTURE. **intermediate r.,** temporary r. **metal-ceramic r.,** a dental restoration in which the procelain is fused directly to a cast alloy crown shell that fits the prepared tooth. Called also *porcelain fused to metal r.* See also ceramic ENAMEL. **overlay r.,** overlay DENTURE. **permanent r.,** one designed to remain in service for not less than 20 to 30 years, usually made of gold casting, cohesive gold, or amalgam. **pin-supported r.,** an amalgam restoration in which stainless steel pins or wires are placed by friction or cemented into holes in the enamel and dentin, and are used to provide retention of the amalgam. The presence of stainless steel in the amalgam is suspected of decreasing its compressive and tensile strength. Called also *pinned amalgam, pin-retained amalgam,* and *pin-supported amalgam.* See also PIN. **porcelain fused to metal r.,** metal-ceramic r. **prosthetic r.,** 1. the replacement of a lost or absent body part with an artificial structure, such as the use of an inlay, crown, bridge, or partial or complete denture or other appliance to replace lost tooth structure, teeth, or oral tissues. 2. any appliance, such as an inlay, crown, bridge, or partial or complete denture used to replace lost tooth structure, teeth, or oral tissue. See illustration. **temporary r.,** a restoration placed for a limited period, from several days to several months, which is designed to seal the tooth and maintain its position until a permanent restoration will replace it. A temporary restoration may be indicated in pulpal lesions as a method of palliative treatment; in cases where a prolonged time is needed for fabrication of the permanent restoration; and in cases of rampant caries after the preparation of the cavity to change the oral

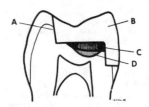

A, Cavity liners. *B,* Permanent restoration. *C,* Intermediate base. *D,* Pulp capping. (From H. W. Gilmore, M. R. Lund, D. J. Bales, and J. Vernetti: Operative Dentistry. 3rd ed. St. Louis, The C. V. Mosby Co., 1977.)

flora and thus arrest caries propagation before the permanent restoration is inserted. Gutta-percha, zinc phosphate cements, silicophosphate cements, and zinc oxide–eugenol cements are the principal materials used in temporary restorations. Called also *intermediate r.* **r. of vertical dimension,** the insertion of artificial structures, such as inlays, onlays, crowns, bridges, and removable appliances that increase the distance between the necks of the maxillary and mandibular teeth when the jaws are closed, in an attempt to restore the lost vertical dimension.

Restryl trademark for *methapyrilene hydrochloride* (see under METHAPYRILENE).

resuscitation (re-sus″ĭ-ta′shun) [L. *resuscitare* to revive] the restoration to life or consciousness of one apparently dead. **cardiopulmonary r.,** the reestablishing of heart and lung action as indicated for cardiac arrest or "sudden death" resulting from cardiovascular collapse, electric shock, drowning, respiratory arrest, and other causes. The technique combines closed cardiac massage and artificial respiration, and is used as an emergency first aid procedure to provide basic life support until more advanced life support is available. Abbreviated *CPR.* See illustration. See also cardiac MASSAGE and artificial RESPIRATION.

resuscitator (re-sus′ĭ-ta″tor) an apparatus for initiating respiration in cases of asphyxia.

ret (ret) [acronym for *rad equivalent therapeutic*] the unit for expressing nominal single dose (see under DOSE).

retainer (re-ta′ner) 1. a device for retaining or keeping something in position. 2. the part of a denture that unites the abutment tooth with the suspended portion of the bridge, such as an inlay, partial crown, or complete crown. See also ATTACHMENT (2). 3. an orthodontic device for maintaining in position the teeth and jaws. 4. any form of clasp, attachment, or any other device used for the fixation or stabilization of a prosthetic appliance. 5. the portion of a fixed prosthesis attaching a pontic to the abutment teeth. **band and spur r.,** one in which a spurlike extension is attached to an orthodontic band to retain adjacent teeth after orthodontic therapy. See illustration. **C & L r.,** C & L ATTACH-

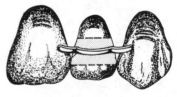

Band and spur retainer. (From T. M. Graber: Orthodontics — Principles and Practice. 3rd ed. Philadelphia, W. B. Saunders Co., 1972.)

MENT. **continuous r., continuous bar r.,** continuous CLASP. **coping r.,** coping. **direct r.,** a clasp or attachment that is a part of a removable partial denture. It retains and stabilizes the prosthesis by attaching it to the abutment teeth; it may be adapted about a tooth or be located in the embrasures of a tooth, or it may rest on and surround the abutment tooth, being either intracoronal or extracoronal. See also CLASP (2). **extracoronal r.,** a direct retainer in which the preparation and its cast restoration lie largely external to the body of the coronal portion of a tooth and complement the contour of the crown. It is a clasp that engages an abutment tooth on its external surface, its arms arising from the minor connector cervically and buccally to the occlusal rest and encircling the buccal and lingual surfaces. One arm is retentive when seated and may be either cast or wrought, the other is reciprocal and is cast in structure. See also

CARDIOPULMONARY EMERGENCY PROCEDURES

Shake or shout to determine unconciousness

If no response

Place patient flat on his back on a hard surface. Send for help if required.

Airway
If unconscious, open airway.
Neck lift. head tilt or Chin lift. head tilt

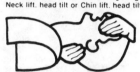
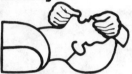

Breathing
If not breathing, begin artificial breathing.
PINCH Nostrils.
OPEN your mouth.
TAKE a deep breath.
SEAL patient's mouth with yours.
4 quick full breaths.
If airway is blocked.
try back blows, abdominal or
chest thrusts and finger probe
until airway is open.

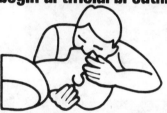

Circulation
Check carotid pulse.
CHECK neckpulse on the side nearest you.
If pulse is present. continue breathing 12 times
per minute (1 each 5 seconds).
Child Infant rate·20 times per minute. (1 each 3 seconds)

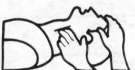

If pulse absent, begin artificial circulation.
Depress sternum 1½ to 2

One Rescuer	Two Rescuers
15 compressions	5 compressions
rate 80 per min.	rate 60 per min.
2 quick breaths	1 breath

Continue uninterrupted until
advanced life support is available

PRESS HERE

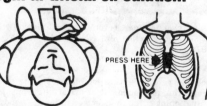

Drugs
Equipment and drugs that should be available.
1. Oxygen and a system to deliver it under positive pressure.

2. Epinephrine.

3. Sodium bicarbonate.

4. Other essential drugs as recommended by local advanced life support unit.

Produced by the American Dental Association and adopted from the American Heart Association CPR Committee

(From Accepted Dental Therapeutics, 38th ed. 1979. Published by American Dental Association.)

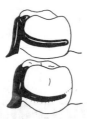

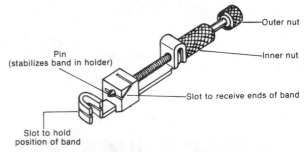

Extracoronal retainer (mirror view). (From D. Henderson and V. L. Steffel: McCracken's Removable Partial Prosthodontics. 5th ed. St. Louis, The C. V. Mosby Co., 1977.)

Tofflemire matrix band holder. Slot is to be placed toward gingivae in all positions. (From H. O. Torres and A. Ehrlich: Modern Dental Assisting. 2nd ed. Philadelphia, W. B. Saunders Co., 1980.)

CLASP (2) and extracoronal ATTACHMENT. See illustration. **Hawley r.,** a removable orthodontic appliance consisting of a removable palatal wire and an acrylic bite plate resting against the palate; used to stabilize teeth after their movement and to serve as a basis for tooth movement by providing an anchorage for wires, elastics, and other attachments. Called also *Hawley appliance.* See also bite PLATE. See illustration. **indirect r.,** a

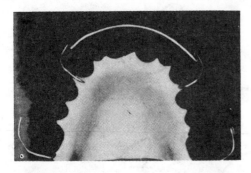

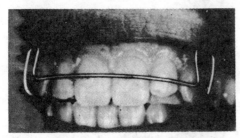

Hawley removable upper retainer. (From T. M. Graber: Orthodontics — Principles and Practice. 3rd ed. Philadelphia, W. B. Saunders Co., 1972.)

part of a removable partial denture which assists the direct retainers in preventing displacement of distal-extension denture bases by functioning through lever action on the opposite side of the fulcrum line. Called also *secondary r.* and *intracoronal rest.* **intracoronal r.,** intracoronal ATTACHMENT. **lingual r.,** lingual ARCH. **matrix r.,** a mechanical device designed to engage the ends of a matrix band or strip and to tighten the matrix around the tooth. Called also *matrix holder.* See illustration. **multiple r's,** two or more attachments approximating each other, used to stabilize teeth with weakened periodotium and for additional abutment support. **precision r.,** precision ATTACHMENT. **screw r.,** a retainer usually consisting of a threaded sleeve within the inner copings and a matched screw that attaches the denture to the coping. **secondary r.,** indirect r. **space r.,** an orthopedic appliance which retains the space created by premature loss of a tooth or the space to be filled by an erupting tooth. See also space MAINTAINER and space REGAINER. **Tach-E-Z r.,** trademark for a spring-loaded plunger used in conjunction with a semiprecision rest for added retention in the intracoronal attachment. Called also *Tach-E-Z attachment* and *Tach-E-Z unit.* See illustration at semiprecision ATTACHMENT.

retardation (re″tar-da′shun) [L. *retardare* to slow down, impede] delay; an abnormal slowness. **mental r.,** subnormal general intellectual development, originating during the developmental period, and associated with impairment of either learning and social adjustment or maturation, or both. It is classified according to intelligence quotient as follows: borderline, 68–83; mild, 52–67; moderate, 36–51; severe, 20–35; and profound, less than 20. Formerly called *feeblemindedness, imbecility, oligophrenia,* and *mental deficiency.*

retarder (re-tar′der) 1. anything that delays or inhibits a process from progressing. 2. a chemical substance that delays or inhibits a chemical reaction from progressing, such as vulcanization or polymerization. See also INHIBITOR. **gypsum r.,** any substance that is capable of retarding the setting time of gypsum products, such as dental plaster. Dried blood, colloidal gels, and borax are the principal gypsum retarders. Sodium chloride and potassium sulfate, while acting as accelerators in low concentrations, may also serve as retarders in high concentrations. See also POISONING of nuclei.

Retasulfin trademark for *sulfamethoxypyridazine.*

retching (rech′ing) a strong involuntary effort to vomit.

Retcin trademark for *erythromycin.*

rete (re′te) [L. "net"] a net or meshwork; used in anatomical nomenclature to designate a network, especially of arteries or veins. **r. cana′lis hypoglos′si,** venous plexus of hypoglossal canal; see under PLEXUS. **r. foram′inis ova′lis,** venous plexus of foramen ovale; see under PLEXUS.

Retens trademark for *doxycycline hyclate* (see under DOXYCYCLINE).

retention (re-ten′shun) [L. *retentio,* from *retentare* to hold firmly back] 1. the act or process of keeping in possession, or of holding in place or position. 2. the persistent keeping within the body of matters normally excreted. 3. denture r. 4. in cavity preparation, the prevention of displacement of a restoration. 5. that period in orthodontic treatment during which the patient is wearing an appliance or appliances to maintain and stabilize the teeth in the position into which they were moved. See also postretention ADJUSTMENT. 6. that part of the insurance premium kept by the insurer to cover his own overhead, administrative costs, commissions, earnings, and other expenses. See also risk CHARGE and WITHHOLD (2). **r. area of tooth,** infrabulge. **r. arm,** retention ARM. **denture r.,** the holding in proper position of a removable denture. Included in the mechanism is the resistance to forces which tend to alter its relation with the teeth and other supporting structures, and the resistance to the movement of a denture from its basal seat in a direction opposite that in which it was inserted. See also *direct r.* and *indirect r.* **denture r., partial,** the fixation of a removable partial denture by the use of clasps, indirect retainers, or precision attachments. **direct r.,** the holding in proper position of a removable denture through the use of attachments or clasps that resist removal from the abutment teeth. See also direct RETAINER. **extracoronal r.,** CLASP (2). **frictional wall r.,** that derived from the parallelism of the surrounding wall of a cavity preparation. **indirect r.,** stabilization of a removable partial denture, whereby retention resists occlusal displacement of a free-end base through the use of an indirect retainer, such as a secondary occlusal rest, lingual plate, embrasure hook, secondary lingual bar, or wide anterior palatal plate. See also indirect RETAINER. **intracoronal r.,** see precision ATTACHMENT. **intracoronal-extracoronal r.,** see Sherer ATTACHMENT. **surgical r.,** retention in the mouth of a dental prosthesis by means of attachments embedded in the oral tissue.

reticular (re-tik′u-lar) [L. *reticularis*] pertaining to or resembling a net.

reticulation (re-tik″u-la′shun) [L. *reticulum* a net] 1. a netlike appearance. 2. a network of wrinkles or corrugations in the emulsion of an x-ray film resulting from sharp temperature differences between processing solutions.

reticulin (re-tik′u-lin) a scleroprotein in the connective tissue of the reticular fibers, which closely resembles collagen. It is resistant to trypsin and pepsin. Its prosthetic groups include polysaccharides and fatty acids.

reticulocyte (re-tik′u-lo-sit″) an abnormal erythrocyte showing a basophilic reticulum appearing as a narrow band transversing the cell. Immature nucleated erythrocytes are usually affected, although mature cells may also contain scattered granules or threads. They are usually somewhat larger than mature normal erythrocytes, and occur in various pathological conditions, such as anemias. Called also *skein cell.*

reticulocytoma (re-tik″u-lo-si-to′-mah) reticulum cell SARCOMA.

reticuloendotheliosis (re-tik″u-lo-en″do-the-le-o′sis) any disease of the reticuloendothelial system, characterized by tumor-like collections of histiocytes. **nonlipid r.,** HISTIOCYTOSIS X. **lipid r.,** a group of diseases of the reticuloendothelial system, including Gaucher's disease, Niemann-Pick disease, Fabry's disease, metachromatic leukodystrophy, and Farber's lipogranulomatosis.

reticulohistiocytoma (re-tik″u-lo-his″te-o-si-to′mah) a small nodule presenting a fibrous tissue stroma containing phagocytic, lipid-laden histiocytes characterized by the presence of numerous bizarre multinucleated giant cells. The nodules appear on various parts of the body, including the lips, tongue, and buccal mucosa, and may be found in persons with gout, rheumatic fever, and rheumatoid arthritis.

reticulohistiocytosis (re-tik″u-lo-his″te-o-si-to′sis) a condition marked by the presence of multiple reticulohistiocytomas. **multicentric r.,** a rare systemic disease, usually affecting women, manifested by polyarthritis of the hands and large joints, frequently leading to crippling absorption of the phalanges, associated with weight loss, bouts of pyrexia, and development of reticulohistiocytomas of the skin and mucous membranes. About half of the patients develop oral lesions, consisting chiefly of papules of the lips and tongue, and less frequently, of the buccal mucosa, gingivae, larynx, and pharynx. Called also *lipid dermatoarthritis.*

reticulosis (re-tik″u-lo′sis) an abnormal increase in cells derived from or related to the reticuloendothelial system. **aleukemic r.,** Letterer-Siwe DISEASE. **benign r.,** cat-scratch DISEASE. **Letterer's r., malignant r.,** Letterer-Siwe DISEASE.

reticulum (re-tik′u-lum), pl. *retic′ula* [L., dim. of *rete* net] 1. a network, especially a protoplasmic network in cells. 2. reticular TISSUE. **agranular r.,** see *endoplasmic r.* **endoplasmic r.,** an ultramicroscopic organelle of nearly all cells of higher plants and animals, consisting of a more or less continuous system of membrane-bound cavities that ramify throughout the cytoplasm of a cell. Two forms have been distinguished: *granular reticulum* (ergastoplasm), which bears large numbers of ribosomes on the outer surface of its membrane and is basophilic, and *agranular reticulum*, which contains no ribosomes and has no distinctive staining properties. Called also *superior protoplasm.* **granular r.,** see *endoplasmic r.* **sarcoplasmic r.,** a form of highly differentiated endoplasmic reticulum of the cells of the striated muscle, comprising a system of longitudinal tubules paralleling the myofibrils, and transverse tubules which pass the muscle fibers from one side of the membrane to the other, and provide a means for transmitting an action potential. **stellate r.,** the soft, middle part of the enamel organ of a developing tooth, situated between the outer enamel epithelium and the stratum intermedium. It constitutes the bulk of the tooth primordium, being made up of cells which have numerous branching and intercommunicating processes. The cells of the reticulum are separated by an increase in the gelatinous intercellular ground substance rich in albumin, which forces the cells apart without breaking the intercellular connections, giving them a stellate appearance and providing protection later for the enamel-forming cells. Called also *enamel pulp.*

Retin-A trademark for *tretinoin.*

retina (ret′ĭ-nah) [L.] the innermost of the three tunics of the eye.

retinol (ret′ĭ-nol) vitamin A. **r.₁,** vitamin A. **r.₂,** vitamin A₂.

retraction (re-trak′shun) [L. *retractio,* from *re* back + *trahere* to draw] 1. the act of drawing back; the condition of being drawn back. 2. distal movement of teeth, usually accomplished with an orthodontic appliance. **clot r.,** 1. contraction of a blood clot, usually with expression of most of the fluid (serum) from the clot. See also HEMOSTASIS. 2. in the process of in vitro blood coagulation, the property of a blood clot to retract and pull away from a glass surface. See also clot retraction TEST and clot retraction TIME. **gingival r.,** the displacement of the marginal gingiva away from a tooth. **mandibular r.,** 1. drawing back or retracting the mandible, accomplished by contraction of the

middle and posterior parts of the temporal muscles and the suprahyoid muscle. 2. the condition of the mandible in which it lies posterior to the orbital plane. Cf. mandibular PROTRACTION (1).

retractor (re-trak′tor) 1. an instrument for maintaining operative exposure by separating the edges of a wound and holding back underlying organs and tissues. 2. any retractile muscle. **Allison r.,** a delicate instrument similar to a hemostat, used for tissue retraction during surgery. Called also *Allison forceps.* See illustration. **Austin r.,** an angled instrument for flap retraction in oral surgery. See illustration. **beaver-tail r.,** a broad-bladed periosteal elevator. **Bishop r.,** a curved instrument for retracting and holding tissue during surgery. See illustration. **Black r.,**

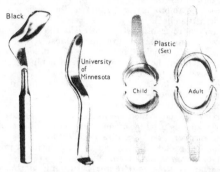

Assorted retractors for the cheek and tongue. (From H. O. Torres and A. Ehrlich: Modern Dental Assisting. 2nd ed. Philadelphia, W. B. Saunders Co., 1980; courtesy of Hu-Friedy Mfg. Co., Inc.)

one for retracting and holding the cheek and tongue during dental or surgical operations. See illustration. **catspaw r.,** an elongated retractor having a looped handle and a three-pronged blade, used in oral surgery. See illustration. **cheek and tongue r.,** one for holding and retracting the cheeks, tongue, or a section of the mucosa during dental and surgical procedures. **Columbia r.,** a wire instrument for retracting the cheek during photography. See illustration. **lip r.,** one for retracting and holding the lip during dental and surgical procedures. **Minnesota r.,** University of Minnesota r. **Moorehead's r.,** one for retracting the lips, cheeks, or margins of a surgical wound. It fits over the crown of the head, being provided with metal buttons, to which shields (or retractors) of desired shapes or sizes may be attached. **rake r.,** a metal instrument with transverse prongs, used for retracting and holding soft tissue. **ribbon r.,** an elongated C-shaped retractor made of a band of steel, used in oral surgery. **Seldin r.,** one used for flap retraction in oral surgery. **Shuman r.,** one for retracting and holding tissue during surgery. See illustration. **University of Minnesota r.,** a curved instrument for retracting and holding the cheek and tongue during oral surgery. Called also *Minnesota r.* See illustration. **vein hook r.,** a metal instrument having a transverse rounded flange for retracting and holding soft tissue. **Wieder r.,** one for tongue retraction in oral surgery.

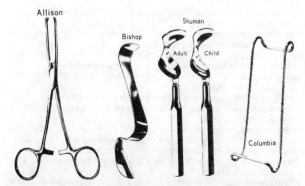

Assorted tissue retractors. (From H. O. Torres and A. Ehrlich: Modern Dental Assisting. 2nd ed. Philadelphia, W. B. Saunders Co., 1980; courtesy of the Hu-Friedy Mfg. Co., Inc.)

retrad (re′trad) [L. *retro* backward] toward a posterior or dorsal part.

retriever (rĭ-tre′ver) a device used to recover or regain something or to draw or bring back. **Caufield r.,** a hand-operated endodontic instrument used to remove silver points from root canals. It has two small prongs at the end with a V-shaped groove in which the point may be engaged and slowly manipulated out of the canal. See also root canal THERAPY. **silver-point r.,** a hand-operated endodontic instrument used for retrieving a silver point from the root canal in endodontic therapy.

retro- [L. *retro* backward] a prefix signifying backward, or located behind.

retroauricular (ret″ro-aw-rik′u-lar) [*retro-* + *auricular*] behind an auricle, or behind the ear.

retrobuccal (ret″ro-buk′al) pertaining to the back part of the mouth near the cheek.

retrocession (ret″ro-sesh′un) [L. *retrocessio*] the act or process of receding or going back; retrogression; relapse.

retroclusion (ret″ro-kloo′zhun) [*retro-* + L. *claudere* to close] closure of a bleeding artery by means of a pin passed over, behind, and under the vessel.

retrocursive (re″tro-kur′siv) [*retro-* + L. *currere* to run] marked by stepping backward.

retrofilling (re″tro-fil′ing) a method of filling the root canal from the apex of the root which has been surgically exposed; zinc-free silver alloy is used most commonly as the filling material. Called also *reverse filling* and *root-end filling.*

retroflexion (ret″ro-flek′shun) [L. *retroflexio*] the act or process of bending of an organ backward.

retrogasserian (ret″ro-gas-se′re-an) pertaining to the sensory (posterior) root of the trigeminal (gasserian) ganglion.

retrognathia (ret″ro-nath′e-ah) [*retro-* + Gr. *gnathos* jaw + *-ia*] retrusion of the lower jaw. See also BRACHYGNATHIA and MICROGNATHIA. Cf. PROGNATHISM. **inferior r.,** mandibular r. **mandibular r.,** a retruded position of the mandible due to its underdevelopment. Called also *inferior r., mandibular retroposition, mandibular retrusion, retrognathic mandible,* and *retruded mandible.* **maxillary r., superior r.,** retroposition of the maxilla, usually associated with retroposition of the middle face, nasal base, and upper lip, such as seen in Crouzon's syndrome. Called also *maxillary retroposition* and *maxillary retrusion.*

retrognathic (ret″ro-nath′ik) pertaining to or characterized by retrognathia. Called also *retrognathism.*

retrognathism (ret″ro-nath′ism) retrognathia.

retrograde (ret′ro-grād) [*retro-* + L. *gradi* to step] going backward or in opposite course; retracing a former course.

retrogression (ret″ro-gresh′un) [*retro-* + L. *gressus* course] degeneration; relapse.

retrojection (ret″ro-jek′shun) [*retro-* + L. *jacere* to throw] irrigation of a cavity by injection of fluid.

retrolingual (ret″ro-ling′gwal) [*retro-* + *lingual*] behind the tongue.

retromandibular (re″tro-man-dib′u-lar) [*retro-* + *mandibular*] behind the mandible.

retromastoid (re″tro-mas′toid) [*retro-* + *mastoid*] behind the mastoid process.

retromolar (ret″ro-mo′lar) distomolar.

retronasal (ret″ro-na′zal) [*retro-* + *nasal*] behind the nose.

retro-ocular (ret″ro-ok′u-lar) [*retro-* + L. *oculus* eye] behind the eye.

retroparotid (re″tro-pah-rot′id) [*retro-* + *parotid*] behind the parotid gland.

retropharyngeal (re″tro-fah-rin′je-al) [*retro-* + *pharyngeal*] situated or occurring behind the pharynx.

retropharyngitis (re″tro-far″in-ji′tis) [*retro-* + *pharyngitis*] inflammation of the posterior portion of the pharynx.

retropharynx (re″tro-far′inks) [*retro-* + *pharynx*] the posterior portion of the pharynx.

retroplasia (ret″ro-pla′se-ah) [*retro-* + Gr. *plasis* formation + *-ia*] retrograde metaplasia; degeneration of a tissue or cell into a more primitive type.

retroposition (re″tro-po-zish′un) [*retro-* + L. *positio* position] backward displacement of an organ. **mandibular r.,** mandibular RETROGNATHIA. **maxillary r.,** maxillary RETROGNATHIA.

retrospective (re″tro-spek′tiv) directed toward the past. See also retrospective STUDY.

retroversion (re″tro-ver′zhun) [*retro-* + L. *versio* turning] 1. the tipping of an entire organ backward. 2. a form of malocclusion in which the teeth or other maxillary and mandibular structures are situated further back than normal. Cf. ANTEVERSION.

Retroviridae (ret″ro-vi′rĭ-de) [*retro-* + *virus* + *-idae*] a family of enveloped, helical viruses whose virions contain linear single-stranded (+)RNA which exists as three or four segments. The genome is enclosed in a helical nucleocapsid, which in turn is enclosed in an icosahedral capsid; this structure is then enveloped by budding through the cell membrane. The virion contains an RNA-dependent DNA polymerase (reverse transcriptase). The diameter of the virion is about 100 nm. No genera have been established, but the family consists of three subfamilies: Oncovirinae, Spumavirinae, and Lentivirinae.

retrovirus (ret″ro-vi′rus) any virus of the family Retroviridae.

retrusion (re-troo′zhun) [*re-* + L. *trudere* to shove] 1. the state of being located posterior to the normal position, as malposition of a tooth posteriorly in the line of occlusion. 2. the act or process of pressing teeth backward. 3. the backward movement or position of the mandible. See RETROGNATHIA. See also closed BITE. **mandibular r.,** mandibular RETROGNATHIA. **maxillary r.,** maxillary RETROGNATHIA.

Retzius, line of, ring of, stria of, zone of [Magnus Gustav *Retzius,* Swedish anatomist, 1842–1919] incremental LINE.

Reudox trademark for *phenylbutazone.*

Reveramine trademark for *mecamylamine.*

Reverdin's graft, needle, operation [Jacques Louis *Reverdin,* surgeon in Geneva, 1842–1929] see epidermic GRAFT, and see under NEEDLE and OPERATION.

Revere, Paul [1735–1818] an American patriot and silversmith, famous for his night horseback ride in 1775 to warn Massachusetts colonists of the coming British troops. He briefly practiced dentistry, specializing in prosthodontics, taking over the practice of John Baker, his preceptor. Revere identified the body of Dr. Joseph Warren by dental work, being the first dentist in America to use dental appliance in the identification of a cadaver.

Reverin trademark for *rolitetracycline.*

reversal (re-ver′s'l) a turning or change in the opposte direction.

reversible (re-ver′sĭ-b'l) capable of going through a series of changes in either direction, forward or backward, as a reversible chemical reaction.

reversion (re-ver′zhun) [L. *re* back + *versio* turning] 1. a returning to a previous condition; regression. 2. in genetics, inheritance from some remote ancestor of a character which has not been manifest for several generations.

review (rĕ′vu) 1. a critical examination, study, or evaluation. 2. to re-examine or to look over or view again. See also SCREENING. **claims r.,** review of insurance claims to determine liability and amount of payment by institutions responsible for payments of benefits. It may include determination of the eligibility of the beneficiary or the provider for the benefit or that the benefit for which payment is claimed is covered in the policy, that the benefit is not payable under another policy, or that the benefit was necessary and of reasonable cost and quality. **continued stay r.,** review during a patient's hospitalization to determine the medical necessity and appropriateness of continuation of his or her stay at a hospital level of care. Called also *extended duration r.* **desk r.,** an examination of a cost report to a third party payer to enable the hospital to receive a tentative payment pending audit and final settlement. **extended duration r.,** continued stay r. **medical r.,** under Medicaid, a review by a team of physicians and other health and social service personnel of the requirements and quality of care delivered to individual inpatients of long-term health care facilities, to insure the adequacy of health care and physical well-being of patients. **peer r.,** 1. in health care delivery, the evaluation by practicing physicians, dentists, or other professionals of the effectiveness and efficiency of services ordered or performed by other practicing physicians, dentists, or other members of the professions. The term frequently refers to the activities of a Professional Standards Review Organization (see under ORGANIZATION), which is required to review services provided under the Medicare, Medicaid, and Maternal and Child Health programs. 2. in dental insurance, a professionally sponsored and operated system for the rendering of professional judgment on disagreements between or among dentists, patients, or third party payers relating to dental fees, quality, or appropriateness of treatment and related matters. **tissue r.,** see hospital tissue COMMITTEE. **utilization r.,** the review and evaluation of the adequacy of use of health services, procedures, and facilities, including the appropriateness of admission to a hospital, services ordered and provided, length of stay, and discharge. It is accomplished by peer review groups, a public agency, a Professional Standards Review Organization, or a hospital utilization review committee. Abbreviated *UR.*

revivification (re-viv"ĭ-fĭ-ka'shun) [re- + L. *vivus* alive + *facere* to make] 1. restoration to life or consciousness. 2. refreshing of diseased surfaces to promote their union.

Revonal trademark for *methaqualone hydrochloride* (see under METHAQUALONE).

Reynier, de see DE REYNIER.

Rf rutherfordium; see ELEMENT 104.

Rh. 1. rhesus factor; see Rh FACTOR, and Rh blood groups, under BLOOD GROUP. 2. rhodium. 3. rhinion.

rhabdo- [Gr. *rhabdos* rod] a combining form meaning rod-shaped or denoting relationship to a rod.

rhabdoid (rab'doid) [Gr. *rhabdo-eides* like a rod, striped looking] resembling a rod; rod-shaped.

rhabdomyoma (rab"do-mi-o'mah) [*rhabdo-* + Gr. *mys* muscle + *-oma*] a benign tumor derived from striated muscle. It occurs very rarely in the oral cavity, usually presenting a firm, nodular, painless mass of the tongue, floor of the mouth, lips, and buccal mucosa. Called also *myoma striocellulare.* **malignant r.**, rhabdomyosarcoma.

rhabdomyosarcoma (rab"do-mi"o-sar-ko'mah) [*rhabdo-* + Gr. *mys* muscle + *sarcoma*] a rare, malignant tumor of striated muscle, which may occur anywhere in the body, but is found most commonly on the lower extremities and trunk. Typically, it presents a rapidly-growing lesion composed of soft, grayish-red tissue resembling fish flesh, which destroys underlying structures. Hemorrhage, necrosis, and cystic softening are common. Histological features vary, but in general, cells resembling normal striated muscle cells are present in all tumors. It is made up of small to large undifferentiated cells with a scant amount of cytoplasm, with no resemblance to muscle cells. The predominant cells are well-defined spindle cells and the cytoplasm is eosinophilic and vacuolated with large amounts of glycogen; they form a syncytial pattern of interlacing bands. The embryonal type of rhabdomyosarcoma arises chiefly from the orbital, facial, and cervical muscles. The soft palate is the most common oral site. Called also *malignant rhabdomyoma.*

Rhabdoviridae (rab"do-vi'rĭ-de) [*rhabdo-* + *virus* + *-idae*] a family of bullet-shaped adenoviruses with virions 130 to 300 nm in length and 60 to 80 nm in diameter; a helical nucleocapsid containing single-stranded, unsegmented RNA genome transcribed by a polymerase into complementary mRNA; and a lipid-containing envelope studded with surface projections. The nucleocapsid matures in the cytoplasm and buds through the cell membrane. Two genera are recognized, *Vesiculovirus* and *Lyssavirus.* Several unaffiliated viruses are also assigned to this family.

rhabdovirus (rab"do-vi'rus) any virus of the family Rhabdoviridae.

rhagades (rag'ah-dēz) [Gr., pl. of *rhagas* rent] fissures or cracks in the skin, especially such lesions around body orifices or regions subjected to frequent movements. For labial rhagades in congenital syphilis, see Parrot's scars, under SCAR. **Parrot's r.**, Parrot's scars; see under SCAR.

rhagadiform (ra-gad'ĭ-form) [Gr. *rhagas* rent + L. *forma* form] fissured; tending to produce fissures; containing cracks.

-rhage [Gr. *rhēgnynai* to burst forth] a word termination meaning a breaking or bursting forth; a profuse flow, as hemorrhage.

rhagiocrine (raj'e-o-krin) [Gr. *rhax* grape + *krinein* to separate] denoting colloid vacuoles in the cytoplasm of gland cells that represent a stage in the development of secretory granules.

-rhaphy [Gr. *rhaphē* a seam] a word termination meaning joining in a seam; suture, as in angiorrhaphy.

Rhazes [A.D. 860–932] an Arabian physician (although born in Persia), who was distinguished for his many writings, his treatise on smallpox and measles being particularly outstanding. His "Al-Fakkir" contains seven chapters on the teeth: *The teeth, Teeth on edge, Decay of the teeth, Looseness of the gums, Suppuration of the gums, Pyorrhea and bleeding gums,* and *Halitosis.* He suggested opium, oil of roses, and honey in the treatment of periodontal disease. To strengthen loose teeth, he recommended astringent mouth washes and dentifrice powders. Rhazes described a procedure of scarification of the gingiva, and the use of counterirritants in the treatment of gingival disease, and recommended filling the carious cavity with a mixture of mastic and alum.

rhe (re) [Gr. *rheos* current] a unit of fluidity, being the reciprocal of the unit of velocity or centipoise.

-rhea [Gr. *rhein* to flow, run, gush] a word termination meaning flow, as in rhinorrhea.

rhenium (re'ne-um) [L. *Rhenus* Rhine] a metallic element. Symbol, Re; atomic number, 75; atomic weight, 186.2; specific gravity, 21.02; melting point, 3180°C; Brinnell hardness number, 250; valences, 1–7, the heptavalent state being the most stable; group VIIB of the periodic table. It has two natural isotopes, 185 and 187; the latter is radioactive with a half life of 10^{11} years. Artificial radioactive isotopes include 177–184, 186, and 188–192. Rhenium occurs as a silvery white solid or gray to black powder, and is attacked by nitric and sulfuric acids, but not with hydrochloric acid. Used in electronics and other technologies. Rhenium is believed to be nontoxic.

rheo- [Gr. *rheos* current] a combining form denoting relationship to an electric current, or to a flow, as of fluids.

rheobase (re'o-bās) [*rheo-* + Gr. *basis* step] the minimum potential of electric current necessary to produce stimulation.

rheology (re-ol'o-je) the science of the deformation and flow of matter, such as the flow of blood through the heart and blood vessels.

rheostat (re'o-stat) [*rheo-* + Gr. *histanai* to place] a device for regulating the resistance and thus controlling the amount of current entering an electric circuit. A variable resistor for regulating the current of an x-ray tube, which on a dental x-ray machine is controlled by the milliampere adjusting knob.

rheumatic (roo-mat'ik) [Gr. *rheumatikos*] pertaining to or affected with rheumatism.

rheumatism (roo'mah-tizm) [L. *rheumatismus;* Gr. *rheumatismos*] any of a variety of disorders marked by inflammation, degeneration, or metabolic derangement of the connective tissue structures of the body, especially the joints and related structures, including muscles, bursae, tendons, and fibrous tissue. It is attended by pain, stiffness, or limitation of motion of these parts. Rheumatism confined to the joints is classified as arthritis. **articular r.**, arthritis. **articular r., acute,** rheumatic FEVER. **articular r., chronic,** rheumatoid ARTHRITIS. **urethral r.,** Reiter's DISEASE.

rheumatoid (roo'mah-toid) [Gr. *rheuma* flux + *eidos* form] resembling rheumatism. See rheumatoid ARTHRITIS.

rhexis (rek'sis) [Gr. *rhexis* a breaking forth, bursting] the rupture of an organ or a vessel.

Rh-Hr see Rh blood groups, under BLOOD GROUP.

rhin- see RHINO-.

rhinalgia (ri-nal'je-ah) [*rhin-* + Gr. *algos* pain + *-ia*] pain in the nose; rhinodynia.

rhinencephalon (ri"nen-sef'ah-lon) [*rhin-* + Gr. *enkephalos* brain] the part of the brain previously believed to be concerned entirely with olfactory mechanisms, consisting of the olfactory bulb, olfactory tract and striae, anterior perforated substance, piriform area, hippocampal formation, paraterminal and parolfactory areas, and fornix. Called also *olfactory brain* and *smell brain.*

rhinencephalus (ri"nen-sef'ah-lus) rhinocephalus.

rhinion (rin'e-on) [Gr., dim of *rhis* nose] the lower end of the internasal suture between the nasal bones.

rhinitis (ri-ni'tis) [*rhin-* + *-itis*] inflammation of the mucous membrane of the nose. **acute catarrhal r.**, acute CORYZA. **allergic r.**, any allergic reaction of the nasal mucosa; it may occur perennially (see *nonseasonal allergic r.*) or seasonally (see hay FEVER). **atopic r.**, nonseasonal allergic r. **atrophic r.**, a chronic form marked by wasting of the mucous membrane and the glands. **r. caseo'sa,** rhinitis with a cheesy, gelatinous, and fetid discharge. **chronic catarrhal r.**, a form characterized by hypertrophy and later by atrophy of the mucous and submucous tissues. **croupous r.**, fibrinous r. **dyscrinic r.**, a form associated with an endocrine disorder. **fibrinous r.**, a form characterized by the development of a false membrane. Called also *croupous r.* See also *membranous r.* and *pseudomembranous r.* **gangrenous r.**, a gangrene-like inflammation of the nasal mucosa. **hypertrophic r.**, a form in which the mucous membrane thickens and swells. **membranous r.**, a chronic form with the formation of a membranous exudate. See also *fibrinous r.* and *pseudomembranous r.* **nonseasonal allergic r.**, allergic rhinitis that may occur continuously or intermittently all year around; it is caused by an allergen to which the individual is more or less always exposed, such as house dust, danders, and food, and is characterized by sudden attacks of sneezing, swelling of the nasal mucosa with a profuse watery discharge, itching of the eyes, and lacrimation. Called also *atopic r.* and *perennial r.* See also hay FEVER. **perennial r.**, nonseasonal allergic r. **pseudomembranous r.**, that in which the inflamed region is covered with an opaque exudation. See also *fibrinous r.* and *membranous r.* **purulent r.**, chronic rhinitis with the formation of pus. **scrofulous r.**, tuberculous r. **syphilitic r.**, syphilitic CORYZA. **tuberculous r.**, a form due to tuberculosis, and associated with ulceration, caries of the nasal bone, and ozena. Called also *scrofulous r.* **vasomotor r.**, 1. a form of nonallergic rhinitis in which transient changes in vascular tone and permeability, with the same symptoms as in allergic rhinitis, are brought on by such stimuli as mild chilling, fatigue, anger, and anxiety. 2. any condition of allergic or nonallergic rhinitis, as opposed to infectious rhinitis.

rhino-, rhin- [Gr. *rhis* nose] a combining form denoting relationship to the nose, or a noselike structure. See also words beginning NASO-.

rhinoantritis (ri″no-an-tri′tis) [*rhino-* + *antrum* + *-itis*] inflammation of the nasal cavity and the antrum of Highmore.

rhinocephalus (ri″no-sef′ah-lus) a fetus exhibiting rhinocephaly. Called also *rhinencephalus.*

rhinocephaly (ri″no-sef′ah-le) [*rhino-* + Gr. *kephalē* head + *-ia*] a developmental anomaly characterized by the presence of a proboscis-like nose above eyes partially or completely fused into one.

rhinocheiloplasty (ri″no-ki′lo-plas″te) [*rhino-* + Gr. *cheilos* lip + *plassein* to form] plastic surgery of the nose and lip.

rhinodynia (ri″no-din′e-ah) [*rhino-* + Gr. *odynē* pain + *-ia*] pain in the nose; rhinalgia.

rhinogenous (ri-noj′ĕ-nus) [*rhino-* + Gr. *gennan* to produce] arising in the nose.

rhinokyphosis (ri″no-ki-fo′sis) [*rhino-* + Gr. *kyphos* hump] the presence of an abnormal hump in the ridge of the nose.

rhinolalia (ri″no-la′le-ah) [*rhino-* + Gr. *lalia* speech] a nasal quality of voice due to some disease or defect of the nasal passages. Called also *rhinophonia.* **r. aper′ta,** that which is caused by undue patency of the posterior nares. Called also *open r.* **r. clau′sa, closed r.,** that which is due to undue closure of the nasal passages. **open r.,** r. aperta.

rhinolaryngitis (ri″no-lar″in-ji′tis) inflammation of the mucous membrane of the nose and larynx.

rhinolith (ri′no-lith) [*rhino-* + Gr. *lithos* stone] a nasal stone or concretion.

rhinolithiasis (ri″no-li-thi′ah-sis) a condition associated with the formation of nasal calculi.

rhinology (ri-nol′o-je) [*rhino-* + *-logy*] the sum knowledge regarding the nose and its diseases.

rhinomycosis (ri″no-mi-ko′sis) [*rhino-* + *mycosis*] fungal infection or mycosis of the nasal mucosa.

rhinopathy (ri-nop′ah-the) [*rhino-* + Gr. *pathos* disease] any disease of the nose.

rhinopharyngeal (ri″no-fah-rin′je-al) nasopharyngeal.

rhinopharyngitis (ri″no-far″in-ji′tis) inflammation of the nasopharynx. **mutilating r.,** a serious complication of yaws, in which an ulcerative lesion progressively destroys the soft tissue, cartilage, and bones of the nose, nasopharynx, and palate, frequently leading to death. Called also *gangosa.*

rhinopharyngocele (ri″no-fah-ring′go-sēl) a tumor, usually an aerocele, of the nasopharynx.

rhinopharyngolith (ri″no-fah-ring′go-lith) [*rhino-* + Gr. *pharynx* + *lithos* stone] a calculus of the nasopharynx.

rhinophonia (ri″no-fo′ne-ah) [*rhino-* + Gr. *phōnē* voice] a nasal quality of the voice; rhinolalia.

rhinophore (ri′no-fōr) [*rhino-* + Gr. *phoros* bearing] a nasal cannula to facilitate breathing.

rhinophycomycosis (ri″no-fi″ko-mi-ko′sis) a fungal infection caused by *Entomophthora coronata,* marked by the development of large polyps in the subcutaneous tissues of the nose and paranasal sinuses; orbital involvement with unilateral blindness may follow. It usually leads to cerebral involvement.

rhinophyma (ri″no-fi′mah) [*rhino-* + Gr. *phyma* growth] a form of acne rosacea characterized by redness, sebaceous hyperplasia, and nodular swelling and congestion of the skin of the nose.

rhinoplasty (ri′no-plas″te) [*rhino-* + Gr. *plassein* to form] plastic surgery of the nose. **Carpue's r.,** Indian r. **English r.,** that in which a nose is formed out of flaps from the cheek. **Indian r.,** that in which the nose is reconstructed by a flap of skin from the forehead, with its pedicle at the root of the nose. Called also *Carpue's r., Carpue's operation,* and *Indian operation.* **Italian r.,** tagliacotian r. **tagliacotian r.,** that in which the nose is reconstructed by a flap of skin from the arm, the flap remaining attached to the arm until union has taken place. Called also *Italian r., Italian operation,* and *tagliacotian operation.*

rhinorrhagia (ri″no-ra′je-ah) [*rhino-* + Gr. *rhēgnynai* to burst forth] nasal hemorrhage; nosebleed; epistaxis.

rhinorrhaphy (ri-nor′ah-fe) [*rhino-* + Gr. *rhaphē* suture] an operation for epicanthus performed by excising a fold of skin from the nose and closing the opening with sutures.

rhinorrhea (ri″no-re′ah) [*rhino-* + Gr. *rhoia* flow] the free discharge from the nose of a thin nasal mucus.

rhinoscleroma (ri″no-skle-ro′mah) [*rhino-* + *sklērōma* a hard swelling] a rare granulomatous disease of the nose and nasopharynx, occurring in Egypt, Eastern Europe, and South America. It is caused by *Klebsiella rhinoscleromatis,* and initially involves the nasal mucosa, from where it may spread to the lips, alveolar process, and hard and soft palates. Plaques or crateriform nodules, forming large hard keloids, are the principal features. Mobility of the tongue may be restricted; adhesions between the palate and posterior palatine arches and oral pharynx may be associated; the palate may undergo scarring; and the teeth frequently become covered with tumorous gingival nodules and often are shed.

rhinoscope (ri′no-skōp) [*rhino-* + Gr. *skopein* to examine] a speculum for use in nasal examinations.

rhinoscopy (ri-nos′ko-pe) [*rhino-* + Gr. *skopein* to examine] the examination of the nasal passages, either through the anterior nares (*anterior r.*) or through the nasopharynx (*posterior r.*). **median r.,** examination of the nasal cavity and the openings of the ethmoid cells, etc., by means of a long nasal speculum.

rhinosporidiosis (ri″no-spo-rid″e-o′sis) a fungal disease caused by infection with *Rhinosporidium seeberi,* characterized by the development of small verrucae or warts which become large pedunculated polypoid growths of oropharynx, nasopharynx, larynx, skin, eyes, and genital mucosa.

Rhinosporidium seeberi (ri″no-spo-rid′e-um se′ber-i) the fungus which causes rhinosporidiosis.

rhinostegnosis (ri″no-steg-no′sis) [*rhino-* + Gr. *stegnōsis* obstruction] obstruction of a nasal passage.

rhinostenosis (ri″no-stĕ-no′sis) [*rhino-* + Gr. *stenōsis* narrowing] narrowing or stenosis of a nasal passage.

rhinotomy (ri-not′o-me) [*rhino-* + Gr. *tomē* a cutting] incision into the nose.

Rhinovirus (ri″no-vi′rus) [*rhino-* + *virus*] a genus of small picornaviruses, about 20–30 nm in diameter, having a core of single-stranded RNA. It includes the human common cold virus, as well as the virus of foot-and-mouth disease in animals and the bovine and equine rhinoviruses. The name was originally used as a designation for a human virus associated with the common cold, classified in the genus *Enterovirus.*

rhinovirus (ri″no-vi′rus) any virus of the genus *Rhinovirus.*

rhizo- [Gr. *rhiza* root] a combining form denoting relationship to a root.

Rhizobiaceae (ri-zo″bĕ-a′se-e) [*Rhizobium* + *-aceae*] a family of gram-negative, aerobic, rod-shaped bacteria found on plant roots, consisting of the genera *Agrobacterium* and *Rhizobium.*

Rhizobium (ri-zo′be-um) [Gr. *rhiza* root + *bios* life] a genus of gram-negative, aerobic rod-shaped bacteria of the family *Rhizobiaceae,* capable of fixing molecular nitrogen and living on plant roots, inciting the production of root nodules.

rhizodontropy (ri″zo-don′tro-pe) [*rhizo-* + Gr. *odous* tooth + *tropos* a turning] 1. the act of rotating a tooth root. 2. the act of attaching an artificial crown to a tooth root by means of a pivot.

rhizodontrypy (ri″zo-don′trī-pe) [*rhizo* + Gr. *odous* tooth + *trypesis* trephination] surgical perforation of a tooth root to provide a channel of egress for a confined fluid.

rhizoid (ri′zoid) [*rhizo-* + Gr. *eidos* form] rootlike; resembling a root.

Rhizopoda (ri-zop′o-dah) [*rhizo-* + Gr. *pous* foot] 1. a class of protozoa of the subphylum Sarcodina. 2. Sarcodina.

Rhizopus (ri-zo′pus) a genus of true fungi of the class Zygomycetes, species of which may cause mucormycosis.

rhizotomy (ri-zot′o-me) [*rhizo-* + Gr. *tomē* a cutting] interruption of the roots of the spinal nerves within the spinal canal. **retrogasserian r.,** transection of the sensory root fibers of the trigeminal nerve for the relief of trigeminal neuralgia. Called also *retrogasserian neurotomy.*

RHN Rockwell hardness number; see under HARDNESS.

rhodium (ro′de-um) [Gr. *rhodon* rose] a rare metallic element of the platinum group. Symbol, Rh; atomic number, 45; atomic weight, 102.9055; melting point, 1966°C; specific gravity, 12.41; valences, 1–6 (1 is most common); group VIII of the periodic table. ^{103}Rh is the sole naturally occurring isotope. Artificial radioactive isotopes include 97–102 and 104–110. It is a silvery white, soft, ductile, malleable metal that is not attacked by acids, including aqua regia. As an alloy with platinum, it is used as an anticorrosive agent. Rhodium is believed to be nontoxic.

rhodo- [Gr. *rhodon* rose] a combining form meaning red.

Rhodotorula (ro″do-tor′u-lah) a genus of deuteromycetous fungi (Fungi Imperfecti), occurring as unicellular budding organisms that may be encapsulated or produce pseudomycelia and contain carotenoid pigments. Many form mycelia on certain mediums. They are common members of the normal human skin flora; rarely an opportunist. **R. glu′tinis,** a common species from air, potatoes, and the skin in seborrhea. The organism is occasionally the cause of opportunistic infections of man and other animals. Called also *Saccharomyces glutinis.* **R. ru′bra,** a skin contaminant which, on rare occasion, may cause pulmonary or systemic infection.

rhomboid (rom′boid) [Gr. *rhombos* rhomb + *eidos* form] shaped like a rhomb, or kite.

rhythm (rith′m) [L. *rhythmus;* Gr. *rhythmos*] a measured movement; the recurrence of an action or function at regular intervals. See also CYCLE and PERIODICITY. **diurnal r.,** see DIURNAL. **circadian r.,** see CIRCADIAN. **nyctohemeral r.,** biologic rhythm in which there is the regular recurrence of activities in cycles during the night and day.

RIA radioimmunoassay.

rib (rib) one of the paired elastic arches of bone, 12 on either side, which extend from the thoracic vertebrae toward the median line on the ventral aspect of the trunk, forming the major part of the thoracic skeleton. The upper seven (true ribs) are connected ventrally with the sternum; the lower five (false ribs) are not. Called also *costa* [NA].

ribbon (rib′un) a flat and narrow closely woven fabric or a similar structure. **r. arch,** ribbon arch APPLIANCE.

ribitol (ri′bĭ-tol) a ribose sugar alcohol derivative.

Ribo-Azauracil trademark for *6-azauridine.*

riboflavin (ri″bo-fla′vin) a water soluble vitamin of the B complex, 7,8-dimethyl-10-(D-ribo-2,3,4,5-tetrahydropentyl) isoalloxazine, occurring as an orange-yellow crystalline powder that is soluble in water, but not in fat solvents, and exhibits green fluorescence under ultraviolet light. Riboflavin is synthesized by plants, bacteria, yeasts, and fungi, but not by animals. In its phosphcrylated form, it is a respiratory enzyme which is not poisoned by carbon monoxide and cyanides, playing a role in the transfer of oxygen from the blood to individual cells and participating in hydrogen transport. It is widely distributed in plants and animals, being an essential cell constituent and is, thus, found in a wide variety of foods, chiefly liver, milk, eggs, vegetables, and fruits. Used mainly in the treatment of riboflavin deficiency (see ARIBOFLAVINOSIS). Relatively large doses of riboflavin are tolerated without toxic effects. Called also *lactoflavin, vitamin B₂* and *vitamin G.* For daily requirements of riboflavin, see table at NUTRITION.

ribonucleoprotein (ri″bo-nu″kle-o-pro′te-in) a nucleoprotein consisting of a conjugate between ribose (RNA) and a protein.

ribonucleoside (ri″bo-nu′kle-o-sĭd) a nucleoside in which the purine or pyrimidine base is combined with ribose. Sometimes called *riboside.*

ribonucleotide (ri″bo-nu′kle-o-tĭd) a nucleotide of RNA, in which a nitrogenous base is combined with D-ribose and a phosphate.

ribose (ri′bōs) a five-carbon aldose that is the carbohydrate component of RNA. It is formed partly from glucose via an aerobic pathway involving essentially oxidative decarboxylation of the phosphorylated hexonic acid and, partly, via a nonoxidative pathway involving the transaldolase-transketolase reactions. Also a component of some coenzymes. See also DEOXYRIBOSE.

riboside (ri′bo-sĭd) a nucleoside which contains ribose as its sugar moiety. See also RIBONUCLEOSIDE. **adenine r.,** adenosine. **guanine r.,** guanosine. **hypoxanthine r.,** inosine. **uracil r.,** uridine.

ribosome (ri′bo-sōm) an intracellular ribonucleoprotein particle, about 140–230 Å, made up of about 40–60 percent ribosomal RNA and of several kinds of basic proteins. Ribosomes are the primary sites of amino acid polymerization during protein synthesis and serve as nonspecific catalysts in the formation of polypeptide chains. They may occur in clusters (*polyribosomes*) joined together by a messenger RNA molecule, or they may be present singly (*monoribosomes*), either bound to membranes or free in the cytoplasm. Those of glandular cells have been called *ergastoplasm,* and those of nerve cells *Nissl bodies.* See also ribosomal RNA.

ribulose (ri′bu-lōs) the 2-ketose isomer of ribose; active in carbohydrate metabolism (the phosphogluconate pathway).

Richards, Dickinson W. [born 1895] American physician; co-winner, with André Frédéric Cournand and Werner Theodor Otto Forssmann, of the Nobel prize for medicine and physiology in 1956, for developing a technique for precise measurement of heart and lung functions.

Richet, Charles Robert [1850–1935] a French physiologist; winner of the Nobel prize for medicine and physiology in 1913, for his work on anaphylaxis.

Richet, Didier Dominique Alfred [French surgeon, 1816–1891] see van der Woude's SYNDROME (Demarquay-Richet syndrome).

Richey condyle marker see under MARKER.

Richmond crown [C. M. *Richmond,* American dentist, 1835–1902] see under CROWN.

rickets (rik′ets) [thought to be a corruption of Gr. *rachitis* a spinal complaint] a metabolic disease of infancy and childhood, in which vitamin D deficiency results in failure of bone calcification, associated with bending of the bones, hypertrophy of the epiphyseal cartilage, delayed closure of the fontanelles, degeneration of the spleen and liver, and pain. Hypoplasia of the enamel and delayed tooth eruption are the most common dental complications. Called also *English disease, Glisson's disease, morbus anglicus,* and *morbus anglorum.* **adult r.,** osteomalacia. **familial r.,** vitamin D–resistant r. **hypophosphatemic vitamin D–resistant r.,** vitamin D–resistant r. **refractory r.,** vitamin D–resistant r., **renal r.,** compensatory hyperparathyroidism due to hypercalciuria and hypocalcemia in renal tubular insufficiency resulting in acidosis, with secondary hyperphosphatemia and deposits of calcium phosphate in the tissue. Disorders of the growth of the mandible are the principal oral manifestations. Called also *renal osteitis fibrosa generalisata.* **r. with renal tubular acidosis,** Lightwood-Albright SYNDROME. **vitamin D–resistant r.,** any form of rickets resistant to vitamin D therapy; specifically, a hereditary metabolic disease, transmitted as an X-linked dominant trait, which occurs predominantly in males. It is characterized by an inability of the renal tubules to reabsorb phosphates, resulting in hypophosphatemia and rickets or osteomalacia which do not respond to vitamin D therapy. Hypophosphatemia without clinical manifestations may occur in children; in adults there may be in addition bowing of the legs, pseudofractures, growth retardation, and skull deformities. Oral manifestations include delayed tooth eruption, wide root canals, pulp chambers with minute pulp exposures, gingival fistulae, large pulp horns and radiolucent microtracts extending through the dentin to the enamel, abscesses, calcification defects of the dentin and enamel, and cracks through the hypoplastic enamel and tooth surface. Called also *familial r., hypophosphatemic vitamin D–resistant r., refractory r.,* and *Albright-Butler-Bloomberg syndrome.* See also Abderhalden-Fanconi SYNDROME and HYPOPHOSPHATASIA.

Ricketts, Howard Taylor [1871–1901] an American physician who first associated spotted fever with *Rickettsia* and who died of typhus contracted in the course of his studies.

Rickettsia (rĭ-ket′se-ah) [named after H. T. *Ricketts*] a genus of bacteria of the tribe Rickettsieae, family Rickettsiaceae, order Rickettsiales, occurring as gram-negative, short rods, about 0.3 to 0.6 by 0.8 to 2.0 μm in size, some species being up to 4 μm prior to cell division, which is pathogenic for man and other animals. Transmission is always mediated by vertebrates, but man and other animals, particularly small rodents, may serve as reservoirs for some species and incidental hosts for others. The organisms are generally found intracytoplasmically or free in the lumen of the gut in lice, fleas, ticks, and mites. Strains fall into three biotypes: typhus, spotted fever, and scrub typhus. **R. akamu′shi,** R. tsutsugamushi. **R. ak′ari,** a species related to *R. rickettsii,* which causes rickettsialpox, being transmitted by the mouse mite. **R. austra′lis,** the etiologic agent of North Queensland tick typhus, believed to be transmitted by ticks and marsupials. It is indistinguishable from *R. conorii* in many respects. **R. burnet′ii,** *Coxiella burnetii;* see under COXIELLA. **R. ca′nada,** a rod-shaped species, 0.4 to 1.6 μm in size, which was originally isolated from ticks in Canada. It belongs to the typhus biotype, but has some properties in common with the spotted fever biotype. In man, it causes a disease similar to Rocky Mountain spotted fever. **R. cono′rii,** a species similar to *R. rickettsii* and *R. sibirica,* which is chiefly a parasite of dog ticks and of dogs. It is the etiologic agent of boutonneuse fever in the Mediterranean region or tick bite fever or tick typhus in other regions. **R. diapor′ica,** *Coxiella burnetii;* see under COXIELLA. **R. nippon′ica,** *R. tsutsugamushi.* **R. orienta′lis,** *R. tsutsugamushi.* **R. pedic′uli,** *Rochalimaea quintana;* see under ROCHALIMAEA. **R. prowaze′kii,** the etiologic agent of epidemic typhus and its recrudescent form, Brill-Zinsser disease, occurring as rods (0.3 to 0.6 by 0.8 to 2.0 μm and often up to 4.0 μm long), singly or in small chains. Man is the primary host and transmission is accomplished by the human louse. Upon recovering from typhus, patients are believed to retain small numbers of the organisms, probably in their lymph nodes, for the rest of their lives. **R. psitta′ci,** *Chlamydia psittaci;* see under CHLAMYDIA. **R. quinta′na,** *Rochalimaea quintana;* see under ROCHALIMAEA. **R. rickett′sii,** the etiologic agent of Rocky Mountain spotted fever, occurring as rods, 1.5 to 2.0 μm in length. The organism is confined to the Western Hemisphere, ticks being its primary reservoirs with rodents playing a role in its dissemination; man is an incidental host. **R. sibir′ica,** a species of the spotted fever biotype, closely related to *R. conorii,* which is the causative agent of Siberian spotted fever. The species occurs mainly in the Asian part of the U.S.S.R.; ticks being the principal reservoir and various domestic animals and rodents playing a role in its dissemination. Called also *Dermacentroxenus sibericus*. **R. tracho′matis**, *Chlamydia trachomatis;* see under CHLAMYDIA. **R. tsutsugamu′shi**, a species, usually occurring as short rods (1.2 μm, sometimes reaching 1.5 μm in length), but diplobacillary forms are seen also. It is an etiologic agent of scrub typhus, transmitted by larval mites and their rodent hosts. Reservoirs of the organism are found in Japan, Southeast Asia, northern Australia, Pakistan, Siberia, the Philippines, and Korea. Called also *Rickettsia akamuski, R. nipponica, R. orientalis*, and *Theileria tsutsugamushi*. **R. ty′phi**, the species causing murine typhus. The rat and other rodents are the primary reservoirs of the organism, the rat flea being responsible for its transmission from rat to rat and to man who is an incidental host; the human flea and louse are believed to be responsible for transmitting the infection from man to man. **R. weig′li**, *Rochalimaea quintana;* see under ROCHALIMAEA. **R. wolhyn′ica**, *Rochalimaea quintana;* see under Rochalimaea.

rickettsia (rĭ-ket′se-ah), pl. *rickettsiae*. A group of generally obligate, small rod-shaped to coccoid intracellular parasitic bacteria, which with rare exceptions are not cultivable on ordinary media but may be grown in tissue cultures. The group comprises the orders Rickettsiales and Chlamydiales.

Rickettsiaceae (rĭ-ket′se-a′se-e) [*Rickettsia* + *-aceae*] a family of the order Rickettsiales, made up of small, rod-shaped, ellipsoidal, coccoid, often pleomorphic or diplococcoid, often pleomorphic bacteria, which frequently occur intracellularly in arthropods, by which they are transmitted to man and other animals, causing disease. It includes the tribes Rickettsieae, Ehrlichieae, and Wolbachieae.

rickettsiae (rĭ-ket′se-e) plural of *rickettsia*.

rickettsial (rĭ-ket′se-al) pertaining to or caused by rickettsiae.

Rickettsiales (rĭ-ket′se-a′lēz) an order of gram-negative bacteria, consisting mostly of small, rod-shaped or coccoid, often pleomorphic cells, occurring as elementary bodies. They are obligate intracellular parasites of certain blood-sucking arthropods (e.g., lice, fleas, ticks, and mites), some of which are pathogenic for man and other vertebrates, being transmitted usually by the bites of the arthropod vectors or by their feces. The pathological changes seen in rickettsial diseases are due to multiplication of the organisms within the endothelial cells of the vascular system throughout the body of the vertebrate host. Most rickettsiae are not pathogenic for the insect vectors that transmit them, and are regarded as essential for the development and reproduction of the host. The order includes the families Anaplasmataceae, Bartonellaceae, and Rickettsiaceae.

rickettsialpox (rĭ-ket′se-al-poks″) a relatively mild, febrile disease first recognized in the Borough of Queens in New York City, caused by *Rickettsia akari*, which is transmitted by the mouse mite. The primary lesion appears at the site of inoculation, 7 to 19 days after the bite of the mite, as a firm red papule, about 1.0 to 2.5 cm in diameter. The papule tends to vesiculate and forms a black eschar with scabs, healing in about two to three days. Fever, chills, sweating, backache, sore throat, and muscular pain are the principal systemic symptoms. Oral symptoms usually include vesicles on the tongue and palate. Called also *Kew Gardens spotted fever*.

rickettsicidal (rĭ-ket′sĭ-si′dal) destructive to rickettsiae.

Rickettsieae (rik′et-si′e-e) a tribe of the family Rickettsiaceae, order *Rickettsiales*, made up of small, pleomorphic, usually intracellular bacteria, found as parasites in arthropods and transmitted to man and other vertebrates, causing disease. The tribe includes the genera *Coxiella, Rickettsia*, and *Rochalimaea*.

rickettsiosis (rĭ-ket″se-o′sis) infection with rickettsiae.

rickettsiostatic (ri-ket″se-o-stat′ik) inhibiting the growth of rickettsiae.

Ricyцline trademark for *tetracycline hydrochloride* (see under TETRACYCLINE).

Ridell's operation see under OPERATION.

rider (ri′der) 1. anything that straddles, rests upon, or is attached to something else. 2. an attachment, addition, or amendment to a document, e.g., in health insurance, an amendment which modifies the protection of a policy, either expanding or decreasing its benefits or excluding certain conditions from policy coverage.

ridge (rij) 1. a projection, or projecting structure. See also CREST and CRISTA. 2. dental r. **alveolar r.**, the bony ridge of the maxilla or mandible which contains the alveoli. **alveolar r., residual**, the bony ridge remaining after disappearance of the alveoli from the alveolar process following removal or loss of the teeth. Called also *edentulous r.* and *residual r.* **anatomic r.**, an impression of the residual alveolar ridge made in a soft impression material, which gives full details of the anatomic configuration of the ridge, including soft and flabby tissues which are not evident in a functional impression. See also *functional r.* and functional IMPRESSION. **basal r.**, cingulum (3). **buccal r.**, a lineal elevation on the buccal surface of the crown of a tooth. **buccocervical r., buccogingival r.**, a ridge or prominence on the buccal surface above the cementoenamel junction of posterior teeth. **center of r.**, the buccolingual midline of the residual alveolar ridge. **cerebral r's of cranial bones**, variable ridges on the inner surface of the cranium, corresponding to the sulci of the brain. Called also *cerebral crests of cranial bones* and *juga cerebralia ossium cranii*. **crest of r.**, the highest prominence of the residual alveolar ridge, but not necessarily the center of the ridge. **cusp r.**, an elevated crest extending both in a mesial and distal direction from the cusp tip, thereby forming the buccal and lingual margins of the occlusal surfaces of the posterior teeth. **dental r.**, any linear elevation on the surface of the crown of a tooth, named according to the surface on which it is located, such as buccal or lingual, or in recognition of some other characteristic. **dermal r's**, ridges of the skin produced by projecting papillae of the corium on the palms or soles, producing fingerprints or footprints that are characteristic of the individual. Called also *cristae cutis* [NA]. **edentulous r.**, alveolar r., residual. **enamel r.**, enamel SPUR. **functional r.**, a residual alveolar ridge when it is supporting a denture base. See also functional IMPRESSION. **genital r.**, the more medial portion of the urogenital ridge, which gives rise to the gonad. **incisal r.**, that portion of the crown of the anterior (incisal) teeth which makes up the actual incisal portion. See also incisal EDGE and incisal SURFACE. **infraorbital r. of maxilla**, infraorbital margin of maxilla; see under MARGIN. **internal oblique r.**, mylohyoid line of mandible; see under LINE. **key r.**, an osteometric landmark, being the lowermost point of the zygomatic bony ridge, situated between the maxillary tuberosity and the canine fossa, seen on the cephalometric roentgenogram. Abbreviated KR. Called also *point KR*. **lingual r.**, a linear elevation on the lingual surface of the crown of a tooth. **linguocervical r., linguogingival r.**, cingulum (3). **longitudinal r. of hard palate**, palatine RAPHE. **r. of mandibular neck**, a blunt, smooth ridge passing obliquely downward and forward from the mandibular condyle on the medial surface of the mandibular neck and ramus, serving as their buttress. **marginal r's**, elevated convex crests which form the mesial and distal borders of the occlusal surfaces of posterior teeth and of the lingual surfaces of anterior teeth. Called also *crista marginalis* [NA]. **mesonephric r.**, the more lateral portion of the urogenital ridge, which gives rise to the mesonephros; see under LINE. **mylohyoid r.**, mylohyoid line of mandible; see under LINE. **r. of nose**, AGGER nasi. **oblique r.**, an elevated crest of variable prominence, comprised jointly of the triangular ridge of the distobuccal cusp and the distal ridge of the mesiolingual cusp, coursing obliquely across the occlusal surface of the maxillary molars to link the apices of the distobuccal and the mesiolingual cusps. **palatine r's, transverse**, palatine folds; see under FOLD. **Passavant's r.**, pharyngeal r., Passavant's BAR. **pterygoid r.**, infratemporal CREST. **r. relation**, ridge RELATION. **residual r.**, residual alveolar r. **semicircular r. of parietal bone, inferior**, temporal line, inferior; see under LINE. **semicircular r. of parietal bone, superior**, temporal line, superior; see under LINE. **sublingual r.**, lingual FRENUM. **supplemental r.**, an abnormal or accessory ridge on the surface of a tooth. **taste r.**, foliate papillae; see under PAPILLA. **transverse r.**, an elevated crest coursing transversely across the occlusal surface of a mandibular premolar to link the apices of the buccal and lingual cusps. It comprises the buccal and lingual cusps and may be an uninterrupted prominence or may be sharply divided at its approximate midpoint by a groove. Called also *crista transversalis* [NA]. **triangular r.**, one which descends from the tips of the cusps of molars and premolars toward the central part of the occlusal surface; so named because the slopes of each side of the ridge resemble two sides of a triangle. Called also *crista triangularis* [NA]. See also *oblique r.* and *transverse r.* **urogenital r.**, a longitudinal ridge or fold in the embryo, which later subdivides into the mesonephric and genital ridges.

ridging (rij′ing) in plastic surgery, a visible line or ridge at the margin of an area that has been surgically planed; occasionally encountered when beveling at the junction of treated and untreated areas has not been performed.

Riedel's thyroiditis (struma) [Moritz Carl Ludwig *Riedel*, 1846–1916] see under THYROIDITIS.

Rieder cell [Hermann *Rieder*, German physician, 1858–1932] see under CELL.

Rieger's syndrome (anomaly, malformation) [Herwigh *Rieger*, Austrian ophthalmologist] see under SYNDROME.

Riehl's melanosis [Gustav *Riehl*, Austrian dermatologist, 1855–1943] jute-spinner's MELANOSIS.

Rietti-Greppi-Micheli syndrome [F. *Rietti*; Enrico *Greppi*; F. *Micheli*, Italian physician] THALASSEMIA minor.

Rifa trademark for *rifampin*.

Rifadin trademark for *rifampin*.

Rifaldin trademark for *rifampin*.

rifampicin (rif-am′pĭ-sin) rifampin.

rifampin (rif′am-pin) a semisynthetic, broad-spectrum macrolide antibiotic, 5, 6, 9, 17, 19, 21-hexahydroxy-23-methoxy-2, 4-12, 16, 18, 20, 22-heptamethyl-8-[*N*-(4-methyl-1-piperazinyl)formimidoxyl-2, 7-(epoxypentadeca[1, 11, 13]-trientimino)naphtho-[2, 1b]-furan-1,11(2*H*)-dione 21-acetate. It inhibits microbial ribonucleic acid synthesis, obtained by reacting 3-formalrifamycin SV with 1-amino-4-methylpiperazine in tetrahydrofuran, occurring as an odorless, red-brown crystalline powder that is unstable in light, heat, and moisture, freely soluble in chloroform, ethyl acetate, and methanol, and slightly soluble in water. It is effective against most gram-positive organisms, including strains of *Streptococcus* and *Diplococcus*, and some gram-negative organisms, including *Haemophilus, Meningococcus, Neisseria,* and *Mycobacterium*. Many bacteria acquire resistance to rifamycin. Some hypersensitivity reactions, including skin rash, thrombocytopenia, and leukopenia; jaundice; and teratogenic reactions in experimental animals have been observed. Called also *rifampicin* and *rifamycin AMP*. Trademarks: Rifadin, Rifaldin, Rimactan, Rimactane.

rifamycin (rif′ah-mi′sin) any of a family of macrolide antibiotics elaborated by *Streptomyces mediterranei*, characterized by the presence of a chromaphoric naphthohydroquinone group spanned by a long aliphatic bridge. They are antibacterial antibiotics which inhibit ribonucleic acid synthesis, being particularly effective against *Mycobacterium tuberculosis*. Rifamycins are designated as AG, B, C, D, E, O, S, SV, and X. **r. AMP,** rifampin.

Riga's aphthae, papilloma [Antonio *Riga*, Italian physician, 19th century] Riga-Fede DISEASE.

Riga-Fede disease [A. *Riga*; Francesco *Fede*, Italian physician, 1832–1913] see under DISEASE.

Riggs' disease [John M. *Riggs*, American dentist, 1811–1885; he developed a method for the treatment of periodontoclasia by scaling and polishing the teeth, followed by trimming the crest of the alveolar process with an instrument inserted into the pocket to the bone. In 1867, he extracted a tooth with the use of anesthesia.] marginal PERIODONTITIS.

rigidity (rĭ-jid′ĭ-te) [L. *rigiditas*] stiffness or inflexibility, chiefly that which is abnormal or morbid; rigor. **arteriosclerotic muscular r.,** see PARKINSONISM. **cadaveric r.,** RIGOR mortis. **cogwheel r.,** rigidity of a muscle which gives way in a series of little jerks when the muscle is passively stretched. **decerebrate r.,** rigid extension of an animal's legs as a result of section of the brain stem; it also occurs as a result of lesions of the upper part of the brain stem. **postmortem r.,** RIGOR mortis.

rigor (ri′gor) [L.] 1. a chill. 2. rigidity. **r. mor′tis,** the stiffening of the skeletal muscles occurring six to ten hours after death. Called also *cadaveric rigidity* and *postmortem rigidity*.

Riley-Day syndrome [Conrad Milton *Riley*, American physician, born 1913; Richard Lawrence *Day*, American physician, born 1905] see under SYNDROME.

rim (rim) a border, or edge. **bite r.,** occlusion r. **occlusion r.,** an occluding border or surface constructed on temporary or permanent denture bases for the purpose of recording the maxillomandibular relation and for positioning the teeth. Called also *bite r., record r., bite-block,* and *biteblock*. **record r.,** occlusion r. **supraorbital r. of frontal bone,** supraorbital margin of frontal bone; see under MARGIN. **supraorbital r. of orbit,** supraorbital margin of orbit; see under MARGIN. **surgical occlusion r.,** an occlusion rim, the base of which has been reduced until it is smaller than the surgical impression tray with which the surgical jaw relation is recorded.

rima (ri′mah), pl. *rimae* [L.] a cleft or crack; a general anatomical term for such an opening. See also FISSURE. **r. glot′tidis** [NA], the elongated fissure between the true vocal cords ventrally, and the bases and vocal processes of the arytenoid cartilages dorsally, which divides the cavity of the larynx into an upper part (*vestibule*) and a lower part (*infraglottic cavity*). It is subdivided into the larger anterior intermembranous and the smaller intercartilaginous parts. In males, its length is about 23 mm and in females 17 to 18 mm; its level corresponding roughly with the bases of the arytenoid cartilages. Width and shape vary with the movements of the vocal cords and arytenoid cartilages during respiration and phonation. Called also *fissure of glottis* and *true glottis*. **r. glot′tidis cartilagin′ea,** the smaller intercartilaginous part of the rima glottidis, between the arytenoid cartilages. Called also *intercartilaginous r., r. respiratoria, glottis respiratoria, interarytenoid space, intercartilaginous glottis,* and *pars intercartilaginea rimae glottidis* [NA]. **r. glot′tidis membrana′cea,** the larger intermembranous parts of the rima glottidis, between the vocal folds. Called also *intermembranous r., r. vocalis, glottis vocalis,* and *pars intermembranacea rimae glottidis* [NA]. **intercartilaginous r.,** r. glottidis cartilaginea. **intermembranous r.,** r. glottidis membranacea. **r. o′ris** [NA], ORIFICE of the mouth. **r. palpebra′rum** [NA], palpebral FISSURE. **r. respirato′ria,** r. glottidis cartilaginea. **r. voca′lis,** r. glottidis membranacea.

Rimactan trademark for *rifampin*.

Rimactane trademark for *rifampin*.

rimae (ri′me) [L.] plural of *rima*.

ring (ring) [L. *annulus, circulus, orbiculus*] 1. a circular line surrounding an object in the center. 2. a circular or annular band. 3. any annular or circular organ or anatomical area. See also ANNULUS and ANULUS. 4. in chemistry, a collection of atoms united in a continuous or closed chain, or circle. **Albl's r.,** a ring-shaped shadow observed in a roentgenogram of the skull, caused by an aneurysm of a cerebral artery. **benzene r.,** the closed hexagon of carbon atoms in benzene (C_6H_6), from which benzene compounds are derived by replacement of the hydrogen atoms. A detailed structure of the benzene ring is shown at the left and commonly used symbols are shown in the middle

and at the right. **Cabot's r.,** a single or double line in the form of a loop or figure-of-eight, appearing in nucleated or non-nucleated erythrocytes in anemias. They stain bright red with Wright's stain. Called also *Cabot's ring body*. **carbocyclic r.,** a chemical ring which includes only carbon atoms. See carbocyclic COMPOUND. 1. a cylinder used as a container for the investment and mold during the process of casting. See illustration at MOLD. 2. refractory FLASK. **cyclopentane r.,** a five-membered ring. Called also *cyclopentane nucleus*. See also *cyclopenta-perhydrophenanthrene r.* and STEROID.

cyclopenta-perhydrophenanthrene r., a tetracyclic ring system consisting of one five-membered (cyclopentane) and three six-membered (perhydrophenanthrene) rings, forming the skeleton of a steroid molecule (see under STEROID). Called also *cyclopenta-perhydrophenanthrene nucleus,* and *perhydrocyclopentanophenanthrene r.* or *nucleus,* and *sterol r.* or *nu-*

cleus. **five-membered r.,** a closed chemical ring having five atoms, such as the furan ring. **furan r.,** a five-membered heterocyclic ring made up of one oxygen and four carbon atoms. **heterocyclic r.,** a chemical ring which includes atoms of different elements. See also heterocyclic COMPOUND. **homocyclic r.,** a chemical ring in which all the members are atoms of the same element. See also carbocyclic COMPOUND. **molding r.,** a band which conforms to the outline of a dental arch and into which plastic material may be packed when making a model or constructing a die. **neonatal r.,** see neonatal LINE. **packing r.,** a cylinder used as a holder for an inlay impression or to withstand pressure exerted during the packing of the amalgam die. **perhydrocyclopentanophenanthrene r.,** cyclopenta-perhydrophenanthrene r. **phenanthrene r.,** a three six-membered ring system which, when fused with the cyclopen-

tane ring, forms the cyclopenta-perhydrophenanthrene ring. Called also *phenanthrene nucleus*. **porphin r.,** SEE PORPHIN. **pyran r.,** a six-membered heterocyclic ring containing one oxygen and five carbon atoms. **pyrrole r.,** see *pyrrole*. **retaining r.,** a ring in an orthodontic appliance that holds the arch wire against the bicuspid bracket to allow free sliding and tipping. **r. of Retzius,** incremental LINE. **six-membered r.,** a closed hexagon of atoms, such as the benzene ring. **split r.,** a three-part casting ring. **sterol r.,** cyclopenta-perhydrophenanthrene r. **Waldeyer's tonsillar r.,** a faucial ring of lymphoid tissue formed by the lingual, pharyngeal, and palatine tonsils. Called also *lymphoid triangle*.

ringworm (ring-worm) a popular name for any of various superficial fungal skin diseases, characterized by the formation of ring-shaped pigmented patches covered with vesicles or scales. Called also *tinea*. **r. of beard,** TINEA barbae. **r. of body,** TINEA corporis. **r. of scalp,** TINEA capitis.

rinse (rins) 1. water or a solution used for washing lightly. 2. to wash lightly. **Janar's acidulated phosphate fluoride r.,** trademark for an aqueous solution containing 0.044 percent sodium fluoride, 0.01 percent orthophosphoric acid, 1.22 percent dihydrogen sodium phosphate, and various amounts of coloring and flavoring agents; used in dental caries prevention. **Janar's sodium fluoride r.,** trademark for a 0.05 percent aqueous solution of sodium fluoride, also containing coloring and flavoring agents; used in dental caries prevention. **Kari r.,** trademark for a 0.05 percent aqueous sodium fluoride solution, also containing preservative, coloring, and flavoring agents; used in dental caries prevention. **mouth r.,** mouthrinse. **NaF rinse,** trademark for a sodium fluoride preparation used in dental caries control, which is available as either a 0.05 percent or 0.2 percent aqueous solution of sodium fluoride, also containing preservative, coloring, and flavoring agents. **Pacemaker Fluorinse,** trademark for a sodium fluoride preparation used in dental caries control, which is available as either a 0.05 percent or 0.2 percent aqueous solution of sodium fluoride, also containing detergents, and flavoring, coloring, and preservative agents. **Phos-Flur oral r. supplement,** trademark for an aqueous solution containing 0.044 percent sodium fluoride, 0.055 percent phosphoric acid, 1.35 percent sodium biphosphate, flavoring agents, and dyes; used in dental caries prevention.

Riogen trademark for *phenylmercuric acetate* (see under ACETATE).

Riolan's muscle, ossicle (bone) [Jean *Riolan*, French physician and anatomist, 1580–1657] see palpebral part of orbicular muscle of eye, under PART, and see under OSSICLE.

Riopan trademark for *magaldrate*.

Risdon approach, wire [F. E. *Risdon*, American oral surgeon] see under APPROACH and WIRE.

Risdon incision see under INCISION.

risk (risk) 1. the chance of harm, injury, or loss. 2. in insurance, the probable amount of loss foreseen by an insurer in issuing a policy. Also, an individual or property insured against loss from some peril or hazard. **absolute r.,** the product of radiation risk times the total population at risk; the number of cases that will result from radiation exposure of a given population. **assigned r.,** a risk which insurance underwriters may not care to insure, such as hypertension, but which, because of a state law or other reasons, must be insured. Insurance of assigned risks is usually handled through a group of insurers. **r. charge,** risk CHARGE.

insurable r., a risk that qualifies for insurance and meets the following criteria: the expected loss by the risk is definable and quantifiable; it belongs to a large homogeneous group of similar risks; the occurrence of loss in individual cases is expected to be accidental or fortuitous; the potential loss may be large enough to the individual to cause hardship; the chance of loss is calculable; it is sufficiently unlikely that loss will occur in many individuals at the same time; the cost of insuring is economically feasible. **preferred r.,** a risk in which the likelihood of a loss for the insurer is below the average and may warrant coverage at a lower than average premium rate.

risorius (ri-so'rius) [L. *risus* laughter] risorius MUSCLE.

Ristella (ris-tel'ah) *Bacteroides*. **R. biacu'ta,** *Bacteroides biacutus*; see under BACTEROIDES. **R. capillo'sa,** *Bacteroides capillosus*; see under BACTEROIDES. **R. corro'dens,** *Bacteroides corrodens*; see under BACTEROIDES. **R. furco'sa,** *Bacteroides furcosus*; see under BACTEROIDES. **R. glutino'sa,** *Fusobacterium glutinosum*; see under FUSOBACTERIUM. **R. melaninogen'ica,** *Bacteroides melaninogenicus*; see under BACTEROIDES. **R. ochra'ceus,** *Bacteroides ochraceus*; see under BACTEROIDES. **R. ora'lis,** *Bacteroides oralis*; see under BACTEROIDES. **R. putre'dinis,** *Bacteroides putredinis*; see under BACTEROIDES.

ristocetin (ris"to-se'tin) an antibiotic substance produced by the fermentation of *Nocardia lurida*, containing both amino and phenolic groups and sugars. Two types are known: ristocetin A and the more active ristocetin B. Used chiefly in the treatment of infections due to gram-positive cocci. Also used in studies on platelet aggregation. Trademarks: Riston and Spontin.

Riston trademark for *ristocetin*.

risus (ri'sus) [L.] laughter. **r. sardon'icus,** a grinning expression produced by spasm of the facial muscles.

Ritalin trademark for *methylphenidate*.

Ritmodan trademark for *disopyramide*.

Ritter's disease, law [Gottfried *Ritter* von Rittershain, German physician, 1820–1883] see under DISEASE and LAW.

Ritter von Rittershain see RITTER.

Rivalta's disease [Sebastiano *Rivalta*, Italian veterinarian, 1852–1893] actinomycosis.

Rivasin trademark for *reserpine*.

Rivet's angle see under ANGLE.

Rivière, Lazare [1589–1655] a French physician who treated toothache by introducing medicines, such as garlic, through the external auditory meatus, believing that the small veins to the teeth pass through the ear. He was also the first to recommend cleaning of the teeth with tobacco ashes.

rivinian (re-ve'ne-an) named after or described by Augustus Quirinus *Rivinus*, as revinian foramen, revinian notch, and incisura Rivini (see tympanic NOTCH).

Rivinus' duct, foramen, gland, incisure, notch [Augustus Quirinus *Rivinus*, Leipzig anatomist and botanist, 1652–1723] see minor sublingual DUCT, sublingual GLAND, and tympanic NOTCH. See also RIVINIAN.

RME rapid maxillary expansion; see maxillary EXPANSION.

RMP regional medical program.

RN registered NURSE.

Rn radon.

RNA ribonucleic acid; a nucleic acid that serves to store and transfer genetic information and to control protein synthesis. It is a macromolecule consisting of nucleotide (ribonucleotide) chains twisted into a single spiral. Its four nucleotides contain purine bases (adenine and guanine) and pyrimidine bases (cytosine and uracil) arranged in a manner similar to the bases in DNA. There are three major types of RNA in cells: *messenger RNA*, which serves in transcription of genetic information from DNA in protein synthesis; *ribosomal RNA*, whose function has not yet been clarified; and *transfer RNA*, which acts as a carrier of specific amino acids during protein synthesis. Messenger RNA is synthesized in the nucleus by enzymatic transcription of a base sequence complementary to that of a single DNA strand. After transcription, messenger RNA enters the cytoplasm, associates with ribosomal RNA, and serves as the template for translating a nucleotide sequence into a specific amino acid sequence during protein synthesis. Called also *ribonucleic acid* and *ribose nucleic acid*. See also DNA, TEMPLATE, TRANSCRIPTION, and TRANSLATION. **adaptor RNA, amino acid RNA,** transfer RNA. **complementary RNA, informational RNA,** messenger RNA. **messenger RNA,** a ribonucleic acid having large molecules of various sizes, which is synthesized with the aid of an enzyme, RNA polymerase, in the nuclei along a single strand of DNA, after the opening of the double helix of the DNA molecule, to produce a template containing the genetic code of DNA, to be translated into the sequence of amino acids in the synthesis of proteins. Called also *comple-*

mentary RNA, informational RNA, mRNA, template RNA, and unstable RNA. See also TRANSCRIPTION. **mRNA,** messenger RNA. **ribosomal RNA,** a form of RNA that comprises about half of the substance of ribosomes and is believed to participate in protein synthesis, although its exact function has not yet been established. Called also *rRNA.* **RNA nucleotidyltransferase,** RNA NUCLEOTIDYLTRANSFERASE. **RNA polymerase,** RNA NU-CLEOTIDYLTRANSFERASE. **rRNA,** ribosomal RNA. **soluble RNA, sRNA,** transfer RNA. **template RNA,** messenger RNA. **tRNA,** transfer RNA. **transfer RNA,** one of some 20 single-stranded RNA varieties of low molecular weight (sedimentation rate of 4S) that represent 10 to 15 percent of the total RNA content in cells and which serve in the translation of the genetic code of DNA into the specific amino acid sequence during protein synthesis. Two or more transfer RNA molecules, specific for both amino acid and template codons, transport information that places the amino acids in their proper position, as determined by the hydrogen bond between the codon and a messenger RNA. Called also *adaptor RNA, amino acid acceptor RNA, soluble RNA, sRNA,* and *tRNA.* See also TRANSLATION (4). **unstable RNA,** messenger RNA. **RNA virus** see under VIRUS.

Roach attachment, clasp see bar CLASP.

rob Robertsonian TRANSLOCATION. See also CHROMOSOME nomenclature.

Robaxin trademark for *methocarbamol.*

Robbins, Frederick C. [born 1916] an American physician; cowinner, with John F. Enders and Thomas H. Weller, of the Nobel prize for medicine and physiology in 1954, for the discovery that poliomyelitis viruses multiply in human tissue.

Robert wiring [César Alphonse *Robert,* French surgeon, 1801–1862] see under WIRING.

Roberts' syndrome [J. B. *Roberts,* American physician] see under SYNDROME.

robertsonian translocation see under TRANSLOCATION.

Robicillin-VK trademark for *penicillin V potassium* (see under PENICILLIN).

Robin's anomalade (syndrome) [Pierre *Robin,* French physician, 1867–1950] see under ANOMALAD.

Robinow's syndrome (dwarfism) [M. *Robinow*] see under SYNDROME.

Robinson's disease [Andrew Rose *Robinson,* American physician, 1845–1924] hidrocystoma.

Rochalimea (ro″kah-li′me-ah) a genus of bacteria of the tribe Rickettsieae, family Rickettsiaceae, the members of which closely resemble those of the genus *Rickettsia.* **R. quinta′na,** a species occurring as gram-negative, short rods, 0.2 to 0.5 by 1.0 to 1.6 μm in size, with a trilaminar cell wall and plasma membrane, similar to those in gram-positive organisms, but lacking flagella or capsules. It is an etiologic agent of trench fever, man being the primary host and transmission being accomplished by the human louse. Called also *Burnetia wolhynica, Rickettsia pediculi, Rickettsia quintana, Rickettsia weigh,* and *Rickettsia wolhynica.*

Rockwell hardness indenter point, hardness number, hardness scale, hardness test see under POINT and HARDNESS.

rod (rod) 1. any slender or elongated straight object or structure. 2. a rod-shaped BACTERIUM. **enamel r's,** enamel prisms; see under PRISM. **Meckel's r.,** Meckel's CARTILAGE. **retinal r.,** specialized cylindrical neuroepithelial cells which, together with visual cones, form the light-sensitive elements of the retina.

Rodiuran trademark for *hydroflumethiazide.*

roentgen (rent′gen) [named after W. C. *Roentgen* (Röntgen)] the international unit of x-rays and gamma rays. It is the quantity of x-rays and gamma rays such that the associated corpuscular emission per 0.001293 gm of air produces in air ions carrying 1 electrostatic unit of electrical charge of either sign. Called also *roentgen unit.* Abbreviated R. **r.-meter,** condenser roentgenMETER.

Roentgen (Röntgen), Wilhelm Conrad [1845–1923] a German physicist who discovered roentgen rays (see x-rays, under RAY) in 1895; winner of the Nobel prize for physics for 1901. See also ROENTGEN.

roentgenogram (rent-gen′o-gram″) a film produced by roentgenography. Called also *skiagram.* See also IMAGE and RADIOGRAPH. **cephalometric r.,** a roentgenogram of the full lateral view of the head, for the purposes of making cranial measurements. Called also *cephalogram.* See also CEPHALOMETRY. **lateral oblique jaw r.,** a roentgenogram of the mandible that unilaterally reveals the mandible from symphysis to condyle. **lateral ramus r.,** a roentgenogram of the mandibular ramus and condyle. **lateral skull r.,** a roentgenogram of the sinuses and lateral aspects of the skeletal structures of the cranium. **maxillary sinus r.,** a roentgenogram of the maxillary sinuses and the zygomas that permits direct comparison of the two sides. Called

also *Water's view r.* **submental vertex r.,** a roentgenogram that permits visualization of the lateral movements of the condyle, lateral displacement of the condyle and/or the coronoid process, and the contour of the zygomatic arches. **Towne projection r.,** a roentgenogram of the mandibular condyles and the midfacial skeleton. **Water's view r.,** maxillary sinus r.

roentgenographic (rent″gen-o-graf′ik) pertaining to or produced by roentgenography.

roentgenography (rent″gen-og′rah-fe) [*roentgen rays* + Gr. *graphein* to write] the making of a record (roentgenogram) of internal structures of the body by passage of x-rays (roentgen rays) through the body to act on specially sensitized film. See also RADIOGRAPHY, x-ray GENERATOR, and x-ray TUBE. **body section r.,** tomography.

roentgenologist (rent″gĕ-nol′o-jist) a physician who has been licensed to practice in roentgenology after successfully fulfilling the requirements for the degree of Doctor of Medicine, completing a 1-year internship and a 3-year residency, and passing medical specialty board examinations. See also RADIOLOGIST. Cf. radiologic TECHNOLOGIST.

roentgenology (rent″gĕ-nol′o-je) [*roentgen rays* + *-logy*] the branch of radiology which deals with the diagnostic and therapeutic use of x-rays (roentgen rays).

roentgenometer (rent″gĕ-nom′ĕ-ter) radiometer.

roentgenometry (rent″gĕ-nom′ĕ-tre) [*roentgen rays* + Gr. *metron* measure] 1. measurement of the intensity of x-rays (roentgen rays). 2. the direct measurement of structures shown in the roentgenogram.

roentgenoscope (rent-gen′o-skōp) fluoroscope.

roentgenotherapy (rent″gen-o-ther′ah-pe) [*roentgen rays* + Gr. *therapeia* therapy] therapeutic use of x-rays (roentgen rays). See also RADIOTHERAPY.

Roger's reflex see under REFLEX.

Roger-Anderson pin see under PIN.

rolitetracycline (ro″li-tet′rah-si′klēn) a semisynthetic tetracycline antibiotic, 4-(dimethylamino)-1,4,4a,5,5a,6,11,12a-octahydro-3,6,10,12,12a-pentahydroxy-6-methyl-1,11-dioxo-N-(1-pyrrolidinylmethyl)-2-naphthacenecarboxamide. It occurs as a light yellow, crystalline powder with a characteristic musty odor, which is very soluble in water, readily soluble in acetone, and slightly soluble in absolute alcohol and ether. Trademarks: Bristacin, Reverin, Superciclin, Syntetrin, Synotodecin, Tetraverin, Transcycline, Velacycline. **r. nitrate,** the nitrate sesquihydrate salt of rolitetracycline, having the same properties as the parent compound. Trademarks: Tetrim, Tetriv, Pyrrocycline-N.

Romanovskii's (Romanovsky's, Romanowsky's) stain (method) [Dimitri Leonidov *Romanovskii,* Russian physician, 1861–1921] see under STAIN.

Romanovsky, Romanowsky see ROMANOVSKII.

Romberg's spasm, syndrome [Moritz Heinrich *Romberg,* German physician, 1795–1873] see under SPASM, and see facial HEMIATROPHY.

Romicil trademark for *oleandomycin.*

Rondar trademark for *oxazepam.*

Rondomycin trademark for *methacycline.*

Rongalite trademark for *sodium formaldehyde sulfoxylate* (see under SODIUM).

rongeur (raw-zhur′) [Fr. "gnawing, biting"] a surgical instrument for cutting tissue, particularly bone, being similar to a forceps, with a spring in the handle and sharp edges on the blade; the blade may be end- or side-cutting. In dentistry, the rongeur is used to remove the sharp edges of the alveolar crest of the bone following tooth extraction. Called also *bone nippers* and *rongeur forceps.* See illustration.

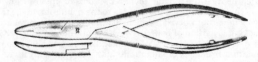

Ronguer. (From H. O. Torres and A. Ehrlich: Modern Dental Assisting. 2nd ed. Philadelphia, W. B. Saunders Co., 1980; courtesy of S. S. White Co.)

Röntgen see ROENTGEN.

roof (roof) a covering structure. See also FLOOR, PARIES, TEGMEN, and WALL. **r. of mouth,** palate. **r. of nasal cavity,** the superior bony structure of the nasal cavity, formed anteriorly by the nasal bone and the spine of the frontal bone; in the middle by the cribriform plate of the ethmoid bone; and posteriorly by the body of the sphenoid bone, sphenoidal concha, ala of the vomer, and sphenoidal process of the palatine bone. **r. of oral cavity,** palate. **r. of orbit,** the superior wall, formed chiefly by the orbital plate of the frontal bone and the orbital surface of the lesser wing of the sphenoid bone. The trochlear fovea for the attachment of the superior oblique muscle of the orbit is situated on its medial aspect. It also lodges the lacrimal fossa for the lacrimal gland. Called also *paries superior orbitae* [NA] and *superior wall of orbit.* **r. of tympanum,** TEGMEN tympani.

room (rōōm) a place in a building enclosed and set apart for occupancy or for performance of certain procedures. See also WARD. **dark r.,** a light-tight room for the processing of x-ray and photographic films. The room is illuminated with safe light filtered by an appropriate filter that allows a certain amount of visibility, filtering out rays that may affect the film. Written also *darkroom.* **emergency r.,** a special site within a hospital where a medical team, utilizing specialized equipment and techniques, is available to handle emergency conditions and to render the necessary medical care, and which is easily accessible to ambulance transport and is self-sufficient in terms of critical care laboratories, x-ray departments, and central supply. In addition, many provide comprehensive medical care to walk-in patients and serve as community health centers. Called also *emergency care facility* and *hospital emergency department.* **intensive care r.,** intensive care UNIT. **operating r.,** a room in a hospital equipped and used for surgical operations. **recovery r.,** a hospital unit usually adjoining operating and delivery rooms, with special equipment and personnel for the care of postoperative or postpartum patients until they may safely be returned to general nursing care in their own rooms or wards.

root (rōōt) [L. *radix*] 1. the lowermost part, or a structure by which something is firmly attached. See also RADIX. 2. r. of tooth. **accessory r.,** a supplementary root of a tooth which is different in size and form and in the direction of the main root. Called also *radiculum appendiciforme.* **accessory buccal r.,** a minute accessory root, similar to a paramolar tubercle, usually found on the mandibular first molars, and sometimes on the second and third molars. Called also *Bolk's paramolar r.* **r. amputation,** root AMPUTATION. **anatomical r.,** that portion of the tooth embedded in the dental alveolus. See *r. of tooth.* **artificial r.,** artificial restoration of a lost root of a tooth. **Bolk's paramolar r.,** accessory buccal r. **r. canal,** root CANAL. **r. canal instruments,** see root canal THERAPY. **r. canal therapy,** root canal THERAPY. **r. of ciliary ganglion, long,** communicating branch of ciliary ganglion with nasociliary nerve; see under BRANCH. **clinical r.,** that portion of a tooth below the clinical crown, being attached to the gingiva or alveolus. Called also *radix clinica* [NA]. See also *physiological r.* **cranial r's of accessory nerve,** four or five delicate roots that emerge from the side of the medulla oblongata, from where they run to the jugular foramen to join the fibers from the spinal roots and thus form the accessory nerve. On leaving the foramen, the cranial root fibers separate again from those of the spinal roots, unite with the vagal nerve proximal to its inferior ganglion, and are distributed by branches of the vagus nerve as motor fibers to the soft palate, constrictors of the pharynx, and larynx. Called also *radices craniales nervi accessorii* [NA]. **facial r.,** NERVE of pterygoid canal. **r. of facial nerve,** fibers passing from the nucleus of the facial nerve to the facial colliculus, and from there to the ventral surface of the pons. Called also *radix nervi facialis.* **hypercemented r.,** hypercementosis. **intra-alveolar r.,** a portion of the root of a tooth that is enclosed in and supported by alveolar bone. **lingual r.,** that root of a posterior tooth, especially a maxillary molar, which is situated nearest the tongue. **locked r's,** roots of upper or lower molars that bow out from the gingiva to the point midway to the apices where they curve toward each other and touch, or nearly so, locking a portion of bone between them, thus complicating tooth extraction. **motor r's of submandibular ganglion,** communicating branches of submandibular ganglion with lingual nerve; see under BRANCH. **motor r. of trigeminal nerve,** the smaller of the two roots of the trigeminal nerve. It consists of motor and proprioceptive fibers to the muscles of mastication, originating from the motor nuclei of the trigeminal nerve, which emerge from the pons to join the mandibular nerve. Called also *masticator nerve, nervus masticatorius, portio minor nervi trigemini,* and *radix motoria nervi trigemini* [NA]. **r. of nose,** the upper portion of the nose which is attached to the frontal bone. Called also *radix nasi* [NA] and *summit of nose.* **physiological r.,** the portion of a tooth proximal to the gingival crevice, or embedded in the dental alveolus. See also *clinical r.* **palatine r.,** that root of a maxillary molar tooth which is situated nearest the palate. **parasympathetic r. of otic ganglion,** petrosal nerve, lesser; see under NERVE. **parasympathetic r. of submandibular ganglion,** a filament connecting the submandibular ganglion with the lingual nerve, consisting of parasympathetic fibers deriving from the intermediate nerve which supply secretory motor innervation to the submandibular, sublingual and lingual glands, and glands in the floor of the mouth. **r. pick,** apical ELEVATOR. **r. planing,** root PLANING. **pyramidal r.,** a single root tapering from the cervix to the apex, usually of the second and third molars. **r. rest,** root REST. **retained r.,** 1. a tooth root, or its part, remaining in the soft tissue or in bone following trauma, extensive caries, or incomplete extraction. 2. an intentionally retained tooth root to prevent resorption of the alveolar process. **sensory r. of trigeminal nerve,** the largest of the three roots of the trigeminal nerve; it consists of a large number of fine sensory bundles emerging from the pons in close association and expanding into a large ganglion, the trigeminal ganglion, from which the ophthalmic, maxillary, and mandibular nerves derive. Called also *portio major nervi trigemini* and *radix sensoria nervi trigemini* [NA]. **r. sheath,** root SHEATH. **spinal r's of accessory nerve,** nerve roots originating from the motor cells of the gray matter of the first five segments of the spinal cord, from where they run along the cord to the foramen magnum into the cranial cavity, cross the occipital bone, penetrate the dura mater as the external branch of the accessory nerve, and enter the jugular foramen. In the foramen, their fibers join the fibers of the internal branch to form the accessory nerve, but upon leaving the foramen, they separate again and run to innervate the sternocleidomastoid and trapezius muscles. Called also *radices spinales nervi accessorii* [NA]. **superior r. of ansa cervicalis,** a long, slender offshoot of the hypoglossal nerve, consisting of fibers of the first or second cervical nerve, descending toward the occipital artery along the surface of the carotid sheath, where they loop to form the ansa cervicalis, and help supply the omohyoid muscle. Called also *radix superior ansae cervicalis* [NA]. **supernumerary r's,** a tooth abnormality characterized by the presence of an excessive number of roots, occurring most commonly in teeth which are normally single-rooted, such as the mandibular bicuspids and cuspids. **sweet r.,** glycyrrhiza. **sympathetic r. of submandibular ganglion,** a filament consisting of sympathetic fibers that passes through the submandibular ganglion without any synaptic connections. Called also *radix sympathica ganglii submaxillaris* and *ramus sympathicus ad ganglion submandibulare* [NA]. **r. of tongue,** the portion of the tongue posterior to the sulcus terminalis, being attached to the hyoid bone by the hyoglossi and genioglossi muscles and the hyoglossal membrane; to the epiglottis by glossoepiglottic folds of the mucosa; to the soft palate by the glossopalatine arches; and to the pharynx by the constrictor pharyngis superiores and the mucosa. Called also *base of tongue* and *radix linguae* [NA]. **r. of tooth,** the part of a tooth from the neck to the apex, embedded in the alveolar process and covered with cementum. A root may be single or divided into several branches, usually identified by their relative position, e.g., *lingual root* or *buccal root.* Single-rooted teeth include mandibular first and second premolars and the maxillary second premolar teeth; the maxillary first premolar has two roots in most cases; maxillary molars have three roots. Called also *anatomical r.* and *radix dentis* [NA].

rope (rōp) a flexible, thick line or cord, usually of braided or twisted strands of fibrous material such as hemp. **foil r., gold foil r.,** a rope made of gold foil for direct filling in dental restorations. See gold FOIL.

rosacea (ro-za′se-ah) ACNE rosacea.

Rose's position [Frank Atcherly *Rose,* British surgeon] see under POSITION.

Rosenbach, Ottomar [physician in Berlin, 1851–1907] see Semon-Rosenbach LAW.

Rosenmüller's cavity, gland, node, recess [Johann Christian *Rosenmüller,* German anatomist, 1771–1820] see pharyngeal RECESS, and palpebral part of lacrimal gland, under PART.

Rosenthal, Curt [German physician] see Melkersson-Rosenthal SYNDROME.

roseola (ro-ze′o-lah, ro″ze-o′lah) [L.] any rose-colored rash. **squamous r.,** PITYRIASIS rosea.

roset (ro-zet′) rosette.

rosette (ro-zet′) [Fr.] any structure or formation resembling a rose, such as (*a*) the clusters of polymorphonuclear leukocytes around a globule of lysed nuclear material, or (*b*) a figure formed by the chromosomes in an early stage of mitosis. Written also *roset.* **EA-r's,** immune rosettes formed by Fc receptors on

B-lymphocytes and macrophages with erythrocytes coated with specific anti–sheep erythrocyte antibody. **EAC-r's,** rosettes formed with erythrocytes coated with specific antibody and complement. **T-r's,** rosettes forming spontaneously when T-lymphocytes from normal individuals are mixed with erythrocytes; used for quantitative determination of T-lymphocytes in peripheral blood.

rosin (roz'in) [L. *resina*] a resin obtained by distilling the volatile oil from the oleoresin obtained from *Pinus palustris* and other species of pine, consisting of 90 percent resin acids and 10 percent neutral matter. Of the resin acids about 90 percent are isomeric with abietic acid and the other 10 percent are a mixture of dihydroabietic and dehydroabietic acid. It occurs as pale yellow to amber, translucent solids with a slight odor and taste of turpentine, which are brittle at room temperature and become fusible on warming. Soluble in ethanol, benzene, ether, glacial acetic acid, oils, carbon disulfide, and solutions of fixed alkali hydroxide, but insoluble in water. Used as a stiffening agent for ointments and plaster. In dentistry, used in cavity varnishes, surgical packs, impression pastes, and pulp capping preparations, together with zinc oxide or eugenol. Called also *abietic anhydride* and *yellow resin*.

rostra (ros'tra) [L.] plural of *rostrum*.

rostrad (ros'trad) 1. toward the rostrum; situated near the rostrum. 2. cephalad.

rostral (ros'tral) [L. *rostralis*, from *rostrum* beak] 1. pertaining to or resembling a rostrum; having a rostrum or beak. 2. rostrad.

rostralis (ros-tra'lis) [L.] rostral.

rostrate (ros'trāt) [L. *rostratus* beaked] having a beaklike process.

rostriform (ros'trĭ-form) [L. *rostrum* beak + *forma* form] shaped like a beak.

rostrum (ros'trum), pl. *rostrums* or *ros'tra* [L. "beak"] a general anatomical term for any beaklike structure. **sphenoidal r., r. sphenoida'le** [NA], a triangular bony spine in the midline of the inferior surface of the body of the sphenoid bone; it articulates with a deep depression between the wings of the vomer.

rot (rot) 1. decay. 2. a disease of sheep, and sometimes of man, caused by the liver fluke *Fasciola hepatica*.

rotameter (ro-tam'ĕ-ter) a flow-rate meter of variable area with a rotating float in a tapered tube; used for measuring the gases in administering an anesthetic.

rotation (ro-ta'shun) [L. *rotatio, rotare* to turn] 1. a turning around a central axis without undergoing any displacement from the axis. See also hinge MOVEMENT. 2. a procedure whereby a malturned tooth is turned into its normal position. 3. malposition due to an abnormal turning of a tooth around its longitudinal axis.

Rotavirus (ro-ta-vi'rus) a tentative genus, comprising naked icosahedral RNA viruses having a virion 70 nm in diameter and 32 capsomers in the virion. Rotaviruses cause diarrhea in human infants and infantile mice, calves, and monkeys. Called also *Duovirus*.

Rothermann attachment see under ATTACHMENT.

Rothia (roth'e-ah) a genus of bacteria of the family Actinomycetaceae, order Actinomycetales, made up of aerobic, grampositive, non–acid-fast, non–spore-forming, nonmotile organisms, which occur in coccoid, diphtheroid, or filamentous forms; filamentous forms are branched, usually 1 μm in diameter, sometimes reaching 5 μm in size. **R. dentocario'sa,** a species consisting of coccoid, diphtheroid, or filamentous forms or mixtures of these, found in the oral cavity of man and primates, particularly in plaque and calculus deposits on the teeth and in carious material. Called also *Actinomyces dentocariosus, Nocardia dentocariosus,* and *N. salivae*.

Rothmund's syndrome [August *Rothmund,* German ophthalmologist, 1830–1906] Rothmund-Thomson SYNDROME.

Rothmund-Thomson syndrome [A. *Rothmund,* Jr.; M. Sidney *Thomson*] see under SYNDROME.

Rotondin trademark for *fenfluramine hydrochloride* (see under FENFLURAMINE).

rotoxamine (ro-toks'ah-mēn) an antihistaminic drug that blocks histamine mediation at the H₁ receptor, (−)-2-[p-chloro-α-[2-(dimethylamino)ethoxy]benzyl]pyridine. Used in the form of the tartrate salt, which occurs as a white crystalline, odorless powder that is soluble in water and methanol, and slightly soluble in ether. Used in the treatment of allergic diseases. Trademark: Twiston.

Rotter-Erb syndrome [Wolfgang *Rotter,* German physician; Werner *Erb,* German physician] see under SYNDROME.

rouge (roozh) [Fr. "red"] 1. any of vrious red cosmetics for coloring the cheeks or lips. 2. ferric OXIDE. **green r.,** chromic OXIDE. **jeweler's r.,** ferric OXIDE.

Rouget cell [Charles Marie Benjamin *Rouget,* French physiologist and anatomist] pericyte.

rouleau (roo-lo'), pl. *rouleaux* [Fr. "roll"] a roll of erythrocytes piled like coins.

Roux, Pierre, Paul Emile [1853–1933] a French bacteriologist who, with Yersin, first described bacterial toxin.

ROW Rendu-Osler-Weber syndrome; see hereditary hemorrhagic TELANGIECTASIA.

Royal alloy see under ALLOY.

Royer's syndrome [Pierre *Royer*] see under SYNDROME.

RPM, rpm revolutions per minute.

-rrhage, -rrhagia [Gr. *rhegnynai* to burst forth] a word termination denoting excessive flow.

-rrhaphy [Gr. *rhaphē* to close by sewing, to suture] a word termination enoting suturing.

-rrhea [Gr. *rhoia* flow] a word termination denoting flow or discharge.

rRNA ribosomal RNA.

RT radiologic TECHNOLOGIST.

RTECS *Registry of Toxic Effects of Chemical Substances;* an acronym for an annual compilation prepared by the National Institute for Occupational Safety and Health, containing acute toxicity data, which is accessible to on-line computer searching.

RTV room temperature VULCANIZATION.

Ru ruthenium.

rubber (rub'er) 1. a highly elastic, solid substance with unique deformation (stretching) properties, which is nearly colorless in its natural state, and is almost insoluble in water, alcohol, and dilute acids and alkali, but dissolves in ether, chloroform, benzene, or carbon disulfide. It is obtained from a variety of trees and shrubs, chiefly *Hevea brasiliensis,* as a milky substance which coagulates into latex. Vulcanization under heat and with sulfur or other cross-linking agents introduces cross links between chains to produce a three-dimensional lattice of improved elasticity, strength, and temperature resistance. The principal chemical component of rubber is *cis*-1,4-polyisoprene. Rubber is also produced synthetically. Called also *India r., natural r., caoutchouc,* and *elastica.* 2. any substance having properties similar to vulcanized rubber. **r. curing,** vulcanization. **heat-vulcanized silicone r.,** heat-vulcanized SILICONE. **India r., natural r.,** rubber (1). **polyether r.,** impression material, polyether; see under MATERIAL. **polysulfide r.,** POLYSULFIDE polymer. **room temperature–vulcanizing silicone r.,** room temperature–vulcanizing SILICONE. **RTV silicone r.,** room temperature–vulcanizing SILICONE. **silicone r.,** a room temperature– or heat-vulcanized silicone having properties and appearance similar to that of natural rubber. See also SILICONE. **synthetic r.,** any of the man-made substances with elastic qualities similar to those of rubber, varying widely in chemical composition and physical properties.

rubber-dam (rub'er-dam) rubber DAM.

Rubberloid trademark for a *reversible hydrocolloid impression material* (see under MATERIAL).

rubefacient (roo″bĕ-fa'shent) [L. *ruber* red + *facere* to make] 1. reddening of the skin. 2. an irritant which acts locally on the skin and mucous membranes to induce hyperemia. Most rubefacients may also exert vesicant effects when applied in high concentrations.

rubella (roo-bel'ah) [L. *ruber* red] an infectious viral disease of childhood, characterized by mild constitutional symptoms, such as a rash similar to that seen in mild measles or scarlet fever. A reddish eruption on the soft palate (*Forchheimer's spots*) is the principal oral manifestation. Complications are rare, except when the infection occurs in women during the first trimester of pregnancy (see congenital rubella SYNDROME). Called also *German measles.* See also rubella VIRUS.

rubeola (roo-be'o-lah, ru″be-o'lah) [L. *ruber* red] measles.

rubescent (roo-bes'ent) [L. *rubescere* to become red] reddish; becoming red.

rubidium (roo-bid'e-um) [L. *rubidus* red] an alkali metal. Symbol, Rb; atomic number, 37; atomic weight, 85.4678; specific gravity, 1.532; melting point, 39°C; valence, 1; group IA of the periodic table. It is an active metal, occurring as a lustrous, silvery white, soft substance that rapidly tarnishes on exposure to air, decomposes water, ignites spontaneously with oxygen, reacts with halogens, and forms solutions with potassium, cesium, and sodium. Used in space technology and electronics. Contact with rubidium causes skin burns.

rubidomycin (ru″bĭ-do-mi'sin) daunorubicin.

Rubinstein-Taybi syndrome [Jack Herbert *Rubinstein,* American physician, born 1925; Hooshang *Taybi,* American physician, born 1919] see under SYNDROME.

Rubivirus (ru″bĭ-vi′rus) a genus of togaviruses, having a virion about 50 nm in diameter, whose only member is the rubella virus.

rubivirus any virus of the genus *Rubivirus.*

Rubner's law [Max *Rubner,* German physiologist, 1854–1932] see under LAW.

rubor (roo′bor) [L.] redness; an area of redness, being one of the cardinal signs of inflammation.

rubricyte (roo′bri-sīt) [L. *rubrum* red + Gr. *kytos* hollow vessel] basophilic NORMOBLAST.

rudiment (roo′dĭ-ment) [L. *rudimentum*] 1. a basic principle or element. 2. a structure in its embryonic state; a vestigial structure. 3. an organ or part having little or no function but which has functioned at an earlier stage of species or individual development. Called also *vestige.* 4. the first indication of a structure in the course of its development; a primordium. Called also *rudimentum* [NA].

rudimenta (roo″dĭ-men′tah) [L.] plural of *rudimentum.*

rudimentary (roo″dĭ-men′tah-re) having the properties of a rudiment; vestigial.

rudimentum (roo″dĭ-men′tum), pl. *rudimen′ta* [L. "a first beginning"] 1. rudiment. 2. [NA] rudiment (4).

Ruffini's corpuscles [Angelo *Ruffini,* Italian anatomist, 1864–1929] lamellar corpuscles: see under CORPUSCLE.

Rufus of Ephesus [c. A.D. 100] a physician and anatomist whose surviving writings are noteworthy, particularly those on anatomy, gout, the pulse, and clinical history taking.

ruga (roo′gah), pl. *ru′gae* [L.] a doubled tissue, or recurved margin; a fold, wrinkle, or crease. **ru′gae palati′nae,** palatine rugae, palatine folds; see under FOLD.

rugae (roo′je) [L.] plural of *ruga.*

rugosity (roo-gos′ĭ-te) [L. *rugositas*] 1. the condition of being wrinkled. 2. a fold, wrinkle, or ruga.

rule (rool) [L. *regula*] a statement of conditions commonly observed in a given situation, or a statement of a prescribed course of action to obtain a result. **Anstie's r.,** in a life insurance examination, the maximum amount of absolute alcohol which can be taken without injury by an adult is 1½ oz. daily. **Bastedo's r.,** the dose of a drug for a child is obtained by multiplying the adult dose by the child's age in years, adding 3 to the product, and dividing the sum by 30. **Cieszynski's r. of isometry,** see bisecting angle TECHNIQUE. **Clark's r.,** 1. the dose of a drug for a child is obtained by multiplying the adult dose by the weight of the child in pounds and dividing the result by 150. 2. (C. A. Clark) a rule for the orientation of structures portrayed in dual or multiple radiographs. **Cowling's r.,** the dose of a drug for a child is obtained by multiplying the adult dose by the age of the child his next birthday and dividing by 24. **discovery r.,** in malpractice, a rule in use in some jurisdictions under which the statute of limitations does not commence to run until the wrongful act is discovered or, with reasonable diligence, should have been discovered. **eligibility r's,** in insurance, the conditions which define who may be entitled to benefits, when persons first become entitled to such benefits, and any provisions which determine how long an individual remains entitled to benefits. **Fried's r.,** the dose of a drug for an infant less than 2 years old is obtained by multiplying the child's age in months by the adult dose and dividing the result by 150. **Lossen's r.,** in

hemophilia, only women transmit the condition; only men inherit it. Called also *Lossen's law.* **Price's r.,** see bisecting angle TECHNIQUE. **Young's r.,** the dose of a drug for a child is obtained by multiplying the adult dose by the age in years and dividing the result by the sum of child's age plus 12.

ruler (roo′ler) a strip of wood, metal, or plastic having a straight edge and gradation in inches and/or centimeters and millimeters, used for measuring objects and drawing lines. Rulers used in dentistry are usually made of plastic or a noncorrosive metal and have the millimeter scale.

Ruminococcus (ru″mĭ-no-kok′us) a genus of anaerobic, gram-positive bacteria of the family Peptococcaceae, occurring as spherical to elongated cocci, which are involved in the fermentation of cellulose in the rumens of cattle and sheep.

rupture (rup′chur) 1. forcible tearing or disruption of tissue. 2. a hernia. **modulus of r.,** flexure STRENGTH.

Russell body cell see under CELL.

Russell index see periodontal disease RATE.

Russell's syndrome (dwarf) [Alexander *Russell,* British physician] see under SYNDROME.

Russell-Silver syndrome [A. *Russell;* Henry F. *Silver,* American physician, born 1918] Russell's SYNDROME.

Rust's disease (syndrome) [Johann Nepomuk *Rust,* German physician, 1775–1840] see under DISEASE.

ruthenium (roo-the′ne-um) [L. *Ruthenia* Russia] a metallic element. Symbol, Ru; atomic number, 44; atomic weight, 101.07; specific gravity, 12.41; melting point, 2310°C; Brinell hardness number, 220; valences, 1–8 (2, 3, and 4 are most common); group VIII of the periodic table. Naturally occurring isotopes include 96, 98–102, and 104; artificial radioactive isotopes include 93–95, 97, 103, and 105–108. It is a silvery white, lustrous metal that is resistant to acids, including aqua regia, and combines with oxygen on heating. Ruthenium forms alloys with platinum, palladium, cobalt, nickel, and tungsten. Used as a substitute for platinum, and as a catalyst in the synthesis of long-chain hydrocarbons.

rutherford (ruth′er-ford) [named after E. R. *Rutherford*] a unit of radioactivity, defined as 10^{10} disintegrations of any radionuclide per second. Abbreviated *rd.* See also CURIE.

Rutherford atom [Ernest R. *Rutherford,* British physicist, 1871–1937] nuclear ATOM. See also RUTHERFORD and RUTHERFORDIUM.

rutherfordium (ruth″er-for′dĭ-um) [named after E. R. *Rutherford*] a proposed name for *element 104* (see under ELEMENT).

Rutherfurd's syndrome [Margaret E. *Rutherfurd,* British physician] see under SYNDROME.

Rx drug prescription DRUG.

Rx Jeneric A trademark for a soft *dental casting gold alloy* (see under GOLD).

Rx Jeneric B trademark for a medium hard *dental casting gold alloy* (see under GOLD).

Rx Jeneric C trademark for a hard *dental casting gold alloy* (see under GOLD).

Rx Jeneric IV trademark for an extra hard *dental casting gold alloy* (see under GOLD).

Rydrin trademark for *nylidrin hydrochloride* (see under NYLIDRIN).

Ryff, Walter Hermann [died c. 1570] a German physician and surgeon, whose book *Nützlicher Bericht,* published in 1545 in German (instead of the then customary Latin), is the first published work dealing with oral hygiene. It has three parts, dealing with the eyes, the teeth, and the first dentition. Ryff noted the relation between dental and ocular diseases.

Ryomycin trademark for *oxytetracycline.*

Rythmodan trademark for *disopyramide.*

S

S 1. siemens. 2. sella (3). 3. Svedberg UNIT. 4. sulfur.

S. abbreviation for L. *sem′is,* half; *sig′na,* mark; *sinis′ter,* left.

s symbol for *satellite* (3). See also CHROMOSOME nomenclature.

Σ the capital of the Greek letter sigma. Symbol for *summation.*

σ, ς the eighteenth letter of the Greek alphabet. See SIGMA. Symbol for *one-thousandth part of a second* and *standard deviation.*

s⁻¹ a symbol for *cycles per second;* see HERTZ.

Sa Sa POINT.

Sabin oral vaccine [Albert Bruce *Sabin,* American virologist, born 1906] poliomyelitis vaccine, live oral; see under VACCINE.

saburra (sah-bur′ah) [L.] foulness of the stomach, mouth, or teeth.

sac (sak) [L. *saccus;* Gr. *sakkos*] a pouch; a baglike organ or structure. **amniotic s.,** amnion. **chorionic s.,** chorion. **dental s.,** a primitive connective tissue which surrounds the developing tooth germ. Called also *odontotheca.* See also dental FOLLICLE. **enamel s.,** a term sometimes used for the enamel organ during the stage in which its outer layer forms a sac enclosing the whole dental germ. **lacrimal s.,** the dilated upper end of the nasolacrimal duct. Called also *dacryocyst, sacculus lacrimalis,* and *saccus lacrimalis* [NA]. **laryngeal s.,** APPENDIX of laryngeal ventricle. **yolk s.,** one of the fetal membranes, forming a pear-shaped sac on the ventral surface of the developing embryo. It arises at the same time as the amniotic cavity, the cuboidal endodermal cells of the embryonic disk providing the basic structure of the primary sac, and attains its average size of 5 mm by the middle of the second month. It provides the primary material from which the tubular primitive gut is formed by folding. In humans, it does not store any yolk, but its role consists of the transfer of nutritive fluid to the embryo from the young trophoblast. A narrow structure connecting the unclosed gut with the sac proper undergoes progessive constriction, becoming the threadlike yolk stalk connecting both structures, which detaches from the gut by the fifth week and degenerates thereafter. After the second month, the sac shrinks and converts into a solid structure containing debris, persisting in this form throughout pregnancy; it may be found in afterbirth. A persistence of its proximal end may produce an abnormal diverticulum (*Meckel's diverticulum*) in the intestinal tract. See illustration at fetal MEMBRANES.

saccharase (sak′ah-rās) β-FRUCTOFURANOSIDASE.

saccharate (sak′ah-rāt) a salt of saccharic acid.

saccharated (sak′ah-rāt″ed) [L. *saccharatus*, from *saccharum* sugar] charged with or containing sugar.

saccharide (sak′ah-rīd) a series of carbohydrates divided into mono-, di-, tri-, and polysaccharides, according to the number of saccharide groups ($C_nH_{2n}O_{n-1}$) composing them.

sacchariferous (sak″ah-rif′er-us) [L. *saccharum* sugar + *ferre* to bear] containing or yielding sugar.

saccharification (sak″ar-ĭ-fĭ-ka′shun) [L. *saccharum* sugar + *facere* to make] conversion to sugar.

saccharin (sak′ah-rin) an artificial nonnutritive, noncaloric, and nonfermentative substance having a sweetening power 300 to 500 times that of sucrose, 1,2-benzisothiazolin-3-one-1,1-dioxide, occurring as a white, crystalline powder with a very sweet taste. It is readily soluble in amyl acetate, ethyl acetate, benzene, and alcohol and is slightly soluble in water, chloroform, and ether. Saccharin is used by those in whom the use of sugar is contraindicated, also being used in drugs and dentifrices. Laboratory studies indicate that feeding experimental animals high doses of saccharin (considerably in excess of that normally consumed by humans) may cause bladder tumors in certain animals. Called also *benzoic sulfimide*, *benzosulfimide*, *o-sulfobenzoic acid*, and *saccharinol*. Trademarks: Glucid, Gluside, Saccharol. **calcium s.,** CALCIUM saccharin. **soluble s., s. sodium,** a saccharin salt, sodium 2,3-dihydro-3-oxobenziosulfonazole, occurring as a white, crystalline solid that has no or little odor and is very soluble in water. Used as a nonnutritive, noncaloric sweetener. Trademarks: Crystallose, Dugutan. Preparations containing soluble saccharin include Sucaryl and Sweet'n Low.

saccharine (sak′ah-rīn) [L. *saccharinus*] sweet; sugary.

saccharinol (sah-kar′ĭ-nol) saccharin.

saccharo- [L. *saccharum*; Gr. *sakcharon* sugar] a combining form denoting relationship to sugar.

saccharobiose (sak″ah-ro-bi′ōs) a disaccharide.

Saccharol trademark for saccharin.

saccharolytic (sak″ah-ro-lit′ik) [*saccharo-* + Gr. *lysis* dissolution] capable of splitting up sugar.

Saccharomyces (sak″ah-ro-mi′sēz) [*saccharo-* + Gr. *mykēs* fungus] a genus of ascomycetous yeasts. **S. cerevis′iae,** a species used in baking bread and making alcoholic beverages (see bakers' YEAST). In very rare cases, it may cause lung disease. **S. glu′tinis,** *Rhodotorula glutinis*; see under RHODOTORULA.

saccharose (sak′ah-rōs) [*saccharo-* + *-ose*] sucrose.

sacci (sak′ki) [L.] plural of *saccus*.

saccular (sak′u-lar) shaped like a sac or bag.

sacculated (sak′u-lāt″ed) characterized by formation of saccules or pouches.

saccule (sak′ul) [L. *sacculus*] 1. a little bag or sac. 2. the smaller of the two divisions of the membranous labyrinth of the vestibule. **laryngeal s.,** APPENDIX of laryngeal ventricle.

sacculi (sak′u-li) [L.] plural of *sacculus*.

sacculus (sak′u-lus), pl. *sac′culi* [L., dim. of *saccus*] saccule. **s. commu′nis,** utricle (2). **s. den′tis,** a fibrous sac in the jaw, the dental follicle (sac), which encloses an unerupted tooth, being connected with the overlying gingiva by the gubernaculum dentis or gubernacular cord. See also dental FOLLICLE and dental SAC. **s. lacrima′lis,** lacrimal SAC. **s. laryn′gis** [NA], APPENDIX of laryngeal ventricle. **s. Morgag′nii,** VENTRICLE of larynx.

saccus (sak′kus), pl. *sac′ci* [L.; Gr. *sakkos*] a sac or pouch; a general anatomical term for such a structure. **s. lacrima′lis** [NA], lacrimal SAC.

Sachs, Bernard [New York neurologist, 1858–1944] see Tay-Sachs DISEASE.

Sacks, Anton see *Clostridium septicum*, under CLOSTRIDIUM (Ghon-Sacks bacillus).

Sacophan trademark for *dextromethorphan hydrobromide* (see under DEXTROMETHORPHAN).

saddle (sad′l) 1. a support whose shape fits the contour of the object resting upon it. 2. denture base s. **denture base s.,** that part of a complete or partial denture which rests upon the basal seat and to which the teeth are attached. See also denture BASE.

Saethre-Chotzen syndrome [Haakon *Saethre*, Norwegian psychiatrist; F. *Chotzen*, German psychiatrist] see under SYNDROME.

Safco 69 trademark for an *amalgam alloy* (see under AMALGAM).

safelight (sāf′lit) safe LIGHT.

Safeway see under DENTIFRICE.

sagittal (saj′ĭ-tal) [L. *sagittalis*, from *sagitta* arrow] 1. shaped like or resembling an arrow; straight. 2. situated in the direction of the sagittal suture; said of an anteroposterior plane or section parallel to the median plane of the body. See under PLANE.

sagittalis (saj″ĭ-ta′lis) [L.] sagittal; a general anatomical term denoting a structure situated in the direction of the sagittal suture. See under SUTURE.

Sagnac rays see under RAY.

St. Apollonia the patron saint of dentistry. A Christian martyr of Alexandria who, in A.D. 249, was persecuted by Roman authorities by having her teeth knocked out, and when threatened with being burned alive, died by leaping into the fire. She was canonized 50 years later. In 1508, the *Utrecht Brevier* was the first to mention her as the patroness of those who suffer from toothache. The custom of guilds and trades to place their members under the protection of a patron saint led medieval dentists to place themselves under the patronage of St. Apollonia.

St. Anthony's fire, St. Francis' fire erysipelas.

Sainton, Raymond see cleidocranial DYSPLASIA (Marie-Sainton syndrome, Scheuthauer-Marie-Sainton syndrome).

Sakati-Nyhan-Tisdale syndrome [N. *Sakati*; William L. *Nyhan*, Jr., American physician, born 1926; W. K. *Tisdale*] see under SYNDROME.

sal (sal) [L.] salt. **s. polychres′tum,** POTASSIUM sulfate. **s. ethyl,** ethyl SALICYLATE. **s. sapien′tiae,** ammoniated MERCURY.

Salamid trademark for *salicylamide*.

salbutamol (sal-but′ah-mol) albuterol.

Sal-Fayne trademark for an analgesic preparation containing aspirin, phenacetin, and caffeine.

Salicain trademark for *salicyl alcohol* (see under ALCOHOL).

salicylamide (sal″ĭ-sil-am′id) the amide of salicylic acid, 2-hydroxybenzamide, occurring as a white, odorless, crystalline powder with a bitter, warm aftertaste, which is soluble in hot water, ethanol, chloroform, and ether. It has pharmacological and toxic properties similar to those of analgesic, antipyretic, and anti-inflammatory salicylates, being less potent than aspirin. Used in certain analgesic mixtures. Trademarks: Acket, Algamon, Algiamida, Benesal, Cidal, Novecyl, Oramid, Salamid, Salrin, Samid, Sylamid.

salicylate (sal′ĭ-sil″āt, sah-lis′ĭ-lāt) any salt of salicylic acid. The term usually refers to a class of analgesic, antipyretic, and anti-inflammatory drugs, aspirin being the prototype, which are esters of salicylic acid obtained by substitution in the carboxyl group, and esters of organic acids in which the carboxyl group of salicylic acid is retained and substitution is made in the OH group. By inhibiting the synthesis of prostaglandins in inflamed tissues, salicylates prevent sensitization of the pain receptors to mechanical stimuli and chemicals, such as bradykinin, which mediate the pain response. By acting on the hypothalamus, they are believed to have central analgesic and antipyretic effects. Salicylates are weak analgesics and are used chiefly in headache, toothache, arthralgia, dysmenorrhea, neuralgia, and myalgia; also used in the treatment of gout, rheumatic fever, and rheumatoid arthritis. In high doses, they may cause central nervous system disorders, acid-base balance disorders with respiratory disturbances, vasomotor disorders, epigastric distress, nausea, vomiting, and blood coagulation disorders. Generally, salicylates are considered as having low toxicity, but poisoning may occur when excessive doses are taken. Mild chronic intoxication (salicylism) due to intake of repeated large doses is usually characterized by headache, vertigo, tinnitus, hearing difficulty, visual disorders, confusion, lassitude, drowsiness, sweating, thirst, hyperventilation, nausea, vomiting, and diarrhea. In acute intoxication, there may be in addition EEG abnormalities, restlessness, incoherent speech, apprehension, tremor, diplopia, delirium, hallucinations, convulsions, symptoms simulating alcoholic intoxication, coma, and death. Acneiform eruption, erythema, and scarlatiniform, pruritic, eczematoid, desquamative, and other skin lesions may occur. Epigastric distress, vomiting, and anorexia are common. Severe cases are also complicated by acid-base balance and plasma electrolyte disorders associated with respiratory disturbances. Hemorrhagic disorders with petechial lesions, occult bleeding, and thrombocytopenic purpura may occur. Toxic encephalopathy is a prominent feature. Hypersensitivity with skin rashes and anaphylaxis may occur. Febrile and dehydrated children are especially prone to intoxication. **ethyl s.,** the salicylic acid ester of ethyl alcohol, occurring as a transparent volatile liquid with a pleasant characteristic odor and taste, which becomes brownish on exposure to light and air, and is slightly soluble in water and miscible with ethanol and ether. Used as a flavoring agent and counterirritant. Called also *sal ethyl, salicylic acid ethyl ester,* and *salicylic ether.* **magnesium s.,** the magnesium salt of 2-hydroxybenzoic acid, occurring as a white or pinkish, odorless, crystalline powder with a faint characteristic odor, which is soluble in water and ethanol. Pharmacological and toxic properties are similar to those of other analgesic, antipyretic, and anti-inflammatory salicylates, except for the hazard of hypermagnesemia in renal diseases. Trademark: Magan. **methyl s.,** a compound, 2-hydroxybenzoic acid methyl ester, occurring as a colorless, yellowish, or reddish liquid with a characteristic pleasant taste and odor of wintergreen, which is soluble in water, ethanol, and glacial acetic acid. It may be obtained from *Gaultheria procumbens* (wintergreen) leaves or produced synthetically. Used as a flavoring agent and as a counterirritant. Used in the past in dentifrices, but discontinued because of its hypersensitizing properties. Toxic when taken internally. Called also *gaultheria oil, oil of betula, oil of wintergreen, sweet birch oil,* and *teaberry oil.* **sodium s.,** the monosodium salt of 2-hydroxybenzoic acid, occurring as white or pinkish powder or scales that are soluble in water, ethanol, and glycerol. Its pharmacological and toxicological properties are similar to those of other analgesic, antipyretic, and anti-inflammatory salicylates. Trademarks: Enterosalicyl, Enterosalil.

salicylism (sal'ĭ-sil″izm) mild chronic salicylate intoxication. See SALICYLATE.

salify (sal'ĭ-fi) to convert into a salt.

Saligenin trademark for *salicyl alcohol* (see under ALCOHOL).

Saligenol trademark for *salicyl alcohol* (see under ALCOHOL).

salimeter (sah-lim'ĕ-ter) [L. *sal* salt + *metrum* measure] a hydrometer for ascertaining the concentration of saline solution.

saline (sa'lēn, sa'lĭn) [L. *salinus,* from *sal* salt] salty; of the nature of a salt; containing a salt or salts; the term is sometimes used alone to mean saline solution.

saliva (sah-li'vah) [L.] a clear, slightly acid, sometimes viscid mixture of secretions of the salivary glands (see under GLAND) and gingival fluid exudate. Human saliva contains 99.42 percent water and 0.58 percent solids; specific gravity 1.003; pH 6.35–6.85; the 24-hour volume is about 1500 ml. Inorganic components include chloride, bicarbonate, and sodium, as well as calcium, sulfate, and phosphate. Organic components include amylase (see also table at ENZYME) and mucin and, in smaller amounts, proteins, urea, glucose, lactic acid, phosphatase, and carbonic anhydrase. The principal functions of saliva are to moisten foods and the mucous membranes and to lubricate the bolus of food for its passage through the esophagus; the secondary function is the digestion of starches and dextrins to maltose by the action of salivary amylase. It also has bactericidal and cleansing functions. Called also *oral fluid.* See also XEROSTOMIA and terms beginning PTYALO- and SIALO-. **artificial s.,** a solution used for irrigating the mouth in xerostomia, such as one of methyl cellulose and mouthwash in distilled water. **s. chor'da,** submaxillary saliva produced in response to stimulation of the chorda tympani nerve, being less viscid and turbid than that of the unstimulated gland. **ganglionic s.,** saliva obtained by irritating the submaxillary gland. **lingual s.,** the secretion of Ebner's glands and other serous glands of the tongue. **parotid s.,** saliva produced by the parotid gland, which is thinner and less viscid than the other varieties. **ropy s.,** saliva which is highly viscid. **sublingual s.,** saliva produced by the sublingual gland, which is the most viscid of all. **submaxillary s.,** saliva produced by the submaxillary gland. **supersaturated s.,** saliva containing excessive amounts of mineral elements; usually involved in calculus formation. **sympathetic s.,** submaxillary saliva produced in response to stimulation of its sympathetic nerves, which is more viscid and turbid than that of the unstimulated gland.

salivant (sal'ĭ-vant) provoking a flow of saliva.

salivary (sal'ĭ-var-e) [L. *salivarius*] pertaining to the saliva. **s. enzymes,** see table at ENZYME.

salivate (sal'ĭ-vāt) to produce an excessive flow of saliva. See also PTYALISM.

salivation (sal″ĭ-va'shun) [L. *salivatio*] 1. the secretion of saliva. 2. ptyalism.

salivator (sal'ĭ-va″tor) an agent that causes salivation.

salivatory (sal'ĭ-vah-to″re) causing salivation.

salivin (sal'ĭ-vin) salivary AMYLASE.

Salk vaccine [Jonas Edward *Salk,* American virologist, born 1914] see under VACCINE.

Sallmann see VON SALLMANN.

Salmonella (sal″mo-nel'ah) [named after Daniel Elmer *Salmon*] a genus of bacteria of the family Enterobacteriaceae, made up of rod-shaped, gram-negative, usually, but not invariably, motile cells set apart from other enteric bacilli by failure to ferment lactose. It includes the typhoid-paratyphoid bacilli and bacteria usually pathogenic for lower animals that are often transmitted to man. The genus is separated into species or serotypes on the basis of O and H antigens, the latter occurring in two phases and identified by antigenic formulae taking the general form: O antigen: phase 1 ⇄ phase 2, in which the O antigens are designated by Roman numerals, the phase 1 antigens by lower case letters, and the phase 2 antigens by Arabic numerals. More than 1000 different serotypes have been described. **S. chol'eraesu'is,** a species pathogenic for animals, including man, which is found as a secondary invader in hog cholera. Called also *Bacillus cholerae-suis.* **S. enteritidis,** a widely distributed parasite of rodents, in whom it may produce an endemic diarrheal disease, and a common cause of gastroenteritis in man. Called also *Bacillus enteritidis.* **S. gallina'rum, S. gallina'rum pullo'rum,** a species causing fowl typhoid, with little or no pathogenicity for man. Called also *Bacillus gallinarum* and *B. pullorum.* **S. hirschfel'dii,** a species causing paratyphoid fever. Called also *S. paratyphi C.* and *bacillus paratyphoid C.* **S. morga'ni,** *Proteus morgani;* see under PROTEUS. **S. paraty'phi A,** a species causing typhoid fever, being pathogenic only for man. Called also *Bacterium paratyphi, B. paratyphi A,* and *B. paratyphi typhus A.* **S. paraty'phi B,** *S. schottmuelleri.* **S. paraty'phi C,** *S. hirschfeldii.* **S. schottmuel'leri,** a species causing paratyphoid fever and food poisoning in man; it is a rare pathogen of other animals. Called also *S. paratyphi B, Bacillus schottmuelleri,* and *Bacterium paratyphi typhus B.* **S. ty'phi,** a species causing typhoid fever, transmitted by water or human feces, and being only pathogenic for man. Called also *S. typhosa, Bacillus typhi, Bacterium typhi,* and *Eberthella typhi.* **S. typhimu'rium,** a species parasitic in rodents, especially mice, which is the causative agent of mouse typhoid and of food poisoning in man. Called also *Bacillus typhi murium.* **S. typho'sa,** *S. typhi.*

salmonella (sal″mo-nel'ah), pl. *salmonel'lae.* Any microorganism of the genus *Salmonella.*

salmonellae (sal″mo-nel'e) [L.] plural of *salmonella.*

salmonellal (sal″mo-nel'al) pertaining to or caused by salmonella.

salmonellosis (sal″mo-nel'lo-sis) infection with any species of the genus *Salmonella.*

salpingion (sal-pin'je-on) a point at the apex of the petrous bone on the lower surface.

salpingopharyngeal (sal-ping'go-fah-rin'je-al) pertaining to the auditory tube and the pharynx.

salpingopharyngeus (sal-ping″go-fah-rin'je-us) salpingopharyngeal MUSCLE.

Salrin trademark for *salicylamide.*

salt (sawlt) [L. *sal;* Gr. *hals*] 1. any compound formed by the reaction of an acid with a base. 2. SODIUM chloride. **basic s.,** any salt with one or more hydroxyl radicals, yielding one or more hydroxyl ions on complete dissociation in water. **bile s's,** a major component of bile, produced from cholesterol (either dietary or synthesized in liver cells), which is converted into cholic and deoxycholic acids. The resultant acids combine with glycine and taurine to form glyco- and tauro-conjugated acids, the salts of which are the bile acids. Their function consists of emulsification (or detergent function), whereby surface tension of fat particles is decreased, thus allowing them to be broken into minute sizes, and also absorbing monoglycerides, cholesterol, and other lipids from the intestinal tract, where they form micelles, to be transported into the venous circulation. See also LIPID metabolism. **bitter s's,** magnesium sulfate heptahydrate; see MAGNESIUM sulfate. **common s.,** SODIUM chloride. **dibasic s.,** a salt formed with displacement of two hydrogen atoms per molecule. **Epsom s's,** magnesium sulfate heptahydrate; see

MAGNESIUM sulfate. **ethereal s.**, ester. **Glauber's s.**, SODIUM sulfate. **iodized s.**, sodium chloride to which minute amounts of iodides have been added; used as a nutritional source of iodine in areas where it is not available from natural sources. **kitchen s.**, SODIUM chloride. **monobasic s.**, a salt formed with displacement of one hydrogen atom per molecule. **quaternary ammonium s's**, quaternary ammonium compounds; see under COMPOUND. **rock s.**, table s. **s. sterilization**, salt STERILIZATION. **table s.**, SODIUM chloride. **s. of tartar**, POTASSIUM carbonate. **tribasic s.**, a salt formed with displacement of three hydrogen atoms per molecule.

salting-out (sawl'ting-owt) the separation of serum or plasma protein fraction in the serum or plasma by precipitation in increasing concentrations of neutral salts; the hydration of the salt progressively added removes water molecules so that each protein fraction becomes dehydrated and consequently less soluble at a different concentration of the salt.

salubrious (sah-lu'bre-us) [L. *salubris*] conducive to health; wholesome.

Salufer trademark for *sodium hexafluorosilicate* (see under SODIUM).

Salunil trademark for *chlorothiazide*.

saluresis (sal"u-re'sis) [L. *sal* salt + Gr. *ourēsis* a making water] the excretion of sodium and chloride ions in the urine.

Saluric trademark for *chlorothiazide*.

Salurin trademark for *trichlormethiazide*.

Saluron trademark for *hydroflumethiazide*.

Salvacard trademark for *nikethamide*.

salvarsan (sal'var-san) arsphenamine.

salve (sav) a thick ointment or cerate; see OINTMENT.

samarium (sah-ma're-um) [mineral samarkite, named after Colonel *Samarski*, a Russian mine inspector] a rare earth of the lanthanide group, occurring as a hard, brittle metal. Symbol Sm; atomic number, 62; atomic weight, 150.4; melting point, 1077°C; specific gravity, 7.5; valences, 2, 3; group IIIB of the periodic table. Its naturally occurring isotopes include 144, 147–49, 150, 152, and 154; ^{147}Sm, which has a half-life of 1.05 × 10^{11} years and emits alpha rays, ^{148}Sm, and ^{149}Sm are radioactive. Artificial radioactive isotopes include 142, 143, 145, 146, 151, 153, and 155–157. Samarium rapidly oxidizes when exposed to air. Used in nuclear technology and metallurgical research.

Samid trademark for *salicylamide*.

sample (sam'p'l) [L. *examplum* example] a representative part taken to typify the whole. **random s.**, a representative part so chosen that each item has an equal chance of being selected.

sand (sand) 1. any gritty particular material. 2. see SILICON dioxide.

Sandedrine trademark for the *l*-form of *ephedrine hydrochloride* (see under EPHEDRINE).

Sandril trademark for *reserpine*.

Sandström's gland [Ivar Victor *Sandström*, Swedish anatomist, 1852–1889] thyroid gland, accessory; see under GLAND.

Sandwith's bald tongue [Fleming Mant *Sandwith*, British physician, 1853–1918] see under TONGUE.

sane (sān) [L. *sanus*] of sound mind.

Sanfilippo's syndrome [Sylvester J. *Sanfilippo*, American physician, born 1926] see under SYNDROME.

sangui- [L. *sanguis* blood] a combining form denoting relationship to blood.

sanitarian (san"ĭ-ta're-an) a person who is expert in matters of sanitation and public health.

sanitary (san'ĭ-ta"re) [L. *sanitarius*] promoting or pertaining to health.

sanitation (san"ĭ-ta'shun) [L. *sanitas* health] the establishment of environmental conditions favorable to health. **environmental s.**, the control of those factors in man's physical environment which exercise or may exercise a deleterious effect on his physical, mental, or social well-being.

sanitization (san"ĭ-ti-za'shun) the process of making or the quality of being made sanitary, whereby the number of microbial contaminants is reduced to a relatively safe level.

Sanorin trademark for *naphazoline*.

Sanotensin trademark for *guanethidine*.

Sansert trademark for *methysergide*.

Santorini, cartilage of, tubercle of [Giovanni Domenico *Santorini*, Italian anatomist, 1681–1737] see corniculate CARTILAGE and corniculate TUBERCLE.

sap (sap) the natural juice of a living organism or tissue. **cell s.**, hyaloplasm (1). **nuclear s.**, karyolymph.

sapo (sa'po) [L. "soap"] 1. soap. 2. castile SOAP. **s. mol'lis**, soft SOAP (1). **s. mol'lis medicina'lis**, green SOAP.

saponification (sah-pon"ĭ-fi-ka'shun) [L. *sapo* soap + *facere* to make] the act or process of converting fats into soaps and glycerol by heating with alkalies. In chemistry, the term now

denotes hydrolysis of an ester by an alkali, resulting in the production of a free alcohol and an alkali salt of the ester acid.

Sappey's fibers, ligament [Marie Philibert Constant *Sappey*, French anatomist, 1810–1896] see under FIBER and LIGAMENT.

sapro- [Gr. *sapros* rotten] a combining form meaning rotten or putrid, or designating relationship to decay or to decaying material.

Sapromyces (sap"ro-mi'sēz) *Acholeplasma*.

Saran trademark for a man-made plastic in which the fiber-forming substance is a long-chain polymer consisting of no less than 80 percent vinylidene chloride. Used in the production of tubings and fabrics that are flameproof and resistant to corrosive substances and rot.

Sarcina (sar-si'nah) a genus of gram-positive bacteria of the family Peptococcaceae, occurring as anaerobic, nearly spherical cocci, about 1.8 to 3.0 μm in diameter, found singly or in groups. The organisms have been isolated from diseased human stomachs, normal rabbit and guinea pig stomachs, and from cereals, soil, and manure. **S. lu'tea**, *Micrococcus luteus*; see under MICROCOCCUS.

sarco- [Gr. *sarx, sarkos* flesh] a combining form denoting relationship to flesh.

Sarcoclorin trademark for *melphalan*.

Sarcodina (sar"ko-di'nah) [Gr. *sarkodes* fleshlike] a subphylum of Protozoa, including all the amebae, both free-living and parasitic, characterized by the ability to produce pseudopodia during most of the life cycle; flagella, when present, develop only during the early stages. It includes class Rhizopoda. Called also *Rhizopoda*.

sarcogenic (sar"ko-jen'ik) [sarco- + Gr. *gennan* to produce] forming flesh.

sarcoid (sar'koid) [sarco- + Gr. *eidos* form] 1. tuberculoid; characterized by noncaseating epithelioid cell tubercles. 2. pertaining to or resembling sarcoidosis. 3. an old term meaning flesh; fleshy. **Boeck's s.**, sarcoidosis. **multiple s.**, benign LYMPHADENOMATOSIS.

sarcoidosis (sar"koi-do'sis) a benign systemic granulomatous disease of young adults, usually involving the liver, spleen, lymph nodes, skin, and lungs. Typically, the lesion is a tubercle with little or no necrosis. *Mycobacterium tuberculosis* and other mycobacteria, beryllium intoxication, and foreign body reaction, are considered as possible etiologic factors. There are no typical oral manifestations, but lesions of the lips may appear as small, papular nodules or plaques, or resemble herpetic lesions or fever blisters, and bleblike lesions containing a clear fluid may appear on the palate. Sarcoidosis associated with parotitis, uveitis, lymphadenopathy, and facial paralysis is known as *Heerfordt's syndrome*. Called also *Besnier-Boeck-Schaumann syndrome, Boeck's sarcoid, granulomatosis benigna, lupus pernio, lymphogranulomatosis benigna*, and *Schaumann's disease*.

L-sarcolysine (sar"ko-li'sin) melphalan.

sarcoma (sar-ko'mah), pl. *sarcomas* or *sarco'mata* [sarco- + -oma] a rapid-growing tumor made up of cells derived from connective tissue, such as bone and cartilage, muscle, blood vessels, or lymphoid tissue, which is often highly malignant and frequently metastasizes. **alveolar soft part s.**, a rare form of sarcoma that may occur in any part of the body, but is located most commonly in the muscles of the extremities, and is also found in the tongue and floor of the mouth. It typically presents as a slow-growing, well-defined mass made up of large cells with a finely granular cytoplasm, arranged in a uniform pseudoalveolar or organoid pattern in numerous endothelial-lined vascular channels and septa. The tumor, having a tendency to metastasize and recur, is often fatal. Called also *malignant granular cell myoblastoma*. **ameloblastic s.**, the malignant counterpart of ameloblastic fibroma, which is very rare and occurs most commonly in children and young adults. It is found more often in the mandible than in the maxilla, presenting a painful, rapid-growing lesion that causes destruction of bone and loosening of teeth. It is made up of cellular connective tissue exhibiting bizarre, pleomorphic cells with hyperchromatic nuclei and mitotic figures, with islands of odontogenic epithelium. Called also *ameloblastic fibrosarcoma* and *malignant ameloblastic fibroma*. **endothelial s.**, Ewing's s. **Ewing's s.**, a primary malignant tumor of bone, usually with a poor prognosis, which never exhibits osteoblastic properties, affecting children, adolescents, and young adults. It is composed of compact, uniform cells with large, round, or ovoid nuclei containing scattered chromatin. Mitotic figures are common; small vascular channels may be present. Long bones are the most common site; the skull, clavicle, ribs, and shoulder and pelvic girdles may be involved. The jaws are frequently involved, with pain, swelling, facial neuralgia, and lip paresthesia being among the early symptoms; the intraoral mass is often ulcerated. A low grade fever and high white blood count may be present. Called also *endothelial s., round cell s., endothelial myoma,* and *Ewing's tumor.* **idiopathic hemorrhagic s., s. idiopath'icum,** Kaposi's s. **Kaposi's s.,** a chronic, idiopathic neoplastic disease of the vascular system, occurring most commonly in old age, associated with the presence of multiple neoplasms of the skin, and manifested by bluish red or dark brown nodules and plaques with an ulcerative tendency. The distal parts of the extremities are most frequently affected; however, visceral lesions may occur. Histological features vary with the age of the lesion: younger lesions are angiomatous; fibrosis and deposits of blood pigment are characteristic of older lesions. Primary involvement of the oral cavity is rare, but secondary lesions may occur on the lower lip, tongue, and buccal mucosa. It has numerous synonyms; among the most common are *idiopathic hemorrhagic s., s. idiopathicum, multiple idiopathic hemorrhagic s., angioreticuloendothelioma, angiosarcoma pigmentosum,* and *Kaposi's angiomatosis.* **large round cell s.,** reticulum cell s. **multiple idiopathic hemorrhagic s.,** Kaposi's s. **neurogenic s.,** malignant SCHWANNOMA. **osteogenic s.,** a malignant tumor of the bone, made up of sarcomatous fibroblastic stroma, in which osteoid and bone are formed. In the sclerosing type there are large amounts of osseous tissue that further cause reactive bone formation to produce dense eburned growths. In the osteolytic type the amounts of osteoid matrix and bone are minimal. Any bone may be involved, but the long bones are affected most commonly. It is relatively uncommon in the jaws, but may occur in the maxilla or mandible, producing swelling and facial asymmetry, and after enlargement, loosening, malposition, and sometimes, exfoliation of the teeth. Called also *osteosarcoma.* **reticulum cell s., retothelial s.,** a lymphoma composed of reticulum cells, which may arise in lymph nodes and in extralymphoidal tissues, such as bones and the central nervous system. Tumors of the lymph nodes exhibit progressive enlargement of the nodes, resulting in the development of solid, grayish nodules up to 5 cm in diameter with obliteration of the normal structures and invasion of the capsule and fusion of nodes into a solid tumor mass. Primary soft tissue oral tumors are uncommon; those found in the oral cavity may be located in the tonsils, pharynx, palate, buccal mucosa, and gingiva. Primary bone tumors occur most frequently in the extremities and less commonly in the jaws. Pain, sometimes present for several months or years, is the most common symptom. Lymphadenopathy, swelling, and bone destruction, accompanied by loosening of the teeth, may follow. Called also *large round cell s., reticulocytoma,* and *reticulum cell lymphosarcoma.* **round cell s.,** Ewing's s.

sarcomatosis (sar″ko-mah-to′sis) a condition characterized by the development of multiple sarcomas. **s. cu′tis,** Kaposi-Spiegler s. benign LYMPHADENOMATOSIS. **Kaposi-Spiegler s.,** benign LYMPHADENOMATOSIS.

sarcomere (sar′ko-mēr) [*sarco-* + Gr. *meros* part] the contractile unit of a myofibril, being a transverse section of a myofibril that, in striated muscle, is characterized by the presence of light and dark bands (I and A bands) separated from each other by the H zones and M and Z lines. See illustration at MUSCLE.

sarcophagization (sar-kahf″ah-ji-za′shun) entombment of the dental pulp by a calcified bridge.

sarcoplasm (sar′ko-plazm) [*sarco-* + Gr. *plasma* anything formed or molded] the intracellular fluid of muscle, which surrounds the myofibrils, and contains glycogen, glycolytic enzymes, adenosine triphosphate, adenosine diphosphate, adenosine monophosphate, phosphate, phosphocreatine, creatine, electrolytes, amino acids, peptides, and other substances necessary for muscle activity.

Sarcoptes scabiei (sar-kop′tēz ska-be′i) an acarid, the itch mite, which produces scabies in humans. Varieties of *S. scabiei* cause mange in domestic animals.

sarcostyle (sar′ko-stīl) [*sarco-* + Gr. *stylos* column] 1. myofibril. 2. Kölliker's COLUMN.

sarcous (sar′kus) pertaining to flesh or to muscular tissue.

satellite (sat′ĕ-līt) [L. *satelles* companion] 1. a celestial body orbiting a larger one. 2. a vein that closely accompanies an artery. 3. a small mass of chromatin attached by a narrow stalk to a short arm of a chromosome. Symbol *s.* Called also *satellite chromosome.*

satiety (sah-ti′ĕ-te) [L. *satis* sufficient + *-ety* state or condition of] sufficiency, or satisfaction, as full gratification of appetite or thirst.

satinite (sat′ĭ-nīt) gypsum.

saturated (sat′u-rāt″ed) 1. soaked or impregnated to the maximum capacity. 2. having all available valence bonds of an atom attached to other atoms. See also saturated COMPOUND. 3. a solution holding the maximum equilibrium quantity of dissolved matter.

saturation (sat″u-ra′shun) [L. *saturatio*] 1. the act or process of soaking or impregnating to the maximum capacity. 2. in chemistry, the state in which all available valence bonds of an atom, especially carbon, are attached to other atoms, paraffin compounds with straight chains being an example of a saturated compound. 3. the state of a solution when it holds the maximum equilibrium quantity of dissolved matter at a given temperature. 4. in radiotherapy, the delivery of a maximum tolerable tissue dose within a short time period and then maintaining this biologic effect for an extended period of time by additional smaller fractional doses. **oxygen s.,** a percentage obtained by dividing the actual oxygen content of the blood by the maximum oxygen content that can be carried by the blood.

saturnine (sat′ur-nīn) [L. *saturninus; saturnus* lead] pertaining to or produced by lead; having the properties associated with lead.

saturnism (sat′ur-nizm) [L. *saturnus* lead] lead poisoning. See LEAD.

saucer (saw′ser) a rounded, shallow depression.

saucerization (saw″ser-i-za′shun) the excavation of the tissue of a wound to form a shallow, saucer-like depression, used in the treatment of osteomyelitis.

saw (saw) a cutting instrument with a cutting blade or serrated edge blade. **Adam's s.,** a small straight saw with a long handle, for osteotomy. **bayonet s.,** a bone saw used for the excision of the nasal dorsal hump. **chain s.,** a surgical saw the teeth of which are set upon links, the saw being moved by pulling upon one or the other handle. **crown s.,** a type of trephine. **Farabeuf's s.,** a saw the blade of which can be set at any desired angle. **Gigli's s., Gigli's wire s.,** a flexible wire with saw teeth, the saw being moved by pulling one or the other handle. Called also *Gigli's wire.* See illustration. **gold s.,** a cutting instrument with

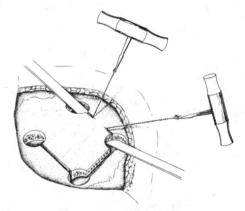

Gigli's wire saw as used in removing segment of the skull. (From Dorland's Illustrated Medical Dictionary. 26th ed. Philadelphia, W. B. Saunders Co., 1981.)

a thin sawlike blade, used for removing surplus metal from the contact area of direct filling gold restorations. **hemp s.,** a hempen cord used in cutting soft tissues. **Hey's s.,** a small saw for enlarging orifices in bones. **hole s.,** trephine. **Joseph's s.,** one used for cutting the ramus of the mandible. **Koeber's s.,** a thin, replaceable blade held in a frame, used to trim foil restorations. **oscillating s.,** an oscillating blade for cutting bone, mounted on a unit driven by electric or gas generated motors. Called also *Stryker's s.* **rotary s.,** a rotary blade for cutting bone, mounted on a shaft in a unit driven by motors powered by gas, air, or electricity. **separating s.,** one for separating teeth. **Shrady's s.,** subcutaneous s. **Stryker's s.,** oscillating s. **subcutaneous s.,** one for cutting bone through a fenestrated cannula that has been introduced alongside the bone by a trocar. Called also *Shrady's s.*

Sb antimony (L. *stibium*).

S-C trademark for a *zinc phosphate cement* (see under CEMENT).

scab (skab) an outer layer of solid matter formed by the drying of a bodily secretion; a crust.

scabies (ska'bēz) [L., from *scabere* scratch] a disease of the skin caused by infestation with the itch mite, *Sarcoptes scabiei,* which bores into the stratum corneum forming cuniculi or burrows, associated with intense itching, together with eczema caused by scratching. **Boeck's s.,** Norwegian s. **Norwegian s.,** a severe form of scabies with crusting, scaling, and suppuration of the face, scalp, and fingers, as well as other parts of the body, and infestation with immense number of mites under the skin. Called also *Boeck's s., Boeck's itch,* and *Norwegian itch.*

scaffold (skaf'ōld) 1. any raised framework. 2. a support, either natural or prosthetic, which maintains the contour of tissue.

scala (ska'lah), pl. *sca'lae* [L. "staircase"] any stairlike structure; applied especially to various passages of the cochlea.

scalariform (skah-lar'ĭ-form) [L. *scalaris* like a ladder + *forma* form] resembling the rungs of a ladder.

scald (skawld) 1. a burn caused by hot liquid or hot, moist vapor. 2. to burn with a hot liquid or steam.

scale (skāl) [Fr. *scale* shell, husk] 1. a thin, compacted, flaky fragment, delicate plate of bone, dried, horny epidermis, or enamel. 2. a thin fragment of tartar or other concretion on the surface of the teeth. 3. [L. *scala,* usually pl. *scalae,* a series of steps] a scheme or device by which some property may be evaluated or measured, such as a linear surface bearing marks at regular intervals, representing certain predetermined units. 4. to remove calcareous deposits from the teeth and from beneath the gingival margin by means of an instrument. **absolute s.,** a temperature scale with 0 at the absolute zero of temperature. See absolute TEMPERATURE. **Brinell s., Brinell hardness s.,** see under HARDNESS. **Celsius s., centigrade s.,** a temperature scale in which the interval between two established points is divided into 100 equal units, with the ice point at 0 and the normal boiling point of water at 100 degrees (100° C). See TEMPERATURE. **Fahrenheit a.,** a temperature scale with the ice point at 32 and the normal boiling point of water at 212 degrees (212° F). See TEMPERATURE. **French s.,** a scale used for denoting the size of catheters, sounds, and other tubular instruments, each unit being roughly equivalent to 0.33 mm in diameter, i.e., 18 French indicates a diameter of 6 mm. Abbreviated *Fr.* **hardness s.,** HARDNESS scale. **Howe's color s.,** a scale in which color changes are indicative of the temperature of a heated body. See table. **Kelvin s.,** an absolute scale on

HOWE'S COLOR SCALE

| Color | Temperature | |
	(°C.)	(°F.)
Lowest visible red	475	890
Dull red	550–625	1020–1150
Cherry red	700	1300
Light red	850	1560
Orange	900	1650
Full yellow	950–1000	1740–1830
Light yellow	1050	1920
White	1150 or above	2100 or above

(From R. W. Phillips: Skinner's Science of Dental Materials. 7th ed. Philadelphia, W. B. Saunders Co., 1973.)

which the unit of measurement corresponds with that of the Celsius (centigrade) scale, but the ice point is at 273.15 degrees (273.15° K). See absolute TEMPERATURE. **Knoop s., Knoop hardness s.,** see under HARDNESS. **Mohs s., Mohs hardness s.,** see under HARDNESS. **Rankine s.,** an absolute scale on which the unit of measurement corresponds with that of the Fahrenheit scale, but the ice point is at 491.67 degrees (491.67° R). See absolute TEMPERATURE. **Réamur s.,** a temperature scale with the ice point at 0 and the normal boiling point of water at 80 degrees (80° R). See TEMPERATURE. **Rockwell s., Rockwell hardness s.,** see under HARDNESS. **scleroscope s.,** a scale used to determine the hardness of material. See scleroscope NUMBER. **temperature s.,** one used for expressing the degree of heat. See TEMPERATURE. **Vickers s., Vickers hardness s.,** see under HARDNESS.

scalene (ska'lēn) [Gr. *skalēnos* uneven] 1. unequally three sided. 2. pertaining to one of the scalene muscles.

scalenectomy (ska"lē-nek'to-me) [*scalenus* + Gr. *ektomē* excision] the operation of resecting a scalenus muscle.

scalenus (ska-le'nus) [L.; Gr. *skalēnos*] uneven; a name given to various muscles of the neck.

scaler (skāl'er) 1. a dental instrument used in removing calculus from the surface of the teeth. See illustration. 2. an electronic instrument for rapid counting of radiation-induced pulses from a Geiger-Müller counter or other radiation detectors. It permits rapid counting by reducing (by a definite scaling factor) the number of pulses entering the counter. See also Geiger-Müller COUNTER. **chisel s.,** periodontal CHISEL. **deep s.,** one used for the removal of the subgingival deposits from the teeth. It is general-

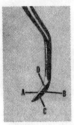

Scaler. The blade has two straight cutting edges (A and B), which terminate at the tip in a point. The flat or slightly convex lateral surface (C) joins the opposing lateral surface at the back of the blade, forming a sharp angle. The facial surface (D) lies between the two cutting edges. (From P. F. Steele: Dimensions of Dental Hygiene. 2nd ed. Philadelphia, Lea & Febiger, 1975.)

ly finer than the superficial scalers and provides accessibility to deep pockets with a minimum of soft tissue damage, having various blade shapes, including sickle-shaped and claw-shaped blades. **double-ended s.,** one having blades on both ends of the handle, one blade for the right side and the other for the left side. **hoe s.,** a single- or double-ended instrument, having the blade bent at a 99° angle; the cutting edge being formed by the junction of the flattened terminal surface with the inner aspect of the blade. The cutting edge is beveled at 45°. The blade is slightly bowed, so that it can maintain contact at two points on a convex surface. The back of the blade is rounded and the blade has been reduced to minimum thickness to permit access to the root of deep pockets without interference from the adjacent tissue. Used for planing and smoothing root surfaces, which entails removal of calculus remnants and softened cementum. See illustration. **Jaquette s.,** one of a set of three scalers: No. 1. has a blade and shank that is in a straight line with the handle; used generally in the anterior part of the mouth. Nos. 2 and 3 are paired with angulated shanks to facilitate accessibility to all tooth surfaces; used in the posterior part of the mouth. The blade of the scaler is triangular in cross

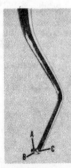

Hoe scaler. The end of the shank is turned at a right angle to form the blade. A, Straight cutting edge; B, Outer surface bevel; C, Lateral surface. (From P. F. Steele: Dimensions of Dental Hygiene. 2nd ed. Philadelphia, Lea & Febiger, 1975.)

section, two lateral surfaces joining the inner surface to form the working edges. The inner surface tapers from a broad base at the shank to form a terminal point. See illustration. **McCall s.,** one in a set of six hoe scalers designed to provide access to all tooth surfaces, each scaler having a different angular relationship between the shank and the handle. **sickle s.,** a scaler for

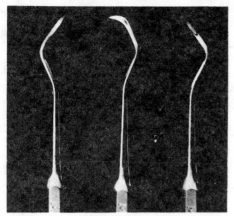

Jaquette scalers. *A*, No. 2. *B*, No. 1. *C*, No. 3. (From F. A. Carranza, Jr.: Glickman's Clinical Periodontology. 5th ed. Philadelphia, W. B. Saunders Co., 1979.)

removing tenacious supragingival or subgingival deposits from the teeth, having a sicklelike blade with flattened sides and a trapezoidal cross section. The inner surface is broad and tapers to a point, the end is rounded to preserve the effectiveness of the instrument when it is reduced by sharpening. See illustration. **superficial s.,** one of several types of scalers designed for removal of supragingival deposits from the teeth. Most are double-ended instruments, having a variety of blade and shank shapes. **ultrasonic s.,** an ultrasonic instrument supplied with a tip for applying high-frequency vibrations of about 25,000 cycles per second, usually accompanied with a stream of water to prevent overheating and to remove adherent deposits from the teeth and bits of inflamed tissue from the walls of the gingival crevice. **wing s.,** a variation of the sickle scaler used in the past, consisting of a short curved blade with a flare at the very edge.

scaling (skāl'ing) removal with the use of a scaler of plaque and calculus from the surface of a tooth. **coronal s.,** removal with a scaler of materia alba, calculus, and other deposits from the coronal surface of a tooth. **deep s.,** subgingival s. **hand s.,** removal of plaque and calculus from the surface of a tooth with the use of hand instruments, such as chisels, hoes, sickle scalers, and files. **root s.,** subgingival s. **rotary s.** removal of debris, plaque, and calculus from the surface of a tooth with a rotary instrument which has six sides on the tapered working surface and is designed to fit into a high-speed contra-angle handpiece. **subgingival s.,** removal of plaque and calculus from the surface of a tooth apical to the gingival margin, usually accumulated in periodontal pockets. Called also *deep s., root s.,* and *subgingival apoxesis.* **supragingival s.,** removal of plaque and calculus from the surface coronal to the gingival margin. **ultrasonic s.,** removal of debris, plaque, and calculus from the surface of a tooth with the use of an ultrasonic scaler, which is a generator containing an electronic unit to energize a handpiece which converts a varying magnetic field into mechanical vibrations (about 25,000/sec) for transmission to an instrument resembling the McCall hand scaler. Water bathes the field for cooling purposes. See also ultrasonic CURETTAGE.

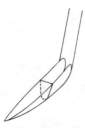

Basic Characteristics of the Sickle Scaler: triangular shape, double cutting edge, and pointed tip. (From F. A. Carranza, Jr.: Glickman's Clinical Periodontology. 5th ed. Philadelphia, W. B. Saunders Co., 1979.)

scalp (skalp) that part of the skin of the head, exclusive of the face and ears, which normally is covered with hair.
scalpel (skal'p'l) [L. *scalpellum*] a surgical knife with an elongated or short pointed blade, used to cut into soft tissue. It may be a solid instrument, or it may have interchangeable blades fitting into a slot of the handle, being locked in position. See illustration.

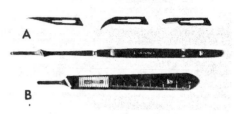

Knife blades nos. 11, 12, and 15 (*A*); handles nos. 7 and 3 (*B*). (From D. E. Waite: Textbook of Practical Oral Surgery. 2nd ed. Philadelphia, Lea & Febiger, 1978.)

scaly (ska'le) [L. *squamosus*] squamous; scalelike or characterized by scales.
scan (skan) a shortened form of *scintiscan.*
Scandicain trademark for *mepivacaine hydrochloride* (see under MEPIVACAINE).
scandium (skaṇ'de-um) [L. *Scandia* Scandinavia] a metallic element, occurring as a silvery white metal that is resistant to moisture and to most acids. Symbol, Sc; atomic number, 21; atomic weight, 44.9559; melting point, 1539°C; specific gravity, 3.989; group IIIB of the periodic table. Sc[45] is the only naturally occurring isotope; artificial radioactive isotopes include 41–44 and 46–50.
scanner (skan'er) something that scans; a scintiscanner. **scintillation s.,** scintiscanner.
scanning (skan'ing) 1. the act of examining visually, as a small area of different isolated areas, in detail. 2. a manner of utterance characterized by somewhat regularly recurring pauses. **radioisotope s.,** the production of a two-dimensional picture (scintiscan or scan), representing the gamma rays emitted by a radioactive isotope concentrated in a specific tissue of the body, such as the brain or thyroid gland, especially after introduction of a substance, labeled with a radioactive isotope, having special affinity for the examined tissue.
scanography (skan-og'rah-fe) a method of making radiographs by the use of a narrow slit beneath the tube in such a manner that only a line or sheet of x-rays is employed and the x-ray tube moves over the object so that all the rays of the central beam pass through the part being radiographed at the same angle.
scapha (ska'fah) [L. "a skiff"] [NA] a long curved depression which separates the helix from the anthelix. Called also *fossa helicis, fossa scaphoidea,* and *scaphoid fossa.*
scapho- [Gr. *skaphē* skiff or light boat] a combining form meaning boat-shaped.
scaphocephaly (ska"fo-sef'ah-le) [scapho- + Gr. *kephalē* head] a condition characterized by an abnormally long and narrow skull.
scaphohydrocephalus (skaf'o-hi"dro-sef'ah-lus) hydrocephalus in which the head assumes a boatlike shape.
scaphoid (skaf'oid) [scapho- + Gr. *eidos* form] shaped like a boat; navicular.
scaphoiditis (skaf"oi-di'tis) inflammation of the scaphoid bone.
scapi (ska'pi) [L.] plural of *scapus.*
scapula (skap'u-lah), pl. *scap'ulae* [L.] [NA] the flat, triangular bone in the back of the shoulder.
scapus (ska'pus), pl. *sca'pi* [L.] a general term for a shaftlike structure.
scar (skar) [Gr. *eschara* the scab or eschar on a wound caused by burning] a cicatrix; the connective tissue union produced by the junction of the lips of a wound. **apical s.,** a well-defined translucent area of the bone surrounding the apex of the root of a tooth that has been treated by root canal therapy or endodontic surgery. The area is generally made up of relatively acellular dense collagen bundles, usually being asymptomatic and nonprogressive. **hypertrophic s.,** one formed by exuberant cicatrization, giving it the appearance of a keloid but without the latter's tendency to progressive extension, and recurrence after excision. **Parrot's s's,** whitish radial cicatrices (rhagades) occurring at the sites of labial fissures, observed in children with

congenital syphilis. Called also *Parrot's cicatrices* and *Parrot's rhagades.*

scarification (skar″ĭ-fĭ-ka′shun) [L. *scarificatio;* Gr. *skariphismos* a scratching up] production in the skin or mucous membrane of numerous superficial scratches or punctures, as for the introduction of smallpox vaccine. The term is sometimes used erroneously for scarring.

scarlatina (skar″lah-te′nah) [L. "scarlet"] scarlet FEVER. **s. angino′sa**, scarlet fever associated with painful pharyngitis, with tonsillar enlargement or peritonsillar abscess. Called also *Fothergill's disease.*

Scarpa's foramen, nerve [Antonio *Scarpa*, Italian anatomist and surgeon, 1747–1832] see under FORAMEN and NERVE.

scarring (skar′ing) the formation of a scar or cicatrix; cicatrization. See also SCARIFICATION.

scatter (skat′er) the diffusion or deviation of x-rays produced by the medium through which the rays pass. Backward diffusion is called *backscatter.* See also scattered rays, under RAY.

scattering (skat′er-ing) 1. the act or process of spreading something over a wide area at irregular intervals. 2. a process that changes the trajectory of a subatomic particle or photon, usually due to collisions with atoms, nuclei, and other particles or by interactions with fields of magnetic force. See also BACKSCATTER and scattered rays, under RAY. **classical s.**, coherent s. **coherent s.**, scattering of x-rays following collision of photons with atoms, associated with deflection of the photon by the nuclear attraction during its passage between the nucleus and electrons in the orbit, but without modifying the energy or wavelength of the photon. Called also *classical s., Thompson s.,* and *unmodified s.* **Compton s.**, incoherent s. **elastic s.**, that in which the scattered particle's internal energy is unchanged in the collision. **incoherent s.**, inelastic scattering of photons interacting with atomic electrons, in which incident photons are scattered with reduced energy, the rest being given to ejection of electrons (recoil electrons). Called also *Compton s.* **inelastic s.**, that in which there is a change in the internal energy. **Thompson s.**, unmodified s., coherent s.

scavenging (skav′inj-ing) 1. the taking or collecting of something from discarded material. 2. the use of a nonspecific precipitate to remove one or more undesirable radionuclides from solution by absorption or coprecipitation. 3. the removal from the atmosphere of radionuclides by the action of rain, snow, or dew. See also FALLOUT.

ScD Doctor of Science.

Schatzmann attachment see under ATTACHMENT.

Schaumann's disease [Jörgen *Schaumann*, Swedish dermatologist, 1879–1953] sarcoidosis.

Schede's operation [Max *Schede*, German surgeon, 1844–1902] see under OPERATION.

schedule (skej′ul) 1. a plan of procedure. 2. a timetable. **allowance s., s. of allowances**, see ALLOWANCE. **s. of benefits**, see under BENEFIT. **fee s.**, see ALLOWANCE. **fixed fee s.**, fixed FEE. **indemnification s.**, see ALLOWANCE. **maximum fee s.**, fixed FEE.

scheelite (skēl′īt) CALCIUM tungstate.

Scheie's syndrome [Harold G. *Scheie*, American physician, born 1909] see under SYNDROME.

schema (ske′mah) [Gr. *schēma* form, shape] a plan, outline, or arrangement; a scheme. **Hamberger's s.**, the external intercostal and the intercartilaginous muscles are inspiratory muscles, the internal intercostal muscles are expiratory.

scheme (skēm) a plan, design, or outline. **occlusal s.**, occlusal SYSTEM.

Schenck's disease [Benjamin Robinson *Schenck*, American physician, 1873–1920] sporotrichosis.

Scherer, Hans J. see van Bogaert-Scherer-Epstein SYNDROME.

Scherofluron trademark for *fludrocortisone 21-acetate* (see under FLUDROCORTISONE).

Scheuthauer-Marie-Sainton syndrome [Gustav *Scheuthauer,* 1832–1894; Pierre *Marie,* French physician, 1853–1940; Raymond *Sainton*] cleidocranial DYSPLASIA.

schindylesis (skin″dĭ-le′sis) [Gr. *schindylēsis* a splintering] a joint or articulation in which a thin plate of bone is received into a cleft or fissure by the separation of two laminae in another bone, as in the articulation of the perpendicular plate of the ethmoid bone with the vomer.

-schisis [Gr. *schisis* cleft, cleavage] a word termination indicating cleft.

schisto- [Gr. *schistos* split] a combining form meaning split or cleft.

schistocyte (skis′to-sīt) [*schisto-* + Gr. *kytos* hollow vessel] a fragment of an erythrocyte, most often in a triangular or elliptical form, and usually resulting as a product of hemolytic processes.

schistosomiasis (shis″to-, skis″to-so-mi′ah-sis) infection with trematode parasites of the genus *Schistosoma.*

schizo- [Gr. *schizein* to divide] a combining form signifying division or splitting.

schizodontism (skiz″o-dont′izm) a form of gemination in which twin teeth derive from a single germ.

schizophrenia (skiz″o-fre′ne-ah) [*schizo-* + Gr. *phrēn* mind + *-ia*] any of a group of severe emotional disorders characterized by misinterpretation and retreat from reality, delusions, hallucinations, ambivalence, inappropriate affect, and withdrawn, bizarre, or regressive behavior. Popularly and erroneously called *split personality.*

Schizoplasma (skiz″o-plaz′mah) *Mycoplasma.* **S. fermen′tans**, *Mycoplasma fermentans;* see under MYCOPLASMA. **S. hom′inis**, *Mycoplasma hominis;* see under MYCOPLASMA. **S. ora′le**, *Mycoplasma orale;* see under MYCOPLASMA. **S. pneumo′niae**, *Mycoplasma pneumoniae;* see under MYCOPLASMA. **S. saliva′rium**, *Mycoplasma salivarium;* see under MYCOPLASMA.

Schlepper (shlep′er) [Ger. "tugboat"] a substance which acts as a carrier for a nonimmunogenic or poorly immunogenic substance and induces a good immune response to the substance by forming a complex with it.

Schlesinger, B. see elfin facies SYNDROME (Fanconi-Schlesinger syndrome).

Schmidt's syndrome [Adolf *Schmidt*, German physician, 1865–1918] see under SYNDROME.

Schmiedel's ganglion, carotid ganglion, inferior; see under GANGLION.

Schmincke's tumor [Alexander *Schmincke*, German pathologist, 1877–1953] nasopharyngeal LYMPHOEPITHELIOMA.

Schmitz bacillus [Karl Eitel Friedrich *Schmitz*, German physician, born 1889] *Shigella dysenteriae* (type 2); see under SHIGELLA.

schmutz pyorrhea marginal PERIODONTITIS.

Schneider, Conrad Victor [1614–1680] a German physician. See SCHNEIDERIAN.

schneiderian (schni-de′re-an) named after Conrad Victor *Schneider,* as schneiderian membrane (see mucous membrane, nasal, under MEMBRANE).

Scholz's syndrome [Willibald Oscar *Scholz*, German neurologist, born 1889] metachromatic LEUKODYSTROPHY.

Schönbein's operation see under OPERATION.

Schönlein's disease [Johann Lukas *Schönlein,* German physician, 1793–1864] Schönlein-Henoch SYNDROME.

Schönlein-Henoch syndrome, (purpura) [J. L. *Schönlein;* Edouard Heinrich *Henoch*, German physician, 1820–1910] see under SYNDROME.

school (skool) 1. any place or institution of learning. 2. a faculty or department of a university devoted to a particular field of study. 3. the body of pupils or followers of a master, system, method, and the like.

Schottky defect see under DEFECT.

Schour-Massler index PMA INDEX.

Schradan trademark for *octamethyl pyrophosphoramide* (see under OCTAMETHYL).

Schreger, lines of (bands, striae, zones) [Bernhard Gottlieb *Schreger*, German anatomist, 1766–1825] see under LINE.

Schroeder van der Kolk's law see under LAW.

Schroetter see SCHRÖTTER.

Schrötter's chorea [Leopold *Schrötter* von Kristelli, Austrian laryngologist, 1837–1908] laryngeal CHOREA.

Schubiger attachment (screw unit), system see under ATTACHMENT and SYSTEM.

Schüller, Artur [Vienna neurologist, born 1874] see Hand-Schüller-Christian DISEASE.

Schultes, Johann [17th century] an Ulm physician, whose book, *Armamentorium Chirurgicum,* gives a description of nine kinds of early instruments used in dental and oral surgery.

Schultz's angina [Werner *Schultz*, German hematologist, 1878–1947] agranulocytosis.

Schultze's cell [Max Johann Sigismund *Schultze*, German biologist, 1825–1874] olfactory CELL.

Schulz, Hugo [German pharmacologist, 1853–1932] see Arndt-Schulz LAW.

Schwalbe's corpuscle [Gustav Albert *Schwalbe*, German anatomist, 1844–1917] taste BUD.

Schwalbe's line, plane see under LINE and PLANE.

Schwann's membrane, sheath of [Theodor *Schwann*, German anatomist and physiologist, 1810–1882] neurilemma.

schwannoma (shwon-no′mah) neurilemmoma. **malignant s.**, a rare malignant neoplasm of the neurilemma, occurring usually as a result of malignant degeneration of neurofibromatosis or as a primary tumor; it is believed that malignant degeneration of the neurilemmoma does not occur. The mandible is the primary site of oral tumors. Pain and paresthesia are the principal symptoms. Histologically, the lesion is similar to fibrosarcoma, and is characterized chiefly by spindle cells and mitotic activity; the cells are arranged in interlacing tightly packed bundles. Called also *malignant neurilemmoma, neurogenic sarcoma,* and *neurofibrosarcoma.*

Schwarz activator, appliance, classification [A. Martin *Schwarz,* Austrian orthodontist] see bow ACTIVATOR, and see under APPLIANCE and CLASSIFICATION.

science (si′ens) [L. *scientia* knowledge] 1. the branch of knowledge or study dealing with a body of facts or truths obtained by the systematic observation of natural phenomena for the purpose of discovering laws governing these phenomena. 2. the body of knowledge accumulated by such means. **applied s.,** that concerned with the application of discovered laws to the matters of everyday living. **behavioral s.,** the group of studies which describes man's reactions to stimuli and to circumstances. Prominent among these sciences are psychology, sociology, and anthropology, but included also are political science and other social sciences. **material s.,** the field of science concerned with the internal structure of materials and with the dependence of properties upon these internal structures, including the principles of physical chemistry, solid state physics, metallurgy, and the like. **pure s.,** that concerned solely with the discovery of unknown laws relating to particular facts.

scientist (si′en-tist) one learned in science, especially one active in some particular field of investigation.

scillaren (sil′ah-ren) a mixture of cardioactive glycosides, scillarens A and B, from fresh squill. Scillaren B is used to induce necrotizing ulcerative gingivitis in experimental animals.

scintillation (sin″tĭ-la′shun) [L. *scintillatio*] 1. an emission of sparks. 2. a subjective visual sensation, as of seeing sparks. See also scintillating SCOTOMA. 3. a flash of light produced in a phosphor by an ionizing event. See also FLUORESCENCE and LUMINESCENCE. **s. scanner,** scintiscanner.

scintiscan (sin′tĭ-skan) a two-dimensional representation (map) of the gamma rays emitted by a radioisotope, revealing its varying concentration in a specific tissue of the body.

scintiscanner (sin″tĭ-skan′er) a system of equipment used in the making of a scintiscan. Called also *scintillation scanner.*

scirro- [Gr. *skirrhos* hard] a combining form meaning hard, or denoting relationship to a hard cancer.

scirrhous (skir′us) [L. *scirrhosus*] pertaining to or of the nature of a hard cancer.

scissel (siz′el) a small piece of metal cut from a plate which is being made into the base of a denture.

scissors (siz′ers) a cutting instrument with two opposed shearing blades, used in oral surgery for removing tabs of tissue during gingivectomy, trimming the margins of flaps, enlarging incisions in periodontal abscesses, and removing muscle attachments. Surgical scissors are available in a variety of types and blade shapes and sizes. **angled s.,** one with angled blades. See illustration. **canalicular s.,** delicate scissors with one of the blades probe pointed; used in slitting the lacrimal canal. **curved s.,** one with curved blades. See illustration. **Fox s.,** delicate, fine-pointed scissors designed to gain access to interproximal areas for the removal of small tissue tabs or slight soft tissue deformities during gingivoplasty or gingivectomy. **gold and crown s.,** sturdy, straight or curved, scissors used to contour preformed crowns or to cut gold foil or matrices. **Lagrange's s.,** a curved type of surgical scissors. See illustration. **Liston's s.,** one for cutting plaster of Paris bandages. **Mayo. s.,** sturdy, either straight or curved, scissors with wide blades and round ends. **Quinby s.,** sturdy, either straight or curved, scissors with wide blades and pointed ends. **straight s.,** one with straight blades. See illustration. **surgical s.,** one used in surgery for cutting tissue. Called also *tissue s.* **suture s.,** one for cutting sutures. **tissue s.,** surgical s.

scissors-bite (siz″erz-bīt′) scissors BITE.

sclera (skle′rah) [L.; Gr. *skleros* hard] the tough white supporting tunic of the eyeball, covering its posterior surface. **blue s.,** a hereditary condition characterized by an unusual blue color of the sclera, due to thinning or to increased transparency, nearly always associated with osteogenesis imperfecta. See also Lobstein's SYNDROME.

scleredema (skle″re-de′mah) a benign chronic disease of unknown cause, characterized by the sudden appearance of diffuse symmetric induration of the skin, which may occur at any age and undergo spontaneous remission within 6 months to 2 years but may occasionally last for decades. The skin shows a hard, nonpitting induration and a loss of the normal skin markings, giving it a shiny or waxy appearance. Only the upper extremities are usually involved, but lesions may spread to other parts, especially the abdominal wall, buttocks, and thighs, and, less frequently, the lower extremities, but not the feet. The tongue and pharynx may be also involved, leading to dysphagia. **s. neonato′rum,** sclerema.

sclerema (skle-re′mah) hardening of the subcutaneous fat in weak premature infants and in term infants with severe systemic, especially diarrheal, diseases. It is characterized by a rapidly spreading waxy, cool, leathery skin with purplish mottling; the skin feels adherent to underlying structures. Called also *sclerema neonatorum* and, erroneously, *scleredema neonatorum.* **s. adulto′rum,** scleroderma. **s. neonato′rum,** sclerema.

sclero- [Gr. *sklēros* hard] 1. a combining form meaning hard. 2. pertaining to the sclera.

scleroderma (skle″ro-der′mah) [*sclero-* + Gr. *derma* skin] a progressive systemic sclerosis involving the collagenous tissue of the skin and other organs. It is characterized by usually sym-

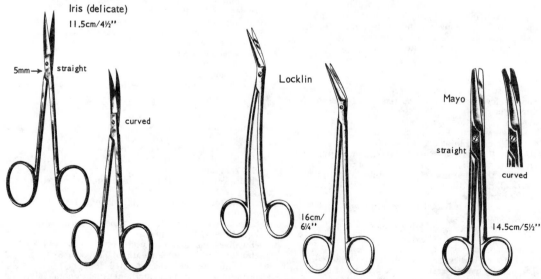

Assorted surgical scissors. (From H. O. Torres and A. Ehrlich: Modern Dental Assisting. 2nd ed. Philadelphia, W. B. Saunders Co., 1980; courtesy of Hu-Friedy Mfg. Co., Inc.)

metrical, leathery induration of the skin, associated with atrophy and pigmentation, followed by fibrotic changes in the muscles, heart, gastrointestinal system, lungs, and, less commonly, other structures of the body. The skin assumes a doughy, edematous appearance, later becoming smooth, shiny and densely bound, and flexion contractures may be present with the affected areas becoming pigmented and ulcerated. The tongue, soft palate, and larynx are the oral structures usually involved, associated with hardening of the tongue, dysphagia, inability to open and close the mouth, speaking and respiratory difficulties, and choking sensation. Rigidity and thinness of the lips is a common symptom. Roentgenographic examination may show widening of the periodontal ligament. Called also *dermatosclerosis, sclerema adultorum,* and *progressive systemic sclerosis*. **circumscribed s., localized s.,** morphea.

scleromyxedema (skle″ro-mik″se-da′mah) [*sclero- + myxedema*] Arndt-Gottron DISEASE.

scleroprotein (skle″ro-pro′te-in [*sclero- + protein*] a simple protein characterized by insolubility in most ordinary solvents and a fibrous structure. Scleroproteins are localized chiefly in connective tissue, bone, hair, skin, and wool. The two major classes of scleroproteins are keratins and collagen. Called also *albuminoid*.

sclerosant (skle-ro′sant) sclerosing AGENT.

scleroscope (skle″ro-skōp) [*sclero- + Gr. skopein to view or examine*] an instrument for determining the hardness of materials according to rebounding of a steel ball dropped from different heights. See also HARDNESS.

sclerosing (skle-rōs′ing) causing or undergoing sclerosis.

sclerosis (skle-ro′sis) [Gr. *sklērōsis* hardness] an induration or hardening of a tissue or an organ. **amyotrophic lateral s.,** degeneration of the anterior horn cells of the spinal cord, Betz cells of the motor cortex, motor nuclei of the medulla oblongata, and fibers of the lateral and ventral portions of the spinal cord, associated with progressive wasting and fibrillation of the muscles of the upper extremities and with weakness and spasticity of the lower extremities. The trigeminal and hypoglossal nerves may also be affected. Indistinct speech and hoarseness, atrophy and fasciculation of the face and tongue, and palatal movement and vocal cord disorders may occur. It occurs most frequently in middle and old age. Syphilis, poisoning, trauma, and genetic factors are suspected as causes. When there is massive involvement of the lower motor neurons with generalized muscular atrophy, it is referred to as *progressive muscular atrophy*. The term *pseudobulbar palsy* applies to spasticity from involvement of the bulbar muscles. Called also *Charcot's s.* and *Charcot's syndrome.* **Charcot's s.,** amyotrophic lateral s. **dentinal s.,** transparent DENTIN. **diaphyseal s.,** progressive diaphyseal DYSPLASIA. **disseminated s.,** multiple s. **familial progressive cerebral s.,** metachromatic LEUKODYSTROPHY. **idiopathic cortical s.,** Garré's OSTEOMYELITIS. **multiple s.,** an acute disorder, usually affecting females between the ages of 20 and 40, characterized by demyelination of the nerves, associated with damage to the brain and spinal cord. Symptoms, which vary in relation to the site of the lesion, include visual disorders, such as blurring of vision, scotoma, double vision, nystagmus, and optic neuritis; vertigo; intention tremor; spastic paraparesis; apoplectiform attacks; bladder and rectal disorders; mental deterioration associated with cheerfulness; fatigability; weakness; stiffness of joints; and facial symptoms, such as facial palsy, facial and jaw weakness, and trigeminal neuralgia. Charcot's triad (nystagmus, scanning speech, and intention tremor) is usually present in advanced stages. Pathologically, it is marked by diffuse or patchy demyelination, usually of the white matter, but sometimes also of the gray matter; axis cylinders may be affected; and glial proliferation with progressive and regressive changes is usually present. The etiology is unknown, but infection and immune mechanisms are suspected. Called also *disseminated sclerosis.* **posterior spinal s.,** TABES dorsalis. **progressive systemic s.,** scleroderma.

sclerotome (skle′ro-tōm) [*sclero- + Gr. tomē a cut*] 1. an instrument used in surgery of the sclera. 2. the area of a bone innervated from a single spinal segment. 3. one of the paired masses of mesenchymal tissue, separated from the ventromedial part of a somite, which develop into the vertebrae and ribs.

scolio- [Gr. *skolios* twisted] a combining form meaning twisted or crooked.

scoliosis (sko″le-o′sis) [Gr. *skoliōsis* curvation] abnormal lateral curvature of the spine. Cf. KYPHOSIS and LORDOSIS.

-scope [Gr. *skopein* to view, examine] a word termination meaning an instrument for examining or observing.

scopolamine (sko-pol′ah-mēn) an antimuscarinic alkaloid from solanaceous plants, especially *Datura metel* and *Scopolia carniolica*, α-(hydroxymethyl)benzeneacetic acid 9-methyl-3-oxa-9-azatricyclo[3,3,1]-non-7-yl ester. It occurs as white crystals or

granular powder that is odorless and slightly efflorescent in dry air and is soluble in water, alcohol, and chloroform. Generally used in the form of the hydrobromide salt as a sedative and tranquilizing depressant. It depresses smooth muscles and secretory glands innervated by parasympathetic nerves, being stronger than atropine in its effects on the ciliary body and salivary, bronchial, and sweat glands, but weaker in its action on the heart, intestinal tract, and bronchi. Used for its sedative effect in preanesthetic medication, and in the treatment of mental disorders and tremor. Side effects and toxicity are similar to those of atropine, including drying of the mouth and mucous membranes, increased intraocular tension, restlessness, tremor, fatigue, motor disorders, skin rash, flushing, vomiting, disorientation, hallucinations, delirium, leukocytosis, shock, and death. Drowsiness and edema of the uvula, glottis, and lips may also occur. Called also *hyoscine.* **s. methylbromide,** METHSCOPOLAMINE bromide. **s. methylnitrate,** METHSCOPOLAMINE nitrate.

Scopolia (sko-po′le-ah) a genus of solanaceous plants, being a source of various alkaloids with antimuscarinic properties, including scopolamine. *S. carniolica* is found in Europe and *S. japonica* and *S. lurida* in Asia.

-scopy [Gr. *skopein* to examine] a word termination meaning the act of examining.

scorbutic (skor-bu′tik) [L. *scorbuticus*] pertaining to or affected with scurvy.

scorbutigenic (skor-bu″tĭ-jen′ik) causing scurvy.

scorbutus (skor-bu′tus) [L.] scurvy.

score (skōr) a rating, usually expressed numerically, based on achievements or the degree to which certain qualities are present. **oral hygiene s.,** oral hygiene INDEX. **periodontal s.,** periodontal INDEX. **periodontal disease s.,** periodontal disease INDEX.

scorings (skor′ingz) small transverse lines caused by increased density of bone, seen in roentgenograms at the metaphysis of growing bones, and due to temporary cessation of growth.

scoto- [Gr. *skotos* darkness] combining form denoting relationship to darkness.

scotoma (sko-to′mah), pl. *scoto′mata* [Gr. *skotōma*] a blind spot or spots in the field of vision, which may be stationary or mobile, sometimes giving the impression that one sees flying insects in front of his eyes. **scintillating s.,** the sensation of a luminous appearance before the eyes, with a zigzag, wall-like outline. Called also *teichopsia.*

scotomata (sko-to′mah-tah) [Gr.] plural of *scotoma.*

Scott, C. I., Jr. see Aarskog-Scott SYNDROME (*Aarskog's syndrome*).

Scott, Henry Harold [British physician] see Strachan-Scott SYNDROME.

Scott attachment [W. R. *Scott*, American dentist] see under ATTACHMENT.

scr scruple (2).

scrap (skrap) chips, fillings, and other remnants left over in producing a dental restoration.

screen (skrēn) 1. a partition, or any movable or fixed device, such as a covered frame, offering shelter or protection. 2. an agent that affords defense against a deleterious influence, such as a substance applied to the skin to protect against the effects of sun rays. See also SCREENING. **fluorescent s.,** 1. the chief component of a fluoroscope, consisting of a sheet of material, such as calcium tungstate or zinc sulfide, which fluoresces upon being irradiated with ionizing radiation. See also FLUOROSCOPE. 2. a sheet coated with a material, such as anthracene, which fluoresces upon being irradiated with ultraviolet rays; used in ultraviolet examination. **s. intensification,** see *intensifying s.* **intensifying s.,** a screen used to intensify the latent image on the x-ray film. It is a thin sheet of celluloid or other radiolucent material, coated on one side with a thin layer of a suspension of dehydrated x-ray excitable phosphors, which is mounted in the cassette, its coated surface being in close contact with the film. The action of x-rays on phosphors causes them to glow with a blue-white light, thus intensifying the generation of the latent image on the film through the added action of light and reducing the exposure time 10 to 40 times. See also screen LAG. **oral s.,** vestibular s. **sun s.,** sunscreen. **vestibular s.,** a removable orthodontic appliance made of acrylic resin, which covers the labial or buccal surface of one or both dental arches, fitting between the oral mucosa and the teeth; used in treating oral habits and to stimulate tooth movement. Called also *oral s.* and *oral shield.*

screening (skrēn′ing) 1. protection from outside influences. 2. selection, sorting out, or evaluation of something according to certain established standards or criteria. See also REVIEW. 3. in dentistry, any examination of individuals, or their records, to ascertain dental needs, assess treatment plans, or evaluate services rendered. See also quality CONTROL, POSTSCREENING, and PRESCREENING. 4. in insurance, a sample survey to determine initial treatment needs of a group seeking coverage under a health insurance plan; used in setting the initial premium. 5. the presumptive identification of an unrecognized disease or defect by the application of tests, examinations, or other procedures which can be applied rapidly. Screening tests sort out apparently well persons who probably have a disease from those who probably do not. **genetic s.**, the presumptive identification of unrecognized diseases or defects, or of healthy heterozygous carriers of mutant genes which may produce children with diseases under appropriate circumstances, but which do not produce significant clinical disease in the heterozygous individual. **mass s.**, the large-scale screening of whole population groups. **medical care s.**, a process of evaluating the delivery of medical care, in which norms, criteria, and standards are used to analyze cases in order to identify those requiring in-depth study. **multiphasic genetic s.**, testing a single sample obtained from a newborn infant for several genetically transmitted diseases. **multiphasic health s., multiple s.**, the simultaneous use of multiple laboratory procedures for the detection of various diseases. Abbreviated *MHS*. **multistep s.**, screening in which the same individual is screened for the same disease by two or more persons at different professional levels. **PKU s.**, testing for phenylketonuria, based on the determination of elevated blood phenylalanine (more than 2–4 mg/100 ml). A disk with several drops of dried blood taken from a newborn infant is placed on a plate containing agar, bacteria, and a specific bacterial inhibitor. Bacterial growth indicates that the concentration of phenylalanine is in excess of 2 mg/100 ml and is considered as a positive test for phenylketonuria. Called also *PKU test.* **selective s.**, the screening of selected high-risk groups of the population.

screw (skroo) a fastener, usually made of metal, having a tapered shank with a helical thread, and topped with a slotted head. See screw RETAINER. **adjustable s.**, a screw that may be accurately adjusted, such as orthodontic screws and jackscrews. **expansion s.**, see *orthodontic s.* **jack s.**, jackscrew. **implant s.**, a small screw used to secure primary retention of a subperiosteal or intraperiosteal implant. **orthodontic s.**, a screw that when turned will drive the parts of an orthodontic appliance apart, such as one used in the expansion plate (see under PLATE). See illustration. See also JACKSCREW. **s. post**, screw-post. **pull s.**, an orthodontic screw whose turning moves a tooth in a desired direction by pulling. **self-taping s.**, one designed to tap its

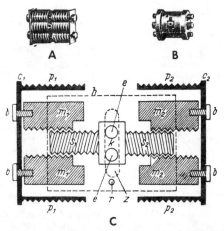

C

Orthodontic screws. *A*, Normal type A (in natural size). *B*, Smaller type B. *C*, Cross-section through type A. The screw is opened to half its maximal expansion. S_1S_2, the screw; k, head of the screw with holes for the key, e; m_1m_2, the nuts (guiding female parts of the screw); h (interrupted line), case with slot, z, and mark r, which indicates the direction in which the screw is to be turned; p_1p_2, casing attached with the tiny screws, b. (From T. M. Graber and B. Neumann: Removable Orthodontic Appliances. Philadelphia, W. B. Saunders Co., 1977.)

corresponding female thread as it is driven, or to cut its own pathway into the bone.

screw-post (skroo′pōst) a threaded post to which a denture is attached with a nut, as in Schubiger's attachment. Also written *screw post.*

scribe (skrīb) to write, score, or mark on metal or any other hard material with a pointed instrument or carbon marker.

Scribonius Largus [1st century A.D.] a Roman physician (probably a freed slave), who wrote *De compositiones medicamentorum*, which contains references to calming the aching tooth with mouthwashes, masticatories, and fumigations, or by direct application of medicines. *Hyoscyamus* seeds scattered over burning charcoal were used as a fumigant (fumigation was expected to cause small worms, which were believed to cause toothache, to be expelled from the mouth). After fumigation, the patient would rinse his mouth with hot water.

scrobiculate (skro-bik′u-lāt) [L. *scrobiculatus*] marked by pits or cavities.

scrobiculus (skro-bik′u-lus) [L. "little trench," "pit"] a small hollow, pit or cavity.

scrofula (skrof′u-lah) [L. "brood sow"] tuberculous infection of the cervical and, sometimes, submandibular lymph nodes, characterized by swelling, abscesses, and draining sinuses discharging necrotic material. The lesion may heal and calcify. The overlying skin is bluish red but the area around the lesion is cool, hence the term *cold abscess*. Draining from the oropharynx may be observed in some cases. Called also *tuberculous cervical lymphadenitis*. See also oral TUBERCULOSIS.

scruple (skroo′p'l) [L. *scrupulus*, dim. of *scrupus* a sharp stone, a worry or anxiety] 1. certain moral or ethical principles that act as a restraining force inhibiting certain immoral or dishonest actions. 2. a unit of mass (weight) of the apothecaries' system, being 20 grains, or the equivalent of 1.296 grams. Symbol ℈ : Abbreviated *scr.* See also *Tables of Weights and Measures* at WEIGHT.

SCS Saethre-Chotzen SYNDROME.

scurvy (skur′ve) [L. *scorbutus*] a nutritional deficiency disease caused by the lack of vitamin C, which was once common, but is now rare. It is characterized by anemia, swollen joints and feet, mucosal hemorrhage, hemorrhage around the hair follicles, ecchymoses, epistaxis, loss of weight, weakness, arthralgia, fractures, beaded ribs, replacement of the bone marrow with connective tissue, and general failure of the body to maintain collagen and supporting structures. Oral manifestations include stomatitis, red swollen gums, gingival ulcers and gangrene, destruction of the periodontal tissue, loose teeth, hemorrhage from the dental pulp, arrest of dentin formation, hypoplasia of the dental enamel, destruction of the periosteum, and exaggerated sensitivity of the oral mucosa to irritants. Called also *scorbutus*. **hemorrhagic s.**, infantile s. **infantile s.**, scurvy sometimes observed in artificially fed infants, caused by vitamin C deficiency and characterized by gingival lesions, hemorrhage, arthralgia, and other symptoms similar to those in adult scurvy. Called also *hemorrhagic s., Barlow's disease, Cheadle's disease, Cheadle-Möller-Barlow disease, infantile hemorrhagic diathesis, Möller's disease*, and *Möller-Barlow disease*.

scute (skūt) [L. *skutum* shield] 1. any squama or scalelike structure. 2. tympanic s. **tympanic s.**, the bony plate which divides the upper part of the tympanic cavity from the mastoid cells.

scutiform (sku′tĭ-form) [L. *scutum* shield + *forma* form] having a shape like a shield.

scyphoid (si′foid) [Gr. *skyphos* cup + *eidos* form] shaped like a cup.

S.D. 1. skin DOSE. 2. standard DEVIATION.

SE sphenoethmoidal SUTURE (2).

Se selenium.

seal (sēl) 1. an emblem, figure, or symbol of authenticity. 2. something that secures or closes tightly. 3. in dentistry, a material, usually a plastic, which hardens in the mouth; used to close the coronal opening in a tooth during endodontic treatment. **S. of Acceptance**, a seal awarded by the Council on Dental Materials and Devices of the American Dental Association (see Appendix) to dental materials and devices evaluated under the provisions of the acceptance program of the Council, based on evidence of safety and usefulness established by biological, laboratory, and/or clinical evaluations. The Seal of Acceptance may be used in advertising, in brochures, and on packages. **border s.**, the contact of the denture border with the underlying or adjacent tissues to prevent the passage of air or other substances. **cavity s.**, 1. the closing of holes in dentin against the toxic agents of restorative materials. 2. the mechanical bonding of enamel and restorative material at the cavosurface margin. 3. the priming or wetting of a cavity surface to improve adaptation of a restorative material. See also cavity lining AGENT. **S. of Certification,** see CERTIFICATION (3). **double s.,** a seal consisting of gutta-percha underneath another material (e.g., temporary cement); used to close the coronal opening during endodontic treatment. **hermetic s.,** the perfect and absolute (air-tight) obstruction of the root canal. **palatal s.,** posterior palatal s. **posterior palatal s., postpalatal s.,** a seal at the posterior border of a denture produced by displacing the soft tissue covering the palate by extra pressure developed in the impression or by scraping a depression in the cast. Called also *palatal s.* See also posterior palatal seal AREA. **Sevriton Cavity S. Primer,** see under PRIMER. **velopharyngeal s.,** closure between the oral and nasopharyngeal cavities, accomplished by the action of the muscles of the soft palate and the superior constrictor muscle.

sealant (se'lant) an agent that protects against access from the outside or leakage from the inside; sealer. **dental s.,** a sealant resin capable of bonding the surface of a tooth and offering protection against outside chemical or physical agents. Called also *dental adhesive.* **fissure s.,** pit and fissure s. **pit and fissure s.,** a dental sealant used to occlude noncarious pits and fissures, thereby preventing caries-producing microorganisms and debris from entering. Several types of resin, filled and unfilled, have been used, including cyanoacrylates, polyurethanes, and the bisphenol-A-glycidal methacrylate. The commercially available sealants are usually based on BIS-GMA resin, being polymerized by means of the amine-peroxide system. Benzoin methyl ester is sometimes used as the initiator with the use of ultraviolet light activation. Sealants are usually applied after treating the enamel with phosphoric or citric acid (acid etching) to create micropores which permit the resin to penetrate the surface of the enamel bonds and form mechanical bonds. The application is performed in a dry field. Called also *fissure s.*

sealer (se'ler) an agent that protects against access from the outside or leakage from the inside; sealant. **endodontic s.,** root canal s. **Kerr S.,** trademark for a *root canal sealer,* prepared by mixing a powder consisting of zinc oxide, precipitated molecular silver, oleoresins, and dithynol iodide and a liquid consisting of oil of cloves and Canada balsam. **ProcoSol s.,** trademark for a *root canal sealer,* prepared by mixing a powder consisting of zinc oxide, precipitated molecular silver, hydrogenated resin, and magnesium oxide with a liquid consisting of eugenol and Canada balsam. **root canal s.,** a substance used for cementing silver and gutta-percha cones to the tooth structure in root canal therapy. Zinc oxide–eugenol cements, chloropercha, and Diaket are the principal types of sealers. Some sealers, such as paraformaldehyde and iodoform preparations, are used for antiseptic and therapeutic purposes, sometimes without cones. Called also *endodontic s., endodontic cement,* and *root canal cement.* Available under various trademarks.

sealing (sēl'ing) closing or securing something tightly or completely.

seam (sēm) a line of union of separate parts of an organ or structure. See also RAPHE.

seat (sēt) 1. something on which one may sit, the part of a chair on which one sits. 2. a part on which the base of something rests. **basal s.,** oral tissues which support a complete or partial denture. See also basal seat OUTLINE and basal SURFACE. **rest s.,** rest AREA.

seater (sēt'er) a device designed to place something firmly in place. **band s.,** an orthodontic instrument designed to assist in placing orthodontic bands on the teeth. See illustration.

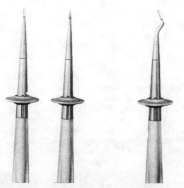

Band seater. (From H. O. Torres and A. Ehrlich: Modern Dental Assisting. 2nd ed. Philadelphia, W. B. Saunders Co., 1980.)

sebaceous (se-ba'shus) [L. *sebaceus*] pertaining to sebum or a sebaceous gland.

seborrhea (seb"o-re'ah) [L. *sebum* suet + Gr. *rhoia* flow] 1. excessive secretion of sebum. 2. seborrheic DERMATITIS.

seborrheic (seb"o-re'ik) pertaining to or affected by seborrhea.

sebum (se'bum) [L.] 1. suet. 2. the secretion of the sebaceous glands; a thick, semifluid substance composed of free fatty acids, esterified fatty acids, and unsaponifiable material, including cholesterol, squalene, alcohols, and higher hydrocarbons. Its function includes furnishing a thin lipoidal film over the stratum corneum of the skin and hair to retard evaporation.

Seckel dwarf, syndrome [Helmut Paul George *Seckel,* born 1900] see under DWARF and SYNDROME.

secobarbital (se"ko-bar'bĭ-tal) a short-acting sedative and hypnotic barbiturate, 5-allyl-5-(1-methylbutyl)barbituric acid, occurring as a white, amorphous or crystalline, odorless, slightly bitter powder that is slightly soluble in water, and readily soluble in alcohol, ether, and alkali hydroxides. It is used in psychoneurotic conditions, cardiac disorders, and preoperative and postoperative medication, including the allaying of apprehension in dental patients. Its side effects are the same as those of other barbiturates. Secobarbital will also produce porphyria in susceptible individuals. It is an addictive drug subject to regulation of the Controlled Substances Act. Called also *quinalbarbitone.* Trademark: Seconal. **s. sodium,** the monosodium salt of secobarbital, occurring as a white, odorless, bitter, hygroscopic powder that is very soluble in water, soluble in alcohol, and insoluble in ether. On exposure to air and moisture, it deteriorates rapidly. Used for short-duration sedation in neuropsychiatry and in allaying apprehension in dental patients. Its indications, contraindications, and adverse effects being similar to those of the parent compound and other barbiturates. Like the parent compound, it is an addictive drug subject to regulation of the Controlled Substances Act. Called also *soluble s.* and *quinalbarbitone sodium.* **soluble s.,** s. sodium.

secodont (se'ko-dont) [L. *secare* to cut + Gr. *odous* tooth] having teeth with sharp molar cusps, as in many carnivores.

Seconal trademark for preparations of *secobarbital.*

second party (sek'und par'te) carrier (5).

secondary (sek'un-der"e) [L. *secundarius, secundus* second] second or inferior in order of time, place, or importance.

secreta (se-kre'tah) [L. pl.] secretion products.

secretin (se-kre'tin) a strongly basic polypeptide hormone secreted by the mucosa of the duodenum and jejunum when acid chyme enters the intestine. Carried by the blood, it stimulates the secretion of pancreatic juice high in salt content but low in enzymes.

secretion (se-kre'shun) [L. *secretio,* from *secernere* to secrete] 1. the process of elaborating a specific product as a result of the activity of an exocrine or endocrine gland for use within the body or on its surface. Cf. EXCRETION. (1). 2. any substance produced by secretion. **antilytic s.,** saliva secreted by the submaxillary gland with nerves intact, as distinguished from that secreted when the nerves are divided. **external s.,** one that is discharged upon the external or an internal surface of the body. See also exocrine GLAND. **internal s.,** one that is not discharged from the gland by a duct, but is given off into the blood and lymph. See also endocrine GLAND.

Secrosteron trademark for *dimethisterone.*

sectio (sek'she-o) pl. sectio'nes [L., from *secare* to cut] 1. an act of cutting. 2. a section; an anatomical term for a segment or subdivision of an organ.

section (sek'shun) [L. *sectio*] 1. the act of cutting. 2. a cut surface. 3. a segment or subdivision of an organ; called also *sectio.* **celloidin s.,** a section cut by a microtome from tissue that has been embedded in celloidin. **end s.,** the distal portion of a twin-wire labial arch wire, consisting of a tube in which the anterior section of the labial arch is engaged.

sectiones (sek"she-o'nēz) [L.] plural of *sectio.*

secundigravida (sek-kun"dĭ-grav'ĭ-dah) [L. *secundus* second + *gravida* pregnant] a woman who is pregnant for the second time; also written *gravida II.*

secundina (se"kun-di'nah), pl. secundi'nae [L. from *secundus* second, following] that which follows.

secundinae (se"kun-di'ne) [L.] plural of *secundina.*

secundipara (se"kun-dip'ah-rah) [L. *secundus* second + *parere* to bring forth, to bear] a woman who has had two pregnancies which resulted in viable offspring; also written *para 2, para II,* and *2-para.*

Sedaform trademark for *chlorobutanol.*

Sedaquin trademark for *methaqualone hydrochloride* (see METH-AQUALONE).

Sedatine trademark for *antipyrine*.

sedation (se-da'shun) [L. *sedatio*] the production of a sedative effect; the act or process of calming. **dental pretreatment s.,** dental PREMEDICATION.

sedative (sed'ah-tiv) [L. *sedativus*] 1. allaying activity and excitement; quieting accompanied by relaxation and rest, without necessarily inducing sleep. 2. any drug that depresses the activity of the central nervous system, reducing cortical excitability without producing sleep. Most sedatives act also as hypnotics and induce sleep when their dosage is sufficiently increased. Because of their common quality of counteracting anxiety, sedatives and hypnotics are often jointly called antianxiety drugs (minor tranquilizers). Sedatives are chiefly used in the management of neuroses and to allay anxiety and apprehension associated with conditions such as hypertension and heart diseases. In dentistry, they are used mainly before dental procedures to relieve nervousness and apprehension and in preanesthetic medication. **barbiturate s.,** barbiturate.

Sédillot's operation [Charles Emmanual *Sédillot*, French surgeon, 1804–1883] see under *operation*.

sediment (sed'ĭ-ment) [L. *sedimentum*] a precipitate, especially one that is formed spontaneously.

sedimentation (sed"ĭ-men-ta'shun) the act of causing the deposit of sediment, especially by the use of a centrifuge. **erythrocyte s.,** the setting of erythrocytes in drawn blood. See *erythrocyte sedimentation* RATE. **s. time,** ERYTHROCYTE sedimentation rate.

seed (sēd) 1. the mature ovule of a flowering plant. 2. semen. 3. a small cylindrical shell of gold or other inert material, used in application of radiation therapy. 4. to inoculate a culture medium with microorganisms. **radiogold s.,** a solid piece of radioactive gold (Au[198]) wire about 2.5 mm long and 0.8 mm thick, used as a permanent interstitial radioactive implant in the treatment of cancer. **radon s.,** a small capsule, about 4 × 1.5 mm in diameter, usually made of gold or glass, which contains radon gas, and is inserted about 1 cm beneath the surface of a tissue for gamma ray therapy of lesions at the base of the tongue, tonsillar pillar, pharynx, and other spaces not readily accessible to other forms of radiotherapy.

seeker (se'ker) one who tries to reach a goal or objective. **bone s.,** a radioisotope that tends to accumulate in the bones when it is introduced into the body, as strontium-90, which behaves chemically like calcium.

Seessel's pouch (pocket) [Albert *Seessel*, American embryologist and neurologist] see under POUCH.

Sefacin trademark for *cephaloridine*.

segment (seg'ment) [L. *segmentum* a piece cut off] a portion of a larger body or structure. **cranial s's,** three segments in which the bones of the cranium may be divided, distinguished as the occipital, parietal, and frontal. **frontal s.,** the anterior of the three cranial segments. **mesoblastic s., mesodermal s.,** somite. **occipital s.,** the posterior of the three cranial segments. **parietal s.,** the central of the three cranial segments.

segmenta (seg-men'tah) [L.] plural of *segmentum*.

segmental (seg-men'tal) pertaining to or forming a segment; undergoing segmentation.

segmentation (seg"men-ta'shun) 1. division into parts more or less similar, such as somites or metameres. 2. cleavage.

segmentum (seg-men'tum), pl. *segmen'ta* [L.] a portion of a larger body or structure; a segment. A general anatomical term for a part of an organ or other structure set off by natural or arbitrarily established boundaries.

segregation (seg"rĕ-ga'shun) 1. the act or process of separating; setting apart. 2. the separation of allelic genes at meiosis as homologous chromosomes begin to migrate to the poles of the cell, so that eventually the members of each pair of allelic genes go to separate gametes. 3. the separation of different elements of a population. 4. the progressive restriction of potencies in the zygote to the various regions of the forming embryo.

seizure (se'zhur) 1. the sudden attack or recurrence of a disease. 2. an attack of epilepsy. See also ICTUS. **jacksonian s.,** Jackson's EPILEPSY.

Seldin retractor see under RETRACTOR.

selection (sĕ-lek'shun) 1. the act or process of choosing in preference to another or others. 2. the play of forces that determines the relative fitness of a genotype in the population. 3. the manner in which kindreds are chosen for study. **adverse s.,** disproportionate insurance of risks who are poorer or more prone to suffer loss or make claims than the average risk. **shade**

s., the determination of the color, hue, brilliance, saturation, and translucency of the artificial tooth or set of teeth to harmonize with the individual characteristics of a given patient. Called also *tooth color s.* **tooth s.,** the determination of the shape, size, and color of the tooth to harmonize with the individual characteristics of a given patient. **tooth color s.,** shade s.

selector (sĕ-lek'tor) one that chooses in preference to another or others. **kilovoltage s.,** an electrical device (see AUTOTRANS-FORMER) which controls the kilovoltage, such as one in an x-ray generator. **milliamperage s., technique s.,** a step-down transformer which controls the milliamperage in the filament circuit of an x-ray tube.

selenic (sĕ-len'ik, sĕ-lēn'ik) a compound of tetravalent or hexavalent selenium.

selenide (sel'ĕ-nīd) a compound containing divalent selenium, =Se.

selenious (sĕ-le'ne-us) a compound containing divalent or tetravalent selenium; selenous.

selenite (sel'ĕ-nīt) a variety of gypsum, found in transparent crystals and foliated masses; the native hydrated form of calcium sulfate; gypsum.

selenium (sĕ-le'ne-um) [Gr. *selēnē* moon] a poisonous nonmetallic element resembling sulfur. Symbol, Se; atomic number, 34; atomic weight, 78.96; specific gravity, 4.79; valences, –2, 4, 6; group VIA of the periodic table. Its naturally occurring isotopes include 74, 76–78, 80, and 82; artificial radioactive isotopes include 70–73, 75, 79, 81, 83–85, and 87. Selenium occurs in an amorphous, crystalline (or red) and a gray (or metallic) form. It is soluble in concentrated nitric acid and in common alkalies and forms binary alloys with silver, copper, zinc, lead, and other elements. In a solid form, it is relatively nontoxic, but its vapors and fumes are highly toxic; exposure may cause pallor, nervousness, depression, garlic-like odor of the breath, and excessive sweating. Increased dental caries incidence is said to occur in areas where the food and water contain high selenium concentrations. Insoluble selenium compounds, such as selenium sulfite or selenium sulfide, are used in the treatment of seborrheic dermatitis, dandruff, and other skin diseases. **s. dilsulfide,** s. sulfide. **s. sulfide,** an antimicrobial agent with mild antifungal properties, SeS$_2$, prepared from H$_2$S and selenious acid. Used in the treatment of seborrhea and pityriasis versicolor. Exposure of mucous membranes, including those of the oral cavity, to selenium sulfide may cause inflammation. Alopecia may also occur. Called also *selenium disulfide.* Trademark: Selsun.

selenodont (se-le'no-dont) [Gr. *selēnē* moon + *odous* tooth] having posterior teeth on which the individual cusps assume a crescenting outline, as in many herbivores.

selenous (sĕ-le'nus) selenious.

self (self) an expression used to denote an animal's own antigenic constituents, in contrast to "not self," denoting foreign antigenic constituents. The "self" constituents are metabolized without antibody formation, whereas the antigens which are "not self" are eliminated through the immune response mechanism. It has been postulated that there exists some mechanism of "self recognition" which enables the organism to distinguish between "self" and "not self." Both soluble factors, such as blocking factors, and T-suppressor cells may be involved in the maintenance of self-recognition and thus the prevention of autoimmune responses.

self-diffusion (self-dĭ-fu'zhun) the changing of position by atoms in solids under equilibrium conditions. See also DIFFUSION (2).

self-insurance (self-in'shur-ans) self INSURANCE.

self-rectification (self"rek"tĭ-fi-ka'shun) rectification in an electric device, without the use of a rectifier. Self-rectification achieved by use of the x-ray tube alone produces half-wave rectification, thereby only half the current impulses are effective in producing x-rays.

sella (sel'ah), pl. *sel'lae* [L.] 1. any saddle-shaped depression. 2. s. turcica. 3. a craniometric landmark, being the mid-point of the sella turcica. Abbreviated S. Also called *point S.* **s. tur'cica** [NA], a small transverse depression in the sphenoid bone in the skull, which houses the pituitary gland.

sellae (sel'e) [L.] plural of *sella*.

sellar (sel'ar) pertaining to the sella turcica.

Selsun trademark for *selenium sulfide.* (see under SELENIUM).

Selye's syndrome [Hans *Selye*, Hungarian-born Canadian physiologist, born 1907] general adaptation SYNDROME.

semen (se'men) [L. "seed"] the thick, whitish secretion of the reproductive organ in the male; composed of spermatozoa in their nutrient plasma, secretions from the prostate, seminal vesicles, and various other glands, epithelial cells, and other constituents.

semi- [L. *semis* half] a prefix signifying one half.

semicanal (sem″e-kah-nal′) a channel or canal which opens on one side. Called also *semicanalis.* See also CANAL and CANALICULUS. **s. of auditory tube,** a small canal in the temporal bone, opening on the inferior surface of the skull just posterior and superior to the foramen spinosum. It constitutes the inferior part of the musculotubal canal and lodges the auditory tube. Called also *semicanalis tubae auditivae* [NA]. **s. of tensor tympani muscle,** a small canal hidden in the temporal bone, constituting the superior part of the musculotubal canal, and lodging the tensor tympani muscle. Called also *muscular sulcus of tympanic cavity* and *semicanalis musculi tensoris tympani* [NA].

semicanales (sem″e-kah-na′lēz) [L.] plural of *semicanalis.*

semicanalis (sem″e-kah-na′lis), pl. *semicana′les* [L.] a channel or canal which opens on one side. See also CANALICULUS, CANALIS. and SEMICANAL. **s. mus″culi tenso′ris tym′pani** [NA], SEMICANAL of tensor tympani muscle. **s. tu′bae auditi′vae** [NA], SEMICANAL of auditory tube.

semicoma (sem″e-ko′mah) [*semi-* + *coma*] a stupor from which the patient may be aroused.

Semih. abbreviation for L. *semiho′ra,* half an hour.

semilunar (sem″e-lu′nar) [L. *semilunaris,* from *semi* half + *luna* moon] half-moon; crescentlike.

semimembranous (sem″ĕ-mem′brah-nus) made up in part of membrane or fascia.

semipermeable (sem″e-per′me-ah-b′l) permitting passage of certain molecules and hindering that of others.

Semken-Taylor forceps see under FORCEPS.

Semon's law [Sir Felix *Semon,* German laryngologist in London, 1849–1921] Semon-Rosenbach LAW. See also Gerhardt-Semon LAW.

Semon-Rosenbach law [Sir F. *Semon;* Ottomar *Rosenbach,* physician in Berlin, 1851–1907] see under LAW.

Senator's angina see under ANGINA.

Sencephalin trademark for *cephalexin.*

Sendoxan trademark for *cyclophosphamide.*

Senear-Usher syndrome [Francis Eugene *Senear,* American dermatologist, 1889—1958; Barney *Usher,* Canadian dermatologist, born 1899] PEMPHIGUS erythematosus.

senescence (se-nes′ens) [L. *senescere* to grow old] the process or condition of growing old; old age; senility. **dental s.,** the gradual deterioration of the teeth and associated structures, associated with advancing age or premature aging processes.

senescent (se-nes′ent) growing old.

senile (se′nil) [L. *senilis*] pertaining to or occurring in old age.

senility (sĕ-nil′ĭ-te) [L. *senilitas*] old age; physical and mental deterioration associated with old age.

sensation (sen-sa′shun) [L. *sensatio*] an impression conveyed by an afferent nerve to the sensorium. **referred s., reflex s.,** a sensation felt at a place other than the point of application of the stimulus. Called also *transferred s.* **transferred s.,** referred s.

sense (sens) [L. *sensus,* from *sentire* to perceive, feel] a faculty by which the conditions or properties of things are perceived. Hunger, thirst, and pain are varieties of sense. **temperature s.,** the ability to recognize heat and cold; thermesthesia.

sensibility (sen″sĭ-bil′ĭ-te) [L. *sensibilitas*] the responsiveness to stimuli; capacity for sensation or feeling. **bone s.,** pallesthesia. **deep s.,** the sensibility to pressure, pain, and proprioception which exists after the skin in an area is made completely anesthetic. It arises from the muscles, tendons, and joints. **epicritic s.,** the ability of skin receptors to discriminate fine tactile and thermal stimuli. See also epicritic PAIN. **protopathic s.,** perception of pain of visual origin that is of low intensity and poorly defined. It is transmitted slowly to the brain by type C nerve fibers. **tactile s.,** sensibility to touch.

sensitinogen (sen″sĭ-tin′o-jen) 1. an antigen capable of producing sensitization, which may be expressed by antibody or immune lymphocyte production. 2. the passive adsorption or coupling of antigen to a cell or particle which renders it sensitive to the action of antibody or an immune cell. See also ALLERGEN and ANAPHYLACTOGEN.

sensitivity (sen″si-tiv′ĭ-te) the state or quality of being sensitive; often used to denote a state of abnormal responsiveness to stimulation or to a drug. **drug s.,** drug REACTION. **s. to percussion,** a condition in which a tooth is abnormally sensitive to percussion, usually indicating the presence of pulpal inflammation. **s. to tactile stimulation,** a condition in which a tooth is abnormally sensitive to touch, usually indicating an exposed root surface due to gingival recession or exposure of the sensitive granulary layer of Tomes, as in scaling. **s. to temperature changes,** a condition in which a tooth is abnormally sensitive to heat or cold, usually indicating exposed root surfaces due to gingival recession or removal of cementum and exposure of the sensitive granular layer of Tomes, as in scaling. **s. threshold,**

absolute THRESHOLD. **tooth s.,** the state of responsiveness of teeth to external stimuli, such as heat, cold, touch, or sweet or sour foods, usually due to diseases of the dental pulp. See also hypersensitive PULPALGIA and hypersensitive TOOTH.

sensitization (sen″sĭ-ti-za′shun) 1. the process or act of being sensitized. 2. the process of rendering a cell sensitive to the action of a complement by subjecting it to the action of a specific amboceptor. 2. the loss of corrosion resistance of an austenitic stainless steel by removal of chromium from the γ-solid solution. See STABILIZATION (2). **protein s.,** anaphylaxis.

Sensival trademark for *nortriptyline hydrochloride* (see under NORTRIPTYLINE).

Sensodyne see under DENTIFRICE.

sensor (sen′sor) something that senses; a device specifically designed to respond to a physical stimulus (light, heat, pressure, etc.) by generating an impulse that can be measured or otherwise interpreted, or used as a control.

sensory (sen′so-re) [L. *sensorius*] pertaining to or subserving sensation.

separation (sep′a-ra′shun) 1. the act or process of forcing apart or keeping apart or dividing. 2. the separation of adjacent teeth having tight contact, as with the separating wire prior to bending in orthodontic therapy. **tooth s.,** the technique of moving a tooth mesially or distally out of contact with its neighbor. **tooth s., gradual,** tooth s., slow. **tooth s., immediate,** separation of teeth accomplished by a mechanical separator that exerts traction or wedging force. Called also *mechanical tooth s.* **tooth s., mechanical,** tooth s., immediate. **tooth s., slow,** separation of the teeth accomplished over a long period of time, usually by the wedging action of materials, such as gutta-percha, orthodontic wire, thread, or fibers. Called also *gradual tooth s.*

separator (sep′ah-ra″tor) [L.] 1. a device for separating one thing from another. 2. a device or instrument for wedging teeth apart, especially proximal teeth having a tight contact, as for the examination of proximal surfaces, finishing a restoration, or before banding in orthodontic therapy. See also space MAINTAINER (2) and separating WIRE. **Ferrier's s.,** a device for separating teeth, consisting of a balanced, double-bowed, adjustable apparatus. **True's s.,** a single-bow separator for wedging teeth apart.

sepsis (sep′sis) [Gr. *sēpsis* decay] the presence in the blood of bacterial toxins; septicemia. **oral s.,** a disease condition in the mouth or adjacent parts, which may affect the general health through the dissemination of toxins. See also focal INFECTION.

Sept. abbreviation for L. *sep′tem,* seven.

septa (sep′tah) [L.] plural of *septum.*

septal (sep′tal) pertaining to a septum; septile.

septan (sep′tan) [L. *septum* seven] recurring every seven (sixth) day, as a fever.

septate (sep′tat) divided by a septum.

septation (sep-ta′shun) division into parts by a septum.

septectomy (sep-tek′to-me) [*septum* + Gr. *ektomē* excision] excision of a portion of a septum, particularly the nasal septum.

septic (sep′tik) [L. *septicus;* Gr. *sēptikos*] relating to or caused by sepsis.

septicemia (sep″tĭ-se′me-ah) [*septic* + Gr. *haima* blood + *-ia*] presence in the blood of bacterial toxins. Called also *blood poisoning* and *sepsis.*

septicemic (sep″tĭ-se′mik) pertaining to, or of the nature of, septicemia.

Septicillin trademark for *penicillin V calcium* (see under PENICILLIN).

septicopyemia (sep″tĭ-ko-pi-e′me-ah) septicemia associated with pyemia.

Septic-Soap see under SOAP.

septile (sep′til) of or pertaining to a septum; septal.

septonasal (sep′to-na′zal) pertaining to the nasal septum.

septoplasty (sep′to-plas′te) [*septum* + Gr. *plassein* to form or mold] plastic reconstruction of the nasal septum.

septotome (sep′to-tōm) an instrument for cutting into the nasal septum.

septotomy (sep-tot′o-me) [*septum* + Gr. *tomē* a cutting] the operation of incising the nasal septum.

Septra trademark for a mixture of *sulfamethoxazole-trimethoprim.*

septula (sep′tu-lah) [L.] plural of *septulum.*

septulum (sep′tu-lum), pl. *sep′tula* [L., dim. of *septum*] a small separating wall or partition; used in anatomical nomenclature to designate such a structure.

septum (sep'tum), pl. *sep'ta* [L.] a dividing wall or partition; a general anatomical term for such a structure. **adipose tissue s.,** a connective tissue septum that separates individual lobules, or groups of fat cells, from each other. **s. alveoli,** 1. interalveolar s. 2. interradicular s. **bony s. of nose,** the bone of the skull interposed between the openings of the nose, consisting primarily of the vomer below and the perpendicular plate of the ethmoid bone. Called also *osseous s. of nose* and *s. nasi osseum* [NA]. **s. cana'lis musculotuba'rii** [NA], s. of musculotubal canal. **s. cartilagin'eum na'si, cartilaginous nasal s.,** cartilaginous part of nasal septum; see under PART. **connective tissue s.,** any septum made of connective tissue; usually referring to a membrane which partitions an organ into territories or lobules. The chief fiber component is collagen, with few cells, such as fibroblasts, leukocytes, and pigment and mast cells, as well as vascular, lymph, and nerve elements being also present. **enamel s.,** enamel CORD. **s. of frontal sinuses,** a thin lamina of bone, in the lower part of the frontal bone, which lies more or less in the median plane and separates the frontal sinuses. Called also *septum sinuum frontalium* [NA]. **gingival s., gum s.,** the part of the gingiva interposed between adjoining teeth. **interradicular s., s. interradicula're,** one of the thin bony partitions separating the crypts of a dental alveolus occupied by the separate roots of a multirooted tooth. Called also *septum alveoli.* See also *interalveolar s.* and *s. septum intra-alveolarium.* **lingual s., s. lin'guae** [NA], the median vertical fibrous part of the tongue, extending throughout its entire length. It is somewhat thicker behind than in front, and sometimes contains a small fibrocartilage. Called also *s. of tongue* and *lyssa.* **s. membrana'ceum na'si,** membranous s. of nose. **membranous s. of nose,** the anterior inferior part of the nasal septum, beneath the cartilaginous part; it is composed of skin and subcutaneous tissues. Called also *s. membranaceum nasi, membranous part of nasal septum,* and *pars membranacea septi nasi* [NA]. **mobile s. of nose, s. mo'bile na'si,** the part of the nasal septum at the apex of the nose, formed by the skin, subcutaneous tissue, and the greater alar cartilage. Called also *pars mobilis septi nasi* [NA]. **s. of musculotubal canal,** the thin lamella of bone that divides the musculotubal canal into the semicanals for the tensor tympani muscle and the auditory tube. Called also *s. canalis musculotubarii* [NA]. **nasal s., s. na'si** [NA], the partition separating the two nasal cavities in the midplane, composed of cartilaginous, membranous, and bony parts. It is formed anteriorly by the crest of the ethmoid bone, posteriorly by the vomer and the rostrum of the sphenoid bone, and inferiorly by the crest of the maxillae and the palatine bone. The septum is frequently deflected to one side (usually to the left). Called also *column of nose, columna nasi,* and *medial wall of nasal cavity.* **nasal s., cartilaginous,** cartilaginous part of nasal septum; see under PART. **nasal s., membranous,** membranous s. of nose. **s. na'si os'seum** [NA], bony s. of nose. **orbital s., s. orbita'le** [NA], a fibrous membrane anchored to the periorbita along the entire margin of the orbit, extending to the tarsal plates of the upper and lower lids. Called also *fascia palpebralis, palpebral fascia,* and *tarsal membrane.* **osseous s. of nose,** bony s. of nose. **partitioning s.,** one that partitions an organ into compartments or lobules, as in the salivary glands or tonsils. **pharyngeal s.,** the partition which separates the mouth cavity from the pharynx in the embryo. **salivary gland septa,** septa which divide lobes of the salivary glands into separate lobules, made up of connective tissue that is less dense than that of the gland capsule, becoming gradually more diffuse with branching until it forms a delicate network of fibers binding the constituents of the lobules. **s. si'nuum fronta'lium** [NA], s. of frontal sinuses. **sphenoidal s., s. of sphenoidal sinuses, s. si'nuum sphenoida'lium** [NA], a thin lamina of bone in the body of the sphenoid bone, lying more or less in the median plane and separating the sphenoidal sinuses. **s. of tongue,** lingual s. **tonsillar septa,** connective tissue septa which branch out from the capsule of the tonsils, dividing the lymphoid mass into lobules.

seq. luce abbreviation for L. *sequen'ti lu'ce,* the following day.

sequel (se'kwel) [L. *sequela*] sequela.

sequela (se-kwe'lah), pl. *seque'lae* [L.] any abnormal condition or lesion which follows a disease or is caused by it either directly or indirectly. See also COMPLICATION.

sequelae (se-kwe'le) [L.] plural of *sequela.*

sequence (se'kwens) [L. *sequens*] a continuous or connected series of things or events following each other.

sequester (se-kwes'ter) [L.; Fr. *sequestrer* to shut up illegally] to detach or separate abnormally a small portion from the whole.

sequestra (se-kwes'trah) [L.] plural of *sequestrum.*

sequestration (se"kwes-tra'shun) [L. *sequestratio*] 1. the formation of a sequestrum. 2. the act or process of separation of something. 3. the isolation of a person or persons. 4. the increase in the quantity of blood within a limited vascular area, occurring physiologically, with forward flow persisting or not, or produced artificially by the application of a tourniquet.

sequestrectomy (se"kwes-trek'to-me) [*sequestrum* + Gr. *ektome* excision] the surgical removal of a sequestrum.

sequestrum (se-kwes'trum), pl. *seques'tra* [L.] a piece of bone that has become separated during the process of necrosis from the sound bone.

Ser serine.

Serapion of Alexandria [c. 280 B.C.] a Greek physician who is believed to have been one of the founders of the Empiric school of medicine (see EMPIRIC).

Serax trademark for oxazepam.

Serenase trademark for *haloperidol.*

Serenid trademark for *oxazepam.*

Seresta trademark for *oxazepam.*

serial (se're-al) arranged in or forming a series.

serialograph (se"re-al'o-graf) an apparatus for making series of radiographs.

series (ser'ez) [L. "row"] 1. a group of related objects or events occurring in succession or arranged in a successive order. 2. an arrangement of the parts of an electric circuit by connecting them successively to form a single path for the current. 3. a taxonomic category subordinate to a subclass and superior to an order. **actinide s., actinium s., actinoid s.,** a group of 15 radioactive elements (metals), starting with actinium (at no 89), and followed by thorium (90), protoactinium (91), uranium (92), neptunium (93), plutonium (94), americium (95), curium (96), berkelium (97), californium (98), einsteinium (99), fermium (100), mendelevium (101), nobelium (102), and lawrencium (103). Those elements in the series with atomic numbers higher than 92 (uranium, tissue), are known as *transuranic* or *transuranium elements.* Called also *actinide, actinoid,* and *actinium group.* **electromagnetic s.,** the array of electromagnetic radiation according to wavelength or photon energy. **lanthanide s., lanthanoid s., lanthanum s.,** rare EARTH.

serine (ser'en) an aliphatic, naturally occurring, nonessential amino acid, 2-amino-3-hydroxypropionic acid. It was first isolated from silk protein and may be biosynthesized from glycine. Used as a dietary supplement and food additive, in biological studies, and in culture media. Serine is also found in the saliva. Abbreviated *Ser.* See also amino ACID. **phosphatidyl s.,** cephalin.

Sernyl trademark for *phencyclidine hydrochloride* (see under PHENCYCLIDINE).

Sernylan trademark for *phencyclidine hydrochloride* (see under PHENCYCLIDINE).

seromucoid (se"ro-mu'koid) seromucous.

seromucous (se"ro-mu'kus) partly serous and partly mucous, such as a seromucous gland.

Seromycin trademark for *cycloserine.*

Serotinex trademark for *clofibrate.*

serotonin (ser"o-to'nin) 5-hydroxytryptamine.

serous (se'rus) [L. *serosus*] 1. pertaining to the serous membrane. 2. pertaining to or resembling serum. 3. producing or containing serum. 4. producing or containing any serous, thin, nonviscous, watery fluid.

serozyme (se'ro-zim) [*serum* + Gr. *zyme* yeast] prothrombin.

Serpasol trademark for *reserpine.*

serpiginous (ser-pij'i-nus) [L. *serpere* to creep] spreading gradually; creeping; pertaining to lesions that spread gradually in an arciform manner, having wavy, serpentine margins.

Serpiloid trademark for *reserpine.*

Serpine trademark for *reserpine.*

serrated (ser'at-ed) [L. *serratus,* from *serra* saw] dentate; resembling a structure or having an edge with teeth projecting like those of a saw.

Serratia (se-ra'she-ah) [named after Serafino *Serrati*] a genus of gram-negative, facultatively anaerobic bacteria of the family Enterobacteriaceae, made up of motile, peritrichously flagellated rods, some strains being capsulated. **S. marces'cens,** a species having red-pigmented varieties, generally occurring as free-living saprophytes and opportunistic pathogens, usually found in water, soil, food, and occasionally in pathologic material. It is sometimes the etiologic agent of bacteremia in hospitalized patients, particularly those with underlying disease or with preceding surgical intervention. Endocarditis caused by *S. marcescens* is often associated with intravenous drug abuse, and hospital-associated pneumonia may be due to contamination of ventilation equipment. Called also *Bacillus marcescens.*

serration (se-ra'shun) [L. *serratio*] 1. a structure or an object having an edge with projecting teeth like those of a saw; a condition of being serrated. 2. a characteristic of the working end of a plugging instrument which, when scored by minute shallow cross-cuts, has a roughened surface that produces an imprint against direct filling gold or amalgam, causing them to attach more readily to the opposite surfaces.

serratus (ser-ra'tus) [L.] serrated.

Serre's operation see under OPERATION.

Serres' angle, gland [Antoine Etienne Reynaud *Serres*, French physiologist, 1786-1868] see metafacial ANGLE, and see under GLAND.

serrulate (ser'u-lāt) [L. *serrulatus*] marked or bordered with small serrations or projections.

Sertan trademark for *primidone*.

serum (se'rum, ser'um), pl. *serums, se'ra, ser'a* [L. "whey"] 1. the clear portion of any animal liquid separated from its more solid elements, especially the blood serum. 2. blood serum from animals that have been inoculated with bacteria or their toxins. Such serum, when introduced into the body, produces passive immunization by virtue of the antibodies which it contains. **s. accelerator,** FACTOR VII. **acute phase s.,** serum collected in the acute phase of an infectious disease. **allergenic s., allergic s.,** serum containing antibodies capable of inducing an allergic response; some of these antibodies may passively transfer the allergic activity of an individual. **anticomplementary s.,** serum which interferes with or destroys the activity of complement. **antilymphocyte s.,** serum containing antibodies to lymphocytic antigens. In the presence of complement, antibodies may kill or lyse lymphocytes. Antilymphocytic sera can be made very specific to specific antigens on subpopulations of T- or B-lymphocytes and are helpful in elaborating the roles of subpopulations of cells. Abbreviated *ALS.* **antireticular cytotoxic s.,** one made by inoculating horses with an extract of spleen and bone marrow; said to have, in small doses, a stimulating effect on the reticuloendothelial system, and in large doses a cytotoxic effect on that system. Abbreviated *ACS.* Called also *Bogomolets' s.* **antivenomous s.,** a serum containing antibodies toward animal venoms, such as the venom of snakes, spiders, or other venomous species. It may be prepared from the blood of animals which have been immunized against the animal venom or obtained from a patient who has recovered from a venomous bite. Called also *Calmette's s.* See also ANTIVENIN. **bacteriolytic s.,** a serum containing antibodies capable of causing lysis of bacteria, usually in the presence of complement. **blood s.,** the clear liquid prepared from the blood plasma after separation of fibrinogen; used in fluid replacement after blood loss. **Bogomolets' s.,** antireticular cytotoxic s. **Calmette's s.,** antivenomous s. **convalescence s., convalescent s., convalescents' s.,** blood serum from a patient who is convalescent from an infectious disease or a toxemia. Such sera were once used as prophylactic injections in such diseases as measles, scarlet fever, whooping cough, etc., but now are prepared from normal serum pools or immunized volunteers in plasmapheresis programs. **heterologous s.,** 1. serum obtained from an animal belonging to a species different from that of the recipient. 2. serum prepared from an animal immunized by an antigen or organism differing from the one that is at issue. **homologous s.,** 1. serum obtained from an animal belonging to the same species as the recipient. 2. serum prepared from an animal immunized by the same antigen or organism that is at issue. **hyperimmune s.,** a serum unusually rich in antibody, obtained by a vigorous course of active immunization. **immune s.,** a serum containing one or more types of antibodies, especially one in which the antibody content has been increased by recovery from a specific infection or by injection with a specific antigen. **inactivated s.,** serum which has been heated to destroy the lytic activity of its complement component; usually accomplished by heating at 56° C for 30 minutes. **monovalent s.,** antiserum containing antibody to only one strain or species of microorganism or to only one kind of antigen. **s. sickness,** serum SICKNESS.

Serv. abbreviation for L. *ser'va,* keep, preserve.

servant (ser'vant) a person who serves others. **borrowed s.,** an employee in a hospital or any medical care institution, temporarily under the control of another. Traditionally, a nurse employed by a hospital, who is assigned to a surgeon in the operating room.

service (ser'vis) 1. an activity or work performed for another person. 2. a contribution to the welfare of other persons. **ancillary s's,** in health care delivery, services other than room and board and professional services provided in a hospital or other inpatient health program. **approved s's,** 1. in health insurance, medical and dental services provided under the plan. In some plans, prior authorization must be obtained before service is provided; other plans make exception for treatment of emergency needs; still others require no prior authorization for any

treatment approved under the program. 2. a medical or dental service which meets quality standards maintained under the plan. **basic s's,** 1. in health care delivery, the minimum supply of health services which should be generally and uniformly available in order to assure adequate health status and protection of the population from disease. Required basic services for Medicaid and health services required of health maintenance organizations include physician services, hospital services, medically necessary emergency care, preventive health services, medical treatment and referral services for drug and alcohol abuse, and radiologic services. 2. in health insurance, one of the two principal categories (the other being the major services) under a health plan. Diagnostic, preventive, and routine restorative dental services are usually included under a dental plan. The plan may provide different deductibles, coinsurance, and maximum for basic vs. major services as an incentive to good dental care. **covered s's,** in health insurance, those services for which benefits are provided under the contract. **Crippled Children's S.,** a federal program, under the Social Security Act, providing health services, including dental services, for crippled children. **dental health s's,** services designed or intended to promote, maintain, or restore dental health, including educational, preventive, and therapeutic services. **donated s.,** the estimated monetary value of services received from persons without compensation or with partial compensation, usually rendered in hospitals by volunteers from auxiliaries, charitable organizations, or religious orders. **extended care s.,** in a skilled nursing facility, a service provided on an inpatient basis for patients who have been discharged from the hospital, including nursing care, bed and board, and physical, occupational, or speech therapy. Medical services are generally provided by an intern or resident of a hospital with which the facility has a transfer agreement. Under Medicare, the extended care services are provided up to 100 days. See also extended care FACILITY. **home health s.,** home health CARE. **hospital ancillary s.,** any diagnostic or therapeutic service performed by a hospital department as distinguished from general or routine patient care such as room and board. **hospital outpatient s.,** ambulatory hospital CARE. **hospital routine s.,** the regular room, dietary, and nursing services, minor medical and surgical supplies, and the use of equipment and facilities for which a separate charge is not customarily made. **Indian Health S.,** the bureau in the Department of Health and Human Services responsible for delivering public health and medical and dental services to American Indians. **industrial health s's,** occupational health s's. **institutional health s's,** health services delivered on an inpatient or outpatient basis in hospitals, nursing homes, or other institutions, such as health maintenance organizations. **major medical s.,** major medical POLICY. **medical s.,** a service performed on behalf of a patient by professional or technical personnel at the direction of or under the direct supervision of a physician. **national health s.,** in the United States, a proposed national system of delivery of health care to recipients; planning, provision, and evaluation of health services (e.g., medical, dental, hospital, and ambulatory care and drugs and appliances); and responsibility for recruitment, education, training, and development of health personnel. See also national health INSURANCE. **occupational health s's,** health services provided by physicians, dentists, nurses, or other health personnel in an industrial setting for the appraisal, protection, and promotion of the health of employees while on the job. Called also *industrial health s's.* **outpatient s.,** ambulatory hospital care. **shared s's,** the coordinated, or otherwise explicitly agreed upon sharing of responsibility for provision of medical or nonmedical services on the part of two or more otherwise independent hospitals or other health programs. **skilled nursing s.,** a type of service that must be provided by or under the direct supervision of licensed nursing personnel and under the general direction of a physician. **visiting nurse s.,** visiting nurse ASSOCIATION.

sesamoid (ses'ah-moid) [L. *sesamoides;* Gr. *sēsamon* sesame + *eidos* form] resembling sesame seed.

sesqui- [L. *sesqui* a half more] a prefix meaning one and a half.

sesquioxide (ses″kwĕ-ok'sīd) a chemical compound of three parts of oxygen and two of another element. **ferric s.,** ferric OXIDE.

sessile [ses'il] [L. *sessilis*] characterized by a direct attachment at the base, not by a stalk or peduncle.

set (set) 1. to put in a particular place, estate, position, or order. 2. to adjust, as of controls on an instrument or device. 3. to fix or calibrate something. 4. to harden, as of dental plaster. 5. a group of similar things that belong or are used together. 6. fixed and rigid; firm. 7. to align bones or bone fragments, as in reducing fractures. **chromosome s.,** 23 pairs of individual chromosomes in the nucleus of a human somatic cell. **s. of teeth,** a full complement of artificial teeth.

Setrol trademark for *oxyphencyclimine hydrochloride* (see under OXYPHENCYCLIMINE).

setting (set′ing) 1. the hardening of a semiliquid mixture on crystallization, as of cement, or organic condensation, as of polymers. 2. the surroundings or environment in which something is found. **s. expansion,** setting EXPANSION. **s. time,** setting TIME.

setup (set′up) 1. organization or arrangement. 2. the arrangement of teeth on a trial denture base. **diagnostic s.,** a procedure involving dissection of teeth from a plaster model and repositioning of the teeth in desired positions to aid in case analysis preliminary to construction of an orthodontic appliance.

Sevriton cavity seal primer see under PRIMER.

sextan (seks′tan) [L. *sextanus* of the sixth] recurring every sixth day; said of fevers.

sextant (seks′tant) [L. *sextus* sixth] in dentistry, one of the six equal sections into which dental arches are sometimes divided.

Sézary's syndrome, [Albert *Sézary,* French dermatologist, 1880–1956] see under SYNDROME.

SH 1. serum hepatitis; see homologous serum HEPATITIS. 2. serum hepatitis (Australia) antigen; see Au ANTIGEN. 3. sulfhydryl.

shadow (shad′o) 1. an attenuated image of an actual object, as a faded or colorless erythrocyte. 2. a figure or image created by the interruption of light or other rays, such as the representation on a roentgenogram of radiopaque structures. **true s.,** see UMBRA.

Shafer's method [Sir Edward Albert Sharpey-*Shafer,* English physiologist, 1850–1935] see artificial RESPIRATION.

shaft (shaft) 1. a long slender part, such as the portion of a long bone between the wider ends or extremities. 2. the handle of a dental instrument. See DENTISTRY.

shank (shangk) 1. a leg, or any leglike part. 2. the tapered portion of a dental instrument which connects the handle and the blade. It may be straight, monoangled, binangled, or triple angled, the angulation providing access to the tooth to be operated upon. See DENTISTRY. **bur s.,** the part of the bur which fits into the handpiece, being tapered, notched, or elongated and smooth in design to fit into a specific handpiece. See BUR.

Shannon bur (drill) see under BUR.

shaping (shāp′ing) the act or process of giving an object an external surface or outline of particular form or pattern; modifying or adapting to fit. **root canal s.,** in root canal therapy, a method, with the use of burs, files, and reamers, aimed at developing a continuously tapering conical form in the root canal preparation; while it remains narrow apically with the narrowest cross-sectional diameter at the terminus, its conical shape is produced in multiple planes, the apical foramen remains as small as practically possible and retains its original position. See also teardrop FORAMEN.

sharpener (shar′pen-er) a device for grinding the edge of a cutting instrument in an effort to make it thin, thereby improving its cutting capability. **electric s.,** a sharpener consisting of a stone wheel driven by a stationary electric motor.

Sharpey's fibers [William *Sharpey,* English anatomist and physiologist, 1802–1880] see under FIBER.

Sharpey-Schafer see SCHAFER.

Shea-Anthony antral balloon sinus BALLOON.

shear (shēr) 1. to cut or cut through with a sharp instrument. 2. to become fractured under a load due to sliding action. 3. an applied force that tends to cause an opposite but parallel sliding motion of the planes of an object. Also, the strain resulting from such force. 4. resistance to a tangential force or a twisting motion. See ultimate shear STRENGTH. 5. shearing STRESS.

sheath (shēth) [L. *vagina;* Gr. *thēkē*] 1. a tubular structure enclosing or surrounding an organ or part. See also THECA and VAGINA. 2. a tube. **carotid s.,** the tubular portion of the cervical fascia enclosing the carotid artery, internal jugular vein, and vagus nerve, which attaches to the visceral, prevertebral, and investing fascia of the sternocleidomastoid muscle. At the root of the neck, it attaches to the sternum and first rib, and fuses with the fascia of the scalenus muscle and with the pericardium. The sheath plays a role in spreading of infection downward. Considered by some to be a part of the fascia, not an anatomic entity. Called also *vagina carotica fasciae cervicalis* [NA]. **connective tissue s.,** a membrane made of connective

tissue, which surrounds a bone, cartilage, muscle, or nerve. **dentinal s., s. of Neumann. enamel prism s., enamel rod s.,** a sheath that completely or partially surrounds each enamel prism, which is less mineralized than the prism itself and is thus less affected by acids. Hydroxyapatite crystals are fewer in the sheath than in the prism substance, with a correspondingly higher organic content in the sheath. Called also *prism s.* and *rod s.* **s. of Hertwig,** root s. (1). **Mauthner's s.,** axolemma. **medullary s.,** myelin s. **myelin s.,** the sheath surrounding the axon of some (myelinated or medullated) nerve fibers, consisting of thin lamellae of myelin (about 100 Å) wrapped around the axon and alternating with the spirally wrapped neurilemma, and giving a whitish appearance to nerves. The sheaths vary in diameter from 2 to 10 μ, with some significant variations present in different nerves. In peripheral nerves, the sheath is interrupted at more or regular intervals of 1 to 2 mm by nodes of Ranvier; in the central nervous system, the nodes occur chiefly at the point of bifurcation. Called also *medullary s.* See also MYELIN. See illustration at NERVE. **s. of Neumann,** an area of interface between peri- and intertubular dental structures demonstrating differences in staining reaction, refractivity, and susceptibility to actions of alkali and acids and mineralization. Called also *dentinal s.* **prism s.,** enamel prism s. **rod s.,** enamel prism s. **root s.,** 1. an epithelial extension of the cervical loop of the enamel organ, consisting of the inner and outer enamel epithelium, and directing the number and morphological growth of the roots. It is bordered externally by the dental sac and internally by developing cementum and root dentin. Upon the terminal stage of apposition, at the time when the formation of enamel and dentin has progressed cervically toward that area which will become the cementoenamel junction, incident to the formation of cementum and root development, ·the sheath turns inwardly toward the developing pulp and becomes the epithelial diaphragm. Called also *s. of Hertwig.* 2. the epithelial portion of the hair follicle, divided into the inner root sheath and the outer root sheath, which gives rise to the sebaceous glands. **s. of Schwann,** neurilemma. **s. of styloid process,** VAGINA processus styloidei. **synovial s. of tendon,** a double-layered, fibrous sheath found usually surrounding a tendon running in an osteofibrous canal, with synovial fluid present between the layers, serving to facilitate the gliding of tendons which pass through fibrous and bony tunnels. Called also *vagina mucosae tendinis* and *vagina synovalis tendinis* [NA].

Sheehan's syndrome [H. L. *Sheehan*] see under SYNDROME.

sheet (shēt) 1. a broad, relatively thin surface, layer, or covering. 2. sheet STRUCTURE.

Sheldon, J. H. [British physician] see craniocarpotarsal DYSTROPHY (Freeman-Sheldon syndrome).

shelf (shelf) 1. a thin slab fixed horizontally. 2. any shelflike structure, normal or abnormal, in the body. **buccal s.,** the surface of the mandible from the residual alveolar ridge or the alveolar ridge to the external oblique line in the region of the lower buccal vestibule; it is covered with cortical bone. **dental s.,** the shelflike epithelial invagination formed by the dental ridge, beneath which the dental papillae are formed. **palatine s.,** 1. palatine process, lateral; see under PROCESS. 2. palatine process, median; see under PROCESS.

shell (shel) any covering or encasement. **electron s.,** see electron ORBIT.

shellac (shĕ-lak′) a natural resin excreted by the insect *Laccifer lacca,* which sucks the juice of various resiniferous trees of India and deposits a sticky substance (stick-lac) on the twigs. The principal component of shellac is a resin which, on hydrolysis, gives a complex mixture of aliphatic and alicyclic hydroxy acids and their polyesters. It occurs as yellowish, transparent, brittle, sheets or pieces or as a powder, soluble in ethanol, ether, benzene, sparingly soluble in turpentine, and insoluble in water. Used in lacquers, varnishes, cements, grinding wheels, and dental impression compounds. Called also *lac, garnet lac,* and *gum lac.*

Sherer attachment see under ATTACHMENT.

Sherman plate see under PLATE.

Sherman unit [Henry Clapp *Sherman,* American biochemist, 1875–1955] 1. Bourquin UNIT. 2. Sherman-Munsell UNIT.

Sherman-Bourquin unit [H. C. *Sherman;* Ann *Bourquin,* American nutritionist, born 1897] Bourquin UNIT.

Sherman-Munsell unit [H. C. *Sherman,* Hazel E. *Munsell,* American nutritionist, born 1891] see under UNIT.

Sherrington's law [Sir Charles Scott *Sherrington,* English physiologist, 1857–1952; co-winner with Edgar Douglas Adrian, of the Nobel prize for physiology and medicine in 1932] see under LAW. See also stretch REFLEX (Liddel and Sherrington reflex).

Shick Sonic-Action trademark for a magnetic stirrer type of denture cleanser (see under CLEANSER).

Shick Ultrasonic trademark for an ultrasonic type of *denture cleanser* (see under CLEANSER).

shield (shēld) any protecting structure, such as one for preventing or reducing the passage of particles or radiation. **Blue S.,** see Blue Shield PLAN, and Association of Blue Shield Plans under ASSOCIATION. **lead s.,** a lead barrier used for protection from ionizing radiation. **lingual s.,** lingual PLATE. **oral s.,** vestibular SCREEN. **radiation s.,** a material used to protect from or reduce the passage of radiation.

shift (shift) a change, as of position or status. **Bennett s.,** Bennett MOVEMENT. **lateral s. of mandible,** Bennett MOVEMENT. **side s. of mandible,** Bennett MOVEMENT.

Shiga's bacillus, toxin [Kiyoshi *Shiga*, Japanese physician, 1870–1957] see *Shigella dysenteriae* (type 1), under SHIGELLA, and see under TOXIN.

Shigella (she-gel′ah) [named after K. *Shiga*] a genus of gramnegative, facultatively anaerobic bacteria of the family Enterobacteriaceae, made up of nonmotile, nonsporogenous, unencapsulated rods. The members ferment carbohydrates with the production of acids but not gas, and usually produce catalase. All species inhabit the intestine of higher animals, including man, and all cause dysentery. The genus is made up of four subgroups, designated A, B, C, and D, each comprising a species: subgroup A is *S. dysenteriae,* B is *S. flexneri,* C is *S. boydii,* and D is *S. sonnei.* With the exception of some strains, subgroup A cannot ferment mannitol; and other subgroups are of the mannitol-fermenting type. **S. boy′dii,** a species corresponding to subgroup C, being the cause of an acute diarrheal disease in man, especially in tropical regions. It is culturally identical with *S. flexneri* but serologically unrelated. The species includes 15 serotypes. **S. dysente′riae,** a species corresponding to subgroup A, and separated into several serotypes. Type 1, the classic Shiga's bacillus, or *S. shigae,* which is set apart from other dysentery bacilli by the production of a potent heat-labile exotoxin (Shiga toxin), is more common in tropical regions and causes severe dysentery. Type 2, Schmitz's bacillus, or *S. schmitzii,* is a non–mannitol-fermenting organism serologically related to *Escherichia coli,* being of limited pathogenicity, but occasionally causing endemic diarrhea in man, and also found in the chimpanzee. Called also *Bacillus dysenteriae, B. shigae, Bacterium dysenteriae, dysentery bacillus,* and *Eberthella shigae.* **S. flexne′ri,** a species corresponding to subgroup B, being one of the most common causes of acute diarrheal disease in man. It occurs in eight serotypes, designated by numbers 1 to 6 and letters X and Y. Called also *S. paradysenteriae* and *Flexner's bacillus.* **S. paradysente′riae,** *S. flexneri.* **S. pseudotuberculo′sis,** *Yersinia pseudotuberculosis;* see under YERSINIA. **S. rettge′ri,** *Proteus rettgeri;* see under PROTEUS. **S. schmit′zii,** *S. dysenteriae* (type 2). **S. shi′gae,** *S. dysenteriae* (type 1). **S. son′nei,** a species corresponding to subgroup D, being one of the most common causes of bacillary dysentery in man in temperate climates. Called also *Bacterium sonnei.*

shigella (she-gel′ah), pl. *shigellae.* Any microorganism of the genus *Shigella.*

shigellae (she-gel′e) plural of *shigella.*

shigellosis (she″gel-lo′sis) infection with any microorganism of the genus *Shigella.*

shim (shim) spacer.

shingles (shin′g′lz) HERPES zoster.

shock (shok) a condition of acute peripheral circulatory failure due to derangement of circulatory control or loss of circulating fluid, and brought about by injury. It is marked by pallor and clamminess of the skin, decreased blood pressure, feeble rapid pulse, decreased respiration, restlessness, anxiety, and sometimes unconsciousness. **allergic s.,** anaphylactic s. **anaphylactic s.,** a violent allergic reaction brought about by a second injection of an anaphylactogenic substance in a sensitized animal. Called also *allergic s.* See ANAPHYLAXIS. **electric s.,** the effects produced by the passage of an electric current through any part of the body. When the current is intense, it may cause (*a*) loss of consciousness or death, owing to effects on the nervous system or heart, (*b*) coagulation of tissue and resultant necrosis due to heat, and (*c*) violent tetanic muscular contractions which may lead to injury. **electrogalvanic s.,** sharp pain in the dental pulp produced by passage of electric current, as in dental galvanism. **endotoxic s., endotoxin s.,** shock associated with circulatory failure, prostration, hypotension, fever, and leukopenia following administration of endotoxin or after infection with endotoxin-producing bacteria. It occurs as the result of the ability of endotoxin to activate complement by the alternative pathway and the lysis of platelets causing disseminated coagulation. **galvanic s.,** pain caused by galvanic current, usually produced by the presence of dissimilar metals in the oral environment e.g. a gold inlay placed opposite or in juxtapo-

sition to a silver amalgam restoration may result in galvanic shock. **hemorrhagic s.,** shock due to vascular collapse brought about by diminished blood volume in hemorrhage. **hypoglycemic s.,** shock due to a rapid drop in the blood sugar content, usually occurring with overdosage of insulin or of the oral sulfonyureas. It is marked by sweating, clamminess of the skin, hypotension, tremor, vertigo, diplopia, convulsions, and collapse. Intermediate-acting insulin may cause hypoglycemia at night, when the only symptoms are nightmares and sweating. Repeated hypoglycemic attacks may cause brain damage, resulting in personality changes, depressed intelligence, cerebral dysrhythmias, and, sometimes, epileptiform convulsions. Called also *insulin s.* and *hypoglycemic attack.* See also diabetic COMA. **insulin s.,** hypoglycemic s. **neurogenic s.,** shock due to abnormal vasodilation brought about by a neurological activity. **traumatic s.,** shock produced by trauma, whether psychic or physical.

shoe (shoo) 1. a covering for the foot. 2. anything that resembles a shoe in form, use, or position. **Neurohr-Williams s., Neurohr-Williams rest s.,** a cast removable partial denture framework, consisting of a lingual bar, the lingual clasp arms, and a male portion of the attachment which engages the prepared abutment tooth. See illustration.

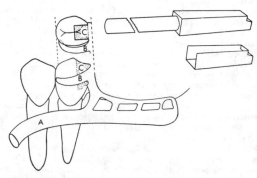

Neurohr-Williams shoe no. 2 with a step and corresponding mandrel and a unilateral view of the skeleton of a lower bilateral distal extension partial denture using the Neurohr shoe as a precision rest. *A,* Lingual bar. *B,* Lingual clasp arm. *C,* Male portion of the attachment, which is cast as part of the skeleton (framework). (From D. Henderson and V. L. Steffel: McCracken's Removable Partial Prosthodontics. 6th ed. St. Louis, The C. V. Mosby Co., 1981; courtesy Williams Gold Refining Co., Inc., Buffalo, N.Y.)

shoeing (shoo′ing) 1. fitting of a human foot with a shoe. 2. placing in position anything resembling a shoe. **s. cusp,** cusp RESTORATION.

Shofu spherical alloy see under ALLOY.

S-H-O-R-T an acronym for *s*hort stature; *h*yperextensibility of joints or hernia (inguinal) or both; *o*cular depression; *R*ieger anomaly; *t*eething delayed. See under SYNDROME.

shortness (short′nes) having little length; not long.

shortstop (short′stop) acid BATH.

shoulder (shōl′der) 1. the upper part of the trunk in man, extending on both sides of the body from the area where the arm articulates with the trunk to the base of the neck. 2. any shoulder-like projection, especially one upon which something else rests. 3. in extracoronal cavity preparations, the ledge formed by the meeting of the gingival wall and the axial wall at the right angle. See illustration. 4. crown LEDGE.

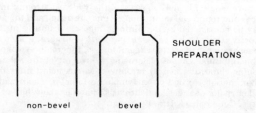

SHOULDER PREPARATIONS

non-bevel   bevel

Shrady's saw [George Frederick *Shrady,* American surgeon, 1837–1907] subcutaneous SAW.

shrinkage (shring′kij) contraction or reduction in size. **casting s.,** thermal shrinkage of a molten metal during solidification in a mold, as of the dental casting gold alloy during the fabrication of dental castings. The shrinkage occurs in three stages: thermal contraction of the liquid metal between the temperature to which it is heated and the liquidus temperature; contraction of the metal inherent in the change from the liquid to the solid state; and thermal contraction of the solid metal which occurs at room temperature. **s. compensation,** compensation TECHNIQUE. **polymerization s.,** the lessening in density during the process of polymerization as of methyl methacrylate which changes from 0.94/1 cm³ to 1.19/1 cm³, resulting in volumetric shrinkage of 21 percent. **thermal s.,** a shrinkage produced by lowering the temperature of a metal, particularly during the change from the molten to the solid state.

Shuman retractor, see under RETRACTOR.

shunt (shunt) 1. to turn to one side; to divert; to bypass. 2. a passage or anastomosis between two natural channels, especially between blood vessels. Shunt may be formed physiologically, or they may be structural anomalies. 3. surgically created anastomosis; also, the operation of forming a shunt. **hexose monophosphate s., oxidative s., pentose s.,** phosphogluconate PATHWAY.

shut (shut) in dentistry, that part of an anterior artificial tooth between the ridge lap and the shoulder in which pins for retaining the tooth in the base material are located.

SI Système International d'Unités; the International System of Units, established in 1960 at the Eleventh General Conference on Weights and Measures. It is an extension and refinement of the metric system (see under SYSTEM) and has been formally accepted in most countries. The seven basic units are the *meter* (length); *kilogram* (mass); *second* (time); *ampere* (electric current); *kelvin* (temperature [absolute]); *candela* (luminous intensity); and *mole* (amount of substance). Supplementary units are *radian* (plane angle) and *steradian* (solid angle). Derived units, which are stated in terms of the basic units, are the *newton* (force); *pascal* (pressure); *joule* (energy); *watt* (power); *volt* (electric potential); *coulomb* (electric charge); *farad* (capacitance); *ohm* (electric resistance); *siemens* (electric conductance); *weber* (magnetic flux); *tesla* (magnetic flux density); *henry* (inductance); *hertz* (frequency); and *degree Celsius* (temperature). See also metric SYSTEM and *Laboratory Reference Values of Clinical Importance* in the Appendix.

Si 1. silicon. 2. Si POINT.

sial- see SIALO-.

sialaden (si-al′ah-den) [*sial-* + Gr. *adēn* gland] a salivary gland.

sialadenectomy (si″al-ad″ĕ-nek′to-me) sialoadenectomy.

sialadenitis (si″al-ad″ĕ-ni′tis) [*sial-* + *adenitis*] inflammation of a salivary gland. Called also *sialoductitis.* See also PAROTITIS. **allergic s.,** swelling of the salivary glands, chiefly the parotid, caused by allergic reactions to food, drugs, or infection. **bacterial s.,** inflammation of a salivary gland due to a bacterial infection, usually involving the pericanalicular and periacinal spaces. **chronic nonspecific s.,** an inflammatory disease of the major salivary glands, characterized by intermittent swelling that may lead to fibrous degeneration, resulting from obstruction of the salivary ducts by calculi, foreign bodies, tumors, or scar formation, with subsequent bacterial invasion. **collagen s.,** a collagen disease of the salivary glands, previously identified with Sjögren's syndrome, now considered a separate entity. It occurs secondarily to a collagen disease, such as dermatomyositis, scleroderma, or lupus erythematosus, affecting most commonly women aged 30 to 40 years, and usually involving the parotid glands. The chief characteristics are xerostomia, generalized debility, rheumatoid pains, fever, bilateral enlargement of the glands, presence of LE cells in the blood, and changes in salivary chemistry; sodium and chloride contents in the saliva are usually increased, while potassium remains at normal levels. Pathologically, the involved glands may show bandlike homogeneous, fibrinoid masses in the widened stromal interstices and round cell infiltration around the ducts, and the acini may be constricted by the fibrinoid masses, resulting in their atrophy. Called also *collagen parotitis.* **retrograde s.,** acute postoperative PAROTITIS. **rheumatoid s.,** Sjögren's SYNDROME. **submandibular chronic sclerosing s.,** swelling of the submandibular gland, marked by atrophy of serous acini, interstitial inflammation, formation of lymphatic follicles, cicatrization, and cirrhotic changes. Sialolithiasis occurs in about half of the cases. Called also *Küttner's tumor.*

sialadenography (si″al-ad″ĕ-nog′rah-fe) roentgenography of the salivary glands and ducts.

sialadenosis (si′al-ad″ĕ-no′sis) [*sial-* + *adenosis*] a disease of a salivary gland. See also PAROTIDOSIS. **diabetic s.,** hormonal sialadenosis involving the parotid and submandibular glands, due to pancreatic insulin insufficiency in diabetes mellitus. **dysproteinemic s.,** sialadenosis in dysproteinemic states, usually characterized by enlargement of the parotid gland. **hepatogenic s.,** sialadenosis due to liver diseases, usually characterized by bilateral, soft, indolent parotid enlargement, depressed salivation, and increased potassium concentration and a normal sodium level in the saliva. **hormonal s.,** a disorder of the salivary glands due to hormonal dysfunctions, characterized by usually bilateral enlargement affecting chiefly the parotid glands, which is not associated with inflammation. Decreased secretion of the saliva and diminished enzyme and protein contents, with increased potassium and unchanged sodium concentrations in the saliva are associated. **malabsorption s.,** sialadenosis due to faulty absorption of nutrients by the intestine, characterized by soft, painless, bilateral enlargement of the parotid gland. **malnutritional s.,** sialadenosis associated with deficiency diseases, most commonly protein deficiency, usually characterized by soft, painless, bilateral enlargement of the parotid gland. See *protein deficiency s.* **neurohumoral s.,** a disorder of the salivary glands secondary to neurohumoral dysfunctions. The peripheral form is usually characterized by excessive salivation without enlargement of the salivary glands, and is most often due to facial paralysis of various origins, hypoglossal neuralgia, and sympathetic disorders. The central form may be characterized by excessive or insufficient salivation, and is due to lesions of the central nervous system, such as neoplasms of the brain, parkinsonism, or cerebral inflammatory diseases. **pancreatogenic s.,** sialadenosis due to a pancreatic disease, usually characterized by bilateral, undulating, painless enlargement of the parotid gland, associated with depressed salivation, increased potassium concentration, and a normal sodium level in the saliva. **protein deficiency s.,** sialadenosis associated with protein deficiency conditions, such as kwashiorkor, characterized by enlargement of the parotid, submandibular, and lacrimal glands, deficient salivary secretion, sialorrhea, and changes in amylase concentrations of the saliva. **thyroid s.,** a disorder of the salivary glands seen in thyroid dysfunctions, usually characterized by enlargement, depressed salivary secretion, and altered viscosity of the saliva.

sialadenotomy (si″al-ad″ĕ-not′o-me) sialoadenotomy.

sialagogic (si″ah-lah-goj′ik) promoting the flow of saliva.

sialagogue (si-al′ah-gog) [*sial-* + Gr. *agōgos* leading] an agent that promotes the flow of saliva; ptyalagogue.

sialectasia (si″al-ek-ta′se-ah) dilatation of a salivary duct.

sialic (si-al′ik) [Gr. *sialikos*] 1. pertaining to the saliva. 2. pertaining to sialic acid.

sialine (si′ah-lēn) [L. *sialinus*] pertaining to the saliva.

sialism, sialismus (si′al-izm; si′al-iz′mus) ptyalism.

sialitis (si″ah-li′tis) [*sial-* + *-itis*] inflammation of a salivary gland or duct.

sialo-, sial- [Gr. *sialon* saliva] a combining form denoting relationship to saliva or to the salivary glands. See also terms beginning PTYALO-.

sialoadenectomy (si″ah-lo-ad″ĕ-nek′to-me) [*sialo-* + Gr. *adēn* gland + *ektomē* excision] excision of a salivary gland. Called also *sialadenectomy.*

sialoadenitis (si″ah-lo-ad″ĕ-ni′tis) sialadenitis.

sialoadenotomy (si″ah-lo-ad″ĕ-not′o-me) [*sialo-* + Gr. *adēn* gland + *tomē* a cutting] incision and drainage of a salivary gland. Called also *sialadenotomy.*

sialoaerophagy (si″ah-lo-a″er-of′ah-je) [*sialo-* + Gr. *aēr* air + *phagein* to eat] the swallowing of saliva and air.

sialoangiectasis (si″ah-lo-an″je-ek′tah-sis) [*sialo-* + Gr. *angeion* vessel + *ektasis* distention] dilation of the salivary ducts.

sialoangiitis (si″ah-lo-an″je-i′tis) inflammation of the salivary ducts.

sialoangiography (si″ah-lo-an″je-og′rah-fe) radiography of the ducts of the salivary glands after injection of radiopaque material.

sialocarcinoma (si″ah-lo-kar″si-no-mah) [*sialo-* + *carcinoma*] a malignant tumor of the salivary glands, characterized by early pain, vascular patterns on the overlying skin, rapid growth, firm consistency, poor demarcation, facial paralysis, infiltration into the surrounding tissue, ulcers, and lymphatic and hematogenous spread.

sialocele (si′ah-lo-sēl) [*sialo-* + Gr. *kēlē* tumor] a salivary cyst or tumor.

sialodochitis (si″ah-lo-do-ki′tis) [*sialo-* + Gr. *dochos* receptacle + *-itis*] inflammation of the salivary ducts.

sialodochoplasty (si″ah-lo-do′ko-plas′te) [*sialo-* + Gr. *dochos* receptacle + *plassein* to form] plastic operation on the salivary ducts.

sialoductitis (si″ah-lo-duk-ti′tis) sialadenitis.

sialogenous (si″ah-loj′ĕ-nus) [*sialo-* + Gr. *gennan* to produce] producing saliva.

sialogogic (si″ah-lo-goj′ik) sialagogic.

sialogogue (si-al′o-gog) sialagogue.

sialogram (si-al′o-gram) [*sialo-* + Gr. *gramma* a mark] a roentgenogram obtained by sialography.

sialography (si″ah-log′rah-fe) [*sialo-* + Gr. *graphein* to write] roentgen examination of the salivary ducts and glands after injection of a radiopaque medium; ptyalography.

sialolith (si-al′o-lith) [*sialo-* + Gr. *lithos* stone] a calcareous concretion or calculus in the salivary ducts or glands, involving most commonly the submaxillary gland and its duct, less frequently the parotid and sublingual glands and their ducts, and seldom the minor salivary glands. It usually presents as a white, yellowish, or tan stonelike concentration, composed mainly of calcium phosphates and carbonates, and also containing iron oxide, sodium chloride, thiocyanates, and magnesium compounds. The salivary duct calculi are usually hard; peripheral salivary gravel is softer. It is typically composed of thin layers around a soft core, giving its cross-section an onion-like appearance. Called also *salivary calculus* and *salivary stone.*

sialolithiasis (si″ah-lo-li-thi′ah-sis) [*sialo-* + *lithiasis*] a condition characterized by the presence of sialoliths. Called also *ptyalolithiasis.*

sialolithotomy (si″ah-lo-li-thot′o-me) [*sialolith* + Gr. *tomē* a cutting] surgical removal of a calculus from a salivary gland or duct. Called also *ptyalolithotomy.*

sialoma (si″ah-lo′mah) a salivary tumor.

sialometaplasia (si″ah-lo-met″ah-pla′ze-ah) metaplasia of the salivary glands. **necrotizing s.,** a benign inflammatory condition of the minor salivary glands, simulating mucoepidermoid and squamous cell carcinoma. Histological findings usually show lobular necrosis and ductal and glandular metaplasia.

sialophagia (si″ah-lo-fa′je-ah) [*sialo-* + Gr. *phagein* to eat] the excessive swallowing of saliva.

sialorrhea (si″ah-lo-re′ah) [*sialo-* + Gr. *rhoia* flow] excessive flow of saliva. Called also *hyperptyalism, hypersalivation, ptyalism,* and *ptyalorrhea.*

sialoschesis (si″ah-los′kĕ-sis) [*sialo-* + Gr. *schesis* suppression] suppression of the salivary secretion.

sialosis (si″ah-lo′sis) [*sial-* +*-osis*] 1. the flow of saliva. 2. salivation. **rheumatic s.,** Sjögren's SYNDROME.

sialostenosis (si″ah-lo-stĕ-no′sis) [*sialo-* + Gr. *stenos* narrow] stenosis of a salivary duct.

sialosyrinx (si″ah-lo-si′rinks) [*sialo-* + Gr. *syrinx* pipe] 1. a salivary fistula. 2. a syringe for washing out the salivary ducts, or a drainage tube for the salivary ducts.

sialozemia (si″ah-lo-ze′me-ah) [*sialo-* + Gr. *zemia* loss] the involuntary flow of saliva.

sib (sib) [Anglo-Saxon *sib* kin] sibling.

sibilant (sib′ĭ-lant) [L. *sibilans* hissing] of a shrill, hissing, or whistling character, said of a type of fricative speech sound, such as *s, z, sh, ch,* and *dg.*

sibling (sib′ling) [Anglo-Saxon *sib* kin + *-ling* a diminutive] any of two or more offspring of unspecified sex of the same two parents. The first generation offspring are designated on genetic records as F_1, the second generation as F_2, etc. Called also *sib.* See also GENERATION, OFFSPRING, PEDIGREE, and PROGENY.

Sibson's fascia see under FASCIA.

Sicard, Jean Athanase [French neurologist, 1872–1929] see Brissaud-Sicard SYNDROME and Collet-Sicard SYNDROME.

siccative (sik′ah-tiv) [L. *siccus* dry] drying, removing moisture from surrounding objects.

siccolabile (sik″o-la′bil) altered or destroyed by drying.

siccus (sik′us) [L.] dry.

sickle (sik″l) 1. a curved, hooklike blade mounted on a short handle; used for cutting grass or grain. 2. sickle SCALER.

sicklemia (sik-le′me-ah) sickle cell ANEMIA.

sickness (sik′nes) any condition marked by pronounced deviation from the normal healthy state; illness. **decompression s.,** a disorder caused by rapid decrease in barometric pressure, occurring in aviators exposed to a sudden loss of cabin pressure when flying at high altitudes and, more frequently, in deep sea divers and caisson workers brought too rapidly to the surface. It is due to bubbles of gases, including nitrogen, escaping from the dissolved state in body fluids to the gaseous state. Symptoms vary from mild joint pain through excruciating arthralgia, abdominal pain, respiratory manifestations, confusion and other neurologic signs, including coma, and skin lesions, to death. Called also *bends* and *caisson disease.* See also DECOM-

PRESSION (2), DYSBARISM, and gas EMBOLISM (2). **radiation s.,** a syndrome following whole-body irradiation (see under IRRADIATION) or exposure of large parts of the body to ionizing radiations, with organs and tissues made up of cells with high reproduction or mitotic activity being most severely affected. Hematopoietic and lymphoid injuries produce lymphopenia, shrinkage of the lymph nodes and spleen, destruction of the lymphocytes, initial increase followed by a decrease in the granulocyte and blood platelet counts, destruction of the bone marrow cells, anemia, and sometimes leukemia. Oral and pharyngeal changes, believed to be due to leukopenia followed by local infection, may include hemorrhagic and necrotizing gingivitis with pseudomembrane formation, tonsillits, and pharyngitis. Gonadal injury produces sterility, spermatogonia, atrophy of the testes, destruction of the ovarian follicles, depressed menstruation, and other reproductive disorders. Gastrointestinal injury produces nuclear and cellular pleomorphism and mitotic abnormalities in the mucosal cells, mucosal edema, hyperemia, ulcers, submucosal atrophy, and fibrosis, leading to intestinal and esophageal strictures. Nervous system injury causes necrosis of the brain and the spinal cord. Symptoms, which vary with the intensity of irradiation, include nausea, vomiting, loss of appetite, bloody diarrhea, fever, thirst, malaise, erythema, alopecia, pigmentation disorders, and coma. Death usually follows. Called also *radiation illness* and *radiation syndrome.* See also radiation INJURY and RADIOSENSITIVITY. **serum s.,** hypersensitivity reaction following the administration of foreign serum or other antigens or certain drugs, and marked by urticaria, edema, adenitis, arthralgia, high fever, and prostration. The acute reaction is attributable to the formation of antibodies against the foreign serum, antigen, or drug, which are usually present in excess at initial antibody production. Soluble antigen-antibody complexes that mediate immunologic injury are deposited in the tissues. In the chronic form, the injury is due to repeated administration of antigen to immune animals with continuous formation of antigen-antibody complexes over a prolonged period, such as in rheumatic fever. Called also *immune-complex disease, serum disease,* and *serum intoxication.*

side (sīd) the lateral (right or left) portion or aspect of the body or a structure. **balancing s.,** the segment of a denture or dental arch on the side opposite to that toward which the mandible is moved. The term pertains to occlusion and bears no relation to masticatory activity. Called also *nonfunctioning s.* **functioning s.,** working s. **nonfunctioning s.,** balancing s. **pressure s.,** the side toward which a tooth is drifting. See also physiologic DRIFT. **safe s.,** the nonabrasive side of a dental disk that protects adjacent teeth during cutting, smoothing, or polishing of the proximal surfaces of teeth. See safe-side DISK. **tension s.,** the side from which a tooth is drifting away. See also physiologic DRIFT. **working s.,** the segment of a denture or dental arch on the same side as that toward which the mandible is moved. The term pertains to occlusion and bears no relation to masticatory activity. Called also *functioning s.,*

side effect (sīd′ ef-fekt′) side EFFECT.

siderinuria (sid″er-ĭ-nu′re-ah) [Gr. *sideros* iron + *ouron* urine + *-ia*] excretion of iron in the urine.

sidero- [Gr. *sidēros* iron] a combining form denoting relationship to iron.

sideroblast (sid′er-o-blast) [*sidero-* + Gr. *blastos* germ] a nucleated erythrocyte containing blue iron granules demonstrated by the Prussian blue reaction; a nucleated siderocyte. **ringed s.,** a sideroblast in which siderocytic granules form a ring around the nucleus.

siderocyte (sid′er-o-sīt) [*sidero-* + Gr. *kytos* hollow vessel] an erythrocyte containing blue iron granules demonstrated by the Prussian blue reaction. Siderocytes are believed to be caused by incomplete iron metabolism and are present in the bone marrow and blood in anemias, except those associated with iron deficiency. The number of siderocytic granules varies in an erythrocyte from 1 to 20; their size being under 2 μ.

sideropenia (sid″er-o-pe′ne-ah) [*sidero-* + Gr. *penia* poverty] iron deficiency; see IRON.

sideropenic (sid″er-o-pe′nik) pertaining to or characterized by sideropenia (iron deficiency); see IRON.

siderophilin (si′der-of′ĭ-lin) transferrin.

siemens (se′menz) the SI unit of electric conductivity, measured by the quantity of electricity transferred across the unit area, per unit potential gradient per unit time. Called also *mho* and *reciprocal ohm.* Abbreviated S. See also SI.

Siemens, Herman Werner [German dermatologist, born 1891] see hypohidrotic ectodermal DYSPLASIA (Christ-Siemens-Touraine syndrome).

sieve (siv) a device having pores or perforations of uniform size used for separating objects or particles from those of different sizes.

Sig. abbreviation for L. *sig'na*, let it be labeled. See SIGNA.

sigh (si) [L. *suspirium*] an audible and prolonged inspiration, followed by an audible expiration.

sigma (sig'mah) σ, ς, Σ, the eighteenth letter of the Greek alphabet.

sigmatism (sig'mah-tizm) the incorrect, difficult, or too frequent use of the *s* sound.

sigmoid (sig'moid) [L. *sigmoides;* Gr. *sigmoeidēs*] 1. shaped like the letter S or the letter C. 2. sigmoid notch of mandible; see under NOTCH. 3. sigmoid COLON.

sign (sīn) [L. *signum*] an indication of the existence of something; any objective evidence of a disease. See also PHENOMENON, SYMPTOM, and TEST. **Aufrecht's s.,** a feeble breathing sound heard just above the jugular fossa, indicative of tracheal stenosis. **Battle's s.,** discoloration in the line of the posterior auricular artery, the ecchymosis first appearing near the tip of the mastoid process; seen in fractures of the base of the skull. **Bespaloff's s.,** in the early stage of measles, the tympanic membrane is red and there is nasopharyngeal catarrh. **Bezold's s.,** an inflammatory swelling below the apex of the mastoid process; an evidence of mastoiditis. **Biederman's s.,** a dark red color (instead of the normal pink) of the anterior pillars of the throat, seen in some syphilitic patients. **Bordier-Fränkel s.,** an outward and upward rolling of the eye in peripheral facial paralysis. **Burton's s.,** lead LINE. **Charcot's s.,** the raising of the eyebrow in peripheral facial paralysis, and the lowering of the same part in facial contraction. **chin-retraction s.,** a sign of the third stage of anesthesia; the chin and larynx move downward during inspiration. **Chvostek's s., Chvostek-Weiss s.,** a spasm of the facial muscles resulting from tapping the muscles or branches of the facial nerve; seen in tetany. **commemorative s.,** any sign of a previous disease. **Corrigan's s.,** copper LINE. **Demarquay's s.,** fixation or lowering of the larynx during phonation and deglutition; a sign of syphilis of the trachea. **Dennie's s.,** Morgan's LINE. **duct s.,** a red spot seen at the orifice of the parotid duct in mumps. **Escherich's s.,** in tetany, percussion of the inner surface of the lips or tongue produces contraction of the lips, tongue, and masseter muscles. **Ewing's s.,** tenderness at the upper inner angle of the orbit; a sign of obstruction of the outlet of the frontal sinus. **Forschheimer's s.,** Forschheimer's spots; see under SPOT. **Granger's s.,** if in the radiograph of an infant two years old or less, the anterior wall of the lateral sinus is visible, extensive destruction of the mastoid is indicated. **Hatchcock's s.,** tenderness on running the finger toward the angle of the jaw in mumps. **Heryng's s.,** an infraorbital shadow produced by fluid or by a hypertrophied, hyperplastic, or neoplastic membrane in the antrum and observable by illumination of the buccal cavity; seen in diseases of the maxillary sinus. **Krisovski's s.,** cicatricial lines which radiate from the mouth in congenital syphilis. **Mirchamp's s.,** when a sapid substance, such as vinegar, is applied to the mucous membrane of the tongue, a painful reflex secretion of saliva in the gland about to be affected is indicative of sialadenitis, e.g., mumps. **Nikolsky's (Nikolskii's) s.,** peeling off of the epidermis similarly to wet tissue paper upon drawing the finger with firm pressure over the surface of the apparently normal skin; symptomatic of pemphigus vulgaris and some other bullous diseases characterized by acantholysis. **objective s.,** one that can be seen, heard, or felt by the diagnostician. Called also *physical s.* **Parrot's s.,** bony nodes on the outer table of the skull of infants with congenital syphilis, giving it a buttock shape. Called also *hot cross bun skull, natiform skull,* and *Parrot's nodes.* **physical s.,** objective s. **rope s.,** acute angulation between chin and larynx, due to weakness of hyoid muscles, noted in bulbar poliomyelitis. **Signorelli's s.,** extreme tenderness on pressure on the retromandibular point in meningitis. **Silex's s.,** furrows radiating from the mouth in congenital syphilis. **Sterling-Okuniewski s.,** the patient is unable to put out his tongue when directed to do so; once considered to be symptomatic of typhus fever. **vital s.,** any evidence of life and vital functions, including blood pressure, pulse, respiration, skin color, consciousness, ability to move the extremities or other parts of the body, reaction to pain, and reaction of the pupils to light.

signa (sig'nah) [L.] mark, or write; Abbreviated *S.* or *Sig.* on prescriptions. See PRESCRIPTION.

signature (sig'nah-chur) [L. *signatura*] that part of a prescription which gives direction as to the taking of the medicine. See PRESCRIPTION.

Signorelli's sign [Angelo *Signorelli,* Italian physician, 1876–1952] see under SIGN.

Sig. n. pro. abbreviation for L. *sig'na nom'ine pro'prio,* label with the proper name.

Silain trademark for *simethicone.*

Silamat trademark for a *mechanical triturator* (see under TRITURATOR), having an operational speed of 4200 rpm.

silane (sī-lān') a silicon hydride, SiH_4, occurring as a gas with a repulsive odor, which is highly toxic and explosive. Called also *silicane, monosilane,* and *silicon tetrahydride.*

silanes (sī-lānz') silicon hydrides with a low degree of polymerization, having Si−Si chains which become thermally unstable when lengths up to Si_6H_{14} are approached. They are gaseous or liquid compounds analogous to alkenes or saturated hydrocarbons with the ability to bond organic polymer systems to inorganic substrates. Silanes SiH_3 is known as *silyl,* Si_2H_5 as *disilanyl,* and SiH_2 as *cyclosilane.* Used as coupling agents. See also SILICONE polymers.

Silastic (sī-las'tik) trademark for a *heat-vulcanized silicone* (see under SILICONE). **S. 382,** trademark for a room temperature–vulcanizing silicone. In its raw state, it has a consistency similar to that of thick honey, and vulcanizes with the use of stannous octoate. Its physical properties are: durometer, 45; tensile strength (psi), 300; elongation (percent), 100; tear (psi), 20. Used in impression materials and maxillofacial prostheses. **S. 399,** trademark for room temperature–vulcanized silicone that was expressly developed for use in maxillofacial prostheses. In its raw state, it resembles petroleum jelly, being nonflowing and easily spatulated. Upon adding a cross-linking agent, the substance becomes milky and remains so without changing consistency for several hours. When catalyst No. 2 is added, it sets up to a translucent rubber in 10 to 15 minutes. Its physical properties are: durometer, 50; tensile strength (psi), 525; elongation (percent), 230; tear (psi), 29. **S. 6508,** trademark for a heat-vulcanized silicone, which, in its raw state, has a consistency similar to that of sticky modeling clay. It is vulcanized at 127°C (260°F) and formed in pressure molds. Its physical properties are: durometer, 26; tensile strength (psi), 785; elongation (percent), 490; tear (psi), 65. Used in impression materials and maxillofacial prostheses.

silent (si'lent) producing no detectible signs or symptoms; noiseless.

silex (si'leks) a refined form of silica powder, which may be mixed with water or a mouthwash solution to form a fine abrasive paste for polishing metal castings.

Silex's sign [Paul *Silex,* German physician, 1858–1929] see under SIGN.

silica (sil'ĭ-kah) [L. *silex* flint] SILICON dioxide.

silicane (sil'ĭ-kān) silane.

Silicap trademark for a *silicate cement* (see under CEMENT).

silicate (sil'ĭ-kāt) a salt derived from silica or silicic acids. **aluminum s.,** ALUMINUM silicate. **s. cement,** silicate CEMENT. **native calcium-magnesium s.,** asbestos. **potassium s.,** POTASSIUM silicate. **zirconium s.,** ZIRCONIUM silicate.

silicious (sī-lish'us) containing silica or a compound of silicon.

silicon (sil'ĭ-kon) [L. *silex* flint] a nonmetallic element occurring in nature as silicon dioxide. Symbol, Si; atomic number, 14; atomic weight, 28.086; melting point, 1410°C; Mohs hardness number, 7; specific gravity, 2.33; group IVA of the periodic table. Its naturally occurring isotopes include 28–30; artificial isotopes include 25–27 and 31–32. It occurs as dark brown powder made up of black to gray, lustrous needle-like crystals. Silicon is soluble in a mixture of nitric and hydrofluoric acids and in alkalies; insoluble in water and nitric and hydrochloric acids. Used in the production of silicones and in various industrial processes. Silicon is nontoxic, but inhalation of its dust may cause respiratory diseases. **s. carbide,** a compound of carbon and silicon, SiC. See CARBORUNDUM. **s. dioxide,** a compound, SiO_2, occurring as transparent, tasteless crystals, or as an amorphous powder, which is insoluble in water or acids, except hydrofluoric acid. It occurs in nature as agate, amethyst, sand, quartz, chalcedony, cristobalite, and flint. It is one of the three major ingredients that make up dental porcelain, providing stiffness and hardness to the product and the framework around which the kaolin and feldspar contract. In granular form, it serves as an abrasive and polishing agent. Called also *silica* and *silicic anhydride.* See also PORCELAIN, SILEX, and TRIPOLI. **eka-s.,** germanium. **s. hydride,** see SILANES. **s. tetrahydride,** silane.

silicone (sil'ĭ-kōn) a chemical compound from a large group of polymers with the siloxane chain, based on a structure consisting of alternate silicon and oxygen atoms with organic radicals attached to the silicon. It may occur as a liquid, semisolid, or solid, depending on molecular weight and degree of polymerization, its properties being determined by the length of the polymer chain and the nature of the side chains; high-molecular-weight polymers are less viscous than corresponding low-molecular-weight hydrocarbon polymers. Polymers may be straight-chain, or cross-linked with benzoyl peroxide or other free radical indicators, with or without a catalyst. Silicones exhibit weathering properties and maintain good physical status over a wide range of temperatures; they may be used as monomers that may be cured either at room temperature or by heat, polymerized with the use of tin octoate, as a catalyst, and alkyl silicate, as a reactor. Silicone preparations are used as adhesives, lubricants, and in the production of a variety of products. In dentistry, they may be used in the production of maxillofacial prostheses and impression materials.

$$-OSi\!\!\begin{array}{c}R\\|\\|\\R\end{array}\!\!-O-\!\!\begin{array}{c}R\\|\\Si\\|\\R\end{array}\!\!-OSi\!\!\begin{array}{c}R\\|\\|\\R\end{array}_n$$

s. catalyst, silicone CATALYST. **s. fluid,** a fluid, dimethylpolysiloxane, occurring as an odorless, clear, almost colorless liquid that is insoluble in water, but is soluble in chloroform, carbon tetrachloride, ethanol, and paraffin oils. Available in a wide range of viscosities, and used in protective creams and lotions. Also used in heat sterilization of dental instruments. Heated to 150°C (300°F.), it will destroy all vegetative microorganisms in 15 minutes; at 125°C (260°F), the organisms will be destroyed in 20 to 30 minutes. **heat-vulcanized s.,** a silicone used in the production of silicone rubber, which is heat-vulcanized with the use of diorganopolysiloxanes, such as polydimethyl siloxane and benzoyl peroxide, as a cross-linking agent. The heating causes the induction of the cross-linking between the polymers through a reaction between methyl radicals in one chain and methyl groups in an adjacent chain, with benzoic acid formed as a byproduct. The rubber silicone thus produced is used in the fabrication of impression materials and maxillofacial prostheses. Called also *heat-vulcanized silicone rubber.* Trademarks: *Silastic,* Silastic 6508. **s. impression material,** impression material, silicone; see under MATERIAL. **s. polymers,** polymers formed by covalent compounds with Si—Si chains, silanes, having a low degree of polymerization and being potentially thermally unstable, or siloxane links,

$$-O-\!\!\begin{array}{c}O\\|\\Si\\|\\O\end{array}\!\!-O-,$$

which are more stable and allow the development of a wide range of polymers, from liquids, through greases and waxes to resins and rubbers. **s. putty,** see impression material, silicone, under MATERIAL. **room temperature–vulcanizing s., RTV s.,** a silicone which is vulcanized at room temperature, consisting of a compound composed of comparatively short chains of silicone polymers which are partially blocked with hydroxyl groups. In liquid form, the silicone condensates with the addition of a catalyst, such as stannous octoate, and a cross-linking agent, such as ethyl orthosilicate, forming a rubbery, somewhat porous substance. Fillers are added to strengthen the final rubber. Used in the production of impression materials and maxillofacial prostheses. Called also *room temperature-vulcanizing silicone rubber* and *RTV silicone rubber.* Trademarks: Silastic 382, Silastic 399.

silk (silk) the soft, lustrous protein filament produced by various silkworms, particularly the species *Bombyx mori.* Dyed and coated with a wax or resin and braided or twisted, it is used as a nonabsorbable suture material.

silkworm-gut (silk'werm-gut) a strand drawn from a silkworm which has been killed when ready to spin its cocoon; less pliable than catgut and nonabsorbable, it is used for retention sutures, which are later removed.

siloxane (sĭ-lok'sān) a straight-chain compound having silicon atoms single-bonded to oxygen with each silicon atom being linked with four oxygen atoms. Some siloxanes have hydrogen

atoms replacing two or more oxygens. The siloxane chain is the basis of the silicone structure. Called also *oxosilane.* See also SILICONE polymers.

$$-\!\!\begin{array}{c}O\\|\\Si\\|\\O\end{array}\!\!-O-\!\!\begin{array}{c}O\\|\\Si\\|\\O\end{array}\!\!-O-\!\!\begin{array}{c}O\\|\\Si\\|\\O\end{array}\!\!-O-$$

s. link, siloxane LINK. **polydimethyl s.,** a siloxane preparation used as a cross-linking agent.

$$H_3C-\!\!\begin{array}{c}CH_3\\|\\Si\\|\\CH_3\end{array}\!\!-O-\!\!\begin{array}{c}CH_3\\|\\Si\\|\\CH_3\end{array}\!\!-O-\!\!\begin{array}{c}CH_3\\|\\Si\\|\\CH_3\end{array}\!\!-O-\!\!\begin{array}{c}CH_3\\|\\Si\\|\\CH_3\end{array}\!\!-O-\!\!\begin{array}{c}CH_3\\|\\Si\\|\\CH_3\end{array}\!\!-O-\!\!\begin{array}{c}CH_3\\|\\Si\\|\\CH_3\end{array}\!\!-CH_3$$

silver (sil'ver) [A.S. *seolfor, siolfur;* L. *argentum*] a metallic element. Symbol, Ag; atomic number, 47; atomic weight, 107.868; specific gravity, 10.53; melting point, 961°C; valences, 1, 2; group IB of the periodic table. Natural silver isotopes include 107 and 109; artificial isotopes are 100–106, 108, and 110–117. It is a white, lustrous, ductile, and malleable metal that resists oxidation, but tarnishes due to reaction with atmospheric sulfur compounds; becomes blackened by ozone; is inert to most acids, but is attacked by nitric, sulfuric, and hydrochloric acids; and is fused by alkalies. Most silver salts are light-sensitive and are thus used in photography. Silver ion combines with biologically important substances, such as amino, imidazole, carboxyl, and phosphate groups; silver salts inhibit sulfhydryl enzymes. Silver attaches to reactive protein groups, increasing their solubility and, sometimes, causing their denaturation. Dietary trace amounts accumulate in the body, but high concentrations occur only as a result of intake of excessively large amounts of silver-containing preparations. Silver compounds are used chiefly as caustic, astringent, germicidal, and antiseptic preparations. In dentistry, silver is used mainly in prostheses, in alloys, in soldering, to neutralize the color imparted by copper in alloys, and as points to obliterate the root canal. In the past, silver was used for purification of drinking water. Silver does not cause serious toxic manifestations, but inhalation of dust may produce adverse reactions and prolonged intake of silver may cause grayish blue skin discoloration (see ARGYRIA). See also terms beginning ARGYR-. **s. amalgam** silver AMALGAM. **s. bromide,** AgBr, pale yellow crystals or powder that darken on exposure to light and are soluble in potassium bromide, potassium cyanide, and sodium thiosulfate solutions, slightly soluble in ammonia water, and insoluble in water. Used as a topical anti-infective and astringent agent. Also used as an x-ray and photosensitive component of photographic and roentgenographic plates and film. **s. chloride,** AgCl, white granular powder which darkens on exposure to light and is soluble in ammonium hydroxide and sulfuric acid, but not in water. Used as an antiseptic and sedative. **s.-copper system,** silver-copper ALLOY. **s. fluoride,** AgF, flexible, hygroscopic leaflets, soluble in water. Used as an antiseptic. Prolonged use may cause mottling of teeth and bone changes. **s. leaf,** a thin sheet of silver; formerly used as a filling material. **liquid s.,** mercury. **s. nitrate,** AgNO₃, prepared by dissolving silver in dilute nitric acid, forming colorless, transparent or white crystals which are readily soluble in water. It has germicidal, astringent, and escharotic properties. Used to cauterize defective enamel, sterilize and detect dental caries, and to reduce tooth sensitivity, in the treatment of gingival diseases and stomatitis, and in root canal therapy. Its use in dentistry has declined because of its toxicity and caustic and staining properties. Called also *lapis imperialis, lapis infernalis,* and *lapis lunaris.* See also ammoniacal silver nitrate SOLUTION. **s. nitrate, fused,** silver nitrate, toughened. **s. nitrate, molded,** silver nitrate, toughened. **s. nitrate, toughened,** white or grayish rods or small cones consisting of about 97 to 98 percent silver nitrate and 2 to 3 percent silver chloride. Used as an escharotic. Called also *fused s. nitrate, molded s. nitrate,* and *lunar caustic.* **s. oxide,** Ag₂O, a brownish-black, odorless powder that is soluble in water and ammonia, but not in alcohol. Used as a topical germicidal and parasiticidal agent. **s.-palladium alloy,** silver-palladium ALLOY. **s. protein, mild,** a preparation containing 19 to 23 percent silver, rendered colloidal by the presence of, or combination with, protein; it occurs as dark brown or almost black scales or granules. Used as a topical anti-infective. It has been responsible for many cases of argyria. **s. protein, strong,** a pale yellowish orange to brownish black powdered compound of silver and protein containing 7.5 to 8.15 percent silver. It is an active germicide with a local irritant and astringent effect. It may cause argyria. **s. solder,** silver SOLDER. **standard s.,** a silver alloy of 900 parts silver and 100 parts copper. **sterling s.,** silver defined legally as an alloy of 925 parts of silver and 75 parts of copper. See silver-copper ALLOY. **sulfadiazine s.,** an antimicrobial agent, C₁₀H₉AgN₄O₂S, combining the antimicrobial properties of sulfadiazine and silver ion. It is particularly effective against *Pseudomonas aeruginosa* and is used in the treatment of burn wounds. **s.-tin alloy,** silver-tin ALLOY. **s.-tin system,** silver-tin ALLOY.

Silver's syndrome [Henry F. *Silver,* American physician, born 1918] see under SYNDROME. See also Russell's SYNDROME (Russell-Silver syndrome).

Silverman, William A. see infantile cortical HYPEROSTOSIS (Caffey-Silverman syndrome).

Silverman needle see under NEEDLE.

Silverman's syndrome [F. N. *Silverman*] battered CHILD.

Silvester's method [Henry Robert *Silvester,* English physician, 1828–1908] see artificial RESPIRATION.

Silvio Negri's syndrome [*Silvio Negri,* Italian physician] retrosphenoidal space SYNDROME.

silyl (sil′il) a silicon hydride, SiH₃; see SILANES.

simethicone (si-meth′ĭ-kōn) a mixture of dimethyl polysiloxanes and silica gel, occurring as a white, viscous, oily liquid that is miscible with chloroform and ether, but not with water. Used as an ointment base, topical drug vehicle, and skin protectant. Also used as an antiflatulent agent for postsurgical patients. Called also *dimethicone* and *dimethyl polysiloxane.* Trademarks: Aeropax, Meteorex, Mylocon, Silain.

Simmonds' syndrome [Morris *Simmonds,* German physician, 1855–1925] see under SYNDROME.

Simpamin trademark for *dextromaphetamine sulfate* (see under DEXTROMAPHETAMINE).

simulation (sim″u-la′shun) [L. *simulatio*] 1. the act of counterfeiting a disease; malingering. 2. the mimicking of one disease by another.

Simulator trademark for an *adjustable dental articulator* (see Granger ARTICULATOR).

sinal (si′nal) pertaining to a sinus; sinusal.

sincipital (sin-sip′ĭ-tal) pertaining to the sinciput.

sinciput (sin′sĭ-put) [L.] [NA] the anterior and upper part of the head.

Sinequan trademark for *doxepin hydrochloride* (see under DOXEPIN).

Sinetens trademark for *prazosin hydrochloride* (see under PRAZOSIN).

sinew (sin′u) the tendon of a muscle.

sing. abbreviation for L. *singulo′rum,* of each.

Singleton-Merten syndrome [E. B. *Singleton;* D. F. *Merten*] see under SYNDROME.

sinister (sin-is′ter) [L.] left; an anatomical term denoting the left-hand one of two similar structures, or the one situated on the left side of the body. Cf. DEXTER.

sinistrad (sin-is′trad) to or toward the left.

sinistral (sin′is-tral) [L. *sinistralis*] 1. pertaining to the left side. 2. a left-handed person.

sinistrality (sin″is-tral′ĭ-te) the preferential use, in voluntary motor acts, of the left member of the major paired organs of the body, as the ear, eye, hand, or leg.

sinistro- [L. *sinister* left] a combining form meaning left, or denoting relationship to the left side.

Sinomin trademark for *sulfamethoxazole.*

Sinophenin trademark for *promazine.*

Sinos trademark for *cyclopentamine hydrochloride* (see under CYCLOPENTAMINE).

Sintecort trademark for *paramethasone acetate* (see under PARAMETHASONE).

sinter (sin′ter) 1. the calcareous or silicious matter deposited by mineral springs. 2. to bring about agglomeration of metallic particles by heating to just below the melting point of the metal, as in the production of mat gold by heating electrolytic gold powder.

sintering (sin′ter-ing) the act or process of solidification in the solid state of powders, including those of metals or earthy substances, by compacting in the presence of temperatures below the melting point, such as that occurring during ceramic firing. The decrease in surface area of agglomerated particles is the principal factor in the mechanism of sintering. See also CERAMIC. **liquid phase s.,** the diffusion between solid surrounded by liquid.

sinuous (sin′u-us) [L. *sinuosus*] bending in and out; winding.

sinus (si′nus), pl. *si′nus, sinuses* [L. "a hollow"] 1. a cavity, or hollow space; used in anatomical nomenclature as a general term to designate such spaces as the dilated channels for venous blood, found chiefly in the cranium, or the air cavities in the cranial bones. 2. an abnormal channel or fistula permitting the escape of pus. **accessory s's of nose,** paranasal s's. **air s.,** an air-containing space within a bone. **s. a′lae par′vae,** sphenoparietal s. **s. aor′tae** [NA], aortic s. **aortic s.,** one of the three dilatations in the wall of the aorta at its origin, just opposite the semilunar cusps of the aortic valve, which gives rise to the coronary arteries. Called also *s. aortae* [NA] and *s. of Valsalva.* **basilar s.,** basilar PLEXUS. **bony maxillary s.,** an air cavity of variable size and shape located in the body of each maxilla, communicating with the middle meatus of the bony nasal cavity on the same side. Called also *s. maxillaris osseus* [NA]. **branchial s.,** an abnormal opening between a branchial groove and its corresponding pharyngeal pouch, homologous with an ancestral gill slit. **Breschet's s.,** sphenoparietal s. **s. carot′icus** [NA], carotid s. **carotid s.,** a slight dilatation at the terminal portion of the common carotid artery and at the internal carotid artery above the bifurcation, containing in its wall pressoreceptors that are stimulated by blood pressure changes and initiate changes in the heart rate and blood pressure to compensate for these changes. Called also *s. caroticus* [NA] and *bulbus caroticus.* See also carotid sinus REFLEX and carotid sinus SYNDROME. **s. caverno′sus** [NA], cavernous s. **cavernous s.,** an irregularly shaped venous space in the dura mater at either side of the body of the sphenoid bone, extending from the medial end of the superior orbital fissure in front to the apex of the petrous bone behind. It receives the ophthalmic vein and empties into the petrosal sinuses. The right and left sinuses communicate across the midline and are traversed by numerous trabeculae. Called also *s. cavernosus* [NA]. **circular s., s. circula′ris,** a venous circle formed by the two intercavernous sinuses and two cavernous sinuses around the pituitary. **cervical s.,** a triangular temporary depression caudal to the hyoid arch, containing the second branchial arch overlapping the next three branchial arches, formed during the sixth week of embryonic development. It is overgrown by the hyoid arch and closes off as the cervical vesicle. **cranial s's,** s's of dura mater. **Cuvier's s's,** ducts of Cuvier; see under DUCT. **s's of dura mater, s. du′rae ma′tris** [NA], large venous channels, situated between the two layers of the dura mater, which drain blood from the brain into the internal jugular vein. They are lined by endothelium, are devoid of valves, do not collapse when drained, and in some parts contain trabeculae. They also drain some diploic and meningeal veins and veins from the orbit, and communicate with superficial veins by small emissary veins. The posterior group includes the superior and inferior sagittal, straight, transverse, and occipital sinuses, and confluence of the sinuses. The anterior inferior group includes the cavernous, intercavernous, superior and inferior petrosal sinuses, and the basilar plexus. Called also *cranial s's* and *venous s's of dura mater.* **ethmoidal s., s. ethmoida′lis** [NA], one of the paired paranasal sinuses located in the ethmoid bone, and communicating with the ethmoidal infundibulum and bullae and with the superior and highest meatuses of the nasal cavity. It consists of numerous thin-walled cavities occupying the ethmoidal labyrinth (ethmoidal cells). **frontal s.,** one of the paired paranasal sinuses located in the frontal bone, and communicating by way of the nasofrontal duct with the middle meatus of the nasal cavity on the same side. They are seldom symmetrical, and the septum separating the right from the left sinus is often situated to one side. Its average size is about 3 cm in height, 2.5 cm in breadth, and 2.5 cm in depth. It is usually present at birth, but it reaches its full size only after puberty. Called also *s. frontalis* [NA]. **frontal air s.,** frontal bony s. **frontal bony s., s. fronta′lis os′seus** [NA], an irregular air sinus situated in the frontal bone on either side, deep in the superciliary arch, separated from its fellow of the opposite side by a bony septum, and communicating with the middle meatus of the bony nasal cavity on the same side. Called also *frontal air s.* **s. fronta′lis** [NA], frontal s. **s. highmori,** maxillary s. **s. interarcua′lis,** tonsillar FOSSA. **s. intercaverno′si**

[NA], intercavernous s's. **intercavernous s's,** either of the two venous channels, the anterior passing anterior to the pituitary gland and the posterior posterior to it, which connect the two cavernous sinuses across the midline. Called also *s. intercavernosi* [NA]. **s. of internal jugular vein, inferior,** inferior bulb of jugular vein; see under BULB. **s. of internal jugular vein, superior,** superior bulb of jugular vein; see under BULB. **laryngeal s.,** VENTRICLE of larynx. **lateral s.,** transverse s. of dura mater. **longitudinal s., inferior,** sagittal s., inferior. **longitudinal s., superior,** sagittal s., superior. **lymphatic s's,** irregular tortuous spaces within lymph nodes through which a continuous stream of lymph passes, to enter the efferent lymphatic vessels. **mastoid s.,** mastoid CELL. **s. maxilla′ris** [NA], maxillary s. **s. maxilla′ris os′seus** [NA], bony maxillary s. **maxillary s.,** one of the paired paranasal sinuses, presenting a large cavity within the body of the maxilla. Its base is directed toward the nasal cavity and its summit extends laterally into the root of the zygomatic process. Its thin walls correspond to the nasal, orbital, anterior, and infraorbital surfaces of the body of the maxilla. It overlies the alveolar process in which the molar teeth are implanted, especially the first and second molars; sometimes it may also overlie the premolars. A layer of bone covered by mucous membrane separates the roots of the teeth and the floor, but projecting into the floor are conical processes corresponding to the roots of the teeth; sometimes they perforate into the sinus. A large aperture communicates with the nasal cavity, but in the articulated skull, the cavity may be partly obliterated by the ethmoid bone, inferior nasal concha, and lacrimal bone. The infraorbital canal usually projects into the sinus. The posterior wall is perforated by the alveolar canals for transmission of the posterior superior alveolar vessels and nerves to the molar teeth. Called also *s. highmori, s. maxillaris, antrum of Highmore, antrum highmori, antrum maxillare,* and *maxillary antrum.* **maxillary s., bony,** bony maxillary s. **s. of Morgagni,** VENTRICLE of larynx. **occipital s., s. occipita′lis** [NA], the smallest of the venous sinuses of the dura mater. It is usually a single sinus, but occasionally there are two. The sinus begins in right and left branches (marginal sinuses) and passes upward along the margin of the falx cerebelli to end in the confluence of sinuses. **oral s.,** stomodeum. **paranasal s's, s. paranasa′les** [NA], a group of air-containing cavities in the cranial bones, having various shapes and sizes, which are lined with ciliated mucous membrane and communicate with the nasal cavity. Their function is uncertain but they are believed to help the nose in circulating, warming, and moistening the air as it is inhaled, and are thought to have a minor role as resonating chambers for the voice. They are arranged in four pairs: the maxillary sinuses, located symmetrically in the maxillae; frontal sinuses, in the frontal bone; sphenoid sinuses, in the sphenoid bone behind the nasal cavity; and ethmoid sinuses, in the ethmoid bone, behind and below the frontal sinuses. Called also *accessory s's of the nose* and *air cells of nose.* **petrosal s., inferior,** a venous sinus arising from the cavernous sinus and running along the line of the petro-occipital synchondrosis to the superior bulb of the internal jugular vein. Called also *s. petrosus inferior* [NA]. **petrosal s., superior,** a sinus arising at the cavernous sinus, passing along the attached margin of the cerebellar tentorium, and draining into the transverse sinus. Called also *s. petrosus superior* [NA]. **s. petro′sus infe′rior** [NA], petrosal s., inferior. **s. petro′sus supe′rior** [NA], petrosal s., superior. **piriform s.,** an elongated fossa in the wall of the laryngopharynx caudal to the lateral glossoepiglottic folds; it is bounded medially by the aryepiglottic fold and laterally by the thyroid cartilage and thyrohyoid membrane. Called also *piriform recess* and *recessus piriformis* [NA]. **s. rectus** [NA], straight s. **sagittal s., inferior,** a small venous sinus of the dura mater, situated in the posterior half of the free margin of the falx cerebri and opening into the upper end of the straight sinus. It receives tributaries from the falx cerebri and occasionally from the medial surface of the brain. Called also *inferior longitudinal s.* and *s. sagittalis inferior* [NA]. **sagittal s., superior,** a venous sinus of the dura mater which begins in front of the crista galli and extends backward in the convex border of the falx cerebri. Near the internal occipital protuberance it ends in a variable way in the confluence of the sinuses. It receives the superior cerebral veins, veins from the nasal cavity, veins from the diploe, and the emissary veins from the pericranium, having numerous anastomoses with veins of the nose, scalp, and diploe. Called also *s. sagittalis superior* [NA] and *superior longitudinal s.* **s. sagitta′lis infe′rior** [NA], sagittal s., inferior. **s. sagitta′lis supe′rior** [NA], sagittal s., superior. **sigmoid s., s. sigmoi′deus** [NA], either of the two venous sinuses within the dura mater that are continuations of the transverse sinuses; each curves downward from the tentorium cerebelli to become continuous with the superior bulb of the internal jugu-

lar vein. **sphenoid air s.,** sphenoidal s., bony. **sphenoidal s.,** one of the paired paranasal sinuses located in the anterior part of the body of the sphenoid bone, and communicating with the highest meatus of the nasal cavity. They are seldom symmetrical due to lateral displacement of the septum. An average sinus is about 2.2 cm in height, 2 cm in breadth, and 2.2 cm in depth. Some large sinuses extend into the roots of the pterygoid processes of the great wings of the sphenoid and may invade the basilar part of the occipital bone. At birth, they present only small cavities and are fully developed only after puberty. Called also *s. sphenoida′lis* [NA] and *sphenoid cell.* **sphenoidal s., bony,** an air cavity of variable size and shape, situated in the anterior part of the body of the sphenoid bone, separated from its fellow of the opposite side by a septum, and opening into the nasal cavity above the superior nasal concha on the same side. Called also *sphenoid air s.* and *s. sphenoidalis osseus* [NA]. **s. sphenoida′lis** [NA], sphenoidal s. **s. sphenoida′lis os′seus** [NA], sphenoidal s., bony. **sphenoparietal s., s. sphenoparieta′lis** [NA], a venous sinus of the dura mater that begins at a meningeal vein next to the apex of the small wing of the sphenoid bone, and drains into the anterior part of the cavernous sinus. Called also *s. alae parvae* and *Breschet's s.* **straight s., tentorial s.,** a venous sinus of the dura mater, situated at the line of junction of the falx cerebri with the tentorium cerebelli, formed by the junction of the great cerebral vein and the inferior sagittal sinus, and ending at the confluence of sinuses. Called also *s. rectus.* **tonsillar s., s. tonsilla′ris,** tonsillar FOSSA. **transverse s. of dura mater, s. transver′sus du′rae ma′tris** [NA], either of two large venous sinuses of the dura mater beginning in a variable fashion at the confluence of the sinuses near the internal occipital protuberance. Each follows the attached margin of the tentorium cerebelli to the petrous temporal, where it becomes the sigmoid sinus. At their origin in the confluence, the right and left sinuses communicate with each other, and with the superior sagittal sinus and the straight sinus. Called also *lateral s. of Valsalva,* aortic s. **venous s's of dura mater,** s's of dura mater.

sinusal (si′nus-al) pertaining to a sinus.

sinusitis (si″nus-i′tis) [*sinus* + *-itis*] inflammation of a sinus. **maxillary s.,** inflammation of the maxillary sinus, usually caused by extension of a dental infection, common cold, influenza, spread of infection from other paranasal sinuses, or traumatic injury. The acute form is characterized by swelling of the tissues overlying the sinus, pain on pressure, often referring to other areas, discharge of pus into the nose, fetid breath, fever, and malaise. In chronic forms symptoms are less pronounced and include a mild discharge of pus into the nose, fetid breath, vague pain, and a stuffy sensation on the affected side.

sinusoid (si′nŭ-soid) [*sinus* + Gr. *eidos* form] 1. resembling a sinus. 2. a form of terminal blood channel consisting of a large, irregular anastomosing vessel, having a lining of reticuloendothelium but little or no adventitia. Sinusoids are found in the liver, adrenals, heart, parathyroid, carotid gland, spleen, hemolymph glands, and pancreas. Called also *sinusoidal capillary.*

sinusotomy (si″nŭ-sot′o-me) [*sinus* + Gr. *tomē* a cutting] incision into a sinus.

Sionit trademark for *sorbitol.*

Sionon trademark for *sorbitol.*

Si op. sit. abbreviation for L. *si o′pus sit,* if it is necessary.

Siqualine trademark for *fluphenazine.*

Siqualon trademark for *fluphenazine.*

Siquil trademark for *triflupromazine hydrochloride* (see under TRIFLUPROMAZINE).

SIR trademark for a *silicone impression material* (see under MATERIAL).

Siris, E. see Coffin-Siris SYNDROME.

-sis a word termination of Greek origin, signifying state or condition. With a combining vowel it usually appears as *-asis, -esis, -iasis,* or *-osis.*

Sistrunk's operation see under OPERATION.

site (sīt) [L. *situs*] a place, position, or locus. **antibody-active s., antigen-binding s.,** combining s. **combining s.,** that portion of the antibody (immunoglobulin) molecule that combines specifically with the antigenic determinants. The antibody specificity is determined by the amino acid sequence that determines the tertiary structure of the Ig molecule and permits its combination with the appropriate antigen. Both heavy and light chains are involved, specifically, the first 110 amino acids from the variable amino-terminal end of each polypeptide chain determine specific antibody activity. Antibody is believed to be due to several hypervariable regions on both light and heavy chains which interact with the determinant on the antigen. Some flexibility of the polypeptide chain of the antibody molecule is required to permit exposure to the antigen of the appropriate contacting amino acids. Called also *antibody-active s.* and *antigen-binding s.* **donor s.,** the site of the body from which a graft, such as skin, bone, tooth, or other tissue, is taken for transplantation. **host s.,** one into which a graft is implanted.

sito- [Gr. *sitos* food] a combining form denoting relationship to food.

situs (si′tus), pl. *si′tus* [L.] site, or position.

Siwe, Sture August [German physician, born 1897] see Letterer-Siwe DISEASE.

size (sīz) the spatial dimensions, proportions, magnitude, or bulk of something. **field s.,** in radiography, the geometrical projection of the x-ray beam on a plane perpendicular to the central ray of the distal end of the limiting diaphragm as seen from the center of the front surface of the source, having the same shape as the aperture of the collimator. It may be determined at any distance from the source.

Sjögren's syndrome [Henrik Samuel Conrad *Sjögren,* Swedish ophthalmologist, born 1899] see under SYNDROME.

Sjögren-Larsson syndrome [Torsten *Sjögren; Tage Larsson*] see under SYNDROME.

SK 1. streptokinase. 2. Sloan-Kettering. Used with numbers to designate various chemical compounds which have been used experimentally in the treatment of cancer at Sloan-Kettering Institute for Cancer Research.

skeleton (skel′ĕ-ton) [Gr. "a dried body," "mummy"] the bony

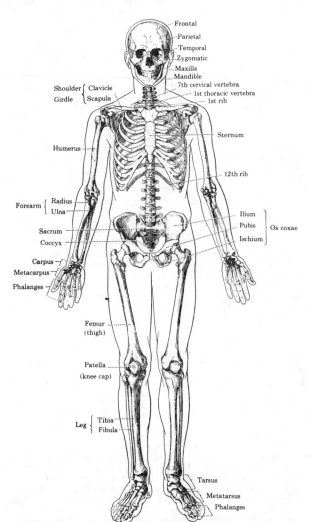

Shoulder { Clavicle
Girdle { Scapula

Frontal
Parietal
Temporal
Zygomatic
Maxilla
Mandible
7th cervical vertebra
1st thoracic vertebra
1st rib

Sternum

Humerus

12th rib

Forearm { Radius
{ Ulna

Sacrum
Coccyx

Ilium
Pubis
Ischium } Os coxae

Carpus
Metacarpus
Phalanges

Femur
(thigh)

Patella
(knee cap)

Leg { Tibia
{ Fibula

Tarsus
Metatarsus
Phalanges

Anterior view of human skeleton. (From Dorland's Illustrated Medical Dictionary. 26th ed. Philadelphia, W. B. Saunders Co., 1981; adapted from King and Showers.)

framework of the animal body. See illustration. **appendicular s.,** the part of the skeleton consisting of the bones of the limbs, shoulder, and hip girdle. **axial s.,** the part of the skeleton, consisting of the skull, spinal column, ribs, and sternum, which protects the major organs of the nervous, respiratory, and circulatory systems. **facial s.,** facial BONES. **masticatory s.,** the masticatory bones; the maxilla and mandible. **visceral s.,** the part of the skeleton which protects the viscera, consisting of the sternum, ribs, and hip bones.

skia- [Gr. *skia* shadow] a combining form denoting reference to shadows, especially of internal structures as produced by roentgen rays.

skiagram (ski′ah-gram) [*skia-* + Gr. *gramma* a writing] a roentgenogram.

skiameter (ski-am′ĕ-ter) [*skia-* + Gr. *metron* measure] an instrument for measuring the intensity of the x-rays, and thus determining how long an exposure is needed.

skin (skin) [L. *cutis;* Gr. *derma*] the outer integument or covering of the body, made up of a tough flexible tissue comprising up to 15 percent of body weight. It provides the anatomical boundary between the body and the environment and protects the internal organs from external noxious influences, such as shock, trauma, poisons, radiant energy, and temperature changes. Other functions include temperature regulation through cutaneous blood vessels and sweat glands; perception of pain, touch, and temperature through its nerves; protection against fluid loss, microorganisms, and heat loss; and secretion through the exocrine glands. The skin contains a variety of exocrine glands, nerves, blood vessels, lymphatic vessels, and muscles, and is stratified into the *epidermis, corium,* and *subcutaneous tissue.* The glandular skin appendages include the apocrine, eccrine, and sebaceous glands; the keratinized or cornified appendages include the hair and nails. Called also *cutis* [NA] and *derma.* See also common INTEGUMENT. **elastic s.,** Ehlers-Danlos SYNDROME. **lax s.,** CUTIS laxa. **mottled s.,** poikiloderma. **scalded s. syndrome,** toxic epidermal NECROLYSIS. **true s.,** corium.

Skinner, Richard C. [18th and 19th centuries] an American dentist who, in 1801, in New York, published *Treatise on the Teeth,* which was the first dental book in the United States. Skinner founded the first dental clinic in the United States.

Skinner's classification [C. N. *Skinner,* American dentist] see under CLASSIFICATION.

Skopyl trademark for *methscopolamine nitrate* (see under METHSCOPOLAMINE).

skull (skull) the bony framework of the head composed of the cranium and the facial bones. The cranium is made up of the occipital, frontal, sphenoid, ethmoid, and pairs of the parietal and temporal bones. The facial skeleton is made up of the vomer and the mandible and pairs of the maxillary, lacrimal, malar, palatine, and inferior turbinate bones. See accompanying illustrations and illustrations at CEPHALOMETRY. See also CRANIUM. **acrocephalic s.,** one with a highly arched cranial vault as seen in an anterior view, having a height-length index of more than 98.0. Called *acrocephaly.* See also *hypsicephalic s.* and OXYCEPHALY. **brachycephalic s.,** a short broad skull, with a cephalic index of 80.0–84.9. Called also *short s., brachycephalia, brachycephalism, brachycephaly,* and *brachycrany.* **brachystaphyline s.,** one with a short, wide palate, having a palatine index of 85.0 or more. **chamecephalic s., chamae-**

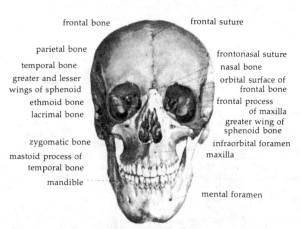

frontal bone
parietal bone
temporal bone
greater and lesser wings of sphenoid
ethmoid bone
lacrimal bone
zygomatic bone
mastoid process of temporal bone
mandible

frontal suture
frontonasal suture
nasal bone
orbital surface of frontal bone
frontal process of maxilla
greater wing of sphenoid bone
infraorbital foramen
maxilla
mental foramen

Skull of adult; anterior aspect (norma frontalis). (From J. Langman and M. W. Woerdeman: Atlas of Medical Anatomy. Philadelphia, W. B. Saunders Co., 1978.)

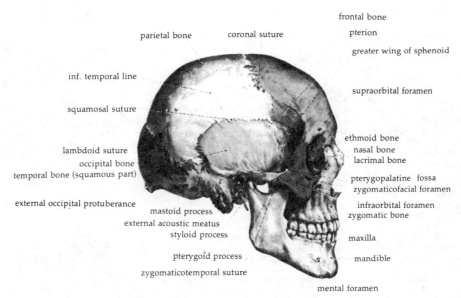

parietal bone
coronal suture
frontal bone
pterion
greater wing of sphenoid
inf. temporal line
supraorbital foramen
squamosal suture
ethmoid bone
nasal bone
lacrimal bone
lambdoid suture
occipital bone
temporal bone (squamous part)
pterygopalatine fossa
zygomaticofacial foramen
external occipital protuberance
infraorbital foramen
zygomatic bone
mastoid process
external acoustic meatus
styloid process
maxilla
pterygoid process
mandible
zygomaticotemporal suture
mental foramen

Lateral aspect of the adult skull (norma lateralis). (From J. Langman and M. W. Woerdeman: Atlas of Medical Anatomy. Philadelphia, W. B. Saunders Co., 1978.)

cephalic s., one with a low cranial vault as seen in profile, having a height-length index of no more than 69.9. Called also *low s., chamaecephaly,* and *chamecephaly.* **chamestaphyline s.,** one with a low-arched palate, having a palatal height index of 27.9 or less. **cloverleaf s.,** a rare congenital form of hydrocephalus resulting from intrauterine synostosis of the coronal and lambdoidal sutures, with bulging through the sagittal and squamosal sutures, giving the skull a flattened, cloverleaf configuration. Low set ears, beaked nose, recessed nasal root, prognathism, exophthalmos, and abnormalities of the facial bones add to the grotesque appearance of the head. Micromelia, spinal deformities, optic atrophy, blindness, and progressive mental deterioration may occur. Called also *trefoil s., cloverleaf skull syndrome, Hottermüller-Wiedemann syndrome, Kleeblattschädel,* and *trefoil skull syndrome.* **dolichocephalic s.,** a long skull having a cephalic index of 70.0–74.9. Called also *elongated s., mecocephalic s., dolichocephalia, dolichocephalism, dolichocephaly.* See also *hyperdolichocephalic s.* and *ultradolichocephalic s.* **dry s.,** the skull of a cadaver that has been cleaned of soft tissue. **elongated s.,** dolichocephalic s. **euryprosopic s.,** one with a low and wide face, having a facial index of 80.0–84.9. See also *hypereuryprosopic s.* **high s.,** see

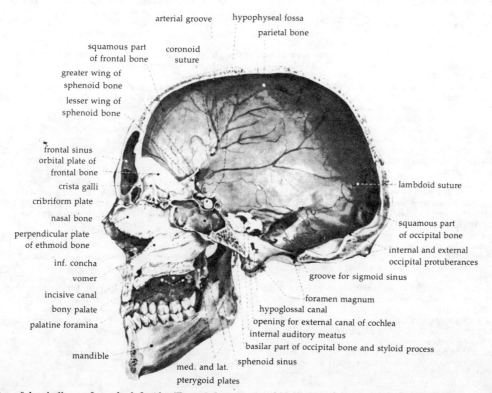

arterial groove
hypophyseal fossa
parietal bone
squamous part of frontal bone
coronoid suture
greater wing of sphenoid bone
lesser wing of sphenoid bone
frontal sinus
orbital plate of frontal bone
crista galli
cribriform plate
nasal bone
perpendicular plate of ethmoid bone
inf. concha
vomer
incisive canal
bony palate
palatine foramina
mandible
lambdoid suture
squamous part of occipital bone
internal and external occipital protuberances
groove for sigmoid sinus
foramen magnum
hypoglossal canal
opening for external canal of cochlea
internal auditory meatus
basilar part of occipital bone and styloid process
med. and lat. pterygoid plates
sphenoid sinus

Median section of the skull seen from the left side. (From J. Langman and M. W. Woerdeman: Atlas of Medical Anatomy. Philadelphia, W. B. Saunders Co., 1978.)

acrocephalic s., hypsicephalic s., and OXYCEPHALY. **hot cross bun s.,** Parrot's SIGN. **hyperbrachycephalic s.,** a very short broad skull, having a cephalic index of 85.0–89.9. **hyperdolichocephalic s.,** a severely elongated skull, having a cephalic index of 65.0–69.9. **hypereuryprosopic s.,** one with a very low and wide face, having a facial index of less than 79.9. **hyperleptoprosopic s.,** one with a very high narrow face, having a facial index of more than 95.0. **hyperprognathous s.,** one characterized by severe protrusion of the lower jaw or prognathism, having total and nasal profile angles of 69.9° or less, and an alveolar profile angle of 60.0°–69.9°. **hypsicephalic s.,** one with a high cranial vault as seen in profile, having a cephalic index of more than 75.0. Called *hypsicephaly.* See also *acrocephalic s.* and OXYCEPHALY. **hypsistaphyline s.,** one with a high-arched palate, having a palatal height index of 40.0 or more. See also HYPSISTAPHYLIA. **hypsistenocephalic s.,** one with a high, curved vertex, prominent cheek bones, and prognathic jaws. See also ACROCEPHALY and OXYCEPHALY. **lacuna s.,** craniolacunia. **leptoprosopic s.,** one with a high narrow face, having a facial index of 90.0–94.9. See also *hyperleptoprosopic s.* and LEPTOPROSOPIA. **leptostaphyline s.,** one with a long narrow palate, having a palatine index of 79.9 or less. **low s.,** chamecephalic s. **low-arched s.,** tapeinocephalic s. **maplike s.,** one marked by irregular tracings resembling outlines on a map; seen in x-ray films of the cranial bones in Hand-Schüller-Christian disease. **mecocephalic s.,** dolichocephalic s. **mesocephalic s.,** one having an average breadth and length and a cephalic index of 75.0–79.9. **mesognathous s.,** one characterized by moderate protrusion of the lower jaw, having a gnathic index of 98–103, total, alveolar, and nasal profile angles of 80.0°–84.9°, and Rivet's angle of 70.0°–72.9°. **mesoprosopic s.,** one with a face of moderate width, having a total facial index of 85.0–89.9. **mesostaphyline s.,** one with a palate of moderate length and width, having a palatine index of 80.0–84.9. **metriocephalic s.,** one with an average cranial height, as seen in an anterior view, having a cephalic index of 92.0–97.9. **natiform s.,** Parrot's SIGN. **orthocephalic s.,** one with an average cranial height and length, having a cephalic index of 70.0–74.9. **orthognathous s.,** one characterized by absence of prognathism or only a minimal protrusion of the lower jaw, having a gnathic index of 98 or less, and total, alveolar, and nasal profile angles of 85.0°–92.9°, and Rivet's angle of 73.0° or more. **orthostaphyline s.,** one with a palate of moderate height, having a palatal height index of 28.0–39.9. **prognathous s.,** one characterized by a protruding lower jaw or prognathism, having a gnathic index above 103, and total, alveolar, and nasal profile angles of 70.0°–79.9°, and a Rivet's angle of 69.9° or less. **short s.,** brachycephalic s. **steeple s., tower s.,** oxycephalic s. **tapeinocephalic s.,** one with a low-arched cranial vault as seen in an anterior view, having a height-breadth index of less than 91.9. Called also *low-arched s.* and *tapeinocephaly.* **trefoil s.,** cloverleaf s. **ultrabrachycephalic s.,** an extremely short broad skull, having a cephalic index of more than 90.0. **ultradolichocephalic s.,** an extremely long narrow skull, having a cephalic index of not more than 64.9. **ultraprognathous s.,** one characterized by extreme protrusion of the jaw (prognathism), having an alveolar profile angle of 59.9° or less. **West's lacuna s., West-Engstler s.,** a honeycomb appearance of the skull in roentgenograms, associated with spina bifida or meningocele and occasionally with encephalocele.

skullcap (skul′kap) 1. a small, brimless, close-fitting cap. 2. a type of headgear used in the past in extraoral orthodontic therapy. See also extraoral APPLIANCE. 3. calvaria.

sleep (slep) a period of rest for the body and mind, during which volition and consciousness are in partial or complete abeyance and the bodily functions partially suspended.

Sleepinal trademark for *methaqualone hydrochloride* (see under METHAQUALONE).

Sleepwell trademark for *methapyrilene hydrochloride* (see under METHAPYRILENE).

slice (slīs) 1. a thin, broad, flat piece cut from something. 2. in cavity preparation, a straight-line cut that removes a thin layer from an axial convexity.

slide (slīd) 1. a glass plate on which objects are placed for microscopic examination. 2. to move along in continuous contact with a smooth surface. **eccentric s.,** a short eccentric jaw movement path that occurs during the bringing of the teeth in contact in centric relation and, simultaneously, squeezing the jaws together into centric occlusion, usually being a combination of forward and lateral movements. **s. in centric,** a short centric jaw movement path that occurs during the bringing of

the teeth in contact in centric relation and, simultaneously, squeezing the jaws together into centric occlusion, usually being a combination of forward and lateral movements.

sling (sling) a bandage or suspensory for supporting all or a part of the body. Also used in anatomy to describe a part of the body which performs a similar function. **s. ligation,** sling SUTURE. **mandibular s.,** a structure formed by the masseter and medial pterygoid muscles; it suspends the mandible and assists in mandibulomaxillary articulation. **sling s.,** sling SUTURE.

slip (slip) 1. to move, pass, or go smoothly or easily; to glide, or slide. 2. a fluid suspension of clay, fluxing material, and water, used to coat ceramics before the glaze stage of firing. 3. the sliding of atoms over one another in a crystal, proceeding most readily along certain crystallographic planes in specific directions. Plastic deformation occurs by atoms sliding along these lines. See also DISLOCATION (2) and slip PLANE. See illustration. **interference s.,** in dental materials, irregularities at grain boundaries that prevent or interfere with the slippage of one grain over another. **s. plane,** slip PLANE.

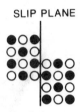

SLIP PLANE

Atomic configuration in a slip occurring in a solid solution.

slit (slit) 1. a long narrow opening or incision. 2. to make a long narrow opening or incision.

Slo-Flo phosphate topical solution see under SOLUTION.

slope (slōp) 1. an inclined plane; a surface which is neither horizontal nor vertical. 2. to deviate from the horizontal and from the vertical plane; said of a surface intersecting the horizontal at an angle between 1 and 90 degrees. **mandibular anteroposterior ridge s.,** lower ridge s. **lower ridge s.,** the slope of the crest of the mandibular residual ridge from the third molar region to its most anterior aspect in relation to the lower border of the mandible as viewed in profile. Called also *mandibular anteroposterior ridge slope.* **mandibular anteroposterior ridge s.,** the slope of the crest of the mandibular residual ridge from the third molar region to its most anterior aspect in relation to the lower border of the mandible as viewed in profile.

slough (sluf) 1. necrotic tissue in the process of separating from viable portions of the body. 2. to shed or cast off.

sloughing (sluf′ing) the formation or separation of a slough.

Sluder's headache, neuralgia, operation [Greenfield *Sluder,* American laryngologist, 1865–1928] see sphenopalatine NEURALGIA, and see under OPERATION.

sludge (sluj) a suspension of solid or semisolid particles in a fluid which itself may or may not be a viscous fluid.

sludging (sluj′ing) the settling out of solid particles from solution. **s. of blood,** intravascular AGGLUTINATION.

Sm samarium.

smallpox (smawl′poks) an acute contagious viral disease, characterized by vomiting, lumbar pain, a papular eruption that becomes vesicular and finally pustular, and fever. Symptoms appear after an incubation period of about 12 days but the eruption occurs the third or fourth day after the prodromal symptoms of chills and fever with the formation of small red spots. Oral manifestations include ulcers of the mucosa and pharynx, sometimes also involving the esophagus and trachea, and swelling and pain of the tongue. Vesicles of the mucous membranes are similar to those of the skin, except instead of developing into pustules they rupture and produce ulcers. Called also *variola.* For specific forms, see VARIOLA. See also variola VIRUS. **black s.,** hemorrhagic VARIOLA.

smear (smēr) a specimen for microscopic study prepared by spreading the material across the glass slide. **blood s.,** BLOOD smear. **Pap s., Papanicolaous's s.,** see Pap TEST.

smell (smel) olfaction; the act or process of perceiving odors. See also olfactory ORGAN and terms beginning OLFACTO-.

Smith, Erwin F. [1854–1927] an American bacteriologist. See ERWININIA.

Smith, Lucian A. [American physician, born 1910] see Achor-Smith SYNDROME.

Smith, Theobald see THEOBALD SMITH.

Smith's resin cement see under CEMENT.

Smith's zinc cement see under CEMENT.

Smith-Lemli-Opitz syndrome [David W. *Smith,* American physician; Luc *Lemli;* John M. *Opitz,* American physician, born 1935] see under SYNDROME.

SMON *s*ubacute *m*yelo-*opticon*europathy (virus); see under VIRUS.

Smyth, Francis Scott see infantile cortical HYPEROSTOSIS (Caffey-Smyth syndrome).

Sn 1. tin (L. *stannum*). 2. subnasale.

snare (snār) a wire loop or noose, such as one used for removing polyps and tumors by encircling them at the base and closing the loop.

SNDA Student National Dental Association.

sneeze (snēz) 1. an involuntary, sudden, and audible act of expulsion of air through the nose, being a mechanism for clearing obstructions from the upper respiratory passages. Sometimes sneezing may be caused by irritation without any obstruction in the air passages, as in hay fever. 2. to expel air suddenly through the nose.

Sn$_{7-8}$Hg α_2-phase of dental amalgam; see α-PHASE.

snoring (snor'ing) noisy breathing in which the inspired or expired air vibrates the uvula and soft palate, usually occurring in sleep in persons who sleep with their mouth open, and in coma. Called also *stertor* and *stertorous respiration.*

snow (sno) a freezing or frozen mixture consisting of discrete particles or crystals, usually of water. **carbon dioxide s.,** dry ice; solid carbon dioxide, formed by rapid evaporation of liquid carbon dioxide; it gives a temperature of about −79°C (−110°F), and is sometimes used in cryosurgery, though it has been almost entirely supplanted by liquid nitrogen.

Snow, George B. [1835–1923] an American dentist who invented the articulator.

SO spheno-occipital SYNCHONDROSIS (2).

soap (sōp) [L. *sapo*] a product of reaction of alkali with animal or vegetable fats. A typical soap is made by reacting sodium hydroxide with a fatty acid. Soaps lower the surface tension of water and, thus, permit emulsification of fat-bearing soil particles in their cleansing action. See also DETERGENT. **antibacterial s.,** a soap containing an antibacterial agent, usually hexachlorophene, triclosan, tribromsalan, or triclocarban. **carbolic s.,** a disinfectant soap containing 10 percent phenol. **Castile s.,** a hard soap, either white or mottled, prepared from olive oil and soda; used in pills, suppositories, plasters, and liniments. Called also *sapo.* **s. clay,** bentonite. **Gamophen antibacterial s.,** a trademark for an antibacterial soap containing 2.0 percent hexachlorophene in a base of sodium stearate and sodium laurate. **Germa-Medica liquid surgical s.,** trademark for a liquid antibacterial soap containing 1.0 percent hexachlorophene in a base of soap prepared from olive oil and coconut oil. **green s.,** a potassium soap made by the saponification of vegetable oils, excluding coconut oil and palm kernel oil, without the removal of glycerin. It is the chief ingredient of green soap tincture. Called also *medicinal soft s., soft s.,* and *sapo mollis medicinalis.* **hard s.,** soda s. **hexachlorophene liquid s.,** a solution of hexachlorophene in a 10 to 13 percent solution of potassium soap, containing in each 100 gm, 225 to 260 mg of hexachlorophene. Used as a topical anti-infective and detergent. **medicinal soft s.,** green s. **mineral s.,** bentonite. **potash s., soft s.** (1). **Septic-S.,** trademark for a liquid antibacterial soap containing 0.25 percent triclosan and various amounts of detergents, wetting agents, ethoxylated lanolin, propylene glycol, preservatives, and coloring and fragrance agents. **soda s.,** a soap made from soda and olive oil. Called also *hard s.* **soft s.,** 1. a liquid soap made from potash and oil. Called also *potash s.* and *sapo mollis.* 2. soda s. **zinc s.,** one containing zinc oxide or zinc sulfate; for use as an ointment or plaster.

soapstone (sop'stōn) native TALC.

Sobril trademark for *oxazepam.*

socia (so'she-ah) [L. "comrade," "associate"] a detached part or exclave of an organ. **s. parot'idis,** parotid gland, accessory; see under GLAND.

Social Security Administration see under ADMINISTRATION.

society (so-si'ē-te) a group of persons with shared interests organized together for various purposes, such as religious, scientific, or benevolent. **American S. for the Advancement of Anesthesia in Dentistry,** a professional dental association whose major tasks and objectives include the promotion and development of modern pain control techniques for use by the dentists. Abbreviation *ASAAD.* **American S. of Dentistry for Children,** a professional dental society having as its aim stimulation of dental care for children, promotion of the foundation of dental departments in children's hospitals, encouragement of research in the field of pedodontics, creation of awareness of children's dental health needs, and contribution to easing access to health care services and prevention of dental diseases. Abbreviated *ASDC.* **American Endodontic S.,** an organization of professional persons in the field of dentistry and allied professions sharing a scientific and clinical interest in root canal therapy, whose objectives include the promotion and provision of educational and scientific programs designed to further knowledge and understanding of the subject of the root canal and endeavoring to preserve the right of the general practitioner to engage in dental procedures for which he is qualified by education and experience. Abbreviation *AES.* **American Equilibration S.,** a professional dental association dedicated to the study of stresses as they apply to or affect the structures and functions of the temporomandibular regions and related parts. Abbreviated *AES.* **American Prosthodontic S.,** a professional dental society having as its objectives the advancement of goals of prosthetic dentistry, including education, research, development of dentures, health and comfort of the patient, ethical and professional standards, and the welfare of the profession and the general public. Abbreviated *APS.* **American S. of Psychosomatic Dentistry and Medicine,** a professional society of physicians, dentists, psychologists, research workers, and teachers in the field of psychosomatic dentistry and medicine, having as its objectives the study of hypnosis in dentistry and medicine and the psychological, psychiatric, and psychopharmacological aspects of patient illness and management, aimed at providing better patient care and better interprofessional relationship and understanding between physician, dentist, and psychologist. Abbreviated *ASPDM.* **American S. for the Study of Orthodontics,** a professional society established to encourage the continuing education of its members, through the medium of lectures, seminars, study clubs, orthodontic clinic affiliations, and demonstration clinics. It was originally established as the *New York Society for the Study of Orthodontics.* **American S. for Testing and Materials,** a national organization for testing and evaluating materials. The American Dental Association is represented in the Society in the Committee F-4 on Medical and Surgical Materials and Devices. The dental profession is also represented in the Society in the Committee F-8 on Protective Equipment for Sports. Abbreviated *ASTM.* **Christian Dental S.,** a society having as its objective the promotion of Christian principles throughout the world, the support of Christian-sponsored mission schools and hospitals with supplies and equipment, and arranging for volunteers to serve tours of service in various countries. Abbreviated *CDS.* **New York S. for the Study of Orthodontics,** former name for the *American S. for the Study of Orthodontics.*

socket (sok'et) a hollow or depression into which a corresponding part fits. **alveolar s.,** dental ALVEOLUS. **dry s.,** a condition sometimes occurring after tooth extraction, particularly after traumatic extraction, resulting in a dry appearance of the exposed bone in the socket, due to disintegration or loss of the blood clot. It is basically a focal osteomyelitis without suppuration and is accompanied by severe pain (alveolalgia) and foul odor. Called also *alveolar osteitis* and *alveolitis sicca dolorosa.* **eye s.,** orbit. **tooth s.,** dental ALVEOLUS.

soda (so'dah) a term applied loosely to sodium bicarbonate (baking soda), sodium hydroxide (caustic soda), or sodium carbonate (washing soda). **s. aluminosilicate,** sodium FELDSPAR. **baking s.,** SODIUM bicarbonate. **s. feldspar,** sodium FELDSPAR. **sal s.,** SODIUM carbonate. **s. soap,** soda SOAP. **washing s.,** SODIUM carbonate.

Soddy see Fajans-Soddy LAW.

sodii (so'de-i) [L.] genitive of *sodium.*

sodium (so'de-um), gen. *so'dii* [L. *natrium*] a metallic element. Symbol, Na; atomic number, 11; atomic weight, 22.990; specific gravity, 0.971; melting point, 97.6°C; valence, 1; group IA of the periodic table. It occurs as one natural isotope (23) and several radioactive ones (20–22, 24–26). Freshly cut sodium is a soft, alkaline, silvery white, lustrous metal, but tarnishes on exposure to air. With a valence of 1, it has a strong affinity for oxygen and other nonmetallic elements, decomposes water on contact, and is soluble in liquid ammonia, but not in organic solvents. Principal physiological functions of sodium include maintenance of water balance and osmotic pressure, acid balance, and neuromuscular irritability, whereby sodium is the chief cation and chloride the chief anion of extracellular fluids, and potassium is the chief cation of intracellular fluids. Sodium deficiency is rare in humans and is almost always associated with chloride deficiency. A prolonged low-sodium diet causes weakness, fatigability, apathy, anorexia, nausea, and muscle cramps. Excessive sweating causes losses of sodium, but, ordinarily, sodium in foods is sufficient for bodily needs. The sodium content of the dental enamel is decreased in caries. It is a highly toxic, caustic, and irritant substance, also presenting a severe fire risk. **s. acid carbonate,** s. bicarbonate. **s. acid sulfite,** s. bisulfite. **s. alkyl sulfoacetate,** $C_{14}H_{27}NaO_5S$, a water-soluble, white powder with a faint odor of coconut. Used as an emulsifier and foaming agent. **s. aluminosilicate,** sodium FELDSPAR. **s. aminosalicylate,** sodium AMINOSALICYLATE. **ampicillin s.,** AMPICILLIN sodium. **s. aurothiomalate,** GOLD sodium thiomalate. **aurothiosulfate s.,** GOLD sodium thiosulfate. **s. benzypenicillinate,** PENICILLIN G sodium. **s. biborate,** s. borate. **s. bicarbonate,** $CHNaO_3$, a white, odorless, crystalline powder with a saline and slightly alkaline taste, which is soluble in water, but not in organic solvents. Used as a gastric antacid, in the treatment of pruritus by local application in the form of a moist paste, to neutralize weak acid solutions, and in a boiling water sterilizer to retard corrosion of steel (but not aluminum) instruments. Because it reacts with hydrochloric acid with the production of carbon dioxide, its gastric antacid action may be complicated by epigastric distress. It has mild abrasive properties and is, thus, used as a dentifrice, either alone or with other materials. A 2 percent sodium bicarbonate solution may be used as a mouthwash. Called also *s. hydrogen carbonate, s. acid carbonate, baking soda,* and *bicarbonate of soda.* **s. bisulfite,** $NaHSO_3$, a white to yellowish granular powder or crystals that are unstable in air and are soluble in water and ethanol. Used as an antioxidant and stabilizing agent for substances such as epinephrine, phenylephrine, and other vasoconstrictors that are readily oxidized. Called also *s. acid sulfite* and *s. hydrogen sulfite.* **s. borate,** $Na_2B_4O_7$, occurring in its anhydrous form as white, efflorescent crystals, powder, or granules that are soluble in water and glycerol, but not in ethanol. Used in industrial processes and as a pharmaceutic alkalizing agent. In dentistry, used as a component of some mouthwashes and to retard the setting action of dental stone. Ingestion by young children may cause vomiting, diarrhea, shock, and death. Called also *s. biborate, s. pyroborate, s. tetraborate,* and *borax.* **s. calciumedetate,** CALCIUM disodium edetate. **s. carbonate,** $Na_2CO_3 \cdot H_2O$, colorless crystals or a white crystalline powder. Used as general cleanser, water softener, and alkalizing agent in pharmaceutical preparations. Therapeutically, used as a bath in the treatment of scaly skin and as a detergent. Also used in developing solution for x-ray films. Excessive exposure may produce a cutaneous reaction and ingestion may cause gastrointestinal corrosion resulting in diarrhea, vomiting, nausea, and, in severe cases, death. Called also *sal soda* and *washing soda.* See also developing SOLUTION. **s. carboxymethylcellulose,** sodium CARBOXYMETHYLCELLULOSE. **s. cellulose glycolate,** sodium CARBOXYMETHYLCELLULOSE. **s. chloride,** NaCl, a white, odorless, salty, hygroscopic powder, crystals, or granules that are soluble in water and glycerol and slightly soluble in alcohol. It is a source of sodium and chloride ions in the body, being absorbed through the intestines and excreted chiefly in the urine and also in sweat and other excretions. Used alone or with glucose as a plasma substitute in physiological solution. Acute excessive intake may cause intoxication with edema: chronic excessive intake may contribute to the development of hypertension. Therapeutically, sodium chloride is used as an electrolyte replenisher, topical anti-inflammatory, and emetic. In dentistry, used as an accelerator of hardening for dental plaster. Called also *common, kitchen, rock,* or *table salt,* and *halite.* See also salt STERILIZATION. **s. citrate,** $C_6H_5O_7Na_3$, occurring in the anhydrous state as odorless, white crystals, powder, or granules with a saline taste, which are soluble in water, but not in alcohol. It has alkalizing, diuretic, expectorant, and sudorific properties. Used in the treatment of chronic metabolic acidosis and as an *in vitro* anticoagulant in blood banks. Some sodium citrate preparations, such as Shohl's solution, may cause irritation of the oral mucous membrane, resulting in necrotic and ulcerative lesions. Called also *trisodium citrate.* Trademarks: Citrosodine, Citnatin. **s. dehydrocholate,** a sodium salt of dehydrocholic acid (see under ACID). Trademarks: Carachol, Decholin Sodium, Dycholium, Dychon, Suprachol. **dibasic s. phosphate,** dibasic sodium PHOSPHATE. **s. dioctyl sulfosuccinate,** DIOCTYL sodium sulfosuccinate. **dodecyl s. sulfate,** s. lauryl sulfate. **s. feldspar,** sodium FELDSPAR. **s. fluoride,** sodium FLUORIDE. **s. fluorosilicate, fluosilicate,** s. hexafluorosilicate. **s. formaldehyde sulfoxylate,** the monosodium salt of hydroxymethanesulfinic acid, occurring as white crystals or crystalline masses with the characteristic odor of garlic, which are soluble

in water, but not in ethanol, benzene, and ether. It is a mercury antidote which combines with mercuric chloride to form insoluble mercurous salts or metallic mercury. Called also *s. hydroxymethanesulfinate, s. methanalsulfoxylate,* and *formaldehyde sodium sulfoxylate.* Trademarks: Aldanil, Rongalite. **s. gentisate,** the sodium salt of gentisic acid. Trademarks: Gentinatre, Gentisod, Legential. **gold s. thiosulfate,** GOLD sodium thiosulfate. **s. hexafluorosilicate,** Na_2SiF_6, a white, odorless, tasteless powder that is slightly soluble in cold and readily soluble in hot water, but not in alcohol. Similarly to other fluorides, it is highly toxic, particularly to the digestive tract on ingestion and to the skin and mucous membranes on contact. Used as an agricultural bactericide, fungicide, and pesticide. In dentistry, it is sometimes used as a topical agent in dental caries control. Called also *s. fluorosilicate, s. fluosilicate,* and *s. silicofluoride.* Trademark: Salufer. See also FLUORIDE. **s. hydrogen carbonate,** s. bicarbonate. **s. hydrogen sulfite,** s. bisulfite. **s. hydroxymethanesulfinate,** s. formaldehyde sulfoxylate. **s. hypochlorite,** NaClO, a strong oxidizing agent, which may be used as a 5 percent aqueous solution without an alkalizing agent or with one such as sodium bicarbonate (*alkaline sodium hypochlorite solution*) for germicidal, bleaching, and deodorizing purposes. It is a clear, yellowish-green solution with a strong odor of chlorine, which deteriorates when exposed to light. In dentistry, it is used as a solvent for pulp tissue and organic debris in root canal therapy and as a cleaning agent for dentures. The solution is caustic and may cause tissue damage. An alkaline solution with sodium hydroxide (Antiformin) has been tried in periodontal therapy, but is believed to cause nonselective tissue injury. A 0.5 percent solution (*diluted sodium hypochlorite solution*), alkalized with sodium bicarbonate, is a light yellowish liquid with faint chlorine odor. It is used as a topical antiseptic for irrigating wounds and in mouthwashes (called also *Carrel-Dakin solution, Dakin's fluid, Dakin's solution, Dakin's modified solution, Labarraque's solution,* and *surgical chlorinated soda solution.* Trademarks: Clorox, Dazzle). Sodium hypochlorite may cause mucous corrosion on ingestion, respiratory disorders on inhalation, and skin and mucous membrane irritation on contact. Sodium bicarbonate is its principal antidote. **s. hyposulfite,** s. thiosulfate. **s. iodide,** NaI, white, odorless, deliquescent crystals or powder with a saline bitter taste. It is soluble in water, alcohol, and glycerol, and, on exposure to air, absorbs up to about 5 percent moisture. Used as an iodine supplement and expectorant. Also used as a source of iodine in various preparations. Trademarks: Anayodin, Ioduril. **s. iodide-**^{131}**I,** s. iodide, radioactive. **s. iodide, radioactive,** a sodium iodide preparation containing a radioactive iodine isotope (^{131}I, which has a half-life of 8 days and emits beta and gamma rays. Used as a tracer in thyroid function tests. Called also *s. iodide-*^{131}*I.* Trademarks: Iodotope, Oriodide. **s. lactate,** the monosodium salt of 2-hydroxypropanoic acid. Used in solution, occurring as a colorless, thick, odorless liquid miscible with ethanol, as an electrolyte replenisher for correction of metabolic acidosis. Trademark: Lacolin. **s. lauroyl sarcosinate,** the sodium salt of *N*-methyl-*N*-(1-oxododecyl)glycine, occurring as a white to yellowish, water-soluble powder. Used in dentifrices as an enzyme-inhibitor, detergent, and foaming agent. Trademarks: Gardol, Medialan. **s. lauryl sulfate,** $NaC_{12}H_{25}SO_4$, a surface-active agent, occurring as small, white or light yellow crystals with a characteristic odor, which are soluble in water, giving an opalescent solution. Used as a wetting agent, emulsifying aid, and detergent in various cosmetic and dermatological preparations. Also used as a toothpaste ingredient. Called also *dodecyl s. sulfate.* Trademark: Irium. **s. metaphosphate,** a compound, $(NaPO_3)_n$, where *n* may range from 3 to 10 for cyclic molecules and larger numbers for polymers. Various forms of sodium metaphosphate are used in water softening, in detergents, as food additives, and as dental polishing agents. **s. methanesulfoxylate,** s. formaldehyde sulfoxylate. **s. monofluorophosphate,** Na_2PFO_3, a fluoride compound, occurring as a white to slightly grayish, odorless powder that is freely soluble in water. Used topically in dental caries control in 6 percent solution for daily application by brushing or in dentifrices. Abbreviated *MFP.* **s. nitrite,** $NaNO_2$, a white to yellowish granular powder or white opaque, fused masses or sticks, which are soluble in water and sparingly in ethanol. Used in the treatment of cyanide poisoning; it produces methemoglobin which combines with cyanide ions and renders them temporarily inactive. Also used in dentistry as a rust inhibitor during the disinfection of instruments. Used in the past as a smooth muscle relaxant. Called also *erinitrit* and *nitrous acid sodium salt.* **s. paraaminosalicylate,** sodium AMINOSALICYLATE. **s. pentachlorophenate,** 2,3,4,5,6-pentachlorophenate, occurring as a buff-colored solid that is soluble in water and alcohol. Used as a disinfectant for instruments and as an industrial bactericide and fungicide. **s. perborate,** $NaBO_3$, a white, odorless, crystalline powder, moderately soluble in water, which is saline to taste, prepared by interaction of boric acid or sodium borate with sodium or hydrogen peroxide. Used in dentistry as a bleaching agent and topical antiseptic in mouthwashes and dentifrices because of its ability to liberate oxygen and its supposed therapeutic effect in gingival diseases caused by anaerobic infections, including necrotic ulcerative gingivitis. Adverse effects may produce chemical burns characterized by erythema of the oral mucosa, sometimes associated with sloughing of the tissue. **s. pertechnetate,** sodium PERTECHNETATE. **phenobarbital s.,** PHENOBARBITAL sodium. **s. pump,** sodium PUMP. **s. pyroborate,** s. borate. **s. ricinoleate,** the sodium salt of ricinoleic acid, occurring as a white odorless powder that is soluble in water and alcohol. Used as a sclerosing agent. It has been tested as a potential plaque and calculus inhibitor. **saccharin s.,** soluble SACCHARIN. **s. salicylate,** SALICYLATE sodium. **s. silicofluoride,** s. hexafluorosilicate. **s. sulfate,** Na_2SO_4, a white, bitter, odorless powder or crystals that are soluble in water and glycerol, but not in ethanol. Used as a saline cathartic. Called also *anhydrous sodium sulfate.* Sodium sulfate occurs in nature as the minerals mirabilite and thenardite. Sodium sulfate decahydrate, $Na_2SO_4 \cdot 10H_2O$, occurs as transparent, efflorescent crystals or granules that are soluble in water and glycerol, but not in ethanol. Called also *Glauber's salt.* **s. sulfite,** $Na_2SO_3 \cdot 7H_2O$, colorless efflorescent crystals that are readily soluble in water. Used in fixing solution in developing x-ray film. Formerly used in the treatment of dyspepsia, and externally in parasitic diseases. **s. tetraborate,** s. borate. **s. thiosulfate,** $Na_2S_2O_3 \cdot 5H_2O$, a colorless, crystalline powder or crystals that are deliquescent in moist air, efflorescent in dry air, and soluble in water, but not in ethanol. Used as an antidote in cyanide poisoning, usually in conjunction with nitrites, forming thiocyanate. Also used as an antidote for iodine compounds. It is a strong antifungal agent that is useful in the topical treatment of certain dermatophytoses. Formerly used in the treatment of arsenic poisoning. It is an antioxidant and preservative of aqueous solutions of epinephrine, phenylephrine, and other vasoconstrictors that are readily oxidized. Also used as a fixative in developing x-ray and photographic film (sometimes referred to as *hypo*). Called also *s. hyposulfite* and *antichlor.* Trademarks: Ametox, Sodothiol, Sulfothiorine. **s. thiosulfate, gold,** GOLD sodium thiosulfate.

Sodothiol trademark for *sodium thiosulfate* (see under SODIUM).

Soemmering, small process of [Samuel Thomas *Soemmering,* German anatomist, 1755–1830] marginal tubercle of zygomatic bone; see under TUBERCLE.

So-Flo phosphate topical gel see under GEL.

Soframycin trademark for *neomycin B.*

softener (sof'ĕ-ner) a substance that promotes or increases softness, smoothness, or plasticity of another substance. **carious dentin s.,** a solution which softens carious dentin, and is used to facilitate its removal.

softening (sof'en-ing) [Gr. *malakia*] the process of becoming soft; a pathologic process of becoming soft. See also MALACIA.

software (soft'wār) any computer program or programming aid, written either in computer language, English, or algebraic formulations, used to simplify computer programming and operations. Cf. HARDWARE.

Sol. solution.

sol (sol) 1. a colloidal solution; see COLLOID (2). See also AEROSOL, ELECTROSOL, and HYDROSOL. 2. the liquid phase of a colloidal solution. **lyophilic s.,** a colloidal system in which the dispersed phase is a liquid and attracts the dispersing medium, such as a hydrocolloid. **lyophobic s.,** a colloidal system in which the dispersed solid, such as a metal, has no attraction for the dispersion medium and tends to separate. **metal s.,** a colloidal dispersion of metals in a liquid. Such dispersions often have catalytic properties similar to those of enzymes and are sometimes called *inorganic enzymes.* Metal sols are lyophobic colloidal systems in which the dispersed solid phase has no attraction for the dispersion medium and tends to separate. **solid s.,** a colloidal system in which both the dispersed phase and the dispersion medium are solids.

sola (so'lah) [L.] plural of *solum.*

Solacin trademark for *tybamate.*

Solamin trademark for *benzethonium chloride* (see under BENZETHONIUM).

Solanaceae (sol"ah-na'se-e) a large genus of widely distributed herbs, shrubs, and trees, including many poisonous species and numerous species that have medicinal properties. *Atropa, Capsicum, Datura, Duboisia, Hyoscyamus, Nicotiana, Scopolia,* and *Solanum* are some of the genera of medical importance.

Solantoin trademark for *phenytoin sodium* (see under PHENYTOIN).

Solanum (so-la'num) [L. "nightshade"] a genus of solanaceous plants, including the potato, tomato, eggplant, several of the nightshades, and many poisonous and medicinal species.

solar (so'lar) [L. *solaris*] 1. pertaining to the sun. 2. denoting the great sympathetic plexus and its principal ganglia; so called because of their radiating nerves.

solarization (so"lar-i-za'shun) a method of making an exact duplicate of a radiograph by exposing the original, with an unexposed film under it, to sunlight. At first, a reversal of the image occurs, but finally the same image as that of the original film will be produced. The same result may be produced with an artificial light source.

Solatene trademark for *β-carotene* (see CAROTENE).

Solaxin trademark for *chlorzoxazone.*

Solbase trademark for *polyethylene glycol* (see under GLYCOL).

Solbrol A trademark for *ethylparaben.*

Solbrol P trademark for *propylparaben.*

solder (sod'er) [L. *solidatio* making solid, fastening] 1. a fusible metal or alloy of metals used to unite pieces of less fusible metals. 2. to fasten together pieces of metal through the use of fusible metals or alloys of metals. **building s.,** a solder that is used to build bulk on certain structures, as in establishing proper contact areas on inlays and crowns with adjacent teeth, without actually soldering parts together. Sticky solder is generally used for building purposes. **gold s.,** a solder having gold as the principal constituent. See table. **hard s.,** a solder having a high fusion point, being stronger and more tarnish resistant than soft solders. Hard solders are the type used in dentistry. **hardened s.,** one that is cooled slowly from a temperature of 450°C (840°F). **silver s.,** a solder having silver as the principal constituent. See table. **soft s.,** a low melting solder, being less resistant to tarnish and weaker than hard solders. Not used in dentistry. **softened s.,** one that is quanched in water from a temperature of 700°C (1292°F). **sticky s.,** one that appears to melt but not flow, usually occurring when large amounts of copper are used at the expense of silver. Generally used as building solders. **white s.,** one in which a white coloration is achieved by replacing the copper with nickel.

soldering (sod'er-ing) the joining of pieces of metal through the use of an alloy which has a lower melting point, usually at least 100°C (180°F) below the fusion temperature of the parts being soldered. Soldering is accomplished by melting the solder which, upon solidifying, joins the parts together, producing a primary (metallic) bonding. In dentistry, soldering is used for joining components of a dental appliance, as in assembling a bridge, joining metals to orthodontic bands, or adding to the bulk of certain structures, such as the establishment of proper contact areas on inlays and crowns with adjacent teeth. See also WELDING.

sole (sōl) [L. *solea; planta*] the bottom of the foot.

COMPOSITION AND MELTING RANGES OF DENTAL GOLD SOLDERS

Solder No.	Gold (%)	Silver (%)	Copper (%)	Zinc (%)	Tin (%)	Melting Range (°C.)	Melting Range (°F.)
A	65.4	15.4	12.4	3.9	3.1	745–785	1375–1445
B	66.1	12.4	16.4	3.4	2.0	750–805	1385–1480
C	65.0	16.3	13.1	3.9	1.7	765–800	1410–1470
D	72.9	12.1	10.0	3.0	2.0	755–835	1390–1535
E	80.9	8.1	6.8	2.1	2.0	745–870	1375–1595

(Adapted from R. W. Phillips: Skinner's Science of Dental Materials. 7th ed. Philadelphia, W. B. Saunders Co., 1973; compiled from R. L. Coleman: National Bureau of Standards Research Paper No. 32.)

COMPOSITION AND FUSION RANGES OF DENTAL SILVER SOLDERS

Solder No.	Silver (%)	Copper (%)	Cadmium (%)	Zinc (%)	Nickel (%)	Melting Range (°C.)	(°F.)
1*	56	22	–	17	–	622–668	1152–1230
2	50	15.5	16	15.5	3	646–688	1195–1270
3	45	15	24	16	–	607–618	1125–1145
4†	67	–	–	‍	–	724‡	1335‡
5	50	15.5	18	16.5	–	630–640	1160–1175
6*	56	22	–	17	–	630–650	1165–1200
7§	42	31	7	20	–	–	–

*Contains 5 per cent tin.
†Contains copper and indium, amounts not specified.
‡Liquidus temperature.
§Experimental solder by P. B. Taylor.
(From R. W. Phillips: Skinner's Science of Dental Materials. 7th ed. Philadelphia, W. B. Saunders Co., 1973.)

solenoid (so′lĕ-noid) [Gr. *sōlen* pipe, gutter, channel + *eidos* shape, form] a coil of wire spaced equally between turns, which acts like a magnet when an electric current is passed through it.

Solevar trademark for *norethandrolone*.

Solganal trademark for *aurothioglucose*.

solid (sol′id) [L. *solidus*] 1. a state of matter in which it assumes a definite shape and volume, having length, breadth, and thickness, and being firm or compact, whereby the relative motion of the molecules has been restricted in a definite fixed position relative to each other, giving rise to a crystalline structure. 2. characterized by firmness; not gaseous or fluid. 3. a substance that is firm, not fluid or gaseous. **α-s.**, α-solid SOLUTION. **β-s.**, β-solid SOLUTION. **covalent network s.**, a solid composed of atoms which are covalently bonded with their neighbors to give a three-dimensional network, forming crystals which may be visualized as giant molecules. The forces between atoms are due to very strong covalent bonds, and result in very high melting points, low vapor pressure, and hardness. Covalent network solids are poor thermal and electric conductors. They include diamond and quartz. **crystalline s.**, a solid characterized by rigidity and by the regular arrangement of its atoms or molecules with respect to one another. **ionic s.**, a solid composed of oppositely charged ions occupying sites in the crystal lattice, each positively charged ion and each negatively charged ion surrounding itself with large numbers of oppositely charged ions at the shortest possible interionic distance. Ionic solids having ions with charges of equal magnitude have crystal lattices determined by the relative sizes of the positive and negative ions. The interionic forces in ionic crystals are strong and result in high melting points and hardness. They include sodium chloride and calcium fluoride. **metallic s.**, a solid composed of metal atoms occupying the lattice sites. Most metallic solids have closed packed structures in which each atom touches its 12 nearest neighbors. They are very good electrical and thermal conductors and their electrons are thought to be responsible for carrying an electric current. They are thought of as a lattice of metal ions which is occupied by electrons that are free to move about in the lattice. Physical properties of metallic solids vary, the hardness ranging from very hard in the case of tungsten to very soft for the alkali metals and the melting point ranging from −38.9°C for mercury to 3370°C for tungsten. **molecular s.**, a solid composed of discrete covalent molecules held together in a lattice by weak intermolecular forces. Solids in this class have the lowest melting points and the highest vapor pressure. They tend to be soft, are poor thermal conductors, and act as electrical insulators. Molecular solids include ice, dry ice, naphthalene, sulfur, and white phosphorus. **s. solution**, solid SOLUTION.

solidification (so-lid″i-fi-ka′shun) changing from the liquid phase to the solid phase; freezing. See also CRYSTALLIZATION. **s. nucleus**, solidification NUCLEUS. **s. temperature**, freezing TEMPERATURE.

solidus (sol′i-dus) a temperature concentration curve of a solution on the phase diagram (see under DIAGRAM), indicating its solid phase; called also *solidus curve* and *solidus line*. Cf. LIQUIDUS.

solitary (sol′i-ter″e) [L. *solitarius*] placed alone; not grouped with others.

Solprin trademark for *calcium acetylsalicylate* (see under CALCIUM).

Solubacter trademark for *triclocarban*.

solubility (sol″u-bil′ĭ-te) the degree to which a solute mixes with a solvent to produce a solution.

soluble (sol′u-b'l) [L. *solubilis*] capable or susceptible of mixing with a solvent (dissolving) to form a solution. Called also *solvable*.

Solucort trademark for *prednisolone sodium phosphate* (see under PREDNISOLONE).

Solu-Cortef trademark for *hydrocortisone sodium succinate* (see under HYDROCORTISONE).

Solu-Dilar trademark for *paramethasone disodium phosphate* (see under PARAMETHASONE).

solum (so′lum), pl. *so′la* [L.] an anatomic term for the bottom or lowest part.

Solu-Medrol trademark for *methylprednisolone sodium succinate* (see under METHYLPREDNISOLONE).

solute (so′loot) in solution, the substance that is dissolved, or if there is doubt as to which substance dissolves the other, the substance present in the lesser amount. See also disperse PHASE. **ionic s.**, electrolyte.

solutio (so-loo′she-o) [L. *solvere* to dissolve] solution.

solution (so-loo′shun) [L. *solutio*] 1. a homogeneous mixture of two or more substances in which the particles are of atomic or molecular size, the substance that is dissolved being called the *solute* and that in which the solute is dissolved, the *solvent*. See DIFFUSION (2). 2. dissolution; the process of dissolving. 3. the process of loosening or separation. **s. No. 220**, merbromin. **acidic s.**, one having a pH of less than 7. **alcoholic s.**, one in which alcohol, especially ethyl alcohol, is used as the solvent. **α-solid s.**, a primary solid solution found at the left extremity of the phase diagram (see under DIAGRAM), being near 100 percent solute concentration. Called also *α-phase* and *α-solid*. **aluminum acetate s.**, Burow's s. **ammonia s.**, see ammonia WATER and AMMONIUM hydroxide. **ammoniacal silver nitrate s.**, an ammonium compound of silver nitrate; used as an antiseptic and in the detection and prevention of dental caries. Because of inflammatory and necrotic tissue reaction, the use of silver nitrate has now declined. Called also *Howe's s.* See also SILVER nitrate. **anisotonic s.**, one that is not isotonic; one having osmotic pressure different from the standard reference, such as the blood serum. See also HYPOTONIC and HYPERTONIC. **aqueous s.**, one in which water is used as the solvent. **basic s.**, one having a pH that is greater than 7. **β-solid s.**, a primary solid solution found at the right extremity of the phase diagram (see under DIAGRAM), being nearly 0 percent solute concentration. Called also *β-phase* and *β-solid*. See also ALLOY. **buffer s.**, one that maintains a nearly constant pH. **Burow's s.**, aluminum acetate solution; used as an astringent, antipruritic, and antiseptic. Ingestion may produce vomiting, nausea, diarrhea, and hematemesis. **Carrel-Dakin s.**, a diluted sodium hypochlorite solution (see SODIUM hypochlorite). **colloid s.**, see COLLOID (2). **concentrated s.**, one containing a large amount of solute in proportion to solvent. **contrast s.**, one of a substance opaque to roentgen rays, used to facilitate roentgen visualization of some organ or structure in the body. **Dakin's s.**, **Dakin's modified s.**, sodium hypochlorite s., diluted. **developing s.**, one containing Metol, hydroquinone, sodium carbonate, potassium bromine, and sodium sulfite, which is used in developing exposed film and converting the latent image to the manifest image. Metol, N-methyl-p-aminophenol sulfate, acts as an activator and hydroquinone removes bromine ions from silver bromide in the film emulsion, leaving black metallic silver, thus giving shape to the image. Sodium carbonate produces a pH of about 11.0, accelerates the reduction, and softens the emulsion. Potassium bromide acts as a restrainer. Sodium sulfate acts as a preservative and slows down oxidation. Called also *film developer.* See also *fixing s.*, acid stop BATH, and water BATH (2). **developing s., rapid,** a developing solution which includes potassium hydroxide as the alkalizing agent for accelerating the developing process. Called also *rapid developer.* **dialyzing s.,** an isotonic aqueous solution used in peritoneal or extracorporeal dialysis, which contains concentrations of sodium, potassium, calcium, magnesium, chloride, bicarbonate, lactate, and glucose that are identical to those in normal blood plasma, but contains no urea, creatinine, or urates. In chemical processes, the fluid used for dialysis may be distilled water or any suitable solution. **dilute s.,** one containing a small amount of the solute in proportion to the solvent. **disclosing s.,** disclosing AGENT. **double-normal s.,** one having double the strength of a normal (1N) solution; designated 2N. See NORMALITY. **fixing s.,** one of sodium thiosulfate, potassium alum, acetic acid, and sodium sulfite, which is used in fixing the manifest image on the exposed film. Sodium thiosulfate serves to dissolve the excess silver bromide salts and to remove them from the emulsion; potassium alum hardens the emulsion by shrinking and tanning action on the gelatin; acetic acid removes fats from the gelatin and acidifies the solution; and sodium sulfite acts as a preservative. Called also *fixer.* See also film FIXATION. **fluoride s., topical,** one of sodium fluoride in distilled water, 100 ml of which contains 2 gm of the fluoride. Also an 8 percent solution of stannous fluoride in distilled water. Used topically in the prevention of dental caries in children. **formaldehyde s.,** see FORMALDEHYDE. **Giemsa s.,** Giemsa STAIN. **hardening s.,** one that increases hardness of the substance to which it is added, such as potassium sulfate, zinc sulfate, or manganese sulfate solutions, which are added to hydrocolloid solutions to increase the hardness of impression materials. **Hartman's s.,** one formerly used to desensitize dentin, consisting of 1¼ part thymol, 1 part ethyl alcohol, and 2 parts sulfuric ether. **Howe's s.,** ammoniacal silver nitrate s. **hundredth-normal s.,** one having one-hundredth the strength of a normal solution; designated N/100 or 0.01 N. **Hurricane topical s.,** trademark for a solution, 100 gm of which contains 20 gm of benzocaine and various flavoring agents in a polyethylene glycol base. **hyperbaric s.,** one having a greater specific gravity than the standard of reference, such as one used for spinal anesthesia having a specific gravity greater than that of the spinal fluid (1.006), causing it to migrate downward and produce anesthesia below the level of injection. **hypertonic s.,** one characterized by increased osmotic pressure; usually referring to a solution having molar concentration greater than that in the erythrocytes in the blood, thereby causing the flow of water across the semipermeable cell membrane out of the erythrocyte. See also *isotonic s.* Cf. *hypotonic s.* **hypobaric s.,** one having a specific gravity less than that of the standard of reference, such as one used for spinal anesthesia having a specific gravity less than that of the spinal fluid (1.006), causing it to migrate upward and produce anesthesia above the level of injection. **hypotonic s.,** one characterized by a decreased osmotic pressure; usually referring to a solution having a molar concentration lower than that in the erythrocytes in the blood, thereby causing the flow of water across the semipermeable cell membrane into the erythrocyte with consequent swelling of its cell and eventual hemolysis. See also *isotonic s.* Cf. *hypertonic s.* **interstitial solid s.,** solid s., interstitial. **iodine s.,** IODINE solution. **iodine s., compound, iodine s., strong,** strong iodine solution; see under IODINE. **iodine disclosing s.,** iodine disclosing AGENT. **Ion Phosphate Fluoride Topical s.,** trademark for an aqueous fluoride solution, 100 ml of which contains 2 gm sodium fluoride, 0.34 gm hydrogen fluoride, and various amounts of preservative, coloring, and flavoring agents, which is acidulated with 1.0 gm phosphoric acid; used in dental caries control. **Iradicav acidulated phosphate fluoride s.,** trademark for an aqueous solution, 100 ml of which contains 2 gm sodium fluoride, 0.35 gm hydrogen fluoride, and various amounts of preservative, flavoring, and coloring agents, which is acidulated with 0.98 gm of phosphoric acid; used in dental caries control. **isobaric s.,** one having the same specific gravity as the standard of reference, such as one used for spinal anesthesia having specific gravity of the spinal fluid (1.006), causing it to remain and produce anesthesia at the level of injection. See also *hyperbaric s.* and *hypobaric s.* **isosmotic s.,** isotonic s. **isotonic s.,** one characterized by equal osmotic pressure; usually referring to a solution having the same molar concentration as the contents of the erythryocytes in the blood. Called also *isosmotic s.* See also *hypertonic s., hypotonic s.,* and *physiologic salt s.* **Karidium phosphate fluoride topical s.,** trademark for an aqueous fluoride solution, 100 ml of which contains 2 gm sodium fluoride and 0.34 gm hydrogen fluoride, which is acidulated with 0.98 gm of phosphoric acid; used in dental caries control. **Labarraque's s.,** diluted sodium hypochlorite solution; see SODIUM hypochlorite. **local anesthetic s.,** a prepackaged solution for dental use made of the hydrochloride salt of a local anesthetic base, being iso-osmotic and acidic with a pH between 3.3 and 5.5, usually containing 1 mg/ml methylparaben as a preservative. Some solutions also contain sympathomimetics and vasoconstrictors and 0.5 mg/ml sodium metabisulfite as an antioxidant. **Lugol's s.,** strong iodine solution; see under IODINE. **Luride topical s.,** trademark for an aqueous fluoride solution, 100 ml of which contains 2 gm sodium fluoride, 0.34 gm hydrogen fluoride, and 0.087 gm potassium sorbate, which is acidulated with 0.98 gm of phosphoric acid; used in dental caries control. **maximum urinary concentration (MUC) s.,** the highest attainable concentration of a solute or of the collective solutes in the urine. **molal s.,** one that contains 1 mole of the solute in 1 kg (1000 gm) of solvent. **molar s.,** one that contains 1 mole of solute in 1 liter (1000 ml) of solution; designated M/1 or 1 M. The concentration of other solutions may be expressed in relation to that of molar solutions as tenth-molar (M/10 or 0.1 M), etc. **molecular disperse s.,** one in which the dispersed particles have a diameter of about 0.1 $\mu\mu$. See also COLLOID (2). **NaFrinse acidulated s.,** trademark for a solution containing 0.044 percent sodium fluoride, 0.055 percent phosphoric acid, 1.35 percent sodium biphosphate, flavoring agents, and dyes; used in dental caries prevention. **neutral s.,** one that is neither basic nor acid, having a pH of 7. **nonaqueous s.,** one in which a liquid other than water is used as the solvent. **normal s.,** one that contains 1 gram-equivalent weight of the solute in 1 liter of solution. Designated N/1 or 1 N. See also *hundredth-normal s., tenth-normal s.,* and *thousandth-normal s.* **Novol-benzocaine s.,** a trademark for an anesthetic solution for topical application, 100 ml of which contains 20 gm benzocaine, 0.3 gm essential oils, and the necessary amount of a water-soluble base. **Pacemaker Nafeen s.,** trademark for a solution, 8 drops (0.5 ml) of which contains 2.20 mg sodium fluoride, being equivalent to 1.0 mg fluoride ion; used in dental caries prevention. **Pacemaker topical fluoride s.,** trademark for an aqueous fluoride solution, 100 ml of which contains 2 gm sodium fluoride, 0.34 gm hydrogen fluoride, and various amounts of flavoring and coloring agents, which is acidulated with 0.98 gm of phosphoric acid; used in dental caries control. **physiological saline s.,** physiological salt s. **physiological salt s., physiological sodium chloride s.,** an isotonic solution of sodium chloride in purified water. Its osmotic pressure is equal on both sides of the semipermeable cell membrane of erythrocytes; thus there is no flow of water across the membrane in either direction, thereby maintaining the physiological condition of the erythrocyte. Called also *physiological saline s.* See also *isotonic s.* **pickling s.,** one used for pickling dental castings for the purpose of removing oxides or other contaminants, usually consisting of 3 oz concentrated sulfuric acid, 3 oz water, and 1 tsp potassium dichromate crystals; 50 percent hydrochloric acid solution is sometimes also used for pickling. **primary solid s's,** solid s's, primary. **Rafluor topical s.,** trademark for an aqueous fluoride solution, 100 ml of which contains 2 gm sodium fluoride and 0.34 gm hydrogen fluoride, which is acidulated with 0.98 gm of phosphoric acid; used in dental caries control. **random solid s.,** solid s., random. **saline s., salt s.,** a solution of sodium chloride in distilled water. See also *physiological salt s.* **saturated s.,** one that contains the maximum dissolved substance for the amount of the solvent and no more solute will dissolve at a given temperature. **sclerosing s.,** one containing an irritant substance that will cause inflammatory changes resulting in fibrosis; used for the treatment of subluxation of the temporomandibular joint, cauterization of ulcers, arresting hemorrhage, and other purposes where obliteration is required. **Slo-Flo phosphate topical s.,** a sodium fluoride solution acidified with orthophosphoric acid for topical application in dental caries prevention, containing in each 100 ml 2 gm sodium fluoride, 0.34 gm hydrogen fluoride, and 0.98 gm orthophosphoric acid. See also sodium FLUORIDE. **sodium fluoride s.,** an aqueous solution containing 1.1, 3.3, 5.5, or 20 mg/ml powdered sodium fluoride; used in dental caries control. **sodium fluoride–orthophosphoric**

acid s., a 1.23 percent aqueous solution of sodium fluoride acidulated with 1 percent phosphoric acid, having a pH between 3.0 and 3.4; used in dental caries control. **sodium hypochlorite s., diluted,** an aqueous solution, 100 ml of which contains 450–500 mg sodium hypochlorite, occurring as a colorless to light yellow liquid with a faint odor of chlorine. It is a deodorant and anti-infective solution used to irrigate suppurating wounds. It also dissolves necrotic tissue and blood clots, thus delaying coagulation, and produces skin irritation. Called also *Carrel-Dakin s., Dakin's modified s.,* and *Dakin's fluid.* **solid s.,** one in which, after solidification, the atoms of the solute are distributed in the space lattice of the solvent, replacing some of its atoms and forming a system that is not separable mechanically and has only one phase. Alloys, such as a palladium-silver alloy, are examples of solid solutions. See also solid solution ALLOY. **solid s., interstitial,** one in which the atoms of the solute occupy interstitial positions in the space lattice. **solid s's, primary,** solid solutions which are found at the extremities of the phase diagram (see under DIAGRAM), being near 100 and 0 percent solute concentrations, designated as *α-solid solution* and *β-solid solution,* respectively. See also ALLOY. **solid s., random,** one having a random configuration of atoms in the space lattice, atoms having little preference to their neighbors and their movement being relatively free at high temperatures. Materials made up of random solid solutions are generally susceptible to dislocations and relatively soft and more ductile than materials of the same system in which the lattice is ordered. **solid s., substitutional,** one in which the atoms of the solute occupy the space lattice positions which normally are occupied by the solvent atoms in the pure metal. **standard s.,** one having a known quantity of the solute, usually expressed in terms of normality (equivalent weight of solute per liter of solution) or molarity (gram molecular weight of solute per liter of solution). **Stohl's s.,** a solution of sodium citrate and citric acid; used in the treatment of chronic metabolic acidosis. It may cause irritation of the oral mucosa, resulting in ulcerative and necrotic lesions. **substitutional solid s.,** solid s., substitutional. **supersaturated s.,** one containing an excess solute over that normally required for saturation at a given temperature. **surgical chlorinated soda s.,** diluted sodium hypochlorite solution; see SODIUM *hypochlorite.* **tenth-normal s.,** one having one-tenth the strength of a normal solution; designated N/10 or 0.1 N. **thousandth-normal s.,** one having one-thousandth the strength of a normal solution; designated N/1000 or 0.001 N. **true s.,** one whose particles are of molecular or ionic dimensions and will not settle out on standing or are less than 1 μ in diameter, are invisible, will pass through filters and membranes, and possess molecular movement. See also COLLOID (2) and SUSPENSION.

solv. abbreviation for L. *sol've,* dissolve.

solvable (sol'vah-b'l) soluble.

Solvan trademark for *diphenadione.*

solvation (sol-va'shun) chemical combination of a solvent with the solute; the energy-releasing solute-solvent interaction.

solvent (sol'vent) [L. *solvens*] in solution, the substance in which the solute is dissolved or, if there is a doubt as to which substance dissolves in the other, that which is present in the greater amount. See also continuous PHASE. **McCall's epithelial s.,** a solution of sodium sulfide; used for the removal of the lateral epithelial wall in pocket eradication.

Soma trademark for *carisoprodol.*

soma (so'mah) [Gr. *sōma* body] 1. the body as distinguished from the mind. 2. the body tissue as distinguished from the germ cells.

Somadril trademark for *carisoprodol.*

somatic (so-mat'ik) [Gr. *sōmatikos*] pertaining to or characterized by the body (soma).

somato- [Gr. *sōma, sōmatos* body] a combining form denoting relationship to the body.

somatometry (so-mah-tom'e-tre) [*somato-* + Gr. *metron* measure] the measurement of the dimensions and proportions of the living human body. See also ANTHROPOMETRY.

somatoplasm (so-mat'o-plazm) [*somato-* + Gr. *plasma* anything formed or molded] the protoplasm of the body cells as distinguished from that of the germ cells.

somatopleure (so-mat'o-ploor) [*somato-* + Gr. *pleura* side] the embryonic wall formed jointly by the somatic mesoderm and ectoderm.

somatoprosthetics (so"mah-to-pros-thet'iks) prosthetic replacement of external parts of the body that are missing or deformed. See also PROSTHESIS.

somatostatin (so"mah-to-stat'in) a cyclic tetradecapeptide isolated from bovine hypothalmic extracts, which inhibits the secretion of immunoreactive growth hormone. At higher concentrations, it also inhibits the secretion of thyroid-stimulating hormone, insulin, glucagon, and gastrin, and inhibits the action of glucagon on the liver and histamine on gastric acid production. Called also *growth hormone release inhibiting factor (GHRIF)* and *somatotropin release inhibiting factor (SRIF).*

somatotropic (so"mah-to-trop'ik) [*somato-* + Gr. *tropē* turning] 1. having an affinity for the body or the body cells; also having an influence on the body. 2. pertaining to somatotropic hormone.

somatotropin (so"mah-to-tro'pin) [*somato-* + Gr. *tropē* a turning] somatotropic HORMONE. **s. release inhibiting factor (SRIF),** somatostatin.

somatotype (so-mat'o-tīp) [*somato-* + *type*] a particular category of body build, determined on the basis of certain physical characteristics. See ECTOMORPH, ENDOMORPH, and MESOMORPH.

Sombulex trademark for *hexobarbital.*

somite (so'mīt) one of the primitive paired segments of mesodermal origin that develop alongside the neural tube. They arise when transverse clefts subdivide the thickened mesoderm next to the midplane into blocklike masses. At the level of any pair lie the primitive kidney tubules and blood vessels arising from the aorta. Individual somites give rise to a muscle mass supplied with spinal nerves; somite pairs jointly produce vertebrae. Each somite differentiates into a dermatome concerned with the development of integumentary tissue, a myotome concerned with muscle development, and a sclerotome concerned with the skeletal development. Segmentation begins about three weeks after fertilization and progresses through the thirty-eighth day, at which time 28 to 30 segments have been formed; in all, about 43 to 44 being formed. Called also *mesoblastic segment* and *mesodermal segment.* See illustration at EMBRYO.

somni- [L. *somnus* sleep] a combining form denoting relationship to sleep.

somnifacient (som"ni-fa'shent) [*somni-* + L. *facere* to make] 1. causing sleep; hypnotic. 2. an agent that induces sleep.

somniferous (som-nif'er-us) [*somni-* + L. *ferre* to bring] inducing or causing sleep.

Somnos trademark for *chloral hydrate* (see under CHLORAL).

sonant (so'nant) a speech sound that has in it a component of tone generated by laryngeal vibration, e.g., *a-a-a* and *z-z-z.*

Sonapax trademark for *thioridazine.*

sonarography (so"nar-og'rah-fe) ultrasonic scanning that provides a two-dimensional image corresponding to clear sections of acoustic interfaces of tissues.

sone (sōn) a unit of loudness, being the loudness of a simple tone of 1,000 cycles per second, 40 decibels above the listener's threshold.

Sonnolin trademark for *nitrazepam.*

Sono-Explorer a trademark for an electronic instrument for measuring the root canal. It determines the length of the canal by measuring the resistance of the oral mucosa during the probing of the root canal, whereby the probe is inserted into the tooth until the resistance is met as indicated by an even tone.

sonorous (so-no'rus) resonant; sounding.

Son-X-Ray trademark for a small-capacity automatic film processor.

Soolingen, Kornelis van [17th century] a Dutch physician who recommended a mixture of mastic and turpentine for stopping carious processes from progressing. He also introduced an emery wheel for grinding the teeth.

sopor (so'por) [L.] sound or deep sleep.

soporific (sop"o-rif'ik, so"po-rif'ik) [L. *soporificus*] 1. causing or inducing profound sleep. 2. a drug or agent which induces sleep.

S. op. s. abbreviation for L. *si o'pus sit,* if it is necessary.

S.Or. supraorbitale.

Soranus of Ephesus [2nd century A.D.] a celebrated Greek physician of the Methodist school, and the most renowned gynecologist and obstetrician of antiquity. He practiced in Alexandria and Rome. His surviving writings on obstetrics, gynecology, and pediatrics are outstanding. See METHODIST.

Sorbicolan trademark for *sorbitol.*

Sorbilande trademark for *sorbitol.*

sorbit (sor'bit) sorbitol.

sorbitan (sor'bi-tan) any anhydride of sorbitol, $C_6H_8O(OH)_4$, the fatty acids of which (*s. monolaurate, s. monooleate, s. monopalmitate, s. monostearate, s. sesquioleate. s. trioleate, s. tristearate*) are surfactants. See also POLYSORBATE.

sorbitol (sor'bi-tol) a crystalline hexahydric alcohol, 1,2,3,4,5,6-hexahydroxyhexane, occurring as a white, odorless, crystalline, hygroscopic powder with a sweet taste, which is soluble in water, glycerol, propylene glycol, alcohols, phenol, and acetamide, but is almost insoluble in organic solvents. It was first found in ripe berries of the tree *Sorbus aucuparia,* and is also found in various berries and fruits. In mammals, sorbitol is formed from glucose and is converted to fructose. Sorbitol is used as a sugar substitute, its sweetening power being about half that of sucrose and equal to glucose. In solution, it is used as a humectant and texturizing agent for drugs, dentifrices, and food products. Also used in the manufacturing of ascorbic acid and in various industrial processes. Sorbitol-containing foods have little or no cariogenic effects. Its toxicity is relatively low. Called also *D-s., D-glucitol, L-gulitol, hexahydric alcohol,* and *sorbit.* Trademarks: Cholaxine, Diakarmon, Karion, Nivitin, Sionit, Sionon, Sorbicolan, Sorbilande, Sorbo, Sorbol, Sorbostyl. **D-s.,** sorbitol.

Sorbitrate trademark for *isosorbide dinitrate* (see under *isosorbide*).

Sorbo trademark for *sorbitol.*

Sorbol trademark for *sorbitol.*

Sorbostyl trademark for *sorbitol.*

sordes (sor'dēz) [L. "filth"] dirt; debris; especially the encrustations and accumulations of food, epithelial matter, and bacteria collected on the teeth and lips during a prolonged fever.

sore (sōr) 1. painful. 2. a wound; a lesion; a popular term for almost any lesion of the skin or mucous membranes. **canker s's,** recurrent aphthous STOMATITIS. **cold s's,** see HERPES simplex. **Kandahar s., Lahore s.,** cutaneous LEISHMANIASIS. **s. throat,** see LARYNGITIS, PHARYNGITIS, septic sore THROAT, and TONSILLITIS.

Sorensen chisel see under CHISEL.

sore throat (sōr thrōt) see LARYNGITIS, PHARYNGITIS, septic sore THROAT, and TONSILLITIS. **epidemic streptococcal s. t., septic s. t., streptococcal s. t.,** septic sore THROAT.

Sormetal trademark for *calcium disodium edetate* (see under CALCIUM).

sorption (sorp'shun) [L. *sorbere* to suck in] the process or state of being sorbed; absorption or adsorption.

Sorquad trademark for *isosorbide dinitrate* (see under ISOSORBIDE).

Sorrin operation see under OPERATION.

sorting (sort'ing) in computer technology, the process of arranging data into a desired order dependent on a key or field contained within each item.

S.O.S. abbreviation for L. *si o'pus sit,* if it is necessary.

Sosigon trademark for *pentazocine.*

Sotacor trademark for *sotalol.*

sotalol (so'tah-lol) β-adrenergic blocking agent, N-[4-[1-hydroxy-2-[(methylenethyl) amino]ethyl] phenyl] methanesulfonamide. Usually used in the form of the hydrochloride salt, which occurs as white crystalline solids, soluble in water and slightly in chloroform. Used as a bronchodilator drug. Trademarks: Beta-Cardone, Sotacor.

Sotos' syndrome [Juan Fernandez *Sotos,* American physician, born 1927] see under SYNDROME.

sound (sownd) [L. *sonus*] 1. the effect produced on the organ of hearing by the vibrations of the air or other medium. 2. mechanical radiant energy, the motion of particles of the material medium through which it travels (air, water, or solids) being along the line of transmission (longitudinal); such energy, of frequency between 20 and 20,000 cycles per second, provides the stimulus for the subjective sensation of hearing. 3. an instrument to be introduced into a cavity to detect a foreign body or to dilate a stricture. 4. a noise, normal or abnormal, heard within the body; for other sounds see under *bruit, fremitus, murmur,* and *rale.* **Souques-Charcot geroderma** [Alexandre Achille *Souques,* French neurologist, 1860–1944; Jean Martin *Charcot,* French neurologist, 1825—1893] see under GERODERMA. **speech s.,** phoneme. **white s.,** that produced by a mixture of all frequencies of mechanical vibration perceptible as sound.

Sovcaine trademark for *dibucaine hydrochloride* (see under DIBUCAINE).

Soxisol trademark for *sulfisoxazole.*

Sp *Sp* POINT.

space (spās) 1. a delimited area. 2. an actual or potential cavity of the body. Called also *spatium.* See also POUCH. 3. the area of the universe beyond the earth and its atmosphere. **apical s.,** a part of the periodontal space between the wall of the alveolus and the apex of the root of a tooth. **s. of body of mandible,** mandibular s. **buccal s., buccinator s.,** a tissue space situated between the buccinator muscle and the masseter muscle; it communicates posteriorly with the pterygomandibular space and superiorly with the postzygomatic space. **s. of Burns,** jugular FOSSA. **cathodal dark s.,** Crookes' s. **Crookes' s.,** a dark space at the cathode of a nearly exhausted x-ray tube through which a

current is being passed. Called also *cathodal dark s.* **Czermak's s's, Czermak's globular s's,** interglobular s's. **dead s.,** 1. space remaining after incomplete closure of surgical or other wounds, permitting the accumulation of blood or serum and resultant delay in healing. 2. space in the respiratory system in which exchange of oxygen does not occur. **denture s.,** that portion of the oral cavity which is occupied or may be occupied by a maxillary and/or mandibular denture, or the space between and around the residual ridges which is available for dentures. **digastric s.,** submandibular s. **s. of Donders,** the space above the dorsum of the tongue and below the hard and soft palates when the mandible is in the respiratory rest position. It is considered to be the lumen of the digestive tract. When swallowing, the lumen is obliterated and the bolus is passed backward; after swallowing, the mandible and the tongue return to the respiratory rest position. **escapement s's,** spaces which permit the escape of material being comminuted between the occlusal surfaces of the teeth, provided by the cusps and ridges, sulci and developmental ridges of the teeth, and the embrasures between the teeth. **Faraday's dark s.,** the dark region separating the negative glow from the positive column in a Crookes' tube. **fascial s.,** tissue s's. **freeway s.,** interocclusal DISTANCE. **geniohyoid s., inferior,** the deep portion of the sublingual space, lying between the geniohyoid and genioglossal muscles. **geniohyoid s., superior,** the superficial portion of the sublingual space, lying between the mylohyoid and geniohyoid muscles. **globular s's of Czermak,** interglobular s's. **haversian s.,** haversian CANAL. **infratemporal s.,** a tissue space bounded anteriorly by the maxillary tuberosity; posteriorly by the lateral pterygoid muscle, condyle, and temporal muscle; laterally by the tendon of the temporal muscle and coronoid process; and medially by the lateral pterygoid plate and inferior belly of the lateral pterygoid muscle. The inferior portion is known as the *pterygomandibular space* and lies between the medial pterygoid muscle and the ramus of the mandible; the *postzygomatic space* extends anteromedially. It contains the pterygoid plexus and veins, maxillary artery, mandibular, mylohyoid, lingual, buccinator, and chorda tympani nerves and pterygoid muscles, and communicates with the submandibular spaces, masticator space, parotid space, and lateral pharyngeal space, thus playing an important role in the propagation of infections. **interarytenoid s.,** RIMA glottidis cartilaginea. **interdental s.,** interproximal s. **interfascial s's,** tissue s's. **interglobular s's,** numerous small irregular spaces on the outer surface of the dentin in the root of the tooth. Called also *globular s's of Czermak* and *spatia interglobularia* [NA]. **interocclusal s., interocclusal rest s.,** interocclusal DISTANCE. **interprismatic s.,** a space between the enamel prisms, which is filled with the cementing substance. See interprismatic SUBSTANCE. **interproximal s., interproximate s.,** a triangularly shaped space between the proximal surfaces of adjoining teeth, normally filled by gingival tissue (gingival papillae); sometimes used to designate especially the space between the proximal surfaces of adjoining teeth that is gingival to the area of contact *(septal s.)* Called also *interdental s., proximal s., proximate s.,* and *interdentium.* See also contact AREA and EMBRASURE. **interradicular s.,** the space between the roots; the entire extent of the space between the roots of a tooth, from apex to base. **interstitial s.,** a small space in a tissue or structure; interstice. **Kiesselbach's s.,** Kiesselbach's AREA. **lateropharyngeal s.,** pharyngeal s., lateral. **leeway s.,** Nance's leeway s. **lymph s.,** any space in tissue occupied by lymph. **s. maintainer,** space MAINTAINER. **mandibular s.,** a tissue space formed by the superficial layer of cervical fascia as it splits medially and laterally at the inferior border of the mandible and becomes continuous superiorly with the alveolar periosteum. It is continuous subperiosteally with the masticator space and contains the anterior part of the ramus of the mandible, mandibular muscle attachments, blood vessels, nerves, and periodontal structures. Dental diseases may result in infections of this space, which sometimes spreads farther, especially to the masticator space at the floor of the mouth. Called also *s. of body of mandible.* **masseter-mandibulopterygoid s., masseteric s.,** masticator s. **masticator s., masticatory s.,** a tissue space formed by the superficial layer of cervical fascia which covers the masseter muscle laterally and the medial pterygoid muscle medially. The space is continuous subperiosteally with the mandibular space, the posterior border of the ramus of the mandible being its posterior boundary, the anterior border of the masseter and the medial pterygoid muscles being its anterior boundary, and the inferior surface of the ramus of the mandible being its inferior boundary. It contains the muscles of mastication, ascending ramus of the mandible, and zygomatic arch. Infections in this space may spread to the temporal space, parotid space, lateral pharyngeal space, and submandibular space. Called also *masseter-mandibulopterygoid s.* and *masseteric s.* **medullary s.**, the central cavity of bone and the intervals between the trabeculae which contain the marrow. **Nance's leeway s.**, the amount by which the space occupied by the deciduous canine and first and second deciduous molars exceeds that occupied by the canine and premolar teeth of the permanent dentition, usually averaging 1.7 mm on each side of the dental arch. Called also *leeway s.* **parapharyngeal s.**, pharyngeal s., lateral. **paravisceral s.**, a tissue space that is a continuation of the lateral pharyngeal space and contains the internal jugular vein and the carotid artery. **perivisceral s.**, a collective name for the lateral pharyngeal space, paravisceral space, retropharyngeal space, retroesophageal space, and pretracheal space, bounded posteriorly by the prevertebral fascia, laterally by the investing fascia, and anteriorly by the infrahyoid fascia. **parotid s.**, a tissue space in the region of the mandibular ramus, containing the parotid gland and all invested associated structures, including the facial nerve, auriculotemporal nerve, posterior facial vein, and external carotid, internal maxillary, and superior temporal arteries. The gland itself is situated outside the masseter muscle, extending posteriorly behind the ramus of the mandible and medially between the masseter and medial pterygoid muscles. The spread of infection usually occurs in a medial direction, into the infraparotid space, masticator space, lateral pharyngeal space, and submandibular space. **peripharyngeal s.**, retropharyngeal s. **periplasmic s.**, see cell WALL. **pharyngeal s., lateral, pharyngomaxillary s., pharyngopterygoid s.**, a tissue space bounded anteriorly by the buccopharyngeal aponeurosis, parotid gland, and pterygoid muscles; posteriorly by the prevertebral fascia; laterally by the carotid sheath; and medially by the lateral wall of the pharynx. It extends from the base of the skull near the petrous part of the temporal bone to the level of the hyoid bone and the attachment of the submaxillary part of the superficial layer of cervical fascia to the coverings of the stylohyoid and digastric muscles. Sometimes it is divided into the anterior prestyloid and posterior poststyloid or restrostyloid compartments. The poststyloid compartment contains the internal carotid artery, the glossopharyngeal, vagus, spinal accessory, hypoglossal, and sympathetic nerves, and the internal jugular vein with its associated lymph nodes. Infection may produce laryngeal edema, thrombosis of the internal jugular vein, and erosion of the internal carotid artery with resulting hemorrhage. Called also *parapharyngeal s., lateropharyngeal s.*, and *pterygopharyngeal s.* **postzygomatic s., pretemporal s.**, the anteromedial part of the infratemporal space. Called also *retrozygomatic s.* and *zygomaticotemporal s.* **pretracheal s.**, a tissue space situated in front of the trachea and formed by the divergence of the pretracheal layer of the cervical fascia and the visceral fascia. **proximal s., proximate s.**, interproximal s. **pterygomandibular s.**, a part of the infratemporal space that lies between the medial pterygoid muscle and the ramus of the mandible. **pterygomaxillary s.**, pterygopalatine s. **pterygopalatine s.**, a tissue space situated below the apex of the orbit, posterior to the maxillary sinus, lateral to the lateral pterygoid plate, and deep to the temporomandibular joint. It communicates with the infratemporal fossa through the pterygomaxillary fissure, and contains the maxillary nerve, sphenopalatine ganglion, and terminal part of the internal maxillary artery. Infections in this space usually originate in the upper molars. Called also *pterygomaxillary s., sphenomaxillary s.*, and *sphenopalatine s.* **pterygopharyngeal s.**, pharyngeal s., lateral. **relief s.**, a slight elevation of a lingual bar type of major connector to allow for a minor degree of settling of a removable partial denture without impinging on the structure over which the bar passes. **retroesophageal s.**, a tissue space that continues downward from the retropharyngeal space. **retromylohyoid s.**, the part of the alveolingual sulcus just lingual to the retromolar pad, bounded anteriorly by the lingual tuberosity, posteriorly by the retromylohyoid curtain, inferiorly by the floor of the alveolingual sulcus, and lingually by the anterior tonsillar pillar. **retropharyngeal s.**, a tissue space bounded anteriorly by the wall of the pharynx, posteriorly by the prevertebral fascia, and laterally by the lateral pharyngeal space and carotid sheath. Called also *peripharyngeal s.* and *retropharyngeal cleft.* **retrozygomatic s.**, postzygomatic s. **septal s.**, the space between the proximal surfaces of adjoining teeth (interproximal s.) that is gingival to the area of contact. See also EMBRASURE. **spheno-**

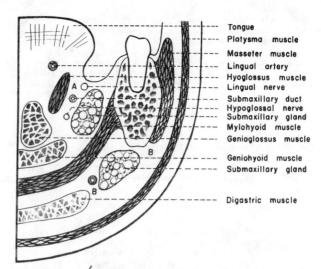

Frontal section through the head in the molar region. *A*, sublingual space; *B*, submaxillary space. (From W. G. Shafer, M. K. Hine, and B. M. Levy: A Textbook of Oral Pathology. 3rd ed. Philadelphia, W. B. Saunders Co., 1974.)

Tongue
Platysma muscle
Masseter muscle
Lingual artery
Hyoglossus muscle
Lingual nerve
Submaxillary duct
Hypoglossal nerve
Submaxillary gland
Mylohyoid muscle
Genioglossus muscle
Geniohyoid muscle
Submaxillary gland
Digastric muscle

maxillary s., sphenopalatine s., pterygopalatine s. **subgingival s.**, gingival CREVICE. **sublingual s.**, a tissue space, considered to be a part of the submandibular space, which is bounded superiorly by the mucosa of the floor of the mouth, inferiorly by the mylohyoid muscle, anteriorly and laterally by the mandible, medially by the median raphe of the tongue, and posteriorly by the hyoid bone. It contains the terminal branches of the lingual artery, sublingual gland, submandibular duct, deep part of the submandibular gland, lingual nerve, and hypoglossal nerve. Sometimes it is divided into the *deep sublingual space*, lying between the geniohyoid and genioglossus muscles, and the *superficial sublingual space*, lying between the mylohyoid and geniohyoid muscles. Because of its continuity with other compartments of the submandibular space, infections spread easily to and from other tissue spaces. A swelling in this space may lead to asphyxiation. It is particularly involved in Ludwig's angina. See illustration. **submandibular s.**, a tissue space formed by a split of the superficial layer of the cervical fascia, and situated under the mandible below the posterior part of the mylohyoid, hyoglossal, and superior constrictor muscles; the superficial layer of the cervical fascia providing the lateral boundary. The posterior boundary is provided by the stylohyoid muscle and the posterior belly of the digastric muscle, and it is limited by the anterior belly of the digastric muscle. It contains the submandibular gland, lymph nodes, and branches of the facial artery and anterior facial nerve. The space is particularly involved in Ludwig's angina. Called also *digastric s.* **submasseteric s.**, a narrow tissue space situated between the masseter muscle and the lateral surface of the mandibular ramus. It is limited anteriorly by the retromolar fossa and posteriorly by the parotid gland. Infections in this space usually originate from the mandibular third molar. See illustration. **submaxillary s.**, submandibular TRIANGLE. **submental s.**, a tissue space of the

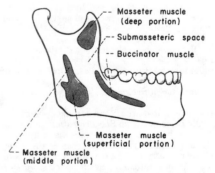

Masseter muscle (deep portion)
Submasseteric space
Buccinator muscle
Masseter muscle (superficial portion)
Masseter muscle (middle portion)

Lateral surface of the mandible showing the location of the submasseteric space. (From W. G. Shafer, M. K. Hine, and B. M. Levy: A Textbook of Oral Pathology. 3rd ed. Philadelphia, W. B. Saunders Co., 1974; redrawn from G. M. Bransby-Zachary: The submasseteric space. Br. Dent. 84:10, 1948.)

submandibular region, located above the hyoid bone, its superior boundary being formed by the mylohyoid muscle and its lower boundary by the superficial layer of the cervical fascia of the suprahyoid region, while the anterior belly of the digastric muscles provides the lateral limits on both sides. It contains the anterior jugular vein and the submental lymph nodes. **suprasternal s.,** jugular fossa of temporal bone; see under FOSSA. **temporal s., superficial,** a tissue space situated between the lateral surface of the temporal muscle and the temporal fascia. Infections in this space usually spread from other areas and fascial spaces. Called also *superficial temporal pouch.* **thyrohyal s.,** the depressed space between the thyroid cartilage and hyoid bone in front. **tissue s's,** potential spaces situated between planes of fascia, forming natural pathways along which infection may spread. Called also *fascial s's* and *interfascial s's.* See also illustration at FASCIA. **zygomaticotemporal s.,** postzygomatic s.

spacer (spās'er) in individual tray construction, a thin layer of wax or other plastic material applied to the surface of edentulous ridges and dental structures before the preliminary application of impression material. After producing the preliminary model, the spacer is discarded, thus providing an equidistant space between the oral structures and the impression tray that allows escape of excess impression material and entrapped air and facilitates manipulation during final impression taking. Called also *shim.*

spano- [Gr. *spanos* scarce] a combining form meaning scanty or scarce.

spar (spar) any of various lustrous, nonmetallic minerals. **light s., satin s.,** gypsum.

spasm (spazm) [L. *spasmus;* Gr. *spasmos*] 1. a sudden, involuntary, usually painful contraction of a muscle or group of muscles. 2. convulsion. 3. a sudden transitory constriction of a passage, canal, or orifice. **clonic s.,** see CLONUS and MYOCLONUS. **clonic facial s., hemifacial s.,** facial MYOCLONUS. **mobile s.,** athetosis. **muscle s.,** see SPASM (1). **Romberg's s.,** spasm of the masticatory muscles supplied by the fifth cranial nerve. **unilateral s.,** hemispasm.

spasmo- [L. *spasmus;* Gr. *spasmos*] a combining form denoting relationship to a spasm.

spasmodic (spaz-mod'ik) [Gr. *spasmōdēs*] of the nature of a spasm.

Spasmodolin trademark for *meperidine hydrochloride* (see under MEPERIDINE).

Spasmolyn trademark for *mephenesin.*

spasmolytic (spaz"mo-lit'ik) [*spasm* + Gr. *lytikos* dissolving] 1. relieving spasm, usually of smooth muscle, as in the arteries, bronchi, intestines, or sphincters, but also of voluntary muscle; antispasmodic. 2. an agent that relieves spasm; usually pertaining to antimuscarinic drugs (see under DRUG).

Spasmomedal trademark for *meperidine hydrochloride* (see under MEPERIDINE).

Spasmophen trademark for *oxyphenonium bromide* (see under OXYPHENONIUM).

spastic (spas'tik) 1. of the nature of or characterized by spasms. 2. hypertonic, so that the muscles are stiff and the movements awkward.

spasticity (spas-tis'ĭ-te) a state of hypertonicity, or increase over the normal tone of a muscle, with heightened deep tendon reflexes.

spatia (spa'she-ah) [L.] plural of *spatium.*

spatial (spa'shal) pertaining to space.

spatium (spa'she-um), pl. *spa'tia* [L.] a space or delimited area; a general anatomical term for an actual or potential open region. See also POUCH and SPACE. **spa'tia interglobula'ria,** interglobular spaces; see under SPACE.

Spatonin trademark for *diethylcarbamazine.*

spatula (spach'ŭ-lah) a flat, blunt, usually flexible instrument, used for mixing and spreading plaster of Paris, cement, dental impression pastes, ointments, etc.

spatular (spach'ŭ-lar) spatulate (1).

spatulate (spach'ŭ-lāt) 1. having a flat blunt end; spatular. 2. to mix or manipulate with a spatula.

spatulation (spat"u-la'shun) 1. the mixing of combined materials to a homogeneous mass by repeatedly scraping them up and smoothing out the mass on a flat surface with a spatula. 2. in condensation of porcelain paste in a matrix prior to firing, rubbing and patting of the paste with a porcelain carver, aimed at removing air bubbles and forcing excess water to the surface to be blotted out. Called also *s. condensation* and *ironing.* **s. condensation,** spatulation (2).

spatulator (spach'ŭ-la'tor) a mechanical device that mixes ingredients to form a homogenous mass.

SPCA serum prothrombin conversion accelerator; see FACTOR VII.

specialist (spesh'al-ist) 1. one who is an expert in and devotes himself to a special field of endeavor. 2. a medical or dental practitioner or another health professional who, by virtue of advanced training, is certified by a specialty board as being qualified to practice in a special field of dentistry or medicine, such as surgery, pathology, or orthodontics. **clinical nurse s., nurse s.,** see under NURSE.

specialization (spesh"al-i-za'shun) 1. the pursuing of a special line of study, activity, or work. 2. the limitation of medical or dental practice to some special field.

specialty (spesh'al-te) something in which one specializes or of which one has special skill or knowledge. In dentistry, a field of practice that calls for special knowledge and skills requiring intensive study and extended clinical and laboratory experience beyond the accepted undergraduate training in order to perform services of an unusual or difficult nature. **s. board,** see under specialty BOARD.

species (spe'shēz, spe'sēz) a taxonomic category subordinate to a genus (or subgenus), and superior to a subspecies or variety, composed of individuals possessing common characters distinguishing them from other categories of individuals of the same taxonomic level. In taxonomic nomenclature, species are designated by the genus name followed by a Latin or latinized adjective or noun.

species-specific (spe'sēz-spe-sif'ik) characteristic of a particular species; see species SPECIFICITY.

specific (spe-sif'ik) [L. *specificus*] 1. pertaining to species. 2. produced by a single kind of microorganism, at the strain, species, genus, or higher level. 3. restricted in application, effect, etc. 4. a remedy specially indicated for any particular disease. 5. pertaining to the special affinity of antigen for the corresponding antibody or antibody for antigen.

specificity (spes"ĭ-fis'ĭ-te) the state or quality of being restricted in application, effect, and the like. **organ s.,** sharing of similar antigenic determinants in organs with similar functions; see organ-specific ANTIGEN. **species s.,** 1. the state or quality of being characteristic of a particular species; having a characteristic effect on, or interaction with, cells or tissues of members of a particular species; said of an antigen, drug, or infective agent. 2. the occurrence of an antigen or other characteristics in a single species alone and not in others. **tissue s.,** organ-specific ANTIGEN.

specimen (spes'ĭ-men) 1. a sample or part of a thing, or of several things, taken to show or to determine the character of the whole, as a specimen of urine. 2. a preparation of tissue for histological, pathological, or chemical examination or analysis.

spectinomycin hydrochloride (spek"tĭ-no-mi'sin) a wide-spectrum antibiotic obtained from cultures of *Streptomyces spectabilis,* decadehydro-4α,7,9-trihydroxy-2-methyl-6,8-*bis*(methylamino)-4*H*-pyrano[2,3-*b*]benzodioxin-4-one dihydrochloride pentahydrate. It occurs as a white, odorless, slightly bitter crystalline powder that is soluble in water, but not in ethanol, chloroform, and ether. Spectinomycin is active against both gram-positive and gram-negative organisms. Used chiefly in the treatment of gonorrhea. Side reactions may include pain at the site of injection, headache, nausea, vomiting, pruritus, and urticaria. Trademarks: Spectogard, Stanilo, Togamycin, Trobicin.

Spectogard trademark for *spectinomycin hydrochloride* (see under SPECTINOMYCIN).

spectrograph (spek'tro-graf) an instrument for photographing spectra on a sensitive photographic plate. **mass s.,** an analytical instrument which identifies a substance by sorting a stream of electrified particles (ions) according to their mass. It consists of a cathode-ray tube containing a trace of the gaseous element to be studied, a perforated cathode with one central opening, electrically charged plates, a magnet, and a continuation of the vacuum chamber in which a photographic plate or an ion detector is placed. In operation, the stream of electrons produces positively charged particles by bombardment of the neutral gas molecules, the positive rays passing through the opening in the cathode and being subjected to electric and magnetic fields. These forces bend the rays out of their straight path into a semicircular path, to the extent that depends on the velocity, the charge, and the mass of the particles, thus sorting them accordingly, before they ultimately strike a photographic plate or photomultiplier tube sensor. Called also *mass spectrometer.*

Spectro-Jel trademark for a soapless skin cleanser containing 0.05 percent acetylpyridinium chloride, 15.0 percent isopropyl alcohol, and various amounts of glycerol, propylene glycol, and dispersing agents in a gel-like base of methylcellulose and glycol polysiloxane.

spectrometer (spek-trom′ĕ-ter) 1. an instrument for measuring the index of refraction by measuring the external angle of a prism of the substance. 2. a spectroscope for measuring the wavelengths of rays of a spectrum. **mass s.,** mass SPECTRO-GRAPH.

spectrophotometer (spek″tro-fo-tom′ĕ-ter) [*spectrum* + *photometer*] 1. an apparatus for measuring the light sense by means of a spectrum. 2. an apparatus for estimating the quality of coloring matter in solution by the quantity of light absorbed (as indicated by the spectrum) in passing through the solution. **absorption s.,** an analytical instrument for comparing the absorption of radiation of a given wavelength against a standard to identify a sample material.

Spectropure trademark for *dental mercury* (see under MER-CURY).

spectroscope (spek″tro-skōp) [*spectrum* + Gr. *skopein* to examine] an optical device used for the analysis of wavelengths in the visible spectrum by separating it into its component rays. It consists of a prism that refracts or a grating that diffracts the rays, with a device for making the rays parallel (collimator), and an eyepiece for enlarging the spectrum.

spectroscopy (spek-tros′ko-pe) observation by means of a spectroscope of the wavelength and intensity of electromagnetic radiation (light) absorbed or emitted by various materials. When excited by an arc or spark, the material emits radiation of certain wavelengths which may be used in the analysis of materials.

spectrum (spek′trum), pl. *spec′tra* [L. "apparition"] a visible display, a photographic record, or a plot of the distribution of the intensity of a given type of radiation as a function or its wavelength, energy frequency, momentum, mass, or any related quantity. See also WAVELENGTH. **acoustic s.,** the distribution of the intensity levels of the various frequency components of a sound. **continuous s.,** a spectrum of electromagnetic radiation that exhibits a gradual variation of wavelengths. See also BREMSSTRAHLUNG. **electromagnetic s.,** the continuous range of electromagnetic energy from cosmic rays to electric waves, including gamma rays, x-rays, ultraviolet rays, visible light, infrared rays, and radio waves. See also electromagnetic RADIATION. **x-radiation s.,** distribution of the intensity of a particular beam of x-radiation over the range of its component wavelengths or photon energies in keV. See also x-rays under RAY.

speculum (spek′u-lum), pl. *spec′ula* [L. "mirror"] an instrument for exposing the interior or a passage or cavity of the body. **ear s.,** one for the examination of the ear. **nasal s.,** one for the examination of the nose.

Spee, curve of (curvature of) [Ferdinand Graf von *Spee*, German embryologist, born 1855] See under CURVE.

speech (spēch) the process of the utterance of vocal sounds conveying ideas, involving activity of the lips, cheeks, tongue, and hard and soft palates. **delayed s.,** failure of speech to develop at the expected age, usually due to slow maturation, hearing disorders, brain injuries, mental retardation, or emotional disorders. **s. sound,** phoneme.

speed (spēd) 1. the rate of motion. 2. a popular name for amphetamine or any compound that is chemically or pharmacologically related to amphetamine. **film s.,** the amount of exposure to light or x-rays required to produce a given image density. It is expressed as the reciprocal of the exposure in roentgens necessary to produce a density of 1.0 above base and fog; films are classified on this basis in six speed groups, between each of which is a two-fold increase in film speed. Commonly, the film speed is classified as slow, medium, and fast (or high); the slow speed requiring the longest exposure time, and the fast speed requiring the shortest time, thereby exposing the patient to the least amount of radiation. **s. of light,** the speed at which the rays of light are traveling; or the speed of 186,284 miles per second. See LIGHT. **linear s.,** the speed at which a point of a moving object travels a given distance. The linear speed of a point on the surface of a rotating wheel (*rotational s.*) is calculated as follows: v = πdn, where *d* = diameter of the wheel, *n* = rpm, *v* = linear speed, and π = the ratio of the circumference of the circle to its diameter, 3.141. **rotational s.,** the speed at which a rotating object is traveling.

Speed liner see under LINER.

sperm (sperm) [Gr. *sperma* seed] 1. the semen or testicular secretion. 2. spermatozoon.

spermaceti (sper″mah-set′e) [Gr. *sperma* seed + *kētos* whale] a waxy substance obtained from the head of the sperm whale, containing chiefly cetyl palmitate, free cetyl alcohol, esters of higher alcohols, and esters of lauric, stearic, and myristic acids. It occurs as translucent, slightly unctuous masses with little odor and no taste, but becomes yellow and rancid on exposure to air, and is soluble in chloroform, ether, carbon disulfide, oils, and boiling alcohol, slightly soluble in petroleum ether, and insoluble in water. Used as a base for ointments, and as a coating of dental floss. Called also *cetaceum.*

spermatid (sper′mah-tid) any of the four haploid cells arising from the secondary spermatocyte by the second division of meiosis, which mature into spermatozoa without further cell division. Called also *spermatoblast.* See also SPERMATOGENE-SIS.

spermato-, spermo- [Gr. *sperma, spermatos* seed] combining form denoting relationship to seed, specifically to the male generative element.

spermatoblast (sper′mah-to-blast″) spermatid.

spermatocyte (sper′mah-to-sit″) [*spermato-* + *-cyte*] any of the sperm mother cells derived from spermatogonia that give rise to a spermatid and, eventually, a spermatozoon. See also SPERMATOGENESIS. **primary s.,** a spermatocyte which, in spermatogenesis, derives from a spermatogonium by mitosis and divides by the first meiotic division into two secondary spermatocytes. **secondary s.,** either of the two cells that derive from the primary spermatocyte by the first meiotic division and divide in turn by the second meiotic division to give rise to the spermatid. Called also *prespermatid.*

spermatogenesis (sper″mah-to-jen′ĕ-sis) [*spermato-* + Gr. *genesis* production] the production of spermatozoa. The process begins in the seminiferous tubules of the testes of the mature male, where the spermatogonia, the earliest cells of the series, are produced. After several series of mitoses, the spermatogonia evolve into the primary spermatocytes. The spermatocytes undergo the first meiotic division to become the secondary spermatocytes and, after the second division, develop into the spermatids. Without further cell division, the spermatids mature into the spermatozoa. See illustration. Cf. OOGENESIS.

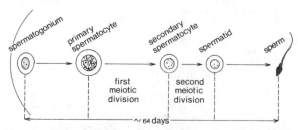

Diagram of human spermatogenesis. (From J. S. Thompson and M. W. Thompson: Genetics in Medicine. 3rd ed. Philadelphia, W. B. Saunders Co., 1980.)

spermatogonia (sper″mah-to-go′ne-ah) plural of *spermatogonium.*

spermatogonium (sper″mah-to-go′ne-um), pl. *spermatogo′nia* [*spermato-* + Gr. *gonē* generation] an immature male germ cell produced in the seminiferous tubules of the testes, which by mitotic division and differentiation gives rise to the primary spermatocyte, and eventually, to the spermatozoon. See also SPERMATOGENESIS.

spermatozoa (sper″mah-to-zo′ah) plural of *spermatozoon.*

spermatozoon (sper″mah-to-zo′on), pl. *spermatozo′a* [*spermato-* + Gr. *zōon* animal] a mature male germ cell which serves to impregnate the ovum in the process of reproduction. Called also *sperm.* See also SPERMATOGENESIS.

spermo- see SPERMATO-.

Speyer no. 18 trademark for a hard *dental casting gold alloy* (see under GOLD).

Speyer no. 21 trademark for a hard *dental casting gold alloy* (see under GOLD).

SPF specific-pathogen free; a term applied to gnotobiotic animals reared for use in laboratory experiments, and known to be free of specific pathogenic microorganisms.

sp. gr. specific GRAVITY.

Sph sphenoidale.

Sphaerocillus bullosus (sfe-ro′si-lus bul-lo′sus) *Fusobacterium bullosum;* see under FUSOBACTERIUM.

Sphaerophorus (sfe-ro′fo-rus) a former genus name for a group of gram-negative, anaerobic bacilli, now assigned to other genera. **S. fusifor′mis,** *Fusobacterium nucleatum;* see under FUSOBACTERIUM. **S. influenzaefor′mis,** *Fusobacterium russii;* see under FUSOBACTERIUM.

sphagitis (sfa-ji'tis) [Gr. *sphagē* throat + *-itis*] a throat inflammation.

sphenia (sfe'ne-ah) [L.] plural of *sphenion*.

sphenion (sfe'ne-on), pl. *sphe'nia* [Gr. *sphēn* wedge + *-on* neuter ending] a craniometric landmark, being the cranial point at the sphenoid angle of the parietal bone.

spheno- [Gr. *sphēn* wedge] a combining form denoting relationship to the sphenoid bone or to a wedge, or meaning wedge-shaped.

sphenobasilar (sfe"no-bas'ĭ-lar) pertaining to the sphenoid bone and the basilar part of the occipital bone.

sphenocephalus (sfe"no-sef'ah-lus) a fetus exhibiting sphenocephaly.

sphenocephaly (sfe"no-sef'ah-le) [*spheno-* + Gr. *kephalē* head] a developmental anomaly characterized by a wedge-shaped appearance of the head.

sphenoethmoid (sfe"no-eth'moid) denoting the curved plate of bone in front of the lesser wing of the sphenoid bone.

sphenofrontal (sfe"no-frun'tal) pertaining to the sphenoid and frontal bones.

sphenoid (sfe'noid) [*spheno-* + Gr. *eidos* form] shaped like a wedge; designating the sphenoid bone.

sphenoidal (sfe-noi'dal) pertaining to the sphenoid bone.

sphenoidale (sfe"noi-da'le) craniometric landmark, being the point of the greatest convexity between the anterior contours of the sella turcica and planum sphenoidale. Abbreviated *Sph*. Called also *point Sph*.

sphenoiditis (sfe"noi-di'tis) inflammation of the sphenoidal sinus.

sphenoidostomy (sfe"noi-dos'to-me) [*sphenoid* + Gr. *stomoun* to provide wih an opening, or mouth] surgical removal of the anterior wall of the sphenoidal sinus.

sphenoidotomy (sfe"noi-dot'o-me) incision into the sphenoidal sinus.

sphenomalar (sfe"no-ma'lar) sphenozygomatic.

sphenomaxillary (sfe"no-mak'sĭ-ler"e) pertaining to the sphenoid and maxillary bones.

spheno-occipital (sfe"no-ok-sip'ĭ-tal) pertaining to the sphenoid and occipital bones.

sphenopagus (sfe"nop'ah-gus) [*spheno-* + Gr. *pagos* that which is firmly set] symmetrical twins conjoined at the sphenoid bone. **s. parasit'icus**, congenital oral TERATOMA.

sphenopalatine (sfe"no-pal'ah-tīn) pertaining to the sphenoid and palatine bones.

sphenoparietal (sfe"no-pah-ri'ĕ-tal) pertaining to the sphenoid and parietal bones.

sphenopetrosal (sfe"no-pe-tro'sal) pertaining to the sphenoid and petrous bones.

sphenorbital (sfe"nor'bĭ-tal) pertaining to the sphenoid bone and the orbit.

sphenosquamosal (sfe"no-skwa-mo'sal) pertaining to the sphenoid bone and the squamous portion of the temporal bone.

sphenotemporal (sfe"no-tem'po-ral) pertaining to the sphenoid and temporal bones.

sphenotic (sfe-not'ik) [*spheno-* + Gr. *ous* ear] denoting a fetal bone which becomes that part of the sphenoid bone which is adjacent to the carotid groove.

sphenotresia (sfe"no-tre'ze-ah) [*spheno-* + Gr. *trēsis* boring] boring of the skull in craniotomy.

sphenoturbinal (sfe"no-tur'bĭ-nal) denoting a thin, curved bone in front of each of the lesser wings of the sphenoid bone, to which bone it becomes fused.

sphenovomerine (sfe"no-vo'mer-in) pertaining to the sphenoid bone and to the vomer.

sphenozygomatic (sfe"no-zi"go-mat'ik) pertaining to the sphenoid and zygomatic bones; sphenomalar.

Spheraloy trademark for an *amalgam alloy* (see under AMALGAM).

sphere (sfēr) [Gr. *sphaira*] a globular body or object; a ball. **attraction s.**, centrosome. **embryonic s.**, morula. **segmentation s.**, 1. blastomere. **vitelline s.**, yolk, s., morula.

spheresthesia (sfe"res-the'ze-ah) [Gr. *sphaira* sphere + *aisthēsis* perception + *-ia*] a morbid sensation of a lump or ball in the throat; globus hystericus.

sphero- [Gr. *sphaira* a ball or globe] a combining form meaning round, or denoting relationship to a sphere.

spherocyte (sfe'ro-sīt) [*sphero-* + Gr. *kytos* hollow vessel] an abnormal erythrocyte which has a globular form, being somewhat smaller but thicker than a normal red cell. Spherocytes are usually found in the blood in spherocytosis and also in other forms of hemolytic anemia. They stain bright red and show no central pallor.

spherocytosis (sfe"ro-si-to'sis) a condition characterized by the presence of spherocytes in the blood. **hereditary s.**, a chronic, hereditary form of hemolytic anemia, characterized by the presence in the blood of spherocytes, which is usually present at birth, but the symptoms may become evident much later in life. Symptoms include increased osmotic fragility of the erythrocytes, high reticulocyte count, icterus, splenomegaly, hyperplasia of the bone marrow, and the presence of urobilinogen in the stools. There also may be a wide variety of complications, such as skeletal, ocular, and dental abnormalities. Roentgenographic examination may show striation and thickening of the frontal and parietal bones, and occasionally oxycephaly. It is transmitted as an autosomal dominant trait; persons of northern European origin are affected most frequently, but it may also occur in other ethnic groups. Called also *acholuric familial jaundice*, *congenital hemolytic anemia*, and *Minkowski-Chauffard syndrome*.

spheroid (sfe'roid) [Gr. *sphaira* a ball or globe + *eidos* form] resembling a sphere; a globular body.

spheroiding (sfe-roid'ing) in occlusal adjustment, the restoration of the original tooth contour, including the buccolingual width of the occlusal surface of the tooth.

spheroidite (sfe-roi'dīt) a mixture of microscopic size particles of cementite spheroids in a matrix of ferrite, formed by heating (tempering) martensite just below the eutectoid temperature. Bainite and pearlite may also be transformed to spheroidite by prolonged heating at a high subeutectoid temperature. Called also *spheroidized cementite*.

Spheromycin trademark for *novobiocin*.

spheroplast (sfer'o-plast) a spherical bacterial or plant cell, produced in hypertonic media under conditions that result in partial removal of the cell wall which no longer serves as a supporting structure.

sphincter (sfingk'ter) [L.; Gr. *sphinktēr* that which binds tight] a ring of muscle fibers, the function of which is the contraction or closing of a natural orifice. Called also *musculus sphincter* [NA] and *sphincter muscle*. **s. of eye**, **s. of eyelids**, orbicular muscle of eye; see under MUSCLE. **s. o'ris**, orbicular muscle of mouth; see under MUSCLE.

sphingolipid (sfing"go-lip'id) [Gr. *sphingein* to bind tight + *lipid*] a lipid containing sphingosine; a fatty acid is attached to the nitrogen atom, and these N-acylsphingosines are called *ceramides*. Sphingolipids are combinations of different compounds with the hydroxyl group of ceramides, e.g., sphingomyelins (with phosphoryl choline), gangliosides (with branched-chain oligosaccharides), and cerebrosides (with glucose or galactose). They occur in membranes and in particularly high concentrations in brain and nerve tissue. Abnormally large concentrations of sphingolipids in glial cells of the nervous system occur in Tay-Sachs disease.

sphingomyelin (sfing"go-mi'ĕ-lin) [Gr. *sphingein* to bind tight + *myelin*] a group of phospholipids containing chiefly sphingolipids and glycolipids, their chief components being fatty acids, phosphoric acid, choline, and sphingosine; some contain the saturated base dihydrosphingosine. Fatty acids are attached to the amino group of sphingosine in the amide linkage. Sphingomyelins are rapidly soluble in benzene, chloroform, and hot alcohol, partially soluble in ether, and insoluble in acetone and water. They are found mainly in the brain and nerves, particularly in the gray and white matter, and are also found in the liver, kidneys, spleen, erythrocytes, blood plasma, and other organs, representing some 5 to 25 percent of the total phospholipids. In the brain, the composition of sphingomyelin fatty acids varies with location and age. In the gray matter, C_{16} and C_{18} acid content is greater than that in the white matter. Being a component of myelin, sphingomyelin plays a role in protecting and insulating nerve fibers. Increased concentration of sphingomyelin in the body occurs in Niemann-Pick syndrome.

sphingosine (sfing'go-sin) a compound, 1,3-dihydroxy-2-amino-4-octadecene, which is a long-chain monounsaturated aliphatic amino alcohol, usually present in certain phospholipids, such as cerebrosides and sphingomyelins.

sphygmo- [Gr. *sphygmos* pulse] a combining form denoting relationship to the pulse.

sphygmograph (sfig'mo-graf) [*sphygmo-* + Gr. *graphein* to write] an instrument for registering the movements, form, and force of the pulse.

sphygmomanometer (sfig"mo-mah-nom'ĕ-ter) [*sphygmo-* + *manometer*] an instrument for measuring arterial blood pressure indirectly by the auscultatory technique. See also blood PRESSURE. See illustration.

spicula (spik'u-lah) [L.] plural of *spiculum*.

spicular (spik'u-lar) pertaining to a spicule.

spicule (spik'ul) [L. *spiculum*] a sharp, needle-like body. **cemen-**

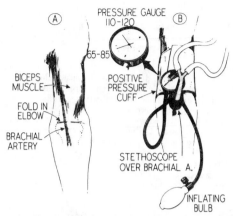

Blood pressure cuff and gauge in place. *A*, Location of artery on inner elbow. *B*, Cuff and gauge in place on arm. (From Emergency Care and Transportation of the Sick and Injured. Committee on Injuries, American Academy of Orthopaedic Surgeons, Chicago, 1971.)

tal s., a projection of calcified cementum extending from the surface of the root of a tooth into the periodontal ligament.

spiculum (spik'u-lum), pl. *spic'ula* [L.] spicule.

spike (spīk) [L. *spica* ear of corn] a sharp-pointed part or projection. **enamel s.,** enamel SPUR.

spillway (spil'wa) 1. a passage or channel through which excess water overflows from a reservoir, lake, etc. 2. embrasure. **axial s.,** a groove that crosses a cusp ridge or a marginal ridge and extends onto the axial surface of the tooth, serving to self-cleanse the tooth and stimulate the investing tissue. **interdental s.,** embrasure. **occlusal s.,** a groove crossing only a cusp ridge or a marginal ridge of a tooth.

spina (spi'nah), pl. *spi'nae* [L.] spine; a thornlike process or projection; used as a general anatomical term for such a structure. See under SPINE. **s. angula'ris,** sphenoidal SPINE. **s. bif'ida,** faulty closure of the bony encasement of the spinal cord, usually associated with protrusion of the meninges (meningomyelocele). **s. fronta'lis,** nasal spine of frontal bone; see under SPINE. **s. mea'tus,** suprameatal SPINE. **s. menta'lis** [NA], mental SPINE. **s. nasa'lis ante'rior maxil'lae** [NA], nasal s. of maxilla, anterior; see under SPINE. **s. nasa'lis os'sis fronta'lis** [NA], nasal spine of frontal bone; see under SPINE. **s. nasa'lis os'sis palat'ini** [NA], **s. nasa'lis poste'rior os'sis palati'ni,** nasal spine of palatine bone; see under SPINE. **s. os'sis sphenoida'lis** [NA], sphenoidal SPINE. **s. palati'na,** palatine SPINE. **s. supramea'tum** [NA], suprameatal SPINE. **s. trochlea'ris** [NA], trochlear SPINE. **s. tampan'ica ma'jor** [NA], tympanic spine, greater; see under SPINE. **s. tampan'ica mi'nor** [NA], tympanic spine, lesser; see under SPINE.

spinae (spi'ne) [L.] plural of *spina.*

spinal (spi'nal) [L. *spinalis*] pertaining to a spine or to the vertebral column.

spinalis (spi-na'lis) [L.] spinal.

spinalgia (spi-nal'je-ah) [*spine* + Gr. *algos* pain + *-ia*] pain in the spinal region.

spinate (spi'nāt) [L. *spinatus*] having spines or thorns, or shaped like a spine or thorn.

spindle (spin'd'l) 1. a round structure with tapered ends or a fusiform structure. 2. the fusiform figure of achromatin in the cell nucleus during mitosis; nuclear spindle. **enamel s's,** club-like structures in the inner third of the dental enamel, believed to be terminals of protoplasmic processes of the odontoblasts which have passed across the dentinoenamel junction. **Kühne's s.,** neuromuscular s. **muscle s.,** neuromuscular s. **neuromuscular s.,** a fusiform end structure found in most voluntary muscles, consisting of parallelly arranged small bundles of three to ten fibers (intrafusal fibers) invested in a capsule, about 0.5 to 5 mm in length, in which the sensory nerve fibers terminate. The axons of the sensory nerves enter the capsule and after losing the myelin sheath, divide into several fibers, each encircling an intrafusal fiber. The spindle is the receptor responsible for the stretch, which responds to passive stretch of the muscle but ceases to discharge if the muscle contracts isotonically, thus signaling muscle length. Called also *Kühne's s.* and *muscle s.*

neurotendinous s., Golgi tendon ORGAN. **nuclear s.,** spindle (2). **tendon s.,** Golgi tendon ORGAN.

spine (spīn) [L. *spina*] 1. any thornlike process or projection. Called also *spina.* 2. vertebral COLUMN. **alar s.,** sphenoidal s. **angular s.,** sphenoidal s. **basilar s.,** pharyngeal TUBERCLE. **Civini's s.,** pterygospinous PROCESS. **ethmoidal s. of Macalister,** sphenoidal CREST. **ethmoidal s. of sphenoid bone,** a bony crest on the intracranial surface of the body of the sphenoid bone, which articulates with the cribriform plate of the ethmoid. **frontal s., external,** nasal s. of frontal bone. **s. of Henle,** suprameatal s. **jugular s.,** jugular PROCESS. **Macalister's ethmoidal s.,** sphenoidal CREST. **mandibular s.,** LINGULA of mandible. **s. of maxilla,** nasal s. of maxilla, anterior. **meatal s.,** suprameatal s. **mental s.,** any of the small bony projections (usually four in number) located on the internal surface of the mandible, near the lower end of the midline, serving for attachment of the genioglossal and geniohyoid muscles. Called also *genial apophysis* and *spina mentalis* [NA]. **mental s., external,** mental PROTUBERANCE. **nasal s., anterior,** 1. nasal s. of maxilla, anterior. 2. a craniometric landmark, being the tip of the anterior nasal spine seen on the lateral roentgenogram (norma lateralis). Abbreviated *ANS.* Called also *point ANS.* See illustration at CEPHALOMETRY. **nasal s. of frontal bone,** a rough and somewhat irregular process of bone projecting downward and forward from the frontal part of the inferior surface of the pars nasalis of the frontal bone and fitting between the nasal bones and the ethmoid bone. Called also *external frontal s., external frontal process, spina frontalis,* and *spina nasalis ossis frontalis* [NA]. **nasal s. of maxilla, anterior,** the sharp anterosuperior projection at the anterior extremity of the nasal crest of the maxilla. Called also *anterior nasal s., s. of maxilla,* and *spina nasalis anterior maxillae* [NA]. **nasal s. of palatine bone,** a small, sharp, backward-projecting bony spine forming the medial posterior angle of the horizontal portion of the palatine bone. Called also *posterior nasal s., spina nasalis ossis palatini* [NA], and *spina nasalis posterior ossis palatini.* **nasal s., posterior,** 1. nasal s. of palatine bone. 2. a craniometric landmark, being the tip of the posterior spine of the palatine bone in the hard palate. Abbreviated *PNS.* Called also *point PNS.* See illustration at CEPHALOMETRY. **occipital s., external,** external occipital PROTUBERANCE. **occipital s., internal,** internal occipital PROTUBERANCE. **palatine s.,** one of the ridges which are laterally placed on the inferior surface of the maxillary part of the hard palate, separating the palatine sulci. Called also *spina palatina.* **pharyngeal s.,** pharyngeal TUBERCLE. **s. of sphenoid bone,** sphenoidal s. **sphenoidal s.,** a bony process directed inferiorly from the inferior aspect of the great wing of the sphenoid bone where the wing projects into the angle between the petrous and squamous portions of the temporal bone; it is just posterior to the foramen spinosum and serves for attachment of the sphenomandibular and pterygospinous ligaments. Called also *alar s., angular s., s. of sphenoid bone, spina angularis,* and *spina ossis sphenoidalis* [NA]. **suprameatal s.,** a small spinous process that sometimes projects from the temporal bone on the anterior border of the suprameatal triangle, at the back of the external acoustic meatus. Called also *s. of Henle, meatal s., spina meatus,* and *spina suprameatum* [NA]. **trochlear s.,** a spicule of bone on the anteromedial part of the orbital surface of the frontal bone for attachment of the trochlea of the superior oblique muscle; when absent, it is represented by the trochlear fovea. Called also *spina trochlearis* [NA] and *trochlear tubercle.* **tympanic s., greater,** a spine of the temporal bone forming the anterior edge of the tympanic notch (deficient part of the tympanic sulcus). Called also *spina tympanica major* [NA]. **tympanic s., lesser,** a spine of the temporal bone forming the posterior edge of the tympanic notch. Called also *spina tympanica minor* [NA].

spinous (spi'nus) [L. *spinosus*] 1. like a spine; acanthoid. 2. pertaining to a spine or to a spinelike process.

spir. abbreviation for L. *spir'itus,* spirit.

spiral (spi'ral) [L. *spiralis* from *spira;* Gr. *speira*] 1. winding about a center like a coil or the thread of a screw. 2. anything coiled or winding about a center.

spireme (spi'rēm) [Gr. *speirēma* coil] the threadlike, continuous or segmented figure formed by the chromosome material during the prophase of mitosis or meiosis.

spirilla (spi-ril'ah) [L.] plural of *spirillum.*

Spirillaceae (spi"ril-la'se-e) [*Spirillum* + *-aceae*] a family of rigid, helically curved rod-shaped, gram-negative bacteria with less than one complete turn to many turns. The cells are motile, swimming in straight lines with a corkscrew-like motion. Some members are aerobic or obligately microaerophilic, others are anaerobic but capable of growing under microaerophilic conditions. They are found in water, some strains being saprophytic or parasitic, and some are pathogenic. It includes the genera *Campylobacter* and *Spirillum*.

Spirillospora (spi-ril″o-spo′rah) [Gr. *speira* a coil + *sporos* seed] a genus of soil bacteria of the family Actinoplanaceae, order Actinomycetales.

Spirillum (spi-ril′um) [L. *spirillum* a small spiral] a genus of rigid, helical, rod-shaped, gram-negative bacteria of the family *Spirillaceae*, made up of cells which form spirals of a portion of a turn to several turns, about 0.25 to 1.7 μm in diameter. S. **bucca′le**, *Treponema buccale*; see under TREPONEMA. S. **chol′erae**, S. **chol′erae-asiat′icae**, *Vibrio cholerae*; see under VIBRIO. S. **coh′nii**, *Treponema buccale*; see under TREPONEMA. S. **den′tium**, *Treponema denticola*; see under TREPONEMA. S. **dutto′ni**, *Borrelia duttonii*; see under BORRELIA. S. **fe′tus**, *Campylobacter fetus*; see under CAMPYLOBACTER. S. **fink′leri**, *Vibrio cholerae* (biotype *proteus*); see under VIBRIO. S. **mi′nor**, S. **mi′nus**, the etiologic agent of the spirillary form of rat-bite fever, occurring as short thick rods, 0.2 to 0.5 μm by 3.0 to 5.0 μm, having two to three windings and polar tufts of external flagella that give the organism a rapid darting motion. It is sensitive to arsenicals, penicillin, and broad-spectrum antibiotics. S. **pal′lidum**, *Treponema pallidum*; see under TREPONEMA. S. **perten′ue**, *Treponema pertenue*; see under TREPONEMA. S. **phosphores′cens**, *Vibrio cholerae* (biotype *albensis*); see under VIBRIO. S. **refrin′gens**, *Treponema refringens*; see under TREPONEMA. S. **vincen′ti**, *Treponema vincentii*; see under TREPONEMA.

spirillum (spi-ril′um), pl. *spiril′la* [L.] 1. a relatively rigid, spiral-shaped bacterium. 2. any microorganism of the genus *Spirillum* or of the family Spirillaceae.

spirit (spir′it) [L. *spiritus*] 1. in pharmacy, an alcoholic solution of a volatile principle, such as camphor or ammonia. 2. any distilled liquid. 3. ethyl ALCOHOL. **s. of ammonia**, s. of ammonia, aromatic. **s. of ammonia, aromatic**, a solution containing 34 gm ammonium carbonate, 90 ml of 10 percent ammonia water, 10 ml lemon oil, 1 ml oil of lavender, 1 ml oil of myristica, 700 ml alcohol, and water; each 100 ml having 1.7 to 2.1 gm ammonia and 3.4 to 4.5 gm ammonium carbonate. Used as a respiratory stimulant in syncope, weakness, or threatened faint. Also available in capsules which are crushed to permit rapid volatilization. Called also *s. of ammonia, aromatic s. of hartshorn*, and *ammonia inhalant*. **s. of camphor**, an alcoholic solution of camphor, 100 ml of which contains 9 to 11 gm camphor; used as a local irritant. **s. of hartshorn**, AMMONIUM hydroxide. **s. of hartshorn, aromatic**, s. of ammonia, aromatic. **s. of turpentine**, turpentine OIL.

Spirochaeta (spi″ro-ke′tah) [Gr. *speira* coil + *chaitē* hair] a genus of gram-negative bacteria of the family Spirochaetaceae, order Spirochaetales, made up of large (up to 500 μm in length) free-living cells, usually found in H₂S-containing mud, polluted water, and sewage. Most of the organisms placed in this genus in earlier nomenclature have been reclassified in other genera. S. **acu′ta**, *Treponema scoliodontum*; see under TREPONEMA. S. **ambig′ua**, *Treponema denticola*; see under TREPONEMA. S. **biflex′a**, *Leptospira interrogans*; see under LEPTOSPIRA. S. **calligy′rum**, *Treponema refringens*; see under TREPONEMA. S. **comando′nii**, *Treponema denticola*; see under TREPONEMA. S. **cunic′uli**, *Treponema paraluis-cuniculi*; see under TREPONEMA. S. **denti′cola**, S. **den′tium**, *Treponema denticola*; see under TREPONEMA. S. **dutto′ni**, *Borrelia duttonii*; see under BORRELIA. S. **herm′si**, *Borrelia hermsii*; see under BORRELIA. S. **hispan′ica**, *Borrelia hispanica*; see under BORRELIA. S. **ic-terog′enes**, S. **icterohaemorrhag′iae**, *Leptospira interrogans*; see under LEPTOSPIRA. S. **inaequa′lis**, *Treponema buccale*; see under TREPONEMA. S. **inter′rogans**, *Leptospira interrogans*; see under LEPTOSPIRA. S. **macroden′tium**, *Treponema macrodentium*; see under TREPONEMA. S. **microden′tium**, *Treponema denticola*; see under TREPONEMA. S. **muco′sa**, *Treponema mucosum*; see under TREPONEMA. S. **nodo′sa**, *Leptospira interrogans*; see under LEPTOSPIRA. S. **obermei′eri**, *Borrelia recurrentis*; see under BORRELIA. S. **orthodon′ta**, *Treponema denticola*; see under TREPONEMA. S. **pal′lida**, *Treponema pallidum*; see under TREPONEMA. S. **pal′lida** var. **cunic′uli**, S. **par′aluis-cunic′uli**, *Treponema paraluis-cuniculi*; see under TREPONEMA. S. **perten′uis**, *Treponema pertenue*; see under TREPONEMA. S. **phagede′nis**, *Treponema phagedenis*; see under TREPONEMA. S. **recurren′tis**, *Borrelia recurrentis*; see under BORRELIA. S. **refrin′gens**, *Treponema refringens*; see under TREPONEMA. S. **skoliodon′tia**, *Treponema scoliodontum*; see under TREPONEMA. S. **vincen′ti**, *Treponema vincentii*; see under TREPONEMA.

Spirochaetaceae (spi″ro-ke-ta′se-e) [*Spirochaeta* + *-aceae*] a family of gram-negative bacteria of the order Spirochaetales, made up of helically shaped cells composed of cytoplasm en-

closed in a cytoplasmic membrane and surrounded by a thin peptidoglycan layer. It includes the genera *Borrelia*, *Leptospira*, *Spirochaeta*, and *Treponema*.

Spirochaetales (spi″ro-ke-ta′lēz) an order of bacteria made up of slender, flexible, helically coiled cells, 3 to 500 μm in length, occurring in chains held together by an outer envelope. The members are motile, do not form endospores, and are aerobic, facultatively anaerobic, or anaerobic, larger ones being gram-negative. Some are pathogenic. The order consists of the family Spirochaetaceae.

spirochetal (spi″ro-ke′tal) pertaining to or caused by spirochetes.

spirochete (spi′ro-kēt) any microorganism of the order Spirochaetales; a spiral bacterium. **Dutton's s.**, *Borrelia duttonii*; see under BORRELIA.

spirochetemia (spi″ro-ke-te′me-ah) [*spirochete* + Gr. *haima* blood + *-ia*] the presence of spirochetes in the blood.

spirocheticidal (spi′ro-ke″ti-si′dal) [*spirochete* + L. *caedere* to kill] destructive to spirochetes.

spirocheticide (spi″ro-ke′ti-sīd) an agent that causes the destruction of spirochetes.

spirochetolysin (spi″ro-ke-tol′ĭ-sin) an agent that causes lysis of spirochetes.

spirochetosis (spi″ro-ke-to′sis) infection with spirochetes.

spirocheturia (spi″ro-ke-tu′re-ah) [*spirochete* + Gr. *ouron* urine + *-ia*] the presence of spirochetes in the urine.

Spirofulvin trademark for *griseofulvin*.

spirography (spi-rog′rah-fe) the graphic measurement of breathing.

spiroid (spi′roid) resembling a spiral.

spirometer (spi-rom′ĕ-ter) [L. *spirare* to breathe + *metrum* measure] an instrument for measuring exhaled and inhaled air. See also breath ANALYZER.

Spironema (spi″ro-ne′mah) [Gr. *speira* coil + *nēma* thread] *Treponema*. S. **bucca′le**, *Treponema buccale*; see under TREPONEMA. S. **den′tium**, *Treponema denticola*; see under TREPONEMA. S. **pal′lidum**, *Treponema pallidum*; see under TREPONEMA. S. **perten′ue**, *Treponema pertenue*; see under TREPONEMA. S. **phagede′nis**, *Treponema phagedenis*; see under TREPONEMA. S. **refrin′gens**, *Treponema refringens*; see under TREPONEMA. S. **vincen′ti**, *Treponema vincentii*; see under TREPONEMA.

spironolactone (spi-ro″no-lak′tōn) a steroid compound, 7α-(acetylthio)-17α-hydroxy-3-oxopregn-4-one-21-carboxylic acid, occurring as a cream-colored to light tan, crystalline powder that is soluble in benzene, chloroform, ethyl acetate, and ethanol, slightly soluble in methanol and fixed oils, and insoluble in water. It is an aldosterone-inhibitor that competes with aldosterone for receptor sites in the tubular epithelial cells and blocks its sodium reabsorption action. Sodium remaining in the tubules acts as an osmotic diuretic. Used in the treatment of hypertension, congestive heart failure, ascites, edema, and nephrotic syndrome. Also used in the diagnosis of aldosteronism. Side reactions may include hyponatremia, hyperkalemia, drowsiness, headache, diarrhea, skin rash, urticaria, confusion, drug fever, ataxia, impotence, hirsutism, deepening of voice, and irregular menses. Trademarks: Aldactone A, Verospiron.

Spiroschaudinnia (spi″ro-shaw-din′e-ah) a proposed generic name for a group of spiral microorganisms, now assigned to the genera *Borrelia* and *Treponema*. S. **bucca′lis**, *Treponema buccale*; see under TREPONEMA. S. **phagede′nis**, *Treponema phagedenis*; see under TREPONEMA. S. **recurren′tis**, *Borrelia recurrentis*; see under BORRELIA. S. **refrin′gens**, *Treponema refringens*; see under TREPONEMA. S. **vincen′ti**, *Treponema vincentii*; see under TREPONEMA.

splanchnic (splank′nik) [Gr. *splanchnikos*; L. *splanchnicus*] pertaining to the viscera.

splanchno- [Gr. *splanchnos* viscus] a combining form denoting relationship to a viscus, or to the splanchnic nerve.

splanchnocranium (splank″no-kra′ne-um) [*splancho-* + Gr. *kranion* cranium] those parts of the skull that are of branchial arch origin.

splanchnopleure (splank′no-ploor) [*splanchno-* + Gr. *pleura* side] the embryonic wall formed jointly by the entoderm and the splanchnic mesoderm.

spleen (splēn) [Gr. *splēn*; L. *lien*] a large, about 125 mm long, glandlike but ductless organ situated in the upper part of the abdominal cavity on the left side and lateral to the cardiac end of the stomach, and surrounded by a connective tissue capsule from which trabeculae extend into the interior. The interior is filled with the white pulp and the red pulp, the white pulp containing lymph nodules and being the chief site of lymphocyte production. The terminal follicles in this region contain B-lymphocytes; the T-lymphocytes being found in the follicles of the periarteriolar sheaths of the white pulp. The arterial blood enters the hilus and follows along the trabeculae until the smaller arteries become surrounded by sheaths or collars of lymphocytes (white pulp), giving off capillaries to the lymph nodules. The blood in the red pulp has reticuloendothelial elements active in phagocytosis. Splenic function, which is not fully understood at present, consists of removing worn-out cells from the circulation, converting hemoglobin to bilirubin, and releasing iron into the circulation for reuse. The spleen is also a part of the peripheral and central lymphoid system, producing lymphocytes and plasma cells, and playing a role in the mediation of specific immunologic events, its function being most important in infancy and childhood. Called also *lien* [NA].

Splendore, A. see South American BLASTOMYCOSIS (Lutz-Splendore-de Almeida disease).

splenomegaly (sple″no-meg′ah-le) [*spleen* + Gr. *megas* large] enlargement of the spleen. **febrile tropical s.**, visceral LEISHMANIASIS.

splint (splint) 1. a rigid or flexible appliance used to maintain in position a displaced or movable part or to keep in place and protect an injured part. 2. the act of fastening or confining with a splint a displaced or movable part, or the support or bracing of such a part. **abutment s.**, adjacent tooth restorations that have been rigidly united at their proximal contact areas to form a single abutment with multiple roots. **acrylic resin bite-guard s.**, a device made of acrylic resin that covers the occlusal and incisal surfaces of the dental arch, designed to immobilize and stabilize the teeth, to eliminate damaging effects of bruxism, and to facilitate the establishment of centric relation. **anchor s.**, one for fracture of the jaw, with metal loops fitting over the teeth and held together by a rod. **Angle's s.**, one for fracture of the mandible. **Asch's s.**, a tube splint for fracture of the nose. **buccal s.**, a material, such as plaster, which after placing on the buccal surfaces of assembled fixed partial denture units, hardens and holds all the components in accurate relation to each other. **cap s.**, a plastic or metallic fracture stabilization device designed to cover the crowns of the teeth and usually cemented in place. **Carter's intranasal s.**, a fenestrated steel bridge, the wings of which are connected by a hinge; used in the bridge splint operation for depressed bridge of the nose. **cast bar s.**, a provisional splint consisting of cast continuous clasps that follow the facial and lingual surfaces of the teeth at the height of contour. It may be cemented in place to the splinted teeth and simultaneously wired in order to bring the clasps into contact with the teeth, or it may not be cemented to serve as a removable cast splint. Called also *Friedman s.* **compressive s.**, one that compresses the splinted organ. Called also *pressure s.* **compressive facial s.**, one of plastic material molded to conform with anatomical details of the head and neck structures, designed to apply constant pressure on the splinted organ to prevent early scar contractures or to promote keloid shrinkage following keloid injection. **continuous clasp s.**, a cast splint used for provisional immobilization of the teeth. **copper band–acrylic s.**, one fabricated from copper bands and acrylic resin. **crib s.**, a device for temporary tooth immobilization, constructed of gold, acrylic resin, chrome-cobalt alloys, or combinations thereof. It consists of a continuous crib clasp covering the facial and lingual surfaces of the splinted teeth. **cross arch bar s.**, one formed by a metal bar that unites one or more teeth of one side of the dental arch to one or more of the opposite side; used to stabilize teeth against lateral tilting forces. **diagnostic s.**, provisional s. **Elbrecht s.**, a temporary or permanent removable cast splint that may be extended around the entire dental arch. **Essig-type s.**, a stainless steel wire passed labially and lingually around a segment of the dental arch and held in position by individual ligature wires around the contact areas of the teeth; used to stabilize fractured or repositioned teeth. **fenestrated s.**, a temporary splint used for short permanent clinical crowns, deciduous teeth when no undercut is available for retention, badly decayed teeth, or cleft palate, consisting of a one-piece device contoured to fit an edentulous maxilla or mandible through fenestrations created for occlusal surfaces of the teeth. See illustration. **fixed s.**, permanent s., fixed. **fixed partial denture s.**, a partial denture used to unite weakened teeth, most frequently applied to stabilize the second premolar when the first premolar and molar are missing. **fracture s.**, 1. any device fabricated of metal or plastic and used to fix segments in the

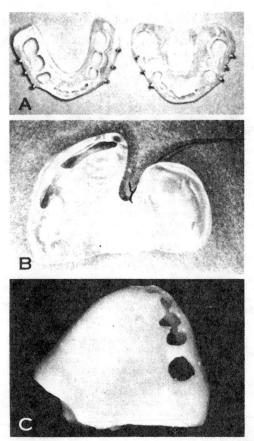

A, Mandibular and maxillary fenestrated splint. B, Fenestrated splint used for child with cleft palate. C, Silicone fenestrated obturator used on heavily radiated teeth. (From V. A. Chalian, J. B. Drane, and S. M. Standish: Maxillo-Facial Prosthetics. Baltimore, Williams & Wilkins, 1971.)

treatment of fractures or facial deformities. 2. a plastic material contoured to the lingual and buccal-labial aspects of the teeth fixed with wire or cement. **Friedman s.**, cast bar s. **Gilmer's s.**, a stainless steel wire fastening for holding the lower teeth to the upper ones in fractures of the mandible. Called also *Gilmer's wire.* **Gunning's s.**, an interdental splint used in fractures of the mandible or maxilla. **Gunning s., one-piece**, one for an edentulous mouth, used to hold together fractured segments of mandibular or maxillary bones and to immobilize the jaws in occlusion, consisting of the upper and lower baseplates joined in a vertical and centric relation with a bite rim, and immobilized by an extraoral Barton bandage or an elastic chin bandage. **Gunning s., two-piece**, one for an edentulous mouth, used to hold together fractured segments of the mandibular or maxillary bones and to immobilize the jaws in occlusion, consisting of separate splints for the maxilla and the mandible, which are interlocked to maintain the proper centric occlusion. See illustration. **Hammond's s.**, a strong gold wire splint used to

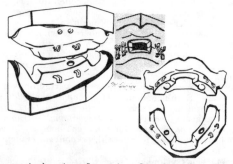

Diagrammatic drawing of two-piece Gunning splint. (From V. A. Chalian, J. B. Drane, and S. M. Standish: Maxillo-Facial Prosthetics. Baltimore, Williams & Wilkins, 1971.)

reduce fractures of the mandible. It is made in one piece and bent to approximate the contact with the labial, buccal, and lingual surfaces of the teeth, and the teeth are then attached to the splint with wire ligatures. **implant surgical s.**, a loosely fitting temporary superstructure without metal clasps or precision attachments, which is inserted immediately after the insertion of the substructure of a subperiosteal or intraperiosteal implant. It serves to maintain occlusion, stabilize the implant, prevent tissue displacement, control hemorrhage, and provide limited chewing capability until the temporary superstructure is installed. Also called *temporary implant superstructure.* **inlay s.**, an inlay casting, consisting of a single casting or two inlays soldered together, designed to give fixation or support to one or more approximating teeth. **interdental s.**, one for fracture of the jaws, held in place by wires passed around the teeth. **Jones' nasal s.**, one for fracture of the nasal bones. **Kazanjian's s.**, one used for nasal fractures, consisting of an oblong metal frame, the lower surface of which is supplied with a round bar. The frame is embedded in a dental compound spread over the forehead, the frame and the compound being held in place with the aid of adhesive tape passed around the head. The horizontal bar is left open for the attachment of a universal joint which can be passed freely along the bar and then held in place near the median line, a vertical bar being attached to the joint. The lower end of the vertical bar consists of a flat base covered with a dental compound pressed against the side of the nose, and elastic bands are used to exert pressure against the side of the nose. See also *nasal fracture s.* **Kingsley s.**, one consisting of a base plate, precisely adapted to the upper dental arch, with stout metal arms that extend out through the mouth and then curve backward along the sides of the cheek to provide fixation to the head cap; used for jaw fractures. See also *trismus* STENT. **labial s.**, an appliance of plastic and/or metal, made to conform to the outer aspect of the dental arch; used in the management of jaw and facial injuries. **labiolingual s.**, one for dentulous or partially edentulous arches, used in reducing jaw fractures, consisting of an acrylic band that fits around the labial and lingual aspects of the teeth, leaving the occlusal surface of the teeth uncovered. The continuity of the two flanges is secured by a stainless steel wire bent to form hinges which are placed bilaterally behind the last posterior teeth. The labial flange is split into two sections from the midline or from another suitable area. Two buttons are used at the labial segment for tightening and immobilizing the splint to the arch with stainless steel wire. The splint is often used with exostosis. See illustration. **lingual s.**, one similar to the labial splint, but conforming to the inner aspect of the dental arch. **molded s.**, one made of a plastic material molded to conform with the anatomical details of an organ. **nasal fracture s.**, a piece of flat, soft, hourglass-shaped metal, bent so that the lower part conforms to the general shape of the nose and the upper part rests flat against the forehead, over which a dental compound is applied. The splint is retained by strips of adhesive tape passing across the forehead at the top, and over the cheeks beneath the eyes at the bottom. See also *Kazanjian's s.* **occlusal s.**, one that overlays the occlusal surfaces of the teeth. One type, made from hard processed acrylic resin, fits over the occlusal and incisal surfaces of the teeth and has a flat occlusal surface, with occlusal contacts in centric relation for all the opposing teeth, being free from any occlusal interferences. An occlusal splint is used sometimes to splint loose teeth, to prevent tooth migration, and to redistribute occlusal stresses over several teeth in conditions where periodontal support is not indicated. Its primary use is to serve as an occlusal guard in treating clenching and bruxism and their sequelae. Another type is the bilateral posterior onlay splint that usually covers the mandibular molars and bicuspids, designed either for increasing the occlusal vertical

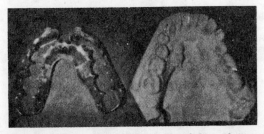

Labiolingual splint and mandibular cast with lingual exostoses over the model. (From V. A. Chalian, J. B. Drane, and S. M. Standish: Maxillo-Facial Prosthetics. Baltimore, Williams & Wilkins, 1971.)

dimension, or for providing bilateral pivot contacts in the first molar area. In the past, onlay splints were made of metal and were often cemented to the teeth; now they are made either of acrylic resin or of metal and may either be cemented or removable. This latter type is used to provide temporary relief from bruxism or muscle or temporomandibular pain. See also Kesling APPLIANCE and occlusal GUARD. **onlay s.**, *see occlusal s.* **permanent s.**, a fixed, semirigid, or removable splint that may be anchored internally or externally to the teeth, used to stabilize teeth that cannot maintain their functional stability. **permanent s., fixed**, a nonremovable restorative prosthesis attached permanently to an abutment, usually with the pin-ledge type of abutment or a horizontal pin, used to stabilize and immobilize teeth. A fixed bridge sometimes serves as a fixed permanent splint. Called also *fixed s.* **permanent s., removable**, one used to stabilize teeth, being most often retained by telescopic crowns and precision attachments. Some types of clasp-supported dentures with continuous lingual bars, embrasure hooks, and other supporting appliances often serve as permanent splints. **pressure s.**, compressive s. **provisional s.**, a temporary splint used in periodontal and occlusal therapy for 3 to 6 months to ascertain whether the teeth can withstand normal functional demands after therapy. It may be made of gold and acrylic resin, acrylic resin alone, or combinations of copper bands and acrylic resin. Called also *diagnostic s.* **temporary s.**, one designed to be worn for limited periods of time, up to 3 years, to reduce occlusal forces following traumatic loosening of teeth, as a supportive measure in the treatment of periodontal diseases, for stabilization of teeth during occlusal reconstruction, to redistribute occlusal forces during restorative procedures in other parts of the mouth, as a protection in faulty oral habits, and for anchorage in orthodontic therapy. **temporary s., external fixed**, a wire-acrylic splint used during periodontal or other dental therapy for periods of 2 to 6 months. The application consists of adaptation singly or doubly of annealed stainless steel wire to the teeth facially, lingually, and slightly gingivally to the contact areas (incisally to the cingulum of anterior teeth), the ends tied together loosely, followed by placing of ligature wires interproximally. A layer of self-curing acrylic resin is then brushed over all the wires. **temporary s., internal fixed**, one used in anticipation of permanent splints at a later date, to be worn 2 to 3 years. Splints of this type include acrylic crowns united as bridges, some having metal cores or bands, or interproximal box preparations with retention grooves and amalgam or acrylic reinforced by wires. **temporary s., removable**, one of a wide variety of splints, including occlusal splints, Hawley's orthodontic appliance, Elbrecht's cast metal splints, or any other splint used when limited stability is required, which may be placed on or removed from the teeth at will.

splinting (splint'ing) 1. application of a splint, or treatment by use of a splint. 2. the tying of two or more teeth together through the use of acrylic resin occlusal guards, orthodontic band splints, wire ligation, provisional splints, fixed prostheses, or other methods joining the teeth. 3. muscle s. **cross arch s.**, the stabilization of weakened teeth against tilting by lateral occlusal loads through the use of a rigid connector projecting to the opposite side of the dental arch where it is attached to one or more teeth. **Essig-type s.**, stabilization and repositioning injured teeth with a stainless steel wire passed labially and lingually around a part of the dental arch and held in position by ligatures around the contact areas of the teeth. **muscle s.**, increased tonus of muscles in which there is resistance to passive movement of a joint, being a protective mechanism whereby injury to a joint is avoided or reduced. **provisional s.**, the interim stabilization of mobile teeth.

split (split) 1. to divide something into parts; to cleave. 2. a tear, crack, or fissure. **intraepithelial s.**, a split in the epithelial attachment crevice.

splitting (split'ing) division in fragments. In chemistry, the separation of a complex substance into two or more simpler substances. **sagittal s. of mandible**, intraoral osteotomy of the ascending mandibular ramus and posterior body of the mandible in the sagittal plane for correction of prognathism, retrognathism, or open bite; an alternative procedure confines the split to the body of the mandible.

Spöndel's foramen see under FORAMEN.

spondylitis (spon"di-li'tis) inflammation of the vertebra. **ankylosing s.**, Bekhterev-Strümpell-Marie SYNDROME.

sponge (spunj) [L., Gr. *spongia*] 1. the elastic fibrous skeleton of certain marine animals; used mainly as an absorbent. 2. an absorbent pad of folded gauze, cotton, or similar material.

Banker's s., a piece of synthetic sponge used to organize root canal files and reamers by inserting them into the sponge vertically, similarly to pins in a cushion. **Bernays' s.,** compressed disks of cotton which expand under moisture; used in checking epistaxis. **fibrin s.,** a spongy form of fibrin, used as a hemostatic. **gelatin s.,** a spongy form of denaturated gelatin used as a hemostatic, especially when wet with thrombin. **gelatin s., absorbable,** a sterile, water-insoluble, gelatin-base sponge, occurring as a light, off-white, nonelastic, though spongy material that, when applied to capillary bleeding, will serve as a framework for fibrin strands and clot formation in arresting hemorrhage. The sponge is completely absorbed 4 to 6 weeks after application. Trademark: Gelfoam.

spongiform (spon'jĭ-form) [L. *spongia* sponge + *forma* shape] resembling a sponge.

spongio- [L.; Gr. *spongia* sponge] a combining form meaning like a sponge, or denoting relationship to a sponge.

spongioid (spun'je-oid) [*spongio-* + Gr. *eidos* form] resembling a sponge in structure or appearance.

spongiosa (spun'je-o"sah) spongy BONE.

Spontin trademark for *ristocetin*.

spool (spool) a tubular surgical instrument around which suture material is usually wound.

spoon (spoon) 1. a utensil consisting of a small, shallow bowl attached to a handle; used for stirring, eating, ladling, or measuring. 2. spoon EXCAVATOR. **s. excavator,** spoon EXCAVATOR. **sharp s.,** a surgical instrument consisting of a spoon with sharp edges for scraping away granulations.

sporadic (spo-rad'ik) [Gr. *sporadikos* scattered; L. *sporadicus*] not widely diffused or epidemic; occurring only occasionally.

sporangia (spo-ran'je-ah) [L.; Gr.] plural of *sporangium*.

sporangiophore (spo-ran'je-fōr) the threadlike stalk which bears at its tip the sporangium.

sporangiospore (spo-ran'je-o-spor) a spore contained in a sporangium.

sporangium (spo-ran'je-um), pl. *sporan'gia* [*spore* + Gr. *angeion* vessel] any encystment containing spores or sporelike bodies.

spore (spore) [L. *spora*; Gr. *sporos* seed] 1. the reproductive element of one of the lower organisms, such as a protozoan or a fungus. 2. bacterial s. **asexual s.,** a spore produced vegetatively, i.e., without involving the union of nuclei in a sexual process. **bacterial s.,** a refractile, oval body formed within the bacterial cell, which is regarded as a resting phase during the life history of the cell, and is characterized by its resistance to environmental changes. It is found both intracellularly and extracellularly. Within the cell, it is an oblate spheroid with its dimensions parallel to the long axis of the bacterium, its breadth being essentially the same as the width of the vegetative cell, or being greater and bulging the vegetative cell wall; the latter appearance is most commonly found in the anaerobic forms. The spore may be located in the center of the vegetative cell (central), or partway between the center and the end of the cell (subterminal), or at the end of the cell (terminal). Sporulation is confined largely to the bacilli; the aerobic spore-forming bacilli making up the genus *Bacillus*, and the obligate anaerobic or microaerophilic, spore-forming bacilli are members of the genus *Clostridium*. **fragmentation s.,** one formed by the breaking up of hyphae into separate cells. **segmentation s.,** one produced by the septation or successive contraction of the protoplasts of the tips of serial filaments.

sporicide (spo'rĭ-sīd) an agent that destroys spores.

Sporiine trademark for *tolnaftate*.

sporo- [Gr. *sporos* seed] a combining form denoting relationship to a spore.

sporoblast (spo'ro-blast) [*sporo-* + Gr. *blastos* germ] one of the bodies developed within the oocyst of the malarial parasite in the mosquito.

sporocyst (spo'ro-sist) [*sporo-* + Gr. *kystis* sac, bladder] 1. any cyst or sac containing spores or reproductive cells, especially in lower eukaryotic organisms. 2. the stage formed from a sporoblast, within the oocyst, in which sporozoites develop; it is differentiated from the sporoblast by the presence of a cyst wall.

sporogenesis (spo"ro-jen'ĕ-sis) [*sporo-* + Gr. *genesis* production] the formation of spores; reproduction by spores; sporulation.

Sporolactobacillus (spo"ro-lak"to-bah-sil'lus) a genus of gram-positive, microaerophilic bacteria of the family Bacillaceae, originally isolated from chicken feed.

sporophore (spo'ro-fōr) [*sporo-* + Gr. *phorein* to bear] that part of an organism that bears spores or spore chains.

Sporosarcina (spo"ro-sar-si'nah) a genus of gram-positive, aerobic, rod-shaped bacteria of the family Bacillaceae.

Sporostatin trademark for *griseofulvin*.

Sporothrix (spo'ro-thriks) [*sporo-* + Gr. *thrix* hair] a genus of deuteromycetous fungi (Fungi Imperfecti), characterized by production of pear-shaped conidia directly from the mycelium on small stems. These arise both laterally and at the tips of delicate conidiophores. After conidiation, the conidiophore may expand sympodially to form another apex and conidiate again. At 37°C it grows as a budding yeast. **S. schenck'ii,** the etiologic agent of sporotrichosis. Formerly called *Sporotrichum schenckii*.

sporotrichosis (spo"ro-tri-ko'sis) a chronic fungal disease caused by *Sporothrix schenckii*. The cutaneous lymphatic form is characterized by papules or nodules at the site of a minor injury, usually on the fingers, followed by lymphatic spread and development of a chain of ulcerating subcutaneous nodules, which heal and form soft pliable scars. In the disseminated form, the muscles, bones, joints, eyes, and gastrointestinal and nervous systems may become involved, usually associated with pain, fever, anemia, weight loss, and leukocytosis. Oral manifestations include nonspecific oronasal and pharyngeal ulcerations, usually associated with lymphadenopathy. Called also *Schenck's disease.*

Sporotrichum (spo-rot'rĭ-kum) [*sporo-* + Gr. *thrix* hair] a genus of deuteromycetous fungi (Fungi Imperfecti), which are common members of the soil flora. **S. schenck'ii,** *Sporothrix schenckii;* see under SPOROTHRIX.

Sporozoa (spo"ro-zo'ah) [*sporo-* + Gr. *zōon* animal] a subphylum of protozoa, characterized by the lack of locomotor organs in the adult stages and by a complex life cycle usually involving an alteration of a sexual with an asexual generation. It includes the malarial parasite, *Plasmodium.*

sporulation (spor"u-la'shun) the formation of spores; sporogenesis. See SPORE.

spot (spot) a circumscribed area or place; a loculus or macula. **aberrant mongolian s.,** Ota's NEVUS. **café-au-lait s.,** a macule having a light brown color of coffee with milk, characteristic of certain skin diseases. **Filatov's s's,** Koplik's s's. **focal s.,** that part of the target on the anode of an x-ray tube which is bombarded by the focused electron stream when the tube is energized. See also x-ray TUBE. **focal s., actual,** the area on the target of an x-ray tube which is actually bombarded by high-velocity electrons from the cathode. See also x-ray TUBE. **focal s., effective,** the apparent dimension and shape of the focal spot when viewed from a position in the useful beam, being somewhat smaller than the actual focal spot with the use of a suitably inclined anode face. **Forchheimer's s's,** reddish eruption on the soft palate in rubella. Called also *Forchheimer's sign.* **Fordyce's s's,** Fordyce's granules; see under GRANULE. **Koplik's s's,** small, irregular, bright red spots on the buccal and lingual mucosa, with a minute bluish white speck in the center of each, which are pathognomonic of beginning measles. Called also *Filatov's s's.* **soft s.,** see FONTANELLE and FONTICULUS. **sore s's,** denture ULCER.

sprain (sprān) a joint injury in which some of the fibers of a supporting ligament are ruptured but the continuity of the ligament remains intact. Called also *luxatio imperfecta.* **temporomandibular joint s.,** injury of supporting ligaments of the temporomandibular joint, occurring in association with its dislocation or subluxation, or as a result of extreme mandibular opening, as in yawning or laughing.

spreader (spred'er) 1. a device or instrument for distributing something over a broader area. 2. root canal filling s. **root canal filling s.,** a hand-operated, smooth, pointed, and tapered metal endodontic instrument; used to compress the filling material laterally against the walls of the root canal, making room for insertion of additional cones in root canal therapy. See illustration at root canal THERAPY. See also root canal filling CONDENSER.

Sprengel's deformity [Otto Gerhard Karl *Sprengel,* German surgeon, 1852–1915] see under DEFORMITY.

spring (spring) 1. the property of rebounding. 2. a piece of resilient metal, such as a hardened coiled steel wire, which will return to its original shape after bending. 3. a resilient wire attached to a denture or other appliance. **auxiliary s.,** a short piece of wire attached to an orthodontic appliance to serve as a lever to apply force to a tooth or teeth. **bow s.,** a loop spring with the shape of a labial bow; used in a removable orthodontic appliance to move teeth. **closed s.,** one having both ends attached. **Coffin s.,** a U-shaped spring connecting the arms of the arch of an orthodontic appliance. See illustration at Bimler APPLIANCE. **coil s.,** a spiral winding of fine wire attached to orthodontic appliances to open or to close spaces between teeth.

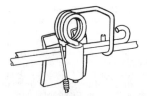

Uprighting spring on an upper left canine tooth. (From P. R. Begg and P. C. Kesling: Begg Orthodontic Theory and Technique. 2nd ed. Philadelphia, W. B. Saunders Co., 1971.)

Called also *helical s.* **finger s.,** one made of stainless steel wire by bending it back to form a finger-like structure; used interproximally as an open spring in removable orthodontic appliances. **free-end s.,** open s. **helical s.,** coil s. **Kesling s.,** a tooth-spacing spring used to gain separation between the teeth to facilitate band placement in fitting orthodontic appliances. **loop s.,** a closed orthodontic spring having a variety of different shapes, from that of a hairpin to that of a bow. See also LOOP. **open s.,** one having free ends. In orthodontic appliances, one having only one end anchored in the active plate. Called also *free-end s.* **paddle s.,** a hairpin-shaped spring used in removable orthodontic appliances, formed of 0.5-mm wire bent to form a paddle. It is activated by bending it toward the tooth. **s. rate,** the ratio between force and deflection, being an index of stiffness. **separating s.,** one placed between the teeth to obtain separation. **split acrylic s.,** split acrylic spring space REGAINER. **uprighting s.,** a coiled spring used for uprighting teeth in orthodontic therapy. See illustration. **Z s.,** one bent in the form of a Z with a coil loop at each end, used to move an individual tooth or group of teeth bucally or labially.

sprue (sproo) 1. a chronic malabsorption disease occurring in both tropical and nontropical forms. 2. in a dental casting, an opening in the investment through which the molten alloy or metal can reach the mold after the wax has been eliminated. It is formed with a metal, resin, or wax that is removed after the mold hardens, leaving a hole through the investment. Called also *ingate.* See also illustration at MOLD. **s. base,** crucible FORMER. **nontropical s.,** celiac DISEASE. **s. pin,** sprue FORMER. **tropical s.,** a malabsorption syndrome of unclear etiology, characterized by metabolic, gastrointestinal, and oral disorders. Initially, it is characterized by fatigue, asthenia, and bulky stools; later, there is weight loss, glossitis, stomatitis, cheilosis, and hyperkeratosis; and finally, anemia, megaloblastosis, steatorrhea, diarrhea, malnutrition, and foul smelling stools occur. The administration of folic acid or vitamin B_{12} produces dramatic improvement, in spite of the absence of any apparent dietary deficiency. Formerly, the disease occurred most commonly in the far East, India, and Puerto Rico, but now it is seen worldwide. Called also *Ceylon sore mouth, Cochin-China diarrhea, psilosis, stomatitis intertropica,* and *stomatitis tropica.*

Spumavirinae (spu"mah-vi'ri-ne) a subfamily of retroviruses, having virions 100 to 140 nm and cores 30 to 50 nm in diameter with electron-lucent centers and core shells contained in envelopes with surface projections 5 to 15 nm long. These viruses are believed to be nonpathogenic. Called also *echinovirus, foamy agent,* and *foamy virus.*

spur (sper) 1. a projecting body, as from a bone. 2. in dentistry, a piece of metal projecting from a plate, band, or other appliance. **cementum s.,** a spiked extension of coronal cementum from the cervical region. **enamel s.,** a tongue-shaped process sometimes found at the margin of the enamel, at the level of the bifurcation of multirooted teeth. Called also *enamel projection, enamel excrescence, enamel ridge, enamel spike,* and *enamel tongue.* **occipital s.,** an abnormal process of bone on the occipital bone behind the posterior process of the atlas.

spurious (spu're-us) [L. *spurius*] simulated; false.

sputum (spu'tum) [L.] matter ejected from the lungs, bronchi, and trachea, through the mouth.

SQ subcutaneous.

squama (skwa'mah), pl. *squa'mae* [L.] 1. a scale or platelike structure. 2. dried, thin, epithelial, horny lamellae, usually resulting from imperfect cornification. **frontal s., s. of frontal bone, s. fronta'lis** [NA], the broad, curved portion of the frontal bone, situated above the supraorbital margin, and forming the forehead. Its convex external surface is crossed vertically in the midline by the remains of the frontal suture which is normally present in infants and sometimes persists into adult life. Rounded elevations on both sides are known as the *frontal eminences;* they are separated by shallow grooves from elevations below (*superciliary arches*). A smooth elevation (*glabella*)

joins the arches. The supraorbital foramina, which perforate the supraorbital notches located above the orbits and below the superciliary arches, transmit veins from the diploë to the supraorbital veins. The internal concave surface presents a vertical groove (*sagittal sulcus*) and ends in the frontal crest; the superior sagittal sinus is lodged in the sulcus. The falx cerebri attaches to the margins of the sinus and the crest. The crest ends in a notch which leads to the foramen cecum. The interior presents depressions for the convolutions of the brain and furrows for the arachnoid granulations. **occipital s., s. occipita'lis** [NA], the largest of the four parts of the occipital bone, extending from the posterior edge of the foramen magnum to the lambdoid suture, its external surface bearing the external occipital protuberance and nuchal lines. Called also *occipital part of occipital bone* and *squamous part of occipital bone.* **temporal s., s. of temporal bone, s. tempora'lis,** the flat, scalelike, anterior and superior portion of the temporal bone, which forms part of the lateral wall of the skull, and contains the articulating surface of the mandible. Its external surface forms the temporal fossa and gives attachment to the temporalis muscle. A projection on the inferior part (*zygomatic process*), gives attachment to the temporal fascia and fibers of the masseter muscle. The anterior edge articulates with the zygomatic bone. Its anterior root ends in the articular tubercle, which forms the boundary of the mandibular fossa, and the posterior root offers attachment to the temporal fascia. A projection at the anterior root provides attachment for the lateral temporomandibular ligament. The interior presents depressions lodging the convolutions of the temporal lobe, with grooves for the branches of the meningeal vessels. Called also *pars squamosa ossis temporalis* [NA], *squamous bone,* and *squamous part of temporal bone.*

squamae (skwa'me) [L.] plural of *squama.*

squamate (skwa'māt) [L. *squamatus,* from *squama* scale] scaly; having or resembling scales.

squame (skwām) [L. *squama*] a scale or scalelike substance.

squamo- [L. *squama* scale] a combining from denoting relationship to a squama or to a scale.

squamofrontal (skwa"mo-fron'tal) pertaining to the frontal squama.

squamomastoid (skwa"mo-mas'toid) pertaining to the squamous and mastoid portions of the temporal bone.

squamo-occipital (skwa"mo-ok-sip'ĭ-tal) pertaining to the occipital squama.

squamoparietal (skwa"mo-pah-ri'ĕ-tal) pertaining to the squamous part of the temporal bone and the parietal bone. Called also *squamosoparietal.*

squamopetrosal (skwa"mo-pe-tro'sal) pertaining to the squamous and petrous portions of the temporal bone.

squamosa (skwa-mo'sah) [L.] scaly or platelike.

squamosal (skwa-mo'sal) squamous.

squamosoparietal (skwa-mo"so-pah-ri'ĕ-tal) squamoparietal.

squamosphenoid (skwa"mo-sfe'noid) pertaining to the squamous part of the temporal bone and to the sphenoid bone.

squamotemporal (skwa"mo-tem'po-ral) pertaining to the squamous portion of the temporal bone.

squamous (skwa'mus) [L. *squamosus* scaly] scaly, or platelike; squamosal.

squamozygomatic (skwa"mo-zi"go-mat'ik) pertaining to the squamous portions of the temporal bone and the zygomatic bone.

Sr strontium.

SRBC sheep erythrocytes (red blood cells).

SRIF somatotropin release inhibiting factor; see SOMATOSTATIN.

SRS-A slow-reacting substance A (see under SUBSTANCE).

S.S. White clamp see under CLAMP.

ss subspinale.

ss. abbreviation for L. *se'mis,* one half.

SSA Social Security Administration; see under ADMINISTRATION.

SSD source-surface DISTANCE.

S.S.V. abbreviation for L. *sub sig'no vene'ni,* under a poison label.

St stomion.

St. abbreviation for L. *stet,* let it stand; or *stent,* let them stand.

Sta staphylion (1).

Stabilex attachment see under ATTACHMENT.

Stabilin V trademark for penicillin V calcium (see under PENICILLIN).

stability (stah-bil'ĭ-te) [L. *stabilitas*] 1. the property of remaining in a fixed position or state; resistance to change. 2. denture s.

denture s., the ability of a denture to withstand pressure, especially a horizontal movement, and remain firmly in a constant position when such a force is applied. **dimensional s.,** the ability of a material to retain a constant shape and dimensions. **occlusal s.,** a state of homeostasis of the masticatory system wherein structural and functional changes are within the normal range for all the components of the system.

stabilization (sta″bil-i-za′shun) 1. the creation of a stable state; making something steady or steadfast. 2. a method for retaining chromium in the γ-solid solution of austenitic stainless steel, thereby preventing loss of its corrosion resistance, as by the addition of titanium. See also SENSITIZATION (2). 3. the seating or fixation of a fixed or removable denture so that it will not tilt or be displaced under pressure.

stabilizer (sta′bi-li″zer) 1. that which holds firm or steadfast. 2. a substance that is added to foods, chemical compounds, or the like to prevent deterioration. 3. a device on an x-ray machine that maintains a constant milliamperage.

stable (sta′b'l) not moving; fixed, firm; resistant to change.

staff (staf) 1. a wooden rod or rodlike structure. 2. the professional personnel of an institution, such as a hospital. See also PERSONNEL. **s. of Æsculapius,** a rod or staff with a snake entwined around it, which always appeared in the ancient representation of Æsculapius, the god of medicine. It is a symbol of medicine and the official insignia of the American Medical Association. **attending s.,** the corps of attending physicians in a hospital. **consulting s.,** the corps of physicians attached to a hospital who do not visit regularly, but may be consulted by members of the attending staff. **house s.,** the resident physicians of a hospital. **medical s.,** all medical physicians and osteopathic physicians holding unlimited licenses, and duly licensed dentists, who are privileged to attend patients in a hospital.

Stafne's cyst, mandibular defect [Edward C. *Stafne*] static bone CYST.

stage (stāj) 1. a period or distinct phase in the course of disease, the life history of an organism, or any biological process. 2. the platform of a microscope on which a slide is placed for viewing of the specimen. **bell s.,** the third (morphodifferentiation and histodifferentiation) stage of odontogenesis, in which the enamel organ undergoes a change in shape from a cap to a bell, and which contains four distinct layers: outer enamel epithelium, stellate reticulum, stratum intermedium, and inner enamel epithelium (preameloblasts). See also enamel CAP. See illustration at ODONTOGENESIS. **cap s.,** the second or proliferative stage of odontogenesis, characterized by cap formation in the tooth germ. It is associated with the organization of the cells into three layers (central stellate reticulum sandwiched between the outer and inner enamel epithelium), and formation of the enamel navel, enamel knot, and enamel cord, which disappear before enamel formation actually begins. See also enamel CAP. See illustration at ODONTOGENESIS. **eruptive s.,** 1. the period during the course of an eruptive fever or exanthem when the rash is present. 2. the period of tooth development characterized by eruption of a tooth, brought about by formation and growth of its root or roots. The eruptive stage may be subdivided into the prefunctional phase, characterized by movements of the tooth which eventually lead to its functional or occlusal position, and the functional phase, characterized by movements which occur to maintain the functional or occlusal position. **lamina-bud s.,** the first incipient stage of odontogenesis, characterized by the development of the dental lamina and initial stages of formation of the tooth bud. See illustration at ODONTOGENESIS. **preeruptive s.,** 1. the stage after infection and before eruption. 2. the period of tooth development, before tooth eruption, characterized by growth of the coronal portion of the tooth, prior to the beginning of the growth of the root. See also tooth ERUPTION. **transitional pulp s.,** a condition of the dental pulp in which chronic inflammatory cells are present but not in sufficient quantities to constitute a typical inflammatory exudate, usually resulting from abrasion, attrition, caries, periodontal disease, or a reaction to a restorative procedure. **ugly duckling s.,** a developmental stage of mixed dentition when the upper central and lateral incisors may be flared, with the crowns distally and with diastema present before the maxillary canine teeth erupt, thus giving a child an ugly duckling appearance.

Stahr's node (gland) [Herman *Stahr*, German pathologist, born 1868] see under NODE.

stain (stān). 1. any dye, reagent, or other material used in producing coloration, such as a substance in coloring tissue or microorganisms. 2. a superficial discoloration, or a colored spot on the skin or mucous membrane. **black s's,** dental stains, usually occurring as a thin black line on the teeth near the marginal gingiva, which are firmly attached, tend to recur after removal, and occur more commonly in women than in men. Apparently, they have no relation to oral hygiene, chromogenic bacteria being suspected as the cause. Black stains may also be caused by inhaling dust containing silver or manganese through the mouth and inhalation of mercury may produce green-black stains. **brown s's,** dental stains, being a thin, translucent, acquired, usually bacteria-free, pigmented pellicle, occurring in individuals who do not brush sufficiently or use a dentifrice with inadequate cleansing action. They are found most commonly on the vestibular surface of the maxillary molars and on the oral surface of the mandibular incisors. **dental s's,** stains on the teeth resulting from the pigmentation of dental cuticles by chromogenic bacteria, food, chemicals, or tobacco. **Feulgen s.,** a specific DNA specific stain, consisting of a solution of concentrated hydrochloric acid (83.5 ml) and distilled water (916.5 ml). See also Feulgen bands, under BAND. **Giemsa s.,** a solution used for histologic staining. The stock solution consists of: azure II–eosin, 3.0 gm; azure II, 0.8 gm; methyl alcohol, 375.0 ml; and glycerin, 125.0 ml. Giemsa working solution consists of Giemsa stain (stock solution), 2.5 ml; methyl alcohol, 3.0 ml; and distilled water, 100.0 ml. Called also *Giemsa solution*. See also R-banding, under BANDING. **green s's,** green or green-yellow dental stains, sometimes of considerable thickness, seen in children, more common among boys than girls, usually on the labial surface of the maxillary anterior teeth, in the gingival half. Their incidence is highest among children with tuberculosis. Fluorescent bacteria and fungi, such as *Penicillium* and *Aspergillus*, are the suspected causative agents. They are sometimes considered to be the stained remnants of the enamel cuticle. Green stains may also be caused by inhaling dust containing copper and nickel through the mouth, and they may be produced by inhalation of mercury. **metallic s's,** dental stains that may be caused by inhalation through the mouth of metal-containing dust, or through orally administered drugs. The stains are usually permanent, metals combining with dental cuticle. Copper produces a green stain; iron, a brown stain; manganese, a black stain; mercury, a green-black stain; nickel, a green stain; and silver, a black stain. **orange s's,** orange dental stains occurring on both the vestibular and oral surfaces of the anterior teeth, believed to be caused by chromogenic organisms, such as *Flavobacterium lutescens* and *Serratia marcescens*. **port-wine s.,** NEVUS flammeus. **Romanovskii's (Romanovsky's, Romanowsky's) s.,** the prototype of the many eosin–methylene blue stains for blood smears and malarial parasites. Called also *Romanovskii's (Romanovsky's, Romanowsky's) method*. **tobacco s's,** brown or black dental stains resulting from coal tar in tobacco smoke and juices penetrating the dental enamel and dentin. **Wright's s.,** a mixture of eosin and methylene blue, used for demonstrating blood corpuscles and malarial parasites.

staining (stān′ing) 1. the artificial coloration of a substance, such as the introduction or application of material to facilitate examination of tissues, microorganisms, or other cells under the microscope. 2. modification of the color of the teeth or denture base to achieve a more lifelike appearance. **acid-fast s.,** see acid-fast bacteria, under BACTERIUM. **Feulgen s.,** a histological technique of staining with Feulgen stain. See also F-BANDING. **Giemsa s.,** G-BANDING. **Gram's s.,** a differential staining procedure consisting of four steps: (1) primary staining with a triphenylmethane dye, such as crystal violet, and containing a mordant, such as ammonium oxalate; (2) the application of dilute (1:15) Lugol's iodine solution; (3) decolorization, most commonly with 95 percent ethanol; and (4) counterstaining with a dye of contrasting color, usually safranin. The bacteria stained by this method are separated into *gram-positive* (those that retain the primary stain and are deep violet in color), and *gram-negative* (those that are decolorized and are lightly stained by the counterstain; pink in the case of safranin). The gram-positive reaction is relatively rare, occurring only among the bacteria, yeasts, and filamentous fungi. Very few biological structures are gram-positive; they include chromosomes of certain species, mitochondria, centrosomes, and centromeres. See also gram-positive bacteria and gram-negative bacteria, under BACTERIUM. **quinacrine s.,** Q-BANDING.

Stainton's syndrome [C. W. *Stainton*] DENTINOGENESIS imperfecta.

Stainton-Capdedont syndrome [C. W. *Stainton;* C. *Capdedont*] DENTINOGENESIS imperfecta.

stalk (stawk) an elongated, more or less slender anatomical structure resembling the stalk of a plant. **allantoic s.,** connecting s. **body s.,** a bridge of mesoderm connecting the caudal end of the young embryo with the chorion and eventually giving passage to the allantois with its accompanying blood vessels. It becomes the connecting stalk. **connecting s.,** a narrow structure formed by differentiation of the body stalk, which connects the embryo with the adjacent portion of the villus chorion, and through which the allantoic circulation is established. It is the precursor of the umbilical cord. Called also *allantoic s.* **pituitary s.,** the upper portion of the posterior lobe of the pituitary gland (see under GLAND), which is an extension of the pars nervosa, and through which the pituitary gland receives nerve fibers from the hypothalamus. Called also *infundibulum* and *infundibulum hypothalami* [NA]. **yolk s.,** a narrow tubular structure connecting the unclosed midgut with the yolk sac in the developing embryo. It detaches from the gut by the fifth week and degenerates shortly thereafter. A persistence of the proximal end may produce an abnormal intestinal diverticulum (*Meckel's diverticulum*). Called also *omphalomesenteric duct, umbilical duct,* and *vitelline duct.*

stammering (stam'er-ing) stuttering.

stamp (stamp) 1. to strike or beat down with a downward force, as with a foot. 2. an impression obtained by such a force. 3. an instrument for shaping or pounding. **cusp s.,** stamp CUSP.

Standalloy trademark for an *amalgam alloy* (see under AMALGAM).

standard (stan'dard) something established as a measure or model to which other similar things should conform. **medical care s's,** professionally developed expressions of the range of acceptable variation in the delivery of medical care.

Stanesco's syndrome [V. *Stanesco*] see under SYNDROME.

Stanide trademark for a preparation of *stannous fluoride* (see under FLUORIDE).

Stanilo trademark for *spectinomycin hydrochloride* (see under SPECTINOMYCIN).

Stanley, Wendell Meredith [born 1904] an American biochemist; co-winner, with James Batcheller Sumner and John Howard Northrop of the Nobel prize for chemistry in 1946, for pioneering work in crystallizing protein.

stannate (stan'āt) a salt of stannic acid.

stannic (stan'ik) pertaining to a compound containing tetravalent tin.

stanniferous (stan-nif'er-us) [L. *stannum* tin + *ferre* to bear] containing tin.

stannous (stan'us) pertaining to or containing divalent tin, Sn^{++}, as in stannous fluoride.

stannum (stan'um) [L.] tin.

stanolone (stan'o-lōn) an androgenic steroid with anabolic properties, 17β-hydroxy-5α-androstan-3-one, occurring as a crystalline substance that is soluble in acetone, ether, ethanol, and ethyl acetate, but not in water. Trademarks: Anabolex, Androlone, Neodrol.

Stanozol trademark for *stanozolol.*

stanozolol (stan'o-zo-lol") an androgenic steroid with strong anabolic and weak androgenic properties, 17-methyl-2H-5α-androst-2-ene[3,2-c]pyrazol-17β-ol. It occurs as a nearly color-less, odorless, crystalline powder, existing either as prisms or needles, which is soluble in dimethylformamide, slightly soluble in ethanol, chloroform, ethyl acetate, and acetone, very slightly soluble in benzene, and insoluble in water. Used to promote nitrogen anabolism and weight gain in cachexia and other debilitating diseases and after serious infections, burns, trauma, or surgery. Also used in osteoporosis. Side effects may include impotence, virilization, sodium retention, edema, hypercalcemia, insomnia, restlessness, hemorrhagic tendency in patients on anticoagulant therapy, acne, liver lesions, and aplastic anemia. Called also *androstanazole.* Trademarks: Stanozol, Winstrol.

staph (staf) a common name for *staphylococcus.*

Staphcillin trademark for *methicillin.*

staphyl- see STAPHYLO-.

staphyledema (staf"il-ē-de'mah) [staphyl- + edema] swelling or edema of the uvula.

staphylematoma (staf"il-em"ah-to'mah) staphylohematoma.

staphyline (staf'ĭ-līn) [Gr. *staphylē* a bunch of grapes] 1. shaped like a bunch of grapes; racemose. 2. pertaining to the uvula; uvular.

staphylinus (staf"ĭ-li'nus) [L.] pertaining to the uvula.

staphylion (stah-fil'e-on) [Gr. "little grape"] 1. a craniometric landmark located at the base of the posterior nasal spine at the median line connecting the most anterior points of the posterior border of the hard palate. Abbreviated *Sta.* See illustration at CEPHALOMETRY. 2. palatine UVULA. 3. a nipple or a nipple-like structure.

staphylitis (staf"ĭ-li'tis) inflammation of the uvula; uvulitis.

staphylo-, staphyl- [Gr. *staphylē* a bunch of grapes] a combining form denoting relationship to the uvula or to staphylococci.

staphyloangina (staf"ĭ-lo-an'ji-nah) a mild form of sore throat, marked by a pseudomembranous deposit in the throat due to staphylococcal infection.

staphylocoagulase (staf"ĭ-lo-ko-ag'u-lās) coagulase produced by staphylococci.

staphylococcal (staf"ĭ-lo-kok'al) pertaining to or caused by staphylococci.

staphylococcemia (staf"ĭ-lo-kok-se'me-ah) [*staphylococcus* + Gr. *haima* blood + *-ia*] the presence of staphylococci in the blood; septicemia caused by staphylococci.

staphylococci (staf"ĭ-lo-kok'si) [L.; Gr.] plural of *staphylococcus.*

staphylococcic (staf"ĭ-lo-kok'sik) pertaining to or caused by staphylococci.

staphylococcide (staf"ĭ-lo-kok'sīd) an agent that is destructive to staphylococci.

staphylococcosis (staf"ĭ-lo-kok-o'sis) [*staphylococcus* + *-osis*] infection caused by staphylococci.

Staphylococcus (staf"ĭ-lo-kok'us) [Gr. *staphyle* bunch of grapes + *kokkos* berry] a genus of pathogenic, gram-positive bacteria of the family Micrococcaceae, occurring as facultatively anaerobic, nonsporogenous, nonmotile, usually unencapsulated cocci, 0.5 to 1.5 μm in diameter, most often found singly or in pairs in irregular clusters. Their metabolism is respiratory and fermentative, using various carbohydrates; lactic acid is produced under anaerobic conditions, and acetic acid and carbon dioxide in the presence of air. They produce several hemolysins (staphylolysins), designated α, β, γ, δ, and ε lysins. Enterotoxins of staphylococci occur as five immunological types, designated A to E; another toxin is exfoliatin, designated A and B. Principal staphylococcal extracellular enzymes include hyaluronidase and staphylokinase, coagulase, and deoxyribonuclease. Most strains are sensitive to antimicrobial agents, such as β-lactam and macrolide antibiotics, tetracyclines, novobiocin, and chloramphenicol (but not polymyxin), and other drugs, including phenols, surface active agents, salicylanilides, carbanilides, chlorine, and iodine, but some types become resistant to antibiotics by acquisition of new strains specifying such resistance, usually by phage transduction. Two phosphorus-containing polysaccharide antigens (teichoic acids), designated A and B, are present in staphylococci. **S. aerog'enes,** *Peptococcus aerogenes;* see under PEPTOCOCCUS. **S. afermen'tans,** *Micrococcus luteus;* see under MICROCOCCUS. **S. al'bus,** *S. aureus.* **S. anaero'bius,** *Peptococcus anaerobius;* see under PEPTOCOCCUS. **S. asaccharolyt'icus,** *Peptococcus asaccharolyticus;* see under PEPTOCOCCUS. **S. au'reus,** a pathogenic species, occurring as spherical cells, about 0.8 to 1.0 μm in diameter, some strains having capsules or slime layers, and forming colonies that are usually orange or yellow in color. They produce acids, both aerobically and anaerobically; enzymes, including proteases, lipases, lipoprotein lipase, phospholipase, esterases, lyases, and acid and/or alkaline phosphatases; and at least three hemolysins (α, β, γ). Coagulases are formed by all strains, and some produce the toxin exfoliatin. The organisms are present on the skin, in some gingival sulci, on the dorsum of the tongue, and in the saliva, nose, throat, and oral cavity; nasal and salivary carriers being the most common source of infection in man. Hair follicles and sweat ducts are the most common routes of infection through intact skin. *S. aureus* may be found in furuncles, boils, infected wounds, carbuncles, paronychia, impetigo, contagiosa, osteomyelitis, endocarditis, meningitis, acne, dermatitis, bronchopneumonia, and other diseases. Infections of the nose and upper lip are particularly dangerous. Occasionally, an infection may assume a fulminant bacteremic form, being often fatal. Transfer of infection from patient to dentist is rare. The organism is also a common cause of food poisoning. *S. aureus* is sensitive to various antibiotics, including penicillin, but some strains produce penicillinase and develop antibiotic resistance. Called also *S. pyogens albus, S. pyogenes aureus, S. pyogenes citreus, Micrococcus aureus, M. citreus, M. pyogenes,* and *M. pyogenes* var. *aureus.* **S. epider'midis,** a potentially pathogenic species, occurring as spheroid cells, about 0.5 to 1.5 μm in diameter, and forming colonies that are usually white or yellow, occasionally orange and, rarely, purple in color. The organisms are coagulase-negative but produce ε-hemolysin and hemolysins corresponding to the α- and β-hemolysins of *S. aureus.* They are residents of the skin and mucosae (including those of the nose and oral cavity) in warm-blooded animals, including man, and many of the strains are pathogens or secondary invaders in various diseases, such as abscesses, infected wounds, subacute bacterial endocarditis, and other diseases. The species is usually sensitive to antibiotics, including penicillin, but may develop resistance. Called also *Albococcus epidermis, Micrococcus epidermidis, M. hyicus,* and *M. violagabriellae.* **S. flavocya'neus,** *Micrococcus luteus;* see under MICROCOCCUS. **S. lac'tis,** *Micrococcus varians;* see under MICROCOCCUS. **S. par'vulus,** *Veillonella parvula;* see under VEILLONELLA. **S. pyog'enes al'bus, S. pyog'enes au'reus, S. pyog'enes cit'reus,** *S. aureus.* **S. ro'seus,** *Micrococcus roseus;* see under MICROCOCCUS. **S. saprophyt'icus,** a usually nonpathogenic species, occurring as spheroid cells, about 0.5 to 1.5 μm in diameter, which usually form compact or loose clusters. They are found in air, dust, dairy products, animal carcasses, and urine, and occasionally cause urinary tract infection in man.

staphylococcus (staf″ĭ-lo-kok'us), pl. *staphylococ'ci.* Any microorganism of the genus *Staphylococcus.* Commonly called *staph.* **coagulase-positive staphylococci,** strains of staphylococci which produce coagulase; the term is generally used synonymously with virulent staphylococci (*S. aureus*).

staphyloderma (staf″ĭ-lo-der'mah) pyogenic infection of the skin caused by staphylococci.

staphylohematoma (staf″ĭ-lo-hem″ah-to'mah) [*staphylo-* + *hematoma*] hemorrhage from a ruptured uvular vessel. Called also *apoplexia uvulea, Bosviel's disease,* and *staphylematoma.*

staphylokinase (staf″ĭ-lo-ki'nās) a lytic factor produced by staphylococci; a kinase which complexes with plasminogen to yield a product with plasmin-like activity and which lyses fibrin clots. The production of staphylokinase is apparently unrelated to the virulence of staphylococci but strains that produce β-staphylolysin do not produce staphylokinase.

staphylolysin (staf″ĭ-lol'ĭ-sin) a hemolysin produced by pyogenic staphylococci. Called also *staphylococcal hemolysin.* **α-s.,** a hemolysin produced by most strains of *Staphylococcus aureus,* acting chiefly against rabbit erythrocytes and, with lesser intensity, against human red cells. It also has dermonecrotic and lethal effects, particularly when tested in rabbits, and it is toxic for rabbit leukocytes. Its production is under the control of a temperate phage. Identical with Neisser-Wechsberg leukocifin. Called also *α-toxin* and *α-lysin.* **β-s.,** a hot-cold hemolysin produced by staphylococci of animal origin, which is more potent than α-hemolysin and acts with greatest intensity against sheep erythrocytes and, with lesser intensity, against human and rabbit red cells. It is enzymatically active as phospholipase C, hydrolyzing sphingomyelin and lysophosphatidyl choline. Cations are required for its activation, cobalt and magnesium being most active. Called also *β-toxin* and *β-lysin.* **γ-s.,** a hemolysin active against a wide variety of erythrocytes, including those of man, sheep, and rabbits; lethal for mice. It requires cations for activation, sodium being most effective. Called also *γ-toxin* and *γ-lysin.* **δ-s.,** a hemolysin with a wide range of lytic activity, hemolyzing human, sheep, rabbit, and monkey red cells with roughly equivalent activity, being less potent than other hemolysins. Suspected modes of action include a surfactant-like behavior, enzymatic mode of action, and phospholipase activity, but the mechanism of action is still not understood. In addition to hemolytic activity, it also exhibits necrotic, leukotoxic, and lethal activities. Called also *δ-toxin* and *δ-lysin.* **ϵ-s.,** a hemolysin which occurs in *Staphylococcus epidermidis.*

staphyloncus (staf″ĭ-long'kus) [*staphylo-* + Gr. *onkos* mass] a tumor or swelling of the uvula.

staphylopharyngorrhaphy (staf″ĭ-lo-far″in-gor'ah-fe) [*staphylo-* + Gr. *pharynx* the throat + *rhaphe* suture] the stitching of the halves of the velum palatini to the posterior wall of the pharynx.

staphyloplasty (staf'ĭ-lo-plas″te) [*staphylo-* + Gr. *plassein* to mold] plastic repair of the soft palate and uvula.

staphyloptosia (staf″ĭ-lop-to'se-ah) [*staphylo-* + Gr. *ptōsis* falling + *-ia*] elongation of the uvula.

staphyloptosis (staf″ĭ-lop-to'sis) staphyloptosia; uvuloptosis.

staphylorrhaphy (staf″ĭ-lor'ah-fe) [*staphylo-* + Gr. *rhaphē* suture] surgical correction of the midline cleft in the uvula and soft palate; cionorrhaphy. See also PALATORRHAPHY.

staphyloschisis (staf″ĭ-los'kĭ-sis) [*staphylo-* + Gr. *schisis* splitting] fissure of the uvula and soft palate, being a form of cleft palate.

staphylotome (staf'ĭ-lo-tōm) [*staphylo-* + Gr. *tomē* a cutting] a knife for cutting the uvula; uvulotome.

star (star) a figure usually having five or six points radiating from a center. **dental s.,** a characteristic deep-yellow spot in the dentin of the incisor teeth of the horse, first appearing at about eight years of age and, thus, being helpful in determining a horse's age.

starch (starch) a polysaccharide made up of glucose units, which is the storage form of carbohydrates in plants. It is composed of ¼ amylose, a chain of glucose molecules connected by α-1,4 linkages and ¾ amylopectin, a branched chain or polymers of glucose with both α-1,4 and α-1,6 linkages. Starch is almost insoluble in water and alcohol and, on hydrolysis by enzymes or by acids, splits into a series of intermediate compounds possessing a small number of glucose units; the product of complete hydrolysis is the free glucose molecule. During digestion in the intestinal tract or in dental plaque, starch yields dextrins (shorter chain polymers of glucose), maltose (the disaccharide of glucose), and ultimately glucose. Starch is the most important source of carbohydrate in the human diet, providing on the average about 50 percent of the carbohydrate content and 20 to 25 percent of the caloric needs in the U.S.A. and greater proportions in cultures dependent on cereals. The terms *starch, sugar,* and *carbohydrate* are sometimes used synonymously. See also CARBOHYDRATE metabolism. **animal s.,** glycogen. **s. cellulose,** amylopectin. **s. gum,** dextrin. **liver s.,** glycogen. **s. syrup,** glucose (1).

Starck see Einstein-Starck LAW.

Stark classification see CLEFT palate.

starvation (star-va'shun) a prolonged deprival of food. See also MALNUTRITION. **oxygen. s.,** see ANOXIA and HYPOXIA.

stasis (sta'sis) [Gr. "a standing still"] 1. a stoppage or diminution of the flow of blood or other body fluid in any part. 2. a state of equilibrium among opposing forces.

Stat. abbreviation for L. *sta'tim,* at once; immediately.

state (stāt) [L. *status*] a condition or situation. See also STATUS. **excited s.,** the condition of a nucleus, atom, or molecule produced by the addition of energy to the system as the result of absorption of photons or of inelastic collisions with other particles or systems; as opposed to the ground state. **ground s.,** the condition of lowest energy of a nucleus, atom, or molecule; as opposed to the excited state. **hemophiloid s. A,** parahemophilia. **hemophiloid s. C,** Christmas DISEASE. **hemophiloid s. D,** FACTOR XI. **transition s.,** in a chemical reaction, an intermediate stage in the transition from reactants to products.

State Board of Dental Examiners, see under BOARD.

statement (stāt'ment) a communication or declaration setting forth facts. **attending dentist's s.,** 1. that portion of the insurance claim form which lists and describes dental services which have been provided. 2. uniform report FORM.

static (stat'ik) [L. *staticus;* Gr. *statikos*] 1. at rest; not in motion; in equilibrium. 2. pertaining to or characterized by a fixed or stationary condition. 3. not dynamic.

Sta-Tic trademark for a *polysulfide impression material* (see under MATERIAL).

statim (sta'tim) [L.] immediately; at once. Abbreviated *stat.*

Statimo trademark for *carbazochrome salicylate* (see under CARBAZOCHROME).

stationary (sta'shun-er″e) [L. *stationarius*] standing still or having a fixed position.

statistics (stah-tis'tiks) numerical facts pertaining to a body of things; also the science which deals with the collection and tabulation of such facts. **vital s.,** statistics relating to births (natality), deaths (mortality), marriages, health, and disease (morbidity). Vital statistics for the United States are collected and published annually by the National Center for Health Statistics of the Health Resources Administration in the Department of Health and Human Services.

Statobex trademark for *phendimetrazine tartrate* (see under PHENDIMETRAZINE).

Stat-Ray trademark for a small capacity automatic film processor.

stature (stat'chur) [L. *statura*] the height or tallness of a person standing.

status (sta'tus) [L.] state or condition. See also STATE. **s. hemicra'nicus,** a state marked by constantly recurring attacks of migraine. **s. lax'us,** excessive relaxation of the internal pores of the body, believed by the Methodists to be one of the causes of disease. **s. stric'tus,** excessive narrowing of the internal pores of the body, believed by the Methodists to be one of the causes of disease.

steapsin (ste-ap'sin) [Gr. *stear* fat + *pepsis* digestion] triacylglycerol LIPASE.

stearin (ste'ah-rin) tristearin.

Stearns, Genevieve [American physician] see Boyd-Stearns SYNDROME.

stearo-, steato- [Gr. *stear, steatos* fat] a combining form denoting relationship to fat.

steato- see STEARO-.

steatorrhea (ste″ah-to-re'ah) [*steato-* + Gr. *rhoia* a flow] excessive amounts of fats in the feces.

steel (stēl) an alloy of carbon and iron, containing less than 2 percent carbon, either in the form of graphite or carbide.

Various types of steel, especially stainless steel, are used in the production of cutting, surgical, and dental instruments, tools, and apparatus. **17-7 PH s.**, a semiaustenitic type of steel containing 17 percent chromium and 7 percent nickel. Solution annealing at 1000°C (1832°F) and quenching to room temperature result in retention of a solid solution of carbon and aluminum in austenite and some Δ-ferrite. The steel strain hardens rapidly during cold working due to the formation of martensite. **18-8 s.**, a type of austenitic stainless steel containing 18 percent chromium and 8 percent nickel, having a very high modulus of elasticity. Used chiefly in the fabrication of orthodontic appliances. **austenitic stainless s.**, a stainless steel containing 16 to 26 percent chromium, 7 to 22 percent nickel, and 0.25 percent (or less) carbon, characterized by a yield strength ranging from 2800 kg/cm² in the annealed state to 3500 to 10,500 kg/cm² in the work-hardened state and a tensile strength ranging from 6700 kg/cm² in the annealed state to 7000 to 12,700 kg/cm² in the work-hardened state. The steel is elastic, ductile with the ability to undergo considerable cold work without breaking; strengthens during cold working; easy to weld; highly resistant to corrosion, and cannot be hardened by heat treatment. There are several austenitic, stainless steels, type 18-8 being the most commonly used in the fabrication of orthodontic appliances. **carbon s.**, an iron alloy containing 2.0 percent or less carbon. An alloy with 0.8 percent carbon is eutectoid, one with 0.8 to 2.0 percent carbon content is hypereutectoid, and one with less than 0.8 percent carbon is hypoeutectoid. **chromium s.**, stainless s. **eutectoid s.**, an alloy consisting of 99.2 percent iron and 0.8 percent carbon, which has been allowed to cool slowly from its molten state. At 1470°C (2678°F) the first solid forms as austenite, and the solidification is complete at about 1390°C (2532°F), the resulting solid being a mixture of ferrite and cementite in 7:1 ratio. **ferritic stainless s.**, a stainless steel containing 11.5 to 27.0 percent chromium and less than 0.2 percent carbon, characterized by high corrosion resistance. It is not readily work hardenable. **hypereutectoid s.**, an iron alloy containing 0.8 to 2.0 percent carbon. The proeutectoid phase which first forms from austenite is cementite and, as the temperature drops, the cementite continues to precipitate until the eutectoid composition of the remaining austenite is reached at the eutectoid temperature (723°C). Then pearlite is formed. Microscopically, the steel shows pearlite nodules surrounded by thin bands of proeutectoid or primary cementite; the higher the carbon content of the steel, the wider the bands, the greater the total content of cementite, and the harder and less ductile the steel. The fraction of primary ferrite in a 0.4 percent carbon steel is about 0.5; in a 1.2 percent carbon steel the fraction of proeutectoid cementite is about 0.07 percent. **hypoeutectoid s.**, an iron alloy containing less than 0.8 percent carbon. Austenite is the first to form and, as the temperature decreases, it changes to ferrite. The carbon content of untransformed austenite is 0.8 percent by the time the eutectoid temperature (723°C) is reached. The remaining austenite, now having a eutectoid composition, is transformed to pearlite. When the transformation of austenite to hypoeutectoid composition to ferrite plus cementite is complete, a microscopic section of steel shows pearlite colonies surrounded by bands of ferrite grains, the lower the carbon content of the steel, the wider the ferrite bands. At 0.02 percent carbon content, only ferrite is present. **manganese substituted austenitic s.**, an austenitic steel in which 5 to 10 percent manganese and 0.25 percent nitrogen replaces some nickel, reducing its content to about 3.5 to 6.0 percent. It is nonmagnetic and hardenable only by cold working. **martensitic stainless s.**, a stainless steel containing 11.5 to 17.0 percent chromium, 0 to 2.5 percent nickel, and 0.15 to 1.20 percent carbon, characterized by a yield strength ranging from 4920 kg/cm² in the annealed state to 18,980 kg/cm² in the heat-treated state and a tensile strength ranging from 7000 kg/cm² in the annealed state to 10,500 to 21,000 in the heat-hardened state. It is less corrosion resistant than other types of stainless steel and its plasticity is limited, causing objects made of it to work harden and fracture when bent. Used in the production of some types of hypodermic needles. **precipitation hardening stainless s.**, a stainless steel that belongs to both the martensitic and austenitic types, which is hardened by precipitation. **stabilized stainless s.**, a stainless steel treated to retain chromium in the γ-solid solution, thereby preventing loss of its corrosion resistance, as by the addition of titanium. See also STABILIZATION (2) and SENSITIZATION (2). **stainless s.**, a steel (an iron-carbon alloy) also containing chromium in excess of 11 percent (generally in the 12 to 30 percent range) and other elements. Room temperature yield strengths of stainless steel may range from 2100 kg/cm² (30,000 psi) to over 17,600 kg/cm² (250,000 psi). The steel is said to be stainless because it is made to resist corrosion and tarnish through the passivating properties of chromium, which produces a thin, transparent, but tough and impervious oxide layer (passivating film or layer) on the surface of the alloy when it is exposed to the oxidizing atmosphere. The passivating layer is a chromic oxide (Cr_2O_3) that provides a mechanical barrier against further oxidation. Rupture of this layer may mean a loss of protection against corrosion. Called also *chromium steel.*

Steele's facing, tooth (interchangeable tooth) see interchangeable FACING, and see under TOOTH.

Steenbock unit [Harry *Steenbock,* American biochemist, 1886–1967] see under UNIT.

stegnosis (steg-no'sis) [Gr. *stegnōsis* obstruction] constriction; stenosis.

Steiger-Boitel attachment (bar) [A. A. *Steiger;* R. H. *Boitel*] see under ATTACHMENT.

Steiger's joint (attachment, connector) [A. A. *Steiger*] see under JOINT.

Stein's operation see under OPERATION.

Steinberg see Landeker-Steinberg LIGHT.

Steinert, Hans [German physician] see myotonic DYSTROPHY (Curschmann-Batten-Steinert syndrome).

Steinmann's pin [Fritz *Steinmann,* Swiss surgeon, 1872–1932] see under PIN.

Stelazine trademark for *trifluoperazine hydrochloride* (see under TRIFLUOPERAZINE).

stellate (stel'āt) [L. *stellatus,* from *stella* star] shaped like a star; arranged in a roset, or in rosets.

stellite (stel'līt) a cobalt-chromium ALLOY. **Haynes s. 21,** ALLOY HS21. **Haynes s. 31,** ALLOY HS31.

stem (stem) an elongated structure, such as a stalk or stem of a plant. See also PEDUNCLE and STALK. **brain s.**, the stemlike portion of the brain connecting the spinal cord with the brain, consisting of the medulla oblongata, pons, and mesencephalon; the diencephalon is considered part of the brain stem by some.

Stemetil trademark for *prochlorperazine dimaleate* (see under PROCHLORPERAZINE).

Stenediol trademark for *methandriol.*

stenia (sten'e-ah) [Gr.] plural of *stenion.*

stenion (sten'e-on), pl. *sten'ia* [Gr. *stenos* narrow + *-on* neuter ending] a craniometric landmark situated at each end of the smallest transverse diameter of the head in the temporal region.

steno- [Gr. *stenos* narrow] a combining form meaning contracted or narrow.

stenobregmatic (sten"o-breg-mat'ik) [*steno-* + Gr. *bregma* the front part of the head] having the upper and anterior portion of the head narrowed.

stenocardia (sten"o-kar'de-ah) [*steno-* + *cardia*] angina pectoris.

stenocephaly (sten"o-sef'ah-le) [*steno-* + Gr. *kephalē* head] abnormal narrowness of the head.

Stenolon trademark for *methandrostenolone.*

stenosis (stĕ-no'sis) [Gr. *stenōsis*] narrowing or stricture of a duct or canal. **cicatricial s.**, that caused by the contraction of a cicatrix. **granulation s.**, stenosis or narrowing caused by the deposit of granulations or by their contraction. **postdiphtheritic s.**, stenosis of the larynx or trachea following diphtheria. **valvular s.**, stenosis affecting any of the valves of the heart, including the aortic, mitral, pulmonary, or tricuspid valve.

stenotic (stĕ-not'ik) [Gr. *stenotēs* narrowness] pertaining to or characterized by stenosis; abnormally narrowed.

Stenovasan trademark for *aminophylline.*

Stensen's canal, duct, foramen, plexus [Niels *Stensen,* Danish physician, anatomist, physiologist, and theologian, 1638–1686] see incisive CANAL, parotid DUCT, and incisive FORAMEN, and see under PLEXUS.

stent (stent) 1. an impression of the mouth and oral structure made of Stent mass. 2. a mold for keeping a skin graft in place, made of Stent mass or an acrylic or dental compound. By extension, used to designate a device or mold of a suitable material, used to hold a skin graft in place or to provide support for tubular structures that are being anastomosed. 3. Stent MASS. **antihemorrhagic s.**, a stent used for controlling postextraction hemorrhage in hemophiliac patients, constructed with methyl methacrylate and lined with a hemostatic agent. The stent is inserted in the mouth immediately after surgery. **drainage s.**, a polyethylene tube constructed on a preexisting partial or complete removable denture or on a specially constructed device, to allow the escape of blood or other fluids in endodontic therapy. **occlusal s.**, a type of bite plate of varied design that may be adapted to either the mandibular or maxillary arch. It is a therapeutic device used in the temporomandibular pain–dysfunction syndrome, to disengage occlusion temporarily and to interrupt existing patterns of muscle function which contribute to painful myospasm, and to assist in repositioning the condylar head in the glenoid fossa which often relieves the acute symptoms. **pedodontic s.,** a methyl methacrylate stent inserted in the mouth to prevent healing of surgically uncovered unerupted teeth and to facilitate their eruption. **periodontal s.,** a labiolingual stent designed to hold dressings in place during the healing phase following periodontal surgery. **periodontal s., labial,** a thin stent dyed to match the color and characteristics of the tissue, used for cosmetic purposes after extensive periodontal surgery in the anterior region of the mouth. **trismus s.,** a modified Kingsley's splint, being a combination of maxillary and mandibular stents with bows extending from the commissures of the mouth to exercise the temporomandibular joint or to open and close the mouth. Called also *dynamic bite opener* and *temporomandibular joint exerciser.*

stephanion (stĕ-fa′ne-on) [Gr. *stephanos* crown + *-on* neuter ending] the point on the side of the cranium at which the superior temporal line cuts the coronal suture.

step-wedge (step′wej) penetrometer.

Sterculia (ster-ku′le-ah) a genus of trees and shrubs, including many species, mostly tropical; some have edible seeds and others are medicinal. See sterculia GUM.

sterculia (ster-ku′le-ah) sterculia GUM.

stereo- [Gr. *stereos* solid] a combining form meaning solid, having three dimensions, or firmly established.

stereoisomerism (ster″e-o-i-som′er-izm) [*stereo-* + *isomerism*] a type of isomerism in which two or more compounds possess the same molecular and structural formulas, but different spatial or configurational formulas, the spatial relationship of the atoms being different, but not the linkages. Stereoisomerism is divided into two branches, *optical isomerism* (which includes *enantiomorphism* and *diastereoisomerism*) and *geometric isomerism*. See structural ISOMERISM, MUTAROTATION, RACEMIZATION, and TAUTOMERISM. Called also *spatial isomerism* and *stereochemical isomerism.*

stereoradiography (ste″re-o-ra″de-og′rah-fe) [*stereo-* + *radiography*] radiography giving an impression of depth as well as of width and height, obtained by the proper mounting and viewing of two very slightly dissimilar exposures of the same structure, and viewed with a stereoscope. It is used for the visualization of structures within the body, the technique making apparent the separation of overlapping structures and/or the depth and shape of a single structure. Called also *stereoscopic radiography.*

stereoscope (ste′re-o-skōp″) [*stereo-* + Gr. *skopein* to examine] an instrument for producing the appearance of solidity and relief by combining the images of two similar pictures of an object. See also STEREORADIOGRAPHY.

sterile (ster′il) [L. *sterilis*] 1. free from living microorganisms; not producing microorganisms; aseptic. 2. not producing young; infertile.

sterility (ste-ril′ĭ-te) [L. *sterilitas*] 1. the state of being free from microorganisms. 2. the inability to produce offspring.

sterilization (ster″ĭ-li-za′shun) 1. the complete elimination of microbial viability. See also DISINFECTION. 2. rendering an individual incapable of reproduction. **boiling water s.,** see boiling water DISINFECTION. **dry heat s.,** sterilization with the use of dry heat. Instruments, such as root canal boxes, blades, and scissors, are usually sterilized with dry heat. They are placed in the oven, after being cleaned, dried, wrapped, and placed in special metal containers, where they are kept for at least 90 minutes at 170°C (340°F) or 120 minutes at 165°C (330°F). See also dry heat OVEN. **flame s.,** placing an instrument in an open flame, such as a Bunsen burner or alcohol lamp, to sterilize it. **glass bead s.,** a method for sterilizing instruments with heated small glass beads (about 1 to 2 mm in diameter). After heating the beads to 218°C to 246°C (424°F to 475°F), root canal instruments are sterilized 15 to 20 seconds, cotton pellets and absorbent points 10 seconds, and metal instruments 20 to 30 seconds. **hot oil s.,** sterilization with heated oils (e.g., mineral oil, silicones, and other synthetic oils) of hand pieces and jointed instruments that are dulled or rusted by moisture. An exposure to 150°C (300°F) for 10 minutes or 121°C (250°F) for 15 minutes will kill all microorganisms, except those which form spores; spore-forming organisms are killed when exposed for 1½ hours to a temperature of 150°C (300°F). **molten metal s.,** a method for sterilizing instruments using a low-fusing alloy, which melts at a temperature of 180°C to 193°C (356°F to 380°F). The metal is placed in a metal cup and melted. Instruments, such as those used in root canal therapy, are placed in the molten metal for at least 10 seconds and removed quickly. The molten metal meth-

od may alter the temper of some instruments and, if the instrument is kept too long, it may become brittle. **root canal s.,** in root canal therapy, irrigation of an empty canal, after extirpation of the pulp, with a germicidal preparation to destroy pathogenic microorganisms and create a sterile environment before filling the root with a sealing agent. Called also *root canal disinfection.* **salt s.,** a method for sterilizing instruments with heated sodium chloride (ordinary salt). After heating salt granules to 218°C to 246°C (424°F to 475°F), root canal instruments are sterilized in 15 to 20 seconds, cotton pellets and absorbent points in 10 seconds, and metal instruments in 20 to 30 seconds. **steam s.,** autoclaving.

sterilizer (ster′ĭ-līz″er) an apparatus for rendering something sterile through the killing of microorganisms. Sterilizers used most commonly in dentistry include those employing steam under pressure, or autoclaves; dry heat ovens; and molten metal, glass beads, and salt. **dry heat s.,** a thermostatically controlled oven used to sterilize surgical instruments and materials. See dry heat OVEN. **glass bead s.,** see glass bead STERILIZATION. **hot oil s.,** a sterilizer for instruments, such as handpieces, in which a silicone base oil is heated. **salt s.,** see salt STERILIZATION. **steam s.,** autoclave.

Sterling-Okuniewski sign see under SIGN.

Stern, W. G. see Guérin-Stern SYNDROME.

Stern attachment (stress-breaker attachment, stress-breaker unit), G/A attachment, gingival latch (G/L) attachment see under ATTACHMENT.

Sternberg, Karl [German pathologist, 1872–1935] see Albright's SYNDROME (Albright-McCune-Sternberg syndrome).

Sterngold 1 trademark for a medium hard *dental casting gold alloy* (see under GOLD).

Sterngold 2 trademark for a hard *dental casting gold alloy* (see under GOLD).

Sterngold 3 trademark for an extra hard *dental casting gold alloy* (see under GOLD).

Sterngold 5 trademark for a hard *dental casting gold alloy* (see under GOLD).

Sterngold B trademark for a hard *dental casting gold alloy* (see under GOLD).

Sterngold G-43 trademark for a low noble metal dental wrought gold wire alloy.

Sterngold Inlay, Sterngold Bridgette Inlay see under INLAY.

Sterngold S trademark for a soft *dental casting gold alloy* (see under GOLD).

Sterngold Supercast trademark for an extra hard *dental casting gold alloy* (see under GOLD).

sterno- [Gr. *sternon* breast] a combining form denoting relationship to the sternum.

sternocleidomastoid (ster″no-kli″do-mas′toid) pertaining to the sternum, clavicle, and mastoid process.

sternocleidomastoideus (ster″no-kli″do-mas′toi-de′us) sternocleidomastoid MUSCLE.

sternohyoid (ster″no-hi′oid) pertaining to the sternum and hyoid bone.

sternohyoideus (ster″no-hi-oi′de-us) sternohyoid MUSCLE.

sternothyroid (ster″no-thi′roid) pertaining to the sternum and to the thyroid cartilage or gland.

sternothyroideus (ster″no-thi″roi′de-us) sternothyroid MUSCLE.

sternum (ster′num) [L.; Gr. *sternon*] [NA] a longitudinal plate of bone forming the middle of the anterior wall of the thorax.

steroid (ste′roid) a class of chemical compounds having in common a structure based on the cyclopenta-perhydrophenanthrene ring (Fig. 1), where the cyclopentane ring (D) is fused to a perhydrophenanthrene ring system (A, B, and C), in which all the carbons are saturated. Substituents and side chains are located by a standard numbering system (Fig. 2). Not all of them possess the $C_{20}-C_{27}$ side chain. The steroids are derivatives of cyclic alcohols of high molecular weight that occur in all living cells, especially cholesterol. They have greatly diver-

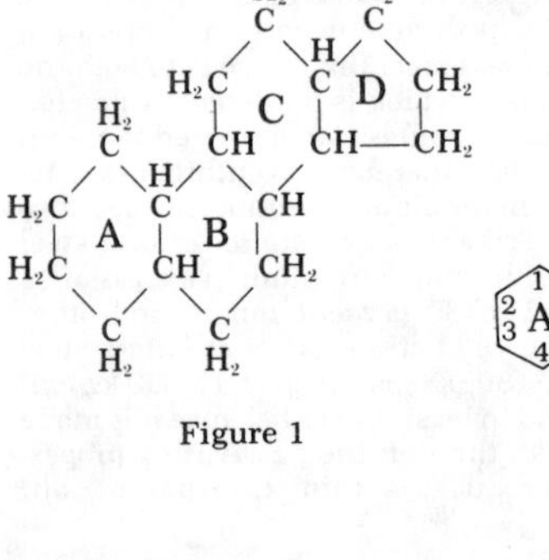

Figure 1 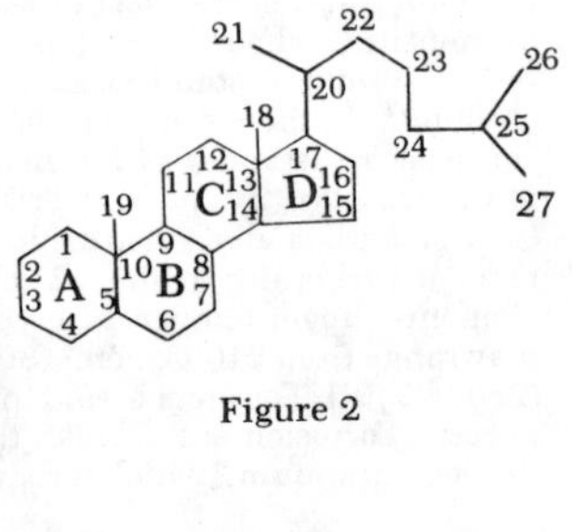   Figure 2

sified physiological properties and include sex hormones, adrenal cortex hormones, vitamin D, bile acids, cholesterol, sterols, saponins, toad poisons, and the nonsugar portion of cardiac glycosides. They may be classed into six main groups in order of increasing complexity of substituents on the ring. They are gonanes, estranes, androstanes, pregnanes, cholanes, and cholestanes, **adrenal cortex s.,** adrenal cortex HORMONE.

sterol (ste'rōl) [Gr. *stereos* solid + *-ol* (L. *oleum* oil)] a steroid alcohol made up of a steroid nucleus and an 8- to 10-carbon side-chain and an alcohol group. Cholesterol is the principal sterol. **s. nucleus,** cyclopenta-perhydrophenanthrene RING. **s. nucleus, s. ring,** cyclopenta-perhydrophenanthrene RING. **s. ring,** cyclopenta-perhydrophenanthrene RING.

stertor (ster'tor) [L.] snoring. **hen-cluck s.,** a respiration sound like a hen's cluck in cases of postpharyngeal abscess.

steth- see STETHO-.

stetho-, steth- [Gr. *stēthos* chest] a combining form denoting relationship to the chest.

stethoscope (steth'o-skōp) [*stetho-* + Gr. *skopein* to examine] an instrument for listening to cardiac, respiratory, pleural, vascular, uterine, intestinal, and other sounds. See also AUSCULTATION. **binaural s.,** one with two adjustable branches, designed for use with both ears. **electronic s.,** an electronic amplifier of sounds within the body; selective controls permit tuning for low or high frequency tones. An auxiliary output permits the recording or viewing of audio patterns. **esophageal s.,** one which is positioned within the esophagus to transmit heart and respiratory sounds.

Stevens-Johnson syndrome [Albert Mason *Stevens*, American pediatrician, 1884–1945] see under SYNDROME.

stheno- [Gr. *sthenos* strength] a combining form denoting relationship to strength.

stibine (sti'bēn) a colorless gas, SbH₃, with disagreeable odor, formed by a reaction of antimony with hydrogen. It is intensely toxic and has been used as a fumigating agent. Called also *antimony hydride*.

stibious (stib'e-us) antimonious.

stibium (stib'e-um) [L.] antimony.

stibophen (stib'o-fen) an antimony compound, pentasodium bis[4,5-dihydroxy-*m*-benzenedisulfonate(4−)]antimonate(5−), occurring as colorless crystals that are soluble in water. Used in the treatment of schistosomal infections and sometimes in acute necrotizing ulcerative gingivitis. It may cause vomiting, albuminuria, arthralgias, and blood dyscrasias, and is contraindicated in liver, kidney, and heart diseases. Trademark: Faudin.

stick (stik) a branch or a slender piece of wood. **bite s., mouth s.,** mouthstick. **compound tracing s.,** compound tracing STICK.

stick-lac (stik'lak) see SHELLAC.

Stickler's syndrome [G. B. *Stickler*, American physician] see under SYNDROME.

Stickstofflost trademark for *mechlorethamine*.

Stieda, palatine foveola of see under FOVEOLA.

stiffness (stif'nes) resistance to elastic deformation; rigidity or firmness. In bending or torsion, stiffness is a measure of the amount of force required to produce a specified deformation, stiffness of an orthodontic wire being proportional to the moment of inertia of its cross section.

Stiglyn trademark for *neostigmine methyl sulfate* (see under NEOSTIGMINE).

Stigmosan trademark for *neostigmine methyl sulfate* (see under NEOSTIGMINE).

stilbestrol (stil-bes'trol) diethylstilbestrol.

Stilbetin trademark for *diethylstilbestrol*.

stilboestrol (stil-bes'trol) diethylstilbestrol.

stili (sti'li) [L.] plural of *stilus*.

Still, Andrew Taylor [1828–1917] the founder of osteopathy.

Stillman's cleft, method, technique [P. R. *Stillman*] see under CLEFT, and see TOOTHBRUSHING.

stilus (sti'lus), pl. *sti'li* [L.] stylus.

Stim-U-Dent trademark for a wooden interdental tip, being small, soft, splinterless, and triangular in cross section, which comes to a point at the working end and which fits into the interdental spaces.

stimulant (stim'u-lant) [L. *stimulans*] 1. producing stimulation. 2. an agent that produces stimulation. **vasomotor s., vascular s.,** an agent that stimulates vasomotor activity. Called also *vasostimulant*.

stimulation (stim"u-la'shun) [L. *stimulatio*, from *stimulare* to goad] the act or process of exciting or producing functional or trophic reaction. **gingival s.,** gingival MASSAGE.

Stimulator trademark for a *Granger articulator* (see under ARTICULATOR).

stimulator (stim"u-la'tor) any agent or device that excites functional activity. **Bimbler s.,** Bimbler APPLIANCE. **Dr. Butler's s.,**

trademark for a device for gingival massage. It is a slender rod curved at one end with a sharp rubber tip for massaging the interproximal gingival papillae. **interdental s.,** a device used to reach the gingivae for papillae massage and cleansing.

Stimulexin trademark for *doxapram*.

stimuli (stim'u-li) [L.] plural of *stimulus*.

Stimulin trademark for *nikethamide*.

stimulus (stim'u-lus), pl. *stim'uli* [L. "goad"] any agent, act, or influence that produces functional or trophic reaction in a receptor or in an irritable tissue. Its two characteristics are intensity and duration, both of which have a threshold value that must be reached to evoke a response. See also THRESHOLD. **subliminal s.,** one below the threshold and, therefore, not producing reaction in a receptor. **supraliminal s.,** one above the threshold and, therefore, producing reaction in a receptor. **s. threshold,** absolute THRESHOLD.

stippling (stip'pling) 1. the appearance of fine light or dark dots, or a spotted appearance. 2. the sprinkling of fine dots in any histological structure exposed to the action of basic stains. 3. gingival s. **basophilic s.,** punctate BASOPHILIA. **gingival s.,** a condition in which the gingiva presents a minutely lobulated surface, like that of an orange peel, having alternate rounded protuberances and depressions on the surfaces of the attached gingivae and the central aspect of the interdental papillae, varying with age and from one individual to another. The papillary layer of the connective tissue projects into the elevations, and both the elevated and depressed areas are covered by stratified squamous epithelium. Stippling is a normal adaptive process of the gingiva and its absence or reduction indicates gingival disease.

Stohl's solution see under SOLUTION.

stoichiometry (stoi"ke-om'ĕ-tre) [Gr. *stoicheion* element + *metron* measure] the study of the numerical relationships of chemical elements and compounds and the mathematical laws of chemical changes; the mathematics of chemistry.

stoke (stōk) a unit of kinematic viscosity, being that of fluid with a viscosity of 1 poise and a density of 1 gram per 1 cm³.

Stokes' law [William *Stokes*, Irish physician, 1804–1878] see under LAW. See also Adams-Stokes DISEASE and Cheyne-Stokes RESPIRATION.

stoma (sto'mah), pl. *stomas, sto'mata* [Gr. "mouth"] any minute opening, or pore, or orifice on a free surface; specifically one of the openings between epithelial cells of the lymph space, forming a means of communication between adjacent lymph channels.

stomacace (sto-mak'ah-se) [*stoma* + Gr. *kakē* badness] ulcerative STOMATITIS.

stomach (stum'ak) [L. *stomachus*; Gr. *stomachos*] the musculomembranous expansion of the digestive system. Gastric glands, which are in the mucous coat of the stomach, secrete gastric juice containing hydrochloric acid, pepsin, and various digestive enzymes into the cavity of the stomach; food mixed with this secretion forms a semifluid substance suitable for further digestion by the intestine. Called also *ventriculus* [NA]. See also terms beginning GASTRO-.

stomata (sto'mah-tah) [Gr.] plural of *stoma*.

stomatalgia (sto"mah-tal'je-ah) [*stoma* + Gr. *algos* pain + *-ia*] pain in the mouth; sore mouth; stomatodynia.

stomatic (sto-mat'ik) pertaining to the mouth.

stomatitides (sto"mah-tit'ĭ-dēz) plural of *stomatitis;* a general term applied collectively to inflammatory conditions of the oral mucosa.

stomatitis (sto-mah-ti'tis), pl. *stomatit'ides* [*stomato-* + *-itis*] any inflammatory disease of the oral mucosa, which may involve the buccal and labial mucosa, palate, tongue, floor of the mouth, and the gingivae. **allergic s.,** stomatitis caused by exposure to allergens; stomatitis occurring as a manifestation of an allergic condition. **angular s.,** superficial erosions and fissuring at the angles of the mouth; it may occur in riboflavin deficiency, in pellagra, or result from overclosure of the jaws in denture wearers. Called also *intertrigo labialis*. **aphthobullous s.,** foot-and-mouth DISEASE. **aphthous s.,** recurrent aphthous s. **arsenical s.,** stomatitis due to chronic arsenic poisoning, characterized by dry, red, and painful mucosa, associated with ulcerations, purpura, and, sometimes, mobility of the teeth. See ARSENIC. **Atabrine s.,** stomatitis due to adverse reactions to Atabrine (quinacrine) with symptoms similar to those seen in lichen planus. **bismuth s.,** stomatitis due to bismuth poisoning, consisting of a thin blue-black line in the marginal gingivae (*bismuth line*), pigmentation of the buccal mucosa, sore tongue, metallic taste, and a burning sensation of the mouth. Called also *bismuth gingivitis* and *bismuth gingivostomatitis*. See also BISMUTH and bismuth PIGMENTATION. **catarrhal s.**, transitory inflammation of the oral mucosa, sometimes also involving the gingivae, associated with erythema, swelling, and, occasionally, epithelial desquamation; believed to be caused by changes in the oral bacterial flora. See also catarrhal GINGIVITIS. **chronic necrotic s.**, PERIADENITIS mucosa necrotica recurrens. **contact s.**, s. venenata. **denture s.**, generalized inflammation of the oral mucosa observed sometimes in patients with new dentures or with old ill-fitting dentures, characterized by redness, swelling, and painfulness of the mucosa coming in contact with the denture. A severe burning sensation, multiple foci of hyperemia, and superinfection with *Candida albicans* may be associated. Called also *denture sore mouth*. See also denture ULCER. **epidemic s.**, **epizootic s.**, foot-and-mouth DISEASE. **erythematopultaceous s.**, uremic s. **s. exanthemat'ica**, stomatitis secondary to an exanthematous disease. **fusospirochetal s.**, necrotizing ulcerative GINGIVOSTOMATITIS. **gangrenous s.**, noma. **gonococcal s.**, gonorrheal s. **gonorrheal s.**, a relatively rare form of gonorrhea of the oral cavity, usually transmitted by orogenital contact, and characterized by a linear or flattened eruption, associated with the presence of intracellular and extracellular neutrophils. Symptoms include redness, itching, and burning of the oral mucosa, and salivation may be depressed. Called also *gonococcal s.* **herpetic s.**, herpes simplex involving the lips and oral mucosa. The primary form occurs in children and young adults, and is characterized by fever, irritability, headache, swallowing difficulty, regional lymphadenopathy, gingivitis, and development of yellowish vesicles on the lips and, less frequently, tongue, buccal mucosa, palate, pharynx, and tonsils. Ruptured vesicles produce ragged, painful ulcers covered by a gray membrane and surrounded by an erythematous halo, which heal in about 7–14 days. In the recurrent or secondary form, which is an attenuated form of the primary infection, the lesions are similar to those seen in the primary infection. It usually occurs in adults, and is often associated with fatigue, pregnancy, emotional problems, exposure to sunlight or ultraviolet rays, and generally reduced resistance of the body. The most significant histological feature is the presence of inclusion bodies. **infectious s.**, a general term for a usually mild infection of the oral mucosa, beginning with a circumscribed red, itchy area. **s. intertrop'ica**, tropical SPRUE. **iodine s.**, see IODINE. **lead s.**, stomatitis due to lead poisoning, marked by a blue-black line along the free gingival margin (*lead line*), pigmentation of the mucous membrane in contact with the teeth, metallic taste in the mouth, excessive salivation, and swelling of the salivary glands. See also LEAD². **s. medicamento'sa**, stomatitis due to an allergic reaction to drugs ingested, absorbed through the skin or mucosa, or given by hypodermic injection. Symptoms are similar to those seen in stomatitis venenata, and include vesicles, erosion, ulcers, erythema, purpura, angioedema, burning, and itching. Some drugs may cause Quincke's edema, edema of the tongue, respiratory obstruction, anaphylactic shock, and death. Many drugs have allergenic properties but those most commonly involved in drug reaction are antibiotics, particularly penicillin, sulfonamides, local anesthetics, salicylates, and barbiturates. See also *s. venenata* and drug REACTION. **membranous s.**, inflammation of the oral mucosa, associated with formation of a false membrane. **mercurial s.**, stomatitis due to acute or chronic mercury poisoning, associated with necrotic and ulcerative lesions and discoloration similar to lead lines (see under LINE) of the gingivae, strong metallic taste in the mouth, foul breath, soreness of gums, excessive salivation, local infections, loosening of teeth, and necrosis of the alveolar processes. See also MERCURY. **mycotic s.**, thrush. **neonatal monilial s.**, a usually subclinical form of candidiasis (moniliasis) of the oral mucosa, due to the presence of *Candida albicans* in the mouth of newborn infants. It may become virulent in sickly infants or under the effect of various factors, such as the use of antibiotics to which *Candida* is virtually insensitive. See also THRUSH. **s. nicoti'na**, a condition believed to be a variant of leukoplakia, observed in smokers, particularly heavy pipe-smokers, characterized by initial redness and inflammation, followed by the appearance on the palate of multiple grayish-white nodules or papules with a red spot in the center of each lesion, representing dilated orifices of accessory palatal salivary glands. Thickening, keratinization, and wrinkling of the epithelium with the development of fissures and cracks may occur in later stages. Called also *palatitis nicotina, pipe-smokers' palate, smokers' palate*, and *smokers' patches*. **nonspecific s.**, inflammation of the oral mucosa occurring in association with other conditions, such as menstrual disorders, diabetes mellitus, or uremia. **Plaut-Vincent s.**, **putrid s.**, acute necrotizing GINGIVITIS. **recurrent aphthous s.**, a recurrent disease of unknown etiology, characterized by the appearance on the oral mucosa of a single or multiple, round or oval ulcers about 2–10 mm in diameter, after prodromal burning and necrotic and erythematous changes. The ulcer is covered by a grayish fibrinous exudate and it is surrounded by a bright red halo. Typical sites of involvement include the mucous membrane of the lips, cheek, tongue, palate, gingivae, floor of the mouth, pharynx, and sometimes the conjunctivae and genital and anal mucosa. Two to eight crops of lesions occur per year; the lesions usually persist for 7 to 14 days and then heal without scarring. Called also *aphthous s., aphthae, canker sores*, and *recurrent aphthous ulcer*. See also PERIADENITIS mucosa necrotica recurrens. **s. scarlati'na**, a condition of the oral mucosa seen in scarlet fever, characterized by fiery red coloration, congestion, and exudate of the throat, strawberry tongue (white coating, fungiform papillae, edema, hyperemia) in the early stages, and raspberry tongue (disappearance of white coating, followed by deep red coloration and glistening smooth surface with hyperemic papillae) in the later stages. Ulceration of buccal mucosa may be present. **s. scorbu'tica**, stomatitis associated with vitamin C deficiency, characterized by red swollen gums, gingival ulcers and gangrene, periodontal destruction, loose teeth, hemorrhage from the dental pulp, hypoplasia of the dental enamel, arrest of dentin formation, and exaggerated sensitivity of the oral mucosa to irritants. See also SCURVY. **syphilitic s.**, inflammation of the oral mucosa in systemic syphilis. **s. trop'ica**, tropical SPRUE. **ulcerative s.**, stomatitis characterized by the appearance of shallow ulcers on the cheeks, tongue, and lips. Called also *stomacace* and *stomatocace*. **uremic s.**, the oral manifestation of uremia, consisting of azotemic odor of the breath, erythema, exudations, ulcerations, pseudomembrane formation, and burning sensation. Called also *erythematopultaceous s., nephritic gingivitis*, and *uremic gingivitis*. **s. venena'ta**, an allergic condition of the oral mucosa resulting from a contact with a substance to which the patient is sensitized, including cosmetics, dentifrices, mouthwashes, and dental materials, as well as drugs applied topically. Inflammation and edema of the mucosa, giving it a shiny, smooth appearance, accompanied by burning and, sometimes, itching are the principal symptoms. Some drugs may cause anaphylactic shock, Quincke's edema, edema of the tongue, respiratory obstruction, and death. Called also *contact s.* See also *s. medicamentosa* and drug REACTION. **Vincent's s.**, acute necrotizing GINGIVITIS. **vulcanite s.**, stomatitis venenata caused by vulcanite dentures.

stomato-, stomo- [Gr. *stoma, stomatos* mouth] a combining form denoting relationship to the mouth or to any mouthlike opening.

stomatocace (sto″mah-tok′ah-se) [*stomato-* + Gr. *kakē* badness] ulcerative STOMATITIS.

stomatodynia (sto″mah-to-din′ē-ah) [*stomato-* + Gr. *odynē* pain + *-ia*] pain in the mouth; sore mouth; stomatalgia.

stomatodysodia (sto″mah-to-dis-o′de-ah) [*stomato-* + Gr. *dysōdia* stench] foul breath; halitosis.

stomatoglossitis (sto″mah-to-glos-si′tis) [*stomato-* + *glossitis*] inflammation of the mucous membrane of the mouth and tongue, observed in nutritional disorders such as pellagra, beriberi, vitamin B complex deficiency, and in infectious diseases and certain other conditions.

stomatography (sto″mah-tog′rah-fe) [*stomato-* + Gr. *graphein* to write] a description of the mouth.

stomatolalia (sto″mah-to-la′le-ah) [*stomato-* + Gr. *lalein* to speak + *-ia*] speaking through the mouth with the nares closed.

stomatologist (sto″mah-tol′o-jist) an expert in or a practitioner of stomatology.

stomatology (sto″mah-tol′o-je) [*stomato-* + *-logy*] the study of the mouth, its diseases, functions, and structure. Called also *oralogy*. See DENTISTRY.

stomatomalacia (sto″mah-to-mah-la′she-ah) [*stomato-* + Gr. *malakia* softness] excessive or abnormal softness of the oral structures.

stomatomenia (sto″mah-to-me′ne-ah) [*stomato-* + Gr. *mēniaia* menses] bleeding from the mucous membrane of the mouth at the time of menstruation.

stomatomycosis (sto″mah-to-mi-ko′sis) [*stomato-* + Gr. *mykēs* fungus] a fungal infection of the mouth.

stomatonecrosis (sto″mah-to-ne-kro′sis) noma.

stomatopathy (sto″mah-top′ah-the) [*stomato-* + Gr. *pathos* suffering] any pathological condition of the mouth.

stomatoplasty (sto′mah-to-plas″te) [*stomato-* + Gr. *plassein* to mold] plastic repair of defects or reconstruction of the mouth.

stomatorrhagia (sto″mah-to-ra′je-ah) [*stomato-* + Gr. *rhēgnynai* to burst forth] hemorrhage from the mouth. **s. gingiva′rum,** hemorrhage from the gingivae.

stomatoschisis (sto″mah-tos′ki-sis) [*stomato-* + Gr. *schisis* split] CLEFT lip.

stomatoscope (sto-mat′o-skōp) [*stomato-* + Gr. *skopein* to examine] an instrument for inspecting the mouth.

stomion (sto′me-on) [Gr. *stomion*, dim. of *stoma* mouth] cephalometric landmark, being the midpoint of the oral fissure when the mouth is closed. Abbreviated *St.* Called also *point St.*

stomo- see STOMATO-.

stomocephalus (sto″mo-sef′ah-lus) [*stomo-* + Gr. *kephalē* head] a fetal abnormality with a rudimentary head and jaws, so that the skin hangs in folds about the mouth.

stomodeal (sto″mo-de′al) pertaining to the stomodeum.

stomodeum (sto″mo-de′um) [*stomo-* + Gr. *hodaios* pertaining to a way] an ectodermal depression at the ventral surface of the primitive gut in the embryo, at the point where later the mouth is formed. The buccopharyngeal membrane, forming its floor, ruptures during the fourth week of embryonic life and allows the stomodeum and the foregut to communicate. Called also *oral fossa, oral sinus,* and *stomodeal pit.*

-stomy [Gr. *stomoun* to provide with an opening or mouth] a word termination denoting the surgical creation of an artificial opening into a hollow organ, as in tracheostomy.

stone (stōn) 1. the hard substance formed from mineral and earth material. 2. a mass of hard and unyielding material. 3. a calculus. 4. an abrading instrument or tool, such as one used for sharpening instruments. 5. a unit of weight recognized in Great Britain as being equivalent to 14 lb, or about 6.34 kg. **Arkansas s.,** stone with special abrasive qualities, used in sharpeners for dental instruments. **black s.,** an abrasive stone of silicon carbide; used for reduction and finishing gold castings. **blue s.,** cupric SULFATE. **Class I s.,** see *dental s.* **Class II s.,** see *dental s.* **dental s.,** dental plaster Types III and IV (for ADA specifications; see dental PLASTER), composed chiefly of the α-hemihydrate of gypsum (see GYPSUM hemihydrate), which occurs as a chalky white, hard, originally white, but colored buff or pastel shades for identification purposes, with various modifiers added to regulate setting time and setting expansion of the stone. Dental stones may be classified according to their particle shape and compactness as Class I stone (Type III plaster, Hydrocal modified α-hemihydrate) and Class II stone (Type IV plaster, Densite, die s., improved s.). The particles of Class II are smaller and more randomly shaped than those of Class I, resulting in a smaller surface area, therefore less water can be used in mixing, and the dry strengths are usually greater than those of Class I. Class I stone is used for the construction of casts, and Class II stone when a very strong and hard stone is required, as in the construction of special casts, such as those for gold castings. Available under numerous trademarks. See table. **diamond s.,** diamond rotary INSTRUMENT. **die s.,** Class II (Type IV) dental stone. **flat s.,** a flat piece of stone, used for sharpening instruments. **gray s.,** an abrasive stone of carborundum and rubber, used for polishing dental restorations. **gray-green s.,** an abrasive stone of silicon carbide, used for polishing metallic dental restorations. **improved s.,** Class II (Type IV)

dental stone. **mounted s.,** an abrasive stone wheel mounted on mandrels which may be placed in a straight handpiece on a belt-driven bench motor; used for sharpening instruments. **pulp s.,** denticle (2). **red s.,** an abrasive stone of garnet, available as plain or impregnated in rubber; used for polishing dental restorations. **salivary s.,** sialolith. **wheel s.,** a small grindstone of carborundum or corundum of various grits, mounted on a mandrel, its thickness varying from 1/2 to 1 inch. See also carborundum WHEEL.

stool (stōōl) an armless and backless piece of furniture with legs or a pedestal for support. **dental s.,** a stool for the dental operator. One type is attached to the dental chair so that it can revolve through 270 degrees around the chair. Its height is adjustable and when not in use, it is retracted close to the chair. The second type is separate from the dental chair, some having a foot-pedal height adjustment and horizontal and vertical back adjustments. The backrest can also be used as a siderest or abdominal rest for the operator. **dental assistant's s.,** a stool for the dental assistant, being 4 to 6 inches higher than the operator's and having a footrest ring.

stop (stop) 1. to come to a halt. 2. to cease, check, discontinue, or arrest. 3. a device that serves to prevent further progression or advancement. 4. a band on arch wire in an orthodontic appliance, designed to limit or prevent its movement through a bracket or tube. 5. a small plastic rubber disk or attachment fitting around the shank or blade of a root canal instrument, such as a broach, file or reamer, to control the depth of its insertion into the root canal. **centric s.,** contact AREA (2). **Krueger s.,** a sliding metal clip that is fastened onto a long-handled root canal instrument and projects forward over the instrument shaft that passes through it; working lengths may be adjusted by sliding the clip along the handle. **occlusal s.,** occlusal REST.

stopbath (stop′bath) acid BATH.

stopping (stop′ing) 1. a substance that stops or interrupts a process. 2. stop (3). **Hill's s.,** a mixture of bleached gutta percha, feldspar, quartz, and quicklime, considered to be the first dependable temporary filling. **temporary s.,** in endodontics, gutta-percha mixed with zinc oxide, wax, and coloring material which softens on heating and rehardens at room temperature; sometimes used beneath another material to provide a temporary double seal in the coronal access opening of the tooth during root canal therapy.

storage (stor′ij) 1. the act or process of placing something for safekeeping. 2. that part of computer hardware which receives data, stores them in the memory bank, and supplies them on command. Called also MEMORY.

storax (sto′raks) a balsam from *Liquidambar orientalis,* a tree of western Asia, or from *L. styraciflua* of North America. Called also *styrax.*

Stout wiring continuous loop WIRING.

Stoxil trademark for *idoxuridine.*

strabismus (strah-biz′mus) [Gr. *strabismos*] deviation of the eye,

SOME PHYSICAL PROPERTIES OF DENTAL STONE

MATERIAL	W/P RATIO	SETTING TIME* (minutes)	SETTING EXPANSION Normal (per cent)	SETTING EXPANSION Hygroscopic (per cent)	COMPRESSIVE STRENGTH Wet† kg/cm²	COMPRESSIVE STRENGTH Wet† psi	COMPRESSIVE STRENGTH Dry‡ kg/cm²	COMPRESSIVE STRENGTH Dry‡ psi
Class I								
A	0.30	5.5	0.16	0.27	250	3,600	720	10,200
B	0.30	7.0	0.09	0.19	240	3,400	670	9,500
C	0.28	8.0	0.18	0.27	330	4,700	710	10,100
Class II								
D	0.23	6.5	0.08	0.13	330	4,700	720	10,300
E	0.24	5.5	0.09	0.15	300	4,300	910	13,000
F	0.24	7.0	0.10	0.14	344	4,900	870	12,400
G	0.24	6.5	0.09	0.13	220	3,200	730	10,400
H	0.23	7.5	0.08	0.16	320	4,500	740	10,500

*Gillmore initial.
†After one hour.
‡After seven days.
(From R. W. Phillips: Skinner's Science of Dental Materials. 7th ed. Philadelphia, W. B. Saunders Co., 1973.)

in which the visual axes assume a position relative to each other different from that required by the physiological conditions. Called also *crossed eyes*.

Strachan-Scott syndrome [William Henry *Strachan*, British physician; Henry Harold *Scott*, British physician] see under SYNDROME.

strain (strān) 1. to overexercise; to use to an extreme and harmful degree; an excessive effort or undue exercise. 2. to filter or subject to colation. 3. a group of organisms within a species or variety, characterized by some particular quality, as rough or smooth strains of bacteria. 4. mechanical s. **engineering· s.,** mechanical s. **s. hardening,** strain HARDENING. **indicator s.,** a strain of organisms used by several groups of investigators *in lieu* of a type of neotype strain. See also NEOTYPE. **mechanical s., nominal s.,** the change of shape (deformation) of an object resulting from external forces acting on it (stress). It is measured in terms of deformation or change in dimension per unit dimension. The formula for calculating strain is as follows: e = $(\Delta l)/l_0$ (e = strain, Δl = specimen length, l_0 = original length). The strain of an orthodontic wire having an original length of 5 cm and having been stretched 0.0015 cm is thus calculated: 0.0015/5 = 0.0003 cm/cm. Called also *engineering s.* See also mechanical STRESS. **reference s.,** a strain of organisms that is used for reference in the production of a specific compound or antigen, or one which appears to meet the description of the type but has not been proposed as a neotype.

strand (strand) a thread or fiber. **lateral enamel s.,** dental lamina, lateral; see under LAMINA.

strangulation (strang″gu-la′shun) [L. *strangulatio*] 1. choking or throttling arrest of respiration, due to occlusion of air passages. 2. arrest of the circulation in a part, due to compression.

strap (strap) 1. a band or slip, as of adhesive plaster in attaching parts to each other. 2. to bind down tightly. **lingual s.,** lingual PLATE. **palatal s.,** a major connector, being a single wide strap crossing the vault of the palate from side to side, which joins two or more bilateral parts of a maxillary removable partial denture.

strata (stra′tah) [L.] plural of *stratum*.

stratified (strat′ĭ-fīd) made up of layers or strata; laminated.

stratigraphy (strah-tig′rah-fe) [L. *stratum* layer + Gr. *graphein* to write] body section radiographic technique accomplished by rotating the body between a stationary x-ray source and the film. See TOMOGRAPHY.

stratum (stra′tum), pl. *stra′ta* [L.] a sheetlike mass of substance of nearly uniform thickness, several of which may be superimposed, one on another. Called also *layer*. **s. adamanti′num** dental ENAMEL. **s. basa′le epider′midis** [NA], **s. cylin′dricum epider′midis** [NA alternative], basal LAYER. **s. cor′neum epider′midis** [NA], horny LAYER. **s. denta′tum epider′midis,** malpighian LAYER. **s. ebo′ris,** dentin. **s. fibro′sum cap′sulae articula′ris,** fibrous membrane of articular cavity; see under MEMBRANE. **s. germinati′vum epider′midis [Malpig′hii],** 1. malpighian LAYER. 2. basal LAYER. **s. granulo′sum epider′midis** [NA], granular LAYER. **s. interme′dium,** a cell layer of the enamel organ, situated between the stellate reticulum and the inner enamel epithelium (preameloblasts). It varies in thickness up to three layers, and consists of small polygonal cells with numerous short protoplasmic processes extending from the cell body. **s. lu′cidum epider′midis** [NA], clear LAYER. **s. malpig′hii,** malpighian LAYER. **s. spino′sum epider′midis** [NA], prickle-cell LAYER. **s. synovia′le cap′sulae articula′ris,** synovial membrane of articular capsule; see under MEMBRANE.

streak (strēk) a line, stripe, or trace. **angioid s′s,** pigmented striae appearing in the retina after hemorrhage. **germinal s.,** primitive s. **primitive s.,** a faint, white trace that appears first as a broad band but later becomes a narrow, well-defined thickening of the primitive ectoderm near the midline of the embryonic disk, which is the earliest evidence of the embryonic axis. It is produced by a medial concentration of ectodermal cells at the beginning of mesoderm formation, which become rounded as they migrate laterally between the ectoderm and endoderm as a mesodermal sheet, while the basement membrane disappears. The lateral sheets of the mesoderm progress anteriorly until they meet and merge near the prechordal plane. A narrow trench along the midline of the streak is known as the *primitive groove*, and a thickening at its anterior terminal is known as *Hensen's node*. Called also *germinal s.* and *primitive line*. See illustration at EMBRYO.

stream (strēm) a current or flow of water or other fluid. **cutting s.,** a stream of abrasive aluminum oxide particles ejected under pressure from the nozzle of the handpiece in the airbrasive

dental technique. **electron s.,** a stream of negatively charged particles (electrons) moving from cathode to anode across a potential difference in a low-pressure gas tube or a vacuum tube. See also cathode rays, under RAY.

streaming (strēm′ing) the act or process of flowing. **cytoplasmic s., protoplasmic s.,** cyclosis.

Streeter's bands see under BAND.

Streiff, E. B. see Hallermann-Streiff SYNDROME.

strength (strength) 1. the quality or state of being able to exert great bodily or muscular power. 2. effective force or potency. 3. the effective or essential characteristic of a beverage or a chemical, as the alcohol content of an alcoholic beverage. 4. in physics, capacity to resist a deforming load without exceeding arbitrary limits of plastic deformation, being proportional to the resiliency of materials and to section modulus of beams. **breaking s.,** ultimate tensile s. **compressive s., crushing s.,** ultimate compression s. **dry s.,** the compression strength of a gypsum product, such as dental plaster, dental stone, or plaster of Paris, when the gauging water has been evaporated and the product is completely dried, being two or more times the wet strength. **flexure s.,** a strength test of a beam supported at each end, under a static load, calculated according to the formula: $S = (3Wl)/(2bd^2)$, where S = flexure strength, l = distance between the supports, b = width of the specimen, d = depth or thickness of the specimen, and W = maximal load before fracture. Called also *modulus of rupture* and *transverse s.* **green s.,** wet s. **impact s.,** the energy required to fracture a material under an impact force. **shear s.,** see *ultimate shear s.* and SHEAR (4). **tensile s.,** see *ultimate tensile s.* **transverse s.,** flexure s. **ultimate s.,** the greatest unit stress that a material may withstand without breaking. **ultimate compression s.,** the maximum resistance of an object to compression stress; the point just before the sample is crushed under increasing loads of compression stress. Called also *compression s.* and *crushing s.* **ultimate shear s.,** the maximum resistance of an object to shear stress. Called also *shear s.* **ultimate tensile s.,** the maximum resistance of an object to tensile stress; the point just before the sample is fractured under increasing loads of tensile stress. Called also *breaking s.* and *tensile s.* See also brittle FRACTURE and ductile FRACTURE. **wet s.,** compression strength of gypsum products, such as plaster of Paris, dental stone, or dental plaster, when gauging water is present, being two or more times less than the dry strength. Called also *green s.* **yield s.,** a stength representing a stress which is slightly higher than the proportional limit. It is a calculated value from the stress-strain curve.

strepto- [Gr. *streptos* twisted] a combining form meaning twisted.

Streptobacillus (strep″to-bah-sil′us) [*strepto-* + *bacillus*] a genus of gram-negative, facultatively anaerobic, unencapsulated, nonmotile, rod-shaped bacteria of uncertain affiliation. They are 0.3 to 0.7 by 1.0 to 5.0 μm in size, with rounded or pointed ends, and usually found in chains and filaments, 0.5 to 0.9 by 10.0 to 150.0 μm long. Their metabolism is fermentative. Formerly called *Haverhillia*. **S. monilifor′mis,** a species that is the etiologic agent of the bacillary form of rat-bite fever, occurring as pleomorphic, nonencapsulated, nonmotile, non–acid-fast, sometimes pathogenic organisms. They are generally sensitive to penicillin and streptomycin but the L₁ form is penicillin resistant. Called also *Actinobacillus muris, Actinomyces muris, A. muris ratti, Asterococcus muris, Haverhillia moniliformis, H. multiformis, Nocardia muris ratti, Proactinomyces muris,* and *Streptothrix muris ratti*.

Streptococcaceae (strep″to-kok-ka′se-e) [*Streptococcus* + *-aceae*] a family of gram-positive, nonmotile, nonendosporogenic, spherical or ovoid bacteria, occurring as cocci in pairs or in chains of varying lengths, or in tetrads. They are fermentative and produce lactic, acetic, and formic acids, and also ethanol and carbon dioxide from carbohydrates. It consists of the genera *Aerococcus, Leuconostoc, Pediococcus,* and *Streptococcus*.

Streptococcus (strep′to-kok′us) [*strepto-* + Gr. *kokkos* berry] a genus of gram-positive bacteria of the family Streptococcaceae, occurring as spherical or ovoid cocci, about 0.8 to 1.0 μm in diameter, in pairs or in chains. They are facultative anaerobic, fermentative organisms that produce D-lactic and other acids. Streptococci represent about half of the viable microorganisms found in the saliva and on the dorsum of the tongue and about one-fourth of those in plaque and the gingival sulcus. They also are found in fissures and proximal caries and in carious dentin, sometimes invading the vital pulp of carious teeth, the route of invasion being along or through dentinal tubules. Most oral streptococci produce their terminal acidity of about pH 3.4 within 24 hours and are thus suspected of being involved in dental caries etiology. Among the various methods of differentiation of streptococci, the most common are: classifying them according to their hemolytic properties (α-hemolytic, β-hemolytic, and γ-hemolytic streptococci, the β-hemolytic group being most virulent); and an immunological method in which a serologically-active carbohydrate (C-substance) is used, with the precipitin technique. **S. agalac′tiae,** a species of β-hemolytic streptococci of group B, which occurs in at least four serotypes. It is a fermentative organism, about 0.6 to 1.2 μm in diameter, which produces lactic acid, and has been isolated from milk and the udder tissue of cows. It has also been associated with various human diseases. Called also *S. mastitidis.* **S. anaero′bius,** *Peptostreptococcus anaerobius;* see under PEPTOSTREPTOCOCCUS. **S. anaero′bius mi′cros,** *Peptostreptococcus micros;* see under PEPTOSTREPTOCOCCUS. **S. angino′sus,** a species consisting of α-, β-, and γ-hemolytic strains, belonging to group F and group G, type 1, the hemolytic strains of which are minute cocci, about 0.3 to 0.5 μm in diameter. The species has been isolated from the human throat, sinuses, abscesses, vagina, skin, and feces. The α- and γ-reacting strains (formerly *S. MG*), are associated with primary atypical pneumonia. **S. bo′vis,** a species of α-hemolytic streptococci of group C, which has been isolated from the gastrointestinal tracts of ruminants and, occasionally, from human feces and in cases of human endocarditis. **S. cremo′ris,** a species belonging to group N, which shows a weak α- and γ-reaction on blood agar, and occurs in milk and dairy products. Called also *S. hollandicus.* **S. e′qui,** a species of β-hemolytic streptococci of group C, occurring as ovoid or spherical cells. It causes a mucopurulent inflammation of the respiratory mucosa in horses; isolated from abscesses in the submaxillary glands and from mucopurulent discharges of the upper respiratory tract in horses. Called also *Bacillus adenitis equi.* **S. equisim′ilis,** a species of β-hemolytic streptococci of group C, having cellular and colonial morphology similar to that of *S. pyogenes,* which has been isolated from the upper respiratory tract of man and animals under normal and pathologic conditions. It sometimes has been associated with erysipelas and puerperal fever. **S. foe′tidus,** *Peptostreptococcus anaerobius;* see under PEPTOSTREPTOCOCCUS. **S. hemolyt′icus,** *S. pyogenes.* **S. hollan′dicus,** *S. cremoris.* **S. lac′tis,** a species of weakly α-hemolytic or nonhemolytic streptococci of group N, occurring as a common contaminant of milk and dairy products. Called also *Bacterium lactis.* **S. lanceola′tus,** *Peptostreptococcus lanceolatus;* see under PEPTOSTREPTOCOCCUS. **S. mastit′idis,** *S. agalactiae.* **S. mi′cros,** *Peptostreptococcus micros;* see under PEPTOSTREPTOCOCCUS. **S. mi′tis,** a species of α-hemolytic streptococci, spherical or ellipsoidal in shape, 0.6 to 0.8 μm in diameter, occurring in long chains. It has been isolated from human saliva, sputum, feces, and dental plaque. **S. MG,** see *S. anginosus.* **S. mu′tans,** a species similar to *S. salivarius,* which is believed to be involved in dental caries etiology. It ferments mannitol and sorbitol and synthesizes dextrans and levans from sucrose. **S. par′vulus,** *Peptostreptococcus parvulus;* see under PEPTOSTREPTOCOCCUS. **S. pneumo′niae,** a species of α-hemolytic streptococci, occurring as ovoid or spherical cells, 0.5 to 1.25 μm in diameter, generally in pairs, and sometimes in short chains or singly, which are fermentative, facultative anaerobes that produce small amounts of lactic acid. *S. pneumoniae* is the most common cause of human pneumonia, and has been isolated from the respiratory tract, inflammatory exudates, and various body fluids associated with pathologic conditions in man. Called also *Diplococcus pneumoniae* and *Micrococcus pneumoniae.* **S. produc′tus,** *Peptostreptococcus productus;* see under PEPTOSTREPTOCOCCUS. **S. putridus,** *Peptostreptococcus anaerobius;* see under PEPTOSTREPTOCOCCUS. **S. pyog′enes,** a species of a β-hemolytic streptococci of group A, occurring as spherical or ovoid, gram-positive, facultative anaerobes, about 0.6 to 1.0 μm in diameter, in pairs or in short to moderately long chains. Some strains form a capsule of hyaluronic acid; in others hyaluronidase production precludes capsule formation. The organisms produce streptolysins O and S, streptokinase, and various other enzymes. *S. pyogenes* causes septic sore throat, blood poisoning, puerperal sepsis, empyema, scarlet fever, rheumatic fever, erysipelas, acute hemorrhagic glomerulonephritis, and many other serious, acute and epidemic diseases in humans. Called also *Streptococcus hemolyticus, S. scarlatinae,* and *Micrococcus scarlatinae.* **S. saliva′rius,** a nonhemolytic species of group K, occurring as spheroid or ovoid cells, 0.8 to 1.0 μm in diameter, in chains of various lengths. It has been isolated from the human tongue, saliva, and feces, being the most abundant species of streptococci in the human oral cavity. **S. san′guis,** a species of α-hemolytic streptococci tentatively identified with group H, occurring as ovoid or spherical cells, about 0.8 to 1.2 μm in diameter, in medium or long chains. It is found in humans in dental plaque, in blood and on heart valves in subacute bacterial endocarditis, and less commonly in saliva

and throat specimens. L-forms are associated with recurrent aphthous stomatitis. It is the most prevalent species of streptococci on tooth surfaces. **S. scarlati′nae,** *S. pyogenes.* **S. u′beris,** a species whose growth on blood agar may be characterized by α- or γ-reaction; it has been isolated from the skin and lips of cows, from the udder in cows with mastitis, and from raw milk. **S. vir′idans,** see ˙α-hemolytic streptococci, under STREPTOCOCCUS.

streptococcus (strep-to-kok′us), pl. *streptococ′ci.* 1. a spherical bacterium occurring predominantly in chains of cells often surrounded by continuous capsular material as a consequence of failure of daughter cells to separate following cell division in one plane. 2. an organism of the genus *Streptococcus.* **α-hemolytic streptococci,** streptococci which produce a zone of greenish discoloration in the medium about the colony, containing disintegrating or disintegrated erythrocytes; outside the green zone is a nearly colorless zone of complete hemolysis. The organisms in this group are normal inhabitants of the human mouth and the upper respiratory and intestinal tracts, regarded generally as having low pathogenicity; but they are opportunists and may produce serious infections, such as subacute bacterial endocarditis and pneumonia *(S. pneumoniae)*. *Streptococcus salivarius* is representative of nonpathogenic α-hemolytic streptococci. Streptococci in this group were formerly included in a single species, *S. viridans.* **β-hemolytic streptococci,** streptococci which produce a clear zone of hemolysis in the red opaque medium immediately surrounding the colony, hemolysis being caused by the presence of streptolysins O and S. The organisms have been divided into groups on the basis of their antigenic variation of cell surface carbohydrate antigen, designated by the letters A through O. β-Hemolytic streptococci comprise the most virulent strains of the genus *Streptococcus; Streptococcus pyogenes* is representative of the pathogenic β-hemolytic streptococci. **γ-hemolytic streptococci,** streptococci which do not produce hemolytic changes in a colony. Called also *nonhemolytic streptococci.* **nonhemolytic streptococci,** γ-hemolytic streptococci.

streptodornase (strep″to-dor′nās) a deoxyribonuclease produced by some hemolytic streptococci, which depolymerizes viscous DNA, being apparently unrelated to the virulence of bacteria. Used for enzymatic wound debridement.

streptokinase (strep″to-ki′nās) an enzyme (kinase) produced by streptococci of the groups A, C, and G and a few from groups B and F and by some staphylococci and clostridia. It is the activator of the proenzyme or plasminogen in serum, converting it into an active enzyme, plasmin, which is involved in lysis of clotted fibrin. It also acts on gelatin, casein, α-lactoglobulin, rennin, hypertension, and prothrombin. According to its antigenic and electrophoretic mobility, streptokinase has been designated A and B. In vitro, it activates plasminogen to plasmin, liberates chondroitin sulfate from collagen, activates complement components, and generates permeability and chemotactic factors. In vivo, it is suspected of being involved in producing arthritis. Formerly called *streptococcal fibrinolysin.*

streptolysin (strep-tol′ĭ-sin) [*streptococcus + hemolysin*] a filterable hemolysin produced by streptococci. **s. O,** a protein containing −S−S− linkages, produced by streptococci from groups A, C, and G, which is stable in the absence of oxygen and at low temperature, and becomes inactivated by oxygen and reactivated by reducing agents. It is also inactivated by high temperatures above 37° C, being reactivated by reduction. In a free state, it has antigenic properties but becomes neutralized by specific antibodieȿ. In vitro, it lyses erythrocytes, leukocytes, tumor cells, mesenchymal cells, and blood platelets by altering membrane permeability; causes systolic contraction of the perfused heart; constricts coronary arteries in the perfused heart; and releases lysosome enzymes. In vivo, it is lethal to mice and rabbits; causes myocardial necrosis; produces intravascular hemolysis; is cardiotoxic; provokes the Shwartzman reaction; and releases acetylcholine. **s. S,** a protein isolated as a lipid-protein complex, produced by all groups of streptococci, each being specific for the group, which induces slowly-progressing hemolysis. It is stable in the presence of oxygen but is sensitive to acids and becomes inactivated by temperatures above 37° C, without being reactivated by reducing agents. In vitro, it lyses erythrocytes, leukocytes, tumor cells, mesenchymal cells, and blood platelets by altering membrane permeability; kills leukocytes; releases enzymes from lysosomes; and inhibits phagocytosis. In vivo, it causes intravascular hemolysis; necrosis of parenchymatous organs; and induces arthritis and renal tubule necrosis. Antigenically, it is a hapten which is mildly antigenic only when present in streptococcal cells.

Streptomyces (strep″to-mi′sēz) [strepto- + Gr. mykēs fungus] a genus of bacteria of the family Streptomycetaceae, order Actinomycetales, separable into several hundred different species, most of which are soil forms but some are parasites of plants and animals. It consists of aerobic, gram-positive organisms, occurring as slender, coenocytic hyphae, about 0.5 to 2.0 μm diameter, with aerial mycelia forming chains of three to several spores. Most strains produce pigments which color the vegetative mycelium, aerial mycelium, and substrate. Many strains produce antibacterial, antifungal, antiviral, antiprotozoal, or antitumor antibiotics. Many are sensitive to antibacterial agents, particularly antibiotics.

Streptomycetaceae (strep″to-mi″se-ta′se-e) [Streptomyces + -aceae] a family of gram-negative, aerobic or facultatively anaerobic bacteria of the order Actinomycetales, consisting mostly of soil forms but some are pathogens. The organisms occur as vegetative hyphae, about 0.5 to 2.0 μm in diameter, producing branched mycelia that do not fragment readily. Reproduction takes place by germination of the aerial spores, sometimes by growth of fragments of the mycelium. It includes various genera, including Streptomyces.

streptomycin (strep″to-mi″sin) an aminoglycoside antibiotic elaborated by Streptomyces griseus, O-2-deoxy-2-(methylamino)-α-L-glucopyranosyl-(1-2)-O - 5 - deoxy - 3 - C -formyl-α-L-lyxofuranosyl - (1-4) - N,N′-bis(aminoiminomethyl)-D-streptamine. It occurs as a white, odorless, hygroscopic powder that is freely soluble in water, slightly soluble in alcohol, and insoluble in chloroform. It acts on the bacterial ribosome, and is bacteriostatic to a broad spectrum of gram-negative and certain gram-positive bacteria. Used in the treatment of various infectious diseases, such as tularemia, bubonic plague, enterococcal infections, brucellosis, and tuberculosis. Malaise, muscle pain, drug fever, hypersensitization, and neurotoxicity may occur. Lesions of the eighth cranial nerve with hearing disorders are the principal complication. Called also streptomycin A. **s. A,** streptomycin. **s. B,** a form of streptomycin, $C_{27}H_{49}N_7O_{17}$. **s. sulfate,** the sulfate salt of streptomycin.

Streptosporangium (strep″to-spo-ran′je-um) [strepto- + Gr. sporos seed + angeion vessel] a genus of soil bacteria of the family Actinoplanaceae, order Actinomycetales. Called also Streptotrix.

Streptothrix (strep′to-thriks) [strepto- + Gr. thrix hair] a proposed generic name for a group of microorganisms, now assigned to the genera Actinomyces, Nocardia, and Streptomyces. **S. eppin′geri,** Nocardia asteroides; see under NOCARDIA. **S. israe′li,** Actinomyces israelii; see under ACTINOMYCES. **S. mu′ris rat′ti,** Streptobacillus moniliformis; see under STREPTOBACILLUS.

Streptotrix (strep′to-triks) Nocardia. **S. asteroi′des,** Nocardia asteroides; see under NOCARDIA. **S. brasilien′sis,** Nocardia brasiliensis; see under NOCARDIA. **S. eppin′geri,** Nocardia asteroides; see under NOCARDIA.

streptozocin (strep′to-zo′sin) streptozotocin.

streptozotocin (strep″to-zo′to-sin) an antibiotic isolated from cultures of Streptomyces achromogenes, 2-deoxy-2-[[(methylnitrosoamino)carbonyl]amino]-D-glucopyranose, occurring as platelets or prisms that are soluble in water, alcohols, and ketones. It is a nitrosourea alkylating agent capable of inhibiting DNA, pyridine nucleotides, and enzymes involved in glyconeogenesis. Used in the treatment of metastatic islet-cell carcinoma and other cancers. Nausea, vomiting, nephrotoxicity, hepatotoxicity, and bone marrow depression with anemia, leukopenia, and thrombocytopenia are the most common adverse reactions. Called also streptozocin.

stress (stres) 1. forcibly exerted influence; pressure. In dentistry, the pressure of the upper teeth against the lower in mastication. 2. general adaptation SYNDROME. 3. mechanical s. **actual s.,** true s. **axial s.,** vertically directed occlusal stress, causing a tooth to press against the periodontal ligament downward. **compressive s.,** compression (2). **s. control,** stress CONTROL. **s. divider,** stress-breaker. **dynamic s.,** a mechanical force applied for a short period of time, such as the forces created by the motion of the mandible against the maxilla during mastication. Called also dynamic force and dynamic load. **engineering s.,** mechanical s. **s. equalizer,** stress-breaker. **lateral s.,** horizontally directed occlusal stress causing a tooth to press against the periodontal ligament on the side opposite to the source of the stress. **mechanical s., nominal s.,** a force (tension, compression, shear, and torsion) applied against an object. It acts on internal

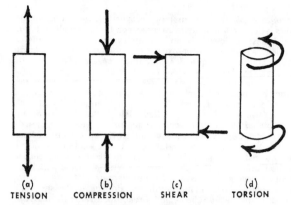

(a) TENSION   (b) COMPRESSION   (c) SHEAR   (d) TORSION

Basic modes of load application. (From E. H. Greener, J. K. Harcourt, and E. P. Lautenschlager. Material Science in Dentistry. Elmsford, New York, Pergamon Press, 1972.)

structures of the objects, particularly on the atoms in the space lattice, displacing them from their original position, with resulting changes in the shape of the object measured across a given area that may be either temporary, whereby the object will spring back to its original shape (elastic deformation), or permanent (plastic deformation). Stress is usually calculated in terms of load units measured as kilograms per square centimeter (kg/cm²); as pounds per square inch (lb/in² or psi); or in international units as newtons per square centimeter (N/cm²) or meganewtons per square meter (MN/m²). The formula for calculating stress is as follows:

$$\sigma = \frac{P}{A_o}$$

where σ = stress, P = load, A_o = original cross section. The load of 10 kg on an orthodontic wire 0.01 cm² in cross section will thus be calculated:

$$\frac{10}{0.01} = 100 \text{ kg/cm}^2$$

Called also engineering s. See also mechanical STRAIN. See illustration. **occlusal s.,** excessive pressure exerted against the teeth. See also occlusal FORCE and occlusal TRAUMA. **residual s.,** forces remaining within the material even after stress relieving procedures. **shearing s.,** the internal force that opposes the sliding of one plane on an adjacent plane or the force that resists a twisting action. The shearing stress is always accompanied by a shearing strain. Called also shear. **static s.,** a mechanical force which is applied constantly for a finite time. Called also static load. **tensile s.,** any induced force that resists elongation of a body in a direction that is parallel to the direction of the stress. Tensile stress is always accompanied by tensile strain. **torsive s.,** torsion (2). **true s.,** stress calculated by dividing the load by the actual cross-section of the specimen at any given instant. Called also actual s.

stress-breaker (stres′brāk-er) a device built into a removable partial denture that relieves the abutment teeth from excessive occlusal loads and stresses. Two basic types are recognized: one consisting of a movable joint between the direct retainer and the denture base (hinge s.), and the other consisting of a flexible connection between the direct retainer and the denture base or using a movable joint between two major connectors. The earliest device of the last type consists of double lingual bars of wrought metal, one supporting the clasps and other components, and the other supporting and connecting the distal extension bases. Called also stress divider and stress equalizer. See also combined ATTACHMENT. **complete s.-b.,** one that eliminates all occlusal stress from the abutment, such as a

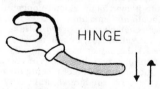

HINGE

Simple hinge stress-breaker (all types function in the same manner). (From S. I. Berger and M. J. Baskas: The use of stress breakers in removable and fixed protheses. Oral Implant. Autumn, 5(2):239.)

Roach attachment. **Crismani s.-b.**, Crismani combined ATTACH-MENT. **hinge s.-b.**, one with a built-in movable joint between the direct retainer and the denture base that permits both vertical movement and hinge action of the distal extension base and serves to prevent some direct transmission of tipping forces of the abutment teeth as the base moves toward the tissue. See also combined ATTACHMENT. See illustration. **partial s.-b.**, one that eliminates only a part of the stress, such as a flexible wire connector. **Stern s.-b.**, Stern ATTACHMENT.

stria (stri′ah), pl. *stri′ae* [L. "furrow," "groove"] 1. a streak, or line. 2. a narrow bandlike structure; used in anatomical nomenclature to designate such longitudinal collections of nerve fibers in the brain. **stri′ae olfacto′riae** [NA], olfactory striae, the extensions of the olfactory tract which join the tissues of the cerebral hemisphere. **s. of Retzius**, incremental LINE. **Schreger's striae**, lines of Schreger; see under LINE. **Wickham's striae**, minute, white to gray elevated dots or lines forming a network on the surface of the papules characteristic of lichen planus.

striae (stri′e) [L.] plural of *stria*.

striated (stri′āt-ed) [L. *striatus*] striped; marked by striae.

striation (stri-a′shun) 1. a stria or streak. 2. the quality of being marked by striae.

stricture (strik′tūr) [L. *strictura*] abnormal contraction or narrowing of a canal, duct, or other passage.

stridor (stri′dor) [L.] a harsh, high-pitched respiratory sound, such as the inspiratory sound heard in acute laryngeal obstruction. See also LARYNGISMUS stridulus. **congenital laryngeal s.**, stridor and dyspnea of the newborn due to an indrawing or infolding of a congenitally flabby epiglottis and aryepiglottic folds during inspiration; the condition is usually outgrown in two years. Called also *laryngeal s.* **s. den′tium**, an old name for BRUXISM. **laryngeal s.**, congenital laryngeal s.

stridulous (strid′u-lus) [L. *stridulus*] attended with stridor; shrill and harsh in sound.

striomuscular (stri″o-mus′ku-lar) pertaining to or composed of striated muscle.

strip (strip) 1. a thin, narrow, comparatively long piece of material. 2. to press the contents from a canal, such as a blood vessel, by running the finger along it. 3. to excise lengths of large veins and competent tributaries by subcutaneous dissection and the use of a stripper. 4. to reduce the mesiodistal width of teeth, usually done to make space to align crowded segments. **abrasive s.**, a linen strip having abrasive material, such as silica or garnet, bonded to one side; used for polishing and contouring of the proximal surface of a tooth or denture. Called also *linen s.* **linen s.**, abrasive s.

stripping (strip′ing) 1. to remove the covering from something; making something bare or naked; decortication; denuding. 2. to excise lengths of large veins by use of subcutaneous dissection. 3. removal of small amounts of surface structures from mesial or distal aspects of the teeth and dental restoration, with the use of abrasive strips. 4. see STRIP (4). **tooth s.**, removal, generally with the use of abrasive strips, of surface tooth structures or restorative material from the mesial or distal surfaces of the teeth, usually to alleviate crowding.

Strobelberger, Johann [17th century] a German physician who recommended that tobacco be used for toothache, believing that smoke causes the flow of saliva from the mouth and mucus from the nose, thus eliminating the morbid humors that provoke the pain. He also recommended the use of mineral waters for toothache by rendering the secretions more active and thus stimulating the elimination of morbid substances from the blood.

stroke (strōk) 1. a simple complete movement, especially one that is repeated. 2. the act or instance of striking. 3. a sudden and severe attack. 4. cerebrovascular ACCIDENT. **circumferential s.**, a stroke used for root and gingival curettage, the blade of the periodontal curet being negotiated mesiodistally while it is in contact with either the root or the inner aspect of the soft tissue wall of the gingival or periodontal pocket. **closing s.**, the part of the masticating cycle in which the mandible is closing, ending in the intercuspation of the teeth. **exploratory s.**, in subgingival root scaling, the stroke in which the curet is held in a featherlike grasp to tactilely ascertain the amount and extent of the accretions on the root surface; the ingress stroke reaching into the pocket area. **opening s.**, the part of the masticating cycle in which the mandible is opening. **power s.**, in scaling, the stroke aimed at splitting or dislodging calculus from the surface of the root of a tooth. It is preceded by the exploratory stroke and is followed by the shaving stroke. **shaving s.**, in scaling, the stroke aimed at smoothing or planing the root surface; it follows the power stroke for dislodging calculus from the root.

stroma (stro′mah), pl. *stro′mata* [Gr. *strōma* anything laid out for lying or sitting upon] the structural element of an organ; used in anatomical nomenclature as a general term to designate the tissue that forms the ground substance, framework, or matrix of an organ or structure, as distinguished from that constituting its functional element or parenchyma. **erythrocyte s.**, the semipermeable membrane of the erythrocyte, forming a biconcave sac in which hemoglobin is held. It represents 2 to 5 percent of the wet weight of the erythrocyte and is composed chiefly of protein and lipids. The semipermeable quality of the stroma permits the passage of cations against the ionic gradient. Potassium is transported across the membrane but not sodium. The stroma carries all the blood group antigens. Called also *erythrocyte membrane* and *red cell membrane*. **s. of thyroid gland, s. glan′dulae thyreoi′deae, s. glandulae thyroi′deae** [NA], the tissue that forms the framework of the thyroid gland.

strontium (stron′she-um) [named after *Strontian*, a town in Scotland] an alkaline earth metal. Symbol, Sr; atomic number, 38; atomic weight, 87.62; specific gravity, 2.54; melting point, 752°C; valence, 2; group IA of the periodic table. Natural strontium is a mixture of four stable isotopes (84, 86, 87, and 88). There are 12 unstable isotopes, ^{90}Sr being of greatest importance. Freshly cut strontium has a silvery appearance, but rapidly yellows when exposed to air. Strontium is soluble in alcohol and acids and decomposes water on contact. In powder form, it is flammable and ignites when heated to above the melting temperature. **s.-90**, a radioactive isotope of strontium, ^{90}Sr, which emits beta rays and has a half-life of 28 years. It is a radioactive poison of the bone-seeking type, present in fallout from nuclear explosions, and readily adsorbed by plants. Used as a source of radiation in the treatment of various diseases, including eye diseases, in radioautography, and in nuclear technology.

strophanthidin (stro-fan′thĭ-din) a toxic aglycone obtained by hydrolysis of glycosides from *Strophanthus kombé*, 3β-5,14-trihydroxy-19-oxo-5β-card-20(22)-enolide. Used in the management of severe cases of congestive heart failure. Called also *corchorin*, *cymarigenin*, and *cynotoxin*.

strophanthin (stro-fan′thin) a very poisonous mixture of glycosides obtained from *Strophanthus kombé*, containing α-glucose, β-glucose, cyramose, and strophanthidin. It occurs as a white or yellowish powder that is photosensitive and is soluble in water and ethanol, but not in chloroform, ether, and benzene. Used in the treatment of severe cases of congestive heart failure. Called also *K-strophanthin*. Trademarks: Combetin, Eustrophinum, Kombetin. **G-s., gratus s.**, ouabain. **K-s.**, strophanthin.

Strovidel trademark for *ouabain*.

structure (struk′chur) [L. *struere* to build] the components and their manner of arrangement in constituting a whole. **closed chain s.**, closed CHAIN. **denture-supporting s.**, the structures, including the residual ridge and the teeth, which provide the support for removable partial or complete dentures. See also rest AREA and denture-bearing AREA. **implant s., intermediate**, a structure of a subperiosteal or endosseous implant, which joins individual components of the implant together, or joins the substructure with the superstructure. Called also *suprastructure*. **open chain s.**, open CHAIN. **ring s.**, closed CHAIN. **sheet s.**, a planar structure in which the tetrahedral units are built in two dimensions forming sheets, as in a compound where each silicon ion is surrounded by two adjacent oxygen ions. Some minerals, such as clays, micas, and talcs have sheet structures. Called also *sheet*. **silicate s.**, a tetrahedral structure, whereby the base of the compound is formed by four oxygen anions in coordination with a silicon ion located at the central interstitial position. It is the basic structure in silicate cements and porcelains. See also TETRAHEDRON (2). **tetrahedral s.**, tetrahedron (2).

struma (stroo′mah) [L.] goiter. **s. lymphomato′sa**, Hashimoto's DISEASE. **Riedel's s.**, Riedel's THYROIDITIS.

Strumazol trademark for *methimazole*.

Strümpell-Leichtenstern encephalitis [Ernst Adolf Gustav Gottfried von *Strümpell*, German physician, 1853–1925; Otto *Leichtenstern*, German physician, 1845–1900] see under ENCEPHALITIS. See also Bekhterev-Strümpell-Marie SYNDROME.

strut (strut) 1. a structural member that provides rigidity and resistance to stresses. 2. connector BAR. **implant substructure s., primary**, one of the main transverse struts that connect the implant neck with the peripheral frame in an implant denture. **implant substructure s., secondary**, one of the additional small, transverse, diagonal, or longitudinal struts that are added in an implant denture when it is necessary to give additional strength and rigidity to the implant, to increase the area of bone support, or to afford additional intermeshing of the mucoperiosteal tissue.

strychnine (strik'nĭn, strik'nēn) an extremely poisonous alkaloid, $C_{21}H_{22}N_2O_2$, obtained chiefly from *Strychnos nux-vomica* and other species of *Strychnos,* occurring as colorless, clear, prismatic crystals or a white crystalline powder, which is odorless and very bitter and is soluble in chloroform, ethanol, ether, and water. It is a central nervous stimulant with no important therapeutic use, employed chiefly in the study of the mode of action of convulsants and as a pesticide. Its effects on the central nervous system consist chiefly of initial stimulation followed by depression of reflexes and enhancement of senses of touch, smell, hearing, and sight. Poisoning is usually manifested by stiffness of the muscles of the neck and face with heightened reflex activity, followed by muscular twitching and convulsions of all voluntary muscles, leading to respiratory failure and death. Opisthotonos, trismus, and risus sardonicus are the typical symptoms.

Stryker's saw oscillating SAW.

Stuart articulator [Charles E. *Stuart*] see under ARTICULATOR.

Stuart defect, factor [named after the person in whom the coagulation factor (X) was first seen] see FACTOR X.

stud (stud) a knob or other protuberance. See also stud ATTACH-MENT.

study (stud'e) the acquisition of knowledge through reading, systematic examination, or other methods. **adequate and well-controlled s's,** the type of investigations, including clinical investigations, which must be conducted by a new drug sponsor to demonstrate that a new drug is effective. **case-control s.,** a study in which two groups of individuals are selected, one group having the disease (cases) and the other not having the disease and serving as controls. Individuals in the two groups are studied and compared for relevant characteristics. **cohort s.,** a study in which a group of persons (the cohort) having a certain common characteristic is chosen and observed over a period of time for the appearance of particular, presumably related characteristics. As, for instance, a study on the appearance of heart failure or stroke in hypertensive persons. **double blind s.,** a method of studying a drug, or other medical procedure, in which both the subjects and investigators are kept unaware (blind to) who actually receives which specific treatment. Called also *double blind technique.* **double-contrast s.,** a radiographic examination in which a contrast medium and air are used simultaneously (or in succession) for the purpose of outlining soft-tissue structures. **Professional Activity S.,** one of the two branches of the Commission on Professional and Hospital Activities. It is a shared-computer medical record information system, containing in its data bank abstracts of hospital records of discharged patients, and producing monthly, semiannual, and annual reports which compare average lengths of stay, number and types of diagnostic tests used, and autopsy rates for a given diagnostic condition of hospitals of similar size and scope of services. Abbreviated *PAS.* See also Medical Audit Program, under PROGRAM. **prospective s.,** an inquiry planned to observe events that have not yet occurred. **retrospective s.,** an inquiry planned to observe events that have already occurred, as a case study.

stupor (stu'por) [L.] any condition characterized by apathy, diminished responsiveness, or partial loss of consciousness.

Sturge-Weber syndrome [William Allen *Sturge,* British physician, 1850–1919; Frederick Parkes *Weber,* British physician, 1863–1962] see under SYNDROME.

stuttering (stut'er-ing) a disturbance of rhythm and fluency of speech by an intermittent blocking, a convulsive repetition, and prolongation of sounds, syllables, words, phrases, or posture of the speech organs. Called also *stammering.* **labiochoreic s.,** labiochorea.

stylet (sti'let) [L. *stilus;* Gr. *stylos* pillar] 1. a wire run through a catheter or cannula to render it stiff or to remove debris from its lumen. 2. a slender probe. Called also *stylus.*

styliform (sti'lĭ-form) [L. *stilus* stake, pole + *forma* form] having a long and pointed form; styloid.

stylo- [L. *stilus* a stake, pole; Gr. *stylos* pillar] a combining form denoting resemblance to a stake or pole, used especially to denote relationship to the styloid process of the temporal bone.

styloglossus (sti"lo-glos'us) styloglossus MUSCLE.

stylohyal (sti"lo-hi'al) stylohyoid.

stylohyoid (sti"lo-hi'oid) pertaining to the styloid process and the hyoid bone.

stylohyoideus (sti"lo-hi-oid'e-us) stylohyoid MUSCLE.

styloid (sti'loid) [*stylo-* + Gr. *eidos* form] resembling a pillar; long and pointed; styliform; pertaining to the styloid process of the temporal bone.

styloiditis (sti"loi-di'tis) inflammation of the styloid process of the temporal bone.

stylomandibular (sti"lo-man-dib'u-lar) pertaining to the styloid process of the temporal bone and the mandible.

stylomastoid (sti"lo-mas'toid) pertaining to the styloid and mastoid processes of the temporal bone.

stylomaxillary (sti"lo-mak'sĭ-ler"e) pertaining to the styloid process of the temporal bone and to the maxilla.

stylomyloid (sti"lo-mi'loid) [*stylo-* + Gr. *mylē* mill + *eidos* form] pertaining to the styloid process of the temporal bone and to the region of the lower molar teeth.

stylopharyngeus (sti"lo-far-in-je'us) stylopharyngeal MUSCLE.

stylostaphyline (sti"lo-staf'ĭ-lĭn) pertaining to the styloid process of the temporal bone and to the velum palatinum.

stylosteophyte (sti-los'te-o-fīt) a pillar-shaped exostosis.

stylus (sti'lus) [L. *stilus*] 1. a stylet. 2. a pencil-shaped medicinal preparation, as a stick of caustic.

styptic (stip'tik) [Gr. *styptikos*] 1. astringent; arresting hemorrhage by means of an astringent quality. 2. an astringent and hemostatic agent. **chemical s.,** one which arrests hemorrhage by causing coagulation through chemical action. **mechanical s.,** one which acts by causing coagulation mechanically, as a pledget of cotton. **vascular s.,** one which acts by producing contraction of injured vessels of small caliber.

styrax (sti'raks) storax.

styrene (sti'ren) a compound, ethenylbenzene, occurring as a yellowish, refractive, oily liquid with a penetrating odor, which on exposure to light and air undergoes polymerization and oxidation. It is a monomer which, on polymerization, forms polystyrene. Exposure may cause lesions of the skin and mucous membranes; in high concentrations, it is narcotic. Called also *cinnamene, cinnamol, phenylethylene, styrol, styrolene,* and *vinyl benzene.* See also POLYSTYRENE.

styrol (sti'rōl) styrene.

styrolene (sti'ro-lēn) styrene.

sub- [L. *sub* under] a prefix signifying under, near, almost, or moderately. See also words beginning with HYPO- and INFRA-.

subacid (sub-as'id) somewhat acid.

subacute (sub"ah-kut) nearly acute; between acute and chronic; said of disease.

subapical (sub-ap'ĭ-kal) situated below an apex.

subarcuate (sub-ar'ku-āt) [*sub-* + L. *arcuatus* arched] somewhat arched or bent.

subaurale (sub"aw-ra'le) an anthropometric landmark, the lowest point on the inferior border of the ear lobule when the subject is looking straight ahead.

subcartilaginous (sub"kar-tĭ-laj'ĭ-nus) 1. situated beneath a cartilage. 2. partly cartilaginous.

subchondral (sub-kon'dral) situated beneath a cartilage; subcartilaginous.

subclavian (sub-kla've-an) situated under the clavicle, as the subclavian artery.

subcranial (sub-kra'ne-al) situated beneath the cranium.

subcutaneous (sub"ku-ta'ne-us) situated or occurring beneath the skin.

subdental (sub-den'tal) [*sub-* + L. *dens* tooth] situated beneath a tooth or teeth.

subdorsal (sub-dor'sal) situated below the dorsal region.

subepiglottic (sub"ep-ĭ-glot'ik) below the epiglottis.

subgemmal (sub-jem'al) [*sub-* + L. *gemma* bud] situated under a taste bud or other bud.

subgingival (sub-jin'jĭ-val) beneath or under the gingiva.

subglenoid (sub-gle'noid) situated under the glenoid fossa; infraglenoid.

subglossal (sub-glos'al) sublingual.

subglossitis (sub"glos-si'tis) inflammation of the lower surface of the tongue. **s. diphtheroi'des,** Riga-Fede DISEASE.

subhyoid (sub-hi'oid) situated under the hyoid bone; infrahyoid.

subiculum (su-bik'u-lum) [L., from *subicere* to raise, lift] an underlying or supporting structure.

subjacent (sub-ja'sent) [*sub-* + L. *jacere* to lie] lying just beneath or underneath.

subjective (sub-jek'tiv) [L. *subjectivus*] pertaining to or perceived only by the affected individual; pertaining to those symptoms and manifestations which are apparent only to the patient, in contradistinction to the objective signs, which may be observed by a person other than the patient.

subjugal (sub-ju'gal) situated below the zygomatic bone.

sublesional (sub-le'shun-al) performed or occurring beneath a lesion.

sublethal (sub-le'thal) not quite fatal; insufficient to cause death.

sublimation (sub"lĭ-ma'shun) in chemistry, the process of molecules leaving the solid state and entering the gaseous state without going through the liquid state.

subliminal (sub-lim′ĭ-nal) [*sub-* + L. *limen* threshold] below the limen, or threshold, of sensation.

sublingual (sub-ling′gwal) located beneath the tongue. Called also *subglossal.*

sublinguitis (sub″ling-gwi′tis) inflammation of the sublingual gland.

subluxation (sub″luk-sa′shun) [*sub-* + *luxation*] a partial or incomplete dislocation. **temporomandibular joint s.,** displacement of the condyle of the mandible in the glenoid fossa, with locking of the temporomandibular joint in positions that do not correspond necessarily to full mandibular opening and without the condyle reaching a position anterior to the articular tuberculum. The condition is usually due to splinting or spastic activity of the jaw muscles, and is commonly associated with a clicking sound in the joint and sprain of the supporting structures. The mandible returns to its normal position after the spasm subsides. See also *temporomandibular joint* DISPLACEMENT.

submandibular (sub″man-dib′u-lar) situated below the mandible; inframandibular.

submarginal (sub-mar′jĭ-nal) situated beneath a margin; inframarginal.

submaxilla (sub″mak-sil′ah) [*sub-* + *maxilla*] the mandible.

submaxillaritis (sub-mak″sĭ-ler-i′tis) inflammation of the submaxillary (submandibular) gland.

submaxillary (sub-mak′sĭ-ler″e) situated beneath the maxilla; inframaxillary.

submedial, submedian (sub-me′de-al; sub-me′de-an) beneath or near the middle.

submembranous (sub-mem′brah′nus) partly membranous.

submental (sub-men′tal) [*sub-* + L. *mentum* chin] situated below the chin.

submersion (sub-mer′shun) [*sub-* + L. *mergere* to dip] the act of placing or the condition of being placed under the surface of a liquid.

submetacentric (sub″met-ah-sen′trik) [*sub-* + *metacentric*] having the center or centromere in an eccentric or submedial location. See submetacentric CHROMOSOME.

submicron (sub-mi′kron) a particle varying in size from 10^{-5} cm to 5×10^{-7} cm. Called also *hypomicron.*

submicroscopic (sub-mi″kro-skop′ik) too small to be visible under the microscope.

submucosa (sub″mu-ko′sah) submucous MEMBRANE. **s. of pharynx,** submucous membrane of pharynx; see under MEMBRANE.

subnasal (sub-na′zal) situated below the nose.

subnasale (sub″na-sa′le) an anthropometric landmark situated at the point where the nasal septum merges with the upper lip in the midsagittal plane. Abbreviated *Sn.* Called also *point Sn* and *subnasion.* See illustration at CEPHALOMETRY.

subnasion (sub-na′ze-on) subnasale.

subnatant (sub-na′tant) 1. situated below or at the bottom of something. 2. the liquid phase situated below a solid phase; it arises when a solid has a lower density than the liquid with which it is in contact.

suboccipital (sub″ok-sip′ĭ-tal) situated below the occiput.

suborbital (sub-or′bĭ-tal) situated beneath the orbit; infraorbital.

subparietal (sub″pah-ri′ĕ-tal) situated below a parietal bone or lobe.

subperiosteal (sub″per-e-os′te-al) situated beneath the periosteum.

subpharyngeal (sub″fah-rin′je-al) situated below the pharynx.

subphyla (sub-fi′lah) plural of *subphylum.*

subphylum (sub-fi′lum), pl. *subphy′la.* a taxonomic category sometimes established, subordinate to a phylum and superior to a class.

subpulpal (sub-pul′pal) below the dental pulp.

subrogation (sub″ro-ga′shun) in insurance, the provision in a policy which requires an insured person to turn over any rights he may have to recover damage from another party to the insurer, to the extent to which he or she has been reimbursed by the insurer.

subscriber (sub-skrib′er) 1. one who assents by or as if by signing his name. 2. one who expresses assent or adhesion to a contract, statement, or plan by or as by signing his name. 3. in group insurance, the person, usually the employee who represents the family unit in relation to the prepayment plan; other family members being known as *dependents.* Called also *certificate holder.* See also BENEFICIARY.

subscription (sub-skrip′shun) that part of the prescription which gives the directions for compounding the ingredients. See PRESCRIPTION.

subserous (sub-se′rus) situated beneath a serous membrane.

subsonic (sub-son′ik) infrasonic.

subsp. subspecies.

subspecies (sub′spe-sēz) a taxonomic category subordinate to a species. Abbreviated *subsp.*

subspinale (sub″spi-na′le) the deepest midline point on the maxilla on the concavity between the anterior nasal spine and prosthion. Abbreviated *A, a,* and *ss.* Called also *point A.*

substance (sub′stens) [L. *substantia*] the material constituting an organ or body. Called also *substantia.* **s. A.,** a blood group substance secreted into body fluids by persons of blood group A who are secretors. **s. ABH,** a group of blood substances secreted into body fluids by persons who are secretors. The substances secreted correspond to the red cell ABO type. **acute phase s.,** a nonantibody substance appearing in the blood plasma after the onset of inflammation due to infection or tissue damage. **adamantine s. of tooth,** dental ENAMEL. **s. B,** blood group substance secreted into body fluids by persons of blood group B who are secretors. **blood group s's,** BLOOD GROUP substances. **carrier s.,** a substance that carries another substance across an obstacle. In diffusion, a substance that combines with substances which are not soluble in lipids, and carries them across the cell membrane in a lipid-soluble state. See also facilitated DIFFUSION. **cement s., cementing s.,** glycocalyx. **chromophil s.,** Nissl bodies; see under BODY. **compact s. of bone,** compact BONE. **cortical s. of lymph nodes,** the outer portion of a lymph node, consisting mainly of dense lymphatic tissue and follicles. Called also *cortex nodi lymphatic* [NA] and *substantia corticalis lymphoglandulae.* **gap s.,** glycocalyx. **gray s.,** the substance of the brain and spinal cord, composed of nerve cells, unmyelinated nerve fibers, and supportive tissue. Called also *gray matter* and *substantia grisea* [NA]. **ground s., of bone,** bone MATRIX. **ground s. of cell,** cytoplasm. **s. H,** a blood group substance secreted into body fluids by persons of blood O who are secretors. **interfibrillar s. of Flemming, interfilar s.,** hyaloplasm (1). **interprismatic s.,** a cementing substance, rarely exceeding 1 μ, which occupies the space between the round or polygonal enamel prisms. X-ray and polarizing microscopic data indicate that the interprismatic substance is softer and more plastic than the enamel prism itself. **intertubular s. of tooth,** dentin. **ivory s.,** dentin. **mediator s.,** transmitter s. **Nissl s.,** Nissl bodies; see under BODY. **proper s. of tooth,** dentin. **receptive s.,** drug RECEPTOR. **slow reacting s. A, slow-reacting s. of anaphylaxis, slow-reactive s. A, slow-reactive s. of anaphylaxis,** a substance capable of producing slow prolonged contraction of certain smooth muscles in anaphylactic reactions or in an isolated muscle, which is not inhibited by antihistaminics. It is believed to be elaborated by mast cells, basophils, and neutrophils, its molecule being an acidic sulfated ester with a molecular weight of less than 500. Abbreviated *SRS-A.* **spongy s. of bone,** spongy BONE. **threshold s.,** any substance in the blood, such as glucose, which is excreted by the kidneys when its concentration exceeds a certain level. See also THRESHOLD (3). **transmitter s.,** a chemical substance that is responsible for conveying impulses across synaptic and neuroeffector junctions. In the parasympathetic nervous system, it is acetylcholine which, upon completing its mission, is destroyed by the enzyme cholinesterase. In the sympathetic nervous system, it is norepinephrine together with small amounts of acetylcholine which, after conveying the impulse, is reabsorbed into the nerve endings and methylated by the enzyme O-methyl transferase. Serotonin and L-glutamic acid are also believed to be transmitter substances. Transmitter substances are usually stored in synaptic vesicles in presynaptic terminals and are released as a result of depolarizing effect of the action potential. Parasympathetic postganglionic nerves liberate acetylcholine and most sympathetic postganglionic nerves liberate norepinephrine, but sympathetic postganglionic fibers to the sweat glands and a few fibers to the vascular beds of the skeletal muscles liberate acetylcholine. Some sympathetic nerves also appear to liberate histamine. The adrenal medulla, innervated by sympathetic preganglionic fibers, liberates mostly epinephrine, believed in the past to be the sympathetic transmitter substance. Called also *mediator s., excitatory transmitter, mediator, neurohumor, neurohumoral transmitter,* and *transmitter.* See also SYNAPSE and neurohumoral TRANSMISSION. **white s.,** the conducting substance of the brain and spinal cord, consisting mostly of myelinated nerve fibers. Called also *substantia alba* [NA] and *white matter.*

substantia (sub-stan′she-ah), pl. *substan′tiae* [L.] material of which a tissue, organ, or body is made up. Called also *substance.* **s. adamanti′na den′tis,** dental ENAMEL. **s. al′ba** [NA], white SUBSTANCE. **s. compac′ta os′sium** [NA] compact BONE. **s. cortica′lis lymphoglan′dulae,** cortical substance of lymph nodes; see under SUBSTANCE. **s. denta′lis pro′pria,** dentin. **s. ebur′nea,** dentin. **s. fundamenta′lis den′tis,** dentin. **s. gris′ea** [NA], gray SUBSTANCE. **s. medulla′ris lymphoglan′dulae,** MEDULLA of lymph node. **s. os′sea den′tis,** cementum. **s. spongio′sa os′sium** [NA], spongy BONE.

substantiae (sub-stan′she-e) [L.] plural of *substantia.*

substituent (sub-stich′u-ent) 1. a substitute; especially an atom, radical, or group substituted for another in a compound. 2. of or pertaining to such an atom, radical, or group.

substitute (sub′stĭ-tūt) a material which may be used in place of another. **blood s., plasma s.,** a fluid, such as a saline or glucose solution, which may be used instead of whole blood or plasma for replacement of circulating fluid in the body. **dentin s.,** intermediary BASE. **tin foil s.,** separating MEDIUM.

substitution (sub″stĭ-tu′shun) [L. *substitutio,* from *sub* under + *statuere* to place] the act of putting one thing in the place of another, especially the chemical replacement of one element or radical by some other. **creeping s. of bone,** the formation of new bone on the surfaces of necrotic trabeculae by osteoblasts, occurring after the revascularization of an area that has been disrupted by fracture.

substrate (sub′strāt) [*sub-* + L. *stratum* layer] a substance upon which an enzyme acts.

substratum (sub-stra′tum) [L.] 1. substrate. 2. a lower layer or stratum.

substructure (sub′struk-chur) 1. a structure which provides a foundation for another structure. 2. a basic underlying or supporting part of an organ or structure. Called also *infrastructure.* 3. implant s. **implant s.,** a framework of metal, usually made of a chromium-cobalt alloy, implanted beneath the mucoperiosteum in contact with the bone, which retains, supports, and stabilizes the superstructural part of an implant denture. Called also *implant framework* and *implant infrastructure.* See also endosseous IMPLANT, implant DENTURE, implant SUPERSTRUCTURE, and subperiosteal IMPLANT.

subsulcus (sub-sul′kus) a sulcus concealed by another.

subterminal (sub-ter′mĭ-nal) situated near an end or extremity.

subthalamus (sub-thal′ah-mus) the ventral thalamus or subthalamic tegmental region of the brain.

subtile (sub′til) [L. *subtilis*] keen and acute.

subtotal (sub-to′tal) nearly but not quite total.

Sucaryl trademark for an artificial, nonnutritive, and noncaloric sweetener containing *soluble saccharin* (see under SACCHARIN).

succedaneous (suk″sĕ-da′ne-us) 1. ensuing; in place of, as succedaneous teeth. 2. of the nature of succedaneum.

succedaneum (suk″se-da′ne-um) [L. *succedaneus* taking another's place] a medicine or material that may be substituted for another of like properties. **royal mineral s.,** former name for *dental amalgam* (see under AMALGAM).

Succicuran trademark for *succinylcholine chloride* (see under SUCCINYLCHOLINE).

Succinal trademark for *ethosuximide.*

succinase (suk′sĭ-nās) an enzyme that catalyzes the hydrolysis of succinic acid or its salts. **arginine s.,** argininosuccinate LYASE.

succinate (suk′sĭ-nāt) any salt of succinic acid containing the group $C_2H_4(COOH)_2$. **s. dimethochloride,** SUCCINYLCHOLINE chloride.

succinimide (suk-sin′ah-mĭd) a hypo-oxaluric agent, 2,5-pyrrolidinedione.

succinylcholine chloride (suk″sĭ-nil-ko′lēn) a depolarizing neuromuscular blocking agent that is rapidly hydrolyzed by cholinesterase, 2,2′-(1,4-dioxo-1,4-butanediyl)bis(oxy)]bis-N,N,N-trimethylethanaminium dichloride. It occurs as a white, odorless, crystalline powder that is soluble in water, ethanol, and chloroform, but not in ether. Used in endoscopy, laryngospasm, and shock therapy, and in anesthesia during various surgical procedures. Excessive salivation, muscle pain, apnea, bradycardia, increased intraocular pressure, fever, and arrhythmia in cardiac patients are the principal side reactions. Called also *succinate dimethochloride* and *suxamethonium chloride.* Trademarks: Anectine, Succicuran.

Succitimal trademark for *phensuximide.*

succorrhea (suk″o-re′ah) [L. *succus* juice + Gr. *rhoia* flow] an excessive flow of a juice or secretion, as in ptyalism.

succus (suk′us), pl. *suc′ci* [L.] any fluid from an animal or plant tissue. See JUICE. **s. gas′tricus,** gastric JUICE.

sucking (suk′ing) the act or process of drawing into the mouth, in which the partial vacuum produced inside the oral cavity through the joint action of the cheeks, lips, and tongue, draws through a narrow opening between the lips air, liquids, or any substance or object, such as a finger. See also SUCKLING. **cheek s.,** the drawing of the buccal tissues toward the center of the mouth. **finger s.,** an infantile oral habit of holding one's finger in the mouth and sucking it as if it were a nipple. According to some authorities, the habit is considered to be normal in infants and children under 4 years of age, but is abnormal in older children. Abnormal finger sucking may lead to malocclusion. **thumb s.,** an infantile oral habit of holding one's thumb in the mouth and sucking it as if it were a nipple. According to some authorities, the habit is considered to be normal in infants and children under 4 years of age but is abnormal in older children. Abnormal thumb sucking may lead to malocclusion. **tongue s.,** the habit of projecting the tongue between the teeth or lips and drawing or sucking air into the mouth.

suckling (suk′ling) 1. nourishing by feeding at the breast. In the suckling activity the gum pads are apart and the tongue is brought forward in plunger-like fashion to produce a partial vacuum thereby drawing the milk or other fluid into the mouth; the tongue and lower lip being in constant contact and the mandible moving up and down rhythmically and forward and backward by virtue of the flat condylar part, as the buccinator mechanism alternately contracts and relaxes. Called also *nursing.* See also SUCKING and EXERCISER (2). 2. an infant or a young animal that is not yet weaned.

sucrase (su′krās) β-FRUCTOFURANOSIDASE.

Sucrets trademark for *hexylresorcinol.*

sucrose (su′kros) [L. *sucrosum*] a disaccharide, α-D-glucopyranosyl-β-D-fructofuranoside, composed of a molecule of glucose joined to a molecule of fructose in such a way that the linkage involves the reducing groups of both sugars (carbon-1 of glucose and carbon-2 of fructose). On hydrolysis, it yields fructose and glucose. Sucrose occurs as hard, white, dry crystals, lumps, or powder that is sweet to taste, odorless, and readily soluble in water, slightly soluble in alcohol, but insoluble in benzene, petroleum, and other organic solvents. Sucrose is obtained chiefly from sugar cane and the sugar beet, and is the ordinary, or table, sugar used as a sweetening agent. It has been directly linked to the etiology of dental caries and is suspected of being involved in certain other human diseases. Called also *saccharose.*

sudomotor (su″do-mo′tor) [L. *sudor* sweat + *motor* move] stimulating the sweat glands.

sudor (su′dor) [L.] sweat.

sudoriparous (su″do-rip′ah-rus) [*sudor* + L. *parere* to produce] secreting or producing sweat.

suffocation (suf″o-ka′shun) [L. *suffocatio*] the stoppage of respiration attended by anoxia and coma; asphyxia.

sugar (shug′gar) [L. *saccharum;* Gr. *sakcharon*] a term generally used synonymously with *carbohydrate* and *starch.* In conventional use, it is restricted to those carbohydrates that are soluble and have a sweet taste. Nutritionally, the term applies to only those carbohydrates that are physiologically assimilable, such as sucrose. **aldehyde-containing s., aldose s.,** aldose. **blood s.,** any sugar or carbohydrate present in the blood. Except immediately after meals, the only monosaccharide present in significant quantities in the blood and interstitial fluid is glucose, its level being controlled by insulin and glucagon. Most sugars are carried from the intestine by the portal circulation to the liver where they are converted to glucose (see CARBOHYDRATE metabolism). The normal glucose concentration in a person who has not eaten a meal within the past 3 to 4 hours is approximately 70 to 90 mg/100 ml of blood (normal fasting level), rarely rising above 140 mg/100 ml of blood after meals, unless the patient has diabetes mellitus. Strenuous exercise or prolonged starvation causes the blood sugar level to decrease, resulting in hypoglycemia. Abnormal increase in the blood sugar level is known as *hyperglycemia.* The terms *blood sugar* and *blood glucose* are sometimes used synonymously. See also lactic acid CYCLE and Embden-Meyerhof PATHWAY. **brain s.,** see GALACTOSE. **bread s.,** dextrose. **corn s.,** dextrose. **fruit s.,** fructose. **grape s.,** dextrose. **ketone-containing s.,** ketose. **malt s.,** maltose. **manna s.,** mannitol. **meat s.,** inositol. **milk s.,** lactose. **ordinary s.,** sucrose. **pectin s.,** arabinose. **simple s.,** monosaccharide. **starch s.,** dextrose. **table s.,** sucrose. **wood s.,** xylose.

suicide (soo′ĭ-sīd) [L. *sui* of himself + *caedere* to kill] the taking of one's own life. **assisted s.,** active voluntary EUTHANASIA.

sulcate (sul′kāt) [L. *sulcatus*] furrowed or marked with sulci.

sulci (sul′si) [L.] plural of *sulcus.*

sulciform (sul′sĭ-form) [*sulcus* + L. *forma* shape] formed like a groove.

sulcoplasty (sul′ko-plas″te) vestibuloplasty.

sulculi (sul′ku-li) [L.] plural of *sulculus.*

sulculus (sul′ku-lus), pl. *sul′culi* [L.] a small or minute sulcus.

sulcus (sul'kus), pl. *sul'ci* [L.] 1. a groove, trench, or furrow; used in anatomy as a general term to designate such a depression, especially one of those on the surface of the brain. See also FISSURE, FURROW, and GROOVE. 2. a linear depression in the surface of a tooth, the sloping sides of which meet at an angle. **alveolabial s.**, the furrow between the dental arch and the lips. **alveolingual s.**, the depression between the dental arch and the tongue. **s. arte'riae occipita'lis** [NA], s. of occipital artery. **s. arte'riae tempora'lis me'diae** [NA], s. of middle temporal artery. **arterial sulci, sul'ci arterio'si** [NA], grooves on the internal surfaces of the cranial bones for the meningeal arteries. Called also *arterial grooves.* **s. of auditory tube,** a furrow on the medial part of the spine of the sphenoid bone; it lodges a portion of the cartilaginous part of the auditory tube. Called also *s. tubae auditivae* [NA], *s. tubae eustachii,* and *groove for eustachian tube.* **s. of auricular branch of vagus nerve,** mastoid CANALICULUS. **basilar s. of occipital bone,** s. of inferior petrosal sinus of occipital bone. **s. canalic'uli mastoi'dei,** s. of mastoid canaliculus. **s. cana'lis innomina'tus,** s. of lesser petrosal nerve. **s. carot'icus os'sis sphenoida'lis** [NA], carotid s. **carotid s.,** a groove along the posterior part of the lateral surface of the body of the sphenoid bone, which lodges the internal carotid artery and the cavernous sinus. Called also *s. caroticus ossis sphenoidalis* [NA], *carotid groove of sphenoid bone* and *cavernous groove of sphenoid bone.* **s. of chiasm, s. chias'matis** [NA], optic GROOVE. **s. col'li mandib'ulae,** s. of mandibular neck. **ethmoidal s. of Gegenbaur,** ethmoid canal, anterior; see under CANAL. **ethmoidal s. of nasal bone, s. ethmoida'lis os'sis nasa'lis** [NA], a groove that extends the entire length of the posteromedial surface of the nasal bone and lodges the external nasal branch of the anterior ethmoid nerve. Called also *ethmoidal groove, nasal groove,* and *groove for nasal nerve.* **s. of eustachian tube,** auditory TUBE. **gingival s.,** a shallow V-shaped space around the tooth, bounded by the tooth surface on one side and the epithelium lining the free margin on the other. The terms *gingival sulcus* and *gingival crevice* are sometimes used synonymously, but some authorities consider them to be two separate and distinct entities. See illustration. **greater palatine s. of maxilla,** the sulcus on the nasal surface of the maxilla which, along with the corresponding one on the perpendicular plate of the palatine bone, forms the canal for the greater palatine nerve. Called also *s. palatinus major maxillae* [NA]. **greater palatine s. of palatine bone,** a vertical groove on the maxillary surface of the perpendicular plate of the palatine bone; it articulates with the maxilla to form the canal for the greater palatine nerve. Called also *s. palatinus major ossis palatini* [NA], *s. pterygopalatinus ossis palatini, pterygopalatine s. of palatine bone, palatine groove of palatine bone, palatomaxillary groove of palatine bone,* and *pterygopalatine fissure of palatine bone.* **s. of greater petrosal nerve,** a small groove in the floor in the middle cranial fossa, running anteromedially from the hiatus of the canal for the greater petrosal nerve to the foramen lacerum, and lodging the greater petrosal nerve. Called also *s. nervi petrosi majoris* [NA], *s. nervi petrosi superficialis majoris, s. of semicanal of vidian nerve,* and *groove of great superficial petrosal nerve.* **s.**

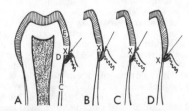

Diagram representing theories of gingival sulcus formation. *A* shows that the sulcus (arrow) is formed as a result of a split which occurs in the intermediate spinous layer of the attached epithelial cuff. The superficial layer remains attached to the enamel while the basal cells rest on the basement membrane. *B* indicates that the sulcus represents the fusion point of the attached and gingival epithelia. *C* suggests that the sulcus is formed at the point at which the attached epithelial cuff is organically bound to the enamel surface. *D* proposes that the sulcus and the crevice are one and the same and, therefore, the sulcus is bordered on the one side by the epithlium of the attached cuff and on the other side by the enamel. Cross-hatched area indicates attached epithelial cuff. Level of sulcus (X), enamel (E), dentin (D), and cementum (C). (From D. V. Provenza: Fundamentals of Oral Histology and Embryology. Philadelphia, Lippincott, 1972.)

ham'uli pterygoi'dei [NA], s. of pterygoid hamulus. **s. of inferior petrosal sinus of occipital bone,** the groove in the floor of the posterior cranial fossa at the line of junction between the basilar part of the occipital and the petrous portion of the temporal bone; it lodges the inferior petrosal sinus. Called also *basilar s. of occipital bone, petrobasilar s., s. petrosus inferior ossis occipitalis,* and *s. sinus petrosi inferioris ossis occipitalis* [NA]. **s. of inferior petrosal sinus of temporal bone,** a groove on the posteromedial edge of the internal surface of the petrous portion of the temporal bone, which, with a corresponding groove on the adjacent basilar part of the occipital bone, lodges the inferior petrosal sinus. Called also *s. petrosus inferior ossis temporalis, posterior petrosal s. of temporal bone,* and *s. sinus petrosi inferioris ossis temporalis* [NA]. **infraorbital s. of maxilla, s. infraorbita'lis maxil'lae** [NA], a groove in the orbital surface of the maxilla, commencing near the middle of the posterior edge of the surface and running anteriorly for a short distance to become continuous with the infraorbital canal. It lodges the infraorbital vessels and nerve. Called also *infraorbital groove of maxilla.* **infrapalpebral s., s. infrapalpebra'lis** [NA], the furrow below the lower eyelid. **s. of innominate canal,** s. of lesser petrosal nerve. **Jacobson's s.,** 1. tympanic s. of temporal bone. 2. s. promontorii cavi tympani. **labiodental s.,** the arched groove in the embryo which separates off the anterior part of the mandibular process, thus helping to form the lower lip. **labiomarginal s.,** a furrow which separates the cheeks from the lower lip in older persons, passing in a posteriorly convex arch close to the corners of the mouth. **lacrimal s. of lacrimal bone,** a deep vertical groove on the anterior part of the lateral surface of the lacrimal bone, which unites with the frontal process of the maxilla to form the lacrimal fossa for the lacrimal sac. Called also *s. lacrimalis ossis lacrimalis* [NA], *groove of lacrimal bone,* and *lacrimal fissure.* **lacrimal s. of maxilla, s. lacrima'lis maxil'lae** [NA], a groove directed inferiorly and somewhat posteriorly on the nasal surface of the body of the maxilla, just anterior to the large opening into the maxillary sinus; it is converted into the nasolacrimal canal by the lacrimal bone and inferior nasal concha. Called also *s. of nasal process of maxilla.* **s. lacrima'lis os'sis lacrima'lis** [NA], lacrimal s. of lacrimal bone. **lateral s. for lateral sinus of occipital bone,** s. of transverse sinus of occipital bone. **lateral s. for sigmoid part of lateral sinus,** s. of sigmoid sinus of parietal bone. **s. of lesser petrosal nerve,** a small groove in the floor of the middle cranial fossa, running anteromedially just lateral to the sulcus for the greater petrosal nerve, and lodging the lesser petrosal nerve. Called also *s. canalis innominatus, s. of innominate canal, s. nervi petrosi minoris* [NA], *s. nervi petrosi superficialis minoris, canaliculus innominatus, canaliculus petrosus, groove of small superficial petrosal nerve, innominate canaliculus,* and *petrous canaliculus.* **s. lim'itans** [NA], a shallow, longitudinal furrow on the inner aspect of the lateral wall of the neural tube, which separates the tube into the dorsal and ventral segments (*alar plates* and *floor plates*). See also intermediate ZONE (1). **lingual s.,** 1. median s. of tongue. 2. terminal s. of tongue. **longitudinal s. of frontal bone,** s. of superior sagittal sinus of frontal bone. **longitudinal s. of occipital bone,** sagittal s. of occipital bone. **longitudinal s. of parietal bone,** sagittal s. of parietal bone. **s. longitudina'lis os'sis occip'itis,** sagittal s. of occipital bone. **mandibular s.,** s. of mandibular neck. **s. of mandibular neck,** the shallow groove between the ridge of the mandibular neck and the line of attachment of the sphenomandibular ligament. Called also *s. colli mandibulae* and *mandibular s.* **s. of mastoid canaliculus,** a small groove in the petrous portion of the temporal bone leading to the mastoid canaliculus. Called also *s. canaliculi mastoidei.* **median s. of tongue, s. media'nus lin'guae** [NA], a shallow groove on the dorsal surface of the tongue, dividing it into two lateral halves, which runs from the apex to the foramen cecum at the root of the tongue. Called also *lingual s.* and *longitudinal raphe of tongue.* **mentolabial s., s. mentolabia'lis** [NA], the depression between the lower lip and the chin. **s. of middle temporal artery,** a nearly vertical groove running just superior to the external acoustic meatus on the external surface of the squamous part of the temporal bone; it lodges the middle temporal artery. Called also *s. arteriae temporalis mediae* [NA] and *groove for middle temporal artery.* **muscular s. of tympanic cavity,** SEMICANAL of tensor tympani muscle. **mylohyoid s. of mandible, s. mylohyoi'deus mandib'ulae** [NA], a groove on the medial surface of the ramus of the mandible, running obliquely downward and forward from the foramen mandibulae, and lodging the mylohyoid artery and nerve. Called also *mylohyoid* *groove of inferior maxillary bone* and *mylohyoid groove of mandible.* **nasal s., posterior,** nasopharyngeal MEATUS. **s. of nasal process of maxilla,** lacrimal s. of maxilla. **nasolabial s., s. nasolabia′lis** [NA], one of two depressions separating the upper lip from the cheeks; they are located on each side of the face, starting at the wings of the nose, from where they diverge at about a 90 degree angle, passing downward at some distance from the corners of the mouth. Called also *nasolabial groove.* **s. ner′vi petro′si majo′ris** [NA], **s. ner′vi petro′si superficia′lis majo′ris,** s. of greater petrosal nerve. **s. ner′vi petro′si mino′ris** [NA], **s. ner′vi petro′si superficia′lis mino′ris,** s. of lesser petrosal nerve. **s. of occipital artery,** the groove just medial to the mastoid notch on the temporal bone, lodging the occipital artery. Called also *s. arteriae occipitalis* [NA] and *occipital groove.* **s. occip′itis,** sagittal s. of occipital bone. **occlusal s.,** a groove or spillway on the occlusal surface of a tooth. **s. olfacto′rius na′si** [NA], olfactory s. of nose. **olfactory s. of nose,** a shallow sulcus on the wall of the nasal cavity, passing upward from the level of the anterior end of the middle concha just above the agger nasi to the lamina cribrosa. Called also *s. olfactorius nasi* [NA]. **optic s.,** optic GROOVE. **palatine s. of maxilla, s. palati′ni maxil′lae** [NA], one of the laterally placed furrows, between the palatine spines on the inferior surface of the hard palate, which lodges the palatine vessels and nerves. Called also *palatine groove of maxilla.* **palatinovaginal s., s. palatinovagina′lis** [NA], the groove on the vaginal process of the pterygoid process of the sphenoid bone that participates in formation of the palatinovaginal canal. **s. palati′nus ma′jor maxil′lae** [NA], greater palatine s. of maxilla. **s. palati′nus ma′jor os′sis palati′ni** [NA], greater palatine s. of palatine bone. **petrobasilar s.,** s. of inferior petrosal sinus of occipital bone. **s. petro′sus infe′rior os′sis occipita′lis,** s. of inferior petrosal sinus of occipital bone. **s. petro′sus infe′rior os′sis tempora′lis,** s. of inferior petrosal sinus of temporal bone. **s. petro′sus supe′rior os′sis tempora′lis,** s. of superior petrosal sinus. **posterior nasal s.,** nasopharyngeal MEATUS. **posterior petrosal s. of temporal bone,** s. of inferior petrosal sinus of temporal bone. **s. promonto′rii ca′vi tym′pani** [NA], a groove in the surface of the promontory of the tympanic cavity, lodging the tympanic nerve. Called also *Jacobson's s.* **s. of pterygoid hamulus,** a smooth groove on the lateral surface of the medial pterygoid plate of the sphenoid bone, in the angle at the base of the pterygoid hamulus; it lodges the tendon of the tensor veli palatini muscle. Called also *s. hamuli pterygoidei* [NA] and *hamular groove.* **pterygopalatine s. of palatine bone, s. pterygopalati′nus os′sis palati′ni,** greater palatine s. of palatine bone. **s. pterygopalati′nus proces′sus pterygoi′dei** [NA], pterygopalatine groove of pterygoid plate; see under GROOVE. **sagittal s. of frontal bone,** s. of superior sagittal sinus of frontal bone. **sagittal s. of occipital bone,** a deep groove on the internal surface of the squama of the occipital bone, generally to the right of the superior division of the cruciform eminence; it lodges the posterior part of the posterior sagittal sinus. The falx cerebri is attached to its margins. Called also *longitudinal s. of occipital bone, s. longitudinalis ossis occipitis, s. occipitis, s. sagittalis ossis occipitalis, s. sinus sagittalis superioris ossis occipitalis* [NA], and *s. of superior sagittal sinus of occipital bone.* **sagittal s. of parietal bone,** a shallow sulcus along the sagittal margin on the internal surface of the parietal bone; with its fellow of the opposite side it forms a groove for the middle portion of the superior sagittal sinus. Called also *longitudinal s. of parietal bone, s. sagittalis ossis parietalis* [NA], and *groove for superior longitudinal sinus.* **s. sagitta′lis os′sis fronta′lis,** s. of superior sagittal sinus of frontal bone. **s. sagitta′lis os′sis occipita′lis,** sagittal s. of occipital bone. **s. sagitta′lis os′sis parieta′lis** [NA], sagittal s. of parietal bone. **s. of semicanal of vidian nerve,** s. of greater petrosal nerve. **sigmoid s.,** s. of sigmoid sinus. **s. of sigmoid sinus,** an S-shaped sulcus beginning on the internal surface of the posteroinferior edge of the parietal bone and continuous with the lateral end of the sulcus of the transverse sinus; it passes onto the internal surface of the mastoid part of the temporal bone, where it bends inferiorly and medially to continue onto the lateral portion of the occipital bone, ending at the jugular foramen. It lodges the sigmoid sinus. Called also *sigmoid s.* and *s. sinus sigmoidei* [NA]. **s. of sigmoid sinus of occipital bone,** the portion of the sulcus of the sigmoid sinus found on the occipital bone. Called also *s. sinus sigmoidei ossis occipitalis* [NA]. **s. of sigmoid sinus of parietal bone,** a short groove on the internal surface of the posteroinferior angle of the parietal bone, continuous with both the sulcus for the sigmoid sinus on the temporal bone and the sulcus for the transverse sinus on the occipital bone; it lodges the superior part of the

sigmoid sinus. Called also *lateral s. for sigmoid part of lateral sinus, s. sinus sigmoidei ossis parietalis* [NA], *transverse s. of parietal bone, s. transversus ossis parietalis,* and *lateral groove for lateral sinus of parietal bone.* **s. of sigmoid sinus of temporal bone, s. sigmoid′eus os′sis tempora′lis,** the portion of the sulcus of the sigmoid sinus found on the temporal bone. Called also *s. sinus sigmoidei ossis temporalis* [NA], *transverse s. of temporal bone, lateral groove for sigmoidal part of lateral sinus, sigmoid fossa of temporal bone,* and *sigmoid groove of temporal bone.* **s. si′nus petro′si inferio′ris os′sis occipita′lis** [NA], s. of inferior petrosal sinus of occipital bone. **s. si′nus petro′si inferio′ris os′sis tempora′lis** [NA], s. of inferior petrosal sinus of temporal bone. **s. si′nus petro′si superio′ris** [NA], s. of superior petrosal sinus. **s. si′nus sagitta′lis superio′ris os′sis fronta′lis** [NA], s. of superior sagittal sinus of frontal bone. **s. si′nus sagitta′lis superio′ris os′sis occipita′lis** [NA], sagittal s. of occipital bone. **s. si′nus sigmoi′dei** [NA], s. of sigmoid sinus. **s. si′nus sigmoi′dei os′sis occipita′lis** [NA], s. of sigmoid sinus of occipital bone. **s. si′nus sigmoi′dei os′sis parieta′lis** [NA], s. of sigmoid sinus of parietal bone. **s. si′nus sigmoi′dei os′sis tempora′lis** [NA], s. of sigmoid sinus of temporal bone. **s. si′nus transver′si** [NA], s. of transverse sinus of occipital bone. **sublingual s.,** the sublingual portion of the oral cavity, bounded by the mandibular gingivae anteriorly and laterally and the ventral lingual mucosa posteriorly. It is lined by a thin and relatively transparent mucous membrane, covered by nonkeratinized stratified squamous epithelium that shows through the rich vascular bed underneath. Called also *floor of oral cavity.* **s. of superior petrosal sinus,** a small posterolaterally directed sulcus that runs along the internal surface of the petrous part of the temporal bone on the angle separating the posterior and middle cranial fossae; it lodges the superior petrosal sinus. Called also *s. petrosus superioris ossis temporalis* and *s. sinus petrosi superioris* [NA]. **s. of superior sagittal sinus of frontal bone,** a median groove on the cerebral surface of the squama of the frontal bone; in the upper part only, it is continuous with the sagittal sulcus of the parietal bone and lodges the anterior portion of the superior sagittal sinus. Called also *longitudinal s. of frontal bone, sagittal s. of frontal bone, s. sagittalis ossis frontalis,* and *s. sinus sagittalis superioris ossis frontalis* [NA]. **s. of superior sagittal sinus of occipital bone,** sagittal s. of occipital bone. **supraorbital s.,** supraorbital INCISURE. **terminal s. of tongue, s. termina′lis lin′guae** [NA], a more or less distinct groove on the tongue, extending from the foramen cecum forward and lateralward to the margin of the tongue on either side, and dividing the dorsum of the tongue from the root. It is marked by a row of vallate papillae. Called also *lingual s.* and *s. of tongue.* **s. of tongue,** 1. median s. of tongue. 2. terminal s. of tongue. **transverse s. of parietal bone,** s. of sigmoid sinus of parietal bone. **s. of transverse sinus,** s. of transverse sinus of occipital bone. **s. of transverse sinus of occipital bone, transverse s. of occipital bone,** a wide groove that passes horizontally, lateralward, and forward from the internal occipital protuberance to the parietal bone, where it becomes continuous with the sulcus of the sigmoid sinus; it lodges the transverse sinus. Called also *lateral s. for lateral sinus of occipital bone, s. sinus transversi* [NA], *s. of transverse sinus, s. transversus ossis occipitalis, lateral groove for lateral sinus of occipital bone,* and *sigmoid fossa.* **transverse s. of temporal bone,** s. of sigmoid sinus of temporal bone. **s. transver′sus os′sis occipita′lis,** s. of transverse sinus of occipital bone. **s. transver′sus os′sis parieta′lis,** s. of sigmoid sinus of parietal bone. **s. tu′bae audi′tivae** [NA], **s. tu′bae eusta′chii,** s. of auditory tube. **tympanic s. of temporal bone, s. tympan′icus os′sis tempora′lis** [NA], a narrow furrow in the medial part of the external acoustic meatus of the temporal bone, into which the tympanic membrane fits. Called also *Jacobson's s.* **sul′ci veno′si** [NA], venous s. **venous sulci,** grooves on the internal surfaces of the cranial bones for the meningeal veins. Called also *sulci veno′si* [NA] and *venous grooves.* **vomerovaginal s., s. vomerovagina′lis** [NA], the groove on the vaginal process of the pterygoid process of the sphenoid bone that helps form the vomerovaginal canal.

sulf- in chemical nomenclature, a prefix used in naming compounds containing sulfur. See also words beginning SULFO- and THIO-.

sulfa (sul′fah) any of a group of compounds containing both sulfur and nitrogen; see SULFONAMIDE.

Sulfabutin trademark for *busulfan.*

sulfactin (sul-fak′tin) dimercaprol.

sulfadiazine (sul″fah-di′ah-zēn) a sulfonamide, 4-amino-4-2-pyrimidinylbenzene-sulfonamide, occurring as a white or yellowish odorless powder that darkens on exposure to light and is sparingly soluble in alcohol and acetone and is freely soluble in mineral acids and potassium solutions. Used in systemic bacterial infections. Adverse reactions may include cyanosis, headache, malaise, loss of appetite, nausea, photosensitization, rash, hypersensitivity, hematuria, anemia, and agranulocytosis. Called also *sulfapyrimidine*. Trademarks: Diazyl, Debenal. **s. silver,** sulfadiazine SILVER.

sulfadimethoxine (sul″fah-di″mĕ-thoks′ēn) a long-acting sulfonamide, 4-amino-*N*-(2,6-dimethoxy-4-pyrimidinyl)benzenesulfonamide, occurring as a white, odorless, crystalline powder that is slightly soluble in ether, chloroform, and alcohol, but is insoluble in water. Used in systemic bacterial infections. Adverse reactions may include cyanosis, headache, malaise, loss of appetite, nausea, photosensitization, skin rash, hypersensitivity, hematuria, anemia, agranulocytosis, and Stevens-Johnson syndrome. Trademarks: Agribon, Diasulfa, Madribol.

sulfadimetine (sul″fah-di′mĕ-tēn) sulfisomidine.

sulfadimidine (sul″fah-di′mĭ-dēn) sulfamethazine.

Sulfadine trademark for *sulfamethazine*.

sulfafurazole (sul″fah-fu′rah-zōl) sulfisoxazole.

sulfaisodimidine (sul″fah-i″so-dim′ĭ-dēn) sulfisomidine.

Sulfalex trademark for *sulfamethoxypyridazine*.

sulfamerazine (sul″fah-mer′ah-zēn) a sulfonamide, 4-amino-*N*-(4-methyl-2-pyrimidinyl)benzenesulfonamide, occurring as a white, bitter, odorless, photosensitive, crystalline powder or yellowish crystals that are readily soluble in mineral acids and hydroxide solutions, slightly soluble in ethanol, and very slightly soluble in water, ether, and chloroform. Used in systemic bacterial infections. Side effects may include crystalluria, hematuria, hypersensitivity, hepatitis, polyarteritis nodosa, lupus, pulmonary eosinophilia, myocarditis, agranulocytosis, aplastic anemia, leukopenia, and thrombocytopenia. Called also *sulfamethyldiazine*. Trademarks: Debenal M, Mesulfa, Methylpyrimal.

sulfamethazine (sul″fah-meth′ah-zēn) a sulfonamide, 4-amino-*N*-(4,6-dimethyl-2-pyrimidinyl)benzenesulfonamide, occurring as a white to yellowish, odorless, bitter, photosensitive powder that is soluble in acetone and slightly soluble in water, ether, and ethanol. Used in systemic bacterial infections. Side effects may include crystalluria, hematuria, hypersensitivity, hepatitis, polyarteritis nodosa, lupus, pulmonary eosinophilia, myocarditis, agranulocytosis, aplastic anemia, leukopenia, and thrombocytopenia. Called also *sulfadimidine*. Trademarks: Azolmetazin, Diazil, Dimezathine, Neazina, Pirmazin, Sulfadine.

sulfamethoxazole (sul″fah-meth-oks′ah-zōl) a sulfonamide, *N*¹-(5-methyl-1-isoxazolyl) sulfanilamide, occurring as a white, odorless, crystalline powder that is soluble in ethanol, acetone, and sodium chloride and sodium hydroxide solutions, but not in water, ether, and chloroform. Used mainly in urinary tract infections. Often used in combination with trimethoprim. Called also *sulfamethoxizole* and *sulfisomezole*. Trademarks: Gantanol, Sinomin.

sulfamethoxizole (sul″fah-meth-oks′ĭ-zōl) sulfamethoxazole.

sulfamethoxypyridazine (sul″fah-meth-ok′sĕ-pi-rid′ah-zēn) a sulfonamide, 4-amino - *N* - (6-methoxy-3-pyridazinyl)benzenesulfonamide, occurring as a white, odorless, photosensitive, crystalline powder with a bitter aftertaste, which is soluble in dilute mineral acids and alkali hydroxide solutions, sparingly soluble in ethanol and acetone, and very slightly soluble in water. Used in the prevention of streptococcal infections in rheumatic fever patients, and in infections of the urinary and respiratory tracts, bacillary dysentery, acne vulgaris, and other infections of soft tissues. Adverse effects may include hypersensitivity, skin rashes, Stevens-Johnson syndrome, and occasional crystalluria, agranulocytosis, and various blood dyscrasias. Trademarks: Davosin, Depovernil, Myasul, Mylosul, Opinsul, Retasulfin, Sulfalex.

sulfamethyldiazine (sul″fah-meth′il-di′ah-zēn) sulfamerazine.

Sulfamidyl trademark for sulfanilamide.

Sulfamylon trademark for *mafenide*.

Sulfan trademark for SULFUR trioxide.

sulfanilamide (sul″fah-nil′ah-mīd) the first synthetic sulfonamide, *p*-aminobenzenesulfonamide, occurring as a fine, white to yellowish, odorless, tasteless powder, and is readily absorbed from the gastrointestinal tract. Used chiefly in the treatment of upper respiratory and gastrointestinal infections, and in the prevention of streptococcal infections, acne, bacillary dysentery, and other bacterial diseases. Adverse reactions may include cyanosis, headache, malaise, loss of appetite, nausea, photosensitization, skin rash, allergic reactions, hematuria, anemia, and agranulocytosis. Most clinically used sulfonamides are sulfanilamide derivatives. Trademark: Sulfamidyl.

sulfanuria (sulf″ah-nu′re-ah) anuria resulting from the use of sulfonamide drugs.

sulfapyridine (sul″fah-pir′ĭ-dēn) a sulfonamide, 4-amino-*N*-2-pyridinylbenzenesulfonamide, occurring as white to yellowish, odorless, photosensitive crystals or granules that are soluble in dilute acids, hydroxide solutions, acetone, ethanol, and water.

It is relatively toxic and may cause leukopenia, agranulocytosis, drug fever, dermatoses, and other disorders. Now largely replaced by other drugs, except for its use in dermatitis herpetiformis. Trademarks: Dagenan, Piridazol, Plurazol, Pyriamid, Sulfidine.

sulfapyrimidine (sul″fah-pi-rim′ĭ-dēn) sulfadiazine.

sulfatase (sul′fah-tās) arylsulfatase.

sulfate (sul′fāt) any salt of sulfuric acid. **calcium s.,** CALCIUM sulfate. **calcium s., dried,** gypsum HEMIHYDRATE. **calcium s. hemihydrate,** gypsum HEMIHYDRATE. **calcium s., native,** the native hydrated form of calcium sulfate; gypsum. **calcium s., precipitated,** the native hydrated form of calcium sulfate; gypsum. **copper s.,** cupric s. **cupric s.,** $CuSO_4 \cdot 5H_2O$, occurring as deep blue crystals or blue crystalline granules or powder; used as an emetic in phosphorus poisoning. Also a component of ascoxal, a plaque and calculus inhibitor. Called also *copper s.* and *bluestone*. **dodecyl sodium s.,** SODIUM lauryl sulfate. **ferrous s.,** $FeSO_4$, occurring as odorless, greenish or yellow-brown crystals or granules that are soluble in water, but not in alcohol; used in the treatment of iron deficiency and as an astringent. Called also *iron s., copperas, green vitriol,* and *iron protosulfate*. Trademarks: Ironate, Irosul. See also IRON. **hydrogen s.,** sulfuric ACID. **sodium s.,** SODIUM sulfate. **iron s., ferrous s. s. of lime, anhydrous,** the natural anhydrous form of calcium sulfate. **potassium s.,** POTASSIUM sulfate. **sodium lauryl s.,** SODIUM lauryl sulfate.

Sulfathalidine trademark for *phthalylsulfathiazole*.

sulfathiazole (sul″fah-thi′ah-zōl) a sulfonamide, *N*′-2-thiazolylsulfanilamide, occurring as a white or yellowish powder, granules, or crystals that are soluble in acetone, diluted mineral acids, and alkali hydroxide solutions, and slightly soluble in water and alcohol. Used for topical application to the nasopharynx and vagina. It may cause hypersensitivity; other potential side reactions include skin rash, low-grade fever, malaise, headache, and anuria. Called also *norsulfazole*. Trademarks: Cibazol, Poliseptil.

sulfatide (sul′fah-tīd) a lipoid substance containing sulfuric acid esters, largely located in the myelinated nerve fibers.

sulfatocobalamin (sul-fa″to-ko-bal′ah-min) a member of the vitamin B_{12} group in which the cyanide group is replaced by a sulfate group. See VITAMIN B_{12}.

sulfhydryl (sulf-hi′dril) the univalent radical, SH. The presence of the sulfhydryl group in a compound is usually indicated by the prefix *mercapto-*, by *thio* in the middle of a chemical name, or by the suffix *-thiol*. Called also *mercaptan* and *thiol*.

sulfide (sul′fīd) any binary compound of sulfur; a compound of sulfur with another element or radical or base. **selenium s.,** SELENIUM sulfide.

Sulfidine trademark for *sulfapyridine*.

sulfimide (sul′fĭ-mīd) a compound containing the group SO_2NH, an imide of sulfuric acid. **benzoic s.,** saccharin.

sulfinic (sul-fin′ik) pertaining to a chemical compound containing the group SO•OH.

sulfinyl (sul′fĭ-nil) thionyl.

sulfinpyrazone (sul″fin-pi′rah-zōn) a strong uricosuric agent, 1,-2-diphenyl-4-[2-phenylsulfinyl)ethyl]-3,5-pyrazolidinedione, occurring as a white powder that is soluble in acetone, sodium hydroxide, ethanol, and dilute alkali, but not in water. Used in the prevention of gout and acute gouty arthritis, having weak analgesic and anti-inflammatory properties. Upper gastrointestinal disorders, skin rash, anemia, leukopenia, agranulocytosis, and thrombocytopenia are the principal side reactions. Trademark: Anturan.

sulfisomezole (sul″fĭ-som′ĕ-zōl) sulfamethoxazole.

sulfisomidine (sul″fĭ-som′ĭ-dēn) a sulfonamide, 4-amino-*N*-(2,6-dimethyl-4-pyrimidinyl)benzenesulfonamide, occurring as a white or creamy-white powder that is soluble in hydrochloric acid and sodium hydroxide solutions, slightly soluble in ethanol and acetone, and insoluble in benzene, ether, and chloroform. Used in systemic bacterial infections. Called also *sulfadimetine* and *sulfaisodimidine*. Trademarks: Domain, Elkosin.

sulfisoxazole (sul″fĭ-sok′sah-zōl) a sulfonamide, 4-amino-*N*-(3,4-dimethyl-5-isoxazolyl)benzenesulfonamide, occurring as a white to yellowish, odorless, crystalline powder that is soluble in dilute hydrochloric acid and boiling ethanol and slightly soluble in water. Called also *sulfafurazole*. Trademarks: Entusil, Gantrisin, Neazolin, Soxisol, Sulfoxol.

sulfite (sul′fīt) a salt of sulfuric acid, M_2SO_3. **sodium acid s., sodium hydrogen s.,** SODIUM bisulfite.

sulfo- a chemical prefix indicating the presence of (*a*) divalent sulfur, or (*b*) the sulfo group. See also words beginning SULF- and THIO-.

sulfocobalamin (sul″fo-ko-bal′ah-min) a compound of the vitamin B₁₂ group, in which the CN is replaced by sulfate. See VITAMIN B₁₂.

sulfocolaurate (sul″fo-co-law′răt) a foaming agent, N-2-ethyllaurate potassium sulfoacetamide, occurring as a white, crystalline powder that is soluble in water and ethanol. Used in dentifrices.

sulfokinase (sul″fo-ki′năs) sulfotransferase.

sulfonamide (sul-fon′ah-mīd) any of a group of compounds having one or more benzene rings and a −SO₂NH₂ group, most being derivatives of p-aminobenzenesulfonamide (sulfanilamide). Sulfonamides were the first drugs found to be effective in human antibacterial therapy. They are antimetabolites which compete with p-aminobenzoic acid metabolism, thus interfering with its incorporation into folic acid in bacterial cells (Woods-Fildes theory). Initially, sulfonamides were believed to be active against only beta-hemolytic streptococci, but later were found to be also effective against gram-positive bacteria (except Enterobacteriaceae), *Haemophilus influenzae*, *Bordetella pertussis*, *Pasteurella*, and certain strains of *Pseudomonas*, *Chlamydia*, *Actinomyces*, *Streptomyces*, *Toxoplasma*, and certain other bacteria and the malarial parasite. Certain sulfonamides are used as antidiabetic drugs. Side effects may include hypersensitivity, headache, anorexia, malaise, hematuria, agranulocytosis, thrombocytosis, jaundice, and stomatitis. Commonly called *sulfa drug*.

sulfonation (sul″fo-na′shun) the introduction of a sulfonic acid (−SO₃H) group into a chemical compound.

sulfone (sul′fōn) any compound having the SO₂ group. All sulfones of medical importance are dapsone derivatives, exerting bacteriostatic effects, particularly against *Mycobacterium tuberculosis* and *M. leprae*. Used in the treatment of leprosy. See also DAPSONE.

sulfonyl (sul′fo-nil) the bivalent radical, −SO₂−.

sulfonylurea (sul″fo-nil-u-re′ah) a group of urea derivatives in which one nitrogen is substituted by a sulfonyl (SO₂) and the other nitrogen is substituted by an alkyl radical. Sulfonylureas have hypoglycemic properties, and are used in the treatment of insulin-resistant diabetes mellitus. Excessive doses may cause hypoglycemic shock (see under SHOCK). The principal sulfonylurea is tolbutamide.

sulfoprotein (sul″fo-pro′te-in) any of a series of albumins containing loosely combined sulfur.

Sulfothiorine trademark for *sodium thiosulfate* (see under SODIUM).

sulfotransferase [E.C.2.8.2] (sul″fo-trans′fer-ăs) a subclass of transferases, the enzymes of which catalyze the transfer of sulfate groups, as from the phosphoadenylsulfates to form adenosine diphosphates. Called also *sulfokinase* and *transsulfurase*.

Sulfoxol trademark for *sulfisoxazole*.

sulfoxone sodium (sul-foks′ōn) an antibacterial drug, disodium[sulfonylbis(p-phenylimino)]dimethanesulfinate, occurring as a white to yellowish powder with a characteristic odor, which is soluble in water and slightly soluble in ethanol. It is converted in the body to dapsone and is used in the treatment of tuberculosis, leprosy, malaria, and dermatitis herpetiformis. Adverse reactions may include hemolytic anemia, methemoglobinemia, gastrointestinal disorders, headache, nervousness, motor neuropathy, blurred vision, paresthesias, pruritus, hematuria, liver lesions, and skin rash. Called also *aldesulfone sodium*. Trademarks: Diasone, Diazon, Novotrone.

sulfur (sul′fer) [L. *sulphurium*] a nonmetallic element. Symbol, S; atomic number, 16; atomic weight, 32.06; specific gravity, 2.06; melting point, 112.8°C; valences, 2, 4, 6; group VIA of the periodic table. Natural sulfur isotopes include 32–34 and 36; artificial radioactive isotopes include 29–31, 35, 37, and 38. Sulfur occurs in nature both in the free state and in combination as sulfides and sulfates. The orthorhombic (cyclooctasulfur or alpha sulfur) occurs as amber-colored crystals that are stable at room temperature; at 94.5°C it becomes opaque. The monoclinic (cyclooctasulfur or beta sulfur) occurs as light-yellow, opaque, brittle, needle-like crystals that change slowly to the alpha form. Both forms are insoluble in water, slightly soluble in alcohol and ether, and readily soluble in benzene, carbon tetrachloride, and other organic solvents. Used in the treatment of scabies, in rubber vulcanization, and in various industrial processes. Exposure to sulfur may cause irritation of the skin and mucous membranes. Called also *brimstone*. Written also *sulphur*. See also terms beginning THIO-. **s. dioxide**, a colorless, nonflammable gas or liquid, SO₂, with a strong pungent odor. It

is soluble in water, alcohol, and ether, and, in aqueous solution, forms sulfurous acid. Used as a disinfectant, bleaching agent, parasiticide, food preservative, and in other processes. Exposure, particularly ingestion or inhalation, may cause lesions of the eyes and mucous membranes of the respiratory tract and oral cavity. Called also *sulfurous anhydride* and *sulfurous oxide*. **s. trioxide**, the anhydride of sulfuric acid, occurring in three solid forms — alpha, beta, and gamma — which combines with water to form sulfuric acid; when dissolved in sulfuric acid, it forms fuming sulfuric acid. Sulfur trioxide is extremely toxic, causing corrosion of tissues on contact and coughing, choking, and extreme discomfort on inhalation of fumes. Called also *sulfuric anhydride*. Trademark: Sulfan.

sulfuric (sul-fyoor′ik) pertaining to hexavalent sulfur, as in sulfuric acid.

sulfurous (sul′fer-us, sul-fyoor′us) pertaining to tetravalent sulfur.

sulph- see SULF-.

sulphur (sul′fur) sulfur.

Sultan topical fluoride gel see under GEL.

Sultanol trademark for *albuterol*.

sulthiame (sul-thi′am) an analeptic agent with carbonic anhydrase inhibitor properties, 4-(tetrahydro-2H-1,2-thiazin-2-yl)benzenesulfonamide. It occurs as a crystalline powder that is soluble in alkalies, slightly soluble in ethanol, acids, and boiling water, and insoluble in cold water. Used in the treatment of epilepsy. Adverse reactions may include tachypnea, anorexia, ataxia, drowsiness, mental changes, weight loss, confusion, and paresthesias. Trademarks: Conadil, Contravul, Elisal.

Sulzberger, Marion Baldur [American dermatologist, born 1895] see Bloch-Sulzberger SYNDROME.

summation (sum-ma′shun) [L. *summa* total] 1. the act or process of adding; obtaining a total of separate numbers or values. 2. the cumulative effect of individual excitatory postsynaptic potentials to elicit an impulse or individual contractions, as in raising the tension developed by a skeletal muscle. **spatial s.**, recruitment (2).

Summer, James Batcheller [1887–1955] an American biochemist; co-winner, with Wendell Meredith Stanley and John Howard Northrop, of the Nobel prize for chemistry in 1946, for pioneering work in crystallizing proteins.

summit (sum′it) [L. *summus*, superlative of *superus*] the highest point. **condyle s.**, condylion. **s. of nose**, ROOT of nose.

Summitt's syndrome [R. L. *Summitt*] see under SYNDROME.

Sumnafac trademark for *methaqualone*.

Sumycin trademark for *tetracycline phosphate complex* (see under TETRACYCLINE).

Sunbeam whirlpool action trademark for a magnetic stirrer type of denture cleanser (see under CLEANSER).

sunburn (sun′bern) injury to the skin and exposed mucous membranes, such as of the lips, associated with erythema, tenderness, and sometimes blistering, following excessive exposure to sunlight, which is produced by ultraviolet rays that are not filtered out by clouds, shade, or sunscreens. Short-term exposure to ultraviolet rays of 290 to 320 nm wavelength is responsible primarily for sunburn and possibly mutagenic and carcinogenic effects. Persons who are light-skinned appear to be particularly susceptible to sunburn. Lip lesions due to excessive exposure to sunlight occur more frequently in males than in females, the lower lip being more frequently involved than the upper one. See also SUNSCREEN.

sunscreen (sun′skrēn) any agent that protects the body from the effects of sunlight, thus preventing sunburn and various diseases of the skin and mucous membranes, including cancer, caused by the effects of sunlight and ultraviolet rays. Chemical sunscreens that block sunlight and act as an opaque mask include zinc oxide paste, talc, titanium dioxide, kaolin, ferric oxide, red petrolatum, and bentonite. Sunscreens which absorb ultraviolet rays in the 290 to 320 nm wavelength range include p-aminobenzoic acid and its esters, cinnamates, and salicylates.

super- [L. *super* above] a prefix signifying above, or implying excess. See also words beginning HYPER- and SUPRA-.

superabduction (su″per-ab-duk′shun) extreme or excessive abduction.

superacidity (su″per-ah-sid′ĭ-te) excessive acidity; hyperacidity.

superactivity (su″per-ak-tiv′ĭ-te) activity greater than normal; hyperactivity.

superacute (su″per-ah-kūt′) extremely acute; hyperacute.

superalimentation (su″per-al′ĭ-men-ta′shun) hyperalimentation.

superaurale (su″per-aw-ral′) an anthropometric landmark, being the highest point on the superior border of the helix of the ear.

superbill (su″per-bil′) a multipart billing form which makes it possible for the patient to fill out his own insurance claim. It includes an itemization of the information necessary to complete the attending dentist's statement portion of the insurance claim form. Called also *E-Z claim* and *instant claim*.

supercentral (su″per-sen′tral) above the center.

supercilia (su″per-sil′e-ah) [L., pl. of *supercilium*] [NA] eyebrow (2).

superciliary (su″per-sil′e-a-re) [L. *superciliaris*] pertaining to the eyebrow.

Superciclin trademark for *rolitetracycline*.

supercilium (su″per-sil′e-um), pl. *supercil′ia* [L.] [NA] eyebrow (1).

superclass (su′per-klas) a taxonomic category sometimes established, subordinate to a phylum and superior to a class.

superconductivity (su″per-kon″duk-tiv′ĭ-te) the phenomenon whereby certain metals, alloys, and various compounds lose both electrical resistance and magnetic permeability near absolute zero.

supercooling (su″per-kool′ing) cooling a liquid to below the freezing point without its solidification. During the period of supercooling, the crystallization begins and the latent heat of fusion brought about by crystal formation causes the temperature to rise to the freezing temperature, where it remains until the crystallization is completed.

Super-Dent topical fluoride gel see under GEL.

superdistention (su″per-dis-ten′shun) excessive distention.

superduct (su″per-dukt′) [*super-* + L. *ducere* to draw] to carry up or elevate.

superextension (su″per-eks-ten′shun) excessive extension.

superficial (su″per-fish′al) [L. *superficialis*] pertaining to or situated near the surface.

superficialis (su″per-fish″e-a′lis) [L.] superficial; used in anatomical nomenclature to designate structures situated near the surface of the body.

superficies (su″per-fish′e-ēz) [L.] an outer surface.

superfunction (su″per-funk′shun) excessive activity of an organ or system; hyperfunction.

superheated (su″per-hēt′ed) a condition of a liquid or gas which has been heated above its boiling point in the liquid state.

superinduce (su″per-in-dus′) to induce or bring on in addition to some already existing condition.

superinfection (su″per-in-fek′shun) a new infection; an infection occurring in addition to one already existing.

superior (su-pe′re-or) [L. "upper"; neut. *superius*] situated above or uppermost; directed upward. Used in reference to a structure occupying a position nearer the vertex.

superjacent (su″per-ja′sent) located immediately above; overlying.

superlattice (su″per-lat′is) in a solid solution, two interpenetrating lattices formed when the solution is heated to a temperature below the lower limit of the melting range (heat treatment) and then is allowed to cool slowly, the atoms from one lattice diffusing and penetrating into the adjoining lattice. It is usually formed within the crystal grain and its presence may result in a localized irregularity in the parent lattice and interruption of slips, thereby increasing the proportional limit, strength, and hardness of the material. The phenomenon of superlattice formation is known as the *solid state reaction*.

superlethal (su″per-le′thal) more than sufficient to cause death.

supermaxilla (su″per-mak-sil′ah) the maxilla.

supermedial (su″per-me′de-al) situated above the middle.

supermotility (su″per-mo-til′ĭ-te) excessive motility.

supernatant (su″per-na′tent) [*super-* + L. *natare* to swim] 1. situated above or on top of something. 2. pertaining to liquid found above the sediment or precipitate.

supernormal (su″per-nor′mal) 1. more than normal; supranormal. 2. a volumetric solution of concentration greater than normal.

supernumerary (su″per-nu′mer-ar″e) [L. *supernumerarius*] in excess of the regular or normal number.

superoccipital (su″per-ok-sip′ĭ-tal) situated above or in the upper portion of the occiput; supraoccipital.

superolateral (su″per-o-lat′er-al) situated above and at the side.

superoxide (su″per-ok′sīd) peroxide.

Superoxol trademark for a 30 per cent hydrogen peroxide solution; see HYDROGEN peroxide.

Superpaste trademark for a *zinc oxide–eugenol impression paste* (see under PASTE).

super-regeneration (su″per-re-jen″ĕ-ra′shun) the development of superfluous tissues, organs, or parts as a result of regeneration.

supersalt (su″per-sawlt′) any salt obtained by reaction with an excess of acid.

supersaturated (su″per-sat′u-rāt″ed) more than saturated, as in a supersaturated solution.

superscription (su″per-skrip′shun) [L. *superscriptio*] the sign ℞ before a prescription. See PRESCRIPTION.

supersecretion (su″per-se-kre′shun) excessive secretion.

supersoft (su″per-soft′) extremely soft; applied to roentgen rays of extremely long wavelength, large absorption coefficients, and low penetrating power.

supersonic (su″per-son′ik) [*super-* + L. *sonus* sound] having a speed greater than the velocity of sound, that is, faster than approximately one-fifth mile per second (or 720 miles per hour) in air. See ULTRASONICS.

supersphenoid (su″per-sfe′noid) situated above the sphenoid bone.

superstructure (su″per-struk′chur) 1. any structure built on something else. 2. the overlying or visible portion of a structure. Cf. SUBSTRUCTURE. **implant s.,** implant denture s., a removable denture that is retained, supported, and stabilized by an abutment post protruding from the substructure of an implanted framework. See also implant DENTURE, implant SUBSTRUCTURE, and subperiosteal IMPLANT. **implant s., temporary,** implant surgical SPLINT. **s. tooth,** superstructure TOOTH.

supervention (su″per-ven′shun) the development of some condition in addition to an already existing one.

supervirulent (su″per-vir′u-lent) extremely virulent.

supervoltage (su′per-vol″tij) very high voltage. In ionizing radiation therapy, it is generally considered to be voltage in the range of 1 to 2 million volts, as contrasted with orthovoltage (30 to 400 kilovolts) and with megavoltage (greater than 2 megavolts).

supine (su′pin) [L. *supinus* lying on the back, face upward] lying with the face upward.

Supirdyl trademark for *pargyline*.

supplement (sup′lĕ-ment) something added to complete a thing. **Phos-Flur oral rinse s.,** see under RINSE.

support (sup-port′) 1. a device or appliance which helps maintain a part in position. 2. the foundation upon which dentures rest, consisting of tooth support, mucosa-ridge support, and combination tooth-mucosa support. 3. abutment TOOTH. 4. to bear or hold up; to serve as a foundation for something. 5. to sustain or withstand weight, pressure or strain. **abutment s.,** abutment TOOTH. **abutment s., multiple,** multiple abutment s. **adequate s.,** a support that is sufficient to bear or hold up indefinitely to stresses and pressures of a denture under the functional conditions of mastication. **cast s.,** an auxiliary device used to support the face-bow fork and the maxillary cast during the mounting operation. **fixed s.,** one that permits no motion, either of translation or rotation, at the support (bar clamped in vise). **free s.,** in a dental prosthesis, support that does not permit translation of the beam perpendicular to its axis and presumably offers no restraint to the tendency of the beam to rotate at the support (knife-edge). **multiple abutment s.,** the use of more than one tooth to retain a restoration, usually consisting of splinting two or more teeth into a single multirooted abutment. **restrained s.,** one that permits no motion perpendicular to the beam axis, but permits some rotation at the support but less than the free support. **rugae s.,** in removable partial dentures, a part of a palatal horseshoe design that provides support for the rugae and indirect retention for the denture. **tooth s.,** abutment TOOTH.

suppression (su-presh′un) [L. *suppressio*] 1. arrest or prevention of a function or activity from occurring, particularly of normal functions, such as growth and development and secretory and excretory activities, or of abnormal phenomena, such as symptoms of diseases. 2. in genetics, the restoration of a lost function by a second mutation either in a gene other than that involved in the primary mutation or within the same gene. **immune s.,** immunosuppression.

suppuration (sup″u-ra′shun) [L. *sub-* + *puris* pus] the formation of pus. **alveodental s.,** periodontitis with the formation of pus.

suppurative (sup′u-ra″tiv) producing pus, or associated with suppuration.

supra- [L. *supra* above] a prefix signifying above or over. See also words beginning SUPER-.

supra-auricular (su″prah-aw-rik′u-lar) situated above the ear.

suprabuccal (su″prah-buk′al) situated above the buccal region or the cheeks.

suprabulge (su′prah-bulj) the surface of the crown of a tooth sloping toward the occlusal surface from the height of contour or survey line. Cf. INFRABULGE.

Suprachol trademark for *sodium dehydrocholate* (see dehydrocholic ACID).

supraclusion (su″prah-kloo′zhun) malocclusion in which the occluding surfaces of teeth extend beyond the normal occlusal plane. Called also *overeruption* and *supraocclusion*.

supracondylar (su″prah-kon′dĭ-lar) situated above a condyle or condyles.

supracranial (su"prah-kra'ne-al) situated on the upper surface of the cranium.

supraepicondylar (su"prah-ep"ĭ-kon'dĭ-lar) situated above an epicondyle.

supraglenoid (su"prah-gle'noid) situated above the glenoid cavity.

supraglottic (su"prah-glot'ik) situated above the glottis.

suprahyoid (su"prah-hi'oid) situated above the hyoid bone, as the suprahyoid muscles.

Supralgin trademark for *phenadoxone hydrochloride* (see under PHENADOXONE).

supraliminal (su"prah-lim'ĭ-nal) [*supra-* + *liminal*] above the limen of sensation; more than just perceptible.

supramalleolar (su"prah-mah-le'o-lar) situated above the malleolus.

supramandibular (su"prah-man-dib'u-lar) situated above the mandible.

supramarginal (su"prah-mar'jĭ-nal) situated above a margin.

supramastoid (su"prah-mas'toid) situated above the mastoid portion of the temporal bone.

supramaxilla (su"prah-mak-sil'ah) the maxilla.

supramaxillary (su"prah-mak'sĭ-ler"e) 1. pertaining to the maxilla or the upper jaw. 2. situated above the upper jaw or the maxilla.

supramaximal (su"prah-mak'sĭ-mal) above the maximum.

suprameatal (su"prah-me-a'tal) [*supra-* + *meatus*] situated above a meatus.

supramental (su"prah-men'tal) [*supra-* + L. *mentum* chin] situated above the chin.

supramentale (su"prah-men-ta'le) in roentgenographic cephalometry, the most posterior midline point in the concavity between the infradentale and pogonium, determined on the lateral head film. Abbreviated *B* and *b*. Called also *point B*.

supranasal (su"prah-na'zal) situated above the nose.

supranormal (su"prah-nor'mal) greater than normal; present or occurring in excess of normal amounts or values; supernormal.

supraoccipital (su"prah-ok-sip'ĭ-tal) situated above the occiput; superoccipital.

supraocclusion (su"prah-ŏ-kloo'shun) supraclusion.

supraorbital (su"prah-or'bĭ-tal) situated above the orbit.

supraorbitale (su"prah-or"bĭ-ta'le) a craniometric landmark, being the uppermost point of the orbital ridge. Abbreviated *S.Or.* Called also *point S.Or.*

suprarenal (su"prah-re'nal) [*supra-* + L. *ren* kidney] situated above a kidney; adrenal.

Suprarenin trademark for *epinephrine*.

suprastructure (su"prah-struk-chur) implant structure, intermediate; see under STRUCTURE.

supratemporal (su"prah-tem'po-ral) situated above the temporal bone; fossa, or region.

supratonsillar (su"prah-ton'sĭ-lar) situated above a tonsil.

supraversion (su"prah-ver'zhun) [*supra-* + L. *versio* a turning] malocclusion in which a tooth or other maxillary or mandibular structure extends further away from the alveolus than normal, the occluding surfaces of the teeth extending beyond the normal occlusal line.

supravital (su"prah-vi'tal) denoting a staining method in which the dye is added to a medium of cells already removed from the living organism.

Supressin trademark for *dextromethorphan hydrobromide* (see under DEXTROMETHORPHAN).

Surbex T trademark for a mixture of vitamins, one tablet of which contains 500 mg sodium ascorbate, 100 mg niacinamide, 20 mg calcium pantothenate, 15 mg thiamine mononitrate, 10 mg riboflavin, 5 mg pyridoxine hydrochloride, and 10 mcg cyanocobalamin.

surdity (ser'dĭ-te) [L. *surditas*] deafness.

Surfacaine trademark for *cyclomethycaine sulfate* (see under CYCLOMETHYCAINE).

surface (ser'fis) the outer part or an external aspect of a solid body. Called also *facies*. **alveolar s. of mandible**, alveolar arch of mandible; see under ARCH. **alveolar s. of maxilla**, alveolar arch of maxilla; see under ARCH. **anterior s.**, 1. the surface which is toward the front of the body, or nearest the ventral aspect in man (called also *facies anterior*), or toward the head in quadrupeds. 2. the proximal surface of a tooth that is closest to the midline of the dental arch. **anterior s. of eyelids**, the external surface of the eyelids. Called also *facies anterior palpebrarum* [NA]. **anterior s. of maxilla**, the surface of the body of the maxilla directed forward and somewhat laterally,

bounded above by the infraorbital margin; medially by the margin of the nasal notch; and posteriorly by the anterior border of the zygomatic process, which has a confluent ridge over the roots of the first molar. The ridge corresponding to the root of the canine tooth is usually the most prominent and is known as the *canine eminence.* Mesial to the canine eminence is the incisive fossa, overlying the roots of the incisor teeth; distal to it is the canine fossa. The zygomatic process projects into the canine fossa, forming a part of its floor. The infraorbital foramen is situated above the canine fossa and below the infraorbital margin. Called also *facial s. of maxilla* and *facies anterior maxillae* [NA]. **anterior s. of petrous part of temporal bone**, the surface of the petrous bone that forms the posterior portion of the floor of the middle cranial fossa. Called also *anterior s. of pyramidal part of temporal bone, facies anterior partis petrosae ossis temporalis* [NA], and *facies anterior pyramidis ossis temporalis.* **anterior s. of premolar and molar teeth**, the contact surface of the premolar and molar teeth that is directed toward the midline of the dental arch. Called also *mesial s. of premolar and molar teeth* and *facies anterior dentium premolarium et molarium.* **anterior s. of pyramidal part of temporal bone**, anterior s. of petrous part of temporal bone. **articular s.**, the surface of a tooth or a bone (*facies articularis ossium* [NA]) which is intended for articulation with another tooth or bone. Called also *facies articularis.* **articular s. of cricoid cartilage**, the surface of the cricoid cartilage that articulates with the thyroid cartilage. Also called *eminentia lateralis cartilaginis cricoideae* and *facies articularis thyroidea cartilaginis cricoideae* [NA]. **articular s. of mandibular fossa**, the articular surface found in the deep part of the mandibular fossa of the temporal bone. Called also *articular s. of temporal bone, facies articularis fossae mandibularis,* and *facies articularis ossis temporalis* [NA]. **articular s. of temporal bone**, articular s. of mandibular fossa. **axial s.**, any surface parallel with an axis; any surface of a tooth that is parallel in direction with the long axis of the tooth, including the labial, buccal, mesial, distal, lingual, and palatal surfaces. **balancing occlusal s.**, occlusal s., balancing. **basal s.**, that surface of a denture the detail of which is determined by the impression and which rests upon the supporting tissues of the mouth. Called also *foundation s.* and *impression s.* **buccal s.**, the vestibular (or oral) surface of posterior teeth, the premolars and molars, which faces the cheek. Called also *facies buccalis dentis.* See illustration. **cerebral s. of frontal bone**, internal s. of frontal bone. **cerebral s. of great wing**, the smooth, concave part of the great wing of the sphenoid bone that forms the anterior part of the floor of the middle cranial fossa, lying in front of the petrous and squamous parts of the temporal bone. Called also *facies cerebralis alae magnae* and *facies cerebralis alae majoris* [NA]. **cerebral s. of parietal bone**, internal s. of parietal bone. **cerebral s. of temporal squama**, the inner surface of the squamous part of the temporal bone, forming the lateral wall of the middle cranial fossa. Called also *facies cerebralis partis squamosae ossis temporalis* [NA] and *facies cerebralis squamae temporalis.* **contact s.**, contact AREA (2). **distal s.**, the proximal surface of a tooth facing away from a line drawn vertically through the center of the face, or the median line of the face. In incisor and canine teeth it is called the *lateral surface;* in molars and premolars, the *posterior surface.* Called also *facies distalis dentis* [NA]. Cf. *mesial s.* **dorsal s.**, 1. posterior s. (1). 2. dorsum (1). **external s. of eyelids**. anterior s. of eyelids. **external s. of frontal bone**, the external surface of the squama of the frontal bone. Called also *frontal s. of frontal bone, facies externa ossis frontalis* [NA], and *facies frontalis ossis frontalis.* **external s. of parietal bone**, a convex, smooth external surface of the parietal bone, marked by the parietal eminence, the temporal lines, and the parietal foramen. Called also *parietal s. of parietal bone, facies externa ossis parietalis* [NA], and *facies parietalis ossis parietalis.* **facial s.**, the surface of a tooth that is directed toward the face (or vestibule of the mouth), including the labial and buccal surfaces, and is opposite the lingual (or oral) surface. The term is used synonymously with *vestibular surface.* See illustration. **facial s. of maxilla**, anterior s. of maxilla. **foundation s.**, basal s. **frontal s. of frontal bone**, external s. of frontal bone. **implant-bearing s.**, a tissue surface upon which an implant rests, such as the surface of a bone selected to support a subperiosteal implant, and which is used to make an impression for the design and fabrication of the implant frame. **impression s.**, basal s. **incisal s.**, the cutting edges of the anterior teeth, the incisors and canines, which come into contact with those of the opposite teeth during the act of protrusive occlusion, in which they assume an edge to edge relationship. See also *occlusal s.* (1). **inferior s.**, that surface which is lower (directed away from the head, in man). Called also *facies inferior* and *undersurface.* **inferior s. of cerebellar** hemisphere, the surface formed by the inferior semilunar lobule, biventral lobule, tonsilla, and flocculus. Called also *facies inferior hemispherii cerebelli* [NA]. **inferior s. of cerebral hemisphere,** the part of the cerebral hemisphere that rests on the tentorium and in the anterior and middle cranial fossae. Called also *facies inferior hemispherii cerebri* [NA]. **inferior s., of cerebrum** the lower, or inferior, surface of the cerebrum. Called also *basis cerebri, basis encephali,* and *facies inferior cerebri* [NA]. **inferior s. of horizontal plate of palatine bone,** palatine s. of horizontal part of palatine bone. **inferior s. of petrous part of temporal bone, inferior s. of pyramid of temporal bone,** the rough and irregular surface that forms the base of the skull. Called also *facies inferior partis petrosae ossis temporalis* [NA] and *facies inferior pyramidis ossis temporalis.* **inferior s. of tongue,** the undersurface of the body of the tongue, which is covered by a simple undifferentiated mucosa. A vertical fold of mucous membrane in its midline (*frenulum linguae*) connects it to the floor of the mouth, and two fimbriated folds on each side run laterally and posteriorly. Called also *facies inferior ·linguae* [NA] and *undersurface of tongue.* **infratemporal s. of maxilla,** posterior s. of maxilla **internal s. of frontal bone,** the vertically situated, concave cerebral surface of the frontal bone; in its midline the sagittal sulcus is seen superiorly and the frontal crest inferiorly. Called also *cerebral s. of frontal bone, facies cerebralis ossis frontalis,* and *facies interna ossis frontalis* [NA]. **internal s. of parietal bone,** the cerebral surface of the parietal bone, presenting depressions corresponding to the cerebral convolutions, and furrows for branches of the middle meningeal vessels. Called also *cerebral s. of parietal bone, facies cerebralis ossis parietalis,* and *facies interna ossis parietalis* [NA]. **interproximal s.,** contact AREA (2). **labial s.,** the vestibular (or oral) surface of anterior teeth, the incisors and canines, which faces the lips. Called also *facies labialis dentis.* See illustration. **lateral s.,** 1. a surface nearer to or directed toward the side of the body. Called also *facies lateralis.* 2. the proximal surface of an incisor or canine tooth that is farthest from the midline of the dental arch. Called also *facies lateralis dentium incisivorum et caninorum* [NA]. See also *distal s.* **lateral s. of zygomatic bone, malar s. of zygomatic bone,** the anterolateral convex surface of the zygomatic bone, perforated by the zygomaticofacial foramen for the passage of the zygomaticofacial nerve and vessels, and giving origin to the zygomaticus major and levator labii superioris muscles. Called also *facies lateralis ossis zygomatici* [NA], and *facies malaris ossis zygomatici.* **lingual s.,** the surface of a tooth that is directed toward the tongue (or oral cavity), and is opposite the vestibular (or facial) surface. The term is used synonymously with *oral surface.* Called also *facies lingualis dentis* [NA]. See illustration. **masticatory s.,** occlusal s., working. **maxillary s. of great wing,** a small surface on the inferior part of the great wing of the sphenoid bone above the pterygoid processes; it is perforated by the foramen rotundum. Called also *sphenomaxillary s. of great wing, facies maxillaris alae majoris* [NA], and *facies sphenomaxillaris alae magnae.* **maxillary s. of perpendicular plate of palatine bone,** the surface of the perpendicular plate which is in relation to the maxilla; posteriorly and inferiorly it contains the greater palatine sulcus, which forms the greater palatine canal with a corresponding groove of the maxilla. Called also *facies maxillaris laminae perpendicularis ossis palatini* [NA] and *facies maxillaris partis perpendicularis ossis palatini.* **medial s.,** mesial s. **medial s. of cerebral hemispheres,** the surface of the cerebral hemisphere parallel to and facing both the median plane and the corresponding surface of the opposite hemisphere. Called also *facies medialis hemispherii cerebri* [NA]. **medial s. of cerebrum,** the surface of the cerebrum parallel to and facing the medial plane. Called also *facies medialis cerebri* [NA]. **medial s. of maxilla,** nasal s. of maxilla. **medial s. of perpendicular plate of palatine bone,** nasal s. of perpendicular plate of nasal bone. **mesial s.,** the proximal surface which faces toward a line drawn vertically through the center of the face, or the median line of the face, or toward the center of the dental arch. Called also *medial s.* and *facies mesialis dentis* [NA]. Cf. *distal s.* **mesial s. of premolar and molar teeth,** anterior s. of premolar and molar teeth. **morsal s's,** the occlusal surfaces of the mandibular and maxillary teeth which make contact in centric occlusion. **nasal s. of horizontal part of palatine bone,** the superior surface of the horizontal part of the palatine bone; it forms the posterior part of the floor of the nasal cavity. Called also *nasal s. of horizontal plate of palatine bone, superior s. of horizontal plate of palatine bone, facies laminae horizontalis ossis palatini* [NA], and *facies nasalis partis horizontalis ossis palatini.* **nasal s. of horizontal plate of palatine bone,** nasal s. of horizontal part of palatine bone. **nasal s. of maxilla,** the surface of the body of the maxilla that helps form the lateral wall of the nasal cavity. It is directed medially toward the nasal cavity and is bordered below by the superior surface of the palatine process and anteriorly by the sharp edge of the nasal notch. Above and anteriorly it is continuous with the medial surface of the frontal process. The lacrimal groove pierces the surface in the posterior area and converts into a canal by articulation with the lacrimal and inferior turbinate bones. The upper area behind the groove corresponds to the medial margin of the orbital surface, and the maxilla articulates here with the lacrimal bone, ethmoid bone, and orbital process of the palatine bone. A groove in its posterior border converts into the posterior palatine canal by articulation with the palatine bone. An opening into the maxillary sinus is situated in the posterosuperior part. The ridged edge anterior to the lacrimal groove articulates with the inferior turbinate bone; the inferior nasal meatus is situated below. The middle nasal meatus is located above the ridge, on the medial side of the nasal process. Called also *medial s. of maxilla* and *facies nasalis maxillae* [NA]. **nasal s. of perpendicular plate of palatine bone,** the medial surface of the perpendicular plate; it articulates with the middle and inferior nasal conchae. Called also *medial s. of perpendicular plate of palatine bone, facies nasalis laminae perpendicularis ossis palatini* [NA], and *facies nasalis partis perpendicularis ossis palatini.* **occlusal s.,** 1. the surface of the posterior natural or artificial teeth which come in contact with those of the opposite jaws during the act of occlusion. In natural teeth, it is restricted to the anatomic surfaces of the posterior teeth that are limited mesially and distally by the marginal ridges and buccally and lingually by the buccal and lingual boundaries of the cusp eminences. Sometimes, by extension, used to designate the incisal surface of the anterior teeth. Called also *facies masticatoria dentis* and *facies occlusalis dentis* [NA]. See also *incisal s.* and *occlusal s., working.* 2. the occluding surface of an occluding rim. **occlusal s., balancing,** the surfaces of the teeth or denture bases that make contact to provide balancing contacts. **occlusal s. of denture,** the surface of artificial teeth in a dental restoration that make contact or near contact with corresponding surfaces of the opposing teeth. **occlusal s., working,** the occlusal surfaces of the teeth, which are engaged in the masticatory activity. Called also *masticatory s.* **oral s.,** the surface of a tooth that is directed toward the surface of a tooth that faces the oral cavity (or tongue), and is opposite the vestibular (or facial) surface. The term is used synonymously with *lingual surface.* See illustration. **orbital s's of frontal bone,** the triangular plates of the frontal bone that form most of the roof of each orbit and the floor of the anterior cranial fossa; they are separated by the ethmoidal notch. Called also *facies orbitalis ossis frontalis* [NA]. **orbital s. of great wing of sphenoid bone,** the quadrilateral surface on the great wing of the sphenoid bone that forms the major part of the lateral wall of the orbit. Called also *facies orbitalis alae magnae, facies orbitalis alae majoris* [NA], and *orbital border of great wing of sphenoid bone.* **orbital s. of maxilla,** a triangular surface of the body of the maxilla that forms the greater part of the floor of the orbit. Its anterior edge corresponds to the infraorbital margin and becomes part of the nasal process; its posterior border coincides with the inferior boundary of the inferior orbital fissure. A notch on its thin medial edge forms the lacrimal groove. Behind the groove, it articulates with the lacrimal bone and, further on, with the thin portion of the ethmoid bone. Posteriorly, it articulates with the orbital process of the palatine bone. Its lateral area is continuous with the base of the zygomatic process. It is traversed by the infraorbital canal, its opening being situated below the infraorbital margin in the anterolateral area, and distally forms a groove. The canal transmits the vessels and nerves to the premolar, canine, and incisor teeth. Called also *superolateral s. of maxilla* and *facies orbitalis maxillae* [NA]. **orbital s. of zygomatic bone,** the part of the zygomatic bone which, together with the orbital surface of the maxilla and the great wing of the sphenoid bone, forms part of the floor and lateral wall of the orbit. It is perforated by two zygomatico-orbital foramina for transmission of the zygomatic branch of the trigeminal nerve and branches of the lacrimal artery. Called also *facies orbitalis ossis zygomatici* [NA]. **palatine s. of horizontal part of palatine bone,** the inferior surface of the horizontal part of the palatine bone; together with the corresponding surface of the opposite bone, it forms the posterior fourth of the hard palate. A ridge near its posterior margin gives attachment for the aponeurosis of the tensor veli palatini muscle. Called also *inferior s. of horizontal plate of palatine bone, facies palatina laminae horizontalis ossis palatini* [NA], and *facies palatina partis* *horizontalis ossis palatini.* **parietal s. of parietal bone,** external s. of parietal bone. **polished s., polished s. of denture,** that portion of the surface of a denture which extends in an occlusal direction from the border of the denture and includes the palatal surface. It is the part of the denture base which is usually polished, and it includes the buccal and lingual surfaces of the teeth. **posterior s.,** 1. a surface nearer or directed toward the back or the dorsal aspect of the body in man (called also *dorsal s., facies dorsalis* and *facies posterior),* or toward the tail in quadrupeds. 2. the surface of a premolar or molar tooth that is farthest from the midline of the dental arch. Called also *facies posterior dentium premolarium et molarium* [NA]. See also *distal s.* **posterior s. of maxilla,** the posterior convex surface of the body of the maxilla, bounded roughly by the inferior orbital fissure, zygomatic process and associated ridge, maxillary tuberosity, and posterior margin of the nasal surface. It is pierced by the apertures of two or more alveolar foramina; these canals are on a level with the lower border of the zygomatic process and are somewhat distal to the roots of the last molar. The lower part of this area is slightly more prominent where it overhangs the roots of the third molar and is called the *maxillary tuberosity.* A sharp, irregular margin situated medially to the tuberosity articulates with the palatine bone. Called also *infratemporal s. of maxilla* and *facies infratemporalis maxillae* [NA]. **posterior s. of petrous part of temporal bone, posterior s. of temporal pyramid,** the surface of the petrous bone that forms part of the anterior portion of the floor of the posterior cranial fossa. Called also *facies posterior partis petrosae ossis temporalis* [NA], and *facies posterior pyramidis ossis temporalis.* **proximal s., proximate s.,** 1. any surface that is nearer to a point of reference. 2. the surface of a tooth facing an adjoining tooth in the same dental arch. The proximal surface facing toward the median line is known as the *mesial surface;* the surface facing away from the median line is known as the *distal surface.* See also contact AREA. **smooth s.,** all surfaces of a tooth other than the occlusal surface, including the mesial, distal, labial, buccal, and lingual surfaces. See illustration. **sphenomaxillary s. of great wing,** maxillary s. of great wing. **subocclusal s.,** a portion of the surface of a tooth which is directed toward but does not make contact with the occlusal surface of its opposite number. **superior s. of horizontal plate of palatine bone,** palatine s. of horizontal part of palatine bone. **superolateral s. of maxilla,** orbital s. of maxilla. **temporal s. of frontal bone,** the slightly concave surface of the frontal bone that forms the upper part of the wall of the temporal fossa and gives attachment to the anterosuperior part of the temporalis muscle. Called also *facies temporalis ossis frontalis* [NA] and *semicircular plane of frontal bone.* **temporal s. of great wing,** the lateral and inferior surface of the great wing of the sphenoid bone, divided by the infratemporal crest into a superior part that forms a portion of

the wall of the temporal fossa, and an inferior part that forms part of the wall of the infratemporal fossa. Called also *facies temporalis alae magnae* and *facies temporalis alae majoris* [NA]. **temporal s. of temporal squama,** the external surface of the squamous part of the temporal bone, the anterior part of which forms a portion of the temporal fossa. Called also *facies temporalis partis squamosae* [NA], *facies temporalis squamosae temporalis,* and *semicircular plane of squama temporalis.* **temporal s. of zygomatic bone,** the internal, concave surface of the zygomatic bone, presenting a rough triangular area which articulates with the maxilla and, laterally, a smooth surface which faces the temporal and infratemporal fossae. It is pierced by the zygomaticotemporal foramen near the center to provide passage for the zygomaticotemporal nerve. Called also *facies temporalis ossis zygomatici* [NA]. **s. tension,** surface TENSION. **vestibular s.,** the surface of a tooth that is directed toward the vestibule of the mouth (or face), and including the labial and buccal surfaces, and is opposite the lingual (or oral) surface. The term is used synonymously with *facial surface.* Called also *facies facialis dentis* [NA alternative] and *facies vestibularis dentis* [NA]. See illustration. **working occlusal s.,** occlusal s., working.

surfactant (sur-fak'tant) any substance capable of reducing interfacial tension between two liquids or between a liquid and a solid, including detergents, wetting agents, and emulsifiers. Surfactants may be classified according to their polar portions because the nonpolar portion is usually made up of alkyl or aryl groups; the major polar groups being divided into anionic, cationic, amphoretic, and nonionic agents. Agents such as demulcents, emollients, protectives, absorbents, and absorbable hemostatics are considered in this category. Also having surface-active properties are astringents, irritants, sclerosing agents, caustics, keratolytics, antiseborrheics, melanizing and demelanizing agents, mucolytics, and certain enzymes. Some surfactants also possess antibacterial properties. Called also *surface-active agent* or *drug.* **amphoteric s.,** any surface-active agent having carboxylate or phosphate groups as the anion and amino or quaternary ammonium groups as the cation, the anion being represented by polypeptides, proteins, and the alkyl betaines, and the cations by phospholipids, such as the lecithins and cephalins. **anionic s.,** one containing substances such as carboxylate, sulfonate, and sulfate ions; those containing carboxylates are soaps. Some have antibacterial properties, acting chiefly against gram-positive organisms, and cause disruption of the lipoprotein structure of the cell membrane. Cationic and anionic surfactants neutralize each other when mixed. **cationic s.,** a surface-active substance containing long-chain cations, such as amine salts and quaternary ammonium compounds. Cationic surfactants have fungicidal and bactericidal properties, being most effective against gram-positive bacteria. They are absorbed into cell membranes in which their positively charged hydrophilic groups associate with the phosphate group of the membrane, resulting in cell lysis. Used chiefly in antimicrobiological preservation of pharmacological preparations; their surface-active use being limited. Cetylpyridinium chloride and benzalkonium chloride are the principal cationic surfactants. Cationic and anionic surfactants neutralize each other when mixed. **nonionic s.,** a class of surface-active agents that include a group of water-insoluble surfactants, including the long-chain fatty acids and their water-insoluble derivatives, and a group of water-soluble agents, consisting of polyoxyethylene compounds.

surgeon (ser'jun) [L. *chirurgio;* Fr. *chirurgien*] 1. a physician who specializes in surgery. 2. the senior medical officer of a military unit.

surgery (ser'jer-e) [L. *chirurgia,* from Gr. *cheir* hand + *ergon* work] 1. that branch of medicine which treats diseases, injuries, and deformities by manual or operative methods. 2. the work performed by a surgeon. **antiseptic s.,** surgery conducted in accordance with antiseptic principles. **aseptic s.,** surgery performed in an environment so free from microorganisms that significant infection or suppuration does not supervene. **clinical s.,** the study of surgical diseases by symptomatic analysis, examination, and observation. **conservative s.,** surgery in which only the lesion is removed and the integrity of surrounding tissues and organs is preserved as much as possible. Cf. *radical s.* **cosmetic s.,** that department of plastic surgery concerned with operations directed at improving the appearance by plastic restoration, correction, removal of blemishes, etc., except when required for prompt repair of accidental injury or for the improvement of the functioning of a malformed organ or part. In health insurance, the term does not apply to surgery in connection with severe burns, repair following a serious automobile accident, or surgery for therapeutic purposes which coincidentally serves some cosmetic purpose. **dental s.,** oral and

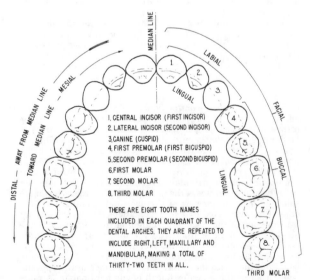

1. CENTRAL INCISOR (FIRST INCISOR)
2. LATERAL INCISOR (SECOND INCISOR)
3. CANINE (CUSPID)
4. FIRST PREMOLAR (FIRST BICUSPID)
5. SECOND PREMOLAR (SECOND BICUSPID)
6. FIRST MOLAR
7. SECOND MOLAR
8. THIRD MOLAR

THERE ARE EIGHT TOOTH NAMES INCLUDED IN EACH QUADRANT OF THE DENTAL ARCHES. THEY ARE REPEATED TO INCLUDE RIGHT, LEFT, MAXILLARY AND MANDIBULAR, MAKING A TOTAL OF THIRTY-TWO TEETH IN ALL.

Smooth tooth surfaces. NOTE: The terms *facial* and *lingual* are sometimes replaced with *vestibular* and *oral,* respectively. (From R. C. Wheeler: Dental Anatomy, Physiology and Occlusion. 5th ed. Philadelphia, W. B. Saunders Co., 1974.)

maxillofacial s. **dentofacial s.,** that branch of surgery dealing with the surgical and adjunctive treatment of diseases, injuries, and defects involving the face and structures of the mouth. **elective s.,** any surgical operation that is subject to the choice of the patient or the physician; one that does not require to be performed immediately or on an emergency basis, because a reasonable delay will not affect its outcome. **galvanic s.,** galvanosurgery. **general s.,** surgery dealing with surgical problems of all kinds. **local s.,** surgery in which only the lesion and area immediate to it are removed. See also *conservative s.* **major s.,** surgery involving the more important, difficult, and hazardous operations, a procedure that requires general anesthesia and involves an amputation of an extremity or includes entering one of the body cavities, such as the abdomen, thorax, or head. Cf. *minor s.* **maxillofacial s.,** oral and maxillofacial s. **minor s.,** surgery restricted to the management of minor problems and injuries, particularly procedures not requiring general anesthesia and not involving amputations or including entering one of the body cavities. Cf. *major s.* **mucogingival s.,** a plastic surgical method for the correction of gingiva-mucous membrane relationships. **operative s.,** the operative or mechanical aspects of surgery; that which deals with manual and manipulative methods or procedures. **oral s.,** oral and maxillofacial s. **oral and maxillofacial s.,** that branch of dental practice which deals with the diagnosis and the surgical and adjunctive treatment of diseases, injuries, and defects of the human mouth and dental structures. Formerly called *dental s.* and *oral s.* **orthognathic s.,** surgical treatment of structural abnormalities of the jaws and resulting facial disharmonies. **physiologic s.,** the indirect treatment of certain diseases by surgically altering normal physiologic functions. **plastic s.,** surgery concerned with the restoration, reconstruction, correction, or improvement in the shape and appearance of body structures that are defective, damaged, or misshapened by injury, disease, or growth and development. Called also *reconstructive s.* and *surgical reshaping.* See also *cosmetic s.* and PLASTY. **preprosthetic s.,** surgical correction of defects and anomalies that may potentially interfere with fitting or wearing of prostheses. **radical s.,** surgery in which the lesion and adjacent parts, as well as natural channels along which the lesion may spread to other organs, such as the lymphatics in cancer, are radically removed, sometimes involving entire organs. Cf. *conservative s.* **reconstructive s.,** plastic s.

surgical (ser′jĭ-kal) pertaining to surgery.

Surgicel trademark for *regenerated oxidized cellulose* (see under CELLULOSE).

Surgi-Cen trademark for *hexachlorophene.*

Surgident trademark for a *reversible hydrocolloid impression material* (see under MATERIAL).

Surital trademark for *thiamylal sodium* (see under THIAMYLAL).

Surofene a trademark for *hexachlorophene.*

survey (ser′va) 1. to inspect, examine, or appraise comprehensively. 2. the act of surveying. 3. a comprehensive or general view. **s. line,** survey LINE. **national health s.,** a continuous survey conducted by the National Center for Health Statistics of the Department of Health and Human Services, established to determine the extent of illness and disability of the population, monitor the use of health services, and gather related information.

surveying (ser-va′ing) 1. the act or process of inspecting, examining, or appraising something. 2. the determination of the exact form, boundaries, position, extent, and other pertinent data through the use of the principles of geometry. 3. the study of the relative parallelism of the teeth and associated structures in selecting the path of insertion for a restoration that will encounter the least tooth or tissue interference and that will provide adequate and balanced retention, and locating the guiding plane surfaces to guide placement and removal of the restoration. 4. the method of locating and delineating the contour and position of the abutment tooth and associated structures before designing a removable partial denture.

surveyor (ser-va′or) 1. one who surveys. 2. a device used to determine the exact form, boundaries, location, size, and other pertinent details of something. **dental s.,** a device for determining the relative parallelism of two or more surfaces of the teeth or other parts of the cast of a dental arch. It may be used for surveying the diagnostic cast, recontouring abutment teeth on the diagnostic cast, contouring wax patterns, measuring specific depth of undercut, surveying ceramic veneer crowns, placing the intracoronal retainers, placing internal rests, machining cast restorations, and surveying the blocking out of the master cast. A standard surveyor usually consists of a platform on which the base is moved; a vertical arm that supports the superstructure; a horizontal arm from which the surveying tool is suspended; a table to which the cast is attached; a base upon

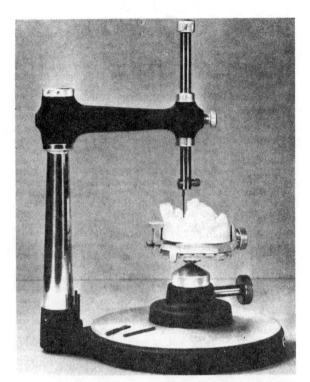

Ney surveyor. (From D. Henderson and V. L. Steffel: McCracken's Removable Partial Prosthodontics. 4th ed. St. Louis, The C. V. Mosby Co., 1977; courtesy of J. M. Ney Co., Hartford, Conn.)

which the table swivels; a paralleling tool or guideline marker; and a mandrel for holding special tools. See also PARALLELOMETER and survey LINE. See illustration. **Jelenko s.,** trademark for a dental surveyor which, in addition to standard components, also contains a spring mounted vertical arm that returns to the top position when released and a swiveling horizontal arm. **Ney s.,** trademark for a standard dental surveyor. **Williams s.,** trademark for a dental surveyor which, in addition to standard components, also contains a gimbal stage table that is adjustable to any desired position, a jointed horizontal arm, and a spring-supported survey rod, as well as a mechanism for locking all components into a desired fixed position.

susceptibility (sus-sep″tĭ-bil′ĭ-te) the state of being readily affected or acted upon.

suspension (sus-pen′shun) [L. *suspensio*] 1. a condition of temporary cessation, as of animation, of pain, or of any vital process. 2. treatment, chiefly of spinal disorders, by suspending the patient by the chin and the shoulders. 3. a liquid having solid or semisolid particles more or less uniformly dispersed through it, which may settle out on standing. Particles in a suspension are more than 100 μ in diameter, are visible to the naked eye, will not pass through filters, and move only by force of gravity. See also COLLOID (2) and SOLUTION.

suspensoid (sus-pen′soid) suspension colloid; see COLLOID (2).

Suteraloy trademark for an *amalgam alloy* (see under AMALGAM).

Sutter antigen (factor) [named after the person in whom antibodies to the Sutter factor (Js^a antigen) were first discovered] see Js^a ANTIGEN and see Kell blood groups, under BLOOD GROUP.

Sutton's disease [Richard L. *Sutton,* Kansas City physician] PERIADENITIS mucosa necrotica recurrens.

sutura (su-tu′rah), pl. *sutu′rae* [L. "a seam"] a type of fibrous joint in which the apposed bony surfaces are closely united by a very thin layer of fibrous connective tissue allowing no movement of united parts; found only in the skull. Called also *suture.* See also FISSURE, RAPHE, SYNCHONDROSIS, and SYNDESMOSIS. **s. corona′lis** [NA], coronal SUTURE. **s. cra′nii,** cranial SUTURE **s. denta′ta,** dentate SUTURE. **s. ethmoidomaxilla′ris** [NA], ethmoidomaxillary SUTURE. **s. fronta′lis** [NA], frontal SUTURE. **s. frontoethmoida′lis** [NA], frontoethmoidal SUTURE. **s. frontolacrima′lis** [NA], frontolacrimal SUTURE. **s. frontomaxilla′ris** [NA], frontomaxillary SUTURE. **s. frontonasa′lis** [NA], frontonasal SUTURE. **s. frontozygomat'ica** [NA], zygomaticofrontal SUTURE. **s. harmo'nia,** flat SUTURE. **s. incisi'va** [NA], incisive SUTURE. **s. infraorbita'lis** [NA], infraorbital SUTURE. **s. intermaxilla'ris** [NA], intermaxillary SUTURE. **s. internasa'lis** [NA], internasal SUTURE. **s. lacrimoconcha'lis** [NA], lacrimoconchal SUTURE. **s. lacrimomaxilla'ris** [NA], lacrimomaxillary SUTURE. **s. lambdoi'dea** [NA], lambdoid SUTURE. **s. limbo'sa,** a suture in which there is interlocking of the beveled surfaces of the bone. **s. nasofronta'lis,** frontonasal SUTURE. **s. nasomaxilla'ris** [NA], nasomaxillary SUTURE. **s. no'tha,** a false suture formed by apposition of the roughened surfaces of the two participating bones. **s. occipitomastoi'dea** [NA], occipitomastoid SUTURE. **s. palati'na media'na** [NA], palatine suture, median; see under SUTURE. **s. palati'na transver'sa** [NA], palatine suture, posterior; see under SUTURE. **s. palatoethmoida'lis** [NA], palatoethmoidal SUTURE. **s. palatomaxilla'ris** [NA], palatomaxillary SUTURE. **s. parietomastoi'dea** [NA], parietomastoid SUTURE. **s. pla'na** [NA], 1. flat SUTURE. 2. simple SUTURE. **s. sagitta'lis** [NA], sagittal SUTURE. **s. serra'ta** [NA], serrate SUTURE. **s. sphenoethmoida'lis** [NA], sphenoethmoidal SUTURE (1). **s. sphenofronta'lis** [NA], sphenofrontal SUTURE. **s. sphenomaxilla'ris** [NA], sphenomaxillary SUTURE. **s. sphenoorbita'lis,** spheno-orbital SUTURE. **s. sphenoparieta'lis** [NA], sphenoparietal SUTURE. **s. sphenosquamo'sa** [NA], sphenosquamosal SUTURE. **s. sphenozygomat'ica** [NA], sphenozygomatic SUTURE. **s. squamo'sa** [NA], squamous SUTURE. **s. squamo'sa cra'nii** [NA], squamous suture of cranium; see under SUTURE. **s. squamosomastoi'dea** [NA], squamosomastoid SUTURE. **s. ve'ra,** true SUTURE. **s. zygomaticofronta'lis,** zygomaticofrontal SUTURE. **s. zygomaticomaxilla'ris** [NA], zygomaticomaxillary SUTURE. **s. zygomaticotempora'lis,** zygomaticotemporal SUTURE.

suturae (su-tu're) [L.] plural of *sutura.*

sutural (su'tu-ral) pertaining to a suture.

suture (su'chur) [L. *sutura* a seam] 1. a type of fibrous joint in which the opposed surfaces are closely united, as in the skull. Called also *sutura.* See also FISSURE, RAPHE, SYNCHONDROSIS, and SYNDESMOSIS. 2. a material used in closing a surgical or accidental wound with stitches. Most commonly used suture materials include catgut, collagen, silk, cotton, metal wire, synthetic materials, and polyglycolic acid. 3. a stitch or series of stitches made to secure apposition of the edges of a surgical or an accidental wound; used also as a verb to indicate the application of such stitches. 4. the act or process of uniting a wound by stitches. **absorbable s.,** a strand of material used for closing wounds which is subsequently dissolved by the tissue fluids. **absorbable surgical s.,** a sterile strand prepared from collagen derived from healthy animals, available in various diameters and tensile strengths, which is capable of being absorbed by living mammalian tissue, but may be treated to modify resistance to absorption. It may be impregnated with a suitable antimicrobial agent, and may be colored by a color additive approved by the federal Food and Drug Administration. **anchor s.,** in periodontal surgery, a technique used to suture one papilla against the interalveolar bone when a flap has been elevated on only one side of the arch. **apposition s.,** a superficial suture used for the exact approximation of the cutaneous edges of a wound. Called also *coaptation s.* **approximation s.,** a deep suture for securing apposition of the deep tissues of a wound. **arcuate s.,** coronal s. **atraumatic s.,** one fused into the end of a small eyeless needle. **basilar s.,** spheno-occipital FISSURE. **bastard s.,** false s. **Bell's s.,** a form of lock-stitch suture in which the needle is passed from within outward alternately on the two edges of the wound. **biparietal s.,** sagittal s. **bolster s.,** one the ends of which are tied over a tiny roll of gauze, cotton, or piece of rubber tubing in order to lessen the pressure on the skin. **bregmomastoid s.,** parietomastoid s. **buried s.,** one placed deep in the tissues and concealed by the skin. **button s.,** one in which the stitch is passed through a button-like disk to prevent the suture material from cutting through the skin. **catgut s.,** an absorbable suture prepared from a strand of the submucosa of the proximal portion of the small intestine of sheep. See also CATGUT. **chain s.,** a continuous suture in which each loop of thread is caught by the next adjacent loop. **circular s.,** one applied to the entire circumference of a hollow viscus to secure closure. **coaptation s.,** apposition s. **cobblers' s.,** one made with suture material threaded through a needle at each end. **continuous s.,** one in which a continuous uninterrupted length of material is used to approximate the cut edges of one or more layers of tissues. Called also *uninterrupted s.* **continuous running s.,** one with a knot at only the beginning and end of a

sutured incision. **continuous sling s., type I,** a suturing technique used when there is a periodontal flap involving many teeth on one surface with another procedure, such as gingivectomy, on the other surface. See illustration. **continuous sling s., type II,** a suturing technique used when there is a periodontal flap involving many teeth on one surface with another procedure, such as gingivectomy, on the other surface. See illustration. **coronal s.,** a transverse line of junction between the frontal and the two parietal bones. Called also *arcuate s., frontoparietal s.,* and *sutura coronalis* [NA]. **cranial s.,** one of the sutures forming the lines of junction between the bones of the cranium, named generally for the specific components participating in their formation. Called also *s. of skull* and *sutura cranii.* **cutaneous s. of palate,** palatine RAPHE. **dentate s.,** a type of suture in which the participating bones are united by interlocking toothlike projecting processes, as in the suture between the parietal bones. Called also *s. dentata.* See also *serrate s.* **double-button s.,** a form of stitch in which the suture material is passed deep across the edges of the wound, between two buttons placed on the surface of the skin, one on either side of the suture line. **ethmoidomaxillary s.,** the line of junction between the orbital lamina of the ethmoid bone and the orbital surface of the maxilla. Called also *sutura ethmoidomaxillaris* [NA]. **everting s.,** a method by which the approximated edges of a wound are everted; used in early blood vessel surgery to achieve apposition. **everting interrupted s.,** an interrupted suture done by inserting the needle into the skin close to the incision line and diverging from the edge of the wound in order to encircle a larger amount of tissue in the lower depths of the skin than at the periphery. **false s.,** a line of junction between apposed surfaces, without fibrous union of bones. Called also *bastard s.* **figure-of-eight s.,** one in which the thread follows the contours of the figure 8. **flat s.,** a suture in which there is simple apposition of the contiguous surfaces, with no interlocking of the edges of the participating bones. Called also *sutura harmonia* and *sutura plana* [NA]. **frontal s.,** the vertical line of junction between the right and left halves of the frontal bone; it is usually transient and disappears after infancy, but the inferior part often persists into adult life. If the entire suture persists, it is called the *metopic suture.* Called also *sutura frontalis* [NA]. **frontoethmoidal s.,** the line of junction in the anterior cranial fossa between the frontal bone and the cribriform plate of the ethmoid bone. Called also *sutura frontoethmoidalis* [NA]. **frontolacrimal s.,** the line of junction between the upper edge of the lacrimal bone and the orbital part of the frontal bone. Called also *sutura frontolacrimalis* [NA]. **frontomalar s.,** zygomaticofrontal s. **frontomaxillary s.,** the line of junction between the frontal bone and the frontal process of the maxilla. Called also *sutura frontomaxillaris* [NA]. **frontonasal s.,** the line of junction between the frontal and the two nasal bones. Called also *nasofrontal s., sutura frontonasalis* [NA], and *sutura nasofrontalis.* **frontoparietal s.,** coronal s. **frontosphenoid s.,** sphenofrontal s. **frontozygomatic s.,** zygomaticofrontal s. **Halsted's s.,** a subcutaneous quilted suture with the strands passing back and forth through the corium. **harelip s.,** a figure-of-eight suture used in the correction of harelip. **hemostatic s.,** one used to control oozing of blood from raw areas or to control bleeding not readily controlled by clamping, tying, or coagulation. **incisive s.,** an indistinct suture sometimes seen extending laterally from the incisive fossa of the space between the canine tooth and the lateral incisor, indicating the line of fusion between the premaxilla and the maxilla. Called also *anterior palatine s., premaxillary s.,* and *sutura incisiva* [NA]. **infraorbital s.,** a suture sometimes seen extending from the infraorbital foramen to the infraorbital groove. Called also *transverse s. of Krause* and *sutura infraorbitalis* [NA]. **interdermal buried s.,** one with a knot placed downward in the lower layers of the dermis. **interendognathic s.,** palatine s., median. **intermaxillary s.,** the line of junction between the maxillary bones of either side, just below the anterior nasal spine. Called also *sutura intermaxillaris* [NA]. **internasal s.,** the line of junction between the two nasal bones. Called also *nasal s.* and *sutura internasalis* [NA]. **interparietal s.,** sagittal s. **interrupted s.,** a suture technique in which each stitch is made with a separate piece of material. **intradermal mattress s.,** mattress s., intradermal. **intradermic s.,** one applied parallel with the edges of the wound, but within the layers of the skin, usually a continuous stitch. **jugal s.,** sagittal s. **Krause's transverse s.,** infraorbital s. **lacrimoconchal s.,** the line of junction between the lacrimal bone and the inferior nasal concha. Called also *sutura lacrimoconchalis* [NA]. **lacrimoethmoidal s.,** the vertical line of junction on the medial wall of the orbit, between the lacrimal bone and the orbital plate of the ethmoid bone. **lacrimomaxillary s.,** a suture on the inner wall of the orbit, between the lacrimal bone and the maxilla. Called also *sutura* *lacrimomaxillaris* [NA]. **lambdoid s., lambdoidal s.,** the line of junction shaped like the Greek letter lambda, which connects the occipital and parietal bones. Called also *occipital s., occipitoparietal s., parieto-occipital s.,* and *sutura lambdoidea* [NA]. **Le Dentu's s.,** for a divided tendon; two stitches are passed on each side, right and left, and are tied in front; a third is taken from right to left above and below the cut, and is tied on one side. **Le Fort's s.,** for a divided tendon; a single loop is passed above the cut, entering at one side, coming out and going in front; it is then passed below the cut at each side, coming out in front, and is there tied. **longitudinal s.,** sagittal s. **longitudinal s. of palate,** palatine s., median. **malomaxillary s.,** zygomaticomaxillary s. **mamillary s.,** occipitomastoid s. **mastoid s.,** occipitomastoid s. **mattress s., horizontal,** a suture method in which the stitches are made parallel with the edges of the wound, the suture material crossing deeply from one side to the other. See illustration. **mattress s., intradermal,** a mattress suture below the level of the skin. **mattress s., right-angle,** mattress s., vertical (II). **mattress s., vertical,** a suture technique used when there is a periodontal flap on the facial surface and another procedure, such as gingivectomy, on the other. See illustration. **mattress s., vertical (II),** a suture method in which the stitches are made at right angles to the edges of the wound, taking both deep and superficial bites of tissue. Called also *right-angle mattress s.* See illustration. **metopic s.,** a name given to the frontal suture when it persists (metopism) in the adult skull. **nasal s.,** internasal s. **nasofrontal s.,** frontonasal s. **nasomaxillary s.,** the line of junction between the lateral edge of the nasal bone and the frontal process of the maxilla. Called also *sutura nasomaxillaris* [NA]. **nerve s.,** uniting a divided nerve by suturing; neurorrhaphy. **nonabsorbable s.,** material for closing wounds which is not absorbed in the body, e.g., silk, cotton, or nylon. **nonabsorbable surgical s.** [USP], a strand of material, either sterile or unsterilized, resistant to the action of living mammalian tissue, which is available in various diameters and tensile strengths. It may be modified with respect to body or texture, or to reduce capillarity, impregnated or coated with an actimicrobial agent, bleached, and colored with a color additive approved by the federal Food and Drug Administration. **occipital s.,** lambdoid s. **occipitomastoid s.,** the line of junction between the occipital bone and the posterior edge of the mastoid portion of the temporal bone, extending into the lambdoid suture. Called also *mamillary s., mastoid s.,* and *sutura occipitomastoidea* [NA]. **occipitoparietal s.,** lambdoid s. **occipitosphenoidal s.,** spheno-occipital FISSURE. **over-and-over s.,** a suture method in which equal bites of tissue are taken on each side of the wound; it may be either interrupted or continuous. **palatine s., anterior,** incisive s. **palatine s., median, palatine s., middle,** the line of junction between the horizontal part of the palatine bones of either side. Called also *interendognathic s., longitudinal s.,* and *sutura palatina mediana* [NA]. See also palatine RAPHE. **palatine s., posterior, palatine s., transverse,** the line of junction between the palatine processes of the maxillae and the horizontal parts of the palatine bone. Called also *sutura palatina transversa* [NA]. **palatoethmoidal s.,** the line of junction between the orbital process of the palatine bone and the orbital lamina of the ethmoid bone. Called also *sutura palatoethmoidalis* [NA]. **palatomaxillary s.,** the suture in the floor of the orbit, between the orbital process of the palatine

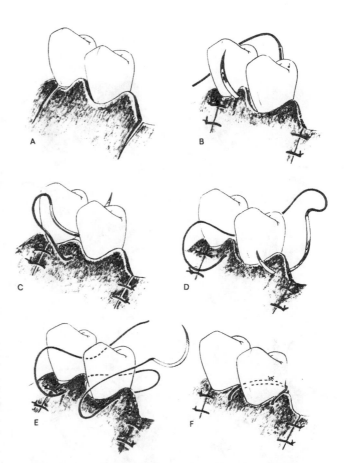

Sling suture. *A,* Tooth with flap on facial surface and gingivectomy on lingual. *B,* Vertical incisions are closed by simple, interrupted sutures. Needle is passed through interdental space from lingual to facial side and pierces flap from its inner aspect. *C,* Needle is returned over edge of flap through same interdental space to lingual side. *D,* Thread is looped around lingual surface of tooth, and needle is passed through adjoining interdental space from lingual side to pierce flap from its inner aspect. *E,* Needle is reversed through same interdental space to lingual side. (Dotted lines show thread on lingual surface.) *F,* Tie is made on lingual surface of tooth (shown in dotted lines). (From F. A. Carranza, Jr.: Glickman's Clinical Periodontology. 5th ed. Philadelphia, W. B. Saunders Co., 1979.)

bone and the orbital portion of the maxilla. Called also *sutura palatomaxillaris* [NA]. **parietal s.,** sagittal s. **parietomastoid s.,** the line of junction between the posterior inferior angle of the parietal bone and the mastoid process of the temporal lobe, merging with the squamosal suture. Called also *bregmomastoid s.* and *sutura parietomastoidea* [NA]. **parieto-occipital s.,** lambdoid s. **petrobasilar s., petrosphenobasilar s.,** petro-occipital SYNCHONDROSIS. **petrospheno-occipital s. of Gruber,** petro-occipital FISSURE. **plastic s.,** a suture method in which a tongue is cut in one lip of the wound and a groove in the other, the tongue and groove then being stitched together, and the ends of the thread tied over a roll of adhesive plaster. **premaxillary s.,** incisive s. **presection s.,** a stitch or a series of stitches placed in the tissues before an incision is made. **primary s.,** prompt surgical closure of a wound. **pterygopalatine s.,** a line of junction separating the lateral pterygoid plate of the sphenoid bone and the pyramidal process of the palatine bone. **quilt s., quilted s.,** a continuous mattress suture. **relaxation s.,** any suture placed to close a wound but so formed that it may be loosened in order to relieve the tension should it become too great. **rhabdoid s.,** sagittal s. **right-angle mattress s.,** mattress s., vertical (II). **sagittal s.,** the line of junction in the midline between the two parietal bones. Called also *biparietal s., interparietal s., jugal s., longitudinal s., parietal s., rhabdoid s.,* and *sutura sagittalis* [NA]. **scaly s.,** squamous s. **seroserous s.,** one which

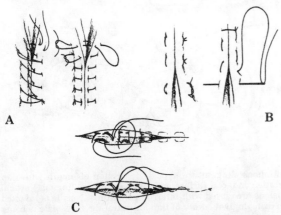

A, Vertical mattress suture (II). *B,* Horizontal mattress suture. *C,* subcuticular suture. (From Dorland's Illustrated Medical Dictionary. 26th ed. Philadelphia, W. B. Saunders Co., 1981; adapted from Nealon.)

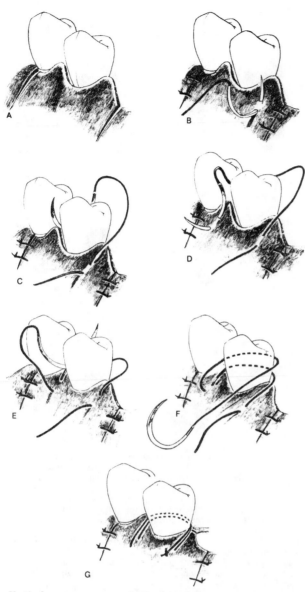

moidalis [NA]. 2. a craniometric landmark, being the most superior point of the sphenoethmoidal suture. Abbreviated *SE*. Called also *point SE*. **sphenofrontal s.,** the line of junction between the orbital part of the frontal bone and the greater and lesser wings of the sphenoid bone. Called also *frontosphenoid s.* and *sutura sphenofrontalis* [NA]. **sphenomaxillary s.,** a suture occasionally seen between the pterygoid process of the sphenoid bone and the maxilla. Called also *sutura sphenomaxillaris* [NA]. **spheno-occipital s.,** spheno-occipital FISSURE. **spheno-orbital s.,** the line of junction between the orbital process of the palatine bone and the body of the sphenoid bone. Called also *sutura spheno-orbitalis* [NA]. **sphenoparietal s.,** the line of junction between the great wing of the sphenoid bone and the parietal bone. Called also *sutura sphenoparietalis* [NA]. **sphenosquamosal s., sphenotemporal s.,** the line of junction between the great wing of the sphenoid bone and the squamous part of the temporal bone. Called also *squamososphenoid s.* and *sutura sphenosquamosa* [NA]. **sphenozygomatic s.,** the line of junction between the great wing of the sphenoid bone and the zygomatic bone. Called also *sutura sphenozygomatica* [NA]. **squamosomastoid s.,** the suture existing early in life between the squamous and mastoid portions of the temporal bone. Called also *sutura squamosomastoidea* [NA]. **squamosoparietal s.,** squamous s. of cranium. **squamososphenoid s.,** sphenosquamosal s. **squamous s.,** a suture formed by overlapping of the broad beveled edges of the participating bones. Called also *sutura squamosa, scaly suture,* and *sutura squamosa* [NA]. **squamous s. of cranium, temporal s.,** the line of junction between the squamous part of the temporal bone and

Vertical mattress suture. *A,* Tooth with facial flap and lingual gingivectomy. *B,* Vertical incisions are closed by simple, interrupted sutures. Mattress suture is started in flap by taking a vertical "bite" with needle. *C,* Needle is then passed through first interdental space, around lingual surface of tooth and through adjoining interdental space in the direction of facial surface. *D,* A vertical "bite" is taken with needle through external surface of flap. *E,* Needle is reversed through second interdental space. *F,* Thread is carried around lingual surface and needle is passed through first interdental space to emerge on facial side. (Dotted lines represent thread on lingual surface.) *G,* Tie is made on facial side. (From F. A. Carranza, Jr.: Glickman's Clinical Periodontology. 5th ed. Philadelphia, W. B. Saunders Co., 1979.)

apposes two serous surfaces. **serrate s.,** a type of suture in which the edges of participating bones are serrated like the teeth of a fine saw, as between the parts of the temporal bone. Called also *sutura serrata* [NA]. See also *dentate s.* **shotted s.,** one in which the two ends of the suture wire are passed through a split or perforated shot, which is then compressed. **simple s.,** one in which the borders of the bones are smooth or nearly smooth. Called also *sutura harmonia* and *sutura plana.* **s. of skull,** cranial s. **sling s.,** a suture technique used for a periodontal flap on one tooth surface, involving two interdental spaces. Called also *sling ligation.* See illustration. See also *continuous sling s. type I* and *type II.* **sphenoethmoidal s.,** 1. the line of junction between the body of the sphenoid bone and the orbital lamina of the ethmoid bone. Called also *sutura sphenoeth-*

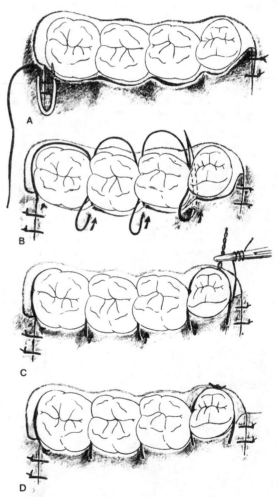

Continuous sling suture, type I. *A,* Section of mouth with flap operation on facial surface and gingivectomy on lingual. Vertical incisions are closed with interrupted sutures. Needle is inverted into distogingival corner of flap for initial tie. *B,* Needle is being returned to lingual side of interdental space, after penetrating flap from its outer aspect. *C,* Loose loop of thread left on the lingual surface of premolar is twisted and tied with other end of suture. *D,* Tie is made on the lingual surface of the premolar. (From F. A. Carranza, Jr.: Glickman's Clinical Periodontology, 5th ed. Philadelphia, W. B. Saunders Co., 1979.)

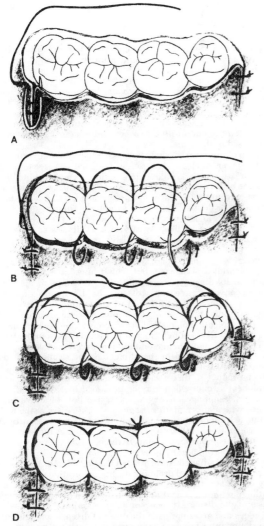

Continuous sling suture, type II. *A*, Section of mouth with flap on facial surface and gingivectomy on lingual. Two vertical incisions are closed with interrupted sutures. Needle has been passed from lingual surface to external surface of facial flap and through distogingival corner of it. One end of thread is left on lingual side. *B*, Thread passes around distal and lingual surfaces and needle is passed through interdental space to facial side. It engages facial flap from its outer aspect and is passed back through same interdental space to lingual. *C*, Suturing is completed on mesial aspect of second premolar and suture is tied with the end of the thread initially left on lingual side. *D*, Lingual tie is completed. (From F. A. Carranza, Jr.: Glickman's Clinical Periodontology. 5th ed. Philadelphia, W. B. Saunders Co., 1979.)

the parietal bone, arching posteriorly from the pterion, and merging posteriorly with the parietomastoid suture. Called also *squamosoparietal s.* and *sutura squamosa cranii* [NA]. **subcuticular s.**, a method of skin closure involving placement of stitches in the subcuticular tissues parallel with the line of the wound; it may be continuous or interrupted See illustration. **superficial s.**, one placed through the superficial fascia only. **temporomalar s., temporozygomatic s.**, zygomaticotemporal s. **transverse s. of Krause**, infraorbital s. **true s.**, a suture in which no movement of the participating bones can occur. Called also *sutura vera*. **uninterrupted s.**, continuous s. **zygomaticofrontal s.**, the line of junction between the zygomatic bone and the zygomatic process of the frontal bone. Called also *frontomalar s., frontozygomatic s., sutura frontozygomatica* [NA], and *sutura zygomaticofrontalis*. **zygomaticomaxillary s.**, the line of junction between the zygomatic bone and the maxilla and, secondarily, the zygomaticotemporal suture and the zygomatic arch. Called also *malomaxillary s.* and *sutura zygomaticomaxillaris* [NA]. **zygomaticotemporal s.**, the line of junction between the zygomatic process of the temporal bone and the temporal process of the zygomatic bone. Called also *temporomalar s., temporozygomatic s., sutura temporozygomatica* [NA], and *sutura zygomaticotemporalis*.

suxamethonium chloride (suk″sah-mě-tho′ne-um) SUCCINYLCHOLINE chloride.
Suximal trademark for *ethosuximide*.
Suzanne's gland [Jean Georges *Suzanne*, French physician, born 1859] see under GLAND.
Svedberg unit [Theodor *Svedberg*, Swedish chemist, born 1884] see under UNIT.
swage (swăj) 1. to shape metal by hammering or by adapting it to a die. 2. to fuse, as suture material to a needle. 3. a tool or form, often one of a pair, for shaping metal by pressure.
swager (swăj′er) a device or apparatus for swaging or shaping metal to a desired form by simultaneous use of pressures from various angles.
swallow (swahl′o) 1. the quantity of food swallowed at one time. 2. the act of swallowing or deglutition.
swallowing (swahl′o-wing) the process of deglutition. It begins with the swallow-preparatory position of the bolus within the mouth, followed by its passage from the mouth to the pharynx, passage through the pharynx, and passage through the hypopharyngeal sphincter. In the first voluntary phase, the chewed food or liquid is placed between the tongue and the anterior teeth and palate, the circumoral and tongue muscles being most active. This preliminary stage is followed by the bolus being propelled posteriorly by the tongue against the palate and into the pharynx and opening of the pharynx, while the hyoid bone is raised by the myohyoid muscles and the soft palate is elevated to allow the palatopharyngeal muscles to constrict so that the passage of the nasal cavity may be closed. While the tongue propels the bolus, the teeth are pressed together and the larynx is raised, with the glottis being closed to interrupt respiration. The bolus is forced over and around the epiglottis through the hypopharynx and into the esophagus. The process is accomplished in about 1 second. The center for swallowing is situated in the floor of the fourth ventricle. **empty s.**, swallowing without any food or liquid being present in the mouth. See also empty MOVEMENT. **infantile s.**, swallowing in infants, in which the facial and circumoral muscles initiate the swallowing and the jaw is braced against the tongue, the gum pads being held separated by the tongue, taking place prior to the establishment of occlusion. Called also *visceral s*. **reverse s.**, the infantile pattern of swallowing in which prior to deglutition the tongue is thrusted forward until it touches the back of the maxillary anterior teeth, or between the upper and lower anterior teeth, resulting sometimes in various orthodontic problems, such as open bite, a narrow maxillary dental arch, or flaring of the front teeth. See also tongue THRUSTING. **somatic s.**, swallowing taking place after eruption of the posterior teeth and the establishment of occlusion, in which the teeth are pressed together, while the tongue propels the bolus posteriorly against the palate and into the pharynx. Called also *teeth-together s*. **teeth-apart s.**, the infantile pattern of swallowing in which the tongue is thrusted between the teeth pushing against the tensed muscles of the lips and cheeks. See also tongue THRUSTING. **teeth-together s.**, somatic s. **traumatic s.**, a swallowing habit in which the tongue is pressed against either mandibular teeth, between the maxillary and mandibular arches, or the maxillary anterior teeth. The tongue collapses during the process and the face shows a grimacing expression. The pressure of the tongue may cause malocclusion in normal dentition or displacement of prostheses in denture-wearers. **visceral s.**, infantile s.
sweat (swet) the perspiration; the clear liquid secreted by the sweat glands (*glandulae sudoriferae*). It consists of about 99 percent water, with a specific gravity of about 1.003; its pH is usually acid, about 5.0 to 7.5. Sweat is a hypotonic solution containing sodium chloride, potassium, calcium, magnesium, and traces of copper, iron and manganese. Organic contents of sweat include chiefly urea nitrogen, lactates, and ammonia. It is sterile but becomes rapidly invaded by bacteria and decomposed after secretion, being especially evident in sweat produced by the apocrine glands, which contains much solid residue after drying and its decomposition results in its specific odor. **apocrine s.**, sweat produced by the apocrine glands in response to emotional stimuli, such as pain, fear, anger, or sexual stimulation. Called also *insensible s*. **eccrine s.**, sweat produced by the eccrine sweat glands, in response to an increase of surface body and blood temperature. Called also *sensible s*. **insensible s.**, apocrine s. **sensible s.**, eccrine s. **unilateral flush s.**, auriculotemporal SYNDROME.
sweating (swet′ing) the act of secreting sweat; perspiration. **gustatory s.**, auriculotemporal SYNDROME.
Sweet's syndrome [R. D. *Sweet*] see under SYNDROME.
sweetener (sweet′en-er) a substance having the taste or flavor characteristic of sugar. **artificial s.**, a substance other than

sugar (sucrose) for sweetening foods, beverages, dentifrices, and mouthwashes, usually, but not necessarily, having no or low caloric content. Some artificial sweeteners are used for dietetic purposes, as in diabetes mellitus or in weight reduction plans. Saccharin is the most commonly used artificial sweetener; other sweeteners include aspartame, mannitol, sorbitol, xylitol, glycerin, and cyclamates.

Sweet'n Low trademark for a noncaloric and nonnutritive artificial sweetener, containing 4 percent soluble saccharin, 94 percent lactose, and 2 percent cream of tartar.

swelling (swel′ing) 1. a transient abnormal enlargement or increase in the volume of a body part or area not caused by proliferation of cells. 2. an eminence, or elevation. **familial fibrous s. of jaws,** cherubism.

Swift's disease [W. *Swift,* Australian physician] acrodynia.

switch (swich) a mechanism or device for turning on or off or directing electric current or connecting or breaking a circuit. **dead man's s.,** dead man's CONTROL.

Sybraloy trademark for a *high copper alloy* (see under ALLOY).

sycosis (si-ko′sis) [Gr. *sykōsis,* from *sykon* fig] 1. a condition characterized by inflammation of the hair follicles. See FOLLICULITIS. 2. a kind of ulcer of the eyelid. **s. bar′bae,** 1. a form of deep folliculitis characterized by follicular pustules pierced by hairs, most commonly affecting the upper lip in men who do not shave. Neglect may lead to impetiginization and crust formation. Called also *barber's itch.* 2. incorrect name for *pseudofolliculitis barbae* (see under PSEUDOFOLLICULITIS).

Sylamid trademark for *salicylamide.*

sym- 1. a prefix indicating symmetry or symmetrical. 2. in organic chemistry, a prefix denoting the structure of a compound in which substituents are disposed symmetrically with respect to the carbon skeleton or to a functional group.

symbiont (sim′bi-ont, sim′be-ont) [Gr. *syn* together + *bioun* to live] an organism that lives in a state of symbiosis.

symbiosis (sim″bi-o′sis) [Gr. *symbiōsis*] the living together or close association of two dissimilar organisms, each of the organisms being known as a *symbiont.*

symbiotic (sim″bi-ot′ik) associated with symbiosis; living together.

symbol (sim′bul) [Gr. *symbolon,* from *symballein* to interpret] 1. a mark or character representing some quality or relation. 2. in chemistry, a letter or combination of letters representing an atom or a group of atoms.

Symmers, Douglas [American pathologist, 1879–1952] see giant follicle LYMPHOMA (Brill-Symmers disease). See also Brown-Symmers DISEASE.

symmetroscope (sĭ-met′ro-skōp) [*symmetry* + Gr. *skopein* to view, to examine] a device for determining right-left symmetry. **Gruenberg s.,** a plastic grid placed over a model, with its central axis overlaying the palatal midline, one transverse line contacting the distal surface of the first permanent molars; used for detecting asymmetry of the dental arch.

symmetry (sim′e-tre) [Gr. *symmetria,* from *syn* with + *metron* measure] the regular or reversed disposition of parts around a common axis, or on each side of any plane of the body. **cubic s.,** arrangement of structural units of the capsid in a virion in the form of the icosahedron (a three-dimensional structure composed of 20 identical sides). Called also *icosahedral s.* **helical s.,** arrangement of structural units of the capsid in a virion in the form of a helix. **icosahedral s.,** cubic s.

sympathetic (sim″pah-thet′ik) [Gr. sympathetikos] 1. pertaining to sympathy. 2. pertaining to the sympathetic nervous system; see under SYSTEM.

sympatholytic (sim″pah-tho-lit′ik) [*sympathetic* + Gr. *lytikos* dissolving] 1. opposing the effects of impulses conveyed by adrenergic postganglionic fibers of the sympathetic nervous system. 2. sympatholytic DRUG. Cf. ADRENOLYTIC.

sympathomimetic (sim″pah-tho-mi-met′ik) [*sympathetic* + Gr. *mimetikos* imitative] 1. mimicking the effects of impulses conveyed by adrenergic postganglionic fibers of the sympathetic nervous system. Called also *adrenomimetic.* 2. sympathomimetic DRUG. **indirectly acting s.,** a sympathomimetic drug which acts on norepinephrine stores in the postganglionic adrenergic nerve terminals.

sympathy (sim′pah-the) [Gr. *sympatheia*] 1. relationship between systems, organs, or parts not in close proximity to each other, shown when changes in one cause similar changes in another. 2. a relation between the mind and the body, causing the one to be affected by the other. 3. the influence exerted by one individual upon another.

symphyocephalus (sim″fe-o-sef′ah-lus) [Gr. *syn* together +

phyein to grow + *kephalē* head] a twin fetus joined at the head.

symphyseal (sim-fiz′e-al) pertaining to a symphysis.

symphyses (sim′fĭ-sēz) [Gr.] plural of *symphysis.*

symphysis (sim′fĭ-sis), pl. *sym′physes* [Gr. "a *growing together,*" "natural *junction*"] a site or line of union; used in anatomical nomenclature to designate a type of cartilaginous joint in which the apposed bony surfaces are firmly united by a plate of fibrocartilage. Called also *fibrocartilaginous joint.* **s. man-dib′ulae, s. men′ti,** the line of fusion of the lateral halves of the body of the mandible, showing a slight ridge at the median line, which splits inferiorly to form the mental protuberance. It shows the junction of the two parts of which the mandible is composed in the fetus.

symptom (simp′tum) [L. *symptoma;* Gr. *symptōma* anything that has befallen one] any functional evidence of disease or of a patient's condition; a change in a patient's condition indicative of some bodily or mental state. See also PHENOMENON, SIGN, and TEST. **cardinal s.,** 1. a symptom of greatest significance to the physician or dentist. 2. [pl.] the symptoms shown in the pulse, temperature, and respiration. **Castellani-Low s.,** a fine tremor of the tongue seen in sleeping sickness. **Colliver's s.,** a peculiar twitching, tremulous, or convulsive movement of the limbs, face, jaw, and sometimes of the entire body, seen in the preparalytic stage of poliomyelitis. **concomitant s.,** a symptom not essential to a disease, but which may have an accessory value in its diagnosis. **consecutive s.,** a symptom appearing during convalescence from a disease, but having no connection with the disease. **constitutional s.,** a symptom indicative of or due to disorder of the whole body. **datum s.,** the tracings on the gnathic projection plane that do not record condyle motions but are distant effects of movements and furnish data indicative of the positions, movements, and motion direction of points in the axes of the condyle of the mandible. **delayed s.,** one which does not appear for some time after the occurrence of the causes which produce it. **direct s.,** one caused directly by the disease. **equivocal s.,** one which may be produced by several different diseases. **esophagosalivary s.,** excessive flow of saliva in patients with cancer of the esophagus. **indirect s.,** one which points to a condition that may or may not be due to a particular disease or lesion. **localizing s.,** one that indicates the location of a lesion. **neighborhood s.,** one produced in an organ by disease in a neighboring organ, as by pressure of a tumor in one organ on an organ adjacent to it. **nostril s.,** dilatation of the nostrils during expiration and dropping during inspiration. **objective s.,** one obvious to the senses of the observer. **passive s.,** static s. **pathognomonic s.,** one that establishes with certainty the diagnosis of the disease. **precursor s., premonitory s.,** one which precedes and gives notice of the onset of disease. **presenting s.,** the symptom or group of symptoms of which the patient complains the most or from which he seeks relief; chief complaint. **reflex s.,** one occurring in a part remote from that which is affected by disease. **static s.,** a condition indicative of the state of some particular organ independent of the rest of the body. Called also *passive s.* **subjective s.,** one perceptible to the patient only. **sympathetic s.,** one due to sympathy, as when pain or other disorder affects a part when some other part is the seat of the disease proper. **withdrawal s.,** one which follows sudden abstinence from a drug to which a person has become addicted.

symptomatic (simp″to-mat′ik) pertaining to or of the nature of a symptom.

syn- [Gr. *syn* with, together] a prefix signifying union or association.

Synadrotabs trademark for *methyltestosterone.*

Synalar trademark for *fluocinolone acetonide* (see under FLUO-CINOLONE).

synalgia (sin-al′je-ah) pain experienced in one place as the result of a lesion in another. See also referred PAIN.

Synalgos trademark for an analgesic preparation, one capsule of which contains 194.4 mg aspirin, 162 mg phenacetin, 30 mg caffeine, and 6.25 mg promethazine hydrochloride.

Synalgos-D.C. trademark for an analgesic preparation, one capsule of which contains 194.4 mg aspirin, 162 mg phenacetin, 30 mg caffeine, 16 mg dihydrocodeine bitartrate, and 6.25 mg promethazine hydrochloride.

Synamol trademark for *fluocinolone acetonide* (see under FLUO-CINOLONE).

Synandrets trademark for *testosterone.*

Synapen trademark for *phenethicillin.*

synapse (sin′aps) [Gr. *synapsis* conjunction, connection] the juncture of two adjacent neurons, consisting of a terminal of the neuron, which conveys impulses toward the synapse (*presynaptic neuron*) and the body of the neuron, which conveys impulses away from the synapse (*postsynaptic neuron*), sepa-

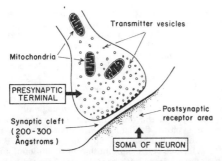

Transmitter vesicles

Mitochondria

PRESYNAPTIC TERMINAL

Synaptic cleft (200-300 Ångstroms)

Postsynaptic receptor area

SOMA OF NEURON

Physiologic anatomy of the synapse. (From A. C. Guyton: Textbook of Medical Physiology. 6th ed. Philadelphia, W. B. Saunders Co., 1981.)

rated from each other by a gap of about 200 Å (*synaptic cleft*). The transmitter substance (see under SUBSTANCE) is stored in vesicles in the presynaptic terminal and released into the cleft by the action potential of an incoming impulse and attaches to a receptor site where it depolarizes or hyperpolarizes the body of the postsynaptic neuron, thus conveying either an excitatory or inhibitory impulse through the synapse. The substance is destroyed immediately after completing its mission, more of it being produced in the knob of the presynaptic terminal. Synaptic function consists of exciting or inhibiting transmission of impulses from one neuron to one or more neurons. Called also *interneuronal junction* and *synaptic junction*. See also neurohumoral TRANSMISSION. See illustration.

synapsis (si-nap′sis) [Gr. "conjunction," "connection"] the pairing off in a point-for-point association of homologous chromosomes from the male and female pronuclei during the second stage (zygotene) of the first division of meiosis.

synaptic (si-nap′tik) pertaining to or affecting a synapse; pertaining to synapsis.

synarthroses (sin″ar-thro′sēz) [Gr.] plural of *synarthrosis*.

synarthrosis (sin″ar-thro′sis), pl. *synarthro′ses* [*syn-* + Gr. *arthrōsis* joint] see fibrous JOINT.

Synasteron trademark for *oxymetholone*.

Syncaine trademark for *procaine hydrochloride* (see under PROCAINE).

Syncelose trademark for *methylcellulose*.

synchondroses (sin″kon-dro′sēz) [Gr.] plural of *synchondrosis*.

synchondrosis (sin″kon-dro′sis), pl. *synchondro′ses* [Gr. *synchondrōsis* a growing into one cartilage] a cartilaginous joint that is usually temporary, the intervening hyaline cartilage ordinarily being converted into bone before adult life. See also FISSURE, SUTURA, SUTURE, and SYNDESMOSIS. **s. arycorniculа′ta**, the cartilaginous union between the upper end of the arytenoid cartilage and the base of the corniculate cartilage. **synchondroses of cranium, synchondro′ses cra′nii** [NA], the cartilaginous junctions between certain bones of the cranium. Called also *synchondroses of skull*. **intersphenoidal s., s. intersphenoiда′lis**, the cartilaginous union of the two halves of the body of the sphenoid bone in the fetus. **intraoccipital s., anterior, s. intraoccipita′lis ante′rior** [NA], the cartilaginous union of the pars basilaris with the partes laterales of the occipital bone in the newborn. **intraoccipital s., posterior, s. intraoccipita′lis poste′rior** [NA], the cartilaginous union of the squama with the partes laterales of the occipital bone in the newborn. **petro-occipital s., s. petrooccipita′lis** [NA], the plate of cartilage in the petro-occipital fissure which helps to unite the basilar portion of the occipital bone and the petrous portion of the temporal bone. Called also *petrobasilar suture* and *petrosphenobasilar suture.* **synchondroses of skull**, synchondroses of cranium. **sphenobasilar s.**, spheno-occipital s. (1). **spheno-occipital s., s. sphenooccipita′lis** [NA], 1. the cartilaginous plate which joins the anterior portion of the basilar part of the occipital bone with the posterior surface of the body of the sphenoid bone. It persists up to the 16th to 18th year of life and serves as a center of growth for the anteroposterior elongation of the base of the skull. Called also *sphenobasilar s., basilar fibrocartilage, fibrocartilago basilaris*, and *petrosphenoid ligament*. 2. in cephalography, the uppermost point of the spheno-occipital synchondrosis. Abbreviated *SO.* Called also *point SO.* **sphenopetrosal s., s. sphenopetro′sa** [NA], the cartilaginous union of the lower border of the great wing of the sphenoid bone with the petrous portion of the temporal bone in the sphenopetrosal fissure. Called also *anterior petrosphenoid ligament* and *petrosphenoid ligament*.

synchronous (sin′kro-nus) [*syn-* + Gr. *chronos* time] occurring at the same time.

Syncillin trademark for *phenethicillin.*

syncope (sin′ko-pe) [Gr. *synkopē*] a faint; a temporary loss of consciousness due to a sudden fall of blood pressure or failure of cardiac systole, resulting in cerebral ischemia, sometimes associated with brief muscle twitching. Serious consequences, such as respiratory failure and shock, may occur, particularly in patients with cardiac diseases, hypertension, or arteriosclerosis. It is one of the most common emergencies in a dental office. **laryngeal s.**, Charcot's VERTIGO. **tussive s.**, brief loss of consciousness associated with vigorous and explosive paroxysms of coughing, usually seen in men. Called also *laryngeal vertigo.*

Syncurine trademark for *decamethonium bromide* (see under DECAMETHONIUM).

syncytial (sin-sish′al) pertaining to syncytium.

syncytiotrophoblast (sin-sit″e-o-trof′o-blast) the outer syncytial layer of the trophoblast, which evolves through proliferative activity and differentiation of the trophoblast. It erodes the endometrium during implantation of the blastocyst within a few days after its formation, and blood from ruptured uterine vessels enters minute cavities (lacunae) within its substance, serving in the nutritive mechanism of the embryo. Called also *syncytial trophoblast* and *syntrophoblast*. See illustration at CLEAVAGE.

syncytium (sin-sish′e-um) [*syn-* + Gr. *kytos* hollow vessel] a multinucleate mass of protoplasm produced by the merging of cells.

syndactyly (sin-dak′ti-le) [*syn-* + Gr. *daktylos* finger] a congenital anomaly marked by webbing between adjacent fingers.

syndesmo- [Gr. *syndesmos* band, ligament] a combining form denoting relationship to connective tissue or particularly the ligaments.

syndesmosis (sin″des-mo′sis), pl. *syndesmo′ses* [*syndesmo-* + *-osis*] a fibrous junction in which the intervening fibrous tissue forms an interosseous membrane, such as one occurring in a fractured tooth. Called also *ligamentous joint*. See also SUTURE and SYNCHONDROSIS.

syndiotactic (sin″di-o-tak′tik) pertaining to a polymer in which the radicals alternate. Cf. ISOTACTIC and ATACTIC (2).

syndrome (sin′drōm) [Gr. *syndromē* concurrence] traditionally, a set of symptoms, usually three or more, which occur together; a group of signs and symptoms characteristic of a morbid condition. In current usage, the term is applied to any condition that cannot be easily defined and is characterized by complex etiology, involvement of several organs, and varied symptomatology. **Aarskog's s., Aarskog-Scott s.**, a hereditary syndrome, inherited as an X-linked recessive trait, consisting chiefly of short stature and craniofacial, acral, genital, and skeletal and orofacial abnormalities. The principal craniofacial anomalies are hypertelorism, antimongoloid palpebral fissures, blepharoptosis, broad nose, anteverted nostrils, dental hypoplasia, malocclusion, long philtrum, dimple inferior to the lower lip, and low-set malformed ears. Acral defects consist chiefly of small broad hands and/or feet, short fifth fingers, mild webbing between fingers, and joint restriction. Inguinal hernia is common. Called also *facial-digital-genital s.* **Aase's s.**, a familial syndrome of unknown etiology, charcterized by hypoplastic anemia, leukopenia, growth retardation, triphalangeal thumbs, mild radial hypoplasia, narrow shoulders, late closure of fontanelles, cardiovascular defects, and hepatosplenomegaly. Cleft lip, cleft palate, webbed neck, and retinopathy may be associated. X-linked inheritance has been suggested. **Abderhalden-Fanconi s.**, osteomalacia, renal glycosuria, aminoaciduria, phosphaturia, and cystine deposits throughout the body. It may begin at the age of 4 to 6 months with failure to grow, vomiting, fever, vitamin D–resistant rickets, acidosis, polyuria, and dehydration. In adults, it presents the same features, although cystine deposits may not be present. Dental symptoms are essentially those of vitamin D–resistant rickets (see under RICKETS). Classified as *Abderhalden-Kaufmann-Lignac syndrome* to designate cystine storage disease and as *Fanconi-De Toni-Debre syndrome* to designate rickets, or osteomalacia, with renal glycoaminophosphaturic diabetes. Called also *De Toni-Fanconi s., Fanconi's s., Lignac's s., Lignac-Fanconi s., cystine diathesis, cystine disease, cystine storage disease, cystinosis,* and *Lignac's disease*. **Abderhalden-Kaufmann-Lignac s.**, see *Abderhalden-Fanconi s.* **Achor-Smith s.**, nutritional deficiency with pernicious anemia, sprue, and pellagra, due to potassium depletion. Severe diarrhea, renal insufficiency, muscular degeneration, achlorhydria, hypochloremic alkalosis, and hypocalcemia are also present. **acro-osteolysis s.**, Hajdu-Cheney s. **acute mucocutaneous-ocular s.**, Fuchs′ s.

Adams-Stokes s., Adams-Stokes DISEASE. **adducted thumbs s.,** flexed, adducted position of the thumbs associated with a syndrome of arthrogryposis, demyelination, craniostenosis, and cleft palate; transmitted as an autosomal recessive trait. **adrenogenital s.,** congenital adrenal hyperplasia in females, resulting in faulty synthesis of adrenal cortical steroids with secondary progressive virilization, hirsutism, precocious puberty, pseudohermaphroditism, growth disorders, obesity, acne, and muscular hypertrophy. Premature eruption of the teeth may occur. It is probably transmitted as a simple autosomal recessive trait. Called also *suprarenal genital s.* **aglossia-adactylia s.,** a nonhereditary syndrome consisting of amelia affecting the upper or all four extremities and frequently associated with micrognathia and aglossia. Called also *Hanhart's s., hypoglossia-hypodactyly s., mandibular dysostosis,* and *peromelia.* **agyria-pachygyria s.,** a congenital syndrome of temporal pachygyria and frontal microgyria or agyria, associated chiefly with microcephaly, various facial abnormalities, feeding difficulty, hypotonia, seizures, abnormal electroencephalogram, and delayed psychomotor development. Called also *lissencephaly s.* **Alajouanine's s.,** symmetric lesions of the sixth and seventh cranial nerves with bilateral facial paralysis and bilateral lateral rectus eyeball palsy, associated with bilateral clubfoot. **Albright's s.,** 1. a combination of fibrous dysplasia of the bone, brown pigmentation of the skin, and endocrine disorders, chiefly precocious puberty in females. All bones may be affected, but the long bones are involved most frequently; bone lesions may be unilateral and there may be multiple fractures. Leontiasis ossium and facial asymmetry occur in some cases due to sclerosis of the base of the skull and facial bones. Distortion of the jaws and disorders in tooth development may be present. Pigmentation of the oral mucosa occurs rarely. Called also *Albright-McCune-Sternberg s., brown spot s., Fuller Albright's s., McCune-Albright s., osteitis fibrosa cystica disseminata, osteitis fibrosa disseminata,* and *osteodystrophia fibrosa.* 2. pseudopseudohypoparathyroidism. **Albright-Butler-Bloomberg s.,** vitamin D-resistant RICKETS. **Albright-McCune-Sternberg s.,** Albright s. (1). **Aldrich's s.,** Wiskott-Aldrich s. **alkalosis s.,** milk alkali s. **Allemann's s.,** double kidney and clubbed fingers, sometimes associated with facial asymmetry and degeneration of various motor nerves. **ambiguospinothalamic s.,** Avellis' s. **aminopterin s.,** fetal aminopterin s. **Andersen's s.,** a triad of cystic fibrosis of the pancreas, celiac disease, and vitamin A deficiency. Called also *Andersen's triad* and *pancreatic infantilism.* **Angelman's s.,** happy-puppet s. **angio-osteohypertrophy s.,** Klippel-Trenaunay-Weber s. **angle tumor s.,** Cushing's s. (2). **anihidrosis-hypotrichosis-anodontia s.,** hypohidrotic ectodermal DYSPLASIA. **anterior bulbar s.,** alternating hypoglossal HEMIPLEGIA. **antibody deficiency s.,** agammaglobulinemia. **Apert's s.,** oxycephaly associated with syndactyly (or polydactyly) of the hands and feet, and often with exstrophy, proptosis, ophthalmoplegia, and visual failure. Oral manifestations may include abnormalities of the hard and soft palates, such as high arched palate, occasionally with a marked median furrow. Posterior cleft palate, bifid uvula, hypoplastic maxilla combined with relative mandibular prognathism, and irregular positioning of teeth may also be present. Called also *acrodysplasia, acrocephalosyndactyly I, acrocraniodysphalangia,* and *ACSI.* **apex of petrous bone s.,** Gradenigo's s. **arachnodactyly s.,** congenital contractural ARACHNODACTYLY. **Arias' s.,** unconjugated hyperbilirubinemia with jaundice of the skin, sclerae, and mucous membranes, transmitted as an autosomal dominant trait with incomplete penetrance and varied expressivity. Signs of liver cell dysfunction and hemolysis are absent. **Ascher's s.,** a combination of blepharochalasis, double lip, and goiter. **Asherson's s.,** a syndrome of dysphagia due to neuromuscular incoordination and achalasia of the cricopharyngeal sphincter with failure of relaxation of the cricopharyngeal muscle during the third stage of swallowing. It causes diversion of liquids into the air passages, precipitating paroxysms of coughing. Called also *cricopharyngeal achalasia s.* **auriculotemporal s.,** sweating, flushing, and a feeling of warmth in the area of sensory distribution of the auriculotemporal nerve, following an injury, lesion, or surgery in the vicinity of the parotid gland, triggered by the eating of foods that produce strong salivary stimulation. Misdirected nerve fiber regeneration is considered the cause. Called also *Frey's s., gustatory sweating,* and *unilateral flush sweat.* **Avellis' s.,** unilateral paralysis of the larynx and soft palate, with loss of the pain and temperature senses on the contralateral side, including the extremities, trunk, and neck. It usually

results from lesions of the nucleus ambiguus and pyramidal tract, but bulbar lesions and mastoiditis have also been implicated. Paralysis of the soft palate produces dysphagia. In the original description, the vagus and glossopharyngeal nerves were involved; concomitant involvement of the neighboring cranial nerves was observed later. Called also *ambiguospinothalamic s.* and *superior laryngeal nerve s.* **Ayerza's s.,** a syndrome of slowly developing asthma, bronchitis, dyspnea, and cyanosis in association with polycythemia, sometimes associated with cardiac complications. Pathologically, there are primary changes in the pulmonary artery, which have been attributed to syphilis. Called also *cardiopathia nigra.* See also ERYTHROCYTOSIS. **Baader's s.,** Stevens-Johnson s. **Babinski-Nageotte s.,** lesions of the pontobulbar or medullobulbar transitional region associated with homolateral Bernard-Horner syndrome, nystagmus, and cerebellar hemiataxia, and with contralateral hemiparesis and disturbance of sensibility. Called also *dorsolateral oblongata s., hemibulbar s.,* and *medullary tegmental paralysis.* **Bäfverstedt's s.,** benign LYMPHADENOMATOSIS. **Bakwin-Eiger s.,** HYPEROSTOSIS corticalis deformans juvenilis. **Baller-Gerold s.,** a relatively rare syndrome combining craniosynostosis and radial aplasia, believed to be an autosomal recessive disorder. Symptoms may include turribrachycephaly, steep forehead, high nasal bridge, long philtrum, prominent mandible, epicanthic folds, ear dysplasia, radial hypoplasia, radial deviation, short ulna, missing carpal bones, fusion of the metopic suture, polymicrogyria, heart defects, and other abnormalities. **Bamatter's s.,** hereditary osteodysplastic GERODERMA. **Bannwarth's s.,** subacute lymphocytic meningitis associated with facial paralysis. **Barré-Liéou s.,** occipital headache, vertigo, tinnitus, vasomotor disorders, and facial spasm due to irritation of the sympathetic plexus around the vertebral artery in rheumatic diseases of the cervical spine. *Bärtschi-Rochain's syndrome* is a variant. Called also *posterior cervical sympathetic s., cervical migraine,* and *vertigo of cervical arthrosis.* **Bartenwerfer s.,** a condition believed to be a variant of Morquio's disease, characterized by disproportionate dwarfism, hypertelorism, high palate, mongoloid palpebral fissures, broad nose, flat vertebrae, lordoscoliosis, flat feet, hip dislocation, and epiphyseal and metaphyseal deformities. **Bärtschi-Rochain's s.,** a variant of Barré-Liéou syndrome, consisting of headache, paresthesia, scotoma, stiffness of the neck, pain on pressure of the cervical vertebrae, and vertigo due to traumatic cerebral artery compression. Called also *cervical vertigo s., cervicoencephalic s.,* and *cervical migraine.* **basal-cell nevus s.,** Gorlin's s. **Bassen-Kornzweig s.,** acanthocytosis. **battered babe s., battered child s.,** battered CHILD. **BD s.,** a congenital syndrome characterized by microbrachycephaly, mental retardation, prominent forehead, hypoplastic midface, mandibular prognathism, apparent midface cleft of the mandible with absence of the lower central incisors, ear and eye abnormalities, growth retardation, and secondary anomalies associated with hypotonia, cerebral palsy, and immobilization. Genetic transmission is unclarified. **Beckwith's s.,** Beckwith-Wiedemann s. **Beckwith-Wiedemann s.,** a congenital syndrome characterized chiefly by macroglossia which regresses over the years, omphalocele or other umbilical cord anomalies, enlarged kidneys, hepatomegaly, facial flame nevus which tends to fade during the first months or years of life, ear lobe anomalies, neonatal hypoglycemia which lasts 1 to 4 months and responds to steroid therapy, neonatal polycythemia, increased birth weight, and subnormal growth during the early months of life, followed by gigantism with increased bone age. Other findings may include mental retardation, muscle hypertrophy, microcephaly, prominent occiput, genital and limb abnormalities, diaphragmatic eventration, and ureteral defects. Hemihypertrophy sometimes develops, and there seems to be an increased risk of adrenal carcinoma, Wilms' tumor, or other intra-abdominal neoplasms. Histological findings may include renal medullary dysplasia, cytomegaly of fetal adrenal cortex, cystic changes in the adrenal cortex, pancreatic hyperplasia, paraganglial hyperplasia, and gonadal interstitial hyperplasia. Most cases are sporadic. Called also *Beckwith's s., EMG s., exomphalos-macroglossia-gigantism s.,* and *macroglossia-omphalocele s.* **Behçet's s.,** a disorder with an onset usually in the third decade, which consists of relapsing ulceration of the mucous membranes of the mouth and pharynx, ulceration of the genitalia, and uveitis with hypopyon. In the early stages, mild iritis or uveitis may be the only symptom, but thrombosis of the central retinal vein and thrombophlebitis of the dural sinus and of the thigh and calf veins are often associated. Oral lesions consist chiefly of aphthae of the lips, tongue, gingiva, buccal mucosa, or palate, which are discrete and usually mild. The blood picture usually shows moderate leukocytosis and increased sedimentation rate. It is chronic, but may become fatal when the nervous system becomes involved. A viral etiology has been suggested, but has not been established. Called also *cutaneomucouveal s.*, *Behçet's aphthae*, *Behçet's disease*, *Behçet's triple symptom complex*, *generalized aphthosis*, and *Touraine's aphthosis*. **Bekhterev-Strümpell-Marie s.**, a progressive chronic inflammatory disease of the joints, usually affecting young males, and characterized by symptoms similar to those seen in rheumatoid arthritis: bilateral swelling, tenderness, pain, and stiffening of the joints. It involves the posterior vertebral, costovertebral, and sacroiliac joints, associated with chronic proliferative changes in the joint capsules and intervertebral ligaments and ossification of the intervertebral disks and overlying ligaments. Bony ankylosis of all affected vertebral joints usually develops. Frequently, there also is involvement of the temporomandibular joint, which may result in ankylosis and cause malocclusion. Extra-articular lesions, such as aortitis and iridocyclitis, may be associated. Called also *ankylosing polyarthritis* and *ankylosing spondylitis*. **Benjamin's s.**, a combination of hypochromic anemia, hypoplastic bone deformities, growth retardation, and mental retardation. The symptoms include dental caries, proportionately small extremities, megalocephaly, and, less frequently, heart murmur, epicanthus, external ear deformities, genital infantilism, and splenic tumors. Called also *Benjamin's anemia*. **Berant's s.**, a syndrome consisting of craniosynostosis of the sagittal suture and radioulnar synostosis, probably transmitted as an autosomal dominant trait. **Bergen s.**, 1. skeletal changes of the face in leprosy, characterized by atrophy of the anterior nasal spine and atrophy and recession of the alveolar process of the maxillae confined to the incisor region. It was originally described in seven leprosy patients in Bergen, Norway. Called also *facies leprosa*. 2. leprogenic changes of the alveolar process of the maxilla with loosening and/or loss of the frontal incisors. **Berlin's s.**, a familial multiple abnormality characterized by short stature bordering on dwarfism; slender build; hyperflexibility of the fingers; sparse eyebrows; small moustache; dark, dry, and abundant hair with a tendency to premature graying; epicanthal folds; saddle nose; thick lips with telangiectases; pale, dry, thin, pliable skin; generalized mottled dyschromia; atrophic scars caused by pyoderma; hyperkeratosis palmaris et plantaris with hyperhidrosis; hyperfunction of the sebaceous glands; delayed dentition; hypodontia; genital infantilism, hypospadias, and testicular atrophy in males, but normal genital development in females; and mental retardation. Pituitary dysfunction is suspected as a probable cause. **Bernard's s.**, acute familial HEMOLYSIS. **Bernard-Horner s.**, a syndrome in which interruption of the sympathetic pathways produces ophthalmoplegia, miosis, ptosis, relative ocular hypotonia, apparent enophthalmos and ipsilateral facial cutaneous hyperemia, anhidrosis, and vasodilatation. It may be produced by lesions, including trauma, neoplasms, thrombosis, substernal thyroid, and syphilitic aneurysm of the brachiocephalic trunk, situated anywhere along the sympathetic pathways, from the hypothalamus to the sympathetic fibers innervating the facial sweat glands. When associated with heterochromia iridis it is known as *Passow's syndrome*, and when associated with trigeminal neuralgia and vasomotor disorders in the area supplied by the trigeminal nerve as *trigeminal nonsympathetic neuralgia. Paratrigeminal syndrome* is an incomplete form of this disorder. See also *Opalski's s.*, *Villaret's s.*, and *Wallenberg's s.* Called also *Claude Bernard's s.*, *Horner's s.*, *oculosympathetic s.*, and *sympathetic ophthalmoplegia*. **Besnier-Boeck-Schaumann s.**, sarcoidosis. **Beuren's s.**, elfin facies s. **Binder's s.**, a syndrome of hypoplasia of the maxillary and nasal bones. Flattening of the nasal spine, apparent elongation of the nose, absence of the angle between the frontal bone and nasal spine, small alae and openings with characteristic semilunar shape, and recession of perinasal structures are the principal nasal anomalies. Maxillary hypoplasia is associated with narrowing of the upper dental arch, gothic palate, and malocclusion. Called also *maxillonasal s.* and *maxillonasal dysostosis*. **Blegvad-Haxthausen s.**, the association of Lobstein's syndrome with atrophy of the skin and zonular cataract. **Bloch-Sulzberger s.**, a congenital ectodermal and mesodermal defect occurring almost exclusively in females. Inheritance is X-linked dominant and lethal in males. The syndrome consists of lesions of the skin, eyes, nails, teeth, and central nervous system; it is considered to be the end-phase of Asboe-Hansen's disease. Patches of vesicles may be present at birth, but they are replaced by a crop of violaceous papules and inflammatory lesions. The inflammatory phase may pass directly to the pigmented stage, or it may blend into a warty or papillomatous phase with subsequent development of pigmented macules. Pigmented areas have a strikingly bizarre configuration in flecks, whorls, spider forms, lines, and patches, which do not follow the lines of cleavage or distribution of nerves or

blood vessels. Chocolate-brown, gray-brown, or slate-colored macules may persist unchanged or may fade, leaving normal depigmented skin. The hair is thin, alopecia of the scalp is frequent, and the nails may be dystrophic. Eye abnormalities usually include strabismus, cataract, optic atrophy, myopia, blue sclera, nystagmus, and microphthalmia. Dental anomalies consist of delayed tooth eruption, pegged or conical crowns, and missing and malformed teeth. The central nervous system complications consist of mental retardation, microcephaly, hydrocephalus, spastic paralysis, and epilepsy. Retarded growth, hearing disorders, hemivertebrae, syndactyly, patent ductus arteriosus, supernumerary ribs and nipples, unilateral breast aplasia, and urachal cysts may also be associated. It is similar to Naegeli's syndrome, except that Naegeli's syndrome occurs in both sexes, does not include an inflammatory phase, and has hypohidrosis and keratosis palmaris et plantaris as features. Called also *incontinentia pigmenti* and *nevus pigmentosus systematicus*. **Bloom's s.**, **Bloom-Torre-Machacek s.**, a hereditary syndrome, transmitted as an autosomal recessive trait, in which telangiectatic erythema of the face, sensitivity to sunlight, and dwarfism are the cardinal features. The eruption appears as erythematous telangiectatic spots, plaques, or patches, or as scattered macular lesions; sun exposure usually causes exacerbation. The birth weight is low, and slow growth becomes evident early. Associated defects may include lichen pilaris, hypertrichosis, café au lait spots, ichthyosis, acanthosis nigricans, pilonidal cysts, syndactyly, absence of a toe, clinodactyly, short lower extremities, pes equinus, absence of upper incisors, prominent ears, hypospadias, and cryptorchidism. **blue sclera s.**, Lobstein's s. **bobble-head doll s.**, a syndrome of rapid flexion-extension of the head and neck on the trunk, associated with third ventricular dilatation from a cyst or hydrocephalus, being strikingly similar to the nodding of a bobble-head doll. Some cases may be associated with stenosis of the ventricular aqueduct. **Bogorad's s.**, gustatory LACRIMATION. **Bonnet's s.**, trigeminal nonsympathetic NEURALGIA. **Bonnevie-Ullrich s.**, an apparently congenital syndrome consisting of pterygium colli, lymphedema of the hands and feet, hypoplasia of the bones and muscles, short stature, syndactyly, skin laxity, nail dystrophy, and cranial nerve disorders. When associated with Klippel-Feil syndrome, the disorder is known as *Nielsen's syndrome*. Considered by some authorities not as a separate entity, but as either *Turner's syndrome* or *Noonan's syndrome*. Called also *pterygolymphangiectasis s.* **Bonnier's s.**, lesions of Deiters' nucleus or vestibular apparatus associated with vertigo, pallor, somnolence, tachycardia, trigeminal neuralgia, locomotor weakness, and a sense of apprehension. Called also *Deiters' nucleus s.* **Böök's s.**, a rare hereditary syndrome, transmitted as an autosomal dominant trait, which consists of premolar aplasia, hyperhidrosis, and canities prematura. Called also *PHC s.* **Boyd-Stearns s.**, rickets beginning during infancy, dwarfism, hypophosphatemia resistant to the usual antirachitic therapy, osteoporosis, and malnutrition, associated with various metabolic disorders, including glycosuria, acidosis, hypochloremia, albuminuria, and hypochloremia. Polyuria and polydipsia, with urine of normal specific gravity, and kidney lesions may be present. **Brachmann-de Lange s.**, de Lange's s. **brachydactyly-spherophakia s.**, Marchesani's s. **Brailsford-Morquio s.**, Morquio's DISEASE. **brain death s.**, irreversible COMA. **branchial arch s.**, first and second branchial arch s. **branchioskeletogenital s.**, a hereditary syndrome consisting of abnormalities of the craniofacial structures, eyes, palate, skeletal system, and genitalia. Its principal features include mental deficiency, broad and flat nasal bones with flared alar cartilages, brachycephalic skull, pectus excavatum, fusion of the spinous processes, hypospadias, hypertelorism, strabismus, blepharoptosis, nystagmus, multiple dentigerous cysts, bifid uvulae with high arched palate, maxillary hypoplasia with relative mandibular prognathism, malocclusion, dental caries, cleft palate, and soft tissue sacs covering some teeth. **Brandt's s.**, ACRODERMATITIS enteropathica. **Brissaud-Marie s.**, hysterical glossolabial HEMISPASM. **Brissaud-Sicard s.**, facial hemispasm associated with contralateral paralysis of the extremities, due to lesions of the pons. **Brocq-Pautrier s.**, median rhomboid GLOSSITIS. **Brown's s.**, a syndrome of congenital analgesia with anhidrosis, characterized by loss of deep and/or superficial pain sensibility; autonomic dysfunction manifested by pupillary abnormalities, neurogenic anhidrosis with otherwise normal sweat glands, and vasomotor instability; aplasia of the dental enamel; meningeal thickening and cystic changes; mild mental retardation; hyporeflexia; blond hair; blue or blue-green eyes;

and fair complexion. An abnormality in the differentiation of the neural crest has been suggested as a cause. Called also *s. of neural crest*. **brown spot s.**, Albright's syndrome (1). **Bürger-Grütz s.**, HYPERLIPOPROTEINEMIA I. **Burnett's s.**, milk alkali s. **Butler-Albright s.**, **Butler-Lightwood-Albright s.**, Lightwood-Albright s. **C s.**, Opitz's trigonocephaly s. **Caffey's s.**, infantile cortical HYPEROSTOSIS. **Caffey-Kempe s.**, battered CHILD. **Caffey-Silverman s.**, **Caffey-Smyth s.**, infantile cortical HYPEROSTOSIS. **campomelic s.**, **campomelique s.**, any of a group of congenital syndromes characterized by bowing of the tibiae; hypoplasia of the vertebral bodies, scapulae, and pelvis; dislocation of the hips, knees, and elbows; short-limb dwarfism; pes equinovarus; pretibial skin dimpling; macrocephaly; prominent forehead with flat face; hypertelorism; micrognathia; cleft palate; laryngotracheal malacia; hydronephrosis; polyhydramnios; hypotonia; and birth weight of less than 6 pounds. Most infants die before the age of 6 months, usually of respiratory disorders. Called also *campomelic dwarfism*. **camptodactyly-muscular hypoplasia-skeletal dysplasia-abnormal palmar creases s.**, Tel Hashomer camptodactyly s. **Camurati-Engelmann s.**, progressive diaphyseal DYSPLASIA. **Capdepont s.**, **Capdepont-Hodge s.**, DENTINOGENESIS imperfecta. **cardioacrofascial s.**, a hereditary syndrome, probably transmitted as an autosomal dominant trait, combining ventricular septal defect and pulmonary stenosis, narrow face with micrognathia, high and narrow nose with a prominent septum, microstomia, earlobes attached to the side of the neck, and minor malformations of the hands and feet. Dolichocephaly, slight mongoloid palpebral fissures, high palate, mandibular prognathism, slender stature, prominent sacrum, and thoracic kyphosis are usually associated. Called also *Rabenhorst s.* **cardiofacial s.**, a syndrome of unilateral facial weakness which may be associated with heart defects. The face appears asymmetric at rest, the mouth being pulled downward to one side when crying (asymmetric crying facies) owing to unilateral partial weakness involving the lip depressor muscle. Cardiovascular abnormalities may include a wide variety of defects, such as patent ductus arteriosus, pulmonary stenosis, or atrial, ventricular, or septal defects. Various abnormalities of the central nervous system, bones, gastrointestinal system, and other organs and systems may be associated. Called also *Cayler's s.* **cardiovocal s.**, Ortner's s. **carotid sinus s.**, a condition resulting from stimulation or pressure applied to the carotid sinus, which causes reflex slowing of the heart rate, vasodilation, and hypotension (carotid sinus reflex). It is associated with the wearing of a tight collar, sudden turning of the head, or manual compression of the neck, presenting as transient attacks of numbness or weakness of the face, arm, or leg, headache, and aphasia, and is sometimes associated with syncope, confusion, and loss of vision. **carpal tunnel s.**, a symptom complex resulting from compression of the median nerve in the carpal tunnel, occurring most commonly in middle-aged women, which is usually precipitated by trauma, rheumatoid arthritis, myxedema, or pregnancy. Symptoms include hypoesthesia, paresthesia, synovitis of the flexor synovialis, and weakness of the thumb. **Carpenter's s.**, an autosomal recessive syndrome consisting principally of an association of craniosynostosis, polysyndactyly of the feet, and short fingers with variable soft tissue syndactyly. The sagittal and lambdoidal sutures are usually involved in the craniosynostosis, with unilateral involvement resulting in cranial asymmetry. Wormian bones may be found. Flat nasal bridge, dystrophia canthorum, microcornea, corneal opacity, epicanthal folds, optic atrophy, blurring of disk margins, low-set ears, short neck, narrow and arched palate, small mandible, and preauricular fistulae may be associated. Clinodactyly, single flexion crease, brachymesophalangy, genua valga, patellar displacement, and other skeletal abnormalities may occur. Growth is retarded, but body weight is increased in most cases; obesity usually involves the trunk, face, neck, and limbs. Congenital heart defects, hydronephrosis, inguinal hernia, and other anomalies may be associated. Mental deficiency is observed in most cases. Called also *acrocephalopolydactylous dysplasia*, *acrocephalopolydactyly*, and *acrocephalopolysyndactyly type II.* **cat-eye s.**, a syndrome due to partial trisomy of chromosome 22. It is characterized by growth and mental deficiency; peculiar facies with coloboma of the iris, hypertelorism, slightly downward slant of palpebral fissures, epicanthic folds, preauricular fistulae, and skin tags; and anal atresia. Microphthalmos, low-set malformed ears, heart defects, hip dislocation, and unilateral kidney aplasia may be associated. **cavernous sinus s.**, ophthalmoplegia and paralysis of the third, fourth, fifth, and

sixth cranial nerves, with bulging of the globe of the eye and proptosis and edema of the eyelids, secondary to lesions of the cavernous sinus. Trigeminal neuralgia may be associated. Called also *Foix's s.* **Cayler's s.**, cardiofacial s. **CCA s.**, congenital contractural ARACHNODACTYLY. **CCM s.**, cerebrocostomandibular s. **s. of cerebellopontile angle**, Cushing's s. (2). **cerebrocostomandibular s.**, a hereditary developmental disorder, transmitted as an autosomal recessive trait, characterized chiefly by costovertebral abnormalities, mental deficiency, and orofacial anomalies, chiefly micrognathia, glossoptosis, palatal defects and dysfunction, and mandibulofacial anomalies. Costovertebral defects may involve segmentation of the ribs and fusion of their dorsal ends to the vertebral bodies. Microcephaly and delayed myelination are the principal neurological components. Called also *CCM s.* **cerebrofaciothoracic s.**, a congenital syndrome consisting of mental retardation; brachycephaly; typical facies, characterized by narrow forehead, bushy eyebrows with synophrys, hypertelorism, broad nose, wide philtrum, maxillary hypoplasia, triangular mouth, short neck, and low hairline; calcified clinoid processes, and multiple bony abnormalities in the upper thoracic vertebrae and sometimes in the cervical region, together with a variety of deformities of the upper ribs. Autosomal recessive transmission is suspected. Called also *cerebrofaciothoracic dysplasia*. **cerebrohepatorenal s.**, a congenital syndrome, transmitted as an autosomal recessive trait, consisting of flat facies, high forehead with shallow supraorbital ridges, inner epicanthic folds, and mild upslanting of the palpebral fissures; liver abnormalities, especially hepatomegaly with cirrhotic changes; albuminuria; renal cysts; cardiac defects, consisting of patent ductus arteriosus and, sometimes, septal defects; brain abnormalities, usually macrogyria and polymicrogyria, and faulty myelinization and sudanophilic leukodystrophy; delayed growth; and hypotonia. A variety of cranial, ocular, and systemic abnormalities may be associated. Excess iron storage has been observed in some cases. Called also *Zellweger's s.* **cerebro-oculofacioskeletal s.**, an autosomal recessive syndrome of craniofacial abnormalities, consisting of relative microcephaly and sloping forehead, high nasal bridge, prominent bony ridge of the nose, large ears, upper lip overhanging the lower, and micrognathia or retrognathia, short neck; and skeletal defects, consisting chiefly of kyphosis and/or scoliosis, hip dislocation, coxa valga, camptodactyly, and flexion contractures. It is usually associated with hypotonia, failure to thrive, osteoporosis, renal abnormalities, oligohydramnios, and wide-set nipples. Called also *COFS s.* **cervical vertigo s.**, **cervicoencephalic s.**, Bärtschi-Rochain's s. **cervicolinguomasticatory s.**, Kulenkampff-Tarnow s. **cervico-oculoacusticus s.**, cervico-oculofacial s. **cervico-oculofacial s.**, a hereditary syndrome characterized by deaf-mutism, retractio bulbi, defective implantation of the hair and teeth, and facial hypoplasia. Subconjunctival neoplasms, status dysraphicus, and facial and cranial asymmetry may occur. Called also *cervico-oculoacusticus s.* and *Wildervanck's s.* **Céstan-Chenais s.**, a variant of *Babinski-Nageotte syndrome* and *Avellis' syndrome*, consisting of unilateral paralysis of the soft palate and vocal cords, ipsilateral ocular signs and contralateral hemiplegia, sensory disorders, and ataxia. It is caused by thrombosis of the vertebral artery at the point of origin of the posterior inferior cerebellar artery. Called also *Céstan's paralysis*. **Chapple's s.**, a syndrome seen in the newborn, consisting of unilateral facial weakness or paralysis associated with a comparable weakness or paralysis of the vocal cord and/or the muscles of deglutition (parts innervated by the recurrent or superior laryngeal nerve) on the opposite side. It is caused by lateral flexion of the head *in utero*, which holds the thyroid cartilage against the hyoid bone or cricoid cartilages with consequent pressure on the laryngeal nerve or its blood supply. **Charcot's s.**, amyotrophic lateral SCLEROSIS. **Charlin's s.**, ciliary NEURALGIA. **Chédiak-Higashi s.**, a hereditary syndrome occurring in infants, characterized by azurophilic leukocytic inclusions, susceptibility to pyogenic infections, photophobia, albinism, and early death. Other features include hepatosplenomegaly, generalized lymphadenopathy, and excessive sweating. The blood shows anemia, neutropenia, with relative lymphocytosis, and thrombocytopenia. The neutrophils contain cytoplasmic inclusions resembling Döhle bodies. **cheilitis-glossitis-gingivitis s.**, plasma cell GINGIVITIS. **Cheney's s.**, Hajdu-Cheney s. **Christ-Siemens-Touraine s.**, hypohidrotic ectodermal DYSPLASIA. **Christian s.**, a syndrome believed to be transmitted as an autosomal recessive trait, consisting of a combination of craniosynostosis, arthrogryposis, and cleft palate. Associated disorders may include microcephaly, prominent occiput, ocular hypertelorism, antimongoloid palpebral slant, ophthalmoplegia, displaced ears, bifid uvula, abducted thumbs, camptodactyly, limited joint extension, pectus excavatus, talipes equinovarus, dysphagia, laryngomalacia, and muscle fibrillation. Central nervous system abnormalities, myelination disorders, and glial proliferation of the white matter are frequent features. **chromosomal s.,** any syndrome caused by a chromosomal defect. **chromosome 4p s.,** Wolf-Hirschhorn s. **chromosome 4p deletion s., partial,** Wolf-Hirschhorn s. **chromosome 4p trisomy s.,** 4p TRISOMY. **chromosome 4q trisomy s., partial,** 4q trisomy, partial; see under TRISOMY. **chromosome 5p s.,** crying cat s. **chromosome 5p deletion s., partial,** crying cat s. **chromosome 5p duplication s.,** TRISOMY 5p. **chromosome 7q duplication s., partial,** 7q trisomy, partial; see under TRISOMY. **chromosome 7q trisomy s., partial,** 7q trisomy, partial; see under TRISOMY. **chromosome 8p deletion s.,** deletion of the short arm of chromosome 8, associated with growth and mental retardation and various combinations of abnormalities, including narrow skull, shallow forehead, prominent occiput, epicanthic folds, flat nasal bridge, malaligned teeth, small mouth with down-turned corners, retrognathism, wide chin, short neck, wide-set nipples, and various cardiovascular anomalies. **chromosome 8 trisomy s.,** TRISOMY 8. **chromosome 9 rings s.,** a hereditary syndrome associated with the presence of ring chromosome 9, characterized by mental deficiency, hypotonia, microcephaly, trigonocephaly, enlarged and arched eyebrows, exophthalmia, upward and outward obliqueness of the palpebral fissures, epicanthus, inward curving nasal wings and out-turned nostrils, long upper lip, down-turned corners of the mouth, retrognathism, and protrusion of the antihelixes. Called also *ring chromosome 9 s.* **chromosome 9 trisomy s.,** TRISOMY 9. **chromosome 9p s.,** partial deletion of the short arm of chromosome 9 distal to band 9p22, characterized by mental retardation, sociable personality, trigonocephaly, low hairline, mongoloid slant of the palpebral fissures, epicanthic folds, flat nasal bridge, anteverted nostrils, long philtrum, low-set abnormal ears, high-arched palate, micrognathia, short and webbed neck, wide-set nipples, cardiac murmurs, omphalocele, square nails, long fingers, and predominance of whorls on fingers. **chromosome 9p monosomy s.,** 9p MONOSOMY. **chromosome 9p tetrasomy s.,** 9p TETRASOMY. **chromosome 9p trisomy s.,** 9p TRISOMY. **chromosome 9q trisomy s., partial,** 9q TRISOMY. **chromosome 10p deletion s.,** deletion of the short arm of chromosome 10, characterized by mental and growth retardation, brachycephaly, and trigonocephaly, antimongoloid palpebral fissures, hypotelorism, epicanthic folds, blepharoptosis, strabismus, dysplastic nose, high-arched palate, microdontia, small low-set posteriorly rotated ears, symmetric thorax, wide-set nipples, and minor abnormalities of hands and feet. Called also *del(10)p autosomal deletion s.* **chromosome 10p duplication s., chromosome 10p trisomy s.,** 10p TRISOMY. **chromosome 10q duplications s., chromosome 10q trisomy s.,** 10q TRISOMY. **chromosome 11p s., partial duplication,** 11p TRISOMY. **chromosome 11q s.,** partial deletion, partial deletion of the long arm of chromosome 11, characterized by growth and mental retardation, scaphocephaly, large square skull, hypertelorism, epicanthus, down- or up-slanting palpebral fissures, short nose, short philtrum, thin upper lip, microretrognathia, low-set malformed ears, short fingers, and hypertonicity. **chromosome 11q s., partial duplication,** 11q TRISOMY. **chromosome 12p s., partial deletion,** partial deletion of the short arm of chromosome 12, characterized by a combination of mental and growth retardation, hypotonia, jaw hypoplasia, microcephaly, narrow forehead, high-arched eyebrows, low-set ears, pointed tip of the nose, protruding occipital bone, downward and outward obliqueness of palpebral fissures, and other abnormalities. Called also *partial chromosome 12p monosomy s., partial 12p monosomy,* and *12p monosomy.* **chromosome 12p monosomy s., partial,** chromosome 12p s., partial deletion. **chromosome 12p trisomy s.,** 12p TRISOMY. **chromosome 13 s.,** Patau's s. **chromosome 13, partial deletion s.,** partial deletion of chromosome 13, frequently associated with ring chromosome, characterized by mental retardation, trigonocephaly, arhinencephaly, microcephaly, prominent nasal bridge, epicanthus, microphthalmos, coloboma, retinoblastoma, protruding maxilla, low-set large ears, cardiovascular defects, renal abnormalities, imperforate anus, thumb aplasia, and genital abnormalities. Death often occurs before six months of life. Called also *partial deletion of chromosome D₁.* **chromosome 13 ring s.,** a hereditary syndrome associated with the presence of the ring chromosome 13, combining mental and growth retardation, microcephaly, premature closure of cranial sutures, asymmetric mongoloid slanting of palpebral fissures, epicanthic folds, broad and prominent nasal bridge, open mouth, short fingers, and abnormal palmar creases. Called also *chromosome D₁₃ ring s.* **chromosome 14q s., partial duplication,** 14q TRISOMY. **chromosome 15, partial duplication of long arm s.,** 15q TRISOMY. **chromosome 18q s.,** deletion of the long arm of chromosome 18, characterized by

mental and growth retardation, associated with skeletal, craniofacial, cardiovascular, genital, ocular, and other abnormalities. Long and usually tapered fingers, supernumerary ribs, hypoplastic genitalia, skin dimples over the subacromion and epitrochlear areas and over the knuckles, glaucoma, strabismus, nystagmus, tapetoretinal degeneration, and optic dystrophy are the most common defects. Craniofacial abnormalities may include midfacial hypoplasia and mild microcephaly with deep-set eyes, small nose, subcutaneous nodule at the site of cheek dimples, carp mouth, deformed ears, and, in some cases, cleft lip and palate. Muscular hypotonia, seizures, and low-pitched voice occur commonly. **chromosome 18, supernumerary isochromosome s.,** a syndrome of multiple anomalies associated with the occurrence of an extra metacentric chromosome, probably an isochromosome, for the short arm of chromosome 18 (+18pi). It is characterized by feeding difficulty, vomiting, frail body habitus, microcephaly, low-set ears, small mouth, narrow high-arched palate, psychomotor retardation, motor neuron disorders, and retinal colobomas. Narrow face, pinched nose, dolichocephaly, absence of flexion creases on fingers, pes planovalgus, poor muscle development, and long thin limbs may occur. **chromosome 18 s.,** TRISOMY 18. **chromosome 18p s.,** deletion of the short arm of chromosome 18, characterized by mental retardation, pterygium colli, lymphedema of the dorsa of hands and feet, shield chest with wide-set nipples, microcephaly, hypertelorism, epicanthal folds, strabismus, blepharoptosis, retraction of midface, broad flat nose, micrognathia, large low-set ears, carp mouth, and other abnormalities. **chromosome 18p deletion s.,** chromosome 18p s. **chromosome 18q deletion s.,** deletion of the long arm of chromosome 18, characterized by midfacial hypoplasia with deep-set eyes; carp mouth; narrow palate; small stature; mental deficiency; hypotonia; poor coordination; nystagmus; conduction deafness; microcephaly; long hands; tapering fingers and short first metacarpal with proximal thumb; simian crease; whorl digital pattern; vertical talus, with or without talipes equinovarus; hypoplastic labia minora; cryptorchidism, with or without small scrotum and penis; eczema; cardiac abnormalities, skin dimples over the acromion; and, less frequently, slanted palpebral fissures, inner epicanthic folds, hypertelorism, ocular abnormalities, cleft palate, wide-set nipples, horseshoe kidneys, supernumerary ribs, and lipomas of the feet. **chromosome 20p, partial duplication s.,** 20p TRISOMY. **chromosome 21q s.,** an abnormality of the long arm of chromosome 21, characterized by mental and growth retardation, hypertonia, nail abnormalities, skeletal malformations, cryptorchidism, hypospadias, inguinal hernia, pyloric stenosis, thrombocytopenia, eosinophilia, and hypergammaglobulinemia. Orofacial defects may include microcephaly, large deformed, low-set ears, antimongoloid slant of the palpebral fissures, blepharochalasis, highly arched or cleft palate, cleft lip, and micrognathia. Called also *antimongolism.* **chromosome 21q deletion s.,** deletion of the long arm of chromosome 21, characterized by antimongoloid slant of the palpebral fissures, redundant eyelids, prominent nasal bridge, large external ears, wide external auditory canals, micrognathia, dysplastic nails, distal axial triradii, hypospadias, pyloric stenosis, thrombocytopenia, retarded bone maturation, low birth weight, and an irregular pattern of other abnormalities. **chromosome D₁₃ ring s.,** chromosome 13 ring s. **Citelli's s.,** loss of power of concentration and drowsiness or insomnia, often associated with intelligence disorders, seen in children with obstructing adenoid tissue in the nasopharynx. **Claude's s.,** inferior nucleus ruber s. **Claude Bernard's s.,** Bernard-Horner s. **cloverleaf skull s.,** cloverleaf SKULL. **CLP-lip pits s.,** van der Woude's s. **Cockayne's s.,** an autosomal recessively inherited syndrome characterized by dwarfism; kyphosis; ankylosis; disproportionately long extremities with large hands and feet; cold blue extremities; lack of subcutaneous fat of the face, prognathism, sunken eyes, and thin nose, giving the patient a prematurely old appearance; mental deficiency; hypersensitivity of the skin to sunlight with pigmentation and scarring; retinal pigmentary degeneration; optic atrophy; cataract; partial deafness; unsteady gait; thickened skull; and dental caries appearing during the second year of life after an apparently normal infancy. Called also *Neill-Dingwall s., progeria-like s.,* and *trisomy 10.* **Coffin-Lowry s.,** an X-linked inherited syndrome of coarse facies, mental retardation, and tapering fingers. Slanting palpebral fissures, bulbous nose due to thickening of the alae and septum, maxillary hypoplasia, and mild hypertelorism, are the principal facial features. Large soft hands with tapering fingers and tufted drumstick roentgenogram appearance to distal phalanges, accessory thenar crease, flat feet, and lax ligaments are the limb defects. Spinal and thoracic anomalies are usually associated. Occasional abnormalities may include thick calvaria and hypoplastic sinuses. **Coffin-Siris s.,** hypoplastic or absent fifth fingers and toenails, growth deficiency, mental deficiency, and variable presence of sparse scalp hair, hypertrichosis, mild microcephaly, coarse facies with full lips, lax joints with radial dislocation at elbows, coxa valga, and small patellae. Blepharoptosis, hypotelorism, preauricular skin tag, hemangioma, cryptorchidism, hernia, short sternum, short forearms, vertebral anomalies, cleft palate, cardiovascular defects, and Dandy-Walker anomaly may be associated. **COFS s.,** cerebro-oculofacioskeletal s. **Collet-Sicard s.,** a variant of Villaret's syndrome unaccompanied by Bernard-Horner syndrome, in which involvement of the ninth, tenth, eleventh, and twelfth cranial nerves produces paralysis of the vocal cords, palate, trapezius muscle, and sternocleidomastoid muscles; secondary loss of taste in the back of the tongue; and anesthesia of the larynx, pharynx, and soft palate. Called also *pharyngolaryngeal paralysis s., posterior laterocondylar space s.,* and *glossolaryngoscapulopharyngeal hemiplegia.* **congenital contractural arachnodactyly s.,** congenital contractural ARACHNODACTYLY. **congenital hyperchloremic acidosis s.,** Lightwood-Albright s. **congenital rubella s.,** a syndrome occurring in infants born to mothers who were infected with rubella during the first trimester of pregnancy. It is characterized by cataracts, heart abnormalities, deafness, mutism, microcephaly, mental deficiency, and, less frequently, microphthalmos, buphthalmos, retinal lesions, talipes equinovarus, syndactyly, hypospadias, muscular weakness, diplegia, cleft palate, and dental abnormalities, including enamel hypoplasia, high caries incidence, and delayed eruption of deciduous teeth. Called also *rubella s.* **congenital webbed neck s.,** Klippel-Feil s. **Conradi-Hünermann s.,** a syndrome, transmitted as an autosomal dominant trait, consisting of growth deficiency; flat facies with variable low nasal bridge, hypoplasia of malar eminences, and down-slanting palpebral fissures; asymmetric shortening of the extremities, punctate mineralization of epiphyses; variable joint contractures; frequent scoliosis; and variable follicular atrophoderma with large skin pores resembling orange peel and sparse, coarse hair. Called also *chondroangiopathia punctata, chondrodystrophia calcificans, chondropathia punctata, dominant chondrodysplasia punctata, punctate epiphyseal dysplasia,* and *stippled epiphyses.* **Cornelia de Lange's s.,** de Lange's s. **Costen's s.,** temporomandibular dysfunction s. **coumadin s.,** fetal warfarin s. **Cowden's s.,** an autosomal dominantly inherited syndrome involving multiple systems, characterized by adenoid facies, hypoplasia of the mandible and maxilla, high-arched palate, hypoplasia of the soft palate and uvula, microstomia, papillomatosis of the lips and oral pharynx, scrotal tongue, thyroid adenomas, thyroid carcinoma, bilateral hypertrophy of the breasts with fibrocystic disease and early malignant degeneration, pectus excavatum, scoliosis, space-occupying lesions in the liver and bone, and abnormalities of the central nervous system. Cowden is the family name of the propositus. **craniometaphyseal dysplasia s.,** craniometaphyseal DYSPLASIA. **Creyx-Lévy s.,** a reverse form of Sjögren's syndrome, in which xerosis is replaced by hypersecretion associated with chlorhydria, chemical changes of the saliva, chloride metabolism disorders, insensitivity to belladonna, and cervical vertebral calcifications. Called also *reverse Gougerot-Sjögren s.* and *ophthalmorhinostomatohygrosis.* **cricopharyngeal achalasia s.,** Asherson's s. **cri du chat s.,** crying cat s. **Crouzon's s.,** craniofacial DYSOSTOSIS. **CRST s.,** a syndrome of calcinosis, Raynaud's phenomenon, sclerodactyly, and telangiectasia, mimicking hereditary hemorrhagic telangiectasia. Telangiectatic lesions appear chiefly on the face, lips, nares, tongue, ears, hands, and feet; subcutaneous calcinosis may be found on the extensor surfaces of the elbows, knees, thighs, fingers, hands, arms, and forearms. Epistaxis and melena sometimes occur. **crying cat s.,** a syndrome of partial deletion of the short arm of one of the chromosomes 5, bands 5p14 and 5p15 being missing. It is characterized by severe mental deficiency, growth retardation, multiple abnormalities, and a peculiar crying sound resembling that of a suffering kitten that disappears within weeks or months after birth. Birth weight is usually less than 2,500 gm and affected infants are hypotonic and fail to thrive. Craniofacial abnormalities usually include microcephaly, round face, hypertelorism, antimongoloid palpebral fissures, epicanthus, large frontal sinuses, broad nasal bones, and low-set ears. Hypertelorism and facial roundness

usually disappear with age and the face becomes thin with a short philtrum. Most patients attain adult height of about 124 to 168 cm. Orodental anomalies may consist of mild micrognathia, malocclusion, and, sometimes, harelip and cleft palate. Premature graying of the hair, strabismus, preauricular skin tags, musculoskeletal anomalies, flat feet, syndactyly, and other defects may be associated. Called also *chromosome 5p s., cri du chat s.,* and *Lejeune's s.* **cryptophthalmos s.,** a congenital syndrome of abnormalities of the eyes, ears, and genitalia, often associated with defects of other organs. The principal features include cryptophthalmos, auricular defects of the ear, and hypospadias and cryptorchidism or bicornuate uterus and vaginal atresia. Associated abnormalities may include a flat nasal bridge, hypertelorism, defects of the lacrimal ducts, palatal defects, partial midfacial cleft, laryngeal stenosis or atresia, syndactyly, atresia of the anus, wide-set nipples, and kidney abnormalities. Called also *Fraser's s.* **Curschmann-Batten-Steinert s.,** myotonic DYSTROPHY. **Cushing's s.,** 1. a syndrome characterized by excessive secretion of cortisone and hydrocortisone, associated with obesity and hypertension, and caused by hyperfunction of the adrenal cortex due to hyperplasia, adenoma, or carcinoma; pituitary hyperfunction due to a basophil or chromophobe adenoma; ectopic production of cortisone; or prolonged excessive intake of glucocorticoids for therapeutic purposes. An abnormal fat distribution giving rise to "buffalo hump" and "moon face" are the principal symptoms. Female patients may show signs of masculinization, with hirsutism, acne, deep and coarse voice, amenorrhea, and enlargement of the clitoris. In males, the external genitalia are usually normal, but evidence of virilization may be present. The metabolic disorders include severe protein depletion with diminution of the muscle mass and calcium disorders with osteoporosis. Fragility of the skin and blood vessels, asthenia, purple striae over the abdomen, thighs, and arms, and increased susceptibility to bruising are also present. Growth retardation may be associated with delayed dentition; osteoporosis seldom involves the jaws; and gingival enlargement may occur. Called also *pituitary basophilism, basophil adenoma,* and *Cushing's basophilism.* 2. nystagmus, tinnitus, deafness, labyrinthine disorders, diminished corneal reflex, hypesthesia of the face, paralysis of the facial and oculomotor nerves, hoarseness, dysphagia, hiccups, vomiting, and headache resulting from interference with the brachium pontis and pressure on the posterior lobe and dentate nucleus in association with involvement of the fifth, sixth, seventh, eighth, ninth, and tenth cranial nerves and the brain stem. A brain neoplasm is a common cause. Called also *angle tumor s.* and *s. of cerebellopontile angle.* **cutaneomuco-oculoepithelial s.,** Fuchs' s. **cutaneomucouveal s.,** Behçet's s. **Danbolt-Closs s.,** ACRODERMATITIS enteropathica. **De Barsy-Moens-Dierckx s.,** a congenital syndrome characterized by mental retardation, dwarfism, dystrophy, progeroid facies, corneal clouding, and cutis laxa, associated with abnormal electroencephalogram, in the presence of no apparent chromosomal abnormalities. **Debré's s.,** cat-scratch DISEASE. **defibrination s.,** a blood coagulation disorder, occurring usually as a complication of various clinical conditions, characterized by symptoms of the underlying disease associated with anemia, hemorrhage, or thrombosis, singly or in combination. Pathologic fibrinolysis complicating therapy of thromboembolism with the use of excessive amounts of an exogenous plasminogen activator is a common cause. Called also *consumptive coagulopathy* and *intravascular coagulation.* **de Gimard's s.,** a form of purpura, most commonly affecting children, in which purpuric lesions become necrosed and healing is accompanied by separation of the resulting sloughs; except for scarring, there are no sequelae. It has been suggested that its etiology may be connected with the Sanarelli-Shwartzman phenomenon. Called also *Martin de Gimard's s., gangrenous purpura,* and *purpura necrotisans.* **Deiters' nucleus s.,** Bonnier's s. **Dejean's s.,** orbital floor s. **Déjérine's s.,** alternating hypoglossal HEMIPLEGIA. **del (10)p autosomal deletion s.,** chromosome 10p deletion s. **de Lange's s.,** a congenital syndrome of unknown etiology, associated with low birth weight after full-term pregnancy; retarded bone maturation; mental retardation; initial hypertonicity; microbrachycephaly; micrognathia; small nose with inverted nostrils; synophrys and long, curly eyelashes; ocular abnormalities; hirsutism; cutis marmorata; hypoplastic nipples and umbilicus; micromelia or phocomelia; syndactyly, oligodactyly, or clinodactyly; simian creases; and flexion contracture of the elbows. The majority of those affected have diminished sucking and swallowing ability. Frequent vomiting results in aspiration pneumonia. Called also *Brachmann-de Lange s., Cornelia de Lange s., Lange's s., Amsterdam dwarf,* and *Amsterdam type.* **Demarquay-Richet s.,** van der Woude s. **dentopulmonary s.,** an association of chronic bronchitis and dental caries, believed to be caused by aspiration of material from carious teeth. Some authorities do not recognize this syndrome as a legitimate entity. Called also *Veeneklaas' s.* **De Toni-Fanconi s.,** Abderhalden-Fanconi s. **De Vries' s.,** a familial congenital condition observed in both sexes, characterized by factor V deficiency, with a tendency to bleed, and syndactyly. **Diamond-Blackfan s.,** a rare refractory aplastic (hypoplastic) anemia of young infants, resulting from defective erythropoiesis and lack of regenerative capacity, with gross deficiency of nucleated erythrocytes in the bone marrow, but normal platelet count and only mild leukopenia. Called also *congenital hypoplastic anemia, Diamond-Blackfan anemia, hypoplastic anemia of childhood,* and *pure red cell anemia.* **DiGeorge's s.,** concurrent congenital absence of the thymus and parathyroid glands, associated with apparently normal levels of immunoglobulins, runting, delayed neurological development, and frequent infections. Cardiovascular complications, particularly aortic arch anomalies and congenital heart defects, may be associated. Oral manifestations are similar to those seen in hypoparathyroidism, including delayed dentition, tooth retention, enamel defects, dentinal dysplasia, and incomplete root formation. **Dilantin s.,** fetal hydantoin s. **Diogenes' s.,** a condition usually observed in the elderly, characterized by gross self-neglect, lack of self-consciousness about personal habits, untidiness, and hoarding of rubbish. It appears to be unrelated to the socioeconomic status of the patient, who is often aloof, suspicious, emotionally labile, aggressive, group-dependent, and reality-distorting. Various nutritional deficiencies are usually associated. The syndrome was named after Diogenes, a Greek philosopher known for his bizarre behavior, who gave up all comforts of life and possessions and lived in an empty wooden tub in order to prove his views and to discredit the social conditions of his times. **dorsolateral medullary s.,** Wallenberg's s. **dorsolateral oblongata s.,** Babinski-Nageotte s. **Down's s.,** a syndrome due to the presence of an extra chromosome 21, usually caused by nondisjunction and, rarely, by translocation. The most common defects consist of mental retardation, short stature, small skull with a flat occiput, fissured tongue, flat nose, and small ears and mandible, giving the appearance of persons of the Mongoloid race. Other symptoms include delayed tooth eruption, short and broad neck, prominent abdomen, short extremities with broad flat hands and small curving fifth fingers, muscular hypotonia, hypogonadism, straight silky pubic hair and delayed development of secondary sex characteristics. Other abnormalities, including cardiovascular defects, may be associated. The patients often exhibit protrusion of the tongue, high-arched palate, malformed teeth, enamel hypoplasia, and microdontia. Called also *mongolism, mongoloid idiocy,* and *trisomy 21.* See also Turner-mongolism POLYSYNDROME. **Dubovitz's s.,** a hereditary syndrome, transmitted as an autosomal recessive trait, characterized principally by low birth weight dwarfism, infantile eczema, microcephaly, mental retardation, hyperactivity, hyperextensibility of joints, peculiar facies, blepharophimosis, broad bridge and tip of the nose, retrognathia, lateral eyebrows, clinodactyly, delayed tooth eruption, and dental caries. **Dubreuil-Chambardel's s.,** dental caries of the incisors, in most instances only the upper incisors. The necrotic processes usually appear during adolescence, and within a few years the teeth are irreparably damaged. Alopecia may be associated. Some authorities do not consider this syndrome a legitimate entity. **dyscraniopygophalangia s.,** Ullrich-Feichtiger s. **Dzierzynsky's s.,** an apparently hereditary form of craniomandibulofacial dysostosis, marked by acrocephaly, scaphocephaly, lordotic curvature at the base of the skull, premature closure of cranial sutures, thickening of the skull, peculiar facies, protruding and straight nose, and thick phalanges, clavicles, and sternum. Called also *dystrophia periostalis hyperplastica familiaris.* **Eagle's s.,** elongation or calcification of the styloid process resulting in two clinically distinct forms: In one form, chiefly affecting persons over 30 years of age, the symptoms occur after tonsillectomy as a dull, nagging pain in the pharyngeal region, which may become stabbing and is aggravated by the act of swallowing. Deglutition disorders and the sensation of a foreign body are usually associated, leading the patient to believe that the surgical wound failed to heal. The constrictor muscles of the upper part of the esophagus and hypopharynx are primarily affected, but pain may be referred to the ear. The second form (called also *styloid process-carotid artery s.*) is caused by pressure exerted by the elongated and medially or laterally deviated process on the carotid artery, causing irritation of the sympathetic nerve fibers. Pain below the level of the eyes and along the routes supplied by the external branches of the artery indicates impairment of the external carotid; pain in the parietal region and along the ophthalmic artery indicates impairment of the inter-

nal carotid. Called also *hyoid s., stylohyoid s., styloid s.,* and *styloid process s.* **ectrodactyly-ectodermal dysplasia-clefting s.,** REEDS s. **eczema-thrombocytopenia s.,** Wiskott-Aldrich s. **Edwards' s.,** TRISOMY 18. **EEC s.,** REEDS s. **Ehlers-Danlos s.,** a congenital syndrome, usually beginning in childhood, most often in males, and transmitted as an autosomal dominant trait. It is marked by hyperelasticity of the skin, excessive susceptibility of the skin to trauma, fragility of the blood vessels, hematomas of the skin at the site of contusion, pigmented granulomatous pseudotumors at the site of injury, and loose joints. Ocular changes may include blue sclera, angioid streaks of the retina, retinal hemorrhage, depigmentation of the choroid, ptosis, eversion of the upper eyelid, strabismus, microcornea, ocular hypertension, keratoconus, and epicanthus. Recurrent dislocation of the temporomandibular joint may be associated. Called also *cutis elastica* and *elastic skin.* **elfin facies s.,** a syndrome of multiple congenital abnormalities, including mental and growth retardation; microcephaly and premature closure of the cranial sutures; peculiar elflike facies, consisting of medial eyebrow flare, short palpebral fissures, depressed nasal bridge, epicanthal folds, periorbital fullness of subcutaneous tissues, blue eyes, stellate pattern in the iris, anteverted nares, long philtrum, prominent lips, and open mouth; hypoplastic nails; hallux valgus; cardiovascular defects, such as supravalvular aortic, pulmonary artery, and pulmonic valvular stenosis, and ventricular and atrial septal defects; and dental abnormalities, which may include oligodontia, enamel hypoplasia, severe caries, microdontia, and abnormally small roots. Cardiac murmurs, muscular hypotonia, hypertension, anorexia, vomiting, hyperphosphatemia, azotemia, albuminuria, low urea clearance, hypertension and high urinary calcium are usually associated, and, to a lesser degree, high urinary phosphates, osteosclerosis, lowered alkaline reserve, and hypercholesteremia. Hypercalcemia is often present, but rarely after the age of one year. The syndrome occurs sporadically. Called also *Beuren's s., Fanconi-Schlesinger s., peculiar facies-vascular stenoses s., supravalvular aortic stenosis s., Williams' s., Williams-Barrat s.,* and *idiopathic hypercalcemia of infancy.* **Ellis-van Creveld s.,** chondroectodermal DYSPLASIA. **Elschnig's s.,** a combination of deformities consisting of extension of the palpebral fissure laterally, displacement of the lateral canthus outward and downward, and ectropion of the lower eyelid and of the lateral canthus. Hypertelorism, cleft palate, and cleft lip are frequently associated. **EMG s.,** Beckwith-Wiedemann s. **Erb-Goldflam s.,** MYASTHENIA gravis. **Estren-Dameshek s.,** a hereditary form of hypoplastic anemia characterized by pancytopenia, pallor, weakness, and a bleeding tendency. **Evans' s.,** autoimmune hemolytic anemia complicated by leukopenia and symptomatic thrombocytopenic purpura. **exomphalos-macroglossia-gigantism s.,** Beckwith-Wiedemann s. **facial-digital-genital s.,** Aarskog's s. **faciocardiorenal s.,** a syndrome of horseshoe kidneys, mental retardation, peculiar facies, and heart defects, transmitted as an autosomal recessive trait. Orofacial abnormalites include malar hypoplasia; broad nasal root; prominent antegonial notch of mandible; poorly developed philtrum, vermilion border, and ala nasi; prominent, relatively inflexible ears; plagiocephaly; cleft palate; and hypodontia. **familial hypercholesterolemia s.,** van Bogaert-Scherer-Epstein s. **Fanconi's s.,** 1. a hereditary, slowly progressive disease of the kidneys. The first symptoms, which become evident at the age of 2 to 3 years, include polydipsia, polyuria, and nycturia, followed by low blood glucose and high electrolyte levels and, later, by signs of glomerular failure marked by increased urinary nitrogen and blood phosphorus. Low blood calcium levels, growth retardation, and osteodystrophy indicate hyperparathyroidism. Other metabolic disorders include a low alkaline reserve and low urinary ammonia excretion. There may be a history of fever and convulsions. The pathological findings include progressive degeneration of the kidney parenchyma, with hyaline changes in the tubules and basal membranes; the collecting tubules are usually atrophied but, on occasion, may be hypertrophied. The anterior pituitary may show eosinophilia, and adenomatous hyperplasia may be found in the parathyroid gland. The bones show fibroid degeneration with excessive production of osteoid tissue. 2. Abderhalden-Fanconi s. **Fanconi-Albertini-Zellweger s.,** a syndrome of congenital heart defect, pachycephalia, calcification of the falx cerebri, peculiar facies, microdontia, albuminuria, leukocytosis and casts in the urine, metabolic acidosis, osteoporosis with spontaneous fractures, curving of the long bones, anemia, cerebrospinal fluid changes and growth retarda-

tion. Called also *osteopathia acidotica pseudorachitica.*
Fanconi-De Toni-Debré s., see *Abderhalden-Fanconi s.*
Fanconi-Petrassi s., a hereditary form of hemolytic anemia
with macrocytosis and hyperchromia. **Fanconi-Schlesinger s.,**
elfin facies s. **Farber's s.,** a congenital form of lipidosis, similar
to Tay-Sachs disease and Niemann-Pick disease, characterized
by infiltration and replacement of normal tissue in the spleen,
heart, liver, and lungs with foam cells, and cerebral changes. It
is marked by a hoarse cry, feeding difficulty, respiratory distress, mental retardation, hepatomegaly, pigmentation of the
skin, subcutaneous nodules, periarticular swelling suggesting
rheumatoid arthritis, and erosion of bones. Called also *disseminated lipogranulomatosis* and *Farber's lipogranulomatosis.*
Fargin-Fayolle s., DENTINOGENESIS imperfecta. **Fegeler's s.,**
NEVUS flammeus, post-traumatic. **Felty's s.,** 1. a syndrome of
splenic neutropenia and rheumatoid arthritis, marked by splenomegaly, myeloid hyperplasia of the bone marrow, leukopenia, granulocytopenia, lymphadenopathy, anemia, weight loss,
weakness, fatigue, and skin pigmentation. Ocular changes may
include keratoconjunctivitis sicca, episcleritis, hypopyon ulcer,
and scleromalacia. Oral changes consist chiefly of recurrent
ulcers of the mucosa, presenting a clean, punched-out lesion
about 2 mm in diameter. 2. congenital NEUTROPENIA. **femoral
hypoplasia–unusual facies s.,** a syndrome of congenital abnormalities, characterized by upslanting palpebral fissures, short
nose, broad nasal tip, narrow nasal alae, long philtrum, thin
upper lip, small mandible, cleft palate, short or absent femurs
and fibulae, clubfoot, mild shortening of humerus, restriction of
elbow movement, and abnormalities of the pelvis, spine, and
ribs. The intelligence of affected persons is normal. **fetal alcohol s.,** a syndrome of infants born to alcoholic mothers,
characterized by growth and mental retardation, short palpebral fissures, poor coordination, tremor, motor disorders, joint
anomalies, heart murmur, and craniofacial defects consisting
of moderate microcephaly, short palpebral fissures, and maxillary hypoplasia. Blepharoptosis, cleft palate, and other abnormalities may be associated. **fetal aminopterin s.,** a syndrome of
cranial dysplasia, foot abnormalities, and other defects occurring in infants of mothers who received aminopterin, as in
attempted induced abortion, particularly during the fourth to
tenth week of gestation. Growth deficiency; microcephaly; hypoplasia of the frontal, parietal, temporal, and occipital bones;
wide fontanelles with synostoses of lambdoid or coronal sutures; upsweep of frontal scalp hair; broad nasal bridge; shallow supraorbital ridges; prominent eyes; epicanthal folds; micrognathia; cleft palate; maxillary hypoplasia; low-set ears;
relative shortness of limbs; talipes equinovarus; and hypodacty-
ly are the principal features. Cleft palate and abnormalities of
the skeletal system and heart may be associated. Called also
aminopterin s. **fetal face s.,** Robinow's s. **fetal hydantoin s.,** a
syndrome occurring in infants whose mothers received hydantoin during pregnancy, consisting of varying combinations of
growth and mental deficiency, wide anterior fontanelles, metopic ridging, hypertelorism, broad depressed nasal ridge, low-set
abnormal ears, broad alveolar ridge, cleft lip and palate, hirsutism, low-set hairline, coarse hair, short neck, wide-set small
nipples, abnormal palmar creases, pilonidal sinus, hernia, hip
dislocation, hypoplasia of phalanges, and rib abnormalities.
Microcephaly, brachycephaly, strabismus, slanted palpebral
fissures, and other abnormalities may be associated. Called also
Dilantin s. and *hydantoin s.* **fetal trimethadione s.,** a syndrome
of infants whose mothers received trimethadione during pregnancy, consisting of growth retardation, speech disorders, V-
shaped eyebrows, epicanthus, low-set ears with anteriorly folded helix, palatal anomalies, and irregular teeth. Microcephaly,
cardiovascular defects, hypospadias, inguinal hernia, simian
creases, and intrauterine developmental retardation may be
associated. Called also *tridione s.* and *trimethadione s.* **fetal
warfarin s.,** a syndrome occurring in infants whose mothers
received warfarin during pregnancy, consisting of growth and
mental deficiency, hypotonia, seizures, optic atrophy, hypoplastic nasal cartilage with a low nasal bridge, upper airway
obstruction, and stippled epiphyses. Called also *coumadin s.*
and *warfarin s.* **Fèvre-Languepin s.,** a hereditary syndrome
characterized by popliteal webbing associated with cleft lip and
palate, fistula of the lower lip, syndactyly, onychodysplasia, and
pes equinovarus. Called also *popliteal pterygium s.* **FG s.,** a
hereditary syndrome, transmitted as an X-linked trait, consisting of mental retardation and multiple congenital abnormalities, including variable growth retardation, disproportionately
large head, craniosynostosis, imperforate anus, hypotonia, py-

loric stenosis, hypoplastic left heart, dilatation of the urinary
tract, and cutaneous syndactyly of third and fourth fingers.
Craniofacial abnormalities consist of a high and prominent
forehead with bifrontal bossing, apparent hypertelorism, slight
mongoloid or antimongoloid slanting of palpebral fissures, and
secondary manifestations of hypotonia, such as elongated philtrum, anteverted nostrils, and abnormal shape of the upper lip.
first and second branchial arch s., a syndrome resulting from
malformation of derivatives of the first and second branchial
arches, characterized by defects of the face, also involving the
primordia of the temporal bone. Dysplasia is usually unilateral;
there is frequency of difference in the expression of abnormalities between the two sides in bilateral cases. It usually involves
the ear or accessory ear tissue and/or asymmetric face, the
parotid gland, middle ear, external ear, zygoma, temporomandibular joint, soft palate, tongue, eye, and vertebrae. Symptoms
include peculiar asymmetric facies, consisting of microtia,
macrostomia, and aplastic or hypoplastic ramus of the mandible. Flattening in the region of the mastoid process, absent ear
canal, lowering of the palpebral fissures on the affected side,
aplasia or hypoplasia on the affected side, growth disorders,
taste aberration, cleft lip and/or palate, high-arched asymmetric palate, and malocclusion may be associated. Called also
*branchial arch s., hemifacial microsomia, intrauterine facial
necrosis, lateral facial dysplasia (LFD), otomandibular dysostosis,* and *unilateral facial agenesis.* **Floating-Harbor s.,** a
congenital syndrome characterized by growth retardation, language development retardation with aphasia, pseudoarthrosis-
like anomaly of the clavicle, short neck, small hands with short
stubby fingers, clinodactyly, incurved toes, limited extension of
elbows, and triangular facies with wide forehead, hypoplastic
maxilla, micrognathia, mandibular overbite, large nose, broad
nasal base, deep-set eyes, narrow palate, hypertrophy of the
maxillary alveolar ridge, and low-set posterior rotated ears. The
intelligence is normal and there are no apparent chromosomal
abnormalities. The syndrome was named after the Boston
Floating and Harbor General Hospitals. **focal dermal hypoplasia s.,** Goltz-Gorlin s. **Foix's s.,** cavernous sinus s. **Foville's s.,** a
syndrome in which, in addition to loss of outward movement of
one eye due to abducens and facial paralysis with contralateral
hemiplegia *(Millard-Gubler s.),* there is loss of inward movement of the other eye in attempting to look toward the side of the
lesion. Called also *peduncular s., hemiplegia abducentofa-
cialis, hemiplegia alternans inferior,* and *hemiplegia alternans inferior pontina.* **fragilitas ossium-blue sclera-
osteosclerosis s.,** van der Hoeve's s. **Franceschetti's s.,** mandibulofacial DYSOSTOSIS. **Franceschetti-Jadassohn s.,** Naegeli's
s. **Fraser's s.,** cryptophthalmos s. **Freeman-Sheldon s.,** craniocarpotarsal DYSTROPHY. **Frey's s.,** auriculotemporal s. **Fuchs' s.,**
a variant of Stevens-Johnson syndrome, a severe form of erythema multiforme, characterized by stomatitis, conjunctivitis, and
macular eruption of the skin, in the absence of fever. The
symptoms disappear gradually in the order of their appearance.
Called also *acute mucocutaneous-ocular s., cutaneomuco-
oculoepithelial s.,* and *mucocutaneous-ocular s.* **Fuller Albright's s.,** Albright's s. (1). G s., a familial syndrome of dysphagia with recurrent aspiration and achalasia, stridorous respiration, and weak, hoarse cry; hypospadias sometimes with a bifid
scrotum; and typical facies, consisting chiefly of low nasal
bridge, hypertelorism, slanted auricles, and prominent parietal
and occipital regions. Cleft palate and larynx and short lingual
frenulum are usually associated. High bifurcation of the trachea, tracheoesophageal fistula, incomplete differentiation of
external genitalia, imperforate anus, duodenal stricture, cardiac defects, absence of the gallbladder, unilateral dysplasia
(including only one lung), or unilateral abnormalities (e.g.,
duplication or bifid renal pelvis) may occur. Familial occurrence is compatible with autosomal dominant inheritance.
Called also *hypospadias-dysphagia s.* and *Opitz-Frias s.* **Garcin's s.,** a rare syndrome with involvement of all or nearly all the
cranial nerves on one side in tumors of the nasopharynx without involving the brain itself. The most common cause is
nasopharyngeal lymphoepithelioma (Schmincke's tumor).
Called also *half-base s.* **Gardner's s.,** a hereditary syndrome,
transmitted as an autosomal dominant trait, characterized by
rectal and colonic polyposis with a tendency to undergo malignant changes; cysts of the skin, usually of the inclusion type;
true compact osteomas in about half the cases; fibrous and fatty
tumors of the skin and mesentery; and oral changes, including
multiple impacted supernumerary teeth, impacted permanent
teeth, and neoplastic changes in the jaws. Called also *hereditary adenomatosis* and *hereditary polyposis and osteomatosis.*
general adaptation s., the sum of reactions to prolonged exposure to stress, including enlargement of the adrenal cortex with
increased production of corticoid hormones, involution of the

thymus and other lymphatic organs, gastrointestinal ulcer, metabolic changes, and variations in the resistance of the organism. The first stage is the alarm reaction, consisting of a shock phase and then a countershock phase, followed by the adaptation stage, in which the resistance to the original stressor is greater, but the resistance to other stressors is decreased. If the stressor is not removed, the exhaustion stage and death follow. Called also *Selye's s.* **geniculate ganglion s.,** Hunt's s. **Gerhardt's s.,** bilateral abductor paralysis of the larynx. **Giedion-Langer s.,** trichorhinophalangeal DYSPLASIA (2). **Gilford's s.,** Hutchinson-Gilford s. **gingivostomatitis s.,** plasma cell GINGIVITIS. **Glanzmann's s.,** a chronic, hereditary hemorrhagic disease in which there is deficient clot retraction and abnormal morphology, but normal or nearly normal bleeding time and platelet count. Purpura, excessive bleeding, and bruising from minor injuries are the main clinical features. Defective pseudopod formation by the blood platelets and the failure of the blood platelets to spread in contact with wettable surfaces may be observed under the electron microscope. Called also *athrombocytopenic purpura, Glanzmann's thrombasthenia, hemorrhagic thrombasthenia,* and *thrombocytopathic purpura.* **glycolysis myopathy s.,** GLYCOGENOSIS V. **Godtfredsen's s.,** oculomotor paralysis, trigeminal neuralgia, and hypoglossal paralysis produced by infiltration of nasopharyngeal tumors into the base of the skull and adjacent structures and compression of the hypoglossal nerve by enlarged retropharyngeal lymph nodes. **Goldenhar's s.,** oculoauriculovertebral s. **Goltz's s.,** Goltz-Gorlin s. **Goltz-Gorlin s.,** a congenital syndrome, probably transmitted as an X-linked dominant trait, lethal in males. It consists of atrophy and linear pigmentation of the skin with occasional papillomatosis, keratosis, and focal aplasia, distributed chiefly on the trunk and limbs; multiple papillomatosis of the labial, oral, and anal mucosae and leukokeratosis of the oral mucosa; occasionally alopecia of the scalp; thin dystrophic nails; hypoplasia of the dental enamel with microdontia and notching of the teeth; thin helix of the ear; coloboma of the iris and choroid with strabismus and microphthalmia; adactyly, syndactyly, or polydactyly; dysplasia of the clavicle; scoliosis; spinal bifida; and frequently mental retardation. Called also *focal dermal hypoplasia s.* and *Goltz's s.* **Gorlin's s.,** a syndrome of multiple nevoid basal cell carcinoma, odontogenic keratocysts of the jaws, ocular hypertelorism, intracranial calcification, ovarian fibroma, lymphomesenteric cysts, and other abnormalities. It is inherited as an autosomal dominant trait with high penetrance and variable expressivity. The cutaneous symptoms include multiple nevoid basal cell carcinoma with calcification, palmar pits, and milia. Orofacial manifestations include multiple jaw cysts, and, rarely, fibrosarcoma of the jaws and ameloblastoma. Various abnormalities of the skeletal system (frontal and temporoparietal bossing, bridging of the sella, and other anomalies); the central nervous system (mental retardation, schizophrenia, congenital hydrocephalus, medulloblastoma, nerve deafness, and other anomalies); the eye (congenital blindness, hypertelorism, sunken appearance, and other defects); the endocrine system; and of other systems and organs are usually present. Called also *basal cell nevus s., Gorlin-Goltz s., multiple nevoid basal cell carcinoma s., naevoid basal cell carcinoma s.,* and *nevoid basal cell carcinoma s.* **Gorlin-Chaudhry-Moss s.,** a syndrome, suspected of being transmitted as an autosomal recessive trait, consisting of craniosynostosis, midfacial hypoplasia, hypertrichosis, and abnormalities of the eyes, teeth, heart, and genitalia. Symptoms may include depressed supraorbital ridges, antimongoloid palpebral slant, inability to fully open or close the eyes, colobomas, microphthalmia, low hairline, and hearing disorders. X-ray examination may show premature synostosis of the coronal suture, brachycephaly, hypoplasia of the maxillary and nasal bones, ocular hypertelorism, and defects of the petrous ridges and lesser sphenoidal wings. Oral changes usually consist of class III malocclusion, narrow high-arched palate, hypodontia, microdontia, and abnormally shaped teeth. Patent ductus arteriosus, umbilical hernia, and hypoplasia of the labia majora may be associated. **Gorlin-Goltz s.,** Gorlin's s. **Gorlin-Holt s.,** frontometaphyseal DYSPLASIA. **Gradenigo's s.,** paralysis of the sixth cranial nerve, with or without involvement of the ophthalmic branch of the fifth nerve, associated with lesions of the apex of the petrous bone and mastoiditis. Transient involvement of the third and fourth cranial nerves may be present, and facial paralysis may also occur. Severe pain of the area supplied by the ophthalmic branch, photophobia, excessive lacrimation, fever, and reduced corneal sensitivity are the principal symptoms. Inner ear infections, trauma, meningitis, extradural abscess, and hemorrhage are possible causes. Called also *apex of petrous bone s.* and *temporal s.* **Gougerot-Houwer-Sjögren s., Gougerot-Sjögren s.,** Sjögren's s. **Gougerot-Sjögren s., reverse,**

syndrome 773

Creyx-Lévy s. **Grob's s.,** see *oral-facial-digital s.* (1). **Guérin-Stern s.,** a congenital syndrome, affecting males more often than females, and believed to be due to prolonged uterine pressure. It is characterized by ankylosis of one or more joints with hypoplasia of the attached musculature and multiple pterygia, in association with dislocation of the hip, smooth and creaseless skin, talipes equinovarus, micrognathia, webbing of the fingers, and various combinations of hand and foot malformations. Typically, the symptoms are present at birth and usually do not progress further. The infants may experience feeding difficulty because of limited movement of the jaw. Called also *amyoplasia congenita, arthrogryposis multiplex congenita, myodystrophia congenita,* and *pterygium universalis.* **Guillain-Barré s.,** polyneuritis, usually following an acute infectious disease, from which the patient may have recovered, and associated with progressive motor paralysis of the extremities. The paralytic stage begins with pain or paresthesia. Weakness of the legs and relative anesthesia in the area of severe weakness follows. Choked disks, paralysis of the facial nerve, paralysis of any of the cranial nerves, and bulbar paralysis may occur. Paroxysmal hypertension is a frequent complication, and high concentrations of proteins in the cerebrospinal fluid are a constant feature. Recovery is usually complete. Called also *acute ascending polyradiculoneuritis, acute infectious polyneuritis,* and *polyradiculoneuritis.* **Gunn's s.,** unilateral ptosis of the eyelid with exaggerated opening of the eye during mastication or movement of the mandible. The etiology is unknown, but a hereditary pattern of transmission is suspected, autosomal dominant inheritance being likely. Called also *jaw winking s., Marcus Gunn's s., Gunn's phenomenon,* and *Marcus Gunn's phenomenon.* **Günther's s.,** erythropoietic PORPHYRIA. **Hajdu-Cheney s.,** a form of osteochondrodysplasia, transmitted as an autosomal dominant trait, with sporadic cases presumably representing fresh gene mutation. It is characterized by short stature augmented by osseous compression, absence of frontal sinuses, elongated sella turcica, basilar impression and bathrocephaly, micrognathia with diminished ramus of the mandible, resorption of the alveolar process with early loss of teeth, kyphoscoliosis with biconcave vertebrae, acro-osteolysis with short distal digits and nails, crowded carpal bones, and joint laxity. Called also *acro-osteolysis s., Cheney's s., acro-osteolysis, arthrodentosteodysplasia (ADOD), cranioskeletal dysplasia,* and *hereditary dysostosis.* **half-base s.,** Garcin's s. **Hallermann-Streiff s.,** a syndrome consisting of birdlike facies, congenital cataract, microphthalmia, micrognathia, and hypotrichosis. The head has an abnormal shape, usually brachycephalic or scaphocephalic; frontal and parietal bones may be enlarged; fontanelles remain open; and cranial vault appears enlarged in proportion to the small face. The mandible is hypoplastic, with a short ascending ramus and absence of the condyle, and the temporomandibular joint may be displaced forward. Thin lips and high-arched palate are usually present. The dental abnormalities may include absence of teeth, persistence of deciduous teeth, malocclusion with open bite, and premature caries. The ears are frequently low set. Nystagmus, strabismus, and other ocular abnormalities may be associated. Called also *François' dyscephaly, mandibulofacial dysmorphia,* and *oculomandibulodyscephaly.* **Hallopeau's s.,** DERMATITIS vegetans. **Handart's s.,** 1. aglossia-adactylia s. 2. Hanhart's NANISM. **happy-puppet s.,** a condition that seems neither familial nor progressive, occurring in seemingly happy and laughing children, and characterized by microbrachycephaly, peculiar facies, mental deficiency, ataxia, and epilepsy. Called also *Angelman's s.* and *puppet child.* **Hayem-Widal s.,** acquired hemolytic JAUNDICE. **Heerfordt's s.,** a manifestation of systemic sarcoidosis characterized by bilateral granulomatous uveitis, parotitis, lymphadenopathy, and facial paralysis, sometimes also involving the submaxillary and submandibular glands. Called also *neurouveoparotitis s., febris uveoparotidea subchronica, uveoparotid fever, uveoparotitic paralysis,* and *uveoparotitis.* See also Waldenström's UVEOPAROTITIS. **hemibulbar s.,** Babinski-Nageotte s. **Herlitz s.,** a form of epidemolysis bullosa characterized by a neonatal onset, absence of milia, pigmentary changes, scarring, and death within the first 3 months of life. Oral manifestations include hemorrhagic bullae at the junction between the hard and soft palates and proliferation of the dental lamina and the inner and outer enamel epithelium in decalcified sections. The latter also shows metaplasia to stratified squamous epithelium. Called also *epidermolysis bullosa letalis.* **Herrmann-Opitz s.,** a congenital syndrome consisting of craniosynostosis, brachysyndactyly of the hands, and absence of the toes. It may be manifested by turribrachycephaly with hypoplastic supraorbital ridges and bitemporal flattening, ocular hypertelorism, prominent eyes, extropia, posteriorly rotated ears with hypoplasia of the helices, micrognathia, high-arched palate, small mastoid sinuses, faulty ossification of the frontal bone, parietal defects, limited extension of the elbows, syndactyly, simian creases, delayed development, and mental retardation. **Herrmann-Pallister-Opitz s.,** a syndrome consisting of craniosynostosis, symmetrical limb malformations, and cleft lip and palate. It may be manifested by microbrachycephaly, synostosis involving chiefly the coronal suture, open sagittal and lambdoidal sutures, patent metopic suture, ocular hypertelorism, occipital capillary hemangioma, protruding ears, deviation of the nasal septum, mental retardation, aplasia of the radius, short ulna, split fingers, congenital hip dislocation, dysplasia of the femoral heads and necks, ankylosis of the knees, cryptorchidism, narrow shoulders and thorax, depression of the sternum, and other abnormalities. **HHHO s.,** Prader-Willi s. **HMC s.,** hypertelorism-microtia-clefting s. **Holtermüller-Wiedemann s.,** cloverleaf SKULL. **Hooft's s.,** familial HYPOLIPIDEMIA. **Horner's s.,** Bernard-Horner s. **Horner's s., incomplete,** paratrigeminal s. **Hughlings Jackson's s.,** Jackson-MacKenzie s. **Hunt's s.,** herpes zoster viral infection of the geniculate ganglion with involvement of the external ear and oral mucosa. Symptoms include facial paralysis; severe pain of the external auditory meatus and pinna *(geniculate neuralgia);* vesicular eruption in the peritonsillar region, oropharynx, and tongue; decreased salivation; hoarseness; loss of sensation in the face; tinnitus; decreased lacrimation; hearing disorders; and vertigo. Called also *geniculate ganglion s., Ramsay Hunt s., herpes zoster auricularis,* and *herpes zoster oticus.* **Hunter's s.,** see *Hunter-Hurler s.* **Hunter-Hurler s.,** the name is applied to two distinct entities, but because of the many overlapping synonyms, both are described here: *Hurler's syndrome* (mucopolysaccharidosis I), transmitted as an autosomal dominant trait, is a systemic mucopolysaccharidosis marked by progressive physical and mental deterioration leading to death before the age of 10 years. The onset follows a few months of normal growth; the early symptoms include lumbar gibbus, stiff joints, and rhinitis. The cornea is usually clear at birth, but shortly thereafter becomes cloudy with an accumulation of gray punctate opacities in the substantia propria, often masking coexisting retinal degeneration. Dwarfism; hepatosplenomegaly due to deposits of mucopolysaccharides in the liver and spleen; hydrocephalus with prominent scalp veins, hypertelorism, flat nasal bridge, snub nose, wide nostrils, thick lips with the upper lip being especially long, and prominent tongue give the face a peculiar coarse appearance (gargoyle-like facies); noisy breathing; and respiratory infection appear later. Mental retardation becomes evident during the second year of life. Mucopolysaccharide deposits in the coronary arteries and heart valves may lead to congestive heart failure. Contractures, clawhand, broad stubby fingers, furrowed thick skin, lanugo, short neck, absence of sexual maturation in spite of apparently normal genitalia, vertebral and skeletal abnormalities, including kyphosis, genu valgum, coxa valga, pes planus, pes equinovarus, and funnel chest, congenital heart defects, and a number of other defects may be present. Oral abnormalities include enlarged maxillary anterior gingiva and alveolar process, small or peg-shaped anterior teeth, spacing between the teeth, delayed root formation, displacement of molars, short and broad mandible, shortening or absence of the ramus, and areas of bone destruction. *Hunter's syndrome* (mucopolysaccharidosis II), transmitted as an X-linked recessive trait, is similar in many respects, except that gibbus and corneal clouding are absent and the symptoms are generally milder, although corneal opacities may appear later in life. Retinitis pigmentosa, nodular skin lesions, hypertrichosis, papilledema, optic atrophy, progressive deafness, and pulmonary hypertension may be present. Death, usually from congestive heart failure, occurs during the third or fourth decade. Called also *gargoylism, Johnie McL.'s syndrome,* and *lipochondrodystrophy.* **Hurler's s.,** see *Hunter-Hurler s.* **Hurler's s., late,** Scheie's s. **Hutchinson-Gilford s.,** a form of progeria characterized by dwarfism in which children fail to gain weight and grow after apparently normal development during the first year of life. A large and prematurely bald head, small face, projecting eyes, absence of eyebrows, beaked nose, receding chin, narrow chest, protruding abdomen, atrophic pigmented skin, and absence of subcutaneous fat give the patients the appearance of premature senility. Arteriosclerosis,

arthritis, anginal attacks, and hemiplegia may also develop. The average age of death is 16 years. Called also *Gilford's s., progeria s.,* and *senilism s.* See also Souques-Charcot GERODERMA. **hydantoin s.,** fetal dydantoin s. **hyoid s.,** Eagle's s. **hyperglobulinemic purpura s.,** Waldenström's s. **hypertelorism-hypospadias s.,** Opitz's s. **hypertelorism-microtia-clefting s.,** a hereditary syndrome, possibly transmitted as an autosomal recessive trait, characterized by growth and mental retardation, hypertelorism, telecanthus, epicanthal folds, ear abnormalities, bifid nose or broad nasal tip, broad nasal root, concave nasal floor, cleft lip and palate, supernumerary teeth, large lips, microcephaly, short mandibular ramus, shortened upper facial height, decreased cranial flexure, abnormal articular surfaces of the occipital bone and first cervical vertebra, syndactyly, and hypoplasia of the thenar eminence. Called also *HMC s.* **hypertrophied frenulum s.,** congenital hypertrophy of the frenulum linguae, associated with pseudocleft of the upper lip, tongue, and palate, mental retardation, tremor, and syndactyly. It is believed to be transmitted as an autosomal dominant trait. **hypoglossia-hypodactyly s.,** aglossia-adactylia s. **hypomelia-hypotrichosis-facial hemangioma s.,** Roberts' s. **hypospadias-dysphagia s.,** G s. **hypotonia-hypomentia-hypogonadism-obesity s.,** Prader-Willi s. **Imerslund-Gräsbeck s.,** a chronic, relapsing, familial form of megaloblastic anemia in children, with the onset occurring any time between the ages of five months and four years. Pallor, weakness, irritability, dyspnea, fever, gastrointestinal disorders with diarrhea and vomiting, lack of appetite, glossitis, jaundice, heart murmurs, and proteinuria are the principal symptoms. Transient neurological disorders, pyoderma, hepatomegaly, hemorrhage, edema, and canities prematura may be present. Urinary tract abnormalities are frequently observed. A metabolic defect, possibly malabsorption of vitamin B_1, is suspected of being the etiologic factor. **inferior nucleus ruber s.,** a condition in which mesencephalic lesions obstruct branches of the paramedian arteries supplying the inferior nucleus ruber, with ipsilateral paralysis of the oculomotor and trochlear nerves and contralateral hemianesthesia. Called also *Claude's s.* and *rubrospinal cerebellar peduncle s.* **intestinal polyposis-cutaneous pigmentation s.,** Peutz-Jeghers s. **Jackson's s.,** Jackson-MacKenzie s. **Jackson-MacKenzie s.,** unilateral paralysis of the soft palate, pharynx, larynx, sternocleidomastoid muscles, tongue, and trapezius muscle as a result of dysfunction of the tenth, eleventh, and twelfth cranial nerves. It is due to cerebral or medullary lesions. *Tapia's syndrome* and *Schmidt's syndrome* are both variants. Called also *Hughlings Jackson's s., Jackson's s., MacKenzie's s., vagoaccessory-hypoglossal s.,* and *hemiplegia alternans hypoglossica.* **Jacobs' s.,** oculo-orogenital s. **Jacod's s.,** retrosphenoidal space s. **Jadassohn-Lewandowski s.,** PACHYONYCHIA congenita. **Jaffe-Lichtenstein s.,** a disease, usually becoming evident during childhood or adolescence, characterized by the development of circumscribed bone-forming fibrous tissue on one (monostotic form) or several (polyostotic form) bones, usually on the femur, tibia, ribs, or facial bones. The lesion usually contains spindle-cell fibrous tissue showing trabeculae of nonlamellar bones and some osteoclasts. About half the patients with the polyostotic form show skull lesions and 15 percent show lesions of the jaws. Fractures and severe deformities frequently occur. Skin pigmentation (café au lait spots) may be present. Called also *fibrous dysplasia of bone, osteitis fibrosa cystica,* and *osteofibrosis deformans juvenilis.* **Jansen's s.,** metaphyseal DYSOSTOSIS. **Jarcho-Levin s.,** a hereditary syndrome, transmitted as an autosomal recessive trait, in which affected children die in infancy. It consists of congenital short trunk, dwarfism, prominent occiput, peculiar facies, short neck with low-growing hair posteriorly, thoracic skeletal anomalies, protuberant abdomen, hernias of various sites, elongated extremities in relation to the trunk, long and thin fingers and toes, and hammer toes. Called also *occipitofacial-cervicothoracic–abdominodigital dysplasia* and *spondylothoracic dysplasia.* **jaw winking s.,** Gunn's s. **Johnie McL.'s s.,** Hunter-Hurler s. **jugular foramen s.,** Vernet's s. **KBG s.,** a syndrome of multiple abnormalities, probably transmitted as an autosomal dominant characteristic. The most common features include mental retardation, shortness of stature, wide biparietal diameter, brachycephaly, wide-arched maxilla with short alveolar ridge, macrodontia, oligodontia, hand abnormalities, syndactyly of the toes, costovertebral abnormalities, delayed bone maturation, and characteristic facies. The face is round with wide eyebrows and synophrys and, often, telecanthus and a short nose with a high bridge and anteverted nostrils; the philtrum is usually long and the upper lip is thin and bow-shaped. Mandibular spurs may be present. The skeletal abnormalities include brachycephaly, biparietal prominence, increased incidence of wormian bones, and cervical ribs. The syndrome has been designated with the original patient's initials. **kinky hair s.**, Menkes' s. **Klein-Waardenburg s.**, a hereditary syndrome, transmitted as an autosomal dominant trait, consisting of lateral displacement of the median canthi and lacrimal points; hyperplastic broad high nasal root; hyperplasia of the median portion of the eyebrows; partial or total heterochromia iridum; congenital deafness or partial (unilateral) deafness; and circumscribed albinism (white forelock). Vitiligo, pigmentary changes of the fundi, and blue irides in Negroes may also be seen. Oral changes may include mandibular prognathism, protruding lower lip, and cleft palate. See also Mende's SYNDROME. **Kleinschmidt's s.**, a type of influenzal infection which begins as acute phlegmonous epiglottitis and spreads to other organs as mediastinitis, pleurisy, pericarditis, and bronchopneumonia. The hematogenous dissemination of the pathogenic agent may result in meningitis, subcutaneous abscesses, and empyema of various joints. Called also *cherry-red epiglottitis* and *Haemophilus influenzae B laryngitis*. **Klinefelter's s.**, a chromosomal abnormality characterized chiefly by male hypogonadism and sterility. The classic form is the XXY syndrome, but variants, such as XXYY, XXXY, and XXXXY syndromes and mosaic patterns, such as XXY/XY, also exist. The XXY syndrome is characterized by small testes, aspermatogenesis, eunuchoid build with female pubic escutcheon, gynecomastia, elevated urinary gonadotropins, decreased 17-ketosteroids, and diminished facial hair. The most severe abnormalities occur in the XXXXY syndrome. They include mental retardation, hypotonia, small penis, cryptorchidism, small testes, and various bone defects. Orofacial abnormalities include microcephaly, ocular hypertelorism, myopia, strabismus, mongoloid palpebral fissures, epicanthus, and short neck with redundant skin on the posterior neck. The rounded face at birth disappears with age and is replaced by retarded midfacial growth with dish face and relative mandibular prognathism. Some patients with XXY and XXYY syndrome exhibit mandibular taurodontism and shovel-shaped incisors. **Klippel-Feil s.**, a congenital syndrome characterized by shortened neck, low hairline, and a reduced number of cervical vertebrae or multiple hemivertebrae fused into a single osseous mass. Associated abnormalities include webbing of the neck and torticollis; spina bifida, meningomyelocele, and syringomyelia; occipital bone defects, Sprengel's deformity, and cervical ribs; hydrocephalus and oxycephaly; scoliosis and lordosis; facial asymmetry, cleft palate, high palate, and micrognathia; mental retardation; deafness, strabismus and nystagmus; spastic quadriplegia; synkinesis and ataxia; anesthesia and paresthesia; and various muscle abnormalities. When associated with Bonnevie-Ulrich syndrome, it is known as *Nielsen's syndrome*. Called also *congenital webbed neck s.* and *brevicollis*. **Klippel-Feldstein s.**, familial hypertrophy of the cranial vault without apparent functional disorders. Called also *simple familial cranial hypertrophy*. **Klippel-Trenaunay-Weber s.**, a syndrome of unilateral hypertrophy of the skeletal and soft tissues, with angiomatosis, nevus flammeus, and varices of the skin. The vascular abnormalities are usually present at birth but may appear in infancy. The skin of the hypertrophied part is warm and may be round and thickened. The nevus flammeus may be located in the area supplied by the second branch of the trigeminal nerve and involve the soft and hard palate. Angiomatosis of the tongue and pharynx, hypertrophy of the orofacial structures, malocclusion, and hypertrophy of the gingiva may be present. Called also *angio-osteohypertrophy s.*, *Parkes Weber's s.*, *Weber's s.*, *hemangiectatic hypertrophy*, and *nevus hypertrophicus*. **Kniest's s.**, Kniest's DISEASE. **Kulenkampff-Tarnow s.**, a combination of spasmodic tension of the muscles of the neck, tongue, floor of the mouth, and pharynx, respiratory disorders, speech disorders, tachycardia, and hypertension, appearing during the first few days of chlorpromazine therapy. Called also *cervicolinguomasticatory s.* and *neck-face s.* **lacrimoauriculodentodigital s.**, a dominantly inherited syndrome of the lacrimal system, teeth, salivary glands, digits, ears, and genitourinary system. Lacrimal defects consist of hypoplasia of the puncta, canaliculus, and tear sac. The incisors are usually peg-shaped and the enamel tends to be dysplastic, with failure of tooth eruption in some cases; the salivary glands show lack of ducts and associated glands. Digital abnormalities usually include finger-like thumb, bifid thumb, polydactyly, preaxial digits, clinodactyly, and other defects. The ears are commonly malformed and deafness is common. Various genitourinary anomalies are noted. Called also *LADD s.* **LADD s.**, lacrimoauriculodentodigital s. **Lange's s.**, de Lange's s. **Langer-Giedion s.**, trichorhinophalangeal DYSPLASIA (2). **Larsen's s.**, a syndrome that seems to be transmitted both dominantly and recessively. It consists of flattened facies, with prominent forehead, depressed nasal bridge, and hyper-

telorism; bilateral dislocation of the elbows, hips, and knees; talipes equinovalgus or equinovarus; cylindrical fingers that do not taper normally; occasionally cleft palate or other palate abnormalities; and sometimes an associated failure of spinal segmentation. **lateral bulbar s.**, Wallenberg's s. **Lawrence's s.**, lipoatrophic DIABETES. **Lejeune's s.**, crying cat s. **lentiginopolypose digestive s.**, Peutz-Jeghers s. **Lenz-Majewski s.**, Lenz-Majewski DWARFISM. **LEOPARD s.**, an acronym for *L*entigines, *E*KG abnormalities, *O*cular hypertelorism, *P*ulmonary stenosis, *A*bnormalities of genitalia, *R*etardation of growth, and *D*eafness. The face is usually triangular, with bilateral bossing, ptosis of the eyelids, epicanthal folds, and low-set ears. Pterygium coli is common. Lentigines are usually found on the skin of the upper trunk and, less densely, on the face, scalp, soles, and genitalia. ECG abnormalities include prolonged P-R and QRS and abnormal P waves. Mental deficiency, mandibular prognathism, café-au-lait spots, unilateral renal and/or gonadal agenesis or hypoplasia, hypogonadism, hypospadias, hyposmia, and subaortic stenosis are occasionally associated. The syndrome is transmitted as an autosomal dominant trait with wide variability in expression, including lack of lentigines in some patients. Called also *multiple lentigines s.* **Leroy's s.**, a congenital syndrome, seemingly transmitted as an autosomal recessive trait, and consisting of retarded growth, high narrow forehead, inner epicanthic folds, low nasal bridge, anteverted nostrils, hypertrophy of the alveolar ridges, limitation of joint movement, kyphosis, broad wrists and fingers, thick tight skin, cavernous hemangiomas, and hepatosplenomegaly. Histologic findings include the presence of unusual cytoplasmic inclusions in the cultured fibroblasts. **Lesch-Nyhan s.**, an X-linked syndrome, consisting of hyperuricemia associated with choreoathetosis, mental retardation, cerebral palsy, and compulsive self-destructive biting of the lower lip; self-mutilation may also involve the upper lip and cheeks and the fingers and hands. The compulsive behavior is associated with faulty purine metabolism caused by a lack of hypoxanthine-guanine phosphoribosyltransferase. Called also *juvenile gout*. See also lip BITING. **Lhermitte-Cornil-Quesnel s.**, slowly progressive pyramidopallidal degeneration, marked by involuntary crying and laughing; hypertonus and rigidity of the locomotor, cervical, and facial muscles; dysarthria; aphonia; dysphagia; abduction of the muscles of the extremities, with the hands held in a position characteristic of paralysis agitans, but without the cogwheel phenomenon and with retention of strength. Inflammation of the basal ganglia and subthalamic region with deposits of calcium-iron salts in the anterior globus pallidus and dentate nucleus are found at autopsy. Called also *progressive pyramidopallidal degeneration*. **Lightwood's s.**, Lightwood-Albright s. **Lightwood-Albright s.**, a syndrome combining metabolic acidosis, hyperchloremia and an inability to acidify urine, hypercalciuria, and hypokalemia. It is attributed to excessive excretion of bicarbonates and an increase in the tubular reabsorption of chlorides. In infants, the symptoms include anorexia, constipation, failure to thrive, wasting, muscular hypotonia, nephrocalcinosis, and vomiting; in older children, the symptoms may be similar but may also include rickets, bone deformities, pathological fractures, and growth retardation. Called also *Butler-Albright s.*, *Butler-Lightwood-Albright s.*, *congenital hyperchloremic acidosis s.*, *Lightwood's s.*, *calcinosis infantum*, *congenital hyperchloremic acidosis*, *evolutive tubular nephropathy*, *idiopathic renal acidosis*, *nephrocalcinosis infantum*, *renal tubular acidosis with rickets*, and *rickets with renal tubular acidosis*. **Lignac s.**, **Lignac-Fanconi s.**, Abderhalden-Fanconi s. **lip pit–cleft lip or palate s.**, van der Woude's s. **lissencephaly s.**, agyria-pachygyria s. **Lobstein's s.**, a hereditary form of osteogenesis imperfecta, associated with blue sclera, transmitted as an autosomal dominant trait. Defects consisting of brittle bones with multiple fractures, spontaneous dislocations, and hypermobility of the joints appear during childhood and adolescence. The blue sclera is present at birth, and cataract, color blindness, and other ocular complications may also be present. Dentinogenesis imperfecta is a common feature. When associated with atrophy of the skin and zonular cataract it is known as *Blegvad-Hazthausen syndrome;* with osteosclerosis and deafness as *van der Hoeve's syndrome*. Called also *blue sclera s.*, *fragilitas ossium tarda*, and *osteogenesis imperfecta tarda*. See also Vrolik's s. **long face s.**, a dentofacial deformity characterized by a long face, with or without dental anterior bite. The upper third of the face is usually within normal limits, but the middle third shows a narrow nose, narrow alar bases, prominent nasal dorsum, and depressed paranasal areas. The lower third usually shows excessive exposure of the maxillary anterior teeth with the lips in repose, exposure of maxillary teeth and gingiva upon smiling, lip incompetency, a retropositioned chin, normal or obtuse nasolabial angle, and long lower third facial height. Class II malocclusion may be associated; a high constricted palatal vault with a large distance between the root apices and the nasal floor and a steep mandibular plane are consistently present. Called also *excessive vertical maxillary height, high angle type, hyperdivergent face, idiopathic long face, long face, skeletal open bite,* and *vertical maxillary excess.* **Louis-Bar s.,** ATAXIA telangiectasia. **Lowry's s.,** a syndrome of craniosynostosis and fibular aplasia, probably transmitted as an autosomal recessive trait. Clinical findings may include a peculiar facies with prominent eyes, low-set ears, short webbed neck, cryptorchidism, short sternum, pilonidal dimple, wormian bones, large posterior fontanelle, and other abnormalities. **Lubarsch's s.,** primary systematized amyloidosis characterized by macroglossia and extensive deposits of amyloid in the skin, tongue, heart, stomach, intestine, and skeletal muscles, with the liver, kidneys, and adrenals being spared. The presence of Bence Jones protein and atypical plasma cells in the bone marrow indicate a relationship to myeloma. **Lyell's s.,** toxic epidermal NECROLYSIS. **3-M s.,** a syndrome that appears to be hereditary, and is suspected of being transmitted as an autosomal recessive trait. It is characterized by low birth weight, proportionate dwarfism, hatchet facies, triangular face, frontal bossing, orodental abnormalities, pointed or pinched mouth and chin, prominent ears, short neck with prominent trapezius, high square shoulders, short thorax, pectus carinatum or excavatum, transverse grooves on the anterior chest, diatasis recti, winging of the scapulae, short fifth fingers, and hyperextensibility of the joints. Orodontal abnormalities usually include V-shaped dental arch, anterior crowding of the teeth, dental caries, malocclusion, and absence of lower second molars. It is similar to Bloom's syndrome and Russell-Silver syndrome. Its name is derived from the first letter of three of the authors' last names (Miller, McKusick, and Malvaux). Called also *MMM s.* **McCune-Albright s.,** Albright's s. (1). **McDonough's s.,** a hereditary syndrome believed to be transmitted as an autosomal recessive trait with minor manifestations in heterozygotes, which combines mental retardation, congenital heart defects, sternal deformity, kyphosis, and craniofacial abnormalities consisting of anteverted auricles, upward slanted palpebral fissures, and squint. **MacKenzie s.,** Jackson-MacKenzie s. **macroglobulinemia s.,** Waldenström's MACROGLOBULINEMIA. **macroglossia-omphalocele s.,** Beckwith-Wiedemann s. **Majewski's s.,** a congenital syndrome characterized by hydropic appearance at birth, narrow thorax, protuberant abdomen, short extremities, polysyndactyly, brachydactyly, short and flat nose, low-set deformed ears, cleft lip and palate, hypoplastic epiglottis, kidney cysts, and cardiovascular and genital abnormalities. Called also *short rib-polydactyly s.* **Marchesani's s.,** a hereditary syndrome, transmitted as an autosomal recessive trait, characterized by brachydactyly, small stature, broad skull, small shallow orbits, mild maxillary hypoplasia, narrow palate, small spherical lens, myopia with or without glaucoma, frequent ectopia lentis, occasional blindness, malformed and malaligned teeth, and cardiac abnormalities in some cases. Called also *brachydactyly-spherophakia s.* and *Weill-Marchesani s.* **Marchiafava-Micheli s.,** a rare disorder, occurring in both sexes, usually in the third decade of life, and marked by chronic hemolytic anemia, with attacks of nocturnal paroxysmal hemoglobinuria that may be precipitated by infection, menstruation, blood transfusion, surgery, vaccination, injection of liver extracts, or administration of iron salts. Weakness, abdominal and lumbar pain, jaundice, with pallor and yellowish discoloration of the skin and mucous membranes, heart murmurs, splenomegaly, and hemosiderinuria are the principal features. Hemolytic crisis also may occur. Pathological findings include systemic venous or portal thrombosis, normoblastic bone marrow hyperplasia, hepatomegaly with necrosis, hemosiderosis, and large iron deposits in the kidneys. Called also *Marchiafava's hemolytic anemia,* and *paroxysmal nocturnal hemoglobinuria.* **Marcus Gunn's s.,** Gunn's s. **Marden-Walker s.,** a congenital syndrome, believed to be transmitted as an autosomal recessive trait, combining failure to thrive, motor and mental retardation, and multiple abnormalities in the form of peculiar facies due to blepharophimosis, blepharoptosis, hypoplastic mandible, and low-set ears, associated with poor muscle

mass, mild congenital joint contractures, pigeon breast, kyphoscoliosis, and arachnodactyly. Cleft palate and cardiac and renal abnormalities may be present. **Marfan's s.,** a syndrome of arachnodactyly, ectopia lentis, and cardiovascular defects, associated with abnormally elongated and thin long bones, disproportionately long extremities, spider fingers, dolichocephaly, high-arched palate, hyperextensibility of joints, pectus excavatum or pectus carinatum, kyphosis or scoliosis, flatfoot, habitual dislocations, and arthrogryposis. Cleft palate or bifid uvula occurs in some cases. The teeth may be long and narrow and malocclusion is common. Lens dislocation may be combined with myopia, strabismus, blue sclera, and nystagmus. The cardiovascular defects usually include aortic aneurysm, heart enlargement, valvular defects, cystic necrosis of the aorta, and aortic regurgitation. It is inherited as an autosomal dominant trait. Called also *arachnodactyly, congenital mesodermal dystrophy, dolichostenomelia, hyperchondroplasia,* and *spider fingers.* **Marie-Sainton s.,** cleidocranial DYSPLASIA. **Maroteaux-Lamy s.,** 1. hereditary systemic mucopolysaccharidosis, transmitted as an autosomal recessive trait, characterized by dwarfism of the trunk and extremities, genu valgum, lumbar kyphosis, anterior sternal protrusion, stiff joints, hepatosplenomegaly, corneal opacities, varying degree of deafness due to recurrent otitis media, and peculiar facies with thick lips and enlarged nose. Radiological examination shows defects of the metaphyses and epiphyses, retarded growth of the carpal and tarsal bones, flattening of the vertebrae, and a wedgelike deformity of the lumbar and thoracic vertebrae. Both polymorphonuclear inclusions and lymphocytic inclusions are found in the blood, and excessive amounts of chondroitin sulfate B in the urine. Called also *mucopolysaccharidosis VI.* 2. a syndrome, probably transmitted as an autosomal recessive trait, consisting of dwarfism, delayed closure of the fontanelles, dysplasia of the skull, hypoplasia of the maxilla and mandible, flattened mandibular angle, cortical density of the bones, predisposition to fractures, short digits with wrinkled skin and nails which override the hypoplastic distal phalanges, partial anodontia, and partial deafness. Frontal bossing, dental caries, double row of teeth, blue sclerae, kyphosis, scoliosis, and mental retardation also may occur. Called also *pyknodysostosis.* **Marshall's s.,** a hereditary syndrome, transmitted as an autosomal dominant trait, characterized by saddle nose, sensorineural hearing loss, high grade myopia, and cataracts. Esotropia, hypertropia, and secondary glaucoma may occur. Radiographic examination may show hypertelorism, enlarged frontal sinuses, small nasal bones, small maxilla, with protruding upper incisors, short ascending ramus of the mandible, dural calcifications, and narrow auditory canals. Hypodontia and hypohidrosis may be present. **Martin-Albright s.,** pseudohypoparathyroidism. **Martin de Gimard's s.,** de Gimard's s. **maxillofacial s.,** maxillofacial DYSOSTOSIS. **maxillonasal s.,** Binder's s. **May-Hegglin s.,** May-Hegglin ANOMALY. **MCA/MR s.,** multiple congenital anomaly/mental retardation s. **median cleft face s.,** frontonasal DYSPLASIA. **Melkersson-Rosenthal s.,** a syndrome, usually beginning during childhood or adolescence, consisting of recurrent facial paralysis and edema, cheilitis granulomatosa with swelling of the lips, and fissured tongue, often associated with migraine. Macroglossia, thickening of the gingiva, leukoplakia of the hard palate, and development of carcinoma may occur. **Melnick-Needles s.,** a hereditary syndrome, transmitted as an autosomal dominant trait, characterized by craniofacial abnormalities consisting of exophthalmos, full cheeks, micrognathia, malalignment of teeth, and high and narrow forehead; bowing of the humerus and tibia with cubitus valgus and genu valgum; and slight shortening of the distal phalanges, most notably of the thumbs. Called also *osteodysplasty.* **Mende's s.,** a congenital familial syndrome similar to Klein-Waardenburg syndrome, consisting of pigmentation disorders, chiefly partial albinism of the scalp, including white forelock and facial and pubic hair, in association with mongoloid habitus and deaf-mutism. Cleft palate, mandibular prognathism, protruding lower lip, external ear abnormalities, and ocular complications may be present. **Ménière's s.,** Ménière's DISEASE. **Menkes' s., Menkes' kinky hair s., Menkes' steely hair s.,** an inborn disorder of copper metabolism, transmitted as a sex-linked recessive trait. It is characterized by peculiar stubby hair, mental retardation, hypothermia, focal cerebral and cerebellar degeneration, widespread arterial tortuosity, convulsions, growth retardation, widening of the metaphyses with formation of lateral spurs which fracture or become fragmented suggesting child abuse, and peculiar facies marked by pallor, lack of expressive movements, pudgy appearance of the cheeks, and horizontal or twisted eyebrows. Low levels of serum copper and ceruloplasmin are present. Called also *kinky hair s., steely hair s.,* and *kinky hair disease.* **Meyenburg-Altherr-Uehlinger** s., chronic atrophic POLYCHONDRITIS. **Meyer-Schwickerath and Weyers s.**, oculodento-osseous DYSPLASIA. **micrognathia-glossoptosis s.**, Robin's ANOMALAD. **microphthalmos s.**, oculodento-osseous DYSPLASIA. **midline cleft s.**, a syndrome of multiple abnormalities, transmitted as an autosomal dominant trait, combining mental retardation; microcephaly; craniofacial anomalies, including cleft lip and anterior cleft palate, hypotelorism, and antimongoloid slant of palpebral fissures; skeletal anomalies, particularly of the foot and spine; and chronic constipation. **Miescher's s.**, familial acanthosis nigricans with progressive evolution of symptoms until the age of 10 years, followed by spontaneous involution, in combination with developmental disorders, including infantilism, mental retardation, cutis verticis gyrata, dental deformities, and diabetes mellitus. **Mikulicz's s.**, bilateral hypertrophy of the lacrimal and salivary glands, associated with xerostomia and decreased or absent lacrimation, which may be caused by tuberculosis, leukemia, lymphosarcoma, poisoning, sarcoidosis, syphilis, or gout. The onset may be associated with upper respiratory tract infection, oral infection, or tooth extraction. Some authorities feel that this disorder and Sjögren's syndrome are identical, but others suggest that it should be considered a separate entity because it does not include rheumatoid arthritis. **milk alkali s.**, a syndrome associated with prolonged excessive intake of milk and absorable alkali, characterized by hypercalcemia without hypercalciuria or hypophosphatemia, normal serum alkaline phosphatase, renal insufficiency with azotemia, mild alkalosis, and calcinosis. Clinical manifestations include dry mouth, anorexia, dizziness, pruritus, polyuria, and manifestations of renal insufficiency. Restriction of milk and alkali intake is usually followed by improvement. Called also *alkalosis s.*, *Burnett's s.*, and *milk poisoning*. **Millard's s.**, Millard-Gubler s. **Millard-Guber s.**, unilateral softening arising from obstruction of the blood vessels of the pons, involving the sixth and seventh cranial nerves and fibers of the corticospinal tract, and associated with paralysis of the abducens and facial nerves and contralateral hemiplegia of the extremities. The muscles of the ipsilateral side of the face are paralyzed, and there is paralysis of outward movement of the eye. If, in addition, there is paralysis of inward movement of the eye, it is known as *Foville's syndrome*. Called also *Millard's s.*, *abducens-facial hemiplegia alternans*, *Gubler's hemiplegia*, *Gubler's paralysis*, *hemiplegia alternans inferior*, and *middle alternating hemiplegia*. **Minkowski-Chauffard s.**, hereditary SPHEROCYTOSIS. **MLNS**, mucocutaneous lymph node s. **MMM s.**, 3-M s. **Möbius' s.**, congenital facial DIPLEGIA. **Mohr's s.**, oral-facial-digital s. (2). **Møller-Christenson's s.**, atrophy of the anterior nasal spine, defects of the pyriform aperture, and atrophy of the maxillary anterior alveolar process developing in advanced cases of lepromatous leprosy. **Morquio's s.**, Morquio-Ullrich s., Morquio's DISEASE. **Mosse's s.**, polycythemia vera associated with liver cirrhosis. Called also *Mosse's polycythemia*. **mucocutaneous lymph node s.**, a disease of unknown etiology, usually affecting infants and young children, which has occurred in significant numbers in Japan since 1960 and, more recently, been reported in North America. It is characterized chiefly by fever, rash, leukocytosis, and cervical lymphadenitis, and complications may include coronary disease, usually aneurysm, with myocardial infarction and death. The fever has a characteristic spiking pattern lasting for at least one to three weeks. Conjunctival involvement, consisting mainly of discrete engorgement of the bulbar conjunctival vessels, is always present. Oral changes include dryness, erythema, and mild fissuring of the lips. The oropharyngeal mucosa is diffusely and deeply erythematous; the tongue assumes an appearance like that of strawberry tongue. The hands and feet become indurated, the skin developing a woody firmness suggestive of scleroderma, and the palms and soles become erythematous, having a deep purple-red or magenta color. An erythematous rash usually occurs, and lymphadenopathy with enlarged nodes in the cervical region is a constant feature. Abbreviated *MLNS*. **mucocutaneous-ocular s.**, Fuchs' s. **multiple congenital anomaly/mental retardation s.**, any syndrome that combines multiple congenital abnormalities and mental retardation. Abbreviated *MCA/MR s.* **multiple lentigines s.**, LEOPARD s. **s. of multiple mucosal neuromas**, multiple mucosal NEUROMAS. **multiple nevoid basal cell carcinoma s.**, Gorlin's s. **Münchmeyer's s.**, progressive myositis ossificans; see under MYOSITIS. **Murk Jansen's s.**, metaphyseal DYSOSTOSIS. **myofacial pain-dysfunction s.**, a disorder of the temporomandibular joint associated with restriction of jaw movement, pain, and eating difficulty. Principal manifestations include pain of the temporomandibular joint, which may either be spontaneous or occur with mastication disorders, otalgia, pain of the mastoid process, neck, and facial region, and headache. Articular crepitus and spasm of the temporal, mas-

seter, and lateral pterygoid muscles are usually associated. Occlusal disharmonies are the usual cause, but neoplasms may also play an etiologic role. **N s.**, a hereditary syndrome transmitted as either an autosomal recessive or an X-linked recessive trait. It combines mental and growth retardation, visual disorders, deafness, dolichocephaly, hypotelorism, scalloped and laterally overlapping upper eyelids, large corneas, abnormal ear auricles, dental dysplasia, generalized skeletal dysplasia, high fingerprint ridge count, cryptorchidism, hypospadias, and spasticity. **Naegeli's s.**, a hereditary syndrome, transmitted as an autosomal dominant trait, and marked by pigmentation similar to that seen in Bloch-Sulzberger syndrome. The symptoms include hypohidrosis, keratosis palmaris et plantaris, dental abnormalities, papillitis, optic atrophy, pseudoglioma, strabismus, and nystagmus. Dental manifestations include chiefly yellowish flecks over surfaces of the teeth. In contrast to Bloch-Sulzberger syndrome, it occurs in both males and females, and it does not include the inflammatory phase. Some authorities feel that the term *incontinentia pigmenti* should be reserved for Bloch-Sulzberger syndrome. Called also *Franceschetti-Jadassohn s.*, *melanophoric nevus*, and *Naegeli's incontinentia pigmenti*. **naevoid basal cell carcinoma s.**, Gorlin's s. **Nager-de Reynier s.**, DYSOSTOSIS mandibularis. **neck-face s.**, Kulenkampff-Tarnow s. **Neill-Dingwall s.**, Cockayne's s. **nephrotic s.**, see NEPHROSIS. **s. of neural crest**, Brown's s. **neurouveoparotitis s.**, Heerfordt's s. **nevoid basal-cell carcinoma s.**, Gorlin's s. **Nielsen's s.**, a condition that combines the symptoms of Bonnevie-Ullrich syndrome and Klippel-Feil syndrome. Called also *dystrophia brevicollis congenita*. **Noonan's s.**, a congenital syndrome characterized by growth and mental retardation; seizures; craniofacial abnormalities, consisting of blepharoptosis, antimongoloid slant of palpebral fissures, inner epicanthal folds, hypertelorism, prominent and fleshy, low-set abnormal ears, high-arched palate, micrognathia, and tooth abnormalities, including malocclusion; neck abnormalities, such as a short or webbed neck and low posterior hairline; shield chest with wide-set nipples; cardiovascular defects; and limb defects, such as cubitus valgus, short stubby hands, and clinodactyly of the fifth fingers. Nerve deafness, kyphoscoliosis, edema of the hands and feet, simian creases, curly hair, skin nevi, keloids, hyperelastic skin, and hypogonadism may be associated. Most cases are sporadic, but an autosomal dominant inheritance has been indicated in some cases. Called also *Turner-like s.* See also *Bonnevie-Ullrich s.* **nucleus amgiguus-hypoglossal s.**, Tapia's s. **oculoauriculovertebral s.**, a syndrome whose principal features include epibulbar dermoid cysts, auricular appendices, pretragal blind fistulae, various vertebral abnormalities, anomalous ribs, and neurological complications, including mental retardation. Ocular complications include conjunctival dermoids and/or lipodermoids, colobomas, and microphthalmia. The skull may be somewhat asymmetric, with frontal bossing, hemifacial microsomia associated with hypoplasia or aplasia of the mandibular ramus and/or condyle, unilateral facial hypoplasia, antimongoloid lid obliquity, macrostomia, low anterior hairline, and atresia of the nostrils. Called also *Goldenhar's s.*, *mandibulofacial dysostosis with epibulbar dermoids*, *oculoauricular dysplasia*, and *oculoauriculovertebral dysplasia (OAV)*. **oculocerebrofacial s.**, a syndrome, transmitted as an autosomal recessive trait, combining mental retardation, microcephaly, mongoloid slant of palpebral fissures, microcornea, strabismus, myopia, optic atrophy, high-arched palate, preauricular skin tags, and small mandible. **oculodentodigital s.**, oculodentodigital dysplasia s., oculodento-osseous dysplasia s., oculodento-osseous DYSPLASIA. **oculo-orogenital s.**, a deficiency disease observed in American prisoners of war in Japanese camps during World War II; more than 75 percent of 8000 Americans after six months of an inadequate rice diet were affected. It is characterized by exfoliating dermatitis of the scrotum, stomatitis, and conjunctivitis, and is thought to be closely associated with pellagra, but is not pellagra per se. It is possibly a result of deficiency of a specific component of the vitamin B complex. Called also *Jacob's s.* and *orogenital s.* **oculosympathetic s.**, Bernard-Horner s. **oculourethroarticular s.**, Reiter's DISEASE. **ODD s.**, oculodento-osseous DYSPLASIA. **OFD I s.**, oral-facial-digital s. (1). **OFD II s.**, oral-facial-digital s. (2). **Opalski's s.**, a combination of pain and temperature hypoesthesia of the face, Bernard-Horner syndrome, and pyramidal paralysis of the extremities on one side of the body, associated with contralateral pain and temperature hypoesthesia of the trunk and extremities. A focal lesion of the sub-bulbar region, involving the spinal segment of the trigeminal nerve, the cerebellospinal zone, and the pyramidal tract, resulting from circulatory disorders of the posterior spinal artery, is the suspected cause. The symptoms of this syndrome are also seen in *Wallenberg's syndrome.* Called also *sub-bulbar s.* **Opitz's s.,** a hereditary syndrome, inherited as an autosomal dominant trait, characterized by ocular hypertelorism and hypospadias in males and only hypertelorism in females. Widow's peak, cryptorchidism, and hernias are usually associated, and mental deficiency, cardiovascular defects, and cleft lip and/or palate occur occasionally.. Called also *hypertelorism-hypospadias s.* **Opitz's trigonocephaly s.,** a syndrome of multiple abnormalities, consisting of a narrow forehead, ridged skull or overriding cranial sutures, hair whorls on the forehead, mongoloid palpebral slant, epicanthic folds, strabismus, short and broad nose, wide mouth, short receding chin, high palate, wide alveolar ridge, attached frenulum, posteriorly rotated ears, short neck, wide-set nipples, short sternum, short limbs, polydactyly, joint dislocation, crepitation, dorsiflexed first toe, ulnar deviation, bridged palmar creases, hemangiomata, redundant skin, syndactyly, deep sacral dimple, neonatal jaundice, and cardiac, renal, and genital defects. Called also *C. s.* and *Opitz's s.* **Opitz-Frias s.,** G s. **oral-facial-digital s.,** 1. a hereditary complex of symptoms characterized by constrictive frena of the upper and lower vestibular sulci that cleave the mandible and maxillary alveolar processes; clefts of the tongue and palate; pseudocleft of the upper lip; dental anomalies, including supernumerary canines and absence of the lower lateral incisors; and finger abnormalities, including osteoporosis, camptodactyly, and syndactyly. Less common are polydactyly, alopecia and dryness of the scalp, seborrheic changes of the facial skin and milia, hypoplasia of columella and alar nasal cartilage, benign tumors of the tongue, lateral palatal tori, mucous pits of the lower lip, dystopia, canthorum and epicanthus, mental retardation, and trembling. Transmission as an incomplete recessive trait was suggested in earlier cases, but it is now believed to be transmitted as an X-linked dominant trait affecting both sexes but lethal to males. *Grob's syndrome* is a variant. Called also *OFD I s., Papillon-Léage* and *Psaume s., dysplasia linguofacialis,* and *orodigitofacial dysostosis.* 2. a congenital syndrome, transmitted as an autosomal recessive trait, consisting of orofacial and digital abnormalities, associated with skeletal defects and conductive deafness and malformed incus. Orofacial abnormalities include lobate tongue, midline cleft of the lip, high-arched or cleft palate, hypertrophied frenula, broad nasal root, broad and bifid nasal tip, dystopia canthorum, micrognathia, and hypoplasia of the zygomatic arch and maxilla. Digital abnormalities include bilateral reduplicated hallux, broad and duplicated medial cuneiform bones, short and broad naviculars and first metatarsals, and brachydactyly, syndactyly, clinodactyly, or polydactyly. Skeletal defects include moderately short stature and metaphyseal irregularity and flaring. Called also *Mohr's s.* and *OFD II s.* **orbital floor s.,** a condition characterized by orbital floor lesions associated with exophthalmos, diplopia, superior maxillary pain, and numbness along the trigeminal nerve branches. Called also *Dejean's s.* **orogenital s.,** oculo-orogenital s. **Ortner's s.,** an association of heart diseases with laryngeal paralysis, due to compression of the recurrent laryngeal nerve. Called also *cardiovocal s.* **otodental** DYSPLASIA. **otopalatodigital s.,** a congenital syndrome combining bone dysplasia, dwarfism, cleft palate, peculiar facies, deafness, and mental retardation. The facial abnormalities include frontal and occipital prominence with a thick frontal bone and thick base of the skull having a steep nasobasal angulation, absence of the frontal and sphenoid sinuses, facial bone dysplasia, hypertelorism, small nose and mouth, and lateral fullness of the supraorbital ridges. Cleft palate, small trunk, pectus excavatum, failure of neural arch fusion, small iliac crest, limited elbow extension, bowing tibia, short broad distal phalanges of thumbs and toes, short nails, short metacarpals, fusion of the hamate and capitate bones, and an accessory ossification center at the base of the second metatarsal are usually associated. Males are severely affected, the syndrome being transmitted as an X-linked semidominant trait; females show mild to almost full expression. Called also *Taybi's s.* **Owren's s.,** 1. hemolytic CRISIS. 2. parahemophilia. **4p s.,** Wolf-Hirschhorn s. **Papillon-Léage and Psaume s.,** oral-facial-digital s. (1). **Papillon-Lefèvre s.,** hyperkeratosis palmaris et plantaris associated with periodontoclasia and premature exfoliation of the teeth. The initial skin lesions usually occur between the ages of one and four years. The periodontosis becomes

evident as soon as the last deciduous tooth has erupted; horizontal bone destruction begins, and the teeth become involved in the sequence in which they erupt. It is inherited in an autosomal recessive mode. **parahemophilia s.,** parahemophilia. **paratrigeminal s.,** a transitory syndrome resembling Bernard-Horner syndrome, most commonly affecting males, usually in the fifth decade, and is due to interruption of the sympathetic pathways. It is characterized by the sudden onset of ptosis and miosis, associated with severe unilateral headache, usually located in and around the eye, or pain in the area of trigeminal distribution. Called also *Raeder's s.* and *incomplete Horner's s.* **parent-infant traumatic stress s.,** battered CHILD. **Parkes Weber's s.,** Klippel-Trenaunay-Weber s. **Parry-Romberg s.,** facial HEMIATROPHY. **partial deletion of chromosome 13 s.,** chromosome 13, partial deletion s. **partial deletion of long arm of chromosome 11 s.,** chromosome 11q s., partial deletion. **partial 12p monosomy s.,** chromosome 12p s., partial deletion. **partial deletion of short arm of chromosome 4 s.,** Wolf-Hirschhorn s. **partial deletion of short arm of chromosome 5 s.,** crying cat s. **partial deletion of short arm of chromosome 12 s.,** chromosome 12p s., partial deletion. **partial duplication 7q s.,** 7q trisomy, partial; see under TRISOMY. **partial duplication 10p s.,** 10p TRISOMY. **partial duplication 10q s.,** 10q TRISOMY. **partial duplication 11p s.,** 11p TRISOMY. **partial duplication 11q s.,** 11q TRISOMY. **partial duplication 14q s.,** 14q TRISOMY. **partial duplication 15q s.,** 15q TRISOMY. **partial duplication 20p s.,** 20p TRISOMY. **Passow's s.,** an association of Bernard-Horner syndrome with heterochromia iridis. **Patau's s.,** trisomy 13 caused usually by primary nondisjunction and, less frequently, by translocation and mosaicism. Birth weight is about 2500 gm; life expectancy is seldom more than 10 years, most infants dying during the first three months of life. It is characterized by multiple abnormalities of the head, brain, ears, eyes, cardiovascular system, spleen, reproductive system, pancreas, and other organs. Microcephaly, sloping forehead, wide sagittal suture and fontanelles, arhinencephaly, cebocephaly, premaxillary agenesis, microphthalmia, single umbilical artery, umbilical hernia, hyperconvex narrow fingernails, capillary hemangiomas, and scalp defects are the most common anomalies. Orofacial defects may include micrognathia and cleft lip and palate. Breath-holding spells, seizures, mental retardation, hypertonicity, deafness, and feeding difficulties are the most common symptoms. Hematological features may include the presence of large amounts of fetal hemoglobin in the blood and sessile and pedunculated nuclear projections in neutrophilic leukocytes. Called also *chromosome 13 s., trisomy 13 s.,* and *trisomy D*$_1$. **Paterson and Brown Kelly s., Paterson-Kelly s.,** Plummer-Vinson s. **peculiar facies–vascular stenoses s.,** elfin facies s. **peduncular s.,** Foville's s. **penta X s.,** XXXXX s. **periodontal s.,** see PERIODONTOSIS. **Petges-Cléjat s.,** poikilodermatomyositis. **Peutz-Jeghers s.,** a hereditary syndrome, transmitted as an autosomal dominant trait, characterized by gastrointestinal polyposis and mucocutaneous pigmentation. Cutaneous pigmentation is usually concentrated about the facial orifices; it may fade after puberty. Mucous lesions, usually of the labial and buccal mucosae, tend to be large and are usually permanent. Complications may include colic, anemia, and intussusception. Called also *intestinal polyposis-cutaneous pigmentation s., lentiginopolypose digestive s.,* and *melanoplakia–small intestinal polyposis.* **Pfeiffer's s.,** a syndrome of craniosynostosis, broad thumbs and great toes, and partial soft tissue syndactyly of the hands and feet. Turribrachycephaly, cranial asymmetry, hydrocephalus, Kleeblattschädel anomaly, Arnold-Chiari malformation, maxillary hypoplasia, relative mandibular prognathism, depressed nasal bridge, beaked nose, ocular hypertelorism, antimongoloid palpebral slant, proptosis, strabismus, high-arched palate, broad alveolar ridges, class III malocclusion, crowded teeth, and epilepsy may occur. Intelligence is usually normal, but mental retardation has been observed in some cases. Supernumerary teeth, gingival hypertrophy, pyloric stenosis, malposed anus, choanal atresia, cryptorchidism, renal abnormalities, congenital heart defects, and a variety of other abnormalities may occur. It has been observed in three generations by Pfeiffer; other pedigrees consistent with autosomal dominant transmission were observed by others; and sporadic cases have been reported. Called also *acrocephalopolysyndactyly type I, Noack's acrocephalosyndactyly* and *Pfeiffer's acrocephalosyndactyly.* See also *Saethre-Chotzen s.* **pharyngolaryngeal paralysis s.,** Collet-Sicard s. **PHC s.,** Böök s. **Pierre Robin's s.,** Robin's ANOMALAD. **Pietrantoni's s.,** mucosal and cutaneous zones of anesthesia and neuralgia of the face and oral cavity, observed in paranasal tumors. **Plummer-Vinson s.,** a syndrome occurring chiefly in middle-aged women suffering from vitamin B deficiency and iron-deficiency anemia. Principal symptoms include cracks or fissures at the corners of the mouth, painful tongue which has a shiny smooth appearance, atrophy of the filiform and later the fungiform papillae, and dysphagia resulting from stenosis or webs of the esophageal mucosa. Lemon-tinted pallor of the skin; spoon-shaped and brittle nails; atrophy and lack of normal keratinization of the mucous membrane of the mouth and esophagus, which often results in carcinoma of the oral cavity, hypopharynx, and upper respiratory tract; and other symptoms of iron deficiency anemia are usually present. Ocular changes may include fissures in the corners of the eyes, blepharoconjunctivitis, keratitis, and hemeralopia. Histological features are similar to those seen in iron deficiency anemia. Called also *Paterson and Brown Kelly s., Paterson-Kelly s., sideropenic s., Paterson-Kelly webs,* and *sideropenic dysphagia.* **Pompe's s.,** GLYCOGENOSIS II. **popliteal pterygium s.,** 1. popliteal web s. 2. Fèvre-Languepin s. **popliteal web s.,** a congenital syndrome consisting chiefly of popliteal webs, cleft palate, lower lip pits, and dysplasia of the toe nails. A wide variety of other abnormalities may be associated, including cleft lip, oral frenula, webs between the eyelids, syndactyly of the fingers and toes, aplasia of the fingers, valgus deformities, hypoplasia of the tibia, bifid or absent patella, hypoplasia of the labia majora, mental retardation, and inguinal hernia. Autosomal dominant inheritance has been demonstrated. Called also *popliteal pterygium s.* **Portsmouth s.,** a hemorrhagic syndrome characterized by platelet dysfunction with generally a prolonged bleeding time, reduced platelet adhesiveness, and an abnormal or absent collagen induced platelet aggregation by normal exogenous ADP-induced platelet aggregation. Named for Portsmouth, England because of the research done there. **postaxial polydactyly–dental–vertebral s.,** a hereditary syndrome either occurring alone as an isolated trait or in association with other abnormalities; it is usually dominantly inherited. It combines craniofacial abnormalities (abnormal ears, webbed neck, low posterior hairline, epicanthus, mandibular prognathism); oral defects (bifid uvula, fusion macrodontia, hypodontia, enamel hypoplasia, dens-in-dente, short roots); cardiovascular disorders; pyelonephritis; hydronephrosis; hand abnormalities (postaxial polydactyly, large lunate bones, brachydactyly); and feet anomalies (postaxial polydactyly, broad toes, syndactyly of the second and third toes). **posterior cervical sympathetic s.,** Barré-Liéou s. **posterior inferior cerebellar artery s.,** Wallenberg's s. **posterior laterocondylar space s.,** Collet-Sicard s. **posterior retroparotid space s.,** Villaret's s. **posttransfusion s.,** cytomegalic inclusion disease due to transfusion of blood contaminated with cytomegalovirus. **Potter's s.,** Potter's DISEASE. **Prader-Willi s.,** a syndrome combining mental retardation, short stature, muscular hypotonia, small hands and feet, obesity, cryptorchidism, and hypogonadism. Associated abnormalities may include ocular hypertelorism, epicanthus, and strabismus; low-set ears and overlapping helix; high-arched palate, micrognathia, microdontia, dental caries, and defective dental enamel; and acromicria and clinodactyly. Most cases have been reported in males. When associated with diabetes mellitus it is known as *Royer's syndrome.* Called also *HHHO s.* and *hypotonia-hypomentia-hypogonadism-obesity s.* **premenstrual salivary s.,** Racine's s. **private s.,** a hereditary malformation syndrome usually occurring in a single individual or members of a single family, in which there is an apparently unique chromosome rearrangement, whereby the probability of occurrence of the same type of arrangement in several families is remote. See also *provisionally private s.* Cf. *public s.* **progeria s.,** Hutchinson-Gilford s. **progeria-like s.,** Cockayne's s. **provisionally private s.,** a hereditary malformation syndrome occurring in two or more siblings, of nonconsanguineous parents and with an apparently normal karyotype in both the patients and parents. It is probably due to a chromosome abnormality that is not detectable with present methods, or a segregating gene mutation. See also *private s.* Cf. *public s.* **pseudo-Crouzon s.,** see *Saethre-Chotzen s.* **pseudothalidomide s.,** Roberts' s. **pterygolymphangiectasia s.,** Bonnevie-Ullrich s. **pterygopalatine s.,** sphenopalatine NEURALGIA. **public s.,** a hereditary malformation syndrome due to a relatively common chromosomal rearrangement which recurs with a specific frequency in a population. Cf. *private s.* and *provisionally private s.* **Puretić's s.,** Puretić-Ishikawa s. **Puretić-Ishikawa s.,** an autosomal recessively inherited syndrome of systemic hyalinosis. It is characterized by contractures of the joints, muscle and/or joint pain, coarse facies, relative macrocephaly, gingival hypertrophy, growth retardation resulting in short stature, osteoporosis, osteolysis of the terminal phalanges, swollen fingers, multiple large subcutaneous nodes, dysseborrheic and sclerodermiform atrophic skin changes, dyspigmentation, and recurrent suppurative infections of the skin, eyes, nose, and ears. Called also *Puretić's s.* **Pyle's s.,** metaphyseal DYSPLASIA. **pyramidohypoglossal s.,** alternating hypoglossal

HEMIPLEGIA. **Rabenhorst s.,** cardioacrofascial s. **Racine's s.,** swelling of the salivary glands and breasts occurring four or five days before menstruation and subsiding with the onset of flow. Called also *premenstrual salivary s.* **radiation s.,** radiation SICKNESS. **Raeder's s.,** paratrigeminal s. **Ramsay Hunt's s.,** Hunt's s. **Raymond-Céstan s.,** a tumor of the cerebral peduncles involving the red nucleus, associated with speech disorders, paralysis of the lateral conjugate gaze, ipsilateral abducens palsy, contralateral hemiplegia, and ipsilateral anesthesia of the face, extremities, and trunk. **REEDS s.,** an acronym for *R*etention of tears; *E*ctrodactyly; *E*ctodermal *D*ysplasia; *S*trange hair, skin, and teeth. A hereditary syndrome believed to be transmitted as an autosomal dominant trait. The principal features, which are variable, are anomalies of the hands and feet, including lobster claw deformity, syndactyly, clinodactyly, and ectrodactyly; severe keratitis, diffuse hypopigmentation of the skin and hair, scanty scalp hair and eyebrows, pili torti, and dystrophic nails; atresia or defects of the lacrimal ducts, associated with tearing, keratoconjunctivitis, blepharitis, blepharophimosis, photophobia, and blue irides; cleft lip and/or palate, anodontia or oligodontia, microdontia, absent permanent central incisors, dental caries, and malar and maxillary hypoplasia. Other abnormalities that may be present include microcephaly, mental retardation, inguinal hernia, kidney and ureteral defects, urinary tract infections, and malformed ears and deafness. Called also *ectrodactyly-ectodermal dysplasia-clefting s.* and *EEC s.* **Reese's s.,** Reese-Blodi s., Reese's DYSPLASIA. **Reichert's s.,** neuralgia of the glossopharyngeal nerve. In the complete form, paroxysms of pain, which start in the tonsillar fossa or base of the tongue radiate deeply into the ear and are associated with salivation, are precipitated by movements of the tongue or throat. In the partial form, the tympanic plexus is involved and the paroxysms of pain in the vicinity of the external auditory canal occur without any movement of the tongue or pharynx. **Rendu-Weber-Osler s.,** hereditary hemorrhagic TELANGIECTASIA. **renofacial s.,** Potter's DISEASE. **retroparotid space s.,** Villaret's s. **retrosphenoidal space s.,** total ophthalmoplegia, optic tract lesions with unilateral amaurosis, and trigeminal neuralgia caused by middle cranial fossa tumors (nasopharyngeal in origin), involving the nerves passing through the foramen ovale, foramen rotundum, and sphenoidal fissure (second, third, fourth, fifth, and sixth cranial nerves). Called also *Jacod's s., Silvio Negri's s.,* and *Jacod's triad.* **reverse Gougerot-Sjögren s.,** Creyx-Lévy s. **Rieger's s.,** a congenital disorder transmitted as an autosomal dominant trait. Principal features include corneal opacities, hypoplastic stroma of the iris, iridotrabecular adhesions, and posterior embryotoxon. Specific ocular findings consist usually of microcornea or megalocornea, cornea plana, aniridia, pupillary defects, coloboma, ectopia or opacities of the crystalline lens, glaucoma, strabismus, and ametropia. Chief extraocular changes consist of dysgnathia, hypodontia of anterior teeth, myotonic dystrophy, hypertelorism, hydrocephalus, cerebral hypoplasia, and mental retardation. When the ocular disorders are present without the associated extraocular changes, it is called *Rieger's anomaly* or *Rieger's malformation.* Called also *posterior marginal dysplasia.* **Rietti-Greppi-Micheli s.,** THALASSEMIA minor. **Riley-Day s.,** a congenital disorder of the autonomic nervous system, suspected of being due to defective metabolism of epinephrine and acetycholine, and probably transmitted as an autosomal recessive trait. Children of Jewish ancestry are affected primarily; few survive beyond adolescence. It is characterized by lack of tears, blotching of the skin, hyperhidrosis, postural hypotension, stress hypertension, indifference to pain, emotional instability, and faulty speech. Oral symptoms include sialorrhea, especially during excitement, and absence or marked diminution of fungiform and circumvallate papillae of the tongue. Called also *familial autonomic dysfunction* and *familial dysautonomia.* **ring chromosome 9 s.,** chromosome 9 ring s. **Roberts' s.,** a hereditary syndrome, transmitted as an autosomal recessive trait, characterized by the presence of a wide range of abnormalities. Principal features include growth and mental retardation, cleft lip and/or cleft palate, prominent maxilla micrognathia, hypertelorism, midfacial capillary hemangioma, thin nares, shallow orbits, prominent eyes, bluish sclerae, malformed ears with hypoplastic lobules, sparse hair that may be silvery-blond, hypomelia of varying degree of severity, absent or malformed thumb, radial aplasia, syndactyly, clinodactyly, talipes deformity, incomplete development of dermal ridges, cryptorchidism, and relatively large penis. Frontal encephalocele, hydrocephalus, short neck, corneal clouding, cataract, heart defects, and kidney and uterus abnormalities may be associated. Called also *hypomelia-hypotrichosis-facial hemangioma s., pseudothalidomide s.,* and SC s. **Robin's s.,** Robin's ANOMALAD. **Robinow's s.,** a syndrome combining unusual facies, forearm shortening, and hypoplastic genitalia. Facial features are midfacial hypoplasia, frontal bossing, apparent ocular hypertelorism, short upturned nose with flat bridge and anteverted nares, triangular mouth, and moderate micrognathia, usually associated with gingival hypertrophy, delayed tooth eruption, and crowding, malalignment, and notching of the teeth. Absence of the uvula and a small midline cleft of the lower lip may be present. The head is disproportionately large; the limbs are short, particularly the forearms, with broad and short hands and feet and clinodactyly of the fifth fingers. Abnormal palmar creases, low-set ears with overhanging helices, small penis, occasional cryptorchidism, and small labia minora are features, and hepatosplenomegaly, renal duplication, and hydronephrosis may occur. Both autosomal dominant and recessive modes of transmission and some sporadic cases have been reported. Called also *fetal face s.,* and *Robinow's dwarfism.* **Romberg's s.,** facial HEMIATROPHY. **Rothmund's s.,** Rothmund-Thomson s., **Rothmund-Thomson s.,** a hereditary syndrome, transmitted as an autosomal recessive trait, characterized by bilateral cataracts, poikiloderma, pigmentation disorders, and hypogonadism. The skin appears normal at birth but, at three to six months of age, bright vermilion erythematous patches appear, followed by hypo- and hyperpigmentation. The cataracts appear between the fourth and seventh years. Proportionate dwarfism, prominent frontal bossing, saddle nose, alopecia, and dental and bone defects are often associated, including small hands and fingers, cystic lesions of the bone, syndactyly, microdontia, malformation of the erupted teeth, and failure of one or more teeth to erupt. Called also *Rothmund's s.* and *poikiloderma congenitale.* **Rotter-Erb s.,** a combination of deformities of the bones, joints, and tendons, marked by dwarfism, brachycephaly, brachymetapody, multiple epiphyseal lesions, loose joints, multiple dislocations, bilateral clubfoot, pterygium colli, vertebral deformities, including kyphoscoliosis and clefting of the vertebral arches, and cleft palate. Some authorities consider this a doubtful entity. **Royer's s.,** an association of diabetes mellitus with Prader-Willi syndrome. **rubella s.,** congenital rubella s. **Rubinstein-Taybi s.,** a combination of congenital disorders consisting of short, broad terminal phalanges of the thumbs and great toes; short stature; skeletal maturation and head circumference that are below average for the age; facial deformities, including high-arched palate and straight or beaked nose; mental retardation; motor retardation; eye abnormalities, including antimongoloid slant, epicanthus, strabismus, cataract, refractive error, high-arched eyebrows, and long lashes; and cryptorchidism. Various other abnormalities and susceptibility to respiratory infections are usually present. **rubrospinal cerebellar peduncle s.,** inferior nucleus ruber s. **Rüdiger's s.,** a hereditary syndrome, probably transmitted as an autosomal recessive trait, characterized by mental retardation, flexion contracture of the hands with thick palmar creases, simian lines, small fingers and nails, ureteral stenosis, hydronephrosis, inguinal hernia, hypoplasia of ear cartilage, cleft palate, coarse facies, and other abnormalities. **Russell's s., Russell-Silver s.,** a congenital syndrome that is similar to, if not identical with, Silver's syndrome. It has a prenatal onset of growth deficiency, and characterized by immature osseous development in early infancy and early childhood, with late closure of the anterior fontanel; small triangular facies with down-turned corners of the mouth; blue sclerae in early infancy; developmental asymmetry, particularly of the limbs; short and/or incurved fifth finger; café-au-lait spots; excessive sweating; and tendency toward fasting hypoglycemia during late infancy and early childhood. Most cases occur sporadically but autosomal dominant inheritance has been implied. An affected individual is known as a *Russell dwarf.* **Rust's s.,** Rust's DISEASE. **Rutherfurd's s.,** an oculodental disorder transmitted as an autosomal dominant trait, consisting of corneal dystrophy, gingival hypertrophy, and failure of tooth eruption. **Saethre-Chotzen s.,** a hereditary syndrome, transmitted as an autosomal dominant trait with incomplete penetrance and variable expressivity, consisting of craniosynostosis, low-set frontal hairline, parrot-beaked nose with deviated septum, ptosis of the eyelids, strabismus, refractive error, tear duct stenosis, dystopia canthorum, brachydactyly, and abnormal dermatoglyphic patterns. Additional symptoms may include facial asymmetry, microcephaly, impaired hearing, optic atro-

phy, amblyopia, ocular hypertelorism, cleft palate, high-arched palate, missing teeth, peg-shaped or anomalous maxillary lateral incisors, spinal anomalies, clinodactyly, syndactyly, hallux valgus, and simian creases. It is sometimes erroneously identified as *pseudo-Crouzon syndrome* or *Pfeiffer's syndrome.* Called also *acrocephalosyndactyly III, ACS III,* and *SCS.* **Sakati-Nyhan-Tisdale s.,** a syndrome consisting of acrocephalosyndactyly, short limbs, congenital heart abnormalities, ear anomalies, and skin defects. Affected patients usually have a large calvaria and a disproportionately small face, synostosis of all cranial sutures, shallow orbits, prominent eyes, low-set dysplastic ears, patchy alopecia, skin atrophy, scarlike lesions of the skin, narrow high-arched palate, maxillary hypoplasia, crowding of the upper teeth, short neck, and low hairline. Abnormalities of the extremities may include short arms, cubitus valgus, short broad hands, fusion of the interphalangeal joints, supernumerary digits, short legs, adducted feet, and polysyndactyly. Roentgenologic examination may reveal coxa valga, bowing of the femurs, hypoplasia of the tibiae, and malformations of the tarsal and metatarsal bones. Wide-set nipples, cryptorchidism, small penis, and inguinal hernia may be associated. **Sanfilippo's s.,** a systemic form of mucopolysaccharidosis, inherited as an autosomal recessive trait, characterized by severe progressive mental retardation, associated with mild forms of dwarfism, stiff joints, skeletal defects, and hepatosplenomegaly. Excessive amounts of heparitin sulfate are found in the urine, and mild corneal opacities may occur. Called also *mucopolysaccharidosis III.* **SC s.,** Roberts' s. **scalded skin s.,** toxic epidermal NECROLYSIS. **Scheie's s.,** systemic mucopolysaccharidosis, transmitted as an autosomal recessive trait, marked by stiff joints, mild bone deformities, clawhand, hirsutism, retinitis pigmentosa, corneal opacities, and broad-mouthed facies. Carpal tunnel syndrome and aortic coarctation occur frequently. Clouding of the cornea, although present at birth in a discrete form, may not become evident until adolescence. Excessive amounts of chondroitin sulfate B are excreted in the urine. Called also *forme fruste of Hurler's s., late Hurler's syndrome,* and *mucopolysaccharidosis V.* **Scheuthauer-Marie-Sainton s.,** cleidocranial DYSPLASIA. **Schmidt's s.,** a variant of Jackson-MacKenzie syndrome, in which unilateral involvement of the tenth and eleventh cranial nerves produces ipsilateral paralysis of the soft palate, vocal cords, and sternocleidomastoid and trapezius muscles. Called also *vagoaccessory s.* **Scholz's s.,** metachromatic LEUKODYSTROPHY. **Schönlein-Henoch s.,** a combination of *Henoch's disease* (purpura associated with abdominal disorders) and *Schönlein's disease* (purpura associated with articular symptoms), characterized by increased permeability of the capillaries, permitting passage of plasma and blood cells, associated with gastrointestinal and articular disorders. It is most often observed in small children, less frequently in adolescents, and rarely in adults. Manifestations include purpura with cutaneous swelling, effusions, diffuse erythema and necrotic areas followed by bullae and ulcers; visceral symptoms, including abdominal pain, vomiting, diarrhea or constipation, and transitory edema of the small intestine; rheumatoid pain and tenderness about the joints with swelling and periarticular edema; and fever. The etiology is unknown, but allergy and upper respiratory infections have been suggested. Called also *allergic nonthrombocytopenic purpura, anaphylactoid purpura, essential athrombopenic purpura, purpura infectiosa acuta, purpura rheumatica,* and *Schönlein-Henoch purpura.* **Schultz's s.,** agranulocytosis. **Seckel's s.,** a syndrome of intrauterine proportionate dwarfism and birdlike facies with a prominent, sometimes beaked nose, micrognathia, high-arched or cleft palate, low-set lobeless ears, prominent eyes, antimongoloid palpebral slant, and epicanthic folds. Bone disorders include multiple dislocations, such as congenital hip dislocation, kyphoscoliosis, sternal defects, absence of the patella, and disorders of bone maturation. There is also clinodactyly, simian creases, increased distance between the first and second toes, cryptorchidism, pancytopenia, and mental retardation. It appears to be transmitted as an autosomal recessive trait. Called also *bird-headed dwarfism, nanocephalic dwarfism,* and *primordial dwarfism.* **secretoinhibitor s.,** Sjögren's s. **Selye's s.,** general adaptation s. **Senear-Usher s.,** PEMPHIGUS erythematosus. **senilism s.,** Hutchinson-Gilford s. **Sézary's s.,** a form of cutaneous reticulosis characterized by exfoliative dermatitis, intense pruritus, generalized erythroderma, keratosis palmaris et plantaris, benign superficial lymphadenopathy, and facial edema. Hepatomegaly, alopecia, nail dystrophy, eversion and thickening of the eyelids, and skin abrasion may occur. **Sheehan's s.,** necrosis of the pituitary gland, associated with functional failure of the anterior lobe and secondary atrophy of the gonads, adrenal cortex, and thyroid gland. Anoxia due to postpartum hemorrhage is believed to be the cause. For manifestations, see *Simmonds' syndrome*. **S-H-O-R-T s.**, a syndrome inherited as an autosomal recessive trait, combining short stature, hyperextensibility of joints or hernia (inguinal) or both, ocular depression, Rieger anomaly, and teething delayed. **short face s.**, a dentofacial deformity due to deficient vertical maxillary growth, presenting a short, square-shaped face, with the maxillary incisors hidden behind the upper lip when the jaw is at rest; a downward curving of the corners of the mouth below the midline; distinct skin folds lateral to the oral commissures when the mandible is in centric occlusion; apparent or actual macrostomia, and an edentulous-like appearance. The upper third of the face tends to be within normal limits, but the middle third usually shows broad nasal alar bases and large nostrils, the posterior part appearing wide because of prominent mandibular angles due to attachment of the masseter muscles to the laterally flared gonial processes. The maxillary and dental arch is broad and the palatal vault is typically flat. Decreased vertical maxillary height, large freeway space, and low mandibular plane are the chief cephalometric findings. Class I or II malocclusion with deep overbite is common. Maxillary buccal cross-bites are frequently associated with interdental spacing. Called also *hypodivergent face, idiopathic short face, low-angle type, short face, skeletal-type deep bite*, and *vertical maxillary deficiency*. **short rib-polydactyly s.**, Majewski's s. **sicca s.**, Sjögren's s. **sideropenic s.**, Plummer-Vinson s. **Silver's s.**, a syndrome usually associated with maternal difficulties during pregnancy, which is similar to, if not identical with, Russell's syndrome. It consists of intrauterine dwarfism, hemihypertrophy, elevated urine gonadotropins, early sexual development, and premature estrogenization of the urethral and vaginal mucosae. Secondary features are café-au-lait areas or other pigmentation disorders of the skin, short in-curved fifth fingers, syndactyly, triangular face, and turned-down corners of the mouth. Catch-up growth occurs by the time of puberty. **Silverman's s.**, battered CHILD. **Silvio Negri's s.**, retrosphenoidal space s. **Simmonds' s.**, a condition occurring in both sexes, in which there is necrosis of the pituitary gland with complete or partial functional failure of the anterior lobe and secondary atrophy of the gonads, adrenal cortex, and thyroid gland. Bradycardia, hypotension, transient diabetes insipidus, hypoglycemia, atrophy of the genitalia and breasts, amenorrhea, anorexia, weight loss, cachexia, loss of body hair, absence of libido, fatigability, depression, coma, hypothyroidism, and adrenal and gonadal insufficiency may ensue. Oral symptoms are nonspecific; they may include xerostomia with associated increased susceptibility of the dental enamel to caries and of the periodontal tissue to inflammatory disease. Anoxia due to hemorrhagic disorders is believed to be the cause. A similar condition due to necrosis of the pituitary in the postpartum period is known as *Sheehan's syndrome*. **Singleton-Merten s.**, a syndrome, possibly transmitted as a recessive trait, combining dental dysplasia, thoracic aortic calcification, osteoporosis, and radiologic changes similar to those seen in severe anemia. Affected patients have muscle weakness appearing during the first or second year of life; general osteoporosis with small bones of the hands and feet, thin cortices of the metacarpal and metatarsal bones, expanded medullary cavities, poorly defined trabeculae, and erosion of the terminal phalanges in the presence of psoriasiform skin lesions; calcific aortic stenosis with systolic murmurs and, in some cases, subaortic stenosis, leading to left heart failure; psoriasis; soft tissue calcification; small stature; eye abnormalities, such as glaucoma and keratitis, in some cases; and dental dysplasia with caries of the deciduous teeth, premature loss of teeth, dysplastic permanent teeth, and delayed eruption. **sinus of Morgagni s.**, Trotter's s. **Sjögren's s.**, xerostomia, keratoconjunctivitis, and rheumatoid arthritis occurring chiefly in postmenopausal women or in young women after artificial menopause. Symptoms include dry conjunctivae, blepharoconjunctivitis, filamentous keratitis, corneal ulcers, oral ulcers, atrophic rhinitis, diarrhea, and dry ichthyotic skin. It is believed that the syndrome is a form of collagen disease. Some authors consider Mikulicz's syndrome to be identical with Sjögren's syndrome; according to others, Mikulicz's syndrome does not include rheumatoid arthritis and, therefore, is a separate entity. It has also been suggested that polymyositis may be substituted for rheumatoid arthritis in the diagnostic triad. Called also *Gougerot-Houwer-Sjögren s., Gougerot-Sjögren s., secretoinhibitor s., sicca s., dacryosialoadenopathia, dacryosialocheilopathy, keratoconjunctivitis sicca, mucoserous dyssecretosis, rheumatic sialosis*, and *rheumatoid sialadenitis*. **Sjögren's s., reverse**, Creyx-Lévy s. **Sjögren-Larsson s.**, a congenital syndrome, transmitted as an autosomal recessive trait, characterized by mental and growth retardation, spastic paralysis, ichthyosis or ichthyosiform erythroderma, and sparse and brittle hair. Occasional anomalies may include tooth enamel dysplasia, hypertelorism, pigmentary degeneration of the retina, hypohidrosis except of the face and dorsum of the hands, and metaphyseal dysplasia with small irregular epiphyses. **Smith-Lemli-Opitz s.**, a recessively inherited syndrome characterized by mental and growth retardation, failure to thrive, muscle tone disorders, microcephaly with narrow frontal area, low-set and slanted ears, blepharoptosis, inner epicanthic folds, strabismus, broad nasal tip with anteverted nostrils, micrognathia, broad maxillary secondary alveolar ridges, simian creases, syndactyly, cryptorchidism, and hypospadias. Seizures, abnormal electroencephalogram, cleft palate, cataract, hip dislocation, dysplasia epiphysealis punctata, and a variety of other abnormalities may be associated. **Sotos' s.**, a syndrome characterized by excessively rapid growth, acromegalic features, and a nonprogressive cerebral disorder with mental retardation. Dolichocephaly, macrocrania, hypertelorism, high-arched palate, and accelerated skeletal maturation in the absence of obvious endocrine dysfunction are usually present. Convulsions are frequent but the electroencephalogram shows only nonspecific abnormalities. Called also *cerebral gigantism*. **Stainton's s., Stainton-Capdepont s.**, DENTINOGENESIS imperfecta. **Stanesco's s.**, a familial syndrome, seemingly transmitted as an autosomal dominant trait, which combines dwarfism and abnormalities of the face, long bones, and teeth. Principal features include brachycephaly, sometimes with depressions at the frontoparietal sutures, lack of pneumatization in the frontal and sphenoid bone, bulging eyes, shallow orbits, narrow maxilla, small mandible with an obtuse angle, crowded and small teeth, enamel hypoplasia, dense and thick cortices of the long bones and relative shortness of the arms and hands. Fractures, exostoses, and flattened palate are sometimes associated. **steely hair s.**, Menkes' s. **Stevens-Johnson s.**, a severe form of bullous erythema multiforme, most often affecting children and young adults during the spring and fall, and usually having a duration of 4 to 6 weeks. Fever and headache are the early signs, followed by ulcerative conjunctivitis, rhinitis, stomatitis, urethritis, and balanitis. Cutaneous eruptions consisting of vesiculobullous and papular lesions over the entire body surface occur within two or three days. Ocular symptoms include keratitis, iritis, uveitis, panophthalmia, and sometimes blindness. Oral lesions, which are sometimes the only presenting symptoms, may be severe and painful, causing difficulty in mastication. Mucosal vesicles or bullae rupture and leave surfaces covered with a thick white or yellow exudate, followed by erosion of the pharynx; the lips may show ulcers with bloody crusting. Staphylococcal septicemia and drug hypersensitivity have been implicated in the etiology. A form consisting of stomatitis, conjunctivitis, and macular eruption, but without fever, is known as *Fuch's syndrome*. Called also *Baader's s., aphthosis generalisata, Baader's dermatostomatitis, bullous malignant erythema multiforme, ectodermosis erosiva pluriorificialis, erythema multiforme exudativum major, generalized aphthosis*, and *Neumann's aphthosis*. **Stickler's s.**, a hereditary disorder transmitted as an autosomal dominant trait, consisting of orofacial abnormalities, including depressed nasal bridge and epicanthal folds, midfacial or mandibular hypoplasia, cleft palate, Pierre Robin's syndrome, and hearing loss; ocular abnormalities, including myopia, retinal detachment, and/or cataracts; and musculoskeletal abnormalities including hypotonia, hyperextensible joints, marfanoid habitus, large joints, joint pains simulating juvenile rheumatoid arthritis, subluxation of the hip, spondyloepiphyseal dysplasia, and narrow shafts of the long bones. Clinical manifestations may show considerable variations in severity of symptoms and organ involvement. Called also *arthro-ophthalmopathy*. **Strachan-Scott s.**, a syndrome associated with nutritional deficiencies, especially deficiency of vitamin B₂, usually observed in its various forms in the malnourished Jamaican poor. The principal symptoms are pain, numbness, and paresthesia of the palms and soles; joint and shoulder girdle pain; symmetrical polyneuritis; dimness of vision, optic neuropathy, and retinal hyperemia; deafness; excoriation of mucocutaneous junctions; and emaciation. Cerebral and spinal pigment deposits are the significant pathological findings. Called also *avitaminosis B₂*. **stroke s.**, cerebrovascular ACCIDENT. **Sturge-Weber s.**, a congenital syndrome characterized by venous angiomas of the leptomeninges; ipsilateral telangiectasia or port-wine nevus of the trigeminal region, including the upper third of the face, eyes, mouth, and nasal mucosa; contralateral hemiplegia; and choroidal changes with late glaucoma. Vascular changes are usually associated with intracranial calcifications, mental retardation, epilepsy, crossed hemiparesis, hydrophthalmia, and hemianopsia. Called also *angiomatosis meningo-oculofacialis, cutaneocerebral angioma,* and *encephalotrigeminal angiomatosis.* **stylohyoid s., styloid s., styloid process s.,** Eagle's s. **styloid process-carotid artery s.,** see *Eagle's s.* **sub-bulbar s.,** Opalski's s. **Summitt's s.,** a combination of craniosynostosis and variable syndactyly, which may be associated with acrocephaly, occipital defects, scaphocephaly, epicanthal folds, strabismus, narrow high-arched palate, delayed dentition, clinodactyly, and brachymesophalangy. An autosomal recessive mode of transmission has been suggested. **superior laryngeal nerve s.,** Avellis' s. **suprarenal genital s.,** adrenogenital s. **supravalvular aortic stenosis s.,** elfin facies s. **Sweet's s.,** a disease resembling erythema multiforme, characterized by raised, dark red plaques occurring most commonly on the face, neck, arms, and legs, in association with fever and neutrophil polymorphonuclear leukocytosis. Histologically, the lesions are characterized by an intense infiltration, mainly of the neutrophil polymorphs, in the absence of signs of infection. **Takahara's s.** acatalasia. **Tapia's s.,** a variant of Jackson-MacKenzie syndrome, in which unilateral involvement of the tenth and twelfth cranial nerves produces ipsilateral paralysis of the tongue and vocal cords. Called also *nucleus ambiguus-hypoglossal s., vagohypoglossal s.,* and *palatopharyngeal paralysis.* **Taybi's s.,** otopalatodigital s. **TDO s.,** trichodento-osseous s. **Tel Hashomer camptodactyly s.,** a syndrome consisting of camptodactyly, distinct facies, muscular hypoplasia, skeletal dysplasia, and abnormal palmar creases, occurring in Jewish families of Moroccan and Arab Bedouin origin. The name derives from Tel Hashomer Hospital near Tel Aviv where the first cases were observed. Principal features include short stature, brachycephaly, prominent forehead and maxilla, broad mandible, asymmetric facies, hypertelorism, small mouth, high-arched palate, increased philtrum length, dental crowding, thoracic scoliosis, winging of scapulae, and various anomalies of the extremities and muscular system. Called also *camptodactyly-muscular hypoplasia-skeletal dysplasia-abnormal palmar creases s.* **temporal s.,** Gradenigo's s. **temporomandibular dysfunction s., temporomandibular joint s., temporomandibular pain–dysfunction s.,** a symptom complex originally described as consisting of partial deafness; stuffy sensation in the ears, especially during eating; tinnitus; clicking and snapping in the temporomandibular joint; dizziness; headache; and burning pain in the ear, throat, tongue, and nose. The cause has been ascribed to lesions of the temporomandibular joint associated with malocclusion with a deep overbite, absence of molar teeth, poorly fitting dentures, or an edentulous state, resulting in impingement of the main branch of the auriculotemporal nerve between the condyle and the postglenoid spine or impingement of the chorda tympani from direct pressure on the ear structures and closure of the eustachian tube. Some researchers feel that the anatomical and physiological evidence to justify this syndrome is lacking. Called also *Costen's s., TMJ s., temporomandibular arthralgia,* and *temporomandibular neuralgia.* **Terry's s.,** osteitis deformans associated with angioid streaks. **9p tetrasomy s.,** 9p TETRASOMY. **thalassemic s.,** Cooley's ANEMIA. **Thornwaldt's (Tornwaldt's) s.,** Thornwaldt's (Tornwaldt's) BURSITIS. **Timme's s.,** a syndrome of thymoadrenopituitary insufficiency, in which the first phase begins before puberty, and is marked by disproportionate bone development, delayed fusion of the epiphyses with the bone shafts, hyperextension of joints, sparsity of body hair, muscle cramps, spasmophilia, hemophilic tendency, delayed dentition, enlarged tonsils and adenoids, hypotension, hypoglycemia, epistaxes, cyanosis of the extremities, fatigability, small sella turcica, enuresis, and low CO_2 coefficiency of the blood. The second phase, beginning at puberty, is characterized by rapid growth, delayed menstruation, genital infantilism, elicitation of an adrenal line, gastric hyperacidity and lack of body hair. The third phase, observed during the third decade, is characterized by enlargement of the sella turcica, acromegaly, drowsiness, confusion, headache, epileptiform attacks, and mental deterioration. **TMJ s.,** temporomandibular dysfunction s. **Tolosa-Hunt s.,** recurrent unilateral retro-orbital pain with extraocular palsies, most often involving the third, fourth, fifth, and sixth cranial nerves, attributed to inflammation of the cavernous sinus, and usually lasting several months to several years. Males and females are equally affected, most commonly during the fifth decade. Diabetes mellitus, intracavernous carotid aneurysm, and nasopharyngeal tumors are the usual causes. Called also *painful ophthalmoplegia.* **tooth-nail s.,** a

syndrome, inherited as an autosomal dominant trait, combining fine hair, oligodontia, and hypoplasia of nails, especially the toenails. **Tornwaldt's s.,** Thornwaldt's BURSITIS. **Treacher Collins' s.,** mandibulofacial DYSOSTOSIS. **trefoil skull s.,** cloverleaf SKULL. **trichodento-osseous s.,** a syndrome, transmitted as an autosomal dominant trait, characterized by kinky hair at birth; small wide-spaced, pitted teeth with poor enamel, and taurodontism; frontal bossing, dolichocephaly, and square jaw; increased bone density, particularly of the skull; and brittle nails. Occasionally, partial craniosynostosis may occur. Called also *TDO s.* **trichorhinophalangeal s.,** trichorhinophalangeal DYSPLASIA (1 or 2). **tridione s., trimethadione s.,** fetal trimethadione s. **trisomy s's,** see also under TRISOMY. **trisomy 8 s.,** TRISOMY 8. **trisomy 9p s.,** TRISOMY 9p. **trisomy 13 s.,** Patau's s. **trisomy 18 s.,** TRISOMY 18. **Trotter's s.,** unilateral neuralgia in the region of the mandible, tongue, and ear due to involvement of the mandibular nerve; ipsilateral middle ear deafness resulting from a lesion of the eustachian tube; preauricular edema caused by neoplastic invasion of the sinus of Morgagni; ipsilateral akinesia of the soft palate secondary to damage of the levator of the palate; and late trismus. Called also *sinus of Morgagni.* **Turner's s.,** a syndrome in which affected patients have only 45 chromosomes, the loss of one of the X chromosomes producing an XO chromosome constitution. Typical features are short stature; infantile development of the vagina, uterus, and breasts; agenesis of the ovaries; pterygium colli; cubitus valgus; low hairline; and sometimes kidney abnormalities, deformed nails and ears, high palatal vault, micrognathia, asymmetry of the facial and cranial bones and alveolar processes, premature dentition, short dental roots, and microdontia. Lymphedema of the extremities, coaractation of the aorta, and deafness may occur. Called also *XO s.* and *gonadal agenesis.* See also *Bonnevie-Ullrich s.* and Turner-mongolism POLYSYNDROME. **Turner-like s.,** Noonan's s. **Ullrich-Feichtiger s.,** a congenital syndrome characterized by multiple abnormalities, including ear deformities, deafness, polydactyly, rudimentary toes, clubfoot, partial atresia of the anus, hypospadias, micrognathia, and masklike facies. Vaginal septa, supernumerary phalanges, and a tendency to develop clefts in various structures, especially the palate, may occur. Called also *dyscraniopygophalangia s.* **Ulysses s.,** a complex of mental and physical disorders which follow the discovery of false-positive results in the course of routine laboratory tests, leading to additional tests and examinations, some physically, mentally, and financially traumatic, before the patient is found to be healthy. It is attributed to a combination of factors in tests and investigations promoted by mass screening, insurance and preemployment examinations, application of unnecessary laboratory tests, physician's hope for a major discovery, patient's neurotic reactions, uncritical interpretation of results, and retention of outdated tests on laboratory forms. The syndrome is named after the Greek epic hero Ulysses (Odysseus), king of Ithaca, who after the Trojan War traveled for 20 years, encountering numerous adventures and perils before returning home. **Urbach-Wiethe s.,** a rare familial and congenital storage disease, characterized by multiple infiltrations that produce waxiness and thickening of the skin and mucous membranes of the mouth, pharynx, larynx, and hypopharynx, resulting in prolonged hoarseness, often from birth. Yellowish ivory or waxy nodules from 1 to several millimeters in size are distributed on the face, neck, hands, and axillary regions, and hyperkeratotic lesions may be found on the knees, elbows, and fingers. Diffuse alopecia is present in some instances. The tongue becomes thickened and may be difficult to move. Intracranial calcifications are common. It has been tentatively identified with the glycoproteinoses, and is probably transmitted as an autosomal recessive trait. Called also *hyalinosis cutis et mucosae, lipoid proteinosis,* and *Urbach's lipoproteinosis.* **vagoaccessory s.,** Schmidt's s. **vagoaccessory-hypoglossal s.,** Jackson-MacKenzie s. **vagohypoglossal s.,** Tapia's s. **Vail's s.,** vidian NEURALGIA. **van Bogaert-Hozay s.,** a syndrome in which there is sudden arrest of growth of the extremities, followed by decalcification and osteolysis of various bones of the hands and feet. Defects of the face, ears, and nose, faulty dentition, micrognathia, astigmatism, and myopia may be associated. **van Bogaert-Nyssen-Peiffer s.,** metachromatic LEUKODYSTROPHY. **van Bogaert-Scherer-Epstein s.,** a slowly progressive familial disorder characterized by hypercholesterolemia, mental retardation, cracked skin, multiple xanthomas, including xanthelasma, dystrophy of the hair, genital infantilism, dental caries, juvenile cataract, spastic disorders of the lower extremities, and labioglossobulbar paralysis. Called also *familial hypercholesterolemia.* **van Buchem's s.,** HYPEROSTOSIS corticalis generalisata. **van der Hoeve's s.,** the association of Lobstein's syndrome with osteosclerosis and deafness. Called also *fragili-*

tas ossium-blue sclera-osteosclerosis s. and *fragilitas ossium hereditaria tarda.* **van der Woude's s.,** a hereditary syndrome, transmitted as an autosomal dominant trait, marked by paramedian pits of the lower lip, cleft lip with or without cleft palate, hypodontia, and missing second premolars. Called also *CLP-lip pits s., Demarquay-Richet s.,* and *lip pit-cleft lip or palate s.* **Veeneklaas' s.,** dentopulmonary s. **Vernet's s.,** a syndrome in which lesions in the region of the jugular foramen produce paralysis of the ninth, tenth, and eleventh cranial nerves with secondary ipsilateral paralysis of the soft palate, larynx, and pharynx and the sternocleidomastoid and trapezius muscles. Symptoms include dysphagia, anesthesia of the soft palate, and loss of sensation and taste in the back of the tongue. Called also *jugular foramen s.* **Villaret's s.,** a syndrome in which lesions of the retroparotid space produce unilateral paralysis of the ninth, tenth, eleventh, twelfth, and occasionally the seventh cranial nerves, resulting in Bernard-Horner syndrome, and in ipsilateral paralysis of the soft palate, pharynx, larynx, and vocal cords. A variant unaccompanied by Bernard-Horner syndrome is known as *Collet-Sicard syndrome.* Called also *posterior retroparotid space s.* and *retroparotid space s.* **von Gierke's s., von Gierke-van Creveld s.,** GLYCOGENOSIS I. **von Willebrand's s.,** Willebrand-Jürgens s. **Vrolik's s.,** a rare and rapidly fatal form of congenital osteogenesis imperfecta, characterized by defective ossification in utero. The symptoms are present at birth and include brittle bones, multiple fractures, micromelia, poor ossification of the cranial vault, small face in proportion to the skull, and short neck. It is considered to be a congenital form of Lobstein's syndrome by some, and as a separate entity by others, because of unproven heredity and the lack of blue sclerae. Called also *o. imperfecta congenita; aplasia ossea microplastica, fetal osteoporosis,* and *fragilitas ossium congenita.* **W s.,** a hereditary syndrome, named for the family in which it was first seen, characterized by prematurity, mental retardation, seizures, slight spasticity, tremor, frontal prominence, anterior cowlick of the hair, hypertelorism, antimongoloid slanting of palpebral fissures, alternating internal strabismus, flat and broad bridge and tip of the nose, incomplete median oral cleft (with medially cleft upper lip, absent upper central incisors, medially cleft maxillary arch, and anterior cleft palate), short and high mandible, cubitus valgus, subluxation at proximal radioulnar joints, short ulnas, lateral bowing of radii, and camptodactyly and clinodactyly. X-linked inheritance with partial expression in females is suspected. **Waardenburg's s.,** a congenital syndrome characterized by dystopia canthorum, hypertelorism, laterally displaced lacrimal points, broad nasal root, lack of frontonasal angle, hypoplasia of the nasal alar cartilage, hyperplasia of the eyebrows, hypoplasia of the iris, white forelock, vitiligo, premature graying of hair, congenital sensorineural deafness, and mandibular prognathism. Associated abnormalities may include epicanthus, square nasal tip, cleft lip and/or palate, spina bifida, and Sprengel's deformity. Autosomal dominant transmission with complete penetrance and variable expressivity has been observed in most pedigrees. **Waldenström's s.,** a chronic disease occurring almost exclusively in women, characterized by high content of gamma-globulin but normal levels of albumins in the blood. Principal clinical features are episodes of purpura of the lower extremities precipitated by exertion, irritation by garments, or infection, leaving areas of brown pigmentation, and xerophthalmia. Moderate hepatosplenomegaly may also occur. Oral manifestations include xerostomia. Called also *hyperglobulinemic purpura s., idiopathic hyperglobulinemia,* and *purpura hyperglobulinemica.* **Wallenberg's s.,** a relatively common vascular disease of the brain stem, usually occurring during the fifth decade, in which occlusion of the posterior inferior cerebellar artery causes ipsilateral loss of the pain and temperature senses of the face, soft palate, pharynx, and larynx; contralateral pain and temperature hypoesthesia of the extremities and trunk; ipsilateral ataxia; muscular hypotonia; ipsilateral Bernard-Horner syndrome; nystagmus; vertigo; nausea; difficulty in swallowing and speaking; and ocular disorders, including miosis, enophthalmos, ptosis, diplopia, and nystagmus. The symptoms of this syndrome are also seen in *Opalski's syndrome.* Called also *dorsolateral medullary s., lateral bulbar s.,* and *posterior inferior cerebellar artery s.* **warfarin s.,** fetal warfarin s. **Waterhouse-Friderichsen s.,** rapidly fulminating meningococcal septicemia characterized by massive purpura, bilateral adrenal hemorrhage, and shock. The onset is sudden with dyspnea, followed in a few hours by abrupt fever, hypotension, rash, collapse, and death. **Weber's s.,** Klippel-Trenaunay-Weber s. **Weber-Cockayne s.,** EPIDERMOLYSIS bullosa. **Weech's s.,** hypohydrotic ectodermal DYSPLASIA. **Weill-Marchesani s.,** Marchesani's s. **Werdnig-Hoffmann s.,** infantile muscular ATROPHY. **Werner's s.,** a rare hereditary condition, transmitted as an

autosomal recessive trait, affecting both sexes, usually beginning during the second or third decade, and characterized by premature aging. It is marked by short stature, cataract, high-pitched voice, early graying and loss of the hair, atrophy of the skin, leg ulcers, vascular disorders, premature loss of the teeth, and endocrine disorders, including diabetes mellitus and testicular atrophy. Other symptoms may include calcinosis, hypertrophic arthritis, dystrophic nails, scleropoikiloderma, osteoporosis, adrenal cortex and pituitary gland hypofunction, thyroid nodules, hyperthyroidism, and hyperparathyroidism. Called also *progeria adultorum.* **Weyers' s.,** 1. iridodental DYSPLASIA. 2. acrofacial DYSOSTOSIS. **Weyers Fülling s.,** DYSPLASIA dentofacialis. **Weyers-Thier s.,** oculovertebral DYSPLASIA. **whistling face s.,** craniocarpotarsal DYSTROPHY. **Wildervanck's s.,** cervico-oculofacial s. **Willebrand's s.,** Willebrand-Jürgens s. **Willebrand-Jürgens s.,** a hemorrhagic disorder, inherited as a simple dominant trait, affecting both sexes. It is characterized by prolonged bleeding time in the presence of normal platelet count, associated with epistaxis and bleeding from the gastrointestinal tract, gums, uterus, and at the sites of surgical operations. Factor VIII deficiency and capillary disorders and blood platelet abnormalities are believed to be the cause. Called also *von Willebrand's s., Willebrand's s., angiohemophilia, constitutional thrombopathy, hereditary hemorrhagic thrombasthenia, pseudohemophilia,* and *vascular hemophilia.* **Williams' s., Williams-Barrat s.,** elfin facies s. **Winchester's s.,** a syndrome combining dwarfism, contractures, corneal opacities, osteoporosis, dissolution of carpal and tarsal bones, joint destruction simulating severe rheumatoid arthritis, and coarse facies with prominent forehead, fleshy large nose, depressed nasal bridge, and thick lips. **Wiskott-Aldrich s.,** a rare and usually fatal hereditary syndrome, transmitted as an X-linked recessive trait. The onset is usually in infancy or early childhood, and is characterized by thrombocytopenic purpura, eczema, bloody diarrhea, and extreme susceptibility to infection (especially otitis media and staphylococcal infections), associated with antibody deficiency and dysgammaglobulinemia. An absence of isohemagglutinins and an increase in serum is found in most cases. Called also *Aldrich's s.* and *eczema-thrombocytopenia s.* **Witkop-Von Sallmann s.,** hereditary benign intraepithelial DYSKERATOSIS. **Wolf's s.,** Wolf-Hirschhorn s. **Wolf-Hirschhorn s.,** a relatively rare syndrome of partial deletion of the short arm of one of the chromosomes 4, characterized by psychomotor and growth retardation and multiple abnormalities. Birth weight is usually low; hypotonia and seizures may be present at birth. Common craniofacial abnormalities include microcephaly, cranial asymmetry, prominent glabella, ocular hypertelorism, antimongoloid palpebral fissures, ptosis of the eyelids, low-set deformed ears with preauricular dimples and sinuses and narrow external canals, and a short philtrum. Down-turned corners of the mouth, cleft palate or lip, and micrognathia are the most prominent oral defects. Bony abnormalities may consist of late ossification of pelvic and metacarpal bones, synostoses, fusion of bony structures, hip dislocation, and pseudohypophyses. Urogenital and cardiovascular abnormalities, simian palmar creases, dermal ridges, strabismus, hydrocephalus, and other defects may be associated. Life expectancy is low, about one-third dying within the first 2 years of life. Called also *4p s.* and *Wolf's s.* **xeroderma-talipes-enamel defect s.,** a congenital syndrome characterized by hypoplasia of the sweat glands, hypohidrosis, xeroderma, evanescent cutaneous bullae, dry coarse hair, nail abnormalities, cleft palate, defective dental enamel, bilateral club foot, hypoplasia of the ocular puncta leading to epiphora and blepharitis, absence of lashes on lower lids, mental deficiency, and abnormal electroencephalogram. In the original cases, the sibs were the product of a consanguineous union. Called also *XTE s.* **XO s.,** Turner's s. **XTE s.,** xeroderma-talipes-enamel defect s. **XXXX s.,** a chromosomal syndrome characterized by mental deficiency and a variable variety of abnormalities, including midfacial hypoplasia, hypertelorism, epicanthic folds, micrognathia, clinodactyly, radioulnar synostosis, narrow shoulder girdle, occasional amenorrhea, and irregular menses. **XXXXX s.,** a chromosomal anomaly characterized by a mental and growth deficiency, mongoloid slant of palpebral fissures, low nasal bridge, short neck, small hands with mild clinodactyly of fifth fingers, and patent ductus arteriosus. Coloboma of the iris, hypertelorism, inner canthal folds, low-set ears, low dermal ridges, simian creases, elbow dislocation, and overlapping toes may be associated. Called also *penta X s.* **XXXXY s.,** see *Klinefelter's s.* **XXXY s.,** see *Klinefelter's s.* **XXY s.,** see *Kline-*

felter's s. **XXYY** s., see *Klinefelter's* s. **XYY** s., a syndrome associated with an extra Y chromosome in males, characterized by a tendency toward a longer body, muscle weakness, a high bridge of the nose, acne vulgaris, and mild facial asymmetry with mandibular deformities, and pectus excavatum. Affected patients may have mild mental retardation and exhibit explosive behavior with a propensity to destroy property, rather than violence against others. **Zellweger's** s., cerebrohepatorenal s. **Zinsser-Engman-Cole** s., DYSKERATOSIS congenita. **Zuelzer-Kaplan** s., 1. familial nonspherocytic hemolytic ANEMIA. 2. thalassemia–hemoglobin C DISEASE. **Zuelzer-Ogden** s., a form of megaloblastic anemia characterized by slowly progressive macrocytic anemia, leukopenia, and thrombocytopenia; megaloblasts in the bone marrow; and gastrointestinal, neurological, and oral symptoms typical of other megaloblastic anemias.

Syndrox trademark for *methamphetamine hydrochloride* (see under METHAMPHETAMINE).

synechia (sĭ-nek′e-ah), pl. *synech′iae* [Gr. *synecheia* continuity] an adhesion or abnormal fusion of parts.

synechiae (sĭ-nek′e-e) plural of *synechia.*

synechotomy (sin″ě-kot′o-me) [*synechia* + Gr. *tomē* a cutting] the cutting of a synechia.

syneresis (si-ner′ě-sis) [Gr. *synairesis* a taking or drawing together] a drawing together of the particles of the dispersed phase of a gel, with the separation of some of the disperse medium and shrinkage of the gel, such as occurs in the clotting of blood.

synergism (sin′er-jizm) the act or process whereby the joint action of separate agents or agencies is greater than the sum of their effects taken independently.

synergist (sin′er-jist) 1. an agent which cooperates with another. 2. synergic MUSCLE.

synergistic (sin″er-jis′tik) acting jointly; enhancing the effect of another force or agent.

synergy (sin′er-je) [L. *synergia;* Gr. *syn* together + *ergon* work] correlated action or cooperation on the part of two or more structures or drugs. In neurology, the faculty by which movements are properly grouped for the performance of acts requiring special adjustments.

synesthesia (sin″es-the′ze-ah) [*syn-* + Gr. *aisthēsis* perception + *-ia*] a secondary sensation accompanying an actual perception; the experiencing of a sensation in one place due to stimulation applied to another place; also the condition in which a stimulus of one sense is perceived as a sensation of a different sense.

synesthesialgia (sin″es-the″ze-al′je-ah) a condition in which a stimulus produces pain on the affected side but no sensation or even a pleasant one on the normal side of the body.

Synestrin trademark for *diethylstilbestrol.*

Synestrol trademark for *dienestrol.*

syngeneic (sin″jě-ne′ik) [*syn-* + Gr. *genos* kind] pertaining to individuals or tissues that have identical genotypes, i.e., identical twins or animals of the same inbred strain, or their tissue. Called also *isogeneic.* Cf. *allogeneic.*

syngenesioplastic (sin″jě-ne″ze-o-plas′tik) [*syn-* + Gr. *genesis* origin + *plassein* to shape] pertaining to transplantation of tissue from one individual to another related individual, as from a mother to her child, or from one twin to another. See also isogeneic GRAFT.

syngenite (sin′jen-īt) a native potassium calcium sulfate, $K_2Ca(SO_4)_2 \cdot H_2O$. Used as an accelerator of the setting time of gypsum products, such as dental plaster, plaster of Paris, and dental stone.

syngnathia (sin-na′the-ah) [*syn-* + Gr. *gnathos* jaw + *-ia*] a congenital condition characterized by the presence of fibrous bands extending from the maxilla to the mandible.

syngraft (sin′graft) [*syn-* + *graft*] isologous GRAFT.

Synkamin trademark for *vitamin K₅ hydrochloride* (see under VITAMIN).

Synka-Vit trademark for *menadiol sodium diphosphate* (see under MENADIOL).

Synkavite trademark for *menadiol sodium diphosphate* (see under MENADIOL).

synkinesia (sin″ki-ne′ze-ah) [*syn-* + Gr. *kinēsis* movement] an associated movement; an unintentional movement accompanying a volitional movement.

synnema (sĭ-ne′mah) a group of parallel hyphae joined together and forming an elongated erect spore-bearing structure.

Synnematin B trademark for *penicillin N.*

synophrys (sin-of′ris) [Gr. "with meeting eyebrows"] growing together of the eyebrows.

synosteology (sin″os-te-ol′o-je) [*syn-* + Gr. *osteon* bone + *-logy*] the field of study concerned with the joints and articulations.

synostosis (sin″os-to′sis), pl. *synosto′ses* [*syn-* + Gr. *osteon* bone] 1. a union between adjacent bones or parts of a single bone formed by osseous matter, such as ossified connecting cartilage or fibrous tissue. 2. fusion of bones that are normally distinct. See also ANKYLOSIS.

synotia (si-no′she-ah) [*syn-* + Gr. *ous* ear] a congenital abnormality characterized by persistence of the ears in their horizontal position beneath the mandible.

Synotodecin trademark for *rolitetracycline.*

synovia (sĭ-no′ve-ah) [L.; Gr. *syn* with + *ōon* egg] synovial FLUID.

synovitis (sin″o-vi′tis) inflammation of a synovial membrane. **tendinous** s., **vaginal** s., tenosynovitis.

Synsac trademark for *fluocinolone acetonide* (see under FLUOCINOLONE).

synstigmin (sin-stig′min) neostigmine. **s. bromide,** NEOSTIGMINE bromide.

Syntarpen trademark for *dicloxacillin sodium* (see under DICLOXACILLIN).

Syntedril trademark for *diphenhydramine.*

synteny (sin′tě-ne) the presence together on the same chromosome of two or more gene loci in such proximity that they may be subject to linkage. See also *linkage.*

Syntetrin trademark for *rolitetracycline.*

synthase (sin-thās) any enzyme, especially a lyase, which catalyzes a synthesis that does not involve the breakdown of a pyrophosphate bond (as opposed to *ligase*).

synthesis (sin′thě-sis) [Gr. "a putting together, composition"] the building up of a chemical compound by the union of its elements or from suitable starting materials.

synthetase (sin′the-tās) ligase. **argininosuccinate** s. [E.C. 6.3.4.5], an enzyme which converts ATP in the presence of L-citrulline and L-aspartate to AMP, pyrophosphate, and L-argininosuccinate. **amide** s. [E.C.6.3.1], a subclass of ligases, the enzymes of which catalyze the linking of an acid and an ammonia group, as in the formation of L-asparagine and L-glutamine. Called also *acid-ammonia ligase.* **fatty acid** s., a multienzyme system involved in the synthesis of fatty acids. **peptide** s. [E.C.6.3.2], a subclass of ligases, the enzymes of which catalyze the linking together of amino acids in peptide synthesis. Called also *acid–amino acid ligase.*

synthetic (sin-thet′ik) 1. pertaining to, of the nature of, or participating in synthesis. 2. produced by synthesis; artificial. 3. synthetic PLASTIC.

Synthomycetine trademark for *chloramphenicol.*

Syntometrine trademark for *ergonovine.*

syntrophoblast (sin-trof′o-blast) synctiotrophoblast.

syphilid (sif′ĭ-lid) a general term for the skin lesions of secondary syphilis, appearing, usually between six weeks and two years after infection, in a series of crops lasting a few days to a few months, and becoming progressively more severe and conspicuous. The serologic test for syphilis is invariably positive. Mucous membrane lesions in this stage are typically teeming with *Treponema pallidum,* and are clinically the most contagious lesions of the disease.

syphilis (sif′ĭ-lis) [*Syphilus* (Ital. *Sifilo*), the name of a herdsman in a poem of Fracastorius published in Latin in 1530, in which the term first appears. Derived probably from Gr. *sys* swine + *philein* to love (hence the name of the herdsman), or from *syn* together + *philein* to love, but the etymology of the term is uncertain] a contagious venereal disease caused by the spirochete *Treponema pallidum,* and transmitted chiefly by coitus; it is transmissible to offspring in utero. It is systemic from the onset, characterized by widespread involvement of the tissues, and associated with a wide variety of symptoms. Lesions of the oral cavity occur most often on the lips, the tongue being the next in frequency of involvement, but the gingivae, palate, pharynx, and buccal mucous membrane may also be involved. The primary stage is characterized by a chancre, initially appearing as a painless, punched out, indurated papule that soon erodes and becomes ulcerated, with cervical lymph nodes becoming enlarged; after two to four weeks, the chancre disappears, leaving a small scar. Oral syphilis is usually transmitted through genito-oral contact. Syphilis is divided into primary, secondary, and tertiary stages (see below). Called also *lues* and *pox.* See also GUMMA, Hutchinson's TEETH and syphilitic OSTEOMYELITIS. **acquired** s., syphilis resulting from exposure, usually sexual contact, including coitus, fellatio, cunnilingus, and kissing, with infected persons. Although sexual contact is the most common route of infection, persons, such as dentists, working with infected individuals may also acquire syphilis. **congenital** s., syphilis acquired in utero, transmitted by infected mothers, characterized by a well-defined pattern of lesions of the skin, bones, oral mucosa, and teeth, which are present at birth or shortly thereafter. The typical cutaneous manifestation is a diffuse, maculopapular, desquamative rash involving most of the body, particularly the palms and soles and about the mouth and anus. Osseous changes, usually occurring at about the end of the fifth month of intrauterine life, may result in destruction of the vomer and collapse of the bridge of the nose, producing the characteristic saddle deformity; perforation of the palate; multiple swellings of the frontal and parietal bones; necrotic changes in the mandible; periosteal nodes; and saber shins. Oral lesions usually consist of acute moist papules with fissuring at the labial commissures and subsequent scarring and formation of rhagades. Hutchinson's teeth with characteristic notching and deformed incisors having a screwdriver shape are the most common dental features. The liver, lungs, cardiovascular and nervous systems, and other organs are often affected. Called also *neonatal s.* and *prenatal s.* **neonatal s., prenatal s.,** congenital s. **primary s.,** the initial stage of syphilis, appearing about three weeks after the infection, and characterized by the development of a chancre at the site of entry, usually the penis, vulva, cervix uteri, or oral cavity. Oral chancres present hard, brownish, painless, ulcerated nodules of the lips, tip of the tongue, tonsils, gingiva, and other parts of the mouth. See also CHANCRE. **secondary s.,** the metastatic stage of syphilis characterized by the appearance, about six weeks after the primary lesion, of diffuse eruptions on the skin and mucous membrane. The oral lesions, most commonly found on the tongue, gingiva, tonsils, and buccal mucosa, are characterized by multiple, painless, grayish white plaques (see mucous patches, under PATCH) overlying an ulcerated surface. All moist lesions of secondary syphilis are highly contagious and may be a source of infection. **tertiary s.,** the late stage of syphilis, which may occur several months or years after the initial infection, characterized by the involvement of the cardiovascular system, bones, and nervous system. Gummata, soft, gummy, grayish lesions of the skin and mucous membranes, liver, testes, and bones, are the chief symptoms; intraoral gummata most commonly involve the tongue and palate. Complications may include osteomyelitis (see syphilitic OSTEOMYELITIS) and diffuse interstitial glossitis. See also TABES dorsalis.

syphilitic (sif″ĭ-lit′ik) [L. *syphiliticus*] affected with, caused by, or pertaining to syphilis.

syphiloma (sif″ĭ-lo′mah) a tumor of syphilitic origin. See GUMMA.

Syr. abbreviation for L. *syrupus,* syrup.

syrigmophonia (sir″ig-mo-fo′ne-ah) [Gr. *syrigmos* a shrill piping sound + *phōnē* voice + *-ia*] a high whistling sound of the voice.

syringe (sĭ-rinj′, sir′inj) [L. *syrinxe;* Gr. *syrinx*] an instrument for injecting liquids into or withdrawing them from any vessel or cavity. It may consist of a glass, plastic, or metal cylinder graduated to show its contents in cubic centimeters or milliliters; a piston within the cylinder which, when withdrawn, causes the liquid to flow into the cylinder and, when pressed, to be ejected from the cylinder; and a hollow needle through which the liquid flows into or out of the cylinder. Also, a rubber bulb with a tube and nozzle at the end, used for irrigation of body cavities. See illustrations. **air s.,** a small syringe connected by a hose to the compressed air tank in the dental unit, consisting of a fine nozzle, a hand grip, a pressure-regulating valve, and a clamp for the attachment of an air tip or a spray bottle; used to direct a current of air into a tooth cavity during excavation, to remove the small chips detached from the tooth, or to dry the cavity. Called also *chip s.* **aspirating s., aspirator s.,** any syringe used for aspirating fluids from a vessel or cavity. **chip s.,** air s. **dental s.,** a small syringe into which is fitted a hermetically sealed cartridge which contains an anesthetic solution. **endodontic s.,** one for forcing semisolid sealers into root canals. Called also *pressure s.* **endodontic irrigating s.,** one for endodontic irrigation, designed to inject a sufficient volume of the solution to the working area, particularly to a fine or tortuous root canal system, aspirate the expended fluid and debris, and prevent the extrusion of either irrigating solution or debris beyond the apical confines of the tooth. It is a disposable 3 ml syringe with an irrigating needle that is blunted and slit for 4 to 5 ml along one side from the tip toward the hub so as to provide an escape for fluids, should it bind in a canal. Another model has the needle passing through the wall and lumen of a polyethylene tube connected to the saliva injection system of the dental unit so as to provide aspiration during irrigation. See also root canal GUN. **Endovage s.,** trademark for an endodontic irrigating syringe that may be used with a variety of needles; aspiration occurs through the irrigating needle once pressure on the plunger is released. **fountain s.,** an apparatus for injecting liquids by the action of gravity. **hand s.,** an air syringe in which the nozzle is connected to a rubber bulb; hand compression forces the air from the bulb through the nozzle. Used to clear debris from desired areas, such as wax patterns. When used to clear debris or dry tooth cavities, the air may be warmed by heating the nozzle. **hydrocolloid s.,** one for the application of

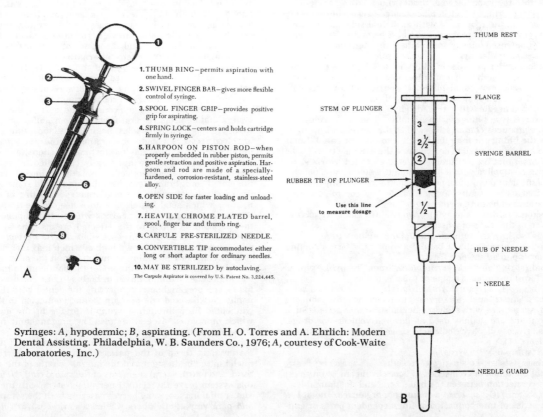

1. THUMB RING—permits aspiration with one hand.

2. SWIVEL FINGER BAR—gives more flexible control of syringe.

3. SPOOL FINGER GRIP—provides positive grip for aspirating.

4. SPRING LOCK—centers and holds cartridge firmly in syringe.

5. HARPOON ON PISTON ROD—when properly embedded in rubber piston, permits gentle retraction and positive aspiration. Harpoon and rod are made of a specially-hardened, corrosion-resistant, stainless-steel alloy.

6. OPEN SIDE for faster loading and unloading.

7. HEAVILY CHROME PLATED barrel, spool, finger bar and thumb ring.

8. CARPULE PRE-STERILIZED NEEDLE.

9. CONVERTIBLE TIP accommodates either long or short adaptor for ordinary needles.

10. MAY BE STERILIZED by autoclaving.

The Carpule Aspirator is covered by U.S. Patent No. 3,224,445.

THUMB REST

STEM OF PLUNGER — FLANGE

3   2½   ②   SYRINGE BARREL

RUBBER TIP OF PLUNGER

Use this line to measure dosage

1   ½

HUB OF NEEDLE

1″ NEEDLE

NEEDLE GUARD

Syringes: *A,* hypodermic; *B,* aspirating. (From H. O. Torres and A. Ehrlich: Modern Dental Assisting. Philadelphia, W. B. Saunders Co., 1976; *A,* courtesy of Cook-Waite Laboratories, Inc.)

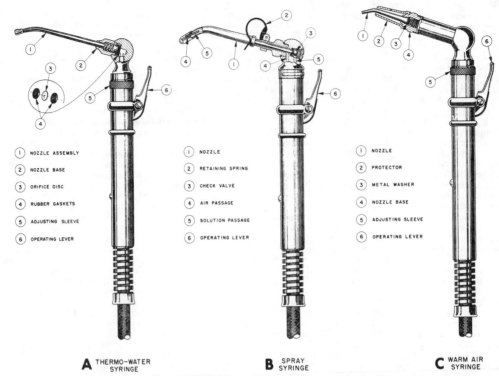

A THERMO-WATER SYRINGE   **B** SPRAY SYRINGE   **C** WARM AIR SYRINGE

Various syringes: *A*, thermowater; *B*, spray; *C*, warm air. (From V. R. Park, J. R. Ashman, and G. J. Shelly: A Textbook for Dental Assistants. 2nd ed. Philadelphia, W. B. Saunders Co., 1975; courtesy of the Ritter Co., Inc.)

hydrocolloid to prepared teeth, having an air valve in the plunger to release trapped air before the material is expelled. **hypodermic s.,** one, usually of small caliber, by means of which drugs in solution or other liquids are injected through a hollow needle into the subcutaneous tissues. **Luer-Lok s.,** trademark for a type of syringe which can be adapted to use a blunt needle for irrigating the root canal with medicinal substances. **pressure s.,** endodontic s. **probe s.,** one whose point may be used also as a probe; used mostly in treating the lacrimal passages. **Pulpdent s.,** trademark for an endodontic syringe for the introduction under pressure of filling materials, especially used for permanent teeth with immature roots or tortuous canals and for retrograde root canal filling. It consists of an internally threaded octagon-shaped syringe barrel, one end receiving a blunt-tipped needle with a threaded hub and the other containing a screw-type plunger with a knurled handle. Turning the plunger produces compression within the barrel and, in turn, forces the filling out from the needle into the root canal. Lines on the handle are used in determining the distance traveled by the plunger and the amount of material extruded. **warm s.,** an air syringe supplied with a heating unit. **water s.,** one, being a part of the dental unit, that permits controlled spraying of water in desired areas, usually having a nozzle, flow control, pressure regulator, and heating element.

syringectomy (sir″in-jek′to-me) [*syringo-* + Gr. *ektomē* excision] excision of the walls of a fistula.

syringitis (sir″in-ji′tis) inflammation of the auditory tube.

syringo- [Gr. *syrinx* tube or fistula] a combining form denoting relationship to a tube or a fistula.

syringoid (si-ring′goid) [L. *syringoides*, from Gr. *syrinx* pipe + *eidos* form] resembling a pipe or tube; fistulous.

syrup (sir′up) [L. *syrupus;* Arabic *sharab*] a concentrated solution of a sugar, such as sucrose, in water or other aqueous liquid, sometimes with some medicinal substance added. Such preparations are usually used as flavored vehicles for drugs. **corn s.,** glucose (1). **hydriodic acid s.,** see hydriodic ACID. **starch s.,** glucose (1).

syrupus (sir′up-us) [L.] syrup.

syssarcosis (sis″sar-ko′sis) [*syn-* together + *sarkōsis* fleshy growth] the union or connection of bones by means of muscles, as the connection between the hyoid bone and the mandible.

system (sis′tem) [Gr. *systēma* a complex or organized whole] 1. a set or series of interconnected or interdependent parts or enti-

ties which function together in a common purpose or produce results impossible of achievement by one of them acting or operating alone. 2. a school or method of practice based on a specific principle. 3. in enzyme nomenclature, a group of enzymes involved in similar activities, as in catalyzing the oxidation of succinate by molecular oxygen, involving succinate dehydrogenase, cytochrome oxidase, and several intermediate cytochrome carriers. **alimentary s.,** the organs concerned with intake of food, digestion, and absorption of nutrients; see *digestive s.* **alloy s.,** ALLOY system. **alternative complement s.,** see PROPERDIN. **arterial s.,** the part of the cardiovascular system which carries the oxygenated blood from the heart to the peripheral tissues, consisting of a network of capillaries, arterioles, arteries, and major arterial trunks. See also systemic CIRCULATION. **autonomic nervous s.,** the part of the nervous system that controls visceral functions, particularly motor activities of the smooth muscles, heart, and glands, thus regulating blood pressure, glandular secretions, urinary output, sweating, body temperature, gastrointestinal functions, and certain other activities that are not totally controlled by voluntary mechanisms. It is a network of neurons that connects centers in the spinal cord, brain stem, hypothalamus, and some parts of the cerebral cortex with visceral organs, consisting of sensory neurons which send impulses from sense organs to the autonomic centers and motor neurons which send impulses from the autonomic centers to the affected organs. The system is divided into two subsystems (see *sympathetic nervous s.* and *parasympathetic nervous s.*), both of which may innervate the same organs, one providing stimulation and the other reciprocal inhibition, but most being under the dominant influence of one system. A neuronal chain in both systems consists of two fibers, one preganglionic, connecting the center with the autonomic ganglia, and one postganglionic, connected to the preganglionic fiber through a synaptic bridge in the ganglion, which innervates visceral organs. The preganglionic fibers of the sympathetic system originate from the centers in the lateral column of the thoracic and upper lumbar segments of the gray matter, and those of the parasympathetic system from the nuclei in the brain stem and the lateral column of the second, third, and fourth sacral segments of the spinal cord. Neurons of this system leave the central nervous system with the spinal and cranial nerves, some nerves carrying both the sympathetic and parasympathetic fibers. Called also *involuntary nervous*

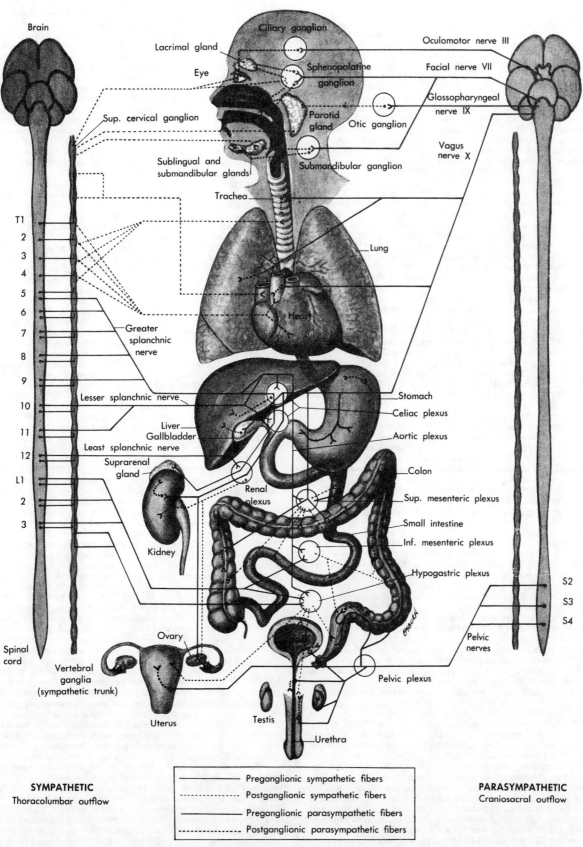

SYMPATHETIC
Thoracolumbar outflow

PARASYMPATHETIC
Craniosacral outflow

————————	Preganglionic sympathetic fibers
- - - - - - - -	Postganglionic sympathetic fibers
————————	Preganglionic parasympathetic fibers
- - - - - - - -	Postganglionic parasympathetic fibers

Autonomic nervous system. (From Dorland's Illustrated Medical Dictionary. 26th ed. Philadelphia, W. B. Saunders Co., 1981.)

s., vegetative nervous s., visceral nervous s., and *systema nervosum autonomicum* [NA]. Formerly called *sympathetic nervous s.* **binary s.,** see binary ALLOY. **biologic s.,** a system composed of living material; such systems range from a collection of separate molecules to an assemblage of separate organisms. **blood group s.,** see BLOOD GROUP. **brunonian s.,** see METHODIST (1). **cardiovascular s.,** the part of the circulatory system concerned with blood circulation, consisting of the heart and the arterial and venous systems. See also systemic CIRCULATION. **centimeter-gram-second s., CGS s., cgs s., cm-g-s s.,** a system of units in which the centimeter, gram, and second are the principal units of length, mass, and time. Abbreviated *CGS* and *cgs.* **central nervous s.,** the part of the nervous system consisting of the brain and spinal cord. It is made up of the gray substance, composed of the neurons, which form connections between each other, the synapses, and the white substance, consisting of the nerve fibers. It controls the activity of tissues and organs through a system of peripheral nerves (*peripheral nervous s.*). Called also *systema nervorum centrale* and *systema nervosum centrale* [NA]. Abbreviated *CNS.* **channel shoulder pin s.,** channel shoulder pin TECHNIQUE. **circulatory s.,** the system consisting of the cardiovascular and lymphatic systems, which is concerned with the circulation of body fluids; transport to the tissues of nutrients, hormones, immune substances, and chemical substances; removal and carrying away of waste products and carbon dioxide; oxygenation of the blood and transport of oxygen to the tissues; maintenance of water-electrolyte balance; equalization of body temperature; and other vital functions. **complement s.,** see COMPLEMENT. **complement activation s., complement priming s.,** see complement activation PATHWAY. **Cooperative Health Statistics S.,** a program of the National Center for Health Statistics for collecting health statistics on the federal, state, and local levels, expected to include data on health manpower, health facilities, hospital care, household interviews, ambulatory care, long-term health care, and vital statistics. Abbreviated *CHSS.* **Coordinated Transfer Application S.,** a program of the American Association of Medical Colleges in which citizens of the United States receiving undergraduate medical education outside the U.S. are evaluated. Students who are found qualified are sponsored for the national board examinations and those who pass the examinations may apply to a U.S. medical school for completion of training with advanced standing. Abbreviated *COTRANS.* **CSP s.,** channel shoulder pin TECHNIQUE. **decimal s.,** a system of counting or measurement, the units of which are powers of 10. See metric SYSTEM. **dentinal s.,** all the tubules radiating from a single pulp cavity. **dermal s., dermoid s.,** the skin and its appendages, including both the hair and the nails. **digestive s.,** a system of organs involved in the intake and digestion of food, absorption of nutrients, and elimination of solid wastes, consisting of the mouth, pharynx, esophagus, stomach, small intestine, large intestine, and rectum, as well as associated organs and glands, such as the pancreas, biliary system, salivary glands, etc. Called also *apparatus digestorius* [NA] and *digestive apparatus.* **eco s., ecologic s.,** ecosystem. **endocrine s.,** the system of glands and other structures that elaborate internal secretions (hormones) that are released directly into the circulatory system and which influence metabolism and other body processes. They include the pituitary, thyroid, parathyroid, pineal, and adrenal glands, and the gonads, islands of Langerhans of the pancreas, and paraganglia. The thymus is no longer considered to perform an endocrine function. **eutectic s.,** one of the intermediate phases of an alloy which may form when the constituent metals are partially soluble in each other. See also eutectic ALLOY. **extrinsic s.,** a blood coagulation mechanism, whereby the process is initiated by interaction of substances in damaged tissue. Called also *extrinsic mechanism.* See blood COAGULATION. **genitourinary s.,** urogenital s. **gold-copper s.,** gold-copper ALLOY. **H-2 s.,** major histocompatibility complex (of mouse); see under HISTOCOMPATIBILITY. **haversian s.,** the basic unit of structure of compact bone, consisting of a haversian canal and its concentrically arranged (haversian) lamellae, forming the osteon. See also haversian CANAL, haversian CANALICULUS, haversian LAMELLA, and OSTEON. **health care s.,** the network of personal health care services, consisting of persons who give services, facilities and resources that support these services, financing mechanisms, the legal framework, and the communications and relationships that link one part of the system to another. **hematopoietic s.,** a system of tissues involved in production of the blood, including the bone marrow and lymphatic tissue. **HLA s., HL-A**

s., see major histocompatibility complex of man, under HISTOCOMPATIBILITY. **hydrodynamic s.,** see *periodontal hydrodynamic s.* **immune s.,** the system responsible for immune responses of the body. It consists of the lymphoreticular tissue, the cellular elements of which are distributed throughout the body; they are found lining the lymphatic and vascular channels, in the blood, lymph nodes, thymus, spleen, and a variety of other organs, including those which are exposed to the external environment, such as the respiratory, gastrointestinal, and genitourinary tracts. See also IMMUNITY. **International S. of Units** (Système International d'Unités), see SI. **international two-digit tooth-recording s.,** a numbering system recommended by the Fédération Dentaire Internationale for the charting and description of human teeth. The first digit indicates the quadrant and the second tooth within the quadrant, numbering from the midline toward the posterior. In the permanent dentition, the maxillary right quadrant is No. 1 (containing teeth numbers 11 to 18); the maxillary left quadrant is No. 2 (containing teeth numbers 21 to 28); the mandibular left quadrant is No. 3 (containing teeth numbers 31 to 38); and the mandibular right quadrant is No. 4 (containing teeth numbers 41 to 48). In the primary dentition, the maxillary right quadrant is No. 5 (containing teeth numbers 51 to 55); the maxillary left quadrant is No. 6 (containing teeth numbers 61 to 65); the mandibular left quadrant is No. 7 (containing teeth numbers 71 to 55); and the mandibular right quadrant is No. 8 (containing teeth numbers 81 to 85). See also dental CHART. **intrinsic s.,** a blood coagulation mechanism, whereby the process is initiated by trauma to the blood itself, as when blood is removed from the body. Called also *intrinsic mechanism.* See blood COAGULATION. **involuntary nervous s.,** autonomic nervous s. **limbic s.,** a group of brain structures common to all mammals (including the hippocampus and dentate gyrus with their archicortex, the cingulate gyrus and septal areas, and sometimes the amygdala), associated with olfaction and other activities, such as autonomic functions and certain aspects of emotion and behavior. It is the portion of the brain that is associated with emotional, affective, motivational behavior, and putative site of antianxiety drug effects. Called also *rhinencephalon.* **lymphatic s.,** a system consisting of a chain of lymphatic capillaries, vessels, nodes, and trunks draining into the venous circulation. It is involved in removing from the interstitial spaces excess fluid, waste substance, and substances leaked out by the blood capillaries. Some diffusible substances re-enter the venous circulation, but large molecules, such as proteins and bacteria, are circulated through the lymph nodes, where they are filtered and bacteria are phagocytized. They are then circulated through the thoracic and right lymphatic ducts, and discharged into the venous circulation through the subclavian veins, to be filtered through the kidneys and removed from the body. By controlling the volume of the interstitial fluid, it also controls the fluid pressure, prevents edema from developing, restores blood volume after hemorrhage, and controls blood protein and electrolyte levels. Its other functions include absorption of nutrients, especially fats from the intestine and proteins from the liver. It is also involved in spreading infection and tumor metastases. The spleen, tonsils, thymus, and adenoids are sometimes considered as parts of this system. Called also *systema lymphaticum* [NA]. See illustration. **lymphoid s.,** a system consisting of (1) a central component involved in the differentiation of the lymphoid stem cells into lymphocytes capable of reacting with antigen (antigen-reactive cells), and (2) a peripheral component in which these cells can subsequently react with antigen. Anatomically, the system includes the bone marrow, the thymus, and a component whose identity is known with certainty only in birds (the bursa of Fabricius) and that in mammals is designated as the *bursal equivalent tissue.* The peripheral segment consists of lymph nodes, spleen, and gut-associated lymphoid tissue. The maturation of lymphoid elements in the central component can occur in the absence of antigen. See illustration. **macrophage s.,** reticuloendothelial s. **masticatory s.,** the organs and structures which function primarily in mastication, including the jaws, teeth with their supporting structures, temporomandibular joint, mandibular muscles, tongue, lips, cheeks, and oral mucosa. Called also *organs of mastication.* **Medicaid Management Information S.,** see MMIS. **meter-kilogram-second s.,** see MKS. **metric s.,** the system of weights and measures based on the decimal system or the meter. Units of length, 1 meter = 10 centimeters = 1000 millimeters; units of mass, 1 kilogram = 1000 grams, 1 gram = 1000 milligrams, 1 milligram = 1000 micrograms; units of volume, 1 liter = 1000 milliliters (or 1000 cubic centimeters), 1 milliliter = 1000 microliters; unit of temperature, 1° Celcius. The multiples and fractions of units uniformly have prefixes derived from Greek and Latin. See

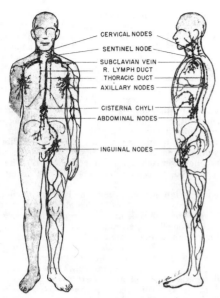

The lymphatic system. (From A. C. Guyton: Textbook of Medical Physiology. 6th ed. Philadelphia, W. B. Saunders Co., 1981.)

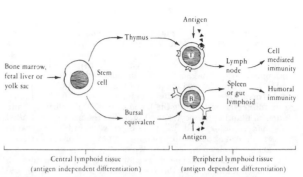

Development of the lymphoid system. (From J. A. Bellanti: Immunology II. Philadelphia, W. B. Saunders Co., 1978.)

table. See also SI and *Tables of Weights and Measures* at WEIGHT. **muscular s.,** the striated, smooth, and cardiac muscles considered collectively. See MUSCLE. **nervous s.,** a system of organs that correlates and integrates the reactions of the body to the internal and external environment. For convenience, it is divided into the central nervous system, comprised of the brain and spinal cord, and the peripheral nervous system, comprised of the nerves, ganglia, and end organs, which connects the central nervous system with the tissues and organs of the body. Called also *systema nervosum* [NA]. See also *autonomic nervous s., central nervous s., parasympathetic nervous s.,* and *sympathetic nervous s.* **occlusal s.,** the form or design and arrangment of the occlusal and incisal units of a dentition or the teeth on a denture. Called also *occlusal scheme.* **parasympathetic nervous s.,** the part of the autonomic nervous system containing preganglionic fibers that originate in the brain stem and the second to fourth sacral segments of the gray matter of the spinal cord. Its neurons leave the central nervous system with the oculomotor, facial, glossopharyngeal, and vagus nerves and enter autonomic ganglia where they transmit to postganglionic fibers through synapses. Parasympathetic nerves supplying the head and neck pass through the ciliary, pterygopalatine, otic, and submandibular ganglia, which give off postganglionic branches supplying individual structures. The sacral portion supplies various thoracic and abdominal structures. Parasympathetic stimulation causes excitation in some organs but inhibition in others, often providing inhibiting stimulation to organs receiving excitatory effects from the sympathetic system. Impulses between the preganglionic and postganglionic

fibers are allowed to pass only when parasympathetic nerve endings secrete acetylcholine, thus providing synaptic bridges. Called also *craniosacral part of autonomic nervous system, parasympathetic part of autonomic nervous system,* and *pars parasympathica systematis nervosi autonomici* [NA]. **periodontal hydrodynamic s.,** a system which resists occlusal forces, consisting of tissue fluid and fluid which passes through small vessel walls and is squeezed into the surrounding areas through foramina in the alveoli. **periodontal pitch s.,** a system, related to the hydrodynamic system, which controls the pitch or level of the tooth in the socket. Called also *pitch s.* **periodontal resilient s.,** a system which causes the tooth to spring back into position when the occlusal forces are removed. Called also *resilient s.* **periodontal vascular s.,** a system of blood vessels which derives from the inferior and superior alveolar arteries and reaches the periodontal ligament from the apical vessels, penetrating vessels from the alveolar bone, and anastomosing vessels from the gingiva. In addition to supplying blood, the system also acts as a shock absorber and takes up strains of sudden occlusal forces. **peripheral nervous s.,** the part of the nervous system consisting of nerve fibers, ganglia, and end organs outside the brain and the spinal cord; it conveys impulses between the end organs and the central nervous system. Called also *systema nervosum periphericum* [NA]. **pitch s.,** periodontal pitch s. **platinum-silver s.,** platinum-silver ALLOY. **PSRO Management Information S.,** a former monitoring program which gathers information needed to evaluate a hospital's performance. Abbreviated *PMIS.* **pyramidal s.,** pyramidal TRACT. **quaternary s.,** quaternary ALLOY. **quinary s.,** see quinary ALLOY. **RE s.,** reticuloendothelial s. **recall s.,** a procedure used in periodically reminding patients to return for examination. **reproductive s.,** the part of the urogenital system consisting of the reproductive organs. The male system consists of the testes, prostate, penis, and a system of ducts; the female system consists of the ovaries, fallopian tubes, uterus, vagina, and external genitalia. **resilient s.,** periodontal resilient s. **respiratory s.,** a system of organs involved in providing oxygen to the cells and tissues and

MULTIPLES AND SUBMULTIPLES OF THE METRIC SYSTEM

Multiples and Submultiples	Prefix	Pronunciation	Symbol
$1{,}000{,}000{,}000{,}000 = 10^{12}$	tera	ter′a	T
$1{,}000{,}000{,}000 = 10^{9}$	giga	ji′ga	G
$1{,}000{,}000 = 10^{6}$	mega	meg′a	M
$1{,}000 = 10^{3}$	kilo	kil′o	k
$100 = 10^{2}$	hecto	hek′to	h
$10 = 10$	deka	dek′a	dk
[The unit = one]			
$0.1 = 10^{-1}$	deci	des′i	d
$0.01 = 10^{-2}$	centi	sen′ti	c
$0.001 = 10^{-3}$	milli	mil′i	m
$0.000\,001 = 10^{-6}$	micro	mi′kro	μ
$0.000\,000\,001 = 10^{-9}$	nano	nan′o	n
$0.000\,000\,000\,001 = 10^{-12}$	pico	pe′co	p
$0.000\,000\,000\,000\,001 = 10^{-15}$	femto	fem′to	f
$0.000\,000\,000\,000\,000\,001 = 10^{-18}$	atto	at′to	a

(From International Committee on Weights and Measures, 1962.)

excreting carbon dioxide and some water wastes from the body. It consists of the nose, paranasal sinuses, nasopharynx, larynx, trachea, bronchi, and lungs. Called also *apparatus respiratorius* [NA] and *respiratory apparatus*. **reticuloendothelial s.**, a functional system that serves in body defense mechanisms; it is composed of phagocytic cells having both endothelial and reticular attributes and the ability to take up particles of colloidal dyes; these cells include macrophages, Kupffer's cells, reticular cells, cells lining the blood sinuses of the pituitary and adrenal glands, monocytes, and probably the microglia. Called also *macrophage,* and *RE.* **Schubiger s.,** Schubiger ATTACHMENT. **silver-copper s.,** silver-copper ALLOY. **silver-tin s.,** silver-tin ALLOY. **skeletal s.,** the bony framework of the animal body. See SKELETON. **somatic nervous s.,** the elements of the nervous system concerned with the transmission of impulses to and from the nonvisceral components of the body, such as the skeletal muscles, bones, joints, ligaments, skin, and eyes and ears. **stomatognathic s.,** the structures of the mouth and jaws, considered collectively, as they subserve the functions of mastication, deglutition, respiration, and speech. See also *masticatory s.* **sympathetic nervous s.,** 1. the part of the autonomic nervous system that forms a network of afferent and efferent (sensory and motor) neurons which derive from the thoracolumbar part of the spinal cord and supply the heart, smooth muscles, and glands. Its preganglionic fibers are axons of cells in the gray matter of the lateral column of the thoracic and lumbar segments of the spinal cord, forming small myelinated fibers that emerge from the cord with the spinal nerves and pass on to the ganglia in the chain of the sympathetic trunk. Most fibers end in the ganglia, transmitting to postganglionic fibers through synaptic connections, but some pass through without synapses and continue to peripheral plexuses. The postganglionic fibers are axons of cells in the chain ganglia, forming unmyelinated long fibers that supply peripheral organs. It is divided into the cephalic, cervical, thoracic, abdominal, and pelvic parts. The cephalic part derives from the superior cervical ganglion and consists of structures and their branches, including the internal carotid, deep petrosal, caroticotympanic, and external carotid nerves; the internal carotid and cavernous plexuses; and branches communicating with the trigeminal and abducent nerves, with the oculomotor, trochlear, and ophthalmic nerves, and with the ciliary ganglion, and branches to the dilator pupillae muscle. The cephalic part consists of the superior cervical ganglion, internal carotid nerve, branches communicating with the cranial nerves, gray rami, branches to the cervical nerves, pharyngeal branches, branches to the external carotid artery, intercarotid plexus, thyroid nerve, middle cervical ganglion, inferior cervical ganglion, stellate ganglion, and branches to the heart. The thoracic, abdominal, and pelvic parts supply their respective organs. Synaptic transmission in the sympathetic nervous system is accomplished through the medium of norepinephrine acting as the transmitter substance. Called also *pars sympathica systematis nervosi autonomici* [NA] and *systema nervosum sympathicum.* 2. former name for *autonomic nervous s.* **T s.,** a system of invaginations of the sarcolemma of muscle fibers forming transverse tubules (T tubules). A T tubule plus the sarcoplasmic reticula of two adjacent cisternae form a triad. Each sarcomere has two triads located at the junctions of the A and I

bands. An action potential depolarizes it and calcium is released at the Z band, causing contraction of the myofibril segment. When the calcium is sequestered by the sarcoplasmic reticulum, the myofibril relaxes. It provides an additional surface for the exchange of metabolites between muscle and the extracellular space. Called also *triad s.* **ternary s.,** see ternary ALLOY. **Threadmate s.,** trademark for self-threading pins. **transport s.,** carrier MOLECULE. **triad s.,** T s. **Universal Numbering S.,** a numbering system adopted by the American Dental Association and used in the charting and description of human teeth. The permanent teeth are numbered 1 to 32, starting with the upper right third molar, working around the maxillary arch to the upper left third molar (number 16); the mandibular left molar is designated number 17, working around the mandibular arch to the lower right third molar (number 32). The primary teeth are lettered, using capital letters A through T, and following the same methodology as for the permanent teeth, starting with the upper right second primary molar (A) and ending with the lower right second molar (T). See also dental CHART. **urogenital s.,** a system of male or female reproductive organs and the organs involved in the production and excretion of urine, consisting of the kidneys, ureters, bladder, and urethra; the male reproductive organs, consisting of the testes, penis, prostate, and a system of ducts; and the female reproductive organs, consisting of the ovaries, fallopian tubes, uterus, vagina, and external genitalia. Called also *genitourinary s., apparatus urogenitalis* [NA], *genitourinary apparatus,* and *urogenital apparatus.* **uropoietic s.,** the part of the urogenital system concerned with the production and excretion of urine, consisting of the kidneys, ureters, bladder, and urethra. Called also *organa uropoët'ica* [NA]. **vascular s.,** the vessels of the body, especially the blood vessels. **vasomotor s.,** the part of the nervous system concerned with controlling the caliber of the blood vessels. **vegetative nervous s.,** autonomic nervous s. **venous s.,** systemic veins; see under VEIN. **visceral nervous s.,** autonomic nervous s. **Zest Anchor s.,** Zest Anchor system ATTACHMENT.

systema (sis-te"mah) [Gr. *systēma* a complex or organized whole] a series of interconnected or interdependent organs which together accomplish a specific function. See also SYSTEM. **s. lymphat'icum** [NA], lymphatic SYSTEM. **s. nervo'rum centra'le,** central nervous SYSTEM. **s. nervo'sum** [NA], nervous SYSTEM. **s. nervo'sum autonom'icum** [NA], autonomic nervous SYSTEM. **s. nervo'sum centra'le** [NA], central nervous SYSTEM. **s. nervo'sum peripher'icum** [NA], peripheral nervous SYSTEM. **s. nervo'sum sympath'icum,** sympathetic nervous SYSTEM. **s. vaso'rum,** the blood and lymph vessels of the body and all their ramifications, considered collectively. See also systemic CIRCULATION and lymph CIRCULATION.

systematic (sis"tĕ-mat'ik) [Gr. *systematikos*] pertaining or according to a system. See also systematic NAME.

systemic (sis-tem'ik) pertaining to or affecting the body as a whole.

systole (sis'to-le) [Gr. *systolē* a drawing together, contraction] the contraction, or period of contraction, of the heart, especially that of the ventricles forcing the blood out of the chambers into the aorta and more distant blood vessels. The stroke volume is about 60 ml of blood. See systemic CIRCULATION. Cf. DIASTOLE.

Szent-Györgi, Albert [born 1893] a Hungarian biochemist in America; winner of the Nobel prize for medicine and physiology in 1937, for his isolation of ascorbic acid and research in muscle contraction.

T

T 1. temperature. 2. tesla. 3. tera-. 4. intraocular TENSION. 5. tritium.

T$_f$ freezing TEMPERATURE.

T$_g$ glass transition TEMPERATURE.

T$_3$ triiodothyronine.

t 1. translocation (2); see also CHROMOSOME nomenclature. 2. temporal.

T life (time).

T½ half-life (time).

Ta tantalum.

tab (tab) a small flap, strap, or any such appendange. **bite-wing t.,** a tab attached to a film used in oral radiography, to be held between the teeth. See bite-wing FILM.

tab. tablet.

tabella (tah-bel'ah), pl. *tabellae* [L.] a medicated tablet or troche.

tabellae (tah-bel'e) [L.] plural of *tabella.*

tabes (ta'bēz) [L. "wasting away," "decay"] any condition characterized by wasting of the body. **cerebral t.,** DEMENTIA paralytica. **t. dorsa'lis,** degeneration of the posterior roots and posterior column of the spinal cord and of the brain stem, marked by attacks of pain; progressive ataxia; loss of reflexes; functional disorders of the bladder, gastrointestinal tract, and larynx; and impotence. It develops as a sequel of tertiary syphilis and appears to affect middle-aged males most frequently. Called also *locomotor ataxia* and *posterior spinal sclerosis.*

tabetic (tah-bet'ik) pertaining to or affected with tabes.

tabification (tab"ĭ-fi-ka'shun) [*tabes* + L. *facere* to make] the process of wasting away.

tablature (tab'lah-chur) the separation of the chief cranial bones into inner and outer tables, which are separated by diploë.

table (ta'b'l) [L. *tabula*] 1. a flat layer or surface. 2. a collection of data (words, numbers, rules, etc.), usually arranged in columns or some other orderly format, to show a desired set of facts in a definite and readily identifiable manner. **t. of allowances,** see ALLOWANCE. **t. clinic,** table CLINIC. **inner t. of bone of skull,** internal lamina of cranial bone; see under LAMINA. **Mendeleev's t.,** periodic t. **occlusal t.,** 1. the occlusal surfaces of the bicuspids and molars; the basic collective topography, including the form of the cusps, inclined planes, marginal ridges, central fossae, and grooves of the teeth. 2. the total surface provided for occlusion by a complete or partial denture, being narrower in unworn dentures than in those whose surfaces have been abraded. **outer t. of bones of skull,** external lamina of cranial bones; see under LAMINA. **periodic t.,** a table of all the currently recognized chemical elements, which is arranged in the form of a chart according to periodic law. Called also *Mendeleev's t.* See ELEMENT (2).

tablespoon (ta'b'l-spoon) a household unit of capacity, approximately equivalent to 4 fluid drams, or 15 milliliters, or 3 teaspoons.

tablet (tab'let) a solid dosage form of varying weight, size, and shape, which may be molded or compressed, and which contains a medicinal substance in pure or diluted form. **buccal t.,** a small, flat, oval tablet to be held between the cheek and gum, permitting direct absorption through the oral mucosa of the medicinal substance contained therein. **Cebefortis t's,** trademark for a mixture of vitamins, each tablet containing 150 mg sodium ascorbate, 5 mg thiamine mononitrate, 5 mg riboflavin, 50 mg niacinamide, 1 mg pyridoxine hydrochloride, 10 mg calcium pantothenate, and 2 mcg vitamin B₁₂ concentrate. **dispensing t.,** a compressed or molded tablet containing a large quantity of a drug, used by dispensing pharmacists in compounding prescription. **enteric-coated t.,** one coated with material that delays release of the medication until after it leaves the stomach. **Flura-T's,** trademark for tablets containing 2.21 mg sodium fluoride equivalent, being equivalent to 1 mg fluoride ion; used in dental caries prevention. **Fluoritab t's,** trademark for tablets containing 2.21 mg sodium fluoride, equivalent to 1 mg fluoride ion; used in dental caries prevention. **hypodermic t.,** one that is dissolved in water, containing a medicinal substance for hypodermic injection. **Karidium t's,** trademark for tablets containing 2.21 mg sodium fluoride (equivalent to 1 mg sodium fluoride ion) and 94.5 mg sodium chloride; used in dental caries prevention. **Luride Lozi-Tabs t's,** a trademark for tablets containing 1.1. and 2.2 mg sodium fluoride, respectively, being equivalent to 0.5 and 1.0 mg of fluoride ion; used for dental caries prevention. **Nargesic t's,** trademark for an analgesic preparation, one tablet of which contains 225 mg aspirin, 160 mg phenacetin, 30 mg caffeine, 25 mg orphenadrine citrate, and excipients. **Nebs analgesic t's,** trademark for an analgesic preparation, one tablet of which contains 325 mg acetaminophen and various excipients. **Nufluor chewable t's,** trademark for tablets containing 2.2 mg sodium fluoride (equivalent to 1 mg fluoride ion), a dye, flavoring agents, and excipients; used in dental caries prevention. **Pacemaker Nafeen t's,** trademark for tablets containing 2.2 mg sodium fluoride (equivalent to 1 mg fluoride ion) and excipients; used in dental caries prevention. **Percogesic t's,** an analgesic preparation, one tablet of which contains 325 mg acetaminophen, 30 mg phenyltoloxamine citrate, and various excipients. **Pfizer-E film coated t's,** trademark for tablets containing erythromycin and excipients. **sublingual t.,** a small, flat, oval tablet to be held beneath the tongue, permitting direct absorption of the medicinal substance contained therein. **Trigesic t's,** trademark for an analgesic preparation, one tablet of which contains 125 mg acetaminophen, 230 mg aspirin, 30 mg caffeine, and various amounts of excipients. **triturate t.,** a small, usually cylindrical, molded disk containing a medicinal substance diluted with a mixture of lactose and powdered sucrose, in varying proportions, with a moistening agent.

tabula (tab'u-lah), pl. *tab'ulae* [L.] table.

tabulae (tab'u-le) [L.] plural of *tabula.*

tabular (tab'u-lar) [L. *tabula* a board or table] resembling or shaped like a table.

Tacaryl trademark for *methdilazine hydrochloride* (see under METHDILAZINE).

tache (tahsh) [Fr.] a spot or blemish.

Tach-E-Z retainer (attachment, unit) see under RETAINER.

tachy- [Gr. *tachys* swift] combining form denoting swift or fast.

tachycardia (tak"e-kar'de-ah) [*tachy-* + Gr. *kardia* heart] abnormally rapid heart beat, usually above 100 beats per minute. **atrial t.,** a rapid heart beat, usually between 160 and 190 contractions per minute, originating from an atrial locus. The electrocardiogram shows a rapid succession of abnormal P waves; QRS complexes are equally rapid but regular and normal in form. **orthostatic t.,** abnormal increase in the heart rate

on rising from a reclining to a standing position. **paroxysmal t.,** an attack of regular but rapid heart action of 100 beats per minute or more, beginning suddenly and lasting from several minutes to several days. Vagal stimulation usually stops the paroxysm completely. **ventricular t.,** an abnormally rapid ventricular rhythm with aberrant ventricular excitation (wide QRS complexes), usually in excess of 150 per minute, which is generated within the ventricle and most commonly associated with atrioventricular dissociation. Minor irregularities of rate may also occur.

tachypnea (tak"ip-ne'ah) [*tachy-* + Gr. *pnoia* breath] rapid breathing or more than 17 breaths per minute. See also RESPIRATION.

tactile (tak'til) [L. *tactilis*] pertaining to the touch.

tactor (tak'tor) a tactile end-organ.

tactual (tak'tu-al) [L. *tactus* touch] pertaining to touch.

tactus (tak'tus) [L.] touch.

Tacumil trademark for a sulfamethoxazole-trimethoprim mixture.

Taenia (te'ne-ah) [L. "a flat band," "bandage," "tape"] a genus of large tapeworms of the family Taeniidae. **T. echinococ'cus multilocula'ris,** *Echinococcus multilocularis* (see under ECHINOCOCCUS). **T. sagina'ta,** a large tapeworm attaining the length of 12 to 25 feet, which infests the human intestine, and is transmitted through consumption of raw or inadequately cooked beef. In its larval stage (*Cysticercus cellulosae*), the parasite infests the soft tissue of various organs (see CYSTICERCOSIS). Called also *beef tapeworm.* **T. so'lium,** a large tapeworm attaining the length of 3 to 6 feet, which infests the human intestine and is transmitted through consumption of raw or inadequately cooked pork. In its larval stage (*Cysticercus cellulosae*), the parasite infests the soft tissue of various organs (see CYSTICERCOSIS). Called also *pork tapeworm.* **T. viscera'lis socia'lis granulo'sus,** *Echinococcus granulosus* (see under ECHINOCOCCUS).

taenia (te'ne-ah), pl. *tae'niae* 1. tenia (1). 2. any individual organism of the genus *Taenia.*

taeniacide (te'ne-ah-sīd") [*taenia* + L. *caedere* to kill] 1. destructive to tapeworms. 2. an agent that destroys tapeworms.

taeniae (te'ne-e) plural of *taenia.*

taeniafuge (te'ne-ah-fuj") [*taenia* + L. *fugare* to put to flight] an agent that expels tapeworms.

taeniasis (te-ni'ah-sis) infestation with tapeworms of the genus *Taenia.*

tag (tag) 1. a small appendage, flap or polyp. 2. label. **auricular t.,** a rudimentary appendage of auricular tissue occurring on the face along the line of union of the first branchial arch. **radioactive t.,** a radioisotope that has been incorporated within a biological chemical by metabolic or other processes.

Taggard's machine, method [William Herbert *Taggard,* American dentist, 1855–1933; he developed a method of casting gold inlays by the invested pattern procedure and made applicable to the casting of gold inlays the principle of disappearing core] see under MACHINE, and see disappearing CORE.

tail (tāl) [L. *cauda;* Gr. *oura*] 1. any slender appendage. 2. the appendage that extends from the posterior trunk of animals.

Takahara's syndrome [Shigeo *Takahara,* Japanese physician] acatalasia.

Talatrol trademark for *tromethamine.*

talbutal (tal'bu-tal) a barbiturate, 5-(1-methylpropyl)-5-(2-propenyl)-2,4,6(1*H*,3*H*,5*H*)-pyrimidinetrione, occurring as a white, odorless, slightly bitter crystalline powder that is soluble in ethanol, ether, chloroform, boiling water, and alkalies, and slightly soluble in cold water. Used as a hypnotic and sedative. Abuse may lead to habituation and addiction. Trademarks: Lotusate, Profundol.

talc (talk) [L. *talcum*] a native hydrous magnesium silicate sometimes containing a small proportion of aluminum silicate. Native talc (soapstone or French chalk) is found in various parts of the world, usually being accompanied by various other minerals. It is a fine, white or grayish, crystalline powder, used chiefly for its desiccant and lubricating properties, either alone or with starch or boric acid, as a dusting powder, excipient, filtering medium, sunscreen, and filler for pills and tablets. When used for dusting surgical gloves, it may cause wound irritation and granuloma. Also used as a filler for impression compounds.

talcum (tal'kum) [L.] talc.

talipomanus (tal"ĭ-pom'ah-nus) [L. *talipes* clubfoot + *manus* hand] clubhand.

talk (tok) 1. to employ speech. 2. utterance of words. **baby t.,** the substitution in speech of sounds similar to those used by a child in the early stages of speech development.

tallow (tal′o) a fat obtained from the bodies of various animals, such as cattle and sheep, which is used in foods, candlemaking, soaps, lubricants, etc. **Japan t.,** Japan WAX.

Talma's disease [Sape *Talma*, Dutch physician, 1847–1918] MYOTONIA acquisita.

Talwin trademark for *pentazocine*.

tampon (tam′pon) [Fr. "stopper, plug"] a pack; a pad or plug made of cotton, sponge, or other material; used variously in surgery to plug the nose and other cavities, for the control of hemorrhage, or the absorption of secretions. **tracheal t.,** an inflatable rubber bag surrounding a tracheotomy tube; used to prevent the entrance of blood into the trachea in operations on the mouth and nose.

tamponade (tam″pon-ăd′) [Fr. *tamponner* to stop up] 1. surgical use of a tampon. 2. pathologic compression of a part.

tan tandem TRANSLOCATION. See also CHROMOSOME nomenclature.

Tanderil trademark for *oxyphenbutazone*.

tang (tang) 1. a strong taste or flavor. 2. a long and slender projection or prong forming part of an object, such as a chisel, fine file, knife, and the like. 3. in dental prostheses, a device that connects rests and direct or indirect retainers to lingual and palatal bars and other parts of denture framework and bases.

Tangier disease (tan-jēr′) [named after *Tangier* Island, a small island in Chesapeake Bay discovered in 1608 by Captain John Smith, where Tangier disease was first observed] see under DISEASE.

Tanicaine trademark for *phenocaine hydrochloride* (see under PHENOCAINE).

tank (tank) an artificial receptacle for liquids.

Tanston trademark for *mefenamic acid* (see under ACID).

tantalum (tan′tah-lum) [named after *Tantalus*, a character in Greek mythology] a metallic element. Symbol, Ta; atomic number, 73; atomic weight, 180.9479; specific gravity, 14.491 or 16.6 (worked metal); melting point, 2996°C; valences, 2, 3, 4, 5; group VB of the periodic table. It occurs as a single natural stable isotope (^{181}Ta) and one radioactive isotope (^{180}Ta with a half-life of 10^{12} years), and several artificial radioactive ones (172–179 and 182–186). Tantalum is a gray, heavy, and very hard metal which, when pure, is ductile and can be drawn into fine wire with a tensile strength up to 130.000 psi. It is insoluble in water and resistant to acids (other than hydrofluoric acid) and alkalies (except fused alkalies). Tantalum is nontoxic and nonreactogenic. Used in surgical and dental instruments, in implants and tissue-staples, as a substitute for platinum, and in a variety of industrial products.

Taoryl trademark for *caramiphen ethanedisulfonate* (see under CARAMIPHEN).

Tapar trademark for *acetaminophen*.

tape (tāp) a long, narrow strip of fabric or other flexible material. **adhesive t.,** a strip of fabric and/or film evenly coated on one side with a pressure-sensitive, adhesive mixture, the whole having high tensile strength; used for the application of dressings and sometimes to produce immobilization. Formerly called *adhesive plaster.* **adhesive t., sterile,** adhesive tape, the adhesive surface of which is covered by strips of a protective material of equal width, and which is sterilized after packaging. Formerly called *sterile adhesive plaster.* **dental t.,** a ribbon of waxed nylon or silk used, similarly to dental floss, for cleansing interproximal spaces and proximal surfaces of the teeth. **floss t.,** a silk tape, often having pumice particles on its surface, used for polishing the proximal surfaces of teeth. **magnetic t.,** a ribbon made from a plastic base, coated on one side (single tape) or both sides (double tape) with a substance containing iron oxide, to make it sensitive to impulses from an electromagnet. Used for recording the voice or to store computer data in the form of magnetically polarized spots.

tapeinocephalic (tap″ī-no-sě-fal′ik) characterized by or pertaining to a low-arched skull. Spelled also *tapinocephalic.* See tapeinocephalic SKULL.

tapeinocephaly (tap″ī-no-sef′ah-le) [Gr. *tapeinos* low-lying + *kephalē* head] a condition characterized by a low-arched skull. Spelled also *tapinocephaly.* See tapeinocephalic SKULL.

taper (ta′per) gradual diminution of width or thickness in an elongated object, such as a cutting instrument.

tapering ta′per-ing) a process of so shaping a clasp arm as to better distribute flexure throughout its length, thus reducing fatigue, strain-hardening, and resultant fracture.

tapeworm (tāp-werm) an intestinal parasite having a flattened,

bandlike form, which is transmitted to man in larval form through consumption of raw or inadequately cooked meat. In their larval form, the parasites may infest various soft tissues, causing cysticercosis. In their adult form, they infest the intestine. The most common tapeworms that are considered parasitic to humans are the beef tapeworm (*Taenia saginata*) and the pork tapeworm (*Taenia solium*). See CYSTICERCOSIS.

tapinocephalic (tap″ī-no-sě-fal′ik) tapeinocephalic.

tapinocephaly (tap″ī-no-sef′ah-le) tapeinocephaly.

tapping (tap′ing) repetitive contacts between opposing teeth or tapping performed to facilitate observation of contact between the teeth for occlusal adjustment.

TAR tissue-air RATIO.

tar (tahr) a dark brown or black, viscid liquid, obtained by heating the wood of various species of pine, or as a by-product of the destructive distillation of bituminous coal. It is a mixture of complex composition, and is the source of a number of substances, such as cresol, creosol, guaiacol, naphthalene, paraffin, phenol, toluene, and xylene. Most tars are irritants, many have antiseptic properties, and some are carcinogenic.

tardive (tahr′div) [Fr. "tardy," "late"] marked by lateness; late; said of a disease in which the characteristic lesion is late in appearing.

Tardocillin trademark for *penicillin G benzathine* (see under PENICILLIN).

target (tahr′get) 1. an object or area toward which something is directed. 2. material subjected to particle bombardment (as in an accelerator) or irradiation (as in a reactor) in order to induce a nuclear reaction, or a nuclide that has been bombarded or irradiated. **x-ray tube t.,** a massive tungsten insert on the end of the face of a copper anode, either stationary or rotating, which is bombarded by high-velocity electrons from a heated cathode. After being suddenly arrested by the target, the electrons give rise to x-rays. See also ANODE (2), ANTICATHODE, and focal spot, actual and focal spot, effective, under SPOT.

tarnish (tar′nish) 1. to dull the luster of a metallic surface. 2. a surface discoloration on the metal part of a denture or dental restoration due to the effect of corrosive substances or galvanic current, which may include some loss of the surface finish and deposits of plaque and calculus. See also CORROSION (2).

Tarnow see Kulenkampff-Tarnow SYNDROME.

tarsadenitis (tahr″sad-ě-ni′tis) inflammation of the tarsus of the eyelid and the meibomian glands.

tarsal (tahr′sal) [L. *tarsalis*] pertaining to the tarsus of an eyelid, or to the instep of the foot.

tarsitis (tahr-si′tis) inflammation of the eyelid; blepharitis, inflammation of a tarsus.

tarso- [Gr. *tarsos* a broad flat surface] a combining form denoting relationship to the edge of the eyelid, or to the instep of the foot.

tarsocheiloplasty (tahr″so-ki′lo-plas″te) [*tarso-* + Gr. *cheilos* lip + *plassein* to mold] a plastic operation upon the edge of the eyelid.

tarso-orbital (tahr″so-or′bĭ-tal) pertaining to the tarsus of the eyelid and to the orbit.

tarsoplasty (tahr″so-plas″te) [*tarso-* + Gr. *plassein* to mold] plastic surgery of the tarsus of the eyelid.

tarsorrhaphy (tahr-sor′ah-fe) [*tarso-* + Gr. *rhaphē* suture] the operation of suturing together a portion of (*partial t.*) or the entire (*total t.*) upper and lower eyelids for the purpose of shortening or closing completely the palpebral fissure. The terms *external, median,* and *internal* are used to indicate the portion of the lids brought together in partial tarsorrhaphy. Called also *blepharorrhaphy.*

tarsotomy (tahr-sot′o-me) [*tarso-* + Gr. *tomē* a cut] 1. surgical incision of the tarsus of the foot. 2. blepharotomy.

tarsus (tahr′sus) [L.; Gr. *tarsos* a frame of wickerwork; any broad flat surface] 1. [NA] the region of the articulation between the foot and the leg. Also the *bony tarsus* (t. osseus [NA], the seven bones, talus, calcaneus, navicular, cuboid, and three cuneiform), constituting the articulation between the foot and leg; the ankle or instep. 2. one of the plates of connective tissue forming the framework of an eyelid; see *t. palpebrae.* **bony t.,** see TARSUS (1). **t. palpe′brae,** the firm framework of connective tissue that gives shape to the upper eyelid (*t. superior palpebrae* [NA]) and lower eyelid (*t. inferior palpebrae* [NA]). Called also *ciliary cartilage, palpebral cartilage,* and *tarsal cartilage.* **t. os′seus** [NA], see TARSUS (1).

tartar (tahr′tahr) [L. *tartarum*; Gr. *tartaron*] 1. sediment of a wine cask; crude potassium bitartrate. 2. dental CALCULUS.

tartarus vitriolatus (tar-tahr′rus ve″tre-o-la′tus) POTASSIUM sulfate.

tartrate (tahr′trāt) [L. *tartras*] any salt of tartaric acid containing $M_2C_4H_4O_6$.

tartrated (tahr′trāted) containing tartar or tartaric acid.

taste (tāst) [L. *gustus*] the sensation caused by the contact of certain soluble substances with the tongue; the sense effected by the taste buds of the tongue, the gustatory fibers of the V, IX, X, and other nerves, and the gustation center. Four primary qualities are distinguished: sweet, sour, salty, and bitter. See also taste BUD, and see terms beginning GUSTO-. **t. center,** gustatory CENTER.

Tauredon trademark for a preparation of *gold sodium thiomalate* (see under GOLD).

taurine (taw'rin) a substance, ethylamine sulfonic acid, found chiefly in bile and, in lesser quantities, in the lungs and muscles. A conjugated form of taurine and cholic acid forms taurocholic acid, the salt of which is one of the bile salts.

taurodontism (taw"ro-don'tizm) [Gr. *tauros* bull + *odous* tooth + *-ism*] a variation in tooth form characterized by prism-shaped molars with large pulp spaces resulting from branching of the root only in the middle (mesotaurodontism), to the apical third, or not at all (hypertaurodontism). It is believed to be caused by a delay in transformation of the enamel organ into several sheaths.

tauto- [Gr. *tautos,* from *to auto* the same] a combining form meaning the same. See also terms beginning ISO-.

tautomeric (taw"to-mer'ik) exhibiting, or capable of exhibiting, tautomerism.

tautomerism (taw-tom'er-izm) [*tauto-* + Gr. *meros* part] a form of stereoisomerism in which the compounds are mutually inconvertible, under normal conditions, forming a mixture which is in dynamic equilibrium. See also ANIONOTROPY, MUTAROTATION, and PROTOTROPY.

taxa (tak'sah) plural of *taxon.*

taxon (tak'son), pl. *tax'a* [Gr. *taxis* a drawing up in rank and file + *-on* neuter ending] a particular group (category) into which related organisms are classified; the main categories are (in ascending order): species, genus, family, order, class, phylum, and kingdom.

taxonomy (tak-son'o-me) [L. *taxinomia;* Gr. *taxis* a drawing up in rank and file + *nomos* law] the orderly classification of organisms into appropriate categories (taxa) on the basis of relationships among them, with the application of suitable and correct names.

Tay-Sachs disease [Warren *Tay,* English physician, 1843–1927; Bernard *Sachs;* New York neurologist, 1858–1944] see under DISEASE.

Taybi's syndrome [Hooshang *Taybi,* American physician, born 1919] otopalatodigital SYNDROME. See also Rubinstein-Taybi SYNDROME.

Taylor see Semken-Taylor FORCEPS.

Taylor, Lucy B. Hobbs [American dentist] the first woman graduate in dentistry, who received a diploma in 1866.

Tb terbium.

TBS trademark for *tribromsalan.*

Tc technetium.

Tcc triclocarban.

TCL total lung CAPACITY.

TCRV total red cell VOLUME.

TDB *T*oxicology *D*ata *B*ank; an acronym for a data base accessible to on-line searching, which contains chemical, pharmacological, and toxicological information extracted from handbooks and text books and reviewed by a peer review group of subject specialists.

t.d.s. abbreviation for L. *ter di'e sumen'dum,* to be taken three times a day.

Te tellurium.

TEA tetraethylammonium.

TEAB TETRAETHYLAMMONIUM bromide.

TEAM *T*raining in *E*xpanded *A*uxiliary *M*anagement; a federally supported program in dental schools, having as its primary goal the training of dental students in the management of extended function dental assistants in the practice of dentistry. See also DAU, and dental assistant, extended function, under ASSISTANT.

team (tēm) a group or body of persons engaged in a joint effort or activity. **dental health t.,** a team consisting of a dentist and various members of the auxiliary dental personnel, such as a dental assistant, dental hygienist, dental laboratory assistant, and expanded duty dental auxiliary. See also team DENTISTRY. **surgical t.,** the operating room staff participating in performing a surgical operation. In oral surgery, the team consists of the dentist (the surgeon), anesthetist, scrub nurse, operating room nurse, and dental assistant, and, in some hospitals, a circulating nurse.

tear[1] (tēr) [L. *lacrima;* Gr. *dakryon*] a drop of the aqueous secretion of the lacrimal glands which serves to moisten the conjunctivae. 2. to exude *tears;* to weep. **crocodile t's,** gustatory LACRIMATION.

tear[2] (tahr) 1. to pull apart or in pieces by force. 2. to wound or injure, especially by ripping apart or rending; lacerate. 3.

laceration. **cemental t., cementum t.,** detachment of a fragment of cementum from the root surface of a tooth, especially that occurring in association with occlusal trauma. It may be complete, with displacement of a fragment into the periodontal ligament, or it may be incomplete, with the cementum fragment remaining partially attached to the root. Called also *cemental* or *cementum fracture.*

teaspoon (te'spōon) a household unit of capacity, approximately equivalent to 5 millimeters, or ⅓ tablespoon.

Tebrazid trademark for *pyrazinamide.*

Techne-Scan PYP trademark for *stannous pyrophosphate* (see under PYROPHOSPHATE).

technetium (tek-ne'she-um) [Gr. *technetos* artificial] an artificial radioactive element. Symbol, Tc; atomic number, 43; atomic weight, 98.9062; melting point, 2172°C; valences, 0, 2, 4–7; group VIIB of the periodic table. Technetium isotopes range from 92 to 107; ^{99m}Tc has a half-life of 6 hours, ^{98}Tc emits beta rays and has a half-life of 1.5×10^6 years, and ^{97}Tc has a half-life of 2.6×10^6 years. Technetium was the first artificial element discovered; it was found in a sample of molybdenum that had been bombarded by deuterons. It is a silvery gray metal that tarnishes in moist air and dissolves in nitric acid, aqua regia, and sulfuric acid, but is insoluble in hydrochloric acid. In medicine, used in scintigraphy and other scanning techniques, particularly of the brain, salivary glands, tissue grafts, and bones. Also used in tracer studies and for corrosion protection of steel in closed systems. Formerly called *masurium.*

technician (tek-nish'an) a person trained in and expert in the performance of technical procedures; a technologist. **dental t., dental laboratory t.,** a person skilled in the fabrication of dental appliances and devices, including complete and partial dentures, as prescribed by a dentist. Traditionally, they were trained on the job, but now training is done usually through formal programs offered by two-year post-secondary educational institutions. Upon completion of an aggregate of 5 years in dental technology training and experience, they are eligible to apply for examination and certification by the National Board for Certification in Dental Laboratory Technology. Called also *dental technologist* and *dental laboratory technologist.* See also DENTURIST. **medical t., medical laboratory t.,** a person trained to be an expert in the performance of a wide range of specialized procedures in a clinical laboratory. The minimum educational requirement for one of several certification programs in medical technology includes a baccalaureate degree with appropriate science course requirements and a 12-month structured American Medical Association approved medical technology program and/or experience. Called also *medical technologist* and *medical laboratory technologist.* **radiologic t.,** radiologic TECHNOLOGIST. **x-ray t.,** radiologic TECHNOLOGIST.

technique (tek-nēk') [Fr.] the manner or method of performing a particular function or field of endeavor. See also METHOD. **1:1 t.,** Eames' t. **angle bisection t.,** bisecting angle t. **aseptic t.,** a technique in which microorganisms have been eradicated from the field of operation, as in root canal therapy. **banding t.,** chromosome BANDING. **Barkann's t.,** a technique for the treatment of periodontal pockets by scaling and curettage, followed by the application of a pheno-camphor coagulating mixture. **Bass' t.,** see TOOTHBRUSHING. **bead t., bead t. filling** see bead technique FILLING. **Begg's t.,** an orthodontic technique, employing a fixed multibanded appliance which incorporates a concept of differential light forces and uses a modified ribbon arch attachment and elastics. The tipping of the crowns of teeth to be moved, rather than moving them laterally, is used in the technique, thereby minimizing the use of orthodontic force. Called also *differential force t.* and *light round wire t.* See also Begg APPLIANCE and Begg's THEORY. See illustration. **bisecting angle t.,** an oral radiographic technique used when the teeth and the film are not parallel with one another. It consists of directing the central ray of the beam at right angles to the plane determined by bisecting the angle formed by (1) the long axis of the tooth or teeth being radiographed and (2) the plane in which the film is positioned behind the teeth. According to *Cieszynski's rule of isometry* (if two triangles have two angles and the included side of one is equal respectively to two angles and the included side of the other, then the triangles are congruent), the normal ray is directed perpendicularly to a plane which lies midway between the plane of the teeth desired and the plane of the film. According to *Price's rule,* the correct position of the x-ray tube is easily ascertained in two ways. It is just half way between the two positions which are at right angles to the long axis of the teeth and to the film. This position is also at right

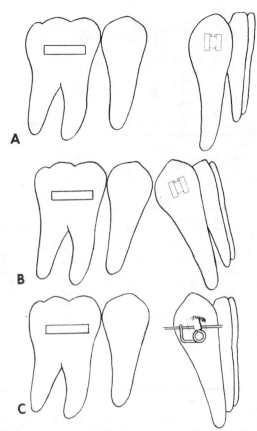

Tooth-moving force values employed in Begg's technique. The brackets used in this technique permit tipping of tooth crowns, but mesial tipping of molar is prevented by the buccal tube. *A*, Position of teeth before force is applied. *B*, 60 to 70 gm or less is optimum for tipping back six anterior teeth with little mesial movement of anchor molar. *C*, One means of preventing anterior from tipping too far distally in mild cases of discrepancy. (From P. R. Begg and P. C. Kesling: Begg Orthodontic Theory and Technique. 3rd ed. Philadelphia, W. B. Saunders Co., 1977.)

angles to a plane half way between that of the long axis of the teeth and the film. Called also *angle bisection t.* and *bisection angle t.* **bisection of angle t.,** bisecting angle t. **Bowles t.,** multiphase APPLIANCE. **Box's t.,** a technique for the treatment of periodontal pockets through the use of scaling and curettage, associated with the application of pressure packs consisting of boracic acid, oil of peppermint, and oxygen in a paraffin base. **brush t. filling,** bead technique FILLING. **bulk t., bulk pack t.,** pressure technique FILLING. **capping t.,** see compression MOLD-ING. **calibrated angle t.,** an intraoral radiographic procedure using a predetermined degree of vertical angulation from the horizontal plane, being a variation of the bisecting angle technique. **Caspersson t.,** Q-BANDING. **channel shoulder pin t.,** a denture attachment method by which the removable section is retained primarily by a series of parallel-sided pins and by the vertical surface of the unit, and is guided into place by retention grooves, fitting over the section that is cemented to an especially prepared tooth. Called also *CSP t., channel shoulder pin attachment* or *system,* and *CSP attachment* or *system.* **Charters' t.,** see TOOTHBRUSHING. **chromosome alkali denaturation and reassociation t.,** see C-BANDING. **compensation t.,** in casting, the enlargement of the mold so that at the time the molten metal is forced into it, the mold space will have been enlarged in an amount equal to the shrinkage of the alloy which occurs during solidification, using: (1) the wax pattern thermal expansion, (2) the investment thermal expansion, and (3) the investment hygroscopic expansion techniques, the last two (or their combination) being most commonly used. The second technique consists of thermal expansion of the investment from

room temperature to a high temperature (700°C) at which the casting is made. The third consists of hygroscopic expansion of the investment; the mold is heated between 427 and 482°C, 482°C being preferred, but some investments give better results at 565 to 593°C. On the basis of their respective mold temperature at the time of casting, the two methods are designated as *high heat* and *low heat casting techniques,* respectively. Called also *shrinkage compensation.* **continuous-gum t.,** a technique patented by John Allen in 1851 whereby artificial teeth are mounted on a platinum base by first soldering the teeth to the base and then fusing around them a porcelain body. No longer used. **controlled water added t.,** a compensation technique in which the shrinkage compensation is controlled by the addition of water during the setting of the investment. **CSP t.,** channel shoulder pin t. **Dental Exposure Normalization T.,** a program of the U.S. Department of Health and Human Services through the Bureau of Radiological Health of the Food and Drug Administration, established for controlling x-ray exposure in dentistry. Under the program, an x-ray exposure card with a thermoluminescent dosimeter is mailed to the dentist, who is instructed to expose the card using his x-ray unit, record certain machine information, and mail it back to the health agency. From the exposed dosimeter, the agency determines the machine output and compares it to the acceptable exposure range. Abbreviated DENT. **differential force t.,** Begg's t. **direct t.,** direct IMPRESSION. **double blind t.,** double blind STUDY. **double pour t.,** see compression MOLDING. **dry field t.,** a technique of tooth preparation, particularly with high-speed rotary instruments, where a fine jet of air removes the debris and prevents the tooth from overheating. See also *washed field t.* **Eames' t.,** in dental alloy preparation, the use of equal amounts of mercury and alloy by weight, thereby preventing residual mercury from accumulating in the plastic mix. Called also *1:1 t.* See also alloy-mercury RATIO. **edgewise t.,** edgewise APPLIANCE. **flow t. filling,** flow technique FILLING. **fluorescent antibody t.,** immunofluorescence. **Fones' t.,** Fones' METHOD. **half-mouth t.,** treatment of the teeth only on one side of the mouth, the untreated side serving as control. **high heat casting t.,** see *compensation t.* **impression t.,** a method employed in making a dental impression. **impression t., dual,** a method by which the anatomic form of the teeth and immediately adjacent structures is recorded and by which the free-end denture foundation areas are registered in their functional form. **indirect t.,** indirect IMPRESSION. **investment hygroscopic expansion t.,** see *compensation t.* **investment thermal expansion t.,** see *compensation t.* **labiolingual t.,** labiolingual APPLIANCE. **Laurell t.,** rocket immunoelectrophoresis used to estimate antigen concentration, in which antigen is placed in wells in decreasing amounts and electrophoresed into an agar layer containing specific antibody. Precipitin patterns form in the shape of cones ("rockets"), the heights of which can be measured to construct a standard curve of heights versus concentration. Inclusion of an unknown quantity of antigen and determination of the height of the rocket permit the estimation of the concentration relative to the standard curve. **light round wire t.,** Begg's t. **lost wax t.,** disappearing CORE. **low heat casting t.,** see *compensation t.* **minimal mercury t.,** see alloy-mercury RATIO. **Nealon's t.,** incremental buildup of autopolymerizing resin in a prepared cavity. **nonpressure t.,** bead technique FILLING. **one-phase subperiosteal implant t.,** subperiosteal implant one-phase t. **one-pour t.,** see compression MOLDING. **open flap t.,** the raising of a mucoperiosteal flap for the multiple extraction of teeth, the removal of a root, or the exposure of any area of bone beneath the flap. **parallel t., paralleling t.,** in intraoral radiography, a technique for producing diagnostic radiographs in which the film is placed parallel with the long axes of the teeth and the central beam is projected at a right angle to the film packet, thus projecting an accurate image of the long axis of the tooth onto the film. Called also *right-angle t.* **porcelain cervical contact and single bake t's,** in anticipating the shrinkage of dental porcelain during firing, direction of the shrinkage toward the shoulder because of a fired bulk of material or a well-condensed band of porcelain lying on the shoulder and in the gingival axial angle of the matrix. **porcelain cervical ditching t.,** in anticipating the shrinkage of dental porcelain during firing, the application of the porcelain so that the initial shrinkage is toward the incisal edge of the matrix, and porcelain is subsequently added in the gingival area to fill and contour the cervical section. **pressure t.,** pressure technique FILLING. **push-back t.,** a surgical procedure designed to reposition the soft palate posteriorly and reestablish velopharyngeal competence. Called also *push-back procedure.* **ribbon arch t.,** ribbon arch APPLIANCE. **right-angle t.,** *parallel t.* **short cone t.,** the use of a short cone distance of 8 inches or less, usually in the bisecting angle technique of radiography. **single-**

pour t., see compression MOLDING. **Stillman's t.,** Stillman's method of TOOTHBRUSHING. **subperiosteal implant one-phase t.,** a technique for the implantation of the framework of an implant denture, which consists of lifting the mucoperiosteum to expose the jaw bone surface and application of a light temporary suture to the surgical wound, followed 12 to 60 hours later by actual implantation of the substructure. The interim period allows for the preparation of an impression of the bone, establishment of surgical jaw relation, and construction of the implant. Called also *one-phase subperiosteal implant t.* **two-pour t.,** see compression MOLDING. **wash t.,** wash IMPRESSION. **washed field t.,** a technique of tooth preparation, particularly with high-speed rotary instruments, where a fine air and water spray constantly bathes the field of operation, removing the debris and keeping tooth temperature at a comfortable level, while the central vacuum removes excess water and debris. See also *dry field t.* **wax pattern thermal expansion t.,** see *compensation t.*

technologist (tek-nol'o-jist) a person trained in and expert in the performance of technical procedures; a technician. **dental t., dental laboratory t.,** dental TECHNICIAN. **medical t., medical laboratory t.,** medical TECHNICIAN. **radiologic t.,** a member of the auxiliary medical staff trained in the performance of technical procedures requiring the use of x-rays and/or radioisotopes that are conducted under the supervision of a physician, dentist, osteopathic physician, or veterinarian. The requirements include a successful completion of specialized courses in a hospital school, a combination of a minimum of four semesters in an accredited college and 2,400 hours of practical experience in a hospital, or completion of an integrated curriculum combining training in a hospital and education in a technical college which includes a minimum of 2,400 hours of practice, and passing the examination given by the American Registry of Radiologic Technologists. Called also *x-ray t., radiologic technician,* and *x-ray technician.* Cf. RADIOLOGIST and ROENTGENOLOGIST. **x-ray t.,** radiologic t.

technology (tek-nol'o-je) [Gr. *technē* art + *logos* treatise] the branch of knowledge or the sum of study of the technical aspects of a branch of science, engineering, or industrial arts. **dental t.,** the fabrication of dental appliances, including dentures, as prescribed by a dentist. See dental TECHNICIAN. **splint t.,** the study of the use of splints in surgery.

Tecodin trademark for *oxycodone hydrochloride* (see under OXYCODONE).

tecquinol (tek'wĭ-nol) hydroquinone.

tectum (tek'tum) [L.] any rooflike structure. See also FLOOR, PARIES, ROOF, TEGMEN, and WALL.

TED threshold erythema DOSE.

teeth (tēth) plural of *tooth* **dead t.,** an erroneous term commonly used to refer to pulpless teeth.

teething (tēth'ing) the entire process which results in the eruption of the teeth.

Teevan's law see under LAW.

Tefacef trademark for *cefazolin sodium* (see under CEFAZOLIN).

Teflon trademark for *polytetrafluoroethylene.*

tegmen (teg'men), pl. *teg'mina* [L. "cover"] a cover or shielding roof; used in anatomical nomenclature to designate any such structure. See also FLOOR, PARIES, ROOF, TEGMEN, and WALL. **t. an'tri, t. tympani. t. cel'lulae, t. mastoideum. t. mastoid'eum,** the bony roof of the mastoid cells. Called also *t. cellulae.* **t. tym'pani** [NA], a thin bony plate on the petrous part of the temporal bone in the floor of the middle cranial fossa, separating the tympanic antrum from the cranial cavity. Called also *roof of tympanum* and *tegmen antri.* See also PARIES tegmentalis cavi tympani.

Tegopen trademark for *cloxacillin.*

Tegosept M trademark for *methylparaben.*

Tegratal trademark for *carbamazepine.*

Tegretol trademark for *carbamazepine.*

teichopsia (ti-kop'se-ah) [Gr. *teichos* wall + *-opsis* vision + *-ia*] scintillating SCOTOMA.

tela (te'lah), pl. *te'lae* [L. "something woven," "web"] any weblike tissue; a general anatomical term for a thin membrane resembling a web. **t. subcuta'nea** [NA], subcutaneous FASCIA. **t. submuco'sa** [NA], submucous MEMBRANE. **t. submuco'sa pharyn'gis** [NA], submucous membrane of pharynx; see under MEMBRANE. **t. subsero'sa** [NA], subserous FASCIA.

telae (te'le) [L.] plural of *tela.*

telangiectasia (tel-an"je-ek-ta'ze-ah) [*tele-*(1) + Gr. *angeion* vessel + *ektasis* dilatation + *-ia*] a condition characterized by dilatation of the capillary vessels and minute arteries, forming a variety of angiomas. **familial hemorrhagic t.,** hereditary hemorrhagic t. **hereditary hemorrhagic t.,** a hereditary disease transmitted as a simple autosomal dominant trait, character-

ized by multiple telangiectatic lesions of the face and body, giving rise to recurrent epistaxis, melena, hematemesis, genital bleeding, and other hemorrhagic complications associated with secondary anemia. The skin of the cheeks and nasal orifices is most commonly affected, and the nail beds, skin of the ears, fingers, toes, and scalp, and the mucosa of the nose, pharynx, gastrointestinal tract, bladder, and genitalia may be involved. Oral manifestations may include involvement of the mucosa of the lips, gingiva, cheeks, palate, tongue, and floor of the mouth. Called also *familial hemorrhagic t., angioma hemorrhagicum hereditaria, hereditary epistaxis,* and *Rendu-Weber-Osler syndrome.*

tele- 1. [Gr. *telos* end] a combining form denoting relation to the end. 2. [Gr. *tēle* far off, at a distance] a combining form meaning operating at a distance, or far away.

telecurietherapy (tel"e-ku"re-ther'ah-pe) [*tele-*(2) + *curietherapy*] radiotherapy with the source of radiation, e.g., radium, being located at a distance from the body.

telemetry (te-lem'ĕ-tre) [*tele-*(2) + Gr. *metron* measure] a method for measuring activities or phenomena from a distance through the use of electronic devices transmitting data via radio waves. **intraoral t.,** a telemetric method for measuring intraoral physiological phenomena, such as the use of miniaturized radio transmitters fitted into artificial dentures which register tooth contacts in the study of occlusion.

Telepaque trademark for *iopanoic acid* (see under ACID).

teleradiography (tel"e-ra"de-og'rah-fe) radiography with the source of radiation being more than 6 feet from the subject, in which rays in the beam are parallel to avoid distortion.

teleradium (tel"e-ra'de-um) a radium source located at a distance from the body.

teleroentgenography (tel"e-rent'gen-og'rah-fe) roentgenography with the x-ray tube 6 1/2 to 7 feet away from the film in order to produce more nearly secure parallelism of the rays. See also parallel rays under RAY.

teleroentgentherapy (tel"e-rent'gen-ther'ah-pe) treatment with x-rays from a source of radiation located at a distance from the body.

telescoping (tel'ĕ-skōp'ing) the sliding of an elongated object into a tubular structure of somewhat larger diameter, as in fitting the primary copings into the secondary ones in telescopic crowns or overlay dentures.

teletherapy (tel"e-ther'ah-pe) [*tele-*(2) + Gr. *therapeia* cure] a form of external radiotherapy in which the source of radiation and radioactive particles is located at least several centimeters from the tissue being treated. Sources may include orthovoltage irradiation, cobalt 60, betatron irradiation, linear accelerator, and neutrons. See also PLESIOTHERAPY and RADIOTHERAPY.

Teleudron trademark for *phthalylsulfathiazole.*

Tel Hashomer camptodactyly syndrome see under SYNDROME.

telo- [Gr. *telos* end] a combining form denoting relationship to an end.

telodendron (tel"o-den'dron) [*telo-* + Gr. *dendron* tree] one of the many fine twiglike terminal branches of a neuron.

telophase (tel'o-fāz) [*telo-* + *phase*] the last of the four stages of mitosis and of the two divisions of meiosis; it begins when the daughter chromosomes reach the poles of the dividing cell and lasts until the two daughter cells take on the appearance of interphase cells.

tellurium (tĕ-lu're-um) [Gr. *tellus* earth] a nonmetallic or metalloid element. Symbol, Te; atomic number, 52; atomic weight, 127.60; Mohs hardness number, 2.3; melting point, 450°C; valences, 2, 4, 6; group VIA of the periodic table. It occurs in eight stable isotopes: 120, 122–126, 128, and 130. Artificial radioactive isotopes include 114–119, 121, 127, 129, and 131–134. It occurs as a grayish white, lustrous (when pure), brittle, crystalline solid or dark gray to brown amorphous powder, and is insoluble in water, benzene, and carbon disulfide and is not attacked by hydrochloric acids. Tellurium reacts with nitric acid and concentrated or fuming sulfuric acids. Used in various alloys, as a secondary rubber vulcanizing agent, as coloring agent, and in various industrial products. It is highly toxic when ingested and inhaled. Called also *aurum paradoxum, metallum paradoxum,* and *metallum problematum.*

telophragma (tel"o-frag'mah) [*telo-* + Gr. *phragmos* a fencing in] Z BAND.

TEM triethylenemelamine.

Temaril trademark for *trimeprazine.*

Temasept IV trademark for *tribromsalan.*

temperature (tem"per-ah-chur) [L. *temperatura*] the degree of heat or cold, or the amount of thermal energy contained by a given quantity of matter, measured on a definite scale. The standard scale in the metric system is the Celsius or centigrade scale, which has 100 gradations (degrees), and is based on the freezing of pure water at sea level as 0 degrees (0°C) and the boiling point at 100 degrees (100°C). According to the Fahrenheit scale, water freezes at 32 degrees (32°F) and boils at 212 degrees (212°F). The formula for converting the Fahrenheit scale to the Celsius or centigrade is: $\dfrac{°F - 32°}{1.8} = °C$. Converting the Celsius scale to the Fahrenheit scale may be done according to the following formula: (°C × 1.8) + 32 = °F. See Table. See also *absolute t.*, and see Howe's color SCALE. **ab-**

TABLE OF EQUIVALENTS OF CELSIUS (CENTIGRADE) AND FAHRENHEIT TEMPERATURE SCALES

CELSIUS	FAHR.	CELSIUS	FAHR.	CELSIUS	FAHR.
Deg.	Deg.	Deg.	Deg.	Deg.	Deg.
−40	−40.0	9	48.2	57	134.6
−39	−38.2	10	50.0	58	136.4
−38	−36.4	11	51.8	59	138.2
−37	−34.6	12	53.6	60	140.0
−36	−32.8	13	55.4	61	141.8
−35	−31.0	14	57.2	62	143.6
−34	−29.2	15	59.0	63	145.4
−33	−27.4	16	60.8	64	147.2
−32	−25.6	17	62.6	65	149.0
−31	−23.8	18	64.4	66	150.8
−30	−22.0	19	66.2	67	152.6
−29	−20.2	20	68.0	68	154.4
−28	−18.4	21	69.8	69	156.2
−27	−16.6	22	71.6	70	158.0
−26	−14.8	23	73.4	71	159.8
−25	−13.0	24	75.2	72	161.6
−24	−11.2	25	77.0	73	163.4
−23	−9.4	26	78.8	74	165.2
−22	−7.6	27	80.6	75	167.0
−21	−5.8	28	82.4	76	168.8
−20	−4.0	29	84.2	77	170.6
−19	−2.2	30	86.0	78	172.4
−18	−0.4	31	87.8	79	174.2
−17	+1.4	32	89.6	80	176.0
−16	3.2	33	91.4	81	177.8
−15	5.0	34	93.2	82	179.6
−14	6.8	35	95.0	83	181.4
−13	8.6	36	96.8	84	183.2
−12	10.4	37	98.6	85	185.0
−11	12.2	38	100.4	86	186.8
−10	14.0	39	102.2	87	188.6
−9	15.8	40	104.0	88	190.4
−8	17.6	41	105.8	89	192.2
−7	19.4	42	107.6	90	194.0
−6	21.2	43	109.4	91	195.8
−5	23.0	44	111.2	92	197.6
−4	24.8	45	113.0	93	199.4
−3	26.6	46	114.8	94	201.2
−2	28.4	47	116.6	95	203.0
−1	30.2	48	118.4	96	204.8
0	32.0	49	120.2	97	206.6
+1	33.8	50	122.0	98	208.4
2	35.6	51	123.8	99	210.2
3	37.4	52	125.6	100	212.0
4	39.2	53	127.4	101	213.8
5	41.0	54	129.2	102	215.6
6	42.8	55	131.0	103	217.4
7	44.6	56	132.8	104	219.2
8	46.4				

(From Dorland's Illustrated Medical Dictionary. 26th ed. Philadelphia, W. B. Saunders Co., 1981.)

solute t., that reckoned from the absolute zero assigned to a hypothetical point where all atomic vibration ceases. In the metric system, it is expressed on the Kelvin scale, which corresponds to the Celsius scale. The absolute zero (−273.09°C) is assigned 0°K, the freezing point of water, 273.15°K, and the boiling point, 373.13°K. On the Rankine scale, which corresponds to the Fahrenheit scale, the absolute zero (−459.67°F) is assigned 0°R, the freezing point, 491.67°R, and the boiling point, 671.67°R. See illustration. **average body t.,** that reflecting the total amount of heat stored in the body, calculated as follows: 0.7 internal or core (rectal) temperature + 0.3 surface (skin) temperature = average body temperature. **body t.,** that of the body, normally about 98.6°F or 37.0°C, remaining constant within ± 1°. Body heat is produced during metabolic processes; on the average, about 55 percent of the energy in the food

ABSOLUTE TEMPERATURE

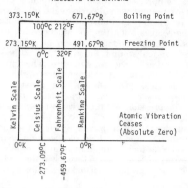

becoming heat during adenosine triphosphate (ATP) formation, with more energy becoming heat as it is transferred from ATP to the functional systems of the cells. It is controlled by the temperature regulating center in the anterior hypothalamus, which receives messages from temperature receptors in the skin and internal organs. Cold-sensitive receptors may also be found in different parts of the hypothalamus, septum, and reticular substance of the midbrain. The circulatory system, particularly the rapid flow of blood and the high specific heat of water, which is the main constituent of blood, tends to equalize the temperature throughout the body, the vasoconstrictor system providing the principal mechanism for heat distribution. Unwanted loss of heat is prevented by vasoconstriction and fatty tissue insulation. Vasodilation and the sweat glands provide a mechanism for releasing excess heat. See illustrations.

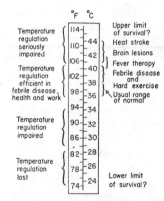

Body temperature. (From E. F. DuBois: Fever and the Regulation of Body Temperature, 1948. Courtesy of Charles C Thomas, Publisher, Springfield, Illinois.)

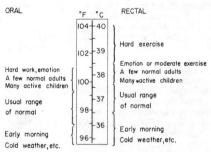

Estimated range of body temperature in normal persons. (From E. F. DuBois: Fever and the Regulation of Body Temperature. 1948. Courtesy of Charles C Thomas, Publisher, Springfield, Illinois.)

See also CALOR, FEVER, and HYPOTHERMIA. **basal t.,** that of the body under conditions of absolute rest. It is subject to diurnal variation, being lowest at about 6 AM and highest about 12 to 14 hours later. **casting t.,** that required to bring about a proper melting of metal to be poured into a refractory mold. **core t.,** internal t. **critical t.,** that below which gas may be liquefied by increased pressure. In heating of steel, the pseudoliquidus temperature that separates the single phase austenite from ferrite plus cementite. For a eutectoid steel this is 723°C (1333°F); for hypoeutectoid steels, the range is 910 to 723°C (1670–1333°F) for compositions from 0.00 to 0.80 percent carbon; and in the hypereutectoid range (0.8–2.0 percent carbon), it is 723 to 1147°C (1333–2097°F). **eutectic t.**, the lowest melting temperature of a eutectic alloy, based on the precise ratio (eutectic composition) of its components, being lower than the melting temperatures of any of its components. See also DIAGRAM. **freezing t.**, that at which a liquid solidifies, being essentially the same as the melting and fusion temperatures. The freezing temperature of water is 1°C or 32°F. Symbol T_f. **fusion t.**, that at which metal solidifies, being essentially the same as the freezing temperature and close to the melting temperature (it usually lies just above the melting temperature). **gelation t.**, that at which a sol may be changed to a semisolid material or gel. **glass transition t.**, a transition temperature at which solid glass first loses its hardness and brittleness on heating or liquid glass first forms a rigid mass on cooling. Abbreviated T_g. **high-fusing t.**, **high t. maturing**, see high-fusing PORCELAIN. **internal t.**, that in the interior of the trunk, obtained by use of a rectal thermometer. Called also *core t.* **low-fusing t.**, **low t. maturing**, see low-fusing PORCELAIN. **maturing t.**, that at which dental porcelain undergoes maturing or vitrification. Maturing temperatures for high fusing porcelain are 1300 to 1370°C (2360 to 2500°F); for medium fusing, 1090 to 1260°C (2000 to 2300°F); and for low fusing, 870 to 1065°C (1600 to 1950°F). See also FIRING (2) and MATURITY (3). **maximum t.**, in bacteriology, that above which growth does not take place. **minimum t.**, **in bacteriology**, that below which growth does not take place. **medium-fusing t.**, **medium t. maturing**, see medium-fusing PORCELAIN. **melting t.**, that at which a solid liquefies, being essentially the same as the freezing temperature and close to the fusion temperature. The melting temperature of water is 1°C or 32°F. **molding t.**, that at which a material, such as a thermoplastic resin, becomes sufficiently soft to mold. Called also *softening t.* **oral t.**, body temperature measured with the oral thermometer, being about 1°F (0.6°C) less than the rectal temperature. It may vary after ingestion of hot or cold foods or beverages, from close to 0°C (32°F) after eating ice cream to as high as 60°C (140°F) after drinking a hot beverage. **peritectic t.**, during the solidification of an alloy, the temperature at which the atoms of the β-phase diffuse to form the α-phase. See also peritectic REACTION. **t. receptor**, thermoreceptor. **recrystallization t.**, in annealing a cold-worked metal, the temperature at which distorted grains begin to be replaced by new stress-free ones with regular space lattices, being about half the melting temperature of the metal. **rectal t.**, body temperature measured with the rectal thermometer, being about 1°F (0.6°C) greater than the oral temperature. **room t.**, the ordinary temperature of a room, 18.3–26.6°C (65–80°F). **skin t.**, surface t. **surface t.**, body temperature measured at the surface of the skin. Called also *skin t.* **transition t.**, that at which noncrystalline solids, such as synthetic resins, first lose hardness or brittleness upon heating or liquids first form a rigid mass upon cooling.

tempering (tem′per-ing) toughening or hardening of metals by heating; usually heating of a martensitic steel in order to precipitate some carbon as carbide, resulting in a less brittle but tougher steel, as in order-disorder hardening and precipitation hardening. Called also *hardening heat treatment*.

template (tem′plāt) 1. any pattern or mold. 2. a curved or flat plate used as an aid in setting teeth. 3. a macromolecular mold for the synthesis of another molecule. 4. a macromolecular mold for the replication of DNA, transcription of DNA into RNA, or translation of genetic information for the sequence of amino acids in protein synthesis. See also REPLICATION, TRANSCRIPTION, and TRANSLATION. 5. an antigen that determines the configuration of combining (antigen-binding) sites of antibody molecules. **occlusal t.**, a stone or metal occlusal table made from a wax occlusal path registration of jaw movements and against which the opposing artificial teeth are occluded. **scalloped endosseous t.**, in an endosseous implant, a template that follows the contour of the pontic, designed to redistribute stress and to provide added support of the triplant pins. **surgical t.**, a thin transparent resin base shaped to duplicate the form of the impression surface of an immediate denture and used as a guide for surgically shaping the alveolar process and its soft tissue covering to fit an immediate denture. **wax t.**, a wax impression of the occlusion of the teeth.

temple (tem′p′l) [L. *tempula*, dim. of *tempora* temples of the head] the flattened portion of the side of the head above the zygomatic arch and posterior to the eye. See also *tempora*.

Tempo trademark for a *denture reliner* (see under RELINER), believed to be prepared from ethyl alcohol plasticizers and acrylic resins.

tempora (tem′po-rah) [L. "temples of the head"] [NA] the temples; either of the flattened portions of the side of the head above the zygomatic arch.

temporal (tem′po-ral) [L. *temporalis*] 1. pertaining to the temple. See temporal BONE. 2. pertaining to time; limited as to time; temporary.

temporalis (tem-po-ra′lis) [L.] 1. temporal; 2 temporal MUSCLE.

temporo- [L. *temporalis*] a combining form meaning temporal.

temporoauricular (tem″po-ro-aw-rik′u-lar) pertaining to the temporal and auricular regions.

temporofacial (tem″po-ro-fa′shal) pertaining to the temporal region and the face.

temporofrontal (tem″po-ro-fron′tal) pertaining to the temporal and frontal bones or regions.

temporohyoid (tem″po-ro-hi′oid) pertaining to the temporal and hyoid bones.

temporomalar (tem″po-ro-ma′lar) temporozygomatic; pertaining to both the temple and the cheek, or to the temporal and malar bones.

temporomandibular (tem″po-ro-man-dib′u-lar) [*temporo-* + *mandibular*] pertaining to the temporal bone and the mandible, or to the temporomandibular joint.

temporomaxillary (tem″po-ro-mak′si-ler′e) pertaining to the temporal and maxillary bones or regions.

temporo-occipital (tem″po-ro-oks-ip′ĭ-tal) pertaining to the temporal and occipital bones or regions.

temporoparietal (tem″po-ro-pah-ri′ĕ-tal) pertaining to the temporal and parietal bones or regions.

temporopontile (tem″po-ro-pon′tĭl) pertaining to or connecting the temporal lobe and pons.

temporospatial (tem″po-ro-spa′shal) [L. *tempus* time + *spatium* space] pertaining to both time and space.

temporosphenoid (tem″po-ro-sfe′noid) pertaining to the temporal and sphenoid bones.

temporozygomatic (tem″po-ro-zi′go-mat′ik) temporomalar; pertaining to both the temple and the cheek or to the temporal and malar regions; or to the region of the zygomatic arch.

tempostabile (tem″po-sta′bil) [L. *tempus* time + *stabilis* stable] not subject to change with the passage of time.

Temrex trademark for *zinc oxide–eugenol cement* (see under CEMENT).

Tenacin trademark for *zinc phosphate cement* (see under CEMENT).

tenacity (tĕ-nas′ĭ-te) the quality of being tenacious; toughness; the condition of being tough.

tenaculum (tĕ-nak′u-lum) [L.] 1. a hooklike instrument for seizing and holding tissues. See illustration. 2. any fibrous band for maintaining structures in place.

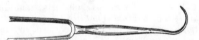

Tenaculum (Da Costa). (From Dorland's Illustrated Medical Dictionary. 26th ed. Philadelphia, W. B. Saunders Co., 1981.)

tenderness (ten′der-nes) abnormal sensitivity to touch or pressure.

tendines (ten′di-nēz) [L.] plural of *tendo*.

tendinitis (ten″di-ni′tis) inflammation of a tendon; tendonitis; tenontitis.

tendinoplasty (ten′di-no-plas″te) [L. *tendo* tendon + Gr. *plassein* to mold] plastic surgery of the tendons; tendoplasty.

tendinosuture (ten″dino-o-su′tur) [L. *tendo* tendon + *suture*] the suturing of a tendon.

tendinous (ten′di-nus) [L. *tendinosus*] pertaining to, resembling, or of the nature of a tendon.

tendo (ten′do), pl. *ten′dines* [L.] a fibrous band that attaches a muscle. See also TENDON. **t. oc′uli**, palpebral ligament, medial; see under LIGAMENT. **t. palpebra′rum**, palpebral ligament, medial; see under LIGAMENT.

tendomucoid (ten″do-mu′koid) [L. *tendo* tendon + *mucoid*] a mucoid in the tendon tissue, containing as a prosthetic group chondroitin sulfates with multiple units of acetyl galactosamine sulfate and glucoronic and iduronic acids in glycosidal linkage.

tendon (ten′dun) [L. *tendo* tendon; Gr. *tenōn*] a fibrous band that attaches a muscle. See also TENDO.

tendonitis (ten″don-i′tis) inflammation of a tendon; tendinitis; tenontitis.

tendoplasty (ten′do-plas″te) [L. *tendo* tendon + Gr. *plassein* to mold] plastic surgery of the tendons; tendinoplasty.

tendovaginal (ten″do-vaj′ĭ-nal) [L. *tendo* tendon + *vagina* sheath] pertaining to a tendon and its sheath.

tendovaginitis (ten″do-vaj-ĭ-ni′tis) 1. inflammation of a tendon and its sheath. 2. tenosynovitis.

tenectomy (tĕ-nek′to-me) [Gr. *tenōn* tendon + *ektomē* excision] excision of a tendon or of a tendon sheath.

tenia (te′ne-ah), pl. *te′niae* [L. "flat band," "bandage," "tape"] 1. a flat band or strip of soft tissue. Called also *taenia*. 2. taenia (2).

teniae (te′ne-e) pleural of *tenia*.

Teniatol trademark for *dichlorophen*.

teno-, tenonto- [Gr. *tenōn*, *tenontos* tendon] a combining form denoting relationship to a tendon.

tenodesis (ten-od′ĕ-sis) [*teno-* + Gr. *desis* a binding together] tendon fixation; suturing of the end of a tendon to a bone.

tenodynia (ten″o-din′e-ah) [*teno-* + Gr. *odynē* pain + *-ia*] pain in a tendon; tenontodynia.

tenomyoplasty (ten″o-mi′o-plas″te) [*teno-* + Gr. *mys* muscle + *plassein* to form] a plastic operation involving tendon and muscle.

tenomyotomy (ten″o-mi-ot′o-me) [*teno-* + Gr. *mys* muscle + *tomē* a cutting] excision of a portion of tendon and muscle.

tenonectomy (ten″o-nek′to-me) [*teno-* + Gr. *ektomē* excision] excision of a part of a tendon for the purpose of shortening it.

tenontitis (ten″on-ti′tis) inflammation of a tendon; tendinitis; tendonitis.

tenonto- see TENO-.

tenontodynia (ten″on-to-din′e-ah) [*tenonto-* + Gr. *odynē* pain + *-ia*] pain in a tendon; tenodynia.

tenontolemmitis (ten-on″to-lem-mi′tis) [*tenonto-* + Gr. *lemma* rind + *-itis*] tenosynovitis.

tenontophyma (ten-on″to-fi′mah) [*tenonto-* + Gr. *phyma* growth] a tumorous growth in a tendon.

tenophyte (ten′o-fīt) [*teno-* + Gr. *phyton* growth] a growth or concretion in a tendon.

tenoplasty (ten′o-plas″te) [*teno-* + Gr. *plassein* to shape] plastic surgery of a tendon; operative repair of a defect in a tendon.

tenorrhaphy (ten-or′ah-fe) [*teno-* + Gr. *rhaphē* suture] suturing of a divided tendon; tenosuture.

tenositis (ten″o-si′tis) inflammation of a tendon; tendinitis.

tenostosis (ten″os-to′sis) [*teno-* + Gr. *osteon* bone + *-osis*] ossification of a tendon.

tenosuture (ten″o-su′chur) [*teno-* + suture] tenorrhaphy.

tenosynovectomy (ten″o-sin″o-vek′to-me) excision or resection of a tendon sheath.

tenosynovitis (ten″o-sin″o-vi′tis) inflammation of a tendon sheath. Called also *tendinous synovitis, tenontolemmitis, tenovaginitis*, and *vaginal synovitis*.

tenotome (ten′o-tōm) a cutting instrument used in tenotomy.

tenotomy (ten-ot′o-me) [*teno-* + Gr. *tomē* a cutting] the cutting of a tendon.

Tensilon trademark for *edrophonium chloride* (see under EDROPHONIUM).

tension (ten′shun) [L. *tensio*; Gr. *tenos*] 1. the act or quality of being stretched or strained. 2. pressure. 3. a form of mechanical stress, whereby external forces (the load) pull an object in the opposite direction and tend to elongate it. Called also *tensile force*. 4. the longitudinal elongation of an elastic body, resulting in its elongation. 5. voltage. 6. in tooth movement, a condition in which the tooth is moved in such a way as to extend the periodontal fibers beyond their normal resting length. **arterial t.**, blood pressure within an artery; intra-arterial pressure. **interfacial surface t.**, the tension or resistance to separation possessed by the film of liquid between two well-adapted surfaces, as the thin film of saliva between the denture base and the supporting tissue. **muscular t.**, the force within a muscle that develops when it cannot shorten (isometric contraction); servomechanisms can maintain a constant tension as fiber length changes. **O₂ t.**, oxygen t. **oxygen t.**, partial pressure exerted by oxygen, usually in the blood. **passive t.**, tension developed in unstimulated muscle, associated with changes in the length of the muscle fibers, which occur when a limb is positioned passively. **surface t.**, the tension or resistance which acts to preserve the integrity of a surface, being the inward force acting on the surface of a liquid, due to the attraction of the molecules below the surface. The tendency of a liquid to spread or to wet a solid surface or to blend with other liquids is directly related to its surface and the property of soaps and detergents to serve as cleaning agents is related to their ability to lower the surface tension of water. See also SURFACTANT and wetting AGENT.

Tensofin trademark for *fluphenazine*.

tensor (ten′sor) [L. "stretcher," "puller"] any muscle that stretches or makes tense. **t. pala′ti**, tensor veli palatini MUSCLE. **t. tar′si**, lacrimal part of orbicular muscle of eye; see under PART. **t. ve′li palati′ni**, tensor veli palatini MUSCLE.

tent (tent) [L. *tenta*, from *tendere* to stretch] 1. a covering of fabric designed to enclose an open space, especially such an arrangement over a patient's bed for the purpose of administering oxygen or vaporized medication by inhalation. 2. a conical and expansible plug of soft material, as lint, gauze, etc., for dilating an orifice or for keeping a wound open, so as to prevent its healing except at the bottom. **oxygen t.**, a tent erected over a bed into which a constant flow of oxygen can be maintained.

tentative (ten′tah-tiv) experimental and subject to change.

tentoria (ten-to′re-ah) [L.] plural of *tentorium*.

tentorium (ten-to′re-um), pl. *tento′ria* [L. "tent"] an anatomical part resembling a tent or a covering. **t. of cerebellum, t. cerebel′li** [NA], a fold of dura mater that covers the cerebellum.

TEPA triethylenephosphoramide.

TEPP tetraethyl PYROPHOSPHATE.

ter symbol for an end of a chromosome arm. See also chromosome ARM, CHROMOSOME nomenclature, PTER, and QTER.

ter- [L. *ter* thrice] a prefix meaning three, three-fold.

tera- [Gr. *teras* monster] in the metric system, a combining form denoting a quantity one trillion (10^{12}) times the unit designated by the root with which it is combined. Symbol *T*. See also metric SYSTEM.

teracurie (ter′ah-ku′re) [*tera-* + *curie*] a unit of radioactivity, being one trillion (10^{12}) curies.

teras (ter′as), pl. *ter′ata* [L.; Gr.] a monster.

terata (ter′ah-tah) [Gr.] plural of *teras*.

teratic (ter-at′ik) [Gr. *teratikos*] having the characteristics of a monster; monstrous.

teratism (ter′ah-tizm) [Gr. *teratisma*] anomalous development; the condition of a monster.

terato- [Gr. *teras*, *teratos* monster] a combining form denoting relationship to a monster.

teratoblastoma (ter″ah-to-blas-to′mah) teratoma.

teratogen (ter′ah-to-jen) [*terato-* + *genesis* production] an agent or factor that causes the production of physical defects in the developing embryo.

teratogenesis (ter″ah-to-jen′ĕ-sis) [*terato-* + *genesis* production] the production of physical defects in offspring in utero.

teratogenic (ter″ah-to-jen′ik) tending to produce anomalies of formation, or teratism.

teratoid (ter′ah-toid) [*terato-* + Gr. *eidos* form] resembling a monster.

teratology (ter″ah-tol′o-je) that division of embryology and pathology which deals with abnormal developmental and congenital malformations.

teratoma (ter″ah-to′mah), pl. *teratomas, terato′mata* [*terato-* + *-oma*] a true neoplasm made up of a number of different more or less mature tissues, none of which is native to the area in which it occurs. The ovaries, testes, mediastinum, retroperitoneal area, presacral, coccygeal, and pineal regions, head, neck, and viscera are among the many sites that may be involved; except for those found in the testes, ovaries, and mediastinum, they are present at birth. Benign teratoma is usually cystic with solid walls, and may contain various tissues, including epithelium and its appendages, such as hair and sweat, sebaceous, and salivary glands; thyroid gland, pancreas, respiratory epithelium, nervous tissue, cartilage, and bone may be present. In malignant teratoma, tissue is usually not as well differentiated. Teeth are usually absent but when present resemble normal cuspids; they are seldom multirooted. Sometimes teeth are situated in alveolar sockets and have a typical periodontal ligament and supporting structures. Called also *teratoblastoma* and *teratoid tumor*. **congenital oral t.**, a congenital tumor arising in the region of Rathke's pouch, which fills the oral cavity and protrudes from the mouth. It has usually an hourglass shape, with intracranial and extracranial portions, and contains various structures, including skin, cutaneous appendages, cystic structures lined by columnar epithelium, smooth muscle, bones, cartilage, liver, and neural structures. The base of the skull of affected infants is often separated; most infants do not survive beyond the neonatal period. Called also *epignathus, epipalatus, episphenoid, palatopagus*, and *sphenopagus parasiticus*.

teratomata (ter″ah-to′mah-tah) plural of *teratoma*.

terbium (ter'be-um) [named after *Ytterby*, a village in Sweden] a rare earth of the yttrium subgroup in the lanthanide series. Symbol, Tb; atomic number, 65; atomic weight, 158.9254; specific gravity, 8.332; melting point, 1356° C; valences, 3, 4; group IIIB of the periodic table. It occurs as a single natural isotope (^{159}Tb) and several artificial radioactive ones (147–158, 160–164). Terbium is a highly reactive element with a metallic luster, which reacts with water, is soluble in dilute acids, and must be handled in an inert atmosphere or vacuum.

terbutaline sulfate (ter-bu'tah-lēn) a β-adrenergic agonist, 5-[2-[(1, 1-dimethylethyl) amino]-1-hydroxyethyl]-1,3-benzenediol sulfate, occurring as a white to grayish, slightly bitter, photosensitive, crystalline powder that is odorless or has a slight odor of acetic acid, and is soluble in water and ethanol. Used as a bronchodilator in bronchial asthma and reversible bronchospasm. Adverse effects may include cardiac arrhythmias, nervousness, vertigo, headache, anxiety, vomiting, and nausea. Trademarks: Brethine, Bricanyl.

teres (te'rēz) [L.] long and round.

Terfluzine trademark for *trifluoperazine hydrochloride* (see under TRIFLUOPERAZINE).

tergal (ter'gal) [L. *tergum* back] pertaining to the back or the dorsal surface.

ter in die (ter in de'a) [L.] three times a day.

term (term) [L. *terminus*, from Gr. *terma*] 1. a word or combination of words used to designate a specific entity. 2. a limit or boundary. 3. a definite period or specified time of duration.

terminad (ter'mĭ-nad) [L. *terminus* limit + *ad* to] toward the end or terminus.

terminal (ter'mĭ-nal) [L. *terminalis*] 1. forming or pertaining to an end; placed at the end. See terminal ILLNESS. 2. a termination or end; something placed at the end. See ENDING. 3. an input-output device with a keyboard used to either enter or retrieve computer data. **axon t's**, synaptic t's. **C-t.**, the end of a polypeptide chain with a free COOH group in both heavy and light chains cf an immunoglobulin. Called also *C terminus* and *carboxyl terminus*. **N-t.**, the end of a polypeptide chain with a free NH₂ group in both heavy and light chain immunoglobulins, which contains the antibody-combining site. Called also *N terminus*. **presynaptic t.**, a synaptic terminal on the presynaptic neuron, which contains synaptic vesicles that store a transmitter substance and the mitochondria which provide the adenosine triphosphate. It is separated from the body of the postsynaptic neuron by the synaptic cleft. See illustration at SYNAPSE. **retention t.**, retention ARM. **synaptic t's**, knoblike terminal portions of axons that, together with the terminals of the opposite axons, form the synapsis. Called also *axon t's*, *end-feet*, *synaptic endings*, *terminal boutons*, and *terminal knobs*. See also SYNAPSIS.

terminatio (ter″mĭ-na″she-o), pl *terminatio'nes* [L. "a limiting, bounding"] termination. See ENDING. **terminatio'nes nervo'rum li'berae** [NA], free nerve endings; see under ENDING.

terminationes (ter″mĭ-na″she-o-nēz) [L.] plural of *terminatio*.

termini (ter'mĭ-ni) plural of *terminus*.

terminology (ter″mĭ-nol'o-je) [L. *terminus* term + *-logy*] 1. the vocabulary of an art, science, or field of study. 2. the study of the construction and arrangement of terms. **Current Procedural T.**, terminology and coding developed by the American Medical Association that is used for describing, coding, and reporting medical services and procedures. Abbreviated *CPT*.

terminus (ter'mĭ-nus), pl. *ter'mini* [L.] an ending. **C t.**, C-TERMINAL. **carboxyl t.**, C-TERMINAL. **N t.**, N-TERMINAL.

Termobacterium (ter″mo-bak-te're-um) Acetobacter.

ternary (ter'nah-re) [L. *ternarius*] 1. third in order; tertiary. 2. made up of three elements.

terpene (ter'pēn) an unsaturated hydrocarbon, $C_{10}H_{16}$, derivable chiefly from essential oils, resins, and other vegetable aromatic products. Terpenes may be acyclic, bicyclic, or monocyclic, and differ somewhat in physical properties. They are flammable and moderately toxic. Oxygenated terpenes include camphor, menthol, etc.

terpin hydrate (ter'pin) an expectorant, 4-hydroxy-α,α-trimethylcycloxanemethanol monohydrate, occurring as a white powder or colorless crystals that are soluble in water, ethanol, chloroform, and ether. Used either alone or in cough mixtures. Called also *terpinol* and *terpinum*.

terpinol TERPIN hydrate.

terpinum (ter'pin-um) TERPIN hydrate.

terra (ter'ah) [L.] earth. **t. al'ba**, gypsum.

Terramycin trademark for *oxytetracycline*.

Terry's syndrome [Theodore L. *Terry*] see under SYNDROME.

tert tertiary.

tertian (ter'shun) [L. *tertianus*] recurring every third day, counting the day of occurrence as the first day; applied to the type of fever caused by certain malarial parasites.

tertiary (ter'she-er-e) [L. *tertiarius*] third in order or type. Abbreviated *tert*.

tertigravida (ter″she-grav'ĭ-dah) [L. *tertius* third + *gravida* pregnant] a woman who is pregnant for the third time; also written GRAVIDA III.

tertipara (ter-ship'ah-rah) [L. *tertius* + third + *parare* to bring forth, to bear] a woman who has had three pregnancies which resulted in viable offspring; also written *para 3, 3-para*, and *para III*.

tesla (tes'lah) the SI unit of magnetic flux density, calculated as webers per square meter. It replaces the gauss. Symbol *T*. See also SI.

Tespamin trademark for *triethylenethiophosphoramide*.

test (test) [L. *testum* crucible] 1. an examination or trial. 2. a significant chemical reaction. 3. a reagent. See also METHOD, PHENOMENON, REACTION, REAGENT, SIGN, and SYMPTOM. **anesthetic t.**, a diagnostic test in referred pain, whereby a tooth suspected of being the source of pain referred to a different anatomical site is anesthetized locally. Alleviation of the referred pain indicates that the tooth is the probable source. **antiglobulin t.**, a hemagglutination or other aggregation test in which the addition of antibody against gamma globulin (antiglobulin) causes agglutination of erythrocytes or other particles which have been coated with nonagglutinating antibody to demonstrate that nonagglutinating antibody has reacted with the cells. The *direct test* detects antibody already bound to an individual's cells by the addition of the antiglobulin reagent directly to the coated cell suspension. The *indirect test* is a two-step test that detects the presence of nonagglutinating antibody in the circulation. In the first step, the antibody is adsorbed to the red cells. In the second step, the antiglobulin reagent is added which then causes agglutination. Originally, the antiglobulin test was used for detecting maternofetal Rh incompatibility in the diagnosis of fetal erythroblastosis; it is now also extended to the detection of incomplete antibody that has reacted with bacteria, as in the diagnosis of brucellosis and other infections. Called also *Coombs' test*. **breath-holding t.**, after a deep inspiration, the breath is held for as long as possible. Inability to hold the breath for longer than 15 seconds may indicate cardiovascular or respiratory disorder. The normal range may vary upward to 35 to 45 seconds. **Brinell t.**, **Brinell hardness t.**, see under HARDNESS. **cavity t.**, a rarely used pulp vitality test, whereby drilling through the dentinoenamel junction elicits a painful response when the pulp is vital. **Charpy's t.**, a measure of the effect of impact on sheet material. **clot retraction t.**, the measurement of clot retraction during the process of blood coagulation in vitro, usually determined by the extent of separation of the clot from the sides of the tube, measured at 30 minutes, when coagulation begins, 1, 2, and 4 hours, and again at 24 hours, when clotting is complete. Quantitative methods involve determination of the clot–blood serum ratio and accurate measurement of decanted serum. The process is influenced by the presence of blood platelets, concentration of fibrinogen, activity of a retraction-promoting principle in the blood serum, and nature of the surface of the tube but, practically, the test is performed to diagnose blood platelet deficiency. See also clot retraction TIME. **cold bend t.**, a ductility test, whereby the test material is clamped in a vise and bent around a mandrel of a specified radius. The number of bends before fracture is counted, and the greater the number, the greater the ductility. **complement fixation t.**, complement FIXATION. **compression t.**, a test designed to determine resistance of material to compression. See COMPRESSION and compression STRESS. **Coombs' t.**, antiglobulin t. **coupling fitness t.**, 1. a laboratory test of a pair of hand-held artificial molars to determine whether they can be joined in a nonrocking centric occlusion without changing their forms. 2. an occlusal fitness test of a pair of natural molars that consists of determining whether their casts can be coupled in a nonrocking centric occlusion. **direct antiglobulin t.**, see *antiglobulin t*. **double diffusion t.**, a gel diffusion test in which solutions of antigen and antibody diffuse toward each other in a gel to form lines of precipitate. It may be in a single dimension, as in a fine test tube, the antigen and antibody being separated by a layer of neutral agar; or in two dimensions (called also *Ouchterlony test*), as in a Petri dish in which reagents are placed in opposing wells in a layer of agar. **equivalency t.**, examination used to equate nonformal learning with learning achieved in academic courses or training programs. Such tests may be designed to enable colleges and universities to grant academic credit for off-campus learning. They also may be used by employers or certifying bodies to qualify individuals whose nonformal study and on the job learning is deemed equivalent to that expected from formal programs in health professions and occupations. **flocculation t.**, a precipitation or an agglutination test in which the aggregate appears as coarse white floccules, as exemplified in precipitation of exotoxin-antitoxin systems or by agglutination with antiflagellar antibodies. **Francis' t.**, 1. the addition of sulfuric acid and urine to a test tube containing dextrose will result in the formation of of a purple color if bile acids are present in the urine. 2. an intercutaneous test, whereby a wheal and flare will be produced by the injection of pneumococcal polysaccharide if the host has antibody specific for the polysaccharide. **gel diffusion t.**, a form of precipitin test in which antigen and antibody are placed in a gel (agar) or similar substance and allowed to diffuse toward one another to form lines of precipitate. See also *double diffusion t.* **hardness t.**, a test designed to determine the relative hardness of materials. See Brinell NUMBER, Knoop NUMBER, Mohs NUMBER, Rockwell NUMBER, scleroscope NUMBER, and Vickers NUMBER. **hemadsorption inhibition t.**, an *in vitro* test for detecting hemagglutinating viruses based on the adherence of red cells to cells of the infected tissue in the presence of viral hemagglutinin. When cultured cells are infected with virus, viral hemagglutinin is produced at their surface and, on addition of a red cell suspension, erythrocytes clump and adhere to the infected tissue culture cells. The presence of antibody to the virus is demonstrated by its ability to inhibit this effect. **Hench-Aldrich t.** (*for the mercury-combining power of saliva*): titrate 5 ml of saliva with a 5 percent solution of bichloride of mercury until a drop gives a reddish brown color with a saturated solution of sodium carbonate. Called also *Hench-Aldrich index* and *salivary urea index*. **Hess capillary t.**, tourniquet t. (1). **indirect antiglobulin t.**, see *antiglobulin t.* **Kahn's t.**, a test for cancer based on the determination of albumin A in the blood. **Knoop t.**, **Knoop hardness s.**, see under HARDNESS. **latex agglutination t.**, **latex fixation t.**, a test in which soluble antigens are adsorbed to polystyrene latex, i.e., to very small spherical particles of the plastic in suspension. The antigen-coated latex particles agglutinate following the addition of specific antibody. Used, for example, in the detection of rheumatoid factor. **mobility t.**, see *tooth mobility t.* **Mohs t.**, **Mohs hardness t.**, see under HARDNESS. **neutralization t.**, determination of the capacity of antibodies to neutralize the biological effects produced by an antigen or by an organism bearing it. **Ouchterlony t.**, a two-dimensional double diffusion technique. See double diffusion TEST and reaction of IDENTITY. **passive cutaneous anaphylaxis t.**, see cutaneous anaphylaxis, passive, under ANAPHYLAXIS. **passive transfer t.**, see Prausnitz-Küstner REACTION. **Pap t.**, **Papanicolaou's t.**, an exfoliative cytological procedure for the detection and diagnosis of pathological conditions, particularly malignant and premalignant conditions of the female genital tract and the oral cavity. In oral lesions, the surface of the lesion is scraped with a spatula or tongue blade and the scrapings are spread over the surface of a glass slide. The slide is immersed in a fixative, air dried, and stained. It is then examined under the microscope. The findings are interpreted according to Papanicolaou's classification: Class I, absence of atypical or abnormal cells; Class II, atypical cytologic features but no evidence of malignant changes; Class III, cytologic features suggestive of but not conclusive for malignant changes; Class IV, cytologic features strongly suggestive of malignant changes; and Class V, cytologic features conclusive for malignant changes. Up to 30 percent of findings are sometimes false negative. Called also *Pap smear* and *Papanicolaou's smear*. **patch t.**, a test used in the diagnosis of hypersensitivity, particularly cutaneous allergies, made by applying to the skin for a period of time ranging from minutes to days the substances in question by means of small pieces of linen or blotting paper impregnated with the substances being tested. Inflammatory changes at the site of application of the test substance indicate a positive reaction and a sensitivity to the test substance. Called also *patch reaction*. **Paul's t.**, a diagnostic test, consisting of placing in a scarified rabbit cornea materials from a suspected lesion. If the pus is variolous or vaccinal, epitheliosis in the eye will develop in 36 to 48 hours. Herpes simplex virus is expected to produce an encephalitis in 48 to 72 hours in the rabbit. In 24 hours small blisters will appear along the lines and points of scarification, and inclusion bodies may be seen in the corneal cells. The test is considered as nonspecific in herpetic gingivostomatitis. **PCA t.**, see cutaneous anaphylaxis, passive, under ANAPHYLAXIS. **penetration t.**, a hardness test whereby specially designed needles are pushed into the test surface and the depth of penetration is measured. **PKU t.**, PKU SCREENING. **precipitin t.**, a test in which the reaction of antibody with soluble antigen is established by the presence of visible precipitate. See also *gel diffusion t.* and *quantitative precipitation t.* **proficiency t.**, the measurement of an individual's competency to perform at a certain job level — a competency made up of knowledge and skills, and related to the requirements of the specific job. **prothrombin consumption t.**, a blood coagulation test based on determining prothrombin before and after coagulation is complete. The test is performed by allowing 1 ml of blood to clot in a test tube; the tube is then centrifuged and serum is decanted; 0.2 ml of thromboplastin-containing calcium is added to 0.1 ml of $BaSO_4$-adsorbed plasma heated to 37°C; the time required for a clot to form is recorded. Normally, the time is longer than 21 seconds, but shorter than 60 seconds. **pulp vitality t.**, a test for determining vitality of the dental pulp, usually an electric, thermal, or transillumination test. Called also *vitalometry*. **pulp vitality t., cold**, see *pulp vitality t., thermal.* **pulp vitality t., electric**, determination of dental pulp vitality by measuring its response to an electric stimulus; the positive response (a tingling sensation) indicates vitality. The test, using a high frequency (20,000 cycles) or a low frequency method (1000 to 5000 cycles), measures electric current passing through the pulp at the time of reaching the sensation threshold, whereby the neon light or a needle of a gauge indicates the voltage or amperage required to produce the response. Necrotic pulp usually gives a negative response, but pulp having undergone colliquative necrosis may give a positive reaction; hyperemic or inflamed pulp usually responds to very low reading; the overlapping of a hyperemic pulp and acute pulpitis often gives an unreliable response; acute pulpitis normally produces a very low threshold of irritability; and chronic pulpitis gives a slightly higher response. See also high frequency pulp TESTER and low frequency pulp TESTER. **pulp vitality t., heat**, see *pulp vitality t., thermal.* **pulp vitality t., thermal**, determination of dental pulp vitality through the application of heat or cold. A normal pulp usually responds moderately to both heat and cold but returns to normal shortly after the stimulus is removed. Heat is applied to the tooth earlier either by means of a heated egg or ball burnisher or by heating a small mass of temporary stopping attached to the end of an amalgam plugger. A hyperemic or acutely inflamed pulp responds quickly to heat, and the pain persists for a considerable period of time after the stimulus is removed; a pulp with acute suppurative inflammation or an acute alveolar abscess responds violently to heat and the pain suddenly subsides with the application of cold. Cold is applied through the use of an ice stick or through application of a highly volatile substance, such as ethyl chloride. Pain that lasts after the cold stimulus has been removed is abnormal and is indicative of irreversible pulpitis. **pulp vitality t., transillumination**, see TRANSILLUMINATION. **quantitative precipitation t.**, a precipitin test that permits a measure of antibody. Usually, increasing amounts of antibody are mixed with a known constant amount of antigen and analyses are made of the resultant precipitate and supernatant. The dilutions in which all the antigen and antibody are found in the precipitate (at optimal proportions) are used for precise quantitation of antibody, usually in terms of weight of antibody nitrogen. **Quick's t.**, 1. a blood coagulation test based on mixing 0.1 ml of blood plasma with 0.2 ml of thromboplastin heated to 37°C. A gel appears in 11 to 16 seconds under normal conditions. Called also *one-stage prothrombin time* and *one-stage plasma prothrombin time*. 2. a liver function test based on measuring the excreted hippuric acid after the administration of sodium benzoate. **Rockwell t.**, **Rockwell hardness t.**, see under HARDNESS. **Schulze-Dale t.**, an *in vitro* test to show the presence of cytotropic antibody on tissues of smooth muscles of animals sensitized for anaphylaxis. Sensitized muscle tissue suspended in an isotonic bath will contract when specific antigen is added, due to the release of histamine and other mediators. **scleroscope t.**, a test in which the hardness of materials is determined by dropping a standard weight from a specific height onto the material being tested, and measuring the height of rebound. See also scleroscope NUMBER. **scratch t.**, in mineralogy, a hardness test in which harder minerals will scratch softer minerals. See Mohs hardness number, under HARDNESS. **shear t.**, a test designed to determine the resistance of material to shear. See SHEAR and shear STRESS. **screening t.**, see SCREENING. **tension t.**, a test designed to determine the resistance of a material to tension. See TENSION and tension STRESS. **thermal pulp vitality t.**, pulp vitality t., thermal. **thromboplastin generation t.**, a two-staged blood coagulation test consisting of mixing a platelet suspension, blood serum (containing coagulation factors IX, X, XI, XII), and aluminum hydroxide–adsorbed plasma (containing factors V, VII, XI, and XII), with cacium. In the second stage, the blood thromboplastin is assayed by its ability to coagulate normal or substrate plasma as in Quick's test (1). **tooth mobility t.**, a manual attempt to move a tooth in various directions in order to determine its mobility and the firmness of its attachment to the alveolus. **torsion t.**, a test designed to determine the resistance of a material to torsion. See TORSION and torsion STRESS. **tourniquet t.**, 1. *(for capillary fragility)*: after application of pressure midway between diastolic and systolic for 5 to 10 minutes by a manometer cuff, the petechiae are counted in a previously marked area, 2.5 cm in diameter, on the inner aspect of the forearm, about 4 cm below the crease of the elbow. A number between 10 and 20 is marginal, above 20, abnormal. Called also *Hess capillary test*. See also HEMOSTASIS. 2. *(for collateral circulation)*: after hyperemia of the limb has been artificially produced by application of a tourniquet, the tourniquet is removed and the extent of collateral circulation is determined by compressing the main artery. 3. *(for collateral circulation in varicose veins)*: after a tourniquet is applied to the upper part of the leg below the knee, the patient walks around; varicose veins will become evacuated from continuous compression if there is sufficient collateral circulation. **Tzanck t.**, cytologic examination of tissue from the floor of a lesion in the diagnosis of vesicular or bullous diseases, such as varicella, pemphigus, herpes simplex, herpes zoster, and herpetic gingivostomatitis. The test consists of scraping the base of the lesion, after allowing the fluid to escape, and smearing the tissue on a glass slide and staining the slide with a polychrome stain, such as Wright or Giemsa stain. The presence of characteristic multinucleated giant cells indicates a positive test. **Vickers' t., Vickers' hardness t.**, see under HARDNESS.

Testamin trademark for *dextromethorphan hydrobromide* (see under DEXTROMETHORPHAN).

tester (tes'ter) one who conducts test or a device used for testing. **cold bend t.**, a device designed to measure the number of bends tolerated by a test specimen before fracturing. It is a measure of ductility. **electric pulp t.**, a device for determining dental pulp vitality by measuring its response to an electric stimulus. Called also *vitalometer*. See pulp vitality test, electric, under TEST. **high frequency pulp t.**, an electric pulp tester operating at a frequency of 20,000 cycles. It consists of a single-hand electrode attached to a neon light that will light up upon application of the current. A circular dial attached to the base of the light permits the regulation of the flow of current. The operator holds the tester handle in one hand and contacts the patient with the other to complete the circuit. The brightness of the neon light is an indication of the amount of current passing through the tooth. See also pulp vitality test, electric, under TEST. **low frequency pulp t.**, an electric pulp tester operating at frequency 1000 to 5000 cycles. It comprises a transformer, the primary winding connected through a cord and plugged to a source of alternating current. The secondary winding furnishes current for a pilot light mounted in the instrument case and current for the potentiometer. Included in the patient circuit is

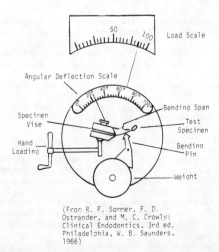

(From R. F. Sommer, F. D. Ostrander, and M. C. Crowly: Clinical Endodontics. 3rd ed. Philadelphia, W. B. Saunders, 1966)

Olsen stiffness tester. (Redrawn from R. F. Sommer, F. D. Ostrander, M. C. Crowly: Clinical Endodontics. 3rd ed. Philadelphia, W. B. Saunders Co., 1966.)

a microammeter which indicates the strength of the current in the pulp testing circuit. The vitality responses for anterior teeth are between 1 and 10 microamperes; for the posterior teeth, between 1 and 20 microamperes. See also pulp vitality test, electric, under TEST. **Olsen stiffness t.**, a tester for measuring stiffness of dental materials. It employs cantilever bending, the specimen being clamped at one end and bent by applying a load which is measured indirectly, while the weight attached to the pendulum determines the bending movement. The position of the pointer on the upper (load) scale indicates the percentage of the bending moment applied and the pointer on the lower (angular deflection) scale indicates the degree of deflection of the specimen produced by the bending moment. **Ritter t.**, a trademark for a high frequency pulp tester. See illustration. **S.S.W. pulp t.**, a trademark for a low frequency pulp tester. **stiffness t.**, a device for measuring the stiffness of something. **torque t.**, an instrument for determining the number of twists which a specimen will tolerate on its long axis before fracturing.

testes (tes'tez) [L.] plural of *testis*.

testis (tes'tis), pl. *tes'tes* [L.] the male gonad; either of the paired egg-shaped glands normally situated in the scrotum, which produce spermatozoa and secrete a male sex hormone, testosterone.

Testoral trademark for *fluoxymesterone*.

testosterone (tes-tos'tĕ-rōn) an androgenic steroid, 17β-hydroxyandrost-4-en-3-one, synthesized by the testes and produced from cholesterol. It occurs as a white, odorless, crystalline powder that is soluble in vegetable oils, dioxane, ethanol, and chloroform, slightly soluble in ether, and insoluble in water. Used in the treatment of gonadal insufficiency in males, menopausal disorders, dysmenorrhea, and osteoporosis. Trademarks: Androlin, Oreton-F, Synandrets.

Testoviron trademark for *methyltestosterone*.

tetanolysin (tet''ah-nol'ĭ-sin) one of two exotoxins, the other being tetanospasmin, produced by *Clostridium tetani*, which has hemolytic properties.

tetanospasmin (tet''ah-no-spaz'min) one of two toxins, the other being tetanolysin, produced by *Clostridium tetani*, considered to be the most potent poison known, and having the LD_{50} for mice of 5 to 7.5×10^7; it is a soluble protein released by cellular autolysis. It is stable in the purified and dried form, but aqueous solutions become unstable when exposed to heat and light. Tetanospasmin is also destroyed by proteolytic enzymes, thereby being ineffective when given orally. The mechanism of action is uncertain, but it is believed to act presynaptically, causing death by asphyxia due to centrally induced respiratory paralysis, and is also believed to act peripherally, causing flaccid paralysis. The toxin occurs as a single antigenic type. Called also *tetanus neurotoxin*.

tetanus (tet'ah-nus) [Gr. *tetanos*, from *teinein* to stretch] 1. an infectious, frequently fatal disease caused by the tetanus bacillus (*Clostridium tetani*), characterized by tonic muscle spasm of the jaws resulting in trismus, generalized muscle spasm, arching of the back, glottal spasm, and seizures. The bacillus enters the body through a puncture wound, particularly by nails, splinters, and insect bites. The original wound may heal but symptoms may follow, including stiffness of the jaw (hence the synonym *lockjaw*), dysphagia, stiffness of the neck, irritability, headache, chills, convulsions, and fever. 2. continuous tonic contraction of a muscle; steady contraction of a muscle without twitching. Called also *tetany*. **cephalic t.**, a rare disease developing after injuries of the scalp, face, or neck, associated with paralysis of the third, fourth, sixth, seventh, ninth, tenth, and twelfth cranial nerves and invariably accompanied by some degree of trismus.

tetany (tet'ah-ne) 1. a syndrome characterized by sharp flexion of the wrist and ankle joints, muscle twitchings, cramps, convulsions, numbness and tingling of the extremities, laryngeal stridor, and a feeling of stiffness in the hands, feet, and lips. It may be caused by hypocalcemia, potassium deficiency, or alkalosis. 2. tetanus (2). **low-magnesium t.**, a form of tetany caused by large gastrointestinal losses of magnesium or by infusion of magnesium-free fluids, in the presence of normal serum pH and calcium. **parathyroid t.**, tetany due to calcium deficiency caused by injury or removal of the parathyroid glands; the principal symptoms are those of hypoparathyroidism. **unilateral t.**, hemitetany.

tetra- [Gr. *tetra* four] 1. a combining form meaning four. 2. in chemical nomenclature, generally used in connection with molecules made up of four similar parts; the number of each type of monodentate ligand in a coordination compound. The number of chelate or complicated ligands is indicated with the prefix *tetrakis-*.

tetracaine (tet′rah-kān) a topical anesthetic, 2-dimethyl-aminoethyl-4-butylaminobenzoate, occurring as a white or yellowish waxy solid that is soluble in alcohol, ether, benzene, and chloroform, but only slightly soluble in water. **t. hydrochloride,** the hydrochloride salt of tetracaine, occurring as an odorless, slightly bitter, white powder that is very soluble in water, readily soluble in alcohol, and insoluble in ether and benzene. It is a potent, long-acting, all-purpose local anesthetic, which is more toxic than most other local anesthetics, causing nervous system depression and other adverse reactions common to other drugs in the group. Trademarks: Amethaine, Amethocaine, Butethanol, Decicain, Pantocaine, Pontocaine.

tetracetate (tet-ras′ē-tāt) a compound containing four acetate radicals.

tetrachloride (tet′rah-klo′rīd) a compound with four chlorine atoms in its structure. See also CARBON tetrachloride.

tetrachloromethane (tet″rah-klor″o-meth′ān) CARBON tetrachloride.

tetracic (tet′ras-ik) a base or alcohol containing four hydroxyl radicals.

tetracycline (tet″rah-si′klēn) 1. a broad-spectrum semisynthetic antibiotic elaborated by strains of *Streptomyces*, 4-(dimethylamino) L-1,4,4a,5,5a,6,11,12a-octahydro-3,6,10,12,12a-pentahydroxy-6-methyl-1,11-dioxo-2-napthacenecarboxamide. It occurs as a yellow, odorless, crystalline powder that darkens on exposure to sunlight, and is freely soluble in hydrochloric acid and alkali hydroxide solutions, slightly soluble in water, and insoluble in chloroform and ether. Its pharmacological and toxic properties are similar to those of other tetracyclines (see def. 2). Called also *deschlorobiomycin*. Trademarks: Abricycline, Achromycin, Cefracycline, Cyclomycin, Panmycin, Polycycline, Tetradecin. 2. any of a group of natural or semisynthetic antibiotics isolated from various species of *Streptomyces*, which are related to tetracycline (see def. 1), and derived from polycyclic naphthacenecarboxamide. Tetracyclines are broad-spectrum antibiotics which inhibit protein synthesis by their action on microbial ribosomes, all having similar toxic and pharmacological properties, differing mainly in their absorption and suitability for various modes of administration. Used in infectious diseases caused by rickettsiae, chlamydiae, and mycoplasmas, *Escherichia coli, Enterobacter, Nocardia, Pasteurella, Leptospira, Actinomyces*, staphylococci, streptococci, and other gram-positive and gram-negative bacteria. Adverse reactions may include hypersensitivity, burning of the eyes, brown or black coating of the tongue, cheilosis, atrophic or hypertrophic glossitis, discoloration of the teeth, pruritus ani and/or vaginae, gastrointestinal disorders, thrombophlebitis, leukocytosis, atypical lymphocytes, thrombopenic purpura, discoloration of nails and onycholysis, phototoxicity, and liver and kidney disorders. **t. hydrochloride,** the hydrochloride salt of tetracycline, occurring as a yellow, odorless, moderately hygroscopic, crystalline powder that darkens on exposure to sunlight and humid air, and is soluble in water and alkali hydroxide and carbonate solutions, is slightly soluble in alcohol, and is insoluble in chloroform and ether. Its pharmacological and toxic properties are similar to those of other tetracyclines. It is also used in the treatment of malaria. Trademarks: Achro, Achromycin, Chromycin V, Diacycline, Dumacyclin, Quatrex, Ricycline, Tetracyn, Tetrosol, Unimycin. **natural t's,** tetracyclines obtained from unmodified cultures of *Streptomyces*. **t. phosphate complex,** a phosphate complex salt of tetracycline, occurring as an odorless, yellow, crystalline powder that is sparingly soluble in water and slightly soluble in ethanol. Its toxic and pharmacological properties are similar to those of other tetracyclines. Trademarks: Sumycin, Tetradecin Novum, Tetrex, Upcyclin. **semisynthetic t's,** tetracyclines elaborated by cultures of various species of *Streptomyces*, to which substances other than culture media components have been added.

Tetracyn trademark for *tetracycline hydrochloride* (see under TETRACYCLINE).

tetrad (tet′rad) 1. a group of four similar or related entities. 2. a group of four chromosomal elements formed in meiosis. 3. a square cell produced by the division into two planes of certain cocci. 4. an atom or group of atoms having the valency of four. 5. a crystal showing four similar faces when rotated 360° about its axis.

Tetradecin trademark for tetracycline (1).

Tetradecin Novum trademark for *tetracycline phosphate complex* (see under TETRACYCLINE).

tetraethoxysilane (tet″rah-eth-ok′sī-lān) ethyl ORTHOSILICATE.

tetraethylammonium (tet″rah-eth″il-ah-mo′ne-um) an antihypertensive drug, *N,N,N*-triethylethanaminium; it is the prototype of ganglionic blocking agents. Abbreviated *TEA*. **t. bromide,** the bromide salt of tetraethylammonium, occurring as deliquescent crystals that are soluble in water, ethanol, chloroform, and acetone and slightly soluble in benzene. It is a ganglionic blocking agent used in the diagnosis and therapy of peripheral vascular disorders. In most types of hypertension it produces a fall in blood pressure, but produces hypertension in the presence of pheochromocytoma. Abbreviated *TEAB*. Trademarks: Etylon, Etambro, Tetranium.

tetraethylpyrophosphate (tet″rah-eth″il-pi″ro-fos′fāt) tetraethyl PYROPHOSPHATE.

tetraethylthiuram disulfide (tet″rah-eth″il-thi′u-ram) disulfiram.

tetraethyoxysilane (tet″rah-eth-e-ok″se-sil′ān) ethyl ORTHOSILICATE.

tetrafluoroethylene (tet″rah-floo″or-o-eth′i-lēn) a substance, $F_2D=CF_2$, occurring as a heavy, colorless gas; used as a monomer which, on polymerization, produces Teflon (polytetrafluoroethylene). Called also *perfluoroethylene*. **t. polymer,** polytetrafluoroethylene.

tetragonum (tet″rah-go′num) [Gr. *tetragonon*] a square or quadrant; a quadrangular area or space.

tetrahedron (te″tra-he′dron) 1. a solid contained by four plane faces; a triangular pyramid. 2. a hypothetical pyramidal structure in the isometric system, such as the basic silicate (SiO_4) structure having a base of four oxygen anions in coordination with a silicon ion located at the central interstitial position. Called also *tetrahedral structure*.

tetrahydrate (tet″rah-hi′drāt) a hydrate containing four molecules of water for every molecule of the other substance in the compound.

tetrahydrocannabinol (tet″rah-hi″dro-kah-nab′i-nol) the active principle of marihuana, tetrahydro-6,6,9-trimethyl-3-pentyl-6*H*-dibenzo[*b,d*]pyran-1-ol, occurring in two isomeric forms: Δ¹-3,4-*trans*- and Δ⁶-3,4-*trans*-. Abbreviated *Thc*.

l-Δ⁹-**tetrahydrocannabinol** (tet″rah-hi″dro-kah-nab′i-nol) a substance believed to be the active component of cannabinoids. Abbreviated Δ⁹-*THC*.

tetrahydroxybutane (tet″rah-hi-drok″se-bu′tān) erythritol.

tetrahydrozoline hydrochloride (tet″rah-hi-dro′zo-lēn) sympathomimetic agent, 2-(1,2,3,4-tetrahydro-naphthyl)-2-imidazoline monohydrochloride, occurring as a white, odorless solid that is soluble in water and ethanol, slightly soluble in chloroform, and insoluble in ether. Used as a local vasoconstrictor and nasal decongestant. Adverse reactions may include dryness and burning of the mucous membranes, sneezing, headache, drowsiness, insomnia, tremor, tachycardia, weakness, cardiac arrhythmias, excessive sweating, respiratory depression, and shock. Prolonged use may produce rhinitis. Trademarks: Tyzine, Visine.

tetrakis- in chemical nomenclature, a prefix indicating the presence of four chelate or complicated similar ligands in a coordination compound. See also TETRA-.

Tetramel trademark for *oxytetracycline*.

tetramethylammonium (tet″-rah-meth″il-ah-mo′ne-um) a compound, *N,N,N*,-trimethylmethanaminium hydroxide, occurring as a corrosive liquid readily absorbing CO_2 from air.

tetranitrol (tet″rah-ni′trōl) ERYTHRITYL tetranitrate.

Tetranium trademark for *tetraethylammonium bromide* (see under TETRAETHYLAMMONIUM).

tetrapeptide (tet″rah-pep′tīd) [*tetra-* + *peptide*] a polypeptide which, on hydrolysis, yields four amino acids.

tetraploid (tet′rah-ploid) [Gr. *tetra* four + *-ploid*] 1. pertaining to or characterized by tetraploidy. 2. an individual or cell having four sets of chromosomes.

tetraploidy (tet′rah-ploi′de) [Gr. *tetra* four + *ploidy*] the presence of four sets of chromosomes.

tetrasomy (tet′rah-so″me) [*tetra-* + Gr. *sōma* body] the presence of two additional chromosomes of one type in an otherwise diploid cell. **9p t.,** tetrasomy of the short arm of chromosome 9, associated with multiple abnormalities, including hydrocephaly, enlarged heart, kidney hypoplasia, hemivertebrae, camptodactyly, thrombocytopenia, myopia, pseudoarthrosis, hand and foot deformities, cleft lip, cleft palate, and other defects. Called also *9p tetrasomy syndrome*.

Tetraverin trademark for *rolitetracycline*.

Tetrex trademark for *tetracycline phosphate complex* (see under TETRACYCLINE).

Tetrim trademark for *rolitetracycline nitrate* (see under ROLITETRACYCLINE).

Tetriv trademark for *rolitetracycline nitrate* (see under ROLI-TETRACYCLINE).

tetrole (tet'rōl) furan.

Tetron trademark for *tetraethyl pyrophosphate* (see under PYROPHOSPHATE).

Tetrosan trademark for *dichlorobenzalkonium chloride* (see under DICHLOROBENZALKONIUM).

tetrose (tet'rōs) a monosaccharide containing four carbon atoms in a molecule, $C_4H_8O_4$.

Tetrosol trademark for *tetracycline hydrochloride* (see under TETRACYCLINE).

Textor's operation see under OPERATION.

TG thioguanine.

Th thorium.

thalamus (thal'ah-mus), pl. *thal'ami* [L.; Gr. *thalamos* inner chamber] [NA] the middle part of the diencephalon, situated deep in the cerebral hemispheres beneath the cortex. It consists chiefly of the gray substance, having a thin layer of white matter on its upper surface, and serves to relay body sensations and to integrate these sensations on their way to the cortex.

thalassemia (thal"ah-se'me-ah) [Gr. *thalassa* sea (because it was originally observed in persons of Mediterranean stock) + *haima* blood + *-ia*] a group of heterogeneous hereditary disorders, manifested in the homozygote by severe anemia or death in utero, and in the heterozygote by relatively mild red cell anomalies. The two major categories are: α-thalassemia and β-thalassemia. **α-t.**, that caused by decreased rate of synthesis of the alpha chains of hemoglobin. **β-t.**, that caused by decreased rate of synthesis of the beta chains of hemoglobin. The homozygous form is *Cooley's anemia*, and the heterozygous form is *thalassemia minor*. **t. C**, thalassemia–hemoglobin C DISEASE. **t.–hemoglobin C d.**, see under DISEASE. **t. ma'jor**, Cooley's ANEMIA. **t. mi'nor**, the heterozygous form of β-thalassemia, most frequently seen in persons of Mediterranean extraction, but also affecting those of other ancestry. It is usually asymptomatic, with mild or no anemia, but with prominent morphologic abnormalities of the erythrocytes, such as microcytosis, hypochromia, stippling, and target cells. Rarely, there is anemia of moderate severity associated with jaundice and splenomegaly. Called also *familial hemolytic hypochromic anemia, familial microcytic anemia, hypochromic familial hemolytic anemia,* and *Rietti-Greppi-Micheli syndrome.* Cf. Cooley's ANEMIA.

thalidomide (thah-lid'o-mīd) a sedative and hypnotic, 2-(2,6-dioxo-3-piperidinyl)-1*H*-isoindole-1,3-(2*H*)-dione. Used commonly in Europe in the late 1950's and early 1960's, its use was discontinued when it was discovered to be the cause of congenital anomalies in the fetus, nobably amelia and phocomelia, when taken by a woman during early pregnancy.

thallium (thal'e-um) [Gr. *thallos* a green shoot or twig (named for its green spectral line)] a metallic element. Symbol, Tl; atomic number, 81; atomic weight, 204.37; specific gravity, 11.85; melting point, 302° C; Brinnel hardness number, 2; valences, 1, 3; group IIIA of the periodic table. It has two natural isotopes (203, 205) and numerous artificial radioactive ones (191–202, 204, 206–210). Thallium is a bluish white soft, inelastic, heavy metal, which is easily fusible, oxidizes superficially on exposure to air, is soluble in nitric and sulfuric acids, but not in water, and forms alloys with other metals, particularly with mercury. It is highly toxic and ingestion or inhalation may cause acute symptoms including vomiting, nausea, diarrhea, polyneuritis, convulsions, coma, and death. Chronic exposure to small doses may cause alopecia, weakness, and polyneuritis.

THAM trademark for *tromethamine*.

Tham-E trademark for *tromethamine*.

Thayer-Doisy unit see under UNIT.

THC tetrahydrocannabinol.

Δ⁹-THC *l*Δ⁹-tetrahydrocannabinol.

Theal trademark for *theophylline*.

thebaine (the-ba'in) an opium alkaloid, 6,7,8,14-tetradehydro-4,5 α-epoxy-3,6-dimethoxy-17-methylmorphinan, occurring as a white crystalline powder that is soluble in water, alcohol, and ether. Unlike other opiates, it is devoid of analgesic action and produces seizures at a relatively low dosage. Called also *paramorphine.*

theca (the'kah), pl. *the'cae* [L.; Gr. *thēkē*] a structure enclosing or surrounding an organ or part. See also SHEATH and VAGINA.

thecae (the'se) [L.] plural of *theca.*

Thecodine trademark for *oxycodone hydrochloride* (see under OXYCODONE).

thecodont (the'ko-dont) [Gr. *thēkē* sheath + *odous* tooth] having the teeth inserted in sockets or alveoli.

Theileria tsutsugamushi (thi-le're-ah soot"soo-gah-moosh'e) *Rickettsia tsutsugamushi;* see under RICKETTSIA.

theine (the'in) an alkaloid of tea leaves, isomeric with caffeine.

thelium (the'le-um), pl. *the'lia* [L.] nipple.

Themison of Laodicea (1st century B.C.) a Greek physician who founded the Methodist school of medicine.

Thenylene trademark for *methapyrilene hydrochloride* (see under METHAPYRILENE).

Thenylpyramine trademark for *methapyrilene hydrochloride* (see under METHAPYRILENE).

Theobald Smith phenomenon [*Theobald Smith*, American pathologist, 1859–1934] see under PHENOMENON.

Theobroma (the"o-bro'mah) [Gr. *theos* god + *broma* food] a genus of sterculiaceous plants; the cacao. See theobroma OIL.

theobromine (the"o-bro'mēn) a xanthine derivative, 3,7-dimethylxanthine, which is an alkaloid of cacao beans and leaves (*Theobroma* spp.), also present in cola nuts and in tea, and is soluble in water, alcohol, and alkali hydroxide. Theobromine is a central stimulant and its pharmacological effects include stimulation of the central nervous system, action on the kidneys resulting in diuresis, stimulation of the cardiac muscle, and relaxation of the smooth muscles. It may counteract the action of sedatives. **methyl t.**, caffeine.

theocin (the'o-sin) theophylline.

Theolix trademark for *theophylline*.

theophylline (the"o-fil'in) [L. *thea* tea + Gr. *phyllon* leaf] a xanthine derivative, 1,3-dimethylxanthine, occurring as a bitter, odorless, white, crystalline alkaloid derived from tea leaves, and synthesized from ethyl cyanoacetate. It is soluble in water, alcohol, and alkaline solutions. Theophylline is a central stimulant and its pharmacological effects include stimulation of the central nervous system, action on the kidneys resulting in diuresis, stimulation of the cardiac muscle, and relaxation of the smooth muscles. Theophylline preparations, usually aminophylline, are used to relax bronchial smooth muscle and to stimulate the myocardium. Used for its bronchodilating, respiratory-stimulating, and hemodynamic actions in the treatment of bronchial asthma and other respiratory disorders. Toxic reactions may include headache, arrhythmia, tinnitus, nausea, hypotension, precordial pain, thirst, convulsions, and vomiting. It may counteract the action of sedatives. Called also *theocin.* Trademarks: Theal, Theolix. **t. cholinate**, oxtriphylline. **t. ethylenediamine**, aminophylline.

theory (the'o-re) [Gr. *theōria* speculation as opposed to practice] 1. the doctrine or the principles underlying an art as distinguished from the practice of that particular art. 2. a formulated hypothesis, or, loosely speaking, any hypothesis or opinion not based upon actual knowledge. **acidogenic t.**, a hypothesis stating that dental caries is a chemicoparasitic process consisting of two stages: the decalcification of enamel, which results in its total destruction and the decalcification of dentin, as a preliminary stage, followed by dissolution of the softened residue. The acid which affects its primary decalcification is derived from the fermentation of starches and sugars lodged in the retaining centers of the teeth. Called also *chemicoparasitic t.* and *Miller's t.* **Begg's t.**, a theory that a light differential force may be used effectively for tooth movement in orthodontic therapy. Called also *Begg's philosophy.* See Begg's TECHNIQUE. **brunonian t.**, brunonianism. **cell t.**, cells are potentially independent organisms and plants and animals are aggregations of these living units arranged according to definite laws. **cellular t. of immunity**, Metchnikoff's t. **chemicoparasitic t.**, acidogenic t. **clonal-selection t. of immunity**, a selective theory of antibody formation, according to which a complement of clones of lymphoid cells capable of reacting with all possible antigenic determinants is present in the normal individual. During fetal life, those clones that react against self-antigens are suppressed on contact with antigen. By contrast, there occurs a change in the response to contact with antigen following maturation of the immune system, when the normal reponse is proliferation, antibody formation, and cell-mediated immunity. Thus, suppression of clones leads to the development of immunological tolerance. If suppressed clones against self-antigens again become active at some time later in life, autoimmune disease may result. **Dalton's atomic t.**, the atom may be considered the smallest unit of an element that can take part in a chemical change and, in chemical changes, the atoms can combine to form small units of compounds, or they can separate or change places in these compounds. Each small unit of a compound contains a definite number of atoms. **Darwin's t.**, **darwian t.**, darwinism. **dimer t.**, the theory that the tooth organ of primates is composed of two halves, each of which is representative of an independent tooth in the lower orders or animals. **Ehrlich's biochemical t.**, the theory that specific chemical affinity exists between the substance of specific living cells and specific chemical substances. **Ehrlich's side-chain t.**, a theory advanced regarding the phenomena concerned in immunity and cytolysis. According to this theory, the protoplasm of the body cells contains highly complex organic molecules, consisting of a tolerably stable central group, to which are attached less stable lateral chains (or side chains) of atoms or atomic groups. The ordinary chemical transformations in the protoplasm are carried on by means of these lateral chains (or *receptors*), the stable center of the molecule remaining unaffected. The lateral chains contain a group of atoms (see HAPTOPHORE), which is capable of uniting with similar groups in toxins, bacterial cells, and foreign cells. **germ-line t.**, a selective theory of antibody formation, which suggests that there are separate genes coding for each type antibody specificity and that the entire collection of genes required for all antibodies is present in each potential antibody-forming cell. It is based on the principle that the population of antibody-forming cells in endowed with a finite number of randomly distributed specific receptor molecules (natural antibodies) that raise spontaneously in the absence of antigens and are released from individual cells; antigen selects these specific receptors, thereby initiating antibody formation (natural selection). See also *clonal selection t.* **hit t.**, target t. **humoral t.**, an ancient theory that the body contains four humors — blood, phlegm, yellow bile, and black bile — health being the result of their proper adjustment, and disease resulting from their imbalance. **Lewis t.**, a chemical bond is polar when an electron passes from one atom to another; nonpolar when two atoms share a pair of electrons equally. **Metchnikoff's t., Mechnikov's t.**, the theory that bacteria and other harmful elements in the body are attached and destroyed by cells called phagocytes, and that the contest between such harmful elements and the phagocytes produces inflammation. Called also *cellular t. of immunity.* **Miller's t.**, acidogenic t. **occupation t.**, only when the receptor is actually occupied by the drug is its function transformed in such a way as to elicit response. See also drug RECEPTOR. **orbital t.**, electrons represent three-dimensional waves that can exist at several levels in relation to the nucleus of an atom and at several energy levels, the level closest to the nucleus having the lower energy level. The electrons are described in terms of probability as cloudlike forms with indefinite boundaries (electron orbital). See also Bohr ATOM, electron ORBIT, and quantum NUMBER. **Planck's t.**, quantum t. **proteolysis-chelation t.**, a hypothesis stating that dental caries is essentially a proteolytic process, whereby keratinolytic microorganisms break down the protein and other organic components of the enamel, thus producing substances which may form soluble chelates with the mineralized components of the tooth and thereby decalcifying the enamel. **proteolytic t.**, a hypothesis stating that dental caries is essentially a proteolytic process: the microorganisms invade the organic pathways of enamel and destroy them through proteolytic processes. **quantum t.**, the theory that the radiation and absorption of energy take place in definite quantities called quanta (E) which vary in size and are defined by the equation $E = h\nu$, in which h is Planck's constant and ν the frequency of the radiation. Called also *Planck's t.* **ratchet t.**, a theory that cross-bridges provide the ratchet mechanism to muscle contraction. At rest, the negative charges of ATP are bound to the cross-bridges of both the myosin and actin filaments, causing the filaments to be repelled from each other. But in the presence of calcium, the negative sites of ATP are bound by the positive calcium ions and the electric field of cross-bridges is thus reversed, causing the filaments to be attracted by the opposite charges and to bind together. Also, while at rest, the repulsion of two negative charges makes the cross-bridges project outwardly away from the myosin filaments, but the subsequent binding of ATP by calcium ions forces the bridges to bend inwardly toward the filaments, sliding the actin filaments alongside the myosin filaments, reducing the size of the sarcomere, and producing muscle contraction. Folding of cross-bridges toward the myosin allows the ATPase activity of myosin to split ATP to ADP, thus breaking the calcium-linked connections between the myosin cross-bridges and the actin. The process is repeated by other groups of cross-bridges, thus a recurrent series of binding, pulling, and separating processes provides the ratchet mechanism for muscle contraction as the actin filaments are pulled past the myosin ones. **sliding filament t.**, see muscle CONTRACTION. **target t.**, the theory advanced to explain some biological effects of radiation on the basis of ionization occurring in a very small sensitive region within the cell, which postulates that one or more ionizing events, or "hits," within the sensitive volume are necessary to bring about the biological end-effect. Called also *hit t.* **template t.**, a theory of antibody formation, whereby antigen directs the formation of antibodies from its precursor molecules by acting as a template which determines the shape and future reactivity of the combining site of the antibody produced by that cell. An *indirect* template theory suggests that antibody specificity is influenced indirectly through the action of antigen on DNA, implying an alteration in the sequence of events in protein synthesis from the usual DNA → RNA → protein, also implying that the antigen can function as a mutagen. In light of current knowledge, this theory has been abandoned. **Woods-Fildes t.**, the theory that the antibacterial activity of some drugs, such as sulfonamides, is due to their competitive inhibitor property, whereby they bear a close structural resemblance to one required for normal physiological functioning and exert their antibacterial effects by interfering with the utilization by bacteria of essential metabolites. See also ANTIMETABOLITE.

Thephorin trademark for *phenindamine.*

Thera-Combex H-P Kapseals trademark for a mixture of vitamins, one tablet of which contains 500 mg ascorbic acid, 100 mg niacinamide, 25 mg thiamine mononitrate, 15 mg riboflavin, 20 mg *dl*-pantothenyl alcohol, 10 mg pyridoxine hydrochloride, and 5 mcg cyanocobalamin.

therapeutic (ther″ah-pu′tik) [Gr. *therapeutikos* inclined to serve] 1. pertaining to therapeutics, or to the art of healing. 2. curative. 3. a term sometimes used to designate a therapeutic agent or drug. **accepted dental t.**, a therapeutic agent which has been evaluated by the Council on Dental Therapeutics of the American Dental Association and for which there is adequate evidence for safety and effectiveness. The accepted agents are described in the *Journal of the American Dental Association* and listed in the *Accepted Dental Therapeutics* (also published by the ADA). The Seal of Acceptance or an authorized statement to that effect may be used in connection with all accepted dental therapeutics. **provisionally accepted dental t.**, a therapeutic agent which has been evaluated by the Council on Dental Therapeutics of the American Dental Association and for which there is reasonable evidence of usefulness and safety, but which lacks sufficient evidence of dental usefulness to justify being accepted. **unaccepted dental t.**, a therapeutic agent which has been evaluated by the Council on Dental Therapeutics of the American Dental Association and for which no substantial evidence of usefulness or for which a question of safety exists.

therapeutics (ther″ah-pu′tiks) 1. the science and art of healing. 2. that branch of medicine which deals with the treatment of disease.

therapist (ther′ah-pist) [Gr. *therapeutēs* one who attends to the sick] one who is skilled in the treatment of disease.

therapy (ther′ah-pe) [Gr. *therapeia* service done to the sick] the treatment of disease. **cold t.**, cryotherapy. **Curie t.**, curietherapy. **endodontic t.**, see *root canal t.* and ENDODONTICS. **enteral t.**, enteral HYPERALIMENTATION. **grid t.**, therapeutic application of ionizing radiations through a metal grid having a pattern of small, evenly spaced perforations. **immunosuppressive t.**, treatment with agents, such as x-rays, corticosteroids, and cytotoxic drugs, which suppress the immune response to antigens; it is used in various conditions, including autoimmune diseases, allergy, multiple myeloma, chronic nephritis, and in organ and tissue transplantation. **inhalation t.**, the use of oxygen, helium-oxygen, and carbon dioxide mixtures in the treatment of some diseases, particularly those involving faulty gas exchange in the cardiopulmonary system. **intraosseous t.**, the infusion of blood or other solutions into the circulation by injection through the bone marrow. **intravenous t.**, the introduction of solutions of therapeutic substances directly into the venous circulation. **myofunctional t.**, training of the orofacial musculature, including modification of habits, in edentulous conditions, malocclusion, or temporomandibular joint disorders. **nonspecific t.**, treatment of infectious diseases by the injection of nonspecific substances, such as immunoglobulins, vaccines, and other therapeutic agents that act on a broad range of pathogenic agents, rather than specifically on the pathogen responsible for the disease from which the patient is suffering. **parenteral hyperalimentation t.**, parenteral HYPERALIMENTATION. **physical t.**, the treatment of disease by physical agents and methods to assist in rehabilitation and restoration of normal bodily functions after illness or injury, including the use of massage and manipulation, exercise, hydrotherapy, and various forms of energy, such as heat or ultrasonics. Called also *physiotherapy.* **pulp canal t.**, root canal t. **radiation t.**, radio-

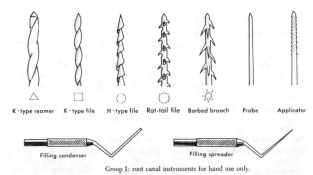

K-type reamer　K-type file　H-type file　Rat-tail file　Barbed broach　Probe　Applicator

Filling condenser　　　　　　　　Filling spreader

Group I: root canal instruments for hand use only.

Group I: root canal instruments for hand use only. (From M. A. Heuer: Instruments and materials. *In* S. Cohen and R. C. Burns (eds.): Pathways of the Pulp. 2nd ed. St. Louis, The C. V. Mosby Co., 1980.)

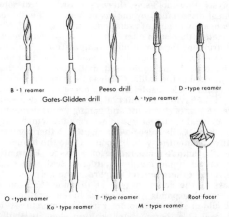

K-type reamer　K-type file　H-type file　Rat-tail file　B-2 reamer　Quarter-turn reamer　Lentulo

Group II: engine-driven root canal instruments, two-part shaft and operative head. (From M. A. Heuer: Instruments and materials. *In* S. Cohen and R. C. Burns (eds.): Pathways of the Pulp. 2nd ed. St. Louis, The C. V. Mosby Co., 1980.)

B-1 reamer　　Peeso drill　　D-type reamer
Gates-Glidden drill　　A-type reamer

O-type reamer　　T-type reamer　　Root facer
Ko-type reamer　　M-type reamer

Group III: engine-driven root canal instruments, one-part shaft and operative head. (From M. A. Heuer: Instruments and materials. *In* S. Cohen and R. C. Burns (eds.): Pathways of the Pulp. 2nd ed. St. Louis, The C. V. Mosby Co., 1980.)

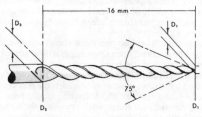

Terminology

Diameters $\{$ = D_1 expressed in hundredths of a mm
　　　　　D_2 = D_1 plus 0.32 mm
Taper　　　　= 0.02 mm per mm
Tip angle　　= 75° · 15° included angle
Tolerance　　= · 0.02 mm
Length blade (D_1 to D_2) = 16.0 mm

Standardized K-type root canal instruments of Group I. (From M. A. Heuer: Instruments and materials. *In* S. Cohen and R. C. Burns (eds.): Pathways of the Pulp. 2nd ed. St. Louis, The C. V. Mosby Co., 1980.)

therapy. **replacement t.,** treatment to replace deficient formation or loss of body products by administration of the natural body products or synthetic substitutes. See also *substitution t.* **roentgen t., deep,** high-voltage roentgen therapy capable of penetrating significantly below the skin level, while sparing the skin and superficial tissues from radiation damage. Called also *deep x-ray t.* **roentgen t., high voltage,** treatment by deeply penetrating x-rays generated by voltage over 300 kilovolts. **root canal t.,** that aspect of endodontics dealing with the treatment of diseases of the dental pulp. It consists of partial (pulpotomy) or complete (pulpectomy) extirpation of the diseased pulp, depending on the pathological changes of the pulp; cleaning and sterilization of the empty canal; enlarging and shaping the canal to receive sealing material; and obturation of the canal with a nonirritating hermetic sealing agent. The instruments used in root canal therapy have been grouped as follows: *Group I,* hand-operated instruments, including K- and H-type files, K-type reamers, rat-tail files, barbed broaches, probes, applicators, and filling condensers and spreaders; *Group II,* engine-driven instruments, with a two-part shaft and operative head, instruments used with a straight handpiece, a contra-angle handpiece, the operative heads being identical with the files, reamers, rasps, or barbed broaches of Group I, or with specially designed instruments, such as a quarter-turn reamer or a lentulo; *Group III,* engine-driven instruments with a one-part shaft and operative head, including the B-1 reamer, Gates-Glidden and Peeso drills, A-, D-, O-, Ko-, T-, and M-type reamers, and root canal facer; and *Group IV,* root canal points, including absorbent and filling points. The K-type instruments of Group I have a standard cutting length and taper and a color code has been provided for identification of different types of instruments. The most commonly used instruments also may be identified by a symbol code. See illustrations and table. See

TERMINOLOGY AND COLOR CODING OF ROOT CANAL INSTRUMENTS*

| Size | Diameter of instrument | | Color | Abbreviation |
	D_1 (mm)	D_2 (mm)		
10	0.10	0.42	Purple	Pur
15	0.15	0.47	White	Wh
20	0.20	0.52	Yellow	Yel
25	0.25	0.57	Red	Red
30	0.30	0.62	Blue	Blu
35	0.35	0.67	Green	Grn
40	0.40	0.72	Black	Blk
45	0.45	0.77	White	Wh
50	0.50	0.82	Yellow	Yel
55	0.55	0.87	Red	Red
60	0.60	0.92	Blue	Blu
70	0.70	1.02	Green	Grn
80	0.80	1.12	Black	Blk
90	0.90	1.22	White	Wh
100	1.00	1.32	Yellow	Yel
110	1.10	1.42	Red	Red
120	1.20	1.52	Blue	Blu
130	1.30	1.62	Green	Grn
140	1.40	1.72	Black	Blk
150	1.50	1.82	White	Wh

*Applies to K-type instruments only.

(From S. Cohen and R. C. Burns: Pathways of the Pulp. 2nd ed. St. Louis, The C. V. Mosby Co., 1980.)

also root canal filling methods, under METHOD. **rotation t.,** in radiotherapy, circular movement of the patient or of the radiation source and beam around a fixed anatomical axis during a treatment exposure. **speech t.,** the use of special techniques for correction of speech and language disorders. **substitution t.,** the administration of a hormone to compensate for deficiency of the gland producing the lacking hormone. See also *replacement t.* **x-ray t., deep,** roentgen t., deep.

therm (therm) [Gr. *thermē* heat] a unit of heat. The word has been used as an equivalent to (a) large calorie; (b) small calorie; (c) 1000 large calories; (d) 100,000 British thermal units (BTU).

therm- see THERMO-.

thermal (ther'mal) pertaining to or characterized by heat, thermic.

thermalgesia (ther″mal-je′ze-ah) [*therm-* + Gr. *algēsis* pain + *-ia*] a condition in which the application of heat produces pain.

thermalgia (ther-mal′je-ah) [*therm-* + Gr. *algos* pain + *-ia*] a condition marked by sensations of intense burning pain. See also CAUSALGIA and GLOSSOPYRA.

thermanalgesia (therm″an-al-je′se-ah) absence of pain on application of heat.

thermanesthesia (therm″an-es-the′ze-ah) [*therm-* + *an* neg + Gr. *aisthēsis* perception + *-ia*] inability to perceive heat (or cold); absence of the sense of heat.

thermesthesia (therm″es-the′ze-ah) [*therm-* + Gr. *aisthēsis* perception + *-ia*] ability to recognize heat and cold; the temperature sense.

thermesthesiometer (therm″es-the″ze-om′e-ter) an instrument for measuring sensibility to varying temperatures, consisting of a metal disk with a thermometer attached for indicating its temperature. It can be used to measure the sensitivity of teeth at various temperatures.

thermhyperesthesia (therm″hi-per-es-the′ze-ah) [*therm-* + Gr. *hyper* above + *aisthēsis* perception + *-ia*] abnormally increased sensitivity to heat.

thermhypesthesia (therm″hi-pes-the′ze-ah) [*therm-* + Gr. *hypo* under + *aisthēsis* perception + *-ia*] abnormally decreased sensitivity to heat.

thermic (ther′mik) of or pertaining to heat; thermal.

thermion (ther′me-on) a particle containing an electric charge emitted by an incandescent substance, such as the electrons emitted from the cathode in an x-ray tube.

thermistor (ther-mis′tor) a thermometer whose impedance varies with the ambient temperature and so is able to measure extremely small changes in temperature.

thermo-, therm- [Gr. *thermē* heat] a combining form denoting relationship to heat.

thermocautery (ther″mo-kaw′ter-e) cauterization by means of a hot wire or point.

thermochemistry (ther″mo-kem′is-tre) the aspect of physical chemistry dealing with heat changes that accompany chemical reactions.

thermochroic (ther″mo-kro′ik) [*thermo-* + Gr. *chroa* color] reflecting some of the heat rays and absorbing or transmitting others.

thermocoagulation (ther″mo-ko-ag″u-la′shun) coagulation of tissue by the action of high frequency currents; used for surgical purposes.

thermocouple (ther″mo-kup″l) a device for measuring high temperatures, based on the electromotive force generated between two dissimilar metals when their junctions are held at different temperatures. One (hot) junction is placed in the furnace or heat source and the other (cold) junction is formed through the pyrometer at room temperature. For a temperature of less than 1093° C (2000° F), alloys of chromium and aluminum are often used; platinum or platinum-rhodium wires are used for higher temperatures. See illustration.

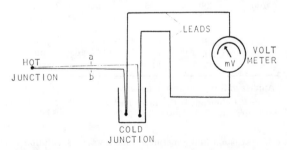

Thermocouple. (From E. H. Greener, J. K. Harcourt, and E. P. Lautenschlager: Materials Science in Dentistry. Elmsford, New York, Pergamon Press, 1972.)

Thermodent see under DENTIFRICE.

thermodiffusion (ther″mo-dĭ-fu′zhun) diffusion under the influence of a temperature gradient.

thermoduric (ther″mo-du′rik) [*thermo-* + L. *durus* enduring] capable of withstanding high temperature.

thermodynamics (ther″mo-di-nam′iks) [*thermo-* + Gr. *dynamis* power] the study of the relations between heat and energy. **equilibrium t.**, that which is concerned with the application of the laws of thermodynamics to systems in equilibrium states, or undergoing transformation between two equilibrium states. **laws of t.**, see under LAW. **nonequilibrium t.**, that which deals with steady states and irreversible processes.

thermoelectricity (ther″mo-e″lek-tris′ĭ-te) electricity generated by heat.

thermogenesis (ther″mo-jen′ĕ-sis) [*thermo-* + Gr. *genesis* production] the production of heat, especially within the animal body.

thermogenic (ther″mo-jen′ik) producing heat.

thermogenics (ther″mo-jen′iks) the science relating to heat production.

thermography (ther-mog′rah-fe) [*thermo-* + Gr. *graphein* to write] a technique wherein an infrared camera is used to photographically portray the surface temperature of the body, based on the self-emanating infrared radiation; sometimes used as a means of diagnosing underlying pathologic processes.

thermohyperalgesia (ther″mo-hi″per-al-je′ze-ah) [*thermo-* + Gr. *hyper* above + *algēsis* pain + *-ia*] a condition in which the application of moderate heat produces severe pain.

thermohyperesthesia (ther″mo-hi″per-es-the′ze-ah) [*thermo-* + Gr. *hyper* over + *aisthēsis* perception + *-ia*] extreme sensitiveness to heat.

thermohypesthesia (ther″mo-hi″pes-the′ze-ah) [*thermo-* + Gr. *hypo* under + *aisthēsis* perception + *-ia*] abnormally diminished sensitivity to heat.

thermoinactivation (ther″mo-in-ak″tĭ-va′shun) destruction of the power to act by exposure to heat.

thermoinhibitory (ther″mo-in-hib′ĭ-tor″e) inhibiting or retarding the production of body heat.

thermolabile (ther″mo-la′bil) easily altered or decomposed by heat; heat labile.

thermoluminescence (ther″mo-lu-mĭ-nes′ens) the property of certain crystalline compounds, e.g., lithium fluoride, to release stored energy as visible light when heated; used in dosimetry.

thermolysis (ther-mol′ĭ-sis) [*thermo-* + Gr. *lysis* dissolution] 1. chemical dissociation by means of heat. 2. the dissipation of bodily heat by means of radiation, evaporation, etc.

thermometer (ther-mom′ĕ-ter) [*thermo-* + Gr. *metron* measure] an instrument for determining temperatures. See also SCALE and TEMPERATURE. **alcohol t.**, a liquid-in-glass thermometer in which alcohol is the liquid used. **axilla t.**, a surface thermometer to be used in the axilla. **Celsius t.**, a thermometer employing the Celsius scale. **centigrade t.**, one employing the Celsius scale, i.e., having the interval between the two established reference points (ice point and boiling point) divided into 100 units. **clinical t.**, one for use in determining temperature of the human body. Called also *fever t.* **depth t.**, a thermometer whose sensitive element may be introduced into the tissue, for registering the actual temperature of a tissue. **Fahrenheit t.**, a thermometer employing the Fahrenheit scale. **fever t.**, clinical t. **Kelvin t.**, a thermometer employing the Kelvin scale. **liquid-in-glass t.**, the common type of thermometer, containing a liquid which expands with increase in temperature. **mercurial t.**, a liquid-in-glass thermometer in which mercury is the liquid used. **oral t.**, a thermometer with an elongated bulb for the mercury, usually employing the Celsius or Fahrenheit scale, which is placed under the tongue to measure body temperature. See also body TEMPERATURE, for comparative values. **Rankine t.**, a thermometer employing the Rankine scale. **rectal t.**, a thermometer with a pear-shaped bulb, usually employing the Celsius or Fahrenheit scale, which is inserted into the rectum to measure body temperature. See also body TEMPERATURE, for comparative values.

thermopenetration (ther″mo-pen″ĕ-tra′shun) application of currents of low tension and high amperage, which produce warmth in the deeper parts of the body.

thermophile (ther′mo-fil) [*thermo-* + Gr. *philein* to love] an organism which grows best at elevated temperatures.

thermoplastic (ther″mo-plas′tik) softening under heat and capable of being molded into shape with pressure, then hardening on cooling without undergoing chemical change, as in a thermoplastic resin.

thermoprecipitation (ther″mo-pre-sip′ĭ-ta′shun) precipitation by heat.

thermoreceptor (ther″mo-re-sep′tor) a sensory receptor (see receptor [6]) that detects changes in temperature, some detecting cold and others, warmth. Thermoreceptors are located in the skin and in the hypothalamus. Called also *temperature receptor.*

thermoresistance (ther″mo-re-zis′tans) the quality of being resistant to heat.

thermoresistant (ther″mo-re-zis′tant) resistant or not greatly affected by heat; heat resistant.

thermosetting (ther′mo-set′ing) rendered hard by heat. See thermosetting RESIN.

thermostabile (ther″mo-sta′bil) unaffected by heat; able to withstand the effects of heat without undergoing change; heat stabile.

thermostasis (ther″mo-sta′sis) [thermo- + Gr. stasis a placing, setting] the maintenance of body temperature in warm-blooded animals.

thermostat (ther′mo-stat) [thermo- + Gr. histanai to halt] a device interposed in a heating system by which the temperature can be automatically maintained at certain levels.

thermosteresis (ther″mo-ste-re′sis) [thermo- + Gr. sterēsis deprivation] the deprivation of heat.

thermotaxis (ther″mo-tak′sis) [thermo- + Gr. taxis arrangement] 1. the normal adjustment of the bodily temperature. 2. the movement of an organism in response to an increase in temperature.

thermotolerant (ther″mo-tol′er-ant) enduring heat; said of bacteria whose activity is not checked by high temperature.

thesaurosis (the″saw-ro′sis) [Gr. thesauros treasure + -osis] a condition resulting from the storing up in the body of unusually large amounts of normal or foreign substance. See storage DISEASE.

thiamin (thi′ah-min) thiamine.

thiamine (thi′ah-min) a water-soluble vitamin of the B complex, 3 - [(4 - amino - 2 - methyl - 5 - pyrimidinyl)methyl] - 5 - (2-hydroxyethyl)-methylthiazolium chloride. Synthesized in higher plants, bacteria, yeasts, and molds, the vitamin is not produced in animals, and its capacity for storage in the body is limited. Found widely distributed in cereals, milk, bread, nuts, eggs, pork, and other foods. It has a role in carbohydrate metabolism, as a coenzyme in the decarboxylation of pyruvic and α-ketoglutaric acids, and in the utilization of pentose in the hexose monophosphate shunt. Used chiefly in the treatment of thiamine deficiency. Usually used as the hydrochloride salt, which occurs as a white crystalline powder or solids that are soluble in water, slightly soluble in glycerol, ethanol, and methanol, and insoluble in ether, benzene, hexane, and chloroform. It is not known to have serious toxic effects, but large doses may produce transient mild dizziness, flushing, and possibly hypersensitivity. Called also vitamin B_1. Spelled also thiamin. Thiamine deficiency is caused by inadequate intake and utilization of thiamine. Mild deficiency may be characterized by loss of appetite, muscular weakness, pain and paresthesias in the limbs, a tendency to edema, hypotension, hypothermia, pallor, weight loss, restlessness, spasticity of the extremities, and other cardiovascular and neurological disorders. Severe deficiency may lead to beriberi and Wernicke's encephalopathy. Deficiency of thiamine triphosphate in the brain occurs in subacute necrotizing encephalomyelopathy. When present, the most common oral symptoms are edematous and red tongue, inflammation of the gingivae, and hypersensitivity of the oral mucosa and tongue. For daily requirements of thiamine, see table at NUTRITION.

thiamizole (thi-am′ĭ-zōl) methimazole.

thiamylal sodium (thi-am′ĭ-lal) an ultrashort-acting barbiturate, dihydro-5-(1-methylbutyl)-5-(2-propenyl)-2-thioxo-4,6(1H,5H)-pyrimidinedione monosodium salt, occurring as a pale yellow, hygroscopic powder with a disagreeable odor. Used as an intravenous anesthetic. Adverse reactions may include respiratory depression, myocardial depression, arrhythmias, somnolence, prolonged recovery, sneezing, coughing, bronchospasm, laryngospasm, and shivering. Trademark: Surital.

-thiazide a word termination of a generic name denoting a benzothiazine, as in chlorothiazide. See benzothiazine DIURETIC.

thickness (thik′ness) the state or condition of being thick. **half-value t.**, half-value LAYER.

Thielemann's principle (formula) see under PRINCIPLE.

Thier, Carl Jorg see oculovertebral DYSPLASIA (Weyers-Thier syndrome).

Thiersch's canaliculus, operation [Karl Thiersch, German surgeon, 1822–1895] see under CANALICULUS and OPERATION.

thiethylperazine (thi-eth′il-per′ah-zēn) an antiemetic agent, 2-(ethylthio)-10-[3-(4-methyl-1-piperazinyl)propyl]phenothiazine. Used in reducing the incidence of nausea and vomiting associated with general anesthetics and with vertigo. **t. maleate,** the maleate salt of thiethylperazine, occurring as a yellowish, crystalline powder with a slight odor and a bitter taste, which is soluble in ethanol, slightly soluble in water, and very slightly soluble in benzene, ether, and chloroform. Its pharmacological properties are similar to those of the parent compound. Trademarks: Torecan, Toresten, Tresten.

thimble (thim′b'l) a small protective cap of metal or plastic worn over the finger that pushes the needle through the fabric in sewing. Also, a device that resembles such a cap. **primary t., coping. secondary t., telescopic t.,** telescopic COPING.

thimerosal (thi-mer′o-sal) an organic mercurial antiseptic, ethyl(2-mercaptobenzoato-S)mercury sodium salt, occurring as a cream-colored crystalline powder with a slight characteristic odor, which is soluble in water and alcohol, but not in ether and benzene, and deteriorates on exposure to light. Used in aerosols, solutions, and tinctures as a bacteriostatic and fungistatic agent, being ineffective against Mycobacterium tuberculosis and spore-forming bacteria. Usually used to disinfect and treat wounds and abrasions of the skin and mucous membranes, including those of the nose and throat. Mercury poisoning may occur from prolonged application to oral or pharyngeal mucosae. Called also mercurothiolate and thiomersalate. Trademarks: Merfamin, Merthiolate, Mertorgan, Merzonin.

thinner (thin′er) a liquid used to dilute or reduce the viscosity of substances, such as varnishes, rubber cements, and the like. Called also body modifier.

thio- [Gr. theion sulfur] in chemical nomenclature, a prefix used in naming compounds in which oxygen is replaced in an acid radical by sulfur having a negative valence. See also words beginning SULF- and SULFO-.

thioglucose (thi″o-glu′kōs) a glucose compound that contains a sulfhydryl group which replaces the oxygen in the aldehyde group. **gold t.,** aurothioglucose.

thioguanine (thi″o-gwah′nēn) an antimetabolite purine analogue, 2-aminopurine-6-thiol, 6-thioguanine which interferes with nucleic acid synthesis. Used in the treatment of cancer, chiefly types of leukemia, and as an immunosuppressive agent in tissue transplantation and in the treatment of nephrosis and collagen diseases. Bone marrow depression with thrombocytopenia, leukopenia, and anemia; predisposition to hemorrhage and infection; gastrointestinal disorders, including ulceration of the mucosa, nausea, vomiting, and diarrhea; and oral disorders, including stomatitis and mucosal ulceration, are the principal side reactions. Abbreviated TG. Trademark: Lanvis.

Thiokol trademark for polysulfide polymer (see under POLYSULFIDE).

thiol (thi′ol) sulfhydryl.

-thiol a suffix indicating the presence of the sulfhydryl group in a chemical compound.

thiolesterase [E.C.3.1.2.] (thi″ol-es′ter-ās) an esterase that catalyzes the hydrolysis of thioester linkages by acting on carboxylic esters of thiols, especially coenzyme A and glutathione.

Thiomerin trademark for mercaptomerin sodium (see under MERCAPTOMERIN).

thiomersalate (thi″o-mer′sah-lāt) thimerosal.

Thio-Mid trademark for ethionamide.

thionyl (thi′o-nil) the bivalent radical SO. Called also sulfinyl.

thiopental sodium (thi″o-pen′tal) an ultrashort-acting barbiturate, 5-ethyl-5-(1-methylbutyl)-2-barbituric acid monosodium salt, occurring as a white or off-white crystalline or yellowish-white hygroscopic powder with a garlic-like odor, which is soluble in water and alcohol, but not in ether, benzene, and other solvents. It is an ultrashort-acting barbiturate central nervous system depressant used for preanesthesia medication or as the sole anesthetic for operations lasting less than 15 minutes. Respiratory depression, myocardial depression, cardiac arrhythmia, coughing, sneezing, drowsiness, laryngospasm, bronchospasm, and shivering are the principal adverse reactions. The drug is contraindicated in liver disorders, cardiac decompensation, respiratory disorders, and porphyria. Thiopental sodium is an addictive drug and subject to regulations of the Controlled Substances Act. Trademarks: Pentothal, Thiopentone.

Thiopentone trademark for thiopental sodium (see under THIOPENTAL).

thioridazine (thi″o-rid′ah-zēn) a phenothiazine tranquilizer with central sedative and minimal antiemetic and extrapyramidal effects, 10 - [2 - (1 - methyl - 2 - piperidyl)methyl]-2-(methylthio)-phenothiazide. Side effects may include drowsiness, some parkinsonian-like reactions, dystonia, dyskinesia, torticollis, involuntary muscle movements, restlessness, hyperreflexia, seizures, cerebral edema, postural hypotension, tachycardia, bradycardia, cardiac arrest, vertigo, agranulocytosis, eosinophilia, leukopenia, thrombocytopenic purpura, pancytopenia, jaundice, hypersensitivity, hypercholesterolemia, xerostomia, constipation, mydriasis, and suppression of cough reflex. Trademarks: Meleril, Mellaril, Sonapax. **t. hydrochloride,** the hydrochloride salt of thioridazine, occurring as a white to yellowish, bitter, photosensitive, granular powder with a faint odor, which is soluble in water, chloroform, and methanol, slightly soluble in benzene, and insoluble in ether. Its pharmacological and toxicological properties are similar to those of the parent compound.

thiorubber (thi″o-rub′er) POLYSULFIDE polymer.

3-thiosemicarbazone (thi″o-sem″ĕ-kar′bah-sōn) methisazone.

thiosulfate (thi″o-sul′fāt) any salt of thiosulfuric acid, $M_2S_2O_3$.

thio-TEPA triethylenethiophosphoramide.

thiothixene (thi″o-thiks′ēn) a tranquilizer, *N*,*N*-dimethyl-9-[3-(4-methyl-1-piperazinyl)propylidine]thioxanthene-2-sulfonamide, occurring as a white to tan, odorless, bitter, photosensitive, crystalline powder that is soluble in chloroform, slightly soluble in acetone, ethanol, and carbon tetrachloride, and insoluble in water. Used in the treatment of mental disorders. Side effects may include drowsiness, parkinsonian-like symptoms, dystonia, dyskinesis, torticollis, involuntary muscle twitching, restlessness, hyperreflexia, seizures, cerebral edema, postural hypotension, tachycardia, bradycardia, cardiac arrest, vertigo, agranulocytosis, eosinophilia, leukopenia, thrombocytopenic purpura, pancytopenia, jaundice, hypersensitivity, hypercholesterolemia, xerostomia, constipation, mydriasis, and suppression of cough reflex. Trademarks: Navane, Orbinamon. **t. hydrochloride,** the hydrochloride salt of thiothixene, occurring as a white, photosensitive, crystalline powder with a faint odor, which is soluble in water, slightly soluble in chloroform, and insoluble in benzene, acetone, and ether. Its pharmacological and toxicological properties are similar to those of the parent compound.

thiouracil (thi″o-u′rah-sil) a thyroid antagonist which prevents iodine from being incorporated into thyroxine, 2,3-dihydro-2-thioxo-4(1*H*)-pyrimidinone. It occurs as bitter crystals that are readily soluble in alkaline solutions, slightly soluble in water, and insoluble in ethanol, ether, and acids. Used in the treatment of hyperthyroidism. Patients receiving thiouracil may exhibit predisposition to parotitis, agranulocytosis, and infections, and ulcerative necrotic lesions of the oral cavity. Trademark: Deracil.

Thipen trademark for *thiphenamil hydrochloride* (see under THIPHENAMIL).

thiphenamil hydrochloride (thi-fen′ah-mil) a tertiary amine with weak antimuscarinic properties, α-phenylbenzeneethanethioic acid *S*-[2-(diethylamino)ethyl]ester hydrochloride, occurring as a white, bitter powder that is soluble in water, and ethanol. Used in the treatment of spasmodic disorders. Side effects may include decreased gastrointestinal motility and gastric secretion, drying of the mucous membranes, mydriasis, urinary retention, decreased sweating, cutaneous flushing, bronchial dilatation, tachycardia, and other disorders associated with antimuscarinic therapy. Trademarks: Thiphen, Trocinate.

Thixokon trademark for *acetrizoate sodium* (see under ACETRIZOATE).

Thom's facing [John *Thom*, English dentist, 19th century] interchangeable FACING.

Thoma-Zeiss counting chamber [Richard *Thoma*, German histologist, 1847–1923; Carl *Zeiss*, German optician, 1816–1888] see under CHAMBER.

Thompson dowel [M. J. *Thompson*, American dentist] see under DOWEL.

Thompson's line see under LINE.

Thompson scattering coherent SCATTERING.

Thomsen's disease [Asmus Julius Thomas *Thomsen*, Danish physician, 1815–1896] MYOTONIA congenita.

Thomson, M. Sidney see Rothmund-Thomson SYNDROME.

Thoraeus filter see under FILTER.

thorax (tho′raks), pl. *tho′races* [Gr. *thōrax*] [NA] that part of the body which lies between the neck and the abdomen and is encased by the ribs; the chest.

Thorazine trademark for *chlorpromazine*.

thorium (tho′re-um) [named after *Thor*, the Norse god of war] a radioactive metallic element. Symbol, Th; atomic number, 90; atomic weight, 232.0381; melting point, 1750°C; specific gravity, 11.72; valence, 4; group IIIB of the periodic table (actinide series). Its longest-lived isotope is ^{232}Th; other isotopes include 224–231 and 233–235. When pure, thorium is a grayish white lustrous metal, which can be cold-rolled, extruded, and welded, and is soluble in acids, but not in alkalies and water. In powder form, it is flammable and explosive. Used in x-ray tubes, alloys, photoelectric cells, and nuclear technology.

Thornwaldt's (Tornwaldt's) bursitis (disease, syndrome), cyst [Gustav Ludwig *Thornwaldt*, German physician, 1843–1910] see under BURSITIS, and see BURSA pharyngea.

thornwalditis (torn″vahlt-i′tis) an old term for Thornwaldt's BURSITIS.

Thr threonine.

thread (thred) a long slender structure, such as a continuous filament of some substance used as suture material.

Threadmate system see under SYSTEM.

threonine (thre′o-nin) an aliphatic, naturally occurring amino acid essential for certain nitrogen metabolic processes in adult humans, 2-amino-3-hydroxybutyric acid. It is also found in the saliva. Abbreviated *Thr*. See also amino ACID.

threshold (thresh′ōld) 1. any place or point of entrance or beginning. 2. that value at which a stimulus just produces a sensation, is just appreciable, or comes just within limits of perception. 3. that degree of concentration of a substance in the blood plasma above which the substance is excreted by the kidneys and below which it is not excreted; such a substance is called *threshold substance*. 4. limen. **absolute t.,** the lowest possible limit of stimulation that is capable of producing sensation. Called also *sensitivity t.* and *stimulus t.* **differential t.,** the lowest limit of discriminative sensibility, permitting two stimuli to be differentiated. **exposure t.,** the minimum radiation exposure that will produce a detectable degree of a specified effect. **photoelectric t.,** in photoelectric emission, the maximum wavelength or a minimum light frequency below which photoelectrons will not be emitted. **renal t. for glucose,** the level of the concentration of glucose in the blood (170 mg/100 ml of blood), above which (hyperglycemia) sugar will be excreted in the urine (glycosuria). Called also *leak point*. **swallowing t.,** the reflex action initiated by minimum stimulation prior to the act of deglutition. **tactile sensibility t.,** the minimum stimulation needed to elicit tactile perception. In the masticatory system, some individuals are capable of perceiving bodies as small as 10 μ between the occlusal surfaces and occlusal force of less than 600 mg exerted on the teeth; bodies of 60 μ in thickness and force of 1.5 gm are detectable by most healthy persons.

thrill (thril) a tremor or vibration felt by palpation.

thrix (thriks) [Gr.] hair.

-thrix [Gr. *thrix* hair] a word termination meaning hair.

throat (thrōt) 1. the cavity which includes the pharynx and larynx and extends from the arch of the palate to the glottis and esophageal opening. Called also *guttur*. See also FAUCES, LARYNX, and PHARYNX. 2. commonly, the front of the neck. **epidemic streptococcal sore t.,** septic sore t. **septic sore t.,** a severe type of sore throat occurring in epidemics, marked by intense local hyperemia with or without a grayish exudate and enlargement of the cervical lymph nodes. It is usually caused by *Streptococcus pyogenes* and sometimes by *S. equisimilis*, and is probably spread largely by droplets or in air, but is also transmitted by direct contact and by food and beverages. Called also *epidemic streptococcal sore t.*, *streptococcal sore t.*, and *streptococcal tonsillitis*. **sore t.,** See *septic sore t.*, LARYNGITIS, PHARYNGITIS, and TONSILLITIS. **streptococcal sore t.,** septic sore t.

Thrombasal trademark for *phenindione*.

thrombase (throm′bās) thrombin (1).

thrombasthenia (throm″bas-the′ne-ah) [*thrombocyte* + Gr. *astheneia* weakness] a functional defect of the blood platelets. **hereditary hemorrhagic t.,** Willebrand-Jürgens SYNDROME. **Glanzmann's t., hemorrhagic t.,** Glanzmann's SYNDROME.

thrombin [E.C.3.4.21.5] (throm′bin) 1. a serine proteinase, formed from prothrombin in the presence of an extrinsic or intrinsic prothrombin. In blood coagulation, it hydrolyzes fibrinogen to fibrin, preferentially cleaving arginine, and removes two low-molecular-weight peptides from each molecule of fibrinogen, forming a molecular of fibrin monomer which polymerizes with other fibrin monomer molecules. During a vascular injury, thrombin alters the platelets to make them bind together irreversibly, thus forming a plug that prevents escape of the blood from a damaged vessel. Called also *fibrinogenase* and *thrombase*. 2. a sterile substance prepared from bovine prothrombin through interaction with added thromboplastin in the presence of calcium. It occurs as a white or grayish, amorphous substance dried from the frozen state. Used as a hemostatic agent to cause the clotting of the blood in the treatment of wounds and injuries associated with bleeding and in surgery to control bleeding. Called also *sterile t.* and *topical t.* **sterile t., topical t.,** thrombin (2).

thrombo- [Gr. *thrombos* clot] a combining form denoting relationship to a clot, or thrombus.

thrombocyte (throm′bo-sīt) [*thrombo-* + *-cyte*] blood PLATELET.

thrombocythemia (throm″bo-si-the′me-ah) [*thrombocyte* + Gr. *haima* blood + *-ia*] a condition, regarded as one of the myeloproliferative disorders, characterized by the presence in the blood of an abnormally high number of blood platelets. It occurs as a primary condition or secondarily to or in association with another disorder. Symptoms include repeated spontaneous hemorrhages from the nose and into the gastrointestinal system, genitourinary system, central nervous system, and skin; venous and arterial thromboses, splenomegaly, and marked hyperplasia of the megakaryocytes. Spontaneous gingival hemorrhage is common, and prolonged bleeding after tooth extraction may occur. Called *piastrinemia* and *thrombocytosis.* **essential idiopathic t.,** hemorrhagic t. **hemorrhagic t.,** that occurring as a primary condition of unknown etiology. Called also *essential idiopathic t., primary t.,* and *megakaryocytic leukemia.* **primary t.,** hemorrhagic t. **secondary t.,** thrombocythemia that may occur in association with another disorder, such as polycythemia vera, chronic myelogenous leukemia, neoplasms, tuberculosis, and sarcoidosis, or after trauma, surgery, or parturition.

thrombocytin (throm″bo-si′tin) 5-hydroxytryptamine.

thrombocytopathy (throm″bo-si-top′ah-the) [*thrombocyte* + Gr. *pathos* disease] a condition characterized by a blood platelet disorder, usually a functional disorder. Called also *thrombopathy.*

thrombocytopenia (throm″bo-si″to-pe′ne-ah) [*thrombocyte* + Gr. *penia* poverty] abnormal decrease in the number of blood platelets due to decreased production of platelets, accelerated platelet destruction, a combination of the two, or abnormal pooling. It occurs in some immunologic conditions, poisoning, splenomegaly and sequestration of the spleen, deficient thrombocytopoiesis, and various diseases resulting in suppression of blood platelets. See also THROMBASTHENIA, thrombocytopenic PURPURA, and Wiskott-Aldrich SYNDROME. **essential t.,** thrombocytopenic purpura, idiopathic; see under PURPURA.

thrombocytopoiesis (throm″bo-si″to-poi-e′sis) [*thrombocyte* + Gr. *poiein* to make] the formation and development of blood platelets.

thrombocytosis (throm″bo-si-to′sis) [*thrombocyte* + *-osis*] a condition characterized by an abnormally high blood platelet count. See also THROMBOCYTHEMIA.

thromboembolism (throm″bo-em′bo-lizm) obstruction of a blood vessel with thrombotic material carried by the blood from the site of origin to plug another vessel.

thromboendarterectomy (throm″bo-end″ar-ter-ek′to-me) [*thrombo-* + Gr. *endon* within + *artēria* artery + *ektomē* excision] removal of an obstructing thrombus together with the inner lining of an obstructed artery.

thrombogen (throm″bo-jen) [*thrombo-* + Gr. *genan* to produce] 1. FACTOR V. 2. prothrombin.

thrombogenesis (throm″bo-jen′ĕ-sis) the formation of thrombin from prothrombin in blood coagulation (see under COAGULATION).

thrombokinase (throm″bo-kin′ās) 1. thromboplastin. 2. FACTOR X.

thrombopathy (throm-bop′ah-the) thrombocytopathy. **constitutional t.,** Willebrand-Jürgens SYNDROME.

thrombophlebitis (throm″bo-fle-bi′tis) [*thrombo-* + Gr. *phleps* vein + *-itis*] a condition in which inflammation of the vein wall has preceded the formation of the thrombus. The presence of a thrombus in a vein without inflammation is called *phlebothrombosis.* **cavernous sinus t.,** cavernous sinus THROMBOSIS.

thromboplastin (throm″bo-plas′tin) 1. a substance involved in both the extrinsic and intrinsic mechanisms of prothrombin activator formation. It is formed when blood comes in contact with injured tissue, which then releases a proteolytic enzyme (*extrinsic t., tissue t., factor III, tissue factor*), leading to the formation of prothrombin activator. Intrinsic thromboplastin begins to form when trauma occurs to the blood itself and collagen in the vascular wall comes in contact with factor XII, causing it to be converted into a proteolytic enzyme, also leading to the formation of prothrombin. Called also *cytozyme.* See also blood COAGULATION and PROTHROMBIN activator. 2. tissue t. **complete t.,** PROTHROMBIN activator. **extrinsic t.,** tissue t. (1). **partial t.,** see thromboplastin time, partial, under TIME. **plasma t.,** a substance found in the blood plasma that, in the presence of calcium ions, brings about activation of prothrombin in blood coagulation. **tissue t.,** a proteolytic enzyme formed when blood comes in contact with injured tissue; see thromboplastin (1). Called also *extrinsic t., factor III, thromboplastin, tissue factor,* and, sometimes, *thromboplastin.*

thromboplastinogen (throm″bo-plas-tin′o-jen) FACTOR VIII.

thromboplastinogenesis (throm″bo-plas-tin′o-jen-ē-sis) the formation of thromboplastin in blood coagulation.

thrombosis (throm-bo′sis) [Gr. *thrombōsis*] the formation of a blood clot (thrombus) within a blood vessel or the heart, producing occlusion of vessels and impairing the flow of the blood, and resulting in ischemic necrosis and infarction of tissue. In thrombosis the blood clot remains stationary, whereas in *embolism* the clot is carried to distant sites. **cavernous sinus t.,** thrombosis affecting the cavernous sinus, causing impairment of vascular drainage of the cerebellum, and characterized by

headache, orbital pain, bulging of the globe of the eye, edema of the eyelids and conjunctiva, proptosis, and frequently nausea, pyrexia, and vomiting. Meningitis is a common complication. It usually follows infection of the eye, face, or nose. About 7 percent of cases are of dental origin. Before antibiotics, the condition was nearly always fatal. Called also *cavernous sinus thrombophlebitis.* **coronary t.,** occlusion of the coronary artery by a thrombus, usually associated with damage of the heart muscle (myocardial infarction) and, sometimes, sudden death. See coronary OCCLUSION. **inferior dental vessel t.,** thrombosis of inferior dental vessel branches or main artery, resulting from breaking of a dental abscess into the bone and marrow spaces of the mandible. Osteomyelitis is a common complication.

thrombus (throm′bus) [Gr. *thrombos*] a plug or clot in a blood vessel or in one of the heart cavities, formed by coagulation of the blood, and remaining at the point of its formation. A dislodged thrombus that is carried by the blood stream to a distant site is known as an *embolus.*

thrush (thrush) candidiasis of the oral mucosa, most frequently involving the buccal mucosa and tongue, but the palate, gingivae, and floor of the mouth may also be affected; in severe cases the entire oral cavity may be involved. It is characterized by the development of creamy, white, slightly elevated plaques made up of soft, creamy or crumbly material resembling milk curds. The plaques are composed mainly of masses of fungal hyphae, which are situated mostly on and not in the tissue; they may be stripped off from the surface of the tissue, leaving a raw bleeding surface. Perlèche is often associated. Formerly common in sick, weak infants and in elderly individuals in poor health; it had been almost eradicated with improved nutrition and hygiene and better medical and oral care, but the incidence is now on the increase due to the widespread use of antibiotics to which *Candida* is almost insensitive. Called also *mycotic stomatitis, oral moniliasis,* and *white mouth.* See also CANDIDIASIS and neonatal monilial STOMATITIS.

thrusting (thrust′ing) suddenly and forcibly pushing or moving forward. **tongue t.,** the infantile pattern of suckling-swallowing in which the tongue is placed between the incisor teeth or alveolar ridges during the initial stages of deglutition, resulting sometimes in anterior open bite, deformation of the jaws, and abnormal function. See also reverse SWALLOWING and teeth apart SWALLOWING.

thulium (thu′le-um) [named after *Thule,* ancient name for an island or region identified as one of the Shetland Islands, Iceland, or Norway] a rare earth of the lanthanide series. Symbol, Tm; atomic number, 69; specific gravity, 9.318; melting point, 1550°C; valence, 3; group IIIB of the periodic table. It has one natural isotope [169]Tm; artificial radioactive isotopes include 152, 154, 161–168, and 170–176. Thulium is a silvery white, easily worked metal, which reacts slowly with water and is soluble in dilute acids.

thumb-sucking (thum-suk′ing) thumb SUCKING.

thymidine (thi′mĭ-dēn) 2,4-dioxy-5-methylpyrimidine; a pyrimidine base and a component of nucleic acids.

Thyloquinone trademark for *menadione.*

Thylose trademark for *sodium carboxymethylcellulose* (see under CARBOXYMETHYLCELLULOSE).

thyme (tīm) [L. *thymus;* Gr. *thymos*] a plant of the genus *Thymus.* *T. vulgaris* (garden thyme) contains a volatile oil, which is aromatic and carminative. It also contains thymol, thymene, and cumene. **t. camphor,** thymol.

thymine (thi′min) a chemical substance, 5-methyluracil, found as a pyrimidine base of DNA but not RNA, occurring as a white, crystalline powder that is slightly soluble in hot water and ether and readily soluble in alkalies. Used in biochemical research.

Thymiode trademark for *thymol iodide* (see under THYMOL).

thymo- 1. [Gr. *thymos* thymus] a combining form denoting relationship to the thymus. 2. [Gr. *thymos* mind, spirit] a combining form denoting relationship to the soul or emotions.

thymocyte (thi′mo-sit) [*thymo-*(1) + *-cyte*] a lymphocyte produced by the thymus, which survives in the circulating blood only for a few days. See LYMPHOCYTE.

thymol (thi′mol) an antibacterial and antifungal phenol derivative, 5-methyl-2-(1-methylethyl)phenol, occurring as colorless crystals or white crystalline powder with a strong pungent odor and caustic taste. It is soluble in water, alcohol, chloroform, olive oil, glacial acetic acid, and alkali hydroxides. Used in the treatment of acne, hemorrhoids, and tinea pedis. Also used in mouthwashes. Called also *m-t.* and *thyme camphor.* **t. iodide,** a mixture of iodine derivatives of thymol, chiefly dithymol diiodide, 4,4′-bis(iodooxy)-2,2′-dimethyl-5,5′-bis(methylethyl)-1,1′-biphenyl, occurring as a reddish-brown or reddish-yellow powder that is readily soluble in chloroform, ether, collodion, oils, slightly soluble in alcohol, and insoluble in water. It loses iodine on exposure to light. It has the pharmacological properties of the parent compound, and is used in dusting powders, in root canal filling materials, and in ointments, usually combined with ethyl aminobenzoate. Trademarks: Aristol, Iodosol, Iodothymol, Thymiode. **m.-t.,** thymol.

thymosin (thi′mo-sin) a family of molecules extracted from the thymus, which have hormonal properties and are capable of restoring T-lymphocyte function to thymus-deficient animals.

thymus (thi′mus) [L.; Gr. *thymos*] [NA] a two-lobed ductless lymphoid organ situated in the anterior mediastinum behind the upper part of the sternum. Its relative size is largest during fetal life and at birth weighs 10 to 15 gm, reaching a maximum of 30 to 40 gm at puberty, and after adolescence, begins to involute. The organ is surrounded by a thin capsule of connective tissue, extending into the substance of the gland, forming septa that partially divide the lobes into lobules. Peripheral portions of the lobule (cortex) are infiltrated with lymphocytes; central portions (medulla) contain fewer lymphocytes but more epithelial elements. Within the substance of the organ are cystic structures containing keratin (Hassall's corpuscles). Its principal functions are believed to be the development of lymphocytes by the cortex and humoral substances (hormones) by epithelial elements; the latter, e.g., thymosin, are believed to be involved in the differentiation of lymphocytes. Lymphocytes from the thymus divide and differentiate into T-lymphocytes and cells that assist (helper cells) or inhibit antibody production (suppressor cells) or destroy target cells (killer cells). Hyperplasia and tumors of the thymus are often associated with myasthenia gravis.

thyratron (thi′rah-tron) a form of discharge tube containing mercury vapor and a multiplicity of electrodes, used as an electric valve to rectify alternating current.

thyreo- see THYRO-.

Thyreostat I trademark for *methylthiouracil.*

Thyreostat II trademark for *propylthiouracil.*

thyro-, thyreo- [Gr. *thyreos* shield] a combining form denoting relationship to the thyroid gland.

thyroadenitis (thi″ro-ad″ĕ-ni′tis) [thyro- + Gr. *adēn* gland + -*itis*] inflammation of the thyroid gland; thyroiditis.

thyroarytenoid (thi″ro-ar″ĭ-te′noid) pertaining to the thyroid and arytenoid cartilages.

thyroarytenoideus (thi″ro-ar″ĭ-te-noi′de-us) thyroarytenoid MUSCLE.

thyrocalcitonin (thi″ro-kal″sĭ-to′nin) calcitonin.

thyroepiglottic (thi″ro-ep″ĭ-glot′ik) pertaining to the thyroid gland or thyroid cartilage and the epiglottis.

thyroepiglotticus (thi″ro-ep″ĭ-glot′i-kus) thyroepiglottic MUSCLE.

thyroglossal (thi″ro-glos′al) pertaining to the thyroid gland and the tongue.

thyrohyal (thi″ro-hi′al) 1. pertaining to the thyroid cartilage and the hyoid bone. 2. greater horn of hyoid bone; see under HORN.

thyrohyoid (thi″ro-hi′oid) pertaining to the thyroid gland or cartilage and the hyoid bone; hyothyroid.

thyrohyoideus (thi″ro-hi-oi′de-us) thyrohyoid MUSCLE.

thyroid (thi′roid) [Gr. *thyreoeidēs*, from *thyreos* shield + *eidos* form] 1. resembling a shield; scutiform. 2. a pharmaceutical preparation obtained from dried and powdered animal thyroid glands, used in replacement therapy in hypothyroid states, low basal metabolism, and obesity. 3. thyroid GLAND. **aberrant t.,** presence of thyroid tissue in an abnormal location.

thyroiditis (thi″roi-di′tis) [*thyroid* + -*itis*] inflammation of the thyroid gland. **Hashimoto's t.,** Hashimoto's DISEASE. **invasive t., ligneous t.,** Riedel's t. **Riedel's t.,** a rare form characterized by an asymmetric hard goiter that is densely adherent to the surrounding tissue. It affects most commonly elderly women, and is manifested clinically chiefly by pressure symptoms. Fibrosis and infiltration of adjacent tissues may suggest carcinoma. Called also *invasive t., ligneous t.,* and *Riedel's struma.*

thyropharyngeus (thi″ro-far-in′je-us) thyropharyngeal MUSCLE.

thyrotropic (thi″ro-trop′ik) [*thyro- + tropic*] 1. having an influence on the thyroid gland. 2. pertaining to thyrotropic hormone.

thyrotropin (thi-rot′ro-pin) [*thyro-* + Gr. *tropē* a turn] thyrotropic HORMONE.

thyroxine (thi-rok′sin, thi-rok′sēn) an amino acid, 3-[4-(4-hydroxy-3,5-diiodophenoxy)-3,5-diiodophenyl]alanine. It is the active principle of the thyroid gland that influences oxygen consumption; growth and tissue differentiation; carbohydrate, lipid, and protein metabolism; reproductive activity; water-electrolyte balance; and temperature sensitivity. The production and secretion of thyroxine is regulated by thyrotropic hormone of the anterior pituitary gland. Its synthesis may be affected by administration of iodine, thiocyanates, and various thyroid antagonists, including those containing a thiocarbamide group (such as thiourea, thiouracil, and related compounds), and those containing aminobenzene groups (such as sulfonamides). DL-Thyroxine occurs as needle-like crystals that are soluble in alkali hydroxide solutions and in the presence of mineral acids or alkalies, in ethanol, but not in water and organic solvents. Used in the treatment of myxedema and simple goiter. The L-form is used as a cholesterogenic agent. Excessive production of thyroxine is known as *hyperthyroidism;* thyroxine deficiency causes *hypothyroidism.*

Ti titanium.

tic (tik) [Fr.] an involuntary contraction or twitching, especially of the facial muscles. **convulsive t.,** spasm of those parts of the face supplied by the seventh (facial) nerve. **t. douloureux** (doo-loo-roo′) trigeminal NEURALGIA. **facial t.,** spasm of the facial muscles. Called also *mimic t.* **mimic t.,** facial t.

Ticonium 44, 50, 100 trademarks for nickel-chromium base-metal crown and bridge alloys, also containing 0.43 to 1.89 percent beryllium. Inhalation of dust and vapors during melting, milling, or grinding may cause beryllium poisoning.

Ticonium TG2 trademark for a medium hard *dental casting gold alloy* (see under GOLD).

Ticonium TG3 trademark for a hard *dental casting gold alloy* (see under GOLD).

Ticonium TG4 trademark for an extra hard *dental casting gold alloy* (see under GOLD).

Ticonium denture Ticonium hidden-lock DENTURE.

t.i.d. *ter in di′e,* three times a day.

Tièche, Max see blue NEVUS (Jadassohn-Tièche nevus).

Tifosyl trademark for *triethylenethiophosphoramide.*

time (tīm) [Gr. *chronos;* L. *tempus*] a measure of duration. **amalgam setting t.,** the period required for the hardening of amalgam. **bleeding t.,** the period of duration of bleeding that follows a skin puncture, measured to determine capillary and platelet function. The test consists of performing three uniform punctures of the skin of the inner surface of the forearm (Ivy method) or a single puncture of the ear-lobe (Duke method). The blood seeping from the punctures is gently wiped with soft filter paper and the period from the puncture to the stoppage of flow is measured. The normal range in the Ivy method is 1 to 9 minutes and 1 to 4 minutes in the Duke method. Prolonged bleeding time is seen in such conditions as thrombocytopenia, von Willebrand's disease, and platelet dysfunction and uncommonly in vascular disorders and rarely in severe coagulation disorders. It may also be abnormal in other conditions, such as acute leukemia, aplastic anemia, liver disease, scurvy, toxic states, and chemical intoxication. **bleeding t., secondary,** the time required to arrest the bleeding when the crust is removed from a traumatized area 24 hours after the original injury; this is generally prolonged in patients with factor VIII deficiency (hemophilia) and with related hemophilioid states. **circulation t.,** the time required for blood to flow between two designated points, as arm-to-tongue time. **clot retraction t.,** the time required for 50 percent of a blood clot (coagulum) to retract from the wall of a glass vessel containing it. Usually the clot begins to retract within a few minutes to 1 hour; prolonged retraction time is indicative of platelet deficiency. See also clot retraction TEST. **clotting t.,** coagulation t. **coagulation t.,** COAGULATION time. **t. of death,** the time of cessation of all vital activities in the body. See somatic DEATH. **dextrinizing t.,** the time required for saliva to convert starch into sugar. **down t.,** downtime. **erythrocyte sedimentation t.,** ERYTHROCYTE sedimentation rate. **exposure t.,** the time during which a person or object is exposed to some effect, such as ionizing radiation. **Gillmore initial and Gillmore final setting t.,** see under *setting t.* **LD 50 t.,** see median lethal t. **median lethal t.,** the time required for the death of 50 percent of the individuals in a large group of organisms following a given exposure to ionizing radiation. Abbreviated *MLT.* Called also *LD 50 t.* **one-stage plasma prothrombin t., one-stage prothrombin t.,** Quick's TEST (1). **partial thromboplastin t.,** thromboplastin t., partial. **plasma prothrombin t., one-stage, prothrombin t., one-stage,** Quick's TEST (1). **plasma recalcification t.,** a blood coagulation test used to measure all coagulation factors based on replacing the calcium of platelet-rich oxalated plasma and determining the clotting time; 4.5 ml of venous blood is mixed with 0.5 ml of 3.8 percent sodium citrate and the mixture is mixed and centrifuged. A tube containing 0.025 M CaCl₂ is warmed to 37°C and 0.2 ml of CaCl₂ solution is placed in the tube containing plasma. The normal clotting time ranges between 90 and 120 seconds. **reaction t.,** the time elapsing between the application of a stimulus and the resulting response. **resin hardening t.,** resin setting t. **resin setting t.,** the time elapsed from mixing the polymer and monomer to the polymerization, measured from the exact time the polymer and monomer have been combined to the time peak temperature is reached. Called also *resin hardening t.* **sedimentation t.,** erythrocyte sedimentation RATE. **setting t.,** the period required for dental cement, dental stone, dental plaster, or plaster of Paris to harden, determined from the time when the powder and water are mixed to the time when the resulting plaster loses its gloss or the time when Vicat's or Gillmore's ¼-pound needles are no longer capable of penetrating its surface (initial setting time, Gillmore initial time), or when Gillmore's 1-pound needle cannot penetrate the surface (final setting time, Gillmore final time). **thromboplastin t., partial,** measuring of the clotting time of recalcified blood plasma in the presence of cephalin (partial thromboplastin). The test is performed by mixing 0.1 ml of plasma with an equal amount of cephalin, heating the mixture to 37°C, and adding to the mixture 0.1 ml of 0.02 M CaCl₂, also warmed to 37°C. The normal clotting time varies from 67 to 83 seconds, with 75 seconds being the average. Partial thromboplastin time of over 100 seconds indicates deficiencies of coagulation factors I, II, V, VIII, IX, X, XI, and XII.

timer (tīm'er) a clock mechanism which may be set to time or to activate or cut off certain other apparatus at the desired time. See also *photo t.* **electronic t.,** one operated by a series of electronic tubes and relays; in an x-ray generator, used for exposures of more than 1/30 of a second. **hand t.,** an x-ray generator timer having an attachment that requires thumb or finger pressure to actuate the timing device. **impulse t.,** one in which a timing device counts the impulses of alternating and half-wave rectified current; used in x-ray generators for exposures of 1/20 or 1/60 to 1/5 second. **mechanical t.,** one operated by a spring-loaded mechanism. **photo t.,** a timing device used in photography and radiography to give a desired exposure. A radiographic photo timer consists of a photomultiplier tube and associated electronic circuitry, designed to terminate exposure of radiographs automatically when a predetermined exposure has been achieved. It usually has a fluorescent screen that, when x-irradiated, gives off a glow which activates the photoelectric cell. The electricity generated in the cell flows to the condenser until it reaches sufficient current to permit discharge; the discharge initiates a series of events that leads to the opening of the relay and termination of the x-ray exposure. Written also *phototimer.* **synchronous t.,** one that operates by a synchronous motor and opens or closes the high-voltage circuit only when the applied voltage is zero; the exposure time being always an integral number of cycles or half-cycles. It is used for exposures of 1/20 second to 20 seconds.

time-sharing (tīm-shār'ing) in computer technology, a method whereby several terminals can access a central computer concurrently.

Timme's syndrome [Walter *Timme,* American physician, 1874–1956] see under SYNDROME.

tin (tin) [L. *stannum*] a metallic element. Symbol, Sn; atomic number, 50; atomic weight, 118.69; specific gravity, (gray tin) 5.75, (white tin) 7.31; Brinell hardness number, 2.9; melting point, 231°C; valences, 2, 4; group IVA of the periodic table. Natural isotopes include 112, 114–120, 122, and 124; artificial radioactive isotopes are 108–111, 113, 121, 123, and 125–132. It is a lustrous, soft, malleable, ductile, silvery metal with a highly crystalline structure. On warming to 13.2°C, gray, or α-tin, changes to white, or β-tin (the ordinary form of the metal); the change is due to impurities and is known as tin pest. Tin is soluble in acids and hot potassium hydroxide solution, but not in water. Used chiefly for plating sheath metal, soldering alloys, and in dental amalgam. Tin alloys include soft solder, pewter, bronze, Babbitt metal, white metal, and die casting alloys. An increase of the tin content of dental amalgam increases the contraction of the alloy, but reduces its strength, hardness, and resistance to corrosion. Tin salts are used as reagents, stains, and in medicines. Although not toxic in pure form, tin salts may be poisonous. See also terms beginning STANN-. **t.-antimony alloy,** tin-antimony ALLOY. **t. ash,** stannic OXIDE. **t. caprylate,** stannous OCTOATE. **t. difluoride,** stannous FLUORIDE. **t. dioxide,** stannic OXIDE. **t. foil,** tin FOIL. **t. foil substitute,** see separating MEDIUM. **flowers of t.,** stannic OXIDE. **t. octoate,** stannous OCTOATE. **t. oxide, white,** stannic OXIDE. **silver-t. alloy,** silver-tin ALLOY. **silver-t. system,** silver-tin ALLOY.

Tinactin trademark for *tolnaftate.*

Tinaderm trademark for *tolnaftate.*

tinct. abbreviation for L. *tinctu'ra,* tincture.

tinctable (tink'tah-b'l) stainable or tingible.

tinction (tink'shun) [L. *tinctura,* from *tingere* to moisten] 1. the act of staining. 2 the addition of coloring or flavoring agents to a prescription.

tinctura (tink-tu'rah), pl. *tinctu'rae* [L.] tincture.

tincturation (tin"chur-a'shun) the preparation of a tincture; the treatment of a drug with a menstruum, such as alcohol or other, for the purpose of preparing a tincture.

tincture (tin'chur) [L. *tingere* to wet, to moisten] an alcoholic or hydroalcoholic solution prepared from drugs from animal, vegetable, or chemical origin. **belladonna t.,** BELLADONNA tincture. **camphorated opium t.,** paregoric. **green soap t.,** a preparation of green soap, lavender oil, and ethanol; used as a skin detergent. Called also *linimentum saponis mollis* and *medicinal soft soap liniment.* **iodine t.,** IODINE tincture. **opium t.,** OPIUM tincture.

tinea (tin'e-ah) [L. "a grub, larva, worm"] any of various superficial fungal skin diseases, which are characterized by the formation of ring-shaped pigmented patches covered with vesicles or scales. Called also *ringworm.* **t. bar'bae,** a fungal infection of the bearded area of the face and neck caused by various species of dermatophytes of the genera *Trichophyton* and *Microsporum.* In the superficial type, there is a low grade scaling lesion surrounded by a vesicular border and the hair is lusterless and brittle, followed by alopecia. In the deep type, there are abscesses, follicular pustules, and draining sinuses. Tinea barbae stimulates various diseases of the face, including pustular dermatitis, impetigo, tertiary syphilis, leprosy, actinomycosis, acne, and the like. Called also *barber's itch* and *ringworm of beard.* **t. cap'itis,** a highly contagious fungal infection of the scalp caused by various species of dermatophytes of the genera *Microsporum* and *Trichophyton,* causing patchy alopecia and dull and friable hair. Called also *ringworm of scalp.* **t. cor'poris,** a fungal infection of the skin of worldwide distribution, caused by species of *Epidermophyton, Trichophyton,* and, sometimes, *Microsporum.* Lesions are usually scaly to granulomatous and itchy, occurring singly or in patches, with a scaly or circumscribed center surrounded by a vesicular and pustular border. Some are moist and crusted. As the lesions develop, a ring of scales forms around each lesion, and new circles form peripherally to the original lesion. *Tinea cruris* is a form that involves the groin and perineal regions. Called also *t. glabrosa* and *ringworm of body.* See also *t. imbricata.* **t. cru'ris,** see *t. corporis.* **t. favo'sa,** favus. **t. glabro'sa,** t. corporis. **t. imbrica'ta,** a form of tinea corporis that is restricted to particular population groups or races of man, occurring in the Pacific, Southeast Asia, and Central and South America. It is characterized by annular lesions with circles of scales in the periphery, attached along one edge, giving rise to large concentric scaling rings; the infection is caused by *Trichophyton concentricum.* **t. versic'olor,** PITYRIASIS versicolor.

tinfoil (tin'foil) tin FOIL.

tingible (tin'ji-b'l) [L. *tingere* to stain] susceptible of being tinged or stained.

tingling (ting'gling) a peculiar pricklike thrill caused by cold, emotional shock, or striking a nerve.

tinnitus (tin'i-tus, ti-ni'tus) [L. "a *ringing*"] a noise in the ears, as ringing, buzzing, roaring, clicking, etc. **objective t.,** a sound originating within the body of the patient, in the region of the ear, which is audible to others than the patient.

tip (tip) a slender or pointed end or extremity of a structure or body part. Called also *apex.* **interdental t.,** a slender tip, sometimes attached to the handle of a toothbrush, used for removing plaque and dislodging food debris from interproximal tooth surfaces which are not accessible to the toothbrush. **rubber t.,** a slender pointed rubber device; usually, a rubber interdental tip.

tipping (tip'ing) 1. causing something to assume a slanted or sloping position. 2. a tooth movement in which its vertical position is altered, either occurring spontaneously or as a result of orthodontic therapy. See also UPRIGHTING. 3. cusp RESTORATION. **t. of cusp,** cusp RESTORATION.

tirebal (tēr-bahl') [Fr.] an instrument resembling a corkscrew, for extracting bullets.

tirefond (tēr-fo') [Fr.] an instrument like a corkscrew, for raising depressed portions of a bone.

Tisdale, W. K. see Sakati-Nyhan-Tisdale SYNDROME.

Tisercin trademark for *methotrimeprazine.*

tissue (tish'u) [Fr. *tissu*] an aggregation of similarly specialized cells and their elaborations, which have been differentiated and organized for the purpose of performing a particular function. A collection of tissues united for the express purpose of executing a specific function in the body, is known as an *organ*. See illustration. See also terms beginning HISTO-. **accidental t.,** a tissue growing in or upon a part to which it is foreign; it is either analogous or heterologous. **adenoid t.,** lymphoid t. **adipose t.,** connective tissue made up of fat cells in a meshwork of areolar tissue. Called also *fatty t.* **analogous t.,** an accidental tissue similar to one found normally in other parts of the body. **areolar t., areolar connective t.,** the principal type of connective tissue, made up largely of a ground substance in which the fibers are loosely arranged. Collagen is its dominant fiber type and reticular fibers are present almost exclusively in areas where it meets another tissue, e.g., the basement membrane, where the connective tissue meets epithelium. Fibroblasts and macrophages are the most common cell types, with mesenchymal and mast cells located near capillaries and leukocytes present only at a site of infection. Support, packing, repair, protection for nerves and blood and lymphatic vessels, and defense against invasion by foreign bodies are among its functions. In the oral cavity, it supports the epithelium of the lips, cheeks, floor of the mouth, palate, tongue, tonsils, and gingivae. Called also *loose connective tissue.* **basement t.,** the substance of a basement membrane, generally comprised exclusively of ground substance and reticular fibers. **bony t.,** bone, whether normal or of a soft tissue, which has become ossified. **bursal equivalent t.,** a component of the lymphoid system, whose identity is not known with certainty, analogous to the bursa of Fabricius in birds, which is considered to be the primary site of the origin of B-lymphocytes and to consist of gut-associated lymphoid tissue, fetal liver, and bone marrow. **cartilaginous t.,** the substance of the cartilages. **cellular t.,** areolar tissue with large interspaces. **chondroid t.,** a transitory type of embryonic cartilage that may persist throughout life to serve as a mechanical support for other structures in higher animals and often occurs in lower vertebrates. It is composed of vesicular cells provided with elastic capsules and having collagenous fibers in its interstitial substance. Called also *pseudocartilage, fibrohyaline t.,* and *vesicular supporting t.* **cicatricial t.,** scar t. **compact t.,** compact BONE. **t. conditioner,** tissue CONDITIONER. **connective t.,** the tissue which binds together and is the support of the various body structures. It is made up of fibroblasts, fibroglia, collagen fibrils, and elastic fibrils, and is derived from the mesoderm, and in a broad sense includes the collagenous, elastic, mucous, reticular, osseous, and cartilaginous tissue. Some also include the blood in this group of tissues. Connective tissue is classified according to concentration of fibers as loose (areolar) and dense, the latter having more abundant fibers than the former. **connective t., areolar** areolar t. **connective t., embryonic,** mesenchymal t. **connective t., loose** areolar t. **critical t.,** the tissue that reacts most unfavorably to radiation or attracts and absorbs specific radioisotopes. **t. culture,** tissue CULTURE. **elastic t., elastic t., yellow** connective tissue made up of yellow, elastic fibers, frequently massed into sheets. **embryonic connective t.,** mesenchymal t. **t. equivalent,** tissue EQUIVALENT. **extracellular t.,** the total of tissues and body fluids outside the cells, including the plasma and all its components, the extracellular fluid and its components, plus the intercellular and extracellular tissue solids, most notably the collagen, cartilage, bone, elastin, and other connective tissues of the body. **fatty t.,** adipose t. **fibrohyaline t.,** chondroid t. **fibrous t.,** the ordinary connective tissue made up largely of yellow or white fibers. **flabby t.,** hyperplastic t. (2). **glandular t.,** an aggregation of epithelioid cells that elaborate secretions. **granulation t.,** young, highly vascularized connective tissue with a component of acute inflammatory exudation, produced in the process of wound healing and forming a scar or cicatrix. It is composed of numerous minute red granules, which are formed in small amounts in wounds that heal by primary union and are more abundant in wounds that heal by secondary union. See also *scar t.* **gut-associated lymphoid t.,** lymphoid tissue associated with the gut, including the tonsils, Peyer's patches, lamina propria of the gastrointestinal tract, and appendix. Abbreviated *GALT*. See also B-lymphocytes, under LYMPHOCYTE, and lymphoid SYSTEM. **hard t.,** any tissue made up of a hard substance, such as bone. In dentistry, the term is often used in connection with the three hard-tissue components of a tooth: the enamel, cementum, and dentin. **hematopoietic t.,** tissue that takes part in

the production of the formed elements of the blood. **homologous t.,** tissue identical with another tissue in structural type. **hyperplastic t.,** 1. tissue affected by hyperplasia. 2. an overgrowth of tissue about the maxilla or mandible that is excessively movable, or more readily displaced than is normal. Called also *flabby tissue.* **indifferent t.,** areolar tissue found in the periodontal ligament in the interstitial spaces between the principal fiber bundles. **interdental t.,** the tissue located between the teeth, consisting of the gingiva, cementum, free gingival and transseptal fibers, and alveolar and supporting bone. See also gingival PAPILLA and interproximal SPACE. **interstitial t.,** the connective tissue between the cellular elements of a structure; the stroma. **intertubular t.,** a term, no longer valid, used to denote the dense tissue of dentin in which the dentinal tubules are embedded. **loose connective t.,** areolar t. **lymphadenoid t.,** tissue resembling that of a lymph node, including the spleen, bone marrow, tonsils, and the lymphatic tissue of other organs and mucous membranes. **lymphatic t.,** lymphoid t. **lymphoid t.,** a latticework of reticular tissue the interspaces of which contain lymphatic lymphocytes; it may be diffuse, or densely aggregated as in lymph nodules and nodes. Called also *adenoid t.* and *lymphatic t.* **mesenchymal t.,** embryonic connective tissue that differentiates into muscle, vascular and lymphatic channels, and other types of connective tissue, including cementum, pulp, and dentin. It is a primitive delicate tissue composed of reticular fibrils, mesenchymal cells, and ground substance. In definitive tissue, it may be found at capillary perithelium. **t. molding,** border MOLDING. **necrotic t.,** tissue undergoing necrosis, which is either dead or dying. **osseous t.,** the specialized tissue forming the bones. **osteogenic t.,** that part of the periosteum adjacent to bone and concerned with the formation of osseous tissue; any tissue capable of generating bone. **osteoid t.,** uncalcified bone tissue. **paraoral t.,** any tissue situated near or around the oral cavity, which is concerned with mastication, speech, respiration, ingestion of food, digestion, the sense of taste, deglutition, protection of the oral cavity, filtering and heating of inspired air, and the sense of smell. **paratransplantal t.,** gingival, periodontal, and alveolar bone tissue that surrounds a transplanted tooth. Called also *transplantal t.* **redundant t.,** fibrous inflammatory HYPERPLASIA. **reticular t.,** connective tissue consisting of reticular cells and fibers, usually occurring in the lymphatic tissue, myeloid tissue, spleen, and in the wall of the sinusoids of the liver. Called also *reticulum.* **scar t.,** the dense fibrous tissue forming a scar or cicatrix and derived from a granulation tissue. Called also *cicatricial t.* See also *granulation t.* **skeletal t.,** the bony, ligamentous, fibrous, and cartilaginous tissue forming the skeleton and its attachments. **soft t.,** any pliable nonosseous tissue. In dentistry, the term is often used to refer to the dental pulp. **subcutaneous t.,** subcutaneous FASCIA. **subcutaneous fatty t.,** PANNICULUS adiposus. **subjacent t.,** the structures that underlie or are in border contact with a denture base. **transplantal t.,** paratransplantal t. **vesicular supporting t.,** chondroid t. **yellow elastic t.,** elastic t.

tissular (tish'u-lar) pertaining to organic tissue.

titanium (ti-ta'ne-um) [named after the *Titans* of Greek mythology] a metallic element. Symbol, Ti; atomic number, 22; atomic weight, 47.90; melting point, 1675°C; specific gravity, 4.54; valences, 2, 3, 4; group IVB of the periodic table. Natural isotopes include 46–50; artificial isotopes include 43–45 and 51. It is a silvery solid or dark gray powder, insoluble in water and resistant to nitric acid, but attacked by hydrochloric and sulfuric acids and alkalies. Used chiefly in alloys, but also in x-ray tubes, chemical equipment, and various industrial products. Titanium alloys are used in dentistry, primarily in implant materials for various orthopedic purposes, having excellent corrosion resistance. Titanium is a nontoxic and bioinert substance, but, in powdered form, presents a serious fire and explosion hazard. **t. dioxide,** the anhydride of titanic acid, occurring as a white powder, TiO_2, which is soluble in sulfuric acid and alkalies, but not in water. Used as a pigment for paints and for artificial dentures, in radioactive decontamination of the skin, as a topical protectant in dusting powder, and in various industrial processes. Also used as a sunscreen for protecting the lips from sunlight. Called also *t. white, titanic anhydride,* and *titanic oxide.* Trademark: Unitane. **t. white,** t. dioxide.

titer (ti'ter) [Fr. *titre* standard] 1. the quantity of a substance required to bring about a reaction with a given volume of another substance, or the amount of one substance required to correspond with a given amount of another substance. 2. in solution, the concentration of a dissolved substance as determined by titration. 3. the solidification point of the fatty acids which have been liberated from the fat by hydrolysis. 4. the

TISSUE CLASSIFICATION AND HISTOGENESIS

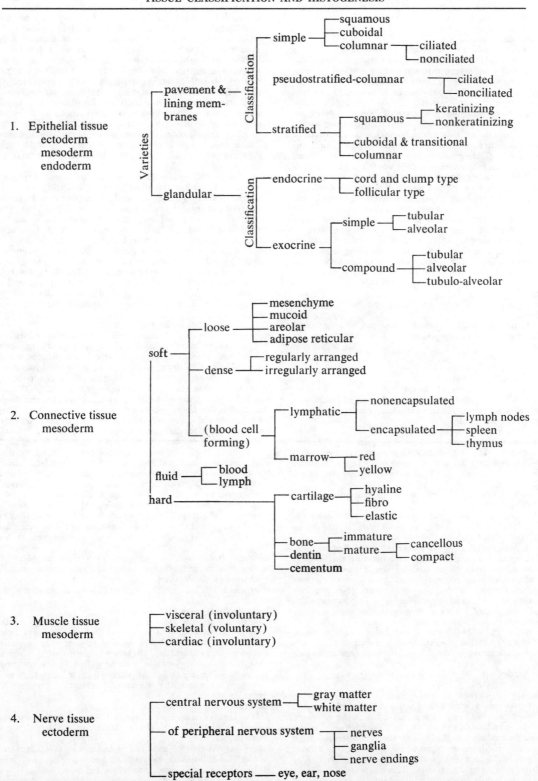

(From D. V. Provenza: Fundamentals of Oral Histology and Embryology. Philadelphia, Lippincott, 1972.)

number of grams of an element or compound in 1 ml of a standard solution. 5. the number of ml/l by which a normal solution differs from a standard. **agglutination t.,** the highest dilution of a serum which causes clumping of microorganisms or other particulate antigens.

title XIX see MEDICAID.

title XVIII see MEDICARE.

titrant (ti′trant) a standard solution used for titration.

titration (ti-tra′shun) [Fr. *titre* standard] the determination of the concentration of a substance through adding a standard solution of known volume and concentration until the reaction is completed, as indicated by color change or some other indicator. **chelatometric t.,** complexometric t. **colorimetric t.,** a method of determining hydrogen ion concentration by adding an indicator to the unknown and then comparing the color with a set of tubes containing this same indicator in solutions of known hydrogen ion concentration. **complexometric t.,** titration of a substance (e.g., the calcium in clear serum) with a complexing agent (e.g., ethylenediaminetetra-acetic acid); the endpoint of the titration is generally observed as a change in color of the solution. Called also *chelatometric t.* **Dean and Webb t.,** a test for measuring antibody in which varying dilutions of antigen are mixed with a constant quantity of antiserum; antibody activity is determined by the dilution in which flocculation occurs most rapidly, i.e., the end point. In this dilution, antigen and antibody are together at a ratio of optimal proportions. **potentiometric t.,** a method of determining hydrogen ion concentration by placing a hydrogen electrode of unknown solution and measuring the potential developed as compared with some standard electrode by means of a potentiometer.

titre (ti′ter) [Fr.] titer.

titrometry (ti-trom′ě-tre) [*titration* + Gr. *metron* measure] analysis by titration.

titubation (tit″u-ba′shun) [L. *titubatio*] the act of staggering. **lingual t.,** stuttering or stammering.

Tl thallium.

TLC total lung CAPACITY.

Tm thulium.

TMJ temporomandibular JOINT.

TMS thread mate system; see TMS PIN.

tobacco (to-bak′o) the dried and prepared leaves of *Nicotiana tabaccum,* a solanaceous plant, containing various alkaloids, the principal one being nicotine.

Tobradistin trademark for *tobramycin.*

tobramycin an antibacterial antibiotic derived from *Streptomyces tenebrarius,* O-3-amino-3-deoxy-α-D-glucopyranosyl-(1→6)-O-[2,6-diamino-2,3,6-trideoxy-α-D-ribohexopyranosyl-(1→4)]-2-deoxy-D-streptamine. Trademarks: Gernebcin, Obramycin, Tobradistin.

toco- [Gr. *tokos* childbirth] a combining form denoting relationship to childbirth, or labor.

tocol (to′kol) a colorless, viscous oil, 2-methyl-2(4,8,12-trimethyltridecyl)-6-chromanol. The tocol ring is the basic structural unit of tocopherols. Used as an antioxidant.

tocopherol (to-kof′er-ol) [*toco-* + Gr. *pherein* to bear + *-ol*] any of a group of compounds containing a hydroxy-bearing ring system and an isoprenoid side chain and having a tocol nucleus. Tocopherols, which have properties similar to those of vitamin E, are found naturally in certain oils and are also prepared synthetically. They occur in several forms: α- (see VITAMIN E), β-, γ-, and δ-tocopherol; all are antioxidants, and are necessary for normal growth and reproduction.

toe-in, toe-out (to′in, to′owt) an arch wire adjustment to cause buccal or lingual rotation of teeth, usually the molars.

Tofranil trademark for *imipramine hydrochloride* (see under IMIPRAMINE).

Togamycin trademark for *spectinomycin hydrochloride* (see under SPECTINOMYCIN).

Togaviridae (to″gah-vi′rĭ-de) [L. *toga* cloak + *virus* + *-idae*] a family of arboviruses with naked icosahedral nucleocapsids that are assembled in the cytoplasm, after which the envelope is acquired by budding through the cell membrane. Virions contain single-stranded (+)RNA and their diameters range from 40 to 60 nm; there are 32 to 42 capsomers in the virion. Four genera are recognized in the family: *Alphavirus, Flavivirus, Rubivirus,* and *Pestivirus.* There are two probable members of the family: the virus causing infectious arteritis of horses and lactic dehydrogenase virus.

togavirus (to″gah-vi′rus) any virus of the family Togaviridae.

toilet (toi′let) cleansing of a wound and the surrounding area. See also DEBRIDEMENT. **cavity t.,** the final step in cavity preparation,

consisting of freeing all angles and surfaces of debris and, often, medication and lining the cavity. The cleaning is usually accomplished with warm water and air or, sometimes, a 3 percent hydrogen peroxide solution alone or with a 5 percent sodium hypochlorite solution. Called also *cavity debridement.*

tolazamide (tol-az′ah-mīd) a sulfonylurea oral hypoglycemic agent, N-[[(hexahydro-1H-azepin - 1 - yl)amino]carbonyl - 4 - methylbenzenesulfonamide, occurring as a white, odorless, crystalline powder that is soluble in chloroform and acetone, slightly soluble in ethanol, and very slightly soluble in water. Used in the treatment of certain types of diabetes mellitus. Trademarks: Diabewas, Norglycin, Tolinase, Tolonase.

tolazoline hydrochloride (tol-az′o-lēn) a vasodilator agent with weak β-adrenergic blocking activity, 4,5-dihydro-2-(phenylmethyl)-1H-imidazole, occurring as a white crystalline powder that is freely soluble in water and ethanol. Its sympathomimetic properties are responsible for heart stimulation associated with some increase of blood pressure. Used chiefly in the treatment of vasospastic diseases. Side reactions may include flushing, tingling, formication, nausea, vomiting, diarrhea, abdominal discomfort, gastric hyperacidity, cardiac arrhythmia, tachycardia, and mydriasis. Trademarks: Benzidazol, Prefaxil, Priscoline, Vasodil.

tolbutamide (tol-bu′tah-mīd) a sulfonylurea oral hypoglycemic agent, 1-butyl-(*p*-tolylsufonyl) urea, occurring as a white, odorless, slightly bitter crystalline powder that is soluble in ethanol and chloroform, but not in water. It stimulates the beta islet cells of the pancreas in the release of insulin and inhibits phosphodiesterase, which preserves cyclic AMP, thus influencing glycogenolysis in certain tissues. Used in the treatment of diabetes mellitus. Gastrointestinal disorders, hypoglycemic shock, headache, tinnitus, paresthesia, hypersensitivity, and alcohol intolerance are the principal side effects. Leukopenia, thrombocytopenia, pancytopenia, agranulocytosis, and cholestatic jaundice may occur. Called also *D-860.* Trademarks: Diabuton, Dolipol, Orinase, Rastinon, Tolbutone, Willbutamide.

Tolbutone trademark for *tolbutamide.*

tolerance (tol′er-ans) [L. *tolerantia*] the ability to endure without ill effect exposure to mental or physical stress or large doses of a drug, and to exhibit decreasing effect to continued use of the same dose of a drug. **high-zone t.,** acquired immunological tolerance due to the presence of supraoptimal concentrations of an antigen that leads to the abolition or reduction in the cellular or humoral response to that specific antigen. **immunologic t.,** a condition in which, under certain conditions, a foreign antigen fails to elicit the formation of antibody or a cellular sensitivity in the recipient to the same antigen; in a normal nontolerant animal the same dose would induce humoral or cell-mediated immunity. It may be a consequence of contact with antigen in fetal or early postnatal life, or may follow the administration of nonoptimal doses of certain antigens to adults. The induction of tolerance to a given antigen does not affect immunological reactions to unrelated antigens. Called also *immunological paralysis.* **low-zone t.,** immunological tolerance due to the presence of suboptimal concentrations of antigens that results in the failure of or in decreased antibody production or cellular hypersensitivity. **self-t.,** immunological tolerance to autoantigens.

tolerogen (tol″er-o-jen) an antigen which is capable of inducing a state of immune tolerance. Called also *tolerogenic antigen.* Cf. immunogenic ANTIGEN.

tolerogenic (tol″er-o-jen′ik) capable of inducing immunologic tolerance.

Tolinase trademark for *tolazamide.*

tolnaftate (tol-naf′tāt) an antifungal agent, methyl-(3-methylphenyl)carbomathioic acid O-2-naphthalenyl ester, occurring as a white, odorless, fine powder that is soluble in acetone and chloroform, slightly soluble in ether, ethanol, and methanol, and insoluble in water. Used in the treatment of superficial mycoses of the skin. Hypersensitization to other drugs is its principal side effect. Trademarks: Sporiine, Tinactin, Tinaderm.

Tolonase trademark for *tolazamide.*

Tolosa-Hunt syndrome [Eduardo *Tolosa,* American physician, born 1936; William E. *Hunt,* American physician] see under SYNDROME.

toluene (tol′u-ēn) an aromatic hydrocarbon, C_7H_8, presenting a colorless, flammable liquid with benzene-like odor, which is obtained from tolu and other resins and from coal tar. Used as a solvent and in the production of various organic compounds. It is somewhat less toxic than benzene, but may cause macrocytic anemia and a necrotic reaction. Called also *methylbenzene* and *toluol.*

toluol (tol′u-ol) toluene.

-tome [Gr. *tomē* a cutting] a word termination signifying (*a*) an instrument for cutting or (*b*) a segment.

Tomes, granular layer of, process of ameloblast [Sir John *Tomes*, English dentist, 1815–1895; he demonstrated the absence of blood circulation in dentin and enamel, proving that inflammatory processes are not involved in dental caries] see under LAYER and PROCESS.

Tomil trademark for *promazine*.

tomo- [Gr. *tomē* a cutting] a combining form denoting relationship to a cutting, or to a designated layer, as might be achieved by cutting or slicing.

tomograph (to'mo-graf) an apparatus for moving an x-ray source in one direction as the film is moved in the opposite direction; thus showing in detail a predetermined plane of tissue while blurring or eliminating detail in other planes. See TOMOGRAPHY.

tomography (to-mog'rah-fe) [*tomo-* + Gr. *graphein* to write] a special radiographic technique whereby the film and x-ray source are rotated in opposite directions in such a way that, while structures lying in a predetermined plane of tissue are shown in detail, the image of tissues and structures in other planes is eliminated or blurred. Various specialized techniques have been developed, including *planigraphy, laminography, stratigraphy,* and *radiotomy.* Called also *body section radiography* and *body section roentgenography.* **circular t.,** that in which the x-ray source and film move in a circular pattern. **elliptical t.,** that in which the x-ray source and the film move in an elliptical pattern. **linear t.,** that in which the x-ray source and the film move in the same plane. **polydirectional-hypocycloidal t.,** that in which the x-ray source and the film move parallel to each other in a three-lobed "pretzel-like" pattern.

Tomsilen trademark for *demecarium bromide* (see under DEMECARIUM).

-tomy [Gr. *tomē* a cutting] a word termination signifying the operation of cutting, or incision.

Tonaril trademark for *tripelennamine*.

tone (tōn) [Gr. *tonos;* L. *tonus*] 1. the normal state of tension of healthy tissue such as muscle. See also TENSION and TONUS. 2. the pitch or character of a sound. **muscle t.,** firmness of skeletal muscles; passive resistance of muscles to stretch.

tongue (tung) [L. *lingua;* Gr. *glōssa*] 1. a movable muscular organ attached to the floor of the mouth and serving as the principal organ of the sense of taste and as an accessory organ of speech, mastication, and deglutition. Its inferior smooth surface is covered by a simple undifferentiated mucosa. A sickle-shaped fold in the midline connects its underside to the floor of the mouth, with two fimbriated folds on each side running laterally and posteriorly. The dorsal surface is divided into two lateral halves by a shallow median sulcus which ends at the root of the tongue in the foramen cecum, from which the sulcus terminalis runs toward the front and sides of the tongue. The vallate papillae cover the superior surface immediately anterior to the foramen cecum and sulcus terminalis; the fungiform papillae are found chiefly on the sides and near the apex; the filiform papillae are present on the anterior two-thirds; and the simple papillae cover the entire surface. The extrinsic muscles include the genioglossus, hyoglossus, chondroglossus, styloglossus, and palatoglossus. The intrinsic muscles include the superior and inferior longitudinalis, transversus, and verticalis. The serous glands (*Ebner's glands*) occur at the back of the tongue, near the taste buds, which are scattered at irregular intervals over the entire surface. The lingual branch of the mandibular nerve, chorda tympani branch of the facial nerve, lingual branch of the glossopharyngeal nerve, superior laryngeal nerve, and hypoglossal nerve provide the innervation. Called also *glossa* and *lingua* [NA]. See also words beginning GLOSSO- and LINGUO-. See illustration. 2. any organ or structure having a shape similar to that of the tongue. See also LINGULA. **adherent t.,** a tongue that is abnormally attached to the sides and floor of the mouth; ankyloglossia. **amyloid t.,** macroglossia due to amyloidosis. **antibiotic t.,** glossitis due to adverse effects of antibiotic therapy. **baked t.,** the dry, brown tongue of typhoid fever. **bald t.,** Möller's GLOSSITIS. **bald t., Sandwith's,** Sandwith's bald t. **bald t. of pernicious anemia,** Hunter's GLOSSITIS. **beefy t.,** erythematous and/or atrophic glossitis, characterized by red, irregular ulcerations on the dorsal surface of the tongue. See also Hunter's GLOSSITIS. **bifid t.,** one divided in its anterior part by a longitudinal fissure, due to faulty fusion. A partially cleft tongue is characterized by a deep groove in the midline of the dorsal surface. Called *cleft t., double t.,* and *diglossia.* **black t.,** a benign condition of the tongue characterized by hypertrophy of the filiform papillae. The color of the elongated papillae varies from yellowish white to brown or black, depending upon staining with tobacco, foods, drugs, etc., resembling stubby hair and giving the tongue a furry appearance. Called also

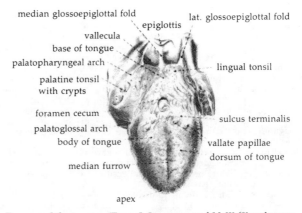

Dorsum of the tongue. (From J. Langman and M. W. Woerdeman: Atlas of Medical Anatomy. Philadelphia, W. B. Saunders Co., 1978.)

hairy t., anthracosis linguae, glossitis parasitica, glossophytia, glossotrichia, hyperkeratosis linguae, keratomycosis linguae, lingua nigra, lingua villosa nigra, melanoglossia, melanotrichia linguae, melanotrichosis linguae, nigrites linguae, and *parasitic glossitis.* **burning t.,** a burning sensation in the tongue. Called also *glossopyrosis.* **cardinal t.,** one whose surface is denuded of epithelium, giving it a bright red appearance. **cerebriform t.,** fissured t. **choreic t.,** a condition characterized by abrupt, snakelike protrusion and withdrawal of the tongue occurring in chorea. **cleft t.,** bifid t. **coated t.,** one covered with a coat of whitish or yellowish material consisting of desquamated epithelium, debris, bacteria, fungi, etc., which is readily removed by scraping. **cobble-stone t.,** a condition marked by interstitial glossitis with hypertrophy of the papillae and a verrucous white coating on the tongue, such as seen in riboflavin deficiency. Formerly used to denote syphilitic glossitis with leukoplakia. **crocodile t.,** fissured t. **curling t.,** a condition characterized by the ability to curl the tip of the tongue, which is observed chiefly in the Caucasian population, and is probably genetically transmitted as a multifactorial trait. See also *tubing t.* **dorsum of t.,** the superior surface of the tongue, having an irregular mucosal covering because of the presence of numerous papillae. Called also *dorsum linguae* [NA]. See TONGUE (1) and illustration. **dotted t.,** stippled t. **double t.,** bifid t. **earthy t.,** one coated with a deposit of rough, calcareous matter. **enamel t.,** enamel SPUR. **encrusted t.,** a heavily coated tongue. **fern leaf t.,** one with a central furrow having lateral branches. **filmy t.,** one marked with symmetrical whitish patches. **fissured t.,** the presence on the dorsal surface of the tongue of numerous furrows, which may radiate outwardly from the median raphe. The condition appears to be transmitted as an autosomal dominant trait. When associated with recurrent facial paralysis and cheilitis granulomatosa, it is known as *Melkersson-Rosenthal syndrome.* Called also *cerebriform t., crocodile t., fluted t., furrowed t., grooved t., plicated t., ribbed t., scrotal t., wrinkled t.,* and *lingua plicata.* **flat t.,** a condition in which the borders of the tongue cannot be rolled, caused by paralysis of the transverse lingual muscle in congenital syphilis. **fluted t.,** fissured t. **furred t.,** one with papillae so changed as to give the mucous membrane the appearance of whitish fur. **furrowed t.,** fissured t. **geographic t.,** benign migratory GLOSSITIS. **glazed t., glossy t.,** Möller's GLOSSITIS. **grooved t.,** fissured t. **t. pressure,** tongue PRESSURE. **hairy t.,** black t. **inflamed t.,** see GLOSSITIS. **lobulated t.,** a congenital condition marked by a secondary lobe arising from the surface of the tongue. **magenta t.,** the magenta-colored tongue seen in riboflavin deficiency. **mappy t.,** see benign migratory GLOSSITIS. **painful t.,** see GLOSSODYNIA. **painful burning t.,** glossopyrosis. **parrot t.,** the dry, horny tongue of low fever, which cannot be protruded. **plicated t.,** fissured t. **raspberry t.,** one exhibiting a deep red color and glistening smooth surface with numerous edematous, hyperemic papillae, seen in the advanced stages of stomatitis scarlatina. **ribbed t.,** fissured t. **Sandwith's bald t.,** an extremely clean tongue sometimes seen in the late stages of pellagra. **scrotal t.,** fissured t. **slick t., smooth t.,** Möller's GLOSSITIS. **smokers' t.,** oral leukoplakia involving the tongue. **stippled t.,** one on which each papilla is covered with a separate white patch of epithelium. Called also *dotted t.* **strawberry t.,** one exhibiting a white coating and small, red, edematous, hyperemic papillae, seen in the early stages of stomatitis scarlatina. **sulcated t., fissured t. t. thrusting,** tongue THRUSTING. **tubing t.,** a condition characterized by the ability to curl the lateral borders of the tongue, which is observed chiefly in the Caucasian population, and is probably genetically transmitted as a multifactorial trait. Information suggests occurrence in identical twins. It may also be learned. See also *curling t.* **varnished t.,** Möller's GLOSSITIS. **white t.,** a condition in which the papillae and epithelium of the tongue have a dull white color. **wooden t.,** actinomycosis. **wrinkled t.,** fissured t.

tongue-tie (tung'ti) restricted movement of the tongue. See ANKYLOGLOSSIA.

tonic (ton'ik) [Gr. *tonikos*] 1. producing and restoring the normal tone. 2. characterized by continuous tension. 3. formerly, a class of medicinal preparations believed to have the power of restoring normal tone to tissue.

tonicity (to-nis'ĭ-te) 1. the normal condition of tone or tension. 2. the ionic concentration of a solution compared to blood plasma.

tono- [Gr. *tonos* tension] a combining form denoting relationship to tone or tension.

tonofibril (ton'o-fi"bril) an organoid made up of microtubular fibrils up to 100 Å in diameter. Their free ends are variously oriented in the cytoplasm of cells, especially epithelial cells, and pass through the protoplasmic projection, ending as spindles or bullous terminals which form desmosomes. Their function is believed to bind the cells together and to serve as the precursor of permanent keratin.

tonofilament (ton"o-fil'ah-ment) a slender threadlike organelle in the cytoplasm of cells. In the basal cells of the epithelium, tonofilaments appear to be diffusely arranged in the cytoplasm, running from the nuclear region to the periphery of the cell; some terminating along the dermoepithelial junctions, others ending in the intercellular bridges. In the prickle-cell layer of the epidermis, some are organized into tonofibrils.

tonometer (to-nom'ĕ-ter) [*tono-* + Gr. *metron* measure] an instrument for measuring tension or pressure.

tonsil (ton'sil) [L. *tonsilla*] a small mass of tissue, especially of lymphoid tissue; specifically, the palatine tonsil. Called also *amygdala* and *tonsilla.* **buried t.,** submerged t. **faucial t.,** palatine t. **lingual t.,** an aggregation of lymphoid tissue on the floor of the oropharyngeal passageway, at the root of the tongue, immediately behind the vallate papillae. There are about 25–30 such aggregations. Each tonsil is an ovoid nodule covered by stratified squamous epithelium with a central crypt on its surface. It usually has a germinal center, and the lymphoid tissue consists of the supporting stroma of reticular fibers and the parenchyma. The cellular component of the lymphoid tissue consists of the lymphocytes, their parent stem cells, mast cells, and, when inflamed, granular leukocytes. Embryologically, it appears at about the fifth month of fetal life, but epithelial invaginations resulting in formation of crypts do not occur until after birth and organization of nodular structures is not completed until the age of five to six years. It is believed to act as a source of phagocytes which destroy oral bacteria. Called also *accessory amygdala, amygdala accessoria,* and *tonsilla lingualis* [NA]. **Luschka's t.,** pharyngeal t. **palatine t.,** one of the two bilateral, almond-shaped structures, about 2.5 cm in length and 1 cm in width, situated in the pharyngeal folds, parallel with the pharyngeal fauces and between the palatoglossal and palatopharyngeal arches. It is made up of lymphoid tissue covered by epithelium. Its surface has a pitted or cribriform appearance due to entrances to excretory ducts and some 25 to 30 crypts, which vary from shallow invaginations to deep and branched terminals; surrounding the entrances to the crypts are mounds of lymphoid tissue (*lymphatic nodules*). The ascending palatine artery, the ascending pharyngeal, descending palatine, and dorsalis linguae arteries, and the tonsillar branch of the facial artery are the principal sources of blood supply. The glossopharyngeal and maxillary nerves provide the innervation. The tonsil is usually divided into 10 or more lobules separated by septa or trabeculae which provide the framework for the blood vessels and nerves. It is believed to act as a source of phagocytes which destroy oral bacteria. Obstruction of lumens in the crypts by cellular debris is the principal cause of infection. Called also *faucial t.* and *tonsilla palatina* [NA]. **pharyngeal t.,** a mass of lymphoid tissue in the roof and posterior wall of the nasopharynx, presenting a fold about 3 cm in length. It is covered by ciliated pseudostratified columnar epithelium similar to that in the respiratory system, but patches

of stratified squamous epithelium may also be present. A 2 mm thick layer of diffuse and nodular lymphatic tissue is found under the epithelium. A thin capsule containing elastic networks separates it from the surrounding tissue. Small glands on the outside discharge their ducts through the lymphatic tissue and empty into the furrows or onto the free surface of the folds. Unlike the lingual and palatine tonsils, no crypts are present. The formation of lymphoid masses begins during the fourth month of fetal life, but its organization is not completed until shortly before birth and, sometimes, not until after birth. Maximum development is reached in childhood and involution begins at the age of 15 years; in adults, it is usually found in an atrophic condition. Formation of new lymphocytes is the only known function. Hypertrophied pharyngeal glands are known as *adenoids.* Called also *Luschka's t., third t., adenoid, tonsilla pharyngea* [NA], and *gland of neck.* **submerged t.,** a palatine tonsil that is shrunken and atrophied and is partly or entirely hidden by the palatoglossal arch. Called also *buried t.* **third t.,** pharyngeal t.

tonsilla (ton-sil'ah) [L.] tonsil. **t. lingua'lis** [NA], lingual TONSIL. **t. palati'na** [NA], palatine TONSIL. **t. pharyn'gea** [NA], pharyngeal TONSIL.

tonsillar (ton'sĭ-lar) [L. *tonsillaris*] pertaining to a tonsil; amygdaline.

tonsillectomy (ton"sĭ-lek'to-me) [tonsil + Gr. *ektomē* excision] surgical removal of a tonsil or tonsils. Called also *amygdalectomy* and *antiotomy.* See also TONSILLOTOMY.

tonsillitis (ton"sĭ-li'tis) [tonsil + -*itis*] inflammation of the tonsils, especially the palatine tonsils; amygdalitis. **caseous t.,** lacunar t. **catarrhal t., acute,** a form associated with acute catarrhal pharyngitis, in which the tonsils are red and swollen. Called also *erythematous t.* **catarrhal t., chronic,** a form attended by permanent hypertrophy, and usually requiring tonsillectomy. **diphtherial t.,** diphtheria. **erythematous t.,** acute catarrhal t. **follicular t.,** that which especially affects the tonsillar crypts (formerly referred to as follicles). Called also *angina follicularis.* **lacunar t.,** a form in which the tonsillar crypts are filled with plugs of caseous matter. Called also *caseous t.* **t. len'ta,** a chronic form associated with prolonged sepsis. **lingual t.,** a form involving the lingual tonsils. Called also *preglottic t.* **mycotic t.,** that due to a fungal infection; tonsillomycosis. **parenchymatous t., acute,** inflammation of the whole substance of the tonsils, associated with suppuration. Called also *suppurative t.* **preglottic t.,** lingual t. **pustular t.,** that associated with formation of pustules. **streptococcal t.,** septic sore THROAT. **superficial t.,** that in which inflammation involves only the mucous membrane over the tonsils. **suppurative t.,** acute parenchymatous t. **Vincent's t.,** that caused by Vincent's organism (*Fusobacterium plauti-vincenti*).

tonsilloadenoidectomy (ton"sil-o-ad"ĕ-noi-dek'to-me) combined tonsillectomy and adenoidectomy.

tonsillolith (ton-sil'o-lith) [tonsil + Gr. *lithos* stone] a concretion or calculus in a tonsil. Called also *amygdalolith.*

tonsillomoniliasis (ton-sil"o-mo"nĭ-li'ah-sis) mycotic tonsillitis due to infection with *Candida (Monilia).*

tonsillomycosis (ton-sil'o-mi-ko'sis) fungal infection of the tonsils; mycotic tonsillitis.

tonsillopathy (ton"sĭ-lop'ah-the) [tonsil + Gr. *pathos* disease] any disease of the tonsils; amygdalopathy.

tonsilloprive (ton"sĭ-lo-prīv) [tonsil + L. *privare* to deprive] having the tonsils removed; due to removal or absence of the tonsils.

tonsillotome (ton-sil'o-tōm) a knife used in tonsillotomy. Called also *amygdalotome.*

tonsillotomy (ton"sĭ-lot'o-me) [tonsil + Gr. *tomē* cutting] incision of a tonsil; the surgical removal of a part of a tonsil. Called also *amygdalotomy.* See also TONSILLECTOMY.

tonus (to'nus) [L.; Gr. *tonos*] tone, specifically muscle tone. See also PRESSURE and TONUS. **decreased t.,** HYPOTONIA and HYPOTONICITY. **increased t.,** HYPERTONIA and *hypertonicity (2).* **muscle t.,** a slight constant tension of a healthy muscle, which serves to maintain constant position of the body or organs and to obviate the muscle taking up slack when it enters contraction.

tooth (tooth), pl. *teeth* [L. *dens;* Gr. *odous*] any of the hard calcified structures set in the alveolar processes of the mandible and maxilla for mastication of food, or a similar structure. Each tooth consists of three parts — the *crown,* the portion exposed above the gingival line, having a central cavity which contains the dental pulp; the *neck,* the constricted region between the crown and the root; the *root,* the portion embedded within the alveolus and attached to the periodontal membrane. The solid part includes *dentin,* forming most of the tooth and resembling true bone; *enamel,* a very hard inorganic substance, covering the crown; and *cementum,* covering the root. The soft tissue,

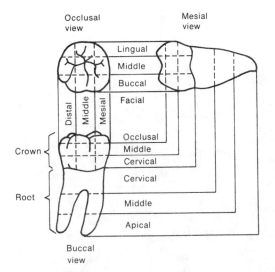

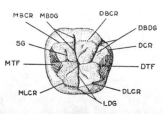

Division into thirds. For descriptive and comparative purposes each tooth surface is divided into imaginary thirds. (From H. O. Torres and A. Ehrlich: Modern Dental Assisting. 2nd ed. Philadelphia, W. B. Saunders Co., 1980.)

Mandibular right first molar — occlusal aspect. *DBCR,* distobuccal cusp ridge; *DBDG,* distobuccal developmental groove; *DCR,* distal cusp ridge; *DTF,* distal triangular fossa (shaded area); *DLCR,* distolingual cusp ridge; *LDG,* lingual developmental groove; *MBCR,* mesiobuccal cusp ridge; *MBDG,* mesiobuccal developmental groove; *MLCR,* mesiolingual cusp ridge; *MTF,* mesial triangular fossa (shaded area); *SG,* a supplemental groove. (From R. C. Wheeler: Dental Anatomy, Physiology and Occlusion. 5th ed. Philadelphia, W. B. Saunders Co., 1974.)

the *dental pulp,* is composed of richly vascularized and innervated connective tissue. Called also *dens.* See also DENTITION. For related terms, see those beginning DENT- and ODONT-. See table of *Chronology of Human Dentition.* See also dental CHART. **t. absence,** anodontia. **abutment t.,** one that has been selected to support a bridge on the basis of the total surface area of a healthy attachment apparatus. Called also *abutment support* and *tooth support.* See ABUTMENT. **accessional teeth,** the permanent molars, so called because they do not supplant deciduous predecessors in the dental arch. Cf. *succedaneous teeth.* **accessory t.,** a supernumerary tooth which does not resemble a normal tooth. **acrylic resin t.,** an artificial tooth made of acrylic resin. **t. adnexa,** tooth ADNEXA. **anatomic teeth,** 1. artificial teeth which duplicate the anatomic forms of natural teeth. 2. teeth which have prominent pointed or rounded cusps on the masticating surfaces and which are designed to occlude with the teeth of the opposing denture of natural dentition. **anchor t.,** see ANCHORAGE (4). **t. angle,** see illustration of *Tooth Angles* at ANGLE. **ankylosed t.,** submerged t. **anterior teeth,** teeth in the anterior portion of each dental arch; the four incisors (two central and two lateral incisors) and the two canines in either jaw. Called also *labial teeth* and *morsal teeth.* **artificial t.,** one fabricated for use as a substitute for a natural tooth in a prosthesis, usually made of porcelain or resin. **avulsed t.,** one that has been abnormally displaced from its alveolar support, usually through trauma. Called also *evulsed t.* **baby teeth,** deciduous teeth. **t. banding,** tooth BANDING. **bicuspid t.,** one having two cusps; see *premolar t.* **blue t.,** see Delta Dental Plans, under PLAN. **t. bonding,** tooth BONDING. **t. brushing,** toothbrushing. **buccal teeth,** posterior teeth. **t. bud,** tooth BUD. **canine t.,** the third tooth to the left and to the right of the midline of either jaw, situated between the second incisor and the premolar teeth. It is a succedaneous tooth, being the strongest and most stable of all teeth, with a single long root and a pointed cusp, resembling the tooth of Carnivora for tearing the flesh of prey (hence the name *canine*). The projec-

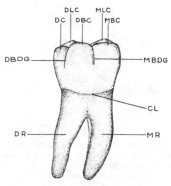

Mandibular right first molar—buccal aspect. *CL,* cervical line; *DBC,* distobuccal cusp; *DBDG,* distobuccal developmental groove; *DC,* distal cusp; *DLC,* distolingual cusp; *DR,* distal root; *MBC,* mesiobuccal cusp; *MBDG,* mesiobuccal developmental groove; *MLC,* mesiolingual cusp. (From R. C. Wheeler: Dental Anatomy, Physiology and Occlusion. 5th ed. Philadelphia, W. B. Saunders Co., 1974.)

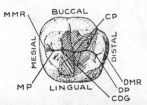

Mandibular right first molar—occlusal aspect. Central fossa (shaded area); *CDG,* central developmental groove; *CP,* central pit; *DMR,* distal marginal ridge; *DP,* distal pit; *MMR,* mesial marginal ridge; *MP,* mesial pit. (From R. C. Wheeler: Dental Anatomy, Physiology and Occlusion. 5th ed. Philadelphia, W. B. Saunders Co., 1974.)

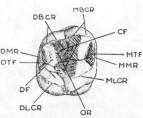

Maxillary right first molar—occlusal landmarks. *CF,* central fossa (shaded area); *DBCR,* distobuccal cusp ridge; *DF,* distal fossa; *DLCR,* distolingual cusp ridge; *DMR,* distal marginal ridge; *DTF,* distal triangular fossa (shaded area); *MBCR,* mesiobuccal cusp ridge; *MLCR,* mesiolingual cusp ridge; *MMR,* mesial marginal ridge; *MTF,* mesial triangular fossa (shaded area); *OR,* oblique ridge. (From R. C. Wheeler: Dental Anatomy, Physiology and Occlusion. 5th ed. Philadelphia, W. B. Saunders Co., 1974.)

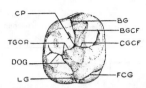

Maxillary right first molar—occlusal aspect—developmental grooves. *BG*, buccal groove; *BGCF*, buccal groove of central fossa; *CGCF*, central groove of central fossa; *CP*, central pit; *DOG*, distal oblique groove; *FCG*, fifth cusp groove; *LG*, lingual groove; *TGOR*, transverse groove of oblique ridge. (From R. C. Wheeler: Dental Anatomy, Physiology and Occlusion. 5th ed. Philadelphia, W. B. Saunders Co., 1974.)

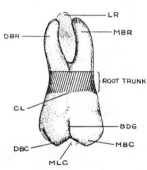

Maxillary right first molar—buccal aspect. *BDG*, buccal developmental groove; *CL*, cervical line; *DBC*, distobuccal cusp; *DBR*, distobuccal root; *MBC*, mesiobuccal cusp, *MBR*, mesiobuccal root; *LR*, lingual root; *MLC*, mesiolingual cusp. (From R. C. Wheeler: Dental Anatomy, Physiology and Occlusion. 5th ed. Philadelphia, W. B. Saunders Co., 1974.)

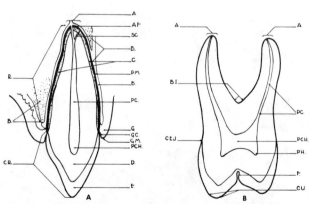

Schematic drawings of cross sections of an anterior and a posterior tooth. *1*, Anterior tooth. *A*, apex; *AF*, apical foramen; *SC*, supplementary canal; *C*, cementum; *PM*, periodontal membrane: *B*, bone; *PC*, pulp canal; *G*, gingiva; *GC*, gingival crevice; *GM*, gingival margin; *PCH*, pulp chamber; *D*, dentin; *E*, enamel; *CR*, crown; *R*, root. *2*, Posterior tooth: *A*, apices; *PC*, pulp canal; *PCH*, pulp chamber; *PH*, pulp horn; *F*, fissure; *CU*, cusp; *CEJ*, cementoenamel junction; *B1*, bifurcation of roots. (From R. C. Wheeler: Dental Anatomy, Physiology and Occlusion. 5th ed. Philadelphia, W. B. Saunders Co., 1974.)

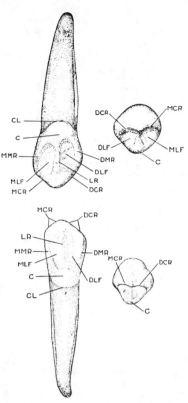

Right canine—lingual and incisal aspects. *Top*, maxillary. *Bottom*, mandibular. *C*, cingulum; *CL*, cervical line; *DCR*, distal cusp ridge; *DLF* distolingual fossa; *DMR*, distal marginal ridge; *LR*, lingual ridge; *MCR*, mesial cusp ridge; *MLF*, mesiolingual fossa; *MMR*, mesial marginal ridge. (From R. C. Wheeler: Dental Anatomy, Physiology and Occlusion. 5th ed. Philadelphia, W. B. Saunders Co., 1974.)

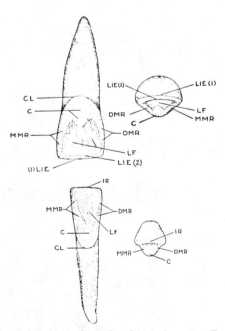

Right central incisor — lingual and incisal aspects. *Top*, maxillary. *Bottom*, mandibular. C, cingulum; CL, cervical line; DMR, distal marginal ridge; IR, incisal-ridge; LF, lingual fossa; LIE (1), labioincisal edge and LIE (2), linguoincisal edge (these [1] and [2] border the incisal ridge); MMR, mesial marginal ridge. (From R. C. Wheeler: Dental Anatomy, Physiology and Occlusion. 5th ed. Philadelphia, W. B. Saunders Co., 1974.)

Right first premolar — mesial and occlusal aspects. *Top,* maxillary. *Bottom,* mandibular. BC, buccal cusp; BCR, buccal cervical ridge; BR, buccal root; BTR, buccal triangular ridge; CDG, central developmental groove; CL, cervical line; DBCR, distobuccal cusp ridge; DLCR, distolingual cusp ridge; DMR, distal marginal ridge; DTF, distal triangular fossa; LC, lingual cusp; LR, lingual root; MBCR, mesiobuccal cusp ridge; MCA, mesial contact area; MDD, mesial developmental depression; MLCR, mesiolingual cusp ridge; MLDG, mesiolingual developmental groove; MMDG, mesial marginal developmental groove; MMR, mesial marginal ridge; MTF, mesial triangular fossa (shaded area). (From R. C. Wheeler: Dental Anatomy, Physiology and Occlusion. 5th ed., Philadelphia, W. B. Saunders Co., 1974.)

tion of the root into the body produces the canine prominence upon the surface of the alveolar arch. Because of their infraorbital situation, the maxillary canines are sometimes referred to as the "eye teeth." The contact areas vary in the mandibular and maxillary canines, the contact being nearer the incisal edge in the mandibular canine. The root of the mandibular tooth is shorter and narrower mesiodistally than that of the maxillary. Their function consists of assisting the incisors and premolars

in cutting and crushing food. Because of their "corner" position in the mouth, they have an important esthetic role. They serve as units of the natural dental arch and sometimes assist in stabilizing replacements for lost teeth in prosthetic dentistry. Called also *cuspid t., canine, cuspid, cynodont,* and *dens caninus.* See illustration. **cheek teeth,** posterior teeth. **cheoplastic teeth,** artificial teeth attached to a cheoplastic base without pins. See CHEOPLASTY. **t. conditioner,** acid ETCHANT. **conical t.,** peg t. **connate t.,** geminate t. **corner t.,** the third incisor on either side of each jaw in the horse. **cross-bite teeth,** artificial posterior teeth designed to accommodate the modified buccal cusps of the maxillary teeth to be positioned in the fossae of the mandibular teeth. **cross-pin teeth,** artificial teeth in which the pins are inserted horizontally. **crowding of teeth,** CROWDING of teeth. **cuspid t.,** canine t. **cuspless t.,** any tooth deprived of a cusp; particularly an artificial tooth designed without cuspal prominences on the occlusal surface. **cutting t.,** incisor t. **t. decay,** dental CARIES. **deciduous teeth,** the 20 teeth of the first dentition, which are shed and replaced by the permanent teeth. They begin to calcify at about the fourth month of fetal life, and near the end of the sixth month they all have begun to develop. The first incisors appear at about the age of six and a half months; they are followed by the second incisors a half month later; and, within one and a half months, by the maxillary incisors. The deciduous molars begin eruption at one year and the deciduous canines approximately four months later. All the deciduous teeth are expected to erupt by the time the child is two and a half years of age. See tables of *Chronology of Human Dentition* and *Measurements of the Deciduous Teeth of Man.* The deciduous dentition formula (one side) is as follows:

$$I\frac{2}{2}\,C\frac{1}{1}\,M\frac{2}{2} = 10$$

where I = *incisor;* C = *canine;* M = *molar.* Called also *baby teeth, first teeth, milk teeth, primary teeth, temporary teeth, deciduous dentition, dentes decidui, first dentition, primary dentition,* and *temporary dentition.* See also illustration at dental CHART. **dead t.,** 1. nonvital t. 2. a term used inaccurately to refer to a pulpless tooth. **t. depression,** INTRUSION (3). **Goslee t.,** an interchangeable tooth attached to a metal base. **devital t.,** 1. nonvital t. 2. a term used inaccurately to refer to a pulpless tooth. **diatoric teeth,** artificial teeth with holes in their base into which the denture base material flows and, when processed, attaches the teeth to the base. Called also *pinless teeth.* **dilacerated t.,** see DILACERATION. **drifting t.,** wandering t. **t. elevator,** dental ELEVATOR. **embedded t.,** one

MEASUREMENTS (in mm) OF THE DECIDUOUS TEETH OF MAN (Averages Only)

Maxillary Teeth	Length Over All	Length of Crown	Length of Root	Mesiodistal Diameter of Crown	Mesiodistal Diameter at Cervix	Labiolingual Diameter of Crown	Labiolingual Diameter at Cervix
First Incisor	16.0	6.0	10.0	6.5	4.5	5.0	4.0
Second Incisor	15.8	5.6	11.4	5.1	3.7	4.0	3.7
Canine	19.0	6.5	13.5	7.0	5.1	7.0	5.5
First Molar	15.2	5.1	10.0	7.3	5.2	8.5	6.9
Second Molar	17.5	5.7	11.7	8.2	6.4	10.0	8.3
Mandibular Teeth							
First Incisor	14.0	5.0	9.0	4.2	3.0	4.0	3.5
Second Incisor	15.0	5.2	10.0	4.1	3.0	4.0	3.5
Canine	17.0	6.0	11.5	5.0	3.7	4.8	4.0
First Molar	15.8	6.0	9.8	7.7	6.5	7.0	5.3
Second Molar	18.8	5.5	11.3	9.9	7.2	8.7	6.4

(Adapted from G. V. Black: Dental Anatomy. Philadelphia, S. S. White Mfg. Co., 1902.)

CHRONOLOGY OF HUMAN DENTITION

	Tooth		Formation of Enamel Matrix and Dentin Begins	Amount of Enamel Matrix Formed at Birth	Enamel Completed	Emergence into Oral Cavity	Root Completed
Primary dentition	Maxillary	First incisor	4 mo. in utero	Five-sixths	1½ mo.	7½ mo.	1½ yr.
		Second incisor	4½ mo. in utero	Two-thirds	2½ mo.	9 mo.	2 yr.
		Canine	5 mo. in utero	One-third	9 mo.	18 mo.	3¼ yr.
		First molar	5 mo. in utero	Cusps united	6 mo.	14 mo.	2½ yr.
		Second molar	6 mo. in utero	Cusp tips still isolated	11 mo.	24 mo.	3 yr.
	Mandibular	First incisor	4½ mo. in utero	Three-fifths	2½ mo.	6 mo.	1½ yr.
		Second incisor	4½ mo. in utero	Three-fifths	3 mo.	7 mo.	1½ yr.
		Canine	5 mo. in utero	One-third	9 mo.	16 mo.	3¼ yr.
		First molar	5 mo. in utero	Cusps united	5½ mo.	12 mo.	2¼ yr.
		Second molar	6 mo. in utero	Cusp tips still isolated	10 mo.	20 mo.	3 yr.
Permanent dentition	Maxillary	First incisor	3–4 mo.		4–5 yr.	7–8 yr.	10 yr.
		Second incisor	10–12 mo.		4–5 yr.	8–9 yr.	11 yr.
		Canine	4–5 mo.		6–7 yr.	11–12 yr.	13–15 yr.
		First premolar	1½–1¾ yr.		5–6 yr.	10–11 yr.	12–13 yr.
		Second premolar	2–2¼ yr.		6–7 yr.	10–12 yr.	12–14 yr.
		First molar	At birth	Sometimes a trace	2½–3 yr.	6–7 yr.	9–10 yr.
		Second molar	2½–3 yr.		7–8 yr.	12–13 yr.	14–16 yr.
		Third molar	7–9 yr.		12–16 yr.	17–21 yr.	18–25 yr.
	Mandibular	First incisor	3–4 mo.		4–5 yr.	6–7 yr.	9 yr.
		Second incisor	3–4 mo.		4–5 yr.	7–8 yr.	10 yr.
		Canine	4–5 mo.		6–7 yr.	9–10 yr.	12–14 yr.
		First premolar	1¾–2 yr.		5–6 yr.	10–12 yr.	12–13 yr.
		Second premolar	2¼–2½ yr.		6–7 yr.	11–12 yr.	13–14 yr.
		First molar	At birth	Sometimes a trace	2½–3 yr.	6–7 yr.	9–10 yr.
		Second molar	2½–3 yr.		7–8 yr.	11–13 yr.	14–15 yr.
		Third molar	8–10 yr.		12–16 yr.	17–21 yr.	18–25 yr.

(Adapted from S. N. Bhaskar (ed.): Orban's Oral Histology and Embryology. 8th ed. St. Louis, The C. V. Mosby Co., 1976; adapted from W. H. G. Logan and R. Kronfeld: Development of the human jaws and surrounding structures from birth to age fifteen. J.A.D.A., 20:379, 1933; modified by McCall and Schour. Copyright by the American Dental Association. Reprinted by permission.)

which is unerupted because of a lack of eruptive force. See also *unerupted t.* **t. eruption**, see under ERUPTION. **t. eruption chronology**, see table of *Chronology of Human Dentition.* **evulsed t.**, avulsed t. **eye t.**, an upper canine tooth. **first teeth**, deciduous teeth. **Fournier teeth**, Moon's teeth. **fused teeth**, union of two or more individual teeth that may be partial, or may involve all portions of the teeth. See also *concrescence* and FUSION (4). **geminate t.**, one with a single root or root canal, but with two completely or incompletely separated crowns, resulting from invagination of a single tooth germ, causing incomplete formation of two teeth. Called also *connate t.* **ghost teeth**, odontodysplasia. **golden t.**, a hoax, whereby a gold tooth was claimed to have erupted in a 7-year-old child in Schiverdnitz, Silesia, in 1593, proved later to be a natural tooth covered with a gold sheath. It is believed to be the first gold crown ever produced. **green teeth**, green-stained teeth usually observed in hyperbilirubinemia. **hag teeth**, upper medial incisors that are widely separated. **hereditary brown opalescent teeth**, AMELOGENESIS imperfecta. **hereditary dark teeth**, hereditary opalescent teeth, DENTINOGENESIS imperfecta. **Horner's teeth**, incisor teeth that are horizontally grooved owing to a deficiency of enamel. **Hutchinson's teeth**, a tooth abnormality seen in congenital syphilis, characterized by convergence of both lateral margins toward the incisal edge, giving the permanent incisors a screwdriver-like shape, sometimes associated with notching of the incisal edges or depressions in the labial surfaces immediately above the cutting edge. When associated with interstitial keratitis and deafness due to eighth cranial nerve lesions, it is known as *Hutchinson's triad.* Called also *Hutchinson's incisors* and *screwdriver teeth.* **hypersensitive t.**, one abnormally sensitive to temperature changes, sweet or sour foods, tactile stimulation, or percussion, due to gingival recession or periodontal or pulpal lesions. See also hypersensitive PULPALGIA. **impacted t.**, one prevented from erupting by a physical barrier. See also *unerupted t.* and dental IMPACTION. **incisive t.**, incisor t. **incisor t.**, any of the eight frontal teeth (four maxillary and four mandibular), having a sharp incisal edge for cutting food and a single root, which occurs in man as both a deciduous and a permanent tooth. Called also *cutting t. incisive t., dens acutus, dens incisivus,* and *incisor.* See illustration. See INCISOR for additional entries. **incisor t., first**, the first tooth to the

left and to the right of the midline in either jaw, having a sharp cutting edge and a single root, with the mesial surfaces of the right and left teeth in contact at the midline. Its function consists of cutting food and producing distinct speech. Because of their central location, they have an important esthetic role. The maxillary first incisor is stronger and larger than its antagonist, the maxillary one being the widest mesiodistally of the anterior teeth, while the mandibular is the smallest of the permanent dentition. The form of the permanent first incisors corresponds to that of their deciduous predecessors. The maxillary first incisor has a single conical root which is usually straight or deflected slightly to the distal side; the root of the mandibular one is usually deflected slightly to the distal side and tends to be slender mesiodistally, being bulky labiolingually and usually as long as that of the maxillary incisor. Called also *central incisor* and *medial incisor.* **incisor t., second**, the second tooth to the left and to the right of the midline in either jaw, situated between the first incisor and the canine tooth; it supplements the first incisor in function and bears a close resemblance to it. The maxillary second incisor is smaller in all dimensions (except in root length) than the first incisor, while the mandibular incisor is somewhat larger than its central neighbor. The form of the permanent second incisors corresponds to that of their deciduous predecessors. Called also *lateral incisor t., lateral incisor,* and *second incisor.* **incisor t., central**, incisor t., first. **incisor t., first**, incisor t. **incisor t., lateral**, incisor t., second. **inferior teeth**, mandibular teeth. **interchangeable t. of Steele**, Steele's t. **kinked t.**, a dilacerated tooth. See DILACERATION. **labial teeth**, anterior teeth. **lateral incisor t.**, incisor t., second. **lower teeth**, mandibular teeth. **malacotic teeth**, teeth that are soft in structure and are abnormally susceptible to caries. **malposed t.**, one out of its normal position. **mandibular teeth**, the teeth of the mandible. Called also *inferior teeth* and *lower teeth.* **maxillary teeth**, the teeth of the maxilla. Called also *superior teeth* and *upper teeth.* **t. measurement**, tooth MEASUREMENT. **metal insert t.**, an artificial tooth, usually of acrylic resin, containing an inserted ribbon of metal or a cutting blade in the occlusal surface, with one edge exposed; sometimes used in removable dentures. **t. migration**, tooth MIGRATION. **milk teeth**, 1. natal teeth. 2. neonatal teeth. **molar teeth**, the most posterior teeth on either side of each jaw, totaling eight in the

MEASUREMENTS (in mm) OF THE PERMANENT TEETH OF MAN (Average Only)

Maxillary Teeth	Length of Crown	Length of Root	Mesio-distal Diameter of Crown°	Mesio-Distal Diameter at Cervix	Labio- or Bucco-lingual Diameter	Labio- or Bucco-lingual Diameter at Cervix	Curva-ture of Cervical Line – Mesial	Curva-ture of Cervical Line – Distal
First Incisor	10.5	13.0	8.5	7.0	7.0	6.0	3.5	2.5
Second Incisor	9.0	13.0	6.5	5.0	6.0	5.0	3.0	2.0
Canine	10.0	17.0	7.5	5.5	8.0	7.0	2.5	1.5
First Premolar	8.5	14.0	7.0	5.0	9.0	8.0	1.0	0.0
Second Premolar	8.5	14.0	7.0	5.0	9.0	8.0	1.0	0.0
First Molar	7.5	b 12 l 13	10.0	8.0	11.0	10.0	1.0	0.0
Second Molar	7.0	b 11 l 12	9.0	7.0	11.0	10.0	1.0	0.0
Third Molar	6.5	11.0	8.5	6.5	10.0	9.5	1.0	0.0
Mandibular Teeth								
First Incisor	9.0†	12.5	5.0	3.5	6.0	5.3	3.0	2.0
Second Incisor	9.5†	14.0	5.5	4.0	6.5	5.8	3.0	2.0
Canine	11.0	16.0	7.0	5.5	7.5	7.0	2.5	1.0
First Premolar	8.5	14.0	7.0	5.0	7.5	6.5	1.0	0.0
Second Premolar	8.0	14.5	7.0	5.0	8.0	7.0	1.0	0.0
First Molar	7.5	14.0	11.0	9.0	10.5	9.0	1.0	0.0
Second Molar	7.0	13.0	10.5	8.0	10.0	9.0	1.0	0.0
Third Molar	7.0	11.0	10.0	7.5	9.5	9.0	1.0	0.0

*The sum of the mesiodistal diameters, both right and left, which gives the arch length, is: maxillary 128 mm., mandibular 126 mm.

†Lingual measurement approximately 0.5 mm. longer.

(Adapted from R. C. Wheeler: Dental Anatomy, Physiology and Occlusion. 5th ed. Philadelphia, W. B. Saunders Co., 1974.)

deciduous dentition (2 on each side, upper and lower), and usually 12 in the permanent dentition (three on each side, upper and lower). They are grinding teeth, having large crowns and broad chewing surfaces. Called also *dentes molares* and *molars*. See illustration. **molar t., first,** the sixth tooth to the left and to the right of the midline in either jaw, situated between the second premolar and the second molar. It is the largest tooth in the dentition, the mandibular one being the larger of the two, having a broad surface for the grinding and crushing of food. It has a well-developed crown, the maxillary molar having four large cusps and a fifth supplemental cusp (cusp of Carabelli), which is often poorly developed and has little physiological significance, and the mandibular molar having five well-developed cusps. The maxillary first molar has three large roots, the lingual being the longest, and the mandibular one has two large, broad roots. Called also *first molar* and *sixth-year molar*. **molar t., second,** the seventh tooth to the left and to the right of the midline in either jaw, situated between the first and third molars. Anatomically and physiologically, it is quite similar to the first molar, except for being somewhat smaller. The maxillary molar may have three or four cusps, but rarely a fifth cusp. The three roots of the maxillary tooth are close together at their apices. The mandibular second molar usually shows four cusps of nearly equal size and two roots which are smaller than those of the first molar, but as well separated at the apices.

Called also *second molar* and *twelfth-year molar*. **molar t., third,** the eighth and last tooth on either side of the dental arch in both the maxilla and mandible, situated behind the second molar. It supplements the second molar in function, being sometimes similar to it in form, but is generally much smaller, having an underdeveloped crown and root. These teeth show more variation in development than any of the other teeth. Most commonly, the crown of the maxillary tooth, when viewed from the occlusal aspect, is heart-shaped, having a very small and poorly developed distolingual cusp; it may have one to eight roots, but they are usually fused together, tapering at the apex and functioning as a single root. The mandibular molar may have four or five cusps, which are not well developed; its roots are fused together but divide near the apex to form two distinct apices. Called also *wisdom t., dens sapiens, dens serotinus,* and *third molar*. **Moon's teeth,** small, domed first molars observed in patients with congenital syphilis. Called also *Fournier teeth* and *Moon's molars*. **morsal teeth,** anterior t. **mottled teeth,** mottled ENAMEL. **mulberry t.,** mulberry MOLAR. **Mummery's pink t.,** tooth resorption, internal; see under RESORP-TION. **natal teeth,** prededuous teeth. **neonatal teeth,** teeth that erupt within the first month of life. Called also *milk teeth* and *neonatal dentition*. **nonanatomic teeth,** artificial teeth the occlusal surfaces of which are especially designed on the basis of engineering concepts, without regard to the features of natural teeth. **nonrestorable t.,** a tooth having a clinical crown damaged by disease processes, trauma, or faulty dental procedures to the point where prosthetic restoration is no longer practical. **nonstrategic t.,** a tooth that is considered as not being essential for denture support in prosthetic restoration. **nonvital t.,** a tooth incapable of response to normal stimuli or clinical testing procedures. Not uncommonly, but inaccurately, used to refer to a *pulpless tooth.* Called also *dead t.* and *devital t.* **peg t., peg-shaped t.,** one having a conical form, whose sides converge or taper together incisally, instead of being parallel or diverging mesially and distally; a condition frequently observed in the maxillary lateral incisor, due to faulty development of the tooth germ, and found in ectodermal dysplasia and other disorders and occasionally in normal children. Autosomal dominant transmission is suspected. Called also *conical t.* **permanent teeth,** the 32 teeth of the second dentition, which begin to appear in man at about six years of age. The first to appear are the first molars, followed by the mandibular central and lateral incisors, maxillary central incisors, maxillary lateral incisors, mandibular canines, first premolars, second premolars, maxillary canines, second molars, third molars. They take their position posterior to the deciduous teeth and erupt in succession, whenever the jaws grow sufficiently to accommodate them. Exfoliation of the deciduous teeth is brought about by resorption of their roots, and the succedaneous permanent teeth take their place. See tables of *Chronology of Human Dentition* and *Measurements of the Permanent Teeth of Man.* The permanent dentition formula (one side) is as follows:

$$I\frac{2}{2}\,C\frac{1}{1}\,P\frac{2}{2}\,M\frac{3}{3} = 16$$

where I = *incisor;* C = *canine;* P = *premolar;* M = *molar.* Called also *dentes permanentes, permanent dentition,* and *secondary dentition.* See also illustration at dental CHART. **t. pick,** toothpick. **pink t., pink t. of Mummery,** tooth resorption, internal; see under RESORPTION. **pinless teeth,** diatoric teeth. **plastic t.,** an artificial tooth constructed of synthetic resins. **t. position,** tooth POSITION. **posterior teeth,** the teeth on either side of each jaw, distal to the canine teeth, including the premolar and molar teeth. Called also *buccal teeth* and *cheek teeth.* **postpermanent teeth,** teeth that have erupted after extraction of permanent teeth. Some result from eruption of retained or embedded teeth and others develop from buds of the dental lamina beyond the permanent tooth germ, thus being identified with the supernumerary teeth. Called also *postpermanent dentition* and *third dentition.* **predeciduous teeth,** teeth that are present at birth. They may be well formed and normal in all respects or may represent hornified epithelial structures without roots, found on the gingivae over the crest of the ridge, arising from accessory buds of the dental lamina ahead of the deciduous buds or from buds of the accessory dental lamina. Called also *milk teeth, natal teeth,* and *predeciduous dentition.* The presence of such teeth is known as *dentia praecox.* **premature teeth,** deciduous teeth that erupt prior to the end of the third month of life, or permanent teeth that erupt prior to the end of the fourth year of life. The presence or eruption of such teeth is known as *dentia praecox.* Called also *precocious* or *premature dentition.* See also *predeciduous teeth.* **premolar teeth,** the eight permanent teeth, two on either side in each jaw, between the canines and the molars, serving for grinding and crushing food; the upper premolars have two cusps (bicuspid) but the lower have from one to three. They are succedaneous to the deciduous molar teeth. Called also *bicuspid teeth, bicuspids, dentes premolars,* and *premolars.* In zoology, they include all teeth which succeed the deciduous molars regardless of the number to be succeeded. See illustration. **premolar t., first,** the fourth tooth on either side of the median line in the mandible and maxilla, whose function consists of grinding and crushing food. It is a succedaneous tooth situated between the canine and the second premolar, being somewhat shorter than the canine and about the same size as the second premolar. Its crown is compressed mesiodistally (anteroposteriorly), and has two cusps, a buccal and lingual, the buccal being larger. The maxillary premolar is usually larger than its antagonist. It usually has two roots and in some instances, a single root with two pulp canals. Called also *first premolar* and *two-pointed premolar.* **premolar t., second,** the fifth tooth to the left and to the right of the median line in either jaw, situated between the first premolar and the first molar teeth. It is somewhat smaller than the neighboring

first molar, both teeth having the same form and function. Called also *second premolar.* **primary teeth,** deciduous teeth. **pulpless t.,** one from which the pulp has been extirpated. Not uncommonly, but inaccurately, called *dead t., devital t.,* and *nonvital t.* **rake teeth,** teeth that are widely separated. **replaced t.,** an artificial tooth which takes the place of a natural one. Called also *supplied t.* **rootless teeth,** dentinal DYSPLASIA. **t. resorption,** tooth RESORPTION. **rotated t.,** one that has been turned on its long axis, having an altered position in relation to the adjacent and opposing teeth and to its basal alveolar process. **sclerotic teeth,** teeth that are hard in structure and resistant to caries. **screwdriver teeth,** Hutchinson's teeth. **sensitive t.,** see *hypersensitive t.* and hypersensitive PULPALGIA. **shell t.,** a condition characterized by dysplasia of the dentin, associated with essentially normal enamel, thus resulting in an extremely large pulp chamber and root canals giving the affected tooth the appearance of a shell. **sickle t.,** a dilacerated tooth. See DILACERATION. **t. size discrepancy,** tooth size DISCREPANCY. **snaggle t.,** one out of proper line with the others. **t. socket,** dental ALVEOLUS. **split t.,** vertical fracture of the crown and/or root of a tooth. Called also *vertical tooth fracture.* **Steele's t., Steele's interchangeable t.,** an artificial tooth, usually a bicuspid or molar, baked with slots of standard sizes, so that a tooth from the same mold may be used as a replacement. Called also *interchangeable t. of Steele.* **stomach t.,** a mandibular canine. **straight-pin teeth,** artificial teeth in which the pins are inserted vertically. **strategic t.,** any tooth considered as essential for denture support in prosthetic restoration. **submerged t.,** a deciduous tooth, usually a second mandibular molar, which has undergone resorption and has become ankylosed to the bone, thus preventing its exfoliation and subsequent replacement by a permanent tooth. It appears to be submerged below the level of occlusion in relation to the adjacent permanent teeth. The cause is unknown but the occurrence of submerged teeth appears to have a familial tendency and is probably a nonsexlinked trait; trauma or infection also has been considered an etiologic factor. Called also *ankylosed t.* **succedaneous t., successional teeth,** the permanent teeth that have deciduous predecessors in the dental arch, compressing the permanent incisors, canines, and premolars. Cf. *accessional teeth.* **superior teeth,** maxillary teeth. **supernumerary t., supplemental t.,** one in excess of the number normally present in the jaw, which usually causes malposition of adjacent teeth or prevents their eruption. Supernumerary teeth may resemble the teeth of the group to which they belong, or may bear little resemblance to them; they may be erupted or impacted. See also MESIODENS, PARAMOLAR, and PREMOLAR. **superstructure t.,** an acrylic, porcelain, or metal artificial tooth retained in the superstructure of a subperiosteal implant, which establishes occlusion with a tooth from the opposite arch. **supplied t.,** replaced t. **temporary teeth,** deciduous teeth. **t. torsion,** tooth TORSION. **tube teeth,** artificial teeth having a vertical, cylindrical aperture from the center of the base up into the body of the tooth, into which a pin may be placed or cast for attachment of the tooth to the denture base. **Turner's t.,** enamel hypoplasia of a single tooth, most commonly one of the permanent maxillary incisors or a maxillary or mandibular premolar, resulting from local infection or trauma. Called also *Turner's hypoplasia.* **twin teeth,** gemination. **unerupted t.,** one that failed to erupt. The presence of multiple unerupted permanent teeth is sometimes referred to as *pseudoanodontia.* See also *embedded t.* and *impacted t.* **upper teeth,** maxillary teeth. **vital t.,** one in which the nerve and vascular supply is intact. **wandering t.,** one that drifts from its normal position in the dental arch, usually into an adjacent edentulous space, or as a result of loss of proximal support, loss of functional antagonists, occlusal traumatic tooth relationship, inflammatory and retrograde changes in the attachment apparatus, and oral habits. Called also *drifting t.* See also tooth MIGRATION. **wandering of t., pathologic,** pathologic tooth MIGRATION. **t. wear,** tooth WEAR. **wisdom t.,** the tooth most distal to the midline on either side in each jaw, so called because it is the last of the permanent teeth to erupt. See *molar t., third.* **t. within a tooth,** DENS in dente. **zero-degree teeth,** artificial posterior teeth having no cusp angles in relation to their horizontal occlusal surfaces.

toothache (tōōth'ak) pain in a tooth; odontalgia. Called also *dentagra.*

tooth-borne (tōōth'born) supported entirely by the teeth; said of a prosthesis or part of a prosthesis entirely supported by the abutment teeth.

toothbrush (tōōth-brush) a brush designed for cleaning the teeth, usually with a brushing surface 1.0″ to 1.25″ long and 5/16″ to 3/8″ wide, two to four rows, five to twelve tufts per row. The bristles are usually made of nylon or hog bristle (natural bristle), and may be grouped in separate tufts in rows or evenly distributed throughout. The surface of the brush may be rounded or cut flat. Bristle hardness is proportional to the square of the bristle diameter and inversely proportional to the square of bristle length. Bristle diameters in common use by adults range from 0.007″ (soft), and 0.012″ (medium), to 0.014″ (hard). **Bass' t.,** a soft toothbrush with a straight handle, nylon bristles 0.007″ in diameter, 13/32″ long, with rounded ends, arranged in three rows of tufts, six evenly spaced tufts per row, with 80 to 86 filaments per tuft. For children, the brush is softer (0.005″) with shorter (11/32″) bristles. Called also *Bass' brush.* **electric t.,** powered t. **interproximal t.,** one so designed that its bristles reach the interproximal tooth areas. Called also *interproximal brush.* **multituft t.,** one in which the bristles are evenly distributed throughout the brush, and containing more bristle than other types. **Oral-B t.,** trademark for a narrow, two-row brush for reaching spaces between the teeth and gingivae in the sulcus area. **powered t.,** one that is electrically powered, having an arcuate motion, or a back-and-forth reciprocal action, a combination of both, or a modified elliptical motion. Called also *electric t.* **t. trauma,** toothbrush TRAUMA.

toothbrushing (tŏŏth-brush′ing) brushing of the teeth, using a toothbrush and dentifrice, for the purpose of cleaning the exposed surfaces of the teeth. **Bass' method of t.,** a method of toothbrushing in which the bristles are pointed apically and directed at a 45° angle to the teeth so that the tips of the bristles enter the gingival sulcus, then the brush is moved with a slight vibratory motion. See illustration. **Charters' method of t.,** the brush is placed on the tooth at a 45° angle with the bristles pointed toward the crown. The brush is then moved along the

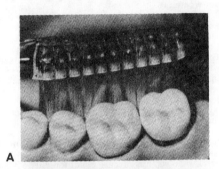

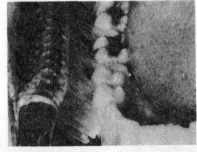

Bass' method of toothbrushing. *A*, Application of the brush to the lingual surface of the mandibular posterior teeth. *B*, Application of the brush on the buccal surface of the mandibular posterior teeth. (From J. F. Pritchard: Advanced Periodontal Disease. 2nd ed. Philadelphia, W. B. Saunders Co., 1972.)

tooth surface until the sides of the bristles engage the marginal gingiva, preserving the 45° angle. The brush is twisted lightly, flexing the bristles so that the sides press on the marginal gingiva, the edges touching the tooth and some bristles extending interproximally. The head of the brush is rotated without dislodging the bristles, maintaining the bent position, while counting to 10. The brush is moved to the adjacent area and the procedure is repeated, continuing area by area on the entire vestibular surface, and then changing to the oral surface. To cleanse the occlusal surface, the bristle tips are forced gently into the pits and fissures and the brush is activated with a rotary motion, without changing the position of the bristles, repeating area by area until all chewing surfaces are cleansed. **crevicular method of t.,** a method of toothbrushing with the ends of the bristles in the gingival crevices. **Fones' method of t.,** the brush is pressed firmly against the teeth and gingiva with the handle of the brush parallel to the line of occlusion and the bristles

perpendicular to the vestibular tooth surface. The brush is then moved in a rotary motion with the jaws closed and the spherical pathway of the brush confined by the limits of the mucobuccal fold. **maxillofacial and facioproximal surface t.,** Bass' method of t. **maxillopalatal and palatoproximal surface t.,** starting with the palatal and proximal surfaces in the maxillary left molar area, brushing continues around the arch to the right molar area. The brush is positioned horizontally in the molar and premolar areas. To reach the palatal surface of the anterior teeth, the brush is inserted vertically and the end bristles are pressed into the gingival sulci and interproximally at about a 45° angle to the long axis of the teeth and the brush is activated with repeated short strokes. If the shape of the arch permits, the brush is inserted horizontally between the canines with the bristles angulated into the gingival sulci of the anterior teeth. **occlusal surface t.,** pressing the bristles firmly on the occlusal surfaces with the ends deep into the pits and fissures, while the brush is activated with short back-and-forth strokes, counting to 10. The brushing advances section by section until all the posterior teeth are cleaned. **physiologic method of t.,** brushing in a manner comparable to the pathway of food in mastication, consisting of gentle sweeping motions, starting on the teeth and progressing over the marginal gingivae and attached gingival mucosa. **scrub-brush technique of t.,** a method in which the bristles are applied at right angles to the teeth over the dentogingival junction and moved back and forth with short, horizontal strokes. **Stillman's method of t.,** the brush is placed with the bristle ends resting partly on the gingiva and partly on the cervical portion of the teeth, being oblique to the long axis of the tooth and directed apically. Pressure is applied laterally against the marginal gingiva so as to produce a perceptible blanching. The brush is removed to permit the blood to return to the gingiva. Pressure is applied several times, and the brush is given a slight rotary motion, with the bristle ends remaining in position. The process is repeated on all the tooth surfaces, starting in the maxillary molar area and proceeding systematically around the mouth. To reach the oral surfaces of the maxillary and mandibular anterior area, the handle of the brush is parallel to the occlusal plane, with two or three tufts of the bristles engaging the teeth and gingiva. The occlusal surfaces of the molars and premolars are cleaned with the bristles perpendicular to the occlusal plane and penetrating deeply into the sulci and interproximal embrasures. **Stillman's method of t., modified,** the brush is placed at the mucogingival line, with the bristles pointed away from the crown and moved with a stroking motion along the attached gingiva, marginal gingiva, and tooth surface. The handle is rotated toward the crown and vibrated as the brush is moved.

Toothkeeper a proprietary program of oral hygiene, based on the teaching of dental health procedures to school children by their teachers who have been especially trained by dentists in modern techniques of preventive dentistry.

toothpaste (tŏŏth-pāst) dentifrice.

toothpick (tŏŏth-pik) any small tapering sliver of wood or other material designed for removing food particles and cleaning the interdental spaces. Written also *tooth pick.*

toothpowder (tŏŏth-pow′der) dentifrice.

topalgia (to-pal′je-ah) [Gr. *topos* place + *algos* pain + *-ia*] localized pain.

topaz (to′paz) a mineral consisting of a silicate of aluminum, $Al_2SiO_4F_2$; a precious stone occurring as colorless or varicolored crystals, having a white, reddish, or yellowish hue. **oriental t.,** corundum.

Topazone trademark for *furazolidone.*

Topco see under DENTIFRICE.

tophi (to′fi) [L.] plural of *tophus.*

tophus (to′fus), pl. *to′phi* [L. "porous stone"] 1. a focal deposit of chalky white urates in tissue, usually surrounded by a zone of inflammatory hyperemia, seen in gout. 2. dental CALCULUS.

topical (top′i-k′l) [Gr. *topikos*] pertaining to or acting upon a particular surface area, as a topical anti-infective applied to a certain area of the skin and affecting only the area to which it is applied.

Topicale liquid, ointment see under LIQUID and OINTMENT.

Topinard's angle, line [Paul *Topinard*, French physician and anthropologist, 1830–1911] see ophryospinal ANGLE, and see under LINE.

Topitracin trademark for *bacitracin.*

topo- [Gr. *topos* place] a combining form meaning place.

Topocaine trademark for *cyclomethycaine sulfate* (see under CYCLOMETHYCAINE).

topography (to-pog'rah-fe) [*topo-* + Gr. *graphein* to write] the description of an anatomical region or of a special part.

Toraloy trademark for preproportioned *dental amalgam* (see under AMALGAM) in disposable capsules, containing 47.25 to 49.53 percent mercury.

torcular (tor'ku-lar) [L. "wine-press"] a hollow, or expanded area. **t. Heroph'ili,** CONFLUENCE of sinuses.

Torecan trademark for *thiethylperazine maleate* (see under THIETHYLPERAZINE).

Toresten trademark for *thiethylperazine maleate* (see under THIETHYLPERAZINE).

tori (to'ri) [L.] plural of *torus*.

Toritron trademark for a variable speed *mechanical triturator* (see under TRITURATOR), operating in the range of 4500 to 7300 rpm.

Tornwaldt see THORNWALDT.

tornwaldtitis (torn"vahlt-i'tis) an old term for Thornwaldt's BURSITIS.

torque (tork) [L. *torquere* to twist] 1. a rotatory force causing a part of a structure to twist about an axis. See also TORSION. 2. the rotation of a tooth on its long axis, especially moving the root apex in a buccal or lingual direction through the application of force produced by torsion within the arch wire.

torquing (tork'ing) the twisting of a tooth into position, as in the correction of malposition.

torr (tor) [named after Evangelista *Torricelli*] a unit of pressure, being 1/760 of 1 atmosphere, or the average pressure exerted by the earth's atmosphere at sea level; a pressure which will support a column of mercury 1 mm high at 0° C and standard gravity in the Torricelli barometer.

Torre, Douglas P. [American physician, born 1919] see Bloom's SYNDROME (Bloom-Torre-Machacek syndrome).

Torricelli barometer [Evangelista *Torricelli*, Italian mathematician, 1608–1647] see under BAROMETER.

torsion (tor'shun) [L. *torsio; torquere* to twist] 1. the act or process of twisting; turning or rotating about an axis. 2. a type of mechanical stress, whereby the external forces (load) twist an object about its axis. Called also *torsive force* and *torsive stress.* See also TORQUE. **negative t.,** rotation in a counterclockwise direction. **positive t.,** rotation in a clockwise direction. **tooth t.,** rotation of a tooth on its long axis in the socket.

torsiversion (tor"si-ver'zhun) [L. *torsio* to twist + *vertere* to turn] the turning or rotation on a perpendicular or long axis; said of a tooth.

torticollis (tor"ti-kol'is) [L. *tortus* twisted + *collum* neck] abnormal twisting of the neck resulting in an unnatural position of the head, due to unequal contraction of the muscles of the neck. Called also *wryneck*. **nasopharyngeal t.,** torticollis in nontraumatic subluxation of the atlas secondary to nasopharyngeal diseases. Synovial effusion is responsible for relaxation of the joint capsule, leading to lesions of the transverse ligament and the atlas. It usually occurs after tonsillectomy or inflammation of the nasal cavity. Called also *Grisel's disease.*

tortua (tor'tu-ah) [L.] agony; torture. **t. fa'cies,** trigeminal NEURALGIA.

tortuous (tor'tu-us) twisted; winding; full of turns.

Torula (tor'u-lah) [L. "roll"] former name for *Cryptococcus.*

toruli (tor'u-li) [L.] plural of *torulus.*

torulopsis (tor'u-lop'sis) European BLASTOMYCOSIS.

torulosis (tor'u-lo'sis) European BLASTOMYCOSIS.

torulus (tor'u-lus), pl. *tor'uli* [L., dim. of *torus*] a small elevation; a papilla.

torus (to'rus), pl. *to'ri* [L. "a round swelling," "protuberance"] 1. a bulging projection, a swelling; used in anatomical nomenclature as a general term to designate such a protuberance. 2. doughnut-shaped surface or solid formed by the revolution of a circle about any axis other than its diameter. **t. fronta'lis,** a protuberance in the middle line of the root of the nose, on the external surface of the skull. **t. levato'rius,** the mucosal fold covering the levator veli palatini muscle in the lateral wall of the nasal part of the pharynx. **t. mandibula'ris,** an exostosis of bone on the lingual surface, probably transmitted as a genetic trait. **t. occipita'lis,** a rounded edge occasionally seen on the occipital bone in the region of the superior nuchal line. **t. palati'nus** [NA], a slowly-growing, flat-based bony protuberance sometimes found in the midline of the hard palate. Varieties of torus palatinus include a flat type with a marked median groove, a lancet- or spindle-shaped type, a large type that fills the palate as far as the alveolar process, and a type that tapers down in front to merge with the palate and may extend behind

on the palatine bone as a distinct knob. It is probably transmitted as a genetic trait. **t. tuba'rius** [NA], the projecting posterior lip of the pharyngeal opening of the auditory tube.

Toryn trademark for *caramiphen ethanedisulfonate* (see under CARAMIPHEN).

Toti's operation [Addeo *Toti*, Italian ophthalmologist, born 1861] dacryocystorhinostomy.

touch (tuch) [L. *tactus*] 1. the sense by which contact with objects gives evidence as to certain of their qualities. 2. palpation or exploration with the fingers or hand.

toughness (tuf'ness) 1. the quality of strength and durability. 2. the ability of a material to resist fracture. Measured by calculating the total area under the total stress-strain curve. See also HARDNESS.

Touraine, Henry [French dermatologist, 1883–1961] see hypohidrotic ectodermal DYSPLASIA (Christ-Siemens-Touraine syndrome).

Touraine's aphthosis [A. *Touraine*] Behçet's SYNDROME.

tourniquet (toor'ni-ket) [Fr.] an instrument for the compression of a blood vessel for the purpose of controlling the circulation and preventing the access of blood to a part. See also tourniquet TEST.

Tourtual's canal palatine canal, major; see under CANAL.

Towne projection, projection, reverse, projection roentgenogram see under PROJECTION and ROENTGENOGRAM.

Townsend ionization avalanche IONIZATION.

toxemia (tok-se'me-ah) [*toxin* + Gr. *haima* blood + *-ia*] 1. a general intoxication sometimes due to the absorption of bacterial products (toxins) formed at a local source of infection. 2. a pathologic condition, usually a metabolic disorder, occurring in pregnant women.

toxic (tok'sik) [Gr. *toxikon* poison] pertaining to, due to, or of the nature of a poison.

toxicity (tok-sis'i-te) the quality of being poisonous, especially the degree of virulence of a toxic microbe or of a poison.

toxico- [Gr. *toxikon* poison] a combining form meaning poisonous or denoting relationship to poison.

toxicologist (tok"si-kol'o-jist) an individual who specializes and is an expert in toxicology.

toxicology (tok"si-kol'o-je) the sum of what is known regarding poisons; the scientific study of poisons, their actions, their detection, and the treatment of the conditions produced by them.

TOXICON Toxicology Information Conversational On-Line Network; see TOXLINE.

toxicosis (tok"si-ko'sis) any disease condition due to poisoning.

toxin (tok'sin) [L. *toxicum* poison, from Gr. *toxikos* of or for the bow] a poison; the term is frequently used to refer specifically to a protein produced by some higher plants (phytotoxin), certain animals (zootoxin), and pathogenic microorganisms, which is highly toxic for other living organisms. Such substances are differentiated from simple chemical poisons and the vegetable alkaloids by their high molecular weight and antigenicity. See also ENDOTOXIN and EXOTOXIN. **α-t.,** α-STAPHYLOLYSIN. **β-t.,** β-STAPHYLOLYSIN. **γ-t.,** γ-STAPHYLOLYSIN. **δ-t.,** δ-STAPHYLOLYSIN. **botulinum t.,** a toxin produced by *Clostridium botulinum.* **exfoliative t.,** exfoliatin. **Shiga t.,** a potent exotoxin produced by *Shigella dysenteriae* (type 1). **tetanus t.,** see TETANOLYSIN and TETANOSPASMIN.

TOXLINE Toxicology Information Online; an acronym for a computerized information storage and retrieval system sponsored by the National Library of Medicine which provides computer on-line access to references published on human and animal toxicity studies, effects of environmental chemicals and pollutants, and adverse drug reactions.

toxo- [Gr. *toxikon;* L. *toxinum*] a combining form denoting relationship to a toxin, or poison.

Toxoplasma (toks"o-plaz'mah) [*toxo-* + Gr. *plasma* anything formed or molded] a genus of sporozoa that are intracellular parasites of many organs and tissues of birds and mammals, including man. See TOXOPLASMOSIS. The only known complete hosts are cats and other Felidae, in which both asexual and sexual developmental cycles occur in the intestinal epithelium, culminating in the passage of oocysts in the feces. The intestinal stages do not occur in other hosts. **T. cunic'uli,** *T. gondii.* **T. gon'dii,** the etiologic agent of toxoplasmosis (q.v.); it also infects cats, swine, dogs, sheep, cattle, and rabbits.

toxoplasmosis (tok"so-plaz-mo'sis) a disease of man caused by the sporozoon *Toxoplasma gondii.* The congenital form is characterized by lesions of the central nervous system, which may lead to blindness, brain defects and death. The acquired form is of two types: the lymphadenopathic type, which closely resembles mononucleosis; and the disseminated type, in which lesions involve chiefly the lungs, liver, heart, skin, muscle, brain, and meninges, and which is characterized by pneumonia, hepatitis, myocarditis, and meningoencephalitis in varying degrees.

TPN 1. total parenteral nutrition; see parenteral HYPERALIMENTATION. 2. triphosphopyridine nucleotide; see nicotinamide-adenine dinucleotide phosphate, under DINUCLEOTIDE.

Tr tragion.

tr. tincture.

trabecula (trah-bek′u-lah), pl. *trabec′ulae* [L., dim. of *trabs,* little beam] a little beam; used in anatomical nomenclature as a general term to designate a fibrous band or septum which unites a capsule to the interior of an organ. **trabec′ulae cra′nii, Rathke's trabeculae,** a pair of longitudinal cranial bars of cartilage in the embryo, bounding the pituitary space that becomes the sella turcica.

trabeculae (trah-bek′u-le) [L.] plural of trabecula.

trabecular (trah-bek′u-lar) pertaining to a trabecula.

trabeculate (trah-bek′u-lāt) [L. *trabecula* a small beam or bar] marked by cross bars or trabeculae.

tracer (trās′er) 1. a dissecting instrument for isolating vessels and nerves. 2. a mechanical device by which the outline of an object or the direction and extent of movement of a part may be graphically recorded. 3. a means or agent by which certain substances or structures can be identified or followed, as a radioactive tracer. **arrow-point t. needle-point t. isotope t.,** radioactive t. **needle-point t.,** a mechanical device used in recording jaw movements, in which the tracing is made on a horizontal plate by a weighted or a spring-loaded needle attached to the jaw. Called also *arrow-point t.* and *stylus t.* See also needlepoint TRACING. **radioactive t.,** a radioisotope replacing a stable chemical element in a compound introduced into the body, enabling the course of its metabolism, distribution, and elimination from the body to be traced by a Geiger-Müller counter or other type of counting instrument. Called also *isotope t., tracer element,* and *tracer isotope.* **stylus t.,** needlepoint t.

trachea (tra′ke-ah) [L.; Gr. *tracheia artēria*] [NA] the cartilaginous and membranous tube descending from the larynx and branching into the right and left main bronchi, which serves as an air passage. Called also *windpipe.*

tracheal (tra′ke-al) [L. *trachealis*] pertaining to the trachea.

trachelo- [Gr. *trachelos* neck] a combining form denoting relationship to the neck or to a necklike structure.

trachelodynia (tra″ke-lo-din′e-ah) [trachelo- + Gr. *odynē* pain + -ia] pain in the neck.

tracheo- [L. *trachea*] a combining form denoting relationship to the trachea.

tracheobronchial (tra″ke-o-brong′ke-al) pertaining to the trachea and bronchi.

tracheogenic (tra″ke-o-jen′ik) [tracheo- + Gr. *gennan* to produce] originating in the trachea.

tracheolaryngeal (tra″ke-o-lah-rin′je-al) pertaining to the trachea and larynx.

tracheolaryngotomy (tra″ke-o-lar″in-got′o-me) incision of the trachea and larynx.

tracheostenosis (tra″ke-o-ste-no′sis) [tracheo- + Gr. *stenōsis* narrowing] contraction or narrowing of the trachea.

tracheostoma (tra″ke-os′to-mah) [tracheo- + Gr. *stōma* mouth] an opening into the trachea through the neck.

tracheostomy (tra″ke-os′to-me) [tracheo- + Gr. *stomoun* to furnish with an opening or mouth] the surgical formation of an opening into the trachea, the edges of the opening being sutured to an opening in the skin of the neck, performed in life-threatening obstruction of the trachea due to foreign bodies, crushing of the air passages, tracheospasm, or by edema or tumors in the hypopharyngeal and supraglottic areas. Also, the opening so created.

tracheotome (tra′ke-o-tōm) an instrument for use in incising the trachea.

tracheotomy (tra″ke-ot′o-me) [tracheo- + Gr. *tomē* a cutting] incision of the trachea through the skin and muscles of the neck, performed in life-threatening obstruction of the trachea due to foreign bodies, crushing of the air passages, tracheospasm, or by edema or tumors in the hypopharyngeal and supraglottic areas. Elective tracheotomy is also sometimes performed for the administration of anesthesia in cases where an intra-oral approach is contraindicated, as in maxillofacial injuries. **inferior t.,** incision of the trachea through the neck, below the isthmus of the thyroid. **superior t.,** incision of the trachea through the cricothyroid (conic) ligament for the introduction of a large lumen needle to provide an airway; usually performed in extreme emergencies. Called also *coniotomy, cricothyrotomy,* and *intercricothyroid laryngotomy.*

trachyphonia (tra″ke-fo′ne-ah) [Gr. *trachys* rough + *phōnē* voice + -ia] roughness of the voice; hoarseness.

tracing (trās′ing) 1. the act or process of drawing by following lines visible through a transparent paper, or producing an exact graphic replica through mechanical means. 2. a record produced through the act of tracing. 3. a record of movements of the mandible produced by a tracer; the shape of the tracing depends on the relative location of the marking point and the tracing plate, and the apex of a properly made tracing is considered to indicate the most retruded unstrained position of the mandible in relation to the maxilla (centric jaw location). 4. cephalometric t. **arrow-point t.,** needlepoint t. **cephalometric t.,** a line drawing of structural outlines of craniofacial landmarks and facial bones, directly from a cephalometric roentgenogram. **extraoral t.,** a tracing of mandibular movements made outside the oral cavity. **Gothic arch t.,** needlepoint t. **intraoral t.,** a tracing of condylar direction made within the oral cavity. **needlepoint t.,** a tracing of the movements of the mandible resembling an arrowhead or a Gothic arch, made by means of a device attached to the opposing arches, the exact shape depending to a large extent on the location of the marking point relative to the tracing table. The apex of the tracing is considered as an indication of the centric relation. Called also *arrow-point t., Gothic arch t.,* and *stylus t.* See also needlepoint TRACER. **stylus t.,** needlepoint t.

tract (trakt) [L. *tractus*] a region, principally one of some length; specifically a collection or bundle of nerve fibers having the same origin, function and termination, or a number of organs, arranged in series, subserving a common function. Called also *tractus.* See also SYSTEM. **ascending t.,** a system of sensory (efferent) neurons which conveys impulses toward the brain. The principal ascending tracts include the ventral spinothalamic tract, which conveys touch and pressure stimuli; the lateral spinothalamic tracts, which convey sensory stimuli for pain, cold, and warmth; and the posterior and anterior spinocerebellar tracts, which convey proprioceptive stimuli. **corticobulbar t's,** descending tracts whose fibers diverge from the corticospinal tracts at the level of the midbrain and terminate in the brain stem in the reticular formation or on voluntary motor nuclei of the cranial nerves (trigeminal, facial, glossopharyngeal, vagus, accessory, and hypophyseal nuclei). **corticonuclear t., corticospinal t.,** pyramidal t. **dead t's,** black zones produced by transmitted light and white zones produced by reflected light in dentin, seen in the ground sections of teeth, due to differences in the refractive indices of the affected tubules. They represent dentinal tubules whose odontoblastic processes have been destroyed, either by strong external stimuli causing death of the odontoblast and its processes, or from deposition of primary and secondary dentin and diminution of the pulp chamber size, resulting in crowding of the odontoblasts and destruction of weaker ones. **descending t.,** a system of efferent (motor) nerves which convey impulses from the brain toward the periphery. Descending tracts include the pyramidal tract, the reticulospinal tracts, the rubrospinal tract, the vestibulospinal tract, the corticobulbar tracts, and other tracts, and descending fibers which exert influence on muscular activity, posture, reflex activity, and voluntary and automatic movements. **fistulous t.,** sinus t. **foraminous spiral t.,** an area on the fundus of the internal acoustic meatus, below the crista transversa and in front of the area vestibularis inferior; it corresponds to the base of the cochlea and consists of a number of small spirally arranged openings for the passage of branches of the vestibulocochlear nerve, which encircle the canalis centralis cochlea. Called also *tractus spiralis foraminosus* [NA]. **hypothalamo-hypophyseal t.,** ends in the neural lobe of the hypophysis which govern the production and release of hormones of the posterior pituitary gland. See OXYTOCIN and VASOPRESSIN. **ionization t.,** ionization PATH. **mesencephalic t. of trigeminal nerve,** the sensory fibers of the entering trigeminal nerve in the midbrain that continue rostrally along the median aspect of the superior cerebellar peduncle, their cell bodies being located in the nucleus of the mesencephalic tract, which accompanies it. Called also *radix descendens* [*mesencephalica*] *nervi trigemini* and *tractus mesencephalicus nervi trigemini* [NA]. **olfactory t.,** a part of the rhinencephalon, forming a narrow band that arises from the olfactory bulb and joins the frontal lobe. It produces a triangular expansion, the olfactory trigone, and extends by dividing into the medial, intermediate, and lateral olfactory striae. Called also *tractus olfactorius* [NA]. **optic t.,** the tract that carries fibers of the optic nerve from the optic chiasm across the surface of the cerebral peduncle to the third ventricle, where it divides into the lateral and medial roots. Called also *tractus opticus* [NA]. **pyramidal t.,** a term applied to two groups of fibers (corticonuclear and corticospinal) arising chiefly in the sensorimotor regions of the cerebral cortex and descending in the internal capsule, cerebral peduncle, and pons to the medulla oblongata, the corticonuclear fibers synapsing with motor nuclei through the brain stem. Most of the corticospinal fibers cross in the decussation of the pyramids and descend in the spinal cord as the lateral pyramidal (lateral corticospinal) tract; most of the uncrossed fibers form the anterior pyramidal (anterior corticospinal) tract; both end by synapsing with internuncial and motor neurons. It is a phylogenetically new tract, most prominent in man, which provides for direct cortical control and initiation of skilled movements, especially those related to speech and involving the hand and fingers. Called also *corticonuclear t., corticospinal t., pyramidal system,* and *tractus pyramidalis* [NA]. **reticulospinal t.,** a descending tract consisting of a system of fibers arising mostly from the medial parts of the reticular formation of the pons and medulla oblongata, which are important to the facilitation and inhibition of reflex activity, voluntary movement, muscle tone, and other functions. Called also *tractus reticulospinalis* [NA]. **rubrospinal t.,** a descending tract consisting of a group of nerve fibers in the lateral funiculus of the spinal cord, arising in the large cells of the red nucleus of the mesencephalon, and exerting influence on the flexor muscle tone. Called also *tractus rubrospinalis* [NA]. **sinus t.,** a tract, usually a nonepitheliated passage, leading from a sinus or abscess to an epithelial surface, such as one leading from a chronic apical abscess to an opening that may be intraoral or extraoral and provides a pathway through which pus is intermittently discharged during active phases of the abscess. It may appear and disappear periodically according to the lapse of time between active phases; elimination of the abscess causes the tract to disappear permanently. Called also *fistulous t.* **spinal t. of trigeminal nerve,** a descending tract of the trigeminal nerve that extends from the level of the entrance of the sensory root of the trigeminal nerve into the pons to the upper cervical segments of the spinal cord, carrying mainly pain and temperature impulses from the face. Called also *tractus spinalis nervi trigemini* [NA]. **spinocerebellar t., anterior,** a group of nerve fibers in the lateral funiculus of the spinal cord, which arise chiefly in the opposite gray matter and are activated by skin, muscle, tendon, and joint endings. They ascend to the cerebellum by way of the anterior part of the lateral funiculus and then the superior cerebellar peduncle. Called also *fasciculus anterolateralis superficialis* and *tractus spinocerebellaris anterior* [NA]. **spinocerebellar t., posterior,** a group of nerve fibers in the lateral funiculus of the spinal cord, which arises chiefly from the nucleus thoracicus and are activated by skin, muscle, tendon, and joint endings. They ascend to the cerebellum by way of the dorsal part of the lateral funiculus and then the inferior cerebellar peduncle. Called also *fasciculus cerebellospinalis* and *tractus spinocerebellaris posterior* [NA]. **spinothalamic t., anterior,** an ascending tract consisting of a group of nerve fibers in the anterolateral funiculus of the spinal cord, which arise in the opposite gray matter, carrying impulses activated by light touch. They ascend to the thalamus, joining the medial lemniscus in the brain stem. Called also *tractus spinothalamicus anterior* [NA]. **spinothalamic t., lateral,** an ascending tract consisting of a group of nerve fibers in the anterolateral funiculus of the spinal cord, which arise in the opposite gray matter, and carry impulses activated by pain and temperature. They ascend to the thalamus, running with the lateral lemniscus in the brain stem. Called also *tractus spinothalamicus lateralis* [NA]. **thyroglossal t.,** thyroglossal DUCT. **trigeminothalamic t.,** fibers from the trigeminal nerve to the thalamus. **vestibulospinal t.,** a descending tract consisting of nerve fibers arising from the lateral vestibular nucleus that descend uncrossed, chiefly in the anterior part of the lateral funiculus, throughout most levels of the spinal cord. They exert a facilitatory influence on the reflex activity of the spinal cord and reflex mechanism controlling muscle tone. Called also *tractus vestibulospinalis* [NA].

traction (trak'shun) [L. *tractio*] 1. any act or process of moving an object by drawing or pulling. 2. use of a pulling force to a fractured bone or dislocated joint in an effort to maintain proper position, or to overcome muscle spasms in musculoskeletal disorders, to lessen or prevent contracture. **elastic t.,** traction by means of an elastic appliance that exerts a pulling force. **external t.,** traction applied by means of a fixed anchorage (as by a headgear) outside the oral cavity; used principally in the management of midfacial fractures. **intermaxillary t.,** maxillomandibular t. **internal t.,** traction applied by using one of the

cranial bones above the point of fracture for anchorage; used in the management of facial fractures. **intramaxillary elastic t.,** the use of intramaxillary elastic (see under ELASTIC). **maxillomandibular t.,** traction applied by means of elastic or wire ligatures and interdental wiring and/or splints. Called also *intermaxillary t.* See also intermaxillary ANCHORAGE. **skin t.,** traction on a body part maintained by an apparatus affixed by dressing to the body surface. **tongue t.,** the pulling forward of the tongue to improve the airway. **weight t.,** traction exerted by means of a weight connected to a pulley mechanism.

tractus (trak'tus), pl. *trac'tus* [L. "a track," "trail"] a tract; a region, principally one of some length; a general anatomical term, especially for a collection or bundle of nerve fibers having the same origin and termination, and serving the same function. See TRACT. **t. mesencephal'icus ner'vi trigem'ini** [NA], mesencephalic tract of trigeminal nerve; see under TRACT. **t. olfacto'rius** [NA], olfactory TRACT. **t. op'ticus** [NA], optic TRACT. **t. pyramida'lis** [NA], pyramidal TRACT. **t. reticulospina'lis** [NA], reticulospinal TRACT. **t. rubrospina'lis** [NA], rubrospinal TRACT. **t. spina'lis ner'vi trigem'ini** [NA] spinal tract of trigeminal nerve; see under TRACT. **t. spinocerebella'ris ante'rior** [NA], spinocerebellar tract, anterior; see under TRACT. **t. spinocerebella'ris poste'rior** [NA], spinocerebellar tract, posterior; see under TRACT. **t. spinothalam'icus ante'rior** [NA], spinothalamic tract, anterior; see under TRACT. **t. spinothalam'icus latera'lis,** spinothalamic tract, lateral; see under TRACT. **t. spira'lis foramino'sus** [NA], foraminous spiral TRACT. **t. vestibulospina'lis** [NA], vestibulospinal TRACT.

trademark (trād'mark) a name (usually capitalized), symbol, or other device used to identify a product, which is usually officially registered with a governmental agency to assure its exclusive use by the owner of the trademark. See also *proprietary.*

tragacanth (trag'ah-kanth) the dried gummy exudation of the plant *Astragalus,* occurring as a white to yellowish-white, amorphous, odorless solid that has an insipid, mucilaginous taste. It is insoluble in alcohol and rapidly absorbs water to form a soft, adhesive paste, without actually dissolving. Used as a suspending agent in lotions, mixtures, and other medicinal preparations, as an emulsifying agent to increase consistency and retard creaming, as a demulcent in sore throat, and alone or combined with other substances, as an adhesive for dentures. Called also *gum t.* **Indian t.,** sterculia GUM.

tragion (traj'e-on) a cephalometric landmark, being the most superior point of the tragus of the ear. Abbreviated *Tr.* Called also *point Tr.*

tragus (tra'gus), pl. *tra'gi* [L.; Gr. *tragos* goat] [NA] the cartilaginous projection anterior to the external opening of the ear.

trait (trāt) 1. any distinguishing quality. 2. visible or detectable expression of a gene; phenotype, as in sickle cell trait. Sometimes used in a specialized sense to mean heterozygous phenotype. 3. character. **autosomal dominant t.,** autosomal dominant CHARACTER. **autosomal recessive t.,** autosomal recessive CHARACTER. **codominant t.,** codominant CHARACTER. **congenital t.,** a trait present at birth, not necessarily genetic. **dominant t.,** see autosomal dominant CHARACTER and X-linked dominant CHARACTER. **genetic t.,** a trait that is determined by genes, not being necessarily congenital. See also entries under CHARACTER and PHENOTYPE. **Hageman t.,** FACTOR XII. **hemoglobin C t.,** a condition characterized by the presence of 28 to 44 percent of hemoglobin C and target cells in the blood, together with normal adult hemoglobin. Anemia is not present and clinical symptoms are rare, but there is reduced osmotic fragility of the erythrocytes. In rare instances, there may be infarction of teeth-bearing bones and renal hematuria. **recessive t.,** see autosomal recessive CHARACTER and X-linked recessive CHARACTER. **sex-limited t., sex-linked t.,** sex-limited CHARACTER. **sickle cell t.,** a benign condition characterized by the presence in the blood of both adult and sickle cell hemoglobin, in which the sickling phenomenon occurs only under the conditions of lowered oxygen tension and reduced pH. See also sickle cell ANEMIA. **X-linked dominant t.,** X-linked dominant CHARACTER. **X-linked recessive t.,** X-linked recessive CHARACTER.

Tral trademark for *hexocyclium methylsulfate* (see under HEXOCYCLIUM).

Tralin trademark for *hexocyclium methylsulfate* (see under HEXOCYCLIUM).

Tramacin trademark for *triamcinolone acetonide* (see under TRIAMCINOLONE).

Trancin trademark for *fluphenazine hydrochloride* (see under FLUPHENAZINE).

Trancolon trademark for *mepenzolate bromide* (see under MEPENZOLATE).

tranquilizer (tran"kwi-līz'er) [L. *tranquillus* quiet, calm + *-ize* verb ending to make + *-er* agent] an agent which acts on the emotional state, quieting or calming the patient without affecting clarity of consciousness. **major t.**, antipsychotic DRUG. **minor t.**, antianxiety DRUG.

trans- [L. *trans* through] 1. a prefix meaning through, across, or beyond. 2. in organic chemistry, a form of geometric isomerism in which the hydrogen atoms attached to two carbon atoms with double bonds are substituted in the opposite location relative to the carbon axis. Usually written in italics and disregarded in alphabetization. See *trans*-ISOMER. 3. in genetics, having one of the two mutant genes of a pseudoallele on each homologous chromosome. Cf. CIS.

transacetylation (trans-as″ĕ-til-a′shun) an enzymatic reaction, occurring in various metabolic processes, which involves the transfer of the acetyl group CH₃—C—.

$$CH_3-\overset{\displaystyle O}{\overset{\|}{C}}-$$

transaminase (trans-am′ĭ-nās) aminotransferase. **glutamic-alanine t.**, alanine AMINOTRANSFERASE. **glutamic-aspartic t.**, aspartate AMINOTRANSFERASE. **glutamic-oxalacetic t.**, aspartate AMINOTRANSFERASE. **glutamic-pyruvic t.**, alanine AMINOTRANSFERASE.

transamination (trans″am-i-na′shun) the conversion of keto acids to amino acids; the enzymatically reversible transfer of an amino group from an amino acid to what is originally an α-keto acid, forming a new amino acid and keto acid, without the appearance of ammonia in the free state. The process is catalyzed by enzymes (*aminotransaminases*). Cf. DEAMINATION.

transcalifornium (trans-kal″ĭ-for′ne-um) pertaining to elements with atomic numbers higher than that of californium. See transcalifornium elements, under ELEMENT.

transcarbamoylase (trans-kar″bah-moi′lās) carbamoyltransferase. **ornithine t.**, ornithine CARBAMOYLTRANSFERASE.

transcription (trans-krip′shun) the process by which genetic information coded in the nucleotide sequence of a DNA molecule is decoded and reproduced on a template which serves as a matrix for the translation of this information into the specific amino acid sequence in protein synthesis. The process involves the opening of the double helix of the DNA molecule, permitting free bases of one of the DNA strands to pair with complementary messenger RNA bases, which are joined with the aid of an enzyme, RNA polymerase. See also messenger RNA, template, and TRANSLATION.

Transcycline trademark for *rolitetracycline*.

transduction (trans-duk′shun) [L. *transducere* to lead across] a method of genetic recombination in bacteria, in which DNA from a lysed bacterium is transferred to another bacterium, thereby changing its genetic constitution.

transfer (trans′fer) [*trans-* + L. *ferre* to carry] the conveyance of something from one place to another. **chain t.**, in a chemical reaction, the process wherein the reactivity of a radical is transferred to another species which would usually be capable of further chain propagation. **heat t.**, the passage of heat energy through solids, occurring by thermal conductivity, or diffusivity, from regions of high temperature to regions of low temperature. **linear energy t.**, see LET.

transferase [E.C.2] (trans′fer-ās) any one in a major class of enzymes involved in the transfer of a chemical group from one substrate to another. See also ENZYME classification. **amino t.**, aminotransferase. **CoA-t.** [E.C.2.8.3], a subclass of transferases, the enzymes of which catalyze the transfer of a CoA group, as from an acetyl group to propionate, oxalate, or malonate.

transferrin (trans-fer′rin) [*trans-* + L. *ferrum* iron + *-in* chemical suffix] a serum protein whose function is to bind and transfer iron, having an electrophoretic mobility of a β₁-globulin, molecular weight of about 88,000, and sedimentation coefficient of 5.0S. It can bind two ferric atoms per molecule; its half life in the blood is 6 to 8 days in adults and 12 days in children. In addition to iron, transferrin can also bind copper and zinc. There are several varieties of transferrin — C, B, D being the most common. Called also *iron-binding β-globulin, iron-binding protein, metal-binding globulin,* and *siderophilin.*

transfix (trans′fiks) [*trans-* + L. *figere* to fix] to pierce through and through.

transformation (trans″for-ma′shun) [*trans-* + L. *formatio* formation] change in form or structure; conversion from one form to another. In oncology, the change that a normal cell undergoes as it becomes malignant.

transformer (trans-for′mer) an electric device that either increases or decreases the incoming voltage. See also AUTOTRANSFORMER. **step-down t.**, one in which the secondary voltage is less than the primary voltage. **step-up t.**, one in which the secondary voltage is greater than the primary voltage.

transfructosylase (trans-fruk″to-sil′ās) fructosyltransferase.

transfusion (trans-fu′zhun) [L. *transfusio*] transfer of blood col-

lected from one or several persons to another, or of any preparation obtained from one blood, such as plasma or serum. In a broader sense, the term also includes infusion of various artificial preparations serving as blood or plasma substitutes. Transfusion is performed to replenish the depleted blood supply caused by hemorrhage, burns, or shock, or to replace incompatible blood, as in fetal erythroblastosis. Transfusion of incompatible blood may cause hemolytic complications (see also BLOOD GROUP). Transfusion of blood from infected persons or use of contaminated equipment may cause such diseases as hepatitis, homologous serum jaundice, syphilis, or malaria. **exchange t.**, **exsanguination t.**, repetitive withdrawal of small amounts of blood and replacement with donor blood, until a large proportion of the blood volume has been exchanged; used in newborn infants with hemolytic disease of the newborn and in patients with severe uremia. Called also *replacement t.* **intravenous t.**, transfusion into the recipient's vein. **t. reaction**, transfusion REACTION. **reciprocal t.**, transfusion of blood from a person recovering from an infectious disease to another person affected with the same disease and, conversely, from the affected to the recovering person, in an effort to provide the affected person with antibodies to combat the infection. **replacement t.**, exchange t.

transglucosylase (trans″gloo-ko-si″lās) glycosyltransferase.

transhexosylase (trans-hek″so-sil′ās) hexosyltransferase.

transhydrogenase (trans-hi′dro-jen-ās) an enzyme in the dehydrogenase group. **decarboxylating isocitrate–PN t.**, isocitrate DEHYDROGENASE. **L-malate–NAD t.**, malate DEHYDROGENASE.

transillumination (trans″ĭ-lu″mĭ-na′shun) the passage of light through an examined object for the purpose of examination of its internal structures. The procedure is sometimes used in the examination of the teeth to identify fractures and of the dental pulp to determine its vitality. Called also *diaphanoscopy* and *diascopy.*

transilluminator (trans-ĭ-lu″mĭ-na′tor) a lamp for passing light through body tissues for examination.

transition (tran-zish′un) a passage or change from a position, state, phase, or concept to another. See also transitional pulp STAGE. **t. state**, transition STATE.

translation (trans-la′shun) [*trans-* + L. *latus* borne] 1. the removal or change of things from one place, state, or form to another. 2. a rendering from one language into another. 3. the second phase (following transcription) of transferring genetic information from DNA in the synthesis of proteins. It consists of decoding on ribosomes, where RNA is used as a template, of a specific amino acid sequence. Two or more molecules of transfer RNA that are specific for both amino acids and template codons, serve for transporting information that places the amino acids in their proper position, as determined by hydrogen bonding between the codon and a messenger RNA molecule. 4. translatory MOVEMENT. 5. movement of a tooth through the alveolar bone without change in inclination. Called also *bodily movement.*

translocase (trans″lok-ās) carrier MOLECULE.

translocation (trans″lo-ka′shun) [*trans-* + L. *locus* place] 1. change of location. 2. a structural chromosome aberration, consisting of the transfer of one segment of a chromosome to a nonhomologous chromosome. It occurs as a result of breakage of both chromosomes, with repair in abnormal arrangement. Translocation, if truly balanced, does not always lead to an abnormal phenotype, but unbalanced translocation between chromosome 21 and another acrocentric chromosome (most often chromosome 13) may result in Down's syndrome. Called also *interchange.* Abbreviated *t.* See also CHROMOSOME aberration and see INSERTION (4). **balanced t.**, translocation which results in no more or no less than the normal diploid or haploid genetic material. **t. of distal segment of long arm of chromosome 8**, see Warkany's SYNDROME. **preeruptive t.**, translocation or migration of the tissue surrounding the tooth, while the tooth itself remains in the same position, occurring during the preeruptive stage. See tooth migration, physiologic, under MIGRATION. **reciprocal t.**, translocation in which two nonhomologous chromosomes exchange broken pieces. Abbreviated *rcp.* **robertsonian t.**, translocation in which the breaks occur at the centromere and whole chromosome arms are exchanged. Abbreviated *rob.* Called also *centric fusion.* **tandem t.**, translocation occurring in one break in the vicinity of the centromere in one chromosome and another break near the end of the second chromosome. Called also *tandem fusion.* Abbreviated *tan.* **unbalanced t.**, see *translocation* (2).

translucency (trans-lu′sen-se) 1. a condition or state of transmitting light, but diffusing it so that objects beyond are not clearly distinguished. 2. a lifelike sheen present in the crowns of teeth with vital pulps.

translucent (trans-lu′sent) [*trans-* + L. *lucens* shining] partially transparent; transmitting light but not a visual image.

transmethylase (trans-meth′ĭ-lās) methyltransferase.

transmissible (trans-mis′ĭ-b'l) capable of being transmitted from one individual or one species to another.

transmission (trans-mish′un) [*trans-* + L. *missio* a sending] a passage or transfer, as of a disease from one individual to another, or of neural impulses from one neuron to another. In genetics, the communication of inheritable qualities to offspring. **horizontal t.,** transmission of infection from one individual to another, usually through contact. **neurohumoral t.,** transmission of an impulse across a synaptic junction through the medium of a chemical substance (transmitter SUBSTANCE). The substance is released from synaptic vesicles in presynaptic nerve terminals as a result of depolarization of the presynaptic terminal by the action potential. Once released, it diffuses across the synaptic cleft, causing increased permeability of the subsynaptic somal membrane, thus allowing sodium ions to flow from the interstitial fluid into the neurons which depolarize it so that the impulse has crossed the synapse. Acetylcholine (in the parasympathetic nervous system) and norepinephrine (in the sympathetic system) are the principal transmitter substances, but serotonin and L-glutamic acid are also believed to be transmitters. Upon conveying the impulse, acetylcholine is destroyed by cholinesterase and epinephrine is absorbed into the nerve tissue and methylated by *o*-methyl transferase. See illustration at SYNAPSE. **synaptic t.,** the transmission of impulses from one neuron to another across a synaptic junction. See also *neurohumoral t.* **vertical t.,** transmission of disease from one generation to another. The term is sometimes restricted to genetic transmission, but some authorities use it for transmission of infection from one generation to another, as by milk or through the placenta

transmitter (trans-mit′er) 1. anything that conveys or passes along. 2. transmitter SUBSTANCE. **excitatory t.,** neurohumoral t., transmitter SUBSTANCE.

transorbital (trans-or′bĭ-tal) performed through the bony socket of the eye.

transoximinase (trans″ok-sim′ĭ-nās) oximinotransferase.

transpalatal (trans-pal′ah-tal) [*trans-* + *palatal*] through the roof of the mouth, or palate.

transparent (trans-par′ent) [*trans-* + L. *parere* to appear] permitting passage of light, so that objects may be seen through substances, as through glass.

transparietal (trans″pah-ri′ĕ-tal) [*trans-* + L. *paries* wall] through or across a wall of an organ or cavity.

transpentosylase (trans-pen″to-sil′ās) pentosyltransferase.

transphosphatase (trans″fos′fah-tās″) phosphotransferase. **ATP gluconate t.,** glucokinase. **ATP glucose t.,** ATP hexose t., hexokinase. **phosphoenolpyruvate-ADP t.,** pyruvate KINASE.

transphosphorase (trans″fos-for′ās) phosphotransferase.

transphosphorylase [E.C.2.7] (trans″fos-for′ĭ-lās) a transferase that catalyzes the transfer of a phosphate group, usually phosphotransferase. **phosphoenol t.,** pyruvate KINASE.

transphosphorylation (trans-fos″for-ĭ-la′shun) the exchange of phosphate groups between organic phosphates, without their going through the stage of inorganic phosphate.

transplant 1. (trans-plant′) to transfer tissue from one part to another. 2. (trans′plant) a piece of tissue or an organ taken from the body for grafting into another portion of the body or into another individual. See also GRAFT. **allogenic t., allogeneic t.,** allogenic GRAFT. **autogenous t., autologous t.,** autogenous GRAFT. **bone t.,** bone GRAFT. **free t.,** free GRAFT. **heterogeneous t., heterologous t.,** heterogeneous GRAFT. **homostatic t.,** homostatic GRAFT. **homologous t., homoplastic t.,** homologous GRAFT. **homovital t.,** homovital GRAFT. **isogenic t., isologous t., syngeneic t.,** isologous GRAFT. **orthotopic t.,** orthotopic GRAFT.

transplantation (trans″plan-ta′shun) [*trans-* + L. *plantare* to plant] 1. the grafting of tissues taken from the same body or from another. See also GRAFT and GRAFTING. 2. tooth t. **autogenous t., autologous t., autoplastic t.,** transplantation of tissue from one site to another in the same individual. See also autogenous GRAFT and AUTOPLASTY. **heterotopic t.,** transplantation of tissue typical of one area to a different recipient site. **homotopic t.,** orthotopic t. **orthotopic t.,** transplantation of tissue typical of one area to an identical recipient site. Called

also *homotopic t.* **syngeneic t.,** transplantation of tissues between animals in the same pure line. **syngenesioplastic t.,** transplantation of tissue from one individual to a related individual of the same species, as from a mother to her child, or from a brother to a sister. **tooth t.,** the insertion, into a prepared dental alveolus, of an autogenous or homologous tooth; it may be a developing tooth germ from the same mouth, a homologous transplant, or a tooth with or without vital pulp, or one having had endodontic treatment, transplanted from one site to another in the same individual or from one individual to another. See also IMPLANTATION and REIMPLANTATION.

transport (trans′port) [L. *transportare* to carry across] in biology, the movement of materials, particularly into and out of cells and across epithelial layers. **active t.,** 1. in thermodynamics, a transport process in which the system gains free energy. 2. unidirectional transport of substances across the cell membrane and epithelial cell layers against electrical, concentration, and pressure gradients through the use of metabolic energy. Forms of active transport include (*a*) a system for extrusion of cellular Na+ and replacement of K+ (see sodium PUMP) through the use of ATP; (*b*) a system for transporting sugars across the epithelial cell layers of the intestine and kidney tubules that appears to be related to active transport of sodium; (*c*) a system for transporting amino acids through the use of the γ-glutamyl cycle. See also facilitated DIFFUSION (3). **homocellular t.,** inward and outward transport of substances across the cell membrane. **intracellular t.,** transport of substances in eukaryotic cells, which allows passing of substances across the membrane of an intracellular organelle. **mediated t.,** facilitated DIFFUSION. **passive t.,** 1. in thermodynamics, a transport process in which the system loses free energy. 2. in biology, the transport of molecules across the cell membrane, whereby the solute crosses the membrane in the direction of decreasing concentration. **t. system,** carrier MOLECULE. **transcellular t.,** a form of homocellular transport that allows inward and outward transport of substances across the entire cell.

transposition (trans″po-zish′un) [*trans-* + L. *positio* placement] 1. displacement of a viscus to the opposite side. 2. the operation of carrying a tissue flap from one situation to another without severing its connection entirely until it is united at its new location. 3. the exchange of position of two atoms within a molecule. 4. alignment of teeth out of their normal sequence in an arch. See *malocclusion*.

transsegmental (trans″seg-men′tal) extending across a segment.

transseptal (trans-sep′tal) through or across a septum.

transsphenoidal (trans″sfe-noi′dal) across or through the sphenoid bone.

transsulfurase (trans-sul′fur-ās) sulfotransferase.

transudate (trans′u-dat) [*trans-* + L. *sudare* to sweat] noninflammatory edema fluid with a low specific gravity (usually below 1.012) and low content of proteins and other colloids. Inflammatory fluid is known as *exudate*.

transuranium (trans″u-ra′ne-um) pertaining to elements having atomic numbers higher than that of uranium. See transuranium elements, under ELEMENT.

transverse (trans-vers′) [L. *transversus*] placed crosswise; situated at right angles to the long axis of a part.

transversion (trans-ver′zhun) eruption of a tooth in the wrong position.

transversus (trans-ver′sus) [L.] transverse. **t. lin′guae, mus′culus t. lin′guae** [NA] transverse muscle of tongue; see under MUSCLE.

Tranxene trademark for *clorazepate dipotassium* (see under CLORAZEPATE).

tranylcypromine sulfate (tran″il-si′pro-mēn) inhibitor, a monoamine oxidase inhibitor, (±)-*trans*-2-phenylcyclopropylamine sulfate, occurring as a white, odorless, crystalline powder that is soluble in water, slightly soluble in ethanol and ether, and insoluble in chloroform. Used in the treatment of mental depression. Adverse reactions may include orthostatic hypotension, vertigo, restlessness, insomnia, drowsiness, weakness, anxiety, agitation, manic symptoms, nausea, vomiting, diarrhea, abdominal pain, constipation, anorexia, xerostomia, impotence, visual disorders, chills, edema, tachycardia, headache, and sometimes fatal cerebral hemorrhage. Trademarks: Parnate, Parnite, Tylciprine.

Trasicor trademark for *oxprenolol hydrochloride* (see under OXPRENOLOL).

trauma (traw-mah), pl. *traumas* or *trau′mata* [L.; Gr.] a wound or injury. **occlusal t., t. from occlusion,** injury to any part of the masticatory system as a result of occlusal dysfunction, including traumatic occlusion, temporomandibular joint dysfunction, temporomandibular joint arthritis, and bruxism. The condition may be brought about by abrupt changes in occlusal force, such as that produced by a restoration or prosthetic appliance, or gradual changes in occlusion produced by tooth wear, drifting and extrusion of teeth, and faulty oral habits. Periodontal changes may include denseness of the periodontal ligament, resorption of the alveolar bone, necrosis, widening of periodontal space, thrombosis, edema, extravasation of blood, tearing of the periodontal ligament and cementum, and loosening of teeth. Pain in the temporomandibular joint, excessive wearing of teeth, and painful spasms of the masticatory muscles may be associated. See also traumatic OCCLUSION. **potential t.**, an alteration in tissue that may occur at any time as a result of an existing dental disharmony. **toothbrush t.**, gingival recession or injury from incorrect toothbrushing methods, usually with a stiff textured brush.

traumata (traw'mah-tah) [Gr.] plural of *trauma*.

traumatic (traw-mat'ik) [Gr. *traumatikos*] pertaining to, occurring as the result of, or causing trauma.

traumatism (traw'mah-tizm) [Gr. *traumatismos*] 1. the physical or psychic state resulting from injury. 2. a wound. **periodontal t.**, traumatic OCCLUSION.

traumato- [Gr. *trauma, traumatos* wound] a combining form denoting relationship to trauma, or to a wound or injury.

traumatogenic (traw″mah-to-jen'ik) [*traumato-* + Gr. *gennan* to produce] 1. caused or due to a wound. 2. capable of causing trauma.

traumatology (traw″mah-tol'o-je) [*traumato-* + *-logy*] the branch of surgery which deals with wounds and disability from injuries.

Trautmann's triangle see under TRIANGLE.

Travelin trademark for *dimenhydrinate*.

tray (tra) a flat-surfaced utensil for the conveyance of various objects or material. **acrylic resin t.**, an impression tray made of acrylic resin. **t. compound**, see impression COMPOUND. **impression t.**, usually a horseshoe-shaped receptacle made of metal or other suitable material used to carry the impression material to the mouth, to confine the material in apposition to the surfaces to be recorded, and to control the impression material while it sets to form the impression.

TRCV total red cell VOLUME.

Treacher Collins' syndrome [E. *Treacher Collins*] mandibulofacial DYSOSTOSIS.

treatment (trēt'ment) the management and care of a patient for the purpose of combating disease or disorder. See also THERAPY. **adjunctive t.**, supplementary or additional therapeutic procedure. **age hardening heat t.**, age HARDENING. **alternate t.**, in health insurance, a contract provision which authorizes the carrier to determine the amount of benefits payable, giving consideration to alternate procedures, services, or courses of treatment that may be performed in order to accomplish the desired results. The attending physician or dentist and the patient have the option for selecting the procedure but payment for the procedure may be based on alternate treatment principles, whereby the amount allowed for the service may be less than the actual fee charged. **Early Periodic Screening Diagnosis T.** see EPSDT. **t. filling**, treatment FILLING. **hardening heat t.**, tempering. **heat t.**, the use of heat in altering physical properties of a material, such as the application of heat to metals to modify their crystalline structure and, therefore, their hardness, brittleness, and other physical characteristics. The process may include: heating the metal to below its melting temperature and allowing it to cool at room temperature to reestablish its crystalline structure after deformation; cooling it slowly in the solid-phase reaction in alloying; or cooling it rapidly (quenching) as in tempering steel. See also ANNEALING and TEMPERING. **heat t., age hardening**, age HARDENING. **heat t., hardening**, tempering. **heat t., homogenizing**, heat treatment to produce uniform composition of a material, as in reestablishing the equilibrium relationship in amalgam alloy. **heat t., softening**, heat treatment of a metal resulting in its softening, as when an alloy is heated in recrystallization. **heat t., solution**, heat treatment of an alloy at high temperature to produce a solid solution, followed by quenching. **homogenizing heat t.**, heat t., homogenizing. **necessary t.**, a procedure or service determined by the doctor to be necessary to either establish or maintain the patient's health. **order-disorder heat t.**, see order-disorder HARDENING. **preventive t., prophylactic t.**, that in which the aim is to prevent the occurrence of the disease; prophylaxis. See also oral PROPHYLAXIS and preventive DENTISTRY. **softening heat t.**, heat t., softening. **solution heat t.**, heat t., solution. **supporting t.**, that mainly directed to sustaining the strength of the patient.

Trecator trademark for *ethionamide*.

tree (tre) 1. a perennial of the plant kingdom characterized by having a main stem or trunk and numerous branches. 2. an anatomical structure with branches resembling a tree. **bronchial t.**, the bronchi and their branching structures. **tracheobronchial t.**, the trachea, bronchi, and their branching structures.

tremor (trem'or, tre'mor) [L. *tremere* to shake] an involuntary trembling or quivering. **coarse t.**, one characterized by slow vibrations. **fine t.**, one characterized by rapid vibrations. **intention t.**, one caused or intensified by a voluntary coordinated movement. **t. lin'guae**, trembling of the tongue, as seen in alcoholism, typhoid fever, and certain neurologic disorders. **trombone t. of tongue**, Magnan's MOVEMENT.

Trenaunay, P. see Klippel-Trenaunay-Weber SYNDROME.

Trendelenburg's position [Friedrich *Trendelenburg*, German surgeon, 1844–1924] see under POSITION.

Treomicetina trademark for *chloramphenicol*.

trepanation (trep″ah-na'shun) [L. *trepanatio*] trephination. **dental t.**, dental TREPHINATION.

trephination (tref″ĭ-na'shun) surgical method for creating a small circular opening in a bone, usually the skull. Called also *trepanation*. See also FENESTRATION. **dental t.**, surgical creation of a fistula by puncturing with a bur or sharp instrument through the soft tissue and cortical bone overlying the root apex to provide drainage. Called also *apical puncture, apicostomy, dental fenestration, dental puncture*, and *dental trepanation*.

trephine (tre-fīn', tre-fēn') [L. *trephina*] 1. a crown saw for removing a circular disk of bone. Called also *hole saw*. 2. to operate upon with a trephine.

Treponema (trep″o-ne'mah) [Gr. *trepein* to turn + *nēma* thread] a genus of anaerobic, motile, gram-negative, slender, flexuous spiral bacteria of the family Spirochaetaceae, order Spirochaetales, made up of cells (0.09 to 0.5 μm in width by 5 to 20 μm in length) with one or more axial fibrils inserted at each end of the protoplasmic cylinder. They are found in the oral cavity, intestines, and genital organs of animals, including man. The genus includes several pathogenic species, as well as parasitic forms of limited or no pathogenicity, such as those found in the mouth. Called also *Microspironema* and *Spironema*. **T. ambig'uum**, *T. denticola*. **T. bucca'le**, a species isolated from the oral cavity. Called also *T. inequale, T. undulatum, Borrelia buccalis, Spirillum buccale, S. cohnii, Spirochaeta inaequalis, Spironema buccale*, and *Spiroschaudinnia buccalis*. **T. calligy'rum**, *T. refringens*. **T. cara'teum**, the etiologic agent of pinta. Called also *Treponema herrejoni, T. pictor*, and *T. pintae*. **T. comando'ni**, *T. denticola*. **T. cunic'uli**, *T. paraluis-cuniculi*. **T. dentic'ola, T. den'tium, T. den'tium-stenogyra'tum**, a species isolated from the oral cavity of man and the chimpanzee, usually found in calculus forming at the gingival margin. Called also *T. ambiguum, T. comandoni, T. microdentium, Spirillum dentium, Spirochaeta ambigua, S. comandoni, S. denticola, S. dentium, S. microdentium, S. orthodonta*, and *Spironema dentium*. **T. genita'lis**, *T. refringens*. **T. herrejo'ni**, *T. carateum*. **T. inequa'le**, *T. buccale*. **T. macroden'tium**, a species isolated from the gingival crevices in man. Called also *Spirochaeta macrodentium*. **T. microden'tium**, *T. denticola*. **T. muco'sum**, a species isolated from the oral cavity in a subject suffering from periodontitis. Called also *Spirochaeta mucosa*. **T. ora'le**, a species found in the gingival crevices of man. **T. pal'lidum**, the etiologic agent of syphilis. Called also *Microspironema pallidum, Spirillum pallidum, Spirochaeta pallida*, and *Spironema pallidum*. **T. pal'lidum** var. **cunic'uli**, *T. paraluis-cuniculi*. **T. paraluis-cunic'uli**, a species causing benign venereal spirochetosis in rabbits, primarily involving the genitalia but cutaneous lesions of the head, ears, nose, and eyes may occur. Called also *Treponema cuniculi, T. pallidum var. cuniculi, Spirochaeta cuniculi, S. pallida var. cuniculi*, and *S. paraluis-cuniculi*. **T. perten'ue**, a species causing yaws in man, which also has been isolated from cases of endemic syphilis. Called also *Spirillum pertenue, Spirochaeta pertenuis*, and *Spironema pertenue*. **T. phagede'nis**, a species believed to be nonpathogenic, which has been isolated from phagedenic ulcer of human external genitalia, and from a case of syphilis. Called also *T. reiteri, Borrelia phagedenis, Reiter's treponema, Spriochaeta phagedenis, Spironema phagedenis*, and *Spiroschaudinnia phagedenis*. **T. pic'tor, T. pin'ta, T. carateum. T. refrin'gens**, a species believed to be nonpathogenic and a part of the normal genital flora in both men and women, which has been isolated from cases of condyloma acuminata and syphilis. Called also *T. calligyrum. T. genitalis, Borrelia refringens, Spirillum refringens, Spiro *chaeta calligyrum, S. refringens, Spiroschaudinnia refringens,* and *Spironema refringens.* **T. reiteri,** *T. phagedenis.* **T. scoliodon′tum,** a species found in the oral cavity in man. Called also *Spirochaeta acuta* and *S. skoliodontia.* **T. undula′tum,** *T. buccale.* **T. vincen′tii,** a species isolated from the human oral cavity. Called also *Borrelia vincenti, Spirillum vincenti, Spirochaeta vincenti, Spironema vincenti,* and *Spiroschaudinnia vincenti.*

treponema (trep″o-ne′mah) a microorganism of the genus *Treponema.*

treponematosis (trep″o-ne-mah-to″sis) an infection with organisms of the genus *Treponema.*

treponeme (trep′o-nēm) a microorganism of the genus *Treponema.* **Reiter's t.,** *Treponema phagedenis;* see under TREPONEMA.

treponemicidal (trep″o-ne-mĭ-si′dal) [*Treponema* + L. *caedere* to kill] capable of destroying organisms of the genus *Treponema.*

Trescatyl trademark for *ethionamide.*

Tresortil trademark for *methocarbamol.*

Tresten trademark for *thiethylperazine maleate* (see under THIETHYLPERAZINE).

tretamine (tre′tah-mēn) triethylenemelamine.

tretinoin (tret′ĭ-noin) a vitamin A derivative, $C_{20}H_{28}O_2$, occurring as a yellow to orange-colored crystalline powder or solids that are photosensitive and are soluble in ethanol and boiling benzene, but not in water. Used as a keratolytic agent in the treatment of keratoses and hyperplastic dermatoses. Called also *retinoic acid* and *vitamin A acid.* Trademarks: Aberal, Retin-A.

tri- [Gr. *treis;* L. *tres* three] 1. a prefix meaning three to trice. 2. in chemical nomenclature, generally used in connection with molecules made up of three similar parts; the number of each type of monodentate ligand in a coordinate compound. The number of chelate or complicated ligands is indicated by the prefix TRIS-.

Tri trademark for *trichloroethylene.*

Tri-Abrodil trademark for *acetrizoate sodium* (see under ACETRIZOATE).

triacetate (tri-as′ĕ-tāt) an acetate which contains three molecules of the acetic acid radical.

triacetyloleandomycin (tri-as″ĕ-til-o″le-an″do-mi′sin) troleandomycin.

triacid (tri-as′id) a base capable of neutralizing three equivalents of monobasic acids.

tri-acid (tri-as′id) tricarboxylic ACID.

triacylglycerol (tri-as′il-glis′er-ōl) triglyceride.

triad (tri′ad) [L. *trias;* Gr. *trias* group of three] 1. a group of three entities or objects. 2. any trivalent element. **Andersen's t.,** Andersen's SYNDROME. **Enslin's t.,** a triad of tower skull due to premature ossification of the coronal sutures, adenoid hypertrophy, and exophthalmos. **Franke's t.,** palatal abnormalities, deviation of the nasal septum, and adenoids. Associated with the triad may be respiration through the mouth, dry lips, and susceptibility to infection. **Hutchinson's t.,** interstitial keratitis, deafness due to lesions of the eighth cranial nerve, and Hutchinson's teeth (see under TOOTH); seen in congenital syphilis. **Jacod's t.,** retrosphenoidal space SYNDROME.

triage (tre-ahzh′) [Fr. "sorting"] 1. the sorting out or screening of patients seeking care in a health care facility, to determine which service is initially required and with what priority. 2. the sorting out and classification of casualties of war or of other disaster, to determine priority of need and proper place of treatment.

trial (tri′al) 1. the examination before a judicial tribunal of the facts put in issue in a cause. 2. an attempt to do something. 3. the act of testing, or putting to the proof. **double-bind t.,** one in which the nature of the treatment being received by a subject at any time is unknown to both subject and observer, as when an active and an inert substance are given during a study on the effectiveness of a drug. **field t.,** an experiment under natural conditions that aims at testing the effectiveness of a method or substance. **random controlled t.,** an experimental prospective study for assessing the effects of a drug or medical procedure in which human or animal subjects are assigned on a random basis to either of two groups, experimental and control, the experimental group receiving the drug or procedure but not the control group. Laboratory tests and clinical studies, usually double-blind studies, determine differences between members of both groups. Abbreviated RCT. **single-blind t.,** one in which one participant, usually the subject, is unaware of the treatment he is receiving, as when an active and an inert substance are given during a study on the effectiveness of a drug.

triamcinolone (tri″am-sin′o-lōn) a synthetic glucocorticoid prepared from hydrocortisone acetate, 9-fluoro-11β,16α,17,21-tetrahydroxypregna-1,4-diene-3,20-dione, occurring as a white, crystalline powder with a slight odor, which is soluble in dimethyl sulfoxide and slightly soluble in water, propylene glycol, ethanol, and chloroform. Used in the treatment of adrenocortical insufficiency and as an anti-inflammatory and antiallergic agent. In dentistry, used in the treatment of sensitive dentin, pulpal reactions to surgery, oral ulcers associated with skin diseases, and arthritic temporomandibular lesions, and in tissue transplantation. Side reactions are those of other glucocorticoids. Trademarks: Aristocort, Kenacort, Tricortale. **t. acetonide,** a triamcinolone derivative that shares its glucocorticoid activity, in which the 16- and 17-hydroxyl groups have formed a ketal by interaction with acetone. It occurs as a white to cream-colored, crystalline powder that is soluble in dehydrated ethanol, chloroform, and methanol, slightly soluble in acetone and ethyl acetate, and insoluble in water. Available in many dosage forms, including dental paste. Trademarks: Aristoderm, Ftorocort, Kenalog, Tramacin, Volonimat. **t. diacetate,** the diacetate ester of triamcinolone, occurring as white crystals with a slight odor and a bitter taste, which are soluble in chloroform, slightly soluble in ether, ethanol, and methanol, and insoluble in water. It has actions and uses identical to those of the parent compound. Available as a dental paste. **t. hexacetonide,** the hexacetonide ester of triamcinolone, occurring as a white odorless, crystalline powder with a slightly bitter taste, which is soluble in methanol and chloroform, but not in water. In the body, it is converted to triamcinolone, thus having identical potential actions, uses, and side effects. Used for injection into inflamed joints and soft-tissue lesions. Trademark: Aristopan.

Triamelin trademark for *triethylenemelamine.*

triangle (tri′ang-g'l) [L. *triangulum; tres* three + *angulus* angle] a three-cornered area. See also ANGLE, TRIGONE, and TRIGONUM. **Assézat's t.,** facial t. **Béclard's t.,** the area lying between the posterior edge of the hypoglossal muscle, the posterior belly of the digastric muscle, and the greater cornu of the hyoid bone. **Bolton's t.,** one formed by drawing a line from the nasion to the sella turcica to the Bolton point. **Bonwill t.,** one formed by a line connecting the centers of the mandibular condyles and lines connecting either center with the mesial contact area of the mandibular medial incisors, each side being approximately 4 inches long. **carotid t.,** the superior part of the anterior triangle of the neck, bounded by the sternocleidomastoid muscle, omohyoid muscle, and posterior belly of the digastric muscle. The hyoglossus, thyrohyoid, and middle and inferior pharyngeal muscles form its floor. Running through it are the external carotid artery, the internal jugular vein, and the vagus, accessory, and hypoglossal nerves, and the cervical part of the sympathetic trunk. Called also *carotid trigone, fossa carotica,* and *trigonum caroticum* [NA]. **carotid t., inferior,** the part of the carotid triangle medial to the omohyoid muscle. Called also *t. of necessity.* **carotid t., superior,** the part of the carotid triangle lateral to the omohyoid muscle. Called also *t. of election, Gerdy's hyoid fossa,* and *Malgaigne's fossa.* **cephalic t.,** one of the anteroposterior planes of the skull, between the lines from the occiput to the forehead and to the chin, and a third line extending from the chin to the forehead. **cervical t.,** t. of neck. **Codman's t.,** a triangular area visible roentgenographically where the periosteum, elevated by a bone tumor, rejoins the cortex of normal bone. **congruent t's,** triangles which coincide when one is placed on the other. See bisecting angle TECHNIQUE. **digastric t.,** submandibular t. **t. of election,** superior carotid t. **facial t.,** a triangular area whose points are the basion, the alveolar point, and the nasion. Called also *Assézat's t.* **Farabeuf's t.,** one in the upper part of the neck, its sides being formed by the internal jugular vein and the facial vein, and its base by the hypoglossal nerve. **frontal t.,** one bounded by the maximum frontal diameter and lines from either end of this diameter to the glabella. **hypoglossohyoid t.,** a triangular area in the subhyoid region, bounded above by the hypoglossal nerve, in front by the posterior border of the mylohyoid muscle, and behind and below by the tendon of the digastric muscle. Called also *Pinaud's t.* and *Pirogoff's t.* **Jackson's safety t.,** a triangular space bounded below by the lower end of the thyroid cartilage, its apex in the suprasternal notch, and its sides the inner edges of the sternocleidomastoid muscle; so called because it marks the limit of the area through which the trachea may safely be incised in tracheostomy. **Lesser's t.,** one bounded by the hypoglossal nerve above and the two bellies of the digastricus muscle on the other two sides. **lymphoid t.,** Weldeyer's tonsillar RING. **Macewen's t.,** suprameatal t. **Malgaigne's t.,** superior carotid t. **t. of necessity,** carotid t., inferior.

t. of neck, one of the triangular areas located in deep structures of the neck, defined by muscular, bony, and cartilaginous landmarks. Called also *cervical t.* **t. of neck, anterior,** a triangular area formed anteriorly by the median line of the neck, superiorly by the lower margin of the mandible, and posteriorly by the sternocleidomastoid muscle. It is divided into the submandibular, submental carotid, and macular triangles, and is separated from the posterior triangle of the neck by the sternocleidomastoid muscle. See also *submandibular t.* and *submental t.* **t. of neck, posterior,** a triangular area bounded anteriorly by the sternocleidomastoid muscle, posteriorly by the trapezius muscle, and inferiorly by the middle third of the clavicle. It is separated from the anterior triangle of the neck by the sternocleidomastoid muscle. Its floor is formed by the prevertebral fascia beneath which are the deep neck muscles, subclavian artery, and cervical and brachial nerve plexuses. **occipital t., inferior,** one formed by lines drawn between three points, two being the mastoid processes and the third the inion. **palatal t.,** one limited by the greatest transverse diameter of the palate and lines from either end of this diameter to the alveolar point. **Pinaud's t., Pirogoff's t.,** hypoglossohyoid t. **retromandibular t.,** retromolar t. **retromolar t.,** a triangular shallow fossa on the mandible posterior to the third molar. Called also *retromandibular t.* **submandibular t., submaxillary t.,** the triangular area of the neck under the mandible, bounded by the stylohyoid muscle, posterior belly of the digastric muscle, and anterior belly of the digastric muscle. The mylohyoid and hypoglossus muscles form its floor. Situated in the triangle are the submandibular gland and duct, beneath them, the lingual and hypoglossal nerves, and the facial artery, which gives off the submental artery, running across the triangle. Called also *digastric t., regio submandibulare, submandibular region, submandibular trigone, submaxillary region, submaxillary space, trigonum submandibulare* [NA]. **submental t.,** the suprahyoid portion of the anterior triangle of the neck, situated between the hyoid bone inferiorly and two anterior bellies of the digastric muscles laterally. The anteromedial portion of the mylohyoid muscle forms its floor. It contains the submental lymph nodes and the beginning of the anterior jugular vein. Called also *suprahyoid t.* **suboccipital t.,** a triangular area lying between the rectus capitis posterior major and the obliquus capitis superior and obliquus capitis inferior muscles of the deep neck. **suprahyoid t.,** submental t. **suprameatal t.,** a small triangular area between the posterior root of the zygomatic arch and the posterosuperior part of the external acoustic meatus. Called also *Macewen's t.* and *mastoid fossa of temporal bone.* **surgical t.,** any triangular area or region in which certain nerves, vessels, or organs are located, established for reference in surgical operations. **Trautmann's t.,** a space with its anterior angle at the prominence containing the labyrinth, bounded behind by the transverse sinus and above by the inferior temporal line. When the bone is removed, the superior petrosal sinus will be encountered at the upper posterior angle of this triangle. **Tweed t.,** one defined by facial and dental landmarks on a lateral cephalometric film, using the Frankfort Horizontal as a base.

triangular (tri-ang′gu-lar) [L. *triangularis*] having three corners or angles; pertaining to a triangle.

triangularis (tri-ang″gu-la′ris) [L.] 1. triangular. 2. triangular muscle; see depressor muscle of angle of mouth, under MUSCLE.

triatomic (tri″ah-tom′ik) [tri- + Gr. *atomos* indivisible] 1. made up of three atoms; pertaining to a molecule containing three atoms, as in triatomic ozone, O_3. 2. pertaining to an acid with three replaceable H atoms. 3. pertaining to a base, alcohol, or phenol with three OH groups.

triaxiality (tri-ax′i-al′i-te) 1. a condition of having three axes. 2. in testing materials under pressure, a condition developing in a material undergoing a compression test, whereby the specimen is not sufficiently lubricated and is thus held in the testing viselike device by friction, preventing free spreading of the material upon deformation. The condition not only produces compression along one axis of compression (uniaxial direction) but also causes lateral compressions in the direction of friction.

triazene (tri′ah-zēn) a chemical group containing three nitrogen atoms with one double bond, NH—N=NR. Some triazenes, such as dacarbazine, have cytotoxic properties.

Triazure trademark for *azaribine.*

tribasic (tri-ba′sik) [tri- + L. *basis* base] having three replaceable hydrogen atoms.

Tribondeau, Louis [French naval physician, 1872–1918] see Bergonié-Tribondeau LAW.

tribromsalan (tri-brom′sah-lan) a bacteriostatic and antifungal agent, 3,5-dibromo-N-(4-bromophenyl)-2-hydroxybenzamide,

occurring as a white, tasteless powder with a slight odor, which is soluble in acetone, ether, ethanol, and benzene, slightly soluble in chloroform, and insoluble in water. Incorporated in antiseptic soaps. Trademarks: TBS, Temasept IV, Tualsal 100.

tributyrase (tri-bu′ti-rās) triacylglycerol LIPASE.

tricalcic (tri-kal′sik) containing three atoms of calcium.

tricalcium orthophosphate (tri-kal′se-um or″tho-fos′făt) CALCIUM phosphate, tribasic.

tricalcium phosphate (tri-kal′se-um fos′făt) CALCIUM phosphate, tribasic.

Trichinella (trik″ĭ-nel′ah) [Gr. *trichinos* a hair] a nematode parasite. **T. spira′lis,** a small nematode which causes trichinosis. The adult male is about 1.4 to 1.6 mm in length, and the female is twice the size of the male. Both the adults and encysted larvae develop within the same host, but two hosts are needed to complete the life cycle. Man and other carnivores, rats, and hogs are the principal hosts. See TRICHINOSIS.

trichinosis (trik″ĭ-no′sis) infection with the nematode *Trichinella spiralis,* usually caused by ingestion of raw or inadequately cooked pork. After ingestion of infected meat, the larvae are released and enter the intestinal mucosa, causing irritation and trauma to the tissues. Within five to seven days, the parasites mature and mate; males are passed out of the intestines and females die after discharging larvae. The migration and burrowing of larvae into the tissues causes muscular pain, tenderness, stiffness, weakness, backache, precordial pain, periorbital edema and swelling of the face, ocular hemorrhage, headache, tinnitus, deafness, delirium, coma, thrombosis, and a variety of other symptoms, depending on the site of invasion. Encapsulation occurs only in the striated muscle, and larvae burrowing into other tissues are eventually destroyed. Leukocytosis, eosinophilia, and increase of serum transaminases are usually present. The parasites are most commonly found in the diaphragmatic, masseteric, intercostal, extraocular, pectoral, deltoid, gluteus, biceps, and gastrocnemius muscles; the tongue and larynx are also common sites of infection.

trichlormethiazide (tri-klor′mě-thi′ah-zīd) a long-acting benzothiazine diuretic with antihypertensive properties, 6-chloro-3-(dichloromethyl) - 3,4 - dihydro-2 H-1,2,4-benzothiazine-7-sulfonamide, occurring as a white, odorless, photosensitive, crystalline powder that is soluble in acetone, ethanol, water, and chloroform. Adverse effects are similar to those associated with other benzothiazide diuretics. Trademarks: Esmarin, Eurinol, Flutra, Gangesol, Metahydrin, Salurin, Triclordiuride.

trichloroethane (tri″klor-o-eth′ēn) trichloroethylene.

trichloroethylene (tri″klo-ro-eth′ĭ-lēn) a compound, CHCl:CCl₂, occurring as a clear, colorless or blue, mobile liquid with a chloroform-like odor, which is miscible with ethanol, chloroform, ether and other organic liquids, but is insoluble in water. It has been used in the past as a general inhalation anesthetic. Sometimes used in treating trigeminal neuralgia and for obstetric analgesia, but is slow in onset of analgesia and is potentially cardiotoxic and hepatotoxic. Called also *ethinyl trichloride* and *trichloroethene.* Trademarks: Chlorylen, Tri, Trilene.

trichlorofluoromethane (tri-klo″ro-floor-o-meth′ăn) a compound, CCl₃F, occurring as a colorless, volatile liquid. Used chiefly as a solvent, fire extinguisher, refrigerant, and aerosol propellant. It may be narcotic in high concentrations. Called also *fluorocarbon 11* and *trichloromonofluoromethane.* Trademark: Freon 11.

trichloromethane (tri″klor-o-meth′ăn) chloroform.

trichloromonofluoromethane (tri-klo″ro-mon″o-floor-o-meth′ăn) trichlorofluoromethane.

Trichloryl trademark for *triclofos sodium* (see under TRICLOFOS).

tricho- [Gr. *thrix, trichos,* hair] a prefix denoting relationship to hair.

Trichomonas (tri-kom′o-nas) [tricho- + Gr. *monas* unit] a genus of protozoa of the subphylum Mastigophora, occurring as pear-shaped cells with four flagella in front, an undulating membrane, and a trailing flagellum. Various species cause disease in animals, including urogenital infection in man. **T. bucca′lis,** *T. tenax.* **T. elonga′ta,** *T. tenax.* **T. hom′inis,** a species that is an intestinal parasite in man. **T. te′nax,** a nonpathogenic species found in the human mouth. Called also *T. buccalis* and *T. elongata.* **T. vagina′lis,** a species parasitizing in the human vagina, which may be transmitted to males.

trichomoniasis (trik″o-mo-ni′ah-sis) infection with *Trichomonas,* usually involving the intestinal and genital tracts, but sometimes also involving the oral cavity.

Trichophyton (tri-kof′ĭ-ton) [*tricho-* + Gr. *phyton* plant] a genus of dermatophytes, species of which cause tinea capitis, tinea barbae, tinea corporis, tinea cruris, and infections of the skin of the feet and nails. **T. concen′tricum,** the etiologic agent of tinea imbricata. **T. schoenlei′nii,** the etiologic agent of favus.

Trichosporon (tri-kos′po-ron) [*tricho-* + Gr. *sporos* seed] a genus of deuteromycetous fungi (Fungi Imperfecti) that reproduces by blastospores and arthrospores, the species of which are normal inhabitants of the respiratory and intestinal tracts in animals. Called also *Trichosporum.* **T. beige′lii, T. cuta′neum, T. gigan′teum,** a species that causes a disease of the hair in which the shafts bear either black or white hard gritty nodular masses of fungi. It is rarely an opportunistic parasite in debilitated patients, causing a fatal systemic infection.

Trichosporum (tri-kos′po-rum) *Trichosporon.*

trichromatic (tri″kro-mat′ik) [*tri-* + Gr. *chrōma* color] 1. pertaining to or exhibiting three colors. 2. able to distinguish only three colors.

tricipital (tri-sip′ĭ-tal) having three heads.

triclocarban (tri″klo-kar′ban) an antiseptic, 3,4,4′-trichlorocarbanilide, occurring as a fine, white to off-white, powder with a slight characteristic odor, which is soluble in acetone, propylene glycol, and dimethyl formamide, but not in water. It is effective against gram-positive and, to a lesser degree, gram-negative bacteria and some fungi, usually incorporated into antiseptic and deodorant soaps, solutions, powders, and ointments. Also used in the treatment of acne. It may cause a photoallergic reaction. Trademarks: Solubacter, TCC.

triclofos sodium (tri′klo-fōs) a hypnotic and sedative agent, 2,2,2-trichloroethanol dihydrogen phosphate monosodium, occurring as a white, odorless, hygroscopic powder with a saline taste, which is soluble in water and ethanol, but not in ether. Used in the treatment of insomnia. It may be habit forming. Trademarks: Triclos, Trichloryl.

Triclordiuride trademark for *trichlormethiazide.*

Triclos trademark for *triclofos sodium* (see under TRICLOFOS).

triclosan (tri′klo-san) an antibacterial agent, 2,4,4′-trichloro-2′-hydroxydiphenyl ether, occurring as a white or off-white crystalline powder with a slight aromatic odor, which is readily soluble in most organic solvents and alkaline solutions and almost insoluble in water. It is ineffective against gram-negative *Pseudomonas.* Used in various cosmetic products and antibacterial soaps. Trademark: Irgasan DP 300.

triconodont (tri-kon′o-dont) [*tri-* + Gr. *kōnos* cone + *odous* tooth] a tooth having three cones in linear arrangement, the central cone being usually the largest.

tricornute (tri-kor′nūt) [*tri-* + L. *cornutus* horned] having three horns, cornua, or processes.

Tricortale trademark for *triamcinolone.*

Tricoryl trademark for *trolnitrate phosphate* (see under TROLNITRATE).

tricresol (tri-kre′sol) cresol.

tricuspal (tri-kus′pal) tricuspid.

tricuspid (tri-kus′pid) [L. *tricuspis*] 1. having three cusps or points, such as a tooth with three cusps; tricuspal. 2. pertaining to the tricuspid valves of the heart.

tricyclic (tri-sik′lik) [*tri-* + Gr. *kyklikos* cyclic] 1. pertaining to or containing a molecule having three rings of atoms, as anthracene. 2. a ring of three atoms.

Tridione trademark for *trimethadione.*

-triene a suffix indicating the presence of three double bonds in a chemical compound.

triethylamine (tri″eth-il-am′in) a compound, *N,N*-diethylethanamine, occurring as a colorless liquid with an ammoniacal odor; used for hardening of polymers and in various chemical processes.

triethylenemelamine (tri-eth″ĭ-lēn-mel′ah-mēn) an alkylating agent with cytotoxic properties, 2,4,6-tris(1-aziridinyl)-*s*-striazine, derived from ethylenimine. It occurs as a white, odorless, crystalline powder with an ammonia-like odor, which is soluble in water, chloroform, ethanol, acetone, benzene, and carbon tetrachloride. Used in the treatment of Hodgkin's disease and other lymphomas, retinoblastoma, and other neoplasms, and in polycythemia vera and mycosis fungoides. Adverse effects include nausea, vomiting, diarrhea, anorexia, abdominal cramps, headache, euphoria, hiccoughs, asthenia, amenorrhea, oligospermia, retrosternal burning sensation, renal damage, hepatic disorders, fetal abnormalities, predisposition to infection, and bone marrow depression with leukopenia, pancytopenia, and thrombocytopenia. Abbreviated TEM. Called also *tretamine.* Trademarks: Persitol, Triamelin.

triethylenephosphoramide (tri-eth″ĭ-lēn-fos-for′ah-mĭd) a poisonous alkylating agent with cytotoxic properties, 1,1′,1″-phosphinylidynetrisaziridine, derived from ethylenimine. It occurs as crystals that are soluble in water, ethanol, ether, and acetone. Used in the treatment of cancer. Also used as a chemosterilant, acaricide, and insecticide, and in various chemical processes. Abbreviated TEPA. Called also *phosphoric acid triethyleneimide.*

triethylenethiophosphoramide (tri-eth″ĭ-lēn-thi″o-fos-for′ah-mĭd) an alkylating agent with cytotoxic properties that is a thio-derivative of triethylenephosphoramide, 1,1′,1″-phosphinothioylidynetrisaziridine. It occurs as white, fine crystalline crystals that are soluble in water, ethanol, chloroform, and ether. Used in the treatment of Hodgkin's disease and other lymphomas, retinoblastoma, and other neoplasms, and in mycosis fungoides. Side effects may include anorexia, nausea, vomiting, headache, fever, neutropenia, predisposition to infection, and bone marrow depression with neutropenia, thrombocytopenia, and anemia. Called also *thio-TEPA.* Trademarks: Tespamin, Tifosyl.

trifacial (tri-fa′shal) [L. *trifacialis*] pertaining to the trigeminal nerve; trigeminal.

trifid (tri′fid) [*tri-* + L. *findere* to split] split into three parts.

trifluoperazine hydrochloride (tri″floo-o-per′ah-zēn) a tranquilizer that is an analogue of chlorpromazine, 10-[3-(4-methyl-1-piperazinyl)propyl]-2-(trifluoromethyl)phenothiazide. It occurs as a white to tan, crystalline powder with a slight characteristic odor, which is soluble in water, ethanol and acetone, but not in ether. Used in the treatment of mental disorders and in controlling apprehension prior to surgical or dental operations. Also used as an adjunct in treating tetanus. Side effects may include drowsiness, parkinsonian-like symptoms, dystonia, dyskinesia, akathisia, hyperreflexia, seizures, cerebral edema, postural hypotension, tachycardia, bradycardia, cardiac arrest, vertigo, agranulocytosis, eosinophilia, leukopenia, hemolytic anemia, thrombocytopenic purpura, and allergy. Trademarks: Eskazine, Stelazine, Terfluzine.

triflupromazine (tri″floo-pro′mah-zēn) a tranquilizer that is an analogue of chlorpromazine, *N,N*-dimethyl-2-(trifluoromethyl)10*H*-phenothiazine-10 propanamine. It occurs as a viscous amber-colored, oily liquid which is insoluble in water and crystallizes on prolonged standing. Used in the treatment of mental disorders and in controlling apprehension prior to surgical or dental operations. Also used as an adjunct in the treatment of tetanus. Side effects may include drowsiness, parkinsonian-like symptoms, dystonia, dyskinesia, akathisia, hyperreflexia, seizures, cerebral edema, postural hypotension, tachycardia, bradycardia, vertigo, cardiac arrest, agranulocytosis, eosinophilia, leukopenia, hemolytic anemia, thrombocytopenic purpura, and allergy. Trademarks: Vesprin, Vetame. **t. hydrochloride,** the hydrochloride salt of triflupromazine, occurring as a white to tan, crystalline powder with a slight characteristic odor, which is soluble in water, ethanol, and acetone, but not in ether. Its pharmacological and toxicological properties are similar to those of the parent compound. Trademarks: Adazine, Fluomazina, Fluorofen, Siquil, Vesprin.

trifunctional (tri-funk′shun-al) 1. having three functions. 2. in chemistry, having three reaction sites; said of a molecule.

trifurcation (tri″fur-ka′shun) [*tri-* + L. *furca* fork] division in three parts or branches, as in a tooth with three roots, such as a maxillary first molar.

trigeminal (tri-jem′ĭ-nal) [*tri-* + L. *geminus* twin] 1. triple. 2. pertaining to the trigeminal nerve.

Trigesic tablets see under TABLET.

triglyceride (tri-glis′er-īd) a glyceride in which all three hydroxyl groups of glycerol are esterified with fatty acids. It is a neutral fat synthesized from carbohydrates for storage in animal adipose cells, being synthesized from glycerol and fatty acids in activated forms. The active form of glycerol is L-glycerol-3-phosphate, which is formed from dihydroacetone phosphate, the product of aldolase reaction in the Embden-Meyerhof pathway of metabolism. The glycerol phosphate reacts with fatty acid CoA derivatives from a diglyceride, which then reacts with another mole of fatty acid CoA to form a triglyceride. Some triglycerides, such as tristearin and tripalmitin, are solids at 20° C; triolein is liquid. Triglycerides are relatively insoluble in water and tend to form highly dispersed micelles. Called also *triacylglycerol.* **blood t's.,** see blood LIPID. **t. hydrolysis,** see LIPOLYSIS. **t. lipase,** triacylglycerol LIPASE. **mixed t.,** one containing two or more different fatty acids. **simple t.,** one containing a single kind of fatty acid in all three positions.

trigona (tri-go′nah) [L.] plural of *trigonum.*

trigone (tri′gon) [Gr. *trigōnon* triangle] 1. a triangle; a triangular area. See also TRIANGLE and TRIGONUM. 2. the first three cusps of a maxillary molar tooth. See METACONE, PARACONE, and

PROTOCONE. **carotid t.,** carotid TRIANGLE. **t. of hypoglossal nerve,** the tapering lower end of the medial eminence of the rhomboid fossa just superficial to the position of the hypoglossal nucleus. Called also *eminentia hypoglossi, trigonum nervi hypoglossi* [NA], and *tuberculum hypoglossi.* **olfactory t.,** a triangular expansion of the olfactory tract, between the diverging striae. Called also *trigonum olfactorium* [NA]. **submandibular t.,** submandibular TRIANGLE. **t. of vagus nerve,** an area in the floor of the fourth ventricle, beneath which lies the dorsal nucleus of the vagus nerve. Called also *eminentia vagi, trigonum nervi vagi* [NA], and *vagal eminence.*

trigonid (tri-gon′id) [*trigone* + *-id*] the triad of three principal cusps (protoconid, paraconid, metaconid) on the elevated moiety of a lower molar of the primitive tuberculosectorial type.

trigonocephaly (tri-go″no-sef′ah-le) [Gr. *trigonon* triangle + *kephalē* head] a deformity characterized by a keel-shaped forehead and wide biparietal diameter of the skull, associated with small nasal septum, premaxilla, and ethmoid plates. It is believed to be due to fusion of the two halves of the frontal bone during fetal development, resulting in the frontal protuberance. **Opitz′ t.,** Opitz′ trigonocephaly SYNDROME.

trigonum (tri-go′num), pl. *trigo′na* [L.; Gr. *trigōnon* triangle] a three-cornered area; a triangle. See also TRIANGLE and TRIGONE. **t. carot′icum,** carotid TRIANGLE. **t. col′li latera′le,** posterior region of neck (2); see under REGION. **t. ner′vi hypoglos′si** [NA], TRIGONE of hypoglossal nerve. **t. ner′vi va′gi** [NA], TRIGONE of vagus nerve. **t. olfacto′rium** [NA], olfactory TRIGONE. **t. submandibula′re** [NA], submandibular TRIANGLE.

trihexyphenidyl hydrochloride (tri-hek″sĕ-fen′ĭ-dil) an antimuscarinic and antispasmodic drug, α-cyclohexyl-α-phenyl-1-piperidinepropanol hydrochloride, occurring as a white crystalline powder with a faint odor, which is soluble in ethanol and chloroform and slightly soluble in water. Used in the treatment of parkinsonism. Side reactions include constipation, dry skin, skin rash, xerostomia, blurred vision, tachycardia, nervousness, headache, muscle weakness, excessive sedation, insomnia, urinary retention, parotitis, vomiting, tinnitus, vertigo, confusion agitation, hallucination, and psychotic episodes. Trademarks: Aparkan, Artane, Cyclodel, Pacitane, Paragit, Parkinsan, Pipanol, Triphenidyl.

Trihistan trademark for *chlorcyclizine.*

trihydrate (tri-hi′drāt) [*tri-* + Gr. *hydōr* water] a hydrate containing three molecules of water for every molecule of other substance in the compound.

trihydroxy- a prefix indicating the presence of three hydroxyl (OH) groups in a chemical compound.

triiodide (tri-i″o-dīd) any binary compound containing three atoms of iodine.

triiodomethane (tri-i″o-do-meth′ān) iodoform.

triiodothyronine (tri″i-o″do-thi′ro-nēn) a thyroid hormone which stimulates metabolic processes, β-[4-(4-hydroxy-3-iodophenoxy)-3,5-diiodophenyl] alanine. Inadequate production of triiodothyronine by the thyroid gland results in hypothyroidism; excessive production results in hyperthyroidism. Used in replacement therapy in hypothyroidism. Symbol T_3. See also thyroid ANTAGONIST.

Trilafon trademark for *perphenazine.*

trilaminar (tri-lam′ĭ-nar) consisting of three layers.

trilateral (tri′lat′er-al) [*tri-* + L. *latus* side] three-sided; having three sides.

Trilene trademark for *trichloroethylene.*

Trilifan trademark for *perphenazine.*

Trimedal trademark for *trimethadione.*

trimeprazine (tri-mep′rah-zēn) a potent antihistaminic drug that blocks histamine mediation at the H₁ receptor, 10[3-(dimethylamino)-2-methylpropyl]phenothiazine. Used therapeutically in the form of the tartrate salt, which occurs as a white to off-white, odorless, crystalline powder that darkens on exposure to light, and is readily dissolved in water and chloroform and is slightly soluble in ether and benzene. It has mild central nervous system depressant, moderate antiemetic, and anticonvulsant properties. Used in the treatment of pruritus and various allergic diseases. Dryness of the mouth and mucous membranes, drowsiness, and gastrointestinal disorders are the potential side effects. Prolonged administration may result in agranulocytosis, hypotension, and parkinsonian-like symptoms. Called also *methylpromazine.* Trademarks: Temaril, Vallergan.

trimer (tri′mer) [*tri-* + Gr. *muros* part] 1. a chemical compound consisting of three monomer molecules reacting to join together to form a single molecule containing three mer. See also POLYMER. 2. a capsomer having three structural subunits.

trimethadione (tri″meth-ah-di′ōn) an antiepileptic drug, 3,3,5-trimethyl-2,4-oxazolidine-dione, occurring as white, crystalline

granules with a camphor-like odor and a burning bitter taste, which are soluble in water, ethanol, ether, and chloroform. Severe side reactions may occur, including hiccups, nausea, vomiting, gastric distress, anorexia, photophobia, diplopia, hemeralopia, vertigo, irritability, insomnia, drowsiness, paresthesia, headache, fatigue, malaise, personality changes, skin rash, petechial hemorrhage, epistaxis, bleeding gingivae, blood dyscrasias, lupus erythematosus–like symptoms, albuminuria, and blood pressure changes. Use in pregnancy may cause fetal trimethadione syndrome (see under SYNDROME). Trademarks: Epidione, Petidon, Tridione, Trimedal, Troxidone.

trimethaphan camsylate (tri-meth′ah-fan) a ganglionic blocking agent, (+)-1, 3-dibenzyldecahydro-2-oxoimidazol[4, 5-*c*] thieno-[1,2-*a*]thiolium 2-oxo-10-bornanesulfonate, occurring as a white powder or white crystals, that are soluble in water, ethanol, and chloroform, but not in ether. Used as a hypotensive drug of very short duration for the induction of brief hypotension, as in surgical operations. It also causes release of histamine. Trademark: Arfonad Camphorsulfonate.

trimethidinium methosulfate (tri-meth″ĭ-din′ĭ-um) a quaternary ammonium ganglionic blocking agent, 1,3,8,8-tetramethyl-3-[3 - trimethylammonio)propyl] - 3 - azoniabicyclo [3,2,1] octane bis(methyl sulfate), occurring as a white, crystalline hygroscopic powder that is odorless or has a slight camphoraceous odor, and is soluble in water and ethanol, slightly soluble in acetone, and insoluble in ether. Used in the treatment of hypertension. Called also *camphidonium.* Trademark: Ostensin.

trimethoprim (tri-meth′o-prim) a broad-spectrum antimalarial and antibacterial drug, 2,4-diamine-5-(3,4,5-trimethoxybenzyl)-pyrimidine, occurring as a white to cream-colored, odorless, bitter, crystalline powder or solids that are soluble in chloroform and ethanol, and slightly in water. It is also a folic acid antagonist. Adverse effects may include nausea, vomiting, diarrhea, malaise, immunosuppression, skin rash, leukopenia, and thrombocytopenia.

trimethylamine (tri″meth-il-am′in) a colorless gas with a fishy, ammoniacal odor, *N,N*-dimethylmethanamine, which is obtained from beet sugar residue and herring brine. In the body, it probably results from the decomposition of choline. In conjugated form, trimethylamine is widely distributed in animal tissue and especially in fish; fishes excrete nitrogen as trimethylamine oxide. It has been reported in menstrual blood and in urine stored at room temperature. Trimethylamine is converted to the free tertiary amine during putrefaction. Used as an insect attractant and in chemical processes. It has been used in the treatment of gout, chorea, and rheumatism.

trimethylene (tri-meth′ĭ-lēn) cyclopropane.

trimmer (trim′er) a device or instrument for shaping something through cutting or clipping the edges. **gingival margin t., (GMT),** margin t. **margin t.,** a cutting instrument having a shaft that is curved and angled in two directions to practice right and left applications for both mesial and distal surfaces; used for believing cavosurface margins. Called also *gingival margin t. (GMT).* See illustration. **model t.,** a device for trimming plaster and stone casts. The casts are held against a large rotating

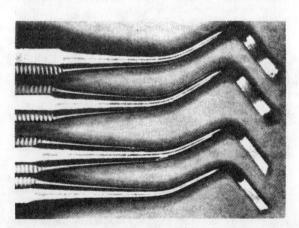

Two sizes of margin trimmers. (From H. W. Gilmore, M. R. Lund, D. J. Bales, and J. Vernetti: Operative Dentistry. 3rd ed. St. Louis, The C. V. Mosby Co., 1977.)

grinding wheel, which is kept wet by a stream of water to keep down dust and keep the cutting wheel clean. Called also *plaster t.* **plaster t.,** model t. **proximal t.,** a delicate file for trimming and smoothing the proximal surfaces of restorations, crowns, etc. **wax t.,** a flat knife for trimming and shaping wax models.

trimming (trim′ing) 1. removing by clipping, paring, or pruning; also, pieces so removed. 2. decorating or embellishing. 3. arranging or shaping. **muscle t.,** border MOLDING.

trimolecular (tri″mo-lek′u-lar) relating to or formed from three molecules.

trinitrate (tri-ni′trāt) a compound containing three nitrate radicals, $(HO_3)_3$. **glyceryl t.,** nitroglycerin.

trinitroglycerin (tri-ni″tro-glis′er-in) nitroglycerin.

trinitroglycerol (tri-ni′tro-glis′e-rol) nitroglycerin.

-trioic a chemical suffix indicating a tricarboxylic acid.

triolein (tri-o′le-in) a triglyceride, $C_{56}H_{104}O_6$, found in various oils and fats; it is a colorless, oily liquid insoluble in water but freely soluble in ether and alcohol. Called also *glyceryl, olein,* and *trioleate.*

Triopac trademark for *acetrizoate sodium* (see under ACETRIZOATE).

triose (tri′ōs) a monosaccharide containing three carbon atoms in a molecule, $C_3H_6O_3$.

trioxide (tri-ok′sīd) a binary compound containing three atoms of oxygen for one atom of another element.

trioxsalen (tri-ok′sah-len) a melanizing agent, 2,5,9-trimethyl-7H-furol[3,2-g][1]benzopyran-7-one, occurring as an off-white, odorless, tasteless, crystalline solid that is soluble in alcohol and chloroform, but not in water. Used to facilitate repigmentation in vitiligo, increase tolerance to sunrays, and enhance pigmentation. The drug promotes pigmentation only in the presence of sunlight and facilitates the action of near ultraviolet light in stimulating melanin formation. Contraindicated in photosensitivity; severe sunburn may occur. The drug may cause gastric irritation and vomiting.

tripalmitin (tri-pal′mĭ-tin) a triglyceride, $C_{51}H_{98}O_6$, obtained from glycerol and palmitic acid, which is insoluble in water and alcohol but is soluble in ether, benzene, and chloroform. It is found in some oils, especially in palm oil. Called also *palmitin* and *tripalmitoylglycerol.*

tripalmitoylglycerol (tri″pal-mĭ-toil-glis′er-ol) tripalmitin.

Tri-Pax trademark for a preparation, 100 mg of which contains 25 mg parachlorophenol, 25 mg metacresyl acetate, and 50 mg camphor; used in root canal therapy and in periapical infections.

tripelennamine (tri″pĕ-lēn′ah-mēn) an antihistaminic agent that blocks histamine at the H_1 receptor, 2-[benzyl[2-(dimethylamino)ethyl]amino]pyridine, used in the treatment of allergic diseases. The citrate salt is a white crystalline powder that is soluble in water and alcohol, slightly soluble in ether, and insoluble in chloroform and benzene; the hydrochloride salt is a white crystalline powder which darkens on exposure to light and is soluble in water, alcohol, chloroform, and acetone. Sedation, occasional central nerve stimulation, and gastrointestinal disorders are the side effects. Trademarks: Azaron, Dehistin, PBZ, Pyribenzamine, Tonaril.

tripeptide (tri-pep′tid) [*tri-* + *peptide*] a polypeptide which, on hydrolysis, yields three amino acids.

triphasic (tri-fa′zik) [*tri-* + Gr. *phasis* phase] 1. occurring in three phases or stages. Cf. DIPHASIC and MONOPHASIC. 2. triply varied or triply phasic; used in describing the electromotive actions of muscles.

Triphenidyl trademark for *trihexyphenidyl hydrochloride* (see under TRIHEXYPHENIDYL).

triphosphatase (tri-fos′fah-tās) adenosinetriphosphatase.

triphosphate (tri-fos′fāt) a salt containing three phosphate radicals. **adenosine t.,** ADENOSINE triphosphate.

triplet (trip′let) 1. one of three individuals produced at the same birth. 2. a combination of three objects or entities. 3. codon.

triplex (tri′pleks) [Gr. *triploos* triple] triple or threefold.

triploidy (trip′loi-de) the presence in humans of 69 chromosomes, or three full sets.

tripod (tri′pod) [Gr. *treis* three + *pous* foot] anything having three feet or supports. **t. of the Empirics,** the three principles on which the Empirics based their theory of medicine: (1) their own chance observation — their own experience; (2) learning obtained from contemporaries and predecessors — the experience of others; and (3), in cases of new diseases, the formation of conclusions from other diseases which they resembled — analogy. See also EMPIRIC.

tripoding (tri″pod-ing) the marking of a cast at three points in the plane as a method for repositioning the cast in the same plane during subsequent procedures.

tripoli (trip′o-le) a granulated white or gray porous siliceous rock that was originally mined near Tripoli in Northern Africa and is presently produced from silica. It occurs as a fine powder consisting of amorphous, soft grains. Tripoli is used as a polishing agent in dentistry and is available in stick form for application to a rag wheel or felt cone for producing a high polish on metal objects, such as dental restorations. It is used following the preliminary polishing with pumice and is followed in turn by the use of rouge, which produces even a higher degree of polish.

triprolidine (tri-pro′lĭ-dēn) an antihistaminic drug that blocks histamine mediation at the H_1 receptor, (*E*)-2-[3-(1-pyrrolidinyl)-1-*p*-tolypropenyl]pyridine, which has a rapid onset and long duration of action. Used in the form of the hydrochloride salt, which occurs as a white crystalline powder with a slight unpleasant odor and a bitter taste, and is soluble in water, alcohol, and chloroform, but insoluble in ether and benzene. Used in the treatment of allergic diseases. Trademarks: Actidil, Actidilon, Pro-Actidil, Pro-Entra.

-tripsy [Gr. *tripsis* a rubbing, friction] a word termination designating a surgical procedure in which a structure is intentionally crushed.

Triptil trademark for *protriptyline hydrochloride* (see under PROTRIPTYLINE).

triquetrous (tri-kwe′trus) [L. *triquetrus*] triangular, three cornered.

TRIS trademark for *tromethamine.*

Tris Amino trademark for *tromethamine.*

tris- in chemical nomenclature, a prefix originally used to indicate three chelates or complicated ligands in a coordinate compound, but generally used in connection with molecules made up of three similar parts.

Trisomin trademark for *magnesium trisilicate* (see under MAGNESIUM).

trismus (triz′mus) [Gr. *trismos* grating, grinding] rigidity of the mandible due to a tonic spasm of masticatory muscles. Called also *lockjaw.* **t. nascen′tium,** the inability to open the jaws sometimes observed in an infant at birth.

trisomy (tri′so-me) the presence of an additional (third) chromosome in an otherwise diploid chromosome complex. **4p t.,** trisomy of the short arm of chromosome 4, associated with a low and flat forehead covered with lanugo; low-set abundant eyebrows dissecting above the nose; aplastic nose with a long and flat saddle, a small tip, and flaring nostrils, resembling a boxer's nose; protruding glabella; horizontal palpebral fissures; blepharophimosis; small eyes and strabismus; and orodental abnormalities, consisting of an elongated upper lip, cleft lip, wide mouth, gothic palate, pointed and recessed chin, and unevenly arranged teeth of diverse sizes, subject to caries. Mortality is relatively high; most infants die during the first few weeks of life. Called also *chromosome 4p trisomy syndrome.* **4q t., partial,** partial trisomy of the long arm of chromosome 4, associated with mental retardation, low birth weight, growth retardation, hypotonia, low life expectancy, and multiple abnormalities. Deformities usually include microcephaly, elongated and open cranial sutures, prominent bridge of the nose that is continuous with a receding forehead, horizontal or slightly oblique palpebral fissures, blepharoptosis, small eyes, low-set and posteriorly rotated malformed ears, a short and sometimes webbed neck, umbilical or inguinal hernia, and a variety of renal, osseous, genital, cerebral, and oral abnormalities. Oral abnormalities usually include short upper lip; elongated philtrum that is bordered by protruding folds and is intersected by a midseam beginning beneath the nasal septum and extending to the middle of the upper lip; protruding lips when the mouth is closed; horizontal dimple in the lower lip; drooping corners of the mouth; straight and receding mandible; pointed chin, and gothic arch. Called also *partial chromosome 4q trisomy syndrome.* **5p t.,** partial duplication of the short arm of chromosome 5, characterized by growth and mental retardation, seizures, an excess of ulnar loops, and characteristic facies with macrocephaly, dolichocephaly, and prominent occiput. Strabismus, hypotonia, hernia, crying difficulty, respiratory disorders, and other complications may occur. Called also *chromosome 5p duplication syndrome* and *trisomy 5p syndrome.* **7q t., partial,** partial duplication of the long arm of chromosome 7, characterized by low birth weight, growth and mental retardation, cleft palate, microretrognathia, small nose, small palpebral fissures, and hypertelorism. Less frequent symptoms include coloboma of the iris, transverse palmar creases, and skeletal abnormalities. Called also *partial chromosome 7q duplication syndrome, partial chromosome 7q trisomy syndrome,* and *partial duplication 7q syndrome.* **t. 8,** a syndrome of a supernumerary chromosome 8, occurring with or without mosaicism, which is characterized by mental retardation, deformed skull, prominent forehead, high-arched palate, low-set and/or dysplastic ears, long and slender trunk, reduced joint mobility, and deep palmar and plantar furrows. Called also *chromosome 8 trisomy syndrome, trisomy C, trisomy C syndrome,* and *trisomy 8 syndrome.* **t. 9,** a syndrome of triplication of chromosome 9, characterized by mental and growth retardation, microcephaly, dolichocephaly, narrow and oblique palpebral fissures, enophthalmos, hypertelorism, large nose, low-set ears, and retromicrognathism. Cerebral, cardiovascular, genital, and osseous abnormalities may be present. Called also *chromosome 9 trisomy syndrome* and *trisomy 9 syndrome.* **9p t.,** trisomy of the short arm of chromosome 9, associated with a syndrome of multiple abnormalities. Principal abnormalities include defects in growth; mental retardation; microcephaly; small, sunken eyes; strabismus; oblique palpebral fissures; moderate hypertelorism; a large nose, especially at the tip, with a nasal bridge that is initially normal but thickens and extends as a thin, protruding subseptum, and with the nostril openings facing downward; short upper lip that permits the incisors and upper canines to be seen, and outward-turned lower lip; large ears; short, sometimes webbed neck; funnel chest; and umbilical hernia. Called also *chromosome 9p trisomy syndrome* and *trisomy 9p syndrome.* **t. 9 mosaicism,** a syndrome characterized by growth and mental retardation, narrow temples, occipital bossing, small palpebral fissures, hypertelorism, enophthalmos, mongoloid palpebral slant, large nose, micrognathia, pouched cheeks, low-set malformed ears, narrow chest, cardiovascular defects, simian creases, and various osseous and genital abnormalities. **9q t., partial,** partial trisomy of the long arm of chromosome 9, associated with mental deficiency, dolichocephaly, sunken eyes, narrow palpebral fissures, flat nose, small mouth, receding chin, and finger deformities. Called also *chromosome 9q partial trisomy syndrome.* **t. 10,** Cockayne's SYNDROME. **10p t.,** duplication of the short arm of chromosome 10, characterized by mental and growth retardation, hypotonia, microsomatia, dolichocephaly, wide sagittal sutures, high prominent forehead, long face, microphthalmia, coloboma, hypertelorism, mongoloid palpebral fissures, arched eyebrows, wide or prominent nasal root, anteverted nostrils, turtle-like mouth, cleft lip or palate, long philtrum, low-set posteriorly rotated ears, micrognathia, and various renal, cardiovascular, pulmonary, genital, and skeletal abnormalities. Called also *chromosome 10p duplication syndrome, chromosome 10p trisomy syndrome,* and *partial duplication 10p syndrome.* **10q t.,** duplication of the distal segment of the long arm of chromosome 10, characterized by mental and growth retardation, microcephaly, high forehead, flat or oval face, antimongoloid palpebral fissures, blepharoptosis, arched and/or spaced eyebrows, epicanthus, blepharophimosis, microphthalmia, small nose with a broad and flat bridge and anteverted nostrils, bow-shaped mouth, prominent upper lip, long philtrum, cleft palate, micrognathia, prominent malar areas, low-set ears, short neck, and various skeletal, cardiovascular, and genital abnormalities. Called also *chromosome 10q duplication syndrome, chromosome 10q trisomy syndrome,* and *partial duplication 10q syndrome.* **11p t.,** partial duplication of the short arm of chromosome 11, characterized by mental and growth retardation, craniofacial developmental disorders, and other abnormalities. A high prominent forehead with frontal upsweep of hair, flat supraorbital ridges and downslanting palpebral fissures; delayed closure of anterior fontanelle; wide glabella; broad short nose with a broad flat bridge; telecanthus and/or hypertelorism; cleft palate; cleft lip; bifid uvula; round full cheeks; strabismus, nystagmus; cryptorchidism; broad fingers and toes; spasticity; and hypotonia are the principal symptoms. Called also *chromosome 11p partial duplication syndrome* and *partial duplication 11p syndrome.* **11q t.,** partial duplication of the long arm of chromosome 11, characterized by growth and mental retardation, microcephalus, short nose, long philtrum, high-arched palate, cleft palate, microretrognathia, retracted lower lip, low-set posteriorly rotated ears, cutix laxa, clavicular defects, cardiovascular defects, hip dislocation, hypotonia, talipes equinovarus, and urogenital malformations. Called also *partial duplication chromosome 11q syndrome* and *partial duplication 11q syndrome.* **12p t.,** trisomy of the short arm of chromosome 12, characterized by mental retardation; flat and round face with a high forehead and protruding occipital bones; horizontal palpebral fissures; bushy and irregular eyebrows; short nose with anteverted nostrils and long and projecting saddle nose; elongated upper lip with a lower lip turning outward; low-set ears; short neck covered with cutaneous folds; distended abdomen; and a variety of skeletal and other abnormalities. Called also *chromosome 12p trisomy syndrome* and

trisomy 12p syndrome. **t. 13, t. 13 syndrome,** Patau's SYNDROME. **14q t.,** partial duplication of the long arm of chromosome 14, associated with mental and growth retardation, seizures, hypertonia, microcephaly, brachycephaly, low hairline, hypo- or hypertelorism, small palpebral fissures, blepharoptosis, microphthalmia, low-set malformed ears, nose with a broad ridge and a prominent tip, cleft palate, high-arched palate, unusual philtrum, mobile mouth, protruding upper lip, micrognathia, short neck, and various skeletal, cardiovascular, and genital abnormalities. Called also *chromosome 14q partial duplication syndrome* and *partial duplication 14q syndrome.* **15q t.,** partial duplication of the proximal segment of the long arm of chromosome 15, characterized by growth and mental retardation, seizures, hyper- or hypotonia, high forehead, prominent occiput, heavy brows, antimongoloid palpebral fissures, epicanthal folds, deep-set eyes, strabismus, cataract, beaked nose with a wide bridge, low or posteriorly rotated malformed ears, high-arched palate, malpositioned teeth, micrognathia, short neck, and skeletal and genital abnormalities. Called also *partial duplication 15q syndrome.* **t. 18,** a syndrome characterized by the presence of an extra chromosome 18, associated with double trisomies, translocation, or mosaicism. Birth weight is about 2300 gm; about one-third of all affected infants die by the age of one month and very few survive past one year of age. Craniofacial defects, the most constant feature, consist of prominent occiput, scaphocephaly, small triangular mouth, micrognathia, blepharoptosis, low-set malformed external ears and, less commonly, cleft lip and palate. Associated defects may include mental retardation, hypertonicity, corneal opacities, failure to thrive, webbing of the neck, shield-shaped chest, short stubby fingers and toes with short nails, overlapping of the index and third fingers, Meckel's diverticulum, and various cardiovascular, gastrointestinal, renal, and skeletal abnormalities. Called also *chromosome 18 syndrome, Edward's syndrome, trisomy E, trisomy 16–18,* and *trisomy 18 syndrome.* **19q t.,** duplication of the long arm of chromosome 19, characterized by low birth weight, microcephaly, flat facial profile, blepharoptosis, glabellar prominence, small upturned nose, downturned angles of the mouth, cleft palate, short neck with redundant skin, shield-shaped chest with wide-set nipples, and clinodactyly. **t. 20,** a syndrome characterized by mental and growth retardation, speech disorders, lethargy, seizures, frequent microcephaly, genital abnormalities, pigmentary dysplasia of the skin, kyphoscoliosis, sacral dimple, thoracic protuberance, hip dislocation, asymmetric breasts with supernumerary nipples, simian creases, atrophic musculature, and coarse facies, particularly telecanthus and hypertelorism, broad nose with comedones at the tip, hirsute forehead, synophrys, broad eyebrows and ectopic eyelashes, mongoloid slanting of the palpebral fissures, ear abnormalities, macrostosmia, macroglossia, and widely spaced teeth. Called also *trisomy 20 syndrome.* **20p t.,** partial duplication of the short arm of chromosome 20, characterized by mental retardation, occipital flattening, round face due to prominent cheeks and short chin, oblique upward slanting palpebral fissures, increased intercanthal distance, epicanthal folds, strabismus, short nose with upturned tip and large nostrils, dental, vertebral, and cardiac abnormalities, coarse hair, poor coordination, and speech disorders. Called also *chromosome 20p partial duplication syndrome* and *partial duplication 20p syndrome.* **t. 22,** a syndrome of mental retardation; turricephaly with apparent increase of vertical skull dimensions; frontal prominence; decreased bifrontal-temporal dimension; semicircular eyebrows merging with the lateral nasal borders; palpebral fissures with decreased transverse and increased vertical dimensions; superior lateral and inferior medial ocular folds; increased philtral length; downturned commissures of the mouth; small lower face with retruded chin; low-set ears with large lobules; and apparent facial asymmetry, most notable in the right ear being more medially positioned. Cleft, high-arched palate, preauricular abnormalities, cardiovascular abnormalities, genital abnormalities, long slender fingers, and finger-like thumbs may be associated. Called also *nonmongoloid trisomy G.* **t. C,** t. 8. **t. D₁,** Patau's SYNDROME. **t. E,** t. 18. **t. G.,** nonmongoloid, t. 22. **partial t.,** trisomy in which only a part of a chromosome, such as one of its arms, has been duplicated. Called also *chromosome arm duplication.*

tristearin (tri-ste′ah-rin) a triglyceride, $C_{57}H_{110}O_6$, occurring as a white powder, insoluble in water but soluble in organic solvents, except ether and cold alcohol, and consisting of glycerol and stearic acid. It is present in vegetable and animal fats, such as butter, cacao, and lard. Used in impression compounds. Called also *glyceryl tristearate* and *stearin*.

Tri-Sweet trademark for *aspartame*.

Triten trademark for *dimethindene maleate* (see under DIMETH-INDENE).

tritium (trit′e-um, trish′e-um) [Gr. *tritos* third] a naturally occurring radioactive isotope of hydrogen that emits gamma rays. Symbol, T or ^{3}H. It has a half-life of 12.26 years, and its isotopic weight is 3.017 (two neutrons and one proton in the nucleus). Tritium occurs as a gas with properties similar to those of hydrogen. Used in thermonuclear technology and as a tracer in biochemical and biological research.

trituration (trich′u-ra″shun) [L. *tritura* the treading out of corn] 1. to grind or rub solid bodies to a powder (usually with a liquid) in a mortar. 2. a triturated drug, especially one rubbed with milk sugar. 3. the mixing of mercury with the dental amalgam alloy (silver-tin alloy with trace amounts of copper and zinc), to form a soft, silvery paste, which is condensed in the prepared cavity where it hardens to form a dental restoration. The reaction between the silver-tin alloy and mercury is as follows:

Silver-tin alloy	+	Mercury	→	Silver-tin alloy	+	Silver-mercury	+	Tin-mercury
Ag₃Sn		Hg		Ag₃Sn		Ag₂Hg₃		Sn₈Hg
(γ-phase)				(γ-phase)		(γ₁-phase)		(γ₂-phase)

See also AMALGAM alloy, dental AMALGAM, and γ-PHASE. **manual t.,** mortar and pestle t. **mechanical t.,** trituration with the use of a mechanical device. Called also *mechanical amalgamation*. See mechanical TRITURATOR. **mortar and pestle t.,** mixing or trituration of dental amalgam alloy with an appropriate amount of mercury in a mortar with the use of a pestle. Called also *manual t., manual amalgamation,* and *mortar and pestle amalgamation.*

triturator (trich′u-ra″tor) an apparatus in which substances can be continuously rubbed, as in the process of amalgamating an alloy with mercury. Called also *amalgam mixer.* **mechanical t.,** a mechanical device for mixing dental amalgam. It consists of an electric motor, timer, speed control, and arms into which a capsule containing a mixture of dental amalgam and an appropriate amount of mercury are placed. The mixture is triturated into a soft, pliable paste by a free-moving cylindrical metal or plastic piston inside the capsule, acting in a manner similar to that of a pestle in a mortar when the capsule is agitated. The amalgam is sometimes triturated without the use of the piston inside the capsule in some high and ultra–high speed triturators operating at speeds of 3000 and 4400 rpm. Available under various trademarks. Called also *mechanical amalgamator.*

trivalent (triv′ah-lent) [*tri-* + L. *valens* powerful] pertaining to or containing an atom or radical capable of replacing three hydrogen atoms.

trivial (triv′e-al) of little importance; common; ordinary. See also trivial NAME.

Trizma trademark for *tromethamine*.

Trobicin trademark for *spectinomycin hydrochloride* (see under SPECTINOMYCIN).

trocar (tro′kar) a cannula with a sharp-pointed obturator for piercing the wall of a cavity.

trochlea (trok′le-ah), pl. *trochʹleae* [L.; Gr. *trochilia* pulley] a pulley-shaped part or structure; a general anatomical term for such a structure.

trochleae (trok′le-e) [L.] plural of *trochlea*.

trochlear (trok′le-ar) [L. *trochlearis*] 1. pertaining to or of the nature of a pulley or trochlea. 2. trochlear NERVE.

trochleariform (trok″le-ar′ĭ-form) pulley-shaped.

trochlearis (trok″le-a′ris) [L.] trochlear.

trochocephaly (tro″ko-sef′ah-le) [Gr. *trochos* wheel + *kephalē* head] a rounded appearance of the head caused by synostosis of the frontal and parietal bones.

trochoid (tro′koid) [Gr. *trochos* wheel + *eidos* form] resembling a pivot or a pulley.

Trocinate trademark for *thiphenamil hydrochloride* (see under THIPHENAMIL).

Trolard's plexus [Paulin *Trolard,* French anatomist, 1842–1910] venous plexus of hypoglossal canal; see under PLEXUS.

troleandomycin (tro″le-an-do-mi″sin) an erythromycin-type macrolide antibiotic, $C_{41}H_{67}NO_{14}$, which is the triacetyl ester of oleandomycin, having properties similar to those of the parent compound. Called also *triacetyloleandomycin*. Trademarks: Cyclamin, Cyclamycin, Oleandocetine.

trolnitrate phosphate (trol-ni′trāt) a smooth muscle relaxant,

triethanolamine trinitrate biphosphate, occurring as a white, crystalline powder that is soluble in ethanol, but not in ether, chloroform, and water. Used as a vasodilator in the prevention of angina pectoris. Trademarks: Angitrit, Bentonyl, Metamine, Nitranol, Ortin, Tricoryl, Vasomed.

tromethamine (tro-meth′ah-mēn) a weak amine base with a pH of 7.8 at body temperature, which is close to pH 7.4 of the plasma, 2-amino-2-hydroxymethyl-1,3-propanediol. It occurs as a white, crystalline powder with a faint sweet, soapy taste, which is soluble in water and the lower aliphatic alcohols, but not in common organic solvents. Used in the treatment of acidosis, asphyxia neonatorum, status asthmaticus, drug intoxication, and other conditions in which pH is low. Also used as an alkalizing agent in the production of surface-active agents, lotions, drugs, and other products. Adverse reactions may include venospasm, thrombosis, slough at the site of extravasation, hemorrhagic liver necrosis, hyperkalemia, hypoglycemia, and respiratory depression. Overdosage may cause alkalosis. Trademarks: Talatrol, THAM, Tham-E, TRIS, Tris Amino, Trizma.

tromexan (tro-mek′san) see ETHYL biscoumacetate.

Tronothane trademark for *pramoxine hydrochloride* (see under PRAMOXINE).

trophic (trof′ik) [Gr. *trophikos* nourishing] pertaining to nutrition.

-trophic, -trophin [Gr. *trophikos* nourishing] a word termination denoting relationship to nutrition. Often confused with *-tropic*.

tropho- [Gr. *trophē* nutrition] a combining form denoting relationship to nutrition, feeding, or supplying with nutrients.

trophoblast (trof′o-blast) [*tropho-* + Gr. *blastos* germ] one of the fetal membranes, consisting of a layer of extraembryonic ectodermal tissue on the outside of the blastocyst, which attaches the ovum to the uterine wall and establishes nutritive and other relations with the uterus. Seven to eleven days after fertilization, its outer stratum enlarges and develops into an outer layer (syncytiotrophoblast) and an inner layer (cytotrophoblast), leading to the development of the chorion. See illustration at CLEAVAGE. **syncytial t.,** syncytiotrophoblast.

trophoneurosis (trof′o-nu-ro′sis) [*tropho-* + *neurosis*] any functional disorder due to faulty nerve supply. **facial t.,** facial HEMI-ATROPHY.

-tropic [Gr. *tropē* a turn] a word termination denoting turning toward, changing, or tending to turn or change. Often confused with *-trophic*.

tropine (tro′pin, tro′pēn) a crystalline alkaloid, $C_8H_{15}NO$, with a smell like tobacco, derivable from atropine and from various plants. **t. mandelate,** homatropine.

tropism (tro′pizm) [Gr. *tropē* a turn] the ability of a nonmotile organism or of one of its parts to turn toward (positive tropism) or away from (negative tropism) a stimulus.

-tropism a word termination denoting a tendency to turn toward; having affinity for.

tropomyosin (tro″po-mi′o-sin) a contractile protein, representing about 10 percent of muscle proteins. Its long and thin molecules have a molecular weight of about 33,000 to 37,000 and are formed by two α-helical polypeptide chains wound around each other. Each coil fits end to end into a groove formed by coiled F-actin filaments, extending toward G-actin monomers, being arranged in such a way that tropomyosin molecules move along the grooves between the F-actin filaments. **t. A,** a contractile protein occurring widely in invertebrate "catch" or tonus muscles. Also called *paramyosin*. **t. B,** a major component of the muscle contraction mechanism, representing 11 per cent of the myofilaments in myofibrils.

troponin (tro′po-nin) a contractile protein, having large globular molecules that are formed by three polypeptide subunits: TN-C (troponin A), TN-I, and TN-T. TN-C is the calcium binding subunit with a molecular weight of 18,000. TN-I is the inhibitory subunit with a molecular weight of 23,000. It has a binding site specific for actin and its function consists of inhibiting the interaction of actin with the myosin head cross bridges. TN-T is the tropomyosin-binding subunit. **t. A.,** the calcium-binding subunit of troponin. See *troponin*.

Trotter's syndrome [Wilfred *Trotter,* British physician, 1872–1939] see under SYNDROME.

Troxidone trademark for *trimethadione*.

troy (troi) a system of weights for precious metals and gems and, formerly, for bread and grain, named after Troyes, France, where it was standard. See troy WEIGHT.

Trp tryptophan.

true (troo) actually existing; not false; real; meeting all the criteria establishing its identity.

True's separator [Harry A. *True,* American dentist] see under SEPARATOR.

truncus (trun′kus), pl. *trun′ci* [L.] 1. the trunk; term used in anatomical nomenclature to designate the main part of the body, excluding the head and extremities. 2. a major portion of a nerve, blood vessel, or lymphatic vessel; used in anatomical nomenclature to designate such a major, usually undivided and usually short, structure. See also TRUNK. **t. brachiocephal′icus** [NA], brachiocephalic TRUNK. **t. costocervica′lis** [NA], costocervical TRUNK. **t. jugula′ris** [NA], jugular TRUNK. **t. linguofacia′lis** [NA], linguofacial TRUNK. **t. pulmona′lis** [NA], pulmonary TRUNK. **t. sympath′icus** [NA], sympathetic TRUNK. **t. thyrocervica′lis** [NA], thyrocervical TRUNK.

trunk (trunk) [L. *truncus* the stem or trunk of a tree] 1. the main part of the body, excluding the head and extremities. 2. a major, usually undivided and usually short, portion of a nerve or of a blood vessel or lymphatic vessel. See also TRUNCUS. **brachiocephalic t.**, the first branch of the aorta which divides into the right common carotid and right subclavian arteries, with distribution to the right side of the head and neck and to the right arm; the inferior thyroid artery may arise from this trunk. Called also *arteria anonyma, arteria innominata, brachiocephalic artery, innominate artery,* and *truncus brachiocephalicus* [NA]. **costocervical t.**, an artery that arises from the subclavian artery, and supplies the vertebral column, upper intercostal spaces, the muscles of the back, and deep muscles of the neck. Called also *truncus costocervicalis* [NA]. **jugular t.**, a lymphatic vessel forming a trunk which unites efferent vessels of the superior and inferior cervical deep lymph nodes. The right side of the trunk joins the junction of the internal jugular and subclavian veins, and the left side empties into the thoracic duct. Called also *truncus jugularis* [NA]. **linguofacial t.**, the common trunk by which the facial and lingual arteries often arise from the external carotid artery. Called also *truncus linguofacialis* [NA]. **pulmonary t.**, the vessel that arises from the right ventricle and divides into the right and left pulmonary arteries. Called also *arterial vein* and *truncus pulmonalis* [NA]. **sympathetic t.**, one of the two symmetrical chains of ganglia interconnected by nerve strands, extending on both sides of the spine from the base of the skull to the coccyx. The upper end is formed by the superior cervical ganglion and continues inside the skull via the internal carotid nerve. The lower ends of both trunks converge and sometimes fuse into a single ganglion. The roots of the chain ganglia are formed by small preganglionic fibers known as the white rami communicantes because of the whitish color of their predominantly myelinated fibers. They derive from the cell bodies in the lateral column of the gray matter of the spinal cord and emerge with the spinal nerves from the twelve thoracic and two lumbar segments of the spinal cord. The postganglionic fibers, known as the gray rami communicantes, are made up of largely myelinated fibers, and serve as the visceral afferent nerves that innervate the smooth muscles, blood vessels, and glands. Called also *truncus sympathicus* [NA]. **thyrocervical t.**, a short arterial trunk that arises from the subclavian artery, dividing into the inferior thyroid artery, supracapsular artery, and transverse cervical artery. Called also *thyroid axis* and *truncus thyrocervicalis* [NA].

trusion (troo′zhun) [L. *trudere* to shove] a former term for malposition; the condition of having been pressed or thrust out of alignment, said of the position of teeth. **bimaxillary t.**, trusion or malposition affecting the teeth of both jaws. **bodily t.**, trusion or malposition of the entire tooth. **coronal t.**, trusion or tipping of the tooth crown, while the root remains in its normal position. **mandibular t.**, trusion or malposition of the mandibular teeth. **maxillary t.**, trusion or malposition of the maxillary teeth.

truss (trus) [Fr. *trousser* to tie up] an elastic, canvas, or metal support for retaining a reduced hernia. **nasal t.**, a trusslike support for fractured nasal bones.

Trycite trademark for *polystyrene.*

try-in (tri′in) a preliminary insertion of a dental prosthetic device or orthodontic appliance to determine its fit and suitability.

trypaflavine (trip″ah-fla′vin) ACRIFLAVINE hydrochloride.

Trypanosoma (tri″pan-o-so′mah) [Gr. *trypanon* borer + *sōma* body] a genus of protozoa of the subphylum Mastigophora. Typically, the adult body is elongate with a whiplike flagellum arising from the posterior end and attached to the cell by a delicate undulating membrane that runs the entire length of the body. Most species live part of their life cycle in the intestines of insect hosts and other invertebrates, where they undergo transformation. Found in the blood and lymph of animals, including man.

trypanosomiasis (tri-pan″o-so-mi′ah-sis) infection with parasites of the genus *Trypanosoma.*

trypsin [E.C.3.4.21.4] (trip′sin) [Gr. *tyrein* to rub + *pepsin*] a serine proteinase that catalyzes hydrolysis of food proteins, particularly peptides, amides, and esters of bonds involving the carboxyl group of L-arginine or L-lysine. It is secreted by the pancreatic acinar cells as an inactive proenzyme, trypsinogen. In the intestine, trypsinogen is activated to trypsin by enterokinase, involving in the process the removal of an acidic peptide from the trypsinogen molecule; also in the intestine, trypsin activates chymotrypsinogen to chymotrypsin. α-Trypsin is derived from β-trypsin by the additional cleavage of peptide bonds, and when the two bonds are cleaved, ψ-trypsin is formed. Trypsin has been isolated from various sources, including man, sheep, turkeys, fish, shrimp, silk moth, bacteria (*Streptomyces*), and a variety of other organisms. That obtained from the pancreas of animals [NF] is a yellow to grayish-yellow powder or crystals, soluble in water, but not in some organic solvents. Used as a debriding (proteolytic) agent. Trademarks: Paraenzyme, Tryptar, Trypure.

trypsinogen (trip-sin′o-jen) [*trypsin* + Gr. *gennan* to produce] a precursor of trypsin secreted by the pancreatic acinar cells as an inactive proenzyme, which is activated to trypsin in the intestine by the enzyme enterokinase.

Tryptar trademark for a preparation of *trypsin.*

tryptophan (trip′to-fān) a heterocyclic, naturally occurring amino acid, 2-amino-3-(3-indole)-propionic acid, which is essential for nitrogen equilibrium in the adult human and for growth in infants. It is also present in the saliva. Adequate levels in the diet may compensate deficiencies of niacin and thus mitigate pellagra. Tryptophan is destroyed during acidic hydrolysis of proteins but may be isolated by enzymic hydrolysis. Abbreviated *Trp.* Formerly called *proteinochromogen.* See also amino ACID.

Trypure trademark for a trypsin preparation.

T.S. test solution.

TSA tumor-specific ANTIGEN.

TSH thyroid stimulating hormone; see thyrotropic HORMONE.

TSTA tumor-specific tissue antigen; see tumor-specific ANTIGEN.

Tualsal 100 trademark for *tribromsalan.*

Tuamine trademark for *tuaminoheptane.*

tuaminoheptane (tu-am″ĭ-no-hep′tān) an indirectly acting sympathomimetic agent, 1-methylhexylamine, occurring as a colorless to yellowish, volatile liquid with an amine-like odor, which is soluble in ethanol, benzene, chloroform, and ether and sparingly in water. Used as a vasoconstrictor in nasal congestion and in the preparation of mucous membranes for surgery to reduce bleeding. Excessive use may cause an increase in blood pressure, tachycardia, mydriasis, and intestinal spasm. Called also *2-aminoheptane* and *2-heptanamine.* Trademarks: Heptamine, Heptedrine, Heptin, Tuamine. **t. sulfate**, the sulfate salt of tuaminoheptane, occurring as a white, odorless powder that is soluble in water and alcohol and sparingly soluble in ether. Its pharmacological and toxicological properties are similar to those of the parent compound.

tuba (tu′bah), pl. *tu′bae* [L. "trumpet"] a tube; an elongated hollow cylindrical organ; used in anatomical nomenclature as a general term for such a structure. See TUBE. **t. acus′tica, t. auditi′va** [NA], auditory TUBE. **t. uteri′na** [NA] fallopian TUBE.

Tubadil trademark for *tubocurarine chloride* (see under TUBOCURARINE).

tubae (tu′be) plural of *tuba.*

Tubarine trademark for *tubocurarine chloride* (see under TUBOCURARINE).

tube (tūb) [L. *tubus*] an elongated hollow cylindrical organ or instrument. Called also *tuba.* **auditory t.**, a channel, about 36 mm long, lined with mucous membrane, which establishes communication between the tympanic cavity and the nasopharynx and serves to adjust the pressure of air in the cavity to the external pressure. It is comprised of a pars ossea, located in the temporal bone, and pars cartilaginea, ending in the nasopharynx. Called also *eustachian t., sulcus of eustachian tube, tuba acustica,* and *tuba auditiva* [NA]. **Bouchut's t's**, a set of tubes for use in the intubation of the larynx. **buccal t.**, end t. **cathode-ray t.**, a vacuum tube in which the cathode rays are accelerated as a beam to form luminous spots on the fluorescent screen. **Chaoul t.**, a low voltage x-ray tube so designed as to permit the anode to be located 2 cm from the body, thus permitting intense but very superficial tissue penetration of the ionizing radiation beam. **Coolidge t.**, x-ray t., hot-cathode. **Crookes' t.**, an early form of vacuum tube by the use of which the x-rays were discovered. **drainage t.**, one used in surgery to facilitate the escape of fluids. **electron multiplier t.**, one in which small electron currents are amplified by a cascade process employing secondary emission. **end t.**, in orthodontic appliance, attachment on the buccal surface of a terminal banded molar; often referred to as a *buccal tube* when using the edgewise arch mechanism. **endotracheal t.,** an inflatable tube which is inserted into the mouth or nose and passed down into the trachea. It is used for the administration of anesthetics and may be left in place after completion of surgery until the patient no longer is in danger of asphyxiation. It may be connected to a mechanical respirator. See also oral AIRWAY. **eustachian t., auditory t. fallopian t.,** one of two slender tubes descending from each ovary to the side of the uterus, which serve to convey ova to the cavity of the uterus and allow passage of spermatozoa in the opposite direction. Called also *uterine t.* and *tuba uterina* [NA]. **gas t.,** early type of x-ray tube in which electrons were derived from residual gases within the tube. **Geiger-Müller t.,** the principal component of the Geiger-Müller counter, consisting of a gas-filled tube with two electrodes. **granulation t.,** a laryngeal intubation tube with a large head which covers any granulations that may have been formed about the wound. **t. head,** tube HEAD. **horizontal t.,** a metal tube attachment placed in a horizontal position on the buccal surface of each anchor molar. **hot-cathode t.,** x-ray t., hot-cathode. **t. housing,** tube HOUSING. **intubation t.,** a breathing tube introduced in the air passage after tracheostomy or laryngostomy. **McCollum t.,** an apparatus for keeping a patient dry when there is a large amount of drainage from a sinus. **molar t.,** a short horizontal tube attached to the molar band to engage and hold in place the arch wire of an orthodontic appliance. **multiple t.,** see multiple-tube INSTALLATION. **neural t.,** an embryonic tube, from which the brain and spinal cord develop. It evolves from the neural plate which appears as a thickening of the ectoderm during the third week of development. The plate invaginates, forming the neural groove which, in turn, is bounded on both sides by the neural folds; the folds continue to thicken until they merge and fuse, thus forming the tube. With fusion, the neural crest develops on the dorsolateral part of the tube. Initially, the plate is made up of undifferentiated proliferative epithelium, one line of its daughter cells becoming the nerve cells and the other becoming the ependymal and neuroglial cells. The plate is at first a single-layered structure consisting of columnar cells but it rapidly becomes many-layered, while the cells lose their sharp outlines. By the sixth week, the neural wall is bounded by the external and internal limiting membranes, and the tube becomes organized into the ependymal, mantle, and marginal layers: the ependymal layer containing the nucleated bodies and ependymal and mitotic cells; the mantle layer becoming the gray substance; and the marginal layer becoming the white substance. **photomultiplier t.,** an electron multiplier tube in which the electrons initiating the cascade originate by photoelectric emission. **salivary t's,** the interlobular ducts of the salivary glands. **tracheotomy t.,** a curved tube to be inserted into the trachea through an opening provided by tracheotomy (or tracheostomy). **uterine t.,** fallopian t. **valve t.,** an electronic tube in which the anode is at a right angle to the cathode, allowing the electron stream to strike the entire anode face. Its function consists of conducting the secondary current of electricity along a predetermined circuit, and it is a component of a rectifier. **vertical t.,** an orthodontic attachment usually placed on the lingual surface of the anchor band to allow for the insertion of the lingual arch wire. **x-ray t.,** an electronic tube used for generation of x-rays (see x-ray GENERATOR). See also *x-ray t., hot cathode.* **x-ray t., hot-cathode, x-ray t., hot-filament,** an x-ray tube consisting of a glass vacuum bulb that encloses a spiral filament of incandescent tungsten and the

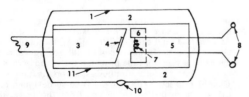

Hot filament x-ray tube: 1. metal shielding; 2. insulating oil; 3. anode; 4. tungsten target; 5. cathode; 6. focusing cup; 7. cathode filament; 8. wire connections to secondary side of filament transformer; 9. anode connection to secondary circuit; 10. port (window) in metal shield; 11. evacuated glass envelope. (From C. A. Jacobi and D. Q. Paris: Textbook of Radiologic Technology. 6th ed. St. Louis. The C. V. Mosby Co., 1977.)

anode (target) of massive tungsten; it may be either stationary or rotating. Electrons traveling at high velocity from a heated cathode are suddenly arrested at target, giving rise to x-rays. In an x-ray generator, the tube is surrounded by a metal shield which prevents the escape of nonuseful rays, and is suspended in oil which fills the space between the glass bulb and the shield. Called also *Coolidge t.* and *hot-cathode t.* See illustration.

tuber (tu'ber), pl. *tubers, tu'bera* [L.] a swelling, protuberance; a general anatomical term for such a structure. See also TUBERCLE, TUBERCULUM, TUBEROSITAS, and TUBEROSITY. **t. fronta'le** [NA], **frontal t.,** frontal EMINENCE. **t. maxil'lae** [NA], **t. maxilla're, maxillary t.,** maxillary TUBEROSITY. **parietal t., t. parieta'le** [NA], parietal EMINENCE.

tubera (tu'ber-ah) [L.] plural of *tuber.*

tubercle (tu'ber-k'l) [L. *tuberculum*] 1. nodule, especially a solid elevation of the skin, larger in size than a papule. 2. any small, rounded nodule produced by the *Mycobacterium tuberculosis.* It is a characteristic lesion of tuberculosis, and consists of a translucent mass, gray in color, made up of small spherical cells which contain giant cells and are surrounded by a layer of spindle-shaped connective tissue cells known as epithelioid cells. Called also *gray t.* 3. a nodule, or small eminence, such as a rough, rounded eminence on a bone. Called also *tuberculum.* See also APOPHYSIS and TUBEROSITY. 4. a small elevation on the crown of a tooth produced by excessive accumulation of enamel, considered to be an abnormal growth. **articular t. of temporal bone,** an enlargement of the inferior border of the zygomatic process of the temporal bone, forming the anterior boundary of the mandibular fossa and part of the anterior root of the zygoma; it gives attachment to the lateral ligament of the temporomandibular joint. Called also *t. of root of zygoma, t. of zygoma, zygomatic t., articular eminence of temporal bone, eminentia articularis ossis temporalis,* and *tuberculum articulare ossis temporalis* [NA]. **Carabelli's t.,** Carabelli CUSP. **condyloid t.,** an eminence on the condylar process of the mandible for attachment of the lateral ligament of the temporomandibular joint. **conglomerate t.,** a mass made up of an aggregation of many smaller nodules. **corniculate t.,** a rounded eminence near the posterior end of the aryepiglottic fold, behind the cuneiform tubercle, corresponding to the corniculate cartilage. Called also *t. of Santorini, tuberculum corniculatum* [NA], *tuberculum corniculatum [Santorini],* and *tuberculum Santorini.* **cuneiform t.,** a rounded eminence in the posterior portion of the aryepiglottic fold, in front of the corniculate tubercle, corresponding to the cuneiform cartilage. Called also *Wrisberg's t., tuberculum cuneiform* [NA], *tuberculum cuneiforme [Wrisbergi],* and *tuberculum Wrisbergi.* **t. of crown of tooth,** cusp (3). **dental t.,** 1. a small elevation of indiscriminate size on some portion of the tooth crown, produced by extra formation of enamel. 2. cusp (3). **epiglottic t.,** a backward projection on the lower part of the posterior surface of the epiglottic cartilage. Called also *cushion of epiglottis* and *tuberculum epiglotticum* [NA]. **genial t.,** mental t. **Ghon's t.,** primary (tuberculous) LESION. **gray t.,** the typical lesion of tuberculosis. See TUBERCLE (2). **intravascular t.,** a tubercle in the intima of a blood vessel. **jugular t. of occipital bone,** a smooth eminence on the superior surface of the lateral part of the occipital bone; it overlays the hypoglossal canal, and is crossed by an oblique groove for the glossopharyngeal, vagus, and accessory nerves. Called also *eminentia jugularis, jugular eminence,* and *tuberculum jugulare ossis occipitalis* [NA]. **labial t., t. of upper lip. lacrimal t.,** a small tubercle situated at the junction of the anterior lacrimal crest with the orbital surface of the frontal process of the maxilla. **lateral orbital t., lateral palpebral t.,** Whitnall's t. **lymphoid t.,** a lesion of tuberculosis consisting of lymphoid cells. **marginal t. of zygomatic bone,** a process on the superior part of the zygomatic bone to which a strong slip of the temporal fascia is attached. Called also *marginal process of malar bone, processus marginalis ossis zygomatici, small process of Soemmering,* and *tuberculum marginale ossis zygomatici* [NA]. **mental t.,** one of the two prominences on both sides of the symphysis menti, on the external surface near the lower border of the body of the mandible. Called also *genial t., mental t. of mandible, tuberculum geniale,* and *tuberculum mentale mandibulae* [NA]. **mental t., external,** mental PROTUBERANCE. **mental t. of mandible,** mental t. **molar t.,** an accessory cusp on a deciduous molar arising from the mesiobuccal ridge prominence, usually on maxillary first molars. **orbital t., lateral, palpebral t., lateral,** Whitnall's t. **paramolar t.,** paramolar. **pharyngeal t.,** an eminence on the inferior surface of the basilar part of the occipital bone, situated about 1 cm anterior to the foramen magnum, for attachment of the fibrous raphe and superior constrictor of the pharynx. Called also *basilar crest of occipital bone, basilar spine, pharyngeal crest of occipital* *bone, pharyngeal spine,* and *tuberculum pharyngeum* [NA]. **pterygoid t.,** pterygoid tuberosity of mandible; see under TUBE-ROSITY. **t. of root of zygoma,** articular t. of temporal bone. **t. of Santorini,** corniculate t. **t. of sella turcica,** a transverse ridge on the upper surface of the body of the sphenoid bone, situated in front of the sella turcica, in back of the optic groove, and between the anterior clinoid processes. Called also *tuberculum sellae, tuberculum sellae ossis sphenoidalis,* and *tuberculum sellae turcicae* [NA]. **thyroid t., inferior,** a more or less distinct tubercle at the inferior end of the oblique line of the thyroid cartilage. Called also *tuberculum thyreoideum inferius* and *tuberculum thyroideum inferius* [NA]. **thyroid t., superior,** a more or less distinct tubercle at the superior extremity of the oblique line of the thyroid cartilage. Called also *tuberculum thyreoideum superius* and *tuberculum thyroideum superius* [NA]. **trochlear t.,** trochlear SPINE. **t. of upper lip,** the central prominence of the upper border in the vermilion zone, marking the distal termination of the philtrum. Called also *labial t., procheilon,* and *tuberculum labii superioris* [NA]. **Whitnall's t.,** a small eminence on the internal aspect of the middle of the orbital surface of the zygomatic bone. Called also *lateral orbital t.* and *lateral palpebral t.* **Wrisberg's t.,** cuneiform t. **zygomatic t., t. of zygoma,** articular t. of temporal bone.

tubercula (tu-ber′ku-lah) [L.] plural of *tuberculum.*

tubercular (tu-ber′ku-lar) pertaining to tubercles or nodules.

tuberculid (tu-ber′ku-lid) a cutaneous papule believed to be caused by allergic reaction in tuberculosis.

tuberculoid (tu-ber′ku-loid) resembling a tubercle or tuberculosis; sarcoid.

tuberculoma (tu-ber″ku-lo′mah) [*tuberculum* + *-oma*] a tumorlike mass resulting from enlargement of a caseous tubercle in tuberculosis. Called also *tuberculous granuloma.* **periapical t.,** tuberculoma situated in the apical area of a tooth, caused by entry of tubercle bacilli through an open cavity and root canal. Called also *periapical tuberculosis.* See also oral TUBERCULOSIS and tuberculous OSTEOMYELITIS.

tuberculosis (tu-ber″ku-lo′sis) an infectious, contagious disease caused by several species of *Mycobacterium* collectively referred to as tubercle bacilli. Human tuberculosis is usually caused by infection with *M. tuberculosis* and, less commonly, *M. bovis.* Nearly all organs and systems may be affected but pulmonary tuberculosis is most common. **acute miliary t.,** miliary t. **avian t.,** tuberculosis of various birds, including chickens and ducks, caused by *Mycobacterium avium,* which is transmissible to man. **bovine t.,** an infection of cattle caused by *Mycobacterium bovis,* transmissible to man, usually through milk. **t. cu′tis lupo′sa,** LUPUS vulgaris. **disseminated t.,** miliary t. **hematogenous t.,** miliary t. **t. of lungs,** pulmonary t. **miliary t.,** an acute, disseminated form of tuberculosis, characterized by the presence of minute tubercles (milia) in various organs, caused by spreading of tubercle bacilli through the blood stream or lymphatic system. Called also *acute miliary t., disseminated t.,* and *hematogenous t.* **oral t.,** a rare condition, usually occurring on the gingiva and tongue, less commonly in the pharynx, and infrequently in other parts of the oral cavity. Lesions are small, crateriform, painless ulcers that bleed readily, surrounded by edema or reddish nodules. There also may be irregular, superficial or deep, painful slow-growing ulcers in any part of the mucosa; nonulcerated lesions with swelling and fissures may also occur. Pathologically, the lesions exhibit foci or caseous necrosis surrounded by epithelioid cells, lymphocytes, and some multinucleated cells. Most forms of oral tuberculosis are secondary and are blood-borne complications of pulmonary tuberculosis. Dentists may become infected by contact with live bacilli in the mouth. See also LUPUS VULGARIS, periapical TUBERCULOMA, SCROFULA, and tuberculous OSTEOMYELITIS. **pulmonary t.,** a chronic tuberculous infection of the lungs caused by *Mycobacterium tuberculosis.* The primary lesion occurs most often in the lungs, and usually involves the apical areas and lower lobes. Pathological changes include formation of tubercles, cavitation, caseation, sloughing, calcification of nodules, and lamination of cavities. Symptoms include loss of weight, nocturnal sweating, chills, malaise, dyspnea, hoarseness, hemoptysis, cough, and fever. A red line on the gingivae (*Thompson's line*) may be present. Complications may include pleurisy, effusions, empyema, pneumothorax, atelectasis, and involvement of the larynx, oral cavity, and other organs. The infection may spread from the lungs to any part of the respiratory tract, oral mucosa, and lips. For oral complications, see *oral t.* Called also *t. of lungs,* and formerly *comsumption.* **osteoarticular t.,** tuberculosis involving the bones and joints. See also tuberculous OSTEOMYELITIS.

tuberculum (tu-ber′ku-lum), pl. *tuber′cula* [L. dim. of *tuber*] a nodule, or small eminence; used as a general term in anatomical nomenclature. Called also *tubercle.* **t. articula′re os′sis**

tempora′lis [NA], articular tubercle of temporal bone; see under TUBERCLE. **t. cornicula′tum** [NA], **t. cornicula′tum [Santorin′i],** corniculate TUBERCLE. **t. coro′nae den′tis,** cusp (3). **t. cuneifor′me** [NA], **t. cuneifor′me [Wrisber′gi],** cuneiform TUBERCLE. **t. epiglot′ticum** [NA], epiglottic TUBERCLE. **t. genia′le,** mental TUBERCLE. **t. hypoglos′si,** TRIGONE of hypoglossal nerve. **t. im′par,** a small tubercle in the midline on the floor of the pharynx of the embryo, between the ends of the mandibular and hyoid arches, which is the primordium of the tongue. **t. jugula′re os′sis occipita′lis** [NA], jugular tubercle of occipital bone; see under TUBERCLE. **t. la′bii superio′ris** [NA], TUBERCLE of upper lip. **t. margina′le os′sis zygomat′ici** [NA], marginal tubercle of zygomatic bone; see under TUBERCLE. **t. menta′le mandib′ulae** [NA], mental TUBERCLE. **t. pharyn′geum** [NA], pharyngeal TUBERCLE. **t. Santori′ni,** corniculate TUBERCLE. **t. sel′lae, t. sel′lae os′sis sphenoida′lis, t. sel′lae tur′cicae** [NA], TUBERCLE of sella turcica. **t. thyreoi′deum infe′rius,** thyroid tubercle, inferior; see under TUBERCLE. **t. thyreoi′deum supe′rius,** thyroid tubercle, superior; see under TUBERCLE. **t. thyroi′deum infe′rius,** thyroid tubercle, inferior; see under TUBERCLE. **t. thyroi′deum supe′rius** [NA], thyroid tubercle, superior; see under TUBERCLE. **t. Wrisber′gi,** cuneiform TUBERCLE.

tuberositas (tu″bĕ-ros′ĭ-tas), pl. *tuberosita′tes* [L.] tuberosity; an elevation or protuberance. Used in anatomical nomenclature for such a structure. Called also *tuberosity.* See also TUBER, TUBERCLE, and TUBERCULUM. **t. pterygoi′dea mandib′ulae** [NA], pterygoid tuberosity of mandible; see under TUBEROSITY.

tuberositates (tu″ber-os″ĭ-tah′tēs) [L.] plural of *tuberositas.*

tuberosity (tu″bĕ-ros′ĭ-te) [L. *tuberositas*] an elevation or protuberance. Called also *tuberositas.* See also APOPHYSIS, TUBER, TUBERCLE, and TUBERCULUM. **malar t.,** the prominence on the zygomatic bone. **maxillary t.,** a rounded eminence at the posteroinferior angle of the infratemporal surface of the maxilla; it becomes prominent after the eruption and growth of the third molars. It is rough on its medial side for articulation with the pyramidal process of the palatine bone and in some cases articulates with the lateral pterygoid plate of the sphenoid bone. The smooth surface above forms the anterior boundary of the pterygopalatine fossa, forming a groove for the maxillary nerve. Called also *maxillary tuber, tuber maxillae* [NA], and *tuber maxillare.* **pterygoid t. of mandible,** a roughened area on the inner side of the angle of the mandible for the insertion of the medial pterygoid muscle. Called also *pterygoid tubercle* and *tuberositas pterygoidea mandibulae* [NA]. **pyramidal t. of palatine bone,** pyramidal process of palatine bone; see under PROCESS.

tuberous (tu′ber-us) covered with tubers; knobby.

tubi (tu′bi) [L.] plural of *tubus.*

Tubliseal trademark for a *zinc oxide–eugenol root canal sealer* (see under SEALER).

tubocurarine chloride (tu″bo-ku-rah′rēn) an alkaloid isolated in the *d*-form from *Chondodendron tomentosum,* 7′,12′-dihydroxy-6,6′-dimethoxy-2,2′,2′-trimethyltubocuraranium chloride, which occurs as a white to yellowish or gray, odorless, crystalline powder that is soluble in water and ethanol, but not in acetone, chloroform, and ether. It is a competitive neuromuscular blocking agent with action typical of curare, its actions being antagonized by cholinesterase inhibitors. Used in conjunction with anesthesia to produce skeletal muscular relaxation during surgery, to relax the laryngeal muscles for endotracheal intubation, to decrease muscle tone in some spastic conditions, in the diagnosis of myasthenia gravis, and during shock therapy. Hyperthermia, certain antibiotics, quinine, ether, and narcotic analgesics potentiate its paralyzant effects. Apnea, cardiovascular collapse, increased salivation, bronchospasm, urticaria, and hypotension due to histamine release are the principal side reactions. Trademarks: Delacurarine, Intocostrin, Tubadil, Tubarine.

tubule (tu′būl) a small tube. Called also *tubulus.* **collecting t's,** see straight t's. **convoluted renal t's,** the convoluted reabsorptive and secretory portions of the renal tubules. **dental t's,** dentinal t's. **dentinal t's,** minute channels in the dentin, which house the odontoblastic processes, extending from the pulp cavity to the enamel or the cementum. In transverse sections, they radiate away from the pulp cavity; in longitudinal sections, they appear to follow a sigmoidally curvilinear course. The curves consist of the outer convex and inner concave segments and are referred to as the *primary curvatures;* lesser curvatures are known as *secondary curvatures.* The diameter of tubules varies from 1 μ in the peripheral dentin to 3–5 μ at the pulp chamber. There are about 15,000 tubules per square millimeter in the periphery and 30,000–75,000 at the pulp chamber. Called also *dental t., canaliculi dentales* [NA], *dentinal canals,* and *dental canaliculi.* **longitudinal t.,** a small tubule of the sarcoplasmic reticulum, arranged parallel with the myofibrils. **mesonephric t's,** the tubules comprising the mesonephros in the embryonic kidney, which originate from the condensed masses of the nephrogenic cords. On one end they are associated with a knot of blood vessels and at the other end open into the mesonephrotic duct. **pronephric t.,** one of several tubules arranged in pairs and arising as dorsolateral sprouts from the longitudinally fused nephrotomes; it is found as the primitive kidney in vertebrates, but is rudimentary in amniotes, including man. **renal t's,** tubules for the passage of urine. Called also *uriniferous t's* and *tubuli renales* [NA]. **straight renal t's,** the excretory or collecting portions of the renal tubules. Called also *collecting t's* and *papillary ducts.* **T t.,** a small tubule of the sarcoplasmic reticulum, which passes the cell membrane from one side to the other, and provides communication from the outside by transmitting an action potential to the interior of the muscle fiber during the process of contraction. Called also *transverse t.* **transverse t.,** T t. **uriniferous t's,** renal t's.

tubuli (tu′bu-li) [L.] plural of *tubulus.*

Tubulitec trademark for a calcium hydroxide suspension in a polystyrene-chloroform solution with a bactericidal agent, dithymoldiiodide, and a fluoride; used as a cavity liner.

tubuloacinar (tu″bu-lo-as′inar) pertaining to or containing both the tubules and acini, as in the tubuloacinar gland. Called also *acinotubular.*

tubulus (tu′bu-lus), pl. *tu′buli* [L. dim. of *tubus*] a tubule or a small tube; used as a general term in anatomical nomenclature for such a structure. **tu′buli rena′les** [NA], renal tubules; see under TUBULE.

tubus (tu′bus), pl. *tu′bi* [L.] tube; used as a general term in anatomical nomenclature.

tuft (tuft) a small clump or cluster; a coil. **enamel t's,** bunches of tuftlike structures extending from the dentinoenamel junction through about one-third the thickness of the enamel, representing defects in mineralization, and confined to the innermost 20 to 30 percent of the enamel. Some believe that only the sheath or the interprimastic substance participates in the formation of the tufts but others think that all enamel structures contribute to their formation; some also believe that they are tubular structures serving as circulatory units for the enamel.

tuftsin (tuft′sin) a gamma globulin capable of stimulating endocytosis of neutrophils.

tugback (tug′bak) in endodontics, the resistance to withdrawal which a fitted gutta-percha cone or silver point should offer when withdrawn from the fully prepared root canal, prior to cementation in the root canal.

tugging (tug′ing) a pulling sensation. **tracheal t.,** the downward tugging movement of the larynx.

tularemia (too-lah-re′me-ah) [*Tulare* a district in California, where the disease was first described] an infectious disease caused by *Pasteurella tularensis,* which may be transmitted from animals, chiefly rabbits, to man. The ulceroglandular form, which is the most common, is characterized by a papule at the site of inoculation which becomes necrotic, forming a depressed lesion with a central ulcer surrounded by an indurated border. Later, the regional lymph nodes become affected and may break down. The less common forms include the glandular variant, in which the lymph nodes are affected but there is no local lesion, and the oculoglandular variant, in which there is ulceration of the conjunctiva, swelling of the eyelids, and involvement of the lymph nodes. In the Japanese form (*Ohara's disease*), the primary lesion is often a small ulcer on the thumb or an ocular and tonsillar lesion. Oral manifestations include necrotic ulcers of the mucosa or pharynx, associated with pain; generalized stomatitis sometimes may occur instead of an isolated lesion. Development of abscesses from nodular lesions may be associated. Lymphatic involvement usually includes the submaxillary and cervical nodes. Called also *deer fly fever, Francis' disease, Pohvant Valley plague,* and *rabbit fever.*

Tulp, Nicolaas [17th century] a Dutch physician who established the importance of diseases of the teeth and their adnexa in the treatment of diseases of the human body. Tulp was the subject of Rembrandt's painting *The anatomy lesson of Dr. Tulp.*

tumefaction (tu″me-fak′shun) [L. *tumefactio*] a swelling; the state of being swollen, or the act of swelling; puffiness; edema.

tumescence (tu-mes′ens) 1. the condition of being tumid or swollen. 2. a swelling.

tumid (tu′mid) [L. *tumidus*] swollen or edematous.

tumor (tu′mor) [L. tumor a swelling] 1. a mass of new tissue which persists and grows independently of its surrounding structures; a neoplasm. 2. a swelling. **Abrikossov's (Abrikossoff's) t.,** myoblastoma. **adenomatoid odontogenic t.,** a tumor of the jaws showing odontogenic epithelium arranged in ductlike structures formed by cuboidal or columnar cells with basal or columnar cells surrounding spaces which are usually empty. It is most common in children and adolescents, and is similar in appearance to ameloblastoma, except it occurs with equal frequency in the mandible and maxilla. The tumor is frequently associated with an impacted tooth or appears to originate in a cyst wall, and it does not seem to recur or metastasize. Called also *adenoameloblastoma.* **Albrecht-Arzt-Warthin t.,** adenolymphoma. **ameloblastic adenomatoid t.,** adenoameloblastoma. **amyloid t.,** a tumorlike lesion caused by deposition of amyloid substance. See also AMYLOIDOSIS. **angle t. syndrome,** Cushing's SYNDROME (2). **basaloid mixed t.,** adenoid cystic CARCINOMA. **benign t.,** a tumor that does not endanger life. It is usually an encapsulated lesion composed of cells that resemble the normal cells of origin, growing slowly and pushing aside the adjacent tissue but without invading it, which does not metastasize and responds to surgical treatment without recurring after excision. Called also *benign neoplasm.* **benign pigmented neuroectodermal t. of infancy,** melanoameloblastoma. **Burkitt's t.,** Burkitt's LYMPHOMA. **calcifying epithelial odontogenic t.,** a slow-growing odontogenic tumor, usually occurring in the mandibular premolar-molar area often in association with an impacted tooth, which is locally invasive and tends to recur. Swelling without pain is an early symptom. It is composed of sheets of packed, polyhedral epithelial cells with outlined cell borders and eosinophilic cytoplasm, associated with considerable intracellular degeneration with spherical spaces filled with eosinophilic material that becomes calcified. The nuclei are pleomorphic with giant nuclei being common. Called also *Pindborg's t.* **compound t.,** one composed of two cell types derived from the same germ layer. **craniopharyngeal duct t.,** craniopharyngioma. **denture injury t.,** fibrous inflammatory HYPERPLASIA. **desmoid t.,** desmoid. **erectile t.,** ANGIOMA cavernosum. **Ewing's t.,** Ewing's SARCOMA. **Küttner's t.,** submandibular chronic sclerosing SIALADENITIS. **malignant t.,** one likely to destroy life, which is usually unencapsulated, composed of embryonic, primitive, or poorly differentiated cells, growing rapidly in a disorganized manner, and expanding to and infiltrating adjacent organs and metastasizing to distant organs. It frequently necroses and becomes ulcerative. Called also *cancer* and *malignant neoplasm.* **mixed t.,** one composed of more than one type of neoplastic tissue; especially a complex embryonal tumor of local origin, which reproduces the normal development of the tissues and organs of the affected part. See also pleomorphic ADENOMA. **mixed t., basaloid,** adenoid cystic CARCINOMA. **mixed t., malignant,** pleomorphic adenoma, malignant; see under ADENOMA. **odontogenic t.,** one derived from odontogenic tissue. See odontogenic CYST, odontogenic FIBROMA, odontogenic FIBROSARCOMA, and odontogenic MYXOMA. **odontogenic adenomatoid t.,** adenoameloblastoma. **peripheral giant cell t.,** giant cell EPULIS. **pigmented anlage t.,** melanoameloblastoma. **Pindborg's t.,** calcifying epithelial odontogenic t. **pregnancy t.,** pregnancy GINGIVITIS. **Rathke's pouch t.,** craniopharyngioma. **retinal anlage t.,** melanoameloblastoma. **Schmincke's t.,** nasopharyngeal LYMPHOEPITHELIOMA. **serous t.,** serous MEMBRANE. **simple t.,** one composed of only one cell type. **soft mixed odontogenic t.,** ameloblastic FIBROMA. **teratoid t.,** teratoma. **true t.,** a neoplasm. **turban t.,** multiple benign epitheliomata of the scalp grouped together so as to cover the entire scalp. **varicose t.,** a swelling, composed of dilated veins. **Warthin's t.,** adenolymphoma.

tumoricidal (tu″mor-ĭ-si′dal) destructive to tumors or cancer cells.

tumorigenesis (tu″mor-ĭ-jen′ĕ-sis) the production of tumors. See also ONCOGENESIS.

tumorigenic (tu″mor-ĭ-jen′ik) giving rise to tumors; said especially of a cell or group of cells capable of producing a tumor; oncogenic.

tumorous (tu′mor-us) of the nature of a tumor.

tungstate (tung′stāt) a salt of tungstic acid.

tungsten (tung′sten) [Swed. *tung sten* heavy stone] a metallic element. Symbol, W (*wolfram*); atomic number, 74; atomic weight, 183.85; specific gravity, 19.3; melting point, 3410°C; valences, 2, 4–6; group VIB of the periodic table. Natural isotopes include 180, 182–184, and 186; artificial radioactive isotopes include 173–179, 181, 185, and 187–189. It is the heaviest of all metals, occurring as a hard, brittle, gray solid, which is resistant to and insoluble in acids, and is attacked superficially by aqua regia and nitric acid. Used to increase the hardness, elasticity, and tensile strength of steels; its alloys are used in various products in space and electronic technology, in dentistry and medicine, and in filaments for electric lamps and x-ray targets. Powdered tungsten is flammable and presents a fire hazard. **t. carbide,** tungsten CARBIDE.

tungstic (tung′stik) pertaining to pentavalent or hexavalent tungsten.

tunic (tu′nik) [L. *tunica*] a covering or coat. See also TUNICA. **muscular t.,** the muscular coat or layer surrounding the submucous tissues in portions of the digestive, respiratory, urinary, and genital tracts. Called also *tunica muscularis* [NA]. **pharyngeal t.,** pharyngobasilar FASCIA. **pharyngobasilar t.,** pharyngobasilar FASCIA. **proper t.,** TUNICA propria.

tunica (tu′nĭ-kah), pl. *tu′nicae* [L.] a coat; covering; used in anatomy to designate a structure covering or lining a part or an organ. Called also *tunic*. **t. adventi′tia** [NA], the outer coat of tubular structures, such as arteries, lymphatic vessels, or the esophagus; specifically, the outer, fibroelastic coat of a blood vessel. Called also the *t. externa vasorum adventitia*. **t. elas′tica inter′na,** t. intima. **t. exter′na vaso′rum,** t. adventitia. **t. fibro′sa** [NA], fibrous tunic or coat; an enveloping fibrous membrane. **t. in′tima, t. in′tima vaso′rum** [NA], the inner coat of the blood vessels, made up of endothelial cells surrounded by elastic fibers and connective tissue. Called also *t. elastica interna*. **t. me′dia, t. me′dia vaso′rum** [NA], the intermediate coat of the blood vessels, made up of transverse elastic and muscle fibers. Called also *media*. **t. muco′sa** [NA], mucous MEMBRANE. **t. muco′sa laryn′gis** [NA], mucous membrane of larynx; see under MEMBRANE. **t. muco′sa lin′guae** [NA], mucous membrane of tongue; see under MEMBRANE. **t. muco′sa na′si** [NA], mucous membrane, nasal; see under MEMBRANE. **t. muco′sa o′ris** [NA], mucous membrane, oral; see under MEMBRANE. **t. muco′sa pharyn′gis** [NA], mucous membrane of pharynx; see under MEMBRANE. **t. muco′sa u′teri** [NA], endometrium. **t. muscula′ris** [NA], muscular TUNIC. **t. muscula′ris pharyn′gis** [NA], the muscular coat of the pharynx, consisting primarily of the pharyngeal constrictor muscles. **t. pro′pria** [NA], a coat or layer of a part, as distinguished from an investing membrane. Called also *proper tunic*. **t. sero′sa** [NA], serous MEMBRANE.

tunnel (tun′el) a hollow tubular passage through a solid body, open at both ends.

Tunol trademark for *cod liver oil* (see under OIL).

turbidity (tur-bid′ĭ-te) [L. *turba* disorder, confusion] cloudiness of a liquid due to the presence of foreign substances. **blood t.,** cloudiness of the blood, usually occurring shortly after meals due to the presence of chylomicrons. Persistent turbidity may be a sign of hyperlipoproteinemia or diabetic acidosis. See also HYPERCHYLOMICRONEMIA.

turbinate (tur′bĭ-nāt) [L. *turbineus*] 1. shaped like a top. 2. pertaining to a turbinate bone (see nasal CONCHA).

turbinectomy (tur″bĭ-nek′to-me) [*turbinate* + Gr. *ektomē* excision] excision of a turbinate bone (nasal concha).

turbinotomy (tur″bĭ-not′o-me) [*turbinate* + Gr. *tomē* a cutting] the surgical cutting of a turbinate bone (nasal concha).

turbulence (ter′bu-lens) 1. the state or quality of being agitated or disturbed. 2. uneven or irregular flow of molten metal into a mold, sometimes resulting in a porous quality of the finished product.

turgescence (tur-jes′ens) [L. *turgescens*] the distention or swelling of a part.

turgid (tur′jid) [L. *turgidus*] swollen and congested.

turgor (tur′gor) [L.] the condition of being turgid; normal or other fullness. **t. vita′lis,** the normal consistency of living tissue.

Türk cell (irritation cell, irritation leukocyte) [Wilhelm *Türk*, Austrian physician, 1871–1916] see under CELL.

Turner's syndrome [Henry Hubert *Turner*, American physician, born 1892] see under SYNDROME. See also Noonan's SYNDROME (Turner-like syndrome).

Turner's tooth (hypoplasia) [Joseph George *Turner*, British dentist, died 1955] see under TOOTH.

turpentine (tur′pen-tīn) [L. *terebinthina*] The concrete oleoresin obtained from *Pinus palustris* and other species of *Pinus*. It contains a volatile oil. **Canada t.,** Canada BALSAM. **spirit of t.,** turpentine OIL.

turret (tur′et) 1. a small tower or tower-like projection, usually one forming part of a larger structure. 2. a pivoted rotating attachment on a lathe for holding tools. **arch t.,** a cylindrical metal form, usually with grooves of various sizes, used for forming an arch wire in an orthodontic appliance.

turricephaly (tur″ĭ-sef′ah-le) [L. *turris* tower + Gr. *kephalē* head] oxycephaly.

Tusilan trademark for *dextromethorphan hydrobromide* (see under DEXTROMETHORPHAN).

tussis (tus′is) [L.] cough.

tussive (tus′iv) pertaining to or due to a cough.

Tweed triangle see under TRIANGLE.

twinning (twin′ing) 1. the production of symmetrical structures or parts by division. 2. the simultaneous production of two or more embryos in the uterus. 3. see GEMINATION.

Twiston trademark for *rotoxamine*.

twitch (twich) a sudden, involuntary, spasmodic contraction of a skeletal muscle elicited by a single maximal volley of impulses in the motor neurons supplying it.

tybamate (ti′bah-māt) a mild tranquilizing agent, butylcarbamic acid 2-[[(aminocarbonyl)oxy]methyl]-2-methylpentyl ester, occurring as a white, crystalline powder or a clear, viscous liquid which may congeal on standing, with a mild characteristic odor and bitter taste. It is soluble in ethanol, acetone, and ether and slightly soluble in water. Used for the relief of anxiety and tension and to induce sleep. Side effects may include drowsiness, vertigo, slurred speech, headache, weakness, paresthesias, visual disorders, euphoria, excitement, overstimulation, nausea, vomiting, diarrhea, cardiac arrhythmias, syncope, hypotension, hypersensitivity, agranulocytosis, aplastic anemia, and thrombocytopenic purpura. Habituation may occur. Trademarks: Benvil, Nospan, Solacin, Tybatran.

Tybatran trademark for *tybamate*.

Tylcasin trademark for *calcium acetylsalicylate* (see under CALCIUM).

Tylciprine trademark for *tranylcypromine*.

Tylenol trademark for *acetaminophen*.

Tylose trademark for *methylcellulose*.

tylosis (ti-lo′sis) [Gr. *tylōs* a knob or callus] the formation of a callus or callosity.

tympanitis (tim″pah-ni′tis) OTITIS media.

tympanohyal (tim″pah-no-hi′al) 1. pertaining to the tympanum and the hyoid arch. 2. a small bone or cartilage at the base of the styloid process; in early life it becomes a part of the temporal bone.

tympanum (tim′pah-num) [L.; Gr. *tympanon* drum] middle EAR.

Tyndall phenomenon (effect) [John *Tyndall*, British physicist, 1820–1893] see under PHENOMENON.

type (tīp) [L. *typus*; Gr. *typos* mark] the general or prevailing character of any particular case of disease, person, or substance. **Amsterdam t.,** de Lange's SYNDROME. **blood t.,** see BLOOD GROUP. **body t.,** the general character of the body structure or constitution; physique. **concave facial t.,** dish FACE. **high-angle t.,** long face SYNDROME. **low-angle t.,** short face SYNDROME. **Wernicke-Mann t.,** Wernicke-Mann HEMIPLEGIA.

typhoid (ti′foid) [Gr. *typhōdes* like smoke; delirious] 1. typhus-like. 2. typhoid FEVER.

typhus (ti′fus) [Gr. *typhos* stupor arising from fever] any of a group of related arthropod-borne infectious diseases caused by species of *Rickettsia*, and marked by malaise, severe headache, sustained high fever, and a macular or maculopapular eruption which appears from the third to the seventh day. In English-speaking countries, the term is often used alone to refer to epidemic typhus (the classic form of typhus caused by *Rickettsia prowazekii*, which is transmitted from man to man by lice), whereas in some European languages, it refers to typhoid fever. **tickborne t.,** Rocky Mountain spotted FEVER.

typing (tīp′ing) determination of the type or category to which an individual, object, or other entity belongs. **blood t.,** determination of the blood groups in one or more blood group systems. See BLOOD matching.

typodont (ti′po-dont) an artificial model that contains artificial teeth or natural teeth that are used for teaching exericises.

Tyr tyrosine.

tyraminase (ti-ram′ĭ-nās) amine OXIDASE.

tyramine (ti′rah-mēn) a decarboxylation product of tyrosine, which may be converted to cresol and phenol; closely related to epinephrine and norepinephrine. **t. oxidase,** amine OXIDASE.

Tyri 10 trademark for *tyrothricin*.

tyrocidine (ti″ro-si′dēn) a crystalline polypeptide antibiotic isolated from cultures of *Bacillus brevis*. Together with gramicidin, it is a component of tyrothricin. It exists as tyrocidines A, B, and C, and the hydrochloride salt (trademarks: Brevicidin, Rapicidin).

Tyroderm trademark for *tyrothricin*.

tyrosine (ti-ro′sin) an aromatic, naturally occurring, nonessential amino acid, 2-amino-3(4-hydroxyphenyl)propionic acid. Found in most proteins and synthesized metabolically from phenylalanine. It is also found in the saliva. Abbreviated *Tyr*. Called also *oxyphenylaminopropionic acid*. See also amino ACID.

tyrothricin (ti″ro-thri′sin) a polypeptide antibiotic isolated from cultures of *Bacillus brevis*, consisting chiefly of gramicidin and tyrocidine (usually as the hydrochloride salt). It is a white to brownish or grayish, odorless, almost tasteless powder that is soluble in alcohol, slightly soluble in acetone, and insoluble in water, chloroform, or ether. Similar to gramicidin, it is active against gram-positive bacteria (except bacilli) and some gram-negative organisms, mainly *Neisseria*. Used topically in the treatment of wounds, ulcers, eye diseases, and pyogenic infections of the nasopharynx and tonsils. Irrigation of the paranasal sinuses with tyrothricin may cause potentially fatal meningitis. It is a potent hemolytic drug; it may also cause occasional anosmia and parosmia. Trademarks: Coltirot, Dermotricine, Hydrotricine, Martricin, Tyri 10, Tyroderm.

Tytin trademark for a *high copper alloy* (see under ALLOY).

Tyzine trademark for *tetrahydrozoline hydrochloride* (see under TETRAHYDROZOLINE).

Tzanck test [Arnault *Tzanck*, Russian dermatologist in Paris, 1886–1954] see under TEST.

U

U 1. unit. 2. enzyme UNIT. 3. uranium.

ubiquinone (u-bik′kwĭ-nōn) a group of related quinones with isoprenoid units in the side chains, occurring in the lipid fractions of mitochondria, and serving in the biological electron transport system responsible for energy conversion in the cell. Ubiquinones function in the terminal system where they act as electron or hydrogen carriers between the flavoproteins and the cytochromes, being involved in the catalysis of the oxidation of succinate and reduced pyridine nucleotides. They are found in most aerobic organisms. Used therapeutically as a cardiovascular agent. Called also *coenzyme Q* and *mitoquinone*.

UCR usual, customary, and reasonable; see under FEE.

UDP URIDINE 5′-diphosphate.

Uehlinger, E. [Swiss pathologist] see chronic atrophic POLYCHONDRITIS (Meyenburg-Altherr-Uehlinger syndrome).

ulaganactesis (u-lag″an-ak-te′sis) [Gr. *oulon* gum + *anganaktēsis* irritation] irritation or itching of the gingivae.

ulalgia (u-lal′je-ah) [Gr. *oulon* gum + *algos* pain + *-ia*] gingivalgia.

ulatrophy (u-lat′ro-fe) [Gr. *oulon* gum + *atrophy*] atrophy of the gingiva associated with its recession and exposure of the root portion of the tooth. **afunctional u.**, that occurring in congenital malocclusion. **atrophic u.**, ischemic u. **calcic u.**, that due to the presence of salivary concretions. **ischemic u.**, that due to deficient blood supply. Called also *atrophic u.* **traumatic u.**, that due to gingival trauma.

ulcer (ul′ser) [L. *ulcus*; Gr. *helkōsis*] a loss of cutaneous or mucous substance with a local excavation of the surface of an organ or tissue, resulting from the sloughing of inflammatory necrotic tissue. Called also *ulceration*. **aphthous u.**, the ulcerative lesion of recurrent aphthous stomatitis. **Chiclero u.**, cutaneous LEISHMANIASIS. **corrosive u.**, noma. **denture u.**, a traumatic ulcer of the oral mucosa due to denture irritation, usually appearing within a day or two after the insertion of a new denture, and may be caused by overextension of the flanges, sequestration of spicules of bone under the denture, or a roughened or high spot on the inner surface of the denture. It is characterized by one or more small, painful, irregular ulcers covered by a delicate gray necrotic membrane, surrounded by an inflammatory halo. Called also *sore spots*. See also denture STOMATITIS. **duodenal u.**, peptic ulcer situated in the duodenum. **gummatous u.**, a broken-down superficial gumma. **peptic u.**, an ulceration of the mucous membrane of the esophagus, stomach, or duodenum. **Plaut's u.**, acute necrotizing GINGIVITIS. **pudendal u.**, GRANULOMA venereum. **recurrent aphthous u.**, recurrent aphthous STOMATITIS. **rodent u.**, ulcerating basal cell carcinoma of the skin. Called also *rodent cancer*. **sublingual u.**, one of the frenum of the tongue. **traumatic u.**, one due to a traumatic injury. Ulcers of the oral mucosa may be caused by biting, denture irritation, toothbrush injury, injuries by sharp tooth edges, or other irritants.

ulcera (ul′ser-ah) [L.] plural of *ulcus*.

ulceration (ul″se-ra′shun) [L. *ulceratio*] 1. the formation or development of an ulcer. 2. ulcer. **Daguet u.**, ulcer of the uvula and other parts of the throat, seen in typhoid fever.

ulcerative (ul′ser-a″tiv) pertaining to or characterized by ulceration.

ulcero- [L. *ulcus*] a combining form denoting relationship to an ulcer.

ulcerogangrenous (ul″ser-o-gang′re-nus) characterized by both ulceration and gangrene; pertaining to a gangrenous ulcer.

ulcerogenic (ul″ser-o-jen′ik) [*ulcero-* + Gr. *gennan* to produce] causing or producing an ulcer.

ulceromembranous (ul″sero-mem′brah-nus) characterized by ulceration and by a membranous exudation.

ulcus (ul′kus), pl. *ul′cera* [L.] ulcer.

ule- see ULO-.

ulectomy (u-lek′to-me) 1. [Gr. *oulē* scar + *ektomē* excision] excision of scar tissue. 2. [Gr. *oulon* gum + *ektomē* excision] excision of the gingiva; oulectomy. See GINGIVECTOMY.

ulemorrhagia (u″lem-o-ra′je-ah) [Gr. *oulon* gum + *rhēgnynai* to burst forth] gingival hemorrhage.

ulitis (u-li′tis) [Gr. *oulon* gum + *-itis*] inflammation of the gums; oulitis. See GINGIVITIS. **aphthous u.**, that associated with the presence of aphthae. **interstitial u.**, that associated with inflammation of the connective tissue around the teeth. **mercurial u.**, that due to mercury poisoning. **scorbutic u.**, that due to scurvy. **ulcerative u.**, that associated with ulcers.

Ullrich, Otto [German physician, 1894–1957] see Bonnevie-Ullrich SYNDROME, Morquio's DISEASE (Morquio-Ullrich syndrome), and Ullrich-Feichtiger SYNDROME.

Ullrich-Feichtiger syndrome [O. *Ullrich*; H. *Feichtiger*] see under SYNDROME.

ulo-, ule- 1. [Gr. *oulē* scar] a combining form denoting relationship to a scar, or cicatrix. 2. [Gr. *oulon* gum] a combining form denoting relationship to the gingiva.

ulocace (u-lok′ah-se) [*ulo-(2)* + Gr. *kakē* badness] ulceration of the gingivae.

ulocarcinoma (u″lo-kar″si-no′mah) [*ulo-(2)* + *carcinoma*] carcinoma of the gingivae.

uloglossitis (u″lo-glos-si′tis) [*ulo-(2)* + Gr. *glōssa* tongue + *-itis*] inflammation of the gingivae associated with glossitis.

uloncus (u-long′kus) [*ulo-(2)* + Gr. *onkos* tumor] a swelling or tumor of the gingivae.

ulorrhagia (u″lo-ra′je-ah) [*ulo-(2)* + Gr. *rhēgnynai* to burst forth] a sudden or free discharge of blood or hemorrhage from the gingivae.

ulorrhea (u″lo-re′ah) [*ulo-(2)* + Gr. *rhoia* flow] an oozing of blood from the gingivae.

ulotomy (u-lot′o-me) 1. [*ulo-(1)* + Gr. *tomē* a cutting] the cutting or division of scar tissue. 2. [*ulo-(2)* + Gr. *tomē* a cutting] incision of the gingivae.

ulotripsis (u″lo-trip′sis) [*ulo-(2)* + Gr. *tripsis* rubbing] revitalization of the gingivae by massage. See gingival MASSAGE.

ultimate (ul′ti-mat) [L. *ultimus* last] the last or farthest; final or most remote.

ult. praes. abbreviation for L. *ul′timum prae′scriptum*, last prescribed.

ultra- [L. *ultra* beyond] a prefix denoting excess, or beyond.

ultrabrachycephalic (ul″trah-brak″e-sĕ-fal′ik) pertaining to or characterized by an extremely broad short skull. See ultrabrachycephalic SKULL.

Ultra Brite see under DENTIFRICE.

Ultracarbon trademark for *activated charcoal* (see under CHARCOAL).

Ultracort trademark for *prednisone*.

Ultracorten trademark for *prednisone*.

ultradolichocephalic (ul″trah-dol″ĭ-ko-sĕ-fal′ik) pertaining to or characterized by an extremely long narrow head. See ultradolichocephalic SKULL.

ultramicroscope (ul″trah-mi′kro-skōp) a special darkfield microscope for the examination of particles of colloidal size, whereby the object is brightly illuminated at right angles to the optical axis to detect particles smaller than 0.1 μ, which appear as dots of bright light.

ultramicrotome (ul″trah-mi′kro-tōm) [*ultra-* + *micro-* + Gr. *tomē* a cut] a microtome for making extremely thin sections of tissue for electron microscopy, using a knife of fractured plate glass or a cleaved and polished diamond.

ultraprognathous (ul″trah-prog-na′thus) [*ultra-* + Gr. *pro* before + *gnathos* jaw] pertaining to or characterized by extreme protrusion of the lower jaw, or prognathism. See ultraprognathous SKULL.

ultrared (ul′trah-red′) infrared.

Ultrasonic trademark for an *ultrasonic denture cleanser* (see under CLEANSER).

ultrasonic (ul″trah-son′ik) [*ultra-* + L. *sonus* sound] pertaining to mechanical radiant energy having a frequency beyond the upper limit of perception by the human ear, that is, beyond about 20,000 cycles per second.

ultrasonics (ul″trah-son′iks) that part of the science of acoustics which deals with the frequency range beyond the upper limit of perception by the human ear (beyond 20 kc/sec), but usually restricted to frequencies above 500 kc/sec. Ultrasonic radiation is injurious to tissues because of its thermal effects when absorbed by living matter, but in controlled doses it is used therapeutically to selectively break down pathologic tissues, as in the treatment of arthritis and lesions of the nervous system, and also as a diagnostic aid by visually displaying echoes received from irradiated tissues, as in echocardiography. In periodontology, instruments producing up to 29,000 vibrations/sec are used. Ultrasonic tips are used for scaling, curettage, root planing, and gingival surgery. When placed against a tooth or soft tissue surface, the instrument mechanically debrides surface accumulations or necrotic tissue, but produces a narrow band of necrotic tissue which strips off from the inner aspect of the pocket.

ultrasonography (ul″trah-son-og′rah-fe) the visualization of deep structures of the body by recording the reflection of ultrasonic waves directed into the tissues.

ultrasound (ul″trah-sownd) mechanical radiant energy (sound) with a frequency greater than 20,000 cycles per second; see ULTRASONICS.

ultrastructure (ul′trah-struk″chŭr) the arrangement of the smallest elements making up a body; the structure beyond the resolution power of the light microscope, i.e., the structure visible only under the ultramicroscope and electron microscope.

Ultratek trademark for a nickel-chromium base-metal crown and bridge alloy, also containing some beryllium. Inhalation of dust during melting, milling, or grinding may cause beryllium poisoning.

ultraviolet (ul″trah-vi′o-let) beyond the violet end of the spectrum; said of ultraviolet rays (see under RAY).

ultravirus (ul″trah-vi′rus) filterable VIRUS.

Ulysseus syndrome [L.; named after the Greek epic hero, *Odysseus*, king of Ithaca] see under SYNDROME.

umbilicus (um-bil′ĭ-kus) [L.] [NA] the navel.

umbo (um′bo), pl. *umbo′nes* [L. "a boss," "a knob"] a round projection; the projecting center of any rounded surface; a knob.

umbonate (um′bo-nāt) [L. *umbo* a knob] knoblike; buttonlike; having a buttonlike, raised center.

umbones (um-bo′nes) [L.] plural of *umbo*.

umbra (um′brah), pl. *um′brae* [L. "shade," "shadow"] an area of high resolution on a radiographic image, representing the true shadow of the examined object. Cf. PENUMBRA.

umbrae (um′bre) [L.] plural of *umbra*.

UMP uridine monophosphate; see uridylic ACID.

uncia (un′se-ah) [L.] 1. ounce. 2. inch.

unciform (un′sĭ-form) [L. *uncus* hook + *forma* form] shaped like a hook.

uncinate (un′sĭ-nāt) hooked or barbed, as the uncinate process.

unconsciousness (un-kon′shus-nes) the condition of being insensible or incapable of responding to sensory stimuli and of having a subjective experience.

unction (ungk′shun) [L. *unctio*] 1. an ointment 2. the application of an ointment or salve; inunction.

underbite (un′der-bīt) a seldom used term variously applied to mandibular underdevelopment or to open bite.

undercut (un′der-kut) 1. that portion of a tooth which lies between the survey line (height of contour) and the gingivae. 2. the contour of a cross-section of a residual alveolar ridge or dental arch which would prevent the insertion of a denture. 3. the contour of flasking stone which interlocks in such a way as to prevent the separation of the parts. **retentive u.,** an area of the abutment surface suitable for the location of a retentive clasp terminal which, to escape the undercut, would be forced to flex and thus generate retention. **soft tissue u.,** an undercut in a residual alveolar ridge or soft tissue covering of a dental arch that would prevent or influence the placement of a removable

denture. **unusable u.,** the area of an abutment tooth or soft tissue across which a unit of the removable partial denture must pass without interference and hence must be blocked out by filling with wax or clay before the master cast is duplicated.

underexposure (un′der-ek-spo′zhur) inadequate exposure of film to light or x-rays resulting in an imperfect image.

undernutrition (un″der-nu-trish′un) malnutrition due to inadequate food supply or to failure to ingest, assimilate, or utilize any or all of the necessary food elements. See table of *Recommended Daily Dietary Allowances* at NUTRITION.

undersurface (un′der-sur′fis) the surface of the inferior portion of something; inferior surface; underside. **u. of tongue,** inferior surface of tongue; see under SURFACE.

underwriter (un″der-ri′ter) carrier (5).

undifferentiation (un″dif-er-en″she-a′shun) absence of normal differentiation; anaplasia.

undulation (un″du-la′shun) [L. *undulatio*] a wavelike motion.

unerupted (un″ē-rup′ted) not having erupted, as an unerupted tooth.

ung. abbreviation for L. *unguen′tum*, ointment.

unguent (ung′gwent) [L. *unguentum*] an ointment, salve, or cerate; see OINTMENT.

unguentum (ung-gwen′tum) [L.] ointment.

uni- [L. *unus* one] a prefix meaning one. See also words beginning MON- and MONO-.

uniarticular (u″ne-ar-tik′u-lar) [*uni-* + L. *articulus* joint] pertaining to a single joint, monarthric.

uniaxial (u″ne-ak′se-al) [*uni-* + axis] 1. having but one axis. 2. developing in an axial direction only.

Unibaryt trademark for *barium sulfate* (see under BARIUM).

unibasal (u″nĭ-ba′sal) [*uni-* + L. *basis* base] having only one base; monobasic.

unicameral (u″nĭ-kam′er-al) [*uni-* + L. *camera* chamber] having only one cavity or compartment.

unicellular (u″nĭ-sel′u-lar) [*uni-* + L. *cellula* cell] pertaining to or made up of but a single cell.

unicentral (u″nĭ-sen′tral) [*uni-* + L. *centrum* center] pertaining to or having a single center.

uniceps (u″nĭ-seps) [*uni-* + L. *caput* head] having one head or origin; said of a muscle.

unicuspid (u″nĭ-kus′pid) a tooth with only one cusp.

unicuspidate (u″nĭ-kus′pĭ-dat) having only one cusp.

unidirectional (u″ni-di-rek′shun-al) flowing in only one direction.

unifocal (u″nĭ-fo′kal) [*uni-* + L. *focus* fire-place] arising from or pertaining to a single focus.

uniforate (u″ni-fo′rat) [*uni-* + L. *foratus* pierced] having only one opening.

unigeminal (u″nĭ-jem′ĭ-nal) [*uni-* + L. *geminum* twin] pertaining to or affecting only one twin of a pair.

uniglandular (u″nĭ-glan′du-lar) pertaining to a single gland.

UniJel trademark for a fast-setting *hydrocolloid impression material* (see under MATERIAL).

unilaminar (u″nĭ-lam′ĭ-nar) having only one layer or lamina.

unilateral (u″ne-lat′er-al) [*uni-* + L. *lateralis*, from *latus* side] one-sided; pertaining to or affecting but one side.

unilobar (u″ne-lo′bar) having only one lobe; consisting of a single lobe.

unilocular (u″ne-lok′u-lar) [*uni-* + L. *loculus*] having but one loculus or compartment.

unimolecular (u″ni-mo-lek′u-lar) pertaining to one molecule. Called also *monomolecular*.

Unimycin trademark for *tetracycline hydrochloride* (see under TETRACYCLINE).

uninuclear (u″nĭ-nu′kle-ar) [*uni-* + *nucleus*] pertaining to a single nucleus. Having but one nucleus; mononuclear.

uninucleated (u″nĭ-nu′kle-āt″ed) [*uni-* + *nucleus*] having but one nucleus; mononucleate.

union (un′yun) [L. *unio*] the process of healing; the renewal of continuity of a broken bone or between the lips of a wound. See HEALING. **faulty u.,** a united fracture; nonunion. See also MALUNION. **fibrous u.,** a union in which the fractured ends of bones are united by fibrous tissue, but there is failure of ossification, sometimes leading to pseudarthrosis. See also fibrous HEALING. **u. by first intention,** primary u. **primary u.,** healing of a wound, usually a clean surgical incision, whereby the union takes place with a minimum of tissue loss and with small amounts of granulation tissue, uncomplicated by bacterial tissue contamination. Called also *u. by first intention, healing by first intention,* and *primary healing.* **secondary u.,**

u. by secondary intention, healing of a wound, usually a large tissue defect, whereby the union is associated with the production of necrotic debris and inflammatory exudate, formation of large amounts of granulation tissue, and production of large scars. Called also *healing by granulation, healing by second intention,* and *secondary healing.* **vicious u.,** malunion of the ends of a fractured bone so as to produce deformity.

Unipen trademark for *nafcillin.*

unipolar (u″nĭ-po′lar) [*uni-* + L. *polus* pole] 1. having but a single pole or process, as a nerve cell. 2. performed with one electric pole.

unit (u′nit) [L. *unus* one] 1. a single thing. 2. a quantity assumed as a standard of measurement. 3. a department or section in an organization, such as a hospital. See also ROOM and WARD. **absolute u's,** a system of units, such as the units of force, work, and power, based on a minimum number of independent units (e.g., mass, length, and time). **acid treating u.,** pickler. **American Drug Manufacturers' Association u.,** one-tenth of the Steenbock unit. **Ångström u.,** the unit of wavelength of electromagnetic and corpuscular radiation, being the wavelength of the red spectrum line of cadmium divided by 6438.4696. It is equal to 10^{-7} mm, 0.1 mμ, or 0.0001 μ. Called also *angstrom* and *international angstrom.* Abbreviated *A, Å,* and *AU.* **Ansbacher u.,** a unit of vitamin K dosage. **antitoxic u.,** a unit for expressing the strength of an antitoxin. The unit of diphtheria antitoxin is approximately the amount of antitoxin which will preserve the life of a guinea pig weighing 250 gm for at least 4 days after it is injected subcutaneously with a mixture of 100 times the minimum lethal dose of diphtheria toxin. Practically, it is the equivalent of a standard unit preserved in Washington. The unit of tetanus antitoxin is approximately 10 times the amount of tetanus antitoxin which will preserve the life of a guinea pig weighing 350 gm for at least 96 hours after injection of a mixture of 100 minimum lethal doses of tetanus toxin. The U.S. Public Health Service unit for scarlet fever antitoxin neutralizes 50 skin test doses of scarlet fever toxin. Abbreviated *AE* (Ger. *Antitoxineinheit*). **atomic mass u. (amu),** a unit of mass equal to one-half the mass of carbon-12, used to measure the masses of elementary particles, such as electrons, protons, and neutrons. 1 amu = 931.4812 MeV, or 1.660531×10^{-27} kg (SI units), or 1.660531×10^{-24} gm (cgs units). Called also *atomic weight u.* **atomic weight u. (awu),** atomic mass u. **Behnken's u.,** a unit of x-rays, being that quantity which, when applied in 1 cc of air at 18° C and 760 mm Hg of pressure, engenders sufficient electric conductivity to equal 1 electrostatic unit, as measured by the saturation current. **Bourquin u.,** that amount of vitamin B$_2$ (riboflavin) which fed daily to a standard test rat for 8 weeks will give a gain of 3 gm per week. Called also *Sherman u.* and *Sherman-Bourquin u.* **British thermal u.,** the quantity of heat required to raise the temperature of 1 pound of water 1° F at its temperature of greatest density (39° F). Abbreviated *BTU.* See also CALORIE and TEMPERATURE. **C & L u.,** C & L ATTACHMENT. **u. cell,** unit CELL. **CGS, cgs u.,** centimeter-gram-second SYSTEM. **combined u.,** combined ATTACHMENT. **coronary care u.,** a specially designed and equipped hospital area with all facilities necessary for constant observation and possible emergency treatment of patients with severe heart disease. See also *intensive care u.* **Crismani combined u.,** Crismani combined ATTACHMENT. **u. of current,** ampere. **Dalbo extracoronal u.,** Dalbo extracoronal ATTACHMENT. **Dalbo stud u.,** Dalbo stud ATTACHMENT. **dental u.,** 1. a masticatory unit consisting of a single tooth and its adnexa. 2. a mobile or fixed article of equipment, which may be combined with a chair in a one-piece unit or a separate piece of equipment, consisting of items and attachments needed for dental examination and operations. It houses the electrical, mechanical, and plumbing facilities needed to operate the equipment and fixtures attached to the unit. See illustration. See also illustration at dental CHAIR. **Dolder bar u.,** Dolder bar unit ATTACHMENT. **electrostatic u's,** that system of units based on the fundamental definition of a unit charge as one which will repel an equal and like charge with a force of 1 dyne when the two charges are 2 cm apart in a vacuum. Abbreviated *ESE* and *esu.* **enzyme u.,** the unit of enzyme activity that converts 1 mole of substrate (the amount of substance of a system that contains as many elementary entities as there are carbon atoms in 0.012 kg of carbon-12) per second. Symbol *U.* See KATAL. **Florey u.,** Oxford u. **Hampson u.,** a unit of roentgen ray exposure; it is ¼ of the erythema dose. **u. of heat,** the quantity of heat required to raise the temperature of 1 kg of water 1° C. See British thermal u. and CALORIE. **Holzknecht u.,** a unit of roentgen ray exposure

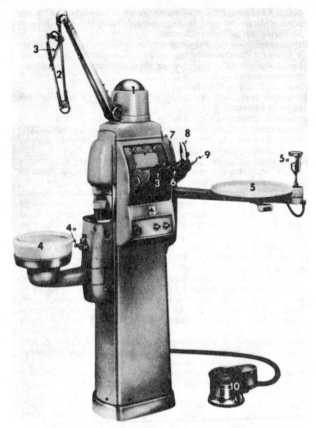

The dental unit. (1) Dome covering dental engine. (2) Engine arm. (3) Handpiece. (4) Cuspidor. (4a) Cuspidor controls. (5) Bracket table. (5a) Attached Bunsen burner. (6) Air syringe. (7) Water syringe. (8) Spray syringe. (9) Pulp vitality tester. (10) Foot controller. (Saliva ejector mouthpiece can be seen immediately to the right of the cuspidor controls.) (From V. R. Park, J. R. Ashman, and G. J. Shelly: A Textbook for Dental Assistants. 2nd ed. Philadelphia, W. B. Saunders Co., 1975; courtesy of the Ritter Co., Inc.)

equal to 1/5 the erythema dose. Abbreviated *H.* **Hruska u.,** Hruska ATTACHMENT. **insulin u., international,** international insulin u. **intensive care u.,** a department in a hospital in which are concentrated special equipment and skilled personnel for the care of seriously ill patients requiring immediate and continuous attention. Abbreviated *ICU.* Called also *intensive care room.* See also *coronary care u.* **international u.,** a unit of biological material, as of enzymes, hormones, vitamins, etc., established by the International Conference for the Unification of Formulas. Abbreviated *IU.* **international insulin u.,** one twenty-second of a mg of the pure crystalline product adopted as the standard. **international u. of penicillin,** the specific penicillin activity contained in 0.6 μg penicillin G sodium. **international u. of vitamin A,** activity equivalent to 0.6 μg of pure beta-carotene. **international u. of vitamin D,** the activity of 1 mg of the international standard solution of irradiated ergosterol (1 mg in 10 ml of olive oil). One mg given daily to rachitic rats for eight consecutive days should produce a wide calcium line. **International System of U's,** see SI. **Ipsoclip u.,** Ipsoclip ATTACHMENT. **Kienböck u.,** a unit of roentgen ray exposure equal to 0.1 the erythema dose. Symbol *X.* **u's of length,** units used for measuring the lengths of objects. See CENTIMETER, INCH, METER, and MILLIMETER. **u's of mass,** units used for measuring the mass (weight) of objects. See KILOGRAM and POUND. **motor u.,** the unit of motor activity formed by a motor nerve cell and the muscle fibers it innervates. **Oxford u.,** that amount of penicillin which, when dissolved in 50 ml of meat extract broth, just inhibits completely a test strain of *Staphylococcus aureus.* Called also *Florey u.* **penicillin u., international,** international u. of penicillin. **peripheral resistance u.,** the unit of resistance to blood flow in a vessel, being the resistance encountered when the pressure gradient between two points in a vessel is 1 mm Hg and the blood flow is 1 ml per second. **power u.,** in an orthodontic appliance, an arch wire configuration with stored forces which are released on appliance activation. **Pressomatic u.,** Pressomatic ATTACHMENT. **projection u.,** projection ATTACHMENT. **quantum u.,** Plack's CONSTANT. **rad u.,** rad. **rem u.,** rem. **roentgen u.,** roentgen. **Schubiger screw u.,** Schubiger ATTACHMENT. **Sherman u.,** 1. Bourquin u. 2. Sherman-Munsell u. **Sherman-Bourquin u.,** Bourquin u. **Sherman-Munsell u.,** that amount of vitamin A which when fed daily just suffices to support a rate of gain of 3 gm per week for 8 weeks in a standard test rat previously depleted of vitamin A. Called also *Sherman u.* **SI u.,** see SI. **smell u., specific,** specific smell u. **specific smell u.,** the smallest amount in substance in gm/liter which can be detected by smell. **Steenbock u. of vitamin D,** the total amount of vitamin D which will produce a narrow line of calcium deposit in the rachitic metaphyses of the distal ends of the radii and ulnae of standard rachitic rats within 10 days. See also *American Drug Manufacturer's Association u.* **Stern stress-breaker u.,** Stern ATTACHMENT. **structural u.,** in a virus, a morphological unit of the capsid that is composed of a single polypeptide chain; the structural unit for the helical capsid. **Svedberg u.,** a protein sedimentation coefficient of 1×10^{-13} sec. Thus, a sedimentation coefficient of 7×10^{-13} sec is denoted 7S. Abbreviated *S.* Called also *Svedberg.* **Tach-E-Z u.,** Tach-E-Z RETAINER. **Thayer-Doisy u.,** a unit of vitamin K activity, being equivalent to the activity of 1 μg of pure vitamin K_1. **USP u.,** one used in the *United States Pharmacopeia* in expressing the potency of antibiotic, pharmacodynamic, and endocrine preparations, as well as most of the sera, toxins, vaccines, and related products, corresponding to units established internationally, by the Food and Drug Administration, or by the National Institutes of Health. **vitamin A. u., international,** international u. of vitamin A. **vitamin A u. of Sherman-Munsell,** Sherman-Munsell u. of vitamin A. **u. of vitamin B₁,** the antineuritic activity of 3 μg of the international standard preparation deposited at the National Institute for Medical Research, Hampstead. **vitamin D u., international,** international u. of vitamin D. **vitamin D u.,** Steenbock u. of vitamin D. **vitamin K u.,** Thayer-Doisy u. **u's of volume,** units used to measure the space occupied by a substance. See LITER and QUART. **u's of weight,** units used for measuring the weight (mass) of objects. See KILOGRAM and POUND. **x-ray u.,** x-ray GENERATOR.

unitage (u'nit-ij) a statement of the unit quantity in any system of measurement.

Unitane trademark for titanium dioxide (see under TITANIUM).

unitary (u'nĭ-tar″e) [L. *unitas* oneness] composed of or pertaining to a single unit.

United States Adopted Name see USAN.

univalence (u″nĭ-va'lens) the state or condition of being univalent.

univalent (u″nĭ-va'lent) [*uni-* + L. *valere* to be strong] having a valence of one; replacing or combining with one atom of hydrogen or its equivalent; monovalent.

unmedullated (un-med'u-lāt″ed) not possessing a medulla or myelin sheath; unmyelinated. Said of a nerve fiber.

unmyelinated (un-mi′ĕ-lĭ-nāt″ed) not possessing a myelin sheath; unmedullated. Said of a nerve fiber.

unorganized (un-or'gan-īzd) not developed into an organic structure; not having organs.

unresponsiveness (un″re-spon'siv-nes) the quality of not responding to a stimulus or influence. **immunologic u.,** a failure of the immune system to respond to antigen, which may include a specific antigenic stimulus in immune tolerance or a variety of antigens in immunologic deficiencies or in artificially produced immunosuppression.

unsaturated (un-sat'u-rāt″ed) 1. not completely soaked or impregnated. 2. in chemistry, a compound in which all the available valence bonds are not satisfied (saturated), the extra bonds being held as double bonds. See also unsaturated COMPOUND. 3. a solution in which more solute may still be added and dissolved under stated conditions.

unsharpness (un-sharp'nes) the lack of sharpness or fuzziness, as of a radiographic or x-ray image. See also image DEFINITION. **geometric u.,** impaired image definition due to the presence of penumbra. See also x-ray beam GEOMETRY.

Upcylin trademark for *tetracycline phosphate complex* (see under TETRACYCLINE).

uprighting (up'rīt-ing) 1. erecting or placing something in a vertical position. 2. tipping inclined teeth to a more vertical axial inclination. See also TIPPING (2) and uprighting SPRING.

upsiloid (up'sĭ-loid) [Gr. *upsilon* + *eidos* form] shaped like the Greek upsilon (v or Y). See HYOID (1) and HYPSILOID.

uptake (up'tak) absorption and incorporation of a substance by living tissue.

UR utilization REVIEW.

uracil (u″rah-sil) a chemical substance, 2,4-dioxypyrimidine, found as a component of RNA (but not DNA) and of the coenzyme uridine diphosphate glucose, occurring as crystalline needles that are soluble in hot water and alkalies. Used in biochemical research. **5-methyl u.,** thymine. **u. mustard,** uracil MUSTARD. **u. riboside,** uridine.

uramustine (u″rah-mus'tēn) uracil MUSTARD.

uranisco- [Gr. *ouraniskos* the roof of the mouth] a combining form denoting relationship to the roof of the mouth or palate. See also URANO-.

uraniscochasma (u″rah-nis″ko-kaz'mah) [*uranisco-* + Gr. *chasma* cleft] CLEFT palate.

uraniscolalia (u″rah-nis″ko-la'le-ah) [*uranisco-* + Gr. *lalia* talking] a speech defect due to cleft palate.

uraniscoplasty (u″rah-nis-ko-plas″te) palatoplasty.

uraniscorrhaphy (u″rah-nis-kor'ah-fe) palatorrhaphy.

uraniscus (u″rah-nis'kus) [Gr. *ouraniskos*, dim. of *ouranos*] palate.

uranium (u-ra'ne-um) [named after the planet *Uranus*] a hard and heavy radioactive metallic element of the actinide series. Symbol, U; atomic number, 92; atomic weight, 238.03; specific gravity, 18.68; melting point, 1132°C; valences, 3, 4, 6. Naturally occurring uranium is composed of three isotopes of mass numbers 234, 235, and 238, respectively. ^{235}U separated from ^{238}U undergoes fission with slow neutrons, giving up neutrons which can join the nucleus of ^{238}U to form neptunium, which in turn decays by beta particle emission to form plutonium. It is a silver-white, lustrous metal that is malleable and ductile, which, on shaking, exhibits luminescence. Uranium and its salts are radioactive poisons causing dermatitis, renal lesions, arterial lesions, and death. Insoluble particles in the lungs may cause cancer long after the initial exposure. Used chiefly in nuclear technology; some compounds are used for medical purposes. **u. X,** protactinium.

urano- [Gr. *ouranos* the roof of the mouth, also the vault of heaven, or sky] a combining form denoting relationship to the palate; sometimes used in reference to the sky, or heaven. See also words beginning PALATO- and URANISCO-.

uranoplasty (u″rah-no-plas″te) [*urano-* + Gr. *plassein* to mold] palatoplasty.

uranoplegia (u″rah-no-ple'je-ah) palatoplegia.

uranorrhaphy (u″rah-nor'ah-fe) palatorrhaphy.

uranoschisis (u″rah-nos'ki-sis) [*urano-* + *schisis*] CLEFT palate.

uranoschism (u-ran'o-skizm) [*urano-* + Gr. *schisma* cleft] CLEFT palate.

uranostaphyloplasty (u″rah-no-staf'ĭ-lo-plas″te) [*urano-* + Gr. *staphylē* uvula + *plassein* to form] plastic repair of a defect of both the soft and hard palate. See also PALATOPLASTY.

uranostaphylorrhaphy (u″rah-no-staf″ĭ-lor'ah-fe) [*urano-* + Gr. *staphylē* uvula + *rhaphē* suture] suture of both the soft and hard palate. See also PALATORRHAPHY.

uranostaphyloschisis (u″rah-no-staf″ĭ-los'kĭ-sis) [*urano-* + Gr. *staphylē* uvula + *schisis* fissure] cleft of both the soft and hard palate. See CLEFT palate.

urari (u-rar'e) curare.

urate (u'rāt) [L. *uras*] a salt of uric acid, found in the blood and urine and in calcareous concretions and tophi.

uratemia (u″rah-te'me-ah) [*urate* + Gr. *haima* blood + *-ia*] the presence of urates in the blood.

uraturia (u″rah-tu're-ah) [*urate* + Gr. *ouron* urine + *-ia*] the presence of an excess of urates in the urine.

Urbach's lipoproteinosis [Erich *Urbach*, 1893–1946] Urbach-Wiethe SYNDROME.

Urbach-Wiethe syndrome [Erich *Urbach*; Camillo *Wiethe*] see under SYNDROME.

Urbasol trademark for *methylprednisolone.*

Urbason-Solubile trademark for *methylprednisolone sodium succinate* (see under METHYLPREDNISOLONE).

URC utilization review committee; see hospital utilization review COMMITTEE.

urea (u-re'ah) a diamide of carbonic acid, $CO(NH_2)_2$. It is a product of protein metabolism, being present in intracellular and extracellular fluids in equal concentrations, in the blood, urine, cerebrospinal fluid, saliva, sweat, and gastrointestinal secretions. Normal blood urea nitrogen level is 10 to 20 mg/100 ml and, in the plasma, 11 to 23 mg/100 ml. It is produced in the liver by a series of reactions involving ammonia, carbon dioxide, and water from the deamination and oxidation of amino acids; from there it is passed into the blood and excreted with the urine. Urea occurs in saliva at levels slightly lower than those in plasma and is degraded by bacteria to ammonia and carbon dioxide. In saliva, it is the main substrate which tends to counteract acid formation from carbohydrates in the production of plaque. Urea is the chief solid component of the urine and impairment of renal secretion is associated with urea retention and symptoms (see UREMIA). Synthetic urea [USP] is produced from ammonia and carbon dioxide. It is a white powder or a solid crystal with a saline taste and having almost no odor, which is readily soluble in water, alcohol, and benzene, slightly in ether, and almost insoluble in chloroform. Used as a diuretic. Called also *carbamide* and *carbonyldiamide*. Trademarks: Aquadrate, Ureaphil. See also SULFONYLUREA. **u. clearance,** blood urea CLEARANCE. **u. hydrogen peroxide,** u. peroxide. **u. peroxide,** a complex of hydrogen peroxide and urea, $CO(NH_2)_2 \cdot H_2O_2$, occurring as white crystals or crystalline powder that decomposes when exposed to moisture and is soluble in water, alcohol, and ethylene glycol. In aqueous solution, it dissociates into urea and hydrogen peroxide. It is an oxygen-liberating agent, used against anaerobic infections, such as acute necrotizing gingivitis. Its continued use may cause hypertrophy of filiform papillae. Also used as an oxidizing agent for bleaching and in the production of drugs and cosmetics. Called also *u. hydrogen peroxide* and *carbamide peroxide*. Trademarks: Hyperhidrit, Hyperol, Ortizon, Perhydrol-Urea.

ureagenetic (u-re″ah-je-net′ik) [*urea* + Gr. *gennan* to produce] forming or producing urea.

Ureaphil trademark for a urea preparation.

ureapoiesis (u-re″ah-poi-e′sis) [*urea* + Gr. *poiein* to make] the formation of urea.

Urecemil trademark for *allopurinol*.

ureide (u′re-īd) a compound of urea and an acid or aldehyde formed by the elimination of water, as alloxan. **cyclic u.,** a compound formed by replacement of one H for each NH_2 by a dibasic acid, as in alloxan or barbituric acid.

uremia (u-re′me-ah) [Gr. *ouron* urine + *haima* blood + *-ia*] the retention of excessive by-products of protein metabolism in the blood due to kidney insufficiency, and the toxic condition produced thereby. The most important effects include generalized edema due to water retention, acidosis resulting from failure of the kidneys to rid the body of normal acidic products, high potassium concentrations resulting from failure of potassium excretion, and high concentrations of nonprotein nitrogens, especially urea, resulting from failure of the body to excrete the metabolic end-products. Symptoms usually include nausea, vomiting, headache, vertigo, dimness of vision, coma or convulsions, parathyroid hyperplasia and abnormal calcium and bone metabolism typical of hyperparathyroidism, a sallow coloration of the skin, and itching and oral symptoms of uremic stomatitis, consisting of azotemic odor of the breath, erythema, exudations, ulcerations, pseudomembrane formation, and burning sensation.

uremic (u-re′mik) pertaining to or characterized by uremia.

ureolysis (u″re-ol′ĭ-sis) [*urea* + Gr. *lysis* a loosing, setting free] the decomposition of urea to carbon dioxide and ammonia.

ureter (u-re′ter) [Gr. *ourētēr*] the fibromuscular tube which conveys the urine from the kidney to the bladder.

urethan (u′rĕ-than) a compound, $CO(NH_2)OC_2H_5$, its structure being typical of the repeating unit in polyurethane resins, prepared by heating urea with ethanol under pressure. It occurs as a white powder or colorless crystalline solids that are odorless and have saltpeter-like taste, and is soluble in water, ethanol, ether, glycerol, chloroform and slightly, olive oil. Used as an intermediate or solvent for drugs, pesticides, and fungicides. Also used as an antineoplastic agent. Called also *urethane*. See also POLYURETHANE.

urethane (u″rĕ-thān) urethan.

urethra (u-re′thrah) [Gr. *ourēthra*] the membranous canal conveying urine from the bladder to the exterior of the body.

urethritis (u″re-thri′tis) inflammation of the urethra.

-uria [Gr. *ouron* urine + *-ia* state] a word termination denoting a characteristic or constituent of the urine, indicated by the stem to which it is affixed, as oliguria and proteinuria.

uric (u′rik) pertaining to the urine. See also uric ACID.

-uric (u′rik) in chemical nomenclature, a word termination used in the names of compounds which were first obtained from uric acid, such as barbituric acid or violuric acid.

Uricemil trademark for *allopurinol*.

uridine (u′rĭ-dēn, u′rĭ-din) a nucleoside, 1-β-D-ribofuranosyluracil, being a component of RNA and some coenzymes, which may be produced by hydrolysis of yeast nucleic acids

with alkali. On hydrolysis, it yields uracil and ribose. Called also *uracil riboside*. **u. 5′-diphosphate,** a nucleotide containing uridine, which participates in glycogen metabolism and in some processes of nucleic acid synthesis. Abbreviated *UDP*. **u. monophosphate (UMP),** uridylic ACID. **u. phosphate,** a nucleotide involved in the growth processes of the body, occurring as the monophosphate (see uridylic ACID), diphosphate (UDP), and triphosphate (UTP). **u. phosphoric acid,** uridylic ACID.

urina (u-ri′nah) [L.] urine.

urinalysis (u″rĭ-nal′ĭ-sis) [*urine* + *analysis*] physical, chemical, or microscopic analysis or examination of urine. For normal values of urine, see table of *Reference Values* in Appendix.

urination (u″rĭ-na′shun) the discharge or passage of urine.

urine (u′rin) [L. *urina;* Gr. *ouron*] the fluid excreted by the kidneys, passed through the ureters, stored in the bladder, and discharged through the urethra. Urine, in health, has an amber color, a slight acid reaction, a peculiar odor, and a bitter, saline taste. The average quantity excreted under ordinary dietary conditions in 24 hours in about 1000 to 2000 ml. Specific gravity, about 1.024, varying from 1.005 to 1.030. One thousand parts of healthy urine contain about 960 parts of water and 40 parts of solutes, which consist chiefly of urea, 23 parts; sodium chloride, 11 parts; phosphoric acid, 2.3 parts; sulfuric acid, 1.3 parts; uric acid, 0.5 part; also hippuric acid, leukomaines, urobilin, and certain organic salts. The abnormal matters found in the urine in various conditions include ketone bodies, proteins, proteoses, bile, blood, cystine, glucose, hemoglobin, fat, pus, spermatozoa, epithelial cells, mucous casts, and crystals of sulfanilamide derivatives (crystalluria). See table of *Reference Values for Urine* in Appendix.

Urinex trademark for *chlorothiazide*.

Urodiazin trademark for *hydrochlorothiazide*.

urokinase [E.C.3.4.99.26] (u″ro-ki′nās) a proteinase that activates plasminogen to form plasmin.

Urokon trademark for *acetrizoate sodium* (see under ACETRIZOATE).

Uronamin trademark for *methenamine mandelate* (see under METHENAMINE).

Uropen trademark for *hetacillin potassium* (see under HETACILLIN).

uroporphyrin (u″ro-por′fi-rin) porphyrin occurring in the urine (but not restricted to it). Chemically, uroporphyrins are tetraacetic, tetrapropionic porphins.

Urosemide trademark for *furosemide*.

urticaria (ur″tĭ-ka′re-ah) [L. *urtica* stinging nettle + *-ia*] a skin disease marked by the transient appearance of wheals or slightly elevated patches which are redder or paler than the surrounding skin and often attended by itching and tingling. Called also *hives* and *nettle-rash*. **cold u.,** edema and whealing occurring at the site of exposure to cold. A severe sloughing of the oral mucosa may occur after placing dry ice in the mouth, and sometimes swelling of the lips and oral mucosa may result from eating ice cream. **u. edemato′sa,** Quincke's EDEMA. **giant u., u. gigan′tea,** Quincke's EDEMA. **u. medicamento′sa,** urticaria caused by drugs taken internally. See DERMATITIS medicamentosa. **Milton's u.,** Quincke's EDEMA.

USAIDR US Army Institute of Dental Research.

USAN United States Adopted Name; a nonproprietary designation for any compound used as a drug (see generic NAME), established by negotiation between the manufacturer of the compound and a nomenclature committee, known as the USAN Council. Controversy concerning the selection of a name is settled by a six-member board, known as the Review Board. The USAN program is sponsored by the American Medical Association, the American Pharmaceutical Association, and the United States Pharmacopeial Convention; a liaison representative of the Food and Drug Administration sits on the Council. The term is currently limited to names adopted by the Council since June, 1961. A compilation of the names selected by the Council appears in the annual publication *USAN and the USP dictionary of drug names*. These names will appear as the monograph titles in the official compendia, *United States Pharmacopeia and the National Formulary*, when and if the respective drugs are admitted to either compendium.

Usher, Barney [Canadian dermatologist, born 1899] see PEMPHIGUS erythematosus (Senear-Usher syndrome).

USMG United States medical graduate.

USMH United States Marine Hospital.

USP The United States Pharmacopeia, a legally recognized compendium of standards for drugs, published by the United States Pharmacopeial Convention, Inc., and revised periodically. It includes also assays and tests for the determination of strength, quality, and purity.

USPHS United States Public Health Service.

uta (oo'tah) mucocutaneous LEISHMANIASIS.

Ut dict. abbreviation for L. *ut dic'tum*, as directed.

Utend. abbreviation for L. *uten'dus*, to be used.

uterus (u'te-rus), pl. *u'teri* [L.; Gr. *hystera*] [NA] the hollow muscular organ in female animals in which the fertilized ovum normally becomes embedded and in which the developing embryo and fetus are nourished.

Uticillin VK trademark for *penicillin V calcium* (see under PENI-CILLIN).

utilization (ut"il-i-za'shun) 1. the act or process of making use of something. 2. a bureaucratic expression frequently used to mean the employment of medical manpower and resources, such as those offered by physicians, dentists, hospitals, and other health professionals and facilities. See also utilization REVIEW. Dental Auxiliary U., see DAU.

UTP uridine triphosphate; see URIDINE phosphate.

utricle (u'tre-k'l) [L. *utriculus*] 1. any small sac, saccule. 2. the larger of the two divisions of the membranous labyrinth, located in the posterosuperior region of the vestibule. Called also *sacculus communis, utriculus* [NA], and *utriculus vestibuli*.

utriculi (u-trik'u-li) [L.] plural of *utriculus*.

utriculus (u-trik'u-lus), pl. *utric'uli* [L., dim. of *uter*] utricle. **u. vestib'uli**, utricle (2).

utriform (u'tri-form) having the shape of a bottle.

uvea (u've-ah) the pigmented middle coat of the eye, consisting of the iris, ciliary body, and choroid.

uveitis (u"ve-i'tis) [*uvea* + *-itis*] inflammation of the uvea.

uveoparotitis (u've-o-par"o-ti'tis) Heerfordt's SYNDROME. **Waldenström's u.**, a disorder related to Heerfordt's syndrome, characterized by bilateral iritis and parotitis. Symptoms vary and may include fever, lethargy, hallucinations, positive Babinski and Oppenheim reflexes, impaired sensitivity in the toes, abolished patellar and Achilles reflexes, facial paralysis, increased level of cerebrospinal albumin, and pleocytosis. In the original description, tuberculosis was the cause.

uviform (u'vi-form) [L. *uva* grape + *forma* form] having the form of a grape; racemose; staphyline.

uvula (u'vu-lah), pl. *u'vulae* [L. little grape] 1. palatine u. 2. any fleshy projection resembling the palatine uvula. See also terms beginning STAPHYLO-. **bifid u.**, bifurcation of the uvula, considered to be an incomplete form of cleft palate. Called also *cleft u., u. fissa, forked u.*, and *split u.* **cleft u.**, bifid u. **u. fis'sa, forked u.**, bifid u. **palatine u.**, a small fleshy projection at the posterior edge of the soft palate above the root of the tongue, comprising the levator and tensor palati muscles and the muscles of the uvula, connective tissue, and mucous membrane. Called also *pendulous p., plectrum,* and *staphylion.* **split u.**, bifid u.

uvular (u'vu-lar) pertaining to the uvula; staphyline.

uvulectomy (u"vu-lek'to-me) [*uvula* + Gr. *ektomē* excision] excision of the uvula; staphylectomy.

uvulitis (u"vu-li'tis) [*uvula* + *-itis*] inflammation of the uvula; staphylitis; cionitis.

uvuloptosis (u"vu-lop-to'sis) [*uvula* + Gr. *ptōsis* falling] a relaxed and pendulous condition of the palate; staphyloptosis; cionoptosis.

uvulotome (u'vu-lo-tōm) an instrument for cutting the uvula; staphylotome.

uvulotomy (u"vu-lot'o-me) [*uvula* + Gr. *tomē* a cutting] the operation of cutting off the uvula or part of it; staphylotomy; cionotomy.

UX uranium X; see PROTACTINIUM.

V

V 1. volt. 2. vanadium.

v 1. volt. 2. symbol for the *rate of reaction catalyzed by an enzyme.*

v. abbreviation for L. *ve'na*, vein.

V$_H$ see variable DOMAIN.

V$_L$ see variable DOMAIN.

VA Veterans Administration.

V/A volt/ampere; see OHM.

Vabrocid trademark for *nitrofurazone.*

vaccination (vak"sĭ-na'shun) [L. *vacca* cow] the inoculation of microorganisms for the purpose of inducing immunity. See also VACCINE. **smallpox v.**, application of smallpox vaccine by multiple punctures, to induce immunity against smallpox. Complications may include vaccinia, erythema multiforme, encephalitis, and bacterial superinfection.

vaccine (vak'sēn) [coined by Louis Pasteur from L. *vacca* in honor of Edward Jenner's contribution toward the prevention of smallpox through developing cowpox (vaccinia) vaccine] a term generally applied to a suspension of attenuated or killed microorganisms (bacteria, viruses, or rickettsiae) containing antigens of one or more pathogenic organisms which, upon administration, will stimulate active immunity against and protect against infection. The term also has been applied to solutions of soluble antigens and suspensions of agents such pollens. **attenuated v.**, a live vaccine containing microorganisms which have lost their virulence and ability to produce disease but retain the capacity to stimulate the production of an immune response. **autogenous v.**, one prepared from killed microorganisms which have been isolated from the lesion of the patient who is to be treated with it. **bacterial v.**, a suspension of attenuated or killed bacteria which is injected subcutaneously, intramuscularly, or intradermally, to increase the patient's immunity to the organisms injected. Certain bacterial vaccines may also be injected for their pyrogenic effects or their ability to induce a nonspecific activation of the defense mechanism. **heterologous v.**, one containing microorganisms that share cross-reacting antigens, which is capable of protecting against pathogens not present in the vaccine, as when cowpox vaccine is used to protect against smallpox. **inactivated v.**, one containing nonreplicating microorganisms that are noninfectious but which retain their protective antigens. Viral vaccines are usually inactivated by agents such as formaldehyde or phenol; bacterial vaccines by heat, acetone, ultraviolet rays, formaldehyde, or phenol. Called also *killed v.* **killed v.**, inactivated v. **live v.**, one prepared from live microorganisms or viruses that have been attenuated and which retain their immunogenic properties; the microorganisms or viruses usually multiply to a limited nonprogressive extent in the host. **mixed v.**, polyvalent v. **poliomyelitis v., live oral** [USP], a preparation of one or a combination of the three types of live, attenuated polioviruses, grown separately in primary cultures of kidney tissue. An active immunizing agent against poliomyelitis, it is administered orally. Called also *Sabin oral v.* **polyvalent v.**, one prepared from cultures or antigens of more than one strain or species. Called also *mixed v.* **Sabin oral v.**, poliomyelitis v., live oral. **Salk v.**, one prepared from three types of killed polioviruses grown in monkey kidney tissue; used intramuscularly in active immunization against poliomyelitis. **smallpox v.**, the living virus of vaccinia (cowpox) that has been grown in the skin of a vaccinated bovine calf or in the membranes of the chick embryo, and is available in liquid or dried form. It is used as an active immunizing agent against smallpox, being administered by multiple punctures with a special instrument, through a suspension applied to the skin. **triple v.**, a polyvalent vaccine prepared from antigens of the cultures of three different species or strains of organisms, such as diphtheria and tetanus toxoids combined with pertussis vaccine. **univalent v.**, one containing a single antigen or only one variety of organism.

vaccinia (vak-sin'e-ah) [L., from *vacca* cow] 1. a viral disease of cattle. See COWPOX. 2. a skin disease in humans, caused by the vaccinia virus; usually a complication of smallpox vaccination. It is characterized by a pustular eruption at the site of inoculation, which may be transmitted to other parts via the bloodstream, by direct contact, or by the fingers after scratching the primary site of inoculation. The lesions are whitish, umbilicated, depressed papules and papulovesicles that pustulate and change into aphthae, which are usually located on the tip or on the dorsum of the tongue, leaving cicatrices after healing. **congenital v.**, infection of the fetus with the vaccinia virus, leading to stillbirth or the appearance of cutaneous lesions shortly after birth, caused by smallpox vaccination or exposure to a vaccinated person during pregnancy. **v. gangreno'sa**, progressive v. **generalized v.**, a benign generalized skin eruption sometimes occurring after smallpox vaccination, due to spreading of viruses by the bloodstream, which may simulate cutaneous eruptions after burns or eczema. **v. necro'sum**, see *progressive v.* **progressive v.**, a complication of smallpox vaccination, characterized by a failure to heal and enlargement of the lesion at the site of vaccination. Initially, there may be no secondary symptoms, but eventually, as the lesion enlarges, there may be localized lymphadenopathy and some inflammatory response. At the first, the lesion presents a soft, rubbery eruption with little scabbing; eventually, it may enlarge extensively and undergo central necrosis associated with formation of a thick, dark eschar (*v. necrosum*). In advanced stages, there may be satellite lesions close to the site of inoculation and viremic lesions at distant sites, such as on the oral mucosa. In cases that are untreated or fail to respond to treatment, the course may last for several months, leading to extensive tissue destruction, bacterial superinfections, septicemia, pneumonia, severe mucosal lesions, and death. Called also *v. gangrenosa.*

Vacudent trademark for a vacuum suction device for removing fluids and debris from the oral cavity during dental operations.

vacuolation (vak″u-o-la′shun) the process of forming vacuoles; the condition of being vacuolated. Called also *vacuolization.*

vacuole (vak′u-ōl) [L. *vacuus* empty + *-ole* diminutive ending] 1. any small space or cavity formed in the protoplasm of a cell. 2. any minute cavity or vesicle in organic tissue.

vacuolization (vak″u-o-li-za′shun) vacuolation.

vacuum (vak′u-um) [L.] a space devoid of air, gas, or any other substance; a space from which the air, gas, or any other substance has been evacuated. **v. firing,** see vacuum FIRING. **v. investing,** vacuum INVESTING.

Vadosilan trademark for *isoxsuprine hydrochloride* (see under ISOXSUPRINE).

vagal (va′gal) pertaining to the vagus nerve.

Vagantin trademark for *methantheline bromide* (see under METHANTHALINE).

vagi (va′ji) plural of *vagus.*

vagina (vah-ji′nah), pl. *vagi′nae* [L.] 1. any sheath, or sheathlike structure; used in anatomical nomenclature as a general term for such a structure. 2. [NA] the canal in the female, extending from the vulva to the cervix of the uterus, being situated between the bladder and the rectum. It receives the erect penis in coitus and serves as a depository for semen during ejaculation, before the semen enters the uterus to fertilize the ovum. During delivery, the vagina dilates to allow passage to the fetus, when it serves as the birth canal. **v. carot′ica fas′ciae cervica′lis** [NA], carotid SHEATH. **v. muco′sae ten′dinis,** synovial sheath of tendon; see under SHEATH. **vagi′nae ner′vi op′tici,** the internal and external meningeal sheaths of the optic nerve within the orbit, continuous with the meninges of the brain. **v. proces′sus styloi′dei,** a ridge on the lower surface of the temporal bone, partly enclosing the base of the styloid process. Called also *sheath of styloid process.* **vagi′nae synovia′les,** double-layered, fluid-filled sheaths, such as those that usually surround tendons running in osseofibrous tunnels. **v. synovia′lis ten′dinis** [NA], synovial sheath of tendon; see under SHEATH. **v. vaso′rum,** a fibrous sheath that encloses certain arteries, sometimes along with their veins and nerves.

vaginae (vah-ji′ne) [L.] plural of *vagina.*

vaginal (vaj′ĭ-nal) 1. of the nature of a sheath; ensheathing. 2. pertaining to the vagina.

vaginate (vaj′ĭ-nāt) [L. *vaginatus* sheathed] provided with a sheath; sheathed.

vagitus (vah-ji′tus) [L.] the cry of an infant.

vagus (va′gus), pl. *va′gi* [L. "wandering"] 1. wandering, as the vagus nerve. 2. vagus NERVE.

vagusstoff (va′gus-stof) [*vagus* + Ger. *Stoff* stuff, substance] a substance liberated by the vagus nerve; the name assigned to acetylcholine by Otto Loewi when he discovered neurohumoral transmission.

Vail's syndrome [H. H. *Vail*] vidian NEURALGIA.

Val valine.

Valacon trademark for a heat-curing denture base acrylic resin.

Valadol trademark for *acetaminophen.*

Valamin trademark for *ethinamate.*

Valamina trademark for *fluphenazine.*

valence (va′βlens) [L. *valentia* strength] the numerical measure of the capacity to combine. In chemistry, it is an expression of the number of atoms of hydrogen (or its equivalent) which oe atom of a chemical element can hold in combination, if negative, or displace in a reaction, if positive. An element is characterized as *univalent* or *monovalent, bivalent* or *divalent, tervalent* or *trivalent, multivalent* or *polyvalent,* according to its valence — one, two, three, many, etc. In immunology, it is an expression of the number of antigenic determinants with which one molecule of a given antibody can combine. Most

antibody molecules possess two combining sites (i.e., two antigen-binding sites) and are said to be divalent, i.e., those belonging to the IgG, IgA, and IgE immunoglobulin classes. The valence of the IgM molecule is frequently found to be 5, although theoretically it should possess 10 combining sites. In like manner, the valence of an antigen may be expressed as the number of antibody combining sites (i.e., antigen-binding sites) with which it can unite. Most large antigen molcules are multivalent, or polyvalent. **biologic v.,** the combining power of molecules of homologous antigen and antibody. See VALENCE. **v. number,** polar NUMBER.

Valentin's ganglion [Gabriel Gustav *Valentin*, German physician, 1810–1883] 1. tympanic ganglion of Valentin; see under GANGLION. 2. INTUMESCENTIA tympanica.

valerian (va-le′re-an) 1. a plant of the genus *Valeriana.* 2. a preparation of the plant *Valeriana,* especially *Valeriana officinalis;* formerly used as an antispasmodic and nerve stimulant. See also valeric ACID.

valine (val′in) an aliphatic, naturally occurring amino acid, 2-aminoisovaleric·acid, which is essential for the growth of infants and certain nitrogen metabolic processes in human adults. It is also found in the saliva. Abbreviated *Val.* See also amino ACID.

Valisone trademark for *betamethasone valerate* (see under BETAMETHASONE).

Valium trademark for *diazepam.*

valla (val′lah) [L.] plural of *vallum.*

vallate (val′āt) [L. *vallatus* walled] having a wall or rim; cupshaped.

vallecula (vah-lek′u-lah), pl. *vallec′ulae* [L., dim. *valles* a hollow] a depression or furrow; used as a general anatomical term. Sometimes used alone to designate the *vallecula epiglottica.* **v. epiglot′tica,** a depression between the lateral and median glossoepiglottic folds on each side. **v. for petrosal ganglion,** petrosal FOSSULA.

vallecular (vah-lek′u-lar) pertaining to a vallecula.

Valleix's point [François Louis Isidore *Valleix,* French physician, 1807–1855] painful POINT.

Vallergan trademark for *trimeprazine.*

vallum (val′um), pl. *val′la* [L. "a fortification"] a mound or wall; a general anatomical term for any such structure.

Valmid trademark for *ethinamate.*

Valoid trademark for *cyclizine hydrochloride* (see under CYCLIZINE).

Valsalva, ligaments of, sinus of [Antonio Maria *Valsalva.* Italian anatomist, 1666–1723] see under LIGAMENT and SINUS. See also DYSPHAGIA valsalviana.

value (val′u) a measure of worth or efficiency; a quantitative measurement of the activity, concentration, etc., of specific substances. **mean clinical v.,** see MCV (2).

valva (val′vah) [L.] valve. **v. aor′tae** [NA], aortic VALVE. **v. atrioventricula′ris dex′tra** [NA], atrioventricular valve, right; see under VALVE. **v. atrioventricula′ris sinis′tra** [NA], atrioventricular valve, left; see under VALVE. **v. trun′ci pulmona′lis** [NA], pulmonary VALVE.

valve (valv) [L. *valva*] a mechanism or structure which controls the flow of liquids and gases, either in one or two directions. Called also *valvula.* **aortic v.,** the valve at the orifice of the aorta in the left ventricle of the heart. It consists of three semilunar cusps (hence the synonym *semilunar v.*), which open when the ventricular pressure exceeds that in the aorta, but close when the pressure is reversed, thus preventing backflow into the ventricle. Called also *valva aortae* [NA]. **artificial v.,** a prosthetic device used to replace a damaged heart valve. **atrioventricular v., left,** the valve in the opening between the left atrium and the left ventricle, usually consisting of two cusps (hence the synonym *bicuspid v.*), but additional small cusps may be present. When blood pressure in the atrium exceeds that of the ventricle, the cusps open and allow the blood to flow into the ventricle; when the ventricular pressure is greater, the cusps close, thus preventing backflow from the ventricle to the atrium. Called also *mitral v.* and *valva atrioventricularis sinistra* [NA]. **atrioventricular v., right,** the valve in the opening between the right atrium and the right ventricle, usually consisting of three cusps (hence the synonym *tricuspid v.*), but additional cusps may be present. When blood pressure in the atrium exceeds that of the ventricle, the cusps open and allow the blood to flow into the ventricle; when the ventricular pressure is greater, the cusps come together, thus preventing the backflow. Called also *valva atrioventricularis dextra* [NA]. **ball-type v.,** an artificial heart valve containing a small free-floating ball that prevents backflow of blood. **bicuspid v.,** atrioventricular v., left. **Hasner's v.,** lacrimal FOLD. **lymphatic v.,** a valve situated in the lymphatic vessels to prevent backflow of lymph and, at the junctions with veins, to prevent the venous blood from entering the lymphatic system. Similar to venous valves, they are situated in pairs and form pockets which allow the lymph to flow in one direction but open on pressure from the opposite direction and prevent backflow. They are made of a thin connective tissue and are covered by a layer of endothelium continuous with the tunica intima. Called also *valvula lymphaticum* [NA]. **mitral v.,** atrioventricular v., left. **pulmonary v.,** the valve at the origin of the pulmonary artery from the right ventricle of the heart. It consists of three semilunar cusps (hence the synonym *semilunar v.*), which open when the ventricular pressure exceeds that in the pulmonary artery, but close when the pressure is reversed, thus preventing backflow into the ventricle. Called also *valva trunci pulmonalis* [NA]. **semilunar v.,** a valve consisting of semilunar cusps. See *aortic v.* and *pulmonary v.* **tricuspid v.,** atrioventricular v., right. **venous v.,** a valve situated in pairs in veins to prevent backflow of blood. The valves are pockets of a thin connective tissue covered by a layer of endothelium that is continuous with the inner lining of the venous wall; they allow the blood to flow freely in one direction by collapsing, but open when the direction of flow changes, thus preventing the backflow.

valvula (val'vu-lah), pl. val'vulae [L., dim. of *valva*] a small valve; used in anatomical nomenclature as a general term to designate a valve. **v. lymphat'icum** [NA], lymphatic VALVE.

vanadate (van'ah-dāt) a salt of vanadic acid.

vanadic (vah-nad'ik, vah-na'dik) pertaining to a compound containing tri- or pentavalent vanadium.

vanadium (vah-na'de-um) [named after *Vanadis*, a Norse deity] a metallic element. Symbol, V; atomic number, 23; atomic weight, 50.942; specific gravity, 6.11; melting point, 1900°C; valences, 2–5; group VB of the periodic table. ^{50}V and ^{51}V are the two natural vanadium isotopes, ^{50}V being radioactive with a half-life of 6×10^{15} years; artificial isotopes include 46–49 and 52–54. It is a silvery white, ductile solid, insoluble in water, resistant to corrosion, attacked by alkali, and soluble in nitric, hydrofluoric, and sulfuric acids. In the metallic form, vanadium is nontoxic, but its pentoxide may cause irritation of the respiratory tract, dyspnea, cough, and cardiac disorders. Used in rust-resistant steels, in targets for x-ray machines, and in various industrial products.

van Bogaert-Hozay syndrome [Ludo van *Bogaert;* Jean *Hozay*] see under SYNDROME.

van Bogaert-Nyssen-Peiffer syndrome [L. *van Bogaert;* René *Nyssen;* Jürgen *Peiffer*] metachromatic LEUKODYSTROPHY.

van Buchem's syndrome [F. S. P. *van Buchem*] HYPEROSTOSIS cortical generalisata.

Vancocin trademark for *vancomycin.*

vancomycin (van'ko-mi"sin) a glycopeptide antibiotic elaborated by cultures of *Streptomyces orientalis.* Used therapeutically in the form of the hydrochloride salt, which occurs as a tan to brown, odorless, bitter powder that is freely soluble in water, moderately soluble in methanol, and insoluble in higher alcohols, acetone, and ether. It acts against bacteria by inhibiting their cell wall synthesis, being most active against gram-positive organisms, including cocci, neisseriae, clostridia, streptococci, micrococci, and pneumococci. Ototoxicity, sometimes with deafness; potentially fatal renal damage with uremia; suprainfection with gram-negative bacteria and fungi; hypersensitivity with skin rashes and anaphylaxis; phlebitis; pain at site of injection; chills; fever; and a shocklike state are the most serious adverse reactions. Trademark: Vancocin.

van Creveld, S. [Dutch pediatrician] see chondroectodermal DYSPLASIA (Ellis-van Creveld SYNDROME) and GLYCOGENOSIS I (van Gierke-van Creveld syndrome).

van der Hoeve's syndrome [J. *van der Hoeve*] see under SYNDROME.

van der Waals forces (bond) [Johannes Diderik *van der Waals,* Dutch physicist, 1877–1923; winner of the Nobel prize in 1910] see under FORCE.

van der Woude's syndrome [A. *van der Woude*] see under SYNDROME.

Vandid trademark for *ethamivan.*

van Hoorne's canal [Jean *van Hoorne,* Dutch anatomist, 1621–1670] thoracic DUCT.

van Leeuwenhoek see LEEUWENHOEK.

Vanobid trademark for *candicidin.*

Vanoxin trademark for *digoxin.*

van Soolingen see SOOLINGEN.

vapor (va'por), pl. *vapo'res, vapors* [L.] an exhalation or gas, especially emitted by a substance that at ordinary temperature is a solid or liquid, forming when the vapor pressure of a substance equals that of the atmosphere. **v. pressure,** vapor PRESSURE.

Vaporale trademark for aromatic ammonia, each 0.33-ml crush-able capsule containing ammonium hydroxide and ammonium carbonate in 35 percent alcohol.

vapores (va-po'rēz) [L.] plural of *vapor.*

vaporization (va"por-i-za'shun) conversion of a solid or liquid into a vapor without chemical change, brought about by heating with subsequent increase of the kinetic energy of the molecules until it is sufficiently large to overcome the intermolecular forces of attraction. Called also *evaporation.* **heat of v.,** HEAT of vaporization.

Vaquez's disease [Louis Henri *Vaquez,* French physician, 1860–1936] POLYCYTHEMIA vera.

Vaquez-Osler disease [L. H. *Vaquez;* Sir William *Osler,* Canadian-born physician and medical educator, 1849–1919] POLYCYTHEMIA vera.

variable (va're-ah-b'l) [L. *variare* to change] 1. changing from time to time. 2. a quality or value subject to change; in statistics, one of the separate numerical values from which a curve of variability can be constructed.

variant (var'e-ant) 1. something that differs in some characteristic from the class to which it belongs, as a variant of a disease, trait, species, etc. 2. exhibiting such variation.

variation (va"re-a'shun) 1. the act or process of changing or altering, as in form, appearance, character, substance, or any other aspect. 2. in genetics, deviation in characters in an individual from those typical of the group to which it belongs; also, deviation in characters of the offspring from those of its parents.

varicella (var"i-sel'ah) [L.] chickenpox.

varicelliform (var"i-sel'i-form) resembling chickenpox (varicella).

varices (var'i-sēz) [L.] plural of *varix.*

variciform (var'is'i-form) [*varix* + L. *forma* form] resembling a varix; varicoid.

varico- [L. *varix*] a combining form denoting relationship to a varix, or meaning twisted and swollen.

varicoid (var'i-koid) [*varico-* + Gr. *eidos* form] resembling a varix; variciform.

varicose (var'i-kōs) [L. *varicosus*] pertaining to a varix; unnaturally distended: said of a vein.

Vari-Mix trademark for a variable speed *mechanical triturator* (see under TRITURATOR), operating in the range of 3400 to 5000 rpm.

variola (vah-ri'o-lah) [L.] smallpox. See also variola VIRUS. **confluent v.,** a severe form of smallpox, characterized by the rapid development of symptoms. Headache, high fever, vomiting, nausea, back pain, and skin eruption are the principal symptoms. The eruption, which may also involve the mucous membranes of the larynx, pharynx, nose, and mouth, may begin on the second day and be fully developed in one to two days, evolving from papules to pustules; confluence occurs only on the face, hands, and feet. Salivation and difficult breathing due to swelling and edema of the mucous membranes are common. **hemorrhagic v.,** a severe and usually fatal form of smallpox, characterized by the development of purpuric lesions, presenting an irregular scarlatiniform eruption on the trunk and extremities, changing to purplish-red lesions, petechiae, and ecchymoses. Hemorrhage from the mucous membranes and death usually follow. Another form *(v. pustulosa hemorrhagica)* is also characterized by hemorrhage from the mucous membranes and death, which follows the development of vesicular and pustular lesions containing blood, intermixed with petechiae and ecchymoses. Called also *v. nigra maligna, v. pustulosa hemorrhagica, black smallpox,* and *purpura variolosa.* **v. ma'jor,** a form of smallpox, such as hemorrhagic variola, characterized by particularly severe symptoms and a high mortality rate. **v. mi'nor,** a relatively mild form of smallpox caused by a virus considered to be virtually indistinguishable from the variola virus, differing from ordinary smallpox by a lesser severity of symptoms and a lower mortality rate. Called also *alastrim.* **v. ni'gra malig'na,** v. pustulo'sa hemorrha'gica, hemorrhagic v.

varioloid (va're-o-loid) a modified and mild form of smallpox occurring in persons partially immune to smallpox, who have had a previous attack or have been vaccinated.

varix (var'iks), pl. var'ices [L.] an enlarged and tortuous vein, artery, or lymphatic vessel. **esophageal v.,** varices of the branches of the azygos vein which anastomose with tributaries of the portal vein in the lower esophagus, occurring in patients with portal hypertension.

varnish (var'nish) 1. a solution of resin or of natural gum, such as copal or rosin, in a suitable solvent, such as acetone, ether, or chloroform, which is capable of hardening into a thin film. 2. cavity v. **Caulk v.,** trademark for a *cavity varnish.* **cavity v.,** a cavity lining agent, consisting of a solution of one or more natural or synthetic resins, gums, and rosin, such as copal or nitrated cellulose, in an organic solvent, such as chloroform, ethanol, acetone, benzene, toluene, ethyl acetate, and amyl acetate; chlorobutanol, thymol, eugenol, and fluorides may be added. After application to the floor and walls of the prepared cavity, the solvent volatilizes, leaving a thin film that forms a semipermeable membrane, which permits penetration of some ions, while restricting others, and also neutralizing acids. Generally used in deep cavities under metallic and acid-containing restorative and cementing materials, but not under acrylic restorations. It also decreases microleakage around amalgam restorations. Trademark: Handi-Liner. **copal v.,** a cavity varnish prepared by mixing 5 gm of copal in 100 ml of chloroform. It sometimes also contains 5 gm of purified talc. Trademark: Copalite. **mastic v.,** a cavity varnish prepared by mixing 30 gm of mastic and 30 ml of balsam of Peru in a sufficient amount of chloroform to make 100 ml. **periodontal v.,** a protective coating applied after scaling and curettage, typically consisting of gum copal, gum mastic, myrrh, ether, and collodion. **rosin v.,** a cavity varnish having rosin as its principal component. Two types are known; *Rosin varnish I,* prepared by dissolving 7 gm of rosin in 100 ml of chloroform; and *Rosin varnish II,* prepared by dissolving 6.7 gm of rosin and 1.7 gm of sodium carbonate monohydrate in 100 ml of acetone.

vas (vas), pl. *va′sa* [L.] any channel for carrying a fluid, such as the blood or lymph; used in anatomical nomenclature as a general term to designate such channels. Called also *vessel.* **vasa afferen′tia,** vessels that convey fluid to a structure or part. **va′sa afferen′tia no′di lymphat′ici** [NA], afferent vessels of lymph node; see under VESSEL. **v. anastomot′icum** [NA], anastomotic VESSEL. **v. capilla′re** [NA], blood CAPILLARY. **v. collatera′le** [NA], collateral VESSEL (1). **va′sa efferen′tia,** efferent VESSELS; see under VESSEL. **va′sa efferen′tia no′di lymphat′ici,** efferent vessels of lymph node; see under VESSEL. **va′sa lymphat′ica profun′da** [NA], lymphatic vessels, deep; see under VESSEL. **va′sa lymphat′ica superficia′lia** [NA], lymphatic vessels, superficial; see under VESSEL. **v. lymphat′icum** [NA], lymphatic vessel. **va′sa nervo′rum,** blood vessels supplying the nerves, being minute arteries which derive from neighboring arteries. **va′sa nutri′tia,** vasa vasorum. **va′sa vaso′rum** [NA], blood vessels supplying larger arteries and veins, being minute arteries which derive from the main vessel or from neighboring arteries and break up into capillaries in the tunica adventitia. In arteries they seldom penetrate into the media, but in veins they may extend nearly to the intima. Called also *vasa nutritia.*

vasa (va′sah) [L.] plural of *vas.*

vasal (va′sal) pertaining to a vas or to a vessel; vascular.

vascular (vas′ku-lar) pertaining to or containing vessels, especially a blood vessel.

vascularization (vas″ku-lar-i-za′shun) the act or process of becoming vascular; or the natural or surgically induced development of vessels in a tissue.

vasculitis (vas″ku-li′tis) [L. *vasculum* vessel + *-itis*] inflammation of a vessel; angiitis.

Vaseline (vas′e-lin) trademark for petrolatum.

vaso- [L. *vas* vessel] a combining form denoting relationship to a vessel. See also terms beginning ANGIO-.

vasoactive (vas″o-ak′tiv) exerting an effect upon a vessel, especially a blood vessel.

Vasocon trademark for *naphazoline.*

vasoconstriction (vas″o-kon-strik′shun) the diminution of the caliber of vessels, especially blood vessels.

vasoconstrictor (vas″o-kon-strik′tor) 1. causing constriction of the blood vessels. 2. an agent (neurological or chemical) that causes constriction of the blood vessels.

vasodentin (vas″o-den′tin) [*vaso-* + L. *dens* tooth] dentin provided with blood vessels, as in the teeth of some fishes.

vasodepression (vas″o-de-presh′un) decrease in vascular resistance with hypotension.

vasodepressor (vas″o-de-pres′sor) 1. having the effect of lowering the blood pressure through reduction in vascular resistance. 2. an agent that causes vasodepression.

Vasodil trademark for *tolazoline hydrochloride* (see under TOLAZOLINE).

Vasodilan trademark for *isoxsuprine hydrochloride* (see under ISOXSUPRINE).

vasodilatation (vas″o-di-lah-ta′shun) the act of process of enlarging the diameter of the blood vessels. Called also *vasodilation.*

vasodilation (vas″o-di-la′shun) 1. dilation of a vessel, especially of a blood vessel. 2. vasodilatation.

vasodilator (vas″o-di-lāt′or) 1. causing dilation of the blood vessels. 2. an agent that causes dilation of the blood vessels.

vasography (vah-sog′rah-fe) [*vaso-* + Gr. *graphein* to write] roentgenography of the blood vessels; angiography.

vasoinhibitor (vas″o-in-hib′ĭ-tor) an agent that inhibits the action of the vasomotor nerves.

Vasomed trademark for *trolnitrate phosphate* (see under TROLNITRATE).

vasomotion (vas″o-mo′shun) [*vaso-* + L. *motio* movement] change in the caliber of a vessel, especially of a blood vessel.

vasomotor (vas-o-mo′tor) [*vaso-* + L. *motor* mover] 1. affecting the caliber of a vessel, especially of a blood vessel. 2. an agent affecting the caliber of a blood vessel.

Vasoplex trademark for *isoxsuprine hydrochloride* (see under ISOXSUPRINE).

vasopressin (vas″o-pres′in) an octapeptide hormone with both pressor and antidiuretic effects. It is believed to be formed in neuronal cells of the hypothalamic nuclei, from where it migrates along the axons and is stored in the nerve cell endings in the posterior pituitary gland. Secretion results in a decrease in urine volume and an increase in urine specific gravity. The secretion of vasopressin is regulated by neurological stimuli through the hypothalamus, osmotic pressure of the blood, volume of body fluids, and various drugs, including nicotine, morphine, anesthetics, etc. Called also *antidiuretic hormone (ADH)* and *pressor principle.* See also DIABETES insipidus and HYPONATREMIA.

vasopressor (vas″o-pres′or) 1. stimulating contraction of the muscular tissue of the capillaries and arteries, thereby reducing their caliber. 2. an agent that so acts.

Vasorbate trademark for *isosorbide dinitrate* (see under ISOSORBIDE).

Vasorome trademark for *oxandrolone.*

vasospasm (vas′o-spazm) spasm of the muscular tissue of the capillaries and arteries, thereby obstructing their lumen.

vasospasmolytic (vas″o-spaz″mo-lit′ik) [*vaso-* + *spasm* Gr. *lysis* dissolution] 1. arresting spasm of the blood vessels. 2. an agent that arrests spasm of the blood vessels.

vasostimulant (vas″o-stim′u-lant) [*vaso-* + L. *stimulans* producing stimulation] 1. stimulating or arousing vasomotor activity. 2. vasomotor STIMULANT.

Vasotonin trademark for *epinephrine.*

vasotonin (vas″o-to′nin) 5-hydroxytryptamine.

Vasotran trademark for *isoxsuprine hydrochloride* (see under ISOXSUPRINE).

vasotribe (vas′o-trib) [*vaso-* + Gr. *tribein* to crush] angiotribe.

vasotripsy (vas′o-trip″se) angiotripsy.

Vasoxyl trademark for *methoxamine hydrochloride* (see under METHOXAMINE).

vastus (vas′tus) [L.] great or vast; description of muscles, as musculus vastus lateralis. A common site for intramuscular injections.

Vater's corpuscles, duct [Abraham *Vater,* German anatomist, 1684–1751] see lamellar corpuscles; under CORPUSCLE, and see under DUCT.

Vater-Pacini corpuscles [A. *Vater;* Filippo *Pacini,* Italian anatomist, 1812–1883] lamellar corpuscles; see under CORPUSCLE.

vault (vawlt) 1. any arched or domelike structure. See also FORNIX. 2. the longest palatal border obtainable through a coronal section of the maxilla. 3. a cavity or a prepared area within the bone for an implant. **cranial v.,** calvaria. **cranial v., high,** see ACROCEPHALY, hypsicephalic SKULL, and OXYCEPHALY. **cranial v., low,** chamecephalic SKULL. **cranial v., low-arched,** tapeinocephalic SKULL. **v. of the palate,** the roof of the mouth. **v. of the pharynx,** the top or archlike roof of the rhinopharynx. Called also *fornix pharyngis* [NA] and *fornix of the pharynx.*

VB Vernochrome Pink trademark for a heat-cured denture base acrylic resin.

VB Vernonite trademark for a heat-cured denture base acrylic resin.

V-Cillin trademark for *penicillin V.*

VD veneral disease.

VDEL Veneral Disease Experimental Laboratory.

VDG venereal disease — gonorrhea.

VDRL Veneral Disease Research Laboratory.

VDS veneral disease — syphilis.

Veau classification see CLEFT palate.

Vebecillin trademark for *penicillin V.*

vector (vek′tor) [L. one who carries, from *vehere* to carry] a carrier, especially an animal, which transfers an infecting agent from one host to another.

Vectrin trademark for *minocycline*.

VEE Venezuelan equine encephalomyelitis (virus); see under VIRUS.

Veeneklaas' syndrome [G. M. H. *Veeneklaas*] dentopulmonary SYNDROME.

vegetative (vej′e-ta″tiv) [L. *vegetatio* growth] 1. pertaining to or concerned with vegetation, or the process of life and growth of plants. 2. possessing the power of, or promoting growth and development, as of a plant. 3. pertaining to the vegetative nervous system. See autonomic nervous SYSTEM. 4. resting; denoting the portion of a cell cycle during which the cell is not involved in replication.

vehicle (ve′ĭ-k′l) 1. any medium through which an impulse is propagated. 2. an inert substance added to a prescription in order to confer a suitable consistency or form to the drug; an excipient.

Veillon, Adrien [1864–1931] a French bacteriologist.

Veillonella (va″yon-el′ah) [named after Adrien *Veillon*] a genus of gram-negative, anaerobic bacteria of the family Veillonellaceae, occurring in culture as nonsporulating, nonmotile, spherical diplococci, about 0.3 to 0.5 μm in diameter. The organisms are parasitic in the mouth, comprising 5 to 10 percent of the cultivable organisms present in human saliva and on tongue surfaces, and less than 1 percent from other sites in the oral cavity. They are also found in the respiratory and intestinal tracts in animals, including man. The members are sensitive to penicillin G, chloramphenicol, chlortetracyclines, oxytetracycline, polymyxin B, and erythromycin. **V. alcales′cens,** a species that decomposes hydrogen peroxide and requires putrescine and cadaverine for growth. It has been isolated from the respiratory tract and oral cavity of man and rodents, and also has been isolated from the blood of patients who have undergone surgical operations. Called also *V. gazogenes, Micrococcus gazogenes,* and *M. lactilyticus.* **V. gazog′enes,** *V. alcalescens.* **V. par′vula,** a species that ferments glucose and produces indole, does not decompose hydrogen peroxide, and does not require putrescine or cadaverine for growth. It has been isolated from the respiratory and intestinal tracts and oral cavity of man and rodents. Called also *Staphylococcus parvulus.*

Veillonellaceae (va″yon-el-a′se-e) [*Veillonella* + *-aceae*] a family of gram-negative, anaerobic, nonmotile, nonflagellated bacteria. The organisms, about 0.3 to 0.5 μm in diameter, occur in pairs, masses, or chains, having diplococcal arrangements in culture. It consists of the genera *Acidaminococcus, Megasphaera,* and *Veillonella.*

vein (vān) [L. *vena*] a hollow vessel that carries blood from peripheral organs and tissues toward the heart. With the exception of the pulmonary veins, a vein transports blood low in oxygen. They usually accompany arteries, but are more numerous and larger than their corresponding arteries. Most veins have three coats: an inner, middle, and outer coat, but their walls are thinner than those of arteries, and they tend to collapse when cut. The boundaries between the individual coats tend to be indistinct, especially those of the middle coat,

which is sometimes indistinguishable. Pairs of pockets in the inner lining of venous walls prevent backflow of blood away from the heart. The smallest veins are in the periphery, where they are formed by merging of several capillaries. At this point, they are about 20 μ in diameter and consist of a layer of endothelium surrounded by a layer of longitudinal collagenous fibers and fibroblasts. Partially differentiated smooth muscle cells appear in veins of more than 45 μ in diameter. Veins over 200 μ in diameter develop well-established coats: an inner coat consisting of endothelium, a middle coat of smooth muscle cells, and an outer coat of scattered fibroblasts and collagenous fibers. Called also *vena.* See also terms beginning PHLEBO-. **accompanying v.,** one that accompanies its homonymous artery, usually enclosed in the same sheath. Called also *vena comitans* [NA]. See also *deep v.* **accompanying v. of hypoglossal nerve,** one formed by the union of the deep lingual and sublingual veins; it accompanies the hypoglossal nerve and empties into the facial, lingual, or jugular vein. Called also *vena comitans nervi hypoglossi* [NA]. **afferent v.,** one that carries blood to an organ. **anastomotic v., inferior,** one that interconnects the superficial middle cerebral vein with the transverse sinus. Called also *vena anastomotica inferior* [NA]. **anastomotic v., superior,** one that interconnects the superficial middle cerebral vein and the superior sagittal sinus. Called also *vena anastomotica superior* [NA]. **angular v.,** a short vein formed between the eye and the root of the nose by the junction of the frontal and supraorbital veins, which continues as the facial vein. It receives the superior and inferior palpebral and external nasal veins. Called also *vena angularis* [NA]. **anonymous v's,** brachiocephalic v's. **anterior cardinal v's,** precardinal v's. **arterial v.,** pulmonary TRUNK. **auricular v., posterior,** one that begins on the side of the head in anastomoses between the occipital and superficial temporal veins, passes down behind the pinna, and joins with the retromandibular vein to form the external jugular vein. It receives tributaries from the back of the ear and the stylomastoid vein. Called also *vena auricularis posterior* [NA]. **brachiocephalic v's [right and left],** the two veins that drain blood from the head, neck, and upper extremities, and unite to form the superior vena cava. Each is formed at the root of the neck by union of the ipsilateral internal jugular and subclavian veins. The right vein passes almost vertically downward in front of the brachiocephalic artery, and the left one passes from left to right behind the upper part of the sternum. Each receives the vertebral, deep cervical, interior thyroid, and internal thoracic veins. The left vein also receives several veins draining the thoracic cavity, as well as the thoracic duct; right one receives the right lymphatic duct. Called also *anonymous v's, innominate v's, venae anonymae,* and *venae brachiocephalicae* [NA]. **Breschet's v's,** diploic v's. **cardinal v's,** embryonic veins that include the precardinal and postcardinal veins, which fuse at the heart where they form the ducts of Cuvier (common cardinal veins). **cardinal v's, anterior,**

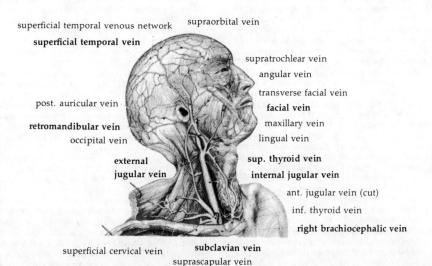

superficial temporal venous network

supraorbital vein

superficial temporal vein

supratrochlear vein

angular vein

transverse facial vein

post. auricular vein

facial vein

maxillary vein

retromandibular vein

lingual vein

occipital vein

sup. thyroid vein

external jugular vein

internal jugular vein

ant. jugular vein (cut)

inf. thyroid vein

right brachiocephalic vein

superficial cervical vein

subclavian vein

suprascapular vein

transverse cervical vein

The veins of the right side of the head and neck. (From J. Langman, M. W. Woerdeman: Atlas of Medical Anatomy. Philadelphia, W. B. Saunders Co., 1978.)

precardinal v's. **cardinal v's, common,** ducts of Cuvier; see under DUCT. **carotid v., external,** retromandibular v. **central v.,** one that occupies the axis of an organ. **cerebellar v's, inferior,** veins from the inferior surface of the cerebellum which empty into the transverse, sigmoid, and inferior petrosal sinuses, or into the occipital sinus. Called also *venae cerebelli inferiores* [NA]. **cerebellar v's, superior,** veins from the upper surface of the cerebellum which empty into the straight sinus and the greater cerebral vein, or into the transverse and superior petrosal sinuses. Called also *venae cerebelli superiores* [NA]. **cerebral v's,** veins that drain blood from the brain. Called also *venae cerebri* [NA]. **common cardinal v's of Cuvier,** ducts of Cuvier; see under DUCT. **condylar emissary v.,** emissary v., condylar. **cutaneous v.,** one found in the subcutaneous connective tissue of the skin. It begins in the papillae of the skin, forming subpapillary plexuses, and opens into larger subcutaneous veins. Called also *superficial v.* and *vena cutanea* [NA]. **deep v.,** one that drains deep structures of the body, frequently accompanying an artery *(accompanying v.),* usually both vessels being enclosed in the same sheath. Called also *vena profunda.* **deep v. of tongue,** lingual v., deep. **diploic v's,** venous channels in the diploë of the cranial bones that have thin walls, made up of endothelium and a layer of elastic tissue, and pouchlike dilatations at irregular intervals. They form sinuses in individual bones and, when sutures between the bones are obliterated, they unite to form large channels. The diploic veins communicate with the meningeal veins and send branches to the external and internal laminae, periosteum, and dura mater, and empty in part inside and in part outside the skull. Called also *Breschet's v's* and *venae diploicae* [NA]. **diploic v., anterior temporal,** one confined to the frontal bone and drains the lateral portion of the frontal and anterior part of the parietal bone, opening internally into the sphenoparietal sinus and externally into the deep temporal vein through an aperture in the great wing of the sphenoid bone. Called also *vena diploica temporalis anterior* [NA]. **diploic v., frontal,** one that drains the frontal bone, emptying externally into the supraorbital vein or internally into the superior sagittal sinus. Called also *vena diploica frontalis* [NA]. **diploic v., occipital,** the largest diploic vein that is confined to and drains the occipital bone and opens either externally into the occipital vein or internally into the transverse sinus or into the confluence of sinuses. Called also *vena diploica occipitalis* [NA]. **diploic v., posterior temporal,** one that drains the parietal bone and empties into the transverse sinus through an aperture at the mastoid angle of the parietal bone or through the mastoid foramen. Called also *vena diploica temporalis posterior* [NA]. **dorsal v's of tongue,** lingual v's, dorsal. **efferent v.,** one that carries blood away from an organ. **emissary v.,** one of the small, valveless veins that pass through foramina and openings of the skull, connecting venous sinuses of the dura mater inside the skull with veins outside the skull. Called also *emissarium* and *vena emissaria* [NA]. **emissary v., condylar,** a small inconstant vein running through the condylar canal in the lateral part of the occipital bone, connecting the sigmoid sinus with the vertebral or the internal jugular vein. Called also *emissarium condyloideum* and *vena emissaria condylaris* [NA]. **emissary v. of foramen of Vesalius,** vesalian v. **emissary v., mastoid,** a small vein passing through the mastoid foramen of the skull and connecting the sigmoid sinus with the occipital or the posterior auricular vein. Called also *emissarium mastoideum* and *vena emissaria mastoidea* [NA]. **emissary v., occipital,** an occasional small vein running through a minute foramen in the occipital protuberance of the skull and connecting the confluence of sinuses with the occipital vein. Called also *emissarium occipitale* and *vena emissaria occipitalis* [NA]. **emissary v., parietal,** a small vein passing through the parietal foramen of the skull and connecting the superior sagittal sinus with the superficial temporal veins. Called also *emissarium parietalis* and *vena emissaria parietalis* [NA]. **ethmoidal v's,** the anterior and posterior ethmoidal veins that follow the anterior and posterior ethmoidal arteries, emerge from the ethmoidal foramina, and empty into the superior ophthalmic vein. Called also *venae ethmoidales* [NA]. **facial v., facial v., anterior,** one draining the superficial structures of the face and usually emptying into the internal jugular vein. It begins at the union of the frontal and supraorbital veins as the angular vein and follows the course of the facial artery, descending along the border of the masseter muscle to the body of the mandible, across which it descends into the neck. Before emptying into the internal jugular vein, it communicates with both the an-

terior and external jugular veins. The trunk formed by the facial and retromandibular veins was formerly called the common facial vein. The facial vein anastomoses with the cavernous sinus through a system of the angular, supraorbital, and superior ophthalmic veins; another system of anastomoses is provided by the deep facial vein, pterygoid plexus, and inferior ophthalmic vein. Through the angular vein it receives the infraorbital, superior and inferior palpebral, and external nasal veins. Called also *vena facialis* [NA] and *vena facialis anterior.* **facial v., common,** the name formerly used for the venous trunk formed by the junction of the facial and retromandibular veins, originating below the angle of the mandible and emptying into the internal jugular vein approximately at the level of the hyoid bone. Called also *vena facialis communis.* **facial v., deep,** one that begins as an anastomosis with the pterygoid plexus and drains into the facial vein. It receives tributaries from the buccinator, zygomaticus, and masseter muscles, and external nasal, superior labial, superior and inferior labial, parotid, external palatine, submental, and submandibular veins. Called also *vena faciei profunda* [NA]. **facial v., posterior,** retromandibular v. **facial v., transverse,** one that passes backward with the transverse facial artery just below the zygomatic arch to join the retromandibular vein. Called also *vena transversa faciei* [NA]. **frontal v.,** supratrochlear v. **frontal diploic v.,** diploic v., frontal. **innominate v's,** brachiocephalic v's. **jugular v., anterior,** one that begins under the chin near the hyoid bone by the confluence of several small superficial submental veins, passes down the neck, and usually discharges into the jugular venous arch. Usually there are two anterior jugular veins, the right and left, but on occasion only one exists. It has no valves and its size varies. It receives tributaries from some laryngeal veins and a small thyroid vein, and discharges laterally to the external jugular vein. The jugular venous arch provides communication between the right and left anterior jugular veins. Called also *vena jugularis anterior* [NA]. **jugular v., external,** one that begins by the junction of the retromandibular and posterior auricular veins in the parotid gland, passes down the neck, and opens into the subclavian, internal jugular, or brachiocephalic veins. It is supplied with two pairs of valves, the inferior at the outlet of the vein, and the superior about 4 cm above. It receives blood from the exterior of the cranium and the deep parts of the face. Tributaries include the occipital, posterior external jugular, transverse cervical, suprascapular, and anterior jugular veins. Called also *vena jugularis externa* [NA]. **jugular v., external posterior,** one that begins in the occipital region and drains the blood from the skin and superificial muscles in the cranial and dorsal parts of the neck. It passes downward and opens into the middle third of the external jugular vein. Called also *vena jugularis posterior.* **jugular v., horizontal,** jugular venous ARCH. **jugular v., internal,** one of the two veins, right and left, draining much of the head and neck, which begins in the sigmoid sinus in the posterior compartment of the jugular foramen at the base of the skull and descends at first with the internal carotid artery and, later, with the common carotid artery, and joins the subclavian vein to form the brachiocephalic vein. It has two slight dilatations, one near the origin (superior jugular bulb) and one near its outlet (inferior jugular bulb). The left vein tends to be smaller than the right; both have a pair of valves near their outlet. Tributaries include the inferior petrosal sinus and the facial, lingual, pharyngeal, superior and middle thyroid, and sometimes occipital veins. The left vein receives the thoracic duct and the right receives the lymphatic duct at its junction with the subclavian vein. Called also *vena jugularis interna* [NA]. **labial v's, inferior,** veins that drain the region of the lower lip into the facial vein. Called also *venae labiales inferiores* [NA]. **labial v., superior,** one that drains the upper lip into the facial vein. Called also *vena labialis superior* [NA]. **laryngeal v., inferior,** one that drains the larynx into the inferior thyroid vein. Called also *vena laryngea inferior* [NA]. **laryngeal v., superior,** one that drains the larynx into the superior thyroid vein. Called also *vena laryngea superior* [NA]. **lingual v.,** a tributary of the internal jugular vein; it drains the tongue and sublingual region, collecting blood from the dorsal, deep lingual, and sublingual veins. Called also *vena lingualis* [NA]. **lingual v., deep,** one that begins near the tip of the tongue with an anastomosis with its fellow of the opposite side and passes as an accompanying vein of the lingual artery to empty into the main lingual trunk. Called also *deep v. of tongue* and *vena profunda linguae* [NA]. **lingual v's, dorsal,** small veins that begin at the dorsum of the tongue and pass posteriorly as accompanying veins of the lingual artery to empty into the main lingual trunk. Called also *dorsal v's of tongue* and *venae dorsales linguae* [NA]. **mandibular articular v's,** temporomandibular articular v's. **mastoid emissary v.,** emissary v., mastoid.

maxillary v., a short vein that begins in the pterygoid plexus and, after passing between the condyle of the mandible and the sphenomandibular ligament, joins the superficial temporal vein to form the retromandibular vein in the parotid gland. Called also *vena maxillaris* [NA]. **median v. of neck**, one formed when the anterior jugular veins unite as they pass down the neck. Called also *vena mediana colli*. **meningeal v's**, the accompanying veins of the meningeal arteries; they drain the dura mater, communicate with the lateral lacunae, and empty into the regional sinuses and veins. Called also *venae meningeae* [NA]. **nasal v's, external**, small ascending branches from the nose that open into the angular and facial veins. Called also *venae nasales externae* [NA]. **nasofrontal v.**, one that begins at the supraorbital vein, enters the orbit, and joins the superior ophthalmic vein. Called also *vena nasofrontalis* [NA]. **occipital v.**, one beginning in a plexus on the posterior part of the vertex in anastomosis with the posterior auricular and superficial temporal veins, from where it follows the occipital artery and the greater occipital nerve into the suboccipital triangle, forming a plexus in the triangle and joining the deep cervical and vertebral veins. In some instances, it empties into the internal jugular or, together with the posterior auricular vein, into the external jugular vein. Called also *vena occipitalis* [NA]. **occipital diploic v.**, diploic v., occipital. **occipital emissary v.**, emissary v., occipital. **ophthalmic v., inferior**, one formed by the confluence of muscular and ciliary branches, running backward either to join the superior ophthalmic vein or to open directly into the cavernous sinus; it sends a communicating branch through the inferior orbital fissure to join the pterygoid venous plexus. Called also *vena ophthalmica inferior* [NA]. **ophthalmic v., superior**, one that begins at the inner angle of the orbit, where it communicates with the frontal, supraorbital, and angular veins. It follows the distribution of the ophthalmic artery, and may be joined by the inferior ophthalmic vein at the superior orbital fissure before opening into the cavernous sinus. Called also *vena ophthalmica superior* [NA]. **ophthalmomeningeal v.**, a small inferior meningeal vein that opens usually into the superior ophthalmic vein, or occasionally into the superior petrosal sinus. Called also *vena ophthalmomeningea*. **palatine v.**, palatine v., external. **palatine v., external**, one that drains the tonsils and the soft palate into the facial vein. Called also *palatine v., vena palatina*, and *vena palatina externa* [NA]. **palpebral v's**, small branches from the eyelids that open into the superior ophthalmic vein. Called also *venae palpebrales* [NA]. **palpebral v's, inferior**, branches that drain the lower eyelids into the facial vein. Called also *venae palpebrales inferiores* [NA]. **palpebral v's, superior**, branches that drain the upper eyelids into the angular vein. Called also *venae palpebrales superiores* [NA]. **parietal emissary v.**, emissary v., parietal. **parotid v's**, small veins from the parotid gland that open into the superficial temporal vein. Called also *posterior parotid v., venae parotideae* [NA], and *venae parotideae posteriores*. **parotid v's, anterior**, parotid branches of facial vein; see under BRANCH. **parotid v's, posterior**, parotid v's. **pharyngeal v's**, veins that drain the pharyngeal plexus and receive some posterior meningeal veins and the vein of the pterygoid canal, and empty into the facial, lingual, superior thyroid, or internal jugular vein. Called also *venae pharyngeae* [NA]. **postcardinal v's**, paired vessels in the embryo, which collect the vascular elements from the areas caudal to the primitive heart, and merge with the precardinal veins to form the ducts of Cuvier (common cardinal veins). **precardinal v's**, paired vessels in the embryo, which collect blood from the cephalic part of the embryo and merge with the postcardinal veins to form the ducts of Cuvier (common cardinal veins.) A segment of the precardinal veins gives rise to the internal jugular veins. Called also *anterior cardinal v's*. **v. of pterygoid canal**, one of the veins that pass through the pterygoid canal and empty into the pterygoid plexus. Called also *vidian v., vena canalis pterygoidei* [NA], and *vena canalis pterygoidei* [Vidii]. **pulmonary v's**, the four veins, two from each lung (the right and left superior and the right and left inferior veins) which carry the oxygenated blood to the left atrium of the heart. Called also *venae pulmonales* [NA]. **retromandibular v.**, one formed in the upper part of the parotid gland behind the neck of the mandible by union of the maxillary and superficial temporal veins; it passes downward through the gland, communicates with the facial vein, and emerging from the gland joins with the posterior auricular vein to form the external jugular vein. Called also *external carotid v., posterior facial v., vena facialis posterior*, and *vena retromandibularis* [NA]. **sternocleidomastoid v.**, one that follows the course of the sternocleidomastoid artery and opens into the internal jugular vein. Called also *vena sternocleidomastoidea* [NA]. **stylomastoid v.**, one that follows the course of the stylomastoid artery and empties into the retromandibular vein.

Called also *vena stylomastoidea* [NA]. **subclavian v.**, one that is the main venous stem of the upper member and joins with the internal jugular vein to form the brachiocephalic vein. Occasionally, it receives branches of the anterior jugular vein. At the angle of junction with the jugular vein, the left subclavian receives the thoracic duct, and the right subclavian the right lymphatic duct. Called also *vena subclavia* [NA]. **sublingual v.**, a small vein that anastomoses with the submental vein and joins the deep lingual vein to form the accompanying vein of the hypoglossal nerve. Called also *vena sublingualis* [NA]. **submental v.**, one that follows the submental artery and opens into the facial vein. Called also *vena submentalis* [NA]. **superficial v.**, cutaneous v. **supraorbital v.**, a vein of the forehead that begins by anastomosing with a frontal tributary of the superficial temporal vein and descends to the root of the nose, where it joins the supratrochlear vein to form the angular vein. Occasionally, the two veins form a single vein in the upper forehead, which bifurcates to join the two angular veins. It forms an anastomosis with the superior ophthalmic vein and receives the frontal diploic veins. Called also *vena supraorbitalis* [NA]. **supratrochlear v.**, one that begins in a venous plexus high up in the forehead and descends to the root of the nose, where it joins with the supraorbital vein to form the angular vein. It communicates with the frontal tributaries of the superficial temporal vein. Occasionally, the supraorbital and supratrochlear veins form a single vein in the upper forehead, which bifurcates to join the two angular veins. Called also *frontal v., vena frontalis*, and *vena supratrochlearis*. **systemic v's**, veins which form a part of the systemic circulation in transporting the blood from the peripheral organs and tissues to the heart. They consist of a network, which begins as small plexuses that receive the blood from the capillaries and unite into larger veins, which eventually unite into venous trunks, gradually increasing in size, until the blood reaches the heart. Called also *venae systemates* and *venous system*. **temporal v's, deep**, veins that drain the deep portions of the temporal muscle and empty into the pterygoid plexus. Called also *venae temporales profundae* [NA]. **temporal diploic v., anterior**, diploic v., anterior temporal. **temporal diploic v., posterior**, diploic v., posterior temporal. **temporal v., middle**, one that arises in the substance of the temporal muscle and descends under the fascia to the zygoma, where it breaks through to join the superficial temporal vein. Called also *vena temporalis media* [NA]. **temporal v's, superficial**, veins that drain the lateral part of the scalp in the frontal and parietal regions, the tributaries forming a single superficial vein in front of the ear, just above the zygoma; this descending vein receives the middle temporal and transverse facial veins and, entering the parotid gland, unites with the maxillary vein deep to the neck of the mandible to form the retromandibular vein. Called also *venae temporales superficiales* [NA]. **temporomandibular articular v's**, small vessels that drain the plexus around the temporomandibular articulation into the retromandibular vein. Called also *mandibular articular v's, venae articulares mandibulae*, and *venae articulares temporomandibulares* [NA]. **thyroid v., inferior**, either of two veins, left and right, that drain the thyroid plexus into the left and right brachiocephalic veins. Called also *vena thyroidea inferior* [NA]. **thyroid v., middle**, one that drains the inferior part of the thyroid gland and emptying into the caudal part of the internal jugular vein, receiving tributaries from the larynx and trachea. Called also *vena thyroidea media* [NA]. **thyroid v., superior**, one that drains the thyroid gland and empties into the internal jugular vein, occasionally in common with the facial vein. It receives tributaries corresponding to the superior thyroid artery and the superior laryngeal and cricothyroid veins. Called also *vena thyroidea superior* [NA]. **transverse facial v.**, facial v., transverse. **tympanic v's**, small veins from the tympanic cavity that pass through the petrotympanic fissure, open into the plexus around the temporomandibular articulation, and finally drain into the retromandibular vein. Called also *venae tympanicae* [NA]. **varicose v.**, a dilated tortuous vein, usually due to incompetency of the venous valves. **vesalian v.**, an emissary vein connecting the cavernous sinus with the pterygoid venous plexus, sometimes passing through an opening in the great wing of the sphenoid bone. Called also *emissary v. of foramen of Vesalius*. **vidian v.**, v. of pterygoid canal.

vela (ve'lah) [L.] plural of *velum*.

Velacycline trademark for *rolitetracycline*.

Velban trademark for *vinblastine sulfate* (see under VINBLASTINE).

Velbe trademark for *vinblastine sulfate* (see under VINBLASTINE).

Velcic trademark for *polyvinyl chloride* (see under POLYVIN-YL).

Veldopa trademark for *levodopa*.

Velonimat trademark for *triamcinolone acetonide* (see under TRIAMCINOLONE).

Velosef trademark for *cephradine*.

velum (ve′lum), pl. *ve′la* [L] a veil, a veil-like structure; a covering; used in anatomical nomenclature for any such structure. **artificial v.,** a rubber or plastic appliance used in prosthetic restoration of the soft palate. **Baker's v.,** an obturator used in cleft palate. **v. pala′ti, v. palati′num,** soft PALATE.

Velvalloy trademark for an *amalgam alloy* (see under AMALGAM).

vena (ve′nah), pl. *ve′nae* [L.] a vessel through which blood passes from various organs or parts back to the heart. See VEIN. **v. anastomot′ica infe′rior** [NA], anastomotic vein, inferior; see under VEIN. **v. anastomot′ica supe′rior** [NA], anastomotic vein, superior; see under VEIN. **v. angula′ris** [NA], angular VEIN. **ve′nae anon′ymae,** brachiocephalic veins; see under VEIN. **ve′nae articula′res mandib′ulae,** temporomandibular articular veins; see under VEIN. **ve′nae articula′res temporomandibula′res** [NA], temporomandibular articular veins; see under VEIN. **v. auricula′ris poste′rior** [NA], auricular vein, posterior; see under VEIN. **ve′nae brachiocephal′icae** [NA], brachiocephalic veins; see under VEIN. **v. cana′lis pterygoi′dei** [NA], **v. cana′lis pterygoi′dei** [Vid′ii], VEIN of pterygoid canal. **ve′nae ca′vae,** the venous trunks which carry systemic blood to the heart. **v. ca′va infe′rior** [NA], the venous trunk which carries the blood from the lower half of the body to the right atrium of the heart. **v. ca′va supe′rior** [NA], the venous trunk, about 7 cm in length and about 2 cm in diameter, formed by the junction of the two brachiocephalic veins, which drains the blood from the upper half of the body. **ve′nae cerebel′li inferio′res** [NA], cerebellar veins, inferior; see under VEIN. **ve′nae cerebel′li supe′rio′res** [NA], cerebellar veins, superior; see under VEIN. **ve′nae cer′ebri** [NA], cerebral veins; see under VEIN. **v. com′itans** [NA], accompanying VEIN. **v. com′itans ner′vi hypoglos′si** [NA], accompanying vein of hypoglossal nerve; see under VEIN. **v. cuta′nea** [NA], cutaneous VEIN. **ve′nae diplo′icae** [NA], diploic veins; see under VEIN. **v. diplo′ica fronta′lis** [NA], diploic vein, frontal; see under VEIN. **v. diplo′ica occipita′lis** [NA], diploic vein, occipital; see under VEIN. **v. diplo′ica tempora′lis ante′rior** [NA], diploic vein, anterior temporal; see under VEIN. **v. diplo′ica tempora′lis poste′rior** [NA], diploic vein, posterior temporal; see under VEIN. **v. emissa′ria** [NA], emissary VEIN. **ve′nae dorsa′les lin′guae** [NA], lingual veins, dorsal; see under VEIN. **v. emissa′ria condyla′ris** [NA], condylar emissary VEIN. **v. emissa′ria mastoi′dea** [NA], emissary vein, mastoid; see under VEIN. **v. emissa′ria occipita′lis** [NA], emissary vein, occipital; see under VEIN. **v. emissa′ria parieta′lis** [NA], emissary vein, parietal; see under VEIN. **ve′nae ethmoida′les** [NA], ethmoidal veins; see under VEIN. **v. facia′lis** [NA], **v. facia′lis ante′rior,** facial VEIN. **v. facia′lis commu′nis,** facial vein, common; see under VEIN. **v. facia′lis poste′rior,** retromandibular VEIN. **v. facie′i profun′da** [NA], facial vein, deep; see under VEIN. **v. fronta′lis,** supratrochlear VEIN. **v. jugula′ris ante′rior** [NA], jugular vein, anterior; see under VEIN. **v. jugula′ris exter′na** [NA], jugular vein, external; see under VEIN. **v. jugula′ris inter′na** [NA], jugular vein, internal; see under VEIN. **v. jugula′ris poste′rior,** jugular vein, external posterior; see under VEIN. **ve′nae labia′les inferio′res** [NA], labial veins, inferior; see under VEIN. **v. labia′lis supe′rior,** labial vein, superior; see under VEIN. **v. laryn′gea infe′rior** [NA], laryngeal vein, inferior; see under VEIN. **v. laryn′gea supe′rior** [NA], laryngeal vein, superior; see under VEIN. **v. lingua′lis** [NA], lingual VEIN. **v. maxilla′ris,** maxillary VEIN. **v. media′na col′li,** median vein of neck; see under VEIN. **ve′nae menin′geae** [NA], meningeal veins; see under VEIN. **ve′nae nasa′les exter′nae** [NA], nasal veins, external; see under VEIN. **v. nasofronta′lis,** nasofrontal VEIN. **v. occipita′lis** [NA], occipital VEIN. **v. ophthal′mica infe′rior** [NA], ophthalmic vein, inferior; see under VEIN. **v. ophthal′mica supe′rior** [NA], ophthalmic vein, superior; see under VEIN. **v. ophthalmomenin′gea,** ophthalmomeningeal VEIN. **v. palati′na, v. palati′na exter′na** [NA], palatine vein, external; see under VEIN. **ve′nae palpebra′les,** palpebral veins; see under VEIN. **ve′nae palpebra′les inferio′res** [NA], palpebral veins, inferior; see under VEIN. **ve′nae palpebra′les superio′res** [NA], palpebral veins, superior; see under VEIN. **ve′nae paroti′deae** [NA], parotid veins; see under VEIN. **ve′nae paroti′deae anterio′res,** parotid branches of facial vein; see under BRANCH. **ve′nae paroti′deae**

posterio′res, parotid veins; see under VEIN. **ve′nae pharyn′geae** [NA], pharyngeal veins; see under VEIN. **v. profun′da,** deep VEIN. **v. profun′da lin′guae** [NA], lingual vein, deep; see under VEIN. **ve′nae pulmona′les** [NA], pulmonary veins; see under VEIN. **v. retromandibula′ris** [NA], retromandibular VEIN. **v. sternocleidomastoi′dea** [NA], sternocleidomastoid VEIN. **v. stylomastoi′dea** [NA], stylomastoid VEIN. **v. subcla′via** [NA], subclavian VEIN. **v. sublingua′lis** [NA], sublingual VEIN. **v. submenta′lis** [NA], submental VEIN. **v. supraorbita′lis** [NA], supraorbital VEIN. **v. supratrochlea′ris,** supratrochlear VEIN. **ve′nae systema′tes,** systemic veins; see under VEIN. **v. tempora′lis me′dia** [NA], temporal vein, middle; see under VEIN. **ve′nae tempora′les profun′dae** [NA], temporal veins, deep; see under VEIN. **ve′nae tempora′les superficia′les** [NA], temporal veins, superficial; see under VEIN. **v. thyreoi′dea i′ma,** occasional vein formed along the inferior pole of the thyroid gland by anastomosing channels of the right and left inferior thyroid veins; it descends in the midline and usually empties into the left brachiocephalic vein. **ve′nae thyreoi′deae inferio′res,** thyroid vein, inferior; see under VEIN. **ve′nae thyreoi′deae superio′res,** 1. thyroid vein, superior; see under VEIN. 2. veins draining the upper thyroid. **v. thyroi′dea infe′rior** [NA], thyroid vein, inferior; see under VEIN. **v. thyroi′dea me′dia** [NA], thyroid vein, middle; see under VEIN. **v. thyroi′dea supe′rior** [NA], thyroid vein, superior; see under VEIN. **v. transver′sa facie′i** [NA], facial vein, transverse; see under VEIN. **ve′nae tympan′icae** [NA], tympanic veins; see under VEIN. **ve′nae vaso′rum,** small veins that return blood from the tissues making up the walls of blood vessels themselves.

venae (ve′ne) [L.] plural of *vena.*

venation (ve-na′shun) [L. *vena* vein] the manner of distribution of the veins in a part.

vendor (ven′dor) 1. a person or agency that sells. 2. in insurance, an institution, agency, organization, or individual practitioner who provides health services; a provider.

veneer (vĕ-nēr′) in the construction of crowns or pontics, a layer of tooth-colored material, usually porcelain or acrylic resin, attached to the surface by direct fusion, cementation, or mechanical retention.

venesection (ven″e-sek′shun) [L. *vena* vein + *sectio* cutting] phlebotomy.

venesuture (ven′ĕ-su″chur, ven″ĕ-su′chur) [L. *vena* vein + *sutura* stitch] phleborrhaphy.

venipuncture (ven′ĭ-punk″chur) puncture of a vein, as in intravenous injections.

venisuture (ven′ĭ-su″chur, ven″ĭ-su′chur) [L. *vena* vein + *sutura* stitch] phleborrhaphy.

Venn diagram [John *Venn*, English logician, 1834–1923] see under DIAGRAM.

veno- [L. *vena* vein] a combining form denoting relationship to a vein or veins. See also terms beginning PHLEBO-.

venography (ve-nog′rah-fe) [*veno-* + Gr. *graphein* to write] phlebography (1). **intraosseous v.,** roentgenography of the veins after injection of the contrast medium into the bone marrow.

venom (ven′um) [L. *venenum* poison] a poison; specifically, a toxic substance normally secreted by poisonous animals. **hornet v.,** a poisonous and stinging secretion of hornets, containing histamine, 5-hydroxytryptamine, kinin, and acetylcholine. **snake v.,** the poisonous secretion of snakes, containing hemotoxins, hemagglutinins, neurotoxins, leukotoxins, and endotheliotoxins. The venoms of various species have been used as hemostatics. **wasp v.,** a poisonous and stinging secretion of wasps, containing histamine, 5-hydroxytryptamine, and kinin.

venomotor (ve″no-mo′tor) pertaining to or producing constriction or dilatation of the veins.

venomous (ven′o-mus) [L. *venenum* poison] poisonous.

veno-occlusive (ve″no-o-kloo′siv) pertaining to obstruction of the veins.

venous (ve′nus [L. *venosus*] pertaining to the veins.

venter (ven′ter), pl. *ven′tres* [L. "belly"] 1. any belly-shaped part; used in anatomical nomenclature to designate a fleshy contractile part of a muscle. 2. the stomach or belly. **v. ante′rior mus′culi digas′trici** [NA], anterior belly of digastric muscle; see under BELLY. **v. fronta′lis mus′culi occipitofronta′lis** [NA], frontal belly of occipitofrontal muscle; see under BELLY. **v. infe′rior mus′culi omohyoi′dei** [NA], inferior belly of omohyoid muscle; see under BELLY. **v. mus′culi** [NA], belly of muscle; the fleshy part of a muscle. **v. occipita′lis mus′culi occipitofronta′lis** [NA], occipital belly of occipitofrontal muscle; see under BELLY. **v. poste′rior mus′culi digas′trici** [NA], posterior belly of digastric muscle; see under BELLY. **v. supe′rior mus′culi omohyoi′dei** [NA], superior belly of omohyoid muscle; see under BELLY.

ventilation (ven″tĭ-la′shun) [L. *ventilatio*] 1. the process or act of supplying a house or a space continuously with fresh air. 2. in respiratory physiology, the process of exchange of air between the lungs and the ambient air. *Pulmonary ventilation* (usually measured in liters per minute) refers to the total exchange; *alveolar ventilation* refers to the effective ventilation of the alveoli, where gas exchange with the blood takes place. See also RESPIRATION.

ventilator (ven″ti-la′tor) an apparatus designed to qualify the air breathed through it or to intermittently or continuously assist or control pulmonary ventilation. Called also *respirator*. See also artificial RESPIRATION.

ventrad (ven′trad) [L. *venter* belly + *ad* to] toward a belly, venter, or ventral aspect.

ventral (ven′tral) [L. *ventralis*] 1. pertaining to the belly or to any venter. 2. denoting a position more toward the belly surface than some other object of reference; anterior.

ventralis (ven-tra′lis) [L.] ventral; a general anatomical term used to designate a position closer to the belly surface. See also ANTERIOR.

ventri- see VENTRO-.

ventricle (ven′trĭ′k′l) [L. *ventriculus*] a small cavity, such as one of the several cavities of the brain, or one of the lower chambers of the heart. Called also *ventriculus*. **fourth v. of cerebrum,** a flattened cavity filled with the cerebrospinal fluid, situated between the medulla oblongata, pons, and cerebellum; it is continuous with the canal of the spinal cord. Called also *ventriculus quatrus cerebri* [NA]. **Galen's v.,** v. of larynx. **lateral v. of cerebrum,** one of the two symmetric cavities in the cerebral hemispheres, filled with the cerebrospinal fluid which flows to the third ventricle through a foramen. Called also *second v. of cerebrum* and *ventriculus lateralis cerebri* [NA]. **left v. of heart,** the lower left chamber of the heart which receives oxygenated blood from the left atrium through the left atrioventricular valve, and pumps it into the aorta and systemic circulation through the aortic valve. Called also *ventriculus sinister cordis* [NA]. **Morgagni's v.,** v. of larynx. **v. of larynx,** a lateral invagination of mucous membrane between the free edge of the vestibular fold, the margin of the vocal fold, and the mucosa covering the thyroarytenoideus muscle. The anterior part leads to a saccule (*appendix of laryngeal ventricle*). Called also *Galen's v.*, *Morgagni's v.*, *laryngeal sinus*, *sacculus Morgagnii*, *sinus of Morgagni*, *ventriculus laryngis* [NA], and *ventriculus Morgagnii*. **right v. of heart,** the lower right chamber of the heart; it receives venous blood from the right atrium through the right atrioventricular valve, and pumps it for oxygenation into the pulmonary circulation through the pulmonary artery and pulmonary valve. Called also *ventriculus dexter cordis* [NA]. **second v. of cerebrum,** lateral v. of cerebrum. **third v. of cerebrum,** a narrow median cleft between the thalami of the two cerebral hemispheres, within the diencephalon. It is filled with the cerebrospinal fluid and communicates with the lateral and the fourth ventricles. Called also *ventriculus tertius cerebri* [NA].

ventricular (ven-trik′u-lar) pertaining to a ventricle.

ventricularis (ven-trik′u-la-ris) ventricularis MUSCLE.

ventriculi (ven-trik′u-li) [L.] plural of *ventriculus*.

ventriculocordectomy (ven-trik″u-lo-kor-dek′to-me) an operation for laryngeal stenosis with bilateral recurrent paralysis, done by excising with the punch forceps the entire ventricular floor anterior to the vocal process and anteroexternal surface of the arytenoid.

ventriculus (ven-trik′u-lus), pl. *ventric′uli* [L., dim. of *venter* belly] 1. [NA] the stomach. 2. a small cavity in an organ. See also *ventricle*. **v. dex′ter cor′dis** [NA], right ventricle of heart; see under VENTRICLE. **v. laryn′gis** [NA], VENTRICLE of larynx. **v. latera′lis cer′ebri** [NA], lateral ventricle of cerebrum; see under VENTRICLE. **v. Morgagnii,** VENTRICLE of larynx. **v. quar′tus cer′ebri** [NA], fourth ventricle of cerebrum; see under VENTRICLE. **v. sinis′ter cor′dis** [NA], left ventricle of heart; see under VENTRICLE. **v. ter′tius cer′ebri** [NA], third ventricle of cerebrum; see under VENTRICLE.

ventro-, ventri- [L. *venter* belly] a combining form denoting relationship to the belly, or to the front (anterior) aspect of the body.

Venturi, G. B. [1746–1822] an Italian physicist.

venturimeter (ven″tu-rim′ĕ-ter) [named after G. B. *Venturi*] an instrument for measuring the flow of liquids, as of the blood in vessels, by relating difference of pressures between a constricted and a nonconstricted portion of a tube through which fluid is flowing. Written also *venturi meter*.

venula (ven′u-lah), pl. *ven′ulae* [L., dim. of *vena* vein] [NA] venule.

venulae (ven′u-le) [L.] plural of *venula*.

venular (ven′u-lar) pertaining to, composed of, or affecting venules.

venule (ven′ūl) [L. *venula*] any of the small vessels that collect blood from capillary plexuses and join to form veins. Called also *venula* [NA]. **postcapillary v.,** a venule in the lymph node cortex having an elongated endothelial cell structure that allows the lymphocytes to pass from the blood to the lymph by the process in which the endothelial cells invaginate and allow lymphocytes to pass directly through. See also recirculating POOL.

Veracillin trademark for *dicloxacillin sodium* (see under DICLOXACILLIN).

Veratrum (vĕ-ra′trum) a genus of poisonous liliaceous plants. **V. al′bum,** European white hellebore, the source of alkaloids used in the treatment of hypertension. See also PROTOVERATRINE. **V. vir′ide,** American or green hellebore; its roots are source of antihypertensive alkaloids.

verbal (ver′bal) [L. *verbum*] consisting of words; pertaining to words or speech.

Verga's lacrimal groove [Andrea *Verga*, Italian neurologist, 1811–1895] see under GROOVE.

Vermillion see oral hygiene index, simplified, under INDEX (Greene-Vermillion index).

vermilionectomy (ver-mil″yon-ek′to-me) excision of the vermilion border of the lip, the surgically created defect being resurfaced by advancement of the undermined labial mucosa.

vernal (ver′nal) [L. *vernalis* of the spring] pertaining to or occurring in the spring.

Vernet's syndrome [Maurice *Vernet*, French neurologist, born 1887] see under SYNDROME.

vernier (ver′ne-er) [named after Pierre *Vernier*] a finely graduated scale accessory to a more coarsely graduated one for measuring fractions of the divisions of the latter.

Vernet's syndrome [Maurice *Vernet*, French neurologist, born 1887] see under SYNDROME.

Vernier, Pierre [1580–1637] a French physicist.

Veronal trademark for *barbital*.

Verospiron trademark for *spironolactone*.

verruca (ver-rooh′kah), pl. *verru′cae* [L.] a small epidermal growth. See also WART. **v. digita′ta,** a wart with finger-like excrescences growing from its surface. Called also *digitate wart*. **v. filifor′mis,** a wart with soft, thin, threadlike projections on its surface. Called also *filiform wart*. **v. pla′na, v. pla′na juveni′lis,** a small, smooth, usually skin-colored or light brown, slightly raised wart sometimes occurring in great numbers on the face, neck, back of the hands, wrists, and knees; seen most frequently in children but also in adults. Called also *flat wart*, *juvenile wart*, and *plane wart*. **v. vulga′ris,** a well-circumscribed, papillomatous, elevated growth with a keratotic surface, most commonly located on the hands, which characteristically contains vacuolated cells and inclusions. It is identified with oral papilloma by some authorities, because of their histomorphological similarities. See also PAPILLOMA.

verrucae (ve-roo′se) [L.] plural of *verruca*.

verrucous (ver′oo-kus) rough; warty.

verruga (vĕ-roo′gah) [Sp.] verruca. **v. peruana,** see BARTONELLOSIS.

Versapen trademark for *hetacillin*.

Versapen K trademark for *hetacillin potassium* (see under HETACILLIN).

Versatrex trademark for *hetacillin*.

versicolor (ver-sik′o-lor) [L. *vertere* to turn + *color*] exhibiting several shades of the same color.

version (ver-zhun) [L. *versio*] 1. a particular form or variant; specifically, situation of an organ or part in relation to an established normal position. See also ANTEVERSION, EXTRAVERSION, INFRAVERSION, INTRAVERSION, RETROVERSION, and SUPRAVERSION. 2. the act or process of turning something.

vertebra (ver′te-brah), pl. *ver′tebrae* [L.] any of the 33 bones of the vertebral column, comprising the seven cervical, twelve thoracic, five lumbar, five sacral, and four coccygeal vertebrae.

vertebrae (ver′te-bre) [L.] plural of *vertebra*.

vertebral (ver′te-bral) [L. *vertebralis*] of or pertaining to a vertebra.

vertebrate (ver′tĕ-brāt) [L. *vertebratus*] 1. having a vertebral column. 2. any animal having a vertebral column.

vertex (ver′teks), pl. *ver′tices* [L.] 1. a summit or top. 2. v. cran′i. **v. of bony cranium,** the highest point on the skull, generally located on the sagittal suture, usually near the midpoint of the suture. Called also *vertex cranii ossei* [NA]. **v. cra′nii** [NA], the top or crown of the head. **v. cra′nii os′sei** [NA], v. of bony cranium.

vertical (ver'tĭ-kal) 1. perpendicular to the horizontal plane. 2. pertaining to the vertex.

verticalis (ver″tĭ-ka'lis) [L.] vertical. **v. lin'guae,** vertical muscle of tongue; see under MUSCLE.

verticomental (ver″tĭ-ko-men'tal) pertaining to the vertex and the chin.

vertigo (ver'tĭ-go; ver-ti'go) [L.] a sensation of loss of equilibrium associated with dizziness. **auditory v., aural v.,** Ménière's DISEASE. **cervical v.,** Bärtschi-Rochain's SYNDROME. **v. of cervical arthrosis,** Barré-Liéou SYNDROME. **Charcot's v.,** a rare condition in which vertigo or syncope caused by an attack of coughing results in laryngeal spasm or closure of the glottis. Called also *laryngeal v., ictus laryngis,* and *laryngeal syncope.* **laryngeal v.,** 1. Charcot's v. 2. tussive SYNCOPE. **objective v.,** a form in which the patient experiences a sensation that the environment is revolving around him. **recurrent labyrinthine v.,** Ménière's DISEASE. **subjective v.,** a form in which the patient experiences a sensation of revolving in space.

vertigraphy (ver-tig'rah-fe) [L. *vertigo* a whirling + Gr. *graphein* to write] a type of tomography accomplished by moving the x-ray source and film in parallel planes to each other and perpendicular to the film surface. See also TOMOGRAPHY.

vesalian (ve-sa'le-an) named after Andreas *Vesalius,* as vesalian vein (see under VEIN).

Vesalius, emissary vein of, foramen of [Andreas *Vesalius,* Flemish anatomist and physician, 1514–1564; he was an eminent anatomist of the 16th century. His great work on anatomy, *De humani corporis fabrica libri septem* (Seven Books on the Structure of the Human Body), is said to be "one of the most remarkable known to science." Vesalius was first to illustrate that teeth had a definite articulation.] see under VEIN and FORAMEN.

Vesamin trademark for *acetrizoate sodium* (see under ACETRIZOATE).

vesica (vĕ-si'kah), pl. *vesi'cae* [L.] a membranous sac or receptacle for a secretion; used as a general term in anatomical nomenclature. Called also *bladder.* **v. fel'lea** [NA], gallbladder. **v. urina'ria** [NA], urinary BLADDER.

vesicae (ve-si'se) [L.] plural of *vesica.*

vesicant (ves'ĭ-kant) [L. *vesica* blister] 1. causing blisters; blistering. 2. an irritant which acts locally on the skin and mucous membranes to induce blister formation (vesication) by causing plasma to escape from the capillaries to form blisters. Many rubefacients may also exert vesicant effects, when applied in sufficiently high concentrations.

vesication (ves″ĭ-ka'shun) 1. the process of blistering. 2. a blistered spot or surface.

vesicle (ves'ĭ-k'l) [L. *vesicula,* dim. of *vesica* bladder] 1. a small bladder or sac containing fluid. 2. a circumscribed, elevated lesion of the skin up to 5 mm. in diameter which contains fluid, such as one seen in herpes zoster. **blastodermic v.,** blastocyst. **cervical v.,** a temporary sac in the cervical region of the foregut formed by the closing of the cervical sinus. It may persist as a branchial or lateral cervical cyst. **micropinocytosis v., pinocytosis v. pinocytotic v.,** any of the minute fluid-filled vesicles found in the cytoplasm during pinocytosis. They are formed by incuppings or invaginations of the cell membrane, the ends of the impocketed membrane moving progressively closer to each other until they fuse; the vesicles then pinch off to become free. Many cells produce these vesicles, but they are particularly numerous in absorption and lining cells of glands and blood vessels. Their function consists of bringing substances into the cell. Called also *micropinocytosis v.* and *pinosome.* See also PIRANKALYSIS. **synaptic v.,** a minute round vesicle in the terminal portion of the presynaptic neuron, which stores a transmitter substance. See also SYNAPSE.

vesico- [L. *vesica* bladder] a combining form denoting relationship to the bladder, or to a blister.

vesicula (vĕ-sik'u-lah), pl. *vesic'ulae* [L., dim. of *vesica*] a small bladder or sac containing liquid; used as a general term in anatomical nomenclature. Called also *vesicle.*

vesicular (vĕ-sik'u-lar) [L. *vesicula* a little bladder] 1. composed of or relating to small, saclike bodies. 2. pertaining to or made up of vesicles.

vesiculated (vĕ-sik'u-lāt″ed) marked by the presence of vesicles.

vesiculation (ve-sik″u-la'shun) the presence or formation of vesicles or blisters.

vesiculobullous (ve-sik″u-lo-bul'us) having the properties of both a vesicle and a bulla.

Vesiculovirus (ve-sik″u-lo-vi'rus) genus of rhabdoviruses, including only the vesicular stomatitis virus.

vesiculovirus (ve-sik″u-lo-vi'rus) any virus of the genus *Vesiculovirus.*

Vespazine trademark for *fluphenazine.*

Vesprin trademark for *triflupromazine.*

vessel (ves'el) any channel for carrying a fluid, such as the blood or lymph. Called also *vas.* See also terms beginning ANGIO- and VASO-. **absorbent v.,** lymphatic v. **afferent v's of lymph node,** lymphatic vessels that carry lymph to a lymph node, entering through the capsule. Called also *collecting lymphatic vessels* and *vasa afferentia nodi lymphatici* [NA]. **anastomotic v.,** a vessel that serves to interconnect other vessels. Called also *vas anastomoticum* [NA]. **blood v.,** any of the vessels conveying the blood, and comprising the arteries, arterioles, capillaries, venules, and veins. **collateral v.,** 1. one that parallels another vessel, nerve, or other structure. Called also *vas collaterale* [NA]. 2. a vessel important in establishing and maintaining collateral circulation. **collecting lymphatic v's,** lymphatic vessels which drain lymphatic capillary plexuses and enter lymph nodes through the capsules. See *afferent v's of lymph nodes.* **coronary v.,** coronary ARTERY. **efferent v's,** vessels that convey fluid away from a structure or part. Called also *vasa efferentia.* **efferent v's of lymph node,** lymphatic vessels that carry lymph away from a lymph node, emerging at the hilus. Called also *vasa efferentia nodi lymphatici.* **great v's,** the large vessels entering the heart, including the aorta, the pulmonary arteries and veins, and the venae cavae. **lymphatic v.,** any vessel which carries lymph, especially one which is greater than 0.2 mm in diameter and is provided with valves. Similar to blood vessels, lymphatic vessels have walls composed of three coats: an internal coat made of a thin, transparent elastic tissue composed of a layer of endothelial cells supported by an elastic membrane; a middle coat made of circular and tangential layers of smooth muscle and elastic fibers; and an external coat made of collagenous and elastic fibers and smooth muscle bundles arranged longitudinally and obliquely, providing a protective covering for the vessel. The function of the lymphatic vessels consists of collecting lymph from the capillaries and carrying it through the filtering system of lymph nodes to the right lymphatic duct and thoracic duct, from where it is discharged into the venous blood. The lymph is propelled by the contractions of surrounding muscles, which compress the vessels and send the fluid through a system of non-return valves toward the thoracic duct and right lymphatic duct. Called also *lymphatic absorbent v.* and *vas lymphaticum.* **lymphatic v., afferent,** one that conveys the lymph to a lymph node. Called also *afferent lymphatic.* **lymphatic v's, deep,** lymphatic vessels which accompany deep veins and are located beneath the deep fascia, communicating with the superficial vessels by perforating the fascia. Called also *vasa lymphatica profunda* [NA]. **lymphatic v., efferent,** one that conveys the lymph away from a lymph node. Called also *efferent lymphatic.* **lymphatic v's, superficial,** lymphatic vessels which accompany the superficial veins and are located immediately beneath the integument, connecting with the deep lymphatic vessels through the deep fascia. Called also *vasa lymphatica superficialia* [NA]. **lymphatic v's of face,** vessels which convey the lymph from the facial region to the lymph nodes: from the eyelids and conjunctiva into the parotid and mandibular nodes; from the posterior part of the cheek into the parotid nodes; from the anterior portion of the cheek, side of the nose, upper lip, and lateral portion of the lower lip into the submandibular nodes; from the temporal and inframtemporal fossae into the deep facial and superior deep cervical nodes; from deep structures of the cheek and lips into the submandibular nodes; and from the central portion of the lower lip into the submental nodes. **lymphatic v's of mouth,** vessels which convey the lymph from the mouth to the lymph nodes: from the gingivae into the submandibular nodes; from the hard palate into the superior deep cervical and subparotid nodes; from the soft palate into the retropharyngeal, subparotid, and superior deep cervical nodes; from the anterior portion of the floor of the mouth into the superior deep cervical and submental nodes; and from the rest of the floor of the mouth into the submandibular and superior deep cervical nodes. **lymphatic v's of nasal cavity,** vessels which convey the lymph from the nasal cavities to the lymph nodes; vessels from the anterior portion draining into the submandibular nodes and vessels from the posterior portion and accessory air sinuses draining into the retropharyngeal and superior deep cervical nodes. **lymphatic v's of neck,** vessels which drain the cervical structures: from the skin and muscle into the deep cervical nodes; from the upper pharynx into the retropharyngeal nodes; from the lower pharynx into the deep cervical nodes; from the upper larynx into the deep cervical nodes; from the lower larynx into the pretracheal and prelaryngeal nodes; from the upper thyroid gland into the superior deep cervical nodes; and from the lower thyroid gland into the pretracheal and paratracheal nodes. **lymphatic v's of palatine tonsil,** about three to five lymphatic vessels which convey the lymph from the palatine tonsil to the tonsillar lymph nodes. **lymphatic v's of scalp,** vessels which convey the lymph from the scalp to the lymph nodes: from the frontal region into the auricular and parotid vessels; from the temporoparietal region into the parotid and posterior auricular nodes; and from the occipital region into the occipital and deep cervical nodes. **lymphatic v's of tongue,** vessels which convey the lymph from the tongue to the lymph nodes: the apical vessels, from the tip of the tongue into the jugulo-omohyoid and submental nodes; the lateral vessels, from the margin of the tongue into the submandibular and superior deep cervical nodes; the basal vessels, from the region of the vallate papillae into the superior deep cervical nodes, especially the jugulodigastric node; and the median vessels, into the superior deep cervical nodes below the digastric muscle. The most median vessels decussate to the opposite side. **nutrient v.,** a vessel that supplies special tissues, such as the walls of blood vessels. See also *vasa vasorum* [NA].

Vestibest 22 Kt inlay see under INLAY.

vestibula (ves′tib-u-lah) [L.] plural of *vestibulum*.

vestibular (ves-tib′u-lar) pertaining to or toward a vestibule. In dental anatomy, the term is used to refer to the surface of a tooth directed toward the vestibule of the mouth (including the buccal and labial surfaces) and opposite the lingual (or oral) surface. Used synonymously with *facial*. See illustration at SURFACE.

vestibule (ves′tĭ-būl) [L. *vestibulum*] a space or cavity at the entrance to a canal. Called also *vestibulum*. **alar v.,** the anterior enlarged portion of the nasal cavity. **buccal v.,** that portion of the vestibule of the mouth which lies between the cheeks and the teeth and gingivae, or the residual alveolar ridges. **labial v.,** that portion of the vestibule of the mouth which lies between the lips and the teeth and gingivae, or residual alveolar ridges. **v. of larynx,** a wide, triangular portion of the laryngeal cavity above the vestibular folds. Called also *atrium glottidis, atrium of glottis, atrium laryngis, atrium of larynx, vestibulum glottidis,* and *vestibulum laryngis* [NA]. **v. of mouth,** the outer part of the oral cavity, forming a horseshoe, which is bounded on the outside by the cheeks and lips and on the inside by the gingivae and teeth, and is lined with mucous membrane and the labial and buccal surfaces of the teeth. It communicates with the outside of the cavity through the orifice of the mouth and with the cavity proper through the spaces between the teeth and an aperture on either side behind the molar teeth. Called also *cavum oris externum, external oral cavity,* and *vestibulum oris* [NA]. **v. of nose,** a slight dilatation of the nasal cavity just inside the aperture of the nostril, limited posteriorly by the limen nasi, laterally by the wing of the nose and lateral crus of the greater alar cartilage, and medially by the medial crus. It is lined by skin containing vibrissae. Called also *vestibulum nasi* [NA]. **v. of pharynx,** 1. fauces. 2. oropharynx.

vestibuloplasty (ves-tib′u-lo-plas″te) [*vestibule* + Gr. *plassein* to form] the surgical modification of the gingival–mucous membrane relationships in the vestibule of the mouth, including deepening of the vestibular trough, repositioning of the frenum or muscle attachments, and broadening of the zone of attached gingiva, after periodontal treatment. Called also *sulcoplasty* and *vestibular extension*.

vestibulum (ves-tib′u-lum), pl. *vestib′ula* [L.] a vestibule; a space or cavity at the entrance of a canal. **v. glot′tidis, v. laryn′gis** [NA], VESTIBULE of larynx. **v. na′si** [NA], VESTIBULE of nose. **v. o′ris** [NA], VESTIBULE of mouth.

vestige (ves′tij) [L. *vestigium*] the remnant of a structure which functioned in a previous stage of species or individual development. Called also *rudiment* and *vestigium*.

vestigia (ves-tij′e-ah) plural of *vestigium*.

vestigial (ves-tij′e-al) of the nature of a vestige, trace, or relic; rudimentary.

vestigium (ves-tij′e-um), pl. *vestig′ia* [L. "a trace"] the remnant of a structure which functioned in a previous stage of species or individual development; used in anatomical nomenclature to designate the degenerating remains of any structure which served as a functioning entity in the embryo or fetus. Called also *vestige*.

Vetalar trademark for *ketamine hydrochloride* (see under KETAMINE).

Vetame trademark for *triflupromazine*.

Veticillin trademark for *penicillin G sodium* (see under PENICILLIN).

VHN Vickers hardness number; see under HARDNESS.

via (vi′ah), pl. *vi′ae* [L.] a way or passage. **vi′ae natura′les,** the natural passages of the body.

viability (vi″ah-bil′ĭ-te) ability to live after birth.

viae (vi′e) [L.] plural of *via*.

vial (vi′al) [Gr. *phialē*] a small bottle.

Vialidon trademark for *mefenamic acid* (see under ACID).

Vialin trademark for *mephentermine*.

vibex (vi′beks), pl. *vi′bices* [L. *vibix* mark of a blow] a narrow linear streak caused by subcutaneous extravasation of the blood.

vibices (vi′bĭ-sēz) [L.] plural of *vibex*.

Vibradox trademark for *doxycycline hyclate* (see under DOXYCYCLINE).

Vibramycin trademark for *doxycycline*.

vibration (vi-bra′shun) [L. *vibratio*, from *vibrare* to shake] a rapid movement to and fro; oscillation. **v. condensation,** vibration CONDENSATION.

vibrator (vi′bra-tor) a device or machine causing a vibratory motion or action. In dentistry, a device used in pouring casts, in flasking dentures, and duplicating models.

Vibrio (vib′re-o) a genus of gram-negative, facultatively anaerobic bacteria of the family Vibrionaceae, made up of short, asporogenous rods with curved or straight axes. They are found in water and in the gastrointestinal tracts of animals, including man. Some species are pathogenic to man and other vertebrates. **V. alben′sis,** V. *cholerae* (biotype *albensis*). **V. alginolyt′icus,** V. *parahaemolyticus*. **V. bub′ulus,** *Campylobacter sputorum* subsp. *bubulus*; see under CAMPYLOBACTER. **V. chol′erae, V. chol′erae-asiat′icae,** a species that is the etiologic agent of cholera. It is made up of short, slightly curved and twisted rods, about 1.5 to 3.0 μm in length and 0.4 to 0.6 μm in width, occurring singly or in chains having the appearance of short spirals or S-shaped forms (two cells); the straight and spiral threads formed in the pellicle of liquid gelatin cultures are regarded as involution forms. The organisms are motile by a single polar flagellum, are nonsporogeneous, and stain readily with aniline dyes. Cholera vibrios occur in a number of differentiable biotypes: 1a, biotype *cholerae*; 1b, biotype *eltor* (El Tor *vibrio, V. El Tor,* named for El Tor lazaret on the Sinai Peninsula where the organism was first isolated from healthy carriers); 1c, biotype *proteus* (V. *metschnikovii,* V. *nordhafen,* V. *proteus, Microspira protea, Microspora finkleri, Pacinia finkleri,* P. *metschnikovi, Spirillum finkleri*); 1d, biotype *albensis* (V. *albensis,* V. *phosphorescens, Microspira albensis, Microspora dunbari, Photobacterium dunbari, Photospirillum dunbari, Spirillum phosphorescens*). Principal toxins of V. *cholerae* are a heat-stable endotoxin, an enterotoxin, a vascular-permeability factor, and a mucinase. In infection, vibrios are believed to adhere to mucosal surfaces where they multiply and secrete the enterotoxin which causes water and electrolyte loss. Called also V. *comma, Bacillus cholerae,* B. *cholerae-asiaticae, Liquidovibrio cholerae, Pacinia cholerae-asiaticae, Spirillum cholerae,* and S. *cholerae-asiaticae*. **V. com′ma,** V. *cholerae*. **V. El Tor,** V. *cholerae* (biotype *eltor*). **V. fe′tus var. intestina′lis,** *Campylobacter fetus* subsp. *intestinalis*; see under CAMPYLOBACTER. **V. fe′tus, V. fe′tus var. venerea′lis,** *Campylobacter fetus*; see under CAMPYLOBACTER. **V. foe′tus-o′vis,** *Campylobacter fetus* subsp. *intestinalis*; see under CAMPYLOBACTER. **V. hepat′icus, V. jeju′ni,** *Campylobacter fetus* subsp. *jejuni*; see under CAMPYLOBACTER. **V. metschnikovii, V. nordhafen,** V. *cholerae* (biotype *proteus*). **V. parahaemolyt′icus,** a halophilic species found in the marine environment, sea food, and feces of patients with acute enteritis. It is responsible for certain outbreaks of food poisoning. Called also V. *alginolyticus, Beneckea parahaemolytica, Oceanomonas alginolytica, O. enteritidis, Pasteurella parahaemolytica,* and *Pseudomonas enteritis*. **V. phosphores′cens,** V. *cholerae* (biotype *albensis*). **V. pro′teus,** V. *cholerae* (biotype *proteus*). **V. sep′ticus,** *Clostridium septicum*; see under CLOSTRIDIUM. **V. sputo′rum,** *Campylobacter sputorum*; see under CAMPYLOBACTER. **V. sputo′rum var. bub′ulum,** *Campylobacter sputorum* subsp. *bubulus*; see under CAMPYLOBACTER.

vibrio (vib′re-o), pl. *vib′rios* or *vibrio′nes*. Any microorganism of the genus Vibrio. **cholera v.,** *Vibrio cholerae*; see under VIBRIO. **v. El Tor,** *Vibrio cholerae* (biotype *eltor*); see under VIBRIO.

vibriocidal (vib″re-o-si′dal) destructive to organisms of the genus *Vibrio*.

vibrion (ve′bre-on) [Fr.] a vibrio. **v. septique,** *Clostridium septicum*; see under CLOSTRIDIUM.

Vibrionaceae (vib′re-o-na′se-e) [*Vibrio* + *-aceae*] a family of gram-negative facultatively anaerobic, rod-shaped bacteria, including the genera *Aeromonas, Lucibacterium, Photobacterium, Plesiomonas,* and *Vibrio*.

vibriones (vib″re-o′nēz) plural of *vibrio*.

vibriosis (vib″re-o′sis) infection with a microorganism of the genus *Vibrio*.

vibrissa (vi-bris′ah), pl. *vibris′sae* [L.] a long coarse hair, such as those occurring about the muzzle of an animal. See also VIBRISSAE.

vibrissae (vi-bris′e) [L.] plural of *vibrissa*. The hairs growing in the vestibular region of the nasal cavity; they arrest foreign substances carried with inspired air. Called also *hairs of nose*.

vicarious (vi-kar′e-us) [L. *vicarius*] acting in the place of another or of something else; occurring at an abnormal site.

Vicat needle see under NEEDLE.

Viccillin trademark for *ampicillin*.

vice (vīs) [L. *vitium*] 1. a blemish, defect, or imperfection. 2. depravity; immorality.

Vickers hardness indenter point, hardness number, hardness scale, hardness test see under POINT and HARDNESS.

vidian (vid′e-an) named after or described by Guido Guidi (L. *Vidius*) as the vidian artery (see ARTERY of pterygoid canal); vidian canal or canalis pterygoideus Vidii (see pterygoid CANAL); vidian nerve (see NERVE of pterygoid canal); and vidian vein or vena canalis pterygoidei [Vidii] (see VEIN of pterygoid canal).

Vidius see GUIDI.

view (vu) an instance of seeing; sight; vision; a range of sight or vision. **roentgenographic v.**, roentgenographic PROJECTION.

viewbox (vu′boks) a lighted device on which radiographs are viewed.

Vildervanck's syndrome [L. S. *Vildervanck*, Dutch physician] cervico-oculofacial SYNDROME.

Villaret's syndrome [Maurice *Villaret*, French physician, 1877–1946] see under SYNDROME.

Villaumite trademark for a preparation of *sodium fluoride* (see under FLUORIDE).

villi (vil′i) [L.] plural of *villus*.

villus (vi′lus), pl. *vil′li* [L. "tuft of hair"] a small vascular process or protrusion, especially such as a protrusion from the free surface of a membrane; a general anatomical term for such a structure. **lingual villi**, filiform papillae; see under PAPILLA. **synovial villi, vil′li synoviales** [NA], slender projections of the synovial membrane from its free inner surface into the joint cavity. Called also *haversian glands, mucilaginous glands,* and *synovial glands*.

Vimicon trademark for *cyproheptadine hydrochloride* (see under CYPROHEPTADINE).

Vinacort trademark for *polyvinyl chloride* (see under POLYVINYL).

vinblastine (vin-blas′tēn) an antineoplastic alkaloid from the plant *Vinca rosea*. Called also *vincaleukoblastine*. **v. sulfate**, the sulfate salt of vinblastine, $C_{46}H_{60}N_4O_{13}S$, occurring as an odorless, white to yellowish powder that is soluble in water. It is a cytotoxic drug that blocks mitosis with metaphase arrest by disrupting microtubules and preventing spindle formation. Used chiefly in the treatment of Hodgkin's disease and certain types of lymphosarcoma, reticulum-cell sarcoma, mycosis fungoides, leukemia, neuroblastoma, Letterer-Siwe disease, and carcinoma of the oral cavity and other organs. Also used as an immunosuppressive agent. Side reactions may include vomiting, headache, paresthesia, diarrhea, ileus, anorexia, stomatitis, malaise, mental depression, loss of deep tendon reflexes, alopecia, and bone marrow depression with thrombocytopenia, leukopenia, and predisposition to infection. Blindness and death sometimes occur. The drug is suspected of being potentially teratogenic. Called also sulfate *vincaleukoblastine*. Trademarks: Exal, Velban, Velbe.

Vinca (vin′kah) a genus of apocynaceous woody herbs, including *V. minor* (common, or lesser, periwinkle) and *V. rosea* (Madagascar periwinkle); the latter contains many cytotoxic alkaloids, including vinblastine and vincristine.

vincaleukoblastine (vin″kah-loo″ko-blas′tēn) vinblastine. **v. sulfate**, VINBLASTINE sulfate.

Vincent's angina, infection, organism, stomatitis, tonsillitis [Henri *Vincent*, French physician, 1862–1950] see under ANGINA and TONSILLITIS, and see acute necrotizing GINGIVITIS, *Fusobacterium plauti* (under FUSOBACTERIUM), and *Borrelia vincenti* (under BORRELIA).

vincristine (vin-kris′tēn) an antineoplastic alkaloid from *Vinca rosea*. Trademark: Leurocristine. **v. sulfate**, the sulfate salt of vincristine, $C_{46}H_{58}N_4O_{14}S$, occurring as an odorless, hygroscopic, white to yellowish powder that is soluble in water. It is a cytotoxic drug that blocks mitosis with metaphase arrest by disrupting microtubules and preventing spindle formation. Used as an antineoplastic agent in Hodgkin's disease and other lymphomas, lymphocytic leukemia, neuroblastoma, Wilms' tumor, rhabdomyosarcoma, and other tumors. Leukopenia is a common side reaction, but bone marrow depression is infrequent. Other complications of therapy may include paresthesia, loss of deep-tendon reflexes, pain, muscle weakness, footdrop, hoarseness, headache, ptosis, double vision, alopecia, fever, polyuria, dysuria, anemia, hyponatremia, and high urinary sodium. Trademark: Oncovin.

vinegar (vin′ĕ-gar) [Fr. *vinaigre* sour wine] a weak solution of acetic acid; especially a sour liquid consisting chiefly of acetic acid, formed by the fermentation of cider, wine, etc., or by the distillation of wood. See acetic ACID.

Vinisil trademark for *povidone*.

Vinson, Porter Paisley [American surgeon, 1890–1959] see Plummer-Vinson SYNDROME.

vinyl (vi′nil) the univalent group $CH_2{:}CH-$. **v. acetate**, a vinyl group to which the monovalent radical CH_3COO- is attached. It is a colorless liquid, stabilized with either hydroquinone or diphenylamine inhibitors. In the presence of a catalyst, vinyl acetate polymerizes to produce polyvinyl acetate, a plastic substance that is stable to light and heat but has a low softening point. On polymerization with vinyl chloride, it forms vinyl chloride–vinyl acetate copolymer; used in producing denture bases and maxillofacial prostheses. Called also *acetic acid ethynyl ester* and *acetic acid vinyl ester*. **v. acetate–v. chloride copolymer**, v. chloride–v. acetate copolymer. **v. chloride**, a vinyl group to which an atom of chlorine is attached, CH_3CHCl. It is a colorless gas which liquefies in a freezing mixture, used in manufacturing plastics and as a refrigerant. In gaseus form, it is suspected of being carcinogenic and causing other disease. When vinyl chloride is spilled on the skin rapid evaporation may cause frostbite. In high concentrations, it may be narcotic. Because of potentially harmful effects, government regulations specify allowable concentrations of vinyl chloride in the air. In the presence of a catalyst, vinyl chloride polymerizes to produce polyvinyl chloride, a hard, tasteless, odorless resin, which darkens when exposed to ultraviolet rays and heat. It is used for producing denture bases and maxillofacial prostheses. On polymerization with vinyl acetate, it forms vinyl chloride–vinyl acetate copolymer. Called also *chloroethene* and *chloroethylene*. **v. chloride–v. acetate copolymer**, a copolymer resin of vinyl chloride (80–95 percent) and vinyl acetate (5–80 percent) forming a plastic material which becomes flexible on exposure to sunlight and aging. It is used for the fabrication of denture bases and maxillofacial prostheses. Called also *v. acetate–v. chloride copolymer*. **v. cyanide**, acrylonitrile. **polymerized v.**, polyvinyl. **v. resins**, resins produced by the polymerization of ethylene monomers; see *v. acetate* and *v. chloride*.

vinylidene chloride (vī-nil′ĭ-dēn-klo′rid) a compound, 1,1-dichloroethylene, occurring as a flammable, oily colorless liquid, which may be copolymerized with vinyl chloride or acrylonitrile to form polymer plastics, such as Saran. It is a toxic substance that may cause lesions of the skin and mucous membranes and is narcotic in high concentrations.

violet (vi′o-let) 1. the hue seen in the most refracted end of the spectrum. 2. a violet-colored dye. **crystal v.**, gentian v. **gentian v.**, a dye, hexamethylpararosaniline chloride, usually admixed with penta- or tetramethyl-pararosanilide chloride, occurring as a green powder or greenish, glistening pieces with metallic luster that are soluble in water and chloroform. It is bacteriostatic and bactericidal to gram-positive bacteria and to many fungi, and as an anthelmintic preparation. It has been used topically in the treatment of various infections, including superficial pyogenic infections, impetigo, irritative skin lesions, and acute necrotizing ulcerative gingivitis, and as an internal anthelmintic. Tattooing and granulation tissue may result from contact with gentian violet. Called also *crystal v., methyl v.,* and *methylrosaniline chloride*. **methyl v.**, gentian v.

viosterol (vi-os′ter-ol) vitamin D_2.

Virchow's angle, law, line [Rudolf Ludwig Karl *Virchow*, German pathologist, 1821–1902] see under ANGLE, LAW, and LINE.

virilization (vir″ĭ-li-za′shun) [L. *virilitas*, from *vir* man] the development of male secondary sex characters, especially in the female.

virion (vi′ri-on) the complete, mature infectious virus particle, with or without an envelope. **defective v's, satellite v's**, satellite viruses; see under VIRUS.

viroid (vi′roid) [*virus* + Gr. *eidos* form] 1. an infraviral agent of infectious diseases, differing from viruses by the absence of a virion and by genomes that are much smaller than those in viruses. Originally, the term was used to describe infectious nucleic acids; presently, it is used to designate a particle of low molecular weight RNA (about 75,000 to 130,000). Introduction of viroid into susceptible hosts leads to autonomous replication of the RNA and, sometimes, disease. Established as a pathogenic agent of diseases in plants, viroids are also suspected of being pathogenic in vertebrates, including man. 2. any biological specific used in immunization (obsolete). 3. a hypothetical, ultramicroscopic organism that is a useful symbiont, occurring universally within cells or larger organisms, and being capable, by mutation, of giving rise to viruses (obsolete).

virucide (vir'u-sīd) an agent capable of destroying viruses.

virus (vi'rus) [L.] any of a group of minute infectious agents. Originally, viruses were set apart by their ability to pass through bacteriological filters, hence the term *filterable virus;* more recently, they were recognized as obligate intracellular parasites (15 to 300 nm in size), considered to be living organisms or borderline entities between living and nonliving, which lack the capacity of independent metabolism and replicate only within living host cells, being able to reproduce with genetic continuity and to mutate. The body of a virus (virion) consists of a single type of nucleic acid, either DNA or RNA, surrounded by a protein coat (capsid), which assumes the form of either a helix or icosahedron; the complex of the nucleic acid and the protein is called the *nucleocapsid.* The capsid is made up of subunits (capsomers), which are composed of multiple polypeptide chains. Subunits formed from a single polypeptide chain are termed *structural units.* Structural units are used to build the helical capsids and capsomers to build the icosahedral capsids. The virion is made up of the nucleocapsid alone or it may be surrounded by an envelope, or limiting membrane, which has spike proteins on the outer surface. Viruses may be grouped into five categories, based on their morphology and nucleocapsid symmetry: naked and enveloped icosahedral viruses, naked and enveloped helical viruses, and complex viruses. Or they may be classified according to their nucleic acid content as DNA viruses and RNA viruses. They may be separated into three subgroups on the basis of host specificity, namely, bacterial viruses, animal viruses, and plant viruses. Viruses may be also classified as to their origin (e.g., reoviruses), mode of transmission (arboviruses, tickborne viruses), or the manifestations they produce (polioviruses, polyoma viruses, poxviruses). Sometimes, they are named for the geographical location in which they were first isolated (e.g., coxsackieviruses). See illustration. **v. 2060,** common cold v. **acute laryngotracheobronchitis (ALTB) v.,** parainfluenza v. type 2; see *parainfluenza v's.* **adenoassociated v's,** a group of parvoviruses, comprising satellite or defective viruses that can replicate in those cells which are concomitantly infected with adenoviruses. The viruses in the group have been isolated from various animals; two types (AAV-2 and AAV-3) have been found in man. Abbreviated *AAV.* **adeno-v.,** adenovirus. **alastrim v.,** variola v. **ALTB (acute laryngotracheobronchitis) v.,** parainfluenza v. type 2; see *parainfluenza v's.* **Amaas v.,** variola v. **Amapari v.,** one of the American hemorrhagic fever viruses isolated in Brazil. **American hemorrhagic fever v's,** a group of arenaviruses, associated with human hemorrhagic fever. The group includes Junin, Tacaribe, Machupo, Amapari, Tamiami, Pi-

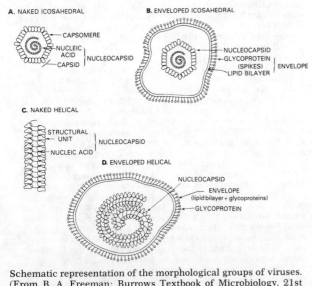

Schematic representation of the morphological groups of viruses. (From B. A. Freeman: Burrows Textbook of Microbiology. 21st ed. Philadelphia, W. B. Saunders Co., 1979.)

chinde, Parana, and Latino viruses. **animal v's,** viruses which parasitize and propagate in animal cells. They have been subdivided into families and genera based on the following criteria: (1) type of nucleic acid in the virion, (2) capsid symmetry, (3) presence or absence of an envelope, (4) sites of capsid assembly and development, (5) size and shape of the virion, and (6) number of capsomers for the icosahedral viruses or diameter of the helix for the helical viruses. Using these criteria, 16 families have been recognized: Adenoviridae, Arenaviridae, Bunyaviridae, Coronaviridae, Herpetoviridae, Iridoviridae, Orthomyxoviridae, Papovaviridae, Paramyxoviridae, Parvoviridae, Picornaviridae, Poxviridae, Reoviridae, Retroviridae, Rhabdoviridae, and Togaviridae. **Apeu v.,** an arbovirus of the C group of the Bunyamwera supergroup of viruses, isolated in Brazil from man, mosquitoes, rodents, and marmosets; suspected of causing febrile diseases in man. **arbor v., arthropodborne v.,** arbovirus. **B v.,** a herpesvirus reported to have caused fatal diseases involving the central nervous system in laboratory personnel dealing with monkeys. **bacterial v.,** bacteriophage. **biundulant meningoencephalitis v.,** tick-borne encephalitis v. (central European subtype). **BK v.,** a polyoma virus believed to occur in man in a latent form. The virus was originally isolated from the urine of a renal transplant patient. It is suspected of being associated with carcinoma of the bladder and possibly other tumors. **bluetongue v.,** a reovirus of the genus *Orbivirus* transmitted by biting flies, which causes hyperemia and edema of the lips, tongue, and oral mucosa of sheep and sometimes cattle. It was first isolated in the southern and eastern parts of Africa, but has now spread to other areas. Called also *ovine catarrhal v.* and *sore mouth v.* **bovine papular stomatitis v.,** a poxvirus of the genus *Parapoxvirus,* producing oral lesions in cattle which resemble those of foot-and-break-mouth disease. **breakbone fever v.,** dengue v. **Bunyamwera v.,** an arbovirus of the Bunyamwera supergroup of viruses. **Bunyamwera group of v's,** a group of arboviruses of the Bunyamwera supergroup of viruses, comprising Bunyamwera, Calovo, Germiston, Guaroa, Ilesha, Tensaw, and Wyeomyia viruses. **Bunyamwera supergroup of v's,** a group of arboviruses of the genus *Bunyavirus,* comprising 10 groups, with the Bunyamwera, Bwamba, C, and California groups being the major ones affecting man. It includes 87 members, 80 of which are in 10 serological groups and seven are unassigned. **Bwamba v.,** an arbovirus of the Bwamba group, Bunyamwera supergroup of viruses, isolated in Africa from mosquitoes and from man in association with febrile illness. **Bwamba group of v's,** a group of arboviruses of the Bunyamwera supergroup of viruses, comprising the Bwamba and Pongola viruses. **C. group of v's,** a group of arboviruses of the Bunyamwera supergroup of viruses, comprising Apeu, Caraparu, Gumbo Limbo, Itaqui, Madrid, Marituba, Murutucu, Nepuyo, Oriboca, Ossa, and Restan. **CA (croup-associated) v.,** parainfluenza v. type 2; see *parainfluenza v's.* **California encephalitis v.,** an arbovirus of the California group Bunyamwera supergroup of viruses, isolated in the United States from man in association with encephalitis. **California group of v's,** a group of arboviruses of the Bunyamwera supergroup of viruses, comprising the California encephalitis, Inkoo, La Crosse, Tahyňa, and Trivittatus viruses. **Calovo v.,** an arbovirus of the Bunyamwera group of viruses, isolated in Central Europe from mosquitoes, and causing febrile diseases in man. **canine oral papillomatosis v.,** a papovavirus of the genus *Papillomavirus,* which causes in young dogs cauliflower-like warts of the lips, spreading to the oral cavity and pharynx. **Caraparu v.,** an arbovirus of the C group, Bunyamwera supergroup of viruses, isolated in Brazil, Guyana, Panama, and Trinidad from man, mosquitoes, rodents, and marmosets; suspected of causing human febrile diseases. **catarrhal jaundice v.,** hepatitis A v. **CELO v.** [chicken-embryonal-*l*ethal *o*rphan + virus], an adenovirus of the genus *Aviandenovirus,* having DNA molecules larger than those of mammalian adenoviruses and a molecular weight of 29 million dl. It is lethal for chicken embryos and induces tumors in newborn and weanling hamsters. **Chagres v.,** an arbovirus of the Phlebotomus fever group, tentatively classified as a bunyavirus, believed to be involved in human febrile disease. **chicken-embryonal-lethal v.** CELO v. **chikungunya v.,** a togavirus of the genus *Alphavirus,* which was formerly classified as a group A arbovirus. It is a mosquito-borne virus originally isolated in Tanzania, which causes chikungunya, an epidemic dengue-like disease. **Colorado tick fever v.,** a reovirus of the genus *Orbivirus,* transmitted by the tick *Dermacentor andersoni,* causing Colorado tick fever. **common cold v.,** a picornavirus of the genus *Rhinovirus,* which causes the common cold in man. It is a small virus about 20–30 nm in diameter, having single-stranded RNA in a continuous segment with a high content of adenylic acid, the RNA being infective. Eighty-nine serotypes are recognized. The common cold virus includes echovirus 28 (virus 2060, JH virus). Called also *coryza v.* or *coryzavirus.* **common wart v.,** human warts v. **complex v's,** a group of viruses with a DNA genome, having virions and envelopes with complex structures, and ranging in diameter from 250 to 300 nm. The viruses in the family Poxviridae and some bacteriophages are included in this group. **condyloma v.,** human warts v. **contagious ecthyma of sheep v., contagious pustular dermatitis of sheep v., contagious pustular stomatitis v.,** orf v. **coryza v.,** common cold v. **cowpox v.,** a poxvirus of the genus *Orthopoxvirus,* which infects the skin, especially of the udders of cows, and may cause lesions of the hands and, sometimes, the arms, face, and eyes of milkers. **Crimean-Congo hemorrhagic fever group of v's,** a group of arboviruses, tentatively classified as bunyaviruses, which are believed to be transmitted by ticks and cause disease in sheep, goats, cattle, and other animals, including man, characterized by severe hemorrhagic manifestations. **croup-associated (CA) v.,** parainfluenza v. type 2; see *parainfluenza v's.* **Coxsackie v., coxsackie v.,** coxsackievirus. **cubic v.,** icosahedral v. **Dandy fever v.,** dengue v. **defective v's, satellite v. dengue v.,** a togavirus that is the type species of the genus *Flavivirus,* formerly classified as a group B arbovirus. Serologic types 1, 2, 3, and 4 are recognized. It is a mosquito-borne virus, which causes dengue. Some strains have been isolated from patients with epidemic hemorrhagic fever. Called also *breakbone fever v.* and *Dandy fever v.* **diphasic milk fever v.,** tickborne encephalitis v. (central European subtype). **DNA v's,** a group of viruses having a DNA genome, consisting of the families *Adenoviridae, Herpetoviridae, Iridoviridae, Parvoviridae,* and *Poxviridae,* ·and several unclassified viruses, including the hepatitis, gastroenteritis, Aleutian disease, Kuru, and spongiform encephalopathy viruses. **Duvenhage v.,** a rhabdovirus of the genus *Lyssavirus,* isolated from a case of human rabies. **eastern equine encephalomyelitis (EEE) v.,** a togavirus of the genus *Alphavirus,* formerly classified as a group A arbovirus. A nonvirulent parasite in several wild animals, the virus is pathogenic to man, horses, and mules, causing encephalomyelitis. The mortality rate in infected equines is about 90 percent. In humans, the mortality rate varies from outbreak to outbreak, being as high as 75 percent. The virus is mosquito-borne and occurs in the eastern United States and Canada, the Caribbean part of Central America, and eastern parts of South America. **EB v., Ebb v.,** Epstein-Barr v. **Ebola v.,** a rhabdovirus isolated in epidemics of human hemorrhage disease in Africa. **ECHO v.,** echovirus. **EEE v.,** eastern equine encephalomyelitis v. **enteric v., enterovirus. enveloped v.,** a virus with a membrane which consists of a lipid bilayer with spike proteins on the outer surface. **enveloped helical v's,** a group of viruses with an RNA genome, whose virions are made up of flexible helical nucleocapsids surrounded by envelopes, or limiting membranes. The virions may appear as rods or spheres and are thus considered pleomorphic. The group may be divided into viruses developing in intracytoplasmic membranes and those developing in surface membranes. Virions of viruses from surface membranes range in diameter from 80 to 300 nm and have helical diameters of between 6 and 18; they include the families Orthomyxoviridae, Paramyxoviridae, and Rhabdoviridae. Virions of viruses from intracytoplasmic membranes range in diameter from 80 to 130 nm and have helical diameters of between 2 and 3; they include the families Coronaviridae and Bunyaviridae. See illustration. **enveloped icosahedral v's,** a group of viruses whose virions consist of icosahedral nucleocapsids surrounded by envelopes, or limiting membranes. Viruses with a DNA genome range in diameter from 100 to 200 nm and their number of capsomers vary from 162 to 1500; this group comprises the families Iridoviridae and Herpetoviridae. Viruses with an RNA genome range in diameter from 40 to 60 nm and their number of capsomers varies from 32 to 42, some genera having an unknown number of capsomers; this group consists of a single family, Togaviridae. See illustration. **epidemic jaundice v.,** hepatitis A v. **epidemic parotitis v.,** mumps v. **Epstein-Barr v.,** a herpesvirus causing infectious mononucleosis, and associated with Burkitt lymphoma and nasopharyngeal carcinoma. Called also *Burkitt lymphoma v., EB v.,* and *Ebb v.* **equine encephalitis v.,** see *eastern equine encephalomyelitis v., Venezuelan equine encephalomyelitis v.,* and *western equine encephalomyelitis v.* **equine papillomatosis v.,** a papovavirus of the genus

Papillomavirus, which causes warts of the nose and lips in horses. **Far East Russian encephalitis v.,** tickborne encephalitis v. (eastern subtype). **filterable v., filtrable v.,** a virus capable of passing through fine filters of diatomite or unglazed porcelain, or through filters capable of retaining most bacteria. Called also *ultravirus.* **fowl plague v.,** the avian subtype of the influenza A virus; see INFLUENZAVIRUS type A. **foamy v.,** Spumavirinae. German measles v., rubella v. **Germiston v.,** an arbovirus of the Bunyamwera group of viruses, isolated in Africa from mosquitoes and rodents; suspected of causing febrile diseases in man. **Guaroa v.,** an arbovirus of the Bunyamwera group of viruses, isolated in Brazil and Central America from man and mosquitoes; suspected of causing febrile diseases in man. **guinea pig salivary gland v.,** guinea pig CYTOMEGALOVIRUS. **Gumbo Limbo v.,** an arbovirus of the C group, Bunyamwera supergroup of viruses, isolated in Florida from mosquitoes and cotton rats. **HA1 v.,** parainfluenza v. type 3; see parainfluenza v's **HA2 v.,** parainfluenza v. type 1; see *parainfluenza v's.* **hand, foot, and mouth disease v.,** a picornavirus which causes hand, foot, and mouth disease. It is variously classified as a coxsackievirus and in a tentative genus *Aphthovirus.* **Heine-Medin disease v.,** poliovirus. **helical v.,** a virus characterized by helical arrangement of the structural units of the capsid. See *enveloped helical v's* and *naked helical v's.* **hemadsorption v. 1 (HA1),** parainfluenza v. type 3; see *parainfluenza v's.* **hemadsorption v. 2 (HA2),** parainfluenza v. type 1; see *parainfluenza v's.* **hemagglutinating v. of. Japan (HVJ),** parainfluenza v. type 1; see *parainfluenza v's.* **hepatitis A v.,** an unclassified virus that causes infectious hepatitis in man. It is a small, nonenveloped virus with an RNA genome, about 27 nm in diameter, and believed to have icosahedral symmetry. Recent information indicates that hepatitis A virus will probably be classified as an enterovirus. Called also *catarrhal jaundice v., epidemic jaundice v.,* and *infective hepatitis v.* **hepatitis B v.,** a virus causing homologous serum jaundice and most frequently transmitted by transfusion of contaminated blood or injections with contaminated unsterilized needles. Recent evidence indicates a low-grade transmission by other nonparenteral routes. Viral particles are spheres 20 nm in diameter, filaments 20 nm wide and of variable length, and Dane particles 40 to 42 nm in diameter (probably the infective virion) with 27-nm cores. The core contains circular double-stranded DNA. The surface coat (which is not an envelope) is 7 nm thick; Australia antigen is associated with the coat. Called also *homologous serum jaundice v., serum hepatitis v.,* and *transfusion hepatitis v.* **hepatoencephalomyelitis v.,** Orthoreovirus. **herpangina v.,** a coxsackievirus, usually of the A group, causing herpangina. **herpes v.,** herpesvirus. **herpes simplex v. type 1,** a herpesvirus that is the most common cause of herpetic infection of the nongenital (labial) type. Viruses may be found in the saliva, conjunctiva, and salivary and lacrimal glands of normal carriers or in persons recovering from infection; exposure to cold or ultraviolet rays, menstruation, emotional stress, or nerve injury may cause the viruses to become active. Members of this group may be associated with cervical cancer. Called also *Herpesvirus hominis type 1* and *human herpesvirus type 1.* **herpes simplex v. type 2,** a herpesvirus that is the most common cause of herpetic infection of the genitals. It is also believed to be associated with cervical cancer. This type can cause a highly fatal infection in the neonate, which is due to contamination during the birth process; the mother may or may not manifest genital lesions. Called also *Herpesvirus hominis type 2* and *human herpesvirus type 2.* **homologous serum jaundice v.,** hepatitis B v. **human warts v.,** a papovavirus of the genus *Papillomavirus,* which produces human warts of the skin. Called also *common wart v., condyloma v., myrmecia v., papilloma v.,* and *verruca vulgaris v.* **HVJ v.,** parainfluenza v. type 1; see *parainfluenza v's.* **hydrophobia v.,** rabies v. **icosahedral v.,** a virus characterized by the arrangement of the structural units of the capsid in the form of an icosahedron. Called also *cubic v.* See *enveloped icosahedral v's* and *naked icosahedral v's.* **Ilesha v.,** an arbovirus of the Bunyamwera group of viruses, isolated in Africa from man and mosquitoes; suspected of causing skin rash and febrile diseases in man. **Ilheus v.,** a togavirus of the genus *Flavivirus,* formerly classified as a group B arbovirus, isolated from mosquitoes and birds in Brazil and Panama. Infection in man may be inapparent, but some cases are associated with encephalitis. **infectious bovine rhinotracheitis v.,** a herpesvirus. **infectious labial dermatitis v.,** orf v. **infective hepatitis v.,** hepatitis A v. **influenza v.** influenzavirus. **Inkoo v.,** an arbovirus of the California group, supergroup of viruses, isolated in Finland from mosquitoes, and from man in association with febrile illness. **iridescent v.,** Iridovirus. **Itaqui v.,** an arbovirus of the C group, Bunyamwera supergroup of viruses, isolated in Brazil from mosquitoes, rodents and marsupials, and from man in association with febrile illness. **Japanese B v., Japanese B encephalitis v.,** a togavirus of the genus *Flavivirus*, formerly classified as a group B arbovirus. The virus is parasitic in birds, and is transmitted by culicine mosquitoes to infect man, especially children. The infection, in most instances, is inapparent, but some cases are complicated by encephalitis, usually associated with paresis. It occurs in Japan and other areas, particularly all over Southeast Asia. Called also *Russian autumn encephalitis v.* **JC v.,** a papovavirus of the genus *Polyomavirus*, suspected of being associated with certain human neoplasms and subacute sclerosing panencephalitis. **JH v.,** common cold v. **Junin v.,** one of the American hemorrhagic fever viruses isolated in Argentina. **JVI v.,** echovirus 20. **Kemerovo v.,** a tickborne reovirus of the genus *Orbivirus*, causing a benign febrile disease in man in Siberia. The term pertains to the specific strain, as well as to a group of viruses, which includes the Kemerovo virus and a large group of antigenically related tickborne viruses isolated in Eastern Europe, Egypt, Sudan, Malaya, Newfoundland, Oregon, California, and Peru. Some strains are believed to also infect horses, cattle, birds, and small mammals. **Kontonkan v.,** a rhabdovirus of the genus *Lyssavirus*, isolated in Nigeria, which may infect humans and domestic animals, and may cause illness in cattle. **Kumba v.,** Semliki Forest v. **kuru v.,** an unclassified virus which causes disease of the central nervous system in the Fore people in Papua, New Guinea. **Kyasanur Forest disease v.,** a togavirus of the genus *Flavivirus*, formerly classified as a group B arbovirus. It is a tickborne virus originally isolated in the Kyasanur Forest in India, and causing a highly fatal infection in man. **La Crosse v.,** an arbovirus of the California group of the Bunyamwera supergroup of viruses, isolated in the United States from mosquitoes, and from man in association with encephalitis. **Lassa fever v.,** an arenavirus that is widespread in West Africa. It is pathogenic to man, the infection being sometimes asymptomatic, but, usually, presenting symptoms similar to those seen in typhoid fever. The multimammate mouse is believed to serve as the reservoir, with human infection occurring as the result of contact with infected rodents, exposure to contaminated dust or urine, or person-to-person contact. **Latino v.,** one of the American hemorrhagic fever viruses isolated in Bolivia. **looping ill v.,** a togavirus of the genus *Flavivirus*, which was formerly classified as a group B arbovirus. It is a tickborne virus, causing a fatal encephalitis in sheep and, less commonly, in cattle, pigs, and horses, which is transmissible to man. Called also *ovine encephalomyelitis v.* **lymphocytic choriomeningitis (LCM) v.,** an arenavirus causing infection in mice, also isolated from man, monkeys, dogs, hamsters, and guinea pigs. In man, infection may be inapparent or present influenza-like symptoms, sometimes associated with meningitis or meningoencephalitis. **lyssa v.,** rabies v. **Machupo v.,** one of the American hemorrhagic fever viruses isolated in Bolivia. **Madrid v.,** an arbovirus of the C group, Bunyamwera supergroup of viruses, isolated in Panama from mosquitoes and rodents, and from man in association with febrile illness. **Maedi v.,** Lentivirinae. **mammary tumor v. (MTV) of mice,** a retrovirus of the subfamily *Oncovirinae*, type B, which is usually latent, but it causes mammary cancers in genetically susceptible strains of mice under appropriate hormonal conditions. Particles resembling those of this virus have been demonstrated in the milk of women with and without cancer, suggesting that they may be associated with breast cancer in humans. Called also *Bittner agent* and *milk factor.* **Marburg v.,** a rhabdovirus occurring as rods 90 to 100 nm in diameter and 130 to 2600 nm in length, with an apparently helical symmetry. It was isolated from infected laboratory personnel who had handled laboratory monkeys. Infection in man has a relatively high mortality rate. Called also *Marburg agent.* **Marituba v.,** an arbovirus of the C group, Bunyamwera supergroup of viruses, isolated in Brazil from mosquitoes and marsupials, and from man in association with febrile illness. **Mayaro v.,** a togavirus of the genus *Alphavirus*, formerly classified as a group A arbovirus, originally isolated in Mayaro county, Trinidad, and in the region of the Gauma River in Brazil. It causes a febrile disease with severe headache. **measles v.,** a paramyxovirus of the genus *Morbillivirus*, causing measles. Called also *morbilli v.* and *rubeola v.* **Middleburg v.,** a togavirus of the genus *Alphavirus*, formerly classified as a group A arbovirus. It is mosquito-borne, and was originally isolated in the Cape provinces in South Africa. **milker's node v.,** paravaccinia v. **molluscum contagiosum v.,** an unclassified poxvirus, occurring as viral particles with nucleoids about 50 to 100 nm in diameter; eccentric nucleoids with single or double membranes surround the particle. The virus parasitizes only human hosts and causes lesions that are confined to the skin. **morbilli v.,** measles v. **mosquito-borne v.,** one transmitted by mosquito bites. See ARBOVIRUS. **mumps v.,** a virus of the genus *Paramyxovirus*, causing mumps. It is transmitted chiefly with the saliva. Called also *epidemic parotitis v.* and *oreillons v.* **Murray Valley encephalitis v.,** a togavirus of the genus *Flavivirus*, formerly classified as a group B arbovirus, believed to be parasitic in birds. It causes encephalitis in man, particularly in children, which resembles Japanese B virus infection. Epidemics occur primarily in Papua, New Guinea, and in northern Australia. **Murutucu v.,** an arbovirus of the C group, Bunyamwera supergroup of viruses, isolated in Brazil from mosquitoes, marmosets, and marsupials, and in man in association with febrile illness. **myrmecia v.,** human warts v. **naked v.,** one not having an envelope, or limiting membrane, surrounding the nucleocapsid. **naked helical v's,** a group of viruses composed of rigid helical nucleocapsids, appearing as long rods, and consisting of an RNA genome intertwined with protein structural units to form a helix. Plant viruses are generally found in this group. See illustration. **naked icosahedral v's,** a group of viruses whose virions consist of icosahedral nucleocapsids, lacking envelopes, or limiting membranes. Viruses with a DNA genome range in diameter from 18 to 90 nm and their number of capsomers varies from 32 to 252; they include the families Parvoviridae, Papovaviridae, and Adenoviridae. Viruses with an RNA genome range in diameter from 20 to 70 nm and their number of capsomers ranges from 32 to 92; they include the families Picornaviridae and Reoviridae. An unaffiliated genus, *Calicivirus*, is also included in this group. See illustration. **Negishi v.,** a tickborne togavirus of the genus *Flavivirus*, formerly classified as a group B arbovirus, which causes encephalitis in Japan. **Nepuyo v.,** an arbovirus of the group C group, Bunyamwera supergroup of viruses, isolated in Brazil and Central America from mosquitoes, rodents, and bats. **newborn pneumonitis v.,** parainfluenza v. type 1; see *parainfluenza v's.* **Omsk hemorrhagic fever v.,** a togavirus of the genus *Flavivirus*, formerly classified as a group B arbovirus. It is a tickborne virus endemic to central USSR, which causes a diphasic hemorrhagic illness in man. **oncogenic v.,** one capable of producing a neoplasm. **oncologic v.,** Oncovirinae. **O'nyong-nyong v.,** a togavirus of the genus *Alphavirus*, formerly classified as a group A arbovirus; it is transmitted by mosquitoes and causes an epidemic dengue-like disease in central and east Africa. **oral papillomatosis v. of rabbit,** a papovavirus of the genus *Papillomavirus*, which produces papillomas of the oral cavity of rabbits. Originally isolated from rabbits in New York, the virus has been found also in Scotland. **oreillons v.,** mumps v. **orf v.,** a poxvirus of the genus *Parapoxvirus*, which causes a highly infectious and sometimes fatal exanthematous disease in lambs and kids and, occasionally, in adult animals. Human lesions of the hands and face may occur as the result of infection. Called also *contagious ecthyma of sheep v., contagious pustular dermatitis of sheep v., contagious pustular stomatitis v., infectious labial dermatitis v., scabby mouth v.,* and *sore mouth v.* **Oriboca v.,** an arbovirus of the C group, Bunyamwera supergroup of viruses, isolated in Brazil, Trinidad, and Guyana from mosquitoes, rodents, and marsupials, and in man in association with febrile illness. **orphan v.,** a virus which has been isolated in tissue culture, but has not been found specifically associated with any illness, such as the echovirus. **Ossa v.,** an arbovirus of the C group, Bunyamwera supergroup of viruses, isolated in Panama from mosquitoes and rodents, and from man in association with febrile illness. **ovine catarrhal v.,** bluetongue v. **ovine encephalomyelitis v.,** looping ill v. **papilloma v.,** 1. papillomavirus. 2. human warts v. **pappataci fever v.,** sandfly fever v. **parainfluenza v's,** a group of paramyxoviruses that cause a large proportion of acute respiratory infections in humans. The group includes four antigenic types. *Type 1:* According to some authorities, this type comprises several subtypes: hemadsorption virus 2 (HA2), Sendai virus, newborn pneumonitis virus, and hemagglutinating virus of Japan (HVJ). The HA2 strain has been isolated only from man, causing acute laryngotracheitis in children and pneumonia in adults. The Sendai strain causes infection in mice and swine. The subtypes are considered by some to be synonymous with parainfluenza virus type 1. *Type 2:* a type associated with croup (acute laryngotracheitis) in infants and young children and with mild upper respiratory disorders in adults. Several strains of simian viruses are sometimes classified as this type. Called also *acute laryngotracheobronchitis (ALTB) v.* and *croup-associated (CA) v. Type 3:* a type associated with pharyngitis, bronchiolitis, and pneumonia in young children. This type has also been isolated from cattle with shipping fever. Called also *hemadsorption v. 1* and *shipping fever v. Type 4:* a type believed to be associated with human respiratory disorders. **Parana v.**, one of the American hemorrhagic fever viruses isolated in Paraguay. **paravaccinia v.**, a poxvirus of the genus *Parapoxvirus*, causing poxlike lesions in man and cattle (usually of the udders). Called also *milker's node v.* and *v. of pseudocowpox.* **Phlebotomus fever v.**, sandfly fever v. **phlebotomus fever group of v's**, a group of arboviruses tentatively classified as a bunyavirus, consisting of 22 viruses, three of which are associated with human disease (sandly fever, Chagres, and Punta Toros viruses). **Pichinde v.**, one of the American hemorrhagic fever viruses isolated in Colombia. **polio v.**, poliomyelitis v., poliovirus. **polyoma v.**, Polyomavirus. **Pongola v.**, a bunyavirus of the Bwamba group of viruses, isolated from mosquitoes in Africa. **pox v.**, poxvirus. **progressive interstitial pneumonia v., progressive pneumonia v.**, Lentivirinae. **v. of pseudocowpox**, paravaccinia v. **pseudorabies v.**, a herpesvirus that causes pseudorabies and may be transmitted by minor trauma of the skin or oral mucosa. **Punta Toros v.**, an arbovirus of the Phlebotomus fever group of viruses, believed to be involved in human febrile disease. **rabies v.**, a rhabdovirus of the genus *Lyssavirus*, causing rabies. Called also *hydrophobia v., lyssa v., rage v., tollwut v.,* and *wut v.* **rage v.**, rabies v. **REO v.**, reovirus. **respiratory syncytial v.**, a paramyxovirus of the genus *Pneumovirus*, causing respiratory infection sometimes involving the lower respiratory tract, which most often affects younger children. **Restan v.**, an arbovirus of the C group, Bunyamwera supergroup of viruses, isolated in Trinidad and Surinam from mosquitoes, and in man in association with febrile illness. **Rift Valley fever v.**, a mosquito-borne arbovirus, tentatively classified as a bunyavirus, causing an often fatal disease in sheep, goats, and cattle in South Africa. Human infection is usually manifested by dengue-like symptoms. In some cases of infection, symptoms are very mild or absent. **RNA v's**, a group of viruses having an RNA genome, consisting of the families Arenaviridae, Bunyaviridae, Calcivirus, Coronaviridae, Orthomyxoviridae, Paramyxoviridae, Picornaviridae, Reoviridae, Retroviridae, Rhabdoviridae, Togaviridae, and the unclassified Marburg virus. **rubella v.**, a togavirus of the genus *Rubivirus*, causing rubella. Meningoencephalitis occurs in some instances. Maternal infection in pregnancy in the nonimmune may result in fetal abnormalities (see congential rubella SYNDROME). Called also *German measles v.* **rubeola v.**, measles v. **Russian autumn encephalitis v.**, Japanese B v. **Russian spring-summer encephalitis v.**, tick-borne encephalitis v. (eastern subtype). **St. Louis encephalitis v.**, a togavirus of the genus *Flavivirus*, formerly classified as a group B arbovirus. The virus infects wild birds and is transmitted by mosquito bites to man, causing a brief febrile illness, frequently associated with encephalitis that may be fatal. The infection was originally described in St. Louis, but now occurs in other parts of the United States. **salivary gland v.**, cytomegalovirus. **salivary gland v. of guinea pig**, guinea pig CYTOMEGALOVIRUS. **sandfly fever v.**, an arbovirus of the Phlebotomus fever group of viruses, consisting of two strains, Sicilian and Naples, which are antigenically distinct from each other and from other arboviruses. The virus is transmitted by sandflies, causing a febrile human disease of short duration with dengue-like symptoms. The virus occurs in Italy and eastwards to Egypt, Iran, and Pakistan. Called also *pappataci fever v.* and *Phlebotomus fever v.* **satellite v's**, a group of viruses that can replicate in cells which are concomitantly infected with other viruses, such as adenoassociated viruses, which must coexist with adenoviruses in order to replicate. Called also *defective v's, defective virions,* and *satellite virions.* **scabby mouth v.**, orf v. **Semliki Forest v.**, a togavirus of the genus *Alphavirus*, formerly classified as a group A arbovirus, originally isolated in the Semliki Forest in Uganda. The virus is believed to cause encephalomyelitis in horses; its natural hosts and vectors are unknown. Called also *Kumba v.* **Sendai v.**, parainfluenza v. type 1; see *parainfluenza v's.* **serum hepatitis v.**, hepatitis B v. **shipping fever v.**, parainfluenza v. type 3; see *parainfluenza v's.* **Sindbis v.**, a mosquito-borne togavirus of the genus *Alphavirus* formerly classified as a group A arbovirus, originally isolated from cows in the Sindbis region of Egypt. The virus may cause infection in man, characterized chiefly by high fever. **slow v.**, any virus causing a disease characterized by a very long preclinical course and very gradual progression once the symptoms appear. **smallpox v.**, variola v. **SMON v.**, subacute myelo-opticoneuropathy v. **sore mouth v.**, 1. vesicular stomatitis v. 2. bluetongue v. 3. orf v. **spongiform encephalopathy v.**, an unclassified virus which

may be the cause of Jakob-Creutzfeldt disease. **v. of subacute myelo-opticoneuropathy (SMON)**, a herpesvirus that causes symmetrical degeneration of the posterior and lateral spinal tracts and peripheral nerves, especially the optic nerves. **submaxillary v.**, guinea pig CYTOMEGALOVIRUS. **swine vesicular v.**, vesicular exanthema v. **Tacaribe v.**, one of the American hemorrhagic fever viruses isolated in Trinidad. **Tahyňa v.**, an arbovirus of the California group, Bunyamwera supergroup of viruses, isolated in Europe and Africa from mosquitoes, and from man in association with febrile illness. **Tamiami v.**, one of the American hemorrhagic fever viruses isolated in Florida. **tanapox v.**, a poxvirus associated with epidemics of a febrile illness accompanied by pocklike skin lesions in children. **Tensaw v.**, an arbovirus of the Bunyamwera supergroup of viruses, isolated in the United States from mosquitoes, dogs, and rabbits; suspected of causing human encephalitis. **tickborne v.**, a virus transmitted by ticks. See ARBOVIRUS. **tickborne encephalitis v. (central European subtype)**, a togavirus of the genus *Flavivirus*, formerly classified as a group B arbovirus. It is transmitted by tick bites or by milk of infected goats, and causes a biphasic febrile disease in man, characterized by an initial afebrile period of four to ten days, followed by the first phase of an influenza-like fever and the second phase of meningitis or meningoencephalitis. The infection with bulbospinal involvement is usually fatal. Some cases are inapparent. Infection occurs predominantly in central Europe. Called also *biundulant meningoencephalitis v.* and *diphasic milk fever v.* **tickborne encephalitis v. (eastern subtype)**, a togavirus of the genus *Flavivirus*, formerly classified as a group B arbovirus. It is transmitted by tick bites and causes encephalitis with flaccid paralysis and muscle atrophy, mortality being about 30 percent. Infection occurs in eastern USSR, sometimes extending west as far as Leningrad and some strains being isolated in Czechoslovakia. Called also *Far East Russian encephalitis v.* and *Russian spring-summer encephalitis v.* **tollwut v.**, rabies v. **transfusion hepatitis v.**, hepatitis B v. **Trivittatus v.**, an arbovirus of the California group, Bunyamwera supergroup of viruses, isolated in the United States from mosquitoes and cotton rats; believed to be associated with human febrile disease. **tumor v.**, Oncovirinae. **v. U**, echovirus 11. **Uruma v.**, a togavirus of the genus *Alphavirus* formerly classified as a group A arbovirus, causing epidemic febrile illness in Colombia. Considered probably to be a strain of the Mayaro virus. **vaccinia v.**, a poxvirus of the genus *Orthopoxvirus*, which is immunologically similar to the variola virus, but causes human lesions which are much less severe than those of variola (smallpox), and is thus used for inoculation against smallpox. Rarely, progressive vaccinia may occur in subjects with immunological deficiency; in these cases, the disease is usually fatal. **varicella-zoster v.**, a herpesvirus causing chickenpox and herpes zoster. **variola v.**, a poxvirus of the genus *Orthopoxvirus*, which causes smallpox and, in its less virulent form, variola minor. Called also *alastrim v., Amaas v., smallpox v.,* and *variola minor v.* **variola minor v.**, see *variola v.* **VEE v.**, Venezuelan equine encephalomyelitis v. **Venezuelan equine encephalomyelitis (VEE) v.**, a togavirus of the genus *Alphavirus*, formerly classified as a group A adenovirus. The virus is found in Venezuela, Colombia, Ecuador, Panama, Trinidad, Brazil, Mexico, Florida, and Texas. Its natural reservoir is unknown, but the virus is transmitted to horses, donkeys, and man by mosquito bites, causing central nervous system disturbance and high mortality. In man, it occasionally causes neurological disorders. The virus is present in the nose, eyes, mouth, urine, and milk of infected horses, and direct-contact infection from horse to horse may occur. **verruca vulgaris v.**, human warts v. **vesicular v.**, vesiculovirus. **vesicular exanthema v.**, a calcivirus, about 35 to 40 nm in diameter, which causes a disease in swine similar to food-and-mouth disease in cattle. It occurs naturally in sea lions. The virus was originally classified as a picornavirus of the genus Enterovirus. Called also *swine vesicular disease v.* **vesicular stomatitis v.**, a rhabdovirus of the genus *Vesiculovirus*, occurring as at least two antigenic types and several subtypes. It causes raised vesicular eruptions, chiefly on the oral mucosa and sometimes on the feet of horses, cattle, sheep, and other animals. Infection in humans may be inapparent or resemble influenza. The virus was originally isolated in the New World, but has spread to Europe and, perhaps, South Africa. Called also *sore mouth v.* **Visna v.**, Lentivirinae. **WEE v.**, western equine encephalomyelitis v. **Wesselsbron disease v.**, a mosquito-borne togavirus of the genus *Flavivirus*, formerly classified as a group B arbovirus. It causes hemorrhage, jaundice, meningoencephalitis, fetal death, and abortion in sheep. The virus also infects man, causing fever and muscular pain. **western equine encephalomyelitis (WEE) v.**, a togavirus of the genus *Alphavirus*, formerly classified as a group A arbovirus, found in most of the United

States and southern Canada, extending to Central and South America. The virus is parasitic in wild birds, and is transmitted by mosquitoes to man and horses, causing encephalomyelitis. It has been isolated from various birds, squirrels, cows, deer, and swine. **West Nile v.,** a togavirus of the genus *Flavivirus,* formerly classified as a group B arbovirus. The virus occurs in various parts of Africa and in Mediterranean countries, Borneo, and the Soviet Union, causing endemic infections in man, chiefly children, and in horses and donkeys. The infection is usually silent, but may also occur with dengue-like symptoms. **wut v.,** rabies v. **Wyeomyia v.,** an arbovirus of the Bunyamwera group of viruses, isolated in Central and South America from man and mosquitoes; suspected of causing human febrile diseases. **yellow fever v.,** a mosquito-borne togavirus of the genus *Flavivirus,* formerly classified as a group B arbovirus, which causes yellow fever.

Viruzona trademark for *methisazone.*

Viscarin trademark for *carrageenan.*

viscera (vis′er-ah) [L.] plural of *viscus.*

visceral (vis′er-al) [L. *visceralis,* from *viscus*] pertaining to a viscus or to the viscera.

viscerocranium (vis″er-o-kra′ne-um) that part of the skull derived from the branchial arches. The components of the cartilaginous viscerocranium represent the cricoid cartilage, thyroid cartilage, greater and lesser horns of the hyoid bone, body of the hyoid bone, styloid process, incus, stapes, and malleus. The components of the membranous viscerocranium represent the mandible, tympanic bone, occipital bone, pterygoid process, vomer, maxilla, premaxilla, nasal bone, lacrimal bone, and petrous part of the temporal and palatine bones.

viscid (vis′id) [L. *viscidus*] glutinous or sticky.

viscidity (vĭ-sid′ĭ-te) the quality of being viscid.

viscoelasticity (vis″ko-e″las-tis′ĭ-te) the quality of materials, whereby they require some time to return to their original shape after removing the source of stress from distorted areas. The phenomenon is considered to be analogous to the behavior of viscous fluid. Called also *anelasticity.*

viscosimetry (vis″ko-sim′ĕ-tre) the measurement of the viscosity of a substance.

viscosity (vis-kos′ĭ-te) [L. *viscum* birdlime made from mistletoe berries] 1. viscidity. 2. the resistance to flow of a liquid due to attraction of adjacent molecules. The ratio of the shear stress to the rate of shear of a fluid. The property of the fluid is glutinous and sticky, the fluid offering resistance to a change of form. Called also *internal fluid friction* and *resistance to fluid flow.* See also Poiseuille's LAW. **absolute v.,** dynamic v. **dynamic v.,** the tangential force per unit area of two parallel planes at unit distance apart, when one plane moves with unit velocity in its own plane relative to the other plane in a space filled with fluid. The unit of viscosity is the *poise.* Called also *absolute v.* **kinematic v.,** the ratio of dynamic viscosity to density of a fluid expressed in stokes.

viscous (vis′kus) [L. *viscosus*] characterized by a high degree of friction between component molecules as they slide by each other; glutinous; sticky; adhesive.

viscus (vis′kus), pl. *vis′cera* [L.] any of the internal organs situated in one of the three great cavities of the body (thoracic, abdominal, and pelvic), or in the visceral compartment of the neck.

Visine trademark for *tetrahydrozoline hydrochloride* (see under TETRAHYDROZOLINE).

vision (vizh′un) [L. *visio,* from *videre* to see] the act or faculty of seeing; sight.

Visotrast trademark for *acetrizoate sodium* (see under ACETRIZOATE).

Visubutina trademark for *oxyphenbutazone.*

vital (vi′tal) [L. *vitalis,* from *vita* life] 1. necessary to or pertaining to life. 2. (pl.) the parts and organs necessary to life.

vitality (vi-tal′ĭ-te) the condition of being alive. **pulp v.,** vital PULP.

Vitallium trademark for a *cobalt-chrome alloy* (see under ALLOY), similar in composition to the alloy HS21; used in prosthetic dentistry, orthopedics, and surgery.

vitalometer (vi″tal-lom′ĕ-ter) electric pulp TESTER. **Burton v.,** a high frequency pulp vitality tester which measures the intensity of electric stimulus in volts.

vitalometry (vi″tal-lom′ĕ-tre) pulp vitality TEST.

vitamin (vi′tah-min) [L. *vita* life + *amine*] any of a number of organic compounds required in trace amounts for normal growth and maintenance of life in animals, being essential for the utilization of energy, in metabolic processes, and for the prevention of nutritional deficiency diseases. Man is unable to synthesize some vitamins and must acquire them from plants in the diet which contain vitamins or their precursors. The term "vitamin" (originally "vitamine") was coined by Kazimierz

Funk, the discoverer of vitamin B_1. For daily requirements of vitamins, see table at NUTRITION. **v: A, v. A_1,** a vitamin, 3,7-dimethyl-9-(2,6,6-trimethyl-1-cyclohexen-1-yl)-2,4,6,6-nonantetraen-1-ol, occurring as a yellowish crystalline solid that is soluble in fats and alcohols, but not in water; is oxidized on exposure to air; and is destroyed by ultraviolet rays. A complex primary alcohol, vitamin A is found in eggs, milk, butter, and fish liver oil. It combines with the protein opsin to form rhodopsin and is involved in the activity of the retina, development and maintenance of epithelial cells, development of bones, synthesis of mucopolysaccharides, production of corticosterone, permeability of membranes, reproduction, and embryonic development. Used in the treatment of oral hyperkeratosis, infections, kwashiorkor, burns, wounds, psoriasis, ichthyosis, and vitamin A deficiency. Called also *anti-infective v., antixerophthol v., antixerophthalmia factor, lard factor, retinol,* and *retinol₁.* Trademark: Axerophthol. Vitamin A deficiency (vitamin A hypovitaminosis) is either due to inadequate intake of vitamin A–containing foods or, more commonly, occurring in chronic diseases affecting fat absorption, such as those of the biliary tract, pancreas, liver, and intestine, or after gastrectomy. The most commonly occurring symptoms are nyctalopia and retarded growth and development. Also occurring may be keratomalacia; respiratory infections due to epithelial changes and mucus secretion; keratinization and drying of the epidermis, sometimes associated with papular eruptions; urinary calculi; sweat gland atrophy and keratinization; gastrointestinal mucosal changes; faulty bone modeling; impaired spermatogenesis; and fetal abnormalities. Oral changes associated with vitamin A deficiency include atrophy and metaplasia of the enamel-forming organ, hypoplasia of the enamel, increased incidence of dental caries, reduced salivary flow, and periodontal lesions. Excessive amounts of the vitamin in the tissues causes vitamin A intoxication (*v. A hypervitaminosis*) (hypervitaminosis A). In chronic cases, usually due to excessive prophylactic vitamin therapy, symptoms may include irritability, vomiting, loss of appetite, headache, dry skin with desquamation, pruritus, fatigue, myalgia, loss of body hair, nystagmus, hepatosplenomegaly, lymph node enlargement, increased intracranial pressure, hyperostoses, and oral lesions, which may include fissures at the corners of the mouth and gingivitis. In acute poisoning, due either to eating polar bear liver or accidental swallowing of vitamins by children, symptoms may include sluggishness, irritability, headache, drowsiness, vomiting, papilledema, and peeling of the skin. Experimental poisoning may result in bone and cartilage resorption, longitudinal bone growth without simultaneous thickening, susceptibility to fractures, anorexia, thickening of the skin, lipid deposits in Küpffer cells, exophthalmos, hypoprothrombinemia, and death. Congenital defects may occur in infants of mothers receiving toxic doses of vitamin A. **v. A_2,** a vitamin A derivative having an additional double bond in the ring at the 3-4 position, 3-dehydroretinol. It has less than half vitamin A biological activity. Called also *retinol₂.* **v. A. acid,** tretinoin. **antiacantinic v.,** p-aminobenzoic ACID. **antihemorrhagic v.,** v. K. **anti-infective v.,** v. A. **antipellagra v.,** nicotinic ACID. **antisterility v.,** v. E. **antixerophthalmia v.,** v. A. **v. B,** any vitamin of the vitamin B complex. The first vitamin B was first discovered on rice polishings by Kazimierz Funk, and was identified as vitamin B_1 (see THIAMINE). See *v. B complex.* **v. B complex,** a class of water-soluble vitamins having common sources, including the liver and yeasts, but characterized by different chemical structures and biological activities. The complex is generally considered to include: B_1 (thiamine), B_2 (riboflavin), B_3 (nicotinamide), B_5 (pantothenic acid), B_6 (pyridoxine, pyridoxal, pyridoxamine), biotin, folic acid, and B_{12} (cyanocobalamin). Inositol, choline, and *p*-aminobenzoic acid are also considered as vitamins B, but there is no general agreement on their being included in the group. **v. B_1,** thiamine. **v. B_2,** riboflavin. **v. B_3,** nicotinamide. **v. B_4,** adenine. **v. B_5,** pantothenic ACID. **v. B_6,** a group of water-soluble vitamins of the vitamin B complex, consisting of pyridoxal, pyridoxamine, and pyridoxine, all having biochemical and pharmacological properties identical to those of pyridoxine. **v. B_c,** folic ACID. **v. B_T,** carnitine. **v. B_x,** *p*-aminobenzoic ACID. **v. B_{12},** 1. cyanocobalamin. 2. a general term for all the cobamides that play a role in human metabolism, i.e., the cobalamins. **v. B_{12a},** a cobalamin in which the CN is replaced by the hydroxyl group; the anhydrous form of vitamin B_{12b}. Called also *hydroxycobalamin.* **v. B_{12b},** a cobalamin in which the CN group is replaced by water. Called also *aquocobalamin.* **v. B_{12c},** a cobalamin in which the CN group is replaced by nitrite. Called also *nitrocobalamin*. **v. C**, ascorbic ACID. **coagulation v.**, v. K. **v. D**, any of several related fat-soluble vitamins (vitamins D_1, D_2, and D_3) that have antirachitic properties, and are produced by ultraviolet irradiation of plant sterols. They act synergistically with parathyroid hormone in controlling calcium and phosphate metabolism, supplying them to bone by stimulating their intestinal absorption, thus participating in the process of bone mineralization. The vitamins also play a still unclarified role in urinary phosphate and calcium excretion. The body requirement for vitamin D can be met by ultraviolet irradiation of the skin without the need for vitamin D–rich foods. Fish liver oil and fortified milk are the principal sources of dietary vitamin D; other dairy products, egg yolk, and fish also contain vitamins D, but their content varies. Deficiency of vitamin D (*v. D hypovitaminosis*) causes rickets in children and osteomalacia in adults. The intake of excessive doses of any vitamin D causes a toxic condition (called *v. D hypervitaminosis*), characterized chiefly by hypercalcemia; symptoms usually include weakness, fatigue, lassitude, headache, nausea, vomiting, diarrhea, polyuria, polydipsia, nocturia, and proteinuria. Chronic hypercalcemia may be also associated with deposits of calcium salts in soft tissue, chiefly the kidneys, with resulting nephrocalcinosis and urinary calculi. Deposits may occur in addition in the heart, blood vessels, lungs, and skin. Infants of mothers receiving excessive doses of vitamin D may exhibit vascular injuries, aortic stenosis, and suppressed parathyroid function. Dental and periodontal lesions may also occur. **v. D_1**, an equimolecular compound of lumisterol and vitamin D_2; used in the treatment of rickets. **v. D_2**, a vitamin, 9,10-secoergosta-5,7-10(19),22-tetraen-3β-ol, occurring as white, odorless crystals that are insoluble in water, but are soluble in oils, organic solvents, and ethanol, and are oxidized in the presence of moist air. Produced by ultraviolet irradiation of ergosterol. Used in the treatment of rickets. Called also *activated ergosterol, calciferol, ergocalciferol, oleovitamin D_2,* and *viosterol*. **v. D_3**, a vitamin, 9,10-secocholesta-5,7,10(19)trien-3β-ol, occurring as white, odorless, and air-sensitive crystals that are soluble in vegetable oils, ethanol, and chloroform and organic solvents, but not in water. It is produced by ultraviolet irradiation of 7-dehydrocholesterol. Used in the treatment of rickets, and may be used in the treatment of hypocalcemic tetany and hypoparathyroidism. Its use is contraindicated in the presence of renal insufficiency and hyperphosphatemia. Called also *activated 7-dehydrocholesterol, cholecalciferol, oleovitamin D_3*. **v. E**, a vitamin, 2,5,7,8-tetramethyl-2-(4′,8′,12′-trimethyltridecyl)-6-chromanol, occurring as a viscous pale, yellow oil that is soluble in oil, fats, acetone, ether, ethanol, chloroform, and other fat solvents, but not in water. Found in high concentrations in wheat germ, corn, sunflower seed, rapeseed, soybean oil, lettuce, and alfalfa. The vitamin appears to be involved in fatty acid metabolism and in the action of various enzymes. Used chiefly as a dietary supplement in the diet of newborn infants, especially premature infants suffering from steatorrhea. Also used in various diseases, including anemia, protein-caloric malnutrition, acanthocytosis, and other conditions, but there appears to be little evidence supporting its effectiveness. Called also *antisterility v., fertility v.*, and *α-tocopherol*. **fertility v.**, v. E. **v. G.** riboflavin. **Goetsch's v.**, v. T. **v. H**, biotin. **v. H′**, *p*-aminobenzoic ACID. **v. K**, a quinone derivative essential for the biosynthesis of blood coagulation factors. Vitamin K substances are fat-soluble and are found in plants, such as alfalfa, and are synthesized in the intestine, from where they are absorbed into the system. They participate in hepatic biosynthesis of prothrombin, proconvertin, plasma thromboplastin component, and the Stuart factor. Antibacterial agents may inhibit their synthesis and intestinal disorders, liver diseases, and biliary obstruction may alter their absorption. Used in the treatment of hemorrhagic states due to vitamin K deficiency. In normal humans, vitamin K is almost free of any pharmacodynamic effects, but a rapid intravenous administration may cause flushing, dyspnea, chest pain, and sometimes, death. Called also *antihemorrhagic v., coagulation v.*, and *prothrombin F*. See also blood COAGULATION. **v. K_1** phytonadione. **v. K_2**, a vitamin, 2-methyl-3-*all-trans*-polyprenyl-naphthoquinone, being a series of compounds (naphthoquinones) in which the phytyl side chain of phylloquinone has been replaced by a side chain of 2 to 13 prenyl units. It occurs in several forms, such as vitamin $K_{2(35)}$, which is 2-(3,7,11,15,19,23,27-heptamethyl-2,6,10,14,18,22,26-octacosaheptaenyl)-3-methyl-1,4-naphthoquinone, or vitamine $K_{2(30)}$, which is 2-difarnesyl-3-

methyl-1,4-naphthoquinone. Originally isolated from petrified fish meal. Called also *menaquinone*. **v. $K_{2(0)}$**, see menadione. **v. K_3**, menadione. **v. K_5**, a vitamin, 4-amino-2-methyl-l-naphthalenol. Its hydrochloride salt occurs as a crystalline powder that darkens on exposure to light and air and is soluble in water, slightly soluble in ethanol, and insoluble in ether. Used as a food preservative and in the treatment of hemorrhagic disorders. Called also *Kayvisyn, Synkamin*. **v. K_6**, a vitamin, 2-methyl-1,4-naphthalenediamine. Its dichloride salt occurs as crystals that are soluble in water. It is a highly toxic antihemorrhagic drug. **v. K_7**, a vitamin, 4-amino-3-methyl-l-naphthalenol. Its hydrochloride salt occurs as crystals that darken on exposure to light and air, and are soluble in water. **v. M**, folic ACID. **v. K-S(II)**, a vitamin, 3/(1,4-dihydro-3-methyl-1,4-dioxo-2-naphthalenyl)thio/proanoic acid, occurring as orange needles that are soluble in benzene and other fat solvents, but not in water. Used in the treatment of hemorrhagic states. **v. L**, a factor believed to be essential for normal lactation. **v. PP**, nicotinamide. **v. T**, a complex of growth-promoting substances isolated from yeasts, fungi, and certain insects. Called also *Goetsch's v.* and *factor T*. **v. U**, a vitamin, (3-amino-3-carboxypropyl)dimethyl sulfonium salt, isolated from cabbage and other green vegetables. Used in the treatment of peptic ulcer and other gastrointestinal diseases.

Vitapulp; Crane Vitapulp a trademark for a battery-operated pulp vitality tester.

vitellin (vi-tel′in) [L. *vitellus* yolk] a phosphoprotein of egg yolk.

vitiligo (vit″ĭ-li′go) [L.] a condition characterized by patches of depigmentation often having a hyperpigmented border, and often enlarging slowly, caused by failure of the skin to form melanin.

vitrification (vi″trĭ-fĭ-ka′shun) the act or process of converting into glass or a glassy substance by heat and fusion. Vitrification of a silicate material is accomplished by heating, whereby the molten substance forms a viscous liquid which hardens on cooling, producing a hard material with a smooth glossy surface; its liquid state being preserved in the solidified state. Glass, the principal product of vitrification, is often referred to as a super-cooled liquid. See also CERAMIC and GLASS (1).

vitriol (vit′re-ol) [L. *vitriolum*] a crystalline form of sulfate. **green v.**, ferrous SULFATE. **oil of v.**, sulfuric ACID. **white v.**, ZINC sulfate. **zinc v.**, ZINC sulfate.

vitrum (vit′rum) [L.] glass.

vivi- [L. *vivus* alive] a combining form meaning alive or denoting relationship to life.

vivisection (viv″ĭ-sek′shun) [*vivi- + section*] the performance of surgical procedures upon living animals for the purpose of research.

VLDL very low density lipoproteins; see prebeta-LIPOPROTEIN.

VNA visting nurse ASSOCIATION.

vocal (vo′kal) [L. *vocalis*, from *vox* voice] pertaining to the voice.

vocalis (vo-kal′is) vocal MUSCLE.

Vogt's angle [Karl *Vogt*, German physiologist, 1817–1895] see under ANGLE.

Vogt's point [Frederick Emmanuel *Vogt*, German surgeon, 1844–1885] see under POINT.

Vogt-Hueter point [F. E. *Vogt*; Karl *Hueter*, German surgeon, 1838–1882] see Vogt's POINT.

voice (vois) [L. *vox* voice] a sound produced by vibration of the vocal cords and uttered by the mouth.

vola (vo′lah) [L.] any concave or hollow surface.

volatile (vol′ah-til) [L. *volatilis*, from *volare* to fly] tending to evaporate rapidly.

Volkmann's canal [Alfred Wilhelm *Volkmann*, German physiologist, 1800–1877] see under CANAL.

Volkmann's cheilitis [Richard von *Volkmann*, German physician, 1830–1889] CHEILITIS glandularis apostematosa.

Volonimat trademark for *triamcinolone acetonide* (see under TRIAMCINOLONE).

volt (volt) [named after Alessandro *Volta*] the SI unit of electric potential being the force necessary to cause 1 ampere of current to flow against 1 ohm of resistance, calculated by dividing watt by ampere. Abbreviated *v* or *V*. See also SI. **absolute v.**, abvolt. **electron v.**, the energy acquired by an electron when accelerated by a potential of 1 volt, being equivalent to 3.82×10^{-20} small calories, or 1.6×10^{-12} ergs; usually expressed in million electron volts, or Mev or MeV. **kiloelectron v.**, a unit of energy equal to 1,000 electron volts, 1.6×10^{-9} ergs, or 3.8×10^{-17} calories. Symbol *keV*. **million electron v's**, see *electron v.*

Volta, Alessandro [Italian physicist, 1745–1827]. See VOLT and VOLTAGE.

voltage (vol′tij) a measure of the electric charge when moving between two points, measured in volts. The voltage measured across a nerve cell membrane is approximately 90 millivolts.

See also VOLT. Called also *potential difference.* **inverse v.,** the negative component of an alternating voltage applied to the anode of an x-ray tube.

Voltane trademark for *brompheniramine maleate* (see under BROMPHENIRAMINE).

voltmeter (volt'me-ter) an instrument for measuring electromotive force in volts.

volume (vol'um) the space occupied by a substance. The standard unit of volume in SI or in the metric system is the liter, or the quart in the avoirdupois system. See also *Tables of Weights and Measures* at WEIGHT. **atomic v.,** the value obtained by dividing the atomic weight of an element by its specific gravity in the solid condition. Abbreviated *at vol.* **blood v.,** BLOOD volume. **body water v.,** the volume of water contained in body fluids. In an average subject of 70 kg there are an estimated 40 liters of water, including about 10 liters in the extracellular fluid, 25 liters in the extracellular fluid, and 5 liters in the blood. **mean corpuscular v.,** see MCV (1). **packed-cell v. (PCV), v. of packed red cells (VPRC),** the number of packed red cells in milliliters per 100 ml of centrifuged blood. **plasma v.,** see BLOOD volume. **stroke v.,** the amount of blood ejected from a ventricle at each beat of the heart. **total red cell v. (TRVC),** the volume of erythrocytes in the circulating blood, usually determined by labeling red cells with radioisotopes of iron, chromium, phosphate, iodine, and the formula

$$TRCV = \frac{Q}{dpm/ml\ RBC_{(t)}}$$

where Q = amount of isotope injection in labeled cells and dpm/ml $RBC_{(t)}$ = amount of isotope in RBC at time t after administration of labeled cells. Determination of total red cell volume may be also used in calculating the blood volume. **v. in volume,** see PERCENT volume in volume.

vomer (vo'mer) [L. *"plowshare"*] [NA] a thin, somewhat quadrilateral, flat bone resembling a plowshare; it forms the inferior and posterior part of the nasal septum and articulates with the sphenoid, ethmoid, palatine, and maxillary bones. Its thick superior border presents a furrow bounded on two sides by wings which articulate with the vaginal process of the pterygoid plate of the sphenoid bone, and with the sphenoid processes of the palatine bone; the furrow receives the rostrum of the sphenoid bone. The inferior border is fused in its superior half with the ethmoid bone and its inferior half presents a groove for the margin of the septal cartilage of the nose. The posterior free border separates the choanae. Called also *vomer bone.*

vomerobasilar (vo"mer-o-bas'ĭ-lar) pertaining to the vomer and to the basilar portion of the cranium.

vomeronasal (vo"mer-o-na'sal) pertaining to the vomer and the nasal bone.

Vomex A trademark for *dimenhydrinate.*

vomiting (vom'it-ing) the forcible expulsion of the contents of the stomach through the mouth. See also REGURGITATION.

Vonamycin trademark for *neomycin.*

von Baelz see BAELZ.

von Bardeleben's prefrontal bone see nasal process of frontal bone, under PROCESS.

von Basedow see BASEDOW.

von Behring see BEHRING.

von Brunn see BRUNN.

von Bunsen see BUNSEN.

von Burow see BUROW.

von Ebner's glands, lines [Victor *von Ebner,* Vienna histologist, 1842–1925] see under GLAND, and see Ebner's lines, under LINE. See also EBNER.

Vonedrine trademark for *phenylpropylmethylamine.*

von Gierke's syndrome [Edgar Otto Conrad *von Gierke,* German pathologist, born 1877] GLYCOGENOSIS I.

von Gierke-van Creveld syndrome [E. O. C. *von Gierke;* S. *van Creveld,* Dutch pediatrician] GLYCOGENOSIS I.

von Gruber, Max [1853–1927] a bacteriologist in Munich who, with Herbert Durham, described in 1896 the agglutination test for bacteria.

von Hebra see HEBRA.

von Hofmann, Georg; von Hofmann-Wellendof, Georg see HOFMANN-WELLENDOF.

von Ihring's line, plane see under LINE and PLANE.

von Kölliker see KÖLLIKER.

von Korff's fibers Korff's fibers; see under FIBER.

von Kupffer's cell [Karl Wilhelm *von Kupffer,* German anatomist, 1829–1902] Kupffer's CELL.

von Langenbeck's pedicle mucoperiosteal flap [Bernhard Rudolf Konrad von *Langenbeck,* German surgeon, 1810–1887] see under FLAP.

von Leyden see LEYDEN.

von Leydig see LEYDIG.

von Ludwig see LUDWIG.

von Mayer, Julius Robert see MAYER, Julius Robert von.

von Meyer, Georg Hermann see MEYER, Georg Hermann von.

von Recklinghausen see RECKLINGHAUSEN.

Von Sallmann, Ludwig [American physician, born 1892] see hereditary benign intraepithelial DYSKERATOSIS (Witkop-Von Sallmann syndrome).

von Spee see SPEE.

von Strümpell see STRÜMPELL.

Vontrol trademark for *diphenidol.*

von Volkmann see VOLKMANN.

von Willebrand's syndrome [E. A. *von Willebrand,* Finnish physician, 1870–1949] Willebrand-Jürgens SYNDROME.

von Zambusch's disease LICHEN sclerosus et atrophicus.

von Zenker see ZENKER.

vowel (vow'el) a speech sound produced by certain positions of the speech organs which offer little obstruction to the air stream and which form a series of resonators above the level of the larynx. Cf. CONSONANT.

vox (voks), pl. *vo'ces* [L.] voice.

VPRC volume of packed red cells; see packed-cell VOLUME.

Vrolik's syndrome [Willem *Vrolik,* 1801–1863] see under SYNDROME.

vs vibration seconds (the unit of measurement of sound waves).

V x s volts by seconds; see WEBER.

Vulcamycin trademark for *novobiocin.*

vulcanite (vul'kan-īt) vulcanized caoutchouc or India rubber; formerly used as a base for artificial dentures. See vulcanite STOMATITIS.

vulcanization (vul"kah-ni-za'shun) change of the tacky, semisolid state of latex into a hard, elastic, and thermostable solid state of rubber by heating and adding a vulcanizing agent, such as sulfur or another cross-linking agent. The process introduces cross links between chains to produce a three-dimensional lattice of improved elasticity, strength, and temperature sensitivity. Vulcanization of silicone rubber may be accomplished by adding a cross-linking agent, such as ethyl orthosilicate, alone without heating. Called also *rubber curing.* **heat v.,** see *vulcanization.* **room temperature v.,** vulcanization of materials, such as silicone rubber, by the addition of a cross-linking agent, such as ethyl orthosilicate, to a silicone composed of comparatively short-chain polymers which are partially end-blocked with hydroxyl groups. Abbreviated *RTV.*

vulgaris (vul-ga'ris) [L.] ordinary; common; of the commonly observed type.

vulnus (vul'nus), pl. *vul'nera* [L.] a wound.

vv. abbreviation for L. *ve'nae* (veins).

v/v PERCENT volume in volume.

Vybak trademark for *polyvinyl chloride* (see under POLYVINYL).

Vycor glass see under GLASS.

W

W 1. watt. 2. wehnelt. 3. tungsten (wolfram).

w watt.

W/A watt/ampere; see VOLT.

WAADA Women's Auxiliary of the American Dental Association (see under AUXILIARY).

Waage, Peter [Norwegian chemist, 1833–1900] see Guldberg and Waage LAW.

Waardenburg's syndrome [P. Johannes *Waardenburg*] see under SYNDROME. See also Klein-Waardenburg SYNDROME.

Wachs paste see under PASTE.

Wagner's line see under LINE.

waiver (wa'ver) relinquishment of an interest, privilege, right, or claim; also, the statement or document that shows such relinquishment. **w. of premium,** a provision in some insurance policies which exempts the insured from paying premiums while he is disabled.

Waldenström's disease, syndrome, uveoparotitis [Jan *Waldenström,* Swedish physician, born 1906] see under DISEASE, SYNDROME, and UVEOPAROTITIS.

Waldenström's macroglobulinemia [Henning *Waldenström,* Swedish physician, born 1877] see under MACROGLOBULINEMIA.

Waldeyer's ring [Heinrich Wilhelm Gottfried von *Waldeyer,* German anatomist, 1836–1921] see under RING.

Walgreen see under DENTIFRICE.

Walker, W. A. see Marden-Walker SYNDROME.

Walker appliance (W. W. *Walker*) Crozat APPLIANCE.

Walker articulator [William E. *Walker,* American dentist, 1868–1914] see under ARTICULATOR.

wall (wawl) a limiting structure enclosing a space, a hollow organ, or a mass of material. Called also *paries.* See also FLOOR, ROOF, TECTUM, and TEGMEN. **axial w.,** a cavity wall approximating the pulp tissue, directed in the long axis of the tooth. Called also *axial floor.* **cavity w's,** the walls of a prepared cavity, named according to the surface of a tooth toward which they are placed, extracoronal walls being named after surfaces that have been reduced, and intracoronal ones after surfaces from which they derive. See illustrations. **cell w.,** a rigid structure that lies just outside of and is joined to the plasma membrane of plant cells and most prokaryotic cells (mycoplasmas lack a true cell wall), which provides protection for the cell and maintains its shape. In gram-positive bacteria, it is usually an amorphous, electron-dense layer surrounding the cell, composed largely of peptidoglycan. Within the wall, or occurring as surface layers, are proteins, polysaccharides, and teichoic acids, some serving as immunologically specific substances. In gram-negative bacteria, the wall is usually an electron-translucent layer of peptidoglycan between the plasma membrane and the double-tract outer membrane, containing significant amounts of lipids, in an enzyme-containing compartment known as the *periplasmic space;* this layer is joined to the outer membrane by lipoproteins. The outer membrane, basically a phospholipid-protein in content, acts as a hydrophobic barrier but does not carry out active transport, and also contains lipopolysaccharides that represent the major surface antigen components of the cell, being responsible for the endotoxic activity of gram-negative bacteria. See illustration at BACTERIUM. See also cell ENVELOPE. **enamel w.,** a cavity wall consisting of tooth enamel, located between the cavosurface margin and the dentinoenamel junction. **gingival w.,** a peripheral cavity wall near the apical end of the crown of the tooth. **w. of heart,** the wall of the muscular sac which forms the heart, consisting of the outer fibroserous layer (pericardium), the middle muscular layer (myocardium), and the inner lining (endocardium). **incisal w.,** a cavity wall in an anterior tooth that is closest to the incisal edge of the tooth. **inferior w. of orbit,** FLOOR of orbit. **lateral w. of nasal cavity,** the

Cavity walls: *A,* occlusal Class I; *B,* interproximal Class II; *C,* Class III. (From H. W. Gilmore, M. R. Lund, D. J. Bales, and J. Vernetti: Operative Dentistry. 3rd ed. St. Louis, The C. V. Mosby Co., 1977.)

lateral bony framework of the nasal cavity, formed anteriorly by the frontal process of the maxilla and the lacrimal bone; in the middle by the ethmoid bone, the maxilla, and the inferior nasal concha; and posteriorly by the vertical plate of the palatine bone and the medial pterygoid plate of the sphenoid bone. The middle part, between the superior and middle nasal conchae, lodges the superior meatus into which ethmoidal cells open; the middle meatus is situated between the middle and inferior conchae; and the inferior meatus is located between the inferior concha and the floor of the nasal cavity. The sphenoethmoidal recess at the superior posterior part of the nasal cavity receives the opening of the sphenoidal sinus. The hiatus semilunaris is situated between the uncinate process and the bulla ethmoidalis; below the bulla is the opening of the maxillary sinus. The inferior orifice of the nasolacrimal canal opens into the inferior meatus. **lateral w. of orbit,** a bony wall which provides the lateral boundary of the orbit, formed by the orbital surface of the great wing of the sphenoid bone, zygomatic bone, and zygomatic process of the frontal bone. It is separated from the roof by the superior orbital fissure and from the floor by the inferior orbital fissure. The oculomotor nerve, trochlear nerve, ophthalmic division of the trigeminal nerve, abducent nerves, filaments of the cavernous plexus, and orbital branches of the middle meningeal artery enter the orbital cavity through the superior orbital fissure. The superior ophthalmic vein and the recurrent branch of the lacrimal artery to the dura mater also leave the orbit through the superior orbital fissure. Called also *paries lateralis orbitae* [NA]. **medial w. of nasal cavity,** nasal SEPTUM. **medial w. of orbit,** a nearly vertical wall of the orbit, formed by parts of the maxillary, lacrimal, ethmoid, and sphenoid bones. It presents the lacrimomaxillary, lacrimoethmoidal, sphenoethmoidal, frontomaxillary, frontolacrimal, frontoethmoidal, and sphenofrontal sutures; the lacrimal groove for the lacrimal sac; the posterior lacrimal crest for attachment of the orbicularis oculi muscle; the dacryon; the anterior ethmoidal foramen for transmission of the posterior ethmoidal nerve and anterior ethmoidal vessels; and the posterior ethmoidal foramen for transmission of the posterior ethmoidal nerve and vessels. Called also *paries medialis orbitae* [NA]. **peripheral w.,** a bounding side wall of a prepared cavity, one side forming a part of the cavosurface angle of the preparation. Called also *surrounding w.* **pocket w.,** the soft tissue side of a periodontal pocket. **pulpal w.,** the cavity wall on the occlusal surface that covers the pulp in a plane at right angles to the long axis of the tooth. Called *pulpal floor.* **subpulpal w.,** the floor of a prepared cavity formed when the pulp is removed and the cavity is extended to include the pulp chamber. **superior w. of orbit,** ROOF of orbit. **surrounding w.,** peripheral w.

Wallenberg's syndrome [Adolf *Wallenberg,* German physician 1826–1949] see under SYNDROME.

Waller's law [August Volney *Waller,* British physician, 1816–1870] see under LAW.

wall-plate (wahl′plāt) an electrical apparatus for giving off a current of low tension and low voltage.

Walton's law see LAW of reciprocal proportions.

wandering (wahn′der-ing) moving about, usually aimlessly. **pathologic tooth w.,** tooth migration, pathologic; under MIGRATION.

Wanscher's mask see under MASK.

Warburg-Dickens-Lipmann pathway [O. H. *Warburg;* Frank *Dickens,* English biochemist, born 1899; Fritz Albert *Lipmann,* German-born biochemist in the United States] nicotinamide-adenine dinucleotide phosphate; see under DINUCLEOTIDE.

ward (ward) a large room in a hospital for the accommodation of several patients. See also ROOM and UNIT. **isolation w.,** a hospital ward for the isolation of persons having or suspected of having infectious diseases. **psychopathic w.,** a ward in a general hospital for temporary reception of psychiatric patients.

WARF [Wisconsin Alumni Research Foundation] warfarin.

warfarin (war′fah-rin) [named after *Wisconsin Alumni Research Foundation*] an oral prothrombopenic anticoagulant, 3-(α-acetonyl-benzyl)-4-hydroxycoumarin, occurring as crystals that are freely soluble in alkaline aqueous solutions, moderately soluble in methanol, ethanol, isopropanol, and some oils, and insoluble in water, benzene, and cyclohexane. Used in the treatment and prevention of thromboembolic disorders. Also used as a hemorrhage-producing rodenticide. Occasional nausea, anorexia, vomiting, purpura, urticaria, and alopecia may occur. Spontaneous gingival bleeding and hemorrhagic complications in surgical patients are the principal adverse reactions. Called also *compound 42* and *WARF.* Trademarks: Athrombine-K, Coumadin. **w. potassium,** the water-soluble potassium salt of warfarin, occurring as a white, odorless, crystalline powder with a slightly bitter taste, which changes color when exposed to light, and is freely soluble in water and ethanol and slightly soluble in chloroform and ether. **w. sodium,** the water-soluble sodium salt of warfarin, occurring as a white, odorless crystalline powder with a slightly bitter taste, which changes color when exposed to light, and is freely soluble in water and ethanol and slightly soluble in chloroform and ether. It has the same properties as the parent compound. Trademarks: Marevan, Prothromadin, Warfilone.

Warfilone trademark for *warfarin sodium* (see under WARFARIN).

warp (worp) to bend or twist out of shape. Torsional change of shape or outline, such as that which may occur in swaging sheet metal, or the change in shape of a plastic denture base which may occur when internal stresses are released by heating.

warranty (wor′an-te) 1. the assurance, guarantee, or promise of something. 2. the assurance, express or implied, by a physician or dentist that a certain procedure may be used safely or will be effective; sometimes used as a ground for legal actions against physicians or dentists.

Warren's fat column [John Collins *Warren*, American surgeon, 1778–1856] fat COLUMN.

wart (wort) [L. *verruca*] a small epidermal growth. See also VERRUCA. **common w.,** VERRUCA vulgaris. **digitate w.,** VERRUCA digitata. **filiform w.,** VERRUCA filiformis. **flat w., juvenile w.,** VERRUCA plana. **mother w.,** a solitary wart that, after a long period of slow growth, appears to give rise to eruption of many new warts. **mucocutaneous w.,** a variant of the common wart (verruca vulgaris), found in the mucocutaneous junctional areas of the genitalia and anus, and occasionally of the nostrils and mouth. **pitch w's,** precancerous, keratotic, epidermal tumors occurring in individuals who work in gas, tar, pitch, or various oils derived from coal. **plane w.,** VERRUCA plana.

Warthin's tumor [Alfred Scott *Warthin*, American pathologist, 1866–1931] ADENOLYMPHOMA.

Warthin-Finkeldey cell see under CELL.

wash (wahsh) a solution used for cleansing or bathing a part, as an eye or the mouth. **w. impression,** wash IMPRESSION. **w. impression material,** impression material, wash; see under MATERIAL. **w. method,** wash IMPRESSION. **mouth w.,** mouthwash. **w. technique,** wash IMPRESSION.

wasting (wa′sting) gradual reduction of fullness or strength of the body. **tooth w.,** a gradual loss of tooth surface characterized by the formation of smooth polished surfaces. Erosion, abrasion, and attrition are the three principal forms of wasting diseases of a tooth.

water (wah′ter) 1. a tasteless, odorless, colorless liquid, H_2O, used as the standard of specific gravity and of specific heat. It freezes at 32°F (0°C) and boils at 212°F (100°C). It is present in all organic tissues. See also hydrogen BOND. 2. aromatic water; the waters for which official standards are promulgated include anise w., fennel w., hamamelis w., orange flower w., peppermint w., rose w., stronger rose w., spearmint w., and wintergreen w. **activated w.,** water in a transient, chemically reactive state, created by absorbed ionizing radiations. **ammonia w.,** AMMONIA water. **ammonia w., stronger,** AMMONIUM hydroxide. **aromatic w.,** see *water* (2). **body w.,** water contained in the body fluids. See body FLUID. **chlorine w.,** a 4 percent aqueous chlorine solution; used as a deodorizer, disinfectant, and antiseptic. **w. of crystallization,** water held in a loose combination in a hydrate and, when the solution is allowed to evaporate slowly, forming part of the crystal. See also HYDRATE. **free w.,** gauging w. **gauging w.,** the excess water (above that necessary to convert hemihydrate back into gypsum) in the water-gypsum hemihydrate mixture in the preparation of dental plaster, plaster of Paris, and dental stone. Called also *free w.* **hard w., permanent,** water containing insoluble salts, such as sulfates or chlorides of calcium, magnesium, or iron, which cannot be removed by heating. The presence of salts prevents water from forming lather with soap. **hard w., temporary,** water containing an inorganic material, such as calcium or magnesium bicarbonate, which may be removed by heating. **heavy w.,** a compound analogous to water, but containing deuterium in place of hydrogen (D_2O or ^2H_2O). It differs from ordinary water in having a higher freezing point (3.8°C) and boiling point (101.4°C), and in the fact that it is incapable of supporting life. Called also *deuterium oxide.* **soft w.,** water that contains little or no mineral matter, readily forming a lather with soap. **stronger ammonia w.,** see AMMONIUM hydroxide.

Water's view roentgenogram see maxillary sinus ROENTGENOGRAM.

waterborne (wah′ter-born″) propagated by contaminated drinking water, said of diseases.

Waterhouse-Friderichsen syndrome [Rupert *Waterhouse*, American neurologist, 1873–1958; Carl *Friderichsen*, Danish physician, born 1886] see under SYNDROME.

Waters projection see under PROJECTION.

Watson, James Dewey [born 1928] an American biochemist; co-winner with Maurice Hugh Frederick Wilkins and Francis Harry Compton Crick, of the Nobel prize for medicine and physiology in 1962, for discovery of the molecular structure of deoxyribonucleic acid.

Watson-Crick helix, model [James Dewey *Watson*, American biochemist, born 1928; Francis Harry Compton *Crick*, English biochemist, born 1916] double HELIX.

watt (wot) [named after James *Watt*] originally, a unit of electric power, being the work done at the rate of 1 joule per second, or the equivalent of a current of 1 ampere under a pressure of 1 volt. In SI, the power of the energy of 1 joule (a unit of potential, kinetic, mechanical, electrical, magnetic, or thermal energy) expended for 1 second. Abbreviated *w* or *W*. See also SI. **absolute w.,** abwatt.

Watt, James [1736–1819] a Scottish engineer. See WATT.

wattage (wot′ij) the power output or consumption of an electrical device expressed in watts.

watt-hour (wot′owr) a unit of electrical work or energy, equal to the wattage multiplied by the time in hours.

wattmeter (wot′me-ter) an instrument for measuring electric activity in watts.

wave (wāv) a uniformly advancing disturbance in which the parts moved undergo a double oscillation. **contraction w.,** the wave of progression of the contraction in a muscle from the point of stimulation. **electromagnetic w's,** the entire series of ethereal waves which are similar in character, and which move with the velocity of light, but which vary in wavelength. The unbroken series is known from the hertzian waves used in radio transmission which may be miles in length (1 mile $= 1.6 \times 10^5$ cm) through heat and light, and ultraviolet rays, x-rays, and the gamma rays of radium to the cosmic rays, the wavelength of which may be as short as 0.0004 Å (4×10^{-12} cm). See also electromagnetic RADIATION. **excitation w.,** an electric wave flowing through a muscle just previous to its contraction. An example is the electrocardiogram or electromyogram. **full w.,** pertaining to a complete wave in a cycle. See full-wave RECTIFICATION. **half-w.,** pertaining to a half of a wave in a cycle. See half-wave RECTIFICATION. **hertzian w's,** electromagnetic waves of long wavelength and low frequency that resemble light waves, e.g., radio waves. **w. length,** wavelength. **light w's,** see LIGHT. **P w.,** see ELECTROCARDIOGRAPHY. **QRS w.,** see ELECTROCARDIOGRAPHY. **radio w's,** electromagnetic radiation of wavelength between 10^{-1} and 10^6 cm and frequency about 10^{11} to 10^4 cps. **short w.,** a wave having a wavelength of 60 meters or less. **sine w.,** the wave form of an alternating current characterized by a rise from zero to maximum positive potential, descending back through zero to its maximum negative value, and then rising back to zero. **sonic w's,** audible sound waves which under certain conditions may be destructive to microorganisms. **supersonic w's,** waves similar to sound waves but of frequencies from 200,000 to 1,500,000 cps; they are highly destructive to some organisms and some chemical substances. **T w.,** see ELECTROCARDIOGRAPHY. **U w.,** see ELECTROCARDIOGRAPHY. **ultrashort w.,** microwave.

wavelength (wāv′length) the distance between corresponding points on successive waves. Radiation of wavelengths of millions of meters is referred to as *electric waves*; radiation of wavelengths about a meter in length is referred to as *radio waves*; radiation of wavelengths between 7700 and 500,000 angstroms is known as *infrared*; radiation of wavelengths between 2900 and 3200 angstroms is known as *ultraviolet*; radiation of wavelengths of about 12 angstroms is known as *x-rays.* See also RADIATION and RAY. **effective w., equivalent w.,** the wavelength of monochromatic x-rays which would undergo the same percentage attenuation in a specific absorber as the heterogeneous beam under consideration. **minimum w.,** the shortest wavelength in an x-ray spectrum.

wax (waks) [L. *cera*] 1. a class of viscous or solid substances of animal, plant, or mineral origin which are composed of fatty acid esters of higher monohydric aliphatic and phytosterol alcohol. Waxes are insoluble in water and have low melting temperatures. 2. beeswax. **adhesive w.,** a dental wax, usually a mixture of beeswax, resins, gum dammar, coloring matter, and other constituents, which becomes sticky on melting and is used in dental laboratories to temporarily hold together small pieces of metallic, plaster, or resinous materials, as when soldering or assembling parts of dentures or dental appliances. Called also *sticky w.* **animal w.,** any wax derived from animal tissue. **barnsdahl w.,** a type of mineral wax used in dental waxes. **base plate w., baseplate w.,** a dental wax containing about 75 percent paraffin or ceresin with additions of beeswax and other waxes and resins, used chiefly to establish the initial arch form in making trial plates for the construction of complete dentures. Base plate waxes are classified into three types: *Type I,* soft; *Type II,* medium, and *Type III,* hard, and are differentiated from each by the percentage of flow at room temperature, at mouth temperature, and at 45°C (113°F); the harder the wax, the less flow at a given temperature. Type I is used for building veneers, Type II is designed for patterns to be tried in the mouth under normal climatic conditions, and Type III is for trial in the mouth in tropical climates. Called also *mouth denture w.* and *try-in w.* **bees w.,** beeswax. **bite w.,** a dental wax used for making an impression of the teeth upon their being brought to closure. **w. bite,** wax BITE. **bleached w.,** white w. **blockout w.,** a processing dental wax used as a blockout material to eliminate undercuts on master casts prior to duplication. See also *blockout* and blockout MATERIAL. **boxing w.,** a type of dental wax used for constructing a wall around a dental impression into which freshly mixed plaster or stone is poured in the fabrication of dental restorations or appliances. Called also *carding w.* See also BOXING (3). **Brazil w.,** carnauba w. **w. burn-out,** wax BURN-OUT. **candelilla w.,** a brownish to yellowish brown, hard, brittle, easily pulverizable plant wax consisting of 40 to 60 percent hydrocarbons containing 29 to 33 carbon atoms, free alcohols, acids, esters, and lactones. It melts at 68 to 70°C, and is soluble in benzene, acetone, carbon disulfide, gasoline, turpentine, chloroform, carbon tetrachloride, and alcohol, but not in water. Obtained from the candelilla plant, *Euphorbia antisyphilitica* and other vegetable sources. Used in dentistry to harden paraffin waxes and to reduce their flow at mouth temperature. **carding w.,** 1. dental wax used as a base for mounting artificial teeth, organized by standard sizes, shades, etc. 2. boxing w. **carnauba w.,** a hard, pale yellow to light brown, moderately coarse powder with a slight pleasant odor, which is freely soluble in warm benzene, chloroform, and toluene, slightly soluble in boiling alcohol, and insoluble in water. It melts at 81 to 86°C. Obtained from the leaves of *Copernicia cerifera,* a South American palm. When used in dentistry, it is combined with paraffin to decrease the flow at mouth temperature. Also used as a polishing agent in the manufacture of coated tablets. Called also *Brazil w.* **casting w.,** a mixture of several dental waxes, usually containing paraffin wax, ceresin, beeswax, resins, and other natural and synthetic waxes, the exact formula of individual casting waxes being trade secrets. Casting wax is used for making patterns to determine the shape of the metallic framework and other parts

COMPONENTS OF DENTAL WAXES

Natural waxes	Synthetic waxes	Additives
Mineral	Acrawax C	Stearic acid
Paraffin	Aerosol OT	Glyceryl
Microcrys-	Castorwax	tristearate
talline	Flexowax C	Oils
Barnsdahl	Epolene N-10	Turpentine
Ozokerite	Albacer	Color
Ceresin	Aldo 33	Natural resins
Montan	Durawax 1032	Rosin
Plant		Copal
Carnauba		Dammar
Ouricury		Sandarac
Candelilla		Mastic
Japan wax		Shellac
Cocoa butter		Kauri
Insect		Synthetic resins
Beeswax		Elvax
Animal		Polyethylene
Spermaceti		Polystyrene

(From F. A. Peyton, and R. G. Craig [eds.]: Restorative Dental Materials. 6th ed. St. Louis, The C. V. Mosby Co., 1980.)

CLASSIFICATION OF DENTAL INLAY CASTING WAXES

Revised Current ADA Specification	Previous ADA Specification	Previous Typical Commercial Designation
Type A – hard	None	
Type B – medium	Type I	"Hard"
Type C – soft	Type II	"Regular"

(From R. W. Phillips: Elements of Dental Materials. 3rd ed. Philadelphia, W. B. Saunders Co., 1977.)

of removable partial dentures. Available in sheets, usually 28- and 30-gauge thick, having ready-made shapes (e.g., round, half-round, half-pear–shaped rods, and rods and wires). **ceresin w.,** ceresin. **corrective w.,** an impression wax, compounded as soft, medium, or hard, generally used as a wax veneer over an original pattern; the medium and hard waxes are used to support the softer wax, which actually contacts and registers the detail of the soft tissues. Most corrective waxes are soft and pliable in the mouth, becoming rigid at room temperature. **dental w.,** a mixture of two or more natural and synthetic waxes, resins, coloring agents, and other additives. Used for pattern making for casting purposes and in the construction of nonmetallic denture bases, for registering jaw relations, and as aids in laboratory work. Beeswax was the original wax used in dentistry. See table. **dental inlay casting w.,** any wax used to make a pattern for an inlay (wax pattern). The composition of individual waxes is a trade secret with manufacturers, but most are known to contain paraffin, carnauba, ceresin, and candelilla waxes, beeswax, and gum dammar; synthetic waxes are sometimes used to replace the carnauba wax. They are classified into three types: *Type A,* a very hard wax with a high melting point, which is rarely used in dentistry; *Type B,* a medium wax, used in the direct technique; and *Type C,* a soft wax and used in the indirect technique. Called also *inlay casting w.* and *inlay pattern w.* Available under various trademarks. See table. **earth w., mineral w. w. expansion,** wax EXPANSION. **fluxed w.,** wax containing flux, used in attaching parts to be soldered in crown and bridgework. **fossil w.,** ozocerite. **grave w.,** adipocere. **Horsley's w.,** a mixture of wax, paraffin, and phenol, used for packing small bone cavities, as in the bones of the skull, for controlling bleeding. **impression w.,** a dental wax used for taking impressions within the mouth. Because of their high flow and low ductility, they distort or fracture readily when withdrawn from undercut areas and are thus restricted to the nonundercut edentulous portions of the mouth. Impression waxes may be classified as corrective waxes and bite wax. **inlay casting w., inlay pattern w.,** dental inlay casting w. **insect w.,** beeswax. **Japan w.,** a fat from the fruit of *Myrica cerifera* and other species of the same genus, occurring as pale yellow flakes with a rancid odor and taste. It melts at 53.5 to 55°C, and is soluble in benzene, carbon disulfide, ether, alkalies, and hot alcohol, but not in water and cold alcohol. Used as a substitute for beeswax in ointments, dental waxes, and other products. Called also *sumac w.* and *Japan tallow.* **Kerr hard w.,** trademark for Type B *dental inlay casting wax.* **Kerr regular w.,** a trademark for Type C *dental inlay casting wax.* **lignite w.,** montan w. **lost w.,** disappearing CORE. **microcrystalline w.,** a wax made up to a large extent of branched-chain hydrocarbons, having 41 to 50 carbon atoms in the average molecule. It is extracted from oil fractions that are heavier than those from which paraffin is made, and occurs as small, tough, flexible plates that melt at 60.0 to 90.5°C (140–195°F). Used similarly to paraffin wax. **mineral w.,** a natural wax obtained from the earth either directly or as a petroleum distillate. Most mineral waxes have as their chief components hydrocarbons ranging from 17 to over 44 carbon atoms. Called also *earth w.* See table. **model denture w.,** base plate w. **montan w.,** a hard, brittle, lustrous white, mineral wax derived from lignite, made up of a mixture of long-chain esters of 40 to 58 carbon atoms, free high-molecular-weight alcohols and acids, and resins. It melts at 80 to 90°C (176–194°F), and is soluble in carbon tetrachloride, benzene, and chloroform, but not in water. Used to improve the hardness and melting range of paraffin-based dental waxes. Also used as a substitute for carnauba wax and beeswax in adhesives and various industrial products. Called also *lignite w.* **Mosetig-Moorhof bone w.,** a mixture of spermaceti, oil of sesame, and iodoform, used for filling sterile bone cavities. Called also *Mosetig-Moorhof filling.* **natural w.,** any wax obtained directly from plant or animal tissues, from petroleum or other fossil material, or produced by insects, such as beeswax. Chemically, natural waxes contain hydrocarbons and esters, some also containing free alcohols and acids. See table. **ouricury w.**, a hard, brittle, plant wax with melting range of 79.0 to 84.5°C (174–184°F), made up of straight-chain esters, alcohols, acids, and hydrocarbons. In dentistry, added to paraffin-based waxes to increase their melting range and decrease the flow at mouth temperature. **paraffin w.**, a white, translucent, tasteless, odorless, somewhat greasy solid, soluble in organic solvents and olive oil, but not in water and various acids. Obtained chiefly from the high boiling point fraction of petroleum, it consists mainly of mixtures of straight-chain saturated hydrocarbons containing 26 to 30 carbon atoms. Paraffin wax melts at 40.5 to 71.0°C (105–160°F), the melting point generally increasing with the molecular weight; oil contamination decreases the melting point. Some waxes undergo crystallization on cooling, 10 to 15 percent contraction occurs during solidification. Used as a component of various dental waxes. Called also *hard paraffin*. **pattern w.**, a dental wax used for producing forms that are used for casting inlays or crowns, the metallic frameworks and parts of removable partial dentures, and base plates for complete denture restorations. **w. pattern**, see under wax PATTERN. **Peck's purple hard w.**, trademark for Type B *dental inlay casting wax*. **plant w.**, a waxy substance, resembling beeswax, derived from various vegetable sources. Called also *vegetable w.* See table. **processing w.**, a mixture of natural and synthetic waxes, used in the fabrication of dental restorations and appliances. Processing waxes include boxing, utility, adhesive, blockout, and setup waxes. **set-up w.**, a processing dental wax used in laboratories for aligning artificial teeth in dentures. **sticky w.**, adhesive w. **sumac w.**, Japan w. **synthetic w.**, any wax produced by chemical synthesis or by chemical alteration of natural waxes. Synthetic waxes include polyethylene, polyoxyethylene glycol, halogenated hydrocarbon, and hydrogenated waxes and wax esters from the reaction of fatty alcohols and acids. See table. **try-in w.**, base plate w. **utility w.**, a soft, pliable, adhesive dental wax consisting chiefly of beeswax, petrolatum, and various soft waxes. It is available in both stick and sheet form, becoming pliable at 21 to 24°C (70–75°F) and flowing at 36.6°C (98°F). Used for a variety of purposes in the dental laboratory, as when giving a desired contour to a perforated tray to be used with hydrocolloids. **vegetable w.**, plant w. **white w.**, the product of bleaching and purifying yellow wax, occurring as a yellowish white, almost tasteless, translucent solid with a faint characteristic odor, which melts at 62 to 65°C (143.6–149.0°F). It is soluble in chloroform, ether, and fixed and volatile oils, partly soluble in cold benzene and cold carbon disulfide, and sparingly soluble in cold ethanol, while boiling ethanol dissolves the cerotic acid and a portion of the myricin; insoluble in water. Used as a stiffening agent for ointments, pastes, and plasters. Called also *bleached w., bleached beeswax, cera alba*, and *white beeswax*. **yellow w.**, purified beeswax, consisting of esters of straight-chain monohydric alcohols with even-numbered carbon chains from C_{24} to C_{36} esterified with straight-chain acids also having even numbers up to C_{36}. Considered to be a mixture of myricin, which consists chiefly of myricyl palmitate and is insoluble in boiling alcohol; cerin or cerotic acid, which dissolves in boiling alcohol and crystallizes on cooling; and cerolein, which is believed to be a mixture of fatty acids and remains dissolved in cold alcoholic liquid. It is a yellow to grayish brown solid with a honey-like odor and a faint characteristic taste, and is brittle when cold but becomes pliable on warming. Yellow wax melts between 62 and 65°C (143.6 and 149.0°F) and is soluble in chloroform, ether, and fixed and volatile oils; partly soluble in cold benzene and carbon disulfide, but becomes soluble when the temperature reaches 30°C (86°F); sparingly soluble in cold alcohol; and insoluble in water. Used chiefly as a pharmaceutic aid in stiffening ointments, plasters, and pastes. Called also *cera flava* and *yellow beeswax*.

waxing (wak'sing) the contouring of a wax pattern or the wax base of a trial denture into the desired shape. Called also *waxing up*.

waxing up (wak̄'sing up) waxing.

wax out (waks owt) blockout.

Wb weber.

Wb/A weber/ampere; see HENRY.

W.B.C. white blood count. See leukocyte COUNT.

Wb/m² webers per square meter; see TESLA.

wear (wār) 1. to carry or to have on one's person. 2. to gradually deteriorate, impair, or diminish in size. 3. the act or process of gradual deterioration, impairment, or diminishing in size, as through use, friction, or abuse; attrition. **compensatory w.**, modification of the curves in root canals through the use of reamers or files in order to obtain a direct approach to the apex. **occlusal w.**, tooth w. **tooth w.**, a loss of tooth substance on the occlusal surfaces through physiological processes of mastica-

tion, or through abnormal oral habits, such as bruxism. Called also *occlusal w.* See also ABRASION.

web (web) 1. a structure or network, such as a woven material. 2. a network of threads, such as one spread by a spider; cobweb. 3. a membrane, such as one connecting the digits in certain water animals. **bind w.**, neuroglia. **laryngeal w.**, the most common congenital malformation of the larynx, which may be a thin, translucent diaphragm or thicker and more fibrotic; it is spread between the vocal folds near the anterior commissure and may cause obstruction, hoarseness, aphonia, and other complications. **Paterson-Kelly w's**, Plummer-Vinson SYNDROME. **terminal w.**, a feltwork of fine filaments in the cytoplasm immediately beneath the free surface of absorption cells of the intestinal epithelium.

Webb see Dean and Webb TITRATION.

weber (web'er) the SI unit of magnetic flux which, linking a circuit of one turn, produces in it an electromotive force of 1 volt as it is reduced to zero at a uniform rate in 1 second. It replaces the maxwell. Symbol *Wb*. See also *SI*.

Weber's gland [Moritz Ignatz *Weber*, German anatomist, 1795–1875] see under GLAND.

Weber's syndrome [Frederick Parkes *Weber*, British physician, 1863–1962] Klippel-Trenaunay-Weber SYNDROME. See also EPIDERMOLYSIS bullosa (Weber-Cockayne syndrome), hereditary hemorrhagic TELANGIECTASIA (Rendu-Weber-Osler syndrome), and Sturge-Weber SYNDROME.

Weber-Cockayne syndrome [F. P. *Weber*; Edward Alfred *Cockayne*, British physician, 1880–1956] EPIDERMOLYSIS bullosa.

Weber-Fechner principle Fechner's LAW.

Weber-Fergusson incision see Fergusson's INCISION.

Wechsberg, Friedrick [German physician] see Neisser-Wechsberg LEUKOCIDIN.

Wedelstaedt chisel see under CHISEL.

wedge (wej) 1. a cuneiform device made of a hard material, wide at one end and tapering to a thin edge at the other end, used for separating or splitting objects apart. 2. any material, such as wood, rubber, tape, or gutta-percha, which, when inserted between the proximal surfaces of adjoining teeth, exerts lateral pressure and forces a separation. **step-w.**, penetrometer.

wedging (wej'ing) the process of separating two adjoining objects, such as teeth, by forcing a wedge between the interproximal surfaces. See also WEDGE and wedging EFFECT.

WEE western equine encephalomyelitis (virus); see under VIRUS.

Weech's syndrome [Alexander A. *Weech*, American physician, born 1895] hypohidrotic ectodermal DYSPLASIA.

Wegener's granulomatosis [F. *Wegener*] see under GRANULOMATOSIS.

wehnelt (va'nelt) the unit of hardness or penetrating ability of roentgen rays. Abbreviated W.

weight (wāt) relative heaviness; the force of attraction exerted by the gravitational field of the earth, being directly proportional to the mass of the object. The standard unit of mass (weight) in SI or in the metric system is the kilogram, or the pound in the avoirdupois and apothecaries' systems of measures. See *Tables of Weights and Measures*. **apothecaries' w.**, a system of weights used in compounding prescriptions based on the grain (equivalent to 64.8 mg). Its units are the scruple (20 grains), dram (3 scruples), ounce (8 drams), and pound (12 ounces). **atomic w.**, the weight of an atom, determined by the sum of the number of protons plus the number of neutrons in its nucleus. The basis for determining atomic weight is the mass of an atom relative to other atoms; the basis of the scale being carbon, the most common element, assigned arbitrarily the atomic weight of 12. The unit of the scale is one-twelfth the weight of the carbon-12 isotope. Abbreviated *At wt* or *at. wt*. **avoirdupois w.**, a system of weights used in most English-speaking countries; its units are the dram (27.344 grains), ounce (16 drams), and pound (16 ounces or the equivalent of 453.6 grams). Abbreviated *Av*. **combining w.**, the relative weight, compared with that of hydrogen (which is considered as 1), of an element that enters into combination with other elements. **equivalent w.**, the weight in grams of a substance which is equivalent in chemical reaction to 1.008 gm of hydrogen. **gram equivalent w.**, gram EQUIVALENT. **gram molecular w.**, mole (3). **molecular w.**, the weight of a molecule of a substance as compared with that of an atom of carbon-12; it is equal to the sum of the atomic weights of its constituent atoms. Abbreviated *Mol wt*. **w. percent, w. percentage**, weight PERCENT. **w. per unit volume**, see *specific w.* **specific w.**, weight per unit volume, normally expressed in units of pounds per cubic feet (pcf). In the metric system,

TABLES OF WEIGHTS AND MEASURES

MEASURES OF MASS
Avoirdupois Weight

GRAINS	DRAMS	OUNCES	POUNDS	METRIC EQUIVALENTS, GRAMS
1	0.0366	0.0023	0.00014	0.0647989
27.34	1	0.0625	0.0039	1.772
437.5	16	1	0.0625	28.350
7000	256	16	1	453.5924277

Apothecaries' Weight

GRAINS	SCRUPLES (Ə)	DRAMS (ʒ)	OUNCES (ʒ)	POUNDS (℔.)	METRIC EQUIVALENTS, GRAMS
1	0.05	0.0167	0.0021	0.00017	0.0647989
20	1	0.333	0.042	0.0035	1.296
60	3	1	0.125	0.0104	3.888
480	24	8	1	0.0833	31.103
5760	288	96	12	1	373.24177

Metric Weight

MICRO-GRAM	MILLI-GRAM	CENTI-GRAM	DECI-GRAM	GRAM	DECA-GRAM	HECTO-GRAM	KILO-GRAM	METRIC TON	EQUIVALENTS	
									Avoirdupois	Apothecaries'
1	...	...	...	...	...	..	...	...	0.000015 grains	
10^3	1	...	...	...	...	...	...	...	0.015432 grains	
10^4	10	1	...	...	...	...	...	...	0.154323 grains	
10^5	100	10	1	...	...	...	...	...	1.543235 grains	
10^6	1000	100	10	1	...	...	...	...	15.432356 grains	
10^7	10^4	1000	100	10	1	...	...	...	5.6438 dr.	7.7162 scr.
10^8	10^5	10^4	1000	100	10	1	...	...	3.527 oz.	3.215 oz.
10^9	10^6	10^5	10^4	1000	100	10	1	...	2.2046 lb.	2.6792 lb.
10^{12}	10^9	10^8	10^7	10^6	10^5	10^4	1000	1	2204.6223 lb.	2679.2285 lb.

Troy Weight

GRAINS	PENNYWEIGHTS	OUNCES	POUNDS	METRIC EQUIVALENTS, GRAMS
1	0.042	0.002	0.00017	0.0647989
24	1	0.05	0.0042	1.555
480	20	1	0.083	31.103
5760	240	12	1	373.24177

MEASURES OF CAPACITY
Apothecaries' (Wine) Measure

MINIMS	FLUID DRAMS	FLUID OUNCES	GILLS	PINTS	QUARTS	GALLONS	EQUIVALENTS		
							CUBIC INCHES	MILLILITERS	CUBIC CENTIMETERS
1	0.0166	0.002	0.0005	0.00013	.....	.....	0.00376	0.06161	0.06161
60	1	0.125	0.0312	0.0078	0.0039	.....	0.22558	3.6967	3.6967
480	8	1	0.25	0.0625	0.0312	0.0078	1.80468	29.5737	29.5737
1920	32	4	1	0.25	0.125	0.0312	7.21875	118.2948	118.2948
7680	128	16	4	1	0.5	0.125	28.875	473.179	473.179
15360	256	32	8	2	1	0.25	57.75	946.358	946.358
61440	1024	128	32	8	4	1	231	3785.434	3785.434

TABLES OF WEIGHTS AND MEASURES (Continued)

METRIC MEASURE

MICRO-LITER	MILLI-LITER	CENTI-LITER	DECI-LITER	LITER	DEKA-LITER	HECTO-LITER	KILO-LITER	MEGA-LITER	EQUIVALENTS (APOTHECARIES' FLUID)
1	...	...	...	...	...	...	...	...	0.01623108 min.
10^3	1	...	...	...	...	...	...	...	16.23 min.
10^4	10	1	...	...	...	...	...	...	2.7 fl.dr.
10^5	100	10	1	...	...	...	...	...	3.38 fl.oz.
10^6	10^3	100	10	1	...	...	...	...	2.11 pts.
10^7	10^4	10^3	100	10	1	...	...	...	2.64 gal.
10^8	10^5	10^4	10^3	100	10	1	...	...	26.418 gals.
10^9	10^6	10^5	10^4	10^3	100	10	1	...	264.18 gals.
10^{12}	10^9	10^8	10^7	10^6	10^5	10^4	10^3	1	26418 gals.

1 liter = 2.113363738 pints (Apothecaries).

MEASURES OF LENGTH
METRIC MEASURE

MI-CRON	MILLI-METER	CENTI-METER	DECI-METER	METER	DEKA-METER	HECTO-METER	KILO-METER	MEGA-METER	EQUIVALENTS
1	0.001	10^{-4}	...	...	...	...	...	...	0.000039 inch
10^3	1	10^{-1}	...	...	...	...	...	...	0.03937 inch
10^4	10	1	...	...	...	...	...	...	0.3937 inch
10^5	100	10	1	...	...	...	...	...	3.937 inch
10^6	1000	100	10	1	...	...	...	...	39.37 inch
10^7	10^4	1000	100	10	1	...	...	...	10.9361 yards
10^8	10^5	10^4	1000	100	10	1	...	...	109.3612 yards
10^9	10^6	10^5	10^4	1000	1000	10	1	...	1093.6121 yards
10^{10}	10^7	10^6	10^5	10^4	1000	100	10	...	6.2137 miles
10^{12}	10^9	10^8	10^7	10^6	10^5	10^4	1000	1	621.370 miles

CONVERSION TABLES
AVOIRDUPOIS—METRIC WEIGHT

OUNCES	GRAMS	OUNCES	GRAMS	POUNDS	GRAMS	KILOGRAMS
1/16	1.772	7	198.447	1 (16 oz.)	453.59	
1/8	3.544	8	226.796	2	907.18	
1/4	7.088	9	255.146	3	1360.78	1.36
1/2	14.175	10	283.495	4	1814.37	1.81
1	28.350	11	311.845	5	2267.96	2.27
2	56.699	12	340.194	6	2721.55	2.72
3	85.049	13	368.544	7	3175.15	3.18
4	113.398	14	396.893	8	3628.74	3.63
5	141.748	15	425.243	9	4082.33	4.08
6	170.097	16 (1 lb.)	453.59	10	4535.92	4.54

METRIC—AVOIRDUPOIS WEIGHT

GRAMS	OUNCES	GRAMS	OUNCES	GRAMS	POUNDS
0.001 (1 mg.)	0.000035274	1	0.035274	1000 (1 kg.)	2.2046

TABLES OF WEIGHTS AND MEASURES (Continued)

APOTHECARIES'—METRIC WEIGHT

GRAINS	GRAMS	GRAINS	GRAMS	SCRUPLES	GRAMS
1/150	0.0004	2/5	0.03	1	1.296(1.3)
1/120	0.0005	1/2	0.032	2	2.592(2.6)
1/100	0.0006	3/5	0.04	3 (1 ℈)	3.888(3.9)
1/90	0.0007	2/3	0.043		
1/80	0.0008	3/4	0.05	DRAMS	GRAMS
1/64	0.001	7/8	0.057		
1/60	0.0011	1	0.065		
1/50	0.0013	1 1/2	0.097(0.1)	1	3.888
1/48	0.0014	2	0.12	2	7.776
1/40	0.0016	3	0.20	3	11.664
1/36	0.0018	4	0.24	4	15.552
1/32	0.002	5	0.30	5	19.440
1/30	0.0022	6	0.40	6	23.328
1/25	0.0026	7	0.45	7	27.216
1/20	0.003	8	0.50	8 (1 ℥)	31.103
1/16	0.004	9	0.60		
1/12	0.005	10	0.65	OUNCES	GRAMS
1/10	0.006	15	1.00		
1/9	0.007	20 (1 ℈)	1.30	1	31.103
1/8	0.008	30	2.00	2	62.207
1/7	0.009			3	93.310
1/6	0.01			4	124.414
1/5	0.013			5	155.517
1/4	0.016			6	186.621
1/3	0.02			7	217.724
				8	248.828
				9	279.931
				10	311.035
				11	342.138
				12 (1 lb.)	373.242

METRIC—APOTHECARIES' WEIGHT

MILLIGRAMS	GRAINS	GRAMS	GRAINS	GRAMS	EQUIVALENTS
1	0.015432	0.1	1.5432	10	2.572 drams
2	0.030864	0.2	3.0864	15	3.858 "
3	0.046296	0.3	4.6296	20	5.144 "
4	0.061728	0.4	6.1728	25	6.430 "
5	0.077160	0.5	7.7160	30	7.716 "
6	0.092592	0.6	9.2592	40	1.286 oz.
7	0.108024	0.7	10.8024	45	1.447 "
8	0.123456	0.8	12.3456	50	1.607 "
9	0.138888	0.9	13.8888	100	3.215 "
10	0.154320	1.0	15.4320	200	6.430 "
15	0.231480	1.5	23.1480	300	9.644 "
20	0.308640	2.0	30.8640	400	12.859 "
25	0.385800	2.5	38.5800	500	1.34 lb.
30	0.462960	3.0	46.2960	600	1.61 "
35	0.540120	3.5	54.0120	700	1.88 "
40	0.617280	4.0	61.728	800	2.14 "
45	0.694440	4.5	69.444	900	2.41 "
50	0.771600	5.0	77.162	1000	2.68 "
100	1.543240	10.0	154.324		

APOTHECARIES'—METRIC LIQUID MEASURE

MINIMS	MILLILITERS	FLUID DRAMS	MILLILITERS	FLUID OUNCES	MILLILITERS
1	0.06	1	3.70	1	29.57
2	0.12	2	7.39	2	59.15
3	0.19	3	11.09	3	88.72
4	0.25	4	14.79	4	118.29
5	0.31	5	18.48	5	147.87
10	0.62	6	22.18	6	177.44
15	0.92	7	25.88	7	207.01
20	1.23	8 (1 fl.oz.)	29.57	8	236.58
25	1.54			9	266.16
30	1.85			10	295.73
35	2.16			11	325.30
40	2.46			12	354.88
45	2.77			13	384.45
50	3.08			14	414.02
55	3.39			15	443.59
60 (1 fl.dr.)	3.70			16 (1 pt.)	473.17
				32 (1 qt.)	946.33
				128 (1 gal.)	3785.32

TABLES OF WEIGHTS AND MEASURES (*Concluded*)

METRIC—APOTHECARIES' LIQUID MEASURE

MILLILITERS	MINIMS	MILLILITERS	FLUID DRAMS	MILLILITERS	FLUID OUNCES
1	16.231	5	1.35	30	1.01
2	32.5	10	2.71	40	1.35
3	48.7	15	4.06	50	1.69
4	64.9	20	5.4	500	16.91
5	81.1	25	6.76	1000 (1 L.)	33.815
		30	7.1		

TABLE OF METRIC DOSES WITH APPROXIMATE APOTHECARY EQUIVALENTS

These *approximate* dose equivalents represent the quantities usually prescribed, under identical conditions, by physicians using, respectively, the metric system or the apothecary system of weights and measures. In labeling dosage forms in both the metric and the apothecary systems, if one is the approximate equivalent of the other, the approximate figure shall be enclosed in parentheses.

When prepared dosage forms such as tablets, capsules, pills, etc., are prescribed in the metric system, the pharmacist may dispense the corresponding *approximate* equivalent in the apothecary system, and vice versa, as indicated in the following table.

For the conversion of specific quantities in converting pharmaceutical formulas, exact equivalents must be used. In the compounding of prescriptions, the exact equivalents, rounded to three significant figures, should be used.

LIQUID MEASURE		LIQUID MEASURE	
METRIC	APPROXIMATE APOTHECARY EQUIVALENTS	METRIC	APPROXIMATE APOTHECARY EQUIVALENTS
1000 ml.	1 quart	3 ml.	45 minims
750 ml.	1 1/2 pints	2 ml.	30 minims
500 ml.	1 pint	1 ml.	15 minims
250 ml.	8 fluid ounces	0.75 ml.	12 minims
200 ml.	7 fluid ounces	0.6 ml.	10 minims
100 ml.	3 1/2 fluid ounces	0.5 ml.	8 minims
50 ml.	1 3/4 fluid ounces	0.3 ml.	5 minims
30 ml.	1 fluid ounce	0.25 ml.	4 minims
15 ml.	4 fluid drams	0.2 ml.	3 minims
10 ml.	2 1/2 fluid drams	0.1 ml.	1 1/2 minims
8 ml.	2 fluid drams	0.06 ml.	1 minim
5 ml.	1 1/4 fluid drams	0.05 ml.	3/4 minim
4 ml.	1 fluid dram	0.03 ml.	1/2 minim

WEIGHT		WEIGHT	
METRIC	APPROXIMATE APOTHECARY EQUIVALENTS	METRIC	APPROXIMATE APOTHECARY EQUIVALENTS
30 Gm.	1 ounce	30 mg.	1/2 grain
15 Gm.	4 drams	25 mg.	3/8 grain
10 Gm.	2 1/2 drams	20 mg.	1/3 grain
7.5 Gm.	2 drams	15 mg.	1/4 grain
6 Gm.	90 grains	12 mg.	1/5 grain
5 Gm.	75 grains	10 mg.	1/6 grain
4 Gm.	60 grains (1 dram)	8 mg.	1/8 grain
3 Gm.	45 grains	6 mg.	1/10 grain
2 Gm.	30 grains (1/2 dram)	5 mg.	1/12 grain
1.5 Gm.	22 grains	4 mg.	1/15 grain
1 Gm.	15 grains	3 mg.	1/20 grain
0.75 Gm.	12 grains	2 mg.	1/30 grain
0.6 Gm.	10 grains	1.5 mg.	1/40 grain
0.5 Gm.	7 1/2 grains	1.2 mg.	1/50 grain
0.4 Gm.	6 grains	1 mg.	1/60 grain
0.3 Gm.	5 grains	0.8 mg.	1/80 grain
0.25 Gm.	4 grains	0.6 mg.	1/100 grain
0.2 Gm.	3 grains	0.5 mg.	1/120 grain
0.15 Gm.	2 1/2 grains	0.4 mg.	1/150 grain
0.12 Gm.	2 grains	0.3 mg.	1/200 grain
0.1 Gm.	1 1/2 grains	0.25 mg.	1/250 grain
75 mg.	1 1/4 grains	0.2 mg.	1/300 grain
60 mg.	1 grain	0.15 mg.	1/400 grain
50 mg.	3/4 grain	0.12 mg.	1/500 grain
40 mg.	2/3 grain	0.1 mg.	1/600 grain

NOTE—A milliliter (ml.) is the equivalent of a cubic centimeter (cc.).

The above *approximate* dose equivalents have been adopted by the Pharmacopeia, National Formulary and New and Nonofficial Drugs, and these dose equivalents have the approval of the federal Food and Drug Administration.

AREA

Square Millimeters	Square Centimeters	Square Inches
1	0.01	0.00155
100	1	0.155
645.2	6.45	1

(From Guide to Dental Materials and Devices, 8th ed. American Dental Association, 1976–1978.)

DENSITY

Grams per Cubic Centimeter	Pounds per Cubic Foot
1	62.428
0.01602	1

(From Guide to Dental Materials and Devices, 8th ed. American Dental Association, 1976–1978.)

PRESSURE

Grams per Square Millimeter	Kilograms per Square Centimeter	Pounds per Square Inch
1	0.1000	1.4223
10	1	14.223
0.703	0.0703	1

(From Guide to Dental Materials and Devices, 8th ed. American Dental Association, 1976–1978.)

specific weight may be expressed in grams weight per cubic centimeter. **troy w.,** a system of weights commonly used for expressing quantities of precious metals and gems and, formerly, for bread, grain, etc., named after Troyes, France, where it was standard. Its units are pennyweight (24 grains), ounce (20 pennyweights), and pound (12 ounces). **w. in volume,** see PERCENT weight in volume. **w. in weight,** see PERCENT weight in weight.

Weil's basal layer (basal zone) [L. A. *Weil*, German dentist, 19th century] see under LAYER.

Weill-Marchesani syndrome [G. *Weill;* Oswald *Marchesani,* 1900–1952] Marchesani's SYNDROME.

Weinberg, Wilhelm [German physician, 1862–1937] see Hardy-Weinberg LAW.

Weisbach's angle [Albin *Weisbach,* Austrian anthropologist, 19th century] see under ANGLE.

Weiss, Nathan [Austrian physician, 1851–1883] see Chvostek-Weiss SIGN.

Welcher's angle sphenoid ANGLE.

welding (weld′ing) the joining or uniting of separate pieces of metal, usually with heat, by compression or fusion without the use of a solder. See also SOLDERING. **arc w.,** see *fusion w.* **cold w.,** union between two pieces of metal taking place at room temperature, as when completely cleaned surfaces of pure gold foil are brought into intimate contact under pressure. **fusion w.,** welding pieces of similar or dissimilar metals by joining the melted parts together which, on solidifying, will fuse by forming the primary (metallic) bond. Depending on the source of heat, fusion welding may be known as *arc, gas,* or *laser w.* **gas w.,** see *fusion w.* **laser w.,** see *fusion w.* **pressure w.,** the joining of two pieces of metal by applying pressure, usually with heat but without melting the metal, whereby the metal recrystallizes across the interface between the pieces. Gold foil can be welded under pressure at room temperature (cold w.), but most other metals require both heat and pressure. Called also *resistance w.* **resistance w.,** pressure w. **spot w.,** welding of localized regions on pieces of metals to be joined, by pressing them together, melting, and cooling under pressure.

Weller, Thomas H. [born 1915] an American physician; co-winner, with John F. Enders and Frederick C. Robbins, of the Nobel prize for medicine and physiology in 1954, for the discovery that poliomyelitis viruses multiply in human tissue.

Wells, Horace [1815–1848] an American dentist and discoverer in 1844 of surgical anesthesia through the inhalation of nitrous oxide gas.

wen (wen) 1. epidermal CYST. 2. sebaceous CYST.

Werdnig's disease [Guido *Werdnig,* Austrian physician] infantile muscular ATROPHY.

Werdnig-Hoffmann syndrome [G. *Werdnig;* Ernst *Hoffmann,* German neurologist, born 1868] infantile muscular ATROPHY.

Werlhof's disease, purpura [Paul Gottlieb *Werlhof,* German physician, 1699–1767] thrombocytopenic idiopathic PURPURA.

Werner's syndrome [Otto *Werner,* German physician] see under SYNDROME.

Wernicke's encephalopathy (disease) [Karl *Wernicke,* German neurologist, 1848–1905] see under ENCEPHALOPATHY.

Wernicke-Mann hemiplegia (type) [K. *Wernicke;* Ludwig *Mann,* German neurologist, 1866–1936] see under HEMIPLEGIA.

West's lacuna skull see under SKULL.

West-Engstler skull West's lacuna SKULL.

Weston crown see under CROWN.

wetting (wet′ing) 1. moistening, or soaking something. 2. covering of the surface of an object with a film or liquid. The liquid, by flowing into irregularities, increases the surface area of an object coming into intimate contact with another, thereby increasing its adhesive properties. Wetting occurs most readily on materials with high surface energy. Close packing of the structural organic groups and the presence of halogens may prevent wetting. Generally measured by determining the contact angle of the adhesive on the adherend.

Weyers' syndrome [Helmut *Weyers,* German physician] 1. irido-dental DYSPLASIA. 2. acrofacial DYSOSTOSIS. See also oculo-dento-osseous DYSPLASIA (Meyer-Schwickerath and Weyers syndrome).

Weyers-Fülling syndrome [H. *Weyers;* Georg *Fülling*] DYSPLASIA dentofacialis.

Weyers-Thier syndrome [H. *Weyers;* Carl Jörg *Thier*] oculovertebral DYSPLASIA.

Wh white; see color coding table at root canal THERAPY.

Wharton's duct [Thomas *Wharton,* English physician and anatomist, 1614–1673] submandibular DUCT.

wheal (wēl) a circumscribed, reddish, more or less transitory elevated lesion of the skin ranging in size from 0.5 to 10 cm, which is surrounded by an areola and accompanied by itching, tingling, or pricking sensation; considered to be a symptom of some allergic diseases.

wheel (wēl) 1. a circular frame or disk designed to revolve around a central axis. 2. a round cutting or polishing dental instrument of various sizes and thickness and made of different materials, which may be uniformly thick or knife-edged. It is mounted on a handpiece or angle mandrel and is driven by the dental engine. See also DISK and wheel BUR. **bristle w.,** a brush in the form of a wheel that is used in the dental lathe or dental engine for cleaning, smoothing, or polishing. **Burlew w.,** trademark for a knife-edged polishing wheel made of rubber impregnated with abrasive particles. Mounted on the mandrel of a dental handpiece, it is used for polishing metallic restorations and tooth surfaces. **carborundum w.,** a cutting wheel whose surface has been impregnated with carborundum (silicon carbide), that may be of medium or coarse grit; it may be rigid or flexible. **chamois w.,** one whose surface has been covered with chamois; used for polishing. **cotton w.,** one of soft cotton cloth; used for polishing. **diamond w.,** a cutting wheel whose surface has been impregnated with diamond chips. **felt w.,** a dental wheel made up of compressed felt, used to polish dentures. See also felt CONE. **grinding w.,** a flat, thick disk with an edge of varied widths, having carborundum or, less frequently, emery, as the abrading medium, which may be fastened to a mandrel and mounted in a handpiece for extensive grinding or cutting of teeth, or mounted on a stationary motor for shaping of dentures. See also dental DISK. **leather w.,** a polishing wheel whose surface is covered with leather. **rag w.,** a dental disk made up of several layers of cloth stitched together and wetted down with pumice; used to polish dentures. Called also *cloth disk.* **rubber w.,** a polishing wheel whose body is made of rubber and whose surface is impregnated with pumice or rouge. **wire w.,** one having short strands of steel or brass wire projecting from its surface; used for cleaning some types of instruments.

wheeze (wēz) a whistling sound made in breathing.

Whip-Mix articulator see under ARTICULATOR.

Whip-Mix Die-Rock trademark for a Class II *dental stone* (see under STONE).

Whip-Mix Microstone trademark for a Class I *dental stone* (see under STONE).

Whip-Mix Quickstone trademark for a Class I *dental stone* (see under STONE).

Whip-Mix Silky-Rock trademark for a Class II *dental stone* (see under STONE).

Whirl-a-Dent trademark for a magnetic stirrer type of *denture cleanser* (see under CLEANSER).

white (wīt) 1. reflecting all the rays of the spectrum; opposite of black. 2. a white dye. **English w.**, prepared calcium carbonate; see CALCIUM carbonate. **mineral w.**, gypsum. **Paris w.**, prepared calcium carbonate; see CALCIUM carbonate. **titanium w.**, TITANIUM dioxide.

White's disease [James Clarke *White*, American dermatologist, 1833–1916] KERATOSIS follicularis.

whitehead (wīt'hed) milium.

Whitehead's operation [Walter *Whitehead*, English surgeon, 1840–1913] see under OPERATION.

whiting (wīt'ing) a purified form of prepared calcium carbonate which has been ground and washed; used for making putty and as a polishing agent for dental materials. See also CALCIUM carbonate.

Whitmore's bacillus, disease [Royal *Whitmore*, American physician] see *Pseudomonas pseudomallei*, under PSEUDOMONAS, and MELIOIDOSIS.

Whitnall's tubercle see under TUBERCLE.

WHO World Health Organization; see under ORGANIZATION.

Wichmann's asthma [Johann Ernst *Wichmann*, German physician, 1740–1802] LARYNGISMUS stridulus.

Wickham's striae [Louis Frédéric *Wickham*, French dermatologist, 1861–1913] see under STRIA.

Widal, Georges Fernand Isidore [French physician, 1862–1927] see acquired hemolytic JAUNDICE (Hayem-Widal syndrome).

widener (wīd'en-er) a device for making something wider or broader. **orifice w.**, a hand-operated or engine-driven endodontic instrument for enlarging the coronal portion of the root canal. The most commonly used engine-driven wideners are the Gates-Glidden drill and Peeso drill. See illustration.

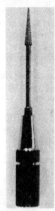

Hand-operated orifice widener. (From S. Cohen and R. C. Burns: Pathways of the Pulp. 2nd ed. St. Louis, The C. V. Mosby Co., 1980.)

Widman flap [L. *Widman*] see under FLAP.

width (width) the measurement of something from side to side; breadth; wideness. See also BREADTH. **anterior arch w.**, the width of the anterior dental arch, being the distance between the first permanent molars. **arch w.**, the width of the dental arch determined by measuring distances between the canines, between the first molars, and between the second bicuspids. **bicanine w.**, the maximum breadth measured at the lateral level of each canine tooth. Called also *bicanine breadth*. **bimolar w.**, the distance measured between the mesial buccal cusps of right and left molars, usually maxillary. Called also *bimolar breadth*. **posterior arch w.**, the width of the posterior dental arch, being the distance between the first molars.

Wiebrecht, Albert T. [American orthodontist] a pioneer in the use of the Crozat appliance.

Wiedemann, Hans Rudolf [German physician] see Beckwith-Wiedemann SYNDROME and cloverleaf SKULL (Holtermüller-Wiedemann syndrome).

Wiener classification, nomenclature [Alexander *Wiener*, American hematologist and immunologist, born 1907; co-discoverer with Landsteiner of the Rh factor] see under FACTOR, and see Rh blood groups, under BLOOD GROUP.

Wien's displacement law see under LAW.

Wiethe, Camillo see Urbach-Wiethe SYNDROME.

Wiggle-Bug trademark for a *mechanical triturator* (see under TRITURATOR).

Wig-l-Bug trademark for a dual speed *mechanical triturator* (see under TRITURATOR], operating at 3400 and 4450 rpm.

Wilde's incision [Sir William Robert *Wilde*, Irish surgeon, 1815–1876] see under INCISION.

Wilding, S. William an English chemist who discovered alginate impression materials (see impression material, irreversible hydrocolloid, under MATERIAL).

wilkinite (wil'kin-īt) bentonite.

Wilkins, Maurice Hugh Frederick [born 1916] an English biochemist; co-winner, with Francis Harry Compton Crick and James Dewey Watson, of the Nobel prize for medicine and physiology in 1962, for discovery of the molecular structure of deoxyribonucleic acid.

Wilkinson 8M trademark for a medium hard *dental casting gold alloy* (see under GOLD).

Wilkinson 9M trademark for a hard *dental casting gold alloy* (see under GOLD).

Wilkinson 2S trademark for a soft *dental casting gold alloy* (see under GOLD).

Willbutamide trademark for *tolbutamide*.

Willebrand's syndrome [E. A. von *Willebrand*, Finnish physician, 1870–1949] Willebrand-Jürgens SYNDROME.

Willebrand-Jurgens syndrome [E. A. von *Willebrand*; Rudolph *Jürgens*, 1898–1961] see under SYNDROME.

Willi, H. [Swiss physician] see Prader-Willi SYNDROME.

Williams, H. see Neurohr-Williams SHOE.

Williams No. 2 trademark for a high noble metal dental wrought gold wire alloy.

Williams No. 4 trademark for a low noble metal dental wrought gold wire alloy.

Williams No. 70 trademark for a low noble metal dental wrought gold wire alloy.

Williams' periodontal probe see Fox-Williams PROBE.

Williams surveyor see under SURVEYOR.

Williams' syndrome [J.C.P. Williams] elfin facies SYNDROME.

Williams-Barrat syndrome [J. C. P. *Williams*] elfin facies SYNDROME.

Willis, nerve of [Thomas *Willis*, English anatomist and physician, 1621–1675] accessory NERVE.

Wilpo trademark for *phentermine hydrochloride* (see under PHENTERMINE).

Wilson's curve CURVE of Wilson.

Wilson's disease [Samuel Alexander Kinnier *Wilson*, English neurologist, 1878–1936] hepatolenticular DEGENERATION.

Winchester's syndrome [Patricia *Winchester*, American physician] see under SYNDROME.

window (win'do) [L. *fenestra*] a circumscribed opening in a plane surface. **beryllium w.**, an opening or window of an x-ray tube, made of beryllium, through which x-rays pass to the outside.

windowing (win'do-ing) surgical creation of an opening in the cortex of a bone. See FENESTRATION.

windpipe (wind'pīp) trachea.

wing (wing) [L. *ala*] 1. the modified anterior appendage of birds, which is the organ of flight. 2. a structure or part resembling the wing of a bird. Called also *ala*. **bite w.**, bitewing. **great w. of sphenoid bone**, a large wing-shaped process arising from the lateral aspect of the posterior part of the body of the sphenoid bone, the posterior part of each wing forming a triangular process fitting in the angle between the squama and the petrous part of the temporal bone. The cerebral (superior) surface provides the anterior part of the floor of the middle cranial fossa and supports convolutions of the temporal lobe. The orbital surface provides the principal part of the lateral wall of the orbit. Its superior serrated edge articulates with the orbital plate of the frontal bone; the inferior border forms the posterior boundary of the inferior orbital fissure; and the lateral border articulates with the zygomatic bone. A grooved surface below the medial part of the superior orbital fissure forms the posterior wall of the pterygopalatine fossa. The margin near the body forms the anterior wall of the foramen lacerum. Called also *lateral w. of sphenoid bone, ala magna ossis sphenoidalis, ala major ossis sphenoidalis* [NA], *ala temporalis ossis sphenoidalis*, and *alisphenoid bone*. See illustration at sphenoid BONE. **Ingrassia's w.**, a small or great wing of the sphenoid bone. **lateral w. of sphenoid bone**, great w. of sphenoid bone. **lesser w. of sphenoid bone**, small w. of sphenoid bone. **minor w. of sphenoid bone**, small w. of sphenoid bone. **orbital w. of sphenoid bone**, small w. of sphenoid bone. **small w. of sphenoid bone**, one of the two thin triangular plates of bone that arise from the superior and anterior parts of the·body of the sphenoid bone and project laterally, ending in sharp points. Its flat superior surface supports parts of the frontal lobe and its inferior surface forms the roof of the orbit and provides the superior boundary of the superior orbital fissure. Its smooth posterior border fits into the lateral fissure of the brain and its medial end forms the anterior clinoid process, giving attachment to the tentorium cerebelli. An opening between the roots, which connects it to the body, is known as the *optic canal* and transmits the optic nerve and ophthalmic artery. Called also *lesser w. of sphenoid bone, minor w. of sphenoid bone, orbital w. of sphenoid bone, ala minor ossis sphenoidalis* [NA], *ala parva ossis sphenoidalis, ensiform process of sphenoid bone, Ingrassia's apophysis, Ingrassia's process,* and *xiphoid process of sphenoid bone.* See illustration at sphenoid BONE.

winking (wingk'ing) quick closing and opening of the eyelids. **jaw w.,** involuntary closing movement of the eyelid occasionally associated with movements of the mandible. See Gunn's SYNDROME.

Winstrol trademark for *stanozolol.*

wintergreen (win'ter-grēn) an ericaceous plant *Gaultheria procumbens,* of North America. **oil of w.,** methyl SALICYLATE.

wire (wīr) 1. a slender, flexible filament of metal or alloy, usually circular but also rectangular, which is produced in a variety of diameters. Used in surgery and dentistry. See also *arch w.* 2. to insert wires into a body structure, as into a broken bone to immobilize the fragments, or into an aneurysm to promote the formation of clots. **arch w.,** an austenitic, stainless steel, orthodontic wire, usually round, ribbon, or rectangular in shape, which has been heat-treated and cold-drawn to its proper shape to give it the required properties of resiliency, toughness, and tensile strength. It is attached to molar bands or an orthodontic appliance, and applied around the dental arch to serve in controlling and forcing the movement of the teeth in orthodontic therapy. Called also *orthodontic w.* **arch w., ideal,** arch wire having a configuration that conforms as closely as possible to the desired ultimate shape of the dental arch for a particular individual. **diagnostic w.,** measuring w. **Gigli's w.,** Gigli's SAW. **Gilmer w.,** Gilmer's SPLINT. **Jelenko super w.,** trademark for a high noble metal dental wrought gold wire alloy. **Kirschner w.,** a surgical steel wire with sharp ends for transfixion of fractured bones and for obtaining traction in fractures; it is inserted through the soft parts of the bone and held tight in a clamp. **ideal arch w.,** arch w., ideal. **labial w.,** a structure of a removable orthodontic appliance made of 0.6-mm stainless steel wire of high tensile strength, its arms coming through the embrasure between the canine and lateral incisors in the maxillary arch, and between the canines and first premolar in the mandibular arch. It serves primarily for moving teeth in the lingual direction, retruding the anterior teeth and closing spaces, having also a vertical component of force. Called also labial bow. **ligature w.,** a soft thin wire used to tie an arch wire to band attachments or brackets in an orthodontic appliance. **measuring w.,** a wire placed in a root canal for the determination of its length; established on the roentgenogram. Called also *diagnostic w.* **Mowrey No. 1 w.,** trademark for a low noble metal dental wrought gold wire alloy. **Mowrey 12% w.,** trademark for a high noble metal dental wrought gold wire alloy. **orthodontic w.,** arch w. **Risdon's w.,** a wire arch bar tied in the midline, used in midline fractures of the mandible. **separating w.,** a brass wire usually threaded between two teeth having tight contact in an effort to wedge them slightly apart before fitting a band in the application of an orthodontic appliance. See also SEPARATION. **twin w.,** twin wire APPLIANCE. **wrought w.,** a wire formed by drawing a cast structure through a die; used for partial dentures and orthodontic appliances.

wiring (wīr'ing) the fixing into position by means of wire, as of segments of a fractured bone. **Baudens w.,** circumferential w. **Black's w.,** a modified method of circumferential wiring around the bone and over a splint in the mouth. A double thread is passed around the bone in two places by means of doubly threaded needle, the thread forming a loop, which is used to draw the wire around the bone. After reduction of the bone fragments, the wire is twisted over the gutta-percha or vulcanite splint. **Buck w.,** interosseous w. **circumferential w., circummandibular w., circumzygomatic w.,** a technique for fixation of mandibular fractures in which wires are passed around a section of bone with the ends exiting into the oral cavity and then around a fixed intraoral splint. Called also *Baudens w.* **continuous loop w.,** wiring of the teeth for the reduction and fixation of jaw bone fractures, by using a single length of wire to form loops on both the maxillary and mandibular teeth, over which intermaxillary elastic can be placed. Called also *Stout w.* and *Stout continuous w.* **craniofacial suspension w.,** wiring of noncontiguous areas of bone (piriform aperture, zygomatic arch, zygomatic process of the frontal bone) for the support of fractured jaw segments. **Gilmer w.,** a method of intermaxillary fixation in which single opposing teeth are wired circumferentially and the wires twisted together. **interosseous w.,** fixation of fractured bones by passing a malleable wire through fractured segments and twisting their ends together. Called also *Buck w.* **Ivy loop w.,** wiring of adjacent teeth in groups of two to provide an attachment for intermaxillary elastics. **perialveolar w.,** the fixing of a splint to the maxillary arch by passing a wire through the alveolar process from the buccal plate to the palate. **piriform aperture w.,** wiring through the maxillary bones at the piriform aperture for the stabilization of fractures of the jaws. **Robert w.,** a modified method of circumferential wiring over a small lead plate. **Stout w., Stout continuous w.,** continuous loop w.

Wiron S trademark for a nickel-chromium base-metal crown and bridge alloy.

Wironium trademark for a high-fusing chromium-cobalt casting alloy.

Wiskott-Aldrich syndrome [Arthur *Wiskott;* Robert A. *Aldrich*] see under SYNDROME.

withdrawal (with-draw'al) 1. a pathological retreat from external reality. 2. abstention from drugs to which one is habituated or addicted. Also, denoting the symptoms occasioned by such withdrawal.

withhold (with-hōld') 1. to hold back; to restrain or check. 2. in dental insurance, an amount which the Delta Dental Plan withholds from payments made to participating dentists for covered services, to raise start-up funds for fulfillment of contracts and to safeguard against other unusual financial circumstances. When the withheld funds are no longer needed, they are phased out. See also CHARGE and RETENTION (6).

Witkop-Von Sallmann syndrome [Carl J. *Witkop,* American dentist, born 1920; Ludwig *Von Sallmann,* American physician, born 1892] hereditary benign intraepithelial DYSKERATOSIS.

Wolff, Kaspar Friedrich [1733–1794] a German anatomist and embryologist. See WOLFFIAN.

Wolff's law [Julius *Wolff,* German anatomist, 1836–1902] see under LAW.

wolffian (woolf'e-an) named after or described by Kaspar Friedrich *Wolff,* as wolffian body (see MESONEPHROS) and wolffian duct (see mesonephrotic DUCT).

wolfram (wool'fram) tungsten.

wood (wood) the hard fibrous substance making up most of the stem and branches of a tree. **w. sugar,** xylose.

Woods-Fildes theory [D. D. *Woods;* P. *Fildes*] see under THEORY.

Woodson elevator see under ELEVATOR.

Wooffendale, Robert [1742–1828] an English-born early American dentist. He served as dentist to King George III before emigrating to the colonies. Wooffendale is believed to be the second American dentist after John Baker.

wool (wool) [L. *lana*] the hair of sheep and lambs; by extension applied to any material existing as fine threads. **w. fat,** lanolin.

Woolco see under DENTIFRICE.

woorali (woo-ra'le) curare.

woorari (woo-rar'e) curare.

work (werk) 1. labor; toil; exertion, effort, or activity, mental or physical, expended to accomplish or produce something. 2. to be handled, processed, or changed into a specified state. **cold w.,** working a metal at room temperature. See strain HARDENING. **w. hardening,** strain HARDENING.

Worm, Olaus [1588–1654] a Danish anatomist. See WORMIAN.

wormian (wer'me-an) described by Olaus *Worm,* as wormian bones (see under BONE).

wound (woond) [L. *vulnus*] an injury to the body caused by physical means, with disruption of the normal continuity of body structures. **aseptic w.,** one which is not infected. **contused w.,** one in which the skin is unbroken. **w. healing,** see HEALING. **incised w.,** one made by a cutting instrument. **lacerated w.,** one in which the tissues are torn or mangled by a dull or blunt instrument. **nonpenetrating w.,** one in which there is no disruption of the skin but there is injury to underlying structures. **open w.,** one that communicates with the atmosphere by direct exposure or with a mucosal or cutaneous surface. **penetrating w.,** one caused by a sharp, usually slender object, such as a nail or ice pick, which passes through the skin into the underlying tissues. Called also *puncture w.* **perforating w.,** a penetrating wound which extends into a viscus or body cavity. **poisoned w.,** one into which septic matter has been introduced. **puncture w.,**

penetrating w. **septic w.,** one that is infected. **seton w.,** one which enters and exits on the same side of the injured part. **subcutaneous w.,** one which involves only the skin and subcutaneous tissue. **surgical w.,** a wound produced by surgical incision. **tangential w.,** an oblique glancing wound which results in one edge being undercut.

W/P ratio see under RATIO.

W-plasty see under PLASTY.

Wright's stain see under STAIN.

Wrisberg's cartilage, tubercle [Heinrich August *Wrisberg*, German anatomist, 1739–1808] see cuneiform CARTILAGE and cuneiform TUBERCLE.

writer (rīt'er) one is engaged in writing, or an instrument or device used for writing or recording. **cusp w.,** a device that simulates mandibular movements and graphically records op-

timum cusp height and angulations which are in harmony with various occlusal determinants.

wrought (rawt) pertaining to a metal shaped by hammering, rolling, or drawing, rather than by casting. See wrought METAL.

wryneck (ri'neck) torticollis.

wt. weight.

w/v PERCENT weight in volume.

w/w PERCENT weight in weight.

Wyamine trademark for *mephentermine.*

X

X 1. see X chromosome, under CHROMOSOME. See also CHROMOSOME nomenclature. 2. Kienbock UNIT.

xanthelasma (zan"thel-az'mah) [*xantho-* + Gr. *elasma* plate] a common type of xanthoma of the eyelids, characterized by yellowish spots or plaques. Called also *xanthoma palpebrarum* and *plane xanthoma.*

xanthine (zan'thēn) [Gr. *xanthos* yellow; named for the yellow color of its nitrates] a compound, 2,6-dioxopurine, occurring as a yellowish, white powder that is soluble in potassium hydroxide, but not in water and acids. Xanthine derivatives are central stimulants and their pharmacological effects include stimulation of the central nervous system, action on the kidneys, resulting in diuresis, stimulation of the cardiac muscle, and relaxation of the smooth muscles. The xanthines include caffeine, theophylline, and theobromine. The stimulating action of xanthines may counteract the effect of sedatives. **x. b's,** *purine* bases; see under BASE. **dimethyl x.,** theobromine. **methyl x's,** methyl xanthine derivatives, including caffeine, theophylline, and theobromine. **trimethyl x.,** caffeine.

xantho- [Gr. *xanthos* yellow] a combining form meaning yellow.

xanthogranuloma (zan"tho-gran"u-lo'mah) a tumor having the histologic characteristics of both granuloma and xanthoma.

xanthoma (zan-tho'mah) [*xantho-* + *-oma*] a nodular yellow or orange tumor, presenting a plaquelike soft elevation containing giant cells, fibroblasts, and nonspecific inflammatory infiltrate. It is usually found on the skin and mucous membranes, most often on the eyelids, in the wrinkles and creases of the body, and over the pressure points, such as the buttocks, elbows, and knees. Xanthoma is not considered a true neoplasm but appears to represent the phagocytosis of circulating lipids by local mesenchymal cells in faulty lipid metabolism; it is usually a symptom of hyperlipemia. See also XANTHOMATOSIS. **craniohypophyseal x.,** Hand-Schüller-Christian DISEASE. **diabetic x., x. diabetico'rum,** eruptive xanthoma occurring in patients with diabetes mellitus, due to faulty carbohydrate metabolism in the liver. **x. dissemina'tum,** a chronic, benign, normolipoproteinemic form of xanthomatosis, characterized by the development of small, yellowish brown papules and plaques appearing chiefly on the flexor surfaces, such as the axillary folds and groin, but also on the face and mucous membrane of the oropharynx and larynx. Mild diabetes insipidus and hepatic complications may occur. Blood cholesterol and total lipids are usually normal or even subnormal. Called also *disseminated xanthomatosis.* **eruptive x.,** xanthomatosis occurring in the presence of severe hyperlipemia, presenting a single or a group of yellowish papules and nodules surrounded by an inflammatory halo; telangiectatic vesicles may appear on the papules. The entire body may be affected but the flexor surfaces of the extremities, trunk, neck, and face are the most common sites. Pruritus is sometimes severe, and arteriosclerosis and coronary complications are frequent. Called also *eruptive xanthomatosis.* **familial x.,** HYPERLIPOPROTEINEMIA II. **x. palpebra'rum, plane x.,** xanthelasma. **x. tubero'sum mul'tiplex,** HYPERLIPOPROTEINEMIA II. **verruciform x.,** a warty lesion of the oral mucosa found most commonly on the lower alveolar ridge, but other parts may be involved. It has either a normal or reddish color and a rough, pebbly surface, with either a sessile or pedunculated base; a typical lesion varies in size from 2 to 15 mm, and is virtually asymptomatic, except for slight tenderness. Histologically, it is covered with a layer of parakeratin of varying thickness, which penetrates into the epithelium, sometimes containing bacterial colonies. The presence of large, swollen foam cells is the typical pathological feature.

xanthomatosis (zan"tho-mah-to'sis) [*xanthoma* + *-osis*] the presence of multiple xanthomas, usually occurring as a complication of lipid metabolism disorders. **disseminated x.,** XANTHOMA disseminatum. **eruptive x.,** eruptive XANTHOMA. **familial hypercholesterolemic x.,** HYPERLIPOPROTEINEMIA II. **normocholesteremic x.,** any condition, such as xanthoma disseminatum, Hand-Schüller-Christian disease, and eosinophilic granuloma, characterized by development of xanthomas in normocholesteremic patients.

Xanthomonas (zan"tho-mo'nas) [Gr. *xanthos* yellow + *monas* unit] a genus of gram-negative, aerobic rod-shaped bacteria of the family Pseudomonadaceae, which produce a yellow pigment; most species are plant pathogens.

xanthosine (zan'tho-sin) a nucleoside, xanthine-9-ribofuranoside, which on hydrolysis yields xanthine and ribose.

xanthosis (zan-tho'sis) [Gr. *xanthos* yellow + *-osis*] a yellowish discoloration; degeneration with yellowish pigmentation. **x. sep'tum na'si,** yellow pigmentation of the mucous membrane of the nose, due to degeneration of the blood after hemorrhage.

Xantopren trademark for a *silicone impression material* (see under MATERIAL).

X-bite crossbite.

Xe xenon.

Xenagol trademark for *phenazocine hydrobromide* (see under PHENAZOCINE).

xeno- [Gr. *xenos* a guest-friend; a stranger or foreigner] a combining form meaning strange, or denoting relationship to foreign material.

xenoantigen (zen"o-an'tĭ-jen) [*xeno-* + *antigen*] xenogeneic ANTIGEN.

xenocytophilic (zen"o-si"to-fil'ik) [*xeno-* + Gr. *kytos* a hollow vessel + *philein* to love] having an affinity for cells derived from a different species, as in xenocytophilic antibodies; see cytotropic ANTIBODY.

xenogeneic (zen"o-jě-ne'ik) [*xeno-* + Gr. *genos* kind] denoting individuals or tissues from different species. Called also *heterogeneic, heterologous,* and *xenogenic.* Cf. ALLOGENEIC.

xenogenic (zen-oj'ě-nik) [*xeno-* + Gr. *gennan* to produce] 1. produced or developed in the host by action on the host's body. 2. originating outside the organism or from material or substance introduced into the organism. Called also *xenogenous.* 3. xenogeneic.

xenogenous (zen-oj'ě-nus) [*xeno-* + Gr. *gennan* to produce] xenogenic.

xenograf (zen'o-graft) [*xeno-* + *graft*] heterologous GRAFT.

xenon (ze'non) [Gr. *xenos* stranger] a noble gas. Symbol, Xe; atomic number, 54; atomic weight, 131.30; density (gas), 5.887 gm/l; specific gravity (liquid at −109°C), 3.52; valence, usually 0; group 0 of the periodic table. Naturally occurring isotopes include 124, 126, 128–132, 134, and 136; artificial radioactive isotopes are 118–123, 125, 127, 133, 135, and 137–144. Xenon is a colorless, odorless, nontoxic gas that is chemically unreactive, but not completely inert. Used experimentally as an anesthetic. **x.-133,** ^{133}Xe, an artificial radioactive isotope of xenon, having a half-life of 5.27 days and emitting beta rays. Used as a radioactive tracer in heart disease diagnosis, blood flow determination, and pulmonary function tests.

xero- [Gr. *xēros* dry] a combining form meaning dry, or denoting relationship to dryness.

xeroderma (ze"ro-der'mah) [*xero-* + Gr. *derma* skin] excessive dryness of the skin. See ICHTHYOSIS.

xeromycteria (ze"ro-mik-te're-ah) [*xero-* + Gr. *myktēr* nose] abnormal dryness of the nasal mucous membrane.

xeroradiography (ze″ro-ra″de-og′rah-fe) [*xero- + radiography*] a dry, photoelectric process for recording x-ray images, produced on a selenium-coated aluminum plate. Selenium becomes photosensitive after exposure to negative or positive electric charges produced by exposure to x-rays. Development of exposed plates is done by blowing a fine electrically charged powder over its surface; the image being formed by the electrostatic attraction and repulsion of the powder particles. Positively charged selenium shows the areas of greatest density as dark blue; the negatively charged plate presents the areas of greatest density as light blue or white. The image transferred to paper may be viewed without translumination.

xerosis (ze-ro′sis) [Gr. *xērosis*] abnormal dryness, as of the eye, skin, or mouth.

xerostomia (ze″ro-sto′me-ah) [*xero- + Gr. stoma* mouth *+ -ia*] dryness of the mouth from salivary gland dysfunction. In severe deficiency or total lack of saliva, the condition may be associated with atrophy of the oral mucosa, cracking of the lips, fissuring of the corners of the mouth, and fissuring, cracking, denudation, and burning sensation of the tongue. When associated with keratoconjunctivitis sicca and rheumatoid arthritis in menopausal women, it is known as *Sjögren's syndrome;* when associated with bilateral hypertrophy of the salivary glands and sometimes the lacrimal glands, as *Mikulicz's disease.*

xiphoid (zif′oid) [Gr. *xiphos* sword *+ eidos* form] shaped like a sword.

XO symbol for the presence of only one sex chromosome, the other X or the Y chromosome being absent.

X-Omat trademark for a large-capacity automatic film processor.

x-ray (eks′ra) see x-rays, under RAY.

XTE xeroderma-talipes-enamel defect syndrome. See under SYNDROME.

xylan (zi′lan) a hemicellulose in trees and industrial wastes.

Xylestesin trademark for *lidocaine.*

xylitol (zi′lĭ-tol) an alcohol derivative of xylose, 1,2,3,4,5-pentahydroxypentane, occurring as a white, odorless, crystalline powder with a sweet taste, having the same caloric content as sucrose. It is readily soluble in water and sparingly in alcohol. Experimental studies in animals and longitudinal studies, in which chewing gums containing sucrose and xylitol were compared in adults, indicate that xylitol may possess non-cariogenic or, possibly, anticariogenic properties, but this view is not generally accepted. Used as a sweetener and osmotic laxative.

Xylocaine trademark for *lidocaine.*

xylol (zi′lol) xylene.

Xylonest trademark for *prilocaine hydrochloride* (see under PRILOCAINE).

xylose (zi′lōs) a pentose (aldose), which is not found in free state but in the form of xylan. It is also found in association with cellulose and as a part of glycosides. Xylose occurs in the mucopolysaccharides of connective tissue and sometimes in the urine. Called also *wood sugar.* See XYLITOL.

Xylotox trademark for *lidocaine.*

xyster (zis′ter) [Gr. *xystēr* a scraper] a surgeon's file or raspatory.

Y

Y 1. yttrium. 2. see Y chromosome, under CHROMOSOME; see also CHROMOSOME nomenclature.

Yankauer's mask see under MASK.

yard (yard) a unit of length, being equivalent to 3 feet, 36 inches, or 86.44 centimeters. Abbreviated *yd.* See also *Tables of Weights and Measures* at WEIGHT.

yato-byo (yah″to-bi′yo) [Japanese *ya* wild, or field *+ to* rabbit, or hare *+ byo* disease] Ohara's DISEASE.

yaw (yaw) a lesion of yaws. **mother y.,** one of the primary cutaneous lesions of yaws.

yawning (yawn′ing) a deep, involuntary inspiration with the mouth open, often accompanied by the act of stretching. Sometimes a cause of temporomandibular joint dislocation.

yaws (yawz) an infectious nonvenereal disease caused by *Treponema pertenue,* characterized by the presence of raspberry-like lesions. Endemic in certain tropical areas, it may begin in childhood. The primary lesions ("mother yaws") are usually formed on the lower parts of the legs by the fusing of several papules into large lesions covered by an amber-yellow crust, which disappear after a few months, leaving atrophic and depigmented areas. In the second stage, the lesions are irregularly disseminated, small reddish papules, which leave furfuraceous patches. The tertiary lesions are characterized by gummatous nodules with deep ulcers. Oral involvement may occur in all three stages; papillomatous lesions and weeping plaques may be found on the oral and labial mucosa, palate, and tonsils. Mutilating rhinopharyngitis, progressively destroying the soft tissue, cartilage, and bones of the nose, nasopharynx, and palate, frequently leading to death, is the most serious complication. Changes in the mandible, maxilla, and other bones also have been reported. Called also *bouba, frambesia, parangi,* and *polypapilloma tropicum.* See also GOUNDOU. **forest y.,** mucocutaneous LEISHMANIASIS.

Yb ytterbium.

yd yard.

year (yēr) a period of 365 or 366 days, in the Gregorian calendar, divided into 12 calendar months and 52 weeks, and beginning on January 1 and ending on December 31. Called also *calendar y.* See also *fiscal y.* **benefit y.,** see benefit PERIOD. **calendar y.,** see *year.* **contract y., policy y., coverage y.,** benefit PERIOD. **fiscal y.,** any 12-month period for which annual accounts are kept, which may begin from any agreed upon date. Abbreviated *FY.* **policy y.,** see benefit PERIOD.

yeast (yest) a general term for a fungus occurring as a unicellular, nucleated organism that usually reproduces by budding, although some yeasts may reproduce by fission, many producing

mycelia or pseudomycelia. On the basis of sexual spore formation, yeasts may be classified in three fungal classes: the basidiospore-forming yeasts (class Basidiomycetes), the ascospore-forming yeasts (class Ascomycetes), and the asporogenous yeasts (certain of the Deuteromycetes [Fungi Imperfecti]). The pathogenic yeasts are deuteromycetes and include the genera: *Candida, Cryptococcus, Geotrichum, Malassezia, Rhodotorula,* and *Trichosporon.* **bakers' y., brewers' y.,** a true fungus, *Saccharomyces cerevisiae,* of the class of Ascomycetes, which produces carbon dioxide and alcohol during fermentation. The organisms occur in two strains, those found in the froth on the surface of the fermenting mixture, which are used for baking bread, and those which sink to the bottom of the mixture, which are used for brewing beer and making alcoholic beverages. **imperfect y's,** single-celled round forms of the Deuteromycetes (Fungi Imperfecti). **perfect y's,** see perfect fungi, under FUNGUS.

Yel yellow; see color coding table at root canal THERAPY.

Yersin, Alexandre Emil Jean [1863–1943] a Swiss bacteriologist who, with Roux, first described bacterial toxin.

Yersinia (yer-sin′e-ah) [named after A. E. J. *Yersin*] a genus of gram-negative, facultatively anaerobic bacteria of the family Enterobacteriaceae, made up of nonencapsulated, nonmotile or motile ovoid cells or rods, about 0.5 to 1.0 μm in length by 1.0 to 2.0 μm in width. **Y. pes′tis,** a species made up of nonmotile, coccoid, oval, or rod-shaped cells with surface slime layers or capsules which render them resistant to phagocytosis; involution forms are common. The organisms are uniformly gram-negative and show a tendency toward polar staining, i.e., heavily stained areas at the ends of the cells separated by a lightly stained area in the center. The species causes plague in man and rats and other rodents, being transmitted from rodent to rodent and from rodent to man by rat fleas. It has been isolated from buboes, blood, sputum, and lung exudate of infected individuals, and also has been isolated from the throats of healthy carriers. Called also *Bacillus pestis, Bacterium pestis, Pasteurella pestis, Pestisella pestis,* and *plague bacillus.* **Y. pseudotuberculo′sis,** a species that is quite similar to the plague bacillus, which causes a fatal disease of rodents. It may cause human infection, most often involving the bowel, often associated with mesenteric lymphangitis, simulating acute appendicitis; also isolated from healthy human carriers. Called also *Bacterium pseudotuberculosis, Pasteurella pseudotuberculosis,* and *Shigella pseudotuberculosis.*

-yl [Gr. *hylē* matter of substance] a chemical suffix signifying a radical, particularly a univalent hydrocarbon radical.

-ylene a chemical suffix used to denote a bivalent hydrocarbon radical.

-yne a chemical suffix used to denote an alkyne.

yogurt (yo′goort) a form of curdled milk, produced by fermentation with organisms of the genus *Lactobacillus*.

yolk (yok) [L. *vitellus*] the stored nutrient of the oocyte (ovum). See also yolk SAC.

Young frame see under FRAME.

Young's rule [Thomas *Young*, English physician, physicist, mathematician and philologist] see under RULE.

Younger-Goode curet see under CURET.

ytterbium (i′ter′be-um) [named after *Ytterby*, a village in Sweden] a rare earth. Symbol, Yb; atomic number, 70; atomic weight, 173.04; melting point, 824°C; specific gravity, 7.01; valences, 2, 3. It has seven naturally occurring isotopes: 168, and 170–176; artificial radioactive isotopes include 154, 155, 162, 164–167, 169, 175, and 177. Ytterbium occurs as a bright silvery lustrous, soft, readily malleable and ductile metal, which is attacked and dissolved by mineral acids and reacts with water. There are two allotropic forms of ytterbium; the alpha form with face-centered cubic modification at room temperature, and the beta form with body-centered cubic form at high temperatures. It is relatively nontoxic and is used in chemical research and as a portable source of x-rays.

yttrium (i′tre-um) [named after *Ytterby*, a village in Sweden] a metallic element found in association with the rare earths. Symbol, Y; atomic number, 39; atomic weight, 88.9059; specific gravity, 4.469; melting point, 1522°C; valence, 3; group IIIB of the periodic table. ^{89}Y is the only naturally occurring isotope; artificial radioactive isotopes include 82–88 and 90–96. It occurs as an iron-gray, lustrous powder that darkens on exposure to light, and is soluble in dilute acids and potassium hydroxide solution and decomposes water. Used in nuclear and electronic technologies, in iron and other alloys, and in various industrial products.

Z

Z 1. atomic NUMBER. 2. impedance.

Zahorsky's disease [John *Zahorsky*, American pediatrician, born 1871] herpangina.

Zambusch see VON ZAMBUSCH.

Zarontin trademark for *ethosuximide*.

Zaroxolyn trademark for *metolazone*.

Zebacem trademark for a *zinc oxide–eugenol cement* (see under CEMENT) reinforced with aluminum oxide.

zein (ze′in) a prolamin obtained from corn. It is a yellowish, tasteless substance, having a molecular weight of about 40,000, which does not contain cystine, lysine, or tryptophan and is soluble in dilute alcohol but not in water and absolute alcohol. Used in producing edible coating for foodstuffs and in various industrial processes.

Zeiss, Carl [German optician, 1816–1888] see Thoma-Zeiss counting CHAMBER.

Zellweger, H. see Fanconi-Albertini-Zellweger SYNDROME.

Zene Artzney the title of the first monographic work, published in 1530 by an unknown author; it was devoted entirely to the subject of dentistry and written in German, instead of the then customary Latin.

Zenker's diverticulum [Friedrich Albert von *Zenker*, German pathologist, 1825–1898] pharyngoesophageal DIVERTICULUM.

Zephiran trademark for *benzalkonium chloride* (see under BENZALKONIUM).

zero (ze′ro) [It. "naught"] 1. the numerical symbol 0; the number between the set of positive numbers and a set of negative numbers. 2. the point on a thermometer scale at which the graduation begins. The zero of the Celsius (centigrade) and Réamur temperature scales (see under SCALE) is the ice point; that of the Fahrenheit scale is 32 degrees below the ice point. **absolute z.,** a hypothetical point where all atomic vibration ceases, being the lowest attainable temperature; it is designated as 0° on the Kelvin and Rankine scales, equivalent to $-273.15°$ C or $-459.67°$ F. See also absolute TEMPERATURE. **0, 00, 000,** designations of the degree of fineness of particles on an abrasive paper; see ABRASIVE (2).

Zest Anchor system attachment (Anchor system) see under ATTACHMENT.

Ziba-Rx trademark for *bacitracin zinc* (see under BACITRACIN).

Zimany's bilobed flap see under FLAP.

Zimmermann, pericyte of pericyte.

zinc (zingk) [Ger. *Zink*; L. *zincum*] a metallic element. Symbol, Zn; atomic number, 30; atomic weight, 65.38; specific gravity, 7.133; melting point, 419.38°C; Mohs hardness number, 2.5; valence, 2; group IIB of the periodic table. Natural zinc isotopes are 64, 66–68, and 70; radioactive isotopes are 60–63, 65, 69, and 71–72. It is a white malleable metal with bluish gray luster, soluble in acids and alkalies, but not in water. Zinc is distributed in plant and animal tissue, being essential to health. In man, it occurs in the prostate, hair, bones, liver, kidneys, muscles, pancreas, gastrointestinal tract, spleen, and blood, the greatest concentrations being in the enamel and dentin. Zinc is involved in metabolism as a component of metalloenzymes and is an activator of other enzymes, and through its influence on the configuration of nonenzyme organic ligands such as α_2-macroglobulin glycoprotein in plasma. It is also believed to be involved in taste sensation. Meat, shellfish, whole grains, and their products are the chief sources of zinc. Teeth of tuberculous patients have an increased zinc concentration. Zinc deficiency may cause growth retardation, delayed sexual maturation, testicular atrophy, and skin lesions. Alcoholic cirrhosis is usually associated with decreased plasma zinc content. Inhalation of zinc fumes may cause vomiting, nausea, fever, cough, muscular weakness, generalized aching, chills, and xerostomia. Zinc is used in various alloys, including those used in dental restorations, in organic chemistry, and in a variety of industrial processes. For daily requirements of zinc, see table at NUTRITION. **z. acetate,** $Zn(C_2H_3O_2)_2$, white crystals or granules with an acetous odor and astringent taste, soluble in water and boiling alcohol and slightly soluble in cold alcohol. Used as an astringent, in low concentrations, and as an irritant, in high concentration. Oral administration causes emesis. Also used as an accelerator in the preparation of zinc oxide–eugenol cement. **z. bacitracin,** zinc BACITRACIN. **z. chloride,** $ZnCl_2$, white, odorless granules, fused pieces, or rods, soluble in water and acetone, but not in alcohol. Used as a topical antiseptic and astringent. In concentrated solutions, used for reducing the sensitivity of dentin; in 8 percent solution, used as an astringent in the treatment of periodontitis. It is a component of many mouthwashes. Excessive use may cause moderate irritation of the skin and mucous membranes. **z. eugenolate,** $Zn(O·C_{10}·H_{11}O_2)_2$. See zinc oxide–eugenol CEMENT. **z. iodide,** ZnI_2, a white, crystalline, hygroscopic powder with a saline taste, which is soluble in water, alcohol, and alkalies, and turns brown on exposure to light or air. Used as a topical antiseptic and astringent and in iodine tincture. **z. ointment,** see *z. oxide*. **z. orthophosphate,** z. phosphate. **z. oxide,** ZnO, a fine, odorless, amorphous, white or yellowish powder, soluble in dilute acids, ammonium carbonate solution, and alkali hydroxide solutions, but not in water and ethanol. Available as an ointment (zinc ointment), containing 20 percent zinc oxide in mineral oil; a paste (Lassar's plain zinc paste, compound paste of zinc oxide), containing 25 percent zinc oxide in white petrolatum; and zinc oxide paste with salicylic acid (Lassar's paste or Lassar's zinc oxide paste with salicylic acid), containing 25 percent zinc oxide and 2 percent salicylic acid in zinc oxide paste. It is a mild astringent agent with protective and antiseptic properties. Also used as a sunscreen. When mixed with phosphoric acid, it forms zinc phosphate cement (see under CEMENT). **z. peroxide,** ZnO_2, a white to yellowish white, odorless powder. Used in pharmaceuticals and, as medicinal zinc peroxide (a mixture of zinc peroxide, zinc carbonate, and zinc hydroxide in a 40 percent solution), as an astringent, deodorant, and topical anti-infective agent. It is an oxygen-liberating agent, and is used most often to treat anaerobic wound infections and oropharyngeal and oral diseases, including necrotizing ulcerative gingivitis. Also used in the treatment of infections caused by certain aerobes, such as hemolytic streptococci. **z. phosphate,** $Zn_3(PO_4)_2$, a white, odorless powder, which is soluble in dilute mineral acids, acetic acid, ammonia, and alkali hydroxide solutions, but not in water or ethanol. Found in nature as the mineral hopeite. Used as a buffering salt added to phosphoric acid to reduce the reaction rate of the setting of zinc phosphate cement. Called also *z. orthophosphate*. **z. polyacrylate,** a polyacrylic acid zinc salt formed through the reaction of zinc oxide and aqueous solution of polyacrylic, being the basic structure of polycarboxylate cement (see under CEMENT). **z. soap,** zinc SOAP. **z. sulfate,** $ZnSO_4 \cdot 7H_2O$, colorless, odorless small needles, prisms, or granular crystalline powder, which is soluble in water and glycerol, but not in alcohol. Used chiefly as an astringent, emetic, and weak antiseptic in ophthalmological therapy, in nasal sprays, in certain skin diseases, in shrinking mucous membranes, and in healing chronic ulcers. Called also z. vitriol, *zinc salt of sulfuric acid,* and *white vitriol.* **z. vitriol, z.** sulfate.

Zinsser-Engman-Cole syndrome [Ferdinand *Zinsser,* German dermatologist, 1865–1952; Martin Feeney *Engman,* dermatologist in St. Louis, 1869–1953; H. N. *Cole,* American physician] DYSKERATOSIS congenita.

zircon (zer′kon) a mineral, $ZrSiO_4$, being the natural form of zirconium silicate.

zirconia (zer-ko′ne-ah) ZIRCONIUM dioxide.

zirconium (zir-ko′ne-um) [Arabic *zergun* gold color] a metallic element. Symbol, Zr; atomic number, 40; atomic weight, 91.22; specific gravity, 5.506; melting point, 1852°C; Brinell hardness number, 85; valences, 2, 3; group IVB of the periodic table. Natural isotopes are 90, 91, 92, 94, and 96; artificial radioactive ones are 81–89, 93, 95, and 99; it occurs as a bluish black, amorphous powder or grayish white metal, soluble in hot concentrated acids, but insoluble in cold acids and water. Zirconium and its salts have low toxicity, but granulomatous lesions of the skin have been reported in users of zirconium-containing deodorants. Used chiefly in nuclear technology and in corrosion-resistant alloys. Also used as a white pigment in dental porcelain and as a whitener for teeth. Chromium impurities may cause it to become yellow. **z. dioxide,** z. oxide. **z. oxide,** ZrO_2, occurring in nature as the mineral baddeleyite. It is a white, heavy, amorphous, odorless, tasteless powder or crystalline solid, slightly soluble in hydrochloric and nitric acids, but not in water. Used therapeutically as a dermatologic agent. Also used as an opaquing agent for dental porcelain and other ceramic processes. Called also *z. dioxide, zirconia,* and *zirconic anhydride.* **z. silicate,** $ZrSiO_4$, found in nature as the mineral zircon in rocks and in beach sand in Florida and South Carolina. It occurs as tetragonal, bipyramidal crystals, which are usually colorless, but may assume the color of impurities. It has the same hardness as quartz (Mohs hardness number, 6.0–7.5). Used as a stabilizer for silicone rubbers and in the manufacture of refractories, ceramics, glazes, and other products. Used as a polishing agent in dental prophylaxis.

Zm zygomaxillare.

Zn zinc.

ZOE zinc oxide–eugenol; see under CEMENT and PASTE.

zoic (zo′ik) [Gr. *zōikos* of or proper of animals] pertaining to or characterized by animal life.

zona (zo′nah), pl. *zo′nae* [L. "a girdle"] 1. an encircling region or area; any anatomical area with a specific boundary or characteristics. Called also *zone.* 2. HERPES zoster. **z. fascicula′ta,** a wide central layer of the adrenal cortex, made up of radially arranged strands of cells, which secretes mostly glucocorticoids, 17-ketosteroids, and estrogens, and is controlled by adrenocorticotropic hormone. **z. glomerulo′sa,** a thin outer layer of the adrenal cortex, made up of short loops of glomeruloid clusters of irregularly arranged cells, which secretes mostly mineralocorticoids and is affected little by adrenocorticotropic hormone. **z. reticula′ris,** a layer of the adrenal cortex, bordering on the medulla, made up of a network of cell cords, which secretes mostly glucocorticoids, 17-ketosteroids, and estrogens, and responds to adrenocorticotropic hormone.

zonae (zo′ne) [L.] plural of *zona.*

zonal (zo′nal) [L. *zona′lis*] pertaining to or of the nature of a zone.

zone (zōn) [Gr. *zōnē* a belt, girdle] an encircling region or area; by extension any area with a specific boundary or characteristics. Called also *zona.* **z. of acceptance, subendosseous,** a noninflammatory area situated anterior or posterior to the site of a previously rejected implant. **apical z.,** a narrow area along the mucous membrane over the apices of the roots of the teeth. **biokinetic z.,** the range of temperatures within which the living cell carries its life activities, lying approximately between 10°C and 45°C. **cell-free z., cell-poor z.,** Weil's basal LAYER. **cell-rich z.,** cell-rich LAYER. **cervical z.,** the third of the coronal zone which is nearest the cervix of the tooth, marked by the cementoenamel junction of crown and root. **combustion z.,** see FLAME (2). **comfort z.,** an environmental temperature between 13 and 21°C (55–70°F) with a humidity of 30 to 55 percent, which is

comfortable if clothing is suitable; 28 to 30°C (82–86°F) is comfortable to the naked body. Neither sweating nor shivering is provoked in these ranges. **contact area z.,** the zone which includes the contact area of adjoining teeth; usually it is in the middle third of the coronal zone between the occlusal and the cervical zone. **dentofacial z.,** the entire lower part of the face; the region of the face overlying the teeth and the alveolar processes of the jaws. **dolorogenic z.,** an area stimulation of which produces pain, or excites an attack of neuralgia. **fatty z. of hard palate,** one of the two anterior parts of the hard palate, separated by the raphe, having irregular communicating compartments between fibrous bands, which are filled with fat globules or mucous glands. Called also *pars corporis adipata.* **glandular z. of hard palate,** one of the two posterior parts of the hard palate, separated by the raphe, having irregular communicating compartments between the fibrous bands, which are filled with the glandular material. Called also *pars corporis glandulosa.* **H. z.,** the central part of the A band of the sarcomere, which is somewhat less dense than the peripheral parts and is bisected by the M band. It represents the distance between the ends of the thin actin filaments. Called also *Engelmann's disk, H band,* and *Hensen's disk.* See illustration at MUSCLE. **hyperesthetic z.,** a region of the body surface marked by abnormal sensibility. **z. of inflammation, subendosseous,** an inflammatory area immediately surrounding the site of implant rejection. **intermediate z.,** 1. the portion of the alar and basal plates of the neural tube of the embryo forming the sulcus limitans. 2. the central zone of the developing periodontal ligament, situated between the pericemental and periosteal zones. Histologically, it is characterized by the presence of collagen fibers in an advanced stage of development, which tend to be organized into bundles. **marginal z. of lips,** vermilion BORDER. **motor z.,** an area of the cerebral cortex which, when stimulated, causes contraction of voluntary muscles. **neutral z.,** the potential space between the lips and cheeks on one side and the tongue on the other, where natural or artificial teeth are subjected to equal and opposite force from the surrounding muscles. **oxidizing z.,** see FLAME (2). **pericemental z.,** the innermost zone of the developing periodontal ligament, which is adjacent to the cementum and structurally and functionally resembles cementum. **periosteal z.,** the peripheral zone of the developing periodontal ligament, which is adjacent to the alveolar bone and functionally and structurally resembles the periosteum. **raphe z.,** the part of the hard palate containing the raphe and the palatine papilla, which extends from the papilla and runs posteriorly for varying distances. Its surface is lined with keratinized or parakeratotic epithelium, long, slender epithelial pegs extending into the underlying connective tissue. Called also *pars corporis raphe.* **red z. of lips,** vermilion BORDER. **reducing z.,** see FLAME (2). **z. of Retzius,** incremental LINE. **rugae z.,** rugae AREA. **z's, of Schreger,** lines of Schreger; see under LINE. **trigger z.,** an area the stimulation of which may precipitate attacks of pain in neuralgia. Trigger zones in trigeminal neuralgia are located on the vermilion border of the lips, alae of the nose, cheeks, and around the eyes. **vermilion z.,** vermilion BORDER. **Weil's basal z.,** Weil's basal LAYER.

Zone Periodontal Pak trademark for a periodontal dressing. In the base, each 100 gm of the preparation contains 3.1 gm polyvinylpyrrolidone-iodine complex, 38.3 gm rosin, 2 gm chlorobutanol, 10 gm mineral oil, 9.3 gm isopropyl myristate, 3.1 mg propylene glycol monoisostearate, 11.1 gm polymers, and 23.1 gm inert fillers. In the catalyst, each 100 gm contains 19.1 gm zinc oxide, 3.2 gm magnesium oxide, 6.6 sodium monolaurate, 8.3 glycerol, 13.7 gm propylene glycol, 36.7 gm inert fillers, and 12.3 mineral and vegetable oils.

zonography (zo-nog′rah-fe) a type of tomography accomplished through narrow-angle (less than 10°) and multidirectional movements of the x-ray tube; used for examination of structures that are at least several centimeters in thickness.

zonula (zon′u-lah), pl. *zon′ulae* [L. dim. of *zona*] a small zone, or zonule. **z. adher′ens,** that portion of the junctional complex of columnar epithelial cells, just deep to the zonula occludens, where the cell membranes diverge to form an intercellular space 150 to 200 Å (15–20 nm) wide and are supported on their inner aspect by moderately dense filamentous material forming a continuous band parallel to the zonula occludens. Called also *intermediate junction.* **z. occlu′dens,** that portion of the junctional complex of columnar epithelial cells, just beneath the free surface, where the intercellular space is obliterated; it extends completely around the cell perimeter, above the zonula adherens. Called also *tight junction.*

zonulae (zon′u-le) [L.] plural of *zonula.*

zonular (zon′u-lar) pertaining to a zonule.

zonule (zon′ul) a small zone; zonula.

zoo- [Gr. *zōon* animal] a combining form denoting relationship to animals.

zoogenous (zo-oj'ĕ-nus) [*zoo-* + Gr. *gennan* to produce] 1. acquired from animals. 2. viviparous.

zooglea (zo''o-gle'ah) [*zoo-* + Gr. *gloios* gum] a colony of bacteria embedded in a gelatinous matrix. See also MICROBIOTA.

Zoogloea (zo''o-gle'ah) [Gr. *zōon* animal + *gloea* jelly] a genus of gram-negative, aerobic, rod-shaped bacteria of the family Pseudomonadaceae, occurring chiefly in water and sewage.

Zoolobelin trademark for *lobeline hydrochloride* (see under LOBELINE).

Zootoxin (zo''o-tok'sin) [*zoo-* + Gr. *toxikon* poison] a toxic substance of animal origin, such as venoms of snakes, spiders, and scorpions. See also TOXIN.

zoster (zos'ter) [Gr. *zōstēr*] a girdle, or encircling structure or pattern. See also HERPES ZOSTER.

Z-plasty Z-PLASTY.

Zr zirconium.

Zsigmondy, Richard Adolf [1865–1929] a German chemist; winner of the Nobel prize in 1925, for his work on colloids; inventor of the ultramicroscope in 1903. See brownian MOVEMENT (brownian-Zsigmondy movement).

Zuberella (zu''ber-el'ah) a proposed generic name for a group of gram-negative, anaerobic bacteria, now assigned to other genera. **Z. pedipe'dis**, *Fusobacterium symbiosum*; see under FUSOBACTERIUM. **Z. plau'ti**, *Fusobacterium plauti*; see under FUSOBACTERIUM.

Zuckerkandl's dehiscences [Emil *Zuckerkandl*, German anatomist, 1849–1910] see under DEHISCENCE.

Zuelzer-Kaplan syndrome [Wolf W. *Zuelzer*; Eugene *Kaplan*] 1. familial nonspherocytic ANEMIA. 2. thalassemia–hemoglobin C DISEASE.

Zutracin trademark for BACITRACIN.

Zy zygion.

zygia (zij'e-ah) plural of *zygion*.

zygion (zij'e-on), pl. *zygia* [Gr.] a craniometric and cephalometric landmark, being the most laterally situated point on either zygomatic arch. Abbreviated *Zy*. Called also *point Zy*. See illustration at CEPHALOMETRY.

zygo- [Gr. *zygon* yoke] a combining form meaning yoked or joined, or denoting relationship to a junction.

zygoma (zi-go'mah) [Gr. *zygoma* bolt or bar] 1. zygomatic process of temporal bone; see under PROCESS. 2. zygomatic ARCH. 3. zygomatic BONE.

zygomatic (zi''go-mat'ik) pertaining to the zygoma (zygomatic arch, process, or bone).

zygomaticofacial (zi''go-mat''ĭ-ko-fa'shal) pertaining to the zygoma (zygomatic arch, process, or bone) and the frontal bone.

zygomaticofrontal (zi''go-mat''ĭ-ko-fron'tal) pertaining to the zygoma (zygomatic arch, process, or bone) and the frontal bone.

zygomaticomaxillary (zi''go-mat''ĭ-ko-mak'sĭ-ler''e) pertaining to the zygoma (zygomatic arch, bone, or process) and the maxilla. Called also ZYGOMAXILLARY.

zygomatico-orbital (zi''go-mat''ĭ-ko-or'bĭ-tal) pertaining to the zygoma (zygomatic arch, process, or bone) and the orbit.

zygomaticosphenoid (zi''go-mat''ĭ-ko-sfe'noid) pertaining to the zygoma (zygomatic arch, process, or bone) and the sphenoid bone.

zygomaticotemporal (zi''go-mat''ĭ-ko-tem'po-ral) pertaining to the zygoma (zygomatic arch, process, or bone) and the temporal bone or region.

zygomaticus (zi''go-mat''ĭ-kus) [L.] zygomatic muscle, greater; see under MUSCLE. **z. ma'jor**, zygomatic muscle, greater; see under MUSCLE. **z. mi'nor**, zygomatic head of quadratus labii superioris; see under HEAD.

zygomaxillare (zi''go-mak'sĭ-ler''e) a craniometric landmark situated at the lowest point of the zygomaticomaxillary suture. See illustration at CEPHALOMETRY.

zygomaxillary (zi''go-mak'sĭ-ler''e) zygomaticomaxillary.

Zygomonas (zi-go'mo-nas) [Gr. *zymē* + *monas* unit] a genus of gram-negative, facultatively anaerobic, rod-shaped microorganisms of uncertain affiliation, found in fermented beverages.

Zygomycetes (zi''go-mi-se'tēz) a class of true fungi of the Phycomycetes group, which is the only class of the group of medical importance. It comprises common fungi of air and soil, including the common bread molds *Mucor, Rhizopus,* and *Absidia*. which are widespread in soil; all of which may cause mucormycosis.

zygote (zi'gōt) [Gr. *zygōtos* yoked together] a diploid cell formed by the fusion of two haploid gametes during fertilization; the fertilized ovum. See also FERTILIZATION.

zygotene (zi'go-tēn) [*zygo-* + Gr. *tainia* ribbon] the second stage of the first prophase in meiosis, characterized by pairing (synapsis) of homologous chromosomes. Called also *synaptic phase* and, sometimes, *amphitene*.

Zyklolat trademark for *cyclopentaloate hydrochloride* (see under CYCLOPENTOLATE).

zylene (zi'lēn) an aromatic hydrocarbon, $C_6H_4(CH_3)_2$, occurring as a clear, mobile, flammable fluid. Commercial xylene consists of a mixture of the three isomers, *ortho-, meta-,* and *para*-xylene. Used as a solvent, in sterilizing catgut, and in the production of various chemicals, including drugs. Xylene is a toxic substance that may be narcotic in high concentrations. Called also *dimethylbenzene* and *xylol*.

Zyloprim trademark for *allopurinol*.

Zymaflour trademark for a preparation of *sodium fluoride* (see under FLUORIDE).

zymo- [Gr. *zymē* leaven] a combining form denoting relationship to an enzyme, or to fermentation.

zymogen (zi'mo-jen) [*zymo-* + Gr. *gennan* to produce] an inactive precursor that is converted to active enzyme by the action of another substance.

zymophore (zi'mo-fōr) [*zymo-* + Gr. *phoros* bearing] the group of atoms in the molecule of an enzyme which is responsible for its specific effects; the active site of an enzyme.

MEDICAL AND DENTAL LEXICOGRAPHY; A BRIEF HISTORICAL NOTE

Stanley Jablonski

As with most things in Western civilization, the art of writing dictionaries and encyclopedias, the two basic forms of lexicography, was probably developed in ancient Greece. Whether there were even earlier models we can not be certain, because the origin of lexicography can not be identified with any single event or work. Speusippos, a Greek scholar of the 4th century B.C.,[1,3,4] is credited with being one of the earliest scientific lexicographers, and his classification of plants and animals is considered as the precursor of the modern encyclopedia. There were many others, however, whose writings could be classified in the same category. Most early scholars attempted in their writings to report on the state of contemporary knowledge, and their works were often encyclopedic in proportion and scope, if not in form. This was especially true of the writings of Hippocrates of Cos, the celebrated Greek physician of the late 5th century B.C.,[2] whose works were later collectively titled *Corpus hippocraticum*; Marcus Terentius Varro, a Roman scholar who lived from 116 to 27 B.C. and wrote the *Disciplinarum libri IX* and the *De forma philosophiae libri II*;[1] Gaius Plinius Secundus (Pliny the Elder, A.D. 23-79), who wrote the *Historia naturalis*, a monumental work in 37 books and 2493 chapters, of which books 7 to 11 and 20 to 32 deal with medical subjects;[1,2] Galen (Latinized to Claudius or Clarissimus Calenus), a Greek physician in Rome who lived from A.D. 129-199 and wrote numerous works and whose teachings dominated the practice of medicine until the Renaissance;[2] and many others. Dentistry was best represented in early encyclopedic works in Al Tasrif (the "Collection") by Albucasis (Abu-l-Kasim), a famous Arabic physician in Cordoba who lived from about 936 to about 1013.[2] It includes the first known detailed illustrations of surgical and dental instruments, a list of rules for tooth extraction, a description of how to cauterize teeth with a red-hot iron as a toothache remedy, and a discussion of dental calculus and its removal.

According to Collison,[1] the first scientific encyclopedia, as we know it, was the anonymous *Compendium philosophiae*, published about 1350.[1] The *Encyclopedia Americana*, however, assigns credit for establishing the encyclopedic form to Francis Bacon, the author of *The great instauration*, published in 1620.[3] The word "encyclopedia" is believed to have been used for the first time by Paul Scalich, a Hungarian nobleman, in his *Encyclopaedia seu orbis disciplinarum tam sacrarum quam prophanum epitome*, published in Basel in 1559.[1,3,4] The encyclopedic form was particularly well suited to inquisitive minds of the educated class during the Renaissance, and it continued to increase in popularity until the 20th century. During the 18th century there was an explosive growth in the number of new encyclopedias, culminating with the publication in 1768 of the first edition of *The Encyclopaedia Britannica*, the world's best known encyclopedia.[4]

The popularity of encyclopedias continues to the present time. Their use, however, is now limited to that of general reference. Scientific encyclopedias began declining in popularity in the late 19th century when it became apparent that, because of their enormous bulk and cost of production, coupled with the explosive development of scientific information, they could not keep up with the pace of discovery or be published economically. Of the numerous large medical encyclopedias that were in existence between the world wars, only the *Bol'shaia meditsinskaia entsiklopediia*, a mammoth work originally published in the Soviet Union in 1928[5] in 36 volumes, is still in publication and is now in its third edition. Otherwise, encyclopedias have been largely replaced by scientific dictionaries--much smaller and, therefore, easier and cheaper to produce, more amenable to frequent up-dating, easier to carry around and, generally, more useful books.

The origin of scientific dictionaries is even more difficult to trace than that of encyclopedias. The format of early dictionaries was sometimes indistinguishable from the encyclopedic form and the word "dictionary" was often used in connection with encyclopedias, thus making differentiation between the two forms difficult. For example, early editions of *The Encyclopaedia Britannica* carried the subtitle, *A dictionary of arts, sciences, literature, and general information.*[4]

Bibliographies of early dictionaries, such as one found in *The Encyclopaedia Britannica*, contain references to works from the pre- and early Christian eras. However, these were largely literature lexicons rather than scientific dictionaries. Moreover, manuscripts of many of these works have been lost, some as early as during the destruction of the library of Alexandria, and their precise characteristics are largely unknown; their similarity to scientific dictionaries as we know them today is a matter for speculation. Some notable examples of early lexicographic works are included in the writings of the Atticists who compiled lists of words and phrases during the second century A.D. in Athens, or Marcus Terentius Varro who wrote the *De lingua Latina* during the first century B.C.,[4] and of Pamphilus of Alexandria, who wrote a lexicon during the first century A.D.[4]

The word "dictionary" is believed to have been used for the first time by John Garland (1202-1252) in his *Dictionarius*.[4] The first medical dictionary so named is probably H. Stephani's *Dictionarium medicum*, published in Paris in 1564.[3] The format of a modern dictionary has its origin in the 18th century.

The most important early medical lexicographic work in English is R. James' *A medicinal dictionary*, published in London in 1743.[6] It is said that Samuel Johnson cooperated in the preparation of this work.[7] The experience thus gained by Johnson must have been essential in writing his famous *A dictionary of the English language*, published 13 years later.[8] James' work was still basically an alphabetically arranged compendium, being somewhat closer in form to an encyclopedia than a dictionary in the modern sense, whereas Johnson's work, using clear, concise definitions, rather than a series of dissertations, as was then customary, was a major landmark in the development of the modern dictionary form. Next in the chain of evolution of medical lexicography, was G. Motherby's *A new medical dictionary or general repository of physic*, published in London in 1801.[9] Motherby's work was still somewhat encyclopedic in form, as the title would indicate, although the author attempted in it to formulate definitions that were more concise than those of his predecessors and contemporaries. Also, he tried to group compound entries on similar subjects through an alphabetical arrangement.

The most rapid progress in the development of medical lexicography occurred in the mid-19th century with a series of dictionaries that began with G. Mayne's *Medical vocabulary*, published in 1836,[10] written while the author was still a medical student. This smallish work (in Mayne's own words, "a thin duodecimo volume") was enlarged to a 1506-page book and published in 1860 as *An expository lexicon of terms, ancient and modern, medical and general science.*[10] In this edition, Mayne established the principles for the scope, typography, and style that were adopted by many later lexicographers. The last in the series was a massive three-volume enlargement of Mayne's original work, *The new Sydenham Society's lexicon of medicine and the allied sciences*, by H. Power and L.W. Sedgwick, published in 1881.[11] This edition, in addition to expanding the scope, also introduced further refinements in style and format.

Probably no one was more knowledgeable on the subject of the language of medicine or more qualified to bring medical lexicography into the twentieth century than John Shaw Billings, an army surgeon and scholar with an enormous range of interests and outstanding achievements. After the Civil War, Billings was assigned to the Army Surgeon-General's Office, where he organized and expanded its small collection of books into an excellent medical library, which eventually evolved into the National Library of Medicine. He also began publishing the world's first significant international bibliography of medical literature, the *Index-Catalogue*, which in time and after a series of modifications, served as the basis for the MEDLARS system, a computerized information system.[12]

The *Index-Catalogue* was a bibliographic masterpiece that, even today, is seldom matched and practically never surpassed in excellence. It was also a major lexicographic landmark. In it, bibliographic references were arranged around a hierarchically structured skeleton made up of a thesaurus of terms serving as subject headings. These were selected according to etymologic and scientific criteria and frequency of use in the literature and tied together by an elaborate system of cross-references.

Thus, the broad area of biomedical sciences was divided into manageable units that would be of specific interest to the user and would also inform him about the existence in the other parts of the bibliography of additional areas of interest. The thesaurus, which was never published separately, was unique in the history of lexicography in that it listed essential terms in the entire field of biomedical sciences and arranged them into a hierarchical classification. The inverting of compound terms under nouns was another lexicographic innovation. In the introduction of the first edition, Billings wrote, "As a rule, substantives rather than adjectives are selected as subject-headings,"[12] and thus laid the foundation for the inverted system now used in most biomedical dictionaries. Under this system, for example, bibliographic references dealing with various types of tuberculosis were clustered under a single heading, *tuberculosis*, rather than being scattered under the adjectives, such as *avian*, *bovine*, *oral*, or *pulmonary*, as would have been done in other bibliographic and lexicographic works of the period.

In 1890, Billings also published *The national medical dictionary*, an elegant two-volume work containing more than 80,000 words that was written in a modified style of British predecessors.[13] One can only speculate on why, after developing a superior lexicographic style of his own, he decided to exclude it from his dictionary. Billings never revised his dictionary, but William A.N. Dorland, a Philadelphia physician, wrote *The American medical dictionary* [14] in 1900 in which he adopted most of Billings' lexicographic ideas, particularly the inverted entry system, typography, capitalization of entry terms, and cross-references. In doing this, he established a format for biomedical lexicography that is standard for most modern medical dictionaries. The title was changed to *Dorland's illustrated medical dictionary* in 1957.

The credit for writing the first important biomedical dictionary in America must go, however, to Chapin Aaron Harris, a dentist. His work, *A dictionary of dental science, biography, bibliography, and medical terminology*,[15] was published in 1849. Its format was traditional, similar to that of the dictionaries of Motherby and early editions of Mayne, and its scope consisted of terms in all branches of dentistry, as well as in those allied areas of science, arts, technology, and biography considered relevant to dentistry--similarly to what would have been done now. Harris attempted to identify subjects that he considered to be of special importance and provided them with a very extensive description--more in the form of a treatise than a definition. For example,

under the term *caries of the teeth*, the definition occupies some 17 columns of print. One of the most amazing aspects of this dictionary is the fact that it was written, edited, typeset, proofread, and printed in less than three years (1846-1849). One must bear in mind that all this was done before the era of typewriters (much less electric ones), word-processors, computerized typesetting, even the electric light, and before adequate library facilities were readily available in America--in not much more time than is now required to negotiate a book contract. Harris' dictionary appeared in five more editions. Its title was changed to *A dictionary of medical terminology, dental surgery, and the collateral sciences*, for the second (1855), third (1867), and fourth (1877) editions, and was again changed to the *Dictionary of dental science and such words and phrases of the collateral sciences as pertain to the art and practice of dentistry* for the fifth (1891) and sixth (1898) editions. Harris died in 1860 and Ferdinand J.S. Gorgas assumed the authorship of the third edition through the sixth and last edition. Gorgas gradually expanded the scope of the book and edited down some of the encyclopedic entries, bringing the style in line with that of other works of the period.

It was not until 1922 that the next dental dictionary appeared, L.P. Anthony's *A dictionary of dental sciences*.[16] The following year, (1923), L. Ottofy published his *Standard dental dictionary*.[17] Neither of these two excellent dictionaries appeared in a second edition.

The next dental dictionary in America was published by W.B. Dunning and S.W. Davenport in 1936, *A dictionary of dental sciences and art*.[18] It was one of the better biomedical dictionaries of the period, having crisp and comprehensive definitions and excellent organizations, scope, and typography. Its major features were quite similar to those of Dorland, except for the approach to inverted entries. Unlike the Dorland, where all compound entries were entered under the nouns, in the Dunning and Davenport, eponymous entries were entered under proper names. Thus, types of crowns, such as *artificial*, *cap*, *collar*, were arranged under the main entry *crown*, but the Richmond crown was to be found under *Richmond*. And, under the main entry *attachment*, there is only one subentry, the "T" attachment, while other attachments were scattered throughout the dictionary under their eponymous entries. Unfortunately, another deficiency of the dictionary--an inadequate cross-reference system--

sometimes made it difficult for the user to locate an appropriate form. Even with these shortcomings, it was an excellent dictionary.

There was another long time gap, this time of some 46 years, before another comprehensive dental dictionary was published, in 1982, the *illustrated dictionary of dentistry* by Stanley Jablonski.[19]

Dental lexicography was not completely dormant during long periods of time between the publication of dictionaries. On the contrary, there appeared to be more activity concerned with vocabulary development, control, and standardization on the part of professional organizations in the field of dentistry than in many other biomedical disciplines, particularly since World War II.

The earliest post-war efforts in the field of dental lexicography were those of the American Dental Association, whose Bureau of Library and Indexing Services sponsored three annual nomenclature conferences in 1952, 1953, and 1954. Three glossaries were generated by these conferences: *Concepts pertaining to occlusion* (1952);[20] *Supplementing the dental dictionary. Terms that have been introduced into the dental vocabulary since 1936* (1953),[21] an effort to update the Dunning-Davenport; and *The troublesome terms* (1954).[22] Thereafter, dental associations assumed responsibility for terminology within their respective disciplines, and a number of specialized glossaries have been produced as the result of these efforts, including glossaries in orthodontics,[23] endodontics,[24] prosthodontics,[25] dental radiology,[26] oral surgery,[27] periodontics,[29,30] and prepaid dental care.[30] These glossaries were produced by specialists and under the supervision of sanctioning professional associations and, thus, had an advantage over conventional dictionaries in that they reflected the official thinking of the profession on the use of dental terms at that particular time. They also had some disadvantages. Fractionation of dentistry into its many specific subfields sometimes resulted in considerable variability of definitions. This sometimes created confusion or, at least, forced the user to consult several glossaries rather than depend on a single source of information, as would be the case with a conventional dictionary. This last problem was remedied to a large degree by Carl O. Boucher who, in 1963, published a cumulation of specialized dental glossaries in a single book, the *Current clinical dental terminology. A glossary of accepted terms in all disciplines of dentistry.*[31] The book was revised and published in a second edition

in 1974 and a third edition in 1982. Two other publications, *Accepted dental therapeutics*[32] and *Dentist's desk reference*,[33] are not glossaries in the true technical sense but must be included here because of their role in vocabulary control of dental pharmacology and material science.

The approach to biomedical lexicography and the methods of preparing and printing dictionaries remains virtually unchanged for more than three quarters of a century. By and large, they have proved to be effective in providing the biomedical community with reference sources that are comprehensive, informative, easy to use, and relatively inexpensive. But, as with everything else in life, that, too, must change. On one hand, we are experiencing an ever increasing growth of terminology, whereby new terms require more complex and longer definitions and many old ones must be redefined and reclassified to conform with new concepts and discoveries. This naturally leads to ever longer and more expensive dictionaries, especially since the accelerating rate of discovery demands that scientific dictionaries should be more detailed and updated more frequently than in the past. Should we continue on this course, the ownership of scientific dictionaries may become a luxury which few of us will be able to afford.

No one knows with any degree of certainty which directions scientific lexicography will take in the future, but one thing is clear, we must find a way to apply modern technology to lexicographic technics. A few decades back, scientific bibliography was drowning in the flood of information. Now, after computerization of major secondary information storage and dissemination systems, bibiographic information may be obtained more efficiently, more rapidly, and more economically than before. The path to follow is well marked.

The author wishes to express his appreciation to Dr. Maria Farkas and Mr. Robert Mehnert of the National Library of Medicine for their cooperation and support in writing this article. Materials from the National Library of Medicine (including the MEDLINE data base) and the American Dental Association were used in preparation of this article.

1. Collison, R. Encyclopaedias; their history throughout the ages. New York, Hafner Publishing Co., 1966.

2. Garrison, F.H. An introduction to the history of medicine. ed.4. Philadelphia, W.B. Saunders Co., 1929.

3. The Encyclopedia Americana. International edition. Danbury, Americana Corp., 1980.

4. The Encyclopaedia Britannica. ed. 15. Chicago, Encyclopaedia Britannica, Inc., 1981.

5. Bol'shaia meditsinskaia entsiklopediia. ed.3, Moskva, Sovetskaia Entsiklopediia, 1981.

6. James, R. A medicinal dictionary, London, 1743.

7. MacNalty, Sir A.S. The British medical dictionary. London, The Caxton Publishing Co., Ltd., 1965.

8. Johnson, S. A dictionary of the English language. London, J. Knapton, 1756.

9. Motherby, G. A new medical dictionary or general repository of physic. ed. 5. Revised by G. Wallis, London, 1801.

10. Mayne, R.G. An expository lexicon of terms, ancient and modern, medical and general science, including a complete medico-legal vocabulary. London, J.Churchill, 1860.

11. Power, H., & Sedgwick, L.W. The New Sydenham Society's lexicon of medicine and the allied sciences. London, The New Sydenham Society, 1881.

12. Index-Catalogue of the Library of the Surgeon-General's Office, United States Army. Washington, Government Printing Office, 1880.

13. Billings, J.S. The national medical dictionary. Philadelphia, Lea Brothers & Co., 1890.

14. Dorland, W.A. The American illustrated medical dictionary. Philadelphia, W.B. Saunders & Co., 1900.

15. Harris, C.A. A dictionary of dental science, biography, bibliography, and medical terminology. Philadelphia, Lindsay & Blakiston, 1849.

16. Anthony, L.P. A dictionary of dental science. Philadelphia, Lea & Febiger, 1922.

17. Ottofy, L. Standard dental dictionary. Chicago, Laird & Lee, Inc., 1923.

18. Dunning, W.B., & Davenport, S.E. A dictionary of dental science and art. Philadelphia, Blakiston Co., 1936.

19. Jablonski, S. Illustrated dictionary of dentistry. Philadelphia, 1982.

20. Concepts pertaining to occlusion. Nomenclature Conference, sponsored by the Bureau of Library and Indexing Services, American Dental Association, Chicago, June 20-21, 1952.

21.Supplementing the dental dictionary. Second Nomenclature Conference, sponsored by the Bureau of Library and Indexing Services, American Dental Association, Chicago, June 10-11, 1953.

22. Troublesome terms. Third Nomenclature Conference, sponsored by The Bureau of Library and Indexing Services, American Dental Association, Chicago, Sept.3-4, 1954.

23. Orthodontic glossary. Compiled by the Council of Orthodontic Education. St. Louis, The American Association of Orthodontists, 1972.

24. An annotated glossary of terms used in endodontics. By the 1971-72 and 1972-73 committees on nomenclature of the American Association of Endodontics. ed. 2. American Association of Endodontics, 1973.

25. Glossary of prosthodontic terms. Edited by the Nomenclature Committee of the Academy of Denture Prosthetics. St. Louis, C.V. Mosby Co., 1977.

26. Glossary of dental radiology. By Nomenclature Subcommitttee. The American Academy of Dental Radiology, 1978.

27. Oral surgery glossary. By the Committee on Hospital Oral Surgery Service. Chicago, American Society of Oral Surgeons, 1978.

28. Glossary of terms. J. Periodontol., Jan. 1977, Suppl.

29. Current procedural terminology for periodontists. ed.3, Chicago, American Academy of Periodontology, p. 1972.

30. Prepaid dental care. A glossary. Bethesda, U.S. Department of Health, Education, and Welfare, 1975. DHEW Publication No. (HRA) 7620.

31. Boucher, C.O. Current clinical dental terminology. A glossary of accepted terms in all disciplines of dentistry. ed. 2. St. Louis, C.V. Mosby Co., 1974. ed. 3. St. Louis, C.V. Mosby, 1982.

32. Accepted dental therapeutics, ed. 39. Chicago, American Dental Association, 1982.

33. Dentist's desk reference. Chicago, American Dental Association, 1981, (formerly Guide to dental materials and devices).